PALLIATIVE MEDICINE

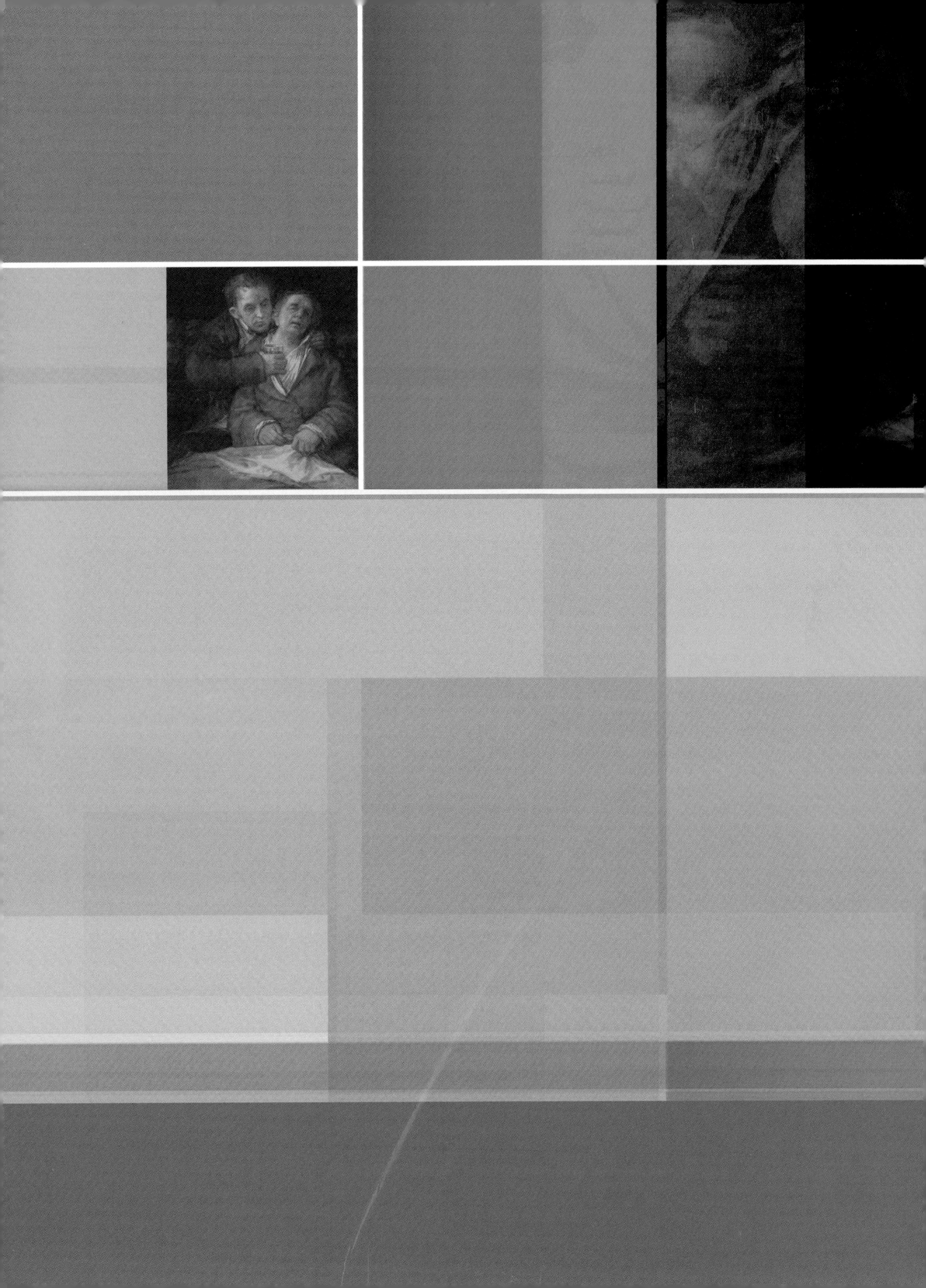

Declan Walsh, MD
Chair
Division of Post-Acute Medicine
Professor and Director
The Harry R. Horvitz Center for Palliative Medicine
Cleveland Clinic
Cleveland, Ohio

PALLIATIVE MEDICINE

Augusto T. Caraceni, MD
Director, "Virgilio Floriani" Hospice Unit
Rehabilitation and Palliative Care Department
National Cancer Institute
Milan, Italy

Robin Fainsinger, MD
Director/Professor
Department of Oncology
Division of Palliative Care Medicine
University of Alberta Faculty of Medicine
Director, Tertiary Palliative Care
Grey Nun's Hospital, Caritas Health Group
Clinical Director
Regional Palliative Care Program
Capital Health
Edmonton, Alberta, Canada

Kathleen Foley, MD
Professor of Neurology, Neuroscience, and
Clinical Pharmacology
Department of Neurology
Weill Medical College of Cornell University
Attending Neurologist
Neurology Pain and Palliative Care Service
Memorial Sloan-Kettering Cancer Center
Medical Director International Palliative
Care Initiative
Network Public Health Program
Open Society Institute
New York, New York

Paul Glare, MB BS, MM, FRACP
Clinical Associate Professor
Department of Medicine
University of Sydney Faculty of Medicine
Sydney, New South Wales, Australia
Head
Department of Palliative Care
Sydney Cancer Centre, Royal Prince Alfred Hospital
Camperdown, New South Wales, Australia

Cynthia Goh, PhD, FRCP, FAChPM
Associate Professor and Centre Director
Lien Centre for Palliative Care
Duke–National University of Singapore Medical School
Senior Consultant and Head
Department of Palliative Medicine
National Cancer Centre Singapore
Republic of Singapore

Mari Lloyd-Williams, MD, FRCP, MRCGP
Professor
Academic Palliative and Supportive Care Studies Group
University of Liverpool
Professor
Liverpool PCT and Royal Liverpool Hospital
Liverpool, United Kingdom

Juan Núñez Olarte, MD
Head
Palliative Care Unit
Hospital General Universitario Gregorio Marañón
Madrid, Spain

Lukas Radbruch, MD
Chair
Department of Palliative Medicine
RWTH Aachen University
Aachen, Germany

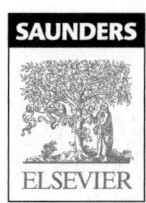

SAUNDERS

ELSEVIER

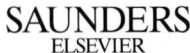

SAUNDERS
ELSEVIER

1600 John F. Kennedy Boulevard
Suite 1800
Philadelphia, PA 19103-2899

PALLIATIVE MEDICINE   ISBN: 978-0-323-05674-8 (Expert Consult)
978-0-323-04021-1 (Expert Consult Premium Ed.)

> **Notice**
>
> Knowledge and best practice in this field are constantly changing. As new research and experience broaden our knowledge, changes in practice, treatment, and drug therapy may become necessary or appropriate. Readers are advised to check the most current information provided (i) on procedures featured or (ii) by the manufacturer of each product to be administered to verify the recommended dose or formula, the method and duration of administration, and the contraindications. It is the responsibility of practitioners, relying on their own experience and knowledge of their patients, to make diagnoses, to determine dosages and the best treatment for each individual patient, and to take all appropriate safety precautions. To the fullest extent of the law, neither the Publisher nor the Editors assume any liability for any injury and/or damage to persons or property arising out of or related to any use of the material contained in this book.

Library of Congress Cataloging-in-Publication Data
Palliative medicine / T. Declan Walsh . . [et al.]. – 1st ed.
    p. ; cm.
    Includes bibliographical references.
    ISBN 978-0-323-05674-8 [Expert Consult]; 978-0-323-04021-1 [Expert Consult
    Premium Ed.]
    1. Palliative treatment. 2. Terminal care. I. Walsh, T. Declan
    [DNLM: 1. Palliative Care. 2. Hospices. 3. Psychology, Social. 4. Terminal
    Care–ethics. 5. Terminal Care. 6. Terminally Ill-psychology. WB 310 P16757 2008]
  R726.8.P3437 2009
  616′.029–dc22   2007040364

Acquisitions Editor: Kim Murphy
Developmental Editor: Catherine Carroll
Developmental Editor: Pamela Hetherington
Associate Developmental Editor: Julia Bartz
Publishing Services Manager: Frank Polizzano
Project Manager: Lee Ann Draud
Design Direction: Ellen Zanolle

Printed in Canada
Last digit is the print number: 9 8 7 6 5 4 3 2 1

Many people influenced me personally and stimulated my interest in palliative medicine.
We have included photographs of some of these individuals and institutions to honor their contribution to the field.
These are not meant to be comprehensive and, by definition, reflect my personal experiences.

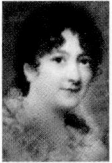

Mary Aikenhead (1787-1858)
Foundress of the Irish Sisters of Charity and Our Lady's Hospice, Dublin, Ireland

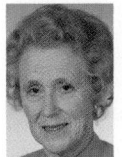

Mary Baines
Joined Dame Cicely Saunders at St. Christopher's Hospice in 1968; started the first Hospice Home Care service in 1969

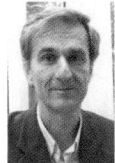

Eduardo Bruera
F. T. McGraw Chair in the Treatment of Cancer, Professor and Chair; Department of Palliative Care and Rehabilitation Medicine, University of Texas M. D. Anderson Cancer Center

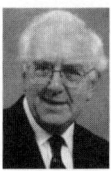

Derek Doyle
Retired Consultant, Senior Lecturer in Palliative Medicine, Edinburgh University. First Chairman of the Association for Palliative Medicine of Great Britain and Ireland

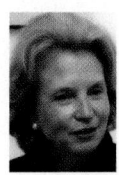

Kathleen Foley
Professor of Neurology, Neuroscience, and Clinical Pharmacology, Weill Medical College of Cornell University; Attending Neurologist; Memorial Sloan-Kettering Cancer Center

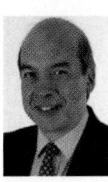

Geoffrey Hanks
Professor, Bristol Oncology Centre, Department of Palliative Medicine, University of Bristol

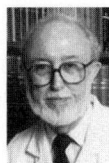

Ray Houde (1916-2006)
Pioneer in the study of clinical analgesics for chronic pain from cancer; Head of the Analgesic Studies Section at Memorial Sloan-Kettering Cancer Center

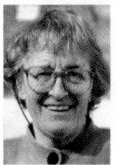

Elisabeth Kübler-Ross (1926-2004)
Psychiatrist, educator, and author of the groundbreaking book *On Death and Dying* (1969)

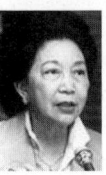

Josephina B. Magno (1920-2003)
Oncologist; founding member of the American Academy of Hospice and Palliative Medicine, and founder of the International Hospice Institute (now the International Association for Hospice and Palliative Care)

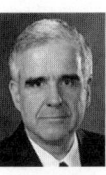

Balfour Mount
Emeritus Professor of Palliative Medicine, Department of Oncology, McGill University

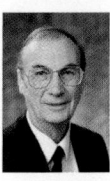

Colin Murray-Parkes, OBE, MD, FRCPsych
Consultant Psychiatrist Emeritus, St. Christopher's Hospice

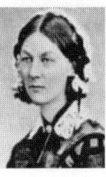

Florence Nightingale (1820-1910)
Pioneer of modern nursing and hospital planning; famous for her care of soldiers during the Crimean War

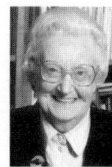

Dame Cicely Saunders (1918-2005)
Founder of the modern hospice movement; founder of St. Christopher's Hospice in 1967

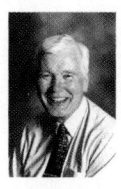

Robert Twycross
Emeritus Clinical Reader in Palliative Medicine, Oxford University

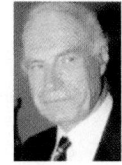

Vittorio Ventafridda
Scientific Director of the Floriani Foundation of Milan; President of the Italian School of Medicine and Palliative Care

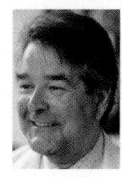

Tom West
Deputy Medical Director, St. Christopher's Hospice, 1973-1985; Medical Director, St. Christopher's Hospice, 1985-1993

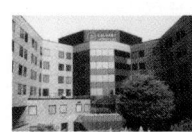

Calvary Hospital
Bronx, New York, and Brooklyn, New York

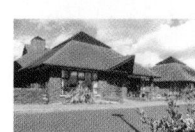

Our Lady's Hospice
Harold's Cross, Dublin, Ireland

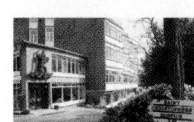

St. Christopher's Hospice
Sydenham, London, United Kingdom

PREFACE

I was first attracted to the concept of a new Palliative Medicine textbook by Elsevier because they are the preeminent international publisher of medical information. The use of a modern, attractive format supplemented by regular chapter updates (rather than a traditional textbook) stimulated my interest. The ability to have book content available and downloadable from the Internet was the deciding factor in my personal involvement. Elsevier's commitment to produce a truly international textbook in scope and stature thus made this a very exciting project. We realized this would be impossible without an expert and diverse group of Associate Editors. I was fortunate to recruit outstanding colleagues to the Editorial Board. We then gathered 403 authors from 23 countries and six continents. This international scope is a tribute to the sophistication of palliative medicine and the growing maturity of the field.

The Editorial Board established several important objectives for the structure and content of the book. One of these was a desire to produce an attractive and useful format not only for physicians, but also for nurses, social workers, and other professionals involved in the discipline of palliative medicine. We also realized that the book (and associated web content) should ideally serve as both a reference and a source of practical information for novices and experts in daily clinical practice in many countries. We endeavored to make the book as user-friendly as possible by extensive cross-referencing. Templates were used to help guide authors to structure their contributions. We wished to address the modern challenges facing medicine in general by directing attention to evidence-based medicine. We also asked authors to identify controversies and priority areas that require further research or other initiatives.

There were many challenges in completing such a large book, one of which is owing to the wide scope of chronic illness inherent in modern palliative medicine and the acuity and complexity of many of the illnesses with which we come into daily contact. Another issue was the inherent tension between evidence-based medicine and the recognition that in many areas of palliative medicine there is no "correct" way to proceed. Accordingly, we have allowed some overlap and repetition of approaches to some common problems in the knowledge that practices do vary internationally. In addition, the evidence base for much of what we do is woefully inadequate in many areas.

Much of our practice is based on the careful and insightful clinical observations of many colleagues from diverse disciplines. In some important areas (such as morphine use), the evidence base of the time did not support their clinical observations and practices, but they persevered and were proven to be correct—a cautionary tale.

I want to express my gratitude to the Editorial Board for all their hard work and commitment. I am grateful to the many distinguished clinicians around the world who have agreed to serve as Consultants to the book and web site. Eoin Tiernan (Dublin) and Ilora Findlay (Cardiff) were involved in the early stages. My colleague, Dr. Mitch Russell, will serve as the web master for the book web site. I am delighted that he has taken on this major responsibility. My thanks must also go to Lisa Clough and Karen Davey for their expert editorial assistance and long hours in helping the project to fruition.

The staff at Elsevier, including Cathy Carroll, Pamela Hetherington, and commissioning editor Kim Murphy, have been most helpful and have made our work much easier. The Editorial Board is most appreciative of their professional assistance throughout. From a national perspective, palliative medicine was finally recognized as a specialty in the United States in 2007; it is appropriate that we celebrate this by the completion of this textbook as the year closes. Palliative medicine has developed rapidly internationally. The time has come for our field to take its place among the major medical specialties in every country throughout the world; my hope is that this book will help that process.

I wish to extend a personal note of thanks to Lois Horvitz and her children, Michael, Peter, and Pam Schneider, for establishing The Harry R. Horvitz Center for Palliative Medicine in memory of her husband and their father, and for their support over so many years.

I would like to dedicate this book to Anne and Tom Walsh, to Cora, Richard, and Rory, and in particular to Conor who has faced a severe, life-long disability with great courage and dignity; he has taught me so much.

DECLAN WALSH

The Harry R. Horvitz Center
for Palliative Medicine
Cleveland, Ohio

INTERNATIONAL ADVISORY BOARD

*The Publisher wishes to acknowledge the following individuals,
who previewed advance materials for this first edition of Palliative Medicine*

CONTRIBUTORS

Judith A. Aberg, MD
Associate Professor of Medicine, New York University School of Medicine; Director of Virology, Bellevue Hospital Center, New York, New York
Complications of Acquired Immunodeficiency Syndrome

Amy P. Abernethy, MD
Assistant Professor of Medicine and Nursing, Duke University School of Medicine; Director, Duke Cancer Care Research Program, Duke University Medical Center, Durham, North Carolina
Evidence-Based Decision Making: Challenges and Opportunities; Modern Supportive Care in Oncology

Janet L. Abrahm, MD
Associate Professor of Medicine, Harvard Medical School; Director, Pain and Palliative Care Program and Palliative Care Fellowship, Dana-Farber Cancer Institute and Brigham and Women's Hospital, Boston, Massachusetts
Nausea, Vomiting, and Early Satiety

Michael Adolph, MD
Assistant Clinical Professor of Medicine and Surgery, Pain and Palliative Medicine Service, James Cancer Hospital and Solove Research Institute, Ohio State University Medical Center, Columbus, Ohio
Cancer Pain: Anesthetic and Neurosurgical Interventions

Michael Aherne, MEd
Director, Initiative Development, The Pallium Project, University of Alberta, Edmonton, Alberta, Canada
Adult Learning

K. Allsopp
Department of Palliative Care, Sydney Cancer Centre, Concord Hospital, Concord, New South Wales, Australia
Consultation Services

Rogelio Altisent, MD
Associate Professor of Bioethics, Faculty of Medicine, University of Zaragoza, Zaragoza, Spain
Making Good Decisions

Carmen Fernandez Alvarez, MD
Radiologist, Hospital General Universitario Gregorio Marañón, Madrid, Spain
Computed Tomography Scanning and Magnetic Resonance Imaging in Palliative Care

Pablo Amigo, MD
Assistant Clinical Professor, Division of Palliative Care Medicine, Department of Oncology, University of Alberta Faculty of Medicine; Tertiary Palliative Care Unit, Grey Nuns Community Hospital, Edmonton, Alberta, Canada
Cough, Hemoptysis, and Bronchorrhea

Wendy G. Anderson, MD, MS
Assistant Professor, University of California, San Francisco, School of Medicine, San Francisco, California
Withholding and Withdrawing Treatment

Sik Kim Ang, MD
Palliative Medicine Clinical Fellow, Cleveland Clinic, Cleveland, Ohio
History and Physical Examination; Tenesmus, Strangury, and Malodor

Tiziana Antonelli, MD
Associate Professor of Pharmacology, Department of Clinical and Experimental Medicine, University of Ferrara School of Medicine, Ferrara, Italy
Psychotropic Drugs

John Armstrong, MD, FRCPI
Professor of Radiation Oncology, University College Dublin; Consultant Radiation Oncologist and Director of Research, St. Luke's Hospital, Dublin, Ireland
Radiation Principles and Techniques

Wendy S. Armstrong, MD
Co-Director of HIV Care, Department of Infectious Diseases, Cleveland Clinic Foundation, Cleveland, Ohio
Acquired Immunodeficiency Syndrome: A Global Perspective

Robert M. Arnold, MD
Professor, Department of Medicine, and Leo H. Criep
Chair of Patient Care, Division of General Internal
Medicine, Section of Palliative Care and Medical
Ethics; Chief, Center for Bioethics and Health Law,
Institute to Enhance Palliative Care, and Institute
for Doctor-Patient Communication, University of
Pittsburgh School of Medicine, Pittsburgh,
Pennsylvania
Withholding and Withdrawing Treatment

Pilar Arranz
Section of Psychology, Service of Hematology and
Hemotherapy, Hospital Universitario La Paz,
Madrid, Spain
Denial and Decision-Making Capacity

Koen Augustyns, Dr. Pharmaceutical Sciences
Professor in Medicinal Chemistry, University of
Antwerp, Antwerp, Belgium
Principles of Pharmacology

Isabel Barreiro-Meiro Sáenz-Diez, MD
Radiologist, Hospital General Universitario Gregorio
Marañón, Madrid, Spain
*Computed Tomography Scanning and Magnetic Resonance Imaging
in Palliative Care*

Pilar Barreto
Madrid, Spain
Denial and Decision-Making Capacity

Debra Barton, PhD, RN
Associate Professor of Oncology, Mayo Clinic,
Rochester, Minnesota
Premature Menopause

Ursula Bates, MA
Occasional Lecturer, College of Human Sciences,
School of Psychotherapy, University College
Dublin; Director of Psychosocial and Bereavement
Services and Principal Clinical Psychologist,
Blackrock Hospice, Dublin, Ireland
Psychiatrists and Clinical Psychologists

Jacinto Bátiz, MD
Director of Palliative Care Unit, Hospital San Juan de
Dios, Bilbao, Spain
Making Good Decisions

Costantino Benedetti, MD
Clinical Professor, Department of Anesthesiology, The
Ohio State University College of Medicine,
Columbus, Ohio
Cancer Pain: Anesthetic and Neurosurgical Interventions

Nabila Bennani-Baiti, MD
Research Fellow, Taussig Cancer Institute, Cleveland
Clinic, Cleveland, Ohio
*Priorities for the Future: The Research Agenda; Bleeding and Clotting
Disorders in Cancer*

Michael I. Bennett, MB ChB, MD, FRCP
Professor of Palliative Medicine, International
Observatory on End of Life Care, Institute for
Health Research, Lancaster University, Lancaster,
United Kingdom
Assessment of Mobility

Kevin Berger, MD, MB BCh
Pediatric Medical Director, Hospice of the Valley;
Partner, Phoenix Pediatrics, Phoenix, Arizona
Hospice and Special Services

Mamta Bhatnagar, MD
Assistant Professor of Medicine, Department of
Medicine, University of Pittsburgh School of
Medicine; Attending Physician, Palliative Medicine,
University of Pittsburgh Medical Center, Pittsburgh,
Pennsylvania
The Frail Elderly

Lesley Bicanovsky, DO
Associate Staff, Department of Obstetrics and
Gynecology, Cleveland Clinic Lorain Family Health
and Surgery Center, Lorain, Ohio
Comfort Care: Symptom Control in the Dying

Lynda Blue, BSc, RGN, SCM, NFESC
Co-ordinator, Glasgow Heart Failure Liaison Service,
Western Infirmary, Glasgow, United Kingdom
Heart Failure

Barton Bobb, MSN, APRN
Department of Hematology/Oncology and Palliative
Medicine, Virginia Commonwealth University
Medical Center, Richmond, Virginia
Fever and Sweats

Jean-Jacques Body, MD, PhD
Professor of Medicine and Head of Department,
Institut Jules Bordet, Université Libre de Bruxelles,
Brussels, Belgium
Drugs for Hypercalcemia

Gian Domenico Borasio, MD, Dip Pall Med
Chair in Palliative Medicine and Head, Motor Neurone
Disease Research Group, Department of Neurology,
University of Munich; Interdisciplinary Center for
Palliative Medicine, Munich University Hospital,
Munich, Germany
Amyotrophic Lateral Sclerosis

Claudia Borreani, PhD
Director, Psychology Unit, National Cancer Institute
Foundation, Milan, Italy
Caregiver Burden

Federico Bozzetti, MD
Head, Department of Surgery, Hospital of Prato, Prato,
Italy
Principles and Management of Nutritional Support in Cancer

Valentina Bozzetti, MD
Department of Pediatrics, Università Vita e Salute, Ospedale San Raffaele, Milan, Italy
Principles and Management of Nutritional Support in Cancer

Jason Braybrooke, MB ChB, FRSCE
Orthopedic Consultant, University Hospitals of Leicester NHS Trust, Leicester, United Kingdom
Palliative Orthopedic Surgery

William Breitbart, MD
Professor of Clinical Psychiatry, Weill Medical College of Cornell University; Chief, Psychiatry Service, Department of Psychiatry and Behavioral Sciences, Memorial Sloan-Kettering Cancer Center, New York, New York
The Desire for Death

Barry Bresnihan, MD, FRCP
Professor of Rheumatology, University College Dublin; Consultant Rheumatologist, St. Vincent's University Hospital, Dublin, Ireland
Musculoskeletal Disorders

Bert Broeckaert, PhD
Coordinator, Interdisciplinary Centre for Religious Study, Catholic University, Leuven, Belgium
Euthanasia and Physician-Assisted Suicide

Eduardo Bruera, MD
Department of Palliative Care and Rehabilitative Medicine, The University of Texas M. D. Anderson Cancer Center, Houston, Texas
Symptom Research

Kay Brune, MD, PhD
Doerenkamp Professor, Department of Experimental and Clinical Pharmacology and Toxicology, Friedrich-Alexander-University, Erlangen-Nuremberg, Germany
Nonsteroidal Anti-inflammatory Drugs

Bradley Buckhout, MD
Kent Institute of Medicine and Health Sciences, University of Kent; Wisdom Hospice, Kent, United Kingdom
Quadriplegia and Paraplegia

Phyllis N. Butow, PhD, MPH
Professor, School of Psychology, and Co-Director, Centre of Medical Psychology and Evidence-Based Decision Making, University of Sydney Faculty of Medicine, Sydney, New South Wales, Australia
Telling the Truth: Bad News

Ira Byock, MD, FAAHPM
Professor of Anesthesiology and Community & Family Medicine, Dartmouth Medical School, Hanover; Director of Palliative Medicine, Dartmouth Hitchcock Medical Center, Lebanon, New Hampshire
Principles of Palliative Medicine

Anthony Byrne, MB, FRCP
Honorary Senior Lecturer, School of Medicine, Cardiff University, Cardiff; Consultant in Palliative Medicine, Marie Curie Cancer Care, Marie Curie Hospice, Penarth, Wales
Design and Conduct of Research and Clinical Trials

Clare Byrne, MSc, RN
Advanced Nurse Practitioner, Hepatobiliary Cancer Service, University Hospital Aintree, Liverpool, United Kingdom
Patterns of Metastatic Cancer

Beryl E. Cable-Williams, MN, RN
Faculty, Trent/Fleming School of Nursing, Trent University, Peterborough, Ontario, Canada
Death in Modern Society

Sarah E. Callin, MB ChB, FRCP
Specialist Registrar in Palliative Medicine, St. Gemma's Hospice, Leeds, United Kingdom
Assessment of Mobility

David Casarett, MD, MA
Associate Professor, University of Pennsylvania School of Medicine; Physician, Philadelphia Veterans Affairs Medical Center, Philadelphia, Pennsylvania
Principles of Bioethics

David Casper
Research Assistant, Department of Psychiatry and Behavioral Sciences, Memorial Sloan-Kettering Cancer Center, New York, New York
Opioid Use in Drug and Alcohol Abuse

Eric J. Cassell, MD
Clinical Professor of Public Health, Weill Medical College of Cornell University, New York, New York; Adjunct Professor of Medicine, McGill University Faculty of Medicine, Montreal, Quebec, Canada
Suffering

Barrie Cassileth, PhD, MS
Chief, Integrative Medicine Service , Memorial Sloan-Kettering Cancer Center, New York, New York
Integrative Medicine: Complementary Therapies

Emanuele Castagno, MD
Attending Physician, Department of Pediatrics, University of Turin; Regina Margherita Children's Hospital, Turin, Italy
Cancer in Children

Carlos Centeno, MD, PhD
Associate Professor of Palliative Care, Faculty of Medicine, University of Nevarra; Palliative Medicine Consultant, University of Nevarra Clinic, Pamplona, Spain
Development of National and International Standards

Walter Ceranski, MD
Kent Institute of Medicine and Health Sciences, University of Kent; Wisdom Hospice, Kent, United Kingdom
Quadriplegia and Paraplegia

Lucas Ceulemans, MD
Department of General Practice, University of Antwerp, Antwerp; General Practitioner and Palliative Consultant, Palliatief Netwerk Mechelen, Mechelen, Belgium
Nutrition in Palliative Medicine

Meghna Chadha, MD
Radiology Institute, Cleveland Clinic, Cleveland, Ohio
Interventional Radiology

Bruce H. Chamberlain, MD, FACP, FAAHPM
Director, Palliative Consultations, and Chief Medical Officer, Harmony Home Health and Hospice, Murray, Utah
Airway Obstruction

Eric L. Chang, MD
Department of Radiation Oncology, The University of Texas M. D. Anderson Cancer Center, Houston, Texas
Vertebral Metastases and Spinal Cord Compression

Victor T. Chang, MD, FACP
Associate Professor of Medicine, University of Medicine & Dentistry of New Jersey, Newark; Senior Attending Physician, Section of Hematology Oncology, Veterans Affairs New Jersey Health Care System, East Orange, New Jersey
Qualitative and Quantitative Symptom Assessment

Harvey Max Chochinov, MD, PhD
Professor, Departments of Psychiatry, Family Medicine (Division of Palliative Care), and Community Health Sciences, and Tier 1 Canada Research Chair in Palliative Care, University of Manitoba Faculty of Medicine; Director, Manitoba Palliative Care Research Unit, CancerCare Manitoba, Winnipeg, Manitoba, Canada
Depression

Edward Chow, MB BS, PhD, FRCPC
Associate Professor, University of Toronto Faculty of Medicine; Radiation Oncologist, Odette Cancer Centre, Sunnybrook Health Sciences Center, Toronto, Ontario, Canada
Palliative Radiation Therapy; Palliative Orthopedic Surgery

Grace Christ, DSW
Professor of Social Work, Columbia University of School of Social Work, New York, New York
Parent and Child Bereavement

Katherine Clark, MB BS, FRACP, FAChPM
School of Medicine, The University of Notre Dame Australia; Senior Lecturer and Senior Staff Specialist, Cunningham Centre for Palliative Care, Sacred Heart Facility, St. Vincent's Master Health, Sydney, New South Wales, Australia
Emergencies in Palliative Medicine

Stephen Clarke, MB BS, PhD, FRACP
Professor of Medicine, University of Sydney Faculty of Medicine; Senior Staff Specialist in Medical Oncology and Head of Pharmacology, Sydney Cancer Centre, Concord, New South Wales, Australia
Clinical Nutrition

Josephine M. Clayton, PhD, MB BS (hons)
Senior Lecturer and Cancer Institute New South Wales Clinical Research Fellow, University of Sydney Faculty of Medicine, Sydney; Head of Department and Staff Specialist, Department of Palliative Care, Royal North Shore Hospital, St. Leonard's, New South Wales, Australia
Telling the Truth: Bad News

James F. Cleary, MD
Director, Palliative Medicine Program, and Program Leader, Cancer Control Program, Paul P. Carbone Comprehensive Cancer Center, University of Wisconsin School of Medicine and Public Health; Palliative Care Program, University of Wisconsin Comprehensive Cancer Center, Madison, Wisconsin
Epidemiology of Cancer

Lawrence J. Clein, MB, BS, FRCSC, ABHPM
Clinical Professor of Family Medicine, University of Saskatchewan College of Medicine, Saskatoon; Medical Director, Palliative Care Services, Regina Qu'Appelle Health Region, Regina, Saskatchewan, Canada
Edema

Katri Elina Clemens, MD, PhD
Department of Science and Research, Centre for Palliative Medicine, University of Bonn; Department of Anesthesiology, Intensive Care, Palliative Medicine and Pain Therapy, Malteser Hospital Bonn, Bonn, Germany
The History of Hospice

Libby Clemens, APN
Symptom Care Team, Blount Memorial Hospital, Maryville, Tennessee
Palliative Sedation

Robert Colebunders, MD, PhD
Professor of Infectious Diseases, Institute of Tropical Medicine and University of Antwerp, Antwerp, Belgium
Fatal and Fulminant Infections; Biology and Natural History of Acquired Immunodeficiency Syndrome

Steven R. Connor, PhD
Vice President for Research and International Development, National Hospice and Palliative Care Organization, Alexandria, Virginia

Palliative Medicine in Institutions

Viviane Conraads, MD, PhD
Professor, Head Lecturer, Department of Medicine, University of Antwerp, Wilrijk-Antwerp; Cardiologist and Deputy Head, Department of Cardiology, University Hospital, Antwerp, Belgium

Cardiac Function Testing

Colm Cooney, MD, FRCPI, MRCPsych
Lecturer, University College Dublin; Consultant Psychogeriatrician, St. Vincent's University Hospital, Dublin, Ireland

The Aging Brain and Dementia

Massimo Costantini, MD
Visiting Professor in Palliative Care, Department of Palliative Care, Policy, and Rehabilitation, King's College, London; Regional Palliative Care Network, National Cancer Research Institute, Genoa, Italy

Health Services Research

Azucena Couceiro, MD, PhD
Professor of Bioethics and History of Medicine, Universidad Autónoma de Madrid, Madrid, Spain

Ethics and Clinical Practice

Holly Covington, PhD, RN, FNP
Advanced Nurse Practitioner, West Slope Mental Health Stabilization Center, Grand Junction, Colorado

Psychological and Psychiatric Approaches

John D. Cowan, MD
Medical Director, Palliative Care Hospice, Blount Memorial Hospital, Maryville; Medical Director, Palliative Care, University of Tennessee Medical Center, Knoxville, Tennessee

Palliative Sedation

Patrick Coyne, MSN, RN
Virginia Commonwealth University Medical Center, Richmond, Virginia

Fever and Sweats

Garnet Crawford, MD, CCFP
Lecturer, Department of Family Medicine, University of Manitoba Faculty of Medicine; Consultant in Palliative Medicine, Winnipeg Regional Health Authority, Winnipeg, Manitoba, Canada

Laxatives

Brian Creedon, MB BCh, BAO, MRCPI
Medical Tutor, University College Dublin and Trinity College Dublin; Medical Tutor, Education and Research Department, Our Lady's Hospice, Dublin, Ireland

Opioid Side Effects and Overdose

Hilary Cronin, MB, BAO, BCh, MRCPI
Senior Lecturer, Medical Gerontology, and Research Fellow, Trinity College Dublin; Senior Lecturer, Medical Gerontology, St. James's Hospital, Dublin, Ireland

Biology and Physiology of Aging

Garret Cullen, MB BCh, MRCPI
Specialist Registrar in Gastroenterology, St. Vincent's University Hospital, Dublin, Ireland

Gastrointestinal Endoscopy

Jennifer E. Cummings, MD
Director, Electrophysiology Research, Cleveland Clinic Foundation, Cleveland, Ohio

Arrhythmias

David C. Currow, B Med, MPH, FRACP
Professor, Department of Palliative and Supportive Services, Flinders University School of Medicine, Adelaide, South Australia, Australia

Emergencies in Palliative Medicine; Evidence-Based Decision Making: Challenges and Opportunities

Paul J. Daeninck, MD, MSc, FRCPC
Assistant Professor, Departments of Internal Medicine and Family Medicine, University of Manitoba Faculty of Medicine; Site Coordinator, Symptom Management Disease Site Chair, Taché Site, CancerCare Manitoba/Winnipeg Regional Health Authority, Winnipeg, Manitoba, Canada

Laxatives

Pamela Dalinis, MA, RN
Director, Education, Midwest Palliative and Hospice CareCenter, Glenview, Illinois

Curriculum Development

Prajnan Das, MD, MPH
Department of Radiation Oncology, The University of Texas M. D. Anderson Cancer Center, Houston, Texas

Vertebral Metastases and Spinal Cord Compression

Mellar P. Davis, MD, FCCP
Director of Research, Palliative Medicine, The Harry R. Horvitz Center for Palliative Medicine, Taussig Cancer Center, Cleveland Clinic, Cleveland, Ohio

Determination of Nutrition and Hydration; Neuropharmacology and Psychopharmacology

Sara N. Davison, MD, MSc, FRCPC
Associate Professor of Medicine, Division of Nephrology and Immunology, University of Alberta Faculty of Medicine, Edmonton, Alberta, Canada

Kidney Failure

Catherine Deamant, MD
Assistant Professor, Rush Medical College of Rush University; Director, Palliative Care Program, John H. Stroger, Jr., Hospital of Cook County, Chicago, Illinois
Curriculum Development

Liliana de Lima, MD, MHA
Director, International Association for Hospice and Palliative Care, Houston, Texas
Program Development: An International Perspective

Conor P. Delany, MD, PhD, FRCSI, FACS
Professor of Surgery, and Chief, Division of Colorectal Surgery, Case Western Reserve University, University Hospitals Case Medical Center, Cleveland, Ohio
Stomas and Fistulas

Peter Demeulenaere, MD
Assistant Teaching, Department of Family Medicine and Palliative Care, University of Antwerp; Medical Staff, Palliative Care Unit, Sint-Augustinus General Hospital, Antwerp, Belgium
Malignant Ascites

Lena Dergham, MD
Hospitalist, Lutheran Hospital, Cleveland, Ohio
Body Image and Sexuality

Noël Derycke, MD
Department of General Practice, University of Antwerp; General Practitioner and Palliative Consultant, Palliatieve Hulpverlening Antwerpen, Antwerp, Belgium
Nutrition in Palliative Medicine

Rajeev Dhupar, MD
Resident, General Surgery, University of Pittsburgh Medical Center, Pittsburgh, Pennsylvania
Palliative Management of Airway Obstruction: Tracheostomy and Airway Stents

Mario Dicato, MD, FRCP (Edin)
Professor of Internal Medicine, Luxembourg Medical Center; Head, Department of Hematology and Oncology, Centre Hospitalier Luxembourg, Luxembourg City, Luxembourg
The Vena Cava Syndrome

Edwin D. Dickerson, PhD, MSc, MBA
Boehringer Ingelheim Pharmaceuticals, Inc., Ridgefield, Connecticut
Interactions, Side Effects, and Management

Andrew Dickman, MD
Senior Clinical Pharmacist, Marie Curie Hospice, Liverpool, United Kingdom
The Role of the Clinical Pharmacist

Maria Dietrich, Diplom-Heilpädagogin, MA
Department of Communication Science and Disorders, University of Pittsburgh School of Health and Rehabilitation Sciences, Pittsburgh, Pennsylvania
Autonomic Dysfunction

Pamela Dixon
Rehabilitation Manager, Physical Medicine and Rehabilitation, Cleveland Clinic, Cleveland, Ohio
Occupational and Physical Therapy

Philip C. Dodd, MB BCh, BAO, MSc, MRCPsych
Lecturer in the Psychiatry of Intellectual Disability, Department of Psychiatry, University of Dublin, Trinity College; Consultant General Adult Psychiatrist, St. Michael's House; Research Associate, Centre for Disability Studies, University College Dublin, Dublin, Ireland
Congenital Intellectual Disability

James T. D'Olimpio, MD
Assistant Professor of Medicine, New York University School of Medicine, New York; Director, Supportive/Palliative Care Programs in Oncology; Cancer Pain and Symptom Management Services; Don Monti Division of Medical Oncology and Division of Hematology, North Shore University Hospital, Manhasset, New York
Physiology of Nutrition and Aging

Per Dombernowsky, MD, DMSci
Emeritus Associate Professor, University of Copenhagen, Copenhagen; Department of Oncology, Herlev University Hospital, Herlev, Denmark
Complications of Chemotherapy

Michael Dooley, BPharm, DipPharm
Professor of Clinical Pharmacy, Department of Pharmacy Practice, Victorian College of Pharmacy, Monash University, Parkville; Director of Pharmacy, Bayside Health, Melbourne, Victoria, Australia
Prescribing

Deborah Dudgeon, MD, FRCPC
W. Ford Connell Professor of Palliative Care Medicine and Professor of Medicine and Oncology, Departments of Medicine and Oncology, Queen's University School of Medicine, Kingston; Director, Palliative Care Medicine Program, Queen's University, Kingston; Provincial Program Head, Palliative Care, Cancer Care Ontario, Toronto, Ontario, Canada
Dyspnea

Geoffrey P. Dunn, MD, FACS
Attending Physician, Department of Surgery; Medical Director, Palliative Care Consultation Service, Hamot Medical Center, Erie, Pennsylvania
Palliative Surgery

David Dunwoodie, MB BS, FRACP
  Consultant Physician, Sir Charles Gairdner Hospital, Perth, Western Australia, Australia

  Antiemetic Drugs

Jane Eades, RN, BA(Hons), DipN
  Clinical Nurse Specialist, Marie Curie Hospice Hampstead, London, United Kingdom

  Rehabilitation Approaches

Badi El Osta, MD
  Department of Palliative Care and Rehabilitative Medicine, The University of Texas M. D. Anderson Cancer Center, Houston, Texas

  Symptom Research

Katja Elbert-Avila, MD
  Medical Instructor, Department of Medicine, Duke University Medical Center, Durham, North Carolina

  Problems in Communication

John Ellershaw, MA, FRCP
  Professor of Palliative Medicine, University of Liverpool; Director, Marie Curie Palliative Care Institute Liverpool, Liverpool, United Kingdom

  Standards of Care

Bassam Estfan, MD
  Clinical Associate, Palliative Medicine Staff, Cleveland Clinic Foundation, Cleveland, Ohio

  Persistent or Repeated Hemorrhage; Antacids; Bronchodilators and Cough Suppressants; Indigestion; Respiratory Failure

Louise Exton, MB BS, MRCP, MSc
  Consultant in Palliative Medicine, Harris HospisCare, Caritas House, Kent, United Kingdom

  Corticosteroids

Alysa Fairchild, BSc, PGDip(Epi), MD, FRCPC
  Assistant Professor, Department of Radiation Oncology, University of Alberta Faculty of Medicine; Clinical Leader, RAPRP, Department of Radiation Oncology, Cross Cancer Institute, Edmonton, Alberta, Canada

  Palliative Radiation Therapy

Matthew Farrelly, PhD, MSW
  Co-ordinator of Social Work and Bereavement Services, St. Francis Hospice, Dublin, Ireland

  Families in Distress

Konrad Fassbender, PhD
  Assistant Professor, Division of Palliative Care Medicine, University of Alberta Faculty of Medicine and Dentistry, Edmonton, Alberta, Canada

  Evidence-Based Economic Evaluation

Jason Faulhaber, MD
  Clinical Instructor, Harvard Medical School; Medical Provider, Fenway Community Health, Boston, Massachusetts

  Complications of Acquired Immunodeficiency Syndrome

Kenneth C. H. Fearon, MB ChB (Hons), MD, FRCS (Glas), FRCS (Ed), FRCS (Eng)
  Professor of Surgical Oncology, Department of Clinical and Surgical Sciences (Surgery), University of Edinburgh, Royal Infirmary, Edinburgh, United Kingdom

  The Anorexia-Cachexia Syndrome

Lynda E. Fenelon, MD, FRCPI, FRCPath
  Consultant Microbiologist, University College Dublin; Consultant Microbiologist, St. Vincent's University Hospital, Dublin, Ireland

  Prevention and Control of Infections

Peter F. Ferson, MD
  Professor of Surgery, University of Pittsburgh School of Medicine; Professor of Surgery, University of Pittsburgh Medical Center, Pittsburgh, Pennsylvania

  Palliative Management of Airway Obstruction: Tracheostomy and Airway Stents

Petra Feyer, MD
  Klinik für Strahlentherapie, Radioonkologie und Nuklearmedizin, Vivantes—Netzwerk fur Gesundheit, Berlin, Germany

  Nuclear Medicine

Marilene Filbet, MD
  Chief, Palliative Care Unit, Centre Hospitalo-Universitaire de Lyon, Hôpital de la Croix Rousse, Lyon, France

  Symptom Management

Pam Firth, CSW, ASW
  Head of Family Support and Deputy Director of Hospice Services, Isabel Hospice, Welwyn Garden City, United Kingdom; Board Member of the European Association for Palliative Care, Milan, Italy

  Spiritual Distress

Susan F. FitzGerald, MD, MPH, MRCPI, MRCPath
  Special Lecturer in Microbiology, University College Dublin; Clinical Microbiologist, St. Vincent's University Hospital, Dublin, Ireland

  Prevention and Control of Infections

Hugh D. Flood MCh, FRCSI
  Consultant Urologist, Department of Urology, Mid-Western Regional Hospital, Limerick, Ireland

  Incontinence: Urine and Stool

Francesca Crippa Floriani, MD
  President, Italian Federation for Palliative Care; President, Associazione Amici Fondazione Floriani, Milan, Italy

  Public Advocacy and Community Outreach

Paul J. Ford, PhD
Assistant Professor, Division of Medicine, Cleveland Clinic Lerner College of Medicine of Case Western Reserve University; Associate Staff (Bioethics and Neurology), Cleveland Clinic, Cleveland, Ohio

Palliative Medicine and the Ethics Consultant

Barry Fortner, PhD
Adjunct, Department of Graduate Psychology, University of Memphis, Memphis, Tennessee; Senior Vice President, Scientific Affairs and Provider Services, P4 Healthcare, Ellicott City, Maryland

Modern Supportive Care in Oncology

Darlene Foth, MA, ATR-BC, LSW
Adjunct Faculty, Ursuline College, Pepper Pike; Art Therapist, University Hospitals of Cleveland, Cleveland, Ohio

Music and Art Therapists

Bridget Fowler, PharmD
Clinical Assistant Professor, Department of Pharmacy Practice, Bouve College of Health Sciences, Northeastern University; Clinical Pharmacy Specialist, Pain and Palliative Care Program, Dana-Farber Cancer Institute, Boston, Massachusetts

Nausea, Vomiting, and Early Satiety

Karen Frame, MB BS, MSc, MRCP, DTM&H
Specialist Registrar, Palliative Medicine, Hospice Africa Uganda, Kampala, Uganda, and Michael Sobell House, Mount Vernon Hospital, Northwood, Middlesex, United Kingdom

Fatal and Fulminant Infections; Biology and Natural History of Acquired Immunodeficiency Syndrome

Thomas G. Fraser, MD, FACP
Assistant Professor of Medicine, Cleveland Clinic Lerner College of Medicine of Case Western Reserve University; Department of Infectious Disease, Healthcare Epidemiology Office, Quality and Patient Safety Institute, Cleveland Clinic, Cleveland, Ohio

Antimicrobial Use in the Dying

Fred Frost, MD
Associate Professor of Medicine, Cleveland Clinic Lerner College of Medicine of Case Western Reserve University; Director of Hospital Rehabilitation Services, Cleveland Clinic, Cleveland, Ohio

Stroke

Michael J. Fulham, MB BS, FRACP
Professor, Department of Medicine, Faculty of Medicine, University of Sydney Faculty of Medicine; Adjunct Professor, School of Information Technologies, University of Sydney Faculty of Medicine; Director, Molecular Imaging, and Clinical Director for Medical Imaging, Royal Prince Alfred Hospital, Sydney, New South Wales, Australia

Positron Emission Tomography

Pierre R. Gagnon, MD, FRCPC
Associate Professor, Laval University Faculty of Pharmacy; Psychiatrist, L'Hôtel-Dieu de Québec; Director of Research, Maison Michel-Sarrazin; and Researcher, Centre de Recherche Université Laval Robert-Giffard, Quebec City, Quebec, Canada

Delirium and Psychosis

Lisa M. Gallagher, MA, MT
Adjunct Faculty, Cleveland Music Therapy Consortium; Music Therapist, The Harry R. Horvitz Center for Palliative Medicine, Cleveland Clinic, Cleveland, Ohio

Music and Art Therapists

Maureen Gambles, BSc
Senior Research Fellow, Marie Curie Palliative Care Institute Liverpool, Liverpool, United Kingdom

Standards of Care

Subhasis K. Giri, MCh, FRCSEd, FRCSI
Senior Specialist Registrar, Department of Urology and Renal Transplantation, Beaumont Hospital, Dublin, Ireland

Incontinence: Urine and Stool

Paul Glare, MB BS, MM, FRACP
Clinical Associate Professor, Department of Medicine, University of Sydney Faculty of Medicine, Sydney; Head, Department of Palliative Care, Sydney Cancer Centre, Royal Prince Alfred Hospital, Camperdown, New South Wales, Australia

Principles of Palliative Medicine Research; Consultation Services; Determining Prognosis; Antiemetic Drugs

Cynthia R. Goh, PhD, FRCP, FAChPM
Associate Professor and Centre Director, Lien Centre for Palliative Care, Duke–National University of Singapore Medical School; Senior Consultant and Head, Department of Palliative Medicine, National Cancer Centre Singapore, Republic of Singapore

Culture, Ethnicity, and Illness

Xavier Gómez-Batiste, MD, PhD
Corporative Director of Education and Training, Institut Català d'Oncologia, University of Barcelona and L'Hospitalet de Llobregat; Director, World Health Organization Centre for Public Health Palliative Care Programmes, Barcelona, Spain

Palliative Medicine—The Global Perspective: Closing the Know-Do Gap; Palliative Medicine: Models of Organization; Program Development: Palliative Medicine and Public Health Services; Acute Palliative Medicine Units

Leah Gramlich, MD
Associate Professor, University of Alberta Faculty of Medicine; Chief, Division of Gastroenterology, Royal Alexandra Hospital; Medical Director, Regional Nutrition Services, Capital Health, Edmonton, Alberta, Canada

The Nutrition Support Team

Luigi Grassi, MD
Professor and Chair of Psychiatry, Section of Clinical
Psychiatry, University of Ferrara School of
Medicine; Director, University Psychiatry Unit, S.
Anna University Hospital, Ferrara, Italy
Psychotropic Drugs

Phyllis A. Grauer, PharmD
Marie Curie Hospice, Liverpool, United Kingdom
The Role of the Clinical Pharmacist

Claire Green, MSc, PhD
Christie Hospital, Manchester, United Kingdom
Good Communication: Patients, Families, and Professionals

Gareth Griffiths
Marie Curie Palliative Care Institute, Marie Curie
Hospice, Liverpool, United Kingdom
Design and Conduct of Research and Clinical Trials

Yvona Griffo, MD
Neurologist, Pain and Palliative Care Service,
Memorial Sloan-Kettering Cancer Center,
New York, New York
Neurological Complications

Hunter Groninger, MD
Assistant Professor, Medical Education, University of
Virginia School of Medicine, Charlottesville,
Virginia; Senior Medical Director, Capital Hospice;
Consulting Physician, Capital Palliative Care
Consultants, Washington, DC
Seizures and Movement Disorders

David A. Gruenewald, MD
Associate Professor of Medicine, Division of
Gerontology and Geriatric Medicine, University of
Washington School of Medicine; Medical Director,
Palliative Care and Hospice Service, Geriatrics and
Extended Care Service, Veterans Affairs Puget
Sound Health Care System, Seattle, Washington
Multiple Sclerosis

Jyothirmai Gubili, MS
Assistant Editor, Integrative Medicine Service,
Memorial Sloan-Kettering Cancer Center,
New York, New York
Integrative Medicine: Complementary Therapies

Terence L. Gutgsell, MD
Cleveland Clinic, Cleveland Ohio
History and Physical Examination; Principles of Symptom Control

Elizabeth Gwyther, MD
Senior Lecturer in Palliative Medicine, University of
Cape Town, Cape Town, South Africa
*Palliative Care for Children and Adolescents with Human
Immunodeficiency Virus/Acquired Immunodeficiency Syndrome*

Paul S. Haber, MD, FRACP, FAChAM
School of Public Health, University of Sydney Faculty
of Medicine; Drug Health Services, Royal Prince
Alfred Hospital, Sydney, New South Wales,
Australia
Alcohol and Drug Abuse

Achiel Haemers, Dr. Pharmaceutical Sciences
Professor of Pharmacology, University of Antwerp,
Antwerp, Belgium
Principles of Pharmacology

Mindi C. Haley, BA
Research Assistant, Pharmacy Practice and Science,
University of Kentucky College of Medicine,
Lexington, Kentucky
Opioid Use in Drug and Alcohol Abuse

Mazen A. Hanna, MD
Associate Staff, Section of Heart Failure and Cardiac
Transplant, Cleveland Clinic, Cleveland, Ohio
Diuretics

Janet R. Hardy, MD, FRACP
Professor in Palliative Medicine, University of
Queensland; Director of Palliative Care, Mater
Health Services, Brisbane, Queensland, Australia
*Principles of Palliative Medicine Research; Opioids; Opioids for
Cancer Pain*

Jodie Haselkorn, MD, MPH
Associate Professor of Rehabilitation Medicine,
University of Washington School of Medicine;
Adjunct Associate Professor of Epidemiology,
University of Washington School of Public Health;
Director, MS Center of Excellence West, Veterans
Affairs Puget Sound Health Care System, Seattle,
Washington
Multiple Sclerosis

Katherine Hauser, MB BS (Hons), FRACGP
Research Fellow, The Harry R. Horvitz Center for
Palliative Medicine, Cleveland Clinic Foundation,
Cleveland, Ohio
*Developing a Research Group; Priorities for the Future: The Research
Agenda; History and Physical Examination; Clinical Symptom
Assessment*

Cathy Heaven, MSc, PhD
Senior Trainer and Manager, Maguire Communication
Skills Training Unit, Christie Hospital, Manchester,
United Kingdom
Good Communication: Patients, Families, and Professionals

Michael Herman, DO
Instructor of Medicine and Fellow in
Gastroenterology, University of South Alabama
Medical School, Mobile, Alabama
Organ Transplantation

Jørn Herrstedt, MD, DMSci
Professor in Clinical Oncology, University of Southern Denmark; Head, Urologic Gynecologic Oncology and Supportive Care, Department of Oncology, Odense University Hospital, Odense, Denmark
Complications of Chemotherapy

Stephen Higgins, MB Bch, BAO, MRCPI
Consultant in Palliative Medicine, Tallaght Hospital and Our Lady's Hospice, Dublin, Ireland
Antidepressants and Psychostimulants

Irene J. Higginson, BMedSci, BMBS, PhD, FFPHM, FRCP
Professor of Palliative Care and Policy, King's College; Honorary Consultant in Palliative Medicine, King's College Hospital; Scientific Director, Cicely Saunders International, London, United Kingdom
Health Services Research

Joanne M. Hilden, MD
Chair, Department of Pediatric Hematology/Oncology; Medical Director, Pediatric Palliative Care, Cleveland Clinic Children's Hospital, Cleveland, Ohio
Neonates, Children, and Adolescents

Kathryn L. Hillenbrand, MA
Faculty Specialist II and Coordinator, Charles Van Riper Language, Speech and Hearing Clinic, Department of Speech Pathology and Audiology, Western Michigan University, Kalamazoo, Michigan
Dysphagia

Burkhard Hinz, PhD
Professor of Toxicology and Pharmacology and Head, Institute of Toxicology and Pharmacology, University of Rostock, Rostock, Germany
Nonsteroidal Anti-inflammatory Drugs

Jade Homsi, MD
Assistant Professor of Medicine, The University of Texas M. D. Anderson Cancer Center, Houston, Texas
Symptom Epidemiology and Clusters

Kerry Hood
Marie Curie Palliative Care Institute, Marie Curie Hospice, Liverpool, United Kingdom
Design and Conduct of Research and Clinical Trials

Juliet Y. Hou, MD
Associate Staff, Cleveland Clinic, Cleveland, Ohio
Durable Medical Equipment

Guy Hubens, MD, PhD
University of Antwerp Faculty of Medicine, Antwerp; Vice-Chairman, Department of Abdominal Surgery, University Hospital of Antwerp, Edegem, Belgium
Principles and Practice of Surgical Oncology

Peter Hudson, MD
Associate Professor, School of Nursing and Social Work, Faculty of Medicine, Dentistry and Health Sciences, University of Melbourne, Carlton; Deputy Director Centre for Palliative Care, St. Vincent's Hospital Melbourne, Fitzroy, Victoria, Australia
Assessing the Family and Caregivers

John G. Hughes, BSc(Hons), PhD
CECo Research Fellow, Academic Palliative and Supportive Care Studies Group, University of Liverpool, United Kingdom
Psychosocial Research

John Hunt, RN
Lead Clinician, Trent Hospice Audit Group (THAG), Trent Palliative Care Centre, Sheffield, United Kingdom
Consultation Services

Craig A. Hurwitz, MD
Clinical Professor of Pediatrics, University of Vermont College of Medicine, Burlington, Vermont; Director, Maine Medical Center for Pain and Palliative Care, Maine Medical Center, Portland, Maine
Neonates, Children, and Adolescents

James Ibinson, MD, PhD
Resident in Anesthesiology, University of Pittsburgh School of Medicine, Pittsburgh, Pennsylvania
Cancer Pain: Anesthetic and Neurosurgical Interventions

Nora Janjan
Professor of Radiation Oncology, Baylor College of Medicine; Radiation Oncologist, The University of Texas M. D. Anderson Cancer Center, Houston, Texas
Vertebral Metastases and Spinal Cord Compression

Birgit Jaspers, MD
Department of Science and Research, Centre for Palliative Medicine, University of Bonn, Bonn, Germany
The History of Hospice

Thomas Jehser
Department of Palliative Medicine, Gemeinschaftskrankenhaus Havelhöhe, Berlin, Germany
Death Rattle

A. Mark Joffe, MD
Royal Alexandra Hospital, Edmonton, Alberta, Canada
Health Care–Acquired Infections

Laurence John, MB BS, MD, MRCP, DTM&H
Specialist Registrar Infectious Diseases and General Medicine, Infectious Disease Institute, Kampala, Uganda
Biology and Natural History of Acquired Immunodeficiency Syndrome

Jennie Johnstone, MD
Clinical Lecturer and Clinical Infectious Disease Research Fellow, University of Alberta Faculty of Medicine, Edmonton, Alberta, Canada

Health Care–Acquired Infections

J. Stephen Jones, MD
Associate Professor of Surgery (Urology), Glickman Urological and Kidney Institute, Cleveland Clinic Lerner College of Medicine of Case Western Reserve University, Cleveland, Ohio

Genitourinary Complications in Palliative Oncology

Javier R. Kane, MD
Director, Palliative Medicine and End-of-Life Care, St. Jude Children's Research Hospital, Memphis, Tennessee

Psychological Adaptation of the Dying Child

Matthew T. Karafa, PhD
Research Associate, Cleveland Clinic Foundation, Cleveland, Ohio

Biostatistics and Epidemiology

Andrew P. Keaveny, MD, FRCPI
Assistant Professor of Medicine, Mayo Clinic College of Medicine, Rochester, Minnesota; Consultant Physician, Mayo Clinic, Jacksonville, Florida

Organ Transplantation

Dorothy M. K. Keefe, MB BS, MD
Department of Medical Oncology, Royal Adelaide Hospital Cancer Centre, Royal Adelaide Hospital, Adelaide, South Australia, Australia

Oral Complications of Cancer and Its Treatment

Catherine McVearry Kelso, MD
Assistant Professor of Internal Medicine, Virginia Commonwealth University School of Medicine; Medical Director, Hospice and Palliative Care, McGuire Veterans Affairs Medical Center, Richmond, Virginia

Drugs for Diarrhea

Rose Anne Kenny, MB BCH, MD
Professor of Geriatric Medicine, Trinity College Dublin, Dublin, Ireland

Biology and Physiology of Aging

Martina Kern, MD
University Lecturer in Palliative Medicine, University of Bonn; Head of Bereavement Service Project for Children and Youth, Center for Palliative Medicine, Malteser Hospital Bonn/Rhein-Sieg, Bonn, Germany

Sexuality and Intimacy in the Critically Ill

Dilara Seyidova Khoshknabi, MD
Research Fellow, The Harry R. Horvitz Center for Palliative Medicine, Taussig Cancer Center, Cleveland Clinic, Cleveland, Ohio

Priorities for the Future: The Research Agenda; Drugs for Myoclonus and Tremors; Muscle Spasms; Sleep Problems and Nightmares

Jordanka Kirkova, MD
Research Fellow, The Harry R. Horvitz Center for Palliative Medicine, Taussig Cancer Institute, Cleveland Clinic, Cleveland, Ohio

Priorities for the Future: The Research Agenda; Measuring Quality of Life

Kenneth L. Kirsh, PhD
Assistant Professor, Pharmacy Practice and Science, University of Kentucky College of Medicine, Lexington, Kentucky

Opioid Use in Drug and Alcohol Abuse

David W. Kissane, MD, MPM, FRANZCP, FAChPM
Alfred P. Sloan Chair and Chairman, Department of Psychiatry and Behavioral Sciences, Memorial Sloan-Kettering Cancer Center, New York, New York

Grief and Bereavement

Eberhard Klaschik, MD, PhD
Department of Science and Research, Centre for Palliative Medicine, University of Bonn; Department of Anesthesiology, Intensive Care, Palliative Medicine, and Pain Therapy, Malteser Hospital Bonn, Bonn, Germany

The History of Hospice

Seref Komurcu, MD
Associate Professor of Medicine, Department of Medical Oncology, Gülhane Military Medical Academy; Head of Medical Oncology Section, Bayindir Hospital, Ankara, Turkey

Biology of Cancer

Kandice Kottke-Marchant, MD, PhD
Chair, Department of Pathology, Cleveland Clinic Lerner College of Medicine of Case Western Reserve University; Chair, Pathology and Laboratory Medicine Institute, Cleveland Clinic, Cleveland, Ohio

Bleeding and Clotting Disorders in Cancer

Kathryn M. Kozell, MScN, ACNP, ET, RN
Associate Professor, University of Windsor Faculty of Nursing, Windsor; Associate Professor, University of Western Ontario School of Nursing; Associate Professor, University of Western Ontario School of Physical Therapy; Coordinator, Disease Site Team/Disease Site Team Council, London, Ontario, Canada

Pressure Ulcers and Wound Care

Sunil Krishnan, MD
Department of Radiation Oncology, The University of Texas M. D. Anderson Cancer Center, Houston, Texas

Vertebral Metastases and Spinal Cord Compression

Deborah Kuban, MD, FACR
Department of Radiation Oncology, The University of Texas M. D. Anderson Cancer Center, Houston, Texas

Vertebral Metastases and Spinal Cord Compression

Damian A. Laber, MD, FACP
Associate Professor of Medicine, University of
Louisville; Scientist, James Graham Brown Cancer
Center, Louisville, Kentucky

Bone Marrow Failure

Ruth L. Lagman, MD, MPH
Director of Clinical Services, The Harry R. Horvitz
Center for Palliative Medicine, Cleveland Clinic
Taussig Center, Cleveland Ohio

*The Business of Palliative Medicine: Quality Care in a Challenging
Environment; Infections in Palliative Medicine*

Rajesh V. Lalla, PhD, BDS, CCRP
Assistant Professor of Oral Medicine, Department of
Oral Health and Diagnostic Sciences, University
of Connecticut School of Dental Medicine; Division
of Oral Medicine, School of Dental Medicine;
Attending Staff, John Dempsey Hospital; Member,
Head and Neck/Oral Oncology Program, Neag
Comprehensive Cancer Center, Farmington,
Connecticut

Oral Symptoms

Deforia Lane, PhD
Resident Director of Music Therapy, University
Hospitals of Cleveland Ireland Cancer Center,
Cleveland, Ohio

Music and Art Therapists

Philip J. Larkin, PhD, RGN
Senior Lecturer in Nursing Studies (Palliative Care),
School of Nursing and Midwifery Studies, National
University of Ireland, Galway, Ireland

Nurses and Nurse Practitioners

Wael Lasheen, MD
Research Fellow, Taussig Cancer Center, The Harry R.
Horvitz Center for Palliative Medicine, Cleveland
Clinic Foundation, Cleveland, Ohio

*Priorities for the Future: The Research Agenda; Kidney and Liver
Disease*

Karen Laurence
Assistant Clinical Professor of Medicine, Case Western
Reserve School of Medicine; Adjunct Professor,
Frances Payne Bolton School of Nursing

*Symptom Management: Symptom Management in Human
Immunodeficiency Virus in Sub-Saharan Africa*

Peter Lawlor, MB Mmed Sc, CCFP(C)
Adjunct Associate Professor, Department of Oncology,
University of Alberta Faculty of Medicine,
Edmonton, Alberta, Canada; Consultant in Palliative
Medicine, Our Lady's Hospice and St. James's
Hospital, Dublin, Ireland

Opioid Side Effects and Overdose

Susan B. LeGrand, MD, FACP
Director, Palliative Medicine Fellowship Program, The
Harry R. Horvitz Center for Palliative Medicine,
Cleveland Clinic Foundation, Cleveland, Ohio

*Anxiolytics, Sedatives, and Hypnotics; Bronchodilators and Cough
Suppressants; Anxiety; Fatigue; Pleural and Pericardial Effusions*

Vincent Lens, MD
Radiology Service, Department of Hematology and
Oncology, Centre Hospitalier Luxembourg,
Luxembourg City, Luxembourg

The Vena Cava Syndrome

Dona Leskuski, DO, MS
Medical Director, Capital Hospice and Capital
Palliative Care Consultants, Leesburg, Virginia

The Speech-Language Pathologist; Communication Devices

Pamela Levack, MB ChB, MSc, B Med Biol, FRCP
Honorary Senior Lecturer, Department of Surgery and
Molecular Oncology, University of Dundee;
Consultant in Palliative Medicine, Ninewells
Hospital, Dundee, United Kingdom

Care of the Dying: Hospitals and Intensive Care Units

Marcia Levetown, MD
Member, American Academy of Pediatrics Ethics
Committee; Chair, American Academy of Pediatrics
Section on Hospice and Palliative Medicine,
Phoenix, Arizona

Hospice and Special Services

Jeanne G. Lewandowski, MD
Medical Director, Pediatrics, Kaleidoscope Kids
Hospices of Henry Ford, and Chair, Michigan
Alliance for Pediatric Palliative Services, Detroit,
Michigan

Neonates, Children, and Adolescents

William R. Lewis, MD
Associate Professor of Medicine, Case Western
Reserve University School of Medicine; Chief,
Clinical Cardiology, MetroHealth Medical Center,
Cleveland, Ohio

Arrhythmias

S. Lawrence Librach, MD
Director, Temmy Latner Centre for Palliative Care,
Mount Sinai Hospital, Toronto, Ontario, Canada

The Specialty of Palliative Medicine

Wendy G. Lichtenthal, PhD
Research Fellow, Department of Psychiatry and
Behavioral Sciences, Memorial Sloan-Kettering
Cancer Center, New York, New York

The Desire for Death; Grief and Bereavement

J. Norelle Lickiss, MD, FRACP, FRCP(Edin)

Clinical Professor of Medicine, University of Sydney Faculty of Medicine, Sydney, New South Wales; Honorary Research Professor, School of Philosophy, University of Tasmania, Hobart, Tasmania; Consultant Emeritus, Royal Prince Alfred Hospital, and Consultant in Palliative Medicine, Royal Hospital for Women, Sydney, New South Wales, Australia

The Human Experience of Illness; The Physician

Stefano Lijoi, MD

Attending Physician, Department of Pediatric Oncohematology, University of Turin; Regina Margherita Children's Hospital, Turin, Italy

Cancer in Children

Edward Lin, MD, FACP

Department of Radiation Oncology, The University of Texas M. D. Anderson Cancer Center, Houston, Texas

Vertebral Metastases and Spinal Cord Compression

Arthur G. Lipman, PharmD, FASHP

University Professor, Department of Pharmacotherapy, College of Pharmacy; Adjunct Professor, Department of Anesthesiology, University of Utah School of Medicine; Director of Clinical Pharmacology, Pain Management Center, University of Utah Health Sciences Center, Salt Lake City, Utah

Development and Use of a Formulary

Jean-Michel Livrozet, MD

Hôpital Edoard Herriot, Lyon, France

Symptom Management

Mari Lloyd-Williams, MD, FRCP, FRCGP

Professor, Academic Palliative and Supportive Care Studies Group, University of Liverpool; Professor of Palliative Medicine, University of Liverpool Hospital, Liverpool, United Kingdom

Psychosocial Research

Richard M. Logan, MDS, PhD

Senior Lecturer and Head of Oral Pathology, School of Dentistry, Faculty of Health Sciences, University of Adelaide; Consultant Oral Pathologist, Division of Tissue Pathology, Institute of Medical and Veterinary Science, Adelaide, South Australia, Australia

Oral Complications of Cancer and Its Treatment

Francisco López-Lara Martín, MD, PhD

Professor of Medicine and Head, Department of Radiology, University of Valladolid Faculty of Medicine; Head, Radiotherapy Oncology Department, Hospital Clínico Universitario de Valladolid, Valladolid, Spain

Natural History of Cancer

Charles L. Loprinzi, MD

Professor of Oncology, Mayo Clinic, Rochester, Minnesota

Premature Menopause

John Loughnane, MB, MSc, MRCGP, MICGP

General Practitioner, Boherbue, Newcastle West, County Limerick, Ireland

Common Medical and Surgical Disorders

Michael Lucey, MB, MRCPI, MBA

Specialist Registrar in Palliative Medicine, Our Lady's Hospice, Dublin, Ireland

Opioid Side Effects and Overdose

Laurie Lyckholm, MD

Assistant Professor and Fellowship Program Director, Department of Hematology/Oncology and Palliative Medicine, Virginia Commonwealth University School of Medicine, Richmond, Virginia

Fever and Sweats

Carol Macmillan, MD, MB ChB, MRCP, FRCA

Consultant in Intensive Care Medicine and Anaesthesia, Ninewells Hospital, Dundee, United Kingdom

Care of the Dying: Hospitals and Intensive Care Units

Frances Mair, MD, DRCOG, FRCGP

Professor of Primary Care Research, Department of General Practice and Primary Care, University of Glasgow Faculty of Medicine, Glasgow, United Kingdom

Heart Failure

Stephen N. Makoni, MD, FACP

Clinical Assistant Professor of Medicine, University of North Dakota School of Medicine and Health Science; Medical Oncologist/Hematologist, Trinity Cancer Care Center, Minot, North Dakota

Bone Marrow Failure

Bushra Malik, MD

Neurologist and Headache Fellow, Cleveland Clinic, Cleveland, Ohio

The Neuropsychological Examination

Kevin Malone, MD, MRCPI, FRC Psych

Professor of Psychiatry, Department of Psychiatry and Mental Health Research, St. Vincent's University Hospital and University College, Dublin, Ireland

Psychiatrists and Clinical Psychologists

Marco Maltoni, MD

Hospice and Palliative Care Unit, Department of Oncology, Valerio Grassi Hospital, Forlimpopoli, Italy

Paraneoplastic Syndromes; Palliative Chemotherapy and Corticosteroids

Aruna Mani, MD
Medical Oncology Fellow, Division of Hematology/
Oncology, Ohio State University Medical Center,
Columbus, Ohio
Bone Metastases

Lucille R. Marchand, MD
Professor of Family Medicine, University of Wisconsin
School of Medicine and Public Health, Madison;
Clinical Director of Integrative Oncology Services,
University of Wisconsin Paul P. Carbone
Comprehensive Cancer Center, Madison; Associate
Medical Director of Integrative Oncology,
ProHealth Care Regional Cancer Center, Waukesha,
Wisconsin
The Plan of Care

Darren P. Mareiniss, MD, JD, MBe
Senior Consultant for Medical and Legal Policy,
University of Maryland Center for Health and
Homeland Security, Baltimore, Maryland
Principles of Bioethics

Anna L. Marsland, PhD, RN
Department of Psychology, University of Pittsburgh
School of Health and Rehabilitation Sciences,
Pittsburgh, Pennsylvania
Autonomic Dysfunction

Joan Marston
University of Cape Town, Cape Town, South Africa
*Palliative Care for Children and Adolescents with Human
Immunodeficiency Virus/Acquired Immunodeficiency Syndrome*

Julia Romero Martinez, MD
Radiologist, Hospital General Universitario Gregorio
Marañón, Madrid, Spain
*Computed Tomography Scanning and Magnetic Resonance Imaging
in Palliative Care*

Isabel Martínez de Ubago
Radiologist, Hospital General Universitario Gregorio
Marañón, Madrid, Spain
*Computed Tomography Scanning and Magnetic Resonance Imaging
in Palliative Care*

Lina M. Martins, ET, MScN, RN
Associate Professor, University of Western Ontario
School of Physical Therapy; Clinical Nurse
Specialist, Enterostomal Therapy Nurse, London
Health Sciences Centre, London, Ontario, Canada
Pressure Ulcers and Wound Care

Timothy S. Maughan, MB, FRCP, FRCR
Professor of Cancer Studies, Cardiff University School
of Medicine; Consultant in Clinical Oncology,
Velindre Hospital, Whitchurch, Cardiff, Wales,
United Kingdom
Design and Conduct of Research and Clinical Trials

Catriona Mayland, MB ChB, MRCP
Honorary Research Associate, University of Liverpool;
Specialist Registrar in Palliative Medicine,
University Hospital Aintree, Liverpool, United
Kingdom
Standards of Care

Susan E. McClement, PhD, MN
Associate Professor, University of Manitoba Faculty of
Nursing; Research Associate, Manitoba Palliative
Care Research Unit, CancerCare Manitoba,
Winnipeg, Manitoba, Canada
Depression

Ian McCutcheon, MD, FACS
Department of Radiation Oncology, The University of
Texas M. D. Anderson Cancer Center, Houston,
Texas
Vertebral Metastases and Spinal Cord Compression

Michael F. McGee, MD
Resident, Department of Surgery, Case Western
Reserve University, University Hospitals Case
Medical Center, Cleveland, Ohio
Stomas and Fistulas

Neil McGill, MB BS, BSc, FRACP
Clinical Senior Lecturer, Department of Medicine,
University of Sydney Faculty of Medicine;
Rheumatologist, Royal Prince Alfred Hospital,
Camperdown, New South Wales, Australia
Common Musculoskeletal Co-morbidities

**Stephen McNamara, MB BS(Hons), BSc(Med), PhD,
FRACP, FCCP**
Clinical Senior Lecturer, Department of Medicine,
University of Sydney Faculty of Medicine, Sydney;
Senior Staff Specialist, Department of Sleep and
Respiratory Medicine, Royal Prince Alfred Hospital,
Camperdown, New South Wales, Australia
Pulmonary Function

Mary Lynn McPherson, PharmD, BCPS, CDE
Professor, University of Maryland School of Pharmacy;
Hospice Consultant Pharmacist, Baltimore,
Maryland
Diabetes Mellitus

Henry McQuay, DM, FRCA, FRCP (Edin)
Nuffield Professor of Clinical Anaesthetics, University
of Oxford; Honorary Consultant, Pain Relief Unit,
Churchill Hospital, Oxford, United Kingdom
Nonopioid and Adjuvant Analgesics

Regina McQuillan, MB BCh, BAO
Medical Director and Consultant in Palliative
Medicine, St. Francis Hospice, Dublin, Ireland
Congenital Intellectual Disability

Robert E. McQuown, AS, RRT, RCP
Respiratory Therapy Manager, Homecare Services, Cleveland Clinic Homecare Services, Independence, Ohio
Respiratory Equipment

Michelle Meiring
University of Cape Town, Cape Town, South Africa
Palliative Care for Children and Adolescents with Human Immunodeficiency Virus/Acquired Immunodeficiency Syndrome

Sebastiano Mercadante, MD
Professor of Palliative Medicine, University of Palermo; Director of Anesthesia and Intensive Care and Pain Relief and Palliative Care Unit, La Maddalena Cancer Center, Palermo, Italy
Intestinal Dysfunction and Obstruction; Challenging Pain Problems

Elaine C. Meyer, PhD
Associate Professor of Psychology, Harvard Medical School; Associate Director, Institute for Professionalism and Ethical Practice, Children's Hospital Boston, Boston, Massachusetts
Family Adjustment and Support

Randy D. Miller, PharmD
Boehringer Ingelheim Pharmaceuticals, Inc., Ridgefield, Connecticut
Interactions, Side Effects, and Management

Yvonne Millerick, BSc, RGN
Heart Failure Liaison Nurse Specialist, Glasgow Royal Infirmary, Glasgow, United Kingdom
Heart Failure

Roberto Miniero, MD
Professor of Pediatrics, University of Turin School of Medicine; Head of Pediatric Unit, Regina Margherita Children's Hospital, Turin, Italy
Cancer in Children

Armin Mohamed
Positron Emission Tomography

Busi Mooka, MB, BCH, BAO, MRCPIS
St. James's Hospital, Dublin, Ireland
Acquired Immunodeficiency Syndrome in Adults

Helen M. Morrison, MB ChB, MRCP(UK)
Specialist Registrar Palliative Medicine, Beatson Oncology Centre Glasgow, Glasgow, United Kingdom
Clinical Practice Guidelines

J. Cameron Muir, MD
Vice President, Medical Services, Capital Hospice; President, Capital Palliative Care Consultants, Falls Church, Virginia
Seizures and Movement Disorders

Fiona Mulcahy, MD, FRCPI
Professor of Medicine and Consultant in Genitourinary Medicine, Trinity College Dublin and St. James's Hospital, Dublin, Ireland
Acquired Immunodeficiency Syndrome in Adults

Hugh E. Mulcahy, MD, MRCPI
Consultant Gastroenterologist, St. Vincent's University Hospital, Dublin, Ireland
Gastrointestinal Endoscopy; Acquired Immunodeficiency Syndrome in Adults

Monica Muller, MD
Bonn, Germany
The Volunteer

H. Christof Müller-Busch, Prof. Dr. Med.
University of Witten/Herdecke, Witten; Humboldt University Berlin, Berlin; Consultant on Palliative Care, Pain Therapy, and Anesthesia, Department of Palliative Medicine, Gemeinschaftskrankenhaus Havelhöhe, Berlin, Germany
Death Rattle

Scott A. Murray, MD, FRCGP, FRCP(Ed)
St. Columba's Hospice Chair of Primary Palliative Care, University of Edinburgh; Family Physician, Mackenzie Medical Centre, Edinburgh, United Kingdom
Illness Trajectories and Stages

Friedemann Nauck, MD
Director, Department of Palliative Medicine, Georg-August-Universität Göttingen, Göttingen, Germany
Opioids; Opioids for Cancer Pain

Katherine Neasham, MB BS
Specialist Registrar, Royal Prince Alfred Hospital, Sydney, New South Wales, Australia
Alcohol and Drug Abuse

Busisiwe Nkosi
University of Cape Town, Cape Town, South Africa
Palliative Care for Children and Adolescents with Human Immunodeficiency Virus/Acquired Immunodeficiency Syndrome

Simon Noble, MB BS, FRCP
Senior Lecturer in Palliative Medicine, Cardiff University School of Medicine, Cardiff, United Kingdom
Deep Vein Thrombosis; Cardiac Drugs

Antonio Noguera, MD
Palliative Care Consultant, Hospital Centro de Cuidados Laguna, Madrid, Spain
Development of National and International Standards

Anna K. Nowak, MB BS, PhD, FRACP
School of Medicine and Pharmacology, University of Western Australia, Nedlands, Western Australia, Australia
Principles of Modern Chemotherapy and Endocrine Therapy

Eugenie A. M. T. Obbens, MD
Professor of Clinical Neurology, Weill Medical College of Cornell University; Neurologist and Acting Chief, Pain and Palliative Care Service, Memorial Sloan-Kettering Cancer Center, New York, New York
Neurological Complications

Tony O'Brien, MB, FRCPI
Clinical Senior Lecturer, National University of Ireland, Cork, School of Medicine; Medical Director, Marymount Hospice, St. Patrick's Hospital; Consultant Physician in Palliative Medicine, Cork University Hospital, Cork, Ireland
Program Development: National Planning

Megan Olden, MA
Predoctoral Research Fellow, Department of Psychiatry and Behavioral Sciences, Memorial Sloan-Kettering Cancer Center, New York, New York
The Desire for Death

Norma O'Leary, MD, MB BCh
Consultant in Palliative Medicine, Gateshead Health NHS Foundation Trust and Marie Curie Cancer Care, Newcastle upon Tyne, United Kingdom
Diagnosis of Death and Dying

David Oliver, MD
Kent Institute of Medicine and Health Sciences, University of Kent; Wisdom Hospice, Kent, United Kingdom
Quadriplegia and Paraplegia

David Oliviere, MD
St. Christopher's Hospice, London, United Kingdom
The Interdisciplinary Team

Aurelius G. Omlin, MD
Senior Lecturer, University of Bern, Bern; Clinical and Research Fellow, Oncological Palliative Medicine, Cantonal Hospital, St. Gallen, Switzerland
Anorexia and Weight Loss

Kaci Osenga, MD
Clinical Instructor, Department of Medicine, University of Wisconsin School of Medicine and Public Health, Madison, Wisconsin
Epidemiology of Cancer

Diarmuid O'Shea, MD, FRCP, FRCPI
Lecturer, University College Dublin; Consultant Geriatrician, Department of Elderly Medicine, St. Vincent's University Hospital, Dublin, Ireland
Syncope and Blackouts; The Aging Brain and Dementia

Christophe Ostgathe, MD
Lecturer and Consultant, Department of Palliative Care, University of Cologne, Cologne, Germany
Brain Metastases

Faith D. Ottery, MD, PhD, FACN
Senior Director, Medical Affairs, Savient Pharmaceuticals, Inc., East Brunswick, New Jersey; President, Ottery & Associates, Oncology Care Consultants, Philadelphia, Pennsylvania
Cancer-Related Weight Loss

Michel Ouellette, PhD
Professionnel de Recherche, Centre de Recherche de l'Hôtel-Dieu de Québec, Maison Michel-Sarrazin, Quebec City, Quebec, Canada
Delirium and Psychosis

Edgar Turner Overton, MD
Assistant Professor of Medicine, Division of Infectious Diseases, Washington University School of Medicine, St. Louis, Missouri
Treatment of Persons Infected with Human Immunodeficiency Virus

Moné Palacios, DDS, MSc
Research Associate, Oncology Department, University of Calgary Faculty of Medicine; Program Manager, Tom Baker Cancer Centre, Centre for Distance Education and Research in Palliative Care, Calgary, Alberta, Canada
Web-Based Learning

Robert Palmer, MD
Head, Section of Geriatric Medicine, Department of Internal Medicine, Cleveland Clinic, Cleveland, Ohio
The Frail Elderly

Teresa Palmer, APN
Symptom Care Team, Blount Memorial Hospital, Maryville, Tennessee
Palliative Sedation

Carmen Paradis, MD
Associate Staff, Bioethics Department, Cleveland Clinic Foundation, Cleveland, Ohio
Research Bioethics

Armida G. Parala, MD
Geriatrics and Palliative Medicine Physician, St. Joseph Mercy Hospital, Ann Arbor, Michigan
Demographics of Aging

Antonio Pascual-López, MD, PhD
Director of the Palliative Care Unit, Hospital Universitari de la Santa Creu i Sant Pau, Barcelona, Spain
Acute Palliative Medicine Units

Steven D. Passik, PhD
Associate Professor, Department of Psychiatry and Behavioral Sciences, Memorial Sloan-Kettering Cancer Center, New York, New York
Opioid Use in Drug and Alcohol Abuse

Timothy M. Pawlik, MD, MPH
Assistant Professor, Department of Surgery and Oncology, Johns Hopkins School of Medicine, Baltimore, Maryland
Pleural and Peritoneal Catheters

Malcolm Payne, MD
Director, Psycho-social and Spiritual Care, and Director, Education, St. Christopher's Hospice, London, United Kingdom
The Interdisciplinary Team

Sheila Payne, PhD
Help the Hospices Chair in Hospice Studies, International Observatory on End of Life Care, Institute for Health Research, Lancaster University, Lancaster, United Kingdom
Qualitative Methodology; Assessing the Family and Caregivers

Silvia Paz, MD
Research Associate, World Health Organization Collaborating Centre for Public Health Palliative Care Programmes, Palliative Care Service, Institut Català d'Oncologia, L'Hospitalet de Llobregat, Barcelona, Spain
Palliative Medicine: Models of Organization; Program Development: Palliative Medicine and Public Health Services

José Pereira, MB ChB, DA, CCFP, MSc
Professor and Head, Division of Palliative Medicine, University of Ottawa Faculty of Medicine; Director, Palliative Care Services, Ottawa General Hospital and Elizabeth Bruyere Palliative Care Program, Ottawa, Ontario, Canada
Adult Learning; Web-Based Learning; Telemedicine

George Perkins, MD
Department of Radiation Oncology, The University of Texas M. D. Anderson Cancer Center, Houston, Texas
Vertebral Metastases and Spinal Cord Compression

Karin Peschardt, MD
Department of Oncology, Herlev University Hospital, Herlev, Denmark
Complications of Chemotherapy

Hayley Pessin, PhD
Clinical Psychologist, Department of Psychiatry and Behavioral Sciences, Memorial Sloan-Kettering Cancer Center, New York, New York
The Desire for Death

Douglas E. Peterson, MD
Professor of Oral Medicine, Department of Oral Health and Diagnostic Sciences, University of Connecticut School of Dental Medicine; Attending Staff, John Dempsey Hospital; Chair, Head and Neck/Oral Oncology Program, Neag Comprehensive Cancer Center, Farmington, Connecticut
Oral Symptoms

Vinod K. Podichetty, MD, MS
Director, Division of Research, Medical Intervention and Surgical Spine Center, Cleveland Clinic, Florida, Weston, Florida
Acupuncture, Transcutaneous Electrical Nerve Stimulation, and Topical Analgesics

Robin Pollens, MS
Adjunct Assistant Professor, Department of Speech Pathology and Audiology, Western Michigan University, Kalamazoo, Michigan
Dysphagia

Eliza Pontifex, MB BS, FRACP
Clinical Research Fellow, St. Vincent's University Hospital, Dublin, Ireland
Musculoskeletal Disorders

Susan Poole, BPharm, DipE
Honorary Research Fellow, Victorian College of Pharmacy, Monash University, Parkville; Pharmacy Research Coordinator, Bayside Health, Melbourne, Victoria, Australia
Prescribing

Josep Porta-Sales, MD, PhD
Head of Palliative Care Service, Institut Català d'Oncologia, L'Hospitalet de Llobregat, Barcelona, Spain
Palliative Medicine: Models of Organization; Program Development: Palliative Medicine and Public Health Services; Acute Palliative Medicine Units

Graeme Poston, MB BS, MS, FRCS
Lecturer in Surgery, University of Liverpool; Chairman, Department of Surgery, and Chief, Hepatobiliary Surgery, University Hospital Aintree, Liverpool, United Kingdom
Patterns of Metastatic Cancer

Ruth D. Powazki, MSW
Clinical Research, Cleveland Clinic, Cleveland, Ohio
Priorities for the Future: The Research Agenda; Qualitative Medicine; The Social Worker

William Powderly, MD
Dean of Medicine, University College Dublin School of Medicine and Medical Science, Dublin, Ireland
Treatment of Persons Infected with the Human Immunodeficiency Virus

Leopoldo Pozuelo, MD
Staff Psychiatrist and Head, Section of Consultation Psychiatry, Cleveland Clinic Health System, Cleveland, Ohio
Neuropharmacology and Psychopharmacology

Eric Prommer, MD
Assistant Professor of Medicine, Mayo Clinic College of Medicine; Director of Palliative Care, Mayo Clinic Hospital, Scottsdale, Arizona
Local and General Anesthetics

Christina M. Puchalski, MD, FACP
Associate Professor of Medicine and Health Sciences, George Washington University School of Medicine and Health Sciences; Associate Professor of Health Management and Leadership, George Washington University School of Public Health; Director, George Washington Institute for Spirituality and Health; Practicing Physician, Medical Faculty Associates at George Washington University Hospital, Washington, District of Columbia

Spiritual Care

Lukas Radbruch, MD
Chair, Department of Palliative Medicine, RWTH Aachen University, Aachen, Germany

Antibiotics; Pain in Cancer Survivors

David F. J. Raes, MD
Staff Member, Department of Cardiology, Sint Augustinus, Wilrijk-Antwerp, Belgium

Cardiac Function Testing

Jane Read, PhD
Dietitian, Sydney, New South Wales, Australia

Clinical Nutrition

Anantha Reddy, MD
Staff, Department of Rehabilitation Medicine, Cleveland Clinic, Cleveland, Ohio

Acupuncture, Transcutaneous Electrical Nerve Stimulation, and Topical Analgesics

Steven I. Reger, PhD
Staff, Cleveland Clinic, Cleveland, Ohio

Durable Medical Equipment

Susan J. Rehm, MD
Department of Infectious Diseases, Cleveland Clinic, Cleveland, Ohio

Infections in Palliative Medicine

Stephen G. Reich, MD
Professor, Department of Neurology, University of Maryland School of Medicine; Co-director, Maryland Parkinson's Disease and Movement Disorders Center, University of Maryland Medical Center, Baltimore, Maryland

Parkinson's Disease

Javier Rocafort, MD, PhD
Manager, Regional Palliative Care Program of Extremadura, Regional Ministry of Health and Dependence, Mérida, Spain

Program Development: Palliative Medicine and Public Health Services

Adam Rosenblatt, MD
Associate Professor of Psychiatry and Director of Neuropsychiatry, Johns Hopkins School of Medicine; Attending Physician, Johns Hopkins Hospital, Baltimore, Maryland

Memory Problems

Cynda Hylton Rushton, PhD, RN, FAAN
Associate Professor of Nursing and Faculty, Johns Hopkins Berman Institute of Bioethics, Johns Hopkins University; Program Director, Harriet Lane Compassionate Care Program, Johns Hopkins Children's Center, Baltimore, Maryland

Pediatric Palliative Care: Interdisciplinary Support

K. Mitchell Russell, MD
Associate Staff, The Harry R. Horvitz Center for Palliative Medicine, Cleveland Clinic Foundation, Cleveland, Ohio

Antiepileptic Drugs

Karen Ryan, MB BCh, BAO, BMed Sc, MRCPI
Consultant in Palliative Medicine, St. Francis Hospice, Mater Misericordiae University Hospital and Connolly Hospital, Dublin, Ireland

Congenital Intellectual Disability

Lisa A. Rybicki, MS
Lead Biostatistician, Cleveland Clinic Foundation, Cleveland, Ohio

Biostatistics and Epidemiology

Paola Sacerdote, PhD
Associate Professor of Pharmacology, Department of Pharmacology, University of Milan School of Medicine, Milan, Italy

Drug Use in Special Populations

Vinod Sahgal, MD
Professor, Case Western University School of Medicine; Cleveland Clinic, Cleveland, Ohio

Durable Medical Equipment

Mary Ann Sammon, RN
Skin/Wound Care Team Manager, Nursing Quality Management, Cleveland Clinic, Cleveland, Ohio

Wound and Stoma Therapists

Dirk Sandrock, MD, PhD
Assistant Professor of Nuclear Medicine, University Medicine of Berlin, Berlin; Head, Clinic of Nuclear Medicine, Chemnitz City Hospital, Chemnitz, Germany

Nuclear Medicine

Mark Sands, MD
Radiology Institute, Cleveland Clinic, Cleveland, Ohio

Interventional Radiology

Denise L. Schilling, PhD
Chair and Associate Professor, Department of Physical Therapy Education, Western University of Health Sciences, Pomona, California

Occupational and Physical Therapy

Valerie Nocent Schulz, MD, FRCPC (Anesthesia), MPH

Assistant Professor, Schulich School of Medicine and Dentistry, and AMS Fellow, End of Life Care Education for General Internal Medicine Residents, University of Western Ontario Faculty of Medicine; Palliative Medicine Consultant, London Health Sciences Centre, London, Ontario, Canada

Pressure Ulcers and Wound Care

Lisa N. Schum, PhD

Postdoctoral Fellow in Pediatric Psychology, St. Jude Children's Research Hospital, Memphis, Tennessee

Psychological Adaptation of the Dying Child

Peter Selwyn, MD, MPH

Professor and Chairman, Department of Family and Social Medicine, Montefiore Medical Center, Albert Einstein College of Medicine of Yeshiva University, Bronx, New York

Consultation Services; Symptom Management

Joshua Shadd, MD, CCFP

Assistant Professor, Departments of Medicine, Family Medicine, and Oncology, Queen's University School of Medicine; Physician Consultant, Palliative Care Medicine Program, Kingston General Hospital, Kingston, Ontario, Canada

Dyspnea

Charles L. Shapiro, MD

Director of Breast Medical Oncology, Division of Hematology/Oncology, Ohio State University Medical Center and Comprehensive Cancer Center, Columbus, Ohio

Bone Metastases

Aktham Sharif, MB BCh, MD

Senior Registrar, Radiation Oncology, St. Luke's Hospital, Dublin, Ireland

Radiation Principles and Techniques

Helen M. Sharp, PhD

Assistant Professor, Department of Speech Pathology and Audiology, Western Michigan University, Kalamazoo, Michigan; Adjunct Assistant Professor (Clinical), Department of Preventive and Community Dentistry, University of Iowa, Iowa City, Iowa

Dysphagia

Kirk V. Shepard, MD

Boehringer Ingelheim Pharmaceuticals, Inc., Ridgefield, Connecticut

Interactions, Side Effects, and Management

J. Timothy Sherwood, MD

Department of Surgery, Johns Hopkins Hospital, Baltimore, Maryland

Pleural and Peritoneal Catheters

Nabin K. Shrestha, MD, MPH

Staff Physician, Departments of Infectious Disease and Clinical Pathology, Cleveland Clinic, Cleveland, Ohio

Urinary Tract Infections

Richard J. E. Skipworth, BSc (Hons), MB ChB, MRSC (Ed)

Surgical Research Fellow, Department of Clinical and Surgical Sciences (Surgery), University of Edinburgh, Royal Infirmary, Edinburgh, United Kingdom

The Anorexia-Cachexia Syndrome

Howard S. Smith, MD

Associate Professor of Anesthesiology, Internal Medicine, and Physical Medicine and Rehabilitation, Albany Medical College; Academic Director of Pain Management, Albany Medical Center Hospital, Albany, New York

Hiccups

Mildred Z. Solomon, MD

Associate Clinical Professor of Social Medicine, Medical Ethics and Anaesthesia, Harvard Medical School, Boston; Vice President, Education Development Center, Inc., Newton, Massachusetts

Advanced Directives

Diego Soto de Prado Otero, MD

Medical Oncology Specialist, Hospital Clínico Universitario de Valladolid, Valladolid, Spain

Natural History of Cancer

Denise Wells Spencer, MD

Associate Medical Director, Hospice of the Bluegrass, Lexington, Kentucky

Inpatient Hospice and Palliative Care Units

Ron Spice, BMedSc, MD, CCFP, FCFP

Clinical Lecturer, Division of Palliative Medicine, and Director, Centre for Distance Education and Research in Palliative Care, University of Calgary Faculty of Medicine; Medical Leader, Regional Palliative and Hospice Care, and Medical Leader, Rural Palliative Telehealth Project, Calgary Health Region, Calgary, Alberta, Canada

Telemedicine

David Spiegel, MD

Jack, Lulu, and Sam Willson Professor and Associate Chair of Psychiatry and Behavioral Sciences, Stanford University School of Medicine, Stanford, California

Counseling

Manish Srivastava, MD

Medical Director, Palliative Care Program, Good Samaritan and Bethesda North Hospital, Cincinnati, Ohio

Community Services

John N. Staffurth, MB BS, MD
Senior Lecturer in Oncology, Cardiff University School of Medicine; Consultant Clinical Oncologist, Velindre Hospital, Cardiff, United Kingdom
Complications of Radiation Therapy

Randall Starling, MD
Section of Heart Failure and Cardiac Transplant, Cleveland Clinic, Cleveland, Ohio
Diuretics

Grant D. Stewart, BSc (Hons), MB ChB, MRSC (Ed)
Surgical Research Fellow, Department of Clinical and Surgical Sciences (Surgery), University of Edinburgh, Royal Infirmary, Edinburgh, United Kingdom
The Anorexia-Cachexia Syndrome

Jan Stjernswärd, MD, PhD, FRCP
Chief, Cancer Emeritus, World Health Organization; Docent, Karolinska Institut, Stockholm, Sweden
Palliative Medicine—The Global Perspective: Closing the Know-Do Gap; Palliative Medicine: Models of Organization; Program Development: Palliative Medicine and Public Health Services

Florian Strasser, MD
Oncology and Palliative Medicine, Section Oncology/Hematology, Department Internal Medicine, Cantonal Hospital, St. Gallen, Switzerland
Anorexia and Weight Loss

Edna Strauss, MD
Professor of Medicine, University of São Paulo; Attending Physician, Hospital das Clinicas, University of São Paulo, São Paulo, Brazil
Liver Failure

Imke Strohscheer
Department of Internal Medicine, Oncology Division, Medical University Graz, Graz, Austria
Prinicples of Medical Oncology

Brett Taylor Summey, MD
Department of Dermatology, Drexel University School of Medicine, Philadelphia, Pennsylvania
Pruritus

Graham Sutton, MRPCI
Specialist Registrar, Department of Medicine for the Elderly, St. Vincent's University Hospital, Dublin, Ireland
Syncope and Blackouts

Nigel P. Sykes, MA, BM BCh, FRCP, FRCGP
Honorary Senior Lecturer in Palliative Medicine, King's College, University of London; Consultant in Palliative Medicine and Medical Director, St. Christopher's Hospice, London, United Kingdom
Constipation and Diarrhea

Alan J. Taege, MD
Co-Director of HIV Care, Department of Infectious Diseases, Cleveland Clinic Foundation, Cleveland, Ohio
Acquired Immunodeficiency Syndrome: A Global Perspective

Marcello Tamburini, PhD*
Formerly in the Psychology Unit, National Cancer Institute, Milan, Italy
Caregiver Burden

Yoko Tarumi, MD
Assistant Clinical Professor, Division of Palliative Care Medicine, Department of Oncology, University of Alberta Faculty of Medicine; Palliative Care Program, Royal Alexandra Hospital, Edmonton, Alberta, Canada
Cough, Hemoptysis, and Bronchorrhea

Davide Tassinari, MD
Supportive and Palliative Care Unit, Department of Oncology, City Hospital, Rimini, Italy
Paraneoplastic Syndromes; Palliative Chemotherapy and Corticosteroids

Martin H. N. Tattersall, MD
Professor of Cancer Medicine and Co-Director, Centre of Medical Psychology and Evidence-Based Decision Making, University of Sydney Faculty of Medicine, Sydney; Medical Oncologist, Royal Prince Alfred Hospital, Sydney, New South Wales, Australia
Telling the Truth: Bad News

Karl S. Theil, MD
Staff Pathologist, Section of Hematopathology, Department of Clinical Pathology, Cleveland Clinic, Cleveland, Ohio
Laboratory Hematology

Keri Thomas, MD
Shrewsbury, United Kingdom
Home Care and Hospice Home Care

Adrian Tookman, MB BS, FRCP
Honorary Senior Lecturer, Royal Free and University College Medical School; Medical Director, Marie Curie Hospice Hampstead; Consultant in Palliative Medicine, Royal Free Hampstead NHS Trust, London, United Kingdom
Rehabilitation Approaches

María P. Torrubia, MD
Coordinator of the Domiciliary Program of Palliative Care, Servicio Aragonés de Salud, Zaragoza, Spain
Making Good Decisions

---

*deceased

Anna Towers, MDCM, FCFP
Associate Professor and Director, Palliative Care Division, McGill University Faculty of Medicine, Montreal, Quebec, Canada

Lymphedema

Daphne Tsoi, MB BS, FRACP
Clinical Fellow, Department of Medical Oncology, Sunnybrook Odette Cancer Centre, Toronto, Ontario, Canada

Principles of Modern Chemotherapy and Endocrine Therapy

Rodney O. Tucker, MD
Assistant Professor, Department of Medicine, University of Alabama at Birmingham School of Medicine; Medical Director, Division of Geriatrics, Gerontology and Palliative Care, University of Alabama at Birmingham Center for Palliative Care, Birmingham, Alabama

Cardiovascular Disorders

James A. Tulsky, MD
Professor, Department of Medicine, Duke University School of Medicine; Director, Center for Palliative Care, Duke University Medical Center, Durham, North Carolina

Problems in Communication

Rachel A. Tunick, PhD
Instructor of Psychology, Department of Psychiatry, Harvard Medical School; Staff Psychologist, Cardiovascular and Critical Care Services, Boston, Massachusetts

Family Adjustment and Support

Claire Turner, MB ChB, MRCP
Specialist Registrar in Palliative Medicine, Princess of Wales Hospital, Bridgend, Wales

Cardiac Drugs

Martha L. Twaddle, MD, FACP
Associate Professor of Medicine, Rush Medical College of Rush University, Chicago; Chief Medical Officer, Midwest Palliative & Hospice CareCenter, Glenview, Illinois

Curriculum Development

Marie Twomey, MB BCh, MRCPI
Consultant in Palliative Medicine, St. Luke's Hospital, Dublin, Ireland

Routes of Administration

Christina Ullrich, MD, MPH
Instructor in Pediatrics, Harvard Medical School; Attending Physician in Pediatric Oncology and Pediatric Palliative Care, Dana Farber Cancer Institute and Children's Hospital Boston, Boston, Massachusetts

Pediatric Pain and Symptom Control

Catherine E. Urch, MD
Honorary Senior Lecturer, University College London; Consultant in Palliative Medicine, St. Mary's and Royal Brompton Hospitals, London, United Kingdom

Pathophysiology of Cancer Pain

Mary L. S. Vachon, PhD, RN
Professor, Departments of Psychiatry and Public Health Science, University of Toronto Faculty of Medicine; Mary L. S. Vachon Psychotherapy and Consulting, Inc., Toronto, Ontario, Canada

Stress and Burnout

Bart Van den Eynden, MD
Professor of Palliative Medicine, Center for Palliative Care Sint-Camillus, University of Antwerp, Wilrijk-Antwerp, Belgium

Cardiac Function Testing; Nutrition in Palliative Medicine; Malignant Ascites

Antonio Vigano, MD
Palliative Care, McGill University Faculty of Medicine; Royal Victoria Hospital, Montreal, Quebec, Canada

Determining Prognosis

Erika Vlieghe, MD
Clinical Infectiologist, Department of Clinical Sciences, Institute of Tropical Medicine, and Department of Tropical Medicine, University Hospital Antwerp, Antwerp, Belgium

Fatal and Fulminant Infections

Angelo E. Volandes, MD
Instructor, Harvard Medical School; Attending Physician, Massachusetts General Hospital, Boston, Massachusetts

Advanced Directives

Raymond Voltz, MD
Senior Lecturer and Head, Department of Palliative Care, University of Cologne, Cologne, Germany

Brain Metastases

Paul W. Walker, MD
Assistant Professor of Medicine, University of Texas M. D. Anderson Cancer Center, Houston, Texas

Hypercalcemia

Sharon Watanabe, MD
Associate Professor, Division of Palliative Care Medicine, Department of Oncology, University of Alberta Cross Cancer Institute, Edmonton, Alberta, Canada

Cough, Hemoptysis, and Bronchorrhea

Michael A. Weber, MD
Professor of Medicine, State University of New York Downstate College of Medicine, Brooklyn, New York

Hypertension

Elizabeth Weinstein, MD
Assistant Professor, University of Pittsburgh School of Medicine, Pittsburgh, Pennsylvania
Withholding and Withdrawing Treatment

Sharon M. Weinstein, MD
Professor, Department of Anesthesiology, University of Utah School of Medicine; Director, Pain Medicine and Palliative Care, Huntsman Cancer Institute, Salt Lake City, Utah
Nonmalignant Pain

Kathryn L. Weise, MD
Staff Physician, Pediatric Critical Care Medicine; Director, Pediatric Palliative Medicine; and Program Director, Cleveland Fellowship in Advanced Bioethics, Cleveland Clinic, Cleveland, Ohio
Research Bioethics

Sherri Weisenfluh, MSW
Associate Vice President of Counseling Services, Hospice of the Bluegrass, Lexington, Kentucky
Parent and Child Bereavement

John Welsh, MB ChB, FRCP, BSc Hons
Professor in Palliative Medicine, Beatson Oncology Centre, Glasgow, United Kingdom
Clinical Practice Guidelines

Clare White, MB BCh, RN
Specialist Registrar, Palliative Medicine, Northern Ireland Hospice Care, Belfast, Northern Ireland
Principles of Palliative Medicine Research

Donna M. Wilson, PhD, RN
Professor, Faculty of Nursing, University of Alberta; Caritas Nurse Scientist, Caritas Health Group, Edmonton, Alberta, Canada
Death in Modern Society

Joanne Wolfe, MD, MPH
Assistant Professor of Pediatrics, Harvard Medical School; Director, Pediatric Palliative Care, Dana Farber Cancer Institute and Children's Hospital Boston, Boston, Massachusetts
Pediatric Pain and Symptom Control

Tugba Yavuzsen, MD
Department of Medical Oncology and Internal Medicine, Dokuz Eylül University Medical Faculty, Izmır, Turkey
Biology of Cancer

Albert J. M. Yee, MD, MSc, FRCSC
Associate Professor, Department of Surgery, University of Toronto Faculty of Medicine; Active Staff and Consultant in Surgical Oncology, Sunnybrook Health Sciences Centre and Odette Regional Cancer Centre, Toronto, Ontario, Canada
Palliative Orthopedic Surgery

Lisa M. Yerian, MD
Assistant Professor of Pathology, Cleveland Clinic Lerner College of Medicine of Case Western Reserve University; Director, Hepatobiliary Pathology, Cleveland Clinic, Cleveland, Ohio
The Role of Pathology

Elena Zucchetti, MD
Documentalist and Educator, Fondazione Floriani, Milan, Italy
Public Advocacy and Community Outreach

CONTENTS

PART I

Principles

Palliative Medicine

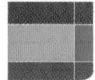

CHAPTER **1**

Palliative Medicine— The Global Perspective: Closing the Know-Do Gap

Jan Stjernswärd and Xavier Gómez-Batiste

K E Y P O I N T S

● More than 30 million people need palliative care today but only a few receive it.

● At least 100 million people worldwide would have improved quality of life if today's great knowledge in palliative medicine could be applied so as to reach all those in need of palliative care.

● Because of the dramatic and rapid aging of the world's populations and a doubling of the cancer rate, the need for palliative care will be significantly greater within the next 50 years.

● Implementing today's knowledge in a rational, public health–oriented manner, so that palliative care becomes part of all countries' health care services, and strengthening the community approach are recommended as the most realistic ways of meeting present and future demands.

● Based on 25 years of experience in developing a public health approach for establishing palliative care as part of national health services, we present some practical, detailed strategies.

THE NEED FOR PALLIATIVE CARE

Background

Palliative care relieves suffering and improves the quality of life of the living and the dying. More than 30 million people suffer unnecessarily from severe pain and other symptoms each year.[1] This is unethical, because simple, effective methods and approaches for palliative care exist that can be applied at the community level and therefore with the possibility of covering all those in need.[1-3] Much is known in palliative medicine, but this knowledge is not benefiting most of those who are in need of it. In spite of all the efforts over the last 2 decades, most people who need palliative care are not getting it.[1] To close the "Know-Do Gap," a public health approach for establishing pallia-

tive care according to World Health Organization (WHO) principles, as a part of countries' National Health Plans and integrated into their Health Care Services, seems to offer the most rational strategy for achieving worldwide coverage. A public health approach in palliative care means improving life through organized efforts of society, such as collective and social actions and involvement of the government's health care systems at all levels, as well as through organized community efforts of the people.

This chapter outlines some simple, practical, and pragmatic approaches to initiating a National Palliative Care Program (NPCP). To ensure that all populations have access to appropriate and cost-effective care, commitments must be demanded from governments and their people. This means developing policies and plans; issuing policies, laws, and regulations; ensuring a competent workforce and drug availability; incorporating palliative care into the health care system at all levels; mobilizing community partnerships; and conducting evaluations and health service research. Since the mid 1980s, WHO has produced guidelines and manuals and has given recommendations to member states on these issues, advising them to establish national programs for palliative care[3] as well as cancer control.[4]

Size of the Need

Estimating the need for palliative care is essential. Table 1-1 indicates the need for palliative care globally, and Box 1-1 shows how one can come up with a rough estimate for purposes of advocacy, health policy, and establishing an NPCP. The need will increase considerably in the coming years, mainly because of the aging of the world's populations. As can be seen from Table 1-1, there will be a dramatic increase in the numbers of the main groups that need palliative care, namely the elderly, the terminally ill, and those with cancer. Because of the aging of the world's populations, the ratio of caregivers (who often are also taxpayers) to care receivers will approach 2:1, something soon to occur in countries such as Japan, Switzerland, and the Nordic countries. An extreme example, but involving one fifth of the world's population, will be China, where, as a consequence of its former "one child to a family" policy, the proportion of caregivers to receivers will be severely distorted.

A country's death rate[5,6] indicates the total number of deaths per year (see Box 1-1). It has been estimated that 60% of all dying patients need palliative care, based on the frequency of major symptoms such as physical pain, anorexia, fatigue, and depression, and also socioeconomic, existential, and spiritual pain. Caring relatives may be included among those whose quality of life will improve

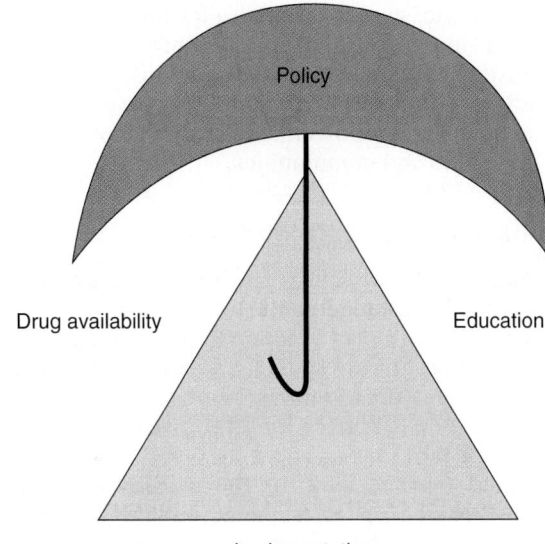

FIGURE 1-1   Foundation measures for establishing a National Palliative Care Program (NPCP).

TABLE 1-1   Projected Annual Need for Palliative Care Worldwide

CATEGORY	NUMBER (IN MILLIONS)
ANNUAL DEATHS	
Globally	58
Developing countries	45
Developed countries	13
Projected increase	
By 2015	64
By 2030	74
NEW CANCER CASES	
2003	10
By 2020	16
By 2050	24
PEOPLE AGED ≥60 YR	
2000	600
By 2025	1200
By 2050	2000
DEATHS FROM AIDS	
2003	3
By 2015	4
By 2030	6

with the provision of palliative care; depending on the local culture, their numbers will vary (see Box 1-1). A global figure of at least 100 million seems reasonable.

Both for advocacy and for convincing health policy makers, it will be important that figures on the size of the problem and unmet needs be presented, as well as outlines for clear solutions.

ACTION: ESTABLISHING A NATIONAL PALLIATIVE CARE PROGRAM

Background

Guidelines and recommendations are available for establishing NPCPs as the most rational approach for imple-

menting the existing wealth of knowledge in a systematic, coordinated way.[3,4] Based on our experience of having initiated or helped countries to establish national initiatives or programs, with both successes and failures,[7-15] we document here an approach that demonstrates some first pragmatic steps to start transforming knowledge into action.

Foundation Measures

Four fundamentally important components need to be established if palliative care is to be incorporated into a country's health care system. Figure 1-1 shows the four foundation measures that must be addressed in a coordinated way for establishing any NPCP.[1,3,5] The first three cost little but will have big effects.

1. *Policies:* Establish policies to integrate palliative care into the national health plan or into any national cancer control program. A major part of needed opiates should be made up of generic, cost-effective, immediate- and slow-release morphine, and key palliative care drugs should be included in the National Essential Drug List.
2. *Drug availability:* Improve availability of and access to opioids and prescription rules for opioids (i.e., who may prescribe sufficient amount and duration); increase the country's International Narcotic Control Board (INCB) quota for opioids.
3. *Education:* Advocate to the public, health professionals, and policy makers with facts and figures; include palliative care in undergraduate and continuing education curricula of doctors, nurses, social workers, clinical pharmacists, and oncologists, as well as volunteer organizations and relevant nongovernmental organizations (NGOs).
4. *Implementation:* Create a critical mass of new clinical palliative care full-time positions, organized around "champions," and the necessary infrastructure for (usually) a first reference center of excel-

lence and state-of-the-art leadership, with services well integrated into the country's Health Care System at all levels, including home care. Organize efforts of society through collective and social actions and empowerment of care-providing family members and communities.

National Palliative Care Workshop

A national workshop offers the most effective way to address the establishment of the four foundation measures and come up with a plan of action for integrating palliative care into the health care system; it brings together the key participants and organizations necessary to accomplish these tasks. Box 1-2 gives the objectives and agenda of such a workshop.

One and one-half days for the workshop should be enough. Breaking up participants into three interactive working groups (Policy, Drugs, and Education) at the end of day 1, and beginning day 2 with the groups' recommendations, has been found useful.

Box 1-3 shows the participants needed. Many times they have not met together previously, but working together will be necessary for establishing the foundation measures and drafting a valid, comprehensive NPCP.

If a champion is not identified, no workshops will result in action. A champion is a person who has charisma, credibility, neutrality, independence, commitment, political awareness, managerial effectiveness, ability to mobilize people and resources, communication skills, and understanding of the health care system.[4]

The Report

The workshop should be followed up with a report including a clear Plan of Action that serves as an outline for the future NPCP or initiative. Box 1-4 is a template for such a report with key points to be covered. An example of a report with details and recommendations[14] is available as it was officialized by the Georgian Parliament, in both

---

Box 1-2 National Palliative Care Workshop: Objective and Agenda

Objective:

To establish a National Palliative Care Program (NPCP), reaching all, through a World Health Organization (WHO) public health approach

Agenda:

Size of Problem
Solutions, State of the Art
Foundation Measures
Policy
Human Right/Responsibility
Ethics
Palliative Care Part of the National Health Care System (HCS)
Palliative Care a Priority
Policies and Legislative Changes Needed
Drug availability
Prescription
Types of Morphine
Essential Drug List
Estimated Future Need: International Narcotic Control Board (INCB)
Specify: 90% of New Quota To Be Generic Immediate-Release (IR) and Slow-Release (SR) Morphine
Education
Trainer of Future Trainers
Undergraduate Curricula Medical
Undergraduate Curricula Nursing
General Practitioners/Family Doctors
Implementation
Future Centers of Excellence, Education, and Bedside Training
Palliative Care in the Whole HCS Including Home Care
Role of Nongovernmental Organizations (NGOs): Identify and Specify
Priorities and Strategy for Implementation
Identify Champion, Coordinator, and Who Will Do What
Financing0

Box 1-3 Participants in National Palliative Care Program Policy Workshop

- Ministry of Health officials
- Other Ministries (e.g., Social Affairs, Higher Education, Women's Affairs)
- International governmental and nongovernmental organizations (e.g., World Health Organization, European Union, International Association for Hospice and Palliative Care [IAHPC], International Union Against Cancer [UICC])
- Directors of cancer, AIDS, and geriatric centers
- Drug regulators
- Chief pharmacist
- Deans of medical schools
- Deans and directors of nursing schools
- Representative family doctors/general practitioners
- Representative social workers
- National NGOs, religious organizations, journalists, advocacy groups
- Relevant leading clinicians, doctors/nurses
- International faculty/resource persons

Box 1-4 Report Template

Objectives
Situation Analysis
Size of Problem
State of the Art
Solutions, Foundation Measures
    Policy
    Drug Availability
    Education and Training
Workshop and Recommendations
Meetings with Key Persons
Action Plan
Follow-Ups
Focal Persons
Time Line
Indicators for Monitoring and Evaluation
Financing
References
Annexes

English and Georgian. Other examples can be found in the reference list.[7-15]

In the Annexes to the report, details are given, such as the WHO foundation measures, WHO recommendations to governments, integration of palliative care into routine cancer care and national cancer control programs, why generic morphine sulphate is optimal, how to estimate future needs of opioids, advocacy, recommendations of participants, or the community approach necessary for palliative care for all.

The planning of the NPCP should be done in the context of the country's socioeconomic profile. The *World Fact Book*[6] is easily accessible, is updated regularly, and provides death rates and other data in country profiles, including information on population, age structure, median age, life expectancy, HIV/AIDS prevalence, religions, literacy, population below poverty line, unemployment rate, household income, communications, and illicit drug use.

Outcomes

Expected outcomes may be divided into immediate, intermediate, and long-term outcomes, as shown in Table 1-2. The countries in Table 1-2 are listed in chronological order of program initiation, from Catalonia in 1989 to Georgia in 2005. In almost all cases, the immediate outcomes are now visible, as well as many of the intermediate ones. It has repeatedly been found that, to be able to close the "Know-Do Gap," three things are essential: finances, manpower, and institutionalization.[16] The workshop often lays a first ground for addressing these points. These

TABLE 1-2 Achievement of Expected Outcomes

OUTCOME	CATALONIA	KERALA	UGANDA	LEBANON	JORDAN	MONGOLIA	GEORGIA
IMMEDIATE							
Awareness/coordination	+	+	+	+	+	+	+
Champion/focal person	+	+	+	−	+	+	+
Action plan	+	−	+	+NGO −MoH	+	+	+
Time line	+	−	+		+	+	+
Indicators	+	?	+	+	+	+	+
INTERMEDIATE							
Legislative changes	+	+	+	+	+	+	+
PC into NHCS	+	+/−*	+		−	+	−
Education/training	+	+	+	+	+	+	+
Drug availability	+	+	+		+	+	+/−
Increased awareness	+	+	+	−	−	−	+
NPCP initiated	+	+	+	−	−	+	+
PC in main CC	+	+	+	+	+	+	+
Starting PC in other CCs−	+	+	−		2/3	+	−
Covering geriatric patients	+	+	−	−	−	−	+
LONG-TERM							
Coverage >80%	+	+ in NNPC	−		−		−
Improved QOL for patients/family	+	+ in NNPC					
DETAILS							
Altered prescription rules	+	+	+	+	+	+	+
Generic morphine available	+	+	+		+	+	+
Cost of IRM, 10-mg tablets (US cents)	18	1-2			14	5	
Cost of SRM, 30-mg tablets (US cents)	43	15	−		NYA	18	12
Cost of oral liquid morphine, 10 mg (US cents)	8		Free†			−	
Morphine consumption increased	+‡	+	+		+	Too soon§	Too soon

+, done, achieved, successful; −, not done, unsuccessful; +/−, incomplete success; CC, care center; IRM, immediate-release morphine; NHCS, National Health Care Service; NGO, nongovernmental organization (in this case, The Lebanese Cancer Society); NNPC, Neighborhood Network in Palliative Care; NPCP, National Palliative Care Program; NYA, not yet available; MoH, Ministry of Health; PC, palliative care; QOL, quality of life; SRM, slow-release morphine; Too soon, not enough time has passed to allow for evaluation.
*PC in the NNPC community and some districts but not in the NHCS.
†The cost of a 3-wk supply of liquid morphine corresponds to the cost of one loaf of bread (<1 US cent). The government provides the morphine free of charge. Qualified palliative care nurses may renew prescriptions and change dosages.
‡Total opioid consumption increased from 3.5 kg per 1 million people in 1990 to 21 kg/million in 2005.
§IRMs and SRMs were not available for the first 3.5 yr of the program.
¶Generic morphine tablets came from HIKMA Pharmaceuticals, Amman, Jordan, and West Coast Pharmaceuticals, Ahmedabad, India, and Nycomed, Denmark; morphine solutions were produced in Kampala, Uganda, from morphine imported from Scotland.

essential factors usually decide whether the program will succeed in its long-term outcomes. Palliative care became a part of the National Health Plan in Catalonia,[7] Uganda,[1,11] Mongolia,[13] and Georgia.[14] It failed in Lebanon[11] and is not yet in place in Jordan.[15] The Indian state of Kerala has successfully integrated palliative care into the health care service and shows the way by its community approach, which is achieving meaningful coverage in the demonstration districts.[17-19]

Unrealistic prescription rules that hindered progress were changed to relevant workable norms, and this was followed in Uganda, Mongolia, and Jordan by the availability of generic morphine. In Uganda, qualified palliative care nurses now can prescribe morphine. The generic oral morphine introduced was so inexpensive that it is now given free of charge. In Mongolia, a prescription previously could be written for only 3 days and only with parenteral application. Now, oncologists and family doctors can prescribe adequate amounts for longer times. Generic morphine tablets[20] are now available in Mongolia and cost US 5 cents per tablet for 10-mg immediate-release morphine (IRM) and 20 cents for 30-mg slow-release morphine (SRM). In Jordan, generic IRM tablets are produced by the leading national pharmaceutical company, HIKMA.[21]

Table 1-3 gives an example of a recommended plan for availability of strong analgesics. Lebanon did not establish a clear drug policy, and nongeneric, expensive transdermal fentanyl patches, costing the equivalent of two-thirds of one month's salary for a nurse for 1 month's supply, took the market. In Lebanon the number of patients seen remains low, as when starting years ago. This example shows that, when establishing morphine availability, it is important to specify in a policy or Ministry of Health resolution that more than 80% of the new INCB quota should be covered by generic IRM and SRM. If this is not done, the market will be taken over by aggressive international pharmaceutical companies when palliative care is being introduced, resulting in availability of only expensive brand name drugs, and the program will not take off.

The Catalonia WHO demonstration project[7-9] was the first to reach the long-term outcomes, having covered 80% of all those needing palliative care in a population of 6 million (now 7 million) and with 15 years of follow-up. Opioid consumption today is 21 kg per million inhabitants per year, and 75% of that amount is morphine (65% tablets, 10% liquid), compared with opioid consumption of 3.5 kg per million population per year in 1990.[9] Box 1-5 shows

how to calculate the amounts of morphine needed in the future.

A key point for success is coordination of the measures taken. Education without availability of drugs will not have the desired effects, nor will adequate drug availability without the necessary education. Introduction of strong opioids without parallel bedside training has usually led to the available drugs' not being used. Many years of work in India never achieved any meaningful pain relief coverage, because morphine availability was not matched with bedside training in palliative care.[22] However, with the combination of morphine availability and bedside training, there was a significant increase in the number of patients treated with opioids and in opioid consumption.[15]

The King Hussein Cancer Centre in Jordan successfully institutionalized palliative care in record time; drug availability was coordinated with intensive bedside training, and national champions emerged.[15] The King Hussein Cancer Centre is now developing into a reference center of excellence, not only nationally but for the region.

PALLIATIVE CARE FOR ALL: THE COMMUNITY APPROACH

The community approach is essential to allow all to benefit from the advantages of palliative medicine and to reach all patients in need of palliative care. The community palliative care projects of the northern Kerala districts, a WHO demonstration project, and the associated Neighborhood Network in Palliative Care[17-19] show a solution to a key worldwide problem: how to achieve meaningful coverage and care for the terminally ill. The majority of India's terminally ill patients reside in its more than 500 districts, and it is in their home districts that patients should receive palliative care, not in the big specialized centers.

Five self-explanatory key points that summarize why this community approach is so important are given in Box 1-6. The Kerala community approach is in accordance with the WHO recommended Public Health and Primary Health approach.

The palliative care specialists in India, fewer than 100 for 1.3 billion people, will not be able to cover the need for palliative care (Fig. 1-2). Their role must inevitably be to train future trainers—to educate the health professionals in the middle part of the triangle in the core competencies of palliative care, so that they can support the large base, the community.

Hopefully, the highly sophisticated palliative medicine establishment will identify with the community palliative

TABLE 1-3 Example of a Drug Availability Plan			
ORAL IRM	**ORAL SRM**	**PARENTERAL**	**OTHER OPIOIDS**
30%	60%	5%	5%
10 mg	30 mg	2 mg/mL	
20 mg	60 mg	10 mg/mL	
	(100 mg)	50 mg/mL	

IRM, immediate-release morphine; SRM, slow-release morphine.

Box 1-5 Estimating Future Amount of Morphine Needed
Based on the average daily dose for control of cancer pain, which is 100 mg/day per patient (in upper range), and assuming an average time of 100 days, a total of 10,000 mg (0.01 kg) will be needed per patient. Therefore, 1 kg of morphine would cover 100 patients.

Box 1-6 Important Points in a Community Approach to Achieving Adequate Coverage (Neighborhood Network in Palliative Care, Kerala, India)

- Succeeded in making palliative care a movement of people taking responsibility and ownership for care of the terminally ill in their society.
- Established high ethical standards, covering most of the terminally ill.
- Demonstrated an alternative to existing overmedicalized, overspecialized, institutionalized, and, in the long run, unaffordable care of the dying.
- Showed financial self-sustainability.
- Showed that social support, psychological support, nursing care, and partial medical management can be done by the community.

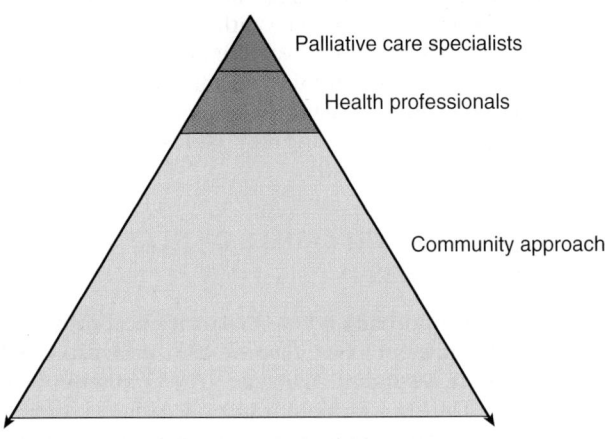

FIGURE 1-2   Palliative Care for All. *(From Stjernswärd J. Community participation in palliative care. Indian J Palliat Care 2005;11:52-58.)*

Future Considerations

- Death is our fate, and palliative care can relieve unnecessary suffering of the terminally ill. Cultural and socioeconomic solutions are as important, and probably more important, than purely medical efforts in achieving a meaningful coverage globally.
- Palliative care should be part of every country's health care system, at all levels, from centers of excellence to palliative home care and home care. A hospice approach alone will not achieve the required coverage.
- Rapid global demographic changes with an increased aging population will in many countries lead to a ratio of caregiver to care receiver of 2:1 or less. China, with one fifth of the world's population, will be the extreme example. Even if palliative care is well established in a country, it is questionable whether it can be sustainable in the present optimal forms, even in the wealthy nations.
- The ethical questions concerning terminal care, death, and dying should be addressed, and education on death as a natural part of a life cycle should be included in curricula for school-aged children.
- The same attention that is given those who are entering life should be given to those who are leaving life, the elderly and terminally ill.
- The community approach, with the active participation of society and caring families, will be critical for achieving meaningfully palliative care coverage.

care approach and continue to help to distill, develop, and provide "methods that are scientifically valid, acceptable and maintainable at community level," similar to the WHO pain ladder.[2]

Some overall considerations are provided in the accompanying box (see "Future Considerations"). For an effective implementation, both the institutionalized, highly specialized palliative medicine centers and the community approaches are needed—they are interdependent and complementary.

REFERENCES

1. Stjernswärd J, Clark D. Palliative medicine: A global perspective. In Doyle D, Hanks G, et cl (eds). Oxford Textbook of Palliative Medicine, 3rd ed. New York: Oxford University Press, 2004, pp 1199-1224.
2. World Health Organization. Cancer Pain Relief: With a Guide to Opioid Availability, 2nd ed. Geneva: WHO, 1996.
3. World Health Organization. Cancer Pain Relief and Palliative Care. WHO Technical Report, Series 804. Geneva: WHO, 1990.
4. World Health Organization: National Cancer Control Programmes: Policies and Managerial Guidelines, 2nd ed. Geneva: WHO, 2002.
5. World Health Organization. Available at http://www.who.int/whr/2003/en/annex2-en.pdf (accessed October 2006).
6. World Fact Book. Available at http://www.cia.gov/cia/publications/factbook/index.html (accessed September 2007).
7. Stjernswärd J. Palliative care: The public health strategy. J Public Health Policy 2007;28:42-55.
8. Gómez-Batiste X, Porta J, Tuca A, et al. Spain: The WHO demonstration project of palliative care implementation in Catalonia. Results at 10 years (1991-2001). J Pain Symptom Manage 2002;24:239-244.
9. Gómez-Batiste X, Porta-Sales J, Nabal M, et al. Catalonia WHO demonstration project at 15 years (2005). J Pain Symptom Manage 2007;33:584-590.
10. Stjernswärd J. Uganda: Initiating a government public health approach to pain relief and palliative care. J Pain Symptom Manage 2002;24:257-264.
11. Daher M, Tabari H, Stjernswärd J, et al. Lebanon: Introducing pain relief and palliative care. J Pain Symptom Manage 2002;3:200-205.
12. Totathathill Z, Kumar S, Stjernswärd J. Report: Kuwait National Palliative Care Programme 2003. Available from dearZiad@lycos.com or janstjernsward@hotmail.com.
13. Stjernswärd J, Odontuya D. Mongolia National Palliative Care Programme, Ulaan Baatar, 2004. Available from d_odontuya@yahoo.com or janstjernsward@hotmail.com; Davaasuren O, Stjernswärd J, Callaway M, et al. Mongolia: Establishing a national palliative care program. J Pain Symptom Manage 2007;33:568-572.
14. Stjernswärd J. Georgia: National Palliative Care Program. Available at http://www.parliament.ge/files/619_8111_336972_Paliativi-Eng.pdf (accessed September 2007).
15. Stjernswärd J. Report: Jordan Pain and Palliative Care Initiative, Amman, 2003. Available from Chairman, Jordan NPCC, S.Khleif@khcc.jo or janstjernsward@hotmail.com; Stjernswärd J, Ferris FD, Khleif SN, et al. Jordan palliative care initiative: A WHO Demonstration Project. J Pain Symptom Manage 2007;33:628-633.
16. World Health Organization. Bridging the Know-Do Gap in Global Health [special issue]. Bulletin WHO 2004:82(10).
17. Neighborhood Network in Palliative Care (NNPC). Work Book: International Workshop on Community Participation in Palliative Care. Manjeri, Malappuram District, Kerala, 26-28 November 2004. Published by NNPC Groups, Department of Community Medicine and Institute of Palliative Medicine, Medical College, Calicut, Kerala, 673008 India.
18. Stjernswärd J. Community participation in palliative care. Indian J Palliat Care 2005;11:52-58.
19. Kumar S. The chronically and incurably ill: Barriers to care. The Commonwealth Health Ministers Reference 2006:2-5.
20. West Coast Pharmaceutical, Ahmedabad, India. Available at http://www.westcoastin.com (accessed September 2006).
21. Hikma Pharmaceuticals, Amman, Jordan. Available at http://www.hikma.com (accessed September 2006).
22. Stjernswärd J. Foreword: Instituting palliative care in developing countries—An urgent needed and achievable goal. In Rajagopal MR, Mazzan D, Lipman AG (eds). Pain and Palliative Care in the Developing World and Marginalized Populations, Binghamton, NY: Haworth Medical Press, 2003, pp xvii-xxiv.

SUGGESTED READING

Gómez-Batiste X, Porta J, Tuca A, et al. Spain: The WHO demonstration project of palliative care implementation in Catalonia. Results at 10 years (1991-2001). J Pain Symptom Manage 2002;24:239-244.

Kumar S. The chronically and incurably ill: Barriers to care. The Commonwealth Health Ministers Reference 2006:2-5.

Stjernswärd J. Community participation in palliative care. Indian J Palliat Care 2005;11:52-58.

Stjernswärd J. Georgia: National Palliative Care Program. Available at http://www.parliament.ge/files/619_8111_336972_Paliativi-Eng.pdf (accessed September 2007).

Stjernswärd J, Clark D. Palliative medicine: A global perspective. In Doyle D, Hanks G, et cl (eds). Oxford Textbook of Palliative Medicine, 3rd ed. New York: Oxford University Press, 2004, pp 1199-1224.

World Health Organization. Cancer Pain Relief and Palliative Care. WHO Technical Report, Series 804. Geneva: WHO, 1990.

World Health Organization. Cancer Pain Relief: With a Guide to Opioid Availability, 2nd ed. Geneva: WHO, 1996.

World Health Organization: National Cancer Control Programmes: Policies and Managerial Guidelines, 2nd ed. Geneva: WHO, 2002.

CHAPTER **2**

Death in Modern Society

Donna M. Wilson and Beryl E. Cable-Williams

KEY POINTS

- Death is often, but inaccurately, portrayed in the media as an unexpected, tragic, and largely preventable phenomenon of youth.

- In modern societies, death commonly occurs in old age as a combined outcome of senescence and the effects of one or more, often chronic illnesses.

- Because dying naturally of old age is not an accepted official cause of death, dying is often subject to efforts aimed at prevention, amelioration, or outright cure.

- The duration and the type of dying process are largely affected by the disease trajectory. A long decline in health is most common; it first leads to functional limitations near death and then to inevitable or unpreventable death.

- Sophisticated life-supporting interventions have prolonged life for many who would not have survived even a short time ago. Questions about the practical and ethical use of resources and the essence of life remain modern challenges.

To judge a society as modern, a standard must exist against which the ideas and methods common to it can be measured for their currency and sophistication. Modernity is thus inherently subjective. In this chapter, modern societies are understood, from an admittedly Western perspective, as being economically and technologically developed. Their progress has been founded largely on science and technology. Beliefs about the cause and cure of illness reflect this orientation, with the relevance of spiritual beliefs and cultural or family resources less evident. Economic prosperity has enabled development and delivery of advanced illness care programs. Markers of a modern approach to illness include the use of leading-edge biomedical knowledge and pharmacological and other technologies. The result is aging populations[1]: staying alive is easier than in less sophisticated conditions.[2] Ironically, it has been suggested that dying is not only delayed in modern societies, but it is also more complex and difficult.[3] In this chapter, the nature of dying and death in modern societies is addressed in terms of the demographics, common causes, disease trajectories or courses of decline at the end of life, and key issues and challenges concerning dying and death.

DEMOGRAPHICS AND CAUSES OF DEATH IN MODERN SOCIETIES

Comparisons of mortality across countries is complicated by inconsistencies in data classification and reporting. Information on Australia,[4] Canada,[5] New Zealand,[6] Switzerland,[7] the United Kingdom,[8] and the United States of America[9] reveal similar trends in life expectancy, leading causes of death, and location of death.

Life Expectancy in Modern Societies

The most remarkable contributor to longer life expectancy has been a major decline in perinatal, infant, child, and maternal mortality, accompanied by a dramatic increase in the likelihood of most adults' surviving past 65 years of age. Death is most common now among seniors, particularly the very elderly[2] (Fig. 2-1). Other major life expectancy trends are shown in Box 2-1.

Improved life expectancy is attributed to technological and social developments that occurred largely in the 20th century.[12] Public health initiatives such as sanitation and immunization were critical for reducing deaths due to infectious diseases before the mid-20th century discovery of antibiotics. Additional life-saving or life-extending interventions, including sophisticated surgical procedures and many pharmacological agents such as antihypertensives and antihyperglycemics, have developed at an unprecedented rate since that time. Communicable diseases such as tuberculosis and smallpox, once the scourge for all ages, are no longer common causes of premature death, even among those most vulnerable, the young and the old. However, the emergence of new and highly virulent pathogens such as those causing sudden acute respiratory syndrome (SARS), the threat of an influenza pandemic, and the rise of antibiotic-resistant strains of bacteria are reminders of human frailty despite modern medicine. Another element of human vulnerability was blazed on the collective consciousness by the September 11, 2001,

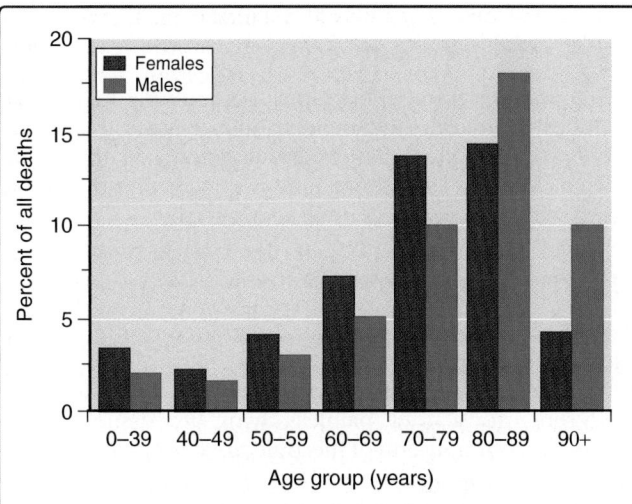

FIGURE 2-1 Distribution of deaths by age in New Zealand in 2004. (From Statistics New Zealand: Deaths—Summary of Latest Trends. Available at http://www.stats.govt.nz/popn-monitor/deaths/deaths-summary-of latest-trends.htm.)

Box 2-1 Common Life Expectancy Trends across Modern Societies

1. Life expectancy increased rapidly and remarkably in the 20th century and continues to do so in the 21st century, although more slowly. In the United States, life expectancy increased from 54 years in 1920 to 77.3 years in 2002.[10] Men born in Australia are expected to live 6 years longer than was true 20 years ago,[4] and in the United Kingdom an increase of 4.8 years in life expectancy occurred for males between 1981 and 2001.[8]

2. Despite gains, men still have a shorter life expectancy than women; men typically live to 75 to 80 years of age, whereas women more often become octogenarians.[10] Women are therefore much more likely to be widowed or single at the end of life and to experience the age-based frailty that is common among the oldest-old.

3. Indigenous people and racial minorities across both genders have significantly shorter life expectancies than their nonindigenous counterparts.[11] The life expectancy for a Maori male in New Zealand is 8 years less than for his non-Maori counterpart.[6]

4. The population subgroup aged 80 to 89 years is the fastest growing demographic group in modern societies. The largest proportion of decedents is from this age-based cohort.[2,3]

---

attacks on the World Trade Center and the Pentagon, events that have become known as "9/11." The remedies for terrorism and its antecedents depend more on manipulation of the sociopolitical determinants of health, such as poverty and cultural oppression, than on medical or health care sophistication.

Common Causes of Death in Modern Society

Despite persistent biological vulnerabilities, the most common causes of death today reflect the impact of improved disease prevention and advanced illness care. As illustrated in Table 2-1, the leading causes of death vary considerably by age. Although childhood deaths are rare, injuries contribute significantly. Deaths from illnesses that are chronic or of long duration, such as circulatory disease, cancer, and respiratory disease, are common at both middle and advanced ages. Cancer, although varying by type, is a leading cause of death across all age groups. Despite many other causes of death, the top three causes (circulatory disease, cancer, and respiratory disease) account for most deaths in modern societies. Early accounts of the preretirement health of the so-called baby boomers, the exceptionally large cohort born in the postwar years of 1946-1966, do not indicate major changes in the leading causes of death.

Interestingly, death from old age is not included in standardized mortality reporting. Rather, all deaths are attributed to pathological processes that might be prevented, ameliorated, or cured. This reflects, as well as contributes to, questions about the acceptability of death, even at advanced age.

Common media portrayals of death involve crime, disaster, mishap, or trauma affecting primarily younger persons. Death is often seen as sudden, untimely, tragic, preventable, and unnecessary. Because it is unexpected, it affords little, if any, opportunity for end-of-life preparation or planning. In reality, death is much more likely to occur in old age, after several years, if not decades, of living with one or more chronic illnesses. These are likely to be protracted and accompanied by increased functional limitations over time.[14] Typical disease trajectories are discussed in more detail in Chapter 3. These trajectories vary with regard to the unexpectedness or expectedness of death and the length of time during which a person is terminally ill or dying. In the first two trajectories, mortal decline is punctuated by one or more illnesses, each pos-

---

TABLE 2-1 Common Causes of Death in Canada by Age Group

AGE (YR)	MOST COMMON	SECOND MOST COMMON	THIRD MOST COMMON
1-14	Injuries	Cancer	Congenital anomalies
15-19	Injuries	Cancer	Circulatory disease
20-24	Injuries	Cancer	Neurological disease
25-44	Injuries	Cancer	Circulatory disease
45-64	Cancer	Circulatory disease	Injuries
65+	Circulatory disease	Cancer	Respiratory disease
All ages	Circulatory disease	Cancer	Respiratory disease

From Child Injury Division. Canadian Injury Data. Bureau of Reproductive and Child Health, Health Protection Branch, Health Canada, 1999.

sibly life-threatening. In another pattern, sometimes called dwindling or lingering, a steady, slow decline is characterized by increasing frailty and dependence.[14] Whereas a lingering death is common, and arguably natural, it is the antithesis of a "good" death in modern society.[12,14]

Kastenbaum[12] recognized in the 1970s that death may be either expected or unexpected and that dying may have a short or long duration. One can expect to live more years in poor health now than would have been the case 20 years ago.[3,8] Increasing support is often needed over several years before life's ending. Caregiver burden is a common outcome. Prolonged, 24 hours per day, 7 days per week caregiving, often provided by only a few primary caregivers—typically, the spouse and/or a daughter—leads to considerable health and other impacts on the caregivers. Worrisome as prolonged decline and disability near death are, acknowledging death as expected creates many opportunities for advanced care planning and more appropriate care provision. This improves support for the primary caregivers as well as for seniors who are single or live alone, particularly in rural or remote areas. It could prevent some of the quandaries that arise with regard to withdrawal of life support and assisted suicide or mercy killing. Improved acceptance by and help for those grieving an impending death, and for those bereaved after the death, are other needed developments.

Location of Death in Modern Society

After World War II, the expansion of hospital-based care contributed to the likelihood that death would occur in hospital, under circumstances categorized as "medicalized."[2,3,12] This largely removed death from the immediacy of family and community and reduced personal experience with death and dying. Common life-saving interventions in hospital, such as artificial nutrition and mechanical ventilation, began to be seen as futile.[15] Decisions about appropriate interventions near death, and earlier in a terminal illness, continue to be problematic, because they affect the quality and quantity of life. Accordingly, the benefits of dying in an institution should be compared to those of dying within the context of home, family, and community. Nevertheless, more deaths occur in institutions than in private residences.[2] Many factors reduce the likelihood of dying at home, particularly for elderly women. Smaller nuclear families, longer lives, and longer dying processes all reduce the availability and caregiving capacity of informal caregivers.

Since its inception in the 1970s, the hospice or palliative care movement has sought to increase comfort-oriented end-of-life care within homes or homelike environments.[15] The emphasis is on comprehensive support and symptom management rather than prolongation of life.[16] Although this movement is laudable, its beneficiaries have typically been younger persons dying of cancer, motor neuron disease, or AIDS, rather than elderly persons experiencing chronic illness and age-based frailty.[17] The latter tend to die shortly after being admitted to hospital or, to a lesser but increasing extent, in nursing homes.[2,3] Concerns about the cost and quality of these and other end-of-life experiences challenge their appropriateness.

Key Issues and Challenges Concerning Dying and Death in Modern Societies

Dying and death occur within a sociocultural milieu that includes commonly held beliefs about dying and death. In this section, modern beliefs about a good death are discussed. Key issues and challenges concerning dying and death in modern societies are also raised.

The Nature of a Good Death

A preference for a peaceful and dignified death at a ripe old age, at the end of a healthful life, is usually expressed by those not imminently facing death.[2,12] Intrinsic is the preference for a brief, painless dying process. However, the most common end-of-life trajectory today is inconsistent with this image. Instead, in most cases, attention to the dying person is required over a period of time, during which living and dying occur together. Achieving a good death is even more challenging. As part of the major American Study to Understand Prognosis and Preferences for Outcomes and Risks of Treatments (SUPPORT), older adults facing the end of life offered insight (Box 2-2) into a good death as they experienced their own dying.[18]

Box 2-2 Elements of Quality End-of-Life Care

1. **Care Related to Symptoms and Personal Care**

   Pain and symptom management
   Being clean
   Having physical touch

2. **Being Prepared for Death**

   Having affairs in order
   Believing family is prepared
   Knowing what to expect
   Communicating treatment preferences and naming a proxy decision maker

3. **Achieving a Sense of Completion**

   Saying good bye to important people
   Recognizing one's own accomplishments
   Resolving unfinished business

4. **Being Treated as a Whole Person**

   Maintaining dignity
   Maintaining a sense of humor
   Not dying alone
   Having someone who will listen

5. **Relating to Family, Society, Care Providers, and the Transcendent**

   Trust in and comfort with physician and nurses
   Being able to discuss personal fears, including dying and death
   Not being a burden to family or society
   Being able to help others
   Coming to peace with God

From Steinhauser KE, Christakis NA, Clipp EC, et al. Factors considered important at the end of life by patients, family physicians and other care providers. JAMA 2000;284:2476-2482.

From another perspective, that of the professional hospice or palliative care provider, the Committee on Care at the End of Life[3] concluded that a good death is "free from avoidable distress and suffering for patients, families, and caregivers; in general accord with patients' and families' wishes; and reasonably consistent with clinical, cultural and ethical standards" (p. 3). The perspectives of seniors who acknowledge their terminal state and those of experts in hospice and palliative care are thus similar. Given that the most common end-of-life trajectory in modern society includes decline over several years, during which death could be expected at any time, it seems possible that health care providers could participate with the terminally ill and their families in the unfolding of a good death. However, this appears to happen infrequently.[15,18] Many ironies complicate the experience of a good death in modern society.

Confident Optimism about Science

Remarkable scientific progress throughout the 20th and into the 21st century has contributed to widespread optimism that all life-threatening conditions can be beaten—particularly if efforts are uncompromised. Imagery of battle and victory over the enemy permeate discourse about diseases that plague modern society. If the battle can be won, then it seems necessary to participate in the fight. Dying people are expected to fight to live, and health care professionals are similarly expected to hold and act on this focus. Even when death is imminent, the fight to preserve life is understood as contributing toward the next breakthrough in knowledge. This may serve to create a meaningful dying process that would otherwise be emotionally painful and bereft of value in a modern society where life is revered above all else.

When dying occurs in hospitals, where the culture and mission are both oriented to saving lives and achieving cures, the inclination to apply aggressive treatment is strong. Accompanying this is the attitude that, if cure is the hallmark of success, death can be construed as failure. The choice to take action rather than to decline or withhold treatment is compelling, even for those whose preference is for an uncomplicated or natural death. Ethical considerations about futility, scarcity of health care resources, and both aging and ageism increasingly complicate decisions near the end of life. Most decisions are made by family or health care providers, with little or no guidance from the dying person. Health care providers and family members moved by loyalty to life and to their loved one may question whether enough is being done. One legacy of the work of Elizabeth Kübler-Ross[19] is the belief that the completion of unfinished business and resolution of life are contingent on the acceptance of impending death. This legacy, coupled with the hospice and palliative care movement, has expanded the idea that, if cure is impossible, terminal symptoms such as pain and nausea must be addressed. Whether fighting and accepting death can be held in creative balance by those who hope for the best and prepare for the worst, is the key question.

Death has not always been viewed as the worst outcome. Many religious traditions believe that death is a passage to something better. As such, desire for death may be understandable, particularly if life has become burden-some from old age or terminal illness. Most often, desire for death is seen as a sign of clinical depression to be treated, rather than personal spiritual transcendence (see Chapters 11 and 12).

Although optimism based on the acquisition and application of science is understandable, trends in the health of Americans suggest that progress in increasing the quantity and quality of life has slowed, or in some cases reversed.[9] The chief concern is the prevalence of risk factors for the leading causes of death, such as obesity and inactivity. Whether medical remedies can be found for diseases that originate in long-term lifestyles, rather than in microorganisms or genetics, remains a challenge.

The Pursuit of Healthy Aging and the Challenge of Prognostication

Healthy aging is often understood in part to involve the personal need for self-integration before death and orchestration of an acceptable relationship between the elderly and society. Interest in healthy aging has increased along with aging of the population.[20] Whether the goal is to avoid suffering or to alleviate the economic and social burdens of chronic illness, the concerns of an aging population and health care planners converge. Independence has become the hallmark of healthy aging. The intent to minimize disability and dependence on others is laudable. However, allegiance to philosophies of restoration, rehabilitation, and social engagement can interfere with recognition and acceptance of unavoidable decline near the end of a long life,[20] particularly if quality of living and palliation are jeopardized.[3]

Imminent death from old age and the presence of one or more chronic illnesses is more difficult to recognize than the rapid, relentless decline that occurs with malignant disease. Oncology-based prognostication models, despite their predominance, are inappropriate for addressing the dwindling decline to death that is common across modern societies. An American study found that, on the day before death, fully half of a group of patients with heart failure were estimated to have a 50% chance of surviving for another 6 months.[21] With such uncertainty, prognostication efforts can detract from high-quality care—care that acknowledges that death will eventually occur.

Recent conceptualizations of healthy aging assist in understanding those who live with an uncertain prognosis. If healthy aging is understood as a process of constructing a meaningful sense of self amid the uncertainties and transitions that accompany serious chronic illnesses and advanced age,[22] there may be little need to establish whether one is living or dying. Instead, the challenge is to provide care that will contribute to an acceptable quality of life whether one is living or dying. This may sound simple, but the consequences include complex social reform in modern societies to support dying well.[21]

The Qualification of Living and the Redefinition of Death

The realization and common understanding that most deaths in modern societies are not sudden, unexpected, nor premature will contribute to a new social construct of death and dying. Reshaping the social construct of death and dying is a paradigm shift that will take considerable time to achieve. The change will derive largely from personal and family understandings that arise from sudden confrontations with mortality. These provide an occasion to weigh quality of life against death, with death often viewed as an acceptable alternative to physical and other suffering. Quality of life considerations have come to affect many of the care decisions in modern societies, in an era in which bodily functions can be sustained regardless of cognitive decline. These decisions are difficult because the distinction between being alive and being dead is now less clear.

The consequences of decisions at the interface between life and death have changed. A short time ago, the implications of these choices were philosophical and spiritual, and they were the business of immediate family members. As a result of advances in organ transplantation, some practical decisions are now based on whether a body is considered alive enough to be sustained or dead enough for organ harvesting. Advocates of organ transplantation have brought decisions of this sort into public policy agendas.

Judgments about quality of life are inseparable from the definition of death. In modern settings, whether in a trauma unit or in long-term care, matters are no longer simply about life and death but about the quality of living and dying (see Chapter 65).

CONCLUSIONS

In this chapter, the impacts of significant scientific and other developments on dying and death in modern societies were highlighted. Less than a century ago, death was more common among the young, due to infection and trauma, and fewer individuals survived to advanced old age than now. Today, early deaths are most commonly the result of injuries or cancer. These deaths can be considered unexpected because they are not timely and not anticipated. They defy the expectations of a medically sophisticated and optimistic society. Death and its prerequisite, dying, are more likely now to occur in old age, from senescence and the chronic effects of one or more progressive health conditions. Although deaths among seniors may be less unexpected, preparation and planning for the end of life are often incomplete. This may be the legacy of a shared optimism in the unending life-saving possibilities afforded by scientific advancements, a strong preference for healthy living rather than healthy dying, and a tendency to rely less on spiritual resources than on science in the face of existential crises. Although death is different in modern societies than in less economically and scientifically developed ones, considerable challenges remain to advance the art and science of end-of-life care. Many changes can also be expected as modern societies face the realities of dying and death along with continued population aging.

REFERENCES

1. United Nations Population Division. World Population Projections to 2150. New York: United Nations, 1998.
2. Northcott HC, Wilson DM. Dying and Death in Canada. Aurora, Ontario: Garamond, 2001.
3. Field MJ, Cassel CK (eds): Approaching Death: Improving Care at the End of Life. Washington, DC: National Academy Press, 1997.
4. Australian Bureau of Statistics. Causes of Death, Australian Preliminary Summary Tables. Government of Australia, 2004. Available at http://www.ausstats.abs.gov.au/Ausstats/subscriber.nsf/o/68D51845F3970A92CA25713000705D3A/$File/33030_2004.pdf (accessed January 2008).
5. Public Health Agency of Canada. Leading Causes of Death and Hospitalization in Canada. Government of Canada, 2000. Available at http://www.phac-aspc.gc.ca/publicat/lcd-pcd97/mrt_mf_e.html (accessed January 2008).
6. Statistics New Zealand. Deaths—Summary of Latest Trends. Available at http://www.stats.govt.nz/popn-monitor/deaths/deaths-summary-of latest-trends.htm.
7. Swiss Federal Statistics Office. Statistical Data on Switzerland 2007: Health—Life Expectancy, 2007. Available at http://www.bfs.admin.ch/bfs/portal/en/index.html (accessed September 2007).
8. National Statistics UK. Health Expectancy: Living Longer, More Years in Poor Health. Government of the United Kingdom Actuary's Department, 2005. Available at http://www.statistics.gov.uk/CCI/nugget.asp?ID=934&Pos=1&ColRank=2&Rank=1000 (accessed January 2008).
9. U.S. Department of Health and Human Services. Health United States, 2005. DHHS Publication No. 2005-1232, Centers for Disease Control and Prevention, 2005. Available at http://www.cdc.gov/nchs/data/hus/hus05.pdf#executivesummary (accessed September 2007).
10. National Center for Health Statistics/ Deaths and Percentage of Total Deaths for the 10 Leading Causes of Death, by Race: United States, 2002. National Vital Statistics Reports November 10, 2004;53(6).
11. Health Canada. Statistical Report on the Health of Canadians. Available at http://www.phac-aspc.gc.ca/ph-sp/phdd/pdf/report/stats/all_english.pdf (accessed January 2008).
12. Kastenbaum R. On Our Way: The Final Passage Through Life and Death. Berkeley: University of California Press, 2004.
13. Child Injury Division. Canadian Injury Data. Bureau of Reproductive and Child Health, Health Protection Branch, Health Canada, 1999.
14. Murray SA, Kendall M, Boyd K, et al. Illness trajectories and palliative care. BMJ 2005;330:1007-1011.
15. Twycross RG. The challenge of palliative care. Int J Clin Oncol 2002;7:271-278.
16. World Health Organization. Definition of Palliative Care. Geneva: WHO, 2002. Available at http://www.who.int/cancer/palliative/definition/en/ (accessed September 2007).
17. Murtagh FEM, Preston M, Higginson I. Patterns of dying: Palliative care for non-malignant disease. Clin Med 2004;4:39-44.
18. Steinhauser KE, Christakis NA, Clipp EC, et al. Factors considered important at the end of life by patients, family physicians and other care providers. JAMA 2000;284:2476-2482.
19. Kübler-Ross E: On Death and Dying. New York: Macmillan, 1969.
20. Agich G. Autonomy and dependence in old age. Cambridge, England: Cambridge University Press, 2003.
21. Lynn J. Learning to care for people with chronic illness facing the end of life. JAMA 2000;284:2508-2511.

Future Considerations

- There is a need to reintegrate into the modern collective conscience the idea that dying is normal and that living and dying occur simultaneously throughout the unfolding of individual life stories.
- Dying people are expected to fight to live. Fostering a willingness to acknowledge and embrace the challenges of dying, regardless of the person's age or cause of death, is needed.
- Fear of pain when dying is common, as are painful deaths. Continued development of more effective pain and symptom management, particularly in nonhospital settings, is needed, along with practice cultures that support its use.
- There is insufficient recognition of the life-threatening nature of chronic illness, and there is a need for appropriate inclusion of end-of-life considerations throughout the entire disease trajectory.
- Decisions about appropriate interventions near death and earlier during a terminal illness are often difficult, because they involve the quality and quantity of life. Considerable research is needed to assist common decisions, such as whether relocating to give or receive care is justified.
- Death is most common among persons aged 80 years or older. End-of-life care planning must consider the advanced age and other sociodemographic factors of the dying person.

22. Chapman SA. Theorizing about aging well: Constructing a narrative. Can J Aging 2004;24:9-18.

SUGGESTED READING

Edwards M. Modern medicine and the pursuit of cure. Med Educ 1999;33:704-706.

Field MJ, Cassel CK (eds). Approaching Death: Improving Care at the End of Life. Washington, DC: National Academy Press, 1997.

Kastenbaum R: On Our Way: The Final Passage Through Life and Death. Berkeley: University of California Press, 2004.

Lynn J: Learning to care for people with chronic illness facing the end of life. JAMA 2000;284:2508-2511.

Northcott HC, Wilson DM: Dying and Death in Canada. Aurora, Ontario: Garamond, 2001.

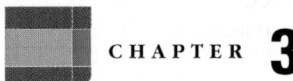

CHAPTER **3**

Illness Trajectories and Stages*

Scott A. Murray

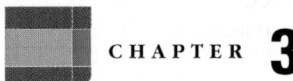

K E Y   P O I N T S

- In the 21st century, chronic illness more frequently precedes death than does cancer.

- Three typical trajectories of physical decline are described in progressive illness: cancer, organ failure, and the frail elderly or dementia trajectory.

- Physical, social, psychological, and spiritual needs may vary according to the trajectory.

- Even if these trajectories cannot be altered, being aware of them may help clinicians plan care to better meet their patient's multi-dimensional needs as the illness progresses toward death and to help patients and carers cope.

- Different models of end-of-life care may be necessary for different conditions.

Deaths in younger people shape the current social construct of dying (see Chapter 2). A century ago, death typically occurred suddenly, as a result of infection, accident, or childbirth. Today, particularly in developed societies, sudden death is less common, as is death before older age. Toward the end of life, most people acquire a serious progressive illness—cardiovascular disease, cancer, and respiratory disorders being the three leading causes—that increasingly interferes with usual activities until death. In a typical population of 2000 patients registered with a U.K. family doctor, there are 20 deaths per annum:

*This chapter was adapted from Murray SA, Kendall M, Boyd K, Sheikh A. Illness trajectories and palliative care. BMJ 2005;330:1007-1011.

whereas 2 of these deaths will be "sudden," 5 patients will die from cancer, 6 from a chronic disease, and 7 after prolonged frailty (Fig. 3-1).

This new demographic of dying poses considerable challenges and opportunities for palliative care services, which have historically focused on cancer. The question, "At what stages of chronic illness should palliative medicine or the palliative care approach be involved?" is vital and may be even more important in chronic diseases other than cancer, because of the longer time scale involved. This chapter highlights and illustrates several typical "illness trajectories" by using patient scenarios to map the various stages of decline in chronic progressive illnesses and frailty.

DIFFERENT TRAJECTORIES FOR DIFFERENT DISEASES

Three distinct illness trajectories have been described for progressive chronic illnesses (see Fig. 3-1).[1-6]

- *Cancer trajectory:* steady progression and, usually, a clear terminal phase
- *Organ failure trajectory* (e.g., respiratory, heart and liver failure): gradual decline, punctuated by episodes of acute deterioration and some recovery, followed by sudden, seemingly unexpected death
- *Frail elderly and dementia trajectory:* prolonged gradual decline

Trajectory 1: Short Period of Decline, Typically Cancer

The cancer trajectory involves a reasonably predictable decline in physical health over weeks, months, or, in some cases, years. This may be punctuated by the positive or negative effects of palliative oncology treatment. Most weight loss, reduction in performance status, and impaired ability for self-care occurs in the last few months. With earlier diagnosis and greater openness about prognosis, there is usually time to anticipate palliative needs and plan for end-of-life care. This trajectory meshes well with traditional specialist palliative care services, such as hospices and their associated community palliative care programs, which provide comprehensive services in the last weeks or months of life for people with cancer. Resource constraints on hospices and their community teams, as well as their association with dying, can limit their availability and acceptability (Box 3-1 and Fig. 3-2).

Trajectory 2: Long-Term Limitations with Intermittent Serious Episodes

With conditions such as heart failure, liver failure, and chronic obstructive pulmonary disease (COPD), patients are ill for many months or years, with occasional acute, often severe, exacerbations. Deteriorations are associated with hospitalization and intensive treatment. Any exacerbation may result in death, and, although patients usually survive many such episodes, a gradual deterioration in health and functional status is typical. The timing of death, however, remains uncertain. Most patients with advanced

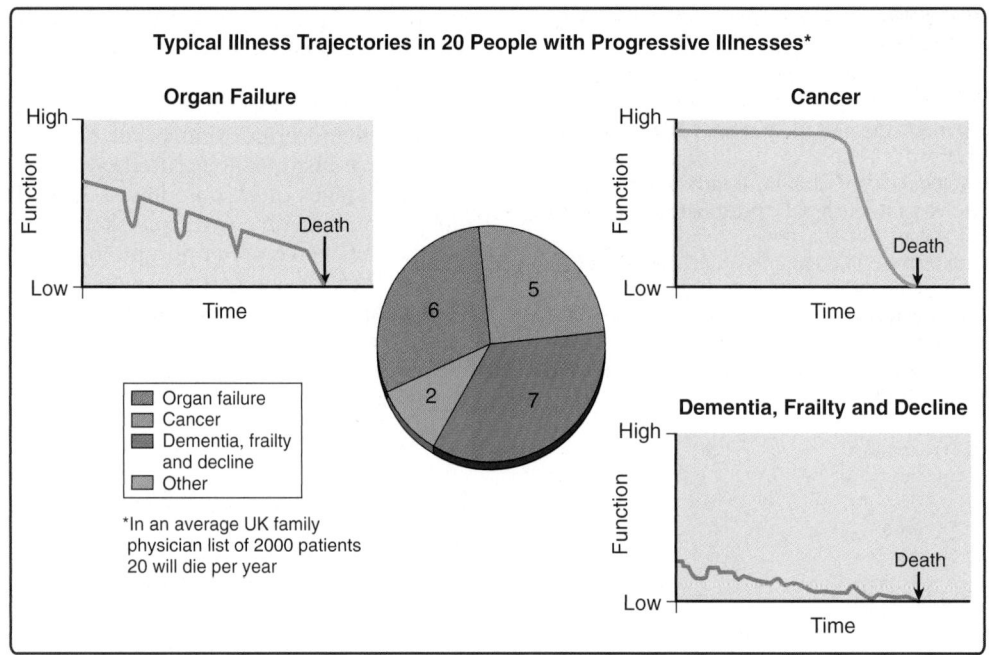

FIGURE 3-1   Typical trajectories of progressive illnesses and number of deaths of each type per year among an average U.K. family physician list of 2000 patients..

Box 3-1 Example of a Cancer Trajectory

JM, a 51-year-old male shop assistant, complained of night sweats, weight loss, and a cough. A radiographic study initially suggested tuberculosis, but bronchoscopy and computed tomography scanning revealed inoperable non–small cell lung cancer.

He was offered and accepted palliative chemotherapy after he had already lost considerable weight (too much to allow him to enter a trial). The chemotherapy may have helped control his breathlessness, but he was subsequently admitted due to vomiting. Looking back, JM expressed regret that he had received chemotherapy:

"If I had known I was going to be like this . . ."

His wife felt they had lost valuable time together during the period when he was relatively well.

JM feared a lingering death:

"I'd love to be able to have a wee turn-off switch, because the way I've felt, there's some poor souls go on for years and years like this and they never get cured; I wouldn't like to do that."

JM's wife, in contrast, worried that her husband might die suddenly:

"When he's sleeping, I keep waking him up, I am so stupid. He'll say, "Will you leave me alone, I'm sleeping." . . . He's not just going to go there and then, I know, but I've got to reassure myself."

JM died at home 3 months after diagnosis, cared for by the primary care team, night nurses, and specialist palliative care services. His death had been openly discussed. He and his wife were confident that nursing, medical, and support staff would be available, which they were.

From Murray SA, Kendall M, Boyd K, Sheikh A. Illness trajectories and palliative care. BMJ 2005;330:1007–1011.

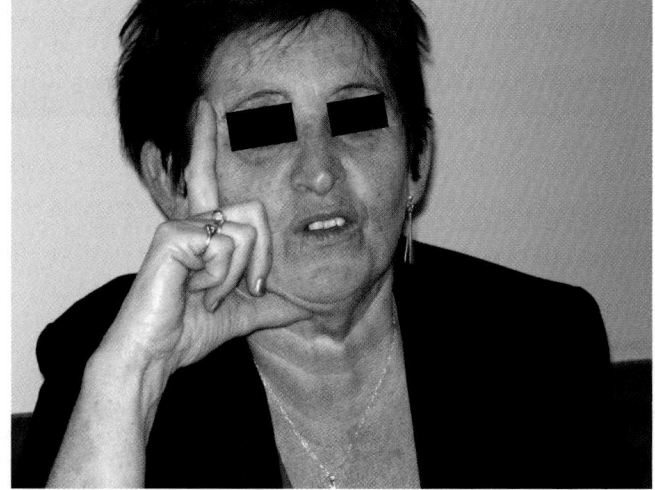

FIGURE 3-2   The wife of Mr. JM, whose decline followed Trajectory 1 (see Box 3-1). (From Murray SA, Kendall M, Boyd K, Sheikh A. Illness trajectories and palliative care. BMJ 2005;330:1007–1011.)

Trajectory 3: Prolonged Dwindling

Those who escape cancer and organ system failure are likely to die at an older age from either brain failure (e.g., Alzheimer's disease or other dementia) or generalized frailty of multiple body systems. This third trajectory is one of progressive disability from an already low baseline of cognitive and/or physical functioning. Patients may lose weight and functional capacity and then succumb to minor events or "hassles" that may in themselves seem trivial, but, when occurring in combination with declining reserves, can prove fatal.[8] This trajectory may be cut short by death after an acute event such as a fractured femur or pneumonia (Box 3-3 and Fig. 3-4).

heart failure die unexpectedly, when they are expected by clinicians to live a further 6 months.[7] Many patients with end-stage heart failure and COPD follow this trajectory, but this may not be true for those with other organ system failures (Box 3-2 and Fig. 3-3).

Box 3-2 Example of an Organ Failure Trajectory

Mrs. AA, a 65-year-old retired bookkeeper, had had a number of hospital admissions with cardiac failure. She was housebound in her third-floor flat and was cared for by a devoted husband, who accepted little help from social work or community nursing. Previously, she had been very outgoing, but she became increasingly isolated. Her major concern was her rapidly deteriorating vision due to diabetes, not her stage IV heart failure. Her treatment included high-dose diuretics and long-term oxygen therapy, and she required frequent blood tests.

She had raised her prognosis indirectly with her general practitioner by mentioning to him that her grandson had asked whether she would be around at Christmas. Prognostic uncertainty is a key issue for heart failure patients and their carers, as illustrated by the following quotations:

"I take one step forward, then two steps back." (84-year-old male, retired engineer, living alone, with several recent hospitalizations)

"I'd like to get better, but I keep getting worse." (72-year-old female, widow, with psoriasis and arthritis)

"Things I used to take for granted are now an impossible dream." (75-year-old male, retired, living with his wife of 50 years and with a large family nearby)

"There were times, last year, when I thought I was going to die." (77-year-old female, widow living alone, with several periods in hospital with acute breathlessness)

"It could happen at any time" (wife and main carer of 62-year-old male, former footballer)

"I know he won't get better, but don't know how long he's got." (wife of 77-year-old male, retired flour mill worker, with severe asthma)

Mrs. AA died on the way home from a hospital admission due to a nosebleed. She had suffered from these occasionally, because she had hypertension and a perforated nasal septum. Attempted resuscitation took place in the ambulance. Her husband later expressed regret that his wife's clear wish not to have her life prolonged was not respected.

From Murray SA, Kendall M, Boyd K, Sheikh A. Illness trajectories and palliative care. BMJ 2005;330:1007–1011.

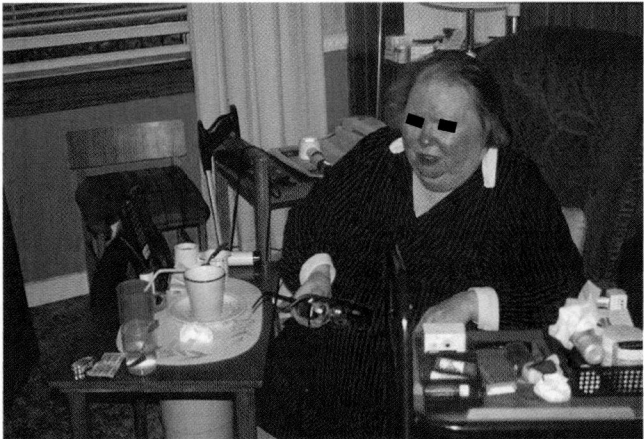

FIGURE 3-3   Mrs. AA, whose husband is her informal carer, illustrates trajectory 2 (see Box 3-2). (From Murray SA, Kendall M, Boyd K, Sheikh A. Illness trajectories and palliative care. BMJ 2005;330:1007–1011.)

Box 3-3 Example of a Frailty Trajectory

Mrs. LC, an 80-year-old widow, lives alone in a ground floor flat in central Edinburgh. Bereaved 6 years ago, she is now housebound due to arthritis and has general physical frailty.

She used to go out occasionally to the shops, but over the years she has felt less able and confident, largely because of a fear of falling. She appreciates the chair and walking aids provided by the occupational therapist, because they provide support and a sense of security at home.

She receives regular visits from friends and local church members and is undemanding of services. Current medications are paracetamol, thyroxine, and bendroflumethiazide (for hypertension).

She has no relatives but is supported by her belief in a God who cares for her. Mrs. LC understands her current trajectory of gradual decline in ability to perform activities and is concerned that she might one day be admitted to a nursing home.

From Murray SA, Kendall M, Boyd K, Sheikh A. Illness trajectories and palliative care. BMJ 2005;330:1007–1011.

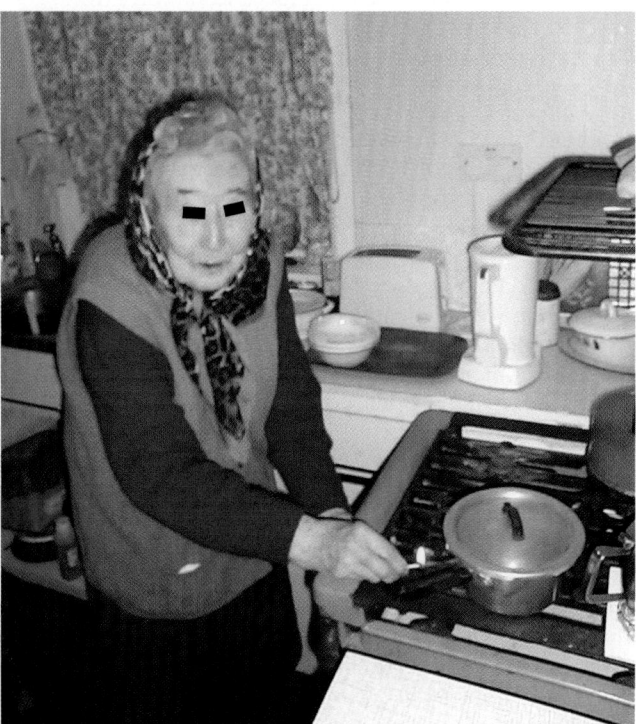

FIGURE 3-4   Mrs. LC, currently on trajectory 3 (see Box 3-3). (From Murray SA, Kendall M, Boyd K, Sheikh A. Illness trajectories and palliative care. BMJ 2005;330:1007–1011.)

CLINICAL IMPLICATIONS

Trajectories Allow Appreciation That "Doing Everything That Can Be Done" May Be Misguided

Optimizing the quality of life leading to a timely, dignified, and peaceful death is the primary aim of palliative care. Understanding and considering the stage of the trajectory may help clinicians understand earlier that progressive deterioration and death are inevitable. Before and even in the final stages of a chronic illness, some professionals may allow the reality of the prognosis to remain unconsidered or unspoken, unwittingly colluding with patients and relatives in fighting death to the bitter end.[9] A realistic outlook

- Concentrating on the physical rather than the dimension of need that is causing most distress
- Doing everything: initiating therapies without fully weighing the pros and cons
- Ignoring opportunities to discuss end-of-life issues with people with chronic illnesses
- Trying to fit patients to services, rather than adapting services to patients' needs and preferences (e.g., having to die in hospital when they wish to die at home)

Box 3-4 Possible Indicators of Need for a Supportive and Palliative Care Approach in Patients with Chronic Disease

- The patient has been discharged from hospital after being admitted for an organ failure disease.
- The patient is housebound.
- The patient has a forced 1-second expiratory volume (FEV_1) of 30 mL or less, stage IV heart failure, or other disease-specific indicators.
- Physicians and nurses, when asking themselves the question, "Would I be surprised if my patient were to die in the next 12 months?" (which could be done during routine consultations or review of a register) determine that the answer is "no."
- See relevant guidance at Gold Standards Framework: http://www. goldstandardsframework.nhs.uk/

on death and expectations may moderate the "technological imperative," preventing unnecessary hospital admissions or aggressive treatments for chronic disease or cancer.[10] A realistic dialogue about the illness trajectory among patient, family, and professional can introduce supportive care, focusing on quality of life and symptom control earlier and more often (see "Common Errors").

Trajectories Allow Practical Planning for a "Good Death"

Dying at home is the wish of approximately 65% of people at the beginning of both cancer and organ failure trajectories, although only about 25% succeed.[11] An appreciation that all trajectories lead to death but that death may be sudden (particularly in trajectory 2) supports advanced planning. Eliciting the "preferred place of care" is now standard in some palliative care frameworks and increases the likelihood that those with cancer may die in their place of choice (see Box 3-1).[12] Some cope by denial or disavowal, making open communication less possible in the earlier stages.[13]

Sensitive exploration can allow issues such as resuscitation status to be clarified and "unfinished business" to be completed for all trajectories. In the case described in Box 3-2, Mrs. AA's death had (unusually for those with heart failure) been planned, but in an emergency she received inappropriate resuscitation. Living wills (advance directives) may be popular, but most health professionals have little experience with them. Directives may be particularly relevant in trajectory 3, in which there may be progressive cognitive decline.

Understanding the Likely Trajectory May Be Empowering for Patient and Carer

Some patients and carers attempt to gain control over illness by acquiring knowledge about how it is likely to progress.[14] In the example described in Box 3-1, JM, who had lung cancer, might have been less worried about a protracted death if he had been aware of his likely course of decline. Similarly, his wife might have been less worried about a sudden death. Both gave clear cues in research interviews that they were concerned about the nature of the death and would welcome sensitive discussion.

Considering the Trajectory Stages May Avoid "Prognostic Paralysis"

"Prognostic paralysis" describes the tendency of clinicians of patients with uncertain illness trajectories to prevari-

Box 3-5 Adopting Patient-Centered Supportive Care: Possible Questions

- What's the most important issue in your life right now?
- What helps you keep going?
- How do you see the future?
- What is your greatest worry or concern?
- Are there ever times when you feel down?
- If things got worse, where would you like to be cared for?

Murray SA, Boyd K, Sheikh A. Palliative care in chronic illnesses: We need to move from prognostic paralysis to active total care. BMJ 2005;330: 611-612.

cate about the end of life.[15] Considering the trajectory stages may help overcome this problem. Quality improvement teams in the United States suggest that, rather than target patients who will die in the next 6 months, clinicians should focus on those who "reasonably might die" now.[1] Possible ways of identifying patients with chronic disease for a supportive and palliative care approach are provided in greater detail in Chapter 119. Box 3-4 provides simple pointers.

Helping Patients and Carers Embrace a More Proactive Approach to Living and Dying with Chronic Illness

Most people with progressive chronic illnesses have already brushed death. They have "competing narratives" in their minds: on the one hand, they hope things will not deteriorate, but on the other hand, they acknowledge that death is inevitable.[16] Greater awareness of these contrasting narratives should make it easier for clinicians to combine active treatment and a supportive approach. Those with disabling, progressive illnesses expect active care, but they also seek comfort, control, and dignity. They need advanced care planning, a whole-patient and -carer approach, symptom control, and therapeutic dialogue. Some questions that can help clinicians and patients explore these issues are listed in Box 3-5.

Clinical Limitations of the Trajectory Approach

Individual patients die at different stages along each trajectory, and the rate of progression varies. Other diseases or social and family circumstances intervene, so that priorities and needs change. Some illnesses follow none, any, or all of the trajectories: a severe stroke may result in sudden death or in an acute decline as in the cancer trajectory; a series of smaller strokes and recovery may mimic trajectory 2; a gradual decline after acquisition of a disability may parallel trajectory 3. Renal failure might represent a fourth trajectory of a steady decline, with the rate depending on the underlying pathology and other patient factors such as comorbidity.[3] Those with multiple disorders may have two trajectories running concurrently, with the more rapidly progressing trajectory taking center stage. This is not uncommon in older patients with slowly progressive cancers.

IMPLICATIONS FOR SERVICE PLANNING AND DEVELOPMENT

One Size May Not Fit All

Different models are appropriate for people with different illness trajectories. The typical cancer palliative care model might not suit a gradual, progressive decline with unpredictable exacerbations. People with nonmalignant disease may have needs that are more prolonged but similar to those of people with cancer. Uncertainty about prognosis should not lead to neglect of these patients and their families by health and social services. A strategic overview of the needs of and services available to patients on the main trajectories leads to development of better policies and services for all people with serious chronic illnesses.

Advanced Care Planning May Prevent Admissions

Advanced care planning and resource provision based on trajectories might help more people with chronic illnesses die where they prefer. For instance, many frail elderly and patients with dementia are admitted to hospital when terminally ill. The use of care pathways in nursing homes is effective in preventing such admissions.[17]

Transferable Lessons

Models of care for one trajectory may inform another. For example, cancer care personnel can learn from the health promotion paradigm within chronic disease management. "Improving Living While Near Death" in North America[18] and "Health-Promoting Palliative Care" in Australia are two examples.[19] These approaches may destigmatize death and maximize cancer patients' quality of life until death. Conversely, patients with organ failure could benefit from ideas in cancer care (such as advanced care planning frameworks and end-of-life pathways)[20-22] to move from a technological to a holistic approach.

There are striking similarities in symptom burden between patients dying of cancer and those dying of nonmalignant cardiorespiratory disease.[23] Hospital palliative care teams, through offering specialist advice and sharing care with other specialists, can improve the care of many noncancer patients.[24]

Research Challenges

Three typical trajectories of physical decline and death have been described. Others may be soon characterized using quantitative and qualitative longitudinal methods. More research is needed to help understand how the insights from these trajectories can be translated into improvements in outcomes for patients and their families. The trajectories considered here relate to physical well-being; other trajectories may exist, such as the spiritual or existential pathway. In cancer patients, spiritual distress and questioning may peak at diagnosis, again at recurrence, and then later during the terminal stage. In contrast, spiritual distress in patients with heart failure may be evident more uniformly throughout the course, reflecting the gradual loss of identity and increased dependence.[25] Psychological and social trajectories may also be mapped. In dementia, the loss of cognitive function may cause parallel loss in activities of daily living, social withdrawal, and emotional distress.

CONCLUSIONS

Estimating prognosis is an inexact science,[10] but uncertainty should not prevent clinicians' talking with their patients about this issue, because a significant number will die suddenly. The key to caring well for those who will die in the (relatively) near future is to understand how they may die and plan appropriately. Because diseases affect individuals differently, prognosis is often difficult. Nonetheless, patients with specific diseases and their carers often have common patterns of experiences, symptoms, and needs as the illness progresses. In Hippocrates' day, the physician who could foretell the course of an illness was highly esteemed even if he could not alter it.[26] Nowadays, physicians can cure some diseases and effectively manage others. Where we cannot alter the course of an illness, we must at least (when the patient wishes) foretell the course sensitively and, together with the patient and family, plan care for better or for worse.

ACKNOWLEDGMENTS

We would like to acknowledge the work of Joan Lynne, Office of Clinical Standards and Quality, The Centers for Medicare and Medicaid Services, who is pioneering work on illness trajectories. The Scottish Executive funded the research that included the case studies.

REFERENCES

1. Lunney JR, Lynn J, Foley DS, et al. Patterns of functional decline at the end of life. JAMA 2003;289:2387-2392.
2. World Health Organization. Palliative Care: The Solid Facts. Geneva: WHO, 2004.
3. Murtagh FEM, Preston M, Higginson I. Patterns of dying: Palliative care for non-malignant disease. Clin Med 2004;4:39-44.
4. Lehman R. How long can I go on like this? Dying from cardiorespiratory disease. B J Gen Pract 2004;54:892-893.
5. Glare PA, Christakis NA. Predicting survival in patients with advanced disease. In Doyle D, Hanks G, Cherny N, Calman K (eds). Oxford Textbook of Palliative Medicine. New York: Oxford University Press, 2004, pp 29-42.
6. Murray SA, Kendall M, Boyd K, Sheikh A. Illness trajectories and palliative care. BMJ 2005;330:1001-1011.
7. Levenson JW, McCarthy EP, Lynn J: The last six months of life for patients with congestive heart failure. J Am Geriatr Soc 2000;48:S101-S109.
8. Williams R, Zyzanski SJ, Wright A. Life events and daily hassles and uplifts as predictors of hospitalisation and out patient visitation. Soc Sci Med 1992;34:763-768.

9. Higgs R. The diagnosis of dying. J R Coll Physicians Lond 1999;33:110-112.
10. Callahan D. Death and the research imperative. N Engl J Med 2000;342:654-656.
11. Murray SA, Boyd K, Sheikh A, et al. Developing primary palliative care. BMJ 2004;329:1056-1057.
12. Higginson I, Sen-Gupta GJA. Place of care in advanced cancer. J Palliat Med 2004;3:287-300.
13. Buetow S, Coster G. Do general practice patients with heart failure understand its nature and seriousness, and want improved information? Patient Educ Couns 2001;45:181-185.
14. Burke SO, Kauffmann E, LaSalle J, et al. Parents' perceptions of chronic illness trajectories. Can J Nurs 2000;32:19-36.
15. Murray SA, Boyd K, Sheikh A. Palliative care in chronic illnesses: We need to move from prognostic paralysis to active total care. BMJ 2005;330:611-612.
16. Murray SA, Boyd K, Kendall M, et al. Dying of lung cancer or cardiac failure: Prospective qualitative interview study of patients and their carers in the community. BMJ 2002;325:929-932.
17. NHS Modernisation Agency. Liverpool care pathway: Promoting best practice for care of the dying. Liverpool: Marie Curie Cancer Care, 2000.
18. Lynn J. Learning to care for people with chronic illness facing the end of life. JAMA 2000;284:2508-2511.
19. Kellehear A. Health-promoting palliative care: Developing a social model for practice. Mortality 1999;4:75-82.
20. Thomas K. Caring for the Dying at Home: Companions on a Journey. Oxford: Radcliffe Medical Press, 2003.
21. Ellershaw JE, Wilkinson S. Care of the dying: A pathway to excellence. Oxford: Oxford University Press, 2003.
22. Casarett DJ, Crowley R, Hirschman KB. Surveys to assess satisfaction with end-of-life care: Does timing matter? J Pain Symptom Manage 2002;25:128-132.
23. McKinley RK, Stokes T, Exley C, Field D. Care of people dying with malignant and cardiorespiratory disease in general practice. Br J Gen Pract 2004;54:909-913.
24. Kite S, Jones K, Tookman A. Specialist palliative care and patients with non-cancer diagnosis: The experience of a service. Palliat Med 2001;15:413-418.
25. Murray SA, Kendall M, Boyd K, et al. Exploring the spiritual needs of people dying of lung cancer or heart failure: A prospective qualitative interview study of patients and their carers. Palliat Med 2004;18:39-45.
26. Cassell E. The nature of suffering. New York: Oxford University Press, 1991.

SUGGESTED READING

Lynn J, Schuster JL, Kabcenell A. Improving Care for the End of Life: A Sourcebook for Health Care Managers and Clinicians. New York: Oxford University Press, 2000.

Lynn J, Adamson DM. Living Well at the End of Life: Adapting Health Care to Serious Chronic Illness in Old Age. Rand Health—White Paper 2003. Available at http://www.medicaring.org/whitepaper/ (accessed September 2007).

WHO Europe. Better palliative care for older people. Copenhagen: World Health Organization, 2004. Available at http://www.euro.who.int/document/E82933.pdf (accessed September 2007).

Thomas K. Caring for the dying at home: Companions on a Journey. Oxford: Radcliffe Medical Press, 2003.

Ellershaw J, Murphy M. Liverpool Care Pathway: Promoting Best Practice for the Care of the Dying. User Guide. Liverpool: NHS Modernisation Agency, 2004. Available at http://www.mcpcil.org.uk/liverpool_care_pathway (accessed January 2008).

ADDITIONAL RESOURCES

Dipex Web site. Allows patients and carers to read and see how cancer and other illnesses have affected other people. Available at http://www.dipex.org/experiences.asp (accessed January 2008).

Growthhouse.org Inc. Patient and professional resources for life-threatening illness and end-of-life care. Available at http://www.growthhouse.org (accessed January 2008).

List of U.K. self-help sites: http://www.ukselfhelp.info (accessed September 2007).

Lynn J, Harrold J. Handbook for Mortals: Guidance for People Facing Serious Illness. New York: Oxford University Press, 1999.

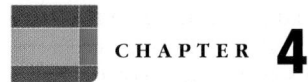

CHAPTER **4**

The History of Hospice

Katri Elina Clemens, Birgit Jaspers, and Eberhard Klaschik

KEY POINTS

- Hospice is primarily a concept of care, not a specific place; it is a philosophy rather than a building or service.
- Modern hospices evolved from the ethical self-obligation of caregivers to fight the deficiencies in the care of the critically ill and dying.
- Unlike conventional medicine, in which death is the ultimate failure, hospice embraces death as a natural part of life.
- Hospice strives to raise public awareness that the taboo on death and dying excludes the dying from society.
- Hospice is a holistic approach (physical, psychological, social, and spiritual), so it uses both volunteers and professionals.

BACKGROUND

Caring for the suffering and dying is part of human history. In the last 25 years, there has been a revolution in the care of the terminally ill and those in pain, primarily due to the work of several individuals whose critical thinking reshaped contemporary views of death. In the second half of the 20th century, medical specialties and subspecialties, new diagnostic tools, and effective therapies emerged as a result of research and unprecedented government funding. There were several cultural consequences: specialists dominated the medical hierarchy; death followed chronic rather than acute illness; the role of the patient changed; and trust between physicians and patients eroded. The emergence of hospice care in the 1960s in England, followed by the United States and Canada in the 1970s, was a reaction to theses changes in medical culture.

Hospice is primarily a concept of care, not a specific place; it is a philosophy of care rather than a type of building or service (see Chapter 5). Hospice philosophy states that there is always something to be done to help patients. The hospice movement has had a major international impact in promoting palliative care and improving care standards in general.

HISTORY

In 6th century BC Greece, medicine was practiced by healers in what we would now call ambulatory clinics—sanctuaries located adjacent to temples of worship—or during home visits.[1] The ill were not housed in a particular location. Until Hippocrates extended the role of the *physikoi* beyond that of a natural philosopher, there was no distinction between science and philosophy, or between body and mind. Physicians diagnosed and treated the whole person rather than just the disease. The link between medicine and religion was inextricable until the Renaissance. Religious societies ran the earliest institutions called hospices, which cared for the ill, primarily people who became ill while traveling. People either recovered and continued traveling or died. The words *hospitality, hotel, hospice, hostel,* and *hospital* are all derived from the same Latin root, *hospes,* meaning "guest."[2] Hospitals as identifiable institutions evolved from these early efforts. For example, St. Bartholomew's Hospital in London was founded in 1123. At the time, there was no practical difference in meaning between *hospital* and *hospice.* Hospitals as institutions for teaching evolved from the observation that the care and study of patients was more convenient for physicians if the patients were assembled in one place. Records from 1544 from St. Bartholomew's Hospital indicate that patients were not to be admitted if they had incurable diseases or conditions.[3] The hospital apparently wanted a reputation for caring for people who could be cured. Subsequently, the term *hospice* was reserved for dedicated places for the care of the incurably ill (and poor). These hospices were mostly administered and staffed by Christian religious orders in France, Ireland, Scotland, and England.[2] In the United States, early examples of hospice care were the Dominican Sisters of Hawthorne and Calvary Hospital, both in New York City.[2]

The first time the term *hospice* was used to describe a place for the terminally ill was in 1842 in Lyon, France. The young widow and bereaved mother Madame Jeanne Garnier formed L'Association des Dames du Calvaire and is credited with establishing an institution there to care for the dying. She died in 1853, but her influence led to the founding of six other establishments for the dying between 1847, in Paris, and 1899, in New York.[4] In the 17th century, a young French priest, St. Vincent de Paul, founded the Sisters of Charity in Paris and opened several houses to care for orphans, the poor, the sick, and the dying. More than a century later, Baron von Stein of Prussia visited these Roman Catholic hospices and was so impressed by the work of the nuns that he encouraged a young Protestant pastor named Fliedner to found the first Protestant hospice, also staffed by nuns, which was located in Kaiserswerth, a small town in Germany at the river Rhine. From this training ground, Mother Mary Aikenhead of the Irish Sisters of Charity, a new Order and the first of its kind in Ireland to be uncloistered, opened St. Vincent's Hospital in Dublin 1834. After years of chronic illness, Mary Aikenhead died in 1858 at nearby Harold's Cross. Fulfilling her ambition, the convent where Mary Aikenhead spent her final years founded Our Lady's Hospice for the care of the dying at Harold's Cross, Dublin, in 1879. In 1900, five members of the Irish Sisters of Charity founded St. Joseph's Convent in the East End of London and started visiting the sick in their homes. In 1902, they opened St. Joseph's Hospice in East London, with 30 beds for the dying poor. Cicely Saunders, then a young physician and previously trained as a nurse and social worker, worked from 1957 to 1967 at St. Joseph's Hospice, studying pain control in advanced cancer (Fig. 4-1). This was the stimulus for her to establish St. Christopher's Hospice in London in 1967 (Fig. 4-2).

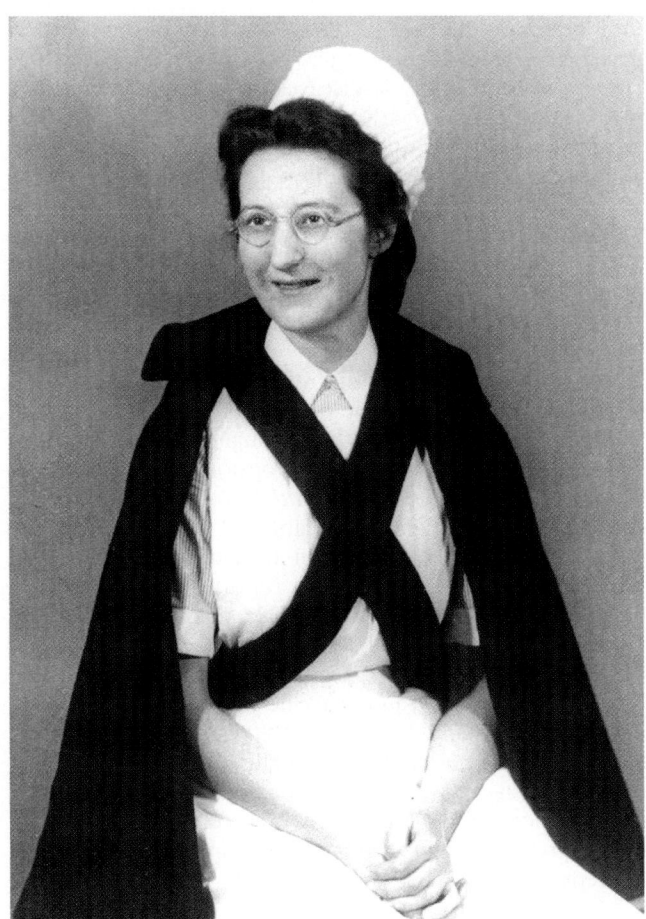

FIGURE 4-1 Dr. Cicely Saunders was first trained as a nurse and a social worker. (Courtesy of St. Christopher's Hospice.)

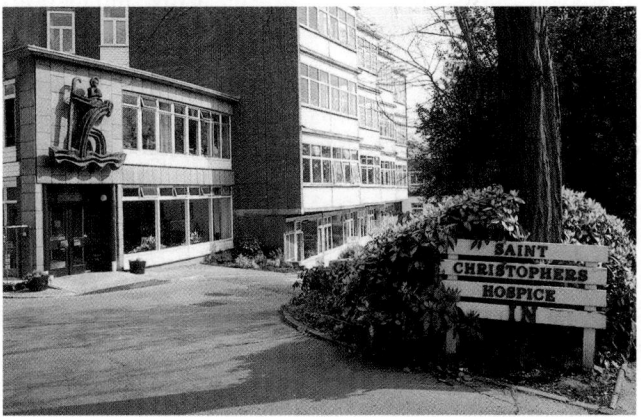

FIGURE 4-2 The entrance of St. Christopher's Hospice, London.

The success of the growing investment in medical research in the first half of the 20th century produced unprecedented scientific discoveries and a change in the pattern of illness in the second half of the century. In the early 1900s, people in the United States usually died of infectious diseases or trauma. The paradigm of the scientific method was successfully applied to the causes of contemporary death, such as pneumococcal pneumonia and infectious diarrhea. By the second half of the century, Americans were living longer, and they were dying primarily of atherosclerotic diseases (myocardial infarctions, stroke, and congestive heart failure) and cancer. Instead of death occurring quickly (within days), there was an increasing period of chronic illness and dying over weeks to years.

Like most jests, the following statement, published in 1975, reflected an uncomfortable reality: "If only patients could leave their damaged physical vessels at the hospital to repair, while taking their social and emotional selves home."[5]

In response, a lively discussion emerged about U.S. attitudes and practices related to death.[6] Empirical research showed that patients with terminal illness wanted to talk about death when given the opportunity.[7] The publication in 1969 of *On Death and Dying* by Dr. Elisabeth Kübler-Ross, a psychiatrist, captured popular attention with a fortuitous combination of media exposure and timely substance. In one widely reported innovation, she interviewed dying patients during teaching sessions and used the information to instruct her students, as with any other medical subject. Another charismatic physician-speaker was Cicely Saunders. She had founded St. Christopher's Hospice after approximately 20 years of direct observation of the care of terminally ill people. St. Christopher's was not the first hospice, but it was the first modern academic hospice at which research and education were conducted as inextricable aspects of meticulous patient care.

The idea of using the hospice as a place to teach and perform research moved from London to the United States. In 1974, with advice from Dr. Cicely Saunders, Florence Wald, then Dean of the School of Nursing at Yale University in New Haven, Connecticut, founded The Connecticut Hospice.[8] Dr. William Lamers, a psychiatrist who pioneered many of the early interactions between hospices and medical schools, was medical director of the second hospice program, Hospice of Marin in California.

In 1974, Balfour Mount, a urologic surgeon, founded the world's first hospital-based palliative care service, at the Royal Victoria Hospital of McGill University in Montreal, Canada (Fig. 4-3), as part of the teaching and research structure. This demonstrated the value of a hospital-based palliative care service (he called it a palliative care unit), especially for research and education on pain control. It was Mount who first used the term *palliative care*. Finally, in New York City, a consulting team began working throughout St. Luke's Hospital in 1974.[9]

On the basis of the St. Luke's model, that of an interdisciplinary palliative care group, its proponents argued as follows[10]:

> Hospice care should be part of the mainstream of American medicine and its institutions. Development of separate facilities for hospice care could be more costly and might result in the public perceiving hospices as nursing homes. Furthermore, hospital care that is caring and curing should be related. A hospice team or consultant in every teaching hospital would enable today's students and tomorrow's health care providers to observe hospice care as an integral part of acute care.

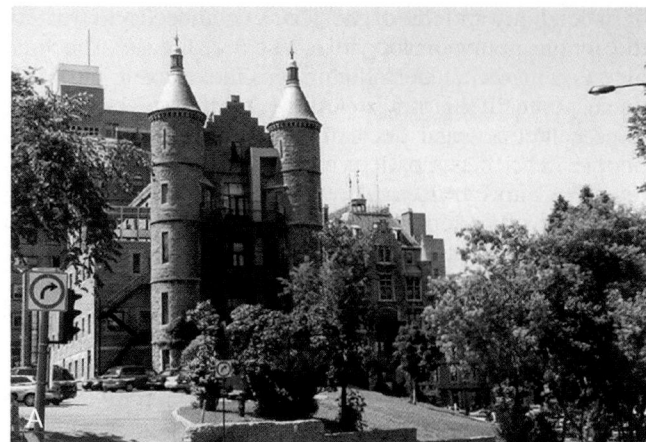
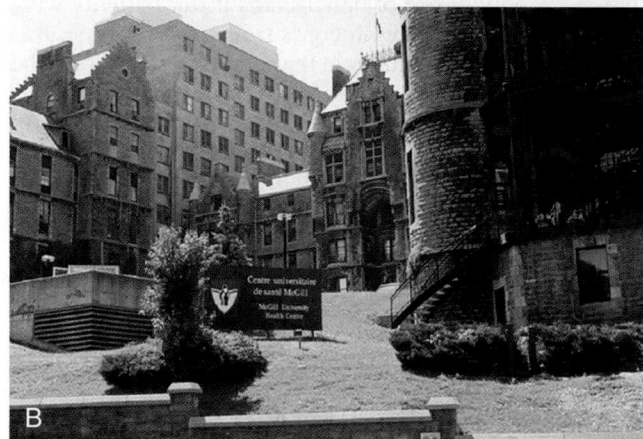

FIGURE 4-3 **A** and **B,** Royal Victorial Hospital, Montreal, Canada. *(Courtesy of Katri Elina Clements.)*

THE LEGISLATIVE ROLE IN HOSPICE AND PALLIATIVE CARE

In 1972, the United States Senate's Special Committee on Aging held hearings on "Death with Dignity." Whereas at first hospice organizers sought to separate hospice from traditional care, the government now became interested in incorporating hospice into traditional institutions. By the late 1970s, interest in the process of dying had become widespread in the United States. Kübler-Ross's book was famous and was the subject of innumerable radio, television, and magazine discussions. Death was impersonal and occurred in sterile institutional settings where modern technological, life-sustaining measures were the primary focus of medicine and health care and individual patient needs were not considered. The credibility of the hospice concept has continued to grow since that time. In 1974, the National Cancer Institute funded the Connecticut Hospice in New Haven, the first U.S. hospice to develop a national demonstration center for home care for the terminally ill and their families. Subsequent U.S. hospices were funded through grants and private donations and relied heavily on lay and professional volunteers. A major impetus for growth of hospice in the United States was rooted in the perception by nurses and families that traditional medical care was failing the dying. Hospice developed as a concept rather than a place. From the beginning, the focus was on care in the patient's home.

The development of hospice paralleled concern for the unnecessary prolongation of life. The 1976 Quinlan decision,[11] which permitted the removal of a ventilator from a comatose young woman, was followed by 15 years of remarkable legal decisions and the evolution of biomedical ethics as a patient care discipline. Most recently, the 1991 Supreme Court Nancy Cruzan decision[12] affirmed the right of patients to have advance directives and to refuse medical care. Interest in death and dying is now focused on the controversial issues of assisted suicide and euthanasia, with forces polarized between the "right to die" and the "right to life." Contemporary palliative care advocates almost universally assert that, if pain and suffering were relieved, requests for assistance in dying would rarely be made. Not all commentators agree, especially when the experience of patients with cancer is compared with that of patients with terminal AIDS, end-stage renal disease, or severe chronic depression.

PHILOSOPHY OF HOSPICE

The modern hospice focuses on the physical and emotional symptoms of the patient and family, rather than on the terminal disease. In addition to controlling symptoms, hospice helps the patient and family confront the issues that accompany dying. An emphasis on "total" pain control, including physical, mental, social, and spiritual aspects, exemplifies the concept of total patient care. Pain control and management of other symptoms (e.g., shortness of breath, anorexia, fatigue, anxiety) provide the primary focus of care based on each patient's needs.

Although hospice serves all those with terminal illnesses, about 75% of hospice patients have cancer.[13] In the United States, hospice care can be appropriate for anyone with a terminal illness that is likely to cause death within approximately 6 months. The patient should eschew futile treatment or treatment aimed at curing the disease, but radiotherapy, chemotherapy, and surgery can have a place in palliative or hospice care if the symptomatic benefits outweigh the risks and if the goal of the therapy is symptom relief.

Similar to palliative care principles (see Chapter 7) and supported by the World Health Organization (WHO), the philosophy of hospice for the terminally ill is based on several concepts[14]:

- Death is a natural part of the cycle of life. When death is inevitable, hospice will not seek to hasten or postpone it.
- Pain relief and symptom control are clinical goals.
- Psychological and spiritual pain are as significant as physical pain, and addressing all three requires an interdisciplinary team.
- Patients, their families, and their loved ones are the unit of care.
- Bereavement care is critical to supporting surviving family members and friends.
- Care is provided regardless of ability to pay.

A primary goal of hospice and palliative care is to promote an alert, dignified, and pain-free life in a manner respectful of individual needs. Hospices have been instrumental in developing new methods of pain management.

Successful hospice techniques have influenced the care of terminally ill patients in conventional settings.

Effective treatment of physical symptoms and of the emotional and spiritual needs of the patient and family requires the diverse skills of physicians, nurses, physiotherapists, social workers, aides, counselors, clergy, and specially trained volunteers. This multidisciplinary team works with the patient and family to develop a plan of care to guide a comprehensive case-management approach. Hospice strongly emphasizes this coordinated approach to enhance the combined skills and sensitivities of caregivers. The frequency of visits to the home is determined by the needs of the patient and family or caregivers. Patients and families often require intensive psychosocial and spiritual support and counseling to cope with the challenges they face as the illness progresses. The needs of those with terminal disease and their families are greater than can be addressed effectively in physicians' offices or outpatient centers or by many current home health care systems.[15]

Several caregivers constitute the core team: the attending physician, hospice physicians with palliative care training, nurses with experience in pain and symptom management and physical assessment, social workers with clinical experience appropriate to the counseling and casework needs of the terminally ill, spiritual counselors with education and experience in pastoral counseling, a volunteer coordinator with skills in organization and communication, and trained volunteers. Additional professionals (e.g., allied therapists, art and music therapists, physiotherapists, dieticians, pharmacists, nursing assistants) may join the team as needed. Each member recognizes and accepts a trusting relationship with the patient and family while also maintaining professional boundaries with them. The team collaborates with the attending physician to develop and maintain a patient-directed, individualized plan of care. This plan addresses the unique physical, social, religious, and cultural needs of the patient and family.

Hospice care also supports family caregivers. Hospice empowers families and considers bereavement care critical to the support of surviving family members and friends. Bereavement services should continue throughout the bereavement period, for at least 1 year, to help the family cope with death-related grief and loss. Survivors with potential pathological grief reactions may be referred to appropriate counseling.

Facilitation of communication is important.[16] Patients have a right to clear information about their condition and the treatment choices available, and hospice strives to improve the level and quality of communication among the patient, the family, and the health care providers. Ideally, decisions affecting patient care are based on adequate information and reflection. Participation by patients in decisions affecting their care is encouraged, and the wishes of patients and families are respected. Hospice also encourages the development of reasonable goals for the relief of pain and other symptoms.

HOSPICE TODAY

Considering that hospice is primarily a concept and not a specific place, it is not surprising that various countries have chosen different types of hospices (see "Common

Common Errors

The following are common misconceptions about hospice care:

- Hospice means ghettoization of the dying.
- Hospice care does not provide appropriate medical treatment.
- Involvement of volunteers is necessary because health care systems refuse to pay for professionals.
- Hospice programs are identical across all countries and in all cultural settings.
- The concept of hospice does not work in developing countries.

Errors"). In the United Kingdom, there are mostly voluntary hospices. An average voluntary hospice consists of an inpatient unit, day care center, home care, and outpatient clinic, as well as a bereavement support service.[17] These different kinds of hospice services have the advantage of being solely oriented toward the needs of the dying and usually provide a homelike atmosphere, in contrast to the rather "sterile" and hectic hospital wards.

Some countries organize palliative care units (PCU) within general hospitals or cancer centers. These units provide good symptom control and usually engage in research. Other services are based on palliative home care teams or hospital support teams. Usually, these teams consist of a doctor and a nurse, both specialized in palliative medicine, but many other medical disciplines and professions (e.g., chaplain, social worker, physiotherapist, music therapist, bereavement counselor) are available as well. Palliative home care teams are suitable for persons who are able to remain at home and prefer to do so.

The types of hospice and their funding vary from country to country. Some hospices have total funding from the national health service, but most rely on voluntary donations for most of their income. There are some privately funded hospices. In 2001, according to the Hospice Information Service at St. Christopher's Hospice, more than 7000 hospices or palliative care services were available in more than 90 countries throughout the world, adapted to suit local needs and culture.[18] In Europe, both the distribution and the type of palliative care services vary. According to a recent study project of the European Association for Palliative Care, most palliative care services are situated in the United Kingdom (total specific resources, 958); other well-developed programs include France, with a provision of 471 services; Poland, providing 362; Germany, 321; Spain, 261; the Netherlands, 138; and Belgium, 121 services.[19] Another research project divided data into inpatient and outpatient services and named the number of beds per 1 million inhabitants: United Kingdom, 54; Netherlands, 40; Belgium, 35; Germany, 22; Poland, 21; France, 17; and Spain, 10.[20]

Even though some studies and articles show that hospice care is developing dynamically, data collection remains difficult. Many countries do not have national databases on the development of hospice care, and, furthermore, naming and definitions of palliative care services vary. Regularly updated international listings of services according to an agreed sample of definitions would not necessarily simplify assessments of the development of hospice care, however, unless there were agreed written quality standards (national and/or international) to be fulfilled by the various types of services.

CHALLENGES FOR THE FUTURE

The roots of hospice care are similar to those of all of contemporary medicine. The modern hospice program, which combines patient care with concern for public health, education, and research, can rightly be called academic. The demographic and economic challenges the world faces highlight the need for more education and research. At a minimum, it would seem obvious that every academic medical center will want to integrate hospice programs in their clinical, teaching, and research activities and networking; at an optimum, some of those academic hospices will further develop into comprehensive centers of competence and serve as liaison institutions for decision makers within the health care system.

Let Dame Cicely Saunders have the last word[2]:

The hospice movement, and the specialty of palliative care that has grown out of it, reaffirms the importance of a person's life and relationships. Focused research, attention to details, and a developing expertise have aimed to avoid the isolation that many have suffered, often increased by inappropriate interventions. If people know they are respected as a part of the human family (and here the developing countries have much to teach us all), the ending of life can be a final fulfillment of all that has gone before.

REFERENCES

1. Lyons A, Petrucelli RJ. Medicine: An Illustrated History. New York: Harry N. Abrams, 1987, 185-194.
2. Saunders CM. Foreword. In Doyle D, Hanks G, Cherny N, Calman K (eds). Oxford Textbook of Palliative Medicine, 3rd ed. New York: Oxford University Press, 2004, pp xvii-xx.
3. Dunlop RJ, Hockley JM. Hospital-Based Palliative Care Teams. New York: Oxford University Press, 1998, pp 1-3.
4. Clark D. Palliative Care History: A Ritual Process. Eur J Palliat Care 2000;7:50-55.
5. Lober J. Good patients and problem patients: Conformity and deviance in a general hospital. J Health Soc Behav 1975;16:213-225.
6. Mor V, Greer DS, Kastenbaum R. The hospice experiment: An alternative in terminal care. In Mor V, Geer D, Kastenbaum R (eds). The Hospice Experiment. Baltimore: Johns Hopkins University Press, 1988, p 6.
7. Aring CD. The Understanding Physician. Detroit: Wayne State University Press, 1971.
8. Wald FS; Zoster Z, Wald HJ. The hospice movement as a health care reform. Nurs Outlook. 1980;28:173-177.
9. O'Neill WM, O'Connor P, Latimer EJ. Hospital palliative care services: Three models in three countries. J Pain Symptom Manage 1992;7:406-413.
10. Torrens PR (ed). Hospice Programs and Public Policy. Chicago: American Hospital Publishing, American Hospital Association, 1985.
11. Beresford HR. The Quinlan decision: Problems and legislative alternatives. Ann Neurol 1977;2:74-81.
12. Life Communications—Volume 1, No. 6, June, 1991. Available at http://www.iclnet.org/pub/resources/text/ProLife.News/1991/pln-0106.txt (accessed September 2007).
13. Mor V, Kidder D. Cost savings in hospice: Final results of the National Hospice Study. Health Serv Res 1985;20:407-422.
14. Standards of a Hospice Program of Care. Arlington, VA: National Hospice Organization, 1993.
15. Kinzbrunner BM. Hospice: What to do when anti-cancer therapy is no longer appropriate, effective, or desired. Semin Oncol 1994;21:792-798.
16. Lamers WM Jr. Hospice: Enhancing the quality of life. Oncology (Huntingt) 1990;4:121-126.
17. Brady D. Hospice and Palliative Care. London: St. Christopher's Hospice, 1996.
18. The Hospice Information Service. Hospice and Palliative Care Facts and Figures 2001. London: St Christopher's Hospice, 2001.
19. Centeno C, Clark D, Roccafort J, Flores LA, Pons JJ. The map of specific resources of palliative care in Europe. Palliat Med 2006;20:316.
20. Jaspers B, Schindler T. Stand der Palliativmedizin und Hospizarbeit in Deutschland und im Vergleich zu ausgewählten Staaten (Belgien, Frankreich, Großbri-

tannien, Niederlande, Norwegen, österreich, Polen, Schweden, Schweiz, Spanien). Im Auftrag der Enquete-Kommission des Bundestages "Ethik und Recht der modernen Medizin," vorgelegt am 30.11.2004. Available at http://www.bundestag.de (accessed September 2007).

SUGGESTED READING

Clark D. Palliative Care History: A Ritual Process. Eur J Palliat Care 2000;7:50-55.

Kübler-Ross E. On Death and Dying: What the Dying Have to Teach Doctors, Nurses, Clergy and Their Own Families. New York: Touchstone Publishing, 1969.

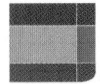 **CHAPTER 5**

Palliative Medicine: Models of Organization

Xavier Gómez-Batiste, Josep Porta-Sales, Silvia Paz, and Jan Stjernswärd

KEY POINTS

- Palliative care is comprehensive, active care of patients with advanced disease or serious illness and their families; it aims to improve quality of life based on patient and family needs, demands, and wishes and is practiced by a competent multidisciplinary team.

- A palliative care service is one that has the aims, values, and structure of such a service (a trained multidisciplinary team being the most relevant feature); is devoted to advanced illness; practices the process of palliative care (evaluation, comprehensive plan, ethical decision making, continuity and liaison, monitoring of results, training, research, and quality improvement); has an independent budget; and is identified as such by users and other services.

- The type, complexity, and location of palliative services are diverse and can involve any element of the health care system.

- Health professionals working in palliative care should pay attention to the opportunities for improvement that usually exist at any level of the palliative care service organization.

- There is strong evidence in support of the effectiveness, efficiency, and satisfaction achieved with palliative medicine.

ORGANIZATIONAL DEFINITIONS

In 1990, the World Health Organization proposed a definition of palliative care.[1] Palliative medicine was first defined in the United Kingdom in 1988, when it was recognized as a medical specialty.[2,3] To define palliative care from a service organization perspective, the following definition is suggested: *Palliative care is the comprehensive care of advanced and terminally ill patients and their families that aims to improve quality of life and promote adjustment to disease based on patients' needs, demands, and wishes and is practiced by a competent multidisciplinary team.*

According to this definition, the principles of palliative care are

- A comprehensive and active approach to end-of-life care
- The patient and family as the unit of care
- Improvement of quality of life and the promotion of dignity
- Effective and efficient care while responding to patients' and families' needs

The characteristics of specialist palliative care include a multidimensional approach using interdisciplinary teamwork, adequate interventions for symptom control, effective communication and emotional support, procedures for ethical decision making, and assessment of the needs and demands of the patient and family.

The methods by which palliative care principles may be achieved include the following:

- Use of systematic needs evaluation to design comprehensive therapeutic plans based on the views of professionals, patients, and families about the care plan
- Development of internal organization (multidisciplinary team, cooperative service network) to perform patient- and family-centered, multidisciplinary care
- Encouragement of education, training, and research activities
- Promotion of strong community links

Palliative care activities can be carried out in various settings, such as home, hospital beds, specialized units, outpatient clinics, day care centers, or bereavement services. *Basic palliative care* includes the actions any health care service would take to improve the care of terminally ill patients and their families. *Specialist palliative care services* are those specifically set up to offer professional care to patients and their families in an independent location with specific managerial, training, and financial resources.

QUALITY

Several elements must be considered when assessing quality of care:

- *Expertise, competence,* and *training* to deal with complex clinical situations
- *Equity* by providing appropriate care according to needs
- *Coverage* as the percentage of people who get appropriate care in relation to the total population cared for
- *Commitment* to patients and families
- *Respect* for patients' and families' values and wishes
- *Accessibility* to palliative care when needed
- *Continuous follow-up* to plan therapeutic strategies and anticipate critical clinical and social situations in which needs and demands increase dramatically. Advance planning is important.
- *Evidence-based effectiveness* and *efficacy* of the specialized service assessed according to the therapeutic aims and objectives, such as symptom control, emotional support, and social adjustment in a given intervention period

- Service *efficiency* by providing effective palliative care at the lowest cost
- *Patients' and families' perceptions* about the type and quality of care received
- *Participation of patients and carers* in care plans
- Respect for patients' *rights to privacy and safety*

To achieve excellence, practitioners should combine all of these elements while adjusting available services according to resource availability. Audits help identify and systemically review deficits and improvements.

The following elements serve as drivers to develop and expand palliative care services:

- A positive attitude toward the discipline
- Systematic evaluation of clinical, functional, and structural results
- Training and research according to available resources
- Quality audit and improvement

DIMENSIONS AND ACTIVITIES OF PALLIATIVE MEDICINE

Palliative care requires a multidimensional approach to design a comprehensive, individualized therapeutic regimen (Box 5-1). Such planning includes both pharmacological and nonpharmacological treatments, emotional aid, social support, education of carers, and bereavement assessment while ensuring appropriate follow-up and accessibility to specialized care.

Carers' perceptions about care should be considered when deciding on therapies or interventions. Patients' and carers' expectations should be systematically explored in a comprehensive therapeutic strategy.

Teamwork is essential for good palliative care. The main principles are communication, advanced training, respect, and organization. These can be furthered by regular team meetings, common activities, development of a team mission, definition of common values, and clear organization of the team structure.

For many patients, ethical problems arise. Services must have decision-making procedures to include the wishes and values of patients and to promote cooperation among families, team members, and other involved professionals.

Systematic needs assessment of patients and families and monitoring of clinical outcomes (e.g., symptom control, psychosocial issues) are crucial. Data on service provision (e.g., patient demographic data, length of stay) help ensure support from political decision makers.

The major resource is professional staff competence, based in advanced specialist training. This allows appropriate responses to complex needs and problems. Education of other nonspecialists is crucial to promote coverage and improve the care of all patients in the health care system. Research helps improve the quality of care and provides credibility to palliative care in mainstream medicine.

Care of the dying is not only a professional but also a social matter, including ethical, economic, social, religious, and cultural elements. Society can be involved through volunteers, and advocacy is needed to help the mission of improving social awareness about life and death.

BASIC PALLIATIVE MEDICINE

Services in oncology, geriatrics, internal medicine, primary care, and other specialties often provide care for patients with life-limiting and far-advanced illness. Not all patients need specialized services, although they might require some palliative care. A rational way to initiate and increase palliative medicine coverage is to provide in nonpalliative services some basic palliative care. This includes multidimensional evaluation, basic protocols for the most prevalent symptoms and problems, and enhanced communication and ethics skills.

In primary care services, basic palliative care should include regular home visits and telephone support. Further improvements include programs for education and support of the family and definition of criteria for access to specialist palliative care services.

In nursing homes and similar service facilities, where most patients are the frail elderly and there is a high prevalence of dementia or advanced chronic illness, basic palliative care knowledge and skills are extremely effective. These include symptom management guidelines and care pathways, grouping of patients by behavioral and cognitive condition, and decision-making protocols for frequently encountered ethical dilemmas, such as withholding of nutrition or hydration.

There are limitations to basic palliative medicine. Organizational difficulties impede care for complex problems. Teamwork may be impossible in the nonspecialist setting. Keeping the balance between cure and care and preventing overtreatment may be difficult in nonpalliative care services. The inherent limits of nonspecialized palliative care teams should be recognized, and criteria should be defined for access to specialist services. Basic palliative care services alone are insufficient and do not obviate the need for specialist resources. Basic and specialist palliative care services should be complementary, cooperative, and synergistic.

SPECIALIST PALLIATIVE MEDICINE

The elements that define and distinguish specialist palliative medicine services are mission, aims, values, leadership, types of patients, structure (skills, documentation, building), process (activities, types of interventions), assessment (tools, training, research), outcomes, outputs, evaluation, and continuous improvement of quality.

Box 5-1 Dimensions of Palliative Care

1. Care of patients and families: evaluation of needs
2. Care of patients and families: comprehensive therapeutic plan
3. Teamwork
4. Ethical decision making
5. Continuity of care and liaison with other services
5. Monitoring of clinical and organizational results
6. Education and training
7. Research
8. Continuous quality evaluation and improvement
9. Links to society

One mission of such a specialist service could be to improve the quality of life and adjustment to advanced disease and loss for those patients and families under their care. In addition, a specialist service strives to achieve appropriate coverage and to improve social and professional awareness about palliative medicine. The aims are to improve the quality of practice, to provide care, and to extend that quality to other services through training and counseling.

The values of palliative medicine teams include competence to respond to patients and families and aiming for the maximum quality of remaining life, through commitment and a comprehensive multidimensional approach. Respect for patient and family beliefs and wishes is one of the essential values.

A palliative medicine service is a specific, independent service devoted to the seriously ill, composed of a competent and specifically trained multidisciplinary team that works according to the principles and methods of palliative care. A palliative medicine team must have a sufficient workload to maintain competence and training to be considered specialized. Specialist palliative care services must be easily identifiable by patients, families, and health care professionals and must have an independent budget.

Palliative medicine services have demonstrated effectiveness, efficacy, efficiency, and satisfaction in most of their structures and locations.[4] Palliative care resources can be versatile, based on individual, specialized nurses or doctors working alone or on multiprofessional teams, which is the ideal. Teams have great variability in their composition. Complete teams incorporate doctors, nurses, social workers, physiotherapists, psychologists and/or psychiatrists, and possibly chaplains, pharmacists, nutrition-ists, and others. Specialist services and resources work in various health care settings (Fig. 5-1), such as acute care hospitals (university, district general, community), rehabilitation centers, subacute and geriatric care facilities, long-term care hospitals, nursing homes, individual hospices, and the community. Programs can include one or more types of resources and may involve cooperation as part of a comprehensive network. According to health care system location, services focus on various types of patients, at varying time points in the disease trajectory, and using various interventions. They influence the quality of care of these patients through local cooperation and networking. Such approaches are usually expressed as service outputs (e.g., mean age, length of stay, mortality) and influence the costs of the service. Outputs are also influenced by the activity of other local palliative care services.

There are several steps or phases in the evolution of palliative medicine services. First is the *project* stage, which features the evaluation of needs, selection and training of specialist professionals, leadership, and design. The *initial* phase of the service focuses on internal team consensus and process building. The *consolidated and advanced* stages involve complex interventions and referrals for clinical, educational, and research activities.

There are three levels of service development (Fig. 5-2):

Level 1—General measures (see "Basic Palliative Medicine")

Level 2—Minimal or complete specialized services (doctor, nurse, and social worker are the minimum for a basic team; more complete teams include other professionals)

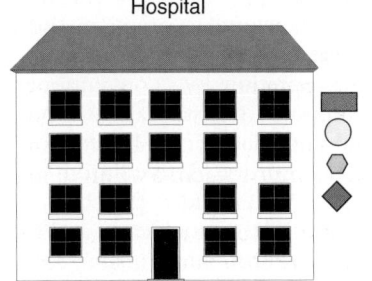
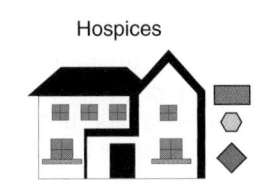
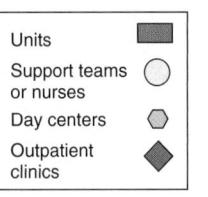
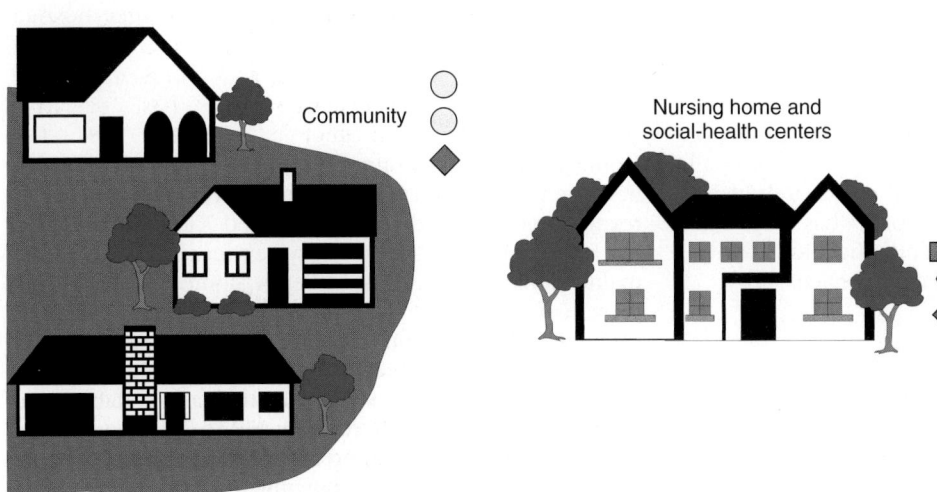

Hospital

Hospices

Units

Support teams or nurses

Day centers

Outpatient clinics

Community

Nursing home and social-health centers

FIGURE 5-1 Types of palliative care and settings in which it is delivered.

Analyze context: Tendencies, scenarios, visions, stakeholders, and strategies	**Define:** Mission, aims, values, leadership	**Dimensions:** Care of patients and families, evaluation, team, ethics, training, research, quality improvement, financing	**FIGURE 5-2** Elements of evaluation, quality improvement, and strategic planning of services.

Patients and Families

Self-evaluation: List strong and weak points, harms and opportunities, and action for every dimension

Team and institution

Actions + indicators: short-, mid-, long-term

Level 3—Referral services (act as referral points for clinical complex situations, training, and research; mainly located in teaching hospitals or comprehensive cancer centers).

TYPES AND LOCATION OF PALLIATIVE MEDICINE SERVICES

Hospices

The modern approach to palliative care was developed initially in British hospices with the establishment of St. Christopher's Hospice in London and extended rapidly into the United Kingdom and most Anglo-Saxon countries (see Fig. 5-1 and Chapter 4). In many countries, a hospice is an independent organization devoted to the care of patients and their families, based in the community, often in a specific, dedicated building. The U.K. hospices built up a new model of care (comprehensive) and a new model of internal organization (multidisciplinary team); both are now considered core aspects of palliative care. Hospices have traditionally displayed a strong orientation toward the needs of patients and families. These concepts and principles have spread into all levels of the health care systems of many countries and have been adapted to diverse organizations (see also Part I, Section F).

The greatest strengths of conventional hospices are the model of care, the multidisciplinary team approach, the high satisfaction of patients and families, and the establishment of strong links to the community. In countries with inadequate health care systems, this approach is important, especially if the political leadership and commitment to develop public health programs are lacking. Although it has been crucial to development of the field, the conventional independent hospice approach also has challenges and controversies. The weaknesses of an approach that locates hospice care in an isolated building include difficulties of coverage, lack of early intervention, lack of rational planning, and the economic difficulties of a small health care structure sited away from the comprehensive public health system. The word "hospice" has a specific meaning in Anglo-Saxon countries, and a hospice is often recognized as a specialist palliative care service.

Specialist Nurses

Home or hospital specialist nurses (of which the best known are the Macmillan nurses) have a good reputation.[5,6] These services work well in developed health care networks or rural areas of developing countries.

Support Teams

A support team is a specialist palliative care multidisciplinary team that acts as a consultation service, without assigned beds. It can work in many places with a limited structure. Usually, it is composed of one or more doctors and nurses, with cooperation of social workers, psychologists, physiotherapists, chaplains, or other professionals. Activities can vary from counseling only to direct involvement in care. The team acts on various intervention levels, according to patients' needs and available resources. The level of intervention needs to be clearly defined as follows: (1) provision of advice for other teams, (2) one-time evaluation of patient and family, (3) on-demand shared care, (4) daily systematic intervention, or (5) complete responsibility for care. Other important activity areas for support teams are resource liaison and education and training.[7]

Hospital support teams have a long tradition for both cancer and geriatric patients.[8] There is evidence of effectiveness, efficiency, and satisfaction.[9] Furthermore, hospital support teams can catalyze the development of a hospital palliative care unit. In everyday practice, these teams are challenged and limited in their interventions by, for instance, the lack of recognition by "conventional" services and the poor acceptance that therapeutic regimens usually recommended in palliative care have among other medical specialists; the burden derived from the enormous hospital needs and demands; the lack of resources for guaranteeing around-the-clock care, and the isolation and vulnerability inherent in small teams. Some of these difficulties are related to the population being cared for (e.g., cancer, noncancer, or mixed patient groups) and the dependence on other bigger hospital services.

Home Care Teams

Home care teams also have had a long tradition since the first one was set up at St. Christopher's Hospice. Home care teams rapidly spread over the United Kingdom and later over the world as a community service. They have been mainly dedicated to cancer patients. Home care teams have proven efficiency, efficacy, and high satisfaction.[10] They are usually composed of one or more doctors and nurses, with other professionals. Their activities are in the home, either alone, or, most often, with primary care collaboration. Home care teams usually care for 250 to 300 new patients per year, for periods ranging from 2 to 12 weeks.[11] Limitations include the need to cooperate with the general practitioner and other primary care services (e.g., in care planning for night and weekend shifts). Home care teams also need close cooperation with local hospitals, hospices, or other institutions to facilitate quick admission when indicated. Small, isolated teams are vulnerable to burnout, so preventative measures should be provided.

Palliative Medicine Units

Palliative medicine units can be defined as independent beds devoted to palliative care. Modern units were initially based in hospices in the United Kingdom and were quickly incorporated into acute hospitals (Royal Victoria Hospital, Montreal, in 1974), community facilities (CESCO, Geneva, in 1986), health centers (Sta Creu Vic, Spain, in 1987), and nursing homes.[12] They can be found in various locations in the health care system, from small independent hospices to large cancer centers. They can be disease specific (e.g., cancer, AIDS, geriatric) or mixed.

Inpatient palliative care units should guarantee privacy and comfort for relatives taking care of the patient, represent a friendly and satisfying place for the team running it, and generate a caring and gentle environment for other professionals and lay people. A minimum of 10 to 12 beds and a maximum of 25 to 30 beds per unit is recommended. Staffing ratio is variable and ranges from 0.5 to 2 nurses per patient, depending on the complexity. Palliative care units can care for specific types of patients or for mixed populations, and they have a wide scope of interventions, outputs, and costs (Table 5-1).[13]

Acute palliative care units are usually based in hospitals or cancer centers and tend to look after younger patients with more complex conditions. A length of stay of less than 10 days, mortality rates of approximately 50%, and more complex interventions are typical. Palliative care units based in health care centers or long-term facilities typically care for older patients, predominantly those with social problems, with lengths of stay longer than 25 days and mortality rates of about 80%. The operating costs of a palliative care unit can be as low as 25% to 50% of those of an acute medical ward.

Outpatient Clinics

Outpatient clinics help improve accessibility by promoting early, flexible, concomitant interventions.[14] They can be run by home or hospital support teams or combined with an inpatient unit. Conceptually, their field of work can range from counseling of other teams to full responsibility for patient care even in urgent situations.[15]

Day Care Centers

Day care centers usually combine medical activities with those of occupational therapy, support groups, rehabilitation, or recreation.[16] In other settings, these centers might address complex situations that require intense interdisciplinary interventions or technical procedures such as titration of intravenous opioids, thoracic or abdominal drainage, or catheter placement.[17]

Comprehensive Palliative Care Systems

Ideally, regional resources should be combined in a comprehensive palliative care network or integrated system. In these organizations, specialist teams and services are available at all levels of health care.[18] This is done in various settings, in combination with case management and support of other teams, but in a comprehensive way. The development of an integrated system depends on consensus and acceptance by other area health resources, leadership, and participation of the health authority. A team's reputation for competence is essential.

OUTCOMES

Outputs and outcomes can be used to compare different services and settings. Outputs are simple, measurable parameters that are used to describe and compare services. Some demographic factors such as age are well-defined parameters of complexity, with younger age suggesting high complexity.[19] Clinical factors include performance status, pain, dyspnea, cognitive failure, and behavioral disorders. Length of treatment may be related to activities and interventions; outpatient clinics and support teams allow earlier and more flexible interventions compared with inpatient units.

For palliative care units, length of stay and mortality are output parameters that depend on the type of patient and the setting. Acute, mid-term, and long-term care units exhibit widely different figures (see Table 5-1).

Place of death has been advocated as an important outcome parameter. As a single parameter, it could cause misunderstandings, because it is affected by resource availability. A home care support team might increase the number of patients that die at home, but the subsequent opening of a palliative care unit could redirect these patients into hospital or hospice beds. Place of death is recommended for use as an output only with other, more longitudinal data. Consumption of resources such as emergency services or phone calls can assess this.

TABLE 5-1	Types of Palliative Care Units		
PARAMETER	ACUTE CARE	MID-TERM CARE	LONG-TERM CARE
Type of patient	Younger (≤60 yr) Complex Acute or subacute	Mixed	Older (>75) Noncomplex Chronic
Mean length of stay (days)	≤15	15-25	25-35
Mortality rate (%)	≤60	60-80	>80
Cost*	40-50	30-40	25-30

*Percentage of the cost of a unit or ward in the same or a similar acute care hospital.

The proportion of scheduled versus emergency calls and the number of hospital admissions are among the most important measures, because it is desirable to have a low utilization of emergency services in crisis situations. Efficacy in symptom control and alleviation of emotional problems are common clinical outcomes. Satisfaction is complex to assess and measure but is considered important.[20]

Cost-efficiency is another major outcome. Support teams have strong evidence of being cost-efficient,[21] because they produce striking changes in the utilization of acute hospital resources and emergency services and reductions in treatments and investigations. Another important result is reallocation of resources from acute wards into palliative medicine beds. Nonmeasurable organizational outcomes could be described as patient-centered care, a comprehensive approach, family involvement, procedures for ethical decision making, and interdisciplinary teamwork.

Social and spiritual outcomes are related to the impact of palliative care and hospice on the public's awareness of death as an integral part of life, and access to information about palliative care to increase quality of life. Palliative care has a tremendous influence on public opinion about the need for, and the right to, the best quality of humanistic care. Although it is difficult to measure, respect for human dignity can be also be defined as a good indicator for any society or organization.

EVALUATION AND QUALITY IMPROVEMENT

The evaluation and improvement of quality and strategic planning is one of the cornerstones of service development and good care (see Fig. 5-2). It requires an open attitude, proper leadership, active participation, and a systematic methodology. The main aim must be to provide the best patient care.

An easy way to evaluate quality improvement is through a systematic, multidisciplinary evaluation of four domains: strengths, weaknesses, threats, and opportunities. Afterward, the areas for improvement can be defined for each dimension and a more detailed list of improvements made. Action plans should include short (0 to 2 years), medium (2 to 5 years), and long-term measures (>5 years) and indicators for monitoring progress.

Evaluation needs the active participation of the team, the institution, and patients. Evaluation requires analysis of context and influences, considering different scenarios, visions, strategies, mission, values, and leadership. Consensus should be established internally and externally among decision makers and stakeholders. Some elements can be improved with internal organizational measures, whereas others require extra resources and external commitment.

DEVELOPMENT TRENDS

The strengths, weaknesses, dilemmas, and tendencies of specific services were described earlier. The culture and practice of the organization should be developed as a key element.

There are several trends in the evolution of palliative medicine services:

1. *Complexity*: After implementation of basic palliative care has been established, most specialist services provide for more complex patients and more complex interventions, either in symptom control or in other dimensions of care. The intervention of specialist teams is related more to the complexity of needs and less to prognosis.
2. *Diversification*: Resources and services are diversified, adjusting to different settings.
3. *Early flexible intervention*: From the original development of the specialty, with an intensive and unique approach to all needs of a few patients in the last few weeks of life, there are now flexible shared patterns of care, offering palliative care earlier in the disease trajectory.
4. *Specialized roles*: Once early flexible intervention patterns are in place, it is important to define the roles of different types of service, distinguishing evaluation from follow-up and case management.
5. *Cooperation*: Specialist palliative care services cooperate in comprehensive networks. In metropolitan areas, there is a tendency to establish networks with different levels of complexity.
6. *Extension of care*: Palliative care should be extended to everyone, so it is worth exploring the most appropriate form of care for different situations and settings.

REFERENCES

1. Available at http://www.who.int/cancer/palliative/definition/en/ (accessed November 28, 2007).
2. Hillier R. Palliative medicine: A new specialty. BMJ 1988;297:873-874.
3. Clark D, Seymour J. Reflections on palliative care: Sociological and policy perspectives. Facing Death Series. Buckingham, UK: Open University Press, 1999.
4. Gysels M, Higginson IJ. Improving supportive and palliative care for adults with cancer. Research evidence. Guidance on Cancer Services. National Institute for Clinical Excellence Guidance on Cancer Services Improving Supportive and Palliative Care for Adults with Cancer: The Manual 2004, Available at http://www.nice.org.uk/nicemedia/pdf/csgspmanual.pdf (accessed March 2008).
5. Clark D, Seymour J, Douglas HR, et al Clinical nurse specialists in palliative care: Part 2. Explaining diversity in the organization and costs of Macmillan nursing services. Palliat Med 2002;16:375-385.
6. Clark D, Ferguson C, Nelson C. Macmillan carers schemes in England: Results of a multicentre evaluation. Palliat Med 2000;14:129-139.
7. Tuca A, Codorniu N. Levels of intervention of a hospital support team. In Third Research Forum of the European Association for Palliative Care, 4-6 June 2004 [Abstracts]. Stressa Lago Maggiore, Italy: EPAC, 2004; and Yennurajalingam S, Zhang T, Bruera E. The impact of the palliative care mobile team on symptom assessment and medication profiles in patients admitted to a comprehensive cancer centre. Support Care Cancer 2007;15:471-475.
8. Evers MM, Meier DE, Morrison RS. Assessing differences in care needs and service utilization in geriatric palliative care patients. J Pain Symptom Manage 2002;23:424-432.
9. Higginson I, Finlay I, Goodwin DM, et al. Do hospital based palliative care teams improve outcomes for patients or families at the end of life? J Pain Symptom Manage 2002;23:96-106.
10. Serra-Prat M, Gallo P, Picaza JM. Home palliative care as a cost saving alternative: Evidence from Catalonia. Palliat Med 2001;15:271-278.
11. Grande GE, Todd CJ, Barclay SI, Farquhar MC. Does hospital at home for palliative care facilitate home death? A randomised controlled trial. BMJ 1999;319:1472-1475.
12. Gomez-Batiste X, Porta J, Tuca A, Stjernsward J. Organizacion de Servicios y Programas de Cuidados Paliativos: Bases de organización, planificación, evaluación y mejora de calidad. ICO Formación Series. Madrid: Aran Ediciones, 2005.
13. Bruera E, Neumann C, Brenneis C, Quan H. Frequency of symptom distress and poor prognostic indicators in palliative cancer patients admitted to a tertiary palliative care unit, hospices, and acute care hospitals. J Palliat Care 2000;16:16-21.
14. Rabow M, Dibble SL, Pantilat SZ, McPhee SJ. The comprehensive care team: A controlled trial of an outpatient palliative medicine consultation. Arch Intern Med 2004;164:83-91.
15. Porta-Sales J, Codorniu N, Gomez-Batiste X, et al. Patient appointment process, symptom control and prediction of follow-up compliance in a palliative care outpatient clinic. J Pain Symptom Manage 2005;30:145-153.

16. Higginson I, Hearn J, Myers K, Naysmith A. Palliative day care: What do services do? Palliat Med 2000;14:277-286.
17. Goodwin DM, Higginson IJ, Myers K, et al. Effectiveness of palliative day care in improving pain, symptom control and quality of life. J Pain Symptom Manage 2003;25:202-212.
18. Nikbakht-Van de Sande CVMV, van der Rijt CC, Visser AP, et al. Function of local networks in palliative care: A Dutch view. J Palliat Med 2005;8:808-816.
19. Izquierdo-Porrera AM, Trelis-Navarro J, Gomez-Batiste X. Predicting place of death of elderly cancer patients followed by a palliative care unit. J Pain Symptom Manage 2001;21:481-490.
20. Avis M, Bond M, Arthur A. Satisfying solutions? A review of some unresolved issues in the measurement of patient satisfaction. J Adv Nurs 1995; 22:316-322.
21. Axelsson B, Christensen SB. Evaluation of a hospital-based palliative support service with particular regard to financial outcome measures. Palliat Med 1998;12:41-49.

CHAPTER **6**

The Specialty of Palliative Medicine

S. Lawrence Librach

KEY POINTS

- Palliative medicine is a specialty.
- Several key factors led to the development of palliative medicine.
- The special knowledge, skills, and attitudes required are being defined.
- Several postgraduate training programs have been developed in Western nations.
- Multiple challenges must be surmounted if palliative medicine is to continue to succeed.

Hospice palliative care is a relatively new addition to the health care system. Although "hospices" have existed for centuries in various forms, usually associated with religious groups (see Chapter 4), the systematic involvement of health care professionals in quality end-of-life care has existed for only about 30 years. The early pioneers believed that we needed to teach pain and symptom management and some other basics of humane end-of-life care to current practitioners and that the need for specialists was limited.[1] However, this view changed as several factors came into play. The result was the development of a new medical specialty, palliative medicine.

DEFINITION OF A MEDICAL SPECIALTY OR MEDICAL EXPERT

Sociologists have identified central characteristics of professions, including the creation, transmission, mastery, and application of formal knowledge. Learning the fundamental concepts, facts, and techniques of a profession and

achieving validated competence in their use takes place through a long process of education, training, and socialization. Finally, professions view themselves as guardians of the knowledge and skills they dispense, a gatekeeping and expert role.[2] Specialists within the wider profession of medicine, for example palliative medicine specialists, stake out and promote a special area of knowledge (palliative care), conduct research to further develop that knowledge base, find ways to support the clinical practice of the discipline, train undergraduate and postgraduate students in the field, and develop the social mechanisms for these functions, including the gatekeeping role, professional organizations, journals, fellowships, and specialty or board certification examinations.[3] Palliative medicine now meets the criteria and can be considered a specialty within medicine.

PALLIATIVE MEDICINE SPECIALISTS

Palliative medicine specialists resemble those in the specialties of family medicine or general internal medicine. Their practice is holistic and broad, requiring knowledge of many different diseases and the ability to assess and manage many symptoms in the physical, psychological, spiritual, and social spheres. The skills are mostly not procedural. There are absolute needs for individual and family counseling and psychoeducational skills. The palliative medicine specialist must also be able to practice within common ethical conundrums at the end of life—advance care planning, end-of-life decision making, family conflict, and physician-assisted dying. Knowledge of patients' experiences in advanced disease spans more than just hospitals and includes home care, long-term care facilities, and day care. The palliative medicine specialist also has to be comfortable with one key issue—dealing with dying and death—that many specialists avoid. Training programs for palliative medicine specialists need to address all of these issues.

DEVELOPMENT OF THE SPECIALTY OF PALLIATIVE MEDICINE

A number of factors have led to the development of the specialty of palliative medicine.

Poor Care for Advanced Disease within Health Care Systems

Given the growth of hospices and palliative care programs in most Western nations, substantial improvements in end-of-life care might be expected. However, experience and data continue to document poor pain and symptom control, lack of access to palliative care programs, poor knowledge among practicing physicians, lack of advance care planning and end-of-life care decision making, and poor education in the care of patients with advanced disease in undergraduate, postgraduate, and continuing education spheres in medicine. Although family physicians and other specialists are expected to have some basic knowledge of palliative care as it is pertinent to their practice, there is a need for opinion leaders and experts in these areas, and palliative medicine physicians can fulfill some of that need.

The Breadth of Knowledge in Palliative Care

A basic competency in palliative care should be expected of every physician (see Chapter 5). The knowledge base in palliative care is expanding. There are at least eight major journals and more research studies. Most research is clinical and not laboratory based. There is a need for "experts" who have a knowledge translation function to improve the care of the dying in the health care system.

The Growing Burden of Aging, Cancer, and Acquired Immunodeficiency Syndrome

The tsunami of aging in developed countries has been discussed extensively. It is the elderly who are dying, and therefore we need palliative medicine specialists to help identify needs for advanced disease care and advocate for system change to meet those needs. The huge epidemics of human immunodeficiency virus (HIV) infection in Africa and Asia require specialists, not so much for care, but for development of health care policy for the dying, advocacy for basic levels of care (e.g., pain control), and development of local practitioners with basic knowledge to improve the quality of dying until pharmaceutical treatment and prevention become more widely effective.

Increasing Complexity of Care Needs of the Dying

As life is extended in those with diseases such as cancer and heart disease, more complex issues and symptoms are created for patients and their families. For instance, pain problems (e.g., neuropathic pain) are now more prevalent and complex in nature, requiring considerable specialized knowledge and management. The increasing presence of comorbid conditions, complex medication regimens, multiple symptoms, and functional disabilities seen in many ill and elderly patients complicates care. Alongside these factors is the requirement to handle intense psychosocial and spiritual needs, complex care planning, and elucidation of goals of care and decision making. Because knowledge, attitudes, and skills in others are inadequate to meet these demands, there is a role for experts or specialists to address these needs across the varied settings in health care—critical care, acute care, chronic care, and home care.

Emphasis on Home Care and Avoidance of Expensive Hospital Care

Most Western nations are trying to de-emphasize expensive and sometimes dangerous hospital care, stimulating the need to provide more comprehensive home care for more patients with complex and acute illnesses. In North America, the diminishing role of family physicians in community care leaves a gap that palliative medicine specialists may fill in both primary and secondary care by working with community interdisciplinary teams.

Defined Practice Standards

Western nations such as Australia, Canada, and the United Kingdom have adopted standards or norms of practice for palliative care. These require upgrading of knowledge and development of interdisciplinary care in which palliative medicine specialists act as medical experts and advocates.

Need for Better Education

All professions are beginning to recognize the need for better education in palliative care for their students and practitioners. Palliative medicine specialists help develop and implement education programs to meet those needs.

Research Needs

Many concerns in palliative care require research to examine all the issues of suffering and ways to respond. The research area for palliative care is broad, ranging from symptoms (physical, psychological, social, and spiritual) to health service delivery and economics of care. Such research crosses many different areas in medicine and other disciplines but requires experts in palliative care in academic centers to further define research questions and participate in this collaborative research.

Program Development

The roles of the specialist include health advocacy and management. In these roles, there is a need for medical specialists who have a more in-depth view of the needs of dying patients and their families to participate in health policy and program development.

Development of Palliative Care Programs and Hospice Units

The rapid growth of specialized palliative care programs or hospices has required medical leadership which well-trained palliative medicine specialists can provide.

Integration of Palliative Care into Mainstream Medicine

The integration of palliative care into mainstream care, for example cancer care, requires specialists to support the primary providers in dealing with more complex issues. Palliative medicine specialists need to be part of the specialist interdisciplinary teams that support this care.

CORE COMPETENCIES OF PALLIATIVE MEDICINE PHYSICIANS

The Royal College of Physicians and Surgeons of Canada, the certification body for medical specialists in Canada, has developed a framework for the core abilities that define each medical specialty, the CanMEDS Physician Competency Framework. This multifaceted framework of physician competence defines core abilities comprising numerous domains. These have been organized thematically around "meta-competencies" or physician roles for CanMEDS. Traditionally, medical education has articulated competence around core medical expertise. In the CanMEDS construct, the role "Medical Expert" is the central integrative role but not the only one (Fig. 6-1). The other six domains of ability cluster around this central role as Medical Expert: Scholar, Professional, Communicator, Collaborator, Manager, and Health Advocate.[4] The

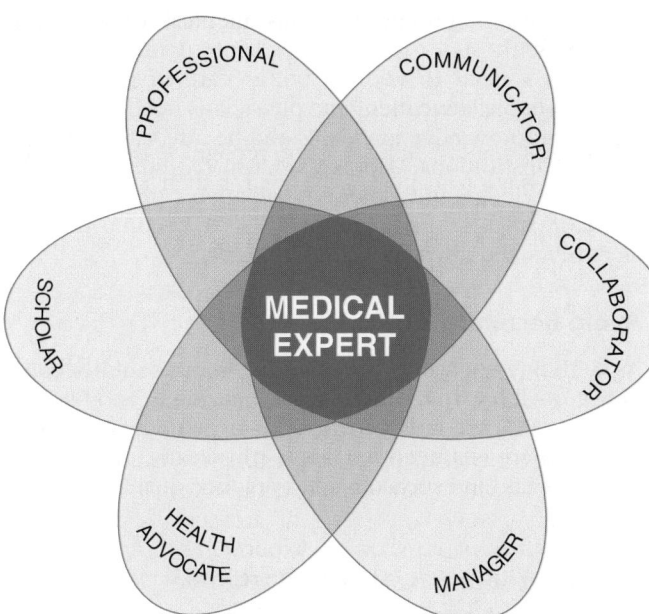

FIGURE 6-1 Framework of Essential Physician Competencies. *(From Frank JR [ed]. The CanMEDS 2005 Physician Competency Framework: Better Standards, Better Physicians, Better Care. Ottawa: The Royal College of Physicians and Surgeons of Canada, 2005, p. 3. Redrawn with permission of The Royal College of Physicians and Surgeons of Canada. © 2001-2006 www.rcpsc.medical.org.)*

CanMEDS Framework defines the competencies or learning outcomes of undergraduate medical education and medical specialty education and frames a process for continuing education and certification in Canada. It has attracted interest from medical educators around the world.

The CanMEDS Framework can be used to define the core competencies of palliative medicine.

Medical Expert

The CanMEDS Physician Competency Framework describes the role of Medical Expert as follows[4]:

Physicians possess a defined body of knowledge, clinical skills, procedural skills and professional attitudes, which are directed to effective patient-centered care. They apply these competencies to collect and interpret information, make appropriate clinical decisions, and carry out diagnostic and therapeutic interventions. They do so within the boundaries of their discipline, personal expertise, the healthcare setting and the patient's preferences and context. Their care is characterized by up-to-date, ethical, and resource efficient clinical practice as well as with effective communication in partnership with patients, other health care providers and the community. The Role of Medical Expert is central to the function of physicians and draws on the competencies included in the roles of Communicator, Collaborator, Manager, Health Advocate, Scholar and Professional (p. 22).

As a Medical Expert, the palliative medicine physician has the following competencies:

1. Assess and manage complex pain and other symptoms.
2. Assess and manage psychosocial and spiritual needs.

3. Assess and manage grief.
4. Describe the elements of suffering in end-of-life care for patients, families, and caregivers.
5. Demonstrate cultural and religious sensitivity in end-of-life care.
6. Function effectively as a consultant to provide optimal, ethical, patient- and family-centered palliative care.
7. Address issues of advance care planning and end-of-life decision making.

Communicator

As a Communicator, the palliative medicine physician has the following competencies:

1. Develop rapport, trust, and ethical therapeutic relationships with dying patients and their families.
2. Participate effectively in patient and family meetings.
3. Develop a common understanding on issues, advance care directives, and goals of care with patients and families, colleagues, and other professionals to develop and implement a shared plan of care.
4. Educate patients and families about end-of-life care issues and pain and symptom management.
5. Convey relevant information and explanations to patients and families, colleagues, and other professionals.

Collaborator

As a Collaborator, the palliative medicine physician has the following competencies:

1. Collaborate effectively as a member of an interdisciplinary team, whether formal or informal.
2. Effectively work with other health professionals to prevent, negotiate, and resolve interprofessional conflict, which is often seen in negotiating the goals of care for dying patients and their families.

Manager

As a Manager, the palliative medicine physician has the following competencies:

1. Describe models of palliative care and assess the amount and efficacy of palliative care community resources.
2. Participate in activities that contribute to the effectiveness of health care organizations and systems.
3. Participate in the development and implementation of standards of palliative care and systematic quality process evaluation and improvement in end-of-life care.
4. Allocate health care resources justly, balancing effectiveness, efficiency, and access with optimal patient care, and advocate for palliative care as cost-effective.
5. Acquire leadership and administrative skills.
6. Develop an understanding of and skills in organizational and health care system change.

Health Advocate

As a Health Advocate, the palliative medicine physician has the following competencies:

1. Respond to individual patient and family needs and issues by developing goals of care.
2. Identify opportunities for advocacy, health promotion, and disease prevention with dying patients and their families.
3. Analyze barriers that inhibit access to palliative care and gaps in care and develop responses to those barriers and gaps in the community.
4. Identify vulnerable or marginalized populations within those served and assist in ways of responding to the special needs of those populations.

Scholar

As a Scholar, the palliative medicine physician has the following competencies:

1. Maintain and enhance professional activities through ongoing learning.
2. Critically evaluate medical information and its sources and apply this information appropriately to practice.
3. Contribute to the development, dissemination, and translation of new knowledge and practices through research and education in palliative care.

Professional

As a Professional, the palliative medicine physician has the following competencies:

1. Self-assess one's own attitudes and beliefs in caring for the dying.
2. Demonstrate self-awareness and self-care in caring for the terminally ill.
3. Participate in the development of professional standards in palliative care with regulatory bodies.
4. Recognize and appropriately respond to ethical issues in palliative care, particularly to the issues involved in physician-assisted dying and withholding or withdrawing therapy.

CHALLENGES FOR PALLIATIVE MEDICINE

Avoid Becoming "Symptomatologists"

There is a concern that palliative medicine specialists will see themselves or be seen as physical symptom control specialists. In some institutions, this has translated into palliative care teams' being called "pain and symptom teams." The loss of identity with the broad issues of dying and death, the psychological and spiritual concerns of patient and family, and the communications and ethical issues that continue to abound in this area of care could be problematic. Quality care must be defined as more than just physical care, and palliative medicine physicians must continue to have broad competencies.

Avoid Becoming Too Hospital Focused

The acute care hospital environment can be challenging for good palliative care, but it also can be comforting and isolating. Nursing homes are just large palliative care institutions, with 30% to 40% of residents dying each year. There is a need to address better care in this setting. Therefore, palliative medicine physicians need to develop pertinent knowledge and skills and be advocates for care in these institutions.[5] Home care also requires some specific knowledge and skills for palliative care. There is a need for palliative medicine specialists to become involved as experts and advocates in that area.

Avoid Becoming Elitist

As with any specialty, palliative medicine could become elitist, pushing out others from providing good-quality primary and secondary care and forgetting community needs. There is a need for family physicians, oncologists, cardiologists, and surgeons who practice quality palliative care.

Avoid Becoming Isolated in Palliative Care Institutions

It would not be in the best interests of palliative medicine for its practitioners to be present only in palliative care or hospice units. They must be present in acute care hospitals and cancer centers, critical care units, pediatric hospitals, and other health care agencies.

Avoid Losing the Advocacy Role in Making Changes

Health care is replete with caring and mostly compassionate people who provide poor end-of-life care that reflects our societal avoidance and depersonalization of dying and death. The new specialty of palliative medicine still has a great role to play in making changes to our approach to dying and death. New palliative medicine specialists need to be trained to be opinion leaders and agents of change.

Avoid Losing the Interdependent Focus of Interdisciplinary Care

Palliative care is at its core interdisciplinary. The multiple needs of patients and their families require special skills that are not served well by any one professional specialist. The need for teams to meet those needs is not completely met by hiring a palliative medicine specialist alone.

PALLIATIVE MEDICINE TRAINING PROGRAMS

Formal specialist training programs in palliative medicine have been established in several countries in association with organizations that have responsibility for postgraduate training and certification.[6-9] The competencies aimed at by all these programs are often similar, but the duration of training differs remarkably, from 4 years in the United Kingdom to 1 year in Canada (beyond core general competency training and/or certification in family medicine or another specialty). Not all programs (e.g., Canada) rely on a final certification examination. In the United States, standards for specialty training in palliative medicine are voluntary,[10] but the American Board of Hospice and Palliative

Medicine is working to standardize training programs.[11] Informal training programs and preceptorships also exist in some countries that produce physicians who have a special interest in palliative care but whose major role is within their root specialties. Informal fellowship programs also exist in local hospital or university programs in the United States and Canada, but these often do not conform to the requirements or curriculum competencies of recognized specialty training programs. Most of the formal training programs are designed to produce physicians with exemplary clinical and some academic skills. It is recognized that physicians destined for academic palliative medicine will require further education in research and areas beyond their specialty training.

CONCLUSIONS

Palliative medicine is a new, growing specialty with a defined role. It is in a developmental stage. Palliative medicine has had some successes but needs to meet a number of challenges (see "Common Errors") to survive and prosper and become part of mainstream medicine.

REFERENCES

1. Librach SL. Defining palliative care as a specialty could do more harm than good! J Palliat Care 1988;4(1&2):23-24
2. Fox RC. The professions of medicine and nursing. In Sociology of Medicine: A Participant Observer's View. Englewood Cliffs, NJ: Prentice-Hall, 1989, pp 38-71.
3. Hayley DC, Sachs GA. A brief history and lessons learned from twin efforts to transform medicine. Clin Geriatr Med 2005;21:3-15.
4. Frank JR (ed). The CanMEDS 2005 Physician Competency Framework: Better Standards, Better Physicians, Better Care. Ottawa: The Royal College of Physicians and Surgeons of Canada, 2005.
5. Miller SC, Teno JM, Mor V. Hospice and palliative care in nursing homes. Clin Geriatr Med 2004;20:717-734.
6. Website of the U.K. Joint Committee on Higher Medical Training, now part of the Joint Royal Colleges of Physicians Training Board. Available at http://www.jrcptb.org.uk (accessed September 2007).
7. Website of the Royal College of Physicians and Surgeons of Canada. Available at http://www.rcpsc.medical.org (accessed September 2007).
8. Website of the Royal Australasian College of Physicians. Available at http://www.racp.edu.au (accessed September 2007).
9. Website of the American Board of Hospice and Palliative Medicine. Available at http://www.abhpm.org (accessed September 2007).
10. Billings JA, Block SD, Finn JW, et al. Initial voluntary program standards for fellowship training in palliative medicine. J Palliat Med 2002;5:23-33.
11. von Gunten CF, Lupu D. Progress for palliative medicine as a subspecialty. J Support Oncol 2005;3:267-268.

CHAPTER **7**

Principles of Palliative Medicine

Ira Byock

KEY POINTS

- Principles articulate fundamental assumptions, values, and goals that motivate and bind a collective endeavor.
- Principles of a profession are distilled through successive processes of discussion, review, and comment.
- Principles of palliative care frame the domains of clinical attention and facilitate evidence-based practice by providing a conceptual structure for measurement, quality assessment, and research.
- The evolution of palliative care principles has been international and multicentered and has involved general clinical disciplines as well as specialty hospice and palliative care organizations.
- Principles of palliative care include both clinical and operational principles.
- Clinical principles of palliative care
  - The unit of care comprises a patient with his or her family.
  - Symptoms must be routinely assessed and effectively managed.
  - Decisions regarding medical treatments must be made in an ethical manner.
  - Palliative care is provided through an interdisciplinary team.
  - Palliative care coordinates and provides for continuity of care.
  - Dying is a normal part of life, and quality of life is a central clinical goal.
  - Palliative care attends to spiritual aspects of patient and family distress and well-being.
  - Palliative care neither hastens death nor prolongs dying.
  - Palliative care extends bereavement support to patients' families.
- Operational principles of palliative care
  - Palliative care preserves and enhances the well-being of clinical and support staff and volunteers.
  - Palliative care engages in continuous quality improvement and research efforts.
  - Palliative care advocates for individual patients and families and advances public policy to improve access to needed services and quality of care.

THE PURPOSE AND FORMATION OF PRINCIPLES

Professional disciplines strive to act by sets of principles that are formally adopted and articulated in published statements by stakeholder organizations. Informally, the principles of a profession may be discerned by the collective actions and work products of the discipline's members. Principles refer to fundamental assumptions, values, and goals that motivate and bind a collective endeavor.

It is common for associations of clinical specialists to adopt and publish formal statements of principles for their field. Such statements complement an association's mission and vision statements in a manner that advances operational objectives for the organization and discipline. Principles enable a clinical specialty to define its focus and scope of practice and, by extension, to define its boundaries. In this way, principles clarify the categorical responsibilities and contributions of a discipline's organizations and individual members within a larger professional or social context. Principles form the basis for clinical practice guidelines and standards of practice. They promote consistency of services and provide a framework for evaluation, quality improvement, oversight, and accreditation (Box 7-1).

Principles published by health care organizations and professional associations emphasize values and goals that guide clinical practice. However, it is also common for them to address the manner in which organizations or members of a field interact with one another and conduct nonclinical, including financial, affairs. Additionally, professional principles can speak to the professional and personal experiences of health care providers and their stresses and satisfactions.

Discussions of principles risk sounding abstract, yet they provide tangible guidance to a field and its members in "real world" practice, particularly during unsettled periods within society or health care. Many organizations routinely begin board meetings, annual meetings, and planning sessions by reading statements of mission and principles to anchor the business conducted in the group's fundamental values and goals.

Formation of Principles of Palliative Care

Key principles of palliative care can be discerned within the early history of the discipline, revealed in the motivations, shared assumptions, and actions of its founding members (see Chapter 4). Formal principles are distilled through successive processes of discussion, review, and comment. Although an essential purpose is to lend stability to a field by grounding it in established values and goals, principles are not immutable. Planned, deliberate review processes by internal and external stakeholders, which for clinical disciplines includes both providers and recipients of care, enable shared assumptions to be challenged and values and goals affirmed, refined, and freshly

---

Box 7-1 Purposes of Principles

- Define the purpose of an endeavor such as an organization or professional field
- Define long-term or ultimate goals of the endeavor or organization
- Guide professional (clinical) actions—both in furtherance of the goals that bind the endeavor and in the process with which the organization and field pursues the goals
- Guide organizational decisions and actions
- Provide basis for standards of practice
- Promote consistency of practice
- Provide framework for evaluation, quality improvement, oversight, and accreditation, including parameters for evaluation and performance indicators

---

applied in rapidly changing and broad-ranging social contexts and practice environments.[1]

Professionals working in hospice and palliative care represent an evolving discipline whose principles will continue to be tested in practice, debated, and refined. This process is ongoing in many countries through the efforts of diverse professional associations and ad hoc groups. This is not an indication of instability of the field, but rather of its vibrancy.

Principles and Evidence-Based Medicine

Published principles of hospice, palliative, and end-of-life care often emphasize the importance of evidence-based medicine to the evolution of palliative care. However, the principles of a clinical specialty are not evidence-based in the current usage of that term.[2]

Although informed by science—particularly anthropology and sociology of illness, caregiving, dying, death, and grief, as well as clinical observation and experimental research—principles are developed through processes from the realm of ethics rather than scientific inquiry.[3] The ethics and science of palliative care are complementary. The principles of palliative care frame the domains of clinical attention and facilitate evidence-based practice by providing a conceptual structure for measurement, quality assessment, and research. Evidence-based medicine is instrumental to fulfilling the principles and accomplishing the goals of palliative care.

Principles of Palliative Care

Although palliative care was once considered almost synonymous with terminal or end-of-life care, contemporary definitions and principles of hospice and palliative care do not confine attention to "dying"—a period that can be as difficult to recognize prospectively as it is to accept emotionally. Of course, many specialties and subspecialties of medicine and nursing and other clinical disciplines share responsibility for people with life-threatening conditions and contribute to both life-prolonging and palliative treatment. Correspondingly, medical, surgical, and nursing organizations have published general principles of palliative and end-of-life care. Some have also published separate statements on specific policies, such as the appropriate use of artificial nutrition and hydration or assisted suicide. Although these statements do not speak for the specialty of palliative care, they do inform palliative domains of practice and root principles of palliative care within encompassing social and clinical contexts of ethics and standards of care.

It is also true that, while exerting no authority over specialists from other disciplines, palliative care organizations can publish principles that seek to establish basic clinical standards applicable to care regardless of the setting or providers' specialties.

The evolution of palliative care principles has been multicentric and international. It has involved the disciplines represented on interdisciplinary teams.

The following delineation of principles of palliative care is drawn from published statements in English and is a distillation of common elements. The published statements by specialty organizations and ad hoc groups in the

United States during the past decade serve as examples of processes occurring in many countries.

The World Health Organization (WHO) first published a seminal definition and statement of the characteristics of palliative care in 1990. The WHO statement has been updated and continues to serve as a common point of reference from which many health care organizations and task forces developed their palliative care principles.[4]

Principles of General Health Care and Clinical Specialty Organizations

In 1996, under the auspices of the Milbank Memorial Fund, Drs. Christine Cassel and Kathleen Foley, two recognized leaders in American palliative care, convened representatives of American medical specialties to review and update "existing or proposed policies concerning decision-making at the end of life and the quality of clinical management of dying patients." A draft set of "Core Principles for End-of-Life Care" was subsequently reviewed and adopted or revised by participating organizations. In 1999, the Milbank Memorial Fund reported that 14 American specialty societies had endorsed or adopted these core principles, either unchanged or with modifications. Additionally, the influential Joint Commission on the Accreditation of Healthcare Organizations formally determined that its standards were well aligned with these principles. In focusing on "end-of-life care," the Milbank Core Principles did not address palliative care during earlier illness and treatment. However, the Milbank process was important for establishing basic palliative principles across multiple specialties (Box 7-2).

In addition to endorsing the Milbank Core Principles, several organizations, such as the American College of Physicians, the American Geriatrics Society, and the American Society of Clinical Oncology (ASCO), expanded their principles to incorporate elements of the specialty of palliative care.[5-8] ASCO's comprehensive statement calls for cancer care programs and providers to address palliative care throughout the illness.[6]

PRINCIPLES OF THE SPECIALTY OF HOSPICE AND PALLIATIVE CARE

During the past 2 decades, organizations with a stake in the care of people with life-threatening conditions have engaged in thoughtful deliberations and published documents that identify and endorse key elements and characteristics of palliative care. The specific mechanisms for developing these have varied, but in general they have conformed to the process described earlier of meetings convened to draft statements, followed by serial reviews and revisions leading to formal adoption of well-considered principles.

In the United States, the National Hospice and Palliative Care Organization (NHPCO) (previously the National Hospice Organization) initially developed Standards of Practice for Hospice Programs in the early 1980s; these were revised and first published in 1987 and have been regularly updated. In addition, in 1997, the organization published *A Pathway for Patients and Families Facing Terminal Illness,* the result of two task forces of the NHPCO Standards and Accreditation Committee.[9] The Pathway document advanced an integrated approach to palliative care by defining salient domains of patient and family experience along with corresponding domains for assessment, care planning, and outcomes measurement.

Last Acts, a nationwide American communications campaign organized under the auspices of The Robert Wood Johnson Foundation, convened an interdisciplinary national task force of thought leaders in palliative care and published the *Precepts of Palliative Care* in 1998.[10] Building on this, Last Acts partnered in 2003 with the National Association of Neonatal Nurses, the Society of Pediatric Nurses, and the Association of Pediatric Oncology Nurses to develop and publish *Precepts of Palliative Care for Children, Adolescents and their Families*[11] (Box 7-3).

In 2000, the Hastings Center, an institute for the study of health care ethics, partnered with the NHPCO and the National Hospice Workgroup to examine the essential elements, underlying values, and roles of hospice and palliative care in society. Meetings involving influential leaders in palliative care, health care philosophy, ethics, and economics convened to draft, circulate, and refine

---

Box 7-2 Milbank Core Principles for End-of-Life Care

Clinical policy of care at the end of life and the professional practice it guides should do the following:

1. Respect the dignity of both patient and caregivers.
2. Be sensitive to and respectful of the patient's and family's wishes.
3. Use the most appropriate measures that are consistent with patient choices.
4. Encompass alleviation of pain and other physical symptoms.
5. Assess and manage psychological, social, and spiritual/religious problems.
6. Offer continuity (the patient should be able to continue to be cared for, if so desired, by his/her primary care and specialist providers).
7. Provide access to any therapy that may realistically be expected to improve the patient's quality of life, including alternative or nontraditional treatments.
8. Provide access to palliative care and hospice care.
9. Respect the right to refuse treatment.
10. Respect the physician's professional responsibility to discontinue some treatments when appropriate, with consideration for both patient and family preferences.
11. Promote clinical and evidence-based research on providing care at the end of life.

Box 7-3 Last Acts Precepts

"Palliative care refers to the comprehensive management of the physical, psychological, social, spiritual and existential needs of patients. It is especially suited to the care of people with incurable, progressive illnesses."

Categorical precepts include the following:

● Respecting patient goals, preferences, and choices
● Comprehensive caring
● Utilizing the strengths of interdisciplinary resources
● Acknowledging and addressing caregiver concerns
● Building systems and mechanisms of support

findings and recommendations. The report, *Access to Hospice: Expanding Boundaries, Overcoming Barriers,* is intended to guide social and governmental policy to affirm and advance positive social values and facilitate access to hospice and palliative care.[12]

In 2002, after a multiyear process, the Canadian Hospice and Palliative Care Association published *A Model to Guide Hospice Palliative Care,* a comprehensive document encompassing foundational concepts, definitions, values, principles of clinical practice, service delivery, and programmatic structure and function.[13]

More recently, five major American palliative care organizations, including the American Academy of Hospice and Palliative Medicine and the Hospice and Palliative Nurses Association, collaborated to form the National Consensus Project for Quality Palliative Care (NCP).[14] The NCP followed an iterative process of drafting, review, and comment by a widely representative advisory committee to develop and publish, in 2004, the *Clinical Practice Guidelines for Quality Palliative Care.* This NCP report defines terms and identifies essential elements of palliative care to promote quality, foster consistency of practice and continuity of care across settings, expand access, and encourage performance measurement and quality improvement.

Principle: The Unit of Care Comprises a Patient with His or Her Family

Serious illness or injury strikes an individual, but it affects everyone to whom the afflicted person matters. This basic human insight gives rise to the fundamental tenet that palliative care attends to the needs and experiences of the patient *with his or her family.* In the contemporary application of this principle, the meaning of family is not restricted to relations of bloodline or marriage; rather, family is understood to comprise a person's relatives and close friends (see Chapter 13). The phrase, "for whom it matters" captures this meaning. For clinical purposes, family can be considered to include the people who most matter to the patient and those for whom the patient matters.

Palliative care teams routinely assess and respond to distress experienced by patients' relatives and close friends, particularly those providing care. Indeed, there are situations in which the family suffers more deeply or acutely than the person whose life is threatened. An elderly woman with advanced dementia who has recurrent pneumonias and little interest in eating may be physically comfortable and content with her surroundings and exhibit no distress while her children struggle with decisions about antibiotics and artificial nutrition, simultaneously resisting and grieving her coming death. Similarly, a 60-year-old man who remains in deep coma after a sudden intracranial hemorrhage may be insensate while his wife, children, and friends experience the agony of sudden loss. These families would benefit from the services of a palliative care team no less than fully conscious patients.

Palliative care for families of dying patients extends beyond alleviating suffering. By listening and becoming familiar with the culture, traditions, and interpersonal style of a seriously ill person's family, palliative care clinicians may offer suggestions for spending time with the ill person, including culturally consonant ways of reviewing and celebrating their relationships and shared lives.

Principle: Symptoms Must Be Routinely Assessed and Effectively Managed

Alleviation of suffering is a central goal and fundamental principle. Too often, however, it has been honored in the breach. The common observation that people were dying in pain was an important impetus for the development of hospice and palliative care. Early in her career, Dr. Cicely Saunders observed that *pro re nata* or "as needed" analgesic orders resulted in patients' having to "earn" their next does of pain medication by suffering. She championed—and studied—the alternative approach of scheduled pain medication: "by the clock" administration to prevent chronic pain from recurring, together with supplemental analgesia for breakthrough pain. This principle has been universally endorsed by palliative care specialty and other clinical specialty organizations.

Suffering from pain and other physical symptoms associated with advanced disease is not inevitable. It is core practice in hospice and palliative care programs to assess each bothersome symptom (see Chapters 63 and 64), considering and (as the patient's condition warrants) investigating potential causes and developing a plan to diminish the discomfort. In advanced illness, multiple physiological problems can contribute to a patient's pain, dyspnea, nausea, fatigue, or other symptoms; not surprisingly, corresponding treatment plans are often multimodal.

Principle: Decisions Regarding Medical Treatments Must Be Made in an Ethical Manner

Honesty and integrity are cornerstones of clinical practice. An overarching principle of health care requires that decisions regarding medical treatments be made in an honest and ethical manner that respects peoples' rights (see Part I, Section C). Patients and their families have a right to accurate information about the patient's condition and treatment options, conveyed in words they can understand and in a manner that respects individual and ethnic cultural values. Truthful information must be offered to patients but need not be imposed. It can be helpful to ask patients how much they wish to know about their condition and prognosis. Some prefer to defer information to a willing relative or friend who can help them make decisions.

Western society acknowledges that, with few exceptions, individuals have primary and final authority over their bodies. Clinicians have a responsibility to educate patients and families and are encouraged to guide them through a shared decision-making process. Ultimately, clinicians must respect the autonomy of individual patients and their right to choose among available options for care or to refuse any indicated treatment offered. If a patient is incapacitated, a formally appointed proxy or, in many jurisdictions, the patient's relatives can assert this right on the individual's behalf. Palliative care clinicians and teams bring their clinical experience, accurate medical information, and communication skills to the difficult and poignant process of decision making, enabling patients and their families to identify valuable, achievable goals and develop a corresponding plan of care.

Autonomy applies to adults with cognitive capacity to understand decisions. Children have partial autonomy that increases in proportion to their growing abilities to comprehend situations and accept responsibility for their decisions. In the *Precepts of Palliative Care for Children, Adolescents and their Families,* the section entitled "Respect for Patients Goals, Preferences, and Choices" states that palliative care "[a]ssists the child and family in establishing goals of care by facilitating their understanding of the diagnosis and prognosis, clarifying priorities and providing an opportunity to collaborate with providers on the creation of a care plan. This process takes into account the child's developmental stage, chronological age and the family's wishes."[11]

Principle: Palliative Care Is Provided through an Interdisciplinary Team

Specialized palliative care programs rely on an interdisciplinary team model of professionals and trained volunteers. Each member brings particular skills and areas of emphasis (see Part I, Section H). Within this interdisciplinary team dynamic, physicians and advanced practice nurses bear primary responsibility for symptom assessment and treatment, as well as for advice and coordination regarding concomitant disease-modifying treatments.

Professionals from many disciplines, including pastoral care, social work, psychology, and clinical pharmacy, contribute to a well-developed interdisciplinary team. Additionally, ostomy and wound specialists can assist with dressing changes in a manner that maximizes comfort and independence. Rehabilitative physical, occupational, respiratory, and speech therapists can help patients adapt to changing functional capacities, and music and art therapists offer nonverbal ways to express feelings and enrich the ill person's days.

Cross-training is encouraged within interdisciplinary palliative care teams. Every member of a clinical team can be alert for physical problems such as uncontrolled pain or constipation, and any member can listen to a patient's or family member's fears or spiritual concerns. By bringing their observations and recommendations to case discussions, team members make the team process collaborative and creative. New, unanticipated clinical strategies may emerge, and the resulting plan of care reflects more than the sum of individual contributions. This process also fosters a coherent approach that can be advanced by all members.

Trained and supervised volunteers from the community are an important component of these teams. Directly or through reports by a coordinator, volunteers contribute observations and insights to care planning. Occasionally, the key to unlocking the suffering of a patient or family comes from the information and perspective a volunteer provides. Simply by being present and keeping company with a seriously ill patient, bearing witness to his or her life and current experience, volunteers demonstrate to people who are ill and struggling with progressive disabilities that they retain their full worth. Volunteers from many walks of life provide pragmatic help to patients and families. Some assist with insurance or governmental forms, others with errands or minor household chores. They are often available to read to patients or to help patients and families review old photographs or record stories as a legacy for future generations. In some programs, a volunteer may offer a manicure or a volunteer masseuse may be available to offer massage, simply to brighten an ill person's day. In all these ways, by their time, efforts, and presence, volunteers remind clinicians of the basic social and community values that hospice and palliative care represent.

In some settings, such as developing countries, isolated rural regions, and disadvantaged inner-city communities, it is impossible to assemble or maintain an interdisciplinary team. Individual clinicians can provide palliative aspects of care from a multidimensional perspective, drawing on the expertise and insights of other pertinent disciplines through consultation by telephone or e-mail and educational meetings.

Principle: Palliative Care Coordinates and Provides for Continuity of Care

Fragmentation of health care has been an unintended consequence of modern medical technical sophistication. As the complexity of diagnostic workups and treatments has increased, health services and settings of care have become ever more specialized. Faced with serious illness, even well-educated and assertive patients can feel lost in a maze of options and complicated plans.[15]

Commonly, processes of oversight and accreditation of health care have been organized by site of care. This makes the problems of fragmentation of care almost invisible to the audit process, difficult to measure or even detect. From the perspective of patients and their families, however, continuity is a critical domain of quality.

Correspondingly, coordination of care is a critical function of palliative practice. Typically in hospice programs, a nurse or social worker is assigned to each patient as a case manager. In a wide variety of innovative palliative care programs serving special populations, often in challenging settings, a common element has been the designation of an individual case manager or care coordinator who functions as the hub for communications and continuity for the team.[16]

The principle of continuity has led to programmatic standards ensuring that there is always a professional on call who is familiar with the patient and family and has timely access to pertinent records and the plan of care.

In some countries and health systems, fragmentation is imposed by payment structures that force choices between curative and palliative care. In the United States, the law establishing the Medicare Hospice Benefit requires a doctor to certify that a patient has a life expectancy of 6 months or less (if the disease runs its natural course) for the patient to be eligible. Corresponding regulations further require that patients (or legal proxies for incapacitated patients) agree to forego future disease-modifying or life-prolonging treatments. These stipulations are inconsistent with the founding principles of palliative care. Many recent organizational and ad hoc statements have called for changes in policy, payment, and health service delivery systems that would enable palliative care to be available early in any illness.[10,11,13,14,17] These statements exemplify circumstances in which a field's principles can inform important public policy statements and actions.

From the perspective of quality improvement in health care, there is strategic value in defining continuity as a distinct domain of quality and incorporating measures of continuity in the evaluation of clinical care and health service delivery.[18] Doing so forces a shift in the perspective of evaluation from the site of care delivery to the experiences of patients and families.

Principle: Dying Is a Normal Part of Life, and Quality of Life Is a Central Clinical Goal

Palliative care regards dying as a normal, albeit inherently difficult, stage within the life of every individual. By extension, death of individuals is understood as normal within the life of every family.

The stipulation by WHO that palliative care "affirms life and regards dying as a normal process" seems self-evident, an acknowledgement that death comes at the end of every life.[4] Many specialty societies have formally endorsed and incorporated these concepts as their own.[6-8] However, during the early development of hospice and palliative care, this stance was a radical departure from the prevailing mainstream of health care and seemed heretical to established practice. Within the predominant professional clinical culture of the mid-20th century, death was regarded as the ultimate negative, and forestalling death was not only the primary but often the exclusive goal of medical practice (Box 7-4).

Hospice and palliative care represented a countercultural view that carried tacit criticisms. The affirmation of life that encompassed dying carried profound and important implications for health care. If dying is part of life, it must not be avoided but must instead be understood. If dying matters, then the quality of a dying person's care

Box 7-4 World Health Organization Statement

Palliative care improves the quality of life of patients and families who face life-threatening illness by providing pain and symptom relief and spiritual and psychosocial support from diagnosis to the end of life and bereavement.

  Palliative care

- Provides relief from pain and other distressing symptoms
- Affirms life and regards dying as a normal process
- Intends neither to hasten or to postpone death
- Integrates the psychological and spiritual aspects of patient care
- Offers a support system to help patients live as actively as possible until death
- Offers a support system to help the family cope during the patient's illness and in their own bereavement
- Uses a team approach to address the needs of patients and their families, including bereavement counseling if indicated
- Enhances quality of life and may also positively influence the course of illness
- Is applicable early in the course of illness, in conjunction with other therapies that are intended to prolong life, such as chemotherapy or radiation therapy, and includes those investigations needed to better understand and manage distressing clinical complications

and quality of life are not merely legitimate but also requisite foci for clinical attention, standards of care, reimbursement, accountability, and research.

Ramifications of this stance continue to distinguish palliative care and represent a seminal contribution of the field to human therapeutics. Prevalent problem-based approaches to care are by nature reactive. Disease-modifying approaches to treatment are by nature limited to correcting pathophysiologies. In contrast, the principles of palliative care are person centered, directing attention to personal experiences and identifying quality of life as a core goal and domain of quality. This shift in focus opens a rich realm of therapeutic opportunities. Further, by design, palliative care is proactive in serious illness. A diagnosis of progressive, incurable disease or a combination of medical problems that causes progressive disability and a limited prognosis is a sufficient indication for referral to palliative care programs and clinicians. A seriously ill patient need not be in acute pain or otherwise suffering to merit clinical time and attention. The person's quality of life intrinsically matters, as does the family's experience related to the person's illness and care. From a palliative care perspective, effective treatment of pain, dyspnea, constipation, and confusion are all important—for alleviating distress, but also for preserving opportunities.

The "treat, prevent, promote" intervention strategy of the NHPCO's Pathway document builds from this core principle. Within salient domains of individual and family experience, hospice and palliative care teams are charged with treating problems that people report or that are uncovered in routine screening and evaluation, preventing crises and foreseeable problems, and promoting a self-determined sense of life closure. Palliative plans of care explore opportunities for each patient and family to accomplish identified goals, such as simply enjoying time together or in solitude, reminiscing and reviewing life, expressing feelings to important people in one's life, and achieving a sense of completion in relationships and life. Faced with the unwanted but inevitable fact of death's approach, many people appreciate anticipatory guidance with these unfamiliar and often difficult tasks of life—completion and closure.

Principle: Palliative Care Attends to Spiritual Aspects of Patient and Family Distress and Well-being

In asserting that improving quality of life is a central clinical goal, the principles of palliative care require clinicians to study and understand the lived experiences of illness and dying as a basis for clinical assessment, care planning, outcomes measurement, and research.

Palliative care brought a "whole person" framework to the clinical assessment and care of patients. Dr. Cicely Saunders introduced the concept of "total pain," in which physical, psychological, social, and spiritual quadrants of an individual's experience contribute to distress. Cassel elaborated that personhood encompasses one's body, one's past and sense of the future, one's innate temperament, one's family of origin and current family, one's ethnic and social cultures, one's social and vocational roles, and one's individual beliefs, habits, preferences, and aversions. For Cassel, suffering involved an impending sense of disintegration of one's self.[19,20]

The principles of palliative care recognize that people have a spiritual or transcendent dimension that derives from an intrinsic human drive to make meaning and an almost universal desire to achieve some sense of one's life in relationship to others and the world. People also have an inner life, involving one's relationship with one's self. In palliative practice, spirituality entails those aspects of a person's experience, beliefs, and relationships that hold inherent importance and a felt connection to something larger than one's self that will endure into an open-ended future. This transcendent construct may involve an individual's sense of God or nature as well as family, community, or country.

This tenet has also been acknowledged by multiple specialty organizations. ASCO states, "Cancer care optimizes quality of life throughout the course of an illness through meticulous attention to the myriad physical, spiritual, and psychosocial needs of the patient and family." Referring to patients who are nearing the end of life, the ASCO statement says, "The dying process creates a myriad of questions and concerns about the meaning of life. People confront and resolve these questions and concerns in their own ways, frequently but not exclusively through religious and philosophical beliefs. Increasingly, those who care for the dying find that spiritual and existential issues are central to the quality of patients' lives as they near death"[6] (see also Chapter 12).

Principle: Palliative Care neither Hastens Death nor Prolongs Dying

Hospice and palliative care was developed in the 1960s and 1970s in response to the perceived pervasive incidence of people dying badly and the related endemic overuse of aggressive and ultimately futile life-prolonging treatments before death. Although generally welcomed by the public and positively portrayed in the press and other media, hospice and palliative care pioneers were careful to distinguish *allowing death* to occur from *killing* and to separate their efforts from assisted suicide or euthanasia. During this time, the phrase "right to die" did not refer to euthanasia or assisted suicide but rather the right to be *allowed to die*. The right to die cases of the day concerned whether and under what circumstances an individual or a surrogate decision maker could refuse or have withdrawn life-prolonging measures such as mechanical ventilation or artificial nutrition.[21]

In the latter part of the 20th century, advocates for legalized physician-assisted suicide, citing growing public support, called for hospice and palliative care organizations to incorporate physician-assisted suicide into their scope of practice. Instead, most palliative care organizations have reaffirmed the principle that palliative care neither hastens death nor prolongs dying, honoring a distinction between acting with the intention of ending life and the palliative practice of providing whatever treatment is necessary for comfort while allowing a person to die of natural causes. Palliative care supports the right of patients to avoid invasive treatments, such as mechanical ventilation, dialysis, and artificial nutrition and hydration (including situations in which a patient has lost interest in or decided to stop eating and drinking), as well as routine treatments, such as antibiotics to treat pneumonia or a urinary infection with bacteremia.[22]

Principle: Palliative Care Extends Bereavement Support to Patients' Families

Palliative care recognizes that the experience of illness does not end with the death of the ill or injured person. As Saunders observed, "How people die remains in the memories of those who live on."[19] This fact is rooted in anthropology and sociology and has been confirmed by an array of psychological and clinical studies.

Clinical principles of palliative care mandate support for a patient's relatives or close friends who are grieving. Perhaps the most effective way to alleviate a family's grief is for them to feel that the person they loved died well. Palliative care programs and clinicians help prevent complicated grief by striving to ensure that each patient is clean and comfortable and that families have a chance to honor and celebrate their loved one during their final days (see Chapter 14).

Palliative principles pertinent to bereavement flow from the mandate to focus on each patient *with his or her family* as the unit of care. In fact, family members' experiences of grief and loss often begin well before the death of their relative or close friend. Therefore, support for grief and loss properly extends to assisting family members during the patient's illness in adjusting to the successive losses that result from progressive disability and growing proximity to death.

Grief is not an illness, but it is an inherently difficult time in life. Particularly during the initial period of grief, people are at high risk for physical and emotional illnesses. Multiple studies have documented an increased risk of illness and death among recently widowed spouses,[23,24] and there is some evidence that palliative care may ameliorate this risk.[25]

In general, principles do not specify a period of time for bereavement support, but it is typically extended through the first anniversary of the person's death. The level of support is also not specified. Bereavement support can entail information about the normal range of experience associated with grief, routine assessment, availability and referral to peer support groups, and referral to individual counseling. At minimum, by maintaining contact with family members of deceased patients, programs can exercise surveillance for complicated grief and intervene as needed by enlisting appropriate health care and community-based services.

OPERATIONAL PRINCIPLES

Several operational principles can be discerned from reviewing prevailing statements of palliative care organizations.

Principle: Palliative Care Preserves and Enhances the Well-being of Clinical and Support Staff and Volunteers

Recently published principles frequently call for attention to the well-being of personnel of hospice and palliative care programs. Palliative care is hard work and can exact an emotional and physical toll from care providers (see

Chapter 15). Hospice and palliative care clinicians and volunteers can best serve patients and families when they are well. Although such statements sound platitudinous— as principles sometimes do—they are intended to formally acknowledge and remind us of important truths. In this case, the implications of preserving the health and well-being of clinical staff can easily be lost in over-busy health systems, within the competitive health care "market-place," and subordinated to the concept that there is nothing more important than taking care of a person who is dying.

Staff well-being has obvious intrinsic importance. The health and well-being of providers has been recognized as a key domain of quality and as a feature of high-functioning microsystems.[18,26]

Principle: Palliative Care Engages in Continuous Quality Improvement and Research Efforts

The founders of hospice in the modern era were committed to the highest standards of medical treatment as a means of enabling people to live as fully as possible for as long as they were able. They understood the importance of careful observation and research to alleviate suffering and recognized the critical need for research to build an evidence base of symptom management. Initially, practice necessarily relied on the empiricism of careful observation and the collected opinions of experienced clinicians. In recent decades, even well-established symptomatic treatments have been tested and either affirmed, rejected, or refined. Studies into the mechanisms of symptom generation and corresponding pharmacological and physical treatments have given rise to innovative approaches to physical discomfort and preserving function in advanced illness. As this textbook reveals, developments in measuring quality of life and its components have opened up active areas of research into psychosocial and spiritual aspects of illness, caregiving, dying, and grief.

Most statements of principles of palliative and end-of-life care in recent years call for efforts to improve the quality and delivery of palliative care across settings.[27] These statements are important given the ethical and methodological challenges inherent in studies involving people with advanced illness and limited prognosis. Careful safeguards and sensitivity are required, but research is essential for advancing the field and improving care for future patients and families. Research must address a range of contexts in which patients live and receive care, including isolated rural and resource-poor communities in developing countries.[27,28]

The commitment to total quality improvement extends to mandates for continuing education of palliative care teams and ongoing efforts to enhance interdisciplinary team dynamics and effectiveness.[1,7,8]

Principle: Palliative Care Advocates for Patients and Families and Advances Public Policy to Improve Access to Needed Services and Quality of Care

Many palliative care organizations and related specialty organizations call for individual patient and family advo-

---

Common Errors

- Palliative care specialists may believe that, once agreed upon, the principles of palliative medicine are set and should not be changed. However, the principles of any profession or discipline can be expected to undergo periodic review and revision in response to changes in the context of practice and the needs of society.
- The importance of evidence-based medicine has led some clinicians to believe that evidence of efficacy is required before an area of practice can be considered valid. In fact, the scope of practice for a discipline is not based on evidence alone; rather, it is developed over time in an iterative process of discussion and agreement. Evidence-based medicine is instrumental to advancing goals within a profession's or a discipline's scope of practice.
- By definition, palliative care is an interdisciplinary team approach to care, but this does not mean that it cannot be practiced by individuals. Individual physicians, nurses, and other clinicians may provide palliative aspects of care in assessing and responding to physical, emotional, social, and spiritual distress or fostering the well-being of patients and their families.

---

cacy within health care systems. Some formally recognize social and public health responsibilities that extend beyond the benefit of individual patients and families, calling for collective social efforts to improve access to services and quality of care for seriously ill people and their families (see Chapter 36).[7,8,29,30]

CONCLUSIONS

Principles are basic to a clinical specialty. The field of palliative care is young and rapidly developing. Palliative care is coming of age during a tumultuous period of health care in Western countries, one that is marked by severe pressures of time, workload, and productivity. The contemporary social context and practice environments are characterized by competition for ever-scarcer resources to meet the needs of an aging population with unprecedented (and growing) burdens of chronic illness, existing unmet needs among many patients and families, and contentious social and political debates over assisted suicide, euthanasia, and discontinuation of artificial nutrition and hydration (see "Common Errors").

The challenges ahead can be only partially anticipated, but the future will assuredly pose difficult decisions for the field. The principles of palliative care will prove invaluable as circumstances become more complex, the stakes ever higher, and economic or political pressures greater. In these situations, the fundamental purpose of principles—to define, guide, and protect the essential elements and scope of a discipline—may be fully revealed. Although they are not immutable, carefully considered, well-seasoned statements of what palliative care values, believes, and exists to achieve can provide a compass during future social storms.

REFERENCES

1. Palliative Care Australia. Standards for Providing Quality Palliative Care for all Australians, Deakin West ACT, Australia: Author, May 2005.
2. Evidence-Based Medicine Working Group. A new approach to teaching the practice of medicine. JAMA 1992;268:2420-2425.
3. Vanderpool HY. The ethics of terminal care. JAMA 1978;239:850-852.
4. World Health Organization. Cancer pain relief and palliative care. Technical Report Series 804. Geneva: WHO, 1990.

5. Cassel CK, Foley KM. Principles for Care of Patients at the End of Life: An Emerging Consensus among the Specialties of Medicine. New York: Milbank Memorial Fund, 1999.

6. Cancer care during the last phase of life. J Clin Oncol 1998;16:1986-1996.

7. Luce JM, Prendergast TJ. The changing nature of death in the ICU. In Curtis RJ, Rubenfeld GD (eds). Managing Death in the Intensive Care Unit. New York: Oxford University Press, 2001, pp 19-29.

8. Mularski RA, Osborne ML. The changing ethics of death in the ICU. In Curtis RJ, Rubenfeld GD (eds). Managing Death in the Intensive Care Unit. New York: Oxford University Press, 2001, pp 7-17.

9. National Hospice Organization Standards and Accreditation Committee. A Pathway for Patients and Families Facing Terminal Disease. Arlington, VA: National Hospice Organization, 1997.

10. Last Acts Task Force. Precepts of Palliative Care. J Palliat Med 1998;1:109-112.

11. Last Acts. Precepts for Palliative Care for Children, Adolescents and their Families. Chicago: Last Acts, 2003.

12. Jennings B, Ryndes T, D'Onofrio C, Baily MA. Access to hospice care: Expanding boundaries, overcoming barriers. Hastings Cent Rep 2003;(Suppl):S3-S7, S9-S13, S15-S21 passim.

13. Ferris F, Balfour H, Bowen K, et al. A model to guide hospice palliative care. Ottawa: Canadian Hospice Palliative Care Association, 2002.

14. National Consensus Project for Palliative Care. Clinical Practice Guidelines for Quality Palliative Care, 2004. Available at http://www.nationalconsensusproject.org (accessed September 2007).

15. Hoffman J. Awash in information, patients face a lonely, uncertain road. The New York Times, August 14, 2005.

16. Byock I, Twohig JS, Merriman M, Collins K. Promoting excellence in end-of-life care: A report on innovative models of palliative care. J Palliat Med 2006;9:137-151.

17. Canadian Palliative Care Association. Palliative Care: Towards Standardized Principles of Practice. Ottawa, Canada: Author, 1995.

18. Clarke EB, Curtis JR, Luce JM, et al. Quality indicators for end-of-life care in the intensive care unit. Crit Care Med 2003;31:2255-2262.

19. Saunders C. A personal therapeutic journey. BMJ 1996;313:1599-1601.

20. Cassel EJ. The nature of suffering and the goals of medicine. N Engl J Med 1982;306:639-645.

21. Zucker MB. The Right to Die Debate: A Documentary History. Westport, CT: Greenwood Press, 1999.

22. Quill TE, Byock IR. Responding to intractable terminal suffering: The role of terminal sedation and voluntary refusal of food and fluids. ACP-ASIM End-of-Life Care Consensus Panel. American College of Physicians-American Society of Internal Medicine. Ann Intern Med 2000;132:408-414.

23. Schulz R, Beach SR. Caregiving as a risk factor for mortality: The Caregiver Health Effects Study. JAMA 1999;282:2215-2219.

24. Parkes CM, Benjamin B, Fitzgerald RG. Broken heart: A statistical study of increased mortality among widowers. BMJ 1969;1:740-743.

25. Christakis NA, Iwashyna TJ. The health impact of health care on families: A matched cohort study of hospice use by decedents and mortality outcomes in surviving, widowed spouses. Soc Sci Med 2003;57:465-475.

26. Donaldson M, Mohr J. Exploring Innovation and Quality Improvement in Health Care Micro-Systems: A Cross-Case Analysis. Washington, DC: Institute of Medicine, The National Academies Press, 2001.

27. European Association for Palliative Care. Adoption of a Declaration to Develop a Global Palliative Care Research Initiative. Available at http://www.eapcnet.org/latestnews/VeniceDeclaration.html (accessed September 2007).

28. Beresford L, Jones A, Person JL, Regas C. Providing Hospice and Palliative Care in Rural and Frontier Areas. Sponsored by the National Hospice and Palliative Care Organization, the Center to Advance Palliative Care, and the National Rural Health Association, 2005.

29. National Association of Social Workers. NASW Standards for Palliative and End of Life Care, 2004.

30. Byock IR, Forman WB, Appleton M. Academy of hospice physicians' position statement on access to hospice and palliative care. J Pain Symptom Manage 1996;11:69-70.

SUGGESTED READING

Ferris F, Balfour H, Bowen K, et al. A Model to Guide Hospice Palliative Care. Ottawa: Canadian Hospice Palliative Care Association, 2002.

Fins JJ. Palliative Ethic of Care: Clinical Wisdom at Life's End. Sudbury, MA: Jones and Bartlett, 2006.

Jennings B, Ryndes T, D'Onofrio C, Baily MA. Access to hospice care: Expanding boundaries, overcoming barriers. Hastings Cent Rep 2003;(Suppl):S3-S7, S9-S13, S15-S21.

National Consensus Project for Quality Palliative Care (NCP). Clinical Practice Guidelines for Quality Palliative Care, 2004. Available at http://www.nationalconsensusproject.org (accessed September 2007).

Randall F, Downie RS. Palliative Care Ethics: A Companion for All Specialities, 2nd ed. New York: Oxford University Press, 1999.

Psychosocial Care

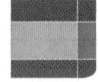

CHAPTER **8**

The Human Experience of Illness

J. Norelle Lickiss

K E Y   P O I N T S

● Illness is a personal, not a medical, reality, and it is part of the human condition.

● A person is a relational reality "not contained between hat and boots" (Whitman) involving environment, history, and inheritance (cultural and biological), with adequate appreciation of process of personal development.

● The seasons of illness need to be differentiated and the challenges of each need to be understood.

● Emotional responses are part of the illness experience and are diverse, sometimes part of global distress or suffering, and associated with accumulated adversity.

● Cancer is increasingly a chronic disease, and the associated concepts are relevant.

Illness is the night side of life, a more onerous citizenship. Everyone who is born holds dual citizenship, in the kingdom of the well and in the kingdom of the sick. Although we all prefer to use only the good passport, sooner or later each of us is obliged, at least for a spell, to identify ourselves as citizens of that other place.

SUSAN SONTAG[1]

WHAT IS ILLNESS?

Illness is a personal, not a medical reality; it is defined usually as a deviation from "health." Adequate definitions of health go beyond medical facts. For example, there is the facet of "potential: "health is a state of well-being characterized by a physical, mental and social potential, which satisfies the demands of a life commensurate with age, culture and personal responsibility."[2]

Although "disease" has some subjective connotations (lack of "ease"), the word refers in the main to an objectively verifiable disturbance of bodily structure or function, whereas "illness" connotes subjective awareness of a state deviating from the normal state of well-being for that individual. Illness is intrinsically experiential, related etymologically to "peril": the experience may be easy or difficult to communicate, describe, or explain. Disease may be manifest in imaging, biochemical studies, histopa-

thology, and the like, in life or in death, but illness is not so demonstrable: the behavioral concomitants of illness may, of course, be observable, but not the illness itself.

It may be worth noting that illness may occur without demonstrable disease, and that also disease may be present without illness. There are many examples of the latter, for example, rising levels of tumor markers heralding recurrence of symptomless ovarian cancer. However, illness may appear, in the form of severe anxiety or depression, simply as a result of the alarming test results.

Illness, as an aspect of the human condition in all places and times, may be looked at through several prisms: history, art, literature, philosophy, sociology, psychology, theology, economics, political science—all the prisms used to refract the light impinging on the human intellect. The study of disease relates medical science to the natural sciences, but the consideration of illness marks medicine as a "human science," requiring understanding of the foundations of the human sciences.[3] For the experience of illness is not marginal to the human condition, nor an aberrant optional extra at the edge of human affairs, but central: illness is core business for a human person, almost always embedded in the pattern of a life.

TOWARD AN ADEQUATE VIEW OF PERSON

Illness is an intensely personal, subjective reality, and a consequence is that medical practice requires an adequate concept of a person, despite age-old difficulty in the definition of the term "person."[4] It has been pointed out that "what medicine lacks is any fundamental notion of the nature of man and any remotely adequate understanding of that to which we refer as a person."[5]

In addition to sacred writings in various traditions addressing the meaning of the human condition, tomes have been written over the centuries, in both East and West, concerning the "nature of man," the "meaning of man," or "images of man," and there are also formal philosophical anthropology studies in a religious framework.[6] Even in a secular world, there needs to be a frame, a way of considering the human person in a manner accessible to medical (and other health) practitioners (and students) who may lack formal philosophical training. They are immersed in the human condition, not merely as individuals living lives but also in the midst of others in need of their skills and often in extreme distress. A simple frame has proved useful in clinical teaching: a frame for the mind and to which may be attached new knowledge and new questions or reflections. A person may be considered from an ecological point of view, with the various components in complex dynamic relationships. A person is a relational reality with respect to the present life situation, but also to a personal past—not only the facts of the past, but also the manner in which the patient understands, incorporates, and interprets the past. All this is of immediate importance to the clinician seeking to restore, rehabilitate, or continue to care for a patient who is deteriorating or approaching death. The inheritance (biological and cultural) of a patient provides the platform on which the personal history has been constructed and may continue to influence the present: it requires respect and clinical attention.

This ecological view of persons applies not just to patients, but also to carers (lay or professional), and it needs to be considered when their distress is evident (see Chapter 15). Fundamental is the conviction that a person is a relational reality. Initially the relation is recognized with the current environment, personal and nonpersonal, in a continuous dialectic. Personal identity is

> defined by the commitments and identifications which provide the frame or the horizon. . . . I am a self only in relation to certain interlocutors: in relation to those conversation partners who were essential to my achieving self definition. . . . A self exists only within 'webs of interlocution.' . . . To ask what a person is, in abstraction, from his or her self-interpretations, is to ask a fundamentally misguided question, one to which there couldn't, in principle, be an answer. . . . We are only selves insofar as we move in a certain space of questions, as we seek and find an orientation to the good.[7]

Walt Whitman remarked, "I am not contained between my hat and my boots,"[8] and Henry James (1892) said, "A man's 'me' is the sum total of all that he can call his, not only his body and his mind, but his clothes and his house, his wife and his children, his ancestors and his friends, his reputation and his works, his lands and horses, his yacht and his bank account."[9] Ernest Becker, who influenced a generation, made the same point.[9]

A NOTE ON PERSONAL DEVELOPMENT

A person is not only an intrinsically relational reality but also a dynamic reality, ever changing perceptibly or not, not merely structurally (e.g., by cell turnover) but as a functioning whole. The self is constantly being fashioned. Developmental psychology reveals that people develop and change.[7,10] Once again, some accessible schema is needed to make sense of the tapestry of personal change and development so that it can be appreciated in everyday clinical practice. It is necessary for a clinician without formal training in psychology or psychiatry to grasp the way people develop, especially in response to life crises, so his or her practice will be facilitatory and not deleterious with respect to personal growth.

The ideas of Erikson have stood the test of time. Erikson considered that human growth takes place by negotiation of developmental tasks through resolution of crisis.[11,12] The growing human is continually faced by options. Each life stage is characterized by options which, although they confront one throughout life, do come to ascendancy in a given stage. For example, the favorable outcome of infancy is an attitude of basic trust, rather than basic distrust, and on this basis the child goes on to be faced with the choice of autonomy or fear of decision.

Analysis of personal growth is sensitive in consideration of the developmental task of the elderly, or the individual of any age who is approaching death. That task is the development of a sense of wholeness, of integrity[12]:

> Only he who in some way has taken care of things and people and has adapted himself to the triumphs and disappointments of being, by necessity, the originator of others and the generator of things and ideas—only he may gradually grow the fruit of the seven stages. I know no better word for it than integrity. . . . It is the acceptance of one's own and only life cycle and of the people who have become significant to it as something that had to be . . . an acceptance of the fact that one's life is one's own responsibility. It is a sense of comradeship with men and women of distant times and of different pursuits, who have created orders and objects and sayings conveying human dignity and love. . . . The lack or loss of this accrued ego integration is signified by despair and an often unconscious fear of death: the one and only life cycle is not accepted as the ultimate of life. Despair expresses the fear that the time is short, too short for the attempt to start another life and to try out alternative roads to integrity. Such a despair is often hidden behind a show of disgust, a misanthropy, or a chronic contemptuous displeasure which (where not allied with constructive ideas and life of co-operation) only signify the individual's contempt of himself.

The shape of the task needs to be understood by those in contact with people approaching death. Patients may vacillate between wholeness and despair and need to be supported gently. They may long and need to try to express their internal states, explore the threat of despair and, through dialogue with significant others, reach out again toward wholeness. If it is the task of each to explore the limits of his or her own possibilities, it is surely the task of the doctor to free a very ill person from obstacles (e.g., pain) to the exploration. Palliative medicine is concerned with the facilitation of a free being, with liberation. The portrayal of the developmental task of the final phase of life as movement toward integrity and away from despair calls for consideration of the clinician's role in the sustaining and reconstruction of hope. No one can live without hope—but in what may hope be anchored, if it is not to be doomed to fail?

No person should die in despair—and the doctor should surely assist the patient to center hope not on what will in the end probably fail (e.g., chemotherapy, radiotherapy, surgery) but in what should not fail, ultimately the physician's commitment to care, the relief of pain, the recognition of dignity, and the value of the patient as a unique and irreplaceable subject of existence.

THE "SEASONS OF ILLNESS"

A physician survivor of cancer, in a landmark paper, coined the term, "seasons of survival."[13] The concept of seasons can also be applied to the different phases of illness, experienced by one person in the course of one disease (e.g., lung cancer), which may or may not prove fatal. The trajectory of chronic disease has definable phases,[14] but until recently the cancer trajectory has not been so considered.

Each phase or season of illness, as the experiential dimension of a disease, has definable although variable features, challenges, and opportunities for influence by carers (lay or professional). The following "seasons" may be delineated: the experience of diagnosis, treatment, surveillance, favorable response, nonresponse, relapse, surveillance, progression, and approaching death.[15] Each phase may include many "perils," such as symptoms, uncertainty, ambiguity, delay, difficulties in decision making, loss of many kinds, relationship stress, and the experience of needing, as one approaches death, to trust "the kindness of strangers."[16]

The "seasons of survival" have been differentiated into "acute survival," "extended survival," and "permanent survival" (surely cure rather than immortality!). An appreciation of the seasons of survival helps both patients and health professionals develop better strategies. Ethicists have highlighted the characteristics of "liminality," a feature recognized[17,18] in other contexts; for example, in the context of chronic pain.[19] Liminality reflects the classic studies of Stonequist (1937) describing the "marginal man," who is "uneasily poised in psychological uncertainty between two (or more) social worlds, reflecting in his soul the discords and harmonies, repulsions and attractions of these worlds, one of which is 'dominant' over the other."[20] Stonequist was concerned with marginality due to ethnicity, but marginality in the sense of Sontag (as described at the beginning of this chapter) appears relevant.

The seasons of survival may be most fruitfully seen as part of this larger spectrum. The needs of survivors and their experience of liminality may be mirrored in other seasons of illness, but we need far more research into such matters. The definable side effects of anticancer treatments such as surgery, chemotherapy, and radiotherapy[21-23] (see also Chapters 246 and 249) are well described. Efforts continue to reduce the price of benefit by technical improvements and better attention to symptom management during therapy. The core competence of palliative medicine practitioners (symptom relief, personal and family support, and clarification of goals) should be available in parallel with all treatment programs, even if curative in intent, in potentially lethal conditions such as lung cancer. Parallel care may bring the benefits of contemporary treatments to patients in such a way that, after the treatment and in survivorship, they do not feel that they resemble a battlefield.

One practical issue is the irresponsibility of introducing potentially toxic or hazardous anticancer treatments into contexts where there is not equal competence in symptom relief (and surveillance) or provision for personal and family support. When decisions are made concerning treatment options in the very ill, such as whether to try further chemotherapy to prolong life, a "carer impact" statement is needed because of the potential to increase caregiver burden (see Chapter 214), and careful consideration must be given to the patient's wishes as well. These wishes preferably will be specified beforehand through advance care planning instituted once it looks possible that the illness might be fatal, not merely after attempts to control it have failed.

Facing death is one of the seasons of illness—the final season indeed. Great literature describes it; Tolstoy, in "The Death of Ivan Ilyich," provided a disturbing (for doctors) literary icon. Medical texts need to be supplemented by the humanities. No empirical medical research can capture the entirety of the experience, any more than can philosophers, or poets, or theologians, or sacred writings. Uncertainties are at the core of human experience, and that aspect of the human experience of illness that involves facing death, although to some extent accessible, remains part of the "riddling essence" of human existence.

PSYCHOLOGICAL RESPONSES TO ILLNESS

Emotions are respectable—and essential! In the consideration of emotional intelligence, emotions shape the landscape of our mental and social lives, intimately related to thought. Proust called the emotions "geological upheavals of thought."[24] Such "upheavals" (which may be related to new knowledge or awareness) are features of the illness of many persons and must be recognized by others as manifestations of underlying tensions, not negative personality features.[25] The changing patterns of emotional responses in the same patient over time, through the different seasons of illness, are less amenable to study than portraits in time in cross-sectional studies; however, there is much value in longitudinal studies. Narrative approaches, more common in qualitative studies, may yield precious information, even if applicability to other patients in other cultures may be limited. The relevance of psychiatry in advanced disease is recognized (see Chapters 159, 164, 165, and 256), and the implications of cognitive failure for palliative medicine are now appreciated (see Chapter 175). The field of psychooncology has developed as a clinical as well as theoretical discipline and is of benefit to those seeking to understand the human experience of illness.[26]

Loss and the responses associated with grieving are to be expected. The self may keenly feel many losses in a serious illness, with the profile of loss changing with the illness: initially, there is loss of time, finance, and capacity for gainful employment, but later one faces loss of mobility and eventually of autonomy—except to express it (the highest exercise of autonomy) in handing over oneself to "the kindness of strangers." There is need, in such serious situations of potential or actual loss, for the professional carer to ensure not only good symptom relief—pain relief is always prominent in research studies as a high priority[27]—but also to facilitate retention of significant personal capacities (e.g., speech, cognition, recognition, continence), even in the last days of life. This is a measurable facet of care[28] which, although simple, may be of more value than complex quality of life indices.

Fear of recurrence of illness is understandable and is amenable to study.[29] The model formulated by Lee-Jones and colleagues proposed that "stimuli, both external and internal, play a role in activating cognitive responses associated with fears of recurrence," which thus comprise cognitions, beliefs, and emotions. They noted that possible consequences of high fears of recurrence include anxious preoccupation, limited planning for the future, and misinterpretation of bodily symptoms.[29] Fear of death has been more extensively considered,[30-32] and indeed has been pondered from time immemorial, but there has been less formal study of other fears spoken of in consulting rooms and even around dinner tables, such as fear of prolonged life (against one's wishes or even in disregard of advance directives), loss of core capacities, pain, and abandonment. Data on these topics are hard to capture, because the context, variability, and diversity may so affect responses that the "truth" may not be findable.

Hope has had more prominence in health research; for example, the relationship between hope and the "will to live"[33] or the concept of hope in nursing in various contexts, from intensive care to palliative care.[34] Some define hope as "a multidimensional life force characterized by a confident yet uncertain expectation of achieving a future good which, to the hoping person, is realistically possible and personally significant."[35] Another approach looks at the implications for nursing practice and identifies the "seven abstract and universal components of hope: a realistic initial assessment of the predicament or threat, the envisioning of alternatives and the setting of goals, a bracing for negative outcomes, a realistic assessment of personal resources and of external conditions and resources, the solicitation of mutually supportive relationships, the continuous evaluation for signs that reinforce the selected goals, and a determination to endure."[36]

The content of hope and its articulation by very ill patients in non-Western and resource-poor countries might differ markedly from that in affluent Western contexts. But humanity is one, and so hope may have some constant components. Expectations of the fulfillment of hopes may vary unless hope is centered on matters that are not contextual, such as enduring love of significant others, nonabandonment, and personal intrinsic worth. What is evident everywhere is that fostering of unrealistic hope (e.g., reassurances that one is cured, that there is no chance of recurrence, or that a new treatment will be successful) may lead to despair. Clinical effort needs to help the patient place hope in things that will not fail and, in the end (if there is nothing else), in his or her own intrinsic dignity.

Distress is a frequent accompaniment of illness, but if it is unrecognized, or if coping mechanisms fail, it may evolve into suffering. Consideration of suffering in health care[37] emphasizes the significance of the relief of suffering (a subjective concept), and improvement in a disease, as a crucial goal for clinical practice. It also provides a useful operational definition of suffering; namely, a sense of impending personal disintegration. This could correspond with the colloquial "feeling about to go to pieces": in an informal study by McCosker, Best, and Lickiss (unpublished data), patients could readily identify a time when they felt like that and an event that triggered the feeling. The identified trigger could involve relationships, a particular loss, an unpleasant investigation, uncontrolled symptoms (especially pain, dyspnea, or nausea), the experience of incontinence, or psychological trauma or poorly communicated "bad news." Clarification of such triggers in an individual is of practical significance, offering opportunities for either reparation, support, or prevention, and certainly must be considered in clinical decision making.

There are other formulations of suffering in recent medical literature; the complexity of the concept of suffering,[38] the relationship of suffering to persisting pain,[39] and the closely associated "demoralization syndrome"[40] have been investigated. Some differentiate the phase of "enduring" from the phase of suffering characterized by emotional release; they point to the need for professional carers to recognize this difference, lest efforts to relieve suffering be misplaced.[41] Welie recently examined the philosophical tradition concerning sympathy in the face of suffering.[42] Further exploration of these issues will be noted elsewhere (see Chapter 9).

The phenomenon of "cumulative adversity" has been recognized in the etiology of psychiatric illness.[43] The adverse events in an eventually fatal illness may add up to an unbearable burden, especially if concurrently there is reduced personal and social support. Observers have concluded that some patients with cancer manifest post-traumatic stress disorder at a higher rate than in the general community.[44] This trait might usefully be studied in relation to measures of "cumulative adversity."

Cancer is increasingly a chronic disease, and the considerable corpus of research concerning the experiences of patients with chronic disease[45-47] is relevant to the understanding of patients with chronic illness related to cancer (see Chapter 3). Perhaps the universe of discourse and research concerning chronic disease needs to be juxtaposed to the conceptual frame within which cancer-as-illness (rather than disease) is considered. Knowledge (concentrated in rehabilitation literature) concerning the relationship among disease, disability, and handicap is relevant, with modes of treatment influencing the resultant disability, but with social and psychological factors largely determining whether a definable disability will lead to a handicap. Such ideas could be readily applied to persons with cancer, from time of diagnosis, not when disability or (worse) handicap is established for want of intelligent preventive measures.

The subjective dimensions of the cancer trajectory need more attention (see "Future Considerations"). In any cancer center, just as much intellectual effort and resources as are expended on anticancer treatment should be brought to bear on the experiential dimensions of cancer: relief of symptoms, personal and family support, and planning for care throughout the course of illness, not only in disease progression with death on the horizon. These ideas echo the recommendations of the World Health Organization, from 2 decades ago, with respect to the distribution of resources in developed or affluent countries (expenditure on palliative care equal to that spent on anticancer treatment) and in developing countries (90% of all cancer expenditures to be for palliative care)[48]— advice disregarded the world over.

CONCLUSION

The experience of serious illness, at any age and in any place, is one of the ordinary elements of the human condition, part of the pattern of life. The philosophical basis of

---

Future Considerations

Seasons of illness justify investigation, to address such questions as

1. What are the definable "perils" of each season (diagnosis, treatment, surveillance, favorable response, nonresponse, relapse, surveillance, progression, and approaching death) for similar diseases?
2. What are definable triggers to a sense of impending personal disintegration ("feeling about to go to pieces") in each of the seasons? Which are preventable?
3. What are the influences of culture (related to ethnicity, occupation, and socioeconomic circumstance) on the experience of seasons of illness?
4. What proportion of resources are expended to address subjective dimensions of cancer (symptom relief and personal and family support) compared with anticancer treatment in each "season," in both affluent and nonaffluent societies?

the duty of care is, in the end, not law or contract but the call of the other, face to face. The required response of physicians involves an unfailing commitment to beneficence (which may imply measures to cure or control disease), to relief of suffering inasmuch as it arises from factors amenable to clinical measures, and respect and guarding of human dignity in every circumstance, especially in the most vulnerable.

REFERENCES

1. Sontag S. Illness as Metaphor. New York: Vintage Books, 1979.
2. Bircher J: Towards a dynamic definition of health and disease. Health Care and Philosophy 2005;8:335-341.
3. Dilthey W. Selected Works: Vol. 1. Introduction to the Human Sciences. (Makkreel RA, Rodi F [eds and transl]). Princeton, NJ: Princeton University Press, 1985. (Original work published 1893).
4. Thomasma DC, Weisstub DN, Hervé C (eds). Personhood and Health Care. Dordrecht, The Netherlands: Kluwer, 2001.
5. Needleman J. The perception of mortality. Ann N Y Acad Sci 1969;164:733-738.
6. Pannenberg W. Anthropology in Theological Perspective. Philadelphia: Westminster Press, 1985.
7. Taylor C. Sources of the Self: The Making of Modern Identity. Cambridge, MA: Harvard University Press, 1989.
8. Whitman W. Song of myself. In Whitman W. Leaves of Grass, 1891-1892 Edition. Philadelphia: David McKay, 1891.
9. Quoted in Becker E. The Birth and Death of Meaning: An Interdisciplinary Perspective on the Problem of Man, 2nd ed. Harmondsworth, UK: Penguin Books, 1971, p. 43.
10. Siegel J. The Idea of the Self: Thought and Experience in Western Europe Since the Seventeenth Century. Cambridge, England: Cambridge University Press, 2005.
11. Erikson EH. The Life Cycle Completed: A Review. New York: Norton, 1982.
12. Erikson EH Identity and Life Cycle: Psychological Issues Monograph. New York: International Universities Press, 1969.
13. Mullan F. Seasons of survival: Reflections of a physician with cancer. N Engl J Med 1985;313:270-273.
14. Corbin JM, Strauss A: A nursing model for chronic illness management based on the Trajectory Framework. Scholarly Inquiry for Nursing Practice 1991;5:155-174.
15. Vachon MLS. The meaning of illness to a long-term survivor. Semin Oncol Nursing 2001;17:279-285.
16. Anderson H. Living until we die: Reflections on the dying person's spiritual agenda. Anaesthesiol Clin North Am 2006;42:213-225.
17. Dow KH. The enduring seasons of survival. Oncol Nursing Forum 1990;17:511-516.
18. Little M. Chronic illness and the experience of surviving cancer. Intern Med J 2004;34:201-202.
19. Honkasalo ML. Vicissitudes of pain and suffering: Chronic pain and liminality. Med Anthropol 2001;19:319-353.
20. Stonequist EV. The Marginal Man: A Study in Personality and Culture Conflict. New York: Charles Scribner's Sons, 1937.
21. Loescher LJ, Welch-McCaffrey D, Leigh S, et al. Surviving adult cancers. Part 1: Physiologic effects. Ann Intern Med 1989;111:411-432.
22. Welch-McCaffrey D, Hoffman B, Leigh SA, et al. Surviving adult cancers. Part 2: Psychosocial implications. Ann Intern Med 1989;111:517-524.
23. Plowman PN, McEwain TJ, Meadows AT. Complications of Cancer Management. Oxford, England: Butterworth-Heinemann, 1991.
24. Nussbaum M. Upheavals of Thought: The Intelligence of Emotions. Cambridge, UK: Cambridge University Press, 2002, p 1.
25. Gibson CA, Lichtenthal W, Berg A, Brietbart W. Psychological issues in palliative care. Anaethesiol Clin North Am 2006;24:61-80.
26. Holland JC. An international perspective on the development of psychooncology: Overcoming cultural and attitudinal barriers to improve psychosocial care. IPOS Sutherland Memorial Lecture. Psychooncology 2004;13:445-459.
27. Steinhauser KE, Christakis NA, Clipp EC, et al. Factors considered important at the end of life by patients, family, physicians, and other care providers. JAMA 2000;284:2476-2482.
28. Turner K, Chye R, Aggarwal G, et al. Dignity in dying: A preliminary study of patients in the last three days of life. J Palliat Care 1996;12:7-13.
29. Lee-Jones C, Humphris G, Dixon R, et al. Fear of cancer recurrence: A literature review and proposed cognitive formulation to explain exacerbation of recurrence fears. Psychooncology 1997;6:95-105.
30. Cicirelli VG. Personal meanings of death. Death Studies 1998;22:713-733.
31. Penson RT, Partridge RA, Shah MA, et al. Fear of death. Oncologist 2005;10:160-169.
32. Spiro HM, McCrea-Curnen MG, Palmer Wandel L (eds). Facing Death: Where Culture, Religion, and Medicine Meet. New Haven, CT: Yale University Press, 1996.
33. Hockley J. The concept of hope and the will to live. Palliat Med 1993;7:181-186.
34. Cutcliffe JR, Herth K. The concept of hope in nursing: 1. Its origins, background and nature. Br J Nursing 2002;11:832-840.
35. Nekolaichuk CL, Bruera E. On the nature of hope in palliative care. J Palliat Care 1998;14:36-42.
36. Morse JM, Doberneck B. Delineating the concept of hope. Sigma Theta Tau International, 1995;27:277-285.
37. Cassell E. The goal of medicine the relief of suffering. N Engl J Med 1982;306:639-645.
38. Cherny NI. The problem of suffering. In Doyle D, Hanks G, Cherny N, Calman K (eds). Oxford Textbook of Palliative Medicine, 3rd ed. New York: Oxford University Press, 2004, pp 7-14.
39. Chapman CR, Gavrin J. Suffering: The contributions of persistent pain. Lancet 1999;353:2233-2237.
40. Kissane D, Clarke DM, Street AF. Demoralisation syndrome: A relevant psychiatric diagnosis for palliative care. J Palliative Care 2001;17:12-21.
41. Morse JM: Toward a praxis theory of suffering. Adv Nursing Sci 2001;24:47-59.
42. Welie JVM. In the Face of Suffering. Omaha, NB: Crighton University Press, 1998, p 125.
43. Turner RJ, Lloyd DA. Lifetime traumas and mental health: The significance of cumulative adversity. J Health Social Behav 1995;36:360-376.
44. Alter CL, Pelcovitz D, Axelrod A, et al. Identification of PTSD in cancer survivors. Psychosomatics 1996;37:137-143.
45. Ironside PM, Schekel M, Wessels C, et al. Experiencing chronic illness: Creating new understandings. Qual Health Res 2003;13:171-183.
46. Delmar C, Boje T, Dylmer D, et al. Achieving harmony with oneself: Life with a chronic illness. Scand J Caring Sci 2005;9:204-212.
47. Thorne SE, Paterson BL: Two decades of insider research: What we know and don't know about chronic illness experience. Annu Rev Nurs Res 2000;18:3-25.
48. World Health Organization Expert Committee Report. Cancer Pain Relief and Palliative Care. Geneva: WHO, 1990.

CHAPTER **9**

Suffering

Eric J. Cassell

KEY POINTS

- Suffering is suffering, a specific kind of distress.
- Suffering is an affliction of the person, not the body.
- Suffering must be recognized before it can be treated.
- Suffering can be relieved even if its source cannot.
- There is more suffering in your patients than you suspect.

The crucial truths about suffering are two: suffering is suffering, its own specific kind of distress, and it is something that happens to persons, not bodies. Medicine, however it is expressed in the diverse cultures in the world, comes into being because human beings suffer. This no less true of Western medicine. In recent centuries, as medicine became solidly grounded on knowledge of diseases and their manifestations, these truths about suffering became obscured. They were hidden by the increasing value placed on objective manifestations of disease and continuation of the stubbornly persistent dichotomy between mind and body, which valued the science of the body and its afflictions and devalued subjective responses of patients. Pain was not treated adequately until recently (and not always even now), because patients' subjective "claims" of distress were not accorded the same validity as objective findings such as x-ray films. The importance of this fact is the enormous power of established ideas to prevent physicians from seeing what is in front of them. To emphasize the point, the pharmacological power to relieve the pain of the dying has been easily available for more than *two centuries*, but it has been an inconstant part of contemporary medicine for only a few decades (and palliative medicine was acknowledged even more recently). If you follow the story of suffering and its relief in an individual patient wherever it takes you, it will profoundly change the way you understand sick patients and the practice of medicine.

SUFFERING VERSUS PAIN

It is necessary first to distinguish *suffering* from *pain*. The magnitude of pain is only one factor in the distress it causes. People will tolerate even severe pain if they know what it is, that it does not portend danger, and that it will end. Pain of lesser degree may be poorly tolerated and lead to suffering if it is considered to have dire meaning or appears to be endless. In a person already suffering with pain, the suffering may be relieved and may stop even if the pain continues. On the other hand, people may suffer because of pain even when it is not present. For example, in patients with successfully treated painful bony metastatic disease, suffering may arise if their consciousness over hours, days, or longer is filled with fear that the pain will recur. People who have had terrible migraines may suffer at the thought, as a wedding or other significant event approaches, that it will be ruined by a migraine headache. This phenomenon is also true of other symptoms, such as dyspnea or diarrhea. People who have no symptoms may suffer as well, for example in the face of the pain of a loved one; especially if they feel helpless, or because of helplessness itself. In all these examples, the word "suffering" is not used in a conversational sense but stands for a specific kind of distress.

CONSTANT FEATURES OF SUFFERING AND A DEFINITION

Suffering has two constant features. First is the place of the future: "If the pain continues, I won't be able to take it." (At that moment, the patient is "taking it.") Another common expression is, "What if the pain recurs and I can't reach you?" The other feature is the constant place of the meaning of the thing causing the suffering: "This pain means that the cancer has recurred." "This pain I have had for so long that no one has diagnosed must mean something bad." "Nobody would leave me on a stretcher in this cold hallway for hours if they weren't just trying to hurt me."

What do these two characteristics tell us? Bodies may have nociception, but bodies do not have a sense of the future, and bodies do not assign meanings. *Bodies do not suffer, only persons do.* Clinical observation suggests a definition of suffering: Suffering is specific distress that occurs when individuals feel their intactness or integrity as persons is threatened and that continues until the threat is gone or intactness or integrity is restored.

Suffering has degrees of severity. It may resolve spontaneously or, if not treated, go on and on. However, once it has happened, it is probably never forgotten.

SUFFERING IS PERSONAL

The Person

What does "person" mean? Person is not mind, although a person has a mind. Person is not body, although a person has a body. The word "self," so commonly used, is not a substitute for person; it is insufficiently inclusive. Personhood, by contrast, can be quite diverse but does not approach total incoherence. It includes a personality, character, a lived past, a family, the family's past, a cultural background, social and professional roles, associations and relationships with others, relationship with itself, and a political being, among others. Persons also do things. Persons have an unconscious (by whatever name or definition), regular behaviors, a body and relationships with the body, a secret life, a perceived future, and a transcendent dimension.[1] For these many reasons—but especially because an individual may contain many selves, but only one person—I distinguish carefully between *self* and *person*.

The Person and Illness

The person is the whole entire being—selves and everything else. It is of importance to physicians to recognize that it is the person who falls ill, the person who is the patient, the person who suffers. It is the person that clinical medicine is all about. Persons are different from other objects of science. Although they are in the here and now, they cannot be understood without knowing about their past and their believed-in future—these represent a historic route of a complex and ever-changing society of parts. Persons cannot be understood by the reductionist methods of science that are successful elsewhere, because, as they are taken down to their parts, they disappear as persons. In fact, persons are of a piece: whatever happens to one part of them happens to the all, and whatever happens to the whole happens to every part. This has enormous consequences for clinicians, yet what it means is only dimly apparent. It certainly means that something done just for the disease or for a diseased part, without thought for what it will mean to the sick person, may cause unintended damage.

The Person and Suffering

In looking at the features that are included in a person, it is important to understand that injury to any one of them may initiate suffering. For example, destruction of a person's believed-in future (which occurs commonly in sickness) may be what cracks the person's integrity and begins the suffering. That often cannot be helped, but physicians can be aware, as the disease progresses, that such a thing may happen and prevent suffering by directly addressing the issue. In some cases, a person's character, although successful while well, may be disadvantageous when sick. The patient with an unbending will of iron may have accomplished great things in life, but in sickness an absence of flexibility in the face of events can destroy his or her intactness. The initiator of suffering in patients with advanced cancer is frequently a belief that physicians and staff have abused them in what they were told or how they were treated.[2,3]

WHAT IS INTEGRITY, AND WHAT IS INTACTNESS?

What is meant, in the definition of suffering, by stating that suffering persons lose their "integrity" (in the sense of wholeness, something undivided, not violated) as persons? In the face of diverse selves, how can one hold that persons have integrity in the first place? The integrity of a person should be understood in functional terms. Persons whose integrity is intact can exercise their purposes, can do the things that intact persons do in private or in the social world, and can know themselves as themselves by what they do, say, or think. To a greater or lesser degree, suffering persons are unable to function as the persons they were in private or in society; they have lost central purpose—that of being or constructing themselves—as their intentions have become diverted to the suffering itself or its perceived sources. Suffering persons no longer know themselves as the persons they were before. An analogy to the skin might be useful. All of us have various cuts, scratches, or lesions; small breeches of the barrier that is the integument, and yet we would not, on that account, say that our skin has lost its integrity, because it still serves its function as a barrier. That function would be lost, however, if the skin had suffered a major burn; in that case, it might be said that the skin had lost its integrity.

ALL SUFFERING IS UNIQUE AND INDIVIDUAL

The identity that the suffering patient feels is now disintegrating did exist in the past and is also projected into the future; something we all do all the time without awareness. That identity is particular—unique to the individual. A suffering person may say, "I'm not myself anymore; I don't know who I am. I don't know what's happening to me, but this mess you're looking at is not me. What's going to happen?" Any of the parts of a person listed earlier may be the locus of suffering. Remember, however, that whatever happens to one part of a person happens to the whole. Even if two persons suffer because of an identical source (e.g., the pain of an expanding lesion), the suffering of each will be unique and particular. This is because suffering occurs not from the insult itself but from its meaning, now and projected into the future, and aspects of meaning are always individual. Why each person suffers (not why each has pain) is individual; related to him or her as a particular person. For example, the neurological deficits of early multiple sclerosis may be a source of intense suffering for a cellist but only moderately distressing for a scholar.

As another example, the sudden appearance of widespread metastatic breast cancer in a 47-year-old single woman that causes her to be hospitalized and near death will result in suffering. But it is not primarily the weakness, profound anorexia, and generalized edema—as distressing as they are—that are the source of her suffering; rather, it is the loss of control and inability to prevent the evaporation of her career whose brilliant promise had finally been realized a few months earlier. The facts and physical consequences of the metastatic disease are something that physicians know, but that the patient does not

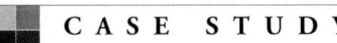

CASE STUDY

The Cause of Suffering

AB is a 64-year-old woman with rapidly progressive metastatic carcinoma from the lung. Her malignancy was initially diagnosed after she developed pain from a pathologic fracture of her left humerus. Within days, she developed one fracture after another, all painful and requiring large doses of analgesics. She was seen one morning and was obviously suffering. "Are you suffering?" her attending physician asked. "Yes," she replied. "What is causing you to suffer?" asked the physician, expecting her to talk about her pain. "It's food," she said. "For years, my husband and I have started each day talking about what we're going to have for dinner. Eating is a really big deal for us. You can't imagine. Now—now, I can't eat. I don't want to even hear about food. And he sits there all day too scared even to talk about eating."

easily comprehend, even if she knows them intellectually. She struggles to understand and suffers most from what has happened to her personal life. It is the increasing awareness of the impact of the physical state on the person, not the physical impairments per se, that causes the suffering.

This does not mean that suffering is psychological, in the sense of affecting or pertaining only to the mental and emotional spheres, as opposed to the physical state of a person. Just as reading, riding a bicycle, or working as a physician may involve any aspect of a person—physical, emotional, or social—so too does suffering, although a psychological insult such as grief may be a precipitating cause (see "Case Study: The Cause of Suffering").

Even in the face of obvious suffering whose source seems evident, it is important to ask questions about the suffering. Understanding how a particular patient feels harmed, deprived, overburdened, or overtaken by fear provides a lever for action tailored to that person's experience.

Suffering Always Involves Self-Conflict

It may at first seem strange to say that suffering always involves self-conflict. Usually the sufferer, as well as others, identifies the source of suffering as *outside* (even if it is a tumor within the patient). This is, after all, what is causing distress. The clue is the fact that meaning enters into suffering. The threat to the person's integrity or intactness lies in the meaning of the distress or beliefs about its consequences, and people are not always of one mind about things. The patient may sincerely want to die or stop living. Yet life is precious; there are still others to care about and responsibilities that have to be met.

Conflict can also be found when suffering occurs as part of chronic illness. It has been known since the 18th century that people have the desires to be approved of by others, to be superior, and to emulate those they admire. The sick person has these same desires, but illness may prevent their realization. This does not stop the desire; it only creates self-conflict. The chronically ill person attempts to meet the standards of the everyday world but often cannot.[4] The standards appear to be external but they are not; they are contained within the verbal categories—mother, doctor, teacher, success, and patient. The result is self-conflict.

Another source is conflict with the body, wherein the patient behaves as though the body is the enemy, an untrustworthy "other" that is seen as actively doing bad things to the patient. Because of bowel and bladder difficulties, for example, the body can be held as an "other" that is trying to humiliate the patient.

All Suffering Involves Loss of or Profound Change in Central Purpose

Purpose is a word that was expunged from science at the end of the 17th century. It carries the theological implication of teleology. In medicine, we have substituted the word *function*—things in the body do not have purposes; they have functions. Persons, however, definitely have purposes—intentions, goals, and the object of doing things. Purpose pervades every moment and every volitional action. These purposes form a hierarchy of actions and behaviors that culminates in central purpose—the purpose of being oneself.

- Purpose is fundamentally not only individual but also social. What one does, wants, acts on, makes, and becomes is ultimately social, because it involves others, takes place in the world, and requires the world for fulfillment. It is important to realize that actions both create a person's world and create the person as he or she is. Withdraw central purpose, and the person is withdrawn from the world.
- In sickness, pain, and suffering, central purpose is lost.[5] Just as attention shifts to the sick parts, so does purpose. The person's focus becomes entirely directed on the self, and all purpose is diverted toward the goal of relief of pain, sickness, and suffering. The more complete and compelling the distress or the sickness, the more complete the redirection of purpose. Further, in suffering, purpose disengages from the social world

Suffering Is Lonely

Loneliness is one of the hallmarks of the suffering patient for two reasons. The first is the individuality of sufferers and the individual origin of their suffering. The second reason is the withdrawal of purpose from social engagement. If suffering is lonely and the sufferer withdraws from the social world, how do we know that he or she is suffering?

RECOGNIZING SUFFERING

As with so many things in medicine, if you do not make the diagnosis of suffering, you will fail to treat it. The problem is that the diagnosis is made by considering the person, not only the body. For the care of the suffering, attending to the person means more than caring about the patient or being compassionate. Often, as one hears physicians talk about dying patients' personal characteristics, details of life and work, and relationships with family, their care and compassion are evident, but suffering is not suspected unless the patient makes it clear. Lack of recognition and treatment of suffering does not come about only because of absence of compassion or concern, whatever our public may believe; it is the result of physicians' *poor diagnostic and therapeutic knowledge and people skills*. That is, there is an inability to focus on the person rather than the disease, the pathophysiology, or the immediate physiological crisis. This blindness to persons may seem strange, because we all know about persons: each of us is one, we live among them all the time, and we care about others and ourselves as persons. But familiarity is not enough; after all, we lived among bodies all the time also (including our own), but we did not know about them *as physicians* until we were trained in how they function and how to examine them, how to gather evidence from them, and how to think about them as part of our work.[6]

To make a diagnosis of suffering requires a high index of suspicion in the presence of serious disease and obviously distressing symptoms. There are five domains of special concern to the dying: inadequate pain and symptom relief, remaining in control, avoiding prolonged dying, relieving others of the burden of their dying, and strengthening personal relationships.[7] If these concerns are evident, suffering should be considered. Suffering should also be suspected whenever pain seems to require inordinately high doses of analgesics.

The most effective way to diagnose suffering is to ask questions such as, "Are you suffering?" "I know you have pain, but are there things that are even worse than just the pain?" "What is causing your suffering?" "Are you frightened by all this?" " What exactly are you frightened of?" "What is the worst thing about all this?" "What do you worry (are afraid) is going to happen to you?" "Do you think this means that your disease is getting worse?" or "Do you think this means that you are dying?" Once such questions are asked, *patients have to be given the time to answer*. The questions are purposely somewhat vague; they tell patients that they have permission to talk about things that usually no one has wanted to hear, and they do not specify what answers are expected. The conversation should be concrete, and abstractions should be avoided.[8]

In the beginning, physicians may find these to be very uncomfortable conversations, because no one enjoys hearing about unrelieved pain, misery, and suffering. Asking the questions and attentively listening to the answers is usually helpful in itself—and the process takes less time than physicians expect. Physicians are also frequently concerned that they will be helpless in the face of the patients' answers. It is often a surprise how easily a patient's concerns are relieved. Attempts should be made to reassure patients even when their worries are correct. Answers should be truthful, even if not the whole truth. In the unusual instance in which a physician feels that he or she should not answer a question, the problem can be solved by changing the subject and focusing on something positive and important: "I know that must be scary, but we are all going to be right here for you no matter what happens." The gratification that commonly follows these interactions more than repays physicians for their discomfort, and with time these conversations become easier.

The Special Meaning of Meaning

It is difficult to overemphasize the importance of meaning in understanding suffering. We usually believe we act or respond because of events, people, circumstances, things, and what is out there in the world, but that really is not true. We act *on the meaning of those things*. The same is true of patients: Almost regardless of the disease, the patient's experience depends on its meaning for that patient. Dyspnea is dyspnea, diarrhea is diarrhea, pain is pain, but how these are experienced and what the patient believes will occur in the future is derived from the meaning assigned by the patient to these symptoms, with or without the physician's influence. Remember, the patient is suffering because of the meaning that he or she has assigned to what is happening and what it portends for the future. We all share some aspects of most meanings, or we could not understand each other. All meanings, however, also have an element particular to an individual. The best way to find out what something means to a patient is to ask. In fact, my favorite and most used question is, "What does that mean?" The other truth is that meanings can be changed, and, when they are, the patient's experience also changes.[1]

Subjectivity

Much information about suffering is subjective and therefore often devalued. In palliative care, we may not able to treat the disease, and that forces us to work with the *person* of the patient if we wish to be effective. As a consequence, subjective information—symptoms and their assessment by the patient, emotions, feelings, beliefs, and concerns—necessarily become the basis for many of our actions. This is uncomfortable for many physicians who were raised on the belief that only objective data, especially measurements, meet the standards for evidence.

Objective knowledge is considered scientific and valuable, whereas subjective information is thought to be second-rate. For relief of suffering, that conflict is not only false but an impediment. Once information about anything has been consciously thought about or converted into words, it has become objective—a thing that can be examined. Subjective information shares the characteristics of all information; it is not merely true or false but probabilistic, more or less probable and existing within confidence limits. This means that the physician's task in making inferences with information, whether data from an x-ray film or the thought that the patient is suffering, is to objectify it in thought, increase the probability of its truth, narrow its confidence limits, and increase its predictive value. Or, put another way, the task with subjective or objective information is to increase its precision, accuracy (reliability), and predictive value. This is accomplished by examining again, looking again, reflecting, listening again, enlarging the scope of inquiry, asking more questions, and thinking about the information.

Because suffering is both personal and individual, knowing the patient has special importance. This is not the knowing of social life, and, in fact, ideas that a person is smart, interesting, bossy, charming, anxious, sexy, and so on—whether correct or not—shut off observation due to premature interpretations. The usual classifications of personality get in the way of a clinicians' knowledge of patients, just as bias and preconceptions not based on what you know about *this patient* are particularly misleading. One wants to be listening to what is said and unsaid, smelling (fear, hygiene, perfume), and watching, always watching, for facial expression and bodily motion as

persons reveal themselves and their suffering becomes increasingly evident.

There is a further important step. Physicians commonly come into a patient's room "all action"—doing things, talking, and then leaving. One has things to do, but it is important to be not just a doer, but also a receiver. Open to the patient: let the patient flow into you as though you had opened a door to your heart or soul. It may sound mushy, but don't be put off. This stance is not something you do as much as something you are. This has sometimes been labeled "sympathetic listening," "empathic communication," or "empathic attentiveness"; it can be taught and learned.[9] Patients will be unaware of what is happening; they will simply experience you as being trustworthy, caring, and understanding. It may seem threatening to you at first, as though your defenses were down. Remember that you are working. It is you, the doctor, doing and being this way, and the role protects you. What will you learn? For one, you will learn what the patient is feeling; ultimately, you can learn to discern patients' feelings even over the telephone. It is important at times to identify those feelings specifically, to name them. For the most part, however, you will not put words to what you learn, in order not to foreclose the experience. Over time, you will come to trust the intuitive thinking that takes place below the level of awareness as your mind continually processes the experience. This intuition is not something magical; it is a kind of nondiscursive thought that is common to experts in many fields.[10] Learning how to do these things will make it possible to diagnose suffering much more frequently.

TREATING SUFFERING

Two facts about suffering are central to understanding its treatment. First, even if the suffering was initiated by, for example, pain or dyspnea, it is a result of the disruptive meaning of that symptom on some aspect of the person. It is an affliction of the person. Second, as a result of its basis in meaning, suffering can be relieved even if the inciting cause cannot be made better, and suffering may continue even if the cause is removed (see "Future Considerations").

Because suffering is a disorder of the person and is related to the particular person, its treatment is a repair of the person. However, symptoms must be relieved as much as possible, and the patient needs to know you are trying and that you mean it. Do not promise what you cannot deliver, but deliver on your promises. Meanings are central to suffering, so your questions are directed at finding out what things mean to the patient and, where those meanings are problematic, attempting to change them. Loneliness is always present in suffering patients,

---

Future Considerations

- Development of measurement indices for suffering
- Sources of suffering
- Prevalence studies of suffering in different settings and different diseases
- Prevalence of suffering in different patient groups
- Treatment and treatment outcomes

and it can be addressed even if you are not certain of the specific wellsprings of the loneliness. To do that, you make a connection to the patient by touch and by assuring the patient that you are there for them and will not abandon them. Central purpose is restored to the degree possible by encouraging other goals—eating, walking, moving, and so on—and by giving larger significance to the patient's distress: "You're going to come out of this stronger." "This [distress] will end and you will see that you were able to overcome." Your words must ring true and should not represent just pie-in-the-sky. Promise yourself that you will relieve a particular patient's suffering and stay with it until you do. Do that, and you will learn about suffering and the meaning of person in medicine.

IS SUFFERING PSYCHIATRIC PATHOLOGY?

Suffering is not a psychiatric condition, and it is not mental illness. David Kissane sees a state that occurs in sick and dying patients that he calls "demoralization" and that he believes is mental illness.[11,12] What he describes has many of the same features as what is here described as suffering. I believe he is wrong. Suffering is part of the human condition and is by no means confined to the physically ill. In fact, suffering may be a response to mental illness, and it can be relieved even in the face of continued mental illness. Chochinov described in detail a therapeutic intervention designed to enhance the dignity of the dying patient that deserves study.[13,14] He also described many of the features of suffering and ascribed them to depression. Depression certainly occurs in suffering patients and deserves treatment, but suffering is not depression. If a dying patient is treated for depression with no response, suffering should be suspected as the problem.

REFERENCES

1. Cassell EJ. The Nature of Suffering and the Goals of Medicine. New York: Oxford University Press, 2004.
2. Daneault S, Lussier V, Monqeau S, et al. The nature of suffering and its relief in the terminally ill: A qualitative study. J Palliat Care 2004;20:7-11.
3. Daneault S, Lussier V, Mongeau S. Souffrance et Medecine. Quebec: Presses de l'Universite du Quebec, 2006.
4. Charmaz K. Loss of self: A fundamental form of suffering in the chronically ill. Sociol Health Illness 1983;5:168-195.
5. Bakan D. Disease, Pain, and Sacrifice. Boston: Beacon Press, 1968.
6. Cassell EJ. Diagnosing suffering: A perspective. Ann Intern Med 1999;131:531-534.
7. Singer PA, Martin DK, Bowman K. Quality end-of-life care: Where do we go from here? J Palliat Med 2000;3:403-405.
8. Cassell EJ, Leon AC, Kaufman SG. Preliminary evidence of impaired thinking in sick patients. Ann Intern Med 2001;134:1120-1123.
9. Platt FW, Keller VF. Empathic communication: A teachable and learnable skill. J Gen Intern Med 1994;9:222-226.
10. Cassell EJ. Doctoring: The Nature of Primary Care Medicine. New York: Oxford University Press, 1997.
11. Clarke DM, Kissane DW. Demoralization: Its phenomenology and importance. Aust N Z J Psychiatry 2002;36:733-742.
12. Clarke DM, Kissane DW, Trauer T, Smith GC. Demoralization, anhedonia and grief in patients with severe physical illness. World Psychiatry 2005;4:96-105.
13. Chochinov HM. Dying, dignity, and new horizons in palliative end-of-life care. CA Cancer J Clin 2006;56:84-103.
14. Chochinov HM, Cann BJ. Interventions to enhance the spiritual aspects of dying. J Palliat Med 2005;8:s103-s115.

SUGGESTED READING

Cassell EJ. The Nature of Suffering, 2nd ed. New York: Oxford University Press, 2004.
Chochinov, Harvey M. Dying, dignity, and new horizons in palliative end-of-life care. CA Cancer J Clin 2006;56:84-103.

CHAPTER **10**

Culture, Ethnicity, and Illness

Cynthia R. Goh

KEY POINTS

- Ethnicity has a bearing on health care in access to services, prevalence of diseases in particular ethnic groups, and how end-of-life decisions are made.
- Cultural and religious backgrounds may influence the understanding of the cause and treatment of a disease and the meaning of the illness to the patient.
- Disclosure of the diagnosis and treatment options should consider different cultural attitudes about treatment decisions and the extent to which and ways in which they are expressed. Decision making by the family may be the norm in some cultures.
- Health care workers should have a working knowledge of the social norms, dietary rules, and religious practices of the different ethnic groups of their patients.
- All people of a particular ethnic group or religion may not have the same beliefs, values, or rituals. There is much variation among individuals, families, dialect groups, sects, and denominations.

Culture can be defined as a "set of distinctive spiritual, material, intellectual, and emotional features of society or a social group that encompass, in addition to art and literature, lifestyles, ways of living together, value systems, traditions, and beliefs."[1] Historians, anthropologists, and sociologists study different aspects of culture. For health professionals, understanding the worldview, values, beliefs, norms, and customs of their patients is essential for good clinical management. It forms the basis for good communication with the patient and the family, which empowers them to make sound decisions about treatment choices.

Ethnicity and race are related concepts that help characterize a social group. Ethnicity refers more to language, religion, culture, and geographical location, whereas race includes genealogy and biological or genetic characteristics. Governments have different ways of characterizing race or ethnicity, which may cause confusion. For example, in the 2001 Census of England and Wales, the word *Asian* denotes people from India, Pakistan, and Bangladesh, but the term does not include Chinese, Japanese, and people from Southeast Asia, who are classified under the heading of *Chinese and others*. In the United States Census, the term *Asian* includes people of East Asia, Southeast Asia, and parts of South Asia.

Ethnicity affects health care in terms of access to services, epidemiology of diseases that may be more prevalent in particular ethnic groups (e.g., sickle cell anemia, hepatitis B carrier state), and in the way decisions on health-related issues are made.

ETHNICITY AND ACCESS

Access to health care services, including palliative care, is often governed by socioeconomic factors.[2-4] Minority ethnic groups, especially if they are more recent immigrants to a country, may have poorer access to health services because of poverty, lack of health insurance, lack of health education, and lower priorities for health. Being unable to speak the language of the dominant ethnic group in a country may form a major barrier to accessing health care.[5] Although health care facilities serving multicultural populations may have arrangements for interpreters, such services also present pitfalls. An interpreter from the same ethnic group may not speak exactly the same dialect as the patient or may not be of the same educational or social class, generating language barriers and nuances that may be lost on a physician or nurse from a different culture. Using family members as interpreters has the advantage of convenience, but accuracy may not be guaranteed, especially in the disclosure of bad news.

PATIENT AUTONOMY AND FAMILY DECISION MAKING

In Anglo-Saxon, North European, and North American cultures, individual autonomy is highly prized. The laws in some of these countries require that the patient be given all his health information, and physicians are trained to give every detail of a medical condition, its treatment, and all the risks associated with each course of action.

In contrast, in many of the cultures of Mediterranean Europe, Latin America, Asia, and Africa, decisions are often made by the family.[6,7] This may reflect the difference in values and the relative importance of self versus the family or social group.

Western-trained doctors are often in a dilemma when the family requests or demands that information about a dire diagnosis be withheld from the patient.[8] Delicate negotiations have to be made to find out exactly how much the patient already knows, how much the patient wishes to know, and how a particular patient or family member makes a decision about treatment.

It is important for the health care team not to make assumptions based on ethnicity, because there is great variation, even among families, in where the power of decision making lies.[9] In some cultures, an elderly, less educated patient may prefer to delegate treatment decisions to a better educated offspring or to the one who will be paying for treatment. Sometimes, the patient may be the decision-making patriarch or matriarch, who does not wish to express his or her views directly to the health care team, preferring to go through a family spokesperson instead.

Language may be a barrier if the patient feels less conversant with the language of the physician or the educated masses. However, if the team suspects that the family is colluding to hide the truth from the patient and this is detrimental to the patient's emotional state, diplomatic persuasion, family counseling, and advocacy on the patient's behalf may be needed.

A patient's wish to defer decision making to the family should be recognized and respected.[10] A wish not to know all the details of his or her condition should also be respected, so that the patient is not bombarded with unsavory and unwanted details of the disease. In some cultures, describing the essential elements of a situation without offering graphic details is the accepted norm.[7,11] It may be less important for a patient to know the name of an illness such as cancer, with all its connotations of a painful death, than to know that he is going to die soon of the illness, especially if he has delegated treatment decisions to his better informed offspring[6,9,12] (see Chapters 17, 19, 116, and 117).

THE SANCTITY OF LIFE AND EUTHANASIA

Most great religions of the world uphold the concept of the sanctity of life. Christians and Muslims believe that all life is in the hands of God, whose will is supreme.[13,14] Hinduism and Buddhism prohibit the taking of life, including one's own. In all these religions, suicide is prohibited, and euthanasia is considered to be deliberate killing, like murder[13-15] (see Chapter 21).

In contrast, there is a secular train of thought from Eastern cultures that a person should not burden the family or society after his usefulness to society is finished.[16] Patients request to die to curtail the suffering associated with ill health and because they wish not to be a burden and waste family or societal resources (see Chapters 9 and 11).

In the West, the humanist tradition has given rise to a strong emphasis on personal autonomy, which extends to the right to die at the time of one's choice and, for some, the right to physician-assisted suicide. There is much controversy in Western society about whether the law should allow this practice.

Understanding about what is futile treatment and about decisions to start or stop life support is greatly affected by culture and religion. In some cultures, the right of the individual to make decisions on life and death may be questioned, whether it is the person's own life or that of a close relative. Filial piety may not allow a decision to forgo treatment, despite the patient's wishes. These are a few examples of the great diversity of views in different cultures regarding decisions on life support.[17,18]

ALTERNATIVE CONCEPTS OF ILLNESS AND DYING

Practitioners of Western allopathic medicine may not be familiar with other systems or views of health and disease. Traditionally, Western medicine practitioners dismiss everything non-Western as quackery or useless. This attitude may not be helpful when caring for the dying. When Western medicine can no longer offer cure for a life-threatening disease, many people seek alternative methods, whether they believe them to work or not. In the presence of disapproval by a Western-trained physician, patients do not let the practitioner know that they are using alternative medicines, which may lead to drug interactions, or they abandon Western medicine altogether.

Some patients and families subscribe to alternative systems of medicine and understanding of how the body functions. The health care team needs to know something about these beliefs, such as the traditional Chinese medicine view of health as a balance between the *Yin* and the *Yang* (i.e., negative and positive), with disease caused by an imbalance of these forces.[19] Different herbs and foods add to the *Yin* or the *Yang*, which often are described as cooling or heating, respectively. Treatment of a disease lies in restoration of the balance. Ayurvedic medicine, commonly practiced in India, also has many food rules.[20] A system that may be more familiar in the West is homeopathy, which posits treating "like with like" by using tiny doses of the same toxin or allergen believed to have caused the disease.[21]

There are many other systems of beliefs about the cause and treatment of illnesses. Traditional healers are found in many societies, ranging from witch doctors to holy men, who heal through rituals such as driving out evil spirits, casting and removal of spells or the evil eye, or prayer, with or without the prescription of holy water, herbs, or stranger items. Although practitioners of Western medicine may dismiss much of these approaches as superstitions, such practices have a significant effect on patients and their families, especially if they cause conflict between family members or for the patient, family, and their health care professionals.

CULTURAL AND RELIGIOUS DIVERSITY

In modern societies, in which there is ready social and physical mobility of persons and of populations, education, language, culture, and religion may differ between generations within a family. In immigrant families, the younger generation may speak the language and take on the norms and values of the society the family has joined. In multiethnic and multireligious communities, children may be educated in mission schools and convert to a different religion from that of the family. This may cause conflicts within the family, especially during a terminal illness (see "Case Study: A Meeting of Cultural and Religious Beliefs in Death and Dying").

Beliefs, Values, and Rituals

The palliative care team must have a working knowledge of the social norms, dietary rules, and religious practices of the different ethnic groups their patients come from. It is important not to assume that all persons or families from one ethnic group or religion must have the same beliefs and values. There may be great differences in social class or caste, between dialect groups, and among the sects and denominations of many of the major religions of the world.[7,9,12] These variations in beliefs and rituals are similar to the differences among Roman Catholic, Orthodox, and Protestant Christians or among Theravada, Tibetan, and Pure Land Buddhism. A family also has its own culture, expressed in the way family members display emotions, in the taboos observed, and how the members cope with stress.

Role of the Team

One of the strengths of an interdisciplinary team is that team members may come from different ethnic groups and have different religions, and they may be able to educate one another. How individuals of different genders greet and speak to one another and other behavioral norms need to be learned. The offering and receiving of food is significant in many cultures, because feeding is a common expression of care. Culturally appropriate advice on food, especially if the patient has special dietary needs because of the illness, is important. It is useful to have some understanding of what constitutes comfort food for a patient, especially for people from diverse backgrounds (Box 10-1).

RELIGIOUS NEEDS IN ADVANCED DISEASE

Religious sensitivities need to be respected (Figs. 10-1 and 10-2). An understanding of the tenets of the major religions represented in a community is useful. This is of practical use in palliative care. Buddhists often need to be lucid at the moment of death,[15] because it is believed that the last thought of a Buddhist must be a good one to achieve the best possible reincarnation. This tenet also holds for Hindus. Terminal sedation should be avoided, and accurate titration of analgesia to achieve a clear mind is necessary. In Pure Land Buddhism, the recitation of the name of Amitabha Buddha at the ear of the dying person is believed to send him or her directly to the Pure Land, where there is no suffering and where the path to *Nirvana* is easier.[22] In modern times, this is often achieved by placing a small tape recorder at the ear of the dying.

For Muslims, being able to continue daily prayers during the final illness is important.[14] It may help to position the bed in the direction of Mecca with the help of a compass. The patient may need help in performing ablutions before

Box 10-1 Dietary Norms		
GROUP	**ACCEPTABLE PRACTICES**	**UNACCEPTABLE PRACTICES**
Hindus	In the caste system, Brahmins usually are vegetarian. Others may be vegetarian on certain days of the week, during festivals, or for certain periods of vows.	They do not eat beef.
Buddhists	Mahayana Buddhist monks and nuns and some lay people are pure vegetarian; many lay people are vegetarian at the new moon and full moon and during certain festivals. Theravada monks and nuns eat everything they are given in their begging bowls, including meat.	Choices depend on which precepts they have adopted. Even nonvegetarians often do not eat beef. They do not smoke. They do not take alcohol, drugs, or intoxicating substances.
Christians	Most Christians have no food taboos.	Some Roman Catholics do not eat meat, except fish, on Fridays and during the season of Lent.
Jews	Strict Jews eat only kosher food.	They do not eat pork. They do not eat seafood without fins and tails. There are many other food taboos.
Muslims	Strict Muslims eat only halal food.	They do not eat pork or lard.

A Meeting of Cultural and Religious Beliefs in Death and Dying

Madam Lee was a 44-year-old Chinese widow with advanced stomach cancer. Her husband had died of stomach cancer 5 years earlier. She had two young children, ages 7 and 11, who were looked after by her mother-in-law. Because there was no one to take care of her when she became bedridden, she was admitted to an inpatient hospice run by some Catholic sisters. Although her physical symptoms were reasonably well controlled, she was greatly grieved by not being able to see her children. Her mother-in-law refused to bring the children to the hospice because she feared that they might contract cancer from their mother. The old lady was convinced that the cancer was infectious, because her son and her daughter-in-law had it. The hospice managed to arrange for volunteers to bring the children to see their mother on occasions when their grandmother allowed such visits.

Later in her illness, Madam Lee expressed the wish to be baptized a Roman Catholic. Although originally Taoist, she had been exposed to Christianity some years earlier but had not made a decision to become a Christian because of her duties as eldest daughter-in-law to look after the family altar and burn incense to the ancestors. Because she could no longer fulfill those duties, she expressed her wish to be baptized and to be buried in the Roman Catholic cemetery. Her mother-in-law was much against this idea because it meant that Madam Lee would be forever separated from her husband and the rest of the family.

The nuns counseled Madam Lee. They said that God looks at the heart and that what she believed in her heart was what mattered. The outward rituals of baptism and where she was buried were not so important, especially if it created so much family conflict. However, Madam Lee was insistent.

After some weeks, when the patient was close to dying, the mother-in-law relented. Perhaps she did not want Madam Lee to die and become a lost soul or "hungry ghost" and come back to haunt her. Madam Lee was baptized and was buried in the Catholic cemetery. Before she died, she told her children that when they grew up and were able to earn their own living, they must not forget the kindness of the nuns who looked after her during her terminal illness. When the children grew up and started working, they visited the hospice and made a donation every year after visiting their mother's grave on the anniversary of her death.

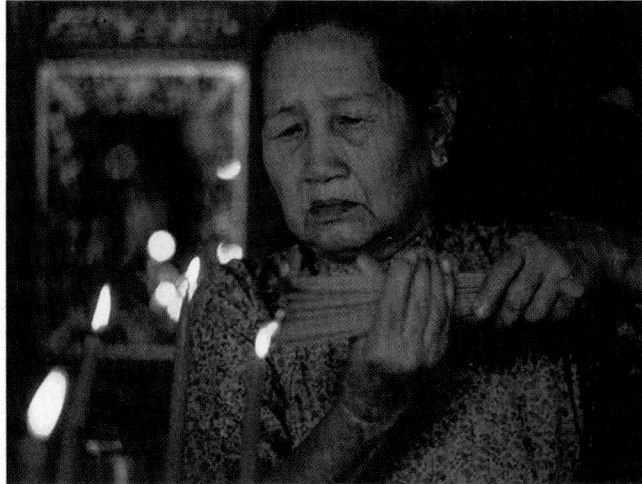

FIGURE 10-1 An elderly Chinese woman lighting joss sticks at a Taoist temple.

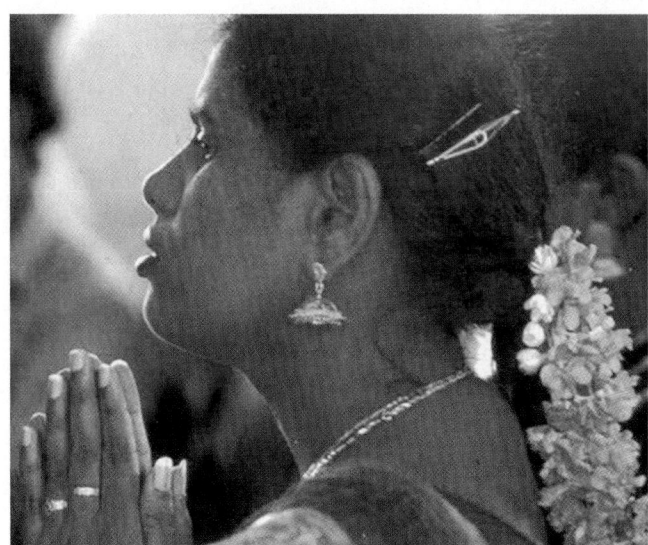

FIGURE 10-2 An Indian woman praying at a Hindu temple.

The timing of bereavement visits should also reflect religious observances and days of remembrance, because certain days are of particular significance to commemorate the dead.[23]

CONCLUSIONS

Culture, ethnicity, and religion have important influences on human behavior and the experience of life and death. The practice of palliative medicine must consider these influences. An understanding of the cultures within which we function is enriching, and it enhances the care we are able to give to our patients and their families.

This is a fertile area for future research. Much work still needs to be done to describe and analyze the differences in attitudes about many issues surrounding death, such as the role of family or the individual in making decisions and the acceptability of starting or withdrawing of life support. Much needs to be learned about how best to address the needs of people from different cultures in

prayers. Someone with a colostomy may think that it would prevent him from being ritually clean for prayers. The advice of a religious teacher on this issue is important to put the patient's mind at ease. Reading the Koran and saying prayers should ideally continue to the moment of death. The presence of a family member, or at least another Muslim, is important at the moment of death, which is why many Muslims wish to die at home.

An understanding of religious rituals after death is important. This information affects handling of the body, the time constraints on death certification and autopsy, and release of the body for burial or cremation (Box 10-2).

Box 10-2 Common Death Rituals	
Hindus	Cremation occurs on a pyre by the river or at a crematorium by the evening of the day of death, and the ashes scattered. Prayers and rituals occur on certain days within the first month. Mourning period is 10 to 30 days.
Taoists (Chinese customs)	Elaborate funeral rituals occur at wakes lasting an odd number of days. Chanting is done by Buddhist or Taoist monks; paper effigies of money, clothes, houses, cars and other items needed in the afterlife are burned. Wealthy are buried in a grand coffin after a funeral procession. Observances or rituals occur at 7, 21, 49, and 100 days. Mourning may last until the end of funeral or for 100 days, 1 year, or 3 years, depending on the individual or family.
Buddhists	Some do not wish the body to be disturbed for 8 hours or longer after death. Buddhists have simpler funerals than Taoists (e.g., no burning of paper effigies). Chanting is provided by Buddhist monks if the family can afford it. Cremation is favored, but burial is acceptable. Ashes may be stored at a columbarium in a temple.
Muslims	Ritual washing is done by family members of the same gender. Burial occurs in a shroud with the body facing Mecca on the day of death before sundown.
Christians	Simple rites are adapted to local custom (e.g., a wake if it is the local practice). Memorial services occur on the nights of the wake; at the funeral, burial, or cremation; and sometimes at a later date. Some Christians advocate burial; otherwise, cremation is done according to local practices. Roman Catholics have funeral masses and prefer burial.

areas such as knowledge of the diagnosis and understanding of the illness.

REFERENCES

1. United Nations Education, Scientific, and Cultural Organization. Universal Declaration on Cultural Diversity. Paris, UNESCO, 2002.
2. Freeman HP, Payne R. Racial injustice in health care [editorial]. N Engl J Med 2000;342:1045-1047.
3. Ahmed N, Bestall JC, Ahmedzai SH, et al. Systematic review of the problems and issues of accessing specialist palliative care by patients, carers and health and social care professionals. Palliat Med 2004;18:525-542.
4. Cintron A, Morrison RS. Pain and ethnicity in the United States: A systematic review. Palliat Med 2006;9:1454-1473.
5. Born W, Greiner KA, Sylvia E, et al. Knowledge, attitudes, and beliefs about end-of-life care among inner-city African Americans and Latinos. J Palliat Med 2004;7:247-256.
6. Blackhall LJ, Murphy ST, Frank G, et al. Ethnicity and attitudes toward patient autonomy. JAMA 1995;274:820-825.
7. Kagawa-Singer M, Blackhall LJ. Negotiating cross-cultural issues at the end-of-life. JAMA 2001;286:2993-3001.
8. Lapine A, Wang-Cheng R, Goldstein M, et al. When cultures clash: Physician, patient, and family wishes in truth disclosure for dying patients. J Palliat Med 2001;4:475-480.
9. Koenig BA, Gates-Williams J. Understanding cultural difference in caring for dying patients. West J Med 1995;163:244-249.
10. Crawley LM, Marshall PA, Lo B, Koenig BA. Strategies for culturally effective end-of-life care. Ann Intern Med 2002;136:673-679.
11. Muller JH, Desmond B. Ethical dilemmas in a cross-cultural context: A Chinese example. West J Med 1992;157:323-327.
12. Hern EH Jr, Koenig BA, Moore LJ, Marshall PA. The difference that culture can make in end-of-life decision making. Camb Q Healthcare Ethics 1998;7:27-40.
13. Rowell M. Christian perspectives on end-of-life decision making: Faith in a community. In Braun KL, Pietsch JH, Blanchette PL (eds). Cultural issues in end-of-life decision making. Thousand Oaks, CA: Sage, 2000, pp 147-163.
14. Sheikh A. Death and dying—a Muslim perspective. J R Soc Med 1998;91:138-140.
15. Keown D. End-of-life: The Buddhist view. Lancet 2005;366:952-955.
16. Goh CR. Challenges of cultural diversity. In Beattie J, Goodlin S (eds). Supportive Care in Heart Failure. New York: Oxford University Press, 2008.
17. Klessig J. Cross-cultural medicine a decade later: The effect of values and culture on life-support decisions. West J Med 1992;157:316-322.
18. Blackhall LJ, Frank G, Murphy ST, et al. Ethnicity and attitudes towards life sustaining technology. Soc Sci Med 1999;48:1779-1789.
19. Traditional Medicine Network (TMN) Philosophy of Chinese Medicine. The causes of disease in Chinese medicine. Available at http://www.traditional-medicine.net.au/chinsynd.htm (accessed November 2007).
20. Dharmananda S. Basics of ayurvedic physiology. Available at http://www.itmonline.org/arts/ayurbasics.htm (accessed November 2007).
21. Vickers A, Zollman C. Homoeopathy. BMJ 1999;319:1115-1118.
22. Pure Land Buddhism. Available at http://en.wikipedia.org/wiki/Pure_Land (accessed November 2007).
23. Firth S. Cross-cultural perspectives on bereavement. In Dickenson D, Johnson M, Samson Katz J (eds). Death, Dying, and Bereavement, 2nd ed. Thousand Oaks, CA: Sage, 2000, pp 339-346.

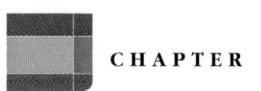

CHAPTER **11**

The Desire for Death

Wendy G. Lichtenthal, Megan Olden, Hayley Pessin, and William Breitbart

K E Y   P O I N T S

- Palliative care patients are at an increased risk of suicide and desire for death.
- Clinical correlates of the desire for hastened death include depression, hopelessness, severe and intractable pain, cognitive dysfunction, low social support, feelings of burden, and loss of dignity or meaning.
- Transitory passive wishes for death are common and should be differentiated from pervasive suicidal ideation that involves a plan and intent.
- Thorough assessment of desire for hastened death and its risk factors should be an essential component of palliative care management.
- Treatments focusing on physical symptoms, psychological distress, and existential concerns may alleviate patients' suffering and alter their attitude toward death.

Desire for hastened death (DHD) is the broad construct that underlies suicidal ideation, requests for assisted suicide, and euthanasia and can identify patients at risk for ending their lives. Clinical severity varies, and those with DHD may exhibit (1) a passive wish (fleeting or persistent) for death without active plans, (2) a request for assistance in hastening death, or (3) an active desire and plan to commit suicide.[1] It is important to differentiate expressions of DHD from suicidal ideation or intent.[2]

PREVALENCE

Epidemiological findings on DHD prevalence depend on how researchers have defined this construct. Occasional, transient suicidal ideation is not uncommon.[3] Forty-five percent of 200 terminally ill patients in one study reported a fleeting desire for death, which was differentiated from a committed wish for hastened death that was found among 9% of patients.[4] High DHD was found among 17% of 92 terminally ill patients assessed in another study.[5] At particularly high risk were depressed patients, who were four times more likely to report high DHD than those who did not meet criteria for major depression.[5] Suicide completion in terminal illness appears rare; in 2004, assisted suicide was the cause of only 0.125% of all deaths in Oregon.[6]

COMMON RISK FACTORS

The most common risk factors[1] for DHD include feeling that one is a burden to others, loss of autonomy and the related wish to control one's death, physical symptoms (e.g., severe pain), depression and hopelessness, existential concerns, and fear of the future, particularly regarding management of physical pain. DHD may change depending on time and circumstance, so frequent reassessments are advantageous. Appreciating the reasons for a desire to die helps the clinician intervene appropriately.

Depression

There is a compelling link between DHD and major depression. Clinicians should determine whether a patient's depressive symptoms reach clinical levels, as opposed to being appropriate feelings of sadness expected among those facing a terminal prognosis. Depression was the strongest predictor of DHD in the study of 200 terminally patients mentioned earlier; 58% of those who reported significant DHD also met criteria for major depression.[4] Similarly, depression was the strongest predictor of DHD in patients with advanced acquired immunodeficiency syndrome (AIDS), although lack of social support, pain intensity, and symptom distress all provided independent contributions.[7]

Hopelessness

Although "hopelessness" was once considered under the umbrella of depressive symptoms, it has emerged as a unique risk factor for DHD among the terminally ill. In addition to depression, hopelessness independently predicts DHD.[5] Several studies have suggested that hopelessness may play an even stronger role than depression in terminally ill patients' wish to hasten death.[8]

Pain

Patients who experience severe intractable physical pain are more likely to report DHD. It is not simply the pain, but more likely its severity, that is associated with DHD. One study found that 76% of patients with moderate to severe pain had significant DHD.[4] Aggressive pain management should be the first line of treatment in such cases.

DHD can be reassessed after effective pain relief has been achieved (see Chapters 253 and 254).

Social Support

Important relationships exist between social support and DHD. Those with less social support are more likely to report DHD.[7] Quality of social support has also been linked with DHD.[7] Because of the influence of interpersonal relationships on DHD, health care providers should include assessment of social support in clinical evaluations.

Cognitive Dysfunction and Delirium

Cognitive impairment has been significantly associated with DHD among hospitalized patients with advanced AIDS.[7] Because delirium and cognitive impairment cloud reasoning ability, they may increase the risk of impulsive behavior and impair the ability to judge long-term consequences of behavior.

Psychiatric History and Personality Factors

Preexisting psychiatric disturbance increases the risk for DHD and suicidal ideation.[3] People with a history of depression, diagnosable personality disorders, or prior suicide attempts should be carefully monitored for suicidality.[9] Factors such as concerns about loss of autonomy or dependency, a strong need to control the circumstances of one's death, or fear of being a burden on caregivers may also be predictors of DHD.[1]

Existential Concerns

Loss of meaning, purpose, or dignity; awareness of incomplete life tasks or regrets; or anxiety about what happens after death and/or the existence of a higher power may be a central struggle for the dying patient and largely contribute to DHD. Terminally ill cancer patients with low spiritual well-being were more likely to acknowledge DHD, hopelessness, and suicidal ideation.[10] Addressing existential and spiritual concerns through access to pastoral care or more secular existential interventions may be helpful (see Chapter 12).

LEGAL AND ETHICAL ISSUES IN ASSISTED SUICIDE

Although a distinction should be drawn between DHD and overt requests for physician assistance with suicide, the controversial nature of assisted suicide is likely to play a role in physicians' assessments of and responses to a patient's wish to die. Oregon is the only state in the United States with legalized physician-assisted suicide. Physicians are permitted to write prescriptions for lethal medication doses for terminally ill Oregon residents who make this request. This practice is also legal in the Netherlands, and similar laws are being considered in California, Vermont, and Great Britain. Those opposed have expressed concern that requests for assistance with suicide are a result of depression, distorted belief that one is a burden, or the other potentially treatable clinical correlates of DHD described earlier.[6] Others have argued that the quality of end-of-life care has improved since assisted suicide was legalized (e.g., providers have increased referrals to hospice and efforts to enhance palliative care knowledge).[11] Regardless of one's position on the issue, comprehensive and detailed assessment is critical to determine whether conditions related to DHD can be modified to enhance quality of life and to verify that the patient is not requesting assisted suicide impulsively (see Chapters 9, 18, and 21).

ASSESSMENT

Clinical Interviews

Clinicians face challenges when a patient makes a desire to die statement. Assessing the intended meaning and underlying cause of the statement quickly and with careful contemplation is crucial for appropriate treatment planning.[2] It is imperative to evaluate the DHD risk factors reviewed earlier, such as depression and severe pain, through detailed interviews and standardized measures (see Chapter 66). Assessment of depression should involve careful consideration of somatic symptoms to determine whether their etiology is psychiatric or organic.[3] This assessment should also include evaluation of suicidal ideation, plan, and intent (Table 11-1).

Appraisals of expressions for DHD that are not overt or explicit can be challenging. The clinician should ask open-ended questions and remain nonjudgmental throughout the assessment[1] (see "Common Errors").

TABLE 11-1 Assessment of Suicidality: Sample Questions

NORMALIZATION

Many patients who are ill have passing thoughts about their death, or even suicide, such as, "If things get really bad, I may . . ." Have you ever had thoughts like that?

It's not uncommon to feel that way. Can you tell me more about that?

FREQUENCY AND INTENSITY

How often do you feel this way?

Do these thoughts come and go, or do you think them all the time?

How strong are the thoughts when they occur?

DESIRE FOR HASTENED DEATH

Do you ever wish you would die sooner instead of later?

Does it seem like death is the only way to relieve your suffering?

SUICIDAL IDEATION

Have you found yourself thinking that you would be better off dead?

Do you ever think about hurting yourself or ending your life?

SUICIDE PLAN

Have you refused treatments or stopped taking care of yourself?

Have you thought about how you would end your life?

Do you have a plan? Have you thought out the details?

Do you have access to the means to carry out your plan?

SUICIDAL INTENT

Do you intend to hurt yourself?

Are you worried you may not be able to stop yourself?

Do you think you would carry out these plans? How likely is it?

Have you made any preparations? (e.g., begun to collect pills, written a suicide note)

Measurement

To improve assessment, researchers have developed scales for DHD, including the Desire for Death Rating Scale (DDRS)[4] and the Schedule of Attitudes toward Hastened Death (SAHD).[12,13] The Hopelessness Scale[14] and the Demoralization Scale,[15] which have been validated in advanced disease, may provide a better understanding of patients' beliefs and feelings about their future. Measures of suicidality that are appropriate for palliative care populations include the Beck Scale for Suicidal Ideation[16] and the Modified Scale for Suicidal Ideation.[17] They assess duration and frequency of ideation, sense of control over making an attempt, deterrents, and amount of actual preparation. Use of standardized measures within a trusting patient–provider relationship can help identify patients' needs and tailor appropriate interventions.

INTERVENTIONS

Although practical suggestions for managing expressions of DHD are available, few have validated their utility.[1] Broad recommendations have included obtaining psychiatric consultation for persons who appear to be at risk for suicide.[1] In fact, decision making should be specific and guided by a thorough assessment. If underlying clinical physical symptoms such as severe pain can be treated, then pharmacological interventions such as analgesics or antidepressants should be applied. Advance care directives may facilitate discussion of end-of-life issues and concerns among patients and their families.[1]

Psychosocial interventions to address modifiable factors related to DHD should also be implemented. For example, if patients feel they are a burden to caregivers, facilitating communication about their relationships might be helpful.[1] Although sadness and grief over losses and challenges may be normalized, cognitive restructuring can be applied to address distorted, unrealistic beliefs that may contribute to hopelessness or demoralization.[18,19] Researchers have conducted empirical investigations of psychosocial interventions that address clinical correlates of DHD, including interventions related to enhancing patients' sense of meaning[20,21] and dignity,[22,23] as well as spiritual and existential concerns.

PROPOSED PRACTICE GUIDELINES

Recommendations and guidelines for managing DHD in palliative care have been proposed.[1] Evaluation of suicidal ideation may be avoided or hindered because of fear of diminishing patients' hope, provoking emotional discussions, or the legal repercussions of possessing knowledge

---

Common Errors

- Assuming that desire for hastened death (DHD) is permanent and not treatable
- Failure to assess in the absence of overt expressions of DHD
- Fearing that assessment of DHD will instigate suicidal ideation or behavior
- Minimizing the role of patient personality characteristics

about patients' suicidality.[2] The guidelines suggest a two-phase approach: Phase I involves assessment and exploration of the expression of DHD to foster a better understanding of underlying factors, and Phase II uses more general background information to apply initial interventions (Table 11-2). These recommendations are intended to be flexible, and they should occur over time and within a trusting relationship. A therapeutic response to DHD includes empathy, active listening, management of realistic expectations, permission to discuss psychological distress, and, if appropriate, referral to a mental health professional.

RESEARCH CHALLENGES AND OPPORTUNITIES

There is ongoing effort to determine the most ethical approaches for balancing a patient's wish to end suffering with a practitioner's commitment to alleviating suffering. As noted earlier, the legalization of physician-assisted suicide has been addressed by the U.S. Supreme Court, and debate continues. High-profile media coverage of individual cases of life support (e.g., Terri Schiavo) illustrates how this topic continues to be emotionally charged and the focus of ethical questions.

There are numerous methodological limitations specific to DHD research. First, the desire to die itself may be dynamic and fleeting, but knowledge of the phenomenon is limited; longitudinal studies that involve multiple assessments may be taxing on dying patients and are often difficult to perform. Few studies have assessed patients who explicitly expressed DHD; most have relied on patients' consideration of the possibility of experiencing DHD in the future or on family and clinician reports.[1] Because family assessments are often conducted after the death, DHD reports may be influenced by grief and by the general effect of time on recall. Additional limitations[1] include the fact that studies usually do not explicitly define factors associated with the desire to die and the homogeneity of study populations, with most consisting of North American cancer patients.

Opportunities for future research include investigation of additional potential DHD predictors, such as demographic and cultural variables, personality factors, social support, cognitive impairment, need for a sense of control, and spiritual concerns.[1] Longitudinal assessments are important to determine how DHD may fluctuate over time and to better identify patients at high risk for DHD. Finally, it is critical to develop interventions to prevent and treat DHD for alleviating suffering at the end of life.

TABLE 11-2 Recommendations for Management of Desire for Hastened Death

BE ALERT TO YOUR OWN RESPONSES
Be open
Be aware of how your response can influence the communication
Monitor your attitude and responses
Demonstrate regard for the patient
Seek supervision

BE OPEN TO HEARING CONCERNS
Gently ask about emotional concerns
Be alert to verbal and nonverbal signs of distress
Encourage expression of feelings
Actively listen without interrupting
Acknowledge desire for death using the patient's own words or language similar to that of the patient
Permit silence and tears
Express empathy verbally and nonverbally
Acknowledge individual differences in patients' responses to illness

ASSESS POTENTIAL CONTRIBUTING FACTORS
Lack of social support
Feelings of burden
Family conflict
Need for additional assistance
Depression
Anxiety
Existential concerns
Loss of meaning or dignity
Cognitive dysfunction
Physical symptoms, including severe pain

RESPOND TO SPECIFIC ISSUES
Acknowledge the patient's or family's fears and concerns
Address modifiable contributing factors
Recommend interventions
Develop a plan to manage more complicated issues

CONCLUDE THE DISCUSSION
Summarize and review important points
Clarify the patient's perceptions
Provide opportunity for questions
Offer assistance with facilitating discussion with others
Provide appropriate referrals

AFTER THE DISCUSSION
Document the discussion in medical records
Communicate to other members of the treatment team

Adapted from Hudson PL, Schofield P, Kelly B, et al. Responding to desire to die statements from patients with advanced disease: Recommendations for health professionals. Palliat Med 2006;20:703-710; and National Health and National Health and Medical Research Council Australia. Clinical Practice Guidelines for the Psychosocial Care of Adults with Cancer. Sydney: National Breast Cancer Centre, 2003.

REFERENCES

1. Hudson PL, Kristjanson LJ, Ashby M, et al. Desire for hastened death in patients with advanced disease and the evidence base of clinical guidelines: A systematic review. Palliat Med 2006;20:693-701.
2. Hudson PL, Schofield P, Kelly B, et al. Responding to desire to die statements from patients with advanced disease: Recommendations for health professionals. Palliat Med 2006;20:703-710.
3. Pessin H, Potash M, Breitbart W. Diagnosis, assessment, and treatment of depression in palliative care. In Lloyd-Williams M (ed). Psychosocial Issues in Palliative Care. Oxford: Oxford University Press, 2003, pp 81-103.
4. Chochinov HM, Wilson KG, Enns M, et al. Desire for death in the terminally ill. Am J Psychiatry 1995;152:1185-1191.
5. Breitbart W, Rosenfeld B, Pessin H, et al. Depression, hopelessness, and desire for hastened death in terminally ill patients with cancer. JAMA 2000;284:2907-2911.
6. Okie S: Physician-assisted suicide: Oregon and beyond. N Engl J Med 2005;352:1627-1630.
7. Rosenfeld B, Krivo S, Breitbart W, Chochinov HM. Suicide, assisted suicide, and euthanasia in the terminally ill. In Chochinov HM, Breitbart W (eds). Handbook of Psychiatry in Palliative Medicine. New York: Oxford University Press, 2000, pp 51-62.
8. Chochinov HM, Wilson KG, Enns M, Lander S. Depression, hopelessness, and suicidal ideation in the terminally ill. Psychosomatics 1998;39:366-370.

9. Breitbart W, Gibson C, Abbey J, Iannarone N. Suicide in palliative care. In Bruera E, Higginson IJ, Ripamonti C, et al (eds). Textbook of Palliative Medicine. London: Hodder Arnold, 2006.

10. McClain CS, Rosenfeld B, Breitbart W. Effect of spiritual well-being on end-of-life despair in terminally-ill cancer patients. Lancet 2003;361:1603-1607.

11. Ganzini L, Nelson HD, Lee MA, et al. Oregon physicians' attitudes about and experiences with end-of-life care since passage of the Oregon Death with Dignity Act. JAMA 2001;285:2363-2369.

12. Rosenfeld B, Breitbart W, Galietta M, et al. The schedule of attitudes toward hastened death: Measuring desire for death in terminally ill cancer patients. Cancer 2000;88:2868-2875.

13. Rosenfeld B, Breitbart W, Stein K, et al. Measuring desire for death among patients with HIV/AIDS: The schedule of attitudes toward hastened death. Am J Psychiatry 1999;156:94-100.

14. Abbey JG, Rosenfeld B, Pessin H, Breitbart W. Hopelessness at the end of life: The utility of the hopelessness scale with terminally ill cancer patients. Br J Health Psychol 2006;11(Pt 2):173-183.

15. Kissane DW, Wein S, Love A, et al. The Demoralization Scale: A report of its development and preliminary validation. J Palliat Care 2004;20:269-276.

16. Beck AT, Steer RA. Manual for Beck Scale for Suicidal Ideation. New York: Pennsylvania Corporation, 1991.

17. Miller IW, Norman WH, Bishop SB, Dow MG. The Modified Scale for Suicidal Ideation: Reliability and validity. J Consult Clin Psychol 1986;54:724-725.

18. Kissane DW, Clarke DM, Street AF. Demoralization syndrome: A relevant psychiatric diagnosis for palliative care. J Palliat Care 2001;17:12-21.

19. Griffith JL, Gaby L. Brief psychotherapy at the bedside: Countering demoralization from medical illness. Psychosomatics 2005;46:109-116.

20. Breitbart W. Reframing hope: Meaning-centered care for patients near the end of life. Interview by Karen S. Heller. J Palliat Med 2003;6:979-988.

21. Breitbart W, Gibson C, Poppito SR, Berg A. Psychotherapeutic interventions at the end of life: A focus on meaning and spirituality. Can J Psychiatry 2004;49:366-372.

22. Chochinov HM. Dignity-conserving care—A new model for palliative care: Helping the patient feel valued. JAMA 2002;287:2253-2260.

23. Chochinov HM, Hack T, Hassard T, et al. Dignity therapy: A novel psychotherapeutic intervention for patients near the end of life. J Clin Oncol 2005;23:5520-5525.

SUGGESTED READING

Breitbart W, Rosenfeld B, Pessin H, et al. Depression, hopelessness, and desire for hastened death in terminally ill patients with cancer. JAMA 2000;284:2907-2911.

Chochinov HM, Wilson KG, Enns M, et al. Desire for death in the terminally ill. Am J Psychiatry 1995;152:1185-1191.

Hudson PL, Schofield P, Kelly B, et al. Responding to desire to die statements from patients with advanced disease: Recommendations for health professionals. Palliat Med 2006;20:703-710.

Mishara BL. Synthesis of research and evidence on factors affecting the desire of terminally ill or seriously chronically ill persons to hasten death. Omega 1999;39(1):1-70.

Rosenfeld B, Krivo S, Breitbart W, Chochinov HM. Suicide, assisted suicide, and euthanasia in the terminally ill. In Chochinov HM, Breitbart W (eds). Handbook of Psychiatry in Palliative Medicine. New York: Oxford University Press, 2000.

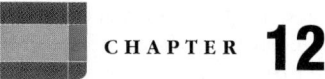

CHAPTER **12**

Spiritual Distress

Pam Firth

KEY POINTS

- Spirituality differs from religion; definitions are complex.
- Spiritual distress is evident in most dying people but is often intertwined with psychosocial distress.
- Spiritual care is part of holistic palliative care. Usually, it is the chaplain's role to offer spiritual care, but most members of the team need to be able to recognize spiritual distress.
- The meaning of the illness is important for the patient and family.
- Reactions to a life-threatening illness will be affected by the belief system of the patient and family. Professional carers need to be aware of their own beliefs, because they can affect their caregiving.

Spiritual care is an important part of the holistic approach offered to patients and families in palliative care, but what distinguishes it from other aspects of care? How our ancestors dealt with loss and suffering provided models, but these models were often lost or denied, particularly in Europe, after the world wars of the 20th century. Traditional societies were preoccupied with the past, but modern societies seem obsessed with the future and do not reflect on loss.[1] For centuries, communities around the world used rituals, prayer, and meditation to bring people together for comfort and strength in times of trauma, crisis, loss, and suffering.[2] Gatherings to memorialize the dead, injured, and bereaved occurred after the attacks on the World Trade Center and the Pentagon in 2001 and people in the United Kingdom gathered for help and support after the bombings in London in 2005. In the face of so much human suffering, helplessness is somewhat countered by feeling connected to others and sharing the experience. Suffering can encompass feelings of injustice, incomprehension, and a sense of being wronged, which are inevitably spiritual issues[3] and are commonly expressed in palliative care.

Spiritual beliefs are a neglected area of research, not only in palliative care but also in psychotherapy; yet people who seek help for emotional problems and interpersonal relationships are often suffering from spiritual distress. As people face the end of their lives, often with fear and anxiety, they review their lives, look at their intimate relationships, examine their values and beliefs, and try to make sense of their situation by ascribing meaning to their suffering. The palliative care approach is to address all areas of pain—physical, social, emotional, psychological, and spiritual. However, unlike other areas, spirituality has had no standard definition, practice, or policy.[4] This is expected to change in the United Kingdom with application of the guidelines produced by the National Institute of Clinical Excellence in 2004, entitled, *Improving Supportive Care for Adults with Cancer.*

DEFINING SPIRITUALITY AND SPIRITUAL DISTRESS

Spirituality has many interpretations. Making sense of human existence is a central preoccupation that is common to all people, whether they have a religious faith or not.[5] Spirituality encompasses an individual's beliefs and attitudes toward God or some higher power. Simply, the spirit is considered to be the essence of a person, but within the context of the life that has been lived. Spirituality is expressed in many ways. Some expressions are easy to articulate, others difficult. Music, literature, and art can provide spiritual resonance. These expressions involve connecting with people, places, and events, so memory is important. It is common for individuals to review their life as they approach middle age. Doing so can stimulate great creativity as people express themselves. Many composers and artists have produced highly meaningful work in midlife.[6] Religion allows people to express their spirituality through organized rituals and practices but also in religious buildings, artifacts, and music. The spiritual domain in the 21st century resembles a diamond that has many facets; its appearance depends on the observer's stance.[7]

Religion and Spirituality

The development of palliative care has seen the separation of religion and spirituality. Most early hospices in Europe were built by Christian communities. Pioneers such as Dame Cicely Saunders and other devout Christians used their beliefs, knowledge, and skills to express love and humanity, to ease the suffering of the dying. This was a creative response based in personal and collective spirituality. Nursing as a profession has strong roots in Christian ideals, particularly from early pioneers such as Florence Nightingale. Social work in the United Kingdom was influenced by Quaker women. Later, social work in both Great Britain and the United States was linked to Freudian psychotherapy, which kept case work and religion separate. Sociological ideas about structural and societal influences on individuals and families moved social work away from religious and spiritual concerns. More recently, there has been greater realization of the importance of culture, which has led the social work profession to focus again on narratives that include religious and spiritual components. Traditionally, Christian chaplains provided the spiritual lead in hospitals and hospices, but the multicultural nature of many communities and the separation of religion from spiritual care is causing changes (see later discussion).

Spirituality

In the 21st century, spirituality is recognized as a more individual experience, one not expressed solely through religion. Religion and spirituality are developed from a mixture of world religions and beliefs and encouraged by the new multicultural nature of families and communities.[2] Palliative care reflects these changes, but structures and services within hospices, hospitals, and nursing homes offering end-of-life care do not always support them. The concern is that spiritual care will become too prescriptive in response to a complex need interpreted in a one-dimensional way.[4] Clinicians need to maintain the concept of the diamond.

Spiritual distress is not always easy to distinguish from emotional, social, or psychological pain. To help people, clinicians must acknowledge that there is a mixture of distress for most individuals and families.[7] When people are upset because of any personal problem, there is always questioning of the meaning and point of the experience as it is perceived. Definitions of spiritual distress encompass the idea that life can lose meaning and that this can lead to diminished problem-solving skills. Because the breakdown of, or threat to, important relationships challenges individual identity, suffering caused by loss and grief always contains an element of spiritual distress. Questions from the bereaved about location of the dead body and spirit are multileveled.

As Viktor Frankel put it[8], "The meaning of life differs from man to man, from day to day and from hour to hour. What matters therefore, is not the meaning of life in general but rather the specific meaning of a person's life at a given moment" (see "Case Study: Spiritual Distress and Personal Narrative").

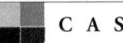 C A S E   S T U D Y

Spiritual Distress and Personal Narrative

John, aged 86 years, was admitted to the hospice dying of lung cancer. He was in great distress because of his breathing. After a few days, he appeared calmer and told the nurses he was feeling safer. Later in the week, the night nurses reported that John had had nightmares in which he was screaming out to be saved. The staff knew little about John and his life except that he was a widower and his two sons were regular visitors. John was encouraged to talk but found the nighttimes too difficult and asked for sleeping pills. However, the nightmares returned whenever he dozed, and John agreed to see a counselor.

John talked about the war. He had been a sailor and was one of only 20 men saved from the sea when his ship was torpedoed. For hours, it seemed, he had hung onto an upturned lifeboat, his friends screaming to be saved from the water, only to watch them drown shortly afterward. He felt guilty at being saved because he was single and they had families. His shortness of breath mirrored the experience of the men in the water. John had learned not to talk about his wartime experiences. He got married and had his own family, but he described feeling diminished, always rather sad. His wife's early death was accepted by John as punishment, and he held a strong belief that when he died he would meet his old friends, who would accuse him of not saving them.

All his adult life, he had strived to work hard, to make something of himself, and the counselor helped him see that this had been a constructive honoring of his friends' memory. They discussed his beliefs concerning retribution and punishment, where had they come from, and why they had so much influence on his life. Although John's narrative was limited by his condition, it was clear that he felt heard. He decided to tell his sons what happened and asked them to stay with him when he died a few days later.

There is increasing awareness that families and caregivers can be negatively affected, both emotionally and physically, by caring.[9] The course of a patient's illness depends on the involvement of family caregivers and how the stress of caregiving and the effects of watching progressive illness and suffering affect carers. Much of a carer's distress may be spiritual.

SPIRITUAL DISTRESS AND BELIEF SYSTEMS

Ideas about the family as a system made up of interacting parts began to emerge about 50 years ago in North America. The concepts focused on patterns of interactions and problem solving. The notion that the illness of a person directly affects other members of the person's family became acceptable with practitioners who were examining common themes in families. Ideas about the ways in which families control interactions and behavior centered on the concept of family beliefs. Family therapy has recognized that families adapt and change as they move through the stages of the family life cycle in distinct but interconnected areas: social, cultural, spiritual, the familial, and the personal.[11] Transitional life cycle points are periods in which individuals and families can be vulnerable to stress, and a terminal illness at this time puts the family system under great strain. There are also life cycle times, such as old age, when concerns about death and dying are more prominent. In general, there is not the outrage and spiritual distress that can accompany the serious illness of a young person.

Beliefs are a mixture from the past and the present, not only ideas from religious teachings. They are an amalgam of myths, past events, and moral teachings; they are built up over time and act as a filter through which the world is viewed (i.e., the individual, the family, and the organization). Beliefs lead to behaviors and actions. They are part of the family blueprint for understanding the world. Sometimes, individuals and families hold on to beliefs that are constraining and prevent adjustment or constructive dialogue. For example, a man diagnosed with bowel cancer that appears to be suitable for treatment might refuse it on the grounds that his father died in agony of bowel cancer 20 years ago after undergoing chemotherapy. Similarly, some people have strongly held cultural and religious beliefs about certain types of cancer that make distress worse. Shame and blame can contribute to secrets and withdrawal.

Studies of the interactions among illness, the patient, the family, and health care professionals' beliefs[3] suggest that suffering is related to the interplay between the professionals' and the family's beliefs.[12] The second case study demonstrates the connections between the patient and staff beliefs (see "Case Study: Working with a Patient's Belief System").

INTERVENTIONS

In both of the case studies presented in this chapter, the patients developed a trusting relationship with practitioners who were reliable, listened, showed concern, had compassion, expressed empathy, and were accepting and nonjudgmental. The professionals also needed to feel competent. The patients were anxious, helpless and

 C A S E   S T U D Y

Working with a Patient's Belief System

Jean was 60 years old and had myeloma. Walking was difficult, and she was miserable. Her doctor referred her to a day hospice. At the day hospice, she was unpopular with the other patients and the nurses because she criticized them and was verbally spiteful. One nurse felt more compassionate toward her and, with her permission, referred her to the social worker. At first, Jean's anger made it difficult to develop a working relationship. This was acknowledged alongside her intense loneliness. Jean was an only child and believed that her conception was a mistake. She had felt unwanted until she met her husband. They had one daughter, Deborah. Jean recounted a happy marriage that had ended 10 years ago when her husband collapsed and died at work. Jean was desperate for several years. She withdrew and also stopped going to church. However, a chance meeting with an old school friend led to her joining an informal walking group of single women. Jean began to live again. She had always enjoyed foreign travel, and she went abroad many times with the group until she became ill. Her walking friends tried to keep in touch, but Jean was jealous of them, and Deborah moved away. Jean believed she was not wanted again and acknowledged that her behavior at the day hospice pushed people away. Much of the material in Jean's sessions with the social worker concerned her self-worth and her belief that everything that was good in her life God took away. However, things began to change: she allowed the nurse to bathe her once a week. The primary care involved in this task—touching, caressing with water, and then the careful drying—made Jean cry. The nurse took great care to buy Jean's favorite soap and shampoo. Jean considered it part of her spiritual care, and bathing was the highlight of her week. The bond between Jean and her nurse was very special. The development of trust had a direct affect on Jean's distress, and she became less hostile.

Later, Jean agreed to go to Lourdes with the local Catholic Church. She had great misgivings and felt sure that her room would be the smallest and that the carers would not bother with her "attitude." She returned a week later and recounted a life-changing experience. She had felt part of something, connected to others and their suffering, and she believed that she would be united with her husband in death. A week later, Jean had a stroke and died. Some of the staff at the day hospice attended her funeral. They recognized that they had believed Jean to be one of the most difficult people to help and that it was her anger and lack of gratitude that made them not want to engage with her. They reflected on their own reasons for working at the hospice and the value of the primary care they provided, recognizing its importance on many levels. Reaching out to another person who is in great need is the essence of holistic palliative care. The team had helped Jean find personal integrity, a sense of meaning, and connection with others through an exploration and understanding of her belief system and through good nursing care.

hopeless, and terrified of dying. One was jealous and angry. Faced with such human suffering, helpers need to be able to stay with emotional pain to act as a safe container of powerful feelings. To do this, they need their own personal and professional support systems, which may include faith systems as well as self-reflection and monitoring. The hospice environment provides a healing setting that includes supervision for the practitioners.

Chaplains use prayer and religious practices for some. Should other professionals who are practicing Christians, Jews, Muslims, Hindus, and so on, disclose their own faith allegiances? Should counselors, doctors, nurses, or social workers pray with their patients or clients? Would it help the relationship if the patient requested it? Would it make the professional feel less helpless?

The debate about professionals' belief systems is beginning to take place. Traditionally, psychotherapy and social work practitioners maintained the need to minimize self-disclosure. However, some family therapists question this approach and ask to what extent spiritual and religious beliefs affect their work. This is partly a response to the growing recognition of spiritual distress and the need to foster resilience. Resilience (the capacity to spring back) is a key transactional process that enables individuals and families to manage critical change and offers a defense against collapse and breakdown. It is also about hope, which has been traditionally linked to religion. Would prayer by other professionals weaken the traditional chaplaincy model (Box 12-1)?

The essential difference between supportive listening, using advanced listening skills, and psychotherapeutic interventions with patients or families is the ability to make safe links and connections. Earlier, it was suggested that beliefs can be constraining. If these are safely challenged, an individual or family can effect change. The importance of the meaning of the illness can be accessed by open questions such as, "What are you thinking about your illness?"

Therapies that use life reviews,[13] reminiscence, and creative writing can help patients to explore beliefs, tell the story of illness, and examine the development of selfhood. The narratives of dying people reveal the therapeutic benefits of writing to make sense of illness and give the authors a sense of purpose in sharing their story.[14] Art projects achieve the same purpose.[15]

RESEARCH AND SPIRITUALITY

There has not been a great deal of palliative care research into the nature of spirituality and interventions that might reduce psychosocial and spiritual distress. The psychotherapy literature is anecdotal and is often discounted by medical colleagues. There can be tension between managers and practitioners in some palliative care units and hospices because of a fear that assessment tools and prescribed action can be limiting. Nevertheless, it is vital to understand what helps, when, and by whom (Box 12-2). Chaplains, social workers, and counselors can find working within a medical model frustrating, but they must recognize and value the rigor and discipline of evidence-based medicine. These professional groups lack power in their workplaces but also in medical research foundations; one way forward is collaboration across disciplines and interdisciplinary education and research. This should not just be left to academics, but practitioners should become involved. Recent articles demonstrate a growing interest in spiritual distress and quality of care.[16,17] The use of a spiritual assessment tool[18] and the availability of on-line text allows readers to learn ways of using the tool.

There is a link between a patient's spirituality and treatment choice.[19] The use of the question, "Are you at peace?" by clinicians begins a dialogue about spiritual and emotional well-being. Empirical data exist concerning the spiritual aspects of the dying experience and interventions to relieve existential suffering.[20] Palliative care must continue to develop responses to spiritual distress that are individual and compassionate. This involves the development of a knowledge and skill base for all disciplines to use to recognize, assess, and meet spiritual and psychosocial needs of dying patients. In-depth qualitative research with 25 dying people at St. Christopher's Hospice London revealed insights into patients' lives and the ways in which they used various media to explore their preoccupation with their forthcoming death using language of spirit, symbols, and metaphors.[15]

CONCLUSIONS

Spiritual distress is an important part of the suffering of most dying people. Defining spirituality is complex, but it

---

Box 12-1 Current Controversies

- Will chaplains remain as the leaders of spiritual care, or will another profession appear as spiritual care leaders? What will their training be?
- Should there be a more rigorous attempt to define spirituality and set quality standards?
- If we do not do this, does it mean that standards will remain low because spiritual care continues to lack scrutiny?
- How is spiritual distress assessed, and should all health care professionals in palliative care be able to do these assessments?
- What skills will be needed?
- Where will funding for research come from?

Box 12-2 Research Challenges

- Research is needed to explore the nature of spiritual distress for patients and for their carers. What is the difference between psychosocial and spiritual distress?
- Further research is needed to understand what specific interventions are effective in reducing spiritual and psychosocial distress.
- The research also needs to look at the timings of interventions and to define the skills needed to assess and then deliver interventions.
- How can clinicians develop skills that are quite complex and do not just mean ticking a series of boxes to show that practitioners are spiritually aware?
- How can professionals in palliative care be encouraged to develop an understanding of their own spiritual concerns and belief systems?
- Interdisciplinary education at the postregistration level could encourage research into spiritual distress and care responses. The subject of spiritual distress could be taught more widely.

is concerned with the essence of people, their spirit. Meaning, connectedness, and personal identity and integrity are all important. When dying people approach their death, their spiritual concerns center on meaning and belief. The development of techniques and interventions that relieve distress are based on assessment. This must include an exploration of the patient's belief systems and those of the family or carers. Professionals should be aware of their own belief systems and how they affect the care they provide. Research in this area is scarce, but there is growing evidence that palliative care is beginning to have more dialogue and interest in spirituality. Individuals are developing their own faith systems, which are often a mixture of religious ideas and reflect our multicultural societies. Hospices and other palliative care units are showing a split between religion and spirituality as they move away, in some cases, from their religious foundations.

REFERENCES

1. Craib I. Reflections on mourning in the modern world. Int J Palliat Nurs 1999;5:87-90.
2. Walsh F. Religion and spirituality. In Walsh F (ed). Spiritual Resources in Family Therapy. New York: The Guildford Press, 2003, pp 3-27.
3. Wright L, Watson WL, Bell JM. Beliefs: The heart of healing in families and illness. New York: Basic Books, 1996.
4. Cobb M. The Dying Soul. Buckingham: Open University Press, 2001.
5. Heyse-Moore L. On spiritual pain in the dying. Mortality 1996;1:297-315.
6. Jacques E. Death and the mid life crisis. Int J Psychoanal 1965;46:502-514.
7. Wright M. Good for the soul? In Payne S, Seymour J, Ingleton C (eds). Palliative Care Nursing. Maidenhead: Open University Press, McGraw-Hill Education, 2004, pp 218-241.
8. Frankel VE. Man's Search for Meaning. London: Hodder and Stoughton, 1987.
9. Smith P. Working with family care-givers in palliative care setting. In Payne S, Seymour J, Ingleton C (eds): Palliative Care Nursing. Maidenhead: Open University Press, McGraw-Hill Education, 2004, pp 312-319.
10. Wright L, Leahey M. Nurses and Families: A Guide to Family Assessments and Interventions, 3rd ed. Philadelphia: F.A. Davis, 2000.
11. Dallos R, Draper R. An Introduction to Family Therapy. Buckingham: Open University Press, 2000.
12. Duhamel F, Dupuis F. Families in palliative care: Exploring family and health care professionals' beliefs. Int J Palliat Nurs 2003;3:113-120.
13. Lester J. Life review with the terminally ill: Narrative therapies. In Firth PH, Luff G, Oliviere D (eds). Loss, Change and Bereavement in Palliative Care. Maidenhead: Open University Press, McGraw-Hill Education, 2005, pp 66-80.
14. Bingley AF, McDermott E, Thomas C, et al. Making sense of dying: A review of narratives written since 1950 by people facing death from cancer and other diseases. Palliat Med 2006;20:183-195.
15. Stanworth R. Recognizing spiritual needs in people who are dying. Oxford: Oxford University Press, 2004.
16. Mount FBM. Existential suffering and the determinants of healing. Eur J Palliat Care 2003;10:40-42.
17. Pronk K. Role of doctor in relieving spiritual distress at the end of life. Am J Hospice Palliat Med 2005;22:419-425.
18. Hallenbeck J. Psychosocial and spiritual aspects of care: A spiritual assessment tool. I Hallenbeck J. Palliative Care Perspectives. Oxford: Oxford University Press, 2003.
19. Steinhauser K, Voils CI, Clipp EC, et al. Are you at peace?: One item to probe spiritual concerns at the end of life. Arch Intern Med 2006;166:101-105.
20. Chochinov HM, Hack T, Hassard T, et al. Dignity therapy: A novel psychotherapeutic intervention for patients near the end of life. J Clin Oncol 2005;23:5520-5525.

SUGGESTED READING

Cobb M. Spiritual care. In Lloyd-Williams M (ed). Psychosocial Issues in Palliative Care. Oxford: Oxford University Press, 2005, pp 135-149.

National Institute for Clinical Excellence. Guidance on Cancer Services: Improving Supportive and Palliative Care for Adults with Cancer. London: Nile, 2004.

Speck P. Spiritual issues in palliative care. In Doyle D, Hanks G, Macdonald N (eds). Oxford Textbook of Palliative Medicine. Oxford: Oxford University Press, 1998, pp 805-814.

Walter T. The ideology and organisation of spiritual care: Three approaches. Palliat Med 1997;11:21-30.

CHAPTER **13**

Families in Distress

Matthew Farrelly

- The family should be considered as more than the traditional legal entity.

- The ethos of the organization providing palliative care significantly influences its approach to working with families in distress.

- Skilled team members can help families address their concerns and fears.

- Not all family conflict and estrangement can be resolved, but when it can, resolution eases distress for the patient and family.

- Assessing family needs may assist in directing limited resources to those who need them, but formal assessments of family functioning may not be appropriate.

A terminal illness is potentially one of the most distressing experiences that a family will ever have to face, bringing changes to its structure and emotional fabric that can threaten its very survival. The role of the palliative care team is to join with the family in providing support to achieve the adaptation that terminal illness and bereavement inevitably demand. Drawing on clinical experience in palliative care and using case studies, this chapter explores common challenges faced by families dealing with terminal illness. How the process of assessment helps the multidisciplinary palliative care team to respond to such challenges is also considered.

WHO IS THE FAMILY?

It is important to consider who is included in the family. Depending on geographical and cultural factors, the identified membership, expectations of roles, patterns of behavior, and rules of emotional expression may vary considerably.[1] Contemporary Western society has seen changes in family structures due to many social factors. These include increased levels of separation and divorce; increased numbers of single-parent families, remarriages, and so-called "blended families"; and increased acknowledgment of same-sex relationships. These factors invite us to view the concept of family through a broader lens, placing the patient within a network of relationships that are not restricted by any rigid definition.

The World Health Organization states that family includes either relatives or other significant people as defined by the patient.[2] It is helpful to think of patients' "social family and carers" as well as their "legal family." Although family membership can have important legal implications in relation to a claim on a deceased person's estate, there is also a clear rationale for including other important relationships and identifying people involved in the patient's care toward the end of life.

Such an approach can alleviate distress, because it helps the patient communicate his or her most significant caring relationships irrespective of legal status. Distress can relate to expectations from others that a particular family member should be a carer for their relative. There may also be associated fear of negative judgment from the palliative care team if the person is not able to carry out this role.[3] Caring for a family member who is terminally ill and coping with the adjustment and stress this brings is acknowledged as one of the major challenges faced by any family.[4] Exploring factors that influence family members' availability as carers, rather than assuming they can perform this role, is essential. The first case study illustrates this issue (see "Case Study: Assumptions about Who Will Provide Care"). This case study illustrates the physical and emotional exhaustion experienced by some caregivers and the pressure they may feel from within the family to undertake a particular role. For some the burden of care can be overwhelming. It also demonstrates how the assessment of patient and family is a shared task, because different team members collaborate in gathering information over time.

ASSESSING FAMILIES IN DISTRESS

A dominant discourse argues that a formal assessment is valuable so that limited resources can be directed to those families that are considered to need them most. This position is reflected in the work of Kissane and Bloch.[5] In their research and development of Family Focused Grief Therapy (FFGT), they used formal assessment tools to develop a typology of family functioning. Three key dimensions of family functioning were identified: "cohesiveness," "conflict," and "expressiveness."

- Cohesiveness describes the family's ability to function together as a team and is considered to be the most important characteristic of a well-functioning family.
- A family's ability to resolve conflict is indicative of "adaptiveness" and is also considered to be an important characteristic.
- "Expressiveness," which is critical, describes a family's ability to share their opinions and feelings with each other.

These three dimensions were used to establish a typology of family functioning that identified five different family types: supportive families, conflict-resolving families, hostile families, sullen families, and intermediate families. The first two categories are considered to be well-functioning units and less vulnerable than the hostile and the sullen categories, which these researchers considered to be dysfunctional and in most need of intervention. Intermediate families, as the term suggests, lie in between.

The association between family type and level of distress is the key,[5] because it provides a means of identifying vulnerable families with whom preventive interventions can be initiated (p. 46). The major goals of FFGT are "to improve family functioning and promote adaptive grieving" (p. 47). The model places responsibility on the team to assess the competence of the family and "actively treat

CASE STUDY

Assumptions about Who Will Provide Care

Mary is a 78-year-old woman admitted to hospice for symptom control. She is a widow with six adult children. During the early days of her admission, she tells nursing staff that her main carers are two neighbors and her unmarried daughter, Julie, who calls every day after work. Two of her children live overseas, and her two other sons and a daughter live in other parts of the country. They visit her occasionally, when work and family commitments allow. Midway through the second week of her admission, a family meeting is proposed by the team to discuss future care.

Mary is enthusiastic about the family meeting and relates that her pain is much better controlled and that she is looking forward to going home. Julie tells nursing staff that family members have not met together since her mother was first diagnosed and is keen for the meeting to be arranged. She also suggests that her mother's two neighbors should be invited to the meeting, because they were providing most of Mary's care before her admission to hospice. As the conversation with the nurse continues, Julie becomes tearful and admits that she is exhausted. She feels unable to tell her mother that she cannot cope with the pressures of working full-time while also playing a major role in her future care. Her perception is that her siblings believe that she is more available for this role because she is unmarried and that she should give up her job to care for her mother. Julie finds work a "distraction" from facing the reality of her mother's pending death and also believes it will help her during her bereavement. She says she is comfortable spending time with her mother but is unable to provide intimate physical care, which her mother now requires.

Over the following days, staff members telephone various family members but find it impossible to arrange a time when more than two family members are able to attend a meeting with the team. Several family members say it is not necessary for them to attend the family meeting because they are happy for their sister Julie to update them and that she is their mother's main carer.

During a team meeting, the social worker reports that Julie has asked her to inform the team that she cannot continue as her mother's main carer. She feels this is a position in which the family have placed her in without appreciating the other responsibilities she has in her life. She has asked the social worker to help her communicate this situation to her mother and to explain that alternative arrangements for her care will have to be made.

it when it is disarrayed" (p. 197). This brings into question the extent of the role of the palliative care team, as well as the level of resources that such an approach might require.

In reality, assessment is a much more informal process that takes place as the unfolding story of the family life is shared with the team over time. In my experience, many families in distress, although open to receiving psychosocial support, do not consent to a formal assessment of family functioning or contract for family therapy. They get to know the team over time and are happy to receive help with particular issues regarding communication, conflict, and enhancing expression of emotion to improve family relations. However, they do not perceive that the palliative care team is responsible for "actively treating" them. Furthermore, family members have contact with the team on a voluntary basis, and there is no obligation for them to seek support or make use of it if offered. Contact with families may be short or long term, varying from a few days or weeks to several months or more than a year. One of the current controversies in this area is the extent of the role of the palliative care team in the provision of long-term therapeutic work with families in distress.

The value of FFGT lies with the identification of the critical factors of cohesion, conflict, and expressiveness, which provide a useful framework for working with families. However, it is helpful to consider alternative approaches. The models that I have found most helpful in working with patients and distressed families are those of Narrative Therapy[6] and structured Life Review work.[7]

Narrative Therapy

Narrative therapy is based on the view that people have many stories by which they live their lives and relationships, occurring simultaneously. The stories about individuals and families are determined by how certain events have been linked together and by the meaning attributed to them.[8] Narrative therapists work with the dominant stories and alternative stories of an individual's or family's life. Alternative stories may be unearthed that stress different behaviors or different aspects of family life not previously told. The dominant story of a family as "dysfunctional" can be challenged by exploring other possible meanings of particular actions that do not fit with this "problem-saturated description." The alternative story can then influence changes in how the individual or family view themselves and how they might choose to act in the future.

Life Review Work

Narrative therapy informs structured Life Review work, which also offers an opportunity to bring about change in interpersonal relationships. As Lester described it,[7] "The basis for a structured Life Review stems from an understanding of life span psychology, which indicates the importance of personal growth and gives particular attention to conflict resolution and the continuing development of a person's coping strategies when facing life crises" (p. 67).

Life Review work enables the patient to review significant life events and to explore happiness, sadness, fear, achievement, and regret. The patient's social and relational history is reviewed, inviting integration of experience and acknowledgment of the values and attitudes that inform his or her actions. It involves bringing to the surface the rich story of a person's life and relationships, to sit alongside the previously dominant story of illness and medical systems. This process may lead to particular actions before death, including attention to family relationships (see "Case Study: Life Review and Reconnection with Family," which features this approach). As Freedman and Combs stated,[9]

> Narrative therapists are interested in working with people to bring forth and thicken stories that do not support or sustain problems. As people begin to inhabit and live out the alternative stories, the results are beyond solving problems. Within

CASE STUDY

Life Review and Reconnecting with Family

John is a 57-year-old man who was admitted to the hospice inpatient unit for terminal care with esophageal cancer. On admission, he reported that he was the last surviving member of his siblings and had had no contact with his wife or two children for more than 25 years, since the breakup of his marriage. His only friends were a married couple, Bernard and Elizabeth, and their two children, who referred to him as "Grand Dad John." He had gotten to know the family some years previously, and they had been caring for him in his apartment for the last few months.

In conversation with the hospice social worker, John began to review major incidents in his life. He spoke about the regrets of his marriage breakup and the loss of contact with his children, which occurred at a time when he had been drinking heavily. At various times, he had considered trying to make contact with his wife and children again, but he was afraid that they would reject him. It was only when the social worker pointed out that his relationship with Bernard and his family had endured for more than 12 years that John began to appreciate his capacity to successfully maintain close personal relationships. Subsequently, the social worker asked him whether he would like her to contact his family, explaining that there would be no guarantee that she would be able to find them or that they would want to meet him. After some days thinking about this, John decided that he would like to trace his family, saying that this was something he would like to do before he died.

Within 2 weeks, the social worker located John's children, who agreed to meet with her. At the meeting, the social worker explained that John was in the hospice and that he had spoken about his desire to meet his children again. His son and daughter, although sad and hurt by what had happened to them in their childhood, agreed that they would meet their father if it would help him before he died. A visit was arranged to the hospice, and, with John's consent, his children were given information by the team about his physical condition to help prepare them for the meeting. The social worker introduced them to their father, and after a few minutes she felt comfortable enough to leave them talking together. John told his children that he had considered tracing them on several occasions over the years but had been fearful that they would reject him because of his past behavior. He apologized to them for the pain of the past and thanked them for coming to visit him.

This tearful reunion was the beginning of a series of visits to John before he died. He was delighted to learn that he had four grandchildren and received a visit from them enthusiastically. After that particular meeting, the social worker visited John and found him smiling broadly. He said he now felt a "sense of security and belonging," knowing that he was in touch with his family again. A week later, he received a visit from his wife in the presence of the social worker and was able to apologize for his part in the breakup of their marriage 25 years earlier. John's family subsequently met his friends, Bernard and Elizabeth and their children. This pattern of visiting by John's family and friends continued over the next month before he died peacefully. They all attended his funeral, and children from all parts of John's "different families" read prayers at his funeral Mass.

the new stories people live out new self images, new possibilities for relationships and new futures.

These alternative or subordinate stories which are not immediately accessible would almost certainly be excluded from any formal assessment of family functioning. Moreover, they may well indicate that the family functions somewhat better than initially thought and has potential to respond positively to the demands of transition. We need to be careful that we do not restrict ourselves with limited views of what a family should look like or how it should function, but rather look for creative ways of working with all kinds of families.

THE NEED FOR INFORMATION: MAINTAINING TRUST

In my experience, many patients do not openly acknowledge the terminal nature of their illness; for those who do, the most commonly expressed fears are those summarized in Table 13-1. Some of these fears are shared by both patient and family members.

Clear information shared sensitively is a prerequisite for families if healthy change and adaptation is to be promoted. The crucial first step in the process should take place during the referral stage, when consent is obtained from the patient to share information about his or her situation with the family and vice versa. Resistance to establishing this feedback loop between patient, staff, and family can indicate blocks in communication. This may provide an entry point for the team to offer an appropriate intervention.

Families require information regarding a range of different issues. The provision of information about disease progress, pain management, and how to provide care is an essential component in helping those who are undertaking the painful transition brought about by the illness

and death of a family member. Whereas some people wish to know a clear prognosis, others prefer to cope with the situation "day-to-day," and it is important to respect difference in this area. Some people have particular fears about how death will actually occur; for example, being worried that the patient may choke or have uncontrollable pain. This may result from perceptions of how somebody died in the past, and it may be possible to alleviate these fears. Other kinds of information may also be needed, such as the availability of social welfare entitlements and how to access services in the community.

Sensitive and skillful communication is essential in maintaining a trusting relationship among the patient, family, and team. Regular team meetings offer an opportunity for ongoing assessment of the family's response to the patient's changing situation and planning appropriate interventions. Although team members communicate with various family members during inpatient visiting or during visits to the patient's home, other meetings are also important. Formal family meetings, organized by the team, provide an opportunity for all family members to gather together to meet representatives from the palliative care team. This allows the family to hear information first hand from team members and to voice concerns and fears. In this way, information is not "filtered" by a family member who may want to protect or exclude another person. During the meeting, family members also hear other people's questions, thus gaining a greater sense of the experience of the whole family. This flow of new information opens communication and also provides an opportunity for shared expression of emotion.

During a family meeting, the team can also explore family members' responses to the illness. Often, people tell stories of past incidents that reveal rich details of family life. It is an opportunity both to normalize various aspects of family responses and to offer additional support to family members if concerns arise; for example, if a

TABLE 13-1 Common Fears and Hopes of Terminally Ill Patients and Their Families	
THE PATIENT	**THE FAMILY**
Fear and experience of pain and other symptoms	Fear that the patient will suffer uncontrolled pain and other symptoms around the time of death
Fear of death; the nature of death (How will I die? Will it be painful?); hope to die peacefully	Worry because the patient is frightened and anxious; hope this will stop, sometimes with unrealistic expectations
Fear of being a burden to family or carers	Inability to carry out the patient's wishes regarding care (patient may want to die at home whereas family members are frightened of this possibility; family members may not want to tell the patient this and may seek admission of their loved one to hospital or hospice or refuse to take the patient home)
Hope to be cared for by family or carers at home	Fear of honest discussion about death with the patient; may want staff not to tell the truth
Spiritual fears (depending on belief system); fear of the unknown, fear that there is no afterlife or fear of punitive judgment by God, loss of faith, anger at God	Worry about the future and the impact of bereavement; loss of the person who is ill (may depend on role, as with the parent of young children)
Anger; sense of injustice; not wanting to die; why me?	Worry about the impact of bereavement on particular family members considered vulnerable
Worry about unresolved conflicts	
Worry about how the family are coping with patient's illness	
Worry about how the family will cope in the future (socially, emotionally, financially)	
Worry about whether he or she will be remembered	

family has particular difficulties in communicating with young children about the illness.

Not all family meetings have positive outcomes. Clinical experience has included angry exchanges between family members and, on one occasion, physical confrontations and violence immediately after the meeting ended.

If an individual or family experience adjustment difficulties, they may require information to be reinforced and repeated several times during different meetings. Other families may resist meeting staff to avoid hearing bad news. A great deal of work by the team may be required to communicate the necessary information, and this can be both time-consuming and frustrating for those involved. Families experiencing high levels of distress should be offered additional support from the multidisciplinary team. The second case study is an example of this approach (see "Case Study: Difficulties of Visitation in Hospice Home Care"). In this case study, the impact of terminal illness on complex family relationships and the role of the palliative care team in giving additional support to the family are demonstrated. In particular, conflict was resolved and Elaine's position was acknowledged. This reduced the very high levels of distress both for the patient and the family.

FAMILY CONFLICT: ESTRANGEMENT AND REUNIFICATION

Distress in families can sometimes be traced back to events or disagreements that took place many years previously. This may have resulted in estrangement of family members, sometimes with people not having seen each other or spoken for many years. It is often a source of considerable distress, because the patient's death will remove any opportunity for reconciliation. Awareness of such estrangements is an opportunity for the team to explore with the patient whether he or she would like to achieve some improvement in the relationship before death. This work often involves extensive efforts to trace people who have not been in contact for many years, but it can be a most valuable aspect of psychosocial support for families in distress.

Assisting patients and family members on a journey of forgiveness and healing can be a critical factor in helping them face death with a greater sense of calm and peace.[10] While recognizing the value of work in this area, it is important to report that not all situations of estrangement can be resolved positively. My experience includes several occasions in which efforts to trace relatives were successful, only to find that they declined any invitation to be reconciled. In order to avoid causing additional distress by building up unrealistic hopes, it is important to be mindful of the possibility that reunification may not be

---

CASE STUDY 2

Difficulties of Visitation in Hospice Home Care

Pat is a 35-year-old man receiving terminal care from the hospice home care team due to his brain tumor. He is the youngest of nine children and up until recently had been living at home with his elderly father. Pat's mother died 5 years ago, and all of his siblings are married with children. For the last 2 months Pat has been living with his brother, Ian, his sister-in-law, Mary, and their three sons, aged 5, 7, and 8, because his father was no longer able to care for him. Pat has been in a long-term relationship with his partner Elaine, and, although they have a son, Damien, age 4, and a daughter, Patricia, age 3, they have never lived together. Although Ian and Pat have always had a close relationship, Ian's wife Mary has never approved of Pat's relationship with Elaine. Some years ago, Ian also fell out with a brother, Tommy; although they meet occasionally at family functions, they do not visit each other's homes. Pat has also been a very significant figure in the lives of his 23 nieces and nephews, who range from 5 to 19 years old.

During a recent home visit, the home care nurse spoke with Mary and Ian and heard that Mary was extremely upset because other family members were arriving on a daily basis to visit Pat without phoning first. A schedule of visiting that had been arranged by Ian had not been maintained, and the previous day Mary had asked one of Pat's sisters to come back later because the family were trying to have a meal together. This led to a row, during which Pat's sister said she would not come back to the house again because she did not feel welcome. Mary also stated that, although she was very happy to care for Pat, she no longer wanted his partner Elaine coming to the family home. During nursing visits, Pat had been quite sleepy and able to participate only in short conversations, but was able to tell the nurse how well he was being cared for and that he did not want to go into the hospice inpatient unit. He said he enjoyed the visits from Elaine, his children, and his father. He told the nurse that he missed his nieces and nephews and would like to see them if they kept their visits short. In addition, he expressed a wish to see Tommy and his wife. He told the nurse that he knew Mary had been very upset the previous day and that there had been an argument with his sister Maura. Pat asked the nurse if she could help his family, because he was worried about them. The hospice nurse discussed the situation in a team meeting the next day, and a family meeting was arranged. This meeting was attended by a total of 18 family members, including Elaine, along with the home care nurse, one of the doctors, and a hospice social worker.

During the meeting, the family were assisted to talk openly about their wishes to see their brother for brief periods at this time. It was acknowledged that Ian and Mary were providing excellent care for Pat. Several family members said that they would not be able to provide this care and were grateful that Ian and Mary could. People spoke about the hurt that had been experienced when some family members felt excluded by others. People also spoke about how Ian and Mary needed a degree of privacy to attend to their own needs as a couple with three young children. Ian and Mary made a clear statement that they wanted to carry out Pat's wishes at this time and acknowledged that people who were important to him, including Elaine, should be able to visit. The family spoke about the bond they shared despite the ups and downs of family life and the disagreements. Tommy crossed the room and embraced Ian and Mary, thanking them for everything they were doing and offering his support. By the end of the meeting, the family were able to make arrangements for visits and assistance for Ian and Mary. The social worker also arranged further counseling sessions for some of the family members.

achieved. If we do not consider this possibility, then we misrepresent the reality of working with families in palliative care.

The third case study is an example of reunification work in a palliative care setting (see "Case Study: Life Review and Reconnecting with Family"). In this case study, the Life Review work (see earlier discussion) unearthed an alternative story of John's life, one that contradicted the dominant story that he was a failure at maintaining close personal relationships. The integration of this reality allowed him to take the risk of seeking reunification with his own family despite the possibility of rejection.

This case study also illustrates the extent to which reunification depends on the openness of all those affected to participate. John's family, despite past hurts, had always lived with the hope of meeting him again. In particular, his wife spoke about forgiveness and how she had brought her children up to believe in this value. In this instance, the level of distress was greatly reduced by reunification. Furthermore, the case study demonstrates the value of having team members who are skilled in working with distressed families.

The ethos of the organization providing the care is critical in determining how much energy and resources are devoted to this type of "whole-person care." According to Kearney,[11] the human experience is multidimensional, and pain in one area of the human experience can affect another. Moreover, human beings are whole persons, and "the most appropriate and effective response this demands is one of attention and care to all aspects of that person's experience, including his or her relationships."[11] In this case study, the approach to caring for John as a "whole person" had a significant impact on relieving his distress and that of his various families. The ethos of the organization can be seen as critical to the approach to working with and supporting families in distress in a palliative care setting.

THE INFLUENCE OF THE TEAM

The way in which the palliative care team responds to a family in distress is critical. The interaction between team and family is the coming together of two different systems engaging in a joint activity to achieve a shared goal; namely, the optimal care of the patient. Systems theory informs us that the palliative care team "as a system has specific attitudes, values, and rules of acceptable behaviors that may vary significantly from not only the patient and family but also from team to team. . . . [U]nder the best circumstances, the optimal result is an effective therapeutic fit between the patient, family, and health care staff."[12] It is important to be mindful of different family structures and cultural norms. An example of this was a case in which a palliative care team was working with an African family living in Ireland. The team wished to communicate directly with the female patient about having an injection for pain, whereas her husband expected communication to be directed through him. This led to a heightened level of distress for both family and team. The patient's family of origin operated within a patriarchal culture with expectations different from those of team members. The team was challenged by the issue of patient autonomy and informed consent, but the patient did not

share their concern. The influence of different cultural norms and family structures was evident. However, it is also important to note that no two families are the same; rather than uniformity, there is often significant variation among families who share similar cultural backgrounds.

The palliative care team will face challenges when patients' or family members' behaviors fall outside the boundaries of what is expected or deemed acceptable. As Altschuler stated, "We may also find ourselves acting in ways that reflect not only our own experiences but also that of the family, as we identify with and 'mirror' different aspects of family relationships."[3] It may also be the case that some patterns of behavior are the result of increased psychological and emotional distress. How a team responds to such situations is very important. If it is possible for a team to model openness to discuss issues that arise, such as conflict between family members and staff, then this may allow families to address difficult issues themselves. Crucially, the behavior of the palliative care team can escalate or reduce patterns of behavior associated with distress by family members.

CONCLUSIONS

Palliative care acknowledges the importance of family relationships and aims to offer support to those affected by the patient's terminal illness. The family includes all significant relationships identified by the patient and is not restricted by legal definition. The process of loss and change with which families must contend is often associated with particular concerns and fears that cause high levels of distress. Although some believe that formal assessments should be carried out on all families to identify and treat those needing long-term help with the process of adaptation, an alternative view has been presented. This approach advocates a more fluid, informal assessment that resists labeling families and incorporates attention to the "alternative story" of the social and relational history of the patient and family. The family are accepted as they are, living their unique experience and responding in ways that make sense to them in their situation. They also choose whether to accept any offer of support. Clinical experience indicates that the ethos of the organization significantly influences the priority the team is able to give to working with families in distress, but it is also important to note that not all attempts to help families are successful. Finally, the value of team members' being trained in systematic family therapy is acknowledged, and the application of such skills should enhance the delivery of psychosocial care.

REFERENCES

1. Carr A. Family Therapy: Concepts, Process and Practice. Chichester, England: John Wiley & Sons, 2000.
2. World Health Organization. Cancer Pain and Palliative Care. Technical Report 804. Geneva: WHO, 1990.
3. Altschuler J. Illness and loss within the family. In Firth P, Luff G, Oliviere D (eds). Loss, Change and Bereavement in Palliative Care. London: Open University Press, 2005, pp 53-64.
4. Carter B, McGoldrick M. The Changing Family Lifecycle: A Framework for Family Therapy, 2nd ed. New York: Gardner, 1989.
5. Kissane DW, Bloch S. Family Focused Grief Therapy. Philadelphia: Open University Press, 2002.
6. White M, Epston D. Narrative Means to Therapeutic Ends. New York: W.W. Norton, 1990.

7. Lester J. Life review with the terminally ill: Narrative therapies. In Firth P, Luff G, Oliviere D (eds). Loss, Change and Bereavement in Palliative Care, 1st ed. London: Open University Press, 2005, pp 66-79.
8. Morgan A. What is narrative therapy? Available at http://www.dulwichcentre.com.au/alicearticle.html (accessed September 2007).
9. Freedman J, Combs G. Narrative Therapy: The Social Construction of Preferred Realities. New York: Norton, 1996.
10. Byock I. The Four Things That Matter Most: A Book About Living. New York: Free Press, 2004.
11. Kearney M. Whole person care: The Irish dimension. In Ling J, O'Síoráin L (eds). Palliative Care in Ireland, 1st ed. Berkshire: Open University Press, 2005, pp 122-133.
12. Loscalzo MJ, Zabora JR. Care of the cancer patient: Response of family and staff. In Bruera E, Portenoy RK (eds). Topics in Palliative Care, Vol 2. New York: Oxford University Press, 1998, pp 209-245.

SUGGESTED READING

Firth P, Luff G, Oliviere D (eds): Loss, Change and Bereavement in Palliative Care, 1st ed. London: Open University Press, 2005.

Kissane DW, Bloch S. Family Focused Grief Therapy. Philadelphia: Open University Press, 2002.

White C, Denborough D (eds). Introducing Narrative Therapy. Adelaide, Australia: Dulwich Centre Publications, 1998.

CHAPTER **14**

Grief and Bereavement

Wendy G. Lichtenthal and David W. Kissane

K E Y P O I N T S

- Bereavement care begins at entry to palliative care services with screening for adverse factors such as family dysfunction and with continued psychosocial care for those at risk.

- Theoretical models of attachment, interpersonal relationships, coping with change, and sociocultural factors influence clinical grief.

- Normal grief is distinguished from morbid grief through lower symptom intensity, symptom resolution over time, and absent maladaptive coping and psychiatric disorders.

- Risk factors for morbid grief include witnessing a difficult death, personal vulnerability, insecure attachment styles, and poor family and social support.

- Preventive grief interventions should be offered only in high-risk situations; if psychiatric disorders complicate bereavement, early psychotherapy and psychopharmacology are indicated.

Mourning typically begins before loss, and knowledge and comfort with expression of grief are critical in palliative medicine. As illness advances, patients and families face multiple losses in physical and mental health, roles, activities, and relationships. The dying patient and his or her family may simultaneously grieve these cumulative losses and mourn the impending death. Continuity of care before and after bereavement is critical because trust in clinicians who cared for their loved one underpins effective support for the family after the loss.

A family-focused approach to care permits clinicians to enhance quality of life for the patient and family, which, in turn, can positively affect bereavement.[1] Specifically, clinicians can facilitate understanding of the dying process, work to temper anxiety-provoking uncertainty before the death, and aid the family in making sense of the loss (see Chapter 13). This support is particularly important after sudden, unexpected deaths, which still occur during palliative care.

The literature uses many terms to indicate reactions to loss, often interchangeably. However, grief theorists maintain specific definitions:

- *Bereavement:* the *state* of loss resulting from death[2,3]
- *Grief:* the distressing *emotional response* to any loss[2]
- *Mourning:* the *process of adaptation,* which includes cultural and social rituals[4]
- *Anticipatory grief:* the *distress* that occurs before an expected loss[4]
- *Pathological, complicated or prolonged grief:* an *abnormal emotional response* to loss involving mental and/or physical health morbidity[5,6]
- *Disenfranchised grief:* hidden grief, typically among individuals who have less social permission to express their response[7]

THEORETICAL MODELS OF GRIEF

Why do we grieve? Observations of mourning among social birds and mammals date back to Darwin. Bonding and social relationships have a functionally adaptive value, but attachment implies a grief experience when separation occurs. Death is universal, but the emotional response to loss is shaped culturally. Theoretical models from multiple disciplines[2,5] guide conceptualization of the clinical phenomena in the bereaved and suggest adaptive tasks facilitated by preventive interventions. Table 14-1 presents an overview of major bereavement theories.

Among the most influential concepts is *attachment theory.* This focuses on interpersonal bonding, which creates a foundation of security and promotion of survival through social support.[8] Exploration of the world and personal individuation flow from this sense of safety. Primary attachments develop between the parents, particularly the mother, and the child but are replaced in adulthood by attachment to the spouse. The initial parent–child relationship affects future attachments. A cornerstone of this theory, based largely on the pioneering work of Mary Ainsworth, is the distinction between secure and insecure attachments. Ainsworth classified insecure attachment styles as anxious, avoidant, or disorganized/hostile.[9] These can be transgenerational, with parents passing down insecure styles to their children. When a loss occurs and bonds are severed, attachment theory posits that mourning is affected by an individual's attachment style.

Another theory is the *psychodynamic theory.*[5] It shares elements with attachment theory but focuses on early life

TABLE 14-1 Theoretical Models of Mourning

MODEL	DEFINING CHARACTERISTICS	MAJOR FIGURES
Attachment theory	The bonds of close relationships are severed by loss	Bowlby, Ainsworth, Parkes, Weiss
Psychodynamic theory	Early relationships lay down a template that guides future relationships	Freud, Klein, Horowitz, Kohut
Interpersonal model	Relational influences are dominant in grief outcome	Sullivan, Shapiro, Bonnano, Horowitz, Benjamin
Psychosocial transition	Changed assumptive world view and related beliefs	Parkes, Janoff-Bulman
Sociological model	Cultural influences shape the form and content of grief	Rosenblatt, Klass, Walter
Family systems theory	Family are the main source of support; family functioning determines outcome	Walsh, McGoldrick, Kissane, Shapiro
Cognitive stress coping theory	Conditioned or learned patterns become entrenched and chronic	Kavanagh, Folkman
Traumatic model	Intrusive aspects of trauma dominate	Horowitz, Pynoos, Prigerson, Jacobs
Ethology	Biological and physiological processes underpin the phenomena across species	Darwin, Lorenz
Dual process coping theory	Oscillation between loss- and restoration-oriented coping tasks	M.S. Stroebe, W. Stroebe, Schut

experiences, development of self-esteem, and the acquired ability to mourn. Object relations theory conceptualizes early relationships as models of interaction that influence the emotions of subsequent relationships. One of the earliest relational templates is when an infant yearns for its mother after separation. Grief and pining are viewed as adaptive coping responses that persist throughout life after separations.

Also rooted in psychoanalytic theory is the *grief work hypothesis*, which asserts that individuals must work through their feelings about loss to sever their bonds with the deceased.[2,5] Freud[10] identified this process as necessary to normal mourning in order to detach libido invested in the loved object; pathological grief is caused by failure to achieve the required tasks. Although the "grief work" hypothesis has been influential, little empirical support for it has emerged.[2,5]

More recently, theorists have examined interpersonal models that complement the psychodynamic approach.[5] Relationship patterns are viewed as expectations based on past experiences; these influence current relationships. A person's identity and associated self schemas develop via interactions with others and roles within these relationships. The stress–response model of grief views these schemas as modifiable, with interventions based on specific principles. Modification of an "ambivalent" schema, which stems from mixed feelings about the deceased, can be identified from current relationships.

Another theory considers psychosocial transitions in *adaptation to loss*. Parkes[3] asserted that critical tasks in adjustment include changing one's belief system, or "assumptive world," to accommodate loss. This involves accepting the inevitability of life changes. Neimeyer,[11] a proponent of a related perspective termed "meaning reconstruction," emphasized a person's need to make sense of loss by organizing his or her understanding into a coherent narrative. Coping through meaning-making can produce positive emotion, which (according to cognitive stress theory and a social-functional perspective), helps sustain well-being, adaptation, and enhanced interpersonal relatedness.[2,5]

The impact of society on individual mourning is the cornerstone of the sociological model (see Chapter 2). Social constructionists assert that emotional expression is largely dictated by culture and social norms.[5] Cultural differences in grieving and related mourning rituals are considerable, influencing emotional expression, practices such as self-mutilation, and public versus private grief. Researchers have emphasized the role of social influences in shaping mourning via specific cultural rituals. These support continuing, not severed, bonds with the deceased; for instance, by revering ancestors and trusting them as spiritual guides.[5] Another means of preserving the relationship is by continuing to speak with or about the deceased.

Other social factors affect the individual grief experience. Social support can reduce isolation and enhance adjustment. Social connectedness is particularly important within a bereaved family (see Chapter 65). The family systems perspective considers the reciprocal relationship between an individual's response to loss and that of their family, which is dependent on family functioning and the role of the deceased.[12] Family dysfunction, poor communication, low cohesion, and increased conflict predict greater psychosocial morbidity after loss (see Chapter 13).[1,13]

Cognitive-behavioral theorists focus on thoughts and behaviors that maintain grief and may prolong mourning.[5,14] Excessive preoccupation with the deceased, such as creating elaborate memorials or chronic weeping at reminders, hinders the bereaved from moving forward. Similarly, avoidant behaviors may prolong grief through negative reinforcement. Avoidant individuals may not process the loss and may deprive themselves of pleasurable, corrective activities.

Some behaviors may help. The Dual Process Theory of coping with bereavement suggests the importance of both approach and avoidance in moderation.[5] This theory posits that both loss-orientation and restoration-orientation tasks are involved in adaptive coping. The former refers to thoughts, emotions, and behaviors centered on the loss; this is how "grief work" is undertaken and the loss confronted. In parallel are coping strategies focused on the world without the deceased; that is, restoring functioning. Positive reappraisal of what the loss means leads to new goals. Oscillation between loss-oriented and restoration-oriented phases permits the bereaved person to actively confront his or her grief for a time and then engage in a period of respite, making efforts to return to premorbid functioning.[2,5]

CLINICAL PRESENTATIONS OF GRIEF

Palliative care providers witness family, carers, and friends navigate the mourning process, from anticipatory distress to acute grief upon learning of the patient's death, to (for a subset of individuals) psychopathology or prolonged grief disorder, previously referred to as complicated grief.

Anticipatory Grief

Families often begin grieving as they understand a patient's terminal condition.[4] Additionally, they may grieve interim losses as overall functioning decreases due to illness and treatment. These can include loss of job, functional family role, independence, leisure activities, physical capacity, and a sense of certainty about the future. Coping with these losses may result in the family's becoming closer and more cohesive as they comfort one another, care for the patient, and adapt to the changes. Anticipatory grief among more dysfunctional families can cause denial, avoidance, withdrawal, or hostility (see Chapter 13). Psychosocial morbidity may manifest as depressive or anxiety disorders. Although theorists suggest that anticipatory grief mitigates the intensity of mourning after death, findings are inconsistent, suggesting that intense anticipatory grief is a risk factor for prolonged grief disorder.[15]

Clinicians can assist adaptive families with anticipatory grief to communicate openly, to honor the patient, and begin to say goodbye by expressing their appreciation and resolving any loose ends. Such deeds create opportunities for positive emotions alongside grief and distress.

Grief at the Time of Death

The experiences around the patient's bed, when family and friends are emotionally charged and pay special attention to the patient's appearance and needs, are often etched into the survivors' memories. Staff interactions with the patient and loved ones require utmost respect and sensitivity. Of particular value is information about the dying process, including the meaning of sounds, secretions, changes in breathing, and level of consciousness. Included is empathy and reassurance about the patient's comfort (see Chapter 181).

If the family is not present, they should be notified when the patient's deterioration is evident or, if death has already occurred, invited to view the body and informed of the sequence of events that preceded death. The palliative care worker must take time to answer questions thoroughly and provide comfort and support. Wishes about autopsy, including any cultural or religious sanctions, warrant respect. Clinicians should facilitate pastoral counseling and encourage religious or cultural rituals, including time alone with the deceased. They should take care not to marginalize grief, for example after an expected death, and to provide survivors with permission to express their sorrow. These considerations prevent disenfranchised grief.[7]

Additional family support may be indicated, although variations in acute grief must be kept in mind. Consultation with a cultural intermediary may assist in understanding responses and how best to provide a space for specific practices. Clinicians may prescribe benzodiazepines and offer support with a follow-up phone call the next day.

Common Errors
• Offering grief interventions to all, rather than respecting resilience and targeting those at high risk • Avoiding the difficult but supporting the likable carers or well-functioning families • Assuming similarity and underestimating differential responses to loss • Being insensitive to culturally specific mourning responses and rituals • Normalizing all grief and not recognizing psychiatric disorders

Expressions of sympathy and direction about how to proceed (e.g., contacting the undertaker) are usually appreciated (see "Common Errors").

Acute Grief after the Death

Because intense negative emotional responses are typical after bereavement, it can be challenging to distinguish normal grief from pathological reactions. The first empirical study of bereavement was done among individuals who lost a relative in a nightclub fire in Boston during 1942. This study found that the bereaved relatives experienced guilt and anger, were preoccupied with memories, and identified with symptoms experienced by the deceased.[5]

Normal grief has characteristic emotional, cognitive, behavioral, and physical symptoms. Common affective responses include sadness, guilt, despair, anger, and anxiety. Memories dominate, with frequent reminiscing about the deceased. Typical behaviors include social withdrawal, efforts to seek social support and comfort, and searching for reminders. Physical symptoms include difficulty sleeping, fatigue, anorexia, mild weight loss, numbness, restlessness, tension, tremors, and sometimes pain.

For years, mourning was conceptualized as a process of emotional stages that needed to be traversed for it to be resolved.[16] However, such stage theories have not been confirmed. Instead, the commonly held view on recovery today is that phases overlap, grief diminishes gradually, but a residual bond to the deceased remains.[5] The initial phase of acute grief is frequently characterized by shock and disbelief. Intense waves of distress, often characterized by a yearning for and triggered by memories of the deceased, may follow. As the pain associated with the absence is felt and realized by the survivors, there may be disorganization characterized by sadness, restlessness, inattention, social withdrawal, and despair; these can persist for months. A phase of reorganization of life without the deceased occurs in time, allowing a new world view and the potential for personal growth and creativity.[2,5,11] This phase can be accompanied by feelings of nostalgia and heightened mood rather than sadness.

There is no definitive time period for grief to resolve. The duration is often proportionate to the strength of attachment to the deceased and may persist for years among the conjugally bereaved elderly. Cultural sanctions also affect duration (see Chapter 2).[7] Some researchers hypothesize that normal and pathological grief are on a continuum and that the latter is an intensification of the former. Another conceptualization of normal grief is the absence of prolonged grief disorder (see later discussion).

Pathological Grief

Distress is expected, and some symptoms of depression, anxiety, and post-traumatic stress disorder (PTSD) may emerge. Prevalence of depressive disorders among the bereaved is highest during the first 2 months but subsequently declines. Zisook and Schuchter[17] found that 24% of bereaved widows in a longitudinal study met criteria for major depression after 2 months and that this figure decreased to 16% by 13 months. Anxiety disorders are prevalent, and individuals may present with separation anxiety, generalized anxiety, and phobic or somatic symptoms. PTSD symptoms may occur after traumatic circumstances, such as gross disfigurement, bedsores, foul odor, or agitated confusion of the patient. PTSD has also been associated with the perception of an insufficient goodbye. In addition, a risk of relapse exists among those with a history of substance use, alcohol use, psychosis, or bipolar disorder.

Mental health clinicians treat bereavement-related psychiatric disorders using standard psychotherapeutic and psychopharmacological approaches (see Chapter 54).[2,5] However, extreme grief responses may benefit from specialized approaches. Pathological grief is a morbid response to loss that is characterized by specific symptoms, many of which resemble normal grief but are intensified and/or prolonged.[6,18] Researchers have identified these symptoms and associated features to better recognize those in need and develop appropriate interventions.

Specifically, researchers have developed diagnostic criteria for "prolonged grief disorder" (formerly referred to as complicated grief) and proposed it is a distinct mental disorder in the standardized diagnostic taxonomy.[2,6,18] Prolonged grief disorder is now conceptualized as a unique cluster of symptoms that are distinct from depression or anxiety symptoms and that are predictive of longer-term physical and mental health problems. These symptoms do not respond to traditional treatments for bereavement-related depression (e.g., interpersonal therapy, tricyclic antidepressants) and may persist for years if left untreated.[6,18] The current empirically derived diagnostic symptom criteria include intense yearning for the deceased, difficulty accepting the death, inability to trust others since the death, excessive bitterness, feeling uneasy about moving on, feeling emotionally numb or detached from others, feeling that life is meaningless without the deceased, feeling that the future holds no prospect for fulfillment without the deceased, avoidance of reminders of the loss, and feeling a diminished sense of self.[6] Symptoms must persist for at least 6 months after the loss. This conceptualization of prolonged grief disorder views the process as a pathological response to both traumatic and nontraumatic events. It occurs in 10% to 20% of the bereaved.[6] There is still substantial debate about the construct validity of prolonged grief disorder and about whether it is a distinct disorder.[5,18]

The lack of consensus on the definition of pathological grief, and accordingly normal grief, has resulted in the use of several terms to describe subtypes of grief.[3,5] For example, *chronic* grief involves persistent, intense distress in approximately 9% of bereaved individuals. *Inhibited* or *delayed* grief is an apparent absence of distress, usually characterized by chronic avoidance of reminders of the deceased, with a prevalence of up to 5%. Persistent avoidance may cause relationship problems or hypomania among individuals with bipolar disorder. Some may not experience heightened grief because of cultural sanctions or the lack of a strong relationship with the deceased.[3,7] Resilience after bereavement is also common.[2,5]

Risk Factors for Pathological Grief

Triaging care to those at risk is important because of limited resources and because most bereaved individuals recover satisfactorily. Clinicians should meet monthly for a multidisciplinary death review to identify family members at risk.[1,5] Risk factors that predict poorer outcome are presented in Table 14-2. Childhood adversity, such as abuse or the death of a parent, has been associated with morbid grief, suggesting that individuals with insecure attachment styles are at greater risk.[6] This may be why close, security-enhancing relationships predict more complicated grief among the conjugally bereaved.[6,18]

Sudden and Unexpected Death

Although palliative medicine does not seek a cure, the patient and family maintain expectations about the time left together. Unexpected deaths arise from sepsis, pulmonary emboli, cardiac events, or hemorrhage. Lack of preparedness for death predicts pathological grief and major depressive disorder; perception of death as violent creates a risk of depression.[2,6] Clinicians should assess the impact of circumstances surrounding the death on the bereaved (see Chapter 65).

Life Cycle and Children's Grief

Expression and understanding of grief is age specific.[4,5] Children may not understand the irreversibility of death

---

TABLE 14-2 Risk Factors for Pathological Grief Outcomes

CIRCUMSTANCES OF DEATH
Untimely within the life cycle (e.g., death of a child)
Sudden and unexpected (e.g., death from septic neutropenia during chemotherapy)
Traumatic (e.g., shocking cachexia and debility)
Stigmatized (e.g., AIDS, suicide)

PERSONAL VULNERABILITY
History of psychiatric disorder (e.g., clinical depression)
Personality and coping style (e.g., intense worrier, low self-esteem)
Attachment style (e.g., insecure)
Cumulative experience of losses

NATURE OF THE RELATIONSHIP WITH THE DECEASED
Overly dependent (e.g., security-enhancing relationship)
Ambivalent (e.g., angry and insecure with alcohol abuse, infidelity, gambling)

FAMILY AND SOCIAL SUPPORT
Family dysfunction (e.g., poor cohesion and communication, high conflict)
Isolated (e.g., new migrant, new residential move)
Alienated (e.g., perception of low social support)

until they have developed the capacity for abstract thinking, by about age 8 to 10 years. Open discussion of the loss, creation of an age-appropriate place to locate the deceased (e.g., in heaven), and support from surviving parents and family facilitate mourning. Clinicians guide parents to facilitate children's grief, including fostering their attendance at rituals and the construction of a memory book about the deceased.

For the very elderly, loss of one's life partner may seem irreplaceable, yet distress may be assuaged by a philosophical acceptance of aging and the inescapable closure of every life.[4,5]

A FAMILY APPROACH TO BEREAVEMENT CARE

Continuity of care between the end-of-life phase and bereavement is meaningful for relatives because it permits them to review the patient's journey of illness and death with the treatment team. Palliative care services should identify those carers and family members who are risk for pathological grief and target preventive support to avoid or minimize a morbid outcome (see Chapter 65). A family-centered approach helps. Kissane and colleagues developed a robust, highly sensitive, and clinically useful measure, the Family Relationships Index, which is a 12-item, validated, pencil and paper (or touch-screen computer) tool to assess a family's relational style.[1,13]

Five types of family functioning have been revealed with screening (Table 14-3). *Supportive* families (33%) are characterized by a high degree of cohesion. *Conflict resolvers* (20%) communicate effectively despite differences of opinion, their mutual respect sustaining high cohesion. These two well-functioning patterns are associated with negligible psychosocial morbidity—such families cope well with bereavement and need minimal clinical services. In contrast, the two dysfunctional types carry high psychosocial morbidity. *Hostile* families (6% to 12%) have a great deal of conflict, decreased cohesiveness, and poor communication. *Sullen* families (9% to 18%) demonstrate similar difficulties but with muted anger and the highest levels of depression. In between the dysfunctional and the well-functioning types lies an *intermediate* family class (20% to 33%) with moderate cohesion but substantial psychosocial morbidity and deteriorated function under the stress of bereavement.[1,13]

Family Focused Grief Therapy (FFGT) is a prophylactic, 6- to 10-session, family-based intervention that begins during palliative care and continues into bereavement for high-risk families (hostile, sullen, or intermediate) to optimize mutual support.[1,13] An initial randomized controlled trial (RCT) of FFGT showed significant reduction in distress at 13 months after death, with largest effects for sullen families. Further dose refinement studies are underway.[13]

EVIDENCE-BASED MEDICINE

Although a standard of care for bereaved relatives and friends has not been established by palliative medicine, follow-up with the family usually involves offering condolences by telephone, sympathy card, or personal visits; attending the funeral; or conducting annual commemoration services. This enhances continuity of care and normalizes grief in a nonintrusive, respectful manner.

In their systematic review of palliative care intervention research for caregivers and the bereaved, Harding and Higginson[19] failed to find benefits of services within the limited evidence base and highlighted the need for more methodologically sound RCTs (see Chapter 30). Similarly, meta-analyses of grief interventions (Table 14-4) highlighted the absence of benefit unless at-risk or symptomatic individuals were targeted.[2,5,20-22] Larson and Hoyt[23] suggested, however, that most of these grief counseling meta-analyses are methodologically limited and that the inefficiency they suggest is an overly pessimistic misrepresentation. In addition to FFGT,[13] potentially efficacious grief interventions include: (1) exposure-based treatments that use guided mourning with systematic desensitization for chronic grief; (2) individual, brief dynamic psychotherapy for ambivalent relationships; (3) short-term psychodynamic group therapy for loneliness and dependent relationships, potentially integrated with art therapy; and (4) religious-oriented psychotherapy when spiritual issues are relevant.[2,5]

Interventions to specifically treat prolonged grief disorder are also being empirically tested. Shear and colleagues[14] compared a manualized treatment for complicated grief (the term formerly used to describe prolonged grief disorder symptoms) to interpersonal psychotherapy in an RCT, with each group receiving 16 sessions of individual therapy. Complicated grief treatment involved psychoeducation about the dual processes of coping and grieving, exposure to the loss through retelling the death story, confrontation of avoided situations, setting personal goals, and exploration of the impact of the loss. Complicated grief symptoms improved more rapidly among participants who received complicated grief treatment compared with interpersonal psychotherapy.[14]

TABLE 14-3	Family Typologies in Palliative Care and Bereavement*		
LEVEL OF FUNCTIONING	**FAMILY TYPE**	**PREVALENCE (%)**	**CHARACTERISTIC FEATURES**
Well functioning	Supportive	33	Strong cohesion; grieve adaptively
	Conflict-resolving	20	Strong cohesion, effective communication; tolerant of difference of opinions
Dysfunctional	Hostile	6-12	Poor cohesion and communication, high conflict; fractured relationships; families resist assistance
	Sullen	9-18	Muted anger; highest levels of depression; families seek assistance
	Intermediate	20-33	Midrange levels of communication, cohesion, and conflict; at risk for deterioration when faced with stressors

*Based on the work of Kissane and colleagues.

TABLE 14-4 Systematic Reviews and Meta-analyses of Bereavement Interventions

AUTHORS AND YEAR	NO. OF STUDIES	STUDY SELECTION	EFFECT SIZE	POSSIBLE CONCLUSIONS
Allumbaugh & Hoyt (1999)	35	Controlled and noncontrolled	0.43	Effects stronger for self-identified participants; low statistical power; moderating variables influence effects
Kato & Mann (1999)	13	Randomized controlled trials; treatment and control groups recruited similarly; post-loss interventions	0.11	Interventions may be ineffective; control groups also improve; may need stronger dose of interventions; methodological problems are common
Fortner & Neimeyer (1999)*	23	Randomized controlled trials	0.13	Greater effects with high-risk populations
Schut, Stroebe, van den Bout, & Terheggen (2001)†	16 Primary 7 Secondary 7 Tertiary‡	Organized help; focused on treating grief; methodologically sound	Low to modest effects	Strongest effects with individuals exhibiting psychopathology or pathological grief; greater effects with self-referred persons
Jordan & Neimeyer (2003)	4	Reviews and meta-analyses	N/A	Generally low efficacy of interventions; intervention may not be necessary for most bereaved; need to develop new approaches; need to improve methodology of studies

*From unpublished work of Fortner and Neimeyer.
†Chapter in reference 24, pp. 705-738.
‡Primary preventive interventions were open to all bereaved individuals. Secondary preventive interventions were open to high-risk individuals. Tertiary preventive interventions were open to individuals with complicated grief or other psychopathology.

Real-world clinical practice often involves supportive-expressive counseling to facilitate emotional expression, but improved coping and cognitive reappraisal are necessary for clinical improvement; simply sharing feelings is unlikely to be therapeutic.[5] Bereavement-related depression should be treated with antidepressants combined with psychotherapy.[2,5]

RESEARCH CHALLENGES

Significant controversies include the distinction between normal and pathological grief, whether expressing grief is therapeutic, whether grief counseling is beneficial,[24] recognition of resilience, and standardization of specific diagnostic criteria for prolonged grief disorder (see "Future Considerations"). Some argue that pathological grief as a distinct entity will lead to overpathologizing of the bereaved. Yet, without standardized diagnostic criteria, clinicians may miss morbid responses and fail to ameliorate suffering.[6,18]

The timeline in which complicated grief symptoms fade has not been established. Prigerson and colleagues[6] suggested a 6-month duration criterion for maladaptive symptoms to ensure that suffering does not persist too long. The trajectory of chronic grief may be distinct from that of depression, the former taking longer to dissipate.

Because continuity of care tends to be the exception and bereavement care is often an afterthought, bereavement research faces unique challenges in recruitment for basic and treatment outcome studies (see Chapter 30). Routine psychosocial screening of patients, carers, and key family members is crucial for recognition of those at risk, with related triage and deployment of targeted services (see Chapters 58 and 65). Finding appropriate ways to integrate the theoretical models underpinning adapta-

Future Considerations

- Integrate theoretical models of adaptation to loss with specific symptom clusters and mediators or moderators of change
- Refine criteria for pathological or complicated grief via empirical research
- Develop efficacious and effective interventions for appropriate populations
- Conduct further research on bereaved children

tion to loss is a challenge that clinicians and researchers alike face. Still, efforts to synthesize the research and bridge the gap between science and clinical practice are under way.[2,5]

CONCLUSION

Numerous theories have been proposed to explain the etiology and course of the various emotional, cognitive, and behavioral responses to bereavement. The grieving experience is complex, and therefore an integrative, biopsychosocial perspective may best inform intervention development. Bereaved individuals often appreciate working with professionals who were witness to the deceased patient's dying experience, and palliative care clinicians can play a unique and important role in providing this kind of continuity of care. Palliative care multidisciplinary teams need to be able to foster resilience and to better recognize those who are most vulnerable before they will succeed in improving outcomes for the bereaved. This may be done through following up with the family informally or by making appropriate referrals for supportive counseling or for more specific psychotherapeutic and psychopharmacological interventions to treat bereavement-related pathological symptoms. Additional research will help our understanding of grief phenomenology and the development of effective treatment approaches.

REFERENCES

1. Kissane DW, Bloch S. Family Focused Grief Therapy: A Model of Family-Centered Care during Palliative Care and Bereavement. Buckingham: Open University Press, 2002.
2. Genevro J, Marshall T, Miller T. Report on bereavement and grief research. Death Studies 2004;28:491-575.
3. Parkes C. Bereavement Studies of Grief in Adult Life, 3rd ed. Madison, CT: International Universities Press, 1998.
4. Raphael B. The Anatomy of Bereavement. London: Hutchinson, 1983.
5. Stroebe M, Hansson R, Stroebe W, Schut H. Handbook of Bereavement Research: Consequences, Coping, and Care. Washington, DC: APA Books, 2001.
6. Prigerson HG, Vanderwerker LC, Maciejewski PK. Prolonged grief disorder as a mental disorder: Inclusion in the DSM. In Stroebe MS, Hannson RO, Schut HA, et al (eds). Handbook of Bereavement Research and Practice: 21st Century Perspectives. Washington, DC: American Psychological Association. In press.
7. Doka K. Disenfranchised grief. In Doka K (ed). Disenfranchised Grief: Recognizing Hidden Sorrow. Lexington, MA: Lexington Books, 1989, pp 3-11.
8. Bowlby J. The making and breaking of affectional bonds: I & II. Br J Psychiatry 1977;130:201-210, 421-431.
9. Ainsworth M, Blehar M, Waters E, Wall S. Patterns of Attachment: A Psychological Study of the Strange Situation. Hillsdale, NJ: Erlbaum, 1978.
10. Freud S. Mourning and Melancholia, Vol 14. In Strachey J (ed. & transl.) The Standard Edition of the Complete Psychological Works of Sigmund Freud. London: Hogarth, 1943-1974.
11. Neimeyer R. Meaning Reconstruction and the Experience of Loss. Washington, DC: American Psychological Association, 2001.
12. Walsh F, McGoldrick M. Loss and the family: A systemic perspective. In Walsh F, McGoldrick M (eds). Living Beyond Loss: Death in the Family. New York: Norton, 1991, pp 1-29.
13. Kissane D, Bloch S, McKenzie M, et al. Family focused grief therapy: A randomized controlled trial in palliative care and bereavement. Am J Psychiatry 2006;163:1208-1218.
14. Shear K, Frank E, Houck PR, Reynolds CR 3rd. Treatment of complicated grief: A randomized controlled trial. JAMA 2005;293:2601-2068.
15. Gilliland G, Fleming S. A comparison of spousal anticipatory grief and conventional grief. Death Stud 1998;22:541-569.
16. Maciejewski PK, Zhang B, Block SD, Prigerson HG. An empirical examination of the stage theory of grief. JAMA 2007;297:716-723.
17. Zisook S, Shuchter SR. Depression through the first year after the death of a spouse. Am J Psychiatry 1991;148:1346-1352.
18. Lichtenthal WG, Cruess DG, Prigerson HG. A case for establishing complicated grief as a distinct mental disorder in DSM-V. Clin Psychol Rev 2004;24:637-662.
19. Harding R, Higginson IJ. What is the best way to help caregivers in cancer and palliative care? A systematic literature review of interventions and their effectiveness. Palliat Med 2003;17:63-74.
20. Allumbaugh D, Hoyt W. Effectiveness of grief therapy: A meta-analysis. J Counseling Psychology 1999;46:370-380.
21. Jordan JR, Neimeyer RA. Does grief counseling work? Death Stud 2003;27:765-786.
22. Kato PM, Mann T. A synthesis of psychological interventions for the bereaved. Clin Psychol Rev 1999;19:275-296.
23. Larson DG, Hoyt WT. What has become of grief counseling? An evaluation of the empirical foundations of the new pessimism. Professional Psychology: Research and Practice 2007;38:347-355.
24. Schut HAW, Stroebe MS, van den Bout J, Terheggen MAMB. The efficacy of bereavement interventions: determining who benefits. In Stroebe MS, Hansson RO, Stroebe W, Schut H (eds). Handbook of Bereavement Research: Consequences, Coping and Care. Washington, DC: American Psychological Association, 2001, pp. 705-737.

SUGGESTED READING

Jacobs S. Pathologic Grief. Maladaptation to Loss. American Psychiatric Press, Washington, DC, 1993.

Kissane DW, Bloch S. Family Focused Grief Therapy. A Model of Family-Centered Care during Palliative Care and Bereavement. Open University Press, Birmingham, 2002.

Parkes CM, Laungani P, Young B (eds). Death and Bereavement Across Cultures. Routledge, London, 1997.

Raphael B. Anatomy of Bereavement. Basic Books, New York, 1983.

Stroebe MS, Hansson RO, Stroebe W, Schut H (eds). Handbook of Bereavement Research. Consequences, Coping, and Care. American Psychological Association, Washington, DC, 2001.

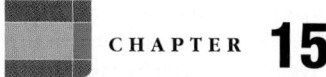

CHAPTER **15**

Stress and Burnout

Mary L. S. Vachon

KEY POINTS

- Health professionals are at increased risk of stress and burnout, but palliative care is not the most stressful specialty.

- Team communication problems, dealing with death and dying, feeling inadequately prepared, and dealing with young patients are associated with stress and burnout in palliative care. Issues with overload may become more of a problem than in the past.

- Burnout may be associated with depression and past history, but it is best viewed within a multidimensional model involving social context and an interpersonal framework.

- Little is known about appropriate interventions to decrease job stress and burnout.

- Job engagement and compassion satisfaction are probably very important in keeping staff involved in palliative care and should be studied. Their association with spirituality and religious beliefs also deserves further research.

DEFINITIONS

Stress

Stress and burnout have been concerns since the early days of palliative care.[1] The European Agency for Safety and Health at Work[2] stated that, "There is increasing consensus around defining work-related *stress* by 'interactions' between employees and (exposure to hazards in) their work environment. Within this model stress can be said to be experienced when the demands from the work environment exceed the employee's ability to cope with (or control) them."

Burnout

Burnout has been characterized as "the progressive loss of idealism, energy and purpose experienced by people in the helping professions as a result of the conditions of their work" (p. 14).[3] "The root cause of burnout lies in people's need to believe that their life is meaningful, and that the things they do—and consequently they themselves—are important and significant" (p. 633).[4]

What has emerged from all this research is a conceptualization of job burnout as a psychological syndrome in response to chronic interpersonal stressors on the job. The three key dimensions of this response are an overwhelming exhaustion, feelings of cynicism and detachment from the job, and a sense of ineffectiveness and lack of accomplishment. The exhaustion component represents the basic individual stress dimension of burnout. It refers to feelings of being overextended and depleted of one's emotional and physical resources. The cynicism (or depersonalization) component represents the interpersonal context dimension of burnout. It refers to a negative, callous, or excessively detached response to various aspects of the job. The component of reduced efficacy or accomplishment represents the self-evaluation dimension of burnout. It refers to feelings of incompetence and a lack of achievement and productivity at work (p. 398).[5]

Exhaustion and cynicism emerge from work overload and social conflict,[6] whereas a sense of inefficacy arises more from insufficient resources to get the work done (e.g. critical information, necessary tools, sufficient time). The combination of variables on the three different dimensions can cause different patterns of work experience and levels of burnout. Research does not support burnout as related to an individual's disposition. Burnout is related to certain demographic characteristics: workers who are single, younger, and male score slightly higher on cynicism than do females. With regard to personality, burnout has been associated with neuroticism and lower levels of hardiness and self-esteem. Research is much stronger for the association between burnout and many job characteristics, including chronically difficult job demands, imbalance between high demands and low resources, and conflict (among people, role demands, or important values).

Compassion Fatigue

A newer concept, compassion fatigue, or secondary traumatic stress disorder,[7,8] has begun to attract attention in palliative care.[9] Compassion fatigue is almost identical to post-traumatic stress disorder, except that it occurs in those emotionally affected by the trauma of another (usually a client or family member).[8] It is also known as secondary or vicarious traumatization.[7,8]

Compassion fatigue[8] describes a syndrome that shares some characteristics with burnout: depression, anxiety, hypochondria, combativeness, the sensation of being on "fast forward," and inability to concentrate. In contrast to one who has burned out, the caregiver with compassion fatigue[10] can still care and be involved. The following are signs[9] of compassion fatigue:

- "No energy for it anymore"
- Feeling emptied, "nothing left to give"
- "Not wanting to go there again"
- "Feeling depleted in every dimension"
- "Too many questions and no answers"
- "Why am I doing this?"

STRESS, DEPRESSION, AND BURNOUT

Specific acute work-related stressful experiences contribute to "depression"; more importantly, enduring "structural" occupational factors, which may differ by occupation, can also contribute to psychological disorders.[11] For physicians, the nature of the specialty and the duration of professional experience were found to influence morbidity.

Low autonomy predicted psychological morbidity in junior doctors, work demands in older physicians. Other factors associated with negative mental well-being included "low task role clarity," routine work administration, job demands, interference with family, and interruptions to work. Among middle-aged physicians, high job demands were associated with both "work dissatisfaction" and psychological disorder (General Health Questionnaire). In regression analysis, lack of control and overwork were independently associated with both dissatisfaction and psychological disorder.[12] Health care workers have psychological morbidity rates higher than those of the general population. In the United Kingdom, the relative risk of disorder was 1.5 and was most marked in direct care staff and women.[13] In that study of 11,000 employees from 19 National Health Service trusts, 27% of health service workers reported significant levels of minor psychiatric disorder, compared with 18% of the general population.

Burnout may be differentiated from depression.[14] The clinical picture of depression seems to reflect a general sense of self-defeat, so individuals high in burnout and low in superiority (i.e., how individuals see themselves compared to others) experience depressive symptoms. Depressive symptomatology was highest among individuals high in burnout who experienced a decline in superiority. "Depression was more strongly related to superiority than emotional exhaustion and depersonalization. In fact, emotional exhaustion, which constitutes the core symptom of burnout, did not have a significant association with superiority"[14] (see "Case Study: Burnout in an Oncologist"). They concluded that "reduced sense of superiority and a perceived loss of status are more characteristic of depressed individuals than for burnt-out individuals. It seems that burnt-out individuals are still 'in the battle' for obtaining status and consider themselves potential winners, while depressed individuals have given up."[15]

Two large European studies examined the issues of depression and burnout. In a Finnish study ($N = 3276$), burnout and depressive disorders were related.[16] The risk of depressive disorders, especially major depressive disorder (12-month prevalence), was greater if burnout was severe. Half of the participants with severe burnout had some depressive disorder. Those with a current major depressive episode experienced serious burnout more often than those who had suffered a major depressive episode earlier.

A Dutch study involved 3385 employees in various work settings; after controlling for background variables, the strongest predictor of all three burnout facets was current depressive symptomatology.[17] Hospital personnel (mostly female) with high interpersonal contacts reported the most depressive symptoms. Independent of background variables and current depressive symptoms, having ever had a depressive episode further predicted current symptoms of two burnout facets: emotional exhaustion and cynicism. A history of depression in close family members independently predicted current emotional exhaustion. A predisposition to depression, from a personal and family history of depression, may increase the risk for burnout (see "Case Study: Unresolved Grief and Burnout in a Physician Working with Patients with AIDS").

Burnout in an Oncologist

I found myself feeling really burned out. I was working 10 to 12 hours a day, and no matter how hard I worked, I had the feeling that I was never on top of it. At the end of a 12-hour day I'd carry home a briefcase that weighed 30 pounds and would then arrive home at night at about 10 o'clock and find myself just too exhausted to begin the work that I had brought home. I came to think that I would be much happier if I could get clear of my workload, but I never felt that I was out from under—I was always backlogged. I was always behind. I'd have problems returning phone calls because I'd have a zillion messages. I'd take these home with me and then think to myself, "Shit, I'll do it tomorrow." When I'd finally get to call a patient, he might say, "Gee, you're hard to get," or "It's nice to finally talk to you." It got so that I just wanted to go somewhere and die. Lots of the phone calls were from family members simply wanting more information. I'd already talked with the patient and felt that I just didn't have time to talk with the family member as well.

One day, it just got to be too much for me. I went into the office of the chief of medicine and said, "I've had it. I quit. I'm leaving and I'm never coming back again." I went home and arrived at my front door at 11 a.m. and said to my wife, "I've had it. I'm leaving work and I'm never going back again." It took me a week of doing absolutely nothing at home, and then I bounced back to the point where my boss said to my wife, "Gee, he bounced back quickly." I've come to realize that I'm probably going to burn out a few times in my life, because I work very hard. I think that it is worth it, though, because I have the feeling that I am better than many of my colleagues. As a result of my yelling and screaming, I got a bit more help than I had before, and so it may be a while before it happens again.

(From Vachon MLS. Occupational Stress in the Care of the Critically Ill, the Dying and the Bereaved. New York: Hemisphere Press, 1987.)

Unresolved Grief and Burnout in a Physician Working with Patients with AIDS

Surrounded by so much suffering and death, especially with the tenuous boundaries I have described between myself and my patients, I became enmeshed in certain ways with their lives; [I had] overinvolvement with work, nightmares and loss of sleep, and feelings of either omnipotence or total vulnerability when patients either survived an episode of illness or died despite all efforts. In other respects, emotionally, I remained somewhat detached. Sometimes detachment is healthy and appropriate for a physician, as long as one does not hide behind it; it is important to maintain appropriate boundaries, for the well-being of both parties. Sometimes, though, detachment—a certain closing off of the heart—can be a sign of one's own unresolved emotional pain, which has been buried under layers of denial, socialization, and professional competence. . . .

One day, [as I was leaving a church after attending a concert, I noticed] a scroll: "In memory of those who have died of AIDS." I stopped and stared at those words, and suddenly everything seemed real in a way that it never had before. At that moment, I felt something opening that had been closed off in me, and I suddenly began to cry for all the patients I had lost, whose faces I could see through the flickering light of the candles. I realized this work was about me and my life in ways that I had not understood. . . . My father died suddenly at the age of 35, when I was 18 months old. . . . My father most likely died by suicide and not, as I had grown up believing, in a bizarre accident in which he inexplicably lost his balance and fell out of a window. . . . It was not until more than 30 years later—when I was confronted with the deaths of all these young men and women whom I could no more save than I could save my father—that I began to come to terms with this primal loss.

(From Selwyn PA. Surviving the Fall. New Haven: Yale University Press, 1998, pp 105-107.)

A MODEL FOR UNDERSTANDING OCCUPATIONAL STRESS

Recent research[5] has focused on the degree of match or mismatch between the person and six job domains: workload, control, reward, community, fairness, and values. The greater the gap or mismatch between the person and his or her environment, the more burnout. The greater the match or fit, the greater the likelihood of engagement with work. Mismatches arise when the process of establishing a psychological contract leaves critical issues unresolved or when the working relationship changes to something the person finds unacceptable.

Burnout arises from chronic mismatches between people and their work settings in some or all of the six areas of work life. Values may play a central mediating role for the other areas, although people may vary in how important each of the six areas is to them. Some may place a higher weight on reward than on values, and some may be prepared to tolerate a mismatch regarding workload if they receive praise and good pay and have good relationships with colleagues.

The literature is somewhat divided as to whether the care of the dying is a major stressor in hospice palliative care.[1,15] Recent burnout research has focused on emotion-work variables (e.g., requirement to display or suppress emotions on the job, requirement to be emotionally empathic) and has found that emotional factors do account for additional variance in burnout scores over and above job stressors.[5,18,19]

JOB SATISFACTION, JOB ENGAGEMENT, AND COMPASSION SATISFACTION

A sense of competence, control, and pleasure in one's work is a major coping mechanism in palliative care,[15] and palliative care workers derive great work satisfaction.[19-21] Researchers have investigated job engagement[5] and compassion satisfaction[22] as the flipsides of burnout and compassion stress or compassion fatigue.

Job engagement is conceptualized as the opposite of burnout. It involves energy, involvement, and efficacy. Engagement involves the individual's relationship with work. It involves a sustainable workload, feelings of choice and control, appropriate recognition and reward, a supportive work community, fairness and justice, and meaningful valued work. Engagement is also characterized by high levels of activation and pleasure.[5]

Others[6] conceptualize job engagement in its own terms, rather than as the opposite of burnout. It is then defined as a persistent, positive motivational state of fulfillment in employees, characterized by vigor, dedication, and absorption. This concept resembles the *vitality* described in palliative care staff.[21]

Compassion satisfaction[22] is derived from helping others. It may be the portrayal of efficacy. Compassion satisfaction may represent happiness with what one can do to make the world a reflection of what one thinks it should be. Caregivers with compassion satisfaction derive pleasure from helping others, such as their colleagues, feel good about their ability to help and make a contribution. There is a balancing act between compassion fatigue and compassion satisfaction.[22] Caregivers in humanitarian settings may experience compassion fatigue yet like their work because they feel positive benefits They believe they are helping others, and the work may even be redemptive. When a person's belief system is well maintained with positive material, personal resiliency may be enhanced.

The compassion of caregivers often catches the attention of others, even at the most difficult times of their lives. Dr. Peter Frost, Professor of Organizational Behavior at the University of British Columbia, was treated for metastatic melanoma and observed the nurses of the British Columbia Cancer Agency, "whose highly professional and empathic behavior caught my attention when I was in their care" (p. ix).[23] Observing and reflecting on their compassion led to his book, *Toxic Emotions at Work: How Compassionate Managers Handle Pain and Conflict*[23]:

> My illness—a trigger for changes, obviously in my personal life—also set in motion my thinking about the kinds of hidden forces that determine our well-being, even to the point of acquiring disease. And in particular, how the behavior of organizations and the people in them can affect the health of certain individuals.... [A] few months after my surgery I found myself at a week-long seminar on health and healing. That is where my ideas about emotional pain in organizations, and its effects on people who try to manage that pain for organizations began to crystallize (p. 2).

The third case study gives an example of the development of compassion satisfaction in a palliative care physician (see "Case Study: Compassion Satisfaction, Meditation, and Healing in a Palliative Care Physician"). Some results of research on stress and burnout in palliative care and oncology are shown in Table 15-1.

THE IMPACT OF RELIGION AND SPIRITUALITY ON BURNOUT

Being religious is associated with less burnout in oncology staff.[25] *Spirituality* may be defined as being "of, or pertaining to, affecting or concerning the spirit or higher moral questions" and the need for caregivers to experience their own inner depths as they care for a patient experiencing

 CASE STUDY

Compassion Satisfaction, Meditation, and Healing in a Palliative Care Physician

I have been a doctor since 1979 and don't recall ever wanting to be anything else. I can't honestly say that compassion was my driving force. On the contrary, I was a high achiever ambitious for success and recognition, driven by self-interest and a fear of failure....

By the end of 1983, my greatest moment was passing the physician's specialist examination. This enabled me to enter specialist training in medical oncology . . . with no more examinations to face....

After 3 months of euphoria, I came to earth. Having satisfied my highest aim, there was nothing left to strive for. I wasn't focused, and I was burning out. There was a lack of discipline in my life, and I had an identity crisis. Without a goal, I felt empty and didn't know myself. I struggled and looked for new mountains to climb.

Fellow high achievers advised me to publish scientific papers, do research, and get a PhD to succeed in medicine. As I thought about this, I discovered a new voice inside me. It was saying, "No, consider others." My ambitions had blinkered me into looking on sick people as problems to solve, rather than opportunities to help and to heal. I began to see beyond this arrogance. People didn't get cancer to further my career; they were suffering, and so were their families. I needed to understand this better and felt angry towards an establishment that seemed academic and out of touch. I started talking to my patients. I explored what it was like to live with cancer, to face death, and to lose someone you love. To my amazement, it really helped them, and I found people were appreciating me in a way I had never experienced before. They were teaching me how to love.

[The turning point was a workshop with Dr. Elisabeth Kübler-Ross.] During the workshop, I had cathartic experience of grief followed by an intense feeling of pure, unconditional love.... At the same time, I felt separated from my physical body and experienced a blissful, unworldly happiness. For the first time in my life, I realized that I was a spirit and that love, peace, and happiness were natural attributes of the soul. When we suppress these attributes, we develop sorrow and disease. I also realized that nobody dies, and that we all eventually rediscover our purity, love, and power....

I began to meditate and to teach meditation to interested cancer patients and their families. Above all, I let down my guard, developed a more open and easy nature, and enjoyed being myself in therapeutic relationships. Having found love, I now discovered that healing is a competency between competency and compassion. Patients benefited most from my knowledge, skills and understanding when I was simply being myself.

(From Cole R. Mission of Love: A Physician's Personal Journey towards a Life Beyond. Port Melbourne, Victoria, Australia: Lothian, 2001, pp xiii-xiv.)

spiritual pain.[26] For many, spirituality is about meaning and connection. The lived experience of Australian palliative care workers, as reported by Webster and Kristjanson,[21] reflected the spiritual belief system some associate with palliative care. Palliative care was described as "a way

POPULATION & REF. NO.	METHOD AND INSTRUMENTS	STRESSORS	STRESS AND BURNOUT	COPING/SOURCES OF SATISFACTION
International convenience sample of 100 hospice caregivers: 38 MD, 42 RN, 13 SW, 17 other[15]	Semistructured interviews, part of a larger study of 581 caregivers to the seriously ill, dying, and bereaved	• System communication problems • Role ambiguity • Team communication • Administration communication • Role conflict	• Staff conflict • Depression, grief, and guilt • Job/home interaction • Feeling helpless	• Team philosophy, support, team-building • Sense of competence, control, and pleasure in one's work • Developing control over practice • Personal philosophy • Increased education • Lifestyle management
All nonsurgical consultant oncologists in the UK (N = 476): 69 med onc, 253 clin onc, and 154 PC specialists; 83% returned questionnaires[20]	Questionnaire survey; *psychiatric disorder* estimated by GHQ-12, *burnout* by MBI	• *Psychiatric disorder* was independently associated with feeling overloaded; treatment toxicity/errors; and low satisfaction from professional status/esteem. • *Burnout* was related to those factors and to high stress and low satisfaction from dealing with patients and low resource satisfaction. • Clinicians who felt insufficiently trained in communication and management had higher distress. • PC specialists had fewer stressors.	• Estimated prevalence of *psychiatric disorder*: 28% • *Burnout* included *emotional exhaustion* (estimated prevalence among PC specialists, 23%; med onc, 25%; clin onc, 38%), *depersonalization* (PC specialists, 13%; med onc, 15%; clin onc, 31%), and *low personal accomplishment* (PC specialists, 25%; med onc, 34%; clin onc, 38%).	• Dealing well with patients and relatives • Having professional status/esteem • Deriving intellectual stimulation • Having adequate resources • PC specialists had significantly more satisfaction from dealing well with patients and relatives, felt significantly more professional status and self-esteem than clin onc, felt significantly less intellectual stimulation than med onc, and felt significantly better resourced than clin onc.
261 house staff, nurses, and med onc at MSKCC and oncologists in outside clinical practice; response rates: 98% of RNs, 97% of house staff, 47% of med onc on staff, 37% of 200 oncologists trained at the center[25]	Questionnaire; life stressors, personality attributes, burnout, psychological distress, physical symptoms, coping strategies, and social support were measured by MBI, *psychological distress* by Psychiatric Epidemiology Research Interview, *physical symptoms* by Hopkins Symptom Checklist, *personality* by Hardy Personality Measure, *social support* by Work Environment Scale and Peer Cohesion Scale, and *methods of relaxing* by the Stress Questionnaire.	• Stressor contributing most to burnout and demoralization was negative work events—high patient deaths or struggling over a DNR decision with another colleague or family member. • Working in a stressful environment while dealing with cancer in a family member led to greater demoralization and increased concerns about personal risk of cancer. • Oncologists perceived significantly less support from others than did nurses or house staff. • "Both house staff and nurses have daily contact with the patients and perform work that requires the greatest physical effort. They deal with the daily details of care and implementation of orders and often must buffer conflicts or differences among the oncologist, the patient, and the family. It is not surprising that they have the highest levels of burnout" (p. 1627). • Nurses' lower sense of accomplishment may be related to feeling overwhelmed by the enormity of patient care or less well supported to meet patient needs, particularly psychological needs. Nurses and house staff complain of doing the "chores" without the bigger picture the oncologist has.	*Burnout* included the following: • *Emotional exhaustion*: group mean (29) was in the high range (>17) and higher than the norm in general medicine (22); house staff had significantly greater emotional exhaustion (mean, 34.03); RNs scored 29.2, med onc 25.1; best predictors of greater emotional exhaustion were (1) being a house officer, (2) more negative work events; (3) using cigarettes, alcohol, or medication to relax; and (4) fewer hardiness traits. • *Depersonalization* (diminished empathy, distancing from patients): total sample scored 10.48, which is above individuals in medicine and near the high score (>12); house staff had higher scores (mean, 14.08) than oncologists (9.92); being a house officer or a nurse, having more negative work events, and using cigarettes, alcohol, or medication to relax contributed most to feeling impersonal or less empathic toward patients. • *Sense of personal accomplishment*: total sample mean (36.22) is almost identical to that of medical population (32.53—reference in original); nurses had significantly lower sense of accomplishment (30.94) than oncologists (36.03); men had a greater sense of accomplishment than women; house officers and nurses had less sense of accomplishment, but hardy	• Peer support significantly decreased psychological distress and demoralization symptoms for the entire group. • Those who considered themselves to be quite a bit or extremely religious had significantly lower scores on diminished empathy or depersonalization than those who were not at all religious; the same held true for significantly lower emotional exhaustion scores; nurses perceived themselves as significantly more religious than other groups. • The four most frequently used relaxation methods were the same across the three groups: talking with someone you know, eating/drinking coffee, watching television, and using humor. • The methods least used to reduce stress were the same across the three groups: taking prescribed medicine, smoking cigarettes, drinking alcohol, using relaxation activities, and prayer or meditation. • Oncologists had a greater sense of personal accomplishment, perhaps based on their understanding of the overall treatment plan of patients, the responsibility for carrying it out, and rewarding interactions with patients and families.

Continued

TABLE 15-1 Stressors, Stress, and Burnout in Palliative Care and Oncology—cont'd

POPULATION & REF. NO.	METHOD AND INSTRUMENTS	STRESSORS	STRESS AND BURNOUT	COPING/SOURCES OF SATISFACTION
		• Nurses and house staff see patients who are the most ill and may be caring for dying people. They don't have the reward of seeing patients get better. • Sense of futility about cancer treatment and feelings of anger and cynicism about limited roles in treatment • Feeling disenfranchised, yet overworked	• personality traits were related to a greater sense of accomplishment; female house staff had the greatest demoralization and least sense of accomplishment. • *Psychological distress/demoralization* (poor self-esteem, anxiety): women had significantly more demoralization symptoms than men (30.08 vs. 24.52); house staff more than oncologists (30.10 vs. 21.63); most significant predictors of demoralization were (1) female gender, (2) being a house officer, (3) more family, social, and residence problems, (4) fewer cathartic means of relaxing and using more cigarettes, alcohol, or medication, (5) fewer hardy personality characteristics, (6) feeling less peer support • *Physical symptoms:* nurses had more headaches, tiredness, and backaches than oncologists or house staff; this was associated with family stressors and negative work stressors.	• Involvement in research was helpful for oncologists.
1016 personnel of the major providers of medical oncology services in Ontario, Canada; response rates: 63.3% of MDs, 80.9% of AHP, 64.5% of support staff[40]	Mailout questionnaire was used to determine job satisfaction and stress, obtain demographic information, and measure consideration of alternative work situations; *burnout* was measured by MBI; *psychological distress* by GHQ-12[40], focus groups with caregivers in the six major cancer treatment centers (N = 108) looked at greatest sources of satisfaction and increased workload[39]	• Conflicting demands on time • Too great an overall volume of work • Disruption of home life by long hours at work • Inadequate staffing to do the job properly • Being involved with the emotional distress of patients[39]	Burnout included the following: • *Exhaustion:* significantly higher among physicians (53%) than among AHP (37%) • *Depersonalization:* 22.1% in MDs vs. 4% in others • *Sense of personal accomplishment:* significantly higher among physicians (48%) and AHP (54%) than among support staff (31%); about one third said they have considered leaving for a job outside the cancer field[39]	• Major sources of job satisfaction stemmed from patient care and contact. • Having good relationships with patients, families, and colleagues were the top three sources of job satisfaction for staff. • Being perceived as doing the job well was the fourth source. • Having variety in one's job was fifth.[39]
89 female hospice nurses from nine hospices in the UK[33]	Questionnaires, MBI, Nursing Stress Scale, Ways of Coping Scale, demographic information	• Death and dying, conflict with staff, and higher nursing grade contributed to *emotional exhaustion.* • Conflict with staff, inadequate preparation contributed to *depersonalization.* • Inadequate preparation and lower professional qualifications contributed to lower levels of *personal accomplishment.* • Overall stressors made the greatest contribution to burnout, and demographic factors the least.	• The level of burnout was low; the mean E and DP scores were low and the PA score was moderate. • Emotional exhaustion: 16% (high) • Depersonalization: 10% (high) • Low personal accomplishment: 31%	• Ways of Coping Scale: accepting responsibility contributed to *emotional exhaustion;* escape and reduced planful problem-solving contributed to *depersonalization;* escape and reduced positive reappraisal contributed to lower levels of *personal accomplishment;* researchers concluded that problem-focused and emotion-focused coping probably simplify the coping–burnout relationship.
60% (23/36) of senior house officers in hospices in the UK[34]	Questionnaire re stressors; perceived stress measured by VAS and psychological stress by GHQ-12	• Many described posts as stressful and cited staff conflict and caring for young patients as particularly stressful.	• Median VAS stress score was 55 mm (range, 0 to 98 mm). • Five respondents (22%) scored for identifiable psychological distress on the GHQ-12.	• Experiential teaching was very positively described.

AHP, allied health professionals; clin onc, clinical oncologists; DNR, do not resuscitate; GHQ-12, General Health Questionnaire 12; MBI, Maslach Burnout Inventory; MD, medical doctor; med onc, medical oncologists; MSKCC, Memorial Sloan-Kettering Cancer Center; PC, palliative care; RN, registered nurse; SW, social worker; UK, United Kingdom; VAS, visual analogue scale.

of living." Vitality—the capacity to live and develop which is associated with energy, life, animation, and importance—is the core meaning of palliative care. The way of living involves unity with self, being touched to the heart, and personal meaning.[21] Crucial to the experience of palliative care was the patient and family, holistic care, and the interdisciplinary team.

Another account of an interdisciplinary palliative care team's struggle to define spirituality included integrity, wholeness, meaning, and personal journeying.[27] For many, their spirituality was inherently relational; it might involve transcendence; it was wrapped up in caring, often manifested in small daily acts of kindness and of love. For some, palliative care was a spiritual calling. A collective spirituality stemming from common goals, values, and belonging surfaced. Further research might explore collective spirituality, including more in-depth study of the relationship between spirituality and tacit skills such as empathy, "being present," and compassion employed by palliative care professionals in caring for the dying. The spiritual belief systems of those in palliative care may protect against burnout and compassion fatigue.

In a study of 230 New Zealand physicians,[28] there was a positive and significant correlation between compassion satisfaction on the Professional Quality of Life–ProQOL Instrument[29] and spirituality. This study examined the relationship between compassion fatigue, compassion satisfaction, and burnout (ProQOL) and resilience, spirituality, empathy, emotional competence, and social support-seeking behaviors. There was also a positive correlation between religion and vicarious traumatization. High scores on the "Relationship with a Higher Power" subscale were related to high scores on the compassion fatigue subscale. There was also a negative and significant correlation between spirituality and burnout.

EVIDENCE-BASED INTERVENTIONS

Burnout

Interpersonal dynamics between the worker and others in the workplace give new insights into the sources of stress, but effective interventions to prevent burnout have yet to be developed.[6] This model suggests that effective interventions for burnout should be framed by the three dimensions of exhaustion, cynicism, and sense of inefficacy (e.g., What changes will reduce the risk of exhaustion? What changes will promote the sense of efficacy?). Interventions may be more effective if they are framed in terms of building engagement rather than reducing burnout.

Stress-Reducing Interventions

A meta-analysis of 48 occupational stress-reducing interventions ($N = 3736$ participants) categorized the studies as cognitive-behavioral interventions, relaxation techniques, multimodal programs (emphasizing both active and passive coping skills), and organization-focused interventions.[30] A small but significant overall effect was found. Cognitive-behavioral and multimodal interventions had a moderate effect; there was a small effect for relaxation; and the effect size for organization-focused intervention

was nonsignificant. Cognitive-behavioral interventions appeared to be effective in improving perceived quality of work life, enhancing psychological resources and responses, and reducing complaints. Multimodal programs showed similar effects; however, they appeared ineffective in increasing psychological resources and responses. There was a marginally significant effect of job status on treatment outcome: those with more job control had a better response to interventions. The cognitive-behavioral interventions with higher job control may have had a relatively large effect because employees profit most when provided with individual coping skills in a job that allows them to use these skills.

Mindfulness is defined as being fully present to one's experience without judgment or resistance. Its emphasis on self-care, compassion, and healing makes it relevant as an intervention for helping nurses. In a study of Mindfulness-Based Stress Reduction on a nursing unit,[31] there had already been work to improve employee satisfaction and retention. A nursing advisory council had been set up, efforts were made to enhance self-governance, and, there was increased opportunity for education and professional development. The treatment group had decreased scores on the Maslach Burnout Inventory, and these lasted 3 months. Specifically, emotional exhaustion and depersonalization were significantly decreased, and there was a trend toward significance in personal accomplishment.

Palliative Care Intervention

A carefully designed training program and staff support activities may enhance personal growth, give emotional support, and help staff deal with death and bereavement.[32] Interventions did not involve mutual collaboration, practical problems, managerial and communication skills, and the skills needed to deliver complex palliative care. Adequate resources, a supportive management structure, an extensive education, and attention to individual needs should accompany support groups. A therapeutic group is fundamentally different from a group that has to work together. Future leaders should perhaps focus on content and process issues.

Teams are one major stressor, the place where much stress is manifested, and also the place for comfort and support.[1,15,25,33,34] Are teams the best way in which to carry out palliative care?[35] The evidence is not there. Good palliative care makes a difference, but is this because of well-functioning teams, or could it be equally well delivered by well-resourced individuals? Practical suggestions include "team or group—spot the difference"; the effect of the setting on the work of the team; user involvement—the patient and carer as team members; leaders and followers; sitting close to death on a palliative care unit; maintaining a healthy team; team building; communication; training; ethical issues; legal issues; and team effectiveness.

Improved Communication

Burnout in oncologists and palliative care specialists is associated with poor communication training.[20] All communication skills training in oncology demonstrates modest improvements (effect sizes, 0.15 to 2.0).[36] Training improves basic communication, but positive attitudes and beliefs are needed to maintain skills over time in clinical practice and to handle emotional situations.

Educational Interventions

Another model for shifting established patterns is being conducted in the European Union with a goal of improving the interaction between mobile palliative care teams (PCMT) and the hospital staff with whom they interact.[37] In this model, recognizing the full range of convictions held by persons in a hospital setting, the concept of palliative care/terminal care has been bolstered by the concept of *continuous care*. Continuous care tends to *articulate* curative and palliative procedures, focusing on holistic care of the patient and family. "'Promoting the integration of continuous care in the hospital' intends to identify the challenges in integrating continuous care through an inventory and analysis of the activity of palliative care mobile teams in several countries of Europe. Competencies for PCMTs have been derived, and based on these, a pilot three phase educational program with PCMTs undertaken and evaluated" (p. 4).[37] One approach to physician awareness includes identifying and working with emotions that may affect patient care.[38] This involves looking at physician, situational, and patient risk factors that can lead to physician feelings and thus influence patient care.

CONCLUSIONS

Despite the fact that stress and burnout are not as significant in palliative care as in other specialties, there are still concerns that these symptoms will increase with current workloads. Although burnout is associated with some personal characteristics (e.g., depression, family history of depression, unresolved grief), burnout is best viewed within a multidimensional model involving the social context and an interpersonal framework. Compassion fatigue has begun to attract attention in palliative care. Researchers are recognizing the importance of looking at what sustains staff, the concepts of job engagement, and compassion satisfaction. Recent work in spirituality in palliative care may be of particular importance for both individuals and teams.

Multidimensional studies involving both social and interpersonal variables are needed. Specific areas to be addressed might be the relationship between burnout and many job characteristics, such as chronically difficult demands, imbalance between high demands and low resources, and conflict (between people, between role demands, or between important values). As there is more pressure, will there be less job satisfaction and more stress and burnout?[6]

The work of the European Commission is relevant. Future research in spirituality and religious belief systems and whether these correlate with job engagement and compassion satisfaction in palliative care would be useful. Bidirectionality in relationships between caregivers and patients in oncology and its correlation to organizational well-being might be relevant to study[39,40] in both oncology and palliative care.

REFERENCES

1. Vachon MLS. Staff stress in palliative/hospice care: A review. Palliat Med 1995;9:91-122.
2. European Agency for Safety and Health at Work. Research on Work-Related Stress, 2000. Available at.http://agency.osha.eu.int/publications/factsheets/8/facts8_en.pdf (accessed September 2007).
3. Edelwich J, Brodsky A. Burn-out: Stages of Disillusionment in the Helping Professions. New York: Springer, 1980.
4. Pines AM. Burnout: An existential perspective. In Schaufeli W, Maslach C, Marek T (eds). Professional Burnout. Washington, DC: Taylor and Francis, 1993.
5. Maslach C, Schaufeli WB, Leiter MP. Job burnout. Ann Rev Psychology 2001;52:397-422.
6. Maslach C. Job burnout: New directions in research and intervention. Curr Dir Psychol Sci 2003;12:189-192.
7. Figley CR (ed). Compassion Fatigue: Coping with Secondary Traumatic Stress Disorder in Those Who Treat the Traumatized. New York: Brunner/Mazel, 1995.
8. Figley CR (ed). Treating Compassion Fatigue. New York: Brunner-Routledge, 2002.
9. Wright B. Compassion fatigue: How to avoid it. Palliat Med 2004;18:4-5.
10. Garfield C, Spring C, Ober D. Sometimes my heart goes numb: Love and caring in a time of AIDS. San Francisco: Jossey-Bass, 1995.
11. Tennant C. Work-related stress and depressive disorders. J Psychosom Res 2001;51:697-704.
12. Johnson JV, Hall EM, Ford DE, et al. The psychosocial work environment of physicians: The impact of demands and resources on job dissatisfaction and psychiatric distress in a longitudinal study of Johns Hopkins Medical School Graduates. J Occup Environ Med 1995;37:1151-1159.
13. Wall TD, Bolden RI, Borrell CS, et al. Minor psychiatric disorder in NHS trust staff: Occupational and gender differences. Br J Psychiatry 1997; 171:519-523.
14. Brenninkmeyer V, Van Yperen NW, Buunk BP. Burnout and depression are not identical twins: Is decline of superiority a distinguishing feature? Pers Indiv Diff 2001;30:873-880.
15. Vachon MLS. Occupational Stress in the Care of the Critically Ill, the Dying and the Bereaved. New York: Hemisphere Press, 1987.
16. Ahola K, Honkonen T, Isometsä E, et al. The relationship between job-related burnout and depressive disorders: Results from the Finnish Health 2000 Study. J Affect Disorders 2005;88:55-62.
17. Nyklicek I, Pop VJ. Past and familial depression predict current symptoms of professional burnout. J Affect Disorders 2005;88:63-68.
18. Selwyn PA. Surviving the Fall. New Haven: Yale University Press, 1998.
19. Vachon MLS, Sherwood C. Staff stress, burnout, compassion fatigue and pleasure in one's work. In Berger AM, Von Roenn JH, Shuster JL (eds). Principles and Practice of Palliative Care and Supportive Oncology, 3rd ed. Philadelphia: Lippincott Williams & Wilkins, 2006.
20. Ramirez AJ, Graham J, Richards MA, et al. Burnout and psychiatric disorder among cancer clinicians. Br J Cancer 1995;71:1263-1269.
21. Webster J, Kristjanson LJ. "But isn't it depressing?" The vitality of palliative care. J Palliat Care 2002;18:15-24.
22. Stamm BH. Measuring compassion satisfaction as well as fatigue: Developmental history of the compassion satisfaction and fatigue test. In Figley CF (ed). Treating Compassion Fatigue. New York: Brunner-Routledge, 2002, pp 107-119.
23. Frost PJ. Toxic Emotions at Work. Boston: Harvard Business School Press, 2003.
24. Cole R. Mission of Love: A Physician's Personal Journey towards a Life Beyond. Port Melbourne, Victoria, Australia: Lothian, 2001.
25. Kash KM, Holland JC, Breitbart W, et al. Stress and burnout in oncology. Oncology 2000;14:1621-1637.
26. Kearney M, Mount B. Spiritual care of the dying patient. In Chochinov HM, Breitbart W. Handbook of Psychiatry in Palliative Medicine. New York: Oxford University Press, 2000, pp 357-373.
27. Sinclair S, Raffin S, Pereira J, et al. Collective soul: The spirituality of an interdisciplinary palliative care team. Palliat Support Care 2006;4:13-24.
28. Huggard PK. Taking Care of the Health Professional. Presentation at the Idaho Conference on Health Care, Health Care 2005: Emerging Issues, Pocatello, Idaho, 27-28 October, 2005, personal communication.
29. Stamm BH. ProQOL R-IV—Professional Quality of Life Scale: Compassion Satisfaction and Fatigue Subscales (Revision IV). Available at http://www.isu.edu/~bhstamm/documents/proqol/ProQOL_vIV_English_Oct05.pdf (accessed September 2007).
30. van der Klink JJL, Blonk RWB, Schene AH, van Dijk FJH. The benefits of intervention for work-related stress. Am J Pub Health 2001;91:270-276.
31. Cohen-Katz J, Wiley SD, Capuano T, et al. The effects of mindfulness-based stress reduction on nurse stress and burnout: A quantitative and qualitative study. Holistic Nurs Prac 2004:18(6):302-308.
32. van Staa AL, Visser A, van der Zouwe. Caring for caregivers: Experiences and evaluation of interventions for a palliative care team. Patient Educ Couns 2000;41:93-105.
33. Payne N. Occupational stressors and coping as determinants of burnout in female hospice nurses. J Adv Nurs 2001;33:396-405.
34. Lloyd-Williams M. Senior house officers' experience of a six month post in a hospice. Med Educ 2002;36(1):45-48.

35. Speck P (ed). Teamwork in Palliative Care. Oxford: Oxford University Press, 2006.
36. Gysels M, Richardson A, Higginson IJ. Communication training for health professionals who care for patients with cancer: A systematic review of effectiveness. Support Care Cancer 2004;12:692-700.
37. European Commission. Promoting the Development and Integration of Palliative Care Mobile Support Teams in the Hospital. Brussels: Directorate-General for Research Food Quality and Safety, 2004.
38. Meier DE, Back AL, Morrison RS. The inner life of physicians and the care of the seriously ill. JAMA.2002;286:3007-3014.
39. Grunfeld E, Zitzelsberger L, Coristine M, et al. Job stress and job satisfaction of cancer care workers. Psycho-oncology 2005;14:61-69.
40. Grunfeld E, Whelan TJ, Zitzelsberger L, et al. Cancer care workers in Ontario: Prevalence of burnout, job stress and job satisfaction. CMAJ 2000;163:166-169.

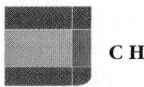

CHAPTER **16**

Body Image and Sexuality

Lena Dergham

KEY POINTS

- Body image and sexuality should be addressed routinely.
- Chronic illness and treatments affect body image and sexuality.
- How to take a good sexual history.
- Patients with chronic illnesses can be helped to improve their body images and sexual life.

Chronic illnesses and their treatments have many negative impacts on psychosocial life, including effects on sexuality and body image. The mechanisms of interference can be neurological, vascular, endocrinological, musculoskeletal, or psychological. Sexuality is a complex phenomenon that involves intricate interactions among biological sex, core identity (sense of maleness or femaleness), gender identity (sense of femininity or masculinity), and gender role behavior (nonsexual and sexual).[1]

Sexual function depends on the neurological, vascular, and endocrine systems and is influenced by many psychosocial factors, including family, religion, sexual partner, and self-esteem.[2] The sexual cycle is affected by chronic medical illness and its treatment. Neurological disorders affect desire, arousal, and orgasm. Some antihypertensive medications negatively affect arousal.

The place and importance of sexuality are influenced by its history. In the 17th century, sexuality was a "shameless discourse." People were open about their bodies and sexual lives.[3] By the 18th century, sex had became a "police matter," which involved controlling sex practices through public discourses. In the 19th century, there was a discourse of silence surrounding sexuality.[3]

Sexuality is also linked to how a person views his or her body, because the body is a sphere of sexuality. In chronic illness, there is usually a change in how a person feels about the body, and this can create problems. The diagnosis of diabetes and consequent lifestyle changes, for example, can have a negative effect on a person's body image.

COMMON DISEASES THAT AFFECT BODY IMAGE AND SEXUALITY

Coronary Artery Disease

Fear and lack of information often prevent those with cardiovascular disease from resuming sexual activity.[4] Acute coronary conditions result in only a temporary prohibition of sexual activity. An expert panel recommended stratifying patients into low-, indeterminate-, and high-risk categories.[2] For low-risk patients, no further workup is required before resuming sexual activity or the treatment of sexual difficulties. For indeterminate and high-risk patients, a cardiology consultation may help. Cardiac rehabilitation may be necessary in persons with indeterminate risk. The panel recommended that high-risk patients defer sexual activity until cardiac function is stable.

Anyone who experiences prolonged palpitations, angina, or fatigue during sexual activity should be evaluated by a physician.

Alternative forms of intimate physical contact can be used until the patient has the necessary strength for sexual activity (e.g., holding hands, kissing, hugging, massage). Many medications for cardiovascular disease can cause sexual dysfunction,[2] and other medications should be substituted if possible.

Human Immunodeficiency Viral Infection

Many patients with human immunodeficiency virus (HIV) infection or AIDS have decreased sexual desire because of fatigue, muscle aches, generalized wasting, paresthesias, pains, and depression. Body image concerns worsen with advanced symptomatic disease.[5] Men with HIV/AIDS usually have low testosterone levels, which can exacerbate existing problems with sexual function, including decreased sexual interest and arousal.[2] Protease inhibitors impair desire and arousal.[2]

HIV-positive patients who do not have a partner may experience problems in establishing a relationship. HIV and AIDS receive much media attention, often accompanied by inaccurate information and wrong beliefs. This emphasizes the important role of physicians as a source of accurate, current information.

Condom use should be emphasized for both partners.[1]

Chronic Respiratory Illness

Chronic respiratory illness can be accompanied by muscle weakness, fatigue, shortness of breath, and poor stamina. The high physiological demand of sexual activity can cause dyspnea and hypoxia.[6] Using an inhaler before sexual activity and changing to less active sexual positions may help. Physical and pulmonary rehabilitation should be considered.

Rheumatoid Arthritis

Rheumatoid arthritis is a chronic, systemic, inflammatory, painful and physically disabling condition. It can affect almost every domain in life, including relationships and sexuality.[7] A questionnaire about sexual problems given to women with rheumatoid arthritis indicated that recently married patients were concerned about pregnancy, the sexual desire of most was diminished, and intercourse had become less frequent and less satisfying; affected hip and knee joints made certain sexual intercourse positions difficult. Those who had unsatisfactory sexual relationships reported less demand for intercourse by their spouses and lower frequency of their own orgasms.[8]

For a fulfilling sexual life, patients should be counseled to adopt a positive attitude toward sexual relationships.[8] A hot shower before sexual activity can help.[1] Placing pillows around the body and joints may ease pain during sex. Trying different sexual positions may help.

Spinal Cord Injury

Substantial changes to both the autonomic and the somatic nervous system occur after spinal cord injury,[9] with varying affects on body image and sexuality.

Because people with spinal cord injury have sensory problems, they should identify body areas that allow sensation and use them to augment sexual expression. Despite sensory problems, erection and vaginal lubrication may be possible through spinal reflexes or through psychogenic reflexes if spinal reflex centers are affected.

If sphincter control has been lost, emptying the bladder and bowels before sexual activity can be helpful. If spasticity of the hips and lower extremities interferes with pleasure and performance, muscle relaxants can be used beforehand.[1]

Bladder and Bowel Problems

Intimacy and privacy focus not only on sexual acts, but also on the body itself. People with bodily anomalies, and their sexual partners, are particularly aware of the contradictions of the body and its exposure in intimate acts.

- People with limited or no bladder or bowel control who use a stoma to manage elimination are sensitive to the proximity of the sites of pleasure and excretion.[10] Pleasurable sex, idealized, involves losing control. People who are incontinent or rely on a stoma, however, must monitor their bladder and bowel, disguising the stoma and bag and controlling their body in sex and other circumstances.
- The need to negotiate bodily boundaries with partners, or to disclose one's imperfections to new sexual partners, causes self-consciousness and social unease, and people need to reconstruct notions of privacy and dignity so that breaches in bodily control do not undermine the sexual relationship. For many, the stoma undermines self-esteem and body image, and its management confuses the status of the individual as "normal" and the partner as lover.[10]

Chronic Renal Failure

Sexual dysfunction is common in those with chronic renal failure. Prevalence estimates run from 9% before dialysis to 60% to 70% afterward in male and female patients. Several somatic factors are implicated.

Sexual dysfunction in men undergoing hemodialysis or peritoneal dialysis is not so much due to erectile failure but to loss of sexual interest, subjectively ascribed to fatigue. Loss of sexual interest was also found in women undergoing these procedures.[11]

Cancer

The trauma of being diagnosed and treated for cancer greatly affects psychosocial functioning, including managing at home, health and welfare services, finances, employment, legal matters, relationships, recreation, and sexuality and body image.[12]

Cancers that potentially have the greatest impact on sexuality, body image, and sexual function are breast, prostate, colorectal, gynecological, testicular, and head and neck cancers.

The disease process itself can affect body image and sexuality in many ways, including the effects of weight loss, muscle loss, anemia, pale skin, anxiety, depression, loss of libido, pain, fatigue, incontinence, neurological impairment, ascites, and loss of sensation.[13]

Chemotherapy has multiple potential side effects that might affect a person's sense of attractiveness, including alopecia of the scalp and body hair, pallor, nausea, vomiting, weight gain or loss, and fatigue.[14] Chemotherapy that causes stomatitis and thrush can results in mouth sores, vaginal irritation, and severe dyspareunia. Alkylating chemotherapy can cause ovarian failure, premature menopause, and low estrogen and testosterone levels. The low testosterone decreases libido.[14] Radiation therapy can cause skin pigmentation, retraction, telangiectasias, erythema, and fibrosis. Fibrosis can affect mobility and limit physical positions during sexual intimacy.

Women given hormonal therapy for breast cancer have low estrogen levels, which can reduce sexual desire and cause vaginal dryness and painful sexual intercourse.

Surgery also affects body image and sexuality. Mastectomy has been described as a mutilation of the body that leads to loss of femininity and attractiveness and makes women feel unacceptable to their partners. Breast conservation has little impact on successful sexual adjustment after breast cancer. Lumpectomy patients may have some advantages in body image and enjoyment of breast caressing, but this does not translate into strong effects on sexual function.[15]

Even with nerve-sparing prostate cancer surgery, impaired sexual function may still be a problem. There is also the risk for urinary incontinence, although this improves over time in most cases.[13]

Psychosocial dysfunction in patients with stomas is higher than in those with intact sphincters.

After surgery for head and neck cancer, those with extensive disfigurement had a significantly higher impact on self image, a worsened relationship with their partner, reduced sexuality, and increased social isolation compared to those with minor disfigurements.[16]

DRUGS COMMONLY USED IN PALLIATIVE MEDICINE WITH EFFECTS ON SEXUALITY AND SEXUAL FUNCTION

Both prescription and over-the-counter medications can alter sexual function.

Opiates

Opiates can cause diminished libido, erectile failure, and retarded ejaculation.[17-19] Loss of sexual function is a primary reason for methadone maintenance program dropout.[20,21] Buprenorphine is a new drug for the pharmacotherapy of opioid dependence. It seems not to suppress plasma testosterone in heroin-addicted men, and it is less frequently accompanied by sexual side effects.[22] Opiate-stimulated prolactin release is thought to be the primary cause of decreased serum luteinizing hormone and testosterone.[17] Decreased serum testosterone and luteinizing hormone levels, along with generalized central nervous system (CNS) depression, decrease libido, whereas the opiate α-adrenergic blocking activity is thought to be the primary cause of retarded ejaculation.[18]

Amphetamines, Cocaine, and Phencyclidine

Amphetamines, cocaine, and phencyclidine can cause erectile and ejaculatory dysfunction.[23,24]

Antihypertensive Medications

Antihypertensive medications interfere with sexual functioning more than any other class of prescription medications. Propranolol, a β-blocker, affects both libido and erectile function.[25-27] Proposed mechanisms include CNS depression, decreased CNS sympathetic outflow, and excessive α-sympathetic tone. Similar sexual dysfunction has been reported with other β-blockers (Nadolol, Timolol).[28,29] The frequency appears to be significantly lower, especially with less lipophilic agents that are more cardioselective (Atenolol, Metoprolol).[30]

Calcium channel antagonists, as a class, are associated with a low incidence of induced erectile dysfunction. There may be differences among the three subclasses, depending on the site of action. Dihydropyridines act primarily in extracardiac sites; therefore, they may have more interaction with the skeletal muscle of the bulbocavernosus and the smooth muscles of the vas deferens and seminal vesicles. This may block semen emission into the urethra, causing ejaculation difficulty.[31]

Clonidine can cause impotence, decreased libido, and gynecomastia.[30]

Spironolactone, a competitive aldosterone inhibitor, may cause decreased libido, impotence, and gynecomastia in men and irregular menses, painful breast enlargement, decreased libido, and decreased vaginal lubrication in women.[30] This occurs because of inhibition of dihydrotestosterone binding to cytosol protein receptors.[32]

Thiazide diuretics may decrease libido and inhibit vaginal lubrication. The mechanism is unclear but may involve vasodilation of vascular smooth muscle, volume depletion, or zinc depletion reducing testosterone production.[31,33]

Psychotropic Agents

Antipsychotics

Drug-induced sexual dysfunction has been reported with most, if not all, antipsychotics. It usually involves ejaculatory or erectile impairment, although decreased libido has been reported. Antipsychotics possess dopamine receptor–blocking, α-adrenergic blocking, anticholinergic, and sedative activities. Ejaculatory failure is a result of α-adrenergic blockade of the pudendal-thoracolumbar spinal sympathetic reflex arc, which is required for emission. Antipsychotic-induced CNS sedation may decrease libido.[34,35]

Antidepressants

Chronic antidepressant treatment (tricyclic antidepressants and monoamine oxidase inhibitors) has caused erectile dysfunction, anorgasmia, or retrograde ejaculation. Selective serotonin reuptake inhibitors (SSRIs) are also reported to cause sexual dysfunction, including decreased libido, delayed orgasm or ejaculation, and anorgasmia.[36] The tricyclic-induced impotence primarily involves blockade of parasympathetic innervation required for erection[34,35]; adrenergic blockade of the thoracolumbar sympathetic innervation is probably also involved.[37] Trazodone is the only antidepressant reported to cause priapism.[38]

Histamine₂ Blockers

Histamine$_2$ blockers (particularly cimetidine) may stimulate prolactin release and secondarily reduce testosterone levels.

Glucocorticoids

High doses of glucocorticoids can cause menstrual irregularities and lower fertility in both men and women. The mechanism is unclear, but inhibition of sex hormone production may contribute.[39]

SEXUAL HISTORY

For many, anxiety about a chronic illness and adjustment to the accompanying changes in sexual function, body image, and intimate relationships can be difficult. There are many challenges to a good sexual history. The person must be made to feel comfortable and safe in self-disclosure. A nonjudgmental, accepting attitude coupled with empathetic statements fosters alignment with the patient. Straightforward inquiries about sexual function, delivered with a sense of comfort, elicit candid responses. The sexual history is best incorporated into the normal medical framework. A full medical history must be taken, including psychiatric and medication history. History taking should proceed from open-ended questions ("How is your sexual functioning?") to specific, sufficiently detailed questions ("Does your partner touch your genitals?").

Examples of general routine questions include the following:

- Are you having sexual relations currently? If not, when did you last have sexual intercourse?
- Are you satisfied with the frequency and quality of your sexual experience?
- How did your partner react to your illness?

Vague answers should prompt more detailed questioning.

Barriers to a Sexual History

There are numerous barriers that may make taking a sexual history difficult[13]:

- Lack of time
- Embarrassment of both physician and patient
- Belief that disfigured bodies are not sexually attractive
- Lack of adequate training and skills
- Lack of privacy or fear of lack of confidentiality
- Cultural issues, age, and gender
- Fear of reminding the patient of a previous sexual assault or difficult relationship
- Fear of legal implications

The PLISSIT Model

The PLISSIT model gives guidance to assist with sexual health issues.[13,14] It has four treatment stages, the first three for the primary care physician:

- *Permission giving (P)* refers to the consent to discuss sexual health (i.e., physician provides the opportunity and initiates discussion about sexuality). The topic should be approached by asking open-ended questions and using normalizing language.
- *Limited information (L)* is the provision of resources regarding sexual health. This includes dispensing relatively basic information, such as books and referral to support groups.
- *Specific suggestions (SS)* include recommendations regarding sexual dysfunction (e.g., to use lubricants for vaginal dryness). Other suggestions to address sexual difficulty include creating a nice atmosphere with candles, scents, and lighting; using medication for hot flashes; and which sexual positions may ease pain and discomfort.
- *Intensive therapy (IT)* should probably be accomplished by a specialist if problems are severe, prolonged, preexisting, or more in-depth.

Medical Therapy

Several medications help with sexual dysfunction, such as lubricants for vaginal dryness; sildenafil, vardenafil, or tadalafil for male sexual dysfunction; and testosterone replacement for low testosterone levels.

Examples of surgical treatment include reconstructive surgery after breast cancer, prosthetics for amputation, and orthodontics after surgery for head and neck cancer.

Psychotherapy helps people process the intense distress of diagnoses and treatment and maintain communication with their partners. Counseling can improve body image, assist in adjusting to life changes, and improve communication skills betweens partners.[14]

Support groups provide the opportunity for each person to share his or her own experience and get support and motivation from other individuals.

CONCLUSIONS

The trauma of being diagnosed and treated for a chronic illness can greatly affect psychosexual functioning and intimate relationships.

The issue of body image and sexuality should be addressed routinely. Simple suggestions may be all that is required for some. More complex situations often require time and further intervention.

Professionals should develop strong, ongoing relationships with their patients and work with them to arrive at creative solutions for their sexual life and body image problems.

REFERENCES

1. Greydanus DE, Rimsza ME, Newhouse PA. Adolescent sexuality and disability. Adolesc Med 2002;13:223-247.
2. Nusbaum MR, Hamilton C, Lenahan P. Chronic illness and sexual functioning. Am Fam Physician 2003;67:347-254.
3. van der Riet P. The sexual embodiment of the cancer patient. Nurs Inquiry 1998;5:248-257.
4. Burke LE. Current concepts of cardiac rehabilitations. Occup Health Nurs 1981;29:41-47.
5. Newshan G, Taylor B, Gold R. Sexual functioning in ambulatory men with HIV/AIDS. Int J STD AIDS 1998;9:672-676.
6. Stockdale-Wooley RS. Respiratory distress and sexuality. In Fogel CL, Lauver D (eds). Sexual Health Promotion. Philadelphia: WB Saunders, 1990, pp 370-383.
7. Hill J, Bird H, Thorpe R. Effects of rheumatoid arthritis on sexual activity and relationships. Rheumatology 2003;42:280-286.
8. Yoshino S, Uchida S. Sexual problems of women with rheumatoid arthritis. Arch Phys Med Rehabil 1981;62:122-123.
9. Elliott SL. Problems of sexual function after spinal cord injury. Prog Brain Res 2006;152:387-399.
10. Manderson L. Boundary breaches: Body, sex, and sexuality after stoma surgery. Social Sci Med 2005;61:405-415.
11. Toorians AWFT, Janssen E, Laan E, et al. Chronic renal failure and sexual functioning: Clinical status versus objectively assessed sexual response. Nephrol Dial Transplant 1997;12:2654-2663.
12. Wright EP, Kiely MA, Lynch P, et al. Social problems in oncology. Br J Cancer 2002;87:1099-1104.
13. Sundquist K, Yee L. Sexuality and body image after cancer. Aust Fam Physician 2003;32:19-23.
14. Bakewell RT, Volker DL. Sexual dysfunction related to the treatment of young women with breast cancer. Clin J Oncol Nurs 2005;9:697-702.
15. Anllo LM. Sexual life after breast cancer. J Sex Marital Ther 2000;26:241-248.
16. Gamba A, Romano M, Grosso IM, et al. Psychosocial adjustment of patients surgically treated for head and neck cancer. Head Neck 1992;14:218-223.
17. Mirin SM, Meyer RE, Mendelson JH, et al. Opiate use and sexual function. Am J Psychiatry 1980;137:909.
18. Cicero TJ, Bell RD, Wiest WG, et al. Function of the male sex organs in heroin and methadone users. N Engl J Med 1975;292:882.
19. Mintz J, O'Hare K, O'Brien CP. Sexual problems of heroin addicts. Arch Gen Psychiatry 1974;31:700.
20. Cushman P, Dole V. Detoxification of rehabilitated methadone maintained patients. JAMA 1973; 226:747.
21. Garbutt G, Goldstein A. Blind comparison of three methadone maintenance dosages in 180 patients. In Proceedings of the Fourth National Conference on Methadone Treatment. New York: National Association for Prevention of Addiction to Narcotics, 1972, p 411.
22. Biesener N, Albrecht S, Schwager A, et al. Plasma testosterone and sexual function in men receiving buprenorphine maintenance for opioid dependence. J Clin Endocrinol Metab 2005;90:203-206.
23. Brock GB, Lue TF. Drug-induced male sexual dysfunction: An update. Drug Saf 1993;8:414-426.
24. Anonymous. Drugs that cause sexual dysfunction. Med Lett Drug Ther 1983;25:73.
25. Burnett WC, Chahine RA. Sexual dysfunction as a complication of propranolol therapy in men. Cardiovasc Med 1979;4:811.
26. Hollifield JW, Sherman K, Vander Zwagg R, et al. Proposed mechanisms of propranolol's antihypertensive effect in essential hypertension. N Engl J Med 1976;295:68.
27. Knarr JW. Impotence from propranolol? Ann Intern Med 1976;85:259.
28. Jackson BA. Nadolol, a once daily treatment for hypertension multi-centre clinical evaluation. Br J Clin Pract 1980;34:211.
29. McMahon CD, Shaffer RN, Hoskins HD, et al. Adverse effects experienced by patient taking timolol. Am J Opthalmol 1979;88:736.
30. Stevenson JG, Umstead GS. Sexual dysfunction due to antihypertensive agents. Drug Intell Clin Pharm 1984;18:113.
31. Barksdale JD, Gardner SF. The impact of first-line antihypertensive drugs on erectile dysfunction. Pharmacotherapy 1999;19:573-581.

32. Loriaux DL, Menard R, Taylor A, et al. Spironolactone and endocrine dysfunction. Ann Intern Med 1976;85:630.
33. Duncan L, Bateman DN. Sexual function in women: Do antihypertensive drugs have an impact? Drug Saf 1993;8:225-234.
34. Aldrige SA. Drug-induced sexual dysfunction. Clin Pharm 1982;1:141.
35. Buffum J. Pharmacosexology: The effects of drugs on sexual function: A review. J Psychoactive Drugs 1982;14:5.
36. Rothschild AJ. New directions in the treatment of antidepressant-induced sexual dysfunction. Clin Ther 2000;22(Suppl A):A42-A61.
37. Shen WW, Mallya AR. Psychotropic-induced sexual inhibition. Am J Psychiatry 1983;140:514.
38. Anonymous. Priapism with trazodone (Desyrel). Med Lett Drug Ther 1984;26:35.
39. MacAdams MR, White RH, Chipps BE. Reduction of serum testosterone levels during chronic glucocorticoid therapy. Ann Intern Med 1986;104:648.

SUGGESTED READING

Cash TF, Pruzinsky T (eds). Body Image: A Handbook of Theory, Research, and Clinical Practice. New York: Guilford Press, 2002.

Lubkin IM, Larson PD. Chronic Illness: Impact and Interventions, 6th ed. Boston: Jones & Bartlett, 2006.

Schover LR, Jensen SB. Sexuality and Chronic Illness: A Comprehensive Approach. New York: Guilford Press, 1988.

ADDITIONAL RESOURCES

American Academy of Family Physicians. Available at: http://www.familydoctor.org (accessed September 2007).

Medline Plus. Health Topics. Available at http://www.nlm.nih.gov/medlineplus/healthtopics.html (accessed September 2007).

UpToDate Patient Information. Available at http://www.patients.uptodate.com (accessed September 2007).

Bioethics

CHAPTER **17**

Principles of Bioethics

Darren P. Mareiniss and David Casarett

KEY POINTS

- End-of-life issues present many difficult decisions for health care providers and patients. The appropriate approach to ethical decision making is essential to provide proper care.

- Within the field of bioethics, there are several ways to approach ethical problems. To understand ethical evaluations, palliative medicine specialists should be familiar with these various approaches.

- Of the factors considered in ethical decision making, patient autonomy has become a predominant consideration. By obtaining proper informed consent, physicians respect such autonomy.

- Palliative medicine specialists must ensure that patients have decision-making capacity before informed consent may be obtained.

- If a patient does not have capacity to make a decision, advance directives such as living wills and health care proxies are mechanisms by which a patient's right to make decisions may be respected.

- Standards for evaluating an incapacitated patient's choice differ depending on whether the patient has lost a prior capacity to choose or never had such a capacity.

The importance of bioethics and ethical decision making within the field of palliative care cannot be overstated. Proxy decision making, pain control, artificial nutrition and hydration, euthanasia, and withholding or withdrawing treatment all raise a variety of difficult ethical issues. Bioethics is a young, multidisciplinary field that focuses on the use of philosophical and principle-based theories to solve dilemmas in medicine and the life sciences.[1] This chapter introduces the basic concepts of bioethics while focusing particular attention on practical ethical decision making at the bedside.

HISTORY OF BIOETHICS

Consideration of the moral obligations a physician has to his or her patient is by no means a recent phenomenon. In fact, medical ethics has existed since the inception of the medical profession itself. More than 4000 years ago, King Hammurabi of Babylon created the Hammurabi Code, which outlined proper conduct for physicians. Fifteen hundred years later, Greek physicians established the Hippocratic Oath, which served as the foundation for medical ethics in Western society and remains influential today.[2] In 1803, the English physician Thomas Percival published one of the first secular works on medical ethics. However, Percival's Code of Medical Ethics, which became an influential guide for Western physicians, was more of a guide to professional etiquette rather than a work focused on ethical decision making. His code employed an attitude of "what was good for the guild was good for the patient" and was guided by a paternalistic view of patient care.[2] In 1847, the American Medical Association borrowed from Percival in creating its Code of Ethics, which remained largely unchanged for more than 100 years.[2] However, this paternalistic view of the patient changed dramatically in the second half of the 20th century as research abuses, publications, social change, technological advances and seminal judicial opinions created a public outcry for greater patient autonomy and heralded the establishment of the field of bioethics.[3,4]

The roots of modern bioethics and the patient autonomy movement may be traced back to the Nuremberg trials of physicians and researchers for human subject research atrocities.[5] These individuals had subjected concentration camp victims and prisoners of war to nonconsensual, harmful, and gruesome human experimentation. As a result of this trial, the first international code of research ethics—the Nuremberg Code—was created.[5] The Code established that patient autonomy and voluntary decision making are integral to ethical human experimentation. Further, the Code stated that human research subjects must participate voluntarily in studies and that they must be fully informed.[5]

Over the next 30 years, the field of bioethics was founded on several key works that included *Morals and Medicine,* by John Fletcher, and *Patient as Person,* by Paul Ramsey. These works focused less on Percival's guild considerations and physician etiquette and more on the ethical justification of decisions, setting the stage for the development of bioethics as an independent field of scholarship.[2]

Key Advances

- In the 1960s, the civil rights movement created an outcry for "patients' rights."[2,4] Adding to the force of this movement was the public disclosure of a series of human subject research abuses. In 1966, Henry Beecher published "Ethics and Clinic Research" in *The New England Journal of Medicine*. This seminal article exposed several human research studies that had endangered subjects without appropriate clinical benefit or disclosure.[5] Several years later, the abuses of the federally funded Tuskegee experiments became public. This long-term study monitored impoverished syphilitic African-American patients in rural Alabama for more than 40 years. Study participants were monitored clinically without the benefit of antibiotics so that the progression of syphilis could be observed in its primary, secondary, and tertiary manifestations.[5] Such abuses struck at the heart of dignity and patient autonomy issues and resulted in public outcry for patient rights.

- As a result of this public condemnation, the U.S. Congress promulgated the National Research Act of 1974.[5] This Act created the National Commission for the Protection of Human Subjects of Biomedical and Behavior Research and mandated independent ethics reviews for all federally funded research. The National Commission subsequently authored the Belmont Report in 1979. This report created the foundations for research disclosure in the United States and set the standards for patient autonomy and voluntary decision making. Before the publication of the Belmont Report, Tom Beauchamp and James Childress published the first edition of their *Principles of Biomedical Ethics* in 1977. This work, like the Belmont Report and the Nuremberg Code, advocated patient participation and autonomy in medical decision making.[6]

- Landmark judicial opinions dealing with the right to refuse care increased public appreciation and support for autonomous decision making in the United States and around the world. In 1976, the New Jersey Supreme Court, in *In re Quinlan,* ruled that a permanently vegetative patient could refuse ventilator support.[7] In 1990, the U.S. Supreme Court, in *Cruzan,* affirmed that patients who can no longer make decisions still retain a constitutional liberty interest and right to refuse care.[8] Although the Court determined that such a right could be exercised through a proxy, it allowed evidentiary restrictions requiring a finding of clear and convincing evidence of a patient's decision. Both of these highly publicized cases reaffirmed a patient's right to refuse treatment.[7,8]

- Technological advancements in medicine during this time created new dilemmas. Innovations in intensive care, ventilator technology, resuscitation, and antibiotic development created additional ethical pressures within medicine, leading to the growth of bioethics.[4] New technologies in medicine were seen as both a blessing and "an oppressive medical technology, unnaturally prolong[ing] dying."[3]

Regulation

Like palliative care, institutional ethics committees and consultation services have seen dramatic growth in the academic and private medical settings. In 1995, the Joint Commission on Accreditation of Healthcare Organizations (JCAHO, now known as The Joint Commission), in recognition of the importance of these considerations, began requiring that hospitals provide ethics committee services.[9] Since then, ethics committees have flourished and are present in 93% of hospitals in the United States.[3] In addition to these committees, there are now numerous centers for

bioethics worldwide, as well as journals of bioethics. Bioethics and palliative care have evolved into multidisciplinary and independent fields, with significant overlap, which share a common approach to decision making.

THEORIES OF BIOETHICS

Within the field of bioethics, there are several ways to approach ethical problems. Religious, philosophical, and principle-based considerations may be used in ethical decision making. To understand such ethical evaluations, it is important to be familiar with each of these various approaches. The following paragraphs provide a brief description of some of these considerations.

Utilitarianism

Utilitarianism is a consequence-based theory that advocates an analysis of the overall good achieved by a given action.[1] The morality of an action is judged solely on its end result. This philosophical analysis had its origins in the writings of Jeremy Bentham (1748-1832) and John Stuart Mill (1806-1873) and advocated for maximizing the "good."[10] For Mill and Bentham, both *hedonistic* utilitarians, the "good" meant maximizing pleasure or happiness. More generally, this theory asserts that all ethical decisions should entail a balancing of the costs and benefits of an action with an eye towards maximizing overall "happiness."

Within this theory, there are two separate utilitarian schools of thought: rule utilitarianism and act utilitarianism.[1] A rule utilitarian operates on precedent. Once it is established that a general rule serves the greater good, they advocate that such a rule should be adhered to regardless of individual consequences. An act utilitarian is more pragmatic. Rather than setting down broad social rules, this type of utilitarian advocates maximizing of the "good" in each separate situation. Thus, an act utilitarian does not adhere to strict rules of general good. For example, a rule utilitarian may advocate that a clinician should always be honest with patients. The justification may be that honesty in the medical profession is an important standard that generates patient trust and results in better patient disclosure and care. However, an act utilitarian may choose not to be honest in a given clinical situation if the beneficial consequences may be maximized by a lie.

Deontology and Kantian Thought

Deontology is a theory that is in almost direct opposition to utilitarian thought. This philosophical theory advocates that actions are morally right if they are consistent with a predetermined moral rule.[1] Immanuel Kant (1724-1804), a German philosopher, established the most famous deontological ethical theory.[11] His theory states that there are absolute moral requirements on actions that can be determined through the use of certain categorical imperatives. These theoretical tests determine the morality of an action. Kant's principle of universality states that one should "act only on the maxim whereby you can at the same time will that it should become a universal law."[11] This moral test requires that an action be applied to all persons in similar situations. If making a rule universal defeats its purpose, it is immoral. In the previous example, if deceiving patients were a universal rule, no patient would believe such deceptions, and any attempt to lie would fail. Therefore, Kant would hold that such an action (i.e., deceiving a patient) is empirically immoral because it cannot be universally applied. The problems with this strict theory are readily apparent. Many actions in the practice of medicine are pragmatic. As a result, it is doubtful that such a strict adherence to this rule would result in beneficial and appropriate results in all situations.

Perhaps the more useful theory for the ethical assessment of medical decision making and patient care is Kant's second categorical imperative: "act in such a way that you treat humanity whether in our own person or in the person of another, always at the same time as an end and never simply as a means."[11] Applying this principle to the practice of medicine requires that clinicians treat patients as ends and not as means. Accordingly, although there may be clinical indications for diagnostic tests, procedures, and medical treatment, the patient's outcome and perspective dictate that objective criteria are secondary to a patient's informed wish. In this sense, the second categorical imperative can be applied to practical clinical decision making and bioethical deliberation. In contrast to both rule and act utilitarian thought, such a consideration appears to put more stock in the patient's perspective.

Principle Theory

Beauchamp and Childress, in *Principles of Biomedical Ethics*, established a model for bioethical decision making that, although not a theory, incorporated some aspects of both utilitarian and deontological thought. This model, principlism, advocated the use of four basic considerations in ethical deliberation: respect for autonomy, beneficence, nonmaleficence, and justice. Each consideration is prima facie binding but may be overridden by another conflicting consideration for good reason. According to this model, clinicians should weigh each of these considerations in determining the appropriate action. This allows clinicians to exercise more discretion in decision making than in the more stringent philosophical models of utilitarian thought and deontology.[6] However, this model does not always provide a single solution. Rather, it provides a checklist of ethical considerations, much like the clinician's review of systems, which helps to ensure that all the relevant issues are considered.

Respect for Autonomy

The word *autonomy* is derived from the Greek *autos* ("self") and *nomos* ("rule") and therefore means "self-rule."[6] Autonomy is defined as an act or decision that a patient undertakes (1) intentionally, (2) with understanding, and (3) in the absence of controlling influences. If a patient acts intentionally, with understanding and without controlling influence, principlism considers this to be an autonomous act that should be respected by a provider.

Beneficence

The principle of beneficence refers to "a moral obligation to act for the benefit of others."[6] Such an obligation is the focus of utilitarian thought. Within principlism, it simply requires consideration of the beneficial outcomes of an action.

Nonmaleficence

The principle of nonmaleficence is closely associated with the well-known medical ethics maxim *primum non nocere*, or "first do no harm."[6] This doctrine has is foundation in the Hippocratic Oath. Essentially, consideration of this principle requires an assessment of the harm that may result from a decision.

Justice

Justice refers to consideration of distributive justice and fairness. Similar to rule utilitarian thought, justice considerations refer to balancing burdens and benefits in resource allocation. Such considerations reflect a desire to use limited medical resources to maximize patient benefit. In other words, the principle of justice requires that medical resources (e.g., costly treatments, scarce hospital beds) be allocated in a way that is based on clear criteria and equity.

Virtue Ethics

Unlike the rule-based, principle-based, and obligation-based theories, virtue ethics emphasizes the pursuit of virtuous characteristics by health care providers. Integrity, fidelity, respect, sympathy, fairness, skill, wisdom, and knowledge are characteristics to be aspired to by providers that guide appropriate behavior.[6] This notion of ideal medical virtues is embodied in the Hippocratic Oath and dates back to Aristotle and Plato.[1] In addition to ancient philosophers, modern medical practitioners such as Pellegrino advocate the importance of virtue ethics in modern biomedical ethics.[4] Of note, this concept focuses on the appropriate motivation of a health care provider. Rather than imposing artificial imperatives, codes, and models, virtue ethics advocates that health care providers adopt virtuous characteristics that will, themselves, serve to guide practitioners to the appropriate ethical decisions.

Casuistry

A casuistic approach to biomedical ethics is a unique case-based consideration of ethical problems. This ethical theory was at its height in medieval and early modern philosophy but has experienced a recent revival.[2] Casuistry uses history, past paradigmatic cases, and factual circumstances to determine appropriate decision making. It favors analogy over deductive reasoning and considers biomedical ethics in terms of past precedent. Like legal case law, a casuistic approach considers the specific facts of an ethical dilemma and compares them to past similar ethical cases in order come to a decision.[1] Theories and rules serve as guidelines for a casuistic review that focuses on practical decision making.

Religious Considerations

An exhaustive treatment of religious beliefs is beyond the scope of this chapter. However, a brief consideration is essential. Of note, the major monotheistic religions—Judaism, Christianity and Islam—have key moral norms that are absolute rules from above.[12] Additionally, most of these religions include some form of the "Golden Rule."[9] The Golden Rule states that you should do unto others as you would have done unto you; that is, a physician should treat patients as he or she would want to be treated in a similar situation. Other religions, such as Buddhism, Hinduism, and Jainism, believe in concepts of karma or a cosmic moral order that create consequences for an action.[12] Clinicians should be aware of cultural and religious beliefs that might influence a patient's actions and decisions and be sensitive to these considerations. Although religious beliefs may appear to be in opposition to logic or appropriate care, they must nevertheless be respected as an autonomous wish.

DECISION MAKING

In recent years, autonomy has emerged as the single most important factor in practical clinical decision making.[9,13] Though principlism remains a useful construct for evaluating the facets of an ethical case in an orderly manner,[4] autonomy has been most emphasized by ethicists, courts, and clinicians.[8,14,15] However, respect for autonomy reflects other ethical philosophies as well. Deontologic concerns for respect of the person are clearly considered by respecting patient autonomy. Additionally, autonomous decision making has aspects of virtue ethics as well. As outlined later, autonomous decisions can occur only when there is full disclosure and open communication. Effective disclosures often require physicians to foster an environment of integrity, fidelity, and trust between themselves and their patients. Such considerations are consistent with the teachings of virtue ethics. Finally, much of a patient's or surrogate's decision making may be guided by religious, faith-based beliefs. As a result, decision making may also encompass religious considerations.

In evaluating decision making, three basic categories of patients must be addressed: patients with the capacity to make medical decisions, patients who have lost that capacity, and patients who never had the capacity. A clinician must make a preliminary determination of the type of patient he or she is dealing with before an analysis may proceed. Once this is established, the clinician must employ a tailored assessment of decision making dictated by the type of patient.

Decision-Making Capacity

A prerequisite to informed consent is a patient's intact *capacity* to make decisions. Evaluation of such capacity is a decision-specific determination that focuses on the patient's ability to understand and communicate a rational decision.[16] In complicated or difficult cases, a neurologist or psychiatrist should be consulted to make this assessment. The key considerations in an assessment of decision-making capacity are the following[17]:

1. *Ability to express a choice:* The person must be able to express his or her choice and communicate that choice.
2. *Ability to understand relevant information:* The person must be able to understand information about the purpose of treatment, remember the

information, and show that he or she can be part of the decision-making process.
3. *Ability to appreciate the significance of the information and its consequences:* The person must understand the consequences of treatment refusal and the risks and benefits of accepting or refusing treatment.
4. *Ability to manipulate information:* The person must be able to engage in reasoning as it applies to making treatment decisions (e.g., use logical processes, weigh treatment decisions, manipulate information about treatment decisions).

It is usually inappropriate to assume that a patient with mental pathology, sedation, or cognitive deficit lacks decision-making capacity. Instead, a formal evaluation is necessary.

Capacity is different from competence. *Competence* is determined by a court of law and uses issues of capacity in evaluating the legal ability to contract, write wills, or conduct one's affairs.[17] Because the standard of competence varies by jurisdiction, an exhaustive discussion of competence is beyond the scope of this chapter.

Patients with Decision-Making Capacity and Informed Consent

As noted earlier, self-determination and respect for a patient's personal choice have become the guiding principles for physicians with regard to ethical issues.[9,13-15] Patients who have decision-making capacity must give informed consent before most treatments or procedures may be performed.[2] This informed consent standard has its roots in the common law of both England and the United States. Treatment of patients without such consent was and is considered a battery. In 1914, Justice Cardozo, in the often cited case of *Schloendorff v. Soc'y of New York Hospital*, stated that "Every human being of adult years and sound mind has a right to determine what shall be done with his own body: and a surgeon who performs an operation without his patient's consent commits an assault for which he is liable."[2] This rule governing consent remains in the American and English common law today.

Within bioethics, respect for autonomy can be traced back to the Nuremberg Code, the Belmont Report, and principlism.[18] Informed consent respects this concept by requiring a patient's authorization of a medical intervention or involvement in research.[6] Informed consent requires three basic elements: (1) disclosure of information, (2) comprehension, and (3) voluntariness. A patient must be informed of the risks, benefits, and alternatives of a procedure, and a clinician must ensure that the patient understands this information.[2] Finally, a patient's decision must be voluntary. Only decisions that are substantially informed and free of constraint or controlling influence are considered autonomous.[6] Of course, no decision is ever truly free of influence or duress.[6] Often, patients feel pressure from family, clinicians, careers, and social situations that influence their ultimate decision making. This is why an autonomous decision requires only that the patient be "substantially free of constraint" and not completely free[6] (See Chapter 18 for a more extensive treatment of practical clinical considerations.)

Patients Who Lose Capacity

If a patient lacks decision-making capacity, other mechanisms for decision making must be explored. Currently, medicine has multiple mechanisms for respecting a patient's autonomy in the face of mental incapacity. Living wills are one such mechanism. These written declarations are a type of advance care directive; they are created in anticipation of incapacity and may dictate which interventions a patient wishes to prevent or have performed[16] (see Chapter 19).

By following the dictates of such documents, a health care provider respects a patient's autonomous wishes. Do not resuscitate (DNR) orders are limited forms of living wills in which patients make decisions regarding future medical care. In addition to living wills, patients may execute durable powers of attorney. These legal documents give a proxy the power to make medical decisions once a patient loses decision-making capacity.[16] Durable powers of attorney and living wills are both advance directives, but they are not mutually exclusive. An individual named under a durable power of attorney may use the patient's living will to guide appropriate decision making.[16] If patients do not have either a durable power of attorney or a living will, health care professionals should consult their local governmental rules and laws regarding appointment of proxy decision makers. In the United States, most states have family consent statutes or common law that specifies the appropriate proxy decision maker.[16]

Surrogate decision makers for previously competent patients exercise patient autonomy by making decisions based on the "substituted judgment" of the incapacitated patient.[8,14,15] Typically, proxies are family members or close friends who are familiar with the incapacitated patient.[13] Such individuals are most likely to understand the incapacitated patient's preferences and accurately predict what the patient would decide if he or she were competent.[13,15] In spite of this thinking, such substituted judgment decisions have been shown to be extremely inaccurate.[19]

However, there is arguably a morally defensible reason for following such surrogate decisions.[13] First, respecting patient proxy decisions indirectly respects patient preference. In the study by Seckler and colleagues of surrogate decision making, 87% of surveyed patients believed that family members would make accurate or fairly accurate decisions.[19] In spite of the poor correlation between surrogate decisions regarding substituted judgment and patient preference, such data imply patient confidence in family members' ability to choose. This confidence may be illustrative of patient desire to transfer decision making to family members. Accordingly, respecting surrogate decision making may indirectly pay respect to an incapacitated patient's preference. Additionally, other factors, such as a family member surrogate's financial responsibility and vested emotional interest in a patient's welfare, argue for respecting these surrogate decisions.[13]

In the United States, substituted judgment with respect to end-of-life issues has received tremendous attention in recent years. Since the landmark *Quinlan* case, two additional judicial opinions—*In re Schiavo* and *Cruzan v. Director, Missouri Department of Health*—have captured public attention and reinvigorated judicial interest in sub-stituted judgment.[15] Both of these cases dealt with surrogate decisions to withdraw nutrition and hydration from patients in a persistent vegetative state. In each case, removal of nutrition and hydration was based on the substituted judgment of the incapacitated patient. In determining the substituted judgment of these patients, the courts required a high standard of evidence to prove that the once-competent patient would have chosen to withdraw care. Arguably, such a high standard was required in these life-and-death decisions to ensure judicial accuracy.[8,15] Although debate remains about the standard of "clear and convincing" evidence required by the courts, there is interdisciplinary consensus among bioethicists, clinicians, and jurists that "substituted judgment" is an appropriate mechanism for decision making on behalf of patients who lose decision-making capacity.[14]

Patients Who Never Had Capacity to Make Medical Decisions

Although the substituted judgment standard is useful if a patient has expressed previous wishes, often these wishes are not known. For instance, mentally retarded and pediatric patients who never had decision-making capacity must be subject to a different surrogate standard. "Substituted judgment" cannot be determined if the patient has never had capacity to make a decision. In these clinical situations, a "best interest" standard has been employed.[20] In such cases, the risks and benefits of care are weighed, and appropriate care is determined by a proxy based on the best interest of the patient.[14]

Mentally Retarded Adults

In the United States, several judicial cases have dealt with never-competent patients.[20] In *Superintendent of Belchertown State School v. Saikewicz*, the Supreme Judicial Court of Massachusetts considered the case of a 67-year-old institutionalized, mentally retarded patient. The patient was suffering from acute myeloblastic monocytic leukemia. In this case, the Massachusetts court decided to forgo chemotherapeutic treatment after weighing the benefits and burdens of treatment.[18] The Court determined that the potential benefit of chemotherapy (i.e., extending the patient's life), did not outweigh the burdens of treatment (i.e., discomfort, side effects). Such an evaluation of benefits and burdens is integral to a proper best interest evaluation. In contrast to substituted judgment, this standard focuses on an objective assessment of what is good for the patient rather than a consideration of what the patient would have wanted done.

One of the factors often considered in these best interest cases is the patient's present quality of life; that is, whether the quality of a patient's life warrants the risks of an intervention. However, such a consideration may be misguided (see "Common Errors"). Lloyd and associates recently published a survey study focused on patient decision making in seriously ill patients.[21] The survey data showed no correlation between a patient's current quality of life and decisions regarding future intensive care. Accordingly, determining whether a never-competent patient would desire a specific treatment based on his or her current quality of life may not be an accurate method of predicting a patient's choice. Additionally, regarding mentally retarded patients, ethicists have noted that it would be difficult for a competent individual to envision the quality of life enjoyed by such a patient. Although the patient's life may appear to be intolerably frustrating to a competent adult, it is unclear how a mentally retarded individual would rate his or her own quality of life.[20]

Pediatric Patients

Traditionally, parents of a pediatric patient have been given significant discretion to make decisions for their children.[20] Minors in the United States are legally incompetent to make health care decisions or enter contracts, regardless of their capacity to understand. As a result, parents typically make their child's health care decisions and wield significant discretion in this process.[20] However, as in the *Saikewicz* case, the benefits and burdens of these decisions should be weighed to determine the best interest of the minor patient.[22] As stated earlier, weighing such benefits and burdens to a patient is the essence of a "best interest" evaluation. Also of importance in such situations, surrogate decision makers must themselves have capacity to make health care decisions for their children. Any concern about the capacity of a surrogate decision maker should prompt investigation and consultation with appropriate hospital personnel. Parents who lack capacity to make a decision are likely also not to be legally competent to make decisions for their child. Finally, although in the case of pediatric decision making parental discretion is significant, it can be overridden. Specifically, parental decisions that clearly are not in a child's best interest may be overruled. A common example is in the case of Jehovah's Witnesses: courts in the United States have ruled that parents may not prevent life-saving transfusions for minors. Such interventions are deemed to serve the best interest of a child and are de facto appropriate regardless of the religious beliefs of a parental surrogate.[20]

CONCLUSION

Bioethics is a young, multidisciplinary field that has become of integral importance to medicine and palliative care. End-of-life issues present many difficult decisions for health care providers and patients. Understanding the appropriate approach to these decisions, while respecting patient preference, is essential to providing proper care. Today, clinicians are expected to know more than the mere physical pathology and treatment of disease. Especially within the field of palliative care, clinicians must grapple with and understand ethical decision making and assist patients or proxies to make appropriate choices. As technology advances, ethical issues will continue to arise in medicine. The astute clinician will seek to learn not only how to correctly approach future ethical issues but also the reasoning behind such approaches. To this end, we hope this chapter has provided some guidance.

REFERENCES

1. Normative ethical theories. In Reich TR (ed). Encyclopedia of Bioethics, revised ed. New York: Simon & Schuster Macmillan, 1995, pp 736-748.
2. Morgan H, Mayo TW. Ethical aspects of neurosurgical practice. In Batjer HH, Loftus CM (eds). Textbook of Neurological Surgery: Principles and Practice. Philadelphia: Lippincott Williams & Wilkins, 2003, pp 3271-3205.
3. Aulisio MP, Chaitin, E, Arnold RM. Ethics and palliative care consultation in the intensive care unit. Crit Care Clin 2004;20:505-523.
4. Pellegrino ED. The metamorphosis of medical ethics: A 30-year retrospective. JAMA 1993;269:1158-1162.
5. Research involving human subjects. In Shapiro MH, Spece RG, Dresser R, Clayton EW (eds). Bioethics and Law, 2nd ed. St. Paul, MN: West Publishing Company, 2003, pp 198-269.
6. Beauchamp TL, Childress JF. Principles of Biomedical Ethics, 4th ed. New York: Oxford University Press, 1994.
7. *In Re Quinlan*, 355 A.2d 647 (N.J. 1976).
8. *Cruzan v. Missouri Department of Health*, 497 U.S. 261 (1990).
9. Iverson KV. Bioethics. In Marx J, Hockberger R, Walls R, et al (eds). Rosen's Emergency Medicine: Concept and Clinical Practice, 5th ed. St. Louis: Mosby, 2002, pp 2725-2734.
10. Mill JS. Utilitarianism (1861). In Sher G (ed). Indianapolis: Hackett Publishing, 1979.
11. Kant I. Grounding for the Metaphysics of Morals (1785). In Ellington JW (ed). Indianapolis: Hackett Publishing, 1987.
12. Religion and morality. In Reich TR (ed). Encyclopedia of Bioethics, revised ed. New York: Simon & Schuster Macmillan, 1995, pp 758-764.
13. Arnold RM, Kellum J. Moral justification for surrogate decision making in the intensive care unit: Implications and limitations. Crit Care Med 2003; 31:347-353.
14. Casarett D, Kapo J, Caplan A. Appropriate use of artificial nutrition and hydration: Fundamental pinciples and rcommendations. N Engl J Med 2005;353: 2607-2612.
15. Mareiniss DP. A comparison of Cruzan and Schiavo: The burden of proof, due process, and autonomy in the persistently vegetative patient. J Legal Med 2005;26:233-259.
16. Kapp MB. Ethical and legal issues. In Duthie EH. Practice of Geriatrics, 3rd ed. Philadelphia, WB Saunders, 1998, pp 31-37.
17. Mufson M. Evaluation of competence in the medical setting. In Samuels MA. Office Practice of Neurology, 2nd ed. Philadelphia: Churchill Livingston, 2003, pp 998-1004.
18. Decisions on life-sustaining treatment. In Shapiro MH, Spece RG, Dresser R, Clayton EW (eds). Bioethics and Law, 2nd ed. St. Paul, MN: West Publishing Company, 2003, pp 960-1086.
19. Seckler AB, Meier DE, Mulvihill M, et al. Substituted judgment: How accurate are proxy predictions? Ann Intern Med 1991;115:92-99.
20. Cantor NL. The bane of surrogate decision-making: Defining the best interest of never-competent persons. J Legal Med 2005;26:155-205.
21. Lloyd CB, Nietert PJ, Silvestri GA. Intensive care decision making in the seriously ill and elderly. Crit Care Med 2004;32:649-654.
22. Rushton CH. Ethics and palliative care in pediatrics: When should parents agree to withdraw life-sustaining therapy for children? Am J Nurs 2004; 104:54-63.

SUGGESTED READING

Beauchamp TL, Childress JF. Principles of Biomedical Ethics, 4th ed. New York: Oxford University Press, 1994.

Cantor NL. The bane of surrogate decision-making: Defining the best interest of never-competent persons. J Legal Med 2005;26:155-205.

Morgan H, Mayo TW. Ethical aspects of neurosurgical practice. In Batjer HH, Loftus CM (eds). Textbook of Neurological Surgery: Principles and Practice. Philadelphia: Lippincott Williams & Wilkins, 2003, pp 3271-3205.

Mufson M. Evaluation of competence in the medical setting. In Samuels MA. Office Practice of Neurology, 2nd ed. Philadelphia: Churchill Livingston, 2003, pp 998-1004.

CHAPTER **18**

Ethics and Clinical Practice

Azucena Couceiro

In a book by Dr. Cicely Saunders, there is a passage that deserves comment, because it expresses ideas widely held by health professionals[1]:

> Health Care Professionals that work day by day with these patients are usually very prudent when they say that, only by listening and reading the works of the moral philosophers they can understand the moral issues that involve their work. And they reach this conclusion because of the existence of a generalized belief that medical ethics is governed by absolute principles—nonmaleficence, justice, autonomy, and beneficence—that we are incapable to understand unless we have certain philosophical knowledge and background. These general principles quickly show their limitation when confronted with the chaotic world of everyday practice. . . . Therefore, the ethics involved in the care of terminally ill patients must be based in the interrelationship that exists between the patient and the team that is delivering the care, as well as in the problems derived by such care. . . . It is better to leave aside the utilization of abstract principles in order to be guided by an ethical model that shows respect for the

people involved in the sanitary relationship. Such model must focus on the conflict between the interests of the patient (self-determination) and those of the physician (paternalism).

In all clinical practice, not only palliative care, physicians must know how to solve conflicts of values. There is no basic contradiction between the interests of physicians and those of patients; rather, one party may give more relevance to some values in the clinical relationship. Medical professionals seek to maintain life and alleviate illness or, if that is impossible, to diminish suffering and provide adequate quality of life.[2] The patient has the same (or similar) objectives but may approach them differently or make decisions that do not coincide with those recommended by the professional. It is in these conflicting situations that bioethical principles help, because adequate knowledge properly applied to each clinical situation allows clinicians to identify ethical problems, analyze them, and propose alternatives.

In 1979, Beauchamp and Childress first formulated the four theoretical principles[3] that became the basis for others developed since. Such theory has been dominant in clinical practice, perhaps because it is directed toward action or because it gives paramount importance to decision making based on rational argument, the same way clinical decisions are made. This normative framework—based on the principles of nonmaleficence, autonomy, justice, and beneficence—seems sufficiently clear until the realities of clinical practice are encountered, in which these principles may conflict. For example, suppose a patient, who is mentally competent, refuses a surgical procedure recommended as part of his palliative care. The medical team has decided that the procedure is indicated to improve the patient's quality of life, but the patient refuses consent. How can such a conflict be resolved? Is autonomy always predominant, even if the patient's psychological ability to make decisions is doubted? Is it actually the family refusing the procedure?

Principles are only a framework within which moral problems in clinical practice can be placed. They are criteria that guide behavior and guarantee that decisions follow a rational process. They are, by themselves, insufficient. Their application is not automatic, because precise behavioral norms cannot be obtained based only on deduction. A deliberative process is needed that allows clinicians to respect these principles in each clinical situation. The principles assist, without eliminating, reflection and deliberation. They are prima facie compulsory[4]; that is, clinicians must deliver correct clinical practices, and respect patient autonomy, within the framework of sanitary justice. What is not known a priori is how this is applied in each case, especially in conflicts. The moral problems are concrete and particular, whereas the principles, by definition, are general and theoretically universal.[5]

As a result, there is a need to introduce into ethical reasoning the concept of the particular or individual approach, because a system based on principles can never be enough by itself. There is an extended and erroneous belief that, to make decisions, knowledge of these principles is sufficient. This is akin to believing that, by knowing the contents of a good palliative care manual, one could become, ipso facto, a good palliative care specialist, without having any practical abilities. Theory and practice go hand in hand.[6] It is incorrect to either undertreat or overtreat, or to oversedate unnecessarily or without authorization.[7] To apply these concepts in individual cases, clinicians must address the fact that not only theoretical principles are important but also the need to harmonize theoretical knowledge with concrete cases.[8] The principles and theoretical considerations are described in Chapter 17.

THE PRINCIPLE OF NONMALEFICENCE OR TECHNICAL CORRECTION

The Problem of Diagnosis and Prognosis

The initial problem is the diagnosis of a terminal illness. *Diagnosis* is a technical word that originated in Hippocratic medicine. The Greeks used two words to design the knowledge of a disease: the verb *diagigizoskeii* ("to discern or distinguish") and a neologism created in the 5th century, the substantive diagnosis. The technical knowledge of a disease is needed to discern it with precision from other diseases. Every diagnosis has an operative character: it is necessary to know in order to act.[9]

If a potentially curable patient is misdiagnosed as terminal, a serious technical mistake with serious ethical consequences has been made. On the other hand, if someone with an incurable disease that has all the characteristics of a terminal condition but is not properly diagnosed, he or she will be subjected to inappropriate therapeutic measures. The choice of a specific treatment must be conditioned by identification of the stage of the disease. Practically, there may be difficulties in identifying the terminal phase or the diagnosis of terminality.[10]

The diagnosis may be erroneous or premature. Good clinical judgment is essential to recognize the terminal stages in cancer; this is even more true in other conditions, such as chronic illnesses associated with malignancy (e.g., a hepatoma in someone with cirrhosis) or noncancerous conditions. In oncology, predictive tools categorize patients by the use of objective factors (functional status, physical symptoms, biological factors) to achieve a prognostic approximation on which therapy can be based.[11] This does not occur in nonmalignant pathologies, whose functional derangement differs from cancer. For example, in congestive heart failure,[12] chronic obstructive pulmonary disease,[13] or advanced dementia, identification of prognostic factors is difficult.[14] Progress in the treatment of some illnesses, such as the use of β-blockers in congestive heart failure, has reduced mortality and sudden death. Such examples certainly move the frontiers between the curative, palliative, and terminal phases, as well as corresponding therapeutic attitudes.

The fundamental element for adequate treatment is recognition of the course of the illness and the correct diagnosis of terminality. It is a technical question but also an ethical obligation, a practical application of nonmaleficence, that affects the clinical decisions proposed to patients and their families.

The Process of Clinical Decisions

Many clinical conflicts arise because patients reject options presented by the professionals. The clinical situations are complex and require the evaluation of many elements. In palliative care, multiple factors influence the evolution of an illness. To make clinical decisions, many factors must be appraised simultaneously, especially in two common clinical scenarios: (1) treatment for an acute complication in the course of an advanced condition and (2) how and when to maintain supportive treatment in a terminal illness.

In an acute complication, many factors, some biological and some biographical, must be integrated. The following factors must be considered to define realistic and reasonable objectives, which must be revised periodically[15]:

- *The illness:* clinical situation, prognosis, possibilities, and general condition of the patient
- *The treatment of the pathological condition:* complexity, efficacy, duration, and possible iatrogenic complications
- *The actual complication:* complexity, prognosis, impact on the general condition, and possible response to treatment
- *A framework of effective symptom control*

The second type of clinical decision refers to vital support measures, the treatments that artificially substitute for essential functions the diseased organism cannot maintain. Mechanical ventilators, peritoneal dialysis, and similar measures were designed to support organic functions in the critically ill so as to gain time until the recovered patient could do it alone, spontaneously or in response to some therapeutic intervention. In terminal illness, patients are neither critical nor able to recover, and these interventions must be contextualized differently. The need for advanced support of vital signs should be rare, and clinical decisions will need to be made about the use of pharmacological agents, less invasive diagnostic procedures (e.g., bronchoscopy), palliative surgery and chemotherapy, and artificial hydration and nutrition.

From the viewpoint of nonmaleficence, ethical reflection can be oriented around three elements: (1) proportionality of the clinical intervention, (2) medical responsibility for the whole process, and (3) goals and objectives. The proportionality of any measure requires integration of many elements: the aggressiveness and inconvenience to the patient, the prognosis (vital and functional), and the possible alleviation of symptoms and improvement of prognosis.

Reservations exist about palliative surgery, whose goal is to avoid local complications from a primary tumor or its metastasis, such as hemorrhage, perforation of a hollow viscus, or blockage of the respiratory or digestive tract. Such complications can cause death long before the expected demise or diminish quality of life. In such cases, the following factors must be analyzed[16]:

- Patient characteristics (poor general condition with associated co-morbidities such as respiratory insufficiency may represent a worse threat to life than the actual cancer)
- The aggressiveness of the tumor and its other biological characteristics

- The existence of a life-threatening clinical emergency (e.g., colostomy in a case of intestinal obstruction resulting from an unresectable colon cancer)
- The magnitude of the intervention, which must accord with the patient's symptoms and interference with quality of life

The concept of proportionality considers the risks and benefits, which can be difficult. For example, a patient with active lymphoma, metastatic dissemination, and multiple associated co-morbidities has a pleural effusion and respiratory insufficiency. Thoracocentesis is followed by recurrence of the effusion. Pleurodesis is then performed. Despite intensive treatment with analgesics, including narcotics, pleurodesis is not well tolerated due to intense pain, fever, and malaise. Chest radiographs reveal pneumonia which is then treated with antibiotics. The pleural effusion recurs, this time with extreme dyspnea and intense pain. On the fourth episode, the medical team studies the options: although thoracocentesis is palliative, it is invasive and impairs quality of life. Given the stage of the disease, it is time to consider exclusively palliative treatment, which is what the patient is in fact demanding.

The health team has the professional and moral responsibility of choosing what they consider to be the more correct options. It is obvious that if a treatment is deemed inadequate, it will not be offered. The selection by the patient is usually made from among choices previously made by the professionals (who have considered and discarded multiple options), which include only those options that avoid malfeasance and are therefore indicated. The limits vary, and the concept of indication must consider the patient as a whole and not any one individual symptom or sign.

Artificial Nutrition and Hydration

Another source of ethical conflicts in terminal patients is artificial nutrition and hydration, which, unlike other therapeutic measures, represents a cultural symbol. Because of the emotions involved, it has been difficult to analyze and rationalize the appropriate use and maintenance of these measures. It is presumed that food and water cannot be denied to anyone. They have acquired the character of elemental means of care and therefore are deemed obligatory.[17] This presumption, however, is incorrect[18,19]; today, it is acknowledged that withholding food and water in certain terminal situations can be the best care.

If one thing characterizes terminal patients, it is anorexia. Inadequate nutrition is associated with many problems, including biochemical conditions (hypercalcemia, uremia, hyponatremia), iatrogenic problems (medications, radiotherapy, chemotherapy), and complications (early satiety, mouth disturbances, constipation, pain). Administration of enteric or parenteral nutrition raises the question of whether the benefits outweigh the risks, inconveniences, and side effects.[20]

From the palliative perspective, it must be determined whether patients experience thirst, hunger, pain, or other unpleasant symptoms when these measures are withdrawn. Many studies suggest that terminally ill patients usually do not experience hunger or thirst.[21] A correlation cannot be made between the sensation of thirst and the level of intravenous fluids given.[22] Symptoms of thirst or hunger cannot be associated with predictive variables such as plasma osmolality or serum sodium or urea levels.[23,24] Nevertheless, hypodermoclysis to hydrate the terminally ill is recommended, as is research to clarify the role of rehydration in symptom control.[25] Dehydration itself can cause complications (renal failure, mental confusion) that also may require treatment. It is necessary to evaluate every case individually to make appropriate therapeutic decisions.[26]

Ethical reflections about nutrition and hydration must consider four aspects:

- Is it medical treatment or basic care?
- The symbolic value
- The possible painful death that may ensue without nutrition and hydration
- Is withholding these measures a synonym of euthanasia?

Is It Medical Treatment or Basic Care?

The question of whether withholding nutrition and hydration constitutes medical treatment or basic care is important and has received much attention. It is difficult to define medical treatment, because there are two fundamental minimum criteria: (1) procedures that require the participation and knowledge of health care providers and (2) administration that implies invasion of the body. According to these criteria, both intravenous hydration and enteric nutrition are medical treatments.[27] The Supreme Court of the United States (*Cruzan* case) demonstrated that no difference exists among various forms of vital support. There is a general conviction among professionals that provision of food and fluids as a maintenance measure when the digestive tract cannot be used (e.g., coma, mental illness, end-stage illness) is basic care and by obligation must be given to anyone who does not refuse.

Cultural Symbolism

The word *symbol* is derived from the Latin word *symbolum*, derived from the Greek *symballo*. The human being is characterized by the capacity to give meaning through original symbolic functions, such as language and myth. To provide food and water is a significant human action that shows respect for the life and care of a fellow human being. As is the case with any symbol, it is directly connected to individual emotions. However, it is one thing to know about cultural symbolism and another to insist that under no circumstances should artificial alimentation and nutrition be withdrawn.

In this situation, there is an obligation that derives from nonmaleficence, to identify situations in which use provides substantial benefit, or not. It is irrelevant how simple, cheap, noninvasive, commonplace, or symbolic a technique might be. The criterion is always whether it is in the best interest of the patient and proportionate and adequate to the biological situation.[28] After acknowledging that these measures are treatments and therefore can be initiated or discontinued, time must be provided to adapt the symbolic value to a new cultural recognition.

Suffering

As discussed earlier, hypothetical suffering has to do with the possible sensations of hunger and thirst. Research of increasing methodological quality supports the belief from clinical practice that loss of appetite is almost consubstantial to terminality, and also that the terminally ill usually do not feel thirsty. If they do, they benefit more from sucking on ice chips to reduce dry mouth or by taking small sips of water, and by applying lip moisturizers and mouth care, without parenteral hydration.

In the moribund patient, opioids in the serum increase with corresponding higher degrees of analgesia. To this is added the ketonemia of fasting, which produces some anorexia. These factors diminish discomfort. However, each case must be analyzed individually to decide what is best. It is unwise to generalize and assume that all patients are experiencing similar suffering.

Does It Constitute Euthanasia?

Many consider withholding of nutrition and hydration to be euthanasia, arguing that not initiating, or discontinuing, these measures causes death. This conclusion is based on a serious conceptual error, which is to consider as euthanasia all actions whose end result is death. To speak about euthanasia (direct, active euthanasia), three elements must be present: (1) the objective element (a grave illness, terminal or irreversible, that causes death or intense suffering); (2) the subjective element (the repeated, reiterated petition by the patient), and (3) action or direct cooperation that causes death.

The criteria of causality is essential, in the sense that, in the terminally ill patient, there is another concomitant and irreversible condition that will cause death. The patient is not dying because of lack of food but rather not eating because he or she is dying. Causality is not linear but multifactorial, even if a direct and deterministic connection were established between the withdrawing of food and water and death. That these measures are not equated with euthanasia does not mean that withholding nutrients is easy. It is a complex decision that must be made in accordance with the principles of proportionality and moral responsibility over the clinical process and the foreseen consequences of the actions.

Within a systematic program of palliative care, nutrition and hydration are not by themselves therapeutic, particularly with malnutrition caused by progression of systemic illness, which often is not amenable to treatment. There is no technical justification for administering hydration and nutrition if the patient will not benefit. From the moral standpoint, there is no distinction between those and other vital treatments. Despite the symbolism involved, clinicians must explain to the patients and their families, in a considered manner, the technical reasons of comfort and beneficence that direct them to modify traditional approaches. In a terminal patient, dehydration, when it provides comfort, is authentic care.[29]

THE PATIENT AND THE EXPRESSION OF AUTONOMY

The second subject of the clinical relationship, the patient, contributes a different principle: autonomy. Professionals are guided by the ethics of indication, patients by the ethics of election. These are not necessarily in conflict, especially if the clinical relation is one of dialogue and joint deliberation.[30] The professional assumes that the patient is a moral subject and brings to the relationship basic skills such as knowing how to establish a therapeutic relationship, how to adequately inform in a timely way using proper manners and forms, and how to communicate and provide emotional support and counseling. If these conditions are provided, decisions can be taken from joint effort and strategy, with both participants (health team and patients) gradually limiting themselves. If these skills are unavailable, conflicts will surface. It is important to establish their causes so that the clinician can determine which elements are present and problems can be solved.

Autonomy means the capacity to realize acts with complete information concerning all of the facts and without internal or external coercion. To achieve this, via informed consent, it is indispensable to have truthful, sufficient, and comprehensive information, as well as the capacity of the patient to understand and evaluate the information and make a voluntary decision. It is a fundamental ethical concept to respect decisions made by competent patients, but this entails a corresponding professional obligation to generate a framework so that the decision can be the product of a mutual dialogue based on an adequate clinical relationship.

From that moment on, diverse conflicts may arise. Examples include the following:

- If a patient makes a decision that is incongruent with previous decisions, this is an alarm signal, indicating the need for re-evaluation of the process and analysis of all the elements discussed earlier.
- If the patient and the family are opposed, the reason for the discrepancy must be sought. Even though the patient's decision prevails, the family are to be considered.
- If the patient makes decisions that are different from those proposed by the health team, the patient's choices must be reanalyzed to see if they are within the indicated measures, even if not those the team would propose.
- If the patient's decisions are not only different but contrary to what has been recommended by the health team, two different situations may arise. In the first, the proposed treatment is refused, and this decision must be respected provided the patient is mentally competent. In the second, a request is made by the patient about something that is absolutely contraindicated, and this decision cannot be respected. The limit to personal autonomy resides in the contraindication.
- In any event, the capacity of the patient to make decisions (i.e., his or her abilities and psychological skills) must always be evaluated.[31,32] If the patient makes a decision that most others would not make, this is not in itself a criterion for incapacity.

Because these patients usually suffer from chronic conditions, it is advisable to prepare in advance a series of decisions that will bring autonomy into practical terms by having the patient express his or her preferences for care and treatments while simultaneously becoming familiar with the process of death.[33] Advance planning tries to establish a plan so that, if the patient loses the capacity to make decisions, choices can be based on the values and desires expressed during the planning.[34] The written advance directive is only one of the steps in this process, and it is valuable for the clinician, because, as a prior record, it can preclude conflicts that arise in decision making after the patient becomes incapacitated.

CONCLUSIONS

The treatment of advanced disease is complex and requires specific professional qualifications. Ethical conflicts may be diverse, because palliative care has to do with life and death and the suffering, fragility, and vulnerability of the patients. These conflicts require rational analysis so that appropriate clinical decisions are made. Ethics and clinical work go hand in hand.[35]

Bioethical principles can be a methodological instrument of immense value, both in the recognition of conflict situations and analysis of causes and in the search for satisfactory responses. What is important is not that conflicts exist but that the path for the patient and the health team can and must be shared. Conflict is a symptom that shows clinicians the need to work with values with the same skill and professional ability with which they handle clinical work.

REFERENCES

1. Saunders CM. In Cuidados en la Enfermedad Maligna Terminal. Barcelona: Salvat, 1980.
2. The Goals of Medicine: Setting New Priorities. Hastings Center Rep 1996;26(Suppl):S9-S14.
3. Beauchamp TL, Childress JF. Principles of Biomedical Ethics. New York: Oxford University Press, 1979.
4. Ross VD. The Right and the Good. Oxford: Clarendon Press, 1930. [Traducción al castellano: Ross WD. Lo Correcto y lo Bueno. Salamanca: Sígueme, 1994.]
5. Couceiro A. Bioética y medicina actual. In Rodés I, Guardia J (eds). Medicina Interna. Barcelona: Masson, 1997; pp 3-7.
6. Couceiro A. Bioética para clínicos. Madrid: Triacastela, 1999.
7. Latimer E. Ethical challenges in cancer care. J Palliat Care 1992;8:65-70.
8. Couceiro A. Problemas éticos en cuidados paliativos. In Torres LM (ed). Medicina del Dolor. Barcelona: Masson, 1997, pp 426-438.
9. Laín Entralgo P. El diagnóstico médico: Historia y teoría. Barcelona: Salvat, 1982.
10. Ashby M, Stoffell B. Therapeutic ratio and defined phases: Proposal of ethical framework for palliative care. BMJ 1991;302:1322-1324.
11. Maltoni M, Nanni O, Pirovano M, et al. Successful validation of the Palliative Prognostic Score in terminally ill cancer patients. J Pain Symptom Manage 1999;17:240-247.
12. Vranckx P, Van Cleemput J. Prognostic assessment of end-stage cardiac failure. Acta Cardiol 1998;53:121-125.
13. Schonwetter RS, Jani CR. Survival estimation in noncancer patients with advanced disease. In Portenoy RK, Bruera E (eds). Topics in Palliative Care, vol 4. Oxford: Oxford University Press, 2000, pp 55-74.
14. Standards and Accreditation Committee, Medical Guidelines Task Force of the National Hospice Organization. Medical Guidelines for Determining Prognosis in Delected Non-cancer Diseases, 2nd ed. Arlington, VA: National Hospice Organization, 1996.
15. Latimer E. Ethical decision-making in the care of the dying, and its applications to clinical practice. J Pain Symptom Manage 1993;6:329-336.
16. Jaurrieta E. Cirugía y otras medidas intervencionistas de carácter paliativo. In Gómez-Batiste X, Planas J, Roca J, Viladiu P (eds). Cuidados Paliativos en Oncología. Barcelona: JIMS, 1996, pp 39-42.
17. Derr P. Why food and fluids can never be denied. Hastings Cent Rep 1986;16(1):28-30.
18. Lynn J, Childress J. Must patients always be given food and water? Hastings Cent Rep 1983;13(5):17-21.
19. President's Commission for the Study of Ethical Problems in Medicine and Biomedical and Behavioral Research. Decide to Forego Life-Sustaining Treatment. Washington DC: Government Printing Office, 1983.
20. Winter SM. Terminal nutrition: Framing the debate for the withdrawal of nutritional support in terminally ill patients. Am J Med 2000;109:723-726.
21. McCann R, Hall W, Groth-Juncker A. Comfort care for terminally ill patients: The appropiate use of nutrition and hydration. JAMA 1994;272:1263-1266.
22. Musgrave CF, Bartal N, Opstad J. The sensation of thirst in dying patients receiving IV hydration. J Palliat Care 1995;11:17-21.
23. Burger FI. Dehydration symptoms of palliative care cancer patients. J Pain Symptom Manage 1993;8:454-464.
24. Vullo-Navick K, Smith S, Andrews M, et al. Comfort and incidence of abnormal serum sodium, BUN, creatinine and osmolality in dehydration of terminal illness. Am J Hosp Palliat Care 1998;15:77-84.
25. Fainsinger RL, MacEachern T, Miller MJ, et al. The use of hypodermoclysis for rehydration in terminally ill cancer patients. J Pain Symptom Manage 1994;9:298-302.
26. Fainsinger R, Bruera E. The management of dehydration in terminally ill patients. J Palliat Care 1994;10:55-59.
27. Musgrave C, Bartal N, Opstad J. Intravenous hydration for terminal patients: What are the attitudes of Israeli terminal patients, their families, and their health professionals? J Pain Symptom Manage 1996;12:47-51.
28. Lynn J (ed). By No Extraordinary Means. Bloomington: Indiana University Press, 1989.
29. De Ridder D, Gastmans C. Dehydration among terminally ill patients: An integrated ethical and practical approach for caregivers. Nurs Ethics 1996; 3:305-316.
30. Emanuel EJ, Emanuel LL. Four models of the physician-patient relationship. JAMA 1992;267:2221-2226. [Traducción al castellano en: Couceiro A (ed). Bioética para clínicos. Madrid: Triacastela, 1999, pp 107-124.]
31. White BC. Competente ton Consent. Washington, DC: Georgetown University Press, 1994, pp 154-184.
32. Grisso T, Appelbaum PS. Assesing Competence to Consent to Treatment: A Guide for Physicians and Other Health Professionals. New York: Oxford University Press, 1998.
33. Singer P, Martin DK, Lavery JV, et al. Reconceptualizing advance care planning from the patient's perspective. Arch Intern Med 1998;158:879-884.
34. Emanuel LL, von Gunten CF, Ferris FD. Advance care planning. Arch Fam Med 2000;9:1181-1187.
35. Couceiro A (ed). Ética en Cuidados Paliativos. Madrid: Triacastela, 2004.

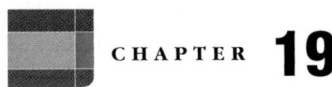

CHAPTER **19**

Advanced Directives

Angelo E. Volandes and **Mildred Z. Solomon**

KEY POINTS

- Advance care planning (ACP) should guide the ongoing care of capacitated patients, as well as care in the future, when patients may lack decisional capacity.

- Physicians should commit to the communication and relational skills needed to share a poor prognosis and establish appropriate goals of care, which should be based on the likely disease trajectory and the patient's values and preferences.

- ACP should focus not only on what treatments patients do not want but also on what treatments and services they need to ensure optimal care.

- Primary care practices, hospitals, nursing homes, and rehabilitation facilities have moral obligations to ensure that ACP is carried out in their care settings and also across institutions as patients travel between settings.

- Advance directives can be useful, but they have serious limitations and should not be the sole means for ensuring ACP. Patient's prior oral expressions of preferences have as much legal and ethical weight as written directives.

DEFINITION OF ADVANCE CARE PLANNING

Advance care planning (ACP) is an ongoing process of communication among physicians, patients and, ideally, families, which ensures that treatment plans are aligned with patients' goals and needs.[1-3] The intent is to develop a treatment plan, and provide care, that ensures the highest quality of life during the final stage of life. Sound ACP equips patients and families to handle the medical, psychosocial, and existential demands of advanced disease. ACP should provide guideposts for future care, when the patient no longer has decisional capacity.

ACP should ensure that a treatment plan brings more benefits than burdens, as patients themselves would evaluate them. ACP should focus not only on what treatments patients do not want but also on what treatments and services they need to ensure optimal care near death. Sound ACP can lead to referrals for so-called "aggressive" treatments that may hold promise for cure (e.g., referrals for assessment for kidney transplantation in end-stage renal dialysis), high-technology interventions that are palliative (e.g., radiation to reduce tumor size), or timely referral to hospice.

Failing to help patients and families plan for dying can impede appropriate pain and symptom management and impose burdensome, ineffective, or marginally beneficial treatments that many might forgo. Inadequate ACP robs people of the opportunity to share their fears and hopes, say farewells, do things that were always desired, and address spiritual concerns and other matters of existential importance.

Individual professionals, particularly physicians, have a professional obligation to ensure that ACP conversations occur. Importantly, institutions also have such obligations. Primary care practices, hospitals, nursing homes, and rehabilitation facilities need to put mechanisms in place, and establish accountabilities, to ensure that ACP is carried out in their care settings and also across institutions as patients travel between settings.

ACP has been promoted by both patient groups and medical associations as important to ensure end-of-life care consistent with individual preferences. The goal is to ensure that all patients, regardless of present health state or disease, discuss their preferences with physicians for the most common future health states, such as dementia and other potentially incapacitating diseases. ACP simultaneously ensures that patients' wishes are respected and that physicians are delivering care consistent with individual values.

HISTORY AND RATIONALE

ACP has evolved in response to seemingly intractable problems in end-of-life care: the imperative to respect patient autonomy; the imposition of burdensome medical interventions on patients who are unlikely to benefit[4,5]; concerns of conscience by clinicians imposing those treatments[5]; unrelieved pain[6,7]; inadequate control of other symptoms that arise in near death; apparently wasteful spending on so-called futile treatments; and under-referral and late referral to hospice. Various ethical and legal guidelines[2,8-10] were based on principles of autonomy (respect for persons and therefore respect for an individual's right to self-determination, including the right to refuse unwanted treatments) and nonmaleficence ("do no harm"; when cure is not possible, provide comfort and alleviate suffering). They underscored the fact that capacitated patients have the right to forgo any kind of medical intervention, including artificial nutrition and hydration, that they deem overly burdensome, and that incapacitated patients maintain these rights even if they can no longer implement them on their own.[2]

Advance Directives in the United States: Important but Limited

Today, all state legislatures in the United States have laws that promote living wills, which are specific treatment directives aimed at clarifying medical interventions that now-capacitated patients would prefer in the future if unable to speak for themselves, and/or durable powers of attorney for health care, which enable capacitated patients to designate a proxy decision maker who can speak for them if they no longer have capacity.[2] In 1990, the U.S. Congress passed the Patient Self-Determination Act, which required that all health care institutions receiving Medicare or Medicaid reimbursement from the federal government notify adult inpatients on admission about their rights under state laws governing advance directives.[11]

There are many barriers to the effective use of advance directives.[12,13] They are weak means of upholding the foundational principles they were meant to safeguard, and they cannot, alone, redress the problems they aim to remedy.[14] First, despite widespread promotion, only 15% to 20% of Americans have executed any advance directive. Vague phrases such as "heroic measures" and "imminent death" in living wills have been criticized as ambiguous and difficult to apply in particular real-life circumstances. Later versions of living wills have attempted to correct this problem by including more end-of-life scenarios and more specific treatments,[15] but some find this type of directive complicated and difficult.[16,17]

Many living wills specifically refer to terminal illness and persistent vegetative states, but these represent only a small percentage of the need. Many end-stage diseases, such as advanced dementia, qualify as being terminal but are not recognized as such.[18] Further, it is often difficult to know whether the circumstances of the incapacitated patient are actually those he or she imagined when providing treatment instructions in the living will. For example, if someone who indicated that he or she never wanted to be placed on a ventilator is now incapacitated and facing a reversible condition that requires only a short time on the ventilator, should the living will pertain? Even when living wills have been executed and are available, using them involves great uncertainty.[14]

Rather than focusing on specific decisions, another strategy has been to encourage patients to designate a decision maker who can represent their interests if they no longer can.[2] Health care proxy statutes authorize the granting of a health care durable power of attorney to someone who can then act as the patient's legal representative for health care decisions (distinct from durable power of attorney for financial matters). A patient may name a family member or friend. A health care proxy avoids uncertain interpretation of living wills by fully empowering the proxy to make medical decisions on the patient's behalf and eliminates the chance for legal conflict over which surrogate is best situated to represent the patient's interests.

For patients who have not formally named a health care proxy, which is usual, state laws provide a default series of family members who may serve as decision maker, and the designated decision maker is referred to as the surrogate decision maker.[2] Surrogate decision making has been considered vital for the decisionally incapacitated. To preserve individual self-determination and autonomy, the surrogate, often a family member, is assumed to know best what the individual would have wanted.

Like living wills, surrogate and proxy decision making are imperfect. Surrogate decision making is inaccurate.[19] Proxies often do not know the patient's preferences and may have been selected for other reasons. Proxies' estimates of patient preferences often are little different from chance. Surrogates sometimes also knowingly disregard patient preferences.

The imperfect nature of surrogacy should not be surprising. Even capacitated patients often make inconsistent decisions due to difficulties assessing risk, misinformation, emotional discomfort, inherent ambivalence about dying, and distrust.[20] Surrogate decisions are complicated by guilt and the desire to avoid being responsible for their loved one's death.

Despite limitations, surrogate decision making is a key component of American end-of-life decision making. There is, indeed, no alternative but to involve those who have been closest to the patient. Unilateral decision making by physicians, ethics committee involvement in every case, or court intervention would undermine patient autonomy even more, would deviate dramatically from current law and ethics guidelines in the United States, and would prove impossibly cumbersome.

Standards for Surrogate and Proxy Decision Making

The goal of surrogate or proxy decision making is to make decisions as the patient would have done.[2] Clinicians often err by asking a surrogate, "What do you think we should do?" Instead, the question should be: "What would your loved one have wanted?" Sometimes, the answer is clear, such as when the patient has had detailed conversations with the surrogate or filled out a living will that anticipated exactly the medical condition at hand. Other times, it is not easy for surrogates to infer what their loved one would do.

Legally in the United States, there are three standards by which surrogate decisions can be made. In the "substituted judgment" standard, the surrogate decides as he or she thinks the patient would have decided, based on the surrogate's knowledge of the patient's past values and preferences. Sometimes it is impossible to infer what the patient would have wanted, and in those cases, surrogates and proxies can rely on the "best interest" standard, which asks what a reasonable person would deem best. A few states require "clear and convincing" evidence; this stricter evidentiary standard requires knowledge that the patient actually indicated his or her preferences in the past, either orally or in writing, about precisely the circumstance the

patient now faces. Whether clear and convincing evidence must be provided or not, in all states the goal is the same: proxy decision makers should ascertain what the patient would have wanted.

ESSENTIAL ELEMENTS OF ADVANCE CARE PLANNING

Most palliative care experts now place their hopes for improvements in end-of-life care, not with advance directives per se, but with the far more robust concept of ACP (Box 19-1), which requires action by the patient's physician. A key ingredient is elucidating the potential treatments that are available toward the end of life. Older advance directives relied on comprehensive lists of interventions potentially available at the end of life, such as cardiopulmonary resuscitation, intubation, ventilators, dialysis, intensive care, antibiotics, intravenous hydration and nutrition, and so on. It may be better to steer away from such lists and focus instead on broad categories of "goals of care," which focus on intentions, broadly conceived, rather than individual treatment choices. For example, in the care of nursing home residents, it may be valuable to think in terms of three different goals: life-prolonging care, limited care, and comfort care.[21]

When considering appropriate goals of care, physicians, patients, and families can be helped to imagine the future and anticipate needs by considering the likely trajectory during the final phase of life. Overall, there are four main trajectories that capture most ways in which Americans die: some die suddenly from an acute cardiac arrest or unforeseen injury; others from a terminal illness such as cancer; still others from chronic organ failure such as congestive heart failure or pulmonary disease; and many from frailty such as Alzheimer's dementia.[22]

BARRIERS THAT IMPEDE ADVANCE CARE PLANNING

The four most important barriers to optimal advance care planning are prognostic uncertainty, physician reluctance to disclose a dire prognosis, inadequate communication skills, and lack of systemic changes that would integrate ACP into the daily routines of health care institutions (see "Common Errors").

Box 19-1 Essential Elements of Advance Care Planning
• Identify patients for whom you "would not be surprised if the patient died in the next year."[25,26]
• Share and discuss the likely prognosis with the patient and family.
• Frame the conversation by acknowledging uncertainty and yet anticipating possible disease trajectories and needs.
• Elicit the patient's (and family's) goals of care, concerns, needs, worries, and hopes.
• Follow through to ensure that care is provided to meet expressed needs and concerns
• Reappraise as the patient's condition and potential treatments evolve.

Prognostic Uncertainty

Prognostication is poor, and most doctors are neither properly trained nor comfortable sharing prognoses.[23] Formal medical education does not place prognostication as a top priority for physicians, and this probably contributes to their unease and uncertainty regarding sharing of prognoses.[23,24] Poor prognostic accuracy further exacerbates the identification of who should be approached for ACP conversations. There is a simple but powerful question for identifying the right target audience. Clinicians should ask themselves, "Would I be surprised if this patient died in the coming year?"[25,26] Whomever is identified in this way is appropriate for an ACP conversation.

Reluctance to Disclose a Dire Prognosis

Even when a poor prognosis seems likely, physicians are often concerned that revealing it might diminish hopes for a cure. This common misconception inadvertently precludes high-quality palliative care. Patients want their physicians to help them understand what they are likely to face in the final stage of their lives.

Framing the conversation as "hoping for the best, but preparing for the worst" allows the clinician to underscore that it is impossible to be certain about prognoses but best to talk together about all contingencies.[27] This framing opens the conversation in a nonthreatening way. Others point out that, as patients' conditions worsen, they can naturally readjust their hopes, which can then focus on the best possible end-of-life period; clinicians can play a vital role in redirecting hope toward life closure goals.[28,29] Most encounters between physicians and patients focus on specific day-to-day clinical issues, such as how to titrate one's insulin or improve laboratory values. This day-to-day focus shifts attention away from sharing of prognostic information which could lead to a discussion of appropriate goals of care.[30]

Failure to communicate prognosis has untoward effects. Sixty-three percent of clinicians treating primarily cancer patients are overly optimistic about prognosis, overestimating the remaining time the death.[24] Systematic overestimation adversely affects the quality of care provided and contributes to late referral for hospice.[24]

Inadequate Communication Skills

Although patients wait for their doctors to initiate these conversations,[31] few do so, in part because of their own emotional distress, and also because there has been little training to help them learn the skills needed. There are three principles for overcoming physicians' emotional, cognitive, and skill barriers: training programs must enable clinicians to manage their own emotional distress; cognitive behavioral principles should help clinicians reshape counterproductive beliefs; and training programs to enhance ACP must provide experiential training in shared decision making and common patient-centered communication skills.[32]

Lack of Systemic Changes and Institutional Routines

Another barrier, particularly in oncology, is "disseminated responsibility": no single health care professional feels responsible for having a conversation with the patient and family about goals of care. To paraphrase an oncologist interviewed in one study: "I knew we were on the wrong path; we spent a lot of time discussing whether she should take the superhighway westward or the back country lanes (whether to do chemo or radiation), but really we should have said, 'Why are you going to Nebraska anyway? It might be better to stay here and finish up what's important to you in the time you have remaining, right where you are.' But she had seen an awful lot of physicians along the way, and I was just one of many. I didn't think it was my place to bring this up, and I guess they didn't either."[33]

RECENT DEVELOPMENTS

There are two kinds of innovations: new decision aids to enhance face-to-face conversations between patients and clinicians and system changes aimed at creating institution- and community-wide interventions to improve ACP.

Innovative Decision Aids

Central to ACP is the patient's understanding of the underlying health state and disease prognosis. Improved modalities for communicating health state and prognosis can help guide end-of-life decision making. In addition to oral discussions, modalities such as video images may improve care. Video can supplement verbal descriptions with illustrations of real people in real circumstances, enabling individuals to better visualize their future.[34] More decision aids have been made widely available by health organizations such as the Foundation for Informed Decision Making (see their Web site at http://www.fimdm.org [accessed September 2007]).[35,36]

Shifts in Institutional Practice

Recently, there have been a number of comprehensive system-wide and community-wide initiatives to enhance ACP. Those that have demonstrated impressive results share certain characteristics:

- A concept of ACP as a process that unfolds over time and that relies on conversations, not documents
- Identification of patients who should be the target of ACP

- Preparation of individual clinicians to hold these conversations
- Establishment of key behaviors and clear protocols, with specific individuals charged with specific accountabilities
- Procedures for documenting conversations and ensuring that the documentation travels across care settings
- Measurable indices of progress

One of the most successful programs is "Respecting Your Choices" (RYC).[37] Originally developed in LaCrosse, Wisconsin, RYC has developed tools and procedures for ensuring family conversations, designation of health care proxies, and more timely referral to hospice.[38] In a rigorous evaluation, RYC was found to have resulted in 81% of decedents in La Crosse having someone designated as their proxy; moreover, the documentation was evident in the medical record as the patient traveled across numerous care settings. This program is now being adapted by many towns and state coalitions.

The Physician Orders for Life-sustaining Treatments (POLST) program does not focus on patient completion of advance directives but rather on ensuring that physicians' orders to use, or to limit, life-sustaining treatments are recorded in the medical record and transmitted from care setting to care setting. In a survey of 151 nursing homes in Oregon, 71% of the facilities reported that they used the POLST form to guide treatment decisions for at least half their residents[39]; another study demonstrated the effectiveness of the program in influencing the response of emergency medical technicians.[40]

Other highly successful programs have included ones that focused on the primary care setting and timely identification and referral of patients to clinical nurse specialists,[26] as well as programs within managed care and comprehensive cancer care. The Web sites listed in "Additional Resources" at the end of this chapter contain descriptions of community- and institution-wide interventions to enhance ACP that have been evaluated and demonstrated to make an impact.

EVIDENCE BASE

There is growing evidence that institutional systems changes are highly effective. Systems approaches have significant impacts on hospice utilization, concordance between spouses' understanding of what patients would want and what patients themselves say they want, number of deaths at home through more appropriate "do not hospitalize" orders, and availability of advance directives when needed (see "Additional Resources" at the end of the chapter).

At the bedside, one study showed the salutary effects of family meetings; less anxiety and depression was found in families who had participated in conversations about treatment.[41] Earlier studies on family meetings, sometimes undertaken as part of ethics case consultation, have shown higher family satisfaction and lower costs, primarily because families learned of the option to forgo treatments that they believed their incapacitated loved ones would not have wanted.[42,43]

CHALLENGES TO ADVANCE CARE PLANNING

There has been one major conceptual challenge to ACP. The argument is that patients should not make decisions for their future selves, because they may have different preferences and different interests later, when they have lost decisional capacity.[44] This philosophical question is about whether the preferences of a previously competent self should have the ability to determine actions that may not be in the best interest of a later, decisionally incapacitated self. Which should take precedence, capacitated persons' concepts of what they think they would want in a future diminished state, or incapacitated persons' best interest as perceived by others?

FUTURE RESEARCH

Future needs include more research on how to design effective ACP processes that reach all appropriate patients; evaluation of programs to determine their impact on patients, families, clinicians, and health care systems; and further research and innovation in how to build ACP programs that are optimally responsive to diverse ethnic and religious groups within our pluralistic society (see "Future Considerations"). Regarding the latter, research suggests that some ethnic groups place less emphasis on Western notions of autonomy and more on values such as family cohesion and filial loyalty.[45] They may find advance directives irrelevant or unfamiliar. African Americans may have different preferences in end-of-life treatments or less trust that their needs will be met by the health care system and may therefore be reluctant to request less treatment.[45]

There is also research suggesting that divergence in attitudes toward end-of-life decisions among minority groups, especially African Americans, may be accounted for more by level of education or "health literacy" than by differences in underlying values.[34] In Latinos, the rates of requests for comfort care were similar to the preferences in Whites after administration of a decision aid.[34] Improved communication should be the focus of ACP discussions, and various novel decision aids (e.g., video) should be used, especially if language barriers exist.

Future Considerations

- Advance Care Planning (ACP) for patients from different populations, such as minority populations, must be culturally sensitive to alternative value frameworks.
- Health literacy and patient educational level may pose barriers to ACP that clinicians must attempt to surmount with improved communication skills.
- Innovative decision aids such as video may have an important role in ACP for more informed decision making at the end of life.
- Community-wide interventions that create institutional protocols, accountabilities, measurable milestones, and easily accessible documentation across care settings need to be established and evaluated.
- The implementation of electronic medical records in hospitals and health care networks may provide improved means of communicating ACP discussions and documentation.

CONCLUSIONS

As the number of elderly persons grows, there will be an increasing need for improved decision making in advanced disease. Although previous efforts to enhance patient and family decision making focused on advance directives, such as living wills and health care proxies, a more expansive formulation of ACP that focuses on patient, family, and health care professional communication, as well as on system-wide changes, should avoid previous pitfalls. Ongoing conversations held early in the patient–physician relationship, before incapacity occurs, ensure that patient autonomy is preserved and that patient and family needs are identified and addressed. Systemic changes bring accountabilities and measurements of progress to ensure that ACP occurs, that patients' wishes and needs are documented, and that documents travel with patients across care settings. To succeed, both physicians and health care institutions must take seriously their obligations to plan for patients' and families' choices and needs.

REFERENCES

1. Emanuel LL, Danis M, Pearlman RA, Singer PA. Advance care planning as a process: Structuring the discussions in practice. J Am Geriatr Soc 1995;43:440-446.
2. Gillick MR. Advance care planning. N Engl J Med 2004;350:7-8.
3. Continuing the Conversation about Advance Care Planning, Parts 1 and 2. Innovations in End of Life Care [E-Journal] 2003;5(2) and 2003;5(3). Available at http://www2.edc.org/lastacts/archives/archivesMarch03/default.asp and http://www2.edc.org/lastacts/archives/archivesMay03/default.asp (accessed September 2007).
4. The SUPPORT Principal Investigators. A controlled trial to improve care for seriously ill hospitalized patients: The Study to Understand Prognoses and Preferences for Outcomes and Risks of Treatments (SUPPORT). JAMA 1995;274:1591-1598.
5. Solomon MZ, O'Donnell L, Jennings B, et al. Decisions near the end of life: Professional views on life-sustaining treatments. Am J Public Health 1993;83:14-23.
6. Morrison RS, Meier DE. Clinical practice: Palliative care. N Engl J Med 2004;350:2582-2590.
7. Butler RN, Burt R, Foley KM, et al. Palliative medicine: Providing care when cure is not possible. A roundtable discussion: Part I. Geriatrics 1996;51:33-36, 42-44.
8. Meisel A, Cerminara KL. The Right to Die, 3rd ed. [Ringbound.] New York: Aspen Publishers, 2004, p v.
9. President's Commission for the Study of Ethical Problems in Medicine and Biomedical and Behavioral Research. Deciding to forego life-sustaining treatment: A Report on the Ethical, Medical, and Legal Issues in Treatment Decisions. Washington, DC: Author, 1983. Available from U.S. Superintendent of Documents, Washington, DC.
10. The Hastings Center. Guidelines on the Termination of Life-Sustaining Treatment and the Care of the Dying. Bloomington: Indiana University Press, 1987.
11. The Patient Self-Determination Act, 42 U.S.C. §§ 1395cc-1396a.
12. Prendergast TJ. Advance care planning: Pitfalls, progress, promise. Crit Care Med 2001;29(2 Suppl):N34-N39.
13. Solomon MZ. The enormity of the task: SUPPORT and changing practice. Hastings Cent Rep 1995;25(6):S28-S32.
14. Fagerlin A, Schneider CE. Enough: The failure of the living will. Hastings Cent Rep 2004;34(2):30-42.
15. Emanuel LL, Emanuel EJ. The medical directive: A new comprehensive advance care document. JAMA 1989;261:3288-3293.
16. Brett AS. Limitations of listing specific medical interventions in advance directives. JAMA 1991;266:825-828.
17. Lo B, Steinbrook R. Resuscitating advance directives. Arch Intern Med 2004;164:1501-1506.
18. Ahronheim JC, Morrison RS, Baskin SA, et al. Treatment of the dying in the acute care hospital: Advanced dementia and metastatic cancer. Arch Intern Med 1996;156:2094-2100.
19. Shalowitz DI, Garrett-Mayer E, Wendler D. The accuracy of surrogate decision makers: A systematic review. Arch Intern Med 2006;166:493-497.
20. Redelmeier DA, Rozin P, Kahneman D. Understanding patients' decisions: Cognitive and emotional perspectives. JAMA 1993;270:72-76.
21. Gillick MR. Choosing medical care in old age: What kind, how much, when to stop. Cambridge, MS: Harvard University Press; 1994.
22. Lunney JR, Lynn J, Hogan C. Profiles of older Medicare decedents. J Am Geriatr Soc 2002;50:1108-1112.

23. Christakis NA. Death Foretold: Prophecy and Prognosis in Medical Care. Chicago: University of Chicago, 1999.
24. Christakis NA, Lamont EB. Extent and determinants of error in doctors' prognoses in terminally ill patients: Prospective cohort study. BMJ 2000; 320:469-472.
25. Pattison M, Romer AL. Improving care through the end of life: Launching a primary care clinic-based program. J Palliat Med. 2001;4:249-254. Also available at http://www.edc.org/lastacts/archives/archivesSept00/fipattison.asp (accessed September 2007).
26. Trandum G. Improving care through the end of life: An interview with Georgeanne Trandum by S.L. Sodickson. Innovations in End of Life Care [E-Journal] 2000;2(5). Available at http://www2.edc.org/lastacts/archives/archivesSept00/fitrandum.asp (accessed September 2007).
27. Back AL, Arnold RM, Quill TE. Hope for the best, and prepare for the worst. Ann Intern Med 2003;138:439-443.
28. Koopmeiners L, Post-White J, Gutknecht S, et al. How healthcare professionals contribute to hope in patients with cancer. Oncol Nurs Forum 1997;24:1507-1513.
29. Tulsky JA. Hope and hubris. J Palliat Med 2002;5:339-341.
30. Davison SN, Simpson C. Hope and advance care planning in patients with end stage renal disease: Qualitative interview study. BMJ 2006;333:886.
31. Johnston SC, Pfeifer MP, McNutt R. The discussion about advance directives: Patient and physician opinions regarding when and how it should be conducted. End of Life Study Group. Arch Intern Med 1995;155:1025-1030.
32. Weiner JS, Cole SA. Three principles to improve clinician communication for advance care planning: Overcoming emotional, cognitive, and skill barriers. J Palliat Med 2004;7:817.
33. Solomon MZ. Research to improve end-of-life care in the United States: Toward a more behavioral and ecological paradigm. In Portenoy RK, Bruera E (eds). Issues in Palliative Care Research. New York: Oxford University Press, 2003.
34. Volandes A, Lehmann LS, Cook EF, et al. Using video images of advanced dementia in advance care planning. Arch Intern Med 2007;167:828-833.
35. O'Connor AM, Stacey D, Rovner D, et al. Decision aids for people facing health treatment or screening decisions. Cochrane Database Syst Rev 2001;(3): CD001431.
36. Barry MJ. Health decision aids to facilitate shared decision making in office practice. Ann Intern Med 2002;136:127-135.
37. Hammes BJ, Rooney BL. Death and end-of-life planning in one Midwestern community. Arch Intern Med 1998;158:383-390.
38. Hammes BJ. The lessons from Respecting Your Choices. In Solomon, MZ, Romer AL, Heller KS (eds). Innovations in End-of-Life Care: Practical Strategies and International Perspectives, Vol. 1, Mary Ann Liebert Publishers, 2001. Also available at http://www2.edc.org/lastacts/archives/archivesJan99/default.asp (accessed September 2007).
39. Hickman SE, Tolle SW, Brummel-Smith K, Carley MM. Use of the Physician Orders for Life-Sustaining Treatment program in Oregon nursing facilities: Beyond resuscitation status. J Am Geriatr Soc 2004;52:1424-1429.
40. Schmidt TA, Hickman SE, Tolle SW, Brooks HS. The Physician Orders for Life-Sustaining Treatment program: Oregon emergency medical technicians' practical experiences and attitudes. J Am Geriatr Soc 2004;52:1430-1434.
41. Lautrette A, Darmon M, Megarbane B, et al. A Communication Strategy and Brochure for Relatives of Patients Dying in the ICU. N Engl J Med 2007;356:469-478.
42. Schneiderman LJ, Gilmer T, Teetzel HD, et al. Effect of ethics consultations on nonbeneficial life-sustaining treatments in the intensive care setting: A randomized controlled trial. JAMA 2003;290:1166-1172.
43. Dowdy MD, Robertson C, Bander JA. A study of proactive ethics consultation for critically and terminally ill patients with extended lengths of stay. Crit Care Med 1998;26:252-259.
44. Dresser R. Missing persons: Legal perceptions of incompetent patients. Rutgers Law Rev 1994;46:609-719.
45. Blackhall LJ, Frank G, Murphy ST, et al. Ethnicity and attitudes towards life sustaining technology. Soc Sci Med 1999;48:1779-1789.

ADDITIONAL RESOURCES

Continuing the Conversation about Advance Care Planning: Part 1. Innovations in End of Life Care [E-Journal] 2003; 5(2). Available at http://www2.edc.org/lastacts/archives/archivesMarch03/default.asp (accessed September 2007).

Continuing the Conversation about Advance Care Planning: Part 2. Innovations in End of Life Care [E-Journal] 2003;5(3). Available at http://www2.edc.org/lastacts/archives/archivesMay03/default.asp (accessed September 2007).

Franciscan Health System West. Improving Care through the End of Life Training Manual. Description available at http://www2.edc.org/lastacts/archives/archivesSept00/fitrandum.asp (accessed September 2007).

Respecting Your Choices and the Respecting Your Choices Advance Care Planning Toolkit. Available at http://www.

gundluth.org/web/ptcare/eolprograms.nsf (accessed September 2007); further information is available at http://www2.edc.org/lastacts/archives/archivesJan99/default.asp (accessed September 2007).

The Physician Orders for Life-Sustaining Treatments (POLST) Program. Available at http://www.ohsu.edu/polst/ (accessed September 2007).

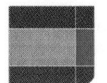

CHAPTER **20**

Withholding and Withdrawing Treatment

Elizabeth Weinstein, Wendy G. Anderson, and Robert M. Arnold

KEY POINTS

- The law follows the ethical consensus on forgoing life-sustaining treatment. These decisions are based on the principle of autonomy.

- Little issue surrounds the choices of a competent patient. If a patient is unable to participate in his or her own care, shared decision making between surrogates and clinicians follows the principle of substituted judgment or best interest.

- It is critical to recognize the importance that religion may have in decisions about forgoing life-sustaining treatment.

- The communication skills needed to discuss forgoing treatment differ from those used in routine clinical decisions in that a large number of clinicians are often involved in the decision making process, surrogates are the primary decision makers, and the discussions are very emotional in nature.

- Implantable cardioverter defibrillators (ICDs) are an increasingly prevalent form of life-sustaining therapy. Palliative care clinicians need to be aware of and discuss ICDs with patients and surrogates.

There are many therapies available to sustain life. Use of these therapies in patients with reversible illness is rarely questioned. In a patient with a terminal illness, the use of these therapies may not be consistent with the patient's wishes. The patient may feel that his or her current quality of life is unacceptable, the expected quality of life after therapy is too low, or the therapy itself is too burdensome. In this situation, the therapy should be withheld or withdrawn (forgone). Medical ethics and the law in most countries allow clinicians to forgo treatment when doing so is consistent with the patient's wishes. This chapter discusses the current status of forgoing therapy, as well as the legal, religious, and ethical principles that support withholding and withdrawing therapy. Finally, the implications of deactivation of an implantable cardioverter defibrillator are reviewed, because this is a new, life-sustaining

therapy that clinicians need to remember to discuss with patients and their families.

CURRENT STATUS OF WITHHOLDING AND WITHDRAWING TREATMENT

Withholding and withdrawing treatment is a common practice in intensive care units (ICUs) in the United States. Data show a significant increase in the number of ICU deaths preceded by limitation of therapy over the past 10 years. In two academic ICUs, the number of deaths preceded by forgoing of life support increased from 51% in 1987-1988 to 90% in 1992-1993.[1] Similarly, in Europe, the Ethicus Study[2] demonstrated that significant numbers of deaths in European ICUs (76%) were preceded by some form of limitation of therapy.

There is, however, wide variation among ICUs in the frequency with which treatment is forgone. A Spanish study showed that rates of withholding or withdrawing life support therapy varied among individual ICUs, ranging from 21% to 56%.[3] A French study similarly demonstrated rates of 0% to 26%.[4]

As expected, patients who have therapy forgone are usually old, sick, and lack decision-making capacity.[3,4] For example, a number of studies showed that three-quarters of patients who forwent therapy lacked decision-making capacity.[4] In attitudinal studies, physicians say they are more likely to forgo treatments in cancer patients, but few data are available from clinical care.

Therapies tend to be forgone in a distinct order. In a U.S. study, the sequence of *withdrawal*, from earliest to latest, was as follows: blood products, hemodialysis, vasopressors, mechanical ventilation, total parenteral nutrition, antibiotics, intravenous fluids, and tube feedings.[5] In a French study, vasopressors and mechanical ventilation were the most frequently withdrawn therapies, whereas withdrawal of intravenous hydration was rare. The most commonly *withheld* treatments are cardiopulmonary resuscitation and mechanical ventilation.[4] These variations reflect health care provider attitudes about the moral acceptability of forgoing specific therapies.[6]

Most patients die shortly after therapy is forgone. The median time to death from the first decision to limit therapy was approximately 15 hours in ICU patients. Following the decision to limit the most active form of therapy, the median time to death was 14.3 hours if the therapy was withheld and 4.0 hours if the therapy was withdrawn. Withholding of life-sustaining therapy resulted in 89% hospital mortality.[2] Interestingly, although clinicians often are concerned that use of opioids and benzodiazepines to palliate dyspnea will cause respiratory depression and thus hasten death, a variety of case-control studies have not found a correlation between opioid or benzodiazepine dose and time to death.[7]

ETHICAL CONSENSUS ON WITHHOLDING AND WITHDRAWING TREATMENT

The increased use of life-prolonging technologies in the ICU in the 1970s led to a debate about the ethics of forgoing these treatments in terminally ill patients. The President's Commission for the Study of Ethical Problems in

Medicine and Biomedical and Behavioral Research published their consensus on this issue in 1983.[8] Their report provided the standard for much of the subsequent literature on the ethics of forgoing life-sustaining treatment. The Commission based its central decision on the principle of *informed consent* and found that, although the consequences of forgoing a life-sustaining treatment may be more serious than those of forgoing other treatments, there is no ethical difference between them.

The Burden/Benefit Ratio

The Commission did not find any moral distinctions "[between] acts and omissions which cause death, [between] withholding and withdrawing care, between an intended death and one that is merely foreseeable, and between ordinary and extraordinary treatment" useful in guiding medical practice.[8] For example, some argued that it was permissible to forgo extraordinary treatments but not ordinary treatments such as intravenous fluids. The problem is that ordinary and extraordinary treatments exist on a continuum and are clinically dependent. For a patient without intravenous access in a small rural hospital, giving fluids may be quite difficult (e.g., extraordinary), whereas administration of vasopressor therapy in a tertiary care hospital may be "ordinary." The Commission argued that what counts is the burden/benefit ratio.[8] The report concluded that the terms *extraordinary* and *ordinary* are "more an expression of the conclusion than a justification" for a treatment. It is the health care institution's and the professional's responsibility to provide the patient with adequate information about treatment options so that he or she can make autonomous decisions concerning the treatment's benefits and burdens.

Surrogates

If a patient is not able to make decisions for himself or herself, the Commission stated that a surrogate should make decisions for the patient.[9] The most powerful argument for surrogate decision making is that it is an extension of the incapacitated person's autonomy. A family member or other surrogate makes decisions based on his or her understanding of what the patient would have wanted; this is termed *substituted judgment.* In the strongest case, the patient has left a written summary of what he or she wanted or has had a clear conversation regarding his or her wishes. If the patient's wishes are unspecified, the family may be most likely to know them. However, the empirical data show that families are only slightly better than chance at predicting a patient's views.[10] A related and empirically stronger justification is that what is being respected is not the substantive treatment decision but the procedural choice of who should make decisions for the patient.

A second justification for surrogate decision making is that a family member (or other designated surrogate) is best suited to make decisions that maximize the patient's best interest. In the "best interest" standard, decisions are made with the goal of achieving what the decision maker perceives to be the patient's best interest.

LEGAL CONSENSUS ON WITHHOLDING AND WITHDRAWING TREATMENT

Legal Consensus in the United States

The legal justification behind withholding and withdrawing treatment in the United States largely mirrors ethical principles and is based on the notions of informed consent, surrogate decision making, and the state's *parens patriae* interest in promoting life.[11,12] These principles are rooted in the common law right to be free from unwanted intrusion on or invasion of bodily integrity. Courts variably refer to this as the "right to privacy," "right to self-determination or autonomy," or "right to control one's own body."[13] The constitutional right to privacy was the basis for the decision in the *Quinlan* case and in many cases until the U.S. Supreme Court's *Cruzan v. Director* decision, wherein the Due Process Clause of the Fourteenth Amendment was used to protect an individual's "liberty" interest (see later discussion).

The legal consensus on forgoing life-sustaining therapy parallels the ethical consensus by allowing competent patients to decide, based on their assessment of burdens and benefits, whether they want to forgo life-sustaining treatment. Courts make no distinction between withholding and withdrawing therapy. They also reject the distinction between "ordinary" and "extraordinary" treatment. The New Jersey Supreme Court in *Conroy,* for example, in referring to ordinary treatment in the context of artificial hydration and nutrition, stated that "the terms [ordinary and extraordinary] . . . have assumed too many conflicting meanings to remain useful."[11]

Incompetent Patients

The way in which courts deal with incompetent patients, although more complicated, largely mirrors the ethical consensus. Some states have determined legislatively the order of surrogates (e.g., wife, then parent, then child) if none has been designated by the patient; others merely declare that the surrogate should be the person who knows the patient best. Although courts also refer to substituted judgment and best interest as the standards surrogates should use to make end-of-life decisions, their application is complicated. Although incompetent patients have the same right as competent persons to forgo life-sustaining treatment, the level of evidence that the surrogate must provide to establish the patient's wishes varies from state to state.

Nancy Cruzan was a young woman in a persistent vegetative state whose parents requested that her feeding tube be withdrawn. The Cruzans lived in Missouri, a state that required "clear and convincing" evidence that an incompetent person would have wanted a treatment withdrawn.[14] The U.S. Supreme Court, while affirming that artificial hydration and nutrition is like all other therapies, determined that states may decide, in their role as *parens patriae,* the level of proof required of a surrogate that a decision is what the patient would have wanted. In Missouri, for example, surrogates may not use the "best interest" standard to forgo life-sustaining treatment in incompetent patients.

Some clinicians are concerned that they may be subject to civil or criminal prosecution if life-sustaining treatment is forgone. However, no clinician has been found liable, provided he or she was acting according to the patient's wishes.[14]

Legal Consensus in Other Countries

There is great variability among the legal systems of different countries in the way in which they address forgoing life-sustaining treatment. The extremes are illustrated by examining the differences between Canada and Japan.

Canada, like most Western countries, values autonomy and informed refusal. Canadian laws protect a competent patient's right to refuse treatment under the common law doctrines of battery or assault. Clinicians may stop treatments "if these contradict the expressed wishes of the patients, or if they are 'therapeutically useless' and not in their [the patients'] best interest."[15] Clinicians are liable for assault if they aggressively treat a patient against the patient's wishes.

Incompetent Patients

How the legal system handles incompetent patients forgoing life-sustaining treatment is more variable, even among Western countries. Canadian provincial law focuses on the substitute decision maker's right to act for an incompetent patient. Patients may designate a proxy while they are competent, or the province will provide a guardian after the patient has become incompetent. Proxies must act in the patient's best interest. If the clinician believes that a proxy's decision to forgo therapy is not in the patient's best interest, he or she can appeal to the courts for the right to provide that treatment.

Self-determination, informed consent, and disclosure are not as important in Japan. It is uncommon for patients to know their diagnosis if they have a life-threatening condition. In one study, 77% of physicians in Japan said they would discuss life-sustaining treatment with a patient's family before discussing it with the patient, even if the patient were competent.[16] Japanese physicians also are less likely to follow a competent patient's wish to forgo treatment.

The Japanese legal system mirrors and supports this clinical practice. Despite the fact that Japanese physicians are comfortable discussing medical diagnoses with patients' families, they are uncomfortable with surrogate decision makers in the matter of forgoing treatment. Although clear living wills are respected, if the patient has not clearly expressed his or her wishes, Japanese physicians tend to adhere to the principles of prolonging life. This is may be due to the fact that "Japanese law does not clearly guarantee relief from criminal responsibility of shortening a patient's life by an act of omission."[17]

Most countries are somewhere between the extremes of Japan and Canada. It is important to be aware of the norms of practice in various cultures, because global travel increases the probability that doctors will see patients from other areas of the world.

RELIGIOUS IMPACT ON WITHHOLDING AND WITHDRAWING TREATMENT

The religious faith of patients and their surrogates may affect their decisions about withholding and withdrawing

TABLE 20-1 Relative Importance of Ethical Concepts in Selected Religions

PRINCIPLE	JUDAISM	CATHOLICISM	ISLAM
Autonomy	+	++	+
Nonmaleficence	++++	+++	+++
Withholding nutrition	+	++	+
Use of advance directives	+	+++	+

+ to ++++, least to most important/acceptable.
From Clarfield AM, Gordon M, Markwell H, et al. Ethical issues in end-of-life geriatric care: The approach of three monotheistic religions—Judaism, Catholicism, and Islam. J Am Geriatr Soc 2003;51:1149-1154.

treatments. For example, Hindu philosophy, Buddhism, Sikhism, and Jainism do not see life on earth as finite, but more as part of a cycle of birth and rebirth. This may explain why only 9% of Hindus have advance directives when the national average in the United States is between 15% and 20%.[18] The lower rate of advance care planning among African Americans and their higher preference for aggressive treatment at the end of life are often attributed to religious beliefs. Knowledge of how various religions approach the ethical issues faced at the end of life can be helpful in caring for patients and their families (see Chapters 10 and 12).

Despite variations in the relative importance of autonomy and sanctity of life, the three most common religions in the United States—Judaism, Islam, and Christianity—all acknowledge that, when a patient is clearly dying, it is acceptable to forgo certain treatments and provide comfort (Table 20-1).[19] In Judaism and Islam, the sanctity of life is paramount and patients are bound to seek healing. For example, artificial hydration and nutrition is required unless the feeding itself causes suffering. Christian bioethics places more priority on patients' weighing the benefit/burden ratio and making autonomous decisions. Catholics have emphasized the distinction between ordinary and extraordinary therapies in their thinking and, until recently, maintained that artificial hydration is not required in terminally ill or comatose patients.[20] This orientation became less clear after the papal statement by John Paul II before his death, which implied that it is unacceptable to withhold artificial hydration and nutrition from patients in a persistent vegetative state.[21]

Although a basic knowledge of the views of organized religions toward forgoing life-sustaining treatment is useful, how any one patient or family interprets them may vary a great deal based on ethnic background, sociocultural status, and personal circumstances. For example, within Judaism, one's beliefs may vary depending on whether one is Orthodox or Reform. A fundamental Christian from one church may see the world differently from someone from another church. What is critical is recognition of the importance that religion may have in the decisions of patients and families and willingness to nonjudgmentally explore these concerns. Further, when issues of religion or spirituality are central to a patient's or family's decision about forgoing therapy, hospital chaplains or clergy are a useful resource.

DISCUSSING THE WITHHOLDING AND WITHDRAWING OF TREATMENT WITH PATIENTS AND THEIR FAMILIES

Although the communication skills needed to discuss forgoing treatment are similar to those used to make any clinical decision,[21] there are differences in emphasis (see Chapter 116).

- These decisions often are made in concert with a number of clinicians, so there are increased opportunities for miscommunication. Therefore, it is important to ask the patient and/or family about their views before giving one's own view, typically by using open-ended questions (e.g., "Tell me what others are saying is going on with your dad").

- Patients are often too sick to participate in these deliberations, so the clinician must talk to the surrogate. The clinician must be able to sensitively ask the surrogate about what the patient would want (e.g., "If your dad were sitting here, what would he say?").

- Because these conversations involve bad news, the clinician must be able to respond empathically to the surrogate's emotional reactions.

A six-step protocol for discussing withholding and withdrawing therapies has been presented previously[22,23] and is summarized in Table 20-2. Several key steps are examined here.

It is necessary to establish or review the overall goals of care (*Step 3*) before discussing forgoing specific thera-

TABLE 20-2	Recommendations for Communicating with Patients and Families about Withholding and Withdrawing Treatment	
STEPS	**TASKS**	**EXAMPLES**
STEP 1: Establish the setting	a. Make sure the right people attend	1. Patient or surrogate 2. Staff 3. Chaplain
	b. Find a comfortable, quiet setting	1. Places for everyone to sit 2. Private 3. Everyone able to see and hear each other
	c. Introduce everyone at the beginning	1. *"Could we start by introducing everyone?"* 2. *"How are you related to Ms. Jones?"*
	d. Introduce the topic for discussion	1. *"I was hoping we could talk about the next steps in your dad's care. I wanted to bring you up-to-date about what was happening, answer your questions, and talk about the future. Was there anything else you want to cover?"*
STEP 2: Review the patient's situation	a. Elicit patient or surrogate understanding	1. *"What have the other doctors told you about your dad's medical situation?"*
	b. Educate as needed	1. *"That's right, the cancer has spread. What that means is that, although there are treatments to control your symptoms, we can't cure the cancer."*
STEP 3: Review overall goals of care	a. Elicit from patient or surrogate	1. *"Did you talk with Dr. Smith about what the goal of your treatments should be?"* 2. *"What would your dad have said if he understood what we are saying about his medical situation?"*
	b. Summarize to confirm	1. *"So, it sounds like the most important thing would be to make sure your father is comfortable."*
STEP 4: Relate your recommendation for withholding or withdrawing treatment	a. Tell the surrogate about what is going to be done to promote the patient's goals	1. *"We will focus on making sure your dad is comfortable. This means we will re-evaluate his pain medicines and increase them to make sure he is not in pain."*
	b. Tell the patient what treatments will not be done because they do not achieve these goals	1. *"If your dad's heart should stop, trying to restart it will not achieve his goal of getting home independently, so we should not do that."*
	c. For treatments you are unsure of, raise the issue and negotiate based on benefits and burdens	1. *"I know your dad did not want to prolong things if we thought he was dying or he needed to be on machines. Unfortunately, sometime we are not sure if non-machine treatments will help him live longer. For example, some people would be willing to be in the hospital for IV antibiotics if they got an infection, but others would not want that. What do you think your dad would say?"*
	d. Offer to discuss what may happen next	1. *"Do you want to hear about what is likely to happen after we turn off the ventilator?"*
STEP 5: Respond to patient or surrogate reaction	a. Show empathy	1. SOLER* 2. NURSE*
	b. Assess concerns	1. *"What questions do you have?"* 2. *"What is your biggest fear/concern at this point?"*
	c. Encourage questions	1. *"I'll be around if you think of things you want to ask me later. Are there questions I can answer now?"*
STEP 6: Summarize and follow-up	a. Summarize	1. *" Good. So we will give you medicines if you get chest pain, and we will turn off your defibrillator."*
	b. Next steps in treatment	1. *"We'll plan on keeping you in the hospital for the next few days and see how things go."*
	c. Next meeting	1. *"I'll see you tomorrow on rounds. Please have your nurse page me if you need anything before then."*

*See text for explanation.
From Evans WG, Hunt S, Chaitin E, Arnold RM. Withholding and withdrawing life-sustaining therapies. In Emanuel L, Librach SL (eds). Palliative Care: Core Skills and Clinical Competencies. Philadelphia, WB Saunders, 2007; and Oncotalk. Available at http://www.oncotalk.info (accessed September 2007).

pies, because the decision about these treatments should be consistent with the overall goals. Whether life should be prolonged depends on the patient's definition of quality of life, the kinds of burdens the patient feels are worth tolerating, and the chance of success that would make a treatment worth undergoing. Patients do not *want* cardiopulmonary resuscitation; they want to live with a certain quality of life.

Given that the clinician is typically talking to a surrogate about this topic, care must be taken to focus the discussion on the patient's values. Asking the surrogate what he or she wants to do often leads to increased guilt or the surrogate's feeling responsible for "killing" the loved one. Moreover, *want* is an ambiguous term that confuses wishes and reality. Therefore, it is important to ask questions such as, "What would your dad say if he were sitting here?" and to continue to focus on the patient's values. Once these values are understood, the clinician can incorporate his or her knowledge of patient preferences and medicine to propose a reasonable plan involving the treatment in question (*Step 4*).

Conversations about forgoing treatment are difficult because of the acknowledgment that death is approaching. Emotional reactions should be expected, and clinicians should be able to recognize and respond to these emotions (*Step 5*). Expressing empathy is the explicit acknowledgment by the clinician of a patient's expression of emotion. The first step in expressing empathy is recognizing when the surrogate or patient is expressing emotion. People express emotion directly by using emotionally laden words such as *worried, frustrated, stressed, concerned, depressed,* and *overwhelmed.* They may also allude to their emotional state without using a word that describes the emotion or nonverbally through tense body posture or facial expressions, sighing, and crying.

The acronym SOLER shows how to exhibit nonverbal empathy[24]: face the patient *squarely;* adopt an *open* body posture; *lean* toward the patient; use *eye contact;* maintain a *relaxed* body posture. Empathy can be shown verbally using the acronym NURSE[25]: *name* the emotion; show that you *understand* what the person is going through; *respect* how well the person has been doing in the face of difficult obstacles; *support* the person's trial and convey nonabandonment; *explore* the emotion.

IMPLANTABLE CARDIAC DEFIBRILLATORS

Although much has been written about withholding and withdrawing artificial hydration and nutrition, hemodialysis, and ventilators, less has been written about implantable cardioverter defibrillators (ICDs) (see Chapter 105). The indications for ICDs have expanded in recent years. In 2002, 96,000 ICDs were implanted in patients in North America.[26] In 2005, it was estimated that 3 million patients would be eligible for an ICD, with approximately 400,000 new patients meeting the criteria each year.[26] ICDs are programmed to deliver shocks for specific arrhythmias, such as ventricular tachycardia and ventricular fibrillation, which would otherwise require external defibrillation. Because this life-sustaining therapy is becoming increasingly prevalent, palliative care clinicians need to understand ICDs, the medical consequences of their being turned off, and how to talk to patients and families about these topics.

The indication for an ICD is a life-threatening ventricular arrhythmia in the setting of severe left ventricular dysfunction. When ICDs are implanted, most conversations between the clinician and the patient focus on efficacy of the device and procedural risks and do not address the option of forgoing the device in the future.

It is important that clinicians discuss deactivating ICDs as patients get sicker. First, given that the patient has had the device placed because of life-threatening ventricular arrhythmias, death from the cardiac condition may be anticipated. In patients for whom continued existence is not desirable, the ICD may result in an unwanted prolongation of life. Second, ICD firing is not benign. ICD shocks are known to lead to anxiety disorders, and they lead to decreased quality of life in 10% to 20% of patients.

Unfortunately, these conversations often do not occur. Even among patients with ICDs who have do not resuscitate (DNR) orders, discussions about deactivating the ICD happen in only 45% of patients.[27] An empirical, retrospective study of patients who had an ICD found that only one quarter of families recalled a discussion about deactivating the device. About three quarters of these conversations occurred within the last few days of the patient's life, with many occurring only hours before death. When the topic was discussed, families typically chose to deactivate the ICD (21 of 27 cases). Disturbingly, 27 of the 100 patients in the study received a shock in the last month of life, and 8 received shocks in the last minutes of life.[27]

Ethically and legally, deactivation of an ICD is equivalent to withdrawal of any other therapy. There is no specific legal precedent addressing whether patients would want their proxies to have authority over decisions pertaining to their ICDs. However, because proxies have authority over a wide variety of life-sustaining interventions, it makes sense to treat ICDs similarly (Box 20-1).

The discussion about deactivating an ICD aims to achieve the same understanding of the patient's overall goals as other conversations about forgoing life-sustaining treatment. Some of the complexity in deciding whether it is appropriate to deactivate an ICD comes from the numerous ways in which the ICD may fit into the patient's situation. The patient's primary life-limiting illness may either be cardiac or noncardiac, and in either case the frequency of device discharge may vary. Finally, irrespective of the historical frequency of device discharge, the metabolic

---

Box 20-1 Research Challenges

- Data are needed to define end-of-life trajectories for patients who have their implantable cardioverter defibrillators (ICDs) left on and for those who have them turned off during the last 6 months of life. Relevant outcomes include neurologic function, quality of life, and family bereavement.

- Data are needed on the best way to discuss ICD deactivation with patients. The best time for these discussions, the information that would be most helpful to patients, and the emotional impact of these discussions need to be ascertained.

- The impact of adapting current DNR forms to address the deactivation of ICDs, to prompt clinicians to discuss this topic with patients, should be investigated.

derangements that occur near the end of life may lead to fatal arrhythmias that would activate an ICD.[28]

Conversations regarding forgoing ICD therapy need to occur even when the patient has a DNR order. If the patient's current quality of life is the basis for the DNR order, then any life-prolonging treatments would be inconsistent with patient wishes, and deactivation of the ICD should be discussed. On the other hand, if postresuscitation quality of life is the basis for the DNR order, external defibrillation outcomes may not be comparable to internal defibrillation outcomes, and deactivation of the ICD may not be appropriate; nevertheless, it should be discussed.[27]

CONCLUSIONS

As technology advances, increasing numbers of life-sustaining therapies become available. It is ethical and legal to withhold or withdraw any therapy, including life-sustaining treatments, based on the principle of autonomy. Decision making for incompetent patients should be done by surrogates who can either represent what the patient would have wanted (substituted judgment) or make a decision based on what they believe is best for the patient (best interest). Although there is variation in how the law treats surrogate decision making in the United States, in general the legal position mirrors the ethical consensus (see "Common Errors").

Decisions to withhold or withdraw therapies should be made jointly between clinicians and patients or their surrogates, based on the patients' values and preferences for medical care. Each decision should be based on the patient's overall prognosis, the effectiveness of the therapy in question, its benefits and burdens to the patient, and the overall goals of care. A structured format for raising the issue, based on the guiding principles of asking before telling, showing empathy, and offering suggestions, may improve the communication process.

Finally, clinicians need to remember that every technological advance requires that they think about when the therapy should be forgone. For example, because of the increasing use of ICDs in patients with ventricular arrhythmias, clinicians need to think about and discuss the discontinuation of this therapy at the end of life. This means understanding the medical facts surrounding use of the therapy, being aware of the need for the discussion, and having the ability to talk about the topic sensitively.

REFERENCES

1. Prendergast TJ, Claessens MT, Luce JM. A national survey of end-of-life care for critically ill patients. Am J Respir Crit Care Med 1998;158:1163-1167.
2. Sprung CL, Cohen SL, Sjokvist P, et al. End-of-life practices in European intensive care units: The Ethicus study. JAMA 2003;290:790-797.
3. Esteban A, Gordo F, Solsona JF, et al. Withdrawing and withholding life support in the intensive care unit: A Spanish prospective multi-centre observational study. Intensive Care Med 2001;27:1744-1749.
4. Ferrand E, Robert R, Ingrand P, et al. Withholding and withdrawal of life support in intensive-care units in France: A prospective survey: Lancet 2001;357:9-14.
5. Asch DA, Faber-Langendoen K, Shea JA, et al. The sequence of withdrawing life-sustaining treatment from patients: Am J Med 1999;107:153-156.
6. Asch DA, Christakis NA. Why do physicians prefer to withdraw some forms of life support over others?: Intrinsic attributes of life-sustaining treatments are associated with physicians' preferences. Med Care 1996;34:103-111.
7. Christakis NA, Asch DA. Biases in how physicians choose to withdraw life support. Lancet 1993;342:642-646.
8. President's Commission for the Study of Ethical Problems in Medicine and Biomedical and Behavioral Research. Deciding to Forego Life-Sustaining Treatment. Washington, DC: Author, 1983. Available from U.S. Superintendent of Documents, Washington, DC.
9. Brock DW. What is the moral authority of family members to act as surrogates for incompetent patients? Milbank Q 1996;74:599-618.
10. Emanuel E, Emanuel L. Proxy decision making for incompetent patients: An ethical and empirical analysis. JAMA 1992;267:2067-2071.
11. *In re Conroy*, 98 N.J. 321, 486 A.2d 1209 (1985).
12. Gostin LO. Deciding life and death in the courtroom—From Quinlan to Cruzan, Glucksberg, and Vacco: A brief history and analysis of constitutional protection of the "right to die." JAMA 1997;278:1523-1528.
13. Meisel A. Nature and sources of the right to die. In Meisel A. The Right to Die, vol. 1, 2nd ed. New York: John Wiley & Sons, 1995, pp 56-66.
14. Luce JM, Alpers A. Legal aspects of withholding and withdrawing life support from critically ill patients in the United States and providing palliative care to them: Am J Respir Crit Care Med 2000;162:2029-2032.
15. Lemmens T. Towards the right to be killed: Treatment refusal, assisted suicide and euthanasia in the United States and Canada. Br Med Bull 1996;52:341-353.
16. Asai A, Fukuhara S, Lo B. Attitudes of Japanese and Japanese-American physicians toward life-sustaining treatment. Lancet 1995;346:356-359.
17. Akabayashi A. Euthanasia, assisted suicide, and cessation of life support: Japan's policy, law and an analysis of whistle blowing in two recent mercy killing cases. Social Sci Med 2002;55:517-527.
18. Deshpande O, Reid MC, Rao AS. Attitudes of Asian-Indian Hindus toward end-of-life care. J Am Geriatr Soc 2005;53:131-135.
19. Clarfield AM, Gordon M, Markwell H, et al. Ethical issues in end-of-life geriatric care: The approach of three monotheistic religions—Judaism, Catholicism, and Islam. J Am Geriatr Soc 2003;51:1149-1154.
20. Address of John Paul II to the Participants at the International Congress. Life Sustaining Treatments and the Vegetative State: Scientific Advances and Ethical Dilemmas. March 20, 2004. Available at http://www.catholicdoctors.org.uk/CMQ/2004/May/Pope_and_PVS.htm (accessed September 2007).
21. Book Review. Field Guide to the Difficult Patient Interview, 2nd ed, by F.W. Platt and G.H. Gordon (Lippincott, 2004). Available at http://www.blackwell-synergy.com/doi/pdf/10.1111/j.1525-1497.2005.01532.x (accessed September 2007).
22. Evans WG, Hunt S, Chaitin E, Arnold RM. Withholding and withdrawing life-sustaining therapies. In Emanuel L, Librach SL (eds). Palliative Care: Core Skills and Clinical Competencies. Philadelphia, WB Saunders, 2007.
23. Oncotalk. Available at http://www.oncotalk.info (accessed September 2007).
24. Egan G. The Skilled Helper: A Problem-Management and Opportunity-Development Approach to Helping. Santa Rosa, CA: Brooks/Cole, 2002.
25. Fischer G, Tulsky J, Arnold R. Communicating a Poor Prognosis. In Portenoy R, Bruera E (eds). Topics in Palliative Care. New York: Oxford University Press, 2000.
26. Harrington MD, Luebke DL, Lewis WR, et al. Implantable cardioverter defibrillator (ICD) at end of life #112. J Palliat Med 2005;8:1056-1057.
27. Goldstein NE, Lampert R, Bradley E, et al. Management of implantable cardioverter defibrillators in end-of-life care: Ann Intern Med 2004;141:835-838.
28. Braun TC, Hagen NA, Hatfield RE, et al. Cardiac pacemakers and implantable defibrillators in terminal care: J Pain Symptom Manage 1999;18:126-131.

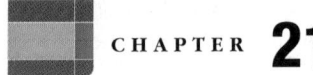

CHAPTER **21**

Euthanasia and Physician-Assisted Suicide

Bert Broeckaert

KEY POINTS

- It is best to limit use of the term *euthanasia* to those cases in which the life of the patient is terminated actively (i.e., by lethal medication) and directly (intentionally).

- Voluntary euthanasia is legalized in two countries, The Netherlands and Belgium. Physician-assisted suicide is allowed in The Netherlands, in Switzerland, and in the U.S. state of Oregon.

- The attitude of world religions toward euthanasia and physician-assisted suicide is predominantly negative.

- There is a sharp distinction between euthanasia and physician-assisted suicide on the one hand and pain control and palliative sedation on the other.

- Requests for euthanasia should always be taken seriously and should cause a thorough evaluation and optimization of the care offered.

The essential ethical dimension of the challenges with which physicians are confronted in care for the terminally ill cannot be ignored. Even though many other ethical questions and problems in palliative care practice are more frequent, euthanasia and physician-assisted suicide are often seen as the foremost ethical problems. This issue provokes much emotion on all sides and can cause major controversy. It is impossible to describe the many facets of the euthanasia debate in just a few pages, so a few important topics are discussed briefly.

DEFINING EUTHANASIA

A meaningful ethical discussion on euthanasia is possible only if we first agree on the terminology. This affects the rest of the discussion. It is of major importance to define euthanasia and physician-assisted suicide in a way that is both sufficiently inclusive and specific but simultaneously links to the language of daily life. Euthanasia literally means "good or mild" (*eu*) "death" (*thanatos*); in the original sense, euthanasia had nothing to do with the actions or interventions of physicians, certainly not in terminating or shortening life. Euthanasia was simply the gentle and natural death almost every human being wanted and wants. When this old term was revisited in the 16th century, the focus shifted to the doctor, even though, at that time, shortening or ending a person's life was not implied. The term referred to what the physician could do to facilitate a gentle death. Euthanasia, thus defined, seems to coincide with what is now called palliative care.

Samuel D. Williams (1870) and Lionel Tollemache (1873), originators of the pro-euthanasia movement, were the first to use the word *euthanasia* in its modern meaning of "mercy killing."[1] From the fierce debate sparked by their ideas, various types of euthanasia were distinguished, and euthanasia became an umbrella term referring to all medical actions or omissions intended to shorten life and/or having a life-shortening effect. Voluntary was distinguished from nonvoluntary euthanasia, active (doing) from passive (withholding or withdrawing), and direct (intentional) from indirect (death accepted but not intended).

Many cling to this broad concept of euthanasia. In contrast, a strict definition of euthanasia has been in use in The Netherlands since 1985, and in Belgium since 1997.[2,3] In these countries, *euthanasia* is defined as "intentionally terminating life by someone other than the person concerned, at the latter's request." Euthanasia is active, direct, and voluntary by definition.

The term *passive euthanasia* does not appear to be expedient. First, it is counterintuitive. Belgium and The Netherlands are said to be the only countries to have legalized euthanasia, but passive euthanasia—withholding or withdrawing life-sustaining treatment—is possible and legal in virtually all countries. Second and most important, it is wrong to imply or suggest that, as a rule, withholding or withdrawing a life-sustaining treatment has a life-shortening effect and implies a life-shortening intention. Therefore, it is best to stop talking about passive euthanasia and assume that euthanasia is active by definition. Many authors share this opinion.[4]

As far as the distinction between *direct* and *indirect euthanasia* is concerned, the same rationale can be followed. First, what is called "indirect euthanasia" is allowed in most countries, so this term also appears to be counterintuitive. Second, when indirect euthanasia refers to pain control with a life-shortening effect, it is (completely erroneously) postulated that pain treatment has an intrinsic life-shortening effect.[5] Moreover, the intention of pain control and direct euthanasia are so different that they cannot be placed under the same heading (euthanasia).

The last of the major classic distinctions is that between *voluntary* and *nonvoluntary* euthanasia. I believe that there are more fundamental similarities than differences between voluntary and nonvoluntary euthanasia, so it is appropriate to maintain this dichotomy. In both cases, the same unusual and controversial act is meant—to actively and directly terminate a life, as painlessly as possible—and for the same reason (i.e., to spare further suffering). Nonvoluntary euthanasia does occur. Even though it is viewed very negatively and often equated with murder, this does not remove the need for a clear terminology.

In conclusion, what is needed is a definition that makes clear (1) that death is the result, not of withholding or withdrawing life-sustaining treatment, but of an active intervention; (2) that there is not only a life-terminating effect but also a life-terminating intention; (3) that the objective is to have a gentle, mild death; and (4) that life-terminating action is undertaken because the patient's incurable condition is considered unbearable. Taking these points into account, I offer the following definitions:

- *Voluntary euthanasia:* The intentional administration of lethal drugs in order to painlessly terminate the life of a patient suffering from an incurable condition deemed unbearable by the patient, at this patient's request.

- *Nonvoluntary euthanasia:* The intentional administration of lethal drugs in order to painlessly terminate the life of a patient suffering from an incurable condition deemed unbearable, not at this patient's request.

The main difference between assisted suicide and euthanasia is that, in the case of assisted suicide and physician-assisted suicide, the patient undertakes the killing act. I suggest the following definitions:

- *Assisted suicide:* intentionally assisting a person, at this person's request, to terminate his or her life
- *Physician-assisted suicide:* a physician's intentionally assisting a patient, at this patient's request, to terminate his or her life

Being for or against euthanasia or assisted suicide does not relieve anyone from their duty to reflect thoroughly on the terminology. Accepting a certain terminology does not mean that one deems the practice defined as acceptable, and certainly not in all circumstances.

LEGAL SITUATION

Until now, only two countries, The Netherlands and Belgium, have legalized voluntary euthanasia. The Termination of Life on Request and Assisted Suicide (Review Procedures) Act came into force in The Netherlands on April 1, 2002; in Belgium, the Act Concerning Euthanasia went into effect on September 23 of the same year. From this and the fact that they are neighboring countries that (partly) share the same language, it cannot simply be concluded that similar social processes are the basis of both laws. This is not the case. In The Netherlands, the euthanasia act is the codification of case law from a broad euthanasia debate and a euthanasia practice that started more than 3 decades ago. In contrast, Belgium was a fairly ordinary European country, as far as euthanasia was concerned, until political debate started in 1999; there was no established euthanasia practice.[6]

The two countries' laws show great resemblance (e.g., allowing voluntary euthanasia in the nonterminal and also on the basis of mental suffering and advance directives), but there are also significant differences. The Belgian Act deals exclusively with euthanasia, the Dutch Act with both euthanasia and physician-assisted suicide. The Belgian Act describes the procedure in minute detail, but the concise Dutch Act does not. In Belgium, euthanasia based on an advance directive is possible only if the patient is irreversibly unconscious; the Dutch Act has no such limitation. The Netherlands allow euthanasia in children older than 12 years of age; the Belgian Act imposes a minimum age of 18 years. The Belgian Act explicitly states that "a serious and incurable disorder *caused by illness or accident*" [italics added] should be at the root of the suffering; the Dutch Act does not mention this medical condition (which could lead to broad interpretations of "hopeless and unbearable suffering" that were, however, rejected by the Dutch Supreme Court in December 2002).[2] In Belgium, 259 euthanasia cases were reported to the national euthanasia commission between September 2002 and December 2003. In 2004 349 cases of euthanasia were reported and in 2005 393 cases.[7] In The Netherlands, 1815, 1886, 1933, and 1923 cases of euthanasia and physician-assisted suicide were officially reported in 2003, 2004, 2005, and 2006, respectively.[8] A study commissioned by the Dutch government indicated that, in 2001, 54% of the actual cases of euthanasia and physician-assisted suicide were officially reported.[9]

Apart from Belgium and The Netherlands, the U.S. state of Oregon, Switzerland, and The Northern Territory of Australia need to be mentioned. In The Northern Territory, the Rights of Terminally Ill Act (1995) was in force for a short time. This act allowed for euthanasia and physician-assisted suicide in competent, terminally ill adults but was revoked by the Australian national parliament in 1997. In Switzerland, assisted suicide is not punishable, provided that this assistance is not given from selfish motives. There is, however, no Swiss law regulating this practice. Euthanasia is illegal. Assisted suicide in Switzerland is only rarely physician assisted; involvement of a physician is neither necessary nor implied.[10] Oregon's Death With Dignity Act came into effect in 1997. It allows physician-assisted suicide (but not voluntary euthanasia) in competent, terminally ill adults. In January 2006, the U.S. Supreme Court upheld this act. In 2003, 2004, 2005, and 2006, respectively, 42, 37, 38, and 46 assisted suicide deaths were officially reported in Oregon.[11] In many other countries, voluntary euthanasia bills have been submitted and debated (e.g., the Assisted Dying for the Terminally Ill bill in Great Britain during 2004, 2005, and 2006), but so far none has had majority support.

Except for The Netherlands, Belgium, the State of Oregon, and Switzerland (which simply decriminalized assisted suicide), there are no countries or states with a legal framework that allows voluntary euthanasia or physician-assisted suicide. Those who perform voluntary euthanasia outside of Belgium and The Netherlands are acting outside the law and risk legal prosecution. Physicians involved in physician-assisted suicide outside of Oregon, Switzerland, and The Netherlands are either breaking the law or at risk. Nonvoluntary euthanasia is not allowed in any country or state and therefore is prone to prosecution everywhere.

PUBLIC OPINION

Data from the European Values Studies (1981, 1990, and 1999-2000) showed that, in virtually all Western European countries, public acceptance of euthanasia (defined as "terminating the life of the incurably ill") has increased.[12] A similar trend can be noticed in the United States. Public opinion, as shown by U.S. figures, is, however, fluctuating and still fluid.[13] The changing public opinion is determined not only by factors such as the waning influence of religion, the greater importance given to autonomy or self-determination, and increasing permissiveness, but also by concrete cases and the ways in which these are portrayed in the media by supporters and opponents of euthanasia.

Based on the most recent data on societal attitudes in 33 European countries, from the 1999-2000 European Values Studies, the average acceptance scores in The Netherlands and in Belgium (on a scale of 1 to 10) are not fundamentally different from those in a number of other European countries. The Netherlands (6.68) does indeed have the highest score, but Denmark (6.61), France (6.16), and Sweden (6.07) all precede Belgium (5.97). The other European countries have scores between 5.63 (Luxembourg) and 2.23 (Malta), with an average European score of 4.71.[14] The reason that Belgium and The Netherlands have euthanasia legislation is clearly not because public opinion in these two countries is significantly different from that in the rest of the world.

Of course, responses to questionnaires on euthanasia and assisted suicide are determined by the ways in which questions are formulated. The image of a terminally ill person, victim to unbearable and indelible physical pain, who requests that his or her life be terminated will find in most Western countries a majority who think that euthanasia not only is morally acceptable but should be legally possible.

FOUR ASSUMPTIONS

Public opinion on euthanasia and physician-assisted suicide is fluid, not rigid. Moreover, it would be a mistake to assume that public opinion on these issues is really *informed;* that is, based on a correct assessment of the actual problems faced by terminally ill patients and the actual possibilities offered by palliative care. Four assumptions are often present in public opinion regarding euthanasia and physician-assisted suicide.

First Assumption: Some People Die an Inhumane Death

Politicians who submit and defend a euthanasia bill often do so from an ethical commitment, a genuine concern for the fate of those who die in inhumane circumstances. Indeed, although great progress has been made in this area, there still are people who are confronted, on their deathbed, with sustained and unbearable suffering. Any family member, friend, acquaintance, or caregiver who has witnessed such dying may, not surprisingly, adopt a positive attitude toward euthanasia and physician-assisted suicide. In any case, the impact of such personal experiences or media stories on attitudes toward euthanasia cannot be overestimated.

Second Assumption: Palliative Care Is Helpless in Such Cases

What is problematic in the reasoning that without euthanasia and physician-assisted suicide some people die an inhumane death is not the fact that incurably ill patients do sometimes end life in degrading circumstances. It is rather the incorrect assumption that they do so because nothing else is possible, because in these tragic cases medicine is powerless and unbearable suffering is simply an unavoidable part of dying. However, even if inhumane deaths do occur, they do not have to.

This assumption underestimates the possibilities offered by specialized and interdisciplinary palliative care. It is almost always possible to allow a humane, dignified death. Pain and other symptoms (e.g., nausea, angst, restlessness) can be handled adequately by specialized palliative care. In extreme cases, it may seem impossible to bring certain physical or psychological symptoms under sufficient control using medication and still leave the patient fully conscious. Palliative care then offers the possibility, in consultation with the patient and the family, to administer palliative sedation, in which consciousness is reduced to the point that refractory symptoms are adequately suppressed. This second assumption is a serious underestimation of the ability of palliative care to free patients from unbearable suffering and to ensure that the reasons for many euthanasia requests simply disappear.

Third Assumption: The Average Physician Has the Necessary Expertise for Palliative Care

The argument that euthanasia and physician-assisted suicide are needed because some people would otherwise die an inhumane death rests on yet another, equally questionable presupposition. This is the idea that people who die inhumanely do so only after their physicians and caregivers have provided all the palliative care possible so as to spare the patient this bitter end. It is a mistake to believe that the average physician, nursing home, or hospital ward possesses the expertise and means for state-of-the-art palliative care. Lessons from the field of pain control—and effective pain control is absolutely essential in palliative care—reveal that the average medical treatment of the incurably ill often exhibits grave shortcomings. Sadly, expert palliative knowledge is not yet generally available.

Fourth Assumption: The Unbearably Suffering Patient Is Making a Free, Autonomous Choice

A fourth, and again questionable, assumption has to do with the putative autonomy of the unbearably suffering patient. A terminally ill patient who suffers intolerable pain and sees no end to the pain will quickly be driven to ask for euthanasia or assisted suicide. In such a case, the patient is not making a free, autonomous choice. The pressure exerted by the degrading circumstances is so great that the patient's own will and convictions scarcely have any influence. In cases like this, the patient's choice cannot be between palliative care on the one hand and euthanasia or physician-assisted suicide on the other. Palliative care is not some exotic or esoteric therapy available to the incurably ill patient as just one possibility. It is, or rather should be, the active and total standard approach with which medicine and health care respond to the terminally ill. In this sense, it is, or should be, more a self-evident point of departure than a conscious and explicit choice made by the patient.

If one really wants to respect autonomy and freedom of choice, it is of the utmost importance that terminally ill patients be treated according to the principles of palliative care. Otherwise, many people will request (and receive) euthanasia for reasons that have more to do with the shortcomings of the health care system than with autonomous will.

Palliative care cannot resolve or prevent every request for euthanasia or physician-assisted suicide. There will always be people who continue to request euthanasia, even with the best palliative measures, and even when the physical and psychological symptoms from which they suffer have been controlled. In many cases, these are people who consider their lives no longer meaningful or people who want to stay in control. It is on the basis of these considerations, the level of meaning rather than purely physical or psychological problems, that their request for euthanasia should be understood. However, regular contact with dying people teaches that only a small minority who request euthanasia belong to these categories. With the vast majority of patients requesting euthanasia, the request vanishes after the beneficial effects of good palliative care (including specific attention to the patient's psychological and spiritual needs) are applied. The vast majority of the terminally ill do not *want* euthanasia; they want to live, even in the final months, weeks, and days. Palliative care is not so much about humane *dying* as it is about humane *living* in the face of death.[15]

WORLD RELIGIONS AND EUTHANASIA

Only a brief overview of how the major religions view euthanasia (as defined earlier in this chapter) and assisted suicide is presented here. Obviously, this says nothing about the various religions' ideas on pain control, palliative sedation, or withholding or withdrawing life-sustaining treatment. All religious traditions share a positive view of palliative care.

Various studies point to a clear link between religious affiliation and a negative attitude toward euthanasia and physician-assisted suicide.[14] This is not surprising. Those who assume that God determines and controls reality and decides on life and death will be reluctant to take such decisions upon themselves. The view of major religions on euthanasia and assisted suicide is predominantly negative. Almost all Jewish rabbinic authors argue against euthanasia and assisted suicide. Even when a person is a *goses* (a person expected to die within 72 hours), it is not allowed to intentionally speed up the process. For this position, orthodox, conservative, and reformist rabbis all refer back to the *halakhah* (the Jewish religious law, consisting of Torah, Talmud, and other texts).[16] Among the various Christian churches, sanctity of life prevails. Life has been given to us by God and it belongs exclusively to Him. Killing an innocent fellow human, even at his or her own request, goes against the biblical command "Thou shalt not kill" and is a denial of the intrinsic value of each human being, made in God's image. The official position of most Christian churches is very much opposed to euthanasia and assisted suicide. Muslims have a similar attitude. Based on the sanctity of life, the idea that human beings are stewards responsible for their bodies, and the prohibition to go against the divine plan that God has for every person, euthanasia and assisted suicide are unacceptable for the Islamic *ulama* (religious authorities).[17]

Euthanasia and assisted suicide violate important Hindu ideals and principles. They clash with the central virtue of *ahimsa* (non-harming) and result in bad *karma* for both the physician (who uses violence) and the patient (who will be faced with suffering again in a next life, because of his or her mistakes in previous lives). On the other hand, it is sometimes argued that helping a patient to die is not a violation of the physician's *dharma* (duty).[18] The principle of *ahimsa* also plays a central role in Bud-

dhism. The first of the Five Precepts, the five fundamental commands for laymen, forbids killing. Based on the aforementioned *karma* doctrine, most Buddhist religious leaders and authors are reluctant to condone euthanasia and assisted suicide. Others, however, point out the major importance of compassion (*karuna*) in Buddhism and, as a result, advocate some openness to euthanasia and assisted suicide.[19] Sikhism offers its followers a general framework (focused on the sacred scripture of the Sikh, the Guru Granth Sahib), but it does not offer concrete guidelines regarding new ethical dilemmas. Sikhism considers life as a gift of God, and God is the one who decides on life and death. Based on these principles, most Sikh denounce euthanasia and assisted suicide.

SLOW EUTHANASIA?

There is much confusion with regard to pain control and sedation among the general public. Medical practice itself is not always unambiguous. Some studies have investigated the incidence of "intensification of the alleviation of pain and suffering *partly with the intention of hastening the patient's death*" [italics added], categorizing this doubtful but regrettably not uncommon practice, no questions asked, as pain and symptom control.[20,21] Sedation, in turn, is sometimes accused of being "slow euthanasia."[22] In any case, ambiguity and abuse put pain control and sedation in a poor light, making them appear similar to euthanasia, and can cause colleagues, patients, and families to fear heavy pain medication or sedation. Undertreatment of serious pain and inhuman suffering can be the tragic consequence.

To avoid misunderstandings and malpractice, I previously introduced the term *palliative sedation* (to replace the ambiguous *terminal sedation*)[23] and offered precise definitions of both pain control ("the intentional administration of analgesics and/or other drugs in dosages and combinations required to adequately relieve pain") and palliative sedation ("the intentional administration of sedative drugs in dosages and combinations required to reduce the consciousness of a terminal patient as much as necessary to adequately relieve one or more refractory symptoms").[23-25] Definitions such as these allow a sharp line between pain control and palliative sedation on the one hand and euthanasia on the other. The essence of both pain control and palliative sedation is that they are forms of symptom control. The physician's intention in both cases is to fight a symptom, not to terminate life. All actions taken need to reflect this intention. In a field where dosages and combinations are crucial (i.e., overdosing can, in fact, shorten life), the dosages and combinations administered should be in proportion to the specific suffering the clinician wants to alleviate. Adequacy and proportionality are at the forefront of what is and should be done on an objective level.

There is, then, this important and threefold distinction: the *intention* (symptom control), the *action* (administering only what is necessary to control the symptom), and the *result* (in the vast majority of cases, no life-shortening effect) are totally different in pain control and palliative sedation versus euthanasia[23-26] (Table 21-1). A physician who claims to carry out pain control or palliative sedation but in fact knowingly overdoses to shorten a patient's life may be administering "slow euthanasia" but is certainly

TABLE 21-1 Distinctions among Pain Control, Palliative Sedation, and Euthanasia

FACTOR	PAIN CONTROL	PALLIATIVE SEDATION	EUTHANASIA AND PHYSICIAN-ASSISTED SUICIDE
Intention	Symptom control	Symptom control	Terminating life
Action	Administering as much medication as needed to control the pain (proportionality)	Administering as much medication as needed to control the symptom (proportionality)	Administering as much medication as needed to terminate life
Result	Shortens life only in very exceptional cases (and may have a life-lengthening effect)	Shortens life only in exceptional cases	Termination of life (by definition)

not performing pain control or palliative sedation. Even more problematic than euthanasia or physician-assisted suicide is euthanasia in disguise.

DEALING WITH REQUESTS FOR EUTHANASIA OR PHYSICIAN-ASSISTED SUICIDE

Caregivers who work with the incurably ill will be confronted with patients who (either in guarded terms or explicitly) ask for euthanasia or assisted suicide or family members who ask to end the suffering of their loved one. Several elements play a pivotal role in an ethically responsible approach to dealing with these questions. Let us assume a legal situation in which both euthanasia and physician-assisted suicide are illegal, although the points discussed are equally important in Belgium, The Netherlands, Oregon, and Switzerland.

Employ Dialogue and Respect

Dialogue and respect are crucial in dealing with requests for euthanasia or assisted suicide. The best chances of a dignified death are through honest dialogue, characterized by openness and respect for the beliefs, emotions, and attitudes of the patient and family as well as those of the physician and other caregivers.

Comply with the Law

In a society in which euthanasia and assisted suicide are prohibited, as a general rule the physician should comply with the law. This principle goes beyond simply avoiding the risk of prosecution and its consequences for the physician and the institution. First of all, physicians are not to put themselves above the law, certainly not in situations of life or death; physicians can and should exert their professional autonomy within the boundaries set by society through its legislative bodies. Second, with illegal euthanasia and assisted suicide, it is likely that procedural safeguards found in euthanasia laws would not be respected; to avoid the risk of prosecution, euthanasia and assisted suicide would be carried out in secret. For this reason, open discussion with the nursing team, with an independent colleague, with the palliative care team, and so forth would not take place. As a result, there is a higher risk that euthanasia or assisted suicide would be performed in cases in which other, much less drastic and problematic measures could have solved the unbearable suffering.

Take the Request Seriously

The fact that what is requested (i.e., euthanasia or physician-assisted suicide) is out of the question, does not imply that the physician should not take the request of the patient or family very seriously. In an open and continued dialogue with the patient and/or the family, the physician should communicate that, although euthanasia and assisted suicide are not an option, the whole team of caregivers will do whatever they can and propose any appropriate palliative treatment (including, if necessary, palliative sedation) to ease suffering.

Discover the Reasons behind the Request

People do not request euthanasia or assisted suicide out of some morbid death wish or because they have always wanted so much to die, but rather because, at a certain moment in their illness, their suffering, and consequently life itself, becomes unbearable. Moreover, will to live and will to die show substantial fluctuation among the dying.[27] Various factors can be decisive in a request for euthanasia or assisted suicide, often in combination; these include fear of what is to come, respiratory difficulties, physical pain, loss of control, increasing weakness and dependence on others, and hopelessness and depression.[28,29] Behind a request for euthanasia or assisted suicide there is always physical, psychological, social, or spiritual suffering that has caused a decline in quality of life. It is the responsibility of the caregiver who receives a request to discover, through successive open and in-depth discussions, the reasons behind the patient's desire to end his or her life. What is it exactly that makes the patient's life no longer bearable?

Re-evaluate and Optimize the Care Offered

How can caregivers alleviate the physical, psychological, social, or spiritual suffering that lies at the origin of requests for euthanasia or assisted suicide? A request to end one's life, even if vague, must always stimulate a thorough evaluation and optimization of the care offered. What might be done to optimize the care (including psychological and spiritual care) even more precisely to the needs of the patient? Is it really impossible to alleviate the suffering? Have we simply reached the limits of our abilities and therefore require specialized advice?

Take an Interdisciplinary Approach

Because it considers patients in their totality, palliative care is interdisciplinary by definition. For this reason, a physician who receives a request for euthanasia or assisted suicide can never act alone. Dealing with such a request responsibly always involves an interdisciplinary approach.

There are diverse and complex motives that can underlie such a request, and various caregivers can offer their own perspectives. For instance, nurses are often close to their patients, both literally and figuratively, and therefore are often in a good position to know the reasons behind the request. Specialized input from various disciplines is frequently necessary to alleviate the patient's suffering.

Consult the Palliative Support Team

Because of the crucial role played by specialized and interdisciplinary expertise, it is strongly recommended that the local palliative support team be consulted whenever a physician or a nurse is confronted with a request for euthanasia or assisted suicide. It is the role of this team to improve the quality of life of the incurably ill and to alleviate their suffering as much as possible, no matter what its nature. These interdisciplinary teams provide palliative expertise; they do not make decisions in the place of the patient, the physician, or the nurse involved but rather inform them about the various palliative options and offer support, especially in very difficult circumstances.

CONCLUSION: A PALLIATIVE FILTER

Euthanasia and physician-assisted suicide are among the most controversial issues in palliative care. There are many aspects of this delicate ethical problem, only a few of which have been briefly discussed here. Interdisciplinary palliative care certainly cannot prevent or give an adequate answer to each and every euthanasia request. What I have called a *palliative filter*[30] can prevent much unbearable suffering as well as the tragedy of euthanasia or physician-assisted suicide associated with false choices resulting from poor palliative care rather than an explicit wish to end one's life.

REFERENCES

1. Emanuel EJ. The history of euthanasia debates in the United States and Britain. Ann Intern Med 1994;121:793-802.
2. Adams M, Nys H. Euthanasia in the low countries: Comparative reflections on the Belgian and Dutch euthanasia act. In Schotsmans P, Meulenbergs T (eds). Euthanasia and Palliative Care in the Low Countries. Paris, Peeters, 2005, pp 5-33.
3. Belgian Advisory Committee on Bioethics. Advice No 1 of 12, May 1997, concerning the desirability of a legal recognition of euthanasia. Available at https://portal.health.fgov.be/portal/page?_pageid=56,512676&_dad=portal&_schema=PORTAL (accessed January 2008).
4. Roy DJ. Euthanasia and withholding treatment. In Doyle D, Hanks G, Cherny N, Calman K (eds). Oxford Textbook of Palliative Medicine, 3rd ed. Oxford: Oxford University Press, 2005, pp 84-97.
5. Bercovitch M, Waller A, Adunsky A. High dose morphine use in the hospice setting: A database survey of patient characteristics and effect on life expectancy. Cancer 1999;86:871-877.
6. Broeckaert B. Belgium: Towards a legal recognition of euthanasia. Eur J Health Law 2001;8:95-107.
7. Federale Controle en Evaluatiecommissie Euthanasie. Eerste verslag aan de wetgevende kamers (22 September 2002-31 December 2003), 22 November 2004. Available at http://www.dekamer.be/FLWB/pdf/51/1374/51K1374002.pdf (accessed September 2007).
8. Regionale toetsingcommissies euthanasie, Available at http://www.toetsingscommissieseuthanasie.nl/Toetsingscommissie/jaarverslag (accessed January 2008).
9. van der Wal G, van der Heide A, Onwuteaka-Philipsen BD, van der Maas PJ. Medische besluitvorming aan het einde van het leven: De praktijk en de toetsingsprocedure euthanasie. Utrecht: De Tijdstroom, 2003.
10. Hurst SA, Mauron A. Assisted suicide and euthanasia in Switzerland: Allowing a role for non-physicians. BMJ 2003;326:271-273.
11. State of Oregon. Death with Dignity Act. Available at http://www.oregon.gov/DHS/ph/pas (accessed January 2008).
12. Cohen J, Marcoux I, Bilsen J, et al. Trends in acceptance of euthanasia among the general public in 12 European countries (1981-1999). Eur J Public Health 2006;16:663-669. Epub 2006 Apr 26.
13. Duncan OD, Parmelee LF. Trends in public approval of euthanasia and suicide in the US, 1947-2003. J Med Ethics 2006;32:266-272.
14. Cohen J, Marcoux I, Bilsen J, et al. European public acceptance of euthanasia: Socio-demographic and cultural factors associated with the acceptance of euthanasia in 33 European countries. Soc Sci Med 2006;63:743-756.
15. Cannaerts N, Dierckx de Casterlé B, Grypdonck, M. Palliatieve Zorg: Zorg Voor Het Leven, een Onderzoek Naar de Specifieke Bijdrage van de Residentiële Palliatieve Zorgverlening. Gent: Academia, 2000.
16. Mackler AL. Introduction to Jewish and Catholic Bio-Ethics: A Comparative Analysis. Washington, DC: Georgetown University Press, 2003, pp 64-84.
17. Brockopp JE. Islamic Ethics of Life: Abortion, War and Euthanasia. (Studies in Comparative Religion.) Columbia: University of South Carolina Press, 2003.
18. Firth S. End-of-life: A Hindu view. Lancet 2005;366:682-686.
19. Keown D. Buddhism and Bioethics. London: MacMillan, 1995.
20. van der Heide A, Deliens L, Faisst K, et al. End-of-life decision-making in six European countries: Descriptive study. Lancet 2003;362:345-350.
21. Seale C. National survey of end-of-life decisions made by UK medical practitioners. Palliat Med 2006;20:3-10.
22. Billings JA, Block SD. Slow euthanasia. J Pal Care 1996;12(4):21-30.
23. Broeckaert B. Palliative sedation defined or why and when sedation is not euthanasia. J Pain Symptom Manage 2000;20:S58.
24. Broeckaert B, Núñez Olarte JM. Euthanasia and physician-assisted suicide. In ten Have H, Clark D (eds). The Ethics of Palliative Care: European Perspectives. Buckingham, Open University Press, 2002, pp 166-180.
25. Broeckaert B. Palliative sedation: Ethical aspects. In Gastmans C (ed). Between Technology and Humanity: The Impact of Technology on Health Care Ethics. Leuven: Leuven University Press, 2002, pp 239-255.
26. Materstvedt LJ, Clark D, Ellershaw J, et al. Euthanasia and physician-assisted suicide: A view from an EAPC Ethics Task Force. Palliat Med 2003;17:97-101.
27. Chochinov HM, Tataryn D, Clinch JJ, et al. Will to live in the terminally ill. Lancet 1999;354:816-819.
28. Chochinov HM. Dying, dignity, and new horizons in palliative end-of-life care. CA Cancer J Clin 2006;56:84-103.
29. van der Lee ML, van der Bom JG, Swarte NB, et al. Euthanasia and depression: A prospective cohort study among terminally ill cancer patients. J Clin Oncol 2005;23:6607-6612.
30. Broeckaert B, Janssens R. Palliative care and euthanasia: Belgian and Dutch perspectives. In Schotsmans P, Meulenbergs T (eds). Euthanasia and Palliative Care in the Low Countries. Paris, Peeters, 2005, pp 34-62.

SUGGESTED READING

Lavi SJ. The Modern Art of Dying: A History of Euthanasia in the United States. Princeton: Princeton University Press, 2005.

Schotsmans P, Meulenbergs T (eds). Euthanasia and Palliative Care in the Low Countries. Paris: Peeters, 2005.

ten Have H, Clark D (eds). The Ethics of Palliative Care: European Perspectives. Buckingham, Open University Press, 2002.

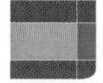

CHAPTER **22**

Research Bioethics

Carmen Paradis and Kathryn L. Weise

K E Y   P O I N T S

- Informed consent is essential for research.
- Risks must be balanced by benefits.
- Research must have scientific validity.
- Placebo use must not result in less than standard quality of care.
- Treating physicians may act as researchers, but care must be taken not to confuse the roles.

Today's research ethics began with the development of international codes after World War II. Individual nations adapted these codes to create their own specific standards. As research experience grew, a more nuanced understanding evolved to ensure that the ethical considerations of beneficence, justice, and respect for persons were safeguarded in research. The use of informed consent attempts to ensure individual respect, the use of equipoise and placebos works to serve beneficence, and inclusivity expresses justice.

RESEARCH ETHICS CODES

Nuremberg Code

The 1947 Nuremberg Code set a standard by which to judge the Nazi human experimentation. It, together with the Helsinki Ethical Principles for Medical Research Involving Human Subjects, developed by the World Medical Association in 1964, forms the basis for the ethical principles many nations have codified to ensure that human research is conducted ethically.

The Nuremberg Code can be divided into two sections: care due to subjects and the scientific attributes of the research. The regulations addressing the care of research subjects are expressions of beneficence and respect for persons[1]:

1. Subjects must voluntarily agree to participate in research, understanding the research's nature, how it is to be conducted, and what that will mean to them in terms of inconveniences and hazards to their health and person.
2. Risks and harms to subjects should be minimized; the degree of allowed risk should be balanced by the value of the knowledge gained.
3. Subjects should be free to withdraw from research during its course.

The regulations regarding the science of research recognize that research that is unlikely to benefit society is unethical because it exposes subjects to unnecessary risk for dubious benefit[1]:

1. Research should be designed with the expectation of yielding results useful to society.
2. Research design should be based on knowledge gained from animal experimentation and/or the natural history of the condition being studied to ensure the results will be useful to society.
3. Research should be conducted by scientifically qualified persons.
4. The scientists in charge must be prepared to terminate research at any point if they believe the risk of harm is too great.

Helsinki Declaration

The Helsinki Declaration of the World Medical Association[2] expresses the same underlying principles as the Nuremberg Code, adding that

1. Special committees, independent of the investigator, should consider, comment upon, and guide research protocols. [In the United States these committees are known as Institutional Review Boards;

in the United Kingdom, Research Ethics Committees; in Canada, Research Ethics Boards.]
2. Risks to subjects should be balanced by potential benefits to the subject or others.
3. Subject privacy should be protected.
4. Researchers must accurately publish their results.
5. Particular care must be taken when obtaining consent if a subject is under duress or in a dependent relationship to the person obtaining the consent.
6. In legal incompetence, whether because of physical or mental incapacity or because the subject is a minor child, informed consent must be obtained from a responsible person in accordance with a nation's laws. If a minor is able to give consent, that consent must be obtained in addition to [that of] the legal guardian.

The Declaration of Helsinki has a special section to address combining medical research with clinical care and nontherapeutic research. It specifies that every patient, including those patients in control groups, must receive the best available standard of care and that refusal to participate in research must not interfere with the physician–patient relationship. It allows the use of a new diagnostic or therapeutic measure if a physician judges that it has the potential to save a life, re-establish health, or alleviate suffering.[2]

Belmont Report

Evolving from both the Nuremberg Code and the Declaration of Helsinki, the 1976 Belmont Report set forth basic ethical principles for research involving humans in the United States.[3] Building on the Helsinki Declaration's caution about dependent subjects, it dealt with the issue of "practice" versus "research." It defined *practice* as "interventions . . . designed solely to enhance the well-being of an individual patient or client, that have a reasonable expectation of success," adding that the purpose of practice is to provide a diagnosis, preventative treatment, or therapy to an individual. *Research* was defined as any activity, described in a formal protocol, that is intended to test a hypothesis or permit conclusions to be drawn to contribute to generalizable knowledge. The Report concluded that it is permissible to carry out research and practice together if the research is designed to evaluate the safety and efficacy of a therapy. It advised that, if there is any element of research in an activity, it should undergo review by an independent committee. Although not every new procedure is to be considered research simply because it is different or untested, if an innovative procedure is thought to potentially have widespread applicability, a research protocol should be developed to test its efficacy and safety. The Belmont Report advised that the same basic ethical principles (respect for persons, beneficence, and justice) that serve as ethical justification to evaluate actions in society should also be used to evaluate research conduct.[3]

Tri-Council Policy Statement

In 1998, Canada developed a Tri-Council Policy Statement which contained many of these same principles, adding respect for human dignity, respect for vulnerable persons, and respect for justice and inclusiveness.

INFORMED CONSENT FOR RESEARCH

Informed consent is essential to honor respect for persons. It is the sine qua non of research involving human subjects, the first directive of the Nuremberg Code and the one with the most detail. It is dealt with in all nations' research codes. Specifically, consent to participate in research must be voluntary and able to be withdrawn at any time. To be able to consent to research, it is necessary to have the capacity to understand the nature, goals, and requirements of the research and its potential benefits and risks of harm to oneself. Lack of such capacity, referred to as decision making capacity (DMC), means that a person lacks the ability to consent to research in an informed way. Persons may have impaired DMC by virtue of diseases such as Alzheimer's dementia or by being too young to have attained sufficient cognitive ability. Duress may impair DMC. Alterations in DMC may be temporary or permanent and may wax and wane with changes in medication and disease progression, especially in advanced disease, when such progression can be rapid (see Chapter 28).

Denying those who lack or have impaired DMC the opportunity to participate in research bars them from the benefits of evidence-based medicine that research produces. Given that the most significant advances in medicine have come from well-designed research, this would be unjust. In addition, such a restrictive policy would prevent these individuals from acting altruistically in the interest of others in their group or society at large. Implying that such persons do not have the ability to contribute to society denotes a lack of respect for them.

To balance these needs of justice and respect for vulnerable persons, guidelines have been developed to allow people with impaired DMC to participate in research. Such individuals should be involved in the consent process to the extent they are able, giving their assent or dissent, while another authorized individual such as a parent, guardian, or designated surrogate gives or withholds permission. Those who act as surrogate decision makers should endeavor to make decisions as they think the subject would, considering the subject's previously expressed desires and actions. DMC should be reassessed if indicated, and, if DMC is present, the individual should then be given the opportunity to voluntarily consent or refuse.

Because children and adolescents are one group not typically considered to have DMC, the American Academy of Pediatrics Committee on Bioethics has specifically addressed the issue of consent among minors. The Committee recommended that minors older than 7 years of age should be engaged in a process of obtaining assent, or agreement, using language commensurate with their development. This approach recognizes that caregivers have a role in helping children develop an active involvement in their own health care. It also recognizes that minors who have been chronically ill may be as capable of understanding illness and the concept of personal mortality as many adults, and in such situations their involvement in decision making is appropriate.[4,5] U.S. regulations require Institutional Review Boards to determine that adequate provisions are made for soliciting permission from parents or guardians and assent from children whose age, maturity, and psychological state allow them to be deemed capable of assenting.[6] This helps ensure that justice is served, by giving children access to the results of research, and that children are accorded the respect they are due as persons while protecting their vulnerability as the situation dictates.

EQUIPOISE

Clinical equipoise allows clinicians to fulfill their therapeutic obligation to provide a patient with the best standard of care and researchers to achieve the goal of advancing generalizable knowledge. To have clinical equipoise, a researcher must have genuine doubt about which intervention is better when research subjects are randomly assigned to one of several interventions. The intent of this requirement is to minimize risk and maximize benefit. In medicine, once a therapy becomes the standard of care, physicians often accept it as providing benefit, even though it may not. This proclivity can be a handicap to a physician-researcher's individual equipoise about a research treatment. Given medicine's history of accepting ineffective treatments (e.g., internal mammary ligation for angina) as a standard of care, it has been recommended that evidence-based knowledge be used as the criterion to determine equipoise. This means that, in general, trials would go forward only if the question of which intervention is better for a particular population had not been answered by well-designed studies.[7] The doubt of clinical equipoise would thus be based on scientific evidence rather than intuition or prevailing practice.

PLACEBOS

The placebo effect occurs when a patient improves with an inactive treatment, the placebo. It is commonly thought that this occurs because people believe that they are being helped, not because of some placebo attribute. There is a great deal of debate about the magnitude of placebo effects. Placebos do appear to have more effect in pain and other subjective symptoms (e.g., quality of life).[8]

Given that changes in quality of life are a significant objective of palliative care research, there is controversy about whether placebos have a place in palliative medicine research with its vulnerable populations. The consensus is that it is ethically permissible to include placebos in randomized, clinical trials (RCTs) if the placebo is additional to the standard of care, if there is no known effective standard of care for the symptom studied, or if subjects are given adequate access to rescue treatment. An essential ethical consideration is that subjects who receive placebo should be no more likely than subjects receiving active treatment to suffer as a result (see Chapter 28).

JUSTICE

Justice means that all persons in a society are due certain benefits and assume burdens in an equitable way. Applied to research, this means that all groups should have equal opportunities to benefit from the scientific evidence generated by research and to assume the burdens that are part

---

Box 22-1 Research Challenges

- Ascertaining that consent is voluntary and sufficiently informed.
- Discriminating between evidence-based and accepted treatment when determining equipoise.
- Separating the roles and responsibilities of the physician and the researcher.
- Ensuring that all societal groups share in research's burdens and benefits equitably.
- Determining how to minimize burdens without jeopardizing scientific validity.

---

of acquiring that knowledge. This does not mean that individuals are obliged to participate in research, but rather that they should be allowed the opportunity. The concern with palliative care subjects is that they may be at increased risk of exploitation because their disease may have made them vulnerable and impaired their DMC. This problem has created perceptual and methodological barriers to conducting such research (see Chapter 28). Too often, patients are subjected to symptomatic treatments with well-documented side effects but unproven benefits.[9] The lack of good evidence in palliative medicine is at least partially, some would say largely, attributable to the perception of the dying as a special class of patients with unique ethical challenges that limit the ability to accumulate research-based evidence. When research with less vulnerable populations can be extrapolated to palliative care, it should be. However, it should be recognized that a dying patient can be unique in terms of physiology and treatment goals, and even quality of life. Research unique to this population must, for justice's sake, be conducted within this population.[10] Similarly, palliative care research in children should be promoted so they can benefit from the evaluation of interventions and models of care.[11]

CONCLUSIONS

Research ethics continues to evolve. Current major controversies center on informed consent, placebo use, defining equipoise, and finding ways to serve the underserved (Box 22-1). Issues in informed consent include how to provide adequate information about sometimes complex concepts, in understandable language, without overwhelming or unduly burdening participants. Placebos are sometimes needed to determine treatments of marginal benefit, but there is concern that their excessive use could cause unnecessary suffering. Arguments still abound about the definition of equipoise, but the consensus is that it must be built on well-designed research evidence to have the greatest likelihood of a favorable balance between risk and benefit. Physicians' struggles with their own beliefs

about what is "best treatment" remain a stumbling block in the application of this concept. The quandary of physician-researchers about executing their differing responsibilities as researcher and as clinician is part of that struggle. As we move into the reality of a global society, we continue to grapple with how to bring the benefits of research to all the world's citizens while making the burdens equitable.

SUGGESTED READING

Jubb AM. Palliative care research: Trading ethics for an evidence base. J Med Ethics 2002;28:342-346.

National Institutes of Health, Office of Human Subjects Research. Nuremberg Military Tribunals: Nuremberg Code, 1947. Available at http://ohsr.od.nih.gov/guidelines/nuremberg.html (accessed September 2007).

National Institutes of Health, Office of Human Subjects Research. The Belmont Report: Ethical Principles and Guidelines for the Protection of Human Subjects of Research. National Commission for the Protection of Human Subjects of Biomedical and Behavioral Research, 1979. Available at http://ohsr.od.nih.gov/guidelines/belmont.html (accessed September 2007).

U.S. Department of Health and Human Services. Code of Federal Regulations, Title 45 Public Welfare, Department of Health and Human Services. Part 46: Protection of Human Subjects. 2005. Available at http://www.hhs.gov/ohrp/humansubjects/guidance/45cfr46.htm (accessed September 2007).

World Medical Association. World Medical Association Declaration of Helsinki: Ethical Principles for Medical Research Involving Human Subjects, 2006. Available at http://www.wma.net/e/policy/63.htm (accessed May 14, 2007).

REFERENCES

1. National Institutes of Health, Office of Human Subjects Research. Nuremberg Military Tribunals: Nuremberg Code, 1947. Available at http://ohsr.od.nih.gov/guidelines/nuremberg.html (accessed September 2007).
2. World Medical Association. World Medical Association Declaration of Helsinki Ethical Principles for Medical Research Involving Human Subjects, 2000. BMJ 1996;313:1448-1449.
3. National Institutes of Health, Office of Human Subjects Research. The Belmont Report: Ethical Principles and Guidelines for the Protection of Human Subjects of Research. National Commission for the Protection of Human Subjects of Biomedical and Behavioral Research, 1979. Available at http://ohsr.od.nih.gov/guidelines/belmont.html (accessed September 2007).
4. Committee on Bioethics, American Academy of Pediatrics. Informed consent, parental permission, and assent in pediatric practice. Pediatrics 1995;95:314-317.
5. Committee on Drugs, American Academy of Pediatrics. Guidelines for the ethical conduct of studies to evaluate drugs in pediatric populations. Pediatrics 1995;95:286-294.
6. U.S. Department of Health and Human Services. Code of Federal Regulations, Title 45 Public Welfare, Department of Health and Human Services. Part 46: Protection of Human Subjects. 2005. Available at http://www.hhs.gov/ohrp/humansubjects/guidance/45cfr46.htm (accessed September 2007).
7. Halpern SD. Evidence-based equipoise and research responsiveness. Am J Bioeth 2006;6:1-4.
8. Krouse RS, Easson AM, Angelos P. Ethical considerations and barriers to research in surgical palliative care. J Am Coll Surg 2003;196:469-474.
9. Arraf K, Cox G, Oberle K. Using the Canadian Code of Ethics for Registered Nurses to Explore Ethics in Palliative Care Research. Nurs Ethics 2004;11:600-609.
10. Jubb AM. Palliative care research: Trading ethics for an evidence base. J Med Ethics 2002;28:342-346.
11. American Academy of Pediatrics. Committee on Bioethics and Committee on Hospital Care. Palliative care for children. Pediatrics 2000;106(2 Pt 1):351-357.

Education

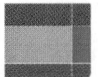

CHAPTER **23**

Curriculum Development

Catherine Deamant, Martha L. Twaddle, and Pamela Dalinis

KEY POINTS

- A curriculum in palliative medicine, although developing, is still inadequate at all levels of training.

- The four phases of curriculum development are needs assessment, curricular design, implementation, and evaluation.

- The curriculum should address the major domains of knowledge, skills, and attitudes concordant with the learner's level of training.

- The curriculum should address competencies common to all disciplines of medicine, nursing, and the health care professions.

- The curriculum should identify the relationship of the learning objectives and educational experiences to the Accreditation Council for Graduate Medical Education (ACGME) core competencies: (1) patient care, (2) medical knowledge, (3) practice-based learning and improvement, (4) interpersonal and communication skills, (5) professionalism, (6) systems-based practice.

The general medical education of physicians is deficient in teaching the care of patients and their families at the end of life. Since the late 1990s, efforts have been made to enhance curricula at all levels to address the identified deficiencies and establish expertise in end-of-life care as a core physician competency. In 1996, the American Board of Internal Medicine set forth standards for internists, and, subsequently, the National Board of Medical Examiners integrated questions pertaining to end-of-life care into licensing examinations. In 1996, the American Board of Hospice and Palliative Medicine offered its first board certification in the specialty. Within academic institutions, attitudinal barriers, the lack of quality educational materials and dedicated faculty, and the frequent lack of a formal curriculum challenge the full integration of end-of-life education and training for medical students and postgraduates.

Students, residents, and faculty perceive end-of-life education as important.[1] Medicine as a culture continues to view death as failure and to focus on cure. A national survey of medical students, residents, and faculty revealed

that few had received formal end-of-life education and that they did not feel prepared to care for the dying. Residents and faculty also felt unprepared to teach others these skills.[1] Medical education deans identified the key barriers to integration of an end-of-life curriculum: a lack of time in the general curriculum, lack of faculty expertise, and inadequate faculty leadership.[2]

Palliative medicine is the medical discipline of the broad therapeutic model known as palliative care. This discipline and model of care are devoted to achieving the best possible quality of life for the patient and family throughout a life-threatening illness by relief of suffering and control of symptoms. This requires the comprehensive assessment and interdisciplinary team management of the physical, psychological, social, and spiritual needs of patients and their families. Palliative care, the interdisciplinary practice of palliative medicine, addresses the end of life but also applies its principles more broadly to the severely and chronically ill. The practice and study of palliative care provides unique educational opportunities for all levels of training that focus on interdisciplinary interaction, learning, enhanced communication skills, and self-reflection, with the rich potential for experiential learning in the home.[3] In June 2006, the Accreditation Council for Graduate Medical Education (ACGME) formally recognized Hospice and Palliative Medicine as a new discipline. Growth of the specialty and development of academic physician leaders will help address curriculum development, integration, and physician training.

CURRICULUM DEVELOPMENT: GENERAL CONSIDERATIONS

Successful curricular change requires dedicated, multilevel efforts. Essential elements include commitment from key institutional and educational leaders within an academic medical center or educational establishment and attention to recommendations by the national accrediting authorities. Knowledge of the institution's educational and practical needs should be based on specific data concerning deficits within current curricula. New curriculum implementation requires effective communication within curriculum committees to discuss and implement change, as well as faculty recruitment and training, resource allocation, and system process improvements for effectiveness.[4-6]

CONTENT AND PROCESS ISSUES IN A PALLIATIVE CARE CURRICULUM

Medical students and residents are influenced by the informal or hidden curriculum of their educational years—

namely, the culture with presiding values and judgments in which they learn medicine.[1] If the prevailing attitude is that end-of-life care is not valued, that the physician's responsibility is to cure and death represents failure, no course work will compensate for the practice and attitudes of key role models and peers.[7] Formal educational efforts regarding end-of-life care reinforce the idea that care for the dying is the physician's responsibility, and empathy, effective communication, and expertise in pain and symptom management are core competencies. Traditionally, there has been little formal opportunity to process the emotional and personal experience of physicians caring for dying patients and their families. Palliative care curricula integrate communication and professionalism and reinforce the knowledge, skills, and attitudes of self-care and reflection as being critically important to practice excellence (Table 23-1).

Curriculum Development: Undergraduate Training

There are no standards for undergraduate training in palliative care in the United States. There are guidelines for palliative care education in the medical school curriculum in both preclinical and clinical years. The curriculum is structured around five basic domains[7]:

1. Understanding psychological, sociologic, cultural, and spiritual issues of patients and families
2. Interviewing and communication skills

TABLE 23-1	Summary of Content and Process Issues in a Palliative Care Curriculum	
PHASE	**CONTENT ISSUES**	**PROCESS ISSUES**
Components of needs assessment	**Assessment of institutional needs**	Literature review
Literature review	Patient/family needs	Patient/family interviews
Assessment of institutional needs	Learner needs	Focus groups
	Resources	Surveys
	Educational	
	Clinical	
	Financial	Interviews with clinicians, administrators,
	Roadblocks	educators, institutional champion
	Denial of death	Interviews with palliative care experts
	Lack of resources	Interviews with educational design
	Political obstacles	experts
	Bureaucracy	
Components of curriculum design	**Curriculum outline**	Developing resources
Curriculum outline	**Goals of the curriculum**	Review of needs assessment
	Core content areas	Further literature review
	Outline of individual units and schedule	Consultation with education expert
	Timing of individual units/total amount of time available	Core curricula from national organizations
		Palliative care curriculum committee
		Grant application
Individual units	**Individual units (for each unit)**	Developing institutional support:
	Goals/objectives	Institutional champion
	Essential content (facts, principles, skills)	Advisory committee
	Instructional strategies	Palliative care curriculum committee
	Evaluation	Follow-up meetings to review needs
	Resources needed	assessment and curriculum outline
	Faculty with expertise	Outside review
	Financial	Internal review
Implementation	**Phased-in implementation**	Meetings with residency director, dean,
Implementation plan	Pilot unit initiation	administrator, institutional champion,
Phased-in implementation	Pilot evaluation	departmental chairs
	Gradual implementation of other curricular units	Administration/secretarial support
		Focus groups about pilot units
Evaluation	**Formative**	Internal review of curriculum
Formative	Focus groups	External review of curriculum
	Individual interviews	Individual interviews with students and
	Feedback forms	teachers
	Objective tests	Pre-test and post-test
	Surveys	Focus groups
Summative	**Summative**	
	Preassessment and postassessment of knowledge, skills	Surveys
	Attitudes by objective written or oral test	Patient feedback forms
	OSCE (Objective Structured Clinical Examination)	Instructor feedback forms
	Presurvey and postsurvey to assess	
	learner self-perception of ability	
	Patient satisfaction surveys	
	Focus groups or interviews to assess cultural change	

From Ury WA, Arnold RM, Tulsky JA. Palliative care curriculum development: A model for a content and process-based approach. J Palliat Med 2002;5:539-548.

3. Management of common symptoms
4. Ethical issues
5. Self-knowledge and reflection

These competencies are not unique to palliative care but are consistent with those necessary for excellence in primary care.[8] Because medical schools are challenged by many competing demands for curricular time allocation, integration of these competencies into other required courses and clinical clerkships is an effective solution.

A method for assessing palliative care education in many curriculum formats is the Palliative Education Assessment Tool (PEAT). It consists of seven domains with specific objectives, skills, and competencies for each[9]:

1. Overview of palliative medicine
2. Pain
3. Neuropsychological symptoms
4. Other symptoms
5. Ethics and the law
6. Patient/family/caregiver perspectives
7. Clinical communication skills

This tool enables schools to identify institution-specific areas in which a palliative care curriculum may be effectively integrated and explicitly taught or is, in essence, already present. This may involve identifying or integrating content in the basic and social-behavioral sciences, patient interview training, or other preclerkship courses. Palliative care content can be identified or formally integrated into current clinical rotations as well as a required experience in a palliative care block format.[9] The PEAT tool facilitates collaboration with existing curricula in the overarching educational objectives.

Basic principles guide best pedagogical practices and curriculum intent. Teaching about palliative care is well received by students, positively influences attitudes, and enhances communication skills.[10] Ideally, teaching about death, dying, and bereavement should occur throughout medical education, and repetition of core competencies should lead to effective integration. Palliative care education can provide a focus to teach many of the core skills, knowledge, and attitudes important for all physicians.[9]

Curriculum Development: Postgraduate Training

Emphasis on patient care is challenged by the demand during residency to educate on many topics, including quality improvement, domestic violence, women's health, and so on. Time constraints limit exposure to these topics to a one-time didactic session. Hospice and palliative medicine constitute a new addition to the residency curricula. Program directors reported that 46% provided formal training in end-of-life care and 31% provided training in hospice, but of the programs that required hospice training, only half included a clinical component.[11]

Since 1998, the National Residency End of Life Education Project has worked with 434 residency programs, including internal medicine, family medicine, surgery, and neurology, to develop curriculum and evaluation of end-of-life care that fulfills ACGME requirements and is tailored to the specific programs and resources. Two to four representatives from each residency program attended a 2-day workshop focused on the processes of educational change and worked to develop instructive techniques specific to palliative care. The workshop focused on five domains[12]:

1. Pain assessment and management and addiction assessment
2. Communication skills and personal reflection
3. Hospice care and prognostication
4. Clinical end-of-life experiences in training
5. Faculty development and institutional change

The teams completed an action plan of educational changes for their residency in the upcoming year. Mentoring by phone and mail contact helped them advance their institutional changes. The experiences of the teams and their programs can guide others to effect formative curriculum change.[12,13]

The National Consensus Conference on Medical Education for Care Near the End of Life proposed that home visits afford an unusually rich opportunity to learn about patients' and families' experiences of severe illness and better appreciate the cultural, spiritual, and practical aspects of care. Academic medical centers should collaborate with hospice and home health agencies to develop this experience.[3]

Curriculum Development: Generalist

Most currently practicing physicians did not receive formal training in palliative care in their residency and must augment their expertise within their work environment and continuing education. The Institute for Ethics at the American Medical Association, with support from The Robert Wood Johnson Foundation, developed a successful curriculum in the 1990s called the Education for Physicians on End-of-life Care (EPEC) project. Now based at the Feinberg School of Medicine at Northwestern University, the project presents a curriculum that covers the core competencies of palliative care that are accessible to essentially all physicians in the United States. In addition, the project uses the train-the-trainer model to further disseminate information and provide access to the educational materials for practicing physicians.[14] In 2005, a new development, cosponsored with the National Cancer Institute (NCI) and American Society of Clinical Oncology (ASCO), expanded the curriculum to specific needs within oncology.

Curriculum Development: Specialist

Palliative medicine has rapidly developed as a medical subspecialty in the United States since the late 1990s. Voluntary program standards were established through collaboration involving directors of fellowship training programs, the American Academy of Hospice and Palliative Medicine, and the American Board of Hospice and Palliative Medicine. Early consultative input from the American Board of Medical Specialties and the ACGME created a training structure for programs that reflected those currently accredited by ACGME.[15] The Palliative Medicine Review Committee was established in 2002 and was modeled after the ACGME residency review committees. This facilitated the rapid recognition of Hospice and

Palliative Medicine as a medical discipline, announced in June of 2006. Subspecialty status was awarded by the American Board of Medical Specialties in September of 2006.

Since the development of Hospice and Palliative Medicine as a specialty, the number of fellowship programs has continued to grow, with 29 programs now accredited by the Palliative Medicine Review Committee. Voluntary program standards require that programs offer a minimum of 12 months of training in the key knowledge and competencies. Training programs must provide fellows the opportunity to care for patients in various settings, including inpatient, community (including Medicare-certified hospices), and ambulatory. Consultation services, longitudinal care, and exposure to bereavement support are also required. These fellowship training programs prepare physicians for a career in either academic or community-based medicine as hospice and palliative medicine specialists. Trainees are required to have already completed training in a primary care specialty, such as internal medicine or family medicine.[15] Currently, seven boards cosponsor the subspecialty of palliative medicine, so trainees from these disciplines are also candidates for fellowships at selected programs.[16]

The curriculum ensures that residents achieve the required knowledge, skills, attitudes, and behaviors. The curriculum of the program must include the following[15]:

1. Epidemiology, natural history, and treatment options for common chronic diseases and life-threatening medical conditions including pediatrics
2. History of palliative medicine
3. Age-appropriate comprehensive assessment, including physical, cognitive, functional, social, psychological, and spiritual domains, using history, examination, and appropriate laboratory evaluation. Assessment of suffering and quality of life should be included.
4. The role, function, and development of the interdisciplinary team and its component disciplines
5. Management of common co-morbidities and complications in life-threatening illness
6. Management of neuropsychiatric co-morbidities in life-threatening illnesses
7. Management of symptoms in palliative care patients, including various pharmacological and nonpharmacological modalities and pharmacodynamics of commonly used agents. Symptom management should include patient and family education, psychosocial and spiritual support, and appropriate referrals for other modalities such as invasive procedures.
8. Palliative care emergencies (e.g., spinal cord compression, suicidal ideation)
9. Management of psychological, social, and spiritual issues of patients and families
10. The natural history, phenomenology, and management of grief and bereavement and the role of the interdisciplinary team in support of bereaved family members
11. Assessment and management in community settings (e.g., home, long-term care)
12. Care of the dying, including managing terminal symptoms, patient/family education, bereavement, and organ donation
13. Economic and regulatory aspects, including national health policy issues and financing mechanisms
14. Ethical and legal aspects, including, but not limited to, those pertinent to infants, children, adults, and geriatric populations
15. Cultural aspects, including geographic location (urban versus rural), ethnicity, and socioeconomic status
16. Communication skills with patients, families, professional colleagues, and community groups
17. Ability to function as a consultant
18. Scholarship, including research methodologies that enable interpretation of the medical literature and are appropriate to palliative care settings and populations
19. Skills in quality improvement
20. Teaching skills
21. Professional self-care (e.g., self-reflection, life-long learning, balancing work and personal interests)

Curriculum Development: Nursing Education

The Hospice Nurses Association was created in 1986 to establish a network and support for nurses in hospice care. In 1998, palliative care was added to reflect and recognize the needs of nurses working not only in hospice but in palliative care settings. The Hospice and Palliative Nurses Association (HPNA) has become a nationally recognized organization providing resources and support for advanced practice nurses, registered nurses, licensed practical nurses, and nursing assistants who care for people with life-limiting and terminal illness. Membership continues to grow, exceeding 9250 in 2007, with members from all 50 states and several foreign countries. As of January 2008, 21% of the organization's membership had advanced degrees (master's or doctorate); 56% had hospice and palliative nursing specialty certification; and 73% described their primary role as clinical (61% indicating that they provided hospice care; 10%, palliative care; and 18%, both).[17]

The mission of the HPNA is to promote excellence by promoting the highest professional standards of hospice and palliative nursing; studying, researching, and exchanging information, experiences, and ideas leading to improved practice; encouraging nurses to specialize in hospice and palliative nursing; fostering professional development; responding to the changing needs of HPNA members and the populations they represent; and promoting hospice and palliative care as essential components of health care.

With a focus on quality in the practice of hospice and palliative nursing, the National Board of Certification of Hospice and Palliative Nurses (NBCHPN) developed and administers national examinations for registered nurses, advanced practice nurses, licensed practical nurses, and certified nurse assistants. The examinations are based on the scope and standards of practice, with corresponding core competencies for each of the disciplines within nursing. The standards, competencies, and credentialing are necessary to meet the goals of fostering quality and consistency and developing hospice and palliative nursing as a nursing specialty.[18]

The core competencies for generalist hospice and palliative nursing are in the following domains[18]:

1. Clinical judgment
2. Advocacy and ethics
3. Professionalism
4. Collaboration
5. Systems thinking
6. Cultural competence
7. Facilitator of learning
8. Communication

In 1997, the International Council of Nurses issued a mandate stating that nurses have a unique and primary responsibility for ensuring a peaceful death. Later that same year, the American Association of Colleges of Nursing convened a group of health care ethicists and palliative care nursing experts, who developed a position paper entitled, "Peaceful Death: Recommended Competencies and Curricular Guidelines for End-of-Life Nursing Care."[19]

Extensive research on the content of end-of-life care in schools of nursing documented the deficiencies in nursing knowledge and attitudes.[20] In particular, there were major deficiencies in nursing textbooks and in knowledge and beliefs of nursing faculty, students, and practicing nurses, and little time was devoted to palliative and end-of-life care. To address these issues, the group developed the End-of-Life Competency Statements (Box 23-1), which

---

Box 23-1 End-of-Life Competency Statements

1. Recognizing changes in population dynamics, health care economics, and service delivery that necessitate improved professional preparation
2. Promoting comfort care to the dying as an active, desirable, and important skill and an integral component of nursing care
3. Communicating effectively and compassionately with the patient, family, and health team about the end of life
4. Recognizing personal attitudes, feelings, values, and expectations about death and the individual, cultural, and spiritual diversity in these beliefs and customs
5. Demonstrating respect for the patient's views and wishes
6. Collaborating with interdisciplinary team members while implementing the nursing role
7. Utilizing scientifically based tools to assess symptoms
8. Utilizing data from symptom assessment to plan and intervene in symptom management using state-of-the-art traditional and complementary approaches
9. Evaluating the impact of traditional, complementary, and technological therapies on patient-centered outcomes
10. Assessing and treating multiple dimensions of patient care, including physical, psychological, social, and spiritual needs, to improve quality at the end of life
11. Assisting the patient, family, colleagues, and one's self to cope with suffering, grief, loss, and bereavement
12. Applying legal and ethical principles in the analysis of complex issues, recognizing the influence of personal values, professional codes, and patient preferences
13. Identifying barriers and facilitators to patients' and caregivers' effective use of resources
14. Demonstrating skill at implementing a plan for improved palliative care within a dynamic and complex health care delivery system
15. Applying knowledge gained from palliative care research

From Ferrell BR, Grant M, Virani R. Strengthening nursing education to improve end-of-life care. Nurs Outlook 1999;47:252-256.

---

every undergraduate nursing student should attain, and made recommendations adopted by the American Association of Colleges of Nursing so these competencies could be addressed.[21-24] These competencies are being incorporated into existing courses, rather than independent palliative care courses. Some of the relevant courses in which to incorporate them are health assessment, pharmacology, psychiatric/mental health, nursing management, ethics, culture, nursing research, professional issues, and health care settings.[26]

The End-of-Life Nursing Education Consortium (ELNEC) project is a national initiative to improve end-of-life care in the United States. The project, launched in 2000, was originally funded by the Project on Death in America from The Robert Wood Johnson Foundation. ELNEC, a train-the-trainer program, provides undergraduate and graduate nursing faculty, continuing education providers, staff development educators, pediatric and oncology specialty nurses, and other nurses with training in palliative care so that they can teach practicing and student nurses. Several threads related to curriculum are integrated throughout the modules. They include the family as the unit of care; the importance of the nurse as advocate; culture as an influence; the need for attention to the needs of special populations, such as children, the poor or uninsured, and the elderly; influence of financial issues; need for interdisciplinary care; and care across all life-defining illnesses and sudden death.[27]

ELNEC courses have been enhanced to include pediatric palliative care and other courses applicable to oncology and critical care. To date, more than 2880 nurses, representing all 50 states, have received ELNEC training. ELNEC trainers are hosting professional development seminars for practicing nurses, incorporating ELNEC content into nursing curricula, hosting regional training sessions to expand the reach into rural and underserved communities, presenting information at national and international conferences, and striving to improve the quality of nursing care in other innovative ways. The ELNEC project is administered by the American Association of Colleges of Nursing and the City of Hope National Medical Center of Los Angeles.[28]

In 2004, through a grant by Project on Death in America, HPNA blended these projects, resulting in an organizational plan to offer nine ELNEC courses over the 3 years (three courses per year in 2004, 2005, 2006). Through a no-cost extension, three additional courses were provided in 2007. Attendees were dyads made up of one chapter nursing member with one long-term care nurse. After the 2-day educational session, participants will be connected as dyads within the local community to ask questions, obtain support and direction, and identify educational resources. More than 450 nursing individuals were educated prior to the end of the grant project. It was the first effort to couple hospice nurses with long-term care nurses to discuss end-of-life nursing care.

Curriculum Development: The Interdisciplinary Team

Hospice and palliative care curricula are being developed in postgraduate social work, and there is also a need to develop core competencies and curricula for other professional studies, including pastoral care and pharmacy.

There are no established competencies for end-of-life education for clergy and chaplaincy. The Florida Clergy End-of-Life Education Enhancement Project served as a statewide model of clergy education on death, dying, grief, and loss. The curriculum began to define competency to train clergy with modules focused on cultural considerations, the dying process, care options, advance directives, the grief process, assisting families, and the role of spiritual care and self-care for clergy.[29]

Formal education for social workers in palliative care and hospice is available. A postgraduate Social Work Fellowship in palliative care is available through the Department of Pain Medicine and Palliative Care at Beth Israel Medical Center.[30] In addition, the New York University School of Social Work offers a Post Master's Certificate in Palliative and End-of-Life Care for practicing social workers.[31] The Social Work End-of-Life Education Project is a 2-day workshop that includes intermediate and advanced social work skills that are crucial to effective social work intervention. This curriculum is based on research supported by a Project on Death in America grant. The format, designed to enhance critical-thinking abilities and to support social workers in their daily practice, includes the following key content areas[30]:

1. Social work role and values specific to palliative care
2. Biopsychosocial spiritual assessment
3. Ethical issues
4. Multidimensional aspects of pain and symptom management
5. Therapeutic interventions, including cognitive behavioral interventions
6. Cultural awareness
7. Self-care, compassion fatigue, secondary trauma
8. Grief and bereavement

RECENT DEVELOPMENTS

The 2004 release by the Clinical Practice Guidelines for Quality Palliative Care by the National Consensus Project (NCP) allowed essential elements of palliative and hospice care in both clinical practice and education to be consistently organized and addressed. The eight domains of the NCP established a guideline for the essential elements and best-quality palliative care[31]:

1. Structure and processes
2. Physical care
3. Psychological and psychiatric care
4. Social aspects of care
5. Spiritual, religious, and existential care
6. Cultural aspects of care
7. Care of the imminently dying
8. Ethical and legal aspects of care upon which standards and policies can be developed

The NCP guidelines develop quality indicators for use by the National Quality Forum and the Joint Commission on Accreditation of Healthcare Organizations (now called The Joint Commission).

CONCLUSIONS

Palliative care education can teach many of the skills, knowledge, and attitudes important and necessary for all physicians. Effective communication, the development of empathy and concern for the patient and family, knowledge of ethics, and expertise in symptom assessment and management, among other areas, are all essential for a good physician regardless of specialty, and therefore they are part of the intended outcome of medical education as a whole. As medical schools are challenged by many competing demands for time allocation and resources, the integration of these competencies into other required courses and clinical clerkships is an effective means to teach all that is necessary for excellence in medicine.

There are many opportunities for curriculum development in hospice and palliative care relevant to subspecialty medicine, such as critical care/trauma, surgery, and gynecology. Challenges exist to educate the practicing physician; possible solutions include professional societies providing or supporting state/regional training with the use of EPEC as an established curriculum.[32] Palliative care curricula are established within nursing, particularly through the work of ELNEC. Substantive curriculum development has occurred in social work and chaplaincy, but much opportunity for growth, expansion, and formalization exists.

The research challenges in palliative medicine education include objective outcome measures to determine whether the curriculum has a long-term impact on the learner's knowledge, skills, and attitudes. Competency-based testing is needed to evaluate learners' ability to perform. There also needs to be an evaluation of the most effective methods of teaching and learning about palliative care and the benefits and pitfalls of interdisciplinary learning.

REFERENCES

1. Sullivan AM, Lakoma MD, Block SD. The status of medical education in end-of-life care: A national report. J Gen Intern Med 2003;18:685-695.
2. Sullivan AM, Warren AG, Lakoma MD, et al. End-of-life care in the curriculum: A national study of medical education deans. Acad Med 2004;79:760-768.
3. Billings JA, Ferris FD, McDonald N, et al. The role of palliative care in the home in medical education: Report from a national consensus conference. J Palliat Med 2001;4:361-371.
4. Wood EB, Meekin SA, Fins JJ, Fleischman AR. Enhancing palliative care education in medical school curricula: Implementation of the palliative education assessment tool. Acad Med 2002;4:285-291.
5. Ury WA, Arnold RM, Tulsky JA. Palliative care curriculum development: A model for a content and process-based approach. J Palliat Med 2002;5:539-548.
6. Ross DD, Fraser HC, Kutner JS. Institutionalization of a palliative and end-of-life care educational program in a medical school curriculum. J Palliat Med 2001;4:512-518.
7. Barnard D, Quill T, Hafferty FW, et al. Preparing the ground: Contributions of the preclinical years to medical education for care near the end of life. Acad Med 1999;74:499-505.
8. Block SD, Bernier GM, Crawley LM, et al. Incorporating palliative care into primary care education. J Gen Intern Med 1998;13:768-773.
9. Meekin SA, Klein JE, Fleischman AR, Finns JJ. Development of a palliative education assessment tool for medical student education. Acad Med 2000;75:986-992.
10. Billings JA, Block S. Palliative care in undergraduate medical education: Status report and future directions. JAMA 1997;278:733-738.
11. Ogle KS, Mavis B, Thomason C. Learning to provide end-of-life care: Postgraduate medical training programs in Michigan. J Palliat Med 2005;5:987-997.
12. Weissman DE, Mullan P, Ambuel B, et al. National residency end-of-life education project: Project abstracts and progress reports. J Palliat Med 2005;8:646-664.
13. End of Life/Palliative Education Resource Center (EPERC). Available at http://www.eperc.mcw.edu (accessed October 2006).
14. Emanuel LL, vonGunten CF, Ferris FD (eds). The EPEC Curriculum: Education for Physicians on End-of-Life Care. The EPEC Project, 1999. Available at http://www.EPEC.net (accessed October 2007).
15. Billings JA, Block SD, Finn JW, et al. Initial voluntary program standards for fellowship training in palliative medicine. J Palliat Med 2002;5:23-33.

16. Cosponsoring boards with the American Board of Internal Medicine of Hospice and Palliative Medicine. Available at http://www.abhpm.org/gfxc_103.aspx (accessed October 2007).

17. Membership and demographics of the Hospice and Palliative Nurses Association (HPNA). Available at http://www.hpna.org/DisplayPage.aspx?Title = Membership%20Demographics (accessed February 2008).

18. Hospice and Palliative Nurses Association. Professional Competencies for the Generalist Hospice and Palliative Nurse, 2nd ed. Dubuque, IA: Kendall/Hunt, 2005.

19. Peaceful Death: Recommended Competencies and Curricular Guidelines for End-of-Life Nursing Care. American Association of Colleges of Nursing. Available at http://www.aacn.nche.edu/education/deathfin.htm (accessed October 2007).

20. Ferrell BR, Verani R, Grant M. Analysis of end of life content in nursing textbooks. Oncol Nurs Forum 1999;26:869-876.

21. Ferrell BR, Verani R, Grant M. Home care outreach for palliative care education. Cancer Pract 1998;6:79-85.

22. Ferrell BR, Verani R, Grant M. Strengthening nursing education to improve end of life care. Nurs Outlook 1999;47:252-256.

23. Ferrell BR, Verani R, Grant M, et al. Beyond the Supreme Court decision: Nursing perspectives on end of life care. Oncol Nurs Forum 2000; 27:445-455.

24. Ferrell B, Verani R, Grant M, et al. Evaluation of the end of life nursing education consortium undergraduate nursing education faculty training program. J Pall Med 2005;8:107-114.

25. Ferrell BR, Grant M, Virani R. Strengthening nursing education to improve end-of-life care. Nurs Outlook 1999;47:252-256.

26. End-of-Life Nursing Education Consortium, American Association of Colleges of Nursing. Available at http://www.aacn.nche.edu/Publications/deathfin.htm (accessed February 2008).

27. Sherman D, Matso M, Rogers S, et al. Achieving quality care at the end-of-life: A focus of the End of Life Nursing Education Consortium (ELNEC) curriculum. J Prof Nurs 2002;18:255-262.

28. The ELNEC project. Available at http://www.aacn.nche.edu/elnec (accessed October 2007).

29. Abrams D, Albury S, Crandall L, et al. The Florida clergy end-of-life education enhancement project: A description and evaluation. Am J Hosp Palliat Med. 2005;223:181-187.

30. Social Work Fellowship in Palliative and End-of-Life Care. Available at http://www.stoppain.org/for_professionals/content/information/s_w_description.asp (accessed October 2007).

31. National Consensus Project of Quality Palliative Care (NCP). Clinical Practice Guidelines for Quality Palliative Care, 2004. Available at http://nationalconsensusproject.org (accessed October 2007).

32. Robinson K, Sutton S, vonGunten CF, et al. Assessment of the Education for Physicians on End-of-life Care (EPEC) Project. J Palliat Med 2004;7:637-645.

SUGGESTED READING

American Academy of Hospice and Palliative Medicine. Hospice and Palliative Medicine Core Curriculum and Review Syllabus. Dubuque, IA: Kendall/Hunt, 1999.

Bland CJ, Starnaman S, Wersel L, et al. Curricular change in medical schools: How to succeed. Acad Med 2000; 75:575-594.

Hospice and Palliative Nurses Association. Core Curriculum for the Generalist Hospice and Palliative Nurse. Dubuque, IA: Kendall/Hunt, 2002.

Lloyd-Williams M, MacLeod RD. A systematic review of teaching and learning in palliative care within the medical undergraduate curriculum. Med Teach 2004;26:683-690.

CHAPTER **24**

Adult Learning

José Pereira and Michael Aherne

K E Y   P O I N T S

- A successful educator must understand how learners learn.
- Learning is a lifelong process of self-directed, continuing inquiry.
- Generally, adults prefer to be involved in decisions regarding the who, what, where, when, why, and how they learn.
- Learning theories and learning styles help clinicians understand learning but have limitations.
- Education aims to change behavior by affecting knowledge, attitudes, and skills; evaluations should capture these domains.

Education is concerned about changing not only knowledge, attitudes, and skills, but also behavior. Educators and learners need to understand learning processes to optimize the experience and to ensure that goals and objectives are achieved. This requires awareness of what motivates adults to learn, how they learn, and which methods are best suited to make this happen.

ADULT LEARNING THEORY

Knowles, a pioneer of modern adult learning theory, identified six major characteristics of adult learners, each with corresponding instructional design considerations (Table 24-1).[1] The term *androgogy* has been used to distinguish adult learning from *pedagogy* (learning in the preadult years). These terms are often used interchangeably.

Knowles proposed seven guidelines for adult learning[1]:

1. Set a comfortable climate.
2. Involve learners in mutual planning.
3. Involve them in diagnosing their own needs.
4. Involve them in formulating their own objectives.
5. Involve them in designing learning plans.
6. Help them carry out their plans.
7. Involve them in evaluating their learning.

There are limitations to Knowles' "theory."[2] It is more a set of principles of good practice, or descriptions of what the adult learner should be like, than a theory. One should not assume that all adults are self-directed learners. Some adults depend on an instructor for structure, whereas some children are independent, self-directed learners. One cannot rely solely on altruistic, intrinsic motivations to learn. Certain life experiences may produce barriers to learning rather than enhancing it. A difficult personal experience with a dying family member may discourage

TABLE 24-1 Knowles' Characteristics of Adult Learners and Instructional Design

CHARACTERISTICS	INSTRUCTIONAL DESIGN CONSIDERATIONS
Autonomous and self-directed	▪ Involve adult participants in learning and serve as facilitators. ▪ Get participants' perspectives about topics and what their interests are. ▪ Show participants how the course will help achieve their learning goals.
Accumulated life experiences and knowledge	▪ Connect learning to this knowledge/experience base. ▪ Draw out participants' experience and knowledge relevant to the topic. ▪ Relate theories and concepts; recognize the value of experience in learning.
Goal orientated	▪ Educational programs should be organized and clearly defined. ▪ Learning goals and course objectives must be made explicit early.
Relevancy orientated	▪ Learning has to be applicable to their work. ▪ Theories and concepts must be related to a familiar setting.
Practical	▪ Focus on aspects most useful in their work. ▪ They may not be interested in knowledge alone; tell learners explicitly how the lesson will be useful in their daily practice.
Need to be respected	▪ Acknowledge the wealth of experiences that adult participants bring. ▪ Treat them as equals in experience and knowledge, and allow them to express their opinions freely.

a clinician from attending palliative care education. Lastly, adult learners are not always aware of what they do not know. This can cause gaps if they establish learning goals independently.

Important Characteristics of Adult Learners

Adults retain the ability to learn, even with aging. Attaining new skills often follows a curve (the learning curve). Success at specific skills increases with practice. There is often a dip in the curve after initial success as learners, having mastered more straightforward cases, attempt difficult cases. Learners vary in their ability to reach a close-to-plateau level, and some take longer than others. Successful performance may fade with time without continual practice. With inactivity, the learning curve falls off over time.

Learning Styles

Learning styles are those approaches that individuals prefer to learn with, and instructors prefer to teach with. Many different style frameworks have been described.

Styles vary from individual to individual, and each has its own strengths and limitations, depending on the learning task. The learning method preferred by a particular individual is presumed to be the style that allows that individual to learn best. It has been proposed that educators should assess the styles of their learners and incorporate learning strategies and exercises that best fit these. It is also useful for learners to know their default styles. Although it is unrealistic to expect every experience to provide for each different learning style, the use of different styles may be guided by six principles[3]:

1. The preferred styles of the instructor and the learner can be identified.
2. Instructors need to guard against using their preferred style exclusively.
3. Instructors are most helpful when they assist learners in identifying and learning through their own style preferences.
4. Learners should have the opportunity to use their preferred style.
5. Learners and instructors should be encouraged to diversify their styles.
6. Instructors can develop specific activities that reinforce each style.

Several instruments can assess learning styles. Two of the best known are Kolb's Learning Styles Inventory[4] and Myers-Briggs Type Indicators (MBTI).[5] The former postulates four phases in the learning cycle: "concrete experience" (CE), "reflective observation" (RO), "abstract conceptualization" (AC), and "active experimentation" (AE). The learning styles that correspond to combinations of these are as follows:

1. Accommodating (CE/AE)
2. Diverging (CE/RO)
3. Assimilating (AC/RO)
4. Converging (AC/AE)

In another, similar model, these four types of learners are classified as activists, reflectors, theorists, and pragmatists, respectively.[6] Reflectors prefer to collect data and think about it carefully before drawing any conclusions. They enjoy observing others and listen to others' views before offering their own. Activists, on the other hand, like new experiences and working with others. Theorists think problems through in a step-by-step way and like to fit things into a rational scheme. Pragmatists want to try things out and like practical concepts.

The MBTI is based on Jung's theory of personality type. It is not a learning style instrument, per se, but measures differences in personality types that affect how individuals behave and interact with others. The MBTI provides data on four sets of preferences (Fig. 24-1). Combinations of these (subtypes) lead to 16 different learning types.

LEARNING THEORIES

A learning theory is a framework of constructs and principles that describe and explain how people learn. Many exist, each with strengths, limitations, interpretations, applications, and level of supportive evidence. They provide conceptual frameworks rather than absolute truths. The principal theories are often categorized into

Subtypes	Commentary	Notes for Educators
Extraversion (E)	Find energy working with people, enjoy group work. Dislike slow-paced learning. Action oriented. Offer opinion without being asked.	Learn by explaining concepts to others. Consider in-class or outside-of-class group exercises and projects.
Introversion (I)	Prefer quiet space. Dislike interruptions. Like working with concepts and ideas and offer opinions only when asked. Want to understand the world. Are concentrators and reflective thinkers.	Want to develop frameworks that integrate or connect the subject matter. To an introvert, disconnected chunks are not knowledge, merely information. Knowledge means interconnecting material and seeing the "big picture." Use concept maps and show learners how to develop these.
Sensing (S)	Detail oriented, practical and realistic. Observant and rely on facts.	Prefer organized, linear structured courses. Identify what must be known in the topic (the essentials), and then build around these. Provide cases to analyze. An opening problem or case should be (1) a familiar context, (2) engage their curiosity, (3) almost solvable; too frustrating if too complex.
Intuition (N)	Trust hunches and intuition. Look for the "big picture" Like something new. Seek out patterns and relationships among the facts gathered.	Encourage learners to take a more active role by a series of questions or problems designed to introduce a concept (discovery learning). This appeals to intuitive learners and teaches sensing learners how to uncover general principles. Combine sensing and intuitive learners.
Thinking (T)	Find ideas and things more interesting than people. Analytical and make decisions based on logic.	Thinking learners like clear learning objectives that are precise and action-orientated.
Feeling (F)	Value harmony and more interested in people than things or ideas. Sympathetic. Make decisions based on human values and needs. Good at persuasion and facilitating differences among group members.	Like working in groups, especially harmonious ones. Enjoy small group exercises. Provide students with guidelines on how to facilitate small group meetings—i.e., group etiquette.
Judging (J)	Plan well in advance, organized, work-orientated, decisive, and disciplined.	Learners do well with the "AOR" Model: In answering essay questions, the learner must first **A**nalyze the question and jot down key ideas, then **O**rganize the ideas into a logical sequence, and finally write the essay (**R**espond). Serve as devil's advocate to suggest other options as learners may seek too rapid conclusions.
Perceptive (P)	Open-ended, flexible, play-orientated, spontaneous, curious, adaptable, spontaneous. They start many tasks and want to know everything about each task, and often find it difficult to complete a task.	Perceptive learners seek information to the last minute (and sometimes beyond). Decompose a complex project or paper into subassignments, with deadlines for each. The deadlines will keep the learner on target. Provide continuous feedback. Provide regular interim feedback.

FIGURE 24-1 Myers-Briggs types and corresponding learning methods.

three traditions: behaviorist, cognitive, and social learning theories. Two others, humanistic learning theory and psychodynamic learning theory, warrant some discussion.

Behaviorist Learning Theories

Behaviorists view all learning as a response to external stimuli without any intention by the learner. They focus on positive reinforcement and repetition to change behavior. A criticism of this theory is that it assumes that learners are relatively passive and easily manipulated. Changed behavior may deteriorate over time.

Cognitive Learning Theories

Cognitive theorists consider cognition (including perceptions, thoughts, memory, calculation, associations, and ways of processing and structuring information) to be the key to learning. They focus on the processes of information acquisition, organization, retrieval, and application. Information is stored in memory as schemas; learning is optimal when new information is hooked onto existing schemas or schemas are modified to adopt the new information. In essence, learning involves perceiving the information, interpreting it based on what is already known, and then reorganizing it into new insights or understanding.[7] Processing and retrieval are enhanced by organizing information and making it meaningful.

Nine steps have been proposed under this theory to activate effective learning[8]:

1. Gain the learner's attention.
2. Inform the learner of the objectives and expectations.
3. Stimulate the learner's recall of prior learning (i.e., retrieve prior knowledge).
4. Present information.
5. Provide guidance to facilitate the learner's understanding (semantic encoding).
6. Have the learner demonstrate the information or skill.
7. Give feedback to the learner.
8. Assess the learner's performance.
9. Work to enhance retention and transfer through application and varied practice.

Metacognition (knowledge of one's own thinking processes and strategies) is an associated concept. It is a salient feature of good self-directed learners. Educators may prompt metacognition by asking people how they believe they learn and by asking them to describe what and how they think as they learn.

Social Learning Theories

Much learning, according to social learning theory, is by observation. Other individuals provide role models for how to think, feel, and act, and their influence should not be underestimated.[9]

Humanistic Learning Theory

Humanistic learning theory assumes that each individual is unique and each has a desire to grow positively. Internal feelings about self, ability to make wise choices, and needs affect learning. A hierarchy of needs may motivate humans.[10] At the bottom are basic needs such as breathing and eating, followed by self-esteem and respect from others at a higher level. At the very top is self-actualization (maximizing one's full potential).

Psychodynamic Learning Theory

Although psychodynamics is not generally considered a learning theory, it stresses emotions rather than cognition and highlights conscious and unconscious forces that guide behavior. Past experiences (including childhood) and internal forces such as emotional conflicts and ego shape motivation and learning.

EMERGING CONCEPTS AND FRAMEWORKS IN ADULT LEARNING

Self-Directed Learning

Self-directed learning (SDL) proposes that professionals are self-motivated, practice self-management and self-monitoring, and are lifelong learners.[11] In SDL, individuals take the initiative and the responsibility for selecting, managing, and assessing their own learning; they set their own goals, locate appropriate resources, decide on which methods to use, and evaluate their own progress. SDL, promoted through problem-based learning (PBL), is embedded in many undergraduate medical curricula.[12]

Several things are known about SDL:

1. Individual learners can become empowered to take increasing responsibility for their own learning.
2. Self-direction is best viewed as a continuum or a characteristic that varies in individuals over time.
3. Self-direction does not mean that learning will be isolated from other forms of learning or replace them.
4. Self-directed study can involve various activities and resources (from self-guided reading to study groups).
5. Educators can nurture SDL using various strategies, including promoting critical thinking.
6. Some educational institutions find ways to support self-directed study (e.g., open-learning programs, individualized study options, nontraditional course offerings).

Several strategies may support SDL. The learner should ask and answer the following three questions at the start of the process:

1. What are the needs, goals, and objectives?
2. What are the methods and the resources required?
3. How will learning be evaluated?

Educators can assist by doing the following:

1. Help the learner ask and answer the three questions just listed.
2. Create a partnership with the learner by negotiating a contract for goals, strategies, and evaluation criteria.
3. Encourage setting of objectives that can be met in several ways, and offer various options for evidence of successful performance.

4. Manage the learning experience, rather than functioning as an information provider.
5. Provide examples of good work.
6. Teach inquiry skills, decision making, personal development, and self-evaluation.
7. Promote learning networks, study circles, and learning exchanges.

Self directed learning is suited to the workplace, and many organizations encourage it.[13] Concerns have been expressed about over-reliance on SDL.[14] Some adults are less self-directed than others. An extreme interpretation of SDL is denial of collective, collaborative learning in favor of focus on the self through independent self-learning. Self-assessment is at the heart of the process, but many learners are poor at self-assessment.[15] People tend to study what they find interesting.

Reflective Practice and Learning

Reflective practice can be seen as consciously thinking about and analyzing what one has done (or is doing); this is known as "critical reflection." Reflection is emphasized to cope with ill-structured, unpredictable, or unexpected situations.[16,17] Reflective practice provides opportunities to identify areas for practice improvement and analyze in-practice decision-making processes. It promotes professional competence by encouraging recognition of mistakes and weaknesses. Strategies for encouraging reflective practice and learning include use of learning journals and portfolios, logs, learning contracts, critical incident analyses, action learning sets, and learning partners.[17] The following elements may be important in reflective writing[18]:

1. Description (What happened?)
2. Feelings (What were you thinking and feeling?)
3. Evaluation (What were the specific strengths and weaknesses?)
4. Analysis (What sense could you make of the situation?)
5. Action plan (What changes in approach are needed?)

Specific elements used in critical incident analysis include the following[19]

1. Description of the incident
2. By whom it was handled?
3. What learning occurred?
4. What were the outcomes of the incident?
5. How has the incident affected one's practice?

Experiential Learning

Experiential learning, or learning by doing, is central to adult learning and closely related to reflective learning. Adults learn most effectively when learning has an experiential active component. Experiential learning enables learners to construct meaning and deep understanding rather than simply record knowledge. The aphorism by Confucius (450 BC), "Tell me, and I will forget; show me, and I may remember; involve me, and I will understand" still holds true. The experiential learning cycle is based on the concept that learners observe and reflect on their experiences so that they can formulate new concepts and action strategies and then experiment with them.[4] To achieve deep learning, learners must practice new behaviors and skills, receive feedback, see the consequences of new behaviors, and integrate new skills into their thoughts and behavior. In experiential learning, experience is used to test ideas and assumptions rather than to practice passively. Educators should encourage learners to observe, think, analyze, synthesize, evaluate, and apply what has been learned.

Transformational (Transformative) Learning

Transformational learning is a process in which the learner goes beyond gaining factual knowledge to be changed by what is learned in a meaningful way.[20] It involves questioning assumptions, beliefs, and values and considering multiple points of view. Both the rational and the affective domains (thoughts and feelings) are important, and instructors must consider how they can help students use both rationality and feelings for reflection and change. The event that triggers the process, or the disorientating dilemma, may be a major experience, a life crisis or life transition, or a gradual accumulation of small experiences over time. Educational programs, with the appropriate design, may trigger the process.

Constructivism

Constructivists believe that learners "construct" their own knowledge based on what they already know. They enter learning with preexisting experiences which can be used to construct new knowledge. Each learner constructs meaning differently based on his or her own experiences. Learners reinterpret what is taught and construct their own meaning from that knowledge. Constructivism transforms the learner from a passive knowledge recipient to an active participant. The instructor is not a transmitter of knowledge but a guide who facilitates learning. Opponents of the theory claim that it fails to provide strong content knowledge. It may work well for professionals with accumulated work-based experiences, but it may be less useful for undergraduates, who have few practical work experiences (but some life experiences). Closely associated with constructivism is the concept of collaborative learning[21] and community of inquiry,[22] wherein learners with different performance levels, skills, or perspectives and different disciplines are grouped together to learn. Proponents claim that the active exchange of ideas within small groups increases interest and promotes critical thinking.

Emerging Concepts

Emerging concepts include situated learning (learning is inherently social),[23] lifelong learning, just-in-time learning (resources available when a learning need and moment arises), informal and incidental learning, and communities of practice (COPS).[24] Most learning derives from informal, everyday opportunities, and learners and educators should recognize and encourage their role. COPS can be particularly useful in exploring tacit knowledge, which is knowledge that an individual has but is unable to fully describe or even unaware that he or she has it. Important job competencies are often tacit, and exploring this information allows one to codify it.

DETERMINANTS OF LEARNING

In addition to learning styles and design frameworks, there are other important determinants of learning, including

1. Motives (many, ranging from chance of promotion and financial gain to satisfying an inquiring mind to licensing requirements)
2. Readiness for learning
3. Reinforcement
4. Retention (through strategies such as repetition, follow-ups, reminders, key points, practice, understanding underlying concepts, use of cognitive schemas, and association of new knowledge with existing schemas)
5. Emotion

Emotion influences learning, both as a motivator and modifier of attitudes and behavior and also by influencing knowledge structure and processes.[17,25] Emotions not directly relevant to the learning may either facilitate or impede it. Journal writing, reflective journals, literature, poetry, movies, art, and narrative can foster emotional responses and connections to learning. At the bedside, encouraging learners to be aware of and express their emotional reactions assists the process.

Adults have many responsibilities (professional, personal, and social), which may not leave much time for learning, particularly formal opportunities. Other barriers include poor awareness of knowledge and skill gaps in a particular field, inadequate financial support, lack of confidence or interest, lack of information about learning opportunities, scheduling problems, limited access to learning opportunities (e.g., rural or remote-based professionals), bureaucratic challenges, and difficulties with child care and transportation. Educators must consider these barriers when designing a course. A course that is disproportionately long for the learning objectives and level of care targeted will discourage many.

COMPETENCY AND ADULT LEARNING

Increasingly, formal learning in the health professions is competency based. Competence has been defined as "the habitual and judicious use of communication, knowledge, technical skills, clinical reasoning, knowledge, emotions, values, and reflection in daily practice."[26] Competence builds on basic clinical skills, scientific knowledge, and moral development and includes cognitive, affective, and psychomotor functions (knowledge, attitudes, and skills). It is therefore an integrated functioning of many attributes that are necessary to successfully and adequately complete tasks required in clinical practice. Several consensus-based competencies have been developed, such as the palliative care competencies for undergraduate and family medicine education in Canadian Medical Schools (available at http://www.afmc.ca/efppec/pages/main.html [accessed October 2007]).

ASSESSMENT AND EVALUATION OF LEARNING IN MEDICINE

The best way of evaluating competencies is a topic of debate. A pyramid model provides a useful framework to consider competency and evaluation of learning.[27] The pyramid base represents the knowledge component of competence ("knows") and application of that knowledge ("knows how"). At a higher level is the demonstration of competence—performance ("showing how") and behavior ("does"). The lower two levels represent the cognitive aspects of competency, and the upper two its behavioral components. "Showing how" does not necessarily predict day-to-day performance ("does"). Students may modify their behavior to score well in a clinical examination but behave differently in real life.

Key considerations and methods in designing assessments and evaluations of clinical competence have been described.[28,29] The competencies and the assessment methods should be planned against learning objectives (blueprinting). Assessment methods should match the competencies learned. The methods for supporting learning should be valid and reliable for the task at hand, should be practical, and should enhance learning. In high-stake evaluations, the minimal standard acceptable for passing should be decided (using one of several methods of standard setting) before the assessment.

The most common method of assessing knowledge ("knows") is the multiple choice question (MCQ) format. Other methods of assessing "know" and "knows how" include true/false tests, single best answer format, extended matching (EMIs), essays, and oral examinations. Essays and oral examinations are time-consuming, and inter-rater reliability may be problematic. Several standardized instruments evaluate attitudes and self-perceived comfort in caring for the dying. Standardized patients can evaluate performance, including objective structured clinical examinations (OSCEs). The assessment of behavior ("does") in real life is challenging. One single assessment method cannot properly assess all the facets of competence. A combination of methods assessing the various levels from "knows" to "does" is optimal, including in-training evaluations (ITERs) and portfolios (sometimes referred to as 360-degree assessments).

CONCLUSIONS

Adult learning is a complex and fluid concept. Many controversies remain (see "Future Considerations"). Despite much activity, understanding of adult learning is far from universal. Several concepts, described in this chapter, can guide understanding and development of educational opportunities. There are many studies that demonstrate the effectiveness of learning events in changing learner behavior when these concepts and guidelines are applied. In essence, learning is a dynamic, lifelong process by which learners acquire new knowledge, skills, and attitudes. It is open to considerable debate as academics and experts attempt to better understand the process of learning, what kinds of experiences and processes facilitate or hinder it, and how to ensure that learning becomes long-term.

SUGGESTED READING

Bastable SB. Nurse as Educator, 2nd ed. Sudbury, MA: Jones and Bartlett, 2003.

Garvin DA. Learning in Action. Boston: Harvard Business School Press, 2000.

Kaufman DM. ABC of learning and teaching in medicine: Applying educational theory in practice. BMJ 2003;326:213-216.

Marsick VJ, Watkins KE. Informal and Incidental Learning in the Workplace. New York: Routledge Press, 1990.

Merriam SB (ed). An Update on Adult Learning Theory. New Directions for Adult and Continuing Education, vol 57. San Francisco: Jossey-Bass, 1993.

Moon J. Reflection in Learning and Professional Development: Theory and Practice. London: Kogan Page, 1999.

Future Considerations

Several questions remain about learning, including the following:

- How do some adults remain self-directed over long periods of time? How does the process change as learners move from novice to expert in subject matter and learning strategies?
- What should be assessed and evaluated, and what constitutes a fair, adequate, and representative assessment and evaluation?
- What exactly is the role of learning theories? Do they still serve a useful purpose, or is it time for a single framework that encapsulates the different elements?
- What is the role of learning styles, and should we continue paying attention to them?
- Why are there gaps between what is taught and what is learned? How much of what is taught is learned?

REFERENCES

1. Knowles MS. The Modern Practice of Adult Education: From Pedagogy to Androgogy, 2nd ed. Chicago: Follet, 1980.
2. Norman GR. The adult learner: A mythical species. Acad Med 1999;74:886-889.
3. Friedman P, Alley R. Learning/Teaching styles: Applying the principles. Theory into Practice 1984;23(1):77-81.
4. Kolb D. Experiential Learning as the Science of Learning and Development. Englewood Cliffs, NJ: Prentice-Hall, 1984.
5. Meyers IB. Introduction to Type. Palo Alto, CA: Consulting Psychologists Press, 1987.
6. Honey P, Mumford A. Manual of Learning Styles. London: Peter Honey Publications, 1982.
7. Bandura A. Social cognitive theory: An agentic perspective. Ann Rev Psychol 2001;52:1-26.
8. Gagne RM. Instruction Based on Research in Learning. J Engineering Educ 1971;61(6):519-523.
9. Bandura A. Social Learning Theory. New York: General Learning Press, 1977.
10. Maslow AH. A theory of human motivation. Psychol Rev 1943;50:370-396.
11. Candy PC. Self-direction for lifelong learning: A comprehensive guide to theory and practice. San Francisco: Jossey-Bass, 1991.
12. Miflin BM, Campbell CB, Price DA. A conceptual framework to guide the development of self-directed, lifelong learning in problem-based medical curricula. Med Educ 2000;34:299-306.
13. Mamary E, Charles P. Promoting self-directed learning for continuing medical education. Med Teacher 2003;25(2):188-190.
14. Schmidt HG. Assumptions underlying self-directed learning may be false. Med Educ 2000;34:243-245.
15. Gordon MJ. A review of the validity and accuracy of self-assessments in health professions training. Acad Med 1991;66:762-769.
16. Schön D. The Reflective Practitioner. San Francisco: Jossey-Bass, 1983.
17. Moon J. A Handbook of Reflective and Experiential Learning: Theory and Practice. London: RoutledgeFalmer Press, London, 2004.
18. Moon J. Reflection in Learning and Professional Development: Theory and Practice. London: Kogan Page, 1999.
19. Ghaye T, Lillyman S. Learning journals and critical incidents: Reflective practice for health care professionals. In Dinton, Wilts. Key Management Skills in Nursing. London: Quay Books, Mark Allen Publishing Group, 1997.
20. Mezirow J. Transformative Learning: Theory to Practice. New Directions for Adult and Continuing Education, vol 74, pp 5-12. San Francisco: Jossey-Bass. 1997.
21. Kearlsey G, Schneiderman B. Engagement theory: A framework for technology-based teaching and learning. Educ Technol 1998;38:20-23.
22. Garrison DR, Anderson T, Archer W. Critical thinking, cognitive presence and computer conferencing in distance education. Am J Distance Educ 2001;15:7-23.
23. Lave J, Wenger E. Situated Learning: Legitimate Peripheral Participation. Cambridge: University of Cambridge Press, 1991.
24. Wenger E, McDermott R, Snyder WM. Cultivating Communities of Practice: A Guide to Managing Knowledge. Boston: Harvard Business School Press, 2002.
25. Taylor EW. Transformative learning theory: A neurobiological perspective of the role of emotions and unconscious ways of knowing. Int J Lifelong Educ 2001;20:218-236.
26. Epstein RM, Hundert EM. Defining and assessing professional competence. JAMA 2002;287:226-235.
27. Miller G. The assessment of clinical skills/competence/performance. Acad Med 1990;65(Suppl):S63-S67.
28. Wass V, Van der Vleuten C, Shatzer J, Jones R. Assessment of clinical competence. Lancet 2001;357:945-949.
29. Newble DI. Assessing clinical competence at the undergraduate level. Med Educ 1992;26:504-511.

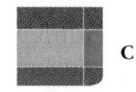 CHAPTER **25**

Web-Based Learning

José Pereira and Moné Palacios

KEY POINTS

- Web-based learning (WBL) includes many technologies and learning activities.
- Increasingly, palliative care instructors are using the World Wide Web for education.
- The adoption of WBL should be guided by well-defined needs.
- Implementation of WBL should be guided by appropriate principles and instructional design.
- Effective WBL requires extensive learner and instructor support and learner–instructor interaction.

The World Wide Web supports education in many different ways. It is already the source of considerable information, and many clinicians use it to address their learning and information needs. Some palliative care educators have already adopted it to support formal learning programs.[1-4]

Web-based learning (WBL) is a generic term for any learning that uses technologies, materials, applications, or communication supported specifically by the Web. It is a subunit of "e-learning," a broader term that also includes learning with the support of other electronic or computer-based technologies. E-learning also embraces other technologies such as personal digital assistants (PDAs), MP3 players, and multimedia compact disc–read-only memory (CD-ROM) or digital video discs (DVD). Combinations of these technologies may be used. It also includes the notion of knowledge management.[5]

KEY CONCEPTS AND TOOLS

"Distance" and "Distributed" Learning

At its most basic, "distance" education takes place when instructors and learners are physically separated. Although distance learning is not new, WBL is revolutionizing not only its delivery but also the associated learning methods. The term "distributed" education is now preferred, to emphasize the increased focus on the learner and the ability to support learning at a place, time, and method of the learner's choosing, whether geographically distant or not.[6]

Synchronous versus Asynchronous Conferencing and Conferencing Tools

Web-based technologies support communication either synchronously or synchronously. Synchronous communication involves real-time interaction between two or more persons, using text, audio, or video (webcams), whereas asynchronous communication is independent of time—participants receive, read, and post messages at times of their own choosing. Applications that support online conferencing, whether text, audio, or video, are referred to as "Web-conferencing" tools, and the process is called "computer-mediated conferencing (CMC)." Although CMC relates to both synchronous and asynchronous conferencing, it is most often used to refer to text-based asynchronous conferencing (aCMC).

Technologies

Technologies that support aCMC include e-mailing, list-servs, bulletin boards, and electronic discussion forums. More recently, "blogs" and "podcasts" have been added. E-mail is the least structured form. Although this technology is familiar to most, the messages related to particular courses or discussions are embedded among all the other messages received, making it difficult to follow the "discussion." Electronic discussion forums, in contrast, organize the postings and keep all those related to a particular discussion together in what is called a *thread* (Fig. 25-1). A learner or instructor posts a message to the discussion board and then logs off. Other participants can then, at a time and place convenient to them, log on, read the previous postings, and respond.

Considerations

Synchronous and asynchronous CMC have their respective advantages and limitations. Synchronous CMC advocates argue that real-time learning activities are critical for creating community; providing a sense of belonging, socialization, and direction for the learners; and providing immediate feedback. The lack of these is a common cause for the high learner dropout rate in distributed learning (up to 30% learner attrition is not uncommon). The logistics of organizing a time convenient for all participants, across time zones in international courses, is limiting. aCMC provides more independence with respect to time and place and may nurture reflection more than synchronous learning.[7] Learners note that the exercise of writing their online responses prompts them to reflect more deeply and pay more attention to their thoughts than in classroom discussions or synchronous CMC.[8] A combina-

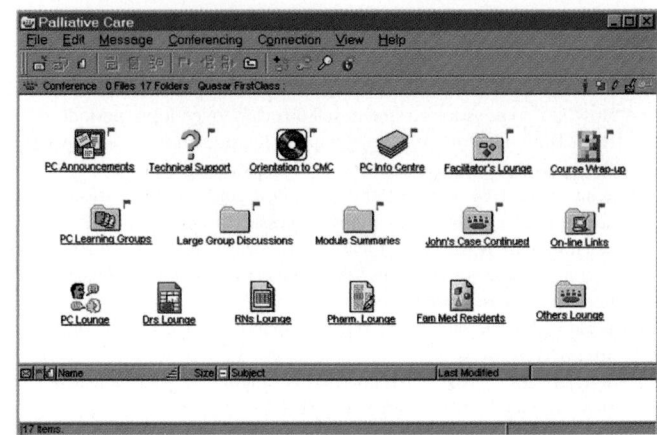

FIGURE 25-1 Example of the home page of an online palliative care course for primary health professionals. The learning management system (LMS) software program is FirstClass (Open Text Corp.). By clicking on each icon, learners entered a different component of the course. "Orientation" contained learning materials, cases, netiquette for the course, course requirements and expectations, and resources about constructive learning and computer-mediated conferencing (CMC). "PC Info" was a conference board where learners could pose any question to content experts on palliative care issues. Facilitator's Lounge was a discussion board open only to facilitators. Facilitators could share experiences in the course and seek advice from one another on content or facilitation issues. Closed discussion boards ("lounges") were also available for physicians, nurses, pharmacists, and family medicine residents in the course. PC Learning Groups contained asynchronous small group discussions (nine groups). The heart of the learning in the course occurred here, through constructive small group learning. Each group completed five modules over 12 weeks. Each module presented new cases and problems. In "Module Summaries," learners selected a representative to summarize the key points from the discussions in their respective small groups and make these summaries available to other groups. John's Case Continued was a single longitudinal case that evolved as the course continued; all learners had access to this discussion forum. "On-line Links" provided a selection of links to useful sites on the Web related to the course. "PC Lounge" was an informal area for participants (learners and faculty) to engage in social interaction through asynchronous CMC.

tion of synchronous and asynchronous CMC can capitalize on the advantages of both (Table 25-1).

Learning Management Systems

Learning management systems (LMS), also referred to as course management systems (CMS), is a broad term for software systems that enable management and delivery of learning content and resources. At a minimum, LMS usually allow for a common space to provide course information and content (text, video, audio, links to other sites), student registration, communication tools, organization of user groups, and tracking of learner and instructor activity. They help faculty create and organize course Web pages, store and manage syllabi and information (including word documents, digital slides such as PowerPoint, audio and video files, images and graphics), track learner and instructor Web site activity (including the number of times each learner has accessed the pages in the LMS and how often each has posted); manage course calendars; and administer online surveys and tests. Discussion forums for asynchronous communication and access to e-mails are often included, but tools to support synchronous text

TABLE 25-1 Examples of Software Programs to Support Asynchronous and Synchronous Communication and Conferencing for E-Learning*

TECHNOLOGY AND SOFTWARE	WEB SITE	SYNC CMC	aCMC	TEXT	AUDIO	VIDEO	DISCUSSION FORUMS	LMS
Not Internet based								
Telephone conferencing		+++			+++			
Video-conferencing		+++				+++		
E-mail			+++	+				
Internet based								
WebBoard	http://webboard.oreilly.com	+	+++	+			+++	
Centra†	http://www.saba.com/products/centra/	++		+	++			
Elluminate†	http://www.elluminate.com	++		+	++			
Moodle	http://moodle.org/	+	++	++			++	+++
WebCT	http://www.blackboard.com/	+	++	++			++	+++
FirstClass	http://www.firstclass.com/	+	++	++			++	+++
BlackBoard	http://www.blackboard.com/	+	++	++			++	+++
Authorware	http://www.adobe.com/products/authorware/		++	+	+	+		+
Click2Learn Toolbook	http://www.toolbook.com/		++	+	+	+		+
Breeze Presenter	http://www.adobe.com/products/presenter/		+++	++	++	+		+
Breeze Meeting	http://www.adobe.com/products/acrobatconnectpro/	+++		++	++	++		
NetMeeting		+++				+++		
Cu-SeeMe		+++				+++		

aCMC, asynchronous computer-mediated conferencing; LMS, learning management system; SYNC CMC, synchronous computer-mediated conferencing.
*Many of these programs are continually being upgraded. Additional functions may have been added since publication of this test. Refer to the specific Web site for more updated information.
†Synchronous sessions can be saved for on-demand viewing asynchronously at a later date.

and audio and video conferencing are becoming more integrated. More sophisticated features include competency management, skills-gap analysis, self-rating quizzes, note-taking and activity planning capabilities for learners, and resource allocation (e.g., venues, rooms, textbooks, instructors). Most systems allow for log-on security through password protection. There are many generic ("off the shelf") LMS available. Moodle is open sourced and therefore available for free downloading and use; most others require licenses. Development of new, custom-built LMS programs de novo is costly and time-intensive and requires expertise.

Online instructors are not restricted to an LMS for WBL. They may forego an LMS and use a program that supports only synchronous conferencing (e.g., Elluminate) or independent self-learning (e.g., Breeze Presenter). Alternatively, they may develop their own Web site using software programs such as Dreamweaver or Frontpage and/or incorporate other asynchronous and synchronous Web-conferencing tools. Audio and video files can be made available to learners through streaming. An alternative if large video files are used (e.g., video vignettes or movies) is to provide learners with copies on CD-ROMs or DVDs.

INSTRUCTIONAL DESIGN CONSIDERATIONS

Several principles are important.[9] The media and technologies chosen for a particular WBL experience cannot be ignored, because their individual characteristics, technologies, and how they are applied influence the learning experience.[10] The learning experience in a Web-based course may be tarnished if Internet access keeps failing, even if the course is impeccably designed.

Instructional Design Processes

The same processes involved in curriculum development in traditional learning, including conducting a needs assessment and establishing learning objectives, should be applied in WBL. However, there are some additional considerations (see Chapter 23).[11] A framework for instructional design consists of four elements[12]: learner autonomy and control, degree of interaction, access, and costs.

Adult Learning

The basic principles of adult learning should be honored (see Chapter 24).

Level of Interactivity

Some WBL programs simply post information and course materials online. Others require significant synchronous and asynchronous discussion between learners and instructors. Programs such as Breeze and Authorware or similar custom-built programs allow instructors to build learning experiences that may incorporate multimedia (text, graphics, audio and video files) and may prompt learners to interact with the programs by, for example, requiring them to review material and respond to quizzes or tests based on the material studied. The design may require that learners first successfully complete a task before being allowed to move on. Graphs, diagrams, and illustrations can facilitate comprehension of ideas presented in text. Software programs such as Hot Potatoes and Zoomerang allow quizzes and tests to be incorporated in online courses, particularly if the LMS being used does not have these functions.

Access

Access to technologies (e.g., high-speed Internet access and firewall issues), preparedness for the technology and learning method, disabilities, culture, and financing are all important instructional design considerations. It is wise to incorporate a technology base that is appropriate for the widest range of students within that program's target audience (the "common denominator" approach).

Costs

Design and development of courses for distributed education has typically been associated with relatively high up-front development costs and variable delivery costs, depending on the technologies being used.[13] Subsequent iterations, provided that not many significant changes are made, decrease in cost. Web site design is relatively inexpensive compared with LMS and Web-conferencing tools; these can be expensive if not provided through institutional support.

Web-Only or Blended Courses

Bonk and Dennen identified 10 levels of integration of WBL into education.[14] These range from using the Web to store and circulate the learning materials of traditional classroom-based courses to courses conducted entirely via WBL (Web-only).[15] Blended or hybrid educational programs combine WBL and traditional classroom-based learning.[4] The WBL component may be minor, or it may constitute the major part of the course. Increasingly, the benefits of hybrid courses are being recognized. Hybrid courses take advantage of the strengths of both approaches, the immediacy of classroom learning and the distributed flexibility of WBL.[16]

Open, Closed, or Paced Courses

Open courses are not time dependent. Learners start and end the course at their convenience. Interaction with other learners is usually limited in these courses. In paced courses, learners must complete the course within a specified time frame. In closed courses, learners enter and finish the courses at preset times. These are usually courses that require a cohort of learners for pedagogical (collaborative and constructive group-based learning) or logistical reasons.

Interface Design and Navigation

Design issues are paramount. Web sites need to be user-friendly, concise, intuitive, and easy to navigate.

Learning Styles

See Chapter 24 regarding learning styles.

Learning Theories

Some learning theories have specific applications in WBL. These include the adult learning theory, constructivism,[17] self-directed learning, communities of inquiry, and communities of practice. Jonassen[18] promoted the idea of using computer-based technologies as cognitive tools for "engaging and enhancing thinking in learners." He contended that students do not learn from computers or their applications, but rather from thinking in meaningful ways, and advocated using technologies as "mindtools." WBL experiences, like their traditional classroom-based counterparts, should include activities that involve active cognitive processes such as creating, problem-solving, reasoning, decision making, and evaluation. Garrison and colleagues proposed a framework, called the *community of inquiry*, within which to develop and study CMC that enhances critical thinking.[19]

Selection of Technologies

Technologies should be selected on the basis of how they will be able to enhance the achievement of the learning objectives, their access, and their costs, among other considerations. Other technologies may also be used to support distributed learning. Plain old telephone conferencing, although considered an "older" technology, can sometimes still be best. See Fig. 25-1 for an example of what the home page of an online palliative care course can look like. In this interdisciplinary course, most of the learning occurred through aCMC.

EFFECTIVENESS OF WEB-BASED LEARNING

The debate as to whether WBL is as effective, more effective, or less effective than traditional learning methods is misguided. WBL is a heterogeneous entity with many different models employing a wide variety of learning activities. Ultimately, its effectiveness depends on both the design and factors such as instructor enthusiasm.

Research that has attempted to compare WBL with traditional learning methods has generally found that, with the appropriate attention to pedagogical and instructional design considerations, WBL is at least as effective as conventional classroom-based courses.[20,21] A systematic review of 700 studies, of which only 19 studies met the inclusion criteria, concluded that "there does not appear to be a difference in achievement between distance and traditional learners."[22] Chumley-Jones and colleagues recently published a review of the evaluation literature in this area.[23] They reviewed several domains, including knowledge changes, learners' attitudes, and efficiency of learning, and concluded that WBL, although useful, does not address all the challenges of medical education. They stated there is no evidence that students learn more from WBL programs than by traditional methods.

The motivation for adopting WBL should not be to replace traditional learning methods, but rather to address barriers to accessing education and to enhance effective traditional learning methods. The heterogeneity of the instructional methods and course designs makes comparisons difficult.

CONCLUSIONS

WBL is a heterogeneous entity that can support a multitude of technologies, learning activities, and levels of interaction. It can be used to enhance traditional classrooms or to offer formal learning programs entirely online. A number of palliative care Web sites offering excellent clinical information are available online (see the list of "Additional Resources"). Given the rapidly expanding role of WBL, several future considerations for palliative care exist (see "Future Considerations").

REFERENCES

1. Irving M. On-line palliative care nursing course. Nurs N Z 2005;11(8):3.
2. Kinghorn S. Delivering multiprofessional web-based psychosocial education: The lessons learnt. Int J Palliat Nurs 2005;11:432-437.
3. Hinkka H, Kosunen E, Metsanoja R, et al. General practitioners' attitudes and ethical decisions in end-of-life care after a year of interactive Internet-based training. J Cancer Educ 2002;17:12-18.
4. Pereira J, Murzyn T. Integrating the "new" with the "traditional": An innovative educational model. J Palliat Med 2001;4:31-38.
5. Chute AG. From Teletraining to e-learning and knowledge management. In Moore MG, Anderson WG (eds). The Handbook of Distance Learning. Mahwah, NJ: Lawrence Erlbaum Associates, 2003, pp 297-313.
6. Holmberg B. Theory and practice of distance education. London: Routledge Press, 1995.
7. Romiszowski A, Mason R. Computer-mediated communication. In Jonassen D (ed). Handbook of Research for Educational Communications and Technology. New York: Macmillan, 1996, pp 438-456.
8. Feernberg A. The written word: On the theory and practice of computer conferencing. In Mason R, Kaye AR (eds). Mindweave: Communication, Computers and Distance Education. Oxford: Pergamon Press, 1989.
9. Clark R. Media will never influence learning. Educ Technol Res Devel 1994;42:21-29.
10. Kozma R. Will media influence learning? Reframing the debate. Educ Technol Res Devel 1994;42:7-19.
11. Clarke D. Getting results with distance education. Am J Distance Educ 1999;12:38-51.
12. Shearer R. Instructional design in distance education: An overview. In Moore MG, Anderson WG (eds). Handbook of Distance Education. Mahwah, NJ: Lawrence Erlbaum Associates, 2003, pp 275-286.
13. Hulsmann T. The costs of distance education. In Harry K (ed). Higher Education through Open and Distance Learning. New York: Routledge Press, 1999, pp 72-84.
14. Bonk CJ, Dennen V. Frameworks for research, design, benchmarks, training and pedagogy in Web-based distance education. In Moore MG, Anderson WG (eds). Handbook of Distance Education. Mahwah, NJ: Lawrence Erlbaum Associates, 2003, pp 331-348.
15. Pereira J. Web-based learning: Comparing two online palliative care courses. In Abstracts of the 2nd Congress of the EAPC Research Network, Lyon, France, May 23-25, 2002.
16. Pereira J, Wedel R, Murray A, et al. Rural family care education: Results of a hybrid distance course for rural family medicine residents [abstract]. J Palliat Care 2005;21:225.
17. Jonassen D, Davidson M, Collins M, et al. Constructivism and computer-mediated communication in distance education. Am J Distance Educ 1995;9(2):7-26.
18. Jonassen DH. Computers in the Classroom: Mindtools for Critical Thinking. Englewood Cliffs, NJ: Prentice-Hall, 1998.
19. Garrison DR, Anderson T, Archer W. Critical thinking, cognitive presence and computer conferencing in distance education. Am J Distance Educ 2001;15(1):7-23.
20. Johnson SD, Aragon SR, Shaik N, Palma-Rivas N. Comparative analysis of learner satisfaction and learning outcomes in online and face-to-face learning environments. J Interactive Learning Res 2000;11(1):29-49.
21. Dusick DM. The learning effectiveness of educational technologies: What does that really mean? Educ Technol Rev 1998;10:10-12.
22. Machtmes K, Asher JW. A meta-analysis of the effectiveness of telecourses in distance education. Am J Distance Educ 2000;14(1):27-46.
23. Chumley-Jones HS, Dobbie A, Alford CL. Web-based learning: Sound educational method or hype? A review of the evaluation literature. Acad Med 2002;77:S86-S93.

SUGGESTED READING

Garrison DR, Anderson T. E-Learning in the 21st Century: A Framework for Research and Practice. London: Routledge-Falmer, 2003.

Holmberg B. Theory and Practice of Distance Education. London: RoutledgeFalmer, 1995.

Salmon G. E-Moderating the Key to Teaching and Learning Online. London: Kogan Page, 2000.

Smith L, Curry M. Twelve tips for supporting online distance learners on medical post-registration courses. Med Teacher 2005;27:396-400.

ADDITIONAL RESOURCES

CLIP online tutorials. Available at http://www.helpthehospices.org.uk/elearning/clip/index.htm (accessed October 2007).

Education for Physicians on End-of-life Care (EPEC) Project. Available at http://www.epec.net/EPEC/webpages/index.cfm (accessed October 2007).

End of Life/Palliative Education Resource Center (EPERC). Available at http://www.eperc.mcw.edu/ accessed October 2007).

International Hospice and Palliative Care Association Manual of Palliative Care, 2nd ed. IAHPC Press. Available at http://www.hospicecare.com/manual/IAHPCmanual.htm (accessed October 2007).

Clinical Management of Neuropathic Pain: A Problem-Based, Interactive Module. Online neuropathic pain course (self-standing and open). Available at http://www.stoppain.org/for_professionals/interactive_module/elearn.asp (accessed October 2007).

Palliative Drugs Online: A community of practice listserv. Available at http://www.palliativedrugs.com/ (accessed October 2007).

Palliative Info. Available at http://palliative.info/ (accessed October 2007).

Research

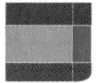

CHAPTER **26**

Principles of Palliative Medicine Research

Clare White, Janet R. Hardy, and Paul Glare

"Palliative care is an art, but it must be based upon science."

— GLIMELIUS, 2000[1]

K E Y   P O I N T S

- Evidence-based medicine forms an essential part of modern medicine.
- Palliative care is not exempt from the need to prove that the interventions employed in everyday practice are not only efficacious and cost effective, but based on scientific evidence.
- Research must be performed in relevant patient groups for it to be clinically applicable.
- Accurate information about the risk/benefit ratio of a treatment or intervention is needed for patients to make informed decisions.
- Palliative care patients are a particularly vulnerable group for whom there is often no 'second chance' to improve care. The idea of allocating patients to less than optimal care is therefore unacceptable
- Randomized, controlled trials have the greatest potential to eliminate bias in research studies.

Innovations in clinical care depend on research. In palliative care, as in other medical specialties, there are many research methodologies including both qualitative and quantitative formats (Tables 26-1 to 26-3). The credibility of research depends on the design chosen by the investigator.[2] The question asked, the characteristics of the patient population under study, the interventions used, and the specific end points all influence the most appropriate trial design[2] (see Chapter 5). The most robust evidence is traditionally considered to come from randomized, controlled trials (RCTs).[3] An RCT is often necessary to validate results from other trial methodologies and is essential in validating new treatments or interventions

against the current standard. However, researchers often have important questions that cannot be answered by a controlled clinical trial or diagnostic study, and in these cases other research methods, such as observational studies, are important.[4] Observational studies form a step in evidence-based medicine, but more trials are usually necessary to validate results (see Chapter 5). Qualitative studies contribute to the depth and richness of knowledge and often generate hypotheses that can then be tested within quantitative methodologies (see Chapter 5).

EVIDENCE-BASED MEDICINE

Evidence-based practice forms an essential part of modern medicine. It is widely accepted that, along with patient preferences, evidence from good-quality research is necessary to guide clinical decision making about practice and service provision. The term *evidence-based medicine* was developed to encourage both practitioners and patients to make use of the best evidence in clinical care. Evidence-based medicine requires integration of individual clinical expertise with the best available clinical evidence based on systematic research.[5] Study designs are ranked in a hierarchy according to their potential to eliminate bias (Table 26-4). Criteria for the rating of evidence have been published by several national research bodies, including the National Health and Medical Research Council in Australia[6] and the Agency for Healthcare Policy and Research in the United States. All are consistent in bestowing the highest rating on meta-analyses of several large, well-designed RCTs and the lowest rating on data from uncontrolled observational studies. There is no consensus for rating qualitative research, and it may be inappropriate to attempt to rate it in the same manner, although the Campbell Collaboration is moving in that direction.[7]

Importance of Evidence-Based Medicine in Palliative Care

Palliative care seeks to enhance quality of life in the face of death by addressing the physical, social, psychological, and spiritual needs both of patients with advanced disease and their families.[8] The range of available treatments has expanded, and patients often receive treatment until death to prevent or control symptoms.[9] To ensure that symptoms are managed in the most appropriate way, a solid body of knowledge must be developed, and that, in turn, depends on good research.[2] Some argue that the need to deliver best-quality care suggests that research in palliative care is a moral imperative[10] (see Chapter 3). The cardinal ethical principles of beneficence, nonmaleficence, autonomy, and justice can be applied to answer this case.[11]

TABLE 26-1 Types of Quantitative Research Trial Design*

TYPE OF RESEARCH	DESCRIPTION
Questionnaire/survey	Can be quantitative or qualitative.
Observational studies	The investigator measures but does not intervene.
Descriptive study (observational)	The investigator describes the health status of a population or characteristics of a number of patients.
Cross-sectional (observational)	Measurement of condition in a representative population (preferably random) at one point in time.
Cohort (observational)	Outcomes are compared for matched groups with and without exposure or risk factors (prospective)
Case-control (observational)	People with and without the outcome of interest are compared for evidence of previous exposure or risk (retrospective).
Randomized, controlled trial (experimental)	Gold standard trial—subjects are randomly allocated to study treatment or standard/placebo treatment; often studies are blind (single or double blind).
Crossover trial (experimental)	The study subjects receive each treatment in a random order; with this type of study, every patient serves as his or her own control.
N of 1 trials (experimental)	Consists of doing a number of crossovers between the study drug and placebo, or between two different drugs in the same patient; the patient serves as his or her own control.
Parallel trials (experimental)	Each patient receives a single treatment.
Systematic review	Review of all the scientific literature on a particular topic to try to answer a research question.

*See chapter 64 for qualitative research.

TABLE 26-2 Qualitative versus Quantitative Research

FACTOR	QUALITATIVE	QUANTITATIVE
Social theory	Action	Structure
Method	Observation, interview	Experimental, survey
Question	What is X? (classification)	How many Xs? (enumeration)
Reasoning	Inductive	Deductive
Sampling method	Theoretical	Statistical
Strength	Validity	Reliability

From Mays N, Pope C. Qualitative Research in Health Care. London: BMJ Publishing Group, 1996.

TABLE 26-3 Clinical Trial Phases

PHASE	DESCRIPTION
I	The experimental drug or treatment is tested in a small number of people (20-80) for the first time to evaluate its safety, determine a safe dosage range, and identify side effects.
II	The experimental drug or treatment is given to a larger group of people (100-300) to determine whether it is effective and to further evaluate its safety.
III	The experimental drug or treatment is given to large groups of people (1000-3000) to confirm its effectiveness, monitor side effects, compare it to commonly used treatments, and collect information that will allow it to be used safely.
IV	Postmarketing studies delineate additional information, including the drug's risks, benefits, and optimal use.

From Brescia F. Pain management as part of the comprehensive care of the cancer patient. Semin Oncol 1993;20(Suppl 1):48-52.

TABLE 26-4 Criteria of the National Health and Medical Research Council (Australia) for Rating Quantitative Evidence

LEVEL OF EVIDENCE	DESCRIPTION
Level 1	A systematic review of all relevant RCTs
Level 2	At least one properly designed RCT
Level 3-1	Well-designed pseudo-RCTs
Level 3-2	Comparative studies with concurrent controls and allocation not randomized, case-control studies, or interrupted time series with a control group
Level 3-3	Comparative studies with historical control, two or more single-arm studies, or interrupted time series without a parallel control group
Level 4	Case series, either post-test or pre-test and post-test

RCT, randomized, controlled trial.
National Health and Medical Research Council. NHMRC Standards and Procedures for Externally Developed Clinical Practice Guidelines. Canberra, 1998. Available at http://www.nhmrc.gov.au/publications/synopses/nh56syn.htm (accessed October 2007).

Beneficence

Research in palliative care must have at its heart a belief that the production of good-quality evidence is a matter of justice and that dying patients and their loved ones, like all patients, deserve to know that the services and inter- ventions they receive are effective.[12] Although the multi- disciplinary nature of palliative care is fundamental, for many patients, drug therapy remains of vital importance in maintaining symptom control and quality of life.[13] Many new drugs and drug formulations are becoming available, and many of the older, established drugs are used on the basis of anecdotal evidence or physician preference alone, without a strong evidence base.[13] The optimal use of these medications often warrants a clinical trial to assess efficacy and safety. Palliative care patients deserve to have the benefits of quality care that research can produce.[14] The converse is that it is potentially unethical not to perform research, because this restricts knowledge of best care.

Nonmaleficence

A priority in palliative care is that the benefits of an inter- vention far outweigh the harms that it might cause. Therefore, one focus of research must be on nonmaleficence—to do no harm. It is essential that the side effects and potential harm that may result from treatments or interventions be known. Although anecdote and observation may highlight some potential problems, many side effects may not be recognized unless formally assessed through high-quality research trials. It is essential that unjustifiable toxicities be avoided.

Autonomy

To respect patient autonomy, information must be made available to allow patients and their loved ones to make informed decisions. To provide accurate information about the risk/benefit ratio of a treatment or intervention, research is needed. This allows patients and their loved ones to maintain autonomy and make informed decisions about the patient's care.

Justice

It is important that a treatment that is effective be available to all those who need it, not just to those fortunate enough to be cared for by a physician who has a preference for the treatment in question. Conversely, if a treatment is ineffective, the patient should not be given it, and the health service provider should not have to fund it. To ensure that resource allocation is fair and appropriate, research evidence is needed to support the development of clinical protocols and best-practice guidelines and to guide service development.[3] Palliative care is not exempt from these conditions.[12,13]

Lack of Evidence in Palliative Care

Many treatments widely used in palliative care have never been proven to be effective, and their use is based on anecdotal evidence and physician preference[15]; examples are benzodiazepines in terminal agitation, antihistamines for opioid-induced nausea, diuretics in malignant ascites, and anticholinergics for retained respiratory secretions (Table 26-5).[16] Although the use of some drugs (e.g., morphine, metoclopramide) is supported by a high level of evidence, that of many others (e.g., midazolam, hyoscine) is not. Moreover, the evidence often comes from trials in specific populations and cannot be generalized to all palliative care patients. For example, the evidence to support the use of tricyclic antidepressants for neuropathic pain has largely come from studies in patients with nonmalignant disease.[17] Similarly, most antiemetic studies have been carried out in cancer patients receiving chemotherapy,[18] and the level 2 evidence supporting the use of haloperidol for delirium was undertaken in patients with human immunodeficiency virus (HIV) disease, not cancer.[19]

Sound evidence is essential to guide palliative care practice.[3] Patients deserve the best care that can be provided, especially when life expectancy is short and there is no "second chance." It is no longer acceptable to use a particular treatment just because a physician believes it is in the patient's best interests.[15] Nebulized morphine in palliative care was once popular, but it has since been demonstrated to be no more effective than placebo.[20] Similarly, diamorphine was once considered a better analgesic than morphine,[21] and a double dose of immediate-release morphine at night was thought to be an acceptable alternative to an early morning dose.[22] In other areas of medicine, treatments that were once common practice have since been overturned, including the use of flecainide after myocardial infarction, corticosteroids for optic neuritis, blood letting, gastric freezing for ulcers, radical mastectomy, and routine tonsillectomy.[15] Practices not based

TABLE 26-5   Levels of Evidence for Commonly Used Drugs in Palliative Care

DRUG	MAIN PALLIATIVE CARE INDICATION	HIGHEST LEVEL OF EVIDENCE
Morphine	Pain	1
Metoclopramide	Nausea and vomiting	1
Paracetamol	Pain	1
Amitriptyline	Neuropathic pain (noncancer)	1
Omeprazole	Dyspepsia	1
Fentanyl	Pain	1
Ranitidine	Dyspepsia	1
Pamidronate	Hypercalcemia	1
Haloperidol	Delirium	2 (in AIDS patients)
Dexamethasone	Anorexia/cachexia	2
Diazepam	Anxiety	2
Lorazepam	Anxiety	2
Chlorpromazine	Delirium	2 (in AIDS patients)
Hyoscine hydrobromide	Excess oropharyngeal secretions	3
Clonazepam	Terminal restlessness	4
Midazolam	Terminal restlessness	4
Cyclizine	Nausea and vomiting	4
Spironolactone	Ascites	4
Promethazine	Nausea/itch	4
Frusemide	Ascites	4

From Good P, Cavenagh J, Currow D, et al. What are the essential medications in palliative care? A survey of Australian palliative care doctors. Aust Fam Physician 2006;35:261-264.

on evidence of effectiveness can be ineffective or even harmful, despite the prevailing "expert opinion."

In palliative medicine, there are wide variations in clinician practice, not only internationally, but within countries and even within departments (e.g., in determining morphine dose-equivalents and opioid conversion ratios). Episodes of inappropriate care and practitioner uncertainty also challenge the credibility of clinical judgment.[23] Well-known examples of controversies in palliative care include the use of opioids for headache associated with increased intracranial pressure, ketamine as a routine adjunct to opioid administration, and metoclopramide for intestinal obstruction.

GENERAL PRINCIPLES OF RESEARCH

To get started in research in palliative care, one needs to begin with an understanding of the research cycle (Fig. 26-1). There is a fundamental distinction between basic research (e.g., How does morphine work?) and clinical questions (e.g., How well does morphine work?). Usually, basic research precedes clinical studies, whereas work that bridges the two is referred to as *translational* research. This chapter considers only clinical research.

Clinical Questions

There are four main types of clinical questions that arise: therapy, diagnosis, prognosis, and harm/etiology. Different types of study design are required to answer these different questions. For studies of therapy or other interventions, it is the randomized trial. For prognosis and harm/etiology, it is the prospective cohort study (retrospective cohorts and case-control studies are alternatives). For diagnostic test evaluation, the cross-sectional study is most appropriate.

Research Ideas

Most often for clinicians, research ideas are generated from clinical issues that arise in day-to-day practice. The first step is to frame an answerable question. Take, for example, the question, "Are 5-hydroxytryptamine 3 (5HT3) antagonists effective in palliative care patients?" This clinical query needs to be reframed as a focused clinical question. Use of the mnemonic PICO (*p*opulation, *i*ntervention/exposure, *c*omparator, *o*utcome) is recom-

mended.[24] In this case, the original, rather vague question becomes, "In patients with advanced cancer [the population], is a 5HT3 antagonist [the intervention] as effective as metoclopramide—or haloperidol, cyclizine, methotrimeprazine, or dexamethasone—[the comparator] in the relief of nausea [the outcome]?" In addition to nausea, toxicity, quality of life, and cost are other important outcomes to be measured.

Literature Search

Having reframed this clinical query as an answerable question, one needs to do a literature search to see where this research topic sits in the research cycle. The search should reveal that there have been a number of case series to support the conjecture that 5HT3 antagonists can be effective,[25] and there was even a multiarm RCT comparing one 5HT3 antagonist with various combinations of metoclopramide, dexamethasone, and chlorpromazine.[18] The research cycle, in this case, generally indicates that a second, similar study needs to be undertaken, so that a meta-analysis can be performed, before a program of research to develop, implement, and evaluate the impact of a clinical practice guideline on the use of 5HT3 antagonists in palliative care is initiated. The latter is a 5- to 10-year research program that should be attractive to a funding agency. On the other hand, another audit of 5HT3 antagonist usage by 50 patients in a single palliative care unit would definitely be irrelevant.

Protocol Development

Whatever research design is undertaken, be it a single-unit audit or a multicenter collaborative RCT, the next step is to develop the protocol. This usually begins as a one-page abstract that can be sent for critiquing by the other researchers who will be involved in the study. This is then expanded into a larger protocol, and finally the full document is submitted to a granting agency and/or Institutional Review Board (IRB) or ethics committee. Irrespective of the stage of development of the document, it is usually structured according to the following headings:

- Purpose of the study: what is already known about the problem, the existing treatments, the rationale for the proposed study
- Aims and objectives: what is to be achieved (aim), what is to be determined (objective), what researchers expect to find (hypothesis)
- Population and setting
- Intervention (if appropriate): nature and method of administration of the drug
- Study design
- Outcomes and measures: outcome measure, end point, measure of effect
- Study procedures and recruitment strategies
- Statistical issues

The co-investigators examining the protocol need to keep in mind two key issues. The first concerns validity, both internal and external, and the second concerns methodological issues (outcomes, measures, statistics). *Internal validity* relates to whether the sample is truly representative of the population in general or whether it is biased. Samples are biased if those patients who receive

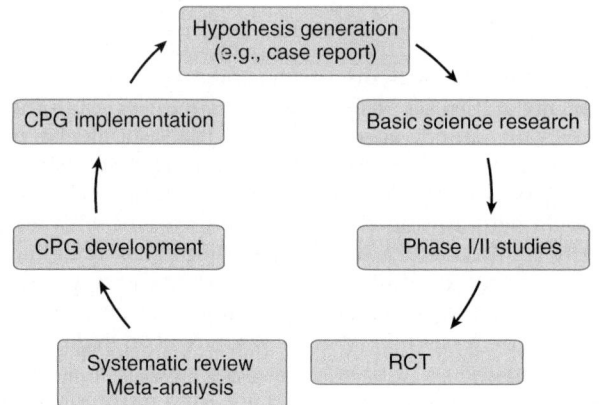

FIGURE 26-1 The research cycle. CPG, clinical practice guidelines; RCT, randomized, controlled trial.

one treatment are systematically (rather than randomly) different from those who receive the other treatment. Bias can artificially make the effects of one treatment look different from those of another when, in fact, no true difference exists (a type I error). This is usually avoided in controlled studies through concealed allocation of randomization and the intention-to-treat analysis; it is harder to avoid in uncontrolled and observational studies. *External validity* refers to the representativeness of the sample and how the results (if internally valid) can be related to other populations. The methodological issues are important because, to add to knowledge, the measures must be clinically relevant and must cover the full range of outcomes of interest. The study needs to be large enough so that the results will be precise and will not miss small but real (and clinically relevant) differences that exist between the treatments (a type II error).

In most situations, studies will be submitted for approval by an ethics committee or IRB. Primarily, the IRB review ensures that persons agreeing to participate in the study are being treated fairly in terms of burden, risks, privacy, and similar issues and that they understand what they are agreeing to participate in. Secondly, most reputable journals now require a study to have IRB approval before they will accept it for publication. Thirdly, the IRB assists the researcher by ensuring that the paperwork and other administrative functions necessary to successfully undertake research are done properly. Clinical research, like any other scientific experiment, needs to be carefully planned and recorded. All types of resources (money, space, equipment, time, and personnel) may be needed. Successful research programs require careful management and a strong commitment from the leader over a prolonged period to see the project through to successful completion.

Clinical Audits

Finally, clinical audit requires some discussion. Increasingly, it is believed that audits should be approved by an ethics committee unless the data are not going to be retained (e.g., on an electronic database) or the results are not going to be disseminated outside the department. Proposals for clinical audits should be worked up using the same outline as for other studies, and the paperwork should be kept just as diligently. A specific type of audit that can be used to improve care is the Plan-Do-Study-Act (PDSA) model, which is perhaps particularly suited to palliative care.[26] The PDSA cycle allows creative ideas and solutions to be tested in small groups of patients, and then used generally to improve on those ideas and to foster even more improvement. The limitation of PDSA projects is that they lack the validity of well-designed clinical trials, and the results cannot easily be generalized to other types of patients. They can sit at the start of the research cycle, however, and from that point more formal evaluations can be undertaken.

ARGUMENTS AGAINST RESEARCH IN PALLIATIVE CARE

Despite the need for more evidence in palliative care, some have argued that research in dying patients is inappropriate[27]:

To research at all into the needs and experiences of this client group could be said to be an affront to the dignity of those people who are terminally ill and an expression of profound disrespect for the emotional and physical state of such patients.

It is often assumed that patients and their families will not want to participate in research, although this view has been challenged.[28,29] The question has been posed whether it is ethically sound to ask patients to participate in research and thus "deprive" them of energy and time that could be spent with family or used to complete "unfinished business."[9] There is also a concern that palliative care patients are psychologically and emotionally vulnerable and may feel coerced into participating. Patients might worry that, if they do not agree to enter a trial, their care may be compromised. Similarly, staff caring for palliative care patients may be concerned about a potential conflict of interest if they are simultaneously recruiting the patients for research trials. Time constraints for health care professionals are another challenging issue: clinical demands are often high, leaving little time for research. There is a fear that time spent researching may detract from patient care. Palliative care practitioners may be reluctant to challenge treatments that they "know" to be effective and may be disinclined to have their assumptions and clinical judgments challenged by research.

Research in the palliative care population is difficult (see later discussion) and, for this reason, it often is not attempted. Many studies have been initiated but never completed, wasting both time and financial resources. Many studies have been grossly underpowered because of number constraints and therefore of dubious value to any evidence base. Few centers have the necessary infrastructure to support large research programs. Palliative care patients, by definition, are likely to be unwell and may by cognitively impaired. They may not be able to provide fully informed consent[22]; this is especially important in countries where proxy consent is not acceptable. Many in the field have chosen to pursue descriptive or qualitative research methodologies as an alternative to clinical research. Although this form of research adds significantly to the richness of knowledge, it is not considered to provide high-level evidence.

ARGUMENTS FOR RESEARCH IN PALLIATIVE CARE

Many of the justifications for undertaking research in palliative care have been discussed earlier. For research to be clinically applicable, it is important that it be performed in relevant patient groups. Clinical trials should be performed in a population that resembles, as much as possible, the population in which the intervention will be used. Patients with advanced disease often present with many severe physical and psychological symptoms. In addition, the nature and intensity of symptoms and the response to treatment change continuously.[2] Clinical studies in cancer are often performed in patients who are at an earlier stage of their illness or in those who are younger or of better performance status. The results are then extrapolated to the terminally ill population.[2] However, these results cannot be automatically applied to patients with advanced illness, who are in a more unstable condition and are often receiving a combination of drugs for pain and other symptoms.[2] It is necessary to perform trials in the population who will be receiving the treatment in order to obtain a good clinical correlation between research and clinical practice.

PROBLEMS WITH RANDOMIZATION IN PALLIATIVE CARE RESEARCH

The concept of randomization carries with it additional concerns. Palliative care patients are a particularly vulnerable group.[22] The idea of allocating patients to less than optimal care is therefore contentious. For a comparative trial to be ethically justifiable, there must be real uncertainty as to whether the new treatment is superior to no treatment or to existing treatments (a concept known as "equipoise"). Even when it exists, it is often difficult to convince others that there is equipoise between trial conditions, because a new treatment, intervention, or service is often perceived to be more desirable by professionals, patients, and their families.[22] There is a need to ensure that any randomization is perceived to be fair and that patients receive, at the very least, good care, regardless of which arm of the study they are randomly assigned to.[22] RCTs in palliative care often compare standard treatment or care (which has proved adequate in the past) with a new form of care (which has not been proven); the value of the new intervention needs to be justified, if only because it may take future resources away from other services.[22] It must be remembered that "new" is not synonymous with "more effective" and that any control group should be cared for with standard comprehensive palliative care.[30]

PROBLEMS IN PALLIATIVE CARE RESEARCH

It is generally acknowledged that it is very difficult to accrue the numbers of patients necessary to perform an RCT in palliative care,[15] and recruitment to trials and research projects is often slow.[13] Specific challenges include difficulties in recruiting patients, small samples, high attrition rates and insufficient events, rapidly changing clinical situations, limited survival times, and gatekeeping by professionals (i.e., a reluctance to refer patients for research studies).[3]

Patients

The course of disseminated cancer is diverse, and patients with advanced disease experience deteriorating health over time, sometimes complicated by acute complications such as bleeding, sepsis, and thromboembolic events.[30] Patients may be too ill and debilitated to provide self-reported data, or their decline during the course of the study may result in large amounts of missing data.[31] Sample attrition is often high, not only because of the patients' declining health but also because patients may die during the course of the research study.[10] Attrition rates of more than 60% have been described.[32] Timing of measurements is crucial for the success of a trial, yet timing in palliative care is often difficult because of the short time between eligibility and death.[3] A study duration longer than 1 month[13] is usually not feasible, because many patients will have died or become too unwell to participate within a 2-month period.

In addition to the declining physical state of patients, their emotional vulnerability makes research difficult.[10] Patients may have debilitating symptoms and emotional distress in the knowledge of impending death and the reality of diminishing time.[14] Cognitive failure is a frequent and serious complication of advanced cancer that can occur several weeks before death.[2] This may be related to the disease process or to medications, and it might adversely affect a patient's ability to consent to or be involved in a trial. In one study, 19% of potentially eligible trial patients had cognitive impairment (Mini Mental State Examination [MMSE] lower than 24/30).[33]

Fatigue is a common symptom in advanced disease and some may also experience "trial fatigue."[15] Terminally ill patients often lack the energy to participate in research,[14] as they often have more pressing concerns and priorities when struggling to cope with daily needs. There is also the ethical concern that patients may be dependent on their health care provider, and therefore may feel coerced into participating in research in order to continue receiving good care.[9]

Families

Patients are often willing to participate in research, but family caregivers may feel protective and try to keep researchers out.[31] Carers may be unwilling to expose the patient to what might be seen as further experimentation,[15] especially for those who have already been involved in oncology trials. Family members may also find it difficult to be involved in research because of the burdens of caregiving, fatigue, and the emotional changes associated with grief and loss.[34] The sheer emotional vulnerability of the carer, and that of the patient, can result in difficult moral and ethical dilemmas.[35] Families may resent the time it takes patients to participate in research, because that time might otherwise be spent with the family.[9]

Health Care Professionals

Gatekeeping that prevents patients from participating in palliative care trials is an important issue. Clinical colleagues are often the source of identification of patients potentially eligible for trials in palliative care. It is therefore essential to gain their support, because lack of (or half-hearted) support can easily undermine a trial.[22] Professionals caring for patients sometimes see themselves as needing to protect the vulnerable from overly demanding research projects.[36] Practitioners may not wish to randomize their patients to treatments in which they lack confidence.[3] In addition, their involvement in research may not be easy in the light of competing clinical and administrative demands.[34]

System

Organizational barriers include a lack of research infrastructure, few trained clinical researchers, prioritization of clinical responsibilities, and funding difficulties (see Chapter 5).[37] Overprotective ethics committees or IRBs can be powerful gatekeepers.[38] Ethics committees might view the palliative care patient as vulnerable because he or she is considered to be a person who is dying, rather than a person who is living with a terminal illness.[34]

Tools

Because palliative care is a relatively new specialty, there are few data collection tools that have been proven to be reliable.[34] Moreover, many of the symptoms being assessed are subjective (e.g., dyspnea, fatigue) and therefore more difficult to measure than an objective end point such as tumor size.

IS RESEARCH IMPOSSIBLE IN PALLIATIVE CARE?

Palliative care is not the only area where research has proved difficult, and many of the issues described here are not unique to palliative care. Difficulties with recruitment to clinical trials have been described in oncology,[40] and it is also often difficult to perform research in patient groups such as children, patients with mental health problems, the elderly, patients from ethnic groupings, patients in intensive care units, and bereaved families.[41] The difficulties discussed earlier do not, therefore, exempt palliative care from seeking to improve care through thoughtful research; rather, they highlight areas that need to be specifically designed to cope with these difficulties.[42]

FACILITATING RESEARCH IN PALLIATIVE CARE

It has been suggested that patients with advanced illness (and their families) may not wish to risk reducing the quality of life of their remaining days in a trial with an uncertain outcome,[3] especially if they are unlikely to receive direct tangible benefits from participation.[14] In contrast, studies have shown that the factors considered most important by dying patients include making a contribution to others.[28] This can be achieved by participation in research trials, even when it is appreciated that the research is unlikely to benefit the individual participating. Moreover, the views of patients regarding research are typically favorable (see later discussion). Gatekeeping, therefore, may not only detract from patient wishes but may also deny patient autonomy by preventing patients from making their own decisions as to whether to enter a trial. Some researchers have solved this problem by employing research officers to approach all patients who are potentially eligible for trials, independent of the treating team.[43]

Trials should be kept short and should employ simple methodology. Assessments should be nontaxing, and follow-up should be as infrequent and nonburdensome as possible (e.g., telephone assessments compared with attending hospital). Short and simple trials may be more acceptable to patients, their families, and health care professionals caring for them. They may also experience less attrition. Brief patient information sheets and consent forms may also ease trial participation; shortened versions of these forms have been accepted by the national ethics committee in the United Kingdom and might set a precedent for future trials.[44]

The development of more acceptable validated tools would ease patient assessment and data collection in a standardized manner, making comparisons between similar trials possible. To facilitate research, new trial designs (e.g., N of 1) have been developed to allow smaller numbers to be recruited but still provide meaningful results; for example, by using the patient as his or her own control. Crossover studies are also useful in reducing the necessary sample size. Trials should have realistic power calculations to detect clinically important but small differences, and attrition should be anticipated when calculating power (see Chapter 5).

Multicenter trials with collaboration among centers may also ease recruitment (see Chapter 5). Research networks should be developed to provide a mechanism to meet the research needs of individual units. Academic centers with the necessary infrastructure may be best equipped to coordinate larger research projects, with support from smaller units. New researchers should be encouraged through interaction with, or exposure to, expertise and leadership of established investigators. New research methods and designs need to be fostered, and training and support need to be available for new researchers. This, in turn, will lead to the development of research networks. The provision of more funding for palliative research would allow the employment of health care professionals and research personnel with designated time for research, thereby reducing pressure on clinicians. Funding may be obtained from governmental agencies, charities, or pharmaceutical companies.

PATIENTS' VIEWS ON PARTICIPATING IN RESEARCH

Studies in patients undergoing more active treatment have shown that they may be more willing to enter trials than might be expected by the doctors and nurses caring for them.[45] Patients near the end of life who are receiving palliative care are not offered any chance of cure by participation in clinical trials, but, like patients at an earlier stage of disease, they might still hope for some therapeutic benefit not available "off trial."[45] In addition, patents with more advanced cancers may seek to find some meaning in their situation through advancement of knowledge and improvements in care for others.[45] People approaching the end of life may want to contribute to service changes that would be put in place after they were no longer alive, seeing this as their legacy to others.[42,46]

CONCLUSIONS

The suggestion that palliative care patients should not be involved in research denies these individuals an active role in living and prevents them from contributing to knowledge about how to improve care for other people.[34] Although palliative care patients have many burdens, as members of our society they have the right to choose whether to participate in an activity that may bring benefit to others, particularly when the research they choose to be involved in poses little risk of harm to them.[34] The voices of the very ill and those at the end of life are in danger of not being heard. Although there are practical, emotional, and conceptual barriers to involving palliative care patients, these should act to spur imaginative thinking rather than serve as an excuse for inaction.[35]

It is a mistake to assume that patients who have crossed a line between active treatment and palliative care are not well enough to take an active part. This stereotyping only serves to mirror the divide that patients themselves often experience when moving from curative anticancer treatment to palliative care.[35] Involvement can confer a sense of empowerment—a sense of being valued and contributing to future care.[35] People with a limited prognosis are still people with decision-making capacity (unless proven otherwise) and, presumably, the same views as others concerning the value to the community of research participation.[9]

The need for more evidenced-based practice is increasing, and simply giving a patient a drug to see whether it works is no longer justified.[1] High-quality care requires an understanding of why and how a particular therapy works.[1] The emphasis in palliative care research needs to be on the development of realistic studies that are practical and achievable in this population with generally poor performance status, and it has been suggested that patients should be involved in the development of protocols and the setting of the research agenda.[13]

There has been a growth in palliative care research, but there is still resistance within the professional community regarding studies in this potentially vulnerable population. Research questions must be asked in areas where answers need to be found; striving for better evidence should result in better care.[47]

REFERENCES

1. Glimelius B, Ekstrom K, Hoffman K, et al. Randomized comparison between chemotherapy plus best supportive care with best supportive care in advanced gastric cancer. Ann Oncol 1997;8:163-168.
2. Bruera E, Neumann CM, Mazzocato C, et al. Attitudes and beliefs of palliative care physicians regarding communication with terminally ill cancer patients. Palliat Med 2000;14:287-298.
3. Aoun S, Kristjanson L. Challenging the framework for evidence in palliative care research. Palliat Med 2005;19:461-465.
4. Mallen C, Peat G, Croft P. Quality assessment of observational studies is not commonplace in systematic reviews. J Clin Epidemiol 2006;59:765-769.
5. Sackett DL, Haynes RB, Guyatt GH, Tugwell P. Clinical Epidemiology: A Basic Science for Clinical Medicine, 2nd ed. Boston: Little, Brown and Company, 1991.
6. National Health and Medical Research Council. NHMRC standards and procedures for externally developed clinical practice guidelines. Canberra, 1998. Available at http://www.nhmrc.gov.au/publications/synopses/nh56syn.htm (accessed October 2007).
7. Campbell Collaboration. Available at http://www.campbellcollaboration.org (accessed September 2007).
8. Saunder C. Foreword. In Doyle D, Hanks GWC, MacDonald N (eds). Oxford Textbook of Palliative Medicine, 2nd ed. Oxford: Oxford University Press, 1998.
9. Addington-Hall J. Research sensitivities to palliative care patients. Eur J Cancer Care 2002;11:220-224.
10. Corner J, O'Driscoll M. Development of a breathlessness assessment guide for use in palliative care. Palliat Med 1999;13:375-384.
11. Gillon R. Medical ethics: Four principles plus attention to scope. BMJ 1994;309:184-188.
12. Hunt J, Keeley VL, Cobb M, Ahmedzai SH. A new quality assurance package for hospital palliative care teams: The Trent Hospice Audit Group model. Br J Cancer 2004;91:248-253.
13. Billings JA. Recent advances: Palliative care. BMJ 2000;321:555-558.
14. Dean R, McClement S. Palliative care research: Methodological and ethical challenges. Int J Palliat Nurs 2002;8:376-380.
15. Hardy J. Placebo-controlled trials in palliative care: The argument for. Palliat Med 1997;11:415-418.
16. Good P, Cavenagh J, Currow D, et al. What are the essential medications in palliative care? A survey of Australian palliative care doctors. Aust Family Physician 2006;35:261-264.
17. McQuay H, Tramer M, Nye B, et al. A systematic review of antidepressants in neuropathic pain. Pain 1996;68:217-227.
18. Mystakidou K, Befon S, Liossi C, Vlachos L. Comparison of the efficacy and safety of tropisetron, metoclopramide, and chlorpromazine in the treatment of emesis associated with far advanced cancer. Cancer 1998;83:1214-1223.
19. Breitbart W, Marotta R, Platt M, et al. A double-blind trial of haloperidol, chlorpromazine, and lorazepam in the treatment of delirium in hospitalized AIDS patients. Am J Psychiatry 1996;153:231-237.
20. Noseda A, Carpiaux J, Markstein C, et al. Disabling dyspnoea in patients with advanced disease: Lack of effect of nebulized morphine. Eur Respir J 1997;10:1079-1083.
21. Twycross R. Choice of strong analgesic in terminal cancer: Diamorphine or morphine? Pain 1977;3:93-104.
22. Grande GE, Addington-Hall JM, Todd CJ. Place of death and access to home care services: Are certain patients groups at a disadvantage? Soc Sci Med 1998;47:565-579.
23. Eddy D. Clinical decision making: from theory to practice: Three battles to watch in the 1990s. JAMA 1993;270:520-526.
24. Craig JC, Irwig LM, Stockler MR. Evidence-based medicine: Useful tools for decision making. Med J Aust 2001;174:248-253.
25. Currow D, Coughlan M, Fardell B, Cooney N. Use of ondansetron in palliative medicine. J Pain Symptom Manage 1997;13:302-307.
26. Lynn J, Schuster JL, Kabcenell A. Improving Care for the End of Life. Oxford: Oxford University Press, 2000.
27. deRaeve L. Ethical issues in palliative care research. Palliat Med 1994;8:298-305.
28. Terry W, Olson L, Ravenscroft P, et al. Hospice patients' views on research in palliative care. Intern Med J 2006;36:406-413.
29. Williams C, Shuster J, Clay O, Burgio K. Interest in research participation among hospice patients, caregivers, and ambulatory senior citizens: Practical barriers or ethical constraints? J Palliat Med 2006;9:968-974.
30. Rinck GC, van den Bos GAM, Kleijnen J, et al. Methodologic issues in effectiveness research on palliative cancer care: A systematic review. J Clin Oncol 1997;15:1697-1707.
31. McMillan S, Weitzner M. Methodologic issues in collecting data from debilitated patients with cancer near the end of life. Oncol Nurs Forum 2003;30:123-129.
32. Jordhoy M, Kaasa S, Fayers P, et al. Challenges in palliative care research; recruitment, attrition and compliance: Experience from a randomized controlled trial. Palliat Med 1999;13:299-310.
33. Bruera E, Spachynski K, MacEachern T, Hanson J. Cognitive failure in cancer patients in clinical trials. Lancet 1993;341:247-248.
34. Lee DS, Austin PC, Rouleau JL, et al. Predicting mortality among patients hospitalized for heart failure: Derivation and validation of a clinical model. JAMA 2003;290:2581-2587.
35. Bradburn J, Maher J. User and carer participation in research in palliative care. Palliat Med 2005;19:91-92.
36. Henderson M, Addington-Hall J, Hotopf M. The willingness of palliative care patients to participate in research. J Pain Symptom Manage 2005;29:116-118.
37. Mitchell G, Abernethy A; Investigators of the Queensland Case Conferences Trial. Palliative Care Trial. A comparison of methodologies from two longitudinal community-based randomized controlled trials of similar interventions in palliative care: What worked and what did not? J Palliat Med 2005;8:1226-1237.
38. Pettit P. Instituting a research ethic: Chilling and cautionary tales. Bioethics 1992;6:90-112.
40. Slevin M, Mossman J, Bowling A, et al. Volunteers or victims: Patients' views of randomised cancer clinical trials. Br J Cancer 1995;71:1270-1274.
41. Stevens T, Wilde D, Paz S, et al. Palliative care research protocols: A special case for ethical review? Palliat Med 2003;17:482-490.
42. Abernethy AP, Shelby-James T, Fazekas BS, et al. The Australia-modified Karnofsky Performance Status (AKPS) scale: A revised scale for contemporary palliative care clinical practice. BMC Palliat Care 2005;4:7.
43. Abernethy A, Currow D, Hunt R, et al. A pragmatic 2 × 2 × 2 factorial cluster randomised controlled trial of educational outreach visiting and case conferencing in palliative care methodology of the Palliative Care Trial. Contemp Clin Trials 2006;27:83-100.
44. Dentith J, Hardy J. Approval by MREC of a modified patient information and consent form: Does this set a precedent for trials in palliative care? [letter to the editor]. Palliat Med 2004;18:484-485.
45. Ross C, Cornbleet M. Attitudes of patients and staff to research in a specialist palliative care unit. Palliat Med 2003;17:491-497.
46. Smale N, Rhodes P. Too Ill to Talk? User Involvement in Palliative Care. London: Routledge, 2000.
47. Cook A, Finlay I, Butler-Keating R. Recruiting into palliative care trials: Lessons learnt from a feasibility study. Palliat Med 2002;16:163-165.

CHAPTER **27**

Developing a Research Group

Katherine Hauser

KEY POINTS

- An experienced mentor helps research career development.
- Research group development involves acquiring personnel, resources, education, and financial support.
- An appropriate research question and detailed protocol are essential components of research methodology.
- Collaborative research can mitigate many of the challenges of palliative medicine research.

Clinical studies often experience problems of inadequate recruitment and difficulties with informed consent and attrition[1-5] (Box 27-1). Problems related to patients, their families, and clinical staff can contribute. Structural issues such as small research groups and the lack of academic chairs, specific research funding, and collaborative groups have hampered research progress. Research training and facilities are lacking in many fellowship programs.[6] National strategies for palliative medicine research exist in Australia, Canada, the United Kingdom, and the United States but have been formulated in few European countries.[2,3] These challenges highlight a need for unique research structure and design. Group work, communication, and collaboration can mitigate some challenges, especially in recruitment and attrition. With creativity, financial support, and hard work, methodologically sound research can be achieved.[7]

MENTORSHIP

Researchers who have an identifiable mentor have higher-self-confidence, more protected research time, and higher publication rates, and they are more likely to receive competitive research grant funding.[8] A chosen mentor should be a successful scientist with a proven publication record and the time and willingness to provide continuing support for the mentee (Box 27-2).

RESEARCH GROUP DEVELOPMENT

Personnel

The research team personnel depend on the type of research (e.g., basic science, clinical, translational, epidemiological, outcomes) and on the questions and goals of the group. Primary and associate investigators may have diverse backgrounds and may include basic scientists, chaplains, nurses, physicians, and social workers.

Statistical expertise is essential. Statisticians can advise about study and database design to generate testable

---

Box 27-1 Challenges of Palliative Medicine Research

PATIENTS

Heterogeneous population
Severely unwell population
Short life expectancy, making longitudinal studies difficult
Renal and hepatic impairment, influencing pharmaceutical studies
Confusion and deteriorating illness, affecting consent

FAMILIES

Distressed group of people

STAFF

Lack of time
Lack of research training
Gatekeeping roles
Structure and politics
Fragmented service provision
Small research groups
Lack of collaborative groups
Lack of academic palliative medicine chairs
Lack of specific funding for palliative medicine research

Box 27-2 Mentorship

ROLE OF THE MENTOR

Help develop independence and self-reliance
Guide education and career development plan
Assist development of professional skills, such as writing, speaking, collaboration, time management, and ethical conduct
Assist in resource procurement

ROLE OF THE MENTORED PERSON

Take control of program, including reading, coursework, and technical skills
Establish and maintain regular communication, including reports of progress, problems, and new data
Contribute knowledge and ideas
Understand mentors' professional pressures and time constraints

Adapted from Johnson D. Mentorship: The art of choosing, using and becoming a mentor. Presented at the Annual Meeting of the American Society of Clinical Oncology, 2007. Available at www.asco.org (accessed November 19, 2007).

---

hypotheses and facilitate data analysis. They calculate sample size and study power, analyze data, and interpret results. Ongoing involvement of a statistician with the research team familiarizes them with the challenges of palliative medicine research. This knowledge can be applied to grant writing strategies and trial design to overcome the challenges of recruitment and attrition.

A research nurse's role may involve screening candidates for clinical trials, confirming eligibility, obtaining consent, and data collection, including questionnaires, compliance information, and an inventory of adverse events. Other personnel may include data, grant, and budget coordinators, administrative workers, and secretarial staff.

Resources

Palliative medicine literature is often difficult to find, especially in general medical journals.[9,10] A librarian trained in Medline and PubMed coding and search strategies enhances the likelihood of a successful search. Automatic literature updates can be generated from both search engines. Online palliative medicine literature databases are available and may list unpublished literature or trials in progress (e.g., CareSearch). Access to computers and the Internet is essential for research. Software should include word processing, data spreadsheets, statistical programs, and reference management packages. Some basic statistical and reference management software is available on the Internet (e.g., EZAnalyze, RefWorks).

The pharmacist's role in clinical trials may include coding and randomization, preparation of placebo, drug storage, dispensing, checking compliance, and disposal of unused medication. Basic science resources may include laboratory space, equipment and chemicals, animal housing and handling, and pharmaceuticals.

Education and Training

Educational needs may be met from several sources (Box 27-3). An experienced mentor can assist with research methods, grant proposals, and article writing. Courses in research methods are available in institutions or universities. Research seminars are often included in international meetings (e.g., European Association for Palliative Care Research Forum, American Society of Clinical Oncology Annual Meeting). The National Institutes of Health provide online training in research ethics. Training in communication and marketing techniques may improve recruitment.

Research Process

Ethical palliative medicine research must ask important (rather than trivial) questions, design methodologically rigorous studies, and use only appropriate and justifiable tests and questionnaires.[11] These factors influence the choice of a research question and protocol preparation. A clear research question defines the research objective,

guides study design, and determines analysis.[12] The research question should be a single question summarizing the problem, intervention, comparison, and outcome (PICO) components.[12]

The research protocol describes what is to be done and how, where, why, and by whom it is done. It includes sections on aims and objectives, study design (including sample size analysis), screening and consent procedures, inclusion and exclusion criteria, data security and analysis (interim and final), and adverse reaction monitoring and reporting. Standardized templates that conform to local Institutional Review Board (IRB), ethics committee, or funding agency requirements save time when preparing multiple protocols.

Recruitment is a major obstacle in palliative medicine research.[7] Study design must consider this issue and institute procedures to ensure that trials proceed appropriately.[13-16] Consent procedures in palliative medicine should include a brief cognitive screen to exclude delirium. Consent may be altered by deteriorating condition or mental status and should be actively revisited throughout a clinical trial.[17,18]

Regular group meetings may discuss planned research questions, protocols, and procedures and review results and upcoming meeting presentations. Interim and final results should be presented to the entire research group for review and discussion. Final results should also be presented to the clinical team involved to ensure feedback and continued support for research. External meeting presentations should be practiced before the group so that audiovisual and spoken content can be revised and perfected and all questions posed before the final presentation.[19] A regular journal club can assist group members' awareness of the literature and promote critical thinking and writing techniques. Manuscripts should be written with a target journal in mind and conform to the requirements of the journal's instructions for authors.[20] The Consolidated Standards of Reporting Trials (CONSORT) group's statement provides guidelines for reporting randomized clinical trials (http://www.consort-statement. org).[21,22]

Budget and Funding

A research budget includes personnel, materials, equipment, travel, clinical tests, laboratory and pharmacy costs, publication costs, and consultants' fees. Many institutions have a grant manager, who understands the process and common errors. Questions also can be directed to the contact person at a granting agency. Funding sources include institutions (i.e., national, public, or private bodies) and the pharmaceutical industry. Funding challenges include limited, specific funding for palliative medicine and limited pharmaceutical funding for off-label uses of established medications or development of new palliative drugs.[5] Palliative medicine research often must compete for funding on the open market, and studies focusing on a single or unique diagnosis, symptom, age group (e.g., geriatric patients), or care setting may open doors to specific grants.[3,7] Internet sites listing grant opportunities include the Community of Science and CareSearch (see "Additional Resources").

Box 27-3 Education and Training Needs for Researchers

- Ethics
- Confidentiality
- Research methods
- Information technology (e.g., spreadsheets, reference management)
- Biostatistics
- Grant writing
- Article writing
- Laboratory procedures, including reagent handling and disposal
- Animal handling and ethics

Data and Records Management

Data management must comply with local privacy standards, which are often dictated by IRBs. Electronic security (e.g., pin numbers, passwords, firewalls) is important, especially with use of spreadsheets and electronic methods of data collection.[23,24] Statisticians can assist with database design, including procedures for handling missing data.[25,26] Clinical trials require procedures for data safety monitoring for serious adverse events.

The U.S. Food and Drug Administration Act of 1997 requires registration of phase II, III, or IV clinical trials of investigational drugs for life-threatening or serious diseases.[27] Registration is also required for publication in several medical journals[28] (see "Additional Resources").

Relationships

A strong relationship with the clinical team is essential for clinical trial recruitment. Regular meetings should discuss upcoming research protocols to avoid excessive gatekeeping by clinical team members.[11,14] Other clinical and research disciplines may provide valuable skills and resources for palliative medicine research. Researchers in diverse fields may contribute other pathophysiologic models (e.g., fatigue in chronic fatigue, multiple sclerosis). Clinicians from disciplines such as cardiology and neurology can facilitate research in advanced, nonmalignant illnesses. Many advanced cancer patients still receive active therapy, and close relationships with oncologists could facilitate their involvement in palliative research studies.

Many IRB members do not understand the challenges and appropriate methods for palliative medicine research, especially qualitative methods.[18] This may result in protectionism and negative attitudes about palliative medicine research.[18] Open and bidirectional dialogue helps these groups become aware of the specific challenges and navigate them in an ethical manner.

COLLABORATIVE RESEARCH: BENEFITS, BARRIERS, AND CHALLENGES

Collaborative research potentially mitigates many challenges of palliative medicine research. Multicenter collaborations enhance clinical trial recruitment and allow adequate sample size for statistical rigor. Collaborations with investigators in other fields (including basic science) may broaden the skill and knowledge set of all investigators involved.

Internationally different service provision models for palliative care impede collaborative research (Box 27-4).

Box 27-4 Barriers to Collaborative Research

- Different and fragmented clinical service delivery models
- Clinical and research funding structures
- Resources
- Communication (e.g., across time zones)
- Different research priorities
- Institutional review board procedures
- Lack of time

Differences may include location, length of stay, providers, and funding. Multicenter studies are impeded by the lack of communication and standardization between different institutional and national ethics bodies and IRBs.[29] Academics may have competing interests and secondary gains to consider.[30]

Collaborative projects require unique funding, including project grants and traveling fellowships. Teleconferencing, Web sites, and arranging group meetings to coincide with international conferences may overcome communication difficulties. Protocol development requires standardization of recruitment, consent, intervention, data collection, and documentation. Methods of review need to be established to ensure quality control. Data from numerous sources must be encoded and entered into a single database. Technology such as visual scanners or secure Web sites can assist this process.[23,24] Guidelines are available for authorship of multicenter collaborative studies. Authorship protocols should be discussed and agreed on before project commencement.[7,31]

Examples of collaborative groups exist at institutional, national, and international levels. Institutional groups may include other clinical or basic science researchers. For example, a proposed central mechanism of cancer-related fatigue was developed and investigated by collaboration between palliative medicine and biomedical engineering researchers in my institution.[32] National research collaborations have been established in Germany, Sweden, the United Kingdom, and other countries.[2,33,34] In the United Kingdom, specific government funding has promoted development of collaborations.[2] In Germany, the implementation of standardized clinical data collection has facilitated research.[33] In the United States, the Study to Understand Prognoses and Preferences for Outcomes and Risks of Treatments (SUPPORT) (funded by a private foundation) recruited a large number of patients and provided many insights into the experience of people dying in hospitals.[35,36] The European Association for Palliative Care (EAPC) Research Network is an international collaboration involving 21 countries. Several projects are being conducted (www.eapc.org/reseacrhNetwork/research-projects.asp), and the results of a large, cross-sectional survey have been published.[37] Research challenges include the following:

- Palliative medicine academic chairs
- Publicly supported international research funding
- Information technology for collaboration
- Research education at palliative care and oncology meetings and in fellowship training programs

CONCLUSIONS

Despite many challenges facing palliative medicine researchers, important research is being performed. Finding and working with a mentor experienced in palliative medicine research is vital to beginning a research career. Many educational resources are available to assist development of a research group. There is a need for more collaborative groups, more specific funding, and national programs for palliative medicine research. The Internet provides an exciting portal to facilitate collaborative research.

REFERENCES

1. Addington-Hall J. Research sensitivities to palliative care patients. Eur J Cancer Care 2002;11:220-224.
2. Hagen NA, Addington-Hall J, Sharpe M, et al. The Birmingham International Workshop on supportive, palliative, and end-of-life care research. Cancer 2006;107:874-881.
3. Kaasa S, Hjermstad MJ, Loge JH. Methodological and structural challenges in palliative care research: How have we fared in the last decades? Palliat Med 2006;20:727-734.
4. Kaasa S, Dale O, for the Pain and Palliation Research Group. Building up research in palliative care: An historical perspective and a case for the future. Clin Geriatr Med 2005;21:viii, 81-92.
5. Sweeney C, Bruera E. Research opportunities in palliative medicine. Tex Med 2001;97:64-68.
6. Stirling LC, Pegrum H, George R. A survey of education and research facilities for palliative medicine trainees in the United Kingdom. Palliat Med 2000;14:37-52.
7. Currow DC, Abernethy AP, Shelby-James TM, Phillips PA. The impact of conducting a regional palliative care clinical study. Palliat Med 2006;20:735-743.
8. Sambunjak D, Straus SE, Marusic A. Mentoring in academic medicine: A systematic review. JAMA 2006;296:1103-1115.
9. O'Leary N, Tiernan E, Walsh D, et al. The pitfalls of a systematic MEDLINE review in palliative medicine: Symptom assessment instruments. Am J Hosp Palliat Care 2007;24:181-184.
10. Sladek R, Tieman J, Fazekas BS, et al. Development of a subject search filter to find information relevant to palliative care in the general medical literature. J Med Libr Assoc 2006;94:394-401.
11. Bruera E. Ethical issues in palliative care research. J Palliat Care 1994;10:7-9.
12. Stone P. Deciding upon and refining a research question. Palliat Med 2002;16:265-267.
13. Cook AM, Finlay IG, Butler-Keating RJ. Recruiting into palliative care trials: Lessons learnt from a feasibility study. Palliat Med 2002;16:163-165.
14. Ewing G, Rogers M, Barclay S, et al. Recruiting patients into a primary care based study of palliative care: Why is it so difficult? Palliat Med 2004;18:452-459.
15. Jordhoy MS, Kaasa S, Fayers P, et al. Challenges in palliative care research, recruitment, attrition and compliance: Experience from a randomized controlled trial. Palliat Med 1999;13:299-310.
16. Steinhauser KE, Clipp EC, Hays JC, et al. Identifying, recruiting, and retaining seriously-ill patients and their caregivers in longitudinal research. Palliat Med 2006;20:745-754.
17. Lawton J. Gaining and maintaining consent: Ethical concerns raised in a study of dying patients. Qual Health Res 2001;11:693-705.
18. Lee S, Kristjanson L. Human research ethics committees: Issues in palliative care research. Int J Palliat Nurs 2003;9:13-18.
19. Sackett DL. On the determinants of academic success as a clinician-scientist. Clin Invest Med 2001;24:94-100.
20. Guyatt GH, Brian Haynes R. Preparing reports for publication and responding to reviewers' comments. J Clin Epidemiol 2006;59:900-906.
21. Moher D, Schulz KF, Altman DG. The CONSORT statement: Revised recommendations for improving the quality of reports of parallel-group randomised trials. Lancet 2001;357:1191-1194.
22. Piggott M, McGee H, Feuer D. Has CONSORT improved the reporting of randomized controlled trials in the palliative care literature? A systematic review. Palliat Med 2004;18:32-38.
23. Marshall WW, Haley RW. Use of a secure internet web site for collaborative medical research. JAMA 2000;284:1843-1849.
24. Quan KH, Vigano A, Fainsinger RL. Evaluation of a data collection tool (TELEform) for palliative care research. J Palliat Med 2003;6:401-408.
25. Fielding S, Fayers PM, Loge JH, et al. Methods for handling missing data in palliative care research. Palliat Med 2006;20:791-798.
26. Palmer JL. Tips for managing data for research studies. J Palliat Care 2002;18:127-128.
27. Zielinski SL. Clinical trials registration efforts gain some ground. J Natl Cancer Inst 2005;97:410-411.
28. De Angelis C, Drazen JM, Frizelle FA, et al. Clinical trial registration: A statement from the international committee of medical journal editors. Ann Intern Med 2004;141:477-478.
29. Kristjanson LJ, Leis A, Koop PM, et al. Family members' care expectations, care perceptions, and satisfaction with advanced cancer care: Results of a multi-site pilot study. J Palliat Care 1997;13:5-13.
30. Rathbun A. The benefits and difficulties of academic collaboration. Am J Hosp Palliat Care 2004;21:337-339.
31. Barker A, Powell RA. Authorship. Guidelines exist on ownership of data and authorship in multicentre collaborations. BMJ 1997;314:1046.
32. Seyidova-Khoshknabi D, Davis M, Siemionow V, et al. EEG frequencies: Evidence of central origin of cancer related fatigue. Presented at the 10th Congress of the European Association for Palliative Care, Budapest, Hungary, June 7-9, 2007.
33. Radbruch L, Nauck F, Ostgathe C, et al. What are the problems in palliative care? Results from a representative survey. Support Care Cancer 2003;11:442-451.
34. Lundstrom S, Strang P, for the Palliative Care Research Network. Establishing and testing a palliative care research network in Sweden. Palliat Med 2004;18:139.
35. A controlled trial to improve care for seriously ill hospitalized patients. The study to understand prognoses and preferences for outcomes and risks of treatments (SUPPORT). The SUPPORT principal investigators. JAMA 1995;274:1591-1598.
36. Phillips RS, Hamel MB, Covinsky KE, Lynn J. Findings from SUPPORT and HELP: An introduction. Study to Understand Prognoses and Preferences for Outcomes and Risks of Treatment. Hospitalized Elderly Longitudinal Project. J Am Geriatr Soc 2000;48(Suppl):S1-S5.
37. Kaasa S, Torvik K, Cherny N, et al. Patient demographics and centre description in European palliative care units. Palliat Med 2007;21:15-22.

SUGGESTED READING

Fielding S, Fayers PM, Loge JH, et al. Methods for handling missing data in palliative care research. Palliat Med 2006;20:791-798.

Guyatt G. Preparing a research protocol to improve chances for success. J Clin Epidemiol 2006;59:893-899.

Guyatt GH, Brian Haynes R. Preparing reports for publication and responding to reviewers' comments. J Clin Epidemiol 2006;59:900-906.

Haynes BR. Forming research questions. J Clin Epidemiol 2006;59:881-886.

Jenicek M. How to read, understand and write 'Discussion' sections in medical articles. An exercise in critical thinking. Med Sci Monit 2006;12:SR28-SR36.

Sackett DL. On the determinants of academic success as a clinician-scientist. Clin Invest Med 2001;24:94-100.

Stone P. Deciding upon and refining a research question. Palliat Med 2002;16:265-267.

ADDITIONAL SOURCES

CareSearch. Palliative medicine literature databases. Available at http://www.caresearch.com.au (also a clinical trial registry) and www.chernydatabase.org (accessed November 2007).

Clinical trial registration. Available at http://www.clinicaltrials.gov and http://www.nci.nih.gov/search/clinicaltrials (accessed November 2007).

Community of Science grant opportunities database. Available at http://www.cos.com (accessed November 2007.)

EZAnalyze statistical software. Available at http://www.ezanalyze.com (accessed November 2007).

RefWorks. Reference management software (subscription required). Available at http://www.refworks.com (accessed November 2007).

Research and bioethics education. Available at http://www.asco.org, http://www.bmj.com, and http://www.nih.gov (accessed November 2007).

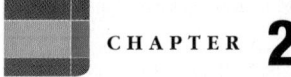

CHAPTER **28**

Design and Conduct of Research and Clinical Trials

Anthony Byrne, Kerry Hood, Gareth Griffiths, and Timothy S. Maughan

---

KEY POINTS

- The clinical impact of research evidence relies on confidence in its quality.
- Palliative care is characterized by complex clinical situations, but clinical trials require simple clinical questions.
- The designs of explanatory and pragmatic trials depend on the clinical research question.
- Choices of study populations and standard comparators influence the generalizability of the study results (i.e., external validity).
- An adequate sample size and low attrition rate influence the reliability of the study results (i.e., internal validity).
- Randomization reduces the risk of bias by overcoming confounding factors.
- Choices of clinically relevant outcome measures and patient populations are crucial for the relevance of palliative care clinical trials.
- Qualitative and other important clinical information can be included in the design of quantitative clinical trials.
- Infrastructural support is essential for adequate recruitment, data management, and research governance.

The purpose of research in palliative care is to provide robust and reliable evidence for clinical practice. This information can be integrated with clinical judgment and patients' values in reaching individual treatment decisions. The evidence must be obtained and reported in a manner that limits bias and allows for consistent interpretation. Evidence-based medicine[1] has built on the logical, quantitative approach to clinical scientific research that evolved throughout the 20th century.[2] This approach aims to reduce information to its most reliable and most easily measured form to aid interpretation. How these data are evaluated encouraged the development of hierarchies of evidence. This suggests levels of reliability for the acceptance into clinical practice of various types of research results.

The influence of this approach is firmly established in the development of clinical guidelines and recommendations.[3] It demands of the researcher a statistical and precise approach to research design. It has championed the role of randomized, controlled trials and systematic reviews as gold standards of evidence. However, simplification of the basis of evidence to fit with a hierarchical approach has created difficulties,[4] especially in interpreting the overall quality of evidence for individual types of clinical questions and setting.[5] The results of a randomized, controlled trial or systematic review of a series of such trials can provide robust evidence of the effectiveness of a particular treatment in a well-defined patient population. However, this approach is unsuited to interventions carried out in a changing population over time.

For a specialty that by definition requires a multidisciplinary approach to complex needs, careful consideration is needed in designing research studies that answer questions of relevance while providing the evidence in an acceptable and interpretable format. Identifying ways of meticulously producing evidence while challenging traditional approaches requires a highly skilled, well-governed, and fully integrated research environment.

THE CHALLENGE OF EVIDENCE

Investigators usually undertake research because of an interest in a particular clinical situation (i.e., patient orientated) or disease process (i.e., disease orientated). Ultimately, the desire is to produce valid, reliable data that can lead to better patient outcomes and be accepted as producing a meaningful change in practice. Whether the driver for this change is at an individual (e.g., patient), organizational (e.g., care provider, commissioner), or strategic (e.g., National Institute for Health and Clinical Excellence, Agency for Healthcare Research and Quality) level, the likelihood of the research influencing care depends on the level of confidence in the quality of the data.[1,6] Convention dictates that methodological factors that reduce confidence include the following[7]:

- Lack of randomization and blinding
- Insufficient sample size
- High attrition rate
- Heterogeneity in study populations and results

These factors point to the need for well-designed and rigorously conducted randomized, blinded, controlled trials and underscore the challenge of assessing palliative interventions in complex patient groups. Research in palliative care has been hampered by underpowered studies, heterogeneous population groups, high attrition rates, and failure to provide definitively reliable results. In producing research outcomes that deliver change, investigators are obliged to comply with established conventions on levels of evidence.[8] This can be achieved through a skilled, multidisciplinary research workforce; focused, coordinated goals; better timing of interventions at an earlier stage of illness; and attitudinal evolution, with research accepted as an integral part of clinical practice.

Useful studies also require organized, purposeful challenges to the status quo to wrestle the focus from statistical comfort zones to the complex needs of advanced illness. Balance is required between the theory that complex study design is an excuse for subjectivity or an "anything goes" approach and the canard that one randomized, controlled trial methodology fits all.

THE RESEARCH QUESTION

Daily clinical interaction in palliative care provides the opportunity for all health care professionals to identify questions concerning best practice and care. This may take the form of a lack of knowledge, gaps in the transition of knowledge to care, or true equipoise in the choice of intervention. Articulating the nature of each challenge is hampered by complexity and heterogeneity. Reducing the complexity of the *clinical* question can maximize the potential of answering the *research* question in a reliable and repeatable manner. To design an effective study, we must be concise in the question we ask and the population within which we ask it. What do we do if the component parts of the clinical question seem unclear or inseparable? What information do we start with as a basis for justifying our aims?

Trials can by their randomization and methodical approach allow an accurate comparison of effects.[2] Encouragement of the meta-analysis of randomized, controlled trials has had a profound impact on assessment of evidence and clinical practice. Availability of this level of evidence is restricted in palliative care and may be lacking in underpinning study aims. This problem appears daunting, but lack of knowledge should not stigmatize research in palliative care but instead be a motivating force[9] that stimulates efforts to harness the information on hand and learn from other areas. Cochrane himself was pragmatic in his approach to clinical questions during his time as a prisoner of war in World War II, and his reflections on care of the dying also testify to his belief in the strength of single observations.[10]

In pursuing robust, large-scale trials, palliative care professionals should not ignore the potential of description, pattern recognition, and sharing of collateral knowledge as vital preludes that help refine the research question.[11] This pathway fits comfortably with the evidence of others that systematic collection and analysis of routine data can enhance our ability to construct questions, investigate effectively, and validate study outcomes.[12,13] It also highlights the need to seek a broad range of views from the multidisciplinary community and patients. In this way, the question is refined, the design is improved, and the study gains greater face validity and cooperation.

Reviewing all available evidence, including well-described clinical observations, can justify the research and focus the research question. A broad clinical question may stimulate interesting debate about a wide range of important options for intervention, but because a research question aimed at numerous outcomes often struggles to succeed, a primary outcome should be identified. This process of refining research goals benefits from well-developed critical appraisal skills[14] and the ability to synthesize qualitative and quantitative data.

Armed with an articulate clinical research question, how can investigators avoid past failures in undertaking a trial? A useful approach is to ask what route the scientific inquiry should take. If a similar question has been asked before in palliative care or other areas of medicine, a systematic qualitative or quantitative review may provide an answer, with the research prompting the opportunity to enhance skills and educate. If further knowledge is required about the question or proposed methodology, a pilot or feasibility study may be required (discussed later). To ensure a robust approach, this may be undertaken in pursuit of an academic qualification, providing useful outcomes in terms of results and a well-trained and skilled researcher. Defining these routes is more productive than a haphazard approach, and it is resource efficient and cost effective in allowing adequate preparation for larger studies (Fig. 28-1).

THE TRIAL DESIGN

The type of study design chosen depends on how the research question has been articulated and on the issue under investigation. Several factors are essential to this process:

- A full appreciation of the evidence already available and knowledge of routine practice
- A clear definition of the intervention and whether it will be compared with anything else
- The exact nature of the patient population to be studied and an understanding of the numbers likely to be recruited
- Availability of validated outcome measures

With this information, it becomes easier to see how the educational or knowledge-based aspects of research and pilot or feasibility data (see Fig. 28-1) feed into the robust design of larger-scale projects. It also underscores the importance of access to appropriate expertise and training. Transforming the research question into a study protocol requires the support of a project group with diverse skills who are engaged at the very beginning of the process.

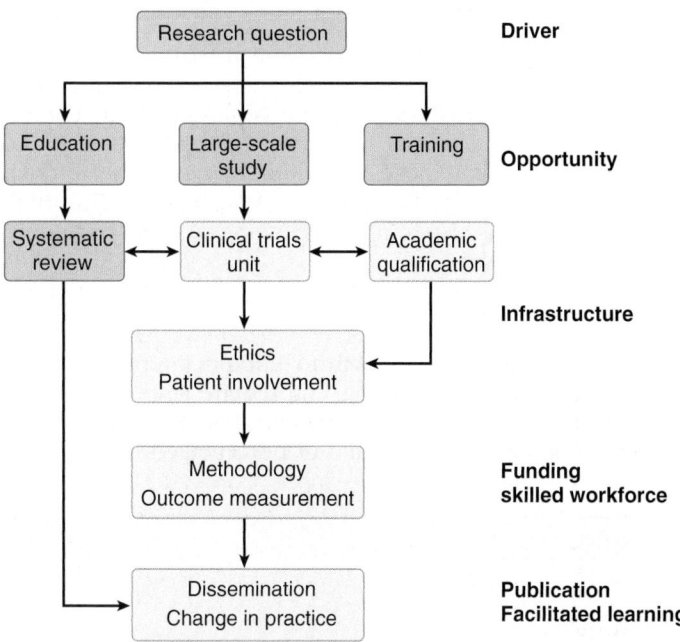

FIGURE 28-1 Algorithm of suggested pathways for research questions. Systematic reviews and feasibility studies provide educational and training outcomes in their own right and contribute to the design of large-scale studies.

In considering study design, it is useful to consider the basic categories of quantitative study that are available. *Descriptive studies* are observational records, including case series or cross sectional studies, that may provide useful exploratory information as outlined earlier. *Longitudinal studies* capture data over time and traditionally include cohort studies and clinical trials. These study types have been described elsewhere,[15,16] and we therefore focus on clinical trials for the remainder of this chapter.

A *clinical trial* is a scientific experiment enrolling humans that differs from other longitudinal studies by being interventional rather than observational. A *controlled trial* is one in which comparisons are made between one or more research arms and a control group (often standard treatment). An experiment on scurvy was credited as the first clinical trial.[17]

Clinical Trial Phases

It is difficult for a single study to answer all of the questions in relation to safety, efficacy, and optimal use of an intervention. Clinical trials are therefore divided into different phases.

- Phase I trials usually involve small patient numbers (≤20) and specifically examine the safety of the intervention and safety range of drug doses (in drug trials).
- Phase II studies assess efficacy of the intervention under consideration and address tolerability and safety. The feasibility of an intervention may be assessed at this stage before a full study. Patient numbers are relatively small (<100).
- Phase III studies are randomized, controlled studies comparing the intervention against standard comparator or placebo. Sufficient patient numbers are required to demonstrate statistical significance (usually in the hundreds).
- Phase IV studies are postmarketing studies exploring the long-term safety and optimal use of an intervention.

The characteristics of the clinical trial are influenced by the desire to produce evidence that is considered reliable (i.e., internal validity) and reproducible in clinical practice (i.e., external validity, or how generalizable the results are). Bias poses a serious threat to the internal validity of a study (Box 28-1). In designing a clinical trial, the factors discussed in the following sections are important to consider.

Randomization

Allocating patients randomly to different interventions can be costly, time consuming, and require large numbers of patients. It is also a process patients find difficult to understand, resulting in a significant percentage refusing entry to the trial because of a preconceived preference for one intervention or the other. In palliative care, such studies have proved difficult to undertake and to complete,[18-20] so why randomize? A randomized, controlled trial overcomes the risk of the *biased selection* of patients for interventions. By extension, it allows estimation of a treatment effect between intervention and control groups by overcoming all confounding factors (Box 28-2).

Nonrandomized Studies

An assessment of the difference between randomized and nonrandomized studies has suggested that nonrandomized, controlled trials may overestimate treatment effects by as much as 40%.[21] Systematic review of transcutaneous electrical nerve stimulation (TENS) for postoperative pain exemplifies the problem of overestimation. Fifteen of 17 randomized, controlled trials found no effect, whereas 17 of 19 nonrandomized, controlled trials suggested analgesic benefit.[22] Blinding patients and researchers to the intervention further reduces the risk of bias in the form of *observer bias*, thereby enhancing study validity.[23] This is particularly important when the primary end point is subjective.

Nonrandomized, controlled trials have a tendency toward smaller sample size and greater patient heterogeneity between studies,[24] which were already identified as problems in palliative care research. There are strong imperatives for randomization, even when the type of question or patient population makes this difficult. Although there may be genuine reasons not to randomize, such obstacles need to be carefully considered and every effort made to avoid compromising the validity of subsequent results.

Randomized Studies

In *crossover randomized trials*, patients receive treatments randomly allocated in sequence. This can allow precise estimation of treatment effect using smaller patient numbers than traditional parallel designs, and it reduces patient heterogeneity by comparison with the same patient. A patient acts as his or her only control; intrapatient variability is much less than interpatient variability, and this approach is frequently employed in palliative care intervention studies.[25-27] A washout period protects against carrying over one intervention into the next treatment period (Fig. 28-2), although changes in the patient over time and other carryover effects can create bias.

Cluster randomization refers to the process of randomizing units such as hospices, clinics, or general practices to create clusters within which individuals are recruited. At that point, informed consent may or may not

---

Box 28-1 Sources of Bias in Clinical Trials
- Lack of randomization
- Lack of blinding
- Heterogeneous sample
- Small sample size
- Patient attrition
- Publication

Box 28-2 Ideal Characteristics of Randomized, Controlled Trails
- Outcomes are predefined.
- Allocation between treatments is random.
- Allocation method is concealed from the researcher.
- Researcher and patient are blind to the treatment given.
- All groups have identical treatment apart from the intervention.
- Patients are analyzed according to allocated group, even if they fail to complete (i.e., analysis by intention to treat).

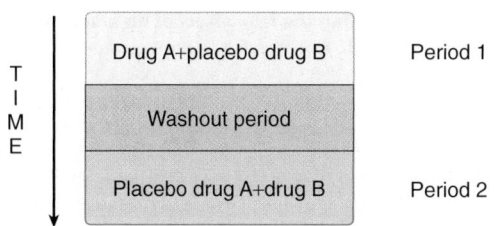

Drug A+placebo drug B	Period 1
Washout period	
Placebo drug A+drug B	Period 2

FIGURE 28-2　Schematic outline of a crossover study. The study duration must be sufficient to allow a treatment effect to occur within each period but not be so long as to allow changes in the patient's condition to alter the treatment effect across the two periods. The washout period should be long enough to allow the biological activity of the drugs to be negated.

be obtained from patients, with the attendant ethical implications of either option (see Chapter 22). This approach may be useful for community-based interventions when consent may be difficult to obtain and when assessing a hospice at home[28] intervention. Its utility[29] in research on the last days of life has been assessed. This approach is methodologically complex and requires careful deliberation in design[30] and interpretation.[31] It requires careful statistical modeling, including determining the appropriate sample size. Because individuals within clusters are not independent of each other (i.e., intracluster correlation), statistical power is reduced, and more subjects must be recruited. However, it is a good example of how consideration of alternative strategies may provide flexibility for the research population while retaining study rigor.

The role of *patient preference* in randomization has gained greater prominence.[32] Patients may not wish to participate in a trial in which they perceive the experimental treatment to be inferior or they feel at risk for harm by not receiving the active intervention. Investigators also may not be inclined to enroll patients in randomized studies about which they have strong opinions or preferences. The introduction of ketamine for neuropathic pain on the basis of descriptive studies is an example of how anecdotal experience can influence clinician preference. These ideas may lead to a lack of participation, poor compliance, and a threat to the internal validity of the trial, and this predicament led to the concept of patient preference or *comprehensive cohort* design. Patients with strong preferences are allowed their treatment choice—a concept opposite to blinding. This approach also implies the opposite of blinding in terms of bias and the risks of confounding[33] and has implications for the size and cost of the study. Cogent arguments have been advanced to avoid losing important information on those who refuse randomization,[34] particularly when patient numbers are limited and recruitment difficult. In this study design, patients are randomized as normal, but those who refuse to be randomized are followed as a cohort for the period of the trial, and their data are then assessed.[33] Monitoring the nonrandomized cohort within the confines of a study and comparing their data with those of the randomized group may produce important additional information.[35,36]

Although this design should be approached with caution, it emphasizes the importance of patient choice in research. The argument to at least prospectively assess patient preferences before study implementation is strong.[37] It draws

attention to the role of understanding patients' knowledge and attitudes in helping to design clinical trials and in shaping the informed consent process.

An alternative is to seek patient consent *after* randomization, which allows patients the opportunity to refuse participation or to switch arms if they are unhappy with the arm to which they have been randomized. This is the Zelen approach, also called *randomized consent*, and it has been much debated.[38] Its use in palliative care research has been limited by preference for alternative approaches.[29]

Randomized discontinuation trials (i.e., enrichment design) involve exposure of all patients to the intervention initially. The design has been most often used in phase II trials of drug interventions.[39] Those whose condition deteriorates despite treatment are then excluded, with those who remain stable subsequently randomized between the intervention and control arms. The variety of options available underlines the importance of the project team and early involvement of a trial statistician.

Placebo and Other Comparisons

In undertaking a controlled trial of an intervention, a key decision is whether to compare this intervention with an established comparator, a placebo intervention, or nothing. The first question to address is whether there is an established standard intervention. There may be several standards, none of which may be fully validated, but all of which may have become established as standard practice in different care settings. Critical evaluation of the data for each of these interventions is required, and a decision then must be made about which to choose as the comparator. Considerations may include which is the best-validated choice, the most widely used option, or the internationally recognized standard.

The use of a placebo is influenced by the practicalities of providing a placebo, the ethical considerations of placebo versus active comparators, and the area under study. The first reaction in a palliative care setting may be that using placebo interventions in a symptomatic population with limited life expectancy is ethically unjust (see Chapter 22). In this setting, an argument can be proposed to alter the question from *why not* to *why*.

The word *placebo* describes an inactive or inert intervention. Its use in clinical trials is advocated in the testing of new interventions to provide an estimate of the true effect of the active arm. By definition, subjects in the placebo group do not receive any treatment, and this may be seen to oppose the Hippocratic code of beneficence and nonmaleficence. However, physicians also have a duty to prove that interventions are effective.

One area for which a placebo arm may be questioned is in pain control. It would be impossible to justify a placebo arm in a study looking at the analgesic efficacy of a new drug for most types of chronic cancer pain. How can the true effect of the new intervention be shown in this case? Ideally, this would be done by using a comparator that is known to have a fixed, certain effect (Fig. 28-3). However, this agent does not exist in real practice. If the two drugs (e.g., new drug E and morphine M as comparator) have similar effects, can we be sure that the effect of drug E is a true effect or a "placebo" effect? When design-

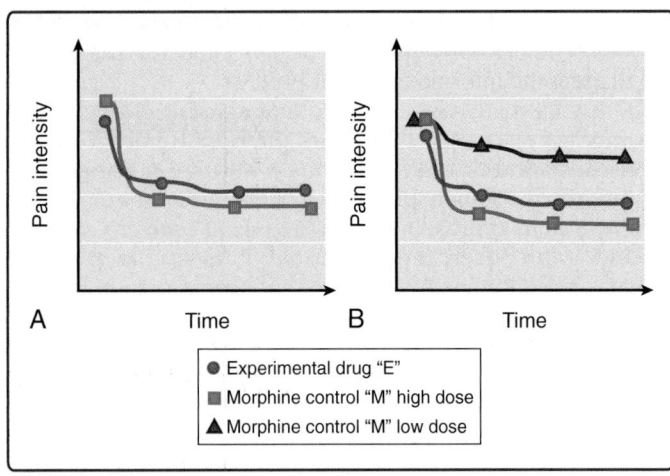

FIGURE 28-3 Defining the true effect of an analgesic in the absence of a control. A, Theoretically, the experimental drug is said to have an effect if the effect of morphine on pain control is fixed and consistent. In practice, we cannot be sure that the effects of both drugs were not the result of chance or a "placebo effect." **B,** A lower dose of morphine is included in this comparison. The difference between the experimental drug and high-dose morphine compared with the lower dose is reassuring in demonstrating the true effect of the experimental drug.

● Experimental drug "E"
■ Morphine control "M" high dose
▲ Morphine control "M" low dose

ing an analgesic study without a placebo, we must look for other ways of defining an internal index of effect. One way is to include a third arm using a lower dose of the comparator drug. If in our example the experimental drug and standard dose of morphine show significantly better analgesic effects compared with the lower dose of morphine, this suggests true benefit. However, even this approach can be ethically challenged. Are the patients receiving the lower dose being denied appropriate treatment? The investigator must be sure that if such a design is used, the lower dose of comparator drug is consistent with known analgesic benefit. This is where previous surveys or uncontrolled trial data may be helpful, as previously advocated.

What is the role of the placebo effect in placebo-controlled trials? This question is relevant to palliative care for several reasons:

- Will it invalidate results by underestimating true effect, particularly if we have small numbers?
- Are we better comparing with nothing rather than placebo?
- What is the role in nondrug interventions?

Much has been written about placebo effects.[40,41] Many issues related to therapeutic effects of placebo remain unclear, although it is certain that the size of the study population is important. The smaller the study population, the greater the potential risk of a placebo effect. The size of effect, however, is unpredictable and does not relate to the size of the effect in the active intervention arm. In our context, in which study sizes are often small, the placebo effect can be relevant.

In clinical practice, physicians find that some interventions that they did not expect to have a therapeutic effect work for what we call placebo reasons. A systematic review of whether placebo interventions outweigh no treatment in clinical trials found no significant differences between the two, except possibly from pain interventions, and even this may be caused by bias.[42] The use of placebos becomes even more interesting in nonpharmacological interventions, for which they may be difficult to construct, have ethical implications (e.g., sham surgery), or be confounded by other factors. A thought-provoking debate[43] on acupuncture argued that such interventions are inherently complex and the characteristic components

responsible for therapeutic effect difficult to define. Trying to construct a placebo or sham intervention for therapies such as acupuncture is risky and may underestimate effect. For example, the interaction between therapist and patient may be an active component but can be present in the intervention and control arms because it is thought to be an incidental part of the intervention.[43] This approach may extend to effects on other aspects of an individual's status by activities present in both arms, such as the impact of an intervention on quality of life. If the treatment under investigation is an analgesic, but patients incidentally have a separate domain of their quality of life improved (e.g., psychological functioning) by a strategy in both arms, the overall quality of life may improve because of this response shift rather than the primary intervention.[44]

In considering how to control for an intervention in palliative care studies, ethical and practical issues (e.g., complexity) are important. Most important are the availability and choice of an established comparator. If using a placebo, the sample size is relevant and can influence the degree of the placebo effect. Patients' understanding and preferences related to placebo-controlled trials and implications for the informed consent process must also be accounted for.

Recruitment and Consent

We have identified the threat to study validity by design and patient population factors prevalent in palliative care, but how should we recruit effectively and ethically (Box 28-3), and how important are the size and makeup of the patient sample? Identifying patients at an earlier, more stable point in their illness—if appropriate to the research question—can improve likelihood of entry into and completion of the trial. Engagement of other stakeholders, particularly professional and caregiver gatekeepers, patient groups, and opinion leaders, through educational and information promotion is essential. Dedicated research staff on the ground and effective mechanisms for data capture maximize identification of eligible patients and minimize the risk of data loss. Underpinning all of these processes are the ability to communicate effectively and honestly with patients and ensuring that if they do agree to participate, it is on the basis of their informed and free choice. The ethical issues regarding consent are explored elsewhere (see Chapter 22), but procedural issues are worthy of reflection.

Structured guidance on the process of gaining informed consent has been issued[45,46] and must be studied and adhered to in seeking approval of ethics or review boards. Key elements[47] in the consent process have been examined, along with how well or poorly they are adhered to. Relevant steps include a clear explanation of the experimental question, open discussion of the degree of equipoise (or uncertainty) relating to the treatment, the rate and sequence in which information is given, and the mode of information giving (e.g., written, verbal, video).[47] In working through these steps, the relevance of patients' knowledge and preferences resurfaces, as does the sensibility of defining these preferences ahead of time and exploring their influence on the whole process of consent.[48] We should explore preferences and patients' views of the consent process to better serve the research process in difficult contexts, such as palliative care. A study of prostate cancer patients suggested that this type of exploration can be enlightening and improve recruitment, and it served as an example of how qualitative research can enrich quantitative studies.[49] Asking "Whose equipoise is it anyway?"[50], Lilford focuses attention on the person who best defines the degree and importance of uncertainty in justifying a randomized, controlled trial design—researcher or patient? A blanket supposition of equipoise regarding a treatment's effects and side effects across a study population has the potential to discourage full discussion and assessment of the benefits and risks for each individual. These effects may vary considerably from patient to patient and should be integral to an informed consent. Supplementing procedural correctness with user involvement in project groups[51] and the use of qualitative methodologies (e.g., in feasibility studies) to assess motivation and preferences will be key to successful recruitment in palliative care studies in future.

This approach is particularly relevant because of the importance of the size of the study. Along with the issues of selection and observer bias, the issue of sample size is critical to study validity, and it has been a major pitfall in palliative care research. Undertaking a study that from the outset cannot provide a true statistical estimate of the effect because of inadequate sample size is ethically questionable. We have also seen its impact on placebo effects.

If an investigator is undertaking a controlled trial, there must be an estimation of sample size at the outset that will provide adequate statistical power to show a difference other than by chance (see Chapter 31). Even with all other things being equal, this random chance can still create significant variability. Some argue that 10 times more patients are needed to show clinical rather than statistical significance.[52] The alternative is to pool the results of several similar, smaller trials in a meta-analysis, provided they have similar designs, populations, and outcome measures.

The rigor of trial design is onerous. Questions should be focused and few in number; patients must be reasonably similar, be enrolled in large number, and remain for the duration of the study; and the type of control may be less obvious than we once thought. As the protocol develops, is there a danger that it becomes too far removed from the clinical starting point and therefore too impractical?

ISSUES OF PRAGMATISM AND COMPLEXITY

Scope of the Study

Studies that are tightly controlled, using narrowly defined interventions under ideal conditions, usually wish to provide evidence of a limited form of efficacy. They often elucidate a scientific principle (e.g., whether a nutritional supplement improves lean body mass) but may not address clinically relevant end points; these are *explanatory trials*.[53] In palliative care, questions of interest may be broader, patients more variable, and interventions more complex, and a refined approach to the randomized, controlled trial may not be possible. For example, a trial evaluating whether a nutritional supplement improves lean body mass does not tell us whether increased lean body mass improves quality of life or mobility or if most patients can take the supplement. An alternative is to use a pragmatic approach[53] by attempting to answer a question in a way that is as relevant as possible to the range of clinical settings and the patient it affects. This allows application of a trial design to a wider range of pharmacological and nonpharmacological interventions and seems particularly suited to a specialty that engages comprehensively with a multidisciplinary approach in varied settings. Other specialties, such as psychiatry, have embraced this approach.[54] It does not eschew the basic principles of the randomized, controlled trial, but it is instead practical in incorporating clinical questions that do not easily enable individual randomization or blinding. Particular attention is paid to ensuring that interventions are compared with clinically relevant alternatives; that diverse, appropriate patient groups are recruited; and that as broad a range of outcomes as possible is incorporated.[55] The outcomes should be directly relevant (e.g., improved mobility) rather than surrogate (e.g., improved muscle strength). This practical strategy promotes a balance between the apparent rigidity of randomized, controlled trial design and the temptation to abandon rigor in the face of complexity. Blinding may not be possible, and the design in accounting for this must ensure strict concealment procedures for randomization (so that researchers cannot predict which arm their patients are randomized to) and diligence in reporting outcomes.

The difficulties faced by researchers in adopting a pragmatic approach to complicated situations are well recognized,[56,57] and attempts are being made to redress the lack of infrastructural and funding support that have hindered practical assessment of complex but important interventions.[55,57]

There is concern that the apparent inflexibility in randomized, controlled trials has led to the abandonment of the approach in some areas of health care to the detriment of patients and the funding of services.[58] Some argue that the complexity of an intervention means that the parts are so interlinked that they cannot be broken down or simplified, defying the probabilistic approach. The Medical Research Council suggests that in approaching such dilemmas, there should be exploratory phases before definitive randomized, controlled trials, rather like phase I and II studies in drug trial design. These phases may use descriptive studies (similar to phase I studies) and qualitative research to better define the elements of the intervention and test the various components in a feasibility study (similar to phase II studies).[56,57] Hawe and colleagues[58] go further in arguing imaginatively for a restructuring of what is standardized within a controlled trial. They suggest that study validity depends on ensuring that key functions are standard rather than process elements—that "integrity defined functionally, rather than compositionally, is the key."[58] Thus, in a study to improve uptake of hospice services, it may be decided that the function is to reach out to minority groups and other nonusers. Traditionally, a set format would be described, such as stakeholder groups using predefined techniques randomized against usual referral practice, perhaps in a cluster randomized fashion. Some argue that the function remains standardized but the format may vary (e.g., steering groups of opinion leaders, outreach information that is adapted to local cultural and learning needs). This allows practical variability without compromising the core function.

Change and Its Measurement

In arguing for clarity and simplicity in asking the research question, we have implied a similar approach to that for outcomes and their measurement. This is particularly the case for the explanatory approach in which biomedical rather than clinical outcomes may predominate. The more outcomes we seek to measure, the more likely one will be significant by chance. We must therefore define outcomes and measurement tools up front and avoid a post hoc data trawl that will be biased.

This argues for a pragmatic approach with a broader range of outcomes measured. These may include societal outcomes using tools to measure health utility or health economic values. However, more outcomes require more patients to avoid random chance, which means that pragmatic studies may be prolonged and expensive and may therefore be difficult to fund.[55]

In a well-established area such as analgesia outcome measurement, it may be possible to pool data from several small trials, assuming the populations were similar and outcome measures were the same or at least capable of cross-interrogation. Sadly, this is not so, even for analgesic studies, and the large amounts of data cannot be ade-

quately interpreted because of a lack of consistency in the type of pain measurement tools used.[59] Other outcomes in palliative care, such as breathlessness,[60] have less developed or validated tools, and a prime function of national and international research agendas must be to ensure proper validation of tools in these areas and consensus on their use.[61] A comprehensive set of recommendations on the use and interpretation of pain measurement tools by an Expert Working Group of the European Association of Palliative Care provides an excellent example of how such guidance and consensus should be approached.[62] In preparing studies, we must make several decisions at the design stage:

- What are the outcomes we must measure, and what is the primary outcome?
- Which tool we will use (this must be validated for the primary outcome and for the population)?
- What will trigger measurement and when?
- What is the effect of the control arm on these outcomes?
- What will constitute a significant clinical, rather than statistical, benefit over the control arm?

CONCLUSIONS ABOUT WHAT MAKES A CLINICAL TRIAL WORK

How do we make a clinical trial happen in reality? Research ideas at an individual level must be harmonized with priorities identified at the national level by bodies such as the National Cancer Research Institute (NCRI) and National Institutes of Health (NIH) to obtain funding (see "Future Considerations"). The opportunities for research as education and research as training must be realized, and academic programs at masters and doctoral levels must be used to produce a skilled workforce. In such programs, students must be allocated supervision from and become embedded within their own local academic structures to ensure that they continue to integrate and develop key collaborative partnerships over time.

This type of development will lead to opportunities for large-scale studies. If studies of sufficient size and integrity are to be completed with such a complex patient group, a robust clinical trial or research collaborative infrastructure is essential. It will allow innovative trial design using a wide range of methodological expertise from broad

---

Future Considerations

- Research priorities should be identified at a national level and reflected in a focused palliative care research portfolio.
- Funding streams must be identified to ensure investment in palliative care research that is proportionate to funding of overall research activity.
- Collaboration between research groups and multidisciplinary clinicians is essential to meet the challenges of complex clinical research questions.
- A structured approach to the involvement of patients and other service users in research design is required.
- Innovative approaches to pragmatic trial design and assessment of complex interventions should form a core part of the research agenda.

strands of health and social care. It can provide the management capacity and information technology for adequate recruitment, data capture, and analysis. It also can provide the quality assurance to guarantee compliance with the demands of Good Clinical Practice (GCP) and the governance structures to deal with the responsibilities of research sponsorship and conduct of trials using medicinal products[63,64] and safety mechanisms for patients being recruited into the trial. The presence of such a framework maximizes the potential for trials of sufficient quality to reach completion and to provide results that will achieve widespread dissemination. The results can be integrated with clinical judgment and patients' values in reaching individual treatment decisions.

REFERENCES

1. Sackett DL, Rosenberg WM, Gray JAM, et al. Evidence based medicine: What it is and what it isn't. BMJ 1996;312:71-72.
2. Cochrane AL. Effectiveness and Efficiency: Random Reflections on Health Services. London: Royal Society of Medicine, 1971.
3. Guyatt G, Gutterman D, Baumann MH, et al. Grading strength of recommendations and quality of evidence in clinical guidelines. Chest 2006;129:174-181.
4. Materia E, Baglio G. Health, science and complexity. J Epidemiol Community Health 2005;59:534-535.
5. Glasziou P, Vandenbroucke J, Chalmers I. Assessing the quality of research. BMJ 2004;328:39-41.
6. Atkins D, Fink K, Slutsky J. Better information for better healthcare: The evidence-based practice center program and the agency for healthcare research and quality. Ann Intern Med 2005;142:1035-1041.
7. Atkins D, Best D, Briggs PA, et al. Grading quality of evidence and strength of recommendations. BMJ 2004;328:1490-1497.
8. Centre for Evidence-Based Medicine. Available at http://www.cebm.net/levels_of_evidence.asp (accessed September 8, 2007).
9. Witte CL, Witte MH, Kerwin A. Ignorance and the process of learning and discovery in medicine. Control Clin Trials 2004;15:1-4.
10. Cochrane AL, Blythe M. One Man's Medicine. London: BMJ Memoir Club, 1989.
11. Dudley HA. The controlled clinical trial and the advance of reliable knowledge: An outsider looks in. BMJ 1983;287:957-960.
12. Lyons RA, Jones S, Kemp A, et al. Development and use of a population based injury surveillance system: The All Wales Injury Surveillance System (AWISS). Inj Prev 2002;8:83-86.
13. Padkin A, Rowan K, Black N. Using high quality clinical databases to complement the results of randomised controlled trials: The case of recombinant human activated protein C. BMJ 2001;323:923-926.
14. Brown P, Brunnhuber K, Chalkidou K, et al. How to formulate research recommendations. BMJ 2006;333:804-806.
15. Hulley SB, Cummings SR. Designing Clinical Research. Baltimore: Williams & Wilkins, 1988.
16. Mayer D. Essential Evidence-Based Medicine. Cambridge: Cambridge University Press, 2004.
17. Thomas DP. Sailors, scurvy and science. J R Soc Med 1997;90:50-54.
18. Rinck GC, Van den Bos GAM, Kleijnen J, et al. Methodological issues in effectiveness research on palliative cancer care: A systematic review. J Clin Oncol 1997;15:1697-1707.
19. Jordhoy MS, Kaasa S, Fayers P, et al. Challenges in palliative care research; recruitment, attrition and compliance: Experience from a randomized controlled trial. Palliat Med 1999;13:299-310.
20. Cook AM, Finlay IG, Butler-Keating RJ. Recruiting into palliative care trials: Lessons learnt from a feasibility study. Palliat Med 2002;16:163-165.
21. Schulz KF, Chalmers I, Hayes RJ, et al. Empirical evidence of bias: Dimensions of methodological quality associated with estimates of treatment effects in controlled trials. JAMA 1995;273:408-412.
22. Carroll D, Tramer M, McQuay H, et al. Randomization is important in studies with pain outcomes: systematic review of transcutaneous electrical nerve stimulation in acute postoperative pain. Br J Anaesth 1996;77:798-803.
23. Schulz KF, Grimes D. Blinding in randomized trials: Hiding who got what. Lancet 2002;359:696-700.
24. Ionnidis JPA, Haidich A-B, Pappa M, et al. Comparison of evidence of treatment effects in randomised and nonrandomised studies. JAMA 2001;286:821-830.
25. Bruera E, Ripamonti C, Brenneis C, et al. A randomized double-blind crossover trial of intravenous lidocaine in the treatment of neuropathic cancer pain. J Pain Symptom Manage 1992;7:138-140.
26. Coluzzi PH, Schwartzberg L, Conroy JD, et al. Breakthrough cancer pain: A randomized trial comparing oral transmucosal fentanyl citrate (OTFC) and morphine sulphate immediate release (MSIR). Pain 2001;91:123-130.
27. Abernethy AP, Currow DC, Frith P, et al. Randomised, double blind, placebo controlled crossover trial of sustained release morphine for the management of refractory dyspnoea. BMJ 2003;327:523-528.
28. Jordhoy MS, Fayers P, Saltnes T, et al. Palliative care intervention and death at home: A cluster randomised trial. Lancet 2000;356:888-893.
29. Fowell A, Johnstone R, Finlay IG, et al. Design of trials with dying patients: A feasibility study of cluster randomisation versus randomised consent. Palliat Med 2006;20:799-804.
30. Jordhoy MS, Fayers PM, Ahlner-Elmqvist M, et al. Lack of concealment may lead to selection bias in cluster randomized trials of palliative care. Palliat Med 2002;16:43-49.
31. Campbell MK, Elbourne DR, Altman DG, for the CONSORT Group. CONSORT statement: Extension to cluster randomized trials. BMJ 2004;328:702-708.
32. King M. The effects of patients' and practitioners' preferences on randomized clinical trials. Palliat Med 2000;14:539-542.
33. Torgerson D, Sibbald B. Understanding controlled trials: What is a patient preference trial? BMJ 1998;316:360.
34. Olschewski M, Scheurlen H. Comprehensive cohort study: An alternative to randomized consent design in a breast preservation trial. Meth Inform Med 1985;24:131-134.
35. Ward E, King M, Lloyd M, et al. Randomised controlled trial of non-directive counselling, cognitive-behaviour therapy, and usual general practitioner care for patients with depression. I. Clinical effectiveness. BMJ 2000;321: 1383-1388.
36. Maughan TS, James RD, Kerr DJ, et al. Comparison of intermittent and continuous palliative chemotherapy for advanced colorectal cancer: A multicentre randomised trial. Lancet 2003;361:457-464.
37. Halpern S. Prospective patient preference assessment: A method to enhance the ethics and efficacy of randomized controlled trials. Control Clin Trials 2002;23:274-288.
38. Altman DG ,Whitehead J, Parmar MKB, et al. Randomised consent designs in cancer clinical trials. Eur J Cancer 1995;31A:1934-1944.
39. Stadler WM, Rosner G, Small E, et al. Successful implementation of the randomized discontinuation trial design: An application to the study of the putative antiangiogenic agent carboxyaminoimidazole in renal cell carcinoma—CALGB 69901. J Clin Oncol 2005;23:3726-3732.
40. Miller FG, Rosenstein DL. The nature and power of the placebo effect. J Clin Epidemiol 2006;59:331-335.
41. McQuay HJ, Moore RA. Placebo. Postgrad Med J 2005;81:155-160.
42. Hrobjartsson A, Gotzsche PC. Is the placebo powerless? Update of a systematic review with 52 new randomized trials comparing placebo with no treatment. J Intern Med 2004;256:91-100.
43. Paterson C, Dieppe P. Characteristic and incidental (placebo) effects in complex interventions such as acupuncture. BMJ 2005;330:1202-1205.
44. Rees J, Clarke MG, Waldron D, et al. The measurement of response shift in patients with advanced prostate cancer and their partners. Health Qual Life Outcomes 2005;3:21-28.
45. Central Office for Research Ethics Committees (COREC). Available at http://www.corec.org.uk (accessed September 8, 2007).
46. Office for Human Research Protections (OHRP). http://www.hhs.gov/ohrp/ (accessed September 8, 2007).
47. Brown RF, Butow PN, Ellis P, et al. Seeking informed consent to cancer clinical trials: Describing current practice. Soc Sci Med 2004;58:2445-2457.
48. Bower P, King M, Nazareth I, et al. Patient preferences in randomized controlled trials: Conceptual framework and implications for research. Soc Sci Med 2005;61:685-695.
49. Donovan J, Mills N, Smith M, et al. Improving design and conduct of randomized trials by embedding them in qualitative research: ProtecT (prostate testing for cancer and treatment) study. BMJ 2002;325:766-770.
50. Lilford RJ. Ethics of clinical trials from a bayesian and decision analytic perspective: Whose equipoise is it anyway? BMJ 2003;326:980-981.
51. Bradburn J, Maher J. User and carer participation in research in palliative care. Palliat Med 2005;19:91-92.
52. Moore RA, Gavaghan D, Tramer MR, et al. Size is everything—large amounts of information are needed to overcome random effects in estimating direction and magnitude of treatment effects. Pain 1998;78:209-216.
53. Schwartz D, Lallouch J. Explanatory and pragmatic attitudes in therapeutic trials. J Chron Dis 1967;20:637-648.
54. Hotopf M. The pragmatic randomized controlled trial. Adv Psychiatr Treat 2002;8:326-333.
55. Tunis SR, Stryer DB, Clancy CM. Practical clinical trials. Increasing the value of clinical research for decision making in clinical and health policy. JAMA 2003;290:1624-1632.
56. Campbell M, Fitzpatrick R, Haines A, et al. Framework for design and evaluation of complex interventions to improve health. BMJ 2000;321:694-696.
57. Medical Research Council. A Framework for the Development and Evaluation of Randomized Controlled Trials for Complex Interventions to Improve Health. London: MRC, 2000.
58. Hawe P, Shiell A, Riley T. Complex interventions: How "out of control" can a randomized controlled trial be? BMJ 2004;328:1561-1563.
59. Caraceni A, Brunelli C, Martini C, et al. Cancer pain assessment in clinical trials. A review of the literature (1999-2002). J Pain Symptom Manage 2005;29: 507-519.
60. Dorman S, Byrne A, Edwards A. Which measurement scales should we use to measure breathlessness in palliative care? A systematic review. Palliat Med 2007;21:177-191.
61. National Cancer Research Institute. Supportive and Palliative Care Research in the UK: Report of the NCRI Strategic Planning Group on Supportive and Palliative care. London: NCRI, 2004.

62. Caraceni A, Cherny N, Fainsinger R, et al. Pain measurement tools and methods in clinical research in palliative care: Recommendations of an Expert Working Group of the European Association of Palliative Care. J Pain Symptom Manage 2002;23:239-255.
63. International Conference on Harmonisation Good Clinical Practice (ICH GCP). Available at emea.eu.int/pdfs/human/ich/013595.en.pdf (accessed September 8, 2007).
64. The Medicines for Human Use (Clinical Trials) Regulations 2004. Available at www.opsi.gov.uk/si/si2004/20041031.htm (accessed September 8, 2007).

SUGGESTED READING

Hulley SB, Cummings SR. Designing Clinical Research. Baltimore: Williams & Wilkins, 1988.
International Conference on Harmonisation Good Clinical Practice (ICH GCP). Available at emea.eu.int/pdfs/human/ich/013595.en.pdf (accessed September 8, 2007).
Mayer D. Essential Evidence-Based Medicine. Cambridge: University Press, 2004.
Medical Research Council. A Framework for the Development and Evaluation of Randomized Controlled Trials for Complex Interventions to Improve Health. London: MRC, 2000.
Tunis SR, Stryer DB, Clancy CM. Practical clinical trials. Increasing the value of clinical research for decision making in clinical and health policy. JAMA 2003;290:1624-1632.

CHAPTER **29**

Biostatistics and Epidemiology

Matthew T. Karafa and Lisa A. Rybicki

K E Y   P O I N T S

- Before starting a research study, it is critical to carefully consider the study questions and determine whether you can collect the appropriate data to answer the questions.

- A **well-developed** study design is more important than the statistical analysis. A complex, sophisticated analysis method cannot compensate for poor design elements.

- Accurate data collection is critical to a successful study. Data need to be checked thoroughly before analysis.

- Many statistical tests are available to analyze data. The choice of an appropriate test depends on an understanding of the data and the underlying assumptions of the statistical tests.

- There are good ways to summarize analysis results—and bad ways. Choose methods that convey important findings in a concise manner.

Broadly defined, biostatistics uses statistical methods to answer questions in medicine and health sciences, whereas epidemiology uses statistical methods to identify risk factors for developing disease. The biostatistical process is not limited to data analysis. It instead begins

with careful assessment of the population to be studied, a well-planned study design, justification of the study size, and accurate data collection and data entry. Only after these steps are completed can analysis begin. This chapter attempts to do the following:

- Define study designs and their advantages and disadvantages
- Define the basic types of data and suggest tabular and graphical ways to summarize them
- Describe common statistical tests and guidelines for their use
- Suggest methods for data collection and cleaning
- Outline steps in conducting a research study

STUDY DESIGNS

Study designs can be experimental or observational. Experimental designs attempt to control for nuisance differences between treatment groups, called *bias* or *confounding*, by randomizing patients to treatment groups.[1] When done correctly, randomized studies yield the strongest evidence of association between treatment and outcome. In contrast, observational studies investigate treatment effects without randomizing patients to treatment groups.[2] These studies can be done when ethical, practical, or financial considerations prohibit a randomized experimental design. In observational studies, confounding and bias are typically addressed in the statistical analysis.

Several observational designs are available, each with advantages and disadvantages. Cohort designs start with patients at risk for a particular outcome and divide them into groups based on their exposure to some treatment or environmental agent. They are then followed over time until the outcome develops. Prospective cohort studies start with current exposure status and follow patients forward. Retrospective cohort studies look back over time (e.g., medical record reviews) to assess past exposure; outcome can be assessed at the current time or some future time. In both designs, the statistical measure of association is called the *relative risk*. The primary disadvantage with cohort designs is cost. Following patients takes time, can be expensive, and is often impractical. Changes in the definitions of the outcome or exposures, or both, can occur over time, adversely affecting inferences that can be made from the study. Differences in treatments can result in differential dropout rates. However, these disadvantages are offset by the ability to make a stronger inference about the outcome. Their prospective nature lets cohort studies directly evaluate the relative risk and creates the correct cause-and-effect relationships.

Case-control designs start with a group with the outcome of interest and a group without it. Prior exposure status is then assessed from medical records, direct interviews, surrogate interviews, or other sources. Case-control studies then assess differences in the exposure of interest that happened before the current time.[3] For such designs, the statistical measure of association is known as the *odds ratio*. For a rare disease (<10% prevalence in the population of interest), the odds ratio is a good approximation of relative risk. The advantages of case-control relative to cohort designs and randomized, controlled trials are that they are typically less costly, easier to manage, and obtain faster results. They are often the only practical method to assess diseases with a long incubation period (e.g., cancer), when the time between exposure and outcome may be decades. The main problem with case-control studies is that of cause and effect. Because we start with diseased and nondiseased groups and retrospectively assign exposure status, there is much potential for confounding associations. Confounding is an association between two exposures that can lead to the erroneous conclusion that an unrelated exposure causes the outcome. Recall bias also can be a problem, because persons with the illness are more likely to recall events than those who are healthy. Although randomized studies are considered to provide the most definitive proof of association between exposure variables and outcomes, well-designed observational studies can also yield valuable evidence of association.

VARIABLE TYPES

There are two basic variable types: categorical and continuous. Categorical variables have values that can be classified into one of two or more categories. Two types of categorical variables are nominal and ordinal. Nominal variables have categories with no natural order, such as gender, race, or cancer primary site. Ordinal variables have categories that have a natural order, such as symptom severity (e.g., none, mild, moderate, severe) or Eastern Cooperative Oncology Group Performance Status. A binary (or dichotomous) variable is a categorical variable with two categories. Categorical variables are summarized as frequency counts and percentages. Percentages should be reported as whole numbers or with one decimal place; any more is excessive. Categorical variables can be graphed using bar charts. The order of categories in the bar chart influences the visual impact. Logical order is best for ordinal variables, and frequency order (i.e., ascending or descending) is best for nominal variables.

Continuous variables are those whose values may be any number within an interval or continuum, such as age or weight. The most common descriptive statistics for continuous variables include the mean, standard deviation, median, interquartile range (25th to 75th percentile), or range (minimum to maximum). The choice of descriptive statistics depends on the statistical test used to analyze the data (discussed later). Continuous variables can be graphed in various ways; the best methods show as much data as possible without being too busy. One good method is the boxplot, which shows the median, interquartile range, and range; boxplots can be done with or without individual data points, depending on the size of the study (Fig. 29-1A). Another common graphical method is disparaged by statisticians as "dynamite" or "detonator" plots; they take up much space to show two descriptive statistics—the mean and a measure of variation, usually the standard deviation (see Fig. 29-1B).

A special case of a continuous variable is one in which all of the values are not observed, such as survival. If all patients in a study are followed until they die, survival is observed for everyone, and survival is a continuous variable. More commonly, patients are followed for a fixed time period; at the end of the study, there is a mix of those

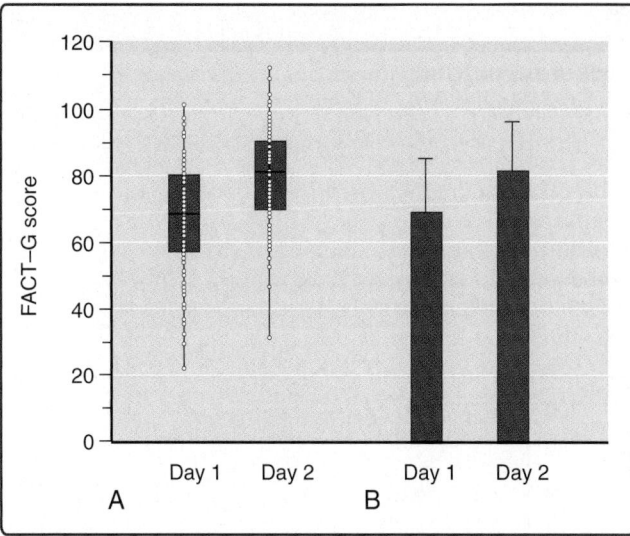

FIGURE 29-1   Quality of life measured by the Functional Assessment of Cancer Therapy–General (FACT-G) instrument at two time points. A, In the boxplots, the boxes indicate the middle 50% of the data, which is the 25th to the 75th percentile or interquartile range. The *thick line* inside the boxes indicates the median. Whiskers indicate the full range of the data. Individual data points are displayed as *circles*. B, Detonator plots. The top of the box indicates the mean, and the *bar* above the box represents one standard deviation.

who have died and those still alive. In this setting, you have actual survival for the people who died and minimum survival for those alive; this is known as *censored data*. A common method for graphing censored data is the Kaplan-Meier curve (Fig. 29-2).

A concept related to all variable types is that of a *probability distribution function* (PDF). A PDF describes the shape of the variable's distribution. The bell-shaped curve or normal distribution is one example of a PDF for continuous variables. Many statistical tests are based on assumptions regarding the underlying PDF, and it is useful to understand the shape of the PDF to decide whether the assumption seems reasonable for your data.

UNIVARIABLE AND MULTIVARIABLE ANALYSIS

The purpose of many analyses is to identify variables associated with some end point. Common names for the end point include dependent variable, outcome variable, response variable, and y variable. Common names for variables that may affect the end point include independent variable, explanatory variable, predictor variable, x variable, prognostic factor, and risk factor. For consistency, we call them outcome and explanatory variables. The choice of an appropriate statistical test to analyze data depends on whether the outcome and explanatory variables are categorical or continuous and whether the underlying assumptions of the statistical test seem reasonable.

Many statistical tests can be classified as parametric or nonparametric. Although both types require assumptions regarding specific aspects of the data, the major difference between the two is that parametric tests are based on assumptions about the underlying PDF of the outcome variable, whereas nonparametric tests are not. Nonparametric tests are also referred to as *distribution-free tests*.

TABLE 29-1	Univariate Analysis of a Continuous Outcome	
USE OF THE OUTCOME	**PARAMETRIC TEST**	**NONPARAMETRIC TEST***
Assess outcome of a single group	One-sample *t* test	Wilcoxon signed rank test
Compare outcomes of two or more independent groups	*t* test (2 groups) Analysis of variance (ANOVA) (3+ groups)	Wilcoxon rank sum test (2 groups) Kruskal-Wallis test (3+ groups)
Compare status before and after treatment in a single group	Paired *t* test	Wilcoxon signed rank test
Assess a linear association of the outcome with another continuous variable	Pearson correlation Simple linear regression	Spearman rank correlation Rank regression

*These tests are also appropriate for ordinal categorical outcomes.

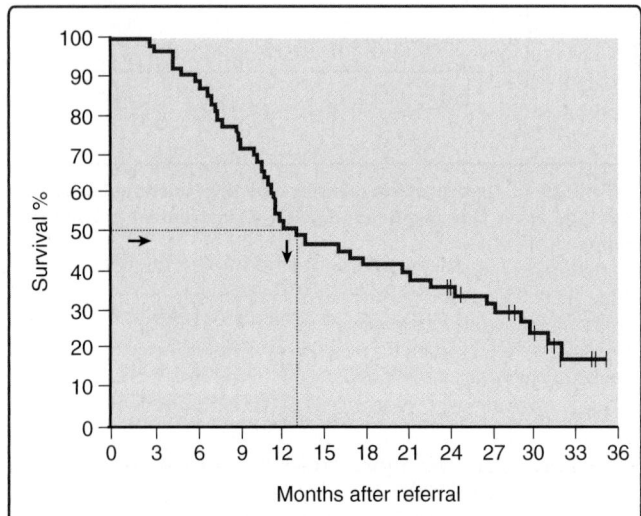

FIGURE 29-2 **Kaplan-Meier survival curve.** *Small vertical lines* on the curve indicate patients who are censored, and drops in the curve indicate deaths. *Arrows* and *dotted lines* are not typically included, but they are shown here to illustrate how an estimate of median survival can be obtained from the curve. To do this, draw a horizontal line from 50% on the survival axis until it intersects the curve, and then draw a vertical line straight down to the time axis. As shown on this curve, median survival is approximately 13 months. Similarly, survival estimates at any given time point can be approximated by starting at that time, drawing a vertical line up until it intersects the curve, and then drawing a horizontal line to the left to see where it intersects the survival axis.

TABLE 29-2	Univariate Analysis of a Censored Continuous Outcome
USE OF THE OUTCOME	**METHOD OR TEST**
Assess outcome of a single group	Kaplan-Meier estimates
Compare outcomes of two or more independent groups	Log-rank test Wilcoxon test Cox regression
Assess association of the outcome with a continuous variable	Cox regression

TABLE 29-3	Univariate Analysis of a Binary Categorical Outcome
USE OF THE OUTCOME	**METHOD OR TEST**
Assess outcome of a single group	Goodness-of-fit test
Compare outcomes of two or more independent groups	Chi-square test, Fisher exact test
Compare the status before and after treatment in a single group	McNemar test
Assess the association of the outcome with a continuous variable	Logistic regression

Univariable (or univariate) analysis examines the association of one explanatory variable with one outcome variable. Multivariable analysis examines the association of multiple explanatory variables with one outcome variable. In the medical literature, multivariable analysis is sometimes (incorrectly) called multivariate analysis. Technically, multivariate analysis examines the association of one or more explanatory variables with multiple outcome variables.

Univariable Analysis Methods

Common statistical tests are described for a continuous outcome (Table 29-1), a censored continuous outcome (Table 29-2), and a binary outcome (Table 29-3), along with suggestions for when these tests can be used. With the exception of paired analyses, notice that all of these tests assume there is one observation per patient. More complex methods exist for situations that involve multiple observations per patient.[4]

Multivariable Analysis

Many statistical methods are available for multivariable analysis. In general, multiple linear regression is used for a continuous outcome, multivariable Cox regression for a censored continuous outcome, and multiple logistic regression analysis for a binary outcome. There are often specific names for the general statistical tests, depending on whether explanatory variables are continuous, categorical, or a combination of the two. Regardless of the name, the underlying idea is to use multiple explanatory variables to develop a statistical model for the association with or prediction of a single outcome.

There are limitations on the number of explanatory variables that can be included in a multivariable model. To prevent overfitting the model, a guideline (sometimes called the *rule of 10*) is to include at most one variable for every 10 observations if the outcome is continuous, one variable for every 10 events if the outcome is censored, or one variable for every 10 patients in the smaller of two categories if the outcome is binary. To illustrate, suppose a 200-patient study assessed three outcomes: quality of life (continuous), response to treatment (binary;

120 patients responded, 80 did not), and survival (censored continuous; 32 patients died). A multiple linear regression model for quality of life should include at most 20 variables. A logistic regression model for response to treatment should include at most 8 variables (not 12), and a Cox regression for survival should include at most 3 variables.

The approach to multivariable analysis depends entirely on the study question. If the purpose is to compare outcome for two treatment groups, statistical adjustment can be made for explanatory variables that differ between groups or variables associated with outcome. If this violates the rule of 10, adjustments should be made for variables that are different between treatments and associated with outcome. If the purpose is to identify prognostic factors for an outcome, only variables that are statistically significant may be included in the final model.

Methods of Analysis

The *one-sample t test* compares the mean with a hypothesized value and assumes the sample was selected randomly from a population with a normal distribution (see Table 29-1). Results are often described with the mean and standard deviation. The *Wilcoxon signed rank test* can be used when the population is not normally distributed; results are often described with the median and range or interquartile range. Both tests are appropriate when the data are paired, such as observations obtained before and after a treatment. In this setting, the difference between each pair of data points is calculated, and one-group tests are applied to those differences. The one-sample t test on paired data is called a *paired t test*.

Analysis of variance (ANOVA) compares means among multiple groups and assumes samples were randomly selected from normally distributed populations with equal variances (see Table 29-1). The *Kruskal-Wallis test* can be used when ANOVA assumptions are violated. Analogous tests for two groups are the t test and Wilcoxon rank sum test.

Pearson correlation assesses the strength and direction of a linear association between two variables (see Table 29-1). Correlation ranges from −1 to +1. Values near 0 indicate little or no linear association, and values close to +1 indicate a strong linear association. Negative values indicate that as values of one variable increase, values of the other decrease; positive values indicate that as values of one variable increase, values of the other also increase. Correlation between two variables is usually depicted as a scatter plot. *Spearman rank correlation* can be used instead of the Pearson correlation when there are outliers (i.e., extreme values) in the data, and it has the same interpretation as the Pearson correlation. Neither test is appropriate if the association between variables is not linear.

Simple linear regression is another method of assessing association between two continuous variables (see Table 29-1). If one of the variables is clearly an outcome and the other an explanatory variable, simple linear regression allows you to predict the outcome for different values of the explanatory variable. *Rank regression,* which is simple linear regression done on the ranked outcome variable, can be used when the outcome is not normally distributed.

The *Kaplan-Meier method*, or product-limit method, is used to estimate the percentage of patients with the outcome at any time within the range of follow-up (see Table 29-2). One-sample tests are available to compare these estimates with a hypothesized value.

The *log-rank test* and *Wilcoxon test* are methods to compare Kaplan-Meier curves between two or more groups (see Table 29-2). The log-rank test, which is most commonly reported in medical literature, is used when the hypothesis involves group differences that exist across the range of follow-up. The Wilcoxon test is used when the hypothesis involves early group differences that may not persist over time. The test of choice should be determined based on the hypothesis that is proposed *before* examining any data. It is not appropriate to perform both tests and choose the one that is more significant. Results are usually presented in tabular form as estimates at selected time points within each group or graphically as Kaplan-Meier curves.

Cox regression, or Cox proportional hazards analysis, is a method to assess the association of categorical or continuous explanatory variables with a censored outcome variable (see Table 29-2). Results are usually presented in tabular format as the hazard ratio (HR), 95% confidence interval for the hazard ratio, and corresponding P value.

The *goodness-of-fit test* is a special case of the chi-square test (see Table 29-3). It tests the observed percentage of events against some prespecified percentage of events.

The *chi-square test* and the *Fisher exact test* compare proportions (percentages) between two or more groups (see Table 29-3). The chi-square test has a variation called the *chi-square test with Yates continuity correction*. Most statistical packages can calculate expected frequencies for a contingency table. Although not all statisticians agree, one rule of thumb is to use the chi-square test if the total study size is more than 40, Yates' continuity-corrected chi-square test for a study size of 20 to 40, and the Fisher exact test for a study size of less than 20 or for a study size of 20 to 40 if any of the expected frequencies are less than 5.

The *McNemar test* is used to compare proportions between two dependent groups (see Table 29-3). This is similar to the concept of a paired t test for a continuous outcome.

Logistic regression assesses the association of a continuous explanatory variable with a binary outcome (see Table 29-3). It can also be used with a categorical explanatory variable, although it is more common to report this with chi-square–type statistics. Results of logistic regression are usually presented in tabular format as an odds ratio (OR), 95% confidence interval for the odds ratio, and corresponding P value.

DATA COLLECTION AND CLEANING

Good statistical analysis cannot be done without good data. There are endless debates about the best tools for data storage. The most commonly encountered methods include text files (i.e., delimited ASCII files), Excel spreadsheets, and databases such as Microsoft Access or Oracle. Data are sometimes recorded first on data collection forms or entered directly into the computerized database or spreadsheet.

Regardless of the data storage method, it is critical to examine the data for accuracy and consistency before analysis. To do this, obtain frequency counts for all study variables. For categorical variables, look for inconsistent coding and invalid values. If frequency counts for gender appear as *M, F, m, f,* and *n,* check the data; *M* and *m* probably represent males, *F* and *f* probably represent females, and *n* may be a typographical error or a code to indicate gender was not available. Because most analysis packages are case sensitive and many do not recognize missing value codes, check the entry *n,* and make the other values all lower or all upper case. If *n* represents a missing value code, remove it, and leave that variable field blank; otherwise, *n* will be analyzed as a third category of gender. Many statisticians recommend using numeric coding for categorical variables to prevent this type of error (e.g., 1 for male and 2 for female), but others believe that data entry will be more accurate if logical codes are used, assuming the codes are used consistently. For continuous variables, look for obvious outliers such as a hemoglobin value of 134 when all of the other values range from 4.2 to 16.9; in this case, 134 probably should have been 13.4. When time intervals need to be calculated, enter the relevant dates, and calculate the intervals using the computer rather than entering a self-calculated interval. Dates should be entered in a format that includes month, day, and four-digit year. Examine individual date ranges and time intervals calculated from these dates to see if they seem reasonable. Intervals such as age or survival should never be negative. In studies that should have one data record per patient, examine frequency counts of the unique study identification number and ensure there are no duplicates. These types of inspection cannot identify data entry errors that are incorrect but fall within a viable range, but they can identify nonsensical data.

STEPS IN CONDUCTING A RESEARCH STUDY

These are five main steps of the biostatistical process:

1. *Define the purpose of the study.* Carefully consider study questions, and identify variables that can reliably be obtained to answer these questions. Write a study proposal that clearly describes the study design, variables to be collected, justification for the study size, and an analysis plan.
2. *Obtain good data.* Good data are compiled from well-defined underlying variables. Carefully collect the data. Enter it into a spreadsheet or database, and check it for obvious errors. After you are confident the data are correct, begin the analysis.
3. *Describe the data.* Use standard descriptive statistics or graphs to summarize the data. For a single group study summarize data for all study subjects. For a study with multiple groups, summarize the data by group.
4. *Analyze the data.* Analyze the data as described in the statistical analysis plan of your study protocol.
5. *Report results.* Provide sufficient information to describe the study design, to justify study size, and to show study findings. Refer to the study protocol

to be sure you answered all of the study questions. Indicate in your report which end points are primary, which are secondary, and which are exploratory. Include tables and graphs to illustrate the main findings. Report *P* values from statistical tests numerically, and include at most three decimal places. A common convention is to report findings with a *P* value greater than .05 to two decimal places, those from .001 to .050 to three decimal places, and those smaller than .001 as $P < .001$. It is never sufficient to report $P > .05$ (or NS for not significant) because the magnitude of the *P* value provides important information about the significance of the findings.

CONCLUSIONS

Because there are many ways to design and analyze a research study, it is best to consult with a biostatistician early. You will never find a biostatistician who knows everything about statistics, just as you will never find a physician who understands all areas of medicine. However, most biostatisticians have specialized training in medical statistics and can provide invaluable assistance with study design, justification of study size, analysis, interpretation, and presentation. If you wait until after the data are collected, you may be dismayed to discover the data cannot be analyzed. There are hundreds of available statistical analysis methods that are based on underlying assumptions; the best analysis depends entirely on which assumptions seem most reasonable for your data. Never try to analyze data without an understanding of the assumptions and the ability to check them. Failure to do so can result in inappropriate usage of statistical tests, which may lead to erroneous conclusions about the data.

Many statistical analysis packages allow you to obtain results for a statistical test regardless of the appropriateness of that test and may yield results that lead you to believe the analysis is valid when it is not. When in doubt, consult a biostatistician. Good design and analysis take time; allow for it.

We recommend simplifying studies as much as possible. This is critical in a palliative medicine setting, which has a fragile patient population, many of whom do not have the energy or ability to participate in lengthy assessments.[5] Many of the best studies are designed to get the minimum data needed to answer the question without placing unnecessary burden on patients. If the study design is too complex and patients are not able to complete the study, the problems of missing data can add a level of complexity to the analysis that may be intractable. Rarely can you answer every question about a given topic in a single study. By designing the study in an appropriate manner, others can use your results and build on them.

REFERENCES

1. Lilienfeld AM, Lilienfeld DE. Foundations of Epidemiology. Oxford: Oxford University Press, 1980.
2. Kelsey JL, Whittemore AS, Evans AS, Thompson WD. Methods in Observational Epidemiology, 2nd ed. Oxford: Oxford University Press, 1996.
3. Kleinbaum DG, Kupper LL, Morgenstern H. Epidemiologic Research: Principles and Quantitative Methods. New York: John Wiley & Sons, 1982.
4. Matthews JN, Altman DG, Campbell MJ, et al. Analysis of serial measurements in medical research. BMJ 1990;300:230-235.
5. Bruera E: Ethical issues in palliative care research. J Palliat Care 1994;10:7-9.

SUGGESTED READING

Daly LE, Bourke GJ. Interpretation and Uses of Medical Statistics, 5th ed. New York: Blackwell Science, 2000.

Gallin JI (ed). Principles and Practice of Clinical Research. New York: Academic Press, 2002.

Glantz SA. Primer of Biostatistics, 5th ed. New York: McGraw-Hill, 2002.

Katz MH. Multivariable Analysis: A Practical Guide for Clinicians. Cambridge: Cambridge University Press, 1999.

Lang TA, Secic M. How to Report Statistics in Medicine: Annotated Guidelines for Authors, Editors, and Reviewers, 2nd ed. Philadelphia: American College of Physicians, 2006.

Norman GR, Streiner DL. Biostatistics: The Bare Essentials, 2nd ed. London: BC Decker, 2000.

van Belle G. Statistical Rules of Thumb. New York: Wiley-Interscience, 2002.

Walker GA. Common Statistical Methods for Clinical Research with SAS Examples, 2nd ed. Cary, NC: SAS Institute, 2002.

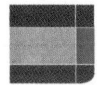

CHAPTER **30**

Symptom Research

Badi El Osta and Eduardo Bruera

KEY POINTS

- Research in symptom control is important because of the paucity of evidence-based therapeutic options.

- Symptom assessment is the first step in symptom research. Validity and reliability of instruments and definition of outcome measures are paramount in building clinical trials.

- There may be specific characteristics of the palliative care population, such as rapidly changing clinical conditions, multiple symptoms, deteriorating cognitive functions, and ethical considerations, that require attention in designing clinical trials.

- The symptoms of advanced illnesses require more emphasis in studies.

Physical and psychosocial symptoms are a major burden for palliative care patients. They are inadequately addressed by conventional medical care, and symptoms can significantly impair patients' quality of life and family dynamics.

Clinical programs in symptom control and palliative care were developed to address the complex, multidimensional, and dynamic nature of the unmet needs of terminally ill patients and their families.[1] However, research in this growing field did not evolve at the same pace as clinical programs or education. In the absence of good-quality evidence to guide our assessment and interventions, clinical practice in symptom control can lead to significant variations in practice, expose patients to futile treatments, and make the outcomes and cost of care unpredictable.

Increased research is important for the overall improvement of palliative medicine, but symptom research in palliative care faces several challenges. The patient population often is extremely ill and therefore unable to complete lengthy questionnaires or undergo complex tests. Patients are affected by many symptoms simultaneously, and the presence of and changes in one symptom can influence the intensity of another symptom. For example, an improvement in pain using an opioid is capable of increasing preexistent nausea, constipation, sedation, and confusion in a given patient. Research designs must control for these variables. Patients frequently suffer changing symptom problems and complications, making lengthy studies impractical because of the large number of dropouts. Most patients become unable to report their own symptoms at some point during the course of their illness. Palliative care patients have difficulty attending ambulatory clinics and frequently require evaluation at home or in inpatient hospice units. A considerable portion of the time of the research assistance is spent trying to identify patients for studies and conducting community-based assessment. The following sections focus on methodological issues in symptom assessment and management research (Box 30-1).

RESEARCH IN SYMPTOM ASSESSMENT

Terminally ill patients develop a number of devastating physical and psychological symptoms[2] that are disease related, treatment related, related to concurrent comorbid illnesses, or a combination of all three. Health care professionals may rely on their professional judgment, may wait until patients spontaneously complain of symptoms, or may be hard pressed to find time to address these symptoms. A priority in symptom research for better management of cancer-related symptoms is to improve the symptom assessment process by testing and standardizing tools that encourage patients to report their symptoms and provide concrete information about the effectiveness and outcomes of symptom control treatments.

Frequency of Cancer-Related Symptoms

The characteristics of a patient's symptom burden are different in each disease. For example, a patient with congestive heart failure may have dyspnea as his main symptom, whereas a patient with bone cancer mainly complains about pain. The patient's symptom burden can be different within the same disease. For example, an asymptomatic patient newly diagnosed with prostate cancer (stage

---

Box 30-1 Difficulties in Palliative Care Research

- Extremely ill patient population
- Symptoms occurring in clusters
- Changes in symptoms and complications
- Symptom changes that influence other symptoms
- Difficulty in attending ambulatory clinics by patients
- Limited number of academic faculty in most universities
- Lack of research funding
- Lack of industry interest in drug development for palliative care

I) starts to complain of back pain when his disease becomes advanced. These characteristics can be different for patients with the same disease status. This is the case for an asymptomatic patient newly diagnosed with metastatic colon cancer who is receiving chemotherapy in the outpatient setting compared with another patient with metastatic colon cancer who is delirious in the palliative care unit.

The frequency of cancer-related symptoms is different in each disease, stage of disease, and setting. Few studies have reported the frequency of cancer-related symptoms. However, more research is needed on specific cancers, on specific inception points in the natural course of cancer, and on specific settings to study the appropriate characteristics of symptom burden of each malignancy at any point in its course.

Some studies[2] have examined the prevalence of symptoms at the end of life. Fatigue was reported to be the most common symptom in different palliative care settings. However, pain, depression, and anxiety were reported to be the most distressing for advanced cancer patients. Other studies[3] reported lack of energy, worry, feeling sad, pain, feeling nervous, drowsiness, and dry mouth as the most frequently reported symptoms in inpatients or outpatients with breast, prostate, colon, or ovarian cancer.

Psychometric Assessment

Any acceptable symptom measure must demonstrate adequate reliability and validity, be able to capture changes over time and give information sufficient for decision-making, and be easy to understand and to complete with minimum response burden for patients and medical staff. *Reliability* refers to the consistency or reproducibility of measurement. *Validity* refers to whether the instrument is measuring what it is designed to measure. We offer some examples of research in this area.

The Edmonton Symptom Assessment System (ESAS)[4] is a nine-item, patient-rated symptom visual analogue scale designed to assess the symptoms of hospice patients. This inventory consists of 10 visual analogue scales (0 to 100 mm) that measure the patient's current level of pain, activity, nausea, depression, anxiety, drowsiness, appetite, sensation of well-being, shortness of breath, and distress. The advantage of the ESAS is that it is easy to administer, it requires minimal effort and concentration from the patient or caregiver, and results can be displayed on a graph in the chart.

Chang and colleagues,[5] in a prospective study, validated the ESAS in a cancer population of the Veterans Administration system. In this group, 240 patients completed the ESAS, the Memorial Symptom Assessment Scale (MSAS), the Functional Assessment Cancer Therapy (FACT) survey, and had their Karnofsky performance status (KPS) assessed. An additional 42 patients participated in a test-retest study. The investigators concluded that the ESAS was a valid instrument for assessing the general cancer population and that test-retest validity was better at 2 days than at 1 week. The ESAS distress score tends to reflect physical well-being. The use of a 30-mm cutoff point on visual analogue scales to identify severe symptoms may not always apply to symptoms other than pain.

Portenoy and colleagues[3] randomly selected 246 inpatients and outpatients with prostate, colon, breast, or ovarian cancer who were assessed using MSAS and a battery of measures that independently evaluate phenomena related to quality of life. They concluded that the MSAS was a reliable and valid instrument for the assessment of symptom prevalence, characteristics, and distress. It provides a method for comprehensive symptom assessment that may be useful when information about symptoms is desirable, such as clinical trials that incorporate quality of life measures or symptom epidemiology.

The Hospital Anxiety and Depression Scale (HADS) is widely used as a tool for assessing psychological distress in patients and nonclinical groups. The HADS is a 14-item scale that requires respondents to endorse a verbal response that is scored as an index of the severity of anxiety or depression. The scores are then summed to produce two subscales corresponding to anxiety (HADS-A) and depression (HADS-D). In addition to the subscale totals, an overall total can be derived to indicate the level of psychological distress. Smith and colleagues[6] investigated the factor structure of the HADS in a large, heterogeneous cancer population of 1474 patients. They concluded that the HADS comprises two factors corresponding to anhedonia and autonomic anxiety, which share a common variance with a primary factor (i.e., psychological distress) and that the subscales of the HADS, rather than the residual scores, were more effective in detecting clinical cases of anxiety and depression.

Screening Performance

Cancer-related symptoms are common. The development of tools with the ability to detect these symptoms early in disease progression is necessary in symptom research. Screening performance using tools with high sensitivity is important, but little research has taken place in this setting.

The ESAS is a concise palliative care assessment tool for many symptoms. It has been widely used in the clinical setting and has been validated for use in patients with advanced cancer.

Vignaroli and colleagues[7] evaluated the screening performance of the ESAS for depression and anxiety compared with that measured by the HADS. The diagnosis of anxiety or depression is made when a patient scores 8 or more on the HADS. For the 216 analyzed cancer patients, Vignaroli and coworkers[7] concluded that the ideal cutoff point of ESAS for the screening for depression and anxiety in palliative care is 2 of 10 or more. Such scores on the ESAS gave a sensitivity of 77% and specificity of 55% for depression and a sensitivity of 86% and specificity of 56% for anxiety.

Symptom Clusters and Correlates of Symptoms

Research is showing that many symptoms share pathophysiology and therefore may occur as genuine clusters that can influence each other or respond to the same intervention. Research on correlates of symptoms will characterize the different roles of the contributing factors (e.g., depression, fatigue). Understanding the relative contribution of these factors will help in developing therapeutic interventions for these symptoms.

The identification of symptom clusters in oncology patients may yield to prioritization of symptoms for assessment and management and provide new avenues for interventions to minimize the impact of symptoms on health-related outcomes.[8] A cross-sectional design is best used to examine how many people in the population of interest have the symptoms at the time the data are collected. To examine the natural history of a symptom cluster, its pattern over time, or relationships among symptoms over time, a longitudinal design is required.

An important factor in symptom research is the clinical context. Although some symptoms are related to cancer, many are related to the treatment that is selected. Treatment-related symptoms are likely to appear, peak, and remain or dissipate at predictable times in relation to treatment. It is important to carefully consider the homogeneity of the sample. The type and stage of cancer may influence the pattern of symptoms. A symptom cluster for patients with lung cancer is likely to be different from that experienced by breast cancer patients.

An important design issue is the timing of symptom measurements. Timing by landmarks becomes more complex in the context of chemotherapy because treatment cycles can vary from 1 to 8 weeks. Innovative approaches to measurement using technology can provide more frequent assessments. Another aspect of the clinical context is the availability and use of symptom management strategies that can confound the measurement of symptoms. It is essential to keep track of symptom management efforts that could alter the expected severity or pattern of a symptom over time. Another issue to consider in an intervention for a symptom cluster is that strategies used to manage or relieve one symptom may exacerbate another. A symptom management intervention for pain that involves the use of opioid analgesics is likely to exacerbate the problems of fatigue and constipation. It may be necessary to compromise optimal management of one symptom (e.g., fatigue) to achieve optimal management of another troubling symptom (e.g., pain). These decisions must be made in the context of the goals of the research and practical and ethical considerations. Another critical issue in the conduct of an intervention for a symptom cluster is the timing of the intervention. An intervention aimed at preventing the development of symptoms must be administered before symptoms occur.

The classic conceptualization of a symptom is that it has several dimensions (e.g., intensity, timing, location). These dimensions potentially increase the complexity of symptom measurement. In the case of a symptom cluster, the easiest approach is to measure one dimension of multiple symptoms. The advantage of this approach is the simplicity and the low response burden, and the disadvantage is that other critical dimensions of the symptom cluster may not be assessed. A thorough measure of symptom clusters would be multidimensional for multiple symptoms. The researcher can minimize the response burden by including the symptoms that are most appropriate for a given clinical context. One way to measure multidimensional symptoms is to select a separate tool for each symptom in the cluster. This approach, using multiple instruments, has the advantage of including all the critical dimensions of each symptom. However, the disadvantages are the complexity of the measures, the use of different methods of scaling responses and time contexts, and higher response burden for study participants. An ideal measure of a symptom cluster would be consistent in measuring parallel dimensions of each symptom within the same time frame and clinical context using the same method of scaling responses to questions with a reasonable response burden.

As the process of measurement becomes more complicated in the case of symptom clusters, it is important to consider the use of technology. Touch-screen computers, hand-held devices, and automated telephone reporting can allow more frequent and more accurate reporting of symptoms than a paper questionnaire or symptom journal. The most common approach to grouping symptoms is factor analysis, which examines the relationships among a number of variables (e.g., symptoms severities) based on the matrix of correlation coefficients between the variables. Factor analysis methods are exploratory and descriptive, examining the underlying structure of a group of symptoms.

Our group conducted a prospective study of 56 patients to test a clinical staging system for cancer pain.[9] We concluded that neuropathic pain, incidental pain, impaired cognitive function, major psychological distress, rapid development of opioid tolerance, positive history for alcoholism, drug addiction, or narcotic exposure were poor prognostic factors for cancer pain control.

Munch and colleagues[10] investigated the correlation between anemia and fatigue intensity in patients with advanced cancer receiving palliative care. Medical charts of 177 consecutive outpatients were reviewed, and information on fatigue intensity and hemoglobin level was collected. Hemoglobin level did not show a significant correlation with fatigue, although there was a trend ($P = .09$). The investigators concluded that anemia is not one of the major contributors to fatigue in patients with cancer receiving palliative care.

To assess the frequency of moderate to severe dyspnea and the correlates of dyspnea in terminally ill cancer patients, our group designed a prospective study[11] in which 135 consecutive patients attending a multidisciplinary pain clinic were tested for respiratory function. Ratings of dyspnea, anxiety, and fatigue were collected from all patients using visual analogue scales. Lung involvement by the tumor was determined from the patient's chart. In the subgroup of patients with moderate to severe dyspnea, multivariate analysis found anxiety ($P = .0318$) and maximal inspiratory pressure ($P = .0187$) to be independent correlates of the dyspnea intensity. The presence of cancer in the lungs, anxiety, and maximal inspiratory pressure are correlates of the intensity of dyspnea in this patient population.

RESEARCH IN SYMPTOM MANAGEMENT

A clinical trial is a research study that answers specific questions about new therapies or new ways of using known treatments. Clinical trials are used to determine whether new drugs or treatments are both safe and effective. Carefully conducted clinical trials are the fastest and safest way to find treatments that work in people. Clinical trials can be subdivided into explanatory and pragmatic trials.

An *explanatory trial* attempts to address the complex pathophysiological or pharmacological issues in a new treatment by providing sophisticated assessment and treatments in a highly selected population. Its great advantage is to help us understand how a certain intervention works in the usual clinical practice.

The *pragmatic trial* has simple aims, interventions, and outcomes. It does not attempt to characterize in great depth the pathophysiology or pharmacology of an intervention rather than asking a very simple question about the role of this intervention in the daily clinical setting.

Explanatory trials are ideal for single institution with sophisticated academic setting. Pragmatic trials are particularly useful in multicentric cooperative trials or community-based practices.

A critical element in designing clinical trials is *validity*, described as whether the results given by the clinical trials represent the truth. An additional measure of the authority of the trial is whether the results can be repeated by different investigators or within another group of similar subjects. This is referred to as *reliability*. A clinical trial design can be reliable but not necessarily valid, and it is important to consider all measures of validity when designing a clinical trial. This helps to maintain the trial's validity in properly assessing the placebo response. The use of placebos (active or inactive) within clinical trials in palliative care is controversial[12,13] despite limited evidence of the effectiveness of many treatments currently used.[14]

Clinical studies can be designed as retrospective studies or prospective trials. Prospective clinical trials can be randomized or nonrandomized. Randomized clinical trials can have single-blinded, double-blinded, or nonblinded (open) formats. Blinded clinical trials can be crossover or parallel studies (Fig. 30-1).

The randomized, controlled trial is the most robust method for evaluating new treatments. It is a technique to ensure that few differences exist between different arms of a trial by giving every patient an equal chance of being allocated to each arm. It allows greater confidence that any effects result from the intervention. Randomiza-

tion does not eliminate confounding variables, but it distributes them equally. This reduces the overall bias in the clinical trial. Randomized, controlled trials are expensive to run, take a long time to conduct, and are carried out on selected patient subsets. The high degree of selectivity may limit the ability of clinical trials to explain the effects of treatments after the treatments are used in more heterogeneous, real-world populations. Despite this disadvantage, conducting randomized, controlled trials with adequate levels of blinding and minimization of other sources of bias provides the highest level of evidence of a treatment effect.

Blinding refers to keeping patients, investigators, and those collecting and analyzing the data unaware of the assigned treatment arm throughout the trial. The term *single blind* means that the patient or the investigator does not know the treatment allocation. In a *double-blind* trial, neither party is aware of the treatment allocation. Blinding is used in palliative care trials to reduce the bias caused by the subjectivity of symptom assessment. This bias may manifest in the decision to withdraw a patient from a study or to titrate the dose of medication, and it can be influenced by knowledge about which treatment group the patient has been assigned to. Blinding is more important in clinical trials assessing symptom management than in trials assessing disease management, for which the response criteria are more objective.

Blinding can be difficult or sometimes impossible to achieve. Single-blind trials (e.g., investigator is not blind to the allocation) are sometimes unavoidable, as are open trials.[15] When blinding treatment is not feasible in a palliative care setting, blind assessment of outcome in ignorance of the treatment received is useful (e.g., effect of transfusion on fatigue in anemic, terminally ill patients).

In parallel designs, patients are allocated to one of the arms and stay with this allocation throughout the trial. In crossover designs, patients are allocated to one arm at the start of the trial and are then swapped to the other arm.

The crossover trial appears to be superior because it reduces the confounding effects of the patients themselves and has more validity and reliability than a parallel trial with the same number of patients. Fewer patients are required in a crossover design. However, the length of the trial is often longer than that of a similar trial with a parallel design, which can be a major problem in a palliative care setting. In this setting, the patient's condition or symptom may undergo natural fluctuations, and by the time of assignment to the second arm, symptoms are naturally better or worse, regardless of which arm they are currently allocated to. The problem in palliative care is that patients are very ill, and their disease can worsen without warning. This can result in increased numbers of dropouts. Another disadvantage of crossover designs is the existence of *order* or *carryover effects*. The effects from the first study arm on the dependent variable persist into and influence the second arm. For example, carryover effects may be mediated by persistence of the drug or its metabolite, a long-lasting change in physiology caused by the treatment, or behavioral effects (e.g., the patient may have less stamina or be less willing to complete outcome measures accurately).

An example of an order effect is illustrated in a clinical crossover trial that examined the effects of the clinician's

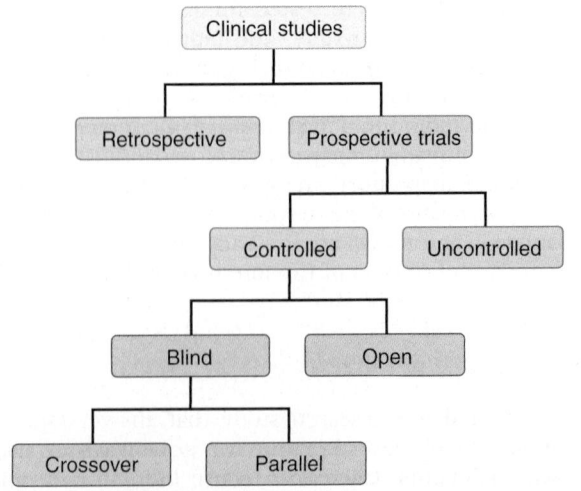

FIGURE 30-1 Clinical trials. Clinical studies may have retrospective or prospective designs. Prospective trials can be modified in several ways.

posture on patients' ratings of compassion while breaking bad news.[16] Patients clearly ranked clinicians who sat as more compassionate than those who stood. For some unexplained reason, they ranked the clinician in the second sequence as more compassionate than the first, regardless of the clinician's posture. Perhaps the patients had had time to adapt to the bad news in the second sequence and therefore thought of the clinician as more compassionate.

In contrast, parallel designs are shorter but require larger numbers of patients. This can result in fewer drop-outs and eliminate carryover effects. Parallel designs are more useful for clinical situations in which the symptom may not be stable or the risk of dropping out is high. This problem was illustrated in one study in which only 12 of 38 palliative care patients who were entered completed a clinical trial lasting only a few days.[17]

The final blinded choice in the case of crossover trial or the global effectiveness in the parallel trial is the patient's balance of the advantageous and inconvenient effects of an intervention. For example, during the evaluation of the effect of mazindol on pain, depression, anxiety, appetite, and activity in terminal cancer patients,[18] the primary outcome of improved analgesia was met, but the final blinded choice of the patient did not favor mazindol, probably because of increased anxiety, anorexia, and fatigue during the mazindol phase. However, the final blinded choice and the primary outcome can be positive, as was found in study that evaluated the effect of methylphenidate to decrease opioid sedation.[19]

CONCLUSIONS

During the past several years, reports from different institutions, including the American Academy of Hospice and Palliative Medicine, have called for substantial investment in palliative care research to address the knowledge gaps in assessment and management of the unmet needs of patients with advanced disease and the needs of their families. However, there has been minimal investment in research that could significantly alleviate these needs. One of the major contributing factors to low levels of research in palliative care is the lack of funding because of the paucity of designated granting agencies and private organizations promoting career awards or funding grants. Other factors are the frail and unstable nature of the patient population, the lack of industry interest in drug development for palliative care, and the limited number of academic faculty in most universities. Studies in the palliative care setting should be short and preferably multicentric, and they should have a simple design with limited outcomes and frequent follow-up.

REFERENCES

1. Saunders C. The evolution of palliative care. J R Soc Med 2001;94:430-432.
2. Bruera E, Neumann C, Brenneis C, Quan H. Frequency of symptom distress and poor prognostic indicators in palliative cancer patients admitted to a tertiary palliative care unit, hospices, and acute care hospitals. J Palliat Care 2000; 16:16-21.
3. Portenoy RK, Thaler HT, Kornblith AS, et al. The Memorial Symptom Assessment Scale: An instrument for the evaluation of symptom prevalence, characteristics and distress. Eur J Cancer 1994;30A:1326-1336.
4. Bruera E, Kuehn N, Miller MJ, et al. The Edmonton Symptom Assessment System (ESAS): A simple method for the assessment of palliative care patients. J Palliat Care 1991;7:6-9.
5. Chang VT, Hwang SS, Feuerman M. Validation of the Edmonton Symptom Assessment Scale. Cancer 2000;88:2164-2171.
6. Smith AB, Selby PJ, Velikova G, et al. Factor analysis of the Hospital Anxiety and Depression Scale from a large cancer population. Psychol Psychother 2002;75(Pt 2):165-176.
7. Vignaroli E, Pace EA, Willey J, et al. The Edmonton Symptom Assessment System as a screening tool for depression and anxiety. J Palliat Med 2006;9:296-303.
8. Barsevick AM, Whitmer K, Nail LM, et al. Symptom cluster research: Conceptual, design, measurement, and analysis issues. J Pain Symptom Manage 2006;31:85-95.
9. Bruera E, MacMillan K, Hanson J, MacDonald RN. The Edmonton staging system for cancer pain: Preliminary report. Pain 1989;37:203-209.
10. Munch TN, Zhang T, Willey J, et al. The association between anemia and fatigue in patients with advanced cancer receiving palliative care. J Palliat Med 2005;8:1144-1149.
11. Bruera E, Schmitz B, Pither J, et al. The frequency and correlates of dyspnea in patients with advanced cancer. J Pain Symptom Manage 2000;19:357-362.
12. Hardy J. Placebo controlled trials in palliative care: The argument for. Palliat Med 1997;11:415-418.
13. Kirkham SR, Abel J. Placebo controlled trials in palliative care: The argument against. Palliat Med 1997;11:489-492.
14. Bell RF, Wisloff T, Eccleston C, Kalso E. Controlled clinical trials in cancer pain. How controlled should they be? A qualitative systematic review. Br J Cancer 2006;94:1559-1567.
15. Ahmedzai SH, Brookes D. Transdermal fentanyl versus sustained-release oral morphine in cancer pain: preference, efficacy, and quality of life. The TTS-Fentanyl Comparative Trial Group. J Pain Symptom Manage 1997;13:254-261.
16. Strasser F, Palmer JL, Castro M, et al. Impact of physician sitting versus standing during inpatient oncology consultations: Patient's preference and perception of compassion and duration: A randomized controlled trial. J Pain Symptom Manage 2005;29:489-497.
17. Reymond L, Charles MA, Bowman J, Treston P. The effect of dexamethasone on the longevity of syringe driver subcutaneous sites in palliative care patients. Med J Aust 2003;178:486-489.
18. Bruera E, Carraro S, Roca E, et al. Double-blind evaluation of the effects of mazindol on pain, depression, anxiety, appetite, and activity in terminal cancer patients. Cancer Treat Rep 1986;70:295-298.
19. Bruera E, Chadwick S, Brenneis C, et al. Methylphenidate associated with narcotics for the treatment of cancer pain. Cancer Treat Rep 1987;71:67-70.

SUGGESTED READING

Kirkova J, Davis MP, Walsh D, et al. Cancer symptom assessment instruments: A systematic review [erratum in J Clin Oncol 2006;24:2973]. J Clin Oncol 2006;24:1459-1473.

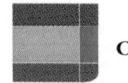

CHAPTER **31**

Health Services Research

Massimo Costantini and Irene J. Higginson

KEY POINTS

- Health services research is important for palliative care because of the complex services required by patients and their families.

- Population-based needs assessment is a dynamic process concerned with how many people need what types of services and interventions at given times and locations. There are three main approaches to needs assessment: corporate, comparative, and epidemiological, which combines approaches from the first two types and includes epidemiological and effectiveness data.

- Health services research provides appropriate strategies and study designs to evaluate services and interventions.

- Choosing appropriate outcome measures is a key issue in the evaluation of services and interventions, but validated outcomes for palliative care are available.

- Systematic literature reviews are important to generate an evidence base and influence practice and policy.

Health services research is the multidisciplinary field of scientific investigation that studies how social factors, financing systems, organizational structures and processes, health technologies, and personal behaviors affect access to health care, the quality and cost of health care, and the health and well-being of patients. Its research domains are individuals, families, organizations, institutions, communities, and populations.[1] This definition, proposed by the American Academy for Health Services Research and Health Policy, covers a broad domain, ranging from needs assessment to quality of care research and economic evaluations.

In palliative care, there are complex services, complex patients and families, complex needs, and complex outcomes.[2] Research is needed to provide an evidence base to ensure the funding, continuation, and development of services and to evaluate and improve specific interventions (e.g., quality improvement, communication, training) offered within these services. Health services research is important in palliative care to aid the development and assessment of services appropriate to the needs of patients and their families (see "Common Errors").

NEEDS ASSESSMENT

Population-based needs assessment starts with a community that requires palliative care, rather than individuals. It is concerned with how many people need various types of services and interventions at certain times and in certain locations. Contributions to the definitions of *need* come from the fields of sociology, epidemiology, health economics, and public health and from clinicians. There may be different types of needs according to who determines these needs and at what level need is experienced (e.g., basic needs for food versus more complex needs).[3,4] In applied health services research, the need for health care has been defined as the population's ability to benefit from health care.[5] Methods for needs assessment, used independently or in combination, include comparative needs assessment, corporate needs assessment, and epidemiological data–based needs assessment.[6]

Comparative needs assessment contrasts the services received by a population in one area with those elsewhere. An example is contrasting numbers of hospice beds, home care nurses, or doctor sessions per million people in two or more regions.

Corporate needs assessment is based on the demands, wishes, and alternative perspectives of interested parties, including politicians. This type of assessment commonly involves surveys of professionals, patients, and the public.

Epidemiological data–based needs assessment compares data on three health dimensions to determine the needs of a community. First, problems are quantified by incidence (i.e., number of new cases arising in a given period) and prevalence (i.e., total number of cases existing at one time). This is supplemented with demographic information on population structure and likely changes to determine the extent and impact of health problems. Second, information on health service effectiveness and cost-effectiveness is generated from literature and local reviews to determine the most effective and cost-effective services in a particular context. This combines local information from a corporate needs assessment with data from systematic literature reviews on effectiveness. Third, information is gathered about supply of the available services. This can include the status of local services and comparison with other areas, as in a comparative needs assessment.

Each approach has drawbacks because of data limitations or because of the comparisons made. Some needs assessments have developed simple formulas to estimate the numbers of patients needing palliative care, based primarily on comparative needs assessments of existing service provision. Using existing national or international service provision as a standard can perpetuate the status quo instead of moving to more appropriately meeting patients' needs. Corporate assessment is affected by the knowledge and prior experiences of those providing information. The epidemiological approach, which incorporates these approaches into a wider assessment, is more robust but more time consuming. Because it often relies on mortality and symptom prevalence data, this approach does not take full account of chronic illnesses that have a long duration (e.g., multiple sclerosis) and that are poorly recorded in death registrations (e.g., dementia). Further it may overlook problems that are poorly reported, especially psychological or social problems. Needs assessment should be a dynamic process that continuously integrates new evidence from health services research and provides more robust estimates of the needs of patients and their families.

EVALUATION OF SERVICES AND INTERVENTIONS

Although health services research uses some of the classic steps when developing a drug, such as test activity, efficacy, and effectiveness, the research also must deal with the complexity of the intervention and the context in which it is delivered.

Scope of an Intervention

Intervention refers to a set of actions with a coherent objective to bring about change or identifiable outcomes. Health professionals and volunteers can carry out interventions. This includes specific therapeutic and clinical interventions for patients or families, such as cognitive behavioral therapy, complementary therapies and counseling, and interventions with professionals or organizations, such as training, education of health professionals,

---

Common Errors

- Developing a palliative care program without a needs assessment
- Implementing innovative palliative care services or programs without testing their activity, efficacy, and effectiveness
- Designing an effectiveness research study without considering the specificity of the palliative care context and all conditions that could contribute to false-negative results
- Using inappropriate design to evaluate a palliative care service, such as failure to consider an appropriate comparison or control group, to understand the intervention, or to select appropriate outcome measures

and specific procedures or methods of communication. Mixed interventions, such as care pathways and clinical audits, combine approaches directed to patients, their families, and health care professionals.

Evaluation Strategies

In palliative care, the outcomes for patients and families are multidimensional, and interventions therefore involve care by many professionals, coordination in different settings, and needs that change over time. Interventions are complex and difficult to evaluate. Systematic reviews have shown serious problems with the evaluation of palliative care interventions and services, including failure to clearly define the intervention; failure to consider the heterogeneity of patients, families, and their needs; and failure to appropriately measure outcomes.[7-10] There often were difficulties in understanding what the intervention did and which staff did what and for whom. The evaluation process must determine the validity of the evaluation method in detecting the success or failure of the intervention, rather than assess the relative success or failure of the intervention itself.

Some newer approaches are highly relevant to the evaluation of palliative care services. One is the Medical Research Council (MRC) framework for the development and evaluation of complex interventions.[11] The MRC evaluation reshapes the classic approach to research for drug development. It uses the model of preclinical and phase I, II, III, and IV studies as found in drug trials, but it also employs study methods from qualitative to randomized, controlled trials and quasi-experimental approaches. Several aspects make it particularly valuable in evaluating palliative care. The MRC framework requires that services be developed using theory about how the interventions may be working and the context in which they are delivered. This can involve psychological, sociological, and anthropological theory about how people and organizations behave to model how the intervention may work. Qualitative phase I studies improve the modeling of the intervention and consider uptake, relationship with other services, acceptability, likely mechanisms, and effects or outcomes. The effect of the service and the evaluation methods are then tested in phase II studies, before a randomized, controlled or quasi-experimental trial (phase III) is conducted. If this is successful, phase IV studies determine the potential to extend the intervention more widely. This process may not be linear. It may be that after phase I, II, or phase III studies, the intervention is remodeled, and even phase IV or observational data may influence how the intervention is modeled.

Appropriate Study Designs

The MRC framework challenges the traditional view of randomized, controlled trials as the only gold standard for the effectiveness of health interventions. It recognizes that all clinical and epidemiological studies, including randomized, controlled trials, are subject to bias, contamination, and confounding.[12] Many sources of bias can affect a randomized study, including bias in the assessment of the outcome, contamination, dropouts, and loss to follow-up. Substantial flaws have been observed in randomization

procedures and blinding. Few randomized, controlled trials can be considered bias free, and their internal validity often is questionable. It is difficult to blind patients, families, professionals, and investigators to the intervention group, thereby affecting uptake and many subjective responses. Randomized trials may be unnecessary, inappropriate, impossible, or inadequate in the assessment of many health care intervetnions.[13]

Such criticism is based on classic randomized, controlled trials in which the intervention is standardized and the individual is the unit of randomization. A better knowledge of the intervention and its context can help to overcome this limitation. Newer approaches to randomized trials take account of some of these complexities. In cluster randomized trials, the unit of analysis is the cluster (i.e., a ward, a service, or a physician, each with a cluster of patients and families).[14] Cluster randomized trials include patient preference trials, in which patients (or families) are randomized only if they do not have strong preferences for or against the intervention.[15] Delay intervention trials in palliative care have been explored, in which all patients (or families) are offered the trial intervention, but one group is offered the intervention only after a delay.[16]

Mixed methods are also important. It is possible in a trial to collect qualitative and quantitative data. Information can be gathered on patients' views of the service, on what worked well or did not, and on aspects that may be improved to understand how the intervention may be working and its effects on outcomes that are difficult to measure.

Observational and quasi-experimental designs can provide, with different degrees of feasibility, validity, and generalizability, useful information for establishing if and to what extent an intervention is effective in health services research. In a quasi-experimental study, an intervention is deliberately introduced to observe its effects (i.e., artificial manipulation of the study factor) without using randomization to create the comparisons from which the effects are inferred.[17] However, like randomized, controlled trials, careful attention must be paid to the design to minimize biases, particularly in patient selection.

Several quasi-experimental study designs have been described.[18] The most important limitation of these designs is that it is impossible to avoid selection bias. The question is how much the selection bias can affect the results. The answer is based on the way participants are assigned to groups and on how much control the investigator has over the independent variable.

Analysis of study design helps determine the internal validity. For example, although popular, results from before-and-after designs are hard to interpret. The investigator measures one or more outcomes before and after the experimental intervention (e.g., a new service, an existing service for different patients). The comparison is made between the pretest and the post-test data. Better study designs use external control groups, and outcomes are measured for the experimental and the control groups before and after the intervention. These designs can be identical to a randomized study, but they proceed without randomization. Internal validity largely depends on the way the subjects are recruited in the experimental and control groups. Designs in which participation of subjects is voluntary are weak, as there is often a relationship between the preference for an intervention and the outcome under study. Other, more robust, designs identify groups based on factors unrelated to their intervention preferences (e.g., geographical area of residence).

Ecological studies are used in health services research and have great value in understanding the factors affecting different communities, especially if palliative care services or other health-related issues vary between communities or over time. In an ecological study, groups are studied rather than single individuals. The groups may be people in a geographical area receiving care from one particular family doctor (or group practice), on one ward, or even one hospital. Independent and dependent variables related to the group are compared. For example, in London[19] and Genoa (Italy),[20] ecological studies analyzing the relationship between community deprivation and the proportion of home deaths found an inverse, remarkably similar relationship between the two variables. These findings were confirmed in a national U.K. study.[21] In an ecological study, associations are found at the level of the group. This does not necessarily mean that the association will hold true for each individual living in those areas. To erroneously make such an assumption is known as the *ecological fallacy*. Ecological studies help to generate hypotheses.

Outcomes

An *outcome* has been defined as any end result that is attributable to health services intervention.[22] It is the change in a patient's current and future health status attributed to antecedent health or social care. If a broad definition of health is used, such as the World Health Organization's (WHO) definition of total physical, mental, and social well-being, improvements in social and psychological function are included.

The selection and measurement of appropriate outcomes in health services research is vital. It is important to choose outcomes that the intervention is expected to change. If we wish to assess a new palliative care service for a specific group of patients (e.g., multiple sclerosis), the outcomes must include symptoms and problems experienced by these patients that the service seeks to alleviate. Measuring commonly used outcomes in earlier stages of illness, such as disability, morbidity, or mortality, is inappropriate.

A multidimensional assessment model is essential to evaluate the complexity experienced by patients and families during advanced and terminal disease. The expression of suffering for each dimension of quality of life is always the product of a complex interaction.[23] Expression of pain cannot be assessed and interpreted per se, but it must include the interaction of the "symptom pain" with all other relevant dimensions of quality of life. There are many appropriate outcome measures validated for palliative care, such as the Palliative Outcome Scale (POS),[24] symptom checklists (e.g., Edmonton Symptom Assessment Scale [ESAS]),[25] and the Memorial Symptom Assessment Scale (MSAS).[26-29]

Bias and Postbereavement Surveys

In palliative care, most outcomes are measured in the same individual on different occasions and viewed in a dynamic perspective over time. As a consequence, researchers deal with several methodological issues, and selection and information biases can compromise the study's validity. Information bias is a particularly sensitive issue in palliative care, because it is difficult to measure without distorting the patient's subjective point of view. Selection bias is difficult to avoid, because it is difficult to prospectively identify representative samples of terminally ill patients; typically, there is uncertainty about the disease course. Outcome assessment over time is constantly biased by missing data due to the progressive decline in performance status.

Retrospective studies have tried to overcome these problems using the after death approach. Information is collected afterward from the caregiver who attended the patient during the last period of life. This design has been used in several influential studies to estimate the multidimensional problems experienced by patients during their last months of life[30,31] or to compare the quality of end-of-life care in different care settings.[32] Representative samples of advanced and terminal disease courses can be evaluated as they are gathered after deaths have occurred. This approach has at least two weaknesses. First, on death certificates, the cause is often unreliable or incomplete, especially for the elderly or noncancer deaths. The assessment of outcomes from bereaved caregivers, usually several months after the death, may distort results.[33] Proxies can reliably report practical and observable aspects of the patient's experience. Validity is reduced for reports on patients' subjective experiences, such as pain and affective states.

Interpretation of Results

The risk of a false-negative result is greater for complex interventions than in clinical trials of drug therapies. In health services research, it is important to distinguish between a failure to demonstrate underlying effectiveness and evidence of ineffectiveness. Negative or positive findings warrant careful exploration. Some crucial factors are not taken into account when considering study results. Any study appraisals should consider the stability of the intervention, the quality of implementation, and the adequacy of the outcomes before a negative result leads to an intervention being dismissed. For positive results, investigators should consider whether this particular complex intervention is the best or definitive solution for a particular problem. To improve pain control in hospitals, a complex intervention may include relatively expensive components, such as trained assessments, education, and clinical care pathways, and cheaper components, such as flagging patients at risk for death.[34] Does the intervention have to include all of these components to be effective? Would it be equally or almost as effective and more cost-effective if only some components of the intervention are present?

Case Studies

In clinical research, a case study reports the changes and events for an individual; in health services research, a case study details the process and activities of a new intervention or service, paying particular attention to the context in which it is delivered and the factors affecting how it works. Outcomes reported in case studies can be particularly helpful in developing a hypothesis about how or which interventions may be effective. However, care should be taken not to draw inappropriate conclusions from the results, particularly regarding an intervention's effectiveness.

Systematic Literature Reviews in Evidence-Based Medicine

Literature reviews use a systematic approach to identify, collate, analyze, and interpret data from published and unpublished scientific research.[35] They are used increasingly to appraise the effectiveness of interventions and services and to compare different care approaches. A systematic method is used of seeking and including studies. The findings are analyzed and compared using reference tables and meta-synthesis or meta-analysis (i.e., results from studies are combined). They are especially useful when there are several small studies that do not individually show a significant effect, but when all studies are combined and if the findings are in a similar direction, a significant effect can be found. Systematic reviews can also estimate the prevalence of problems affecting patients and families[36] or identify factors affecting care. For example, in analyzing factors affecting place of death, a systematic review identified 17 significant common reliable factors that affect the place of death for cancer patients.[37]

DEVELOPMENTS IN PALLIATIVE CARE RESEARCH

A few examples demonstrate the global amount of evidence for the effectiveness of palliative care accumulated over past decades. The Evidence-Based Guidelines for Improving Supportive and Palliative Care for Adults with Cancer was produced by the National Institute for Clinical Excellence.[38] Through a systematic review of the scientific literature until 2003,[39] the Guidelines aimed at ". . . determining the current state of the evidence on interventions to improve service configurations for the supportive and palliative care for those affected by cancer."[38] For 13 relevant domains, the Guidelines provided[20] evidence-based key recommendations to help ". . . health care professionals or the structure in which health care professionals deliver their care to improve the support and palliative care for cancer patients."[38]

Two other publications, promoted and supported by the WHO Regional Office for Europe, promote awareness of comprehensive palliative care services and examine the implications for aging populations.[2,40] The two publications, written primarily for policy makers, summarize the best available evidence on the impact of palliative care. These documents would have been impossible without an increasing quantity and quality of health services research in palliative medicine.

CONCLUSIONS AND FUTURE CHALLENGES

Populations in all developed countries are aging, and more people are living with the effects of serious chronic illness near the end of life. Meeting their needs is a public health challenge, but health services research should provide policy makers with more evidence-based estimates of the palliative care needs of patients and families. Different countries have various approaches, and the quality of assessments is often poor. Moreover, most available evidence is for cancer. A global, evidence-based approach for needs assessment in palliative care, particularly for noncancer patients, is necessary.

Health services research is needed for expanding the evidence available on the effectiveness of care solutions. The core aspects of palliative care have been shown to be effective for cancer, and there is preliminary evidence for this model for people with other illnesses. Expanding expert international collaboration supported by appropriate investment in research can encourage innovative health service research in palliative care, with the aim to help people with serious chronic disease live well and die well.

Although management of patients is expected to be evidence-based care, interventions or programs aimed at improving the quality of care often are implemented on the basis of expert beliefs, paradigms, or schools of thought.[41] That is the case of palliative care improvement programs; some focus on changing professionals and others on changing organizations, but the evidence of their effectiveness is limited or, more often, not studied at all.

The development and implementation of new care pathways to improve the quality of end-of-life care provide an example. The objective is relevant, and the methodology is promising. Clinical pathways are effective in delivering a better quality of care at lower cost for many health conditions. The proposed care pathways for dying patients are complex interventions. They are expensive and time consuming, and the evidence for their effectiveness is limited to a few observational or quasi-experimental study designs.[42-44]

The challenge to design and implement high-quality experimental studies to assess the effectiveness of such important programs should be a priority for health services research. The theoretical model of assessment may be the MRC framework,[11] although for this new field of health services research, the optimal methodology is unclear.

REFERENCES

1. Lohr KN, Steinwachs DM. Health services research: An evolving definition of the field. Health Serv Res 2002;37:15-17.
2. Davies E, Higginson IJ (eds). Palliative care. The solid facts. Geneva: World Health Organization, 2004. Available at http://www.euro.who.int/document/E82931.pdf (accessed September 16, 2007).
3. Bradshaw JS. A taxonomy of social need. In McLachlan G (ed). Problems and Progress in Medical Care, 7th series. Oxford, UK: Oxford University Press, 1972.
4. Zalenski RJ, Raspa R. Maslow's hierarchy of needs: A framework for achieving human potential in hospice. J Palliat Med 2006;9:1120-1127.
5. Stevens A, Raftery J. Health care needs assessment. In Stevens A, Raftery J (eds). The Epidemiologically Based Needs Assessment Reviews. Oxford, UK: Radcliffe Medical Press, 1994, pp 11-30.
6. Higginson IJ, von Gunten CF. Population-based needs assessment for patient and family care. In Bruera E, Higginson IJ, Ripamonti C, von Gunten C (eds). Textbook of Palliative Medicine. London: Hodder Arnold, 2006, pp 251-258.
7. Goodwin DM, Higginson IJ, Edwards AG, et al. An evaluation of systematic reviews of palliative care services. J Palliat Care 2002;18:77-83.
8. Harding R, Higginson IJ. What is the best way to help caregivers in cancer and palliative care? A systematic literature review of interventions and their effectiveness. Palliat Med 2002;17:63-71.

9. Higginson IJ, Finlay IG, Goodwin DM, et al. Is there evidence that palliative care teams alter end-of-life experiences of patients and their caregivers? J Pain Symptom Manage 2003;25:150-168.

10. Harding R, Easterbrook PE, Karus, D, et al. Does palliative care improve outcomes for patients with HIV/AIDS? A systematic review of the evidence. Sex Transm Infect 2005;81:5-14.

11. Campbell M, Fitzpatrick R, Haines A, et al. Framework for design and evaluation of complex interventions to improve health. BMJ 2000;321:694-696.

12. Delgado-Rodriguez M, Llorca J. Bias. J Epidemiol Community Health 2004;58: 635-641.

13. Black N: Why we need observational studies to evaluate the effectiveness of health care. BMJ 1996;312:1215-1218.

14. Murray DM, Varnell SP, Blitstein JL. Design and analysis of group-randomized trials: A review of recent methodological developments. Am J Public Health 2004;94:423-432.

15. Howard L, Thornicroft G. Patient preference randomised controlled trials in mental health research. Br J Psychiatry 2006;188:303-304.

16. Higginson IJ, Vivat B, Silber E, et al. Study protocol: delayed intervention randomised controlled trial within the Medical Research Council (MRC) framework to assess the effectiveness of a new palliative care service. BMC Palliat Care 2006;5:7.

17. Kleinbaum DG, Kupper LL, Morgenstern H (eds). Epidemiologic Research. New York: Van Nostrand Reinhold, 1982.

18. Shadish WR, Cook TD, Campbell DT (eds). Experimental and Quasi-experimental Designs. Boston: Houghton Mifflin, 2002.

19. Higginson IJ, Webb D, Lessof L. Reducing hospital beds for patients with advanced cancer. Lancet 1994;344:47.

20. Costantini M, Fusco F, Bruzzi P. Uno studio epidemiologico a Genova dal 1986 al 1990 sul luogo di decesso per neoplasia. Inf Med Oncol 1996;5,21-24.

21. Higginson IJ, Jarman B, Astin P, Dolan S. Do social factors affect where patients die: An analysis of 10 years of cancer deaths in England. J Public Health Med 1999;21:22-28.

22. Donabedian A. The definition of quality and approaches to its assessment. In Donabedian A (ed). Explorations in Quality Assessment and Monitoring. Chicago: Health Administration Press, 1996.

23. Vignaroli E, Bruera E. Multidimensional assessment in palliative care. In Bruera E, Higginson IJ, Ripamonti C, von Gunten C (eds). Textbook of Palliative Medicine. London: Hodder Arnold, 2006, pp 319-332.

24. Hearn J, Higginson IJ. Development and validation of a core outcome measure for palliative care: The palliative care outcome scale. Qual Health Care 1999;8:219-227.

25. Bruera E, Kuehn N, Miller MJ, et al. The Edmonton Symptom Assessment System (ESAS): A simple method for the assessment of palliative care patients. J Palliat Care 1991;7:6-9.

26. Portenoy RK, Thaler HT, Kornblith AB, et al. The Memorial Symptom Assessment Scale: An instrument for the evaluation of symptom prevalence, characteristics and distress. Eur J Cancer 1994;30A:1326-1336.

27. Edwards B, Ung L. Quality of life instruments for caregivers of patients with cancer. Cancer Nurs 2002;25:342-349.

28. Salek S, Pratheepawanit N, Finaly I, et al. The use of quality of life instruments in palliative care. Eur J Palliat Care 2002;9:52-56.

29. MAPI Research Trust. Patient-Reported Outcome and Quality of Life Instruments Database (ProQOLID). Available at www.proqolid.org (accessed January 4, 2007).

30. Addington-Hall JM, McCarthy M. The regional study of care for the dying: Methods and sample characteristics. Palliat Med 1995;9:27-35.

31. Costantini M, Beccaro M, Merlo F. The last three months of life of Italian cancer patients. Methods, sample characteristics and response rate of Italian Survey of the Dying of Cancer (ISDOC). Palliat Med 2005; 19:628-638.

32. Teno JM, Clarridge BR, Casey V, et al. Family perspectives on end-of-life care at the last place of care. JAMA 2004;291:88-93.

33. McPherson C, Addington-Hall J. Judging the quality of care at the end of life: Can proxies provide reliable information? Soc Sci Med 2003;56:95-109.

34. Morrison RS, Meier DE, et al. Improving the management of pain in hospitalised adults. Arch Intern Med 2006;166:1033-1039.

35. Hearn J, Feuer D, Higginson IJ, et al. Systematic reviews. Palliat Med 1999;13:75-80.

36. Murtagh FE, Addington-Hall J, Higginson IJ. The prevalence of symptoms in end-stage renal disease: A systematic review. Adv Chronic Kidney Dis. 2007;14:82-99.

37. Gomes B, Higginson IJ. Factors influencing death at home in terminally ill patients with cancer: systematic review. BMJ 2006;332:515-521.

38. National Institute of Clinical Excellence (NICE): Improving Supportive and Palliative Care for Adults with Cancer: The Manual. London: National Institute of Clinical Excellence, 2004. Available at www.nice.org.uk (accessed January 4, 2007).

39. Gysels M, Higginson IJ, Rajasekaran M, et al. Improving supportive and palliative care for adults with cancer. London: National Institute of Clinical Excellence, 2004. Available at www.nice.org.uk (accessed January 4, 2007).

40. Davies E, Higginson IJ (eds). Better Palliative Care for Older People. Geneva: World Health Organization, 2004. Available at http://www.euro.who.int/document/E82933.pdf (accessed September 16, 2007).

41. Grol R, Baker R, Moss F (eds). Quality Improvement Research. Understanding the Science of Change in Health Care. London: BMJ Publishing Group, 2004.

42. Ellershaw J, Ward C. Care of the dying patient: The last hours or days of life. BMJ 2003;326:30-34.

43. Bookbinder M, Blank AE, Arney E, et al. improving end-of-life care: Development and pilot-test of a clinical pathway. J Pain Symptom Manage 2005;29: 529-543.

44. Bailey FA, Burgio KL, Woodby LL, et al. Improving processes of hospital care during the last hours of life. Arch Intern Med 2005;165:1722-1727.

SUGGESTED READING

Davies E, Higginson IJ (eds). Better Palliative Care for Older People. Geneva: World Health Organization, 2004. Available at http://www.euro.who.int/document/E82933.pdf (accessed September 16, 2007).

Davies E, Higginson IJ (eds). Palliative Care. The Solid Facts. Geneva: World Health Organization, 2004. Available at http://www.euro.who.int/document/E82931.pdf (accessed September 16, 2007).

Higginson IJ, von Gunten CF. Population-based needs assessment for patient and family care. In Bruera E, Higginson IJ, Ripamonti C, von Gunten C (eds). Textbook of Palliative Medicine. London: Hodder Arnold, 2006, pp 251-258.

The National Institute for Clinical Excellence (NICE). Improving Supportive and Palliative Care for Adults with Cancer. London: NICE, 2002 Available at http://www.nice.org.uk (accessed September 16, 2007).

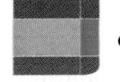

CHAPTER **32**

Psychosocial Research

John G. Hughes and **Mari Lloyd-Williams**

KEY POINTS

- Psychosocial research attempts to address the multifactorial issues that can affect the quality of life of those affected by terminal illness.

- A range of methodologies can be used for researching psychosocial issues within palliative care.

- All methodological approaches are associated with inherent strengths and weaknesses.

- "Good" psychosocial research is that which chooses a methodology appropriate for the aims of the study, considers the practical and ethical problems associated with researching within the field, and is executed in a rigorous manner.

- Continued research into the psychosocial needs of those affected by terminal illness is paramount to ensure that those affected receive the optimal support possible.

In 1997, the National Council for Hospice and Specialist Palliative Care Services,[1] a palliative care umbrella organization of professionals from various disciplines involved with the care of the terminally ill, defined psychosocial care as concerned with the psychological and emotional well-being of patients and their families and caregivers, including issues of self-esteem, insight into adaptation to the illness and its consequences, communication, social functioning, and relationships.

Psychosocial care addresses the psychological experiences of loss and facing death for patients and their families, friends, and caregivers. It encompasses the values, culture, and spiritual beliefs of those concerned and social factors that influence their experiences, such as financial issues, housing, and aids to daily living. Psychosocial care also encompasses the health professionals caring for the dying, who may also require support to deal with their experiences.[2]

Psychosocial research attempts to explore the views, feelings, and concerns of those affected by terminal illness and evaluate interventions to improve the psychological and emotional well-being of those affected by terminal illness. Psychosocial research within palliative care has burgeoned over the past 4 decades. Good-quality psychosocial research within palliative care includes the seminal qualitative study that explored the experiences of dying cancer patients and identified the central importance of communication and awareness of dying for cancer patients.[3] Another example was the randomized, controlled trial that found services coordinated by a nurse had little impact on patient or family outcomes in terms of symptoms or satisfaction with services.[4]

Psychosocial research within palliative care is not methodologically specific to the discipline. It can encompass all methodological approaches. Research is distinguished as psychosocial by its attempt to address the multifactorial issues that affect quality of life for the patient, family and friends, or caregivers.

At the inception of any research, the methods chosen must be appropriate for the question being investigated. The researcher has to clarify the specific aims of the research and must possess an appreciation and knowledge of the scope of methodological approaches available. Many methodological approaches are suitable for psychosocial research within palliative care, and each has inherent strengths and weaknesses. Within palliative care research, it is important to consider practical and ethical issues when choosing a methodological approach. The following sections describe some of the main methodological approaches, including surveys, observational studies, controlled clinical trials, and qualitative studies.

SURVEYS

Surveys gather information on the views and perspectives of those affected by terminal illness. They have been the most frequently used methodological approach for psychosocial research in palliative care. Examples of good-quality surveys within palliative care include assessments of the views of bereaved family and friends about the experience of terminally ill patients[5] and an appraisal of senior house officers' experience of a 6-month hospice post that identified their sources of stress and their support needs.[6]

Typically, surveys generate data through a series of closed questions or Likert or visual analogue scales to aid data collection and statistical analysis. Some also contain open questions that allow the respondent to answer a question freely and that can be analyzed by various methods, typically content or thematic analysis. Surveys are administered as face-to-face interviews with the respondent, as telephone interviews, or by self-completion of postal questionnaires. Each has certain advantages and disadvantages.

- Face-to-face interviews provide respondents with an opportunity to clarify any misunderstandings or ambiguities with the survey and are associated with the highest completion rates of the three types, but they are the costliest to administer and the most susceptible to interviewer bias.
- Telephone interviewing reduces cost compared with face-to-face surveys. Completion rates are lower, they cannot be used for nonaudio information, respondents may not give as much attention to a telephone survey as to a face-to-face survey, and the researcher loses nonverbal cues that can help detect that the respondent has not understood the question.
- Self-completion postal surveys are the cheapest of the three and have less risk of interviewer bias because the respondent and researcher have no direct contact. This also means there is no guarantee that the person completing the survey is the intended respondent, and even if the intended person does complete the survey, he or she may not answer questions accurately because there is no opportunity to clarify its contents with the researchers. Self-completion postal surveys can be associated with low completion rates, which reduce the validity of the findings.

For all approaches, surveys have difficulties in obtaining representative samples and with respondents providing accurate data. It can be difficult to obtain a representative sample of patients accessing palliative care, and those with a specific interest in the research question or with personal agendas they wish to advance are most likely to complete the survey. The problem of a representative sample is compounded by the number of patients too ill to complete it, resulting in most palliative surveys having a skewed sample. Patients with the most problems are the least likely to be included in data collection. Some surveys have exclusions, such as for patients unable or unwilling to accept their diagnosis or prognosis or patients dying of noncancer causes, and these exclusions skew samples. There can be difficulties in acquiring accurate information from those completing the surveys; patients may be reluctant to criticize their care for fear of repercussions.[7]

Some palliative care researchers have attempted to obtain a more representative sample by conducting their survey by proxy after the patient's death. Relatives or the patient's caregivers are asked for their views on the services received. This enables the researcher to collect data on the whole period leading up to the patient's death. It is also associated with various problems. Numerous studies found that patients and their relatives or caregivers can have divergent views on symptom control and service satisfaction.[8] Bereavement itself also may influence the views of those completing the survey, or negative memories of the patient's care may be more prominent during the period of sadness likely to accompany this period of bereavement.[7]

OBSERVATIONAL STUDIES

The term *observational research* describes several approaches in which the researcher does not control the treatment or care received by those taking part in the study and in which the participants are observed or certain outcomes are measured. This broad range of methods includes cohort studies, in which the researcher follows participants from their initial treatment to assess the incidence of outcomes and identify predictors, and case-control studies to collect information on patients with terminal illness and those without it to compare factors across groups. A prospective, observational study was exemplified by the evaluation of a comprehensive, adaptable, life-affirming, longitudinal intervention in cases of life-threatening cancer, cardiac illness, respiratory conditions, or dementia.[9]

Observational designs are particularly useful in studying palliative care, for which ethical concerns exist about controlled clinical trials, because they do not deny or affect the treatment of those participating. It is impossible to establish causality from observational studies. Positive outcomes identified may result from factors not specifically related to the palliative care treatments or services administered. It is impossible to rule out, for instance, chance and natural remission of the illness influencing results. Patients' responses to the outcome criteria may have been influenced by beliefs about, attitude toward, and expectations of the treatment or by the beliefs or expectations of health professionals. Findings may be skewed by the Hawthorne effect (i.e., additional attention from participation in an observational study may lead to feelings of gratification and reward, resulting in patients reporting better effects from treatment, regardless of any change from the treatment itself).

CONTROLLED CLINICAL TRIALS

If a researcher does wish to conduct research to establish causality, the controlled clinical trial, particularly the randomized, controlled clinical trial, is considered the gold standard. Controlled clinical trials attempt to exert control over variables that can affect outcome. They compare the intervention under investigation with a control (typically a placebo, no intervention, or waiting list group) or with another intervention (typically one regarded as the best standard therapy).

Advantages

The main advantage of controlled clinical trials is that the methodological rigor of the trial is higher than that of the observational study, because controlled trials reduce the likelihood of results being caused by a placebo effect or other confounding variable. The reliability and validity of a clinical trial are issues not specific to palliative care, but they require some discussion. *Validity* refers to the degree to which the research findings accurately reflect what was assessed, and it can be further divided into internal and external validity. *Internal validity* refers to the extent to which causal statements are supported by the findings. *External validity* is the extent to which the findings can be generalized to the whole population or other settings. In quantitative research, *reliability* refers to the ability to obtain the same findings on all occasions, regardless of which researcher collected or analyzed the data. The rigor of a clinical trial is also higher if participants are randomized to the various treatment arms as this

eliminates study bias. Nonrandomized, controlled trials using matched controls are more common within palliative care, but they do have flaws compared with randomized trials. For instance, there may be fundamental differences between patients who select different care packages, such as those who choose hospice rather than routine care. As the perspectives of patients, health care professionals, and researchers can all bias a clinical trial, the rigor of a trial can be further enhanced by the blinding of the patient (single blind), those administering treatments or services (double blind), and those collecting and analyzing the data (triple blind).

Disadvantages

Despite controlled clinical trials being the gold standard for effectiveness, they are rarely conducted because of a number of methodological and ethical difficulties in palliative care research. Practical challenges for clinical trials in palliative care include the fact that few palliative care services have sufficiently large numbers of patients to recruit the samples necessary to detect statistically significant effects. If researchers are unable to recruit a large sample, it is often advisable to employ stratified randomization to increase the chance of compatibility between groups. Random assignment is done within groups defined by participant characteristics, such as condition severity, to ensure a better balance of these factors across intervention groups. There is also difficulty obtaining patients representative of those receiving palliative care services because of attrition resulting from disease progression or death. The problem of trial samples being unrepresentative of the general population of patients receiving palliative care is exacerbated by unnecessarily excluding patients from the study because of factors such as age or mental status. These complications raise the risk of selection bias (i.e., the characteristics of the sample may be different from those of the wider population receiving palliative care).

Clinical trials in palliative care that rely on self-reported outcome measures have the additional problem that the findings may be biased by those surveyed not giving accurate responses. Some palliative care patients and their relatives find it difficult to be critical of their care, and they want to give favorable reports on those caring for them. Others may understate their symptoms to avoid unpleasant therapeutic repercussions or admission to hospital, and some may exaggerate problems in the hope of altering the services they are receiving. The problem of eliciting accurate responses is not confined to patients. Staff may be reluctant to reveal their psychosocial problems for fear that they will be perceived as weak and unsuited for the job or promotion.[10]

The choice of outcome measures in palliative care clinical trials can be problematic. Few outcome measures have been specifically designed for those affected by terminal illness, raising questions about their validity and reliability when used with these patients. Some outcome measures appear sensitive to the setting in which they are used. Examples include scales for depression that are valid when used for psychiatric patients but that appear invalid for the terminally ill because the outcome measure is sensitive to changes in biological functioning (e.g., sleeping, eating, activity levels), and results are frequently impaired by illness and treatment. Even if outcome measures valid for the patient population are used, patients may be too sick or in too much pain, or their cognitive functioning may be impaired to such a degree that answering questions becomes difficult. If clinical trials use quality of life measures, findings may be distorted by the response shift, sometimes referred to as *positive adjustment*. There is still a dearth of research that has investigated how terminally ill patients perceive their life and judge which aspects of their life are important. Available research suggests patients adjust their standard for quality of life throughout their illness.[10] The purpose of most quality of life instruments is to measure the impact of an intervention in a relatively stable situation. It is debatable whether these instruments are applicable to palliative care, for which the focus of the intervention is on achieving the best possible quality of life in a situation in which known deterioration will occur. Research has found that cancer and noncancer patients report similar levels of life satisfaction, but that non–health-related domains have a greater contribution to quality of life in cancer patients.[11]

To avoid some of the problems associated with attrition, clinical trials have used relatives or caregivers to complete outcome measures by proxy, similar to the approach of some surveys. Considerable evidence suggests that relatives and health care professionals have divergent perceptions to the patient.[12-14] Despite the inherent possibility that relatives or caregivers will have different perspectives from those of the patient, it is sometimes necessary to adopt this approach in palliative care research. The psychosocial self-assessment of the severely ill, for example, can be contaminated by effects of the underlying disease, medication, or treatment.

QUALITATIVE STUDIES

Qualitative methodologies have also been extensively used in palliative care research. These studies typically use open questions in face-to-face interviews with those affected by terminal illness or conduct focus groups with patients, relatives, or caregivers. They can provide a deeper understanding of the views and perspectives of those affected and determine how these views influence and are influenced by their behavior or experiences. Qualitative studies can be particularly suited to topics that participants may find sensitive or personal. Palliative care research has largely allocated a passive role to those affected by terminal illness, responding to questionnaires and measures of quality of life.[15] By their design, qualitative research can provide an opportunity for a more active role, which may help empower those taking part and permit the research to be more directed by the participants' needs and concerns.[16] Within qualitative research, rigor is often assessed in terms of trustworthiness and credibility.[17,18]

As with all methodological approaches within palliative care, qualitative studies have certain ethical concerns that should be considered before undertaking the research. Qualitative approaches to research have intruded on the lives of those affected, raised false hopes, and elicited painful and difficult emotions.[19] Several researchers thought that some patients participating in qualitative research benefited from "telling their story."[20] This raises another ethical question about what happens to the

patient and these therapeutic benefits after the research has been completed and the patient is no longer interacting with the researcher.[19]

RESEARCH DIFFICULTIES

There are generic problems with any psychosocial research methodology used in palliative care. One example is the ethics of including patients with terminal illness. Debate continues about the ethics of involving people who are dying, particularly whether the gain from improving the quality of palliative care in general outweighs the additional demands placed on those taking part.[19,21,22] Investigators agree that palliative care studies must ensure the research questions and designs are relevant and rigorous. "There is an absolute requirement to ensure that such studies are carefully designed to reduce burden to a minimum and to make optimal use of the data collected."[21]

Many researchers can find it difficult to gain access to patients and their relatives. Obtaining approval from research ethics boards can be problematic for studies that involve this population.[23] This difficulty is pronounced for patients perceived by ethics committees as vulnerable, such as those with learning difficulties or mental illness in addition to terminal disease. Gatekeepers, typically health professionals directly caring for the patients, also can impede access. Many investigators have documented the barriers experienced in gaining access to the terminally ill.[24,25] Gatekeeping issues are one of the biggest barriers to recruitment. Health professionals admitted in focus groups that although they believed research was important, they were uneasy approaching individuals for fear of burdening them or in case they said no or got angry with them for asking, believing them to already "have plenty on their plate."[26]

Although the motives for ethics committees and gatekeepers denying access may be justifiable (e.g., concerns about the extra time, effort, and discomfort for patients or their relatives), denying patients the option to participate suggests a paternalistic attitude. Unnecessary exclusion of vulnerable groups from research in palliative care poses a threat to research validity and raises questions about the civil rights of these patients. Even when access is permitted, bias can be introduced by the gatekeeper. Health professionals may choose individuals with positive attitudes about their illness and the care they are receiving or who appear likely to want to participate in research.[26]

Exposure to the distress of patients with a terminal illness may affect the people conducting research. Most palliative care research involves direct contact with the terminally ill, which may raise fears and anxieties about the researcher's own mortality or his or her family and friends.[27] This reaction can be exacerbated by the altruistic nature of the patients or family members participating.

CONCLUSIONS

A range of methodologies can be used for researching psychosocial issues within palliative care. Good research considers the practical and ethical issues in this field and matches the aims of the project with appropriate methods. The study should be rigorous and open in carrying out the research and in dissemination of the findings afterward. All methodological approaches have their own strengths and weaknesses. It is the appropriateness of the methodology and the rigor with which the research is conducted that dictates whether research is good or bad. A rigid distinction between various methodological approaches may be unhelpful, and the triangulation of data through the concurrent use of more than one methodological approach is frequently acknowledged as the most rigorous approach to research.

Most psychosocial research in palliative care has centered on small, unicenter issues. Future research needs to improve the evidence base within the discipline. More longitudinal studies should be conducted to identify how the psychosocial needs of patients, their families, and their caregivers change. Research into methodological approaches and outcome instruments should evaluate their appropriateness for the study of palliative care.

Collaborative research groups within and between academic and service organizations may address some of these issues and increase the number and quality of psychosocial studies in palliative care, particularly for multicenter clinical trials. Collaborative research of this nature may also help alleviate some difficulties associated with research in palliative care. Funding of the Cancer Experiences Collaborative by six partner organizations through the U.K. National Cancer Research Institute is one example. The Cancer Experiences Collaborative is an equal partnership between researchers at five U.K. universities, various clinical organizations, and user representatives, whose purpose is to make substantive progress in research capacity and quality in supportive and palliative care over the next 5 years in a way that ensures that progress is maintained thereafter.[28]

Psychosocial research is essential to ascertain the psychosocial needs of patients with terminal illness. The support and treatments offered require rigorous evaluation to ensure those affected receive optimal support. Psychosocial research also places the user at the center, representing a way of conducting research that retains the holistic approach of modern palliative care.

REFERENCES

1. National Council for Hospice and Specialist Palliative Care Services. Feeling better: Psychosocial care in specialist palliative care. Occasional paper no. 13. London: National Council for Hospice and Specialist Palliative Care Services, 1997.
2. Jeffrey D. What do we mean by psychosocial care in palliative care? In Lloyd-Williams M (ed). Psychosocial Issues in Palliative Care. Oxford, UK: Oxford University Press, 2003, pp 1-12.
3. Glaser BG, Strauss AL. Awareness of Dying. Chicago: Aldine, 1965.
4. Addington-Hall JM, MacDonald LD, Anderson HR, et al. Randomised controlled trial of effects of coordinating care for terminally ill cancer patients. BMJ 1992;305:1317-1322.
5. Addington-Hall JM, MacDonald LD, Anderson HR, et al. Dying from cancer: The views of bereaved family and friends about the experience of terminally ill patients. Palliat Med 1991;5:207-214.
6. Lloyd-Williams M. Senior house officers' experience of a six month post in a hospice. Med Educ 2002;36:45-48.
7. Addington-Hall JM, McCarthy M. Survey research in palliative care using bereaved relatives. In Field D, Clark D, Corner J, et al (eds). Researching Palliative Care. Buckingham, UK: Open University Press, 2001, pp 27-36.
8. Curtis AE, Fernester J. Quality of life of oncology hospice patients: A comparison of patients and primary caregivers' reports. Oncol Nurs Forum 1989;16:49-53.
9. London MR, McSkimming S, Drew N, et al. Evaluation of a comprehensive, adaptable, life-affirming, longitudinal (CALL) palliative care project. J Palliat Med 2005; 8:1214-1225.
10. Courtens A. Instruments to assess quality of palliative care. In Abu-Saad H (ed). Evidence-Based Palliative Care across the Life Span. London: Blackwell Scientific, 2001, pp 103-115.
11. Kreitler S, Chaitchik S, Rapoport Y, et al. Life satisfaction and health in cancer patients, orthopedic patients and healthy individuals. Soc Sci Med 1993;36:547-556.
12. Cohen SR, Mount BM, Bruera E, et al. Validity of the McGill Quality of Life Questionnaire in the palliative care setting: A multi-centre Canadian study demonstrating the importance of the existential domain. Palliat Med 1997;11:3-20.
13. Sprangers MA, Aaronson NK. The role of health care providers and significant others in evaluating the quality of life of patients with chronic disease: A review. J Clin Epidemiol 1992;45:743-760.
14. Higginson I, Wade A, McCarthy M. Palliative care: Views of patients and their families. BMJ 1990;301:227-281.
15. Payne S. Are we using the users [guest editorial]?. Int J Palliat Nurs 2002;8:212.
16. Gott M, Stevens T, Small N, et al. User Involvement in Cancer Care: Exclusion and Empowerment. Bristol, UK: Policy Press, 2000.
17. Guba EG, Lincoln YS. Fourth Generation Evaluation. Thousand Oaks, CA: Sage, 1989.
18. Lincoln YS, Guba EG. Naturalistic Inquiry. Thousand Oaks, CA: Sage, 1985.
19. Wilkie P: Ethical issues in qualitative research in palliative care. Palliat Med 1997;11:321-324.
20. Newman S, Morton R. Research in palliative care nursing. In Kinghorn S, Gamlin R (eds). Palliative Nursing: Bringing Hope and Comfort. London: Baillière Tindall, 2001.
21. Field D, Clark D, Corner J, et al (eds). Researching Palliative Care. Buckingham, UK: Open University Press, 2001.
22. De Raeve L. Ethical issues in palliative care research. Palliat Med 1994;8:298-305.
23. Lee S, Kristjanson L. Human Research ethics committees: Issues in palliative care research. Int J Palliat Nurs 2003;9:13-18.
24. Addington-Hall J. Research sensitivities to palliative care patients. Eur J Cancer Care 2002;11:220-224.
25. Janssens R, Gordijn B. Clinical trials in palliative acre: An ethical evaluation. Patient Educ Couns 2000;41:55-62.
26. Kennedy L, Lloyd-Williams MA, Gabbay M. Children's experiences when a parent has advanced cancer [unpublished PhD thesis, University of Liverpool, submitted 2008].
27. Clark D, Ingleton C, Seymour J. Support and supervision in palliative care research. Palliat Med 2000;14:441-446.
28. Bailey C, Wilson R, Addington-Hall J, et al. The Cancer Experiences Research Collaborative (CECo): Building research capacity in supportive and palliative care. Prog Palliat Care 2006;14:265-270.

SUGGESTED READING

Field D, Clark D, Corner J, et al. Researching Palliative Care. Buckingham, UK: Open University Press, 2001.

Lloyd-Williams M. Psychosocial Issues in Palliative Care. Oxford, UK: Oxford University Press, 2003.

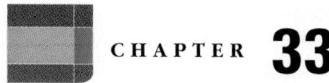

CHAPTER **33**

Qualitative Methodology

Sheila Payne

KEY POINTS

- Qualitative research methodologies are based on a range of theories of knowledge that affect how data are collected, how data are regarded during analysis, what claims are made for the findings, and how the different methods are evaluated.

- There are two major types of qualitative research: experiential (i.e., focuses on how people understand their world) and discursive (i.e., focuses on how language is used to construct the world).

- Qualitative data collection seeks to obtain talk, texts, observations, images, and artifacts using techniques such as interviews, focus groups, and observation.

- There are multiple methods of qualitative data analysis that are rigorous, but most do not transform data into numbers.

- There are several criteria for judging the value of qualitative research that are compatible with the range of theories on which they are based.

Features of Qualitative Methods

A range of rigorous research methods
A heterogeneous group of methods
Suitable to be used alone or in conjunction with quantitative methods
Suitable for examining how things work in context, allowing for attention to the detail, nuances, richness, and complexity of the social world
Suitable for understanding many perspectives
Techniques to collect textual rather than numerical data
Capable of producing explanations, arguments, and theories
Capable of transferability

Incorrect Assumptions about Qualitative Methods

Soft science
A single method in contrast to quantitative research
A preliminary technique before real quantitative research methods are used
Testing preconceived ideas in restricted conditions
Journalism
A tool kit
Merely descriptive
Idiosyncratic accounts

There has been increasing emphasis on evidence-based health care, and within the field of palliative care, qualitative research has been important in providing this.[1] Qualitative methods are among the most useful and frequently used in palliative care research.[2] They concentrate on the richness, diversity, depth, context, complexity, and many perspectives of real life. Their popularity may suggest that they are simple (see "Common Errors"), but the assumptions on which they are based ensure ? that research questions, data collection, and analysis are congruent. Qualitative research is exciting and challenging because it requires intellectual engagement at all stages, especially in data analysis and interpretation. This chapter offers an introduction to the design, conduct, and interpretation of qualitative research. It provides a broad overview that can be supplemented by specialist textbooks for specific methodological procedures and advice from experienced researchers before embarking on research projects.

One widely respected international definition of qualitative research has been proposed[3]:

It is a situated activity that locates the observer in the world. It consists of a set of interpretive, material practices that make the world visible. These practices transform the world. They turn the world into a series of representations, including field notes, interviews, conversations, photographs, recordings, and memos to the self (p. 3).

Qualitative methods draw on a theoretical range that has implications for how data are collected and from whom, how data are regarded during analysis, what claims are made for the findings, and how different methods should be evaluated. These methods are often regarded as different from quantitative methods, but alternatively, they may be conceptualized as varying in several dimensions ? such as researcher control. Qualitative research focuses on contextualized examinations of particular situations and celebrates diversity rather than combining data to make generalizations about populations. Qualitative research methods represent a broad range of approaches to data collection and analysis. There are two major types: experiential, which focuses on how people interpret and understand their world, and discursive, which focuses on how language shapes and constructs the world.[4] Experiential approaches are widely used in palliative care research, and they use analytical methods, such as grounded theory, interpretive phenomenological analysis, and thematic analysis. They are based on the assumption that it is possible to make inferences about experience from verbal accounts. Discursive approaches are less commonly used in palliative care research. They employ analytical methods such as discourse analysis, some types of narrative analysis, and ethnomethodology. They are based on the assumption that language actively shapes the world in which people live. Language is not regarded as a transparent medium for the relay of information. Discursive approaches do not assume it is possible to draw direct inferences about how people feel or think from their verbal accounts.[5] Instead, there is attention to how language is used as a social behavior (e.g., people may use language to threaten, cajole, persuade, or appeal).

Broad approaches to research design that may use quantitative and qualitative methods are called mixed methods designs:

- Ethnography originally was developed in the fields of anthropology and sociology to investigate cultural practices in populations and social groups.
- Action research aims to develop, implement, and evaluate cycles of action (i.e., interventions) using a participatory approach to real world contexts.
- Formative evaluation methodology assesses service and other evaluations, taking account of many perspectives and changing social dynamics.
- Case study methodology focuses on one or more case organizations or social entities (this should not be confused with clinical case studies) to examine phenomena in real world contexts and capture many perspectives.

In the following sections, we consider specific qualitative methodologies. We examine the sequential stages faced by researchers in designing a study, including identifying appropriate research questions for qualitative studies, approaches to data collection, techniques for capturing and transforming data, brief accounts of key methods of analysis, and ways to ensure the quality of qualitative studies. We then comment on the contribution of qualitative research to palliative medicine, provide examples of research using different qualitative methods, and discuss the challenges and opportunities these methods offer to palliative medicine.

DEVELOPMENTS IN QUALITATIVE RESEARCH METHODOLOGY

Qualitative research methodology has a long, rich tradition in social science.[3] It is therefore not new or any less scientific than research in the natural sciences and medicine. However, these methods may be less well known and accepted by some who have backgrounds purely in the biomedical sciences. In the United Kingdom, health services research has increasingly adopted mixed or qualitative methods to address some research questions.

Use of Qualitative Methods

All good research should address specific research questions or hypotheses. Qualitative research tends to answer research questions rather than hypotheses because these designs are often exploratory rather than designed to test predictions. There is a need to identify the intellectual puzzle[6] at the heart of each study to ensure qualitative research is more than descriptive. The wording of the research question should make it clear what, who, when, and how will be researched (Box 33-1). Certain qualitative methods, such as grounded theory analysis, allow refinement and refocusing of questions during the research process.[7,8] In Box 33-1, several research questions relevant to palliative medicine and possible methods of answering them are presented. Research studies designed to explore processes or meanings using questions that ask why lend themselves to qualitative methods. If the research is predominantly concerned with questions that ask how many or how often, these studies may be better suited to

---

Box 33-1 Research Questions and the Types of Qualitative Methods That May Be Used to Answer Them

1. What are informal caregivers' experiences of social care services in specialist palliative care units?
    This question could be answered by conducting interviews to elicit caregivers' understanding and experience using a grounded theory analysis.
2. How do counselors conceptualize psychological support?
    This question could be answered by interpretative phenomenological analysis of interview data.
3. How do doctors' interactions with patients invoke emotional support?
    This question could be answered by using transcripts of medical clinic consultations in a discourse analytic study.
4. How do earlier experiences of loss and life transitions influence adaptation to cancer?
    This question could be answered by asking participants for biographical accounts and using narrative analysis to explore relationships between cancer and loss and life changes.
5. What are the attitudes and beliefs about euthanasia expressed by advanced cancer patients?
    Semistructured interviews may be used to collect data and then analyzed by content analysis.

Box 33-2 Examples of Qualitative Research Designs

As a prelude to using quantitative methods: A study may start by doing a few interviews to clarify the issues before constructing a questionnaire or structured measure. The use of qualitative methods is designed to benefit the quantitative research, which tends to be regarded as the real research.

Concurrently with quantitative methods: Described as mixed methods designs, they have advantages gained by combining approaches. They may help to explain counterintuitive results or offer multiple perspectives (i.e., triangulation). However, they increase the burden of data collection on patients.

After using quantitative methods: Qualitative methods may be used to supplement a quantitative study.

Alone: Qualitative methods may be used as a stand-alone design. The advantage is that the methods of sampling, data collection, and analysis are congruent within the selected epistemological position. This chapter predominantly refers to this type of research design.

---

quantitative designs. Quantitative and qualitative research methods may be used synergistically or separately (Box 33-2).

Types of Sampling

The experiential category is based on investigations of naturalistic contexts in which there is no intention to control variables or manipulate interventions. This may be because it is unethical; for example, it is impossible to randomly allocate people to die or not. Qualitative researchers are interested in how people behave in real world situations, such as caring for a dying person at home. Unlike quantitative research, in which randomization ensures samples represent defined populations to minimize bias and provide the rationale for generalization, qualitative samples are selected on the basis of purposeful intent. This approach may use predefined criteria, such as gender, age, and diagnosis, which are known to differ in the topic of interest. Alternatively, purposeful sampling may be guided by theoretical considerations that emerge during the analysis, such as in grounded theory methods.[7] As in quantitative methods, convenience sampling is the weakest type. Qualitative researchers should describe their sample characteristics in sufficient depth for readers to understand any potential recruitment anomalies.

Qualitative designs collect extensive data about relatively few people, because the analysis focuses on a range of features in the data and considers various nuances that provide the social context of that data set (see Chapter 34). This detailed engagement with understanding, interpreting, and processing textual data is why qualitative methods are so time consuming. There are no established formulas about sufficient sample sizes. Researchers must explain in their reports why their sample is adequate. The following points indicate the usual sample sizes:

- Fewer than 10 people may be appropriate in some types of phenomenology, interpretive phenomenological analysis, and narrative analysis.
- Between 11 and 50 people may be the best sample size in grounded theory and thematic analysis.
- More than 50 people may be used in content analysis.

Types of Data Collected

Most data collection methods are not inherently quantitative or qualitative.[9] Different theoretical positions regard data in different ways. At a simple level, realist researchers regard phenomena as being unproblematically and objectively "out there" in the world and available for collection (albeit with correct measurement tools), whereas an alternative social constructionist stance rejects this possibility. They argue that phenomena are socially defined and shaped within the interaction between the researcher and researched person. In this position, researchers are regarded as being part of the process of data generation and are not independent of it.

Box 33-3 lists different types of data that may be collected for qualitative analysis. The way in which the data are collected and transformed renders them suitable for

qualitative analysis. Some data are *elicited* specifically for the research, such as interviews and focus group discussions, and other data occur *naturally,* such as policy documents and political speeches. Generally, experiential approaches use data that have been specifically collected for the purpose, such as information gathered by interviewing patients to ask them about their experiences with a new service. Discursive approaches prefer spontaneously occurring data for reasons that are described later in "Data Analysis."

In the following sections, we describe common data collection methods that focus on language and text. These are not exclusively used by qualitative researchers because textual data can be transformed into numbers. Each has advantages and disadvantages, and researchers need to consider these features in making choices.

Interviews

The most common way to access data for qualitative analysis is interviews.[10] Interviews vary in the extent to which they are controlled by the researcher's agenda. In *structured interviews,* the researcher asks closed questions requiring yes or no answers or provides predetermined answers that respondents are invited to endorse or reject. The interview is prepared like a questionnaire, and interviewers are often carefully trained to ensure consistency in asking and responding to questions. This approach to interviewing is unsuitable for qualitative analysis. *Semi-structured interviews* predefine to some extent the research topics but enable the interviewee's freedom to present a range of views and offer insights. Interview schedules may be loosely specified (e.g., list of topics). *Unstructured interviews* are open ended and typically invite participants to talk about a topic or tell a story with minimal prompts. Research interviews are different from clinical interviews but build on similar communication skills to encourage respondents to feel comfortable and relaxed and to talk freely.[11] Interviews can be conducted face to face or by telephone. Some qualitative research concentrates on spontaneous talk, such as recording medical consultations, public meetings, or broadcast media such as radio and television.

Focus Groups and Group Discussions

Sometimes, researchers collect data from groups engaged in discussions or debates. In focus groups, the purpose is to encourage interaction between participants so a range of views may be elicited and discussion generated. Decisions must be made at the outset whether group participants should be homogeneous or heterogeneous. The choice is likely to relate to the research question and topic area, and it should consider existing group dynamics. For example, asking unqualified care assistants to discuss work in the presence of their managers may limit data because of preexisting power relationships. Focus groups usually are run by a facilitator, whose role is to introduce topics, encourage participation, and address respondent comfort and safety issues, while an observer records the nature and type of participation by the group. The number of participants varies from 6 to 12, depending on the topic and group. It is a balance between the desire to have a range of views represented and the difficulties of a

---

Box 33-3 Examples of Data That Can Be Used in Qualitative Research

Language in the form of spoken words: These data may be collected during interviews, focus groups, or group discussions.

Language in the form of written text: These data may be collected from written accounts, diaries, newspapers, or policy documents.

Observations of behaviors and environments: These data include behaviors such as talk and nonverbal interactions and environmental factors such as the social organization of space and territories in ethnographic approaches.

Images: These data may be dynamic events (e.g., captured digitally as videos or films), photographs, drawings, or paintings.

Artifacts: These data may include objects and symbols such as sculptures, jewelry, or clothing.

large group and making sense of the resultant audio recording.

Observation

Researchers may wish to observe social interaction. If they do this without being involved directly, it is called *non-participant observation*, and if they are involved (e.g., a nurse working in the observed environment), it is called *participant observation*. Whatever methods are used, observations are systematically recorded as *field notes.* Technological developments mean it is also possible to record behavior using digital cameras more unobtrusively than in the past.

Ethnography emphasizes observation as a key part of data gathering.[12] Observation of human interaction raises important ethical and practical issues. For example, is it ethical to conduct research within sensitive environments such as hospices and with dying patients? Researchers need to consider to what extent behavior and organizational practices are changed by the presence of an observer.

Documentary Data Sources

Written information may be collected. Sources include official documents (e.g., patients' medical records, information leaflets for patients, government policy reports), public media (e.g., newspapers, magazines), private documents (e.g., diaries, essays, biographies), and electronic information (e.g., Web sites, blogs).

Images and Artifacts

Researchers may collect elicited or spontaneous images and artifacts. Sources include drawings, objects, photographs, and paintings (e.g., patients' artwork, family photographs).

DATA CAPTURE AND TRANSFORMATION

Most of the previously described methods of data collection rely on spoken words or behaviors. These are ephemeral phenomena and need to be captured by the researcher writing field notes (i.e., contemporaneous written accounts) or, more commonly, by audio or visual recording. If the analysis is concerned with linguistic performance, the latter techniques must be used because it is difficult to write down conversations. Field notes are acceptable if the researcher wants to capture complex social situations and record general behaviors, but they are prone to bias because of selective attention and recall.

When data are captured electronically as an audio or video recording, they usually require transcription to written text. Although this work is often delegated to a secretary, choices about the level and type of transcription involve analytical decisions that depend on the nature of the analysis to be conducted.[13] For example, if a grounded theory analysis is planned, it is important to transcribe the speech of the interviewer and interviewee, but it is not usually necessary to transcribe prosodic, paralinguistic, or extralinguistic elements. Discourse analysis requires more complete and detailed transcriptions because the researcher is often concerned with what is said and how it is said. The most detailed and therefore time-consuming transcription procedures are necessary for conversation analysis where specific and precise notation systems are available.

One key feature of qualitative analysis is that it does not start by transforming non-numerical phenomena into numbers, although in some approaches, researchers may use counts of categories or themes to support their arguments. A practical problem in most qualitative research is that it quickly generates large amounts of data that need consistent and reliable data storage systems. This ensures data can be retrieved when required during analysis and provides an audit trail, which is part of the quality process. There are several qualitative data analysis software packages, with characteristic advantages and disadvantages. They are useful for facilitating the manipulation, indexing, and retrieval of data, but they do not alter the need for sustained and intensive engagement with the data during the intellectual process of coding and interpretation. The disadvantage of some packages is that they are labor intensive during data input and coding, and they may inadvertently structure data analysis in prescribed ways, such as hierarchical or linear structures.

DATA ANALYSIS

Having collected and transformed words, texts, and images, the next step facing the researcher is to make sense of and interpret the data. There are many ways to do this, and this is a brief introduction to common approaches. More information can be obtained from specialist sources and experts before embarking on analysis. Research methods are dynamic and open to modification, but they must be logically coherent with the research purpose (i.e., expressed in the research question) and with the theoretical position taken. A selection of analytical methods is presented to reflect the diversity of approaches (Table 33-1).[14]

Content Analysis

The purpose of content analysis is to group data into categories and establish frequency counts. It can be used alone or in combination with quantitative analysis.[15] It is a highly structured approach that involves mutually exclusive, predetermined categories. These can be single words, such as vomiting or nausea, or tightly defined conceptual categories, such as types of coping behavior. Considerable effort is expended in defining the categories before examining the data, because this perhaps enhances rigor. The data are then searched and instances identified. Counts of the frequencies of the categories in the interview transcripts or documents are made. Alternatively, in inductive content analysis, the categories are derived directly from the material to be analyzed rather than applied a priori. This is most suitable when there is a desire to combine qualitative and quantitative data. An advantage is that there are clear analytical procedures, and it is possible to achieve good inter-rater reliability between coders. However, it tends to decontextualize data by segmenting it, and evidence of greater frequency alone cannot be taken to infer importance. There may be many reasons why particular words occur more or less frequently.

TABLE 33-1   Key Features of Common Qualitative Research Methods of Analysis

METHOD	TYPES OF DATA	SAMPLE SIZE	FEATURES OF CODING	RESULTS OF ANALYSIS
Content analysis	Open-ended questions in questionnaires, structured interviews, documents	Larger data sets	Predetermined categories, mutually exclusive	Frequency counts
Thematic analysis	Semistructured interviews, focus groups, written texts, images	Medium to smaller data sets	Inductive categories, including manifest and latent themes	Descriptive accounts summarizing common phenomena across individuals
Grounded theory analysis	Semistructured or unstructured interviews, focus groups	Smaller data sets, theoretical sampling	Inductive coding, constant comparative analysis, theoretical saturation	Generation of new theory, analytic and complex accounts of the data
Narrative analysis	Stories from verbal accounts (e.g., oral histories) and written accounts (e.g., diaries, autobiographies, biographies)	Smaller data sets	Experiential: focus on life changes, events, and meaning Discursive: focus on linguistic features, employment	Experiential: descriptive and analytical account of stories and experience Discursive: account of the way language is used to create a story, moral accounts that convey messages
Phenomenology	Unstructured in-depth interviews and accounts	Smaller data sets	Practical strategies to gain access to essence of phenomenon	Exploring the lived experience, detailed insight into the life world of participants; in-depth interpretation of phenomena
Discourse analysis	Naturally occurring or spontaneous text (e.g., medical records) or talk (e.g., public speeches)	Medium to smaller data sets	No specific procedures but include reading, coding, interpenetration, writing	Discursive approach: detailed accounts of how language is used in shaping social interaction Foucauldian discourse analysis: detailed analytic accounts of role of language in the social construction of reality

Adapted from Payne S. Qualitative methods of data collection and analysis. In Addington-Hall J, Higginson I, Bruera E, Payne S (eds). **Research Methods in Palliative Care.** Oxford: Oxford University Press, 2007.

Thematic Analysis

Thematic analysis identifies commonalities in transcripts, documents, and other types of data.[15] Thematic analysis refers to a group of methods similar to content analysis but without necessarily the intent of converting the data into frequencies or imposing a priori categories. Coding of themes may focus on manifest content (e.g., specific phrases such as dying at home) or may include identification of latent content (e.g., coding segments of text, making references to place of death even when this actual phrase is not used). One example is framework analysis,[16] which offers distinct, interconnected steps involving familiarization, identifying a thematic matrix, indexing, charting, mapping, and interpretation. Thematic analysis is popular because it appears to represent the subtlety and complexity of qualitative data, and it results in intuitively coherent accounts. It allows researchers to group apparently similar responses across individuals and capture meanings. It has the advantage of being less time consuming than methods such as grounded theory analysis. Thematic analysis should be considered when the aims of analysis are descriptive accounts that summarize phenomena across individuals.

Grounded Theory Analysis

The purpose of grounded theory analysis is to develop new inductive theory, not merely describe data. Several versions have developed,[7,8] and there are lively debates about what should be regarded as the essential principles

and procedures. Analysis involves careful reading, followed by allocating labels (i.e., categories) to segments of text (i.e., meaningful units). Coding is based on constant comparative analysis, in which the coding of each transcript is compared with previous codes, and they are modified by new insights as they are "discovered." Analysis, coding, and sampling are concurrent and iterative, rather than sequential. Some key features of grounded theory analysis include theoretical sampling and theoretical coding, because the aim is to develop explanatory theory, not merely describe data. The disadvantages are that this process is time consuming, and by segmenting text, it decontextualizes data.

Narrative Analysis

Narrative analysis examines the stories people tell about their lives. Narrative analysis represents methodological approaches that can focus on interpreting the meaning of life events and transitions through biographical stories, or it can examine the linguistic structure, plot, and function of stories.[17] Analysis usually aims to maintain the integrity of the account by focusing on features of the story as told by each participant, rather than making comparisons among several individuals. Narrative analysis is appropriate if the research is interested in life transitions.

Phenomenology

The purpose of using a phenomenological approach is to gain an in-depth understanding of the lived experience of another person and an insight into their world. Phenomenology is a philosophy that conceptualizes human experience, and various analytical procedures have been developed from this approach. Perhaps the most useful is interpretative phenomenological analysis (IPA), which offers clear guidance on analyis.[18] The advantages are that these analytical procedures emphasize the meaning given to events and experiences. This approach does not impose external categories or theories, but it is complex and time consuming.

Discourse Analysis

The purpose of discourse analysis is to identify (i.e., decontextualize) ways of talking or writing (i.e., discourses). For example, dying patients may be described as medical failures, as heroes (i.e., fighting cancer), or as victims. These descriptions imply different representations or perceptions of people. There are many methods of analysis that focus on how everyday social interactions are negotiated and managed or that examine how language constitutes social and psychological experience.[5] Analysis includes careful reading, coding, interpretation, and writing while continually questioning the text to focus on how language is used rather than on what people are saying. Discursive analysis may help if the researcher is interested in how different versions of reality are produced, negotiated, and evoked in normal conversation and texts. These powerful techniques challenge ways of knowing that are taken for granted, and they can reveal competing power positions in society.

ASSESSING THE QUALITY OF QUALITATIVE RESEARCH

Criteria have been published for the quality of general and specific methods used in qualitative research.[19] The following techniques depend on the analytical method used:

- Maintaining an audit trail
- Triangulation
- Respondent validation
- Reflexivity

Qualitative researchers tend to address credibility, trustworthiness, and transferability rather than use the quantitative terminology of validity, reliability, and generalizability to establish rigor.

Qualitative studies have provided evidence for many common practices that underpin contemporary palliative medicine. For example, the open disclosure of diagnostic information in cancer care and open awareness arise from research on dying people in hospitals conducted in the United States in the 1950s.[20] Qualitative data collection techniques, such as interviewing and the narrative interview, were developed in the work of Dame Cicely Saunders and Elisabeth Kübler-Ross. Both produced seminal work based on carefully listening to and analyzing the accounts of individual patients.

Developments in this field include the emergence of narrative medicine, in which careful attention is paid to understanding the life and perspectives of patients in formulating agreed plans of care, and the growing focus on user involvement and attempts to elicit the views and preferences of patients and families to guide service development. Research about dying people using ethnographic techniques has revealed, challenged, and shaped our understanding of palliative care.

CONCLUSIONS

Qualitative research methods include diverse techniques and approaches that can contribute to the development of an evidence base in palliative medicine. These techniques, which celebrate the complexity and richness of the social world, are useful for dealing with the multifaceted organizational and sociopolitical contexts of palliative care services. Many of the techniques of data collection, such as interviewing, are acceptable to patients, even in the advanced stages of illness. Critiques of quantitative research designs, particularly randomized, controlled trials, in palliative medicine highlight the advantages of qualitative studies and research using mixed methods.[1] Although participatory and mixed methods designs offer advantages, there remain substantial practical and ethical hurdles. Further advances in systematic review methodology are required to enable the inclusion and synthesis of qualitative designs. Clark[21] has argued that qualitative methods are more than a tool kit; they require intellectual engagement, innovation, ethical sensitivity, reflexivity, and the ability to write.

REFERENCES

1. Aoun S, Kristjanson IJ. Challenging the framework for evidence in palliative care research. Palliat Med 2005;19:461-465.
2. Bailey C, Froggatt K, Field D, Krishnasamy M. The nursing contribution to qualitative research in palliative care 1990-1999: A critical reflection. J Adv Nurs 2002;40:48-60.
3. Denzin NK, Lincoln YS. Handbook of Qualitative Research, 2nd ed. Thousand Oaks, CA: Sage, 2000.
4. Reicher S. Against methodolatry: Some comments on Elliott, Fischer and Rennie. Br J Clin Psychol 2000;39:1-6.
5. Willig C. Introducing Qualitative Research in Psychology. Buckingham, UK: Open University Press, 2001.
6. Mason J. Qualitative Researching, 2nd ed. London: Sage, 2002.
7. Strauss A, Corbin J. Basics of Qualitative Research: Grounded Theory Procedures and Techniques. Newbury Park, CA: Sage, 1990.
8. Glaser BG. Emergence vs Forcing: Basics of Grounded Theory Analysis. Mill Valley, CA: Sociology Press, 1992.
9. Payne S. Selecting an approach and design in qualitative research. Palliat Med 1997;11:249-252.
10. Kvale S. InterViews: An Introduction to Qualitative Research Interviewing. London: Sage, 1996.
11. Payne S. Interview in qualitative research. In Memon A, Bull R (eds). Handbook of the Psychology of Interviewing. Chichester, UK: John Wiley, 1999, pp 89-102.
12. Denzin NK. Interpretive Ethnography. Thousand Oaks, CA: Sage, 1997.
13. Ingleton C, Seymour J. Analysing qualitative data: Examples from two studies of end-of-life care. Int J Palliat Nurs 2001;7:227-234.
14. Payne S. Qualitative methods of data collection and analysis. In Addington-Hall J, Higginson I, Bruera E, Payne S (eds). Research Methods in Palliative Care. Oxford, UK: Oxford University Press, 2007.
15. Joffe H, Yardley Y. Content and thematic analysis. In Marks D, Yardley L (eds). Research Methods for Clinical and Health Psychology. London: Sage, 2004, pp 56-68.
16. Ritchie J, Spencer L. Qualitative data analysis for applied policy research. In Bryman A, Burgess R (eds). Analyzing Qualitative Data. London: Sage, 1994.
17. Reissman C. Narrative Analysis—Qualitative Research Methods, series 30. London: Sage, 1993.
18. Smith JA, Osborn M. Interpretative phenomenological analysis. In Smith JA (ed). Qualitative Psychology: A Practical Guide to Research Methods. London: Sage, 2003.
19. Appleton J. Analyzing quantitative data: Addressing issues of validity and reliability. J Adv Nurs 1995;22:993-999.
20. Glaser BG, Strauss AL. Awareness of Dying. New York: Adeline Publishing, 1965.
21. Clark D. What is qualitative research and what can it contribute to palliative care? Palliat Med 1997;11:159-166.

SUGGESTED READING

Addington-Hall J, Higginson I, Bruera E, Payne S (eds). Research Methods in Palliative Care. Oxford, UK: Oxford University Press, 2007.

Denzin NK, Lincoln YS. Handbook of Qualitative Research, 2nd ed. Thousand Oaks, CA: Sage, 2000.

Mason J. Qualitative Researching, 2nd ed. London: Sage, 2002.

Sliverman D. Doing Qualitative Research. London: Sage, 2000.

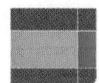

CHAPTER **34**

Priorities for the Future: The Research Agenda

Katherine Hauser, Nabila Bennani-Baiti, Jordanka Kirkova, Wael Lasheen, Ruth Powazki, and Dilara Seyidova-Khoshknabi

KEY POINTS

- The gold standard for evidence-based medicine is the randomized, controlled trial, but these studies have been difficult to conduct in palliative medicine, and some authorities have suggested alternative strategies for finding and classifying evidence.

- Gold standards require agreement on definitions of symptoms, syndromes, and quality of life.

- Practice guidelines are often based on clinical experience and extrapolation of evidence from other conditions. Even when good evidence exists, gaps remain in dissemination and implementation.

- Research priorities indicated by patients include communication, service provision, and caregiver support more often than symptom research.

- Patients are more willing to participate in disease-modifying trials than those for symptom-related therapy.

- Qualitative or mixed (i.e., qualitative and quantitative) methods may be especially relevant for evaluation of communication, coping, preferences, satisfaction, services, and support.[28]

Palliative medicine has been a recognized medical specialty in the United Kingdom since 1987. Specialty recognition also has been achieved in Australia, Canada, and the United States. To justify the distinction of palliative care as a unique form of clinical practice, we need a supporting evidence base. The gold standard for evidence-based medicine is the randomized, controlled trial. In palliative medicine, randomized, controlled trials have been difficult to conduct, and some authorities have suggested alternative strategies for finding and classifying evidence.[1-3]

THE EVIDENCE BASE

Epidemiology of Needs and Symptoms

Much is known about symptom epidemiology of advanced cancer in palliative medicine, but little is understood about the symptoms of oncology patients receiving active treatment. The literature suggests that patients with advanced noncancer conditions (including human immunodeficiency virus [HIV] infection) experience a high symptom burden and have psychosocial needs in hospital or community settings.[4,5] Few prospective studies describe the symptom burden in children with advanced cancer. Information is lacking about the symptom burden in children with advanced nonmalignant diseases (e.g., neurological conditions) and the longitudinal course and impact of symptoms.[6] Despite the high symptom burden in advanced disease, the lack of symptom recognition remains an issue.[7,8]

Symptom Mechanisms and Pathophysiology

Much is known about the pathophysiology of pain, nausea, vomiting, and anorexia-cachexia, but less is understood about other symptoms, such as depression, delirium, fatigue, and memory loss. It has been suggested that many cancer symptoms cluster and may originate from common mechanisms (e.g., inflammation).[9]

Assessment

Reviews of available assessment instruments for pain, other symptoms, and quality of life have been published (Table 34-1). Although many validated instruments are available, head-to-head comparisons (Box 34-1) and gold standards are lacking. Gold standards require agreement on definitions of symptoms, syndromes, and quality of life. For example, fatigue may be defined as a unidimensional symptom or a multidimensional syndrome (including mood, sleep, and cognitive problems). Quality of life instruments are often based on definitions by experts rather than on the situation as perceived by an individual. Consensus is lacking about the format of a gold standard instrument (e.g., how many symptoms, dimensions, time frame).

Interventions and Outcomes

The Cochrane Pain, Palliative, and Supportive Care Group was established to produce systematic reviews.[10] Many published systematic reviews (see Table 34-1) were unable to find any randomized trials. Practice guidelines are often based on clinical experience and extrapolation of evidence from other conditions (e.g., diabetic peripheral

> **Box 34-1 Methodological Issues in Palliative Medicine Clinical Trials**
>
> - Small numbers
> - Nonrandomized, nonblinded trials
> - Insufficient follow-up
> - Lack of standardized outcomes and reporting

TABLE 34-1   Selected Systematic Reviews in Palliative Medicine

TOPIC	STUDY	RCT EVIDENCE	CONCLUSIONS
SERVICE PROVISION			
Palliative care teams	Hearn and Higginson, 1998[38] Higginson et al, 2002[39]	5 RCTs 13 others	Increased satisfaction, reduced hospital days and cost Overall small positive effect Standardized outcome measures needed Need comparisons of different models of care provision
Communication skills training for cancer professionals	Fellowes et al, 2004[40]	3	Training effective in some areas of communication
Palliative care for HIV/AIDS	Harding and Higginson, 2003[41]	1	Lack of standardized outcomes Further studies needed
ASSESSMENT INSTRUMENTS			
Pain*	Caraceni et al, 2002[42]	NA	Summarizes psychometrics of instruments and gives recommendations for research use
Quality of life (as outcome measure in clinical trials)†	Kaasa and Loge, 2002[43]	17	Attrition high in randomized studies Need definitions of clinically significant changes Various instruments used; no agreement on number or type of domains
Symptoms (cancer)	Kirkova et al, 2006[44]	NA	Wide variety of instruments Consensus lacking on number of symptoms, scales, dimensions, and time frame Need guidelines on validation
INTERVENTIONS			
Anorexia, cachexia	Yavuzsen et al, 2005[45]	29 on progestins 6 on corticosteroids Others	Evidence supports progestins and corticosteroids, not hydrazine Other interventions with mixed results Universal outcome measures needed
Anxiety	Jackson and Lipman, 2004[46]	None met criteria	Insufficient evidence RCTs needed
Bisphosphonates, bone metastases	Wong and Wiffen, 2002[47]	30	Evidence supports bisphosphonates for some delayed pain relief
Caregivers	Harding and Higginson, 2003[41]	2 RCTs 3 Observational	Lack of standardized outcomes Alternative research designs needed Limited evidence for effectiveness
Complementary therapy†	Ernst, 2001[48]	NA	Preliminary evidence supports many complementary therapies Need trials comparing complementary and traditional approaches (e.g., antiemetics)
Constipation	Miles et al, 2006[49]	4	Inadequate evidence Need RCTs comparing different classes and combinations
Depression	Rodin et al, 2007[50]	7 Pharmacologic 4 Nonpharmacologic	Limited evidence RCTs needed, especially for newer agents
Delirium	Keeley, 2007[51]	4 (3 HIV)	Few RCTs, methodologically weak Some evidence for haloperidol, but little evidence for artificial hydration, barbiturates, benzodiazepines, opioid switching
Dyspnea and opioids	Jennings et al, 2001[52]	18 (9 nebulized, 9 not nebulized)	Evidence supports oral or parenteral, not nebulized opioids Numbers small; larger trials needed
Fatigue (cancer related)	Lawrence et al, 2004[53]	11	Only 1 in advanced disease (weekly support group) Majority small trials ($N < 100$)
Insomnia	Hirst and Sloan, 2002[54]	0	Insufficient evidence RCTs needed
Malignant bowel obstruction (medical management)	Mercadante et al, 2007[55]	5	Small numbers and methodological problems Octreotide more effective than hyoscine butylbromide, corticosteroids debatable
Nausea	Glare et al, 2004[56]	7 RCTs 12 Observational	Response rates higher in observational studies than RCTs Evidence supports metoclopramide for dyspepsia and corticosteroids for malignant bowel obstruction Evidence conflicting or lacking for other therapies
PAIN			
Opioids for breakthrough pain	Zeppetella and Ribeiro, 2006[57]	4	All oral transmucosal fentanyl citrate studies No trial evidence for other opioids
Ketamine	Bell et al, 2003[26]	2 (2 others had inappropriate designs)	Insufficient evidence Need RCTs

TABLE 34-1 Selected Systematic Reviews in Palliative Medicine—cont'd

TOPIC	STUDY	RCT EVIDENCE	CONCLUSIONS
Methadone	Nicholson, 2004[58]	8	Evidence supports analgesic efficacy similar to morphine Most single-dose or short-term studies No evidence for role in neuropathic pain
Morphine	Wiffen et al, 2003[59]	45	Unable to perform meta-analysis Most trials small ($N < 100$)
NSAIDs or paracetamol	McNicol et al, 2005[60]	42	NSAIDS superior to placebo Combination with opioid inconclusive
Opioid switching	Quigley, 2004[61]	0	Observational evidence supports opioid switching Randomized studies needed for effectiveness, conversion ratios, and order of opioids
Psychosocial Interventions	Uitterhoeve et al, 2004[62]	10	Evidence supports behavior therapy in advanced cancer
RADIOTHERAPY			
Bone metastases (single vs. multifraction)	McQuay et al, 2000[63] Wai et al, 2004[64]	20 11	Number needed to treat for complete pain relief at 1 mo = 4.2 Duration of relief = 12 weeks No difference in pain relief or spinal cord compression Higher retreatment and pathological fracture rates with single fraction
Brain metastases	Tsao et al, 2006[65]	8	No benefit (survival, symptoms, neurological function) for altered dose vs. standard schedule

*Expert Working Group Recommendations.
†Clinical nonsystematic review.
HIV/AIDS, human immunodeficiency virus infection/acquired immunodeficiency syndrome; NA, not available; NSAIDs, nonsteroidal anti-inflammatory drugs; RCT, randomized, controlled trial.

TABLE 34-2 Anorexia Research Agenda

TOPICS	HIGH PRIORITIES	LOW PRIORITIES
Definition	Standard definition of anorexia Symptom or syndrome? Unidimensional or multidimensional?	
Assessment	Validated tools to assess response to intervention Validated severity grading Screening: part of routine practice? Nausea and vomiting: part of anorexia assessment?	
Pathophysiology	Origins: central or peripheral, or both? Anorexia: part of cachexia or separate? Correlations between anorexia and cachexia Translational studies: involvement of neurohormones in human eating Role of cytokines and hormones (e.g., ghrelin, leptin) Mechanisms of orexigenic drugs	Prevalence in cancer Prevalence in advanced cancer Role of therapeutic (e.g., opioids, antitumor) modalities in pathogenesis
Intervention and outcomes	Prevention: nutritional counseling Management: clinical guidelines Therapeutics: metoclopramide, cannabinoids, ghrelin, thalidomide, nutritional counseling	Therapeutics: hydrazine sulfate, enteral nutrition, corticosteroids, progestins

neuropathy for neuropathic pain). Few interventions have been subjected to cost-benefit analysis. When good evidence does exist, gaps remain in dissemination and implementation. For example, despite evidence supporting hypofractionated radiotherapy for symptom palliation, it is not routinely practiced.[11]

TOPICAL RESEARCH AGENDAS

Challenges of research in symptom and quality of life assessment include a lack of agreed definitions (e.g., unidimensional versus multidimensional symptoms). Lengthy questionnaires are difficult to complete, and studies comparing them struggle with attrition and missing data. *Quality of life* is a multidimensional construct, and choosing the right instrument is challenging. Many instruments have determined domains of assessment, which may not always comply with individual quality of life. Individualized assessments seem attractive; however, there are no standard statistical methods to compare with standardized quality of life instruments. Challenges in advanced disease include involving caregivers in the assessment of a very individual perception such as quality of life and symptoms. Future research should determine the quality of life domains and assessment methods that can provide the most reliable data (Tables 34-2 to 34-8).

TABLE 34-3   Cachexia Research Agenda

TOPICS	HIGH PRIORITIES	LOW PRIORITIES
Definition	Standard definition Symptom or syndrome? Unidimensional or multidimensional? Different diseases: same definition?	
Assessment	Guidelines for assessment Screening tools Validated severity grading Body compartment assessment Role of imaging in screening, detection, assessment	
Pathophysiology	Comparison in different diseases Predictors: What are they? Clinical utility? Inflammation Correlation with tumor type, stage, therapy Markers (e.g., CRP) for detection, follow-up, prognosis	Prevalence studies
Intervention and outcomes	Prevention: preventive measures in at-risk populations, nutritional counseling Management: clinical guidelines Therapeutics: anti-cytokine therapy, NSAIDs, nutritional management, combination therapies (e.g., NSAIDs and progestins), ghrelin, omega-3-fatty acids, cannabinoids, physical training Outcomes: cost-benefit analysis of intervention (e.g., survival, quality of life, reduced toxicities)	Therapeutics: enteral nutrition, progestins, corticosteroids

CRP, C-reactive protein; NSAIDs, nonsteroidal anti-inflammatory drugs.

TABLE 34-4   Fatigue Research Agenda

TOPICS	HIGH PRIORITIES	LOW PRIORITIES
Definition	Language of fatigue (i.e., comparing fatigue, weakness, tiredness)	
Assessment	Validation of 1-item fatigue screen Incorporate bioelectrical impedance analysis (BIA) and body fat index (BFI) to determine correlation between lean body mass, phase angle, and fatigue Association of fatigue, sleep-awake cycle, and depression (to create data on sleep habits and fatigue) Ecological momentary assessment (EMA) and subjective assessment of fatigue plus distress	Assessing only subjective fatigue (different questionnaires measuring sensitivity of fatigue and their correlation to different symptoms) Validation of different lengthy instruments (specificity and sensitivity)
Pathophysiology	Screening algorithm predicting response to different medications based on pharmacogenetics	
Intervention and outcomes	Pharmacological: psychostimulants (large, placebo-controlled trials with subjective and objective assessment), vitamin D (placebo-controlled studies), L-carnitine, gabapentin with neuromuscular testing Nonpharmacological randomized, controlled trails: exercise incorporated with changes of immune function, sleep therapy, cognitive behavioral therapy, nutritional counseling	

TABLE 34-5   Pain Research Agenda

TOPICS	HIGH PRIORITIES	LOW PRIORITIES
Definition	Universal classification to facilitate communication and devise treatment guidelines	
Assessment	Consensus on assessment instruments to allow comparison and meta-analysis Characteristics in advanced noncancer diseases	Comprehensive pain assessment instruments
Pathophysiology	Screening algorithm predicting opioid response based on pharmacogenetics	
Intervention and outcomes	Complementary therapy: acupuncture, art, music, hypnosis, and aromatherapy Adjuvants: adjuvants and coanalgesic for use in cancer pain (e.g., nonsteroidal anti-inflammatory drugs for neuropathic pain) Opioids: evidence-based route of conversion and drug rotation potency ratio tables, long-term (>7 days) safety evaluation of methadone, evidence-based protocols for dose adjustment after active interventions (e.g., radiotherapy, surgery) Other interventions: role of chemotherapy and radiotherapy for pain control, guidelines for use (e.g., indications, contraindications, dosing, timing)	Comparative efficacy studies Multiple opioids simultaneously Utility in patient-controlled analgesia

TABLE 34-6   Psychosocial Research Agenda

TOPICS	HIGH PRIORITIES	LOW PRIORITIES
Definition	Psychosocial model of care: What is psychosocial research? How is research organized? Who decides?	
Assessment	Patient's needs: Identify differences in needs between gender and age. Family's needs: How to meet needs? Do they cluster? Survey of needs of patient and family. Caregiver's needs: self-identify needs, user involvement Spiritual or existential meaning of illness: identify patient-preferred discussion (three questions in every consult).	
Processes and interventions	Communication: family conferences, how to enable family care, guidelines to ensure comprehension when discussing transitions in life-threatening illness Boundaries and termination: identify relationship termination styles as effective work with families; self-awareness of relationship boundaries Interdisciplinary teams: collaboration and integration of medical and psychosocial information Decision making and advance care planning: patient and family styles (passive, active, collaborative)	
Outcomes	Patient and family satisfaction: overall satisfaction with emotional and social care, reduced burden of care and bereavement, enhanced family functioning Enhanced or optimized use of resources: discharge planning (length of stay)	

TABLE 34-7   Symptoms Research Agenda

TOPICS	HIGH PRIORITIES	LOW PRIORITIES
Definition	Compare symptoms at the end of life for cancer and noncancer diseases	

Assessment	Randomized, controlled trials for different assessment elements:
	  Structure (self-assessment vs. medical records)
	  Raters (observers vs. self-assessment) in specific conditions: delirium, dementia, poor performance status, end of life
	  Scales (e.g., visual analogue, numerical, categorical)
	  Longitudinal symptom assessment
	  Minimally clinically important difference determined for different symptoms and scales
	  Determine how to equate scales and instruments
	  Computerized adaptive testing for comprehensive assessment
	  Determine dimension (e.g., severity, distress, relief) most sensitive to change for a single-item scale
		Develop new questionnaires; current existing are not ideal
		Prevalence studies, which provide important epidemiology information and epidemiology changes with advances of treatment

Intervention and outcomes	The role of feedback of symptom assessment in improving treatment outcomes Factors that influence assessment and possibly outcomes: compliance, clear explanation, attrition	

TABLE 34-8   Quality of Life Research Agenda

TOPICS	HIGH PRIORITIES	LOW PRIORITIES
Definition	Quality of life (QOL) of caregivers and patients; QOL of the family QOL and patient needs	Overall QOL of patients from caregiver's perspective
Assessment	Randomized, controlled trials to compare summary indexes from individualized QOL, standard instruments and single overall QOL questions QOL and personality traits (e.g., coping skills, demographics)	QOL with interventions with lack of control for compliance, learning, personality traits Many studies showed minimal improvement, or results were negative.
Intervention and outcomes	Longitudinal trials to determine response shift and areas to intervene QOL and services of care, disposition compared with subjective QOL QOL-adjusted years (QUAY) for patients on antitumor treatment QOL as secondary outcome in every clinical trial	QOL as a primary outcome in a clinical trial

Symptom research encounters similar challenges, including a lack of standardization, agreed-on definitions, and consistent outcome measures. Placebo-controlled trials (especially in studying pain) face ethical dilemmas. Clinical studies comparing active treatments face recruitment challenges and are often underpowered to definitively answer clinical questions. Longitudinal studies are challenged by attrition because of short survival. Development of appropriate animal models to study advanced disease (e.g., anorexia-cachexia) is also challenging.[12] Different models are needed for the same symptom in different diseases (e.g., anorexia-cachexia) and different cancer stages (e.g., fatigue during treatment versus survival versus advanced disease). Lack of research funding specifically for palliative medicine hampers clinical trials of expensive investigations and treatments.

Delivering, assessing, and evaluating psychosocial care is challenged by fragmentation. Primary psychosocial care providers include social workers, psychologists, psychiatrists, nurses, health care chaplains, and providers of complementary care. Each profession has a different skill set and approach to care. Psychosocial interventions are difficult to standardize and describe in the research studies evaluating them.

PATIENT, FAMILY, AND CONSUMER RESEARCH AGENDAS

Despite ethical concerns about asking dying patients to participate in research, many are interested in doing so and have opinions about what is important. Research priorities indicated by patients include communication, service provision, and caregiver support more often than symptom research.[13] Patients are more willing to participate in disease-modifying trials than studies of symptom-related therapy.[14] Complementary therapies also attract support. Trials involving venipuncture and daily symptom diaries are less attractive.[15] Encouraging user participation in research may improve study design and recruitment.

FUTURE DIRECTIONS

Research Methods

Basic science research is needed in symptom pathophysiology in animal models and in humans for various conditions (e.g., cachexia in cancer, heart failure). Randomized trials of interventions are needed in palliative medicine (Box 34-2), but they are difficult, and attention to design is important. Randomized trials in palliative medicine must be pragmatic; involve clinically relevant, diverse populations and practice settings (e.g., limited exclusion criteria, multiple sites); and incorporate a wide range of outcomes, including satisfaction, quality of life, and costs.[16] Drawbacks of these designs include large sample size, long duration, and expense. Data collection should be minimized. Control arms should be active or best standard care, rather than placebo (i.e., comparisons of two clinically reasonable alternatives or standard versus complementary therapy). These trials require much time and money. Multicenter collaboratives may facilitate randomized trials, but more specific funding is needed. Trial design should aim for adequate statistical power for definitive results. This requires larger sample sizes, and recruitment methods need to be addressed (Box 34-3).[17-20] Standardized outcomes and definitions of intervention response are needed to allow meta-analysis in the future. Alternative research designs (e.g., crossover designs, cluster randomized, factorial designs, N of 1 trials) need to be considered and may improve the ability to complete a clinical trial.[19,21,22]

Past efforts to perform randomized trials in palliative medicine have resulted in frustration and high costs (time and money) for minimal returns.[3] Meta-analyses suggest that for selected clinical questions, observational studies provide reliable answers that can later be confirmed by

---

Box 34-2 Future Directions in Palliative Medicine Research

Basic Science

Symptom pathophysiology
Comparison of pathophysiology of symptoms between diseases

Randomized, Controlled Trials

Pragmatic trials
Multicenter collaborations

Alternative Research Designs

Crossover designs
Before and after intervention or practice change
N of 1 trials
Mixed methods (qualitative and quantitative)
User participation in research design

Populations

Noncancer
Pediatric
Minorities or indigenous people
People of developing nations

Policy and Funding

Increased funding for specific palliative medicine research
Funding encouraging collaborations

Dissemination of Evidence

Evidence-based clinical guidelines
Strategies for implementation of guidelines

Box 34-3 Improving Recruitment in Palliative Medicine Clinical Trials

- Participation of stakeholders (e.g., clinical staff, nurses, community leaders)
- Recruitment officer separate from clinical team
- Eligible patients identified by clinical criteria rather than clinician's referral
- Inclusion criteria minimized but ensure adequate survival in longitudinal studies
- Minimize data collection
- Recruitment letters and brochures
- Matched-ethnicity interviewers

---

randomized trials.[23-25] Reviews concluding that there is insufficient evidence to make recommendations provide little clinical guidance and risk "throwing the baby out with the bath water."[26,27] Standards are needed for assessing observational evidence so it contributes to clinical practice while randomized trials are developed.

Qualitative or mixed (i.e., qualitative and quantitative) methods may be especially relevant for evaluation of communication, coping, preferences, satisfaction, services, and support.[28] Mixed methods enable evaluation of an individual's experiences from physical to inner being and measure the process and outcomes of care. A rating system for evaluating qualitative evidence has been developed.[1]

Populations

Several subgroups are underrepresented in palliative medicine research. Research agendas for pediatric and HIV patients have been published.[29,30] Minority and indigenous communities underuse palliative medicine services. Research must address this issue and strive to include these groups in clinical trials.[31] Research has documented the symptom burden of people with advanced noncancer conditions. Questions remain about how these groups benefit from palliative medicine and how to integrate symptom and psychosocial support and advanced care planning with life-prolonging therapy. Research is also needed in the end-of-life education needs of other specialist and general physicians.

Policy and Funding

Funding initiatives specifically for palliative medicine, especially encouraging collaborative research efforts, are needed. Comparisons of service delivery models and cost-benefit analyses are needed to inform policy on service provision. Where evidence exists, proven techniques for dissemination and implementation are needed, along with studies following the outcomes resulting from these policies.

Research Developments

Randomized trials designed to answer pharmaceutical and psychosocial questions have been successfully completed and published.[32-35] Although many are small, single-site studies, the ability to complete them provides lessons for larger, multicenter trials. National and international research collaboratives have been formed. They will provide the infrastructure for multicenter clinical trials (see "Common Errors").

CONCLUSIONS AND CONTROVERSIES

Palliative medicine is a relatively new specialty in need of an evidence base. Randomized trials suggest acquisition of evidence is possible, but it requires considerable effort. Alongside efforts to perform large, randomized, controlled trials, the use and recognition of alternative research

methods, such as qualitative or mixed-method designs, needs expansion. Basic science research is needed to provide pathophysiologic mechanisms for symptoms to better target therapeutic efforts. Agreement about definitions and outcomes is needed among the members of the research community. Research efforts into communication and service provision are highly valued by patients and caregivers. Qualitative or mixed methods are ideal for investigating these multifaceted issues, and they provide information about diverse outcomes.

REFERENCES

1. Aoun SM, Kristjanson LJ. Evidence in palliative care research: How should it be gathered? Med J Aust 2005;183:264-266.
2. Grande GE, Todd CJ. Why are trials in palliative care so difficult? Palliat Med 2000;14:69-74.
3. Storey CP Jr. Trying trials. J Palliat Med 2004;7:393-394.
4. Solano JP, Gomes B, Higginson IJ. A comparison of symptom prevalence in far advanced cancer, AIDS, heart disease, chronic obstructive pulmonary disease and renal disease. J Pain Symptom Manage 2006;31:58-69.
5. Walke LM, Gallo WT, Tinetti ME, Fried TR. The burden of symptoms among community-dwelling older persons with advanced chronic disease. Arch Intern Med 2004;164:2321-2324.\
6. Hockenberry M. Symptom management research in children with cancer. J Pediatr Oncol Nurs 2004;21:132-136.
7. Stromgren AS, Groenvold M, Pedersen L, et al. Does the medical record cover the symptoms experienced by cancer patients receiving palliative care? A comparison of the record and patient self-rating. J Pain Symptom Manage 2001;21:189-196.
8. Stromgren AS, Groenvold M, Sorensen A, Andersen L. Symptom recognition in advanced cancer. A comparison of nursing records against patient self-rating. Acta Anaesthesiol Scand 2001;45:1080-1085.
9. Cleeland CS, Bennett GJ, Dantzer R, et al. Are the symptoms of cancer and cancer treatment due to a shared biologic mechanism? A cytokine-immunologic model of cancer symptoms. Cancer 2003;97:2919-2925.
10. Wiffen PJ. Evidence-based pain management and palliative care in issue one for 2006 of the Cochrane library. J Pain Palliat Care Pharmacother 2006; 20:77-78.
11. Lutz ST, Chow EL, Hartsell WF, Konski AA. A review of hypofractionated palliative radiotherapy. Cancer 2007;109:1462-1470.
12. Bennani-Baiti N, Davis M, Walsh D. Experimental models for cancer cachexia: What are the options? Support Care Cancer 2007;15:773.
13. Perkins P, Barclay S, Booth S. What are patients' priorities for palliative care research? Focus group study. Palliat Med 2007;21:219-225.
14. Crowley R, Casarett D. Patients' willingness to participate in symptom-related and disease-modifying research: Results of a research screening initiative in a palliative care clinic. Cancer 2003;97:2327-2333.
15. Ross C, Cornbleet M. Attitudes of patients and staff to research in a specialist palliative care unit. Palliat Med 2003;17:491-497.
16. Tunis SR, Stryer DB, Clancy CM. Practical clinical trials: Increasing the value of clinical research for decision making in clinical and health policy. JAMA 2003;290:1624-1632.
17. Cook AM, Finlay IG, Butler-Keating RJ. Recruiting into palliative care trials: Lessons learnt from a feasibility study. Palliat Med 2002;16:163-165.
18. Jordhoy MS, Kaasa S, Fayers P, et al. Challenges in palliative care research; recruitment, attrition and compliance: Experience from a randomized controlled trial. Palliat Med 1999;13:299-310.
19. Currow DC, Abernethy AP, Shelby-James TM, Phillips PA. The impact of conducting a regional palliative care clinical study. Palliat Med 2006;20:735-743.
20. Steinhauser KE, Clipp EC, Hays JC, et al. Identifying, recruiting, and retaining seriously-ill patients and their caregivers in longitudinal research. Palliat Med 2006;20:745-754.
21. Fowell A, Russell I, Johnstone R, et al. Cluster randomisation or randomised consent as an appropriate methodology for trials in palliative care: A feasibility study [ISRCTN60243484]. BMC Palliat Care 2004;3:1.
22. Mazzocato C, Sweeney C, Bruera E. Clinical research in palliative care: Choice of trial design. Palliat Med 2001;15:261-264.
23. Benson K, Hartz AJ. A comparison of observational studies and randomized, controlled trials. N Engl J Med 2000;342:1878-1886.
24. Concato J, Shah N, Horwitz RI. Randomized, controlled trials, observational studies, and the hierarchy of research designs. N Engl J Med 2000;342:1887-1892.
25. Ioannidis JP, Haidich AB, Lau J. Any casualties in the clash of randomised and observational evidence? BMJ 2001;322:879-880.
26. Bell R, Eccleston C, Kalso E. Ketamine as an adjuvant to opioids for cancer pain. Cochrane Database Syst Rev 2003;(1):CD003351.
27. Jackson K, Ashby M, Goodchild C. Subanesthetic ketamine for cancer pain. By insisting on level I/II evidence, do we risk throwing the baby out with the bath water? J Pain Symptom Manage 2005;29:328-330.
28. Wallen GR, Berger A. Mixed methods: In search of truth in palliative care medicine. J Palliat Med 2004;7:403-404.

Common Errors

- Use of nonvalidated instruments
- Lack of prespecified response criteria in clinical studies, especially for pain and other symptom relief studies
- Insufficient clinical information (e.g., pain type, classification, time frame of intervention)[36]
- Poor description of psychosocial interventions, preventing reproduction of study
- Lack of distinction between intervention and control[37]
- Inappropriate outcome measures, especially lack of quality of life and satisfaction measures[37]

29. Davies B, Steele R, Stajduhar KI, Bruce A. Research in pediatric palliative care. In Portenoy RK, Bruera E (eds). Issues in Palliative Care Research. New York: Oxford University Press, 2003:355-370.

30. Jones K, Breitbart W. Palliative care research in human immunodeficiency virus/acquired immunodeficiency syndrome: Clinical trials of symptomatic therapies. In Portenoy RK, Bruera E (eds). Issues in Palliative Care Research. New York: Oxford University Press, 2003:371-401.

31. Crawley LM. Racial, cultural, and ethnic factors influencing end-of-life care. J Palliat Med 2005;8(Suppl 1):S58-S69.

32. Abernethy AP, Currow DC, Hunt R, et al. A pragmatic $2 \times 2 \times 2$ factorial cluster randomized controlled trial of educational outreach visiting and case conferencing in palliative care-methodology of the palliative care trial [ISRCTN 81117481]. Contemp Clin Trials 2006;27:83-100.

33. Kissane DW, McKenzie M, Bloch S, et al. Family focused grief therapy: A randomized, controlled trial in palliative care and bereavement. Am J Psychiatry 2006;163:1208-1218.

34. Mercadante S, Villari P, Ferrera P, et al. Transmucosal fentanyl vs intravenous morphine in doses proportional to basal opioid regimen for episodic-breakthrough pain. Br J Cancer 2007;96:1828-1833.

35. Norton SA, Hogan LA, Holloway RG, et al. Proactive palliative care in the medical intensive care unit: Effects on length of stay for selected high-risk patients. Crit Care Med 2007;35:1530-1535.

36. Caraceni A, Brunelli C, Martini C, et al. Cancer pain assessment in clinical trials. A review of the literature (1999-2002). J Pain Symptom Manage 2005;29:507-519.

37. Rinck GC, van den Bos GA, Kleijnen J, et al. Methodologic issues in effectiveness research on palliative cancer care: A systematic review. J Clin Oncol 1997;15:1697-1707.

38. Hearn J, Higginson IJ. Do specialist palliative care teams improve outcomes for cancer patients? A systematic literature review. Palliat Med 1998;12:317-332.

39. Higginson IJ, Finlay I, Goodwin DM, et al. Do hospital-based palliative teams improve care for patients or families at the end of life? J Pain Symptom Manage 2002;23:96-106.

40. Fellowes D, Wilkinson S, Moore P. Communication skills training for health care professionals working with cancer patients, their families and/or carers. Cochrane Database Syst Rev 2004;(2):CD003751.

41. Harding R, Higginson IJ. What is the best way to help caregivers in cancer and palliative care? A systematic literature review of interventions and their effectiveness. Palliat Med 2003;17:63-74.

42. Caraceni A, Cherny N, Fainsinger R, et al. Pain measurement tools and methods in clinical research in palliative care: Recommendations of an expert working group of the European Association of Palliative Care. J Pain Symptom Manage 2002;23:239-255.

43. Kaasa S, Loge JH. Quality-of-life assessment in palliative care. Lancet Oncol 2002;3:175-182.

44. Kirkova J, Davis MP, Walsh D, et al. Cancer symptom assessment instruments: A systematic review. J Clin Oncol 2006;24:1459-1473.

45. Yavuzsen T, Davis MP, Walsh D, et al. Systematic review of the treatment of cancer-associated anorexia and weight loss. J Clin Oncol 2005;23:8500-8511.

46. Jackson KC, Lipman AG. Drug therapy for anxiety in palliative care. Cochrane Database Syst Rev 2004;(1):CD004596.

47. Wong R, Wiffen PJ. Bisphosphonates for the relief of pain secondary to bone metastases. Cochrane Database Syst Rev 2002;(2):CD002068.

48. Ernst E. Complementary therapies in palliative cancer care. Cancer 2001;91:2181-2185.

49. Miles CL, Fellowes D, Goodman ML, Wilkinson S. Laxatives for the management of constipation in palliative care patients. Cochrane Database Syst Rev 2006;(4):CD003448.

50. Rodin G, Lloyd N, Katz M, et al. The treatment of depression in cancer patients: A systematic review. Support Care Cancer 2007;15:123-136.

51. Keeley P. Delirium at the end of life. BMJ Clin Evid 2007;6:2405.

52. Jennings AL, Davies AN, Higgins JP, Broadley K. Opioids for the palliation of breathlessness in terminal illness. Cochrane Database Syst Rev 2001;(4):CD002066.

53. Lawrence DP, Kupelnick B, Miller K, et al. Evidence report on the occurrence, assessment, and treatment of fatigue in cancer patients. J Natl Cancer Inst Monogr 2004;32:40-50.

54. Hirst A, Sloan R. Benzodiazepines and related drugs for insomnia in palliative care. Cochrane Database Syst Rev 2002;(4):CD003346.

55. Mercadante S, Casuccio A, Mangione S. Medical treatment for inoperable malignant bowel obstruction: A qualitative systematic review. J Pain Symptom Manage 2007;33:217-223.

56. Glare P, Pereira G, Kristjanson LJ, et al. Systematic review of the efficacy of antiemetics in the treatment of nausea in patients with far-advanced cancer. Support Care Cancer 2004;12:432-440.

57. Zeppetella G, Ribeiro MD. Opioids for the management of breakthrough (episodic) pain in cancer patients. Cochrane Database Syst Rev 2006;(1):CD004311.

58. Nicholson AB. Methadone for cancer pain. Cochrane Database Syst Rev 2004;(2):CD003971.

59. Wiffen PJ, Edwards JE, Barden J, McQuay HJ. Oral morphine for cancer pain. Cochrane Database Syst Rev 2003;(4):CD003868.

60. McNicol E, Strassels SA, Goudas L, et al. NSAIDS or paracetamol, alone or combined with opioids, for cancer pain. Cochrane Database Syst Rev 2005;(1):CD005180.

61. Quigley C. Opioid switching to improve pain relief and drug tolerability. Cochrane Database Syst Rev 2004;(3):CD004847.

62. Uitterhoeve RJ, Vernooy M, Litjens M, et al. Psychosocial interventions for patients with advanced cancer—a systematic review of the literature. Br J Cancer 2004;91:1050-1062.

63. McQuay HJ, Collins SL, Carroll D, Moore RA. Radiotherapy for the palliation of painful bone metastases. Cochrane Database Syst Rev 2000;(2):CD001793.

64. Wai MS, Mike S, Ines H, Malcolm M. Palliation of metastatic bone pain: Single fraction versus multifraction radiotherapy—a systematic review of the randomised trials. Cochrane Database Syst Rev 2004;(2):CD004721.

65. Tsao MN, Lloyd N, Wong R, et al. Whole brain radiotherapy for the treatment of multiple brain metastases. Cochrane Database Syst Rev 2006;3:CD003869.

SUGGESTED READING

Cleeland CS. Cross-cutting research issues: A research agenda for reducing distress of patients with cancer. In Foley KM, Gelbon H (eds). Improving Palliative Care for Cancer. Washington, DC: National Academy Press, 2001, pp 233-274.

Ferrell BR, Grant M. Nursing research. In Ferrel B, Coyle N (eds). Textbook of Palliative Nursing, 2nd ed. New York: Oxford University Press, 2006.

Kissane D, Street A. Research into psychosocial issues. In Doyle D, Hanks G, Cherny NI, Calman K (eds). Oxford Textbook of Palliative Medicine, 3rd ed. Oxford, UK: Oxford University Press, Oxford, 2004, pp 154-163.

Kramer BJ, Christ GH, Bern-Klug M, Francoeur RB. A national agenda for social work research in palliative and end-of-life care. J Palliat Med 2005;8:418-431.

National Hospice and Palliative Care Organization. Development of the NHPCO research agenda. J Pain Symptom Manage 2004;28:488-496.

National Institutes of Health. State of the Science Conference on Improving End of Life Care, Bethesda, MD, 2004. Available at http://consensus.nih.gov/2004/2004EndOfLifeCare.505024PDF.pdf (accessed November 10, 2007).

Portenoy RK, Bruera E (eds). Issues in Palliative Care Research. New York: Oxford University Press, 2003.

Rubenfeld GD, Curtis JR, for the End-of-Life Care in the ICU Working Group. End-of-Life care in the intensive care unit: A research agenda. Crit Care Med 2001;29:2001-2006.

Teno JM, Byock I, Field M. Research agenda for developing measures to examine quality of care and quality of life of patients diagnosed with life-limiting illness. J Pain Symptom Manage 1998;17:75-82.

Administration

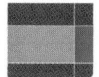

CHAPTER **35**

Program Development: An International Perspective

Liliana de Lima

KEY POINTS

- Palliative care programs vary internationally. They have adopted different models of care because of differences in socioeconomic conditions, health policies, and needs of patients and families.

- Palliative care in developing countries is provided mostly through hospices and programs with limited connections to public health care.

- Institutionalizing palliative care is a strategy that may increase recognition of the field as a component of care in addition to prevention, diagnosis, and treatment.

- Limitations in funding and personnel in developing countries hinder the ability of institutions to develop and implement palliative care programs.

- Strategies to provide financial and technical support to institutions in developing countries willing to implement palliative care programs need to be developed by funding organizations.

Palliative care programs around the world follow different models, ranging from multidisciplinary teams in tertiary facilities to care at home by trained volunteers and families (see "Common Errors"). These differences usually are caused by a lack of recognition of palliation as an integral component of care, the different needs of patients and families, insufficient education of health care providers, and inadequate policies on how to legislate and regulate palliative care.

Development of palliative care programs in countries with limited resources faces additional challenges: poverty, inadequate infrastructure, poor administration, limited access to medications, bureaucracy, restrictive laws and opioid regulations, insufficient support from national health authorities, and little political will to establish palliative care programs.[1]

Some locations have implemented successful volunteer-based palliative care programs that rely on home and community for the provision of care. Examples include the Neighborhood Palliative Care Initiative, Kerala, India[2]; South Coast Hospice in KwaZulu-Natal, South Africa[3]; the volunteer program from the Liga Argentina de Lucha Contra el Cancer (LALCEC) in San Nicolas, Argentina[4]; and Hospice Uganda in Africa.[5] They have been effective and efficient in caring for patients at home and in maximizing resources. Most programs in resource-limited countries have developed as islands of excellence without health care system integration and with limited impact on physician and nursing knowledge.

INSTITUTIONALIZATION OF PALLIATIVE CARE

Palliative care programs continue to be adopted in institutions around the world. The American Hospital Association reported that 22% of all U.S. hospitals have palliative care programs. Organizations such as the Center to Advance Palliative Care (CAPC) have been a strong force behind this change in the United States.[6]

The development of palliative care programs in institutions has several advantages:

1. There is a greater chance of becoming part of the health care system, with allocation of resources from the institutional budget and designation of space and human resources.
2. An institutional palliative care program offers greater potential to expand and influence the general population than if palliative care is provided in isolation.
3. The program is integrated as a component of medical care, along with prevention, diagnosis, and active treatment, in a continuum of care for incurable, progressive diseases.
4. Institutions can drive the development and maintenance of palliative care by structure, systems, and policies to support the demand and offer palliative care services.
5. In academic institutions, a palliative care program allows bedside teaching of residents and undergraduate students, and it establishes the discipline within the medical community.
6. An institutional program facilitates research in palliative care. Most information and treatment protocols are developed in wealthy countries and may not be applicable in poor settings lacking resources. A palliative care research agenda to address the specific needs in these locations is easier in academic settings, where most resources are located.

The Faculty Scholars Program, implemented in 1994 by Project Death in America (PDIA), has been successful with a major impact in institutionalizing palliative care in North

TABLE 35-1   Beneficiaries of the IAHPC Faculty Development Program

INSTITUTION	LOCATION	FACULTY PHYSICIAN	IAHPC MONITOR OR MENTOR PHYSICIAN
Unidad de Cuidados Paliativos*	Rosario, Argentina	Hugo Fornells	Eduardo Bruera (United States)
Amrita Institute of Medical Sciences†	Kochi, India	Gayatri Palat	M. R. Rajagopal (India)
Ocean Road Cancer Institute	Dar es Salaam, Tanzania	Msemo Diwani	Elizabeth Gwyther (South Africa)
West China Fourth Hospital of Sichuan University	Chengdu, China	Jinxiang Li	K. S. Chan (Hong Kong)
Universidad Catolica	Santiago, Chile	Maria Alejandra Palma	Roberto Wenk (Argentina)

*This program was implemented in 2003 as a 2-year pilot program.
†Because of administrative changes at the Amrita Institute of Medical Sciences, this grant was suspended. The faculty position and the teaching activities are still active in the institution.
IAHPC, International Association for Hospice and Palliative Care.

Common Errors

- A single model is not applicable in all countries and regions of the world.
- Institutionalization does not lead to dehumanization of palliative care.
- Establishing models with limited or no connection to the health care system will continue to isolate palliation from mainstream care.
- Implementing programs without strong public support from top institutional managers and administrators is likely to fail.
- Adoption of a defensive and hostile attitude in newly established faculty within an institution reduces the political support needed for survival.

America. PDIA has supported 78 faculty scholars through 67 awards, representing 50 medical schools (including 4 in Canada) and 3 nursing schools.[7] There are no data available on developing countries, and most publications reporting results come from developed countries.[8-12] The level of institutionalization of palliative care in developing countries is low. In response, the International Association for Hospice and Palliative Care (IAHPC) adopted a program called IAHPC Faculty Development Program,[13] which was modeled after the PDIA Scholars Program.

International Association for Hospice and Palliative Care Faculty Development Program

The goal of the IAHPC Faculty Development Program is to promote and help implement palliative care in institutions in developing countries. The program funds faculty positions in palliative care for nurses or physicians for 5 years. It requires identifying and selecting an appropriate institution and candidate, an application and selection process, a program mentor or monitor, and periodic reports on the progress and challenges faced. The IAHPC Board can identify and select outstanding candidates and institutions. The institutions should be recognized teaching centers and academic hospitals. Candidates should have completed formal training in hospice or palliative care in a recognized program and have the intention to return to their home country (if they are abroad) and develop a hospice or palliative care program. After the candidate and an institution are selected, they are invited to begin the application process. If approved, an agree-ment is signed between IAHPC and the institution for 5 years. During this time, the employee is required to comply with mastering clearly defined goals in clinical develop-ment, administrative, educational, and research areas. Funding is contingent on achievement in specific goals in these four domains. IAHPC identifies a mentor or monitor physician for each program from its Board who ideally should be in the same region as the program. The mentor is responsible for training, technical support, site visits, and brief reports to the IAHPC office. His or her role is helping the institution and candidate complete the objec-tives and goals set at the beginning of the program.

Program Results

The program requires substantial funds to cover costs during the full agreement. Since the start of the program in 2003, IAHPC has received donations from the Joy McCann Foundation, the National Hospice and Palliative Care Organization (NHPCO), the Open Society Institute (OSI), the U.S. Cancer Pain Relief Committee, and private donors. These sources have been crucial to the program and the organization's ability to promote it.

IAHPC has provided grants to five institutions in devel-oping countries in Africa, Asia, and Latin America (Table 35-1). Of these, the Unidad de Cuidados Paliativos (UCPAR) in Argentina completed the term of the agreement, and the program at the Amrita Institute of Medical Sciences (AIMS) was terminated early due to institutional adminis-trative changes. The faculty position and teaching activi-ties in AIMS remain active.

Progress reports about each program are received peri-odically, and mentors perform site visits at least once yearly to each institution. The reports from the institu-tions and mentors show that all five programs face similar challenges (Table 35-2), including lack of recognition and credibility among colleagues, inadequate health care poli-cies, limited economic resources, and administrative and regulatory barriers. Since the start of the program and the creation of the faculty positions in palliative care, they all report significant advances in their ability to provide patient care within their institutions.[14-18] None has a research agenda, and most activities have focused on service provision, classroom instruction, and bedside teaching.

It is too early to determine long-term outcomes or success, and continuous monitoring and follow-up are

TABLE 35-2 Challenges Faced by Institutions and Benefits Resulting from the Faculty Development Program

INSTITUTION	CHALLENGES OF INSTITUTIONAL PALLIATIVE CARE PROGRAMS	BENEFITS RESULTING FROM FACULTY DEVELOPMENT PROGRAMS
Unidad de Cuidados Paliativos	Lack of recognition of palliative care as a discipline	Educational sessions implemented on a weekly basis
	Lack of a physical space to house the palliative care clinic and team	Ability to dedicate full time to palliative care tasks
	Large geographical area to be covered by home care services and the large volume of patients	Bus rounds started and palliative care ambulatory clinics set in community clinics
	Lack of trained personnel to form a multidisciplinary palliative care group	Gave credibility to the discipline and the position as one recognized and supported by an international organization
Ocean Road Cancer Institute	Palliative care not included in the health care policy	Palliative care included as a component of the cancer control program presented to the government for approval
	Lack of adequately trained personnel	Bedside teaching implemented
		Provides credibility and helpful in getting other funders interested
		Program helped push the palliative care agenda to a national level
		A formal agreement of collaboration established for Ocean Road Cancer Institute, Muhimbili University College of Health Sciences, and University of Cape Town in South Africa through the mentor of the program
Amrita Institute of Medical Sciences	No postgraduate palliative care education programs in the country	Implemented a postgraduate palliative care diploma at Amrita Institute
	Lack of recognition from other disciplines	Developed a palliative care fellowship program for graduate students
		Increase organizational credibility
Sichuan University	Lack of recognition by other medical specialties	Implemented a palliative care program to teach physicians and nurses in China; more than 30 workshops given since the program's start
	Lack of institutional support	The palliative care team in the wards and in home care gradually accepted and welcomed by patients with cancer and their relatives
	Lack of knowledge about palliative care	Approach of combining Western medicine with traditional Chinese medicine for pain relief established
	Myths concerning use of analgesics and progress of disease and death	
	Frequent requests for euthanasia from patients and relatives	
Universidad Catolica*	Lack of awareness about the needs of patients with advanced conditions	Faculty of medicine at Universidad Catolica (a leading academic institution in Latin America) with the potential to influence local and regional levels of care
	Lack of comprehensive palliative care education	Program serves as a model to other medical schools in the country
	Limited resources for faculty positions	Faculty position created and adopted by the Universidad Catolica
		Increased awareness among the other faculty members about palliative care

*This program began in August 2006.

needed. The true measure would be if such programs were successful in establishing palliative care within the institutions long term, affect the quality of care provided, implement teaching for nurses and doctors, and conduct research on treatment protocols and guidelines tailored to the population's needs. After the grant term is completed, IAHPC will maintain close contact with the institutions and carry out surveys when appropriate to help determine long-term results and outcomes.

CONCLUSIONS

Many people are still dying with unnecessary suffering around the world. Policy makers and most of the international philanthropic community have underestimated the importance of investing in palliative care (see "Future Considerations"). Palliative care needs to be part of national health care policies to ensure continuity and financial stability, especially in developing countries. Efficient allocation of funds and greater resource mobilization

Future Considerations

- Identify and support centers of excellence.
- Institutionalize palliative care in teaching hospitals.
- Include palliative care training in undergraduate and graduate curricula.
- Motivate palliative caregivers to become institutional agents of change.
- Establish collaborative agreements between organizations starting new programs and those with existing, successful ones.

are needed, including identification of strategies with the highest probability of success. One example is the institutionalization of palliative care in teaching hospitals and academic settings. This should lead to greater integration of the discipline into mainstream patient care. Palliative care providers must be the driving force, and they must reach out to policy makers and administrators to make this happen. Stakeholders should learn from the success of institutions that have implemented palliative care and instruction of physicians and nurses. Ultimately, the relief of unnecessary pain and suffering will improve the quality of life of patients and families and be a more effective use of health care resources.

REFERENCES

1. De Lima L, Hamzah E. Socioeconomic, cultural and political issues. In Bruera E, Wenk R, de Lima L (eds). Palliative Care in Developing Countries: Principles and Practice. Houston: IAHPC Press, 2004.
2. Kumar S, Numpeli M. Neighborhood network in palliative care. Indian J Palliat Care 2005;11:6-9.
3. Defilippi K. Integrated community-based home care: Striving towards balancing quality with coverage in South Africa. Indian J Palliat Care 2005;11:34-36.
4. Wenk R, Bertolino M, Pussetto J. Direct medical costs of an Argentinean domiciliary palliative care model. J Pain Symptom Manage 2000;20:162-165.
5. Merriman A. Uganda: Current status of palliative care. J Pain Symptom Manage 2002;24:252-256.
6. Meier D, Sieger C. The Case for Hospital Based Palliative Care, vol 3. New York: Center to Advance Palliative Care, 2005.
7. Aulino F, Foley K. The project on death in America. J R Soc Med 2001;94:492-495.
8. Pan CX, Morrison RS, Meier DE, et al. How prevalent are hospital-based palliative care programs? Status report and future directions. J Palliat Med 2001;4:315-324.
9. Pantilat S, Billings A. Survey of palliative care programs in United States teaching hospitals. J Palliat Med 2001;4:309-314.
10. Higginson IJ, Finlay I, Goodwin DM, et al. Do hospital-based palliative teams improve care for patients or families at the end of life? J Pain Symptom Manage 2002;23:96-106.
11. Llamas K, Pickhaver A, Piller N. Mainstreaming palliative care for cancer patients in the acute hospital setting. Palliat Med 2001;15:207-212.
12. Glare PA, Auret KA, Aggarwal G, et al. The interface between Palliat Med and specialists in acute-care hospitals: Boundaries, bridges and challenges. Med J Aust 2003;179(Suppl):S29-S31.
13. International Association for Hospice and Palliative Care (IAHPC) Faculty Development Program. Available at http://www.hospicecare.com/faculty/ (accessed September 12, 2007).
14. Fornells H. Final Report to IAHPC—Faculty Development Program, UCPAR, Argentina (working document). Houston: IAHPC Press, 2005.
15. Rajagopal M. Progress Report to IAHPC—Faculty Development Program, AIMS, India (working document). Houston: IAHPC Press, January 2006.
16. Diwani M. Progress Report to IAHPC—Faculty Development Program, ORCI, Tanzania (working document). Houston: IAHPC Press, September 2006.
17. Li J. Progress Report to IAHPC—Faculty Development Program, Sichuan University, China (working document). Houston: IAHPC Press, September 2006.
18. Wenk R, Nervi F. Initial Visit Report to IAHPC—Faculty Development Program, Universidad Catolica, Chile (working document). Houston: IAHPC Press, September 2006.

SUGGESTED READING

Lorenz KA, Shugarman LR, Lynn J. Health care policy issues in end-of-life care. J Palliat Med 2006;9:731-748.

Morrison RS, Maroney-Galin C, Kralovec PD, Meier DE. The growth of palliative care programs in United States hospitals. J Palliat Med 2005;8:1127-1134.

Ross DD, Fraser HC, Kutner JS. Institutionalization of a palliative and end-of-life care educational program in a medical school curriculum. J Palliat Med 2001;4:512-518.

Weissman DE, Block SD, Blank L, et al. Recommendations for incorporating palliative care education into the acute care hospital setting. Acad Med 1999;74:871-877.

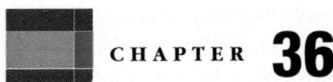

CHAPTER 36

Program Development: National Planning

Tony O'Brien

KEY POINTS

- Palliative care is a vital and integral part of national health and social care policy. Provision must be made for its development and integration into health and social services in all countries.

- Development of palliative care programs involves a detailed needs assessment to quantify the scale of unmet need. Each country should identify actual and potential barriers to comprehensive palliative care services for all those in need.

- Informed by the needs assessment study, each country should produce an implementation plan with assessments of needed funding and time frames and with regard for the needs of patients and families. The plans address issues of infrastructure, education and training, personnel, and quality assurance.

- The ultimate aim is to ensure that patients have access to high-quality care, delivered in a setting, at a time, and in a style that best meets their individual needs and preferences.

- Capital and revenue funding of palliative care services should be adequate, fair, and equitable and should be settled in advance with funding agencies.

- All palliative care providers must have an explicit and quantifiable commitment to the provision of a comprehensive and equitable range of services, delivered in an efficient and professional manner to the highest possible standards.

Almost 40 years have elapsed since John Hinton focused on the level of unmet needs experienced by patients with advanced and progressive disease.[1] Inspired by the pioneering work of Dame Cicely Saunders and others, we have witnessed a welcome renaissance in our understanding of the needs of palliative care patients and their families. Across the world, many service models have evolved.[2] Commonly, services focus on the needs of patients in a particular institution or within a narrowly defined geographical region. They often have developed in a reactive fashion, with little formal prospective planning. Although such services undoubtedly make a valuable contribution to a select group of patients and families, insufficient attention is paid to those unable to access care. This inequality can best be addressed by a formal process of strategic planning and integration.

A comprehensive national plan for palliative care is an unambiguous statement by national governments, health care providers, and communities of a shared commitment to address the needs of the seriously ill. In many societies, palliative care is viewed in a somewhat negative context. It may be seen purely as end-of-life care and interpreted as "giving up" on a patient or failing to try to preserve life.

The need for a basic attitudinal change was identified by Dr. Michael Kearney when he wrote, "Patients with incurable disease must no longer be viewed as medical failures for whom nothing more can be done. They need palliative care, which does not mean a hand-holding, second-rate soft option, but treatment that most of us will need at some stage in our lives, and many from the time of diagnosis, demanding as much skill and commitment as is normally brought into preventing, investigating and curing illness."[3]

International experience suggests development of services often predates any formal national planning by many years. Although such pioneering services may achieve much in a comparatively short time, their overall impact is limited. Typically, they operate in relative or absolute isolation from established medical services. They focus on a small and clearly defined population. Although they may provide high-quality care to this select population, many others are prevented from accessing appropriate care. Lack of resources often results in all available resources being focused on direct patient care. Education, training, and research tend to suffer (Box 36-1). The preferred way to proceed is through a structured planning process that involves input from all of the relevant stakeholders, including patients and families.

PALLIATIVE MEDICINE AS A SPECIALTY

Palliative medicine was first recognized as a specialty in the United Kingdom in 1987 and in Ireland in 1995. Since then, several countries have added palliative medicine to their medical specialties. For palliative medicine to be recognized as a specialist area, regulatory authorities must be satisfied that there is a distinct corpus of knowledge specific to the specialty. They also must be satisfied that there is a cohort of professionals to oversee the new specialty, including curriculum development and training of future specialists. After this core principle is approved, effort can focus on developing and implementing a strategy that can best serve the needs of the national population.

The recognition of palliative medicine as a distinct specialty is an important step in its development and integration. It formally recognizes the distinct corpus of knowledge unique to palliative medicine. It puts an onus on palliative medicine professionals to develop and implement an agreed curriculum to undergraduate and postgraduate students. It also creates an opportunity to develop programs of education for nonspecialist colleagues from other disciplines. It facilitates the introduction and development of services in all settings, including specialist units and hospital and community settings. It helps to create a culture of critical assessment, research, and quality assurance.

COUNCIL OF EUROPE REPORT

In November 2003, the Committee of Ministers of the Council of Europe formally adopted the report of the expert committee on the organization of palliative care.[4] This clear and comprehensive series of recommendations reinforces the core principles of palliative care and encourages member states to "adopt policies, legislative and other measures necessary for a coherent and comprehensive national policy framework for palliative care."[4] Although this is not legally binding on any of the 46 member states, it is an important statement regarding the duties and responsibilities of national governments in terms of palliative care. Best results can be achieved by a cooperative effort involving many different governmental and nongovernmental agencies. The Council of Europe report identified key principles for member states when developing palliative care policy (Box 36-2).

Box 36-2 Council of Europe's Key Principles for Developing Palliative Care Policy

- Palliative care is a vital and integral part of health services. Provisions for its development and functional integration should be incorporated into national health strategies.
- Any person who is in need of palliative care should be able to access it without delay in a setting that is as consistent with his or her needs and preferences as reasonably feasible.
- Palliative care has as its objective the achievement and maintenance of the best possible quality of life for patients.
- Palliative care seeks to address physical, psychological, and spiritual issues associated with advanced disease. It requires a coordinated input from a highly skilled and adequately resourced interdisciplinary and multiprofessional team.
- Acute intervening problems should be treated if the patient wishes, but they should be left untreated while the best palliative care continues to be provided if the patient prefers.
- Access to palliative care should be based on need, and it must not be influenced by disease type, geographical location, socioeconomic status, or other such factors.
- Programs of palliative care education should be incorporated into the training of all health care professionals.
- Research aimed at improving the quality of care should be undertaken. All palliative care interventions should be supported to the greatest possible extent by relevant research data.
- Palliative care should receive an adequate and equitable level of funding.
- As in all sectors of medical care, health care providers involved in palliative care should respect patients' rights, comply with professional obligations and standards, and act in the best interest of individual patients.

Box 36-1 Consequences of Inadequate Service Planning

- Poor integration with existing health care services in hospital and community settings
- Professional isolation
- Focus on a single domain of care, usually community
- Focus on unidisciplinary care, usually nursing
- Poorly defined roles and governance structures
- Excessive reliance on fundraising activities
- Lack of professionalism
- Tendency to be reactive rather than proactive in service delivery
- Little or no quality assurance and performance indicators
- Narrowly defined geographical focus
- Absence of clearly defined policies and structures
- Limited scope

NATIONAL STRATEGY FOR PALLIATIVE CARE

National Palliative Care Committee

The initial step in formulating a strategy requires a national palliative care committee, who employ detailed and explicit terms of reference (Box 36-3). The terms should be sufficiently detailed to focus the committee but not so restrictive that the members lose the ability to respond to new and unforeseen issues. The role of chairperson is essential in guiding the committee through its work.

A national palliative care strategy group is required to produce detailed recommendations on the organization and integration of a comprehensive national palliative care program. It needs to draw on a broad range of expert opinions. If the group is too large and diverse, it will be more difficult to develop and maintain an appropriate sense of urgency and commitment. If it is too small, it may lack the necessary expertise and insights. It may be preferable to limit membership to a maximum of 12 individuals but allow for the option of using consultants with particular expertise on an as-required basis.

Members must understand they are invited to contribute because of their particular expertise. However, they are primarily charged with representing the best interests of patients and families. Occasionally, members may seek to selectively promote their own institutions, geographical regions, or professional groups. This introduces a destructive dynamic and must be identified and addressed at the earliest opportunity. Clear terms of reference may help, but ultimately, the chairperson must ensure the committee members undertake their work in a professional and equitable fashion and in accordance with the agreed terms of reference.

Members who agree to serve on a national committee must ensure that they devote sufficient time and energy to the process. This involves a commitment to attend meetings regularly and to undertake the necessary work and research between meetings. The committee must be supported by motivated and enthusiastic administrative and secretarial personnel. The appointment of a suitably qualified medical writer who takes responsibility for producing the various drafts and final report is strongly recommended.

Definitions

The palliative care literature is littered with many terms that lack precise definition. For example, the term *hospice* may describe a highly complex program of care, requiring input from a broad range of medical and allied professionals in an internationally renowned tertiary referral hospital. The same term also may be used to describe a volunteer companion offering to sit with a patient to allow the main caregiver to take a short break. It is important to discuss and agree on definitions, encompassing all terms used in the committee's work. This includes terms such as palliative care, specialist palliative care, hospice care, terminal care, end-of-life care, family, multidisciplinary team, interdisciplinary team, degrees of specialization, and bereavement care. It also is helpful to define the patient groups who may benefit from specialist palliative care and the settings where such care will be provided. The Statement of Definitions document produced by the National Council for Hospice and Specialist Palliative Care Services offers useful guidance in this regard.[5]

Timescale

At the outset, the committee should agree on a realistic program of work, with defined dates of completion for each of the different phases. Committees require a sense of urgency to function efficiently. The work schedule should be realistic to achieve the approved objectives. However, it must not be so generous that momentum is lost.

Every effort should be made to support the committee in its work. This includes the provision of good-quality secretarial and administrative support. Much of the work is conducted between formal meetings. This process is facilitated by telephone conferencing, video conferencing, and electronic communication systems. Nevertheless, regular formal meetings are still required to facilitate face-to-face discussion and debate. It is a function of the chairperson to ensure that all views are equally heard and respected.

Principles

Before detailing service development and integration, it is helpful to agree on core principles and objectives. After the principles are accepted, the committee can focus on the issues involved in planning the necessary measures to ensure that the key principles are satisfied. In essence, key principles identify the ultimate destination, and the committee's report will detail the road map that must be followed. A recurring theme in all of the published national strategies for palliative care is the importance of providing choice. In Australia, for example, this aspect has been well captured: "The National Strategy for Palliative Care respects the central importance of choice for people who are dying and their families—choice regarding the setting of care and the manner and type of care provided. This requires that options be available to meet a wide range of medical, social, cultural, linguistic, and spiritual needs. It

---

Box 36-3   Reference Terms for a Palliative Care Committee

- Membership
- Definitions
- Timescale and work schedule, including date for report completion
- Essential principles (i.e., what we want to achieve)
- Needs assessment study data
- Places of care (i.e., integrated models of service provision)
- Team (i.e., range of professionals and numbers required)
- Infrastructural requirements
- Manpower planning
- Education, training, and research
- Barriers
- Integration
- Funding (i.e., capital and revenue)
- Implementation plan, prioritization, and timescale
- Benchmarks for best practice
- Governance issues

also requires that people understand the nature of palliative care and can access the service they need."[6]

Individual countries produce their own key principles based on their unique set of needs and circumstances. In Ireland, the Department of Health and Children published a Cancer Strategy in 1996 (Box 36-4).[7] In the United Kingdom, reports over the past 25 years have proposed key principles (Box 36-5).[8-10] The Council of Europe report includes a section devoted to "guiding principles" that may prove useful in the production of a national strategy (Box 36-6).

Measuring the Scale of the Deficit: Needs Assessment Data

In an ideal world, strategic planning would always predate service development. However, in many instances, some service provision is established before any formal planning is undertaken. The established services may be severely limited in their availability, accessibility, and integration. One of the challenges facing service planners is to ensure established services are encouraged and enabled to integrate successfully with new and evolving services. It is important that they adopt standard policies and procedures and operate fully within the system. Otherwise, a parallel system may develop that cannot support high-quality care.

Detailed needs assessment is an essential element in a national strategy for specialist palliative care. There are three key elements[11] of a comprehensive health needs assessment study:

- Gathering and interpretation of epidemiological and demographic data
- Estimation of the views of the major stakeholders, including service providers, service users, and purchasers or planners
- Collection and collation of comparative data relating to outputs, outcomes, and costs

Epidemiological data about the population under review involve estimating the incidence and prevalence of conditions likely to require specialist palliative input such as cancer and other progressive, nonmalignant diseases. This does not give direct information on need, but it does describe the burden of disease within a population.[12] Incidence and mortality rates for cancer and other progressive nonmalignant diseases may be applied to projected population figures to estimate expected deaths from a specific disease in the future.

In the same context, it is useful at this stage to identify the groups of patients likely to benefit from palliative care. Traditionally, palliative care services have focused on patients suffering from advanced cancer. The need to extend palliative care services to patients with nonmalignant disease is recognized.[13] Practice has lagged behind the rhetoric. Motor neuron disease (i.e., amyotrophic lateral sclerosis) was the dominant nonmalignant condition associated with hospice care in the United Kingdom.[14] In 1995, a regional study of care for the dying identified many patients dying from nonmalignant diseases, such as congestive heart failure, chronic obstructive pulmonary disease, and stroke, who had significant unmet health and social care needs.[14] In many countries, the proportion of palliative care patients with nonmalignant disease is less

---

Box 36-4 Cancer Strategy of Ireland's Department of Health and Children, 1996

- Patients should be encouraged to express their preferences about where they wish to be cared for and where they wish to spend the last period of their lives
- Services should be sufficiently flexible and integrated to allow movement of patients from one care setting to another, depending on their clinical situation and personal preferences.
- The ultimate aim should be for all patients to have access to specialist palliative care services when they are required.

Box 36-5 Principles for Palliative Care Collected in the United Kingdom, 1983 to 2008

- Palliative care is an important part of the work of most health care professionals, and all should have knowledge in this area and feel confident in the core skills required.
- Primary health care providers in the community have a central role in and responsibility for the provision of palliative care and accessing specialist palliative care services when required.
- Specialist palliative care should be seen as complementing, not replacing, the care provided by other health care professionals in hospital and community settings.
- Specialist palliative care services should be available to all patients in need, wherever they are and whatever their disease.
- Specialist palliative services should be planned, integrated, and coordinated and should assume responsibility for education, training, and research.

Box 36-6 Council of Europe's Guiding Principles for Palliative Care

- Palliative care is a vital and integral part of health service provision. It is not a luxury add-on item.
- All persons who require palliative care must be able to access an appropriate level of palliative care expertise at a time and in a setting that is consistent with their individual needs and personal preferences.
- Specialist palliative care services must be established and integrated across all care environments, including specialist palliative care in-patient units, day care and out-patient facilities, hospitals, and all community settings, including residential care and nursing homes.
- Services must be sufficiently coordinated and integrated to allow easy movement of patients from one care setting to another in response to changing clinical needs or personal preferences.
- Access to specialist palliative care services must be based on need and must not be subject to the lottery of postal address or histological subtype.
- Actual and potential barriers to optimal service provision must be identified and addressed at the earliest opportunity.
- Adequate and equitable funding must be made available to support vital specialist palliative care services.
- All funds raised or allocated to support specialist palliative care services must be applied solely and exclusively to specialist palliative care purposes and at the earliest opportunity.
- Systems of quality assurance must be developed and implemented across all specialist palliative care settings.

than 10%, although this figure is somewhat higher in the United States. Other groups may become marginalized and find that available palliative care services are difficult to access or are less responsive and sensitive to their needs (Box 36-7).

Another aspect of policy formation is the timing of the introduction of palliative care services. In many instances, palliative care is involved only in the final stages of disease. This model of service provision is ethically bankrupt and devoid of any logic or humanity. Access to core services must not be influenced by a crude and probably inaccurate assessment of a likely prognosis. Access to care must be determined by need alone, encompassing the physical, emotional, social, and spiritual aspects of the human condition.

Places of Care

Ideally, a patient should be able to access care in various inpatient and community-based settings. Services must be sufficiently integrated to allow movement of patients from one care setting to another, depending on their needs and personal preferences. This may prove difficult, and it requires a degree of flexibility and responsiveness not typically associated with many health care programs. Patients with palliative care needs cannot afford to join lengthy waiting lists for investigative or therapeutic procedures. They should be fast tracked when they need attention at the emergency room. This integrated model of care requires services to become more sensitive and responsive to the needs of patients and families and less restricted by cumbersome and ineffective administrative structures.

Team

Specialist palliative care services require input from many medical and allied professionals in hospital and community settings. Team members should behave in a cooperative and collaborative fashion, and they should always act in the best interests of patients and families. This is best achieved if individual members are confident and competent in their own skills and have a willingness to involve other professionals as appropriate. When producing a national strategy, it is necessary to specify the range and numbers of the various disciplines required. In inpatient settings, the minimum and desired ratios may be defined according to bed numbers. In community settings, the ratios are usually defined according to populations of 100,000. These ratios enable accurate accounting. This is achieved by selecting the midpoint on the salary scale for

each of the various staff members identified and including an agreed percentage to cover nonpay elements.

Having quantified and financially assessed the total number of health care professionals required to service the palliative care needs of a defined population, the next step is to review current personnel. If the funding is immediately available, are these professionals ready to take up their posts? In most instances, a significant investment in education and training is required, and there is typically a considerable delay involved. Personnel planning and investment in education and training are vital elements of a national palliative care strategy.

Infrastructure

An infrastructural needs assessment study can yield useful information on the specific accommodation needs of all aspects of the service, including specialist inpatient beds, community-based services, rehabilitation services, day care facilities, and educational and research facilities. These elements are interdependent and must not be considered in isolation. It is futile to estimate the needs for inpatient beds unless there is clarity about community- and hospital-based services. The availability and accessibility of one element of the program affects the demands for another element.

A population-based needs assessment study can yield useful information on the number of specialist palliative care beds required to meet the needs of a specific population. When planning the location of these beds, the current and projected population distributions should be considered. Other factors include the proximity of cancer-related and other services, established referral patterns, ease of access in transport and parking, construction costs and difficulties, and projected time to completion. Although it is desirable that patients are able to access specialist palliative care services as close as possible to their own homes, this presents logistical difficulties in areas of low population density. All specialist palliative care services should have a sufficient critical mass of activity to ensure economic viability and to ensure that the skill level of the specialist staff is maintained.

Integrated Planning Process

Specialist palliative care services have various dimensions, and each must be considered in the planning process. Ultimately, we must deliver an integrated program of high-quality, patient-focused care that is sensitive and responsive to the individual needs of patients and families. At the national level, health planning and administration are frequently fragmented and focused on particular channels of decision making and budgetary routing. The difficulty for palliative care providers is that they are involved in all of these diverse areas. Some mechanism must be found to ensure that the administrative structures support and do not impede the development of services.

Benchmarks for Best Practice

All specialist palliative care services must have a commitment to providing a high-quality service that offers best value for money. This must be robustly and explicitly

---

Box 36-7 Groups Who Have Difficulty Accessing Palliative Care Services

- Children
- Adolescents
- Very elderly
- Prisoners
- People with learning difficulties
- People with physical and sensory handicaps
- Illegal immigrants
- Intravenous drug users
- Alcohol-dependent individuals

TABLE 36-1 Specialist Palliative Care Services

SERVICE AVAILABILITY	Benchmark		
	Structure	**Process**	**Outcome**

Cancer
    Baseline: 50% of all cancer deaths to access SPCS
    Desired: 70% of all cancer deaths to access SPCS
	Integrated data collection system for each SPCS that allows accurate data on patients accessing services to be generated
	Staff trained in coding of diagnosis and data collection and entry
		Accurate data kept on numbers of patients accessing SPCS and their diagnostic group
		Generation of statistics on percent of patients dying of cancer who access SPCS
		Comparison of data on access by cancer patients of SPCS with death certificate statistics on cancer deaths
			Patients accessing SPCS services on the basis of need

Nonmalignant diseases
    Baseline: 5% of patients with nonmalignant disease
    Desired: 25% of patients with nonmalignant disease
	Integrated data collection system for each SPCS
	Staff trained in coding of diagnosis and data collection and entry
		Accurate data kept on numbers of patients accessing SPCS and their diagnostic group
		Generation of statistics on percent of patients with nonmalignant disease
			Patients accessing SPCS services on the basis of need

SPCS, specialist palliative care services.

measured and demonstrated. At the national level, it is necessary to define clear measures of quality. The temptation is for services to measure what is easy to measure, even though it may not provide the most useful or relevant data. There is also a temptation to measure aspects of service provision concerned with the process of delivery, rather than with the outcome or product. The International Expert Advisory Group Report on Palliative Care (Marymount Hospice and The Atlantic Philanthropies) has produced benchmarks for specialist palliative care services.[15,16] The group agreed on the following framework:

- Benchmarks are defined in terms of structure, process, and outcome.
- Where applicable, benchmarks are defined in terms of a baseline level, which is the absolute minimum standard that must be achieved, and a desired level, which is the optimal standard in terms of excellence.
- These levels do not remain static but are revised and redefined at regular intervals.
- Benchmarks are produced for each domain of specialist palliative care activity. One example is illustrated in Table 36-1.

The Irish Health Services Accreditation Board produced a detailed framework to aid service providers in identifying their strengths and opportunities for quality and safety improvements.[17] The ultimate objective of the exercise is to support organizations in the continuous improvement of their services to patients and families.

Implementation, Priorities, and Timescale

The completion of a national strategy for palliative medicine is an important milestone, but it is just the beginning. Informed by the national strategy, strategic planners and service providers must work together to produce a realistic program of implementation. It is informed by the strategy document and undertaken on a national or regional basis. The national strategy should describe the administrative structures that best support the development and implementation of the agreed strategy. The ultimate index of the success of the strategy will be the extent to which the palliative care needs of the community are identified and addressed.

REFERENCES

1. Hinton JM. Dying. Harmondsworth, UK: Penguin Books, 1967.
2. Addington-Hall JM & Higginson IJ. Introduction. In Addington-Hall JM, Higginson IJ (eds). Palliative Care for Non-Cancer Patients. Oxford, UK: Oxford University Press, 2001, p 7.
3. Kearney M. Palliative care in Ireland. Jr Ir Coll Physicians Surg 1991;20:170.
4. Recommendations Rec (2003) 24 of the Committee of Ministers to Member States on the Organisation of Palliative Care. Strasbourg: Council of Europe, 2003.
5. National Council for Hospice and Specialist Palliative Care Services. Specialist Palliative Care: A Statement of Definitions. Occasional Paper 8. London: National Council for Hospice and Specialist Palliative Care Services, 1995.
6. National Palliative Care Strategy: A National Framework for Palliative Care Service Development. Canberra: Commonwealth of Australia, 2000.
7. Department of Health. Cancer Services in Ireland: A National Strategy. Dublin, Department of Health, 1996.
8. Wilkes E, for the Standing Medical Advisory Committee. Terminal Care: Report of a Working Party. London: HMSO, 1980.
9. Department of Health. Joint Report of the Standing Medical Advisory Committee and Standing Nursing and Midwifery Advisory Committee. The Principles and Provision of Palliative Care. London: Department of Health, 1992.
10. Department of Health. A Policy Framework for Commissioning Cancer Services: A Report by the Expert Advisory Group on Cancer to the Chief Medical Officers of England and Wales (the Calman-Hine Report). London: HMSO, 1995.
11. Clark D, Malson H. Key issues in palliative care needs assessment. Prog Palliat Care 1995;3:53-55.
12. Williams R, Wright J. Epidemiological issues in health needs assessment. BMJ 1998;316:1379-1382.
13. Saunders C, Baines M. Living with Dying: The Management of Terminal Malignant Disease. Oxford, UK: Oxford University Press, 1983.
14. O'Brien T, Kelly M, Saunders C. Motor neurone disease—a hospice perspective. BMJ 1992;304:471-473.
15. Addington-Hall JM, McCarthy M. The regional study of care for the dying: Methods and sample characteristics. Palliat Med 1995;9:27-35.
16. International Expert Advisory Group Report on Palliative Care. Cork, Ireland: Marymount Hospice and the Atlantic Philanthropies, 2006.
17. Palliative Care Accreditation Scheme: A Framework for Quality and Safety. Dublin: Irish Health Services Accreditation Board, 2005.

SUGGESTED READING

International Expert Advisory Group Report on Palliative Care. Cork, Ireland: Marymount Hospice and the Atlantic Philanthropies, 2006.

National Palliative Care Strategy: A National Framework for Palliative Care Service Development. Canberra: Commonwealth of Australia, 2000.

Palliative Care Accreditation Scheme: A Framework for Quality and Safety. Dublin: Irish Health Services Accreditation Board, 2005.

Recommendations Rec (2003) 24 of the Committee of Ministers to Member States on the Organisation of Palliative Care. Strasbourg: Council of Europe, 2003.

Report of the National Advisory Committee on Palliative Care. Dublin: Department of Health and Children, 2001.

CHAPTER **37**

Program Development: Palliative Medicine and Public Health Services

Xavier Gómez-Batiste, Josep Porta-Sales, Silvia Paz, Javier Rocafort, and Jan Stjernswärd

---

K E Y   P O I N T S

- There is a growing need for palliative care for patients with advanced chronic diseases and for the elderly.

- Palliative care services and measures must be incorporated in public health plans globally, particularly in the management of cancer, acquired immunodeficiency syndrome (AIDS), geriatric disorders, and other diseases.

- The main aims of public health–oriented palliative care plans are coverage, equity, quality, community orientation, and empowerment of families and informal caregivers.

- Defined elements of rational public health plans include service implementation, education and training, and drug availability.

- The best results are achieved with clear leadership from health administrators and health care organizations.

Since the 1970s, pioneering palliative care physicians such as Eric Wilkes in the United Kingdom, Jan Stjernswärd at the World Health Organization (WHO) Cancer Unit, and Vittorio Ventafridda in Italy have stated that palliative medicine should be an essential part of any national health service.[1] There is evidence for the effectiveness and efficiency of palliative care services in providing adequate care by lessening unnecessary suffering and satisfying the needs and demands of patients and families in the setting of advanced disease.[2] The WHO palliative care demonstration projects and similar initiatives developed as part of a rational plan to implement palliative care within the public health sector have been highly effective in responding to people's needs. As a consequence, the right for good-quality care in the management of advanced disease has been recognized in law in several countries.[3]

Palliative care provides innovation in the public health care system in several ways:

- Provides a comprehensive approach to care
- Provides patient- and family-centered care
- Promotes multidisciplinary team work
- Facilitates service integration and network collaboration
- Underscores ethics-based clinical decisions that respect the values of patients and families
- Engenders esteem for the social and cultural dimensions of palliative care
- Promotes debate on the respect for quality of life and dignity in the provision of care for the dying

PRINCIPLES AND AIMS OF A PUBLIC HEALTH APPROACH

Each palliative care program within the public health sector should provide at least three basic elements (Fig. 37-1):

1. Education and training
2. Availability of opioids and other medications to control symptoms
3. Implementation of service (i.e., specialist services)

National policies on palliative care provide the framework in which these elements interact.[4]

Robust public palliative care programs should establish several principles:

- To guarantee coverage to reach most people in need of specialized care
- To ensure equity so care can be provided to all terminally ill patients, regardless of gender, age, social class, type of disease, or economic situation
- To be accessible so the most complex clinical cases are cared for by experienced palliative care teams
- To secure good quality in service provision by effectiveness and efficiency

Crucial to culturally meaningful palliative care is systematic exploration of the views of patients and caregivers to empower them to make informed decisions. Successful implementation of palliative care within the public health sector will ultimately rely on strong leadership; collaboration and support obtained from health administrators, health care organizations, and other health professionals; and links with established, experienced groups. Palliative care programs developed by all public health administrations, including the WHO demonstration projects, should regularly disseminate their results and cooperate with newly established services.

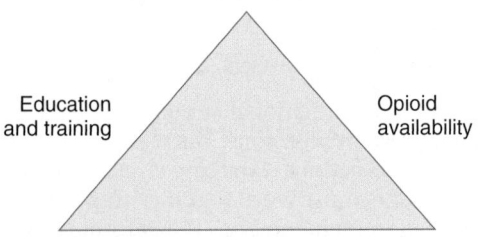

FIGURE 37-1   Three major elements of a global policy. Each palliative care program within the public health sector should provide education, pain control, and services by specialists.

COMBINED METHODS FOR IMPLEMENTING PROGRAMS

Developing and implementing a global palliative care program require a combination of strategies and a clear understanding of public programs, including clear aims, strong leadership, professional consensus, and a rational public health approach.[5] Rational, stepwise implementation of new services and policies is advised. It is useful to reallocate preexisting service resources, promote organizational changes, optimize conventional services, and start with catalytic measures such as the use of support teams. All changes should be planned and designated as short-, medium-, and long-term measures. Systematic assessments of needs and outcomes are strongly advised.

ELEMENTS OF RATIONAL PLANNING

Assessment of Needs

The first step in planning is to assess needs (Box 37-1).[6] It is crucial to identify epidemiological data, such as mortality rates, incidence and prevalence of cancer, dementia, AIDS, or other target conditions, and to accrue demographic information on the aging population.[7] This information should be combined with data from local or population studies on physical and emotional symptom frequency and the consumption of health care resources (e.g., place of death, hospital mean stay, emergency room use). It is also important to assess the perceptions of needs of health professionals, patients, and families.

This information is preferably obtained in various settings, such as oncology services, emergency units, geriatric centers, and homes. Data about place of death may not be reliable, because it is greatly affected by the available resources and by social and demographic variables. In developed countries, especially in urban areas in which palliative care has not been implemented, 60% to 80% of deaths occur in acute hospitals. In these circumstances, the implementation of palliative care resources has impressive results, reducing hospital bed use and emergency room visits and allowing care and death at home.

Leadership

Leadership is fundamental for innovation. Culture changes generate considerable resistance, and combating this requires specific skills. Experiences in different communities in which palliative care has been developed rapidly indicate that success can be explained by synergistic work from a relevant and visible technical leadership, along with strong support from institutional politicians and health care organization managers. In countries with relatively destructed governments, nongovernmental organizations (NGOs) have had an important role in model programs and initial projects.[8] Their more difficult challenge is propelling projects and resources into public health services for long-term viability.

Implementation of Specialist Palliative Care Services

Implementation of specialist palliative care services can be done in several ways (Box 37-2).[9] It may be reasonable to start by implementation of palliative care services in key places such as main hospitals, in nursing homes, or in the community. A good start may be promotion of at least one specific service in different key places, such as a hospital or care at home. This identifies reference services, builds appropriate leadership, and forms a core of pioneering teams. The selection of where and which kind of service should be set up can be considered on the basis of need and according to the feasibility (e.g., real capacity, availability) and the opportunity, personalities, restructuring possibilities, or local leadership.

We recommend starting with a *basic support team* that is appropriate in terms of initial size, flexibility, effectiveness, and efficiency.[10] Support teams usually provide consultation, outpatient care in clinics, and home-based health care. The decision to implement units with beds needs to be developed rationally, and most beds can come from reallocation of preexisting beds. To avoid misunderstandings, some basic items and standards should be defined before palliative services begin, such as the kind of patients to be cared for, the type of team, activities and aims, and planned evaluations over the short, middle, and long term.

Directories and national databases are useful in this initial phase to improve visibility and promote benchmarks. Many different palliative care models in hospitals or the community have been described, reflecting the heterogeneity of health care resources around the world and the need to adapt the services to each place to best serve people.

Specialist Nurses

The use of Macmillan nurses at home in the United Kingdom and specialist nurses in hospitals has shown excellent results.[11] This approach could be applied in

---

Box 37-1 Components of Public Health Planning

- Needs assessment
- Unambiguous aims
- Clear leadership
- Implementation of specific services
- Measures of conventional resources
- Legislation and standards
- Availability of opioids
- Funding and purchasing
- Training strategies
- Research strategies
- Implementation of short-term, mid-term, and long-term plans
- Monitoring of outcomes

Box 37-2 Suggested Resources in Developed Countries

- One support team available per district (i.e., 100,000 to 200,000 people)
- Eighty to 100 beds per million people for acute, mid-term, long-term, and hospice care
- One support team available in each hospital
- Services in cancer institutes and university hospitals

developing countries, where primary care nurses might undertake this role.

Support Teams

A palliative care support team is a multidisciplinary team with specialized training that operates as a consultation team without specific beds or units in the community, in hospital, or through a comprehensive network. Its basic structure includes at least one physician, one nurse, and the assistance of a social worker or psychologist. The most relevant factor is advanced training, which makes team members highly effective and efficient in the care of cancer patients and their families and in caring for the elderly with chronic diseases. In hospitals, support teams can be the initial resource of a program that later implements a unit with beds and achieves an agreement with the related services, such oncology, geriatrics, or primary care.[12]

Specialist Units

Basic questions arise about the number of beds, type of patients, and architecture of the setting. Based on our experience, we recommend between 80 and 100 beds per 1million inhabitants as optimal if noncancer patients are to be included. Experience indicates that 20% to 30% of beds should be in acute hospitals, 50% to 60% in the social health sector (e.g., intermediate-stay centers), and another 20% to 30% in nursing homes or rest homes for the elderly. The size and numbers of units depend on the sector or district served; for instance, in a small sector (<50,000 inhabitants), it is not essential to have specific beds for palliative care. For individual projects, the number of beds depends on various factors (e.g., architecture, organization of the nurses, cost), but a reasonable number is 12 to 25 beds per unit.

Depending on their location, palliative care units provide care to a wide range of patients, with differences in hospital stay, age, mortality, and costs. Some units may be devoted exclusively to cancer, but others care for patients with other chronic diseases. Other units can deal with acute and complex cases and some stable patients who do not have the possibility of home care.

The physical structure of a palliative care unit should promote privacy and comfort for the patients, the company of family members (enabling nighttime rest, allowing total accessibility, and providing a kitchenette), and workplace comfort for health professionals. The number of beds per room depends on economic aspects and the institutional structure.

Outpatient Clinics and Day Care Centers

An outpatient clinic is an optimal resource for generating accessibility and enhancing coverage of the palliative care program, especially in promoting early interventions shared with other specialties.[13] It can be carried out by a hospital or home support team or as part of the activity of a more comprehensive hospital palliative care service.

Comprehensive, Integrated Systems

Comprehensive, integrated systems operate in a sector in an integrated manner and with a team involved in all aspects of care and with a methodology focused on case management.[14]

Demographic and Sector Models

It is useful to define models by different demographic scenarios and construct the ideal model of service organization and its future placement for the long term, defining in advance short-term and mid-term measures.

Quality Improvement or General Measures in Conventional Nonspecialist Resources

To maximize coverage, it is crucial to promote improvement measures in all contexts of the health care system. Important and inexpensive improvements include better documentation, treatment protocols for the most prevalent symptoms, improved accessibility, continuous care of patients and families, increased care for family members, and better availability of opioids. Other areas for quality improvement include training personnel in symptom control, communication skills, clinical ethics, and teamwork.

Legislation, Guidelines, and Standards

Palliative care providers need to be aware of relevant health system legislation, including laws, decrees, and ministerial orders. Palliative care should be an essential element in health care planning, and it is vital to insert it into the national, regional, and local plans for the management of cancer, geriatric illness, and other diseases. Incorporating palliative care in general health plans helps to promote the adoption of measures in all contexts.

Palliative care standards and guidelines encourage consensus among professionals, managers, policy makers, and patients about the quality of any service. The standards must be defined before implementation. Standards for services include definitions, types of patients, mission, values, structure (e.g., staffing, documentation, architecture), process or activities, and the main outcomes and outputs. A clear definition of the scope of the specialist palliative care service, as well as its expected level of complexity, distinguishes palliative care from other specialist services. Levels of complexity of palliative care services depend very much on the resources available and on the type and the needs of the population to be cared for (see Chapter 5).

Availability and Accessibility of Opioids

There are numerous barriers to opioid availability. In countries where palliative care has developed, laws regulate and promote drug availability and access to opioids without limits of dose or frequency. This is an essential requirement for palliative care; opioids must be available in every setting, including community pharmacies, hospitals, and nursing homes. Many palliative care teams have developed systems to improve accessibility, including providing them from their own team prescriptions or persuading the hospital pharmacy to supply home care patients.

Systems of Funding and Purchasing

In initial phases of palliative care programs implementation, we need catalytic funding, so that a little expenditure can have a major impact.[15] Many parameters have been used, particularly those for activity (e.g., number of hospital stays, number of hospital discharges, number of outpatients), for structure (e.g., number of beds, staffing), or a combination of activity and structure constraints.

One innovation consists of purchasing services based on case mix, patient complexity, or type of intervention. Mechanisms of payment or incentives based on quality parameters (e.g., interdisciplinary work, time between demand and visit even in an outpatient clinic or home) help. All purchase systems have strengths and weaknesses, and all are evolutionary, normally from the structure to the activity and from the activity to the process. Sophisticated measures are based on outcomes plus incentives for quality. Capitation systems of funding benefit palliative care because they are efficient, especially in integrated systems. Private or NGO service funding is important in the early phases, but this approach has long-term problems because funding agencies change priorities.

Strategies for Training and Research

Training in palliative care can be described according to level, objectives, targets, advisable methods, type of provider, or degree of priority. If we consider training requirements at the start of programs or services, we can define different priorities and actions (Table 37-1).

The initial priority is to create a nucleus of teams that will lead clinical and training implementation. One method consists of a postgraduate course (e.g., master's degree) in addition to a stay in a reference palliative medicine center or service. Once consolidated, wider coverage is achieved when these teams develop and execute their own training programs. They serve as local references for successive teams until broad coverage is achieved.

Along with training, research is a cornerstone of improvement of palliative care. Research includes a wide range of topics, and the methodology used can be quantitative or qualitative.[16] Easy descriptive studies to start can be informative and provide the basis for further studies. Research should be stated as one of the activities of any palliative care program.

Marketing, Advocacy, and Social Interaction

Palliative care is effective and efficient, and it generates high levels of satisfaction among users, which can be used for further promotion of these services. There is a need to develop specific measures to involve different sectors and stakeholders, health professionals, administrators, planners, financers, politicians, and journalists while avoiding conflicts. Some are natural allies, such as nurses, quality-improvement services, bioethicists, NGOs, and patient organizations. We should rationally evaluate resistance as caused by human nature, cultural habits, difficulty in confronting death, changes in organizational culture (e.g., cure to care), or maintenance and use of power.[17]

Implementation of Plans in the Short, Middle, and Long Term

Smooth implementation of a palliative care program depends on strong leadership and clearly defined objec-

TABLE 37-1 Dilemmas in Palliative Care Programs	
DILEMMA	**RECOMMENDATION**
Coverage	Cancer: 60% to 70% of total patients
	Cancer to noncancer needs ratio of 1:2.5 to 1:3
	Cancer to noncancer ratio of 90:10 in initial phases; 30:70 subsequently
Appropriate location	General measures in all resources, especially target resources with high prevalence to consider resources needed for each location (e.g., hospital, cancer institutes, social health centers, residences, community)
	Each resource influences its context and health care of different patients
	Bed location: 30% to 40% in acute hospitals, 40% to 60% in intermediate hospitals, 10% to 30% in nursing homes
Specific resources	Number of beds: 80 to 100 per million inhabitants
	Home care teams: 1 basic team per 100,000 to 200,000 inhabitants, with sectorization crucial for efficiency
	Specialist physicians: 25 to 30 per 1 million inhabitants
	Minimum of 1 team in every hospital
Mixed or disease-specific problems	Specific: cancer institutes or university hospitals with high prevalence or for specific aspects of health care (e.g., pediatrics, AIDS patients in prisons)
	Mixed: community (e.g., home care support teams) and integrated systems in small or middle-sized areas
Initial measures	Support teams (as a good start)
	Re-assignment of beds
	Clinical and organizational training for core leaders
	Local and ministerial leadership (crucial for feasibility)
Teams, units, and health care centers	Avoidance of competition between different settings
	Independent hospices as a way for nongovernmental organizations to start, with insertion into the public health care network being a challenge
	Support teams used as the initial service in many settings
	Units needed in different settings
	Services needed long term within the national public health care system at all levels
General measures or specialist services	Both are needed and are synergistic
	General measures in conventional services have limits because the complexity or prevalence is high
	To maintain training, specialist teams are needed

tives for the short, middle, and long term, which need to be formalized with an independent budget. Having a visible leader responsible at the health administration level is recommended. In the early phase of development, common aims include evaluating needs, defining objectives, naming leadership at the health administration level, selecting the core initial projects, defining core standards, adapting legislation, and creating funding models.

The short-term (0 to 2 years) aims include starting and consolidating core initial reference services (e.g., home care, hospital units, heath care centers) or specific services (e.g., cancer, geriatrics, AIDS), promoting appropriate leadership and training for the core initial projects, and measuring and publishing results. At the mid-term period (2 to 5 years), efforts should be devoted to the consolidation and extension of initiatives, sharing and disseminating experience and reproducible evidence, promoting benchmarks, and training trainers. The long-term (>5 years) aims are to reach the highest possible coverage for the various types of needs and services and for all levels of training.

Monitoring Outcomes

Monitoring should choose metrics that are easy to obtain, such as the number of specific services, population coverage, geographical coverage, accessibility, continuity of care use, consumption of opioids, place of death, and use of resources by patients with advanced or terminal disease. Indicators of specialized services include clinical results (e.g., pain control), mean length of stay, mean intervention time, clinical population pattern (e.g., function, survival, pain prognostic index), patient feedback, mortality, estimates of coverage, satisfaction of the patient and family (i.e., external clients) and of related teams (i.e., internal clients), and costs.

SUCCESSFUL PALLIATIVE CARE EXPERIENCES

Under the leadership of the WHO Cancer Unit and following the principles of rational planning, several initial projects were established in the 1990s. In Edmonton, Canada, a rational strategy was implemented, and it achieved excellent results in caring for dying cancer patients.[18] For 7 million people in Catalonia, Spain, a systematic WHO demonstration project developed many resources (i.e., 70 home care teams, 52 units, and 34 hospital support teams), achieving high coverage, effectiveness, and efficiency for cancer and geriatric patients.[19] Many European countries have established laws and services. In Eastern Europe, countries such as Hungary and Slovenia are developing palliative care plans based on the experience gained in Poland.

DILEMMAS AND CONTROVERSIES

Problems are common in the design of palliative care programs, including size, location, and starting resources (see Table 37-1). Additional dilemmas relate to the definition of the appropriate coverage and whether the resources should be new or reassigned.

Palliative care teams risk burnout as they attend to difficult clinical situations. Organizational factors contribute enormously, and managers have a responsibility to deal with the risk of burnout. Work overload, isolation, overcommitment, and organizational difficulties can cause burnout.[20] Recommended measures to reduce the risk are to enhance formal and informal support within the team, define reasonable clinical and organizational goals, recognize the limits of intervention with patients, and develop better coverage and programs.

FUTURE TRENDS

In the developed world, with a rising tide of geriatric patients, the most relevant short-term challenge is to develop palliative care for the elderly and for patients with chronic diseases. Palliative care should be incorporated in most public health care systems and be available at all levels of care through appropriate coverage for patients with the most common advanced or progressive diseases. Training should occur early in the pregraduate level of health sciences education (e.g., medicine, nursing, psychology, social work) and continue at the specialty or subspecialty level. Research in palliative care has grown enormously, but there is still room for improvement.

In less developed countries, palliative care as geriatric care offers challenges and opportunities to facilitate changes in the values and organization of health care. In the developing world, broad-coverage palliative care is needed for the enormous numbers of patients with advanced illness and their families.

Palliative care is essential for relieving this suffering. Community-based care with empowerment of families and nurses and easy access to cheap opioids can ensure success.

REFERENCES

1. Stjernswärd J, Colleau SM, Ventafridda V. The World Health Organization Cancer Pain and Palliative Care Program: Past, present and future. J Pain Symptom Manage 1996;12:65-72.
2. Gysels M, Higginson IJ. Improving supportive and palliative care for adults with cancer: Research evidence. Guidance on Cancer Services. The National Institute for Clinical Excellence (NICE), 8 October 2003. Available at http://www.nice.org.uk/pdf/SupportivePalliative_Research_Evidence_SecondCons.pdf (accessed January 2006).
3. Bakitas M, Stevens M, Ahles T, et al. Project ENABLE: A palliative care demonstration project for advanced cancer patients in three settings. J Palliat Med 2004;7:363-372.
4. Gómez-Batiste X, Fontanals de Nadal MD, Via JM, et al. Catalonia's five-year plan: Basic principles. Eur J Palliat Care 1994;1:45-49.
5. Gómez-Batiste X, Fontanals MD, Roca J, et al. Rational planning and policy implementation in palliative care. In Clark D, Hockley J, Ahmedzai S (eds). New Themes in Palliative Care. Buckingham, UK: Open University Press, 1997, pp 148-169.
6. Franks PJ. Salisbury C, Bosanquet N, et al. The level of need for palliative care: A systematic review of the literature. Palliat Med 2000;14:93-104
7. Tebbit P. Population-Based Needs Assessment for Palliative Care: A Manual for Cancer Networks. London: The National Council for Palliative Care, May 2004.
8. International Observatory on End of Life Care. Palliative care developments in developing regions of the world. Available at http://www.eolc-observatory.net/global_analysis/index.htm (accessed January 2006).
9. Sepulveda C, Marlin A, Yoshida T, Ullrich A. Palliative care: The World Health Organization's global perspective. J Pain Symptom Manage 2002;24:91-96.
10. Cheng WW, Willey J, Palmer JL, et al. Interval between palliative care referral and death among patients treated at a comprehensive cancer center. J Palliat Med 2005;8:1025-1032.
11. Douglas HR, Halliday D, Normand C, et al. Economic evaluation of specialist cancer and palliative nursing: Macmillan evaluation study findings. Int J Palliat Nurs 2003;9:429-438.
12. Axelsson B, Christensen SB. Evaluation of a hospital-based palliative support service with particular regard to financial outcome measures. Palliat Med 1998;12:41-49.
13. Porta-Sales J, Codorniu N, Gómez-Batiste X, et al. Patient appointment process, symptom control and prediction of follow up compliance in a palliative care outpatient clinic. J Pain Symptom Manage 2005;30:145-153.

14. Nikbakht-Van de Sande CVMV, van der Rijt CC, Visser AP, et al. Function of local networks in palliative care: A Dutch view. J Palliat Med 2005;8:808-816.
15. Walsh D. The business of palliative medicine. Part 4. Potential impact of an acute-care palliative medicine inpatient unit in a tertiary care cancer center. Am J Hosp Palliat Med 2004;21:217-221.
16. Hopkinson JB, Wright DN, Corner JL. Seeking new methodology for palliative care research: Challenging assumptions about studying people who are approaching the end of life. Palliat Med 2005;19:532-537.
17. Stevens T, Wilde D, Hunt J, Ahmedzai SH. Overcoming the challenges to consumer involvement in cancer research. Health Expect 2003;6:81-88.
18. Bruera E, Neumann CM, Gagnon B, et al. Edmonton Regional Palliative care program: Impact on patterns of terminal cancer care. CMAJ 1999;161:290-293.
19. Gómez-Batiste X, Porta-Sales J, Pascual A, et al. Catalonia WHO palliative care demonstration project at 15 years (2005). J Pain Symptom Manage 2007;33:584-590.
20. Aoun SM, Kristjanson LJ, Currow DC, Hudson PL. Caregiving for the terminally ill: At what cost? Palliat Med 2005;19:551-555.

SUGGESTED READING

Fassbender K, Fainsinger R, Brenneis C, et al. Utilization and costs of the introduction of system wide palliative care in Alberta, 1993-2000. Palliat Med 2000;19:513-520.
Gómez-Batiste X, Porta J, Tuca A, Stjernswärd J (eds). Organización de Servicios y Programas de Cuidados Paliativos. Bases de organización, planificación, evaluación y mejora de calidad. ICO Formación Series. Madrid: Aran Ediciones, 2005.
Stjernswärd J. Uganda: Initiating a government public health approach to pain relief and palliative care. J Pain Symptom Manage 2002;24:257-264.

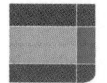

CHAPTER **38**

Consultation Services

Paul Glare, John Hunt, Peter Selwyn, and K. Allsopp

KEY POINTS

- Up to 25% of patients in acute care hospitals need palliative care.
- Consultation services aim to transfer the skills learned in hospice into the acute care hospital setting, and they are the fastest growing sector of palliative care.
- The structure of consultation services and their level of involvement in patient management vary among countries and institutions.
- The main functions of the consultation services are assessment and management of physical symptoms, assisting patients in the identification of personal goals for end-of-life care, family support, and discharge planning.
- Consultation services can be a focus of education and research within the hospital.
- Audit tools and standards have been developed to evaluate the effect of consultation services on patient outcomes.
- Controlled studies have documented the improvements in care that a consultation service can make.
- The maintenance of an effective consultation service depends on sound leadership from an experienced and trusted clinician, adequate funding, and good communication at all levels.

In this era of rapid expansion in medical knowledge and increasing medical specialization, consultation services are becoming common in all branches of medicine where a specialist in one area offers advice to generalists or specialists from a different area. Consultation services can be provided by traditional specialties, such as cardiology, surgery, or psychiatry, or by newer specialties, such as ethics, genetics, and transcultural mental health. Palliative care can be added to this list. Consultations can be provided to patients while they are in the hospital, which is the main focus of this chapter, or they can be provided to patients in ambulatory outpatient clinics or at home.

Although most terminally ill patients indicate a preference to die at home, national statistics for the latter half of the 20th century show a trend toward death in institutions, with more than 60% taking place there, and most of these deaths occur in acute care hospitals. Many studies have documented the deficiencies of care at the end of life in hospitals. Audits of patients on general medical wards of hospitals in the United Kingdom and New Zealand have indicated that up to 25% of patients are receiving only palliative care.[1] Hospital-based palliative care teams have been established to transfer the skills learned in hospice into the hospital setting to assist the doctors and nurses primarily in charge of the patient's care.

HISTORY

There is some historical irony in the development of hospital-based palliative care services. One of the main drivers behind the emergence of the hospice movement in Britain in the 1960s was the reaction to the inadequacies of care for patients dying in hospitals. Although care of the dying had always been a fundamental task of physicians, progress in modern medicine over the past 150 years brought about changes in this role. In some cases, it led to physicians concentrating on aggressively trying to cure patients rather than give up on them. In other cases, physicians said to dying patients, "There is nothing more that can be done for you." This created the perception that the patient was being abandoned by the health care system. As a result, hospices were set up: inpatient facilities in the United Kingdom, which were charity funded and run outside the mainstream system, and home-based services in the United States, which were paid for by Medicare.

The growth of palliative care consultation services within hospitals in the past 10 to 20 years has refocused the health care system on the needs of dying patients while they are hospitalized. The first hospital palliative care services were set up in the United Kingdom at St. Thomas's Hospital in 1977 and in Australia in the early 1980s. The first U.S. hospital-based palliative care program was begun at the Cleveland Clinic in 1987, and it was partly driven by perceived inadequacies of the hospice system in caring for the seriously ill and dying in acute care hospitals.

By 2005, there were more than 1200 hospital palliative care teams in the United States and almost 300 in the United Kingdom. Most Australian hospitals now have consultation teams. Local differences in health care service delivery, type of hospital, and history of the consultation team's establishment have resulted in differences in the provision of palliative care consultation services internationally.[2]

STRUCTURE

Palliative care consultation services in acute care hospitals, also referred to as *hospital palliative care teams* (HPCTs), may or may not be associated with an inpatient unit for palliative care in the hospital. The staff may be part of the hospital staff or provide an in-reach service from a palliative care facility off site. The HPCT may stand alone, may be established by a visionary at an institution, or may be part of an integrated palliative medicine program,[3-5] interfacing with other components of the program (e.g., inpatient facility, home care team, ambulatory clinic, day hospital) and with other services addressing similar issues (e.g., cancer multidisciplinary teams, ethics consultation services).

HPCT staffing depends on local factors. In Britain, many HPCTs are led by nurses, whereas in the United States and Australia, they are usually led by physicians. In 2000, the U.K. National Council for Hospice and Specialist Palliative Care Services (NCHSPCS, which later became the National Council for Palliative Care) identified the core and extended members of an HPCT (Box 38-1). Funding for HPCTs varies from country to country, which affects team composition. In the United Kingdom and many other countries, all palliative care is offered free to patients and their families through the U.K. National Health Service or through charities working in partnership with the local health services. Palliative care services in the United States are financed by philanthropic sources, fee-for service mechanisms, or direct hospital support.

As with other forms of palliative care service delivery, training and development are important for staff members of HPCTs. Service organization and management, including development and use of protocols and information systems, are essential. HPCTs are dynamic entities, and their ongoing development depends on needs assessments and performance assessments. In the United Kingdom, HPCTs have not escaped the demands of the clinical governance agenda of the National Health Service, which requires a rigorous review of systems, policies, and procedures; documentation; and the adoption of appropriate quality measures to assist the evidence base for clinical effectiveness.[6] In the United States, there have been some publications on the business aspects of providing an HPCT service.[5]

PROCESS AND FUNCTIONS

Many articles have described the establishment and functioning of HPCTs in the United States,[7,8] Canada,[9] the United Kingdom,[10,11] and Australia,[12,13] and they indicate that HPCTs vary according to their case mix of patients, the country they work in, the type of institution, the referring services who use them, the patients' diagnoses, and the mode of separation of the patient from hospital (i.e., death, discharge home, or transfer to another institution). The common thread in this variability is the transfer of the principles of hospice care into the acute care setting. Most studies report the workload or case mix of the HPCTs, and a few have tried to measure the effectiveness of their interventions. Findings show that HPCTs can carry out clinical and nonclinical functions.

Clinical Functions

The core clinical functions of a palliative medicine consultation have been described (Box 38-2).[14] Although the initial consultation question focuses on one issue, it is typical for there to be a host of related issues that must be identified, if not resolved, before arriving at the optimal management program. For example, Canadian investigators reported that less than 50% of referrals to their HPCT were known to have untreatable cancer at the time of their admission to hospital a few days earlier.[9]

Symptom control is a major focus of HPCT work because symptoms are more common in hospitalized patients than nonhospitalized persons, although in a U.S. study,[8] consultation about the prognosis and goals of care was the most common intervention undertaken. A member of the team should see all referrals within 24 hours. After the assessment of the patient and family, the HPCT typically makes three or four recommendations. Strategies to ensure implementation of the recommendations include establishing personal contact with involved parties (e.g., family members, nurse, primary physician, house staff) rather than relying on notes in the medical chart and seeking permission to directly implement certain critical interventions promptly to prevent unnecessary suffering.[8] Unlike the consultations provided by many other specialties, palliative care consultations are intense and time consuming, address many sensitive issues, and involve a large number of interventions, often requiring visits more than

---

Box 38-1 Membership of Hospital Palliative Care Teams in 2000 According to the U.K. National Council for Hospice and Specialist Palliative Care Services

- One or more nurses who hold or who are working toward a specialist practitioner recordable qualification in palliative care
- A consultant in palliative medicine supported by other medical staff, including junior staff members who may be on rotations
- Secretarial and administrative support
- Extended teams with expertise in chaplaincy, social work, psychology, and pharmacy
- Access to specialist pain management
- Access to specialists in physiotherapy, occupational therapy, and dietetics

---

Box 38-2 Core Functions of a Palliative Medicine Consultation Service

- Assessment and management of physical symptoms
- Assisting patients in the identification of personal goals for end-of-life care
- Documentation of advanced directives
- Assessment and management of psychological and spiritual needs
- Assessment of the patient's support system
- Assessment and communication of the estimated prognosis
- Assessment of discharge planning issues

once each day, sometimes for symptom management but more often because of ongoing discussions about goals and plans of care. The high implementation rate of palliative care interventions reported in surveys indicates an acknowledgment that the HPCT provides a service that is not part of usual hospital care.

A feature of all consultation services is their level of involvement in the care of the patient. Interaction with the patient can range from giving phone advice to formal transfer of care in the case of physician-led HPCTs, with one-time contact with the patient or ongoing interaction with the patient and family for the duration of the admission as intermediate levels of involvement. Contact may even continue after the patient is discharged if the HPCT staff provides an ambulatory clinic. Another issue that varies is whether the HPCT carries out the interventions or merely makes recommendations. The results of a randomized, controlled trial of phone interviews are compared with face-to-face consultations in the "Evidence-Based Medicine" section.

Nonclinical Functions

Publications about the role and function of HPCTs in Britain indicate that the emphasis is as much on influencing the ward team and fostering the development of knowledge, skills, and practice within the hospital setting as on providing direct clinical care to individual patients and their families.[11] Frequently, these services develop symptom control guidelines and other educational materials, hold ward-based teaching sessions, and promote one-to-one education by means of case discussion. They can also undertake research about relevant clinical, programmatic, and health services issues in palliative care.

Several studies have described the function of their service, with or without outcome data. Because of a lack of uniformity in the way these HPCTs work and differences in what the audits report, the studies are hard to compare. Selected items are summarized in Table 38-1 to illustrate some of the differences and challenges between the processes of the HPCT and hospice, such as the following:

- The time in contact with patient and family is typically short (1 to 2 weeks).
- Only a few referrals die during the admission process.
- The focus is on relief of symptoms, improving insight, and discharge planning.

- The team has incomplete control over their recommendations being carried out.

OUTCOMES

As its name suggests, the focus of our specialty is on care, and it depends on the process as much as the outcome. In certain jurisdictions, particularly the United Kingdom, clinical governance mandates that palliative care services—including HPCTs—should be focused on outcomes. The outcomes of HPCTs can be evaluated in different ways. For clinical processes, there can be evidence for the effectiveness of interventions, which may or may not involve the use of validated outcome measures. Two validated tools developed in the United Kingdom are the Support Team Assessment Schedule (STAS), with standard and extended forms (E-STAS), and the Palliative Care Assessment (PACA) (Box 38-3).[15-17]

U.S. and Australian tools have concentrated on clinical outcomes. They have shown a high degree of compliance with recommendations, and one study indicated that these

---

Box 38-3 Palliative Care Outcome Tools

Core items of the 3.1 STAS[28]: Rated 0 to 4 by the Observer (Definitions Provided)

Pain control
Other symptom control
Patient anxiety
Family anxiety
Patient insight
Family insight
Communication between patient and family
Communication between professionals
Communication from professionals to the patient and family
Additional items: planning, practical aid, financial advice, wasted time, spiritual values, professional anxiety, professional advice, and team anxiety

Core items of the 3.2 PACA[16]: Rated by the Observer (Definitions Supplied)

Symptom controlled or not: graded 0 to 3
Insight of patient or relatives, full or not: graded 1 to 5
Placement decided and organized: graded 1 to 4

PACA, Palliative Care Assessment; STAS, Support Team Assessment Schedule.

TABLE 38-1 Studies Describing Hospital-Based Palliative Medicine Consultation Services

STUDY	AGE*	MALE PATIENTS (%)	PATIENTS WITH CANCER (%)	SYMPTOM CONTROL (%)	DAYS FROM CONSULT TO DISCHARGE	RECOM. PER PATIENT	COMPLIANCE (%)	DIED IN HOSPITAL (%)
Ellershaw et al,[16] 1995	68	54	100	62	10	4	NS	26
Jenkins et al,[9] 2000	67	55	100	NS	8	NS	89	20
Manfredi et al,[8] 2000	71	54	57	75	5	4.2	91	39
Virik and Glare,[13] 2002	58.5	50	80	44	NS	3	NS	NS
Penrod et al,[19] 2006	72	100	50	NS	13	NS	NS	100

*Average age (years) of patients.
RECOM., recommendations; NS, not stated.

interventions improved patient care in up to 90% of cases.[13] British studies using STAS and PACA have shown significant improvements in symptoms and in the insight of patients and families as a result of the involvement of the HPCT.[16,17]

The outcome of nonclinical functions can also be assessed. British studies have looked at educational outcomes, including demonstration that improvements in hospital-wide analgesic prescribing patterns followed the creation of an HPCT.[18] U.S. studies have begun reporting financial outcomes, and as for other settings, patients receiving palliative care in the hospital cost less. A study of per diem direct costs of deceased patients from two Veterans Administration medical centers found that the patients seen by the HPCT cost $239/day less than those who were managed in other settings.[19] Another study suggested savings on length-of-stay and ancillary charges for patients referred to the palliative care service compared with those who were not referred.[20]

DEVELOPMENTS IN THE USE OF HOSPITAL PALLIATIVE CARE TEAMS

The most notable development in the use of HPCTs has been the rapid growth of this type of service delivery in American acute care settings, with more than 600 HPCTs now in existence. To support this growth, the Center for the Advancement of Palliative Care (CAPC) has developed a number of resources, including *A Guide to Building a Hospital-Based Palliative Care Program*, a manual for starting a successful HPCT. Using examples and tools from thriving palliative care programs, the *Guide* shows how to develop the financial case for the HPCT, obtain institutional support, operate and implement a program, and use customizable clinical, management, and administrative tools. The *Guide* can be purchased from CAPC (www.capc.org).

In countries such as Britain and Australia, the financial pressures for HPCTs are a different type from those in the United States. Although the state government pays for HPCTs in these locations, the teams are in competition with all other services for part of the hospital budget. There has been no formula to determine the appropriate level of funding needed to provide optimal staffing configurations. In 2003, Palliative Care Australia published clinical staffing guidelines for specialist palliative care services. The guidelines are based on a number of assumptions and estimates about the number of deaths that occur per 100,000 people, the percentage of those patients to be referred for specialist palliative care, and the amount of work that can be done. The clinical staffing levels recommended for an HPCT providing no direct patient care are shown in Table 38-2 and amount to more than four full-time HPCT staff members per 100 beds in the hospital.

The work done by HPCTs to improve symptom control, patient and family insight, and the discharge plan varies in complexity. This raises a fundamental philosophical question about the role and function of an HPCT: Does the HPCT exist to substitute for the primary caring team or to empower it? A U.K. group has developed operational definitions for basic and specialist level palliative care in each of the domains that an HPCT receives referrals for:

TABLE 38-2 Australian Recommendations for Staffing Levels of Hospital Palliative Care Teams per 125 Hospital Beds	
POSITIONS	**NUMBER OF FULL-TIME STAFF**
MEDICAL	
Physician	1.5
Registrar	1.0
Liaison psychiatrist	0.25
NURSING	
Consultant	0.75
ALLIED HEALTH	
Social work	0.25
Pastoral care	0.25
Pharmacist	0.25
Dietician	0.2
Physiotherapist	0.2
Occupational therapist	0.2
Speech pathology	0.2
Bereavement support	0.1
Psychology	0.1

pain control, other symptoms, psychological support, insight of the dying patient, and discharge planning. The primary caregiving team is expected to be responsible for the basic management of simple problems, with the advice, if necessary, of the HPCT, whereas complex problems are appropriate for direct patient contact from the HPCT. Preliminary data from two hospitals indicate that 25% to 50% of referrals were in the simple category, identifying unnecessary clinical work for the HPCT while allowing for strategic service delivery and focused education initiatives regarding empowerment of generic staff in these areas to be developed.[21]

Trent Hospice Audit Group Standards

The U.K. Trent Hospice Audit Group (THAG) has been working in the field of specialist palliative care since 1990 to translate hospice philosophy into quality measures for use in different settings. The quality measures are audit tools based on self-assessment, which have been validated. The THAG HPCT package covers the organizational aspects of the HPCT work in addition to clinical assessment, care planning, and monitoring the effectiveness of care. THAG uses a structure-process-outcome approach, with criteria under each heading related to the breadth of HPCT activities. The HPCT audit tool contains a management documentation questionnaire, a review of patient records (10 sets of notes should be reviewed), and a staff questionnaire (to be applied on two wards, with a minimum of two members of staff).

Evidence-Based Medicine

Higginson and colleagues[22] published a systematic review of the effectiveness of palliative care and hospice teams. Of 44 studies published before 2000, only 9 assessed solely HPCTs; other studies evaluated combined home and hospital care (4 studies) or integrated teams (6 studies).[22] Only one of the HPCT studies had an experimental design (i.e., comparator group but nonrandomized [level II evidence]), allowing it to be included in the formal meta-analysis; none of the others had comparator groups (i.e., level III evidence). The one controlled study showed a benefit for patient outcomes in favor of the HPCT, similar to the overall finding of the meta-analysis.[11] Since that analysis, several other evaluations of HPCTs have been published. Most have been level III studies and would not have been included in the review by Higginson and associates.[22]

Results of the ImPaCT study,[23] a randomized, controlled trial designed to evaluate the impact of an HPCT, were published in 2002. This study assessed the effectiveness of a U.K. HPCT on physical symptoms and health-related quality of life. The patient, family caregiver, and primary care professional reported satisfaction with the care received and the health service resources used. The full package of advice and support provided by a multidisciplinary specialist palliative care team (designated as full-PCT in the study) was compared with limited telephone advice (telephone-PCT, which was the control group). The trial recruited 261 out of 684 new inpatient referrals. A 2:1 randomization design was used, with 175 patients allocated to full-PCT and 86 to telephone-PCT. One hundred ninety-one (73%) participants could be assessed at 1 week. There were highly significant improvements in symptoms, health-related quality of life, mood, and "emotional bother" with full-PCT at 1 week, and improvements were maintained over the 4-week follow-up. A smaller effect was seen with telephone-PCT, although the differences between the two treatment groups were not significant. Satisfaction with care in both groups was high, and there was no significant difference between the two types of intervention. The investigators interpreted this negative result as a study design issue, reflecting the generally high standard of care of patients dying in the hospital where the study was undertaken as a consequence of the HPCT having worked there for many years.

Common Errors

Little has been written on error within palliative care and whether interventions made or recommended by palliative care staff ever contribute to morbidity and mortality.[24] In assessing the effects of HPCTs, iatrogenic disease would be hard to detect because of the complex nature of the interventions and the number of clinicians involved. In one study in which the impact of HPCT interventions on outcomes was graded from "deleterious" to "very positive," two of 150 recommendations were graded negatively.[13]

Much has been written on the threats to survival of HPCTs, including the short life of one British HPCT that was disbanded after 18 months.[25] The work of HPCTs is difficult because much of the activity involves eliciting and giving information and providing counseling, requiring an extraordinary investment of time. Lessons learned over the past 20 years indicate that to survive and grow, HPCTs need sound leadership from an experienced and trusted clinician, adequate funding, and good communication at all levels. Strategies for growing an HPCT and handling the hazards of excessive growth have been formulated by CAPC.[26]

RESEARCH CHALLENGES

HPCTs are being established at a growing pace around the world as the advantages of transferring the knowledge learned in hospices into the acute care setting are realized. Despite differences in the structure and function of HPCTs in different countries, there is evidence that they can improve outcomes for the patient and family and, where relevant, save the hospital money. How they fulfill these functions varies from place to place.

It has been suggested that the success of HPCTs may have unintended negative outcomes, such as deskilling of hospital staff in end-of-life care and even "patient abandonment" by primary physicians.[27] *Abandonment* in this setting refers to the primary physician's deciding to withdraw from the continuing care of the patient. This can occur because of formal takeover of care by the HPCT or, more insidiously, because the primary team remains nominally in charge but gradually ceases having direct contact with the patient or family. The situation causes problems for all concerned if a change in focus of care delivery is not communicated by the primary care team to the patient and family. This raises several issues:

- What is the moral obligation of the primary team to provide continuity of care to dying patients?
- Is end-of-life care something that all physicians should be competent in?
- Is it a specialized area that is outside the scope of some subspecialties?
- Does it make a difference whether the patient's or the family's end-of-life issues are straightforward or complex?
- What are the primary team's motivations for withdrawing from continuing care?

Guidelines are available to help HPCTs avoid promotion of patient abandonment and reinforcement of narrow professional roles for physicians that exclude providing end-of-life care (see Box 38-2). Developments in the United Kingdom, for example, show how an HPCT can empower other teams. They are providing leadership and support in the rollout of the Liverpool End of Life Care Pathway in hospital services, and they have a role in advising other specialist services, such as cardiac and renal departments, as palliative care becomes a component of the National Service Frameworks (NSFs) for chronic, progressive illnesses.

Unless they are particularly innovative, more studies describing the structure and function of HPCTs are not needed. The use of telemedicine for palliative care consultations is an example of an innovation. Well-designed studies comparing interventions by an HPCT with a control arm, such as the ImPaCT study, are needed, as are studies of the health economic implications of HPCTs.

The failure of the ImPaCT study to demonstrate the benefits of direct patient contact over telephone advice emphasizes the many issues in study design that need to be taken into account when trying to evaluate HPCTs. In addition to the usual problems of patient recruitment and retention in the study, there are many biases operating in the context of routine service delivery that are difficult to gauge (Box 38-4).

> ### Box 38-4 Strategies for the Hospital Palliative Care Team to Prevent Patient Abandonment and Deskilling of the Primary Team
>
> - Palliative care specialists should resist taking over primary care responsibilities for dying patients.
> - Palliative care specialists should attempt to communicate directly, frequently, and consistently with clinicians who request their services.
> - Physicians' withdrawal from further care of their dying patients should be planned and communicated clearly among clinicians, consultants, patients, and families.
> - Palliative care specialists should seek ways to partner proactively and constructively with physicians in greatest need of assistance.

REFERENCES

1. Skilbeck J, Small N, Ahmedzai SH. Nurses' perceptions of specialist palliative care in an acute hospital. Int J Palliat Nurs 1999;5:110-115.
2. O'Neill WM, O'Connor P, Latimer EJ. Hospital palliative care services: Three models in three countries. J Pain Symptom Manage 1992;7:406-413.
3. Weissman DE, Griffie J. Integration of palliative medicine at the Medical College of Wisconsin 1990-1996. J Pain Symptom Manage 1998;15:195-207.
4. Lickiss N, Glare P, Turnewr K, et al. Palliative care in central Sydney: The Royal Prince Alfred Hospital as catalyst and integrator. J Palliat Care 1993;9:33-42.
5. Walsh D, Gombeski WR Jr, Goldstein P, et al. Managing a palliative oncology program: The role of a business plan. J Pain Symptom Manage 1994;9:109-118.
6. Hunt J, Keeley VL, Cobb M, Ahmedzai SH. A new quality assurance package for hospital palliative care teams: The Trent Hospice Audit Group model. Br J Cancer 2004;91:248-253.
7. Weissman DE, Griffie J. The Palliative Care Consultation Service of the Medical College of Wisconsin. J Pain Symptom Manage 1994;9:474-479.
8. Manfredi PL, Morrison RS, Morris J, et al. Palliative care consultations: How do they impact the care of hospitalised patients? J Pain Symptom Manage 2000;20:166-173.
9. Jenkins CA, Schulz M, Hanson J, Bruera E. Demographic, symptom and medication profiles of cancer patients seen by a palliative care consult team in a tertiary referral hospital. J Pain Symptom Manage 2000;19:174-184.
10. Hockley J. The development of a palliative care team at the Western General Hospital, Edinburgh. Support Care Cancer 1996;4:77-81.
11. McQuillan R, Finlay I, Roberts D, et al. The provision of a palliative care service in a teaching hospital and subsequent evaluation of that service. Palliat Med 1996;10:231-239.
12. Lickiss JN, Wiltshire J, Glare PA, et al. Central Sydney Palliative Care Service: Potential and limitations of an integrated palliative care service based in a metropolitan teaching hospital. Ann Acad Med Singapore 1994;23:264-270.
13. Virik K, Glare P. Profile and evaluation of a palliative medicine consultation service within a tertiary teaching hospital in Sydney, Australia. J Pain Symptom Manage 2002;23:17-25.
14. Weissman DE. Consultation in palliative medicine. Arch Intern Med 1997;157:733-737.
15. Higginson I, McCarthy M. Measuring symptoms in terminal cancer: Are pain and dyspnoea controlled? J R Soc Med 1989;82:264-267.
16. Ellershaw JE, Peat SJ, Boys LC. Assessing the effectiveness of a hospital palliative care team. Palliat Med 1995;9:145-152.
17. Edmonds PM, Stuttaford JM, Penny J, et al. Do hospital palliative care teams improve symptom control? Use of a modified STAS as an evaluation tool. Palliat Med 1998;12:345-351.
18. McQuillan R, Finlay I, Branch C, et al. Improving analgesic prescribing in a general teaching hospital. J Pain Symptom Manage 1996;11:172-180.
19. Penrod JD, Deb P, Luhrs C, et al. Cost and utilization outcomes of patients receiving hospital-based palliative care consultation. J Palliat Med 2006;9:855-860.
20. O'Mahony S, Blank AE, Zallman L, Selwyn PA. The benefits of a hospital-based inpatient palliative care consultation service: Preliminary outcome data. J Palliat Med 2005;8:1033-1039.
21. Ellershaw JE, Murphy D, Glare P. A referral criteria model for hospital palliative care teams to inform education and service delivery. Presented at the Seventh Congress of the European Association for Palliative Care. Palermo, Italy, 2001.
22. Higginson IJ, Finlay IG, Goodwin DM, et al. Is there evidence that palliative care teams alter end-of-life experiences of patients and their caregivers? J Pain Symptom Manage 2003;25:150-168.
23. Hanks GW, Robbins M, Sharp D, et al. The ImPaCT study: A randomised controlled trial to evaluate a hospital palliative care team. Br J Cancer 2002;87:733-739.
24. Hargreaves P. Palliative medicine: Too easy to bury our mistakes? Palliat Med 2005;19:503.
25. Herxheimer A, Begent R, MacLean D, et al. The short life of a terminal care support team: Experience at Charing Cross Hospital. Br Med J (Clin Red Ed) 1985;290:1877-1879.
26. Meier DE. Planning for the mixed blessing of unexpected growth. J Palliat Med 2005;8:906-908.
27. Han PK, Arnold RM. Palliative care services, patient abandonment, and the scope of physicians' responsibilities in end-of-life care. J Palliat Med 2005;8:1238-1245.
28. Higginson I, McCarthy M. Validity of the Support Team Assessment Schedule: Do staffs' ratings reflect those made by patients and their families? Palliat Med 1993;7:219-228.

SUGGESTED READING

Case for hospital-based palliative care. Available at http://www.capc.org/support-from-capc/capc_publications/making-the-case.pdf (accessed September 16, 2007).

Glickman M for the Working Party on Palliative Care in Hospital. Occasional Paper 10: Palliative Care in the Hospital Setting. London: National Council for Palliative Care, October 1996, pp 1351-9441.

Palliative Care Australia. Palliative Care Service Provision in Australia: A Planning Guide 2003, 2nd ed. Available at http://www.pallcare.org.au/ (accessed September 16, 2007).

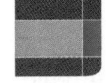

CHAPTER **39**

Acute Palliative Medicine Units

Josep Porta-Sales, Xavier Gómez-Batiste, and Antonio Pascual-López

> **KEY POINTS**
>
> - Acute palliative care units (APCUs) are effective within a comprehensive palliative care network.
> - APCUs should be combined with other palliative care resources in the same hospital, such as an outpatient clinic and consultation team.
> - The units provide expert and intensive multidimensional care for complex cases.
> - Easy access to high-tech diagnostic and therapeutic procedures is essential.
> - The need for an APCU is an indicator of the maturity and complexity of a particular palliative care system.
> - The outputs of APCUs and the complexity of intervention can be defined.

From a historical perspective, early hospice care in Great Britain was provided in inpatient facilities, mostly located outside acute care hospitals. Despite the development of home care and hospital support teams, inpatient care has always had a central role in the network of palliative care. Some palliative care programs were started in acute care settings, such as the support team in St. Thomas' Hospital in London (1975) or the Palliative Care Unit at the Royal Victoria Hospital in Montreal (1976).[2] In the 1970s and

1980s, most countries developed and implemented palliative care programs. Some provided in-home care, as in the United States or Italy, and others developed more comprehensive models, as in Great Britain, Canada, or Catalonia, Spain. Not until the 1990s were palliative care services integrated into acute care hospitals, and most of them served as support teams or consultation services with a positive effect on the care of patients and families.[1,2]

DEFINITION AND CHARACTERISTICS

Published data about the range of acute palliative care units (APCUs) provide no unifying concept or definition (see Chapter 5). Even so, the canonical principles of palliative care are always present: comprehensive care of physical, emotional, social, and spiritual aspects of patients; interdisciplinary teamwork; and an adaptable organization to fulfill their mission. The main differences from traditional palliative or hospice units in long-term facilities arise from the localization and acuity of the problems treated, which heavily influence the APCU's activity and outcomes.

One model of an APCU is characterized by an inpatient facility staffed by registered nurses with volunteer support, and the medical input is provided by the previous attending physicians in a homelike environment.[3] Others provide a more comprehensive hospital service (Table 39-1), with some combination of an inpatient unit, an outpatient clinic, and a consultation or support team (see Chapter 5). It is staffed by its own physicians and nurses, with various degrees of input from psychosocial and spiritual professionals. Patients admitted to these units have acute and complex physical and emotional problems that need intensive evaluation and high-tech treatment, occasionally with invasive procedures. Architecturally, these units are not necessarily homelike but rather more like traditional, technologically driven, shared hospital rooms.[4] Between both models, a great range of programs may be found, such as the comprehensive models of the M. D. Anderson Cancer Center (Houston, Texas),[5] the Institut Català d'Oncologia (Barcelona, Spain),[6] the Cleveland Clinic (Cleveland, Ohio),[7] and the Hospital General Universitario Gregorio Marañón (Madrid, Spain).[8] These institutions offer full palliative care services (Box 39-1) with an acute inpatient unit, an outpatient clinic, a consultation or hospital support team, and academic links with the local universities.

APCUs can be conceptualized as follows:

- They provide inpatient facilities.
- They usually are located on the premises of an acute care hospital.
- They are dedicated to acute, severe, complex, and unstable physical or psychosocial problems.
- They care for patients with far-advanced and terminal diseases.
- They provide diagnostic precision, close monitoring, and intensive treatment.
- Care is provided by an advanced, highly specialized, multidisciplinary palliative care team.

RATIONALE

APCUs are needed for several reasons. They are essential for advanced and terminal patients who have acute problems. Another reason is the inadequate approach to the management of advanced cancer and noncancer patients with unfulfilled clinical needs in acute care settings, as shown by European,[9] American,[10] and Australian studies.[11] Although physicians recognize the inappropriateness of dealing with the needs of patients with advanced disease and dying patients in acute care hospitals, most cancer patients are first diagnosed, treated, and followed in hospital hematology-oncology services. Patients and families may experience abandonment after referral to other settings. "Palliative care programs should be developed within tertiary hospitals and comprehensive cancer centers to provide the appropriate treatment for control of difficult symptoms occurring during the entire onco-

---

Box 39-1 Main Characteristics of Acute Palliative Medicine Units

- Low mortality rate (≤60-75%)
- Short length of stay (<14 days)
- Maximal symptom complexity
- Research oriented
- Advanced teaching level
- Early referrals
- Supported by ancillary services needed for management of difficult symptoms

---

TABLE 39-1 Outcomes from Acute Palliative Medicine Units

INSTITUTION	LOCATION	STUDY	YEAR UNITS BEGAN	MORTALITY RATE (%)	PATHOLOGY	MEAN AGE (YEARS)	MEAN LENGTH OF STAY (DAYS)
Northwestern Memorial Hospital	Chicago, Illinois	Kellar et al[3]	1986	59	Mixed (45% cancer)	67	6
H. R. Horvitz Center, Cleveland Clinic Foundation	Cleveland, Ohio	Walsh[14]	1991	27	Cancer	62	11.3
Institut Català d'Oncologia	L'Hospitalet-Barcelona, Spain	Gómez-Batiste et al[6]	1995	50	Cancer	66	9.3
Hospital General Universitario Gregorio Marañón	Madrid, Spain	Directorio Sociedad Española de Cuidados Paliativos (SECPAL) 2004	1990	78	Cancer	63	15
M. D. Anderson	Houston, Texas	Bruera12	2002	23	Cancer	57	9.6

logical life . . . regardless of the stage of disease."[4] Others think that APCUs should "provide an appropriate bridge to community hospice programs and home care . . ."[12] and "need to have strong links with home support teams and other units based in community health centers or hospices to create comprehensive district networks."[6] The existence of a consultation or palliative support team in an acute hospital does not exclude an APCU in the same hospital, because they are complementary. Data from a well-known palliative care network indicate that 11% of the patients after a consultation assessment need to be transferred from a tertiary teaching hospital to an APCU.[13]

Although APCUs should be part of a wider palliative network, their perceived need indicates maturity in the network and increasing clinical complexity. Patients in APCUs have acute and complex health problems.[14] The San Diego Severity Index[15] was proposed as an assessment tool to identify the acuity of patients and help transitions among acute care hospitals, home care, and long-term care. Differences between APCUs[16] and hospices have been found; patients are younger, have higher symptom scores, have worse pain prognosis, and are less cognitively impaired in the APCU. Patients with the most complex and symptomatic conditions are admitted to APCUs. They have higher symptom scores, and their medical conditions are more complicated. Expectations of success of the attending team are higher than for those treated by home care teams.[17]

In tertiary hospitals and cancer centers, research is a major activity. Far-advanced cancer patients are enrolled in phase I antitumor trials. Those enrolled in phase I or II trials are incurable and have the same or even more physical and psychosocial difficulties than nonparticipants. Palliative care can help patients recruited for phase I or II trials.[18] Including palliative care in cancer research increases the opportunities for the recruited patients to obtain better symptom control and overall emotional support while performing the trial, and a palliative care team ensures better continuity of care.

Developing palliative medicine services, including APCUs, in the settings where most cancer patients are diagnosed, treated, followed, and researched is a rational approach. In Alberta, Canada, acute care consultation was the activity with the greatest increase, whereas APCU activity remained steady because the number of beds available was static.[19] The increase of consultation and care in acute units, including APCUs, can help palliative medicine

move into the early stages of cancer treatment, which fits the World Health Organization's vision on palliative care (Fig. 39-1).

Locating APCUs in teaching hospitals and cancer centers will be most valuable in spreading palliative knowledge and skills into other specialties, with benefit provided for the health care system and society. Courses and books on symptom palliation, communication, ethics, and other aspects of palliative medicine are widely available. Few APCUs teach by modeling. Residents of different specialties should learn side by side with experienced physicians to manage difficult symptoms, upgrade communication skills, or learn genuine team working and organization. The same teaching value is applicable for other professionals, such as nurses, social workers, psychologists, and physiotherapists.

Further support for APCUs may come from directives of health authorities when palliative care networks achieve the sophistication that sustains widespread acceptance of the philosophy of comprehensive care. A common language is key for concept expansion and an essential preliminary step toward recognition by health administrators. For example, the concept of APCUs is far advanced in Spain and reflected in numerous policy papers by national and regional health authorities. Palliative care did not start in Spain as a grassroots movement; it was instead promulgated within the existing health system. After the Spanish authorities embraced the concept of APCUs, it became easier to implement new units in the European public system. Similar efforts at conceptualization may not be as immediately effective as in Spain in other health environments, such as the United States.

ISSUES BEYOND THE SCOPE OF ACUTE PALLIATIVE MEDICINE UNITS

Intervention of an experienced and specific palliative medicine team is indicated when problems are beyond the palliation expertise of the primary team (see "Common Errors"). The palliative medicine or palliative care team may be needed at any disease stage and wherever the patient is, such as at home, in a long-term care facility, or in the hospital.

APCUs have achieved their position within the wider palliative medicine network. If the APCU is the only palliative resource in a particular health sector, functional failure can occur. Wherever a comprehensive network for palliative medicine develops, especially in metropolitan

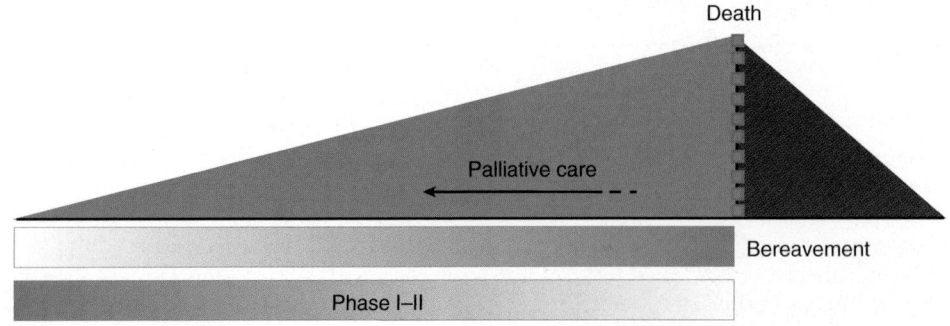

FIGURE 39-1   Direction of palliative care in acute settings. This type of care can help patients recruited for phase I or II trials, which fits the World Health Organization's paradigm for palliative care.

Common Errors
• Insufficient planning and staff training
• Isolation from palliative and other health resources
• Poor staffing and physician input
• Scattered beds
• Low psychosocial and paramedical input
• Architecturally inappropriate settings
• Competition with other hospital services and departments
• No research or teaching

CASE STUDY

Prostate Cancer

A 51-year-old man with prostate cancer and many bone, retroperitoneal, and pulmonary metastases was admitted to the oncology ward with pelvic pain and a decline in his general condition. After oncologic assessment, he was advised that there was no effective treatment for his tumor. He reported inadequate pain control despite opioid rotation. Magnetic resonance imaging of his spine excluded epidural cord compression. He was admitted to the acute palliative care unit (APCU) for symptom management.

At the initial assessment in the APCU, he had nociceptive somatic pain (numerical rating scale [NRS] basal score of 4/10, crisis score of 8/10 × 4 per day, and average score of 6/10) caused by bone metastases and pelvic soft tissue infiltration and classified as bad prognosis pain. The patient was bedridden at admission. He had a low palliative performance status score (PPS = 40), was moderately dependent (Barthel index = 45), and had an intermediate prognosis (palliative prognostic [PaP] score = 6.5). Other distressing symptoms were anorexia (6/10), insomnia (7/10), constipation (8/10), and dry cough (4/10). Emotional distress was evident, as were persistent irritability, cognitive decline, and fear (anxiety score of 9/10). He identified his emotional distress as related to the recent loss of his autonomy and his sense of abandonment by his oldest son.

Intensive psychosocial intervention with the family was started to address the feelings of the eldest son related to his father's suffering and predicted death. Concurrently, intravenous opioid titration and pharmacological management for the patient's physical and emotional symptoms and support from a physiotherapist allowed him to obtain adequate pain relief and a reduction in his emotional distress. After 10 days in the APCU, the patient was discharged to his home with a greater sense of autonomy and improved performance status. A home follow-up visit was arranged by the home palliative support team.

tertiary hospitals, there is a tendency to establish different levels of palliative medicine specialist resources in different settings of the health system. Comprehensive acute palliative services (e.g., unit, outpatient, support teams) can intervene earlier and in acute, complex situations, and they act as reference services for other hospital services and other community palliative care services. In those circumstances, the roles and the outputs of APCUs are clearly defined.

APCUs deal with acute and severe problems, and inside those units, a specialist team is expected to deal with physical and psychosocial crises. These units should have their own staff, including physicians. Dedicated staff members also affect the unit's teaching and research roles. Low medical input is a therapeutic disadvantage and provides an opportunity for criticism. An APCU should be a unit where treatments and care can be delivered in a congruent therapeutic atmosphere. Scattered acute palliative medicine beds prevent this. Conflicting therapeutic goals in a mixed pathology and acute care ward engender divergent actions by team members, challenging the therapeutic results.

The clinical equipment and routines should match the intense and complex clinical needs of APCU patients. Because these patients usually are transferred from other acute care units or wards, they may perceive a dramatic break in clinical routines, which can be emotionally damaging and clinically inopportune. It is advisable to create a gentle therapeutic atmosphere while avoiding the pitfall of a nonclinical or low-level clinical setting. A homelike atmosphere may be interpreted as a death ward, which can be fatal for the whole palliative medicine program.

The APCU is a well-defined resource designed to handle patients with far-advanced disease and their families. It should not be confused with or run as a low-level oncological or internal medicine ward. Competition for patients and resources with other specialties should be avoided, promoting a mood of honest and open cooperation with the rest of the hospital or center services.

CONCLUSIONS

Despite early initiatives, APCUs are a recent addition to the palliative care repertoire. Most information about palliative medicine in the acute care hospital setting comes from research on support or consultation teams. APCU studies usually are based on low levels of evidence, are descriptive, and rely on the opinions of reputed professionals and highly experienced teams. APCUs are the result of a rational and reasonable implementation of resources to fit the needs of patients with complex, far-advanced cancer and their families in a setting where the patients are diagnosed and treated, allowing early referral into a wider palliative care program. APCUs are exceptional places for learning, teaching, and research. In any comprehensive palliative care program, it is useful to have an APCU in each sector to offer specialized care for the more complex cases that cannot be treated at home or in long-term facilities and for patients who benefit from high-tech and palliative care incorporating holistic attitudes and values (see "Case Study: Prostate Cancer").

It is unclear whether it is better to start a palliative care program from an APCU in a teaching hospital and disseminate knowledge to other hospitals, long-term facilities, and home care or begin the opposite way. Our experience supports both approaches. One way to start is establishing support teams at home and in hospitals and using beds in long-term facilities, because the first referrals are dying patients, who usually are elderly and do not have complex symptoms. As the team's reputation increases, early acute-setting referrals begin, and setting up an APCU seems to be the next logical step. This stepwise approach can avoid the known difficulties and tensions between palliative medicine and the other specialties. The opposite approach is also reasonable, and it has been successful if the caregiving team keeps in mind the advantages of networking and the dangers of isolation.

Although there is strong evidence about the effectiveness and efficiency of home care and support teams in acute care settings, this information is lacking for APCUs, which provides a great opportunity for research. Experience more than evidence supports the recommendation to set up APCUs in tertiary hospitals and cancer centers, but many questions remain unanswered, such as how many acute palliative medicine beds are needed per million inhabitants and what determines the appropriate size, staffing, and outputs of APCUs. Efficiency, efficacy, and satisfaction should be investigated to sustain implementation, and early information from this research should be made available.[20]

REFERENCES

1. Virik K, Glare P. Profile and evaluation of palliative medicine consultation service within a tertiary teaching hospital in Sydney, Australia. J Pain Symptom Manage 2002;23:17-25.
2. Ryan A, Carter J, Lucas J, et al. You need not make the journey alone: Overcoming impediments to providing palliative care in a public urban teaching hospital. Am J Hosp Palliat Care 2002;19:171-180.
3. Kellar N, Martinez J, Finis N, et al. Characterization of an acute inpatient hospice palliative care unit in U.S. teaching hospital. J Nurs Adm 1996;26:16-20.
4. Mercadante S, Villari P, Ferrera P. A model of acute symptom control unit: Pain relief and palliative care unit of La Maddalena Cancer Center. Support Care Cancer 2003;11:114-119.
5. Elsayem A, Swint K, Fisch MJ, et al. Palliative care inpatient service in a comprehensive cancer center: Clinical and financial outcomes. J Clin Oncol 2004;22:2008-2014.
6. Gómez-Batiste X, Porta J, Tuca A. Palliative care at the Institut Català d'Oncologia, Barcelona. Eur J Palliat Care 2003;10:202-205.
7. Zhukovsky DS. A model of palliative care: The palliative medicine program of the Cleveland Clinic Foundation: A World Health Organization Demonstration Project. Support Care Cancer 2000;8:268-77.
8. Morch MM, Neuenschwander H, Bruera E, et al. From roots to flowers: Challenges of developing a sustainable palliative care program. J Palliat Care 2003;19:58-62.
9. Toscani F, Di Giulio P, Brunelli C, et al. How people die in hospital general wards: A descriptive study. J Pain Symptom Manage 2005;30:33-40.
10. Fins JJ, Miller FG, Acres CA, et al. End-of-life decision making in the hospital: Current practice and future prospects. J Pain Symptom Manage 1999;17:6-15.
11. Middlewood S, Gardner G, Gardner A. Dying in hospital: Medical failure or natural outcome. J Pain Symptom Manage 2001;22:1035-1041.
12. Bruera E, Sweeney C. The development of palliative care at the University of Texas M.D. Anderson Cancer Center. Support Care Cancer 2001;9:330-334.
13. Jenkins CA, Schulz M, Hanson J, et al. Demographic, symptom, and medication profiles of cancer patients seen by a palliative care consult team in a tertiary referral hospital. J Pain Symptom Manage 2000;19:174-184.
14. Walsh D. The business of palliative medicine. Part 4. Potential impact of acute-care palliative medicine inpatient unit in tertiary care cancer center. Am J Hosp Palliat Care 2004;21:217-221.
15. Staruse L, Herbst L, Ryndes T, et al. A severity index designed as an indicator of acuity in palliative care. J Palliat Care 1993;9:11-15.
16. Bruera E, Neumann C, Brenneis C, et al. Frequency of symptom distress and poor prognostic indicators in palliative cancer patients admitted to a tertiary palliative care unit, hospice, and acute care hospitals. J Palliat Care 2000;16:16-21.
17. Núñez Olarte JM, Santos Miranda JA, Cuesta Alvaro P. Estudio transversal europeo de cuidados paliativos de la EAPC: Analisis estadistico de variables. Med Pal (Madrid) 2006;13(Suppl 1):1-5.
18. Meyers FJ, Linder J, Beckett L, et al. Simultaneous care: A model approach to the perceived conflict between investigational therapy and palliative care. J Pain Symptom Manage 2004;28:548-556.
19. Fassbender K, Fainsinger R, Brenneis C, et al. Utilization and costs of the introduction of system-wide palliative care in Alberta, 1993-2000. Palliat Med 2005;19:513-520.
20. Davis MP, Walsh D, LeGrand SB, et al. The financial benefits of acute inpatient palliative medicine: An inter-institutional comparative analysis by all patient refined-diagnosis related group and case mix index. J Support Oncol 2005;3:313-316.

SUGGESTED READING

Bosanquet N, Salisbury C (eds). Providing a Palliative Care Service: Towards an Evidence Base. Oxford, UK: Oxford University Press, 1999.
Gómez-Batiste X, Porta J, Tuca A, Stjernswärd J (eds). Organización de Servicios y Programas de Cuidados Paliativos [Palliative Care Services and Programs Organization]. Madrid: Arán, 2005.

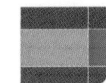

CHAPTER **40**

Inpatient Hospice and Palliative Care Units

Denise Wells Spencer

KEY POINTS

- The many administrative considerations involved in developing an inpatient unit are critical to the effectiveness of the unit.
- In addition to delivering the highest-quality patient care possible, hospitals often have a financial incentive to be closely affiliated with an inpatient hospice unit.
- Clinical aspects of the unit, such as criteria for admission, should be determined before opening the unit.
- The environment within the unit—the colors, furnishings, amenities, and restrictions—is a comfort or hindrance to the clinical, emotional, and spiritual processes of the patient and family.

The development of a financially sound, efficiently run inpatient hospice or palliative care unit is a formidable task. The operational and administrative infrastructure is the foundation on which the clinical program rests. The physical and caregiving environments created within such an inpatient unit set the emotional tone for patients and their families. There is no single clinical model that is best; each hospice unit must be tailored to the needs of the patient population to be served while coexisting with staffing, logistic, and budgetary constraints. This chapter provides an overview of major aspects to consider when planning the development of an inpatient hospice unit.

STARTING A SPECIALIZED UNIT

The first step in the development of a specialized unit is deciding which model works better for the target patient population, given available staffing and budget constraints coupled with the needs and desires of the hospital administration. There are two basic models to serve hospice patients and palliative care patients who are not yet enrolled in hospice: a dedicated inpatient palliative care unit or an inpatient hospice unit.

Typically, palliative care units do not serve hospice patients. Palliative care beds are licensed and approved for acute hospital care, and hospitals are reimbursed for palliative care patients as they are for any other hospitalized patient. Those reimbursements depend on standard Medicare and Medicaid regulations, private insurance, and managed care contracts. Palliative care patients typically have complex medical profiles. They need more and costlier care than the usual hospice patient. Studies demonstrate that having these patients in a dedicated unit or being cared for by a full palliative care team when no dedicated unit is available results in shorter length of stays, better clinical outcomes, and higher patient and family satisfaction. Chapter 41 provides a more detailed discussion of inpatient palliative care units.

Hospitals caring for hospice patients without the benefit of formal hospice oversight that a dedicated hospice unit provides are at risk for financial loss, poor clinical outcomes, and patient and family dissatisfaction. The contracted hospital receives payment for patient care at the standard hospice per diem rate, which is generally at a lower reimbursement rate than for the nonhospice patient. Payment provides for diagnostic procedures, therapeutic treatments, and room and board at the usual rate. If the hospice patient is cared for in a nonhospice fashion by nonhospice clinicians, the per diem payment may not cover the patient's cost to the hospital, nor do the patient and family typically receive the specialized care that is standard for a hospice unit. The nonhospice focus of care may be one of altering disease process rather than holistic care for the patient and family. However, if the patient is admitted to a dedicated hospice unit, the hospice organization receives the daily per diem payment, and the hospice team becomes directly responsible for the cost of providing care. With a hospice plan of care and a dedicated hospice team in place, providing excellent care can be accomplished in a relatively budget-neutral fashion. The hospital has a clear interest in developing a close working relationship with its local hospice in developing such a unit.

A strong home-based hospice team providing oversight for the care of a hospitalized hospice patient may achieve the same benefits described for hospice patients admitted to hospice units; however, patient care outcomes and costs are directly related to the oversight the team is allowed to provide and to the willingness of the treating nonhospice physicians to accept hospice suggestions. Box 40-1 lists the administrative and clinical advantages of having a dedicated inpatient hospice unit.

The disadvantages of an inpatient hospice unit are few. The public may see the separate unit as marginalizing the terminally ill or perceive it to be a place where people no longer receive care. In some hospitals, the inpatient hospice unit may become known as the "death ward," with those who work there closely associated with death. This stigma may be especially true of a free-standing hospice. However, these misconceptions quickly dissipate with community education, which is achieved largely through the services provided at the center itself. Table 40-1 compares the freestanding hospice model and the model of a hospice within a hospital.

Box 40-1 Advantages of an Inpatient Hospice Unit

For the Hospital

- The hospital contracts with the local hospice to lease the space for the inpatient unit.
- The local hospice uses the hospital's ancillary, diagnostic, pharmaceutical, and environmental services at a negotiated rate.
- The hospital is not responsible for the Joint Commission for the Accreditation of Healthcare Organizations' (JCAHO) approval of the hospice unit because the unit is a "hospital within a hospital," operating under a license obtained by the hospice.
- The hospital has ready access to hospice beds for easy transfer of hospice-appropriate patients. Transferring patients to an inpatient hospice unit results in the following:

  Increased throughput by opening acute care beds to patients with a new diagnosis-related group

  Decreased average length of stay because transfer to an inpatient hospice unit is essentially a discharge from one hospital and admission to another

  Decreased average cost per day because hospitals are often not getting reimbursed for services rendered to hospice patients

  Decreased number of inpatient deaths (many patients who die in the inpatient hospice unit would have died in the main hospital)

- The inpatient hospice unit is a powerful marketing tool that accentuates the range of services provided within the hospital.
- The presence of a palliative medicine consultation service within the hospital further streamlines efficiency by facilitating the transfer of appropriate patients sooner.
- The presence of palliative medicine or hospice care directly affects a hospital's rating as a comprehensive cancer center, top 100 heart hospital, or other such medical center.

For the Hospice

- All ancillary, diagnostic, pharmaceutical, environmental, and full consultative services are readily available.
- The hospice has control of hiring staff and determining staffing ratios.
- Staff members who are specially trained in clinical and interpersonal or communication aspects can be concentrated in one unit and focus on one patient population.
- A dedicated interdisciplinary team (e.g., physician, nurses, social worker, chaplain, and volunteer) can be assembled.
- Having patients in one location is convenient.

For Patients and Families

- The environment is tailored to the special and specific needs of patients and their families.
- Continuity of care is accentuated by consistent staffing of nurses and the interdisciplinary team.

ADMINISTRATIVE CONSIDERATIONS

After the space is allotted and contracts are signed, there are staffing and administrative questions to address, including efficient use of the space and a budget appropriate to the needs of the unit. Box 40-2 provides a list of considerations before starting an inpatient hospice unit.

A major decision facing the hospice-unit administrators is the number of beds to make available for specialized hospice care. At start up, it would be ideal for a new hospice unit to have the entire component of beds avail-

TABLE 40-1   Advantages and Disadvantages of Freestanding Hospice and a Hospice within a Hospital

HOSPICE WITHIN A HOSPITAL	FREESTANDING HOSPICE
Direct access to ancillary, diagnostic, pharmaceutical, and consultative services	Limited access to hospital services or must provide on-site services
Access is greater for that hospital	Access is equal for all hospitals in the referral area
Somewhat institutionalized atmosphere remaining after renovation of the unit	Specially designed structure for the unique needs of hospice patients and their families
Creates visibility for the sponsoring hospital	Creates visibility for the sponsoring hospice organization
Perception of patient marginalization within the hospital	Perception of patient marginalization within the entire community
Often how an inpatient unit is started	Transitions to a freestanding hospice after firm establishment within a hospital

---

Box 40-2 Administrative Considerations of Creating an Inpatient Hospice Unit

- Number of beds
- Physician and nurse practitioner full-time equivalents
- Staff of registered nurses versus staff of registered nurses plus licensed practical nurses (will a certified hospice and palliative nurse be required?)
- Clinical director of the unit (registered nurse or physician)
- Administrative director of the unit (registered nurse or physician)
- Charge nurse
- Nurse-to-patient ratio
- Nursing assistant–to-patient ratio
- Unit clerk full-time equivalent
- Social work full-time equivalent
- Chaplain full-time equivalent
- Use of volunteers
- Use of students
- Physician access to the unit
- On-call coverage

Box 40-3 Staffing a 20-Bed Inpatient Hospice Unit

- Physicians: 1.5 full-time equivalents
- Nurse practitioner (Monday to Friday): 1.0 full-time equivalent
- Registered nurses and licensed practical nurses: 16.0 full-time equivalents
- Certified nursing assistants: 10.0 full-time equivalents
- Registered nurse administrative director (Monday to Friday): 1.0 full-time equivalent
- Unit clerks: 2.8 full-time equivalents
- Social workers: 2.0 full-time equivalents
- Chaplain: 1.0 full-time equivalent

TABLE 40-2   Pros and Cons of Exclusive and All-Inclusive Physician Access

EXCLUSIVE TO HOSPICE ACCESS	ALL-INCLUSIVE ACCESS
May marginalize the unit	Creates image of openness
Hospice physicians good stewards of the per diem	No way to ensure that laboratory tests, medications, and radiographic studies ordered are in the hospice plan of care
Consistent hospice philosophy practiced and taught	May send mixed message about hospice philosophy by multiple nonhospice physicians practicing end-of-life palliative medicine

---

able that satisfies its ultimate goal. However, only a portion of those beds may be activated for patient care. If it is anticipated that a unit eventually will run at a capacity of 12 beds, plans may allow for the initial use of four of the 12 until staffing and use is better determined. This pilot approach allows the unit to work out systemic problems that surely exist but cannot be known before opening the full-scale unit. Opening a unit without a pilot period can cause frustration for staff and provide less that optimal patient care.

After the number of beds has been determined, staffing equivalents and ratios must be addressed. This decision is based largely on the staff needed to deliver quality patient care while remaining within budgetary guidelines, which governs every aspect of planning and executing a dedicated unit. Box 40-3 shows an approximation of full-time equivalents (FTEs) needed for a 20-bed inpatient hospice unit. The seriousness of the nursing shortage in the area and the pool of nurses who have a particular interest in hospice care affect hiring practices for the unit, such as hiring registered nurses rather than a mix of registered nurses and licensed practical nurses for primary patient care.

Physicians' access is key to establishing a successful hospice unit. It is assumed that any hospice organization opening an inpatient hospice unit has a trained physician available to care for patients in that unit. However, non-hospice physicians in the hospital or community may request to follow their patients in the unit, a situation that holds advantages and disadvantages. Unit administrators may wish initially to limit access to outside physicians during the pilot stage of the unit to avoid confusion for staff, patients, and families and to support administrative and clinical trouble-shooting within the unit. This controlled phase also allows time for cultural changes to occur within the institution regarding hospice education and changes in attitudes about hospice care. After the pilot phase of the unit is complete, access may be granted to all physicians, because after the culture of the institution has been established, nonhospice physicians will better understand how the unit functions and will likely adapt to the unit rather than the unit having to educate many nonhospice physicians. Over time, most nonhospice physicians ask the hospice physician to assume care of their patients (Table 40-2).

CLINICAL CONSIDERATIONS

The first clinical consideration is to determine the criteria for admission to the hospice unit. Having admission criteria in place greatly assists the nursing staff and referring physicians in understanding what the unit has to offer patients and their families. The patient must be a hospice patient. Beyond that, there are normally four basic criteria for admission to an inpatient hospice unit (Table 40-3). These criteria are general guidelines for practice, because each admission is judged on an individual basis. A general rule is to admit patients who are likely to have their needs met within 7 to 14 days. Although some patients have needs that cannot be met within this target period, having this guideline in place allows for enough time to serve the patient and family fully while creating an environment where the average length of stay maximizes access to all patients at any time.

Advocates for *open access* seek to influence admission criteria and treatment plans, and some encourage relatively aggressive diagnostic, surgical, pharmaceutical, and radiological services. The question about limiting access arises in all hospice units. Access to laboratory testing and diagnostic services and to therapies such as chemotherapy and blood transfusions is increasingly being requested. The level of access a hospice can offer depends on the number of patients served and the specific plan of care within that hospice's philosophy. It is highly desirable for the hospice to have protocols in place that define levels of clinical access offered to patients before establishing an inpatient hospice unit to reduce confusion about care issues among the hospice staff, referring physicians, patients, and families.

ENVIRONMENTAL CONSIDERATIONS

The ambience within a hospice unit is of the utmost importance. The décor, creative use of space, lighting, and furnishings are significant considerations in reflecting immediately the environment of an inpatient hospice unit. Providing all the services and safety features needed to care properly for the patient within a deinstitutionalized, homey atmosphere can put the patient and family at ease. Seeking personal items for the room, such as photographs, quilts, and favorite music, can add to the comfortable surroundings and encourage the hospice staff to recognize and to celebrate the unique life lived by the person for whom they are caring at the end of life. Minimal restrictions on the patient and family during their stay humanize and soften the experience of being in a hospice unit. Box 40-4 lists ideas and amenities that make the inpatient hospice unit more inviting.

The ideal inpatient hospice unit would take exceptional care of its patients and provide for professional care of the staff. Providing care to the terminally ill and dying is a highly rewarding endeavor. However, staff members can become emotionally and physically drained by the very act of caring. If this psychic and physical loss is not replenished, staff burnout will occur. Staff should have a retreat, an area beyond a standard break room that offers a serene atmosphere. Such a space should offer music with headphones, comfortable furniture, a pleasant view, or a treadmill. Creative group exercises during interdisciplinary team meetings can promote collegiality and relieve stress. Box 40-5 provides ideas for group exercise.

TABLE 40-3   Criteria for Admission to an Inpatient Hospice Unit

REASON FOR ADMISSION	DEFINITION
Terminal care	Care of the dying patient who cannot be cared for at home and his or her family
Symptom management	Management of symptoms that cannot be managed in setting where the patient resides (e.g., home, hospital, nursing home); the patient is expected to go home, but admission may be for terminal care
Transition from hospital to home	Care of the hospitalized patient who is new to hospice and is expected to go home; allows for time to optimally manage symptoms (symptom needs are requisite) and evaluate the patient's psychosocial and spiritual needs and plan accordingly
Respite	Admission to give the patient's caregivers time off from their caregiving duties; assumes no active symptom issues; reimbursed at a home per diem rate; usually limited to 5 days

---

Box 40-4 Creating a Homelike Setting in an Inpatient Hospice Unit

- Visiting hours: 24 hours/day, 7 days/week
- Allowing pets to visit
- Providing access to television, video cassette recording (VCR), and a digital video disc (DVD) player
- Providing access to a compact disc (CD) player
- Kitchen available for visitor use
- Family room available for visitor use
- Shower and restroom available for visitor use
- Fold-out chair or sofa in patients' rooms for family to sleep on at night
- Color, lighting, furnishings, and wall décor to create homelike atmosphere
- Large, private rooms
- Conference room for family conferences
- Access to a quiet garden or sun patio
- Access to an approved smoking area for patients who continue to smoke

---

Box 40-5 Group Exercises to Promote Professional Self-Care and Collegiality

- Read an encouraging passage that relates to this type of work or self-care.
- Open the discussion to problems or questions that individual staff members have had regarding patient care, ethical dilemmas, or other topics. Discussion in a forum is often therapeutic.
- Have each person tell what he or she does to "recharge," thereby giving ideas to others.
- Do positive visualization exercises.
- Have people disclose interesting facts about themselves that would not otherwise come up in conversation. This often generates laughter and a greater sense of camaraderie.

Box 40-6 Research Challenges and Opportunities

• Inpatient hospice units are a significant resource for conducting clinical research.
• A survey reports that terminally ill patients and their families would like to participate in clinical investigations to maintain autonomy, to find a sense of value, and for altruistic reasons.
• Pooled patient populations in multicenter studies can add strength to the evidence revealed by such studies.
• A national database is needed for available patient populations, current and upcoming research studies, and active researchers and their particular interests. It could link investigators, research projects, and subjects, resulting in the strongest evidence-based results, rapid growth of the palliative medicine literature, and improved patient care.

Hospice inpatient units are ideal settings for research on end-of-life topics. However, conducting research on terminally ill patients and grieving families is complex and fraught with logistical and ethical problems. Nonetheless, with the rapidly growing hospice and palliative care movement and the development of dedicated inpatient hospice and palliative care units, there are opportunities for doing groundbreaking research. Box 40-6 briefly enumerates the challenges and opportunities.

SUGGESTED READING

Carey DA. Prerequisites for planning the inpatient hospice unit. J Palliat Care 1989;5:47-49.
Fischberg D, Meier D. Palliative care in hospitals. Clin Geriatr Med 2004;20:735-751.
Herbst L. Hospice care at the end of life. Clin Geriatr Med 2004;20:753-765.
Kilburn L. Hospice for the next century. In Hospice Operations Manual. National Hospice and Palliative Care Organization. Dubuque, Iowa: Kendall/Hunt Publishing, 1997.
Medland J, Howard-Ruben J, Whitaker E. Fostering psychosocial wellness in oncology nurses: Addressing burnout and social support in the workplace. Oncol Nurs Forum 2004;31: 47-54.
Terry W, Olsen LG, Ravenscroft P, et al. Hospice patients' view on research in palliative care. Intern Med J 2006;36: 406-413.

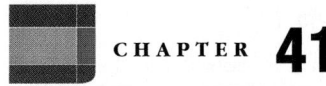

CHAPTER **41**

Palliative Medicine in Institutions

Stephen R. Connor

KEY POINTS

• Palliative care has limited availability outside of acute care settings.
• Hospice care is being delivered more commonly in nursing and residential care facilities.
• Lack of specialized reimbursement for interdisciplinary palliative care before hospice has limited availability in other institutions.
• Increased and ongoing palliative care education and training are needed to facilitate the provision of palliative care in all institutional settings where care is needed.
• Although some institutions have embraced palliative care, resistance to palliative and hospice care remains a barrier to patients and families receiving competent palliative care in institutions.
• The field of palliative medicine is still emerging and has had limited impact in health care institutions outside of the acute care setting.

PALLIATIVE CARE IN NURSING FACILITIES

Nursing facilities have become a major part of the U.S. health care system. Approximately 25% of all U.S. deaths occur in these facilities, and the number is growing.[1] The median survival of those admitted to nursing facilities is estimated to be 18 months.[2] An argument can be made that virtually all patients admitted for chronic care to nursing facilities could likely benefit from palliative care.

In the United States, hospice care is the most reliable way to deliver palliative care to nursing facility residents; however, they must meet Medicare hospice criteria to receive such services. Criteria include a physician-estimated prognosis of 6 months or less (if the disease runs its normal course) and the patient's consent for receipt of palliative rather than curative care. Legal surrogates can consent for the patient to receive hospice care.

Estimates of hospice use provided by the National Hospice and Palliative Care Organization projected that as many as 185,000 nursing home residents died under hospice care in 2005. This represented about 30% of all nursing home deaths. Several studies of hospice care in nursing facilities have found positive outcomes for nursing home residents[3]:

• Hospice patients had superior pain assessments, and hospice patients in daily pain are twice as likely to receive strong pain relievers as are nonhospice residents in daily pain.
• There is a 93% increased likelihood that patients in daily pain will have some attempt made at managing their pain.

- Lower proportions of hospice patients compared with nonhospice patients had invasive procedures, such as physical restraints, intravenous feeding, or feeding tubes.
- There is less likelihood of return of hospice patients to acute care facilities.

The more hospice use a nursing facility had, the more likely these outcomes, especially death at the nursing facility rather than in an acute care hospital, would occur.[4] Further studies demonstrated improved outcomes for hospice nursing home collaboration, including improved management of pain,[5,6] increased likelihood of having an advanced directive,[7] and reduced cost for Medicare.[8]

Although collaboration between nursing homes and hospices appears to be good for both, many patients who could benefit still do not receive palliative care. Increased use of hospice for nursing home patients is desirable; however, a general increase in the capacity of nursing home staff to deliver general palliative care, especially for those who do not qualify for hospice, is also needed. Achieving improved competence in nursing facilities to deliver palliative care is challenging. The American Health Care Association (AHCA) reports annual turnover rates of 50% for all nurses and 71% for certified nursing assistants.[9] The proportion of U.S. nursing facility deaths is expected to increase significantly in the next 30 years.

There is a need to instill palliative care principles and practices in all nursing facilities and provide continuous training of the facility staff.[10] One approach is to expand hospice nursing home relationships to add ongoing training and consultation services. In this model, hospices would provide traditional hospice services and be a vendor to provide ongoing training and clinical consultations to help the facility staff develop prehospice palliative care. Palliative care capacity and competence vary considerably among hospices and nursing facilities in the United States; many nursing facilities already provide excellent general palliative care services to residents.

In the future, it would be desirable to see a health care system that facilitates patients living in the setting of their choice as death approaches. Not all people have familial or financial resources to live independently until their death. There will continue to be a need for facilities to provide long-term care for chronic and life-threatening illnesses or conditions. The current long-term care environment is not conducive to person-centered care.

PALLIATIVE MEDICINE CONSULTATION AND OUTPATIENT CLINIC SERVICE

Expansion of palliative medicine and palliative care usually begins with a consultation service. A physician or nursing professional with training and expertise in palliative medicine often initiates a service, usually in an acute care setting. Chapter 40 provides more details on hospital-based palliative care services. These services can be expanded to include home-based palliative care (see Chapter 42) and, in more highly developed services, include a mobile palliative care consultation service that can be provided in other settings, including nursing facilities, assisted living facilities, personal residences, and when patients have sufficient mobility, in outpatient clinic settings.

Outpatient palliative care clinics are rare. One was initiated by Hospice and Palliative Care of the Bluegrass (HPCB) in Lexington, Kentucky. The HPCB Center opened in 1999. It is a multiphysician office practice with an interdisciplinary team. It is closely linked with consultation teams that see patients in acute care settings and with the community-wide hospice and palliative care program. It is the hub of the palliative program. Hospitals in this community have palliative care teams staffed from two sources. The HPCB Center supplies the physician and nurse practitioner, and the hospital provides other staff members, including registered nurses, social workers, and chaplains. All of these hospitals refer patients to the clinic for follow-up after hospitalization. Patients are seen Monday through Friday in the clinic. Each staff physician practices 1 day in the clinic. The HPCB Center gets about one third of its referrals from area physicians for patients not seen in the hospital. The clinic also sees a small number of usually ambulatory hospice patients being evaluated for continued appropriateness of pain control, and patients from surrounding hospices are seen in the clinic.

The clinic acts as a home base for palliative care. The director of the HPCB palliative care program's office is there. Palliative nurse case managers are based in the clinic, as is a part-time social worker. The clinic does not yet cover its costs. Five to 12 patients are seen daily, and visits are complex and lengthy. Billing by physicians, nurse practitioners, and licensed clinical social workers does not cover the clinic's operating, administrative, and general costs.

The clinic has been invaluable in giving HPCB an identity in the medical community and providing an identity separate from hospice. Many patients are seen to help identify their goals of care, and many have just learned that they will probably not be cured. They are followed on an ongoing basis, and many eventually are referred to hospice.

The HPCB Center is one of the Center to Advance Palliative Care's six palliative care leadership centers. People from all over the United States go there to receive training and technical assistance in the development of palliative care services. Participants who are accepted pay a fee to receive a year-long, comprehensive curriculum that focuses on the operational aspects of starting and building palliative care programs. The curriculum includes needs assessment, financing, staffing models, community partnerships, palliative care education, marketing, and implementation strategies.

RESIDENTIAL CARE

Residential care facilities include assisted living, group homes, board and care, congregate living health facilities, and life care communities. A growing number of hospice-run residential facilities provide care for hospice patients who cannot live independently. Other than hospice-run facilities and hospice care delivered to those living in residential care, there are no organized palliative care services provided by residential care facilities.

In the 1980s and 1990s, a significant number of residential care facilities specialized in people living with acquired immunodeficiency syndrome (AIDS). These AIDS hospices provided various degrees of palliative care to residents dying of AIDS. The need has dropped significantly, and there are now only a few in the United States (i.e., Maitri and Zen Hospice in San Francisco and Broadway House in New Jersey).

It is likely that there will continue to be significant growth in the residential care industry, in part as an alternative to nursing facility care. The original model for residential care did not allow patients to remain there when they became nonambulatory. The congregate living health facility model, developed primarily for AIDS patients, allows dying patients to remain in place until death.

More than 200 hospice freestanding facilities provide residential care beds. Many are mixed-use facilities that provide general hospice inpatient care and residential care. There is a growing need for this kind of care, although the availability is uneven and usually requires subsidization. The first were developed in more affluent areas, where funds could be raised for capital costs. Many of the patients who reach the point of needing supervised care have limited income and cannot afford the full cost.

As in nursing facilities, there is a growing need for greater palliative care competency in residential care. Residential care facility staff members need to have a basic knowledge of palliative care principles and practices. One of the few resources for the development of palliative care in residential care is the book *Developing Hospice Residences* (http://iweb.nhpco.org/iweb/Purchase/Product-Detail.aspx?Product_code=820284).

PROGRAMS FOR ALL-INCLUSIVE CARE OF THE ELDERLY

Programs for All-inclusive Care of the Elderly (PACE) are now covered under Medicare. PACE is a capitated benefit that features a comprehensive service delivery system and integrated Medicare and Medicaid financing. The program is modeled on the system of acute and long-term care services developed by On Lok Senior Health Services in San Francisco, California. This was tested through the Centers for Medicare and Medicaid Services (CMS) (then called the Health Care Financing Administration [HCFA]) demonstration projects in the mid-1980s. For most participants, the comprehensive service package enables them to continue living at home while receiving services rather than be institutionalized. Capitated financing allows providers to deliver all services participants need, rather than be limited to those reimbursable under the Medicare and Medicaid fee-for-service systems.

An interdisciplinary team of professional and paraprofessional staff assesses PACE participant needs, develops care plans, and delivers integrated services for seamless provision of total care. PACE programs provide social and medical services primarily in an adult day health center, supplemented by in-home and referral services in accordance with the participant's needs. The PACE service package must include all services covered by Medicare and Medicaid and other services determined necessary by the interdisciplinary team for the PACE participant.

Palliative care is considered part of the PACE program, but the model has had a difficult time spreading. To become an approved PACE provider, a complex set of requirements must be met, and applicants must meet large capital requirements. Some hospices have added PACE services. In some respects, PACE is a natural extension of hospice to provide a comprehensive seamless continuum of care (http://www.cms.hhs.gov/PACE/Downloads/PACEFactSheet.pdf).

OTHER SETTINGS FOR PALLIATIVE CARE

Palliative medicine and palliative care are needed in other specialized settings, including prisons and facilities that care for the developmentally disabled. Several models have been developed to deliver hospice and palliative care in a correctional setting.[11] Tougher sentencing laws have increased the prison population. In the middle of 2000, state, federal, and private correctional facilities held 1,305,253 inmates, a 28% increase from the number held in 1995.[12] Between July 1, 1999, and June 30, 2000, 3175 inmates died in prison, with illness or natural cause accounting for 85% of deaths in federal prisons, 75% of deaths in state prisons, and 66% of deaths in private facilities. AIDS was the second most common cause of death, accounting for 7% in federal, 10% in state, and 13% in private facilities.

Although prisoners are entitled to health care commensurate with community standards, most inmates dying in prison do not have access to palliative care that meets these standards. Efforts have been made to improve hospice and palliative care for inmates.[13,14] However, several challenges remain, such as reconciling incarceration practices with hospice practices, providing palliative care that complies with correctional goals, administering adequate pain management in an environment lacking of trust between inmate and staff,; and involving family within the confines of visitation restrictions.

At one time, most of the developmentally disabled population lived in specialized inpatient facilities and died at relatively early ages. Today, only those with the most profound disabilities are institutionalized, and many are living to older age and dying of the usual chronic diseases. One percent of the general population is developmentally disabled, and most now live independently or in group homes. Professionals working with the developmentally disabled have limited knowledge of palliative care principles, and palliative professionals have limited knowledge of the special challenges of care for the developmentally disabled (http://www.nhpco.org/i4a/pages/index.cfm?pageid=4733).

STATUS OF PALLIATIVE CARE AND RESEARCH OPPORTUNITIES

Thirty percent of nursing home decedents in the United States were cared for under the Medicare hospice benefit in 2005. In 2006, 1240 U.S. hospitals provided palliative care programs, compared with 632 programs in 2000, which is a 5-year increase of 96%.

The Center to Advance Palliative Care coordinates training programs at their six palliative care leadership centers, where participants learn all aspects of developing palliative care in their communities. Recognition of hospice and palliative medicine as a subspecialty in 2006 should lead to more physician involvement in palliative care in the United States. The initial conflict between hospice and palliative medical providers in the United States has turned to increased cooperation as palliative medicine increases referrals to hospice care.

Major problems continue to exist, especially the lack of evidence for palliative care. Research funding is limited for palliative medical research, and major private foundations are retreating from support for palliative and hospice care. Funding for interdisciplinary palliative care in institutions is limited to existing billing mechanisms, used mostly for evaluation and management by physicians and, where allowed, nurse practitioners. Licensed clinical psychologists and licensed clinical social workers can also bill for some services independently.

REFERENCES

1. Brown University. Facts on dying. Available at http://www.chcr.brown.edu/dying/2001DATA.htm (accessed January 6, 2007).
2. Rothera IC, Jones R, Harwood R, et al. Survival in a cohort of social services placements in nursing and residential homes: factors associated with life expectancy and mortality. Public Health 2002;116:160-165.
3. Miller SC, Gozalo P, Mor V, et al. Outcomes and utilization for hospice and non-hospice nursing facility decedents. U.S. Department of Health and Human Services. March 2000. Available at http://aspe.hhs.gov/daltcp/reports/oututil.htm (accessed January 18, 2007).
4. Miller SC, Gozalo P, Mor V. Hospice enrollment and hospitalization of dying nursing home patients. Am J Med 2001;111:38-44.
5. Miller SC, Gozalo P, Wu N, et al. Does receipt of hospice care in nursing homes improve the management of pain at the end of life? J Am Geriatr Soc 2002;50:507-515.
6. Miller SC, Mor V, Teno J. Hospice enrollment and pain assessment and management in nursing homes. J Pain Symptom Manage 2003;26:791-799.
7. Parker-Oliver D, Porock D, Zweig S, et al. Hospice and nonhospice nursing home residents. J Palliat Med 2003;6:69-75.
8. Miller SC, Intrator O, Gozalo P, et al. Government expenditures at the end of life for short- and long-stay nursing home residents: Differences by hospice enrollment status. J Am Geriatr Soc 2004;52:1284-1292.
9. American Health Care Association. Results of the 2002 AHCA Survey of Nursing Staff Vacancy and Turnover in Nursing Homes. February 12, 2003. Available at http://www.ahca.org/research/rpt_vts2002_final.pdf (accessed January 18, 2007).
10. National Hospice and Palliative Care Organization. Hospice care in nursing facilities (2 CD set).
11. Maull FW. Issues in prison hospice: Toward a model for the delivery of hospice care in a correctional setting. Hosp J 1998;13:57-82.
12. U.S. Department of Justice, Bureau of Justice Statistics. Census of State and Federal Correctional Facilities, 2000. Washington, DC: Bulletin NCJ 198272, 2003.
13. Craig EL, Craig RE. Prison hospice: An unlikely success. Am J Hosp Palliat Care 1999;16:725-729.
14. Yampolskaya S, Winston N. Hospice care in prison: General principles and outcomes. Am J Hospice Palliat Care 2003;20:290-296.

SUGGESTED READING

Assistant Secretary for Planning and Evaluation, U.S. Department of Health and Human Services. Reports on hospice care in nursing facilities. Available at http://aspe.hhs.gov/daltcp/reports/oututil.htm (accessed September 16, 2007).
Center to Advance Palliative Care. Available at http://www.capc.org (accessed September 16, 2007).
Liebhaber RW. Developing Hospice Residences. Available at http://iweb.nhpco.org/iweb/Purchase/ProductDetail.aspx?Product_code=820284 (accessed February 1, 2007).
National Hospice and Palliative Care Organization. Available at http://www.nhpco.org (September 16, 2007).
National Quality Forum. A National Framework and Preferred Practices for Palliative and Hospice Care Quality. Available at http://www.qualityforum.org/pdf/reports/palliative/txPHreportPUBLIC01-29-07.pdf (accessed September 16, 2007).
Programs for All-inclusive Care of the Elderly (PACE). Available at http://www.npaonline.org (accessed September 16, 2007).
Sampson-Katz J, Peace S (eds). End of Life in Care Homes: A Palliative Care Approach. New York: Oxford University Press, 2003.

CHAPTER **42**

Home Care and Hospice Home Care

Keri Thomas

KEY POINTS

- Home is where patients spend most of their time and where most would prefer to die. However, current community provision can be inadequate, leading to patient and family distress, crises, unwanted admissions, and excessive expenditure.

- Achieving an excellent quality of home care is of major importance if we are to fulfill patients' wishes to remain living at home and to die at home, if this is their preference.

- Reliable home care can reduce unnecessary hospital admissions and costs. This requires a preplanning approach, flexible care provision, and cross-boundary collaboration, with a focus on coordinating reliable quality care in the community.

- Key factors in improving home care include early identification of patients approaching the final stage of life, anticipation of likely needs, coordination of customized care, anticipatory prescribing, and specialist and community staff and resources available full time to the patient, family, and other caregivers.

- The provision of hands-on care at home is a key support for patients and families, and numerous good-practice models are used in different countries and settings, although they usually are less available for patients with noncancer illnesses.

- Use of good-practice models to optimize the care given by generalist providers has been shown to improve the quality of home care by better planning and coordination, decreasing hospital admissions and increasing the number of people dying where they choose.

IMPORTANCE OF GOOD HOME CARE

Few things in health care are more important and more rewarding than enabling a patient to die peacefully in a place of choice, usually at home. Care of the dying is an important and intrinsic part of the work in family medicine. Challenges exist for the elderly, who have many comorbidities, complex needs, and distinctive social issues.[1] A large number of elderly live and die in care homes or nursing homes, where end-of-life care and support can be inadequate. As we extend palliative care services to include end-of-life care to an aging population, the challenge is to build on good-practice models in cancer and palliative care services and develop new models appropriate to the needs of patients dying from all conditions, especially those with organ failure and the frail elderly with comorbidities. Getting end-of-life care right, particularly care at home, is one of the greatest challenges faced by the health care industry as the baby boomers reach old age.

Primary care teams contribute knowledge of context and community and continuing, supportive and long-term relationships with patients and their families that extend into bereavement. In many countries, primary caregivers deliver most palliative care to patients, and they do this in a sound and effective way, especially when backed by appropriate specialist support.[2] Others use primary care less as a first port of call, although it is still relevant, and in some areas, specialist palliative caregivers take over the care of identified patients. In the 21st century, people are living longer with advanced, irreversible illnesses. Because 90% of the final year of life is spent at home, providing good community-based care is vital, regardless of where a patient eventually dies.

Sensitively facing the reality of dying and making a plan for the final stage of life is as important in "antemortem" or end-of-life care as planning for pregnancy and labor is in antenatal or early-life care. However, pre-emptive planning is often neglected, resulting in a tendency toward reactive, crisis-led care that does not always meet the needs of dying patients. Thorpe's paradoxes[3] summarize the urgent need to get this right—that "most dying people would prefer to remain at home, but most of them die in institutions, and that most of the final year of life is spent at home, but most are admitted to hospital to die."

Home for most people is a special place. Being at home is a frame of mind. It is where we can most be ourselves and be in touch with our deepest sense of being. It represents life, continuity, activity, self-determination, and retaining control, rather than illness, passivity, and the "patient mode" of inpatient care. The strong instinct to return home to die, the so-called salmon instinct, is demonstrated in our society by an old grandmother returning to Pakistan or the deep longing of many hospital or hospice inpatients to see their homes again. It is a cruel consequence of our medical advances that dying patients may feel grateful for their care but imprisoned in an artificial environment and long to reconnect with all that makes them most human.

Maintaining a sense of control is even more important during a time of crisis. As Neuberger[4] said, "Where the locus of care is the home, more will be enabled to retain control." Spilling[5] added, "Home is where we have chosen to live, and the surroundings of our home will encourage us to live while dying. The decision to move a terminally ill patient from home should be made in the knowledge that in addition to loss of familiarity and freedom, an element of hope will be lost."

Experiences of living and dying at home do vary, and some patients and their families prefer other settings as the most healing environments, or they find a death at home impossibly difficult. A consistent research finding is the preference for a home death as the first option for most people.[6,7] Some providers work on the principle that every admission indicates a failure in community care,[8] and most national policies affirm the importance of shifting more care to the community.[9] Still, the home death rate is falling. Ensuring high-quality, reliable home care is important and becoming a greater priority because getting it right is important for us all.

CONSEQUENCES OF INADEQUATE HOME CARE

Many inappropriate hospital admissions result from unresolved symptom control or a breakdown in home care service provision, such as a lack of nursing or night-time caregivers, lack of caregiver support, and difficulties in communication or coordination.[10] Key factors in enabling cancer patients to remain at home have been clarified in a systematic review as intense, sustained, reliable home care provision, self-care or public education, support for families and caregivers, advance care planning and risk assessment, and training of practitioners.[7]

Many more patients prefer to die at home than are able to do so, and a hospital death is more likely for some groups of patients, particularly the poor, the elderly, solitary women, and those with a long illness.[11] Many choose to die in inpatient units such as hospices (only about 17% of cancer patients and 4% of all patients in England die in inpatient hospices), but the outstanding issue is the excess of preventable hospital deaths occurring when home care is not possible (Fig. 42-1). In Great Britain, this is causing a growth of activity in admission avoidance and encouraging improvement of community services. Cost-effectiveness is a reality, and there is some evidence that improved community care is more cost-effective in the long term than overuse of hospitals[12] and that better use of appropriate hospital resources for curative measures rather than comfort care may reduce the hospital mortality ratios.[13]

One of the most significant challenges we face in health care provision is to enable more people to live well and die well in the place and in the manner of their choosing. Within community palliative care, there is a pressing need for active anticipatory management, coordination, and orchestration of services to optimize the quality and reliability of palliative home care services and enable good home care for the dying.

GOOD END-OF-LIFE CARE FOR ALL

Almost 1% of the population dies each year in the United Kingdom, or about 600,000 deaths. For most general practitioners or family physicians with an average number of patients, this means about 20 deaths each year. Lynn's disease trajectories help us understand the three typical

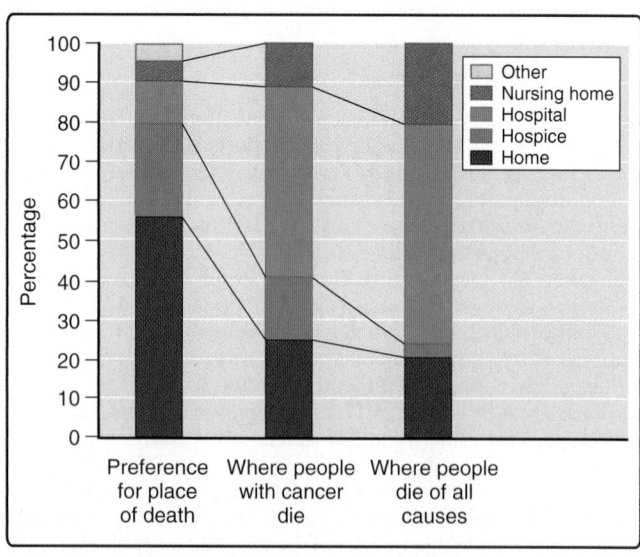

FIGURE 42-1 Preferred and actual places of death. *(From Higginson I. Priorities for End of Life Care in England, Wales, and Scotland. London: Cicely Saunders Foundation, Scottish Partnership for Palliative Care, and the National Council for Hospice and Specialist Palliative Care Services, 2003.)*

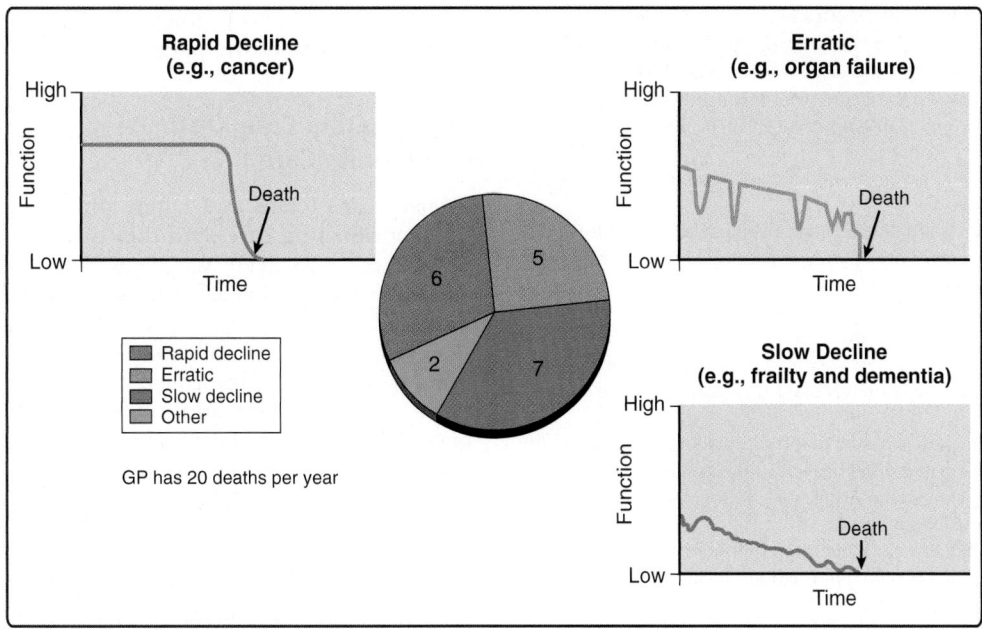

FIGURE 42-2   Three trajectories of dying. *(Adapted from Lynn J, Adamson DM. Living Well at the End of Life: Adapting Health Care to Serious Chronic Illness in Old Age. Arlington, VA; Rand Health, 2003.)*

ways of dying (Fig. 42-2).[14] About one fourth are deaths of cancer patients after a relatively predictable, progressive course, often with rapid deterioration in the final weeks, to which palliative and hospice care has responded appropriately and focused most resources. About one third die of organ failure and have a more erratic, unpredictable course. Most people dying are elderly, frail patients with many comorbid conditions. They typically die more slowly, with gradual deterioration and waning resilience. As people live longer and acquire more comorbid conditions, the situation becomes complicated by likely concomitant degrees of dementia causing decreased resistance to otherwise treatable conditions. As illnesses become more chronic and treatments extend lifespans, this will be the most common end-of-life model in the future, rather than that of death from single diseases or organ failure. These patients already represent the largest group of Medicare-funded patients in the United States.

Home-based care presents a more holistic and less biomedical approach to care, with the general practitioner or family doctor as the lead clinical decision maker who is consulted frequently and who considers the broader context of the patient's illness. Tinetti and Fried[15] argue that as we attempt to care for more patients with accumulated comorbidities, the time has come to abandon disease as the focus of medical care and move to the attainment of individual goals and modifiable factors. They posit that this holistic, integrated model is the only one able to cope with the looming onslaught of aging baby boomers.[15]

One of the challenges is to reframe palliative or end-of-life care to include all those with advanced, progressive, life-limiting conditions in the final year or so of life and to meet their needs appropriately. Different patient needs require different responses, and there are considerable challenges for those in community care to meet these needs appropriately. Home care for each type of patient should be enhanced to ensure excellence for all.

The needs of different groups vary. The needs of patients in rapid decline (typically, cancer patients) are often related to symptom control, family support, intense appropriate home care, continuity of relationships, life closure, and adaptability to rapid changes. The needs of those with organ failure or an erratic course of decline are related to preplanning for urgent situations, prevention of exacerbations, decisions about benefits of low-yield treatments, life closure, family preparation for sudden death, and support at home. The needs of patients with a gradual decline in health or the frail elderly are related to endurance, long-term home care service and supervision, keeping skin intact, helping caregivers understand underlying reasons for certain behaviors, finding moments of joy and meaning, avoiding unnecessary suffering, and protecting themselves from too much intervention and hospitalization.

People's needs can also change with time, and more intensive care may be required for some periods. Toward the end of life, the pace of change may be very rapid, and without good planning and proactive management, the speed of events and domino effects can rapidly become disastrous, despite the best efforts. Enabling patients to remain at home near the end of their lives involves a close collaboration of many people, services, and agencies, involving generalists and specialists and an agreed, proactive, managed plan of care (Box 42-1).

MEETING THE CHALLENGE: KEY SOLUTIONS TO ENABLE GOOD HOME CARE

Preparation: Identify Patients, Assess Needs, and Plan Care

By identifying early the patients with life-limiting disease, estimating their likely illness trajectory and estimated prognostic stage, and discussing their needs and preferences, there is greater likelihood of providing the most

Box 42-1 Key Components of Best Practice in Community Palliative Care

1. Patients with needs for palliative care are identified according to agreed criteria, and a management plan is discussed by the multidisciplinary team.
2. Patients and their caregivers are regularly assessed using agreed assessment tools.
3. Anticipated needs are documented, planned for, and addressed.
4. Patient and caregiver needs are communicated within the team and to specialist colleagues, as appropriate.
5. The preferred place of care and place of death are discussed and documented, and measures are taken to comply when possible.
6. Coordination of care is orchestrated by a named person in the practice team.
7. Relevant information is passed to those providing care during off hours, and anticipated drugs are left in the home.
8. A protocol for care in the dying phase is followed, such as the Liverpool Care Pathway for the Dying Patient.
9. Caregivers are educated, enabled, and supported, which includes the provision of specific information, financial advice, and bereavement care.
10. Audit, reflective practice, development of practice protocols, and targeted learning are encouraged as part of personal, practice, and primary care organization or National Health Service Trust development plans.

Data from National Institute for Health and Clinical Guidance. NICE guidance on supportive and palliative care. Available at www.nice.org.uk (accessed March 2004).

appropriate care at the right time. The Prognostic Indicator Guidance of the Gold Standards Framework[16] and a question (i.e., would you be surprised if the patient were to die in the next year?) are commonly used. This approach does not focus on tight prognostication. It is instead a key to practical preparation. For instance, if the patient's death is not a surprise, what preparatory measures should be made to ensure that he or she lives well and dies well?

Use of assessment guidance and tools can clarify the patient's symptoms, concerns, and needs. After these issues are identified, planning includes two areas: within clinical management teams and among patients, families, and caregivers. Clinical management plans can be developed, preferably at multidisciplinary case conferences, leading to improved communication and continuity of care. Practical anticipation of possible symptoms and their treatment leads to better symptom control and crisis management when needed (e.g., a "just-in-case" box kept in the home with standard drugs such as diamorphine for pain, haloperidol for nausea and vomiting, midazolam for agitation, and hyoscine for secretions).

Discussions about advance care planning with patients and families include clarifying preferences, fears, and anticipated needs. This is not easy against the common backdrop of shock, denial, ignorance, and sometimes inappropriate hopefulness. Increasingly, it is thought that having these difficult discussions with patients earlier rather than later is important to plan the best care, adjust expectations, support fuller living, and enhance hope.[17] This approach enables a greater sense of self-determination and control, enhances coping strategies and adjust-

ment behaviors, and enables better practical planning of care in response to the patient's needs.

Coordinating Care: Optimizing Primary and Community Care

Primary care teams and family physicians are crucial in this coordinating care, and they should be supported to work most effectively with specialist hospice providers and community clinical nurse specialists. Models such as the Gold Standards Framework can formalize good practice and enhance collaboration (www.goldstandardsframework.nhs.uk). Improved coordination is required in cases of emergency and off-hours services to ensure maximal continuity of care, and developments in one-stop coordination centers are proving valuable in some areas.[18] The provision of end-of-life care in care homes or nursing homes, where about one fifth of all people die, is an important area. Although there are many excellent examples of good care, there can be variability in provision and medical support, inconsistent practice, and high turnover rates of staff caring for highly dependent patients with complex comorbidities. Our concepts of palliative care must be expanded to include all with life-limiting illness, moving to proactive rather than reactive care (as in the Gold Standards Framework), increasing recognition of the particular needs of the elderly (especially those with dementia), and reframing care to help people live their final years of life as well as possible.

Provision of Home Care: Hospice at Home and Other Programs

Many hospice home care teams extend support to the community to deliver hands-on care for patients in their home. In England, district nurses (i.e., registered nurses) form the mainstay of nursing care in the home, and they are supported by specialist nurses, nighttime sitters, and care assistants. Lack of such support is a key factor in the breakdown of home care. Access to pre-emptive respite and crisis care (e.g., rapid response teams) is required to ensure the kind of reliable home care that avoids the knee-jerk reaction of hospitalization when under stress. The use of hospice programs is increasing in the United States, but hospice still supports only a minority of cancer patients for limited time and even fewer patients with noncancer illnesses. In most countries, supportive care at home is a key area for improvement, requiring increased resources and extension to all those in need.

Enablement: Caregiver Support and Self-Care Empowerment

Most dying patients are part of a family or care system, and the prevention of breakdown of this support system is essential to ensure the stability of home care. The role of family and other caregivers should be enhanced, and primary care and hospice care can offer families support.[19] Caring for a loved one dying at home can place enormous strains on most families and caregivers, leading to increasing morbidity and mortality. Support into the bereavement period is another vital element. Self-care and patient empowerment are growing ideas within palliative care. The Expert Patient and Carer Programs in England[20] and equivalent programs in other countries are encouraging the patient's voice in care planning, and they will become more important in the future.

Underpinnings: Education and Public Awareness

End-of-life care involves all health care professionals and is enhanced by expert specialist advice and support. The most effective strategies involve many staff members and medical practitioners, enabling the best-practice model to become formalized and incorporated as part of routine care. Education, training, and aids to life-long learning such as use of reflective practice (e.g., significant event analysis), are essential for optimizing care. Awareness of these methods and goals must be raised within the public domain if we are to reduce the element of luck in the way we plan end-of-life care and overcome the taboo of talking about death. This means discussing issues of death and dying as part of public health agendas, considering these topics as related to pensions and life insurance when we plan our lives, and destigmatizing the process to enable easier conversations. Creating greater involvement and encouraging public debate and awareness are important if we are to make progress.

DEVELOPMENTS IN END-OF-LIFE CARE

In England, the National Health Service (NHS) End-of-Life Care Programme (www.endoflifecare.nhs.uk) supported three established models of generalist care for all patients. England is now developing an NHS End-of-Life Care Strategy to mainstream improvements in end-of-life care to ensure high-quality, equitable care that is cost-effective and enables greater choice by patients. The Canadian end-of-life care strategy has made progress in the delivery of good end-of-life care in Canada, but all acknowledge the size of the challenge.[21]

The Gold Standards Framework[22] is a common-sense, systematic approach to optimizing the care delivered by primary care teams for any patient nearing the end of life in the community. It has been used by thousands of U.K. practices during the past 8 years. The aim is to develop a framework for each practice or team that will enable the members to deliver the best (gold standard) care consistently for every patient. Adopting the Gold Standards Framework has been found to affirm good practice, improve consistency of care so that fewer patients slip through the net,[23] and improve the experience of care for patients, caregivers, and staff; it has also increased the home death rate. This work is underpinned by the best available evidence and fully evaluated. It is recommended by the National Institute for Health and Clinical Excellence,[24] the Royal College of General Practitioners, and others. It has been modified and further developed for use in care homes in a separate Gold Standards Framework in Care Homes Program, which is used by hundreds of care homes (e.g., nursing homes) and has demonstrated an improvement in quality of care and a reduction in hospital admissions.[25]

The framework is based on the principles of identifying the patients in need of palliative or supportive care, (e.g., using the Prognostic Indicator Guidance of the Gold Standards Framework and a surprise question or other suitable criteria); assessing their needs, problems, and preferences; and planning care, with an agreed management plan discussed at the team meeting and using an advance care plan. At each stage, communication is improved within and between teams and with the patients and families. A list of key tasks, the 7 Cs, is introduced, beginning with inclusion of patients on a supportive care register and holding a team meeting to discuss their proactive care. Details are provided in typified case histories (Box 42-2) and can be found at the Gold Standards Framework Web site (www.goldstandardsframework.nhs.uk). Care in the final days of life can be improved using an integrated care pathway for the dying, such as the Liverpool Care Pathway.[26] This generic tool enables greater consistency of care, standardization, and benchmarking, and it is used in several countries and for patients with different conditions.[27]

Advance care planning has been used extensively in many countries, and these discussions underpin all end-

---

Box 42-2 Reactive and Proactive Patient Journeys

Mr. B: A Reactive Patient Journey without the Gold Standards Framework

- Ad hoc arrangements with the physician and nurse; no preferred place of care discussed or anticipated
- Problems with symptom control because of anxious or frightened caregiver
- Crisis call after normal daytime hours; no plan or drugs available in the home
- Admitted to hospital
- Dies in hospital
- Caregiver given minimal support in grief
- No reflection by team on care given
- Possibly inappropriate use of hospital bed

Mrs. W: A Proactive Patient Journey Using the Gold Standards Framework

On supportive care register; discussed at team meeting (C1)*
Benefits, advice, and information given to the patient and caregiver (i.e., home pack) (C1, C6)
Regular support, visits, and phone calls part of proactive care (C1, C2)
Assessment of symptoms; partnership with palliative care specialists to give customized care to the needs of the patient and caregiver (C3)
Caregiver assessed, including psychosocial needs (C3, C6)
Preferred place of care recognized and organized (C1, C2)
Handover form issued; care plan and drugs issued for home (C4)
End-of-life pathway, Liverpool Care Pathway, or minimum protocol used (C7)
Patient dies in preferred place; bereavement support for staff and family; audits of service to improve care and knowledge (C5, C6)

The 7 Cs of the Gold Standards Framework are communication (C1), coordination of care (C2), control of symptoms and ongoing assessment (C3), continuing support (C4), continued learning (C5), caregiver and family support (C6), and care in the final days (C7).

of-life care strategies. Advance care planning discussions with patients promote choice, offer a realistic degree of hopefulness,[17] communicate decisions to others, and ensure more patient-focused care. Various examples are used, and there is much development in this area.[28] Various forms of written refusal of treatments or advance directives or decisions exist in England with guidance from the Mental Capacity Act,[29] and together with preference-based advance statements, they can guide physicians and planners in providing the most appropriate care.[30] Failing to plan is planning to fail! Despite inherent difficulties, this is a crucial area for future development.

CONCLUSIONS

Within health care systems and society as a whole, there are gradual moves toward the recognition that quality care of the dying is a measure of our success, rather than a sign of failure. Some degree of "death denial" is pervasive, but in their attempts to offer best care for patients, health care professionals can be overly optimistic in prognostication, become focused on curing at all costs, and become too aggressive in management. A balance of "hoping for the best while preparing for the worst" may ensure we are better able to anticipate and cope with the issues that arise at the end of life and the complex range of services that are required. The excellent services of palliative care units and hospices are challenged by broadening the scope to include more noncancer patients, whose clinical, emotional, and practical needs are as great as those of cancer patients. Good home care is vital in this situation.

We now must address the new situation of a population growing old and becoming unwell more slowly than in previous generations. With the demographic changes of aging populations, better treatments that can prolong the later stages of chronic illnesses, fewer inpatient beds, and rising costs, the need to provide good home care for all seriously ill patients is urgent.

A death dominated by fear, crises, inappropriate hospital admissions, overmedication, and poor communication can be a tragedy, and it represents a failure of our medical system. Enabling a peaceful death at home can be a great accomplishment for all concerned. The most significant challenge we face in end-of-life care provision is to enable more people to live well until they die, and improving home care is central to this challenge. "Palliative care at home embraces what is most noble in medicine: sometimes curing, always relieving, supporting right to the end."[31]

REFERENCES

1. Davies E, Higginson IJ. Better Palliative Care for Older People. Geneva: World Health Organization, 2004.
2. Mitchell GK. How well do general practitioners deliver palliative care? A systematic review. Palliat Med 2002;16:457-464.
3. Thorpe G. Enabling more dying people to remain at home. BMJ 1993; 307:915-918.
4. Neuberger J. Palliative care. Palliative Care Congress, University of Warwick, 2000.
5. Spilling R. Terminal Care at Home. General Practice Series. Oxford, UK: Oxford University Press, 1986.
6. Higginson I. Priorities for End of Life Care in England, Wales, and Scotland. London: Cicely Saunders Foundation, Scottish Partnership for Palliative Care, and the National Council for Hospice and Specialist Palliative Care Services, 2003.
7. Gomes B, Higginson IJ. Factors influencing death at home in terminally ill patients with cancer: A systematic review. BMJ 2006;322:515-518.
8. Ham C, York N, Sutch S, Shaw R. Hospital bed utilisation in the NHS, Kaiser Permanente, and the US Medicare programme: Analysis of routine data. BMJ 2003;327:1257. Available at http://www.pubmedcentral.nih.gov/articlerender.fcgi?artid=286244 (accessed September 25, 2007).
9. Department of Health. Our health, our care, our say: A new direction for community services. London: Department of Health, 2006. Available at http://www.dh.gov.uk/PublicationsAndStatistics/Publications/PublicationsPolicyAndGuidance/PublicationsPolicyAndGuidanceArticle/fs/en?CONTENT_ID=4127453&chk=NXIecj (accessed September 25, 2007).
10. Thomas C, Morris SM, Clark D. Place of death: Preferences among cancer patients and their carers. Soc Sci Med 2004;58:2431-2444.
11. Higginson IJ, Astin P, Dolan S. Where do cancer patients die? Ten year trend in the place of death of cancer patients in England. Palliat Med 1998;12:353-363.
12. Taylor D, Carter S. Valuing Choice—Dying at Home. A Case for the More Equitable Provision of High Quality Support for People Who Wish to Die at Home. An economic and social policy opinion commissioned by Marie Curie Cancer Care. London: School of Pharmacy, University of London, 1998. Available at http://www.campaign.mariecurie.org.uk/NR/rdonlyres/646C31D0-49C1-42C5-8BFE-D1A8F3F3A499/0/campaign_valuing_choice.pdf (accessed September 25, 2007).
13. Jarman B, Gault S, Alves B, et al. Explaining differences in English hospital death rates using routinely collected data. BMJ 1999;318:1515-1520.
14. Thomas K from Lynn J, Adamson DM. Living well at the end of life. Adapting health care to serious chronic illness in old age, White Paper, RAND Health, 2003 (http://www.medicaring.org/whitepaper/).
15. Tinetti M, Fried T. The end of the disease era. Am J Med 2003;116:179-184.
16. Gold Standards Framework. Prognostic Indicator Guidance. Available at http://www.goldstandardsframework.nhs.uk/content/gp_contract/Prognostic%20Indicators%20Guidance%20Paper%20v%2025.pdf (accessed September 25, 2007).
17. Davison S, Simpson C. Hope and advance care planning in patients with end stage renal disease: Qualitative interview study. 2006;333:886-887.
18. Marie Curie Cancer Care. Marie Curie Delivering Choice Programme. Available at http://deliveringchoice.mariecurie.org.uk (accessed September 25, 2007).
19. Simon C. Informal carers and the primary care team. Br J Gen Pract 2001;51:920-923.
20. Expert Patient Programme Community Interest Company. Expert patient and carer programmes in England. Available at http://www.expertpatients.co.uk/public/default.aspx (accessed September 25, 2007).
21. Carstairs S. Still Not There—Quality End-of-Life Care. A Progress Report. Ottawa, Ontario: Canadian Hospice Palliative Care Association, 2005.
22. Thomas K. Caring for the Dying at Home: Companions on the Journey. Oxford, UK: Radcliffe Medical Press, 2003.
23. King N, Thomas K, Martin N, et al. Now nobody falls through the net. Practitioners perspectives on the Gold Standards Framework for community palliative care. Palliat Med 2005;19:619-627.
24. National Institute for Clinical Excellence. Guidance on Cancer Services: Improving Supportive and Palliative Care for Adults. London: National Institute for Clinical Excellence, 2004.
25. Badger F, Thomas K, Clifford C. Raising standards for elderly people dying in care homes. Eur J Palliative Care, in press.
26. Marie Curie Palliative Care Institute, Liverpool. Improving patient care through palliative care research, development and education. Available at http://www.mcpcil.org.uk (accessed September 25, 2007).
27. Ellershaw J, Wilkinson S. Care of the Dying: A Pathway to Excellence. Oxford, UK: Oxford University Press, 2003.
28. Lets Talk. Available at http://www.fraserhealth.ca/Services/HomeandCommunityCare/AdvanceCarePlanning/Pages/default.aspx (accessed November 10, 2007).
29. Department for Constitutional Affairs. Mental Capacity Act of 2005. Available at http://www.dca.gov.uk/legal-policy/mental-capacity/index.htm (accessed September 25, 2007).
30. Murray S, Aziz S, Thomas K. Advance care planning in primary care [editorial]. BMJ 2006;333:868-869.
31. Gomas JM. Palliative care at home: A reality or mission impossible? Palliat Med 1993;7(Suppl 1):45-59.
32. National Institute for Health and Clinical Excellence. NICE Guidance on Supportive and Palliative Care. Available at www.nice.org.uk (accessed September 25, 2007).

SUGGESTED READING

Aitken PV Jr. Incorporating advance care planning into family practice. Am Fam Physician 1999;59:605-614, 617-620. Available at http://www.aafp.org/afp/990201ap/605.html (accessed September 25, 2007).

Aging with Dignity. Five Wishes. Available at www.agingwithdignity.org/5wishes.html (accessed September 25, 2007).

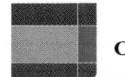

The Business of Palliative Medicine: Quality Care in a Challenging Environment

Ruth L. Lagman

> **KEY POINTS**
>
> - The care of individuals with advanced illness is inadequate.
> - Palliative medicine provides comprehensive and holistic care.
> - Palliative medicine is cost-effective.
> - Communication is key and warrants a well-versed interdisciplinary team.
> - Delivering quality care is a challenge given the realities of health care.

Individuals are living longer with more chronic illnesses. Diseases, specifically cancer, with fatal diagnoses in the past have been transformed into chronic illnesses by disease-modifying agents. Patients have more symptoms and use health care resources more intensively. The physical, psychosocial, and financial toll on them and their families cannot be underestimated.

Palliative medicine is being recognized as an important clinical service in many countries, and it has been accredited as a subspecialty in the United States. Patients with advanced, incurable diseases have always existed in the health care setting, but their medical and psychosocial needs were never clearly defined.

Historically, the care of these patients has been fragmented, and their symptoms and complications have been managed by different specialties, often with no clear definition of goals of care until the patient's death. When diagnosed with a terminal illness, the patient was often transitioned to hospice care with little or no involvement of the physician. Modern palliative medicine offers an alternative model of care for this unique patient population. It is not hospice care, but it incorporates most of its concepts. This model allows individuals to have palliative treatment for their life-limiting illness through chemotherapy, irradiation, or surgery, which may alleviate their symptoms and improve their quality of life. Palliative medicine is involved earlier in the disease trajectory, ideally at the time of diagnosis, until death. The demand to establish palliative medicine programs has surged.

THE BUSINESS PLAN

To be successful and guarantee longevity, a new program should conduct itself in a business-like manner given the realities of the health care industry. Although recently accredited, the specialty is a relatively new concept in health care. Any new program is scrutinized more closely than existing specialties. A business plan is imperative and should have the following characteristics:

- Forward-looking strategy
- Proposal written in the decision-maker's language
- Detailed outline of operational and financial projections
- Program objectives that are in line with the goals of the institution
- Involvement of individuals with various skill sets[1,2]

An environmental analysis is the initial step in determining strengths, weaknesses, and opportunities. Medicare has been the predominant payer for palliative medicine in the United States and hospice services, and reimbursement has been favorable. Because fee structures are legislated, there is always a possibility of decreased reimbursement in the future. Private insurers and other third-party payers often follow Medicare and may mandate the best outcomes in terms of resource use.[2] Despite the growth of hospice and palliative medicine programs, patients are still referred late. There has been a significant increase in enrollment since 1992, but the median length of stay in hospice decreased from 34 days in 1992 to 22 days in 2003, with 37% dying within 7 days of enrollment.[3] These figures have financial and emotional implications for hospice personnel because the greatest intensity of service delivery (e.g., nursing, psychosocial care, delivery of medications, durable medical equipment, oxygen) is at the beginning and end of care.[4]

PROGRAM DEVELOPMENT

Definitions

The distinction between palliative medicine and hospice should be clear, and the goals of care should be defined after patients are admitted to either program. Modern palliative medicine has its roots in hospice. Although the overall philosophy of care is similar, there are differences. Using both terms interchangeably (at least in the United States) causes confusion for patients, families, and professional staff in terms of what services are being delivered and what services can be reimbursed by insurance.

Although both deal with life-limiting illnesses, these patients are in different phases of dying. Metastatic cancer, depending on the primary site and performance status, has been transformed into a chronic illness with the use of disease-modifying agents. These patients may be undergoing palliative treatment for their tumor (e.g., irradiation, chemotherapy, surgery). The hospice philosophy in the United States is not in line with these life-prolonging interventions and favors less aggressive care. Most patients in hospice have exhausted antitumor options.

Palliative medicine should distinguish itself from end-of-life care and should start at the diagnosis of any advanced disease. There is no time line for the care of these patients; some can be given care for many years even though they have metastatic disease and are undergoing palliative chemotherapy and irradiation. Because of the nature of their illness, they can have symptoms (e.g., pain, nausea, vomiting) that need immediate attention and have complications (e.g., hypercalcemia, infections, pathologic fractures) that may be palliated in the interim to alleviate symptoms and improve quality of life. Congestive heart failure and individuals with chronic obstructive pulmonary disease are managed for a long time, often in a palliative mode; they may have exacerbations of their symptoms but are never referred to as patients receiving end-of-life care.[5] This should be the model for palliative medicine. It is a seamless collaborative model from the beginning, rather than a dichotomous and discontinuous care plan that often is involved only at the terminal stage and therefore warranting the term *end-of-life care.*

To use both terms interchangeably has several adverse effects:

● Patients and families misunderstand what service is being provided.
● Instead of educating and enlightening professional staff about the difference, careless terminology perpetuates misconceptions.
● Insurance companies may lower reimbursements because they think less aggressive care (i.e., hospice or end-of life care) is being delivered.

A service may follow a palliative medicine model or a hospice model in a given institution, in line with its own culture, mission statement, and goals. In certain instances, a consultation service may be sufficient; in others, a consultation service with a dedicated hospice unit is needed. A comprehensive, integrated program that can offer several product lines is the model that guarantees financial feasibility and longevity. It is also the most difficult to establish because it needs careful planning and years to accomplish. More importantly, it requires more scarce trained and experienced professional staff as the program expands.

The Acute Care Setting

Many patients die in a hospital, which is a significant culture change from the 1900s, when individuals were cared for and died at home. Most people prefer to die at home, and 50% do so[6] for several reasons, including more intensive symptom control, rapid clinical deterioration, and caregiver breakdown. There is a cultural perception that death can be resisted, postponed, or avoided.[7] More than 90% of Medicare beneficiaries are hospitalized in the last 12 months of life.[8] More than one third of decedents in an academic medical center died in an intensive care unit.[9] In a New York hospital, 47% received invasive palliative treatments during the final few days of life, with 51% of dementia patients and 11% of cancer patients on enteral tube feeding at the time of death.[10] Although a poor prognosis was documented in 75% of charts, life-prolonging treatment (e.g., intravenous antibiotics, transfusions, intravenous fluids, cardiac monitoring, ventilator use) was still being implemented within 24 hours of death because some physicians viewed palliative medicine as abandonment.[11] Curative treatment was aggressively pursued because of miscommunication among physicians, patients, and families and because of the insistence for such care by family members.[11]

The growth of hospices has been explosive, but many are unable to access this care. Although the care during

terminal illness is more clearly defined, there is still a subset of individuals with advanced illnesses who are in the acute care setting whose physical, psychosocial, and spiritual needs are not being addressed.

The emphasis on the acute medical care system is driven by technology and specialists who focus on diagnosis, treatment, and cure of acute illness.[12] A multi-institutional study showed that 50% of patients dying in hospitals suffered uncontrolled pain; the wishes of patients and their families were often unmet and incongruent with the physician's plan of care.[13] A study of barriers in acute care palliative medicine showed the following:

● The emphasis on treatment overshadowed the discussion of goals of care, which were dictated by usual and routine practice.
● Palliative care was not seen as a viable alternative and was often viewed negatively because it was not considered to be proactive.
● Patient's preferences and goals of care were not considered to be important and were not followed.[14]

Hospitals use most resources for chronic illnesses (cancer included) without the prospect of cure.[15] Exploring patients' preferences and treatment options earlier enables better care planning in the event that all palliative treatment modalities have been exhausted.[14]

Palliative medicine consultation commonly occurs near the time of discharge (median of 5 days before discharge). Patients may clinically deteriorate during hospitalization, and this precipitates a palliative medicine consultation.[16] For patients with nonphysical concerns, the charges were higher because of difficult decision-making issues. A highly skilled interdisciplinary team is essential in the overall care of a palliative medicine patient because no one individual can address the psychosocial and spiritual care of these individuals. It is unreasonable to expect physicians and nurses with no background in psychosocial and spiritual assessment to assist and fulfill all these needs. Third-party payers do not reimburse holistic care.[16]

Acute care palliative medicine is a relatively new concept of care for patients with life-limiting diseases. It should be part of the acute care system in any hospital. It is not hospice care. One model uses a separate acute care inpatient palliative medicine unit solely to serve patients with advanced illness.[17,18] This approach is no different from that of any medical-surgical floor in the hospital and is judged by the same standards.[19] In this unit, the typical patient population is older, 71% have co-morbid conditions, 91% get laboratory tests, 64% have radiologic interventions, 96% receive intravenous fluids, 19% have blood transfusions, 14% receive radiation therapy and chemotherapy, and 44% undergo therapeutic interventions.[18]

Palliative medicine physicians provide primary care for these patients while they are in the hospital. There are several advantages:

● Physicians have control of decision making in terms of ordering medications and diagnostic and therapeutic interventions.
● The goals of care are continually evaluated for benefit from palliative chemotherapy and irradiation, and the patient is assessed for hospice care, leading to more efficient coordination of care.

- A well-versed interdisciplinary team providing holistic care to patients and families is readily available.
- Nurses and support staff have physicians readily available.
- Physicians conserve valuable time and energy by physically staying on one floor.[20]

The unit is financially viable.[19] Compared with institutions with acute care palliative medicine units, the pharmacy and nursing costs are lower. Radiologic costs are about 33% higher than in peer institutions.[21] The philosophy is an aggressive but judicious approach to palliate symptoms and manage complications as necessary to improve the patient's quality of life. Such palliative medicine is part of the fabric of the acute care system. This means every patient has access to any available modern technology, similar to any other patient in a medical-surgical department.[17,18] Some patients are discharged to hospice care. Palliative procedures such as radiation therapy, stents, and venting gastrostomies may be done in the acute care setting before hospice enrollment because these procedures may pose financial constraints on any hospice given the capitated reimbursement structure.

This patient population has high acuity after all co-morbidities and complications are considered. Patients with lower acuity require less care and are subject to care over a longer period, whereas patients with higher acuity require more intense care over a shorter period. Current reimbursement in terms of the diagnosis-related group (DRG) may have pitfalls and may be inaccurate. The all-patient refined–diagnosis-related group (APR-DRG) may more accurately reflect acuity of this patient population. After we more accurately and completely documented co-morbidities and complications, our patients' acuity closely approximated the average acuity in our institution.[22]

The implication is significant. When individuals are admitted to a palliative medicine unit, there is a perception by patients, relatives, and some physicians and nurses that patients receive less care. The reality is that the acuity of these patients is high to start. The challenge is to deliver quality medical care with desirable outcomes in symptom control by using inexpensive but proven medications for symptom control, judicious and thoughtful diagnostic or therapeutic interventions that may improve the quality of life and is in line with their plan of care.[22] While the medical condition is being managed, a discharge plan is assembled. This process must start early because it often takes time to talk to patients' families and caregivers. Patients need to go home with the appropriate service, whether hospice or home care.[17,18]

A model that can work for palliative medicine in an acute care setting requires an institutional response that encourages this service for patients and their families.[11] Barriers to end-of-life discussion include the following:

- Discomfort in talking about death
- A sense of failure by the treating physician
- Time constraints in discussing treatment plans
- Absence of goals of care
- Legal ramifications of withholding aggressive treatment
- Financial incentives that encourage curative options[11]

Hospice

Some institutions may allocate beds for hospice. When goals of care have changed to comfort care and the patient has entered the actively dying phase, it is logical to transfer the individual from another part of the institution (e.g., intensive care units to a hospice inpatient unit). After admission to this unit, stopping all medications and diagnostic and therapeutic interventions that do not add to the patient's comfort is warranted, because the patient's outcome or survival is not affected. Medicare defines this category of care in hospice as general inpatient (GIP) and reimburses at a fixed cost (capitated) on a daily basis, not according to a specific DRG. The financial implications necessitate the day-to-day operations of this unit in terms of bed allocation, staffing, medications used, and laboratory and radiologic interventions allowed.

DELIVERY OF CARE

A physician trained in palliative medicine is the cornerstone of the program.[20] The physician's skills are essential to the care of this unique patient population. The skill set includes the following:

- Communication
- Symptom control
- Management of complications
- Psychosocial care
- Coordination of care
- Decision making
- Care of the dying[5,23]

When palliative medicine is involved, patient care and the institution benefit by assisting the referring team to develop a plan of care. Complex management problems are shared with the referring team, and the team members help to address the common clinical and financial goals of the institution.[24]

The ultimate goal of a palliative medicine program in acute care is to have desirable outcomes of improved symptom control and excellent patient satisfaction within fixed reimbursement. This includes judicious resource use and decreasing length of stay, which are goals of any institution.[25] Quality medical care takes precedence over cost savings. When clinical outcomes are satisfactory, financial benefits usually follow because of increased marketing, patient feedback, and customer satisfaction.

Cost saving is not easy. It requires care to be comprehensive and integrated. Close communication with the family member to discuss the goals of care, discharge planning, and appropriate care after discharge is essential to lower costs. Dedicated interdisciplinary team members communicating with the patient and family for care planning is mandatory. This is a particular skill set needed in managing patients with life-limiting illnesses because most experience clinical deterioration and eventual death. A dedicated social worker experienced in palliative medicine may assist with the financial, psychosocial, and spiritual burdens.[18] The social worker is essential in procuring background information, identifying decision makers, and structuring family meetings. Communication between physicians and family members often is inadequate, leading to limited knowledge about the patient's condition, difficulty in getting information, insufficient explanations about procedures, and the erroneous perception that the death of a loved one was unexpected.[11]

Because communication is important, a family meeting is mandatory for every patient admitted to the acute inpatient palliative medicine unit.[18] The meeting helps to educate the families about expectations for care after the patient is discharged and about how they can seek help if the patient's condition worsens. Simultaneously, a dedicated nurse case manager reviews options for discharge planning that can be presented to the patient and family. Often, these patients cannot be left alone and need 24-hour care at home or at an inpatient facility. When appropriate, hospice care or palliative medicine outpatient follow-up is recommended, and a 24-hour telephone hotline is provided.[20]

FINANCIAL FEASIBILITY

Costs and Benefits

Palliative medicine in the inpatient setting is commonly delivered by a consultation service and has some cost benefit.[26] The consultation team affects the goals of care when recommendations are implemented by the requesting physicians, and there are fewer admissions to the intensive care unit.[27] Because care delivered is often terminal care, interventions inconsistent with the goals of care at the time of consultation are withdrawn. Significant decreases occur in the direct and ancillary costs (i.e., radiology and laboratory), but not in pharmacy costs. Patients sometimes are assumed to be less ill than those getting standard care, which may explain the lower costs. Costs and acuity are different in these settings.[21,22] Hospital charges are lower 5 days after an inpatient palliative medicine consultation.[14] A multidisciplinary inpatient palliative care team improved the quality of care and symptoms and decreased inpatient and outpatient costs for individuals with less than 1-year survival times.[28]

A retrospective review of inpatient palliative medicine consultation showed that more than 90% of the interventions recommended were implemented by the primary care team and that 87% of individuals experienced symptom improvement.[29] Ancillary and ventilatory charges were decreased after palliative care consultations, and for those being referred to hospice, the length of hospital stay decreased. Managed care patients had fewer charges for emergency room visits and future hospitalizations after palliative medicine consultations. The median number of ancillary tests dropped from four to none. The median number of ventilator charges dropped from six to two after palliative medicine consultations.[29]

A high-volume, specialist care palliative medicine unit reduced daily charges and costs by 66% overall and by 74% for other charges (i.e., medications and diagnostics) after transfer to the palliative care unit.[30] Although treatment goals may be different, the costs outside the palliative medicine unit were higher for 57 case-matched individuals. Sometimes, referring teams did not know how to adjust care, because expensive interventions such as tube feeding, intravenous antibiotics, total parenteral nutrition, and hemodialysis were probably not going to change the outcome for someone who is dying.[30] Mean daily charges

were 38% lower in a palliative care unit in a comprehensive cancer center compared with patients treated outside the inpatient unit.[31]

After implementation of a comprehensive palliative medicine outpatient program,[32] deaths in acute care facilities declined from 84% to 55%. There was an increase in the number of terminally ill individuals receiving palliative care from 23% to 71%, and the cost savings was $1.7 million. There was a decrease in hospital costs for terminal care after an outpatient, integrated palliative medicine program was implemented.

Medicare spending for hospice care increased 60%, from $3.5 billion in 2001 to $5.9 billion in 2003, as hospice programs grew 8%, from 2266 in 2001 to 2454 in 2003.[33] Hospices can provide care and still be profitable by maintaining a high daily patient census, streamlining care, and increasing length of stay.[34]

Comprehensive Integrated Program

To ensure financial viability of any palliative medicine program, the key is a comprehensive, integrated program. Having a consultation service first may be a reasonable and logical step to establishing a program, but it may not be enough. Although a consultation service in the hospital improves patient care, the risk is that recommendations may not be implemented.[35] The Cleveland Clinic has a comprehensive and integrated program consisting of the acute care inpatient unit, inpatient consultation, outpatient clinic, and a home hospice or home care program. There are several advantages:

- The patient can enter the program at several access points.
- An individual can traverse each product line, depending on his or her disease trajectory, keeping the revenues within the program.
- Palliative medicine physicians follow these individuals at each access point and provide continuity of care.[20]

The danger of presenting palliative medicine or hospice as a cost-saving program is the expectation that it will and should continue to do this, which will eventually doom the program. Delivering quality care overrides cost savings.[4]

Palliative medicine is a cognitive specialty, but the reimbursement climate in the United States favors technical expertise. It is challenging to provide quality care in the setting of fixed DRG reimbursements in acute care or in hospice. To provide holistic quality care for patients with advanced illnesses requires an experienced interdisciplinary team (e.g., physicians, nurses, social worker, pastor). Financial viability can be ensured in an acute care specialty unit or a hospice inpatient unit by using inexpensive older but proven medications for symptom control, selectively ordering diagnostic and therapeutic interventions in accordance with the patient's plan of care, and maintaining a high occupancy rate to offset the high costs, particularly for labor.[4]

CONCLUSIONS

There are several models of palliative medicine. A comprehensive and integrated program helps financial viability. It helps to offset the financial challenges in delivering care under fixed reimbursement. Acute care palliative medicine provides appropriate care for the individual's disease trajectory and should be reimbursed according to the resources used. A business plan is mandatory for any nascent or existing program.

REFERENCES

1. Walsh D, Gombeski WR, Goldstein P, et al. Managing a palliative medicine oncology program: The role of a business plan. J Pain Symptom Manage 1994;9:109-118.
2. Walsh D. The Harry R. Horvitz Center for Palliative Medicine, the Cleveland Clinic Foundation. Millbank Memorial Fund, 2000, pp 51-72.
3. National Hospice and Palliative Care Organization. Facts and figures on hospice care in America. Arlington, VA: National Hospice and Palliative Care Organization 2003.
4. Lagman RL, Walsh D. The business of palliative medicine: Business planning, models of care and program development. In O'Mahony S, Blank A (eds). Choices in Palliative Care. New York: Springer Publications, 2007, pp 184-197.
5. Davis MP, Walsh D, LeGrand SB, Lagman R. End-of-life care: The death of palliative medicine? J Palliat Med 2002;5:813-814.
6. National Center for Health Statistics. New study of patterns of death in the United States. Available at http://www.cdc.gov (accessed November 2007).
7. Clark D. Between hope and acceptance: The medicalisation of dying. Br Med J 2002;324:905-907.
8. Pritchard RS, Fisher ES, Teno JM, et al. Influence of patient preferences and local health system characteristics on the place of death. SUPPORT Investigators. J Am Geriatr Soc 1998;46:1242-1250.
9. Lagman R, Walsh D, Davis MP, et al. Deaths in an academic medical center. J Palliat Med 2006;9:1260-1263.
10. Ahronheim JC, Morrisson RS, Baskin SA, et al. Treatment of the dying in the acute care hospital: Advanced dementia and cancer. Arch Intern Med 1996;156:2094-2100.
11. Jacobs LG, Bonuck K, Burton W, Mulvihill M. Hospital care at the end of life: An institutional assessment. J Pain Symptom Manage 2002;24:291-298.
12. Strauss A, Fagerhaugh S, Suczek B, Wiener C. Social Organization of Medical Work. Chicago: University of Chicago Press, 1985.
13. SUPPORT Principal Investigators. A controlled trial to improve care for seriously ill hospitalized patients. The study to understand prognoses and preferences for outcomes and risks of treatments (SUPPORT). JAMA 1995;274:1591-1598.
14. Cowan JD. Hospital charges for a community inpatient palliative care program. Am J Hosp Palliat Med 2004;21:177-190.
15. Willard C, Luker K. Challenges to end of life care in the acute hospital setting. Palliat Med 2006;20:611-615.
16. Ahmedzai S, Walsh D. Palliative medicine and modern cancer care. Semin Oncol 2000;27:1-6.
17. Lagman R, Walsh D. Acute care palliative medicine—the Cleveland model. Eur J Palliat Care 2007;14:17-20.
18. Lagman R, Rivera N, Walsh D, et al. Acute inpatient palliative medicine in a cancer center: Clinical problems and medical interventions—a prospective study. Am J Hosp Palliat Med 2007;24:20-28.
19. Davis MP, Walsh D, Nelson KA, LeGrand SB. The business of palliative medicine—part 2. The economics of acute inpatient palliative medicine. Am J Hosp Palliat Care 2002;19:89-95.
20. Lagman R, Walsh D. Integration of palliative medicine into comprehensive cancer care. Semin Oncol 2005;32:134-138.
21. Davis MP, Walsh D, Lagman R, et al. The financial benefits of acute inpatient palliative medicine: An inter-institutional comparative analysis by all patient refined-diagnosis related group and case mix index. J Support Oncol 2005;3:1-4.
22. Lagman R, Davis MP, Walsh D, Young B. All patient refined-diagnostic related group (APR-DRG) and case mix index in acute care palliative medicine. J Support Oncol 2007;5:145-149.
23. Weissman DE. Consultation in palliative medicine. Arch Intern Med 1997;157:733-737.
24. Glare PA, Auret KA, Aggarwal G, et al. The interface between palliative medicine and specialists in acute care hospitals: Boundaries, bridges and challenges. Med J Aust 2003;179(Suppl):S29-S31.
25. Meier DE. Palliative care programs: What, why, and how? Physician Exec 2001;27:43-47.
26. Morrison RS, Maroney-Galin C, Kralovec PD, Meier DE. The growth of palliative care programs in United States hospitals. J Palliat Med 2005;8:1127-1134.
27. Penrod JD, Deb P, Luhrs C, et al. Cost and utilization outcomes of patients receiving hospital-based palliative care consultation. J Palliat Med 2006;9:855-860.
28. Richardson RH. Outcomes of a randomized controlled trial of a multidisciplinary inpatient palliative care service. Am Acad Hosp Palliat Med Bull 2006;3:5-15.
29. O'Mahony S, Blank A, Zallman L, Selwyn PA. The benefits of a hospital-based inpatient palliative care consultation service: Preliminary outcome data. J Palliat Med 2005;8:1033-1039.
30. Smith TJ, Coyne P, Cassel B, et al. A high-volume specialist palliative care unit and team may reduce in-hospital end-of-life care costs. J Palliat Med 2003;5:699-705.
31. Elsayem A, Swint K, Fisch MJ, et al. Palliative care inpatient service in a comprehensive cancer center: Clinical and financial outcomes. J Support Oncol 2004;22:2008-2014.
32. Bruera E, Neumann CM, Gagnon B, et al. The impact of a regional palliative care program on the cost of palliative care delivery. J Palliat Med 2000;3:181-186.
33. Medicare Payment Advisory Commission (MedPac). Hospice care in Medicare: Recent trends and a review of the issues. In Report to Congress: New approaches to Medicare. Available at http://www.medpac.gov (accessed November 2007).
34. McCue MJ, Thompson JM. Operational and financial performance of newly established hospices. Am J Hosp Palliat Med 2006;23:259-266.
35. Cowan JD, Burns D, Palmer TW, et al. A palliative medicine program in a community setting: 12 points from the first 12 months. Am J Hosp Palliat Care 2003;20:415-433.

Quality

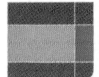

CHAPTER **44**

Development of National and International Standards

Carlos Centeno and Antonio Noguera

K E Y   P O I N T S

- The most widely accepted standards in the field of palliative care focus on organizational or structural dimensions of care provision.
- National organizational standards may be used as a starting point for national change and improved palliative care. The Canadian standards are a good example.
- Clinical standards have been developed. The Liverpool Care Pathway and the Gold Standards Framework are good models for improving the quality of palliative care.
- Although international standards on palliative care are not available, a number of documents from international organizations and certain indicators on the provision of services obtained by means of comparative studies may be valid for reference purposes.

STANDARDS AND QUALITY IN PALLIATIVE CARE

Standards of palliative care are developed to ensure and improve the quality of care. A standard is a normative criterion. It establishes a norm for what may be considered the desired outcome of each resource or process. A *standard statement* is a declaration of desired performance that defines a required or essential condition that should be achieved or maintained. In their formulations, standards are more about how something must be than about how the things must be done. The standard statement is different from guidelines. *Guidelines* are systematically developed statements that assist in making decisions about appropriate health care interventions for specific clinical conditions. The definitions of standards and guidelines often lead to imposing particular methods of auditing or evaluation to determine the degree of compliance of the norms, recommendations, or standards for individual cases or for whole systems.

Defining and proposing standards of quality, developing guidelines, and undertaking audits are three ways of enhancing quality and of ensuring the application of the

principles of palliative care and the hospice movement. There is an increasing demand to establish indicators of quality and effectiveness specific to palliative care, and it is important that the process of developing standards is followed by creating ways to measure the impact made by the standards.

The very existence of standards may serve as an agent for change in the direction of improved care. The interest in designing standards usually is the result of an intention to promote positive development in palliative care. Minimum standards may be put forward to establish a framework with the aim of obtaining funding from a particular health care system or insurance company. The standards also may ensure accreditation for professionals or centers that provide specialized care. The legal implications of particular standards depend on their recognition by the corresponding authority.

Typically, standards are distributed in printed documents, which frequently are available on the Web sites of institutions. Definitions, goals, and the design of existing documents on standards are often different and sometimes unclear. A survey by Lunder and colleagues[1] was carried out in Europe with the aim of reviewing existing documents on standards to gain a deeper understanding of the different quality indicators, standards, and perspectives used for quality improvement in palliative care. Most of the palliative care standards provided criteria that were quantifiable across a variety of settings. Most standards are applicable to all patients, including those with nonmalignant diseases, but few include pediatric palliative care. A small number have proposed practical assessment tools for peer review or audits. To what extent and for what purposes standards are used were not studied in the review.[1] Despite the remarkable work in producing these documents, the study[1] found great variations in documents concerning aims, target groups, areas covered, and structure. There was no common format for a standard, and the terminology used in the documents was often confusing.

CLASSIFICATION AND TYPES OF STANDARDS

Table 44-1 shows some of the types of standards that have been used. In palliative care, development of standards usually has been more focused on the organizational or structural dimensions of care provision. Some organizational standards may concern structural features (i.e., staff, structure, and physical organization of the resource), the processes or activity of providing care, or the results of clinical intervention.[2] Professional standards describe how particular groups of professionals should participate in the care process. These standards may be viewed as a subtype

TABLE 44-1 Standards Used in Palliative Care

AMBIT OF APPLICATION	TYPES OF STANDARDS	STANDARD SUBTYPES	MAIN ISSUES AND COMMENTS
National standards (for provision of palliative care in a country or region)	Organizational standards of practice	Structural standards	Structure of palliative care services, process of providing care, clinical outcomes to achieve
		Standards for professional conduct	Professional acts and competencies
		Minimum standards	Characteristic for access to funds, to use denomination of services, or to accredit professionals in palliative care
	National clinical standards		Address any concrete point of the process of care adopted by the health authority (e.g., home care at the end of life)
	National standards for training	Standards for any professional palliative care worker	Contents of advanced training in palliative care that may be considered as specialist areas in a country
International standards (applicable in any nation or setting)	International standards for palliative care provision	General standards	Some recommendations to governments or international organizations considered as general standards
	Clinical standards		Address any concrete point of the process of care (e.g., last 2 days of life)
	International standards for training		Main characteristic and contents of the process of training in palliative care

of process standards. Some standards define nursing care, the tasks of social workers or hospice chaplains, or the work of palliative care centers.

Clinical standards are focused on defining certain aspects of patient care. A particular clinical process may have great efficiency, become accepted and generalized, and be adopted as standard clinical procedure by others. One example is the Liverpool Care Pathway (discussed later). Other definitions of standards depend on specific aspects of the task, such as standards for training or research in palliative care. For example, the European Association for Palliative Care (EAPC) has made proposals for nursing training.[3]

Broad application of the standards has been proposed. The standards can be subdivided into national and international categories for the purpose of evaluating them.

The Process of Defining Standards

After an organization has established the type of standard to be developed, an approach to working toward it must be outlined. A suitable starting point is a formal review on the definition and mission of the institution. There must also be a clear statement about the target of the standards and about the justification of this goal. After the framework has been decided on, one working method may be the choice of a suitable model of palliative care provision and the adaptation of that model's standards to the individual setting. In other cases, when the group is sufficiently mature or when the work being undertaken involves newer topics, independent development may be attempted.

The definitions of standards are frequently trusted to groups of experts. The methodologies of developing standards vary from dedicated workshops, which last only a few days and draw on the results of prior preparatory working groups, to more formal consensus processes, such as the Delphi method or others, which may be operative over longer periods, possibly lasting several years. It is customary in palliative care to form multidisciplinary groups with experts representing all those who are involved in the process under discussion. During the defi-

nition process, consensus among experts is vital, and it will increase the possibilities of later acceptance. The participation of colleagues from other specialties, diverse scientific associations, policy makers, managers, and the users or beneficiaries of palliative care services is recommended during part or all of the definition process or at the end of the process as part of the review procedure. Because the standards proposed should be as widely accepted as possible, their dissemination should be as broad as possible.

NATIONAL STANDARDS

Developing Standards of Palliative Care in Different Countries

We speak of *national palliative care standards* when the norms or recommendations on quality are proposed for the resources of one particular nation. No one common standard can be designed for application in different countries. When comparing various national standards, we find a common basis for principles and common roots in the methodology applied, but there are great differences in the methods for developing palliative care structures or programs. There is a logical basis for adapting and localizing general principles of palliative care because each cultural, political, and geographical setting possesses individual features that influence care. Although palliative care is applied more and more universally, individual disparities in definitions remain. For example, *hospice* in Scotland has a very different meaning from the same term in California. In many Mediterranean countries, *hospice* as a term is devoid of meaning, but the palliative resources found in one country are very similar to those seen at a nursing home in Holland. For this reason, developing norms or standards for hospice or palliative care in each country is recommended.

Standards to be applied on a national scale usually are proposed by institutions, scientific associations, national palliative care organizations, or specific professional groups. Each body defines its interest as achieving a specific degree of development in palliative care in its own setting. The health care authorities of a country often collaborate in the development of standards of quality. This support is evident in the backing given to the definition process or to the final results. Sometimes, collaboration is limited to the diffusion of information. Standard design has been an efficient measure for the good, quick development of palliative care. It is worth citing countries such as Germany or Holland, which in less than a decade have set up extensive networks of quality care services for the terminal-stage patient, or many countries of Eastern Europe, which have adopted the implementation of basic standards as key goals for the development of palliative care.[4]

National standards reflect the degree of palliative care development in individual countries and the particular concerns of health care systems within the same settings. As an example, in many countries in Western Europe, decision making must be carried out with the patient. In Eastern Europe, palliative standards are based more on equality by developing an appropriate care network that allows access to this type of assistance by the entire population within a country.

International cooperation may be a determinant in developing a country's standards. For example, the standards of the Romanian Society of Palliative Care were developed in collaboration with experts from the United States and with Romanian palliative care professionals. This process is described later. Organizations such as the National Hospice and Palliative Care Organization (NHPCO) or Help the Hospices[5] offer a range of different programs to support the development of palliative care in developing countries. The EAPC organized the Eastern European Task Force[6] to promote the development of palliative care in the countries of that region.

The study on national standards in different countries may be a valuable source of information to define or review particular standards. Table 44-2 compares the standards adopted by national bodies and indicates the name, language, year of publication, and Web site addresses. An attempt was made to identify documents available in English, but in some cases, the documents are available in other languages.

Standards of organization have undergone more thorough development in countries with longer traditions in palliative care, especially in the Anglo-Saxon community. Most of the current standards have been established over the past 5 years. In the United Kingdom, different standards are used in Wales, Scotland, and England. Most standards have been developed by scientific or professional bodies, but some have been developed by wider-ranging initiatives, such as the Joint Commission in the United States. In some countries, different bodies provide diverse views, and specific standards have been adopted for specific professional groups (e.g., nursing practitioners) or for specific activities (e.g., home care, bereavement).

When a country enacts quality standards, a process of change automatically begins. The efforts employed in the process give rise to new needs. To respond to these needs, new standards directed at more precisely defined areas of intervention are established. This trend has been observed in countries with a longer tradition of palliative care, where ongoing development has led to continuous review of existing standards.

Models of National Structural Standards

Standards for Providing Quality Palliative Care for All Australians

Standards for providing quality palliative care recognize and reflect the considerable effort and success that some sectors have had in developing and implementing coordinated, network-based approaches to service development and delivery.[7] The methodology represents a great change with respect to the 1999 publication of the standards for palliative care for Australians, which was based on the holistic approach closely linked to palliative care, which had a greater philosophical bias, and in which each group of affirmations related to the different aspects of care: physical, psychological, social, and spiritual.

The new edition of the Australian standards is the product of efforts to promote greater coordination between the different levels of care and to identify the aims at each level for each standard. Care is divided into four levels, with the lower one defined as primary care and the three upper levels characterized by the presence of palliative care specialists. In primary care, a preliminary assessment is performed, together with the selection and evaluation of the need for specific support. The first specialist level includes health care attention for complex patients and the evaluation of the primary care teams. At the second and third specialist levels, as well as care for complex patients, there is ongoing training of other specialists and the training of new palliative care specialists, respectively.

The Australian standards emphasize social solidarity between neighbors, increasing social awareness about the growing problem of chronic disease and the rising number of frail patients. They recognize the need for an accurate social focus to promote dignified support for the Aborigine population, respecting their way of life.

National Organizational Standards as a Focus for National Change and Improved Palliative Care in Canada

In the late 1980s, several individuals and organizations across Canada recognized that there was no common language and no widely accepted standards to guide hospice or palliative care practice. From 1989 to 2002, a precedent-setting, iterative, consensus-building process involved thousands of stakeholders. In 2002, after more than 75% agreement was reached, a nationally accepted *Model to Guide Hospice Palliative Care*[8] was published by Canadian Hospice Palliative Care. It included definitions for many commonly used terms, and it suggested values, principles, and norms of practice to guide organizational development and care delivery.[8]

Since the *Model to Guide Hospice Palliative Care* was published in 2002, it has been endorsed by all of the major hospice palliative care associations and several national medical organizations in the country. It is being adopted and adapted by many individual hospice palliative care providers, and it forms the basis for many health care initiatives to expand palliative care services and for many educational, research, and advocacy activities. It is being adapted to produce companion standards of practice for nurses (through the Canadian Nurses Association), social

TABLE 44-2 Standards Available on Internet

COUNTRY	ORGANIZATION	DOCUMENT	YEAR	LANGUAGE	WEB SITES*
Australia	Palliative Care Australia	Standards for Providing Quality Palliative Care for All Australians	2005	English	http://www.pallcare.org.au/Portals/46/docs/Standards%20Palliative%20Care.pdf
Austria	Hospiz Oesterreich	Sozialarbeit im Bereich Palliative Care	2003	German	http://www.hospiz.at/
Canada	Canadian Hospice Palliative Care Association	The Pan-Canadian Gold Standard for Palliative Home Care	2006	English, French	http://www.chpca.net/home.htm
		A Model to Guide Hospice Palliative Care: Based on National Principles and Norms of Practice	2005		http://www.chpca.net/marketplace/national_norms/national_norms_of_practice.htm
		Hospice Palliative Care Nursing Standards of Practice	2002		http://www.chpca.net/marketplace/nursing_norms/Hospice_Palliative_Care_Nursing_Standards_of_Practice.pdf
Czech Republic	Asociace Poskytovatelu Hospicové Paliativní Péce	Standardy Hospicové Paliativní Péce	2006	Czech	http://www.asociacehospicu.cz/download/standardy.doc
Germany	Deutsche Gesellschaft für Palliativmedizin e.V.	Palliative Care Lehren, Lernen, Leben (i.e., Nurse Standards)		German	http://www.dgpalliativmedizin.de/
	Der Hospize-Verlag	HOPE 2006 (i.e., Standard Documentation System)			http://www.hospizverlag.de/index.php?bef=menue&menue=12&art=13
		SORGSAM—Qualitätshandbuch für stationäre Hospize (i.e., Hospice Standards)			www.palliativmed.org/asset/33124/1/33124_1.pdf
Norway	Norsk Forening for Palliativ Medisin	Standard for Palliasjon	2004	Norwegian	
United Kingdom	National Health System	Gold Standards Framework (GSF) for Palliative Care	2001	English	http://www.goldstandardsframework.nhs.uk/advanced_care.php
	Association of Hospice and Palliative Care Chaplains	Standards for Hospice & Palliative Care Chaplaincy	2006		http://www.ahpcc.org.uk/pdffiles/AHPCC%20Standards%202006.pdf
United States	National Hospice and Palliative Care Organization	Standards of Practice for Hospice Programs		English	www.nhpco.org/marketplace

Continued

TABLE 44-2 Standards Available on Internet—cont'd

COUNTRY	ORGANIZATION	DOCUMENT	YEAR	LANGUAGE	WEB SITES*
	Joint Commission on the Accreditation of Healthcare Organizations (JCAHO)† Quality Palliative Care	Crosswalk of JCAHO Standards and Palliative Care with Palliative Care Policies Procedures and Assessment Tools	2004		http://www.capc.org/support-from-capc/capc_publications/JCAHO-crosswalk.pdf
	National Association of Social Workers (NASW)	NASW Standards for Palliative and End-of-Life Care	2004		http://www.socialworkers.org/practice/bereavement/standards/default.asp
	American Nurses Association	Scope and Standards for Hospice and Palliative Nursing Practice	2002		http://www.hpna.org/Publications_HPN22.aspx
Poland	Polish Association for Palliative Care	Standard of Medical Service Provision: Palliative Medicine—Materials for Service Providers and Payers	1999	English	http://health.osf.lt/downloads/news/Luczak-Polish%20PALLMED%20standards.doc
Portugal	Asociação Nacional de Cuidados Paliativos	Critérios de Qualidade para Unidades de Cuidados Paliativos	2006	Portuguese	http://www.apcp.com.pt/index.php?sc=vis&id=229&cod=68
Romania	Asociata Nationala de Ingrijiri Paliative	Standarde Nationale Îngrijirea Paliativa	2002	Romanian, English	http://www.nhpco.org/files/public/national_standards.doc
Scotland	Scottish Partnership for Palliative Care	Making Good Care Better (national practice statements for general palliative care in adult care homes in Scotland)	2006	English	http://www.palliativecarescotland.org.uk/publications/
		NHS Quality Improvement Scotland	2004		
		Palliative Care in Community Hospitals in Scotland: A Framework for Good Practice	2003		
		Clinical Standards for Specialist Palliative Care	2002		
		Palliative Care for Young People Aged 13-24	2001		
		National Care Standards: Hospice Care	2002		http://www.scotland.gov.uk/Resource/Doc/1095/0001719.pdf
Switzerland	Swiss Society for Palliative Care	Standards für Palliative Medizin, Pflege und Begleitung in der Schweiz	2001	German, French, Italian	http://www.palliative.ch/de/index.php

*Web sites were accessed September 26, 2007.
†The Joint Commission on the Accreditation of Healthcare Organizations (JCAHO) is now called The Joint Commission (JC).

workers, counselors, and volunteers; for pediatric health care; for provincial and national norms of practice for hospices; and for hospital and long-term care accreditation (through the Canadian Council on Health Services Accreditation). All of this activity strongly suggests that the process of developing national standards can provide a significant focus, the content, and the energy needed to motivate policy makers, regulators, administrators, and clinicians to change palliative care delivery for patients and families.[8]

National Palliative Care Standards in Romania

The National Palliative Care Standards in Romania (Standarde Nationale Îngrijirea Paliativa) are the fruit of cooperation between the Hospice Casa Sperantei and the National Hospice and Palliative Care Organization (NHPCO), with funding provided by the U.S. Agency for International Development (USAID).[9] The document describes the need to provide palliative care to all patients in need of it, and it establishes the fundamental bases for the way in which palliative care should be provided in a hospice. It outlines the need for development of different kinds of teams, which should be assembled to create a complete palliative care network.

The document focuses on the pediatric population. In Romania, this group has been identified as requiring special attention. It identifies international support as an indispensable source of obtaining funds to permit the maintenance of this kind of care, and it mentions the need for centers of excellence, where professionals can be trained. It is a good example of the establishment of basic standards as a function of the current situation and needs of the country, which leads to the development and evolution of palliative care.

Several Standards of Palliative Care in the United States

Examples of U.S. standards for palliative care promoted by diverse bodies are shown in Table 44-3. The earliest standards for hospice care were formulated in 1974 by a committee of the International Work Group on Death and Dying.[10] In 1981, the W. K. Kellogg Foundation awarded a grant to the Joint Commission for the Accreditation of Healthcare Organizations (JCAHO) (now called The Joint Commission [JC]) to investigate the status of hospice in the United States and to develop standards for accreditation.[11] Since then, widely accepted norms and standards of practice based on the needs and expectations of patients and families have been developed. These models can be used to guide programs as they develop their own standards of practice.

In 2006, the Standards of Practice for Hospice Programs were updated.[12] They are organized around the components of quality in hospice care: rights and ethics, crosswalk of standards, hospice inpatient facilities, human resources, interdisciplinary teams, leadership, and governance. These standards are intended for self-assessment and ongoing use in performance improvement and national hospice quality initiatives. A specific self-assessment tool was developed to evaluate each group of standards. After each group of standards is a set of practice examples, which are intended to teach various ways of implement-

TABLE 44-3 Standards of Palliative Care or End-of-Life Care Available in the United States

INSTITUTION	STANDARD
American Association of Colleges of Nursing	Competencies and Curricular Guidelines for End-of-Life Nursing Care
American Geriatrics Society (AGS)	Position Statement: The Care of Dying Patients
American Society of Clinical Oncology (ASCO)	Cancer Care During the Last Phases of Life.
Children's Hospice International (CHI)	Standards for Hospice Care for Children
Grace Project	End-of-Life Care Standards of Practice for Inmates in Correctional Settings
Joint Commission on the Accreditation of Healthcare Organizations*	Pain Standards 2001
Last Acts	Compendium of Guidelines and Position Statements
	Precepts of Palliative Care
Milbank Memorial Fund	Principles for Care of Patients at the End of Life
National Hospice and Palliative Care Organization	Hospice Standards of Practice

*The Joint Commission on the Accreditation of Healthcare Organizations (JCAHO) is now called The Joint Commission (JC).
Modified from Von Guten CF, Ferris FD, Poetenoy RK, Glajchen M (eds). How to Establish a Palliative Care Program. New York: Center for Advance Palliative Care, 2001. Available at http://64.85.16.230/educate/content/elements/normsofpractice.html (accessed September 26, 2007).

ing the standards. The practice examples are not intended to be requirements or descriptions of the best or only way to meet the standards. They are examples from practice that can be imitated or used to spur ideas and creativity. This is a way to set benchmarks for a hospice and to assess the services it provides. The monograph includes appendices on hospices in nursing facilities and hospice inpatient facilities, and it is consistent with the standards of Medicare, JCAHO, and the Community Health Accreditation Program (CHAP).

Models of Good Practice in Palliative Care Achieved through Development of Clinical Standards

The Gold Standards Framework: Optimizing the Care Delivered by Primary Care Teams in the United Kingdom

The Gold Standards Framework (GSF) is a systematic approach to optimizing the care delivered by primary care teams in the United Kingdom for any patient nearing the end of life in the community.[13] It was developed from within primary care for primary care by Keri Thomas, a physician with a special interest in palliative care and the National Health Service (NHS) clinical lead for generalist palliative care (formerly a Macmillan general practitioner facilitator), and it was supported by a multidisciplinary reference group of specialists and generalists to improve palliative care provided in the community by the patient's usual health care team. It was piloted in West Yorkshire in 2001 with 12 practices and was then expanded to another 78 practices in 18 areas, followed by a national phased program supported by Macmillan and the Cancer Services Collaborative.

GSF is now part of the NHS End-of-Life Care Program, which posits that the care of the dying must be raised to the level of the best because improving the reliability and quality of home care is a basic step in improving end-of-life care for all patients. The GSF is a common sense approach to formalizing the best practice standards, so that good care becomes standard for all patients every time. The GSF is a tested group of strategies, tasks, and enabling tools to help primary care teams deliver the best possible care for people nearing the end of their lives (Box 44-1). GSF is a generic improvement tool. It was developed initially for the primary care of cancer patients by primary care practitioners, but it is now used for any patient with a life-limiting illness and in other settings such as care homes.

The Liverpool Care Pathway: A Minimum Clinical Standard for the Dying

Integrated care pathways (ICPs) provide a method of recording and measuring outcomes of care in the last days. The ICP document replaces all previous documentation and is a multiprofessional record of patient care.

The aim of the Liverpool Care Pathway for the Dying Patient (LCP) was to implement an ICP in an inpatient hospice setting to set standards of care for symptom control in the dying phase of a patient's life.[14] The LCP is an evidence-based document that acts as a guide for health care professionals when caring for patients in the last days of their lives. It is a multiprofessional document providing an evidence-based framework for the dying phase. The LCP starts when the multiprofessional team agrees that the patient is dying and two or more of the following descriptions apply: bed bound, semicomatose, only able to take sips of fluid, and no longer able to take tablets. Then the framework of LCP includes three stages: initial assessment and care, ongoing care, and care after death, with physical, psychosocial, and spiritual care as a goal of care in each stage. These stages act as prompts. If it is more appropriate to manage a patient in a different way, notes are recorded on a variance sheet with the justification for the change.

The LCP provides an evidence-based framework for the dying phase. The LCP specifies treatment and care for a given condition based on nationally accepted guidelines, standards, and protocols. It provides a consistent standard of documentation and provides the basis for an ongoing audit. It ensures a consistently good standard of care, even when the professional changes or has a different background or experiences. The LCP was developed to transfer the hospice model of care into other care settings. Widely used in hospitals, it also has been adopted for use in hospices, in nursing homes, for pediatric terminal care, and for the care of noncancer patients.

The Pan-Canadian Gold Standard for Palliative Home Care

The Pan-Canadian Gold Standard for Palliative Home Care was developed to ensure equitable access to high-quality hospice palliative and end-of-life care at home.[15] The starting point was the recognition that Canadians prefer to spend their final days at home. Faced with this need, the public health care system encountered two problems to

---

Box 44-1 The Gold Standards Framework

One Aim

There is one chance to aim for the best care for all, one gold standard to aspire to for all patients nearing the end of life, whatever the diagnosis, stage, or setting.

Three Processes

The processes of the Gold Standards Framework (GSF) all involve improved communication:

1. Identify patients in need of palliative or supportive care toward the end of life.
2. Assess patients' needs, symptoms, preferences, and any issues important to them.
3. Plan care around patients' needs and preferences, and enable these requirements and requests to be fulfilled; particularly, allow patients to live and die where they choose.

Five Goals

GSF goals are to provide high-quality care for people in the final months of life in the community:

1. Symptoms of patients are as controlled as possible.
2. Patients are enabled to live well and die well in their place of choice.
3. Security and support include better advanced care planning, information, less fear, and fewer crises and admissions to the hospital.
4. Caregivers are supported, informed, enabled, and empowered.
5. Staff confidence, communication, and co-working are improved.

Seven Key Tasks

The GSF standards (www.goldstandardsframework.nhs.uk) include 7 Cs that detail specific tasks and suggest means to achieve them:

C1 Communication
C2 Coordination of care
C3 Control of symptoms and ongoing assessment
C4 Continuing support, including during off hours
C5 Continued learning
C6 Caregiver and family support
C7 Care during the dying phase

From www.goldstandardsframework.nhs.uk.

be resolved: that patients in need of palliative care do not have access to 24 hours-per-day, 7 days-per-week caregiving if they are looked after in their own homes and that there are problems of access to specific material and medicines needed for full care provision in the home. To provide a solution to these problems, the GSF adopted a number of measures that aim to provide to all patients full-time, round-the-clock specialist nursing care, to ensure that the nurse attending these patients has the support and advice of a multidisciplinary palliative care team, and to create a list of essential material and medications for the treatment and care of these patients that should be available at all times from any pharmacy and be financed entirely by public funding.

INTERNATIONAL STANDARDS

International standards are statements that define a required or essential condition to be achieved or maintained in a specific group of countries or in all countries. There are several reasons why international standards for palliative care do not exist as they do for national or more localized standards. Transnational professional organizations are in their earliest stages, and the difficulties of defining various aspects of palliative care are experienced on an international level. International bodies do not normally have the responsibility for the provision of health care services; they are instead concerned with health care policies.

In the absence of international standards of organization, we can refer to important recommendations on palliative care that have been issued by various international bodies. Some authorities consider these documents to be the general standards for palliative care internationally.[16] Some indicators of the provision of palliative care obtained from international studies also can be used for reference when comparing developments in a particular country.

Recommendations by International Organizations for the Development of Palliative Care Services

Diverse international organizations have shown their interest in palliative care and have issued declarations or recommendations to governments concerning the "way things should be" for the care of dying patients. World Health Organization (WHO) publications on palliative care stand out because of the importance of the body behind them, their widespread distribution, and their importance in the 1990s, the early years in the development of palliative care in many countries.[17,18] Later, the WHO again raised the issue of the development of palliative care with two important documents. *Palliative Care for Older People*[19] recognizes that the elderly have traditionally received less palliative care than younger people and that services have focused on cancer. The booklet is part of the WHO Regional Office for Europe's work to present evidence for health policy and decision makers in a clear and understandable form. It describes the needs of older people, the different trajectories of illnesses they suffer, evidence of underassessment of pain and other symptoms, their need to be involved in decision making, evidence for effective palliative care solutions, and issues

for the future. The second publication is a companion booklet entitled *Palliative Care—The Solid Facts,*[20] and it considers how to improve services and educate professionals and the public.

In Europe, widespread dissemination has taken place of the declaration "Recommendation 24 (2003) of the Committee of Ministers to Member States on the Organization of Palliative Care and Explanatory Memorandum."[21] The document, which has been translated into many languages, makes four main recommendations to governments:

- Adopt policies, legislative tools, and other measures necessary for a coherent and comprehensive national policy framework for palliative care
- When feasible, take the measures presented in the appendix of this recommendation, taking account of particular national circumstances
- Promote international networking among organizations, research institutions, and other agencies that are active in the palliative care field
- Support active, targeted dissemination of this recommendation and its explanatory memorandum, accompanied by a translation where appropriate

An internationally relevant body, the EAPC, has released a number of recommendations on the training of nurses in palliative care[3] that have been widely distributed.

Indicators on the Provision of Palliative Care in Different Countries

No single country has achieved the gold standard of palliative care compared with others. Nevertheless, the development of palliative care in several, more-developed countries may be useful for comparison. Valid, reliable data are needed on how patients requiring palliative care are being looked after. Many governments do not know whether their citizens are receiving appropriate care, whether the programs launched are improving the situation, and whether the results are comparable to those of other countries in similar geographical settings. Despite difficulties in measuring how patients are treated at the end of their lives, certain strategies should be adopted by all countries in the future.[22]

Although making policies about palliative care on a European level remains elusive, some studies and initiatives have been designed to create an evidence base for what is occurring on the national level. Some work has been done to generate comparative analyses of countries and contexts.

The EAPC Task Force on the Development of Palliative Care in Europe began its work in 2003, reporting in full by the end of 2006. Led by the EAPC, the collaboration included members of the EAPC, the International Observatory of End-of-Life Care (IOELC), Help the Hospices, and the International Association for Hospice and Palliative Care. This survey represents the most cooperative effort ever done. Tables 44-4 and 44-5 show some results, with several indicators of the development of palliative care in Western European countries. Since the late 1990s, the evidence base for palliative care in Europe has improved, and several facts and figures are shown in the tables.

TABLE 44-4   Provision of Specific Palliative Care Resources

COUNTRY	INPATIENT UNITS	HOSPICES	HOSPITAL SUPPORT TEAMS	HOME CARE TEAMS	TOTAL SPECIFIC RESOURCES	POPULATION (MILLIONS)	SERVICES/ MILLION PEOPLE
Iceland	2	0	1	3	6	0	20
United Kingdom	63	158	305	356	882	60	16
Sweden	40	5	10	50	105	9	12
Belgium	29	0	77	15	121	10	12
Ireland	8	0	22	14	44	4	9
Luxemburg	1	0	1	2	4	0	9
Netherlands	4	84	50	—	138	16	8
France	78	0	309	84	471	61	8
Norway	12	2	16	1	31	5	7
Austria	18	7	10	17	52	8	6
Spain	95	0	27	139	261	43	6
Switzerland	12	5	7	14	38	7	5
Finland	2	4	10	10	26	5	5
Germany	106	129	56	30	321	83	4
Italy	5	90	—	143	238	59	4
Israel	5	4	3	14	26	7	4
Denmark	1	6	6	5	18	5	3
Cyprus	0	1	0	2	3	1	3
Malta	0	0	1	0	1	0	3
Portugal	3	1	1	3	8	10	1
Greece	0	0	20	9	29	11	1
Turkey	10	1	10	0	21	74	0.3

TABLE 44-5   Provision of Specialist Palliative Care Beds and Estimates of Full-Time Physicians in 19 Countries

COUNTRY	TOTAL DEDICATED PALLIATIVE CARE BEDS	RATIO OF DEDICATED BEDS TO POPULATION	TOTAL FULL-TIME PHYSICIANS	RATIO OF FULL-TIME PHYSICIANS TO POPULATION
Luxemburg	39	86	—	—
Sweden	650	72	300	1:30,147
Iceland	17	58	1	1:294,947
United Kingdom	3180	53	442	1:135,496
Norway	220	48	—	—
Netherlands	716	44	10	1:1,632,258
Ireland	147	37	40	1:100,683
France	1615	27	361	1:167,922
Austria	209	26	35	1:232,251
Spain	1098	25	492	1:88,283
Germany	2034	25	—	—
Belgium	216	21	14	1:745,929
Cyprus	18	19	2	1:475,474
Italy	1095	19	1000	1:58,609
Denmark	90	17	12	1:450,966
Finland	75	14	10	1:524,692
Israel	78	11	10	1:698,664
Portugal	53	5	6	1:743,862
Turkey	241	3	—	—

Comparative studies help to advance policy making to promote palliative care in Europe. Such work should be rooted in public health and social science models and should consider the provision of palliative care within the wider milieux of health and social care policies and many social, ethical, and cultural factors. The work should recognize the complex character of palliative care provision in many countries and the combination of statutory, voluntary, and civil society organizations that are involved. There are encouraging signs of productive alliances that can produce important research evidence in a context in which high-quality data can be hard to obtain. Interest in studying palliative care development at the world level has never been greater.[23]

RESEARCH OPPORTUNITIES IN PALLIATIVE CARE

Sharing definitions for all possible palliative care services and resources would help in developing standards of care and allow comparisons between regions or countries. Future research projects should include measurement of the impact of structural standards in developing palliative care in various countries.

Consensus among scientific societies and international organizations of professionals working in palliative care should be encouraged to develop international structural standards. International comparative studies can greatly advance policy making to promote palliative care in Europe and other regions of the world.

CONCLUSIONS

The development of standards in palliative care is a first step toward ensuring the quality of care administered. These standards are important for all who work directly with patients and for policy makers and health care providers. Some clinical standards are becoming accepted, which is an encouraging sign that the importance of quality palliative care is being more widely appreciated.

REFERENCES

1. Lunder U. Palliative care standards. Presented at the Palliative Care Policy Development Conference, Budapest, October 16-18, 2003. Available at http://health.osf.lt/en/archive/2003/index.php?id=1287&no=0&gid=(accessed October 4, 2007).
2. Glickman M, for the Working Party on Standards. Making Palliative Care Better: Quality Improvement, Multiprofessional Audit, and Standards. Occasional paper no. 12, March 1997. London: National Council for Palliative Care, 1997.
3. Vlieger M, Gorchs N, Larkin PJ, et al. Palliative nurse education: Towards a common language. Palliat Med 2004;18:401-403.
4. Wright M, Clark J, Greenwood A, et al. Palliative care policy development in Central and Eastern Europe and Central Asia: An Open Society Institute initiative. Conference Report: Palliative Care Policy Development, Budapest, October 16-18, 2007. Available at http://health.osf.lt/en/archive/2003/index.php?id=1287&no=0&gid= (accessed October 4, 2007).
5. Help the Hospices. Grants. Available at http://www.helpthehospices.org.uk/grants/index.asp (accessed October 4, 2007).
6. Fürst CJ. The European Association for Palliative Care Initiative in Eastern Europe. J Pain Symptom Manage 2002;24,134-135.
7. Palliative Care Australia. A Guide to Palliative Care Service Development: A Population Based Approach. Canberra: Palliative Care Australia, May 2005. Available at http://www.pallcare.org.au/Portals/46/docs/Standards%20Palliative%20Care.pdf (accessed October 4, 2007).
8. Ferris FD, Balfour HM, Bowen K, et al. A Model to Guide Hospice Palliative Care: Based on National Principles and Norms of Practice. Ottawa, Ontario: Canadian Hospice National Care Association, 2002; updated 2005. Available at http://www.chpca.net/marketplace/national_norms/national_norms_of_practice.htm (accessed October 4, 2007).
9. Standarde Naţionale Îngrijirea Paliativa [National Standards in Palliative Care]. Asociata Nationala de Îngrijiri Paliative, 2002. Available at http://www.nhpco.org/files/public/national_standards.doc (accessed October 4, 2007).
10. Kastenbaum R. Toward standards of care for the terminally ill: What standards exist today? Omega 1975;6:289-290.
11. McCann B: JCAH hospice project: Proposed standards. Caring 1983;2:15-27.
12. National Hospice and Palliative Care Organization. Standards of Practice for Hospice Programs, 2006. Available at http://iweb.nhpco.org/iweb/Purchase/ProductDetail.aspx?Product_code=711077 (accessed October 4, 2007).
13. Thomas K. Improving the delivery of palliative care in general practice: An evaluation of the first phase of the Gold Standards Framework. Palliat Med 2007;21:49-53.
14. Ellershaw J, Smith C, Overill S, et al. Care of the dying: Setting standards for symptom control in the last 48 hours of life. J Pain Symptom Manage 2001;21:12-17.
15. Canadian Hospice Palliative Care Association. The Pan-Canadian Gold Standard for Palliative Home Care. Ottawa, Ontario: Canadian Hospice Palliative Care Association, December 2006. Available at http://www.chpca.net/home.htm (accessed October 4, 2007).
16. Robbins M. Evaluating Palliative Care. Establishing the Evidence Base. New York: Oxford University Press, 1998, pp 29-59.
17. World Health Organization (WHO) Regional Office for Europe. Palliative cancer care: Policy statement based on the recommendations of a WHO consultation, Leeds, February 10-11, 1987. Copenhagen: WHO Regional Office for Europe, 1989.
18. World Health Organization (WHO). Cancer pain relief and palliative care: Report of a WHO Expert Committee. Geneva: WHO Technical Report Series 804, 1990.
19. Davies E, Higginson IJ (eds). Better palliative care for older people. Copenhagen: WHO, 2004.
20. Davies E, Higginson IJ (eds). Palliative care: The solid facts. Copenhagen: WHO, 2004.
21. Recomendación Rec 24 (2003) del Comité de Ministros Sobre la Organización de los Cuidados Paliativos, CM 130, Addendum 15, Octubre 2003. Documentos CM6.3. Comité Europeo de Salud (CDSP), 2003.
22. Casaret DJ: How should nations measure the quality of end-of-life care for older adults? Recommendations for an international minimum data set. J Am Geriatr Soc 2006;54:1765-1771.
23. Clark D. Palliative care in Europe: An emerging approach to comparative analysis. Clin Med 2006;6:197-201.

SUGGESTED READING

Ellershaw JE, Wilkinson S. Care of the Dying: A Pathway to Excellence. Oxford, UK: Oxford University Press, 2003.

Ferris FD, Balfour HM, Bowen K, et al. A Model to Guide Hospice Palliative Care: Based on National Principles and Norms of Practice. Ottawa, Ontario: Canadian Hospice National Care Association, 2002. Available at http://www.chpca.net/marketplace/national_norms/national_norms_of_practice.htm (accessed October 4, 2007).

Glickman M, for the Working Party on Standards. Making Palliative Care Better: Quality Improvement, Multiprofessional Audit, and Standards. Occasional paper no. 12, March 1997. London: National Council for Palliative Care, 1997.

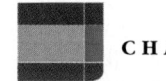

CHAPTER **45**

Clinical Practice Guidelines

Helen M. Morrison and John Welsh

K E Y   P O I N T S

- There is great variation in the quality of practice guidelines, and quality can be improved by rigorous methodology, such as that in the AGREE instrument.
- Guidelines should be based on a validated, systematic review of the evidence.
- Evidence should be graded, and recommendations should be explicitly linked to the evidence.
- Dissemination and implementation strategies are crucial to change practice and improve outcomes.
- High-quality guidelines are facilitated by an increased evidence base.

Practice guidelines, defined as systematically developed statements to assist decisions of practitioners and patients about appropriate health care for specific clinical circumstances,[1] have been produced since the late 1970s. The past decade has seen a dramatic increase in the number produced worldwide. This expansion was driven by evidence-based medicine and an increasing need for health care purchasers to base spending on proven effective measures. Guidelines usually aim to improve consistency of care and cost-effectiveness. Where there is variation in practice, explicit guidelines improve clinical practice.[2]

Historically, guidelines were derived from consensus or experts based on opinion, experience, and available evidence. Currently, the explicit methods used are based on systematic review of the evidence. In the United Kingdom, professional bodies backed by the National Health Service are producing evidence-based guidelines. For example, the Scottish Intercollegiate Guideline Network aims to reduce variations in practice by national evidence-based guidelines that are adapted locally.[3] Similarly, in the United States, there is effectively a substantial guideline industry, but there is wide variation in the rigor of the process, and many guidelines are still based on opinion or consensus.[4] The potential to improve practice depends on the quality of the guideline, and the generation of palliative care guidelines is hampered by insufficient evidence.

GUIDELINE DEVELOPMENT

There are three main methods: informal consensus, formal consensus, and evidence linked. Informal consensus is inexpensive and rapid, but the decision-making criteria are ill defined, and recommendations are based on experience and opinion, not evidence. This approach is likely to be employed by local guideline developers. Formal consensus methods include consensus development conferences and the Delphi technique. Although these are more structured, recommendations are still not linked to evidence quality. The evidence-linked method requires explicit linkage of recommendations to evidence. It is the best method for producing credible, valid guidelines.[5]

The development process is crucial to ensure valid guidelines, and it must overcome potential biases.[6] International collaboration led to the Appraisal of Guidelines for Research and Evaluation (AGREE) instrument as a standard for appraising guidelines, but it is also useful for guideline developers (e.g., Scottish Intercollegiate Guidelines Network [SIGN]). The instrument consists of six domains, each with subheadings and with criteria for good-quality practice guidelines (Box 45-1).[7]

Scope and Purpose

The initial step, choosing the topic, requires careful consideration (see "Common Errors"). The topic should be important to the delivery or outcome of patient care. It is often chosen because of unexplained or considerable practice variations, or it is a national priority (e.g., coronary heart disease, cancer). The objectives must be specific and detailed, usually better patient outcomes (e.g.,

Box 45-1 Appraisal of Guidelines for Research and Evaluation in Europe (AGREE) Instrument

Scope and Purpose

The overall guideline objectives are specifically described.
The clinical questions covered by the guideline are specifically described.
The patient population affected is specifically described.

Stakeholder Involvement

The guideline development group includes people from all relevant professional groups.
Patients' views and preferences are sought.
The target users of the guideline are clearly defined.
The guideline has a pilot test among targeted users.

Rigor of Development

Systematic methods were used to search for evidence.
The criteria for evidence selection are clearly described.
Methods used for formulating recommendations are clearly described.
Health benefits, side effects, and risks are considered in the recommendations.
There are explicit links between the recommendations and the supporting evidence.
The guideline has been externally reviewed by experts before publication.
A procedure for updating the guideline is provided.

Clarity and Presentation

The recommendations are specific and unambiguous.
The different options for management of the condition are clearly presented.
Key recommendations are easily identifiable.
The guideline is supported with tools for application.

Applicability

Potential organizational barriers to applying the recommendations have been discussed.
Potential cost implications of applying the recommendations have been considered.
The guideline identifies key review criteria for monitoring and audit purposes.

Editorial Independence

The guideline is editorially independent from the funding body.
Conflicts of interest of guideline development members have been recorded.

From The AGREE Collaboration. The Appraisal of Guidelines for Research and Evaluation (AGREE) Instrument, 2001. London: The AGREE Research Trust. Available online www.agreetrust.org (accessed March 10, 2008).

reducing skeletal events caused by bone metastases from breast cancer) or delivery of care. The clinical questions must be specific to ensure that recommendations are evidence based and the target population is carefully defined. Without these constraints, it is difficult to synthesize evidence and formulate recommendations.

Common Errors
Guideline Development
• Failure to address specific questions • Failure to involve all relevant stakeholders • Failure to perform systematic review • Failure to explicitly link recommendations to the level of evidence
Dissemination and Implementation
• Inadequate dissemination strategies (e.g., lack of educational strategies) • Lack of implementation strategies
Interpretation
Uncritical application of guidelines in patient management Misconception that guidelines diminish the role of the physician

Box 45-2 Hierarchy of Evidence of the Agency for Health Care Policy and Research
1. Systematic reviews and meta-analyses of randomized, controlled trials 2. Randomized, controlled trials 3. Nonrandomized intervention studies 4. Observational studies 5. Nonexperimental studies 6. Expert opinion

From United States Department of Health and Human Services, Agency for Health Care Policy and Research. Acute Pain Management: Operative or Medical Procedures and Trauma. Clinical practice guideline no. 1, AHCPR publication no. 92-0023. Rockville, MD: U.S. Department of Health and Human Services, 1993.

Stakeholder Involvement

The composition of a development group influences credibility. Teams should be multidisciplinary and representative of all professional groups who will use the guideline (i.e., the stakeholders), avoiding any party being overrepresented or underrepresented.[6] If one group feels underrepresented, the guideline may not be implemented because of the lack of participation.

The composition includes patients' experiences and opinions, which are important in a valid and credible guideline. Patient or caregiver groups often are represented on guideline development panels. If their direct involvement is inappropriate or impossible, relevant information should be sought from patient interviews and research into patients' experiences.[7]

Multidisciplinary involvement can result in large teams. Balance must be achieved between representation of all stakeholders and team function. An international survey of 18 guideline programs showed that groups typically have 10 to 20 members; many included epidemiologists, and patients were represented in 61%.[8] As with any team, leadership and the skill mix are crucial; members need adequate skills, time, and motivation.[9] Administrative and technical supports are vital. Multidisciplinary teams require resources, and smaller organizations and societies may have difficulties. To determine the individual relevance of a guideline, target users should be defined by validation through a pilot process.

Rigor of Development

Synthesis of Evidence

Evidence can be obtained in three ways: expert opinions, unsystematic literature reviews, and systematic literature reviews. Expert opinion is likely to be biased, strongly influenced by personal beliefs and experience. Unsystematic literature reviews obtain evidence, but the approach is not systematic, and results are likely to be biased by the reviewer. Systematic review is "an efficient scientific technique to identify and summarize evidence on the effective-

ness of interventions and to allow the generalizability and consistency of research findings to be assessed and data inconsistencies to be explored."[10] A systematic review is the most crucial step in evidence-based guidelines because it can identify all the evidence for the specific clinical question. The strategies for obtaining evidence should be detailed in a guideline, and sources likely include electronic databases (which have revolutionized searches), databases of systematic reviews, and journal searches. Explicit criteria should be used for inclusion and exclusion of evidence related to each key question posed, and these criteria should be carefully detailed.

Evaluating Evidence

A systematic review identifies the evidence, but assessment of the quality is also necessary for conclusions and recommendations. Recommendations must be graded to differentiate strong from weak evidence. Grading systems developed in the past decade are often based on a hierarchy of evidence such as that by the U.S. Agency for Health Care Policy and Research (Box 45-2).[11]

This hierarchy has been criticized for its focus on effectiveness. Randomized, controlled studies are most robust in this setting, but they are not always practical or appropriate. In palliative care, randomized, controlled trials can be fraught with difficulties (e.g., recruitment, ethics, patient numbers, attrition rates), and other studies are more appropriate in certain circumstances.[12] This approach has been criticized for failing to address study quality. For example, a poor-quality, biased randomized, controlled trial can be graded the same as a well-conducted trial with low bias.[13] As a result, grading systems have attempted to judge quality. Harbour and Miller[12] describe the SIGN process, in which methodological evaluation combines study type with a separate quality rating. After synthesis of the evidence, a judgment is made about relevance and applicability to the target population, consistency of evidence, and likely clinical impact. A grade is then assigned to a recommendation according to the strength of the evidence.[12] The latest development in grading evidence quality has been by the Grading of Recommendations Assessment, Development, and Evaluation (GRADE) Working Group,[14] an informal collaboration in which reviewers consider four key elements regarding evidence:

1. *Study design.* Studies are limited to randomized trials and observational studies that include cohort studies, case-control studies, and interrupted time series analyses.
2. *Study quality.* Criteria appropriate to a study type (randomized or observational) are used to assess quality. For example, in a randomized study, important criteria include allocation and blinding.
3. *Consistency.* Reviewers assess whether study results are consistent with those of other studies. If there is consistency of results in several studies, recommendations based on such evidence are likely to be more robust. Important inconsistencies result in downgrading of the level of evidence.
4. *Directness.* Reviewers assess whether the subjects, interventions, and outcomes are similar to those of interest in the target population.

The four elements can be combined to give a grade (Box 45-3). The combined elements provide a high rating (i.e., further evidence unlikely to change confidence in the estimate of effect), moderate rating (i.e., further evidence likely to impact confidence in the estimate of effect and may change the estimate), low rating (i.e., further evidence very likely to impact confidence and likely to change the effect), or very low rating (i.e., any estimate of effect is very uncertain).

Guideline development panels must grade evidence and make specific clinical recommendations on the level of evidence. Using the GRADE system, the panel considers quality of the evidence, how evidence translates into practice, and the trade-offs versus net benefits. Judgments about these factors produce simplified recommendations of *do it or do not do it* and *probably do it or probably do not do it.*[14] In contrast to previous systems, this system aims to make the recommendations more straightforward for the target users.

The place of qualitative research in grading evidence is unclear. Grading systems have been concerned mainly with quantitative research, and qualitative research does not fit these models. Much of palliative care research is qualitative, and guideline development therefore is hampered by a lack of evidence and by the difficulties in assessing available evidence.

Clarity and Presentation

The GRADE system is the latest system for grading evidence, but whatever system is adopted by guideline producers, the key is to make recommendations explicitly linked to evidence. If a recommendation is based on weak evidence, this must be acknowledged. Recommendations should be specific and unambiguous. For example, a guideline for managing patients with lung cancer recommends that patients with lung cancer and symptomatic bone metastases should be treated with a single 8-Gy fraction of palliative radiotherapy, and it specifies that this recommendation is based on the highest level of evidence.[15] When evidence is lacking, it may be impossible to make recommendations, and these areas should be highlighted for further research. Key recommendations should address specific clinical questions asked in the guideline—usually those most important in patient care. These key recommendations are usually summarized and highlighted within the guideline. Whether the guideline is addressing clinical care or service delivery, the options should be presented and recommendations made based on the level of evidence.

Applicability

Organizational barriers and potential resource implications must be considered in the development of guidelines. Recommendations may have significant impacts on staffing, equipment, or drug budgets. For example, based on the highest level of evidence, a guideline on lung cancer recommends that patients having radical radiotherapy should be given continuous hyperfractionated accelerated radiation therapy as 54 Gy in 36 fractions over 12 days rather than 60 Gy in 30 fractions over 6 weeks."[15] However, the resource implications of this recommendation have impeded using it as standard therapy in many centers. National and regional guideline panels should consider how guidelines could be incorporated locally. Local guideline development groups can economize by identifying appropriate national guidelines and adapting them for local use.[6]

Guidelines should be peer reviewed before dissemination. Specific criteria derived from the key recommendations can be used in auditing adherence to guidelines and evaluating patient outcomes. Guidelines usually are reviewed after a defined period to incorporate the ever-changing evidence base.

Editorial Independence

Professional societies, governmental organizations, and academic institutions may be involved in national and

---

Box 45-3 Criteria for Assessing Grade of Evidence

Types of Evidence

Randomized trial: high grade
Observational study: low grade
Any other evidence: very low grade

Factors that Decrease Grade

Serious (−1) or very serious (−2) limitation to study quality
Important inconsistency (−1)
Some (−1) or major (−2) uncertainty about directness
Imprecise or sparse data (−1)
High probability of reporting bias (−1)

Factors that Increase Grade

Strong association: significant relative risk of >2 (<0.5) based on consistent evidence from two or more observational studies with no plausible confounders (+1)
Very strong association: significant relative risk of >5 (<0.2) based on direct evidence with no major validity threats (+2)
Evidence of a dose-response gradient (+1)
All plausible confounders would have reduced the effect (+1)

From GRADE Working Group: Grading quality of evidence and strength of recommendations. BMJ 2004;328:1490-1494.

regional guideline development. Conflicts of interest arise when members of development panels have relationships with the pharmaceutical industry or government. It is inevitable that some members will have industry links, especially if they are experts in the field, but this does not necessarily impact guideline validity or necessitate exclusion of the expert from the panel. Nevertheless, there should be complete disclosure of potential or actual conflicts of interest, and development groups must decide whether a member's relationship with industry may produce significant bias.[16]

DISSEMINATION AND IMPLEMENTATION

Evidence suggests guidelines are effective in changing practice and improving patient outcomes.[2] Scientifically valid guidelines are developed to produce a specific health gain, and to achieve this, they must have effective dissemination and implementation. Health gains cannot be achieved if target users are unaware of or unfamiliar with a guideline. Research has shown that dissemination can be achieved by journal publication, postal distribution to target users, didactic lectures, and conferences; passive dissemination alone is unlikely to be successful. Dissemination backed by educational programs and initiatives (e.g., seminars) achieves greater success.[9,17] The international survey of 18 guideline programs revealed that most employ educational strategies and conferences in dissemination.[8]

Implementation strategies facilitate change in clinicians' practice using the guideline. Grimshaw and Russell[17] distinguish strategies as those that operate during a consultation with a patient (e.g., patient-specific reminders attached to clinical notes), general guideline reminders in consultation rooms, and those that operate outside the consultation. Methods include aggregated feedback of compliance and specific marketing and financial incentives or disincentives. Strategies operating within the consultation seem more effective.[17] In palliative care and other specialties, there is growing interest in the dissemination and implementation of guidelines by their incorporation into integrated care pathways, which are increasingly used clinically.

QUALITY OF CLINICAL PRACTICE GUIDELINES

The profusion of guidelines in the past 20 years has caused concerns about quality and conflicting advice. In the United States, the Agency for Health Care Policy and Research (AHCPR), which was renamed the Agency for Healthcare Research and Quality (AHRQ), had a development program that produced 17 guidelines between 1990 and 1996. When the program ended, it was credited with improving the quality of guideline development. However, there is still much variation in quality.[18] In Europe, Grilli and colleagues[19] demonstrated many guidelines that were being produced with inadequate information about stakeholders or how evidence was identified; most do not use explicit criteria to grade evidence.[19] The AGREE instrument resembles an international standard to increase the rigor of guideline development, but it is used more in Europe than the United States.

RISKS AND BENEFITS

The most important potential benefit of clinical practice guidelines is improved consistency of care and patient outcomes by means of better decisions by health care professionals. The guidelines help to keep practitioners abreast of current evidence and clarify which interventions work. Strategically, guidelines may improve efficiency and value for money. However, much depends on guideline quality. Poor quality (e.g., scientific evidence is lacking, recommendations are influenced by personal experience and opinions) can produce ineffective or harmful practices and waste valuable resources.[4] There is still professional skepticism, which mostly centers on physicians feeling that guidelines diminish their role in decision making.[20]

Concerns have been expressed that the evidence from clinical trials used in guidelines may not represent the relevant patient population; for example, the elderly are underrepresented in clinical trials. Many patients have complex problems that may not easily fit into a guideline algorithm. Palliative care patients may have complex psychological, social, and spiritual needs in addition to physical symptoms. However, guidelines must not be viewed as a set of orders and applied uncritically. They should be regarded as "the best advice about the most effective intervention in a particular clinical situation"[13] to help decision making. Physicians must apply clinical judgment in applying a guideline and incorporate their knowledge about individual patients. The patient's role must not be neglected; clinicians must be sensitive to patients' wishes regarding sharing of information and involvement in decision making, and they should tailor the approach to the individual. This patient-centered approach, familiar to all working in palliative care, does not preclude use of clinical guidelines.

PRACTICE GUIDELINES AND PALLIATIVE CARE

As in other specialties, there has been a trend to produce clinical practice guidelines over the past 2 decades in palliative care. The specialty can claim one of the most widely used guidelines: The World Health Organization's analgesic ladder.[21] However, it has been acknowledged that the evidence for the ladder is weak. Concerns have been expressed about evidence for its effectiveness.[22] As with many palliative care guidelines, it was developed by consensus and would not fit current rigorous methodology. A randomized, controlled trial to provide evidence for the three-step ladder is neither feasible nor ethical. This situation illustrates the challenges facing the specialty and guideline developers; much of clinical practice is based on evidence lacking in quantity and quality. Researchers intending to carry out randomized, controlled trials in palliative care face difficulties with recruitment, randomization, attrition, and outcome measurement. There is a need to improve the evidence base but not necessarily through randomized, controlled trials alone; observational studies may be more appropriate in certain circumstances, and good-quality cohort studies and case series can provide valuable evidence. The most important factor is the quality of study design, methodology, and reporting, which is reflected in the latest systems for grading evidence. The narrative approach of qualitative research lends itself to palliative care. A significant amount of palliative care research is qualitative, but it does not fit current hierarchies for grading evidence.

Despite the difficulties of lack of evidence, there has been a drive to produce guidelines relevant to palliative care. The Association of Palliative Medicine of Great Britain and Ireland[23] has a program of guideline development through task forces that appraise all available evidence about a specific clinical question (e.g., bisphosphonates to control pain of bone metastases, use of antimuscarinic drugs for death rattle). In the United States, the National Consensus Project for Quality Palliative Care produced "Clinical Practice Guidelines for Quality Palliative Care" through the collaboration of the major palliative care organizations.[24] These guidelines are probably more appropriately regarded as standards for multidisciplinary palliative care, but they emphasize the increasing prominence of guidelines in the specialty.

In addition to guidelines for specific symptoms and conditions, there is a need to incorporate the principles and practice of palliative care into guidelines for chronic, incurable conditions. Surveys of medical textbooks dealing with chronic, incurable disease have highlighted the lack of information about palliative care. One study demonstrated alarming paucity of information regarding end-of-life issues (e.g., pain, ethics, distress) in nationally developed guidelines for chronic, incurable conditions. Most failed to recommend palliative care services despite the obvious palliative needs of the patients.[25] In response, the Palliative Care Guidelines Group of the American Hospice Foundation devised a template for integration of palliative care into chronic disease guidelines. The guidelines should contain recommendations regarding when palliative care involvement is appropriate and which palliative services can be harnessed. Recommendations can be made regarding assessment of the whole patient; discussions about illness, limitations, and prognosis; and goal setting and bereavement.[26]

PROGRESS IN GUIDELINE DEVELOPMENT AND RESEARCH OPPORTUNITIES

Practice guideline development is evolving along with the evidence base for clinical practice. Frameworks such as the AGREE instrument and more refined systems for grading evidence such as the GRADE system should result in more reliable, scientifically valid, and applicable clinical practice guidelines. Guideline programs are increasingly using an evidence-based approach; national and regional programs are producing guidelines that can be adapted and adopted locally. There is a desire for increased international collaboration in guideline production.[8]

Modern medicine is increasingly evidence based, and care should be the best and most appropriate for the clinical circumstance. Health care purchasers also demand evidence of effectiveness for clinical interventions as medical advances compete for health care budgets. Guidelines provide a mechanism to facilitate evidence-based medicine to improve consistency of care. They also assist clinicians in keeping abreast of current evidence pertaining to their practice. Several challenges remain in palliative care:

- Production of high-quality evidence in palliative care to increase the evidence base
- Increased numbers of good-quality, randomized, controlled trials in palliative care
- Incorporation of qualitative research into hierarchies of evidence or development of a specific hierarchy
- National and international collaboration on producing guidelines
- Production of national, high-quality guidelines that can be adopted locally

CONCLUSIONS

Clinical practice guidelines can be effective in improving consistency of care and patient outcomes. Although there is much variation in the quality of guidelines, more rigorous methodology is used by many guideline development programs, including addressing specific questions, involving all relevant stakeholders, systematically reviewing evidence, using systems to grade evidence, and making explicit recommendations linked to the evidence. Guidelines produced using rigorous methodologies are more likely to be valid, applicable, and reliable. They should not be viewed as a cookbook approach to medicine. Individual clinicians must always use judgment in their interpretation and application of guidelines for individual patients. Palliative care faces the challenge of producing guidelines from a weak evidence base, and more good-quality research is needed.

REFERENCES

1. Field MJ, Lohr KN (eds): Clinical Practice Guidelines: Directions for a New Program. Washington, DC: National Academy Press, 1990.
2. Grimshaw JM, Russell IT: Effect of clinical guidelines on medical practice: A systematic review of rigorous evaluations. Lancet 1993;342:1317-1322.
3. Scottish Intercollegiate Guidelines Network (SIGN). Available at http://www.sign.ac.uk (accessed October 9, 2007).
4. Woolf SH, Grol R, Hutchinson A, et al. Clinical guidelines: Potential benefits, limitations and harms of clinical guidelines. BMJ 1999;318:527-530.
5. Grimshaw J, Russell I. Achieving health gain through clinical guidelines. I. Developing scientifically valid guidelines. Qual Health Care 1993;2:243-248.
6. Grimshaw J, Eccles M, Russell I. Developing clinically valid practice guidelines. J Eval Clin Pract 1995;1:37-48.
7. AGREE Collaboration. Appraisal of Guidelines Research and Evaluation in Europe (AGREE) Instrument. London: St. George's Hospital Medical School, September 2001. Available online http://www.agreecollaboration.org (accessed October 9, 2007).
8. Burgers JS, Grol R, Klazinga NS, et al. Towards evidence-based clinical practice: An international survey of 18 clinical guideline programs. Int J Qual Health Care 2003;15:31-45.
9. Thomson R, Lavender M, Madhok R: How to ensure that guidelines are effective. BMJ 1995;311:237-242.
10. Woolf SH: Practice guidelines—a new reality in medicine. II. Methods of developing guidelines. Arch Intern Med 1992;152:946-952.
11. U.S. Department of Health and Human Services, Agency for Health Care Policy and Research. Acute Pain Management: Operative or Medical Procedures and Trauma. Clinical practice guideline no. 11993, AHCPR publication no. 92-0023. Washington, DC: U.S. Department of Health and Human Services, ••.
12. Harbour R, Miller J. A new system for grading recommendations in evidence based guidelines. BMJ 2001;323:334-336.
13. Keeley PW. Clinical guidelines. Palliat Med 2003;17:368-374.
14. Atkins D, Best D, Briss PA, et al, for the GRADE Working Group. Grading quality of evidence and strength of recommendations. BMJ 2004;328:1490-1494.
15. Scottish Intercollegiate Guidelines Network (SIGN). SIGN 80: Management of patients with lung cancer. Edinburgh: SIGN, February 2005. Available at http://www.sign.ac.uk (accessed October 9, 2007).
16. Choudhry NK, Stelfox HT, Detsky AS. Relationships between authors of clinical practice guidelines and the pharmaceutical industry. JAMA 2002;287:612-617.
17. Grimshaw JM, Russell IT. Achieving health gain through clinical guidelines. II. Ensuring guidelines change medical practice. Qual Health Care 1994;3:45-52.
18. Hasenfeld R, Shekelle PG. Is the methodological quality of guidelines declining in the US? Comparison of the quality of US Agency for Health Care Policy and

Research (AHCPR) guidelines with those published subsequently. Qual Saf Health Care 2003;12:428-434.

19. Grilli R, Magrini N, Penna A, et al. Practice guidelines developed by specialty societies: The need for a critical appraisal. Lancet 2000;355:103-106.
20. Lubbe AS. Risks and misconceptions of guidelines in medicine and palliative medicine in particular. Prog Palliat Care 2002;10:275-279.
21. World Health Organization. Cancer Pain Relief. Geneva: WHO, 1986.
22. Reid C, Davies A. The World Health Organization three step analgesic ladder comes of age. Palliat Med 2004;18:175-176.
23. Bennet M, Ahmedzai S. Evidence based clinical guidelines for palliative care: The work of the APM Science Committee. Palliat Med 2000;14:453-454.
24. National Consensus Project for Quality Palliative Care. Clinical practice guidelines for quality palliative care: Executive summary. J Palliat Med 2004; 7:611-627.
25. Mast KR, Salama M, Silverman G, et al. End of life content in treatment guidelines for life-limiting diseases. J Palliat Med 2004;7:754-773.
26. Emmanuel L, Alexander C, Arnold R, et al. Integrating palliative care into disease management guidelines. J Palliat Med 2004;7:774-783.

SUGGESTED READING

AGREE Collaboration. Appraisal of Guidelines Research and Evaluation in Europe (AGREE) Instrument. London: St. George's Hospital Medical School, September 2001. Available online http://www.agreecollaboration.org (accessed October 9, 2007).

Atkins D, Best D, Briss PA, et al, for the GRADE Working Group. Grading quality of evidence and strength of recommendations. BMJ 2004;328:1490-1494.

Grimshaw J, Eccles M, Russell I. Developing clinically valid practice guidelines. J Eval Clin Pract 1995;1:37-48.

Grimshaw JM, Russell IT. Achieving health gain through clinical guidelines. II. Ensuring guidelines change medical practice. Qual Health Care 1994;3:45-52.

Keeley PW. Clinical guidelines. Palliat Med 2003;17:368-374.

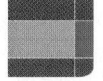

CHAPTER **46**

Evidence-Based Economic Evaluation

Konrad Fassbender

KEY POINTS

- Sustainability of health care reform requires that decisions be made on the basis of evidence in accordance with the stated objective (i.e., better health at lower cost).

- Economic evaluation is concerned with tabulating the clinical and economic consequences of adopting a new technology. The consequences of an alternative or comparator are also considered.

- As an aid to decision making, economic evaluation is designed to provide valuable information: identification of comparators, systematic measurement and valuation of costs and consequences, and construction of an efficiency ratio.

- In the case of primary health care reform, the study question needs to address whether a proposed procedure, service, or program is worth providing as an alternative to the standard (existing) practice.

Canada's expenditure on health care (10.3% of the gross domestic product [GDP] in 2006) is characteristic of a country that embraces technological advancement in medicine. Canadians expect the highest level of medical technology when they, their families, or friends become ill. This demand for medical technology is supported and encouraged by a third-party payment system. The increasing health care expenditures are perceived as problematic by the public (i.e., taxpayers). As a result, cost-containment policies are an integral element of health care reform. However, adoption of health care reforms takes place largely in the absence of evidence demonstrating its effectiveness. Demand for economic evaluations is a recent development in the health industry; evaluations of new technologies have been historically limited to safety and efficacy.

The recent popularity of economic evaluations reflects the fact that policy makers perceive expenditures on technology as highly mutable. In Canada, health care reform has targeted hospital and capital expenditures, resulting in a shift from public to private financing of total health care services.[1] Capital expenditure reductions include postponing construction of facilities and purchases of equipment necessary for high-technology procedures. As a consequence, spending on other institutions has increased. Administration costs related to regionalization and restructuring of health care services, public health, and health research program expenditures have increased. Professional care and drug expenditure growth has also remained above average. In addition to hospital reimbursement, health reform has variously targeted pharmaceutical costs, home care, and primary health care. Primary health care reform, for example, is characterized by de-institutionalization, team-oriented decision making, prevention, earlier intervention, and introduction of incentive-based reimbursement. Until recently, the rhetoric has been limited to cost containment.

Economic evaluation, or "the pursuit of efficient practice,"[2] is not merely about reducing costs. Sustainability of health care reform requires decisions to be made on the basis of evidence in accordance with the stated objective (i.e., better health at lower cost). Economic evaluation in its broader context is synonymous with the terms *cost-effectiveness analysis* and *efficiency evaluation*. In North America, *economic evaluation* and *cost-effectiveness* encompass cost-benefit, cost-utility, cost-effectiveness, cost-minimization, and cost-consequence analyses. It is a method used to ask whether deployment of health care resources is worthwhile. The relevant question is whether a proposed health service intervention yields favorable clinical and economic outcomes compared with some alternative, often stated as the status quo.

Economic evaluation is used to inform decision makers of all consequences after adoption of a technology. It is not a substitute for decision making; it is an input to the decision-making process. Decisions usually employ value judgments made from a particular perspective. Incorporation of value judgments into a decision-making framework requires valuation of health consequences, such as lives saved, pain avoided, or quality of life improvements. Consensus on how to value health has not been achieved, and the topic continues to be controversial.

Valuation of costs and consequences are made from a particular perspective. Use of a particular technology or intervention often requires several decisions to be made. Patients, physicians, and regional health planners, for example, experience different consequences from the introduction of the same technology. In these cases, it is useful to compare these evaluations with each other to understand the incentives for adoption of technology.

Incorporation of evidence generated from economic evaluation is not a well-defined process in most cases. A notable exception occurs when pharmaceutical companies are required by governments to submit evidence on cost-effectiveness to states and provinces that pay for prescription drugs for the elderly and economically disadvantaged. In this case, pharmaceutical companies follow guidelines that structure the methodological approach and reporting of the analysis. When other technologies are adopted, the process of incorporating economic consequences into the decision-making process is not as clear. As the public begins to accept the idea that budgetary restrictions influence health care decisions, economic evaluation will become more acceptable as an input into the decision-making process for procedures and programs. Some evidence for this shift is observed in reimbursement for procedures, development of medical and public health guidelines, and development of public and private benefit packages.

The remainder of this chapter addresses the technical aspects of economic evaluation. Various types of economic evaluation are described. I then consider the generation and integration of this information in a decision-making framework. The uniqueness of technological interventions in health care and the challenge that this poses for economic evaluation are considered. An evidence-based guide is provided for readers to evaluate economic evaluations.

ECONOMIC EVALUATION

The relevant elements of an economic evaluation are described in this section. Excellent introductions to economic evaluation,[3-7] guides to reading and understanding the economic evaluation literature,[8-10] guides for conducting an economic evaluation,[11,12] and discussions about the need to implement evidence[13-15] can be found elsewhere.

Economic evaluation is concerned with improving the decision-making process. It is a technical methodology based on economic principles intended for decision makers. Health economists, as practitioners of the "black art," tend to use terms such as *efficiency*, *equity*, *opportunity cost*, and *marginal*. Analyses are published in medical journals, public health journals, and policy journals and presented as health technology assessment working papers. Decision making, however, is the purview of many: taxpayers, purchasers, planners, public health practitioners, clinicians, medical advisory boards, hospital pharmacy and therapeutics committees, and technology assessment panels. The challenge is to communicate the methods and language of economic evaluation to this wide audience.

History of Economic Evaluation

Although there is evidence that Benjamin Franklin used principles of economic evaluation, credit for the first writings on the subject goes to the French economist Jules Dupuit[16] and Italian social scientist Vilfredo Pareto. British economists Nicholas Kaldor and Sir John Hicks were the first to make significant contributions to the underlying principles in the 20th century.[17,18]

In 1939, legislation was introduced in the United States that required maximization of "benefits to whomsoever they may accrue in excess of the estimated costs."[19] The U.S. federal budget grew substantially over the next 2 decades due to the large investments in managing water resources (e.g., hydroelectric facilities), health, education, and defense (e.g., Vietnam War). This led the U.S. federal government (during the Johnson Administration) to adopt the planning programming budgeting system (PBBS) in 1965, which was adapted from a version developed a few years earlier in Robert McNamara's Department of Defense. It outlined an attempt to standardize methods of weighing benefits and costs of programs compared with alternate activities. Substantial difficulties in implementation of the guidelines resulted in adoption of cost-containment measures over the next 12 years (primarily during the Nixon Administration). In 1977, however, the Office of Management and Budget (OMB) adopted a revised version of the PBBS called zero-based budgeting (ZBB), which originated with Jimmy Carter while he was Governor of Georgia.

The application of economics to health began with the seminal work of Kenneth Arrow.[20] At the same time, economic evaluation methods were beginning to be applied to health problems. For example, in the late 1960s and early 1970s, studies included bacillus Calmette-Guérin (BCG) vaccination, cervical cancer screening, preventative fluoride application, and methadone programs. Health economic evaluations were criticized similar to those completed previously because the monetary valuation of benefits was controversial. As a result, economic evaluation of health technologies evolved and focused on nonmonetary valuation of consequences. Economic evaluations of health care programs remained an academic exercise throughout the 1970s and 1980s.

In 1992, Australia was the first country to develop and implement guidelines for economic evaluation.[21] The province of Ontario and the governments of Canada and the United Kingdom soon followed.[22-24] These early efforts were limited to the adoption of pharmaceuticals. In 1993, the U.S. Public Health Service convened the Panel on Cost-Effectiveness in Health and Medicine. The panel surveyed delivery of state-of-the-art care and provided recommendations that were published in 1996.[25] This effort, however, did not resolve all areas of controversy among the experts and did not represent a consensus. As a compromise and in accordance with the earlier guidelines, the recommendations attempted to introduce uniformity among the studies at the expense of conforming to principles of underlying economic theory.

This brief history demonstrates that economic evaluation is recognized as being important for decision making by governments and the health care industry. Because of the complexities of the methodology, mandated acceptance of economic evaluation has not been forthcoming.

With the exception of pharmaceuticals, governments have largely relied on tried (but not true) cost-containment methods.

Elements of an Economic Evaluation

Economic evaluation is defined as "the comparative analysis of alternative courses of action in terms of their costs and consequences."[26] Economic evaluation is concerned with tabulating the clinical and economic consequences of adopting a new technology. The consequences of an alternative or comparator are also considered. Evaluating a technology and a comparator emphasizes the fact that *choice* faced by decision makers is a central tenet. As illustrated in Figure 46-1,[27] economic evaluation aids the decision-making process and provides information on the tradeoffs between resources and outcomes associated with decisions. When making a decision, two choices are available: A or B. Choosing A, for example, entails the use of resources as measured by cost (A) and commensurate health consequences (A).

The choice of a comparator (i.e., alternative or comparison therapy) is a central consideration in economic evaluations.[28] The status quo or existing therapy is often recommended but not easily identified. Recommendations sometimes consider a do nothing approach or use of a placebo. Doing nothing does not imply an absence of consequences. Additional considerations are required to identify an appropriate comparator. Is it ethical to compare against a placebo when there exists an established standard? Is established therapy cost-effective?

What if the costs and consequences of alternatives are not considered? Table 46-1 classifies studies on the basis of whether alternatives are considered and whether costs and consequences are considered.[29] Many studies claiming to be economic evaluations do not assess all health costs and consequences.[30] Health care technologies often generate health benefits and cost savings, but much of the economic evaluation literature ignores improvements in health and recommends programs that save costs. One study demonstrated that 60% of studies claiming to be economic evaluations did not adequately consider consequences.[31] Another review stated that less than 10% of the articles adhered to major methodological criteria.[32] Studies that do not adhere to methodological guidelines may provide useful information, but they should not be called economic evaluations.

Economic evaluation is synonymous with efficiency analysis and cost-effectiveness analysis. As applied to health, it comprises five analytic techniques (discussed later). An economic evaluation results in the construction of an efficiency ratio and is thereby differentiated from other study designs. An efficiency ratio is a summary indicator of costs and consequences of alternatives. The efficiency ratio (ER) for the decision between the two choices in Figure 46-1 is calculated as follows:

$$ER = (C^B - C^A)/(E^B - E^A)$$

In the equation, C refers to costs, E refers to the consequences, and the superscripts refer to the two choices, A and B. Suppose the consequences are measured in terms of survival probabilities, in which case this ratio would be expressed in units of dollars per lives saved. Because the ratio is obtained by comparing *additional* costs to *additional* benefits, the ratio is sometimes called an *incremental* or *marginal* efficiency ratio. These ratios should not be confused with the *average* efficiency ratio, C^A/E^A. Marginal ratios are used to make resource allocation decisions, whereas average ratios are used for budgeting purposes. Calculation of average efficiency ratios does not require alternatives, and they are strictly considered cost-outcome descriptions (see Table 46-1).

Economic evaluation comprises five analytic techniques: cost-minimization analysis (CMA), cost-consequence analysis (CCA), cost-effectiveness analysis (CEA), cost-utility analysis (CUA), and cost-benefit analysis (CBA). Cost-minimization analysis assumes that the consequences for two alternatives are identical. Cost-consequence analysis considers alternatives, costs, and consequences but stops short of calculating an efficiency ratio. Information provided in this manner may be familiar to readers of *Consumer Reports*. For example, repair records, crash test results, fuel economy, style, and handling are important considerations when purchasing a vehicle. The remaining three techniques result in the estimation of efficiency ratios proper and differ only in the units of measurement of the consequences. Cost-effectiveness consequences are expressed in natural units, such as lives saved, life-years

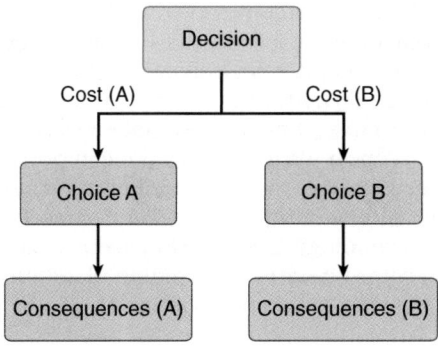

Figure 46-1 Decision-making process.

TABLE 46-1	Study Designs when Considering Alternatives, Costs, and/or Consequences		
ALTERNATIVES	**Are Costs and Consequences Considered?**		
	No		**Yes**
Alternatives are not considered	Only consequences examined = outcome description	Only costs examined = cost description	Cost outcome description
Alternatives are considered	Only consequences examined = efficacy analysis	Only costs examined = cost analysis	Economic evaluation

saved, or reduction in blood pressure in millimeters of mercury (mm Hg). Cost-utility consequences are measured in units called quality-adjusted life years (QALYs), and cost-benefit consequences are expressed entirely in dollar terms.

CBA differs from the other analytic techniques in several aspects. Converting health benefits to dollars is considered controversial by many decision makers. From a governmental perspective, CBA can be used to compare health interventions with programs in other sectors, such as social services or education. CEA and CUA are restricted to comparisons with similar health outcome measures. CBA can be used to measure *process utility*, such as the satisfaction arising from knowledge that a diagnostic test provides.[33] This satisfaction can be valued by an individual's willingness to pay. Health costs and benefits from treating an individual are not always confined to that individual. For example, immunization of a child reduces the probability of other children becoming infected. These effects are referred to as *externalities*, and they are best considered by CBA.

All five analytic techniques require that a perspective or viewpoint to be adopted when an economic evaluation is performed. A perspective can usually be identified by asking who is affected by the costs and consequences. The perspectives of society, the ministry of health, industry, and patients are the most commonly adopted. A societal perspective is obtained by summing all costs and consequences, regardless to whom they apply. Suppose, for example, that a new treatment resulted in fewer days of recuperation for the patient. This may enable the patient to resume normal activities and therefore is a benefit to the patient. In this example, the societal perspective includes all identified costs and benefits. A ministry of health perspective is restricted to the direct medical costs reimbursed by the government. Time costs accruable to the patient are included in the patient's perspective. This does not imply that the government does not care about the patient's well-being. Most governmental guidelines state that policies should be developed while adopting a societal perspective.

An economic evaluation is robust but can also be used to evaluate atypical situations. For example, a new treatment may result in higher initial costs and slightly increased quality of life over a long period. The fact that costs and health consequences accrue at different rates requires discounting. Another situation occurs when information used to conduct an economic evaluation may be uncertain or lacking altogether. In these cases, statistical and mathematical modeling techniques may be employed to determine a range of efficiency ratios. The economic evaluation includes techniques that enable analysis of most imaginable technologies. If performed improperly, however, economic evaluations generate results that are difficult to accept (an application of the adage "garbage in—garbage out"). Appropriate training, knowledge of theory, and use of guidelines are therefore important considerations in undertaking an economic evaluation.

Importance of an Economic Evaluation

Would you buy a package without knowing its contents? Economic evaluation is important in the decisions that

people make every day. For example, when purchasing a toaster, a person evaluates the decision based on price and other characteristics, such as how many slices it toasts at one time. How toasted bread impacts utility (i.e., happiness) is also considered. Other decisions are more complex. When purchasing a house, a person may need a real estate agent, appraiser, banker, and lawyer to understand the relevant consequences of any decision. Health care usually involves even more complex decisions and therefore demands greater complexity in the analysis of decisions. Because of the limits of human thought, economic evaluation can be considered beneficial in such circumstances.

Systematic economic evaluation is a specialized, expensive, and lengthy undertaking. As a result, it is often overlooked in program evaluation. Although some of the criticism is warranted, economic evaluation is considered by many to be important in the consideration of provision and financing of health care by organizations, regional authorities, and provincial and national governments.

Economic evaluation is considered to be an important dimension in the health care program decision-making framework. It is not a complete decision-making process, nor is it intended to replace decision making. Economic evaluation instead is considered an aid in decision making. As an aid to decision making, it is designed to provide valuable information: identification of comparators, systematic measurement and valuation of costs and consequences, and construction of efficiency ratios.

Budget allocation processes typically involve making decisions on one or a few programs at a time. Economic evaluation can be used to examine all programs simultaneously, once or periodically. CBA results in an efficiency ratio (denominated entirely in dollars) and can be used to inform decision makers about the relative merits of health compared with nonhealth technologies. Ultimately, CEA and CUA require valuation of benefits in dollar terms as part of the decision-making process, not the analytic process. As a result, these techniques may be viewed as equivalent because outcomes eventually require valuation in dollar terms.[34]

In summary, economic evaluation provides superior information compared with alternative approaches. For example, the most common alternative decision-making process is to repeat what has been done in previous years. Decision makers rely on cost-minimization and conveniently ignore the health and private consequences of adopting a technology. The decision makers need to trade-off the benefits and costs of obtaining of additional information yielded by economic evaluation.

GUIDANCE FOR CONDUCTING AN ECONOMIC EVALUATION

The mechanics (i.e., what) and justification (i.e., why) for conducting economic evaluations have been discussed. This section deals with who, where, and when. Given the technical nature of economic evaluation, it may appear that it is best performed with an academic team (e.g., health economist, epidemiologist, statistician). Including planners, providers, and recipients or payers is consistent with a community-based, participatory research approach.[35] Including the users in the process allows them to ask appropriate questions and helps in the collection of necessary data. They also play an important role in the generation and interpretation of results. They may be responsible for making the final decisions.

Economic evaluation therefore results in an efficiency ratio and embodies an ongoing process by a research team. This process is briefly reviewed, followed by a discussion of the relationship between formal economic evaluation and this process. How is this process initiated? How do analysts conduct formal economic evaluations? What standards are used to incorporate evidence into practice?

Processes and Outcomes of Economic Evaluations

Economic evaluation can be described in terms of the processes individuals or organizations use to arrive at decisions. Economic evaluation is a technique used to calculate an efficiency ratio that is used at a single point in time, and it refers to an ongoing process of determining the best use of resources given current technologies and circumstances. To best describe this process, it is important to recognize that there are two types of analyses: summative and formative. Summative evaluations ask if something is worth doing. Formative evaluations ask if something is worth doing better.

If we consider that health is the only output for CEA and CUA, least-cost measures of producing health are explored. Economists refer to this as *technical efficiency* (i.e., doing something better). Patients, physicians, and health care organizations tend to maximize health and therefore are more likely to conduct formative economic evaluations. CBA can compare health with nonhealth outcomes. CBA can be used to assess *allocative efficiency*, or the manner in which deployment of resources yields the highest value (across health and nonhealth uses). Government and academics are likely to conduct summative economic evaluations. The process describes the need for different types of analysis over time and suggests whom the resulting analysis benefits.

Consider the role of economic evaluation in health care reform. Major initiatives are undertaken with a strong belief that they are cost-effective. Hospital reform, home care, pharmaceutical care, and primary health care describe successive initiatives undertaken by governments and other third-party payers. In each case, substantial increases in resource allocation were predicated on the summative assumptions of their cost-effectiveness. Demonstration projects and academic research are periodically conducted to ascertain the validity of these assumptions. On a day-to-day basis, organizations and individuals strive to improve efficiency within the broad confines of funding and policy. Formative economic evaluation therefore can be viewed as conducting everyday business.

To illustrate the formative process, consider a finance department executive of a health authority attempting to reduce costs. At the same time, physicians (acting as agents on behalf of patients and their families) attempt to improve the patients' quality of life. Through dialogue and consensus building, a middle ground or best practice is identified. Formative economic evaluation can result from the complex process of conducting everyday business.

Economic evaluation processes cannot always be categorized so neatly. In some cases, progressive individuals and organizations conduct formative economic evaluations directly. This is best observed when hospital or regional formulary committees decide which drugs and doses are prescribed on a routine basis. The disaggregated model of formative economic evaluations described here is not always expected to result in optimal resource allocations. It therefore becomes necessary to periodically conduct summative economic evaluations.

Initiating and Conducting an Economic Evaluation

Economic evaluation always begins with formulation of a question by planners, providers, recipients, or payers—not by health economists. In the case of primary health care reform, the question needs to address whether a proposed procedure, service, or program is worth providing as an alternative to the standard (existing) practice. It would be helpful to concentrate on what is unique to the particular setting. What is proposed that should reduce costs and improve health? This question is intrinsic to conducting the business of providing health care.

Economic evaluation is not required for all new procedures, services, and programs. This may appear to be confusing at first glance, but consider a procedure that is more costly and less effective. In this case, it is self-evident that formal analysis is not necessary to conclude that the procedure should not be adopted. The converse is true for a new service that increases health at a lower cost. Formal economic evaluations are required when a new technology increases cost and increases benefits. Without formal evaluation, it would be difficult to determine whether the benefits outweigh the costs. Economic evaluation can quantify the tradeoff (when one exists) between the economic and non-economic consequences.

In Canada, health economists use the Canadian Agency for Drugs and Technologies in Health (CADTH) guidelines when conducting economic evaluations.[36] The primary purpose of these guidelines has been to standardize reporting of summative economic evaluations to provincial governments for reimbursement of pharmaceuticals. These and other guidelines outline the basic requirements of an economic evaluation acceptable to most audiences. Widespread adoption of these guidelines has occurred because they have been written in a format comprehensible to anyone with a basic understanding of elementary economics.

Standards for Adoption of New Technologies

An efficiency ratio is required when both costs and benefits are demonstrated to improve as the result of introduction of a new technology. Then what? What does $150,000 per life saved mean? There is no clear consensus about how this information can be incorporated into a decision-making framework. Perhaps the most influential (and most refuted) guideline is the $20,000 to $100,000 per QALY rule proposed by Laupacis and colleagues.[37] This rule states that technologies costing less than $20,000 per QALY should be automatically adopted and that those costing more than $100,000 per QALY should not be adopted. Those falling between the two QALY figures should be considered on a case-by-case basis.

Although this rule has been challenged by colleagues,[38,39] its incorporation into practice continues to be widespread. Some argue that this approach assumes that technology prices remain stable with increased use and ignores quality improvements commensurate with use. Other arguments include the fact that these ratios reflect average utilities and do not consider the fact that the technology may be cost-effective for a subset of patients. There is no guidance proposed that deals with the quality of underlying studies. Many argue that QALYs are not the gold standard, because there are many issues with the measurement of utility, and some say it cannot be done. Despite the absence of clear delineation about how the thresholds should be set and despite formidable objections, continued use of standards persists.

DEVELOPMENTS AND OPPORTUNITIES

The application of economic evaluation is intrinsically challenging. However, the nature of health care and describing technological innovation also prove to be difficult. This difficulty is compounded when the technological innovation is complex.

The need for economic evaluations is great. Health economists are scarce, and noneconomists are therefore often directed to conduct such evaluations. In part, guides such as provided in this chapter provide resources that encourage this practice. There remain, however, a large number of decision makers who are limited to requesting and reading economic evaluations. An evidence-based guide is provided to enable assessment of the economic evaluations themselves.

Technological Innovation and Economic Evaluations

Victor Fuchs, a leading health economist, wrote, "Technologic change is the most important force behind the escalation of health care expenditures." *Technology,* however, has become a catchword, and its meaning is often limited to product innovations (e.g., diagnostic machines, pharmaceuticals). Primary health care includes process and organizational innovations that allow us to distinguish innovations that decrease costs (i.e., old procedures done more efficiently) from those that increase costs (i.e., additional procedures, existing or new). These characteristics create problems in conducting economic evaluations of many innovations.

Defining *technology* is difficult. It has been portrayed in popular literature such as Alvin Toffler's *Future Shock* and Aldous Huxley's *Brave New World*. Derived from the Greek words *tekhne* ("art"), and *tecknologia* ("systematic treatment"), it is defined in the Oxford dictionary as a science or practical or industrial art and as the application of science and technique as a mechanical skill or art. More broadly, it is a descriptor for equipment, knowledge, and skills. This definition is likely derived from Ellul's classic reference[40] to tools, machinery, and matter; technology as a form of knowledge; and technology as a complex set of human activities or procedures.[40]

This definition is encapsulated in a comprehensive framework of technological innovation used by health economists.[41] In this framework, three types of innovation are considered: product, process, and organizational. Product innovation refers to a good or service acquiring additional or novel attributes. This results in higher costs. Pharmaceuticals are the best example of product innovations. Process innovation results in increased productivity or lower production costs. For any given level of labor and capital investment, increased output levels are possible. Organizational innovation refers to the reorganization of activities of production, including administration of those activities.

A major limitation, magnified in the context of health care, is that technology must be identifiable. Comprehensive descriptions of competing alternatives are not easily identified. There are several reasons for this. Consider the fact that process and organizational changes are intrinsically more complicated than product changes. Consider also that the process and organizational innovations may not be considered replicable or generalizable to other jurisdictions. An inability to define an innovation leads to an inability to calculate the relevant costs.

Several additional aspects of this framework cause difficulties. There is no single decision maker. Consumption, innovative, and medical care expenditures are governed by different objective functions. Health insurance is not considered, and extra welfare considerations may be present. For example, health care providers may be forced to provide a minimum level of medical care to achieve a desired health status according to medical norms. It is difficult to forecast the costs of services under these circumstances.

The increased difficulty of adequately describing health care technologies applies equally to formative and summative economic evaluations. Successful implementation of economic evaluations requires telling who did what to whom, where, and how often. High-quality evidence on the efficiency of new health care technologies is sparse, and evaluations of new technologies have been historically limited to safety and efficacy. Demand for evidence on efficiency is a recent development, and it has been primarily concerned with the evaluation of drugs and devices. Evidence for process and organizational innovations in health care are needed and should result in improvements in conducting economic evaluations of all technologies.

Reading and Evaluating Economic Evaluations

The bedside clinician, the minister of health, and all those between them can be described as decision makers. Many of these decision makers are limited to requesting or reading economic evaluations, and a summary set of indicators is proposed to help them evaluate or grade the level of evidence.

A set of indicators is proposed to aid in the initiation and evaluation of economic evaluation processes (Box 46-1). These questions are adapted from the critical appraisal literature by Drummond and colleagues[42] and grouped into five sets of questions. The first set asks whether an evaluation question has been posed. Formulation of a question requires reference to standardized elements of economic evaluation. The second set addresses data requirements. The point is whether the data are being collected to answer these questions. Third, recognition of the decision-making context is required. Fourth, plans should be generated to acquire or generate evidence. The fifth set of questions asks how the resulting information will be incorporated.

These indicators should not be evaluated without some background or preparation, as provided in this chapter. There is no established scoring algorithm, and a minimum acceptable quality threshold has not been described for an economic evaluation. These indicators are therefore helpful in situations comparing more than one evaluation. They can also be used to formulate requests for proposal and evaluation criteria in assessing the performance of those who conduct economic evaluations (see Box 46-1).

Box 46-1 Economic Evaluation Indicators

1. Are well-defined questions posed in answerable form?
   1.1. Do the questions address both costs and effects of the services or programs?
   1.2. Do the questions involve a comparison of alternatives?
   1.3. Is a viewpoint stated?
   1.4. Are comprehensive descriptions of the competing alternatives given (i.e., can you tell who did what to whom, where, and how often)?
   1.5. Are important alternatives omitted?
2. Which data (i.e., outcomes and costs) are anticipated for each question?
   2.1. Are all the important and relevant consequences for each alternative identified (some guidelines suggest generic, specific, and utility-based quality of life measures in addition to relevant physical measures)?
   2.2. Are consequences to be measured accurately in appropriate physical units (e.g., self-rated or interviewed health-related quality of life or utility instruments)?
   2.3. Are consequences to be valued credibly (e.g., quality-adjusted life years for utility, contingent valuation techniques, willingness to pay, hedonic pricing for dollars)?
   2.4. Are all the important and relevant costs identified for each alternative (e.g., direct: medications, laboratory, office visit, inpatient, rehabilitation; indirect: out-of-pocket costs, externalities)?
   2.5. Are costs measured accurately in appropriate physical units (e.g., may include diaries, questionnaires, interviews)?
   2.6. Are costs valued credibly (e.g., charges or prices, cost-to-charge ratios, relative value units, activity-based costs or microcosting)?
3. What is the decision-making context?
   3.1. Who makes the decisions, and how are the decisions being made?
   3.2. How are the relevant services financed and provided?
   3.3. Are incentives congruent with decisions?
4. What plans are being made to acquire evidence?
   4.1. Are the cost and outcome data reported in a useable format? Is the data being used to calculate cost-effectiveness ratios?
   4.2. Are there plans to tender the study questions? Are applications to funding agencies being made or supported to study these questions?
5. How is the evidence to be incorporated into practice (evidence-based decision making)?

REFERENCES

1. Health Canada. The public and private financing of Canada's health system. Presented at the National Forum on Health, September 1995.
2. Maynard A. Logic in medicine: An economic perspective. BMJ 1987;295:1537-1541.
3. Weinstein MC. Economic assessment of medical practices and technologies. Medical Decis Making 1981;1:309-330.
4. Warner KE, Luce BR. Cost-benefit and cost-effectiveness analysis in health care: Growth and composition of the literature. Medical Care 1982;18:1069-1084.
5. Luce BR, Elixhauser A. Standards for socioeconomic evaluation of health care products and services. Berlin: Springer-Verlag, 1990.
6. Gold MR, Siegel JE, Russell LB, Weinstein MC (eds). Cost Effectiveness in Health and Medicine. New York: Oxford University Press, 1996.
7. Drummond MF. Principles to Economic Appraisal in Health Care. Oxford, UK: Oxford University Press, 1997.
8. Drummond MF, Richardson WS, O'Brien BJ, et al. Users' guides to the medical literature. XIII. How to use an article on economic analysis of clinical practice. A. Are the results of the study valid? JAMA 1997;277:1552-1557.
9. O'Brien BJ, Hayland D, Richardson WS, et al. Users' guides to the medical literature. XIII. How to use an article on economic analysis of clinical practice. B. What are the results and will they help me in caring for my patients? JAMA 1997;277:1802-1806.
10. Stoddart GL, Drummond MF. How to read clinical journals. VII. To understand an economic evaluation (parts A and B). Can Med Assoc J 1984;130:1428-1434, 1542-1549.
11. Canadian Coordinating Office for Health Technology Assessment. A guidance document for the costing process, version 1.0. Ottawa: Canadian Coordinating Office for Health Technology Assessment, 1996.
12. Canadian Coordinating Office for Health Technology Assessment. Guidelines for economic evaluation of pharmaceuticals: Canada, 2nd ed. Ottawa: Canadian Coordinating Office for Health Technology Assessment, 1997.
13. Grahame-Smith D: Evidence-based medicine: Socratic dissent. BMJ 1995;310:1126-1127.
14. Evidence-based medicine, in its place. Lancet 1995;346:785.
15. Evidence-based medicine. Lancet 1995;346:1171-1172.
16. Dupuit J. On the Measurement of the Utility Of Public Works. International Economic Papers, 1952 [French translation of the 1844 version].
17. Kaldor N. Welfare Propositions of Economists and Interpersonal Comparisons of Utility. September 1939.
18. Hicks J. The valuation of social income. Economica 1940.
19. U.S. Flood Control Act of 1939.
20. Arrow K. Uncertainty and the Welfare Economics of Medical Care. Am Econ Rev 1963;53:941-973.
21. Australia Department of Health. Guidelines for the Pharmaceutical Industry on Preparation of Submissions to the Pharmaceutical Benefits Advisory Committee. Canberra, Australia: AGPS, 1992 (revised November 1995).
22. Ontario Ministry of Health. Ontario Guidelines for Economic Analysis of Pharmaceutical Products. Toronto: Ontario Ministry of Health, Drug Programs Branch, 1994.
23. Canadian Coordinating Office for Health Technology Assessment. Guidelines for Economic Evaluation of Pharmaceuticals. Ottawa: Canadian Coordinating Office for Health Technology Assessment, 1994 (revised November 1997).
24. United Kingdom Department of Health. Guidance on Good Practice in Conduct of Economic Evaluations of Medicines. London: PharmacoResources, 1994.
25. Gold MR, Siegel JE, Russell LB, Weinstein MC (eds). Cost Effectiveness in Health and Medicine. New York: Oxford University Press, 1996.
26. Drummond MF. Principles to Economic Appraisal in Health Care. Oxford, UK: Oxford University Press, 1997.
27. Drummond MF. Principles to Economic Appraisal in Health Care. Oxford, UK: Oxford University Press, p 9.
28. O'Brien B. Economic evaluation of pharmaceuticals: Frankenstein's monster or vampire of trials? Med Care 1996;34:DS99-DS108.
29. Drummond MF. Principles to Economic Appraisal in Health Care. Oxford, UK: Oxford University Press, 1997, p 10.
30. Ganiats TG, Wong AF. Evaluation of cost-effectiveness research: A survey of recent publications. Fam Med 1991;23:457-462.
31. Zarnke KB, Levine MA, O'Brien BJ. Cost-benefit analyses in the health-care literature: Don't judge a study by its label. J Clin Epidemiol 1997;50:813-822.
32. Smith WJ, Blackmore CC. Economic analyses in obstetrics and gynecology: A methodologic evaluation of the literature. Obstet Gynecol 1998;91:472-478.
33. Donaldson C, Shackley P. Does "process utility" exist? A case study of willingness to pay for laparoscopic cholecystectomy. Soc Sci Med 1997;44:699-707.
34. Phelps CE, Mushlin AI. On the (near) equivalence of cost-effectiveness and cost-benefit analyses. Int J Technol Assess Health Care 1991;7:12-21.
35. Viswanathan M, et al. Community-based Participatory Research: Assessing the Evidence. AHRQ evidence report/technology assessment no. 99, publication no. 04-E022-2, 2004.
36. Canadian Agency for Drugs and Technologies in Health (CADTH). Guidelines for the Economic Evaluation of Health Technologies: Canada, 3rd ed. Ottawa: Canadian Agency for Drugs and Technologies in Health, 2006.
37. Laupacis A, Feeny D, Detsky AS, Tugwell PX. How attractive does a new technology have to be to warrant adoption and utilization? Tentative guidelines for

using clinical and economic evaluations [see comments]. CMAJ 1992;146:473-481.

38. Naylor CD, Williams JI, Basinski A, Goel V. Technology assessment and cost-effectiveness analysis: misguided guidelines [see comments]? CMAJ 1993;148:921-924.

39. Gafni A, Birch S. Guidelines for the adoption of new technologies: A prescription for uncontrolled growth in expenditures and how to avoid the problem. CMAJ 1993;148:913-917.

40. Ellul J. The Technological Society. New York: Vintage Books, 1964.

41. Zweifel P, Breyer F. Health Economics. New York: Oxford University Press, 1997.

42. Drummond M. Critical assessment of economic evaluation. In Drummond M, O'Brien B, Stoddart GL, Torrance GW (eds). Methods for the Economic Evaluation of Health Care Programmes, 2nd ed. Oxford, UK: Oxford University Press, 1997, pp 27-51.

Health Professions, Family, and Volunteers

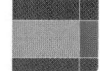

CHAPTER **47**

The Interdisciplinary Team

Malcolm Payne and David Oliviere

KEY POINTS

- Interdisciplinary teamwork seeks to provide holistic care by coordinating the contributions of different professional disciplines.

- Disciplines are branches of knowledge associated with education and research that produce systematic, well-organized behavior, and in health and social care, they are associated with professions that focus on different areas of a shared field of knowledge.

- Interdisciplinary teams are work groups of people with a shared identity and shared aims of high-quality work and innovation. These people adapt their professional roles to coordinate their work with others.

- Providing palliative care through interdisciplinary teamwork is more effective than using other forms of organization. There is little evidence for the value of particular team formations or ways of working, but methods of team building include improving understanding of tasks and how to manage knowledge, refining the contributions and social relationships of the group, and instituting joint training.

- Palliative care attempts to be holistic in two ways—by seeing patients as people within networks of social relationships and service provision, rather than as health care patients with a particular prognosis or diagnosis, and by providing care that integrates different professional perspectives and disciplines into one service delivered in the patient's preferred place of care.

In palliative care, an interdisciplinary team is the main instrument by which holistic service is provided. An interdisciplinary team is a group of professional and other service providers who work together by adapting their practice to each others' contributions to achieve shared objectives in providing innovative and high-quality palliative care. The implication of *interdisciplinary* work is that it requires this adaptation of individuals to each other, as opposed to the mere presence of people from different disciplines in the same organization, a situation implied by *multidisciplinary* work.

DISCIPLINE AND PROFESSION

A *discipline* is a branch of knowledge and the education and research associated with it that produces systematic, well-organized behavior. In health and social care, disciplines are associated with professional groups, including allied health professions (e.g., art, music, and occupational therapy; physiotherapy), chaplaincy, counseling, medicine, nursing, psychology, and social work. However, there is a significant shared field of knowledge within which these professions operate. Different professions focus on different aspects of knowledge within that field, and some also incorporate disciplines not usually associated with health and social care.

Medicine and nursing, the leading professions in palliative care, are primarily associated with biomedical disciplines. Clinical psychology, art and music therapies, and counseling draw strongly on psychology, and some also use the humanities. Social work is associated with the broader social sciences, especially sociology and social policy. The discipline of social work incorporates significant elements of psychology and counseling. This is less prominent in some countries, such as in many parts of Europe, where social workers are predominantly engaged in the management and provision of public welfare services. In palliative care, chaplains, as ordained ministers, are primarily educated in theological studies, and the ministerial training and specialist training that some undertake in preparation for chaplaincy roles includes elements of pastoral care and counseling.

Because discipline is closely associated with profession in health and social care, understanding how professions function is an important aspect of undertaking interdisciplinary work. *Professions* are occupational groups that have gained a particular social status that is associated with an altruistic lack of self-interest. Traditional research on professions[1,2] focused on the traits or characteristics of occupations that were recognized as professions and tried to distinguish them from other occupations. Among the traits examined were the existence of codes of conduct, the nature of the work of professions, the moral values they demonstrated in their practice, their knowledge base, and the nature of professional education and control of it by the profession. Research also examined qualifying organizations and their regulation of professions.

This approach has been criticized for being focused on the aspirations of occupational groups and failing to take into account alternative perspectives. The classic critique is that they operate in their own interests rather than those of the people they serve, that their control of knowledge disempowers users of their services,[3] and that self-regulation does not control the failings in treatment that make matters worse. Examples are medical iatrogenesis and social workers' creation of dependence on services rather than independence.

Later research on professions focused on processes of professionalization and deprofessionalization and the interactions among professions and other social groups. The research identified several features:

- The capacity of professional groups to gain and maintain control over admission to, education for and within, knowledge and research about, and regulation of their profession[2]
- The high social status associated with some professional roles, such as medicine and the law, which may inhibit effective communication and interaction with service users and other professions and occupational groups
- The extent to which professions operate in the public interest, in the interests of service users, or in their own interests[4]

TEAMS AND TEAMWORK

The definition of a team outlined in the introduction to this chapter contains several elements. First, a team is a group of people. This implies that there are interpersonal relationships among them, that those relationships continue for a period of time, and that they have a shared identity and expectations that they will work together on behalf of their organization. Second, interdisciplinary team members adapt their professional roles and disciplinary understanding to respond to the involvement of other team members. This requires communication, passing work and responsibility among them, differentiating their various tasks, and developing roles and boundaries between them that reflect their cooperation. Third, they have or will develop shared objectives that involve a concern for high-quality work and innovation. The purpose of organizing work is to do it as well as possible, and that involves creativity and innovation. To organize it in a team implies that this form of organization should achieve the best outcomes for professionals and for the patients, caregivers, and families that they work with; otherwise, it would be organized in another way.

Much of the literature on teamwork focuses on three elements:

- Improving interpersonal relationships and group development
- Devising systems for cooperation among team members
- Identifying shared aims and ways of improving the quality and innovation of work

A nonsystematic but extensive review of the literature on the concepts of teams and teamwork in management and health and social care[5] identifies a number of common themes:

- Clear and common purpose
- A sense of belonging, openness, good cooperation, informal atmosphere, mutual support, participation in good group relations, and synergy (i.e., the team is more than the sum of its parts)
- Clear roles and responsibilities
- Sound procedures and regular review of practice
- Appropriate leadership
- Effective external relationships
- Creativity

Achieving these goals offers an agenda for successful teamwork practice in palliative care. Teamwork is a continuum of practices considering the task to be undertaken, the people doing it, and the group relations between them. A continuum of practices is described in Table 47-1.

The sports analogy in Table 47-1 is instructive. It draws attention to how teams representing their country or university have to work in different ways because of the requirements of their sports. The kind of teamwork a hockey or football team needs to achieve—all present on the field and wanting to win against an opposition that confronts them—is very different from that of an athletics team, who may be involved in different sports in different places, often competing against the clock.

Some of the literature on health care teams assumes that the main focus should be on the group and how it seeks to improve relationships between members and increase understanding of their roles within the group. For example, Tuckman's[6] account of small group development, often applied directly to teamwork, is based mainly on laboratory research into small groups. It identifies five stages of team development:

- *Forming*, in which members deal tentatively with getting to know each other and anxieties about what the group is going to be like
- *Storming*, in which members try to assert their understanding of their own role and needs
- *Norming*, in which members gain experience of working together and build norms of shared practice
- *Performing*, in which members are able to implement the norms as a matter of course
- *Adjourning*, in which members deal with closure, with major losses in their membership, and with changes in functioning

TABLE 47-1 Types of Teamwork			
TYPE OF TEAMWORK	**SPORTS ANALOGY**	**DESCRIPTION**	**PALLIATIVE CARE EXAMPLE**
Coordinating	Hockey, football	All members work as a group, doing similar things but with different roles.	Nursing team on an inpatient ward
Cooperative	Tennis	All members do similar things in similar roles but act separately.	Professional team (e.g., doctors, nurses, social workers)
Networking	Gymnastics	All members do different things, acting separately in different places.	Interdisciplinary home care team

Behind this analysis is the assumption that teams naturally progress through these stages, as laboratory groups do, or that they may become hung up at one stage or another and need to be helped to move to the next stage. It also assumes that the main purpose of the exercise is to create groups that perform.

An alternative perspective focuses on the task and person, rather than the group. The contingencies affecting a team and creating the situation in which it operates affect the kind of teamwork it needs to use. This is understood by exploring three factors: types of teams and their relationships, team building, and teamwork difficulties.

Understanding a Team

An important step in interdisciplinary practice for any professional is clarity in understanding the teams that they are involved in. There are several types:

- A professional team, such as medical, nursing, social work, or spiritual care teams
- An organizational team, such as the ward or home care team
- A patient or case team, whose members work with a particular patient or who are working on a case
- A functional team, whose members are brought together to carry out a particular function, such as a computer records working group or an area adult protection committee

Some of these teams are part of an organization's system; others involve links across organizations. Because all professionals are part of several teams, it is important to identify the focal team for any particular purpose. For example, a ward team may be the focus for nurses planning to meet the care needs of patients, but a ward round that includes several professional groups may be the focus for strategic decision making about the treatment plan for the patient.

A helpful way of understanding the range of teams involved uses systems[7] ideas that see them as interlocking groups. This avoids focusing on organizational hierarchies. Figure 47-1 shows a common form of team organization[8]: the core and periphery team. All organizational structures present their own difficulties. Core and periphery teams have to deal with a tendency for core team members to form a tighter group and, in doing so, to exclude peripheral members from particular kinds of decisions, communications, or work. Figure 47-1 shows the staff members who are part of the core team (i.e., the focal team for this analysis) for a hospice inpatient ward. Some staff personnel, such as a physiotherapist or social worker, constitute the periphery of team members associated with the ward. However, these professionals regularly attend the weekly multiprofessional team meeting for all the patients on the ward. The team for each patient includes a doctor and a primary nurse, and it may include some of the noncore team members.

Drawing diagrams of such systems is a helpful way of perceiving the relationships between interdisciplinary team members. It is useful to start by asking team members to list whom they see as members of the team and to explore differences in their views. Clerical or cleaning staff and volunteers may be excluded by some team

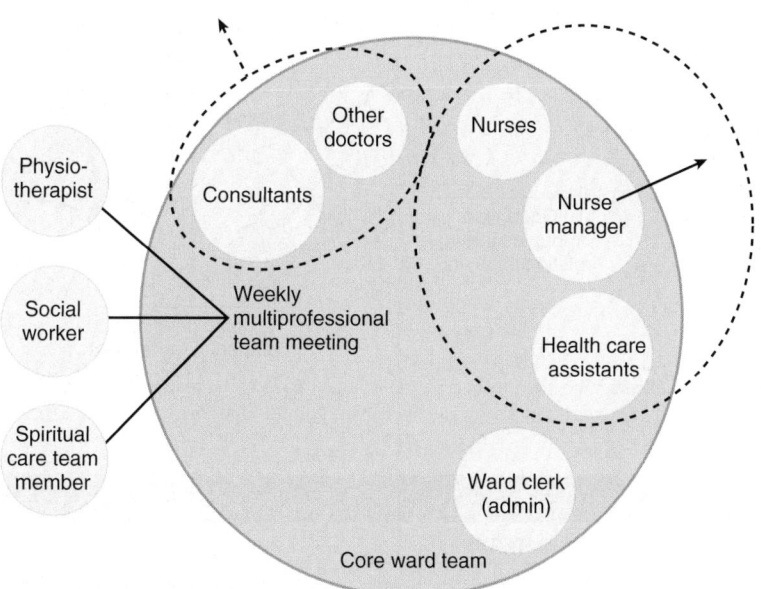

FIGURE 47-1 Core and periphery teamwork. Within the *green circle* are the several groups of staff who are part of the core team for an inpatient ward in a hospice. In addition to the ward clerk, two groups of professionals are identified: (1) doctors and (2) nurses and paraprofessional health care assistants. Within the team, the doctors have their own hierarchy of a senior doctor and others; the senior doctor has overall independent medical responsibility for the patients on the ward. The *dashed arrow* shows that there is a connection with the wider team of doctors outside this ward, within which planning and support of medical care throughout the hospice is organized. The nursing group also has an internal hierarchy within the ward, with different grades of nursing staff and a manager. However, the hierarchy is outside the ward *(solid arrow)* from the manager to a more senior manager, rather than the more collective responsibility of the doctors, and the diagram shows the direction of responsibility inside a group that extends to more senior people outside the ward team. Some staff, such as a physiotherapist, social worker, and spiritual care team member, regularly work with or are attached to the ward *(solid lines)*, but do not provide medical or nursing care for inpatients.

members. In these cases, attempting to draw a diagram that everyone can agree on can be a useful exercise in shared understanding.

Another important factor in understanding a team is how it relates to external groups. Figure 47-2 draws attention to the fact that an important aspect of teamwork is planning its contacts with the outside world. The open team[5] sees itself as part of a wider network. In addition to improving internal group relations, it coordinates and develops external relationships by sharing responsibilities among its members to form relationships with individuals and groups elsewhere in the local organization and outside of it. Being a group or a network team is increasingly not a choice; the effective team should be both. A useful exercise for a team may be identifying and codifying its external links and contacts and having a periodic audit to update the information.

Team Building

Team building is the process of developing teamwork in a team. Several approaches to team building exist (Table 47-2). These approaches are not mutually exclusive, and a combination of them is likely to be required, changing the focus of the team in particular circumstances. For example, when an organization is set up or is experiencing major change, organization development may be a useful approach to achieve overall strategic aims in designing a pattern of teamwork that covers several teams of the whole organization. As teams are established, work on group relations may be useful, and teamwork may be maintained by everyday team building. Within this analysis of approaches, however, group relations and contingency or situational approaches reflect the alternative models of teamwork discussed previously.

Group relations in team building often focus on interpersonal roles that people accept in the team. Two well-known systems for analyzing these roles include questionnaires and scales, which help identify and stimulate discussion about roles. Research[9] on groups of commercial managers identified nine roles that people assume in teams because of expertise, experience, and personal preference and because the configuration of the team presses them to accept a role. Examples are resource

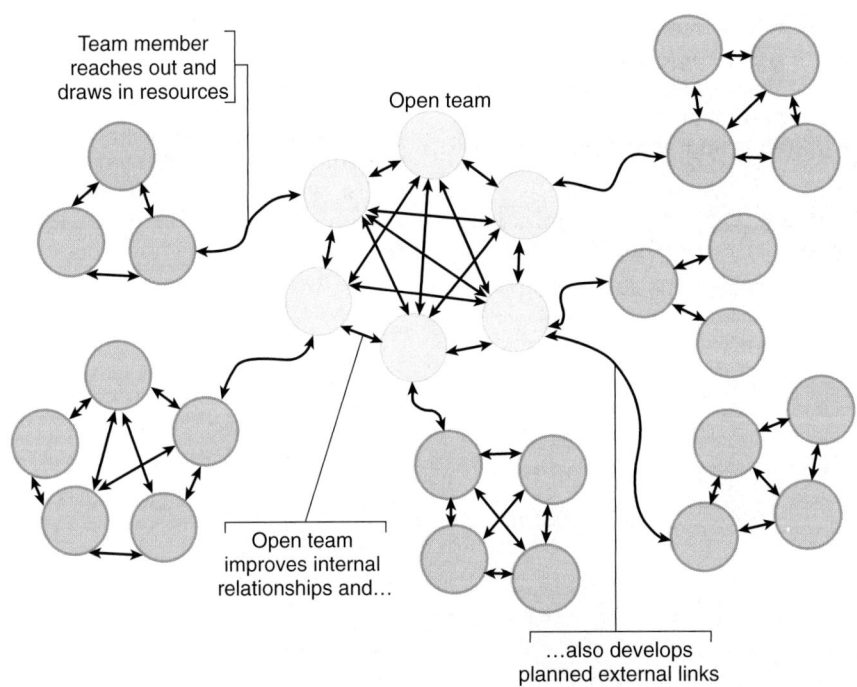

FIGURE 47-2 Open team with external links. The open team is part of a wider network. The team develops and coordinates external relationships by sharing responsibilities among its members to form relationships with individuals and groups outside itself.

TABLE 47-2 Approaches to Team Building		
APPROACH	**STRATEGY**	**CRITIQUE**
Organization development	Plan an organizational structure, including teams that meet organizational objectives.	Top-down approach assumes that organizational priorities are most important factors in teamwork.
Group development	Improve interpersonal and group relations.	Approach focuses on relationships of the team, encouraging "navel gazing."
Contingency or situational team building	Identify team members' preferences, types of work done, and organizational imperatives, and develop teamwork accordingly.	Approach responds to needs and wishes of team members and their work, and it focuses on tasks rather than people.
Everyday team building	Identify and tackle team issues continuously in every aspect of work, and use team projects to develop team resources.	Approach is practical and relevant to everyday tasks, but it may be difficult to meet strategic, organizational, and change objectives.

investigators, who are good at identifying new resources that the team can use to users' advantage; monitor evaluators, who are good at reviewing effectiveness; and complete finishers, who like to complete tasks consistently. In such formulations, the interaction of the individual and the group is the main focus of thinking. Another frequently used analysis, the Myers-Briggs type indicator (MBTI),[10] is derived from Jungian psychological theory and claims that different personality types, such as extraversion, introversion, thinking, feeling, judging, and perceiving, may be identified by a personality scale. As with many self-report personality scales, Belbin's and Myers-Briggs's scales are not well validated[11] and have been criticized, but they have been valued in team building and management consultancy because they stimulate useful debate.

Teamwork Difficulties

Difficulties often arise in teamwork (see "Common Errors"). Table 47-3 identifies areas of team functioning in which problems may occur, indicates the kind of issues that arise, and suggests some strategies for dealing with them through activities in the team (see "Case Study: Team Disputes").

DEVELOPMENTS AND RESEARCH OPPORTUNITIES

The most significant development in teamwork is the emergence of a knowledge management approach, which focuses on the individual rather than group and task and which argues that disciplinary and professional knowl-

---

Common Errors

- Friendly interpersonal or intergroup relationships are insufficient for effective teamwork, but interpersonal support may improve team members' mental health and work effectiveness.
- Leadership does not always reside with an appointed or assumed leader or key worker. It may move to others in some cases or for particular tasks. Clarity in leadership is crucial in all cases.
- In the absence of serious problems, team building does not require conferences outside the work setting with external facilitation. It should be undertaken through everyday attention to team processes and by internal leadership of team projects and knowledge about management mechanisms.
- It is unnecessary to pass specialized or complex work to another professional. It may be better to plan for the specialist to act as consultant or co-worker to increase the flexibility and skill of the primary worker.

TABLE 47-3 Common Teamwork Difficulties

DIFFICULTIES	ISSUES	RESPONSES
Individual development	People's personal development neglected	Appraisal
		Training and career plans
		Confidence building
		Swapping jobs to gain experience
		Knowledge building, courses
Strategic development	Unclear vision and mission	Write a press release explaining vision or mission
		Draw a badge for the team
		Devise a team motto
Work flow	Problems in getting work and passing on responsibility	Referrals audit (i.e., what do referrers think?)
		Hand over audit
		Forms audit
		Ward rounds or case conference audit
Communication	People not participating	Goldfish bowl (i.e., team meetings observed by outsiders)
		External feedback
		Assessing audio or video tape of team interactions
		Counting who says what, who is quiet
		Tallying who participates by gender or ethnicity
		Sociograms
Task differentiation	Identifying tasks and skills	Skills audit
		Define skills for different professions
Role integration	Specifying roles	Boundary drawing
		Interlocking circles
		Concentric circles
Problem solving	Long-running problems not resolved	Force field analysis of issues preventing or helping resolution
		Getting ideas and filtering them to plan solutions
Decision making	Unable to agree on decisions	Audit of difficult decisions
		Getting ideas and filtering them to plan solutions
		Review of all contributions and reasons for rejections
Conflict	Frequent conflict	Agree on rules of behavior
		Agree when and where difficult issues will be resolved
		Identify and resolve barriers to communication
		Focus on situations in which parties to conflict often work together

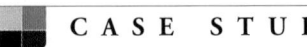

CASE STUDY

Team Disputes

A multiprofessional team works in a suburban area and provides home care. Mrs. M is a 50-year-old patient with breast cancer and bone metastases. She complained to the specialist nurse that she was feeling increasingly tired. She has managed to carry her shopping uphill to her home and to perform the household tasks despite her edematous arm.

Several team members became increasingly enraged by Mrs. M's plight and were particularly infuriated by the presence of Mr. M and two adult children in their 20s who lived at home. The children were unemployed but continued to be waited on by their mother. Some female members of the team voiced the claim that female abuse was occurring and demanded the social worker take action to change family members' attitudes. The male medical staff resisted inpatient admission to resolve these family problems. The multiprofessional team became increasingly divided over care plans and in their work with the M family.

edge is incorporated into the personal identity of individual members. Rather than wearing a professional badge, colleagues join together to deal with a complex human situation. Shared work focuses on the knowledge that is used together and applied to the patient, not organizational or professional divisions. The team task is to allow members to express their particular knowledge and skills and use them to complete the task. Individual members have their own specialist tasks to complete, but the work of individuals is combined to complete the shared task.[12]

In this model of teamwork, successful task completion is a process of shared learning. Team members can use this process to move closer together personally, gain a better understanding of what each can offer, and through understanding, value all the different contributions more highly. In this way, each incorporates the shared learning of the team; the members become a community of practice.[13] Communities of practice build up their approach to their work by incorporating their shared learning into the members' way of practicing and therefore into the members' professional identities. To each task, chaplains, doctors, nurses, and social workers bring their professional identities; their specialist identities as palliative care workers; their organizational identities as health care workers, hospice workers, or palliative care team workers; and their community of practice identities. All of these identities are implemented in the particular palliative care team.

Knowledge management approaches focus strongly on everyday team building. Several strategies are important:

- Regular case discussion, including team functioning
- Event reviews, after a particularly significant event or error has occurred
- Reviews when communication or decision making has been difficult

The evidence base for interdisciplinary teamwork is provided by research and practice in four areas:

- Management studies in industrial, commercial, and public sector organizations
- Social psychological research into group and team behavior[14]
- Interdisciplinary work in health care and social care
- Coordination of public sector organizations[8]

The most extensive review of outcome evidence relevant to interdisciplinary teamwork in palliative care was carried out for the U.K. National Institute for Health and Clinical Excellence (NICE),[15] incorporating seven systematic reviews. It found that the evidence (i.e., grade Ia and lower levels of evidence) strongly supported specialist palliative care teams working in the home, hospitals, and inpatient units or hospices as a means of improving outcomes for cancer patients (e.g., pain control, symptom control, satisfaction) and of improving care more widely. The benefit has been demonstrated quantitatively and qualitatively in studies and in systematic reviews of studies.

Because of the variety of interventions by teams, more work is needed to test the specific components of palliative care team activity (e.g., compare different types of hospital or hospice teams, test specific ways of working within their practice).[15] Studies are needed to discover whether a different skill mix or set of interventions performed by the team is more effective than others.[15]

A large study of 500 U.K. health care (but not palliative care) teams[16] who were mainly community based found four factors relevant to successful outcomes:

- Clear team objectives
- Participation
- Commitment to quality
- Support for innovation

Because research shows that interdisciplinary teamwork is effective in palliative care, palliative care professionals should enhance the form of teams in any particular service by seeking to achieve these objectives by available means. This provides an opportunity for research on the best modes and organization of teamwork that can achieve the coordination objectives of interdisciplinary palliative care practice. There is considerable evidence that joint education at a qualifying level and in continuing professional development enhances cooperation and coordination in health care.[8]

Despite these developments, several research challenges remain:

- To identify the most successful formation of work teams to enhance interdisciplinary practice
- To identify economical and effective methods of team building to enhance interdisciplinary teamwork
- To identify methods of practice within teams that enhance the quality of service to patients

CONCLUSIONS

Interdisciplinary teamwork is accepted as the best way of delivering holistic palliative care. Health care teams who are eager to participate, have clear objectives, and focus on improving quality and innovation are effective. Particular team formations and methods of team development are controversial and require further research. Although developing group and interpersonal relationships in a team is an accepted form of team development, there is interest in knowledge management techniques as a way of creating shared understanding in communities of practice that focuses on how knowledge is used within teams.

REFERENCES

1. Freidson E. Professionalism Reborn: Theory, Prophecy and Policy. Cambridge, UK: Polity, 1994.
2. Hugman R. Power in the Caring Professions. Basingstoke, UK: Macmillan, 1991.
3. Wilding P. Professional Power and Social Welfare. London: Routledge & Kegan Paul, 1982.
4. Saks M. Professions and the Public Interest: Medical Power, Altruism and Alternative Medicine. London: Routledge, 1994.
5. Payne M. Teamwork in Multiprofessional Care. Basingstoke, UK: Macmillan, 2000.
6. Tuckman RW. Developmental sequence in small groups. Psychol Bull 1965;63:384-399.
7. Anderson RE, Carter I, Lowe GR. Human Behavior in the Social Environment, 5th ed. New York: Aldine de Gruyter, 1999.
8. Miller C, Freeman M, Ross N. Interprofessional Practice in Health and Social Care: Challenging the Shared Learning Agenda. London: Arnold, 2001.
9. Belbin RM. Management Teams: Why They Succeed or Fail. London: Heinemann, 1981.
10. Myers IB, McCaulley MH. A Guide to the Development and Use of the Myers-Briggs Type Indicator. Palo Alto, CA: Consulting Psychologists Press, 1985.
11. Gardner WL, Martinko MJ. Using the Myers-Briggs type indicator to study managers: A literature review and research agenda. J Manage 1996;22: 45-83.
12. Opie A. Thinking Teams/Thinking Clients: Knowledge-based Teamwork. New York: Columbia University Press, 2003.
13. Wenger E. Communities of Practice: Learning, Meaning and Identity. Cambridge, UK: Cambridge University Press, 1998.
14. West MA. Effective Teamwork: Practical Lessons from Organizational Research, 2nd ed. Oxford, UK: BPS Blackwell, 2004.
15. Gysels M, Higginson I. Improving Supportive and Palliative Care for Adults with Cancer: Research Evidence. London: National Institute for Clinical Excellence, 2004, p 215.
16. Borrill CS, Carletta J, Carter CS, et al. The Effectiveness of Health Care Teams in the National Health Service, 2001. Available at http://homepages.inf.ed.ac.uk/jeanc/DOH-final-report.pdf (accessed October 10, 2007).

SUGGESTED READING

Gysels M, Higginson I. Improving Supportive and Palliative Care for Adults with Cancer: Research Evidence. London: National Institute for Clinical Excellence, 2004.

Payne M. Teamwork in Multiprofessional Care. Basingstoke, UK: Macmillan, 2000.

Speck P (ed). Teamwork in Palliative Care. Oxford, UK: Oxford University Press, 2006.

West MA. Effective Teamwork: Practical Lessons from Organizational Research, 2nd ed. Oxford, UK: BPS Blackwell, 2004.

CHAPTER **48**

The Physician

J. Norelle Lickiss

KEY POINTS

- The task of health care involves more than physicians, and the overall role of physicians in the 21st century should be reconsidered, with recognition of their diagnostic and analytic responsibilities.
- Sustaining concepts of medical practice include an awareness of personal dimensions and an adequate view of persons.
- Sustainable medical practice avoids flat-of-the-curve medicine.
- Clinical decision making may benefit from a more comprehensive approach, involving explicit awareness of the relationships of persons, of values, and of medical facts and the legal context.
- The idea of human dignity can focus the efforts of physicians; human dignity should be understood, restored, and safeguarded.

We may say that at this moment, as in the time of Galileo, what we most urgently need is many fewer new facts (there are enough and even embarrassingly, more than enough of these in every quarter) than a new way of looking at the facts and accepting them. *A new way of seeing, combined with a new way of acting—that is what we need.*

— TEILHARD DE CHARDIN[1]

"Medical theories always represent one aspect of the general civilization of a period, and in order to understand them fully, we must be familiar with the other manifestations of that civilization, its philosophy, literature, art, music."[2] This view is challenging to anyone reflecting on the role of a physician in the early years of the 21st century. Why should it be appropriate to reflect on the physician in a palliative medicine textbook? Medical histories document patterns of evolution of medical practice, the writings and teachings of notable clinicians, and the impact of medical practice on humankind. Examinations of the history of ideas within the Western medical tradition have been published.[3,4] Many focus on the history of hospitals, one of the more tangible signs of medical activity within a society. The social roles of physicians have evolved over the past millennium, and modern clinicians play a critical but difficult role in mediating the tension between health care as a commodity and as a human right.[5-7] As the history of modern palliative medicine continues to be documented,[8,9] it is recognized that palliative medicine and palliative care (a larger activity) are embedded in the health care systems and communal practices of all societies. Watson[10] encapsulated this development:

It seems obvious to me that, once we get away from the terrible calamities that have afflicted our century, once we lift our eyes from the horrors of the past decades, the dominant intellectual trend, the most interesting, enduring, and profound development, is very clear. Our century has been dominated intellectually by a coming to terms with science. . . . [S]cience has changed how we think.

The dominant trend of the first decade of the 21st century already might have shifted to dealing with terrorism, including its roots, its manifestations, the moral dilemmas it engenders, and the responses of people to the uncertainty and violence. What does this mean for medicine and for physicians, who are privileged by education and by their roles as persons with access and responsibility deep in the recesses of the human condition? Does this situation urge medical practice to go far beyond the dramatic scientific advances that changed medical practice in the 20th century and refocus on the foundations of the practice of medicine and on the moral and ethical principles that sustain individual physicians in all contexts (e.g., administration, hospitals, community)? This in a time when the previously sustaining grand narratives and verities appear to be giving way in the face of violence done to people, institutions, and ideas (e.g., weakening of the prohibition of torture, traditionally abhorred by physicians). Palliative medicine, often concerned with the most vulnerable persons in society, may be the appropriate place for such considerations of medicine in an age of violence and terror. "If we are entering a post-scientific age . . . the new millennium will see as radical a break as any that has occurred since Darwin produced 'the greatest idea, ever.' "[10]

Extreme distress, violence, and inhumanity are not novel contexts for physicians. Camus portrayed the key role of a physician in his allegorical novel, La Peste, which described a city afflicted by plague. In it Dr. Rieux concluded, as might an experienced palliative medicine practitioner, that there was more good in men than evil to despise. In a nonfictional setting, Sir Edward "Weary" Dunlop, a young Australian surgeon (his face is on Australian coins), was immersed in distress and practiced sensitive palliative care in harsh conditions on the Burma Road in World War II. He comforted his soldiers as they died and maintained morale and a belief in humanity. Medical heroes abound, but there also have been occasions when physicians have become purveyors of distress, not because science or resources failed them, but because of thought patterns that betrayed the core principles of medical practice. An observer at the 1948 Nuremberg trials, seeking to understand the tragic inhumanity in which high-ranking physicians and leading academics participated, concluded that, "The infinitely small, wedged-in lever from which this entire trend of mind received its impetus was the attitude toward the non-rehabilitatable sick."[11]

The link with palliative medicine is poignant, reinforcing the view that the reexamination of the root concepts and principles of palliative medicine may be timely. Palliative medicine is core business in any health system and a barometer of the moral health of society. It is not only terror that causes fear and distress. Distinguished scientists pointed out that in the face of brilliant medical advances, people were afraid. Such fears are perceived by doctors not insulated by aberrant hospital or health system culture, excessive work load, fatigue, or even affluence from mainstream life. The elderly frequently are afraid of their future, not merely the availability of care, but especially of life prolonged beyond their wishes, with disregard for what they have expressed and for the directives given. A physician may insist on life-prolonging measures for a patient of any age near the end of life, even at great cost in resources or distress and in the face of a directive to do otherwise. At issue is a perception of what is the "good" to be sought or done.

The philosophical issues about the merits of prolonging life need focus. Shakespeare confronted the issue as King Lear, slipping in and out of sanity, was dying (King Lear, Act V, Scene iii) in the presence of his bastard son, Edgar, and the Duke of Kent:

Edgar: He faints. My lord, my lord!
Lear: Break, heart, I prithee break.
Edgar: Look up, my Lord!
Kent: Vex not his ghost: O, let him pass! He hates him much
That would upon the rack of this tough world
Stretch him out longer.

Physicians share the experiences and fears of their patients. Some distinguished medical authorities have been articulate in their criticism of care and specifically of physicians with respect to their competence as decision makers, comforters, and humble and wise practitioners. Do these contributions receive the attention they merit? Where do such anecdotes of core deficiencies fit in the spectrum of medical evidence? Recognition of the power of error as a tool for the advancement of learning may regard such testimonies as more important than countless expressions of gratitude confirming that care is satisfactory; outcome evaluations based on searches for errors may yield more than measures of praise, even in busy hospital practices.[12]

There is a need to avoid flat-of-the-curve medicine, in which the benefits are not proportional to the huge costs.[13] For the patient, who is the critical judge of benefit and cost, this approach spells disaster, with opportunities multiplying for physicians to increase rather than alleviate suffering. For the physician, who often has great enthusiasm but little time, activities with a high benefit-to-cost ratio (e.g., pain relief for cancer patients) must not be neglected in favor of measures at the flat of the curve (Fig. 48-1) There is room for more research to establish measures of benefit and cost and for efforts in clinical practice to reduce cost (e.g., by less toxic therapies) and maximize benefit (e.g., good care, symptom relief throughout treatment, rehabilitation). Care to reduce the "price of benefit" should involve all physicians in contact with patients with probably eventually fatal illnesses.

Global distress related to medical practice goes beyond violence and aberrant practices in affluent countries. There continues to be global inequity in access even to basic health care. One nation may seek to provide heart transplants or expensive anticancer drugs, whereas in a nearby country, there may be no basic cancer pain relief programs. How can 21st century physicians and medical organizations endure such inequities? Burnout statistics, suicide rates, and other empirical evidence attest to the deep personal pain of physicians. A renewal program may

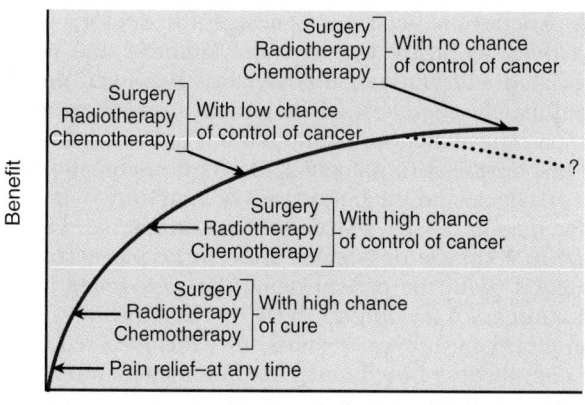

FIGURE 48-1 Cost-benefit analysis of medical care for patients with cancer.

be a timely objective for individual physicians and for the community, which may look to them again for sustenance. Studies and reviews of the roles of physicians in palliative care[14] support the initiative of finding ways to support these professionals in the complex situations in which they practice in affluent and emerging nations. In less affluent countries, medical developments in palliative medicine often need to be guided by homegrown wisdom, not imitation of other social and health care systems.

SUSTAINING CONCEPTS OF MEDICAL PRACTICE

Medical Practice as an Interpersonal Activity

In the 17th century, Sydenham commented on Hippocrates: "His system led him to assist nature, to support her when enfeebled, and to the coercion of her when she was outrageous." However, the physician is not caring for nature, but for persons experiencing illness, and the activity of physicians needs to be seen in the context of interpersonal relationships. "What medicine lacks is any fundamental notion of the nature of man and any remotely adequate understanding of that which we refer to as a person."[15]

Has thinking within society and medicine advanced since Needleman wrote these words 40 years ago? We are much more aware of the relational quality of persons; we exist within webs of interlocution.[16] Philosophers have said that our relationships with others are constitutive of self. Ideas of such complexity are needed within medical practice, but they need translation to be useful; a grasp of the relational nature of persons is critical for physicians. An ecological model of person has been useful in thinking, clinical activity, and teaching (see Fig. 8-1 in Chapter 8).[17] The concept of person needs to be accompanied by a sound view of personal development and the role of crises (e.g., illness) in fostering such development. A view of the opportunities[18] and the tasks[19] of the last phase of life, at any age, may add depth to a physician's medical practice. When individual differences are blurred—this is philosophically regarded as the core of terrorism[20]—it is the privilege of the physician to celebrate difference and uniqueness, especially in palliative medicine. The blurring of difference by randomization in trials for the purpose of advancing knowledge requires a counterbalance of the difference and distinctiveness in knowledge garnered in such trials.[21] The objectification (even in outcomes) of what is properly subjective is a trend to be observed with concern and understanding. An adequate concept of person is needed to enable the physician to understand the patient and his or her experience of illness and to prioritize medical activity accordingly. It is also needed for physicians to understand and care for themselves[22] and for colleagues if necessary.

The Tasks of Medicine

Sigerist, the eminent medical historian, wrote: "The scope of medicine is broad, and it always includes infinitely more than the physician's actions. The task of medicine may be outlined under the following four headings:

- Promotion of health
- Prevention of illness
- Restoration of health
- Rehabilitation"[23]

The care of persons with fatal illnesses in the setting of the family and community should include all four dimensions, although they are not always considered in practice. Health promotion and preventive medicine are clear objectives, especially for community-based physicians. Psychological and spiritual rehabilitation have long been recognized by practitioners within hospice,[24] but formal involvement in rehabilitation programs to improve quality of life also is a worthy goal after treatment and for progressive disease.[25] Restoration of health for the patient and caregivers is possible, especially with good symptom relief as the starting point[19] for significant recovery of function and comfort, even in patients with progressive disease. The canvas is large, and meaningful medical practice is possible in situations of both affluence and poverty.

How do physicians approach these tasks, and what are their roles and strategies? Physicians have a large charter, and fulfilling the four medical tasks previously listed requires many significant activities:

- Comprehensive diagnosis
- Clinical decision making
- Management of disease processes proportionate to the benefit (i.e., avoiding flat-of-the-curve medicine)
- Relief of symptoms
- Relief of distress and suffering
- Advocacy for the weak in society
- Recognition and use of opportunities for prevention and rehabilitation

The role of physicians can be regarded as primarily analytic or diagnostic. What is the current problem of this person? What is the cause of this situation? What intervention, if any, should be undertaken for the benefit of this person? Who should intervene? What preventive measures can be undertaken and in what order of priority? How can the success or failure of any intervention be evaluated? This analytic or diagnostic activity is based on fundamental principles:

- A person is a relational reality (not a mere individual).
- Beneficence is the overriding incentive for action.
- Other persons may be needed to improve the quality of the diagnosis or assessment.

All enlightened clinicians recognize that a patient is more than his or her disease. The disease exists only in relation to this person, and this person is characterized by relationships with other persons in the past and present that are fundamental, historical, and embedded in a cultural matrix. This is the truth and richness of the human condition, the stuff of suffering and joy, fear, meaning, and hope. Ideas such as these are the substrate on which clinical understanding and diagnoses can be built; the physician as diagnostician logically precedes any notion of the physician as healer.

Diagnostic activity involves recognition of the patient's priorities, which may be focused on a particular symptom or on one aspect of care. It is far more respectful and efficient for the patient to volunteer the perceived needs than for a physician or colleagues to intrude into unnamed territories. This is a significant issue when complex issues such as demoralization, distress, suffering, or spirituality are considered. The only assistance the patient may ask for is pain relief, and any attempt to introduce other matters into a consultation by a primary or specialist physician may be inappropriately invasive. However, data indicate that some patients may appreciate the assistance of a competent physician in such matters. Physicians need to ponder such issues deeply, be prepared to modify their roles in various circumstances, and recognize the limits of their competence. Lack of sensitivity to adapt to the patient's needs can seriously compromise the benefit of a physician's intervention and increase the distress of a vulnerable patient and family.

Analytic activity includes unraveling layers of causes, options available for altering the course of the disease, and improving symptoms whether the disease can be controlled or not. A solid understanding of disease pathogenesis and pathophysiology should assist in assessing the next likely problems. What is on the horizon? Are acute complications to be expected? What can be anticipated? What distress can be prevented?

Cultural matters should be considered. Are there cultural implications or components of the current situation that need particular attention, or are they likely to occur in the future? Culture includes ethnicity, historical facts (e.g., trauma in war, imprisonment), the current geographic situation, economic hardship, and occupational factors. The culture gap between doctor and patient may be broad in terms of social and economic status; lifetime personal experience; world view; understanding of life, illness, death, and suffering; perception of the cosmos or ultimate reality; and appraisal of relevant personal responsibilities. The interpersonal gap between a competent, young physician, who is intent on providing excellent care and perhaps on establishing a family, and an elderly person facing fragility or death, who has different goals, may be unbridgeable by the best empathy training. The gap can be addressed by recognition while searching for a sense of common humanity. The occasional situation of a physician who is also a patient brings profound culturally determined ingredients into the care situation, a fact that must be considered sensitively but clearly by the treating physician. The literature abounds in stories of compromised care experienced by patients, physicians, and their families.

An idealized view may consider the physician to be a partner or, as in earlier times, to be a servant of the ill.

The patient may be seen as guest in the doctor's sphere of activity to be treated with the kindness and respect associated with traditional hospitality. However, the physician may be the guest in the patient's presence, invited to a place in which he or she is alien but welcome, with the responsibility to recognize the status and responsibilities of a guest and the boundaries of a mystery, which the other person always remains. What difference would it make to a clinical or hospital ward if the physician were the guest, with the patient being the welcoming host in the context of a complex web of relationships? Rather than glorifying power or autonomy, this idea recognizes the complexity of the human condition and another facet of human interdependence.

Diagnostic activity includes the assessment of needs, and it requires specialists with complementary skills. The primary physician is responsible for specifying the needs as precisely as possible to determine the correct referrals. The competence of colleagues in nursing, physiotherapy, social work, and other cognate professions ordinarily far exceeds the physician's competence in specific matters. The physician needs to ensure sensible goals and methods to evaluate the progress, leaving the specific strategies to be formulated by the relevant nonmedical colleagues.

Is referral to a palliative medicine specialist desirable? If one is not available in the vicinity (i.e., acute hospital, nursing home, or home), what is the next best alternative? Is telephone assistance reliable? Would it be in the patient's interest to arrange attendance at a palliative medicine clinic or seek admission to a special facility? An aspect of the competence expected of all physicians is to recognize poor symptom relief and not accept poor pain relief as inevitable or to be treated merely by antidisease strategies. Anticancer therapy is not usually the primary solution to pain in cancer. Analgesic treatment is mandatory even if antidisease strategies are available and appropriate. Palliative care can be given by a variety of persons, and it is not to be equated with specialist palliative care services (Fig. 48-2), which are not available in many situations globally or even in countries where widespread availability of consultative services is the national goal.

How do the activities of physicians relate to the actions of the others involved in achieving the goals of palliative care? The Hippocratic tradition (aphorisms) declared: "The physician must not only be prepared to do what is right himself, but also to make the patient, the attendants, and externals cooperate." Hippocrates saw the physician as a regulator or controller of the whole enterprise. This may not fit the ethos of modern interdisciplinary teams and families. The community physician has advantages in several dimensions of medical practice. The breadth of opportunities and the comprehensive knowledge of the community-based practitioner sometimes must be supplemented by the less comprehensive but more focused competence of a hospital-based palliative medicine specialist.

The physician who is a specialist in palliative medicine and other persons in a specialist palliative care team are envisaged at the pointed end at the base of the care pyramid (see Fig. 48-2). Their role is seen as supporting the whole enterprise, available if the more visible and usual means of care prove insufficient or inadequate. The team members have no claim to moral high ground or

The Care Pyramid

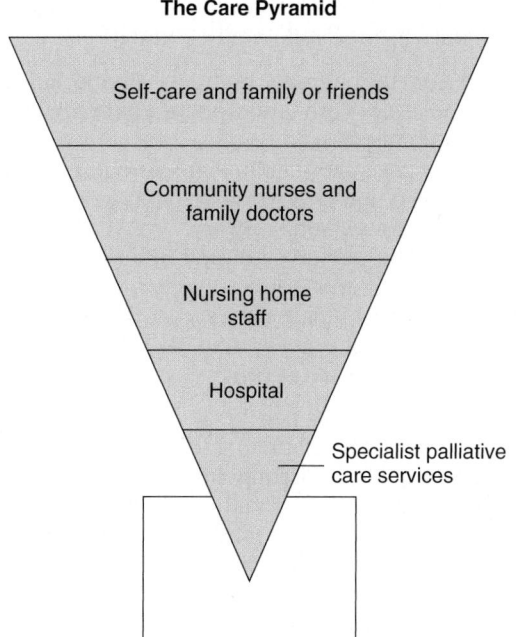

FIGURE 48-2   The care pyramid. Levels of care are shown for patients who have fatal illnesses, especially when approaching death.

Concepts and Values

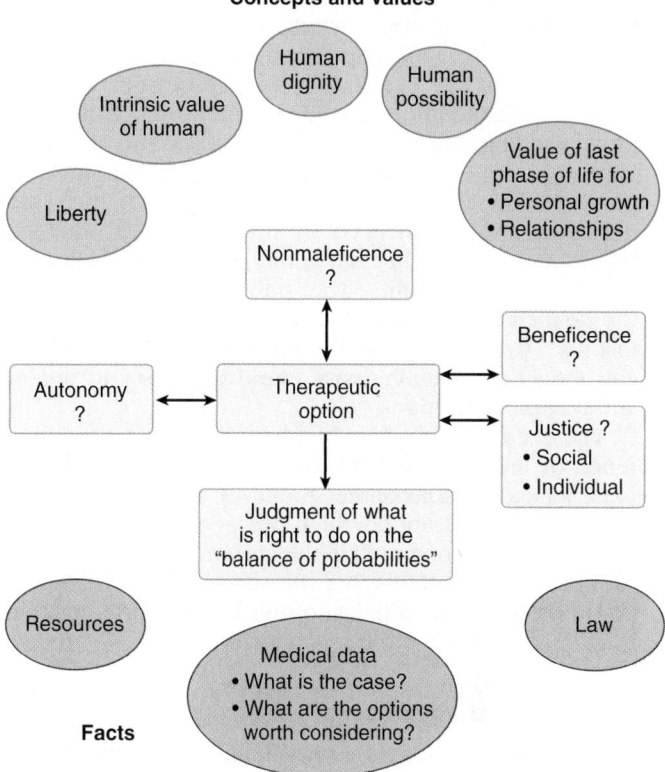

FIGURE 48-3   An ecological view of decision making.

excellence in communication, but they are charged with having higher levels of critically needed knowledge and skills, such as relief of major symptoms, help with existential distress, or resolution of complex ethical situations. This way of considering the complexity of care accords well with the *mixed management* called for in the landmark report of the Institute of Medicine.[26] The ramifications are far reaching for the physician's self concept and for medical education, clinical practice, administration, funding, and research.[27]

Approaching Clinical Decision Making

Diagnosis underpins clinical decisions, which usually involve a choice of wisest options in the face of several alternatives. There may be value in outlining approaches by physicians charged with navigating difficulties, often in emotionally charged circumstances. Clinicians are faced with many difficult decisions every day and frequently late at night and in emergency situations. Decision making is facilitated by internalization of relevant philosophical, legal, and ethical concepts so that a balanced approach becomes intuitive. Sound clinical decision making and practice may then contribute to human flourishing throughout life, especially at critical periods, and community cohesiveness may be enhanced. An ecological framework for decision making may be of practical assistance in assisting physicians to be aware of the context in which they strive to reach wise decisions. They are not alone; they have the legacies of human thought and experience embedded in a rich stream of human activity and compassion. In the care of those approaching death, the traditional Jewish ethic of "affirming life but not obstructing death" is a wise guideline.

An ecological approach to clinical decision making has been developed (Fig. 48-3). It is based in the following ideas:

- Cost-benefit analysis, with recognition of the complexity of the costs and benefits under scrutiny
- An adequate anthropology, with an ecological view of the person that takes into account the environment (including the personal field), personal history (more than medical facts), and inheritance (biological and cultural)
- An amalgam of some features of ethical traditions, notably principle-based, rule-based, and utilitarian, with the incorporation of the core notions of virtue ethics

Note is taken of prevailing values (so conditioned by historical and cultural factors) and of the relevant facts (medical, including evidence base, relevant law, and resource limitations). Careful analysis is undertaken of the implications of autonomy, beneficence, non-maleficence, and justice (individual and social). The central task remains that of making a decision on the balance of probabilities (as in a civil case) by the exercise of wisdom. Such an ecological portrayal of the process of decision-making emphasizes the complexity of the personal. This approach appears to be welcomed by medical students and graduates. The model needs to become intuitive if it is to be a practical clinical tool.

Appraisal may demonstrate the fruitfulness of exploring the interface of philosophy and medicine to facilitate human flourishing by understanding complexity. Awareness of the law is necessary in clinical decision making to clarify the limits of possibility and facilitate accuracy in analysis of factors pertaining to the human good.

Particular issues such as decisions on behalf of incompetent patients are seen as part of life narratives, not as arguments to be won by set procedures or principles. Uncertainty is part of the whole dynamic. We cannot be sure of all of the facts, judgments, perspectives, or consistent wishes of any person, but we can be sure whether every reasonable effort has been made to reach the best understanding. Many far-reaching decisions in everyday clinical practice must be made quickly. The classic situation is making decisions in the emergency room, but rapid decisions also are needed in hospital wards, nursing homes, homes, and the community, such as while driving a car in heavy traffic. The only sound approach is the deliberate internalization by physicians of an ethical instinct ("traffic sense") through painstaking education and reflection, enabling wise, rapid responses in urgent and complex situations.

The exercise of wisdom by physicians implies the existence of lines in the sand that ethical, beneficent, and experienced persons agree should be there and beyond which we should not go. Such precarious circumstances are not often encountered in the current context of caring for seriously ill patients, but the situation may change in the future through technical options for life prolongation that are considered ethically abhorrent.

A Focus for the Passion of Physicians

Michel Foucault[28] wrote, "What counts in the things said by men is not so much what they may have thought or the extent to which these things represent their thoughts, as that which systematizes them from the outset, thus making them thereafter endlessly accessible to new discourses and open to the task of transforming them."

There is talk about the passion of the Western mind, an idea so powerful that it sustains in dark times. What is the passion of the medical mind? Is it curiosity about the causes, treatment, and prevention of disease? Intellectual curiosity is a powerful medical driver, but it must be tempered by compassion for people. Rather than law or contract, the philosophical basis for the duty of care is the "call of the other," an instinctive response to someone in need or distress. For physicians, there is an imperative to relieve suffering.[29] The desire to preserve human dignity may foster such responsiveness. Can danger to life, distress (e.g., pain, rape, torture), or other harm be subsumed under threats to human dignity, with physicians charged in society to be guardians of human dignity? Can human dignity be safeguarded or maintained, even in horrendous suffering?

Legal documents, political documents, advocacy statements, the media, and common discourse address respect for and violation of human dignity. In 2006, the United Nations Educational, Scientific, and Cultural Organization (UNESCO) produced the New Universal Declaration on Bioethics, which highlights such matters. Philosophers write about human dignity from diverse perspectives, and religious documents (e.g., Vatican Council) extol it as derived from a divine source. Physicians and nurses have in the past decades paid attention to human dignity in clinical contexts and research.[30-32] Dying with dignity is not a slogan for the glorification of autonomy or a corrupted synonym for a deliberately accelerated death.[33] Logically, an adequate concept of human dignity should relate to a suitable concept of person. If the ecological concept discussed in Chapter 8 is the starting point, human dignity has the following connotations:

- Respect for the human body in all circumstances, before and after death and especially when vulnerable, and its basic needs
- Respect for personal relationships, such as bonds with family, friends, and fellow citizens
- Respect for the person's history
- Respect for the person's cultural inheritance
- Respect the person's hopes and even secret dreams
- Respect for the human capacity to transcend the self and to extend to others or to the absolute other in prayer or through other rituals

All of these objectives may be systematically violated in torture, in inhumane imprisonment, in public policies (e.g., regarding illegal immigrants), or in some social systems in which the most vulnerable in society are systematically neglected. The complexity of the term *human dignity* mandates interdisciplinary consideration. Some view the term as a useless or vague concept,[34] but even vague ideas can set the world on fire.[35]

What does it mean for physicians, especially palliative medicine practitioners, to be advocates for the weak in society[36] and guardians of human dignity? It implies more concentration on public policies and health care strategies and a greater focus on the quality of medical practice with regard to individual patients. It may also unify a fragmented profession by recognized participation in a critical human project of high relevance in the 21st century.

CONCLUSIONS

Clinical science, the basis of the care of others by physicians (usually in a team), needs to be recognized as a human rather than a natural science. In the 18th and 19th centuries, knowledge was compartmentalized into natural and human sciences. The foundation of the human sciences was in the historicity of humankind.[37] This was also the basis of medical science. Elements of the natural sciences provide a strategy for increasing human personal good by increasing the well-being of whole persons and whole communities, and there may be need for reappraisal of medicine in relation to the humanities. Palliative medicine may have the capacity for building bridges between the natural and human sciences. Palliative medicine should recognize the need for medical practice to be more scientific, with goals clarified in light of the view of a person as a relational reality and strategies defined by a sound grasp of the relevant natural sciences. Mortimer[38] said, "The task of medicine is to emancipate man's interior splendour."[38] In this millennium, the meaning of that splendor may be discerned, even in the ruins wrought by violence, as a source of hope for rebuilding the human edifice and with physicians guarding it.

REFERENCES

1. Teilhard de Chardin P. Activation of Energy. London: Collins, 1970, p 294-295; quoted in Kearney MA. Place of Healing: Working with Suffering in Living and Dying. Oxford, UK: Oxford University Press, 2000, p 15.
2. Sigerist HE. A History of Medicine, vol 1. Primitive and Archaic Medicine. New York: Oxford University Press, 1951, p 11.
3. Conrad LI, Neve M, Nutton V, et al. The Western Medical Tradition 800 BC to AD 1800. Cambridge, UK: Cambridge University Press, 1995.

4. Grmek MD (ed), Shugaar A (transl). Western Medical Thought from Antiquity to the Middle Ages. Cambridge, UK: Harvard University Press, 1998.
5. Geraghty KE, Wynia MK. Advocacy and community: The social roles of physicians in the last 1000 years. Part I. MedGenMed 2000;2(4):E29.
6. Geraghty KE, Wynia M. Advocacy and community: The social roles of physicians in the last 1000 years. Part II. MedGenMed 2000;Nov 6:E28.
7. Geraghty KE, Wynia M. Advocacy and community: The social roles of physicians in the last 1000 years. Part III. MedGenMed 2000;Nov 13:E27.
8. Bruera E, Higginson IJ, Ripamonti C, von Gunten CF. Textbook of Palliative Medicine. London: Hodder Arnold, 2006, pp 49-57.
9. Lewis M. Medicine and the Care of the Dying: A Modern History. Oxford, UK: Oxford University Press, 2006.
10. Watson D. A Terrible Beauty: The People and Ideas that Shaped the Modern Mind. A History. London: Phoenix, 2000.
11. Alexander L. Medicine under dictatorship. N Engl J Med 1949;241:40-47.
12. Glare PA, Lickiss JN. Quality Assurance in Palliative Care [letter]. Med J Aust 1992;157:572.
13. Enthoven AC. Cutting cost without cutting the quality of care (Shattuck lecture). N Engl J Med 1978;298:1229-1238.
14. Farber SJ, Egnew TR, Herman-Bertsch JL. Defining effective clinical roles in end-of-life care. J Fam Pract 2002;51:153-158.
15. Needleman J. The perception of mortality. Ann N Y Acad Sci 1969; 164:733-738.
16. Taylor C. Sources of the Self: The Making of Modern Identity. Cambridge, MA: Harvard University Press, 1989.
17. Lickiss JN. The human experience of illness. In Walsh TD, Fainsinger R, Foley KM, et al (eds). Palliative Medicine. Philadelphia: Elsevier, 2008.
18. Byock IR. Caring for the dying. In Morgan JD (ed). Readings in Thanatology. New York: Amityville, 1997, pp 181-195.
19. Anderson H. Living until we die: Reflections on the dying person's spiritual agenda. Anesthesiol Clin North Am 2006;24:213-225.
20. Borradori G. Philosophy in a Time of Terror: Dialogues with Jurgen Habermas and Jacques Derrida. Chicago: University of Chicago Press, 2003, p 7.
21. Feinstein AR. Clinical judgment revisited: The distraction of quantitative models. Ann Intern Med 1994;120:799-805.
22. Meier DE, Back AL Morrison RS. The inner life of physicians and the care of the seriously ill. JAMA 2001;286:3007-3014.
23. Sigerist HE. A History of Medicine, vol 1. Primitive and Archaic Medicine. New York: Oxford University Press, 1951, p 7.
24. Kearney M. Mortally Wounded: Stories of Soul Pain, Death and Healing. Dublin: Mercier Press, 1996.
25. Gerber LH. Cancer Rehabilitation into the future. Cancer 2001; 92(Suppl):975-979.
26. Institute of Medicine, Committee on Care at the End of Life. Approaching Death: Improving Care at the End of Life. Washington, DC: National Academy Press, 1997.
27. Glare PA, Virik K. Can we do better in end of life care? The mixed management model and palliative care. Med J Aust 2001;175:530-533.
28. Foucault M. The Birth of the Clinic: The Archeology of Medical Practice. New York: Vintage Books, 1993.
29. Cassell E. The Nature of Suffering and the Goals of Medicine. N Engl J Med 1982;306:639-645.
30. Turner K, Chye R, Aggawal G, et al. Dignity in dying: A preliminary study of patients in the last three days of life. J Palliat Care 1996;12:7-13.
31. Street A, Kissane D. Constructions of dignity in end-of-life care. J Palliat Care 2001;17:93-101.
32. Chochinov HM. Dignity and the essence of medicine: The A, B, C, and D of dignity conserving care. BMJ 2007;335:184-187.
33. Roy DJ. To die with dignity [editorial]. J Palliat Care 1986;2:3-5.
34. Macklin R. Reflections on the human dignity symposium: Is dignity a useless concept? J Palliat Care 2004;20:212-216.
35. Malpas J, Lickiss JN (eds). Perspectives on Human Dignity: A Conversation. Dordrecht: Stringer, 2007.
36. Lickiss JN. On the care of our aged: Privilege and responsibility. Aust Rehabil Rev 1982;2:51-57.
37. Dilthey W, Betzanos RJ (transl). Introduction to the Human Sciences. Detroit, MI: Wayne State University Press, 1988 (originally published in 1923).
38. Mortimer K. The impossible profession: The doctor-priest relationship. Proc Aust Assoc Gerontol 1974;2:81-82.

CHAPTER **49**

Nurses and Nurse Practitioners

Philip J. Larkin

KEY POINTS

- Nursing has contributed significantly to early concepts of palliative care.
- The evidence base for specialist palliative nursing is weak, particularly in relation to measurable outcomes.
- Palliative nursing must be vigilant regarding the potential impact of a biomedical model on nursing practice, particularly at the specialist level.
- Good palliative nursing should reflect a healthy balance between self (i.e., practitioner) and others (i.e., patient, family, and team) to be clinically effective.
- Palliative nurses in practice need to embrace a stronger research agenda.

The contribution of nursing to palliative care is well founded. Cicely Saunders[1] validated the strategic role that nursing played in her concept of the care of the dying in her early letters (1959-1999), in which she contends that her approach to individual patient suffering is possible only through "individual and careful nursing."[1] Modern palliative nursing faces two main challenges: negotiating the interface between palliative care and hospice care (the former is considered an evolution of the latter) and the broadening of a "palliative care for all" reality. Pioneers' values and aspirations are set against the demands of a society that increasingly seeks technological solutions to health problems. As higher levels of specialist practice develops, palliative nursing practitioners must ground themselves further in fundamental nursing practice to complement the new skills from the traditional biomedical model, rather than become overwhelmed by them.[2] Only then can nurses meet the full range of challenges in palliative nursing.

PALLIATIVE NURSING

Many patients receive good palliative nursing care from nurses who do not claim any specialist knowledge. The shift in The World Health Organization's definition of palliative care from *specialty* to *approach*[3] questions the extent to which palliative care should be a set of transferable principles for best practice or a specialty. Definitions of palliative nursing often highlight the generic rather than specialist nature of practice: "The role of palliative care nursing is therefore to assess needs in each of these areas and to plan, implement, and evaluate appropriate interventions. It aims to improve the quality of life and to enable a dignified death."[4]

Palliative care nurses need to be clear about how their specific contributions[5] to care differ from those of other nursing colleagues. For example, a supportive care model for Ann (see "Case Study: Nursing Contribution to Palliative Care") frames holistic palliative nursing as shown in Table 49-1. Analysis of these core values identified that palliative nursing "encompasses several dimensions, but the skill of providing comprehensive family care was seen to be based on knowledge, wisdom, and personal strengths."[6]

Further refinement clarified clinically relevant concepts such as comfort, empathy, and hope.[7] Their global applicability needs to be considered carefully within the cultural context. Specialist palliative nursing is featured in the U.K. and U.S. literature, with only limited global application to nurses elsewhere for whom such specialist roles are aspirational.

How can specialist palliative nursing lead to measurable outcomes? This can best be achieved through a clinical practice that enables continual proximity to patients and families and that is supported by sound theoretical preparation and more research. This ideal is increasingly

evident as academic nursing is developed. However, the dominant medical culture has raised concern among palliative nurses that medicine defines palliative care. This challenges palliative nursing to articulate its position as a co-contributor to care that is intended to be multidisciplinary.[8]

KEY CONSTRUCTS WITHIN PALLIATIVE NURSING

One well-apportioned analysis of the constituents of palliative nursing regrettably reveals the somewhat weak evidence base for some of the elements in palliative nursing.[7] Caring and its "emotional labor" for nurses are well explored.[9] Other dimensions, such as comfort and empathy, are less well delineated. The meaning of referral to palliative nursing services for support lacks clarity.[10] The multifaceted nature of nursing support in the clinical case of Ann requires Julie, the palliative care nurse specialist, to define the aims, objectives, and boundaries of her practice with Ann. The expansion of palliative care to patients with nonmalignant diseases has become a critical element in contemporary palliative nursing, reflecting shifting roles, the autonomy of practice, and the clinical capacity of the nurse to provide care. The key issues are presented in the interaction between Julie as specialist nurse practitioner and Ann and her family as care recipients. The term *practitioner* is used in a generic sense rather than the clinical role notable in the United States, United Kingdom, and Australia. This distinction only complicates the debate.

DEVELOPMENTS AND OPPORTUNITIES IN PALLIATIVE NURSING

Roles and Functions

Given the limited empirical evidence about what Julie does, it is no less complicated to consider who Julie is. Titles rarely reflect function and are used arbitrarily. Within the titles possible (i.e., clinical nurse specialist, nurse practitioner, advanced nurse practitioner, and nurse consultant), efforts continue to delineate roles and functions of the specialist nurse and avoid competing agendas.[11] Randomized, controlled trials suggest that specialist nursing can deliver and change the experience and quality of care, although conclusive evidence of effectiveness, outcome measures, or patient benefit is less robust.[12,13] Julie's specialist role was created more because of organizational expediency than professional nursing development, reflecting a failing health service and the patient demands for greater choice and accessibility.[14] Julie encounters resistance to specialist nursing within and outside the profession, manifested in restrictive practice guidelines and a lack of consensus on the scope of practice. Nurse prescribing (where permitted) is one example where Julie, acting on her clinical assessment, can respond effectively to Ann's need for immediate symptom relief. However, regulatory constraint may limit her ability to act within the full capacity of her skills and knowledge.

Autonomous Nursing Practice

Increasing clinical autonomy appears to define the scope of the nurse practitioner (Box 49-1). Although nursing

CASE STUDY

Nursing Contribution to Palliative Care

Ann is a 76-year-old woman with end-stage chronic obstructive pulmonary disease. She is a widow, and she lives alone on the family farm, supported by her daughter and two sons. She has chosen to stay at home for her end-of-life management under the supervision of the local palliative care team. Their main point of contact is Julie, the palliative care nurse specialist who visits twice weekly. Julie has 15 years of clinical experience in oncology and palliative care. Ann's key symptoms are increasing breathlessness and fatigue. She has a limited prognosis. The option of a hospice bed has been discussed with the family, but it was declined at that time.

TABLE 49-1	Supportive Care Model for a Patient
CONCEPT	**ACTION**
Valuing	Being aware of the events that have shaped patient Ann's life and her recent health history
Connecting	Sensing the family dynamic and the role of the specialist nurse for Ann and her family
Empowering	Enabling Ann to care for herself as much as possible and becoming an active agent in her decision making
Doing for	When beyond family capacity, intervening appropriately through clinical judgment, such as enhanced comfort measures or oxygen therapy
Finding meaning	Being open to the broader context in which Ann experiences her end-of-life care and what may affect her interpretation of that experience
Preserving integrity	The ability to invest and withdraw from Ann's care in a fashion that does not cause the family to feel abandoned nor the nurse to feel compromised professionally or emotionally

Adapted from Davies B, Oberle K. Dimensions of the supportive role of the nurse in palliative care. Oncol Nurs Forum 1990;19:763-767.

TABLE 49-2	Proposed Levels of Palliative Nurse Education		
CHARACTERISTICS	**LEVEL A**	**LEVEL B**	**LEVEL C**
Target group	Basic undergraduate, basic postgraduate	Advanced postgraduate	Specialist, postgraduate
Aim (core practice competencies)	Promoting a palliative care approach	Key referent persons (e.g., community nurse)	Specialist practitioner

Adapted from DeVlieger M, Gorchs N, Larkin P, Porchet F. A Guide to the Development of Palliative Nurse Education in Europe. Report of the European Association for Palliative Care (E.A.P.C.) Taskforce on Palliative Nurse Education. Milan, Italy: European Association for Palliative Care, 2004, p 9.

Box 49-1 Increasing Clinical Autonomy for the Nurse Practitioner

Role extension: A particular skill or practice not previously associated with a nursing role (e.g., phlebotomy to ascertain the patient's blood gas values)

Role expansion: Clinical management of referred cases, prescription, and re-referral to the senior clinician (e.g., nurse's use of the physician as a second level of clinical advice)

Role development: Highest level of clinical autonomy that involves diagnosis and eventual discharge or independent referral to another agency (e.g., nurse refers the patient to the radiography department for a radiograph)

Adapted from An Bord Altranais. Scope of Nursing and Midwifery Practice Framework 2000. Dublin: An Bord Altranais, 2000.

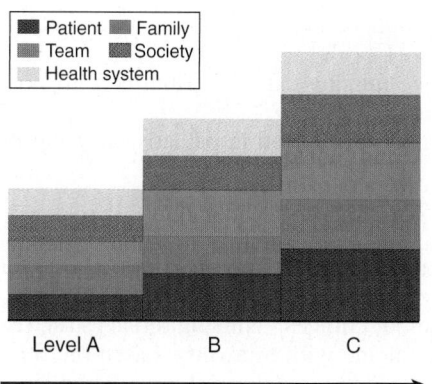

FIGURE 49-1   Dimension of the palliative care learning process. Learning levels should reflect the foci of clinically complex palliative nursing. *(Adapted from DeVlieger M, Gorchs N, Larkin P, Porchet F: A Guide to the Development of Palliative Nurse Education in Europe. Report of the European Association for Palliative Care (E.A.P.C.) Taskforce on Palliative Nurse Education. Milan, Italy: European Association for Palliative Care, 2004, p 20.)*

roles differ considerably in autonomy, comparative studies highlight the similarity in expertise.[11] Empirical studies support the positive impact of specialist nursing compared with medical provision. Specialist nurses consistently provide higher continuity of care, greater cost-effectiveness, increased patient satisfaction, higher outcome indicators, and reduced waiting times.[12] Statistically significant improvements in emotional and cognitive functioning[15] follow intervention by a specialist nurse, with positive outcomes reported for 55% of patients. Theoretically, Ann should find her needs met by Julie working from this specialist framework.

In palliative nursing, rapid expansion and limited evidence to demonstrate role effectiveness have led to increasing concern about the benefit and cost implications. Role evaluation in palliative nursing is particularly difficult because of the changing complexity of need. Research into the impact and efficiency of specialist nursing roles is sparse and has not determined how much effectiveness can be demonstrated. Future research must examine tangible evidence of the value and contribution of palliative nursing.

CONTROVERSIES AND RESEARCH OPPORTUNITIES

Specialization—An Ongoing Debate

The risk that a narrow focus on specialist practice may prevent innovative approaches to palliative care indicates that a public health approach may offer a better structure for palliative care practice. There is a need to refocus palliative nursing practice on a wider range of care provision than only cancer, and this will be a challenge for the future. Many services still focus on the "safety net" of oncology, even though it is clear that the nurse specialist's applied knowledge can benefit noncancer patients' life quality and symptom management.

Education

Equally challenging is the nursing knowledge required for quality palliative care.[16] Guidelines recommend an incremental approach (Table 49-2) from basic to specialist levels, noting key areas for learning and core practice competencies. Significantly, the guidelines make specific reference to level B practitioners, for whom palliative care comprises only one part of their daily clinical work beyond the specialist dimension. As palliative nursing develops, it will be important to see how the dissemination of knowledge affects the quality of patient care.

These learning levels should reflect the foci of clinically complex palliative nursing (Fig. 49-1). In Ann's case, Julie must identify and act on the levels of knowledge required regarding Ann, her family, team involvement, her changing life role, and her increasing needs from the health system as her illness progresses. This includes shared working (e.g., with the community nurse) to enhance the care plan offered.

Challenges in Practice and Research

The vision[5] of caring as a condition and goal of palliative nursing practice, especially given the importance nurses place on personal relationships with patients, is based on an ideal of nursing as a "moral practice."[17] There are four potential challenges to contemporary palliative care nursing: clinical integrity, intuition, emotional authenticity, and diagnostic reasoning. The holistic nature of practice means they should not be considered as discrete entities.

Research is warranted in several areas:

- Studies that measure the outcomes of palliative nursing interventions
- Studies of the costs and benefits of specialist nursing roles
- Application of clinical nursing judgment in palliative care
- Palliative nursing care for patients with nonmalignant diseases
- The value of intuition in palliative nursing practice

Clinical Integrity

Nurses function from a holistic model that offers a broad framework within which to make diagnostic decisions and treatment choices.[2] Nursing replaces the risk of paternalistic medicine with mutuality, based on "a relationship that is collaborative, reciprocal, negotiated, and participatory."[2] Nurses need to balance biomedical knowledge with a view that focuses on patients' distress, suffering, and vulnerability. In the Case Study, it is important that Julie as a palliative nurse specialist does not abandon her nursing foundation in search of a decontextualized, technologically focused symptom approach that distances her from Ann. Her unique contribution includes a transitional role, guiding the family and patient through the facets of curative, palliative, and terminal care. Within this framework, symptom management and emotional support figure highly, and clinical judgment is often about balancing the two dimensions. As the closest practitioner to Ann as death approaches, Julie needs to impart news that requires comprehension of physical deterioration and family readiness to accept those consequences. Palliative nursing can be a struggle against a professional ideal based on science, in which expertise is defined in terms of medical technology that manages dying as efficiently as possible but risks the essence of caring. This continual shift in priorities demands of Julie a high level of responsiveness and the capacity to deal with uncertainty.

Emotional Authenticity in Relationships

Relationship seems key to the success or failure of quality palliative nursing care. Mutual trust in the clinical relationship enables nursing excellence through the personal qualities and skills the nurse brings to that relationship. Being continually available to the needs of patients and families has its own consequences. The emotional burden of palliative nursing suggests that sustaining relationships leads to loss and emotional distress when death occurs. The family model of care creates a framework in which emotion, intimacy, and authenticity can be shared, but it can be hard for nurses to set limits to preserve themselves from loss. Retreat into the safe zone of technical expertise can diminish the holistic nature of palliative nursing. If emotional authenticity is to function in Ann's case, formal support systems that enable Julie to share and validate her experiences need to be enacted. Clinical supervision is valuable for palliative nursing,[18] particularly using a multidisciplinary approach that offers greater potential for solidarity in palliative care practice.

Intuition

Intuition is one facet of the complexity of nursing knowledge, complementing empirical science, aesthetics, and moral knowledge. Given the shift toward evidence-based practice, it is surprising that more research into this aspect of palliative nursing has not been done. There are counterarguments against intuition as the basis for nurses' decision making; intuitive decisions cannot be made explicit and therefore limit transparency and patient participation.[19] However, Julie has a responsibility to respond to Ann as a person and a patient. This is possible only by blending intuitive and empirical ways of knowing.

Diagnostic Reasoning

Diagnostic reasoning is "the hallmark of an expert nurse practitioner."[21] It is a combination of analytical and intuitive thinking that favors discretionary judgment. It is about "understanding the illness experience, in contrast to knowing the disease."[21] Julie's ability to reason effectively requires melding empirical and aesthetic knowledge. Her clinical effectiveness is based on adaptability to diverse clinical situations. Julie must combine technical knowledge and creative care with practical wisdom to elicit positive outcomes for Ann and her family. Palliative nursing may be uniquely able to respond to tangible aspects of living that palliative patients fear losing as disease progresses: time, connections to their world, and companionship. As an effective diagnostician, Julie should reflect this responsive nursing paradigm at all times and not lose sight of the greater good—care where cure is no longer possible.

CONCLUSIONS

Palliative nurses face challenges in their professional practice, particularly the need to be vigilant to the effect of biomedicine on the structure and function of palliative nursing practice. The historical contribution of nursing to palliative care is a legacy current practitioners should uphold, given the value placed on it by Cecily Saunders. Refinement of the World Health Organization's definition of palliative care offers a wealth of possibilities to nurses for whom care of advanced disease is an integral part of their clinical practice. This does not preclude the ideal of extended practice within a specialist framework.

Nurses must expand palliative nursing practice beyond an isolationist, cancer-driven policy to demonstrate its intrinsic value. There are great opportunities for research in palliative nursing, but only if a structured application to education linked to practice is enacted. The future of a palliative nursing expert such as Julie will be determined by the combined efforts of nurse practitioners, educators, and managers to promote a deeper understanding of clinical nursing expertise in their unique contribution to the care of incurable and advanced disease.

REFERENCES

1. Clark D (ed). Cicely Saunders, Founder of the Hospice Movement: Selected Letters, 1959-1999. Oxford, UK: Oxford University Press, 2002.
2. Chase SK. Clinical Judgment and Communication in Nurse Practitioner Practice. Philadelphia: FA Davis, 2004, p 5.
3. World Health Organization (WHO): Definition of palliative care, 2002. Available at http://www.who.int/cancer/palliative.definition/en/ (accessed October 11, 2007).
4. Lugton J, Kindlen M (eds). Palliative Care: The Nursing Role. Edinburgh: Churchill Livingstone, 1999.
5. Davies B, Oberle K. Dimensions of the supportive role of the nurse in palliative care. Oncol Nurs Forum 1990;19:763-767.
6. Wilson-Barnett J, Richardson A. Nursing research and palliative care. In Doyle D, Hanks GWC, MacDonald N (eds). Oxford Textbook of Palliative Medicine. Oxford, UK: Oxford University Press, 1995, p 101.
7. Seymour J. What's in a name? A concept analysis of key terms in palliative care nursing. In Payne S, Seymour J, Ingleton C (eds). Palliative Care Nursing, Principles and Evidence for Practice. London: Open University Press, 2004, pp 55-74.
8. Payne S, Sheldon F, Jarrett N, et al. Differences in understanding of specialist palliative care amongst service providers and commissioners in South London. Palliat Med 2002;16:395-402.
9. Aranda S. The cost of caring. Surviving the culture of niceness, occupational stress and coping strategies. In Payne S, Seymour J, Ingleton C (eds). Palliative Care Nursing, Principles and Evidence for Practice. London: Open University Press, 2004, pp 620-635.
10. Skilbeck J, Corner J, Bath P, et al. Clinical nurse specialists in palliative care. I. A description of the Macmillan nurse caseload. Palliat Med 2002;16: 285-296.
11. Roberts-Davis M, Read S. Clinical role clarification using the Delphi method to establish similarities and differences between nurse practitioners and clinical nurse specialists. J Clin Nurs 2001;10:33-43.
12. Mundinger MO, Kane RL, Lenz ER, et al. Primary care outcomes in patients treated by nurse practitioners or physicians: A randomized trial. JAMA 2000;28:59-68.
13. Venning P, Durie A, Roland M, et al. Randomized controlled trial comparing cost effectiveness of general practitioners and nurse practitioners in primary care. BMJ 2000;320:1048-1053.
14. Daly W, Carnwell R. Nursing roles and levels of practice: A framework for differentiating between elementary, advanced and specialist nursing practice. J Clin Nurs 2003;12:157-166.
15. Blackford J, Street A. The role of the palliative care nurse consultant in promoting continuity of end-of-life care. Int J Palliat Nurs 2001;7:273-278.
16. Corner J, Halliday J, Haviland J, et al. Exploring nursing outcomes for patients with advanced cancer following intervention by Macmillan specialist palliative care nurses. J Adv Nurs 2003;41:561-574.
17. De Vlieger M, Gorchs N, Larkin P, Porchet F. A Guide to the Development of Palliative Nurse Education in Europe. Report of the European Association for Palliative Care (E.A.P.C) Taskforce on Palliative Nurse Education. Milan, Italy: European Association for Palliative Care, 2004.
18. Georges JJ, Grypdonck M, Direckx de Casterlé B. Being a palliative care nurse in an academic hospital: A qualitative study about nurses' perceptions of palliative care nursing. J Adv Nurs 2002;11:785-793.
19. Jones A. Some benefits experienced by hospice nurses from group clinical supervision. Eur J Cancer Care 2003;12:224-232.
20. Lamond D, Thompson C. Intuition and analysis in decision making and choice. J Nurs Scholarsh 2000;32:411-414.
21. Ritter BJ. An analysis of expert nurse practitioners' diagnostic reasoning. J Am Acad Nurse Pract 2003;15:137-141.

SUGGESTED READING

Morse JM, Johnson JL. The Illness Experience: Dimensions of Suffering. Newbury Park, CA: Sage, 1991.

Payne S, Seymour J, Ingleton C. Palliative Care Nursing, Principles and Evidence for Practice. London: Open University Press, 2004.

Rasmussen BH, Norberg A, Sandman PO. Stories about becoming a hospice nurse: Reasons, expectations, hopes and concerns. Cancer Nurs 1995;18:344-354.

Skilbeck JK, Payne S. End of life care: A discourse analysis of specialist palliative care nursing. J Adv Nurs 2005;51: 325-334.

Walsh K, Kowalko I. Nurses' and patients' perceptions of dignity. Int J Nurs Pract 2002;8:143-151.

CHAPTER **50**

The Social Worker

Ruth D. Powazki

KEY POINTS

- Social work roles include clinical practice, education, consultation, advocacy, and research.
- Social workers function in varied practice settings in an interdisciplinary context.
- Social workers are skilled in age-appropriate, life-stage, and multidimensional assessment of individuals and their families.
- Social workers design and implement psychosocial interventions to help individuals and their families accommodate to illness.
- Social workers are trained how to access systems that people must navigate as they cope with the impact of illness.

During the 1960s in the United States and the United Kingdom, social workers began to publish their concerns about the pain, suffering, and unmet needs of cancer patients and their families. Lack of communication about diagnosis and prognosis was identified as a key barrier to timely and appropriate discharge from the hospital, and it prevented continuity of care.[1]

Research and experience have since shown that social workers' knowledge and skills are essential to provide palliative care that meets the complex needs of patients and their families in various practice settings: hospitals, outpatient clinics, nursing homes, home care, and hospice.

The social worker is aligned with other health professionals in providing palliative care to patients and families. The 21st century social worker collaborates in consultation and education with other team members regarding appropriate psychosocial intervention; educates and advocates within the health care setting and community at large; and participates in research to establish best practices in palliative care.

FUNCTION OF SOCIAL WORK

Social work in palliative care focuses on psychosocial care delivered to the patient and his or her family through assessment, communication, and interventions of education and counseling. Psychosocial care is multidimensional and addresses the impact of illness on the patient and family in terms of physical and cognitive limits, social and emotional needs, and cultural, spiritual, religious, and ethical values and beliefs.[2]

Assessment

Psychosocial care for the patient begins with the assessment. The primary assessment requires an understanding of the illness, including the diagnosis and prognosis; an ability to make decisions; a grasp of the influence of functional and cognitive decline on continuity of care; and a capacity for adaptation and resilience.

Secondary assessment requires an understanding of family values, structure, and function (especially of the primary caregiver for any adverse function). This information guides interventions to improve understanding, accommodation, and support to ensure the patient's comfort and symptom control in the home. Further secondary assessment identifies unmet needs and potential barriers to care, including mental health, employment, legal, and financial issues; a history of loss; dependent family members; caregiver strain; and the ability to participate in the plan of care.

Communication

The overall function of the social worker is to assess family function and provide counseling and referrals to resources for managing those risks.[3] As illness progresses, the involvement of family becomes an added focus of care. Many family members with frequent questions (who do not always share the information received within the family circle) can create excess demands on the treatment team. If the patient's needs are changing, it is distressful when the family appears to be receiving conflicting information. This can be minimized if patients identify their significant family members and designate a family spokesperson. Although usually the primary caregiver, the spokesperson may be a different family member, such as one who is more articulate about medical issues.

The content of conversations requires the social worker to be familiar with the language used by the patient, family, and professionals to convey the transitions from aggressive to supportive care and to approaching death. Achieving congruence and reciprocity in this communication is necessary to establish a consensus about goals of care. A family's values, ethics, and religious views can give insight to its decision making.[4] Some may have significant communication challenges due to illiteracy, language deficits, or a different primary language, requiring specialized translators.

A family is dynamic and greater than the sum of its parts, creating a powerful system. Understanding communication from the perspective of the family system is valuable for appreciating the impact of closed system communications (i.e., prevents penetration) on patients with a life-limiting illness. For example, in a closed system, the patient is aware of the poor prognosis and has extensive knowledge but does not communicate with anyone. The family has basic information from the physician that is supplemented by other sources. This information is distorted and reinterpreted in conversations among family members. The physician and palliative care interdisciplinary team have their own system of communication based on medical facts. They are influenced by emotional reactivity to the family and within the staff[5] (Fig. 50-1).

Obstacles, such as desire for more treatment without benefit, resistance to transition, family dysfunction, and emotional volatility of patients and families, can block communication among the team, patient, and family.

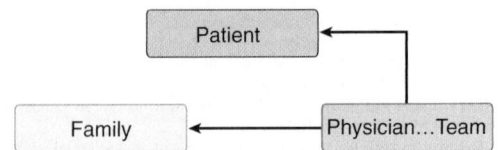

FIGURE 50-1 Communication in a closed system. The patient often does not communicate with anyone else in the closed system. The family receives basic information from the physician that may be supplemented by other sources. The physician and palliative care interdisciplinary team communicate based on medical facts.

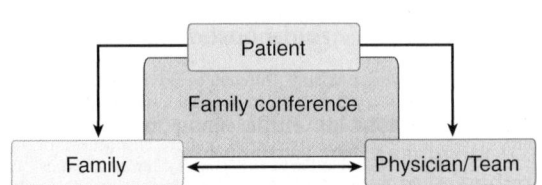

FIGURE 50-2 Communication in an open system. Information is exchanged among all parties in an open system. Using interventions to support the patient and family promotes good communication with all concerned. In palliative medicine, the structured family conference is a comprehensive communication intervention.

Common Errors
• Social work remains too peripheral in team discussions, and psychosocial issues are not integrated into decision making.
• Individual psychology receives too much focus, and the influence of family and social issues is minimized.
• Medical issues are misconstrued as psychosocial issues.
• Information is given before the plan of care is clarified (e.g., decision on code status pursued too aggressively)
• Information is given to the wrong person, who is not the designated spokesperson.

These issues must be managed to ensure quality and continuity of care (see "Common Errors").

A structured family conference can enhance the communication of the team with the patient and family. Developing and using interventions to support the patient and family promotes good communication with all concerned, and the family conference may be the best practice format for good communication (Fig. 50-2).

In palliative medicine, the structured family conference is a comprehensive communication intervention. Its twin goals are to integrate medical and psychosocial information within a specific agenda and engage the patient and family. It is an educational and supportive meeting attended by at least one family member or patient-designated spokesperson; the patient, when able to participate; and two members of the multidisciplinary team (usually the physician and social worker).

Having one person coordinate the family conference minimizes confusion, and the social worker who has been collaborating with the family is the best person to do this. The greatest integration of the medical and psychosocial information occurs when the physician and social worker both facilitate the family conference. Communication centers on essential information such as diagnosis, prognosis, advanced directives, performance status, mental status, illness course, likely complications as the disease progresses, and recommended plan of care (Table 50-1).[6]

Family conferences promote mutual understanding and trust among the patient, family, and the team; encourage compliance with medical recommendations; and support discharge planning in a timely fashion and continuity of care. The structure, content, and process of the family conference can benefit the patient and family, especially regarding transition and adaptation.

ROLES OF SOCIAL WORKERS

Functions of the social worker may include accessing practical services, developing programs, creating and presenting educational programs, and research. During the transition into palliative care, a range of services is needed to help the patient and family cope with the illness. The social worker can link entitlement programs, home care needs, equipment, and supportive services for the patient and family.

Social workers provide specialized services within palliative medicine, such as psychosocial rounds to address psychosocial practice themes. This can focus on complex and challenging needs of the patient and family and the demands that impede medical management.

Social workers share their expertise in education within the work setting and with colleagues in other health care settings and in the community. They participate in the clinical supervision of fellows and residents as they learn the skills of family conferences. In cooperation with graduate schools of social work, social workers train master's level social workers. They participate in research advances, palliative care as evidence-based practice, and social work practice in the improvement of standards of care.

Job Description

A palliative care social worker has the following background:

- Master's level education in basic social work and the advanced skill set to be effective with patients, families, and the interdisciplinary team in palliative care (Box 50-1)
- Experience in one or more areas, such as oncology, geriatrics, degenerative diseases (e.g., amyotrophic lateral sclerosis [ALS]), and chronic illnesses
- At least 2 years of supervised counseling and therapy with individuals and families

Generalist or Specialist Status

Although some efforts have been launched to credential palliative care as a specialty in social work, controversy remains. Many propose that a generalist approach is best for social work across the entire spectrum. As of 2006, only a few formal certificate programs for social workers have specialization in palliative care.[7] Continuing education courses, on-the-job supervision, and mentoring are the primary ways that knowledge and skills in this area are shared.

Continuing education courses provide the best opportunity to gain the knowledge and skills needed. Collaborative education and training experiences in conjunction with medical schools, residency programs, and physician continuing education activities can help all disciplines improve their competency in the psychosocial and other dimensions of palliative care and can enhance their ability to participate effectively in interdisciplinary patient care.[8]

Key Responsibilities

Social workers in palliative care settings have five key responsibilities:

1. They must be guided by the ethics and values of social work and demonstrate an attitude of compassion and sensitivity.
2. They must understand the theoretical perspectives that encompass basic knowledge about individual function and family systems and about the norma-

TABLE 50-1	Agenda for the Family Conference
SESSION LEADER	**TOPICS AND ACTIONS***
Physician, who is prepared to educate about a variety of issues	Discusses diagnosis, extent of disease, illness course
	Explores family's understanding of illness
	Explains medical findings for this admission; uses drawings and films to clarify
	Encourages questions and clarification
	Explains treatment of symptoms
	Describes complications and interventions
	Facilitates patient's expression of quality of life
	Describes nutritional needs and limitations
	Discusses medications, side effects, and issue of sedation
	Educates about performance status and mental status
	Explains prognosis
	Outlines goals of care in collaboration with the patient and family
	Educates about death
	Discusses the discharge date, location, and follow-up with health caregiver
Social worker, who integrates medical and psychosocial issues	Assesses comprehension, education, coping of patient and family
	Addresses unrealistic goals to patient's care needs and illness course
	Provides crisis intervention
	Explores how family intends to organize care in home
	Discusses discharge options (e.g., home care, hospice, hospital inpatient)
	Reviews management of emergencies
	Identifies caregiver stress, plan of respite, impact of grief
	Addresses unfinished business
	Provides recommendations for continuity of care as needs change
	Develops backup caregiving plan

*Not all elements are needed for every meeting.

Basic Skills and Knowledge

- Advocacy and respect for self-determination
- Biopsychosocial approach of assessment
- Clarification of goals of care
- Cultural competence
- Enhancement of patient and family problem-solving and coping capacities
- Knowledge of theoretical perspectives in individual and family functioning
- Knowledge of insurance, entitlements, and financial issues
- Knowledge of the law as it applies to at-risk populations and protective services
- Linkage to resources
- Promotion of effective use of systems that provide resources and services
- Support of discharge planning and continuity of care

Specialized Skills and Knowledge

- Collaboration and integration as interdisciplinary team members
- Crisis intervention, debriefing, and family counseling
- Effective termination of work with families
- Knowledge of basic bioethical principles
- Knowledge of conceptual and theoretical perspectives in family systems, family life cycle, communication, and grief and loss
- Ongoing education in psychosocial issues and emerging concepts
- Organization and facilitation of family conferences, enabling family care
- Participation in addressing team concerns
- Prevention of undue hardship or caregiver burden
- Self-reflection about consultation and supervision
- Understanding of physical systems
- Understanding of the dying process
- Understanding of extent of disease and functional impact
- Understanding of surrounding systems (e.g., family, physician, self)
- Understanding of pain and symptom management
- Understanding of impact of illness on the individual and family (i.e., children and grandchildren)
- Understanding of congruence and reciprocity of language for illness progression

tive psychosocial demands of health problems over the course of an illness.

3. They advocate for the needs of patients with chronic, life-limiting illness and specialized needs at the end of life; encourage patient-centered decision making; and uphold the rights of patients and families.

4. They develop and implement interventions that enhance and support the patient and family in decision making, adaptation, and accommodation to a life-threatening illness.

5. They document all practice with the patient and family.

DEVELOPMENTS AND RESEARCH OPPORTUNITIES

Social workers in the United Kingdom have a shared perspective with those in the United States on their roles.

Qualitative research in the 1990s captured the essence of the social work role as perceived by those carrying it out. Themes were grouped and a conceptual framework developed. The resulting categories were family focus, influencing the environment, being a team member, managing anxiety, values and valuing, and knowing and working with limits.[9] When symptoms are managed with good palliative care, nonmedical goals emerge. The patient and family are freed to address emotional, spiritual, and practical issues. From this situation, the social work role evolves.[10]

An interdisciplinary palliative care team allows the full expression of each member's expertise. It is important for social workers to be skilled in communicating psychosocial care; otherwise, social workers may be more comfortable at the interface between team and the patient-family system.[11]

In the United States in 2002, social workers from clinical, academic, and research settings met for a national Social Work Leadership Summit on End-of-Life and Palliative Care. Summit participants developed a consensus statement for their work role by identifying the knowledge competencies, skills for assessment, treatment planning, interventions, interdisciplinary teamwork, supervision, training, values, and attitudes essential in social work practice in end-of-life and palliative care.[12] Participants proposed a national agenda for social work research in continuity in care, diversity, financing, mental health, individual and family care needs, communication, quality of care and services, decision making, family conferencing, grief and bereavement, pain and symptom management, and curriculum development.[13] Concurrently, the National Association of Social Work identified standards for social work practice in palliative and end-of-life care (www.naswdc.org).[14]

Social workers are now more likely to be in an acute care setting that incorporates the medical discipline of palliative medicine as part of the broad therapeutic model known as palliative care. The medical model focus is "quality of life for persons facing a life-threatening illness and for their families."[15]

The term *palliative care* is used extensively in the literature and often is linked or used interchangeably with *end-of-life care*. Concern has been expressed that end-of-life care implies time-defined care and lacks hope, whereas palliative care practice in the broad context requires a complex skill set of communication, decision making, management of complications, symptom control, psychosocial and spiritual support, care of the dying, bereavement support, interdisciplinary teamwork, and coordination of care.[16,17]

For a social worker within palliative medicine, the full range of palliative care can begin when treatment has limited benefit, and it extends to the actively dying stage and death. The social work skills in palliative care complement the skills of others and evolve with the illness trajectory. As palliative medicine expands its role across the continuum of care, social workers will be challenged to broaden their skill set to address the chronic needs of those with ongoing illness and the specialized needs of people approaching death.

Evidence is emerging regarding the impact of social work on health care. For example, increased social work

CASE STUDY

Psychosocial Assessment

John is 44 years old. He was diagnosed with metastatic lung cancer and was admitted to the Acute Care Palliative Medicine Unit for symptom management. In the initial morning report, he was described as living on the street and having no family. It is agreed this will be an easy discharge because he can go to one of the local hospices that cares for cancer patients without resources.

The social worker completed a psychosocial assessment and then learned that John had sisters and brothers who were relieved to hear that he was in the hospital. They understood his prognosis was several months. In a family conference, the siblings asked for reconciliation and an opportunity to be near their brother. John agreed to be placed in a care facility close to his siblings so they could visit and share in the last months of his life. Financial resources were applied for that allowed this plan to occur.

involvement is significantly associated with lower hospice costs.[18] Additional benefits included better team functioning, more issues addressed by the social worker on the team, reduced medical services, and fewer visits by other team members. Expert psychosocial interventions from the beginning ensure that all options are explored before less-effective, higher-cost options. For example, studies showed that social work and psychological and educational interventions delay nursing home placement for patients with Alzheimer's disease by about 1 year compared with conventional care.[19]

Identifying the social worker as the skilled professional for managing family issues, a study assessed interdisciplinary education for physicians and social workers to participate in professional socialization.[20] A pilot intervention showed increased openness and confidence in skills needed to conduct a family conference.[20]

Multiple viewpoints influence social work practice in palliative care. It is hoped that the research agenda proposed can help apply a meaningful conceptual framework and develop a consensus on the facets of the social work role. Including the patient and family in research will add a much-needed perspective to establish the best practices in palliative care for the social work practitioner.

REFERENCES

1. Saunders C. Social work and palliative care—the early history. Br J Soc Work 2001;31:791-799.
2. Powazki RD, Walsh D. Acute care palliative medicine: Psychosocial assessment of patients and primary caregivers. Palliat Med 1999;13:367-373.
3. Powazki RD, Palcisco C, Richardson M, et al. Psychosocial care in advanced cancer. Semin Oncol 2000;27:101-108.
4. Foster LW, McLellan LJ. Translating psychosocial insight into ethical discussions supportive of families in end-of-life decision-making. Soc Work Health Care 2002;35:37-51.
5. Bowen M. Family reaction to death. In Bowen M (ed). Family Therapy in Clinical Practice. New York: Jason Aronson, 1978, pp 321-335.
6. Miller RD, Krech R, Walsh TD. The role of a palliative care service family conference in the management of the patient with advanced cancer. Palliat Med 1991;5:34-39.
7. Walsh-Burke K, Csikali EL. Professional social work education in end of life care: Contributions of the Project on Death in America's Social Work Leadership Development Program. J Soc Work End Life Palliat Care 2005;1:11-26.
8. Field MJ, Cassel CK (eds). Approaching Death: Improving Care at the End of Life. Washington, DC: National Academy Press, 1997, pp 231-232.
9. Sheldon FM. Dimensions of the role of the social worker in palliative care. Palliat Med 2000;14:491-498.
10. Monroe B. Social work in palliative medicine. In Doyle D, Hanks G, Cherny NI, Calman K (eds). Oxford Textbook of Palliative Medicine, 5th ed. Oxford, UK: Oxford University Press, 2004, pp 1007-1017.
11. Oliviere D. The social worker in palliative care—the "eccentric" role. Prog Palliat Care 2001;6:237-241.
12. Gwyther LP, Altilio T, Blacker S, et al. Social work competencies in palliative and end-of-life care. J Soc Work End Life Palliat Care 2005;1:87-119.
13. Kramer BJ, Christ GH, Bern-Klug M, et al. A national agenda for social work research in palliative and end of life care. J Palliat Med 2005;8:418-431.
14. National Association of Social Workers. NASW Standards for Social Work Practice in Palliative and End of Life Care. Available at www.socialworkers.org (accessed October 2, 2007).
15. Billings JA, Block SD, Finn JW, et al. Initial voluntary program standards for fellowship training in palliative medicine. J Palliat Med 2002;5:23-33.
16. Davis MP, Walsh D, LeGrand SB, et al. End-of-life care: The death of palliative medicine? J Palliat Med 2002;5:813-814.
17. Blacker S. Palliative care and social work. In Berzoff J, Silverman PR (eds). Living with Dying. New York: Columbia University Press, 2004, pp 409-423.
18. Reese DJ, Raymer M. Relationships between social work involvement and hospice outcomes: Results of the National Hospice Social Work Survey. Soc Work 2004;49:415-422.
19. Mittelman MS, Ferris SH, Shulman E, et al. A family intervention to delay nursing home placement of patients with Alzheimer disease: A randomized controlled trial. JAMA 1996;27:1725-1731.
20. Fineberg IC. Preparing professionals for family conferences in palliative care: Evaluation results of an interdisciplinary approach. J Palliat Med 2005;8:857-866.

SUGGESTED READING

Berzoff J, Silverman PR (eds). Living with Dying: A Handbook for End-of-Life Care Practitioners. New York: Columbia University Press, 2004.

Doyle D, Hanks G, Cherny NI, Calman K (eds). Oxford Textbook of Palliative Medicine. Oxford, UK: Oxford University Press, 2004.

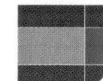

CHAPTER 51

The Nutrition Support Team

Leah Gramlich

KEY POINTS

- Specialized nutritional support has a role to play in the care of patients with terminal illness.
- The complexity of specialized nutritional support is related to nutritional assessment, nutritional support access, the nutrition prescription, monitoring, and psychological and social considerations.
- Nutrition support teams facilitate excellent nutritional care for short-term and long-term management.
- The role of nutritional support team members is to identify and optimize specialized nutritional support, thereby targeting the right therapy for the right patient and the right outcome.
- Optimal nutrition requires broad expertise, including nursing, dietetic, pharmacological, and medical knowledge.
- The nutritional care plan evolves with the patient's status.
- Without a nutritional support team, it is important to ensure that the staff members providing specialized nutritional support are competent.

Specialized nutritional support by enteral and parenteral nutrition has been integrated into patient care since the 1970s. Optimal nutrition in terminal illness may include specialized nutritional support for the short term during therapy for the illness or longer term in the home setting. Although nutritional support can prolong life and may enhance the quality of life, it has significant complications. They can be reduced by an interdisciplinary nutritional support team (NST) or, without a team, by specially trained individuals.

SPECIALIZED NUTRITIONAL SUPPORT DURING ADVANCED DISEASE

Specialized nutritional support includes enteral nutrition (EN) and parenteral nutrition (PN). EN is indicated when someone cannot meet his or her nutrient needs with oral intake and when the gastrointestinal tract is functional (e.g., cancers of the head and neck or esophagus, stroke or other central nervous system lesion causing transfer dysphagia). PN is indicated when an individual cannot meet his or her nutrient needs with oral intake and the gastrointestinal tract is nonfunctional (e.g., bowel obstruction, ileus, malabsorption, diarrhea).

In patients with newly diagnosed, unresectable cancers, gastrointestinal symptoms, including abdominal fullness, taste change, constipation, nausea, and vomiting, are common.[1] The frequency of weight loss and malnutrition in cancer ranges from 31% to more than 80%, depending on the tumor.[2] Cancer therapy, including surgery, chemotherapy, and irradiation, has nutritional implications. Malnutrition correlates with poor wound healing, risk of infection, impaired physical function, and longer hospital stays. Specialized nutritional support is indicated for patients with cancer at high nutritional risk (i.e., weight loss >10% of usual weight).[3] In these cases, EN is favored over PN.[4]

The use of home nutritional support (called home artificial nutrition [HAN] in European countries) is growing for patients with terminal illnesses. Adult cancer patients account for 5% to 57% of home PN in European and North American centers.[5] Home PN benefits the quantity and quality of life for some patients.[5] It is a positive alternative to hospital nutritional support or the crisis that occurs when a patient cannot eat.[6] Home EN also is becoming more widespread and often is an adjunct to cancer care, particularly for cancers of the head and neck.[7]

Specialized nutritional support in the home is expected to grow. It is important to consider the goals of home PN and EN in conjunction with the overall palliative care goals, including withdrawal of nutritional support if patients are near death (see "Common Errors").

RATIONALE FOR THE TEAM APPROACH TO SPECIALIZED NUTRITIONAL SUPPORT

Specialized nutritional support is complex and requires appropriate and safe access for supplying nutrients and an individual nutritional prescription that considers the medical condition, comorbidities, and medications as they relate to nutritional support (Table 51-1). During palliative care, the patient's response to nutritional therapy should be regularly reassessed as the underlying disease progresses.

The composition of the NST reflects the diverse expertise required. NSTs consist of a registered nurse (RN), registered dietitian (RD), pharmacist (RPh), and a physician (MD). Each discipline plays a unique role

TABLE 51-1	Considerations in Specialized Nutritional Support	
FEATURES	**ENTERAL NUTRITION**	**PARENTERAL NUTRITION**
Nutritional assessment	Functional gastrointestinal tract	Nonfunctional gastrointestinal tract
	Individual at high nutritional risk	Individual at high nutritional risk
	Unable to meet nutrient needs by mouth	Unable to meet nutrient needs by mouth
	Anticipated survival > 6 wk	Anticipated survival > 6 wk
Nutrition support access	Intragastric: PEG, surgical (G tube)	PICC
	Intrajejunal: PEJ, surgical (J tube)	Broviac/Hickman
Complications	Infection	Infection
	Malposition	Malposition
	Obstruction	Obstruction
Nutrition prescription	Commercial products or other	Patient-specific TPN or other
	Disease-specific products	TNA versus 2 : 1
Complications	Intolerance	Electrolyte imbalances
	Constipation or diarrhea	Hyperglycemia
	Metabolic effects	Liver disease
		Bone disease
Monitoring	Response to therapy	Response to therapy
	Complications	Complications
Psychosocial issues	Medicalizes care and feeding	Medicalizes care and feeding
	Relatively simple	Complex
	Costly	Very costly

PEG, percutaneous endoscopic gastrostomy; PEJ, percutaneous endoscopic jejunostomy; PICC, peripherally inserted central catheter; TNA, total nutrient admixture; TPN, total peripheral nutrition.

- Misidentification of individuals who may benefit from nutritional support
- Failure to establish realistic goals for nutritional therapy
- Inadequate anticipation of complications of nutritional support in a proactive and timely fashion
- Miscommunication among care providers and the patient, who is at the center of the team

Box 51-1 Goals of Nutritional Support Team

- Nutrition support should be indicated.
- The route of administration should be appropriate.
- The patient should benefit from therapy.
- The incidence of complications should be low.
- The patient should understand the risks and benefits of therapy.
- The proper quantity of nutritional substrate should be ordered.
- The proper quantity of nutritional substrate should be administered.
- The patient should not experience a detrimental interaction between drugs and nutrients.
- The patient should receive nutritional support in a timely manner.

TABLE 51-2 Membership and Role in Nutrition Support Team

TEAM MEMBER	ROLES
Registered nurse (RN)	Assess adequacy of access for nutrition support
	Psychosocial assessment of patient
	Initiate and manage EN and PN
	Patient education
	Complications of EN and PN
Registered dietitian (RD)	Nutritional assessment
	Determine energy and protein needs
	Deliver appropriate route of feeding
	Assess adequacy of access for nutrition support
	Initiate and manage EN and PN
	Nutritional prescription, transition feeding
Pharmacist (RPh)	Optimize nutritional (PN) prescription
	Identify drug and nutritional indications
	Coordination of home TPN and prescriptions
Physician (MD)	Nutritional assessment
	Determine energy and protein needs
	Determine approval route of feeding
	Assess and obtain access for nutritional support
	Initiate and manage EN and PN
	Psychosocial assessment of patient

EN, enteral nutrition; PN, parenteral nutrition; TPN, total parenteral nutrition.

(Table 51-2). Standards of care and guidelines for nutritional support are facilitated by the interdisciplinary NST (Box 51-1).[8] During palliative care, the team evaluates the nutritional support for a given individual to maintain ongoing quality improvement. NSTs represent a system of specialized nutritional support to ensure that treatment decisions optimize outcomes and do not compromise patients' safety.[9]

Before NSTs, there were high rates of catheter-related complications and metabolic complications.[10] NSTs reduce line infection rates, metabolic abnormalities (including electrolytes, glucosuria, and hyperglycemia), mortality,[11,12] and costs[13,14] in adult and pediatric populations.[13,15]

NST members add their expertise to education in palliative care, and they influence other professionals about nutritional support. They study and evaluate nutritional support in various disease states.[16] NSTs also are in a position to advocate for support—whether financial or intellectual—with other care providers. These value-added benefits of NSTs may not typically be assumed by other members of the health care team, but they represent an important aspect of care that allows the field of nutrition to advance (see "Case Study: Benefits of a Nutrition Support Team").

NUTRITIONAL SUPPORT TEAMS: ESTABLISHMENT, ORGANIZATION, AND FUTURE CONSIDERATIONS

NSTs do not represent the norm in hospital pharmacies.[17,18] In the United States and Europe,[19] between 33% and 65% of hospitals have an NST. In a multicenter study of NSTs in Germany, Austria, and Switzerland, NSTs had been established at only 3.2% of the hospitals studied.[20] Seventy-one percent of the physicians, 40% of the nurses, and 69% of the dietitians held an additional nutrition-specific qualification. The main team activities identified included creating nutritional regimens, education, and monitoring therapy.

Despite the imperative to optimize nutritional care and reduce the complications of nutritional support, it is noteworthy that NSTs do not represent the standard of care. Without an NST, it is important to ensure that staff members are competent to provide specialized nutritional support (see Table 51-2) and that a system exists to monitor patient outcomes. Physicians, dietitians, and nurses who offer specialized nutritional support within designated program areas without NSTs must adopt a coordinating, collaborative, and integrating role to optimize nutrition.

Goals for incorporating NSTs in palliative care include the following:

- Standardizing the approach and goals of nutritional support
- Evaluating specialized nutritional support in the home in palliative care
- Prioritizing creation of NSTs to optimize complete care

CONCLUSIONS

Specialized nutritional support has a role in caring for patients with advanced and terminal illness. Ideally, this

CASE STUDY

Benefits of a Nutrition Support Team

Mrs. AS is a 42-year-old woman who has been diagnosed with metastatic cervical cancer. She has undergone palliative chemotherapy and radiation therapy. She has had recurrent bowel obstruction caused by many factors, including adhesions, intra-abdominal tumor, and radiation injury to the small bowel. An ileostomy was created to reduce the symptoms of bowel obstruction, but the problem has persisted. Her main symptoms are nausea, vomiting, and weight loss of 17 pounds over the preceding 4 months (i.e., loss of >10% of usual body weight).

Mrs. AS is still able to perform most of the activities of daily living, including participation in the school-related activities of her children (12 and 8 years old) and in food preparation for the family. Her supports in the home are good. Her Karnofsky Performance Status (KPS) score is 90. Her main concerns are about the fatigue and weakness that accompany her dehydration, and she is worried that she will not live out the rest of the school year because of her rapid weight loss. Pain management is not an issue at this time. Her family members are fearful that they are watching her "starve to death."

Recent computed tomography showed relative stability for the intra-abdominal tumor burden. The home total parenteral nutrition (TPN) program was contacted by Mrs. AS's oncologist and the palliative care team, who thought that parenteral nutrition was needed because her gastrointestinal tract was unusable because of the obstructive disease.

Mrs. AS was evaluated by the nutritional support team. Results indicated that death from starvation and dehydration would likely precede death caused by metastatic tumor. Based on her (good) functional status and potential to benefit from home parenteral nutrition, the patient was accepted into the home TPN program.

Before initiating formal teaching about the program, a discussion is undertaken with Mrs. AS and her husband to ensure that they are aware that they may stop parenteral nutrition at any time if they feel the therapy is too burdensome. The nurses on the nutritional support team arrange for insertion of a central venous access device, and they teach Mrs. AS and her husband (3 to 5 days) about the therapy while she is in the hospital. The dietitian writes the parenteral nutrition prescription and monitors for refeeding syndrome. The patient's electrolytes are stabilized.

A prescription for home TPN is written and communicated to the local distributor, who ensures that the parenteral nutrition is delivered to the patient's home. The patient's status is reviewed by the nutritional support team on an ongoing basis by phone conversations and by periodic visits, and the TPN formula is revised as needed. Mrs. AS has no complications associated with home TPN, such as line-related thrombosis or infection, and her metabolic status is stable, requiring only minor modifications to the TPN prescription.

Six months later, Mrs. AS is continuing to do relatively well and remains in her home, although she is experiencing increasing pain and has developed edema. Her KPS score is 60. The local palliative care nurse leads a discussion with the patient and her husband, and they decide to continue the TPN but agree to review this decision on an ongoing basis. The palliative care nurse communicates this information to the nutritional support team. Mrs. AS died of her illness 7 months after initiation of TPN.

complex care is provided by a coordinated, interdisciplinary NST that works with the palliative care team for patient-centered care. Without a formal NST, excellence in nutrition can be achieved through committed staff members who have expertise in nutritional support that is based on established standards of care and who collaborate with the patient care team.

REFERENCES

1. Grosvenor M, Bulcavage L, Chlebowski RT. Symptoms potentially influencing weight loss in cancer population. Cancer 1989;63:330-334.
2. Dewys WD, Begg C, Lavin PT, et al. Prognostic effect of weight loss prior to chemotherapy in cancer patients. Eastern Cooperative Oncology Group. Am J Med 1980;69:491-497.
3. Klein S, Koretz RL. Nutrition support in cancer: What do the data really show. Nutr Clin Pract 1994;9:87-89.
4. Bozzetti F, Braga M, Gianotti L, et al. Postoperation enteral vs. parenteral nutrition in malnourished patients with gastrointestinal cancer: A randomized multicentre trial. Cancer 2001;358:1487-1492.
5. Bozzetti F, Cozzaglio L, Biganzoli E, et al. Quality of life and length of survival in advanced cancer patients on home parenteral nutrition. Clin Nutr 2002;21:281-288.
6. Orrevall Y, Tishelman C, Herrington MK, Permert J. The path from oral nutrition to home parenteral nutrition: A qualitative interview study of the experiences of advanced cancer patients and their families. Clin Nutr 2004;23:1280-1287.
7. Hebuterne X, Bozzetti F, Moreno Villares JM, et al. Home enteral nutrition in adults: A multicentre study in Europe. Clin Nutr 1999;18(Suppl 1):21.
8. Schneider PJ, Bloth A, Bisognano M. Improving the nutritional support process: Assuring that more patients receive optimal nutritional support.. Nutr Clin Pract 1999;14:189-194.
9. Schneider P. Nutrition support teams: An evidence-based practice. Nutr Clin Pract 2006;21:62-67.
10. Kaminski MV, Stolar MH. Parenteral hyperalimentation: A quality of care survey and review. Am J Hosp Pharm 1974;31:228-235.
11. Nehme AE. Nutritional support of the hospitalized patient. JAMA 1980;243:1906-1908.
12. Trujillo EB, Young LE, Chertow GM. Metabolic and monetary costs of avoidable parenteral nutrition use. JPEN J Parenter Enteral Nutr 1999;23:109-113.
13. Jonkers CF, Prins F, Van Kempen A, et al. Towards implementation of optimum nutrition and better clinical nutrition support. Clin Nutr 2001;20:361-366.
14. Howard P. Organizational aspects of starting and running an effective nutritional support service. Clin Nutr 2001;20:367-374.
15. Agostoni C, Axelson I, Colomb V, et al. The need for nutrition support teams in pediatric units: A commentary by the ESPGHAN committee on nutrition. J Pediatr Gastroenterol Nutr 2005;41:267-271.
16. Puoane T, Sanders D, Ashworth A, et al. Improving the hospital management of malnourished children by participatory research. Int J Qual Health Care 2004;16:31-40.
17. Holcombe BJ, Thorn BD, Strausberg MS. Analysis of the practice of nutrition support pharmacy specialists. Pharmacotherapy 1995;15:806-813.
18. Ebiasah RP, Schneider PJ, Pedersen CA, Mirtallo JM. Evaluation of board certification in nutrition support pharmacy. JPEN J Parenter Enteral Nutr 2002;26:239-247.
19. Maisonneuve RD, Raguso CA, Paolini-Giacobino A. Parenteral nutrition practices in hospital pharmacies in Switzerland, France and Belgium. Nutrition 2004;20:528-535.
20. Shang E, Hasenberg T, Schlegel B, et al. An European survey of structure and organization of nutrition support teams in Germany, Austria, and Switzerland. Clin Nutr 2005;24:1005-1013.

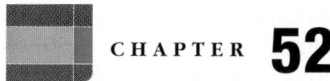

CHAPTER **52**

Occupational and Physical Therapy

Denise L. Schilling and Pamela Dixon

KEY POINTS

- The health care team should be informed about the professional abilities and expertise of occupational and physical therapists.

- The major goals of occupational and physical therapists should be discussed with other members of the palliative medicine team.

- Occupational and physical therapy practice models in palliative medicine should be identified.

- Palliative occupational and physical services have eligibility and reimbursement requirements.

- Occupational and physical therapy research and resources should be expanded in palliative medicine.

Death is not the greatest loss in life. The greatest loss is what dies inside us while we live.

—NORMAN COUSINS

OCCUPATIONAL AND PHYSICAL THERAPY DEFINED

Occupational therapists and physical therapists are critical members of the palliative medicine team. They are trained with a set of skills and knowledge that promote independence and enhance the quality of life for all individuals. This philosophy and skill set apply to the living seeking rehabilitative care, health, and to the dying seeking to maintain maximal function and dignity until the end of life.

Occupational therapy (OT) is defined as the therapeutic use of self-care, work, and play and leisure activities to increase independent function, enhance development, and prevent disability. OT also may include the adaptation of task or environment to achieve maximum independence and enhance the quality of life.[1] Occupational therapists are acutely aware that people have a vital need for occupation[2] and that they should be allowed to and encouraged to participate in desired activities and roles for them to achieve meaning and quality of life.

Physical therapy (PT) services aim to prevent the onset of or to slow the progression of conditions resulting from injury, disease, and other causes.[3] PT includes developing plans that focus on preservation, development, and restoration of optimal physical function.

GOALS OF OCCUPATIONAL THERAPY AND PHYSICAL THERAPY IN PALLIATIVE MEDICINE

OT and PT in palliative medicine take a positive approach and broaden services to maximize function, increase comfort, and ensure patient and caregiver safety through education.[4] Palliative OT assists patients to make a contribution and achieve their preferred occupational roles in the time that remains.[5] Palliative PT assists in maintaining independence through an ongoing analysis of patients' abilities in relation to their environment and personal goals.[6] Focus is placed on strengths, skills, and goals instead of weaknesses and deficits, promoting and facilitating living until death. Types of services may include pain management, positioning, mobility re-education, training in activities of daily living for energy conservation and safety, treatment of secondary health risks such as edema and wound management, equipment recommendations, home modifications, and education of patients and caregivers.

MODELS OF OCCUPATIONAL THERAPY AND PHYSICAL THERAPY SERVICE DELIVERY IN PALLIATIVE MEDICINE

The key components of successful service delivery are ongoing assessment coupled with compassionate listening that facilitates patient-therapist communication that leads to the joint development of functional, realistic, and patient-valued goals. Factors considered in selecting an appropriate service delivery model include the patient's medical status, goals of the patient and family, the practice setting, and reimbursement options. There are six models for PT service delivery[7]:

- Traditional rehabilitation
- "Rehab light"
- Rehabilitation in reverse
- Case management
- Skilled maintenance
- Supportive care

These models are equally applicable to OT service delivery. Traditional rehabilitation and rehab light are commonly employed medical models based on regularly scheduled treatments; the latter occurs less frequently and has an emphasis on a home exercise program. Case management is the Medicare-supported model in which direct care service usually is delivered in the home, the focus is on caregiver education, and it occurs on an intermittent basis. Less common is the skilled maintenance model, in which unskilled caregivers are trained in the delivery of physical therapy. Supportive care is most common in hospice care, and patient comfort is the primary goal. The rehabilitation in reverse model is designed to address the needs of the patient whose condition and skills are progressively deteriorating, and this model aligns most intimately with palliative care. In anticipation of the patient's deteriorating condition, assessment occurs frequently, short-term goals address each level of decline, and new skills are taught, or old ones are retrained. Mobility training for each level of decline may proceed in the following order:

1. Gait training with no assistive device
2. Use of an assistive device (e.g., cane, walker)
3. Use of a manual wheelchair
4. Use of a power wheelchair
5. Bed mobility

Although the rehabilitation in reverse model may be most frequently used in palliative medicine, any one of the six models is appropriate. The key components of successful service delivery (regardless of the model selected) are ongoing assessment, team communication, compassionate listening to the needs of patients and caregivers, and development of realistic, patient-driven, jointly agreed goals.

REIMBURSEMENT FOR OCCUPATIONAL THERAPY AND PHYSICAL THERAPY SERVICES IN PALLIATIVE MEDICINE

A concern frequently raised regarding referral to and delivery of OT and PT services is reimbursement. Traditional and rehab light services are reimbursed as skilled interventions. OT and PT services in the case management model are covered under the U.S. Medicare hospice benefit. OT and PT can be used 1 day each week and reimbursed in lieu of a nursing visit. Education of family members can decrease the need for home health aides, providing long-term savings for the individual and insurer.[8] The skilled maintenance model of service delivery can be reimbursed under the Medicare home health guidelines. Supportive OT and PT services also are covered by per diem hospice benefits in the United States.

EVIDENCE-BASED PRACTICE

OT and PT are relatively new in palliative medicine, and research is limited. Many studies are qualitative and focus on the experiences and perspectives of therapists regarding palliative care.[9-11] One single-subject qualitative study[12] and a small 10-subject qualitative study[13] examined patient outcomes, and they determined that patients valued improvement in social relationships and quality of life, not traditional values such as independence or rehabilitation.

Pain is one of the most disabling conditions addressed in palliative medicine.[14] Occupational and physical therapists are trained in various techniques to assess and address pain, including massage, relaxation strategies, and modalities such as transcutaneous electrical nerve stimulation (TENS). Relaxation training and TENS help patients with chemotherapy-induced nausea and vomiting.[15-17]

Three observational studies[18-20] and one small qualitative study[12] examined PT needs in palliative care. Two of the three observational studies used components of the Functional Independence Measure (FIM).[19,20] Both studies demonstrated that therapy services improved FIM motor scores. The third study used the Barthel Index.[18] Patients in this study also demonstrated improved scores after therapy.

Occupational and physical therapists need to expand this limited but promising body of knowledge. Research will not only contribute to evidence-based practice, but it will be valuable in advocating for increased availability and affordability of OT and PT services in palliative medicine.

CONCLUSIONS

As members of the palliative medicine interdisciplinary team, occupational and physical therapists help to promote and support activities that are valued by patients and that contribute to patients' independence and quality of life. Accomplishment of tasks that seemed impossible can mean the difference between existing from day to day to feeling truly alive. Death comes to all of us. Therapists provide the support needed to live each day to its fullest potential.

REFERENCES

1. American Occupational Therapy Association. Available at http://www.aota.org (accessed April 2008).
2. Reilly M. Occupational therapy can be one of the great ideas of 20th century medicine. Am J Occup Ther 1962;16:1-9.
3. American Physical Therapy Association. http://www.apta.org (accessed April 2008).
4. Prizzi MA, Briggs R. Occupational and physical therapy in hospice. Topics Geriatr Rehabil 2004;20:120-130.
5. Marcil WM. The hospice nurse and occupational therapist: A marriage of expedience. Home Health Care Manage Pract 2006;19:26-30.
6. Robinson D. The contribution of physiotherapy to palliative care. Eur J Palliat Care 2000;7:95-98.
7. Briggs R. Models for physical therapy practice in palliative medicine. Rehabil Oncol 2000;18:18-21.
8. Reis E. A special place: Physical therapy hospice and palliative care. PT Magazine 2007;March:42-47.
9. Hasselkuss B. Death in very old age: A personal journey of caring. Am J Occup Ther 1993;47:717-723.
10. Prochnau C, Lui L, Boman J. Personal-professional connections in palliative care occupational therapy. Am J Occup Ther 2003;57:196-204.
11. Rahlman H. Journey of providing care in hospice: Perspectives of occupational therapists. Qual Health Res 2000;10:806-818.
12. Mackey KM, Sparling JW. Experiences of older women with cancer receiving hospice care: Significance for physical therapy. Phys Ther 2000;80:459-468.
13. Bye R. When client's are dying: Occupational therapy perspectives. Occup Ther J Res 1998;18:3-24.
14. Abrahm JL. Update in palliative medicine and end-of-life care. Annu Rev Med 2003;54:53-72.
15. McMillian CM, Dundee JW. The role of transcutaneous electrical stimulation of Neiguan anti-emetic acupuncture point in controlling sickness after cancer chemotherapy. Physiotherapy 1991;77:499-502.
16. Morrow GR, Morrell C. Behavioral treatment for the anticipatory nausea and vomiting induced by cancer chemotherapy. N Engl J Med 1982;307:1476-1480.
17. Redd WH, Andrykowski MA. Behavioral intervention in cancer treatment: Controlling aversion reactions to chemotherapy. J Consult Psychol 1982;50:1018-1029.
18. Yoshioka H. Rehabilitation for the terminal cancer patient. Am J Phys Med Rehabil 1994;73:199-206.
19. Marciniak CM, Sliwa J, Spill G, et al. Functional outcome following rehabilitation of the cancer patient. Arch Phys Med Rehabil 1996;77:54-57.
20. Cole RP, Scialla SJ, Bednarz L. Functional recovery in cancer rehabilitation. Arch Phys Med Rehabil 2000;81:623-627.

SUGGESTED READING

Frost M. The role of physical, occupational, and speech therapy in hospice: Patient empowerment. Am J Hosp Palliat Care 2001;18:397-402.

Marcil W. The hospice nurse and occupational therapist: A marriage of expedience. Home Health Care Manage Pract 2006;19:26-30.

Santiago-Palma J, Payne R. Palliative care and rehabilitation. Cancer 2001;92:1919-1925.

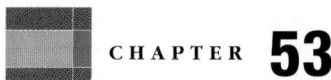

CHAPTER **53**

The Speech-Language Pathologist

Dona Leskuski

K E Y P O I N T S

- The speech-language pathologist is an expert in evaluation and management of multiple aspects of communication disorders and swallowing.

- Communication is a complex, multimodality process that can sustain breakdowns arising from multiple causes.

- Even subtle speech, language, and cognitive-linguistic disturbances can be devastating to patients and families.

- Dysphagia has a major impact on caregiving and quality of life. The goals of care should guide swallowing evaluation and management.

- Research is needed in the areas of evaluation and treatment efficacy in all aspects of speech-language pathology.

A speech-language pathologist (SLP) is a specialist serving communication and swallowing needs across the lifespan.[1] Most SLPs in the United States hold a state license to practice and a Certificate of Clinical Competence awarded by the American-Speech-Language-Hearing Association, but some SLPs working in the school systems are not required to be licensed. The training of SLPs provides a well-rounded education that allows for experience with all populations (Box 53-1). Post-baccalaureate education leads to a master's degree for clinical practice. In addition to academic coursework, the master's degree education includes supervised clinical practica. All candidates must pass a national board examination and then complete a clinical fellowship year before receiving the Certificate of Clinical Competence. Coursework leading to a doctoral degree prepares for a research-centered career.[2] Because the scope of practice is broad, many practitioners develop specialized clinical skills with certain populations or disorders. This can be done in the work setting with continuing education courses or specifically designed academic experiences.

DISORDERS OF LANGUAGE

Disorders of language can arise from delay in development or be acquired after normal development. Acquired language disorders have many causes, including stroke, tumor, radiation effects, degenerative neurological disorders, hypoxia, and traumatic brain injury.[3] Devastating communication breakdowns can arise from even mild language impairment. The goal of the SLP is to reduce frustration while maximizing communication. Aphasia is an acquired disorder of symbolic representation of language, with problems in reading, writing, listening, and speaking.

Box 53-1 Roles and Responsibilities of Speech-Language Specialists

Assessments of abilities
  Language
  Cognitive-linguistic skills
  Speech intelligibility
  Voice
  Swallowing safety
Development of greatest chance for compensation of deficits
Education of caregivers, family, and medical team
Rehabilitation to the extent possible

Areas of the brain that sustain injury determine the deficit profile. The broadest categories of aphasia classification are expressive and receptive aphasias. Each is associated with predictable deficits, although there may be wide variations among affected individuals.

Expressive Aphasia

For patients with expressive aphasia, language production is halting with the use of many content words (nouns or verbs), and patients visibly struggle as they try to produce the desired word. Writing is often similarly impaired and therefore cannot be substituted successfully for speech. Time pressure and emotional messages increase the difficulty. Comprehension and error awareness can be good even when expression is severely impaired. This fuels frustration, because an individual may be aware of an error while the family urges him or her to "say it right." Because repetition can be impaired, well-meaning attempts by caregivers to model words they expect the patient to repeat causes frustration.

Receptive Aphasia

The greatest impairment in receptive aphasia is auditory comprehension. It reduces understanding of others along with awareness of the patient's own speech production errors. Speech is often fluent, with few signs of struggle. Unfortunately, output often consists of low-content words (e.g., "the thing," "the place") and few definitive nouns. The patient may make sound and word substitutions, making speech seem garbled. Like expressive aphasia, repetition can be impaired, and writing output mirrors speech production. This can cause much frustration for the caregiver, because it is difficult to get messages to the patient and equally difficult to understand messages the patient intends to convey. Patients become frustrated because they may not be aware the message was not received.

If there is confusion in *yes* or *no* responses, perseveration of words or behaviors, or fluctuations in concentration, these communication difficulties are magnified, compounding social isolation and frustration. When appropriate communication is essential to decision making and establishing goals of care, patients and families find themselves in a vicious cycle of misunderstanding and stress about the inability to communicate.

In these situations, the SLP can assess the patient's language profile and train caregivers in techniques with the best chance of communicative success. With severe language impairments, remedies may be limited, but they are still important for meeting daily needs. Even the most basic communication, a reliable yes or no response, can facilitate the patient's communication about wants and needs. The SLP can provide valuable insight into the deficits for the medical team and caregivers, which helps in discussions regarding the goals of care. This profile can also help other professionals evaluating the patient's competence to make decisions. In cases deemed amenable to remediation, a rehabilitation program can be designed and implemented unless limited life expectancy makes this impractical (see "Case Study: Role of a Speech-Language Pathologist in Palliative Care").

DISORDERS OF COGNITIVE-LINGUISTIC SKILLS

Disorders of cognition impair communication. Common challenges are reductions in insight, orientation, memory, attention, and concentration (see "Common Errors"). The patient also may be affected by concrete thinking, poor problem-solving skills, and impulsivity. Difficulties in these areas pose significant barriers to appropriate care and end-of-life discussions.[4] When these deficits are subtle or when the patient's behavior is otherwise socially appropriate, it may be difficult to detect cognitive-linguistic deficits until

 CASE STUDY

Role of a Speech-Language Pathologist in Palliative Care

BW was a 79-year-old woman with a medical history of hypertension and metastatic lung cancer who had a stroke in the hospital. The stroke left her with profound deficits in language and right-side paralysis. She initially produced only one word: *bathroom*. She often produced this word, frowned, and then tried again without success. Her concerned family tried to correct her speech. They brought in picture books and unsuccessfully tried to get her to repeat the words they said. She demonstrated frustration by hitting and crying. Because of these behaviors, her family thought they could not care for her after discharge from the hospital.

A speech-language pathology evaluation revealed good understanding of simple questions and commands. Using head gestures for *yes* and *no* allowed the patient to answer questions about her immediate wants and needs. The family was educated about the type of problems the patient was experiencing and how to ask questions to elicit a yes or no response, rather than using an open-ended format. The speech-language pathologist worked with the patient and her caregivers during activities of daily living and was able to make practical suggestions for improving communicative success. The course of therapy lasted approximately 5 days.

After the patient and her family began practicing the prescribed techniques, the hitting behavior ceased. The patient still cried when frustrated, but the family was able to accept this behavior, and they agreed to take her home. The patient transitioned to hospice and was cared for in her home by family members until her death approximately 8 weeks later.

a problem occurs. Often, a patient who appears normal is unsafe to be home alone, administer drugs, drive, work, or care for children. In these cases, the SLP can assess the deficit profile and help in several ways:

● Assist the medical team coordinate a safe discharge plan
● Help families understand what they are observing and its implications for the future, because cognitive-linguistic reductions can be frightening for caregivers
● Suggest compensation strategies such as memory notebooks listing important phone numbers or calendars for orientation

DISORDERS OF SPEECH PRODUCTION AND VOICE

Poor articulation, altered anatomy, or respiratory difficulties may prevent successful messages. Cognitive-linguistic skills may be negatively judged based on reduced speech clarity.[5] The severity may require the SLP to assess the need for augmentative or assistive communication devices. Ventilators pose special challenges. An oral endotracheal tube severely impairs articulation and renders voicing impossible. If an individual is ventilator dependent for an extended time, he or she is often tracheostomized. The SLP can train with an assistive device, such as a tracheostomy speaking valve or electrolarynx, to achieve voicing.

Laryngectomy patients face initial challenges similar to those of tracheostomized patients. Preoperatively, the SLP assesses language skills, answers questions about changes in communication, and develops a long-term communication plan. Immediately after surgery, the individual may need a communication board. Later, as healing takes place, the patient may be trained in esophageal speech, use of an electrolarynx, or use of a voice prosthesis with a transesophageal puncture. The transesophageal puncture is a surgically created tract between the trachea and esophagus that allows diversion of air into the esophagus on exhalation.[6,7] The procedure is usually done at the time of the laryngectomy, but it can be preformed later. The SLP works with the otolaryngologist to fit the voice prosthesis and then trains the individual in air diversion to achieve a voice.

Common Errors

● Underestimating frustration and social isolation a person experiences when communication breaks down
● Underestimating overall comprehension (e.g., someone with severe language impairment may get the general idea of what is said)
● Assuming an individual whose behavior is socially appropriate has intact cognitive-linguistic skills
● Judging cognition or linguistic competence by the clarity of speech
● Assuming that nothing can be done to improve safe oral intake in dysphagia

SWALLOWING DISORDERS

A major aspect of the SLP's responsibilities involves evaluation and management of swallowing disorders.[8-12] Patients and families become distressed when there is a breakdown of swallowing safety. Although the gravest risk of airway compromise is occlusion, aspiration risk and pneumonia lead to discussions regarding alternate means of nutrition delivery. These decisions should not be embarked on without a thorough evaluation of swallowing and input from the SLP about recommendations for practical and safe eating procedures. The initial swallowing evaluation should be done by the SLP at the bedside. This is essential to gain an understanding of the problems observed. If indicated, it can be followed by an instrumental assessment of swallowing mechanics and airway protection.

The videofluoroscopic modified barium swallow study is administered by the SLP with a radiologist in most settings. It is a dynamic identification of points of breakdown, airway protection during eating or drinking, and effectiveness of compensatory techniques to maximize eating safety. It is a useful eating safety assessment tool and should not be ordered only to "look for aspiration."

Another instrumental dysphagia assessment is fiberoptic endoscopic evaluation of swallowing (FEES), in which a nasopharyngolaryngoscope is fed through one nasal passage to the superior pharynx to assess for airway penetration and pharyngeal residue after the swallow. SLPs must have adequate training to perform the procedure and must work with a physician. Less commonly performed forms of instrumental assessments for dysphagia include pharyngeal manometry, manofluorography, ultrasonography, and scintigraphy.

When there is difficulty swallowing, some may believe that nothing can be done to improve the situation and that the only recourse is a feeding tube. Swallowing safety can often be improved by alterations in diet texture, presentation, rate control, or postural maneuvers. The SLP is an invaluable resource to the medical team as an expert who performs a thorough evaluation, translates the results into practical recommendations, and trains caregivers. This is especially important for people nearing the end of life, because food has such strong symbolism with satisfaction and caring. Often, eating is the last pleasure a person has, and success with even small amounts food or liquid can greatly enhance the quality of life.

Because the palliative medicine population has many diagnoses and prognoses, the SLP may devise swallowing safety plans for patients along a continuum from anticipation of cure and recovery to end-of-life care. Treatment plans are individualized and may include therapy with rehabilitation intent or compensation for fixed deficits. The SLP should join with the medical treatment team in making swallowing decisions. This includes sharing medical information on longevity and the goals of care with the SLP before the initial swallowing evaluation takes place. Ultimately, the decision about whether to continue oral nutrition is a medical one, but when consulting an SLP for dysphagia, requests should be made for the most conservative and the best chance for safety with eating recommendations. This approach can provide practical information and help cope with the situation when the caregiver gets a "failed the swallow" report.

DEVELOPMENTS AND OPPORTUNITIES IN RESEARCH

Use of Speech-Language Pathologists in Palliative Care

Traditionally, speech-language pathology caseloads rarely included hospice and palliative medicine patients. With heightened awareness about the importance of communication and swallowing decisions at the end of life, SLPs are now more often included.[13-15] Specialized training prepares the SLP for the roles of consultant, educator, and communication coordinator. This may appear to depart from the traditional rehabilitative tract of therapy, but the SLP has always functioned in these roles. In palliative care, however, limited life expectancies and hospice funding have caused underuse of SLPs. As the focus on quality of life expands, consultative and educational visits by the SLP to improve overall functional communication and swallowing safety are gaining popularity.

Evidence-Based Medicine

Study designs vary, with case reports, case-control, and cohort studies making up most of the literature.[16-20] Randomized, controlled trials are few but have been reported in the aphasia and dysarthria literature. A 1996 review of aphasia treatment efficacy suggests that "for people who become aphasic because of a single, left hemisphere thromboembolic stroke and who receive speech and language therapy at least 3 hours weekly for 5 months make significantly more improvement than people with aphasia who are not treated."[17] Likewise, similar examination of treatment efficacy for dysarthria in 1996 found that "important changes in speech can be obtained many years post-onset of traumatic brain injury."[18] Others point to the intensity of therapy as having greater benefit than duration. A challenge to well-constructed trials has been the heterogeneity of deficit profiles among patients, even among those with common causes. Single-subject treatment has emerged as a method for assessing the magnitude of treatment effect, and it offers a means to compare treatment approaches addressing specific processes. As understanding of single-subject treatment outcomes increases, routine calculation of effect sizes will help to promote evidence-based practices.

There are many opportunities for research:

- Efficacy of therapeutic techniques to improve language skills and speech clarity
- Optimization of duration and intensity of treatment
- Generalization of aphasia therapy
- Timing of therapy initiation for all disorders
- Cost effectiveness
- Epidemiological dysphagia studies
- Longitudinal studies of dysphagia intervention
- Studies of quality of life improvement after communication and swallowing interventions
- Investigational studies of new interventions
- Cultural considerations for treatment planning

CONCLUSIONS

It is the role of the SLP to work with the patient, family, physician, nurse, allied health professional, and any other person or group member who interacts with the patient to maximize success in communication and safe eating. Appropriate care in advanced disease must take projected longevity, patient endurance, and, in some cases, hospice funding into account. This approach results in a shift from traditional goals that are mostly geared toward restoration to a greater emphasis on compensation and caregiver training. As experts in communication and swallowing across the lifespan, SLPs provide valuable input to patient management. By assessment of problems, educating the medical team and families, and advising about compensatory techniques for areas of breakdown, SLPs can enhance quality of life for the hospice and palliative medicine population.

REFERENCES

1. American Speech-Language-Hearing Association. Scope of Practice in Speech-Language Pathology. Rockville, MD: American Speech-Language-Hearing Association, 2001, p I-25.
2. Logemann JA. Preparation of speech-language pathologists in the United States: The master's degree. Folia Phoniatr Logop 2006;58:55-58.
3. Goodglass H, Kaplan E, Barresi B. The Assessment of Aphasia and Related Disorders, 3rd ed. Philadelphia: Lippincott Williams & Wilkins, 2000.
4. Salt N, Robertson SJ. A hidden client group? Communication impairment in hospice patients. Int J Lang Commun Disord 1998;33(Suppl):96-101.
5. Fox A, Pring T. The cognitive competence of speakers with acquired dysarthria: Judgments by doctors and speech and language therapists. Disabil Rehabil 2005;27:1399-1403.
6. Kasperbauer JL, Thomas JE. Voice rehabilitation after near-total laryngectomy. Otolaryngol Clin North Am 2004;37:655-677.
7. Perry AR, Shaw MA, Cotton S. An evaluation of functional outcomes (speech, swallowing) in patients attending speech pathology after head and neck cancer treatment(s): Results and analysis at 12 months post-intervention. J Laryngol Otol 2003;117:368-381.
8. Langmore SE. Issues in the management of dysphagia. Folia Phoniatr Logop 1999;51:220-230.
9. Langmore SE, Terpenning MS, Schork A, et al. Predictors of aspiration pneumonia: How important is dysphagia? Dysphagia 1998;13:69-81.
10. Logemann JA. Evaluation and Treatment of Swallowing Disorders, 2nd ed. Austin, TX: Pro-Ed, 1998.
11. Martin-Harris B, Logemann JA, McMahon S, et al. Clinical utility of the modified barium swallow. Dysphagia 2000;15:136-141.
12. Robbins J, Langmore S, Hind JA, Erlichman M. Special report: Dysphagia research in the 21st century and beyond. Proceedings from the Dysphagia Experts Meeting, August 21, 2001. J Rehabil Res Dev 2002;39:543-547.
13. Eckman S, Roe J. Speech and language therapists in palliative care: What do we have to offer? Int J Palliat Nurs 2005;11:179-181.
14. Salt N, Davies S, Wilkinson S. Communication. The contribution of speech and language therapy to palliative care. Eur J Palliat Care 1999;6:126-129.
15. Pollens R. Role of the speech-language pathologist in palliative hospice care. J Palliat Med 2004;7:694-702.
16. Beeson PM, Robey RR. Evaluating single-subject treatment research: Lessons learned from the aphasia literature. Neuropsychol Rev 2006;16:161-169.
17. Holland AL, Fromm DS, DeRuyter F, Stein M. Treatment efficacy: Aphasia. J Speech Hear Res 1996;39:S27-S36.
18. Yorkston KM. Treatment efficacy: Dysarthria. J Speech Hear Res 1996;39:S46-S57.
19. Miller RM, Langmore SE. Treatment efficacy for adults with oropharyngeal dysphagia. Arch Phys Med Rehabil 1994;75:1256-1262.
20. Thompson CK. Single subject controlled experiments in aphasia: The science and the state of the science. J Commun Disord 2006;39:266-291.

SUGGESTED READING

Fox A, Pring T. The cognitive competence of speakers with acquired dysarthria: Judgments by doctors and speech and language therapists. Disabil Rehabil 2005;27:1399-1403.

Pollens R. Role of the speech-language pathologist in palliative hospice care. J Palliat Med 2004;7:694-702.

Salt N, Robertson SJ. A hidden client group? Communication impairment in hospice patients. Int J Lang Commun Disord 1998;33(Suppl):96-101.

CHAPTER **54**

Psychiatrists and Clinical Psychologists

Ursula Bates and Kevin Malone

KEY POINTS

- Psychiatry and clinical psychology have significant roles in palliative medicine.
- Mental health issues are underdiagnosed and remain untreated in palliative care.
- Patients with significant distress are best treated by a combination of medication, psychological therapy, and milieu management.
- Resilience and promotion of dignity may protect against psychological distress.
- Research is needed into the effectiveness of psychological and psychopharmacological interventions in palliative medicine.

The National Cancer Comprehensive Network (NCCN) guidelines on distress management[1] recommends the use of the word *distress* in the field of psychosocial care because it is less stigmatizing and more amenable to definition and self-report than other terms. It defines distress as a multifactorial, unpleasant emotional experience of a psychological (e.g., cognitive, behavioral, emotional), social, or spiritual nature that may interfere with the ability to cope effectively with cancer and with its physical symptoms and its treatment.

Distress ranges from common normal feelings of vulnerability, sadness, and fear to disabling problems such as depression, anxiety, panic, social isolation, and existential and spiritual crisis.[1] Over the past decade, our knowledge of psychological responses to illness from psycho-oncology, combined with medical advances and longer survival, has focused attention on quality of life. Throughout an illness, intervention may be required at several points: diagnosis, treatment, recurrence, and end of life. The transition to palliative care is a significant adjustment for patients and their families. Although it is distressing, it is also an opportunity to engage in anticipatory loss and closure. The psychosocial needs of palliative patients are complex and can require the assessment and intervention of many disciplines. "Referrals to health care professionals with specialized skills in age-appropriate psychological and psychiatric management are made available when appropriate (e.g., psychiatrists, psychologists, and social workers). Identified psychiatric comorbidities in family and caregivers are referred for treatment."[2]

Liaison psychiatry has been an integral part of a multidisciplinary approach since the inception of palliative care. Clinical psychologists are becoming a part of comprehensive end-of-life services. With the expansion of palliative care services in acute hospitals and the community, the patient population increasingly includes those with special needs, previous mental health issues, learning disabilities, and trauma, all of which benefit from specialized services. Clinical psychology and psychiatry play critical roles in our understanding and treatment of palliative care patients.

The National Institute for Clinical Excellence[3] (NICE), in its document "Improving Supportive and Palliative Care for Adults with Cancer 2004," based its recommendation for the inclusion of psychiatric and clinical psychology services on the severity of distress, unidentified mental health needs, underestimation of the benefits of psychological and pharmacological treatments, and the needs of patients with previous or ongoing psychological problems (Box 54-1).

Colin Murray Parkes, Elizabeth Kübler-Ross, Jimmie Holland, Davis Kissane, and others contributed significantly to the development of psychosocial care in oncology and palliative care. The growth of liaison psychiatry within palliative care began in the 1970s and remains the recommended model of best practice. "Where specialist mental health management is required, it is best if this is delivered by a liaison psychiatric service, which should include liaison nurses, clinical psychologists, and social workers in addition to consultant and trainee psychiatrists."[4]

Clinical psychology developed its contribution to the care of the medically ill in primary care and the acute general hospital.[5] Psychological interventions include relaxation training, stress and pain management, individual therapy for anxiety and depression, and family and group psychotherapy. These interventions improve patient satisfaction, reduce distress, increase compliance with medical treatment, and enhance patients' sense of control. Psychological expertise[6] should be regarded as a core component of psychosocial care.

PSYCHOLOGICAL DISTRESS IN PALLIATIVE CARE

Between 10% and 50% of palliative care patients have significant anxiety and depression, 35% have unmet emotional needs, and 20% to 70% have inadequate pain relief.[7] The prevalence depends on the stage of the illness, level of disability, and degree of pain. These needs include many comorbid mental health disorders (often undetected), complex bereavements, and end-of-life issues[8] (Boxes 54-2 and 54-3). "Active listening, supportive interventions, trust, and respect are the most important elements of psychotherapeutic work with patients suffering from advanced illness."[9]

Box 54-1 Objectives of the National Institute for Clinical Excellence 2004 Guidelines

- Patients and caregivers are offered psychological support that is appropriate to their needs, and those experiencing particular distress are referred to specialists.
- The psychological needs of the staff caring for patients and caregivers facing difficult circumstances are adequately met.

Clinical Psychology

Psychology as a discipline aims to reduce psychological distress and promote psychological well-being. Psychological assessments in palliative care include assessment of reactions to illness, levels of anxiety and depression, grieving and coping strategies, cognitive functioning, and existential concerns. Comprehensive psychological assessment includes consideration of the mental health and coping strategies of the family and caregivers. Clinical psychologists understand the complex theoretical models, developmental perspectives, and organizational development skills that enhance end-of-life care for patients and staff[10] (Boxes 54-4 and 54-5).

Because most clients in palliative care are older than 65 years, knowledge about geriatric psychological assessment is beneficial. Assessment requires attention to the physical causes of symptoms, iatrogenic effects of medica-

Box 54-2 Generic Functions of Psychiatrists and Clinical Psychologists

- Assessment and treatment of the patient
- Assessment and treatment of the caregivers and family
- Staff consultation and debriefing
- Teaching and training
- Research and clinical audits
- Advocating policies

Box 54-3 Generic Psychological and Psychiatric Interventions

- Establish a relationship that reduces the sense of isolation experienced in terminal illness.
- Help patients face their experience.
- Assist patients to find the language for their experience in word, poetry, story, and image.
- Review life narratives, and assist the patient with reframing and the search for meaning.
- Find expression for and treat unbearable affect with pharmacology and other therapies.
- Explore issues of separation and loss.
- Acknowledge uncertainty and the experience of the unknown.
- Assist caregivers in managing difficult conditions.

Box 54-4 Specialist Psychological Assessment

- Anxiety disorders, including adjustment disorders, phobias, and panic attacks
- Depression, including adjustment disorders and recurrent depression
- Grief reactions to loss of role and identity
- Coping style and control
- Cognitive impairment, including memory loss, functional difficulties
- Pain and symptom management
- Communication barriers
- Beliefs about symptoms, self, the world, and the future
- Resilience and wellness

tions, and psychological distress. It often benefits from multidisciplinary case conferences because of the complexity of presentations in palliative care. Younger clients suffer considerable social isolation, ruptures in identity and body image, and sexuality difficulties that benefit from skilled intervention. The purpose of assessment is to produce a formulation of a client's specific concerns and needs, which informs multidisciplinary care planning and specific psychotherapeutic interventions (Box 54-6).

Psychotherapeutic interventions may include individual or group approaches, depending on the needs of the client and the theoretical orientation of the psychologist. Psychology is theory driven; psychologists are trained in various therapeutic orientations, including cognitive, meta-cognitive, psychodynamic, and psychoanalytic approaches. Psychologists bring expertise in qualitative and quantitive research methodology to their clinical work and are well placed to design and implement research, clinical audits, and outcome evaluations. Psychologists also offer supervision to clinical psychology interns and palliative care staff.

Role of the Liaison Psychiatrist

The role of the liaison psychiatrist has a strong clinical focus on the assessment, diagnosis, and treatment of mental illness. Recommended treatments usually include a combination of medication and psychotherapy.

Training in psychiatry usually consists of 4 years of postgraduate study, within which students can specialize, such as in geriatric or forensic psychiatry. Most training includes psychotherapy supervision. Adult psychiatric liaison services within a general hospital or community setting are the most common source of services for palliative care teams and hospices in the United Kingdom and Ireland. Liaison psychiatry at the interface of palliative care and mental health is well placed to act as an agent for social change in end-of-life care. Liaison psychiatrists contribute to teaching and training in palliative care and have contributed extensively to research on mental health in the field.

Accurate diagnostic assessment is critical for identification of mental health difficulties and decisions about treatment plans. Common comorbid conditions, including depression, iatrogenic complications, psychotic features, alcohol abuse, and behavioral disturbances, often warrant psychopharmacological and psychosocial interventions. The most frequently referred conditions for evaluation are depression, dementia, delirium, and suicidal risk[11] (Box 54-7).

Because polypharmacy is common, reactions to psychotropic drugs need to be monitored. Compromised renal and hepatic function can affect antidepressant medications, and these functions must be assessed before treatment. The timing of antidepressant medication (when required) needs to be considered in those who may have only weeks to live. Effective psychiatric treatments include a combination of psychotherapy and medication.

As patients live longer and actively participate in decisions about care, issues about competency arise. This complex and challenging situation requires skilled evaluation of cognition, affect, and personality limitation. Liaison psychiatry is uniquely skilled to undertake and communicate such assessments to colleagues and families. Support for the primary physician and medical colleagues in such cases reduces the emotional burden on the care team. The psychiatrist can educate the family by providing a greater understanding of the patient's difficulties, thereby reducing distress. Effective psychiatric treatments include a combination of psychotherapy, medication, and electroconvulsive therapy (Box 54-8).

The American Psychiatric Association has identified the reduction of stigma associated with mental illness and increased awareness that such conditions are treatable as primary goals of psychiatry. The psychiatrist in palliative care has an educational role in countering reluctance to refer patients and the excessive normalization of depression in the terminally ill (Box 54-9).

PROVISION OF PSYCHOLOGICAL AND PSYCHIATRIC CARE

Slightly more than one half of the general hospitals in the United Kingdom have access to a multidisciplinary palliative care team. In a survey of 160 hospices in 1999,[12] 97 services had an annual referral rate to psychology or psychiatry professionals of 0 to 64 patients. The referral rate was directly related to service access. When a liaison psychiatrist was available, approximately 10% of patients were referred annually. The study concluded, "It appears that support for the hospice services from psychologists and psychiatrists is very haphazard."[12]

A report on inpatient referrals to clinical psychology in a hospice setting[13] over a 2-year period showed that 11% of the 648 patients admitted were referred to the clinical psychologist. There was no gender bias in the group referred, and their medical diagnoses were similar to those of the overall hospice population. The most common reasons for referral were depression (32%), anxiety (16%), and pain (11%), with a few referrals made to assess confusion, family issues, aggression, and dementia. Most interventions were brief, involving one to two sessions. The overall aim of the consultation was for the psychologist to contribute to the care plan. Clients seen more frequently had significant marital and family stressors on admission. Their behavior often posed significant management challenges and communication difficulties for the general palliative care staff, who became a target for the patients' unresolved distress.

Models of Service Delivery

The necessary basis for good psychosocial care is a mutually respectful relationship between the patient and his or her team. This can be challenging because most palliative care patients display fluctuating levels of defense and denial in their dynamic adaptation to terminal illness. Clinical psychologists and psychiatrists are uniquely placed to model, explore, and teach the basics of creating and maintaining effective therapeutic relationships. Best-practice psychological and psychiatric interventions enhance and empower the patient's relationship with the primary care team. Respect for the individual's defensive structure should guide clinical interventions at every stage of service delivery.

Multidisciplinary teams are usually recommended for psychosocial care, and in most policy documents, the range and complexity of care are described by division in levels of care of increasing complexity and skill. In 2004, NICE recommended and described four levels of psychosocial care.[14] These classifications are efforts to ensure that patients are adequately assessed, that their needs are met with appropriate expertise at appropriate times in their disease journey, and that intervention is evaluated for effectiveness (Table 54-1) (see "Case Study: Brief Psychological Interventions").

Promoting Psychological Wellness in Palliative Care

Research Advances

Mental health is not just the absence of pathology but also the presence of wellness. The 2007 NCCN palliative care guidelines remind us that palliative care provides a different kind of hope from that of anticancer therapy. The guidelines describe a hope for closure and a hope for growth at the end of life.[1]

Psychological theory in the fields of mental health and gerontology focus on psychopathology and on normal development, adjustment resilience, and growth in old age.[15] Research on positive mental health in old age addresses people's capacity to flourish and adjust to life's adversities. Protective factors that support resilience from a multidisciplinary perspective include biological, social, and psychological resources. Psychological well-being is determined by six factors, which have been identified by well-researched and validated instruments. The six dimensions are purpose in life, environmental mastery, self-acceptance, positive relationships, autonomy, and personal

---

Box 54-9 Roles of a Psychologist in Palliative Care

Job Description

- Senior clinical psychologist in the psycho-oncology and palliative care service of St. Vincent's University Hospital, Dublin, Ireland

Principal Duties and Responsibilities

- Setting up and developing a multidisciplinary psycho-oncology service within St. Vincent's Health Care Group
- Coordination of psycho-oncology services of assessment and therapeutic intervention with people with cancer and their families
- Assessment and follow-up of all referrals
- Writing case notes, reports, and all documents pertaining to the delivery of a complete psycho-oncology service
- Supporting other health care professionals in providing psychological support for patients with cancer and for their caregivers
- Cooperation and regular communication with other clinicians and professionals as part of the multidisciplinary team caring for patients within the hospital and in the community
- Communication with the director of the cancer support center as required
- Incorporation of international best-practice strategies in psycho-oncology into the St. Vincent's Health Care Group multidisciplinary oncology support program

Other Duties: Education, Audits, and Research

- Participation in the training, supervision, and education of professional staff in all disciplines involved in the care of oncology patients and their families
- Development of a program of audits and service evaluations
- Conducting research within the field of psycho-oncology

LEVEL	PROFESSIONAL GROUP	ASSESSMENT TYPE	INTERVENTION
1	All health and social care professionals	Recognition of psychological needs	Information Compassionate communication General psychological support
2	Health and social care professionals with additional expertise	Screening for psychological distress	Psychological coping techniques
3	Trained and accredited professionals	Assessment for psychological distress, diagnosis of some pathology	Counseling Psychological interventions, relaxation, and anxiety management delivered according to an explicit theoretical framework
4	Mental health specialties	Diagnosis of psychopathology	Specialist psychological and psychiatric interventions Psychotherapy Psychopharmacology Cognitive behavior therapy

TABLE 54-1   Levels of Psychological Assessment and Treatment

Adapted from National Institute for Clinical Excellence. Guidance on Cancer Services: Improving Supportive and Palliative Care for Adults with Cancer. London: National Institute for Clinical Excellence, 2004. www.nice.org.uk (accessed October 2, 2007).

CASE STUDY

Brief Psychological Interventions

A 44-year-old woman, who was the main caregiver of a young man with lung cancer, was severely distressed and preoccupied with family problems and existential worries about the meaning of her brother's life. After the therapist listened carefully and allowed the woman to express her distress, a number of therapeutic techniques were employed, including cognitive reframing, the skills, strengths, and resources exercise, to help her reflect on her brother's life and on the resources the family members were bringing to bear on his illness. She did not follow up on the offer of future appointments. Three months after her brother's death, she wrote the following note to her therapist:

I wish to thank you sincerely for the help you gave me when I needed it. Your words comforted me so much when my brother P was ill, especially when you told me he would die knowing that he was loved. Well, that is exactly what happened.

We took him home 3 weeks before the end, and every single member of the family was there for him. P had never discussed dying with us, but a week before he died, he gave me a big hug and told me that he loved me, for which I will be forever grateful. Then, when we were all gathered around his bed, he said that Mary (our late sister) and our father and Uncle Mick would all be waiting for him. It was such a special time. He asked me to play Roy Orbison, his favorite singer, and I promised him that I would think of him every time I did. He died at home at 12.45 AM on Friday, October 14, and we were all with him.

Surprisingly, I've been fine ever since. It was as if I had done all my grieving while he was alive, and it's okay. I feel that you helped me get through that despair, and now he has given me the strength to move on.

Yours Truly,

C

growth.[16] We need to consider how best to support the development and maintenance of these factors, which buffer the adverse reactions to life's stressors in palliative populations.

Therapeutic Advances

Dignity-conserving care[17] places the maintenance of dignity at the center of end-of-life care. It outlines a framework for the exploration of dignity, which examines the meaning, strengths, resilience, and personal control that the person brings to bear on his or her illness. This biopsychosocial model guides the clinician in sensitive bedside interventions, and the written record generated strengthens ties with caregivers and family members.

Mindfulness-based stress reduction is a well-defined and systematic patient-centered educational approach. It is an 8-week outpatient group session with guided exercises on breathing, gentle stretching, and home assignments that encourage daily practice and the extension of mindfulness to everyday activities. It aims to establish a more compassionate, harmonious relationship between mind and body. This approach has been applied to many physical conditions with significant results. Five studies of oncology outpatient populations have been completed, with promising results in lowering stress levels, improving immunological markers, and reducing mood disturbances[18] (see "Case Study: Day Hospice Mindfulness Group").

There is merit in training all members of the palliative team to recognize the early signs and symptoms of depression to rapidly ameliorate symptoms and unnecessary psychological suffering, which can seriously reduce the quality of life during precious end-of-life care. Few randomized, controlled trials have been conducted on the use of modern antidepressant agents for depression in palliative care.[19]

Some clinicians tend to favor a tricyclic agent such as amitriptyline as an antidepressant because of its sedative and possibly analgesic effects (for neuropathic pain). However, the doses prescribed are rarely in the therapeutic range, and the antidepressant response is frequently modest. Modern selective serotonin reuptake inhibitors (SSRIs) such as fluoxetine, paroxetine, sertraline, and

CASE STUDY

Day Hospice Mindfulness Group

Blackrock Hospice in Ireland provides nursing care, physiotherapy, hydrotherapy, and psychological care to outpatients receiving palliative care. Nineteen patients, who were between 55 and 94 years old and who had a variety of terminal conditions, completed a pilot mindfulness-based stress reduction program and were interviewed by the psychology intern. It emerged that 79% were highly satisfied, and 21% were satisfied with the 6-week group, and they made the following comments:

- When I catch myself becoming depressed, I try to do the breathing exercises, and I notice I feel less tense and more relaxed.
- If you did not care about anything before the group, it brings home to you why you are here. Once you come to terms with it, you can enjoy what you have left.
- I surprised myself; seeing others open up emotionally made it easier for me to do the same.
- Sometimes, a stranger can open a door a family member cannot and correct you or give you hope.
- I did not want to miss any of the weeks, even though I didn't know what to expect beforehand.
- It makes me feel less like an ill person and more in line with life.
- On each seat [in the group], I could see a vision of myself.

citalopram usually are well tolerated, have fewer side effects, and have a greater likelihood of being prescribed within the therapeutic range, increasing the chances of a clinical antidepressant response. Anecdotal evidence supports the use of the psychostimulant methylphenidate in conjunction with antidepressant pharmacotherapy, especially when lethargy is a prominent symptom in the psychological profile.

Transient and brief psychotic episodes and delirium can occur in palliative care, with subtle symptoms becoming more prominent near evening. Training all palliative team staff to understand and be watchful for early symptoms can facilitate early detection and prevent full-blown psychotic episodes and their attendant impact on quality of life. Early symptoms include increased early evening restlessness or agitation and an increased vigilance about and hesitancy to take evening medications or fluids by patients (e.g., delusions that staff are trying to poison them). Second-generation antipsychotic agents are effective for these symptoms and need only small doses for effect, reducing the likelihood of side effects such as unnecessary drowsiness that typically is associated with the older neuroleptics[20] (see "Psychological and Psychiatric Care by a Multidisciplinary Team").

Evaluation of Psychological and Psychiatric Interventions

Direct evaluation of and evidence for the efficacy of psychological and psychiatric interventions in palliative care are limited, relying mainly on single-case studies. This deficit reflects the developmental stage of psychosocial care in the field and the ethical problems in evaluating a

CASE STUDY

Psychological and Psychiatric Care by a Multidisciplinary Team

Mrs. E was a 62-year-old patient with ovarian cancer and paraneoplastic cerebellar syndrome. She presented with despair and a persistent wish to die.

The psychiatric assessment confirmed cognitive ataxia and eliminated psychotic features. On assessment, Mrs. E had a Mini-Mental State Examination score of 25, and she was referred for therapy in combination with day hospice and antidepressant medication. The clinical interview and reports from the palliative care consultant, hospice staff, and family led to the diagnosis of major depression with inhibited processing of loss and withdrawal from social contact. This previously independent woman had developed an anxious, clinging attachment style that left her emotionally dependent on her husband, who was her main caregiver.

When first assessed, Mrs. E sat hunched in her wheelchair and mostly silent, with intermittent episodes of sobbing and heart-rending questions about when she would get well again. Because her speech was indistinct, her husband attended all sessions. Mrs. E's position was that she would work intensively at rehabilitation and get well again. Her previous coping style was one of immense competence and hard work, which had led to a successful career as a manager in the fashion industry combined with rearing four able children. Beneath this public style was the significant effect of the loss of her mother when Mrs. E was 10 years old, followed by years of foster care, which she managed by "being good." Cognitively, she was negatively evaluating all aspects of her life and was not able to assimilate limited progress. Her emotional range was limited, and she lacked the language to express her feelings.

Treatment consisted of antidepressant medication combined with couples sessions twice each month for a year, two family meetings, and attendance at mindfulness-based stress reduction group in the latter half of the year. Her processing of affect was validated and encouraged in every session. Behavioral interventions included psychological education on coping styles and adjustment to illness to enable Mrs. E to reduce her tense striving and to work from her current baseline so that she could value her progress, no matter how limited. Cognitive therapy helped her make connections between her thoughts and feelings, and it reduced her personalization, all-or-nothing thinking, and self-blame. Her family used the sessions to express their grief about her limitations, learn how to manage her intense affect, and reassess the family's myth that "bad things do not happen to good people."

By the end of treatment, her anxiety and depression were at moderate levels. Mrs. E was better able to communicate her feelings, and her husband was more comfortable and accepting of her. As she became less striving and tense, her speech improved, and she engaged with her day hospice group. Gradually, she accepted caregivers into her home and was able to trust the staff sufficiently to separate from her husband for respite care. Her husband reported that the modeling of and learning about listening and validation of feelings had been the most valuable aspect of the sessions. He felt less pressured to fix her pain and more able to be present.

Common Errors

- Inadequate assessment of the interaction of complex comorbidities, medications, and existential concerns
- Underestimation of the value of brief psychotherapy for patients older than 65 years, even in the last weeks of life
- Lack of risk assessment for complicated grief reactions in bereaved relatives
- Assumption that psychiatric symptoms (e.g., depression) are a natural reaction to illness
- Hesitancy in asking about psychological and psychiatric symptoms, leading to delay in treatment intervention

vulnerable population. There is a need for a review of the efficacy of all psychological and pharmacological treatments for depression in the palliative care setting.[19]

Advocacy Role

Psychiatrists and psychologists work with other health care professionals to advocate for ongoing discussions in the media, among community teams, and within professional groups to overcome the stigma of mental illness and to promote the best practice in care of the dying. There are considerable gaps in medical undergraduate and postgraduate education among psychologists, particularly in the areas of chronic illness, death and dying, and palliative care. Awareness needs to be raised among all professionals about the mental health treatment possibilities for distressed patients. In highlighting psychosocial needs, professionals can ensure marginalized groups, such as those with chronic mental health needs and personality difficulties, have adequate care at the end of life and equity of access to palliative care (see "Common Errors").

CONCLUSIONS AND FUTURE DIRECTIONS

The mental health needs of palliative patients are challenging areas of service development. Disciplines need to draw on lifespan developmental models of aging and current theories to identify factors that promote and support mental wellness. Clinical psychologists and psychiatrists are underrepresented in palliative care. Their education, research, and experience are needed to understand and support the intrapsychic life of the elderly. These patients can be helped to engage creatively with the end of their lives.

Assessment of mental health should be grounded in empirical research and in qualitative studies that address human values and the struggle for meaning at the end of life. There is an urgent need for well-designed clinical trials of antidepressant and antipsychotic pharmacotherapy in palliative medicine. Common psychosyndromes such as depression and transient psychosis need a strong evidence base for determining which agents work best in

this setting and for assessing their effects on quality of life. Palliative mental health issues should be included in the training of professionals in all areas of medicine, psychology, and social work to meet the demands of an aging population.

REFERENCES

1. National Comprehensive Cancer Network (NCCN). Clinical Practice Guidelines in Oncology: Distress Management, version 1, 2007. Available at www.nccn.org (accessed October 2, 2007).
2. National Consensus Project for Quality Palliative Care. Domain 3: Guideline 3.1, 2004. Available at www.nationalconsensusproject.org (accessed October 2, 2007).
3. National Institute for Clinical Excellence. Guidance on Cancer Services: Improving Supportive and Palliative Care for Adults with Cancer. London: National Institute for Clinical Excellence, 2004. www.nice.org.uk (accessed October 2, 2007).
4. Joint Working Party of the Royal College of Physicians and the Royal College of Psychiatrists. The Psychological Care of Medical Patients: A Practical Guide, 2nd ed. London: Royal College of Physicians and the Royal College of Psychiatrists, 2003.
5. Brown R, Freeman W, Brown R, et al. The role of psychology in health care delivery. Prof Psychol Res Pract 2002;33:536-545.
6. Paine S, Haines R. The contribution of psychologists to specialist palliative care. Int J Palliat Nurs 2002;8:401-406.
7. Bradley EH, Fried TR, Kasl SV, et al. Quality of life trajectories of elders in the end of life. Ann Rev Gerontol Geriatr 2002;20:64-96.
8. National Council for Hospice and Specialist Palliative Care Services (NCHSPCS). Definition of Supportive and Palliative Care. Briefing paper 11. London: NCHSPCS, September 2002.
9. Tremblay A, Breitbart W. Psychiatric dimensions of palliative care. Neurol Clin 2001;19:949-967.
10. Haley W, Larson D, Kasl-Godley J, et al. Roles for psychologists in end-of-life care: Emerging models of practice. Prof Psychol Res Pract 2003;34:626-633.
11. Breitbart W, Chochinov HM, Passik SD. Psychiatric symptoms in palliative medicine. In Doyle D, Hanks G, Cherny N, Calman K (eds). Oxford Textbook of Palliative Medicine, 3rd ed. New York: Oxford University Press, 2004, pp 746-771.
12. Lloyd-Williams M (ed). Psychosocial Issues in Palliative Care. New York: Oxford University Press, 2003.
13. Alexander P. An investigation of inpatient referrals to a clinical psychologist in a hospice. Eur J Cancer Care 2004;13:36-44.
14. Holland JC (ed). Psycho-Oncology. New York: Oxford University Press, 1998.
15. Lomranz J (ed). Handbook of Aging and Mental Health: An Integrative Approach. New York: Plenum Press, 1998.
16. Ryff CD, Singer BH. Psychological well-being: Meaning, measurement, and implications for psychotherapy research. Psychother Psychosom 1996;65:14-23.
17. Chochinov HM. Dignity-conserving care—a new model for palliative care. JAMA 2002;287: 2253-2260.
18. Speca M, Carlson LE, Mackenzie MJ, et al. Mindfulness-based stress reduction (MBSR) as an intervention for cancer patients. In Baer R (ed). Mindfulness-Based Treatment Approaches: Clinician's Guide to Evidence Based Applications. New York: Academic Press, 2006, pp 239-257.
19. Lan Ly K, Chidgey J, Addington-Hall J, Hotopf M. Depression in palliative care: A systemic review. Palliat Med 2002;16:279-284.
20. Billings JA. Recent advances: Palliative care. BMJ 2000;321:555-558.

SUGGESTED READING

Chochinov HM, Breitbart W (eds). Handbook of Psychiatry in Palliative Medicine. Oxford, UK: Oxford University Press, 2000.

Kabat-Zinn J. Full catastrophe living: How to cope with stress, pain, and illness using mindfulness meditation. New York: Delacorte, 1990.

Lloyd-Williams M (ed). Psychosocial Issues in Palliative Care. New York: Oxford University Press, 2003.

Lomranz J (ed). Handbook of Aging and Mental Health: An Integrative Approach. New York: Plenum Press, 1998.

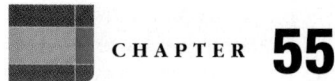

CHAPTER **55**

Spiritual Care

Christina M. Puchalski

K E Y   P O I N T S

- Spirituality is essential to compassionate care.

- Two theoretical models support the inclusion of spirituality in health care: patient-centered care and the biopsychosocial-spiritual model.

- Spiritual care involves all members of the interdisciplinary health care team.

- Chaplains, spiritual directors, and pastoral counselors are trained spiritual care professionals who are responsible for more in-depth spiritual work.

- Spiritual care involves a compassionate presence with patients and awareness of the health care professional's own spiritual beliefs and values.

- The extrinsic aspect of spiritual care involves communicating with patients about spiritual issues, recognizing patients' spiritual distress or spiritual resources of strength, making referrals to chaplains or other spiritual care professionals, and incorporating patients' spiritual practices into the treatment or care plan as appropriate.

Health care is focused on a disease-centered model of care in which primary attention is given to the illness. Patients' satisfaction with this type of care has decreased. Fifty-five percent of Americans are "dissatisfied with the quality of care in this country."[1] Many patients believe that compassion is lacking.[1]

Some models support compassionate systems of care rather than a strictly disease-centered approach to care. They include patient-centered care[2] and the biopsychosocial-spiritual model.[3] In the patient-centered model, the patient's illness or disease is diagnosed and treated within the context of the whole person (i.e., values and beliefs, family and culture, and world view). Outcomes are superior if patients' wishes are respected, if their beliefs and values are integrated into their care, and if there is a larger community of caregivers, such as family and church members. The biopsychosocial-spiritual model defines four dimensions of care of the whole person, echoing the precepts of the patient-centered care model. In this model, attention is equally focused on physical, psychological, social, and spiritual needs.

HOLISTIC MODELS OF CARE

Holistic models have as their focus a more compassionate approach to patients. When the focus is only on the disease or illness, the patient's experience may be lost and not integrated into how he or she understands and therefore copes with the illness. For example, if a patient with diabetes remembers an uncle who died a miserable death after many amputations, the patient will think of his own illness in that context. The approach to diabetes may be altered by this memory, and health care professionals need to understand the patient's views. Similarly, in a disease-focused model, a patient's suffering may not be confronted or even recognized. Pain as a physical symptom may be treated, but existential or spiritual suffering may not be addressed.

There are distinctions among fixing, helping, and serving. "Helping, fixing, and serving represent three different ways of seeing life. When you help, you see life as weak. When you fix, you see life as broken. When you serve, you see life as whole. Fixing and helping may be the work of the ego and service the work of the soul."[4] In a disease-oriented model, the caregiver tends to focus on the fix, whereas in the more holistic models, the focus is on the compassionate care of the whole person and on service.

Biopsychosocial-Spiritual Model of Care

In whole-person or patient-centered care, all of the four dimensions—physical, emotional, social, and spiritual— are intertwined, and how a person is doing in one area can affect the others. All four dimensions affect quality of life. The World Health Organization (WHO) has said that this model of care is important for good patient outcomes. WHO also stated that spirituality is an important dimension of quality of life.[5] Spiritual distress can influence physical pain and emotional angst. All dimensions must be addressed (Table 55-1) to provide the best medical care (see "Case Study: Biopsychosocial-Spiritual Care").

Spiritual Care: Compassion in Action

Spirituality has been defined by consensus of academic medical educators and clinicians as what gives ultimate meaning to a person's life. This meaning can be expressed in many ways, including religion; relationship with God, the divine, or the sacred; a transcendent belief system; through family; and by means of naturism, rationalism, or humanism and the arts. Spirituality is fundamentally relational. For example, the spirituality of the health care professional underlies the relationships formed with patients and their families.[6] By integrating spirituality more fully into the care of patients, care can become more compassionate.

Compassion is essential in the care of patients and their families. Compassion comes from two Latin words: *cum*, which means "with," and *pati*, which means "to suffer."[7] The act of compassion is to suffer with another. The Dalai Lama defines compassion as "a state of mind that is nonviolent, nonharming, and nonaggressive. It is a mental attitude based on the wish for others to be free of their suffering and is associated with a sense of commitment, responsibility, and respect toward the other."[8] Compassion is an attitude, a way of approaching the needs of others, and a way of helping others with their suffering. It is also a way of being, a way to be of service to others, a spiritual practice, and act of love.

Many organizations, such as the American Medical Association (AMA), the Association of American Medical

TABLE 55-1   Jamie's Biopsychosocial-Spiritual Assessment and Plan

ASPECT	SIGNS AND SYMPTOMS	ACTION
Physical	Pain, constipation, decreased appetite (may be from $MgSO_4$), insomnia	Adjust pain medications, add Colace, senna, massage
Emotional	Depression exacerbation, grief may be contributing to loss of appetite and insomnia	Increase visits with patient's psychiatrist, adjust antidepressant dose, use counseling
Social	Financial fears, job loss	Encourage talking with a supervisor; encourage to work with a friend from church to help manage her finances
Spiritual	Sense of abandonment by God	Refer to a chaplain for spiritual counseling; encourage patient to talk with her priest, with whom she has always been close and who is a guide to her; use prayer, meditation, guided imagery (help with insomnia)

CASE STUDY

Biopsychosocial-Spiritual Care

Jamie is a 57-year-old woman with a history of bipolar illness, which has caused many difficulties in relationships and work. Her faith has helped her cope. Her beliefs provide support in the middle of life's stresses, and her church offers her social support and structure.

Jamie struggled all her life to find the right job, and at age 50, she found a good position, found joy for the first time, and developed supportive relationships. At age 57, a breast mass was detected during an examination, and she was diagnosed with breast cancer. She had complications after surgery and required more time off work. Some friends have not been supportive.

Jamie has had pain, constipation, and decreased appetite. She is thinking about stopping chemotherapy because she thinks she should die. She is sure that she will be fired from her job and that her friends will abandon her. Jamie feels hopeless and wonders where God is.

In approaching Jamie, health care professionals need to focus on her pain and other symptoms and on the psychosociospiritual issues that she faces. Encouraging her to talk to people at work and to seek support at her church may help Jamie with some of her concerns. Referral to a chaplain can help Jamie work on the spiritual issues she faces, such as a sense of abandonment by God and others. Table 55-1 shows how the biopsychosocial-spiritual framework can be used to form an assessment and plan for Jamie from this model.

Colleges (AAMC), the American College of Physicians (ACP), and the American Nursing Association (ANA), hold their professionals accountable to be compassionate and altruistic in their interactions with patients. Compassion and altruism are spiritual values. Historically, U.S. hospitals were founded on these spiritual values. The Joint Commission (formerly called the Joint Commission on Accreditation of Healthcare Organizations), which accredits U.S. hospitals, requires that pastoral care be available to all patients who request it.

PRACTICAL TOOLS FOR HEALTH CARE PROFESSIONALS

A consensus conference developed guidelines for spiritual care.[9] Important among the guidelines was the idea that

clinicians should create environments where patients feel they can trust their clinician and share their concerns, including spiritual concerns. The first step in spiritual care is to communicate a genuine interest and compassion for the patient. By creating an atmosphere of compassion and having a willingness to be open to whatever concerns the patient, the interaction becomes focused in a patient-centered model. A patient's understanding of illness can be influenced by many factors, including spiritual and religious beliefs and practices.[2] Defining spiritual care as intrinsic and extrinsic helps to see care as stemming from what the clinician brings to the encounter and what that clinician does for the patient.

Intrinsic and Extrinsic Spiritual Care

All medical care has intrinsic aspects (i.e., behavior, attitudes, and values health care professionals bring to the encounter) and extrinsic aspects (i.e., knowledge and skills applied in the encounter). The relationship-centered aspect of medical care is the intrinsic and essential aspect of all care, from which extrinsic care emanates, including physical, emotional, and social care. Spiritual intrinsic care refers to the intention of presence, and spiritual extrinsic care refers to the ability to integrate spiritual issues as they manifest in the health care problem or situation. Spiritual care includes recognizing patients' inner resources of strength or a lack of those resources. Once assessed, clinicians incorporate patients' spirituality into the care plan if appropriate to the clinical situation.

Everyone on the interdisciplinary health care team practices spiritual care, but the specifics of how it is delivered depend on the context. A chaplain provides spiritual care in the context of his or her training as a spiritual counselor in a health care setting. Clergy provide spiritual care in a religious setting, and a nurse and physician practice spiritual care of patients in a spiritual health care situation (e.g., hospital, clinic, patient visits, education). Although the relationship-centered and caring aspects are similar, how patients' spiritual issues and problems are dealt with depends on the professional's level of training and the context. Chaplains and clergy work primarily with spiritual issues and spiritual problems in depth, but not necessarily in relation to health and illness. They may secondarily be aware of and interface with social, emotional, and physical issues, but they deal with them more in a supportive way. Nurses and doctors are trained primarily to address the physical issues of patients. However, emotional, social, and spiritual issues may affect or be related to the physical issue. Physicians, nurses, social workers, counselors, and physical, occupational, and other therapists recognize, support, and triage spiritual issues appropriate to the spiritual care of these professionals (Box 55-1).

Compassionate Presence

To engage in spiritual care, health care professionals need training on how to be intentionally open, willing, and accepting of mystery. This means that the clinician brings his or her whole being to the encounter and places full attention on the patient, not allowing distractions to interfere. They must be attentive to all dimensions of the lives of patients and their families. Some clinicians suggest that current medical practices do not allow time for this type of care, but being wholly present is not time dependent. It requires the physician's intention to be fully present for patients. The caregiver becomes fully present when he or she approaches the patient with deep respect that stems from a commitment to honoring the whole person.

Spiritual Self-Care

To be fully available to the patient, health care professionals must be aware of their own values, beliefs, and attitudes and recognize how those viewpoints influence their understanding of life, health, and illness. Clinicians should be aware of what spiritual issues may be elicited in themselves in response to their patients so as to not impose their personal spiritual conflicts or issues on patients.

Box 55-1 Characteristics of Spiritual Care

Compassionate Presence

- Intention to being fully present for patients
- Being fully attentive to patients
- Comfort with mystery
- Relationship-centered care
- Partnership
- Care not agenda driven
- Listening to patients' fears, hopes, dreams, meaning

Spirituality of Health Care Professional

- Awareness of own spirituality
- Awareness of own mortality
- Reflection on meaning and purpose in profession (i.e., calling)
- Awareness of own spiritual issues that may be raised in response to patients' spiritual issues
- Spiritual coping skills for self-care
- Having a spiritual practice

Extrinsic Spiritual Care

- Taking a spiritual history
- Recognizing patients' spiritual issues
- Recognizing patients' spiritual problems or spiritual pain
- Recognizing patients' resources of inner strength or lack of resources
- Incorporating patients' spirituality into treatment or care plans (e.g., presence, referral, rituals, meditation)

They also need to reflect on what gives their professional life meaning and how their call to serve others is practiced in their daily lives. Many health care professionals speak of their own spiritual practices and how they help them deliver good spiritual care and good medical care.[10] To practice spiritual care effectively, health care professionals need to be aware of and be supported in their spiritual needs and journey.

Communicating with Patients about Spiritual Issues

Communicating with patients about spiritual issues includes several key elements:

- Responding to spiritual themes
- Recognizing spiritual clues
- Taking a formal spiritual history

The patient in conversation with the health care professional may bring up spiritual issues, such as the following examples:

- Why is this happening to me?
- I deserve to die; God is punishing me.
- My life is meaningless.
- I feel alone and unloved.
- I need to be forgiven before I die.
- I feel despair, hopelessness, and a lack of peace.

The first step in communicating is to listen for spiritual themes and then offer the patient the opportunity to discuss the issues more fully. This requires open-ended questions, respect for the inherent dignity of each person, and openness to a diversity of belief systems and values. Open-ended questions (e.g., What do you think is happening?) invite patients to discuss whatever is on their minds—physical, spiritual, or existential issues.

Patients may wear religious jewelry or have spiritual or religious readings at the bedside or with them in the office. The health care professional can refer to these items to assess the importance of the symbols or reading material in their lives. Sometimes, a patient may respond with religious expressions when the health care professional breaks bad news: "Oh God, help me. Lord, have mercy." The health care professional can respond, "You seem upset. Is God important to you as you face what we are talking about?"

THE SPIRITUAL HISTORY

A spiritual history refers to formal questioning about spiritual beliefs and practices. Listening to themes alone cannot elicit all the information needed for good medical care. Specific questions need to be asked to target specific areas, such as depression, social support, domestic violence, sexual preferences, and spiritual beliefs and practices. Patients may not volunteer information unless they are invited to share that particular area. This is particularly true of spirituality. Although patients are interested in having spirituality integrated into their care, it is not a common practice to have physicians and other health care professionals address spiritual issues.

A spiritual history is a set of targeted questions aimed at inviting patients to share their spiritual or religious

TABLE 55-2   Taking a Spiritual History

FICA DIMENSIONS	QUESTIONS	COMMENTS
Faith and belief (F)	"Do you consider yourself spiritual or religious?" "Do you have spiritual beliefs that help you cope with stress?"	If the patient responds, "No," the physician may ask, "What gives your life meaning?" Sometimes patients respond with answers such as family, career, or nature.
Importance (I)	"What importance does your faith or belief have in your life?" "Have your beliefs influenced how you take care of yourself in this illness?" "What role do your beliefs play in regaining your health?"	
Community (C)	"Are you part of a spiritual or religious community?"	Communities such as churches, temples, and mosques or a group of like-minded friends can serve as strong support systems for some patients.
	"Is this of support to you and how?" "Is there a group of people you really love or who are important to you?"	
Address in care (A)	"How would you like me, your health care provider, to address these issues in your health care?"	It is often unnecessary to ask this question, but it is important to think about which spiritual issues should be addressed in the treatment plan. Examples include referral to chaplains, pastoral counselors, or spiritual directors; journaling; and music or art therapy. Sometimes, the plan may be to listen and support the person on his or her journey.

© Puchalski CM, 1996.

beliefs if desired. Several tools have been developed for spiritual history taking. These include FICA (Table 55-2),[11,12] SPIRIT,[13] and HOPE questions.[14] A spiritual history can be done as part of a social history during the intake examination or annual history and physical examination. It has several goals:

- To invite the patient to share spiritual and religious beliefs if they choose to
- To learn about the patients' beliefs and values
- To assess for spiritual distress (e.g., meaninglessness, hopelessness) and spiritual sources of strength (e.g., hope, meaning, purpose, resiliency, spiritual community)
- To provide an opportunity for compassionate care whereby caregivers connect to the patient in a deep and profound way
- To empower the patient to find inner resources of healing and acceptance
- To learn about patients' spiritual and religious beliefs that may affect health care decision making

The questions are meant to guide the discussion about spiritual issues. Spiritual history taking is normally done during the social history section of the patient's medical history and physical examination. While asking about the patient's living situation and significant relationships, the clinician can transition into how the person cares for himself or herself. Questions about exercise and dealing with stress and difficult situations are asked because these issues are an important part of self-care. In this context, the clinician then asks whether spiritual beliefs and practices are important.

The spiritual history is patient centered. The clinician should not force the questions if the person does not wish to discuss spirituality. Proselytizing is not allowed because it violates the trust that patients place in clinicians. There is a power differential between clinicians and patients.

Patients may feel vulnerable with their clinicians, and that feeling needs to be honored.

Clinicians usually are not trained spiritual care providers. Chaplains, clergy, pastoral counselors, and spiritual directors are trained to work specifically with spiritual issues. Chaplains are certified by chaplaincy organizations to work specifically in health care. Chaplains are also trained to participate in and lead important rituals and to facilitate connections with the patients' clergy. Chaplains work with patients of any religious or nonreligious background. Clergy are ordained, trained in religious care, and usually work predominantly with patients from their religious denomination. Pastoral counselors have master's or doctoral level training. One half of their training is in how spiritual and religious issues affect the manifestation of and coping with symptoms. Spiritual directors are not counselors; they are trained to assist people in their spiritual journey by helping them discern how God or the divine is working in their lives.

CONCLUSIONS

For more compassionate systems of care, the biopsycho-social-spiritual model of care should be implemented across the lifespans of all patients. Spirituality is an integral part of the model, in which patients' spiritual beliefs and values are respected, they are treated with dignity, and health care professionals are fully attentive to the suffering their patients encounter. Spiritual care can be practiced by all health care professionals; more intense spiritual care can be done by trained spiritual care professionals such as chaplains, pastoral counselors, and spiritual directors. Ultimately, spiritual care is about providing warmth and connection to those who face stress and suffering.

"When people are overwhelmed by illness, we must give them physical relief, but it is equally important to encourage the spirit through a constant show of love and compassion. It is shameful how often we fail to see that what people desperately require is human affection. Deprived of human warmth and a sense of value, other forms of treatment prove less effective. Real care of the sick does not begin with costly procedures, but with the simple gifts of affection, love, and concern."[15]

REFERENCES

1. Sanghavi DM. What makes for a compassionate patient-caregiver relationship? J Qual Patient Saf 2006;132:283-291.
2. Institute for Alternative Futures. Patient-Centered Care 2015: Scenarios, Vision, Goals & Next Steps. Alexandria, VA: Picker Institute, 2004.
3. Sulmasy DP. A biopsychosocial-spiritual model for the care of patients at the end of life. Gerontologist 2002;42:24-33.
4. Remen R. Kitchen table wisdom: Stories that heal. New York: Riverhead Books, 1996.
5. WHOQOL Group. The WHO Quality of Life Assessment (WHOQOL) Position Paper from the World Health Organization. Soc Sci Med 1995;41:1403-1409.
6. Association of American Medical Colleges (AAMC). Report III—Contemporary Issues in Medicine: Communication in Medicine. Medical School Objectives Project (MSOP). Washington, DC: Association of American Medical Colleges, 1999. Available at http://www.aamc.org/meded/msop/msop3.pdf (accessed June 14, 2006).
7. Berube M (ed). Webster's II: News college dictionary. Boston: Houghton Mifflin, 2001.
8. Dalai Lama, Cutler H. The Art of Happiness. New York: Riverhead Books, 1998, p 114.
9. Puchalski CM, Anderson MB, Lo B, et al. Washington, DC: Association of American Medical Colleges, in preparation.
10. Sulmasy DP. The Healer's Calling: A Spirituality for Physicians and Other Health Care Professionals. New York: Paulist Press, 1997.
11. Puchalski CM, Romer A. Taking a spiritual history allows clinicians to understand patients more fully. J Palliat Med 2000;3:129-137.
12. Puchalski CM. Spiritual assessment in clinical practice. Psychol Ann 2006;36:150-155.
13. Maugans TA. The SPIRITual history. Arch Fam Med 1996;5:11-16.
14. Anandarajah G, Hight E. Spirituality and medical practice: Using the HOPE questions as a practical tool for spiritual assessment. Am Fam Physician 2001;63:81-88. Available at http://www.aafp.org/afp/20010101/81.pdf (accessed July 7, 2006).
15. Dalai Lama. Foreword. In Puchalski CM (ed). Time for Listening and Caring: Spirituality and the Care of the Chronically Ill and Dying. New York: Oxford University Press, 2006.

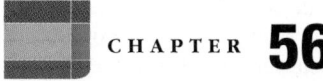

CHAPTER **56**

The Role of the Clinical Pharmacist

Andrew Dickman and Phyllis A. Grauer

KEY POINTS

- The clinical pharmacist has extensive pharmaceutical and therapeutic skills that have many applications in hospice and palliative care.

- The clinical pharmacist is an integral member of the interdisciplinary team and plays a critical role in formulary and protocol development, research, education, and training.

- The role of the clinical pharmacist continues to expand with new responsibilities such as prescribing medicines.

Thirty years ago, the traditional pharmacist's role consisted of procurement, formulation, and dispensing of medicines without input into the medication decision process. This changed near the end of the 20th century with the adoption of pharmaceutical care and the introduction of inpatient unit-based, patient-focused activities, referred to as *clinical pharmacy services*. The traditional roles are increasingly performed by pharmacy technicians and other support staff, and pharmacists are encouraged to use their pharmaceutical and therapeutic skills. In the United Kingdom, this has been taken a step further, and suitably trained pharmacists can prescribe a whole range of medications independently or under the supervision of a medical practitioner.

Research is providing new drugs and changing existing drugs and dosage formulations. Engaging a competent, specialized palliative care pharmacist allows physicians, nurses, and other health care team members to tap into an invaluable resource to assist them in providing optimal patient care in a cost-effective manner. By incorporating traditional dispensing and expanded clinical roles, pharmacists assist in providing cost-effective pharmacotherapy in all types of hospice and palliative care practice settings in a variety of ways (Boxes 56-1 and 56-2).

PHARMACOTHERAPEUTIC ADVICE

Professional-Centered Duties and Advice

Although palliative care has adopted a holistic approach to treatment, medication-driven pain and symptom management arguably form the critical aspect of care. Pharmacological therapy can be extremely complex because the

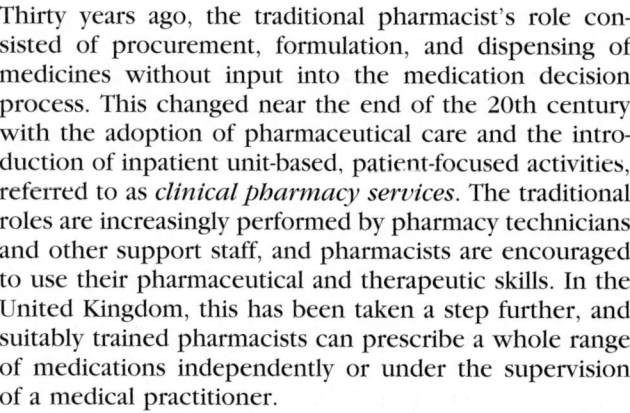

Box 56-1 Definitions of Clinical Pharmacy and Pharmaceutical Care

Clinical pharmacy is the part of the practice of pharmacy that contributes directly to patient care and develops and promotes the rational and appropriate use of medicinal products and devices.
Pharmaceutical care is the person-focused care relating to medication, which is provided by a pharmacist and the pharmacy team with the aim of improving the outcomes of therapy.

Box 56-2 Pharmacists' Responsibilities in Hospice and Palliative Care According to the American Society of Health-System Pharmacists

- Assessing the appropriateness of medication orders and ensuring the timely provision of effective medication for symptom control
- Counseling and educating the hospice team about medication therapy
- Ensuring that patients and caregivers understand and follow the directions provided with medication
- Providing efficient mechanisms for extemporaneous compounding of nonstandard dosage forms
- Addressing financial concerns
- Ensuring safe and legal disposal of all medications after death
- Establishing and maintaining effective communication with regulatory and licensing agencies

patients often have medical conditions coexisting with symptoms caused by their terminal disease. More often than not, patients require several medicines to control their symptoms and may have medicines prescribed for coexisting conditions. The resulting polypharmacy increases the risk of undesirable effects and interactions, and it can reduce the effectiveness of treatment through poor patient compliance or poor patient-provider concordance.

Pharmacists receive comprehensive training in all aspects of medicines, including physiology, pathology, pharmaceutics, pharmacology, and therapeutics. They have specialist knowledge of drug interactions, undesirable effects, cautions, and contraindications, including use in patients with liver or renal impairment, availability of products or formulations, and associated costs. Using this knowledge and expertise, they can devise individual pharmaceutical care plans and advise on cost-effective drug therapy to achieve an acceptable balance between benefit and harm, thereby improving the patient's quality of life. The pharmacist can also apply this knowledge on a wider scale in medication management with the development of evidence-based treatment guidelines and local formularies (discussed later).

Pharmacists may attend interdisciplinary team meetings or inpatient unit rounds, or both, and they frequently have been described as being valuable members of the palliative care team.[1-3] Successful integration into the interdisciplinary team affords clinical pharmacists access to vital information that will be necessary to devise a pharmaceutical care plan, such as current and past medical history; biochemical, hematological, and pharmacokinetic parameters; and allergies and conditions of the patient. The response to drug therapy can vary because a palliative care patient's condition is often unstable, particularly as the disease progresses.

Off-Label Use of Medicines

Although the use of unapproved, unlicensed medicines in palliative care is rare, the use of approved medicines outside the labeled indication is common and necessary, and the practice usually is encountered on a daily basis. One study reported the off-label use of medicines represented 15% of prescriptions written in a palliative care unit.[4] The pharmacist has a duty of care to the patient and is in a prime position to be able to advise the prescriber by assessing the potential benefit and harm of using a medicine in an off-label manner.

Medication Errors

Prescribing errors occur for many reasons, including inadequate knowledge of the medicine, factors related to the patient and his or her condition, calculation errors, illegible handwriting, nonstandard abbreviations, drug name confusion, and poor history taking. Prescribing in palliative care can be a demanding activity, especially given the relatively high incidence of complex therapy and off-label use of medicines. Attendance at interdisciplinary team meetings and inpatient unit rounds places the clinical pharmacist in a position to be able to intervene at the point of prescribing, thereby identifying problems at an early stage and avoiding some altogether.

Patient-Centered Responsibilities and Advice

The pharmacist is the ideal health care professional to confirm medication histories. Potential benefits of the pharmacist taking a medication history include knowledge of over-the-counter preparations and herbal supplements, the ability to identify medicines, identification of actual and potential drug-related problems (e.g., undesirable effects, drug interactions), and continuity of therapy.

The patient may have practical difficulties in taking certain medicines, such as an inability to read the label or difficulty opening the medicine container. The pharmacist can identify such problems and arrange for compliance aids to be made available. Before discharge, the pharmacist can counsel and educate patients and caregivers about the prescribed medicines. This may include the reasons for needing each medicine, instructions on how and when to take them, and a discussion of possible undesirable effects.

Verbal advice should be supplemented with patient information leaflets, although they can be misleading, confusing, and distressing if the medicine has been prescribed for an off-label use. In such circumstances, the patient needs to be informed about and agree to the off-label use. The clinical pharmacist can produce specific patient information leaflets for off-label medicines to allay fears and aid compliance.

If a patient has been prescribed complex treatment that has an involved or complicated ordering process, the pharmacist can collaborate with the patient's elected community pharmacist to ensure continuity of care.

Formulary and Protocol Development

Because palliative care may be required at various stages of an illness, designing a stock drug formulary is inappropriate and ineffective. A more realistic approach is to develop drug therapy protocols and associated formularies based on the current and anticipated functional status and prognosis of patients. In hospice care, emphasis is placed on symptom control rather than managing underlying disease states. The rationale for medication use when patients have years to live may or may not be appropriate in the final months of life. Patients with end-stage disease usually begin discontinuing medications that are intended to prevent long-term disease progression. For example, medications that lower cholesterol in patients who have weeks to live may add an unnecessary financial burden and the risk of drug interactions and side effects. However, if a patient has years to live, prematurely discontinuing this medication would be inappropriate. When designing protocols, criteria for drugs used to manage the disease must be linked to the functionality and anticipated life span of the patient.

The pharmacist has several roles in the development of patient care protocols or guidelines:

- To provide supportive literature to substantiate the use of medications
- To extrapolate pharmacokinetic and pharmacodynamic principles to support appropriate use of medication in end-of-life care that may be less acceptable in mainstream health care

- To provide medication information and to ensure that the formulary reflects the most therapeutically appropriate and cost-effective drugs

Traditional Pharmacy Services

The traditional activities of the pharmacist include procuring, dispensing, and compounding pharmaceuticals. Although rarely involved in this activity, the clinical pharmacist involved in hospice and palliative care collaborates with colleagues who provide these services to ensure patients receive a timely supply of medicines. The liaison is particularly important when patients are prescribed products that are known to be difficult to obtain commercially or require extemporaneous preparation.

PRACTICES OF PHARMACISTS

Pharmacist Practice Models

The practice models of U.K. and U.S. pharmacists differ widely, as do the respective health care systems. Despite this, there are a few similarities. The logistics of incorporating a pharmacist within the palliative care interdisciplinary team depends on the practice setting. With health care budgets tightening, the additional cost of adding a pharmacist must make financial sense. Because clinical pharmacy services are not revenue generating, the cost savings and improved patient outcomes resulting from the participation of a pharmacist in the care of patients justifies their involvement. Historically, provision of drug information and medication counseling by pharmacists has been considered by the public and health care community to be a free service in the outpatient or community setting and a non–revenue-generating service in hospitals.

- In the United Kingdom, a clinical pharmacist associated with a hospital typically provides the palliative care pharmacy service to the hospital and local hospice. In a decreasing number of situations, the pharmaceutical service for a hospice may be obtained from a local retail pharmacy. Although costs are important, the expertise of the pharmacist is a recognized necessity, and the service is funded by the government through the National Health Service.
- In the United States, the 1987 Omnibus Reconciliation Act (OBRA) and the Medicare Prescription Drug, Improvement, and Modernization Act of 2003 (MMA) provide justification and validation of the value of clinical pharmacists' involvement and associated reimbursement in health care.

Research, Education, and Training

Pharmacists are regularly involved in patient counseling and education. Increasingly, more experienced pharmacists are becoming involved in the education of students and health care professionals about various aspects of medicines. Palliative care is a relatively new specialty, and it frequently involves the use of complex pharmacotherapeutic options. It is not surprising that the pharmacist is seen as a valuable resource for such activity.

Undertaking palliative care research is becoming an important part of the pharmacist's role. Involvement may range from provision of information about medications to the development and implementation of research protocols.

Developing Roles

In the United Kingdom, the Medicines Act 1968 defined the legal right to prescribe medicines; this was limited to doctors, dentists, and veterinary surgeons. Thirty-five years later, the legislation was amended, and in 2003, pharmacists were among a group of health care professionals granted the authority to become supplementary prescribers. As of May 2006, qualified pharmacists became independent prescribers, who can legally prescribe any licensed medicine for any medical condition within their area of practice. Supplementary and independent means of prescribing are collectively called *nonmedical prescribing* (Box 56-3).

In the United States, the rights and responsibilities of a pharmacist are dictated by state legislative and regulatory agencies (Table 56-1 and Boxes 56-4 and 56-5). Collabora-

---

Box 56-3 Nonmedical Prescribing

Supplementary prescribing is a voluntary partnership between an independent prescriber (e.g., doctor, dentist) and a supplementary prescriber to implement an agreed patient-specific clinical management plan with the patient's agreement.

Independent prescribing is prescribing by a practitioner responsible and accountable for the assessment of patients with undiagnosed conditions and for decisions about the clinical management required, including prescribing.

Box 56-4 Functions of the Pharmacist in Hospice and Palliative Care

- Participation in multidisciplinary team meetings and ward rounds
- Taking patients' drug histories
- Advising on symptom control
- Providing information about medicine, highlighting potential undesirable effects, interactions, and the suitability of treatments for patients with comorbidities
- Coordinating with other health care professionals to ensure safe, effective, and economic use of medicines
- Nonmedical prescribing
- Monitoring treatment regimens, ensuring treatment protocols, guidelines, and standards are adhered to
- Counseling patients and caregivers about all prescribed medicines, including the purpose for each medicine and potential undesirable effects
- Communicating effectively with the patient's chosen community pharmacist to ensure continuity of care
- Writing guidelines for use of medicines in the hospital, hospice, or local area
- Providing financial information with respect to expenditure for medicines
- Contributing to education of health care professionals
- Undertaking research and development

TABLE 56-1   Clinical Pharmacy Services Models for Hospice Programs

PHARMACIST EMPLOYER	REIMBURSEMENT STRUCTURE	PROS	CONS
Independent clinical consultant as pharmacist service provider	Fee for clinical services based on patient census and clinical services provided	Focus is on needs of the hospice Not tied to dispensing; no conflict of interest for profitability	Requires added communication time by hospice staff with clinical and dispensing pharmacy services May be off site
Retail dispensing pharmacy	Built into cost of prescriptions dispensed Fee for clinical services used	One-stop shopping for dispensing and clinical consultation Reduces hospice staff time Off site or on site	Difficult to balance cost containment needs of hospice with profitability needs of dispensing pharmacy Lack of time to provide consultation Lack of palliative care expertise Generally off site
Specialized pharmacy benefit manager with or without prescription dispensing providers	Fee included in cost of each prescription dispensed Fee for clinical services Per diem fee covering medications dispensed and clinical services	Provides clinical pharmacist availability when needed based on patient census and clinical services use	Difficult to balance cost containment needs of hospice with profitability needs of the service provider Usually off site
Hospice	Salary and benefits provided by the hospice	Focus is solely on the needs of the hospice and the patient Pharmacist integration within the hospice team On site	Difficult to staff adequately for 24-hour service without overstaffing Usually feasible only in a large hospice program

---

Box 56-5 Current Procedural Terminology (CPT) Codes for Pharmacists

0115T: Initial face-to-face assessment or intervention with the patient; 1 to 15 minutes

0116T: Subsequent face-to-face assessment or intervention with the patient; 1 to 15 minutes

0117T: Each additional 15 minutes of face-to-face consultation with the patient; used in addition to 0115T or 0116T

---

tive practice agreements among a pharmacist, prescriber, and patient are emerging in many states, each with its own set of rules. In a study[5] of executive directors of boards of pharmacy published in 2003, of the 48 states responding to the survey, "32 (66%) had existing pharmacist collaborative practice laws; 23 states (48%) allowed pharmacists to initiate and modify therapy, whereas 9 (19%) allowed only modification of therapy. Most state laws applied to hospital, long-term care, and community settings."

These changes may revolutionize the services a pharmacist can provide in the palliative care setting. Pharmacists' roles within the palliative care setting continues to evolve, but there is no doubt about the valuable contribu-

tion that this group of professionals provides to the overall quality of patient care.

REFERENCES

1. Lucas C, Glare PA, Sykes JV. Contribution of a liaison pharmacist to an inpatient palliative care unit. Palliat Med 1997;11:209-216.
2. Gilber P, Stefniuk K. The role of the pharmacist in palliative care: Results of a survey conducted in Australia and Canada. J Palliat Care 2002;18:287-292.
3. Austwick A, Brooks D. The role of the pharmacist as a member of the palliative care team. Prog Palliat Care 2003;11:315-320.
4. Atkinson CV, Kirkham SR. Unlicensed uses for medication in a palliative care unit. Palliat Med 1999;13:145-152.
5. Punekar Y, Lin S-W, Thomas J III. Progress of pharmacist collaborative practice: Status of state laws and regulations and perceived impact of collaborative practice. J Am Pharm Assoc 2003;43:503-510.

SUGGESTED READING

Doyle D, Hanks G, Cherny N, Calman K (eds). Oxford Textbook of Palliative Medicine, 3rd ed. Oxford, UK: Oxford University Press, 2003.

Lipman AG, Jackson KC, Tyler LS. Evidence-Based Symptom Control in Palliative Care: Systematic Reviews and Validated Clinical Practice Guidelines for 15 Common Problems in Patients with Life-Limiting Disease. Binghamton, NY: Pharmaceutical Products Press, 2000.

Twycross R, Wilcock A. Hospice and Palliative Care Formulary USA. Nottingham, UK: Hospice Education Institute, 2006. Available at Palliativedrugs.com (accessed October 18, 2007).

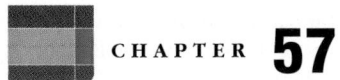

CHAPTER **57**

Palliative Medicine and the Ethics Consultant

Paul J. Ford

KEY POINTS

- Clinical ethics consultation focuses on good decision making and good process.

- Several consultation models are available; they usually are connected with a hospital ethics committee in collaboration with other disciplines.

- Ethics consultants can be a resource for conflict resolution among health care providers, patients, and families concerning contentious decisions and can help to resolve moral distress.

- The palliative medicine service can be an important resource for the ethics consultant dealing with a patient not yet on the palliative medicine service.

- Ethics consultants can assist in research ethics and policy questions.

Clinical ethics consultation provides a specialized service for health care providers, patients, and families in complex situations in which genuine differences of judgment exist about deeply meaningful decisions. These moral disagreements often exist between various people within the treatment context and within a single individual. Although controversy exists concerning when an ethics consultant should be involved, disagreement about how to choose between values frequently causes significant moral distress. A balance of values plays an important role in the decision for a patient to accept palliative treatment and in implementation of treatment. An example can be found in the debate about when, how, and if antimicrobials should be used in the terminally ill.[1] How to maximize the values of comfort, longevity, public health, individual choice, and fiscal responsibility can be particularly complex given the dearth of precise outcome data. Good communication can resolve some conflicts through better understanding or by making values apparent. Sometimes, a clinical ethicist or a small ethics committee group can maximize good process when genuine moral disagreement occurs.

Clinical ethics consultants are rarely needed in cases in which palliative medicine physicians already have been involved and accepted by patients and families. Although there are differences in approaches between ethics and palliative service, there are also many similarities.[2] This is especially true when clergy and social work have been used by the palliative medicine service. The skills of an ethics consultant for conflict resolution and understanding the implications of values are largely shared with many disciplines. The relationships between palliative medicine and ethics consultation are bidirectional. Palliative medicine physicians often play a formal role in ethics consultation services at many hospitals. In complex cases, the clinical ethics consultant can be of great assistance to palliative medicine services, and palliative medicine services can aid clinical ethics consultants.

HISTORICAL BACKGROUND

Formal clinical ethics consultation services have arisen in the past 30 years. As treatment choices increased, patient autonomy became more prominent, and greater attention was paid to research, the utility of a service specializing in resolving moral dilemmas became apparent. Legal cases regarding withdrawal of life support, such as the Quinlan case, stimulated more formalized ethics reviews for certain end-of-life choices. In the 1970s, ethics consultation emerged as a discrete field.[3] There are few formal standards.[4] Traditionally, individual ethics consultants come from varied backgrounds, including theology, philosophy, and medicine. The expertise and skill sets vary, and there is no formal accreditation or certification for an ethics consultant. Tension exists in bioethics concerning the role and method of practical involvement an ethicist should have in patient care decisions.[5]

Prompted by law and accreditation organizations, most hospitals have formalized multidisciplinary ethics committees, which are responsible for ethics consultation support for the institution. Theoretically, these groups are available from any ethics committees. However, they often suffer from inactivity, lack of education, and an inability to respond quickly. Most often, committees are composed of dedicated volunteers who have not been provided significant resources to undertake the various tasks. Large academic medical centers often employ specialized individuals to provide ethics consultation support and ethics education. They usually have more institutional mission support, but they may not have the same access to the health care culture of ethics committee members.

ROLE AND MODELS OF ETHICS CONSULTATION

When ethics consultants are called into a case, they may have any one of several roles, depending on the need. Most commonly, an ethics consultant assists in balancing values or principles articulated by the interested parties to assist in the best possible decision.[6,7] Ethics consultants are often asked to provide mediation when a value conflict can be identified. Attempting to find the best solution raises the question of whether the ethics consultant plays the role of an advocate. The ethics consultant advocates for good transparent process and articulates the ethical boundaries given the contingencies of a case. As a secondary goal, the consultant provides the tools for clinicians to address similar cases in the future. If the consultation is well done, this should reduce similar consultations in the future from the same service because the service should understand the tools used to resolve the situation.[8] The ethics consultant is best used in innovative or especially complex cases and not as a lever to convince a party nor as a simple formality.

Ethics consultation may involve a single, highly trained individual or a group of consultants, depending on the circumstances of the case and the institution.[9] As a rule, an individual or small ethics committee can convene more quickly in response to needed consultations. When a patient is already cared for by a palliative medicine team, the ethics consultant may be of assistance when there is disagreement among the patient, family, and health care providers regarding requests for therapies inconsistent with a particular care plan. An individual consultant may be useful to a physician who wishes to be sure his or her reasoning for a nonstandard approach is well considered. A larger, multidisciplinary group provides useful diversity. For questions in cases that do not yet involve palliative medicine, a larger group may be useful when the topic is futility of aggressive measures. In this consultation, the palliative medicine physician may be called on to provide expertise about the diversity of options available. Palliative medicine providers may consult bioethics consultants or vice versa about a good process. In the first case, the palliative services may request an ethics consultation to help their moral deliberations or find a solution to a value conflict between parties. In the second, palliative medicine provides a service and perspective to the ethical deliberations of the ethics consultant.

Although difficult ethical issues in palliative medicine go beyond those addressed previously, the examples highlight the service an ethics consultation can provide. These services are not intended to be medically directive; they instead support the patient, physician, nurse, and others in the best care that respects the values at stake for all involved (see "Case Study: Consultation about a Feeding Tube"; "Case Study: Consultation about Anti-infective Therapy"; and "Case Study: Consultation about Palliative Sedation").

DEVELOPMENTS AND RESEARCH OPPORTUNITIES

Although advance directives, living wills, and health care proxy documents were advertised as making end-of-life decisions easier, they have not lived up to this expectation.[13] The need for ethics consultation remains despite increasing use of these documents because of their vagueness and the propensity for patients to change their mind. Ethics consultants increasingly are asked to help in cases in which a patient loses cognitive capacity and contradicts previously expressed wishes.

Empirical research about ethics consultation is difficult and challenging. Some studies have viewed the end point of ethics consultation as reduction of "unwanted" therapies or decreased length of stay in the intensive care

 C A S E   S T U D Y

Consultation about a Feeding Tube

The attending physician in palliative medicine consults the ethics consultation service. She describes her patient as a 60-year-old man with terminal cancer. His family pressured the man into accepting a feeding tube and demanded placement by the team.

The medical judgment is that the feeding tube will provide little or no benefit in life extension and that it may complicate good symptom relief. The question in this case is how to respect the patient's autonomous choices and his value of his family while honoring the consistent philosophy of palliative medicine.

The consultant meets with the patient alone and finds him awake and cognitively intact. The patient expresses a desire to avoid having a feeding tube placed and a desire to die peacefully. However, he is worried about the spiritual consequences of not accepting artificial nutrition because of his religious beliefs. He also is concerned that he will disappoint his family.

The consultant makes explicit for the patient his competing value interests, suggests avenues such as clergy to clarify the spiritual issues, and then brings the patient, team, and family back together to find a best solution for the set of now clearly articulated values. The consultant is helpful in facilitating communication, mediating between parties who placed different weights on particular values, and creating a framework for what is ethically permissible.[10]

 C A S E   S T U D Y

Consultation about Anti-infective Therapy

A palliative medicine physician consults the ethics service about a 75-year-old woman whose prognosis for survival is less than a week. This young physician asks whether it would be appropriate to initiate anti-infective treatment for a curable infection at the request of the family. The patient is unable to participate in making the decision.

In this case, the ethics consultant focuses on assisting the young physician in considering whether withholding this "standard" therapy for the infection would be ethically permissible.[1] The value of the family's wishes, maximizing the patient's comfort, the efficacy of treatment in the context of the larger health care goals, and the obligations of a physician are highlighted for consideration.

 C A S E   S T U D Y

Consultation about Palliative Sedation

A relatively young patient with a terminal prognosis requests palliative sedation because he is tormented by the thought of dying. The indications for palliative sedation continue to be debated internationally.[11,12] The clinical ethicist can assist the treating team in evaluating this case and assist in developing the broader policies for the institutional indications for palliative sedation.

Part of the assistance in the individual case may be to talk with the patient and family to uncover the patient's values that supersede the one on which she has focused. In interacting with the medical team in the individual case, there may be a need to outline the limits of medical obligation. On the policy issue, the ethics consultant may be helpful in generalizing the problem and in articulating how a policy can account for the diversity of value judgments of patients, physicians, and nurses.

unit.[14,15] Another suggested endpoint has been satisfaction of patients, families, and health care providers. Although clinicians and patients may express appreciation in some cases, the most appropriate decision may not satisfy all parties. If ethics consultation is about good process, these measures may be inadequate, and there may be few ways of testing whether ethics consultation is useful.[16] Creating some benchmarks is important.

For palliative medicine programs, ethics consultation may be useful for research protocols or to create robust policies given the significant challenges of the population.[17,18] In these cases, the ethics consultant moves away from a role in clinical ethics consultation into research ethics or policy ethics consultation. This is an emerging service area many believe can be undertaken because of the experience and skill set of clinical ethics consultants. Several areas of research remain:

- How can quality improvement be undertaken in ethics consultation?
- Is there a need for accreditation of consultation services?
- What are the practice limits for ethics consultants?
- Which model of ethics consultation is superior?

CONCLUSIONS

A clinical ethics consultation service can be useful in complex decisions that involve the necessary loss of one value to preserve another. These services are not intended to replace careful consideration by health care providers, patients, or families. Rather, they should be used to empower good processes and decision making. Ethics consultants usually contribute their skill of identifying which values are in conflict, and they facilitate communication from outside the patient-physician dyad. The palliative medicine service also provides an important contribution to an ethics consultation. The ethics consultant provides an additional service to enhance the palliative medicine system.

REFERENCES

1. Ford PJ, Fraser TG, Davis MP, et al. Anti-infective therapy at the end of life: Ethical decision making in hospice eligible patients. Bioethics 2005;19:380-392.
2. Aulisio MP, Chaitin E, Arnold RM. Ethics and palliative care consultation in the intensive care unit. Crit Care Clin 2004;20:505-523.
3. Branson R. Bioethics as individual and social: The scope of a consulting profession and academic discipline. J Relig Ethics 1975;3:111-139.
4. Society for Health and Human Values and the Society for Bioethics Consultation (SHHV-SBC) Task Force on Standards for Bioethics Consultation. Core Competencies for Ethics Consultation. Glenview, IL: American Society for Bioethics and Humanities, 1998.
5. Faden R. Bioethics. A field in transition. J Law Med Ethics 2004;32:276-278.
6. Beauchamp TL, Childress JF. Principles of Biomedical Ethics, 5th ed. New York: Oxford University Press, 2001.
7. DeMarco JP, Ford PJ. Balancing in ethical deliberation: Superior to specification and casuistry. J Med Philos 2006;31:1-15.
8. Orr RD. Who does the ethics consultation serve? Lahey Clin Med Ethics 2004;11:10-11.
9. Smith ML, Bisanz AK, Kempfer AJ, et al. Criteria for determining the appropriate method for an ethics consultation. HEC Forum 2004;16:95-112.
10. Orr RD, Genesen LB. Requests for "inappropriate" treatment based on religious beliefs. J Med Ethics 1997;23:142-147.
11. Jansen LA, Sulmasy DP. Proportionality, terminal suffering and the restorative goals of medicine. Theor Med Bioeth 2002;23:321-337.
12. Davis MP, Ford PJ. Palliative sedation definition, practice, outcomes, and ethics. J Palliat Med 2005;8:699-710.
13. Fagerlin A, Schneider CE. Enough. The failure of the living will. Hastings Cent Rep 2004;34:30-42.
14. Dowdy MM, Roberston C, Bander JA. A study of proactive ethics consultation for critically and terminally ill patients with extended length of stay. Crit Care Med 1998;26:252-259.
15. Schneiderman LJ, Gilmer T, Teetzel HD. Impact of ethics consultations in the intensive care setting: A randomized, controlled trial. Crit Care Med 2000;28:3920-3924.
16. Craig JM, May T. Evaluating the outcomes of ethics consultation. J Clin Ethics 2006;17:168-180.
17. Janssens MJPA, Gordijn B. Clinical trials in palliative care: An ethical evaluation. Patient Educ Couns 2000;41:51-62.
18. Burns JP. From case to policy: Institutional ethics at a children's hospital. J Clin Ethics 2000;11:175-181.

SUGGESTED READING

Aulisio MP, Arnold RM, Youngner SJ (eds). Ethics Consultation: From Theory to Practice. Baltimore: Johns Hopkins University Press, 2003.

Dubler NN, Liebman CB. Bioethics Mediation: A Guide to Shaping Shared Solutions. New York: United Hospital Fund, 2004.

Fletcher JC, Spencer EM, Lombardo P (eds). Introduction to Clinical Ethics. Hagerstown, PA: University Publishing Group, 2005.

Zaner RM: Ethics and the Clinical Encounter. Englewood Cliffs, NJ: Prentice Hall, 1988.

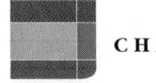

CHAPTER **58**

Music and Art Therapists

Lisa M. Gallagher, Deforia Lane, and Darlene Foth

KEY POINTS

- Music therapy is effective in managing symptoms of advanced disease.
- Art therapy helps people reduce symptoms, focus on positive thoughts, express themselves, share their wishes, gain independence, and obtain comfort on their journey.
- Art is a process, and anyone who has used art media can substantiate the power of imagery.
- Music and art therapists use the arts for therapeutic objectives.
- Expressive arts play significant roles in improving physical and mental health.

HISTORICAL BACKGROUND

Music therapy has been used throughout history to assist healing. It became a formal profession at the end of World War II, when music therapists assisted in veterans' hospitals. In 1950, the National Association for Music Therapy was formed, and in 1971, the American Association for Music Therapy was created. These two organizations united to form the American Music Therapy Association (AMTA) in 1998. The AMTA now has more than 3500 members.[1]

Art therapy has its roots in prehistory, when people drew images on cave walls to express their world. In the early 20th century, psychiatrists became interested in the art created by patients who had mental illness. By the middle of the 20th century, rehabilitation centers, hospitals, and various clinical settings began to incorporate art therapy into their treatment programs to improve health, coping skills, emotional expression, recovery, and wellness. It began to be recognized as a profession in the 1940s, and in 1969, the American Art Therapy Association (AATA) was established. The AATA has more than 4500 members.[2]

DEFINITION AND QUALIFICATIONS

According to the 2005 AMTA Member Sourcebook, "Music therapy is the clinical and evidence-based use of music interventions to accomplish individualized goals within a therapeutic relationship by a credentialed professional who has completed an approved music therapy program."[1] Along with practical experience, music therapists receive training in music, psychology, treatment models, therapeutic approaches, and anatomy. In the United States, on completion of the bachelor's level coursework, the individual completes a 6- to 10-month internship and then must take and pass the board certification examination. The Certification Board for Music Therapists (CBMT) grants board certification, which is maintained through continuing education.

Art therapy combines the fields of art, psychology, and counseling. It uses art media, imagery, and the creative art process to help people explore personal potential, problem solving, and verbal or visual expression. It is based on the premise that the creative process, not the product, is healing. According to AATA, "Art therapists need to hold a master's degree in art therapy and counseling."[2] The Art Therapist Registered (ATR) and Art Therapist Registered Board Certified (ATR-BC) are the recognized credential standards for the field of art therapy and are conferred by the Art Therapy Credentials Board (ATCB). In addition to educational requirements, an individual must complete a minimum of 1000 direct client contact hours after graduation to become an ATR. After registration, the art therapist becomes board certified by taking and passing the ATCB's examination and then maintaining it through continuing education.

MUSIC AND ART THERAPY

Function

Music therapy has been used to address physical, emotional, social, and spiritual needs; provide distraction from treatments and procedures; improve quality of life; and promote closure at the end of life. It has specifically been used for the following: pain, anxiety, depression, shortness of breath, mood, nausea, fear, agitation, restlessness, insomnia, anger, confusion, stress, comfort, relaxation, coping, withdrawal, communication, family dynamics, self-expression, and actively dying.

Art therapy provides a means for people to come to terms with their illness and their lives; to develop coping skills; to reduce fear, anxiety, and stress; to increase self-awareness; to distract from pain; to express emotions; and

to provide a sense of control. Images are a "bridge between body and mind or between the conscious level of information processing and the physiological changes in the body."[3] In palliative care, "art therapy is one effective way to identify and subsequently explore fears, anxieties, loss of control, and feelings of helplessness and hopelessness."[4] It can also decrease depression, decrease pain, assist in dealing with body changes, reduce anxiety, increase a sense of autonomy, build self-esteem, increase coping skills, help maintain self identity, increase quality of life, and provide a means of leaving something of themselves behind for family or friends (see Case Study: "Providing Medical and Psychosocial Care").

Responsibilities of Therapists

Music and art therapists are trained to work with various populations. There are no formal specializations for either profession at this time, but many individuals prefer to focus on gaining experience and knowledge with one population. Although many programs use volunteer musicians and artists, hiring music and art therapists who hold the appropriate credentials ensures quality training and professional organizations with established standards of practice and codes of ethics.

It is important for art therapists and music therapists to work in an interdisciplinary team with doctors, nurses, social workers, and psychologists. They often attend team

---

 C A S E   S T U D Y

Providing Medical and Psychosocial Care

An example of how an interdisciplinary team can work together to provide comprehensive medical and psychosocial care is seen in the case of Elizabeth, a 42-year-old wife and mother of two girls (ages 8 and 12 years) and a patient with stage IV breast cancer. She was referred to music and art therapy to increase her coping skills, to reduce pain perception and anxiety, to normalize the environment, and to encourage communication with her children and husband.

With the guidance of the music and art therapists, Elizabeth composed and recorded original songs expressing her hopes and dreams for each member of her family, and she created a book and illustrated stories for each of her children. As Elizabeth became less able to interact with her family and eventually lapsed into coma, the children were given the opportunity to write songs for their mother. Their lyrics focused on what they loved most about her. They recorded their songs, and they found comfort in knowing that their mother could listen to them sing, even when they could not be present. The art therapist helped the daughters create a collage of family photos, which was hung near the patient's bed. This evoked compliments from the staff to the children while providing a glimpse into the patient's life.

On the day Elizabeth died, her family gathered in the intensive care unit. As the hours dragged on, Elizabeth's daughters asked if they could sing, and a surprised and exhausted family was treated to the sweet voices of two little girls singing the songs they created for their mother.

Common Errors

- Playing music constantly until patient is overstimulated
- Insensitivity to the music's emotional effect on the patient
- Inattentiveness to the patient's physical response (i.e., autonomic or central nervous system) to the music and an inability to reverse it (i.e., increased heart rate, blood pressure, respiration rate, or galvanic skin response)
- Choosing music without regard for the patient's preferences
- A limited musical repertoire
- Inability to build on or re-create positive experiences
- Inability to avoid the negative reactions of music or re-create positive experiences
- Inability to use music to establish a hierarchy of goals or objectives
- Thinking artistic or musical talent is necessary to engage in therapy
- Believing an art therapist can interpret an image by looking at it
- Believing anyone can do art therapy or music therapy without proper education, training, and credentials
- Thinking art therapy will regress a patient's emotional state
- Believing art therapy is only for children

---

meetings to obtain information, and they share the results of the therapy sessions with team members. The therapists are responsible for assessing patients, conducting sessions, and documenting results. The music therapist first performs an assessment to determine the patient's needs. After this is completed, individualized goals, objectives, and interventions are designed. Various strategies, techniques, and interventions may be used, depending on the needs; the therapist's training and philosophy of music therapy; and the patient's age, culture, and religion. Common strategies include listening to live and recorded music, playing an instrument, singing, instrumental or vocal improvisation, musical entrainment, music-assisted relaxation, guided imagery plus music, writing songs, musical life review, choosing songs, lyric analysis, verbal processing or communication, participation in musical experiences, and planning funeral or memorial service music (see "Common Errors").

Data may be collected to determine whether progress has been made. Session notes are made in the patient's chart so that other team members can see the effects of music therapy. Recommendations for the future may also be included. Family members, who are integral to the patient's experience, may also be included if they are present during music therapy sessions.

Assessment is the goal of the initial art therapy session. One art therapist uses the Mind, Body, Spirit Mandala, which she developed to assess the patient's emotional, physical, and spiritual aspects, as well as motor, visual, cognitive, and psychological functioning. Throughout the sessions, the therapist observes what media the patient chooses because each medium has different psychological effects. Tapping into the client's strengths and integrating what occurs during art therapy helps increase the patient's coping skills (see Case Study: "Art Therapy for a Breast Cancer Patient").

Music and art therapists function as team members while providing clinical interventions for patients and their families. They also provide education about how

CASE STUDY

Art Therapy for a Breast Cancer Patient

Kate was a 34-year-old, white, single female with breast cancer that had metastasized to her abdomen and lungs. She was referred to art therapy because she wanted something to do between chemotherapy sessions.

During her first art therapy session, she completed the mind, body, and spirit mandala. This was a large circle divided into three equal pieces. In the upper left section of the mandala, she was instructed to "draw how you're feeling today as a weather condition." Her image was of a storm with lightning bolts on one side and a sun with blue sky on the other side. Kate explained that this image indicated her anger, sadness, and peace. She was angry at the cancer that was taking her life away too soon. She was sad to leave her family because she loved them so much, but she believed she would find peace in a new life in heaven.

In the upper right side of her mandala, she was instructed to "draw a tree that represents you." She drew a picture of a young tree with a saw lying next to it on the ground. Kate explained she felt like that young tree that was growing tall and strong until someone called cancer came and cut her life short.

For the last image, she was instructed to "draw where you get your life spirit or energy from." Kate's image included a gold cross, her family, and a Bible. She spoke about how difficult her illness and impending death were for her family, especially her mother. She also spent several art therapy sessions creating cards or notes for people who sent her gifts, visited, and phoned.

Kate continued to participate in art therapy sessions at home. This allowed her to be independent of her illness, and it met her emotional, spiritual, and psychological needs. During one of the last sessions, she created an abstract color tissue paper image in which she saw the image of a man whom she identified as Jesus (Fig. 58-1). She said he would be coming soon to take her to heaven, and she died a week later. She instructed her family members to go into her room after she was gone and take an item that would remind them of her. The artwork was the first to be taken.

music and art can continue to be used after a patient goes home. On discharge of the patient, the therapists may provide services in the home or act as a consultant to the patient. Many also have a role in conducting research that helps further the development and evidence base of these professions.

DEVELOPMENTS AND DEBATES IN PALLIATIVE CARE

As hospice and palliative medicine have continued to grow and develop, so has the use of music therapy. Several books have been published.[5-8] Research is being done on what works best, various approaches to music therapy, specific techniques, and the effects on the various needs of patients and their families.

Throughout the development of art therapy, books were published that created an interest in art therapy and provided history and information on this field.[9,10] Research

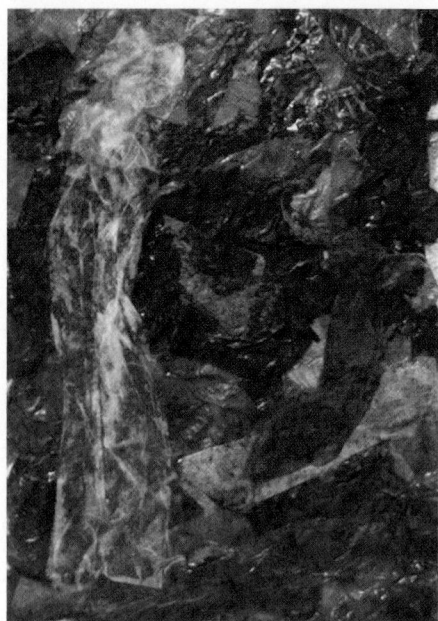

FIGURE 58-1   Kate's abstract image.

is being done to evaluate techniques and theories, and case studies have been written to share the therapists' work. In Great Britain, research has focused on issues relating to the professional development in the field or exploration of clinical practice.[11] In the United States, research has concentrated on developing diagnostic indicators in patients' artwork. Research has demonstrated physical and emotional improvements and decreased heart rate, blood pressure, and respiration rates for those who have engaged in art therapy. Potential research with art therapy includes reducing anxiety levels, improving recovery time, decreasing hospital or outpatient treatment stays, comparing different therapy effectiveness, and treatment time.

Several topics remain controversial, such as conducting clinical research on this patient population and determining whether the collection of data is intrusive to the therapeutic process. Another problem with research in this area is eliciting discomfort because of the powerful feelings that may surface during the sessions. Expression of these feelings is considered part of the healing process, and the therapist's job is to allow these emotions to be safely explored and appropriately expressed.

Although many qualitative studies and case studies have been published, the medical profession has demanded more evidence-based research. Studies have demonstrated that music therapy is effective for the following: pain,[12-14] comfort and relaxation,[13] mood,[14] anxiety,[14] quality of life,[15] and shortness of breath.[16] The largest study in which results were statistically significant is a retrospective study of 200 palliative care patients.[16] A review of empirical data in music therapy in hospice and palliative care has also been published.[17] Many case studies and qualitative studies on art therapy have been published, and one quantitative study demonstrated that art therapy was effective in reducing various symptoms in cancer.[18]

CONCLUSIONS

Art and music are an intrinsic part of every culture, and they are embedded in tradition, ceremony, and celebration. The arts give expression to thoughts, feelings, and values. Art therapists and music therapists add another dimension to this inherent beauty and meaning by skillfully structuring the use of the arts to accomplish therapeutic gain.

Art and music help patients give voice to what cannot be expressed any other way, but measuring the mechanism that causes the change is not simple. Educating health care professionals, patients, and families about the benefits of music and art therapy is imperative. Many are still unaware of the significant roles the expressive arts can play in physical and mental health. Quantitative and qualitative research exists, but more is needed to explore and expand the understanding of theoretical models, clinical applications, and appropriate biological and psychosocial measures.

The two case reports illustrate the power of music and art therapy in the lives of these patients and their families. Although the effects may resist the confines of empirical data, the impact can be meaningful and often profoundly beyond measure.

REFERENCES

1. American Music Therapy Association. AMTA Member Sourcebook. Silver Spring, MD: American Music Therapy Association, 2005.
2. American Art Therapy Association. Art therapy news. Available at www.art-therapy.org (accessed October 18, 2007).
3. Lusebrink V. Imagery and Visual Expression in Therapy. New York: Plenum Press, 1990.
4. Trauger-Querry B. Art Therapy. Alexandria, VA: National Hospice and Palliative Care Organization, 2001, pp 1-11.
5. Munro S. Music Therapy in Palliative/Hospice Care. St. Louis: MMB Music, 1984.
6. Aldridge D. Music Therapy in Palliative Care: New Voices. London: Jessica Kinsley Publishers, 1999.
7. Dileo C, Loewy JV (eds). Music Therapy at the End of Life. Cherry Hill, NJ: Jeffrey Books, 2005.
8. Hilliard RE. Hospice and Palliative Care Music Therapy: A Guide to Program Development and Clinical Care. Cherry Hill, NJ: Jeffrey Books, 2005.
9. Prinzhorn H, von Brocdorff E (transl). Artistry of the Mentally Ill. New York: Springer-Verlag, 1972.
10. Junge MB, Asawa PP (eds). A History of Art Therapy in the United States. Alexandria, VA: American Art Therapy Association, 1994.
11. Gilroy A, Lee C (eds). Art and Music: Therapy and Research. London: Routledge, 1995.
12. Curtis SL. The effect of music on pain relief and relaxation of the terminally ill. J Music Ther 1996;23:10-24.
13. Krout RE. The effects of single-session music therapy interventions on the observed and self-reported levels of pain control, physical comfort, and relaxation of hospice patients. Am J Hosp Palliat Care 2001;18:383-390.
14. Gallagher LM, Steele AL. Developing and using a computerized database for music therapy in palliative medicine. J Palliat Care 2001;17:147-154.
15. Hilliard RE. The effects of music therapy on the quality and length of life of people diagnosed with terminal cancer. J Music Ther 2003;40:113-137.
16. Gallagher LM, Lagman R, Walsh D, et al. The clinical effects of music therapy in palliative medicine. Support Care Cancer 2006;14:859-866.
17. Hilliard RE. Music therapy in hospice and palliative care: A review of the empirical data. Evidence Based Complement Alternat Med 2005;2:173-178.
18. Nainis N, Paice JA, Ratner J, et al. Relieving symptoms in cancer: Innovative use of art therapy. J Pain Symptom Manage 2006;31:162-169.

SUGGESTED READING

Gallagher LM, Lagman R, Walsh D, et al. The clinical effects of music therapy in palliative medicine. Support Care Cancer 2006;14:859-866.

Hilliard RE. Music therapy in hospice and palliative care: A review of the empirical data. Evidence Based Complement Alternat Med 2005;2:173-178.

Hilliard RE. The effects of music therapy on the quality and length of life of people diagnosed with terminal cancer. J Music Ther 2003;40:113-137.

Krout RE. The effects of single-session music therapy interventions on the observed and self-reported levels of pain control, physical comfort, and relaxation of hospice patients. Am J Hosp Palliat Care 2001;18:383-390.

Nainis N, Paice JA, Ratner J, et al. Relieving symptoms in cancer: Innovative use of art therapy. J Pain Symptom Manage 2006;31:162-169.

CHAPTER **59**

Wound and Stoma Therapists

Mary Ann Sammon

KEY POINTS

- Wound ostomy continence (WOC) nursing is a specialized field.

- WOC nurses are certified to manage surgical, diabetic, and cancer-related wounds; pressure ulcers, vascular ulcers, and burns; and incontinence, stomas, and fistulas.

- WOC nurses educate patients, caregivers, and nurses.

- WOC nurses offer palliative care through assessment and appropriate use of advanced wound care products.

Wound ostomy continence (WOC) nursing started in 1958, when a young patient named Norma Gill was treated by a Cleveland Clinic doctor, Rupert B. Turnbull, Jr., for ulcerative colitis. Their doctor-patient relationship led to the development of enterostomal therapy, the progenitor of WOC nursing.[1]

Norma Gill, although not a medical professional, asked ostomy product manufacturers to produce more advanced equipment to replace the awkward rubber bag for her ileostomy. Realizing patients would have to be schooled in managing these new stoma products, Dr. Turnbull enlisted Norma Gill to do this in 1961. With an office at the Cleveland Clinic, Norma Gill began teaching ileostomy and colostomy patients how to handle their pouches and how to cope psychologically. Soon afterward, she began educating nurses and doctors in the art of treating stomas, and the specialized field of enterostomal therapeutic nursing started; it later became WOC nursing. Through research and experience, WOC nurses use scientific principles to assess wounds, stoma care, and incontinence problems, and they recommend solutions to best treat the problem and provide pain relief in palliative care.[1]

WOUND AND STOMA THERAPY

WOC nursing is a specialized field of health care. Because of distinct study and training, nurses are certified to treat sustained surgical, diabetic, or cancer-related wounds, pressure ulcers, or skin maladies from vascular failure or burns. They are uniquely qualified to provide medical care to skin problems from fistulas, incontinence, percutaneous tubes, and urinary or fecal diversions known as stomas (i.e., ostomies).

WOC nurses are skilled in assisting those with colon or rectal cancers surgically fitted with stomas and to assess their equipment to determine whether it is suitably palliative. They also educate principal caregivers (e.g., family, friends, hospice nurses) in buying and applying ostomy equipment and about the function of the intestine as death nears. Areas addressed at this stage are the irrigation of colostomies necessitated by iatrogenic constipation and changes in the type or size of flange dictated by loss of weight or abdominal swelling.

WOC nurses palliate patients by securing and pouching draining fistulas. Pouching protects the surrounding skin by containing the drainage, and it eliminates odor. They have been trained to ease discomfort from nausea and vomiting by using nasal tube holders that can better secure nasogastric tubes. They can outfit the patient requiring percutaneous endoscopic gastrostomy (PEG) tubes or biliary tubes, which decrease discomfort when held securely with a horizontal tube holder (Hollister, Libertyville, IL). Adhesive pouches, dressings, and devices can be held in place, and the skin is protected by a nonalcoholic skin preparation (Cavilon No Sting Barrier Film, 3M, London, Ontario, Canada) (Box 59-1).

STAFF EDUCATION

Besides specialized care, WOC nurses educate hospital nursing staffs about risk assessments such as the Braden, Norton, and Gosnell scales,[7] which allow the nurse to determine the risk of pressure ulcers. *Pressure ulcers* are defined as localized areas of tissue necrosis that develop when soft tissue is compressed between a bony prominence and an external surface for a prolonged time.[2,7]

Pressure ulcers are a concern in advanced disease because of immobility, increased pain, moisture, compromised nutrition status, and a tendency to be immunocompromised. Appropriate specialty beds provide pressure redistribution and comfort. Nursing interventions prevent pressure ulcers from developing by recommending advance wound care dressings that heal pressure ulcers when possible or that provide comfort while preventing worse ulceration (Box 59-2).

ADVANCED WOUND CARE

Advanced wound care modalities can assist persons undergoing radiation therapy and chemotherapy or who are

---

Box 59-1 Scope of Practice of Wound Ostomy Continence Nurses

- Stomas
- Surgical wounds
- Fistulas
- Incontinence
- Pressure ulcers

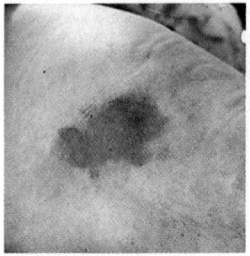
Stage I Pressure Ulcer

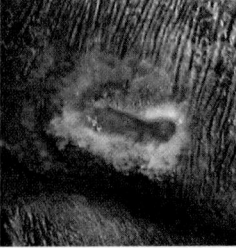
Stage II Perineal Wound

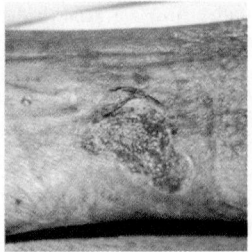
Partial Thickness Wound

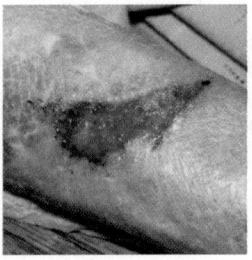
Skin Tear

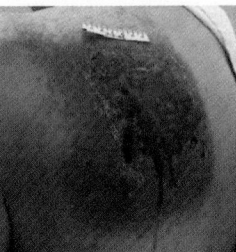
Radiodermatitis

FIGURE 59-1   Use of Xenaderm ointment can help heal and protect difficult-to-dress wounds.

> **Box 59-2 Staff Education Points**
>
> • Pressure ulcer prevention, including risk assessment with instruments such as the Braden scale
> • Treatment, including advanced wound care

> **Box 59-3 Tips for Handling Skin Damage from Chemotherapy and Irradiation**
>
> • Use of products to decrease pain
> • Use of products to decrease odor
> • Use of products to contain diarrhea

suffering with skin and odor problems from cancer (usually fungating tumors). Radiotherapy technique and technologies continue to improve, but radiation burns still occur at the site of the therapy, and skin reactions and complications distress patients.[3] Combined chemotherapy and irradiation to shrink tumors increases the cytotoxic effect of radiation on the skin.[4] Because radiation effects are not restricted to malignant cells, a reaction may develop that progresses from erythema to dry and moist desquamation.[5]

Another problem in palliation is *radiation recall*. This occurs when a chemotherapeutic agent produces a tissue reaction in a previously irradiated field.[6] Because management of these skin reactions can be inconsistent, WOC nurses have been trained to administer the most practical, soothing, and cost-effective dressings and ointments for individual needs. Chemical débriding agents include those containing chlorophyll (Panafil, Healthpoint, Fort Worth, TX), healing ointments (Xenaderm, Healthpoint), and odor-controlling ointments (Fig. 59-1).

WOC nurses may recommend a gel sheet (Vigilon, Bard Medical, Covington, GA) to alleviate erythematous, blistering skin burns from radiation treatment. There are also ointments; some contain lidocaine that provides comfort and pain relief (e.g., EMLA cream) (Box 59-3 and Fig. 59-2). Silicone dressings (Mepitel, Mölnlycke, Newtown, PA) provide pain-free application and removal while promoting healing.

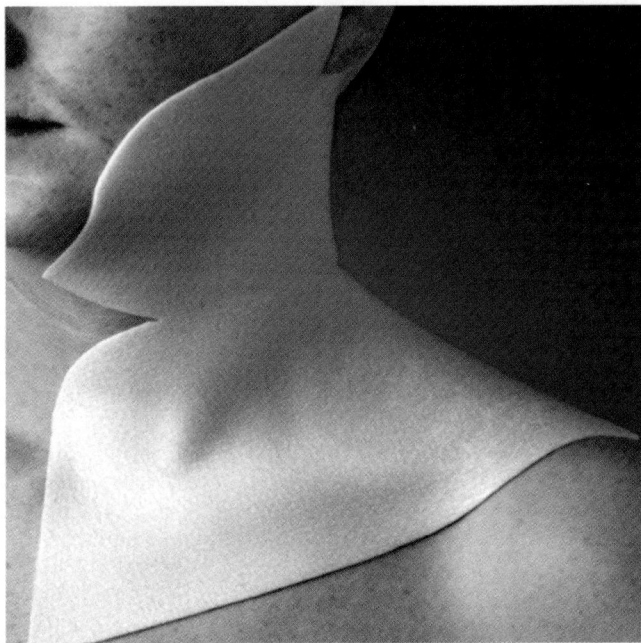

FIGURE 59-2   Management of wounds. Mepilex Lite is designed for the management of a wide range of non-exuding to low-exuding wounds, such as leg and foot ulcers, pressure ulcers, partial-thickness burns, radiation skin reactions, and epidermolysis bullosa. Mepilex Lite can also be used as protection for compromised or fragile skin. *(Courtesy of Mölnlycke Health Care, Göteborg, Sweden, 2006.)*

Patients undergoing chemotherapy or radiation therapy may suffer from diarrhea, which often results in a fungal rash or severe, painful injury to the perianal epidermis. Ointments and powders can provide comfort and healing to the sensitive areas. Several fecal management systems can ease the discomfort of severe diarrhea (Fig. 59-3).

CONCLUSIONS

WOC nurses are indispensable resources for the care of palliative patients suffering with end-of-life issues, including skin and wound problems. WOC nurses have the training and skill to intervene, and they have up-to-date

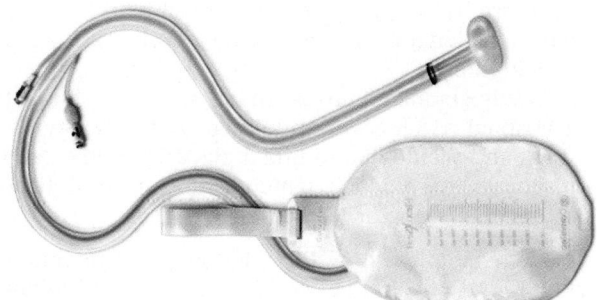

FIGURE 59-3 Incontinence care with a fecal management system. The Flexi-Seal fecal management system is a temporary containment device that is indicated for bedridden or immobilized patients who are incontinent with liquid or semi-liquid stools. It diverts fecal matter, protects the patient's wounds from fecal contamination, and reduces the risk of skin breakdown and spread of infection. This system includes a silicone catheter, syringe, and collection bag. *(Courtesy of ConvaTec, Bristol-Myers Squibb, Princeton, NJ, 2006.)*

knowledge of the most effective wound care products to alleviate pain and suffering.

REFERENCES

1. Erwin-Toth P, Krasner D. Enterostomal Therapy Nursing—Growth and Evolution of a Nursing Specialty Worldwide. A Festschrift for Norma N. Gill-Thompson, ET. Baltimore: Halgo, 1996, pp 1-11, 167-180.
2. National Pressure Ulcer Advisory Panel. Pressure ulcers prevalence, cost and risk assessment: Consensus development conference statement. Decubitus 1989;2:241.
3. Lopez AP, et al. What is your diagnosis? Wounds 1998;10:132.
4. Margolin SG, Brenemaqn JC, Denman DL, et al. Management of radiation-induced moist skin desquamation using hydrocolloid dressings. Cancer Nurs 1990;13:71.
5. British Columbia Cancer Agency. Guidelines for Radiation Therapy: Cancer Management Manual, 1998.
6. Schweitzer VG, Juillard GJ, Bajada CL, Parker RG. Radiation recall dermatitis and pneumonitis in a patient treated with paclitaxel. Cancer 1995;76:1069.
7. Bryant RA: Acute and Chronic Wounds: Nursing Management, 2nd ed. St. Louis: Mosby, 2000.

SUGGESTED READING

Ayello E, Baranoski S. Wound Care Essentials: Practice and Principles. Philadelphia: Lippincott Williams & Wilkins, 2004.
Bryan RA. Acute and Chronic Wounds: Nursing Management, 2nd ed. St. Louis: Mosby, 2000, pp 17-40, 85-124, 387-400.

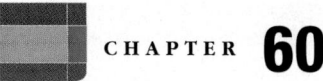

The Volunteer

Monica Muller

KEY POINTS

- Institutional and outpatient services may refuse to cooperate with volunteers.
- Voluntary services are mentioned in daily meetings, but the support from voluntary staff may be disregarded as a cornerstone in palliative care.
- Volunteers may become surrogate family members.
- Some volunteers may have negative opinions about the administrative process and feel that administrative necessities such as documentation are incompatible with their role as informal and empathic caregivers.
- Individuals interested in volunteer work resign because their efforts are unappreciated.
- Volunteers may suffer from helper's disease.
- Volunteers may be abused as substitutes for professional staff.
- Voluntary organizations sometimes refuse to cooperate with professionals.
- Some voluntary organizations believe that only the experience of a similar kind of suffering qualifies volunteers to support the persons concerned. For example, the "Compassionate Friends" organization is made up of bereaved parents.

CONTRIBUTIONS OF VOLUNTEERS

In theory, volunteers are an indispensable part of palliative care. The hospice movement and palliative medicine regard voluntary support as important. This contribution should not be mistaken as an economy measure to meet the challenges of changing political and social conditions (Box 60-1). Volunteers are not to be regarded as substitutes when professional staff can no longer be afforded. Their role in caring for the dying in the health care system represents a complementary but independent contribution that "ensures that the care for the dying is not entirely left to professionally educated people, but stays within the community."

Most palliative care literature mentions volunteers. Volunteers are the subject of conference agendas and relevant textbooks. Publications by volunteers are rare, and they usually describe the process and challenges of volunteer work from an emotional viewpoint. Nonetheless, hospice and palliative services strongly rely on volunteer support and cannot achieve their social and political aims without them.

The problems of voluntary work should be identified. There is a gap between theory and reality. The practice of voluntary work shows a less ideal picture.

Box 60-1   Volunteers' Contributions, Needs, and Roles

Contributions

Personality
Openness to self-reflection
Dependability
Identification with the practical concept of care
Willingness to serve and cater to another person's needs
Personal strength and life experience not limited to the process of helping
Acceptance of training and documentation

Needs

Trust and respect
Competent, sensitive, tutelary, and/protective coordinators
Continuing training, work assistance, and supervision

Roles

Voluntary actions
Reliability
Work for no material gains
Public service
Cooperation
Supportive function
Responsible and autonomous behavior
Giving despite limited time and resources

From Relf M. The effectiveness of volunteer bereavement support: Reflections from the Sobell House Bereavement Study. Presented at the Internationale Konferenz über Trauer und Verlust in der heutigen Gesellschaft (Swedish National Association for Mental Health), Stockholm, 1994.

CHARACTERISTICS, ROLES, AND DUTIES OF VOLUNTARY WORKERS

Personalities

Volunteers have a variety of backgrounds and goals:

- A 48-year-old woman's children have left home, and she is looking for another meaningful occupation. Having been a housewife, she would like to take up "some kind of social work" and care for others in a different way. She also longs for social contact and interaction.
- A 62-year-old widow volunteers. Two years ago, her husband died of cancer after a long period of suffering. During the course of his illness, she had a very bad time and thought she had little support. In response to this, she made up her mind to work toward a more appropriate culture of dying.
- A man in his mid-50s is a highly esteemed member of his community. He is endowed with organizational talent and has many connections. He wants to perform his social responsibilities, and he likes being asked for advice and seeing his authority exerted a little. He will provide perfect material for a committee chairman!
- A young mother of two children has temporarily neglected her career for her children's sake and lost touch with her former profession. She hopes that working as a volunteer can earn her some additional qualification and references and increase her chances

to return to her profession of a social worker. She also feels challenged and is interested in her personal development.

- A freshly graduated physician has started his first job at a hospital. He feels disappointed by the reality of his work and would like to find a place where he can put his ideals into practice, which had been the motivation to become a doctor in the first place.

These examples show the wide range of people who can be found in volunteer services. Our idea of voluntary work may be too simple a conception. Because there is no such thing as a stereotypical dying person, why should there be a stereotypical volunteer? People who offer their work in volunteer services have many different personalities and motivations.

What do these people with different sets of motivations and reasons have in common? Is there a common denominator? Is the education of volunteers completely different from that of professionals? It is not so much training that they need, but rather support and a refinement of the interpersonal qualifications and skills they already possess.

Commonalities of Volunteers

Could the status of a layperson be the link for the five volunteers described? No; the doctor is not a layperson, and the four others bring along their life experience, emotional maturity, and compassion. This indicates a core competence not reflected in the term *layperson*.

Honorary post is a historical term with many promising connotations. However, where is the honor, and does a post really exist? When making comments such as "This is what you do in your spare time? I couldn't do this kind of job!" outsiders, acquaintances, and friends may still bear a rather colorful idea of the term's historical meaning in mind. A post or a job usually follows clearly defined descriptions of its content, which is not true for voluntary work. Whatever needs to be done depends on the wishes and needs of those who require support. The volunteer has to meet these requirements and the schedule set up by the coordinator.

The term *voluntary work* is ambiguous. A person may start voluntary work but still has to meet commitments and work on a fixed schedule. This is not unlike the situation a professional faces when going to work every morning.

Volunteers are not paid for their work. This seems to be the common bond between them, but the term "*unpaid work*" may diminish the huge commitment of the many people who do it. There are other terms for a volunteer's work:

- Charity (describing a personal obligation to do social good)
- Solitary action
- Informal care
- Nonprofit work
- Acts of social and civil responsibility

These terms are vague and unhelpful in defining a common denominator of volunteers. If there is no exemplary volunteer, there is no ideal role. Their roles seem as individual as the volunteers themselves. The roles are determined by the volunteers' various approaches and individual wills, and they follow diverse cultural, social, religious, and political considerations, which vary in each country and cultural context.

"The point of reference for volunteer's" contributions and commitments is the needs of the dying person and the needs of his or her family. Addressing these needs is what is required of volunteers beyond the medical control of pain and symptoms, palliative nursing care, and the social support of professional staff. From the viewpoint of a dying person and his or her relatives, a volunteer is expected to have chameleon-like qualities.

Volunteers should not have aims, ideas, or needs of their own. They cannot act according to their will or wishes, because the services offered should fit exactly the expectations of those in need of support. In practice, their commitment is centered in ability, not inclination.

Who makes a good volunteer, and who is going to decide? Who is going to place volunteers with certain families according to their individual abilities? A very important part is played by coordinators. They organize information and events. People willing to begin volunteer work take part in qualification courses. This early stage is the cornerstone of future commitment. It is the key to future success or disappointment. If this early chance to create mutual trust, solidarity, cooperation, and openness to honest self-appraisal is mishandled, the first step to regressive development is already taken. The aims and qualification content need to be considered in advance. The same applies to education and the role model represented by the coordinator.

Volunteer Skills

Communication with Self

Professional caregivers must employ a twofold attitude toward the suffering of human existence. They need to identify the reasons for suffering to remedy or reduce other people's pain. Caregivers also are expected to provide practical and affirmative support for existential and physical ailments.

Caregivers must accept their own existential suffering as an indispensable part of human nature and live in harmony with the knowledge of their own inevitable mortality. In working with people facing death, caregivers must reflect on their own lives and evaluate their attitudes about mortality. Otherwise, true support is impossible.

An important aspect of courses for trainees is autobiographical reflection and self-assessment. Participants learn about the influence of previous experiences of death and dying on their expectations regarding their own death. Every experience has left its mark on a person's idea of what death should or should not be.

As a student, I worked at the University Clinic of Bonn during term break. One day, I found myself involved in caring for an old patient, who—even on his deathbed—continued to act like a despot with his family members, and none of them came to see him. Fearing his death would be a lonely experience, I tried to make up for his behavior. He sensed what I was up to and fortunately was not too weak to stop me by saying, "Don't even think of dragging my family to my bedside when I'm going to die. This is a moment I will celebrate on my own." I learned a lot from that man. There is a danger of transferring a personal concept of death to a person cared for, which does not allow him or her an individual experience of death.

Motivation

The reasons for the social involvement of voluntary workers should be examined. This is not mistrust; it is the first and most important step toward truly autonomous and responsible action. A volunteer must answer several questions. What am I doing? For whose benefit are my actions? What are my intentions?

Some people do what they do because it was the only possible role within their family. They might have been loved only because they cared for others. Some people volunteer because they feel less important, even invisible, in their ordinary life, and they may strengthen their self-esteem through a position of "being in charge." None of these reasons is bad, but it is important that volunteers and coordinators are aware of their motivations so that they do not become counterproductive and a burden to a patient or cause burnout.

People caring for the dying are often described by others as brave, strong, selfless, empathic, compassionate, kind, warm-hearted, ready to help, and altruistic. Before accepting these descriptions as self-evident, volunteers should ask themselves whether the adjectives match the attitudes behind their contributions. They should reflect on whether some selfish reasons—something neither unusual nor forbidden—might determine their actions. To do so, volunteers need family support from the early stages of their involvement.

Attitude

A concept in which the wishes and needs of the dying person and his or her family are a priority stresses certain attitudes rather than techniques. If the principal aim was to learn a couple of techniques, it would indicate that the persons cared for were objects, not subjects. A dying person needs human care and concern, not methods.

The wishes and needs of the dying person and his or her relatives must be introduced to the volunteer and, if unclear, be carefully evaluated. The persons concerned may be under immense physical and emotional stress, and it may be difficult for them to clarify what they want.

Volunteers cannot assume that the wishes and needs of the dying and their families follow certain patterns. Volunteers should be taught to listen carefully to what is being transmitted by the persons concerned and to understand nonverbal messages.

During a supervised session, a volunteer described an aphasic patient to whom she recited a prayer at the end of her visits. After the death, when preparing for the funeral, she learned from the daughter that the patient had not been a member of any church for many years. Looking back, the volunteer felt insecure about her approach. When asked why she believed that the patient would have appreciated a prayer, she said she had assumed this to be the case. In a role-playing session, she took the position of the patient, and reflecting on all the gestures she had observed, it became obvious that the patient showed signs of disapproval and distancing. The volunteer's assumptions did not allow her to detect those signs. This example demonstrates the importance of including the policy of unprejudiced attention to the patient in the volunteer qualification course. Training volunteers how to perceive situations is essential.

The Mature Volunteer

A mature volunteer described her role: "It is not only us who are in need of training. It is as well those who coordinate our services and the institutions and services relying on our support that must be enabled to work alongside us volunteers. It is not our responsibility to find out what these services regard as targets of voluntary support. Therefore, services must clearly define their roles before they are in a position to develop training standards for us."

Services and institutions should ask themselves several questions. What should our volunteers do? Where should they do it? With whom should they cooperate, and whom should they complement?

Institutions and services, not volunteers, are responsible for sensibly connecting professional and voluntary work. Care is largely influenced by professional attitudes, and when volunteers are part of care, professionals must adjust routines. Cooperation with volunteers must regard changing needs and contexts.

INTEGRATION

The patient's care needs a holistic approach. The division of professional and voluntary contributions is artificial. Reducing voluntary work to "holding hands" in contrast to the proper treatment and supplementary care given by professionals is demeaning and does not reflect reality. To create a trusting atmosphere that is fully attentive to the patient, volunteers need to be involved in the early stages of care. Volunteer involvement is not a last resort to compensate for less attention by professionals. Volunteers are a complementary social service of everyday care based on its own qualifications. Together, professional staff and volunteers must find appropriate ways to join forces effectively.

REFERENCES

1. Doyle D (ed). Volunteers in Hospice and Palliative Care. A Handbook for Volunteer Service Managers. Oxford, UK: Oxford University Press, 2002.
2. Rosenkranz D, Weber A. Freiwilligenarbeit-Einführung in das Management von Ehrenamtlichen in der Sozialen Arbeit. Weinheim, Germany: Juventa, 2002.
3. Müller M. Ausbildung" für Ehjrenamtliche. In Aulbert E, Nauck F, Radbruch L (eds). Lehrbuch der Palliativmedizin. Stuttgart, Germany: Schattauer, 2007, p 1318.
4. Müller M. Handbuch für Multiplikatoren, 3rd ed. Bonn, Germany: Pallia Med Verlag, 2005.
5. Müller M. Dem Sterben Leben Geben. Gütersloh, Germany: Gütersloher Verlagshaus, 2004.

CHAPTER **61**

History and Physical Examination

Katherine Hauser, Sik Kim Ang, and Terence L. Gutgsell

K E Y   P O I N T S

- History and physical examination serve several purposes in palliative medicine, including evaluation of symptoms and underlying causes, medication review, and assessment of psychosocial and family functioning.
- Information is elicited to determine the needs of the patient and family.
- Data gleaned from evaluation of the patient are used to define the goals of care, to develop a treatment plan, and to calculate the prognosis.

The palliative medicine consultation involves much more than a diagnosis. Goals and priorities of the patient, the family or caregivers, and the physician must be considered. A thorough history and examination provide the backbone of the consultation. Good communication during the history and examination facilitates a trusting therapeutic relationship. This relationship allows exploration of "the big picture," including psychosocial functioning and concerns, coping, grief, dignity, spirituality, sexuality, and care priorities.

The classic medical history consists of the presenting problem, medical and surgical history, medication history, family and social history, and a systems review. Each component needs to be tailored to the palliative approach (see "Common Errors"). Information may need to be elicited over several consultations, particularly if acute distress requires immediate action. The examination should be systematic and focused. Many clinical signs can be obtained from careful bedside observation. Many diagnoses can be made based on history and examination thus relieving patients of unnecessary, burdensome investigations.

GOALS OF THE HISTORY AND EXAMINATION

The history and examination in palliative medicine is aimed at eliciting the priorities and needs of the patient and caregivers. The physician's goal is to attend to these priorities and gather information needed to provide care for the patient and family throughout the disease trajectory.

Patient's Priorities

Patients may have diverse expectations about a consultation with a palliative medicine physician. Poorly controlled pain and other symptoms may be the main priorities. Other priorities may be medication management, psycho-

---

How to Avoid Common Errors

History

- Listen to the patient, caregiver, nurse, and other team members.
- Clarify—What do you mean by that? How is that affecting you?
- Prioritize—What is most important at this time?
- Review medication, including exact dosages and schedules and the patient's compliance.
- Medication allergies and interactions—Ask about smoking, alcohol, nonprescription or recreational drugs, and complementary drugs and therapies.

Examination

- Wash your hands.
- Ensure privacy—Does the patient want family members present or not?
- Look (inspect) before touching.
- Screen for delirium.
- Perform a rectal examination, especially if cord compression is suspected.
- Get the patient out of bed and walking, if possible.

Box 61-1 Psychosocial Assessment: The Big Picture

Support

    Family
    Friends
    Financial (e.g., insurance, benefits)
    Physical environment
    Church, synagogue, mosque
    Other resources

Information Needs

    Moods, coping style, grief
    Function (e.g., activities of daily living, mobility, falls)
    Spirituality
    Sexuality

Future Plans and Wishes

    Goals of care
    Advance directives
    Designated spokesperson or health care proxy
    Desired place of death
    Death rituals (e.g., cultural, religious)

Caregiver Needs

    Information
    Emotional support, grief education and support
    Physical support
    Practical and financial support
    Family function

---

logical support, or a need for information (e.g., prognostication, available services, future planning).

Family's Priorities

Families and caregivers may have very different priorities for the consultation. Symptoms observed by the family might be different from those reported by the patient. For example, changes in mood, appetite, weight, and appearance may by very distressing for family members. Symptoms of delirium (e.g., hallucinations, agitation) may be reported by caregivers but not patients.[1] The information needs of the family and caregivers may be different from those of patients. As illness progresses, caregivers may need specific information about the dying process and how to provide physical and emotional care.[1]

Physician's Priorities

The physician's goal is to prioritize the most important current issues and predict future issues. Medical priorities may include the following:

- Screening for treatable symptoms or urgent conditions (e.g., spinal cord compression, gastrointestinal obstruction, infection, bone or brain metastases, depression or anxiety)
- Optimizing and simplifying medications and screening for side effects, compliance, and drug interactions
- Eliciting prognostic information and predicting future problems, such as symptoms with prognostic significance, signs of imminent death, and lesions likely to hemorrhage or obstruct (e.g., large gastrointestinal tumors, head and neck tumors)
- Determining the role or necessity of investigations
- Developing goals of care
- Eliciting and responding to the information needs of the patient and family

The physician's estimation of patient's prognosis, although not exact, is important, and families often ask for and expect some prognostic information.[1,2] This estimation is also important when considering the goals of care and relevance of investigation or treatment options. Investigations may be avoided if the diagnosis is evident from the history and results of the examination.

The Big Picture

An overview of the patient's medical and social situation may evolve over several consultations and is often contributed to by many care team members, such as nurses, social workers, chaplains, physical therapists, and occupational therapists (Box 61-1). Team members may also provide important symptomatic information not elicited in the initial consultation. Communication may be assisted by the use of a prompt list.[3] A list of potential questions may be provided in a brochure when the patient first meets the palliative care team. Topics may include the role of the palliative care team, physical symptoms, future expectations, and caregiver needs.[3]

CLINICAL HISTORY

Assessing Current Status

The physician should ask open-ended questions: What has been troubling you recently? What led to you to come in today?

Characteristics of the current problem should be elicited, such as time course, onset, pattern, site and radiation, character, severity, aggravating and relieving factors, and associated symptoms. The meaning and impact (e.g., psychological, existential) of the symptom are important. Interpretations of symptoms are highly individual and can influence treatment success. Pain may be interpreted as a challenge, punishment, weakness, or a sign of progressive disease or impending death.[4,5] Coexistent depression may alter the interpretation of pain.[6]

Many patients underreport symptoms,[7] whereas others may give an exhaustive list. Asking the patient to prioritize may help to identify the most urgent problems to be addressed if time is limited: What is the most important thing we can help you with today?

Underreported symptoms include fatigue, sleep problems, depression, and symptoms of delirium, such as hallucinations (especially visual), paranoia, and agitation. Caregivers may more reliably report some of these symptoms. Routine use of symptom assessment instruments can improve detection.

Review of Symptoms

A systems review should begin with general screening questions: How is your breathing? How are your bowels? A positive answer to any of the screening questions prompts thorough questioning about that system (Box 61-2).

Medical History

The history of the advanced illness includes the diagnosis, previous treatments, cancer histology, sites of recurrence, and any systemic or local treatment. Other medical conditions are important and must be managed alongside care of the advanced illness. For example, hypertension, diabetes, airways disease, cardiac disease, or renal or hepatic impairment are common, and these conditions influence management plans and medication regimens.

Medication History

A thorough medication history includes all prescribed and nonprescribed substances, including those for symptoms, disease modification, and co-morbidities, and complementary medicines. Medications for co-morbidities need review; for example, antihypertensive and lipid-lowering medications may be inappropriate for patients with advanced disease. Compliance with medications and side effects experienced should be evaluated. The medication list should be analyzed for potential drug interactions.

Questions should determine the use of recreational drugs, alcohol, and tobacco. Dependence on any of these substances may cause symptoms, affect treatment, or be associated with withdrawal in the hospital or during the terminal phase. Alcohol dependence is common and usually overlooked without specific screening.[8] Brief screening for alcohol dependence can be done using the CAGE questions:

C: Have you ever felt you ought to *cut down* on your drinking?
A: Have people *annoyed* you by criticizing your drinking?
G: Have you ever felt bad or *guilty* about your drinking?
E: Have you ever had a drink first thing in the morning to steady your nerves or get rid of a hangover (i.e., *eye opener*)?

Cigarette smokers may need nicotine replacement when physically unable to smoke.

Family History

A genogram of family members, their names, and other relevant details helps the team communicate and care for the family (Fig. 61-1). Family members may be at risk for certain cancers or other conditions, and they may need referral for genetic counseling.

Psychosocial Assessment

Psychosocial issues are important to patients, and they expect physicians to be comfortable discussing them. A full psychosocial assessment may take place over many consultations and be contributed to by other team members. Issues include mood, coping, support, functioning, family, spirituality, sexuality, financial burdens of illness, and end-of-life preferences (Box 61-3).

Screening for depression can be accomplished with a single question that is sensitive and specific: Are you

---

Box 61-2 Review of Systems: Topics of Screening Questions
• Aches, pain, and headache
• Energy
• Eating and appetite
• Bladder and bowel
• Breathing
• Sleep
• Mood, depression, and anxiety
• Mental status, including confusion, hallucination (especially visual), disorientation, and memory
• Function and mobility

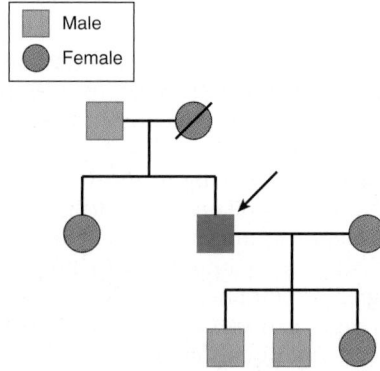

FIGURE 61-1 Family tree diagram. The married male patient *(arrow)* has three children and one sister, and his mother is deceased. The diagram can be labeled with names, ages, diagnoses, and locations. The symbols for any relatives affected by the same condition are also shaded.

Box 61-3 Symptoms of Prognostic Significance
• Anorexia
• Absence of depressive mood
• Cognitive impairment
• Delirium
• Dry mouth
• Dysphagia
• Dyspnea
• Nausea
• Change in performance status
• Significant weight loss

Box 61-4 Signs Evident from the Bedside
• Alertness, mental status, affect, memory, orientation, speech
• Pain, distress, dyspnea, abnormal respirations
• Nutrition, hydration, wasting
• Bruising, pressure areas, pallor, or jaundice of skin
• Mouth (e.g., ulcers, nutrition, thrush, hygiene, breath), tongue, and teeth (e.g., ill-fitting dentures)
• Tremors, flaps, myoclonus

depressed? Other questions can be used to assess mood and social functioning:

- Questions about helplessness and hopelessness: Do you feel hopeless about the future? Do you feel you have enough help from family, friends, health care workers, and yourself (i.e., internal strength)?
- Questions about decision making: Are you having trouble making decisions?
- Questions about emotions: Are you crying more, and are the tears from a place of deep sadness or from a place of peace? Do you feel unhappy or sad much of the time?
- Questions about pleasure: Have you lost pleasure in the things that have brought you joy in the past?
- Questions about psychosocial functioning: How are you coping? How is your family coping? Is there someone you can talk to?
- Questions about activity and mobility: How are you managing to take care for yourself? How is your mobility? Have you had any falls?

Financial Issues

Chronic, life-threatening conditions are often associated with loss of income for the patient and caregiver. The emotional stress of role loss is compounded by the financial burden of medical and pharmaceutical costs. Questions should be asked about medical and pharmaceutical insurance and about employment, sickness, and disability benefits.

Spirituality

Spirituality is important to patients at the end of life, and it influences physical and emotional health. Physicians often feel uncomfortable initiating a discussion about spirituality. Two frameworks for a spiritual history that are useful in palliative medicine are FICA[9] and HOPE[10]:

F: What is your *faith* or belief?
I: What is its *importance* or *influence*?
C: Are you part of a religious *community*?
A: How would you like me to *address* this in your care?

H: Sources of *hope*, meaning, comfort, strength, peace, love, and connection
O: *Organized* religion
P: *Personal* spirituality and *practices*
E: *Effects* on medical care and *end of life*

The spiritual history includes beliefs and rituals regarding end-of-life practices, such as care of the body and timing of burial. These ideas may vary according to cultural or religious beliefs.

Sexuality

Sexuality is important at the end of life and should be discussed by physicians.[11] Several questions may be used: What does sexuality mean to you? How important is your sexuality? How do you express your sexuality? Has your sexuality changed since being ill?

CARE PLANNING

Information should be sought about advance directives, power of attorney, living wills, and resuscitation status. These instructions may already be in existence, or information may be needed to enable preparation before death. Cultural preferences regarding health care information and decisions should be elicited. In Western cultures, information is usually provided to the individual, who is responsible for his or her own decisions. In some Asian, African, Latin American, and Eastern European cultures, health care decisions are made by a family spokesperson rather than the patient. In all families, a designated spokesperson should be sought, and patients should be questioned about who should make medical decisions on their behalf if they are incapacitated.

A complementary method of psychosocial evaluation is the dignity model.[12] This model involves evaluation of physical and psychological distress (e.g., illness-related concerns), personal resources for maintaining dignity (e.g., acceptance, autonomy, hopefulness, legacy, pride, resilience), and social dignity (e.g., burden, privacy, support, aftermath) (Table 61-1).

EXAMINATION

Observation of the patient while the history is taken provides several clinical clues. Evidence of distress from pain or dyspnea (e.g., facial grimace, writhing in bed, rapid respirations) indicates the need for a brief history and focused examination so treatment can be initiated quickly. Neurological status can be evaluated by observing alertness, speech patterns, and evidence of tremors or myoclonus. Nutritional and fluid status may be evident from the bedside; loose clothing, skin, or dentures and muscle wasting are all evidence of weight loss. Fluid overload may be evidenced by edema or abdominal distention due to ascites.

Systems examination should be focused (Boxes 61-4 to 61-8). Complete history taking defines the systems that

TABLE 61-1 A Model of Dignity and Dignity-Conserving Interventions for Patients Nearing Death		
FACTORS OR SUBTHEMES	**DIGNITY-RELATED QUESTIONS**	**THERAPEUTIC INTERVENTIONS**
ILLNESS-RELATED CONCERNS		
Symptom distress		
Physical distress	"How comfortable are you?" "Is there anything we can do to make you more comfortable?"	Vigilance to symptom management Frequent assessment Application of comfort care
Psychological distress	"How are you coping with what is happening to you?"	Assume a supportive stance Empathetic listening Referral to counseling
Medical uncertainty	"Is there anything further about your illness that you would like to know?" "Are you getting all the information you feel you need?"	Upon request, provide accurate, understandable information and strategies to deal with possible future crises
Death anxiety	"Are there things about the later stages of your illness that you would like to discuss?"	
Level of independence		
Independence	"Has your illness made you more dependent on others?"	Have patients participate in decision making, regarding both medical and personal issues
Cognitive acuity	"Are you having any difficulty with your thinking?"	Treat delirium When possible, avoid sedating medication(s)
Functional capacity	"How much are you able to do for yourself?"	Use orthotics, physiotherapy, and occupational therapy
DIGNITY-CONSERVING REPERTOIRE		
Dignity-conserving perspectives		
Continuity of self	"Are there things about you that this disease does not affect?"	
Role preservation	"What things did you do before you were sick that were most important to you?"	Acknowledge and take interest in those aspects of the patient's life that he/she most values
Maintenance of pride	"What about yourself or your life are you most proud of?"	See the patient as worthy of honor, respect, and esteem
Hopefulness	"What is still possible?"	Encourage and enable the patient to participate in meaningful or purposeful activities
Autonomy/control	"How in control do you feel?"	Involve patient in treatment and care decisions
Generativity/legacy	"How do you want to be remembered?"	Life project (e.g., making audio/video tapes, writing letters, journaling) Dignity psychotherapy
Acceptance	"How at peace are you with what is happening to you?"	Support the patient in his/her outlook Encourage doing things that enhance his/her sense of well-being (e.g., meditation, light exercise, listening to music, prayer)
Resilience/fighting spirit	"What part of you is strongest right now?"	
Dignity-conserving practices		
Living in the moment	"Are there things that take your mind away from illness, and offer you comfort?"	Allow the patient to participate in normal routines, or take comfort in momentary distractions (e.g., daily outings, light exercise, listening to music)
Maintaining normalcy	"Are there things you still enjoy doing on a regular basis?"	
Finding spiritual comfort	"Is there a religious or spiritual community that you are, or would like to be, connected with?"	Make referrals to chaplain or spiritual leader Enable the patient to participate in particular spiritual and/or culturally based practices
SOCIAL DIGNITY INVENTORY		
Privacy boundaries	"What about your privacy or your body is important to you?"	As permission to examine patient Proper draping to safeguard and respect privacy
Social support	"Who are the people that are most important to you?" "Who is your closest confidante?"	Liberal policies about visitation, rooming in Enlist involvement of a wide support network
Care tenor	"Is there anything in the way you are treated that is undermining your sense of dignity?"	Treat the patient as worthy of honor, esteem, and respect; adopt a stance conveying this
Burden to others	"Do you worry about being a burden to others?" "If so, to whom and in what ways?"	Encourage explicit discussion about these concerns with those they fear they are burdening
Aftermath concerns	"What are your biggest concerns for the people you will leave behind?"	Encourage the settling of affairs, preparation of an advanced directive, making a will, funeral planning

From Chochinov HM. Dignity-conserving care—a new model for palliative care: Helping the patient feel valued. JAMA 2002;287:2253-2260.

Box 61-5 Interpretation of Clinical Signs

Skin

Decreased skin turgor (i.e., dehydration)
Pressure ulcers, bruises (i.e., poor performance status)
Scratch marks (i.e., pruritus from renal or hepatic failure, opioids)

Hands

Clubbing
   Cardiovascular disease
      Congenital heart disease
   Gastrointestinal disease
      Inflammatory bowel diseases
   Pulmonary disease
      Bronchiectasis
      Interstitial lung disease
      Lung cancer
      Pulmonary hypertension
Tremor
   Intention (i.e., cerebellar pathology)
   Postural (e.g., essential tremor, thyroid disease)
   Resting (i.e., parkinsonism)
Palmar erythema
   Normal
   Liver disease
   Portal hypertension
   Thyrotoxicosis
Asterixis (i.e., flapping tremor)
   Organ failure
      Brain
      Respiratory system
      Cardiovascular system
      Renal system
Ipsilateral muscle wasting
   Pancoast (apical lung) tumor

Eyes

Sclera icterus
   Hyperbilirubinemia

Sclera pallor
   Anemia
Chemosis
   Carbon dioxide retention
Horner's syndrome (i.e., apical lung tumor with ptosis, miosis, anhidrosis)

Neck

Virchow nodes (supraclavicular)
   Abdominal malignancy

Respiratory Disease

Percussion
   Dull (e.g., pneumonia, pleural effusion)
   Hyperresonance (e.g., chronic obstructive pulmonary disease)

Gastrointestinal Disease

Spider nevi (i.e., central arteriole with radiating small vessels—liver disease)
Sister Joseph's nodule (i.e., palpable nodule in the umbilicus [see Fig. 61-4]—metastatic gastric cancer)
Ascites (i.e., congestive heart failure, liver disease, peritoneal carcinomatosis)

Lower Extremities

Bilateral swelling (e.g., malnutrition)
Unilateral swelling (e.g., deep vein thrombosis, pelvic lymphadenopathy)

Neurological Disease

Babinski sign (i.e., upgoing plantar reflex indicating an upper motor neuron lesion)
Myoclonus (i.e., rapid, brief, irregular muscle jerking—opioid toxicity)

Box 61-6 Signs of Death within Hours to Days

Mental status
   Drowsiness
   Unconscious
   Delirium
Respiratory status
   Ataxic breathing (i.e., irregular timing and depth)
   Cheyne-Stokes breathing (i.e., periods of apnea alternate with hyperpnea)
   Respiratory secretion (i.e., death rattle)
   Shallow respiration
Cardiovascular status
   Weak pulse
Skin
   Cold extremities
   Diaphoresis
   Mottling
Miscellaneous signs
   Reduced urine output

need thorough examination. The site of pain should be inspected palpated, percussed, and auscultated (if in the chest or abdomen). Knowledge of the patterns of referred pain (Figs. 61-2 and 61-3) directs the examination. For example, pain in the shoulder tip may indicate local bony metastases, underlying Pancoast tumor of the lung apex, or diaphragmatic irritation (e.g., from liver metastases). Pain radiating down limbs or around the chest may indicate involvement of spinal nerve roots or plexuses. Neurological examination of motor and sensory function may locate the lesion to specific nerve roots. Delirium is common in patients with advanced cancer and palliative medicine inpatients. Because it is often missed with the basic history and examination, every patient should be screened systematically. A brief, reliable instrument for palliative medicine is the Bedside Confusion Scale[13] (Table 61-2).

If possible, gait, mobility, falls risk, and activities of daily living should be assessed (see Chapter 68). Simple

Box 61-7 Upper Limb Myotomes

FUNCTION	MYOTOMES
Power	
Shoulder	
Abduction	C5, C 6
Adduction	C 6, C7, C8
Elbow	
Flexion	C5, C6
Extension	C7, C8
Wrist	
Flexion	C6, C7
Extension	C7, C8
Fingers	
Flexion	C7, C8
Extension	C7, C8
Abduction	C8, T1
Reflexes	
Biceps jerk	C5, C6
Triceps jerk	C7, C8
Brachioradialis jerk	C5, C6
Finger jerks	C8

Box 61-8 Lower Limb Myotomes

FUNCTION	MYOTOMES
Power	
Hip	
Flexion	L2, L3
Extension	L5, S1, S2
Knee	
Flexion	L5, S1
Extension	L3, L4
Ankle	
Plantar flexion	S1, S2
Dorsiflexion	L4, L5
Inversion or eversion	L5, S1
Reflexes	
Knee jerk	L3, L4
Ankle jerk	S1, S2
Plantar reflex	L5, S1, S2

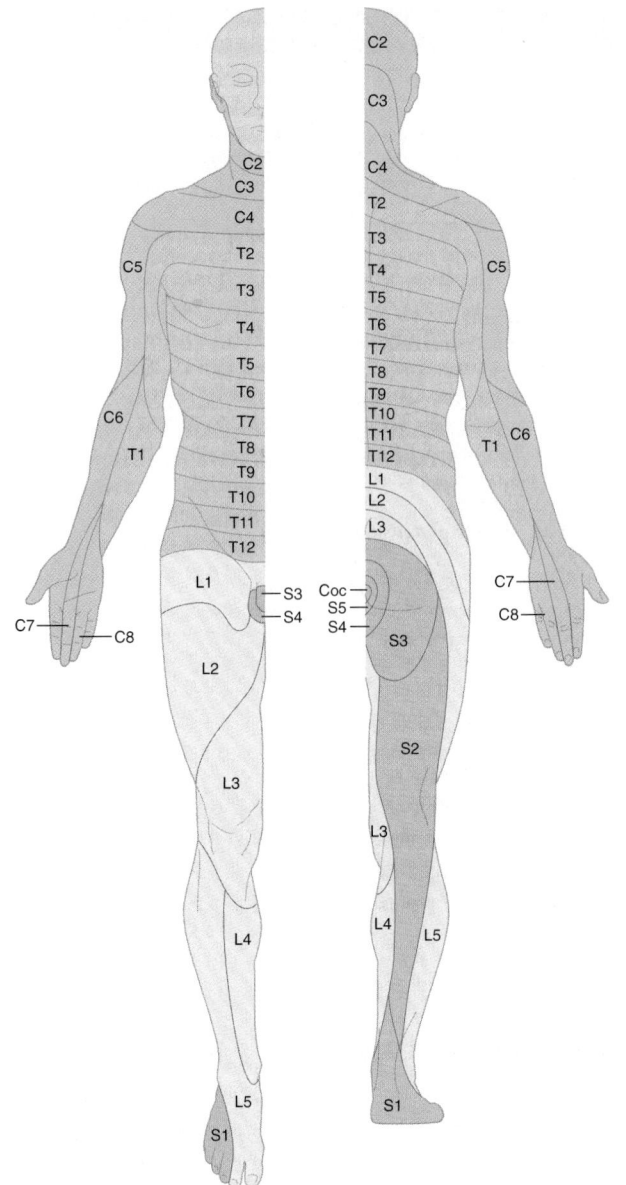

FIGURE 61-2 Sensory dermatomes.

tasks such as walking, rising from a chair, and Romberg's test (i.e., standing with feet together and eyes closed) provide information about safety and the needs for physical or occupational therapy or home aids and modifications.

NUTRITIONAL ASSESSMENT

Gastrointestinal symptoms such as anorexia and weight loss are common in patients with advanced cancer and other nonmalignant conditions.[14,15] Cachexia is a frequent complication of advanced cancer and other illnesses, and it indicates a poor prognosis. Weight loss commonly has many causes, which may include poor oral intake due to symptoms or treatment complications (e.g., oral problems, taste changes, anorexia, nausea, early satiety) combined with catabolic effects of the disease. Secondary vitamin and nutrient deficiencies may contribute to fatigue, skin problems, and susceptibility to infection. Vitamin D deficiency is common in hospitalized patients and is associated with muscle weakness and falls.[16] Vitamin K deficiency is common in palliative medicine patients and may lead to problems with bleeding.[17] Zinc deficiency has been associated with abnormalities of taste and magnesium deficiency with anorexia, weakness, and parasthesia.[18,19]

A thorough history is an important part of the nutritional assessment (Box 61-9). Complaints of nausea or lack of appetite may mean many things: bloating, early satiety,

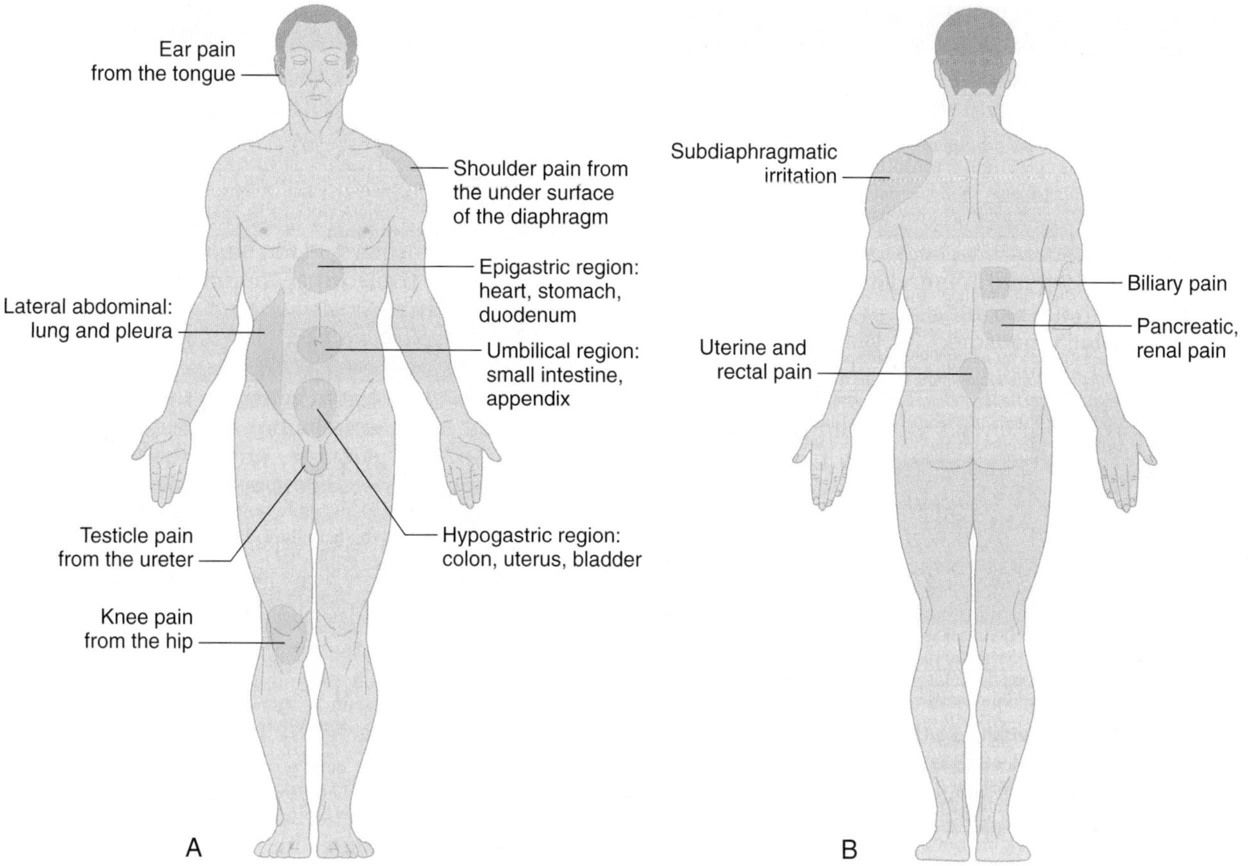

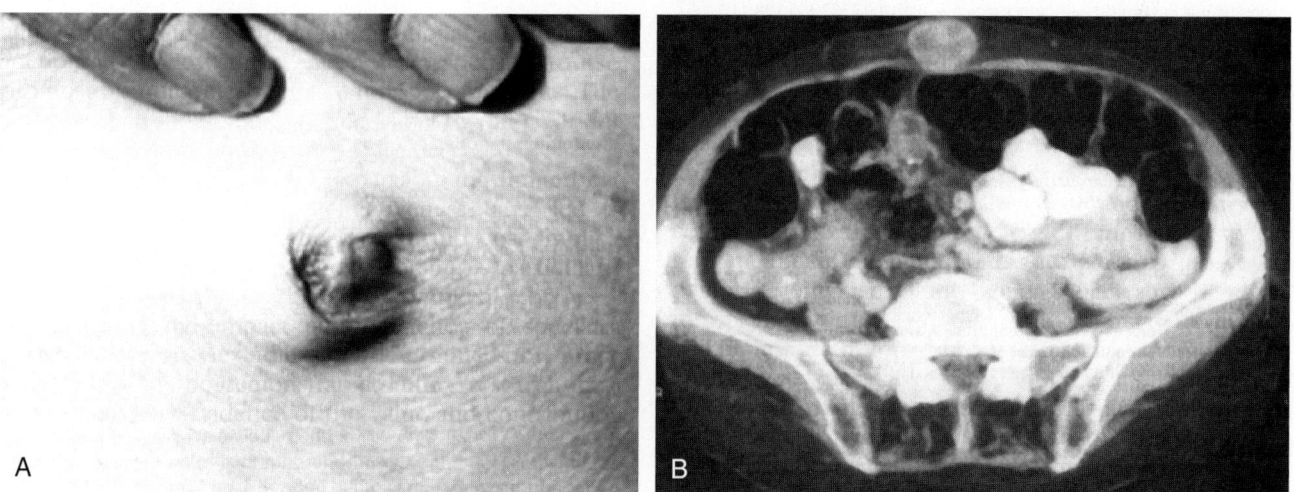

FIGURE 61-3 **A** and **B,** Knowledge of patterns of referred pain directs the examination.

FIGURE 61-4 **A,** Sister Joseph's nodule. **B,** Computed tomography shows an umbilical subcutaneous nodule *(arrow)*, which is Sister Joseph's nodule. (**A** *from Leow CK, Lau WY. Sister Joseph's nodule. Can J Surg 1997;40:167;* **B** *from Moll S. Images in clinical medicine. Sister Joseph's node in carcinoma of the cecum. N Engl J Med 1996;335:1568.)*

dysphagia, and dry or painful mouth. Taste and smell changes are common in cancer patients and influence the type and amount of food consumed.[20] Examination includes inspection of the mouth for signs of infection (e.g., thrush) and nutrient deficiencies.

CONCLUSIONS

A thorough history and examination are diagnostic and therapeutic tools. Many symptoms are unreported without specific questioning. All patients should be screened for depression, delirium, and alcohol dependence.

TABLE 61-2   Bedside Confusion Scale

PARAMETER	LEVEL	SCORING*
Assess level of alertness	Normal	0
	Hyperactive	1
	Hypoactive	1
Test of attention: a timed recitation of the month of the year in reverse order	Normal	0
	Delay >30 seconds	1
	1 omission	1
	2 omissions	2
	≥2 omissions, reversal of task, or termination of task	3
	Inability to perform	4

*Total score is the sum of the scores for both parameters: 0 = normal, 1 = borderline, ≥2 = confused.
Adapted from Sarhill N, Walsh D, Nelson KA, et al. Assessment of delirium in advanced cancer: The use of the bedside confusion scale. Am J Hosp Palliat Care 2001;18:335-341.

A thorough psychosocial assessment of the patient and caregiver is essential. Spirituality and sexuality are important to patients and often avoided by physicians.

REFERENCES

1. Parker SM, Clayton JM, Hancock K, et al. A systematic review of prognostic/end-of-life communication with adults in the advanced stages of a life-limiting illness: Patient/caregiver preferences for the content, style, and timing of information. J Pain Symptom Manage 2007;34:81-93.
2. Glare P, Virik K, Jones M, et al. A systematic review of physicians' survival predictions in terminally ill cancer patients. BMJ 2003;327:195-198.
3. Clayton J, Butow P, Tattersall M, et al. Asking questions can help: Development and preliminary evaluation of a question prompt list for palliative care patients. Br J Cancer 2003;89:2069-2077.
4. Barkwell DP. Ascribed meaning: A critical factor in coping and pain attenuation in patients with cancer-related pain. J Palliat Care 1991;7:5-14.
5. Spiegel D, Bloom JR. Pain in metastatic breast cancer. Cancer 1983;52:341-345.
6. Cleeland CS. The impact of pain on the patient with cancer. Cancer 1984;54(Suppl):2635-2641.
7. Homsi J, Walsh D, Rivera N, et al. Symptom evaluation in palliative medicine: Patient report vs systematic assessment. Support Care Cancer 2006;14:444-453.
8. Bruera E, Moyano J, Seifert L, et al. The frequency of alcoholism among patients with pain due to terminal cancer. J Pain Symptom Manage 1995;10:599-603.
9. Puchalski C, Romer AL. Taking a spiritual history allows clinicians to understand patients more fully. J Palliat Med 2000;3:129-137.
10. Anandarajah G, Hight E. Spirituality and medical practice: Using the HOPE questions as a practical tool for spiritual assessment. Am Fam Physician 2001;63:81-89.
11. Lemieux L, Kaiser S, Pereira J, Meadows LM. Sexuality in palliative care: Patient perspectives. Palliat Med 2004;18:630-637.
12. Chochinov HM. Dignity-conserving care—a new model for palliative care: Helping the patient feel valued. JAMA 2002;287:2253-2260.
13. Sarhill N, Walsh D, Nelson KA, et al. Assessment of delirium in advanced cancer: The use of the bedside confusion scale. Am J Hosp Palliat Care 2001;18:335-341.
14. Solano JP, Gomes B, Higginson IJ. A comparison of symptom prevalence in far advanced cancer, AIDS, heart disease, chronic obstructive pulmonary disease and renal disease. J Pain Symptom Manage 2006;31:58-69.
15. Teunissen SC, Wesker W, Kruitwagen C, et al. Symptom prevalence in patients with incurable cancer: A systematic review. J Pain Symptom Manage 2007;34:94-104.
16. Thomas MK, Lloyd-Jones DM, Thadhani RI, et al. Hypovitaminosis D in medical inpatients. N Engl J Med 1998;338:777-783.
17. Harrington DJ, Western H, Seton-Jones C, et al. A study of the prevalence of vitamin K deficiency in patients with cancer referred to a hospital palliative care team and its association with abnormal haemostasis. J Clin Pathol 2007 [Epub ahead of print].

Box 61-9 Nutritional Assessment

History

Patient's medical history
  Previous abdominal operations
  Severity or extent of disease
  Dietary history
Gastrointestinal symptoms
  Anorexia
  Dysphagia
  Early satiety
  Loss of appetite
  Taste and smell changes
  Dry mouth
  Nausea
  Vomiting
  Diarrhea or steatorrhea
  Weight loss
Social history
  Activities of daily living, instrumental activities of daily living
  Caregiver role, food preparation, food beliefs

Physical Examination

Body mass index
Loose clothing
Folds of loose skin
Oral hygiene (relevant deficiencies)
  Atropic papillae (folate, iron, vitamins B_2, B_3, and B_{12})
  Angular stomatitis (iron, vitamin B_2)
  Cheilosis (vitamin B_2)
  Glossitis (folate and vitamins B_2, B_3, B_6, and B_{12})
  Dentition, loose dentures
Lower extremities edema (i.e., protein deficiency)
Muscle bulk

Laboratory Tests

Serum levels of albumin and prealbumin
Serum level of blood urea nitrogen
Iron studies
Serum levels of folate and vitamin B_{12}
Serum level of vitamin D

18. Ripamonti C, Zecca E, Brunelli C, et al. A randomized, controlled clinical trial to evaluate the effects of zinc sulfate on cancer patients with taste alterations caused by head and neck irradiation. Cancer 1998;82:1938-1945.
19. Brogan G, Exton L, Kurowska A, Tookman A. The importance of low magnesium in palliative care: Two case reports. Palliat Med 2000;14:59-61.
20. Comeau TB, Epstein JB, Migas C. Taste and smell dysfunction in patients receiving chemotherapy: A review of current knowledge. Support Care Cancer 2001;9:575-580.

SUGGESTED READING

Anandarajah G, Hight E. Spirituality and medical practice: Using the HOPE questions as a practical tool for spiritual assessment. Am Fam Physician 2001;63:81-89.

Chochinov HM. Dignity-conserving care—a new model for palliative care: Helping the patient feel valued. JAMA 2002;287:2253-2260.

Clayton J, Butow P, Tattersall M, et al. Asking questions can help: Development and preliminary evaluation of a question prompt list for palliative care patients. Br J Cancer 2003;89:2069-2077.

Comeau TB, Epstein JB, Migas C. Taste and smell dysfunction in patients receiving chemotherapy: A review of current knowledge. Support Care Cancer 2001;9:575-580.

Hordern AJ, Currow DC. A patient-centered approach to sexuality in the face of life-limiting illness. Med J Aust 2003;179(Suppl):S8-S11.

Lemieux L, Kaiser S, Pereira J, Meadows LM. Sexuality in palliative care: Patient perspectives. Palliat Med 2004;18:630-637.

McMahon K, Decker G, Ottery FD. Integrating proactive nutritional assessment in clinical practices to prevent complications and cost. Semin Oncol 1998;25(Suppl 6):20-27.

Parker SM, Clayton JM, Hancock K, et al. A systematic review of prognostic/end-of-life communication with adults in the advanced stages of a life-limiting illness: Patient/caregiver preferences for the content, style, and timing of information. J Pain Symptom Manage 2007;34:81-93.

Puchalski C, Romer AL. Taking a spiritual history allows clinicians to understand patients more fully. J Palliat Med 2000;3:129-137.

Sarhill N, Mahmoud FA, Christie R, et al. Assessment of nutritional status and fluid deficits in advanced cancer. Am J Hosp Palliat Care 2003;20:465-473.

Sweeney MP, Bagg J. The mouth and palliative care. Am J Hosp Palliat Care 2000;17:118-124.

Talley NJ, O'Connor S. Clinical Examination: A Systematic Guide to Physical Diagnosis, 3rd ed. Sydney, Australia, MacLennan & Petty, 1996.

PART II

The Patient

Patient Evaluation

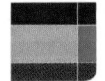

CHAPTER **62**

Assessing the Family and Caregivers

Sheila Payne and Peter Hudson

K E Y   P O I N T S

● Caregiving usually is provided by family members and those in close social and emotional relationships.

● Caring for a dying family member is unpredictable, with an uncertain duration and nature.

● Most family care provided to those near the end of life is provided by women, spouses, and those in the same generation, and in developed countries, many caregivers are elderly.

● Providing care has positive aspects, including greater emotional closeness, fulfilling duty, and negative impacts such as increased risk of physical illness and injury, psychological distress, social isolation, and financial demands.

● Assessment of caregiving should examine positive and negative aspects.

● Supportive interventions include education, information provision, respite care, stress management, and relaxation.

Historically and currently in most societies, families and neighbors have cared for the young, the old, the sick, and the dying. In most cultures, there are powerful norms, and caregiving within kinship networks are obligations that most people fulfill out of duty, filial piety, and reciprocal altruism. An evolutionary perspective suggests that caregiving has survival value for the family unit and individual members. However, it is not a role to which most people aspire. In caring for people with advanced disease and those who are dying, the evidence supports it as both demanding and fulfilling.[1] The paradox of this social role and the effects of the role on those who provide care is the focus of this chapter. Caring for a dying family member is unpredictable and uncertain in duration and nature.

DEFINITIONS

Family

The notion of family is contested and changes over time. We offer the following broad definition drawn from the United Kingdom.[2] *Family* includes "those related through committed heterosexual or same-sex partnerships, birth and adoption, and others who have strong emotional and social bonds with a patient."[2]

Family life has changed markedly in many developed countries during the past 50 years, with high rates of divorce, marital separation, serial marriage, step-parenting, single parenting, and co-habitation becoming common. Increased longevity may result in more people enjoying being grandparents or great-grandparents and increasing the possibility of the loss of or distancing from family members in late old age. In many developed countries, there is a declining birth rate, with some people remaining childless (approximately 10% of women in the United Kingdom), and the normal family size has declined to one or two children per partnership. In countries such as China, one-child families have been imposed by government policy. This reduces the potential number of people related by kinship available to offer care near the end of life. Combined with changing work patterns with increased female employment outside the home, greater geographical mobility, more job insecurity, part-time and casual working, this means that assumptions about the availability of women to provide unpaid care need to be reconsidered. Same-sex partnerships are formally and legally recognized in many parts of the world, giving these people the same rights and obligations to provide care, along with or instead of other family members. In the African context, the devastating acquired immunodeficiency syndrome epidemic caused by human immunodeficiency virus (HIV/AIDS) has affected traditional family structures, with many children being raised by siblings, grandparents, or more distant kin.[3] Complex webs of social change affect family structures, economic viability, and the sense of cohesion. For some, technological developments such as the mobile telephone and Internet have offered new ways to maintain family relationships and support even when geographically apart. Although families may be sources of support, comfort, attachment, care, and love, they can also be conflict ridden, abusive, and exploitive. A full account of the complexity of family function is beyond this chapter, but all should be aware of these background issues.

Caregiver

From the same source,[2] we offer a definition of caregiver. "Carers, who may or may not be family members, are lay people in a close supportive role who share in the illness experience of the patient and who undertake vital care work and emotion management."[2]

The terminology of caregiving is potentially confused with several terms used in various situations, countries, and the research literature.[4] The following terms are widely used: carer, caregiver, informal caregiver, care taker, relative, companion, and significant other. We use the term *caregiver*. Although health and social care professionals may ascribe this term to family members, they may not identify themselves as a caregiver. We may assume that there is a main caregiver to whom we direct communication, instructions, and advice. The reality is that in many families, there is a network of support and care from people who may or may not be co-located. These people are crucially important in the lives of those facing the end of life, but they are often relegated by health and social care professionals and even in health care policy to marginal status.

Palliative care philosophy has considered the patient and family to be the unit of care.[5] Capable and willing caregivers make possible options and choices such as being cared for and dying at home. The absence of caregivers limits care options and choices and may contribute to more institutional deaths. We explore to what extent reality matches the rhetoric of palliative care.

Much of the general literature on caregiving has been derived from caring for frail older people, especially those with dementia[6] or those with acquired conditions such as stroke,[7] but this literature has not examined the final phase of life. There is now literature on caregivers of people with cancer[8,9] and for those in the end of life.[1] Because there are few comparative studies on caregivers of those with different advanced conditions or those receiving different services, it is difficult to make definitive statements about the relative challenges of caring for people in differing contexts or with different conditions.

In most end-of-life care, an assumption is made that family members are willing and able to undertake caring. Caregiving may be taken on in a crisis or through default; rarely is it a carefully considered decision. Unlike other types of caregiving, there is no opportunity to correct things later or to have a second chance. Many caregivers take on the role with little understanding of what it involves. The predominant model of caregiving in the psychological and health care literature is that of arduous work and burden. This represents caregivers as physically and psychologically overwhelmed by the tasks of care and having personal deficits or needs. This view has arisen from a focus on negative outcomes such as psychological morbidity and from enumerating predominantly physical care tasks. This observation presents a bleak picture and constructs caregivers as vulnerable. An alternative model recognizes that caregiving has positive and negative elements and that many people take it on willingly and derive benefits from caring. This model emphasizes resilience, mastery, and empowerment.[8] Although it is important not to romanticize the caregiver role, the different perspectives on caregiving are considered in terms of how well they accord with caregivers' accounts[8] (Box 62-1).

> **Box 62-1 Perspectives of Caregivers on Their Role**
>
> "Caring for a terminally ill person produces an unrelenting strain. The key is to understand that it is natural to experience stress while recognizing that you, too, need help coping before matters get out of hand."*
>
> "I felt the burden—as the one who thought something was wrong with myself, as the one who seemed to be held responsible by others, and after all, as the oldest daughter in the family, the one who saw him most—to do something."†
>
> "The greatest hardship for anyone during this time and later was for those who had to be absent. It was a solace to sit quietly in that room, holding her hand or just looking at her when she was asleep, wondering about the dreams that brought a smile to her face and unintelligible remarks to her lips."‡
>
> "Despite the pain and confusion, it was also a time of intense loving for the two of us."§

*Floyd M. Caretakers: The Forgotten People. Phoenix, AZ: Eskualdun Publishers, 1988, p 102.
†Miller S. The Story of My Father. London: Bloomsbury, 2003, p 29.
‡Taylor J. Brigie—A Life. London: Hodder & Stoughton, 1984, p 110.
§Jesudasan U. I Will Lie Down in Peace. Madras: East West Books, 1998, p 67.

> **Box 62-2 Factors Influencing Caregivers**
>
> **Sociodemographic Characteristics**
>
> Gender
> Age
> Relationship with person cared for
>
> **Material and Social Resources**
>
> Income
> Education
> Culture
> Housing
> Community
>
> **Personal and Family Resources**
>
> Mastery
> Meaning
> Self-concept
> Resilience
> Health and fitness
> Supportive family or kinship networks
>
> **Circumstances of Care**
>
> Type of disease or condition
> Nature and pattern of dying trajectory
> Timeliness and expectedness of dying
> Nature of relationship with cared-for person
> Information and communication
> Access to health and social care services
> Nature of health and social care services
> Adverse events and concurrent stressors

FACTORS INFLUENCING CAREGIVERS

In this section, we discuss factors that may influence the experience of caregiving (Box 62-2). There are no reliable international data on the number of people in caregiving relationships with dying people. It has been estimated by the charity Help the Hospices that at any one time, there are about 500,000 people providing care to people with terminal illness in the United Kingdom. This estimate is from data in 2000 in England and Wales,[10] where there were approximately seven million caregivers of all types. Analysis of hours of unpaid care work per week indicate that 3.5 million of them provide 1 to 19 hours, about one-half million provide 20 to 49 hours, and more than one million provide more than 50 hours of unpaid care. This definition of caring work is limited by its emphasis on direct physical care work, which inadequately recognizes the volume of anticipatory, emotional, and social care provided. Within palliative care contexts, many families provide supportive care throughout the illness, and they only gradually become engaged in direct physical care during the dying phase.

Gender

Although we know little about the numbers of people who provide care for dying people, we know that caregiving is a gendered role, with care predominantly provided by women. In the United Kingdom, more women (approximately 4.0 million) than men (2.9 million) provide general care.[10] Data indicate that most caregivers are in the age range 50 to 59 years, but older people (>65 years) increasingly are involved in caring for their spouses and parents, who may live into late old age (>85 years).[10] Older people who take on the role of caregivers may also have health care problems and impairments associated with aging, such as visual difficulties and deafness. In palliative care, there is more likely to be within-generational than cross-generational caregiving, which is different from other types of caring. Children may be the receivers and providers of care within palliative care. There are few data on the extent to which children provide care. In the United Kingdom, it has been estimated that approximately 51,000 young people (<16 years) are involved in care for other ill or disabled family members, only a small number of whom are dying.[10] Segal and Simkins[11] documented the impact on children of being involving in providing care for parents with chronic neurological conditions such as multiple sclerosis, including restriction on social activities, additional responsibilities, and less attention to educational achievement.

Material, Social, and Personal Resources

The material and social resources that caregivers can call on influence their performance of this role and ability to sustain caregiving at home until the death of the person.[12] Caring for a terminally ill person places heavy financial demands on the family. The costs of medical care, transport to hospital appointments, additional equipment or home adaptations, laundry, heating, clothing, and special food are rarely acknowledged. A U.K. end-of-life care initiative[13] that aims to provide patient choice and facilitate more care at home and home deaths may inadvertently increase the hidden costs of caring. At this time, families are likely to be experiencing reduced income, especially if the main wage earner is the ill person. Caregivers may be faced with difficult choices about employment, reducing working hours, or leaving, with short-term loss of income but long-term consequences for careers, pensions, and social contact. In a comprehensive review of the literature on caregiver employment in palliative care, only eight studies addressed this topic.[14] The study authors concluded that helpful strategies included flexible working practices, back to work training, and extended leave arrangements. Caregivers from poorer backgrounds, who were doing low-paid and manual work, were most adversely affected because they had few reserves. Other income supports may be required for those who leave employment, such as that pioneered by the Canadian government. Expectations about caregiving being largely a female occupation likely limit more flexible working[15] opportunities for men.

Caregivers bring their own personal resources to their role. Caregivers' written accounts[9] (see Box 62-1) have highlighted the demands of psychosocial care rather than the physical burden but this may be an artefact of retrospective published material. The diversity of responses[16] from caregivers can be understood based on a transactional model of coping, in which caregivers make cognitive appraisals about how current caring demands exceed their capacity to cope. In this way, caregiving is not seen as inherently stressful but depends on individual internal coping resources such as feelings of mastery and competence and on external resources such as supportive neighbors or sufficient income to purchase additional help. This model celebrates the capacities and skills that people bring to caregiving. It recognizes that people differ in their personal coping styles, such as being optimistic or pessimistic, and personality traits, such as hardiness and resilience. Self-appraisals of caregiving that find meaning in the caring relationship that enhances self-esteem, such as feelings of love, duty, moral obligation, and social approval, are more likely to be sustained. If the caregiver has a sense of mastery, self-efficacy, perceived competence, and perceived control, he or she is more likely to benefit from it. This may come from previous life experiences as a caregiver of other dependents or from professional backgrounds such as nursing.

Providing care is physically and emotionally demanding. Caregivers may have different levels of fitness and health before giving care. Many are older and have their own health problems. Caregiving affects health because of exhaustion. Lifting may cause back injury, and health care behaviors such as screening, exercise, and relaxation may be neglected. The rate of psychological morbidity is high,[17] and caregivers may experience more distress than the ill person.[18]

Families collectively differ in their responses to a dying member, as do individual family members.[19] They also differ in the degree to which they are enmeshed and can resolve conflict. Families who can resolve conflict[19] and are emotionally engaged are more supportive of each other. Although the availability of social support and an extended social network are associated with better outcomes, families may exhibit conflict and unsupportive behaviors.[20] Conflict may be more intense in small kinship networks. Heavy demands occur on a few people compared with larger, more diverse social networks with more resources, for which the potential for overloading individuals is less.

CIRCUMSTANCES OF CARE

Typical dying trajectories propose that certain diseases are associated with recognizable patterns of decline,[21] such as the prolonged trajectory of dying in late old age compared with the more precipitous decline in those with cancer. This suggests that caregiving may be highly influenced by factors such as the duration of dying, level of dependency of the cared-for person, and complex and difficult symptoms clusters such as refractory pain or incontinence. A further consideration is the extent to which symptoms are amenable to medical interventions and the resources available to purchase necessary medication or services. Vicarious suffering by families, who witness intractable pain or distressing breathlessness, may influence feelings of competency and subsequent bereavement.

In many societies, there are shared norms for the timeliness of dying in the life cycle. For example, dying is anticipated and acceptable in late old age but not in young adulthood, when it is generally regarded as a tragedy. In the United States,[22] most people view all deaths, except those of the very old, as personal tragedies. This view, combined with relatively few but intense personal relationships, means that caring for a dying spouse is often highly emotional and unlikely to build on previous experiences of caregiving.

Attachment theory[23] suggests the closer the relationships between caregiver and cared-for person, the greater the impact. Caregiving relationships that are conflicted or ambivalent or relationships in which there is marked dependency may also be problematic.

The social circumstances of caregiving are important. Caregivers require access to suitable health and social care services for themselves and for the cared for person. First, they need information about the types and methods of accessing services. They also require communication with service providers in a style and pace appropriate to their wishes about the ill person, and they need to know how to address their own concerns, which may be different. In a study[24] of 524 older people with end-stage heart failure in the United Kingdom, less than one fourth had contact with social care services in the previous 2 years. Even for patients and caregivers who reported contact, most found services limited or unsuitable, or they did not qualify because they did not have terminal cancer. Some who had applied for means-tested grants and been rejected when their condition was less severe were reluctant to apply again.

Caregiving may take place within wider family and social disruption, such as refugees or asylum seekers or living in environments of social unrest, famine, or war. In these circumstances, normal kinship obligations and supports may not function. For example, social links with extended family members may be unavailable because they remain in the place of origin or are displaced by social change. In these families, concurrent stressors may be overwhelming and prevent engaging with caring. For example, in Sierra Leone, palliative care services largely deal with deaths from HIV/AIDS, and their model has to consider orphaned and vulnerable children whose parents die in the hospice.[3]

ASSESSING THE FAMILY CAREGIVER EXPERIENCE

Those involved in palliative care must consider the family caregiver's needs. Despite frameworks and principles for assessing family caregiver needs,[2,5] it is important to acknowledge specific assessment-related issues. This may lead to more effective application of the frameworks and principles:

1. Caregivers' needs in end-of-life care are likely to change from day to day, and ongoing assessment therefore is recommended.
2. Determining whose needs to assess may pose a dilemma. Although palliative care standards in many countries promote support for the entire family, the reality is that in many circumstances this is inhibited by insufficient resources. Rather than health professionals attempting to support the entire family, the focus of support should be determined by the person with the advanced, incurable illness. We should ask the patient to determine the person (or persons) whom they consider to be the most important support to him or her. In keeping with definitions outlined earlier, this support person does not have to be related to the patient. Professionals should then seek permission to share the patient's medical and health care information with the family caregiver.
3. In considering family assessment, it is necessary to consider the distinction between the needs and satisfaction of the caregiver. These concepts are related, but assessment of the caregiver's needs should be the basis for support at the most immediate level. The caregiver's satisfaction may serve as a valuable means to determine the utility of service delivery.
4. Family members may not self-identify as caregivers; they may need prompting to articulate their concerns for their needs to be assessed. They may not see their needs as legitimate, and they may not feel comfortable expressing them in the company of their cared-for relative or friend.[25]
5. The needs of family caregivers may be incongruent with the patient's needs, making it challenging to discern whose needs should take priority.[26]
6. Working with family caregivers is a new and difficult role for some health care professionals, such as nurses. Without a tradition of practice in this area and lacking relevant training, some experience difficulties in assessing the needs of the family caregiver and in making appropriate responses.[6,26]

Tools for Assessing the Caregiver Experience

The increasing number of tools (instruments) validated in palliative care populations is encouraging. In considering their use in the family caregiver experience, the first issue is the purpose of the assessment. Is it used to assess the family caregiver's current needs or satisfaction with service delivery, or is the information used for research? If the assessment focuses on the caregiver's needs, administration of the tool should be followed by a discussion. In other words, assessment should not be undertaken in isolation; rather, it should serve as the basis for a more detailed discussion of the caregiver's needs.

If the purpose of the assessment tool is research (and ultimately to guide practice), careful consideration about the number of tools to be used and the specific reason for them is warranted. It should be determined whether the rationale for the assessment is to describe the caregiver experience, to describe the quality of relationship between the family caregiver and the patient (or other family members), or to evaluate the utility of interventions or service delivery. A comprehensive review of this topic and the psychometric properties of several related tools has been provided by Hudson and Hayman-White.[16]

Regardless of the rationale for tool selection, the usual checks for reliability and validity are essential. The administration process also warrants careful consideration. For example, is it intended that the tool be a self-report (i.e., completed by the family caregiver)? Will the assessment take place in the home, by mail, or by telephone?

Box 62-3 provides examples of tools for measuring the family caregiver experience and relevant references. The purpose is to highlight relevant examples, not to describe every tool.

Evidence Base for Assessing and Responding to Caregiver Needs

Although family caregivers are valid service recipients in standard definitions of palliative care, they have largely unmet needs. Support for family caregivers is often crisis driven, resulting from our assumptions that normally they are "coping well." Current evidence barely supports the claim that palliative care services provide effective support for family caregivers.[27]

We have a basic understanding of the family caregiver experience but limited grasp of the effectiveness of strategies to support family caregivers.[26] More longitudinal studies are required.[28] Additional research is needed about the experience for caregivers of noncancer patients and for children in the caregiving role. Further studies should include other family members; most studies have focused on the primary family caregivers. There is a significant gap in our understanding of the caregiver experience for new immigrants, those who do not speak English, and those in resource-poor countries. The influence of spirituality and religious belief related to the caregiver experience also is underreported.[29]

Some standard approaches related to family support lack a suitable evidence base. Family meetings, for example, are commonly promoted as a useful means for discussing end-of-life issues; however, their utility has not been well researched. Respite services, an almost standard support approach offered by specialist palliative care services for family caregivers, also warrant more attention.[30,31]

The other significant gap related to assessing the family caregivers' needs is how to discern which family caregivers are prone to psychological distress. Screening methods to identify family caregivers most at risk are required for targeted interventions.[32] Although several studies have explored factors predictive of adverse psychological outcome after bereavement,[32] few have explored psychological functioning in family caregivers at the commencement of and during caregiving.[33]

Given existing research, do we know what family caregivers want? According to consistent findings, it is evident that family caregivers desire information that prepares them for what is involved. This includes discharge planning, how to provide patient comfort, practical care needs, and how to minimize their own physical, psychological and social burdens.[34]

In addition to information, there is evidence identifying what most family caregivers value in an optimal end-of-life experience. Families expect their relative's symptoms be controlled; that they will receive emotional, social, and spiritual support; that treatment decisions will be respected; that they will have access to respite care and bereavement support; and that the preference for the site of death will be upheld.[35]

Evidence-Based Interventions for Family Caregivers

Despite significant gaps in knowledge about the family caregiver, we recommend more intervention research so we can ascertain what helps family caregivers. This is important to meet families' needs and to ensure resources are used wisely.[36] Research is also important to show that current supportive strategies are helpful and not harmful.

Box 62-4 provides examples of interventions for supporting family caregivers. As with family caregiver tools (see Box 62-3), this is not comprehensive; the selections exemplify topics addressed in studies and initiatives. Most of the interventions could benefit from further testing. We have not included studies of bereavement. A more comprehensive description of family caregiver interventions is given in an article by Hudson.[26]

There are several challenges to the evidence base for assessing family caregivers. They are not insurmountable and should not detract from the aim of improving assessment and support for family caregivers in end-of-life care. Caregivers are central to enhancing the remaining life of

---

Box 62-3 Tools for Measuring the Family Caregiver Experience

Family inventory of needs scale (FIN)
Preparedness for caregiving scale
Caregiver competence scale
Rewards of caregiving scale
Social support questionnaire (30SSQ)
Caregiver self-efficacy
Caregiver reaction assessment (CRA)
Life orientation test
Caregiver mutuality instrument
FAMCARE—satisfaction
Family strain questionnaire
Family functioning
Brief assessment scale
Caregiving at life's end questionnaire
Caregiver quality of life index

Box 62-4 Evidence-Based Interventions for Family Caregivers

- Group education program
- One-to-one psychoeducational program
- Problem solving
- Family therapy
- Depression reduction
- Burden reduction for caregivers of people with dementia
- Social care

the patient. Although their role is challenging, they should emerge from their experience with a sense of well-being, not feeling overwhelmed, guilty, and exhausted. Future research to support caregivers may focus on the effects of practical, cognitive, behavioral, and social interventions on outcomes such as quality of life, well-being, and financial status.

REFERENCES

1. Payne S, Ellis-Hill C (eds). Chronic and Terminal Illness: New Perspectives on Caring and Carers. Oxford, UK: Oxford University Press, 2001.
2. National Institute for Clinical Excellence. Improving supportive and palliative care for adults with cancer. In Services for Families and Carers, Including Bereavement Care: The Manual. London: National Institute for Clinical Excellence, 2004, p 155.
3. Kwaka J. The hospice model in Sierra Leone. Int J Palliat Nurs 2006;12:157.
4. Payne S. Carers and caregivers. In Oliviere D, Monroe B (eds). Death, Dying and Social Differences. Oxford, UK: Oxford University Press, 2004, pp 181-198.
5. Ferrell BR, Coyle N (eds). Textbook of Palliative Nursing. Oxford, UK: Oxford University Press, 2006.
6. Nolan M, Grant G, Keady J (eds). Understanding Family Care. Buckingham, UK: Open University Press, 1996.
7. Low JTS, Payne S, Roderick P. The impact of stroke on informal carers: A literature review. Soc Sci Med 1999;49:711-725.
8. Thomas C, Morris S, Harman JC. Companions through cancer: The care given by informal carers in cancer contexts. Soc Sci Med 2002;54:529-544.
9. Clark D, Thomas C, Lynch T, Bingley A, for the International Observatory on End of Life Care. What Are the Views of People Affected by Cancer and Other Illnesses about End of Life Issues? Lancaster, UK: Lancaster University, 2005.
10. Mather J, Green H (eds). Carers 2000 Office of National Statistics. London: The Stationery Office, 2002.
11. Segal J, Simkins J (eds). My Mum Needs Me: Helping Children with Ill or Disabled Parents. London: Penguin Books, 1993.
12. Gomes B, Higginson I. Factors influencing death at home in terminally ill patients with cancer: A systematic review. BMJ 2006;332:515-521.
13. Department of Health. NHS End of Life Care Programme Progress Report, March 2006. Leicester, UK: Department of Health, 2006.
14. Smith P, Payne S, Ramcharan P, et al. Carers of the Terminally Ill and Employment Issues: A Comprehensive Literature Review. Report to Help the Hospices. Sheffield, UK: University of Sheffield, 2006.
15. Lee C, Owens G (eds). The Psychology of Men's Health. Buckingham, UK: Open University Press, 2002.
16. Hudson P. A conceptual model and key variables for guiding supportive interventions for family caregivers of people receiving palliative care. Palliat Support Care 2003;1:353-365; and Hudson P, Hayman-White K. Measuring the psychosocial characteristics of family caregivers of palliative care patients: Psychometric properties of nine self-report instruments. J Pain Symptom Manage 2006;31:215-228.
17. Payne S, Smith P, Dean S. Identifying the concerns of informal carers in palliative care. Palliat Med 1999;13:37-44.
18. Harding R, Higginson I. What is the best way to help caregivers in cancer and palliative care? A systematic literature review of interventions and their effectiveness. Palliat Med 2003;17:63-74.
19. Kissane DW, Bloch S (eds). Family Focused Grief Therapy. A Model of Family-Centred Care during Palliative Care and Bereavement. Buckingham, UK: Open University Press, 2002.
20. Nuefeld A, Harrison MJ. Unfulfilled expectations and negative interactions: Non-support in the relationships of women caregivers. J Adv Nurs 2003; 41:323-331.
21. Lunney JR, Lynn J, Hogan C. Profiles of older medicare decedents. J Am Geriatr Soc 2002;50:1108-1112.
22. Lofland LH. The social shaping of emotion: A case of grief. Symbol Interact 1985;8:171-190.
23. Bowlby J (ed). Attachment and Loss, vol 3. Loss: Sadness and Depression. London: Hogarth Press, 1980.
24. Gott M, Barnes S, Payne S, et al. Patient views of social services provision for older people with advanced heart failure. Health Soc Care Community 2007; 29:872-890.
25. Hudson P, Aranda S, Kristjanson L. Meeting the supportive needs of family caregivers in palliative care: Challenges for health professionals. J Palliat Med 2004;7:19-25.
26. Harding R, Higginson I. What is the best way to help caregivers in cancer and palliative care? A systematic literature review of interventions and their effectiveness. Palliat Med 2003;17:63-74; and Hudson P. A critical review of supportive interventions for family caregivers of palliative stage cancer patients. J Psychosoc Oncol 2004;22:77-93.
27. Harding R. Carers: Current research and developments. In Firth P, Luff G, Oliviere D (eds). Facing Death: Loss, Change and Bereavement in Palliative Care. Buckingham, UK: Open University Press, 2005:150-166.
28. Grunfeld E, Coyle D, Whelan TJ, et al. Family caregiver burden: Results of a longitudinal study of breast cancer patients and their principal caregivers. CMAJ 2004;170:1795-1801.
29. Allen RS, Haley WE, Roff LL, et al. Responding to the needs of caregivers near the end of life: Enhancing benefits and minimising burdens. In Werth JL, Blevins D (eds). Psychosocial Issues Near the End of life: A Resource for Professional Care Providers. Washington, DC: American Psychological Association Books, 2005, pp 183-201.
30. Payne S, Ingleton C, Scott G, et al. A survey of the perspectives of specialist palliative care providers in the UK of inpatient respite. Palliat Med 2004; 18:692-697.
31. Skilbeck JK, Payne SA, Ingleton MC, et al. An exploration of family carers' experience of respite services in one specialist palliative care unit. Palliat Med 2005;19:610-618.
32. Kelly B, Edwards P, Synott R, et al. Predictors of bereavement outcome for family carers of cancer patients. Psychooncology 1999;8:237-249.
33. Hudson P, Hayman-White K, Aranda S, Kristjanson LJ. Predicting family caregiver psychosocial functioning in palliative care. J Palliat Care 2006;22:133.
34. Hudson P, Aranda S, Kristjanson L. Information provision for palliative care families: Moving toward evidenced based practice. Eur J Palliat Care 2004;11: 153-157.
35. Howell D, Brazil K. Reaching common ground: A patient-family-based conceptual framework of quality EOL care. J Palliat Care 2005;21:19-26.
36. Calman K, Hanks G. Clinical and health services research. In Doyle D, Hanks G, Macdonald N (eds). Oxford Textbook of Palliative Medicine, 2nd ed. Oxford, UK: Oxford University Press, 1998, pp 159-165.

SUGGESTED READING

Hudson P. A conceptual model and key variables for guiding supportive interventions for family caregivers of people receiving palliative care. Palliat Support Care 2003;1: 353-365.

Payne S, Ellis-Hill C (eds). Chronic and Terminal Illness: New Perspectives on Caring and Carers. Oxford, UK: Oxford University Press, 2001.

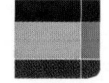

CHAPTER **63**

Clinical Symptom Assessment

Katherine Hauser

KEY POINTS

- Palliative medicine patients are polysymptomatic.
- Most symptoms are not volunteered, even if they are distressing.
- Symptom distress is not always in proportion to severity.
- Pain, fatigue, depression, anorexia and early satiety, and delirium are often underevaluated.
- Systematic recording of symptoms improves recognition and treatment.

Symptoms (Box 63-1) are subjective physical or psychological experiences. Advanced cancer patients are polysymptomatic, experiencing a median of 10 to 13 symptoms. On average, they report only one symptom when asked an open-ended question. People with advanced nonmalignant diseases have a similar symptom burden.[1] Symptoms affect physical, emotional, and social functioning and quality of life. In patients with advanced cancer, symptoms such as anorexia, weight loss, xerostomia, dysphagia, dyspnea, and confusion are prognostic.[2]

Symptoms commonly unreported include fatigue, anorexia, early satiety, dry mouth, drowsiness, insomnia, and weight loss.[3] Symptom reporting to physicians is influenced by many factors:

- Perception about what is important to the physician
- Belief that symptoms (e.g., fatigue) are inevitable
- Not wanting to complain
- Fear of distressing the family
- Fears about potential side effects of treatment (e.g., opioids)
- Fear that symptoms represent progression of disease

Physician's barriers to adequate symptom assessment include lack of time, language and cultural differences, and inadequate knowledge and training. For these reasons, systematic evaluation and documentation of symptoms are important to optimize quality of life and functioning.

SYMPTOMS THAT SHOULD BE ASSESSED

Symptoms are multidimensional. Symptoms are experienced in terms of severity, frequency, distress, and interference with function. Meaning is attributed to symptoms by patients and their families. Distress is not necessarily proportional to symptom severity.[4] Some symptoms, such as nausea, limited activity, or difficulty thinking, even when rated as mild or moderate may be distressing. More severe symptoms, such as fatigue or anorexia, may be rated less distressing.[4] Symptoms most frequently identified as priorities by patients include pain, fatigue, physical function, loss of appetite, nausea, vomiting, dyspnea, and depression.[5]

Prevalence and Severity

Symptom prevalence varies by diagnosis, stage of disease, age, gender, and performance status.[6,7] The most common advanced cancer symptoms include pain, fatigue, weakness, anorexia, dry mouth, constipation, early satiety, dyspnea, and weight loss.[8] These tend to be the most severe despite different primary sites. Reports of symptom prevalence in advanced noncancer illnesses vary, although pain, dyspnea, and fatigue are consistently reported in more than 50%.[9]

Clusters

Cancer symptoms occur in clusters or groups. For example, depression clusters with anxiety and sleep prob-

lems.[10] The occurrence of one symptom should trigger an inquiry about the others in the cluster.

CLINICAL SYMPTOM ASSESSMENT

The flow chart outlines a systematic approach to symptom assessment in palliative medicine. Clinical assessment focuses on eliciting symptoms, their underlying causes, and contributing or treatable factors (Fig. 63-1).

History and Examination

The history should start with open-ended questions about perceived problems and move to more specific screening questions (see Chapter 61). Each symptom elicited should be thoroughly described. Symptom characteristics include quality, quantity, timing, exacerbating and relieving factors, and interference with activities such as mobilization, sleep, eating, and work. A thorough review of systems is important to elicit symptoms not volunteered. Exploring the meaning attributed to a symptom by the patient and family is essential. New symptoms may be attributed to recurring or progressing cancer or to treatment side effects, or they may be interpreted as a sign of impending death.

Medication History

A history of treatments tried in the past, their effects, and particularly their side effects is essential. Many symptoms such as constipation are side effects of many common medications. Screening for medications and anticancer therapy side effects may elicit symptoms assumed to be normal and acceptable. Common adverse effects of chemotherapy and radiotherapy include nausea, vomiting, mucositis, diarrhea, skin reactions, alopecia, fatigue, and menopausal symptoms. Complementary medicines, herbal agents, and vitamins are commonly used and may interact with prescription medicines and with chemotherapy.

Psychosocial Screens

Anxiety, depression, sleep, and family problems may contribute to or be caused by other symptoms. Many patients do not report them unless specifically asked. Asking simple questions (e.g., Are you depressed?) quickly screens for psychological distress.[11]

Goals of Care

Goals of care, performance status, and life expectancy influence appropriate investigations and interventions. Invasive investigations are less appropriate for a patient with a life expectancy of hours to days than for an ambulatory patient receiving active treatment with a life expectancy of months.

Documentation

Systematic documentation is essential for review, especially in a team environment. Documentation should include a summary of symptoms and their characteristics, the proposed cause, and intervention, and it should

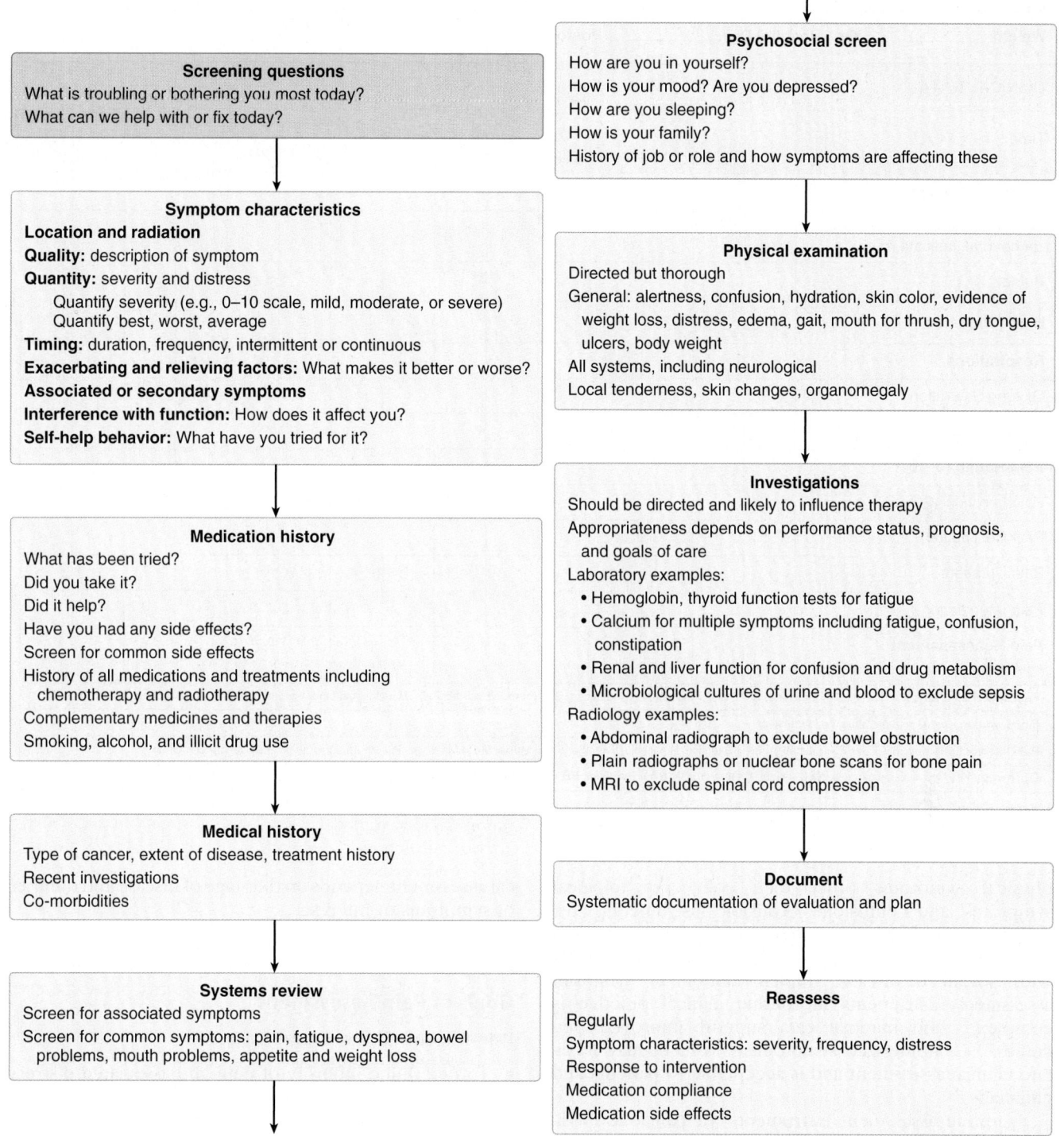

FIGURE 63-1   Flowchart for clinical symptom assessment.

prompt further review. Examples of systematic documentation include the Cleveland Clinic Foundation vital signs chart (Fig. 63-2) and palliative medicine problem list.[12]

Reassessment

Symptoms should be reassessed regularly. Appropriate time intervals depend on symptom severity and patient's location (i.e., inpatient or outpatient). Outpatients may require follow-up by telephone. Reassessment includes symptoms already detected, their response to treatment, and screening for new symptoms and medication side effects. Outpatients need detailed information about after-hours support—who to call and specific instructions about when to call.

SYMPTOM ASSESSMENT INSTRUMENTS

Symptom assessment instruments detect more symptoms than a clinical evaluation. This is especially the case for

Date _____   Page _1 of 12_____

Weight _____ Kg Hospital Day: _____ Postop Day: _____

IMPRINT / LABEL

CLINICAL DATA													
Time / Initials													
I.D. Band Present													
Temperature (if not oral, indicate route)													
Pulse													
Blood Pressure													
Respirations													
Oxygen Saturation / %													
Oxygen Therapy													
Pain Rating (0–10)													
Pain Location													
Pain Description													
Pain Duration													
Pain Intervention													
Pain Reassessment (0–10)													

Pain Description Key: **B** = Burning, **C** = Crushing, **D** = Dull, **I** = Incision, **R** = Radiating, **S** = Sharp, **ST** = Stabbing, **SU** = Surgical/other than incision pain, **T** = Throbbing, **O** = Other

Pain Duration Key: **C** = Continuous, **I** = Intermittent

Pain Interventions Key: **C** = Cold, **E** = Education, **EX** = Exercise, **H** = Heat, **I** = Imagery, **M** = Music, **MA** = Massage, **P** = Pharmacology, **R** = Relaxation, **O** = Other

O₂ Therapy Key: **NC** = Nasal cannula, **NRB** = Nonrebreather mask, **RA** = Room air, **RB** = Rebreather mask, **SM** = Simple mask, **TC** = Trach collar, **VM** = Venti mask

FIGURE 63-2 Vital signs chart at the Cleveland Clinic Foundation.

physical symptoms other than pain, psychological symptoms, and confusion.[13] Available instruments have significant problems, including incomplete symptom lists[14] and completion difficulties, especially for patients with advanced disease. Implementation of symptom assessment instruments in routine clinical practice is complex,[15] and minimal data support improved outcomes.[16] Computerized symptom assessment may facilitate clinical assessment and is acceptable to patients and clinicians.[17,18]

Symptom assessment instruments for palliative medicine include the Edmonton Symptom Assessment System (ESAS), M.D. Anderson Symptom Inventory (MDASI), Memorial Symptom Assessment Scale (MSAS), Rotterdam Symptom Checklist (RSCL), and Symptom Distress Scale (SDS).[19] The length of these instruments ranges from 9 (ESAS) to 32 items (MSAS). Some assess only symptom severity (e.g., ESAS, MDASI); others are multidimensional (e.g., MSAS). The ESAS and MSAS are validated for completion by family or staff caregivers. The ESAS, RSCL, MDASI, and MSAS assess global symptom distress, and the MDASI assesses interference from symptoms. Long, multidimensional instruments may be difficult for patients with advanced disease to complete. Instrument choice for clinical assessment depends on the stage of disease and number of symptoms of interest.

PAIN

Goals of Pain Assessment

Pain is assessed for several reasons:

- To determine intensity of pain and associated distress and interference
- To formulate a differential diagnosis of cause and contributing factors
- To formulate an appropriate plan of investigation and management
- To communicate the plan to the patient, family, and other team members
- To document and reassess the nature or degree of pain

Pain Classification

Pain in cancer is usually persistent and related to the cancer (Table 63-1). Pain attributed to anticancer treatment or noncancer causes is less common.[20] Most patients with cancer pain have two or more different types of pain. Classification of pain as nociceptive or neuropathic provides clues to the underlying pathophysiology and possible response to opioid and adjuvant analgesics. Many pain syndromes have mixed nociceptive and neuropathic qualities.

History

Pain is a subjective experience. It is essential to listen to and believe the patient. Each pain syndrome should be assessed separately. A body diagram helps document many sites of pain. Pain severity should be quantified. Categorical or numerical scales are easiest to administer, and they can be verbal or written. A simple question can be used to quantify pain: How would you rate your pain on a scale of 0 to 10, where 0 is no pain, and 10 is the worst pain you can imagine? Pain should be rated in the present and at its worst, best, and average levels.

Pain characteristics identify the likely source and pathophysiology (Table 63-2). Referred pain is common in visceral (e.g., shoulder tip pain of liver lesions) or neuropathic pain syndromes. Neuropathic pain is often referred along the distribution of the affected nerve. Bone or muscle pain may be worsened or precipitated by movement; visceral pain may improve. The time course of pain is important. New or rapidly escalating pain suggests progressive disease or an emergent complication (e.g., spinal cord compression). Visceral or neuropathic pain may be associated with autonomic effects (e.g., nausea, vomiting, sweating, pallor, altered pulse and blood pressure).

Breakthrough pain is associated with more severe and frequent background pain, more pain-related functional impairment, and worse mood.[21] Breakthrough pain may be related to movement, end-of-dose failure, or inadequate background analgesia.

Contributing factors in poorly controlled pain are described in Box 63-2. These factors should be screened for, especially noncompliance and psychosocial issues, including depression and sleep problems.

The medication history includes background dosage and the time and the number of as-needed (i.e., pro re nata [PRN]) doses in a 24-hour period. Timing of PRN doses may indicate end-of-dose failure of around-the-clock medication. Compliance, side effects, and benefit should be assessed for all medications. Common opioid side effects include dry mouth, sedation, nausea, constipation, and myoclonus.[22] Itch, urinary retention, vomiting, delirium, and respiratory depression are less common.

Examination

Focused examination of a painful site or system includes observation, palpation, percussion, auscultation, passive and active movement, and a neurological examination.[23] Signs on observation include skin changes (e.g., pallor, erythema, sweating, breakdown), deformity of bone or joint, muscle wasting, and abnormal posture. Palpation may elicit tenderness, mass, organomegaly, or distended bowel loops. Percussion differentiates distention due to gas from fluid accumulation. Percussion of vertebrae or bony prominences may elicit localized tenderness. Auscultation may reveal hyperactive bowel sounds due to obstruction or reduced or absent bowel sounds in a patient with ileus. Passive and active movement may reproduce pain. Gait should be observed for abnormalities and risk of falls.

A thorough neurological examination includes mental status, cranial nerves, power, sensation, coordination, and reflexes. Signs elicited in neuropathic pain include allo-

Box 63-2 Poorly Controlled Pain: Contributing Factors
Patient Related
Emotional distress, anxiety, depression, sleep problems
Delirium
Medication Noncompliance
Medication side effects
Fear of opioid addiction, tolerance
Neuropathic pain
History of drug or alcohol dependency
Financial, spiritual, or social concerns
Physician Related
Inappropriate assessment and prescribing
Concern about addiction and tolerance

TABLE 63-1 Pain Classification	
Nociceptive pain	Pain due to activation of nociceptors located in skin, mucous membranes, bones, joints, muscles, (somatic) or solid or hollow organs (visceral)
Neuropathic pain	Pain due to abnormal activation or injury to central or peripheral nervous system
Breakthrough pain	Transient pain occurring on a background of stable pain
Incident pain	Pain due to movement or weight bearing

TABLE 63-2 Clinical Pain Syndromes				
FEATURE	SUPERFICIAL SOMATIC	DEEP SOMATIC	VISCERAL	NEUROPATHIC
Source	Skin, mucosa	Muscles, joints, bones	Solid and hollow organs, tumor masses	Nerve damage
Description	Hot, sharp, stinging	Dull, aching throbbing	Deep, dull, throbbing, cramping	Stabbing, shooting. hot, searing, electric shock, tingling, burning, numbness
Localization	Well localized	Well localized	Poorly localized	Nerve or dermatome distribution
Adapted from Therapeutic Guidelines: Palliative Care, version 2. North Melbourne, Australia: Therapeutic Guidelines Limited, 2005.				

dynia (i.e., pain due to nonpainful stimuli such as light touch) and sensory or motor signs in a nerve or dermatomal distribution.

Investigations

Potential treatment options, prognosis, and goals of care must be considered before investigations begin. If an investigation is unlikely to alter the treatment plan, it may be inappropriate. Recent serum renal and liver function test results may influence the appropriateness of medications metabolized by these systems. Radiological investigations may determine causes of pain, such as plain radiographs and a bone scan for musculoskeletal pain, computed tomography for visceral pain, and magnetic resonance imaging for neuropathic pain.

Clinical Pain Syndromes

Spinal cord compression is a palliative medicine emergency. Clinicians should be alert to this possibility in patients with known vertebral metastases and metastatic cancer at time of diagnosis.[24] It is characterized by new-onset or severe middle or upper back pain. Pain may radiate to upper or lower limbs or occur as a band around the chest or abdomen. Pain may be worsened by lying supine or by a Valsalva maneuver. The history should screen for bladder or bowel problems, limb weakness, and sensory changes. A full neurological examination, including perianal sensation and anal tone, is essential.

Bone pain is common in patients with advanced cancer. Pain is worse with movement or weight bearing; it is well localized, dull, aching, or throbbing. Examination may reveal skin changes, muscle wasting, deformity, tenderness, pain reproduced by movement, and gait abnormalities.

Pain Assessment Scales and Instruments

Routine use of pain scales improves detection of pain, even in cognitively impaired elderly people.[25] Systematic pain evaluation in hospitalized patients reduces pain intensity.[26] Inpatient pain charts should include a record of intervention and reassessment[27] (see Fig. 63-2). For outpatients, twice-daily recording in a pain diary has good compliance, and it improves coping skills and communication.[28] Pain diaries also promote recording of regular and breakthrough medication doses, facilitating review of compliance and overall pain control.[29] A choice of pain scales (e.g., faces, categorical, numerical) is ideal because the ability to complete them varies.[30]

Multidimensional pain assessment instruments for clinical use include the Memorial Pain Assessment Chart (MPAC)[31] and Brief Pain Inventory (BPI).[32] The MPAC has visual analogue scales for pain severity, pain relief, and mood and a verbal pain-rating scale. The BPI has numeric scales (0 to 10) for pain at its worst, least, and average levels and for right now, and it has seven questions about pain interference with activity, mood, walking, work, relationships, sleep, and enjoyment of life. A body diagram and pain relief scales are included.

FATIGUE

Fatigue frequently is not reported because patients consider it "inevitable, unimportant, and untreatable."[33] Physicians are often reluctant to screen for fatigue, because it is a complex symptom with no single treatment option. Definitions of cancer-related fatigue vary. The National Comprehensive Cancer Network (NCCN) defines fatigue as "a persistent, subjective sense of tiredness related to cancer or cancer treatment that interferes with usual functioning." Proposed ICD-10 criteria highlight the multidimensional nature of fatigue.[34] The criteria specify significant fatigue over a 2-week period plus five other symptoms, including weakness, insomnia, concentration difficulties, reduced motivation, emotional reactivity, memory problems, and post-exertional malaise. Specific causes of fatigue are unknown. Contributing factors include advanced disease, anticancer therapy or other medications (e.g., opioids, antidepressants, antiemetics, antihistamines), anemia, biochemical abnormalities, endocrine abnormalities, organ failure, and psychosocial factors.

History

All palliative medicine patients should be screened for fatigue with questions.[34] Do you get tired for no reason? Are you experiencing any fatigue? Severity also can be quantified by a question. How would you rate your tiredness or fatigue on a scale of 0 to 10? A score of 4 or greater indicates need for further evaluation.[35]

Fatigue should be evaluated using the schema for symptom evaluation. The character of fatigue may include tiredness, weakness, exhaustion, or problems with mood, concentration, and motivation. Exacerbating and relieving factors should be documented. The temporal pattern of fatigue includes onset, duration, daily pattern, response to the treatment cycle, and activity. Fatigue affects activity, social functioning, and work.

Nutritional status, weight loss, activity level, and physical fitness should be assessed. Restricted physical activity (e.g., due to angina, arthritis) may affect treatment recommendations. Contributing factors, including poorly controlled symptoms such as pain, depression, anxiety, and sleep disturbance, should be thoroughly assessed (Box 63-3). Medications and co-morbidities, including cardiac or respiratory failure and thyroid dysfunction, may contribute to a patient's fatigue. Co-morbidities may result from anticancer chemotherapy or radiotherapy.

Examination and Investigations

The examination should be a thorough review of all systems, including body weight, temperature, pallor, muscle wasting and strength, gait, and functional status.

Laboratory screening tests should include hemoglobin; electrolytes, including sodium, potassium, magnesium, and calcium; and glucose, renal, liver, and thyroid function if not recently performed.

Assessment Instruments

Fatigue, lack of energy, and tiredness subscales are included in the ESAS, MDASI, and MSAS. The Brief Fatigue

Poorly controlled symptoms, e.g., pain
Psychological: depression, anxiety, or sleep problems
Anorexia, cachexia
Immobility, muscle wasting
Anemia
Electrolyte abnormalities: sodium, calcium
Medications

- Opioids
- Sedatives

Anticancer treatment

- Chemotherapy
- Radiotherapy

Co-morbidities

- Cardiac failure
- Respiratory
- Endocrine: thyroid, gonadal
- Renal
- Hepatic

Inventory (BFI) is a multi-item instrument for clinical assessment.[36] Questions evaluate fatigue right now, usually, and at its worst on numerical scales of 0 to 10. Interference with activity, mood, walking, work, relationships, and enjoyment of life are rated on separate numerical scales.

SPECIAL POPULATIONS

Non–English-Speaking Groups

Non–English-speaking patients may receive inferior symptom assessment and management because of communication problems and cultural differences.[37] Professional interpreters should be used rather than family members. This avoids additional distress and burden for the family and facilitates accurate translation of medical information.[38] Multilingual symptom assessment tools include the BPI, BFI, ESAS, and MDASI.

Elderly or Confused Patients

Elderly or confused patients are at risk for underdiagnosis of pain. Contributing factors include communication difficulties, reluctance to report pain, belief that pain is normal in old age, and fears of opioid addiction and side effects. Systematic use of pain scales by nursing home residents with mild to moderate dementia increases the frequency of a pain diagnosis.[25,39] Instrument completion rates vary, and simultaneous use of several scales (e.g., faces, categorical, numerical) is recommended. Simple categorical scales are the easiest to complete, especially for symptoms other than pain.[39,40] Visual analogue scales are especially problematic for the elderly.[39] Patients with severe dementia who are unable to complete any verbal scale should be assessed with a behavioral scale (e.g., Abbey Pain Scale).[41] An extended version of the ESAS has been used to detect symptom burden in community-dwelling elderly with advanced, chronic conditions.[4]

Children

Children dying in hospitals have a high symptom burden and distress.[42,43] Symptoms are similar to those in adults: fatigue, pain, dyspnea, drowsiness, psychological distress, poor appetite, nausea, vomiting, constipation, and diarrhea. Symptoms are often not documented and infrequently treated successfully.[42]

Toddlers and preschoolers may use words other than pain (e.g., ouch, hurt, booboo). They cannot comprehend abstract concepts and therefore may not describe pain characteristics. Young children may be able to draw the location of pain on a body diagram. Many pediatric pain scales are available. Most instruments were developed to evaluate acute or procedural pain.[44,45] Children younger than 3 years are assessed using a behavioral scale (e.g., Face, Legs, Activity, Cry, and Consolability [FLACC] scale). Children older than 3 years may be able to use a faces pain scale (e.g., Oucher Scale, Poker Chip Scale). The Oucher Scale combines six photographs depicting facial expressions ranging from no hurt to biggest hurt with a scale of 0 to 10. It is available in several ethnic versions. The Poker Chip tool asks children to quantify their pain between 0 (no hurt) and 4 (most hurt) chips. School-age children may be able to understand numerical, categorical, or modified visual analogue scales (e.g., thermometer). For multiple symptoms, a modified MSAS is validated for children with cancer who are older than 7 years.[46]

Advanced Noncancer Diagnoses

Patients with advanced noncancer diagnoses have symptom burdens similar to those of cancer patients, but they less frequently receive palliative services.[1] This may reflect uncertainty about the prognosis and natural history. Pain, breathlessness, and fatigue affect more than 50%.[9] Noncancer patients have more dyspnea and cough and have rates of fatigue and psychological symptoms similar to those of cancer patients. Cachexia is common in patients with human immunodeficiency virus (HIV) infection, heart failure, or renal failure. Anxiety, depression, and insomnia are common in all these conditions.[9] Patients with advanced motor neuron disease experience symptoms from chronic muscle wasting and weakness. These include spasticity, fasciculations, cramps, and contractures. Respiratory muscle weakness results in chronic hypoventilation symptoms, including sleepiness, fatigue, poor concentration, and headaches. More than 50% have uncontrollable episodes of laughing or crying due to pseudobulbar affect.[47] A thorough symptom assessment should be based on the same schema as for cancer symptoms. The MSAS is validated in noncancer patients and may improve systematic symptom assessment.[1]

CONCLUSIONS AND RESEARCH CHALLENGES

Palliative medicine patients experience many symptoms, but symptoms often are not reported to physicians (see "Common Errors"). A thorough history is essential to identify the symptom burden.

Quantification of symptom severity, especially pain, improves treatment outcomes. Use of systematic symptom assessment instruments increases symptom reporting.

Common Errors

- Communication—not listening to the patient and family
- Failure to evaluate treatable causes of symptoms, leading to blind prescribing
- Not screening for medication compliance and side effects
- Failure to evaluate psychosocial factors contributing to symptom distress
- Poor documentation and lack of review

Symptom assessment instruments are validated for cancer and noncancer patients, children, and the elderly, and they are available in many languages.

Research challenges remain. For example, we need to know how to incorporate systematic symptom assessment into routine clinical practice and whether systematic symptom assessment alters clinical outcomes.

REFERENCES

1. Tranmer JE, Heyland D, Dudgeon D, et al. Measuring the symptom experience of seriously ill cancer and noncancer hospitalized patients near the end of life with the Memorial Symptom Assessment Scale. J Pain Symptom Manage 2003;25:420-429.
2. Glare P. Clinical predictors of survival in advanced cancer. J Support Oncol 2005;3:331-339.
3. Homsi J, Walsh D, Rivera N, et al. Symptom evaluation in palliative medicine: Patient report vs systematic assessment. Support Care Cancer 2006;14:444-453.
4. Walke LM, Byers AL, McCorkle R, et al. Symptom assessment in community-dwelling older adults with advanced chronic disease. J Pain Symptom Manage 2006;31:31-37.
5. Stromgren AS, Sjogren P, Goldschmidt D, et al. Symptom priority and course of symptomatology in specialized palliative care. J Pain Symptom Manage 2006;31:199-206.
6. Donnelly S. The symptoms of advanced cancer. Semin Oncol 1995;22:67-72.
7. Walsh D. The symptoms of advanced cancer: Relationship to age, gender, and performance status in 1,000 patients. Support Care Cancer 2000;8:175-179.
8. Donnelly S. The symptoms of advanced cancer: Identification of clinical and research priorities by assessment of prevalence and severity. J Palliat Care 1995;11:27-32.
9. Solano JP. A comparison of symptom prevalence in far advanced cancer, AIDS, heart disease, chronic obstructive pulmonary disease and renal disease. J Pain Symptom Manage 2006;31:58-69.
10. Walsh D. Symptom clustering in advanced cancer. Support Care Cancer 2006;14:831-836.
11. Chochinov HM, Wilson KG, Enns M, et al. "Are you depressed?" screening for depression in the terminally ill. Am J Psychiatry 1997;154:674-676.
12. Walsh D. Communication in palliative medicine: A pilot study of a problem list to capture complex medical information. Am J Hosp Palliat Care 2004;21:365-371.
13. Stromgren AS, Groenvold M, Pedersen L, et al. Does the medical record cover the symptoms experienced by cancer patients receiving palliative care? A comparison of the record and patient self-rating. J Pain Symptom Manage 2001;21:189-196.
14. Stromgren AS, Groenvold M, Pedersen L, et al. Symptomatology of cancer patients in palliative care: Content validation of self-assessment questionnaires against medical records. Eur J Cancer 2002;38:788-794.
15. Bourbonnais FF. Introduction of a pain and symptom assessment tool in the clinical setting—lessons learned. J Nurs Manage 2004;12:194-200.
16. Hoekstra J, de Vos R, van Duijn NP, et al. Using the symptom monitor in a randomized controlled trial: The effect on symptom prevalence and severity. J Pain Symptom Manage 2006;31:22-30.
17. Berry DL, Trigg LJ, Lober WB, et al. Computerized symptom and quality-of-life assessment for patients with cancer. Part I. Development and pilot testing. Oncol Nurs Forum 2004;31:E75-E83.
18. Mullen KH. Computerized symptom and quality-of-life assessment for patients with cancer. Part II. Acceptability and usability. Oncol Nurs Forum 2004;31:E84-E89.
19. Kirkova J, Davis MP, Walsh D, et al. Cancer symptom assessment instruments: A systematic review. J Clin Oncol 2006;24:1459-1473.
20. Grond S, Zech D, Diefenbach C, et al. Assessment of cancer pain: A prospective evaluation in 2266 cancer patients referred to a pain service. Pain 1996;64:107-114.
21. Portenoy RK. Breakthrough pain: Definition, prevalence and characteristics. Pain 1990;41:273-281.
22. Glare P. The adverse effects of morphine: A prospective survey of common symptoms during repeated dosing for chronic cancer pain. Am J Hosp Palliat Med 2006;23:229-235.
23. Portenoy RK. The physical examination in cancer pain assessment. Semin Oncol Nurs 1997;13:25-29.
24. Lu C, Gonzalez RG, Jolesz FA, et al. Suspected spinal cord compression in cancer patients: A multidisciplinary risk assessment. J Support Oncol 2005;3:305-312.
25. Kamel HK, Phlavan M, Malekgoudarzi B, et al. Utilizing pain assessment scales increases the frequency of diagnosing pain among elderly nursing home residents. J Pain Symptom Manage 2001;21:450-455.
26. Faries JE, Mills DS, Goldsmith KW, et al. Systematic pain records and their impact on pain control. A pilot study. Cancer Nurs 1991;14:306-313.
27. Bercovitch M. Pain and symptom management. Multidimensional Continuous Pain Assessment Chart (MCPAC) for terminal cancer patients: A preliminary report. Am J Hosp Palliat Care 2002;19:419-425.
28. de Wit R, van Dam F, Hanneman M, et al. Evaluation of the use of a pain diary in chronic cancer pain patients at home. Pain 1999;79:89-99.
29. Maunsell E, Allard P, Dorval M, et al. A brief pain diary for ambulatory patients with advanced cancer: Acceptability and validity. Cancer 2000;88:2387-2397.
30. Jensen MP. The validity and reliability of pain measures in adults with cancer. J Pain 2003;4:2-21.
31. Fishman B, Pasternak S, Wallenstein SL, et al. The Memorial Pain Assessment Card. A valid instrument for the evaluation of cancer pain. Cancer 1987;60:1151-1158.
32. Cleeland CS. Pain assessment: Global use of the brief pain inventory. Ann Acad Med Singapore 1994;23:129-138.
33. Stone P, Richardson A, Ream E, et al. Cancer-related fatigue: Inevitable, unimportant and untreatable? Results of a multi-centre patient survey. Cancer Fatigue Forum. Ann Oncol 2000;11:971-975.
34. Portenoy RK. Cancer-related fatigue: Guidelines for evaluation and management. Oncologist 1999;4:1-10.
35. National Comprehensive Cancer Network. Clinical Practice Guidelines in Oncology: Cancer-Related Fatigue, version 2, 2005. Available at http://www.nccn.org/professionals/physician_gls/PDF/fatigue.pdf (accessed November 2007).
36. Mendoza TR, Wang XS, Cleeland CS, et al. The rapid assessment of fatigue severity in cancer patients: Use of the Brief Fatigue Inventory. Cancer 1999;85:1186-1196.
37. Chan A. Comparison of palliative care needs of English- and Non–English-speaking patients. J Palliat Care 1999;15:26-30.
38. Searight HR. Cultural diversity at the end of life: Issues and guidelines for family physicians. Am Fam Physician 2005;71:515-522.
39. Closs SJ, Barr B, Briggs M, et al. A comparison of five pain assessment scales for nursing home residents with varying degrees of cognitive impairment. J Pain Symptom Manage 2004;27:196-205.
40. Radbruch L, Sabatowski R, Loick G, et al. Cognitive impairment and its influence on pain and symptom assessment in a palliative care unit: Development of a minimal documentation system. Palliat Med 2000;14:266-276.
41. Abbey J, Piller N, De Bellis A, et al. The abbey pain scale: A 1-minute numerical indicator for people with end-stage dementia. Int J Palliat Nurs 2004;10:6-13.
42. Wolfe J, Grier HE, Klar N, et al. Symptoms and suffering at the end of life in children with cancer. N Engl J Med 2000;342:326-333.
43. Drake R. The symptoms of dying children. J Pain Symptom Manage 2003;26:594-603.
44. Franck LS, Greenberg CS, Stevens B. Pain assessment in infants and children. Pediatr Clin North Am 2000;47:487-512.
45. National Comprehensive Cancer Network. Clinical Practice Guidelines in Oncology: Pediatric Cancer Pain, version 1, 2005. Available at http://www.nccn.org/professionals/physician_gls/PDF/pediatric_pain.pdf (accessed November 2007).
46. Collins JJ, Devine TD, Dick GS, et al. The measurement of symptoms in young children with cancer: The validation of the Memorial Symptom Assessment Scale in children aged 7-12. J Pain Symptom Manage 2002;23:10-16.
47. Borasio G. Palliative care in amyotrophic lateral sclerosis. Neurol Clin 2001;19:829-847.

SUGGESTED READING

Davis MP, Walsh D. Cancer pain: How to measure the fifth vital sign. Cleve Clin J Med 2004;71:625-632.

Franck LS, Greenburg CS, Stevens B. Pain assessment in infants and children. Pediatr Clin North Am 2000;47:487-512.

National Comprehensive Cancer Network. Clinical Practice Guidelines in Oncology: Adult Cancer Pain, version 2, 2005. Available at http://www.nccn.org/professionals/physician_gls/PDF/pain.pdf (accessed November 2007).

National Comprehensive Cancer Network. Clinical Practice Guidelines in Oncology, version 1, 2006, Cancer-Related Fatigue. Available at http://www.nccn.org/professionals/physician_gls/PDF/fatigue.pdf (accessed November 2007).

National Comprehensive Cancer Network. Clinical Practice Guidelines in Oncology, version 1, 2005, Pediatric Cancer Pain. Available at http://www.nccn.org/professionals/physician_gls/PDF/pediatric_pain.pdf (accessed November 2007).

Portenoy RK. The physical examination in cancer pain assessment. Semin Oncol Nurs 1997;13:25-29.

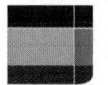

CHAPTER **64**

Qualitative and Quantitative Symptom Assessment

Victor T. Chang

KEY POINTS

- The subjective assessment of symptoms is based on specific psychometric theories.

- Symptom assessment instruments need to be valid and reliable.

- For assessing a specific symptom, an instrument needs to have been specifically validated for that purpose.

- In palliative medicine, symptoms are the common language shared by clinicians, patients, and caregivers, and they are classified as patient-reported outcomes.

PRINCIPLES OF ASSESSMENT AND MEASUREMENT

Symptoms are biological phenomena, such as temperature or blood pressure, and they can fluctuate over time. Unlike temperature or blood pressure, symptoms are reported by the patient. The idea that symptoms can be measured in a rigorous way has gained acceptance only recently. Psychophysics and psychometrics have provided a way of conceptualizing symptoms. Psychophysics relates an external stimulus to a perceived sensation. An important contribution of psychophysics is the concept of the *just noticeable difference* (JND), defined as the smallest change in the stimulus that changes perception. The goal of psychometrics is to make intrinsically coherent and scaled measurements of abstract concepts, such as pain. Symptom assessment instruments have been developed with classic test theory, and in the future, they may be developed with item response theory.

Classic Test Theory

The classic test theory underlies the development and construction of currently available instruments. These instruments are derived from the theory underlying education tests, originally developed to measure abstract concepts such as intelligence or aptitude. Based on answers to the same set of questions, the respondent's level of intelligence (or symptoms) is estimated from the sum of the answers. The interpretation of the score is sample dependent, and scores from one population may not be generalizable to another. Depending on the population, all the respondents may answer no to a question (i.e., floor effect) or yes (i.e., ceiling effect).

Item Response Theory

In the item response theory, the response to a test item is characterized as a probability of answering an item as a function of the item's level of difficulty, the respondent, and how the slope of the response curve varies with the severity of the symptom. With these three parameters characterized, an item bank can be developed, and items from the bank are used to select or construct questionnaires with predictable psychometric properties for the population and question at hand. This approach ultimately provides more flexibility, much shorter questionnaires, and a more statistically precise assessment of the answers. It allows comparisons of answers from responses to different instruments and avoids problems with floor and ceiling effects. However, it is unclear whether the questions selected will be the best ones, especially if the examiner is trying to capture the extremes of experience. The development process is resource intensive. A large effort has been funded by the National Institutes of Health (NIH) to develop and test items for symptom assessment in several chronic conditions. Information about the Patient-Reported Outcomes Measurement Information System (PROMIS) can be found online (http://www.nihpromis.org).

The goal of clinimetrics is describing a clinical phenomenon. The Apgar score is usually cited as a good example. It is empirical, not based on a single concept, and useful. Another example is the Karnofsky Performance Status, a mixture of functional and physical descriptors. Unlike psychometrics, clinimetrics is not restricted to a conceptually pure approach. Clinimetric instruments may seem messy to psychometricians, but they can be quite useful to health care providers.

Dimensions of Symptom Assessment

The same symptom can affect the patient and family in different ways. A severe symptom can make a patient bedridden (i.e., functional effect), depressed (i.e., emotional effect), isolated (i.e., social effect), and unpleasant (i.e., behavioral effect). The nature of the symptom can be expressed as severity, frequency, distress, or in other ways. Patients respond in different dimensions when asked about how severe a symptom is. One symptom is thought to occur frequently, and another symptom is unpleasant because it interferes with the activities of daily living. This variety is reflected in the concept of multiple dimensions, in which one dimension is unaffected by other dimensions, but all are relevant to understanding the effect of the symptoms. Instruments vary in which dimensions are selected and how the choices for answers are provided. In one study that compared dimensions of intensity and frequency of fatigue, both dimensions were equivalent.[1]

Quantitative instruments ask the respondent to give a number or a rating of a symptom or an aspect of a symptom. The number can be between 0 and 10 (or 100), derived from a mark on a 10-cm line (i.e., visual analogue scale) or a Likert rating (e.g., not at all, a little bit, somewhat, quite a bit, very much). Qualitative instruments may ask about categories. For example, a patient is asked whether his pain is burning or stabbing or is asked to describe how his breathing feels to him. Behavioral and functional aspects may also be cataloged this way.

What is the perfect assessment instrument? Ultimately, this depends on what is desired of the instrument (see "Applications"). Symptom instruments, like other scientific instruments, are required to be valid, reliable, responsive to change, and precise. Instrument validity means that the instrument measures what it is supposed to measure. Commonly accepted forms of validity for instruments include face validity, content validity, criterion validity, and test-retest validity. Face validity means that the item seems relevant to the symptom under study. Content validity means that the kinds of questions seem adequate to the person who plans to use the instrument in describing the symptoms and to the patient. In criterion validity, the instrument is compared with other accepted measures obtained concurrently. With the use of correlation coefficients, symptom scores are correlated in sign and magnitude with other accepted measures. Test-retest validity compares measurements at two points in time.

Instruments are different from physical scientific devices in that they are based on constructs, a concept about the symptom measured. The symptom, which can be perceived only by the patient, is described as a latent variable. Construct validity refers to the degree to which measurements of the instrument reflect the variability of the symptom as they are arranged on the continuum of the construct. Construct validity applies to the meanings and interpretations of the instrument scores, not of the instrument itself, and it is estimated using bivariate correlations and multivariate regression models. On one level, an instrument may be valid, but on a more abstract level, the same instrument may not be valid because it may not conceptually capture the symptom to be measured.[2]

Reliability means that the measurement does not change if the measured symptom has not changed (e.g., test-retest, paired correlation coefficient), and the standard threshold is 0.70. Internal reliability means that responses to statements about the symptom are internally consistent (e.g., Cronbach's alpha). Responsiveness means that if the symptom changes, the change will be detected by the instrument. Instruments that are reliable may not be responsive to change, and this has led to the development of "transition items" to capture change. Criteria have been proposed for assessment of transition changes.[3] For scales with continuous numbers, evidence is accumulating that one half of a standard deviation (MID) can provide an estimate of the clinically significant difference,[4] and this may provide a new way to analyze data from symptom instruments. Other potentially important features are discussed later (see "Applications").

Principles of Symptom Assessment Tool Development

Assessment instruments are made up of items. An item is a question. Current thinking about how the item should be written posits a context, stem, and response options. The context provides a time frame, which may be a day, a week, or at most a month. Shorter time frames such as 1 day are less likely to suffer from patient recall bias. However, because patients have good days and bad days, answers may be skewed if a 24-hour period is stipulated. A 7-day period is thought to represent a good balance between what patients can recall and an adequate sampling period. For an instrument that is used frequently, such as three times each day, no time frame is stipulated.

The stem is the statement or question itself (e.g., I have been feeling sad). The words in the question are often determined by the definition of the symptom employed or related experiences that are thought relevant. Symptoms are easy to recognize and difficult to define. Most definitions of symptoms (e.g., hot flashes) are consensus statements by medical specialty groups.[5] Another feature of the stem is that negative statements or questions can confuse patients (e.g., I have not been feeling sad).

The format of the response may be different. In a quantitative scale, the answer is a rating by number, category, or on a visual analogue scale. Choices can be ordered or ranked by increasing or decreasing levels (e.g., categorical answers, such as a little bit, somewhat, quite a bit, or very much), or they can be continuous numbers (e.g., 0 to 10, visual analogue scale). An important detail is the anchor, which is the words used to describe the two ends of the visual analogue or numerical scale. Another detail is the direction of the scale. Is it from least to greatest or greatest to least? Frequent changes in direction can confuse patients. When compared, visual analogue and numerical scales show good agreement.[6] Categorical scales are sometimes easier for patients to answer and for scoring, and the optimal number of categories ranges from five to seven. For analysis, work with patients who have pain suggests that it may not make much difference whether patients answer with a numerical rating scale, a category, or a visual analogue scale.[7]

In qualitative symptom assessment, the answers sought are more descriptive, such as "Tell me how it feels to you." This is what clinicians and patients are used to. For example, with pain assessment, the questions may be the quality of the pain, aggravating and relieving factors, and conditions of pain relief. In a qualitative scale, the patient is asked to choose from a collection of descriptors or to supply symptom descriptors. This approach has been used most extensively in assessing neuropathic pain or dyspnea.

To obtain the items, the developers of the instrument may survey patients, caregivers, and health care professionals for candidate items. After an item pool is developed, the items are reviewed for redundancy by the developers. Multivariate statistical analysis may be performed at this point, including factor analysis or cluster analysis. A draft instrument is then produced and administered to the population of interest along with other accepted tools or measures. The subject responses to the instrument are checked for self-consistency, and they are compared with the responses to the other measures. If there is a reasonable correlation, the tool is deemed usable. These aspects often require multivariate statistical analysis. The development of a summary score has proponents and critics. Proponents point to the advantages of a summary measure in statistical analyses, but critics are concerned that the score may mask important details. The instrument should then be studied in similar populations to verify its psychometric properties.

A related issue is determining whether symptoms have changed: "Are you better or worse?" Responses are often categorical and bidirectional, ranging from much worse to much better. The concept of a clinically significant difference is important for bedside assessment, symptom instrument development, and clinical trial design. An important theoretical consideration is the possibility of response shift. This results from physiological adaptation as circumstances change. If perception changes as patients adapt, symptom change may be underestimated or overestimated. From a patient-centered approach, this is what clinicians have to live with. On a research basis, it is an active area of interest in quality of life studies,[8] and it may be relevant to symptom assessments.

CLINICAL EVALUATION AND DIAGNOSIS

Symptom instruments can aid in clinical evaluation by identifying the presence of unreported symptoms and by providing patients' ratings of severity. Clinicians often underestimate the presence of symptoms and symptom distress.[9]

Assessment Tools

Several Web sites provide access to symptom assessment tools. These include the American Thoracic Society (http://www.atsqol.org), the Center to Advance Palliative Care (http://www.capc.org), the International Hospice Association (www.hospicecare.com), the Mapi Research Institute (www.mapi-research-inst.com; www.qolid.org), the Edmonton Regional Palliative Care Program (http://www.palliative.org), the Robert Wood Johnson Promoting Excellence in End of Life Care (http://www.promotingexcellence.org), the TIME: Toolkit of Instruments to Measure End-of-life Care (http://www.chcr.brown.edu/pcoc/Physical.htm), and the Oncology Nurse Society (http://www.ons.org/outcomes/measures; http://painconsortium.nih.gov/symptomresearch).

Symptom Tools in Specific Categories

Pain

Ratings of pain by patients can be rigorously analyzed to demonstrate analgesic effects.[10] Among the first formal symptom instruments was the McGill Pain Questionnaire. Developed to quantify pain, the pain descriptors in the instrument showed there were specific kinds of pain syndromes associated with descriptors. Since then, multiple instruments have been developed for pain. One hundred twenty-six pain instruments have been used in cancer pain studies.[11] A consensus has been reached on six core outcome domains for pain studies for chronic pain, which may also help development of future instruments for assessing pain in palliative medicine.[12,13] It has been suggested that a verbal five-category response is optimal.[14] An evidence review selected a 20-mm difference on a visual analogue scale or a 30% decline in pain intensity as clinically significant.[15] A 2-point change on the scale of 0 to 10 for pain is also clinically significant in assessing chronic pain.[16] A new generation of instruments has been developed for neuropathic pain.[17] The relevance of pain instrument content to palliative medicine remains a topic for investigation.

Fatigue

Fatigue can be difficult to study because of the lack of clear definitions. Unlike many other symptoms, it can be highly distressing, even when not severe. *Fatigue* can have different meanings for patients and physicians; it may imply muscular weakness, lethargy, sleepiness, mood disturbance (e.g., depression, difficulty concentrating), or other disturbances. Many instruments have been developed; some are unidimensional, and others are multidimensional.[18,19]

Depression

Depression refers to a symptom and a psychiatric diagnosis. The definition of depression in the *Diagnostic and Statistical Manual* (DSM) is depressed mood or loss of interest or pleasure in most activities for a period of at least 2 weeks and the presence of associated symptoms. Efforts to develop symptom instruments for depression have centered on implementation of the DSM criteria for depression. The problem is the applicability of diagnostic criteria to patients who are chronically ill with advanced illnesses and for whom many symptoms of depression overlap with those of underlying illnesses. Neither the Edmonton Symptom Assessment Scale (ESAS) nor the Hospital Anxiety and Depression Scale (HADS) is particularly sensitive for screening in palliative medicine. The NIH 2004 State of the Art Conference recommended currently available instruments for screening and medical interviews for diagnosis.[20,21]

Appetite

Visual analogue scales have been widely used in appetite research. Combinations of visual analogue scale items related to appetite can account for much of the variance. Visual analogue scale ratings of appetite predict feeding but not energy intake. The ratings may be most useful for within-subject comparisons because intersubject differences can account for much of the variance in experiments.[22]

Appetite assessment in oncology has been stimulated by research in the use of progestational agents such as megestrol acetate. These include the Mayo instrument, a series of visual analogue scales, and the Functional Assessment of Appetite Cachexia (FAACT). Single items, such as distress from lack of appetite, have also appeared. In a group of veterans, the FAACT, the Mayo instrument, and the single appetite item showed significant correlations with each other, with quality of life as measured by the sum of Functional Assessment of Cancer Therapy subscales (FACT SUMQOL), and with specific symptoms.[23]

Confusion

Instruments have been based on the DSM definition of delirium, which emphasizes reversible cognitive changes. Many original instruments were developed for psychiatric populations, and instruments such as the Confusion Assessment Method have been developed for medical patients.

Dry Mouth

The patient's perception of dryness and related symptoms, as indicated on a numerical or visual analog scale, has been used to assess xerostomia.[24] In one study, symptom relief did not correlate well with measures of salivary output.[25] This finding highlights the importance of subjective reporting of distress in interpreting results of a therapeutic intervention.

Dysphagia

Most studies have used an ordinal scale for measuring dysphagia in five categories: no symptoms, can take some solids, can take semisolids only, can take liquids, cannot swallow at all. Many studies do not specify whether the dysphagia scale was patient rated or observer rated. Improvements with stent placements have been on the order of 1 or 2 points, with most starting in the middle categories. Newer instruments developed for esophageal cancer provide more opportunities for patient-rated experiences (Table 64-1).

Respiratory Symptoms

Current methods for assessing dyspnea have been based on studies of tasks and effort in asthma and cardiac disease. Although many scales for dyspnea have been developed and validated,[26] few have been used in palliative care, and of these, the visual analogue scale is the most common. Patient-rated scales have been based on psychophysical descriptions of the relationship between work and perceived exertion. Three patient-rated scales include the Borg scale, the vertical visual analogue scale,[27] and the numerical rating scale.[28] Qualitative approaches with descriptors of dyspnea have led to the concept of a "language of dyspnea."[29] The descriptors may not be specific enough to regularly guide the differential diagnosis or therapy.[30] For dyspnea, a change of 1 point on the Borg scale and of 10 to 20 points on a visual analogue scale is likely clinically significant.[31] Assessment of cough has been reviewed.[32]

Nausea and Vomiting

Nausea has been described as an unpleasant sensation with an urge to vomit, retching as an effort to vomit, and vomiting as the expulsion of contents from the stomach.[33] Although nausea and vomiting cluster closely together,

clinicians prefer to maintain a distinction between the two.

The visual analogue scale has been widely used for patient-rated nausea assessments. In one study of ovarian cancer during cisplatin-based chemotherapy, there was good correlation between ratings on visual analogue scales and categorical scales, with a change of 20 mm on the visual analogue scale for each change in category. The visual analogue scale was thought to be more sensitive for individual changes and the categorical scale more sensitive for studying groups.[34] The methodology for assessment of nausea and vomiting in chemotherapy-associated nausea and vomiting is well developed, with primary and secondary end points for emesis set.[35] The definition of a *clinically significant* visual analogue scale change remains unclear.

Multiple Symptoms

Patients with advanced illnesses have many symptoms, which prompted the development of multisymptom tools. The ESAS was one of the first. The ESAS and other symptom instruments (Table 64-2) fill an important practical need in palliative medicine.[36]

DEVELOPMENTS AND CONTROVERSIES IN ASSESSMENT

Use and Evaluation of Instruments

Patient-based symptom scores are a standard method for assessment in palliative care. Garyali and colleagues[37] used the ESAS to evaluate the frequency of errors in interpretation of items and response scales by patients. They concluded that vigilance was required in reviewing the scores derived by the patients, particularly for the symptoms of sleep, appetite, and pain.[37] Errors were likely if doctors or nurses did not routinely check the way patients completed the assessment form. The study authors think more research is needed to determine the best way to teach patients how to minimize errors in self-reporting of symptoms.

Several research challenges remain:

- Comparing instruments derived from item response theory with older instruments
- Development of symptom instruments for symptoms that are less well studied
- Establishing clinically significant difference for other symptoms
- Determining cut-off points for different symptoms if a scale of 0 to 10 is used
- Computerized or automated assessment of symptoms
- Demonstration that symptom instruments improve delivery of health care
- Ways to display and interpret the data from symptom instruments
- Comparing the data from different symptom instruments
- Symptom assessment in special populations

As the final item indicates, more information is needed about the application of assessment tools to special groups of patients. A review of available instruments for pain concluded that no ideal instrument is available for the

TABLE 64-1 Chart of Patient-Rated Scales

SYMPTOM OR DISEASE	INSTRUMENT	NUMBER OF ITEMS	SUBSCALES	TYPES OF RESPONSES	TIME FRAME	ORIGINAL POPULATION	USE IN PALLIATIVE MEDICINE
Pain	VAS	1	None	Numerical	Not specified	Different populations	
	McGill Pain Questionnaire[42]	22	Pain rating index, number of words, present pain intensity	Yes/no	Not specified	Different groups of pain patients	
	Short Form McGill Pain Questionnaire[43]	17	3 pain scores	Likert, VAS	Not specified	Surgical inpatients	
	Brief Pain Inventory[44]	22	Severity Relief Interference	0-10 Multiple choice Descriptors	Past week	Cancer	
	Brief Pain Inventory–Short Form	4 1 7	Severity Relief Interference	0-10 0-100 0-10	24 hours	Cancer	
	Memorial Pain Assessment Card[45]	4	Pain severity, mood, relief	VAS, severity descriptors	Not specified	Cancer	
Fatigue	Brief Fatigue Inventory[46]	9	Severity, interference	0-10	Past week	Anemic cancer patients	
	FACIT-F[47]	13	None	Likert	Past week	Anemic cancer patients	Yes
	Schwartz Cancer Fatigue Scale[48]	28	Physical, emotional, cognitive, temporal	Likert, 0-4	Past 2-3 days	Cancer patients	
Confusion	Confusion Assessment Method[49]	10	None	Yes/no	Not specified	Geriatric patients	
	CAM-ICU[50]	11	None	Yes/no	Not specified	ICU patients	
	DSR-R-98[51]	10	None	0-3	Any time frame	Medical center psychiatric patients	Psychiatrist
	Memorial Delirium Assessment Scale[52]	10	None	0-3	Past several hours	Cancer patients	
	Bedside Confusion Scale[53]	2	None	NA	Not specified	Palliative medicine patients	
Cough	BCSS scale[54]	3	None	Likert, 4 points	None	COPD patients, clinical trial	
	Cough Quality of Life[55]	28	6	Likert, 4 points	None	COPD patients	

Continued

TABLE 64-1 Chart of Patient-Rated Scales—cont'd

SYMPTOM OR DISEASE	INSTRUMENT	NUMBER OF ITEMS	SUBSCALES	TYPES OF RESPONSES	TIME FRAME	ORIGINAL POPULATION	USE IN PALLIATIVE MEDICINE
	Leicester Cough Questionnaire[56]	19	3	Likert, 7 points	2 weeks	Chronic cough patients	
Dyspnea	VAS[57]	1	None	NA	Variable	COPD, hospice	Yes
Appetite	VAS	1	VAS	NA	Variable	Variable	
	NCCTG[58]	7 plus quality of life item	VAS	Categorical	Past week	Cancer cachexia	
	FAACT[59]	12	Likert	0-4	Past week	HIV cachexia	
Dysphagia	Ordinal scale	1	Likert	0-4	Variable	Esophageal cancer	
	FACT-E[60]	17	Likert	0-4	Past week	Esophageal cancer	
	EORTC Esophageal Module (OES18)[61]	18	Likert	1-4	Past week	Esophageal cancer	
Nausea	VAS	1	0-100		Variable	Hospice, chemotherapy	
Constipation	Constipation Assessment Scale[62]	8	None	Likert, 0-2	Past 3 days		
Sadness	VAS	VAS					
	Two-item scale[63]	2					
	CES-D[64]	20	None	Likert	Past week	Psychiatric patients	
	Beck Depression Inventory[65]	21	None	Likert	None	Various	
	Hospital Anxiety Depression[66]	14	Anxiety, depression	Likert	Past week	Physically sick patients	
	Geriatric Depression Scale[67]	15	None	Yes/no	Past week	Age > 55 years	
	Zung Depression Self-Assessment Test[68]	20	None	Likert	Now	Various	Yes
Itch	Eppendorf Itch Questionnaire[69]	111 descriptors, body map, VAS scale		Likert, 0-4	Not specified	Atopic dermatitis	
	Singapore Itch Questionnaire[70]	6 sensations, 4 affective descriptors, body map, VAS scale	Severity, descriptors, affect	Likert, 0-3	Not specified	Psoriasis, uremia, atopic dermatitis	

BCSS, Breathlessness, Cough, and Sputum Scale; CAM-ICU, Confusion Assessment Method for the Intensive Care Unit; CES-D, Center for Epidemiologic Studies Depression Scale; COPD, chronic obstructive pulmonary disease; DRS-R-98, Delirium Rating Scale-Revised-98; EORTC, European Organization for Research and Treatment of Cancer; FAACT, Functional Assessment of Anorexia/Cachexia Therapy; FACIT-F, Functional Assessment of Chronic Illness Therapy-Fatigue; FACT-E, Functional Assessment of Cancer Therapy-Esophageal; HIV, human immunodeficiency virus; ICU, intensive care unit; Likert, type of psychometric response scale; NA, not applicable; NCCTG, North Central Cancer Treatment Group; VAS, visual analogue scale.

TABLE 64-2	Multisymptom Instruments				
INSTRUMENT	**ITEMS**	**SUBSCALES**	**RESPONSE SCALE**	**TIME FRAME**	**ORIGINAL POPULATION**
Edmonton Symptom Assessment Scale[71]	9	None	VAS, NRS	Not specified	Hospice patients
Symptom Distress Scale[72]	15	None	Likert, 1-5	Today	Cancer patients
Rotterdam Symptom Checklist[73]	30 plus 7 ADL items	Psychological distress, physical distress	Likert	Past 3 days or past week	Cancer patients
MSAS[74]	32	4 subscales, 3 dimensions	Likert	7 days	Cancer patients
MSAS Short Form[75]	32	4 subscales, 1 dimension	Likert	7 days	Cancer patients
MSAS Condensed[76]	14	3 subscales, 2 dimensions	Likert	7 days	Cancer patients
Lung Cancer Symptom Scale[77]	9 5	Patient rated Observer rated	VAS, categorical	Past day	Cancer patients
M. D. Anderson Symptom Inventory[78]	19	2 dimensions: severity (13), interference (6)	0-10	Past 24 hours	Cancer patients
RAI-PC[79]	21	9 pain items 8 nonpain symptoms 4 cognitive items	Categorical, 0-2	Daily	Nursing home patients

ADL, activities of daily living; Likert, type of psychometric response scale; MSAS, Memorial Symptom Assessment Scale; NRS, numerical rating scale; RAI-PC, Resident Assessment Instrument for Palliative Care; VAS, visual analogue scale.

cognitively impaired.[38] A review of pain scales for pediatric patients[39] found that one instrument can be used for many symptoms in children.[40] Specialized instruments may be needed for multicultural assessments and intensive care unit patients.

Interpretation of Data

It is important to ensure that the patient understands and answers all the questions. Patient stamina is the rate-limiting factor. Formal interpretation of the answers to symptom instruments has advanced significantly, especially for pain. Work based on interference with function caused by pain suggests that the division of the 0-to-10 scale into mild (1 to 4), moderate (5 or 6), and severe (7 to 10) is true for different types of pain. This also may apply to other symptoms, but the cut points may be different. As with any other clinical test, bedside interpretation relies on the overall clinical picture and combination with other data gathered by the clinician.

Choosing an Instrument

Many instruments are available for assessing pain, fatigue, depression, and dyspnea. However, many have not been used in palliative medicine. Most were developed for cancer patients. The choice of an instrument depends on the intended application and the resources available. As with the use of medical tests, Alvin Feinstein would ask what the investigator was trying to prove and what the researcher intended to do with the results. Some symptoms have too many instruments, and some symptoms do not have enough instruments, prompting questions about when to make a new one and when to stick with what is available. Available symptom instruments should be obtained and reviewed for content, psychometric data, previous applications, and appearance.[41] Researchers are interested in psychometric data regarding reliability and validity. The developer should be contacted regarding questions. An investigator who has few resources and is interested in clinical applications is best advised to start with a short, accepted instrument and to add experimental items that reflect the clinician's interest. Mixing and matching items from different instruments is not recommended. Researchers at major medical centers are limited only by the stamina of their patients, but they will want to include one widely used instrument to allow comparison with other studies.

Applications

Symptom instruments have been used for screening purposes, usually with one item per symptom. Requirements for instruments in these settings are brevity, ease of understanding by patients, and ease of interpretation by clinicians. Single items may be adequate. Many symptom instruments have been developed for screening, and they should be evaluated for this type of application with sensitivity and specificity measurements. A third application has been to monitor symptoms over time. This may occur on a palliative care ward, or the instrument may be used to record the effects of palliative care interventions. Demonstration of symptom control is an important goal of palliative care programs. Clinical trials have been the major motivator for the development of symptom instruments as researchers determine whether their interventions had any effect on the symptom. The concept of symptoms as a primary outcome of clinical trials in cancer has further stimulated interest in symptom instruments, as have patient-reported outcomes, by the U.S. Food and Drug Administration (FDA) as a basis for the approval of new drugs. A guideline is being drafted by the FDA regarding the use of symptoms and quality of life instruments for trials.

Symptom instruments have many applications.. General areas include epidemiology, health care services research, and symptom research. The goal of research may be explanatory or pragmatic. Single-symptom instruments may be used to study several topics:

- Validity of symptom concepts, such as components of neuropathic pain
- Hypotheses regarding symptoms and other aspects of the patient's status (e.g., survival, quality of life)
- Validity of the instrument in a new population of patients
- Validity of new symptom instruments

For multisymptom instruments, data from symptom surveys can clarify the epidemiology and symptom burden experienced by patients, can determine relationships between symptoms, and can be used to derive symptom clusters. Qualitative approaches can help answer questions about the meaning of symptoms to patients and their caregivers and be used to develop hypotheses about how sensory information is processed. Information from symptom instruments can be important for other health professionals. For health service researchers, symptom assessment instruments may provide a way to relate symptom burden to the use of health care resources. These instruments may be useful in evaluating quality of care by providing a way to document whether measures to reduce symptoms improve patient outcomes. Related areas that merit further research include proxy ratings, communication issues, symptom assessment, quality of life, and symptom control.

REFERENCES

1. Chang CH, Cella D, Clarke S, et al. Should symptoms be scaled for intensity, frequency, or both? Palliat Support Care 2003;1:51-60.
2. Sechrest L. Validity of measures is no simple matter. Health Serv Res 2005;40(Pt 2):1584-1604.
3. Guyatt GH, Norman GR, Juniper EF, Griffity LE. A critical look at transition ratings. J Clin Epidemiol 2002;55:900-908.
4. Norman GR, Sloan JA, Wyrwich KW. Interpretation of changes in health-related quality of life: The remarkable universality of half a standard deviation. Med Care 2003;41:582-592.
5. Sloan JA, Loprinzi CL, Novotny PJ, et al. Methodologic lessons learned from hot flash studies. J Clin Oncol 2001;19:4280-4290.
6. Hollen PJ, Grall RJ, Kris MG, et al. A comparison of visual analogue and numerical rating scale formats for the Lung Cancer Symptom Scale (LCSS): Does format affect patient ratings of symptoms and quality of life? Qual Life Res 2005;14:837-847.
7. Jensen MP. The validity and reliability of pain measures in adults with cancer. J Pain 2003;4:2-21.
8. Schwartz CE, Rapkin BD. Reconsidering the psychometrics of quality of life assessment and appraisal in light of the response shift and appraisal. Health Qual Life Outcomes 2004;2:16-27.
9. Stephens RJ, Hopwood P, Girling DJ, Machin D. Randomized trials with quality of life endpoints: Are doctors' ratings of patients' physical symptoms interchangeable with patients' self ratings? Qual Life Res 1997;6:225-238.
10. Houde RW, Wallenstein SL, Rogers A. Clinical pharmacology of analgesics: A method of assaying analgesic effect. Clin Pharmacol Ther 1960;1:163-174.
11. Carr DB, Goudas LC, Balk EM, et al. Evidence report on the treatment of pain in cancer patients. J Natl Cancer Inst Monogr 2004;32:23-31.
12. Turk DC, Dworkin RH, Allen RR, et al. Core outcome domains for chronic pain clinical trials: IMMPACT recommendations. Pain 2003;106:337-345.
13. Turk DC, Dworkin RH, Burke LB, et al. Developing patient-reported outcome measures for pain clinical trials: IMMPACT recommendations. Pain 2006;125:208-215.
14. Littman GS, Walker BR, Schneider BR. Reassessment of verbal and visual analog scales for pain relief. Clin Pharmacol Ther 1985;38:16-23.
15. Carr DB, Goudas LC, Balk EM, et al. Evidence report on the treatment of pain in cancer patients. J Natl Cancer Inst Monogr 2004;32:23-31.
16. Farrar JT, Berlin JA, Strom BL. Clinically important changes in acute pain outcome measures: A validation study. J Pain Symptom Manage 2003;25:406-411.
17. Bennett MI, Attal N, Backonja MM, et al. Using screening tools to identify neuropathic pain. Pain 2007;127:199-203.
18. Lawrence DP, Kupelnick B, Miller K, et al. Evidence report on the occurrence, assessment, and treatment of fatigue in cancer patients. J Natl Cancer Inst Monogr 2004;32:40-50.
19. Jacobsen PB. Assessment of fatigue in cancer patients. J Natl Cancer Inst Monogr 2004;32:93-97.
20. Pirl WF. Evidence report on the occurrence, assessment and treatment of depression in cancer patients. J Natl Cancer Inst Monogr 2004;32:32-39.
21. Trask PC. Assessment of depression in cancer patients. J Natl Cancer Inst Monogr 2004;32:80-92.
22. Stubbs RJ, Hughes DA, Johnstone AM, et al. The use of visual analogue scales to assess motivation to eat in human subjects: A review of their reliability and validity with an evaluation of new hand-held computerized systems for temporal tracking of appetite ratings. Br J Nutr 2000;84:405-415.
23. Chang VT, Qi X, Kasimis B. The Functional Assessment of Anorexia/Cachexia Therapy (FAACT) Appetite Scale in veteran cancer patients. J Support Oncol 2005;3:377-382.
24. Oneschuk D, Hanson J, Bruera E. A survey of mouth pain and dryness in patients with advanced cancer. Support Care Cancer 2000;8:372-376.
25. Johnson JT, Feretti GA, Nethery WJ, et al. Oral pilocarpine for post-irradiation xerostomia in patients with head and neck cancer. N Engl J Med 1993;329;390-395.
26. Bausewein C, Farquhar M, Booth S, et al. Measurement of breathlessness in advanced disease: A systematic review. Respir Med 2007;101:399-410.
27. Gift AG. Validation of a vertical visual analogue scale as a measure of clinical dyspnea. Rehabil Nurs 1989;14:323-325.
28. Gift G, Narasvage G. Validity of the numeric rating scale as a measure of dyspnea. Am J Crit Care 1998;7:200-204.
29. Scano G, Stendardi L, Grazzini M. Understanding dyspnea by its language. Eur Respir J 2005;25:380-385.
30. Wilcock A, Crosby V, Hughes A, et al. Descriptors of breathlessness in patients with cancer and other cardiorespiratory diseases. J Pain Symptom Manage 2002;23:182-189.
31. Ries AL. Minimally clinically important difference for the UCSD Shortness of Breath Questionnaire, Borg Scale, and Visual Analogue Scale. COPD 2005;2:105-110.
32. Irwin RS. Assessing cough severity and efficacy of therapy in clinical research. Chest 2006;129:232S-239S.
33. Rhodes VA. Criteria for assessment of nausea, vomiting, and retching. Oncol Nurs Forum 1997;24(Suppl):13-19.
34. Borjeson S, Hursti TJ, Peterson C, et al. Similarities and differences in assessing nausea on a verbal category scale and a visual analogue scale. Cancer Nurs 1997;20:260-266.
35. Hesketh PJ, Gralla RJ, duBois A, et al. Methodology of antiemetic trials: Response assessment, evaluation of new agents and definition of chemotherapy emetogenicity. Support Care Cancer 1998;6;221-227.
36. Kirkova J, Davis MP, Walsh D, et al. Cancer symptom assessment instruments: A systematic review. J Clin Oncol 2006;24:1459-1473.
37. Garyali A, Palmer JL, Yennurajalingam S, et al. Errors in symptom intensity self-assessment by patients receiving outpatient palliative care. J Palliat Med 2006;9:1059-1065.
38. Herr K, Bjoro K, Decker S. Tools for assessment of pain in non-verbal older adults with dementia. A state of the science review. J Pain Symptom Manage 2006;31:170-192.
39. Stinson JN, Kavanagh T, Yamada J, et al. Systematic review of the psychometric properties, interpretability and feasibility of self-report pain intensity measures for use in clinical trials in children and adolescents. Pain 2006;125:143-157.
40. Collins JJ, Devine TD, Dick GS, et al. The measurement of symptoms in young children with cancer: The validation of the Memorial Symptom Assessment Scale in children aged 7-12. J Pain Symptom Manage 2002;23:10-16.
41. Turner RR, Quittner AL, Parasuraman BM, et al. Patient-reported outcomes: Instrument development and selection issues. Value Health 2007;10(Suppl 2):S86-S93.
42. Melzack R. The McGill pain questionnaire. Major properties and scoring methods. Pain 1975;1:277-299.
43. Melzack R. The short-form McGill Pain Questionnaire. Pain 1987;30:191-197.
44. Daut RL, Cleeland CS, Flanery RC. Development of the Wisconsin Brief Pain Questionnaire to assess pain in cancer and other diseases. Pain 1983;17:197-210.
45. Fishman B, Pasternak S, Wallenstein SL, et al. The Memorial Pain Assessment Card. A valid instrument for the evaluation of cancer pain. Cancer 1987;60:1151-1158.
46. Mendoza TR, Wang XS, Cleeland CS, et al. The rapid assessment of fatigue severity in cancer patients: Use of the Brief Fatigue Inventory. Cancer 1999;85:1186-1196.
47. Yellen SB, Cella DF, Webster K, et al. Measuring fatigue and other anemia-related symptoms with the Functional Assessment of Cancer Therapy (FACT) measurement system. J Pain Symptom Manage 1997;13:63-74.
48. Schwartz AL. The Schwartz Cancer Fatigue Scale: Testing reliability and validity. Oncol Nurs Forum 1998;25:711-717.
49. Inouye S, van Dyck CH, Alessi CA, et al. Clarifying confusion: The Confusion Assessment Method. A new method for detection of delirium. Ann Intern Med 1990;113:941-948.
50. Ely EW, Inouye SK, Bernard GR, et al. Delirium in mechanically ventilated patients: Validity and reliability of the Confusion Assessment Method for the Intensive Care Unit (CAM-ICU). JAMA 2001;286:2703-2710.
51. Trzepacz PT, Mittal D, Torres R, et al. Validation of the Delirium Rating Scale-Revised-98: Comparison with the Delirium Rating Scale and the Cognitive Test for Delirium. J Neuropsychiatry Clin Neurosci 2001;13:229-242.
52. Breitbart W, Rosenfeld B, Roth A, et al. The Memorial Delirium Assessment Scale. J Pain Symptom Manage 1997;13:128-137.
53. Sarhill N, Walsh D, Nelson KA, et al. Assessment of delirium in advanced cancer: The use of the bedside confusion scale. Am J Hospice Palliat Care 2001;18:335-341.

54. Leidy NK, Rennard SI, Schmier J, et al. The breathlessness, cough and sputum scale: The development of empirically based guidelines for interpretation. Chest 2003;124:2182-2191.

55. French CT, Irwin RS, Fletcher KE, Adams TM. Evaluation of a cough-specific quality-of-life questionnaire. Chest 2002;121:1123-1131.

56. Birring SS, Prudon B, Carr AJ, et al. Development of a symptom specific health status measure for patients with chronic cough: Leicester Cough Questionnaire. Thorax 2003;58:339-343.

57. Corli O, Cozzolino A, Battaiotto L, et al. A new method of food intake quantification: Application to the care of cancer patients. J Pain Symptom Manage 1992;7:12-17.

58. Loprinzi CL, Sloan JA, Rowland KM Jr. Methodologic issues regarding cancer anorexia/cachexia trials. In Portenoy RK, Bruera E (eds). Research and Palliative Care: Methodologies and Outcomes. New York: Oxford Press, 2003, pp 25-40.

59. Ribaudo JM, Cella D, Hahn EA, et al. Re-validation and shortening of the Functional Assessment of Anorexia/Cachexia Therapy (FAACT). Qual Life Res 2000;9:1137-1146.

60. Darling G, Eton D, Sulman J, et al. Validation of the functional assessment of cancer therapy esophageal cancer subscale. Cancer 2006;107:854-863.

61. Blazeby JM, Conroy T, Hammerlid E, et al. EORTC gastrointestinal and quality of life groups. Clinical and psychometric validation of an EORTC questionnaire module, the EORTC QLQ-OES18, to assess quality of life in patients with esophageal cancer. Eur J Cancer 2003;39:1383-1394.

62. McMillan SC, Williams FA. Validity and reliability of the Constipation Assessment Scale. Cancer Nurs 1989;12:183-188.

63. Whooley MA, Avins AL, Miranda J, Browner WS. Case-finding instruments for depression. Two questions are as good as many. J Gen Intern Med 1997;12:439-445.

64. Radloff LS. The CES-D scale: A self-report depression scale for research in the general population. Appl Psychol Meas 1977;1:385-401.

65. Beck AT. An inventory for measuring depression. Arch Gen Psychiatry 1961;4:53-61.

66. Zigmond A, Snaith RP. The Hospital Anxiety Depression Scale. Acta Psychiatric Scand 1983;67:367-370.

67. Yesavage JA, Brink TL, Rose TL, et al. Development and validation of a geriatric depression screening scale: A preliminary report. J Psychiatr Res 1982-83;17:37-49.

68. Zung WWK. A self-rating depression scale. Arch Gen Psychiatry 1965; 12:63-70.

69. Darsow U, Scharein E, Simon D, et al. New aspects of itch pathophysiology: Component analysis of atopic itch using the "Eppendorf Itch Questionnaire." Int Arch Allergy Immunol 2001;124:326-331.

70. Yosipovitch G, Goon A, Wee J, et al. The prevalence and clinical characteristics of pruritus among patients with extensive psoriasis. Br J Dermatol 2000; 143:969-973.

71. Bruera E, Kuehn N, Miller MJ, et al. The Edmonton Symptom Assessment System (ESAS): A simple method for the assessment of palliative care patients. J Palliat Med 1991;7:6-9.

72. McCorkle R, Young K. Development of a symptom distress scale. Cancer Nurs 1978;1:373-378.

73. De Haes JCJM, van Knippenburg FCE, Nejit JP. Measuring psychological and physical distress in cancer patients: Structure and application of the Rotterdam Symptom Checklist. Br J Cancer 1990;62:1034-1038.

74. Portenoy RK, Thaler HT, Kornblith AB, et al. The Memorial Symptom Assessment Scale: An instrument for the evaluation of symptom prevalence, characteristics and distress. Eur J Cancer. 1994;30A:1326-1336.

75. Chang VT, Hwang SS, Feuerman M, et al. The Memorial Symptom Assessment Scale Short Form (MSAS-SF): Reliability and validation. Cancer 2000;89:1162-1171.

76. Chang VT, Hwang SS, Kasimis B, Thaler HT. Shorter symptom assessment instruments. The Condensed Memorial Symptom Assessment Scale (CMSAS). Cancer Invest 2004;22:477-487.

77. Hollen PJ, Gralla RJ, Kris MG, et al. Measurement of quality of life in patients with lung cancer in multicenter trials of new therapies. Psychometric assessment of the Lung Cancer Symptom Scale. Cancer. 1994;73:2087-2098.

78. Cleeland CS, Mendoza TR, Wang XS, et al. Assessing symptom distress in cancer patients: The MD Anderson Symptom Inventory. Cancer 2000;89:1634-1646.

79. Steel K, Ljunggren G, Topinkova E, et al. The RAI-PC: An assessment instrument for palliative care in all settings. Am J Hosp Palliat Care 2003;20:211-219.

SUGGESTED READING

Lipscomb J, Gotay CC, Snyder C. Outcomes Assessment in Cancer. Measures, Methods, and Applications. Cambridge, UK: Cambridge University Press, 2005.

McDowell I. Measuring health. A Guide to Rating Scales and Questionnaires, 3rd ed. New York: Oxford University Press, 2006.

Portenoy RK, Bruera E (eds). Issues in Palliative Care Research. New York: Oxford University Press, 2003.

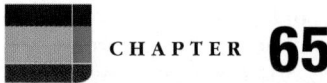

CHAPTER **65**

Measuring Quality of Life

Jordanka Kirkova

K E Y   P O I N T S

- Quality of life is a multidimensional construct. Assessing many dimensions reveals the multifaceted character of quality of life.

- Single-item quality of life measurement better reflects overall quality of life and is appropriate for very sick patients and follow-up.

- Simple, easily completed and interpreted, validated instruments should be applied in palliative medicine.

- Quality of life is an individual experience, and self-assessment is recommended.

- Individualized assessments better reflect important quality of life domains and possible response shifts that occur with chronic and life-threatening illnesses.

- When self-assessment is impossible, caregivers can provide information about physical symptoms and function.

QUALITY OF LIFE: DEFINITION AND STRUCTURE

Determining what constitutes quality of life (QOL) has led to a debate with economical, philosophical, sociological, psychological, and medical implications. Theories of how to describe and weigh life values have historically led to different criteria for how good is good and how bad is bad. More than 2000 years ago, happiness was the measure of the good life or well-being for Plato and Aristotle. According to Plato, an individual whose passions and reason are balanced is happy or content and satisfied.[1] According to Aristotle, happiness is "to live and do well."[2] Aristotle also mentioned that "people tend to value what they are missing," and he was one of the first to link QOL with the difference between a person's life experience and expectations.[2]

QOL is a broader concept than mere happiness. Economic welfare as a part of QOL was discussed in the early 20th century.[3] Reconsideration of health as a main determinant of QOL led to a rapid boom in articles on QOL, from 8 in 1974 to 1209 in 1994.[4] The World Health Organization (WHO) defines health as "not merely the absence of disease, but the presence of physical, mental, and social well-being."[5] The WHO group defines QOL as the "individual's perception of his or her position in life in the context of culture and value systems" and stresses its multidimensionality.[6] The multidimensional nature of QOL is assumed to be a number of domains or dimensions, which are combined to define QOL as a whole, but there is no consensus on the most appropriate domains or their relative importance.[3] Six main QOL domains are consistently recognized by the WHO group. These reflect physical, psychological, material, and social (i.e., family and professional relationships) well-being; the environment; and the level of independence. Additional domains involve specific populations such as "living in vulnerable conditions" or "suffering from chronic diseases."[6] Figure 65-1 represents the most appropriate domains for palliative medicine QOL according to the WHO definition.

Objective components of QOL include the use of services related to these domains, whereas subjective components relate to happiness, satisfaction, and well-being.[3] A definition similar to that of the WHO includes a subjective sense of well-being, which has physical, psychological, social, and spiritual dimensions.[7] Objective indicators (e.g., functional ability, performance status) may outweigh QOL assessment only if individuals are unable to determine subjectively their QOL.[7] According to the gap theory, QOL is the difference between an individual's hopes and ambitions and current reality, with both modulated by past experience and personality[8]; this includes satisfaction, contentment, happiness, and fulfillment with life. Reality and personal expectations fluctuate, and the greater the gap is between the two at any given moment, the lower the QOL.[8] Reducing the gap improves the QOL. Ways to improve the QOL include lowering the expectations or increasing activities that achieve goals (Fig. 65-2).

A QOL definition that combines elements from the gap theory involves four constructs of individual QOL: social utility, happiness as an emotional state, life satisfaction measured as the difference between expectations and reality, and functional status (i.e., physical, psychological, social, and spiritual factors).[9]

Quality of Life and Well-Being

Some QOL instruments (e.g., Edmonton Symptom Assessment System [ESAS])[10] measure *well-being*, and others (e.g., European Organization for Research and Treatment

of Cancer Core Questionnaire QLQ-C30 [EORTC QLQ-C30])[11] use the term *quality of life*. Well-being is related to specific, subjective aspects of QOL. A sense of well-being or improved overall QOL may involve better symptom control and satisfaction of the patient and caregiver.[12] QOL refers to more global perspectives than well-being, and it is commonly regarded as combining subjective and objective components.[3]

Health-Related Quality of Life

There is no uniform definition of health-related QOL. Some see health-related QOL as the effect of disease on the physical functioning and subjective well-being of the patient, and health therefore is a major determinant of QOL. Health-related QOL is expressed as a continuum between the extremes of death and excellent health.[13] Karnofsky performance status is considered one of the first measures of health-related QOL in cancer patients.[14] Unfortunately, health status, functional status, well-being, and QOL are used interchangeably, but QOL is broader than any of the other terms.[3] Functional status, for example, is not equated with QOL, because people with disabilities can enjoy good QOL.[15]

Quality of Life in Palliative Medicine

A discrepancy exists in using the term *health-related QOL* in terminal illness.[16] A shift in personal values to transcendence, spirituality, security, conformity, and tradition are self-preserving mechanisms in patients with advanced cancer or amyotrophic lateral sclerosis (ALS) who maintain QOL despite fading health.[4,17] At the end of life, QOL may shift from focusing on health to restoring healing connections through ameliorating existential anguish and enhancing meaning.[18] Meaning and spiritual well-being correlate with QOL to the same extent as physical and emotional well-being.[19] People with greater spiritual well-being reported that they enjoy life despite pain and fatigue.[19] Spirituality in the context of a person's beliefs

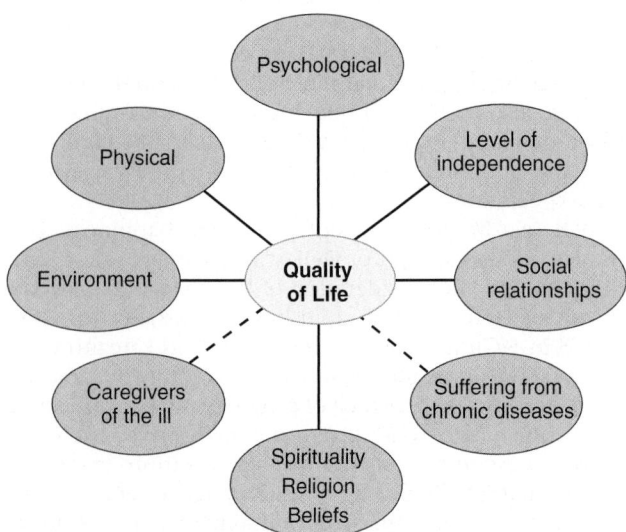

FIGURE 65-1 Six main and two additional quality of life domains applicable to palliative medicine as defined by the World Health Organization group. *(Adapted from World Health Organization. World Health Organization Quality of Life Assessment (WHOQOL): Position paper from the World Health Organization. Soc Sci Med 1995;41:1403-1409.)*

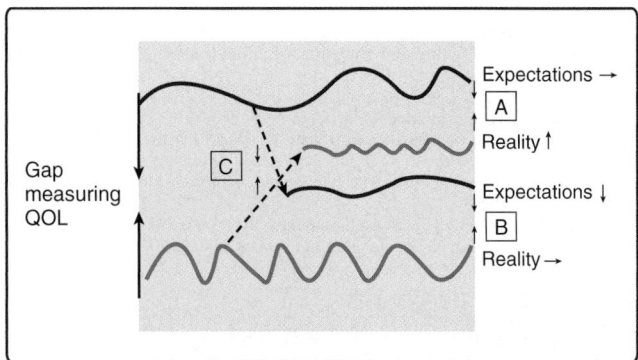

FIGURE 65-2   The gap theory for quality of life (QOL). The person's activities in real life (Reality) are fluctuating, as are his Expectations. The bigger the gap between them, the lower the QOL. There are three possible ways to improve QOL by reducing the gap between Expectations and Reality: the level of Reality increases, and Expectations stay the same (A); the level of Expectations decreases, and the level of Reality stays the same (B); or both the level of Expectations (decreases) and Reality (increases) change (C). *(Adapted from reference 8.)*

about transcendence and ultimate meaning is a more important QOL domain at the end of life.

Response Shift in Quality of Life

Response shift refers to a change in the meaning of a person's self-evaluation of a target construct, such as QOL.[20] Several factors can influence a response shift:

- A change in internal standards used to measure the construct (i.e., scale recalibration in psychometric terms)
- A change in values or changes in the priorities of domains (i.e., importance of component domains constituting the target construct)
- A redefinition of the target construct or changes in the content of the domains (i.e., reconceptualization)

Response shift phenomena may explain why the overall QOL stays stable despite health decline and fades with the progression of chronic and life-threatening diseases. Response shift may lead to an increase in overall QOL when the shift occurs from a less positively rated to a more positively rated domain, whereas the opposite shift can lead to diminishing QOL.[21] In terminally ill cancer patients, response shift was greater in reconceptualization and a change in values, and it occurred more frequently in those with worse QOL.[22] Individual QOL remained stable and was even higher than observed in advanced cancer outpatients.[23] A clearer response shift is observed with ALS (Fig. 65-3) compared with advanced cancer.[15,24] Slow deterioration allows for better adjustment through a change in value systems and reconceptualization, which keeps the overall level of QOL high. Response shift may be best captured using whole domains rather than single questions regarding QOL. There is almost a universal agreement that QOL has a multidimensional characteristic that depends on the values of the individual and a dynamic nature in that domains shift over time in terms of content and importance.[25]

PRINCIPLES OF ASSESSMENT AND MEASUREMENT

Reasons for Measuring Quality of Life

Improving QOL in chronic and debilitating illnesses is one of the most important goals in palliative care.[9] QOL assessments help to screen and prioritize problems, facilitate communications, and monitor changes in response to treatment.[26]

Objective and Subjective Measures

Objective measures in health-related QOL include mortality, health service use, and the level of provision of these services. Subjective measures of QOL are symptom control and the patient's preferences, satisfaction, and concerns, which are captured by questionnaires.[27] Modes of administration and completion of the questionnaires include self-completed, interviewer administered, and observer rated.

The objective and subjective measures may interact differently, and they reveal different aspects of QOL. Low

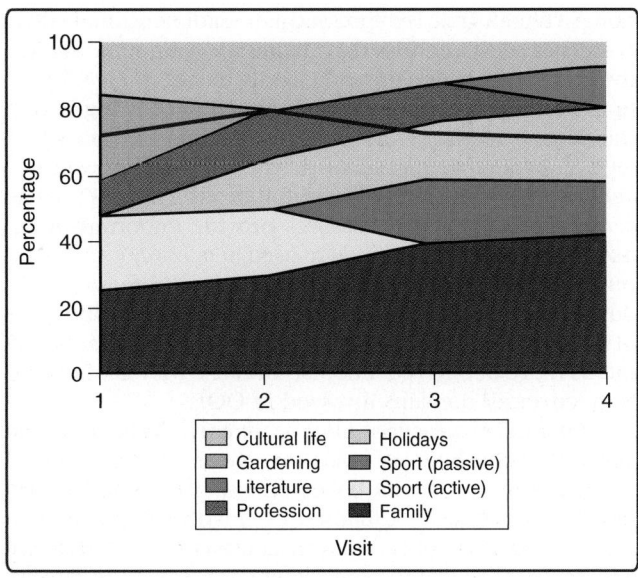

FIGURE 65-3 The response shift in individualized quality of life of a patient with amyotrophic lateral sclerosis was measured by the Schedule for the Evaluation of Individual Quality of Life–DW (SEIQoL-DW)[69] and the Sickness Impact Profile (SIP).[71] The distribution and relative weight of the patient-selected domains are shown for visit one to visit four; the interval between visits was 2 months. The family *(bottom area)* was the most important domain from the beginning, and its relative weight increased further with time. Up to the second visit, the 53-year-old man was able to dive and hike (i.e., active sport); from the third visit on, he was able only to follow sports on TV (i.e., passive sport) Holidays became more important over time, and profession became less significant and eventually disappeared. Gardening, a heavy physical activity, was dropped after the first visit, and literature turned up at the last visit. The importance of cultural life decreased, probably because of the patient's reduced mobility. Overall, there is a trend from active QOL domains to more passive ones as the disease progressed, which is reflected in the SIP values from 62 to 56 *(not shown)*. In contrast, the SEIQoL-DW total score *(purple line)* showed no decrease over the 6-month period. *(From Neudert C, Wasner M, Borasio GD. Patients' assessment of quality of life instruments: A randomised study of SIP, SF-36, and SEIQoL-DW in patients with amyotrophic lateral sclerosis. J Neurol Sci 2001;191:103-109.)*

QOL may predict shorter survival, but social functioning (i.e., social QOL domain) does not differ in those with shorter or longer survival.[28] Subjectively rated QOL is less predictive of survival in palliative cancer patients compared with clinical variables.[29]

Multidimensional and Unidimensional Measures

A multidimensional construct should be separated into its domains, and the separate domains then are aggregated for an overall QOL measure.[27,30] Another way of presenting multidimensional QOL is reporting separate domains as profiles.[27,30] Instruments such as the Spitzer Quality of Life Index (Spitzer QLI) aggregate scores in five domains and create a composite single score.[31] Profile scores of nine subscales are provided in the EORTC QLQ-C30.[11] The McGill Quality of Life (MQOL) questionnaire has profile and aggregated scores.[32]

Overall QOL can best be captured by an " imprecise holistic" means, such as a self-assessed global single question.[33] Overall QOL is expressed as a unidimensional single construct with anchors that define a continuum. Subjective assessments ask the individuals to rate their satisfaction with life as a whole or their overall well-being within the range from the "worst possible," to the "best possible" QOL.[33] Objective measures of the global QOL employ anchors of death (rated 0) and full health (rated 1).[13] The single unidimensional measures provide important information for overall QOL and are used in economic analyses, but the improvement or deterioration in different QOL domains is missed by single questions.[13] The proponents of single scale measures consider multidimensional instruments more or less reductionist, because they cannot possibly cover all domains involved in QOL.

QOL can be measured in psychometric and clinimetric ways. Psychometric methods involve the statistical level of significance for data collected using designed instruments and scales. Clinimetrics involves quantitative methods in the collection and analysis of data that are compared. The main requirement for scientific quality using clinimetric methods is a consistent, reproducible process of observation and expression of the clinical variables.[34,35]

Several methods can be used to measure the response shift in QOL, and two are quite popular:

- Individualized assessments: measuring and weighing elicited by patients' QOL domains at each time of assessment and comparing the change in domain values, or reconceptualization
- Then tests: comparing patient's perspectives at time of assessment (i.e., now) with how they felt before (i.e., then)[20]

The then test is relatively sensitive and easy to perform, but it may involve recall bias or inaccuracy due to interval reconceptualization.[20] Individualized QOL instruments such as the Schedule for the Evaluation of Individual Quality of Life (SEIQoL)[23,36] prioritize specific domains of patients' QOL and are considered to provide a patient-centered approach.[20] Computerized assessments, especially computerized adaptive testing (CAT) with cueing of the most appropriate questions for the individual, may provide more accurate individual QOL assessments.[26]

INSTRUMENTS

QOL instruments vary and can be divided into different groups based on several criteria. One division is based on profiles to measure and population.[13] These instruments can be divided into two groups:

- Generic instruments, with subgroups of health profiles and utility measures
- Instruments that are specific for disease, function, or population[13,16]

Generic health profiles assess different domains of quality of life, and they can be applied to the general population and different diseases. An example is the Medical Outcome Studies Short Form-36 (MOS SF-36).[37] Preference or utility instruments calculate quality-adjusted life years and assess the value of QOL to the patient, excluding time with the side effects from treatment.[13] Utility measures are less frequently used in palliative medicine. Specific instruments are developed for certain diseases, such as the EORTC QLQ-C30[11] in cancer, or are disease and site specific, such as the Lung Cancer Symptom Scale (LCSS) for lung cancer.[38] Instruments may be symptom or domain specific,[39] such as the Brief Pain Inventory (BPI), which was developed and validated for cancer and later validated for noncancer pain.[40,41] Disease- or population-specific measures should minimally assess clinically important changes in longitudinal studies as they are validated for such populations.[13] Symptom-specific instruments provide a more comprehensive assessment of the impact of the given symptom on QOL, which is appropriate for research but may be burdensome for the very sick.[42] Symptom-specific instruments are limited in specific areas of physical or psychological well-being and cannot be compared with generic QOL instruments.

Standardized instruments can be multidimensional or single, overall QOL questions. Multidimensional questionnaires use a single question or multiple questions per domain. The standardized multidimensional QOL instruments differ by domains and language, and the outcomes measured by overall QOL, when it is determined by aggregating separate domains in two instruments, may differ. Instruments should possess reliability and validity (Table 65-1).[43]

TABLE 65-1 Basic Concepts of Reliability and Validity

CONCEPTS	TYPE	EXPLANATION
Reliability	1. Internal consistency 2. Interrater 3. Intrarater or test-retest	1. Consistency of the scale to measure a certain construct (e.g., physical, psychological) 2. Concordance of different raters assessing a respondent with the same instrument 3. Correlation between two assessments of the same rater in the same population
Validity	1. Content or face 2. Construct factor 3a. Criterion concurrent 3b. Criterion predictive 4. Construct convergent or divergent 5. Group differences or sensitivity 6. Responsiveness to change	1. Adequacy of the questionnaires to assess the designed measure 2. Description of the underlying conceptual framework of the instrument, usually through factor analysis 3. Correlation of the instrument to a gold standard at one time (3a) or with future outcomes (3b) 4. Correlation of items, scales, or total scores with similar questionnaires that measure the same or unrelated constructs at the same time* 5. Ability of the instrument to distinguish between respondents (e.g., well and sick, different treatment groups, different performance status) 6. Ability of the instrument to capture small changes over time

*Criteria for good validity and reliability vary, but correlation coefficients should be greater than 0.7 for good reliability and validity. Correlation coefficients range from worst (0) to best possible (1).
Data from McDowel I. The Theoretical and Technical Foundations of Health Measurement. Measuring Health: A Guide to Rating Scales and Questionnaires, 3rd ed. Oxford, UK: Oxford University Press, 2006, pp 10-54.

Based on the goal of assessment, QOL instruments can be divided into screening and outcome instruments. The screening instruments must be sensitive enough to detect people with high or low quality of life. These tools should have a high sensitivity and specificity. The outcome instruments should have a high responsiveness to change as determined by the minimally important change that has a clinical significance of interest.[13]

Types of Quality of Life Instruments

The QOL instruments used in palliative care (Table 65-2) can be divided into two groups: instruments that are specially developed for palliative medicine and those adopted from general populations or cancer patients. Historically, palliative medicine was developed for symptom management of cancer, but it has expanded to care for patients with chronic, degenerative, nonmalignant diseases. Most of the instruments used initially were introduced from cancer QOL measures.[4] In palliative medicine, QOL instruments need to assess specific domains of QOL, such as existential issues, that are not included in the instruments for cancer or other diseases.[39,44] QOL instruments in palliative medicine are also considered outcome instruments.[45] The relationship between QOL and outcome instruments is vague. Satisfaction, improved symptom control, and overall QOL are subjective outcome measures. The Palliative Outcome Scale (POS)[46] and the Support Team Assessment Schedule (STAS)[47] have included subjective and objective measures, whereas the other QOL instruments target patient well-being.

Generic Instruments

MOS SF-36 is one of the earliest QOL instruments developed for the general population.[37] The most popular 36-item version, developed from the original MOS QOL instrument, measures dichotomously and on 3- to 6-point Likert-type scales with eight QOL domains[48]:

1. Physical functioning and well-being
2. Role limitations due to physical problems
3. Bodily pain
4. Social role and well-being
5. Mental health
6. Role limitations due to emotional problems
7. Vitality, energy, or fatigue
8. General health

Functioning is defined as the ability to perform daily activities, and *well-being* is a more subjective internal state not observable by others, such as symptoms or feelings. There are shortened versions (12 and 8 items) that reflect the scale profile of the original instrument. However, the 36-item questionnaire continues to be used extensively, and it has a greater precision.[9] The MOS SF-36 has been validated by other QOL and symptom assessment instruments in ALS with a good reliability (i.e., internal consistency and test-retest).[49] The MOS SF-36 can be used in palliative medicine, but the length of the instrument and the floor effect (i.e., patients tending to score on the lower end of the scale) are issues. It was less responsive to change compared with instruments specifically developed for ALS.[49]

Disease-Specific Instruments

The EORTC QLQ-C30 is a self-completed, disease-specific QOL questionnaire that measures the impact of disease and treatment on physical health, psychological symptoms, and social functioning in cancer patients.[11] Its 30 questions include 9 multi-item scales on a 4-point Likert-type format: 5 functional (i.e., physical, role, cognitive, emotional, and social), 3 symptom scales (i.e., fatigue, pain, nausea, and vomiting), and a global health and QOL scale on a 7-point numerical format with anchors at "worst possible" (1) and "best possible" (7). The time frame is "over the past week." The instrument gives profile scores based on the domains. The instrument has good validity, overall reliability, responsiveness to change, and cross-cultural reliability. It has been used in palliative medicine, but it is inappropriate for very sick individuals and has a floor effect. The European Organization for Research and Treatment of Cancer Quality of Life Questionnaire Core-15 Palliative Care (EORTC QLQ-C15-PAL) is a 15-item, shortened version developed for palliative medicine.[50] The initial content was validated by the item response theory (IRT) through expert and patient participation.[50] Further testing of reliability, validity, and feasibility is needed. The EORTC QLQ-C30 and its shortened version are appropriate for QOL screening and follow-up.

Instruments Designed for Palliative Medicine

Many assessment instruments in palliative medicine involve some individualized assessment, which includes questions of importance or weighing the items. The Hospice Quality of Life Index (HQLI) is a self-report, multidimensional measure of QOL, which has 28 items graded on a numerical rating scale (NRS) of 1 to 10. The physical, functional, social, spiritual, psychological, and financial well-being QOL domains are assessed with an additional total aggregated score.[51,52] The instrument showed a good internal consistency, and validity was confirmed by factor analysis. The instrument is able to discriminate between hospice patients and healthy volunteers, and it can be used for screening and follow-up of QOL in hospice patients.[51,53] Further validation is needed.

The MQOL was developed for assessing advanced cancer patients and further revised and tested in patients with acquired immunodeficiency syndrome (AIDS).[32,54] QOL is broadly defined as "subjective well-being."[54] A single QOL question measures overall QOL, followed by 16 items, graded with an NRS of 1 to 10. The instrument covers four domains: physical (patients i.e., volunteer three troublesome symptoms), psychological, existential, and support. A total score is derived from the mean of all four domains. The instrument correlates well with the MQOL Single-Item Scale (SIS) for overall QOL assessment and with the Spitzer QLI.[32] The SIS is considered by its authors to be a measure that best expresses patients' meaning of QOL.[32] The instrument is appropriate for assessment of QOL in palliative medicine, for identifying existential well-being of the patients, and for evaluating interventions aimed to affect different domains of QOL in research or clinical practice.[54]

The McGill Quality of Life Questionnaire–Cardiff Short Form (MQOL-CSF) was developed and validated against

TABLE 65-2   Scales for Assessment of Quality of Life and Quality of Care Applied in Palliative Medicine and Advanced Cancer Cases

INSTRUMENTS* ORIGINAL DESIGN		O'BOYLE[4]	DONNELLY[6,44]	HEARN[4]	BRULEY	KAASA[3]	MASSARO[4]	OTHER SOURCES
				SOURCE				
Spitzer Quality of Life Index[31]	QOL	Yes	Yes				Yes	
Spitzer Uniscale	QOL	Yes	Yes					
Linear Analogue Self-Assessment (LASA) Scale	QOL	Yes	Yes					
Functional Living Index–Cancer (FLIC)	QOL	Yes	Yes					
McGill Quality of Life (MQOL) Questionnaire[32]	QOL	Yes	Yes	Yes	Yes	Yes	Yes	
Life Evaluation Questionnaire (LEQ)	QOL	Yes	Yes			Yes		
McMaster Quality of Life Scale (MQLS)[56]	QOL	Yes	Yes	Yes		Yes	Yes	
MacAdam Scale	QOL	Yes						
Support Team Assessment Schedule (STAS)[47]	OUT	Yes		Yes				
Quality of Life Index (QLI)	QOL	Yes			Yes			
Life Satisfaction Questionnaire	QOL	Yes						
Hospice Quality of Life Index (HQLI)[51]	QOL	Yes	Yes		Yes		Yes	
Schedule for the Evaluation of Individual Quality of Life (SEIQoL)[36]	QOL	Yes	Yes	Yes		Yes		
Schedule for the Evaluation of Individual Quality of Life–Direct Weighting (SEIQoL-DW)	QOL	Yes	Yes					
Assessment of Quality of Life at the End of Life	QOL		Yes					
Global Quality of Life Assessment (how is life?)[66]	QOL		Yes					
Functional Assessment Cancer Therapy–General (FAACT-G)	QOL		Yes			Yes		
Rotterdam Symptom Checklist (RSCL)	QOL		Yes	Yes				
European Organization for Research and Treatment of Cancer Core Questionnaire (EORTC QLQ-C30)[11]	QOL		Yes	Yes	Yes	Yes		
Edmonton Symptom Assessment System (ESAS)[10]	S			Yes		Yes		
Hebrew Rehabilitation Center for Aged Quality of Life (HRCA-QL) Index	QOL			Yes				
Palliative Care Assessment (PACA)	OUT			Yes				
Palliative Care Core Standards (PCCS)	OUT			Yes				
Symptom Distress Scale (SDS)	S			Yes				
Medical Outcome Studies Short Form–36 (MOS SF-36)[37]					Yes			
Missoula-Vitas Quality of Life Index (MVQOLI)[57]	QOL				Yes	Yes	Yes	
Therapy Impact Questionnaire[64]	QOL					Yes		
Palliative Outcome Scale (POS)[46]	OUT							Yes
McGill Quality of Life Questionnaire–Cardiff Short Form (MQOL-CSF)[55]	QOL							Yes
European Organization for Research and Treatment of Cancer Quality of Life Questionnaire Core-15 Palliative Care (EORTC QLQ-C15-PAL)[50]	QOL							Yes
Patient-Evaluated Problem Score (PEPS)[61]	QOL							Yes
Palliative Care Quality of Life Instrument (PQLI)[83]	QOL							Yes
Target population†		Palliative medicine	Advanced cancer	Palliative care	Palliative care	Palliative care	Palliative care	Palliative medicine
Psychometric properties reported		No	Yes	Yes	Yes	Yes	Yes	Yes

*Citations for some instruments refer to the chapter's reference list. Unreferenced instruments can be identified from the relevant review papers.
†Target populations were defined by the researchers.
OUT, outcome; QOL, quality of life; S, symptom.

the original MQOL instrument.[55] It consists of eight questions (i.e., one global QOL item, three physical, two psychological, and two existential), and it employs an NRS of 1 to 10. The MQOL-CSF has a good (preliminary) reliability. The MQOL-CSF and MQOL questionnaires have moderate to good reliability and validity.[55] The MQOL-CSF can be used in palliative settings (i.e., inpatients, outpatients, and hospice clients) as a routine QOL assessment and for follow-up. It may be insensitive for capturing support, treatment, and pain compared with the original instrument.

The McMaster Quality of Life Scale (MQOLS) has 32 questions to assess physical, emotional, social, and spiritual domains on a 7-point NRS.[56] Important items are rated by patients. The instrument correlates well with the Spitzer QLI.[56] Patients' and caregivers' ratings of the patient correlate moderately, but the instrument authors recommend that QOL should be assessed by patients whenever possible. Interviewer bias accounted for some differences between self-assessed and interviewer-rated QOL.[56] The questionnaire may be burdensome because of its length. There are additional forms for family and staff.

The Missoula-VITAS Quality of Life Index (MVQOLI) is a self-completed questionnaire that defines QOL as "the subjective experience of an individual living with the interpersonal, psychological, and existential or spiritual challenges that accompany the process of physical and functional decline and the knowledge of impending demise."[57,58] The instrument includes 25 questions to assess symptoms, function, interpersonal interactions, well-being, and transcendence; responses are graded on a 5-point NRS. Satisfaction and importance within each separate domain are assessed. It has a summary score with a weighted sum of the importance of each domain. MVQOL has been validated in cancer and noncancer hospice patients. It shows a good test-retest reliability and responsiveness to change over time, but it was not found to be psychometrically robust. The instrument has been used to measure QOL successfully in terminally ill hospice cancer patients.[59] A cross-cultural validation has been performed in AIDS patients in Uganda.[60]

The Patient-Evaluated Palliative Score (PEPS) was designed as a self-assessment QOL instrument suitable for use in the seriously ill. QOL is "the level of well-being or of global satisfaction in several life domains."[61] PEPS is a composite measure of traditional nurse or physician assessments and an individualized patient self-assessment. First, the individualized assessment consists of patient–selected problems (e.g., physical, emotional, social, spiritual) that are measured on a 3-point Likert scale. Second, patients rate their function on the WHO function scale. In another study, patients elicited problems by a prompt list of symptoms.[62] Third, a single question on an NRS of 1 to 10 measures overall QOL. MQOL and PEPS correlated well, and they were found to be valid and acceptable for assessing advanced cancer patients, but the greater preference was for MQOL (60% vs. 28%).[62] PEPS captured more psychological problems. PEPS can be an appropriate measure for individualized patient assessment in practice when the emphasis is on psychological issues. PEPS needs more extensive testing of validity and reliability to be used as an outcome instrument.

The Quality of Life at the End of Life Measure (QUAL-E) is a self-completed questionnaire that was developed with expert, patient, and family participation. It was validated to measure QOL at the end of life in cancer and noncancer patients.[63] QOL is globally defined as "patients' direct subjective experience" at the end of life.[63] The instrument was tested initially in patients with advanced cancer, end-stage congestive heart failure, chronic obstructive pulmonary disease (COPD), or renal failure. The questionnaire has 25 items graded on a 5-point Likert-type scale, which includes four QOL domains: life completion, symptom impact, relationship with health care provider, and preparation for the end of life. Patients initially volunteer three bothersome symptoms and are then asked to evaluate the importance of the contribution of each domain to their QOL. Comparison with Functional Assessment of Chronic Illness Therapy (FACIT), FACIT-Spiritual, and MVQOL showed moderate convergent validity. The instrument is appropriate for assessment and evaluation of the interventions to improve QOL the end of life. It needs further validation, especially in patients with nonmalignant diseases because of the small validation samples.

The Therapy Impact Questionnaire (TIQ) was designed to assess the influence of therapy on the QOL of patients with advanced cancer.[64] A 4-point Likert-type scale is used to measure four QOL domains: physical symptoms (24 items), functional status (3 items), emotional and cognitive factors (6 items), and social relationships (2 items). A global single item assesses feeling well.[64] In a large, national Italian study, the instrument was found to be accurate to describe symptoms and QOL of palliative cancer patients over time.[65] The instrument creates a summary score, which can be used to follow QOL over time as an outcome measure.

A single question may be used for a global QOL assessment. Many instruments, such as the EORTC QLQ-C30 and MQOL questionnaire, have a single question on QOL in addition to the multidimensional assessment.[11,54] A frequently used global QOL question is the Spitzer uniscale.[31] A single, overall QOL question was easy to complete and repeat in patients with advanced cancer over time and had validity comparable to that of multi-item questionnaires.[66,67] The QOL uniscale is reliable and has the greatest sensitivity to change over time compared with summated scores from multi-item questionnaires.[68] A single QOL question can be recommended when the outcome is overall QOL and when it will be followed longitudinally. Its use is feasible in the very sick, when lengthy multi-item questionnaires are impossible to complete. However, the multiple domains of QOL are lost.

Individualized Quality of Life Instruments

The Schedule for the Evaluation of Individual Quality of Life (SEIQoL) was developed for individual assessment of the QOL of patients with noncancer diseases, and it was later tested in patients with cancer, AIDS, or ALS.[15,23,36] In a semi-structured interview, patients elicit the five most important areas of their QOL. Patients further weight the five areas according to their relative importance. A simpler form (Schedule for the Evaluation of Individual Quality of Life–Direct Weighting (SEIQoL-DW) that directly weights patients' domains decreases the assessment burden.[69] Five color-laminated, circular discs are rotated to form a pie chart. The weighted domains are combined to give a QOL index. SEIQoL-DW was found valid and reliable in assessing patients with advanced cancer or ALS and was acceptable in seriously ill lung cancer patients.[15,22,23,70] Pitfalls include a possible assessment burden in evaluating the seriously ill and in routine practice and an interviewer bias from nominating QOL domains to help patients.[70] Comparing the SEIQoL-DW with other QOL instruments is difficult. The instrument individualizes assessments into self-determined QOL and is able to follow response shifts throughout the trajectory of illness (Table 65-3).

Ideal Measures of Quality of Life

Instrument designers and critics are always looking for an ideal measure of QOL. An ideal QOL instrument is unlikely to be constructed. Certain recommendations about how to choose the right instrument for research or clinical practice can be made based on the objectives of QOL assessment (Fig. 65-4).

CLINICAL EVALUATION: STRUCTURE OF ASSESSMENT

QOL scores have been used predominantly as secondary measure of outcomes in cancer research.[16] In the clinical

setting, measuring QOL should be done in addition to measuring treatment response and symptom relief.[26] Function, disabilities, and needs should be considered with QOL for the patient's well-being and quality of care.[26] QOL instruments in clinical practice should be easy to understand and complete, and they should be easily incorporated in clinical protocols.[26] The instruments should be

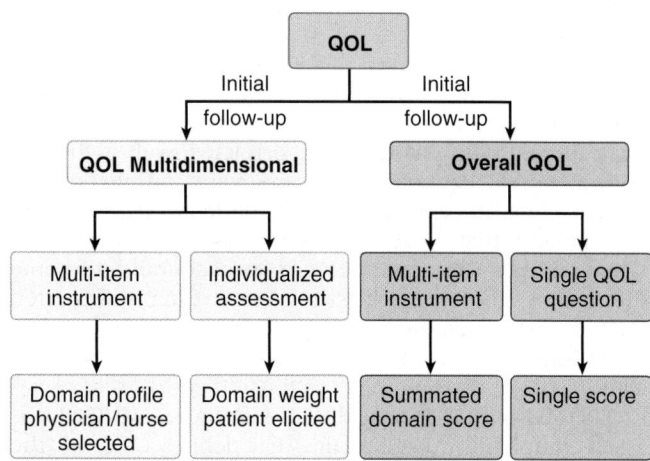

FIGURE 65-4 Selecting a quality of life (QOL) instrument for research or clinical practice based on the assessment goal.

TABLE 65-3 Multi-item, Self-Completed Quality of Life Instruments Developed for Palliative Medicine							
INSTRUMENT COMPONENTS	**HQOL[5,51]**	**MQOL[6,32,54]**	**MQOL-CSF[55]**	**MVQOLI[5,57]**	**EORTC QLQ-C15-PAL[5]**	**PEPS[6,61]**	**PQLI[8]**
Domains	Physical Psychological Social Spiritual	Physical Physical well-being Psychological Existential well-being Support Global QOL	Physical Psychological Existential well-being Global QOL	Global Symptom Functional Social Well-being (satisfaction) Spiritual	Physical F Emotional F Symptoms Overall QOL	Volunteered: Physical Emotional Social Spiritual Activity Global QOL Nurse or physician-elicited problems graded by patients	Functional[2] Symptom Choice of treatment Psychological Overall QOL
Number of items	28	17	8	25	15	—	28
Scale	0-10 NRS Profile scores Total score	0-10 NRS Profile scores Total score	0-10 NRS Profile scores	5-point NRS Profile scores Total score	4-point Likert 7-point NRS Profile scores	4-point Likert 0-10 NRS	3,5-point Likert 0-10 NRS
Time frame	Not specified	Past 2 days–hospice Past 7 days–outpatient	Past 2 days–hospice Past 7 days–outpatient	Not specified	Past week	Not specified	Not specified
Completion time (min)	Not reported	10-30[6]	3 (range, 1-8)	15-20[6]	Not reported	3-8[6]	8
Reliability*	Good	Good	Moderate or good	Moderate or good	Not tested	Moderate or good	Good
Validity*	Moderate	Moderate or good	Moderate or good	Moderate	Content	Moderate or good	Moderate or good
Responsiveness to change	Not tested	Not tested	Not tested, small numbers	Moderate or good	Not tested	Not tested	Not tested

*Criteria for reliability and validity are based on reported correlation coefficients. Factor analysis was considered as an additional method that strengthens validity. Criteria: good > .70; moderate = .40 to .70; poor < .40. Factor analysis was considered as an additional method that strengthens validity.
EORTC QLQ-C15-PAL, European Organization for Research and Treatment of Cancer Quality of Life Questionnaire–Core 15–Palliative Care; HQLI, Hospice Quality of Life Index; Likert, type of psychometric response scale used in questionnaires; MQOL, McGill Quality of Life Questionnaire; MQOL-CSF, McGill Quality of Life Questionnaire–Cardiff Short Form; MVQOLI, Missoula-Vitas Quality of Life Index; NRS, numerical rating scale; PEPS, Patient-Evaluated Problem Score; PQLI, Palliative Care Quality of Life Instrument; QOL, quality of life.

interpretable to be clinically useful. Barriers to QOL instruments include complexity of many QOL instruments and scales, cost, time burden in collecting and analyzing findings, and clinical interpretation of data.[16,27]

The structure of QOL assessment is rarely discussed, and it usually follows the structure of standard instruments. Different instruments list domains in the order of importance to the developers. The order in which domains are assessed or whether questions should be mixed is unknown. Some questionnaires, such as the Sickness Impact Profile (SIP)[71] that has been used for patients with ALS,[24,71] mix scales and reverse the direction of scales (i.e., positive to negative items) to prevent examinees from mechanically circling items in consecutive order. Whether overall QOL assessment should be an initial or ending question influences the score; the overall QOL level was higher when assessed at the beginning.[32] For this reason, some instruments, such as the MQOL, have adopted an initial overall QOL assessment.[32] At the end of life, when existential suffering is more important, the initial question (How can we help you in your suffering?) may elicit existential issues. Another approach is initial individualized assessment, which can identify areas of priority derived from the patient's QOL to be further explored and managed.

DEVELOPMENTS, DEBATES, AND RESEARCH

Evidence-Based Medicine

Research underlying evidence-based medicine has demonstrated several trends[12]:

- Psychosocial counseling improved depression, life satisfaction, and self-esteem, but the remaining symptom burden was not positively influenced.
- Improvement in care was better for hospice patients than home care patients.
- Home visits by nurses and physicians decreased concerns about certain symptoms (e.g., nausea, itching).
- Hospital-based home care programs did not influence survival.
- Health-related QOL did not differ between ambulatory and inpatient palliative medicine units.
- Better QOL was identified for chemotherapy plus supportive care compared with supportive care alone, but there was no significant difference for specific symptom effects, except for pain.
- Improved QOL was associated with longer survival.
- Caregivers were more satisfied and had less anxiety when they were involved in care.
- Improving patients' QOL did not reduce the caregiver's burden or improve their QOL.[72]

A possible explanation for the lack of evident efficacy for the holistic palliative medicine approach on symptoms and QOL is disease progression with an increasing symptom burden that is difficult to manage only with supportive care. The multidimensional character of the QOL precludes simultaneous positive influences on multiple dimensions.[12] The evidence for improving QOL assessment is sparse. Regular QOL assessments (Box 65-1) in oncology can improve patient and physician communications.[73]

Box 65-1 Recommendations for Improving Quality of Life Assessments in Palliative Medicine

- Determine main areas affecting QOL based on QOL definition and intervention.[30]
- When possible, measure self-assessed QOL.[30]
- Use proxy ratings for function and physical symptoms when self-assessment impossible.[76]
- Define a clinically important difference applicable to the QOL instrument.[13]
- Choose instruments with validity and reliability adequate for the population, research, or clinical question.[13]
- Trained interviewers are necessary to avoid interviewer-induced bias with individualized assessments (e.g., SEIQoL).[70]
- Use separate global ratings for overall QOL and for overall health-related QOL. Rate the severity and the importance of the problem.[30]
- A single question can better represent overall QOL.[33]
- A single question for overall QOL is an appropriate measure at the end of life.[66]
- At the end of life, consider instruments with a greater emphasis on spirituality.[18,54]

QOL, quality of life; SEIQoL, Schedule for the Evaluation of Individual Quality of Life.

Problems Linked to Measuring Quality of Life

Assessing Patients' Needs

Assessing the patient's needs, similar to assessing the quality of care, is linked closely to QOL. Health-related QOL tools can identify specific and general health needs.[74] The limitations of measuring QOL with the available instruments, especially near death, should be acknowledged, as well as the challenges posed by the need to document the impact of palliative care on the patient's QOL (see "Common Errors").

Quality of Life of Caregivers

Although the patient's QOL has been extensively studied from the patient's and the caregiver's perspective,[75-77] the research on the QOL of caregivers is limited. The relation may be bilateral—the patient's QOL influences the QOL of the family and vice versa. The Quality of Life in Life-Threatening Illness—Family Carer (QOLLTI-F) is a specific instrument that was developed with initial validation.[78] Thirty specific and two global QOL items are included for a time frame within the past 2 days. Domains included are the caregiver's own state, relationships, outlook, and quality of care and the patient's condition, finances, and environment.

Research Opportunities

Extreme variability in the content and validity of assessment instruments and interpretation of QOL results makes comparisons between studies difficult. The multidomain nature of instruments requires large sample sizes to determine differences in outcomes.[12]

Interpreting QOL changes is difficult and may be inaccurate on population level. QOL is strongly influenced by individual medical, environmental, and sociocultural factors. Genetic factors also influence QOL assessed as a symptom experience.[80]

1. QOL self-assessment is considered the gold standard. Surrogate assessments reduce the accuracy of assessment. However, in advanced disease, QOL may be measured by a caregiver with some reliability. Instruments such as the ESAS, STAS, MQOL, and PEPS have included caregivers to different degrees in assessment. Patient and observer score congruency varies for symptoms and QOL, and the correlation is moderate.[56,61,76] Proxy reports of more observable domains, such as physical function and cognition, are closer to patient reports compared with symptoms or overall QOL.[76] The congruity for different pairs varies; it is higher for nurse and patient than for patient and caregiver or physician and patient pairs, most likely because of more time spent by nurses with patients.[76,77] Multiple raters improve the reliability of assessment.[76]

2. Using single items from or shorter versions of validated questionnaires is attractive to clinicians for routine assessments. However, extrapolations from original versions may not be a valid substitute for the full versions. In a similar fashion, single items or subscales measuring symptoms such as pain and fatigue need to be tested for responsiveness, discriminating properties, and validity against the full instrument.[13]

3. Without consensus for what is meant by QOL, investigators should define or adopt a definition of QOL equivalent to the instrument's definition.[30] If overall QOL is not differentiated from overall health-related QOL, nonmedical factors may overinfluence or underinfluence the global score, and health outcomes may be undervalued.[30]

4. Instruments adopted from other disciplines have questions inappropriate for patients at the end of life. An example is the question concerning "difficulties with a long walk" from the EORTC QLQ-C30. These scales show a "floor effect" when used for severely impaired patients.[9,13,44] Using instruments with scales with a significant floor effect provides little relevant information. The time frame of assessment is important for accuracy. Assessing QOL with lengthier time frames (1 week or more) may be inappropriate at the end of life, but assessment at 2 days using the MQOL was found by patients to be a period that was too short to demonstrate a change in QOL.[55] QOL instruments for palliative medicine usually employ a categorical or numerical format. QOL instruments with visual analogue scales, although assumed to be more precise, are difficult to complete, especially in the last days of life.[10,79]

EORTC QLQ-C30, European Organization for Research and Treatment of Cancer Core Questionnaire; ESAS, Edmonton Symptom Assessment System; MQOL, McGill Quality of Life Questionnaire; PEPS, Patient-Evaluated Problem Score; QOL, quality of life; STAS, Support Team Assessment Schedule.

Palliative medicine studies have high dropout rates, which leads to missing data. Missing data influence the QOL outcomes. QOL may appear to improve or stabilize as those with poor QOL drop out over time (Box 65-2).

Individualized instruments such as the SEIQoL determine areas of QOL important to patients, but they do not assess specific symptoms, which require a separate symptom instrument. Palliative medicine patients are polysymptomatic, and appropriate symptom management is a significant part of improving their QOL. The EORTC QLQ-C30 has 12 common symptoms, which is an advantage compared with other QOL instruments.[81] Symptoms can be underreported if not asked in a systematic way.[61,82] Common symptoms such as pain were underreported by patients and were selected only after being mentioned by the staff caregivers.[61] However, the problems of patients and caregivers are different, with psychological issues being more important to patients and patient function and mobility being more important to caregivers.[61] Individualized questionnaires miss symptoms and QOL domains important to patient. Research is needed to determine the balance between assessment burden and comprehensiveness and to identify an unbiased way of prompting patients with individualized assessments.[70] Statistical methods that compare these measures need to be researched.[26]

Cultural differences are important in determining QOL. Belief systems, economics, and the quality of medical care influence QOL and should be considered in the assessment. Cultural differences and translation may influence understanding QOL instruments.[13,44]

Many instruments have aggregated scores, but important information is lost. Using total scores from generic questionnaires may give misleading results for overall QOL. For patients with ALS, despite a decline in function and general health-related QOL as measured by the MOS SF-36, individual QOL measured by SEIQoL remained stable.[15] QOL is more than physical function and physical health, and an emphasis on these factors cannot reflect overall QOL. Lack of knowledge about the minimal clinical difference of a QOL change measured by different instruments can confound interpretation of the results. Whether a summary score or overall QOL score better represents QOL is unclear. The variability of a single QOL question increases responsiveness to change over time, which is valuable in longitudinal assessments and interventional trials.[68]

CONCLUSIONS

Quality of life is a multidimensional and strongly individual construct. Assessing the individual can help in understanding the experiences of the patient and family and in conserving important values throughout the life-threatening disease. Assessing QOL by subjective and objective measures helps to determine its multifaceted nature and reflects important outcomes. Proxy information about physical symptoms can be important at the end of life, when self-assessment is impossible. Simple, understandable, and easy-to-interpret instruments can improve measuring QOL outcomes in palliative medicine. Regular QOL assessments improve communication between the patient and caregivers. Assessing the family along with the patient represents a holistic approach to care.

REFERENCES

1. Plato, Cornford FM (ed). The Republic of Plato. New York: Oxford University Press, 1972, pp 139-143.
2. Aristotle, Ross WD (ed). Ethica Nicomachea. Oxford, UK: Clarendon Press, 1925, pp 1095a-1095b.
3. Sirgy MJ, Michalos AC, Ferris AL, et al. The quality-of-life (QOL) research movement: Past, present, and future. Soc Indicators Res 2006;76:343-466.
4. O'Boyle CA, Waldron D. Quality of life issues in palliative medicine. J Neurol 1997;244(Suppl 4):S18-S25.
5. Preamble to the Constitution of the World Health Organization as adopted by the International Health Conference, New York, June 19-22, 1946; signed on July 22, 1946 by the representatives of 61 states and entered into force on April 7, 1948. Official Records of the World Health Organization, no. 2. Geneva, World Health Organization, 1948, p 100.
6. World Health Organization. World Health Organization Quality of Life Assessment (WHOQOL): Position paper from the World Health Organization. Soc Sci Med 1995;41:1403-1409.
7. Haas BK. A multidisciplinary concept analysis of quality of life. West J Nurs Res 1999;21:728-742.
8. Calman KC. Quality of life in cancer patients—an hypothesis. J Med Ethics 1984;10:124-127.
9. Bruley DK. Beyond reliability and validity: Analysis of selected quality-of-life instruments for use in palliative care. J Palliat Med 1999;2:299-309.
10. Bruera E, Kuehn N, Miller MJ, et al. The Edmonton Symptom Assessment System (ESAS): A simple method for the assessment of palliative care patients. J Palliat Care 1991;7:6-9.
11. Aaronson NK, Ahmedzai S, Bergman B, et al. The European Organization for Research and Treatment of Cancer QLQ-C30: A quality-of-life instrument for use in international clinical trials in oncology. J Natl Cancer Inst 1993;85:365-376.
12. Kaasa S, Loge JH. Quality-of-life assessment in palliative care. Lancet Oncol 2002;3:175-182.
13. Guyatt GH, Feeny DH, Patrick DL. Measuring health-related quality of life. Ann Intern Med 1993;118:622-629.
14. Karnofsky DA, Burchenal JH. The clinical evaluation of chemotherapeutic agents in cancer. In Macleod CM (ed). Evaluation of Chemotherapeutic Agents. New York: Columbia University Press; 1949, pp 191-205.
15. Neudert C, Wasner M, Borasio GD. Individual quality of life is not correlated with health-related quality of life or physical function in patients with amyotrophic lateral sclerosis. J Palliat Med 2004;7:551-557.
16. Velikova G, Stark D, Selby P. Quality of life instruments in oncology. Eur J Cancer 1999;35:1571-1580.
17. Fegg MJ, Wasner M, Neudert C, Borasio GD. Personal values and individual quality of life in palliative care patients. J Pain Symptom Manage 2005; 30:154-159.
18. Mount BM, Boston PH, Cohen SR. Healing connections: On moving from suffering to a sense of well-being. J Pain Symptom Manage 2007;33:372-388.
19. Brady MJ, Peterman AH, Fitchett G, et al. A case for including spirituality in quality of life measurement in oncology. Psychooncology 1999;8:417-428.
20. Schwartz CE, Sprangers MA. Methodological approaches for assessing response shift in longitudinal health-related quality-of-life research. Soc Sci Med 1999;48:1531-1548.
21. Sharpe L, Butow P, Smith C, et al. Changes in quality of life in patients with advanced cancer: Evidence of response shift and response restriction. J Psychosom Res 2005;58:497-504.
22. Echteld MA, Deliens L, Ooms ME, et al. Quality of life change and response shift in patients admitted to palliative care units: A pilot study. Palliat Med 2005;19:381-388.
23. Waldron D, O'Boyle CA, Kearney M, et al. Quality-of-life measurement in advanced cancer: Assessing the individual. J Clin Oncol 1999;17:3603-3611.
24. Neudert C, Wasner M, Borasio GD. Patients' assessment of quality of life instruments: A randomised study of SIP, SF-36 and SEIQoL-DW in patients with amyotrophic lateral sclerosis. J Neurol Sci 2001;19:103-109.
25. Haas BK. Clarification and integration of similar quality of life concepts. Image J Nurs Sch 1999;31:215-220.
26. Higginson IJ, Carr AJ. Measuring quality of life: Using quality of life measures in the clinical setting. BMJ 2001;322:1297-1300.
27. Rogerson RJ. Environmental and health-related quality of life: Conceptual and methodological similarities. Soc Sci Med 1995;41:1373-1382.
28. Lundh Hagelin C, Seiger A, Furst CJ. Quality of life in terminal care—with special reference to age, gender and marital status. Support Care Cancer 2006;14:320-328.
29. Toscani P, Brunelli C, Miccinesi G, et al. Predicting survival in terminal cancer patients: Clinical observation or quality-of-life evaluation? Palliat Med 2005;19:220-227.
30. Gill TM, Feinstein AR. A critical appraisal of the quality of quality-of-life measurements. JAMA 1994;272:619-626.
31. Spitzer WO, Dobson AJ, Hall J, et al. Measuring the quality of life of cancer patients: A concise QL-index for use by physicians. J Chronic Dis 1981;34:585-597.
32. Cohen SR, Mount BM, Bruera E, et al. Validity of the McGill Quality of Life Questionnaire in the palliative care setting: A multi-centre Canadian study

demonstrating the importance of the existential domain. Palliat Med 1997;11:3-20.
33. Bernheim JL. How to get serious answers to the serious question: "How have you been?": Subjective quality of life (QOL) as an individual experiential emergent construct. Bioethics 1999;13:272-287.
34. Feinstein AR. Clinimetric perspectives. J Chron Dis 1987;40:635-640.
35. Wright JG, Feinstein AR. A comparative contrast of clinimetric and psychometric methods for constructing indexes and rating scales. J Clin Epidemiol 1992;45:1201-1218.
36. O'Boyle CA, McGee H, Hickey A, et al. Individual quality of life in patients undergoing hip replacement. Lancet 1992;339:1088-1091.
37. Ware JE Jr, Kosinski M, Gandek B. SF-36 health survey: Manual and interpretation guide. Lincoln, RI: Quality Metric, 2003.
38. Hollen PJ, Gralla RJ, Kris MG, Potanovich LM. Quality of life assessment in individuals with lung cancer: Testing the Lung Cancer Symptom Scale (LCSS). Eur J Cancer 1993;29A(Suppl 1):S51-S58.
39. Kaasa S, Loge JH. Quality of life in palliative care: Principles and practice. Palliat Med 2003;17:11-20.
40. Cleeland CS, Ryan KM. Pain assessment: global use of the Brief Pain Inventory. Ann Acad Med Singapore 1994;23:129-138.
41. Keller S, Bann CM, Dodd SL, et al. Validity of the brief pain inventory for use in documenting the outcomes of patients with noncancer pain. Clin J Pain 2004;20:309-318.
42. Massaro T, McMillan SC. Instruments for assessing quality of life in palliative care settings. Int J Palliat Nurs 2000;6:429-433.
43. McDowel I. The Theoretical and Technical Foundations of Health Measurement. Measuring Health: A Guide to Rating Scales and Questionnaires, 3rd ed. Oxford, UK: Oxford University Press; 2006, pp 10-54.
44. Donnelly S. Quality-of-life assessment in advanced cancer. Curr Oncol Rep 2000;2:338-342.
45. Hearn J, Higginson IJ. Outcome measures in palliative care for advanced cancer patients: A review. J Public Health Med 1997;19:193-199.
46. Hearn J, Higginson IJ. Development and validation of a core outcome measure for palliative care: The palliative care outcome scale. Palliative Care Core Audit Project Advisory Group. Qual Health Care 1999;8:219-227.
47. Higginson IJ, McCarthy M. Validity of the support team assessment schedule: Do staffs' ratings reflect those made by patients or their families? Palliat Med 1993;7:219-228.
48. Ware JE Jr, Sherbourne CD. The MOS 36-item short-form health survey (SF-36). I. Conceptual framework and item selection. Med Care 1992;30:473-483.
49. Bourke SC, McColl E, Shaw PJ, Gibson GJ. Validation of quality of life instruments in ALS. Amyotroph Lateral Scler Other Motor Neuron Disord 2004;5:55-60.
50. Groenvold M, Petersen MA, Aaronson NK, et al. The development of the EORTC QLQ-C15-PAL: A shortened questionnaire for cancer patients in palliative care. Eur J Cancer 2006;42:55-64.
51. McMillan SC, Mahon M. Measuring quality of life in hospice patients using a newly developed Hospice Quality of Life Index. Qual Life Res 1994 Dec;3:437-447.
52. McMillan SC, Weitzner M. Quality of life in cancer patients: Use of a revised Hospice Index. Cancer Pract 1998;6:282-288.
53. McMillan SC, Small BJ. Symptom distress and quality of life in patients with cancer newly admitted to hospice home care. Oncol Nurs Forum 2002;29:1421-1428.
54. Cohen SR, Mount BM, Tomas JJ, Mount LF. Existential well-being is an important determinant of quality of life. Evidence from the McGill Quality of Life Questionnaire. Cancer 1996;77:576-586.
55. Lua PL, Salek S, Finlay I, Lloyd-Richards C. The feasibility, reliability and validity of the McGill Quality of Life Questionnaire-Cardiff Short Form (MQOL-CSF) in palliative care population. Qual Life Res 2005;14:1669-1681.
56. Sterkenburg CA, King B, Woodward CA. A reliability and validity study of the McMaster Quality of Life Scale (MQLS) for a palliative population. J Palliat Care 1996;12:18-25.
57. Byock IR, Merriman MP. Measuring quality of life for patients with terminal illness: The Missoula-VITAS quality of life index. Palliat Med 1998;12:231-244.
58. Schwartz CE, Merriman MP, Reed G, Byock I. Evaluation of the Missoula-VITAS Quality of Life Index-revised: Research tool or clinical tool? J Palliat Med 2005;8:121-135.
59. Steele LL, Mills B, Hardin SR, Hussey LC. The quality of life of hospice patients: Patient and provider perceptions. Am J Hosp Palliat Care 2005; 22:95-110.
60. Namisango E, Katabira E, Karamagi C, Baguma P. Validation of the Missoula-Vitas Quality-of-Life Index among patients with advanced AIDS in urban Kampala, Uganda. J Pain Symptom Manage 2007;33:189-202.
61. Rathbone GV, Horsley S, Goacher J. A self-evaluated assessment suitable for seriously ill hospice patients. Palliat Med 1994;8:29-34.
62. Pratheepawanit N, Salek MS, Finlay IG. The applicability of quality-of-life assessment in palliative care: Comparing two quality-of-life measures. Palliat Med 1999;13:325-334.
63. Steinhauser KE, Clipp EC, Bosworth HB, et al. Measuring quality of life at the end of life: Validation of the QUAL-E. Palliat Support Care 2004;2:3-14.
64. Tamburini M, Rosso S, Gamba A, et al. A therapy impact questionnaire for quality-of-life assessment in advanced cancer research. Ann Oncol 1992;3:565-570.

65. Paci E, Miccinesi G, Toscani F, et al. Quality of life assessment and outcome of palliative care. J Pain Symptom Manage 2001;21:179-188.
66. Donnelly S, Rybicki L, Walsh D. Quality of life measurement in the palliative management of advanced cancer. Support Care Cancer 2001;9:361-365.
67. Donnelly S, Walsh D. Quality of life assessment in advanced cancer. Palliat Med 1996;10:275-283.
68. Huschka MM, Mandrekar SJ, Schaefer PL, et al. A pooled analysis of quality of life measures and adverse events data in north central cancer treatment group lung cancer clinical trials. Cancer 2007;109:787-795.
69. Hickey AM, Bury G, O'Boyle CA, et al. A new short form individual quality of life measure (SEIQoL-DW): Application in a cohort of individuals with HIV/AIDS. BMJ 1996;313:29-33.
70. Westerman M, Hak T, The AM, et al. Problems eliciting cues in SEIQoL-DW: Quality of life areas in small-cell lung cancer patients. Qual Life Res 2006; 15:441-449.
71. Bergner M, Bobbitt RA, Kressel S, et al. The sickness impact profile: Conceptual formulation and methodology for the development of a health status measure. Int J Health Serv 1976;6:393-415.
72. Clark MM, Rummans TA, Sloan JA, et al. Quality of life of caregivers of patients with advanced-stage cancer. Am J Hosp Palliat Care 2006;23:185-191.
73. Velikova G, Booth L, Smith AB, et al. Measuring quality of life in routine oncology practice improves communication and patient well-being: A randomized controlled trial. J Clin Oncol 2004;22:714-724.
74. Asadi-Lari M, Tamburini M, Gray D. Patients' needs, satisfaction, and health related quality of life: Towards a comprehensive model. Health Qual Life Outcomes 2004;2:32-41.
75. Lobchuk MM. The memorial symptom assessment scale: Modified for use in understanding family caregivers' perceptions of cancer patients' symptom experiences. J Pain Symptom Manage 2003;26:644-654.
76. Nekolaichuk CL, Maguire TO, Suarez-Almazor M, et al. Assessing the reliability of patient, nurse, and family caregiver symptom ratings in hospitalized advanced cancer patients. J Clin Oncol 1999;17:3621-3630.
77. Kutner JS, Bryant LL, Beaty BL, Fairclough DL. Symptom distress and quality-of-life assessment at the end of life: The role of proxy response. J Pain Symptom Manage 2006;32:300-310.
78. Cohen R, Leis AM, Kuhl D, et al. QOLLTI-F: Measuring family carer quality of life. Palliat Med 2006 Dec;20:755-767.
79. Hauser K, Walsh D, Davis MP, et al. The pitfalls of visual analogue scales in palliative medicine. Eur J Cancer 2007;14:99-102.
80. Sloan JA, Zhao CX. Genetics and quality of life. Curr Probl Cancer 2006; 30:255-260.
81. Stromgren AS, Groenvold M, Pedersen L, et al. Symptomatology of cancer patients in palliative care: Content validation of self-assessment questionnaires against medical records. Eur J Cancer 2002;38:788-794.
82. Homsi J, Walsh D, Rivera N, et al. Symptom evaluation in palliative medicine: Patient report vs systematic assessment. Support Care Cancer 2006;14:444-453.
83. Mystakidou K, Tsilika E, Kouloulias V, et al. The "Palliative Care Quality of Life Instrument (PQLI)" in terminal cancer patients. Health Qual Life Outcomes 2004;2:8-19.

SUGGESTED READING

Donnelly S. Quality-of-life assessment in advanced cancer. Curr Oncol Rep 2000;2:338-342.

Higginson IJ, Carr AJ. Measuring quality of life: Using quality of life measures in the clinical setting. BMJ 2001;322: 1297-1300.

Kaasa S, Loge JH. Quality of life in palliative care: Principles and practice. Palliat Med 2003;17:11-20.

O'Boyle CA, Waldron D. Quality of life issues in palliative medicine. J Neurol 1997;244(Suppl 4):S18-S25.

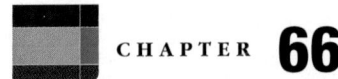

CHAPTER **66**

The Neuropsychological Examination

Bushra Malik

K E Y   P O I N T S

- The neuropsychological examination is useful in discriminating between psychiatric and neurological symptoms.
- Tests focus on the psychometric assessment of cognition and behavior.
- The neuropsychological assessment is unique in its ability to address functional abilities
- Repeated neuropsychological evaluation is invaluable for monitoring cognitive change over time.

Clinical neuropsychology is an applied science concerned with the behavioral expression of brain dysfunction. It deals with the classic problems of psychology, attention, learning, perception, cognition, personality, and psychopathology. Techniques include the methods of experimental psychology, test construction, and the psychometric assessment of cognition and behavior. Neuropsychological assessment can discriminate between psychiatric and neurological symptoms, distinguish different neurological conditions, and provide behavioral data for localizing the site or at least the hemisphere of a lesion.

CLINICAL EVALUATION

The primary goal of neuropsychological assessment is to identify and describe cognitive strengths and weaknesses and to characterize impairments and deficits. Assessment of neuropsychological functioning often detects subtle cognitive deficits undetected by electrophysiological tests or neuroimaging.[1] Other goals of the clinical evaluation are differentiation of intellectual changes associated with brain damage, cognitive and behavioral impairments resulting from psychiatric illness, and cognitive changes caused by normal aging. Indications for neuropsychological assessment include the following:

- Inadequate situational explanations for changes in emotions or cognitive functioning
- A medical condition or injury suspected to have affected brain health (i.e., compromised circulation, chronically poor nutrition, or drug toxicity)
- Sudden, unexpected, and unexplained mental or cognitive performance changes that affect work or daily function
- Gradual or sudden onset of unusual physical, sensory, or motor changes (medical examination is always indicated)
- Failure to improve with special educational or therapeutic interventions for a specific mental or cognitive problem

- Screening examination positive for a brain disorder
- A known brain injury or disease (comprehensive understanding of functional impact is desired)
- A suspected brain injury or disease is suspected (comprehensive neurofunctional characteristics desired to complement the neurological examination and diagnosis)
- Comprehensive diagnostic and functional nature of brain injury or disease needed for rehabilitation and lifelong planning
- Comprehensive diagnostic, functional, and causative nature of brain injury or disease needed for forensic application

Complex diagnostic efforts require careful, objective, and often serial measurement of neurofunctional performance across cognitive domains. In addition to offering information regarding the diagnosis and neuroanatomical localization of dysfunction, the neuropsychological assessment is unique in its ability to address functional abilities. Neuropsychologists often are called on to assess a person's ability to make financial and health care decisions, drive a car, and live independently. These decisions can also determine when someone is able to return to work after injury or what type of job he or she is suited for. A neuropsychological assessment may determine appropriate adjustments to treatment and recommendations about activities of daily living.[2]

Neuropsychological data can help families and caregivers understand the strengths and weaknesses of their loved ones and cope with patients who may suffer from challenging limitations of independent functioning. Beleaguered family members are less likely to be angry with a patient when they understand that the symptoms that appear to be related to motivation or personality instead result from a disease. An understanding of the prognoses of the illness can be invaluable to families who must plan their use of finances and future care.[3]

Neuropsychological deficits can be insidious and difficult to describe, even for sophisticated clinicians. An understanding of the patient's capabilities can help the clinician assess the degree to which he or she will comply with treatment and medications and the extent to which the patient or the patient's family may need continued supervision after discharge.

Repeated neuropsychological evaluation can monitor cognitive change over time. Repeated assessments can track cognitive decline in a progressive illness, such as dementia or multiple sclerosis, or monitor recovery after acute injury. Evaluating the effectiveness of medical procedures and neurological surgery also entails repeated, comprehensive cognitive assessments. Comparison of pretreatment and post-treatment data offers information about changes in the level of functioning after medical intervention[3] (Box 66-1).

COMPONENTS OF THE NEUROPSYCHOLOGICAL ASSESSMENT

The neuropsychological assessment usually involves a clinical interview, review of the patient's records, test selection, test administration and scoring, test interpretation, diagnosis, and recommendations for treatment and rehabilitation.

Box 66-1 Goals of Neuropsychology

- To describe and identify changes in psychological functioning
- To determine the biological correlates of test results
- To decide whether changes are associated with neurological disease, psychiatric conditions, developmental disorders, or neurological conditions
- To assess changes over time and develop a prognosis
- To offer guideline for rehabilitation, vocational, and educational planning
- To provide guidelines and education to the family and caregivers
- To plan for discharge and treatment implementation

Adapted from Hebben N, Milberg W. Essentials of Neuropsychological Assessment. New York: John Wiley, 2002.

The clinical interview may vary in length according to the presenting concerns. A complete interview typically covers developmental background, personal medical and psychiatric history, family medical history, academic performance, vocational achievements, psychosocial functioning, and activities of daily living. Information obtained from collateral sources such as caregivers or spouses about the patient's medical and psychosocial history often is critical. Behavioral observations during the examination are an important source of information that can influence test selection and the interpretation of test scores.[2]

ASSESSMENT TOOLS

The Mini-Mental State Examination

Before neuropsychological referral, the physician typically has clinical or historical evidence of cognitive concerns. The ability to rapidly and reliably assess the nature and extent of cognitive impairments is important. Although a variety of standardized mental status examinations have been used,[3] some are used more widely.[4] One popular mental status examination is the Mini-Mental State Examination, an 11-item standardized method assessing orientation, attention, immediate and short-term recall, naming, and the ability to follow simple verbal and written commands (Fig. 66-1).

Test Selection

Different tests may be appropriate in individual cases, and the test selection process is essential in gathering meaningful information. Some neuropsychologists prefer fixed test batteries such as the Halstead-Reitan battery or the Luria-Nebraska battery for all. These tests include a wide range of cognitive functions, and advocates believe that all functions must be assessed in everyone to avoid diagnostic bias or failure to detect subtle problems. The more common approach is to use a flexible battery based on hypotheses generated through a clinical interview, patient observation, and medical record review. Although this approach is more prone to bias, it prevents unnecessary testing. Because patients often find neuropsychological testing stressful and fatiguing, which can negatively influence performance, advocates of the flexible battery approach argue that tailoring test batteries to particular patients can provide more accurate information.[5]

Maximum score	Score	
		Orientation
5	( )	What is the: (year) (season) (date) (day) (month)
5	( )	Where are we: (state) (county) (town) (facility) (floor)
		Registration
3	( )	Name three objects and have person repeat them back. Give one point for each correct answer on the first trial.
		Attention and Calculation
5	( )	Serial 7's. Count backward from 100 by serial 7's. One point for each correct answer. Stop after 5 answers. [93 86 79 72 65] Alternatively spell "world" backward. [D - L - R - O - W]
		Recall
3	( )	Ask for the names of the three objects learned above. Give one point for each correct answer.
		Language
9	( )	Name: a pen (1 point) and a watch (1 point) Repeat the following: "No ifs, ands, or buts" (1 point) Follow a three-staged command: "Take this paper in your [non-dominant] hand, fold it in half, and put it on the floor." (3 points) [1 point for each part correctly performed] Read to self and then do: "Close your eyes" (1 point) copy design [5 sided geometric figure; 2 points must intersect] (1 point)

Score: _____ /30

Close your eyes

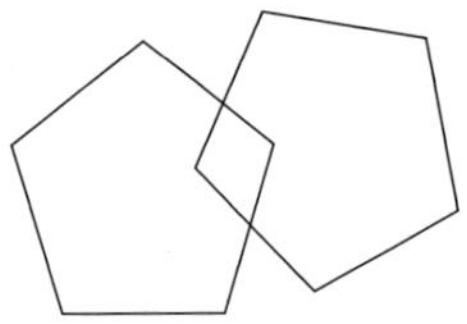

Sentence:

FIGURE 66-1   Mini-Mental State Examination. *(From Broshek DK, Barth JT. The Halstead-Reitan neuropsychological test battery. In Groth-Marnat G (ed). Neuropsychological Assessment in Clinical Practice: A Guide to Test Interpretation and Integration. New York: John Wiley & Sons, 2000.)*

Test Batteries

The test is selected based on the reason for referral. The examiner entertains hypotheses about possible deficits and chooses the test that can elicit and measure deficiencies in expected areas. Consideration of age and education plays a role in test selection, and in some cases, language and cultural history may determine test choice. It is usually necessary to measure intelligence to establish a baseline against which other tests will be compared to confirm discrepancies between skills. The clinician must assemble a test battery that permits assessment of the same cognitive domain with multiple measures to explore deficits reliably. A test battery usually needs to include various measures of attention; executive functions such as reasoning, planning, organization, set establishment, and maintenance; and measures of verbal and visual learning and memory. A test battery usually includes language and perhaps academic skills and visual, tactile, and motor abilities. In many cases, testing must address issues of motivation, effort, and emotional function. The number of tests is determined partly by items available for testing and the patient's stamina.[3] The particular test battery used is the choice of the neuropsychologist and often reflects personal preferences.

Fixed Battery

In the fixed battery approach, the same tests are given to everyone in a standardized manner. One of the most commonly used is the Halstead-Reitan battery.[5] It consists of tests that examine language, attention, motor speed, abstract thinking, memory, and spatial reasoning, and it is often used to produce an overall score that identifies the probability of brain dysfunction. An advantage is that the information gathered is comprehensive and systematically assesses multiple domains of cognitive functioning. The battery also provides useful information regarding the cause of damage (e.g., closed head injury, alcohol abuse, Alzheimer's disease, stroke), which part of the brain was damaged, whether the damage occurred during childhood development, and whether the damage is getting worse, staying the same, or getting better. If repeated assessments are available, test scores can be directly compared with baseline information. Drawbacks of the fixed battery approach include its length (typically 8 hours), because it may be too long for some to tolerate, and its cost and limited reimbursement schedules in managed care.[6] A comprehensive assessment may not be necessary to address the referral question.

Flexible Battery

The flexible (or hypothesis-driven) approach tests intellectual ability, attention, memory, language function, visuoperceptual function, abstract reasoning, and fine motor skills. In contrast to fixed batteries, the number or the type of tests selected within each category depends on the referral question, the history, and results of the clinical interview. A brief set of basic tests is initially administered, and additional tests of more specific abilities are used to meet each patient's needs.

REFERENCES

1. Corral M, Rodriguez M, Amenedo E, et al. Cognitive reserve, age, and neuropsychological performance in healthy participants. Dev Neuropsychol 2006; 29:479-491.
2. Paulsen JS, Ferneyhough-Hoth K. Neurology in clinical practice. In Bradley WG, Daroff RB (eds). Neuropsychology, 4th ed. London: Butterworth, 2000, pp 675-678.
3. Hebben N, Milberg W. Essentials of Neuropsychological Assessment. New York: John Wiley, 2002.
4. Folstein MF, Folstein SE, McHugh PR. Mini-Mental State: A practical method for grading the cognitive state of patients for the clinician. J Psychiatr Res 1975;12:189-198.
5. Lezak MD, Howieson DB, Loring DW. Neuropsychological Assessment, 4th ed. New York: Oxford University Press, 2004.
6. Broshek DK, Barth JT. The Halstead-Reitan neuropsychological test battery. In Groth-Marnat G (ed). Neuropsychological Assessment in Clinical Practice: A Guide to Test Interpretation and Integration. New York: John Wiley & Sons, 2000.

SUGGESTED READING

Anastasi A. Psychological Testing, 4th ed. New York: Macmillan, 1976.
Garvis PE, Barth JT. The Halstead-Teitan Neuropsychological Battery: A Guide to Interpretation and Clinical Application. Odessa, FL: Psychological Assessment Resources, 1994.
Grant I, Adams KM. Neuropsychological Assessment of Neuropsychiatric Disorders, 2nd ed. New York: Oxford University Press, 1996.
Heaton RK, Grant I, Mathews CG. Comprehensive Norms for an Expanded Halstead-Reitan Battery. Odessa, FL: Psychological Assessment Resources, 1991.
Heilman KM, Valenstein E. Clinic Neuropsychology, 3rd ed. New York: Oxford University Press, 1993.
Kaplan RM, Saccuzzo DP. Psychological Testing: History, Principles, and Applications, 4th ed. Boston: Allyn & Bacon, 2001.
Spreen O, Tisser AH, Edgell D. Developmental Neuropsychology. New York: Oxford University Press, 1995.

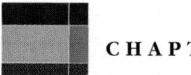

CHAPTER **67**

Sexuality and Intimacy in the Critically Ill

Martina Kern

> **KEY POINTS**
> - People with a life-limiting illness continue to be sexual beings.
> - Patients and partners should be given space and privacy to facilitate closeness.
> - Many critically ill patients need support to develop appropriate strategies for sexual activity.
> - A caregiver whom the patient trusts and with whom he or she wants to talk needs to accept the role and be prepared to discuss sexual issues.
> - The caregiver's ability to communicate about sexuality depends on knowledge, empathy, and self-reflection.

Sexuality often is not addressed in the care for the critically ill. Caregivers struggle to accept that people with a life-limiting illness, particularly older individuals, are still sexual beings and that their intimacy should be respected. This important aspect of human existence is often neglected when dealing with the critically ill and the dying, even though the approach of palliative care is holistic by definition (see "Common Errors").

DEFINITIONS OF SEXUALITY

A widely used German medical lexicon defines sexuality as follows: "Genetic, morphologic, and functional differentiation of a species into two—in some lower organisms even more—sexes and their mutual functional relation with regard to reproduction."[1] How sexuality is addressed or neglected in palliative care probably reflects this rather biological and functional understanding of sexuality.

> **Common Errors**
> - Critically ill people, particularly older people, are no longer interested in sexual activity.
> - Caregivers should never address sexual issues, except when asked to do so.
> - Sexual issues are to be discussed with a gynecologist, urologist, or psychologist (e.g., family therapist) but not with palliative care physicians or nurses.
> - If a patient has a serious disease-related sexual problem, he will talk about it.
> - Loss of sexual activity is a self-evident and unavoidable result of a life-limiting advanced illness.

The World Health Organization defines human sexuality as "a central aspect of being human throughout life [encompassing] sex, gender identities and roles, sexual orientation, eroticism, pleasure, intimacy, and reproduction. Sexuality is experienced and expressed in thoughts, fantasies, desires, beliefs, attitudes, values, behaviors, practices, roles, and relationships."[2]

SEXUALITY AND SOCIETY

In Western societies, sexuality is widely discussed by the media. So-called information about normal habits creates a climate of pressure to succeed in terms of intercourse frequency and multiple orgasms. Almost without exception, sexuality is associated with youth and beauty. A truly sexual being is dynamic, athletic, thin, and healthy. Sexuality in the context of illness is taboo.

As an example, a workshop on sexuality in the critically ill begins with an introduction of the participants. At first, they are asked to name their favorite dish and describe it in detail. The atmosphere is playful, and there is a variety of dishes and descriptions. Although the participants had never met, they quickly make close contact and want to learn more about the other participants' likings. The workshop leader then announces this was only a warm-up and that they would now have to talk about their sexual preferences. There is dead silence. After letting the uncomfortable silence linger, the leader says, "Okay, I only wanted to show you how it is to be confronted with a taboo."

As expected, the participants feel relieved and start to discuss how it feels having to talk about their own sexuality. They express dismay, shame, feeling dumbstruck, fear of not meeting expectations suggested in the media, and anger at having others look into their private lives. Talk about sexuality is a taboo, and this often makes it impossible for caregivers to address the subject with patients and their families.

SEXUALITY AND SEXUAL NEEDS OF THE CRITICALLY ILL

"People who have cancer are people. They have sexual identity, and although varied from each other in most aspects, they have one thing in common: a need for love and intimacy and are entitled to have those needs met."[2] There is hardly a difference in the meaning of sexuality for healthy or ill persons. Sexuality is a dominant drive of human nature. The wish to experience intimacy, warmth, closeness, safety, empathy, and relationships is universal and independent of age and of health or illness. Sexual identity in terms of femininity and masculinity affects all aspects of life. Sexual expression is associated with the feeling of being alive.

Self-esteem and self-confidence are related to how comfortable an individual feels in his or her gender role and sexual identity. Most critically ill patients have a history of health; they experienced sexual intimacy and bad or good sexual relationships.

A serious illness causes major life changes, a process of destabilization, and changed priorities. The disease itself and therapeutic interventions may have a serious impact on organ functions. Patients are often in pain and are limited in daily routines by compromised physical functioning. Whereas the main interest of patients newly diagnosed with a life-limiting disease is survival, their remaining quality of life will be considered after the first shock. Patients may ask others or ask themselves questions about their relationships. In which way will the disease alter my body or my looks? How will the others react? Will they still accept me as I am? Will they still love me?

Assuming that sexuality is as important for sick as for healthy persons, a severe, function-limiting disease is bound to affect self-esteem and self-confidence. Any disorder or dysfunction of the body may have an impact on sexuality and libido (i.e., on sexual function, reaction, and fulfillment). Physical disorders may be associated with emotional problems. Uncertainty, fear, strain, loneliness, shame, guilt, and depression affect vitality, self-esteem, and the feeling of being in control.

It is unusual for critically ill individuals to be perceived as persons with a sexual identity. The focus of attention is the disease. Critically ill persons need to be reassured that talking about sexual or intimate issues is permitted. They need information, space, and support. Otherwise, the feeling of loneliness and exclusion may increase further. It is not uncommon among couples for the healthy person to withdraw from the sick partner.

THE MEANING OF SEXUALITY FOR CAREGIVERS

Caregivers may feel insecure and too ashamed to address sexuality. Communication with patients about the subject is rarely covered in their education. They may believe that asking patients about whether the disease affects their sexuality is intrusive. That patients rarely take the initiative to address the subject is widely seen as proof they do not wish to talk about it. Caregivers may feel uneasy about raising the issue, because they may have to communicate openly and react. Under the false assumption that silence means consent not to address a taboo, patients get the message caregivers have more important tasks to fulfill and that it is inappropriate to broach a private subject.

Inhibitions to talk about sexuality, however, are rarely based on not wanting to disrupt a patient's privacy. Other tasks of caregivers, such as catheter or thermometer insertion, are intimate.[3] Problems in addressing sexual issues are comparable with the difficulties caregivers experience in talking about death and dying. Caregivers' inabilities and fears are mostly responsible for excluding these topics during communication with patients. It is of utmost importance for caregivers of critically ill and dying patients to look into these subjects. With regard to sexuality, intimacy, and tenderness, this includes improvement of knowledge and communication skills and self-reflection. Without this, a more comfortable and empathic approach to dealing with these needs cannot be achieved.[4]

For example, patients often ask their nurse, "Nurse, look at me, at what I look like. Do you think I will be getting better? If the nurse perceives the message of only the last sentence, she will think that the patient's wish is to talk about diagnosis and prognosis. However, if the nurse focuses on the patient's self-esteem, she may hear the hidden invitation to talk about the patient's altering body and her problems with it. The nurse may reply "Sometimes, you are no longer familiar with your own body or your looks, are you?" In this way, she would give a hint that she accepts the invitation to talk about physical changes and, probably later on, the impact of these changes on the patient's sexual identity.

COMMUNICATION PROBLEMS

Verbal communication, an art in itself even under favorable terms, becomes difficult under pressure. Disrupted or failed communication may cause misunderstandings, irritation, frustration, disappointment, and retreat. Failed communication may lead to total loss of sexual practice and therefore quality of life (Fig. 67-1) Good and empathic communication, however, may help patients realize that they can learn to live with their losses and focus on the positive aspects of what is still possible. They can look for new and alternative ways of finding satisfaction and sexual feeling. Creativity and imagination are the keys to further integration of sexuality in the patients' lives.

INTERVENTIONS

What support and which interventions do critically ill patients need for sexuality, intimacy, and tenderness? It is best to let them speak for themselves. They communicate their needs in various unequivocal ways. They want respect. They want to be seen as human beings, as individuals. When exposed to others in their nakedness, they may have to relinquish the protective covering of their clothes, but not their dignity, individual values, opinions, wishes, and longings. They have the right to information about any intervention or development that concerns their condition, body, and health and therefore their quality of life.

The PLISSIT Model

In 1976, the American psychologist Jack Annon developed a simple model based on the fact that most people with sexual problems do not need intensive therapy. He used the acronym PLISSIT for four basic forms of sex therapy:

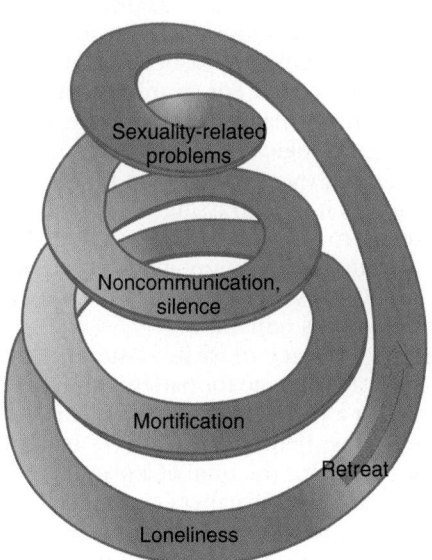

FIGURE 67-1 Spiral of loneliness.

permission, limited information, specific suggestions, and intensive therapy.

Permission

Permission means acknowledging that patients, at any age or condition, have sexual identity and needs. These should be given legitimacy, discussed, and met.

Many sexual dysfunctions are caused by anxiety, feelings of guilt, or inhibition. When patients are given the permission to express their feelings and are being told these feelings are normal, no further intervention may be needed. If a therapist using his or her professional authority gives permission to do what the patient is already doing, it can alleviate much unnecessary suffering (e.g., guilt and anxiety about masturbation).

Patients often suffer from fear of failure. Fear of failure leads to avoidance of sexual contact. It is mostly men who become victims of their own high sexual standards. When they are with a woman, they are intimidated by negative thoughts (e.g., Will I have a proper erection? Will I be able to keep it?) These concerns cause anxiety and tension and act as a self-fulfilling prophecy. The next intimate situation increases tension and distress and creates sexual problems, a vicious cycle of fear of failure and sexual dysfunction. This most likely leads to sexual retreat and the associated avoidance.[5]

A 28-year-old patient with testicular cancer was asked whether his disease affected his relationship. He answered that he was about to split up with his partner because the relationship had become increasingly difficult. When asked to tell more about the difficulties, he said, "It no longer worked." Since he underwent surgery, he had erectile dysfunction. Being with his partner felt increasingly tense, even though she said that she could cope. They gave up having sex. For him, the situation was unbearable, and he would rather dissolve the relationship than have his partner stay out of pity.

The first step was to explain to the patient that is normal to have such feelings and that it is normal for unexpressed anxiety, fear, and inhibition to lead to introversion. The patient realized how important it was to talk with his partner in more detail about the problem, because it affected both of them. When the couple discussed the issue, she admitted that it had bothered her to no longer have a sexual relationship. Nevertheless, she wanted to stay because she loved him, not because she pitied him. She had kept her distance because she did not want to increase the distress he already had trying to cope with his disease.

After talking openly, the couple was able to try other forms of sexual contact, such as enjoying caressing each other without feeling under pressure to perform sexual intercourse. The information that the patient's erectile disorder probably was intermittent was also of great importance in this case.

Limited Information

Giving limited information provides correct anatomical and physiological information to help patients understand body functions. Well-chosen and well-presented information leads to appropriate expectations and reduces fear. For example, it is important to inform a patient that after a medication for cystitis, the urine will be red. It should be routine to tell patients that certain interventions and the disease itself may suppress menstruation and cause early menopause, that loss of pubic hair from genital radiotherapy is irreversible, or that libido and sexual potency are negatively affected by certain medications. Nevertheless, explanations of serious side effects of treatments are often neglected, probably because caregivers believe such information can lead to rejection of a proposed intervention.

A patient with severe burning pain caused by his cancer was given low-dose antidepressants for pain. When asked, he stated that he suffered from severe erectile dysfunction as a consequence. His pain was substantially reduced, but he wanted to discontinue the medication because of its other physical effects, which he found unacceptable.

Specific Suggestions

Specific suggestions offer explicit information. General statements minimize the problem and are not helpful. Examples of specific suggestions are that dyspareunia from vaginal dryness due to hormone therapy responds to lubricating gel and that irrigation or use of a safety pouch, deodorant, or gas filter should be used before sexual intercourse for those with a colostomy.

Even though some of these suggestions may seem obvious and are often intuitively implemented by some patients, they should be mentioned. It is always helpful to verbalize practical suggestions, even if they match the ideas of the patients. Helpful suggestions may shorten the time for finding a solution or reassure the patient about his or her own solution. The more specific the information, the easier it may be put into practice by a patient and the partner.

A patient with advanced cancer and ascites was regularly admitted to a palliative care unit for ascites drainage and pain control. She mentioned to her nurse that she found her swollen belly intrusive. Later, she said that she no longer had sexual intercourse with her husband because of her belly but that she would like to. "This belly is like being pregnant," she said thoughtfully. When the nurse asked her whether she had sexual intercourse during her pregnancy, the patient answered, "Well, of course we had; we just chose a different position." The nurse also mentioned that the patient's belly usually was rather flat immediately after ascites drainage.

Intensive Therapy

Intensive therapy requires long-term intervention for complex problems. These cases are uncommon. Nevertheless, caregivers should be able to recognize when patients need intensive therapy and refer them to specialists.

Addressing Sexuality and Intimacy in Palliative Care

Facilitating Communication

Not every critically ill patient wants to talk about sexuality, and carefully placed words will not solve every problem. Progressive diseases cause irreversible changes, and from some point in the course of disease onward,

patients no longer have the same sexuality as in their healthy days. Avoiding these issues does not make it easier for patients. An invitation to talk creates a climate of normality. The message is that it is normal to have sexual needs and to fulfill them. Patients and their partners may be enabled to change or abandon the possibilities of earlier days and find new ways to seek fulfillment and intimacy.

The beginning of this process is usually accompanied by strong grief reactions. Talking about this grief, if only among the partners, is a precondition for acknowledging the new situation and developing strategies to cope.

Developing New Forms of Sexuality and Intimacy

Sexuality is more than sexual intercourse. Coitus is one expression of a loving relationship, but it is not the only one. Many couples confronted with physical restrictions of sexual activity cancel any trial of sexual intercourse and any physical contact and closeness. They overlook the fact that the whole body responds to a tender and arousing touch[5]; partners often feel insecure about how and when to do this. Careful instruction can overcome shyness and clumsiness and develop new, creative sexual activity.

Instructions may include massage techniques, such as foot massage. Giving and receiving a massage can be a first step to getting into touch again, and it may reactivate the experience of being a couple in a sexual relationship.

Preconditions for Good Communication

Several elements can facilitate a discussion about sex. The first is the role of the caregiver. It is indispensable to reflect on the caregiver's own role and adhere to this. The work of nurses includes many tasks in which patients are exposed, naked, and defenseless, often in a way they would never expose themselves to their partners (e.g., ulcerating wounds). Patients are intimately touched by nurses (e.g., washing of genitals, application of ointments in genital areas). Some patients find this extremely embarrassing, or they exhibit an automatic reaction of arousal, which probably leads to misunderstandings and more embarrassment.

In intimate caregiving situations, it is important to act in a matter-of-fact way with business-like action. Talk about sexuality in situations that can lead to misunderstandings (e.g., while being washed by a nurse) is neither helpful nor professional. For example, Mrs. G was very nervous because she had to see a new gynecologist for her regular gynecological checkup after her old doctor retired. During the examination, she told the doctor that she always found it embarrassing to go to a gynecologist and that having to see a new doctor made her feel even more uneasy. The doctor complimented her on her youthful looks. Mrs. G. was utterly distressed and did not know what to make of this remark.

The patient's privacy must be ensured. Talking about sexual issues is a challenge for patients and, as experience shows, for most caregivers. It takes sensitivity and attentiveness. It is most helpful if caregivers make provisions not to be disturbed for the time of a planned conversation with patients and their partners (i.e., no phone calls or interruptions). As in all conversations, it is good to allow some time for discussing a subject but the duration should be limited. The capacity of the critically ill to concentrate is often underrated; the length of a conversation is not necessarily proportional to its effectiveness.

The patient must be respected. When a patient invites a caregiver to talk about an issue of individual importance, this must be respected and taken seriously. Their problems must not be belittled or denied. Patients should be encouraged to use their own language about sexual issues. Caregivers should reflect on their own behavior in distressing conversations. For most caregivers, it may make things easier to keep their distance by using professional or medical terminology. Patients, however, may feel insecure when they get the impression they must use medically correct terms about sexual issues.

Development of a helpful attitude needs self-reflection. The preconditions for a good conversation about sexual issues are not different from other thematic caregiver-patient conversations. Caregivers need an empathic, professional, and matter-of-fact approach to create an atmosphere in which patients and their partners can talk about private matters and fears. A caregiver whom the patient trusts and with whom he or she wants to talk, however, needs to accept the role and have a clear opinion of what healthy sexuality is. Caregivers should also know about physiological, pharmacological, pathological, and other aspects of the disease and have good communication skills.

SEXUAL COUNSELING

Patients expect that effects on their sexuality will be treated with the same respect as other effects of their illness, such as sleep disorders. They assume that caregivers know what needs to be done, but they do not understand that caregivers may be too shy, inhibited, or insecure to bring up the issue because of lack of education, expertise, or communication skills. Patients may believe their caregivers have no interest when the subject is not addressed. Patients may believe that they are expected to take care of it or that there is no solution and therefore no reason to talk about it.

In complex cases in which a specialist is needed, physicians should be careful to make the referral themselves and pass on relevant information. This spares the patient embarrassing questions and situations. Patients with a clearly defined physical disorder need not be referred to a psychologist. Instead, the physical problem needs to be treated.[3] It is rarely necessary to refer critically ill patients to specialist counselors. Instead, the situation needs open communication, empathy, and self-reflection, and it requires respect for patients and their partners as human beings with sexual identities and needs.

REFERENCES

1. Roche Lexikon der Medizin, 3rd ed. Munich: Urban & Schwarzenberg, 1993.
2. Von Eschenbach AC, Schouer LR. Sexual rehabilitation of the cancer patient. Cancer Nurs 1984;12:10-15.
3. Yaniv H. Sexualität und Intimität. In Allbert E (ed). Lehrbuch der Palliativmedizin Sexualität und Intimität. Stuttgart: Schattauer, 1997, pp 780-788.
4. Schover L, Jensen S. Sexuality and chronic illness. New York: Guilford Press, 1988.
5. Zettl S, Hartlapp J. Krebs und Sexualität. Berlin: Weingärtner Verlag, 2002.

SUGGESTED READING

Deutsches Krebsforschungs-Zentrum. Krebspatienten und Sexualität. Heidelberg: Krebsinformationsdienst (KID), 1998.

Dunde SR. Handbuch Sexualität. Weinheim: Deutscher Studien Verlag, 1992.
Johnson D. Touch—Die Berührung. Paderborn: Junfermann Verlag, 1994.
Kockott G. Männliche Sexualität. Stuttgart: Hippokrates Verlag, 1988.
Müller M. Dem Sterben Leben Geben. Bonn: Gütersloher Verlaghaus, 2004.
Rosemeier HP, Höfert HW, Göpfert W (eds). Intimität und Sexualität. Berlin: Quintessenz Verlag, 1993.

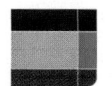

CHAPTER **68**

Assessment of Mobility

Sarah E. Callin and Michael I. Bennett

> **K E Y   P O I N T S**
>
> - Being independently mobile is a key component of quality of life in advanced disease.
> - Assessment of mobility is best viewed as an assessment of performance across a range of tasks.
> - Several tools are commonly used, including Karnofsky Performance Status Scale, Eastern Cooperative Oncology Group Performance Status Scale, and the Barthel Index.
> - Accurate assessment of mobility informs decisions about prognosis and the place of care.
> - Maintaining mobility is important because it prevents deconditioning and delays dependency on others.

PRINCIPLES OF ASSESSMENT

The ability to move or mobilize independently is taken for granted by healthy people. However, during ill health or after permanent injury, being independently mobile is a significant component of quality of life. For people facing life-threatening disease, assessment and maintenance of mobility are key areas to focus on.

Assessment of mobility is best viewed as assessment of performance across a range of tasks. Maintaining mobility is important because it prevents deconditioning and delays dependency, which influences the place of care, such as the home or an institution. Even low-intensity exercise or rehabilitation can reduce the symptom burden.

Reduced mobility or disability (i.e., inability to perform a certain task) is not the same as handicap. The latter is defined as the consequences of the disability that limits or prevents fulfillment of a significant role (e.g., mother, lover, worker, independent adult). Someone may be disabled but does not necessarily perceive herself or himself as handicapped.

ASSESSMENT TOOLS

The science of assessing mobility began in the middle of the 20th century. Most initial development and testing of tools occurred between 1950 and 1990. Many such tools are in regular use in oncology, elderly medicine, and rehabilitation.

Karnofsky Performance Status Scale

The original Karnofsky Performance Status (KPS) Scale was developed to measure the impact of cancer and its treatment on function in lung cancer patients given nitrogen mustard therapy.[1] The KPS scale has been widely used in clinical practice and research within cancer and palliative care, and it is considered a gold standard method of quantifying the functional status of cancer patients.

Uses

The KPS scale provides more accurate prognosis than clinical estimation for the terminally ill,[2] and it is used to stratify and select patients in chemotherapeutic trials.[3] It is used with other measures to evaluate the response to and impact of treatments and disease progression in individuals.[4]

Structure

In its original form, the KPS scale consists of 11 categories, with scores divided into deciles ranging from 100 (i.e., asymptomatic, normal function) to 0 (i.e., death). Each category combines information on the ability to function, ability to work, severity of symptoms, and need for care (Table 68-1). It provides a global assessment of mobility by assessing ability to carry out normal activity. The KPS scale does not record information regarding specific mobility impairment or the ability to carry out particular activities of daily living (ADLs). Information to determine which category best describes the performance status can be collected by interview, observation, examination, or a combination of these methods. It is quick and easy to complete. Modified versions have been developed, and they include condensed and expanded versions. The original form remains the most widely used (see Table 68-1).

Validity and Reliability

The KPS scale is reliable and valid for the assessment of physical functioning in cancer.[5-7] Early studies raised questions about reliability.[8] The main cause for poor reliability outcomes was lack of guidance for those completing the assessments about how to assign a given level of function. Further studies using standardized assessment and structured training have shown good interrater agreement.[5,6] These validation studies have established that KPS scores are closely correlated with deterioration in function and that the tool correlates well with other independent measures of physical functioning. The ability of the KPS scale to monitor change is less certain, and scores for terminal cancer patients cluster[9] at the low end of the scale (≤30), limiting its sensitivity to change (Table 68-2).

Eastern Cooperative Oncology Group Performance Status Scale

In 1960, an alternative measure, the Eastern Cooperative Oncology Group Performance Status Scale (ECOG-PS)

TABLE 68-1	Karnofsky Performance Status Scale	
SCORE	**CRITERIA**	**DEFINITION**
100	Normal: no complaints, no evidence of disease	Able to carry on normal activity and to work; no special care needed
90	Able to carry on normal activity, minor symptoms	
80	Normal activity with effort, some symptoms	
70	Cares for self, unable to carry on normal activities	Unable to work; able to live at home and care for most personal needs; various degrees of assistance needed
60	Requires occasional assistance, cares for most needs	
50	Requires considerable assistance and frequent care	
40	Disabled: requires special care and assistance	Unable to care for self; requires equivalent of institutional or hospital care; disease may be progressing rapidly
30	Severely disabled: hospitalized but death not imminent	
20	Very sick: active supportive care needed	
10	Moribund: fatal processes are progressing rapidly	
0	Dead	

TABLE 68-2	Strengths and Limitations of the Karnofsky Performance Scale
STRENGTHS	**LIMITATIONS**
Widespread use in cancer and palliative care	Provides a global assessment of mobility with difficulty separating out impact of mobility from that of symptoms
Reliable when used in cancer patients with structured guidelines	
Good validity demonstrated in cancer patients	
Required information can be collected by interview, observation, or examination	
Compact and not time consuming	Less sensitive to change due to limited number of categories
Minimal training required although improved reliability with structured training employed	
Simple scoring system	
Scores easily communicated	Ordinal measure
Metric scoring system convenient for statistical analysis	

was developed for cancer.[10,11] It assesses how the disease affects ADLs.

Uses

As with the KPS, it is widely used in cancer and palliative care to compare functional outcome after cancer treatment, to select patients for clinical trials, and to predict survival. Many trials include minimum ECOG-PS scores as part of their eligibility criteria.

Structure

The ECOG-PS consists of six categories that measure the ability to function (at work and home) and the ability for self-care, with a focus on activity (Table 68-3). Total scores range from 0 (i.e., fully active) to 5 (i.e., dead). As with the KPS scale, the ECOG-PS provides a global assessment of function. It includes reference to level of ambulation, including the percentage of time confined to bed, and general ability to carry out self-care, but it does not provide a detailed assessment of mobility or ability to carry out any single ADL. The ECOG-PS is self-explanatory and easy to complete, requiring no formal training.

Validity and Reliability

The ECOG-PS has good validity and reliability in assessing cancer patients.[7,12] It is reliable as a self-assessment tool.[13,14] Comparisons of the ECOG-PS with the KPS scale have described them as comparable, but the former had lower interrater variability and greater predictive validity[12] (Table 68-4).

Barthel Index

The Barthel Index, used in clinical practice since 1955 as the Maryland Disability Index, was first published in 1965.[15] It was originally developed to monitor functional independence in self-care and mobility during inpatient rehabilitation.

Uses

Use of the Barthel Index has been extended to patients with different conditions, including cancer, and to those receiving palliative care. Moderate to severe functional disability in stroke and elderly patients as measured by the Barthel Index predicts hospital mortality, prolonged hospital stay, discharge destination, early emergency hospital readmission, use of home health care services, later social functioning, and mortality within 6 months of discharge.[16-20] The rate of change of the Barthel Index is an important indicator of survival in hospice.[21]

The Barthel Index measures independent function in ADLs and the need for care. The main aim is to establish some independence from any help, physical or verbal. Use of independence aids is allowed, but supervision renders the patient not independent. Versions of the Barthel Index include the original 10-item form,[15] the expanded 15-item version,[22] and the Modified Barthel Index (MBI).[23]

Structure

In its original form, the Barthel Index contained 10 items scored on a 3-point scale (Table 68-5). Two items can be described as purely mobility related (i.e., walking or propelling a wheelchair on a level surface and ascending and descending stairs) and eight as self-care activities requiring

---

TABLE 68-3 Eastern Cooperative Oncology Group Performance Status Scale

GRADE	PERFORMANCE STATUS
0	Fully active; able to carry on all predisease performance without restriction
1	Restricted in physically strenuous activity but ambulatory and able to carry out work of a light or sedentary nature (e.g., light housework, office work)
2	Ambulatory and capable of all self-care but unable to carry out any work activities; up and about more than 50% of waking hours
3	Capable of only limited self-care; confined to bed or chair more than 50% of waking hours
4	Completely disabled; cannot carry on any self-care; totally confined to bed or chair
5	Dead

TABLE 68-4 Strengths and Limitations of the Eastern Cooperative Oncology Group Performance Scale

STRENGTHS	LIMITATIONS
Widespread use in cancer and palliative care	Less sensitive to change because of the small number of categories
Reliable scale for use in cancer patients	Ordinal measure
Good validity demonstrated in cancer patients	
Simple to understand	
Quick and easy to complete	
Minimal or no formal training required	
Simple scoring system	
Scores easily communicated	

TABLE 68-5 Original Barthel Index

ITEMS	UNABLE TO PERFORM TASK	WITH HELP	INDEPENDENT
Feeding (if food needs to be cut = help needed)	0	5	10
Moving from wheelchair to bed (includes sitting up in bed)	0	5-10	15
Personal toilet (e.g., wash face, comb hair, shave, clean teeth)	0	0	5
Getting on and off toilet (e.g., handling clothes, wipe, flush)	0	5	10
Bathing self	0	0	5
Walking on a level surface (or if unable to walk, propel wheelchair)	0 (0)	10 (0)*	15 (5)*
Ascend and descend stairs	0	0	10
Dressing (includes tying shoes, fastening fasteners)	0	5	10
Controlling bowels	0	5	10
Controlling bladder	0	5	10

*Score only if unable to walk.

various degrees of mobility (i.e., feeding, transfer from chair to bed and back, grooming, toileting, bathing, dressing, and bowel and bladder continence). Items get arbitrary weightings, and those considered more important for independence, including ambulation and transfers, are weighted more heavily than less important items such as bathing and personal hygiene. The scoring system for the original 10-item form ranges from 0 (i.e., fully dependent) to 100 (i.e., fully independent). The original 10 items were modified and a different scoring system[24] proposed because a score of 100 could lead to a misleading impression of accuracy. Scores were modified for each item and the scoring converted to 1-point increments, for a maximum possible total score of 20.

The 15-item version[22] extended the index to 15 topics using 4-point response scales for most items, with overall scores from 0 to 100. The latest adaptation was developed[23] to improve sensitivity to change. It retains the original 10 items and provides scores up to a maximum of 100, but it has five instead of three levels of dependency (Table 68-6). There is no consensus about which is the definitive Barthel Index, but the original, whether scored to 100 or 20, appears to be the most widely used.

Reliability and Validity

The Barthel Index is simple and easy. The information to complete the score can be obtained through interview, observation, examination, or a combination of these methods.[24] It is quick to complete and the scoring straightforward, although it requires calculation by adding individual ADL subscores. Unlike the KPS scale and the ECOG-PS, there is a risk of inaccurate scoring if items are incomplete. Assessors need to be trained.

The Barthel Index has been widely tested for reliability and validity.[22-27] The main use remains in specialist rehabilitation units, and most reliability and validity tests are done in this context. Published studies use different versions of the Barthel Index.

Studies have demonstrated the reliability of different versions and confirmed high interrater agreement, good internal consistency, and test-retest reliability. Concordance[24] exists among the four ways of administering the original scale: self-report, clinical observation, nurse examination, and physiotherapist examination. Telephone scoring with the help of relatives is reliable.[25]

Validity testing showed the Barthel Index correlated highly with other outcome measures at a particular point in time and as a measure of improvement over time. High predictive validity correlates well with clinical judgment and predicts mortality and place of discharge after strokes.[26,27] The Barthel Index, particularly the MBI, may provide greater sensitivity than other measures because it has more measuring tiers within its multi-item scale.[23]

Drawbacks

The major criticism of the Barthel Index has been scoring. Although the original is easy to use and focuses on physical limitations, interpreting the middle dependency categories and what defines *requiring assistance* is difficult and can be inconsistent. The different approaches to scoring, along with their suggested guidelines, have helped to overcome this problem (Table 68-7).

Other Measures of Physical Functioning

Although the KPS scale, the ECOG-PS, and the Barthel Index are the most widely used measures of physical functioning used in palliative care, many other indices are available. Some are different versions of tools already discussed. The World Health Organization Performance Status Scale (WHO-PS) and the New York Heart Association (NYHA) classification are widely used and replicate the ECOG-PS. Both measure ability to carry out normal activity and describe limitations in function imposed by symptoms, with deterioration recorded as the percentage of time restricted to bed. The WHO-PS scale is specific to cancer patients and refers to "tumor manifestations," and

TABLE 68-7 Strengths and Limitations of the Barthel Index	
STRENGTHS	**LIMITATIONS**
Compact and not time consuming	Formal training required
Sensitive to changes over time	(although reported to be
Provides detailed information about	quick)
individual activities of daily living,	Risk of incomplete scores
including pure mobility activities	Patients not fully cooperating
Total score easily communicated	may be inaccurately scored
Metric score convenient for statistical	
analysis	

TABLE 68-6 Modified Barthel Index					
ITEMS	UNABLE TO PERFORM TASK	ATTEMPTS TASK BUT UNSAFE	MODERATE HELP REQUIRED	MINIMAL HELP REQUIRED	FULLY INDEPENDENT
Personal hygiene	0	1	3	4	5
Bathing self	0	1	3	4	5
Feeding	0	2	5	8	10
Toilet	0	2	5	8	10
Stair climbing	0	2	5	8	10
Dressing	0	2	5	8	10
Bowel control	0	2	5	8	10
Bladder control	0	2	5	8	10
Ambulation (wheelchair)	0 (0)	3 (1)	8 (3)	12 (4)	15 (5)
Chair-bed transfers	0	3	8	12	15

the NYHA classification is used for assessing congestive heart failure.

Other available measures are used less and have limited validity and reliability data. Direct comparison of the Barthel Index with two other ADL indices—the Katz Index and the Kenney Care Index—found that all were valid and reliable but that there were no benefits gained from the Katz and Kenney Indices and that the Barthel Index had more extensive supportive data.[26]

ADL measures such as the Edmonton Functional Assessment Tool (EFAT) were specifically developed for and tested in palliative care patients, and they include assessment of psychosocial activities and physical ADLs.[9] They may be useful when more comprehensive ADL assessments are required. However, when the focus is on physical functioning, it can be difficult to separate relevant information, and psychosocial functioning may distort the outcome. Quality of life instruments that contain various degrees of physical functional assessment and varied weighting between tools create similar difficulties.

Sometimes, it may be appropriate to do a more detailed assessment of mobility. Subitems of ADL scales cannot detect small differences in mobility. In these situations, pure mobility measures may help, and several are available. The Rivermead Mobility Index (RMI) is one.[28] It was developed from the gross function section of the Rivermead Motor Assessment and is a 15-item scale that assesses mobility disability through a range of fundamental activities from turning over in bed to running. It has been tested only in patients with neurological impairments.

CONCLUSIONS AND RESEARCH OPPORTUNITIES

The KPS scale and ECOG-PS are performance status scales with established reliability and validity for use in cancer. Direct comparison has shown the ECOG-PS minimizes differences between observers and has greater predictive validity. The ECOG-PS and KPS scale provide a general overview of performance status and therefore of physical function but not specific mobility impairments. The Barthel Index is an ADL measure with more extensive subcategory information for recording specific ADLs. It has predominantly been used in and shown to be reliable and valid in specialist rehabilitation, and further research is needed to support its use in palliative care. The KPS scale, the ECOG-PS, and the Barthel Index provide an overview of physical function and therefore may not detect low-level disability. Pure mobility measures, such as the RMI, include more detailed assessments but are suitable only in certain circumstances. For most palliative care patients, assessment of mobility is a key step to determine their ability to maintain independence.

Research is needed in the following areas:

- Determining the impact of routine assessment of mobility should be a core function of palliative care teams or units.
- More evidence is needed to support the use of established mobility assessment tools in noncancer palliative care populations (e.g., patients with respiratory or heart failure), and different tools may be needed.
- Deterioration in ADL performance (or rate of change) may serve as an early marker of increasing disease burden and shorter prognosis, but more evidence is needed to quantify this correlation.

REFERENCES

1. Karnofsky DA, Abelmann WH, Craver LF, et al. The use of the nitrogen mustards in the palliative treatment of carcinoma. Cancer 1948;1:634-656.
2. Evans C, McCarthy M. Prognostic uncertainty in terminal care: Can the Karnofsky index help? Lancet 1985;1:1204-1206.
3. Ainser J, Hansen HH. Current status of chemotherapy for non-small cell lung cancer [commentary]. Cancer Treat Rep 1981;65:979-986.
4. Berry WR, Laszlo J, Cox E, et al. Prognostic factors in metastatic and normally unresponsive carcinoma of the prostate. Cancer 1979;44:763-775.
5. Schag CC, Heinrich RL, Ganz PA: Karnofsky performance status revisited: Reliability, validity, and guidelines. J Clin Oncol 1984;2:187-193.
6. Mor V, Laliberte L, Morris JN, et al. The Karnofsky performance status scale: An examination of its reliability and validity in a research setting. Cancer 1984;53:2002-2027.
7. Roila F, Lupatteli M, Sassi M, et al. Intra- and interobserver variability in cancer patient's performance status according to Karnofsky and ECOG scales. Ann Oncol 1991;2:437-439.
8. Hutchinson TA, Boyd NF, Feinstein AR. Scientific problems in clinical scales as demonstrated in the Karnofsky index of performance status. J Chronic Dis 1979;32:661-666.
9. Kaasa T, Loomis J, Gillis K, et al. The Edmonton Functional Assessment Tool: Preliminary development and evaluation for use in palliative care. J Pain Symptom Manage 1997;13:10-19.
10. Zubrod CG, Scheiderman M, Frei E, et al. Cancer—appraisal of methods for the study of chemotherapy of cancer in man: Thiophosphoramide. J Chronic Dis 1960;11:7-33.
11. Oken MM, Creech RH, Tormey DC, et al. Toxicity and response criteria of the Eastern Cooperative Oncology Group. Am J Clin Oncol 1982;5:649-655.
12. Buccheri G, Ferrigno D, Tamburini M. Karnofsky and ECOG performance status scoring in lung cancer: A prospective, longitudinal study of 536 patients from a single institution. Eur J Cancer 1996;32:1135-1141.
13. Conill C, Verger E, Salmero M. Performance status assessment in cancer patients. Cancer 1990;65:1864-1866.
14. Loprinzi CL, Laurie JA, Wieland HS, et al. Prospective evaluation of prognostic variables from patient completed questionnaires. J Clin Oncol 1994;12:601-607.
15. Mahoney FI, Barthel D. Functional evaluation: The Barthel Index. Md State Med J 1965;14:56-61.
16. Bohannon RW, Lee N. Association of physical functioning with same-hospital readmission after stroke. Am J Phys Med Rehabil 2004;83:434-438.
17. Bohannon RW, Lee N, Maljanian RRN. Post admission function best predicts acute hospital outcomes after stroke. Am J Phys Med Rehabil 2002;81:726-730.
18. Thomassen B, Bautz-Holter E, Laake K. Predictors of outcome of rehabilitation of elderly stroke patients in a geriatric ward. Clin Rehabil 1999;13:123-128.
19. Alarcon T, Barcena A, Gonzalex-Montalvo JI, et al. Factors predictive of outcome on admission to an acute geriatric ward. Age Ageing 1999;28:429-432.
20. Chu LW, Pei CKW. Risk factors for early emergency hospital readmission in elderly medical patients. Gerontology 1999;45:220-226.
21. Bennett M, Ryall N. Using the modified Barthel index to estimate survival in cancer patients in hospice: Observational study. BMJ 2000;321:1381-1382.
22. Granger CV, Greer DS. Functional status measurement and medical rehabilitation outcomes. Arch Phys Med Rehabil 1976;57:103-109.
23. Shah S, Vanclay F, Cooper B. Improving the sensitivity of the Barthel index for stroke rhabilitation. J Clin Epidemiol 1989;42:703-709.
24. Collin C, Wade DT, Davies S, Horne V. The Barthel ADL index: A reliability study. Int Disabil Stud 1988;10:61-63.
25. Shinar D, Gross CR, Bronstein KS. Reliability of the activities of daily living scale and its use in telephone interview: A modified Barthel Index. Arch Phys Med Rehabil 1987;68:723-728.
26. Gresham GE, Phillips TF, Labi ML. ADL status in stroke: Relative merits of three standard indexes.Arch Phys Med Rehabil 1980;61:355-358.
27. Wylie CM, White BK. A measure of disability. Arch Environ Health 1964;8:834-839.
28. Collen FM, Wade DT, Robb GF, et al. The Rivermead mobility index: A further development of the Rivermead motor assessment. Int Disabil Stud 1991;13:50-54.

Investigations

CHAPTER **69**

Nuclear Medicine

Dirk Sandrock and Petra Feyer

KEY POINTS

- Bone scintigraphy with technetium 99m–labeled phosphonates is a sensitive but not specific tool for detecting bone disease.

- Nuclear medicine provides a variety of different radiopharmaceuticals for special cancer entities, such as iodine 131 for thyroid cancer.

- Nuclear medicine provides radionuclide therapy for metastatic bone pain.

- ^{18}F-fluorodeoxyglucose positron emission tomography (FDG-PET) is a sensitive tool for detecting cancer.

- FDG-PET can detect other diseases with increased glucose metabolism, such as inflammatory diseases.

BONE SCINTIGRAPHY

Characteristics and Applications

Bone scintigraphy is the cornerstone of skeletal nuclear medicine imaging, and it is highly sensitive for bone disease, often providing earlier diagnosis or demonstrating more lesions than conventional radiology. Primary bone tumors are uncommon in adults, whereas bone metastases are common (i.e., breast, prostate, lung, head, and neck cancers). Phosphate analogues labeled with Tc-99m are used for bone imaging because of good skeletal localization and rapid soft tissue clearance Phosphonates concentrate in the mineral phase of bone, almost two thirds in hydroxyapatite crystals and one third in calcium phosphate. Blood flow and extraction efficiency control this and depend on factors such as capillary permeability, acid-base balance, and parathyroid hormone levels. About 50% of activity injected accumulates in the skeleton. Maximum bone accumulation occurs 1 hour after injection and remains constant up to 72 hours. Bone scintigraphy images the distribution of this skeletal radioactive tracer. It can be performed in several ways:

- Limited bone scintigraphy or spot views (i.e., planar images of a selected portion of the skeleton)
- Whole-body bone scintigraphy (i.e., planar anterior and posterior images of the entire skeleton)
- Single photon emission computed tomography (SPECT) (i.e., tomographic image of a portion of the skeleton)
- Multiphase bone scintigraphy (i.e., immediate and delayed images to study blood flow)

In assessing cancer patients, the standard technique of bone scintigraphy is the whole-body scan. Limited bone scintigraphy or spot views are indicated only where a specific clinical problem is detected on whole-body imaging. SPECT has higher diagnostic specificity than planar imaging and is preferable in cases of diagnostic uncertainty. Multiphase bone scintigraphy is more useful when trauma or musculoskeletal inflammation or infection is suspected.

The most commonly used diphosphonates are methylene diphosphonate (MDP), hydroxymethylene diphosphonate (HMDP), and hydroxyethylene diphosphonate (HDP or HMDP). The average activity for bone scintigraphy by single intravenous injection should be 500 MBq (300 to 740 MBq). The activity for children should be a fraction of the adult activity (calculated from body weight according to the European Association of Nuclear Medicine Paediatric Task Group). In children, a minimum activity of 40 MBq is necessary for quality images. Unless contraindicated, patients should be well hydrated and instructed to drink one or more liters of water (4 to 8 glasses) between the injection and the imaging. They should void frequently between the injection and delayed imaging and immediately before the scan. The estimated adsorbed effective radiation dose is 3.24 mSv per bone scintigraphy in adults (natural annual radiation exposure is 1 to 5 mSv). Routine images are usually obtained as whole-body scans 2 and 5 hours after injection, and they take about 20 minutes. In people with severe pain for whom two visits to the nuclear medicine department would be uncomfortable, the injection can be done at the bedside.

When evaluating bone scan images and reports, two ideas are important. First, the bone scan is sensitive for localization of skeletal metastases or tumors, but the specificity is low. It must be interpreted with all available information, especially patient history, physical examination, other test results, and comparison with previous studies. Second, symmetry in the representation of right and left sides of the skeleton and homogeneity of tracer uptake within bone structures are important normal features. Particular attention should be paid to left-right asymmetries and heterogeneity of tracer uptake.

Treatment of Metastatic Bone Pain

Intravenous beta-emitting therapy agents (i.e., ^{89}Sr chloride, ^{153}Sm lexidronam pentasodium, and ^{186}Re etidronate) are approved in Europe for bone pain from osteoblastic metastases. They have no place in managing acute or chronic spinal cord compression or pathological fractures. The treatment facility must have appropriate personnel, radiation safety equipment, waste handling procedures, contamination procedures, and personnel monitoring for accidental contamination and controlling contamination spread.

Practical Considerations

Patients will have undergone recent (≤8 weeks) bone scintigraphy documenting increased osteoblastic activity at painful sites. Radiographs demonstrating osteosclerotic lesions are inadequate because increased bone density does not always increase uptake on radionuclide imaging. Abnormalities on bone scintigraphy must be correlated with appropriate physical examination results to exclude other causes of chronic pain unlikely to respond to bone-seeking radiopharmaceuticals. Neuropathic pain and pathological fracture should be specifically excluded.

Treatment can be combined with local field external beam radiotherapy. Wide-field (hemibody) radiotherapy within 3 months of radionuclide therapy increases myelosuppression and is relatively contraindicated. Long-acting myelosuppressive chemotherapy (e.g., nitrosourea) should be discontinued at least 4 weeks before administration and withheld for 6 to 12 weeks afterward to avoid concomitant myelosuppression. A full hematological and biochemical profile should be obtained within 7 days of proposed treatment. Recent bisphosphonate therapy may reduce uptake by bone metastases and reduce the effectiveness of pain palliation. An interval of at least 48 hours is recommended between bisphosphonate administration and treatment. Radionuclide therapy is inappropriate for patients with a life expectancy of less than 4 weeks.

^{89}Sr chloride, ^{153}Sm lexidronam, and ^{186}Re etidronate should be given by slow injection through an indwelling intravenous butterfly catheter or cannula, followed by a 0.9% saline flush. Care should be taken to avoid extravasation. Recommended administered activities have been described:

- ^{89}Sr chloride: 150 MBq
- ^{153}Sm lexidronam: 37 MBq/kg
- ^{186}Re etidronate: 1295 MBq

Imaging after therapy (^{153}Sm lexidronam or ^{186}Re etidronate also have a gamma emission) may be useful for individual patient dosimetry.

Patients should be advised to observe rigorous hygiene to avoid contaminating groups at risk using the same toilet. They should be warned to avoid soiling underclothing or areas around toilet bowls for 1 week after injection, and significantly soiled clothing should be washed separately. A double toilet flush is recommended after urination. Patients should wash their hands after urination. Incontinent patients should be catheterized before radiopharmaceutical administration. The catheter should remain for 3 to 4 days. Catheter bags should be emptied frequently. Gloves should be worn by staff caring for catheterized patients.

Treatment may be repeated at more than 12-week intervals for recurrent pain, assuming adequate bone marrow

reserve. The response rate for second and subsequent treatments may be lower: 60% to 80 % benefit from ^{89}Sr chloride, ^{153}Sm lexidronam, or ^{186}Re etidronate. Radionuclide therapy is palliative and cannot cure metastatic cancer. There is a risk of temporary increase in bone pain (i.e., pain flare).

Other Tracers

Iodine 123 metaiodobenzylguanidine (^{123}I MIBG) may be used. Somatostatin receptor scintigraphy is used to detect uptake in the neurosecretory granules of indium 111 pentetreotide, a ^{111}In-DTPA-D-Phe-conjugate of octreotide, which binds to somatostatin receptors. It is used in detection, localization, staging, and follow-up of neuroendocrine tumors and their metastases, functioning and nonfunctioning gastroenteropancreatic tumors, pheochromocytomas, neuroblastomas, ganglioneuroblastomas, ganglioneuromas, paragangliomas, carcinoid tumors, medullary thyroid cancers, and Merkel cell tumors.

Radioiodine (^{131}I) may be used for thyroid cancers because of the iodination in thyroid cells. The use of ^{131}I allows staging and follow-up of differentiated thyroid cancers.

Treatment of Malignant Effusions

Respiratory distress due to fluid in the chest and abdomen are among the most difficult symptoms. Systemic chemotherapy and external beam radiation are rarely effective. Local antitumor agents, such as nitrogen mustard, are effective but toxic. The mode of action of antineoplastic agents is their ability to cause pleural sclerosis and obliterate the pleural space. Instillation of a cytotoxic agent such as bleomycin after drainage of the malignant effusion is the standard procedure, because it is effective in preventing recurrence of the effusion, is usually free from systemic effects, and can be given to myelosuppressed patients or those already undergoing systemic cytotoxic therapy. Colloidal radioactive gold (^{198}Au) has been replaced by a pure beta emitter, colloidal chromic phosphate (^{32}P) or yttrium (^{90}Y). Instillation of a colloidal suspension of radioactive phosphorus is effective for managing malignant effusion.

POSITRON EMISSION TOMOGRAPHY
Characteristics and Applications

Positron emission tomography (PET) is a noninvasive diagnostic tool that provides tomographic images and quantitative parameters of perfusion, cell viability, proliferation, and metabolic activity of tissues (see Chapter 71). These images result from the use of different substances of biological interest (e.g., sugars, amino acids, metabolic precursors, hormones) labeled with positron-emitting radioisotopes (i.e., PET radiopharmaceuticals). ^{18}F-fluorodeoxyglucose positron emission tomography (FDG-PET) can reveal the presence of a tumor when conventional morphological diagnostic modalities (i.e., radiography, CT, magnetic resonance imaging, and ultrasound) do not detect any evident lesions. Because FDG uptake in tumors correlates with tumor growth and viability, the PET scan and the possible metabolic quantification may provide useful information about tumor characterization, patient prognosis, and the response to anticancer therapy.

The present clinical indications of FDG-PET in oncology are diagnosis of malignant lesions, evaluation of the extent of disease (i.e., staging or restaging), differentiation of recurrent or residual malignant disease from therapy-induced changes, grading of malignant lesions, evaluation of tumor response to chemotherapy or radiotherapy, and planning of radiotherapy with therapeutic and palliative intent.

Practical Considerations

The patient must fast for 6 hours before a PET scan but drink water (with no carbohydrates) to ensure hydration and promote diuresis. For brain tumors, the patient should wait in a quiet dark room before and after FDG administration. Because of the short half-life of 110 minutes, precise timing is essential.

The injected activity of FDG to obtain good imaging with a full-ring PET scanner should be 6 MBq/kg (for adults, 111 to 555 MBq). A 60-minute interval between FDG injection and the scan is usually enough to obtain adequate FDG biodistribution. During this time, the patient should drink up to 1 liter of water to promote diuresis. Hydration and voiding is advised to limit radiation exposure to the urinary tract. The estimated effective absorbed radiation dose for 370-MBq injection of FDG is 7 mSv in an adult (natural annual radiation exposure is 1 to 5 mSv) (Fig. 69-1).

Depending on the scanner, the image acquisition time is 30 to 90 minutes. The FDG-PET images are analyzed by looking for local differences of FDG uptake in the regions imaged. PET evaluation should be compared with morphological studies to better localize the lesion. The standard uptake value (SUV) can be calculated for a semi-quantitative estimate of tumor metabolism. SUVs should be calculated in the hottest part of the lesion because cancer tissues have a heterogeneous FDG uptake distribution. SUV may guide the differential diagnosis between a benign lesion and malignancy; this seems more reliable in the evaluation of treatment response. False-positive results can be artifacts (e.g., urine), sites of physiological uptake (e.g., muscular activity, myocardial uptake, uptake in the stomach and intestine), post-therapy uptakes (e.g., bone marrow, spleen, thymus [in young patients]), or inflammatory sites (in oncology patients).

DEVELOPMENTS AND RESEARCH OPPORTUNITIES

Several areas of controversy require further research:

- Does the combined use of functional imaging (e.g., PET) and anatomic imaging (e.g., CT) increase sensitivity and specificity?
- Which radiopharmaceutical is appropriate for which tumor?
- Can nuclear medicine predict therapy response?
- Will nuclear medicine develop more radionuclide therapies (e.g., radioimmunotherapy) for other cancer entities?

SUGGESTED READING

Balon HR, Goldsmith SJ, Siegel BA, et al. Procedure guideline for somatostatin receptor scintigraphy with (111)In-pentetreotide. J Nucl Med 2001;42:1134-1138.

Blodgett TM, Meltzer CC, Townsend DW. PET/CT: Form and function. Radiology 2007;242:360-385.

Bombardieri E, Maccauro M, De Deckere E, et al. Nuclear medicine imaging of neuroendocrine tumours. Ann Oncol 2001;12: S51-S61.

Bourguet P, Group de Travail SOR. Standards, options and recommendations 2002 for the use of Positron Emission Tomography with (18)F-FDG (PET-FDG) in cancerology (integral connection). Bull Cancer 2003;90:S5-S17.

Cook GJ, Fogelman I. The role of nuclear medicine in monitoring treatment in skeletal malignancy. Semin Nucl Med 2001;31: 206-211.

Croll MN, Brady LW. Intracavitary uses of colloids. Semin Nucl Med 1979;9:108-113.

van Dalen JA, Vogel WV, Corstens FH, et al. Multi-modality nuclear medicine imaging: Artefacts, pitfalls and recommendations. Cancer Imaging 2007;28:77-83.

De Klerk JMH, Zonnenberg BA, Blijham GH, et al. Treatment of metastatic bone pain using the bone seeking radiopharmaceutical Re-186 EDP. Anti Cancer Res 1997;17:1773-1778.

Faulhaber PF, Mehta L, Echt EA, et al. Perfecting the practice of FDG-PET: Pitfalls and artefacts. In Freeman LM (ed). Nuclear Medicine Annual. Philadlephia: JB Lippincott, 2002, pp 149-214.

Gambhir SS, Czernin J, Schwimmer J, et al. A tabulated summary of the FDG PET literature. J Nucl Med 2001;42:1S-93S.

Hain SF, Fogelman I. Nuclear medicine studies in metabolic bone disease. Semin Musculoskelet Radiol 2002;6:323-329.

International Commission on Radiological Protection (ICRP). Radiation Dose to Patients from Radiopharmaceuticals. ICRP publication 80. Annals of the ICRP. Oxford, UK: Pergamon Press, 1998, p 3.

International Commission on Radiological Protection (ICRP). Radiological Protection in Biomedical Research. ICRP publication 62. Annals of the ICRP. Oxford, UK: Pergamon Press, 1991, p 3.

International Commission on Radiological Protection (ICRP). Radiation Dose to Patients from Radiopharmaceuticals. ICRP publication 53. Annals of the ICRP. Oxford, UK: Pergamon Press, 1987, pp 1-4.

Krenning EP, Kwekkeboom DJ, Bakker WH, et al. Somatostatin receptor scintigraphy with [111In-DTPA-D-Phe1]- and [123I-Tyr3]-octreotide: The Rotterdam experience with more than 1000 patients. Eur J Nucl Med 1998;20:716-731.

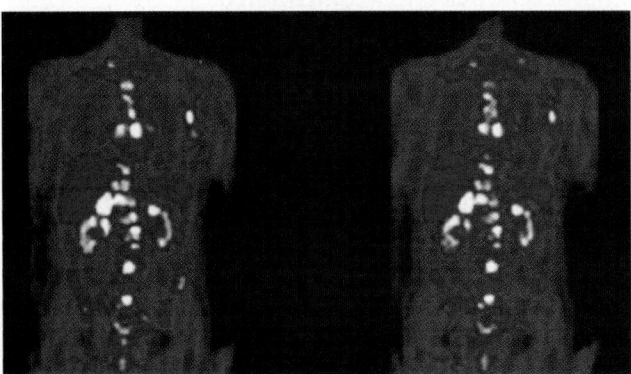

FIGURE 69-1 ^{18}F-fluorodeoxyglucose positron emission tomography (FDG-PET) of a patient with lung cancer shows many bone and soft tissue metastases.

Kwekkeboom DJ, Krenning EP. Radiolabeled somatostatin analog scintigraphy in oncology and immune disease: An overview. Eur Radiol 1997;7:1103-1109.

McEwan AJ, Porter AT, Venner PM, et al. An evaluation of the safety and efficacy of treatment with strontium-89 in patients who have previously received wide field radiotherapy. Antibody Immunoconj Radiopharm 1990;3:91-98.

Olivier P, Colarinha P, Fettich J, et al. Guidelines for radioiodinated MIBG scintigraphy in children. Eur J Nucl Med Mol Imaging 2003;30:B45-B50.

Ostrowski MJ, Halsall GM. Intracavitary bleomycin in the management of malignant effusions: A multicenter study. Cancer Treat Rep 1982;66:1903-1907.

Reisinger I, Bohuslavizki KH, Brenner W, et al. Somatostatin receptor scintigraphy in small-cell lung cancer: Results of a multicentric study. J Nucl Med 1998;39:224-227.

Resche I, Chatal JF, Pecking A, et al. A dose-controlled study of Sm-153 EDTMP in the treatment of patients with painful bone metastases. Eur J Cancer 1997;33:1583-1591.

Sandrock D, Munz DL. Primary and secondary neoplasias of the skeleton. Nuklearmedizin 2002;25:230-237.

Spaepen K, Stroobants S, Dupont P, et al. ^{18}F-FDG-PET monitoring of tumour response to chemotherapy: Does ^{18}F-FDG uptake correlated with the viable tumour cell fraction? Eur J Nucl Med Mol Imaging 2003;30:682-688.

Wong TZ, Paulson EK, Nelson RC, et al. Practical approach to diagnostic CT combined with PET. AJR Am J Roentgenol 2007;188:622-629.

Zuetenhorst JM, Hoefnagel CA, Boot H, et al. Evaluation of (111)In-pentetreotide, (131)I-MIBG and bone scintigraphy in the detection and clinical management of bone metastases in carcinoid disease. Nucl Med Commun 2002;23:735-741.

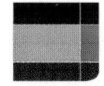

CHAPTER **70**

Computed Tomography Scanning and Magnetic Resonance Imaging in Palliative Care

Carmen Fernandez Alvarez, Isabel Barreiro-Meiro Sáenz-Diez, Julia Romero Martinez, and Isabel Martínez de Ubago

KEY POINTS

- The use of sophisticated imaging is increasing in medical practice in general, and in palliative medicine in particular.

- Both CT and MRI provide information that cannot be obtained in any other way.

- The procedures are in general well-tolerated, provided patients are carefully selected and the indications for the imaging thoughtfully considered.

- CT and MRI independently have strengths and weaknesses in identifying specific pathological conditions; it is important that the ordering physician is aware of their strengths and limitations.

- A major question is how will the information obtained change disease management or therapeutic decision-making.

- The major uses of both CT and MRI are diagnostic, but they are also important in assessing response to therapy, particularly in oncology.

Radiodiagnostic services are a faithful reflection of the other medical and surgical services of care centers, and the activities of these services usually evolve in tandem. There has been a progressive increase in the requests for computed tomography (CT) for palliative care patients, which parallels a broader offering of management options for this group.

Terms such as *palliative* and *terminal* should not be confused. Terminal patients are in the last stage of their disease, and only limited care that alleviates and eases the situation can be offered. Palliative care patients do not receive curative treatment, but they are offered a range of therapeutic alternatives that can improve quality of life and prolong it.

Imaging tests frequently are used in the management of palliative care patients. It is not always possible to reach a diagnosis or rule out pathological conditions without using CT or magnetic resonance imaging (MRI), a test that may be considered a last resort among diagnostic examinations. The number of CT and MRI studies performed in palliative care units has increased because the techniques are easily accessible. CT has become the diagnostic technique of choice in following oncology patients because of the information it supplies. It causes little discomfort for the patient, and radiation exposure is not a critical problem for this group of patients.

COMPUTED TOMOGRAPHY

The use of CT in palliative care continues to increase. In our area during the 2006, 40 CT scans were requested from the palliative care unit. The studies requested from other services were not included, although they could have been for incurable patients, nor does the figure include cranial CT scans, which were performed using other equipment. In the first 10 months of 2007, 44 CT scans were performed, 4 more than during the previous 12 months. The estimated final count was expected to yield an increase of about 20% to 30% in the number of studies, and this degree of increase has been the tendency in recent years (Fig. 70-1).

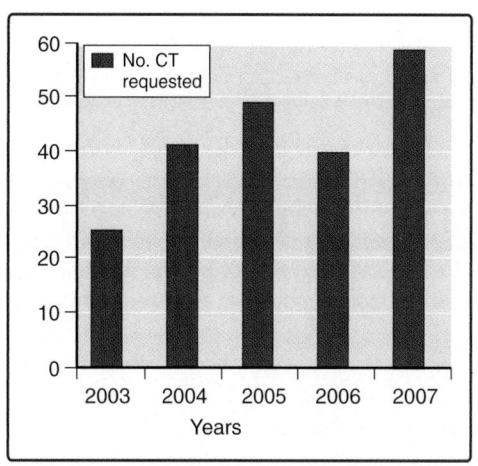

Figure 70-1 Evolution of the requests for computed tomography studies for 2003 through 2007. There was a significant increase from 2003, with the growth tendency more or less sustained during subsequent years. The 2007 data was inferred from the first three trimesters.

The most frequent origins of tumors are shown in Table 70-1. The two most common sites (coinciding with the two most common tumors) account for almost one half of the requested studies.

CT studies are requested for many reasons, but the most common is to follow the progress of patients after treatment begins (Table 70-2). We consider this is an acceptable reason for requesting a CT scan. All other reasons depend on the patient's status and the intent to treat symptoms.

Cranial and Spinal Computed Tomography

Cranial and spinal CT scans are requested less often than studies of the thoracic and abdominal areas. There are four main reasons for obtaining cranial and spinal CT scans:

- Suspicion of nondiagnosed brain metastasis
- Clinical suspicion of intracranial hemorrhage
- Diagnosis of hydrocephalus
- Vertebral pain and cord compression

MRI or isotopic tests also may be performed, especially in the case of cord compression.

These four clinical situations can be very serious for the patient, and CT is the diagnostic method of choice. If these clinical conditions are identified, they can be treated.

Thoracic Computed Tomography

Typical reasons for requesting thoracic CT are to follow the progression of disease and to identify urgent situations that warrant treatment. CT scans may identify causes of vascular compromise such as superior vena cava syndrome that are produced by obstruction or extrinsic compression (Fig. 70-2) and may diagnose pulmonary thromboembolism. For these conditions, CT has become the diagnostic modality of choice.

Many of the less common reasons for requesting CT scans can be resolved with conventional radiographs or thoracic ultrasound scans. The use of CT is warranted when occult, concomitant pathology is suspected, as in the case of pulmonary infections and pleural hemorrhage. It can be difficult to determine the volume and location of the pleural hemorrhage in a patient with an invasive pulmonary mass, which can be studied only with the patient in the supine decubitus position. CT can guide the selection of the ideal site for draining the pleural hemorrhage and help to establish whether the patient's symptoms are caused by the hemorrhage (and therefore will disappear on evacuation of the fluid) or are caused by tumoral growth and invasion.

CT may be used to identify obstructions of the esophagus in the thorax. Esophageal obstruction usually is confirmed by means of a barium meal study. This study is used for making the diagnosis, before placing an esophageal endoprosthesis, and before resuming the normal diet. CT is performed only in exceptional cases, and it has the advantage of not being limited to the esophagus. It can be used to perform extensive studies beyond the targeted organ. For example, CT scans can evaluate the growth of tumor beyond the esophageal walls, invasion of the neighboring organs, and pulmonary metastasis.

Abdominal Computed Tomography

Abdominal CT may be used to follow the progress of the patient's disease and for other reasons:

1. Obstructions of any part of the digestive tract. Abdominal CT can be used for the placement of an endoprosthesis, surgery, or other type or treatment. It is therefore necessary to know the cause of the obstruction, the degree of its extension, and its loca-

TABLE 70-1 Requested Computed Tomographic Studies According to Tumor Origin (2007)	
SITE OF TUMOR	**NUMBER OF CT SCANS REQUESTED**
Lung	11
Colon, rectum	10
Pancreas	2
Melanoma	2
Bladder	2
Other site	4
Not determined	13

TABLE 70-2 Requested Computed Tomographic Studies in Hospital General Universitario Gregorio Marañón, 2007	
REASON	**NUMBER OF CT SCANS REQUESTED**
Monitoring progression, follow-up	16
Intense pelvic pain	3
Superior vena cava syndrome	2
Intra-abdominal abscess	2
Intestinal perforation	1
Intestinal obstruction	1
Necrotizing fasciitis	1
Localization of pleural hemorrhage for drains	1

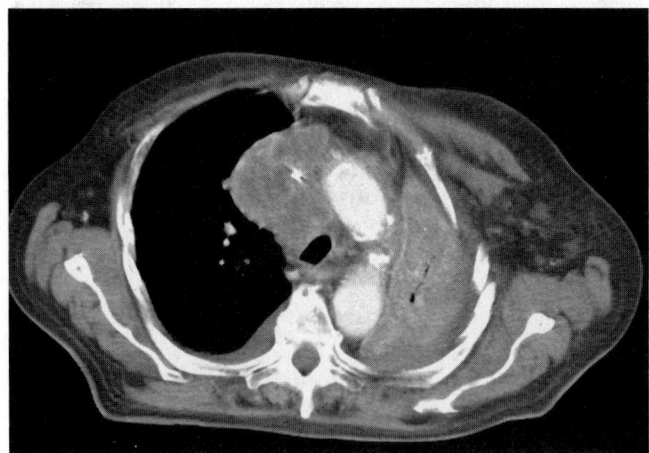

Figure 70-2   Superior vena cava syndrome. Superior vena cava syndrome in a patient with a left pulmonary tumor. The superior vena cava was obstructed by a right paratracheal ganglionic conglomerate that compromised and obliterated the light. Other findings include left pulmonary atelectasis by a left hilar mass, mediastinal adenopathies, and right pleural hemorrhage.

tion as precisely as possible and to know whether the patient has a single or several obstructed areas. Barium studies are still commonly used, but when studying the small intestine and when considering surgery as alternative, a CT scan is indicated.

2. Obstructive jaundice. The initial diagnostic technique is ultrasound, but it may be necessary to obtain a CT scan when the information yielded by ultrasound is insufficient or associated pancreatic pathology is suspected.

3. Obstruction of the urinary tract. Ultrasound usually is sufficient to detect an obstruction, but intravenous urography also may be employed. However, the most precise information about the cause, size of the obstruction, and its location is provided by CT (Fig. 70-3).

4. Vascular complications, such as thromboembolism of the intra-abdominal arteries. Tumors predispose patients to thromboembolic disease, which can be detected by CT.

5. Acute abdomen. CT can be used to detect causes such as intestinal perforation (Fig. 70-4).

6. Malignant psoas syndrome. CT frequently helps to diagnose this syndrome.

Skeletal Computed Tomography

CT is indicated in the study and diagnosis of bone metastasis when conventional radiography and bone gammog-raphy are not sufficient. CT scans also are used for diagnosing fractures caused by metastasis, nonmalignant disease, or injuries.

Overview of Computed Tomography Use

CT and MRI frequently are used in managing palliative care patients. It is not always possible to make a diagnosis or rule out pathology without resorting to these studies. CT has become the diagnostic technique of choice for following oncology patients because of the information it supplies, the accessibility of the technology, and the minimal discomfort for the patient. Protection against radiation exposure is not a critical problem for this group of patients.

The number of CT and MRI studies performed has increased in general practice and in palliative care units, and the increase seems to be reasonable. Re-evaluation of patients is not always possible by means of clinical assessment or other diagnostic tests, such as conventional radiography and ultrasound. When capable of modifying the treatment or when there is no other diagnostic alternative, a CT study is necessary and its request is justified. However, when all the therapeutic possibilities have been exhausted, a more extensive diagnostic evaluation cannot modify management. In this case, a request for CT scans may not be warranted.

MAGNETIC RESONANCE IMAGING

Utility, Advantages, and Inconveniences

Because MRI can differentiate tissues, it is useful for diagnosing tumors, identifying masses of soft tissue associated with tumors, and defining tumors' extensions. MRI can determine with great precision compromised structures such as nerve roots and medulla, indicating the degree of vertebral compression and the existence of associated myelopathy through analysis of the signals obtained in different sequences.

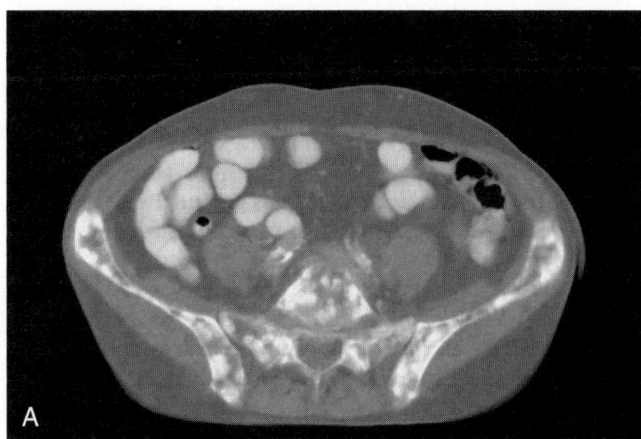
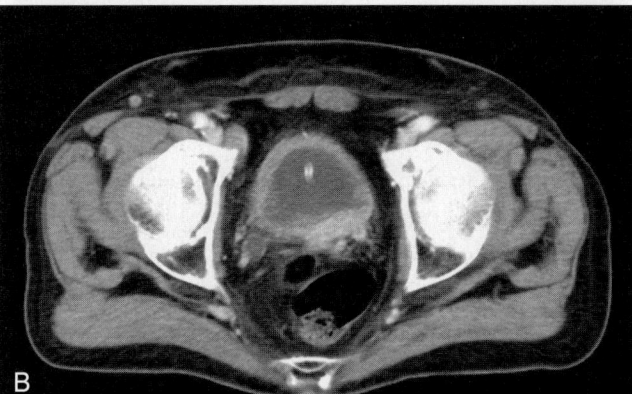

Figure 70-3   Obstruction of the urinary tract. A, Hydronephrosis caused by blastic metastasis. **B**, Bilateral hydronephrosis caused by vesical infiltration in a patient with prostatic recidivation and blastic bone metastasis.

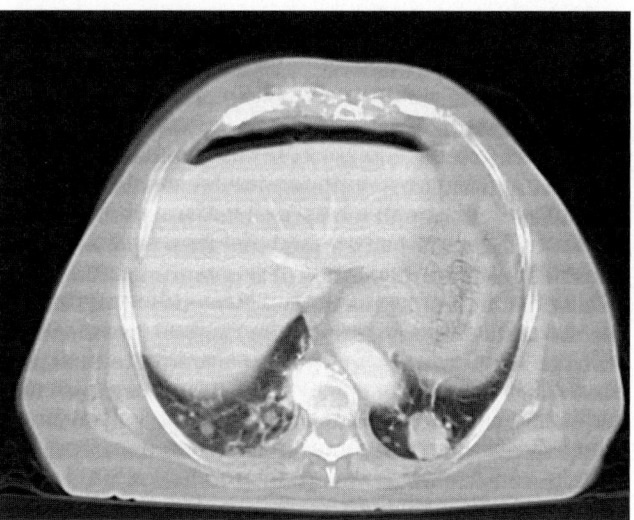

Figure 70-4   Intestinal perforation and pulmonary metastasis. Pneumoperitoneum caused by intestinal perforation and pulmonary metastasis.

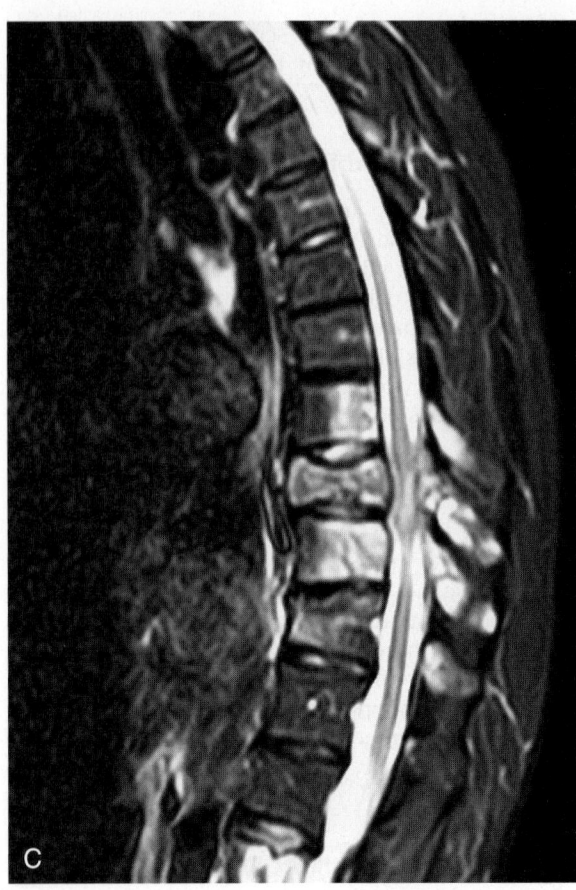

Figure 70-5 **A**, Cord compression (T1-weighted MRI). **B**, Cord compression (TSE T2-weighted MRI). **C**, Cord compression (short tau inversion recovery [STIR]).

Disadvantages of this technique include the high cost and the duration of testing. Although the time to complete the sequences is shorter with the latest MRI technology, the process is usually slower for palliative care patients because of their clinical characteristics, intense pain, and significant limitations in mobility. These difficulties sometimes inhibit cooperation, which is necessary to perform the examination and achieve images of maximum quality and therefore facilitate the diagnostic.

Indications

The indications for MRI studies of patients with advanced-stage cancer in a palliative care service are few. Common indications include studies of the vertebral column resulting from the advanced-cancer patient's symptoms and clinical findings. Spinal cord or radicular compressions may result from surgery or radiotherapy. Less common entities capable of producing compression of the neural structures include lymphoma, myeloma, and primary vertebral tumors. The MRI exploration should be performed as soon as the cord compression is suspected to improve the effectiveness of treatment (Fig. 70-5). MRI is also indicated to identify leptomeningeal metastatic dissemination, which can change the choice of treatment.

Overview of Magnetic Resonance Imaging Use

Appropriate criteria for requesting MRI studies must be followed because unnecessary and arbitrary use of

these tests means discomfort for palliative care patients. Although excess MRI studies do not affect treatment, they cause work overloads, increase the costs of health departments, use a significant amount of resources, and impede the access of other patients to a diagnosis in an acceptable time frame.

Cooperation among oncologists, radiologists, radiotherapists, and surgeons is essential in managing resources to perform the most efficient examinations. The criteria for requesting diagnostic MRI tests for palliative care patients should include the significance of the study, the effect of the treatment, and the benefit to the patient.

SUGGESTED READING

Mauricio C, Smith JK, Mukherji SK. Spine. In Lee JK, Sagel SS, Stanley RJ, Heiken JP (eds). Computed Body Tomography with MRI Correlation, 3rd ed. Madrid: Marban, 1999, pp 1473-1475.

Kenney PJ, McClennan BL. Pelvis. In Lee JK, Sagel SS, Stanley RJ, Heiken JP (eds). Computed Body Tomography with MRI Correlation, 3rd ed. Madrid: Marban, 1999, pp 1218-1225.

Núñez Olarte JM. Palliative care. In Diagnostic Treatment Guide for Malignant Tumors, 2nd ed. Madrid: University General Hospital Gregorio Marañón, 2003, p xvii.

Sagel SS, Slone MRI. Lung. In Lee JK, Sagel SS, Stanley RJ, Heiken JP (eds). Computed Body Tomography with MRI Correlation, 3rd ed. Madrid: Marban, 1999, pp 355-380.

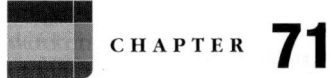

CHAPTER **71**

Positron Emission Tomography

Michael J. Fulham and Armin Mohamed

TABLE 71-1 Common Positron Emitters

POSITRON EMITTER	DESIGNATION	APPROXIMATE HALF-LIFE
Fluorine 18	^{18}F	108 min
Carbon 11	^{11}C	20 min
Ammonia 13	^{13}N	10 min
Oxygen 15	^{15}O	2 min
Rubidium 82	^{82}Rb	76 sec
Gallium 68	^{68}Ga	68 min

KEY POINTS

- ^{18}F-fluorodeoxyglucose (FDG) uptake is increased in high-grade malignant tumors by virtue of expression of the glucose transporter and inefficient respiration; well-differentiated or low-grade tumors have mildly increased FDG uptake. Certain benign conditions may display increased FDG uptake.

- FDG positron emission tomography (PET) and computed tomography (CT)—PET/CT—provide functional and anatomical information that is invaluable in the assessment (staging and restaging) of a variety of malignancies. CT improves localization of glucose-avid lesions and therefore facilitates staging.

- FDG uptake reflects cellular glucose metabolism except in the brain, where it mainly reflects synaptic activity.

- Nonpathological patterns of increased FDG uptake can be seen because of normal physiological effects, with prostheses and pacemakers, and may result from misregistration of PET and CT data.

- Combined PET/CT can assess the response to therapy before there are any changes on conventional structural imaging (CT and magnetic resonance [MR] imaging) and may influence patient management by the detection of a lack of response early in the course of treatment.

Positron emission tomography (PET) is a functional imaging modality. It can image and measure aspects of human tissue metabolism in vivo.

Positron emission refers to the physical event whereby a positron, which is a positive electron, is emitted from the nucleus of an unstable (PET) radioisotope so that the molecule can return to a stable electronic state. Positron emitters have an excess number of protons and a positive charge. Common positron emitters are shown in Table 71-1. Positron emitters are produced in medical cyclotrons. A cyclotron is a compact linear accelerator, which accelerates charged particles to high velocities and energies. These particles are then directed to bombard a target (i.e., gas or solid), and a nuclear reaction is induced within the target, producing the positron emitter. The positron emitter can then be incorporated into a compound (i.e., tracer or radiotracer, indicating that it is radioactive) after a series of synthetic radiolabeling steps, which usually are performed in automated radiochemistry modules. The ubiquitous nature of the positron emitters allows them to be inserted into a large variety of physiological substrates, compounds, and drugs. The end product undergoes a series of quality control steps to ensure that it has the

appropriate chemical characteristics of the intended compound, and it can then be injected intravenously into or inhaled (i.e., gas) by a patient. The term *radiotracer* is used because it is injected or inhaled in minute quantities, which are able to participate in the process of interest (e.g., glucose metabolism) but not perturb it.

The radioactive decay process occurs after the positron emitter is produced in the cyclotron. This process continues within the patient, where the emitted positron travels a small (millimeters) distance in tissue before it collides with an electron and both particles are annihilated with the production of two gamma rays (i.e., photons with energies of 511 keV), which are emitted 180 degrees apart. The PET scanner, which has a circumferential array of detectors or scintillation crystals and associated electronic circuits, is able to detect the resulting gamma rays. Through sophisticated electronics and software reconstruction algorithms, the scanner provides a three-dimensional display of the distribution of the radiotracer. The most widely used PET radiotracer in clinical practice is ^{18}F-fluorodeoxyglucose (FDG). Deoxyglucose is an analogue of glucose, and FDG-PET therefore provides a noninvasive measurement of glucose metabolism.

PET was developed in the late 1970s in a research environment, and for many years, it was mainly restricted to the neurosciences. In this setting, it provided insights into many aspects of normal and abnormal brain function by parameters such as glucose and oxygen metabolism, blood flow, pH, status of the blood-brain barrier, amino acid uptake, presence or concentration of receptors, and the pharmacokinetics of delivery of chemotherapeutic agents. Early PET scanners were crude, had a limited scan extent (i.e., field of view [FOV]), were often made locally in the research institution, and had long data acquisition times and poor resolution (i.e., ability to detect small structures). There were progressive improvements in scanner and detector technology over the subsequent decades. Resolution improved, and more efficient scintillation crystals such as lutetium oxyorthosilicate (LSO) and gadolinium oxyorthosilicate (GSO), which had greater and faster light output, were incorporated into the detectors. In 2001, the first PET and computed tomography (CT) scanners were introduced into the clinic. The PET/CT scanner, which combines a helical CT scanner and a PET scanner in one device, is the most important advance in medical imaging in the past decade.[1] The addition of a CT scanner to a PET scanner provided two immediate advantages: a solution to the accurate measurement of photon attenuation by the body in a very short time (<1 minute) using the CT scan compared with existing methods and a mechanism to accurately localize the PET findings with the underlying anatomy available through the CT scan, with good registration between these data sets in one examination.

However, what was not anticipated initially was the impact of the anatomical data on image interpretation and the shortening of scan time and increased patient throughput as the faster electronics and detectors (i.e., LSO and GSO) replaced older detector materials such as bismuth germanate (BGO) and sodium iodide (NaI). The ability to accurately localize the abnormal foci of increased FDG uptake with the aid of CT has finessed scan interpretation and improved staging.[2] Accurately localizing foci of metastatic disease in a variety of malignancies affects patient management. In our experience, we have moved from performing nine patient studies on a PET scanner with BGO detectors in a 12-hour day to carrying out 20 to 24 PET/CT scans on an LSO PET/CT in a 10-hour day (Fig. 71-1). We performed the same number of scans in 3 years with a PET/CT scanner that previously took a decade with a PET-only scanner (Fig. 71-2). PET-only devices have become essentially obsolete. The immediate future is PET/CT, for which the continued advances in CT technology are being incorporated into the scanner with improvements in PET instrumentation (e.g., extended FOV), electronics, and software (e.g., time-of-flight, reconstruction algorithms). In 2001, when the first PET/CT scanners were used clinically, the helical CT could provide one to four slices, whereas the state-of-the-art PET/CT scanner in 2007 is a 64-slice helical CT combined with a PET scanner with LSO or GSO detectors (Fig. 71-3).

TECHNIQUE

The ^{18}F-fluorodeoxyglucose Method

The application of FDG to the measurement of glucose metabolism is based on the [^{14}C]deoxyglucose method described by Sokoloff and colleagues[3] to study cerebral glucose metabolism in the albino rat brain in 1977. Sokol-

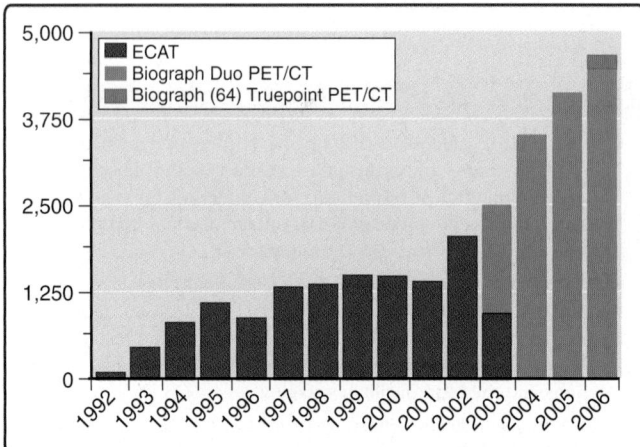

FIGURE 71-2 Serial histograms from commencement of scanning at our institution in 1992 show the yearly patient throughput. Initial scanner (ECAT 951) had bismuth germanate (BGO) detectors and was replaced by our first PET/CT scanner in 2003. This PET/CT has lutetium oxyorthosilicate (LSO) detectors, and more than 13,000 patients were scanned with it in just over 3 years. The LSO Biograph Truepoint was installed in late 2006.

Wed, 16 Aug 2006					**Technologist Schedule** **Data & Co-ord**						
	Age/Sex	**Ht/Wt**	**Study Type**	**# Beds**	**Arms**	**Booked** **to Arrive**	**Cannulate** **by**	**Inject**	**On** **Bed**	**Delay**	**Off** **Bed**
1	34/M	185/78	WB Soft_tissue	8 @ 3 min	down	7:00	7:15	7:27	8:27	9 min	9:00
2	71/M	180/90	WB Lung	8 @ 3 min	up	7:10	7:35	8:05	9:08	0 min	9:30
3	74/M	163/72	WB Lung	7 @ 3 min	down	7:30	8:06	8:36	9:36	0 min	9:57
4	26/M	175/80	WB Hem	7 @ 3 min	down	7:40	8:33	9:03	10:03	0 min	10:24
5	56/M	170/107	WB H&N	2 @ 3 min	down	8:10	9:00	9:30	10:03	-3 min	10:33
6	56/M	170/107	WB H&N	3 @ 4 min	up	8:15	9:09	9:39	10:39	0 min	10:51
7	*17/F	188/82	WB Hem	6 @ 2 min	down	8:45	9:27	9:57	10:57	2 min	11:11
8	22/M	/	Neuro Hem	1 @ 30 min		8:50	9:57	10:27	11:17	4 min	11:51
9	34/M	180/78	WB Soft_tissue	7 @ 3 min	down	9:00	10:27	10:57	11:57	0 min	12:18
10	52/M	180/79	WB Off	7 @ 3 min	down	9:00	10:27	10:57	11:57	0 min	12:18
11	*19/F	161/80	WB Soft_tissue	6 @ 2 min	down	9:45	11:21	11:51	12:51	0 min	13:03
12	22/M	/	Neuro Ref_Epi	1 @ 10 min		10:00	11:49	12:19	13:09	0 min	13:19
13	72/M	168/65	WB Lung	7 @ 3 min	down	11:00	11:55	12:25	13:25	0 min	13:46
14	50/Fe	158/57	WB Hem	6 @ 2 min	down	11:15	12:22	12:52	13:52	0 min	14:04
15	*50/Fe	173/45	WB H&N	5 @ 2 min	down	11:45	12:40	13:10	14:10	0 min	14:20
16	*23/Fe	160/89	WB Hem	6 @ 2 min	down	12:15	12:56	13:25	14:26	0 min	14:38
17	54/M	163/75	WB H&N	6 @ 3 min	down	12:45	13:14	13:44	14:44	0 min	15:02
18	70/Fe	/	Neuro Brain Tumor	1 @ 10 min		12:50	13:84	14:18	15:08	0 min	15:18
19	52/Fe	155/80	WB Off	6 @ 2 min	down	13:00	13:54	14:24	15:24	0 min	15:18
20	51/Fe	149/44	WB Hem	6 @ 2 min	down	13:29	14:12	14:42	15:42	4 min	15:58
21	55/M	172/90	WB Hem	7 @ 3 min	up	13:45	14:34	15:04	16:04	0 min	16:25
22	*47/M	180/85	WB Lung	7 @ 3 min	down	14:10	15:01	15:31	16:31	0 min	16:52
23	53/Fe	165/69	Cardiac	1 @ 10 min	down	14:30	15:28	15:58	16:58	0 min	17:08

*Check pregnancy

FIGURE 71-1 Patient scanning schedule for a day in 2006. The patient details have been eliminated, but height and weight (in cm and kg) are shown because they determine the extent of the study, except for neurological scans (nos. 8, 12, 18). The isotope injection time is listed. The scan duration is time from "on-bed" to "off-bed" or the number of beds multiplied by the time per bed position indicated in the # Beds column.

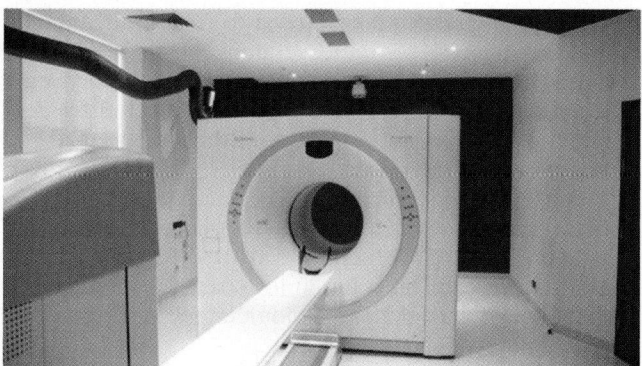

FIGURE 71-3 The 64-slice Biograph Truepoint positron emission tomography and computed tomography (PET/CT) scanner with an extended PET field of view of 22 cm.

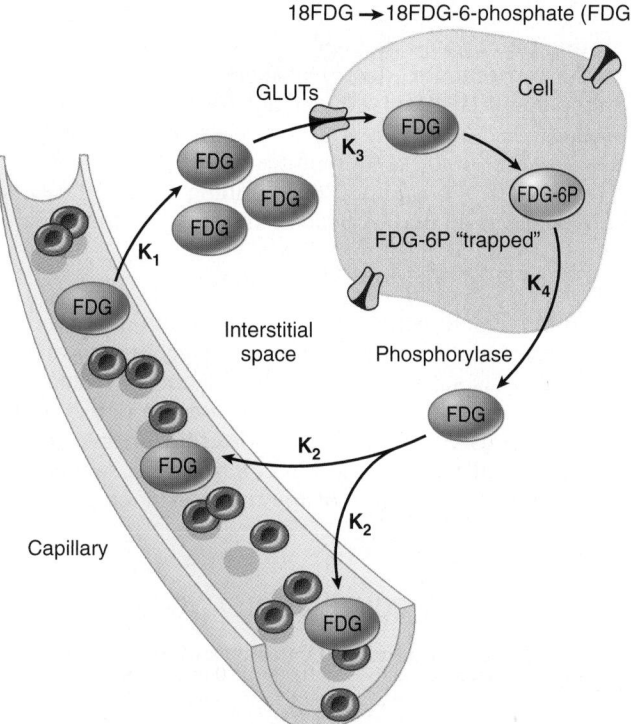

FIGURE 71-4 Schematic representation of ^{18}F-fluorodeoxyglucose (FDG) uptake. Rate constants describe the movement of FDG from the capillary to the interstitial space and back to the capillary. K3 describes entry of FDG into the cell by means of the glucose transporters (GLUTs), where it is trapped and phosphorylated to FDG-6-phosphate. K4 describes the dephosphorylation of some of the FDG-6-phosphate.

off and associates provided a mathematical model with rate constants to estimate glucose use in terms of milligrams of glucose per 100 g of tissue per minute. FDG is taken up by cells by one of the glucose transporters, which are overexpressed in malignant tumors. FDG is then phosphorylated by hexokinase to fluorodeoxyglucose-6-phosphate (FDG-6-P), but the FDG-6-phosphate cannot participate in other steps of the glycolytic cycle and is effectively trapped in the cell (Fig. 71-4). Phosphorylation of FDG to FDG-6-P therefore reflects cellular glucose use. The glycolytic cycle is an inefficient method of energy production but is favored by malignant tumors.

A general principle of using FDG-PET in oncology is that malignant tumors have increased FDG uptake, but well-differentiated tumors (e.g., low-grade gliomas and prostate cancer) have minimal FDG uptake.[4] FDG-PET is not a good method to determine the extent of well-differentiated tumors. There are some other important considerations or exceptions:

- The brain can metabolize only glucose for energy use, and a cerebral FDG scan shows avid tracer uptake into the brain. The glucose metabolism is localized at synaptic terminals rather than in the cell soma, which is important to remember in the interpretation of PET scans of the brain, in which remote effects from disruption of long axons can be evident.
- Acute (e.g., pneumonia) and chronic inflammatory conditions can display markedly increased FDG uptake where the glucose uptake is localized to macrophages.
- In some benign conditions (e.g., bowel polyps, pigmented villonodular synovitis, pilocytic astrocytomas, nonsecretory pituitary macroadenomas), there is increased FDG uptake similar to the degree seen in malignant tumors.
- Less marked FDG uptake can be seen in degenerative changes in the vertebral column in facet joints and in other joints.

Techniques for Positron Emission Tomography and Computed Tomography in Clinical Practice

The application of PET/CT in clinical practice for palliative care patients usually is restricted to the use of FDG. PET ligands (e.g., ^{11}C-carfentanil, ^{18}F-cyclofoxy) that target opioid receptors have been used in the experimental setting in studying focal epilepsy and pain states, but they do not have a proven clinical role.

FDG-PET/CT studies can be separated into whole-body and neurological scans. All scans are performed after the intravenous injection of FDG (the injected dose depends on the patient's weight) and after an uptake period has elapsed. The uptake period is the time from the injection of the PET tracer to the performance of the scan. During the uptake period, the tracer circulates throughout the body and is preferentially localized in specific tissues. FDG is excreted by the kidneys and then pools in the bladder.

Patient preparation and scanning technique may vary slightly from center to center. Our procedures, which have been used with slight modifications for more than 27,000 patient studies (PET and PET/CT) are described in the following sections.

Whole-Body Scanning

Our technique for whole-body scanning is as follows:

- Patients fast for 6 hours before isotope injection.
- The study is explained to the patient; a short history and informed consent are obtained; and metal objects are removed because they can induce an artifact in the CT scan.

- An intravenous cannula is inserted into a peripheral vein for isotope injection, and vein patency is maintained by heparinized saline. The blood sugar level is measured; elevated blood sugar is not treated, and a decision to continue with the study is made by the attending physician.
- Oral sedation (typically 2.5 to 5.0 mg of diazepam) may be given if the patient is anxious, nervous, or claustrophobic.
- The patient is injected with 350 MBq of FDG while resting quietly in a recliner or in a bed. The patient is asked not to talk and to remain still during the uptake period.
- The uptake period is 60 minutes. Just before being positioned on the scanner bed, the patient is asked to empty the bladder.
- Patients are positioned on the scanning palette and asked to remain still. They are scanned with their arms above the head if the weight exceeds 90 kg; otherwise, patients are scanned with their arms at the side, which is more comfortable for the patient.
- The scan extent generally extends from the vertex to the upper thighs (approximately 90 cm) and is measured in beds; a *bed* indicates the *z*-axis length of the FOV of the scanner and is typically 16 cm, except in the Biograph Truepoint (see Fig. 71-3). Lower limbs are scanned if the tumor is located in the lower limbs or if there is a clinical indication.
- When the scan commences, the CT scan is done first over scan extent. This typically takes less than 60 seconds.
- PET acquisition follows the CT scan from the head to the upper thighs, which is important for claustrophobic patients because the head begins to move out of the scanner gantry early in the course of the scan.
- The scan duration depends on the patient's weight and typically varies from 16 to 30 minutes.
- On completion of the scan, the venous cannula is removed. Patients are encouraged to drink fluid over the subsequent 4 to 6 hours.

The radiation exposure is in the range of 12 to 15 mSv. Diabetics are not excluded, but hyperglycemia results in a poor signal-to-noise ratio because FDG competes with circulating glucose for uptake into tissues. The end result is decreased cerebral FDG uptake and "noisy" images because the tracer dose of FDG competes with glucose for facilitated uptake.

Neurological Scanning

Our technique for neurological scanning is as follows:

- Patients fast for 6 hours before isotope injection.
- The study is explained to the patient. The patient is also asked about claustrophobia, but claustrophobia is less of an issue because of the short duration of the scan. A short history and informed consent are obtained.
- An intravenous cannula is inserted into a peripheral vein for isotope injection. Vein patency is maintained by heparinized saline. A second venous cannula may be inserted into a distal peripheral vein in a heated upper limb for blood sampling (i.e., arterialized venous sam-

pling), which can then be used to obtain quantitative data (milligrams of glucose/gram of tissue/minute) about cerebral glucose metabolism. The blood sugar level is measured; elevated blood sugar is not treated, and the decision to continue with the study is made by the attending physician.

- Video electroencephalographic data may be obtained before the study and during the uptake period for patients with a history of seizures. Seizure activity before the scan can result in focal regions of increased metabolism and glucose hypometabolism in the completed study.
- Sedation is not given because most sedatives reduce cerebral glucose metabolism. In the exceptional circumstance in which sedation is required, a short-acting anesthetic is given with full anesthetic support at the completion of the uptake period and just before the patient proceeds onto the scanning palette.
- The patient is injected with 350 MBq of FDG while resting quietly in a recliner or in a bed. The eyes and ears are patched to decrease sensory stimulation, and the patient is asked not to talk during the uptake period.
- The uptake period is 45 minutes.
- The patient is positioned on scanning bed, and head movement is limited by head restraint. CT is done first, and PET data acquisition follows.
- The total scan duration is 8 minutes.

Head movement can result in misregistration between CT and PET data, which can result in image artifacts. The PET/CT analysis software allows the CT and PET data to be overlaid or fused, and this can be used to detect and correct for misregistration. Corticosteroids result in a marked, generalized reduction in cerebral glucose metabolism, which is independent of any effect on blood glucose levels.

INDICATIONS AND CONTRAINDICATIONS

FDG-PET/CT has general indications and those for the palliative care setting.

General Indications

Although PET was developed in the neurosciences and was then applied to the assessment of viable cardiac muscle before coronary artery bypass grafting, the main indication for PET/CT is the staging and restaging of cancer.[5,6] In our center, more than 90% of the PET/CT studies are undertaken in the context of cancer. However, the local application of PET/CT is influenced to some extent by funding arrangements (e.g., health insurance, Medicare reimbursement), local expertise, availability of PET isotopes (e.g., FDG), local oncology expertise, and the demographics of the local population.

The term *oncology* is a misnomer to the extent that with the exception of lymphomas, the main role of PET/CT in our center has been in the surgical oncology setting. In our experience, the PET/CT scan result often determines whether a patient undergoes surgery, and it is therefore imperative that the interpretation of these studies is accurate. This information is needed to provide an individual with beneficial surgery and to avoid futile and morbid surgery and chemoradiotherapy in a patient with incurable disease (Fig. 71-5).

In our experience over the past decade, PET/CT has played a major role in the presurgical evaluation and staging of the following conditions:

- Non-small cell lung cancer (NSCLC) and solitary pulmonary nodules
- Lymphomas (i.e., Hodgkin's lymphoma and non-Hodgkin's lymphoma)
- Metastatic melanoma before major surgery
- Head and neck cancers
- Metastatic colorectal cancer when local recurrence or hepatic and pulmonary metastases are suspected
- Carcinoma of the esophagus, stomach, gallbladder, biliary tree, or pancreas

- Soft tissue and bony sarcomas
- Primary cervical cancer
- Anorectal carcinoma
- Carcinoma of an unknown primary
- Suspected primary brain tumors

Combined PET/CT has been used to evaluate suspected tumor recurrence in the following conditions:

- Urogenital malignancies, including testicular and transitional cell carcinomas
- Ovarian, uterine, and cervical cancers
- Head and neck cancers, including thyroid cancer
- Soft tissue and bony sarcomas
- Breast cancer
- NSCLC

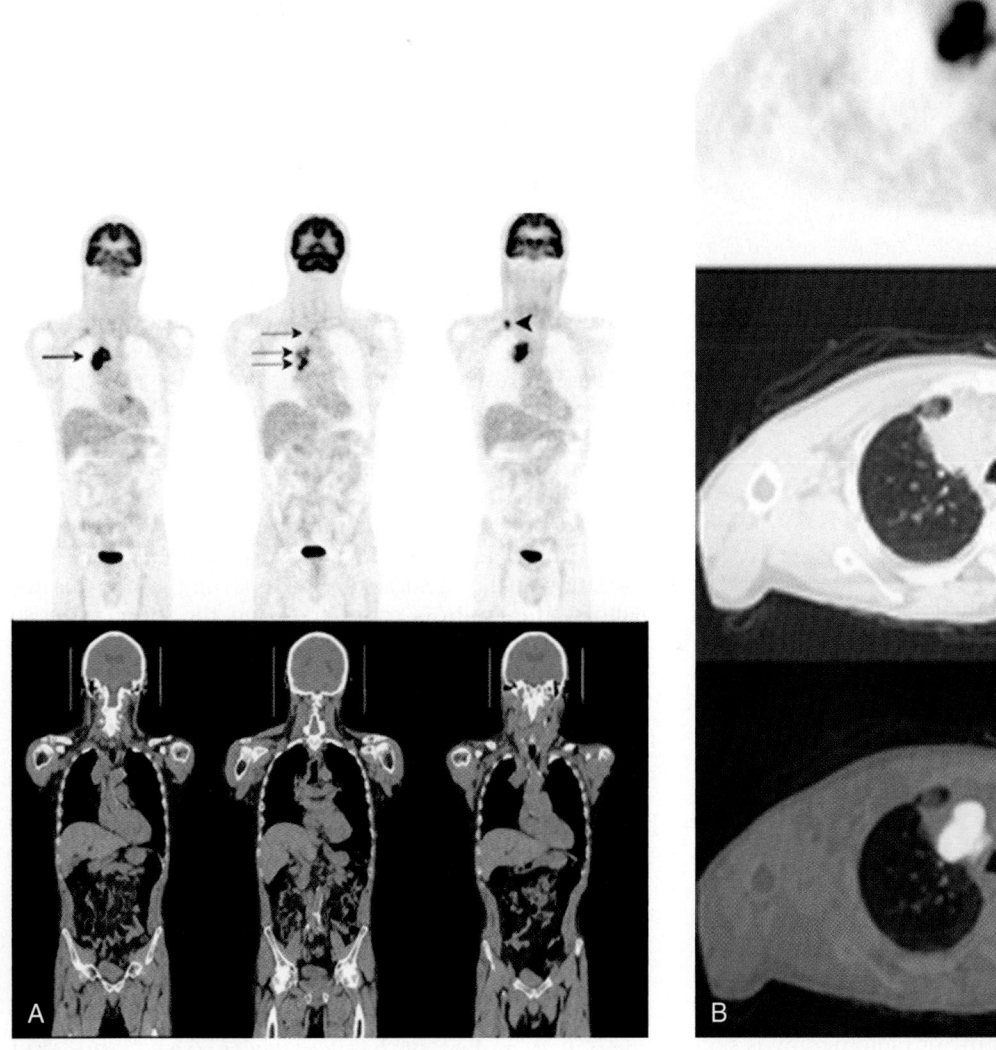

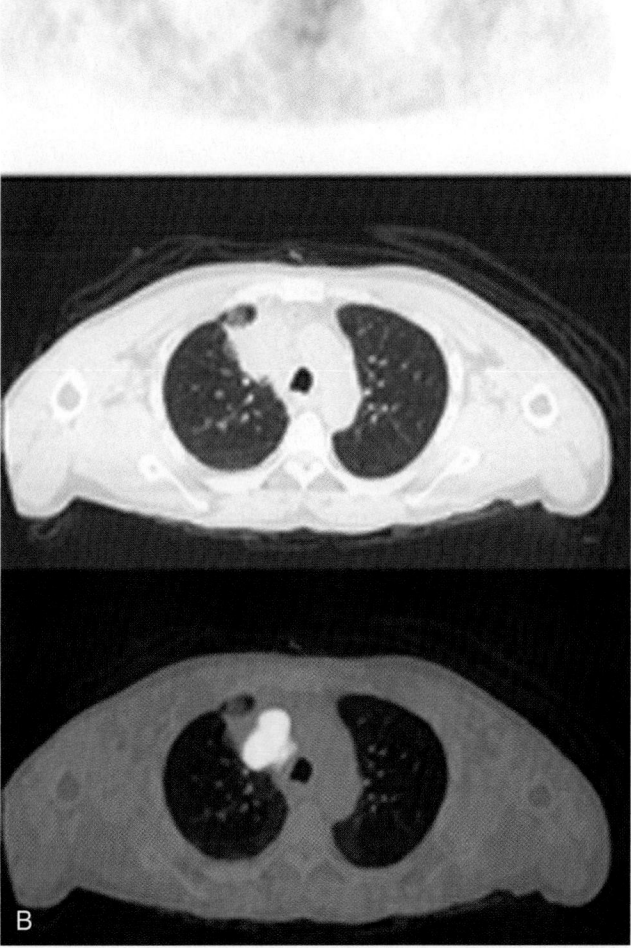

FIGURE 71-5 A 60-year-old man had newly diagnosed non–small cell lung cancer (NSCLC) in the upper lobe of his right lung. The suspected T4 tumor was studied on the Biograph Truepoint combined positron emission tomography and computed tomography (PET/CT). The PET/CT findings indicate extensive nodal involvement and cerebral metastases consistent with stage IV disease. **A,** Coronal ¹⁸F-fluorodeoxyglucose PET (FDG-PET) *(top row)* and CT images with soft tissue window settings *(bottom row)* show the markedly glucose-avid tumor in the right upper lobe and extension into mediastinum *(single arrow)*; adjacent mediastinal nodal disease in subcarinal, paratracheal, and para-esophageal regions *(dashed arrows)*; and right supraclavicular nodal disease *(arrowhead)*. The overall findings are consistent with T4N3 disease (stage IIIB). **B,** Transaxial FDG-PET *(top row)*, CT with lung window settings *(middle row)*, and fused PET/CT images *(bottom row)* show the mass extending directly into the mediastinum with compression of the superior vena cava, findings consistent with a T4 tumor.

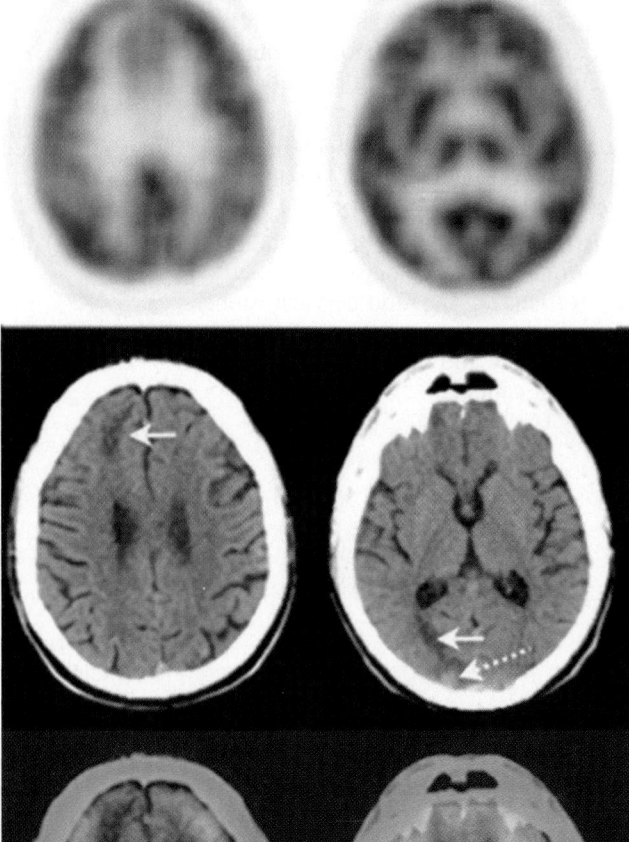

FIGURE 71-5, cont'd **C,** Transaxial FDG-PET *(top)*, CT *(middle)*, and fused PET/CT *(bottom row)* of the brain show white matter vasogenic edema in the right frontal and occipital lobes *(solid arrows)* due to cerebral metastases; the *dashed arrow* shows occipital metastasis on uncontrasted CT. Findings were confirmed on magnetic resonance imaging. Cerebral metastases are often small and necrotic and not visible on FDG-PET.

- Lymphomas
- Brain tumors

PET/CT studies have been used to assess treatment responses and the extent of residual tumor. This is best illustrated with the lymphomas and gastrointestinal tumors (GISTs), but any tumor that displays markedly increased FDG uptake before chemotherapy or radiotherapy is suitable for a post-treatment evaluation with FDG-PET/CT. Combined PET/CT has been used to assess patients with previous malignancies and elevated tumor markers (e.g., carcinoembryonic antigen, cancer antigen 125, alpha-fetoprotein).

In the neurosciences, PET/CT studies have been used to evaluate refractory epilepsy before surgery. The modal-ity also is useful in the diagnosis of neurodegenerative conditions, including dementia, diffuse Lewy body disease, progressive supranuclear palsy, multiple system atrophy, frontotemporal dementia, and prion diseases. PET/CT aids the preoperative assessment of proven or suspected primary cerebral tumors and the differentiation of recurrent tumor from radiation necrosis after a primary brain tumor has been treated (Fig. 71-6).[4,5]

For patients with heart disease, PET is the gold standard for the accurate identification of viable myocardium. The common clinical context is when intervention (e.g., bypass grafting) is being considered.

Indications in the Context of Palliative Care Patients

In our clinical experience, the number of referrals we receive from palliative care physicians is small, which suggests that this is relatively uncharted territory. However, we suggest that PET/CT should be considered in the palliative care setting for several conditions:

- Accurate staging of a malignancy to identify sites of disease
- Intractable pain (e.g., pelvic, bony, brachial plexus)
- Assessment of bony metastatic disease
- Assessment of response or lack of response to therapy

Contraindications

There are no true contraindications to performing FDG-PET/CT scans. There have been no reported side effects or allergies resulting from FDG.

Hyperglycemia is a relative contraindication to scanning because as the blood sugar rises, the signal-to-noise ratio progressively decreases. In many PET studies reported in the literature, diabetics are excluded because of the poor technical quality of the scan. In our experience, unless the blood sugar level is very high (>18 mmol/L), the study quality is sufficient for reporting. If it is unsatisfactory, the study is repeated when the blood glucose level is lower. We do not attempt to reduce the glucose level with insulin before the scan because this increases FDG uptake into muscle.

COMPLICATIONS

PET/CT scans are safe procedures, and there have never been any adverse events reported during or after the performance of a PET/CT scan. Increasingly, attention is focused on radiation exposure related to imaging studies, and although this is not a cause for concern in the palliative care population, the exposure with our approach is between 8 and 9 mSv for a neurological study and is 12 to 15 mSv for a whole-body study, depending on whether the CT is a dual or 64-slice device (see "Pearls and Pitfalls").

FUTURE CONSIDERATIONS

PET radiotracers that are more specific for the molecular substrates of malignancy and pain generation will be available in the future. Instrumentation (e.g., CT slices increased

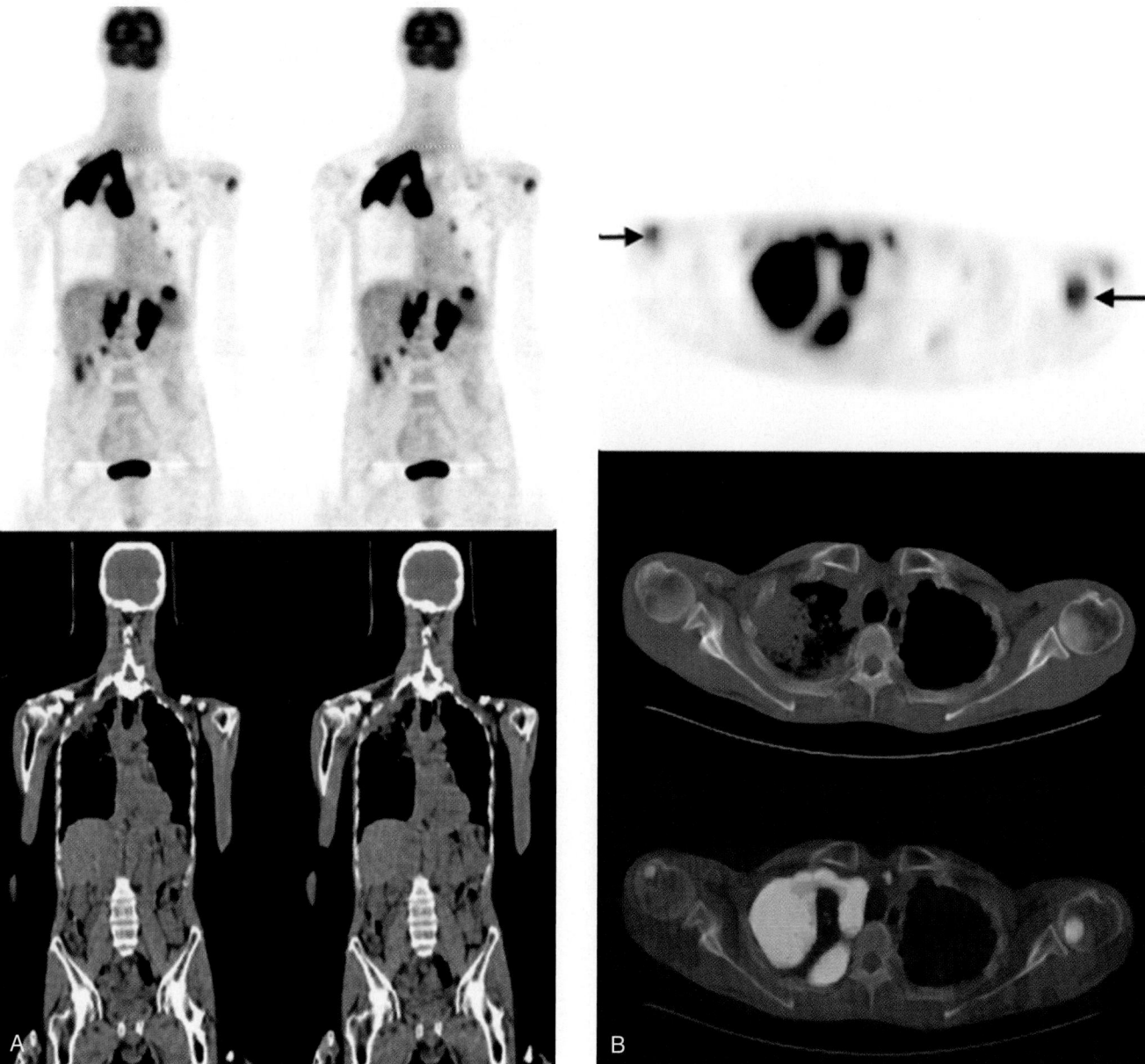

FIGURE 71-6   A 66-year-old man had a suspected recurrence of diffuse, large B-cell non-Hodgkin lymphoma (NHL) in his right lung. Fused positron emission tomography and computed tomography (PET/CT) findings show disseminated, unsuspected disease. **A,** Coronal ^{18}F-fluorodeoxyglucose PET (FDG-PET) *(top row)* and CT images with soft tissue window settings *(bottom row)* show many, markedly glucose-avid foci involving the apex of the right lung, the lung fields, both proximal humeri, and nodes and viscera in the upper abdomen. There is normal FDG uptake into the brain, and there is pooling of FDG in the pelvis in the bladder. **B,** Transaxial FDG-PET *(top)*, CT with bone window settings *(middle)*, and fused PET/CT images *(bottom row)* at the level of the apex of the lungs show the very extensive involvement of the lung and adjacent pleura and the focal bone marrow involvement *(arrows)* of both proximal humeri.

Pearls and Pitfalls

- There is no substitute for extensive experience in the accurate interpretation of ^{18}F-fluorodeoxyglucose (FDG) positron emission tomography and computed tomography (PET/CT) studies.
- Misregistration between PET and CT data is not uncommon, and it should be identified because overreliance on fused images can be misleading. Misregistration can have several causes:
  Physiological—at the lung-liver interface due to respiratory motion, FDG excretion in ureters and pooling in the bladder as the PET study is acquired, in the bowel due to peristalsis
  Caused by motion—head movement or trunk and limb movement during the scan acquisition, causing misalignment between the CT and PET that can result in errors in the reconstructed image

- Normal and physiological, markedly increased FDG uptake can be seen in many tissues:
  Symmetrically in soft tissues of posterior neck, both supraclavicular fossae, superior mediastinum, costovertebral junctions posteriorly, axillae (i.e., "brown fat uptake" in anxious patients)
  In bowel in the abdomen
  As an artifact after oral iodinated contrast in the bowel (CT related)
  In relation to a prosthesis as an artifact (CT related)
  In muscles due to exertion before the study and if the patient was not fasting before the study
- Increased FDG uptake can be seen in hilar and mediastinal lymph nodes due to granulomatous inflammation (e.g., silicosis, sarcoidosis) and in other sites due to inflammation.

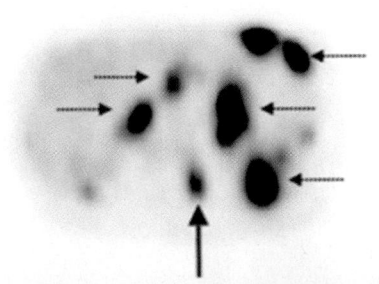

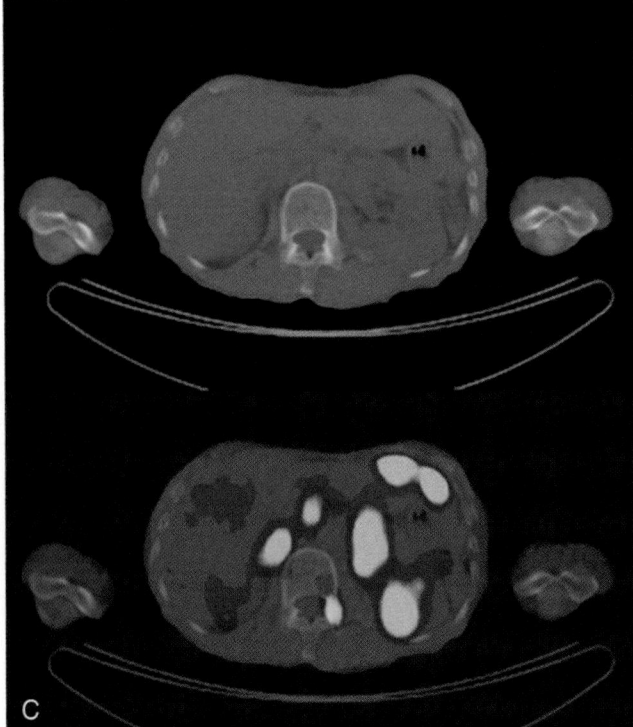

FIGURE 71-6, cont'd **C,** Transaxial FDG-PET *(top)*, CT with bone window settings *(middle)*, and fused PET/CT images *(bottom)* at the level of the upper abdomen show many foci involving the liver, spleen, and upper abdominal nodes *(dashed arrows)* and the focal involvement of the left pedicle of a thoracic vertebral body.

to 128, extended FOV) and software (e.g., time-of-flight data acquisition, three-dimensional reconstruction algorithms) developments will improve image resolution, shorten scan time, and improve patient throughput. Combined PET/MR scanners are being developed.

REFERENCES

1. Beyer T, Townsend DW, Brun T, et al. A combined PET/CT scanner for clinical oncology. J Nucl Med 2000;41:1369-1379.
2. Czernin J (ed). PET/CT in cancer patient management. J Nucl Med 2007;48(Suppl 1):S1-S88.
3. Sokoloff L, Reivich M, Kennedy C, et al. The 14C-deoxyglucose method for the measurement of local cerebral glucose utilization: Theory procedure and normal values in the conscious and anesthetized albino rat. J Neurochem 1977;28:897-916.
4. Di Chiro G. Positron emission tomography using [18F]fluorodeoxyglucose in brain tumors: A powerful diagnostic and prognostic tool. Invest Radiol 1987;22:360-371.
5. Fulham MJ, Di Chiro G. Positron emission tomography and 1H-spectroscopic imaging. In Berger MS, Wilson CB (eds). The Gliomas. Philadelphia: WB Saunders, 1999, pp 295-317.
6. Ell PJ. The contribution of PET/CT to improved patient management. Br J Radiol 2006;79:32-36.

 CHAPTER **72**

Cardiac Function Testing

David F. J. Raes, Bart Van den Eynden, and Viviane Conraads

KEY POINTS

- Cardiac disease is common in palliative medicine.
- Clinical presentation is often nonspecific.
- Diagnosis is important because cardiac disease causes significant morbidity and mortality.
- The electrocardiogram and echocardiogram are well-tolerated, noninvasive screening tests that are not time consuming and provide pertinent information.
- Other cardiac function tests are performed for specific indications.

Cardiac function is the ability of the heart to maintain adequate circulation in all conditions. Cardiac dysfunction often manifests with signs and symptoms that are nonspecific in the palliative setting: dyspnea and edema, fatigue and hypotension, and chest pain and palpitations.

Cardiovascular disease has high morbidity and mortality rates and is prevalent in palliative care (see Chapter 184). Cardiovascular disease is common, cancer treatment can cause cardiac disease, and the heart may be part of a malignant process (e.g., malignant pericardial effusion, metastatic lesions). For all these reasons, early and proper detection in this population is important. Many cardiac function tests are available, but not all are equally relevant in palliative medicine. The following questions can provide guidance in the choice of an appropriate test for a particular clinical situation:

- Does the test contribute to palliation? It does only if it leads to a treatment that alleviates symptoms.
- Which cardiac disease is treatable and likely to be found? How does it manifest, and how do we test for it? For which symptom should we perform which test?
- Does the test contribute to the prognosis? The answer depends on the treatment options and on the general prognosis. Typically short in the hospice setting, the prognosis can be much longer for someone with metastatic breast cancer. In this case, a revascularization procedure with percutaneous coronary intervention (PCI) can make sense. Approaching life's end, the focus shifts from prognostic to symptomatic treatment. The same cardiac function test that is useful and meaningful in early palliation becomes senseless in the terminal stage. The distinction between symptomatic and prognostic treatment is not straightforward and changes

dynamically over time. The choice of cardiac function test changes in conjunction.

- Is the test well tolerated or harmful? What is the complication rate?
- Is the test expensive? Is the test available, or do we have to move the patient? Is there a waiting list?

What are we looking for, when and how do we test for it, and what can we do about it? The following pathologies are frequent, detectable, and treatable:

- Heart failure, such as that caused by chemotherapeutic toxicity, can manifest as dyspnea and edema (see Chapter 79). Echocardiography quickly provides a diagnosis and helps differentiate heart failure from pulmonary embolism (see Chapter 185). Medication gives fast alleviation of symptoms and even prognostic benefit.
- Cardiac tamponade by a malignant pericardial effusion can manifest as dyspnea and hypotension. Echocardiography easily diagnoses it. Immediate pericardial puncture is lifesaving and palliative.
- Atrial fibrillation and other arrhythmias can manifest as palpitations, heart failure, or angina (see Chapter 80). The electrocardiogram provides an easy bedside diagnosis. Medication can quickly alleviate symptoms.
- Angina pectoris and cardiac ischemia are common in the elderly, but they can be caused by cancer treatment (e.g., 5-fluorouracil). Coronary disease in palliative medicine is a complex matter with many tests and therapies, ranging from noninvasive to invasive and from symptomatic to prognostic. The test of choice is different in each case.

THE TESTS

The following sections describe test selection. Techniques may be noninvasive and well tolerated, semi-invasive or less well tolerated, or invasive. Table 72-1 shows the status of these tests.

Electrocardiography

Electrocardiogram

The electrocardiogram (ECG) is a basic cardiac examination. Skin electrodes attached to specific locations on the thorax and extremities detect the changing electrical field of the heart during contraction and relaxation. The signal is transferred to an electrocardiograph (Fig. 72-1). This is a graphic display of voltage versus time, also known as the classic 12-lead ECG (Fig. 72-2). The ECG is used to diagnose pericarditis, acute coronary syndromes, and rhythm and conduction disturbances. It does not assess contractility.[1]

Indications for an ECG include suspected arrhythmia (i.e., palpitations or bradycardia, tachycardia, and irregularity), a suspected cardiac cause of chest pain or dyspnea, and syncope and shock. Contraindications include severe and open skin disease. Radiation dermatitis and recent surgical wounds are relative contraindications (i.e., they limit the number of leads). Uncontrollable movement and tremor limit quality and make the results more difficult to interpret, but they are not contraindications.

Electrocardiographs are portable. There is no special preparation, but the thorax must be free of clothing, bandages, and tapes. The procedure only takes a few minutes (see "Pearls and Pitfalls"). There are no significant complications.

Pearls and Pitfalls

1. Incorrect electrode position produces false disease patterns.
2. Incorrect calibration of the time scale of the recording paper produces false bradycardia or tachycardia.
3. Tremor can produce false major arrhythmias.
4. Breathing movements can cause undulation of the baseline and false signs of ischemia.
5. Anyone can perform the test, but trained doctors must interpret the results.

TABLE 72-1 Invasiveness of Tests			
TEST	**NONINVASIVE AND WELL TOLERATED**	**SEMI-INVASIVE OR LESS WELL TOLERATED**	**INVASIVE**
Electrocardiogram	Yes		
Exercise electrocardiogram		Yes	
Electrocardiographic Holter monitoring	Yes		
Echocardiography	Yes		
Transthoracic echocardiography	Yes		
Transesophageal echocardiography		Yes	
Stress echocardiography			
Myocardial perfusion imaging, resting images	Yes		
Myocardial perfusion imaging, stress images		Yes	
Radionuclide ventriculography	Yes		
Cardiac magnetic resonance		Yes	
Coronary computed tomography		Yes	
Invasive coronary and ventricular angiography			Yes

The ECG remains a core cardiac function test. It is noninvasive and well tolerated, and it yields useful information in the palliative care setting. It is widely available at the bedside, and it is inexpensive.

Exercise Electrocardiogram

The exercise ECG is registered during stress imposed by walking on a treadmill or exercising on a cycle ergometer (Fig. 72-3). Both require the use of both legs, adequate equilibrium, and a minimum of exercise tolerance. It provides information on coronary perfusion and total cardiovascular performance.[2]

Indications include chest pain suggesting angina pectoris (once stable), assessment of ischemia or exercise tolerance before palliative surgery, evaluation of dyspnea on exertion or fatigue when a cardiac cause is probable, and evaluation of arrhythmia and syncope when they are effort induced.

Contraindications include any unstable patient (e.g., acute coronary syndrome, critical valve disease, and pulmonary embolism). Certain conditions hamper interpretation of the ECG, such as ventricular pacing, complete left bundle branch block, preexisting abnormality of repolarization, and some drugs (e.g., digoxin). These conditions are relative contraindications because they lower diagnostic accuracy.

There is no special preparation for an exercise ECG. Blood pressure is monitored during the test, but the cuff of the sphygmomanometer should not be placed on an arm with lymphedema. The test must be performed under continuous medical supervision by skilled personnel.

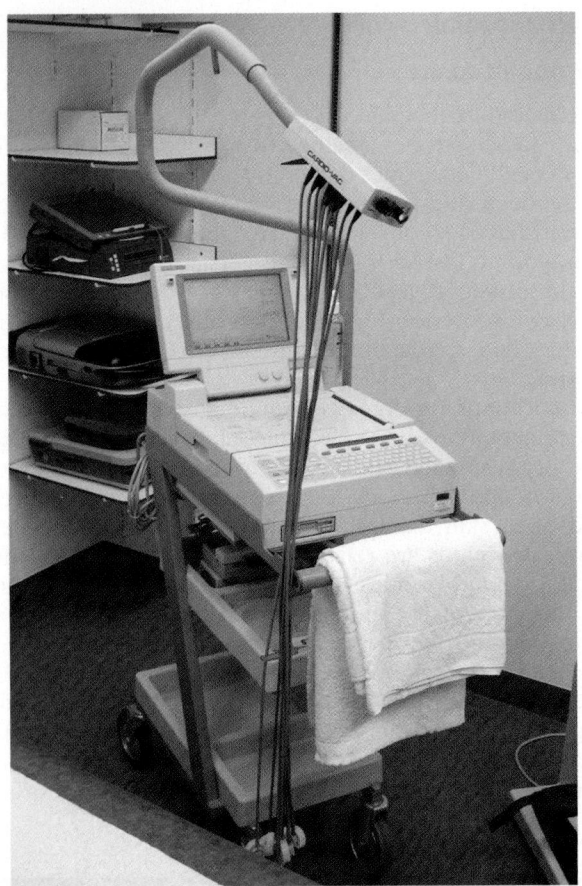

FIGURE 72-1 An electrocardiograph and skin electrodes are used to record a graphic display of voltage versus time: The electrocardiogram.

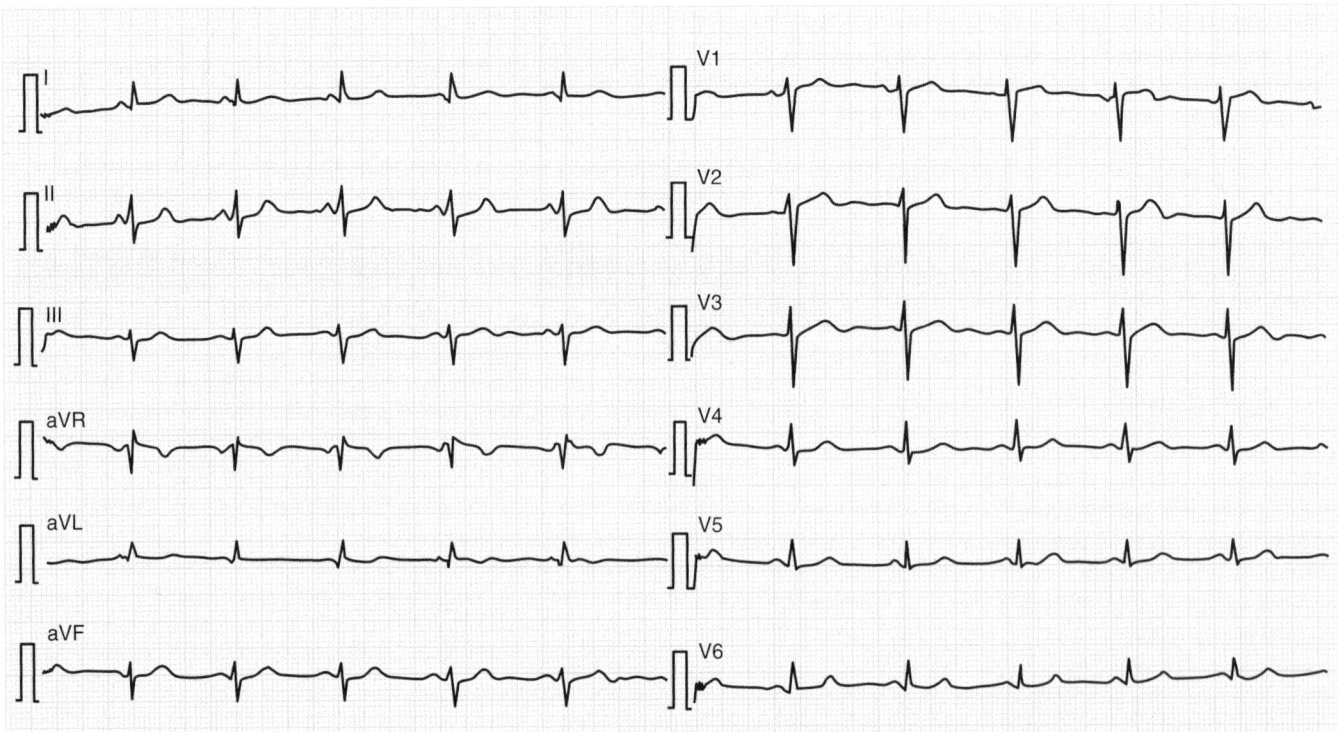

FIGURE 72-2 The classic 12-lead electrocardiogram is a basic cardiac examination. It represents the voltage that the heart is producing during contraction and relaxation.

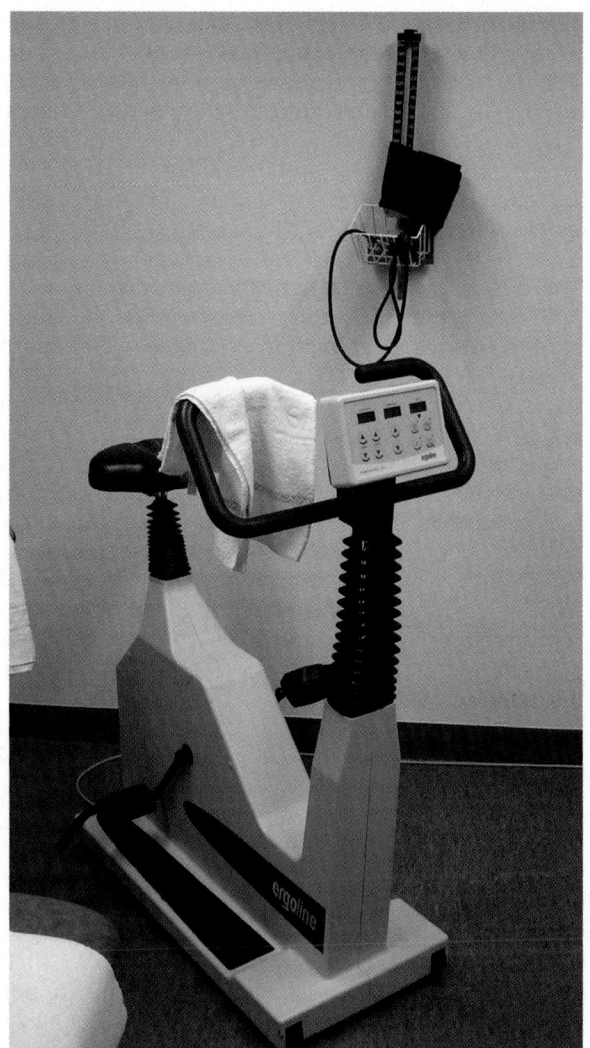

FIGURE 72-3 The cycle ergometer is used for performing an exercise electrocardiogram. This test gives information on coronary perfusion and on cardiovascular performance as a whole.

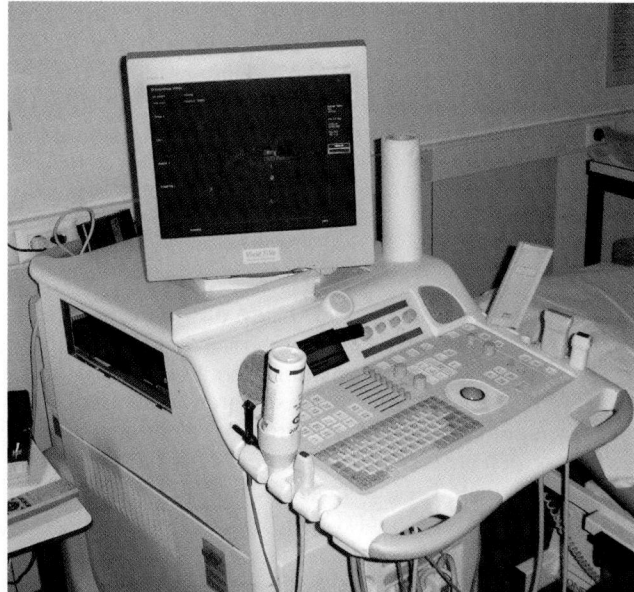

FIGURE 72-4 The echocardiograph is a dedicated processor that provides real-time images of the beating heart, based on ultrasonic waves that are projected on tissue and reflecting waves that are collected with a transducer or probe.

Electrocardiographic Holter Monitoring

A dedicated portable recorder registers the ECG continuously during a prolonged period, usually 24 hours. It allows diagnosis of transient disturbances of rhythm and conduction.

Indications include arrhythmia, syncope, and palpitations. Contraindications include severe skin disease and the need for intensive hygiene, because the system is not waterproof, and it is not possible to take a shower or a bath.

Holter monitoring requires no special preparation. The patient remains ambulatory during the test.

The test itself has no monitoring or alarm function. Artifacts of motion or tremor can mimic major arrhythmia, such as ventricular fibrillation or asystole, also. If an arrhythmia is found with prognostic relevance, the physician needs to balance the pros and cons of treatment with a pacemaker or a defibrillator against the general prognosis. In hospice care, there is no place for implanting defibrillators.

Complications are rare. Self-adhesive skin electrodes can cause skin irritation.

Twenty-four hour Holter monitoring is a noninvasive test that is generally well tolerated. The results can guide treatment of symptomatic arrhythmia.

Cardiac Imaging Techniques

Echocardiography

In echocardiography, ultrasonic sound waves are projected on tissue, and reflecting waves are collected with a transducer or probe. An echocardiograph (Fig. 72-4) uses the signals to reconstruct an image that is still or moving. Velocity of blood and tissue can be measured with the Doppler principle and displayed as a color or

The interpretation of a stress ECG is specialized. Predictive accuracy depends on the clinical pretest probability for coronary heart disease.[3] The exercise ECG is the first of a group of cardiac function tests that have greater sensitivity and specificity but are more expensive, less available, or more invasive. They are performed for specific indications, and a cardiologist should choose which test is indicated. The complications for an exercise ECG are the same as for the ECG plus syncope, myocardial infarction, and sudden cardiac death (<1 in 10,000).[4]

The exercise ECG remains a core and first-line cardiac function test for ischemia. It is noninvasive and usually well tolerated but can rarely be hazardous. It is widely available and inexpensive. It is the responsibility of a cardiologist or specialized doctor to decide if the test is indicated and to do the interpretation. In the palliative setting, the physician has to consider in advance if exercise testing will lead to a treatment with a benefit and whether this outweighs the possible discomfort. It may be wiser to do another type of stress test or none at all.

time graph.[5] If images are recorded through the chest wall, the method is transthoracic echocardiography (TTE), which is the main technique used. Transesophageal echocardiography (TEE) is the method used if images are recorded through the esophagus with a probe that looks like an endoscope (Fig. 72-5). Image resolution is usually better because of the proximity of the heart and the esophagus.

TRANSTHORACIC ECHOCARDIOGRAPHY

Images and measurements are made of the beating heart and its valves, great vessels, and pericardium. Blood flow is studied to obtain information about cardiac output, valve function, and pressure estimates. One important measurement is the left ventricular ejection fraction (LVEF), which is used as a parameter of cardiac contractility. It is calculated using the end-diastolic volume (EDV) and end-systolic volume (ESV). The formula is LVEF = (EDV − ESV)/EDV.[6]

Indications are broad and include any suspicion of cardiac disease. Indications for TTE include cardiac murmur; chest pain with characteristics of angina; symptomatic hypotension, syncope, or shock; fever without explanation with suspicion of endocarditis; and suspicion of heart failure.[7] Heart failure is suspected in case of signs and symptoms of heart failure with cardiomegaly on the chest radiograph and signs and symptoms of heart failure with elevation of B-type natriuretic peptide (BNP) or N-terminal-pro-brain natriuretic peptide (NT-pro-BNP). BNP and NT-pro-BNP are serologic markers produced by the cardiac ventricles. Serum levels are elevated in cases of left and right ventricular dysfunction. The markers have a high sensitivity and negative predictivity.[8]

Signs and symptoms of heart failure can be dyspnea, orthopnea, third heart sound, neck vein distention, edema, pleural effusion, liver enlargement, or fatigue and exercise intolerance. Contraindications include interfering disease of the left thorax wall, such as recent surgery, severe radiation dermatitis, or local painful metastasis, and an inability to adopt a dorsal or left decubitus position.

TTE requires no special preparation, but it must be performed by skilled personnel. The left anterior thoracic wall must be free of clothes, bandages, or tapes. Its takes up to 45 minutes, but the procedure can be paused if the patient needs it. Information can be processed offline. Some conditions may affect the imaging:

- There is a significant loss in image quality in cases of pulmonary hyperinflation (e.g., ventilation support, chronic obstructive pulmonary disease) and morbid obesity.
- A low LVEF is not the same as heart failure. Heart failure is a syndrome diagnosed based on clinical presentation and additional test information. Echocardiography can provide multiple parameters of heart failure other than LVEF, such as cardiac filling properties and cardiac output. Echocardiography can also detect causes of heart failure, such as infarction or valve lesions. The LVEF assessed by echocardiography is less accurate and reproducible than that measured with other techniques. Echocardiography is easy and provides additional information.
- Pericardial effusion is not the same as pericardial tamponade. Echocardiography allows differentiation of the conditions.

Complications are few, but the transducer pressure on the chest wall can cause pain. TTE is a noninvasive, well-tolerated, and harmless test. It is widely available, fast, and can be performed at the bedside. It provides much information relevant in the palliative care setting (e.g., heart failure, tamponade). TTE is a first-line cardiac function test in palliative medicine.

TRANSESOPHAGEAL ECHOCARDIOGRAPHY

In TEE, a specially designed transducer is inserted into the esophagus (see Fig. 72-5). The left atrium lies beside the esophagus and provides a good window for ultrasound with no interference from bone, fat, or air. This gives more detailed morphological information than TEE.

Indications include the suspicion of a cardiac source of emboli, endocarditis (if TTE cannot exclude it), cardiac invasion by tumor, and pathology of the aorta. Contraindications include narrowing of the esophagus by a tumor or stricture, Zenker's diverticulum, severe dyspnea, and an unstable patient.

The patient must be fasting, well informed, and relaxed. An intravenous line must be in place for sedation, if needed. Dental prostheses must be removed.

Complications are rare but include insertion of the probe into the trachea, damage to the esophagus (if diseased), and damage to teeth.[9] TEE is a semi-invasive test that is generally well tolerated in experienced hands. It is less widely available, but it can be done at the bedside. It is not a first-line test. It is done when a more detailed image is needed than can be obtained with TTE.

STRESS ECHOCARDIOGRAPHY

Stress echocardiography is essentially TTE combined with physical exercise (i.e., adapted cycle ergometer) or, more

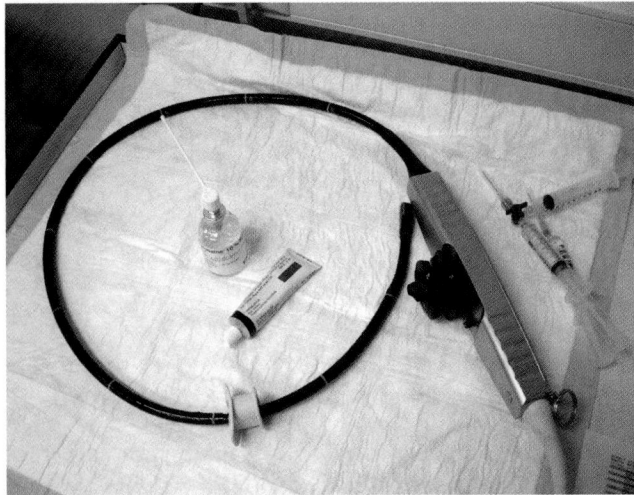

FIGURE 72-5 The images of transesophageal echocardiography (TEE) are recorded through the esophagus close to the heart with a probe that looks like an endoscope. Image resolution is usually better because there is only a thin layer of tissue between the probe and heart.

often, with pharmacological stress (i.e., dobutamine or adenosine).[10] We discuss only the dobutamine stress echo test. Dobutamine is administered intravenously according to a graded protocol. It stimulates contractility and heart rate and elevates oxygen consumption. In cases of inadequate coronary perfusion, ischemia is induced and detected on echocardiography as wall motion abnormalities even before detection by electrocardiographic changes. Dobutamine stress echo is more sensitive than the exercise ECG.

Indications include evaluation of angina pectoris to detect and localize ischemia and assessment of known coronary artery disease with symptoms or before palliative surgery. Dobutamine stress echocardiography can be used as a second line test in cases of equivocal stress ECG testing, when higher sensitivity and specificity are necessary. It is the first-line test when the patient is unable to do a regular exercise test or the ECG is not interpretable.

Contraindications include instability and bad TTE image quality. Dobutamine is contraindicated in patients with tachyarrhythmia or pheochromocytoma.

For the test, β-blockers must be stopped because they counteract dobutamine. Interpretation of regional wall movement requires thorough training. The test takes about 45 minutes and can cause palpitations, anxiety, and dyspnea. Recovery occurs swiftly after cessation of dobutamine. Complications of dobutamine are the induction of angina, arrhythmia, and hypotension. The indication, procedure, and interpretation are specialized.

Dobutamine stress echo provides noninvasive information on coronary perfusion with a higher diagnostic accuracy than classic exercise testing. It is more complex and has limited indications in palliative medicine.

Nuclear Imaging

The most important nuclear imaging tests (see Chapter 69) are myocardial perfusion imaging (MPI) and radionuclide ventriculography (RVG). The former visualizes coronary perfusion of the heart, and the latter determines LVEF. They require a fully equipped department of nuclear medicine. These techniques are more expensive and less available than ECG testing and echocardiography, and they must be performed by dedicated personnel.

RESTING AND STRESS MYOCARDIAL PERFUSION IMAGING

Resting and stress myocardial perfusion imaging tests are based on visualization of a radioactive-labeled substance that distributes in the myocardium proportionate to coronary perfusion. Imaging can be done with the patient resting and under physical stress with an ergometer or pharmacological stress. Myocardial ischemia is recognized as a perfusion defect induced by stress that is absent while resting. Scar tissue is visualized as a perfusion defect at rest and under stress. The most frequently used tracers are thallium 201 (^{201}Tl)- and technetium 99m (^{99m}Tc)-labeled agents such as ^{99m}Tc sestamibi. MPI has a higher sensitivity and specificity than regular exercise ECG, comparable to the dobutamine stress echo test.[11]

Indications are the same as for dobutamine stress echo testing. Contraindications to pharmacological stress are instability or hypotension (e.g., adenosine, dipyridamole, dobutamine) and atrioventricular conduction disease (e.g., adenosine). Contraindications to physical stress are the same as for exercise ECG testing.

MPI requires an intravenous line. In cases of pharmacological stress, patients must abstain from caffeine-containing foods and theophylline-containing drugs. The timing must be respected. Depending on the technique, scanning starts immediately or 30 to 60 minutes after injection, and the patient is scanned for 15 to 30 minutes. The procedure and interpretation is specialized and requires knowledge about auto-absorption, diaphragm attenuation, breast superposition, and liver artifacts.

There is no special aftercare, except for limited radioprotection measures. The radiation dose is low. Complications are rare. The resting scan is well tolerated. Pharmacological and physical stress testing can harm or cause discomfort. Pharmacological stress can cause bronchial constriction, atrioventricular block, hypotension, or nausea and flushing, depending on the substance used.

Nuclear MPI provides noninvasive information on coronary perfusion, is well tolerated, and has higher diagnostic accuracy than classic exercise testing. It is more expensive, time consuming, and less available. It requires specialized staff and equipment, and it has limited indications in palliative medicine.

RADIONUCLIDE VENTRICULOGRAPHY

RVG, or multiple-gated cardiac blood pool imaging, measures LVEF with high accuracy and reproducibility. The technique uses labeling and gating methods.

A radioactive substance labels red blood cells. Continuous measurement of radioactivity over the heart is performed with a scanner. The measured radioactivity is proportional to the volume of the heart at any time during the cardiac cycle.

By electrocardiographic gating, the cardiac cycle is divided in time frames, and systole and diastole are determined. This provides end-diastolic and end-systolic volumes, and the LVEF can be calculated as described earlier. This LVEF value is more accurate than that produced by echocardiography, and it is comparable to that obtained by left ventricular angiography.[12]

Indications include determining LVEF when echocardiography is impossible or gives equivocal information, signs and symptoms of heart failure (e.g., dyspnea, orthopnea, edema, fatigue), and detection and follow-up of anthracycline-induced cardiomyopathy. Contraindications include an inability to achieve dorsal decubitus positioning (e.g., pain, uncontrolled movement), severe claustrophobia, and arrhythmia (e.g., great irregularity of the RR interval) or tachycardia. Some correction can be done with software.

For RVG, gating, labeling, and positioning of the camera must be done by skilled personnel. Scanning takes no more than 10 minutes, and postprocessing is done offline.

The technique provides an LVEF value that is highly accurate, with good correlation with the value produced by invasive ventriculography. It is not operator dependent, given good camera positioning, and it is independent of body size, unlike TTE. A stable heart rhythm is needed, and the examiner must remember that a low LVEF is not the same as heart failure.

Complications for RVG are the same as for ECG. The radiation dose is low and does not produce complications. Nuclear RVG is noninvasive and well tolerated. It provides a more accurate LVEF than echocardiography. Echocardiography remains the test of first choice because it gives much more pertinent information in the palliative medicine setting.

Cardiac Magnetic Resonance

Cardiac magnetic resonance (CMR) is mentioned here (see Chapter 70) because it is noninvasive, well tolerated, gives highly detailed images of almost any cardiac structure, and is evolving rapidly. The test and equipment are expensive, and the test is not widely available and has limited use in palliative medicine.

The advantages of CMR include high-resolution images of tumor invasion in cardiac structures, accurate LVEF values, and image quality independent of body mass index or of pleura or chest wall pathology. The disadvantages include patient positioning in a narrow tunnel and sedation in case of claustrophobia or uncontrolled movement. Electrocardiographic gating makes the technique vulnerable to arrhythmia and tachycardia. Breath-holding is necessary and troublesome for patients with dyspnea. Gadolinium contrast is given intravenously and can be problematic in volume overload. More severe adverse reactions occur if kidney function is damaged.[13] Moreover, implanted metal objects diminish image quality because of scatter, and they are mobilized by the huge magnetic fields. Cardiac pacemakers and defibrillators are a contraindication; prosthetic heart valves not recently implanted are not a contraindication.

Radiological Techniques

CORONARY COMPUTED TOMOGRAPHY

Coronary computed tomography (CT) (see Chapter 71) provides fast and noninvasive information on coronary anatomy. It is well tolerated but can cause side effects. The contrast medium can produce volume overload, kidney toxicity, possible allergic reactions, and thyroid dysfunction. It requires gating (troublesome in cases of arrhythmia and tachycardia) and breath-holding (troublesome in cases of dyspnea). Information on coronary anatomy is inferior to that provided by invasive coronary angiography. Coronary CT is expensive and not widely available. Coronary CT still has limited use in palliative medicine.

In the future, we may have the one-stop shop for chest pain and dyspnea. One thorax CT scan provides information on coronary anatomy and on pulmonary embolism, aortic dissection, pericardial pathology, pleural pathology, pulmonary pathology, and abnormalities of chest wall and vertebrae.

INVASIVE CORONARY AND VENTRICULAR ANGIOGRAPHY

Invasive coronary and ventricular angiography is still the gold standard imaging mode for coronary anatomy, but its use is limited in palliative medicine because of its invasive character. A peripheral artery is punctured to provide access through which special catheters are inserted into the aorta. They are manipulated to position their distal end in the ostium of the coronary arteries. A radiopaque contrast medium is injected through the catheter directly into the coronary artery, and conventional images are obtained with cine-angiography.

Possible complications include bleeding at the arterial puncture, complications of the contrast medium (i.e., volume, kidney, thyroid, and allergy), angina, ischemia, and arrhythmia and hemodynamic instability with possible fatal consequences.

Use of this modality is limited to specific settings in which the possibility of immediate percutaneous coronary angioplasty or stenting is anticipated and judged beneficial. They include palliation of highly symptomatic angina that interferes with daily life and is resistant to full medical therapy and therapy for significant ischemia before palliative surgery. In the latter case, an endovascular stent must be avoided because of the need for antiplatelet medication for several weeks, which makes surgery impossible.

FUTURE CONSIDERATIONS

The ideal cardiac function test in palliative medicine is noninvasive, harmless, well tolerated, and fast. It is independent of body mass and chest wall pathology. It should be available at the bedside and inexpensive. The test should be highly informative because it is highly predictive, accurate, and reproducible.

Few tests approach this ideal. In the future, we expect evolution in cardiac imaging that will revolutionize the possibilities. In palliative medicine, coronary diagnostic testing will remain limited as long as revascularization requires invasive strategies.

REFERENCES

1. Goldberger AL, Goldberger E. Clinical Electrocardiography: A Simplified Approach. St. Louis: Elsevier/Mosby, 2006.
2. Gibbons RJ, Balady GJ, Bricker JT, et al. ACC/AHA 2002 guideline update for exercise testing: summary article: A report of the American College of Cardiology/American Heart Association Task Force on Practice Guidelines (Committee to Update the 1997 Exercise Testing Guidelines). Circulation 2002;106:1883.
3. Gianrossi R, Detrano R, Mulvihill D, et al. Exercise-induced ST depression in the diagnosis of coronary artery disease: A meta-analysis. Circulation 1989;80: 87.
4. Stuart RJ, Ellestad MH. National survey of exercise testing. Chest 1980;77:94.
5. Feigenbaum H. Instrumentation. In Feigenbaum H (ed). Echocardiography. Philadelphia: Lea & Febiger, 1994, pp 1-67.
6. Folland ED, Parisi AF, Moynihan PF, et al. Assessment of left ventricular ejection fraction and volumes by real-time, two-dimensional echocardiography. A comparison of cineangiographic and radionuclide techniques. Circulation 1979;60:760.
7. Guidelines for the Diagnosis and Treatment of Chronic Heart Failure: Executive Summary (update 2005). The Task Force for the Diagnosis and Treatment of Chronic Heart Failure of the European Society of Cardiology. Eur Heart J 2005;26:1115.
8. McCullough PA, Nowak RM, McCord J, et al. B-type natriuretic peptide and clinical judgment in emergency diagnosis of heart failure: Analysis from Breathing Not Properly (BNP) multinational study. Circulation 2002;106:416.
9. Daniel WG, Erbel R, Kasper W, et al. Safety of transesophageal echocardiography: A multicenter survey of 10,419 examinations. Circulation 1991;83:817.
10. Roger VL, Pellikka PA, Oh JK, et al. Stress echocardiography. Part I. Exercise echocardiography: Techniques, implementation, clinical applications, and correlations. Mayo Clin Proc 1995;70:5.
11. Garber AM, Solomon NA. Cost-effectiveness of alternative test strategies for the diagnosis of coronary artery disease. Ann Intern Med 1999;130:719.
12. Burow RD, Strauss HW, Singleton R, et al. Analysis of left ventricular function from multiple gated acquisition cardiac blood pool imaging. Comparison to contrast angiography. Circulation 1977;56:1024.
13. Kuo PH, Kanal E, Abu-Alfa AK, et al. Gadolinium-based MR contrast agents and nephrogenic systemic fibrosis. Radiology 2007;242:647.

SUGGESTED READING

Baim DS, Grossman W. Cardiac catheterization, angiography and intervention. Baltimore: Williams & Wilkins, 1996.

Braunwald E, Zipes DP, Libby P (eds). Heart Disease. Philadelphia: WB Saunders, 2004.

Feigenbaum H. Echocardiography. Philadelphia: Lea & Febiger, 1994.

Froelicher VF. Manual of Exercise Testing. St. Louis: CV Mosby, 1994.

Zaret BL, Beller GA. Clinical nuclear cardiology. Philadelphia: Mosby, 2005.

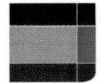

CHAPTER **73**

Pulmonary Function

Stephen McNamara

KEY POINTS

- Pulmonary function tests reliably and objectively evaluate an individual's respiratory system.

- The results should be compared with predicted normal values for the subject being tested.

- Spirometry is a simple bedside or office test that can provide great insight into significant respiratory impairment.

- More detailed measurements of lung function require expensive, laboratory-based equipment. Such tests can be invaluable in a detailed assessment of impairment.

- Measuring arterial blood gases is the most accurate way of assessing gas exchange. Sound knowledge of the normal values for the parameters measured in blood gas analysis is required to interpret results.

Objective assessment of pulmonary function can provide valuable information about the severity of respiratory impairment. These tests can help in understanding the pathophysiology involved in respiratory system illness, especially when disease processes have been gradual and when the patient has become tolerant of the effects of the condition. Physicians see patients with advanced lung disease who seem comfortable at rest but have profound derangements in arterial blood gas values or severely impaired spirometric results. Objective testing reveals the true severity of the condition.

SPIROMETRY

Spirometry measures the volume of air exhaled during a maximal forced expiratory maneuver. This provides important information about lung function. Spirometry is easy to carry out at the bedside or clinic using simple, portable equipment[1] (see Chapter 102).

For meaningful results, spirometry must be performed correctly and reproducibly. Those performing the test need to provide unambiguous instructions. The subject makes a maximal inspiratory effort, completely filling the lungs to the total lung capacity (TLC). Before exhaling, the subject must have his or her mouth sealed tightly around the spirometer's mouthpiece. The subject then exhales as rapidly as possible through the mouthpiece into the spirometer, until he or she has exhaled completely (i.e., to residual volume [RV]). It is essential that the expiratory effort during the test is maximal and that all the exhaled air is captured in the spirometer. This test is usually repeated at least three times, with at least two measurements for each spirometric parameter being within 150 mL of each other, to ensure reproducibility. The best value is recorded as the test result.[2]

Various spirometric devices are used in clinical practice. Originally, spirometers were large, barrel-shaped devices. Portable office spirometers providing a paper trace on touch-sensitive paper have been in widespread use during the past 40 years. Handheld and desktop electronic spirometers are available. They calculate exhaled volume using a pressure transducer at the mouthpiece rather than measuring the volume of exhaled air into a reservoir. Whatever device is used, regular calibration is important for reliable results.

The results of spirometry are usually reported as the forced expiratory volume in 1 second (FEV_1) and forced vital capacity (FVC) (Fig. 73-1A). Sometimes, in advanced obstructive airways disease, there may be merit in also measuring slow vital capacity (SVC). The examiner asks the patient to exhale fully from TLC into the spirometer but at a slower (rather than maximal) rate. The SVC may be larger than the FVC because of the effects of dynamic airway narrowing during a forced expiratory maneuver.

The absolute values of the FEV_1 and FVC are compared with predicted values, which are obtained from a nomogram or provided by the software in electronic spirometers. Predicted values vary with sex, age, height, and racial background. The normal range is 80% to 120% of predicted values.

The ratio of the FEV_1 to the FVC is also calculated. Normally, 80% of the forced expiratory volume is exhaled in the first 1 second of expiration. An FEV_1/FVC ratio less than 0.78 indicates airflow obstruction, but it is not often of clinical significance until the value is less than 0.70. In severe airflow obstruction, this ratio can be greatly reduced (see Fig. 73-1B). This pattern is typical of obstructive lung diseases, such as smoking-related lung disease, asthma, and bronchiectasis. In contrast, FEV_1/FVC ratios of more than 0.90 occur in restrictive lung diseases (see Fig. 73-1B). Restrictive lung diseases cause stiffening of the lung interstitium (e.g., pulmonary fibrosis), limit chest wall movement (e.g., kyphoscoliosis), or include respiratory muscle weakness. Although caused by different pathological processes, pulmonary disorders are often labeled as restrictive or obstructive lung diseases based on their spirometric function pattern. Serial spirometry tests provide an objective guide to disease progression and treatment effects.

With low FEV_1 and FVC values and a reduced FEV_1/FVC ratio, spirometry may be repeated after an inhaled bronchodilator (e.g., salbutamol). Significant reversibility (i.e.,

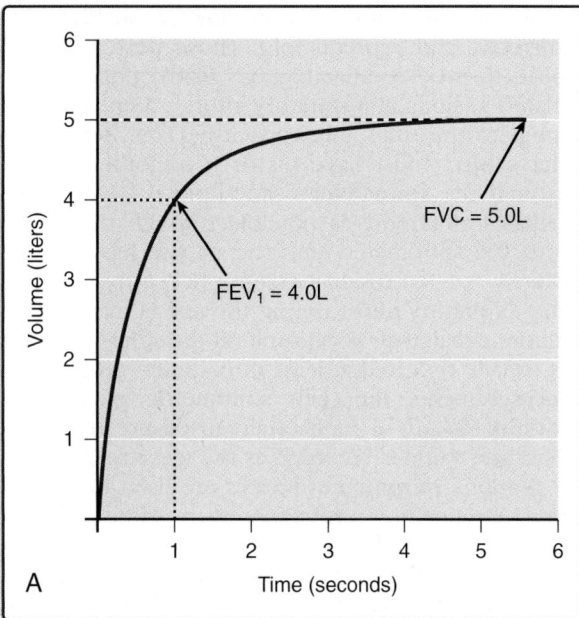
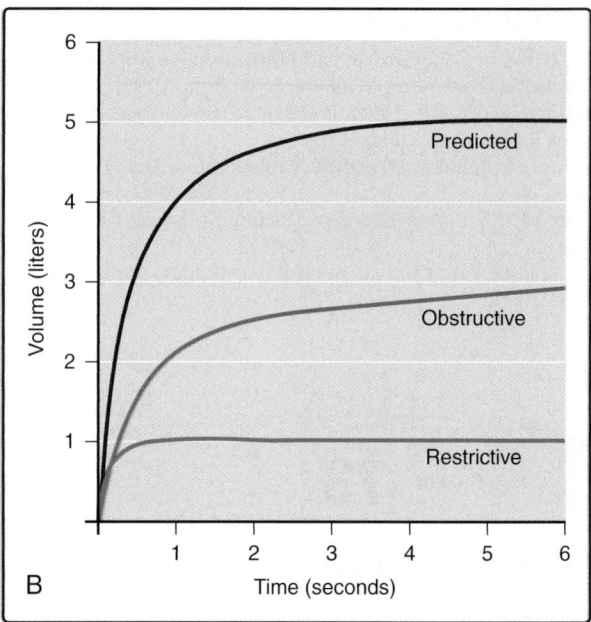

FIGURE 73-1   Spirometry.   A, A normal spirometric tracing of volume versus time for a 40-year-old white man (height of 176 cm). The forced expiratory volume in 1 second (FEV$_1$) and the forced vital capacity (FVC) are measured as shown. These absolute results are compared with predicted values for the patient, and the ratio of the two results is calculated. **B,** Typical tracings for obstructive spirometry *(dotted line)* and restrictive spirometry *(solid line)*. Predicted values are also shown *(dashed line)*.

improvement in FEV$_1$ of 15% or more) is diagnostic of asthma and has obvious management implications.

FLOW-VOLUME LOOPS

Measuring the flow rate (rather than volume) of air during maximal forced expiration and rapid inspiration can provide further information. Tracing airflow versus lung volume generates the flow-volume loop. Most electronic spirometers also obtain flow-volume information during spirometry.

A normal flow-volume loop has a characteristic appearance (Fig. 73-2A). Typically, lung volume is represented on the abscissa and flow rate on the ordinate of the graph. The subject's TLC is on the left of the abscissa, with the RV to the right. Expiration is shown above the abscissa and inspiration below.

In normal lungs, the expiratory flow rate reaches a maximum (i.e., peak flow rate) early in maximal expiration, when the lungs are at high volume. It then falls linearly as an airway flow limitation develops as the lung volume falls. At RV, the expiratory flow stops. During rapid inspiration, the flow-volume loop has a smooth, saddle-shaped appearance. Normally, the negative flow rate at mid-inspiration (i.e., halfway between RV and TLC) about equals the positive flow rate at mid-expiration.

Characteristic flow-volume loops are seen in certain pathologies (see Fig. 73-2B to 2D). Obstructive lung disease, such as that from smoking, has a typical scooped-out appearance in the expiratory limb as expiratory flow rates fall below predicted values at low lung volumes. Restrictive lung diseases, such as pulmonary fibrosis, also have a typical flow-volume loop profile, with small lungs but increased expiratory flow rates relative to lung volume.

Although they are not primary diagnostic tools, flow-volume loops can help identify the level of airway obstruction. Typical loops occur in variable intrathoracic obstruction (e.g., tracheal tumor), variable extrathoracic obstruction (e.g., laryngomalacia, vocal cord dysfunction), and fixed obstruction (e.g., tracheal stenosis).

PEAK FLOW READINGS

Whereas spirometry measures the volume of exhaled air during forced expiration, the maximal flow rate during this period can also provide lung function information. The maximal flow rate is referred to as the peak expiratory flow rate. It is usually expressed in liters per minute or liters per second. The peak flow rate is achieved early in expiration at relatively high lung volumes and before flow limitation occurs as the lungs fall to lower lung volumes. It provides a guide to the caliber of the larger airways.

As with spirometry, it is important that the maneuver to measure peak expiratory flow rate is performed correctly and reproducibly. Most electronic spirometers automatically record peak expiratory flow rate during a spirometric maneuver. Inexpensive handheld peak flow meters are commonly used. The subject makes a maximal inspiratory effort to reach TLC and then exhales as forcefully as possible through the mouthpiece of the peak flow meter. This is repeated at least three times, and the best of the three values is recorded as the test result.

The values for peak flow rate are compared with predicted values from a nomogram. Reduced peak flow rates are seen in patients with obstructive airway disease. In restrictive lung disease, the absolute peak flow value may be reduced compared with the predicted value, but when measured against lung volume, it may be normal or increased.

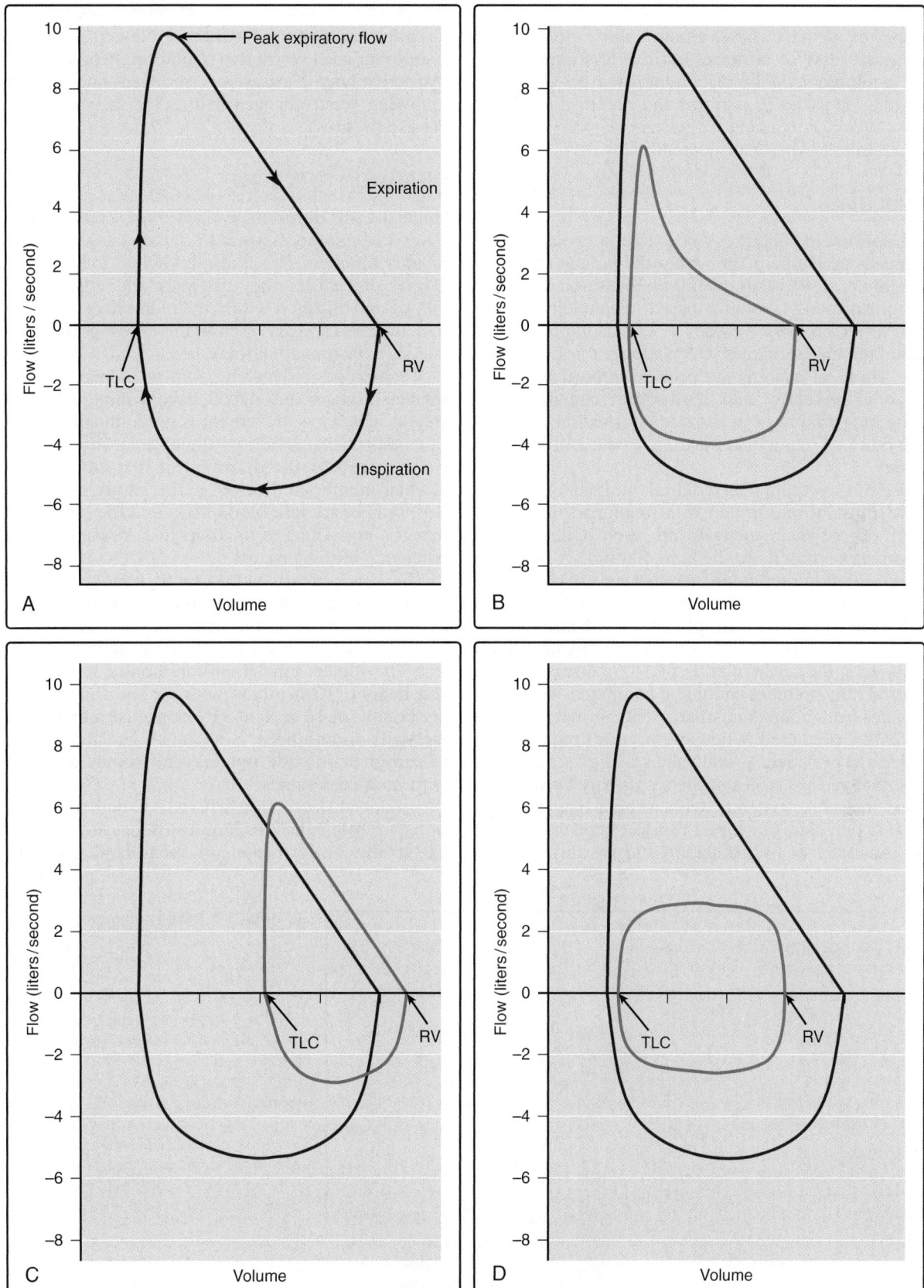

FIGURE 73-2 Flow-volume loop. A, A normal expiratory and inspiratory flow-volume loop. **B**, A characteristic flow-volume loop as seen in a patient with severe chronic airflow limitation caused by smoking. Notice the deeply scooped-out appearance of the expiratory limb of the curve, reflecting the pronounced flow limitation occurring at low lung volumes (predicted flow-volume loop in the *red line*). **C**, A characteristic flow-volume loop in a patient with severe lung restriction from pulmonary fibrosis. Notice the patient's relatively small lung volumes. Compared with predicted values, flow rates are relatively increased in relation to lung volume (predicted flow-volume loop in the *red line*). **D**, A characteristic flow-volume loop in a patient with a fixed tracheal stenosis (predicted flow-volume loop in the *red line*). TLC, total lung capacity; RV, residual volume.

Although it does not provide as much information as spirometry or detailed flow-volume loops, peak flow recordings are easy to perform and use less expensive, portable equipment. In some conditions (e.g., asthma), patients may be asked to perform and record their own peak flow readings to monitor their airways disease and assist them in following management plans.

LUNG VOLUMES

Although spirometry measures forced expiratory capacity, there remains a volume of air within the lung at the end of expiration (i.e., RV) that cannot be measured without more sophisticated, laboratory-based technology. Measurement of RV provides a means of calculating the TLC. The same technique allows calculation of other lung volumes. These measurements provide important information about restrictive and obstructive lung diseases. Measuring lung volumes can provide information about a mixed picture of combined restrictive and obstructive pathologies.

Because of the equipment required, lung volume measurements must be performed in a pulmonary function laboratory. Three main methods are used. One uses a simple principle based on helium dilution. A second popular gas dilution method is the nitrogen washout procedure. The third common technique makes calculations using whole-body plethysmography; this is the most accurate and the least susceptible to the effects of impaired gas mixing in some severe obstructive lung diseases.[2,3]

Measured lung volumes should be compared with predicted values from nomogram charts. The normal range is 80% to 120% of predicted. When interpreting lung volume results, we are provided several values that give a profile of lung size at various stages of the respiratory cycle (Fig. 73-3). For instance, someone with asthma may have a normal TLC but high functional residual capacity (FRC) and RV, indicative of hyperinflation and gas trapping in this condition. Another patient with obstructive airways disease from smoking may have a reduced TLC, suggesting a superimposed restrictive condition. People with severe restrictive lung diseases have reduced lung volumes, and following serial changes in the TLC accurately assesses disease progress.

DIFFUSION CAPACITY

Single-breath diffusion capacity for carbon monoxide (DLCO) is commonly used in detailed assessment of pulmonary function. This is also known as the transfer factor (TLCO). It reflects the dynamics and efficiency of gas mixing and diffusion within the pulmonary tree and across the alveolar-capillary membrane. It is potentially influenced by factors at all these levels.[1-3]

Whereas gas movement is linear in larger airways, the smaller airways and alveoli have a large cross-sectional area in which gas movement is predominantly from diffusion. Gas exchange across the alveolar-capillary interface is influenced by the dynamics of that diffusion process, alveolar membrane thickness, the nature of the capillary bed, pulmonary tree blood flow, and the blood hemoglobin content. DLCO is an objective measurement of the efficiency of this process.

The single-breath DLCO test is relatively simple. For accurate results, the subject must have an FEV_1 value of more than 1.5 liters. It is also necessary for supplemental oxygen to be stopped for about 20 minutes before the test. The subject inhales carbon monoxide (usually 0.3%) and helium (10%) mixed with air and then holds his or her breath for 10 seconds. He or she then exhales quickly through a mouthpiece, allowing a calculation to be made of carbon monoxide uptake. The results are compared with predicted values.

A reduced DLCO value may reflect ventilation and perfusion ($\dot{V}A/Q$) inequalities, not just impairment of gas transfer at the alveolar-capillary membrane. Patients with

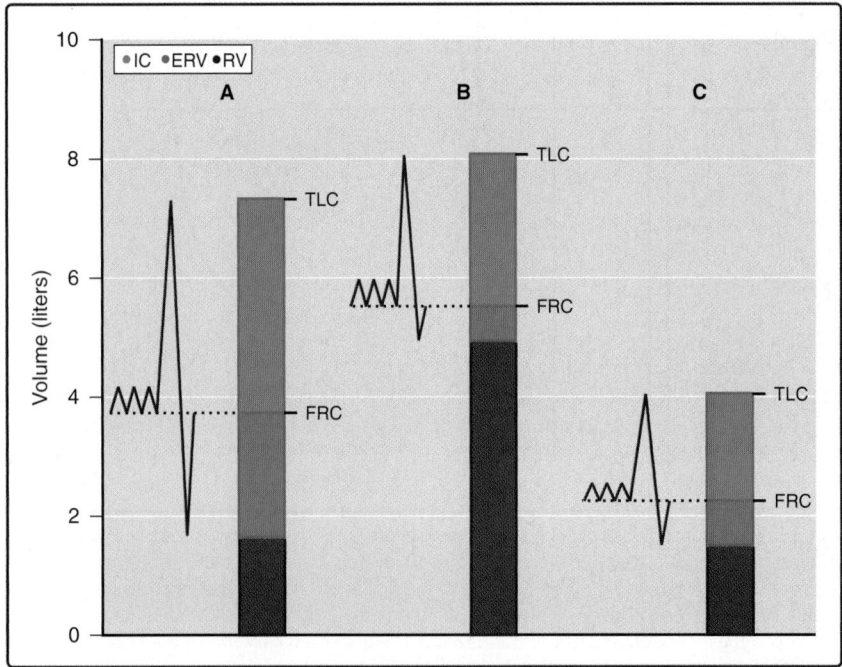

FIGURE 73-3 Lung volumes. The leftmost tracing (A) shows a typical breathing pattern in a normal subject, including the change in lung volumes associated with maximal inspiration (to total lung capacity [TLC]), followed by maximal expiration to residual volume (RV). Using techniques described in the text, lung volume measurements can allow accurate calculation of the RV, TLC, and the other components of lung volume, including the functional residual capacity (FRC), inspiratory capacity (IC), and the expiratory reserve volume (ERV). Also shown are typical lung volume profiles of a patient with severe asthma with hyperinflation and gas trapping (B) and a patient with restrictive lung disease causing severe reduction in lung volumes (C).

smoking-related airways disease usually have a reduced D_{LCO} value, whereas those with asthma and similar $\dot{V}_A/\dot{Q}$ abnormalities do not. This reflects the emphysema and other alveolar capillary membrane abnormalities in smokers. The D_{LCO} value is reduced in conditions affecting pulmonary blood flow, such as thromboembolic disease or pulmonary hypertension. Relatively few conditions cause increased D_{LCO} values. Important among these is pulmonary hemorrhage and polycythemia. The D_{LCO} value is increased with left-to-right intracardiac shunts.[2]

CHALLENGE TESTS

Despite suggestive symptoms and a strong clinical suspicion of asthma, initial spirometric testing may not be diagnostic. Challenge tests (e.g., bronchoprovocation testing) may be performed in the respiratory function laboratory to seek evidence of bronchial hyperresponsiveness, which is considered diagnostic of asthma.[2]

Various challenge agents have been used, including methacholine, hypertonic saline, and mannitol. The procedure is similar with all agents. It begins with spirometry. The subject is then exposed to a known dose of the challenge agent, and after a standard time, spirometry is measured again. If the FEV_1 has fallen by 15% to 20% or more, the test result is considered positive; if that has not occurred, the subject is given a second dose of the challenge agent, and the process is repeated. The test is continued with further doses of challenge agent until the subject reaches the end of a standardized protocol or a positive result occurs.

In addition to being a helpful diagnostic tool for bronchial hyperresponsiveness, challenge tests can guide the effectiveness of treatment for asthma. The test should not be performed on patients with an FEV_1 of less than 1.2 liters or an FEV_1 less than 80% of predicted.

ARTERIAL BLOOD GAS DETERMINATIONS

Direct sampling of arterial blood with measurement of the pH and partial pressures of oxygen (Pao_2) and carbon dioxide ($Paco_2$) provides critical information about the lungs' most important function—gas exchange. Although sampling is a relatively simple test, difficulties often arise in interpreting results, particularly when mixed metabolic and respiratory problems are present.

The analysis is performed from arterial blood taken directly from a peripheral artery. The most commonly accessed artery is the radial; it is important to ensure there is adequate collateral arterial supply from the ulnar artery before performing the test. The sample should be taken with the subject at rest in a steady state, breathing a known concentration of oxygen (or air) for at least 10 minutes. This allows accurate interpretation of gas exchange. The arterial blood is collected in a heparinized syringe and analyzed in a device using electrochemical sensors. Standard information includes measurement of the pH, $Paco_2$, and the Pao_2. The blood gas analyzer also calculates the base excess (BE) and bicarbonate (H_2CO_3) concentration, and it measures arterial oxyhemoglobin saturation (Sao_2) if the machine incorporates an oximeter.

Interpreting the results relies on knowledge of the normal values.[4] Oxygenation is easily appreciated from

the Pao_2; the normal range is 80 to 100 mm Hg (i.e., breathing air at sea level). A Pao_2 value of less than 60 mm Hg is critical and definitive of respiratory failure, and cell and organ functions are compromised if this degree of hypoxia is sustained (see Chapters 159 and 185). Because of the shape of the oxyhemoglobin dissociation curve, a Pao_2 value of 60 mm Hg correlates with an Sao_2 of 90% when the oxyhemoglobin dissociation curve is normally positioned.

The blood pH (normal range is 7.35 to 7.45) provides information about the acid-base status. If the pH is abnormal, the physician must decide whether it is from a primary metabolic or primary respiratory condition. The subject's $Paco_2$, BE, and H_2CO_3 values help. In general, if the pH is acidic and the $Paco_2$ is high (normal range is 35 to 45 mm Hg), the likely condition is a primary respiratory acidosis. If the pH is acidic and the BE (and H_2CO_3) values are low, the problem is likely a primary metabolic acidosis. If the pH is alkaline and the $Paco_2$ are low, the likely condition is a primary respiratory alkalosis. If pH is alkaline and the BE (and H_2CO_3) are high, the problem is likely to be a primary metabolic alkalosis. From that point, the degree of compensation (partial or complete) should be assessed from other reported parameters.

Pulse oximetry is a widely used, noninvasive means for obtaining information about the oxygen level.[5] It is a measure of the Sao_2 (not Pao_2). None of the detailed information from blood gas measurements (e.g., $Paco_2$) is provided by the oximeter. However, oximetry can be invaluable in monitoring oxygenation rapidly and continuously to allow titration of oxygen therapy. Oximetry is also useful for monitoring trends in the oxygen level during sleep.

TESTS OF RESPIRATORY MUSCLE STRENGTH

Weakness of the respiratory muscles can be subtle and difficult to appreciate on clinical assessment. Patients with weak respiratory muscles may complain of exertional dyspnea but have only minimal or no measurable abnormality detected by bedside spirometry. If respiratory muscle weakness is suspected, measurement of the maximal inspiratory and expiratory mouth pressure is a simple, helpful test.

The measurement is made by having the subject breath at rest through a mouthpiece that can be closed quickly at any time, thereby creating a sealed system. To measure the maximal inspiratory pressure (PI_{max}), the subject inhales as deeply and as strongly as possible from the FRC against a closed mouthpiece. The negative pressure within the closed mouthpiece reflects the force generated by the inspiratory muscles. A similar maneuver, performed by exhaling as forcefully as possible from the TLC, measures the maximal expiratory pressure the subject is able to generate (PE_{max}). The positive pressure reflects the force generated by the expiratory muscles. The results are compared with predicted normal values. Recognition of reduced respiratory muscle strength may direct further investigations for neuromuscular disorders or consideration of the potential contribution of muscle weakness to the clinical picture (see Chapter 193).

This is a very technique-dependent test, and cooperation and a clear understanding of the required maneuver is essential. Those performing the test should be experienced with this methodology and able to judge the subject's compliance with instructions.

Another test for assessing suspected weakness of the diaphragm is to compare vital capacity in an upright and supine posture. A fall of 20% (or more) in the supine position is evidence of significant diaphragmatic weakness.

In generalized weakness of advanced malignancy or systemic illness, tests of respiratory muscle strength (combined with arterial blood gas tensions) can be helpful in determining the cause of tachypnea or dyspnea. Although individual circumstances influence the decision to perform any investigation, tests of respiratory muscle strength are relatively simple and may identify potential areas of management and palliation, such as noninvasive pressure support. Similarly, respiratory muscle weakness as a cause for hypoventilation should always be considered in any patient who is hypercapnic.

CONCLUSIONS

These tests represent the common clinical investigations of pulmonary function to assess respiratory status and explore the cause of respiratory symptoms. As with any clinical investigation, ordering pulmonary function tests must be made with a clear pretest question in mind. The interpretation of results must always be made using the information from the pretest history and physical examination.

REFERENCES

1. Crapo RO. Pulmonary function testing. N Engl J Med 1994;331:25-30.
2. American Thoracic Society. Lung function testing: Selection of reference values and interpretative strategies. Am Rev Respir Dis 1991;144:1202-1218.
3. Guidelines for the measurement of respiratory function. Recommendations of the British Thoracic Society and the Association of Respiratory Technicians and Physiologists. Respir Med 1994;88:165-194.
4. Williams AJ. ABC of oxygen—Assessing and interpreting arterial blood gases and acid-base balance. BMJ 1998;317:1213-1216.
5. Hanning CD, Alexander-Williams JM. Pulse oximetry: A practical review. BMJ 1995;311:367-370.

SUGGESTED READING

West JB. Pulmonary Pathophysiology—The Essentials, 6th ed. Philadelphia: Lippincott Williams & Wilkins, 2003.
West JB. Respiratory Physiology—The Essentials, 7th ed. Philadelphia: Lippincott Williams & Wilkins, 2004.

CHAPTER **74**

Laboratory Hematology

Karl S. Theil

KEY POINTS

- The classification of blood disorders begins with a complete blood cell count and differential leukocyte count.
- Peripheral blood smear review can be an essential component of proper patient care because it can result in a timely diagnosis and improved patient management.
- Bone marrow aspirates and biopsies provide complementary information in the evaluation of hematologic disorders and metastatic disease.
- Body fluid samples sent to the hematology laboratory for a routine cell count and differential count include morphological review that can suggest infection, reactive changes, or neoplasia.
- An elevated C-reactive protein level correlates with an unfavorable prognosis in advanced cancer.

The complete blood cell count (CBC) with a differential cell count provides hemoglobin and hematocrit values, red blood cell (RBC) count, mean corpuscular volume (MCV), mean corpuscular hemoglobin (MCH), mean corpuscular hemoglobin concentration (MCHC), red cell distribution width (RDW), white blood cell (WBC) count and differential count, platelet count, and mean platelet volume (MPV). The RDW is a measure of variability of RBC size (i.e., anisocytosis) that may aid in the differential diagnosis of anemia. The MPV is inversely proportional to the platelet count, and its value in evaluating thrombocytopenia is controversial. If abnormal findings are found in the CBC, careful review of the peripheral blood smear is helpful.

Peripheral blood smear review may be triggered by predefined laboratory indicators or a physician's request. Automated hematology analyzers have significantly decreased manual peripheral blood smear reviews. Review of the peripheral smear to integrate clinical information with morphologic findings can facilitate the diagnosis of anemia, thrombocytopenia, and leukopenia, which commonly affect cancer patients.

Bone marrow evaluation is performed on a case-by-case basis after review of the CBC and peripheral blood smear. The need for special diagnostic studies, such as extra aspirate smears or core biopsies for protocol studies or clinical staging, cytochemical stains, flow cytometry, bone marrow cultures (e.g., bacterial, fungal, mycobacterial), cytogenetics, or molecular analysis, should be anticipated before the procedure.

Body fluid analysis in the hematology laboratory consists of a gross examination, determination of WBC and RBC counts per cubic millimeter, and evaluation of cellular morphology with a differential count. Cerebrospinal, pleural, pericardial, peritoneal, bronchoalveolar lavage, and synovial fluids are processed similarly, as soon as possible after collection to prevent cell lysis. Samples may also be submitted for ancillary studies, including total protein, specific gravity, glucose level, protein level, and microbiologic studies. Flow cytometry can be useful when a hematologic malignancy is suspected.

C-reactive protein (CRP), an acute phase reactant, is most often used as a nonspecific but sensitive screening test for inflammatory conditions, infections, tissue injury, and neoplastic diseases. It was first isolated in 1930 and is so named because the protein binds to the "C" polysaccharide of *Pneumococcus* sp. The same protein was later found in association with many inflammatory and infectious conditions. CRP is a member of the pentraxin family of proteins and is composed of five identical, noncovalently associated protomers arranged around a central pore. Although CRP binds to various proteins and phospholipids (including phosphatidyl choline found on the surface of microorganisms and in damaged cell membranes), serves as an opsonizing agent, and can activate complement through the classic pathway, its exact biological function is unknown.[1]

INDICATIONS AND CONTRAINDICATIONS

Complete Blood Cell Count

The CBC with a differential count is one of the most commonly ordered laboratory tests. It is indicated in the evaluation of any blood disorder or to screen for a blood disorder.

Peripheral Blood Smear Review

Peripheral blood cellular morphology is assessed in a hierarchical manner, beginning with an automated hematology analyzer. Automated hematology analyzers perform leukocyte differential counts and erythrocyte morphological evaluations with greater precision and accuracy than manual assessment of blood smears.[2] Abnormal samples on automated screening are flagged for manual review by a technologist or physician. Results on samples that fulfill predetermined criteria may be accepted, validated, and released without human review. Although analyzers are efficient at differentiating normal from abnormal cells, manual smear review is still required to confirm certain abnormal results and establish a specific diagnosis. Common indications[2] for manual review include the following:

- Leukopenia (WBC $< 2.5 \times 10^9$/L)
- Leukocytosis (WBC $> 20 \times 10^9$/L)
- Thrombocytopenia (PLT $< 80 \times 10^9$/L)
- Thrombocytosis (PLT $> 800 \times 10^9$/L)
- Anemia (Hb < 8.0 g/dL)
- Polycythemia (Hb > 18.0 g/dL)
- Erythrocytopenia (RBC $< 2.0 \times 10^{12}$/L)
- Erythrocytosis (RBC $> 7.0 \times 10^{12}$/L)
- Microcytosis (MCV < 70 fL)
- Macrocytosis (MCV > 105.1 fL)

Indications for physician review of the peripheral blood smear are determined by specific clinical practice (Table 74-1).[3] Many morphological abnormalities cannot be specifically identified by automated hematology analyzers, but they are encountered during manual review for

TABLE 74-1 Indications for Physician Review of Peripheral Blood Smear

ABNORMALITY	REASON FOR REVIEW
Lymphocytosis >5.0 × 10⁹/L (if not within age-specific reference range)	Rule out lymphoproliferative disorder, reactive lymphocytosis
Reactive lymphocytes (>10%)	Rule out viral infection or drug effect
Atypical cells	Rule out lymphoma, hairy cell leukemia, myeloma, metastatic carcinoma, endothelial cells, myelodysplastic syndrome, acute or chronic leukemia, drug effect (e.g., ATRA, arsenic therapy)
Blasts	Rule out myelophthisic process, myelodysplastic syndrome, chronic myeloproliferative disorder, myelodysplastic or myeloproliferative disease, acute leukemia
Auer rods	Rule out acute myeloid leukemia or myelodysplastic syndrome
Myelodysplastic changes (i.e., hypogranular or pelgeroid neutrophils or megakaryocyte fragments)	Rule out myelodysplastic syndrome, myelodysplastic or myeloproliferative disease, acute leukemia, Pelger-Huët anomaly
Abnormal cytoplasmic granulation	Rule out Alder-Reilly anomaly, Chédiak-Higashi syndrome, May-Hegglin anomaly
Spherocytes (>5/HPF)	Rule out hereditary spherocytosis, autoimmune hemolytic anemia
Sickle cells	Rule out hemoglobinopathy
Red cell fragments	Rule out microangiopathic hemolytic anemia, disseminated intravascular coagulation, thrombotic thrombocytopenic purpura, metastatic carcinoma, vasculitis, drug effect, burn, aortic aneurysm, vascular malformation, cardiac valve defect, intravascular device
Bite cells	Rule out glucose-6-phosphate deficiency, unstable hemoglobin, drug-induced hemolysis
RBC agglutination	Rule out cold agglutinin, lymphoproliferative disorder, immune hemolytic anemia
Microorganisms and toxic vacuoles	Rule out sepsis due to bacterial or fungal infection, malaria, babesiosis, borreliosis, ehrlichiosis
MCV > 109.9 fL with hypersegmented or dysplastic neutrophils	Rule out drug effect, megaloblastic anemia or myelodysplastic syndrome
Abnormal platelet morphology (e.g., giant platelets, oval platelets, hypogranular platelets)	Rule out myeloproliferative disorder, post-splenectomy state, hereditary platelet disorder, myelodysplastic syndrome
Thrombocytopenia or thrombocytosis	Rule out spurious thrombocytopenia, myeloproliferative disorder

ATRA, all-*trans* retinoic acid; HPF, high-power field; MCV, mean corpuscular volume.

another abnormal finding. These include basophilic stippling, sickled cells, elliptocytes, target cells, teardrop cells, Heinz bodies, hemoglobin crystals, rouleaux, Howell-Jolly bodies, Pappenheimer bodies, malarial parasites, fungal organisms, bacteria, toxic granulation, Döhle bodies, Pelger-Huët anomaly, Chédiak-Higashi anomaly, dysplastic features in granulocytes (including nuclear segmentation defects and hypogranular cytoplasm), megakaryocyte fragments, and hypogranular platelets. Low numbers of circulating blasts also may not be flagged as abnormal by automated hematology analyzers. When there is high clinical suspicion for any of these abnormalities, manual peripheral smear review can be diagnostic.

Bone Marrow Evaluation

General indications[4] for bone marrow examination include the following:

- To establish a primary diagnosis of a hematologic neoplasm
- To further investigate abnormalities identified in peripheral blood
- To evaluate for possible infectious diseases
- To determine stage of hematologic and nonhematologic neoplasms
- To evaluate fever of unknown origin
- To investigate suspected lymphoproliferative disorders
- To monitor the response to therapy or assess unexpected changes in hematologic findings
- To evaluate splenomegaly
- To evaluate for uncommon diseases (e.g., metabolic bone disease, storage diseases, mast cell disease)
- To assess for residual disease before bone marrow transplantation

Before a decision to perform this invasive procedure is made in the palliative setting, the clinician should balance the need to know against the anticipated value of the information gained in guiding future treatment. For patients with isolated anemia, secondary erythrocytosis, toxic neutrophilia due to a known disease process, and reactive thrombocytosis, peripheral blood findings alone may be sufficient to establish a diagnosis and guide therapy. In certain patients with acute leukemia, definitive diagnostic studies, including ancillary flow cytometry and genetic testing, can all be performed on peripheral blood, making a bone marrow examination optional.

Bone marrow examination, including aspiration and biopsy, can be safely performed on most patients. Relative contraindications include acquired or congenital coagulation deficiencies and thrombocytopenia. Patients with hemophilia require factor replacement to levels above 50% of normal levels before the procedure. Diamino-D-arginine vasopressin (DDAVP) can increase levels of factor VIII and stimulate platelet function in von Willebrand disease (other than type IIB) or chronic renal failure. Patients receiving warfarin or heparin should have prothrombin time (PT) or activated partial thromboplastin time (aPTT) values, respectively, within the therapeutic range.[5] Isolated thrombocytopenia should not be a contraindication, and platelet transfusions usually are not required if the procedure is properly performed and tech-

nical difficulties are not encountered.[5] Localized skin infection or previous irradiation at the biopsy site may preclude posterior iliac crest sampling, and poor patient cooperation may prevent obtaining aspiration and biopsy samples. Sternal aspiration should not be attempted in young children and in myeloma or bone resorptive process because of the possibility of sternal perforation and potentially fatal cardiac complications.[4,5] The major contraindication to bone marrow examination is failure to meet appropriate indications for the study.[4]

Body Fluid Analysis

Indications for obtaining cerebrospinal fluid can be divided into diagnostic (e.g., suspected meningitis or encephalitis, intracranial hemorrhage, demyelinating disorder, Guillain-Barré syndrome) and therapeutic (e.g., administration of chemotherapy or antimicrobial agents, cerebrospinal fluid drainage in benign intracranial hypertension). Meningitis may be acute (e.g., bacterial, viral), subacute (e.g., fungal, tuberculous, neoplastic) or chronic (e.g., granulomatous, neoplastic). Contraindications include elevated intracranial pressure due to a mass lesion or obstructive hydrocephalus, local skin or epidural infection, and bleeding diathesis.

Normally, serous cavity body spaces (i.e., pleural, pericardial, and peritoneal) and joint spaces (i.e., synovial) do not contain aspirable fluid, and the presence of an effusion at these sites can indicate a pathologic process. Contraindications are related to the presence of local skin infections. Bronchoalveolar lavage is useful to evaluate interstitial and alveolar pulmonary infiltrates and pulmonary infiltrates in immunocompromised patients.

C-Reactive Protein

CRP levels are routinely used as an indicator of infection and inflammation. CRP also has been used as a prognostic marker in advanced cancer, for which an acute phase response, defined as an elevated CRP level and decreased serum albumin concentration, correlates with a poor prognosis.[6] Increased CRP levels also are associated with the anorexia-cachexia syndrome in advanced cancer, and they correlate with increased levels of interleukin-6.[6] Because CRP assays are widely available and interleukin-6 assays are less well standardized and expensive, CRP is the preferred marker for assessing inflammation in patients with advanced cancer. An elevated CRP level may reflect cytokine production by the tumor or tumor-associated inflammation that induces increased production of CRP.

The association between elevated CRP levels and inflammation prompted the development of high-sensitivity CRP (hsCRP) assays, which have a role in assessing risk for acute coronary syndromes, atherosclerosis, peripheral vascular disease, and stroke. An elevated hsCRP finding is considered a biomarker of chronic inflammation that is important in atherosclerosis. Whether the elevated CRP is causally linked to or merely associated with atherosclerosis remains controversial. The hsCRP assay result predicts risk for cardiovascular disease. Those with baseline hsCRP levels in the highest quartile have a twofold to threefold risk for subsequent vascular events compared with patients in the lowest quartile. Patients most likely to benefit from hsCRP screening include those with a moderate risk estimate of coronary heart disease using standard risk factors. Universal hsCRP screening of adults is not warranted.

TECHNIQUES

Complete Blood Cell Count

The proper sample is venous blood anticoagulated with potassium EDTA (K_2 or K_3 EDTA), and use of a filled collection tube is important to prevent clotting. If platelet clumping is a concern, blood may be collected into a sodium citrate tube, but counts must be corrected for a dilution factor (1:9). Heparin is unacceptable as an anticoagulant because of the potential for platelet clumping and suboptimal staining when slides are prepared for differential counts.

CBCs are performed in automated hematology analyzers. Different manufacturers use various methods for cell enumeration, differential counting, and quantitation of hemoglobin. Fluorescent dyes that bind to cytoplasmic RNA can quantitate reticulocytes and reticulated platelets, which is useful in anemia and thrombocytopenia. Manufacturers are incorporating cytochemical stains, monoclonal antibodies for lymphocytes (e.g., CD3, CD4, CD8) and platelets (e.g., CD41, CD61), and fluorescent dyes for hematopoietic progenitor cells.

Peripheral Blood Smear Preparation

The basic elements of blood film preparation and analysis have not changed for more than a century.[7] A drop of blood placed near the edge of a clean glass slide is spread manually across the length of the slide to create a sufficiently large area for viewing where red cells are barely touching. Air-dried slides are fixed in absolute methanol, stained with Romanowsky dyes (i.e., Wright stain), and examined under a light microscope with an oil immersion objective. In a manual differential count, 100 consecutive leukocytes typically are classified, observing the morphology of erythrocytes and platelets encountered during the process.

Bone Marrow Evaluation

The posterior iliac crest is the preferred site for marrow aspiration and biopsy in adults. Alternate sites include anterior iliac crest (i.e., children and adults), anterior tibial plateau (i.e., infants only), and sternum (i.e., adults only and aspirate only). Sternal aspirates should not be attempted by a novice, and sternal biopsies are contraindicated due to the risk of bony perforation. The preferred type of needle, technique, and sequence of obtaining bone marrow aspirate and biopsy vary.[4,5]

The first pull of the aspirate should be used to prepare smears for morphologic examination. Subsequent small aspirations reduce peripheral blood contamination when obtaining specimens for ancillary studies. The remaining aspirated material can be allowed to clot, then wrapped in tissue paper, and placed in fixative to prepare a histological section of the clot. Imprint preparations may be prepared from the core biopsy before placing it in fixative.

Subsequent biopsies are obtained for special studies, as needed, using a new biopsy needle. When no aspirate is obtainable, an attempt can be made to tease cells from an extra biopsy specimen before fixation to obtain material for flow cytometry or cytogenetics. After it is received in the laboratory, additional processing is required to decalcify the biopsy and embed it in paraffin before preparing multiple thin histological sections for examination. The clot is processed and sectioned similarly, but it does not require decalcification.

Body Fluid Analysis

Specimens are obtained under sterile conditions. The sample volume submitted varies with the type and site of fluid. For cerebrospinal fluid, a minimum of 1 mL of fluid is placed into each of three sterile, capped containers. The first is used for chemistry analysis (e.g., protein, glucose, serology), the second is used for microbiology (e.g., Gram stain, culture, antigen tests), the third is used for the cell count and differential count.

Pleural fluid is collected by thoracentesis. Samples are sent for cell count and differential count (i.e., EDTA tube); chemistries, including total protein and lactate dehydrogenase (i.e., clot tube); Gram stain and microbial cultures (i.e., heparinized); and cytology (i.e., heparinized). Peritoneal fluid is collected by paracentesis, with samples handled similar to those for pleural fluid. Pericardial fluid is collected by pericardiocentesis, with samples sent for cell count and differential count (i.e., EDTA tube), cytology (i.e., heparinized), and Gram stain and microbial cultures (i.e., heparinized). To distinguish whether the effusion is a transudate or an exudate, venous blood (i.e., clot tube) is sent for total protein and lactate dehydrogenase identification; this sample is used to calculate the fluid-to-serum lactate dehydrogenase and protein ratios. Flow cytometry can be performed, if necessary, using the remainder of the sample sent for the cell count and differential count or cytology.

Synovial fluid is collected under sterile conditions using a syringe rinsed with sodium heparin, and samples are sent for a cell count and differential count, wet mount for crystals, and Gram stain and microbial cultures. Bronchoalveolar lavage fluid is obtained during bronchoscopy, and the lavage fluid is sent for a cell count and differential count, Gram stain and microbial cultures, cytology, and when indicated, flow cytometry to quantitate and phenotype T and B lymphocytes.

Cell counts are performed using a hemacytometer chamber, and differential counts are performed on cytospin or similar preparations. Cytospin preparations are made using a cytocentrifuge, a device that concentrates the cells in the sample directly onto the surface of a glass slide. The air-dried cytospin slides are stained with a Romanowsky stain for differential counting. A 100-cell differential count typically includes assessment of all cellular elements in the sample, including leukocytes, mesothelial cells, macrophages, plasma cells, squamous and respiratory epithelial cells, ependymal cells, synovial cells, malignant cells, and others. Because the cellular morphology is identical to that in peripheral blood smears or bone marrow aspirates, these slides are ideal for evaluating hematological malignancies involving body fluids. Even if the fluid cell count is zero, the cytospin preparation permits recovery of at least some cells for a differential count.

C-Reactive Protein

Standard CRP assays may be performed using nephelometry, precipitations, radioimmunoassay, or enzyme immunoassay. When used as a marker of chronic inflammation or infection, standard CRP assays that have a detection limit of 3 to 8 mg/L are satisfactory. When used to assess risk of cardiovascular disease, hsCRP assays with a detection limit of less than 0.3 mg/L are required. The hsCRP assays are performed by automated immunonephelometry or immunoturbidimetry. The increased sensitivity of hsCRP assays compared with standard CRP assays is obtained by linking a latex particle to a specific anti-CRP antibody; this larger antigen-antibody complex has greater light scattering properties that permit a lower detection threshold. Standardization of hsCRP assays is important, because more than 30 types of hsCRP assays are commercially available.

INTERPRETATION OF RESULTS

Complete Blood Cell Count

The CBC results are used to classify disorders of RBC, WBC, and platelets. CBC results should always be interpreted in the context of the clinical findings. In palliative medicine, the most frequent clinical problems involve workups for anemia, neutropenia, and thrombocytopenia. Anemia is defined as a hemoglobin level less than 12 g/dL in women and less than 13.5 g/dL in men. Neutropenia is defined as an absolute neutrophil count less than 1500/μL, and thrombocytopenia is defined as a platelet count less than 150,000/μL.

Anemia

One popular approach to the classification of anemia is to examine the MCV and RDW; six categories of anemia can be recognized (Table 74-2).[8] This scheme has some overlap between categories, and the classification of anemia of chronic disease can be problematic. Anemias can be further evaluated using the reticulocyte count as a measure of functional erythropoietic reserves. Anemias due to decreased red cell survival with a normal marrow proliferative response show a normal or elevated reticulocyte count; those from hypoproliferative responses or erythropoietic production defects are associated with a low reticulocyte count. Anemia in cancer may be multifactorial.

Microcytic anemias associated with an elevated RDW commonly include iron-deficiency anemia, anemia of chronic disease, thalassemia, and sideroblastic anemias. These causes can usually be distinguished on the basis of iron studies, including serum iron level, total iron binding capacity, percent saturation, serum soluble transferrin receptor, and bone marrow storage iron; free erythrocyte protoporphyrin and hemoglobin electrophoresis may be useful (Table 74-3). Some patients with early iron deficiency may lack the microcytosis and hypochromia that characterizes severe deficiency. Iron-deficiency anemia and anemia of chronic disease may occur together.[9] For microcytic anemias with a normal RDW, consider anemia of chronic disease, thalassemia minor, and some hemoglobinopathies (e.g., hemoglobin E trait).

Normocytic anemias associated with an elevated RDW include early or partially treated iron or vitamin B_{12} or folate deficiency, sickle cell anemia, or sickle cell disease. Normocytic anemias associated with a normal RDW include anemia of chronic disease, hereditary spherocytosis, acute bleeding, some hemoglobinopathies, and dilutional anemia. Other causes of normocytic anemia include aplastic anemia, storage disorders, neoplasms, renal disease, human immunodeficiency virus (HIV) infection, and hypothyroidism.

Macrocytic anemias associated with an elevated RDW include vitamin B_{12} or folate deficiency, myelodysplastic syndromes, chemotherapy effect (e.g., hydroxyurea), autoimmune hemolytic anemia, cold agglutinin disease, liver disease, alcohol effect, and thyroid disease. In the presence of a low reticulocyte count, the likelihood of vitamin B_{12} or folate deficiency (i.e., megaloblastic processes) increases with increasing MCV. A high reticulocyte count suggests a peripheral destructive process, and direct antiglobulin test and antibody screen can point to an immune-mediated hemolytic anemia. Macrocytic anemias associated with a normal RDW include aplastic anemia and myelodysplastic syndromes. Pancytopenia is often present, and bone marrow evaluation is required for diagnosis.

Neutropenia

The absolute neutrophil count is calculated by multiplying the total WBC count by the percent of band and seg-

---

TABLE 74-2 Classification of Anemia Based on Red Blood Cell Size and Distribution Width

CELL SIZE	NORMAL RDW	HIGH RDW
Microcytosis (MCV < 70 fL)	Thalassemia minor, anemia of chronic disease, some hemoglobinopathy traits	Iron deficiency, hemoglobin H disease, some anemia of chronic disease, some thalassemia minor, fragmentation hemolysis
Normocytosis	Anemia of chronic disease, hereditary spherocytosis, some hemoglobinopathy traits, acute bleeding	Early or partially treated iron or vitamin deficiency, sickle cell anemia or sickle cell disease
Macrocytosis (MCV > 100 fL)	Aplastic anemia, some myelodysplasias	Vitamin B_{12} or folate deficiency, autoimmune hemolytic anemia, cold agglutinin disease, some myelodysplasias, liver disease, thyroid disease, alcohol

MCV, mean corpuscular volume; RDW, red cell distribution width.
From Perkins S. Diagnosis of anemia. In Kjeldsberg CR (ed). Practical Diagnosis of Hematologic Disorders, 4th ed. Chicago: ASCP Press, 2006, p 7. © 2006 American Society for Clinical Pathology.

TABLE 74-3   Differential Diagnosis of Microcytic Hypochromic Anemias by Laboratory Tests

TEST	IRON DEFICIENCY ANEMIA	ANEMIA OF CHRONIC DISEASE	THALASSEMIA MINOR	SIDEROBLASTIC ANEMIA
Peripheral blood smear	Normocytic to microcytic hypochromic RBCs, pencil cells	Normocytic to microcytic hypochromic RBC	Normocytic to microcytic hypochromic RBC, target cells, basophilic stippling	Dimorphic RBCs (microcytic hypochromic and macrocytic), basophilic stippling, Pappenheimer bodies
RDW	Increased	Near normal	Normal	Increased
Serum iron	Reduced	Reduced	Normal to increased	Normal to increased
Transferrin	Increased	Reduced to normal	Reduced to normal	Reduced to normal
Saturation (%)	Reduced	Reduced	Normal to increased	Increased
Soluble serum transferrin receptor	Increased	Normal	Variable	Variable
FEP	Increased	Increased	Normal	Normal to increased
Hemoglobin electrophoresis	Normal	Normal	Increased Hb A_2 in β-thalassemia, normal in α-thalassemia	Normal
Bone marrow storage iron	Absent	Increased	Normal to increased	Increased, + ringed sideroblasts

FEP, free erythrocyte protoporphyrin; Hb A_2: hemoglobin A_2; RBC, red blood cell; RDW, red cell distribution width.

mented neutrophils. Patients with a low absolute neutrophil count are at increased risk for bacterial infections. The cause for absolute neutropenia should be determined. Drug effects are commonly implicated, but ethnic variation in neutrophil counts and primary marrow disorders should be ruled out. Aged or improperly stored samples can cause a spurious diagnosis of neutropenia.

Thrombocytopenia

Thrombocytopenia may be related to bone marrow production defects (e.g., hematologic malignancy, metastatic carcinoma, drug effect, chemotherapy, radiation therapy) or increased peripheral destruction (e.g., sepsis, disseminated intravascular coagulation, splenomegaly, drug effects, immune-mediated disorders, thrombotic thrombocytopenic purpura, hemolytic uremic syndrome). Low platelet counts obtained by automated hematology analyzers are typically verified in the laboratory to avoid reporting spurious identification of thrombocytopenia (e.g., platelet clumping, platelet satellitosis, clotted specimen).

Peripheral Blood Smear Review

Review of the peripheral blood smear is useful in anemia or thrombocytopenia. For example, microcytic hypochromic anemias are associated with iron-deficiency anemia (Fig. 74-1), thalassemia minor, sideroblastic anemias, lead poisoning, anemia of chronic disease, and some hemoglobinopathies (e.g., CC, EE). Microangiopathic hemolytic anemia (Fig. 74-2) with thrombocytopenia suggests possible disseminated intravascular coagulation, thrombotic thrombocytopenic purpura, hemolytic uremic syndrome, metastatic carcinoma, vasculitis, malignant hypertension, drug effect (e.g., mitomycin C, cyclosporine), or other condition. Spherocytes are associated with immune-mediated hemolytic anemias and transfused RBCs. Rouleaux (Fig. 74-3) may be observed with serum monoclonal proteins and in inflammatory processes with elevated

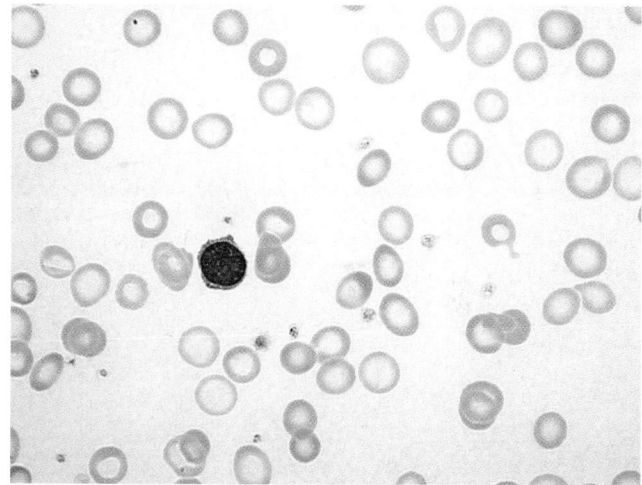

FIGURE 74-1   Iron deficiency anemia. Erythrocytes are microcytic (compare size with lymphocyte nucleus) and hypochromic, with an enlarged area of central pallor (more than one third) (×1000).

levels of fibrinogen and gamma globulins. Red cell agglutination (Fig. 74-4) may or may not be associated with anemia, and it can point to a diagnosis of autoimmune hemolytic anemia, cold agglutinin disease, or underlying lymphoproliferative disorder. Macrocytosis (Fig. 74-5) can suggest vitamin B_{12} or folate deficiency, liver disease, thyroid disease, or a chemotherapy effect (e.g., hydroxyurea, methotrexate). Neutrophilic leukocytosis with toxic changes and left shift in maturation (Fig. 74-6) suggests sepsis, but it may be seen with granulocyte colony-stimulating factor (G-CSF) therapy. A careful search for bacterial (Fig. 74-7) or fungal (Fig. 74-8) organisms may be revealing and can point to a diagnosis before the availability of culture results. Circulating cells derived from nonhematopoietic malignancies can occasionally be found in peripheral blood smears (Fig. 74-9). Dysplastic changes include

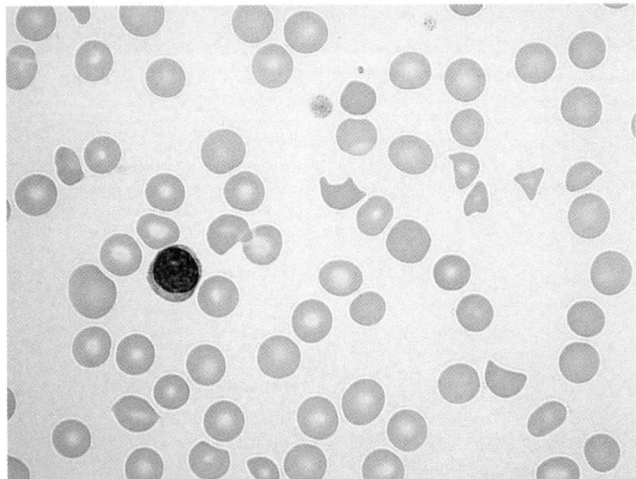

FIGURE 74-2   Microangiopathic hemolytic anemia. Fragmented erythrocytes (i.e., schistocytes) are evidence of intravascular trauma causing hemolysis. Associated thrombocytopenia raises concern about disseminated intravascular coagulation, thrombotic thrombocytopenic purpura, and metastatic carcinoma, among other conditions (×1000).

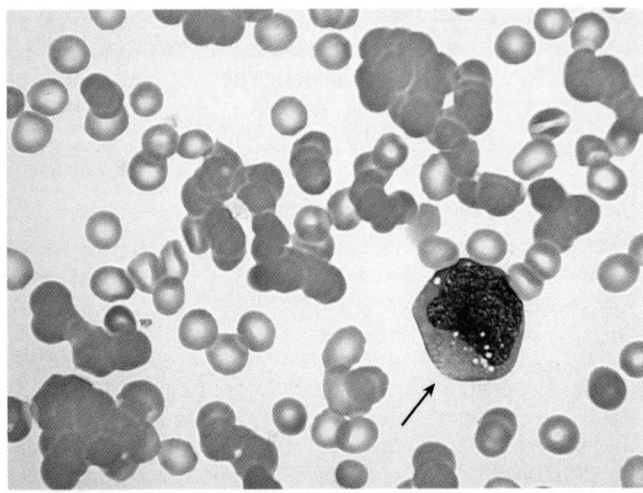

FIGURE 74-4   Cold agglutinin. Erythrocytes form irregular clumps, often in the presence of an IgM antibody. The presence of circulating lymphoma cells in this case *(arrow)* prompted a diagnosis of non-Hodgkin's lymphoma with an associated monoclonal IgM serum paraprotein (×1000).

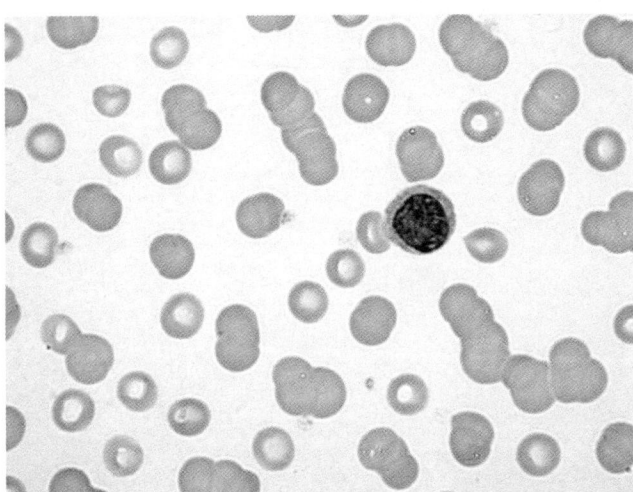

FIGURE 74-3   Rouleaux. Erythrocytes form "stacks of coins" that are composed of four or more cells. The condition often is related to increased positively charged plasma proteins (i.e., fibrinogen and gamma globulins) (×1000).

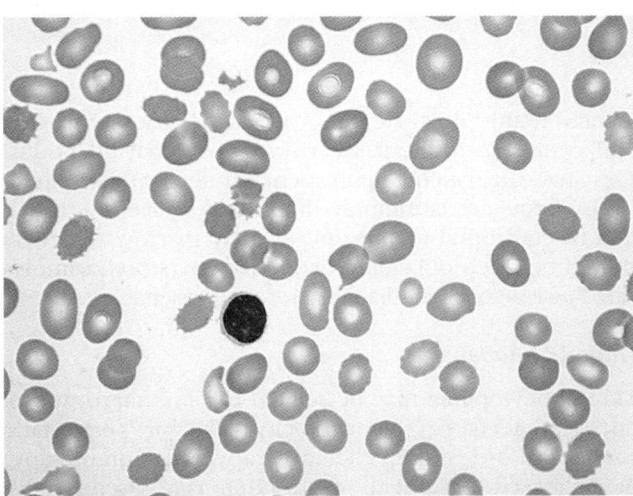

FIGURE 74-5   Oval macrocytes. Oval macrocytes are larger than normal erythrocytes, lack polychromatophilia, and have nonparallel sides. Oval macrocytes are a pathologic finding associated with megaloblastic anemias (×1000).

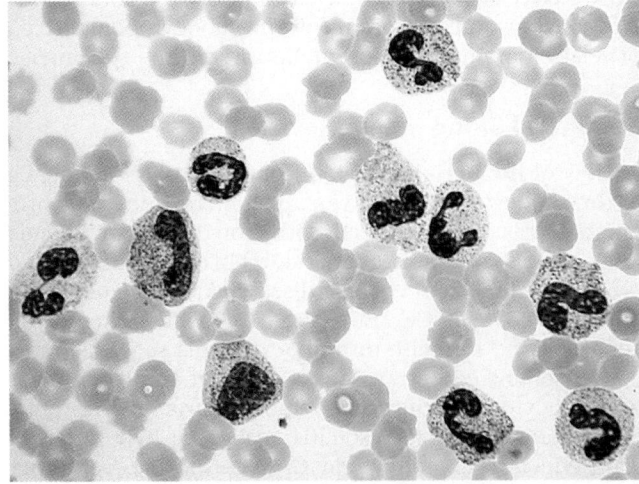

FIGURE 74-6   Leukocytosis with left shift and toxic changes. Increased segmented neutrophils with left shift (i.e., band forms and myelocytes) show prominent cytoplasmic granulation that suggests an infectious or inflammatory process (×1000).

hypogranular neutrophils (Fig. 74-10), pelgeroid nuclei, megaloblastoid nucleated RBCs, and giant or hypogranular platelets. Dysplastic changes suggest a possible myelodysplastic process and are an indication for marrow evaluation. The presence of blasts (Fig. 74-11) is always abnormal; circulating blasts may be seen in benign conditions (e.g., marrow regeneration, G-CSF therapy) and in neoplastic disorders (e.g., myelodysplastic or myeloproliferative disease, acute leukemia, metastatic carcinoma). Leukoerythroblastic changes, defined as the presence of circulating immature myeloid cells and nucleated RBCs, suggest a marrow replacement process such as myelofibrosis, metastatic solid neoplasm, myeloma, myeloproliferative disease, lymphoma, leukemia, or storage disorder. Benign conditions including hemolysis may also cause a leukoerythroblastic appearance. Platelet clumping (Fig. 74-12)

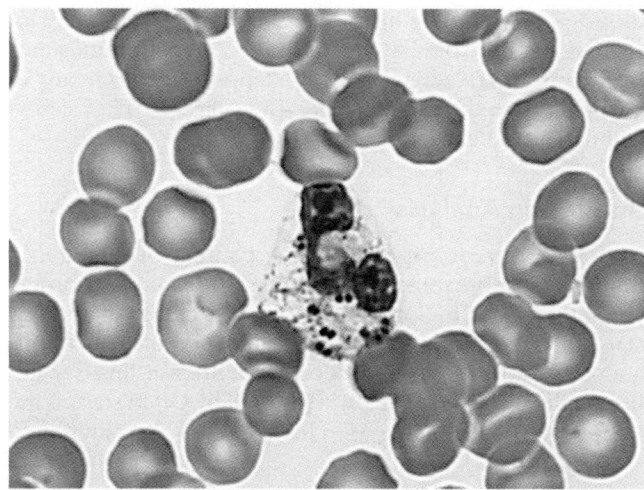

FIGURE 74-7 Bacteria. Peripheral blood smear shows a neutrophil with phagocytized bacteria (i.e., diplococci) that were subsequently identified as *Neisseria meningitidis*. Morphologic identification with Gram stain enables rapid institution of antibiotic therapy before availability of culture results (×2000).

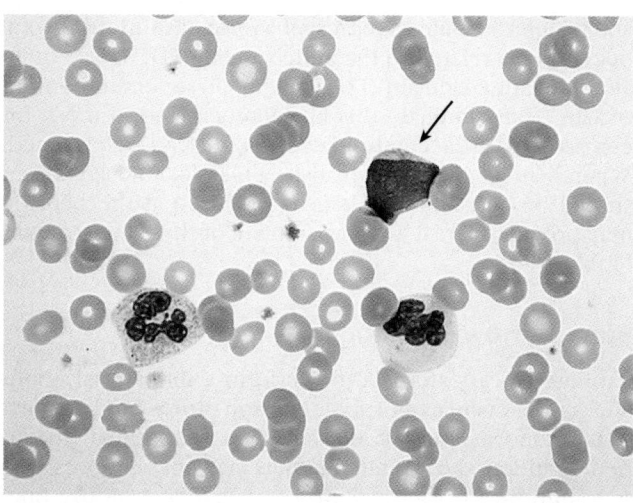

FIGURE 74-10 Myelodysplastic syndrome. The presence of a circulating blast *(arrow)* and dysplastic hypogranular neutrophil *(right)* raises concern about myelodysplasia. Notice the difference in cytoplasmic granulation between a normal neutrophil *(left)* and dysplastic neutrophil *(right)* (×1000).

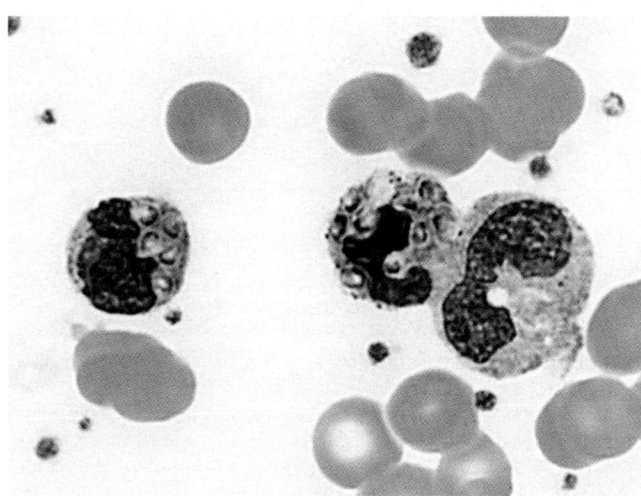

FIGURE 74-8 Disseminated histoplasmosis. Neutrophils contain phagocytized, small yeast forms. A careful search of the smear is usually required to identify the organisms (×2000).

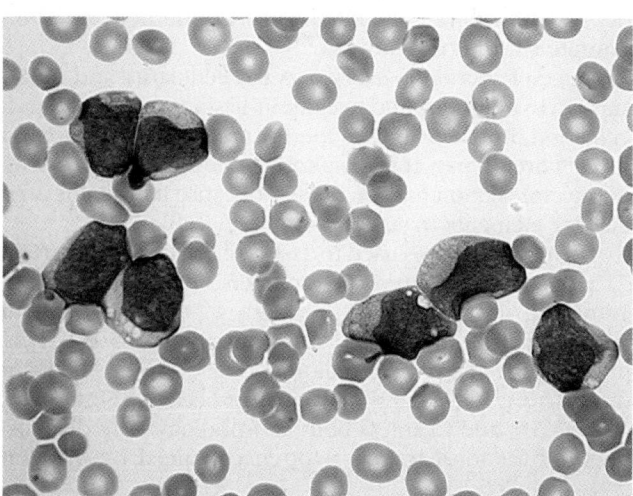

FIGURE 74-11 Acute myeloid leukemia. Blasts have high nuclear to cytoplasmic ratios, agranular to sparsely granular cytoplasm, and nuclei with prominent nucleoli and open chromatin in this case of acute myeloid leukemia. Identification of blasts in a peripheral blood smear should prompt further investigation (×1000).

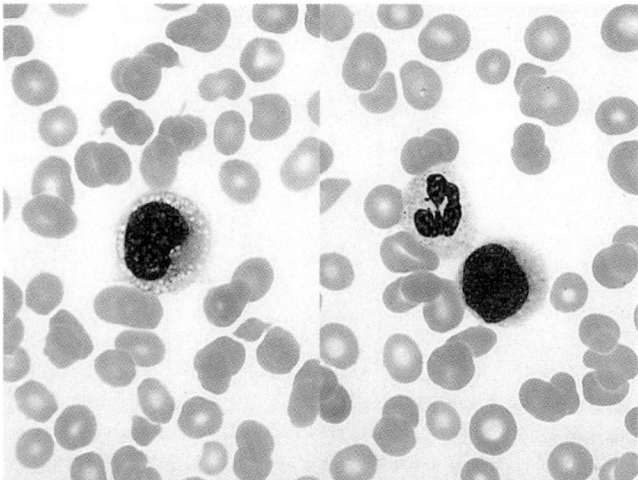

FIGURE 74-9 Carcinocythemia. Circulating malignant cells in this case of breast cancer resemble monocytes, but they have atypical nuclear chromatin, irregular nuclear outlines, and cytoplasmic vacuolization (×1000).

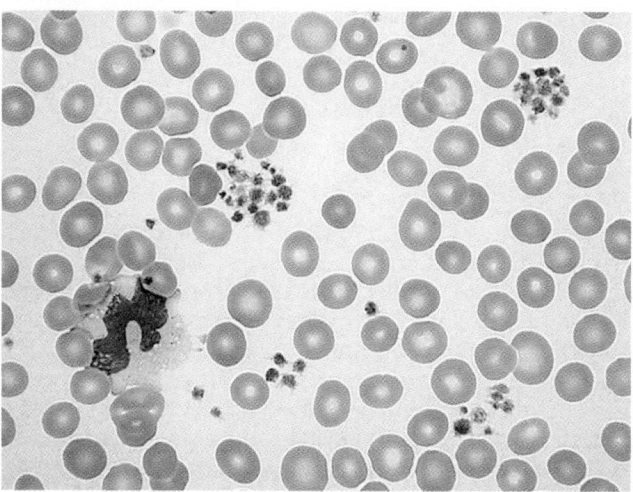

FIGURE 74-12 Platelet clumping. Aggregates of platelets form in vitro in the EDTA-anticoagulated sample used for cell counting. This may result in spurious identification of thrombocytopenia (×1000).

and platelet satellitosis represent a form of spurious thrombocytopenia related to the anticoagulant EDTA. Use of an alternate anticoagulant (i.e., sodium citrate or ammonium oxalate) can eliminate this interference, and in most circumstances, an accurate platelet count can be obtained. When platelet clumping persists, a platelet cold agglutinin should be considered. A smear prepared at the bedside may provide at least a visual estimate of the platelet count (Table 74-4).

Bone Marrow Evaluation

Aspirate smears are used to perform a differential count and assess cellular morphology, iron stores, and maturational abnormalities. If the smear is suboptimal due to hemodilution, the aspirate findings may not be representative. Imprint preparations may better reflect biopsy findings, especially when the aspirate is unsuccessful, and can facilitate rapid diagnosis of metastatic disease. Compared with a well-made aspirate smear, cellular morphology in an imprint can be compromised by cell smudging and blood contamination. Various cytochemical stains used in the classification of acute leukemia can be performed on aspirate smears or imprints.

The clot section is used to assess cellularity and megakaryocyte numbers, and because it has not required decalcification, it may provide superior morphology compared to the core biopsy. If the aspirate is suboptimal, the utility of the clot section may be limited because it contains only cellular elements that were aspirable (Table 74-5).

The core biopsy is used to assess overall cellularity (Fig. 74-13) and megakaryocyte numbers; to evaluate topographical organization of the marrow; to look for focal lesions such as metastatic carcinoma (Fig. 74-14), lymphoma (Fig. 74-15), or granulomas (Fig. 74-16); to evaluate the marrow stroma and infiltrative processes (Figs. 74-17 and 74-18); and to assess bone morphology. The diagnostic yield for focal lesions is often enhanced by bilateral biopsies and multiple histologic sections of each. The clot section and core biopsy can be studied with immunostains to further characterize cell populations, and they are of particular use after chemotherapy (Fig. 74-19) to assess cellularity and detect residual disease.

Body Fluid Analysis

Test results are interpreted in the context of the clinical findings. Cerebrospinal fluid findings in selected disorders are summarized in Table 74-6. Acute bacterial meningitis (Fig. 74-20) is marked by a predominance of neutrophils and elevated protein and decreased glucose levels, with intracellular bacteria usually identified by Gram stain. Viral or aseptic meningitis is characterized by increased

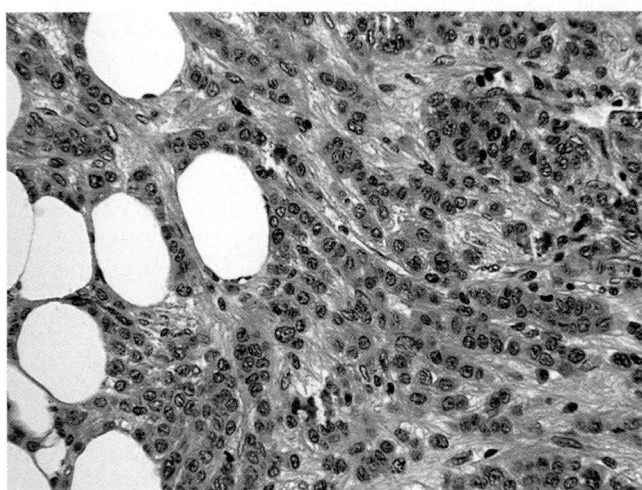

FIGURE 74-14 Metastatic carcinoma. Normal hematopoietic elements are replaced by clusters of malignant cells and associated stromal fibrosis in the bone marrow biopsy of metastatic breast cancer. Marrow fibrosis may result in a "dry tap" (×400).

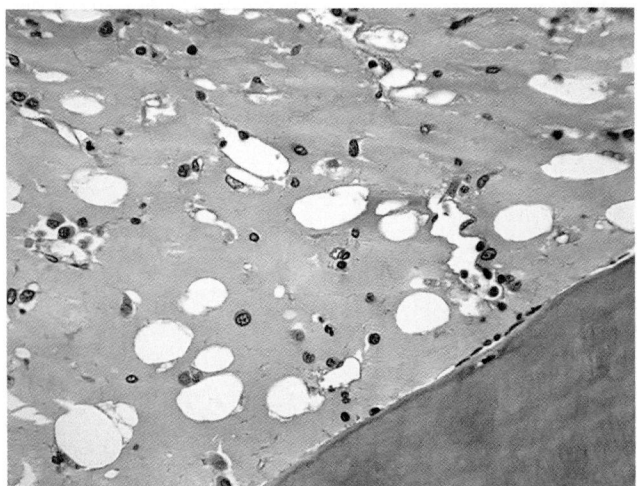

FIGURE 74-13 Hematopoietic hypoplasia. The bone marrow biopsy from a patient with pancytopenia due to anorexia nervosa shows markedly reduced cellularity. The marrow stroma (pink intercellular material) shows serous atrophy of fat. Serous atrophy may be associated with severe malnutrition, chronic renal disease, malabsorption, and disseminated malignancy (×400).

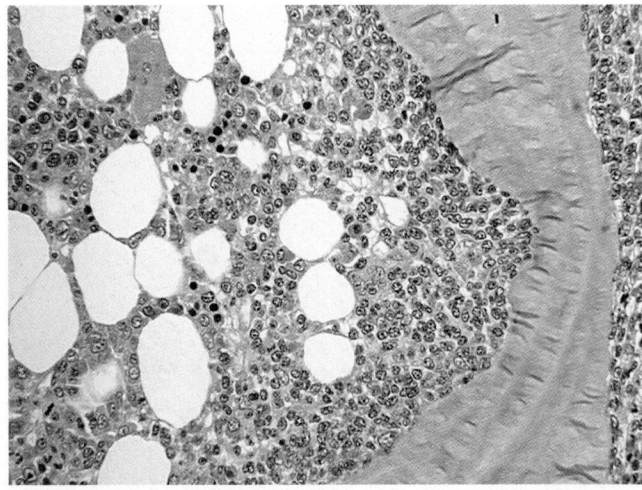

FIGURE 74-15 Non-Hodgkin's lymphoma. Follicular lymphoma typically shows a cellular infiltrate that runs adjacent to bony trabeculae. As a result, the lymphoma cells may not be well represented in aspirate smears or flow cytometry samples (×400).

TABLE 74-4 Abnormal Findings in Peripheral Blood Smears and Disease Correlations

ABNORMALITY	DISEASE ASSOCIATIONS	KEY FINDINGS	USEFUL LABORATORY TESTS	EXAMPLES
Microcytic, hypochromic erythrocytes	Iron deficiency anemia, thalassemia minor, anemia of chronic disease, lead poisoning, sideroblastic anemias, hemoglobin E trait	Small, hypochromic RBCs with or without target cells, pencil cells associated with iron deficiency anemia, coarse basophilic stippling associated with sideroblastic anemias and lead poisoning, target cells associated with thalassemia	Serum iron, TIBC, transferrin, ferritin to rule out iron deficiency or anemia of chronic disease; hemoglobin electrophoresis and Hb A$_2$ quantitation for thalassemia and Hb E trait; FEP and lead level for sideroblastic anemias	Figure 74-1
Fragmented cell (schistocyte)	DIC, TTP, HUS, vasculitis, metastatic carcinoma, damaged heart valve, severe burns, drug effect (e.g., cyclosporine, clopidogrel, mitomycin C), aortic aneurysm, malignant hypertension	Irregular cell shape and absence of central zone of pallor; variants include helmet cells, triangulocytes, schistocytes, and keratocytes	PT, aPTT, fibrinogen and D-dimer to rule out DIC; BUN and creatinine to look for renal disease in TTP and HUS; increased LDH and decreased haptoglobin in intravascular hemolysis	Figure 74-2
Rouleaux	Elevated fibrinogen (e.g., chronic infection, inflammation) or serum immunoglobulin levels (e.g., multiple myeloma, monoclonal gammopathy, chronic liver disease)	RBCs appear as "stack of coins" with linear arrangement of 4 or more cells; non-artifactual rouleaux appears in the thin area of the smear	Serum protein electrophoresis, quantitative immunoglobulins, immunofixation to rule out monoclonal protein (as necessary)	Figure 74-3
Red cell agglutinates	Cold agglutinin with or without anemia, lymphoma, myeloma, paroxysmal cold hemoglobinuria (PCH)	RBCs appear as a three-dimensional cluster of overlapping cells; may be associated with elevated MCV and RDW	Direct antiglobulin test positive for anti-complement in AIHA; monoclonal IgM in lymphoma or myeloma; anti-P antibody in PCH	Figure 74-4
Macrocytosis	Oval: vitamin B$_{12}$ and folate deficiency, alcoholism, chemotherapy, myelodysplasia (MDS), aplastic anemia Round: liver disease, post-splenectomy, thyroid disease	MCV > 100 fL; may be oval or round in shape; cytoplasm is not polychromatophilic	Serum vitamin B$_{12}$ and folate levels to rule out megaloblastic anemia; bone marrow aspirate and biopsy to rule out MDS	Figure 74-5
Neutrophil with toxic changes	Infection, trauma, burns, growth factor therapy (e.g., G-CSF)	Prominent cytoplasmic granularity with increased primary granules; vacuolization and Döhle bodies may be present; seek left shift in maturation	Blood cultures, C-reactive protein	Figure 74-6
Bacteria	Bacterial infection; *Neisseria* sp, *Streptococcus* sp, and *Staphylococcus* sp most common	Organisms may be intracellular or extracellular; seek toxic changes in neutrophils and post-splenectomy changes as a risk factor; rule out colonized intravascular catheter	Gram stain, blood cultures	Figure 74-7
Fungi	Disseminated *Candida* or *Histoplasma* infections; *Pityrosporum* sp in TPN lines; colonized intravascular catheter	Organisms may be intracellular or extracellular; seek for toxic changes in neutrophils	Gram stain, blood cultures	Figure 74-8
Metastatic carcinoma	Nonhematopoietic neoplasm	Large, pleomorphic cells that tend to clump; leukoerythroblastic changes may be present, rarely observed in peripheral blood	Bone marrow aspirate and biopsy	Figure 74-9
Dysplastic neutrophils	MDS, MDS/MPD, AML, drug effect	Decreased cytoplasmic granulation, nuclear segmentation defects (e.g., hyposegmentation, bizarre hypersegmentation)	Bone marrow aspirate and biopsy, flow cytometry, cytogenetics	Figure 74-10
Blasts	Metastatic carcinoma, marrow fibrosis, MDS, MPD, MDS/MPD, acute leukemias, myeloma, lymphoma, growth factor therapy, marrow regeneration	Leukoerythroblastic changes (e.g., left shift, circulating erythroid precursors, teardrop cells) may be present in myelophthisic conditions; seek dysplastic features or Auer rods in MDS and AML	Bone marrow aspirate and biopsy, flow cytometry, cytogenetics	Figure 74-11
Platelet clumping	None	Platelets clumped when collected in EDTA anticoagulant, resulting in spurious thrombocytopenia	Use blood collection tube with alternate anticoagulant (e.g., sodium citrate) to eliminate clumping	Figure 74-12

AIHA, autoimmune hemolytic anemia; AML, acute myeloid leukemia; aPTT, activated partial thromboplastin time; BUN, blood urea nitrogen; DIC, disseminated intravascular coagulation; EDTA, ethylene-diamine tetra-acetic acid; FEP, free erythrocyte protoporphyrin; G-CSF, granulocyte colony-stimulating factor; Hb, hemoglobin; Hb A$_2$: hemoglobin A$_2$; HUS, hemolytic uremic syndrome; LDH, lactate dehydrogenase; MCV, mean cell volume; MDS/MPD, myelodysplastic or myeloproliferative disease; PT, prothrombin time; RBC, red blood cell; RDW, red cell distribution width; TIBC, total iron binding capacity; TTP, thrombotic thrombocytopenic purpura.

TABLE 74-5 Bone Marrow Findings in Selected Disorders

ABNORMALITY	DISEASE ASSOCIATIONS	KEY FINDINGS	CAVEATS	EXAMPLE
Hypoplasia	Chemotherapy, drug effect, toxin, viral or other infection, radiation therapy, aplastic anemia, paroxysmal nocturnal hemoglobinuria, anorexia nervosa	Cellularity varies inversely with patient age; subcortical zone in older adults may be hypocellular; requires adequate biopsy	Rule out hypocellular acute myeloid leukemia, MDS, or hairy cell leukemia	Figure 74-13
Metastatic carcinoma	Lung, breast, prostate, melanoma, gastrointestinal tract, and renal primaries in adults; neuroblastoma, rhabdomyosarcoma, Ewing's sarcoma, and osteosarcoma in children	Seek cell cohesiveness and pleomorphism, nuclear molding, prominent nucleoli; immunostains used to establish cell lineage	Metastatic lobular carcinoma of breast can be cytologically bland and may require immunostains to detect	Figure 74-14
Lymphoma	Non-Hodgkin's and Hodgkin's lymphoma	Lymphoid infiltrates, abnormal cellular morphology; ancillary studies often required	Differentiate from reactive lymphoid aggregates and granulomas	Figure 74-15
Granulomas	Infections (e.g., bacterial, fungi, viruses, *Rickettsia*); neoplasms, sarcoidosis, autoimmune disease, drug reactions, BCG therapy	Differentiate lipogranuloma from epithelioid granuloma, seek necrosis; special stains may help identify organisms	Correlate with marrow cultures and serology	Figure 74-16
Acute leukemia	Acute myeloid leukemia, acute lymphoblastic leukemia, acute leukemia of ambiguous lineage	≥20% blasts in blood or marrow; establish lineage with flow cytometry, cytochemical stains	Cytogenetics and molecular analysis required for definitive classification	Figure 74-17
Myeloma	Plasma cell myeloma and variants, including POEMS syndrome and plasma cell leukemia	Increased plasma cells, often cytologically atypical; demonstrate monoclonality by immunostains or other method	Differentiate from other lymphoproliferative disorders with plasma cell differentiation; expect poor recovery of plasma cells in flow cytometry studies	Figure 74-18
After chemotherapy	Hematologic or nonhematologic neoplasm	Cellular necrosis, stromal hemorrhage and edema, microvesicular fat, scattered lymphocytes and plasma cells, hemosiderin-laden macrophages	May be difficult to differentiate persistent leukemia from marrow regeneration by morphology alone	Figure 74-19

BCG, bacillus Calmette-Guérin; MDS, myelodysplastic disease; POEMS, polyneuropathy, organomegaly, endocrinopathy, M protein, skin changes.

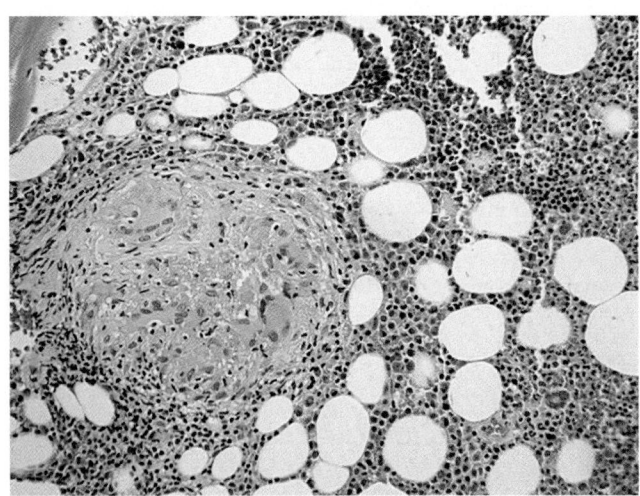

FIGURE 74-16 Granuloma. A small, circumscribed, noncaseating granuloma composed of lymphocytes, histiocytes, and multinucleate giant cells is shown in the bone marrow biopsy. The differential diagnosis for marrow granulomas typically includes infections (e.g., fungal, mycobacterial, viral, parasitic), sarcoidosis, autoimmune disease, and drug reactions (×200).

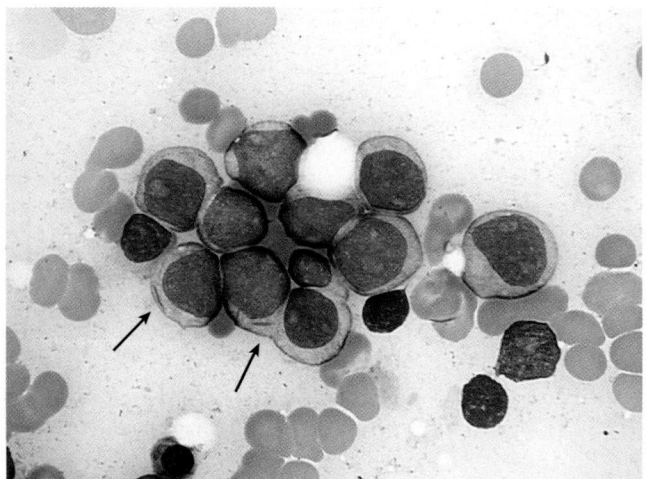

FIGURE 74-17 Acute myeloid leukemia. Bone marrow aspirate smear shows a cluster of blasts, some of which contain Auer rods *(arrows)*. Aspirate smears are used for evaluation of cellular morphology and cytoplasmic differentiation (×1000).

TABLE 74-6	Cerebrospinal Fluid Findings in Selected Disorders				
CONDITION	**GROSS EXAMINATION**	**CELL COUNTS**	**MORPHOLOGY**	**OTHER**	**EXAMPLE**
Normal (adult)	Clear, colorless, watery fluid	WBC: 0-5/μL RBC: 0-5/μL	Lymphocytes: 40-80% Monocytes: 15-45% Neutrophils: 0 6%	Glucose: two thirds of serum value Protein: 15-45 mg/dL	
Bacterial meningitis	Turbid, may clot	WBC: 100-10,000/μL	Neutrophils predominate	↓ Glucose ↑↑ Protein	Figure 74-20
Viral meningitis	Clear or slightly turbid	WBC: 10-500/μL	Lymphocytes predominate	Glucose: normal ↑ Protein	Figure 74-21
Fungal meningitis	Clear or slightly turbid	WBC: 0-500/μL	Variable	Glucose: varies ↑ Protein	Figure 74-22
Hemorrhage	Bloody or xanthochromic	RBC: increased	Numerous RBC, ± erythrophagocytosis	↑ Protein	Figure 74-23

RBC, red blood cell; WBC, white blood cell; ↓, decreased; ↑, increased; ↑↑, very increased.

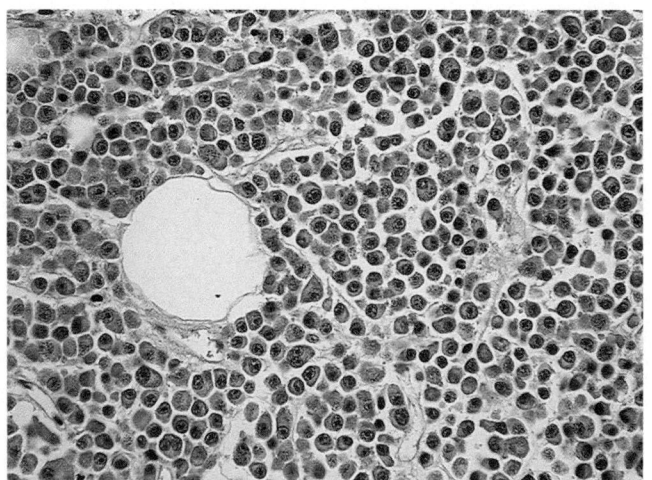

FIGURE 74-18 Plasma cell myeloma. The bone marrow biopsy shows virtual replacement of normal hematopoiesis by sheets of plasma cells. Immunostaining for kappa and lambda cytoplasmic immunoglobulin (not shown) can help define a clonal proliferation of plasma cells (×400).

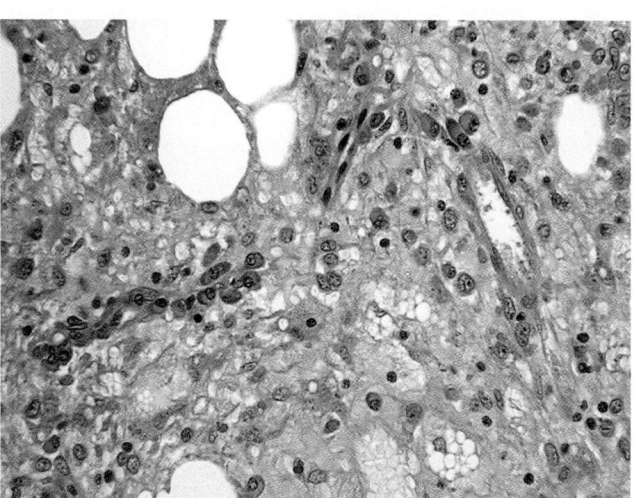

FIGURE 74-19 Postchemotherapeutic changes. The bone marrow biopsy obtained at day 14 after chemotherapy for acute leukemia shows markedly reduced cellularity, stromal edema and hemorrhage, scattered lymphocytes and plasma cells, and hemosiderin-laden macrophages. No residual leukemic blasts are identified (×400).

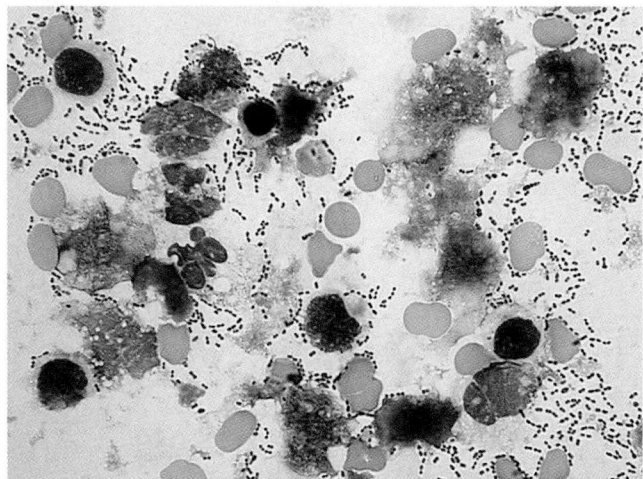

FIGURE 74-20 Bacterial meningitis. Acute inflammation with numerous bacteria (i.e., diplococci) is shown in this case of overwhelming *Streptococcus pneumoniae* meningitis (×1000).

numbers of reactive lymphocytes (Fig. 74-21), increased protein levels, and normal glucose concentrations. Findings for fungal meningitis depend on the organism and immune status of the host. Identification of widely spaced encapsulated yeast forms of various sizes with narrow-based buds in cytospin preparations can point to cryptococcal meningitis (Fig. 74-22). Macrophages with erythrophagocytosis (Fig. 74-23) and hemosiderin pigment point to prior hemorrhage into the cerebrospinal fluid.

Serous body cavity fluids can be classified as transudates or exudates, which can narrow the differential diagnosis. Features associated with transudates include a clear, straw-colored gross appearance, specific gravity less than 1.016, WBC less than 1000/μL, fluid-to-serum protein ratio less than 0.5, and fluid-to-serum lactate dehydrogenase ratio less than 0.6. Transudates are caused by protein or hemodynamic abnormalities, and the differential diagnosis includes congestive heart failure, cirrhosis, nephrotic syndrome, and hypoproteinemia. Features associated with

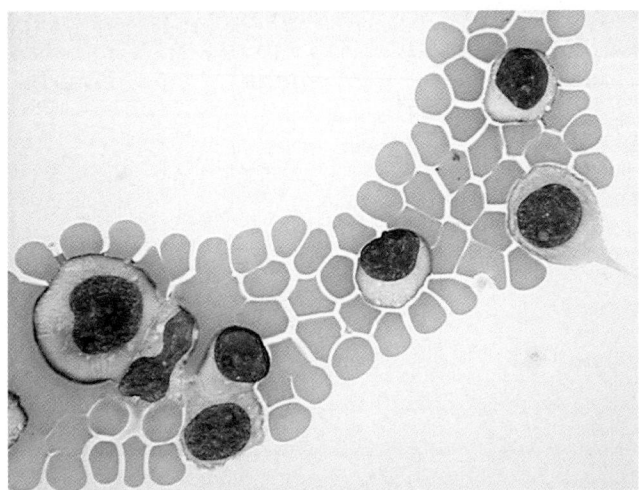

FIGURE 74-21 Viral meningitis. Lymphocytes with reactive changes and plasmacytoid forms predominate. The differential diagnosis includes fungal meningitis, demyelinating disorders, and partially treated bacterial meningitis (×1000).

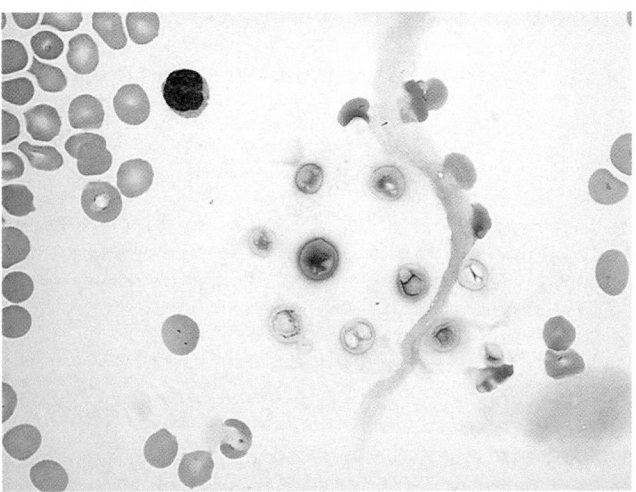

FIGURE 74-22 Cryptococcal meningitis. Clusters of widely spaced, encapsulated yeast of various sizes are a hallmark of cryptococcal meningitis. Unlike bacterial meningitis, the inflammatory response may be absent or minimal (×1000).

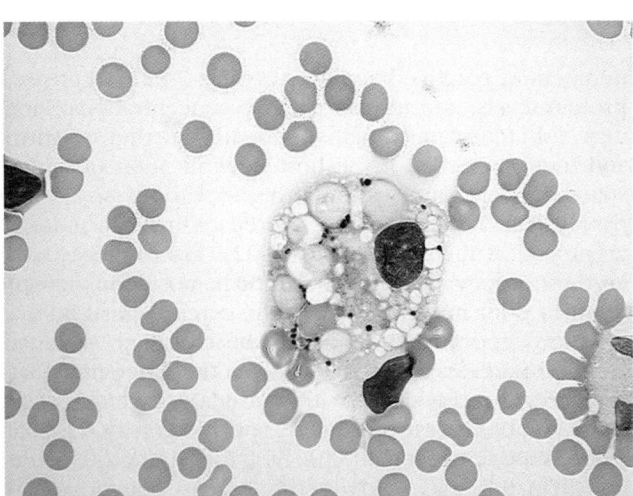

FIGURE 74-23 Central nervous system hemorrhage. Hemorrhagic fluid is seen with a macrophage showing erythrophagocytosis and hemosiderin pigment. Erythrophagocytosis implies the presence of blood in the cerebrospinal fluid for at least several hours (×1000).

exudates include turbid, bloody, or purulent gross appearance; specific gravity higher than 1.016, WBC higher than 1000/μL, fluid-to-serum protein ratio more than 0.5, and fluid-to-serum lactate dehydrogenase ratio more than 0.6. Exudates are caused by a localized pathologic process, including bacterial infection, infarct, neoplasm, autoimmune disorder, pancreatitis, or trauma. Originally developed for pleural effusions, these tests found application in ascitic fluids.

Pleural fluid may show metastatic carcinoma (Figs. 74-24 and 74-25). Bronchoalveolar lavage may reveal evidence of *Pneumocystis jiroveci* (Fig. 74-26) or cytomegalovirus (Fig. 74-27) in immunocompromised patients. Synovial fluid should be evaluated for crystal-induced arthritis, septic arthritis, hemorrhage, inflammation, and noninflammatory conditions.

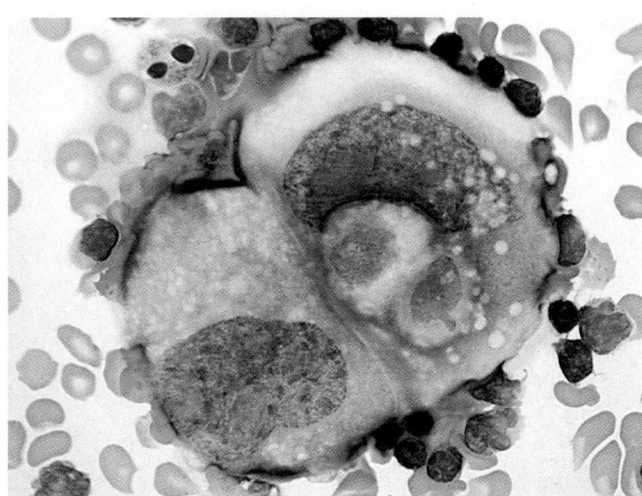

FIGURE 74-24 Metastatic adenocarcinoma. This hemorrhagic pleural fluid contains clusters of large, atypical cells with clumped chromatin, irregular nuclear outlines, and atypical cytoplasmic vacuolization (×1000).

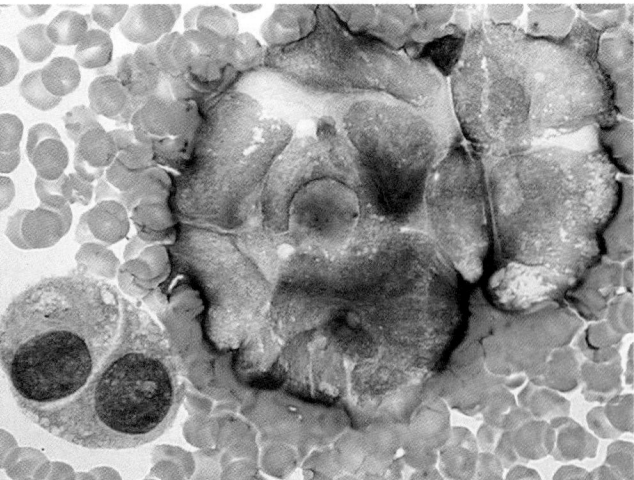

FIGURE 74-25 Metastatic small cell carcinoma. The hemorrhagic pleural fluid contained reactive mesothelial cells *(lower left)* and large clusters of malignant cells that show nuclear molding typical of small cell carcinoma of the lung (×1000).

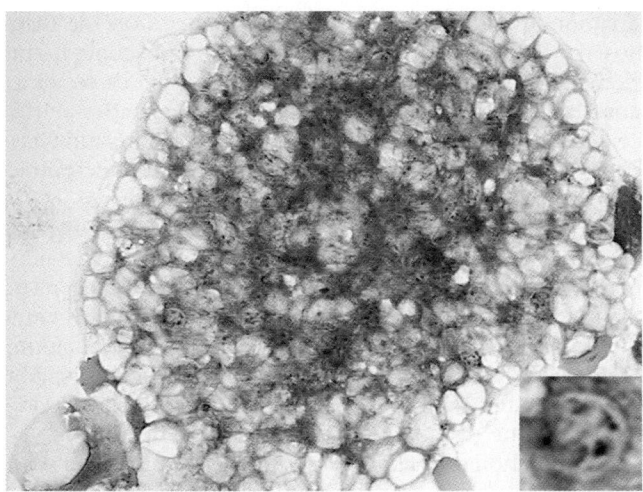

FIGURE 74-26 *Pneumocystis* pneumonia. A foamy alveolar cast composed of many small, round, thin-walled cysts with central trophozoites (*blue dots in inset*) is present in this bronchoalveolar lavage (×1000).

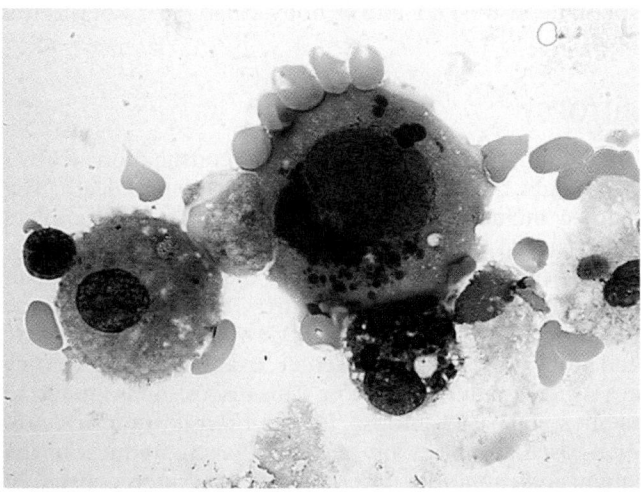

FIGURE 74-27 **Cytomegalovirus infection.** Bronchoalveolar lavage contains enlarged cells (compare with the alveolar macrophage on the left) with smudgy nuclear outlines and nuclear and cytoplasmic inclusions (×1000).

C-Reactive Protein

The CRP level rises rapidly in response to acute inflammation (6 to 10 hours) and peaks at approximately 36 to 50 hours. CRP has a short half-life (19 hours) and is not subject to diurnal variation. CRP is synthesized in the liver and is induced by pro-inflammatory cytokines, including interleukin-6 and, to a lesser extent, interleukin-1 and tumor necrosis factor-α. In acute inflammation or infection, CRP levels increase 100- to 1000-fold over normal levels, reflecting increased synthesis by hepatocytes as part of the acute phase response.

When monitoring for cardiovascular risk in healthy men and women, hsCRP levels of less than 1, 1 to 3, and more than 3 mg/L differentiate those at low, intermediate, and high risk, respectively. The hsCRP levels should be averaged from two specimens drawn 2 or more weeks apart. If the levels are less than 10 mg/L, the average value

Pearls and Pitfalls

- Leukoerythroblastic changes in the peripheral blood of patients with metastatic malignancy are highly correlated with marrow involvement.
- Spurious thrombocytopenia resulting from platelet clumping or satellitosis may be observed when blood is collected in EDTA. Blood should be collected in an alternate anticoagulant (i.e., sodium citrate or ammonium oxalate) to obtain an accurate platelet count. If clumping persists, consider a platelet cold agglutinin.
- When the marrow aspirate is a dry tap, it may be possible to isolate cells from an unfixed core biopsy to provide material for flow cytometry, cytogenetics, or molecular analysis.
- Wright-stained cytospin preparations of body fluids in the hematology laboratory are ideal for evaluating involvement by hematologic malignancies.
- Standard C-reactive protein (CRP) assays are not affected by diurnal variation or fasting status; they are inexpensive and widely available. An elevated level is an unfavorable prognostic finding for patients with advanced cancer. High-sensitivity CRP assays should be requested only when assessing the risk for coronary artery disease, stroke, or peripheral vascular disease.

should be used to calculate risk. If a level of more than 10 mg/L is found, a search should be undertaken to rule out subclinical infection or inflammation, and the test should repeated when the patient is stabilized.

CRP levels may have a role in monitoring cardiovascular disease. Interventions such as weight loss and adoption of a healthy lifestyle are associated with a decline in CRP. Similarly, anti-inflammatory and antiplatelet agents, lipid-lowering agents, β-adrenoreceptor antagonists, angiotensin receptor blockers, and antioxidants reduce serum levels of CRP. It is not known whether a decreased hsCRP level is associated with reduced risk of subsequent vascular events.

In critically ill patients and those with cancer, CRP levels can assess nutritional status and prognosis as a component of the prognostic inflammatory and nutritional index (PINI).[10] The index is calculated by dividing the product of two acute phase reactants by the product of two serum proteins:

$$PINI = \frac{[\alpha_1\text{-acid glycoprotein (mg/L)}] \times [\text{CRP (mg/L)}]}{[\text{serum albumin (g/L)}] \times [\text{prealbumin (g/L)}]}$$

The PINI should be less than 1 in normal, healthy people; in an acute phase response, the index is more than 1. Significantly elevated scores have been found for patients with advanced cancer, anorexia, and weight loss. Because the CRP level rises higher than other acute phase proteins, it contributes significantly to the elevated PINI and may be the most important value in this setting.

There is a statistically significant association between those with an elevated CRP level and an unfavorable prognosis in advanced cancer who survive for less than 90 days.[11] An elevated CRP level has prognostic significance independent of age, sex, and stage of disease in some studies (see "Pearls and Pitfalls").

REFERENCES

1. Black S, Kushner I, Samols D. C-reactive protein. J Biol Chem 2004;279:48487-48490.

2. Novis DA, Walsh M, Wilkinson D, et al. Laboratory productivity and the rate of manual peripheral blood smear review: A College of American Pathologists Q-probes study of 95,141 complete blood count determinations performed in 263 institutions. Arch Pathol Lab Med 2006;130:596-601.

3. Peterson P, Blomberg DJ, Rabinovitch A, Cornbleet PJ. Physician review of the peripheral blood smear: When and why. An opinion. Lab Hematol 2001;7: 175-179.

4. Foucar K. Bone marrow examination: Indications and techniques. In Foucar K (ed). Bone Marrow Pathology, 2nd ed. Chicago: ASCP Press, 2001, pp 30-49.

5. Riley RS, Hogan TF, Pavot DR, et al. A pathologist's perspective on bone marrow aspiration and biopsy. I. Performing a bone marrow examination. J Clin Lab Anal 2004;18:70-90.

6. Mahmoud FA, Rivera I. The role of C-reactive protein as a prognostic indicator in advanced cancer. Curr Oncol Rep 2002;21:250-255.

7. Houwen G. Blood film preparation and staining procedures. Clin Lab Med 2002;22:1-14.

8. Perkins S. Diagnosis of anemia. In Kjeldsberg CR (ed). Practical Diagnosis of Hematologic Disorders, 4th ed. Chicago: ASCP Press, 2006, pp 3-16.

9. Weiss G, Goodnough LT. Anemia of chronic disease. N Engl J Med 2005;352: 1011-1023.

10. Nelson KA, Walsh D. The cancer anorexia-cachexia syndrome: A survey of the prognostic inflammatory and nutritional index (PINI) in advanced disease. J Pain Symptom Manage 2002;24:424-428.

11. Maltoni M, Caraceni A, Brunelli C, et al. Prognostic factors in advanced cancer patients: Evidence-based clinical recommendations. A study by the steering committee of the European Association for Palliative Care. J Clin Oncol 2005;23:6240-6248.

SUGGESTED READING

Foucar K: Bone Marrow Pathology, 2nd ed. Chicago: ASCP Press, 2001.

Galagan KA, Blomberg D, Cornbleet PJ, Glassy EF (eds). Color Atlas of Body Fluids: An Illustrated Field Guide Based on Proficiency Testing. Northfield, IL: College of American Pathologists, 2006.

Glassy EF (ed). Color Atlas of Hematology: An Illustrated Field Guide Based on Proficiency Testing. Northfield, IL: College of American Pathologists, 1998.

Vajpayee N, Graham SS, Bem S. Basic examination of blood and marrow. In McPherson RA, Pincus MR (eds): Henry's Clinical Diagnosis and Management by Laboratory Methods. 21st ed. Philadelphia, Saunders/Elsevier, 2007, pp 457-483.

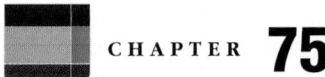

CHAPTER **75**

The Role of Pathology

Lisa M. Yerian

KEY POINTS

- The purpose of pathologic analysis is to provide information about the diagnosis and extent of disease.

- An autopsy is a postmortem gross and microscopic examination that provides information about the diagnosis, extent of disease, and events leading to death.

- A biopsy is a small tissue sample procured to establish a diagnosis.

- Frozen sections are used for rapid diagnosis, but they are limited by artifacts and the inability to perform specialized analyses.

- Cytology analyzes individual cells that are aspirated by a needle or exfoliated.

Anatomic pathology is the field that focuses on the diagnosis of disease by means of gross and microscopic tissue examination. The information provided includes the diagnosis of disease (or absence thereof); determination of the cell type and, if possible, the body site of origin; and characterization of other relevant prognostic or therapeutic factors.

Pathologists use various techniques to identify and describe many inflammatory, reactive, infectious, and neoplastic conditions. The postmortem autopsy is the most comprehensive examination, involving a complete review of clinical data, external and internal gross examination, microscopy, and other laboratory tests. It provides insight into the extent and nature of disease, co-morbid conditions, and the events ultimately leading to death.

Examination of selected tissues may be performed with a biopsy, which is a small sample of the patient's tissue. Surgical pathologists interpret thinly sectioned, whole tissue samples from biopsies or surgical resection specimens. If an urgent diagnosis is required, a frozen section may be performed. Cytology involves analysis of cells from the aspiration of a lesion, brushing of a body surface, or spontaneously shed into a body cavity (e.g., peritoneal fluid).

AUTOPSY

The autopsy is a comprehensive consultation with a pathologist to determine the events leading to death. The autopsy includes review of the medical history, complete external and internal physical examination, documentation of findings, and analysis of the consequences surrounding the individual's death. The findings include integrated data gathered from review of the clinical history and from gross and microscopic examinations, and they are issued as a written report. This discussion is limited to the hospital-based autopsy. Unlike forensic autopsies, hospital-based autopsies are performed at the request of the family and cannot be ordered without written consent of the next of kin.

Autopsy rates have been declining for many years. Frequently cited reasons include improved imaging and diagnostic testing, such that clinicians (and often loved ones) feel they understand the disease and know why the patient died. However, studies show that 49% of deceased patients were clinically misdiagnosed and that more than one half of these errors were missed major diagnoses.[1] Medical lawsuits may also contribute to the decline. Physicians may be hesitant to suggest an autopsy for fear that the results may elicit information that may be used in a lawsuit. An autopsy more frequently reveals information that patients died of causes unrelated to the standard of care; failure to perform an autopsy, however, may allow speculation about events leading to the death and create greater distrust from an impression that physicians wish to hide mistakes.

Despite the decline in autopsy rates, the procedure carries great benefits for the survivors, physicians, and society. It helps provide closure for the family by answering questions about the nature and extent of the disease and the events ultimately leading to the patient's demise. In selected cases, the autopsy may uncover evidence of an inherited condition, allowing family members to seek treatment or surveillance. The autopsy provides information to the clinicians, helping advance their clinical knowledge. The autopsy is a critical part of the training of medical students and residents about autopsy technique and the anatomy, histology, and pathology of human disease. For society, the autopsy helps gauge the quality of medical care, inform future care standards, and build public trust in medicine.[2]

Indications and Contraindications

Because the autopsy offers many benefits, a discussion about autopsy is always indicated. The major indication is when the major disease diagnosis or the cause of death is unknown. Many diseases require tissue evaluation for diagnosis, and tissue often is not or cannot be obtained before the death. Certain neurological diseases may be suspected in life (e.g., Alzheimer's disease, Lewy body dementia), but definitive diagnosis requires tissue analysis that can be obtained only by postmortem examination of the brain. An autopsy is particularly desirable when the primary diagnosis or the sequence of events leading to death is unclear. The autopsy can detect previously undetected conditions that might have contributed.

The only contraindication to an autopsy is the objection of the next of kin, because hospital-based autopsies cannot be performed without written consent. The next of kin may place restrictions on the extent of the autopsy or request that the examination's scope is limited. Typical limitations include examination of the brain only (for neurological disease such as Alzheimer's), no examination of the brain, examination of the chest or abdomen only, examination and sampling of organs without removal, and return of organs to the body before burial (Box 75-1).

Features of the Procedure

The key to maximizing the benefits of an autopsy is a thoughtful, considerate, and informative conversation with the survivors. It is the clinician's responsibility to request permission to perform an autopsy, and the most successful clinicians are informed about autopsies. The clinician must be prepared to explain how an autopsy is performed and how the procedure will benefit the survivors, the clinicians involved, and the field of medicine. The physician must be prepared to answer logistical questions related to the procedure, some of which depend on the particular institution. Typical questions address the actual procedure (detailed previously), cost, timing, and funeral concerns (Box 75-2). A complete autopsy in the United States typically costs $1500 to $2000. This expense is not covered by Medicare or private payers, and it is typically borne by the hospital, especially in teaching hospitals, or by the family. In Europe and in any countries where there is a national public health system, autopsy costs are irrelevant. Physicians must understand the procedure in their institutions.

Families often ask whether they will be able to have an open-casket funeral after an autopsy. The autopsy-related skin incisions include a Y-shaped incision on the chest and abdomen and an incision at the back of the head that will be invisible at the funeral. Incisions or other alterations of the face and hands are strictly prohibited, except in rare circumstances and with express written permission. Most hospitals retain the organs for a minimum of 3 months after the autopsy report. Physicians must check with the autopsy director at their institutions for local protocols. At the family's request, the organs can be returned to the body after examination and sampling. It is a good idea to keep the name and contact information for the director of autopsy service at the hospital, because this person will be most familiar with the hospital's autopsy procedures, costs, timing, and when a completed written report may be expected. There remain several areas of debate:

- Role of autopsy as a source of information and knowledge for the decedent's family members, pathologists, and clinical caregivers
- The impact of declining autopsy rates on medical education, resident training, and medical knowledge
- Viability of autopsy practices in an increasingly payer-driven health care industry

BIOPSIES

A biopsy is a small sample of tissue procured for investigation. Typically, the procedure is done for primary histological diagnosis, but other analyses (e.g., molecular, cytogenetic) can be performed. Analysis may be performed on biopsy specimens from essentially any body part, and the indications, techniques, and risks vary with the biopsy site. Endoscopic biopsies are common and can

---

Box 75-1 Steps in a Complete Autopsy Examination

- Review of the medical history and the events leading to the patient's death
- External physical examination
- Photographing and documentation of external findings
- Procurement of samples for culture and analysis (see Chapter 74)
- Internal physical examination
- Removal of organs
- Examination of organs: measuring, weighing, sectioning, examination, and procurement of samples for histologic analysis
- Photographing and documentation of internal findings
- Histologic examination
- Review of laboratory testing data (culture results, chemistry) (see Chapter 74)
- Written report detailing pertinent positive and negative findings, including diagnoses and immediate cause of death

---

Box 75-2 What Clinicians Should Know about Autopsies before Speaking with the Family

- Basic steps of the examination and procedures used at the institution
- Benefits to the family, the clinicians, and medical knowledge
- Cost: $1500 to $2000, which is payable by the hospital or the patient's family, or no charge in a public national health system
- Timing: when autopsies are typically performed and when the family can expect a written report
- The name and contact information for the autopsy director at the institution

be performed on localized lesions under direct visualization. Needle biopsies are done by placing a hollow needle in the tissue or lesion of interest and obtaining a small core of tissue. Open biopsies are performed in the operating room.

Biopsy specimens can be transported to the surgical pathology laboratory fresh or in tissue fixative. Fresh biopsies should be slightly moistened with saline or moist gauze to prevent desiccation, which encourages specimen adherence to the container and can negatively affect the morphological examination. Fresh biopsies should be transported to the laboratory quickly, because autolysis (decomposition) begins immediately after the specimen is removed from the body. Fixative stabilizes the tissue and prevents decomposition. Various tissue fixatives are available; the most frequently used is formalin. Others are preferred for certain specimen types to accentuate certain morphological features. Some analyses cannot be performed on fixed tissues (e.g., flow cytometry, cytogenetics, some immunostains). When in doubt, a telephone call to the surgical pathology laboratory can save the patient from a nondiagnostic procedure and the need for a repeat biopsy.

Indications and Contraindications

A biopsy is indicated when a tissue diagnosis is required to document malignancy, stage a known disease, or initiate a treatment or palliative care plan. Contraindications include risk factors specific to the patient or the specific biopsy site. A hypocoagulable state (e.g., liver failure, anticoagulative drugs) is a relative contraindication to certain biopsies and requires special precautions.

Equipment

The equipment varies with the site and type of biopsy. Core biopsies are performed with hollow needles that remove a thin cylinder of tissue. Biopsies obtained intraoperatively during an open or laparoscopic procedure may consist of a small wedge sample or a thin sample acquired with a needle. All biopsies should be placed in a container labeled with the patient's name, patient identifying number, and biopsy site. Tissue may be submitted in fixative (typically formalin) for routine processing or fresh for special studies. Prefilled specimen containers are available. For small specimens submitted fresh, a few drops of saline or a piece of saline-soaked gauze help prevent the specimen from drying out (Boxes 75-3 and 75-4).

Special Stains for Histochemistry and Immunochemistry

In some cases, specialized tissue or cell stains can add information to that from the hematoxylin and eosin–stained slide alone. Immunohistochemistry or immunocytochemistry can provide information that is a helpful adjunct to routine microscopic examination. These methods are based on the application of specific antibodies to the cells on a cytologic preparation or a tissue section. If the antigen of interest is present on the cells, the antibody will bind to the cells in a site-specific fashion.

Box 75-3 Biopsy Specimen Technique

- In surgical pathology, all specimens are examined grossly and placed in tissue cassettes, small plastic cages that hold tissue specimens during processing.
- Processing is usually performed in a machine that bathes the tissue in heated formalin for fixation, dehydrates the tissues, and infuses paraffin wax.
- Tissue is embedded in a small cake of wax to enable cutting of very thin slices (4- to 5-μm sections for most tissues, 2-μm sections for some bone marrow and lymphoid specimens).
- Tissue sections are mounted on glass slides.
- Mounted sections are stained with hematoxylin and eosin.
- Coverslips are placed over the slides.

Box 75-4 Performance of a Biopsy

- A biopsy is carried out for histologic diagnosis.
- Specimen submission requirements should be known for the analysis required.
- Specimens for routine processing may be submitted fresh or in fixative, but if lymphoma is suspected, the specimen should not be submitted in fixative.
- Histochemical stains, molecular techniques, and immunohistochemical analyses can help identify and classify a newly diagnosed or metastatic neoplasm.

A detection system is applied, and a positive reaction may be visualized. Many immunohistochemical and immunocytochemical stains are available to characterize the cell type (e.g., actin for muscle cells, cytokeratins for epithelial cells) and to evaluate prognostic features (e.g., proliferative indices using Ki67, proliferating cell nuclear antigen [PCNA]).

Histochemical stains can identify many tissue components. They are particularly useful for identifying normal and abnormal intracellular (e.g., iron) or extracellular (e.g., amyloid, collagen) substances or organisms. The Gomori methenamine silver (GMS) or periodic acid–Schiff (PAS) stains are common stains for fungi, and mycobacteria are identified using various acid-fast stains (e.g., Fite, Ziehl-Neelsen). Tissue Gram stains can be performed, but determination of a specific bacterium on tissue sections can be difficult. Given the many stains available and the technical expertise required to perform and interpret them, physicians should seek the advice of the hospital's pathologist and histotechnologist about which stain works best for answering a specific question. All stains should be interpreted only with appropriate control stains.

The applications of immunohistochemistry and immunocytochemistry have expanded because of the increasing number of available antibodies, multiplex staining in a single reaction, enzyme metallography, and development of new prognostic markers. Immunohistochemistry can be used to diagnose genetic and inherited diseases (e.g., mismatch repair protein analysis for hereditary nonpolyposis colorectal cancer).

Postoperative Care and Complications

The postoperative care for a biopsy depends on the biopsy site. Patients should be observed or instructed to watch for signs of bleeding or infection.

Complications are similar to those for other invasive procedures and include pain, bleeding, and infection. An increased risk of bleeding should be recognized for those on anticoagulant medications or who have liver failure. Additional risks related to the specific biopsy site should be evaluated on an individual basis.

FROZEN SECTION

A frozen section is performed during a surgical procedure when the immediate course of the treatment depends on the tissue sample diagnosis. When the time required to prepare a routine tissue section is unacceptable, a frozen section can be requested by the clinician.

The technique for a frozen section is similar to that described for a biopsy, except that the specimen is embedded in a freezing compound (i.e., optimal cutting temperature [OCT] compound) and rapidly frozen. Sectioning is performed in an enclosed freezing microtome (i.e., cryotome).

To prepare histologic slides more rapidly, the tissue is rapidly frozen, and thin sections (approximately 4 to 5 µm) are cut in a chilled container. The sections can usually be cut, fixed rapidly in formalin, stained, and interpreted in less than 20 minutes. Frozen sections are most frequently used for intraoperative consultations (while the patient is anesthetized) to assist the surgeon in determining the best course of action. Occasionally, frozen section may be used for evaluation of tissue adequacy for a diagnosis or for rapid diagnosis when the histology laboratory is closed.

Tissue for frozen section analysis must be submitted to the laboratory fresh (not in fixative). After the tissue is in the fixative, a frozen section cannot be performed. The major limitation is the artifacts from the freezing process. Certain tissues do not section well when frozen (e.g., fatty tissue), and some cannot be sectioned at all (e.g., bone requires decalcification). Many ancillary procedures (e.g., special stains, immunohistochemistry) cannot be done, reducing the full benefit of all available diagnostic tools.

The diagnostic accuracy of frozen sections is up to 95%, with the exact percentage varying with the specimen type and clinical question.[3,4] In certain clinical scenarios, it is an essential tool for patient care.

Indications and Contraindications

A desire to provide results quickly is not an indication for frozen section, because the diagnostic accuracy, although high, is not as high as that produced through routine processing. Small biopsies may be depleted during frozen sectioning, leaving no tissue for routine processing or ancillary studies. In some cases, small specimens (e.g., needle core biopsies) can be processed on a rush protocol, yielding a diagnosis in hours. Although this takes longer than a frozen section, it may yield a better diagnostic result, and it preserves tissue for ancillary studies. If unsure about whether a frozen section is indicated, the

physician should speak with a pathologist. Several ideas should be considered when deciding whether to employ a frozen section (Box 75-5).

Box 75-5 Features Affecting the Choice of Frozen Section

- Frozen section results are typically reported within 20 minutes.
- A specimen submitted for frozen section must be submitted fresh (i.e., no fixative).
- Frozen section interpretation is limited by freezing and sectioning artifacts, and specialized analyses (e.g., special stains, immunohistochemistry) usually are not available for frozen sections. Such studies often can be performed after further processing of the specimen.
- Some tissue types are not amenable to frozen sectioning. Bone or bony lesions cannot be cut in the fresh-frozen state, and frozen sections of fatty tissues are difficult to cut, making interpretation difficult or impossible.
- Frozen sections can determine whether lesional tissue is present. A distinction between benign and malignant lesions usually can be made, and neoplasms often can be classified by tissue type (i.e., adenocarcinoma versus squamous cell carcinoma). Precise determination of the primary site, however, is usually not possible on frozen section in the absence of additional clinical information.

Equipment

Some basic equipment is needed for the procedure:

- Liquid nitrogen or aerosolized freezing spray, or both
- OCT embedding compound
- Cryotome
- Glass slides
- Slide fixation and staining solutions
- Microscope for interpretation

CYTOLOGY

Cytology, or cytopathology, focuses on obtaining a diagnosis through evaluation of individual or small groups of cells on a slide, rather than complete tissue sections. Cytologic specimens may be derived from fine-needle aspiration or exfoliative specimens. Rapid interpretation is available in some locations to determine specimen adequacy and sometimes to provide a preliminary diagnosis.

The two major specimen types are exfoliative and aspiration (Box 75-6). In exfoliative cytology, the specimen includes spontaneously shed cells and those scraped or brushed from bodily surfaces. Examples include fluid specimens (e.g., ascitic fluid, cerebrospinal fluid, bronchial washings) and brushings (e.g., Papanicolaou test, endoscopic brushings). Fine-needle aspiration entails the insertion of a small needle (typically 21 to 27 gauge) into an organ to sample cells. This may be done percutaneously by palpation (e.g., breast lesions, lymph nodes, subcutaneous masses), under radiographic guidance (i.e., ultrasound or computed tomography), or endoscopically.

For aspiration cytology, the cells aspirated into the bore of the needle are forced out onto a glass slide or placed

Box 75-6 Aspiration and Exfoliation Techniques

Aspiration Technique

- Slides, needle, and needle holder are prepared and labeled.
- The lesion is identified by palpation.
- The skin surface is cleaned with alcohol.
- The needle is placed in the lesion.
- If suction technique is used, the syringe is drawn up to create a vacuum.
- The needle is moved up and down in a cutting motion.
- Aspirated material (i.e., cells and matrix) is forced out of the needle and onto glass slides.
- The material is smeared across the slide with a second slide.
- The needle is rinsed in cytology fixative solution to obtain any residual material. This solution is taken back to the cytology laboratory, and the contents used to make additional slides.

Exfoliation Technique

- A brush or spatula is applied to the surface to be sampled.
- Surface cells adhere to the brush or spatula.
- The sampling device is dragged across a glass slide or rinsed in cytology fixative, from which cells are collected and dropped onto glass slides.

in a fixative to be centrifuged later and placed on glass slides. The cytology preparations are then stained and evaluated under a microscope. For aspiration cytology, rapid staining and evaluation can be performed for determination of specimen adequacy and sometimes to provide a preliminary diagnosis.

Indications and Contraindications

As with a biopsy, cytology is indicated for diagnosis or prognostication. In many cases, cytology and histological examination of a biopsy specimen are complementary, with maximum sensitivity and specificity achieved by combining the techniques. For palpable lesions such as subcutaneous masses, lymph nodes, or breast lesions, there are specific advantages of aspiration over biopsy. Aspiration is quick and can be done in the clinic, and adequacy interpretations are often available so additional sampling can be performed before the patient leaves.

Equipment

The equipment consists of a needle and syringe; some prefer to use a needle holder for greater control. Slides labeled with the patient's name or specimen number should be prepared. A fixative spray is usually applied to the slides. Cell samples may be obtained through fluid sampling with a needle (i.e., paracentesis) or by sampling a surface with a brush or spatula. Staining reagents and a microscope are required for all types of cytologic analysis.

Postoperative Care and Complications

Postoperative care consists of pressure to the aspiration site to control bleeding, which usually is minimal. No specific postoperative care is required for the brushing or scraping exfoliative procedures.

The complications resemble those of a needle biopsy, but a smaller (thinner) needle is used. For exfoliative cytology, the complications vary with the specimen type. Discordant histologic and cytologic results may be obtained from the same diagnostic procedure, and the physician should know how to handle this situation in a clinical setting. The use of ancillary techniques (e.g., immunocytochemistry, fluorescent in situ hybridization [FISH]) on cytology specimens yields greater diagnostic information.

REFERENCES

1. Bayer-Garner IB, Fink LM, Lamps LW. Pathologists in a teaching institution assess the value of the autopsy. Arch Pathol Lab Med 2002;126:442-447.
2. Crawford JM. Evidence-based interpretation of liver biopsies. Lab Invest 2006;86:326-334.
3. Rakha E, Ramaiah S, McGregor A. Accuracy of frozen section in the diagnosis of liver mass lesions. J Clin Pathol 2006;59:352-354.
4. Stewart CJ, Brennan BA, Hammond IG, et al. Intraoperative assessment of ovarian tumors: A 5-year review with assessment of discrepant diagnostic cases. Int J Gynecol Pathol 2006;25:216-222.

SUGGESTED READING

DeMay RM (ed). The Art and Science of Cytopathology. Chicago: American Society of Clinical Pathologists, 1996.

Kumar V, Abbas AK, Fausto N (eds). Robbins and Cotran's Pathologic Basis of Disease, 7th ed. Philadelphia: Elsevier Saunders, 2005.

Lester SC (ed). Manual of Surgical Pathology. Philadelphia: Churchill Livingstone, 2001.

Prayson RA. Autopsy: Learning from the Dead. A Cleveland Clinic Guide. Cleveland, OH: Cleveland Clinic Press, 2006.

Co-morbidities

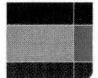

CHAPTER 76

Common Medical and Surgical Disorders

John Loughnane

PEPTIC ULCER DISEASE

Peptic ulcer disease is an ulcer of the gastrointestinal mucosa in or near an acid-producing area. Ulcers are most commonly found in the proximal duodenum, but they may also involve the stomach and esophagus.

Epidemiology and Prevalence

Peptic ulcers affect 15% of the population at some time. Duodenal ulcers are more common than gastric ulcers, which are more common than esophageal ulcers. Duodenal ulcers are more common in men. Duodenal and gastric ulcers are more common in the elderly.

Pathophysiology

Peptic ulcers develop when aggressive factors (e.g., *H. pylori* infection, acid, nonsteroidal anti-inflammatory drugs [NSAIDs]) predominate over protective factors (e.g., prostaglandins, mucus, bicarbonate) and interrupt mucosal integrity. The main aggressive factor is *H. pylori* infection. About 4% of NSAID users develop a peptic ulcer.

Clinical Manifestations and Treatment

The most common presenting symptom is epigastric pain. If the ulcer is located posteriorly, the pain may radiate to the back. Pain is often described as a burning or gnawing sensation. Nighttime pain is common. Duodenal ulcer pain may begin 2 to 3 hours after eating and be relieved by food or milk. Gastric ulcer pain is frequently precipitated by food and may be associated with nausea, vomiting, and weight loss.

Upper gastrointestinal endoscopy can demonstrate duodenal ulcer, gastric ulcer, and esophagitis. In patients with upper gastrointestinal symptoms, endoscopic results often are normal. Distinguishing ulceration from esophagitis is not very useful in management. An alternative strategy suggests[1] that those with alarming symptoms and those who have not responded to treatment should be referred for endoscopy. Alarming symptoms are dysphagia, persistent vomiting, weight loss, abdominal mass, evidence of gastrointestinal bleeding or iron deficiency anemia, and symptoms occurring in patients older than 55 years. Others are tested for *H. pylori* infection without endoscopy. The ^{14}C-urea breath test and the stool antigen test are most widely used. If infection is confirmed, 1 week of the following eradication therapies is prescribed:

- A proton pump inhibitor (PPI) plus 1 g of amoxicillin plus 500 mg of clarithromycin, all given twice daily
- In case of penicillin allergy, a PPI plus 400 mg of metronidazole plus 250 mg of clarithromycin, all given twice daily

Eradication doses of PPIs (all given twice daily) are 20 mg of omeprazole, 30 mg of lansoprazole, 40 mg of pantoprazole, 20 mg of rabeprazole, and 20 mg of someprazole (*S*-isomer of omeprazole). In patients with liver disease, the dose of PPI should be halved. Omeprazole and esomeprazole may potentiate warfarin. A PPI is continued for 1 month if endoscopy has identified a gastric ulcer or a complicated or large duodenal ulcer.

GASTROESOPHAGEAL REFLUX DISEASE

Gastroesophageal reflux disease (GERD) has been defined as reflux of gastric contents into the esophagus, reflux symptoms sufficient to impair quality of life, or risk long-term complications.[2] Many with reflux are asymptomatic and have normal endoscopic findings. Gastroesophageal reflux becomes a disease when it impairs the quality of life or causes distal esophageal mucosal damage. The degree of damage does not correlate with symptom severity.

Epidemiology and Prevalence

In Western populations, 25% of adults have heartburn at least once monthly.[3]

Pathophysiology

The main mechanism of reflux is transient relaxation of the lower esophageal sphincter. The cause is unknown. Hiatal hernia does not cause reflux but may exacerbate an existing tendency. *H. pylori* infection is negatively associated with GERD.

Clinical Manifestations

Heartburn and regurgitation are the main symptoms of GERD. Heartburn is a feeling of retrosternal burning or discomfort that may radiate to the neck. Regurgitation is effortless passage of stomach contents into the pharynx. Absence of heartburn does not exclude GERD. Dysphagia and odynophagia may be present. Gastropharyngeal reflux can cause cough, sore throat, and hoarseness.

Differential Diagnosis

In palliative medicine, combining upper gastrointestinal symptoms under the label of dyspepsia is useful because investigation is likely to be limited and treatment directed by symptoms. Dyspepsia may be caused or exacerbated by smoking, abdominal distention, esophageal candidiasis, upper gastrointestinal stenting, or drugs such as steroids, NSAIDs, bisphosphonates, opioids, metronidazole, nitrates, calcium channel blockers, and theophyllines.

Treatment

Advice to reduce smoking and alcohol intake, avoid tight clothing, and avoid stooping often is given, although it has little evidence base. Antacid-containing alginates (10 to 20 mL every 8 hours) may help reflux symptoms, but they have no effect on esophagitis. Although H_2-receptor antagonists and PPIs are effective in treating esophagitis, PPI therapy is superior. Prokinetic drugs such as metoclopramide and domperidone may relieve reflux symptoms, but they have little efficacy in esophagitis. Most patients with GERD experience recurrent symptoms on stopping treatment. Continuous, standard-dose PPI use is the most effective therapy to prevent recurrence. Intermittent, on-demand therapy with PPIs and H_2-receptor antagonists is more effective in preventing recurrence than placebo.

CELLULITIS

Cellulitis is a noncontagious skin infection. It is common in palliative medicine patients, who frequently require admission for intravenous antibiotics.

Pathophysiology

Most erysipelas is caused by *Streptococcus pyogenes* and by *Staphylococcus aureus*, alone or in combination with *Streptococcus*. The most common infection site is the lower limb. Bacteria gain entry through a break in the skin surface (e.g., varicose ulcers, trauma, tinea pedis, eczema, intravenous drug abuse). Diabetes, lymphedema, obesity, and peripheral vascular disease are risk factors.

Clinical Manifestations and Complications

Cellulitis is a spreading bacterial infection of the lower dermis and subcutaneous tissues giving rise to tender inflammation. Erysipelas is more superficial, involving the dermis and upper subcutaneous tissues. Erysipelas manifests with a raised, distinct border. The advancing border of cellulitis is more difficult to define. In practice, it is difficult to tell how deep the skin involvement is, and it is therefore probably best to consider erysipelas as a superficial cellulitis. In early infection, complaints are of pain and of feeling generally unwell. Infection tends to progress rapidly, with malaise, rigors, listlessness, and confusion. Examination reveals swelling and redness that is tender and hot. Lymphangitis (i.e., tender, red swelling of the lymphatics) may be present, and there may be tender regional lymphadenopathy. The diagnosis is essentially clinical.[4]

Septicemia may complicate cellulitis. Cellulitis damages the lymphatic drainage system. Up to 7% of people develop chronic edema after one episode of leg cellulitis. Once established, lymphedema predisposes to further episodes of cellulitis.

Differential Diagnosis

The diagnosis of cellulitis is usually obvious. However, if there is a possibility of deep vein thrombosis, an ultrasound scan should be obtained.

Treatment

A high index of suspicion, prompt diagnosis, and treatment are vital. Appropriate antibiotics at adequate dosage and for sufficient time should be given systemically. Those who are not systemically unwell and do not have significant co-morbidities can be managed at home. The patient should rest and elevate the affected limb, which reduces swelling and pain.

Paracetamol (1 g every 6 hours) may be used for pain. Avoid NSAIDs because they risk development or aggravation of necrotizing fasciitis. Antibiotic treatment is empirical. The chosen antibiotic should cover staphylococcal and streptococcal infections. High-dose flucloxacillin covers streptococci and penicillinase-resistant staphylococci. Flucloxacillin (1 g every 6 hours) used alone is recommended as initial treatment. Some recommend combining flucloxacillin with amoxicillin (1 g every 8 hours) or phenoxymethylpenicillin (500 mg every 6 hours). Tissue penetration of phenoxymethylpenicillin is poor. In patients with penicillin allergy, use 500 to 1000 mg of erythromycin every 6 hours. Staphylococcal resistance to erythromycin is becoming prevalent. Clindamycin is an alternative for patients allergic to penicillin. Antibiotics should be continued for at least 10 days. Patients should then be reviewed and treatment continued if signs of infection persist. Antibiotics may need to be continued for up to 4 weeks.

Because of the high risk of recurrence, prophylactic antibiotic therapy should be considered. Phenoxymethylpenicillin (500 mg every 12 hours for 1 month, followed by 500 mg daily indefinitely) is advised. Use erythromycin (500 mg daily) if the patient is allergic to penicillin.

ROTATOR CUFF INJURY

The shoulder joint is held together by a fibrous capsule reinforced by muscle and tendons that form the rotator cuff. The cuff is formed anteriorly by the subscapularis, posteriorly by the infraspinatus, and superiorly by the supraspinatus. Inflammation of the rotator cuff causes tendinitis (e.g., supraspinatus tendonitis). Inflammation of the shoulder capsule causes adhesive capsulitis (i.e., frozen shoulder syndrome). The most common cause of shoulder pain and stiffness in palliative care patients is adhesive capsulitis from prolonged immobility.

Epidemiology and Prevalence

Three percent of people develop adhesive capsulitis some time in their life. Women are affected more frequently than men. Up to 20% of diabetic and neurosurgical patients develop capsulitis.

Pathophysiology and Clinical Manifestations

The most consistent finding in established disease is fibrotic thickening of the anterior capsule of the shoulder joint. Initially, there tends to be gradual rather than acute onset of diffuse shoulder pain over some months. Improvement is gradual and may take many years. As pain lessens stiffness gets worse. Pain is often worse at night, causing considerable sleep disturbance.

The main finding on examination is marked limitation of active and passive shoulder movements. In capsulitis, all shoulder movements are affected, whereas in tendinitis, restriction is limited to the movement generated by the affected tendon (e.g., abduction in supraspinatus tendinitis). The supraspinatus is the tendon most frequently involved, giving rise to tenderness as it runs anterior to the shoulder joint.

Differential Diagnosis

In the palliative medicine setting, shoulder pain may result from cervical radiculopathy or bronchogenic carcinoma in the lung apex. Metastatic spread of disease to bone in the shoulder area also should be considered. Radiographic examinations of the cervical spine, chest, and shoulder may be indicated.

Treatment

The aim is to relieve pain and increase mobility. Rest should be advised, and a sling may be worn because too rapid a return to normal function may worsen pain and stiffness. As soon as pain permits, exercises to improve range of motion should be started with a physiotherapist. Analgesia should be prescribed according to World Health Organization pain ladder. NSAIDs may be added if pain persists.

Steroid injection into the shoulder joint capsule is widely employed in treating rotator cuff lesions. Although there is little difference in long-term outcomes for steroid injection, physiotherapy, or NSAIDs, the rapid relief of pain and stiffness with injection is a significant advantage.[5] Steroid injection is better than other treatments at improving the range of movement.[6] Steroid injection should be avoided if there is any suggestion of bacterial infection in the joint.

Oral prednisolone is as effective as injected steroids. The starting dose should be 40 to 50 mg each morning, with tapering of the dose every 3 days, depending on the response. To place an injection within the capsular space, the lateral (subacromial) approach is the most popular (Fig. 76-1).

PREVENTIVE MEDICINE

Preventive medicine grows apace with other approaches. Prevention is classified as primary, secondary, or tertiary. Primary prevention aims to prevent a disease occurring. Secondary prevention involves controlling a disease early in its course to prevent complications. Tertiary prevention involves management of symptomatic disease to prevent further complications.

In palliative medicine, progressive disease and polypharmacy place patients at increased risk for drug interactions and toxicity.[7] The benefits of preventive interventions are measured in populations over many years. Patients with limited life expectancies are unlikely to obtain any benefit from preventive drugs during the remainder of their lives. Drug regimens need to be reviewed and modifications discussed with each patient. Great care needs to be taken in discussing possible changes with patients because many will see it as a further indication of their poor prognosis. The patient's life may seem less worthwhile and somewhat devalued. However, drugs have side effects, and the number of medications taken by palliative medicine patients imposes a considerable burden.

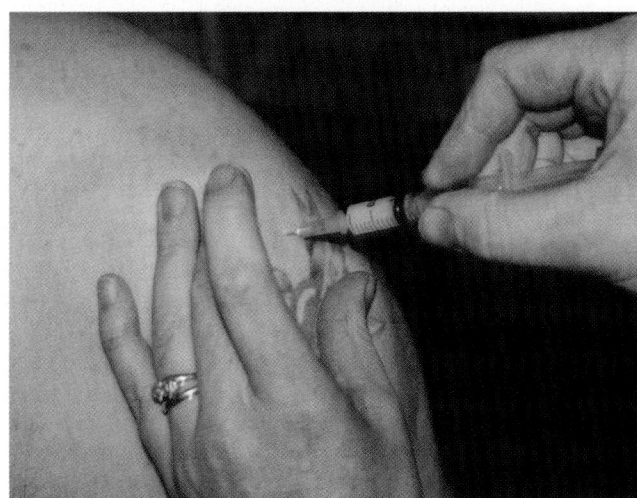

FIGURE 76-1 Injecting the subacromial bursa. Use aseptic technique and single-use ampules of steroid in a size G needle. The patient sits with the arm hanging loosely at the side. The acromion is the most lateral point of the shoulder; about 0.5 inch below this point, an indentation is felt. The needle is inserted at this point and advanced horizontally and slightly posteriorly under the acromion. Inject the steroid when the needle has been advanced to a depth of 1 inch.

TABLE 76-1	Preventive Drugs Whose Continued Use Should Be Reviewed	
DRUG	**INDICATION**	**COMMENT**
Statins and other lipid-lowering drugs	Primary and secondary prevention of cardiovascular and cerebrovascular disease	
Antihypertensives	Primary and secondary prevention of cardiovascular and cerebrovascular disease	Some medications may be needed to relieve symptoms in angina and cardiac failure.
Antiplatelet drugs (e.g., aspirin, clopidogrel, dipyridamole)	Primary and secondary prevention of cardiovascular and cerebrovascular disease	Drugs may be needed to control symptoms of angina and peripheral vascular disease.
Antidiabetic drugs	Secondary prevention of complications of diabetes	Dose may be reduced or stopped as less tight control of disease is indicated.
Warfarin	Secondary prevention of deep vein thrombosis or pulmonary embolus; stroke prevention in atrial fibrillation	If continued anticoagulation is deemed necessary, consider low-molecular-weight heparin.

Drugs affecting bone metabolism
   Bisphosphonates (e.g., alendronic acid, risedronate)
   Vitamin D and calcium
   Strontium ranelate
   Hormone replacement therapy
	Primary prevention of osteoporosis	Hormone replacement may be needed to control flushing or hot sweats.

Anti-obesity drugs (e.g., orlistat, sibutramine)	Prevention of obesity	

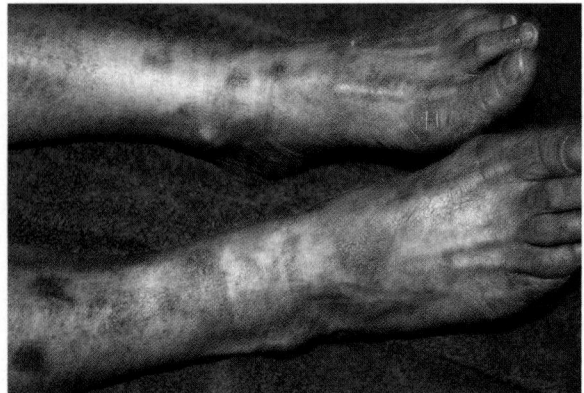

FIGURE 76-2 Eczema of both lower limbs with itchy, dry, scaly, erythematous patches.

ECZEMA

Eczema is inflammation of the skin. The terms *eczema* and *dermatitis* are synonymous (Fig. 76-2).

Pathophysiology

Eczema is caused by constitutional (endogenous) or external (exogenous) factors. External factors are allergens or irritants giving rise to allergic contact eczema or irritant contact eczema. In palliative medicine, most external agents are irritants. Endogenous eczemas include atopic eczema, seborrheic eczema, asteatotic eczema, discoid eczema, and varicose eczema. Eczema often results from a combination of endogenous and exogenous factors. A common scenario is someone whose skin is constitutionally dry, with a low lipid and water content, leading to a compromised skin barrier. Further damage on exposure to external irritants (e.g., cleansing agents, urine or feces, secretions around a feeding tube, ostomy, or fungating wound) results in eczema.

Clinical Manifestations

Acute eczema manifests with erythema, papules, vesicles, oozing, and crusting. Chronic eczema also manifests with erythema, but it is dry, thickened, and scaly (see Fig. 76-2).

Treatment

The cornerstone of management is irritant avoidance and regular emollient use. Irritants such as soap, bubble baths, and shampoos should be avoided. Moisturizers are formulated as lotions, creams, or ointments, depending on their lipid content. Lotions have the lowest lipid content, creams have intermediate content, and ointments have the highest lipid content. Generally, the greasier the emollient, the better. For dry skin, use an ointment, whereas a cream or lotion may be more acceptable for less affected skin. An emollient bath involves a soak for 20 minutes in moderately warm water to which an emollient has been added. A soap substitute, such as aqueous cream, is used for washing. Skin saturated with water looks pale and wrinkled. After a bath, a person has 3 minutes to trap this water in the skin because it rapidly evaporates. An emollient, such as an emulsifying ointment, is applied rapidly over water-saturated skin. It is easier to apply emollient to wet skin. Emollients should also be applied to the skin outside of bath time as often as necessary to keep skin soft and comfortable.

When eczema is active and itchy, a topical steroid should be applied. For chronic, dry eczema, use ointments. For acute, oozing eczema, use creams. A potent steroid such as betamethasone is acceptable and produces a prompt response (Table 76-1).

REFERENCES

1. Gillen D, McColl KE. Does concern about missing malignancy justify endoscopy in uncomplicated dyspepsia in patients less than 55? Am J Gastroenterol 1999;94:75-79.
2. Dent J, Armstrong D, Delaney B, et al. Symptom evaluation in reflux disease: Workshop background, processes, terminology, recommendations, and discussion outputs. Gut 2004;53:1-24.

3. Moayyedi P, Axon ATR. Gastro-oesophageal reflux disease: The extent of the problem. Aliment Pharmacol Ther 2005;22(Suppl 1):11-19.
4. Swartz MN. Cellulitis. N Engl J Med 2004;350:904-912.
5. Winters JC, Sobel JS, Groenier KH, et al. Comparison of physiotherapy, manipulation and steroid injection for treating shoulder complaints in general practice: A randomized single blind study. BMJ 1997;314:1320-1325.
6. Green S, Buchbinder R, Glazier R, et al. Systematic review of randomized controlled trials of interventions for painful shoulder: Selection criteria, outcome assessment, and efficacy. BMJ 1998;316:354-360.
7. Field TS, Gurwitz JH, Avorn J, et al. Risk factors for adverse drug events among nursing home residents. Arch Intern Med 2001;161:1629-1634.

SUGGESTED READING

Moayyedi P, Talley NJ. Gastro-oesophageal reflux disease. Lancet 2006;367:2086-2100.

Silver T. Joint and Soft Tissue Injection. Oxford, UK: Radcliffe Medical Press, 2002.

Swartz MN. Cellulitis. N Engl J Med 2004;350:904-912.

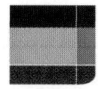

CHAPTER **77**

Common Musculoskeletal Co-morbidities

Neil McGill

KEY POINTS

- Nonsteroidal anti-inflammatory drugs (NSAIDs) and cyclooxygenase 2 (COX-2) inhibitors have increased toxicity in severe concurrent disease, especially if impaired renal function or fluid retention is present.
- Rheumatoid synovitis often responds to low-dose corticosteroid (e.g., prednisone 10 mg daily).
- Methotrexate is the foundation of disease-modifying therapy in rheumatoid arthritis.
- Biological therapies, especially anti-tumor necrosis factor (anti-TNF) agents, have an established role in rheumatoid arthritis, although a history of malignancy is a contraindication.

MUSCULOSKELETAL CHRONIC PAIN DISORDERS WITHOUT PHYSICAL PATHOLOGY

Fibromyalgia

The syndrome of diffuse pain and tenderness, sleep disturbance, and depressed or anxious mood is common. When these symptoms are present without physical disease, recognition is usually straightforward. Explanation, reassurance, regular exercise, and low-dose antidepressants are standard approaches, but many patients continue to report symptoms. The detection and management of physical disease in fibromyalgia is often difficult. The risks of dismissing the significance or severity of symptoms or, conversely, exposure to toxicity through

use of more potent therapies that are not required are both real. Communication with a clinician who has had a long-term relationship with the patient should be part of the assessment.

DEGENERATIVE JOINT, TENDON, AND BONE DISEASES

Osteoarthritis

Functional capacity in the elderly relates closely to muscle strength, and efforts to maintain or improve muscle strength and endurance should be encouraged in patients with osteoarthritis. Available medications produce only modest improvements in pain and function. Glucosamine, chondroitin, and paracetamol are safe.

Nonsteroidal anti-inflammatory drugs (NSAIDs) and cyclooxygenase 2 (COX-2) inhibitors produce greater short-term symptom control but are more toxic. Intercurrent illness produces an environment in which NSAID-induced peptic ulceration or renal impairment are more common. Chronic use of some COX-2 inhibitors increases stroke and cardiac risk; it is unclear whether that risk is shared by NSAIDs. All NSAIDs and COX-2 inhibitors increase blood pressure. In elderly patients with renal or cardiovascular disease and in intercurrent illness, NSAID and COX-2 inhibitor therapy should be avoided or used with caution and monitoring.

Joint replacement is effective at reducing pain, but the discomfort and risks associated with surgery make it appropriate only if life expectancy is greater than 1 year. Potent opioid analgesia has a relatively small role in osteoarthritis but can improve mobility and is appropriate if simple analgesia and a walking stick or frame prove insufficient and joint replacement is impossible or inappropriate.

Degenerative Spinal Disease

Well-controlled twin studies (comparing identical and nonidentical pairs) have shown the dominant genetic effect in the severity of cervical and lumbar spine degenerative disc disease. Invasive therapy (corticosteroid injection, surgery) has a role for persistent symptomatic neural compression but is usually inappropriate in other circumstances.

Rotator Cuff Disease

Degeneration of the rotator cuff tendons (often aggravated by impingement of the humeral head upward against the subacromial bursa and the cuff during abduction of the arm) represents the most common cause of shoulder pain. Muscle wasting caused by systemic disease aggravates impingement due to strength imbalance between the deltoid (which pulls the humeral head upward) and the infraspinatus and subscapularis (which stabilize the humeral head with downward force). Patients in bed often use the upper limbs to lift themselves and can aggravate rotator cuff symptoms. Acute pain flares can respond to a subacromial bursa corticosteroid injection. Specific exercise programs reduce impingement but usually need to be continued for a few months to achieve benefit.

Surgery is useful but must be followed by conscientious physical therapy.

OSTEOPOROSIS

Loss of bone mineral and strength produces clinical effects only when a fracture occurs. Vertebral fractures may occur without a recognized acute event, and then they manifest as a gradual progression of kyphosis or loss of height. The risk of fracture is influenced by bone density, likelihood of falling, corticosteroid therapy (additive to its effect on bone density), and whether a minimal trauma fracture (e.g., due to a fall from standing height) has occurred previously. A bone mineral density T score worse than −2.5 warrants therapy, which usually involves a bisphosphonate, calcium supplementation, and maintaining normal vitamin D levels. The oral bisphosphonates alendronate and risedronate must be used correctly to be safe and effective. Patients with concurrent illness, and particularly those confined to bed, are often unable to take the medication as directed—on an empty stomach, with tap water, and remaining erect (sitting or standing) to avoid reflux for at least 30 minutes and until eating. Intravenous bisphosphonates such as pamidronate and zoledronate do not have this limitation. Proof of fracture reduction exists for alendronate, risedronate, and zoledronate. Osteonecrosis of the jaw may occur, usually after tooth extraction, but most reported cases have occurred in patients with malignancy who were taking higher doses of bisphosphonate than used for osteoporosis. Raloxifene reduces vertebral fracture rates but has an increased risk of venous thromboembolism and stroke mortality.

CRYSTAL-INDUCED ARTHRITIS

Gout

The formation of monosodium urate monohydrate crystals, the critical step in the pathogenesis of gout, occurs over months and years. The acute attack, typically in the great toe metatarsophalangeal, midtarsal, ankle, or knee joint, occurs from rapid escalation of the inflammatory response to the crystals in the synovial membrane and synovial fluid. Changes in surface characteristics and in the protein coating of the urate crystals influence the intensity of the interaction between the inflammatory system, especially neutrophils, and the crystals. These changes most likely account for the propensity of gouty attacks to occur with sudden reduction of the serum uric acid level (e.g., when commencing allopurinol) and with intercurrent illness or surgery.

Bacterial infection and acute crystal-induced arthritis produce similar clinical features. Diagnosis requires synovial fluid aspiration and examination by polarized microscopy, Gram stain, and culture. Inflammatory markers, serum uric acid level, other blood tests and radiographs may assist management but do not replace synovial fluid analysis.

Treatment first consists of controlling the acute attack and later assessing whether hypouricemic drug therapy (usually a lifelong undertaking) is warranted. Management of the acute attack depends on the presence or absence of concurrent disorders. For an otherwise healthy indi-vidual, full-dose NSAID therapy for 1 to 3 weeks may suffice. Intra-articular or systemic corticosteroid therapy is effective and is usually safe and well tolerated. Low-dose colchicine (0.5 mg twice daily) prevents recurrence in the medium term. High-dose colchicine is rarely warranted, because better tolerated and safer options are available. Provided that life expectancy is greater than 12 months, measures to reduce the uric acid level below 0.36 mmol/L, 6 mg% are indicated in the presence of recurrent attacks not responding rapidly to safe therapy, tophi; erosions visible on radiographs, uric acid renal calculi, renal impairment, or symptoms persisting between attacks.

Weight reduction and decreased alcohol intake are important lifestyle variables. Allopurinol (xanthine oxidase inhibitor that decreases uric acid production) and probenecid (uricosuric that increases renal clearance of uric acid) are the common drug options.

Patients with malignancies that cause high cell turnover are likely to be hyperuricemic, but only those with chronic hyperuricemia (e.g., in myeloma, chronic lymphatic leukemia, myeloproliferative disorders) are at risk for gout. Acute severe hyperuricemia can cause uric acid nephropathy from tubular obstruction, but there is insufficient time for urate crystals to form. Allopurinol inhibits metabolism of azathioprine, and the combination should be avoided.

Calcium Pyrophosphate Deposition Disease

Calcium pyrophosphate dehydrate (CPPD) crystal deposition is common in the elderly, particularly in fibrocartilage such as the knee menisci, triangular fibrocartilage of the wrist, pubic symphysis, and intervertebral discs. If the patient is younger than 55 years of age, a search for an underlying disorder is worthwhile. Hemochromatosis (iron studies, ferritin); hyperparathyroidism (calcium, parathyroid hormone); hypomagnesemia, usually from renal wasting (magnesium); and hypophosphatasia (alkaline phosphatase) should be excluded, because the first three diagnoses influence management.

CPPD crystals can often be seen on radiographs (chondrocalcinosis), although the absence of chondrocalcinosis on radiography does not exclude CPPD as a potential cause of joint symptoms. The crystals can be found in patients with advanced age (without joint disease), osteoarthritis, previous trauma such as meniscectomy, chronic "pseudorheumatoid" synovitis, destructive arthritis resembling neuropathic arthropathy, and acute synovitis. It is the acute "pseudogout" presentation that is of greatest importance to the ill patient with concurrent disease. As in gout, synovial fluid aspiration for polarized microscopy, Gram stain, and culture is the key diagnostic investigation. Because CPPD crystals are more difficult to identify than urate crystals, prompt examination of the fluid by an experienced observer is valuable. Sepsis can coexist with pseudogout and, less commonly, with gout, and inflammatory synovial fluid should be cultured even if crystals have been identified.

Treatment involves settling the acute inflammatory episode with intra-articular corticosteroid, NSAID, or systemic corticosteroid. Prophylaxis is only rarely required (low-dose colchicine). If frequent recurrent attacks of pseudogout occur, a careful search for coexistent urate crystals (i.e., coexistent gout) is worthwhile.

RHEUMATOID ARTHRITIS

Rheumatoid arthritis affects 1% to 2% of the population, with a female preponderance. Knowledge of the pathogenesis and treatment of this most common chronic inflammatory synovitis has improved. Chronic synovial inflammation is characterized histologically by prominent perivascular T lymphocytes, plasma cells, and macrophages, driven by cytokines such as tumor necrosis factor (TNF) and interleukin-1 (IL1). This leads to the formation of pannus, a hyperemic, fibrovascular granulation tissue that invades and destroys cartilage and subchondral bone. Although joints bear the brunt, the disorder is systemic and, when active, typically causes malaise, lethargy, anemia, thrombocytosis, and hypoalbuminemia. Systemic involvement can include dry eyes and mouth (sicca symptoms), pulmonary fibrosis, pleural effusions, vasculitis (Fig. 77-1) with neuropathy, digital ischemia and leg ulceration, splenomegaly and lymphadenopathy, and amyloidosis (usually with proteinuria).

Although corticosteroids and, to a lesser extent, NSAIDs and COX-2 inhibitor drugs can provide symptomatic

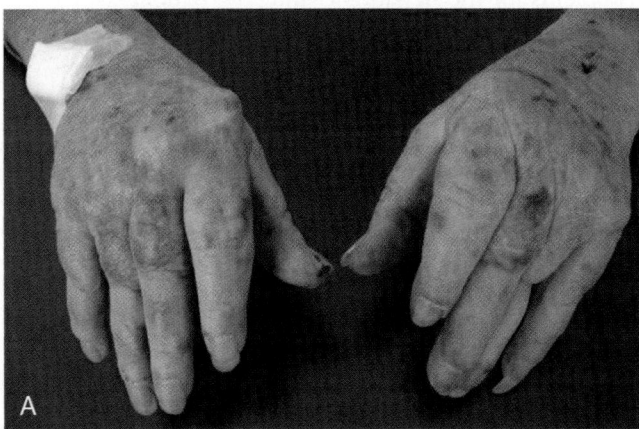

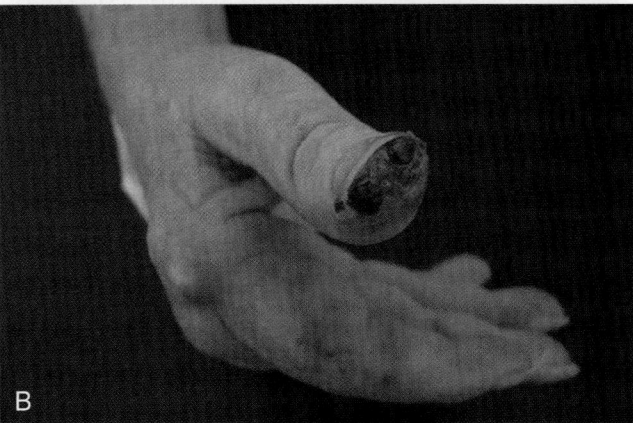

FIGURE 77-1 A and **B,** Rheumatoid arthritis with vasculitis. This 51-year-old woman with a 20-year history of rheumatoid arthritis developed vasculitis after withdrawal of immunosuppressive therapy because of an episode of pneumonia. Assessment of disease activity can be difficult in the presence of severe joint deformities; it is easy to underestimate activity in what appears to be "burnt out" chronic disease.

benefit, disease-modifying antirheumatic drugs (DMARDs) are the cutting edge of therapy. Remission on therapy is now a realistic and appropriate aim. Methotrexate, a folic acid antagonist, given weekly, either orally or subcutaneously, remains the foundation stone. The maintenance dose is usually 15 to 25 mg per week. Single-agent therapy with sulfasalazine (which is relatively weak and of low toxicity) or leflunomide (a pyrimidine antagonist with efficacy and toxicity similar to methotrexate) may be sufficient in some patients. Combinations that been proved to be more effective than methotrexate alone include methotrexate, sulfasalazine, and hydroxychloroquine; methotrexate and leflunomide; and methotrexate and cyclosporin.

Biological therapies, particularly anti-TNF agents such as etanercept (a fusion protein of human immunoglobulin G [IgG] and two p75 TNF receptors), infliximab (chimeric human/mouse IgG1 monoclonal antibody) and adalimumab (humanized IgG1 antibody), have improved the therapeutic options. The anti-TNF agents work better with methotrexate than as sole therapy; they improve symptoms, signs, function, and quality of life and reduce radiological evidence of joint damage.

Injection site and infusion reactions can occur, but the major drawbacks are infection (particularly reactivation of tuberculosis, frequently extrapulmonary) and expense. The risks of lupus-like syndromes, demyelination (multiple sclerosis, optic neuritis), and lymphoproliferative disease increase. A history of malignancy within 10 years, except for fully resected basal cell carcinoma treated more than 5 years ago, is a contraindication to anti-TNF therapy.

Other biological therapies, such as the anti–B cell antibody, rituximab, have an important role. Many other biological options are being investigated.

Potent drug therapy is appropriate only in active disease. Assessment of activity is usually simple in early disease but can be difficult with marked joint deformity, particularly if concurrent diseases might raise inflammatory markers. Careful assessment incorporating history, physical signs, and laboratory markers of inflammation is required, sometimes with a trial of (increased) DMARD therapy.

When patients become ill due to concurrent disease, especially if renal function becomes compromised, previously well tolerated and stable therapy can produce toxicity. If bone marrow suppression is likely due to malignancy or chemotherapy, it is usually prudent to retreat to single DMARD therapy, often at reduced dose. However, complete cessation of methotrexate often leads to rheumatoid reactivation, and frequent monitoring is often the appropriate strategy unless marrow suppression occurs; in that case, corticosteroid therapy becomes the best option, particularly if life expectancy is months rather than years.

SPONDYLOARTHROPATHIES

Among the spondyloarthropathies, ankylosing spondylitis, psoriatic spondyloarthropathy, reactive arthritis (Reiter's syndrome), and spondyloarthropathy associated with inflammatory bowel disease are the main entities. The spinal component of these diseases is managed similarly. Disease activity is characterized by prominent early morning stiffness and pain, which often forces patients out of bed early; improvement with activity; elevated inflammatory markers; and usually a substantial response to full-dose NSAIDs. Physical activity improves symptoms and function. Immobilization, such as during concurrent illness, increases pain. Enabling activity may reduce analgesic requirements. Ankylosing spondylitis with substantial symptoms from disease activity (not fixed spinal immobility) often warrants anti-TNF therapy, usually without concurrent methotrexate or other DMARD, in contrast to its use for rheumatoid arthritis.

Psoriatic arthritis can present several different patterns, including dactylitis (diffuse swelling of a finger or toe), distal interphalangeal joint involvement, oligoarthritis, and severe destructive synovitis (arthritis mutilans). Although benefit from DMARD therapy has been harder to demonstrate than in rheumatoid arthritis, the approach is similar, including the use of anti-TNF agents, which help both skin and joint manifestations.

CONNECTIVE TISSUE DISEASES

The management of systemic lupus erythematosus (SLE), scleroderma (Fig. 77-2), and overlap connective tissue diseases depends on which organ systems are involved rather than the diagnostic label. Assessment includes seeking esophageal, lung, pulmonary, vascular, muscle, and renal involvement. Skin, joint, or peripheral vascular (Raynaud's) involvement is usually obvious. Specific treatment options are complex but can include proton pump inhibitor therapy for esophagitis, hydroxychloroquine for skin and joint involvement and prevention of SLE flares, and calcium channel blockers for Raynaud's disease. Digital ischemia complicating scleroderma is common in the cold months of the year (Fig. 77-3) and can be treated with intravenous vasodilators such as prostaglandin. Glomerulonephritis, interstitial pneumonitis, and myositis often require aggressive corticosteroid and immunosuppressive therapy.

INFECTION AND THE MUSCULOSKELETAL SYSTEM

Septic Arthritis

Although septic arthritis can cause rapid severe joint damage, there are major advantages in obtaining all appropriate specimens (at least from the joint and blood) before antibiotic therapy is initiated. Oral antibiotics are almost never sufficient but can complicate and delay effective therapy by making isolation of the organism more difficult. Particularly in ill patients, sepsis involving the vertebral column, sacroiliac, and hip joints can be difficult to detect. Magnetic resonance imaging is the most useful imaging method, but aspiration remains the key diagnostic step.

Human Immunodeficiency Virus Infection

In addition to an increased risk of bacterial septic arthritis, human immunodeficiency virus (HIV) infection can be associated with aggressive reactive arthritis and with lightening limb pains without arthritis.

Hepatitis C Infection

Rheumatoid factor is present in up to 75% of hepatitis C–positive patients. Differentiating the nonerosive, usually mild and fluctuating inflammatory synovitis of hepatitis C from the threatening synovitis of rheumatoid arthritis can be difficult. In patients with rheumatoid arthritis, concurrent hepatitis C infection requires more careful monitoring of DMARD therapy. Although caution is warranted, thus far anti-TNF therapy appears not to cause additional problems for the hepatitis C–infected patient.

Hepatitis B Infection

Immunosuppressive therapy, such as that used to treat for rheumatoid arthritis or SLE, can allow increased hepatitis B viral replication. When immunosuppressive therapy is withdrawn, a severe flare of liver inflammation and damage can result. Prophylactic antiviral agents with activity against hepatitis B should be considered in the presence of ongoing viral replication before, during, and after immunosuppressive therapy.

MALIGNANCY-ASSOCIATED MUSCULOSKELETAL DISORDERS

Dermatomyositis in adults is associated with malignancy in about 30% of cases. Removal of the tumor can, but does

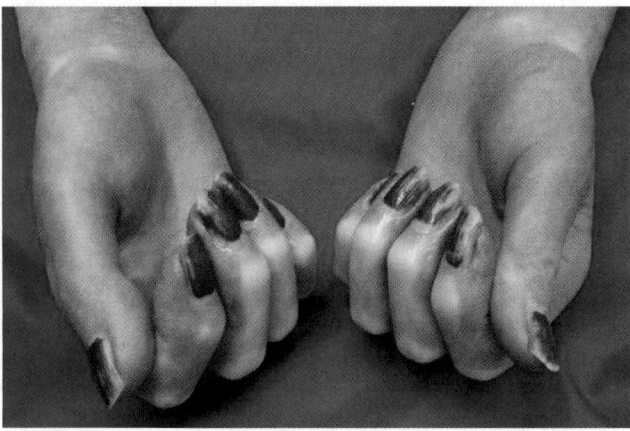

FIGURE 77-2 Scleroderma. This 75-year-old woman had a 15-year history of Raynaud's disease and progressive loss of hand mobility over the last 5 years. She is trying to make a tight fist.

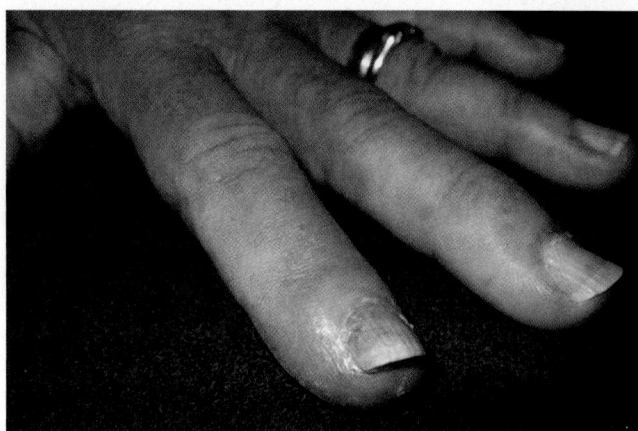

FIGURE 77-3 Digital ischemia complicating scleroderma during winter.

not always, result in remission. Diagnostic investigations include creatine kinase, nailfold capillaroscopy, electromyography, and muscle biopsy.

Hypertrophic pulmonary osteoarthropathy is associated with clubbing in most patients. It occurs most commonly in non–small cell lung cancer but also in pulmonary fibrosis, bronchiectasis, right-to-left cardiac shunts, severe liver disease, bacterial endocarditis, and some other disorders. Symptoms resolve if the offending cause can be removed or cured. NSAIDs, corticosteroids, and anticholinergic agents provide symptom relief.

SUGGESTED READING

Herrick AL. Advances in palliative care for the patient with scleroderma. Curr Opin Rheumatol 1996;8:555-560.

Hochberg MC, Silman AJ, Smolen JS, et al (eds). Rheumatology, 3rd ed. Edinburgh: Mosby, 2003.

Kavanaugh A, Tutuncu Z, Catalan-Sanchez T. Update on anti-tumor necrosis factor therapy in the spondyloarthropathies including psoriatic arthritis. Curr Opin Rheumatol 2006;18: 347-353.

Scott DL, Kingsley GH. Tumor necrosis factor inhibitors for rheumatoid arthritis. N Engl J Med 2006;355:704-712.

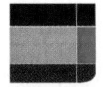

CHAPTER **78**

Diabetes Mellitus

Mary Lynn McPherson

KEY POINTS

- Diabetes mellitus is growing in prevalence in the general population and is a common co-morbid condition in patients with advanced illness. Most of these patients have type 2 diabetes mellitus, and an even larger percentage have prediabetes.

- The goal of care for diabetes at the end of life is to primarily prevent symptoms of blood glucose excursions (hyperglycemia and hypoglycemia). Blood glucose control can be liberalized to 140 to 300 mg/dL provided the patient remains asymptomatic.

- The diet should be liberalized in the terminally ill; the patient and family should be reassured that this does not represent "giving up," but rather a shift in the goals of care.

- Patients with type 1 diabetes will likely continue to require insulin therapy until close to death to prevent diabetic ketoacidosis. Many achieve adequate control with once- or twice-daily injections of intermediate- or long-acting insulin.

- Patients with type 2 diabetes may not require pharmacotherapeutic management as their appetite lessens and oral intake declines. Practitioners should avoid drug therapy options that worsen co-morbid conditions or symptoms.

- Corticosteroid-induced diabetes is a common finding at the end of life; the primary metabolic finding is postprandial hyperglycemia.

Diabetes mellitus is a metabolic syndrome characterized by hyperglycemia due to insufficient insulin secretion, insufficient insulin action, or both. The incidence continues to grow, and some experts claim a worldwide epidemic. Reasons include the aging population; obesity resulting from a high-carbohydrate, high-fat diet; and a culture that promotes overeating and discourages exercise. Given the increased diabetes in the general population, palliative care practitioners will increasingly be required to address this chronic condition. Patients are not usually admitted to hospice or palliative care with a terminal diagnosis of diabetes per se, but diabetes-related complications can cause death. More commonly, diabetes is a co-morbid condition in patients with life-limiting illnesses.

Despite guidelines on diagnosis and management from the American Diabetes Association and other groups, there is little guidance on managing diabetes at the end of life. Focus groups and surveys of practitioners who care for patients with diabetes and advanced disease have failed to reach consensus.[1,2]

EPIDEMIOLOGY AND PREVALENCE

The American Diabetes Association estimates that almost 21 million children and adults in the United States have diabetes mellitus (about 7% of the population); of these, 6.2 million are undiagnosed. About 1.5 million new cases were diagnosed in people 20 years of age or older in 2005, and about 54 million people are estimated to have "prediabetes," in which glucose levels are higher than normal, but not enough to be diagnostic.[3] Among people 60 years of age or older, 10.3 million, or almost 21%, have diabetes. There are differences in prevalence by race and ethnicity: high-risk groups include Asian Americans and Pacific Islanders, American Indians and Alaska Natives, Hispanic Latino Americans, and non-Hispanic blacks.

Diabetes in Advanced Disease

People with life-limiting illnesses are more likely to have diabetes than the general population. In 2005, four out of five hospice patients were 65 years of age or older, and one third were 85 years or older.[4] Diabetes is more prevalent in older populations, as are life-limiting illnesses. More than 1.2 million patients received hospice care in 2005; if 21% had diabetes, the importance of appropriate management at the end of life is clear. The National Hospice and Palliative Care Organization (NHPCO) also reported that approximately 50% of patients who received hospice services in 2005 had a primary diagnosis of cancer.

Classification

There are two broad categories of diabetes, as well as several additional minority categories.[5] The two primary classifications are type 1 and type 2 diabetes mellitus. Type 1 diabetes represents about 4% to 5% of the cases and is characterized by autoimmune destruction of the beta pancreatic cells. These patients are dependent on exogenous insulin administration for survival, having little or no endogenous insulin secretion.

Type 2 diabetes accounts for about 90% to 95% of the cases, and the pathogenesis includes insulin resistance and a relative lack of insulin production. Therapeutic strategies aim at improving insulin sensitivity and action and enhancing insulin secretion. Most patients do not require exogenous insulin administration initially and may never require insulin for survival. There are many possible causes of type 2 diabetes, but it probably is not caused by autoimmune processes. In the large population with undiagnosed diabetes (mostly undiscovered type 2 diabetes), hyperglycemia develops gradually and symptoms may not be recognized.

BASIC SCIENCE

Glucose homeostasis is complex, involving extensive neuroendocrine processes and hormones. The aroma of food sends signals to the gut to prepare by increasing digestive juices containing gastric acid and digestive enzymes. Incretin peptides secreted from the distal stomach and proximal small intestine (e.g., glucagon-like peptide-1 [GLP-1], glucose-dependent insulinotropic peptic [GIP]) stimulate insulin release from the pancreas and facilitate glucose uptake by peripheral tissues.

In response to a meal, insulin is secreted from the beta pancreatic cells in two phases. The first phase is a rapid burst over about 10 minutes; this comes from storage granules close to the cell membrane surface. This burst of insulin inhibits liver glucose production, which maintains euglycemia during fasting. After a meal, hepatic glucose production (glycogenolysis) is no longer needed. The second phase of insulin secretion facilitates glucose uptake by peripheral tissues. By binding to cell surface receptors, insulin mediates the following:

- Storage of glucose as glycogen in the liver and muscles (glycogenesis)
- Synthesis of fatty acids and triglycerides and their storage in adipose tissue (lipogenesis)
- Incorporation of amino acids into proteins
- Inhibition of fat breakdown (lipolysis) and of formation of ketones (ketogenesis)

Later, the blood glucose level falls, and the body shifts to producing glucose from glycogen in muscles and the liver (glycogenolysis), from amino acids and lactate (gluconeogenesis), and, if necessary, from fat (lipolysis). Glucagon and other counter-regulatory hormones (e.g., cortisol, epinephrine, growth hormones) increase blood glucose levels. During this period, a small amount of insulin is continuously secreted, to facilitate glycolysis (entry of glucose into the cells to serve as an energy substrate). During a 24-hour period, about 50% of the insulin secreted is "basal" insulin (i.e., secreted around the clock); the remainder is in response to meals and snacks.

PATHOPHYSIOLOGY

Type 1 diabetes mellitus is predominantly an autoimmune disease, with destruction of 90% or more of the beta pancreatic cells. Patients usually have circulating islet cell antibodies and autoantibodies against insulin and islet cell proteins. People with type 1 diabetes have an absolute lack of insulin production (insulinopenic) and require insulin replacement for both basal and bolus needs. Amylin, a beta cell hormone cosecreted with insulin after meals, is also absent in type 1 diabetes. Amylin has several glucoregulatory actions that complement insulin in glucose disposi-

tion. Those with type 1 diabetes may or may not receive an "amylinomimetic" agent during therapy.

There are about twice as many people with "prediabetes," or impaired glucose tolerance, as there are people with diabetes mellitus. They frequently have metabolic syndrome (insulin resistance, hyperinsulinemia, obesity, hypertension, and dyslipidemia). Impaired glucose tolerance may remain stable, improve (with weight loss, exercise, and removal of medications that increase blood glucose), or deteriorate to frank diabetes.

Impaired glucose tolerance usually progresses to type 2 diabetes. Patients are usually obese (primarily abdominal obesity) and physically inactive. Insulin resistance, defined as a diminished ability of peripheral tissues to respond to insulin, results in hyperinsulinemia. Insulin is less effective at suppressing hepatic glucose production and facilitating glucose uptake by muscle and adipose tissue. This may be caused by downregulation of insulin receptors or by defects in the glucose transporter protein. Over time, patients with type 2 diabetes are unable to supply the insulin needed to overcome insulin resistance, and insulin production diminishes. Initially, only the first phase of insulin secretion is affected, but eventually both phases become impaired. The impaired ability to suppress hepatic glucose production worsens hyperglycemia. Those with type 2 diabetes also have diminished secretion of amylin and incretin hormones. Pharmacologic interventions in type 2 diabetes aim at improving insulin sensitivity and action and enhancing or mimicking the secretion of insulin, amylin, and incretin hormones.

CLINICAL MANIFESTATIONS

Usually, diabetes predates the need for palliative care services, but this is not always the case. For example, if a patient with impaired glucose tolerance is started on a corticosteroid for palliative purposes, blood glucose control may worsen and precipitate frank diabetes. Most patients with diabetes remain undiagnosed (Box 78-1), probably because the symptoms are not recognized as abnormal. Symptoms include the following: frequent uri-

---

Box 78-1 Criteria for the Diagnosis of Diabetes Mellitus

1. Symptoms of diabetes plus casual plasma glucose concentrations >200 mg/dL. Casual is defined as any time of day without regard to time since last meal. The classic symptoms of diabetes are polyuria, polydipsia, and unexplained weight loss.
   OR
2. Fasting plasma glucose ≥126 mg/dL. Fasting is defined as no caloric intake for at least 8 hours.
   OR
3. Two-hour postloading glucose ≥200 mg/dL during an oral glucose tolerance test (OGTT). The test should be performed as described by the World Health Organization (WHO), using a glucose load containing the equivalent of 75 g anhydrous glucose dissolved in water.

Note: In the absence of unequivocal hyperglycemia, these criteria should be confirmed by repeat testing on a different day. The third measure (OGTT) is not recommended for routine clinical use.

Adapted from American Diabetes Association. Diagnosis and classification of diabetes mellitus. Diabetes Care 2007;30(Suppl 1):S42-S47

nation (including nocturia), excessive thirst, extreme hunger, increased fatigue, irritability, unusual weight loss, and blurred vision. Patients at the end of life rarely present acutely with confusion, altered consciousness, or hyperglycemic emergencies (diabetic ketoacidosis or hyperglycemic, hyperosmolar nonketotic syndrome).

In life-limiting illness, it can be difficult to differentiate symptoms of glucose intolerance from those of the terminal illness. For example, nausea and vomiting may be caused by poorly controlled diabetes or by advanced disease. Patients with diabetes experience altered utilization of glucose, with mobilization of protein and fat stores, which frequently causes weight loss, weakness, and lethargy; these are also common symptoms of advanced disease. Although this point is controversial, diabetes doubles the odds of co-morbid depression, which is also a common co-morbid condition in advanced disease.[6] Even over the short term, worse blood glucose control has been associated with lower quality of life, cognitive function, and general perceived health; these complaints are highly consistent with the end-of-life experience as well.[7] It is equally important to recognize complaints suggestive of hypoglycemia, a significant risk to patients with diabetes at the end of life. Symptoms include hunger, nervousness and shakiness, dizziness or lightheadedness, sweating, sleepiness, confusion, difficulty speaking, weakness, and anxiety. Again, these symptoms may be consistent with other end-of-life diagnoses.

DIFFERENTIAL DIAGNOSIS

Diabetes mellitus may be classified as primary or secondary, although the principles of management are similar for both. Primary diabetes includes both types 1 and 2 diabetes. Patients with type 1 tend to be close to ideal body weight at diagnosis and are typically younger than those with type 2 diabetes. Type 2 patients are usually overweight with a sedentary lifestyle. Use of the terms insulin-dependent diabetes mellitus (IDDM) and non–insulin-dependent diabetes mellitus (NIDDM) to indicate type 1 and type 2 diabetes, respectively, is no longer recommended. Although patients with type 2 diabetes may not strictly be "dependent" on insulin, as type 1 patients are, for survival, they account for most of the insulin use in the United States. It is helpful to know whether the patient has type 1 or type 2 diabetes, because this determines the absolute versus relative need for insulin.

Diabetes may develop secondary to pancreatic disease (e.g., cancer, pancreatectomy, chronic pancreatitis) or an endocrine disorder (e.g., Cushing's disease, acromegaly); it may be nutrition induced (enteral or parenteral nutrition products) or drug induced. More than 100 medications can cause hyperglycemia. Examples commonly used in palliative care include diuretics, β-adrenergic blocking agents, antipsychotic agents, antidepressants, octreotide, and corticosteroids.

Corticosteroids (e.g., dexamethasone, prednisone) are commonly used in palliative care. A prospective study of dexamethasone in a palliative care unit showed that only 2 of 83 patients experienced hyperglycemia (one mild, one moderate) during a median treatment duration of 21.5 days.[8] Others have shown a much higher incidence of steroid-induced hyperglycemia (40% to 55%) during short-duration steroid treatment and an adjusted odds ratio of 2.31.[9-11] The mechanism is probably multifactorial. Glucocorticoids increase gluconeogenesis and cause insulin resistance, probably by interfering with intracellular glucose metabolism, decreasing glucose transport, and/or effects on insulin receptor binding.[12,13] The result is postprandial hyperglycemia. It is important not to rely on fasting glucose determinations for potential steroid-induced hyperglycemia, but to check the 2-hour postprandial glucose level.

TREATMENT

Goals of Care

The Diabetes Control and Complications Trial (DCCT) demonstrated that intensive insulin therapy (multiple daily injections or an insulin pump) can delay the onset and slow the progression of retinopathy, nephropathy, and neuropathy in type 1 diabetes.[14] Similarly, for every 1% reduction in glycosylated hemoglobin (HbA1c), there was a 37% reduction in microvascular complications and a 21% reduction in risk of any end point related to diabetes.[15,16] Glycosylated hemoglobin measures longer-term blood glucose control (e.g., 2 to 3 months). The American Diabetes Association has offered metabolic goals designed to decrease and delay diabetes-related complications. These include an HbA1c level of less than 7.0% (or even 6.0% if possible), a preprandial capillary plasma glucose level of 90 to 130 mg/dL, a peak postprandial capillary plasma glucose level of less than 180 mg/dL, and other goals for blood pressure and lipids.[17]

Goals in Advanced Disease

Although these goals are appropriate for patients not facing a life-limiting illness, they do not make as much sense for those with a limited life expectancy. One guideline emphasizes[18] the importance of individualized goals, and states, "For frail older adults, persons with life expectancy of less than 5 years, and others in whom the risks of intensive glycemic control appear to outweigh the benefits, a less stringent target such as 8% [HbA1c] is appropriate."

When dealing with advanced disease, the HbA1c value may no longer be useful, and the patient's stress may be increased by trying to achieve an inappropriate target. Even the preprandial and postprandial plasma glucose goals are less meaningful in life-limiting illness. Every intervention for the palliative care patient should be preceded by the question, "Will this make the patient more comfortable?" Continuing to strive for blood glucose goals designed to curtail long-term complications will not improve comfort and may render the patient more uncomfortable from the increased risk of hypoglycemia and the suffering associated with painful blood glucose monitoring.

In the absence of evidence-based or consensus guidelines, it seems reasonable to establish the following goals of care for diabetes in life-limiting illness:

- Prevent symptoms of hyperglycemia
- Prevent symptoms of hypoglycemia
- Target a blood glucose range of 140 to 300 mg/dL during the last weeks of life (unless there is symptomatic hyperglycemia)

Blood glucose monitoring should be performed as clinically indicated. For example, in someone not close to death, it would be reasonable to continue monitoring blood glucose as usual. For patients considerably closer to death, it may be reasonable to discontinue blood glucose monitoring altogether. Blood glucose monitoring in 18 terminally ill patients with type 2 diabetes who stopped receiving diabetic treatment at the onset of the terminal phase of their illness showed that blood glucose levels did not rise in dying patients with type 2 diabetes, even when their pharmacologic therapies were discontinued.[19]

Nondrug Measures

The initial management of type 2 diabetes is lifestyle modification, including medical nutrition therapy and physical activity. People with life-limiting illnesses are unlikely to participate in a physical activity program. Their diet should also be liberalized, although many patients and families or caregivers may perceive this as "giving up." It is important to discuss with them that this change is not "giving up" but rather a shift in the goals of care. As patients decline, their appetite naturally abates, and failure to recognize this fact increases the risk for drug-induced hypoglycemia.

Pharmacotherapeutic Options

Insulin

Insulin products (Table 78-1) are used in various combinations to provide both basal and bolus insulin action in type 1 and advanced type 2 diabetes. About 50% of the insulin secreted over a 24-hour period is "basal" insulin. Basal insulin delivery can be replicated with a continuous infusion via insulin pump or with injections of intermediate-acting insulin (e.g., NPH, Lente) twice daily or long-acting insulin (e.g., glargine, detemir) once or twice daily. Glargine insulin is virtually peakless insulin; it usually is administered once a day at bedtime. Short- and rapid-acting insulins are used as "bolus" insulins. One popular combination regimen is regular plus NPH insulin taken before breakfast and before dinner. The intent is that the prebreakfast regular insulin will cover breakfast, and the NPH will cover lunch. Similarly, the predinner regular insulin will cover that meal, and the predinner NPH will cover the overnight period. Unfortunately, once administered, insulin cannot be removed. A prebreakfast NPH insulin dose (intended to cover lunch), in a very sick patient who decides he cannot eat lunch, is a recipe for disaster.

Oral Hypoglycemic Agents

Patients with type 2 diabetes are usually treated with oral medications (Table 78-2) if lifestyle modification is insufficient. There is a consensus algorithm for the initiation and adjustment of therapy for hyperglycemia in type 2 diabetes.[20] Principles that guided this algorithm include medication effectiveness, extraglycemic effects, safety profiles, tolerability, and expense. Metformin is one of the most widely used oral antidiabetes medications, and it is a step 1 agent in this consensus. A biguanide, metformin acts primarily by decreasing hepatic glucose output, and lowering fasting glucose. It is well tolerated, with gastrointestinal upset being the most common adverse effect. Metformin is unlikely to cause hypoglycemia as monotherapy. Very rarely (1 in 100,000 cases), lactic acidosis may occur. Metformin is best avoided when accumulation

TABLE 78-1 Insulin and Injectable Products

GENERIC NAME	TRADE NAME	ONSET OF ACTION	PEAK ACTION	EFFECTIVE DURATION
RAPID-ACTING INSULIN				
Lispro	Humalog	5-15 min	30-90 min	3-5 hr
Aspart	NovoLog	5-15 min	30-90 min	3-5 hr
Glulisine	Apidra	5-15 min	30-90 min	3-5 hr
SHORT-ACTING INSULIN				
Regular	Humulin R Novolin R	30-60 min	2-3 hr	5-8 hr
INTERMEDIATE-ACTING INSULIN				
NPH	Humulin N Novolin N	2-4 hr	4-10 hr	10-16 hr
Lente	Humulin L Novolin L	3-4 hr	4-12 hr	12-18 hr
LONG-ACTING INSULIN				
Glargine	Lantus	2-4 hr	Peakless	20-24 hr
Detemir	Levemir	2-4 hr	6-14 hr	16-20 hr
COMBINATION INSULIN PRODUCTS				
70/30 (70% NPH/30% regular)	Humulin 70/30 Novolin 70/30	30-60 min	Dual	10-16 hr
50/50 (50% NPH/50% regular)	Humulin 50/50	30-60 min	Dual	10-16 hr
Lispro mix 75/25 (75% NPL/25% lispro)	Humalog Mix 75/25	15-30 min	Dual	10-16 hr
Lispro mix 50/50 (50% NPL/50% lispro)	Humalog Mix 50/50	15-30 min	Dual	10-16 hr
Aspart mix 70/30 (70% aspart protamine/30% aspart)	NovoLog Mix 70/30	15-30 min	Dual	10-16 hr

TABLE 78-2   Noninsulin Antidiabetic Agents

GENERIC NAME	TRADE NAME	Dosage		COMMENTS
		SD	MDD	
SULFONYLUREAS (2nd GENERATION)				
Glyburide	DiaBeta, Micronase	1.25-5 mg qd	20 mg in 1-2 divided doses	Administer qd doses with breakfast or first main meal. Intermediate to long duration of action, active metabolites.
Glyburide, micronized	Glynase	0.75-3 mg qd	12 mg in 1-2 divided doses	Administer qd doses with breakfast or first main meal. Long duration of action, active metabolites.
Glipizide	Glucotrol	2.5-5 mg qd	40 mg in 2 divided doses	Administer qd doses 30 min before breakfast or first main meal. Doses >15 mg/day should be divided and given bid. Short to intermediate duration of action, inactive metabolites.
Glipizide, extended release	Glucotrol XL	5 mg qd	20 mg qd	Administer with breakfast. Intermediate duration of action, inactive metabolites.
Glimepiride	Amaryl	1-2 mg qd	8 mg qd	Administer with breakfast or first main meal. Intermediate to long duration of action, active metabolites.
MEGLITINIDES				
Repaglinide	Prandin	*If hypoglycemic, agent naïve, or HbA1c <8%:* 0.5 mg tid *If previously treated with hypoglycemics or HbA1c >8%:* 1-2 mg tid	16 mg/day	Administer within 15–30 min of each meal (consider administering after a meal for patients with erratic oral intake).
Nateglinide	Starlix	60 mg tid	180 mg tid	
BIGUANIDES				
Metformin	Glucophage	500 mg bid or 850 mg every morning	2550 mg in 3 divided doses	Administer with meals. Contraindicated if creatinine >1.5 (males) or 1.4 (female); hold for patients with congestive heart failure requiring pharmacological treatments.
Metformin, sustained release	Glucophage XR	500 mg every evening; then 500 mg/day/wk	2000 mg qd	
α-GLUCOSIDASE INHIBITORS				
Acarbose	Precose	25 mg tid	*If >60 kg:* 100 mg tid *If ≤60 kg:* 50 mg tid	Administer with first bite of each main meal. If patient skips a meal, hold dose.
Miglitol	Glyset	25 mg tid	100 mg tid	
THIAZOLIDINEDIONES				
Rosiglitazone	Avandia	4 mg qd or 2 mg bid	8 mg qd or 4 mg bid	May be given without regard to meals. May cause fluid retention and weight gain; may worsen heart failure.
Pioglitazone	Actos	15-30 mg qd	45 mg qd	May be given without regard to meals; 45 mg dose studied only as monotherapy. May cause fluid retention and weight gain; may worsen heart failure.
DIPEPTIDYL PEPTIDASE-4 (DPP-4) INHIBITOR				
Sitagliptin	Januvia*	100 mg qd	100 mg qd	Take with or without food. Adjust dose with renal impairment.
INCRETIN MIMETIC				
Exenatide	Byetta†	5 µg bid	10 µg bid	Injected SQ within 60 min before morning and evening meals. Do not administer WITH meals.
AMYLINOMIMETIC				
Pramlintide	Symlin	*Type 1 DM:* 15 µg before major meals *Type 2DM:* 60 µg before major meals	*Type 1 DM:* 60 µg before major meals *Type 2DM:* 120 µg before major meals	Inject SQ immediately before a major meal (defined as ≥250 kcal or ≥30 g carbohydrate)

*Januvia home page. Available at http://www.merck.com/product/usa/pi_circulars/j/januvia/januvia_pi.pdf (accessed October 2007).
†Byetta home page. Available at http://pi.lilly.com/us/byetta-pi.pdf (accessed October 2007).
DM, diabetes mellitus; MDD, maximum daily dose; SD, starting dose.

may occur, such as in renal impairment (serum creatinine ≥ 1.5 mg/dL for men, ≥ 1.4 mg/dL for women; creatinine clearance ≤ 60 mL/min and age ≥ 80 years are relative contraindications), hepatic impairment, or chronic heart failure. Metformin either does not affect body weight or causes some weight loss, which is beneficial in most type 2 patients, but not necessarily in the terminally ill.

If lifestyle modification and metformin therapy are insufficient, the consensus recommends a step 2 agent such as insulin, a sulfonylurea, or thiazolidinedione. Sulfonylureas act by enhancing insulin secretion from beta pancreatic cells. They are very effective at lowering blood glucose. Their major adverse effect is hypoglycemia, which can be severe in patients with impaired hepatic and/or renal function. First-generation agents (e.g., chlorpropamide, acetohexamide, tolazamide, tolbutamide) are rarely used now. The pharmacokinetic characteristics of the sulfonylureas influence decision making in advanced disease. All sulfonylureas are metabolized by the liver. They should be avoided in hepatic impairment, or, alternatively, a short-acting sulfonylurea (e.g., glipizide) should be used, starting at a low dose and titrating slowly. Similarly, short-acting glipizide is probably the best sulfonylurea for patients with renal impairment, because it is metabolized to inactive products.

Thiazolidinediones (pioglitazone, rosiglitazone) are "insulin sensitizers." They serve as agonists for peroxisome proliferator–activated receptor-γ (PPAR-γ), increasing glucose uptake in skeletal muscle, liver, and fat cells. Secondarily, the thiazolidinediones may also suppress liver gluconeogenesis, lowering hepatic glucose output. The thiazolidinediones are not as effective as metformin or the sulfonylureas at lowering blood glucose. Adverse effects include edema (first noted with combination rosiglitazone and insulin therapy), which may exacerbate chronic heart failure; weight gain; anemia; headache; myalgias; and hepatotoxicity (troglitazone was taken off market several years ago). The thiazolidinediones are unlikely to cause hypoglycemia when used as monotherapy. Reports of an increased risk of myocardial infarction and all-cause cardiovascular mortality with rosiglitazone exist.[21] The mechanism is uncertain but may be related to the adverse effect of rosiglitazone on the lipid profile. Some claim it is too early to draw definitive conclusions, but it is best to avoid thiazolidinediones in patients with heart failure.

Patients with type 2 diabetes who are taking one, two, or perhaps even three oral antidiabetes medications who have not achieved adequate blood glucose control may benefit from the addition of basal insulin (once- or twice-daily NPH, detemir, or glargine).

Supplemental Agents

The consensus guidelines also list "other drugs" for type 2 diabetes should step 1 and step 2 agents be insufficient. These include the α-glucosidase inhibitors (acarbose and miglitol), exenatide, pramlintide, and the glinides (repaglinide and nateglinide). The α-glucosidase inhibitors reduce polysaccharide digestion in the small intestine, lowering postprandial glucose levels. The most common adverse effect is increased gas production and gastrointestinal symptoms, which a significant number of patients

find unacceptable. Exenatide is a GLP-1 agonist and stimulates insulin secretion. Administered by subcutaneous injection twice daily, exenatide primarily reduces postprandial glucose. The primary adverse effects are gastrointestinal (e.g., nausea, vomiting, diarrhea) and affect up to 45% of patients. Sitagliptin is a dipeptidyl-peptidase inhibitor; it blocks the enzyme that inactivates and degrades incretin hormones (GLP-1 and GIP). Sitagliptin is administered once daily and has an adverse effect profile similar to placebo (primarily gastrointestinal effects and hypoglycemia). Pramlintide is an amylin agonist that is administered subcutaneously before meals. It slows gastric emptying, inhibiting glucagon production and decreasing postprandial glucose. About one third of patients experience nausea with pramlintide, and it may cause weight loss.

The oral antidiabetes medications referred to as "glinides" deserve special mention. The glinides stimulate pancreatic insulin secretion, similar to the sulfonylureas, but they bind to a different site within the sulfonylurea receptor. Repaglinide and nateglinide are the only available agents; they have a much shorter half-life than sulfonylureas, and they are administered more frequently (e.g., with each meal). Because they increase insulin secretion, they may cause hypoglycemia, although less frequently than the sulfonylureas.

DRUGS OF CHOICE AND SUPPORTIVE CARE

The management of diabetes in palliative care ranges from usual and customary care and no intervention at all, depending on the patient's prognosis, quality of life, and degree of symptomatology. Those who are still active and have an acceptable quality of life should continue their usual diabetes therapy if it is not too burdensome; blood glucose monitoring should be continued, at a longer but sufficient interval, to ensure that the patient is stable and symptom free. On the other end of the spectrum, persons who are within days of death (and may be unconscious) probably will not receive any antidiabetes therapy or blood glucose monitoring. It is the scenarios that fall between these two extremes that are problematic for practitioners, patients, families, and caregivers. First, it is important to remember the goals of care (see earlier discussion). Most would agree that long-term blood glucose control and the prevention of chronic complications is not important for terminally ill patients, but that it is important to prevent symptoms related to blood glucose excursions.

Some data suggest that tight blood glucose control in patients in intensive care units (ICUs) reduces morbidity and mortality in the short term, and a parallel has been drawn to patients with advanced illness. Patients admitted to an ICU (most after cardiac surgery) with hyperglycemia were randomized to conventional versus intensive insulin infusion therapy.[22] A team of ICU nurses and a study physician adjusted the insulin every 1 to 4 hours to maintain blood glucose between 80 and 110 mg/dL. Results showed that mortality was reduced by about 40%, and in-hospital mortality by more than 30%, in the intensively treated group. The incidence of hypoglycemia (blood glucose ≤ 40 mg/dL) was 5.1% in the intensively treated group and 0.8% in the conventionally treated group. Hypoglycemia based on the American Diabetes Association definition (blood glucose ≤70 mg/dL) was not reported. These data are intriguing but not uniformly applicable to palliative care. If a patient with diabetes is receiving inpatient palliative care services and is expected to return to a good quality of life, extra efforts to maintain blood glucose in a "tighter" range may be appropriate. Most end-of-life patients do not have a team of ICU nurses and physicians caring for them. The care required for tight blood glucose control is not feasible or even appropriate for most terminally ill patients. In fact, given the sixfold higher incidence of hypoglycemia in the ICU study, this approach in a patient with advanced life-limiting illness could be detrimental or even fatal. Rather, blood glucose control should be guided by symptoms of both hyperglycemia and hypoglycemia in this population.

There are four primary symptom groupings of hyperglycemia[23]:

- *Agitation*—feeling tense, irritability, restlessness, poor concentration
- *Osmotic*—thirst, dry mouth, need to urinate, not feeling right, sweet/funny taste, weakness

- *Neurological*—dizziness, blurred vision, lightheadedness, weakness
- *Malaise*—headache, nausea

Many of these symptoms are seen in terminally ill patients even without glucose intolerance, and it is difficult to determine causality without blood glucose monitoring (Tables 78-3 and 78-4).

Type 1 Diabetes Mellitus

It is likely that patients with type 1 diabetes will continue to require insulin to prevent ketoacidosis. For those who experience a general decline in appetite with weight loss, it may be useful to forgo the prandial insulin component and switch entirely to basal insulin (NPH, detemir, or glargine once or twice daily). The insulin dosage should be adjusted to provide a fasting glucose on the low end of the suggested therapeutic range (e.g., <200 mg/dL), so that postprandial glucose will be unlikely to exceed the recommended upper range (e.g., 300 mg/dL). This strategy should allow once-daily insulin dosing with minimal

TABLE 78-3   Management of Type 1 Diabetes Mellitus and Fully Insulin-Dependent Type 2 Diabetes Mellitus

PATIENT CLINICAL STATUS	TREATMENT RECOMMENDATIONS	BLOOD GLUCOSE MONITORING RECOMMENDATIONS
Stable nutritional status with good quality of life	Maintain current therapy with basal and bolus insulin.	Three times weekly if stable and largely asymptomatic
Consistent but declining appetite (anorexia) accompanied by weight loss	Consider changing to once- or twice-daily intermediate- or long-acting insulin.	One to two times daily until stable, then every 3 days if stable and largely asymptomatic
Patient experiencing nausea, vomiting, erratic oral intake, weight loss, and anorexia	Lower basal dose of insulin; administer rapid-acting insulin after meals, using rough carbohydrate counting to determine insulin dose.	Twice daily to assess insulin/carbohydrate ratio, then every 3 days once stable and largely asymptomatic
Patient symptomatic and/or blood glucose values >250–300 mg/dL	Continue intermediate- or long-acting insulin, titrating to acceptable fasting blood glucose levels; if necessary, add rapid-acting insulin to cover meals.	Two to three times daily until stable, then every 3 days if stable and largely asymptomatic
Actively dying (days to 1 week before death)	Consider discontinuing insulin therapy.	If insulin therapy is discontinued, cease blood glucose monitoring.

Data from Poulson J. The management of diabetes in patients with advanced cancer. J Pain Symptom Manage 1997;13:339–346.

TABLE 78-4   Management of Type 2 Diabetes Mellitus

PATIENT CLINICAL STATUS	TREATMENT RECOMMENDATIONS	BLOOD GLUCOSE MONITORING RECOMMENDATIONS
Stable nutritional status with good quality of life	Maintain current therapy. Monitor for drug-induced adverse effects.	Three times weekly if stable and largely asymptomatic
Consistent but declining appetite (anorexia) accompanied by weight loss	Consider discontinuing all diabetes therapies. Reduce dose of hypoglycemic agents (sulfonylureas, glinides, insulin) by 50%. If using sulfonylureas, consider use of glipizide. Consider use of glinide administered postprandially based on carbohydrate intake.	One to two times daily until stable, then every 3 days if stable and largely asymptomatic
Patient experiencing nausea, vomiting, erratic oral intake, missed meals	Discontinue medications while patient is symptomatic with nausea, vomiting. Consider discontinuing all diabetes therapies. Consider use of glinide administered postprandially based on carbohydrate intake.	One to two times daily, then every 3 days once stable. Increase monitoring if patient resumes diabetes therapy.
Patient symptomatic and/or blood glucose values >250–300 mg/dL	Consider use of glinides or rapid-acting insulin. If hyperglycemia continues, consider addition of, or shift to, intermediate- or long-acting insulin.	Two to three times daily until stable, then every 3 days if stable and largely asymptomatic
Actively dying (days to 1 week before death)	Discontinue therapy.	If therapy is discontinued, cease blood glucose monitoring.

Data from Poulson J. The management of diabetes in patients with advanced cancer. J Pain Symptom Manage 1997;13:339–346.

blood glucose monitoring and should keep the patient asymptomatic.

For patients with type 1 diabetes who are experiencing nausea, vomiting, erratic oral intake, weight loss, and anorexia, continuing just basal insulin may be sufficient. However, if hypoglycemia occurs with this regimen, it may be more prudent to lower the daily basal insulin dose and consider covering meals with rapid- or short-acting insulin, dosed according to an approximation of carbohydrate intake (e.g., 1 unit of insulin for every 15 g of carbohydrate ingested).

The timing of rapid- or short-acting insulin administration is critically important in patients with erratic oral intake. Because regular insulin has an onset of 30 to 60 minutes, it is usually administered at least 30 minutes before a meal. Rapid-acting insulin (e.g., lispro, aspart, glulisine) is administered up to 15 minutes before the meal. Patients who have erratic oral intake (despite their best intentions) may take advantage of the rapid-acting characteristics of these newer insulin analogues and administer an appropriate dose after the meal, instead of before the meal. For example, if the patient anticipated eating a meal containing 30 g of carbohydrates for lunch but had early satiety and consumed only 10 g of carbohydrates, a dose of insulin administered before the meal would most likely cause hypoglycemia. By waiting until after the meal, the patient or caregiver could administer a lower, more appropriate insulin dose, thereby avoiding hypoglycemia. The delayed onset of action is an acceptable consequence to avoid postprandial hypoglycemia.

People who become symptomatic or have large blood glucose swings (e.g., >250–300 mg/dL) may benefit from full basal insulin therapy plus rapid- or short-acting insulin to cover meals, again dosed after the meal. If the blood glucose concentration is consistently 300 mg/dL or higher, it may be beneficial to perform urine ketone testing, to avoid diabetic ketoacidosis. Those who are actively dying (days before death) may discontinue insulin therapy and blood glucose monitoring altogether.

Patients with type 1 diabetes may be receiving pramlintide (Symlin), an amylin analogue that lowers postprandial glucose. In type 1 diabetics, concurrent use of pramlintide resulted in a 3.6% lowering of rapid- or short-acting insulin but a 1.9% increase in long-acting insulin at 6 months. The long-term effect of pramlintide is a placebo-adjusted decrease in the HbA1c by 0.33%. These effects are negligible in someone with advanced disease, and there is also a 30% incidence of nausea; therefore, this medication can probably be discontinued.[24] Minor adjustments to the insulin regimen may or may not be required.

Type 2 Diabetes Mellitus

For people with an acceptable quality of life, good oral intake, and stable blood glucose values, management of type 2 diabetes should continue as usual. Regardless of oral intake, the development of symptoms or co-morbid conditions that are contraindications to antihyperglycemic therapies should be noted and adjustments made as appropriate (Table 78-5).

If the patient has anorexia accompanied by weight loss, consider discontinuing all diabetes therapies and evaluate for signs and symptoms of hyperglycemia. If continued treatment is required, use lower doses of hypoglycemia agents (sulfonylureas, glinides, insulin); if a sulfonylurea is used, consider a short-acting agent such as glipizide. If pharmacological treatment is required to control symptomatic hyperglycemia but appetite is sporadic, consider prescribing a glinide to be taken after a meal containing at least 30 g of carbohydrate.

TABLE 78-5   Influence of Symptoms and Co-morbid Conditions in the Treatment of Type 2 Diabetes

SYMPTOM/CO-MORBID CONDITION	CAUTIONS FOR DIABETES MEDICATIONS
History of frequent hypoglycemia or hypoglycemic unawareness	Hypoglycemia is caused/worsened by sulfonylurea agents, glinides, and insulin.
Early satiety, anorexia, poor oral intake, weight loss	Patient is at increased risk for hypoglycemia (sulfonylurea agents, glinides, insulin). Anorexia and early satiety are worsened by metformin, pramlintide, and exenatide. α-Glucosidase inhibitors should not be taken by patients who are not eating. Sitagliptin inhibits the enzyme that degrades incretin hormones; may contribute to early satiety. If a meal is skipped, glinide should not be taken.
Nausea, vomiting, gastrointestinal (GI) distress	Although any medication can cause or worsen nausea or vomiting, the following cause a high incidence of nausea, vomiting, and GI distress: metformin, exenatide, pramlintide, sulfonylurea agents, glinides, and α-glucosidase inhibitors. α-Glucosidase inhibitors cause GI distress and are contraindicated in patients with a history of GI tract problems such as inflammatory bowel disease, colonic ulceration, intestinal obstruction, or chronic intestinal diseases.
Liver impairment	The following diabetes medications are relatively contraindicated: metformin, thiazolidinediones, sulfonylurea agents (minimally, choose a shorter-acting agent such as glipizide), α-glucosidase inhibitors.
Renal impairment	The following diabetes medications are relatively or absolutely contraindicated: metformin, sulfonylurea agents (consider glipizide; its metabolites are inactive, causing less problems), miglitol (an α-glucosidase inhibitor), repaglinide, sitagliptin (requires dosage adjustment), and exenatide.
Heart failure	The following diabetes medications are relatively or absolutely contraindicated: metformin and thiazolidinediones.
Edema	Thiazolidinediones may worsen fluid retention (particularly if taken with insulin). First-generation sulfonylureas may cause syndrome of inappropriate antidiuretic hormone (SIADH).

Patients with nausea and/or vomiting are unlikely to have a robust appetite or oral intake; therefore, diabetes therapies should be withheld while the gastrointestinal upset resolves, and possibly for the duration of care. If the patient does require a glucose-lowering agent once the gastrointestinal upset resolves but oral intake is sporadic, consider administration of a glinide after a meal that contains at least 30 g of carbohydrate. Occasionally, patients have large blood glucose swings; in such cases, a glinide taken before or after meals or a rapid-acting insulin may be useful, particularly if the oral intake and blood glucose values are inconsistent. Patients who are actively dying will most likely not require any diabetes therapy. The newer agents (sitagliptin, exenatide, and pramlintide) are of less value at the end of life. They primarily act to lower the postprandial glucose. Exenatide and pramlintide cause frequent nausea and early satiety, and they have only a small insulin-sparing effects. They can be discontinued in most people with advanced disease.

Patients with type 2 diabetes frequently take insulin as part of their therapy. If the patient is receiving only basal insulin, this may be sufficient to control blood glucose, and oral agents can be discontinued. At some point, the basal insulin dose may also require reduction. Many patients with type 2 diabetes require full insulin therapy (basal and bolus); their therapy should be assessed and managed as described for type 1 diabetes.

Corticosteroid-Induced Hyperglycemia

Corticosteroids are used frequently in palliative care. They can cause hyperglycemia in a previously nondiabetic patient or worsen diabetes control. Practitioners need to be aware of this risk and monitor patients for hyperglycemia. The primary glucose abnormality is postprandial hyperglycemia. Therapies that would most specifically treat this condition include the glinides before or after each meal, rapid-acting insulin, or short-acting insulin. If all blood glucose values are elevated, other medications to treat type 2 diabetes may be considered, assuming there are no risk factors that contraindicate therapy. Diabetes mellitus is a prevalent chronic condition in a significant number of patients with advanced illness. It is important that practitioners provide sufficiently aggressive, yet not overly aggressive, diabetes management to minimize patient stress while preventing and relieving symptoms.

REFERENCES

1. Quinn K, Hudson P, Dunning T. Diabetes management in patients receiving palliative care. J Pain Symptom Manage 2006;32:275-286.
2. Ford-Dunn S, Smith A, Quin J. Management of diabetes during the last days of life: Attitudes of consultant diabetologists and consultant palliative care physicians in the UK. Palliat Med 2006;20:197-203.
3. American Diabetes Association. Total prevalence of diabetes and pre-diabetes. Available at http://diabetes.org/diabetes-statistics/prevalence.jsp (accessed October 2007).
4. National Hospice and Palliative Care Organization. NHPCO's Facts and Figures—2005 Findings. Available at http://www.nhpco.org/files/public/2005-facts-and-figures.pdf (accessed October 2007).
5. American Diabetes Association. Diagnosis and classification of diabetes mellitus. Diabetes Care 2007;30(Suppl 1):S42-S47.
6. Anderson RJ, Freedland KE, Clouse RE, Lustman PJ. The prevalence of comorbid depression in adults with diabetes. Diabetes Care 2001;24:1069-1078.
7. Testa MA, Simonson DC. Health economic benefits and quality of life during improved glycemic control in patients with type 2 diabetes mellitus: A randomized, controlled, double-blind trial. JAMA 1998;280:1490-1496.
8. Hardy JR, Rees E, Ling J, et al. A prospective survey of the use of dexamethasone on a palliative care unit. Palliat Med 2001;15:3-8.
9. Uzu T, Harada T, Sakaguchi M, et al. Glucocorticoid-induced diabetes mellitus: Prevalence and risk factors in primary renal diseases. Nephron Clin Pract 2007;105:c54-c57.
10. Hailemeskel B, Dutta A, Daftary MN, et al. Corticosteroid-induced adverse reactions in a university teaching hospital. Am J Health Syst Pharm 2003;60:194-195.
11. Blackburn D, Hux J, Mamdani M. Quantification of the risk of corticosteroid-induced diabetes mellitus among the elderly. J Gen Intern Med 2002;17:717-720.
12. Dunning T. Corticosteroid medications and diabetes mellitus. Practical Diabetes Int 1996;13:186-188.
13. Hoogwerf, Danese RD. Drug selection and the management of corticosteroid-related diabetes mellitus. Rheum Dis Clin North Am 1999:25:489-505.
14. Diabetes Control and Complications Trial Research Group. The effect of intensive treatment of diabetes on the development and progression of long-term complications in insulin-dependent diabetes mellitus. N Engl J Med 1993;329:977-986.
15. United Kingdom Prospective Diabetes Study (UKPDS) Group. Intensive blood-glucose control with sulphonylureas or insulin compared with conventional treatment and risk of complications in patients with type 2 diabetes (UKPDS 33). Lancet 1998;352:837-853.
16. Stratton IM, Adler AL, Neil HA, et al. Association of glycaemia with macrovascular and microvascular complications of type 2 diabetes (UKPDS 35): Prospective observational study. BMJ 2000;321:405-412.
17. American Diabetes Association. Standards of medical care in diabetes—2007. Diabetes Care 2007;30(Suppl 1):S4-S41.
18. California Healthcare Foundation/American Geriatrics Society Panel on Improving Care for Elders with Diabetes. Guidelines for improving the care of the older person with diabetes mellitus. J Am Geriatr Soc 2003;51(5 Suppl):S265-S280.
19. Ford-Dunn S, Smith A, Quin J. Blood glucose levels in diabetic patients during the terminal phase: Is continuation of treatment necessary? Poster presentation. Proceedings of the 5th Palliative Care Congress, University of Warwick, United Kingdom, 2004, p 161.
20. American Diabetes Association and the European Association for the Study of Diabetes. Management of hyperglycemia in type 2 diabetes: A consensus algorithm for the initiation and adjustment of therapy. Diabetes Care 2006;29:1963-1972.
21. Nissen SE, Wolski K. Effect of rosiglitazone on the risk of myocardial infarction and death from cardiovascular causes. N Engl J Med 2007;356:2457-2471. Epub 2007 May 21. Erratum in: N Engl J Med. 2007;357:100.
22. Van Den Berghe G, Wouters P, Weekers F, et al. Intensive insulin therapy in critically ill patients. N Engl J Med 2001;345:1359-1367.
23. Warren RE, Deary IJ, Frier BM. The symptoms of hyperglycemia in people with insulin-treated diabetes: Classification using principal components analysis. Diabetes Metab Res Rev 2003;19:408-414.
24. Symlin home page. Available at http://www.symlin.com/PDF/HCP/SYMLIN-pi-combined.pdf (accessed October 2007).

SUGGESTED READING

McCoubrie R, Jeffrey D, Paton C, et al. Managing diabetes mellitus in patients with advanced cancer: A case note audit and guidelines. Eur J Cancer Care 2005;14:244-248.

Poulson J. The management of diabetes in patients with advanced cancer. J Pain Symptom Manage 1997;13:339-346.

Quinn K, Hudson P, Dunning T. Diabetes management in patients receiving palliative care. J Pain Symptom Manage 2006;32:275-286.

Stevenson J, Abernethy AP, Miller C, et al. Managing comorbidities at the end of life. BMJ 2004;329:909-912.

CHAPTER **79**

Heart Failure

Frances Mair, Lynda Blue, and Yvonne Millerick

K E Y   P O I N T S

- The prognosis of heart failure is worse than that of most common cancers.

- Prognostication in heart failure is challenging.

- Greater emphasis must be placed on ensuring that patients with advanced heart failure are aware of their prognosis and participate in treatment choices. The views of patients should be paramount.

- Patients with terminal heart failure are less well served than similar patients with cancer in terms of symptom control, communication, and support mechanisms, and they frequently experience fragmented treatment.

- As with cancer care, end-of-life needs should be an integral component of the multidisciplinary care offered; much of the good practice with cancer patients should be transferable to heart failure. Clear guidelines aimed at the specific management of end-stage heart failure are urgently needed.

EPIDEMIOLOGY

Heart failure is a common disorder that affects up to 4% of the general population and 8% to 10% of the elderly[1-4] —more than 20 million people worldwide,[5] including 5 million in the United States alone.[6] The lifetime risk for heart failure is 1 in 5 for both men and women.[7] Although the incidence has been static over the last 2 decades,[8] it poses a major public health problem in developed countries. This is because of high prevalence but also because of the associated morbidity, because patients with heart failure often experience frequent hospital stays. Although the incidence may not be increasing, the overall disease burden may, because of increased survival. Recent studies from both the United States and the United Kingdom confirm this improved survival,[9,10] with reasons ranging from improved treatment effectiveness to earlier diagnosis, resulting in lead-time bias. The high morbidity is demonstrated by high utilization of secondary care inpatient and outpatient services. For example, in the United States, hospital discharges for heart failure rose from 399,000 in 1979 to 1,093,000 in 2003 (a 174% increase),[6] and outpatient contacts in excess of £3 million annually are recorded in the United Kingdom.

The societal costs are high. By 2000,[11] the total direct cost of heart failure in the United Kingdom was estimated to be £905 million, equivalent to 2% of total National Health Service expenditures, mostly for hospitalization. In the United States in 2006, the combined direct and indirect costs of heart failure were $29.6 billion.[6]

Heart failure is a terminal condition. Except for lung cancer, heart failure is as "malignant" as many common cancers and is associated with similar expected life-years lost.[12] This poor prognosis is under-recognized. After their first hospital admission, patients with heart failure have a median survival time of 16 months, with only 25% of men and women surviving to 5 years.[12-14] It is only recently that discussion of the needs of patients with end-stage heart failure has received any significant attention, and the implications from the patient perspective have been relatively neglected compared to those of other illnesses.

PATHOPHYSIOLOGY

Heart failure is a complex clinical syndrome that has been defined in numerous ways, most recently as any structural or functional cardiac disorder that impairs the ability of the ventricle to fill with or eject blood.[15] It may result from disorders of the pericardium, myocardium, endocardium, or great vessels.[15] Coronary artery disease remains the most common, potentially reversible cause.[15]

Other underlying causes include hypertension, dilated cardiomyopathy, valvular disease, and alcohol abuse. Heart failure may also be idiopathic. There are several rare causes, including multisystem disorders such as hemochromatosis, amyloidosis, and collagen vascular disorders; occasionally, it is drug induced. Anemia and thyroid dysfunction can also precipitate heart failure. It can be associated with reduced left ventricular systolic dysfunction, diastolic dysfunction, or both.

DIAGNOSIS AND MANAGEMENT

The major symptoms of heart failure are fatigue, exercise intolerance, exertional dyspnea, orthopnea, paroxysmal nocturnal dyspnea, and dependent edema. These symptoms resemble those of many other diseases. For example, exertional dyspnea is common but has many other causes, including chronic obstructive pulmonary disease, interstitial lung disease, asthma, respiratory infection, deconditioning, and obesity. Many people with impaired left ventricular function have no obvious symptoms. The patient's past medical and medication history contributes to the overall clinical assessment. Physical findings that may support a diagnosis include raised jugular venous pressure, peripheral edema not due to venous insufficiency, a third heart sound, gallop rhythm, laterally displaced apical impulse, tachycardia, and pulmonary crepitations that do not clear with coughing. No one clinical feature can accurately predict heart failure.[16] Therefore, the history and physical examination alone, although important and valuable, are insufficient to confirm a diagnosis in most patients. Recommended initial tests for those with signs or symptoms of heart failure include a full blood count, serum electrolytes, glucose, serum creatinine, serum albumin, liver function tests, possibly natriuretic peptides, urinalysis, electrocardiography, chest radiography (Fig. 79-1), and echocardiography (Fig. 79-2).[16]

TREATMENT

Standard therapies include the following:

- General advice and nonpharmacological measures (e.g., salt avoidance)

Pulmonary vascular congestion

Pulmonary vascular congestion

Pulmonary border enlargement

FIGURE 79-1 Chest radiograph of a patient with pulmonary edema. *(Courtesy of L. Blue.)*

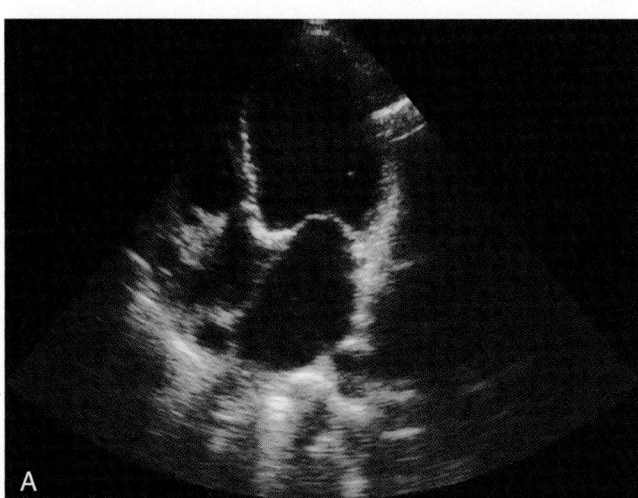

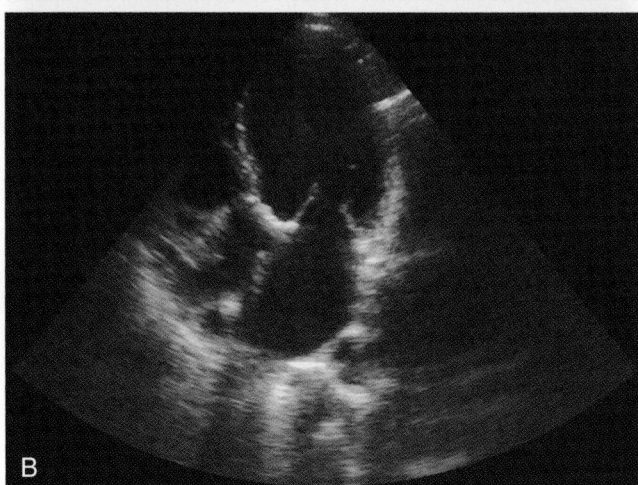

FIGURE 79-2 Echocardiograms showing left ventricular systolic dysfunction in systole (**A**) and diastole (**B**). *(Courtesy of Dr. Derek Connelly, Glasgow Royal Infirmary.)*

- Pharmacological therapy: diuretics, angiotensin-converting enzyme inhibitors, β-blockers, aldosterone antagonists, angiotensin II receptor blockers, digoxin, and other drugs (e.g., anticoagulants, vasodilators)
- Devices: cardiac resynchronization therapy (CRT), implantable cardioverter defibrillators (ICDs)

Modern therapies and most cardiovascular guidelines aim at preventing death and improving quality of life. It is important when considering management of heart failure to move the focus from what can be done to what should be done (see "Impacts of Progressive Heart Failure").

CLINICAL MANIFESTATIONS

The case study illustrates some clinical manifestations of end-stage heart failure that can be wide ranging. Some manifestations are readily associated, such as dyspnea and edema (Fig. 79-3), but many other common difficulties are often less well noted, including cough, pain, fatigue, sleep problems, anorexia, nausea and vomiting, early meal satiety, cachexia, abdominal fullness, ascites, constipation, dry mouth, skin problems, pruritus, and mental health problems, particularly lowered mood and anxiety.

MANAGEMENT

A holistic approach is necessary, taking into account the physical, psychological, spiritual, and social needs of the patient (see "Common Therapeutics"). Prognostication is particularly difficult because of the numerous pathological scenarios, unpredictable treatment responses, and the possibility of sudden death.[17] Deterioration of heart failure may result from eversible causes, and a combination of agents such as inotropes, vasodilators, and diuretics may initiate a remission.[17] There is no definitive way to ascertain the terminal phase. Even the 1996 criteria of the U.S.

CASE STUDY

Impacts of Progressive Heart Failure

The following case report outlines the progressive nature of chronic heart failure. It examines the impact on both the patient living with the disease and the professionals responsible for providing patient care and highlights some important issues.

Background

Mrs. Y is 72 years old; she has been widowed for 7 years and lives alone in a one-bedroom flat. A home help worker visits twice weekly and has proved to be invaluable during times of need. Referral to the heart failure service began 10 months ago, after admission to hospital with symptoms of dyspnea, bilateral thigh edema, and increased lethargy. Echocardiography confirmed a diagnosis of heart failure secondary to moderately impaired left ventricular systolic dysfunction. After hospital discharge, Mrs. Y was visited by the heart failure liaison nurse service. Optimization of evidence-based therapy proved difficult due to episodes of heart failure decompensation, symptomatic hypotension, and renal impairment. Eventually, however, optimal tolerated doses of both angiotensin-converting enzyme inhibitor and β-blocker therapy were achieved.

Approximately 4 months ago, Mrs. Y's health status started to deteriorate, with worsening symptoms of dyspnea, peripheral edema, and fatigue. These symptoms proved difficult to treat and required increasing doses of both loop and thiazide diuretics. Maintaining Mrs. Y in her own home had been made possible by regular visits (usually once weekly) from the heart failure liaison nurse. The main purpose of these visits was symptom management and monitoring of renal function. Hospital admission had been kept to a minimum of two visits for intravenous diuretic therapy. However, the impact of progressing from New York Heart Association (NYHA) class III to class IV was clearly distressing and very limiting, both for Mrs. Y and for health professionals trying to provide a high standard of quality care.

What Are the Main Issues?

Patient Perspective

Every day Mrs. Y is inconvenienced by a complicated medication regimen, with adherence leading to restriction of activities and frequent toilet visits. Adherence is vital, however, if she wants to keep her condition at a manageable level, even though she knows that "manageable" still means suffering the symptoms.

Symptoms

Mrs. Y is breathless all day, every day, during minimal exertion. On a good day, she might manage to wash and dress without too much discomfort, but on a bad day she needs to pause for breath during normal conversation. Paroxysmal nocturnal dyspnea and orthopnea often result in only 2 to 4 hours of quality sleep per night. This lack of sleep, coupled with progressive muscle changes, increase her symptoms of fatigue and lethargy. Bilateral ankle edema generally means that Mrs. Y is having a good day. Typically, however, she is 3 kg over her dry weight, leading to bilateral calf edema that restricts her choice of clothes and shoes and limits her daily activities, not to mention the pain and discomfort associated with heavy, tight legs filled with fluid that may or may not lead to weeping and inflammation. It is hardly surprising that Mrs. Y also has symptoms of fear, depression, anorexia, and generalized pain.

Professional Perspective

For many professionals, providing care for patients with heart failure can be difficult. The patients' symptoms present a major challenge and often lead to a juggling act between medication adjustment and minimizing the effect this may have on impaired renal function. Prognosis is difficult to predict and is rarely discussed until the very end, when death is imminent. Mrs. Y was relatively well until 4 months ago; now her condition has deteriorated. But discussion of prognosis in this situation can be challenging. Professionals may wonder whether her prognosis should now be described to her as poor, or whether this might be delivering bad news too soon. Most nurses have witnessed the recovery of patients who were previously thought to be on the brink of death and may well be concerned about what would happen if Mrs. Y were informed of a "poor" prognosis but subsequently made a good recovery and remained well for a long period thereafter. Would this cause her to lose confidence in the health professionals, and would it adversely affect the nurse–patient relationship? These are all common concerns.

Communication issues have become difficult because Mrs. Y is not responding to medication changes. Treatment options within the specialty of heart failure are now limited. The health professional may feel uncomfortable because of an inability to help the patient feel better but also because of concerns that the patient will ask about her prognosis.

The Challenge

- Is Mrs. Y approaching end of life? This seems likely based on the history.
- Or, is there a precipitant for this period of instability—and, if so, is it treatable and will she recover?
- Has every possible treatment been considered?
- Does the patient know how ill she is and her prognosis?
  What would she want to happen if the end were near? (For example, what would be her preferred place of care, and what should be her resuscitation status?)

What Do We Know?

- Mrs. Y is on maximum tolerated evidence-based therapy.
- She is taking increasing doses of combined diuretics (symptoms are now resistant to previously effective lower doses).
- Mrs. Y requires increased contacts for monitoring and symptom control by the heart failure nurse.
- Renal function is deteriorating.
- Symptoms are progressing, so the patient is moving from NYHA class III to class IV.
- Quality of life is poor—Mrs. Y very rarely gets outside the house.

What Can Be Done Based on What We Know?

Symptom Management

Symptom management guidelines would encourage heart failure professionals to think outside the cardiology box. Opiates are underused in patients with heart failure, and yet it is known that low doses of opiates can reduce dyspnea and promote a regular sleep pattern. If the patient is getting proper rest and sleep, then perhaps the level of edema will also reduce.

Coordination of Care

Accessing advice from other specialties, such as palliative care, will encourage heart failure specialists to learn from others' expert knowledge and skills. Mrs. Y and other patients like her will benefit from the coordination and continuity of care that this interprofessional work can provide.

Communication

Mrs. Y should be given the opportunity to discuss end-of-life care issues. Breaking bad news is never easy, but this should not deter heart failure professionals from providing important information. Most patients are given their diagnosis, but very few actually know their prognosis. Acknowledgment that skills and knowledge in this role need to be supported and updated will hopefully lessen the taboo associated with breaking bad news.

Where Do We Go from Here?

Until now, we have been very proactive at treating the disease; we now need to start being proactive at treating the patient.

Palliative Care

Mrs. Y's journey began with her diagnosis. Good palliative care should begin here and continue throughout her journey. Prognosis is only a small part of that journey, and not knowing exactly when the end of life is likely should not deter the delivery of good-quality health care.

Communication

Patients need to have access to information about their heart failure condition. How much information is provided should depend on their personal information needs, which can be determined only through in-depth, open, and honest discussion. Some patients do not wish to know everything, and this is their prerogative; others want to know as much detail as possible. Mrs. Y already had some idea that she might not get any better and was keen to know what symptoms would trouble her most and what could be done about them. She also made it clear that she did not wish to be readmitted to hospital for further treatment and that her preferred place of care would be at home.

Symptom Management

Mrs. Y remained on tolerated doses of evidence-based heart failure medication. Oramorph was also added, in response to symptoms of dyspnea, pain, and poor-quality sleep, with desired effect.

Social Care Services

Mrs. Y gave consent for a social services referral. She lived alone and was extremely unwell, leaving her feeling quite vulnerable. Therefore, it was important that structures to support her personal, cleaning, and shopping needs be put in place and that they be flexible and sensitive enough to respond to change as needed.

Psychological Care

Psychological distress is a natural response to any life-threatening situation, although Mrs. Y appeared to be coping well.

Mrs. Y, like most patients, wished for a dignified death in her own home. However, like so many, she died in hospital after an emergency admission with decompensation of heart failure. Her death occurred 3 weeks after commencing Oramorph and 1 week after increased social care input.

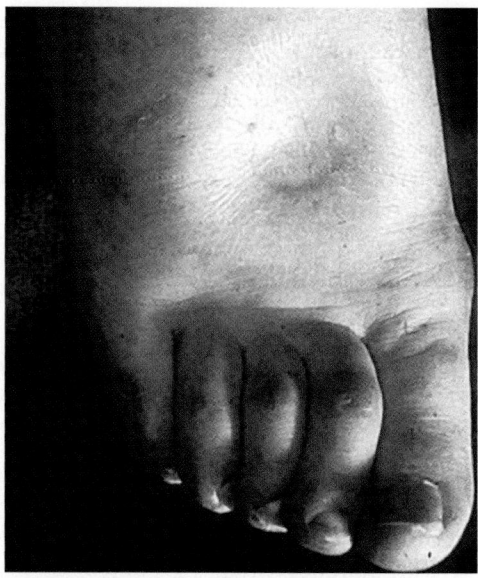

FIGURE 79-3 Pitting edema. *(Courtesy of L. Blue.)*

Common Therapeutics

- Breathlessness. One of the most distressing symptoms is dyspnea. The value of opioid therapy for dyspnea is widely accepted, but it remains underutilized.[17] Nebulized saline with or without bronchodilators has also been advocated and can sometimes help those with cough, as may cough suppressants such as codeine linctus or low-dose sustained-release morphine.
- Pain. Paracetamol is effective for generalized pain, and in particular for leg ache from peripheral edema. Opioids are useful to control pain that is unresponsive to simpler measures.
- Nausea or vomiting. If this is problematic, iatrogenic causes should be sought first. If none are present, then various medications may help, such as haloperidol or, if related to meals or to early satiety, metoclopramide or domperidone. Low-dose levomepromazine has also been used and may have the added benefit of an anxiolytic effect.
- Constipation is common, secondary to immobility and poor diet associated with anorexia and fatigue. Treatment with stool softeners or stimulant laxatives, or both, should be considered, depending on patient requirements.
- Psychological issues. Depression and anxiety are common. Antidepressants may be used. There is uncertainty about the best agent, but selective serotonin reuptake inhibitors are preferred to tricyclics because they are less cardiotoxic. Anxiolytics may also be necessary.

National Hospice and Palliative Care Organization (NHPCO) for admission of heart failure do not provide a good prediction of 6-month mortality.[18]

> For many heart failure patients the day that they die they will probably appear no more ill than any other day. This is in sharp contrast to patients who die from cancer as they are most likely to be the most ill they have ever been on the day of death.
>
> — M. CONNOLLY[19]

Clinical guidelines stress that reversible causes of heart failure must not be overlooked and that all reasonable treatment options must be considered. Without identifiable or reversible precipitants, the presence of the following situations should help identify those patients who require a palliative approach:

- Worsening symptoms despite optimally tolerated evidence-based therapy
- Combined loop and thiazide diuretics—requiring frequently increased doses
- NYHA class IV
- Deteriorating renal function
- Need for multiple home visits and/or hospital admissions

In such circumstances, the views of patient and carer on the merits of continuing active treatment should be sought.[17] Symptom control should continue, along with active cardiological management, with standard agents such as diuretics and angiotensin-converting enzyme inhibitors as long as these remain appropriate. Optimal palliation of symptoms often depends on compliance, especially with diuretics.

An effective management plan to ease the suffering associated with end-stage heart failure has several elements:

- A mechanism to communicate and document management to relevant health and social care professionals after hospital discharge, ensuring clarity about the management plan
- Good coordination and continuity of care by a single physician to determine whether the patient experiences periodic severe heart failure due to other extraneous factors (e.g., nonadherence to treatment) or is simply experiencing the natural history of his or her particular form of heart failure
- An adequate package of care whenever the patient is discharged from hospital
- If discharged to hospice care established communication with heart failure expertise to support nursing and medical staff in managing care
- An updated management plan included in the general practice and hospital case notes (e.g., to make all clinicians aware of the patient's desire to avoid active resuscitation in the event of cardiorespiratory arrest)

Pharmacological Therapies

Continuation of heart failure medication, except diuretics, in advanced heart failure can differ for each patient (see "Pearls and Pitfalls"). Rationalization of drug therapy minimizes side effects from existing medications, some of which may no longer be required, and also decreases the overall medication burden, which is a particular issue in heart failure. In addition, drugs for palliative purposes may interact with existing medications, and it is essential to decrease the potential for such interactions. For example, medications such as statins are unnecessary in the terminal phases of heart failure. The thinking behind such medication changes needs to be fully discussed with patients, and treatment goals must be agreed on and transparent to all involved.

Nondrug Measures

Involvement of all members of the multidisciplinary team, including the physiotherapist, occupational therapist,

---

Pearls and Pitfalls

- Oral diuretics should be continued, if possible, to minimize distress or anxiety from fluid overload.
- Paroxetine has been used successfully for intolerable itch. Begin with the lowest dose, and increase accordingly. Ondansetron and paracetamol have also proved successful in these patients.
- Anecdotal evidence suggests that some patients benefit psychologically from nebulized saline and that it has reduced dyspnea.
- Those patients with coexisting airways disease may benefit from nebulized salbutamol, but caution should be used in ischemic heart disease, because this may precipitate angina.

Future Considerations

- Prognostication remains difficult and needs further exploration.
- The evidence base supporting many approaches to symptom control in terminal heart failure remains poor, and further research should be supported.
- Nebulized medication and oxygen for the palliation of dyspnea in advanced heart failure is worthy of further investigation.
- The role, if any, of specialist palliative care nurses for end-stage heart failure merits further evaluation.
- The use of subcutaneous furosemide to help ameliorate intractable peripheral edema merits investigation in randomized controlled trials.
- Educational initiatives, aimed at the health professionals dealing with this patient group and focusing on terminal care needs and practical approaches to management, are urgently required.

---

social worker, psychologist, and chaplain, may be appropriate. Patients with advanced failure have many support needs. For example, physiotherapists may provide patients and carers with invaluable advice on mobility that can maximize independence and decrease complications. Occupational therapists can help the patient undertake routine activities by providing appropriate home modifications and advice. General advice should be offered on positioning, use of fans, relaxation, breathing control, pacing of activities. and coping strategies. Spiritual support should also be addressed. Alternative therapies, such as reiki, massage, and relaxation, may help and should be considered in addition to medication for relief of symptoms and optimal well-being. As with pharmacological therapies, it is important to identify what is appropriate management (e.g., to achieve symptom relief and pain control) and also to identify what is inappropriate (e.g., the use of central lines). Communication is key to ensuring that the needs of patients and their carers are met effectively. Patients' views should be paramount, and their perspectives on topics such as overall management and preferred location for end-of-life care must be explored and respected. Sensitive issues such as resuscitation status and withdrawing or withholding treatment need to be fully discussed with the patient and documented accordingly (see "Future Considerations").

An increasingly common issue is the presence of implantable cardioverter defibrillators (ICD) and the indications for their withdrawal. The use of such devices in heart failure is becoming more common. Their purpose is to extend life, and the shocks from such devices can be painful and may be considered unsuitable in patients with heart failure when death is imminent. Furthermore, a functioning ICD is incompatible with a coexisting do not resuscitate (DNR) order. The issue of when to deactivate an ICD needs to be fully discussed with both cardiologist and patient. Patients also need to know that turning off the ICD does not mean instant death and is not painful; it does mean that the device will no longer be functioning to provide life-saving treatment in a fatal arrhythmia.[20]

There are many barriers to high-quality palliative care for patients in serious heart failure. Common difficulties include the following:

- Inadequate staffing for support services in the community and hospital. Nurses in medical and cardiac wards may be frustrated because they can barely meet the physical needs of patients with end-stage heart failure, let alone have time to provide more holistic, patient-centered care.[21]
- Perceived barriers to effective interdisciplinary working among acute care staff, community, and palliative care teams. These perceptions can cause fragmented care and adversely affect quality.[21]
- Differences in opinion between professionals as to when to transition from life-sustaining treatment to palliative care. For example, nurses' ability to address and implement orders for end-of-life care can be influenced by a reluctance of physicians to issue "not for resuscitation" orders.
- The lack of innovative care models for terminal heart failure. This lack of progress diminishes the ability of professionals to meet the needs of patients in end-stage heart failure and permits overzealous treatment in advanced disease.

REFERENCES

1. Davies MK, Hobbs FDR, Davis RC, et al. Prevalence of left-ventricular systolic dysfunction and heart failure in the Echocardiographic Heart of England Screening study: A population based study. Lancet 2001;358:439-444.
2. Mair FS, Crowley TS, Bundred P. Prevalence, aetiology and management of heart failure in general practice. Br J Gen Pract 1996;46:77-79.
3. McDonagh TA, Morrison CE, Lawrence A, et al. Symptomatic and asymptomatic left-ventricular systolic dysfunction in an urban population. Lancet 1997;350:829-833.
4. Mosterd A, Hoes AW, de Bruyne MC, et al. Prevalence of heart failure and left ventricular dysfunction in the general population: The Rotterdam Study. Eur Heart J 1999;20:447-455.
5. Tendera M. The epidemiology of heart failure. JRAAS: Journal of the Renin-Angiotensin-Aldosterone System 2004:5(Suppl):S2-S6.
6. Thom T, Haase N, Rosamond W, et al. Heart disease and stroke statistics—2006 update: A report from the American Heart Association Statistics Committee and Stroke Statistics Subcommittee. Circulation 2006;113:e85-e151.
7. Lloyd-Jones DM, Larson MG, Leip EP, et al. Lifetime risk for developing congestive heart failure: The Framingham Heart Study. [See comment.] Circulation 2002;106:3068-3072.
8. Roger VL, Weston SA, Redfield MM, et al. Trends in heart failure incidence and survival in a community-based population. JAMA 2004;292:344-350.
9. Levy D, Kenchaiah S, Larson MG, et al. Long-term trends in the incidence of and survival with heart failure. N Engl J Med 2002;347:1397-1402.
10. Stewart S, MacIntyre K, Capewell S, McMurray JJ. Heart failure and the aging population: An increasing burden in the 21st century? Heart 2003;89:49-53.
11. Stewart S, Jenkins A, Buchan S, et al. The current cost of heart failure to the National Health Service in the UK. Eur J Heart Fail 2002;4:361-371.
12. Stewart S, MacIntyre K, Hole DJ, et al. More "malignant" than cancer? Five-year survival following a first admission for heart failure. Eur J Heart Fail 2001;3:315-322.
13. Jaagosild PM, Dawson NVM, Thomas CB, et al. Outcomes of acute exacerbation of severe congestive heart failure: Quality of life, resource use, and survival. Arch Intern Med 1998;158:1081-1089.
14. Lowe JM, Candlish PM, Henry DA, et al. Management and outcomes of congestive heart failure: A prospective study of hospitalised patients. Med J Aust 1998;168:115-118.
15. Hunt SA, American College of Cardiology, American Heart Association Task Force on Practice Guidelines. ACC/AHA 2005 Guideline Update for the Diagnosis and Management of Chronic Heart Failure in the Adult: A Report of the American College of Cardiology/American Heart Association Task Force on Practice Guidelines (Writing Committee to Update the 2001 Guidelines for the Evaluation and Management of Heart Failure). J Am Coll Cardiol 2005;46:e1-e82.
16. Mair FS, Lloyd-Williams F. Evaluation of suspected left ventricular systolic dysfunction. J Fam Pract 2002;51:466-471.
17. Ward C. The need for palliative care in the management of heart failure. Heart 2002;87:294-298.
18. Reisfield GM, Wilson GR. Prognostication in heart failure #143. J Palliat Med 2007;10:245-246.
19. Lynn J, Harrell F Jr, Cohn F, et al. Prognoses of seriously ill hospitalized patients on the days before death: Implications for patient care and public policy. New Horizons 1997;5(1):56-61.
20. Harrington MD, Luebke DL, Lewis WR, et al. Implantable cardioverter defibrillator (ICD) at end of life #112. J Palliat Med 2005;8:1056-1057.
21. Wotton K, Borbasi S, Redden M. When all else has failed: Nurses' perception of factors influencing palliative care for patients with end-stage heart failure. J Cardiovasc Nurs 2005;20(1):18-25.

SUGGESTED READING

Goodlin SJ, Hauptman PJ, Arnold R, et al. Consensus statement: Palliative and supportive care in advanced heart failure. J Card Fail 2004;10:200-209.

Harrington MD, Luebke DL, Lewis WR, et al. Cardiac pacemakers at end of life #111. J Palliat Med 2005;8:1055-1056.

Harrington MD, Luebke DL, Lewis WR, et al. Implantable cardioverter defibrillator (ICD) at end of life #112. J Palliat Med 2005;8:1056-1057.

Ward C. The need for palliative care in the management of heart failure. Heart 2002;87:294-298.

Wotton K, Borbasi S, Redden M. When all else has failed: Nurses' perception of factors influencing palliative care for patients with end-stage heart failure. J Cardiovasc Nurs 2005;20:18-25.

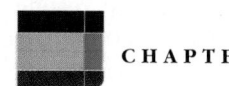

CHAPTER **80**

Arrhythmias

William R. Lewis and **Jennifer E. Cummings**

KEY POINTS

- Hypoxia, electrolyte abnormalities, age, and preexisting cardiac disease predispose seriously ill patients to cardiac arrhythmias.
- Many drugs, including antibiotics, antiarrhythmic medications, and antipsychotic therapies, can precipitate malignant ventricular arrhythmias and must be administered carefully.
- Treatment of many arrhythmias can improve quality of life and may be considered comfort care.
- Atrial arrhythmias often respond to drugs that slow conduction, such as β-blockers and calcium channel blockers.
- Implantable cardioverter defibrillator (ICD) shocks are painful and inconsistent with comfort care. Withdrawal of shock therapy should be considered in advanced disease after careful counseling.

Although cardiac arrhythmias are often misdiagnosed or ignored in the terminally ill, they are important in palliative medicine; recognition and understanding can improve quality of life. Arrhythmias may occur independently of the terminal illness, may be directly related to the disease, or may be secondary to treatment. In some patients, diagnosis and treatment of arrhythmias may assure comfort. In others, arrhythmias may allow the very ill to succumb to their illness painlessly and require no treatment.

EPIDEMIOLOGY AND PREVALENCE

Although arrhythmias in advanced disease may occur secondary to the disease or its treatment, they also can be independent of the terminal process. Susceptibility to cardiac arrhythmias depends on several factors, including age, organic heart disease, and hypertension. Age is directly related to several arrhythmias, including atrial fibrillation, sinus node dysfunction, and symptomatic bradycardia. These are more frequent in patients 65 years of age or older. Preexisting organic heart disease (e.g., cardiomyopathy, valvular heart disease, coronary artery disease) increases the risk of more dangerous arrhythmias such as ventricular tachycardia (VT) and ventricular fibrillation (VF).

PATHOPHYSIOLOGY

The most important determinant is underlying structural heart disease. Prior myocardial infarction, hypertension, valvular heart disease, and congestive heart failure increase the risk of VT, VF, bradycardia, and atrial fibrillation. Derangement of the cardiac substrate by co-morbidities in advanced disease may develop or worsen cardiac arrhythmias. Hypoxia and electrolyte imbalance often contribute. For example, potassium abnormalities alter the resting part of the action potential, which causes cardiac arrhyth-

mias.[1] Hypoxia slows heart conduction, increasing susceptibility to VT and bradycardia.[2] Treatment of these underlying conditions often terminates or minimizes these arrhythmias.

CLINICAL MANIFESTATIONS

Atrial Fibrillation and Atrial Flutter

Atrial fibrillation is the most common arrhythmia and is seen in 2.2 million Americans.[3] It is most common in the elderly (>9% of individuals aged 80 years or older).[4] It is increased in electrolyte imbalances and hypoxia, which are common in patients with serious illnesses. Atrial fibrillation (Fig. 80-1) is a chaotic heart rhythm in which the atria beat rapidly (up to 300 beats/min) and irregularly. Atrial flutter (Fig. 80-2) is another rapid atrial rhythm, but it is regular because it follows a defined reentry circuit path. Although it is not as chaotic as atrial fibrillation, it creates many of the same problems. These rapid atrial impulses from both fibrillation and flutter attempt to conduct to the ventricle through the atrioventricular (AV) node. Conduction occurs as quickly as possible, leading to an irregularly irregular ventricular rhythm. The ventricular rate during atrial fibrillation or flutter can be fast or slow, depending on AV node conduction ability. Because the atria are beating so rapidly, they are unable to fill the ventricle and may lower cardiac output. Additionally, disorganized atrial systole causes atrial stasis of blood with thrombus formation and subsequent stroke. Anticoagulation to prevent this stroke is standard treatment in atrial fibrillation or flutter. Warfarin therapy can be difficult in patients with advanced diseases. Although anticoagulation significantly lowers the risk of stroke in atrial fibrillation or flutter,[5] it also significantly increases the risk of hemorrhage.[6] Serious illnesses such as cancer with intracranial lesions or gastrointestinal malignancy increase the risk of hemorrhage. The benefits of antico-

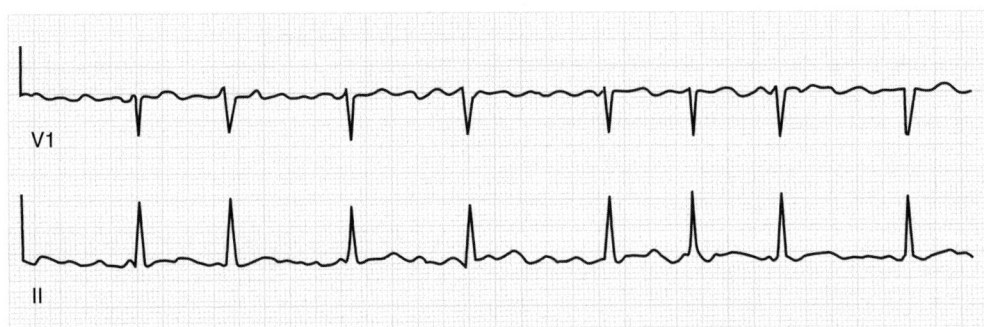

FIGURE 80-1   An example of atrial fibrillation. The baseline is chaotic, and there is no regular P wave denoting sinus node firing. This rhythm is irregular and at times may be very rapid.

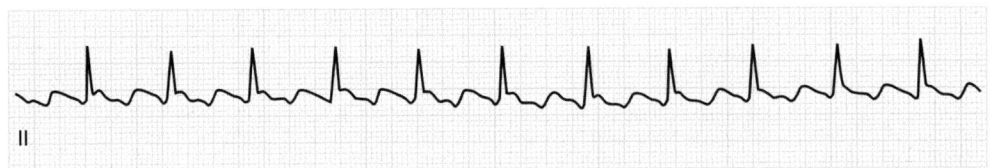

FIGURE 80-2   An example of atrial flutter. In contrast to atrial fibrillation, atrial flutter is regular. The baseline has a sawtooth shape. In most patients, as in this example, the ventricular rate is very rapid. Here, atrial flutter is conducting at a 2:1 rate (i.e., two atrial beats for every single ventricular conduction).

agulation in atrial fibrillation must be weighed against the risks in each individual. In contrast, warfarin may prevent other thrombotic complications because of hypercoagulable states secondary to neoplasm.

Patients with atrial fibrillation or flutter may also experience palpitation, syncope, dizziness, dyspnea, and fatigue. The treatment of these arrhythmias in advanced disease focuses on symptom relief. Many of these symptoms reflect the fast and sometimes irregular ventricular rate during the arrhythmia. Control of the ventricular rate should be the first goal of therapy. β-Blocking drugs can control the ventricular response but may cause fatigue. Calcium channel blockers also may be used, but can cause constipation or worsening of congestive heart failure. Digoxin may not be very effective, because it is less useful with enhanced sympathetic tone, as in fever or anxiety. In some patients, maintaining normal sinus rhythm may be the only means of obtaining acceptable rate control and improved cardiac output. Antiarrhythmic medications such as amiodarone may help. Converting to sinus rhythm often requires electrical cardioversion. This is a relatively safe and brief intervention that administers current through the heart to convert it to sinus rhythm, but sedating anesthesia should be used. This requires a complete understanding of the medical condition, an estimate of the likelihood of maintaining sinus rhythm, and knowledge of the potential risks and benefits. For example, in a severely ill patient with multiple medical problems, sinus rhythm is less likely to be maintained. In such cases, the amount of medical intervention required would be relatively high and the likelihood of improving comfort low.

Ventricular Tachycardia

VT is a rapid, regular heartbeat from an ectopic focus or reentry circuit within the ventricle. The rate is often very rapid, and the heart is unable to pump blood to the body, leading to hypotension, hypoxia, and degeneration into VF. VF is an even more rapid and chaotic ventricular rhythm that results in no circulation (sudden cardiac death). Ventricular arrhythmias usually occur in patients with preexisting organic heart disease, such as congestive heart failure or coronary artery disease. Because it is life-threatening, the questions of when, how, and whether to treat it must be carefully considered in the context of comfort care. Some VT may be stable enough to not degenerate to VF, but it is typically symptomatic. This rapid rhythm and subsequent hypotension cause dizziness, syncope, and shortness of breath. Electrical conver-

sion to normal sinus rhythm can be a comfort care measure. Medical treatments to slow or convert the rhythm are unlikely to be successful acutely.

Short runs of VT, termed nonsustained ventricular tachycardia (NSVT), can predict sustained, life threatening arrhythmias. The symptoms and the degree of risk from these rhythms depend on the duration and rate of the NSVT episodes. When this arrhythmia is first observed, evaluation of electrolytes, oxygenation, and signs and symptoms of coronary ischemia is warranted. Both the treatment and the instigating condition require assessment of the near-term prognosis. Some patients might elect drug therapy to suppress the rhythm if their quality of life is acceptable. In others, treatment may not be indicated.

One variety of VT, torsades de pointes (Fig. 80-3),[7] occurs with electrolyte abnormalities (hypokalemia, hypomagnesemia) or drug administration (antipsychotics, antibiotics). Those patients with preexisting heart disease are at increased risk. QT interval prolongation is often associated with torsades de pointes. Unlike monomorphic VT, this rhythm is characterized by a polymorphic VT: Each QRS complex is different in appearance. On the electrocardiogram, the rhythm often appears to be twisting, like a strand of DNA (hence the name, *torsades de pointes*, "twisting on a point"). The immediate treatment of this life-threatening arrhythmia is defibrillation. However, this condition is often incessant, requiring multiple shocks and other interventions to interrupt it. Intravenous magnesium is the adjuvant temporary treatment of choice for recurrent torsades de pointes. It can often be prevented with electrolyte repletion and removal of the offending drug.[8] This rhythm is usually iatrogenic, and it is critical to prevent it in a population likely to have do not resuscitate (DNR) orders preventing defibrillation.

Sinus Bradycardia and Atrioventricular Block

Sinus bradycardia and AV block can occur from the aging process, electrolyte imbalance, structural heart disease, or infiltrative heart disease. Symptoms of significant bradycardia include shortness of breath, lightheadedness, fatigue, and syncope. Other than correction of electrolytes or withdrawal of bradycardic drugs, medical therapy for sinus bradycardia or AV block is inadequate. Pacemakers are the mainstay for bradycardia. Pacemaker therapy is invasive and requires careful thought in patients with advanced disease. In those who are able to tolerate it,

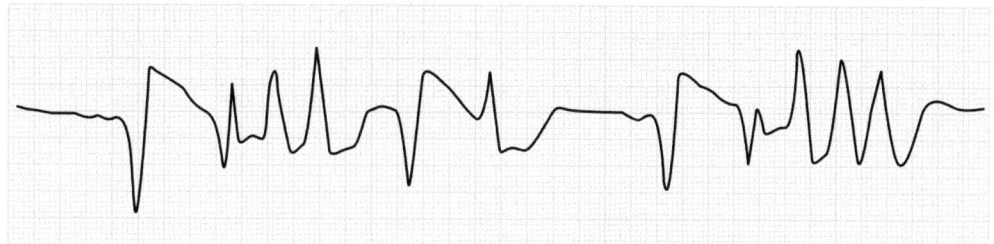

FIGURE 80-3 An example of torsades de pointes. Two bursts are seen in this example. In the first beat of each burst, the QT interval is prolonged. Additionally, this rhythm is pause dependent: Each burst occurs after a pause in the cardiac rhythm. These arrhythmias are "polymorphic," which means that the QRS sequences differ from each other.

pacemaker implantation may reduce symptoms and improve quality of life. Continuation of pacing in the terminally ill does not, however, prolong life compared with discontinuation of pacing,[9] most likely because myocardium, when critically ill and acidotic (hypoxia, lactic acidosis), cannot contract even with artificial electrical stimuli.

WITHDRAWAL OF IMPLANTABLE CARDIOVERTER DEFIBRILLATOR AND PACEMAKER THERAPY

Implantable cardioverter defibrillators (ICDs) monitor and terminate ventricular arrhythmias with a shock. They are effective in prolonging life in people at risk of arrhythmic death but are not indicated in terminal illness. Current cardiology guidelines state that placement of an ICD in someone with a prognosis of less than 6 months is contraindicated. Many patients may have had ICDs implanted previously. With the indications for implantation expanding, implant numbers have grown exponentially. Because ICDs reduce sudden cardiac death, patients with these devices live longer and are more likely to develop other, nonarrhythmic diseases such as cancer, lung disease, advanced dementia, and congestive heart failure.

ICD shocks are physically painful and psychologically stressful,[10] and the psychological consequences increase with multiple shocks.[11] As patients approach the final phase of their disease, they may change their goals from prolongation of life to comfort care. At that point, ICD shocks no longer serve a purpose and may be contraindicated. It is critical for physicians to counsel patients with serious diseases about withdrawal of ICD shock therapy. Such counseling should occur early after the diagnosis of a potentially life-threatening illness and not wait until death is imminent. Patients and their families may not approach medical personnel to discuss ICD shock withdrawal. They may feel that approaching the physician may be a sign of "giving up," or they may not know that the terminal illness may increase susceptibility to ventricular or atrial arrhythmias resulting in ICD shocks. In general, those who elect to avoid aggressive life-saving therapy should be considered for ICD shock therapy withdrawal. Physicians and medical personnel who care for the terminally ill should ask about ICD therapy as a routine part of history taking and should broach the subject of withdrawal of shock therapy. They should develop a relationship with their electrophysiology (cardiac rhythm) team to streamline the counseling and withdrawal of shock therapy.

Pacemakers elevate the heart rate in bradycardia or AV block. Pacemakers are implanted for various reasons. Many patients have prophylactic pacemakers implanted because of intermittent profound arrhythmias. Others are pacemaker dependent: Without pacing, their cardiac rhythm would not sustain life or would result in serious symptoms such as syncope or congestive heart failure. Occasionally, patients and families approach medical personnel to turn off a pacemaker. They may believe that the pacemaker will keep the heart beating and artificially prevent death. With the electrolyte imbalances, hypoxia, and acidosis at the end of life, pacemakers cannot capture the myocardium and will not keep the heart beating endlessly. Continuing pacing therapy is usually a comfort care measure that can prevent the symptoms of congestive heart failure or syncope but is unlikely to prevent death.[9]

CONCLUSIONS

The treatment of cardiac arrhythmias in advanced disease should be focused on symptom management and not on increased longevity. Some life-threatening arrhythmias can be treated with simple measures such as electrolyte repletion and medications such as β-blockers or digoxin. Awareness of ICD and pacemaker therapy is important in palliative medicine. Appropriate withdrawal of ICD shock therapy is essential when comfort care is elected. Medical teams that care for patients with serious illnesses should be aware of any underlying heart disease and risk of cardiac arrhythmias, because they may directly affect palliative care.

REFERENCES

1. Janse M. Reentrant arrhythmias. In Fozzard HA, Haber EA, Jennings RB, et al (eds). The Heart and Cardiovascular System. New York: Raven, 1992, pp 2055–2094.
2. Furuta T, Kodama I, Shimizu T, et al. Effects of hypoxia on conduction velocity of ventricular muscle. Jpn Heart J 1983;24:417–425.
3. Fuster V, Ryden LE, Asinger RW, et al. ACC/AHA/ESC Guidelines for the Management of Patients with Atrial Fibrillation: Executive Summary. A Report of the American College of Cardiology/American Heart Association Task Force on Practice Guidelines and the European Society of Cardiology Committee for Practice Guidelines and Policy Conferences (Committee to Develop Guidelines for the Management of Patients with Atrial Fibrillation): Developed in Collaboration with the North American Society of Pacing and Electrophysiology. J Am Coll Cardiol 2001;38:1231–1266.
4. Go AS, Hylek EM, Phillips KA, et al. Prevalence of diagnosed atrial fibrillation in adults: National implications for rhythm management and stroke prevention. The Anticoagulation and Risk Factors in Atrial Fibrillation (ATRIA) Study. JAMA 2001;285:2370–2375.
5. Hart RG, Benavente O, McBride R, Pearce LA. Antithrombotic therapy to prevent stroke in patients with atrial fibrillation: A meta-analysis. Ann Intern Med 1999;131:492–501.
6. Hart RG, Tonarelli SB, Pearce LA. Avoiding central nervous system bleeding during antithrombotic therapy: Recent data and ideas. Stroke 2005;36:1588–1593.
7. El-Sherif N. Polymorphic ventricular tachycardia. In Podrid PJ KP (ed). Cardiac Arrhythmia: Mechanisms, Diagnosis, and Management. Baltimore, MD: Williams and Wilkins, 1995, pp 936–950.
8. Information from Sudden Arrhythmia Death Syndromes Foundation. Available at http://www.sads.org/ (accessed October 2007).
9. Lewis WR, Luebke DL, Johnson NJ, et al. Withdrawing implantable defibrillator shock therapy in terminally ill patients. Am J Med 2006;119:892–896.
10. Schron EB, Exner DV, Yao Q, et al. Quality of life in the antiarrhythmics versus implantable defibrillators trial: Impact of therapy and influence of adverse symptoms and defibrillator shocks. Circulation 2002;105:589–594.
11. Sears SE Jr, Conti JB. Understanding implantable cardioverter defibrillator shocks and storms: Medical and psychosocial considerations for research and clinical care. Clin Cardiol 2003;26:107–111.

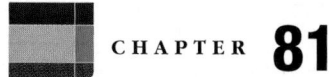

CHAPTER **81**

Hypertension

Michael A. Weber

Hypertension affects about one quarter of the adult population, so inevitably it will be a common finding in palliative care. The main concern with hypertension is its consequences, including stroke, myocardial infarction, and heart failure, which clearly would add substantially to the complexity of dealing with the other major underlying problems.

It is appropriate to evaluate and manage hypertension in palliative care patients in much the same way as in other patients. Even so, there may be some important differences in palliative care, particularly the lifestyle changes typically recommended. Strategies such as weight loss, reduced sodium intake, and aerobic exercise should obviously be individualized, considering the needs of the patient and the effects of other co-morbid diseases. Extra consideration should be given to the choice of antihypertensive drugs, including diuretics, that may alter fluid balance.

PATHOPHYSIOLOGY

Hypertension can be defined in various ways. First, it can be described almost entirely in terms of blood pressure. Second, it can be considered as part of a syndrome of cardiovascular risk factors, including high blood pressure, with evidence for underlying vascular abnormalities. Finally, it is empirically a high-risk condition in which cardiovascular prognosis can be improved by appropriate therapies.

The Blood Pressure Approach

Since early actuarial data showing the connection between blood pressure and cardiovascular events were reported,

prospective clinical observations have supported the importance of this relationship. Long-term follow-up of a large cohort of young and middle-aged men recruited for a study known as the Multiple Risk Factor Intervention Trial showed that both systolic and diastolic blood pressures were highly predictive of subsequent strokes and cardiovascular outcomes.[1] A meta-analysis of 1 million people defined the link between blood pressure and major outcomes.[2] Regardless of age, blood pressure is clearly a major determinant of coronary and stroke mortality (Fig. 81-1). For every 20 mm Hg increment in systolic blood pressure, there is approximately a doubling of the risk of events. Age is also a major determinant of outcomes.[2,3]

Clinical trials of the importance of reducing blood pressure in patients with high-risk hypertension arrived at similar conclusions. Hypertensive patients treated with more aggressive as compared with less aggressive blood pressure–lowering therapy, particularly those who were also diabetic, had significantly fewer clinical events.[4] Tighter compared with less tight control of blood pressure was significantly more effective at preventing cardiovascular and diabetic clinical end points.[5] Meta-analysis of hypertension clinical trials supported the conclusion that the clinical effects of antihypertensive therapy could be explained mainly by their effects on blood pressure.[6] The clinical effects of a systolic blood pressure goal of less than 140 mm Hg,[7] using either valsartan or amlodipine (Fig. 81-2), sharply reduced the incidence of cardiac events, stroke, and mortality.

For these reasons, the 2003 report (Fig. 81-3) of the Joint National Committee on the Prevention, Detection and Treatment of High Blood Pressure (JNC 7) adopted a blood pressure–focused approach toward defining and treating hypertension.[8]

Staging of Hypertension

The JNC recommended that a diagnosis of hypertension should be made when blood pressure is 140/90 mm Hg or higher. As long as either the systolic or the diastolic criterion is met, the diagnosis is established. Hypertensive patients whose blood pressures are lower than 160/100 mm Hg are considered to be in stage 1, whereas those with blood pressures at or above this level are in stage 2. The main exception to the 140/90 mm Hg diagnostic threshold is for patients with diabetes or chronic kidney disease, in whom the diagnosis should be made and treatment begun if blood pressure is 130/80 mm Hg or higher. The goal is to reduce blood pressures to less than these threshold levels.

Prognosis is progressively better at levels of systolic blood pressure down to 115 mm Hg, or possibly lower (see Fig. 81-1). Why was 140 mm Hg chosen as a diagnostic criterion? Most evidence has come from trials that used treatment targets of approximately 140/90 mm Hg. A systolic goal of less than 140 mm Hg is associated with dramatic reductions in clinical events (see Fig. 81-2).[9] Clinical trial evidence that aims even lower in an attempt to actually improve outcomes in hypertensive patients is still awaited.

The JNC suggested a category called prehypertension, which encompasses blood pressures between 120/80 and 139/89 mm Hg (Table 81-1). They did not recommend

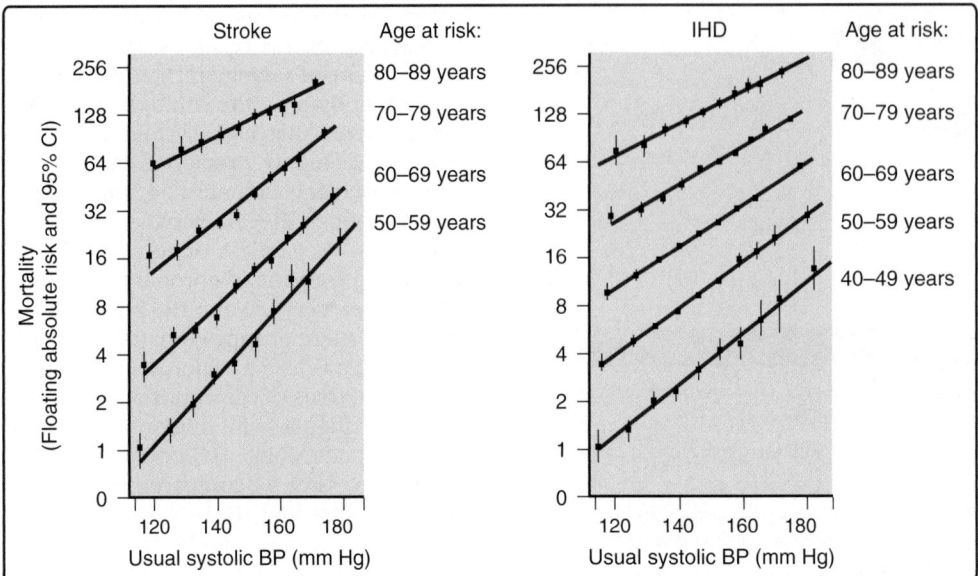

FIGURE 81-1 Relationships between systolic blood pressure and stroke or coronary heart disease mortality, according to deciles of age, derived from a meta-analysis of 1 million people. BP, blood pressure; CI, confidence interval; IHD, ischemic heart disease. *(Redrawn from Lewington S, Clarke R, Qizilbash N, et al. Prospective Studies Collaboration. Age-specific relevance of usual BP to vascular mortality: A meta-analysis of individual data for one million adults in 60 prospective studies. Lancet 2002;14:1903-1913.)*

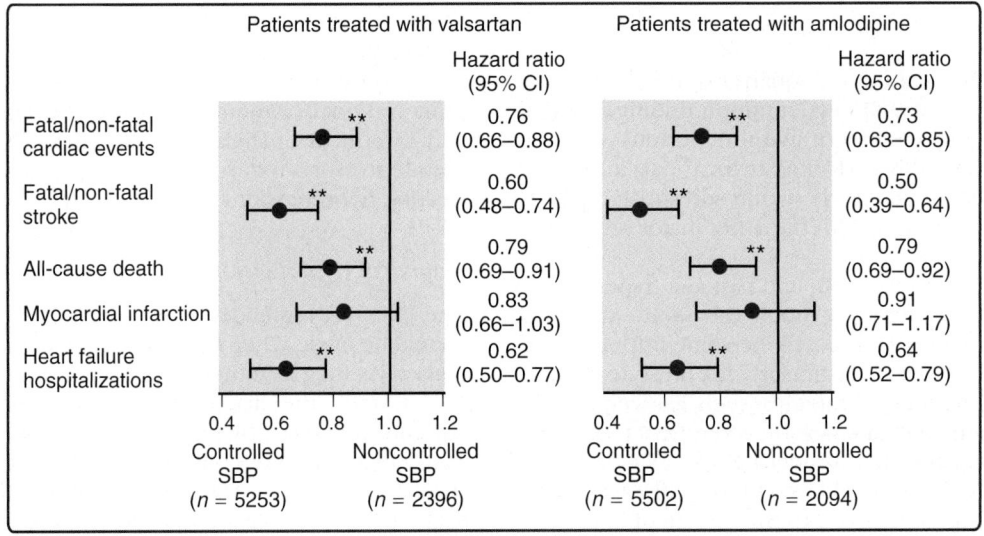

FIGURE 81-2 Effects on major clinical outcomes or mortality of blood pressure control (SBP <140 mm Hg), compared with noncontrol, at 6 months in high-risk hypertensive patients treated with either valsartan- or amlodipine-based antihypertensive therapy. **, *P* = .01. CI, confidence interval; SBP, systolic blood pressure. *(Redrawn from Weber MA, Julius S, Kjeldsen SE, et al. Blood pressure dependent and independent effects of antihypertensive treatment on clinical events in the VALUE trial. Lancet 2004;363:2049–2051.)*

treatment for patients with prehypertension (except for diabetics with renal disease) but suggested lifestyle modifications that could slow the usual age-related increase in blood pressure and delay the onset of clinical hypertension.

The Risk Factor Approach and the Metabolic Syndrome

Hypertension commonly clusters with other cardiovascular risk factors, including lipid abnormalities, glucose intol-erance, and obesity. This is referred to as the metabolic syndrome, syndrome X, or the hypertension syndrome.[10] None of these descriptions is satisfactory, for there is variability in the clinical picture. Moreover, because evidence for cardiovascular and renal changes are often part of this constellation of findings, limited terms such as "metabolic" do not suffice. Evidence for this syndrome can appear early in life. Normotensive offspring of parents with hypertension can have early metabolic changes and microalbu-minuria, early changes in the structure and function of the left ventricle, and stiffening of the arteries.[10] It is uncertain whether these familial findings reflect a genetic tendency or simply the effects of a commonly shared environment. Because the definition of the metabolic syndrome is arbitrary,[10] it may not truly represent a condition with a single underlying etiology.[11]

Despite these controversies, there is no doubt that a number of metabolic, cardiovascular, and renal changes are commonly associated with hypertension and almost certainly affect total cardiovascular risk. The official guidelines of the European Society of Hypertension differ sharply from the JNC guidelines in taking these co-morbidities into account.[12] The Society advocates earlier and more aggressive therapy in hypertensive patients who have concomitant risk factors, even if blood pressure is only modestly elevated; this also allows a more deliberative and protracted period of observation before starting treatment in hypertensive patients who do not have other risk factors.

One thing is clear. All the guidelines agree that every patient should be evaluated for all known cardiovascular risk factors, and, when these are found, they should be dealt with. In one important example of this approach, there is compelling evidence that statin therapy in hypertensive patients, even when in those whose low-density lipoprotein (LDL)-cholesterol levels do not reach traditional therapy criteria, reduces adverse cardiovascular outcomes.[13]

A More Fundamental Definition

Finally, a more fundamental paradigm sees hypertension as a disease affecting the structure and function of arteries and myocardium, together with other underlying abnormalities of renal and neuroendocrine mechanisms.[9] In this construct, there is a heterogeneity of causes leading to high blood pressure and an assumption that hypertension, although important, should also be interpreted as a diagnostic sign of underlying abnormalities. This sets the stage for anticipating that hypertension ultimately will be regarded as a set of varying conditions that, once carefully described, might respond optimally to different therapeutic strategies.

EVALUATION OF HYPERTENSION

Evaluating and diagnosing hypertension, although relatively straightforward, has long-term implications. In general, elevated blood pressure is all that is required to make a diagnosis, but the impact is considerable. Regular medical visits, lifestyle changes, and medication administration are now necessary to control the disease. Clinicians must communicate to patients that cardiovascular events, strokes, and other serious outcomes can result if hypertension is not well treated. It is critical to provide encouragement that the diagnosis should not adversely alter patients' long-term outlook, provided they make sensible commitments to their own care.

Measuring Blood Pressure

Blood pressure readings should be confirmed on two or three occasions, preferably days apart.[8] Some advocate

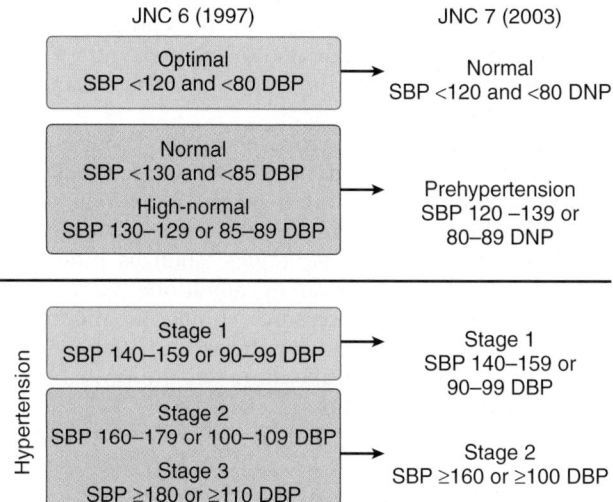

FIGURE 81-3 The change in classification of blood pressure between the two most recent reports of the Joint National Committee on Prevention, Detection, Evaluation, and Treatment of High Blood Pressure (JNC), indicating the recent adoption of a simplified classification in which the concept of prehypertension was proposed for the first time. All measurements are in millimeters of mercury (mm Hg). DBP, diastolic blood pressure; SBP, systolic blood pressure. *(Redrawn from The Seventh Report of the Joint National Committee on Prevention, Detection, Evaluation, and Treatment of High Blood Pressure: The JNC 7 report. JAMA 2003;289:2560–2572.)*

TABLE 81-1	Hypertension Writing Group: Definition and Classification of Hypertension*			
PARAMETER	**NORMAL**	**STAGE 1 HYPERTENSION**	**STAGE 2 HYPERTENSION**	**STAGE 3 HYPERTENSION**
BP pattern and CVD status	Normal BP or rare elevations AND No identifiable CVD	Occasional or intermittent BP elevations OR Risk factors suggesting early CVD	Sustained BP elevations OR Evidence of progressive CVD	Marked and sustained BP elevations OR Evidence of advanced CVD
Cardiovascular risk factors	None	≥1 risk factor present	Multiple risk factors present	Multiple risk factors present
Early disease markers	None	0-1	≥2	≥2 present with evidence of CVD
Target organ damage	None	None	Early signs present	Overtly present with or without CVD events

*Classification of hypertension proposed by a working group of the American Society of Hypertension that, in addition to blood pressure levels, takes into account concomitant risk factors as well as evidence for cardiovascular structural or functional changes in determining the status of hypertensive patients.
BP, blood pressure; CVD, cardiovascular disease.
Adapted from Giles TD, Berk BC, Black HR, et al; on behalf of the Hypertension Writing Group. Expanding the definition and classification of hypertension. J Clin Hypertens 2005;7:505-512.

ambulatory blood pressure monitoring if "white coat hypertension"—high blood pressure in the clinical setting but normal pressure at most other times—is suspected. This can be useful, but is probably unnecessary if other clinical findings, particularly other risk factors or cardiovascular or renal changes, suggest the need for antihypertensive therapy. Home blood pressure readings by patients are interesting, but blood pressures measured at home typically are lower than those in the clinic, because they are often taken at times when blood pressures are expected to be lower.

Investigations

Laboratory studies[8,12] should evaluate lipids, glucose, electrolytes, renal function, and liver function. Fasting tests diagnose diabetes and identify the lipid profile. Microalbuminuria should be sought as an important prognostic factor; likewise, an electrocardiogram (or echocardiogram, if feasible) should be obtained to check for left ventricular hypertrophy or other evidence of cardiac involvement.

TREATMENT

Most patients require antihypertensive drugs, but there is evidence that nonpharmacologic strategies (lifestyle modifications) are also effective. Stage 1 hypertension (pressures between 140/90 and 159/99 mm Hg) in motivated patients warrants a trial of up to 3 or even 6 months of nonpharmacological strategies (JNC 7 guidelines favor a shorter period). A decision should then be made about drug therapy. Patients with stage 2 hypertension require immediate drug therapy.

An alternative is to start drug treatment and lifestyle modification simultaneously, with a promise that successful lifestyle strategies could enable drug treatment to be reduced or discontinued if blood pressure remains well controlled. In any case, appropriate dietary and other lifestyle measures should be a continuing part of hypertension management.

Lifestyle Modifications

Perhaps the most compelling results (Table 81-2) in terms of blood pressure reduction occur in overweight people

TABLE 81-2 Lifestyle Modifications*

MODIFICATION	APPROXIMATE RANGE OF SBP REACTION
Weight reduction	5-20 mm Hg for every 10 kg weight loss
Adoption of DASH eating plan	8-14 mm Hg
Dietary sodium reduction	2-8 mm Hg
Increased physical activity	4-9 mm Hg
Moderation of alcohol consumption	2-4 mm Hg

*Recommended nonpharmacological strategies that potentially can provide meaningful blood pressure reductions in hypertensive patients. Citations for these differing approaches are listed in the JNC 7 Report.
DASH, Dietary Approach to Stop Hypertension; SBP, systolic blood pressure.
From The Seventh Report of the Joint National Committee on Prevention, Detection, Evaluation, and Treatment of High Blood Pressure: The JNC 7 report. JAMA 2003;289:2560–2572.

who successfully lose weight.[8] Blood pressure often falls after small early weight reductions, suggesting that the metabolic and neuroendocrine factors that mediate the hypertension of obesity[14] are promptly responsive to reduced caloric intake.

The DASH (Dietary Approach to Stop Hypertension) diet encompasses increased intake of fruits and vegetables and reduction in dietary fat. This diet is effective in blood pressure reduction, particularly in African Americans, but may be difficult to follow at home. The benefits of this diet were based on professionally prepackaged meals; it is not yet established whether the costs and effort involved in assembling such a diet privately allow long-term compliance. A low-sodium diet can also reduce blood pressure; this may not be true for everyone, but for those who have some form of sodium sensitivity, it helps. For people who consume large amounts of alcohol, a meaningful reduction helps reduce blood pressure. Although modest consumption of alcohol appears to be cardioprotective, consumption of more than two drinks a day often raises blood pressure, apart from other possible deleterious health effects.

Exercise, particularly aerobic exercise, reduces blood pressure. One virtue is that those who successfully take up an exercise program often persist for a long period. Moreover, those who exercise consistently are more likely to follow other lifestyle strategies, such as monitoring caloric intake. One final strategy, albeit one that does not directly reduce blood pressure, should be mentioned: smoking cessation. Many hypertensive patients smoke regularly, which dramatically increases the probability of cardiovascular complications.

Starting Drug Treatment

The objective of drug treatment is to reduce blood pressure to less than 140/90 mm Hg in most patients, and to less than 130/80 mm Hg in high-risk groups such as patients with diabetes or chronic kidney disease (Fig. 81-4).

The JNC 7 Algorithm

Patients can be divided into three groups: those with compelling indications (concomitant conditions that dictate the use of certain drugs appropriate for those conditions and for hypertension); those with stage 1 hypertension (blood pressures between 140/90 and 159/99 mm Hg); and those with blood pressures of 160/100 mm Hg or higher. These designations lead to three different strategies.

COMPELLING INDICATIONS

Hypertensive patients often have other conditions (Table 81-3) that require specific therapies. For example, those with diabetes or renal disease should receive renin-angiotensin blockers such as angiotensin-converting enzyme (ACE) inhibitors or angiotensin receptor blockers (ARBs), which are the treatments of choice for both the concomitant condition and the hypertension; likewise, β-blockers or calcium channel blockers are treatments of choice in patients with angina pectoris.

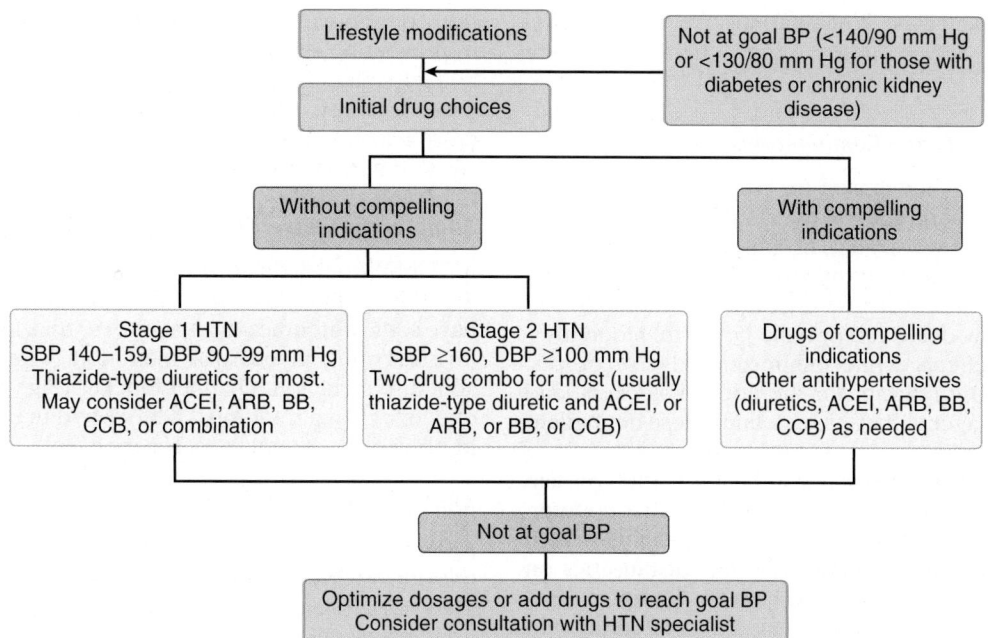

FIGURE 81-4   Recommendations of the Joint National Committee on the Prevention, Detection, and Treatment of High Blood Pressure (JNC 7) for diagnosis, setting of treatment goals, therapeutic strategies, and drug selection in patients with hypertension. ACEI, angiotensin-converting enzyme inhibitor; ARB, angiotensin II receptor blocker; BB, β-blocker; BP, blood pressure; CCB, calcium channel blocker; DBP, diastolic blood pressure; HTN, hypertension; SBP, systolic blood pressure. *(Redrawn from The Seventh Report of the Joint National Committee on Prevention, Detection, Evaluation, and Treatment of High Blood Pressure: The JNC 7 report. JAMA. 2003;289:2560–2572.)*

TABLE 81-3 Compelling Indications for Individual Drug Classes*		
COMPELLING INDICATION	**INITIAL THERAPY OPTIONS**	**CLINICAL TRIAL BASIS**
Heart failure	THIAZ, BB, ACEI, ARB, ALDO ANT	ACC/AHA Heart Failure Guideline, MERIT-HF, COPERNICUS, CIBIS, SOLVD, AIRE, TRACE, ValHEFT, RALES
Postmyocardial Infarction	BB, ACEI, ALDO ANT	ACC/AHA Post-MI Guideline, BHAT, SAVE, Capricorn, EPHESUS
High CAD risk	THIAZ, BB, ACEI, CCB	ALLHAT, HOPE, ANBP2, LIFE, CONVINCE

*A summary of possible drug selections in hypertensive patients whose concomitant cardiovascular or other conditions can be treated with drugs that are also appropriate for the management of high blood pressure. Further details on the use of these drugs and citations for the studies from which these recommendations are derived are provided in the JNC 7 report.

ACC/AHA, American College of Cardiology/American Heart Association; ACEI, angiotensin-converting enzyme inhibitors; AIRE, Acute Infarction Ramipril Efficacy; ALDO ANT, aldosterone antagonist; ALLHAT, Antihypertensive and Lipid-Lowering Treatment to Prevent Heart Attack Trial; ANBP2, Second Australian National Blood Pressure Study; ARB, angiotensin receptor blocker; BB, β-blocker; BHAT, β-Blocker Heart Attack Trial; CAD, coronary artery disease; Capricorn, Carvedilol Post-Infarct Survival Control in Left Ventricular Dysfunction; CCB, calcium channel blocker; CIBIS, Cardiac Insufficiency Bisoprolol Study; CONVINCE, Controlled Onset Verapamil Investigation of Cardiovascular End Points; COPERNICUS, Carvedilol Prospective Randomized Cumulative Survival Study; EPHESUS, Eplerenone Post-Acute Myocardial Infarction Heart Failure Efficacy and Survival Study; HOPE, Heart Outcomes Prevention Evaluation Study; LIFE, Losartan Intervention for Endpoint Reduction in Hypertension Study; MERIT-HF, Metoprolol CR/XL Randomized Intervention Trial in Congestive Heart Failure; MI, myocardial infarction; RALES, Randomized Aldactone Evaluation Study; SAVE, Survival and Ventricular Enlargement Study; SOLVD, Studies of Left Ventricular Dysfunction; THIAZ, thiazide diuretics; TRACE, Trandolapril Cardiac Evaluation Study; ValHEFT, Valsartan Heart Failure Trial.

From The Seventh Report of the Joint National Committee on Prevention, Detection, Evaluation, and Treatment of High Blood Pressure: The JNC 7 report. JAMA 2003;289:2560–2572.

STARTING TREATMENT IN STAGE 1 HYPERTENSION

The major guidelines for patients with stage 1 hypertension recommend therapy with one drug.[12,15] The JNC 7 guidelines[8] are biased in favor of thiazide diuretics but acknowledge that other drug types may be considered. Clinical trials have found diuretics to be useful, compared with placebo, in preventing major clinical events. One study compared a thiazide-like diuretic, chlorthalidone, with the ACE inhibitor, lisinopril, and the calcium channel blocker, amlodipine, on clinical outcomes in high-risk hypertension.[16] There were no differences among the three drugs on the primary study end point, fatal and

nonfatal coronary events, but the diuretic appeared to be better than the ACE inhibitor in preventing strokes, and better than the calcium channel blocker in preventing heart failure. The results are still under debate.[17-19]

STARTING TREATMENT IN STAGE 2 HYPERTENSION

Those requiring blood pressure reductions of at least 20/10 mm Hg should have their treatment started with combination therapy. The rationale is that, because most of these patients will eventually require more than one drug, starting with a combination accelerates treatment and makes timely achievement of blood pressure targets more likely.[7] Fixed-dose combinations are more convenient, require fewer doses, and often are more cost-effective.

The Growing Use of Drug Combinations

Efficacy is not the only reason for using combinations of agents. Side effects and adverse events also can be reduced. This occurs in two ways. First, because the dose-response characteristics of most antihypertensive agents provide much of their efficacy at low doses, the combination of two agents in low doses can provide powerful blood pressure-lowering effects while minimizing adverse events. This is particularly relevant for diuretics, β-blockers, and centrally acting agents that have definite dose-dependent side effects.

The second way in which combination therapy can reduce adverse effects is in the use of drugs that counteract each other's unwanted actions. Renin–angiotensin blockers attenuate the unwanted actions of diuretics on potassium, glucose, and other metabolic findings. Similarly, ACE inhibitors or ARBs may be combined with calcium channel blockers; the peripheral edema caused by the calcium channel blockers can be largely offset by blockers of the renin–angiotensin system.

Choice of Agent

The abundance of antihypertensive agents can cause confusion. Drugs that interrupt the renin–angiotensin system should probably be part of most antihypertensive regimens.

Calcium Channel Blockers

Both dihydropyridine and nondihydropyridine agents are equal to the other major drug classes in preventing major clinical outcomes and mortality.[20,21] Amlodipine, in patients with minimally raised blood pressures (prehypertension) and coronary disease, was effective in reducing the need for coronary revascularization and hospitaliza-

tion for angina.[22] Amlodipine was as effective as an ARB in preventing strokes, coronary events, and mortality, but less effective in preventing heart failure.[7] Amlodipine-based therapy was as effective as therapies based on diuretics or ACE inhibitors in preventing coronary events, strokes, and mortality.[16]

Angiotensin-Converting Enzyme Inhibitors

ACE inhibitors are similar to other drug classes in preventing major clinical outcomes.[23] ACE inhibitors appear to have some outcome advantages over thiazides, particularly in preventing myocardial infarction.[24] An ACE inhibitor added to a calcium channel blocker (Fig. 81-5) was more effective than a traditional β-blocker/diuretic combination in preventing mortality, coronary events, and strokes.[25,26]

Angiotensin Receptor Blockers

ARBs are the newest of the major classes; they are effective in lowering blood pressure and are well tolerated. They are at least as effective as other antihypertensive drug classes (Fig. 81-6) in preventing major cardiovascular events.[27] Like ACE inhibitors, they are also indicated for congestive heart failure. In hypertension and diabetes with nephropathy, the ARBs prevent progression to end-stage renal disease.[28,29]

In high-risk hypertensive patients (with left ventricular hypertrophy on electrocardiography), losartan was 25% more effective than a β-blocker in reducing stroke.[30] After ischemic strokes, eprosartan had blood pressure effects identical to those of a dihydropyridine but reduced recurrent stroke events by 25%.[31] When compared with a β-blocker in patients who had hypertension with left ventricular hypertrophy, losartan was more effective in preventing new-onset atrial fibrillation despite equal blood pressure effects.[32] In patients with atrial fibrillation pharmacologically or electrically converted back to sinus rhythm who were prescribed amiodarone, the addition of irbesartan was more effective than placebo in preventing atrial fibrillation recurrence.[33]

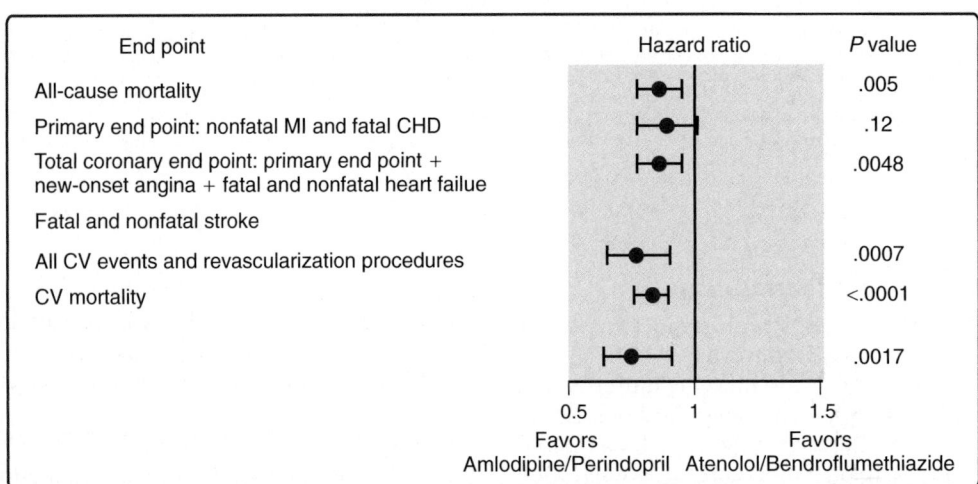

FIGURE 81-5 Hazard ratios (relative benefits) for major clinical outcomes and mortality in high-risk hypertensive patients being treated with either an older antihypertensive drug combination (atenolol/thiazide) or a newer drug combination (amlodipine/perindopril). CHD, coronary heart disease; CV, cardiovascular; MI, myocardial infarction. *(Redrawn from Dahlof B, Sever PS, Poulter NR, et al; for the ASCOT Investigators. Prevention of cardiovascular events with an antihypertensive regimen of amlodipine adding perindopril as required versus atenolol adding bendroflumethiazide as required, in the Anglo-Scandinavian Cardiac Outcomes Trial–Blood Pressure Lowering Arm [ASCOT-BPLA]: A multicentre randomized controlled trial. Lancet. 2005;366:895-906.)*

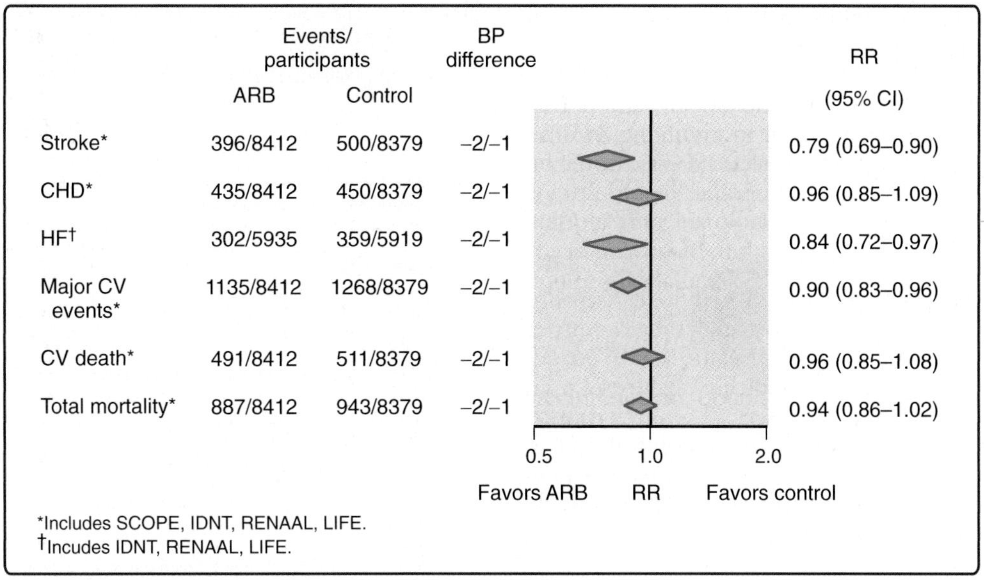

	Events/ participants		BP difference			RR
	ARB	Control				(95% CI)
Stroke*	396/8412	500/8379	–2/–1			0.79 (0.69–0.90)
CHD*	435/8412	450/8379	–2/–1			0.96 (0.85–1.09)
HF†	302/5935	359/5919	–2/–1			0.84 (0.72–0.97)
Major CV events*	1135/8412	1268/8379	–2/–1			0.90 (0.83–0.96)
CV death*	491/8412	511/8379	–2/–1			0.96 (0.85–1.08)
Total mortality*	887/8412	943/8379	–2/–1			0.94 (0.86–1.02)

*Includes SCOPE, IDNT, RENAAL, LIFE.
†Incudes IDNT, RENAAL, LIFE.

FIGURE 81-6   A comparison of the effects of angiotensin receptor blocker (ARB) regimens and control regimens (drugs other than ARBs or angiotensin-converting enzyme inhibitors) on major clinical outcomes or mortality in hypertensive patients included in a large-scale meta-analysis. BP, blood pressure; CHD, coronary heart disease; CI, confidence interval; CV, cardiovascular; HF, heart failure; IDNT, Irbesartan Diabetic Nephropathy Trial; LIFE, Losartan Intervention for Endpoint Reduction in Hypertension Study; RENAAL, Reduction of Endpoints in Non-Insulin Dependent Diabetes Mellitus with the Angiotensin II Antagonist Losartan Study; RR, relative risk; SCOPE, Study on Cognition and Prognosis in the Elderly. *(Redrawn from Blood Pressure Lowering Treatment Trialists' Collaboration. Effects of different blood pressure lowering regimens on major cardiovascular events: Second cycle of prospectively designed overviews. Lancet. 2003;362:1527-1535.)*

Inadequate Adherence

Some hypertensive patients simply do not fill their drug prescriptions; and even when they do, there is often little attempt to remain with the recommended treatment regimen. Explanations for this so-called poor compliance are not entirely satisfactory. Drug side effects certainly can be a factor in poor treatment compliance, but the newer drug classes are usually well tolerated. Cost also can be a reason, but in health systems where drugs are provided, compliance is not much better than in the community in general. Certainly, in cases of poor treatment response, the possibility that the prescribed medications have not been taken should be actively considered.

Common Errors

Perhaps the single most common error made in putting together treatment combinations is the omission of a diuretic. Most patients eat diets with excessive sodium, which mitigates against the efficacy of many drug classes. If the patient will not modify his or her diet, a diuretic (e.g., hydrochlorothiazide in a dose of 25 mg daily) should be strongly considered.

A number of drug classes used for indications other than hypertension can raise blood pressure and interfere with blood pressure–lowering agents. Among the most common are the nonsteroidal anti-inflammatory drugs (NSAIDs). These drugs, which are frequently prescribed for arthritis and pain, often cause some degree of sodium and water retention and increase blood pressure. This applies both to the conventional drugs and the newer cyclooxygenase 2 (COX 2)–selective inhibitors. It may be necessary to add or increase the dose of a diuretic and to reduce sodium intake to minimize this interaction. Corti-

costeroids, often prescribed in palliative care, similarly can cause volume expansion.

Oral contraceptives can increase blood pressure. Various cold remedies, particularly those containing sympathomimetic agents and antihistamines, can raise blood pressure. Typically, such treatments are used only for short-term symptomatic relief; once the drug is discontinued, its adverse blood pressure effects disappear promptly. Some dietary agents raise blood pressure and should be asked about if blood pressure responses to treatment seem inadequate.

Secondary Hypertension

Secondary hypertension is worth considering if blood pressure control deteriorates rapidly or there is rapid onset of hypertension. The full workup and diagnosis of secondary hypertension usually involve specialists and sophisticated laboratory and imaging techniques.

Hypertensive Emergencies and Urgencies

True hypertensive emergencies usually require hospital care. A hypertensive emergency is not defined solely on the basis of high blood pressure but requires evidence of acute blood pressure–related effects. Encephalopathy, pulmonary edema, and hematuria are examples. Such emergencies require closely monitored, aggressive therapy, usually based on intravenous therapy selected according to the presumed underlying cause and clinical features of the crisis.

Very high blood pressure (systolic values >180 mm Hg) without acute concomitant clinical findings is sometimes referred to as a hypertensive urgency. Oral treatment is acceptable but should employ drugs with long durations of action. Clonidine, ACE inhibitors, ARBs, β-blockers, and long-acting calcium channel blockers often bring blood pressure to acceptable levels within 1 to 4 hours. Use of a combination of two agents should be strongly considered, but even if the initial result is gratifying, prompt follow-up visits should ensure that blood pressures remain acceptable.

EFFECTIVENESS

Hypertension management in the United States is probably more successful than in almost all other countries. Even so, data from the National Health and Nutrition Examination Survey (NHANES) indicate that results are disappointing.[34] About three quarters of all hypertensive people know they have this condition, but only about half are receiving therapy, and barely one third have acceptable blood pressure control. A variety of social, emotional, and financial reasons contribute.[35]

SUPPORTIVE CARE

High blood pressure responds to weight loss and fluid depletion, both of which are common in the terminally ill. Under these circumstances, it often becomes necessary to taper and then discontinue antihypertensive drugs. Diuretics add directly to fluid depletion and potentially unwanted changes in potassium and other electrolytes, so they should be discontinued early in the tapering process. If β-blockers are being used, their doses should be progressively reduced over a 7- to 10-day period to avoid the risk of coronary events. Most other modern antihypertensive agents can be stopped without the danger of returned hypertension.

REFERENCES

1. Neaton JD, Wentworth D; for the Multiple Risk Factor Intervention Trial Research Group. Serum cholesterol, blood pressure, cigarette smoking, and death from coronary heart disease. Overall findings and differences by age for 316,099 white men. Arch Intern Med 1992;152:56-64.
2. Lewington S, Clarke R, Qizilbash N, et al. Prospective Studies Collaboration. Age-specific relevance of usual BP to vascular mortality: A meta-analysis of individual data for one million adults in 60 prospective studies. Lancet 2002;14:1903-1913.
3. Weber MA. Is there more to life than blood pressure? J Clin Hypertens 2005;7:149-151.
4. Hansson L, Zanchetti A, Carruthers S, et al; for the HOT study group. Effects of intensive blood-pressure lowering and low-dose aspirin in patients with hypertension: Principal results of the Hypertension Optimal Treatment (HOT) randomized trial. Lancet 1998;351:1755-1762.
5. U.K. Prospective Diabetes Study Group. Tight blood pressure control and risk of macrovascular and microvascular complications in type 2 diabetes: UKPDS 38. BMJ 1998;317:703-713.
6. Staessen JA, Gasowski J, Wang JG, et al. Risks of untreated and treated isolated systolic hypertension in the elderly: Meta-analysis of outcomes trials. Lancet 2000;104:865-872.
7. Weber MA, Julius S, Kjeldsen SE, et al. Blood pressure dependent and independent effects of antihypertensive treatment on clinical events in the VALUE trial. Lancet 2004;363:2049-2051.
8. The Seventh Report of the Joint National Committee on Prevention, Detection, Evaluation, and Treatment of High Blood Pressure: The JNC 7 report. JAMA 2003;289:2560-2572.
9. Giles TD, Berk BC, Black HR, et al; on behalf of the Hypertension Writing Group. Expanding the definition and classification of hypertension. J Clin Hypertens 2005;7:505-512.
10. Weber MA. Cardiovascular and metabolic consequences of obesity. In Topol EJ (ed). Textbook of Cardiovascular Medicine. New York: Lippincott Williams & Wilkins, 2006.
11. Kahn R, Buse J, Ferrannini E, Stern M. The metabolic syndrome: Time for a critical appraisal. Joint statement from the American Diabetes Association and the European Association for the Study of Diabetes. Diabetologia 2005;48:1684-1699.
12. 2003 European Society of Hypertension—European Society of Cardiology Guidelines for the Management of Arterial Hypertension. J Hypertens 2003;21:1011-1054.
13. Sever PS, Dahlof B, Poulter NR, et al; for the ASCOT Investigators. Prevention of coronary and stroke events with atorvastatin in hypertensive patients who have average or lower-than-average cholesterol concentrations, in the Anglo-Scandinavian Cardiac Outcomes Trial—Lipid Lowering Arm (ASCOT-LLA): A multicentre randomized controlled trial. Lancet 2003;361:1149-1158.
14. Weber MA. The metabolic syndrome. In Antman EM (ed). Cardiovascular Therapeutics. Philadelphia: Elsevier, 2006.
15. Douglas JG, Bakris GL, Epstein M, et al. Management of high blood pressure in African Americans: Consensus statement of the Hypertension in African American Working Group of the International Society on Hypertension in Blacks. Arch Intern Med 2003;163:525-541.
16. The ALLHAT Officers and Coordinators for the ALLHAT Collaborative Research Group. Major outcomes in high-risk hypertensive patients randomized to angiotensin-converting enzyme inhibitor or calcium channel blocker vs diuretic. The Antihypertensive and Lipid-Lowering Treatment to Prevent Heart Attack Trial. (ALLHAT). JAMA 2002;288:2981-2997.
17. Weber MA. The ALLHAT Report: A case of information and misinformation. J Clin Hypertens 2003;5:9-13.
18. Julius S. The ALLHAT study: If you believe in evidence-based medicine, stick to it! J Hypertens 2003;21:453-454.
19. McInnes GT. Size isn't everything: ALLHAT in perspective. J Hypertens 2003;21:459-461.
20. Brown MJ, Palmer CR, Castaigne A, et al. Morbidity and mortality in patients randomized to double-blind treatment with a long-acting calcium-channel-blocker or diuretic in the International Nifedipine GITS study: Intervention as a Goal in Hypertension Treatment (INSIGHT). Lancet 2000;356:366-372.
21. Vasan RS, Beiser A, Seshadri S, et al. Residual lifetime risk for developing hypertension in middle-aged women and men: The Framingham Heart Study. JAMA 2002;287:1003-1010.
22. Nissen SE, Tuzcu EM, Libby P, et al; for the CAMELOT Investigators. Effect of antihypertensive agents on cardiovascular events in patients with coronary disease and normal blood pressure. The CAMELOT study: A randomized controlled trial. JAMA 2004;292:2217-2226.
23. Blood Pressure Lowering Treatment Trialists' Collaboration. Effects of ACE inhibitors, calcium antagonists and other blood pressure lowering drugs: Results of prospectively designed overviews of randomized trials. Lancet 2000;355:1955-1964.
24. Wing LMH, Reid CM, Ryan P, et al; for the Second Australian National Blood Pressure Study Group. A comparison of outcomes with angiotensin-converting-enzyme inhibitors and diuretics for hypertension in the elderly. N Engl J Med 2003;348:583-592.
25. Dahlof B, Sever PS, Poulter NR, et al; for the ASCOT Investigators. Prevention of cardiovascular events with an antihypertensive regimen of amlodipine adding perindopril as required versus atenolol adding bendroflumethiazide as required, in the Anglo-Scandinavian Cardiac Outcomes Trial-Blood Pressure Lowering Arm (ASCOT-BPLA): A multicentre randomized controlled trial. Lancet 2005;366:895-906.
26. Poulter NR, Wedel H, Dahlof B, et al; for the ASCOT Investigators. Role of blood pressure and other variables in the differential cardiovascular event rates noted in the Anglo-Scandinavian Cardiac Outcomes Trial-Blood Pressure Lowering Arm (ASCOT-BPLA). Lancet 2005;366:907-913.
27. Blood Pressure Lowering Treatment Trialists' Collaboration. Effects of different blood pressure lowering regimens on major cardiovascular events: Second cycle of prospectively designed overviews. Lancet 2003;362:1527-1535.
28. Brenner BM, Cooper ME, DeZeeuw D, et al; for the RENAAL study investigators. Effects of losartan on renal and cardiovascular outcomes in patients with type 2 diabetes and nephropathy. N Engl J Med 2001;345:861-869.
29. Lewis EJ, Hunsicker LG, Clarke WR, et al; for the Collaborative Study Group. Renoprotective effect of the angiotensin-receptor antagonist irbesartan in patients with nephropathy due to type 2 diabetes. N Engl J Med 2001;345:851-860.
30. Lindholm LH, Ibsen H, Dahlof B, et al for the LIFE study group. Cardiovascular morbidity and mortality in patients with diabetes in the Losartan Intervention For Endpoint Reduction in Hypertension study (LIFE): A randomized trial against atenolol. Lancet 2002;359:1004-1010.
31. Schrader J, Luders S, Kulschewsli A, et al; for the MOSES Study Group. Morbidity and mortality after stroke, eprosartan compared with nitrendipine for secondary prevention: Principal results of a prospective randomized controlled study (MOSES). Stroke 2005;36:1218-1226.
32. Wachtell K, Lehto M, Gerdts E, et al. Angiotensin II receptor blockade reduces new-onset atrial fibrillation and subsequent stroke compared to atenolol: The Losartan Intervention For End Point Reduction in Hypertension (LIFE) study. J Am Coll Cardiol. 2005;45:712-719.
33. Madrid AH, Bueno MG, Rebollo JM, et al. Use of irbesartan to maintain sinus rhythm in patients with long-lasting persistent atrial fibrillation: A prospective and randomized study. Circulation 2002;106:331-336.
34. Burt VL, Cutler JA, Higgins M, et al. Trends in the prevalence, awareness, treatment and control of hypertension in the adult US population: Data from the health examination surveys, 1960 to 1991. Hypertension 1995;26:60-69.
35. Weir MR, Maibach EW, Bakris GL, et al. Implications of a healthy lifestyle and medication analysis for improving hypertension control. Arch Intern Med 2000;160:481-490.

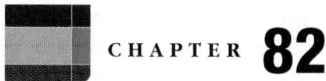

CHAPTER **82**

Kidney Failure

Sara N. Davison

AGE (YR)	Time on Dialysis			
	1 yr	**2 yr**	**3 yr**	**5 yr**
20 29	94.0	90.6	85.8	81.8
30-39	91.8	85.4	79.9	70.2
40-49	89.0	81.0	73.2	60.0
50-59	85.9	74.6	64.6	46.7
60-64	81.1	68.0	55.7	35.6
65-69	76.9	62.6	48.5	27.3
70-79	69.6	51.9	37.3	18.4
80+	58.9	37.8	23.9	8.4
All	78.2	65.2	53.7	37.7

TABLE 82-1 Unadjusted Survival Probabilities (%) for Incident ESRD Patients*

*The incident cohorts are determined at the time of ESRD treatment initiation (dialysis or renal transplantation) with the 60-day stable modality and 90-day survival.
ESRD, end-stage renal disease.
Data from U.S. Renal Data System, National Institutes of Health, and National Institute of Diabetes and Digestive and Kidney Diseases. 2005 Annual Report: Atlas of End-Stage Renal Disease in the United States. USRDS 2005. Bethesda, MD: U.S. Renal Data System, 2005.

Chronic kidney disease (CKD) is a major public health problem; end-stage renal disease (ESRD), requiring renal replacement therapy such as dialysis or renal transplantation, affects more than 500,000 patients in the United States.[1] The prevalence of ESRD is projected to double in the next decade. ESRD patients are typically elderly: the average age of patients starting chronic dialysis in North America is 63 years. Patients older than 70 years of age are the fastest-growing group of patients starting long-term dialysis, with 38,711 incident cases in 2003; 13,839 of them more than 80 years old.[1] CKD patients also have much co-morbidity. More than 40% are diabetic, and 80% are hypertensive; cardiomyopathy, peripheral and cerebral vascular disease, arthropathies, and psychiatric conditions are common and contribute significantly to symptoms.

It is not surprising that, despite technological improvements, more than 82,588 ESRD patients die yearly in the United States, for an unadjusted annual death rate of 20% to 25%.[1] The risk of death of a 45 -year-old starting dialysis is 20 times that of someone the same age without CKD (Table 82-1). These mortality rates rival those of acquired immunodeficiency syndrome (AIDS) and most cancers. In North America, approximately 15% to 25% of the annual mortality among patients with ESRD results from decisions to discontinue dialysis, and this is the second leading cause of death after cardiovascular disease. The need for advance care planning and open discussions concerning end-of-life issues is great. It is increasingly recognized that CKD patients are among the most symptomatic of any patients with chronic disease, and growing evidence suggests that the quality of the dying experience is suboptimal.[2] These issues have made caring for patients with ESRD a unique challenge. Many have called for the implementation of modern palliative care into this field.

EPIDEMIOLOGY AND PREVALENCE

Pain and other symptoms are common in CKD, due to concurrent co-morbidity (e.g., diabetic neuropathy, peripheral vascular disease), primary renal disease (e.g., polycystic kidney disease), or disease caused by renal failure itself (e.g., calciphylaxis, renal osteodystrophy, dialysis-related amyloidosis [DRA]). Such symptoms are also related to management of renal failure with dialysis (e.g., ischemic neuropathies from arteriovenous fistulas dialysis-related cramping) or with renal transplantation (e.g., avascular necrosis).

Little is known about the epidemiology of pain and other symptoms in CKD and only recently has this subject become a research focus. At least 50% of patients undergoing long-term dialysis experience chronic pain; for 82%, of them pain is moderate to severe.[3] Even in the last day of life after withdrawal of dialysis, pain is present in 42%. Causes are diverse and often multifactorial. It appears that musculoskeletal pain is the most common type, as in the general population. Joint symptoms such as stiffness, pain, decreased range of motion, effusions, crepitus, and deformity have been described in up to 69% to 82% of ESRD patients. The causes are different from those in the general population, however, and chronic musculoskeletal pain is more likely to be attributed to causes such as acute monoarthritis or polyarthritis resulting from periarticular calcification, pseudogout or gout, septic arthritis, carpal tunnel, or ruptured tendon. These symptoms are often present with renal osteodystrophy or dialysis-related amyloidosis (DRA). Musculoskeletal pain in CKD is equal in severity to neuropathic or ischemic pain. After renal transplantation, patients continue to experience troublesome symptoms, of which pain is one of the most common; 59% of these patients report headaches, and 30% report bone pain.

Dialysis itself is "palliative." There is no cure for ESRD; although dialysis sustains life, concurrent co-morbidities progress. Diabetic complications such as gastroparesis, enteropathy, autonomic neuropathy, diabetic ulcers, and cardiovascular disease need to be dealt with. Medical literature that addresses these topics specifically in patients with CKD is sparse, so care is often extrapolated from the nonrenal setting. These disease entities are discussed elsewhere[2] and in other chapters of this book. Drug kinetics and side effects in CKD are dealt with later in this chapter.

Intradialytic symptoms related to dialysis itself are common, and patients with high co-morbidity have more of them. These symptoms include symptomatic hypotension, cramps, nausea, vomiting, pruritus, and pain from arteriovenous fistulas. Approximately 40% of dialysis treatments are associated with symptoms, and more than 80% of dialysis patients experience them at least once a week. These symptoms are routinely handled by the dialysis staff and often are related to a lack of appropriate vasoconstriction as fluid is removed.

ESRD patients have been evaluated using a modified version of the Edmonton Symptom Assessment System (to which pruritus was added). Comparisons with other patient populations, such as patients with cancer, can therefore be made. The most frequently reported symptoms are tiredness (92%), decreased well-being (92%), anorexia (83%), and pruritus (73%), although the most severe were pain, pruritus, and fatigue.[4] Insomnia is also distressing and is reported by 50% to 90% of dialysis patients. Many have specific primary sleep disorders such as sleep apnea, periodic leg movement disorder, and restless legs syndrome. Depression is also seen in 15% to 50% of ESRD patients. Depression and insomnia in ESRD are significantly associated with symptom burden.[5] The number and severity of these reported symptoms resemble those reported by patients hospitalized in palliative care settings with cancer. Symptom burden is highly predictive of all domains of health-related quality of life (HRQL), and change in burden is highly predictive of change in HRQL.[4] Symptom burden and HRQL, however, are not well correlated with objective clinical assessments, including biochemical parameters such as dialysis adequacy, serum albumin, hemoglobin, or calcium and phosphorous parameters. This highlights the importance of efforts to improve symptom burden to optimize clinical care and maximize HRQL.

PATHOPHYSIOLOGY

The discussion of pathophysiology in this chapter is limited to the pathophysiology of the painful syndromes encountered in CKD.

Renal Osteodystrophy

Changes in mineral metabolism and bone structure are almost universal in patients with CKD. There are three major types of bone disease (collectively called renal osteodystrophy) in advanced CKD.

Osteitis Fibrosa

Osteitis fibrosa is characterized by increased bone turnover due to secondary hyperparathyroidism. As the glomerular filtration rate decreases, phosphorous is retained. Three major and not mutually exclusive theories have been proposed to explain how hyperphosphatemia promotes release of parathyroid hormone (PTH): (1) hypocalcemia; (2) decreased formation of active vitamin D and decreased responsiveness of bone to vitamin D; and (3) a direct effect of hyperphosphatemia to increase PTH gene

expression. Over the long term, hyperparathyroidism is maladaptive, producing bone disease and calcium phosphate precipitation into arteries, joints, soft tissues, and the viscera. The prevalence of osteitis fibrosa among dialysis patients has decreased; currently, it affects approximately 20% of patients with CKD.[6]

Osteomalacia

Osteomalacia is characterized by decreased bone turnover, reductions in the number of bone-forming (osteoblastic) and bone-resorbing (osteoclastic) cells, and increased volume of unmineralized bone (osteoid) with increased osteoid seam thickness. This is usually caused by aluminum deposition in bone due to aluminum in dialysis water and aluminum-containing phosphate binders.

Adynamic Bone Disease

Adynamic bone disease is characterized by decreased bone turnover and decreased osteoblastic and osteoclastic cells. In contrast to osteomalacia, there is no increase in osteoid formation or unmineralized bone. Adynamic bone disease has become more frequent in the past decade and currently represents the major bone lesion in both peritoneal dialysis and hemodialysis patients, affecting 20% to 60%, depending on geographic region.[6] Adynamic bone disease is probably caused by suppression of PTH release induced by the use of calcium carbonate and calcitriol. This may be exacerbated by malnutrition. Some patients develop adynamic bone disease despite persistent hyperparathyroidism, suggesting that calcitriol itself may directly suppress osteoblastic activity and contribute to adynamic bone disease.[7]

Dialysis-Related Amyloidosis

DRA commonly develops in patients undergoing long-term dialysis and involves deposition of amyloid in bone, joints, and synovium. The amyloid is composed primarily of β_2-microglobulin and resembles other forms of amyloid in staining with Congo red and exhibiting apple-green birefringence under polarized light. β_2-Microglobulin may have a high affinity for collagen, which could explain the predominance of joint and bone disease. The incidence of DRA is closely linked to the duration of dialysis. A prospective postmortem study found joint amyloid deposition in 21% of patients requiring hemodialysis for less than 2 years, in 50% of those at 4 to 7 years, in 90% at 7 to 13 years, and in 100% at more than 13 years.[8] By comparison, the clinical prevalence of disease is zero at 5 years but increases to 50% at 12 years and almost 100% by 20 years.[9]

Calcific Uremic Arteriolopathy

"Calciphylaxis" is the clinical presentation of metastatic soft tissue calcification and necrosis in the skin and visceral organs. The term has been misleadingly used by physicians to describe a relatively rare but serious disorder seen almost exclusively in ESRD that is characterized by tissue ischemia and painful violaceous mottling of the skin that can progress to ulcers and eschar formation. The pathogenesis and histology of the two disorders are different. In the original animal model, calcification was found in the subcutaneous tissues without vessel calcification, which is the hallmark of calciphylaxis in humans. Therefore, a more appropriate term for the disorder in ESRD is calcific uremic arteriolopathy (CUA), because it represents the underlying pathohistology. The incidence of CUA appears to be increasing, partly because of the current practice of treating hyperparathyroidism with high-dose calcium and calcitriol; the rate has been reported to be as high as 4.5 per 100 patient-years.[10]

The pathogenesis of CUA remains unclear. It appears to result from multiple predisposing and/or sensitizing events commonly present in the uremic milieu, including elevated PTH, increased calcium and phosphate product, and increased prescribed vitamin D compounds. Female gender, morbid obesity, and Caucasian ethnicity also appear to be risk factors. Precipitating influences are thought to initiate the process and may include intravenous albumin, recent severe weight loss, local trauma or local injection, a hypercoagulable state, warfarin, and use of corticosteroids and other immunosuppressants. The established risk factors carry different relative risks for CUA.[11] Intimal fibrosis with the calcifications, massive mural calcifications of the arterioles, and thrombus formation within venules may account for the ischemic changes associated with CUA.

Polycystic Kidney Disease

Pain is common in autosomal-dominant polycystic kidney disease (PCKD), afflicting about 60% of patients. The sensory and autonomic innervation to the kidneys and pathophysiology of pain have been reviewed.[12] The painful syndromes associated with PCKD are discussed later.

CLINICAL MANIFESTATIONS
Renal Osteodystrophy

Symptoms caused by renal osteodystrophy generally do not occur until the patient is receiving dialysis therapy and disease is advanced. Patients with osteitis fibrosa present with bone and joint pain on exertion in skeletal sites subject to biomechanical stress. Pain at rest, localized pain, pathological fractures, or bone deformities suggest other problems such as osteomalacia, amyloid, adynamic bone disease, or concomitant osteoporosis. Osteitis fibrosa can be associated with red-eye syndrome due to conjunctival deposition of calcium. Soft tissue calcium deposition, proximal myopathy, ruptured tendons, pseudogout (calcium pyrophosphate dehydrate crystals), pseudoclubbing (from erosive loss of the ends of bones), and CUA may all be seen with osteitis fibrosa. Osteomalacia presents with bone pain (which can be localized) and fractures. Those with adynamic bone disease are prone to bone and joint pain both at rest and with exertion, fractures, skeletal deformities, and hypercalcemia. The incidence of hip fracture is 14 times greater for men with ESRD than in the general population, and 17 times greater for women.[13]

Dialysis-Related Amyloidosis

Tissue amyloid deposition occurs earlier than any clinical or radiographic manifestations. The major clinical manifestations are carpal tunnel syndrome, bone cysts, spondyloarthropathy, pathologic fractures, and swollen painful joints, especially scapulohumeral periarthritis. Amyloid deposition can also occur in subcutaneous tissues and skin, and less frequently in rectal mucosa, liver, spleen, and blood vessels.

Calcific Uremic Arteriolopathy

CUA is characterized by ischemic necrosis in the dermis, in subcutaneous fat, and sometimes in muscle. Painful violaceous skin mottling (livedo reticularis) can progress to painful, well-demarcated nonulcerating plaques (believed to represent early, potentially preventable disease) but may be misdiagnosed as cellulitis.[10] If not treated, most progress to ulcer and eschar formation that often become superinfected (Fig. 82-1) Multiple subcutaneous tender nodules represent subcutaneous calcium deposits. Mortality is high if lesions become ulcerated. Sepsis and ischemic events are the two main causes of death. Even with aggressive therapy, as many as 60% to 89% of CUA patients die from sepsis. Prognosis can be influenced by the location of skin lesions. Proximal lesions over the abdomen, thigh, or buttock have a poorer prognosis than lesions in distal sites such as hands, fingers, elbows, or below the knees. Distal lesions may mimic atherosclerotic peripheral vascular disease.

Polycystic Kidney Disease

Both acute and chronic pain syndromes are common in PCKD. Infected cysts can cause sudden diffuse unilateral or bilateral pain with fever. The pain stays in one area, without radiation or relief with change in position. Because cysts may not communicate with the urinary tract, urine cultures may be negative. Cyst rupture can cause acute, localized pain with or without gross hematuria. Referred pain to another location in the abdomen or shoulder can occur with hemorrhage into a larger cyst. Pain from cyst rupture usually resolves spontaneously over 2 to 7 days. If a surface kidney cyst ruptures, hemorrhage can produce a subcapsular hematoma. The patient may then experience a mild, steady pain until the hematoma has been reabsorbed. Renal colic from kidney stones occurs in 20% to 30% of patients with PCKD due to anatomic deformity and urinary stasis. This may cause sudden, severe pain typical of renal colic with radiation into the groin.

Chronic pain may result from increased abdominal girth due to enlarged cysts, with accompanying lumbar lordosis and accelerated spinal degenerative changes. Patients may develop spinal stenosis and radiculopathies. Cysts may also cause chronic pain due to compression on surrounding tissues or distention of the renal capsule. This chronic, steady pain is well localized (often to anterior abdominal area rather than the lower back) and is often exacerbated by standing and walking.[12]

DIAGNOSIS
Renal Osteodystrophy

Dual x-ray absorptiometry (DEXA) is widely used to measure bone mineral density. The role in the assessment of bone disease in CKD is not well established. DEXA

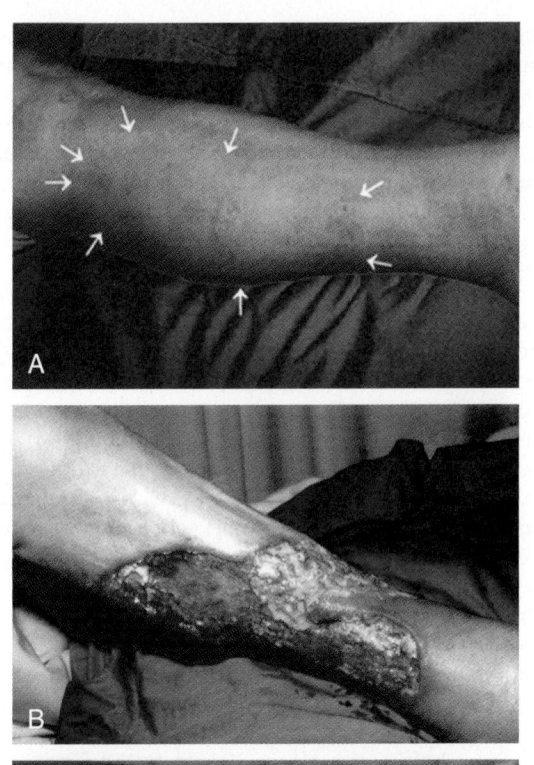

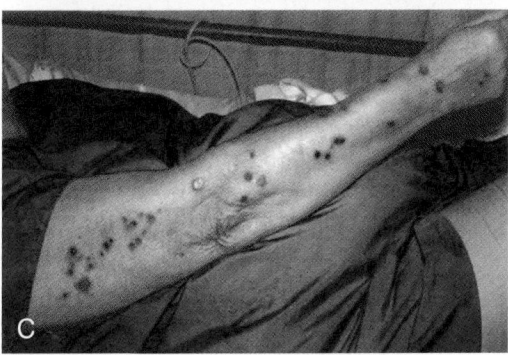

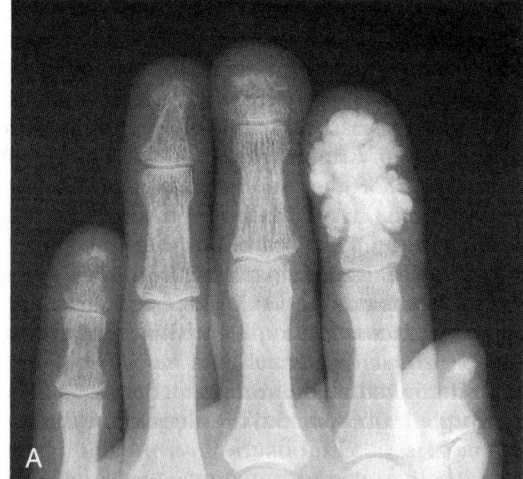

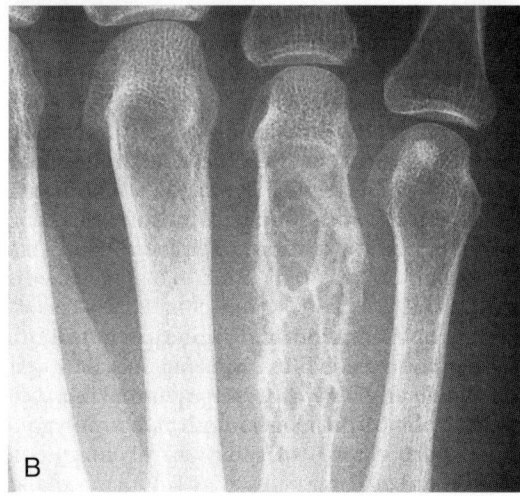

FIGURE 82-2   Radiographic findings in osteitis fibrosa. **A**, Acro-osteolysis of the terminal phalanges and periarticular calcifications. **B**, Brown tumor in the hand (*arrow*). *(Photographs courtesy of Dr. Robert Lambert.)*

FIGURE 82-1   Calcific uremic arteriolopathy (calciphylaxis). **A**, Confluent calf plaques (borders shown with arrows). Parts of the skin are erythematous, which is easily confused with simple cellulitis. **B**, Gross ulceration in the same patient 3 months later. The black eschar has been surgically débrided. **C**, Calciphylactic plaques, a few of which are beginning to ulcerate. *(Photographs courtesy of Dr. Adrian Fine.)*

provides information on overall bone mineral content or density but not on bone turnover or bone architecture, the principal abnormalities in renal osteodystrophy. Circulating intact PTH levels predict the presence and severity of hyperparathyroidism but may not predict underlying bone disease. Bone radiographs can provide important information. Recommended sites are the hands, shoulder, skull, spine, and pelvis. Accelerated bone resorption and bone deposition is seen with osteitis fibrosa. Subperiosteal resorption, resorptive loss of acral bone (terminal phalanges, distal ends of clavicles, and skull), resorption within cortical bone (longitudinal striation), endosteal resorption (cortical thinning), and brown tumors may all be present (Fig. 82-2). Osteosclerosis in the upper and lower thirds of the vertebra may lead to a "rugger jersey spine." Soft tissue (vascular, periarticular, and bursa) calcifications are common. Unlike osteitis fibrosa, radiographic changes of adynamic bone disease usually appear after clinical signs

and symptoms. In any case, radiographic findings will not establish the type of bone disease. Bone biopsy is the gold standard for establishing the type of renal bone disease, because no combination of biochemical parameters is accurate. Controversy exists regarding the exact indications for biopsy.

Dialysis-Related Amyloidosis

The diagnosis is dependent on the typical clinical features supported by documented tissue deposition of amyloid (via synovial biopsy or aspirate of joint effusions) or the characteristic radiographic picture of multiple bone cysts. Cysts typically occur at the ends of long bones. They contain amyloid, enlarge with time, and may be associated with pathological fractures of the carpal bones, fingers, femoral and humeral heads, acetabulum, tibial plateau, or distal radius. They may be mistaken for the brown tumors of osteitis fibrosa. DRA can also be confirmed in extra-articular tissues by subcutaneous fat pad aspiration, rectal submucosal biopsy, and two-dimensional echocardiography. Skin biopsy is usually negative. Ultrasonography may be of use in DRA of the shoulder. It can detect increased rotator cuff thickness and a thickened synovial sheath of the long head of the biceps.

Calcific Uremic Arteriolopathy

There is no diagnostic laboratory test for CUA. High plasma PTH, phosphate, and calcium concentrations are consistent, but all of these abnormalities are not always present. The diagnosis is usually suggested by characteristic ischemic skin lesions. CUA is more difficult to diagnosis when it manifests with nonulcerating plaques that may be misdiagnosed as cellulitis or with peripheral gangrene without skin lesions. In the latter setting, atherosclerosis, atheroemboli, and vasculitis must be excluded. Those affected typically lack other signs of vasculitis and, in contrast to atherosclerosis, have intact peripheral pulses and frequent upper extremity involvement. Roentgenographic studies may exhibit ectopic calcification of the soft tissue. The diagnosis can be confirmed by skin biopsy. Skin biopsy reveals arteriolar medial calcification, intimal hyperplasia and/or proliferation, thrombosis, adipocyte calcification, and subcutaneous ischemic necrosis without vasculitis. Affected subcutaneous arterioles commonly range from 30 to 600 μm (average, about 100 μm). Skin biopsy can be hazardous, because ulceration often develops in the biopsy incision within 2 to 6 weeks. Most cases can be confirmed by bone scan, which shows abnormal uptake in areas of calcium deposition. Transcutaneous oxygen tension (TCPO$_2$) is abnormally low, revealing arterial insufficiency, even if the skin is intact.

Polycystic Kidney Disease

The diagnosis of autosomal-dominant PCKD is supported by a positive family history and large kidneys with multiple cysts on ultrasonography or CT scanning. However, 25% to 40% of new cases have a negative family history.[14] Criteria are used to modify for age to minimize false-negative and false-positive results.[15] In patients younger than 30 years of age, at least two cysts (unilateral or bilateral) are required. Simple renal cysts are uncommon in these patients and are rarely multiple or bilateral. In patients aged 30 to 59, at least two cysts in each kidney must be present to make the diagnosis of PCKD. The requirement for bilateral involvement helps distinguish PCKD from the less common localized cystic disease of the kidney, which is unilateral and not associated with progressive renal failure. In patients older than age 60, four or more cysts in each kidney are required, as multiple simple cysts are relatively common in these patients. The presence of cysts in the liver, pancreas, and spleen and/or enlarged kidneys helps establish the diagnosis of PCKD in problem cases.

TREATMENT

Barriers to Pain Assessment and Management

Current management of physical and psychological symptoms in patients with CKD is inadequate. This is especially true for pain. Inadequate management is not unique to nephrology, and, as with other patient populations, patient-related factors are a major issue. ESRD patients may not seek medical attention until pain becomes severe. They may believe that they need analgesics, especially strong opioids, only "when absolutely necessary." Fear of addiction is common. There is a lack of training in pain assessment and management in nephrology nurse and physician training programs.

In addition, there are unique barriers that must be overcome in CKD. There is a lack of recognition by the medical community of the extent and severity of symptom burden and, hence, a lack of clinical and research focus. The high incidence of co-morbidity, polypharmacy, and an elderly population complicate pain management due to increased toxicity and adverse effects of analgesics. In addition, adverse effects may be mimicked by uremic symptoms, resulting in the inappropriate withdrawal of analgesia. One of the largest obstacles is the altered pharmacokinetics and pharmacodynamics of analgesics in ESRD and the increased risk for toxicity. This has led to reluctance to prescribe analgesics, especially opioids, in this patient population. Despite an increasing prevalence of chronic pain, analgesic use has decreased over the last few years. The Dialysis Outcomes and Practice Patterns Study (DOPPS) compared analgesic use in 1997 to 2000 for 3749 patients in 142 facilities in the United States.[16] The percentage using any analgesic decreased from 30% to 24%. Narcotic use decreased from 18% to less than 15% and acetaminophen use from 11% to 6%. In this study, 74% of those with pain that interfered with work had no analgesic prescription. These findings are consistent with other reports, in which 35% of hemodialysis patients with chronic pain were not prescribed analgesics despite the fact that most were experiencing moderate or severe pain; fewer than 10% of the patients were prescribed strong opioids.[3]

Pharmacological Management of Pain

Given the lack of pharmacokinetic and pharmacodynamic data, it is difficult to confidently advocate specific algorithms for pain management in ESRD. The World Health Organization (WHO) analgesic ladder for malignant pain management is now advocated also for nonmalignant chronic pain; it can be adapted and integrated with the management of chronic pain from CKD. Analgesics must be selected with care, taking into account the altered pharmacokinetics and pharmacodynamics.

Most of the information about opioid use in ESRD comes from experience with morphine. Clinical data suggest that patients with renal failure are particularly susceptible to the toxic effects of morphine. Nausea, vomiting, myoclonus, and seizures, as well as prolonged and profound analgesia, sedation, and respiratory depression, have been reported with morphine use in patients with renal failure. There are several hypotheses to account for this, including increased enterohepatic circulation of morphine and accumulation of the active metabolites morphine-6-glucuronide (M6G) and morphine-3-glucuronide (M3G). Because of these adverse effects, alternative strong opioids are typically recommended. It has been suggested that hydromorphone, methadone, and fentanyl are better tolerated in this patient population (Table 82-2). However, data remain limited with these opioids, and the evidence is anecdotal.[17] As in the nonrenal setting, adjuvants may be used for specific indications (e.g., neuropathic pain), but caution must be used in the setting of CKD (Table 82-3).

Systematically tested protocols for symptoms other than pain are also lacking in CKD. Commonly used symptom management techniques in ESRD are presented in Table 82-4. Considerations for specific pain syndromes in CKD are described here.

TABLE 82-2   Analgesics in Chronic Kidney Disease

CLASS OF DRUG	RENAL HANDLING	COMMENTS
NONOPIOID ANALGESICS		
Nonsteroidal anti-inflammatory drugs (NSAIDs)	Eliminated via reual excretion	Exacerbate sodium and water retention, hypertension, hyperkalemia, and further loss of kidney function in CKD. Increased gastrointestinal toxicity in CKD. Not recommended for chronic use in CKD, although effective for acute pain management.
Acetaminophen	Metabolized in liver; 2-5% is excreted unchanged in the urine.	No dose adjustment required in CKD. Accumulation of inactive metabolites in CKD. Analgesic of choice for mild to moderate pain in CKD.
Tramadol	Metabolized by liver. Active metabolites are excreted in the urine; 30% is excreted unchanged in the urine.	Dose adjustment required in CKD. Maximum dose with a creatinine clearance of <30 mL is 100 mg bid. Associated with a lower seizure threshold in CKD. Use with extreme caution.
WEAK OPIOIDS		
Codeine	Metabolized in liver to form morphine and norcodeine; conjugated to form glucuronides and sulfates. Metabolites are excreted in the urine and accumulate in CKD.	Several case reports of prolonged narcosis in CKD. Profound toxicity can be delayed and has occurred after trivial doses. Some patients can tolerate well. Use with extreme caution in CKD.
Dextropropoxyphene	Renally excreted, with decreased elimination and accumulation of active metabolites in CKD.	Associated with central nervous system and cardiac toxicity in CKD. Not recommended for use in CKD.
STRONG OPIOIDS		
Morphine	5-10% is excreted unchanged in the urine. Metabolized by liver to active metabolites (morphine 3- and 6- glucuronides) that are excreted in the urine and accumulate in CKD.	Chronic administration not well tolerated in CKD and not recommended. Use with caution for acute pain management.
Hydromorphone	Metabolized in liver to hydromorphone-3-glucuronide; conjugates excreted in the urine and accumulate in CKD.	Better tolerated than morphine in CKD. May be a safer, effective analgesic for use in CKD if carefully monitored.
Methadone	Excreted mainly in the feces; ~20% excreted unchanged in the urine. No evidence of accumulation in CKD.	May be a safer, effective analgesic for use in CKD if carefully monitored.
Fentanyl	Rapidly metabolized in liver; 5–10% excreted unchanged in the urine. Conflicting data, although accumulation in CKD appears to be minimal in most studies.	The transdermal patch may be a safer, effective analgesic for use in CKD if carefully monitored.
Oxycodone	Eliminated mainly by metabolism in the liver; <10% excreted unchanged in the urine. Despite this, accumulation of parent compound and metabolites in CKD.	Use with extreme caution in CKD. Consider another opioid.
Pethidine	5% excreted unchanged in the urine. Metabolized by liver to active and inactive metabolites that are excreted in the urine and accumulate in CKD.	Not recommended for use in CKD due to accumulation of norpethidine and the associated neuroexcitatory effects and risk of convulsions.

CKD, chronic kidney disease.

Dialysis-Related Amyloidosis

Analgesics help with periarticular and bone pain. Because DRA is a progressive disease, early surgical correction of complications such as carpal tunnel syndrome is warranted. Other interventions include

- Arthroscopic or open surgery of the joint (e.g., shoulder) with removal of synovium infiltrated by amyloid
- Curettage and bone grafting of amyloid cysts in the femoral neck to relieve hip pain
- Replacement of a diseased joint with a prosthesis
- Successful renal transplantation. This reduces plasma β_2-microglobulin levels to normal, and joint pains resolve quickly. There may also be regression in the amyloid deposits. Bone cysts resolve more slowly.

Calcific Uremic Arteriolopathy

The optimal therapy for CUA is prevention—eliminating known sensitizing or precipitating factors. This includes

maintaining normal calcium phosphate product and parathyroidectomy if appropriate. Given the high mortality rate, especially with ulcerated lesions, early recognition and treatment are essential. No definitive treatment regimens are available, owing to the unidentified pathogenetic mechanisms. The largest published single-center experience recommended a therapeutic trial of steroids for non-ulcerating disease. Once ulceration develops, mortality increases dramatically. Most sources recommend normalization of serum calcium, phosphorous, and PTH levels. This often includes cessation of vitamin D supplementation, a low-calcium dialysate and non–calcium-containing phosphorus binders, and surgical parathyroidectomy for markedly elevated PTH refractory to calcitriol. Aggressive systemic antibiotics and repeated débridement of necrotic tissue are required for secondary infection of nonhealing skin ulceration. Successful hyperbaric oxygen therapy to elevate the $TCPO_2$ has been reported. Consideration should be given to the withdrawal of immunosuppression in the renal transplantation patient who demonstrates progressive or persistent CUA despite these measures. There is a

TABLE 82-3   Adjuvant Drugs for Pain and Symptom Management in Chronic Kidney Disease

CLASS OF DRUGS	RENAL HANDLING	DOSE SCHEDULE	COMMENTS
TRICYCLIC ANTIDEPRESSANTS			
Amitriptyline	Metabolized in the liver (cytochrome P-450), <5% excreted unchanged in the urine.	10-100 mg od	Dose alteration not usually necessary in CKD, but may be poorly tolerated due to common anticholinergic side effects. Lowers seizure threshold.
Desipramine	Metabolized in the liver as above.	10-150 mg od	Less sedating and fewer anticholinergic side effects, therefore, may be better tolerated than amitriptyline in CKD.
ANTICONVULSANTS			
Carbamazepine	Metabolized by the liver.	200 mg od, increasing weekly to effectiveness or toxicity or a maximum dose of 1600 mg	No dose adjustment required in CKD. Effect may occur within 2-3 days. Plasma concentrations reduced by other anticonvulsants.
Valproic acid	Metabolized by liver and eliminated via the kidneys.	200 mg od, increasing to pain control or a maximum dose of 1000 mg.	Well tolerated. Interaction with other anticonvulsant.
Gabapentin	Excreted unchanged by the kidney. Accumulates in renal impairment.	100-300 mg after dialysis or qhs	Accumulation of gabapentin and cases of neurotoxicity in CKD have been reported when using >300 mg daily. Used for neuropathic pain and restless legs syndrome.
Benzodiazepines	Avoid long-acting benzodiazepines in CKD.		No dose adjustment required for most benzodiazepines in CKD.
Temazepam		7.5-15 mg qhs	Used for insomnia.
Flurazepam		15-30 mg qhs	Used for insomnia.
Lorazepam		0.5-1.0 mg od	Used for insomnia.
			Manufacturer does not recommend in ESRD.
Oxazepam		10-30 mg tid-qid	Used for insomnia and anxiety.
Clonazepam		0.5-2.0 mg od	Used for anxiety and restless legs.

CKD, chronic kidney disease; ESRD, end-stage renal disease; od, once daily; tid, three times daily; qid, four times daily; qhs, at bedtime.

growing interest in intravenous sodium thiosulfate as an adjunctive treatment in patients with debilitating calciphylactic necrotic lesions. Prospective studies are needed to assess its safety and efficacy before sodium thiosulfate can be recommended as a standard of care. The response to any therapeutic regimen is never assured, and the prognosis associated with CUA remains poor.

Polycystic Kidney Disease

Drugs with good cyst-penetrating ability, such as trimethoprim-sulfamethizole, metronidazole, and fluoroquinolones, are required for infected cysts. Renal prostaglandins may be a major contributing factor in renal colic: acute ureteral obstruction by a stone can increase renal pressure with release of prostaglandins, causing vasodilation of the afferent arterioles and inhibition of antidiuretic hormone, with a resultant diuresis and further increase in renal pressure. Prostaglandin inhibitors such as NSAIDs would seem to be the obvious choice in renal colic and may be as efficacious as opioids. However, opioids remain the cornerstone of analgesic therapy for acute renal colic, even though they do not influence renal prostaglandins. Because of the compressed and distorted renal calices, treatment modalities such as ureteroscopy and extracorporeal shock wave lithotripsy are more difficult in PCKD and may not be as efficacious. For that reason, patients may have prolonged and repeated renal colic while undergoing medical management. Treatment of lower back pain has been covered elsewhere, and modalities such as physical therapy, transcutaneous electrical nerve stimulation (TENS), trigger point injections, acupuncture, and autonomic plexus blockade can all be tried. However, if conservative measures fail, surgical intervention such as laparoscopic cyst decortication (unroofing and collapse of cysts) and marsupialization may be required. This is typically reserved for severe pain attributed to cysts greater than 5 cm in diameter. For some patients approaching or with ESRD, nephrectomy may be the only option for pain control.[12]

DRUGS OF CHOICE

The properties of available analgesics and adjuvant drugs for control of pain and other symptoms are described in Tables 82-2 through 82-4.

SUPPORTIVE CARE

Given the significant burden of physical and psychological symptoms and the compromise in HRQL, withdrawal from dialysis is one of the most common causes of death in ESRD. It is well accepted that, for some, the benefits of dialysis are outweighed by physical and psychological suffering and an unacceptable HRQL. Depression is also a complicating factor in 15% to 50% of the patients. Most

TABLE 82-4 Guidelines for Management of Symptoms in Chronic Kidney Disease

SYMPTOM	TREATMENT	DOSAGE	COMMENTS
Cramps	Quinine	300–600 mg PO od	Dose before dialysis.
	Vitamin E	400 IU PO od	Dose before dialysis.
	Benzodiazepines	See Table 82-3	Dose before dialysis.
	Carnitine	1-2 g IV during dialysis	3-mo trial; also used for cardiomyopathy and refractory anemia.
Restless legs	Benzodiazepines	See Table 82-4	
	Carbidopa/Levodopa	25/100-100/400 mg qhs prn	Can be given in divided doses over the day.
	Pergolide	0.10-1.00 mg qhs	
	Gabapentin	100 mg od-tid prn	Also used for neuropathic pain.
	Clonidine	0.1-0.2 mg qhs or bid	
	Opioids	See Table 82-3	Can be effective in severe and resistant cases.
Pruritus	Hydrourea cream	bid-qid	
	Capsaicin cream	bid-qid	
	Hydroxyzine hydrochloride	25 mg tid	Increased effect when used in conjunction with narcotics and sedatives; also used for nausea.
	Ketotifen	1-2 mg PO bid	Limited trials.
	Ondansetron	4-8 mg PO bid	Limited trials; no accumulation in CKD.
	Cholestyramine	5 mg PO bid	Effective, but can interfere with absorption of other medications.
	UVB ultraviolet light	3 times a week	Effective but inconvenient.
Anorexia	Megestrol	40-400 mg PO od has been used in CKD	Limited data.
	Dronabinol	2.5-5 mg PO bid/tid	Limited data.
	Prednisone	10-20 mg PO od-bid has been used in ESRD	Limited data.
Lethargy, fatigue	Methylphenidate	5-10 mg PO qam and noon	Psychostimulant.
Insomnia	Benzodiazepines	See Table 82-3	This may be a long-term measure so use drugs with a short duration of action and reduced potential for addiction.
	Zopiclone	7.5 mg qhs	Signs and symptoms of depression could be intensified.
Nausea	Metoclopramide	5 mg qid	Increased extrapyramidal side effects in CKD.
	Hydroxyzine hydrochloride	25 mg tid	Increased effect when used in conjunction with narcotics and sedatives; also used for pruritus.
	Ondansetron	4-8 mg PO bid	Also used for pruritus in CKD.

bid, twice daily; CKD, chronic kidney disease; ESRD, end-stage renal disease; IU, international units; IV, intravenous; od, once daily; PO, by mouth; prn, as needed; tid, three times daily; qam, every morning; qid, four times daily; qhs, at bedtime.

experience a significant loss of control from dialysis and the associated physical and dietary restraints. Therefore, comprehensive care of ESRD requires not only expertise in all the medical and technical aspects of maintaining dialysis, including pain and symptom management, but also advance care planning (ACP) and attention to ethical, psychosocial, and spiritual issues related to starting, continuing, withholding, and stopping dialysis. ACP allows patients and families to prepare for death and facilitates communication of values, goals, and beliefs about the end of life among the patient, family, and staff. However, ACP is not occurring routinely in dialysis units: only 6% to 35% of dialysis patients have advance directives, and these tend to outline limited treatment options. Few dialysis patients choose a do not resuscitate (DNR) order, despite the low chance of survival after cardiopulmonary resuscitation. Patients often do not know that they have the option to withdraw from dialysis, and even the few who have an advance directive do not usually consider withdrawal of dialysis. Dialysis patients typically do not view themselves as having a terminal illness, and many assume they can be

kept alive indefinitely on dialysis. Denial and similar coping mechanisms are used commonly to adapt to life on dialysis. Most dialysis patients appear to either deny or be unaware of the unpleasant reality of their dependency on a life-sustaining treatment and possible imminent death. Denial may be an effective coping mechanism early in the illness, when the diagnosis is overwhelming and there has been insufficient time to adapt. Ongoing denial may present a barrier to effective communication and prevent ACP from having the desired effect of enhancing care at the end of life. The end result is that issues related to death and dying are commonly avoided until late in the illness, when suffering is common and patients may no longer be competent to make decisions. New tools for facilitated ACP in CKD are available and have been shown to positively enhance (rather than diminish) patients' hope.[18] A clinical practice guideline has been developed to address withholding and withdrawing dialysis.[19] It is informed by ethical principles, case and statutory law, and a systematic review of the literature and provides excellent guidance to health care providers, including the options to forego initiation of dialysis or to choose a time-limited trial of dialysis.

A model of supportive care that embraces disease-specific therapy to halt the progression of disease while embracing the principles of palliative care to maximize HRQL needs to be established for ESRD (see "Future Considerations"). This will require the incorporation of aggressive management of physical and psychological symptoms, ongoing ACP, and routine assessment of HRQL so that patients' perspective of their well-being can be integrated into the evaluation of care.

REFERENCES

1. U.S. Renal Data System, National Institutes of Health, and National Institute of Diabetes and Digestive and Kidney Diseases. 2005 Annual Report: Atlas of End-Stage Renal Disease in the United States. USRDS 2005. Bethesda, MD: U.S. Renal Data System, 2005.
2. Chambers EJ, Germain M, Brown E (eds). Supportive Care for the Renal Patient, 1st ed. New York: Oxford University Press, 2004, pp 1-267.
3. Davison SN. Pain in hemodialysis patients: Prevalence, cause, severity, and management. Am J Kidney Dis 2003;42:1239-1247.
4. Davison SN, Jhangri GS, Johnson JA. Cross sectional validity of a modified Edmonton symptom assessment system in dialysis patients: A simple assessment of symptom burden. Kidney Int 2006;69:1621-1625.
5. Davison SN, Jhangri GS. The impact of chronic pain on depression, sleep and the desire to withdraw from dialysis in hemodialysis patients. J Pain Symptom Manage 2005;30:465-473.
6. Martin KJ, Olgaard K, Coburn JW, et al. Diagnosis, assessment, and treatment of bone turnover abnormalities in renal osteodystrophy. Am J Kidney Dis 2004;43:558-565.
7. Coen G. Adynamic bone disease: An update and overview. J Nephrol 2005;18:117-122.
8. Jadoul M, Garbar C, Noel H, et al. Histological prevalence of beta 2-microglobulin amyloidosis in hemodialysis: A prospective post-mortem study. Kidney Int 1997;51:1928-1932.
9. Koch KM. Dialysis-related amyloidosis. Kidney Int 1992;41:1416-1429.
10. Fine A, Zacharias J. Calciphylaxis is usually non-ulcerating: Risk factors, outcome and therapy. Kidney Int 2002;61:2210-2217.
11. Wang HY, Yu CC, Huang CC. Successful treatment of severe calciphylaxis in a hemodialysis patient using low-calcium dialysate and medical parathyroidectomy: Case report and literature review. Ren Fail 2004;26:77-82.
12. Bajwa ZH, Gupta S, Warfield CA, et al. Pain management in polycystic kidney disease. Kidney Int 2001;60:1631-1644.
13. Coco M, Rush H. Increased incidence of hip fractures in dialysis patients with low serum parathyroid hormone. Am J Kidney Dis 2000;36:1115-1121.
14. Gabow PA. Medical progress: Autosomal dominant polycystic kidney disease. N Engl J Med 1993;329:332.
15. Ravine D, Gibson RN, Walker RG, et al. Evaluation of ultrasonographic diagnosis criteria for autosomal dominant polycystic kidney disease I. Lancet 1994;343:824.
16. Bailie GR, Mason NA, Bragg-Gresham JL, et al. Analgesic prescription patterns among hemodialysis patients in the DOPPS: Potential for underprescription. Kidney Int 2004;65:2419-2425.
17. Dean M. Opioids in renal failure and dialysis patients. J Pain Symptom Manage 2004;28:497-504.
18. Davison SN, Simpson C. Hope and advance care planning in patients with end stage renal disease: Qualitative interview study. BMJ 2006;333:886.
19. Shared Decision-Making in the Appropriate Initiation of and Withdrawal from Dialysis. Washington, DC: Renal Physicians Association and American Society of Nephrology, 2000.

CHAPTER **83**

Alcohol and Drug Abuse

Paul S. Haber and Katherine Neasham

KEY POINTS

- Brief screening for alcohol and substance misuse, particularly prescription drug misuse, should be part of basic history taking.
- Recognition of substance misuse, abuse, and dependence in a palliative care population can be difficult.
- Alcohol, benzodiazepine, and nicotine withdrawal are common causes of agitated delirium.
- It is usually possible to negotiate a reasonable goal for substance and alcohol use with patients in the palliative care context.
- Palliative care patients on maintenance pharmacotherapy programs (e.g., methadone) may be managed successfully by both prescriber and palliative care teams concurrently.

Alcohol and drug abuse are becoming more frequently encountered problems in palliative medicine. Harmful use or misuse is a pattern of substance use with damage to health. Harmful use commonly, but not invariably, has adverse social consequences. The *Diagnostic and Statistical Manual of Mental Disorders* (DSM-IV)[1] defines diagnostic criteria for abuse and dependence. *Abuse* is a maladaptive pattern of use leading to clinically significant impairment or distress resulting in one or more of the following problems: a failure to fulfill major role obligations at work, school, or home; recurrent use in situations in which it is physically hazardous; legal problems; and social or interpersonal problems. This definition applies to all substances, including alcohol.

Over time, abuse may progress to *dependence,* in which drug-seeking, drug use, and recovery from drug use become self–perpetuating dominant behaviors, displacing other activities. To meet the criteria for dependence, three or more of the following must be manifested over a 12-month period: tolerance, withdrawal, dose escalation, loss of control of use, inability to cut down, spending a great deal of time in activities related to substance or alcohol use, losing important social and occupational function as a result of use, and continued substance use despite evident harm (e.g., continued drinking despite advanced liver cirrhosis and a variceal bleed). Although the terms "addiction" and "alcoholism" are commonly used in both lay and scientific circles, neither is a diagnostic term in either the DSM-IV or the *International Classification of Diseases* (ICD). These terms stigmatize patients.

One problem in relying on the formal definitions in a palliative medicine setting is that they are derived from populations without medical illness. It is vital that behaviors be interpreted in context. For example, motivation for aberrant drug-taking behavior in a cancer patient may be inadequate pain relief. This "pseudoaddiction"[2] typically settles with the provision of adequate pain relief. Tolerance and withdrawal are key components of dependence. However, both are normal physiological phenomena after continuous use of various drugs for medical purposes.[3] Many patients seen in a palliative care setting have some degree of tolerance to prescribed medications (e.g., opiates, benzodiazepines) and also experience withdrawal if they are discontinued. In the absence of biopsychosocial and behavioral problems, it is inappropriate to diagnose dependence or "addiction" in such patients (see "Pathophysiology"). Distinguishing addiction from physiological tolerance is an important task for both doctor and patient.

EPIDEMIOLOGY AND PREVALENCE

General Population

Patterns of substance use (including alcohol use) in communities vary over time in relation to social trends, availability, and the law. The highest rates of substance abuse and dependence are in the 18- to 25-year age group and then decline with age. Almost 10% of the American adult population were classified with substance abuse or dependence in the past year, and 50% are current drinkers of alcohol (7% heavy drinkers).[4]

Substance Abuse in Palliative Care

The available data are conflicting and indicate the need for more studies (Table 83-1). The explanation for this conflict is unclear. Perhaps it reflects a combination of under-reporting in an outpatient setting and selection bias, because patients with alcohol and substance abuse issues are less likely to be referred to tertiary referral centers. Various methods are used to detect dependence in individual studies, and the data do not include results for those who fall into the categories of misuse and abuse.

The prevalence of substance misuse varies across palliative care settings according to the underlying pathology. Hepatocellular carcinoma complicating hepatitis C cirrhosis is an increasing problem. The most common cause for hepatitis C in many communities is injectable drug use, often with opioid dependence. Advanced hepatocellular carcinoma is likely to occur in those patients with active or past opioid dependence. Challenges with pain management and other sequelae of opioid dependence are common in this setting.

BASIC SCIENCE

Drug addiction is a chronic, relapsing disorder. There is now neurobiological evidence for abnormalities that sustain continuing drug use. It is proposed that there is dysregulation and subsequent hypersensitization in the brain "reward" system, which is located in the mesolimbic system and regulated by dopamine (Fig. 83-1). This leads to compulsive drug-seeking behavior independent of withdrawal symptoms and difficulty in decision making. All the major drugs of abuse increase mesolimbic dopaminergic transmission. Each acts by different and specific mechanisms. Opioids act on opioid receptors that indirectly increase dopamine release from the nucleus accumbens. This is mediated by other neurotransmitters, possibly γ-aminobutyric acid (GABA). The effect of opioids on mood, and the desire for continuing opioid use, appear to result from changes in this region. Analgesia results from

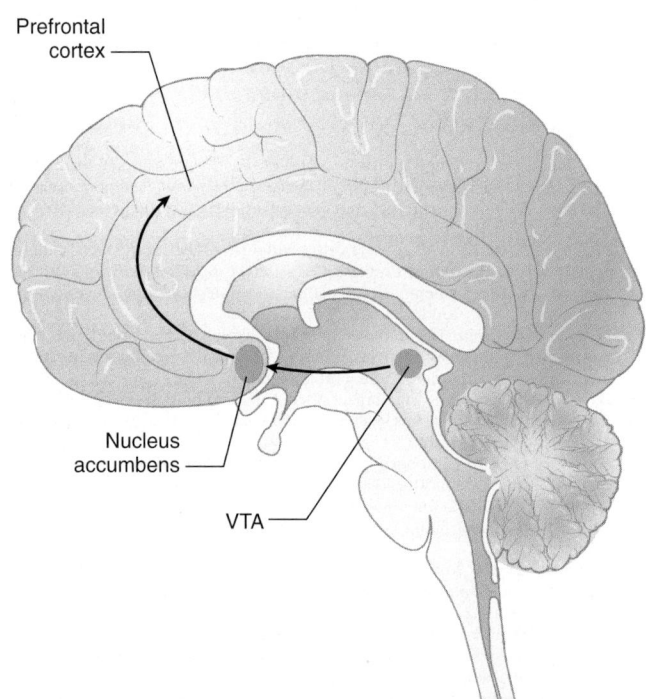

FIGURE 83-1 The reward pathway. Major structures involved in psychological reward include the ventral tegmental area (VTA), the nucleus accumbens, and the prefrontal cortex and connections. Major drugs of abuse, food, and sex all activate the reward system via increasing dopamine neurotransmission, even though the rewarding stimuli act by different mechanisms.

TABLE 83-1	Studies on Substance Abuse in Palliative Care		
STUDY	**STUDY POPULATION**	**METHOD**	**RESULTS**
Derogatis et al, 1983[5]	Ambulatory cancer patients in tertiary care hospitals	Structured clinical interviews	5% of 215 patients met DSM criteria for dependence
Bruera et al, 1995[6]	Patients admitted to palliative care unit	CAGE questionnaire, multidisciplinary interviews	28% patients in 1989 and 27% patients 1992 diagnosed with alcoholism

DSM, *Diagnostic and Statistical Manual of Mental Disorders.*
From Derogatis LR, Morrow GR, Fetting J, et al. The prevalence of psychiatric disorders among cancer patients. JAMA 1983;249:751-757; Bruera E, Moyano J, Seifert L, et al. The frequency of alcoholism among patients with pain due to terminal cancer. J Pain Symptom Manage 1995;10:599-603.

action at the thalamus. Clinically, it is possible to distinguish among the desires to use opioids for analgesia, to influence mood, or to relieve withdrawal. These effects appear to be mediated by the action of opioids on different parts of the brain: thalamus, nucleus accumbens, and locus ceruleus, respectively. Drug addiction is a complex problem, and even though there are emerging neurobiological theories, they cannot completely explain all aspects of addictive behavior (see Chapter 122).

PATHOPHYSIOLOGY

The changes in function caused by substance use are determined by several factors and manifest in different ways. Personality traits and psychiatric disorders are major conditioning factors in substance misuse and dependence. Genetic factors that influence metabolism and effects of drugs also contribute.[7] Other risk factors include adolescence, male gender, a history of psychiatric disorder, social disadvantage, and genetic factors. Factors beyond individual control contribute significantly to substance abuse. The pharmacological properties of substances influence how they are consumed recreationally. Drugs that quickly reach high levels in the brain are preferred, because they have a rapid, intense effect. Routes of administration that cause rapid rises in blood levels, namely injection and smoking, promote rapid intoxication or a "hit." A short half-life produces a more intense withdrawal than a prolonged half-life does.

Substance use, misuse, abuse, and dependence exist along a continuum, and in some cases it can be difficult to confidently classify an individual. Misuse or harmful use can manifest in a person who is having complications while intoxicated but may not lead to abuse. Tolerance and withdrawal reflect physiological adaptation but are neither necessary nor sufficient for a diagnosis of dependence. Tolerance is a reproducible pharmacological effect of regular opioid use. The key features are that higher doses are required for the same effect, or the same dose has a lesser effect. The clinical consequences of tolerance, without any evidence of addiction, are

- Dose escalation
- Fear of unrelieved pain
- Fear of becoming addicted
- Fear of being labeled as a "drug addict"

The concerns of patients who are already drug-tolerant are described in the case study (see "Case Study: Concerns of Drug-Dependent Patients Entering Palliative Care").

CLINICAL MANIFESTATIONS

Assessment and Evaluation

Several challenges are posed in diagnosing alcoholism and substance abuse in palliative care populations. Alterations to physical and psychosocial functioning may be caused by medical illness and its treatment and cannot be relied upon to diagnose abuse. Aberrant drug-seeking behaviors can exist along a continuum, and not every episode of drug-related harm reflects a continuing disorder. For example, a patient may use excessive alcohol or sedatives intermittently, representing misuse and possibly associ-

CASE STUDY

Concerns of Drug-Dependent Patients Entering Palliative Care

A 48-year-old woman maintained on a stable dose of methadone for several years presented to an addiction medicine specialist at a regional center. She had recently been diagnosed with hepatocellular carcinoma and expected increasing pain as her disease progressed. She was intelligent and cognitively intact but held a belief that, because of her long-term methadone use, she would be unable to respond to analgesics adequately. This made her afraid of suffering severe unrelieved pain.

She also expressed a worry that health care professionals would stigmatize her because of her background of substance abuse and would be reluctant to prescribe her medication due to a belief that she was "drug seeking." Simple explanation reassured her and helped to relieve her anxieties. Her beliefs reflect common emotions among this population.

ated with some harms (such as a fall), without meeting diagnostic criteria for abuse or dependence. On the other hand, patients often disguise signs of a stigmatizing disorder such as alcoholism, and if this concealment is successful, it can complicate diagnosis. Every person must be assessed individually, and there are several ways in which this can be accomplished. Of first importance is a thorough history and examination (see later discussion). Validated questionnaires for alcohol use disorders are quick, cheap, and more sensitive than "routine" history taking. The most commonly used questionnaires are CAGE and AUDIT, but they are less accurate than a comprehensive clinical assessment. CAGE is an acronym for four simple questions:

- Have you felt you should *C*ut down your drinking?
- Have people *A*nnoyed you by criticizing your drinking?
- Do you feel *G*uilty about your drinking?
- Have you ever had an *E*ye-opener?

It is 93% sensitive at detecting dependence if more than two answers are positive but is less sensitive for abuse without dependence.[8] The Alcohol Use Disorders Identification Test (AUDIT) questionnaire was developed by the World Health Organization (WHO) as a simple method of screening for hazardous and harmful patterns of alcohol consumption. It has the advantage of screening for misuse, abuse, and dependence.[9]

The first person to suspect a history of drug abuse or problematic drug taking should alert the palliative care team. A thorough assessment process should begin, and it should be empathic and nonjudgmental. Obtaining information over a series of consultations usually is advised, because it builds trust and a therapeutic relationship. This can be a difficult subject, and there is a fear of offending patients with preconceived ideas and judgments. At times, an external consultant provides both expertise and independence, so that conflicts that arise during assessment can be kept separate and not impair the therapeutic relationship with the palliative care team.

The initial history and examination should cover the following points:

1. Drug use history, including quantity, frequency, duration, and route of administration for each drug used. Begin with prescribed medications, move to tobacco and alcohol, and then ask about illicit drug use, commencing with cannabis.
2. Drug- or alcohol-related harms
3. Clinical features of dependence
4. Formulation of a substance use diagnosis
5. Co-morbidity, including mental health and relevant physical health
6. Insight, motivation, and goals with respect to substance use

It is also useful to obtain information regarding a person's drug and alcohol use from other sources. Family members, friends, and the patient's general practitioner may all contribute valuable information to assemble a full clinical picture.

Investigation

There is no diagnostic test for addiction, and laboratory investigation plays a limited role. Investigations can provide relatively objective markers of drug use and toxicity. Measures of alcohol in breath, urine, and blood confirm alcohol use if the patient denies recent drinking. Liver function tests (particularly γ-glutamyl transferase levels) may be checked to determine whether they parallel the self-reported trend in alcohol use. Urinary drug screens are valuable markers of drug use but not of quantity, toxicity, or misuse. Other limitations include the inability to distinguish between prescribed and nonprescribed sources of the same drug, metabolism of one drug to another, the potential for urine testing to become a degrading experience, and tampering with specimens.

Importance of Alcohol and Drug Abuse Management in Palliative Care

Some may ask why they should bother to address and manage such issues in a population whose life expectancy is short. Addressing addiction is not about depriving people of pleasure. Addiction is a self-destructive pattern of behavior that involves continued use of a substance despite physical harm and impaired social functioning. Addiction causes suffering, to both patients and families, and it impairs the capacity for other palliative care measures to relieve symptoms. If this problem is addressed, other symptoms can be managed more effectively, and suffering can be reduced.[10]

It is always important to use a "common sense" approach. As an analogy, how assertively ought one to address cigarette smoking in a patient with lung cancer? To answer this question, the stage of the illness, any adverse physical and social consequences if the patient continues to smoke, and the patient's attitude and goals are considered. There is no easy answer, but most physicians would agree that a "harm reduction" approach involves nicotine replacement therapy and explanations of the effects of continued smoking in terms of symptoms and prognosis. The difficulty of stopping smoking given the considerable distress of the diagnosis of lung cancer should also be evaluated.

Recognition of Addiction to Prescribed Medication

In palliative medicine, there is a need to identify those patients using prescription medications in a way that would imply substance abuse. In practice, this can be difficult, especially in patients with an incurable illness. Consideration of the following indicators of abuse of prescribed analgesics[11] may assist in defining such behaviors; when observed, they should be a indication to monitor more closely and reassess treatment plans

- Use for indications not prescribed
- Use outside prescribed amounts
- Excessive amounts per day
- Use of nonprescribed drugs (black market, family member)
- Drug seeking
- Breaches of therapeutic relationship
- Lying to get scripts (scripts/pills lost, stolen, and so on)
- Doctor shopping
- Tampering with prescriptions

Misuse of analgesics is common. It is important to ask, "Do you sometimes take pain-killers when you do not have any pain?" In certain patients, aberrant drug taking may be suspected but never confirmed. As long as the principles of safe prescribing are followed and the patient is not coming to harm as a result of this behavior, it must be accepted that a patient's pattern of substance use cannot always be established.

Recognition of Intoxication and Withdrawal

When patients are admitted to a palliative care unit, staff may be reluctant to enquire about previous alcohol and substance misuse. Withdrawal phenomena can cause considerable distress in advanced medical illness, and it is important to recognize it particularly as a cause of delirium.[12]

The most commonly encountered withdrawal in palliative medicine is from alcohol and nicotine (Table 83-2). Diagnosis may pose a challenge in patients with delirium, who may have multiple other causes (e.g., brain metastases, metabolic disturbance). In these instances, an assessment on admission of alcohol and drug use would be helpful.

MANAGEMENT

Goal Setting

The clinician's primary goal is to ensure patient safety and prevent diversion of medications while remaining respectful to the patients' needs and not undertreating symptoms (Fig. 83-2). A key step is to set pragmatic treatment goals collaboratively with the patient. These must be tailored to the individual and will most likely be negotiated over a series of consultations. Goals and motivation may change and be influenced by many factors at different stages in a person's illness and also are influenced by the clinician and carers. Ongoing communication and careful assess-

TABLE 83-2	Signs of Intoxication and Withdrawal	
DRUG	**INTOXICATION**	**WITHDRAWAL**
Alcohol	Relaxation, disinhibition, impaired judgment and coordination, decreased concentration, slurred speech, ataxia, vomiting	Delirium, terminal restlessness, autonomic hyperactivity, tremor, insomnia, nausea, vomiting, hallucinations, psychomotor retardation, anxiety, grand mal seizures
Benzodiazepines	Disinhibition, sedation, drooling, incoordination, slurred speech, low blood pressure, dizziness	Restlessness, anxiety, sweating, tremors, agitation, delirium, seizures
Opiates	Pupil constriction, itching, sedation, low blood pressure and pulse rate, hypoventilation	Rhinorrhea, sneezing, yawning, lacrimation, abdominal cramps, leg cramps, piloerection, nausea, vomiting, diarrhea, dilated pupils
Stimulants	Hyperactivity, restlessness, agitation, sweating, tremor, elevated blood pressure and pulse rate	Dysphoria, excessive sleep, hunger, severe psychomotor retardation
Cannabis	Relaxation, decreased concentration, impaired balance	Irritability, anxiety, insomnia, anorexia, headaches

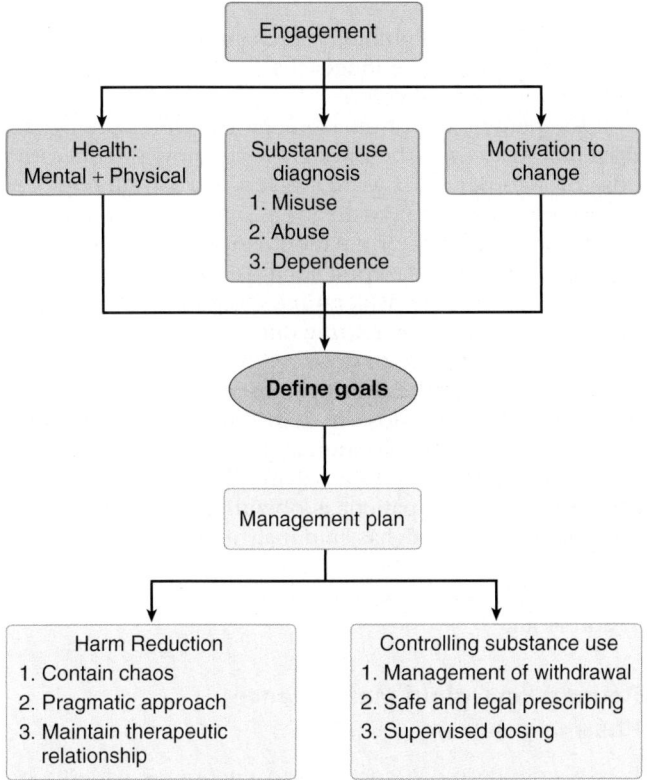

Common Errors

- Dismissive attitude
- Inadequate analgesia in drug dependence
- Under-recognition of alcoholism and substance abuse problems
- Turning a blind eye
- Belief that addressing dependence unreasonably deprives the patient of enjoyment

FIGURE 83-2 Management of drug and alcohol problems in a palliative care context is always challenging. This is a useful guide to follow. The aim of the initial assessment is to diagnose substance use and to assess motivation in addition to defining health issues. This is followed by definition of treatment goals, a management plan to achieve these goals, and periodic monitoring of outcomes with restatement of goals or revisions to the management plan.

amounts. Supply may be contained via regular dispensing by pharmacy or carer. The regularity of dispensing may be negotiated and depends on practical issues and the risk of adverse consequences, ranging from daily dispensing for the most unstable through to monthly supplies (see Chapter 123).

A Pragmatic Approach

Typically, opiates are used relatively liberally in palliative medicine. There is a widespread reluctance to receive opioid medications for pain. Indeed, opiophobia is a greater problem than opioid abuse. More often than not, the palliative care physician encourages use of opioids. Risk factors for substance misuse, if present, mandate more care with prescribing. When the question of medication abuse arises, it is often difficult, despite assessment, to reach a clear diagnosis. Careful attention to responsible prescribing guidelines should be made, and clinical progress should be carefully but nonjudgmentally monitored. The cause of some misunderstanding may become evident, after which there may be no further difficulties with medication. In some patients, careful medication monitoring establishes that there is a problem of medication misuse. Occasionally, the doubt is never removed. If symptoms are well controlled and there is no opioid toxicity or withdrawal, the outcome may be considered satisfactory without a clear diagnosis (see "Common Errors").

Treatment of Intoxication and Withdrawal

Evidence suggests that nicotine replacement therapy (NRT) in a patch or inhaler can be effective at treating withdrawal (Table 8-3). The dose should be titrated according to symptoms. Benzodiazepines are the primary medications for alcohol withdrawal. Diazepam and lorazepam

ment of an individual's concerns are essential to adhere to goals and maintain a therapeutic relationship. A good clinician must also have flexibility in changing management plans, adopting a nonjudgmental stance while setting reasonable limits on medication use and behavior.[13] For example, one patient may be willing to cease harmful benzodiazepine use, another may agree only to moderate the dose, and still another may not recognize any problem with drug use, in which case the best management would be a containment strategy that limits supply to safe

TABLE 83-3 Pharmacological Treatment of Withdrawal	
DRUG	**TREATMENTS**
Nicotine	Nicotine replacement therapy
Alcohol	Benzodiazepines, oral diazepam or infusional midazolam
	Phenobarbitone
	Neuroleptic agents
	Gabapentin, dexamethasone
Benzodiazepines	Benzodiazepines
	Neuroleptic agents
Opiates	Symptomatic therapy
	Opiates if required for analgesia
Stimulants	Symptomatic therapy

TABLE 83-4 Dose Equivalents of Common Benzodiazepines	
Diazepam	10 mg
Alprazolam	0.5-1 mg
Chlordiazepoxide	25 mg
Clonazepam	0.5 mg
Flunitrazepam	1 mg
Lorazepam	1 mg
Midazolam	5 mg
Nitrazepam	5 mg
Oxazepam	20 mg
Temazepam	20 mg

Modified from Hulse G, White J, Cape G. Management of Alcohol and Drug Problems. Melbourne, Australia: Oxford University Press, 2002, Table 1.1.

Box 83-1 Nondrug Measures

- Nonjudgmental therapeutic relationship
- Reassurance that symptom relief can be achieved despite coexisting drug dependence
- Counseling
- Managing challenging behavior appropriately
- Nursing in reassuring, calm environment

are both effective oral therapy but, in the terminal phase, bolus parenteral midazolam or a continuous infusion may be most appropriate. Agitation and restlessness can be difficult to control in alcohol withdrawal, and phenobarbitone is helpful and has anticonvulsant properties. Neuroleptic agents (olanzapine or risperidone is preferred) may be combined with benzodiazepines to treat delirium; as monotherapy, they can lower the seizure threshold.[14] Gabapentin and dexamethasone may decrease neuronal activity in acute alcohol withdrawal, but evidence is limited[15,16] (Box 83-1) (see Chapters 132 and 156).

Patients admitted to a palliative care unit who are taking prescribed opiates will usually continue on this medication. Opiate withdrawal may occur if doses are rapidly reduced (e.g., after a good symptomatic response to radiotherapy). Withdrawal may also occur in patients who are using more than prescribed amounts of opioids and are admitted to hospital or who discontinue use of illicit opioids such as heroin. Management should include monitoring for withdrawal and closely supervised use of long-acting opiates such as methadone. Input from an addiction medicine specialist is advised.

Benzodiazepines

Benzodiazepines are commonly prescribed in palliative medicine but are substances that can be abused. Benzodiazepine withdrawal can be difficult to diagnose because of the nonspecific symptoms and lack of objective signs. It is a cause of delirium and in this event can be treated with neuroleptic agents combined with a low-dose benzodiazepine.

Withdrawal onset is usually 1 to 10 days after cessation or major reduction of intake, depending on the half-life, and may last for 1 to 2 weeks. Withdrawal severity is related to dose and duration of treatment. For those who have been taking benzodiazepines for less than 3 months,

withdrawal is usually mild, if present at all. If treatment has been continued for longer than 1 year, symptoms tend to be moderate to severe.

If the patient and physician negotiate to reduce benzodiazepine use, then the options are to slowly reduce the dose by 10% per week or to convert to a long-acting benzodiazepine of equivalent dose (e.g., diazepam) and reduce by the same amount. If a patient is using more than one short-acting benzodiazepine and is experiencing withdrawal symptoms, consideration should be given to converting to a regular long-acting one, usually diazepam. For the final 25%, the rate or dose reduction schedule should be reduced to half the previous dose reduction. It is usual to try to reduce the dose to zero, but some benefit may be obtained from stabilization at a low dose (e.g., equivalent of diazepam 5 mg twice daily) if this is not possible (Table 83-4). If the patient is obtaining medication from multiple doctors and has minimal motivation to control drug use, it may not be possible to contain drug use. In such difficult cases, it may be best not to prescribe medication at all.

Patients on Opioid Maintenance Pharmacotherapy

It is becoming more common to encounter patients on methadone or buprenorphine programs who are diagnosed with a terminal illness. Many challenges are posed (see Chapters 138 and 251). First, there is the stigma of a treatment program and a history of substance misuse. Attempts to obtain strong analgesia may be labeled as drug-seeking behavior. Second, patients with a history of opioid use have tolerance to these drugs, requiring careful titration and monitoring of analgesic effect in higher doses than usual. Third, the distress of coping with a terminal disease in a person with a history of substance abuse may lead to relapse of aberrant drug-taking behavior. Finally, patients may fear that, because of their past behavior, they will not receive appropriate treatment.

Usually, these cases are comanaged with the addiction medicine team. General guidelines (listed at the end of this section) apply to all of these patients, and close communication between prescribing teams is vital. The equivalent doses for the various opioid drugs in a single dose for acute pain differ from those required for continuing

TABLE 83-5 Dose Equivalence of Opioid Drugs				
DRUG	**Single-Dose Analgesic Equivalence**		**Maintenance Dose Equivalence (Total Daily Dose)**	
	Subcutaneous (mg)	**Oral (mg)**	**Subcutaneous (mg)**	**Oral (mg)**
Morphine	10	60	40	100
Heroin	4	—	16	—
Methadone	10	20	10	20
Buprenorphine	0.3	1 (sublingual tablet)	1	2 (sublingual tablets)
Codeine	120	200	—	600

Modified from An Overview of Opioids and Treatment Approaches. New South Wales Health Department. North Sydney, Australia, 2001.

treatment of chronic pain (Table 83-5). This may be due to differing bioavailability after oral treatment, potency, and duration of action. In addition, much higher doses are usually required in the face of opioid tolerance. After repeated dosing, the half-life of methadone is approximately 24 hours. It takes four to five half-lives to achieve a steady state, so at least 1 week is required to determine the clinical effect of a change in a daily dose. Buprenorphine has a high μ-receptor affinity but low intrinsic activity. Because of the former property, it may displace or compete with full opioid agonists when administered concurrently. Usually, higher doses of short-acting opioid analgesia are required for desired effect.[17]

The following may be used as a general guide:

1. Continue methadone; verify the dose with clinic or physician.
2. Add analgesia as needed, using established guidelines (transition from nondrug methods, to nonopioid drugs, to low-potency opioids, and finally to high-potency opioids).
3. Opioids are usually required in higher doses due to tolerance.
4. Initiate with parenteral opioids if patient is distressed.
5. If continuing pain is present, increase methadone.
6. Similar principles may be followed for buprenorphine. May need to switch to methadone if analgesia is difficult to achieve. Caution must be taken when stopping buprenorphine, because theoretically increased sensitivity to full agonist may occur.
7. If patient is vomiting acutely, convert methadone to parenteral administration (approximately one-half to one-third of the oral dose).

Clinical Trials

There is little evidence from clinical trials looking at substance abuse and alcoholism in palliative care. Prevalence data are conflicting; management of the problems previously discussed is mainly extrapolated from principles established in non–palliative care patients.

Alternative Therapies

Complementary and alternative therapies such as hypnosis, relaxation training, acupuncture, homeopathy, and herbal preparations are usually considered with skepticism by physicians because of the lack of scientific validation. American consumers spent an estimated $27 billion on alternative therapies in 1997 and may wish to look at alternative options combined with other, more traditional therapies.

Controversies and Future Challenges

Liver cirrhosis from hepatitis C is increasing in prevalence, and the numbers of patients with a history of substance abuse and subsequent liver failure and/or hepatocellular carcinoma who require palliative care services will increase.

There are significant regulatory and legal obstacles to the use of tetrahydrocannabinol (THC) and other cannabinoid treatments for medical purposes. Some evidence suggests they are useful in the treatment of symptoms such as anorexia and nausea. Some believe that cannabis is beneficial, but clinical trials are available only for pharmaceutical preparations that are less clinically appealing. The challenge is to develop these treatments for safe therapeutic use with minimum side effects.[18]

REFERENCES

1. American Psychiatric Association. Diagnostic and Statistical Manual of Mental Disorders, Fourth Edition (Text Revision) DSM-IV-TR Arlington, VA: American Psychiatric Publishing, Inc., 2000.
2. Weissman DE. Pseudoaddiction. J Palliat Med 2005;8:1283–1284.
3. Kirsh KL, Whitcomb LA, Donaghy K, et al. Abuse and addiction issues in medically ill patients with pain. Clin J Pain 2002;18:S52–S60.
4. Substance Abuse and Mental Health Services Administration. Results from the 2004 National Survey on Drug Use and Health: National Findings. Office of Applied Studies, NSDUH Series H-28, DHHS Publication No. SMA 05-4062. Rockville, MD: Substance Abuse and Mental Health Services Administration, 2005.
5. Derogatis LR, Morrow GR, Fetting J, et al. The prevalence of psychiatric disorders among cancer patients. JAMA 1983;249:751–757.
6. Bruera E, Moyano J, Seifert L, et al. The frequency of alcoholism among patients with pain due to terminal cancer. J Pain Symptom Manage 1995;10:599–603.
7. Cami J, Farre M. Drug addiction. N Engl J Med 2003;349:975–986.
8. Bernadt M, Mumford J, Taylor C, et al. Comparison of questionnaire and laboratory tests in the detection of excessive drinking and alcoholism. Lancet 1982;1:325–328.
9. Babor TF, Higgins-Biddle JC, Saunders JB, Monteiro MG. AUDIT: The Alcohol Use Disorders Identification Test, 2nd ed. Geneva: World Health Organization, 2001.
10. Passik SD, Theobald DE. Managing addiction in advanced cancer patients: Why bother? J Pain Symptom Manage 2000;19:229–234.
11. Wesson DR, Ling W, Smith DE: Prescription of opioids for treatment of pain in patients with addictive disease. J Pain Symptom Manage 1993;8:289–296.

12. Irwin P, Murray S, Bilinski A, et al. Alcohol withdrawal as an underrated cause of agitated delirium and terminal restlessness in patients with advanced malignancy. J Pain Symptom Manage 2005;29:104–108.

13. Passik SD, Kirsh KL. Managing pain in patients with aberrant drug-taking behaviours. J Support Oncol 2005;3:83–86.

14. Mayo-Smith M. Pharmacological management of alcohol withdrawal: A meta-analysis and evidence based practice guideline. JAMA 1997;278:144–151.

15. Pol S, Nalpas B, Berthelot P. Dexamethasone for alcohol withdrawal. Ann Intern Med 1991;114:705–706.

16. Myrick H, Malcolm R, Brady KT. Gabapentin treatment of alcohol withdrawal. Am J Psychiatry 1998;155:1632.

17. Alford DP, Compton P, Samet JH. Acute pain management for patients receiving maintenance methadone or buprenorphine therapy. Ann Intern Med 2006;144:127–134.

18. Hall W, MacDonald C, Currow D. Cannabinoids and cancer: Causation, remediation, and palliation. Lancet Oncol 2005;6:35–42.

SUGGESTED READING

Graham AW, Schultz TH, Mayo-Smith MF, et al. Principles of Addiction Medicine, 3rd ed. Chevy Chase, MD: American Society of Addiction Medicine, 2003.

Holland JC (ed). Psycho-Oncology. New York: Oxford University Press, 1998.

Hulse G, White J, Cape G. Management of Alcohol and Drug Problems. Melbourne, Australia: Oxford University Press, 2002.

Koob GF, Moal M. Neurobiology of Addiction. Philadelphia: Elsevier, 2006.

Complications of Advanced Disease

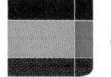

CHAPTER **84**

Liver Failure

Edna Strauss

Liver failure, or hepatic insufficiency, may be acute or chronic. Acute liver failure (ALF) is rapid deterioration of liver function in previously healthy individuals without chronic liver disease. Also known as fulminant hepatitis, it is rare and unpredictable and requires skilled, careful management. Chronic liver failure is linked to cirrhosis and manifests as hepatic encephalopathy (HE), often with multiple organ dysfunctions. A new concept is to differentiate end-stage liver disease (little prospect of recovery) from "acute-on-chronic liver failure" (ACLF). An acute injury to a chronically diseased liver can cause a clinical picture similar to that of terminal liver failure, but the patient may recover.

CHRONIC LIVER FAILURE

The slow deterioration of liver function as a result of etiological agents that damage the hepatic parenchyma evolves without symptoms for years or decades. Whatever the cause, architectural liver changes and cirrhosis develop, frequently complicated by portal hypertension. Some chronic liver diseases compromise the excretory pole of the hepatocyte, the canaliculi, and the biliary ducts, producing cholestasis. The clinical manifestations of chronic cholestasis can also appear gradually over many years, sometimes before cirrhosis.

The large functional liver reserve is compatible with long survival, and the many complications that occur in cirrhosis are associated more with portal hypertension than with hepatocellular failure. Important complications in cirrhosis, such as digestive hemorrhage, ascites, bacterial infections, hepatorenal syndrome, and hepatopulmonary syndrome, are not directly related to hepatocellular insufficiency. Any of these can be more severe and can have a worse prognosis in patients with lower hepatic functional reserve. Quantifying the reserve represents a major clinical challenge.

The condition most commonly associated with chronic liver failure is HE (Table 84-1). Usually, in cirrhosis, there is combined hepatocellular insufficiency and portal hypertension.

CHRONIC CHOLESTASIS

Biliary secretion is a complex process influenced by several factors. Any impediment to bile flow, whether hepatocyte secretory failure or an obstruction in the bile ducts, can result clinically, biochemically, and histologically in cholestasis. Retention of bile acids, bilirubins, and other substances causes the clinical manifestations of jaundice, pruritus, choluria, and acholic stool, which characterize cholestasis. Chronic cholestasis is reflected histologically by retention of bile pigments in hepatocytes, canaliculi, and Kupffer cells. Besides increased bilirubin, some enzymes, such as alkaline phosphatase, γ-glutamyl transferase (GGT), and 5′-nucleotidase, are characteristically elevated.[1]

Cholestasis can be caused by established cirrhosis, or it may be a primary manifestation of chronic cholestatic diseases such as primary biliary cirrhosis or primary sclerosing cholangitis. Various other cholestatic diseases may be diagnosed in chronic liver disease. The common denominator in most is progressive loss of bile ducts, the vanishing bile duct syndrome, which is common in children but is also present in adults.

TABLE 84-1 Chronic Liver Failure Syndromes: Main Clinical Manifestations

CHOLESTASIS	PORTAL HYPERTENSION	HEPATOCELLULAR INSUFFICIENCY
Jaundice	Gastrointestinal bleeding	Hepatic encephalopathy
Choluria	Ascites	Multiple organ failure
Pruritus	Spontaneous bacterial peritonitis	
Acholic stools	Hepatorenal syndrome	
Elevated GGT and alkaline phosphatase	Hepatopulmonary syndrome	

GGT, γ-glutamyl transferase.

The initial dilemma, given a clinical picture of cholestasis, is separating the mechanical/obstructive causes from parenchymal ones. Because the clinical and biochemical manifestations are identical, imaging procedures are performed. Once obstructive causes are excluded, liver biopsy is often needed to clarify the etiology and stage the liver injury.

One of the main symptoms of chronic cholestasis is pruritus. The medication for pruritus is cholestyramine, a bile-acid chelating agent, in 4-g doses two to six times a day. Antihistamines are not indicated, but other drugs, such as ursodeoxycholic acid, rifampicin, phenobarbital, and opiate antagonists (e.g., naltrexone), can be used.[2] Ondansetron, a serotonin receptor antagonist, was of no benefit in a recent controlled trial.[3]

In primary biliary cirrhosis, particularly in early disease, ursodeoxycholic acid is recommended. This is a natural hydrophilic bile acid that is cytoprotective and immunomodulatory in chronic cholestasis. In primary sclerosing cholangitis, several other medications (methotrexate, corticoids, cyclosporin) have been used in addition, without convincing therapeutic efficacy. In vanishing bile duct syndromes, ursodeoxycholic acid has been used successfully.[4]

CLINICAL COMPLICATIONS OF PORTAL HYPERTENSION

Clinical complications of portal hypertension derive from the formation of collateral veins and from hyperdynamic splanchnic and systemic circulation. The most characteristic complication is undoubtedly hemorrhage from ruptured esophageal varices.

In cirrhosis, ascites is the most frequent complication of portal hypertension.[5] Incorrect management (e.g., excessive diuresis) may promote more serious complications: hepatorenal syndrome or HE. Spontaneous bacterial peritonitis (SBP) develops in cirrhosis with ascites because of the immunodeficiency due to liver insufficiency, which favors infections, and the portal hypertension, which activates vasoactive substances that interfere with physiological defense mechanisms.

SBP develops in 30% of patients with cirrhosis and ascites, with high morbidity and mortality. Impairment of immune defense mechanisms in advanced cirrhosis, over-growth of intestinal flora, and bacterial translocation from the intestinal lumen to mesenteric lymph nodes contribute. Clinical manifestations vary from severe to mild or absent. SBP is diagnosed when the ascitic fluid neutrophil count is greater than 250 cells/mm³ with or without a positive bacterial culture result. Enterobacteria are the main agents, with *Escherichia coli* being most common. Early diagnosis and antibiotic treatment reduce mortality. Intravenous third-generation cephalosporins are effective in 70% to 95% of the cases. Recurrent SBP is common and can be prevented by oral norfloxacin, improving survival. Bacterial resistance has led to the search for new prophylactic choices; probiotic therapy remains promising but requires further evaluation.[6] Short-duration primary prophylaxis is recommended in cirrhotic patients with ascites during acute upper digestive hemorrhage.[7]

Hyperdynamic circulation causes hypervolemia, increased cardiac output, and a drop in arterial pressure. The clinical manifestations of this become relevant only in decompensated or end-stage cirrhosis. They may worsen with time or develop after digestive hemorrhage, bacterial infection, or some medications (e.g., nonsteroidal anti-inflammatory agents).[8] The most serious consequences of hyperdynamic circulation are hepatorenal syndrome[9] and hepatopulmonary syndrome. The latter is different from portopulmonary hypertension, which is less common but also associated with portal hypertension.[10]

HEPATIC ENCEPHALOPATHY

HE is most characteristic of chronic liver failure. It is usually a terminal process with a poor prognosis and little effective therapy. There are three types[11]:

Type A: Encephalopathy with ALF
Type B: Encephalopathy with a portosystemic shunt
Type C: Encephalopathy with cirrhosis and portal hypertension.

Type C has three different clinical forms:
Episodic HE: Precipitated, spontaneous, and recurrent
Persistent HE: Mild, severe, and treatment-dependent
Minimal HE: This category covers preclinical manifestations, which require special diagnostic methods and replaces previous terminology.

Physiopathology and Clinical Diagnosis

Encephalopathy results from intoxication of the brain when nitrogenous substances, usually from the intestine, are not metabolized by the liver. This occurs because of shunting of portal blood by the intrahepatic or extrahepatic collateral circulation or because of hepatocellular insufficiency. Those patients with extensive collateral circulation are more likely to develop spontaneous or precipitated encephalopathy from exogenous factors.

Although the physiopathology is controversial, ammonia is considered the main agent[12] of cerebral intoxication, with astrocyte swelling the only morphological marker of encephalopathy (Fig. 84-1). Hyperammonemia has toxic synergy with all the metabolic changes of HE.[13] Ammonia is produced mainly in the intestines but also in the kidneys; it is metabolized to urea or glutamine in the liver (Fig. 84-2) as well as in brain and muscle. Clinical diagnosis is

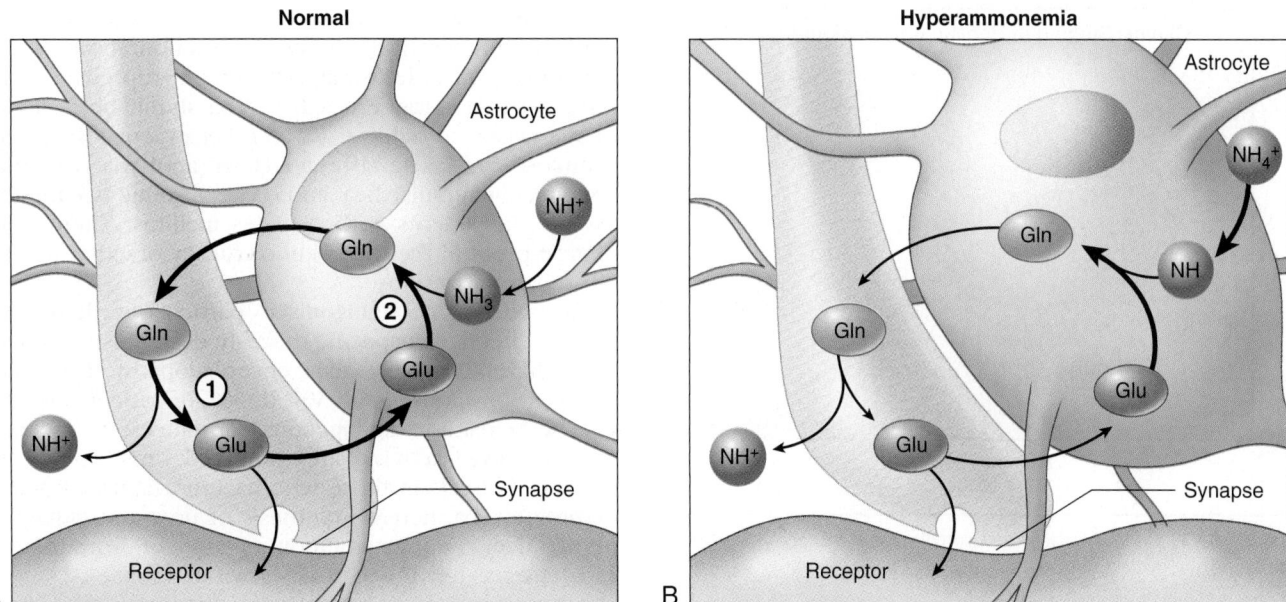

FIGURE 84-1 Metabolic cerebral disturbances caused by ammonia overload of the astrocytes. 1, glutaminase activity; 2, glutamino synthetase activity; Gln, glutamine; Glu, glutamate.

Detoxification of Ammonia

Periportal Hepatocyte

Perivenous Hepatocyte

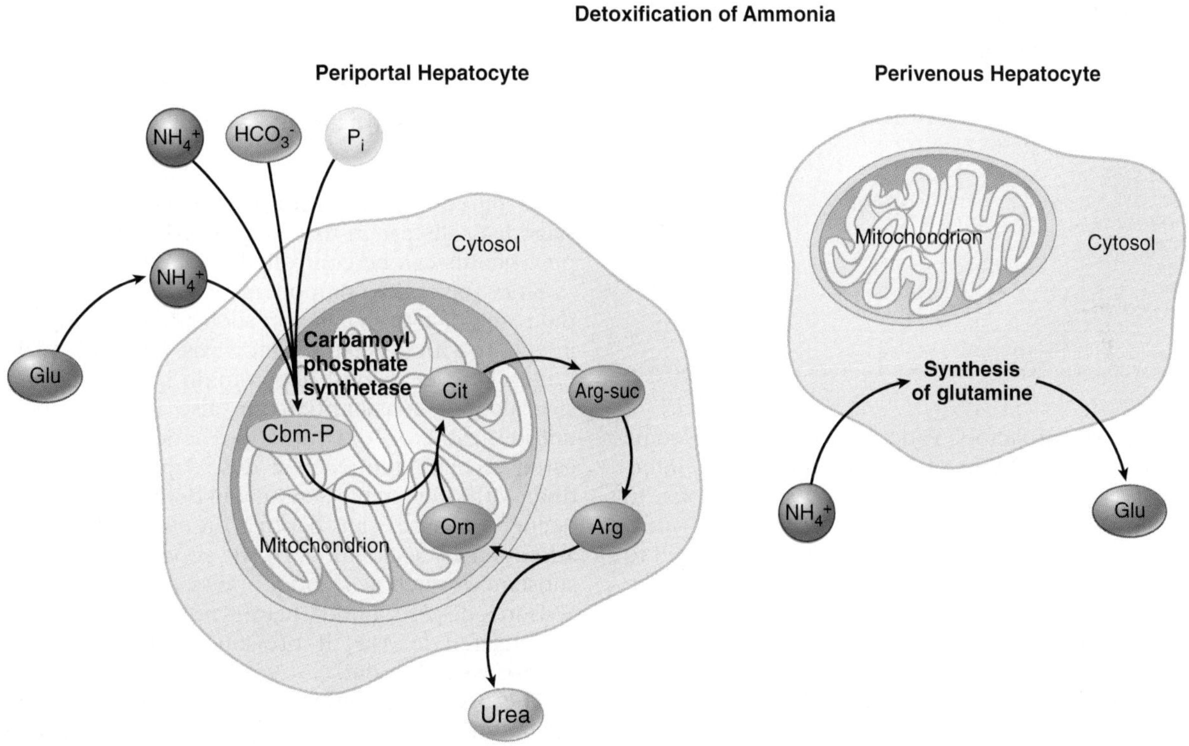

FIGURE 84-2 Two different metabolic pathways in hepatocytes can detoxify ammonia. In periportal hepatocytes, ammonia is metabolized to urea via the Krebs cycle, and in perivenous hepatocytes, ammonia is metabolized to glutamine (as occurs also in muscle and brain). Arg, arginine; Cit, citruline; Gln, glutamine; Glu, glutamate; Orn, ornithine.

relatively easy but subjective, because it depends on observer experience in characterizing the various phases, from stage 1 (disorientation) through lethargy and semi-stupor to hepatic coma (Fig. 84-3).

The main precipitants of HE are digestive hemorrhage and bacterial infections. Common precipitants in cirrhotic patients are intestinal obstipation and dehydration or water/electrolyte imbalance from diuretics. Elimination of precipitants alone may revert the encephalopathy without specific medication.

General and Specific Therapeutic Measures

General measures include protein restriction (more vegetable proteins or branched-chain amino acids) and intestinal cleansing along with diagnosis and treatment of

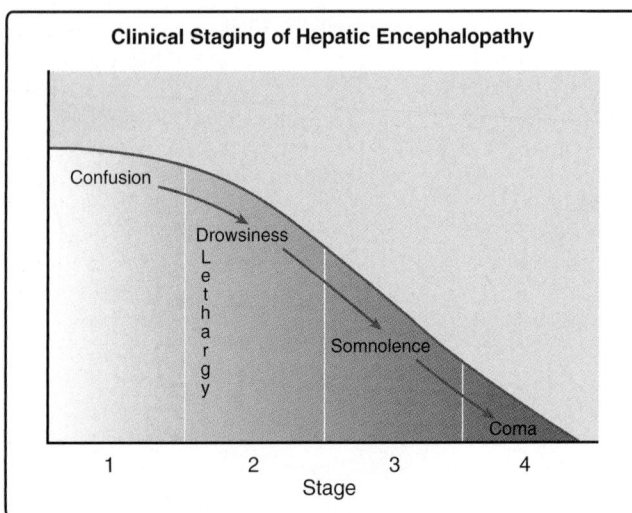

Clinical Staging of Hepatic Encephalopathy

FIGURE 84-3 In clinical practice, staging of hepatic encephalopathy in the classic four grades is very useful.

TABLE 84-2 Treatment of Hepatic Encephalopathy in Chronic Liver Disease		
MEASURES TARGETING THE INTESTINES	**MEASURES TARGETING THE BRAIN**	**MEASURES TARGETING THE LIVER**
Oral nonabsorbable antibiotics (e.g., neomycin)	Rebalancing of plasma amino acids → BCAA-enriched solutions	↑ Synthesis of urea and glutamine: zinc; L-ornithine, L-aspartate as substrates
Disaccharides (e.g., lactulose)	Benzodiazepine antagonists (especially flumazenil)	Liver transplantation
Intestinal cleansing		

BCAA, branched-chain amino acid.

possible precipitant factors. Patients in precoma or coma need intensive care (Table 84-2), with attention to infection prophylaxis and respiratory and renal functions. In hepatic coma, unlike other types of coma (especially neurological), death is usually quicker, because it is linked to hepatic insufficiency. Because the potential regenerative liver capacity cannot be known, maintenance of life awaiting a possible recovery must be the rule.

Medications that target the intestine aim to reduce ammonia both by inhibiting production and by either reducing absorption or increasing elimination. Neomycin sulfate and other oral antibiotics with limited absorption were adopted to sterilize the colon. Neomycin sulfate was recommended in doses of 4 to 6 g daily, reduced by 2 g every day as the condition improved. Because of side effects such as nephrotoxicity and/or ototoxicity, it is no longer recommended for chronic treatment. Added to lactulose, it has little additional effect because the antibiotic needs an alkaline pH (pH > 8), and lactulose makes the colon acidic (pH < 6). Two studies compared neomycin with a placebo, and neither found significant differences.[14]

Lactulose and other disaccharides that cannot be broken down by digestive enzymes (lactitol, and lactose itself in lactase-deficient individuals) produce acidification of the colon and, theoretically, lower production/absorption of ammonia. Lactulose is a sweet-tasting syrup given in 15-mL doses two to four times daily. This should be increased or decreased to achieve two bowel evacuations a day. Lactulose can cause taste aversions, anorexia, vomiting, abdominal pain, diarrhea, and rectal burning. It should be avoided in patients with diabetes mellitus. There is no clinical proof of the therapeutic efficacy of either neomycin sulfate or lactulose.[15]

Benzodiazepine antagonists, particularly flumazenil, may be effective in specific cases. In drug poisoning from benzodiazepines or stage 4 encephalopathy, flumazenil restores consciousness in 30% to 50% of patients, but this can be transitory. Endogenous substances with benzodiazepine-like activity are inhibited, explaining the beneficial effects in those who have not ingested benzodiazepines. To increase synthesis of urea and glutamine in the liver, supplementation of zinc or L-ornithine–L-aspartate has been used,[16] as shown in Table 84-2.

Liver transplantation is undoubtedly the definitive treatment, not only for encephalopathy but also for the underlying disease, which is usually cirrhosis (Fig. 84-4). Every patient who recovers from HE must be assessed for liver transplantation.

ACUTE-ON-CHRONIC LIVER FAILURE

Definition, Precipitating Factors, and Prognosis

ACLF differs from the chronic decompensation of end-stage liver disease in that ACLF is potentially reversible if precipitants can be controlled.

First, the acute component of the liver injury may be the result of a known factor, such as a superimposed viral infection with a hepatotropic virus, hepatitis A, or hepatitis B. Drug reactions, hepatotoxin ingestion, and excessive alcohol consumption are also factors. Drugs with unforeseeable or idiosyncratic reactions must be investigated. Acetaminophen is a dose-dependent hepatotoxic drug with predictable action, and both ALF and ACLF may occur.[17] Misuse can happen intentionally (in suicide attempts), by accident, or by the concomitant use of other substances, such as alcohol.[18] Less common causes (e.g., Wilson's disease, Budd-Chiari syndrome) also need to be investigated in ALF, if previous signs of chronic liver disease were present.

The liver injury may also be caused by precipitating factors such as variceal bleeding or sepsis. ACLF manifests through altered functioning of all organ systems, most notably the liver, circulation, brain, and kidneys. Hyperbilirubinemia with clinical jaundice is prevalent. Reduction of hepatic synthetic function produces hypoalbuminemia with edema and increasing ascites. Decreased clotting factor production, sometimes with thrombocytopenia (from hypersplenism), may cause a hemorrhagic diathesis.

The prognosis can be determined by organ-failure scoring systems such as the Sepsis-related Organ Failure Assessment (SOFA) or the Acute Physiological And Chronic Health Evaluation (APACHE), or even by using a modified Model for End-Stage Liver Disease (MELD) score.[19]

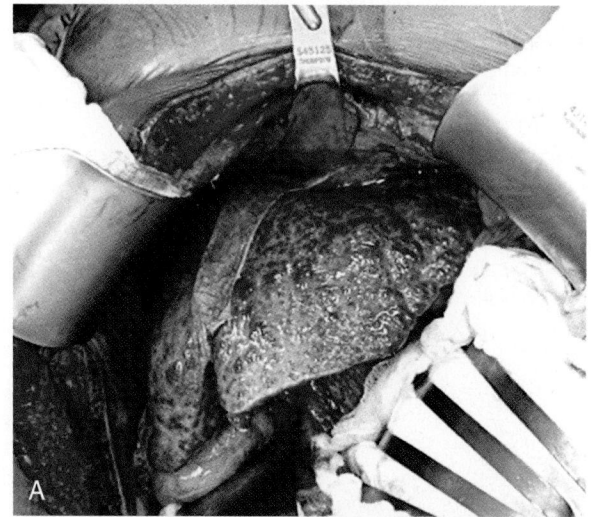

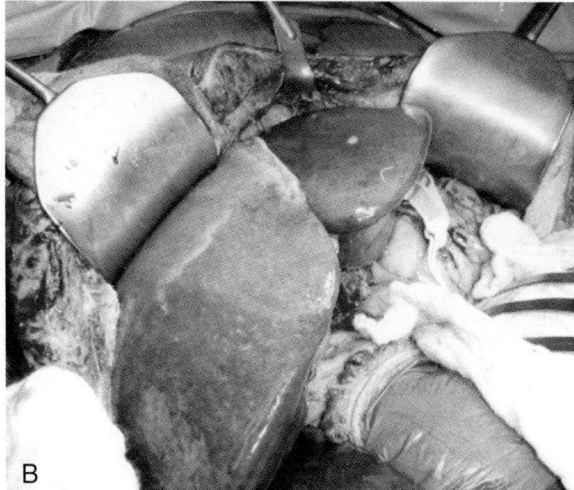

FIGURE 84-4   For chronic liver failure and for acute-on-chronic liver failure, when spontaneous recovery fails, the best therapy is liver transplantation.

The MELD is a continuous staging system with no ceiling or floor scores, derived statistically so that appropriate weights are given to variables according to their relative importance. It considers renal function and is reliable for predicting outcome in decompensated cirrhosis, with predicted 3-month mortality of 27% at a score of less than 20 to 76% at a score of 20 or higher.[20] The National Hospice and Palliative Care Organization (NHPCO) uses the same criteria for end-stage liver disease, namely Child-Pugh scores and MELD. The most suitable scoring system for ACLF is the SOFA scoring system, which includes parameters representing the respiratory, cardiovascular, and central nervous systems as well as coagulation and renal and liver functions (Table 84-3).[21] A score of 8 seems to be a suitable cutoff value, with predicted hospital mortality being 4% with a score lower than 8 and 88% with a higher score. Mortality (both at hospital discharge and at 6 months) increases dramatically when the number of organ failures increases.

Complications

Cerebral edema, although frequently a cause of death in ALF, is rare in ACLF. If intracranial pressure exceeds 30 mm Hg, the patient may have intermittent or sustained arterial hypertension, bradycardia, and irregular respiration (Cushing's triad). Later, decerebrate posture, pupillary dilation with poor response to light, papilledema, headache, vomiting, and opisthotonus occur.[22]

Infections are more common in cirrhosis due to malfunctioning Kupffer cells, intestinal bacterial translocation, leukocyte dysfunction, reduced opsonization with complement activation, and the release of immunosuppressive endotoxins and cytokines. Invasive procedures are an important point of entry for infections.[23] Any bacterial infection, especially SBP, can enhance HE. Early diagnosis and prompt treatment may prevent ACLF.

Multiple organ failure increases mortality and is also one of the main contraindications for liver transplantation. This manifests as hypotension with peripheral vasodilation, pulmonary edema, acute tubular necrosis, and disseminated intravascular coagulation. Renal insufficiency is common in liver failure. It can be difficult to differentiate between mere intravascular volume depletion and acute tubular necrosis, which is characteristic of multiple organ failure. Circulatory changes are part of the manifestation of the condition itself. Any alteration in hepatic perfusion in a chronically diseased liver may cause acute decompensation. Reversible depression of myocardial function suggests that the circulatory derangement of ACLF may be different from that occurring with liver dysfunction alone.[24]

Hepatorenal syndrome develops during progressive liver function deterioration, with poorly controlled ascites and marked alterations in splanchnic and systemic hemodynamics. It is unclear whether renal dysfunction in ACLF is merely an aggravation of the circulatory disturbance from cirrhosis or whether there are different elements more amenable to intervention. Apart from jaundice, HE is probably the most apparent major manifestation in ACLF. The pathophysiological basis of HE in ACLF is probably similar to that in ALF.

Management

Careful examination of the patient's history, laboratory tests, and even a liver biopsy may identify the superimposed liver injury. Distinguishing among alcoholic hepatitis, drug reaction, and infection may aid in deciding whether to treat with immunosuppressors such as corticosteroids or with anti-tumor necrosis factor (TNF) drugs. Viral screening to exclude superimposed infection is crucial, and hepatitis B reactivation can be treated promptly with potent specific oral antivirals (e.g., lamivudine, entecavir). Bacterial infections, such SBP, pneumonia, or urinary tract infections, should be aggressively managed. Control of gastrointestinal bleeding is essential, because the prognosis for uncontrolled bleeding is poor. Supportive measures for ACLF resemble those already described for ALF in regard to circulatory changes, renal dysfunction, HE, coagulopathy, nutrition, and extracorporeal liver support (Table 84-4).

RESEARCH ADVANCES

We need new drugs for chronic HE tested against a placebo, because no clear benefit has been linked to classic lactulose therapy.

TABLE 84-3   The Sequential Organ Failure Assessment (SOFA) Scoring System for Acute-on-Chronic Liver Failure

SOFA SCORE	0	1	2	3	4
RESPIRATION					
PaO_2/FIO_2 (mm Hg)	>400	≤400	≤300	≤200	≤100
				—— with respiratory support ——	
COAGULATION					
Platelets × $10^3/mm^3$	>150	≤150	≤100	≤50	≤20
LIVER					
Bilirubin					
(mg/dL)	<1.2	1.2-1.9	2.0-5.9	6.0-11.9	>12.0
(μmol/L)	(<20)	(20-32)	(33-101)	(102-204)	(>204)
CARDIOVASCULAR					
Hypotension	No hypotension	MAP <70 mm Hg	Dopamine ≤5 or dobutamine (any dose)*	Dopamine >5 or epinephrine ≤0.1 or norepinephrine ≤0.1*	Dopamine >15 or epinephrine >0.1 or norepinephrine >0.1*
CENTRAL NERVOUS SYSTEM					
Glasgow Coma Score	15	13-14	10-12	6-9	<6
RENAL					
Creatinine					
mg/dL	<1.2	1.2-1.9	2.0-3.4	3.5-4.9	>5.0
(μmol/L)	(<110)	(110-170)	(171-299)	(300-440)	(>440)
or urine output				or <500 mL/day	or <200 mL/day

*Adrenergic agents administered for at least 1 hr (doses given are in μg/kg/min).
FIO_2, fractional inspired oxygen; MAP, mean arterial pressure; PaO_2, arterial oxygen tension.
From Vincent JL, Moreno R, Takala J, et al. The SOFA (Sepsis-related Organ Failure Assessment) score to describe organ dysfunction/failure. On behalf of the Working Group on Sepsis-Related Problems of the European Society of Intensive Care Medicine. Intensive Care Med 1996;22:707-710.

TABLE 84-4   Management of Acute-on-Chronic Liver Failure

COMPLICATION	THERAPEUTIC MANAGEMENT
Hepatic encephalopathy	Hypoprotein diet (BCAA or vegetable proteins)
	Avoid sedatives
	Intestinal lavage
	Lactulose (?)—*avoid in cases of cerebral edema*
Cerebral edema	Monitor intracranial pressure
	Avoid movement
	Avoid nasotracheal aspiration
	Head of bed at 45 degrees
	Mannitol
Hypoglycemia	Constant glycemia control
	Continuous intravenous glucose infusion
Renal insufficiency	Dialysis
	Hemofiltration
Respiratory insufficiency	Monitor arterial gases
	Orotracheal intubation
	Mechanical ventilation
Hypotension	Dopamine
Infection	Frequent cultures
	Antibiotic therapy
Hemorrhage	Fresh plasma/platelets
	Blood clotting factors
	Histamine₂ blockers/proton pump inhibitors

BCAA, branched-chain amino acid.

An active search for precipitants of ACLF may lead to its control. Prognosis should be determined using an effective scoring system, such as SOFA.

REFERENCES

1. Perez Fernandez T, Lopez Serrano P, Tomas E, et al. Diagnostic and therapeutic approach to cholestatic liver disease. Rev Esp Enferm Dig 2004;96:60-73.
2. Bergasa NV. Medical palliation of the jaundiced patient with pruritus. Gastroenterol Clin North Am 2006;35:113-123.
3. O'Donohue JW, Pereira SP, Ashdown AC, et al. A controlled trial of ondansetron in the pruritus of cholestasis. Aliment Pharmacol Ther 2005;21:1041-1045.
4. Paumgartner G. Medical treatment of cholestatic liver diseases: From pathobiology to pharmacological targets. World J Gastroenterol 2006;12:4445-4451.
5. Sandhu BS, Sanyal AJ. Management of ascites in cirrhosis. Clin Liver Dis 2005;9:715-732, viii.
6. Strauss E, Caly WR. Spontaneous bacterial peritonitis: A therapeutic update. Expert Rev Anti Infect Ther 2006;4:249-260.
7. Bernard B, Cadranel JF, Valla D, et al. Prognostic significance of bacterial infection in bleeding cirrhotic patients: A prospective study. Gastroenterology 1995;108:1828-1834.
8. Westphal JF, Brogard JM. Drug administration in chronic liver disease. Drug Saf 1997;17:47-73.
9. Cardenas A, Arroyo V. Hepatorenal syndrome. Ann Hepatol 2003;2:23-29.
10. Hoeper MM, Krowka MJ, Strassburg CP. Portopulmonary hypertension and hepatopulmonary syndrome. Lancet 2004;363:1461-1468.
11. Ferenci P, Lockwood A, Mullen K, et al. Hepatic encephalopathy—Definition, nomenclature, diagnosis, and quantification: Final report of the working party at the 11th World Congresses of Gastroenterology, Vienna, 1998. Hepatology 2002;35:716-721.
12. Shawcross DL, Damink SW, Butterworth RF, Jalan R. Ammonia and hepatic encephalopathy: The more things change, the more they remain the same. Metab Brain Dis 2005;20:169-179.
13. Mas A. Hepatic encephalopathy: From pathophysiology to treatment. Digestion 2006;73(Suppl 1):86-93.
14. Strauss E, Tramote R, Silva EP, et al. Double-blind randomized clinical trial comparing neomycin and placebo in the treatment of exogenous hepatic encephalopathy. Hepatogastroenterology 1992;39:542-545.

15. Als-Nielsen B, Gluud LL, Gluud C. Non-absorbable disaccharides for hepatic encephalopathy: Systematic review of randomised trials. BMJ 2004;328:1046.
16. Kircheis G, Wettstein M, Dahl S, Haussinger D. Clinical efficacy of L-ornithine-L-aspartate in the management of hepatic encephalopathy. Metab Brain Dis 2002;17:453-462.
17. Ostapowicz G, Fontana RJ, Schiodt FV, et al. Results of a prospective study of acute liver failure at 17 tertiary care centers in the United States. Ann Intern Med 2002;137:947-954.
18. Zimmerman HJ, Maddrey WC. Acetaminophen (paracetamol) hepatotoxicity with regular intake of alcohol: Analysis of instances of therapeutic misadventure. Hepatology 1995;22:767-773.
19. Sen S, Williams R, Jalan R. The pathophysiological basis of acute-on-chronic liver failure. Liver 2002;22(Suppl 2):5-13.
20. Kamath PS, Wiesner RH, Malinchoc M, et al. A model to predict survival in patients with end-stage liver disease. Hepatology 2001;33:464-470.
21. Vincent JL, Moreno R, Takala J, et al. The SOFA (Sepsis-related Organ Failure Assessment) score to describe organ dysfunction/failure. On behalf of the Working Group on Sepsis-Related Problems of the European Society of Intensive Care Medicine. Intensive Care Med 1996;22:707-710.
22. Lee WM. Acute liver failure. N Engl J Med 1993;329:1862-1872.
23. Rolando N, Harvey F, Brahm J, et al. Prospective study of bacterial infection in acute liver failure: An analysis of fifty patients. Hepatology 1990;11:49-53.
24. Fernandez J, Navasa M, Garcia-Pagan JC, et al. Effect of intravenous albumin on systemic and hepatic hemodynamics and vasoactive neurohormonal systems in patients with cirrhosis and spontaneous bacterial peritonitis. J Hepatol 2004;41:384-390.

SUGGESTED READING

Als-Nielsen B, Gluud LL, Gluud C. Non-absorbable disaccharides for hepatic encephalopathy: Systematic review of randomised trials. BMJ 2004;328:1046.

Mas A. Hepatic encephalopathy: From pathophysiology to treatment. Digestion 2006;73(Suppl 1):86-93.

Sen S, Williams R, Jalan R. The pathophysiological basis of acute-on-chronic liver failure. Liver 2002;22(Suppl 2):5-13.

Shawcross DL, Damink SW, Butterworth RF, Jalan R. Ammonia and hepatic encephalopathy: The more things change, the more they remain the same. Metab Brain Dis 2005;20: 169-179.

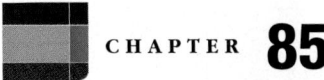

CHAPTER **85**

Deep Vein Thrombosis

Simon Noble

K E Y   P O I N T S

- Venous thromboembolism is common in advanced malignancy.
- Concurrent pathological conditions make accurate diagnosis challenging.
- Cancer patients have a higher rate of bleeding and recurrent thrombosis than do noncancer patients.
- Low-molecular-weight heparin (LMWH) appears to be safer and more efficacious than warfarin in cancer patients.
- The evidence suggests that LMWH is better than warfarin in cancer patients, but there is limited research in the palliative care setting.

An association between cancer and venous thromboembolism (VTE) has been recognized since at least 1865.[1] Those with clinically evident malignant disease or occult cancer have an increased risk of VTE, and necropsy studies document an increased risk of thrombosis in visceral cancers.[2,3] Fifteen percent of all cancer patients have a thromboembolic event, and one in five of all episodes of deep vein thrombosis (DVT) and pulmonary embolism (PE) occur in patients with known cancers.[4] Although the management of VTE in the general population is well established, the diagnosis and subsequent treatment in cancer patients raise several problems, especially in advanced metastatic disease.

CLINICAL EVALUATION AND DIAGNOSIS

DVT is a common medical condition in which a thrombus forms in the venous system. It most frequently occurs in the lower limbs, manifesting as a hot, painful, swollen, red leg, but is sometimes asymptomatic or with atypical symptoms. As well as causing pain and impaired mobility, thrombus from the leg veins can embolize to the lungs, resulting in PE. Like DVTs, PEs have a range of symptoms and signs. Some are asymptomatic, chronically causing shortness of breath and right-sided heart failure; others manifest classically with pleuritic chest pain, shortness of breath, and hemoptysis. Large PEs can cause cardiovascular collapse and instant death.

The incidence of VTE in the cancer population is at least 15% but increases with disease progression. In the palliative care population, more than 50% of inpatients may have undiagnosed DVT, with up to 30% developing symptoms.[5]

The increased prothrombotic risk is multifactorial:

- *Stasis*—Many patients are bedridden due to general debility, lethargy, neurological deterioration, cord compression, or terminal disease. Local vessel stasis is common in pelvic malignancy, and leg edema may cause external compression with local stasis.
- *Endothelial perturbation*—This may occur after surgery or because of local tumor infiltration.
- *Hypercoagulable state*—Procoagulants, including tissue factor and thrombin–antithrombin complex, are increased in certain cancers.
- *Iatrogenic*—Venous indwelling catheters are prothrombotic in the cancer patient. Modifications in catheter design and tip position have decreased the risk of VTE. Some chemotherapeutic agents are prothrombotic, and this effect may increase if multiple agents are used.

DIFFICULTIES IN THE MANAGEMENT OF VENOUS THROMBOEMBOLISM

There are difficulties in both assessment and treatment of suspected VTE in the palliative care setting. Although VTE is common in advanced cancer, it is often not considered as a cause of symptoms, because many other aspects of the pathology common to cancer patients manifest similarly. Investigations with a high sensitivity and specificity in the general population are not always useful in cancer patients, and other definitive tests may be inappropriate or impractical in the palliative care environment.

Specialist palliative care units (SPCUs) are unlikely to investigate suspected VTE unless the investigation is accessible, noninvasive, accurate (given the multiple pathologies in this patient group), acceptable to the patient, and likely to alter management.

Not all patients will be considered suitable for anticoagulation, and investigation is unlikely unless the patient is a candidate for warfarin or low-molecular-weight heparin (LMWH). Transfer of a patient with suspected DVT from the SPCU to a neighboring hospital for a Doppler ultrasound study is too arduous for many, even more so for an invasive investigation such as contrast venography. Suspected PEs are even harder to diagnose radiologically. Ventilation/perfusion scans are often not considered, because other lung pathologies, common in advanced cancer, make them unreliable.

The treatment of VTE can be problematic, because cancer patients have a higher incidence of recurrent thromboses (despite adequate anticoagulation). In addition, there is an increased incidence of bleeding during anticoagulation, and anticoagulants such as coumarins have significant drug interactions with commonly prescribed medicines.

PRESENTATION AND DIAGNOSIS OF DEEP VEIN THROMBOSIS

In a noncancer patient, leg swelling and pain raise a high index of suspicion of DVT. However, painful, swollen legs are common in the palliative population and may have other causes. Although many conditions mimic DVT, the presence of one such diagnosis does not negate concurrent thrombosis. Cellulitis or stasis from pelvic disease, for example, may increase the prothrombotic state and the likelihood of undiagnosed VTE.

The diagnosis of DVT of the lower limb by clinical signs is unreliable. Individual signs and symptoms are of little value, and Homan's sign of no value (Table 85-1; Fig. 85-1).

D-Dimers

Plasma D-dimers are specific cross-linked fibrin derivatives produced when fibrin is degraded by plasmin. Concentrations are raised by thrombolysis. They are highly sensitive

for VTE but insufficiently specific for diagnosis, because they occur in other disorders (e.g., infections, cancers) and in postoperative states.[6,7] D-dimer levels are now accepted as an important exclusionary test for VTE, with a negative predictive value close to 100%. Their use in cancer patients is limited, and they have no role in the palliative care setting.

Imaging Techniques

There are several imaging techniques available for lower limb DVT. Each has advantages and disadvantages, including different degrees of sensitivity, specificity, operator dependence, cost, accessibility, and invasiveness. Radiological diagnosis will depend on local practice and availability of investigations.

Doppler ultrasonography is the most widely available, cheap, noninvasive test and has largely replaced venography. A recent meta-analysis suggested that the sensitivity of ultrasonography is 89% overall for symptomatic DVT and 97% for above-knee thrombus. Problems with ultrasonography include poor sensitivity for asymptomatic disease, difficulties diagnosing DVT recurrence, and limited visualization in the pelvis[8,9] (Fig. 85-2).

Impedance plethysmography is also commonly used but has similar limitations in recurrent thrombosis, asymptomatic DVT, and DVT below the knee or in the pelvis.[8,9]

Venography is the reference standard diagnostic test, but it has been replaced by noninvasive tests.[8-11] In prac-

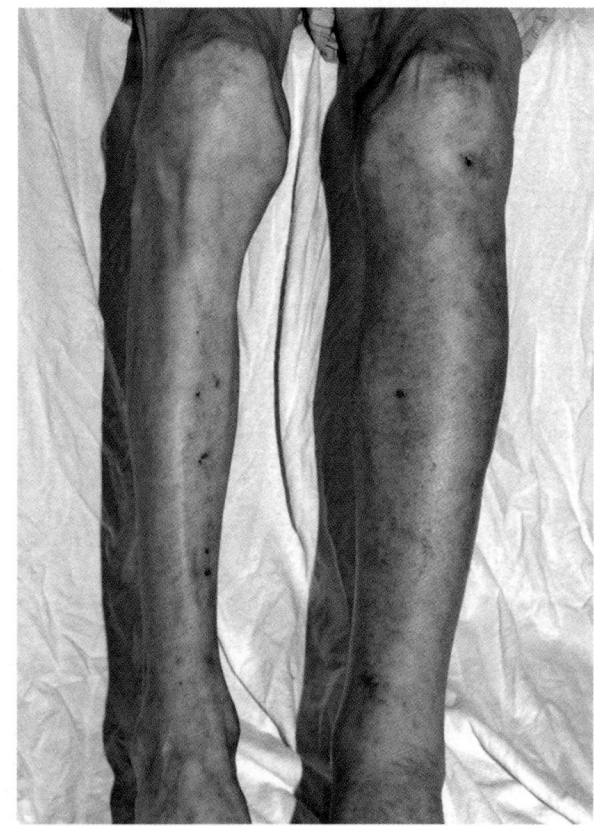

FIGURE 85-1   Patient with swollen left leg secondary to deep vein thrombosis.

TABLE 85-1   Common Causes of Swollen Legs in the Palliative Care Patient

UNILATERAL SWELLING
- Deep vein thrombosis
- Cellulitis
- Nodal disease in groin
- Lymphedema

BILATERAL SWELLING
- Deep vein thrombosis
- Hypoalbuminemia
- Heart failure
- Medicines (e.g., steroids, nifedipine)
- Lymphedema
- Pelvic disease causing reduced venous outflow

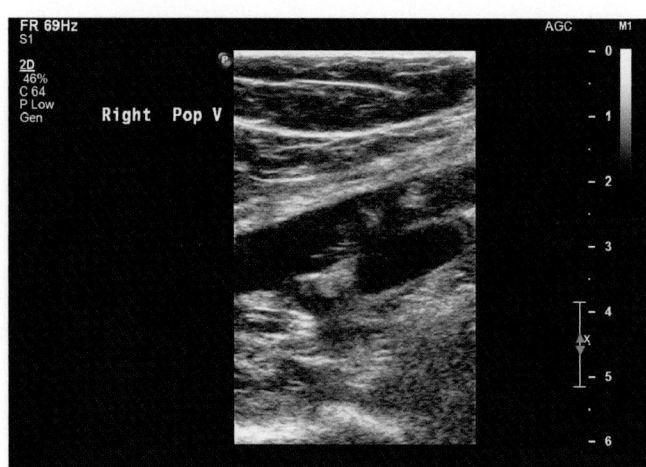

FIGURE 85-2 Doppler ultrasound image showing thrombus in the right popliteal vein.

Box 85-1 Common Causes of Dyspnea in Advanced Cancer

- Pneumonia
- Pulmonary edema
- Pleural effusion
- Anemia
- Lung metastases
- Lymphangitis
- Muscle fatigue
- Concurrent pulmonary illness
  - Chronic obstructive pulmonary disease
  - Emphysema
  - Interstitial lung disease
  - Congestive cardiac failure

Box 85-2 Presenting Features of Pulmonary Embolus

- Dyspnea (80%)
- Tachypnea (70%)
- Pleuritic chest pain (52%)
- Cough (20%)
- Syncope (19%)
- Substernal chest pain (12%)
- Hemoptysis (11%)
- Pleural effusion (usually blood-stained transudate)

tice, it is the most reliable test for asymptomatic thrombus and for thrombus within the calf or pelvis. It involves injection of intravenous contrast material.

PRESENTATION AND DIAGNOSIS OF PULMONARY EMBOLUS

Postmortem studies suggest that PEs may occur in up to 50% of patients with advanced cancers.[3,4] The incidence clinically is lower, suggesting that PEs are underdiagnosed. The most frequent presenting symptom, breathlessness, is commonly present in advanced cancer. Dyspnea may also be caused by any of several coexistent conditions, of which PE is one.

Recognized clinical features of PE (Box 85-1) do not narrow the differential diagnosis of breathlessness in cancer. Many are present in causes of dyspnea (Box 85-2).

Sudden-onset dyspnea may be the only symptom of a PE, and those patients with preexisting pulmonary or cardiac disease may notice only a worsening of preexisting dyspnea. Likewise, a PE sufficient to cause cardiovascular compromise or hypoxia may manifest as a worsening of other medical conditions such as angina and heart failure or induce arrhythmias such as atrial fibrillation. A large central PE may manifest with syncope or sudden hemodynamic collapse, oliguria, acute right-sided heart failure, and peripheral vascular shutdown. Sudden death in palliative care is often attributed to embolic phenomena.

Practically, a physician is likely to exclude and treat conditions such as infection, pulmonary edema, and anemia before considering the diagnosis of PE. Clearly, confirmation of PE first requires the diagnosis to be considered. Secondly, the clinician must decide whether a positive diagnosis of PE would alter management. In a specialty in which the balance of quality of life and active treatment is paramount, one must consider the burden of radiological confirmation (which may need to be obtained at a site away from the SPCU). In addition to the burden on the patient, one must also consider whether treatment is safe and feasible. Anticoagulation of someone who is at high risk of hemorrhage would be inappropriate, as it would in someone who is actively dying, in whom other symptom control measures could be instigated.

Imaging of Suspected Pulmonary Embolus

Investigations used in the diagnosis of PE in the non–palliative care setting have little role here other than identifying other pathology (Box 85-3).

Imaging tests available for PE include ventilation/perfusion lung scintigraphy (V/Q scan), pulmonary angiography, spiral computed tomographic pulmonary angiography (CTPA), and magnetic resonance angiography. However, all imaging techniques have limitations, and access may vary between SPCUs.

Pulmonary Angiography

Pulmonary angiography is the reference standard, but it is technically demanding and invasive.[12,13] It is unlikely to be the investigation of choice in palliative care unless the patient is robust enough to undergo the test. It has a major complication rate of 0.5% and a mortality rate of 0.1%.

Ventilation/Perfusion Scan

V/Q scans are relatively simple and noninvasive but alone can be nondiagnostic in up to 70% of suspected PEs.[14] In advanced cancer, concurrent lung pathology makes interpretation challenging. Better results have been obtained by combining clinical probability with V/Q scan interpretation, but the role of this modality in the palliative setting is limited.[15]

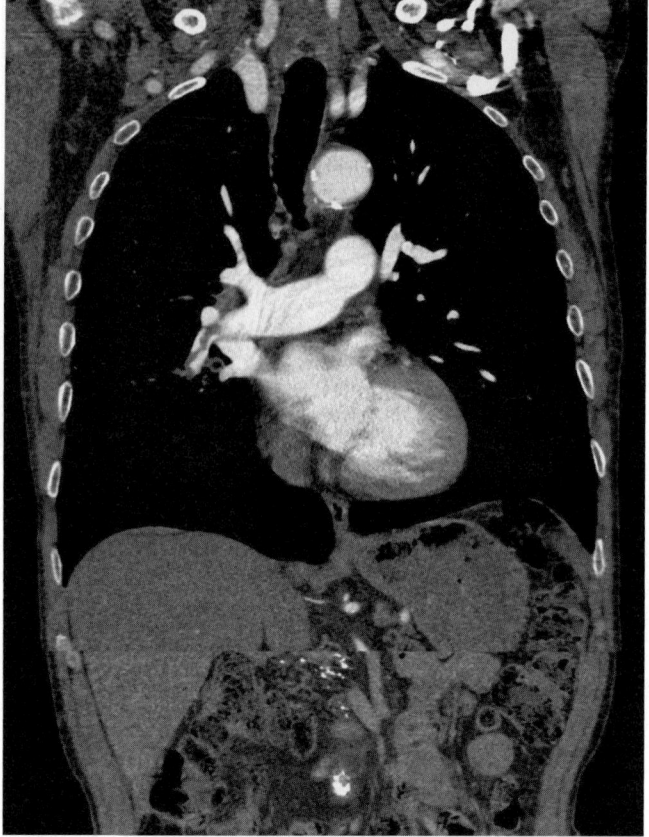

FIGURE 85-3 Spiral computed tomographic pulmonary angiograph (CTPA) demonstrating pulmonary embolus in the right pulmonary artery.

TABLE 85-2 Utility of Investigations for Pulmonary Embolism (PE) in the Palliative Care Setting

INVESTIGATION	ACCURACY IN DIAGNOSING PE	BURDEN ON PATIENT	USEFULNESS IN PALLIATIVE CARE
Pulmonary angiography	++++	++++	++
Ventilation/perfusion (V/Q) scan	++	+	+
Spiral computed tomographic pulmonary angiography (CTPA)	+++	+	+++

Spiral Computed Tomographic Pulmonary Angiography

CTPA is readily available in most hospitals and is well tolerated. Although it is excellent for central or lobar PEs, it cannot exclude isolated subsegmental PEs. Meta-analyses have suggested that CTPA has a sensitivity of about 70% and a specificity of 90% for PE.[16] A negative result does not exclude a diagnosis in 30% of patients. Despite these limitations, CTPA is likely to be the most appropriate diagnostic tool for PE in palliative care (Table 85-2; Fig. 85-3).

ACUTE MANAGEMENT

The current treatment for confirmed VTE is initial anticoagulation with LMWH for 4 to 6 days, followed by long-term warfarin.[17]

Although warfarin is the mainstay of long-term anticoagulation for VTE, several studies showed higher rates of bleeding in cancer patients compared with other patients receiving oral anticoagulation (22% in one study).[18,19] The bleeding risk in palliative care patients is greater. An audit of anticoagulation in a Scottish SPCU reported 15 bleeding episodes in 17 patients; the rate improved to 11 episodes in 18 patients with stringent international normalized ratio (INR) monitoring.[20] There is a resultant tendency to maintain the INR at subtherapeutic levels in advanced cancer.[21]

In addition to bleeding, cancer patients are more likely than noncancer patients to develop further thrombotic events while taking warfarin.[18,22] Studies have shown that up 27% of cancer patients develop secondary VTE despite therapeutic treatment with warfarin. The incidence is probably higher in advanced malignancy, because prothrombosis increases as the malignancy advances and because subtherapeutic anticoagulation is often maintained to minimize bleeding.

Evidence suggests LMWH is the drug of choice in the long-term management of VTE.[23] One qualitative study suggested that LMWH is acceptable in palliative care and, for some, preferable to warfarin. LMWH has several benefits over warfarin in cancer patients:

- Dose is calculated by patient weight, so there is no need to monitor anticoagulation.
- Efficacy is unaltered by nutritional status.
- Efficacy is unaffected by absorption problems or poor oral intake.
- Efficacy is unchanged by new medicines.

Although several trials have addressed long-term therapy for VTE with oral anticoagulant versus LMWH, only three have investigated patients with cancer. One study randomized patients with cancer and VTE to 3 months of either LMWH enoxaparin (1 mg/kg) or warfarin.[24] The composite outcome of major bleeding and recurrent VTE was observed in 15 (21%) of 71 patients receiving warfarin, compared with 7 (11%) of the 67 receiving LMWH ($P = .09$). The Long-term Innohep Treatment Evaluation (LITE) trial randomized 737 patients with acute VTE to either unfractionated heparin followed by warfarin for 84 days at a targeted INR of 2.5 or LMWH tinzaparin (175 IU/kg) for 85 days.[25] In a subgroup analysis of the 167 cancer patients, the rate of recurrent VTE was 6% in the LMWH group and 12% in the warfarin group ($P = .03$).

The Comparison of Low-Molecular-Weight Heparin versus Oral Anticoagulant Therapy for the Prevention of Recurrent Venous Thromboembolism in Patients with Cancer (CLOT) trial was a large, multicenter trial that compared LMWH dalteparin with oral anticoagulant in active cancers with acute DVT.[2] A total of 338 patients were enrolled into each arm and were well matched for gender, age, outpatient treatment, and performance status. Twenty-seven of those in the LMWH group experienced recurrent VTE, compared with 53 in the oral anticoagulant group. Patients receiving long-term LMWH had a lower cumulative risk of recurrent VTE at 6 months than did those receiving long-term oral anticoagulant (9% versus 17%; 52% risk reduction; $P = .0017$). Major bleeding was seen in 19 (6%) of the 338 patients receiving LMWH compared with 12 (4%) of the 338 in the oral anticoagulant group ($P = .27$). Corresponding data for "any bleeding" were 14% and 19% respectively ($P = .09$).

Although no studies have been conducted specifically in palliative care, one prospective cohort study in metastatic cancer (brain or liver) and VTE investigated low-dose dalteparin. A total of 203 patients received a 7-day course of dalteparin according to body weight, followed by a fixed dose of 10,000 IU dalteparin once daily for at least 3 months.[26] Eleven patients (5%) developed major bleeding complications (6 fatal) during the 3-month study period, and 18 patients (9%) had VTE recurrences (2 fatal). Complication rates were no different in liver versus brain metastasis.

COMMON ERRORS

The most common errors are underdiagnosis or underappreciation of the risk of VTE in the palliative care population. There is a view that "a large PE is a good way to go." This is nonsense, because, as one study suggested, most deaths from PE take up to 4 hours and do not occur suddenly, as some would believe.

RESEARCH CHALLENGES

The research challenges in management of VTE are vast. Because the palliative care patient population is so broad (ranging from those with incurable disease to those in the last hours of life), developing guidelines for all palliative care patients is difficult.

The emphasis on research needs to focus on identifying the true scope of the problem, assessing the real impact on patients, and developing effective strategies for managing VTE in the most appropriate way for this patient population.

REFERENCES

1. Trousseau A. Phlegmasia alba dolens. In Clinique Medicale d'Hotel-Dieu de Paris, Vol 3. Paris: JB Balliere et Fils, 1865, pp 654-812.
2. Bick RL. Alterations of haemostasis with malignancy. Semin Thromb Hemost 1978;5:1-26.
3. Sproul EE. Carcinoma and venous thrombosis: The frequency of association of carcinoma in the body or tail of the pancreas with multiple venous thrombosis. Am J Cancer 1938;34:566-585.
4. Ambrus JL, Ambrus CM, Pickren JW. Causes of death in cancer patients. J Med 1975;6:61-64.
5. Johnson MJ, Sproule MW, Paul J. The prevalence and associated variables of deep venous thrombosis in patients with advanced cancer. Clin Oncol (R Coll Radiol) 1999;11:105-110.
6. Kelly J, Hunt BJ. Role of D-dimers in diagnosis of venous thromboembolism. Lancet 2002;359:456-458.
7. Kelly J, Rudd A, Lewis RR, Hunt BJ. Plasma D-dimers in the diagnosis of venous thromboembolism. Arch Intern Med 2002;162:747-756.
8. Kearon C, Julian JA, Newman TE, Ginsberg JS. Noninvasive diagnosis of deep venous thrombosis. McMaster Diagnostic Imaging Practice Guidelines Initiative. Ann Intern Med 1998;128:663-677.
9. Fraser JD, Anderson DR. Deep venous thrombosis: Recent advances and optimal investigation with US. Radiology 1999;211:9-24.
10. Rose SC, Zwiebel WJ, Nelson BD, et al. Symptomatic lower extremity deep venous thrombosis: Accuracy, limitations and role of color duplex flow imaging in diagnosis. Radiology 1990;175:639-644.
11. Lensing AW, Prandoni P, Prins MH, Buller HR. Deep vein thrombosis. Lancet 1999;353:479-485.
12. Nilsson T, Carlsson A, Mare K. Pulmonary angiography: A safe procedure with modern contrast media and technique. Eur Radiol 1998;8:86-89.
13. Hudson ER, Smith TP, McDermott VG, et al. Pulmonary angiography performed with iopamidol: Complications in 1,434 patients. Radiology 1996;198:61-65.
14. The PIOPED Investigators. Value of the ventilation/perfusion scan in acute pulmonary embolism. Results of the Prospective Investigation Of Pulmonary Embolism Diagnosis (PIOPED). JAMA 1990;263:2753-2759.
15. Hull RD, Hirsh J, Carter CJ, et al. Diagnostic value of ventilation-perfusion lung scanning in patients with suspected pulmonary embolism. Chest 1985;88:819-828.
16. Remy-Jardin M, Remy J, Deschildre F, et al. Diagnosis of pulmonary embolism with spiral CT: Comparison with pulmonary angiography and scintigraphy. Radiology 1996;200:699-706.
17. Noble SIR. Anticoagulation in advanced malignancy: Pitfalls, dangers and future developments [abstract]. Palliat Med 2004;18:161.
18. Hutten BA, Prins MH, Gent M, et al. Incidence of recurrent thromboembolic and bleeding complications among patients with venous thromboembolism in relation to both malignancy and achieved international normalized ratio: A retrospective analysis. J Clin Oncol 2000;18:3078-3083.
19. Prandoni P. Antithrombotic strategies in patients with cancer. Thromb Haemost 1997;78(Suppl):141-144.
20. Johnson MJ. Problems of anticoagulation within a palliative care setting: An audit of hospice patients taking warfarin. Palliat Med 1997;11:306-312.
21. Johnson MJ, Sherry K. How do palliative physicians manage venous thromboembolism? Palliat Med 1997;11:462-468.
22. Lee AY, Levine M, Baker RI, et al. Low-molecular-weight heparin versus a coumarin for the prevention of recurrent venous thromboembolism in patients with cancer. N Engl J Med 2003;349:146-153.
23. Noble SI, Finlay IG. Is long-term low molecular weight heparin acceptable to palliative care patients in the treatment of cancer related venous thromboembolism? A qualitative study. Palliat Med 2005;19:197-201.
24. Meyer G, Marjanovic Z, Valcke J, Lorcerie B. Comparison of low-molecular-weight heparin and warfarin for the secondary prevention of venous thromboembolism in patients with cancer. Arch Intern Med 2002;162:1729-1735.
25. Hull RD, Pineo GF, Mah AF, Brant RF; for the LITE study investigators. A randomised trial evaluating long-term low molecular weight heparin therapy for three months versus intravenous heparin followed by warfarin sodium [abstract]. Blood 2002;100:556.
26. Monreal M, Zacharski L, Jimenez JA, et al. Fixed-dose low-molecular-weight heparin for secondary prevention of venous thromboembolism in patients

with disseminated cancer: A prospective cohort study. J Thromb Haemost 2004;2:1311-1315.

SUGGESTED READING

Lee AY. Management of thrombosis in cancer: Primary prevention and secondary prophylaxis. Br J Haematol 2005; 128:291-302.

Lugassy G, Falanga A, Kakkar AK, Rickles FR (eds). Thrombosis and Cancer. London: Taylor & Francis Publishing 2004. ISBN: 1841842877.

CHAPTER **86**

Persistent or Repeated Hemorrhage

Bassam Estfan

KEY POINTS

- Hemorrhage is common in advanced cancer. Recurrent hemorrhage can be distressing physiologically and psychologically.

- Hemorrhage in advanced disease has multiple causes. A multimodal management strategy is frequently required for hemostasis.

- Hemodynamic support with intravenous fluids and blood products is an essential fist step.

- Interventional treatments are frequently needed in addition to conservative measures. Examples include endoscopy, surgery, and interventional radiology.

- Nonmedical interventions are essential at the end of life and when specific therapy is not feasible. Examples include patient and family emotional support, education, preparation for death, and dark towels to hide blood.

Abnormal visible hemorrhage is alarming and is a common reason for doctor visits. Pathological bleeding from the respiratory, gastrointestinal, genitourinary, or other systems is serious; it may be the first manifestation of an occult malignancy or a serious hematological disease, and it frequently complicates advanced disease. People get frightened at the unexpected or recurrent sight of blood; they may associate bleeding with disease recurrence, disease progression, management failure, and possible impending death. The more severe the bleeding, the higher the apprehension and the risks.

Bleeding in advanced disease and near death, especially with advanced cancer, is not uncommon. Massive or intractable hemorrhage is a medical emergency and can be fatal. Not only are the physiological effects of bleeding dangerous, but so are the psychological effects: bleeding

may cause panic among patients and their caregivers. All bleeding should be dealt with meticulously, especially if it is recurrent and intractable to conventional management. Intractable, recurrent, or persistent bleeding resistant to conventional measures challenges medical staff, patients, and caregivers because of the possibility of death.

BASIC SCIENCE

Hemostasis physiology is complex and maintains blood inside the circulatory system. When a blood vessel injury occurs, three main mechanisms prevent further blood loss.[1] First, after vessel wall injury, vascular wall contractions cause vasoconstriction. This is mediated by thromboxane A_2 released by platelets and by nervous reflexes after trauma. These contractions require normal vessel anatomy and structure.

Second, damaged vessel walls activate circulating platelets and consequently undergo structural and physiological changes. This allows platelets to attach to severed vascular walls. This initiates a cascade of similar changes in other platelets, causing a platelet plug to form and prevent further bleeding. This is important for hemostasis in smaller vessels.

Clot formation is the third and most important mechanism. It involves activation of coagulation factors via an extrinsic or an intrinsic pathway. Multiple coagulation factors are activated in a cascade to activate prothrombin to form thrombin, which then releases fibrin threads from fibrinogen. Fibrin filaments form the final clot that blocks bleeding sites. The clot is maintained through a balance between procoagulant and anticoagulant factors until repair of the damaged vessel. Vitamin K and calcium are essential in producing and activating clotting factors. In summary, maintenance of hemostasis relies on intact vessel walls, functional and sufficient platelet count, and normal coagulation factor levels.

EPIDEMIOLOGY AND PREVALENCE

In advanced cancer, bleeding can occur in up to 10% of patients, mostly from acquired causes.[2] Hemorrhage caused 50% of deaths in acute leukemia before the availability of platelet transfusions. Thrombocytopenia (of various origins) is the leading cause of bleeding in cancer. Tumor invasion and disseminated intravascular coagulation (DIC) are other common causes in cancer.[2] Recurrent bleeding can be a major feature in some genetically predisposed individuals, but this is rare. Genetic mutations responsible for inherited coagulation disorders lead to recurrent and persistent bleeding (see Chapter 230). These mutations may affect coagulation factors (e.g., hemophilia A and B) or platelet function and aggregation (e.g., Glanzmann's thrombasthenia).

PATHOPHYSIOLOGY

Hemorrhage in advanced and terminal illnesses is predominantly from acquired causes. It is more common in cancer, in end-stage liver diseases (decreased production of clotting factors, esophagogastric varices), and in acquired platelet disorders.

Box 86-1 Causes of Bleeding in Advanced Illness

- Thrombocytopenia (various causes)
- Disseminated intravascular coagulation
- Bone marrow failure (e.g., metastatic infiltration, hematological malignancies)
- Direct tumor spread and invasion
- Malnutrition (e.g., procoagulant depletion, vitamin K deficiency)
- Drug-induced (e.g., NSAIDs, corticosteroids, anticoagulants)
- Radiation therapy (mucosal hemorrhage, bone marrow toxicity)
- Chemotherapy toxicity
- End-stage cirrhosis (variceal bleeding, procoagulant depletion)
- Advanced hematological diseases (e.g., myelodysplasia, aplastic anemia, idiopathic thrombocytopenic purpura)

TABLE 86-1 Differential Diagnosis according to Bleeding Site

Bronchial	Neoplasms (e.g., invasion, vessel erosions)
	Infections (e.g., tuberculosis, bronchitis)
	Bronchiectasis
	Immunological (e.g., Goodpasture's syndrome)
Upper gastrointestinal	Variceal bleeding (esophageal, gastric)
	Mucosal ulceration (benign, malignant, postradiation)
	Neoplasm
	Esophageal tears (severe emesis after chemotherapy)
Lower gastrointestinal	Massive upper gastrointestinal bleeding
	Diverticular bleeding, arteriovenous malformations
	Inflammatory bowel disorders
	Postradiation proctitis
	Rectal or colonic ulceration (benign, malignant)
Uterine	Menstrual disorders
	Uterine cancer
	Leiomyomas
Urinary	Postradiation cystitis
	Mechanical irritation (catheters)
	Mucosal ulcerations
	Neoplasms
Cutaneous	Malignant fistulating masses
	Deep ulcers

Reasons for severe bleeding in advanced disease are many (Box 86-1); a combination of factors may contribute.[3] In cancer, new vessel formation nourishes neoplastic masses. Malignant neovascularization is chaotic, lacks the normal structure of healthy vessels, and lacks the capability for normal hemostasis. Some cancers are known for more bleeding; these include renal cell carcinomas and melanomas. Tumors may invade or fistulate into skin or adjacent cavities (e.g., bronchial tree, gastrointestinal tract). Because abnormal vascular formation is easily disrupted, spontaneous or induced bleeding may occur easily, allowing recurrent superficial or cavitary bleeding. Cavitary bleeding can manifest as massive hemoptysis, hematemesis, hematuria, or lower gastrointestinal tract bleeding. Internal bleeding may occur into enclosed areas such as pleural or abdominal cavities.

Platelet-related hemorrhage is caused by abnormal platelet count or function. Severe thrombocytopenia is important in recurrent bleeding and is a common cause of hemorrhage in cancer. It is usually a result of malignant bone marrow infiltration or chemotherapy- or radiation-induced bone marrow toxicity.[4] Bone marrow failure may result from other hematological diseases, such as myelodysplasia. The risk of bleeding increases with a platelet count lower than 50,000/μL; counts lower than 10,000/μL are associated with more severe or spontaneous bleeding.[5] In advanced renal insufficiency, uremia contributes to platelet function abnormalities.

Hemorrhage due to coagulation factor disorders in advanced illness is usually from acquired decreased production. Procoagulant levels decrease in advanced liver disease and malnutrition, which is frequently present in patients with terminal illnesses (e.g., vitamin K deficiency).

CLINICAL MANIFESTATIONS

Detailed history and physical examination are important, including any history of previous similar episodes. In the event of active bleeding, attention should be focused on vital signs, airway maintenance, and hemodynamic stability. Hemorrhage may be acute and catastrophic, recurrent, or chronic. Internal hemorrhages may go unnoticed and should be suspected in the case of hemodynamic instability or shock in someone with a higher tendency to bleed. Visible hemorrhage easily directs clinicians to the site of origin; nevertheless, uncertainties may arise, especially in distinguishing bronchial from upper gastrointestinal bleeding.

Common sites for visible recurrent bleeding, especially in advanced cancer, are the bronchial tree, upper and lower gastrointestinal tracts, uterus, urinary bladder, and skin. Recurrent bleeding is an indirect indicator of disease extension and the need for repetitive therapeutic interventions or new management modalities.

Useful laboratory tests include complete blood count (CBC), coagulation profile (prothrombin time [PT], partial thromboplastin time [PTT], and international normalized ratio [INR]), blood type, metabolic profile, DIC panel (fibrinogen, fibrin degradation products, D-dimers [see Chapter 85]), and liver function tests. Computed tomographic (CT) scan imaging with contrast may diagnose active occult bleeding. Angiography of suspected arteries can be simultaneously diagnostic and therapeutic; it detects active bleeding at a rate of 1 mL/min. Nuclear imaging with technetium-labeled red cells can detect active bleeding of as little as 0.1 mL/min but is anatomically less accurate than angiography.[6] If hemorrhage is suspected to be of pulmonary, gastrointestinal, or genitourinary origin, endoscopy is an essential tool for diagnosis and treatment.

DIFFERENTIAL DIAGNOSIS

Identification of the bleeding site narrows the differential diagnosis (Table 86-1). Clinical presentation and past medical history may readily lead to the proper diagnosis.

In the absence of a related underlying pathology, medications or hematological abnormalities may be the leading cause. A prolonged INR or PT may suggest DIC, warfarin therapy, or liver pathology (cirrhosis, liver metastasis), especially with abnormal liver function tests. Decreased platelet count is usually related to chemotherapy if it is consistent with the drug nadir for thrombocytopenia. Otherwise, in cancer, it may represent bone marrow failure from radiotherapy or metastatic infiltration. Review of medications[7] is critical to exclude possible offending drugs affecting platelet function or count (Box 86-2).

TREATMENT

Management is multimodal and may require various interventions and subspecialty involvement. A surgical consultation is essential in all cases of active or massive intractable bleeding, in case emergency intervention is indicated. If a bleeding event has already stopped spontaneously, hemodynamic stabilization is a priority; if bleeding is active, cessation of hemorrhage is the first priority.

General Measures

Vital signs should be closely monitored. Initial hemodynamic stability is achieved with intravenous saline solution (regardless of the specific cause or planned future interventions), given abnormal vital signs or symptoms and signs of hypovolemic shock. A careful review of current medications should be done. Possible offending drugs should be stopped and replaced with others that have similar therapeutic effects but do not cause thrombocytopenia and lack bone marrow toxicity. In massive hemoptysis, airway maintenance with bronchoscopy or intubation and suction should be done quickly. Oxygen therapy helps hypoxia with anemia.

Transfusion

Volume repletion with blood products can follow intravenous fluids. The main goal is maintenance of vital signs with reversal of anemia and thrombocytopenia. Packed red blood cells should be transfused to maintain the hemoglobin concentration at greater than 9 g/dL for adequate oxygenation. Platelet transfusion should be considered if active bleeding is associated with a platelet count lower than 50,000/μL and prophylactically with counts lower than 10,000/μL.[5] Patients with persistent thrombocytopenia and recurrent bleeding can be serially tested for platelet count and prophylactically transfused. Platelet count should be 6,000 to 10,000/μL after a single-unit transfusion; the usual transfusion contains six units. Platelets have a short half-life of 7 days, even shorter in transfused platelets, so once- or twice-weekly transfusions will be required for patients with intractable thrombocytopenia (see Chapter 230). Fresh-frozen plasma transfusion can help restore coagulation in those taking warfarin. Stopping anticoagulants can be difficult if a balance between anticoagulation and hemostasis cannot be safely maintained. This is especially true in patients with recent or active thrombotic illnesses such as deep venous thrombosis or pulmonary embolism. Frequently, a family meeting is required to discuss the risk/benefit ratio and alternatives to anticoagulation (e.g., inferior vena cava filters).

Local Measures

Persistent cutaneous bleeding is usually related to deep local ulcerations or openings of malignant fistulas, especially surgical sites or fistulating tumor masses. Surgical management should be sought whenever possible. Sterile packing of open wounds can achieve hemostasis. Packing may be effective in nose, vaginal, and rectal bleeding. Special surgical dressings such as absorbable gelatin are useful because they form local clots through fibrin activation. Fibrin sealant dressings soaked with coagulation factors may achieve local hemostasis with topical pressure.[8] Local formalin may stop recurrent bleeding in radiation-induced cystitis and proctitis. Good ulcer and wound care (see Chapter 88) should minimize and prevent future bleeding.

Topical sucralfate has been successfully used in recurrent hemorrhagic proctitis resulting from local radiation therapy. It is most effective in grades 1 and 2. Two grams of sucralfate are dissolved in 20 mL of water and given as rectal enemas three times daily until response. It is ineffective in preventing or ameliorating acute postradiation bleeding.[9] Topical adrenaline or epinephrine is useful in topical endoscopic management of repeated hemorrhages (bronchoscopy, upper and lower endoscopy). They exert their effects through locally constricting bleeding vessels and enhancing platelet aggregation.

Endoscopy

Persistent and active gastrointestinal or bronchial bleeding requires emergency endoscopy for diagnosis and management. Upper gastrointestinal endoscopy assists in treating bleeding esophageal varices with sclerosing agents or clips in advanced liver disease.[5] Aberrant arteries in bleeding benign or malignant ulcers can be cauterized (neodymium-yttrium-aluminum garnet [Nd-YAG] laser or heat therapy) or treated with local epinephrine or adrenaline to stop and prevent rebleeding episodes; these techniques can also be used in lower gastrointestinal bleeding with colonoscopy. Bronchoscopy in hemoptysis allows identification of the bleeding site.[10] Temporary control may be obtained with bronchial iced saline lavage. Topical epinephrine and laser photocoagulation help visible bleeding bronchial lesions. Isolating a bleeding segment by tamponading it can be done temporarily to prevent blood aspiration into other segments.

Radiotherapy

Radiotherapy has a double effect. First, organs with mucosal lining exposed to radiation may be subject to recurrent bleeding because of inflammation (e.g., hemorrhagic cystitis or proctitis after pelvic radiation). Second, radiotherapy can be useful in bleeding from bronchial, uterine, vaginal, rectal, and bladder hemorrhages,[11] which is believed to be a result of tumor and vessel necrosis altering tumor vascular supply. Radiotherapy is of limited use in emergencies, because its effect is delayed and latent. But when applied successfully, it can be valuable in recurrent bleeding, especially in the case of an inoperable lesion or a patient who is not a good surgical candidate.

Surgery

Active, uncontrolled bleeding, especially if recurrent, may require emergency surgery. This may involve resection of the bleeding site (e.g., partial gastrectomy, hysterectomy, hemicolectomy), artery ligation, surgical débridement of wounds, or fistula repair. Persons with advanced illnesses may be poor surgical candidates. A careful decision should be made, taking into account the risks, benefits, clinical status, performance status, and patient or family wishes.

Interventional Radiology

Angiography can be both diagnostic and therapeutic. Regular or super-selective angiography can identify leaking artery branches, allowing for arterial coil embolization, especially in recurrent hemoptysis[12] or gastrointestinal or gynecological hemorrhage. It has considerable success in stopping active arterial bleeding (see Chapter 101). Embolization is minimally invasive and is an option in selected patients who are poor surgical candidates (e.g., instead of hemicolectomy in recurrent diverticular hemorrhage).

DRUGS OF CHOICE

Some adjunctive drugs can help control or minimize bleeding and possibly reduce the need for blood product transfusion.[13] Some are controversial in cases of general bleeding, because they are usually used for specific indications.

Antifibrinolytics

Aminocaproic acid and tranexamic acid are two lysine analogues of the antifibrinolytics class. They bind to plasminogen, preventing plasminogen activator–plasminogen compound from degrading fibrin filaments and thereby preventing clot lysis. Antifibrinolytics are specifically effective in mucosal bleeding from sites rich in plasminogen activator, such as bladder and oral mucosa. They are usually indicated for confirmed hyperfibrinolysis but are used liberally sometimes. The main use for antifibrinolytics has been perioperative blood conservation in cardiac surgery and, to a lesser extent, in other surgeries such as in advanced cirrhosis. Tranexamic acid is 10 times more potent than aminocaproic acid. Both are available in oral and parenteral forms but have been used topically on

occasion. The usual parenteral dose of tranexamic acid is 10 to 15 mg/kg administered three to four times daily; aminocaproic acid is usually primed with a loading dose over 1 hour, followed by 50 to 60 mg/kg administered four times daily. Side effects are mainly gastrointestinal (nausea, vomiting, diarrhea); rarely, thrombotic events may occur. Chronic high-dose aminocaproic acid can cause myopathy.[14]

Vasopressin Analogues

Desmopressin is indicated in hemophilia A and von Willibrand's disease. It is also used in variceal bleeding caused by portal hypertension. It is useful in qualitative platelet disorders resulting from cirrhosis and uremia. Desmopressin dosage is 0.1 to 0.4 μg/kg given subcutaneously or intravenously.

Activated Recombinant Factor VII

Activated recombinant factor VII (rFVIIa) was originally used for bleeding in hemophiliacs with inhibitors. It has been successfully used off-label for severe or intractable and persistent hemorrhage. It is thought to act by potentiating the normal coagulation process and is currently undergoing intensive investigation for use in general bleeding. The usual dose is 90 μg/kg intravenously every 2 hours until hemostasis is achieved.[15]

Vitamin K

Phytonadione, a lipophilic vitamin, is used for the correction of hemorrhages related to vitamin K deficiency (e.g., warfarin use). Coagulation factors II, VII, IX, and X are vitamin K–dependent and are reduced in deficiency. In cancer patients, supertherapeutic anticoagulation levels with warfarin may occur, increasing bleeding tendency. In the absence of active bleeding and with only moderate increase in INR, cessation of warfarin until normal or desired values return may suffice. With very high INR values or active bleeding, parenteral or oral vitamin K is indicated. An initial dose of 2.5 to 10 mg is customary and may need to be repeated.

SUPPORTIVE CARE

Massive bleeding is psychologically traumatic for patients and families, especially when it leads to death. If interventions such as transfusions, endoscopy, and surgery are not feasible, indicated, or desired, careful support should be directed to patients and their families. Emotional support provided by social workers, hospital, or hospice personnel is important in preparing for future events, the consequences of recurrent bleeding, education regarding handling of further hemorrhage episodes, and the dying process. Taking care of a bleeding person, or one who is at high risk of bleeding, can be difficult at home and is often best done in an inpatient setting. Inpatient hospices can be an invaluable resource. Hospitalization and hospice at home are other alternatives (see "Future Considerations").

Conservative measures in recurrent, possibly fatal, bleeding include the use of dark towels at the bedside.

Future Considerations

- The general use of fibrinolytics and other antihemorrhagic drugs in hemorrhage needs investigation, especially in advanced diseases.
- The effect of hemorrhage on patients and family has not been well documented in palliative medicine. Information collected after death due to hemorrhage concerning family and patient experiences could be invaluable.
- There is a need to publish palliative medicine bleeding management guidelines and to conduct appropriate related research.
- It is unclear whether fractionated or single-fraction radiotherapy is superior in controlling hemorrhage. The answer to this question would help in caring for many patients in the least aggressive yet effective way.

Dark-colored towels (e.g., green, navy blue, black) mask the sight of blood by altering its color and help prevent panic. In hemoptysis or hematemesis, turning the patient to one side allows for minimum spread of blood around the patient and may help prevent aspiration and asphyxiation, especially when bleeding is massive. Patients may panic during massive or recurrent bleeding. It is helpful to have readily available a large dose of a tranquilizer such as chlorpromazine, or a benzodiazepine, in an injectable form for sedation.[16]

REFERENCES

1. Guyton AC. Hemostasis and blood coagulation. In Guyton AC (ed). Guyton Textbook of Medical Physiology, 8th ed. Philadelphia: Saunders, 1991, pp 390-399.
2. Belt RJ, Leite C, Haas CD, et al. Incidence of hemorrhagic complications in patients with cancer. JAMA 1978;239:2571-2574.
3. DeSancho MT, Rand JH. Bleeding and thrombotic complications in critically ill patients with cancer. Crit Care Clin 2001;17:599-622.
4. Johnson MJ. Bleeding, clotting and cancer. Clin Oncol (R Coll Radiol) 1997;9:294-301.
5. Avvisati G, Tirindelli MC, Annibali O. Thrombocytopenia and hemorrhagic risk in cancer patients. Crit Rev Oncol Hematol 2003;48S:S13-S16.
6. Imbesi JJ, Kurtz RC. A multidisciplinary approach to gastrointestinal bleeding in cancer patients. J Support Oncol 2005;3:101-110.
7. George JN, Raskob GE, Shah SR, et al. Drug-induced thrombocytopenia. Ann Intern Med 1998;129:886-890.
8. Neuffer MC, McDivitt J, Rose D, et al. Hemostatic dressings for the first responder: A review. Mil Med 2004;169:716-720.
9. Gul YA, Prasannan S, Jabar FM, et al. Pharmacotherapy for chronic hemorrhagic radiation proctitis. World J Surg 2002;26:1499-1502.
10. Dweik RA, Stoller JK. Flexible bronchoscopy in the 21st century: Role of bronchoscopy in massive hemoptysis. Clin Chest Med 1999;20;89-105.
11. Hoegler D. Radiotherapy for palliation of symptoms in incurable cancer. Curr Probl Cancer 1997;21:129-183.
12. Yoon W, Kim JK, Kim YH, et al. Bronchial and nonbronchial systemic artery embolization for life-threatening hemoptysis: A comprehensive review. Radiographics 2002;22:1395-1409.
13. Mannucci PM. Hemostatic drugs. N Engl J Med 1998;339:245-253.
14. Dean A, Tuffin P. Fibrinolytics inhibitors for cancer-associated bleeding problems. J Pain Symptom Manage 1997;13:20-24.
15. Mahdy AM, Webster NR. Perioperative systemic hemostatic agents. Br J Anaesth 2004;93:842-858.
16. Pereira J, Phan T. Management of bleeding in patients with advanced cancer. Oncologist 2004;9:561-570.

SUGGESTED READING

Davis MP. Hematology in palliative medicine. Am J Hospice Palliat Med 2004;21:445-454.
Pereira J, Phan T. Management of bleeding in patients with advanced cancer. Oncologist 2004;9:561-570.

CHAPTER **87**

Lymphedema

Anna Towers

KEY POINTS

- Lymphedema is a common yet often unrecognized and undertreated complication of cancer treatment and recurrence.
- Combined decongestive therapy (CDT) comprises active reduction (manual lymph drainage, compression bandaging) followed by a maintenance phase consisting of skin care, compression garments, specific remedial exercise, and maintenance of normal body weight. CDT can be adapted for palliative settings.
- Treatments should be started early and should emphasize self-management. Interdisciplinary collaboration is essential.
- Policymakers should ensure that these treatments are covered by medical insurance.
- University training programs for health professionals should include lymphedema management.

Chronic lymphedema is swelling caused by failure of the lymphatic system to drain fluid and proteins from the interstitial space. It results in accumulation of protein-rich fluid, usually in a limb, as an iatrogenic complication of cancer treatment or as part of the clinical picture accompanying cancer recurrence.[1] It cannot be cured, and the swelling may result in disability or impaired function. Early detection is essential for effective control through physiotherapy. Lymphedema is also commonly seen in palliative care, often exacerbated by other causes of edema prevalent in advanced disease.

The recent development of physical treatments has increased interest in lymphedema; nevertheless, the condition is often unrecognized. A patient with lymphedema may present to emergency or casualty departments with cellulitis and undergo inpatient admission for antibiotic therapy, only to be discharged with the cause undiagnosed and untreated. Although the technology for physical treatment exists, few services are available. There is a lack of knowledge and interest by physicians and a belief that "nothing can be done." There is little research,[2,3] and few cancer rehabilitation programs address this problem (see "Common Errors").

Increased cancer incidence, reduced mortality, and prolonged life expectancy indicate that more persons will face survivorship issues, including lymphedema. Surgery, lymph node dissection, and radiation therapy can all have long-term, negative effects on limb function and cause pain, lymphedema, and limited motion. More knowledge is needed about the incidence, etiology, and degree of impact lymphedema has on patients' lives. Progress will require interdisciplinary collaboration between medicine, physiotherapy, kinesiology, nursing, and nutrition and appropriate cancer rehabilitation programs.

EPIDEMIOLOGY AND PREVALENCE

Lymphedema is most common after breast cancer but may also be seen whenever lymph nodes are ablated by surgery or included in radiotherapy fields, such as in melanoma, prostate, gynecological, or anorectal tumors. The incidence varies widely (13% to 63%), depending on the definition used, differences in measurement techniques, extent of surgery, radiotherapy doses, and length of follow-up.[1,4,5] Conservative therapies such as lumpectomy and sentinel node biopsy may also result in lymphedema in 14% to 28% of cases.[4,6] The arm may feel tight and heavy, and the associated nerve injuries, venous obstruction, and ligament strain may cause pain. Without treatment, loss of limb function and chronic infections occur.[7,8] The risk of infection is believed to be partly caused by accumulation of protein-rich interstitial fluids.[10] Lymphedema can cause psychological distress that may profoundly affect quality of life.[8-10] (Figs. 87-1 and 87-2).

Secondary lymphedema related to cancer treatment is not the only type of lymphedema. Filariasis as a cause of secondary lymphedema is an important cause of suffering and disability in tropical countries. Primary lymphedema is a genetically influenced condition caused by impaired lymph vessel or lymph node development.[1] It is less common than secondary lymphedema and usually affects the lower extremities, but any part of the body may be involved.

Risk factors for lymphedema include the following:

- Cancer recurrence
- Extent of surgery
- Extent of radiotherapy
- History of local infections/cellulitis
- Obesity
- Preexisting venous insufficiency
- Reduced muscle tone from lack of exercise

PATHOPHYSIOLOGY

The pathophysiological consequences of chronic lymphostasis are many. With time, edema that is initially pitting will become hard and difficult to reduce. The protein-rich interstitial edema produces fibrosis, sclerosis, and an increased risk of cellulitis in the affected limb (Fig. 87-3). There are changes to blood vessels in the form of vasculitis, as well as alterations to ligaments, tendons, and joints (lymphostatic arthropathy).[1] Malignant degeneration is a rare complication of lymphedema.

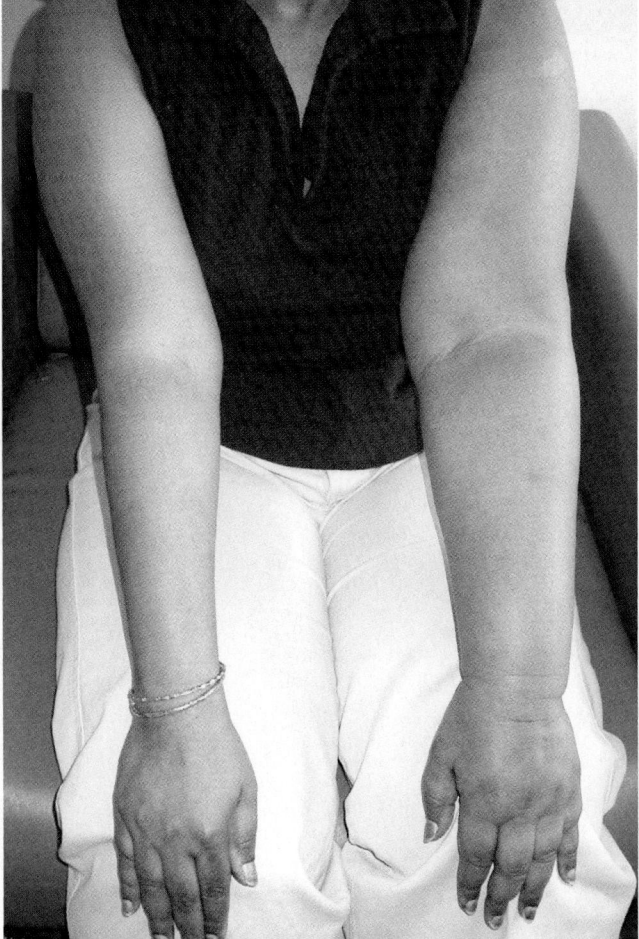

FIGURE 87-1 Lymphedema after breast cancer.

CLINICAL MANIFESTATIONS

Lymphedema is defined clinically as a difference in limb girth of at least 2 cm at any standard measurement point.[11] For research purposes, a volume difference of 10%[12] or 200 mL[13] is used. It can be characterized in terms of stages (stage I, soft and pitting; stage II, nonpitting with skin changes) and severity (mild, moderate, severe).[14]

Lymphedema is also often associated with neuropathic pain syndromes after cancer treatment. Although lymphedema is not believed to be a painful condition per se, pain syndromes after surgery or radiotherapy pain syndromes may coexist with lymphedema and may also have a significant impact on cancer survivors' lives. Like lymphedema, these pain syndromes have been understudied.[15]

DIFFERENTIAL DIAGNOSIS

Because the onset of lymphedema may signal a recurrence of carcinoma, it is essential that the treating physician or oncologist exclude this possibility. With unilateral limb swelling, it is important to consider the presence of either a deep venous thrombosis or cellulitis. In addition, in the palliative care setting, lymphedema may coexist with edema from other causes, such as hypoalbuminemia or a blocked inferior vena cava.

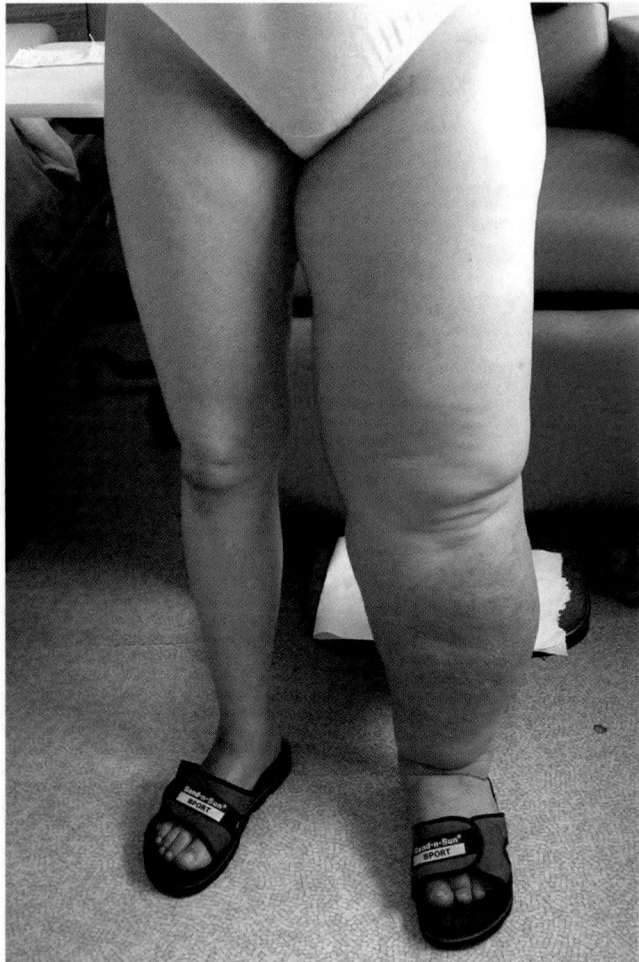

FIGURE 87-2   Lymphedema after endometrial cancer.

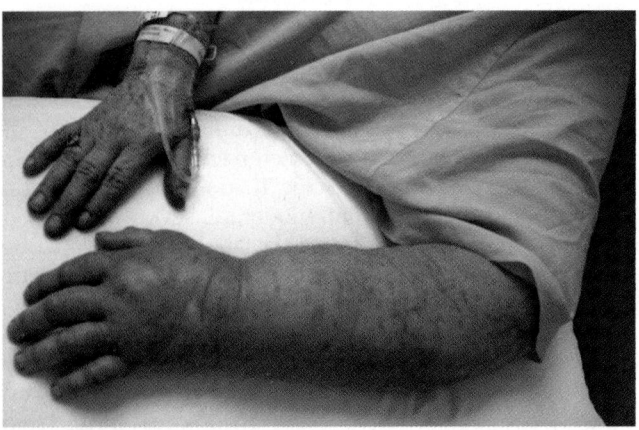

FIGURE 87-3   Cellulitis.

TREATMENT

Combined Decongestive Therapy

The current recommended treatment for chronic lymphedema is combined decongestive therapy (CDT), which aims to improve lymph drainage through existing lymphatic vessels and to encourage collateral circulation (Box 87-1).[3,14,16] It can be subdivided into two treatment phases:

1. An edema reduction phase of approximately 1 month that involves specific light massage techniques (manual lymphatic drainage) and application of low-stretch bandages for 5 days per week. Electric pneumatic compression machines may also be used in this stage of treatment.[2]

2. A maintenance phase, which is a lifelong commitment to wearing a graduated pressure elastic garment during the day (Fig. 87-4; Box 87-2) and to performing daily specific remedial exercises. Additional manual lymph drainage and bandaging can be performed as needed during the maintenance phase in those with more severe degrees of lymphedema. Skin care to try to reduce the incidence of cellulitis is an important component of the maintenance routine.

CDT is administered by a specially trained lymphedema therapist—a physiotherapist, nurse, kinesiologist, or massage therapist with specific approved extra training. Lymphedema associations and schools can provide a list of appropriately trained individuals.

Drug treatments are not effective for chronic lymphedema.[5] Therefore, research into physical treatments and methods of self-management are of primary importance in this chronic, lifelong condition.

Although the level of evidence to date is weak (case series), exercises are recommended in the maintenance phase of lymphedema by international consensus statement.[14,17,18] No randomized, controlled clinical trials (RCTs) have yet been published to ascertain the effectiveness of exercise in the control of lymphedema. From the available evidence, it appears that neither low-intensity strength training[19] nor vigorous exercise in the form of dragon boat training[18,20] exacerbates existing lymphedema. While awaiting the results of RCTs, clinical experience suggests that exercise is beneficial.[5] Videos and digital video discs (DVDs) of specific remedial exercises are available through lymphedema associations and schools.

Drug Management

Diuretics are ineffective in chronic lymphedema, because the increased interstitial oncotic pressure exerted by the protein-rich fluid causes rapid reaccumulation of the edema.[2] Diuretics may cause untoward effects such as hypotension and electrolyte imbalance. However, in the palliative care setting, where lymphedema can be severe and can threaten skin integrity, diuretics in combination with physical treatments may be necessary to try to prevent skin breakdown.

Other Considerations in the Palliative Care Setting

Ongoing palliative oncological treatments such as chemotherapy, steroids, and radiotherapy may help reduce tumor mass and thus reduce the lymphedema. All of the elements of CDT can be adapted in the face of advanced cancer. Here the treatment aim changes: the goal is not to obtain a normal limb, but rather to minimize edema, improve function, prevent skin breakdown, and generally support a patient who may be undergoing frightening bodily changes. If patients are introduced to CDT earlier in their cancer trajectory, they will adapt most readily to the adjustments required of them during the palliative phase. In the case of leg lymphedema, often both legs become affected in the last months of life. With the variable edema often present in this phase, compression garments are no longer suitable and one may have to resort to 24-hour bandaging of the most affected limb. The newer, padded sleeves and stockings with Velcro attachments may help. Physical treatments such as massage and bandaging, provided either by a professional or by a family member, will go a long way toward making the patient feel secure, in control, and not abandoned. Continuing visits by a familiar therapist, either at home or in the hospital or hospice environment, should be encouraged.

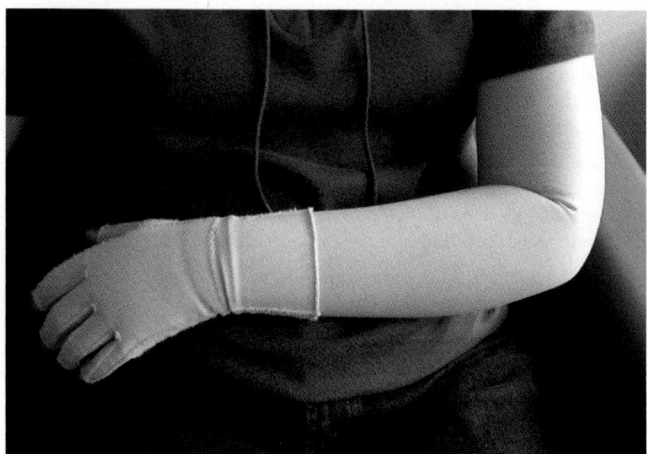

FIGURE 87-4   Compression garments.

Box 87-2 How to Prescribe Lymphedema Compression Garments

Classification of Compression Garments

- Class I: 20-30 mm Hg compression (generally inadequate for treating lymphedema; use only in older individuals who may be unable to tolerate a class II garment)
- Class II: 30-40 mm Hg (use for arm lymphedema)
- Class III: 40-50 mm Hg (use for leg lymphedema)
- Class IV: >50 mm Hg (use for severe leg lymphedema)

Garments should be flat-knit to provide a low resting pressure and a high working pressure. They are usually worn during the day and taken off at night.

Upper Limb Lymphedema

- If wrist is involved, prescribe a sleeve and gauntlet.
- If hand is involved, prescribe a sleeve and an open glove.
- If shoulder is involved, add a shoulder piece.

Lower Limb Lymphedema

- Prescribe a full-length stocking.
- If groin or abdomen is involved, prescribe stocking(s) and integral panty.

General Considerations

Garments should be replaced every 4 to 6 months.

Consider costs of garments. Use the most experienced fitter available. Counsel and support patients in obtaining insurance reimbursements.

Future Considerations

- Policymakers must accept responsibility for promoting the area of cancer rehabilitation and must provide adequate insurance coverage so that sufferers are not subject to financial stresses or unavailability of treatment resources.
- Specific lymphedema treatment modules should be developed in the training of physiotherapists, kinesiologists, nurses, and related professionals.
- Basic information about lymphedema should be provided in undergraduate and postgraduate medical curricula. Interdisciplinary collaboration should be encouraged.
- Patient advocacy groups can do much to help increase awareness of this condition and to provide peer support.

EVIDENCE-BASED MEDICINE

Much needs to be learned concerning the incidence, risk factors, and prevention of cancer-related lymphedema (see "Future Considerations"). RCTs are urgently needed to determine which elements of CDT are the most effective, with an emphasis on the evaluation of self-management techniques.[2,3,5]

REFERENCES

1. Weissleder H, Schuchhardt C (eds). Lymphedema: Diagnosis and Therapy. Koln: Viavital Verlag GmbH, 2001.
2. Harris SR, Hugi MR, Olivotto ML. Clinical practice guidelines for the care and treatment of breast cancer: 11. Lymphedema. Can Med Assoc J 2001;164:191-199.
3. Kligman L, Wong RKS, Johnston M, Laetsch NS. The treatment of lymphedema related to breast cancer: A systematic review and evidence summary. Supportive Care Cancer 2004;12:421-431.
4. Pain SJ, Purushotham D. Lymphoedema following surgery for breast cancer. BJ Surg 2000;87:1128-1141.
5. Towers A. Lymphoedema. In MacDonald N, Oneschuk D, Hagen N (eds). Palliative Medicine: A Case-Based Manual, 2nd ed. New York: Oxford University Press, 2005, pp 349-358.
6. Querci della Rovere G, Ahmad I, Singh P, et al. An audit of the incidence of arm lymphoedema after prophylactic level I/II axillary dissection without division of the pectoralis minor muscle. Ann R Coll Surg Engl 2003;85:158-161.
7. Bosompra K, Ashikaga T, O'Brien PJ, et al. Swelling, numbness, pain and their relationship to arm function among breast cancer survivors: A disablement process model perspective. Breast J 2002;8:338-348.
8. Voogd AC, Ververs JMMA, Vingerhoets JJM, et al. Lymphoedema and reduced shoulder function as indicators of quality of life after axillary node dissection for invasive breast cancer. Br J Surg 2003;90:76-81.
9. Beaulac SM, McNair LA, Scott TE, et al. Lymphedema and quality of life in survivors of early-stage breast cancer. Arch Surg 2002;137:1253-1257.
10. Tobin MB, Lacey HJ, Meyer L, Mortimer PS. The psychological morbidity of breast cancer related arm swelling: Psychological morbidity of lymphedema. Cancer 1993;72:3248-3252.
11. Erickson VS, Pearson ML, Ganz PA, et al. Arm edema in breast cancer patients. J Natl Cancer Inst 2001;93:96-111.
12. Box RC, Reul-Hirche HM, Bullock-Saxton JE, Furnival CM. Shoulder movement after breast cancer surgery: Results of a randomised controlled study of post-operative physiotherapy. Breast Cancer Res Treat 2002;75:35-50.
13. Andersen L, Hojris I, Erlandsen M, Anddersen J. Treatment of breast-cancer-related lymphedema with or without manual lymphatic drainage. Acta Oncol 2000;39:399-405.
14. International Society of Lymphology Consensus Document: The Diagnosis and Treatment of Peripheral Lymphedema. Lymphology 2003;36:84-91.
15. Kwan W, Jackson J, Weir LM, et al. Chronic arm morbidity after curative breast cancer treatment: Prevalence and impact on quality of life. J Clin Oncol 2002;20:4242-4248.
16. Cheville AL, McGarvel CL, Petrek JA, et al. Lymphedema management. Semin Radiat Oncol 2003;13:290-301.
17. Lasinski B, Boris M. Comprehensive lymphedema management: Results of a 5-year follow-up. Lymphology 2002;35(Suppl):301-304.
18. Harris SR, Niesen-Vertommen SL. Challenging the myth of exercise-induced lymphedema following breast cancer: A series of case reports. J Surg Oncol 2000;74:95-99.
19. McKenzie DC, Kalda AL. Effect of upper extremity exercise on secondary lymphedema in breast cancer patients: A pilot study. J Clin Oncol 2003;21:463-466.
20. McKenzie DC. Abreast in a boat: A race against breast cancer. Can Med Assoc J 1998;159:376-378.

SUGGESTED READING

Casley-Smith Judith R, Casley-Smith JR (eds): Modern Treatment for Lymphoedema, 5th ed. Adelaide: University of Adelaide Press, 1997.

Harris SR, Hugi MR, Olivotto ML. Clinical practice guidelines for the care and treatment of breast cancer: 11. Lymphedema. Can Med Assoc J 2001;164:191-199.

International Society of Lymphology Consensus Document: The Diagnosis and Treatment of Peripheral Lymphedema. Lymphology 2003;36:84-91.

Weissleder H, Schuchhardt C (eds). Lymphedema: Diagnosis and Therapy, 2nd ed. Koln: Viavital Verlag GmbH, 2008.

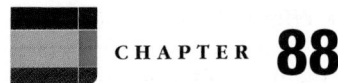

CHAPTER **88**

Pressure Ulcers and Wound Care

Valerie Nocent Schulz, Kathryn M. Kozell, and Lina M. Martins

KEY POINTS

- Comprehensive care for wounds requires the attention of an interdisciplinary wound care team and a pressure ulcer prevention program.

- The management of wounds in the palliative context combines evidence-based wound care principles and best practice, which includes patients' experience and perception of the wound and their social, emotional, and functional status.

- The dynamics of pressure is multifaceted: intensity and duration of pressure, friction, shearing, and moisture cause the seriously ill to be particularly vulnerable to pressure ulcers.

- Some adjunctive therapies have high-level evidence as effective treatment for pressure ulcers. These therapies must be the responsibility of the entire interdisciplinary team and must be evaluated for contraindications or side effects.

- In some cases, the goal of wound healing is inappropriate. Modification of goals to comfort, prevention, protection, and control can still optimize the quality of life and patient dignity.

Seriously ill patients are susceptible to wounds including pressure ulcers. Despite awareness of the internal and external factors that predispose to pressure ulcer development, prevalence remains high. This indicates the need to identify patients at risk and institute interdisciplinary prevention strategies. When life expectancy is limited, the goals of care often shift from wound healing to symptom and quality of life management.

BASIC SCIENCE

The Skin

The skin is the body's largest organ and performs multiple functions: protection, thermoregulation, metabolism, sensory transmission, storage, and esthetic communication. It has two major layers, the epidermis and the dermis.

The four zones of the epidermis are the basal/suprabasal, spinous, granular, and stratum corneum. The stratum corneum, comprised mostly of keratin, prevents dehydration by moderating transepidermal water loss to 2 to 5 g/hour/cm^2 and paces normal desquamation. Biochemical barriers in the acidic mantle maintain protein and lipid production and have an antifungal/bacterial effect. Dead keratinized cells shed normally every 4 to 6 weeks. This is a natural defense against infection. Biosensory feedback from the epidermis to the deeper tissue layers triggers healing in response to injury.[1]

The dermis contains microvascular blood vessels, lymphatics, hair follicles, and sebaceous and sweat glands. Fibroblasts form collagen, ground substance, and proteins. Collagen bundles anchor the dermis to the subcutaneous supporting structures of bone, fascia, and muscle.[2]

EPIDEMIOLOGY AND PREVALENCE

The reported prevalence of pressure ulcers in hospitalized patients ranges from 10% to 28%.[3,4] In Canada, data from 1990-2003 suggest that pressure ulcers are a significant concern in all health care settings, with an estimated prevalence at 26.0% (95% confidence interval: 25.2% to 26.8%)[5] (Table 88-1).

The best approach to pressure ulcers is to institute an interdisciplinary wound care team and a pressure ulcer prevention program. Incidence is the best indicator of effective prevention.[6] Further analysis will identify specific areas for program improvement. As patient acuteness increases, pressure ulcers are more common and represent a health care system dilemma.

PATHOPHYSIOLOGY

Dynamics of Pressure

Pressure ulcer development is influenced by several factors, the primary cause being sustained compression of the cutaneous and subcutaneous tissue between bony prominences and support surfaces.[7] Sustained pressure obstructs blood vessels, leading to ischemia and tissue necrosis. Shearing, friction, and moisture modulate tissue tolerance when subjected to mechanical forces.[8] The dynamics of pressure refers to intensity and duration. Pressure and duration are inversely related: higher pressure causes tissue damage in a shorter time. Capillary closure occurs[9] when sustained arterial pressure exceeds 32 mm Hg. The traditional 2-hour repositioning time interval is not supported by scientific literature.[10] The recommended 2-hour time interval should be only a starting point; it should be decreased or extended depending on patient susceptibility.[2]

Chronic Wound Healing—Pressure Ulcers

Wound healing is a complex process of cellular and chemical actions. The physiological phases are hemostasis, inflammation, proliferation, and maturation. Normal healing is sequential and predictable. Chronic wound healing is delayed; the wounds fail "to progress through a normal, orderly, and timely sequence of repair" or "pass through the repair process without restoring anatomic and functional results."[11] Pressure ulcers are chronic wounds that stagnate along the healing curve. Inflammation begins healing. Pressure ulcers that fail to respond to the inflammatory phase must be converted to an "acute wound" to initiate the inflammatory, biochemical healing response. If the prognosis is shorter than the time required to heal the wound, symptom management becomes the primary goal (see "Case Study: Pressure Ulcer Care in a Patient with Alzheimer's Dementia").

CLINICAL MANIFESTATIONS

Pressure Ulcer Staging

The modified staging classification by the National Pressure Ulcer Advisory Panel is a universal clinical standard.[12] This pertains only to pressure ulcers. The depth of tissue damage is a unidimensional process, with deep tissue injury progressing from stage 1 to stage 4. Stage 1 manifests as intact, nonblanchable, erythematous skin. Stage 2 is a partial-thickness injury of the epidermis and/or dermis, a superficial ulcer, or an intact blister. Stage 3 is a full-thickness injury of the subcutaneous tissue to fascia. Stage 4 is extensive, full-thickness injury through the fascia to muscle, bone, and other supporting structures. A pressure ulcer can have multiple stages at once. Stage X or "Stage Unknown" relates to a pressure ulcer that cannot be assessed accurately due to eschar. Wounds heal with granulation tissue composed of endothelial cells, fibroblasts, collagen, and extracellular matrix, leading to scarring. Reverse staging for pressure ulcers, from stage 4 to stage 1, is incorrect.[2,12] The European Pressure Ulcer Advisory Panel has images of pressure ulcer grading.[13]

DIFFERENTIAL DIAGNOSIS

Accurate diagnosis of an ulcer presentation is necessary to plan treatment. If an ulcer does not demonstrate healing in 6 to 12 weeks, the wound should be biopsied, the diagnosis confirmed, and the treatment plan revised.[14] Referring to chronic wounds, the following are the differential diagnoses[15]:

1. *Pressure ulcer:* external pressure-induced ischemia and necrosis. *Ulcer:* red, blistered, partial- to full-thickness cutaneous erosion, or necrotic eschar. *Location:* typically over bony prominences like the sacrum, ischial tuberosity, trochanter, posterior heel, scapula, elbow, and occipital area
2. *Arterial ulcer:* inadequate arterial blood perfusion causing lower-extremity ischemia. *Ulcer:* round, punched-out appearance, ischemic wound bed, necrotic, gangrenous, partial- to full-thickness injury, ischemic pain secondary to intermittent claudication. *Location:* typically the distal foot and toes
3. *Venous ulcer:* venous insufficiency, venous hypertension due to incompetent perforator valves and inadequate pump muscle action of the lower leg. *Ulcer:* partial-thickness, irregularly shaped, flat surface, surrounded by white atrophic skin with tiny blood vessels, red, edematous, high exudate

TABLE 88-1	Prevalence of Pressure Ulcers in Canadian Health Care Settings			
PARAMETER	ACUTE CARE	NONACUTE CARE	MIXED	COMMUNITY CARE
No. of settings	18	23	19	5
No. of patients	4831	3390	4200	1681
Estimates of prevalence (%)	25	30	22	15

From Woodbury G, Houghton P. Prevalence of pressure ulcers in Canadian healthcare settings. Ostomy Wound Manage 2004;50:22-24, 26, 28.

CASE REPORT

Pressure Ulcer Care in a Patient with Alzheimer's Dementia

Mr. HL was an 82-year-old man with progressive Alzheimer's dementia. He had been living at home with his wife. He presented to the emergency department with fever and failure to cope and thrive. The history revealed that Mr. HL's condition had declined over the past year, with short- and long-term memory loss; he had become bedridden and was unable to perform self-care tasks. His intake was reduced, and he had a decreased level of consciousness. The assessment revealed frailty, temperature of 38.0° C, blood pressure of 95/55 mm Hg, regular heart rate at 110 beats/min, respiratory rate of 18 breaths/min, no apnea spells, decreased level of consciousness, and a Palliative Performance Scale score of 30%. Auscultation of the chest revealed coarse crackles in the right upper lung region. Heart sounds were normal; the abdomen was soft and nontender; and bowel sounds were normal. He was incontinent of strong-smelling urine and had smearing of stool near his rectum.

Examination of skin and extremities revealed a 3 × 2 × 1.5 cm pressure ulcer over the coccyx with excoriation of the periwound skin, odor, and moderate green-brown exudate. The Braden Scale for predicting risk for pressure ulcers demonstrated the following:

Sensory perception—2 (very limited, communicating discomfort with restlessness)

Moisture—1 (constantly moist)

Activity—2 (with severely limited ability to walk)

Mobility—2 (very limited ability to change body position)

Nutrition—2 (rarely eats a complete meal and coughs while eating)

Friction and shearing—1 (frequent assistance with repositioning needed and slides in the bed)

Total Braden Score—10

Socially, the couple had three children; two of whom assisted in Mr. HL's care; his wife was devoted but exhausted. Mr. HL was admitted with severe Alzheimer's dementia, dehydration, pneumonia, and a stage 3 pressure ulcer. The initial goals of care determined by the health care providers and family were rehydration, antibiotics, and treatment of the pressure ulcer. The family tried to accept that Mr. HL had end-stage Alzheimer's disease.

Pressure ulcer management consisted of symptom management, odor reduction with antibiotics, and containment of exudate with an antimicrobial silver hydrofiber primary dressing covered with a secondary foam dressing. The periwound skin was protected with a non–alcohol-based liquid skin barrier. Pain was managed with low-dose morphine. After treatment for pneumonia, the interdisciplinary team and family decided to transition Mr. HL's care to end-of-life hospice/palliative care.

Location: the medial malleolus or lower leg after infection or trauma
4. *Neurotrophic ulcer* (associated with diabetes): polyneuropathy causing motor, sensory, and proprioceptive abnormalities; skin surface insensate, developing abnormal gait, joints and increased pressure points over bony support structures. *Ulcer:*

Box 88-1 Adjunctive Therapies for Pressure Ulcers

Level of Evidence A

- At least two randomized, controlled trials (RCTs) as part of a quality body of evidence
- *Example:* Electrical stimulation therapy (EST) is recommended for pressure ulcers.

Level of Evidence B

- Well-constructed trials but no RCTs
- *Examples:* Consider platelet-derived growth factor, topical negative pressure, electromagnetic fields, therapeutic ultrasound, normothermia, ultraviolet light C, and larval débridement for stimulating closure of nonhealing pressure ulcers.

Level of Evidence C

- Expert opinion, indicating absence of applicable studies
- *Examples:* Limited evidence supports the use of laser, oxidized regenerated cellulose/collagen, skin equivalents, and hyperbaric oxygen for treatment of nonhealing pressure ulcers.

---

partial- to full-thickness, punched-out appearance, with hyperkeratotic callus over pressure point. *Location:* first and fifth metatarsal heads, middle weight-bearing surface of the arch, heel
5. *Skin cancer:* nonhealing induration, nodules, subcutaneous spread, fungating, ulcerating, mixed wound appearance, bleeding wound, granulation tissue, pigmented, punched-out, exudating. *Location:* anywhere on the skin

TREATMENT

Principles and key recommendations for pressure ulcer prevention, assessment, and treatment are shown in Table 88-2. Figure 88-1 shows a flow chart for wound care in the palliative setting.

FUTURE CONSIDERATIONS

Complementary and Therapeutic Modalities

Other medical modalities used for pressure ulcers are surgical revision, topical antimicrobials, growth factors, bioengineered skin, hyperbaric oxygen, and negative-pressure vacuum-assisted closure. Physical modalities are electrical stimulation, ultrasound, ultraviolet light C, pneumatic compression, hydrotherapy, normothermia, laser, and electromagnetic fields. Multiple treatments, complementary or medicinal, are a responsibility to be shared with caution by all interdisciplinary members. The following is a summary of the latest recommendations for adjunctive therapies for pressure ulcers[27] (Box 88-1).

For patients with advanced disease and their families, modalities such as nutrition, relaxation, aromatherapy, yoga, and reflexology address alternative treatments in the management of multidimensional, chronic wounds. Healing can be affected by economic factors such as the cost of treatment products, social factors such as access

TABLE 88-2 Pressure Ulcer Prevention, Assessment, and Treatment: Principles of Wound Care

PRINCIPLES	KEY RECOMMENDATIONS
Prevention	Conduct a head-to-toe skin assessment on admission, and daily for those at risk for skin breakdown.
	Use the Braden Scale for Predicting Pressure Sore Risk to ensure that individual risk factors are systematically identified and evaluated.[16]
	Occupational and physical therapists assess for and reduce the risk of pressure, friction, and shearing injuries. The three most important risk factors for pressure ulcers in a palliative care setting are physical activity, mobility, and age.[17,18]
	Implement pressure support surfaces or devices to offload and redistribute pressure from bony prominences and/or to manage pain.[19]
	Promote skin integrity and protect from excessive moisture and incontinence (e.g., hydration, pH-balanced skin and perineal cleansing products, lubrication, protective padding).
	Develop and deliver a patient-centered educational plan for patient/family and health care professionals about pressure ulcer prevention.
	Refer to RNAO Best Practice Guideline, Risk Assessment and Prevention of Pressure Ulcers.[20]
Etiology	Conduct a history to understand the etiology of the wound.
	Consult and collaborate with the interdisciplinary team.
	Correct co-morbidities (if possible).
	Shift goals of care from healing to palliation when necessary.
	Conduct risk assessment for pressure ulcer development.
Interdisciplinary team	Share the vision of care.
	Create an interdisciplinary team (i.e., patient/family, physician, nurse, dietitian, occupational therapist, physical therapist, enterostomal therapy nurse, social worker, spiritual care worker, palliative care consultant).
	Deliver evidenced-based standards and best practice.
	Develop educational programs for professionals and for the patient and family.
	Build organizational resource commitment (e.g., financial, personnel).
Psychosocial functional assessment	Consult and collaborate with interdisciplinary team (e.g., social work, psychology, spiritual care).
	Assess patient/family perception of needs, goals, ability to understand and adhere to plan.
	Assess quality of life, values, cultural factors, financial factors, social support.
Pressure ulcer assessment	Assess and monitor characteristics of the wound bed and periwound: stage, size, depth, location, odor, bleeding, edema, exudate.
	Perform complete assessment weekly to determine treatment effectiveness.
	Lower-extremity ulcers should be assessed for vascular viability before treatment or débridement.
	Refer to Bates-Jensen Wound Assessment Tool.[21]
Nutrition	Consult dietician for assessment and/or maintenance of nutrition.
	Healing wounds demand high caloric intake. Nutritional supplementation should be considered (e.g., vitamin C, zinc, enteral feeding, parenteral feeding).[22]
Pain	Assess pain related to the pressure ulcer or treatment. Determine the patient's ability to describe or sense pain.
	Determine pain associated with location, frequency of dressing changes, body positioning, time of day.
	Consider local or systemic analgesia,[23] type of dressing product, diversional therapy, and the patient's ability to participate in care.
	Refer to RNAO Best Practice Guideline: Assessment and Management of Pain.[24]
Support surfaces	Pressure ulcers will not heal if the causative factors of pressure, shearing, and friction are not removed or minimized (see Prevention).
	Implement support surface: "A specialized device for pressure redistribution designed for management of tissue loads, microclimate, and/or other therapeutic functions (i.e., mattresses, mattress replacement, seat cushion or overlay)."[19]
	Assess support surface needs using the Braden Scale for Predicting Pressure Sore Risk[16] and the Risk and Related Interventions in RNAO Best Practice Guideline, Risk Assessment and Prevention of Pressure Ulcers.[18,20]
Débridement	Débride healable wounds using one or a combination of débridement modalities (e.g., surgical, autolytic, enzymatic, hydrotherapy).
	Nonhealable wounds should have only nonviable tissue removed; active débridement to bleeding tissue is contraindicated.
Wound cleansing	Cleanse wounds with normal saline, Ringer's lactate, sterile water, or noncytotoxic wound cleansers.
	Reserve topical antiseptics for nonhealable wounds or cases in which the local bacterial burden is greater than the wound's ability to heal.
	Safe and effective irrigation pressure against the wound is 4-15 psi.[2]
Infection	Assess for infection or persistent inflammation.
	Use nonsensitizing topical antibacterial agents for local symptoms and signs of infection.
	Use systemic antibiotics if symptoms or signs of infection extend beyond wound margins or to bone.[25,26]
Wound dressing	Maintain moisture balance with appropriate dressings. When selecting a dressing, consider the following: type of wound, patient response and need, location, size, depth, exudate (type and amount), infection, type of tissue exposed, phase of healing, frequency of dressing changes, comfort and esthetics, and who is providing care.
	Refer to Wound Care for the Palliative Patient (see Fig. 88-1).
Nonhealing wound	Consider surgical intervention if appropriate. With delayed healing, adjunctive therapies may be considered.
	Although a wound may not heal, if comfort, protection, prevention, and control are achieved, there is wound care success.

RNAO, Registered Nurses Association of Ontario.

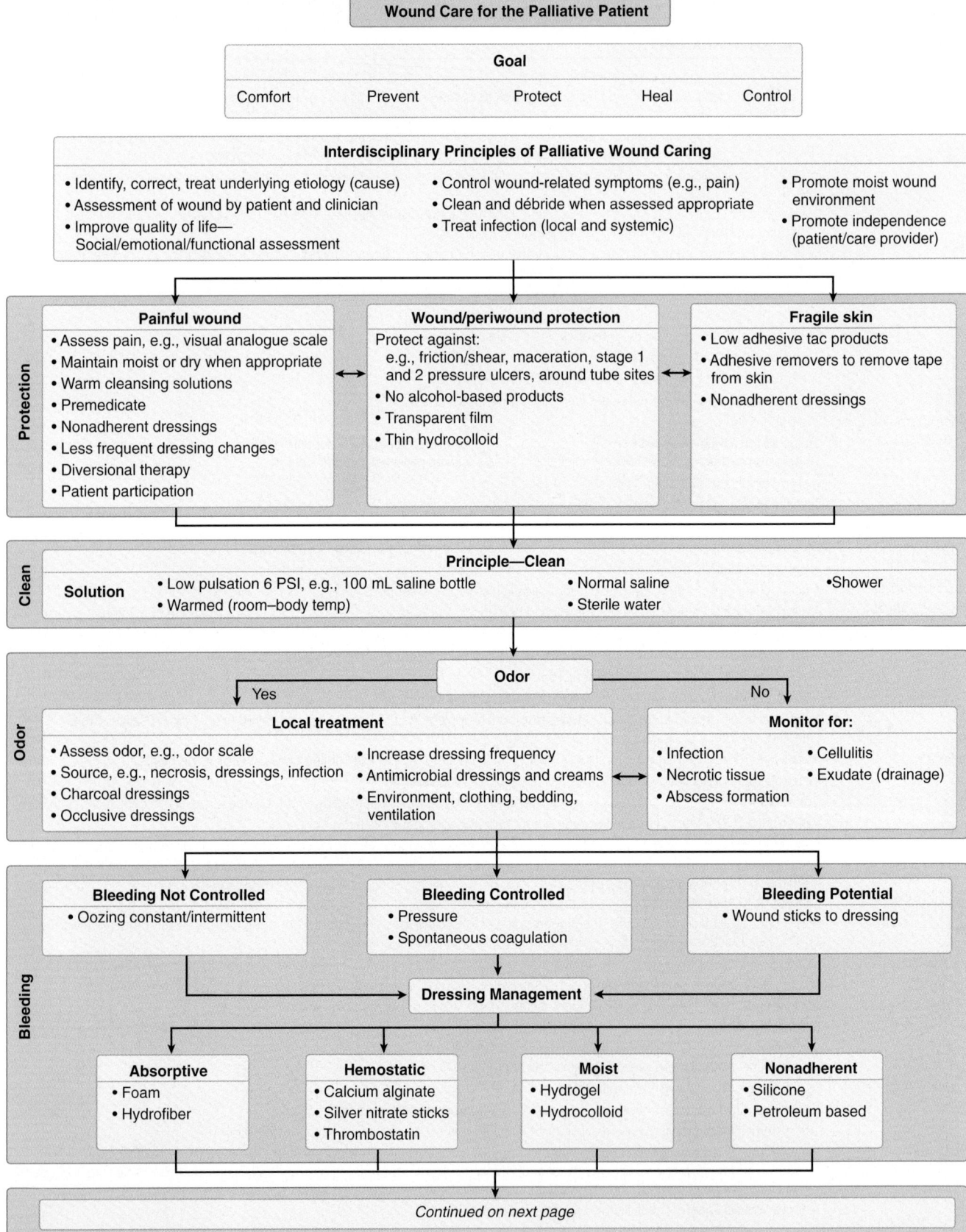

FIGURE 88-1 Wound care for the palliative patient. *(From Poteete V. Case study eliminating odours from wounds. Decubitus 1993;4:43-46; Visual Analogue [VAS] Assessment and Management of Pain, November 2002, available at http://www.rnao.org [accessed October 2007]; modified with permission from the C7 Oncology Education Working Group, Victoria Hospital, London Health Sciences Center, London, Ontario, Canada, 2006.)*

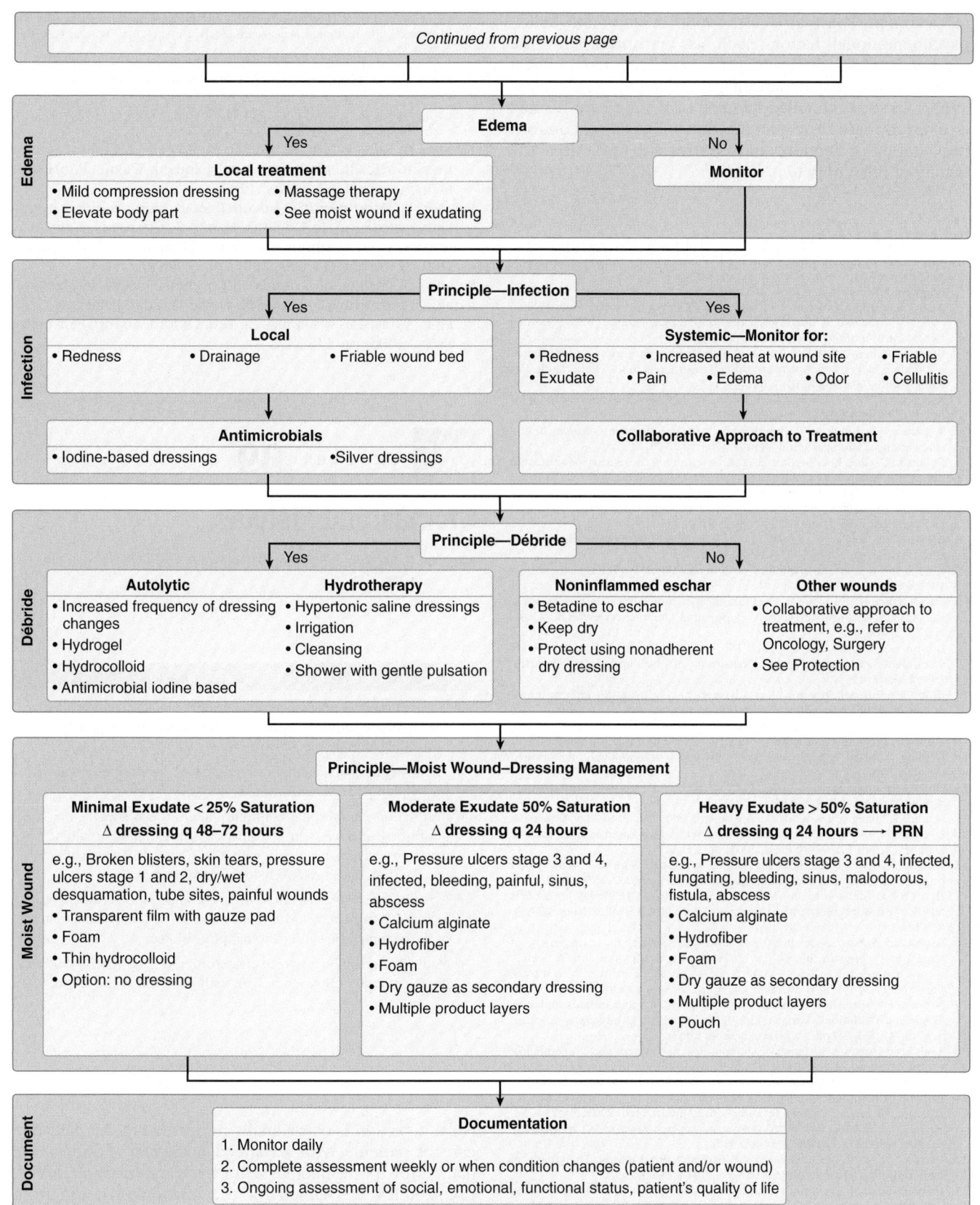

FIGURE 88-1, cont'd

to treatment, spiritual factors found in hope and belief, psychoemotional factors such as motivation and the "caring attitude" of health care providers, and political factors in the cost or advantage of having health insurance.[28] In some patients, the goal of wound care healing is inappropriate. The modification of goals to comfort, prevention, protection, and control still optimizes the quality of life and patient dignity.

REFERENCES

1. Fore-Pfliger J. The epidermal skin barrier: Implications for the wound care practitioner. Part 1. Adv Skin Wound Care 2004;17:417-424.
2. Registered Nurses Association of Ontario. Nursing Best Practice Guideline: Assessment and Management of Stage I to IV Pressure Ulcers, August 2002. (Online). Available at http://www.rnao.org/Storage/29/2371_BPG_Pressure_Ulcers_I_toIV.pdf (accessed October 2007).
3. Bours G, Halfens R, Abu-Saad H, et al. Prevalence, prevention, and treatment of pressure ulcers: Descriptive study in 89 institutions in the Netherlands. Res Nurs Health 2002;25:99-110.
4. Redelings MD, Lee NE, Sorvillo F. Pressure ulcers: More lethal than we thought? Adv Skin Wound Care 2005;18:367-372.
5. Woodbury G, Houghton P. Prevalence of pressure ulcers in Canadian healthcare settings. Ostomy Wound Manage 2004;50:22-24, 26, 28.
6. Robinson C, Gloeckner M, Bush S, et al. Determining the efficacy of a pressure prevention program by collecting prevalence and incidence data: A unit based effort. Ostomy Wound Manage 2003;49:44-51.
7. Flam E, Raab L. Dynamics of pressure ulcer management: Interaction of load and duration. J Enterostom Ther Nurs 1991;18:184-189.
8. Bergstrom N, Braden B, Laguzza A, et al. The Braden scale for predicting pressure sore risk. Nurs Res 1987;36:204-210.
9. Koziak M. Etiology and pathology of ischemia ulcers. Arch Phys Med Rehab 1959;40:60-69.
10. Buss I, Halfens R, Abu-Saad H. The most effective time interval for repositioning subjects at risk of pressure sore development: A literature review. Rehab Nurs 2002;27:59-66, 77.
11. Lazarus GS, Cooper DM, Knighton DR, et al. Definitions and guidelines for assessment of wounds and evaluation of healing. Arch Dermatol 1994;130:489-493.
12. Black JM; National Pressure Ulcer Advisory Panel. Moving toward consensus on deep tissue injury and pressure ulcer staging. Adv Skin Wound Care 2005;18:415-421.
13. European Pressure Ulcer Advisory Panel. The EPUAP Guide to Pressure Ulcer Grading. (Online). Available at http://www.epuap.org/grading.html (accessed October 2007).
14. Sibbald RG. An approach to leg and foot ulcers: A brief overview. Ostomy Wound Manage 1998;44:28-35.
15. Schulz VN. Malignant wounds and pressure ulcers. In MacDonald N, Oneschuk D, Hagen N, Doyle D (eds). Palliative Medicine: A Case-Based Manual, 2nd ed. Oxford: Oxford University Press, 2005, pp 333-347.
16. Barbara Braden: Braden Scale for Predicting Pressure Sore Risk. Available at http://www.bradenscale.com/bradenscale.htm (accessed October 2007).
17. Henoch I, Gustafsson M. Pressure ulcers in palliative care: Development of a hospice pressure ulcer risk assessment scale. Int J Palliat Nurs 2003;9:474-484.
18. Registered Nurses Association of Ontario. Assessment and management of stage I to IV pressure ulcers. Part 2: Positioning techniques and devices in wound management, August 2002 (Online). Available at http://www.rnao.org/Storage/11/551_BPG_Pressure_Ulcer.pdf (accessed October 2007).
19. National Pressure Ulcer Advisory Panel. Support Surface Standards Initiative, Terms and Definitions, Version 08/29/2006. Available at http://www.npuap.org/NPUAP_S3I_TD.pdf (accessed October 2007).
20. Registered Nurses Association of Ontario. Risk Assessment and Prevention of Pressure Ulcers, March 2005. (Online). Available at http://www.rnao.org/Storage/29/2371_BPG_Pressure_Ulcers_I_toIV.pdf (accessed October 2007).
21. Barbara Bates-Jensen. Quality Indicators for Prevention and Management of Pressure Ulcers in Vulnerable Elders. Ann Intern Med 2001;135:744-751. (Online). Available at http://www.rand.org/pubs/authors/b/bates-jensen_barbara_m.html (accessed October 2007).
22. Harris C, Fraser C. Malnutrition in the institutionalized elderly: The effects on wound healing. Ostomy Wound Manage 2004;50:54-63.
23. Evans E, Gray M. Do topical analgesics reduce pain associated with wound dressing changes or debridement of chronic wounds? J Wound Ostomy Continence Nurs 2005;32:287-290.
24. Registered Nurses Association of Ontario. Assessment and management of pain. August 2002 (Online). Available at http://www.rnao.org/Storage/11/543_BPG_assessment_of_pain.pdf (accessed October 2007).
25. Sibbald G, Orstead H, Coutts P, et al. Best practice recommendations for preparing the wound bed: Update 2006. Wound Care Can 2006;4:15-29.
26. Gardner F, Troia E, MacDonald B, et al. A tool to assess clinical signs and symptoms of localized infection in chronic wounds: Development and reliability. Ostomy Wound Manage 2001;47:40-47.
27. Keast D, Parslow N, Houghton P, et al. Best practice recommendations for the prevention and treatment of pressure ulcers: Update 2006. Wound Care Can 2006;4:31-43.
28. Popoola M. Complementary therapy in chronic wound management: A holistic caring case study and praxis model. Holistic Nurs Pract 2003;17:152-158.

SUGGESTED READING

Krasner D, Kane D (eds). Chronic wound care: A Clinical Source Book for Healthcare Professionals, 2nd ed. Wayne, PA: Health Management Publications, 1997.

Pearson IC, Mortimer PS, Grocott P, et al. Skin problems in palliative medicine. In Doyle D, Hanks G, Cherny N, Calman K (eds). Oxford Textbook of Palliative Medicine, 3rd ed. Oxford: Oxford University Press, 2005, pp 618-640.

Schulz VN. Malignant wounds and pressure ulcers. In MacDonald N, Oneschuk D, Hagen N, Doyle D (eds). Palliative Medicine: A Case-Based Manual, 2nd ed. Oxford: Oxford University Press, 2005, pp 333-347.

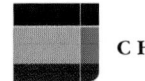

CHAPTER **89**

Stomas and Fistulas

Michael F. McGee and Conor P. Delaney

KEY POINTS

- Stoma surgery is necessary for a variety of conditions in palliative care patients, and it is usually performed on an emergency basis or for palliation of specific symptoms.

- Trained enterostomal nursing support is of paramount importance for helping patients with stomas.

- Restoration of intestinal continuity after stomal surgery may be performed selectively in fit palliative care patients, usually if the patient is having problems with the stoma or if the patient is expected to have a relatively long survival time.

- External enteric fistulas can have catastrophic physical and psychological consequences and are best managed with the collaboration of a surgeon and/or enterostomal professional.

- Many fistulas can be managed conservatively (parenteral hydration, nutrition, and local wound care), with predictable closure rates.

STOMAS

Fecal diversion is occasionally performed in the palliative care of patients with advanced malignancy. Stomas are named for the respective segment of exteriorized bowel. Colostomies are named for the portion of colon from which they are fashioned—sigmoid, descending, transverse, ascending colon, or cecum. Ileostomies and jejunostomies are formed when respective segments of ileum or jejunum are mobilized and externalized through the abdominal wall.

Several stoma configurations may be created, each with unique advantages tailored to suit specialized purposes

(Fig. 89-1). An end stoma is created when a segment of intestine is divided (with or without concomitant bowel resection) and the proximal end is exteriorized, allowing complete diversion of fecal effluent outside the abdomen. Loop stomas are created by exteriorizing an entire loop of bowel, without ligation or division, and incising and maturing the antimesenteric surface of the bowel to the skin. This looped configuration preserves the integrity of bowel conduit but effectively diverts effluent through the stoma site. The loop stoma typically as intended for temporary diversion, with staged reanastomosis as planned at a later date; however, in patients with an unresectable distal bowel obstruction, a loop stoma is an excellent option that avoids a "closed-loop" obstruction in the segment of bowel between the ostomy and the obstructing lesion.

Specialized forms of colostomies and ileostomies are occasionally helpful in complicated cases in which bowel cannot be mobilized adequately to reach the skin. An end-loop ileostomy allows slightly better reach than a straight end-ileostomy, facilitating stoma construction in obese and difficult reoperative patients. In some cases, large-bore tubing may be used as a conduit to bridge from the fixed bowel segment out through the tube, forming a tube colostomy or ileostomy, although these stomas are often very difficult to manage and can cause significant skin problems. Additionally, stomas may be used for non-digestive purposes for a variety of urinary diversion procedures.

ROUTINE CARE

Although several different stoma configurations exist, care for all stomas types is similar and adheres to core tenets.[1] Ideally, the best postoperative care starts with preoperative meetings involving the patient, surgeon, enterostomal professional, and important family members or caregivers (see Chapter 59). At this meeting, the indications with

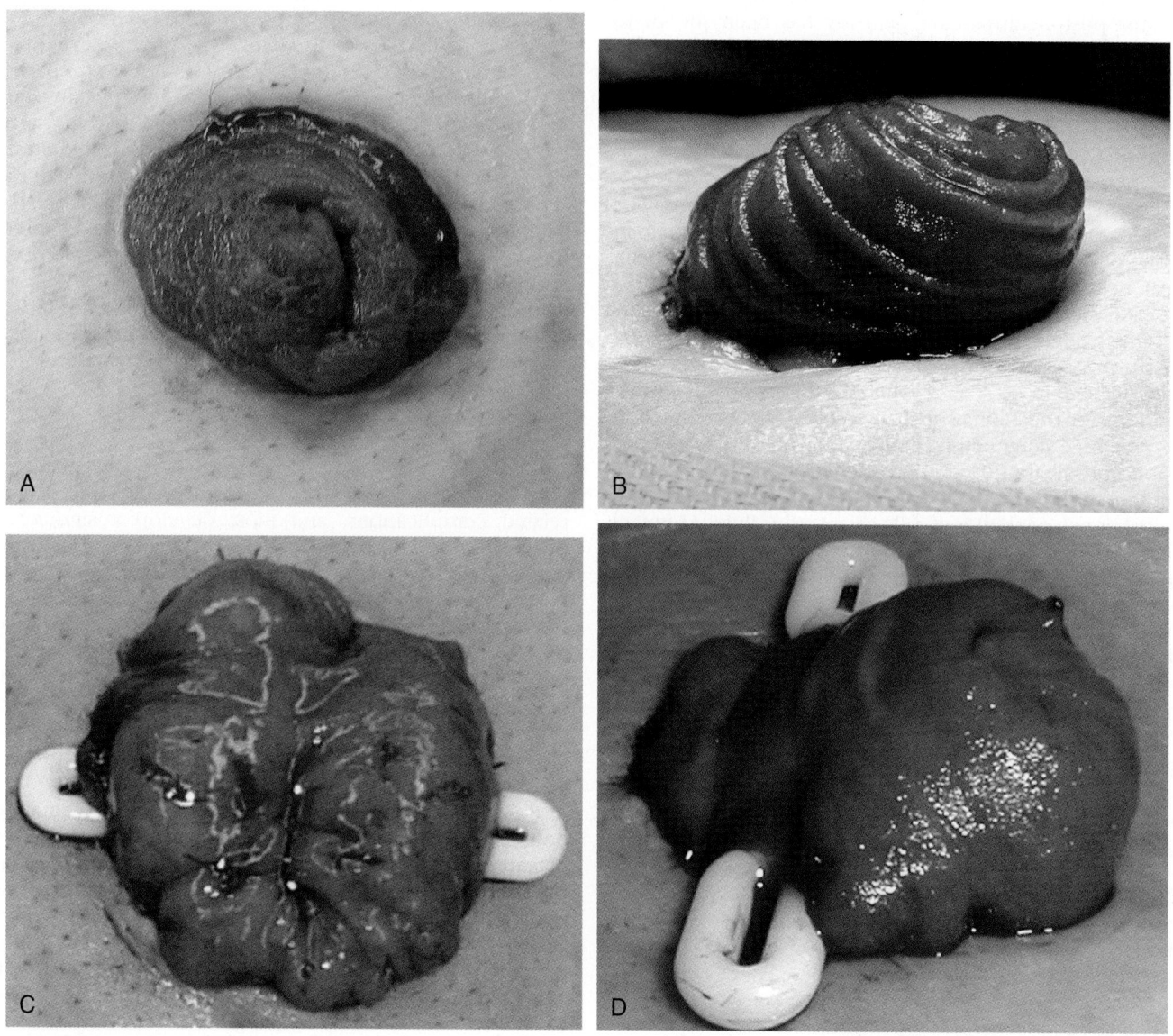

FIGURE 89-1 Stoma configurations. **A**, End colostomy; **B**, end ileostomy; **C**, loop colostomy; **D**, loop ileostomy. The loop stomas are fashioned initially with a temporary supportive retaining bar placed between the afferent and efferent aspects of each stoma.

relevant intestinal anatomy and physiology should be reviewed to educate the patient regarding the necessity of the stoma. The patient can be introduced to the appliances and routines required for proper stoma care and should be encouraged to ask questions. The meeting should include stoma site marking, which enables optimal placement of the stoma site with respect to skin folds, waistline, pannus, and prior incisions in standing, sitting, and supine positions. Preoperative site marking has been shown to decrease patient complications and improve patient satisfaction postoperatively.

If possible, palliative ostomies are performed using laparoscopic surgical approaches. In many cases, this permits the largest wound to be only 1 cm long, which greatly reduces postoperative pain and scarring and also reduces the incidence of many complications.[2,3] Laparoscopic surgical approaches also tend to reduce hospital stay and costs of hospitalization.[2,4]

In the immediate postoperative period after stoma formation, inpatient care is focused on ensuring viability of the stoma, pain control, awaiting return of bowel function, and enterostomal education. Incorporation of a formal postoperative care pathway has been shown to accelerate the recovery of the patient from surgery, and it is important that the enterostomal therapist be involved as early as the first postoperative day.[2] The initial pouch placed in the operating room is usually a two-piece device. The first piece applied is an adhesive wafer attached to the peristomal skin, which should be trimmed to allow for a small gap between stoma and wafer aperture. The wafer, in turn, accepts a sealed, clear, plastic snap-fit pouch. A proper stoma site typically ensures an adequate seal between the peristomal skin and the device; this helps to eliminates leakage, odor, and skin breakdown.

On the first postoperative day, the stoma should be visually assessed for viability. Pink, glistening, moist mucosa should be seen throughout the externally visible portions of the stoma. Any suggestion of dusky mucosa, retraction, or lengthening of the stoma merits expeditious surgical evaluation. Attention should be paid to the contents of the stoma pouch in the early postoperative period. Initial pouch content is usually clear serous fluid. As bowel function returns, flatus and stool accumulate, and this may happen immediately in patients who have laparoscopic surgery. Ileostomies often function within the first 48 hours after surgery, whereas colostomies often take up to 96 hours.[1]

Examination of the stoma on the first postoperative day provides an excellent opportunity for the enterostomal nurse to discuss appliance changes with the patient. During the first few appliance changes, each step is carefully described to the patient. Some patients are capable of changing the device under supervision of the surgeon or enterostomal professional on the second day, although many patients take significantly longer to learn this process. Also during the second postoperative day, the entire pouch assembly should be removed (including adhesive wafer) to enable full examination of the surrounding peristomal skin. The adhesive wafer should be carefully removed with the use of a wet, warm washcloth, minimizing direct shearing trauma to the skin. After removal of the wafer, the skin should be cleaned with a gentle soap and warm water and examined for evidence of discoloration, mucocutaneous separation, or stoma retraction.

By the third postoperative day, the goal is for the patient to be able to change his or her own appliance autonomously. If the patient is unable to provide self-care, then the educational process should include the appropriate caregiving proxies responsible for the patient. For many patients in a palliative care situation, home or skilled nursing resources must be made available. If a loop stoma has been constructed over a supporting rod, the rod is usually removed on the third postoperative day.

Once bowel function returns, the pouch should be regularly emptied on becoming one-half to two-thirds full. Timely emptying of the device reduces the weight and associated forces that would otherwise cause separation of the device from the skin. Rather than be discarded, the pouch may be reused several times with the assistance of a bulb-syringe rinse after every bag emptying. Usually, the pouch and appliance are changed to a new system every 48 to 72 hours. Once the patient has recovered from the initial postoperative period, an opaque pouch device may be applied in lieu of the clear plastic pouch that is typically used in the immediate postoperative period.

As the patient learns to change the pouch device and care for his or her own stoma, attention turns to preparing for the outpatient issues, such as integrating stoma hygiene into the patient's daily activities. Showers may be taken with or without the pouch device. Mild soaps should be used and harsh or caustic detergents or antibacterial agents avoided. A variety of commercially available adjuncts can ease stoma care routines while enabling freedom and the transition back to a normal schedule. Specialized underwear is a helpful adjunct that can secure the pouch assembly and conceal the bulky contents. Other devices, such as one-piece nonadhesive pouches, can ameliorate problems with adhesive pouch systems for intolerant patients.

TREATMENT

One or two of every three ostomates develop stoma-related complications, and most develop a significant degree of psychosocial sequelae.[5,6] Eighty percent of patients with enteric stoma require lifestyle adjustments pertaining to stoma care and hygiene, and more than 40% of these patients have difficulty in subsequent sexual relations (see Chapter 16). Patients often feel embarrassed or ashamed of their altered body image. The degree of resultant social restriction is related to the number of stoma care complications. Much of the psychosocial stress associated with stoma creation can be minimized with proper stoma-care education.

Peristomal skin irritation develops in approximately one half of ostomates and constitutes the most frequent reason patients seek advice from an enterostomal therapist.[7,8] Chemical irritation, fungal colonization, local trauma during appliance changes, contact dermatitis, and allergy frequently contribute to localized irritation. Effluent contact, adhesives, and chronic dampness can further exacerbate irritation to the surrounding skin and provide a fertile environment for fungal growth.[8] Skin irritation is most commonly seen in older and larger patients (body mass index >25).[8] Ileostomies, compared with colostomies, are more prone to skin irritation, due to the liquidity and reactivity of the effluent. Aside from the constant presence of pain and irritation, skin irritation undermines the seal between the device and the stoma, which promotes further leakage and intensification of ongoing irritation. Local skin care and maintenance of skin integrity, beginning in the immediate postoperative period, is of paramount importance in treating peristomal skin irritation. Peristomal skin should be bathed and dried routinely with gentle soaps, as described earlier, with avoidance of caustic agents. Nystatin powder may be applied to rashes consistent with fungal etiology; these rashes usually display characteristic satellite lesions. For allergic or contact dermatitis, a trial period of a topical steroid often proves beneficial once a new pouch device is selected. Fever, fluctuance, undermined or painful ulcer, or rapidly progressive erythema should alert the patient to seek surgical evaluation. Some patients develop peristomal pyoderma gangrenosum, which is difficult to treat and requires knowledge of a variety of different techniques and medications (Fig. 89-2).

Inadequate sealing of the stoma–device interface is a common problem that leads to odor and leakage and can further exacerbate the psychosocial distress that occurs in almost one third of ostomates.[7] The key to ensuring a proper seal with stoma devices is preoperative site marking by an experienced surgeon or enterostomal professional. The emergent nature of a stoma surgery may preclude proper site marking and necessitate stoma placement at the discretion of the surgeon. If leaks are refractory to optimal enterostomal care, viscous pastes and putty-like sealing adjuncts may be used to fill skin folds that enable leakage to occur. With the help of an experienced enterostomal professional, satisfactory seals are almost always attainable.

Herniation of bowel or omentum adjacent to the fascial defect used to create the stoma can occur in up to 48% of ostomates.[9] Like other types of abdominal wall hernias, parastomal hernias are associated with malnutrition, corticosteroid use, malignancy, old age, and wound sepsis, as well as other causes of elevated intra-abdominal pressure, such as chronic obstructive airways disease and obesity.[9] Most parastomal hernias are asymptomatic; however, as with any hernia, complications ranging from mild discomfort to obstruction or strangulation can occur. Digital stoma exploration may reveal the presence and location of the hernia sac with respect to the fascial trephine, although these hernias are often difficult to palpate and diagnose, particularly in obese patients. Computed tomographic (CT) imaging may be a useful adjunct to aid diagnosis if symptomatic herniation is suspected. Many parastomal hernias can be managed conservatively, whereas obstruction or suspicion of intestinal strangulation should merit expeditious surgical consultation and exploration. The options for surgical correction of parastomal hernia are numerous and are specific to the type and clinical constellation surrounding each patient. Surgical options include local fascial repair, stoma relocation, and a variety of synthetic mesh placements. Conservative management of a parastomal hernia may be obtained with specially fitted stoma hernia belts, which are fitted to apply pressure directly over the hernia defect to keep the hernia sac reduced.

Stoma prolapse is a complication whereby the ostomy protrudes out from the anterior abdominal wall; it occurs in an estimated 3% to 22% of ostomates (Fig. 89-3). Stomal prolapse should not be confused with parastomal herniation: the former involves lengthening of an intact stoma, whereas the latter involves inappropriate passage of abdominal viscera adjacent to the facial trephine. Stoma prolapse, as well as parastomal herniation can compromise blood flow to the prolapsed intestine, which can cause ischemia, infarction, and necrosis. On discovery of a prolapsed stoma, a full examination of the stoma should be performed by removal of the pouch device and wafer to inspect the color of the mucosa. Mucosal areas of duski-

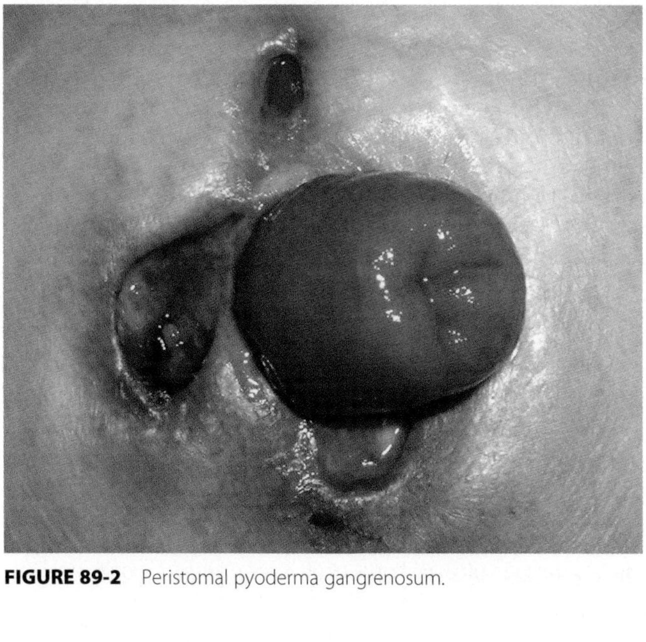

FIGURE 89-2 Peristomal pyoderma gangrenosum.

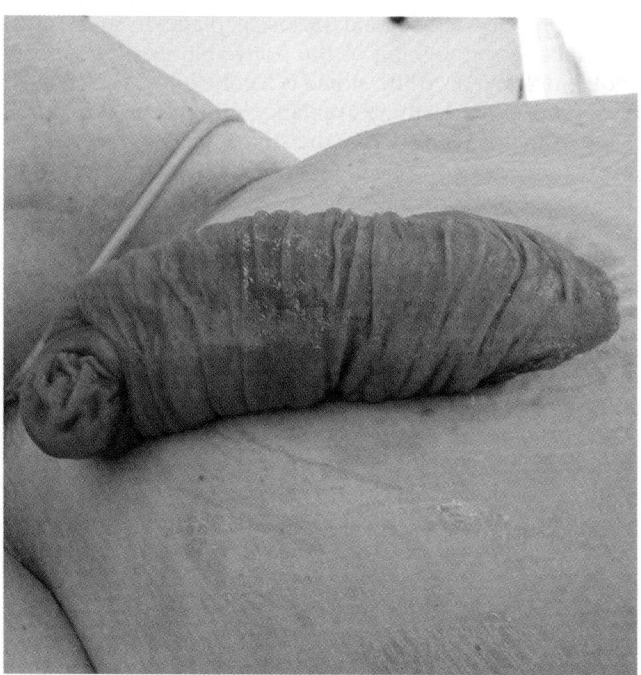

FIGURE 89-3   Stoma prolapse. A prolapsed transverse loop colostomy.

ness prompt concern for inadequate blood flow and should merit expeditious surgical consultation. If the prolapsed stoma elicits no concern for ischemia, gentle bedside reduction may be attempted. Occasionally, prolapse impairs venous return to the prolapsed segment of bowel, causing edema and venous engorgement that may hinder reduction efforts. In experienced hands, warm or cold compresses may be applied directly to the prolapsed bowel to assist with reduction. Moreover, small amounts of ordinary table salt or sugar may be applied directly to the prolapsed bowel to further assist with manual reduction by reducing the extent of edema fluid. If stoma ischemia, incarceration, or frequently recurring prolapse is encountered, surgical stoma revision is warranted. This can often be performed with a small peristomal incision, permitting a more expeditious recovery for the patient.

After stoma creation, inadequate blood supply may cause ischemic changes to the tissue that can complicate both short- and long-term recovery. This complication may be caused by extreme illness and hypotension in some emergency cases, but is most commonly a technical problem of surgery. A well vascularized stoma should demonstrate pink, glistening, mucosa free from dusky, cyanotic, or blanched mucosal surfaces. Approximately 5% to 22% of stomas exhibit some degree of clinical necrosis in the postoperative period.[10,11] Proper bedside evaluation of the stoma should include a thorough visual exploration of the stoma site with determination of the extent of ischemia. A glass or plastic blood sampling tube can be passed into the stoma and used (with the aid of a flashlight) to determine the level of demarcation between pink, viable mucosa and dusky or necrotic tissue. Alternatively, a rigid anoscope or proctoscope may be used to evaluate the recessed portions of the stoma. Superficial mucosal ischemia is managed expectantly. If the line demarcating healthy from ischemic tissue is superficial to the fascial plane, the stoma may be observed. Serial examinations are performed to ensure that the ischemic area has not progressed beyond the fascial plane. In such cases, full-thickness sloughing of the nonviable portions of the stoma may occur. If the stoma is a colostomy, this may be observed, with a stoma appliance applied at skin level. Such ischemic retraction of the stoma occurs in 5% to 25% of ostomates, complicating appliance attachment and increasing peristomal skin irritation. If the stoma is an ileostomy, retraction renders the stoma flush with skin level, making pouching very difficult. Therefore, surgical stoma revision is required in all but the sickest of patients. If ischemia is suspected to extend deep to the fascia, emergent surgical revision is required.

In some cases, scarring, contraction, and stenosis of the stoma orifice causes obstructive symptoms (Fig. 89-4). This may occur particularly in patients who have distended or obstructed bowel during surgery and in those who have experienced stoma ischemia. If obstruction is suspected, digital examination of the matured stoma will indicate the level of obstruction or, in some cases, dislodge impacted stool that may be causing obstruction. Surgical revision of the stoma may be necessary. This can usually be performed with local surgical approaches without laparotomy. Dilation of the stenotic stoma may provide temporary relief of stoma stenosis in patients who

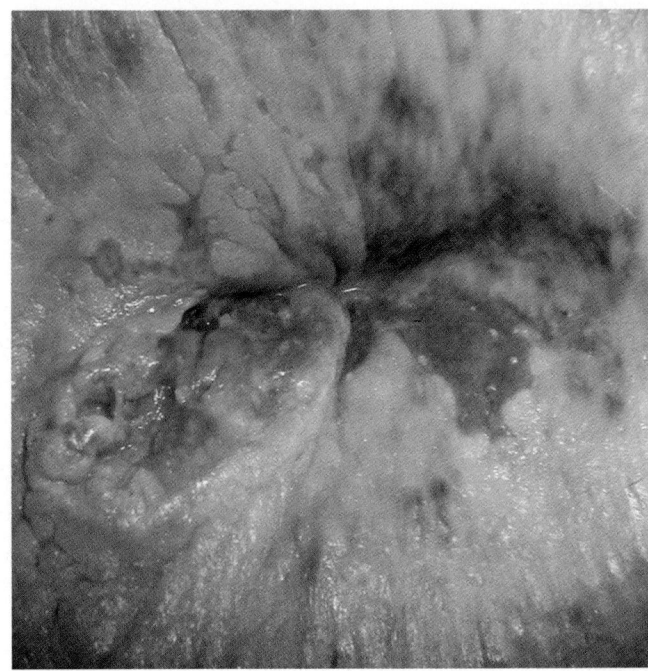

FIGURE 89-4 Stomal retraction. Chronic ischemia and scarring can result in stomal retraction, with the stomal orifice withdrawn below the skin level.

are poor candidates for surgical revision but they may be prone to recurrence.

Dehydration and electrolyte imbalances may occur in patients with an ostomy, and this is directly related to how far proximally the stoma has been placed in the intestine. As a compensatory reaction, ileostomy patients have increased levels of circulating aldosterone to adjust for excessive sodium and free water losses. In time, ileostomy patients attain a euvolemic state; however, periodic dehydration may require treatment with supplemental fluid and salt administration. During the body's adaptive period, ileostomy outputs typically begin high (1000 to 1800 mL/day) and gradually approach normal outputs of 400 to 700 mL/day. Supplemental fiber may be added to the diet to control persistent high-output ileostomy. If high outputs persist in the face of optimal dietary control, Kaopectate, Imodium, or, lastly, diphenoxylate hydrochloride and atropine (Lomotil) may be used to control ileostomy outputs. In our practice, Imodium and Lomotil are added in stepwise fashion to control output and are prescribed as 1 to 2 pills after each meal and before bedtime. Patients with rapid transit, very high-volume output, or proximal stomas (jejunostomies) may be given these medications as syrups to improve absorption. Tincture of opium may also be added at 1 mL orally after each meal and before bedtime in difficult cases as needed. High-output ileostomy patients are at an increased risk of developing uric acid renal calculi due to their chronic dehydrated state.

FISTULAS

A fistula (based on the Latin word for "pipe") is an abnormal communication between two epithelial-lined surfaces. Fistulas are usually classified by anatomical type, magnitude of output, and degree of complexity. Anatomical descriptions describe the segmental anatomy adjacent to the afferent and efferent ends of the fistula tract. Specific types of fistulas, such as enterocutaneous (between bowel and skin), enteroenteric (small bowel to small bowel), colovaginal (between colon and vagina), or colovesical (between colon and urinary bladder) are the most often encountered anatomical types; however, fistulization may occur between any two adjacent organs.

Fistulas may be described as internal if there is an intracorporeal connection between two hollow organs, or as external if they drain onto external skin. External fistulas are further divided into those producing high outputs (>500 mL/day), moderate output (200 to 500 mL/day) or low output (<200 mL/day). Internal fistulas tend to be occult and are less likely to become clinically apparent than external fistulas. This section focuses on external fistulas, because they have a larger clinical impact than internal fistulas.

Fistulization occurs most commonly as a complication of surgery, and these surgeries are usually performed for resection of malignancy, resection of inflammatory bowel disease, or lysis of intra-abdominal adhesions. Anastomotic leak, inadvertent enterotomy, or surgical adjuncts such as mesh, sutures, clips, and other foreign bodies may serve as a nidus of fistula formation. Postoperative, or secondary, fistulas represent 85% of external fistulas encountered.[12] Spontaneous, or nonsurgical, fistulas caused by inflammation are most often seen in the setting of Crohn's disease or resolving diverticulitis; however, they may also be caused by locally advanced cancers. External beam irradiation may predispose to their development.[12]

PATHOPHYSIOLOGY

The associated mortality and morbidity of patients with external fistulas can be very high, reflecting the devastating course of the disease in conjunction with either typically poor preoperative health or chronic inflammatory disease. Historically, the development of enterocutaneous fistula was associated with mortality rates as high as 50% to 65%; more recent case series report rates between 4% and 11%, which is most likely attributable to the ease and availability of parenteral nutrition. Other contributions that have improved mortality rates in fistula include improvements in antimicrobial therapy, imaging, and drainage procedures and understanding of the pathophysiology. High-output fistulas convey a fourfold increase in mortality when compared with low-output fistulas,[13] with an overall mortality rate ranging between 13% and 50% The classic triad of sepsis, malnutrition, and electrolyte imbalance is responsible for the gravity of this condition. As a fistula is formed, intraperitoneal extravasation of luminal contents can cause infection, abscess, or frank sepsis. Indeed, sepsis is the most frequently implicated cause of death in patients with enterocutaneous fistulas, accounting for more than 76% of deaths in case series and increasing the likelihood of death 22-fold.[13]

Inappropriate loss of enteric fluids causes significant swings in fluid and electrolyte states of patients with external fistula. Proximal or upper gastrointestinal sources of fistula can deplete the body of free water, hydrogen, bicarbonate, and chloride, with resultant compensatory changes producing hypokalemic, hypochloremic, and metabolic alkalosis. Additional fluid shifts caused by co-morbid sepsis, ileus, adrenal deficiency, or hypertonic resuscitative fluids can exacerbate already existing electrolyte imbalances. Fistulas involving the distal gastrointestinal tract are less likely to manifest dehydration or electrolyte imbalance.

Whether neoplastic, inflammatory, or postsurgical, fistulas typically manifest with local erythema, swelling and pain, leukocytosis, fever, and purulent drainage. Over the next several days, drainage changes consistency and ultimately progresses to contain enteric contents. Most secondary fistulas manifest within 2 weeks after surgery, whereas primary fistulas are typically more insidious and may develop over months to years. Fistulization involving foreign bodies, such as mesh, prosthetic vascular conduits, and nonabsorbable suture lines, may develop slowly.

TREATMENT

Management of external fistulas can be an intense endeavor requiring adequate resuscitation, assessment of the fistula tract and associated abscesses, control of the source of sepsis, and evaluation and supplementation of nutritional status. Once the patient and the fistula have been fully investigated, a long-term management plan is developed. Ensuring adequate resuscitation of the septic or unstable patient is the first priority, and this may require assistance from a surgery-based intensivist team. Patients should be placed on nothing by mouth (NPO) status and appropriately resuscitated. Although central venous access is not immediately required, it may later be required to deliver nutritional support. Initial attempts to address electrolyte imbalances should be undertaken concomitantly with resuscitation (see Chapter 109). Once stable, septic patients are investigated to determine the source of sepsis.

After excluding the presence of peritoneal signs that would mandate urgent surgical intervention, CT is typically used to evaluate for an intra-abdominal source of sepsis or concomitant abscess. Triple-contrast CT scans are usually performed with oral, intravenous, and rectal contrast. Although the fistulous site may be identified, this is not really necessary, because it usually does not change management. Intra-abdominal abscesses are best treated with CT-guided drainage procedures, particularly if they are larger than 4 cm. If an abscess is present and less invasive means to control sepsis are not available, surgical drainage of the abscess may be required. Use of other imaging modalities to define the fistula tract, including retrograde fluoroscopic fistulography, Gastrografin upper-gastrointestinal studies, and Gastrografin enemas, is never urgent and rarely changes clinical management unless surgical intervention is being planned. The presence or absence of distal obstruction or abscess is determined in most cases, because treatment of these conditions may permit spontaneous fistula closure.[12]

Crucial in the early management of enterocutaneous fistulas is protection of the surrounding skin. Enterostomal nursing support is enlisted to control leakage, improve hygiene, and ease nursing care for the patient with an external fistula. Small, low-output fistulas may be controlled with dressing changes, but collecting appliances are usually superior by virtue of the reduced need for nursing care. Higher-output fistulas mandate more effective drainage control. If dressings quickly become saturated and require frequent changes, a collecting system is required to protect the surrounding skin (Fig. 89-5).[14] Many fistula sites can be controlled with a simple pouch attachment, similar to colostomy, ileostomy, or urostomy collection systems. Because fistulas are often in close association with wounds, these sites may require advanced pouching or tubing techniques and may benefit from consultation with an enterostomal professional. One useful adjunct is a vacuum-assist closure device (VAC, Kinetic Concepts Incorporated, San Antonio, TX), which controls fistulous drainage while concomitantly promoting wound healing (Fig. 89-6).[15] A more economical alternative to the costly VAC system is to place a drain close to the fistula, surrounded by gauze and covered with a large occlusive transparent dressing (Tegaderm Transparent Dressing, 3M, St. Paul, MN). These dressings are removed periodically to examine the wound.

Colovaginal and enterovaginal fistulas pose a more complex problem, because no pouching system can be applied, and local discomfort and skin breakdown are extremely disabling for the patient. Although a combination of therapeutic fasting coupled with total parenteral nutrition may reduce drainage, these types of fistula often require surgical intervention.

Nutritional support is required in most patients with enterocutaneous fistula, in part because of poor nutritional status, unabsorbed nutritional losses of fistulous effluent, and the fact that patients are often kept fasting to minimize fistulous drainage. Because malnutrition is present in 55% to 90% of patients with enterocutaneous fistulas, nutritional assessment is important for all patients.[16] Serum albumin levels, absolute white blood cell count, retinol-binding protein, and prealbumin levels in patients with fistulas provide surrogate markers for evaluating both long- and short-term nutritional status (see Chapter 105). A variety of validated equations, such as the Harris-Benedict equation, may be used to empirically target baseline nutritional needs, which should later be adjusted according to indirect calorimetry or laboratory surrogates of nutritional status. The ideal modality of supplemental nutrition depends on the anatomical location, volume of fistula output, and hepatic function. Generally speaking, high-output fistulas respond best to reduction of oral intake through fasting and supplementation with total parenteral nutrition, whereas low-output fistulas can be managed with oral dietary supplements or enteral feeding formulas. In the case of a proximal fistula, enteral feeds may be tolerated via insertion of a feeding tube through the fistula and resumption of enteral feeds through the remainder of bowel distal to the fistula.

In the palliative care patient, fistulas present a delicate situation to be discussed with the patient, family, and associated caregivers. As with stoma creation, the shock of an enterocutaneous fistula may be psychologically disturbing to the patient and family members. Spontaneous closure of the tract is the ideal long-term goal in a patient with a fistula. Rates of spontaneous closure vary depending on the anatomical location of the fistula and the output volumes. Uncomplicated, low-output, secondary fistulas that are amenable to enteral feedings are more likely to demonstrate spontaneous closure. Moreover, fistulas involving the duodenum or biliopancreatic tract are 1.5 to 2 times more likely to heal than those of colonic origin.[13] Fistulas involving radiation-induced bowel injury or malignant gastrointestinal lesions are not likely to close spontaneously. Moreover, colovesicular, colovaginal, and

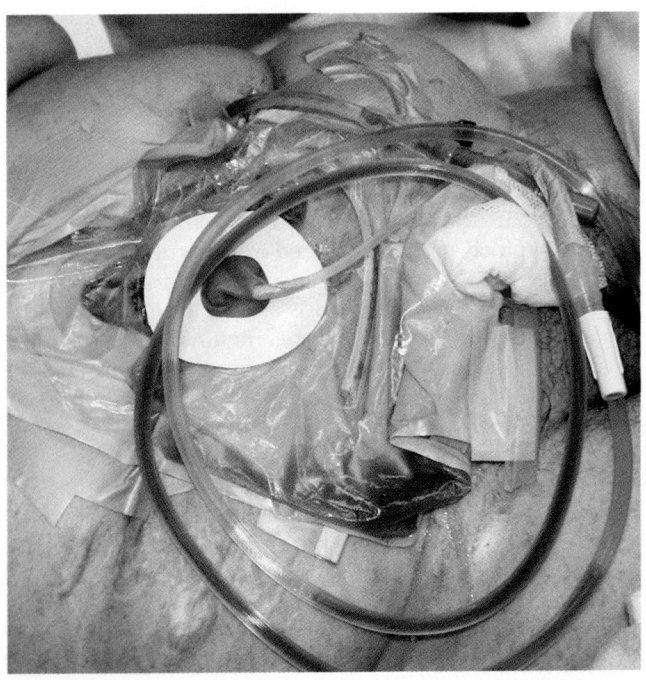

FIGURE 89-5 High-volume enterocutaneous fistulas may require collecting systems to protect surrounding skin and wounds and to promote healing.

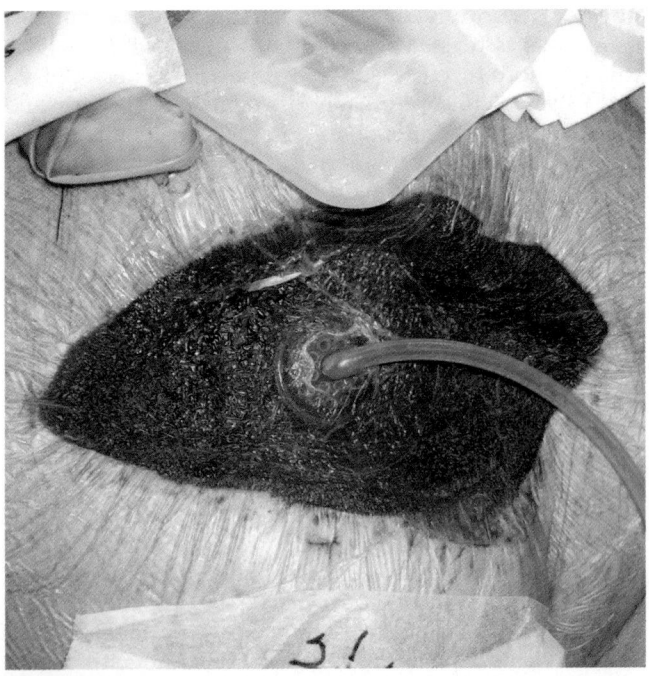

FIGURE 89-6 A vacuum-assisted closure device can be a useful adjunct in the management of enterocutaneous fistulas.

enterovaginal fistulas are not likely to heal without surgical diversion and definitive repair, because pouching and external control is not attainable.

Ideally, enterocutaneous fistulas that persist despite optimal management are resected and repaired. However, surgical resection of a fistula may not be a desirable option in palliative care patients because of the complexity of surgical correction, the rate of recurrence, and the uncertain long-term benefit to the patient.[17] In such cases, the benefits of resection require careful deliberation in light of the risks of the surgery and possible subsequent complications and the diminished long-term benefit that is absent from palliative care patients. A proximal diverting stoma may be required for control of a complex fistula for which reparative surgery would be too severe for the palliative care patient or in the case of an unresectable tumor causing fistulization. Patients with colovaginal or enterovaginal fistulas also frequently need surgery because of inability to control the drainage. Surgical options in the palliative care patient include resection and primary bowel repair, proximal diversion alone, and forms of exclusion bypass of the fistulous segment.

CONCLUSIONS

Judicious use of ostomies can provide excellent palliation of symptoms, but stoma care is complex for these patients and requires support from the surgical team and enterostomal nursing care professionals. Patients with fistulas present challenging management problems and require a coordinated effort between the palliative care and surgical teams to provide optimal management (see "Future Considerations"). Supportive care to maintain nutrition, hydration, and treat sepsis is crucial, as is attention to wound or skin care. Operative intervention is selectively used, depending on the exact clinical situation.

REFERENCES

1. Rosenthal M, Rosenthal D. Stomal care. In Wilmore D, Laurence Y, Cheung AH, et al (eds). ACS Surgery: Principles and Practice. New York: WebMD Professional Publishing, 2003, pp. 1655-1670.
2. Delaney CP, Kiran RP, Senagore AJ, et al. Case-matched comparison of clinical and financial outcome after laparoscopic or open colorectal surgery. Ann Surg 2003;238:67-72.
3. Abraham NS, Young JM, Solomon MJ. Meta-analysis of short-term outcomes after laparoscopic resection for colorectal cancer. B J Surg 2004;91: 1111-1124.
4. Senagore AJ, Delaney CP. A critical analysis of laparoscopic colectomy at a single institution: Lessons learned after 1000 cases. Am J Surg 2006;191: 377-380.
5. Arumugam PJ, Bevan L, Macdonald L, et al. A prospective audit of stomas: Analysis of risk factors and complications and their management. Colorectal Dis 2003;5:49-52.
6. Cheung MT. Complications of an abdominal stoma: An analysis of 322 stomas. Aust N Z J Surg 1995;65:808-811.
7. Nugent KP, Daniels P, Stewart B, et al. Quality of life in stoma patients. Dis Colon Rectum 1999;42:1569-1574.
8. Hellman J, Lago CP. Dermatologic complications in colostomy and ileostomy patients. Int J Dermatol 1990;29:129-133.
9. Carne PW, Robertson GM, Frizelle FA. Parastomal hernia. Br J Surg 2003;90:784-793.
10. Park JJ, Del Pino A, Orsay CP, et al. Stoma complications: The Cook County Hospital experience. Dis Colon Rectum 1999;42:1575-1580.
11. Duchesne JC, Wang YZ, Weintraub SL, et al. Stoma complications: A multivariate analysis. Am Surg 2002;68:961-966; discussion 966.
12. Evenson AR, Fischer JE. Current management of enterocutaneous fistula. J Gastrointest Surg 2006;10:455-464.
13. Campos AC, Andrade DF, Campos GM, et al. A multivariate model to determine prognostic factors in gastrointestinal fistulas. J Am Coll Surg 1999;188: 483-490.
14. Dearlove JL. Skin care management of gastrointestinal fistulas. Surg Clin North Am 1996;76:1095-1109.
15. Goverman J, Yelon JA, Platz JJ, et al. The "Fistula VAC," a technique for management of enterocutaneous fistulae arising within the open abdomen: Report of 5 cases. J Trauma 2006;60:428-431; discussion 431.
16. Berry SM, Fischer JE. Classification and pathophysiology of enterocutaneous fistulas. Surg Clin North Am 1996;76:1009-1018.
17. Lynch AC, Delaney CP, Senagore AJ, et al. Clinical outcome and factors predictive of recurrence after enterocutaneous fistula surgery. Ann Surg 2004;240: 825-831.

SUGGESTED READING

Evenson AR, Fischer JE. Current management of enterocutaneous fistula. J Gastrointest Surg 2006;10:455-464.

MacKeigan J. Stomas. In Nicholls R, Dozois R. Surgery of the Colon and Rectum, 1st ed. Edinburgh: Churchill Livingstone, 1997.

Rosenthal M, Rosenthal D. Stomal care. In Wilmore D, Laurence Y, Cheung AH, et al (eds). ACS Surgery: Principles and Practice. New York: WebMD Professional Publishing, 2003, pp 1655-1670.

CHAPTER **90**

Emergencies in Palliative Medicine

Katherine Clark and David Currow

- Acute pulmonary embolus (PE)
  - Acute PE is associated with high mortality; most cases of PE are diagnosed post mortem.
  - Approximately 10% of PE cases are fatal within 1 hour of onset, and the overall 3-month mortality is 15%.
  - Patients in shock have increased mortality.
  - Patients who survive are at increased risk of morbidity: recurrent PE, recurrent deep vein thrombosis (DVT), post-thrombotic syndrome, pulmonary hypertension.
- Acute pneumonia
  - Pneumonia accounts for approximately 5 million deaths per year worldwide.
  - Pneumonia tends to be more serious in the very young, the very old, and those with severe underlying illnesses.
  - Poor prognostic features include age greater than 60 years, hypoxia, decreased total white blood cell count, neutrophilia greater than 20,000, abnormal urea and creatinine, low albumin, confusion, and intercurrent illness.
- Hypoproteinemic edema
  - Albumin is the body's predominant protein that maintains plasma fluid oncotic pressures.
  - Low albumin levels may cause edema.
  - Low albumin levels are associated with significant morbidity and mortality.
- Seizures and status epilepticus
  - Seizures may occur at the end of life.
  - Status epilepticus is persistent seizure activity or a failure to regain consciousness for more than 5 minutes after a witnessed seizure.
  - Seizures are classified according to the origin of the focus.
  - Seizures are frightening for both patients and families and require prompt attention.
- Acute myocardial infarction
  - Acute myocardial infarctions form one end of the spectrum of acute coronary syndromes, which include acute myocardial infarctions associated with electrocardiographic (ECG) ST-segment changes, acute myocardial infarction without ECG changes, and angina.
  - All these syndromes represent disruptions to coronary artery blood flow, and the clinical presentation depends on the degree of flow disruption and on the permanence of tissue damage.
- Sepsis
  - *Sepsis* refers to a state of inflammation from infection.
  - The inflammatory response is called *systemic inflammatory response syndrome* (SIRS).
  - When SIRS is severe, patients are shocked and suffer hypoperfusion of organs.

- Septic shock carries an extremely poor prognosis, especially in palliative medicine.
- Family crisis
  - Serious illness and impending death are traumatic events that may place great stress on an individual and family unit.
  - This stress may cause an imbalance between the demands placed on a family and the capabilities they possess to deal effectively with the problem, a situation considered a crisis for this family.
  - The best outcomes for families are conversation and conflict resolution. It is imperative for families to be made aware that the multidisciplinary team shares concern for the patient, and this extends to the family unit.

ACUTE PULMONARY EMBOLUS

- PE is a common problem encountered more frequently in hospitalized patients than in the community.
- The presenting symptoms are common to numerous other conditions, so a high index of suspicion is needed.
- Investigations depend on the previously estimated prognosis of the affected individual.

Basic Science and Pathophysiology

PE occurs when a more distal venous thrombus dislodges and passes through the venous system, through the right side of the heart, and to the pulmonary circulation. The size of the embolus dictates its severity and reflects the degree of obstruction to pulmonary artery flow and the ability of the right ventricle to compensate (Fig. 90-1).

Epidemiology and Prevalence

PE is common in hospitalized patients, and 7% to 10% of patients who die of PE are hospitalized patients. Most people have no symptoms. The causes of venous thrombus and PE may be acute, resulting from a change in physical circumstances, or secondary to an underlying chronic predisposition (Table 90-1 and Case Study: Pulmonary Embolus).

Clinical Manifestations

The most common presenting symptoms are as follows:

- Acute dyspnea
- Pleuritic chest pain
- Cough
- Hemoptysis
- Palpitations
- Diaphoresis
- Syncope
- Shock
- Sudden, unexplained death

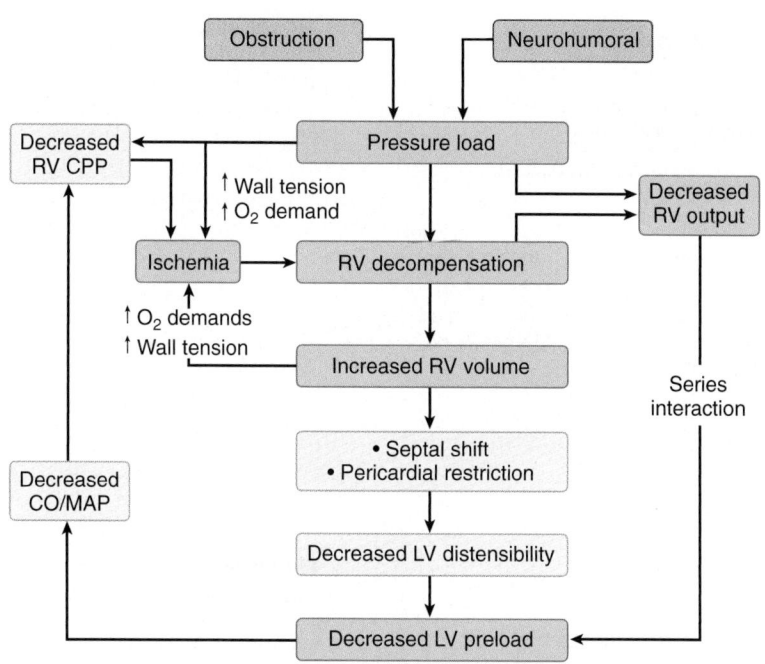

FIGURE 90-1 Physiological changes associated with PE. CPP, cerebral perfusion pressure; LV, left ventricular; MAP, mean arterial pressure; RV, right ventricular.

TABLE 90-1	Venous Thromboembolism Risk Factors

ACUTE RISK FACTORS

Hospitalization
Surgical procedures
Limb fracture
Long-distance travel
Relative hypovolemia
Estrogen
Intravascular devices

CHRONIC PREDISPOSITION

Inherited
Protein C deficiency
Protein S deficiency
Antithrombin III deficiency
Factor V Leiden

Acquired
Major medical illness
Cancer
Previous thromboembolic disease
Increasing age
Obesity

CASE STUDY

Pulmonary Embolus

Ms. A is 70-year-old woman with metastatic rectal cancer. As a result of general weakness, she was admitted under the hospital palliative care team. Overnight, she had acute onset of shortness of breath. Her physical examination was unremarkable. The electrocardiogram showed tachycardia with right-sided heart strain. Results of the computed tomography pulmonary angiogram were consistent with a diagnosis of multiple pulmonary emboli.

Therapeutic intravenous heparin was commenced. A long-term plan was made for a maintenance regimen of low-molecular-weight heparin.

Differential Diagnosis

The extent of investigations and interventions depends on (Fig. 90-2) the following considerations:

- The patient's prognosis before the onset of this problem guides diagnostic investigations and interventions.
- The likelihood that the combination of symptoms and signs is the result of a PE is determined by considering the pre-test PE probability.
- Both the prognosis and the probability of a PE must be considered, and investigations should be tailored appropriately. A score equal to or greater than 6 indicates a high pre-test probability of PE (Fig. 90-3 and Table 90-2).

Investigations

Pulse Oximetry Arterial Blood Gases

Patients may not be hypoxic and may therefore have normal arterial blood gas values. Assessment of hypoxia is still indicated, and patients who are hypoxic require oxygen. Hypoxic patients have larger emboli and a poorer prognosis.

Electrocardiography

ECG findings may be normal. More commonly, tracings show nonspecific changes of tachycardia or right-sided strain. The classic $S_I Q_{III} T_{III}$ change is found in approximately 20% of patients. Predominantly, ECG study eliminates other cardiac causes of chest pain and dyspnea. In patients too unwell for more intensive investigations, a positive ECG finding is useful to steer management.

Chest Radiography

The most common finding on the chest radiograph is atelectasis. Other findings may include a well-defined

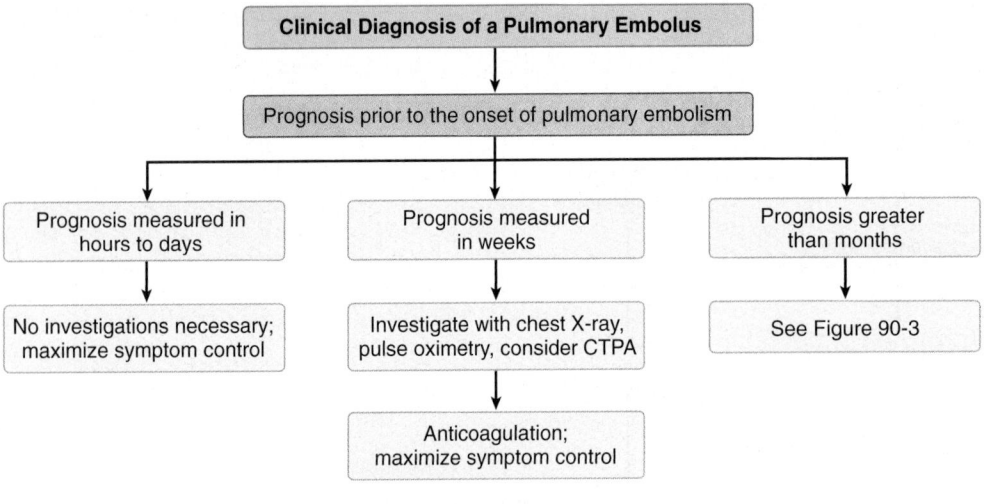

FIGURE 90-2 Management flow chart based on prognosis of pulmonary embolism. CTPA, computed tomography pulmonary angiography.

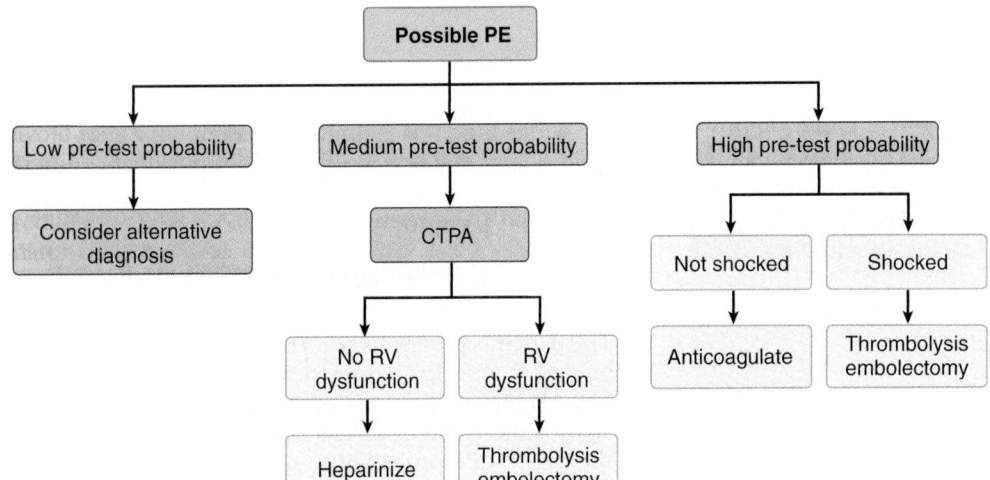

FIGURE 90-3 Management flow chart for patients with reasonable performance status before the onset of pulmonary embolism (PE). CTPA, computed tomography pulmonary angiography; RV, right ventricular.

TABLE 90-2	Calculating the Pre-test Probability of a Pulmonary Embolus	
FACTOR	**PRE-TEST PROBABILITY**
Clinical signs and symptoms of deep vein thrombosis	3.0
Tachycardia >100 beats/min	1.5
Immobility >3 days	1.5
Surgical procedures <4 weeks earlier	1.5
Previous thromboembolism	1.5
Hemoptysis	1.0
Cancer	1.0
Pulmonary embolus as likely or more likely than any other diagnosis	3.0

translucency and an abrupt cutoff of vascular markings. Pleural effusion may accompany pleural infarct. The main use of chest radiography is to exclude other pulmonary causes of chest pain, dyspnea, and cough.

Ventilation/Perfusion Scans

Ventilation/perfusion lung scintigraphy (V/Q scan) is an important diagnostic aid, but it is most reliable when the pre-test probability is moderate to high.

Helical Computed Tomography

Helical computed tomography (CT pulmonary angiography) scanning is the investigation of choice for PE. The investigation is readily available and provides rapid results. Fewer false-positive results occur than with the V/Q scan. Small, peripheral changes may not be well imaged.

Pulmonary Angiography

Pulmonary angiography is the gold standard investigation for PE.

Treatment

Drugs of Choice

● Unfractionated heparin and low-molecular-weight heparin

Anticoagulation with either unfractionated heparin or low-molecular-weight heparin is administered according to protocols laid down by individual health care centers.

● Warfarin

Patients with a life expectancy longer than months should receive long-term warfarin therapy. This therapy

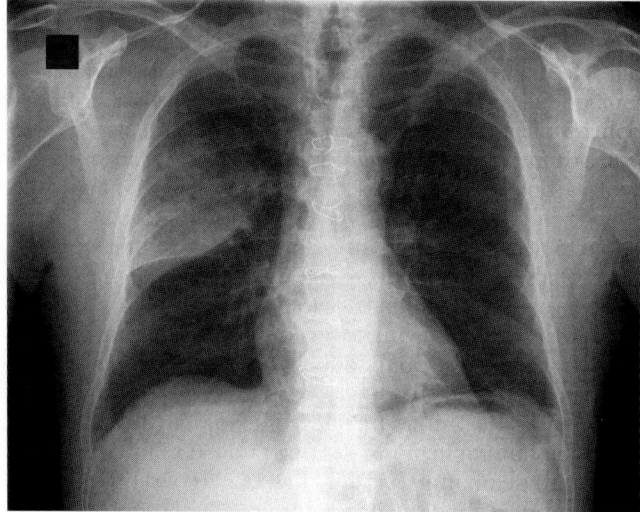

FIGURE 90-4   Right upper lobe pneumonia.

TABLE 90-3   Causes of Acute Onset of Chest Pain and Dyspnea

SYMPTOM	CAUSES
Acute dyspnea	Pulmonary embolus
	Exacerbation of airway disease
	Pulmonary edema
	Pneumothorax
	Pneumonia
	Airway obstruction
Acute chest pain	Coronary artery disease (angina, myocardial infarction)
	Pulmonary embolism
	Aortic dissection
	Pneumothorax
	Esophageal rupture or esophageal spasm

needs to be titrated using the prothrombin time according to the local guidelines.

- Thrombolysis

Thrombolysis may be considered when the patient's previously established prognosis was measured in months to years. Although long-term improvements in overall mortality have not been demonstrated, patients who are initially hemodynamically unstable may improve with thrombolysis. An urgent echocardiogram and cardiology consultation are indicated.

ACUTE PNEUMONIA

Pneumonia is either an acute or a chronic infection, associated with inflammation of the terminal bronchioles and alveoli. This condition causes consolidation, evident both clinically and radiologically. The type of pneumonia, the previous prognosis, and the patient's current clinical state dictate the appropriate individual investigations and interventions (Fig. 90-4).

Pneumonia tends to be divided into the following three main groups:

- Hospital acquired
- Compromised host
- Community acquired

Epidemiology and Prevalence

Pneumonia causes 4 million deaths per year worldwide. Approximately one third of patients with pneumonia will require hospitalization, and mortality for hospitalized patients with pneumonia is approximately 20% (Table 90-3).

Pathophysiology

The lungs become infected with organisms, either inhaled or aspirated. Normally, host defenses maintain a sterile lung environment. A failure of normal host defenses, both anatomical and cellular, leads to clinical pneumonia (Table 90-4 and "Case Study: Pneumonia").

Clinical Manifestations: Evaluation, Tests, and Laboratory Findings

Symptoms Associated with Pneumonia That Require Consideration

- Dyspnea
- Delirium
- Pleuritic chest pain
- Cough
- Hemoptysis
- Fevers or rigors

Patients may present with acute fever, cough productive of purulent sputum, and pleuritic chest pain. Other presenting features may include dry cough or a flulike illness with fatigue, myalgias, and arthralgias.

Physical examination may reveal an extremely unwell patient, with fever, tachycardia, and perhaps hypotension. Mental obtundation may be present, and patients may also

TABLE 90-4   Causes of Pneumonia

TYPE OF PNEUMONIA	CAUSES
Community acquired	*Streptococcus pneumoniae* *Haemophilus influenzae* *Mycoplasma pneumoniae* *Staphylococcus aureus* *Legionella* species Viruses
Nosocomial	*Pseudomonas* species Gram-negative enterobacteria *Staphylococcus aueus* *Pseudomonas* *Klebsiella*
Aspiration	Anaerobes Chemical pneumonitis Immunocompromised status
Immunocompromise related	*Streptococcus pneumoniae* *Haemophilus influenzae* *Staphylococcus aureus* *Mycoplasma pneumoniae* *Pneumocystis jiroveci* (formerly *Pneumocystis carinii*) Gram-negative bacilli

TABLE 90-5   Investigations of Pneumonia

INVESTIGATIONS	EXPECTED FINDINGS
Pulse oximeter	<92% suggesting severe hypoxia
Arterial blood gases	Poor prognosis with acidosis, hypoxia
Full blood cell count	Bacterial pneumonia and aspiration pneumonia: Elevated white blood cell count, anemia, and thrombocytosis Leukopenia in sick patients Viral pneumonia: lymphocytosis
Sputum examination	Likely to identify an organism in >50% of bacterial and aspiration pneumonias
Blood cultures	Positive in ~40%
Chest radiograph	**Bacterial pneumonia** Air bronchogram Cavitations Consolidation Pleural effusion **Aspiration pneumonia** Infiltrates Air bronchogram Changes most common in upper lobes **Viral pneumonia** Patchy or diffuse infiltrates
Serology	Atypical organisms in acute illness
Urea, creatinine, electrolytes, liver function tests	Hyponatremia possible indication of syndrome of inappropriate diuretic hormone or *Legionella* pneumonia Renal function possibly impaired, suggesting a poor prognosis Hypoalbuminemia possible indication of a poorer prognosis

CASE STUDY

Pneumonia

Mr. SB is a 60-year-old man with a past history of smoking, now complicated by chronic bronchitis. He is normally breathless on minimal exertion but presented with increasing shortness of breath at rest, associated with sharp chest pain on coughing. Associated with this finding, Mr. SB had become more unwell and confused, and his level of function had deteriorated acutely.

At presentation, Mr. SB was febrile (38° C) and tachycardic, and his oxygen saturations were 86% on room air. Chest examination revealed bronchial breath sounds at the right base. A clinical diagnosis of pneumonia was made.

have central cyanosis (lips or ear lobes) with significant respiratory compromise. Physical examination may be remarkable for decreased expansion of the affected lung, with decreased percussion note and vocal resonance and air entry with coarse crackles. Bronchial breath sounds may be audible over the affected area. In less typical presentations of pneumonia, abnormal physical findings may be minimal. Table 90-5 lists the expected findings of diagnostic tests for pneumonia.

Differential Diagnosis

Table 90-6 is a list of possible diagnoses in patients with acute dyspnea, productive cough, fever, and pulmonary infiltrates.

Treatment

Therapeutics

Optimal management of pneumonia requires prompt diagnosis and antibiotics tailored to the patient and in accordance with local guidelines (Fig. 90-5).

TABLE 90-6   Differential Diagnoses of Acute Dyspnea, Productive Cough, Fever, and Pulmonary Infiltrates

SIGN OR SYMPTOM	POSSIBLE CAUSES
Acute onset of dyspnea	Pneumonia Exacerbation of chronic airway disease Coronary artery disease or heart failure Pulmonary embolus Pneumothorax
Cough	Pneumonia Upper respiratory tract infection Exacerbation of chronic airway disease Chronic aspiration Malignant disease (primary lung cancer, secondary metastases) Airway obstruction
Production of sputum	Pneumonia Infective exacerbation of chronic airway disease Bronchiectasis Malignant disease leading to obstruction
Fever	Infections Malignant disease Connective tissue disease Medications (antibiotics, interferon, anticonvulsants, anticholinergics, serotonin syndrome, malignant hyperthermia)
Pulmonary infiltrates	Lung infections Heart failure Pulmonary embolus Atelectasis Malignant disease Vasculitis

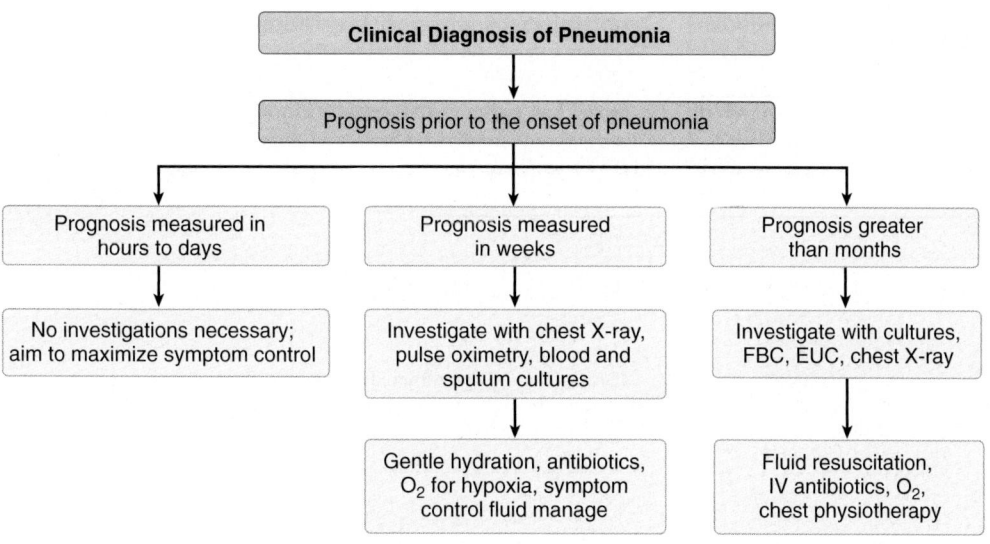

FIGURE 90-5 Management flow chart for pneumonia based on prognosis. EUC, electrolytes, urea, and creatinine; FBC, full blood cell count; IV, intravenous.

Pearls and Pitfalls

- Patients with pneumonia require prompt diagnosis and initiation of antibiotics.
- Patients may be highly symptomatic, and attention to symptom control is imperative.
- Even toward the end of life, consideration of intravenous antibiotics may be appropriate.
- Aspiration pneumonia usually causes significant chemical inflammation with the risk of secondary infection.

Rational Management Plan for Pneumonia

- Commence antibiotic treatment quickly.
- Antibiotic treatment should be guided by Gram staining.
- Modify the prescription based on microbiological results.
- Prolonged treatment does not prevent recurrence.
- Patients with chronic airway disease should receive coverage for *Pseudomonas*.
- The specific course of antibiotics should be tailored to the patient's previous antibiotic exposure.
- Local guidelines must be considered, adhered to, and updated on a regular basis for the patterns of pathogens likely to be encountered.

HYPOPROTEINEMIC EDEMA

Edema results from an imbalance between the physiological forces that balance intravascular volumes and the extravascular interstitial spaces. This change usually results in an outward shift of intravascular fluid that leads to an abnormal accumulation of interstitial fluid. The fluid distribution may be localized to a body part, or it may be generalized (anasarca). Other specialized forms of edema include pleural effusions, pericardial effusions, and ascites (fluid in the peritoneal space).

TABLE 90-7 Causes of Hypoproteinemic Edema

FINDING	CAUSES
Increased plasma volume (relative albumin deficiency)	Heart failure Renal failure Pregnancy Medications
Increased protein loss	Malabsorption Protein-losing enteropathy Nephrotic syndrome Cachexia of malignancy Burns
Decreased protein synthesis	Cirrhosis Liver failure Malabsorption Thiamine deficiency

Epidemiology and Prevalence

Hypoalbuminemia occurs most commonly in frail elderly and severely ill patients (e.g., those with advanced cancer or burns) (Table 90-7).

Pathophysiology

- Decreased or defective synthesis
  Decreased protein intake
  Ineffective hepatocyte function
- Inadequate albumin secretion from the hepatocyte
  Decreased oxygen secondary to impaired blood supply to the hepatocyte in cirrhosis
- Increased albumin excretion or destruction
  Inflammatory states (acute, chronic)
  Burns
  Nephritic or nephrotic syndrome
  Protein-losing enteropathy
- Hemodilution
  Heart failure
  Renal failure (see "Case Study: Hypoproteinemic Edema")

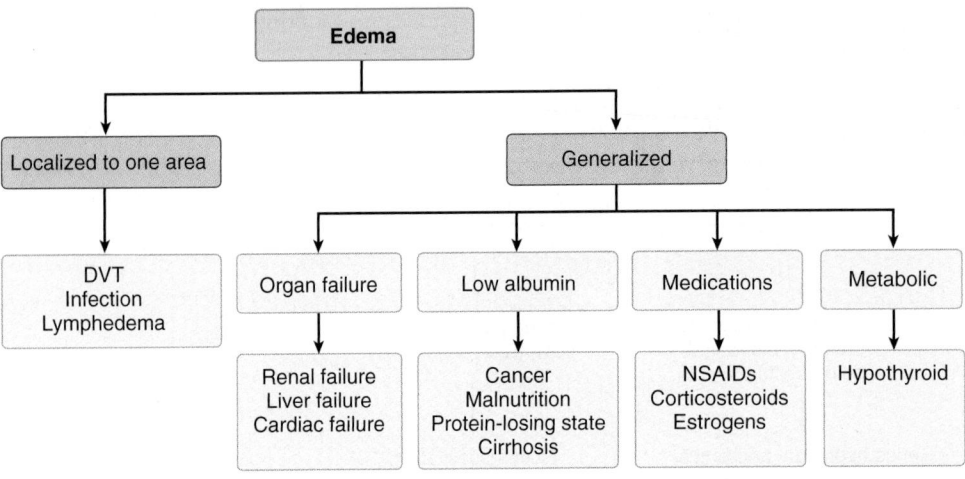

FIGURE 90-6   Differential diagnosis of swelling. DVT, deep vein thrombosis; NSAIDs, nonsteroidal anti-inflammatory drugs.

 C A S E   S T U D Y

Hypoproteinemic Edema

Ms. PO is a 36-year-old woman with metastatic adenocarcinoma of the cervix. She presented with gross lower limb edema bilaterally.

Diagnostic investigations were remarkable for a serum albumin concentration of 22 mmol/L. Further investigations revealed a large pelvic mass with bilateral hydronephrosis. The patient's edema was deemed multifactorial, with identified causes including hypoalbuminemia, lymphedema, and renal dysfunction.

Clinical Manifestations

Because the causes of hypoproteinemic edema are multiple, findings will differ depending on the origin. The most important to consider are the following:

- Medical history, especially of malignant disease, renal or liver disease, medications, and malabsorption
- Dietary history
- Any inflammation, acute or chronic

Physical examination is most commonly remarkable for peripheral edema.

Differential Diagnosis

Figure 90-6 shows the differential diagnosis of swelling.

Treatment

Optimal management depends on correct identification and reversal of the cause. As with all problems in palliative care, the extent of investigations and management depends on the prognosis of the patient and on his or her ability to tolerate interventions.

SEIZURES AND STATUS EPILEPTICUS

- The extent of investigations depends on the patient's overall condition and prognosis.
- The need to intervene depends on the type and duration of the seizure.

Pearls and Pitfalls

- Bed rest and supportive stockings may help to reduce lower limb edema.
- Diuretics may also help to reduce peripheral and pulmonary edema and ascites:
  - Loop diuretics
  - Spironolactone
- Referral to a dietitian may be of benefit.
- Other symptoms associated with hypoalbuminemia include the following:
  - Pain or discomfort
  - Breathlessness
  - Early satiety
  - Constipation
  - Reflux
- Drainage of gross collections of fluid in the peritoneal or pleural cavities may promote comfort.

Future Considerations

- Research to define the best way to prevent hypoalbuminemia in patients with cancer is necessary.
- The role of albumin replacement in patients with cancer is unclear.
- The role of diuretics in patients with peripheral edema resulting from hypoalbuminemia remains to be determined.
- Clinicians need a way to ascertain which patients with ascites are likely to respond to diuretics.

- Any witnessed grand mal seizure should prompt anti-seizure therapy.
- Status epilepticus is a medical emergency that requires prompt recognition and initiation of treatment. Untreated, it has a mortality of approximately 25%.

Epidemiology and Prevalence

- Seizures may develop at any age, and the prevalence of epilepsy is estimated at 1 to 4 individuals per 1000.
- The risk factors of trauma, infections, and tumors occur across all age groups. Among individuals more than 60

years of age, the most likely underlying cause of new seizures is cerebrovascular disease.

- Status epilepticus is most common in either very young or elderly persons.
- The onset of seizures increases the likelihood of sudden death, trauma, pneumonia, and fractures (Table 90-8).

Pathophysiology

A seizure is a transient collection of symptoms that results from excessive brain neuronal activity. In adults, the cause may be structural change, metabolic disorders, or drug-related conditions. Status epilepticus is prolongation of this abnormal state (see "Case Study: Focal Seizure," "Case Study: Generalized Seizure," and "Case Study: Status Epilepticus").

Differential Diagnosis

When considering a diagnosis of epilepsy, the following must be considered (Fig. 90-7 and Tables 90-9 and 90-10):

- The appearance of the incident
- Precipitating factors

CASE STUDY

Focal Seizure

Mrs. CC is a 50-year-old woman with new onset of headaches and intermittent episodes of blurred vision. She presented with new-onset nausea and headaches. A cerebral computed tomography scan revealed a large mass, with an appearance typical of a glioblastoma of the occipital region. A diagnosis of focal seizures secondary to newly diagnosed glioblastoma was made.

CASE STUDY

Generalized Seizure

Mr. GW is an 80-year-old man with known metastatic melanoma. He presented with a new onset of witnessed generalized tonic-clonic seizure. Investigations revealed a large hemorrhagic mass in the patient's right frontal lobe. A regimen of dexamethasone and phenytoin was commenced.

CASE STUDY

Status Epilepticus

Despite adequate loading with anticonvulsants, approximately 1 week later, Mr. GW suffered a marked deterioration in his level of consciousness again. The nursing staff reports were of constant jerking movements in a man unable to be roused. A diagnosis of status epilepticus was made.

TABLE 90-8 Causes of Seizures in Palliative Medicine

CATEGORY	CAUSES
Physical	Trauma
	Space-occupying lesion
	Cerebrovascular disease
	Malignant hypertension
	Vascular malformations
	Autoimmune diseases (systemic lupus erythematosus, sarcoidosis)
Infectious	Meningitis
	Encephalitis
	Cerebral syphilis
	HIV infection
Metabolic	Alcohol withdrawal
	Electrolyte abnormalities
	Hypoglycemia
	Hyperglycemia
	Hyponatremia
	Hypernatremia
	Hypocalcemia
	Uremia
	Liver failure
	Medications (benzodiazepine withdrawal)
	Hypoxia
Inherited	Benign rolandic epilepsy
	Juvenile myoclonic epilepsy
	Temporal lobe epilepsy
Preexisting seizures Iatrogenic reduction in seizure threshold	Inability to take medications because of progressive illness
	Tricyclic antidepressants, theophylline, antipsychotic medications, anticonvulsants

TABLE 90-9 Diagnosis of Seizure Type Based on Pattern of Activity

SEIZURE TYPE	ACTIVITY PATTERN
Generalized seizures (seizures that cannot be localized to one hemisphere, with associated loss of consciousness as activity crosses the midline)	Absence Tonic-clonic Myotonic Atonic Flaccid
Partial seizures (features that may be localized to one hemisphere)	Focal (simple) Focal (complex)
Status epilepticus	Generalized (tonic-clonic, myotonic, atonic, flaccid) Focal (simple, complex)

FIGURE 90-7 Differential diagnosis of unexpected temporary loss of consciousness.

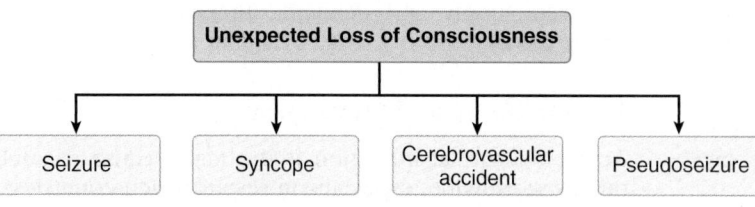

TABLE 90-10 Investigations of Seizures	
TYPE OF TEST	**SPECIFIC INVESTIGATIONS OR INDICATIONS**
Blood tests	Serum urea, creatinine, Sodium, potassium, calcium, blood glucose Liver function tests Full blood cell count Coagulation studies Drug levels
Scans	Computed tomography Magnetic resonance imaging or magnetic resonance angiography
Lumbar puncture	If patient has no evidence of raised intracranial pressure, lumbar puncture helpful in diagnosis of infectious causes of seizures
Electroencephalography	Not required when overt seizure activity is visible; in patients presenting with no obvious cause of altered consciousness, an electroencephalogram possibly helpful in defining seizure activity
Electrocardiography	Indicated for any patient who presents with a history of falls and a loss of consciousness

TABLE 90-11 Seizure Therapeutics	
INDICATION	**REGIMENS**
Seizure arrest	Diazepam: 10 mg IV or rectally (use a mixing tube) Midazolam: 5 mg SC/SL/IV
Maintenance therapy in the dying	Clonazepam: 0.5-1.0 mg SL or SC bid or 2-4 mg infused SC over 24 hr Midazolam: 20 mg infused SC over 24 hr Phenobarbitone: 100 mg SC immediately and then 200 mg/day infused SC, a particularly useful regimen in difficult cases when sedation is required
Maintenance therapy for focal seizures (longer prognosis)	Sodium valproate: initially 400-600 mg/day and titrate to response Carbamazepine: initially 200 mg/day in divided doses and titrate to response
Maintenance therapy for generalized seizures (longer prognosis)	Sodium valproate: initially 400-600 mg/day and titrate Phenytoin: 4-5 mg/kg/day loading by slow infusion IV or orally and titrate up to 300 mg as a maintenance dose

bid, twice daily; IV, intravenously; SC, subcutaneously; SL, sublingually.

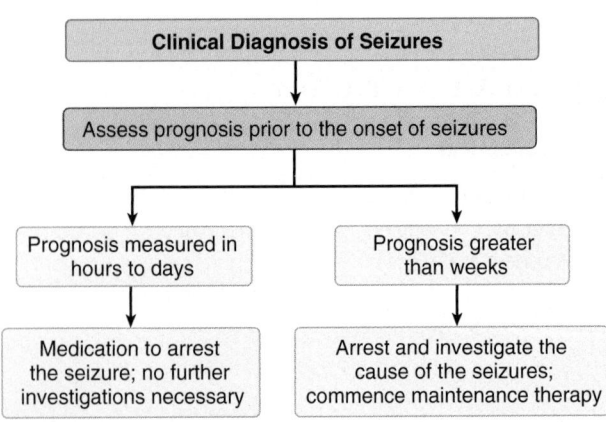

FIGURE 90-8   Management flow chart for seizures.

Common Therapeutics

- Isolated seizures may not require any intervention.
- Repeated seizures require prompt intervention to arrest the seizure and to prevent further seizure activity.
- Midazolam is readily available and may be given by a variety of routes including subcutaneously (SC), intramuscularly (IM), intravenously (IV), or buccally; start with 2.5 to 5.0 mg and repeat as necessary.
- Alternative benzodiazepines include the following:
  - Clonazepam: SC or sublingually (SL); start with 0.5 to 1.0 mg and repeat if necessary
  - Diazepam: IV, IM (2 to 5 mg), or rectally (10 mg)
  - Lorazepam: SL or IV (2 to 4 mg)

- The duration of the incident and the recovery phase
- The patient's previous history of seizures or temporary loss of consciousness
- Past history of substance abuse or head injury

Management of Status Epilepticus

Status epilepticus is a medical emergency (Fig. 90-8 and Table 90-11), and treatment is as follows:

- Protect the airway (positioning, oral airway, intubation).
- Administer oxygen, and establish intravenous access.
- Check the patient's full blood cell count, electrolytes, urea, and creatine, and blood glucose.
- Administer 100 mg thiamine intravenously (IV).
- Give 50 mL of 50% dextrose if the patient has low blood glucose, but thiamine must always be given first.

- Commence diazepam (5 to 10 mg IV) or lorazepam (1 to 2 mg), clonazepam (0.5 to 1 mg IV), or midazolam (2.5 to 5.0 mg IV or SC).
- Initiate phenytoin therapy with 4 to 5 mg/kg/day in two to three divided doses, and assess plasma levels.

ACUTE MYOCARDIAL INFARCTION

Myocardial infarctions result from impaired blood supply to the myocardium. The impaired blood supply may be transient, as in angina, or the more serious case of myocardial infarction, with irreversible heart muscle necrosis. The most common cause of myocardial infarction is thrombus that occludes a narrowing previously caused by atherosclerotic plaque. Other causes to be considered in low-risk patients include prothrombotic states, a mismatch between supply and demand (anemia), and coronary artery vasospasm.

Epidemiology and Prevalence

Acute myocardial infarction is the major cause of adult deaths worldwide, especially in resource-rich countries.

CASE STUDY

Acute Myocardial Infarction

Mr. DW is a 74-year-old man with multiple myeloma. He presented with an acute deterioration in his level of function, associated with increasing severity and frequency of chest pain and dyspnea. His physical examination was remarkable only for basal crackles at both his lung bases.

Investigations included a chest radiograph, which revealed increased lung markings consistent with early pulmonary edema, and an electrocardiogram, which revealed ST-segment elevation across the inferior leads. A diagnosis of inferior myocardial infarction was made.

Pathophysiology

The most common cause of myocardial infarction is a thrombus aggravating a narrowed segment of coronary artery resulting from atherosclerosis. The thrombus typically occurs when platelets aggregate over an area of ruptured plaque.

Other causes of myocardial infarction include the following:

- Coronary artery vasospasm
- Prothrombotic states (cancer [see "Case Study: Acute Myocardial Infarction"] disseminated intravascular coagulopathy, infectious and endocarditis)
- Mismatch between supply and demand (severe anemia)
- Vasculitis

Clinical Manifestations

The following are clinical features of patients with myocardial infarcts:

- Chest pain
  - Often central pain that typically radiates to the neck, left shoulder, and left arm
  - Often described as heavy
  - May occur on exertion or at rest
- Shortness of breath
- Palpitations
- Diaphoresis
- Sense of impending doom

Differential Diagnosis

Table 90-12 lists possible diagnoses based on the patterns and characteristics of acute chest pain.

Treatment

The degree of investigations and interventions depends on the overall prognosis of the patient before the development of the problem (Table 90-13). Regardless of prognosis, the immediate clinical aims are as follows:

TABLE 90-12	Differential Diagnosis of Acute Chest Pain
DISORDER	**CHARACTERISTIC PAIN PATTERN**
Angina or myocardial infarction	Classically central, dull chest pain radiating to the jaw or left arm
Pericarditis	Sharp central chest pain that may worsen with inspiration and lessen with sitting forward
Aortic dissection	Distressing tearing pain that may radiate to the back
Pneumonia	Dull pain over the site of disease, often with a sharp, well-localized component
Esophageal spasm	Possibly difficult to differentiate from myocardial pain except more typically radiates to the throat than to the left arm

TABLE 90-13	Investigations of Chest Pain
TYPE OF TEST	**SPECIFIC INVESTIGATIONS OR INDICATIONS**
Blood tests	Cardiac enzymes: creatine kinase MB isoenzyme, troponin Full blood cell count Coagulation studies Serum creatinine, urea, and electrolytes
Electrocardiography	Least invasive and most useful investigation for new-onset chest pain
Radiology	Chest radiography Cardiac angiography
Echocardiography	Less invasive than angiography and therefore useful in palliative medicine because it may display regional ventricular wall motion abnormalities

- Pain reduction
  - Opioid analgesia with morphine (2.5 to 5.0 mg subcutaneously or IV)
  - Nitrates (sublingual or topical) for vasodilation and reduction of preload
- Restoration of the imbalance between oxygen supply and demand in the myocardium
  - Oxygen (to maintain saturations >94%)
  - Aspirin (100 mg immediately PO)
  - Heparin (use low-molecular-weight heparin if non–ST-segment elevation acute myocardial infarction or angina; otherwise, commence heparin infusion, and ensure normal renal function)
  - Patients considered to have a good prognosis beforehand require consideration of thrombolysis or coronary artery stenting.
- Minimizing of complications
  - β-Blocker
  - Angiotensin-converting enzyme inhibitor or angiotensin II receptor blocker

SEPSIS

Sepsis is a complex response to infection. It is clinically characterized by tachycardia, tachypnea, either hyperthermia or hypothermia, and usually an elevated or occasionally suppressed white blood cell count. Sepsis occurs in older patients with significant co-morbidities and has a poor prognosis.

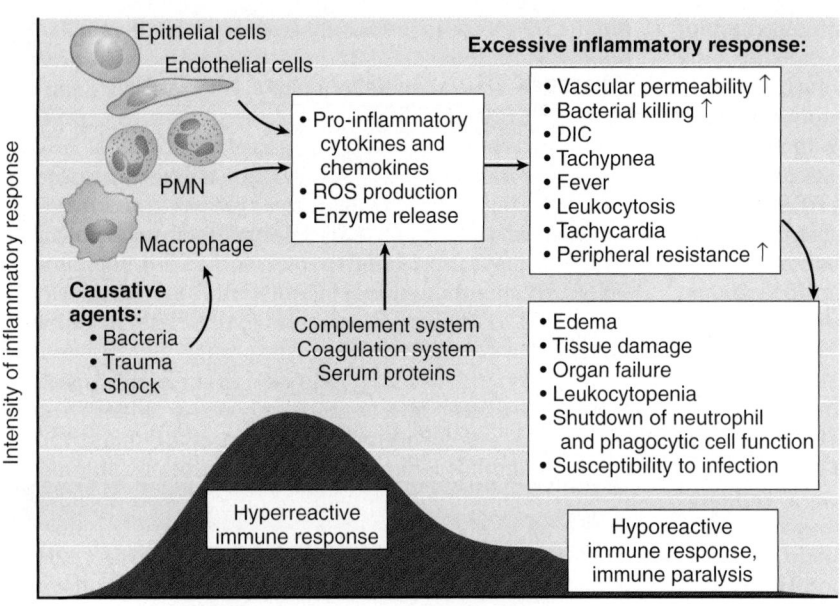

FIGURE 90-9   Excessive inflammatory response leads to severe immune paralysis. DIC, disseminated intravascular coagulation; PMN, polymorphonuclear leukocyte; ROS, reactive oxygen species.

Dynamic time-course of the inflammatory response during sepsis

---

Common Therapeutics

- Pain
  - Morphine
  - Topical or sublingual nitrates
  - Oxygen
- Breathlessness
  - Oxygen to maintain saturations >94%
  - Morphine
  - Diuretics if patients are clinically in pulmonary edema
- Anticoagulation
  - Low-molecular-weight or unfractionated heparin, regardless of stage of life, if no contraindications exist

---

Epidemiology and Prevalence

The incidence of sepsis, severe sepsis, and septic shock seems to be increasing. The incidence is approximately 50 to 100 cases per 100,000 population per year. This increase may reflect an aging population, together with the use of more indwelling devices, invasive procedures, and immunosuppression in at-risk groups who may not previously have been offered these interventions. Mortality is high, 25% to 50%, depending on co-morbidities.

Pathophysiology

Sepsis results from a complicated series of events initiated by the interaction of pathogens with host defenses. The most significant immediate response by the host is cytokine release, which sets up an inflammatory cascade. This process changes the endothelium: capillaries become more permeable, vasodilation occurs, and coagulation changes lead to thrombi and organ ischemia (Fig. 90-9 and "Case Study: Sepsis").

CASE STUDY

Sepsis

Mr. PS is a 77-year-old man with metastatic renal cell carcinoma who had been coping independently at home. He presented acutely unwell, with delirium, incontinence of urine, and vomiting. On examination, he was hypothermic (35° C), tachycardic (pulse, 120 beats/min), and hypotensive (blood pressure, 85/60 mm Hg). He was incontinent of malodorous urine.

Despite his advanced disease, Mr. PS was resuscitated with 0.9% sodium chloride fluid. Based on the premise that a renal tract infection was responsible for this presentation, a combination of ceftriaxone and metronidazole was administered. Gentamicin was not given because of the patient's known underlying renal impairment.

Clinical Manifestations

Presenting problems of sepsis include the following:

- Fevers or rigors
- Nausea or vomiting
- Fatigue
- Confusion
- Dyspnea
- Localizing symptoms:
- Dysuria
- Cough
- Abdominal pain
- Headache
- Sore throat

Diagnosis of Systemic Inflammatory Response Syndrome

At least two or more of the following signs are necessary to confirm the diagnosis of SIRS:

- Tachypnea
- Tachycardia (>90 beats/min)
- Either hyperthermia (>38° C) or hypothermia (<36° C)
- White blood cell count either elevated (>12,000/mL) or reduced (<4000/mL)

Investigations must be tailored to the estimated prognosis of the individual before the onset of this problem (Table 90-14).

Differential Diagnosis

The following serious medical conditions may mimic sepsis:

- Cardiogenic shock
- Extensive myocardial infarction
- Saddle PE
- Major hemorrhage
- Hypoadrenal crisis
- Acute pancreatitis
- Diabetic ketoacidosis

Treatment

Treatments must be tailored to the overall prognosis. In some patients, measures to ensure only comfort are appropriate. Patients with a previously good prognosis require immediate consultation from intensive care services.

Immediate Management

- Identification and elimination of the septic foci
  - Removal of infected catheters or venous access devices
  - Identification and drainage of abscess
  - Débridement of infected tissue
- Fluid resuscitation guided by vital signs (including central venous pressure) and urine output
- Broad-spectrum antibiotics (based on the particular risk factors for infection) and assessment of the patient's immune state
- Supportive care and management of other symptoms:
  - Oxygen, to keep saturations greater than 90 mm Hg
  - Treatment of delirium with haloperidol
  - Treatment of nausea and vomiting
  - Ensuring that pain is considered and addressed appropriately

Drugs of Choice

- Fluid resuscitation
  - A crystalloid fluid should be the initial choice of intravenous fluid (either 0.9% sodium chloride or 4% dextrose with N/5 saline).
- Antibiotics need to be broad spectrum and tailored to the patient's risk factors. All patients should receive coverage for gram-positive, gram-negative, and anaerobic bacteria. Special consideration should be given in the following situations:
  - Patients with central access devices should receive staphylococcal coverage.
  - Patients with burns should receive coverage for *Pseudomonas*.
  - Local guidelines for treatment of infectious diseases should be consulted.

Evidence-Based Medicine

- Recombinant human activated protein C and low-dose corticosteroids may improve mortality in some patients.
- Patients with a previously good prognosis and evidence of lung injury should be ventilated.
- Patients with a hemoglobin value lower than 90 g/dL should be transfused.
- All patients should receive DVT and stress ulcer prophylaxis.

FAMILY CRISIS

Traumatic events are those associated with actual or threat of injury or death. For the individual and those associated

TABLE 90-14	Investigations of Sepsis and Expected Results
TESTS	**EXPECTED FINDINGS AND INDICATIONS**
Full blood cell count	Hemoglobin < 10 g/dL Platelets may be elevated, reflecting inflammation; platelets reduced in DIC White cell count usually elevated but sometimes suppressed
Coagulation studies	Elevated prothrombin time, activated partial thromboplastin time, D-dimer or fibrinogen degradation products in DIC, decreased fibrinogen levels in DIC
Renal function tests	Abnormal in hypoperfusion renal failure
Liver function tests	Helpful in localizing sepsis; consider biliary sepsis, especially in elderly patients with no obvious localizing signs
Blood cultures	Three sets of cultures must be obtained in all patients before administration of antibiotics
Urine cultures	Part of the diagnostic workup for sepsis
Lumbar puncture and cerebrospinal fluid examination	Performed after cerebral computed tomography in suspected meningitis; antibiotics should *not be* withheld until after cerebrospinal fluid is obtained
Imaging	
Chest radiography	May provide diagnostic and prognostic information
Abdominal ultrasound	Noninvasive and well tolerated investigation especially for suspected intra-abdominal or biliary sepsis or upper urinary tract infections
Computed tomography	Provides both diagnostic information and may also guide treatment when abscess is the septic focus

DIC, disseminated intravascular coagulation.

Future Considerations

- Whether all patients should receive corticosteroids or whether only those patients with suppressed adrenal function as measured by cortisol levels should be given these agents has not been determined.
- The optimal method of preventing the development of sepsis in patients at risk is not yet clear.
- The role of melatonin and of tumor necrosis factor blockade in the treatment of sepsis will require further examination.

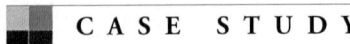

CASE STUDY

Family Crisis

Mrs. ED is a 32-year-old woman with a recent diagnosis of hepatocellular cancer. She and her husband have been advised of the seriousness of the situation, the lack of interventions available to change the behavior of the cancer, and her very limited prognosis. During the conference at the hospital, more family members appeared. They demanded further information and became abusive to Mrs. ED's husband and the staff.

with that individual, these events may generate fear, helplessness, or horror that may lead to a crisis. Family members in this situation require support, comfort, information, assurance, and proximity to the sick individual. A family's relationship of trust with the professionals involved will reduce or prevent displays of anger and frustration, which impair the relationships of the individual, the family, and the health care staff.

Epidemiology and Prevalence

Families may be categorized into different classes based on their functional capacity. Cohesiveness, family conflict, and anger are characteristics that lead families to be at greater risk of crisis and complicated bereavements. Approximately 10% to 15% of families in palliative medicine fall into this category (see "Case Study: Family Crisis").

Interventions

Intervening in family crisis includes the following steps:

- Early identification of families likely to be at risk of dysfunctional behaviors is important.
- Ensure that family members have been offered or involved in a well-run family conference.
- When a crisis occurs, listen to the family.
- Ensure that an advocate is nominated for the family.
- If necessary, enlist the skills of an independent counselor who is not involved with the direct care of the patient (e.g., patient representative, hospital ethics committee).

SUGGESTED READING

Annane D, Bellissant E, Cavaillon JM. Septic shock. Lancet 2005;365:63-78.

Chao S, Atwood E. Peripheral edema. Am J Med 2002; 113:580-586.

Covey A. Management of malignant effusions and ascites. J Support Oncol 2005;3:169-178.

Cunha BA. Sepsis and its mimics. Intern Med 1992;13:48-55.

Cunha BA. The atypical pneumonias: Clinical diagnosis and importance. Clin Microbiol Infect 2006;12(Suppl 3):12-24.

Currow D, Clark K. Emergencies in Palliative and Supportive Care. Oxford: Oxford University Press, 2006.

Duncan J, Sandar J, Sisoidyia J, Walker M. Adult epilepsy. Lancet 2006;367:1087-1100.

File TM. Clinical implications and treatment of multiresistant *Streptococcus pneumoniae* pneumonia. Clin Microbiol Infect 2006;12(Suppl 3):31-41.

Fox K. Update on acute coronary syndromes. Heart 2004; 90:698-706.

Goldstein JA. Cardiac tamponade, constrictive pericarditis and restrictive cardiomyopathy. Curr Probl Cardiol 2004; 24:503-567.

Gullo A, Bianco N, Berlot G. Management of severe sepsis and septic shock: Challenges and recommendations. Crit Care Clin 2006;22:489-501.

Ho W, Hankey G, Lee C, Eikelboom J. Venous thromboembolism: Diagnosis and management. Med J Aust 2005;182: 476-481.

Katalaris P. Chest pain: Differentiating GIT from cardiac causes. Aust Fam Physician 2001;30:847-851.

Kissane D, McKenzie M, Bloch S, et al. Family focused grief therapy: A randomised, controlled trail in palliative care and bereavement. Am J Psychiatry 2006;7:1208-1218.

Laird A, Driscoll P, Wardrope J. The ABC of community emergency care: Chest pain. J Emerg Med 2004;21:226-232.

Nguyen HB, Rivers EP, Abrahamian FM, et al., Emergency Department Sepsis Education Program and Strategies to Improve Survival (ED-SEPSIS) Working Group. Severe sepsis and septic shock: Review of the literature and emergency department management guidelines. Ann Emerg Med 2006;48:28-54.

Patterson J, Garwick A. Levels of meaning in the family stress theory. Fam Process 1994;33:287-304.

Pendleton R, Wheeler M, Rodgers G. Venous thromboembolism prevention in the acutely ill medical patient: A review of the literature and focus on special populations. Am J Hematol 2005;79:229-237.

Phillip J, Gold M, Schwarz M, Komesaroff P. Anger in palliative care: A clinical approach. Intern Med J 2007;37:49-55.

Prandoni P, Falanga A, Piccioli A. Cancer and venous thromboembolism. Lancet Oncol 2005;6:401-410.

Rahimtoola A, Bergin J. Acute pulmonary embolism: An update on diagnosis and management. Curr Probl Cardiol 2005; 30:61-114.

Rahman NM, Chapman SJ, Davies RJ. Pleural effusions: A structured approach to care. Br Med Bull 2004;72:31-47.

Rello J, Diaz E, Rodriguez A. Advances in the management of pneumonia in the ICU: Review of current thinking. Clin Microbiol Infect 2005;11(Suppl 5):30-38.

Sessler CN, Perry JC, Varney KL. Management of severe sepsis and septic shock. Curr Opin Crit Care 2004;10:354-63.

Shiozaki M, Morita T, Hirai K, et al. Why are bereaved family members dissatisfied with specialist inpatient palliative care service? A nationwide qualitative study. Palliat Med 2005; 19:319-327.

Soler-Soler J, Sagirista-Sauleda J, Permanyer-Mirala G. General cardiology: Management of pericardial effusions. Heart 2001;86:235-240.

Surven R, Waterhouse E. Management of status epilepticus. Am Fam Physician 2005;68:469-476.

Syren S, Saveman B-I, Benzein E. Being a family in the midst of living and dying. J Palliat Care 2006;22:26-32.

Warrell D, Cox T, Firth J (eds). Oxford Textbook of Medicine. Oxford: Oxford University Press, 2003.

Watson M, Lucas C, Hoy A, Back (eds). Oxford Handbook of Palliative Care. Oxford: Oxford University Press, 2005.

Infections

CHAPTER 91

Infections In Palliative Medicine

Ruth L. Lagman and Susan J. Rehm

KEY POINTS

- Infections are common in non-neutropenic individuals with advanced illness, and they are a significant cause of mortality and morbidity.

- Mild to life-threatening urinary and respiratory tract infections are common.

- Anti-infectives are often initiated based on clinical evaluation alone (i.e., signs and symptoms on presentation) without laboratory and other diagnostic confirmation.

- The decision to start an anti-infective drug in the palliative care patient population is controversial, because ethical considerations of providing comfort in advanced disease versus prolonging suffering and the dying process often arise.

- There are no guidelines to assist physicians about when to treat infections in this patient population. The research is limited and often difficult to conduct.

Pneumonia is called the "old man's friend" because if left untreated, patients often succumb peacefully.[1] Infections are common in palliative medicine and are a common cause of morbidity and mortality. People with advanced illness brought to the attention of their physicians with signs and symptoms of lethargy, fever, and delirium often present a dilemma. Is this a reversible or irreversible infection? What are the goals of care? What does this patient want? If the patient is unable to make decisions, what does his or her spokesperson want? How much diagnostic intervention should be done? Should antibiotics even be given? If so, how long? How do the potential costs—both financial and in terms of adverse events—stack up against the potential benefits? These are the questions palliative medicine physicians face daily.

INCIDENCE

The prevalence of infections in advanced illness may be difficult to discern. The distinction, for example, between palliative medicine and hospice patients is not always clear. What will likely guide their management is their status within the disease trajectory and the overall goals of care. There are sparse data published, and the study authors often are not specific about the population treated. Published data suggest that the proportion of palliative care patients treated for infection ranges from 36% to 88%.[2-6]

Infections in patients with hematological malignancies have been extensively investigated, but there have been few studies of infections in non-neutropenic patients with solid tumors.[7] Infections are a common cause of morbidity and mortality in advanced metastatic disease. This is also true in nonmalignant, life-limiting illnesses, such as dementia. The proportion of patients with advanced cancer who developed infections (29%) resembled that of patients admitted to an acute care palliative medicine unit (27%). In both populations, *Escherichia coli* was the most common pathogen, causing 19% of infections.[3,4]

In one study, 88% of palliative medicine patients, including people with dementia and advanced cancer, admitted because of an acute medical condition were treated empirically with antibiotics. Dementia patients were more likely to receive antibiotics than patients with advanced cancer.[5] A large, retrospective review of Medicare patients hospitalized for community-acquired pneumonia (CAP) demonstrated the following:

- Mortality from CAP was directly proportional to age and the number of co-morbidities.
- Individuals with malignancies and with liver and renal dysfunction had the highest mortality rates.
- Fifty percent of these individuals were more likely to die within a few months, even if they survived their hospitalization for CAP.[8]

CONTRIBUTING FACTORS

Older individuals who have more co-morbidities are more susceptible to infections (Table 91-1).[9] Those who have altered anatomical barriers (i.e., skin, mucosa, airways, and viscera) lose their normal defenses. When performance status declines, they are more likely to have aspiration pneumonia and decubitus ulcers. They are often multisymptomatic, with a median number of 11 symptoms (range, 1 to 23),[10] leading some to polypharmacy. Most of these drugs predispose to dry mouth. Corticosteroids are also commonly used in this population. Xerostomia and steroids can cause oral thrush. Opioids may cause immunosuppression, but the clinical significance of this phenomenon remains unclear.[11]

TABLE 91-1 Factors Contributing to Infection

DISRUPTION OF ANATOMICAL BARRIERS
Skin
Mucosae
Respiratory tract
Viscera

POOR PERFORMANCE STATUS

DRUGS
Opioids
Corticosteroids

SYMPTOMS
Dry mouth
Intractable nausea or vomiting

POOR NUTRITIONAL STATUS
Anorexia
Cachexia

IMMUNOSUPPRESSION
Hypogammaglobulinemia

COMPLICATIONS OF ADVANCED ILLNESS
Ascites

PALLIATIVE TREATMENT
Radiation
Chemotherapy

CYTOKINES
Transforming growth factor-β (TGF-β)
Interleukin-2 (IL-2)
Tumor necrosis factor-α (TNF-α)

INVASIVE DEVICES
Urinary catheters
Long-term venous access devices

Box 91-1 Common Invasive Devices Used in Palliative Medicine

Indwelling urinary catheter
Central venous catheter (tunneled and nontunneled)
Peripherally inserted central catheter (PICC)
Subcutaneous port
Biliary stent
Ureteral stent
Gastrostomy tube
Transesophogeal gastrostomy tube
Pleurx catheters

The nutritional status of individuals with advanced age, malignancies, and other chronic conditions is often poor. They may be anorexic and cachectic, resulting in hypogammaglobulinemia. Some may be neutropenic, but most individuals with advanced cancer or other nonmalignant, life-limiting illness are not.

Some individuals have prosthetic devices or appliances (i.e., stents, tubes, catheters, central venous catheters, or ports) that may become infected or obstructed (Box 91-1). Although venous access devices are usually not a factor in

the care of hospice patients, they significantly increase the risk for bloodstream infections. In one study, 34% of cancer patients with a tunneled central venous catheter developed bacteremia or fungemia.[12] The risk for device-related infection varies by device. A retrospective analysis of patients admitted to an acute care palliative medicine unit demonstrated no significant difference in the rate of urinary tract infections among those with or without an indwelling urinary catheter.[3]

Cytokines such as transforming growth factor-β (TGF-β), interleukin-2 (IL2), and tumor necrosis factor-α (TNF-α) may play a role in susceptibility and reaction to infection.[13] Most patients referred to hospice have exhausted their antitumor treatment options (i.e., chemotherapy and irradiation) and face progressive disease. In some cases, the sequelae from previous therapy, including bone marrow insufficiency, immunosuppression, tissue fibrosis, and fistulas, may predispose to infection.

SIGNS AND SYMPTOMS OF INFECTION

Fever, often the cardinal sign of infection, is common but nonspecific in the palliative medicine population. Among hospitalized patients with advanced disease who were not in intensive care units, 66% were febrile.[14] In many, the fever was caused by infection. Medications, blood transfusions, atelectasis, and allergic reactions contributed.[14] Among cancer patients, particularly those with solid tumors, fever may result from the malignancy.

Fever may be absent. Other systemic symptoms (i.e., malaise, anorexia, confusion, and weight loss) commonly associated with infection are frequently related to the underlying condition.[15] Leukocytosis may be absent; when present, it may represent a leukemoid reaction from the malignancy or corticosteroid therapy rather than an infection. Because patients are multisymptomatic, they may be taking adjuvant analgesics for pain (i.e., nonsteroidal anti-inflammatory drugs [NSAIDs], acetaminophen, and corticosteroids), all of which may mask fever. Other symptoms that may represent manifestations of the underlying condition or harbingers of impending infection include pain, cough, dysuria, and diarrhea.

Clinicians rely on patients' and caregivers' knowledge of baseline medical status and their sensitivity to changes in symptoms and signs. Cultures of indwelling catheters or drains often represent colonization rather than active infection. Because the clinical presentation in advanced cancer can be nonspecific, antibiotics are often initiated empirically for presumed infection without confirmatory diagnostic tests. Changes in symptoms, rather than the symptoms themselves, may be most helpful in determining the need for empirical antimicrobial therapy.

DIAGNOSTIC TESTS

The use of diagnostic tests for patients with advanced illness is controversial (Table 91-2). Data to support evidence of infection are sparse and difficult to find for this patient population. The treatment setting also influences the decision to order confirmatory diagnostic tests. If a patient is brought to an acute care hospital to treat a presumed infection, basic laboratory and radiologic procedures may be done routinely. Some are admitted to

TABLE 91-2 Diagnostic Tests for Infections
CULTURES
Urine
Sputum
Blood
Wound
IMAGING
Ultrasonography
Computed tomography
Magnetic resonance imaging

inpatient hospices that may or may not have laboratory or radiographical resources. A positive culture does not establish the diagnosis of infection. For example, the urine samples of all patients with long-term indwelling urinary catheters are colonized with bacteria, leading to a positive urine culture; however, this usually represents asymptomatic colonization rather than infection.[16] Likewise, culture of an established drainage device (e.g., chest tube, biliary T tube) is likely to result in positive cultures irrelevant to the acute infection.

Patients often are treated empirically based on clinical signs and symptoms alone. In a retrospective study, 88% of patients who died with advanced dementia or metastatic cancer during hospitalization at a large New York City teaching hospital were treated empirically with antibiotics during admission.[5] Therapeutic trials with antibiotics are common, and diagnostic tests often are not performed. If there is a suspected infection, antibiotics will be started empirically, regardless of the results of laboratory tests.

COMMON INFECTIONS IN ADVANCED ILLNESS

In two retrospective studies in palliative medicine units,[3,4] urinary tract infection, septicemia, and pneumonia were among the more common infections treated in an acute care setting. In one study involving palliative medicine patients, chest infections were more common than urinary tract infections (52% versus 29%), perhaps related to differences in the definition of infection.[17] People admitted to a hospice develop the same types of infection.[2,18] This is significant because infections are often correlated with typical microbiological isolates in addition to clinical symptoms. Less frequently observed infections in palliative medicine and inpatient hospice settings are skin, soft tissue, or wound infections and oral infections.[2-4]

Common organisms isolated from hospice and palliative medicine patients include *E. coli*, *Klebsiella pneumoniae*, *Staphylococcus* species (i.e., *S. aureus* and coagulase-negative staphylococci), and enterococci.[2-4,18] *Pseudomonas aeruginosa*, a pathogen feared because of its virulence and potential for antimicrobial drug resistance, has been a surprisingly uncommon isolate. *P. aeruginosa* was the causative organism in approximately 10% of urinary tract infections, bacteremias, pneumonias, and miscellaneous infections in an acute care palliative medicine unit.[3]

TREATMENT OF INFECTIONS IN ADVANCED ILLNESS

Despite the high incidence of infections in patients with advanced disease, there are no clear guidelines for the initiation and continuation of anti-infective medications in this setting. Most commonly, empirical anti-infective therapy is based on clinical judgment rather than culture or radiographical findings. In a large, retrospective study involving palliative medicine patients in an inpatient setting, gentamicin, ticarcillin, vancomycin, and ceftazidime were the most frequently prescribed antibiotics.[3] Because it was an acute care setting, 82% of individuals were treated with parenteral antibiotics, and sometimes, two or three agents were administered. The median time of treatment in this unit was 11 days, and the median duration of hospital stay was 12 days (range, 1 to 84 days). In another palliative medicine inpatient unit, 72% of patients were treated with antibiotics: trimethoprim-sulfamethoxazole, ciprofloxacin, or amoxicillin. In contrast to the previous study, oral preparations were used in 72% of the episodes. Patients were treated for an average of 6.4 ± 3.3 days (median of 7 days; range, 1 to 21 days).[4]

A retrospective study involving palliative care patients admitted to a district hospital showed that antibiotics were administered empirically to 61% of those with presumed infective episodes; the types of antibiotics were not specified.[17] In one of the few studies that measured outcomes of infections, antibiotic use in an inpatient palliative medicine unit was monitored for 13 months, during which only 41 of 913 patients were treated with antibiotics. Sixty-two percent had "helpful" outcomes, 19% were unhelpful, and another 19% could not be assessed. The mean duration of parenteral antibiotic administration was 2.3 days, and the maximum length of therapy was 9 days.[19]

A Dutch prospective cohort study of patients with Alzheimer's disease demonstrated that treatment of pneumonia improved quality of life (i.e., reduction in signs and symptoms) and increased average survival by 3 months.[20] Use of antibiotics for hospice and palliative medicine patients with possible infection may vary according to the local practice setting and various cultural influences. In a comparative study of Alzheimer's patients who developed lower respiratory infection in the Netherlands or in Missouri, individuals in the United States were more likely to be hospitalized, intravenously hydrated, and given parenteral antibiotics (i.e., second- and third-generation cephalosporins as opposed to amoxicillin in the Netherlands).[21] Eighty-four percent of terminal cancer patients in Korea were hospitalized and given antibiotics for presumed infection.[6]

CONTROVERSIES

There are no generally accepted guidelines for treatment of infections in patients with advanced illness. In a retrospective study involving 1256 individuals in an extended care facility, the mortality rate was high for those not treated with antibiotics and hospitalized compared with those treated (59% versus 9%).[22] This controversial study showed that physicians often made clinical judgments regarding those they believed would benefit from anti-infective therapy compared with those who would not. Later retrospective studies of treatment of infections in patients with advanced illness showed that 36% to 88% were treated for infections.[2-6]

Prognostication, the ability to predict an individual's life expectancy based on objective information, is often inaccurate. The decision to treat a presumed infection is based on clinical symptoms, extent of underlying disease, and performance status in conjunction with the individual physician's past experience in treating these individuals.

Hospice patients treated with antibiotics seemed to have a longer survival time than those who were not.[23] Often, the argument is made that intervening with antibiotics only postpones the inevitable and causes unnecessary suffering by prolonging dying.[24] However, antibiotics are often used until the time of death in palliative care units.[6,25]

The possibility of antibiotic side effects impacts the risk-benefit equation when empirical antimicrobial therapy is contemplated. Adverse events related to antimicrobials run the gamut of severity, but compromised patients are often unable to tolerate side effects that would otherwise serve as little more than an annoyance. Antibiotic-associated anorexia, taste disturbances, rashes, oral thrush, intertrigo, and loose stools may be devastating for a compromised patient. Diarrhea is a particular concern because of the potential for rapid dehydration in frail patients. It is also important, but clinically difficult, to distinguish between simple antibiotic-associated diarrhea and illness due to toxin production by *Clostridium difficile*.

The rate of *C. difficile* infection is increasing[26] and may be attributable to the use of fluoroquinolones,[27,28] the use of broad-spectrum antimicrobials, and the use of multiple agents.[29] The emergence of a particularly virulent strain of *C. difficile* has led to excess morbidity and mortality, particularly among the elderly.[30] Even with aggressive hydration and use of oral metronidazole or vancomycin, or both, many patients experience severe colitis, leading to colectomy in some.

Individuals with advanced illness are usually polysymptomatic and have multiple co-morbidities. Polypharmacy is common. Drug interactions play a significant role in the use and choice of anti-infective therapy.[31] Certain antibiotics may produce significant organ toxicity (e.g., hematological, renal, hepatic) and affect the use of other therapeutic agents.[31]

With each decision to use antimicrobial therapy, a risk-benefit and cost-benefit analysis takes place. Although clinicians usually focus on the impact of these decisions on the individual, societal risks, benefits, and costs should also be considered. Societal implications are difficult to measure. Regardless of the practice setting, widespread use of antibiotics leads to microorganism resistance. The Infectious Diseases Society of America's guidelines on antibiotic stewardship emphasize the need for responsible antimicrobial therapy.[32]

Ethical considerations in the treatment of infections[33] in advanced disease include the following:

- Delay in hospice enrollment until a parenteral antibiotic regimen is completed because the cost of these antibiotics may be prohibitive

- Economic impact of parenteral antibiotic therapy to hospice services in a capitated reimbursement system
- Possible contribution of antimicrobial therapy to prolongation of the dying process
- Dilemmas in determining criteria for institution or discontinuation of antibiotics when goals of care are defined for a patient's comfort
- The impact of unnecessary treatment of infections on drug resistance

Measuring outcomes of anti-infective therapy can be difficult.[19] Available studies are inconsistent in the parameters used to determine outcomes, and formal risk-benefit analyses are lacking. The measurement of outcomes with anti-infectives will continue to be a challenge for several reasons:

- The population is diverse and in different stages of their disease trajectories.
- Goals of care may not be clearly defined at the time infection is recognized.
- Resource use, particularly in the hospice population, will continue to present some limitations on how many diagnostic and therapeutic interventions can be performed in those with advanced illness.
- The uncertainty of duration of survival in this population with chronic and often fatal disease will always be a factor.

CONCLUSIONS

Infections are common in non-neutropenic individuals with advanced illness. Urinary and respiratory tract infections are the most common types. In the absence of established treatment guidelines, patients are often treated empirically with antimicrobial agents based on their clinical signs and symptoms.

Because of general frailty and preexisting organ dysfunction, palliative medicine and hospice patients may be particularly vulnerable to adverse clinical events and laboratory abnormalities associated with antibiotic use. The initiation of anti-infective medication in this patient population remains controversial because of economic and ethical implications.

Although infections are a major cause of mortality, research in this area is sparse. Future efforts should focus on prospective studies of practice guidelines with risk-benefit and cost-benefit analyses along with outcome measurements. These are challenging tasks for most palliative medicine specialists. The current fragmented system of medical care delivery does not encourage clear communication and defined goals of care for individuals with advanced illness.

REFERENCES

1. Osler W. Principles and Practice of Medicine Designed for the Use of Practitioners and Students of Medicine, 3rd ed. Edinburgh: Young J. Pentland, 1898, pp 108-137.
2. Vitetta L, Kenner D, Sali A. Bacterial infections in the terminally ill hospice patients. J Pain Symptom Manage 2000;20:326-334.
3. Homsi J, Walsh D, Panta R, et al. Infectious complications of advanced cancer. Support Care Cancer 2000;8:487-492.
4. Pereira J, Watanabe S, Wolch G. A retrospective review of the frequency of infections and patterns of antibiotic utilization on a palliative care unit. J Pain Symptom Manage 1998;16:374-381.

5. Ahronheim JC, Morrison RS, Baskin SA, et al. Treatment of the dying in the acute care hospital: Advanced dementia and metastatic cancer. Arch Intern Med 1996;156:2094-2100.
6. Oh DY, Kim JH, Kim DW, et al. Antibiotic use during the last days of life in cancer patients. Eur J Cancer Care 2006;15:74-79.
7. Rossini F. Prognosis of infections in elderly patients with haematologic diseases. Support Care Cancer 1996;4:46-50.
8. Kaplan V, Clermont G, Griffin MF, et al. Pneumonia: Still the old man's friend? Arch Intern Med 2003;163:317-323.
9. Pawelec G. Immunity and ageing in man. Exp Gerontol 2006;41:1239-1242.
10. Donnelly S, Walsh D, Rybicki L. The symptoms of advanced cancer: Identification of clinical and research priorities by assessment of prevalence and severity. J Palliat Care 1995;11:27-32.
11. Budd K. Pain management: Is opioid immunosuppression a clinical problem? Biomed Pharmacother 2006;60:310-317.
12. Groeger JS, Lucas AB, Thaler HT, et al. Infectious morbidity associated with long-term use of venous access devices in patients with cancer. Ann Intern Med 1993;119:1168-1174.
13. Elliot RL, Blobe GC. Role of transforming growth factor beta in human cancer. J Clin Oncol 2005;23:2078-2093.
14. Bodey GP. Infection in cancer patients: A continuing association. Am J Med 1986;81:11-26.
15. McClure CL. Common infections in the elderly. Am Fam Physician 1992;45:2691-2698.
16. Warren JW, Tenney JH, Hoopes JM, et al. A prospective microbiologic study of bacteriuria in patients with chronic indwelling urethral catheters. J Infect Dis 1986;146:719-723.
17. Lam PT, Chan KS, Tse CY, Leung MW. Retrospective analysis of antibiotic use and survival in advanced cancer patients with infections. J Pain Symptom Manage 2005;30:536-543.
18. White PH, Kuhlenschmidt HL, Vancura BG, Navari RM. Antimicrobial use in patients with advanced cancer receiving hospice care. J Pain Symptom Manage 2003;25:438-443.
19. Clayton J, Fardell B, Hutton-Potts J, et al. Parenteral antibiotics in a palliative care unit: Prospective analysis of current practice. Palliat Med 2003;17:44-48.
20. Van der Steen JT, Ooms ME, vanderWal G, Ribbe MW. Pneumonia: The demented patient's best friend? Discomfort after starting or withholding antibiotic treatment. J Am Geriatr Soc 2002;50:1681-1688.
21. Van der Steen JT, Kruse RL, Ooms ME, et al. Treatment of nursing home residents with dementia and lower respiratory tract infection in the United States and the Netherlands: An ocean apart. J Am Geriatr Soc 2004;52:691-699.
22. Brown NK, Thompson DJ. Nontreatment of fever in extended care facilities N Engl J Med 1979;300:1246-1250.
23. Chen LK, Chou YC, Hsu PS, et al. Antibiotic prescription for fever episodes in hospice patients. Support Care Cancer 2002;10:538-541.
24. Nagy-Agren S, Haley H. Management of infections in palliative care patients with advanced cancer. J Pain Symptom Manage 2002;24:64-70.
25. Oneschuk D, Fainsinger R, Demoissac D. Antibiotic use in the last week of life in three palliative care settings. J Palliat Care 2002;18:25-28.
26. Blossom DB, McDonald LC. The challenges posed by reemerging *Clostridium difficile* infection. Clin Infect Dis 2007;45:222-227.
27. Muto CA, Pokrywka M, Shutt K, et al. A large outbreak of *Clostridium difficile*-associated disease with an unexpected proportion of deaths and colectomies at a teaching hospital following increased fluoroquinolone use. Infect Control Hosp Epidemiol 2005;26:273-280.
28. Gaynes R, Rimland D, Killum E, et al. Outbreak of *Clostridium difficile* infection in a long-term care facility: Association with gatifloxacin use. Clin Infect Dis 2004;38:640-645.
29. Bignardi GE. Risk factors for *Clostridium difficile* infection. J Hosp Infect 1998;40:1-15.
30. McDonald LC, Killgore GE, Thompson A, et al. An epidemic, toxin gene-variant strain of *Clostridium difficile*. N Engl J Med 2005;353:2433-2441.
31. Bernard SA. The interaction of medications used in palliative care. Hematol Oncol Clin North Am 2002;16:641-655.
32. Dellit TH, Owens RC, McGowen JE Jr, et al. Infectious Diseases Society of America and the Society for Healthcare Epidemiology of America guidelines for developing an institutional program to enhance antimicrobial stewardship. Clin Infect Dis 2007;44:159-177.
33. Ford PJ, Fraser TG, Davis MP, Kodish E. Anti-infective therapy at the end of life: Ethical decision-making in hospice-eligible patients. Bioethics 2005;19:379-392.

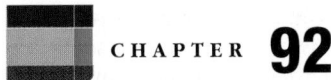

Prevention and Control of Infections

Susan F. FitzGerald and Lynda E. Fenelon

KEY POINTS

- The routine application of basic infection control practices should be integral to the delivery of palliative care, in all care settings, for the safety and well-being of patients and staff.

- Effective hand hygiene is the single most effective way of preventing transmission of infection.

- Correct handling and disposal of sharps is essential to prevent transmission of bloodborne viruses such as hepatitis and the human immunodeficiency virus (HIV).

- Indwelling devices should be appropriately managed to reduce the risk of associated infection.

- Infections with multidrug-resistant organisms can cause considerable morbidity and mortality, so every care should be taken to prevent their occurrence and subsequent spread.

The population served by palliative medicine is diverse, with a wide range of chronic and terminal conditions. Many patients have factors that predispose them to infection, such as indwelling devices, chronic wounds and pressure sores, and suppression of immune function due to their disease, its treatment, or both. Infection can manifest with many different symptoms, which increase patient discomfort, cause additional morbidity, and hasten death. Prevention of infection and the spread of infection is vital for both patients and health care workers.

Palliative care patients may receive care in various places, including acute care settings, hospices, and the home. Most infection control standards have been devised for acute care facilities, and some recommendations may not be easily translated to, or indeed necessary in, other settings. However, the basic principles of infection prevention and control should be applied at all times in palliative medicine to ensure that services are delivered in an environment that is safe for patients and staff.

All organizations providing palliative care services should have in place a system in which the corporate lines of responsibility for prevention and control of infection are defined and provide clear and regularly updated policies relevant to local needs. These should be evidence-based and consistent with scientific knowledge and expert consensus. All staff should receive education and training in infection control practices when starting work and at regular intervals thereafter.

BASIC PRINCIPLES OF INFECTION CONTROL

For infection to occur, several elements are required. These include a microorganism capable of causing infection, a reservoir of that organism (e.g., human, equipment, environment), a route of transmission, and a susceptible host. Interventions aimed at these elements can reduce the potential for infection or prevent its transmission. In general, multiple or "bundled" interventions have more success than a single intervention.

Basic infection control precautions should be applied to the care of all patients to reduce transmission of microorganisms from recognized and unrecognized sources. These are termed "standard precautions" and are aimed at all patients, regardless of their diagnosis or presumed infectious status.[1] They include hand hygiene, personal protective equipment (e.g., gloves, aprons, eyewear), correct handling and disposal of sharps and clinical waste, cleaning and decontamination of equipment and the environment, and appropriate patient placement (Box 92-1).

HAND HYGIENE

The hands of health care workers are the most likely vector for the transfer of microorganisms between patients, and effective hand hygiene is the single most important method of preventing transmission of infection.

Microorganisms on the hands may be resident or transient organisms. Resident organisms are normal skin flora, such as *Staphylococcus epidermidis*, and are infrequently implicated in infection. Removal of resident hand flora is indicated only before invasive procedures into normally sterile body sites. Transient organisms are those acquired during contact with patients, objects, or the environment. They include most of the organisms responsible for cross-infection, such as gram-negative bacilli, *Staphylococcus aureus*, and viruses. They are not part of the normal flora but survive on the hands for a limited time. Transient flora can be easily removed by effective hand hygiene. This can be achieved by hand washing with soap or detergent and water, or by an alcoholic hand rub on visibly clean hands. Alcoholic hand rubs may be particularly useful in home care, where there may not be ready access to hand washing facilities. Health care organizations should ensure adequate hand hygiene facilities for patients and staff (Fig. 92-1).

Optimal hand hygiene should be performed when hands are visibly soiled; before and after every patient contact, including handling of invasive devices and dressing of wounds; when moving from a contaminated area (e.g., wound) to a clean area of the same patient; after contact with blood, body fluid, clinical waste, or used laundry; after removal of gloves; after using the toilet; and before and after meals (Box 92-2).[2]

PERSONAL PROTECTIVE EQUIPMENT

Personal protective equipment (PPE) should be used as necessary, to protect the skin and mucous membranes from exposure to blood and body fluids and to prevent contamination of clothing, thus reducing the potential spread of organisms from patient to patient. The level of risk associated with a particular care activity or intervention must be assessed to decide whether PPE is indicated and, if so, what PPE is appropriate. PPE includes gloves, aprons and gowns, protective eyewear, and facemasks.

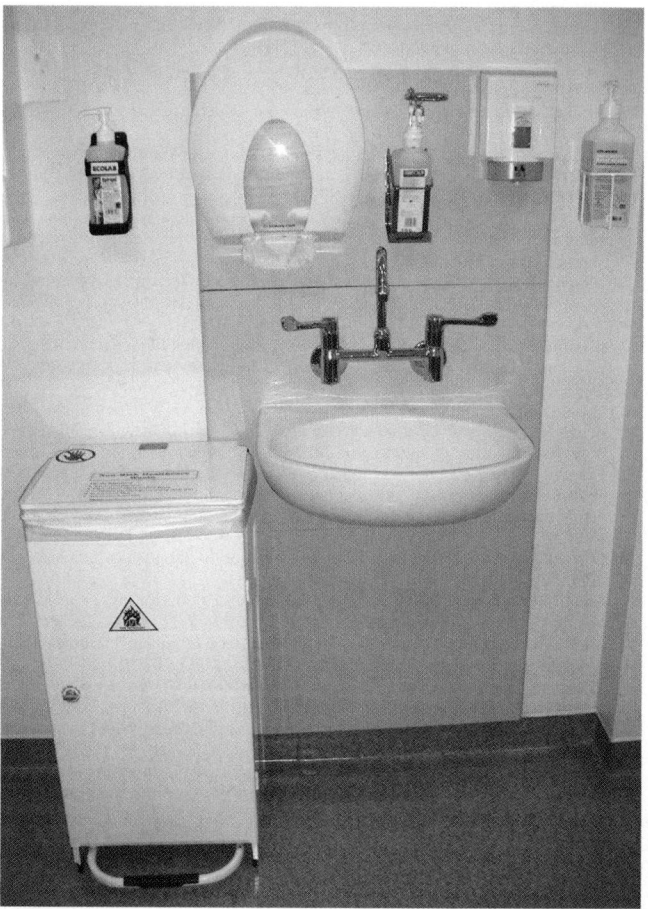

FIGURE 92-1 Adequate hand hygiene facilities should be provided in all health care settings.

Box 92-1 Basic Principles of Infection Prevention and Control

- Hand hygiene
- Personal protective equipment
- Isolation precautions
- Safe handling and disposal of sharps
- Safe handling and disposal of clinical waste
- Cleaning and decontamination of equipment
- Cleaning and disinfection of the environment

Box 92-2 Indications for Hand Hygiene

- When hands are visibly soiled
- Before and after patient contact
- When moving from a contaminated to a clean area of the same patient
- After removal of gloves
- After contact with
  - Blood or body fluid
  - Nonintact skin
  - Equipment contaminated with body fluid
  - Clinical waste
  - Used laundry
- After using the toilet
- Before leaving the clinical area
- Before and after meals

Gloves

Gloves should be worn for any activity during which blood or body fluid may contaminate the hands. Sterile gloves are indicated for aseptic procedures, nonsterile gloves for all other procedures. Gloves should be changed after each patient contact and between separate procedures on the same patient. They should also be changed if punctured or torn. Washing of single-use gloves between patients or procedures is unacceptable. Because the hands may become contaminated during glove removal, they must be decontaminated after gloves are used. Gloves contaminated with blood or body fluid must be considered as clinical waste and disposed of appropriately. Gloves are not a substitute for hand hygiene.[1]

Aprons and Gowns

Aprons are recommended during care activities when there is the potential that staff clothing may be contaminated by blood or body fluids and when caring for a patient who is colonized with an organism that has the potential for subsequent transmission to other patients or the environment. Single-use disposable plastic aprons are suitable for general use and should be removed immediately after use and discarded appropriately. Hand hygiene must be performed after removal of aprons.

For procedures likely to expose staff to spraying or splashing of blood or body fluids, a nonsterile, water-repellent gown should be worn. This should be disposed of appropriately after use, and the hands should be decontaminated after removal.

Protective Eyewear and Facemasks

Protective eyewear (glasses, goggles, or face-shields) prevent exposure of the mucous membranes to blood or body fluids splashed into the face during certain procedures. Eye protection and a facemask should be worn during procedures that are likely to generate droplets of blood or body fluid. Masks are not indicated for routine procedures. A surgical or procedure mask should be worn when within 1 m (3 feet) of patients with meningococcal disease, adenovirus, or influenza.[3] A particulate respirator (N95) is recommended in confirmed or suspected pulmonary tuberculosis.[4]

ISOLATION PRECAUTIONS

Physical isolation may be employed to prevent the spread of infection. When making a decision as to the type of isolation, it is important to consider the needs of the individual patient, the route of transmission of the infection in question, its potential severity, and the level of risk of spread to other patients and staff. There are two types of isolation precautions: (1) *source isolation*, in which the aim is to prevent the transmission of infection (known or suspected) to other patients or staff, and (2) *protective isolation* to prevent infection in severely immunocompromised patients who are at risk of infection from other patients or staff and the environment.

With regard to source isolation, a two-tier approach is recommended by the Centers for Disease Control and Prevention (CDC).[1] Standard precautions (see Box 92-1) should be applied to all patients, regardless of diagnosis or presumed infection status. Additional, "transmission-based" precautions supplement standard precautions and are grouped into categories depending on the route of transmission of infections. The main categories are airborne, droplet, and contact precautions.

Airborne Precautions

Airborne precautions should be applied to known or suspected infections caused by pathogens such as tuberculosis and varicella-zoster virus (chicken pox or disseminated varicella infection). Airborne transmission occurs by dissemination of small airborne droplet nuclei of 5 μm or less, or dust particles containing the microorganism, dispersed widely by air currents. If these particles are inhaled by a susceptible host and reach the alveoli, they can cause infection. Patients should be isolated in a negative-pressure ventilation room; the door must be kept closed at all times.

Droplet Precautions

Droplet precautions reduce transmission of infections by large particle droplets (>5 μm), including influenza, measles, mumps, and rubella. Droplet transmission occurs when such particles contact the conjunctivae or the mucous membranes of the nose or mouth of a susceptible person. These droplets are generated from the source patient during coughing, sneezing, or talking and during certain clinical procedures such as suctioning of the airway and bronchoscopy. For transmission, close contact is required with the infected person, because droplets travel only short distances. These patients should be nursed in a single room. No special ventilation is required.

Contact Precautions

Contact precautions should be applied to prevent infection from patients who are known or suspected to be infected or colonized with microorganisms transmitted by direct or indirect contact. These include methicillin-resistant *Staphylococcus aureus* (MRSA), vancomycin-resistant enterococci (VRE), *Clostridium difficile*, and respiratory syncytial virus (RSV). Direct contact transmission involves the physical transfer of microorganisms from an infected or colonized patient to a susceptible host by skin-to-skin contact or via the hands of a health care worker. Indirect contact spread occurs when a susceptible patient comes into contact with a contaminated object, such as a commode.

HANDLING AND DISPOSAL OF SHARPS

"Sharps" are any medical items or devices, contaminated with blood or high-risk body fluids, that can cause a laceration or puncture wound. They are frequently implicated in injuries sustained by health care workers and may transmit bloodborne viruses such as the human immunodeficiency virus (HIV), hepatitis B (HBV), and hepatitis C (HCV) (see "Bloodborne Viruses"). Sharps injuries are mainly caused by needles and are associated with veni-puncture, intravenous medications, or resheathing of needles. Health care organizations should ensure that staff personnel are trained in the correct handling and disposal of sharps.

Sharps usage should be avoided if possible, and needle-less systems should be used. If sharps must be used, safety devices should be provided. Needles should never be resheathed but should be disposed of immediately after use into a sharps container.[5] Sharps boxes should be readily available wherever sharps are used and securely closed when three-quarters full.

WASTE HANDLING AND DISPOSAL

The handling and disposal of any potentially infectious medical waste should be in accordance with local rules and legislation, to minimize the risk of transmission of infection. Organizations providing health care services should have appropriate policies and procedures in place, and all staff should be instructed in their application.

CLEANING AND DECONTAMINATION

Environment

Effective cleaning of the environment is important, because contaminated surfaces may act as reservoirs of potential pathogens. Transfer of microorganisms from environmental surfaces to patients occurs mainly via hand contact with the contaminated surface. Surfaces should be cleaned with detergent and water regularly, with high-touch areas (door handle, light switch, bed rail) cleaned more often than areas with less frequent hand contact. Disinfection is required for pathogens that can survive for a prolonged period, such as MRSA, VRE, and the spores of *C. difficile*.

Spills of blood and blood-containing body fluids should be cleaned promptly, and the surface should be disin-fected with sodium hypochlorite.[6]

Equipment

Medical equipment can be classified as noncritical (items in contact with intact skin), semicritical (close contact with intact mucous membranes or nonintact skin), or criti-cal (close contact with a break in skin or mucous mem-brane, or introduced into a sterile body space).

Noncritical items, such as stethoscopes, blood pressure cuffs, and syringe drivers, pose little risk and should be cleaned with detergent when visibly soiled and between each patient use (Fig. 92-2). Semicritical items, such as thermometers and sigmoidoscopes, require disinfection, which removes all microorganisms but not bacterial spores. Critical items, such as surgical instruments, require sterilization, which destroys spores and microorganisms.

Single-use medical equipment must never be reused.

IMMUNIZATION OF PATIENTS

Immunization of palliative care patients and health care staff (see "Protection of the Health Care Worker") against vaccine-preventable diseases is important. Patients with

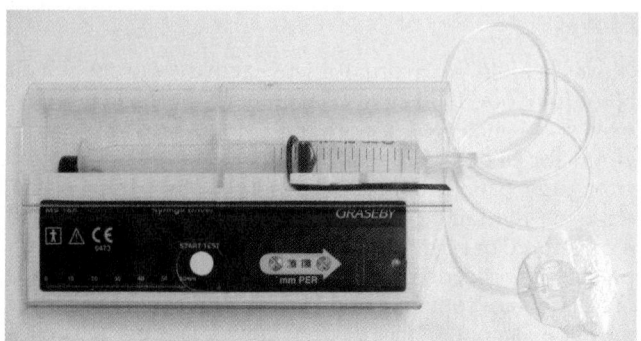

FIGURE 92-2 Noncritical medical equipment should be cleaned and disinfected after each patient use.

malignancy or HIV infection, those receiving immunosup-pressive therapies (including long-term high-dose cortico-steroids), and those with chronic heart, lung, or liver disease should be vaccinated annually against influenza. They should also be immunized against *Streptococcus pneumoniae* (pneumococcus), and the pneumococcal vaccine should be repeated once after 5 years in those who have impaired immune function (malignancy, HIV) or are undergoing immunosuppressive therapies.[7]

PREVENTION OF DEVICE-RELATED INFECTION

Palliative care patients may have indwelling devices, such as urinary catheters or intravascular catheters. These are associated with an increased risk of infection and there-fore must be managed appropriately.

Intravascular Catheter Infection

The infections associated with intravascular catheters include infection of the catheter insertion site and blood-stream infections. Coagulase-negative staphylococci are the most frequent isolates from catheter-related blood-stream infections (CRBSI), followed by *S. aureus*, entero-cocci, and, less commonly, gram-negative bacteria and *Candida* spp. Commonly used central venous catheters (CVC) in palliative care include tunneled CVCs (Hickman catheters), which have a lower rate of infection than non-tunneled CVCs because the cuff inhibits migration of organisms into the catheter tract, and totally implanted CVCs, which have the lowest risk for CRBSI and the advan-tage of not requiring local catheter-site care.

Intravascular catheter infections can be minimized by adherence to aseptic technique during catheter insertion and manipulation and by good care of the insertion site (Fig. 92-3).

Catheter sites should be monitored regularly by inspec-tion or palpation for signs of inflammation or infection. Hand hygiene should be observed before palpation of the insertion site and also before accessing or dressing the catheter. For dressing changes, clean or sterile gloves should be worn, and clean skin should be disinfected with an appropriate antiseptic, ideally a 2% chlorhexidine-based preparation. Catheter sites should be dressed with sterile gauze or a sterile, transparent, semipermeable dressing. Tunneled CVC sites that are well healed may not require dressings.

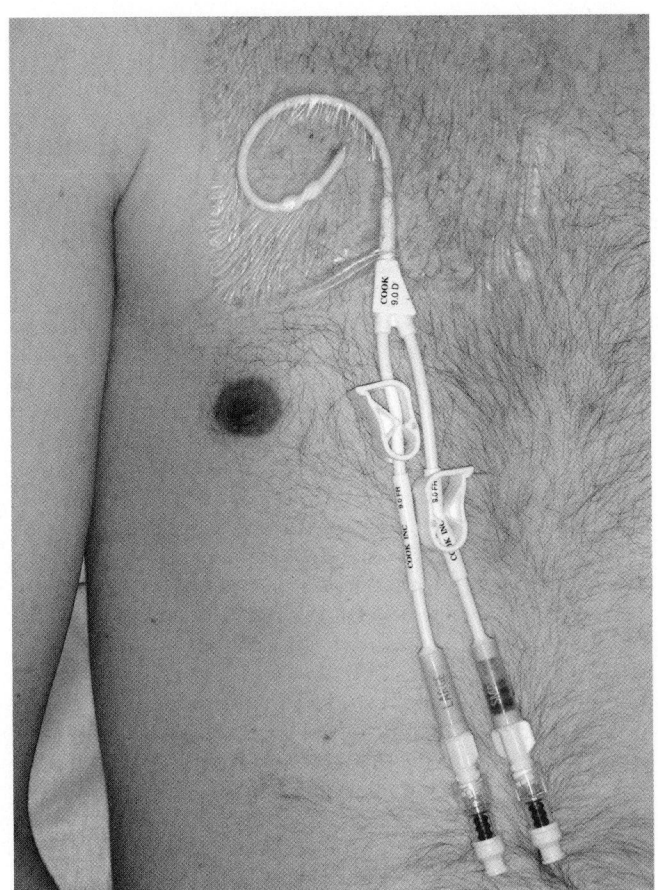

FIGURE 92-3 Adherence to aseptic technique during catheter manipulation and good care of the insertion site are vital in the prevention of catheter-related infection.

The aseptic management of the catheter hub, connection ports, and administration sets is vital to prevent contamination of the system and subsequent infection. Administration sets should be replaced at 72-hour intervals, unless catheter-related infection is suspected or documented. Needleless components and caps should be changed at the same frequency. Access ports should be wiped with an appropriate antiseptic before use and should be accessed only by sterile devices.[8] The use of multidose vials should be avoided because of the potential for contamination of the vial contents and subsequent transmission of infection.

Urinary Catheter Infection

The urinary tract is the most common site of health care infections, and most are associated with urinary catheterization. Infection may be complicated by prostatitis, epididymitis, pyelonephritis, or gram-negative bloodstream infection. Many urinary tract infections (UTIs) could be prevented by proper management of the indwelling catheter.

Hand hygiene should be observed before and after manipulation of the catheter and apparatus. Aseptic technique and sterile equipment should be used during catheter insertion. The smallest catheter diameter that allows free flow of urine should be chosen. A continuously closed sterile drainage system should be maintained, and drainage bags should be positioned to prevent the backflow of urine, because reflux is associated with infection. The drainage bag should be emptied regularly, and a separate container should be used for each patient, avoiding contact between the drainage tap and the container. Gloves should be worn when emptying the bag. Specimens should be aspirated using a sterile needle and syringe from the sampling port, which should first be disinfected. There is no indication for routine replacement of urinary catheters at fixed intervals.[9] Bacteriuria will be present in almost all patients with long-term urinary catheters. Antimicrobial treatment is indicated only in symptomatic patients.

WOUND MANAGEMENT

The correct management of wounds in palliative care is essential to promote healing, prevent wound infection, and minimize transmission of organisms to other patients and staff. Wounds quickly become colonized with various organisms, which may lead to infection. Infecting organisms may be acquired endogenously, from the patient's own flora, or exogenously, from the environment or the hands of health care workers.

Hand hygiene should be performed before dressing of wounds. Clean gloves should be worn, and an apron should be worn if there is the risk of contamination of the clothing. Dressings that promote wound healing should be used. All clinical waste generated should be disposed of appropriately. Gloves and apron should be discarded, and hands disinfected, after wound dressing.

MULTIDRUG-RESISTANT ORGANISMS

Multidrug-resistant organisms (MDROs) such as MRSA, VRE, and multidrug-resistant gram-negative bacteria (MDR-GNB) are prevalent. Many palliative care patients have had prolonged exposure to health care services and are at risk of being infected or colonized with an MDRO. Infection with one of these microorganisms can be difficult to treat and may cause morbidity and death. It is important to prevent the occurrence and reduce the risk of spread of these organisms within the palliative care patient population, if possible. Potentially modifiable risk factors for the acquisition of MRSA and VRE include prior antimicrobial exposure and indwelling devices. Antimicrobial agents should be used judiciously, and use of indwelling devices should be minimized. Standard infection control precautions should be used routinely for all patients, whether or not they are known to harbor an MDRO.

Further infection control management depends on the setting of care. In acute care facilities, contact precautions should be instituted for all those known or suspected of being infected or colonized with these organisms. A gown and gloves should be worn for all interactions that may involve patient contact or contact with potentially contaminated areas in the patient's environment. Noncritical patient equipment, such as stethoscopes and blood pressure cuffs, should be dedicated to each patient, or single-use disposable items should be used. Infected or colonized patients should be source isolated, in a single room or cohort unit.

In long-term care facilities, the clinical situation of each patient with an MDRO should be considered, along with the prevalence of MDRO in the particular facility, when making the decision to implement or modify contact precautions. For patients who are mainly independent in activities of daily living, standard precautions should be used, ensuring that gloves and gowns are used for contact with uncontrolled secretions and wounds. Contact precautions should be instituted for dependent patients and for those whose secretions or drainage cannot be well controlled. If single rooms are available, priority should be given to patients with known or suspected MDRO infection, particularly those whose conditions may facilitate transmission, such as uncontained secretions or excretions.

In home care, standard precautions should be followed, ensuring the use of gloves and gowns for contact with wounds, excretions, and uncontrolled secretions. The amount of reusable patient equipment brought into the home should be limited, and ideally the equipment should remain there until the patient no longer requires home care services. Otherwise, noncritical equipment should be cleaned and disinfected before removal from the home.[10]

TUBERCULOSIS

Tuberculosis (TB) is an infection caused by the *Mycobacterium tuberculosis* complex. Many primary infections are asymptomatic, and most people who are infected become latent carriers. The risk of developing active disease when first exposed, or of reactivating latent infection, is higher in people with impaired immune function, especially HIV infection.

TB is usually transmitted by small droplet nuclei (≤5 μm), which are produced by the patient with "open" pulmonary TB during coughing and sneezing. These particles can remain airborne for a considerable time because of their small size, and they may become widely dispersed by air currents. If inhaled, they can travel to the alveoli, where they may cause infection, either latent or active. Transmission of TB to other patients has occurred in acute care and long-term care facilities, and transmission to health care workers has occurred in acute, long-term, and home care settings.

A patient with known or suspected to have smear-positive pulmonary TB should be cared for in a single room with negative-pressure ventilation (also known as an airborne infection isolation room, or AII). The door should be kept closed at all times. Staff entering the room should wear a particulate respirator (N95) that has been fitted for them and tested. The patient should leave the room only for necessary procedures and should wear a surgical or procedure mask during that time.[4]

In confirmed TB, isolation precautions may be discontinued after the patient has received standard multidrug anti-TB treatment, has clinically improved, and has had three consecutive acid-fast bacillus (AFB)-negative smear results of sputum samples taken 8 to 24 hours apart, at least one of which was an early morning specimen.[11] Patients with known or suspected infectious TB may remain in a long-term care facility if adequate administrative and environmental controls (including airborne precautions capabilities) are in place. If not, they should be transferred to a facility in which they can receive appropriate care.

If a patient with known or suspected infectious TB is cared for in the home, the health care worker should wear an N95 mask and should not perform any aerosol-generating procedures. Sputum collection should take place outdoors, away from other persons, windows, and ventilation intakes.[4]

VARICELLA ZOSTER VIRUS

Primary infection with varicella-zoster virus (VZV) causes chickenpox, which is usually a mild disease in childhood. However, in adults, it may be complicated by pneumonia, which can cause severe disease, and immunocompromised patients can develop disseminated infection, which can be fatal. Zoster ("shingles") is a local manifestation of reactivation of the latent varicella infection in the dorsal root ganglia and usually is confined to one dermatome. Disseminated zoster can occur in immunosuppressed patients. Nonimmune individuals can develop chickenpox after contact with either zoster or chickenpox.

VZV is spread from person-to-person by direct contact or by the respiratory route from secretions from the respiratory tract or vesicle fluid. To minimize transmission to nonimmune patients and staff, patients with chickenpox or disseminated zoster should be cared for in a single room, ideally with negative-pressure ventilation, and both contact and airborne precautions should be applied.[12] Patients with localized zoster should be nursed in a single room if there is potential exposure to nonimmune or immunocompromised individuals, and contact precautions should be observed.

Immunocompromised patients are at risk for severe complications of varicella infection. Administration of varicella-zoster immunoglobulin (VZIG) is recommended for nonimmune immunocompromised patients who have had significant exposure to VZV. Direct contact exposure is defined as more than 1 hour of contact with an infectious person while indoors; substantial exposure for hospital contacts involves sharing the same hospital room with an infectious patient or prolonged, direct, face-to-face contact with an infectious person. The administration of VZIG within 96 hours of significant contact may prevent or modify VZV infection.[12] Exposed nonimmune patients who are in a health care facility should be cared for in a single room with appropriate infection control measures from 10 days after their earliest varicella exposure until 21 days after their most recent exposure. This isolation period should be extended to 28 days after the most recent exposure for patients who have received VZIG. All susceptible health care workers should be immunized against VZV, and immunization is also recommended for family contacts of immunocompromised patients.[13]

PROTECTION OF THE HEALTH CARE WORKER

Because of their contact with patients and infective material from patients, many health care workers may be at risk of exposure to and possible transmission of infectious diseases. Providers of health care have a responsibility to ensure that the risk to the worker of an infectious disease through occupational exposure be minimized. Transmissible infections in health care workers must be identified promptly, so that the risk of subsequent transmission to patients or other staff can be reduced.

Measures to protect health care workers from infection include immunization, education and training, and reporting of illnesses and accidents. All health care workers should be immunized against vaccine-preventable diseases, including hepatitis B, influenza, measles, mumps, rubella, and varicella-zoster. In addition, baseline testing for latent TB infection should be performed.[13]

All staff must receive appropriate education and training in infection control before starting work, and this should be reinforced at least annually through a continuing education program. Health care workers should be trained in the basic principles of infection control, including hand hygiene, use of PPE, handling and disposal of sharps and wastes, and the cleaning and decontamination of equipment and the environment. Staff should be aware of local infection control policies and guidelines. Adequate facilities for hand hygiene should be available to all staff, and appropriate PPE should be provided when indicated.

Staff illnesses should be reported to the line manager, so that workers with an infection potentially transmissible to the patients for whom they care may be removed from the workplace until no longer infectious. All sharps injuries should be reported immediately, so that evaluation of the need for postexposure prophylaxis may be carried out promptly (see "Bloodborne Viruses").

BLOODBORNE VIRUSES

Bloodborne viruses are viruses that are transmitted by contact with infected blood or body fluids. They include HIV, HBV, and HCV. In health care, the risk of acquisition of a bloodborne virus as a consequence of a sharps injury depends both on the prevalence of infection in the population served and the likelihood of inoculation incidents during procedures. The risk of infection after percutaneous exposure to blood from an HBV-infected individual is 5% to 30%; from an HCV-infected person, 0% to 7%; and from an HIV-positive person, 0.3%.

Several factors have been associated with an increased risk of bloodborne viral infection after percutaneous injury, including the type and quantity of blood or body fluid inoculated, the type of needle involved, the nature of the injury, and the infectivity of the source patient.

If a health care worker sustains a sharps injury, the wound should be encouraged to bleed and then washed with soap and water. The incident should be reported according to organizational guidelines, and evaluation of the exposure by a designated physician should occur as soon as possible, to determine the need for HBV and/or HIV postexposure prophylaxis.[14]

All health care organizations should have prevention programs to reduce the risk of occupational transmission of bloodborne viruses that include the routine immunization of all health care workers against HBV, the use of needleless devices, and the management of sharps injuries.

SURVEILLANCE

Surveillance is a key component of good infection control practice. Surveillance is the systematic monitoring of the

Future Considerations

- A frequent criticism is that infection control precautions for MDROs have a negative impact on the psychosocial well-being of the terminally ill patient and therefore are not in keeping with the holistic model of palliative medicine. However, MDROs can cause significant infection and death, so reduction of their transmission is important. The needs of the individual patient should be considered in each instance and balanced against the setting in which care is being delivered and the risk to other patients.
- Surveillance is a key activity in infection control. Limited information is available regarding the incidence of infection and the outcome of infection control practices in the home care setting. This deficit should be addressed in the future to inform the development of targeted interventions for implementation in the home.

occurrence of disease in a population; it involves the collection, recording, analysis, and interpretation of data. The main objectives are to establish infection rates, reduce infection rates by feedback of results, identify outbreaks of infectious disease, facilitate comparison of infection rates among health care organizations, and evaluate the control measures that are in place. Surveillance is "information for action," so it is vital that the information collected be provided to those who can influence practice. Standard definitions and methods of collection should be agreed on a regional or national level so as to allow valid comparisons of data.

HOME CARE

There has been a substantial expansion of home care. Most infection control practice guidelines are specifically designed for the acute care setting, and many recommended practices are unnecessary or inappropriate in home care. Infection control practices in home care often may not be derived from scientific evidence. There is a need to establish surveillance of home care–related infections, to study the effect of various infection control interventions on the incidence of these infections, and to devise clear, evidence-based guidelines for infection control in home care[15] (see "Future Considerations").

REFERENCES

1. Garner JS; and the Hospital Infection Control Practices Advisory Group. Guideline for Isolation Precautions: Preventing Transmission of Infectious Agents in Healthcare Settings, 2007. Available at http://www.cdc.gov/ncidod/dhqp/gl_isolation.html (accessed October 2007).
2. Centers for Disease Control and Prevention. Guideline for hand hygiene in healthcare settings: Recommendations of the Healthcare Infection Control Practices Advisory Committee and the HICPAC/SHEA/APIC/IDSA Hand Hygiene Taskforce. MMWR 2002;51(RR-16):1-45.
3. Centers for Disease Control and Prevention. Guidelines for preventing healthcare-associated pneumonia, 2003: Recommendations of CDC and the Healthcare Infection Control Practices Advisory Committee. MMWR 2004;53(RR-3):1-36.
4. Centers for Disease Control and Prevention. Guidelines for preventing the transmission of *Mycobacterium tuberculosis* in healthcare settings, 2005. MMWR 2005;54(RR-17):1-141.
5. National Institute for Occupational Safety and Health. Preventing Needlestick Injuries in Health Care Settings. Available at http://www.cdc.gov/niosh/pdfs/2000-108.pdf (accessed October 2007).
6. Centers for Disease Control and Prevention. Guidelines for environmental infection control in healthcare facilities: Recommendations of CDC and the Healthcare Infection Control Practices Advisory Committee (HICPAC). MMWR 2003;52(RR-10):1-44.

7. Advisory Committee on Immunization Practices. Recommended adult immunization schedule—United States, October 2006–September 2007. MMWR 2006;55(40):Q1-Q4.

8. Centers for Disease Control and Prevention. Guidelines for the prevention of intravascular catheter-related infections. MMWR 2002;51(RR-10):1-29.

9. Wong ES. Guideline for prevention of catheter-associated urinary tract infections. Am J Infect Control 1993;11:28-36.

10. Siegel JD, Rhinehart E, Jackson M, et al. Management of Multidrug-Resistant Organisms in Healthcare Settings, 2006. Available at http://www.cdc.gov/ncidod/dhqp/pdf/ar/mdroGuideline2006.pdf (accessed October 2007).

11. Centers for Disease Control and Prevention. Controlling tuberculosis in the United States: Recommendations from the American Thoracic Society, CDC and the Infectious Diseases Society of America. MMWR 2005;54(RR-12):1-81.

12. Centers for Disease Control and Prevention. Prevention of varicella: Recommendations of the Advisory Committee on Immunization Practices (ACIP). MMWR 1996;45(RR-11):1-36.

13. Centers for Disease Control and Prevention. Immunization of healthcare workers: Recommendations of the Advisory Committee on Immunization (APIC) and the Healthcare Infection Control Practices Advisory Committee (HICPAC). MMWR 1997;46(RR-18):1-42.

14. Centers for Disease Control and Prevention. Updated U.S. Public Health Service Guidelines for the management of occupational exposures to HBV, HCV and HIV and recommendations for postexposure prophylaxis. MMWR 2001; 50(RR-11):1-52.

15. Rhinehart E. Infection control in home care. Emerg Infect Dis. 2001; 7:208-211.

SUGGESTED READING

Damani NN. Manual of Infection Control Procedures. London: Greenwich Medical Media, London, 2003.

Rhinehart E, Friedman MM. Infection Control in Home Care. Boston: Jones and Bartlett, 2005.

Wilson J. Infection Control in Clinical Practice. London: Bailliere Tindall, 2001.

CHAPTER **93**

Urinary Tract Infections

Nabin K. Shrestha

KEY POINTS

- Urinary tract infections (UTIs) are among the most common infectious complications associated with the use of indwelling urinary catheters.

- The basic laboratory tests for diagnosis are a urinalysis and urine culture, but both may be misleading if an indwelling urinary catheter is in place.

- Significant bacteriuria often indicates a UTI, but if *Staphylococcus aureus* is isolated, it is more likely to be secondary to bacteremia.

- Initial empirical therapy should be tailored down to narrow-spectrum antibiotics once culture and susceptibility data become available.

- Indwelling urinary catheters should be used only when necessary, removed promptly after they are no longer needed, and removed or changed promptly if a UTI is suspected.

The term *urinary tract infection* (UTI) describes infection in any part of the urinary tract. *Bacteriuria* is bacteria in the urine detected in the laboratory and does not necessarily mean that a UTI is present. More than 10^5 bacteria per milliliter of urine is defined as significant bacteriuria and exceeds that expected to be present from contamination from the distal urethra. Lower UTIs include infections of the bladder (cystitis), urethra (urethritis), prostate (prostatitis), and associated structures (e.g., epididymoorchitis). Upper UTIs include infections of the renal parenchyma and pelvis (pyelonephritis). *Urosepsis* is septicemia caused by a UTI.

BASIC SCIENCE

For UTI to occur, a microorganism must have the opportunity to interact with the host, must colonize the uroepithelium, and must stimulate and survive the host's immune defenses. Anatomical abnormalities pose an added difficulty for the host's immune response and favor the microorganism in its struggle to establish infection.

Escherichia coli is the most common cause of UTIs. It is also one of the important microorganisms that constitute the normal colonic flora, in which situation it is not causing disease. *E. coli* strains from the urine of patients with UTI adhere better in vitro to uroepithelial cells and periurethral epithelial cells than do strains from feces of healthy individuals.[1,2] Cell surface structures on bacteria called type 1 fimbriae mediate attachment of the bacteria to uroepithelial cells.[3-6] More than 95% of all isolates of *E. coli*, irrespective of origin, express type 1 fimbriae. Epidemiological studies do not show evidence of differential distribution of type 1 fimbriae between uropathogenic isolates and fecal isolates from healthy individuals.[7] Type 1 fimbriae are composed of a major structural subunit (FimA) and several minor subunits (including the adhesion FimH) encoded by the *FIM* gene cluster. The FimH protein is at the fimbrial tip and interspersed along its shaft.[8] Phenotypic variation in FimH influences a microorganism's ability to bind to uroepithelium and thereby cause UTI.[9] It is not the type 1 fimbriae alone but their composition that influences a microorganism's ability to adhere to uroepithelial cells and cause UTI.

Several other virulence factors have been described for *E. coli*. Perhaps the most well-characterized are the P fimbriae, which are bacterial cell surface structures that can bind to glycolipids containing a terminal or internal Gal(α1-4)Galβ moiety (Gal-Gal).[10,11] Gal-Gal–containing glycolipids are the predominant glycolipids in human renal epithelial cells.[12] P fimbriae are strongly associated with the ability to cause pyelonephritis.[13-15] At a structural level, P fimbriae are composed of a major subunit (PapA) and several minor subunits (including PapG) encoded for by the *PAP* gene cluster. The PapG subunit is at the tip of the P fimbria, and its phenotypic variation influences a microorganism's ability to cause pyelonephritis, analogous to the influence of FimH variation on attachment to uroepithelium in type 1–fimbriated *E. coli*.

The host response to uropathogens depends on recognition by the host of the presence of bacteria and the defenses engaged to prevent them from causing harm. Recognition of uropathogens depends on both toll-like receptor 4 (TLR4)-dependent mechanisms (through recognition of lipopolysaccharide) and TLR4-independent mechanisms.[16,17] Epithelial cells respond to uropathogenic *E. coli* by secreting interleukin 8 (IL8).[18] Anti-IL8 antibodies block neutrophil migration across infected epithelial cell layers, and recombinant IL8 therapy supports this process in the absence of bacteria.[18] Antibody treatment blocks the passage of neutrophils into the urine and causes them to accumulate under the kidney and bladder epithelium.[19] IL8 mediates its biological activity through the G protein–coupled receptors CXCR1 and CXCR2. Its effect on neutrophil chemotaxis is mostly through CXCR1.[20] People with CXCR1 deficiency have increased UTI susceptibility, supporting the idea that IL8 plays an important role in the host inflammatory response to UTI.[21] The host response in UTI consists of recognition of pathogens (possibly involving TLR4) and recruitment of neutrophils to the urinary tract (secretion of IL8 by uroepithelial cells and IL8-mediated neutrophil chemotaxis).

EPIDEMIOLOGY AND PREVALENCE

UTIs are common; 150 million people are diagnosed annually.[22] Catheter-associated UTIs are the most common nosocomial infections, accounting for 40% of all hospital-acquired infections.[22] More than 95% of UTIs are monomicrobial. *E. coli* is the most common microorganism (Box 93-1).[23]

PATHOPHYSIOLOGY

There are two major routes by which bacteria reach the urinary tract. The more common is the ascending route, whereby bacteria colonizing the periurethral region access the urinary tract. The second is hematogenous seeding of the kidney during bacteremia. Ascending UTIs are often associated with predisposing factors that facilitate UTI (Box 93-2).

Box 93-1 Common Causes of Urinary Tract Infections

- *Escherichia coli*
- *Klebsiella pneumoniae*
- *Enterobacter* spp.
- *Pseudomonas aeruginosa*
- *Proteus* spp.
- *Morganella* spp.
- *Providencia* spp.
- *Enterococcus* spp.
- *Candida* spp.

Box 93-2 Conditions That Predispose to Ascending Urinary Tract Infections

- Female gender
- Obstruction or stasis in the urinary tract
- Vesicoureteric reflux
- Preexisting renal lesions such as scarring
- Nephrolithiasis
- Diabetes mellitus
- Pregnancy
- Instrumentation of the urinary tract

The first step in ascending UTI is colonization of the periurethral region and distal urethra by pathogenic bacteria. This is followed by introduction of bacteria into the urinary bladder, a process that is facilitated by the presence of an indwelling catheter. The next step is multiplication in the bladder, which is helped by urinary stasis and incomplete bladder evacuation. The next step is ascent to the ureters and renal pelvis, aided by vesicoureteric reflux and pregnancy. From the renal pelvis, bacteria access the renal parenchyma through intrarenal reflux, most commonly in the upper and lower poles of the kidneys (see Box 93-2).

Biofilm formation is important in the pathogenesis of catheter-associated UTIs. Biofilms are composed of Tamm-Horsfall protein, struvite and apatite crystals, bacterial products, and living bacteria.[22] Biofilms provide a safe haven for microorganisms, where they are protected from immune effector cells, cytokines, and antibiotics.[24]

Bacteremic seeding occurs when bacteria are filtered out in the kidney glomeruli. This is the pathogenesis of renal abscesses from *Staphylococcus aureus* and *Candida* species. UTI caused by gram-negative bacilli is usually a result of ascending infection, not hematogenous seeding.

Congenital anomalies and postsurgical anatomical changes that result in urinary tract obstruction or urinary stasis, fistulous communications involving the urinary tract, spinal cord diseases that result in bladder stasis, nephrolithiasis, chronic indwelling urinary catheters, and frequent instrumentation are important causes of recurrent UTIs.

CLINICAL MANIFESTATIONS

Symptoms vary between upper and lower UTI. Pyelonephritis usually manifests with high-grade fever with chills and rigors, flank pain, and sometimes diarrhea. Lower UTIs are usually characterized by dysuria, urgency, frequency, and sometimes suprapubic discomfort and low-grade fever. UTIs may be complicated by septicemia. Elderly patients may present only with confusion. Any elderly patient presenting with acute confusion, especially if an indwelling urinary catheter is present, should be evaluated for UTI. Complications of UTI include pyonephrosis, renal abscess, perinephric abscess, chronic prostatitis, and septicemia.

DIAGNOSIS

Diagnosis is made by clinical features and laboratory tests. The laboratory tests that help are a urinalysis and urine culture. Urinalysis usually reveals pyuria. Leukocyte esterase may be positive, as may nitrites. Leukocyte esterase reflects the presence of leukocytes in the urine. Detection of nitrites is a marker of nitrate-reducing bacteria in the urine. Patients with pyuria may or may not have infection.[25] Urine culture reveals microorganisms, identifies them, and provides antimicrobial susceptibility data. If urine culture is positive but the urinalysis is normal, the positive culture may represent bladder or catheter colonization or contamination at collection. Those patients with chronic indwelling catheters may have pyuria because of the irritation and consequent low-grade inflammation induced by the catheter. They may also have chronic bladder colonization without infection. Therefore, laboratory tests should not be the sole basis on which a diagnosis is made. The information from these tests should be used along with the clinical picture in making a diagnosis. There are no accurate laboratory tests that distinguish between upper and lower UTIs. That determination is best made on the basis of the clinical features. Isolation of *S. aureus* in the urine should always lead to investigation for *S. aureus* bacteremia.

TREATMENT

Guidelines for acute cystitis and uncomplicated pyelonephritis in women have been published by the Infectious Diseases Society of America.[26] Evidence has shown that short courses of antibiotics are effective. Treatment should be based on culture results and susceptibility data whenever possible. Antimicrobial resistance is increasingly recognized in UTI.[27]

Higher cure rates occur when UTI is treated with an antimicrobial to which the offending microorganism is susceptible in vitro.[28] With complicated UTIs, successful treatment hinges not only on selection of the appropriate antimicrobial but also on the alleviation of other factors that predispose to or perpetuate infection. This may include removal or changing of infected indwelling catheters, treatment of obstructing or nonobstructing renal stones, and removal or replacement of drugs that slow bladder emptying.

The choice of antibiotic is best made with an understanding of the microbiology of UTIs and drug pharmacokinetics. Most ascending infections are from enteric microorganisms, and empirical therapy should be directed against enteric gram-negative bacteria. Trimethoprim-sulfamethoxazole and ciprofloxacin are favorites because of their broad range of antimicrobial activity (against enteric flora) and convenient pharmacokinetic properties that allow oral dosing. When choosing among antibiotics, it may be wiser to choose one predominantly excreted by the kidneys over one predominantly excreted by the liver. This is especially valuable in palliative care, where it may be preferable to avoid an intravenous line. UTI may be treated with an oral antimicrobial, like ciprofloxacin, despite reduced susceptibility on in vitro testing, because antimicrobial levels in the urine of normally functioning kidneys are substantially higher than in blood.

Asymptomatic bacteriuria usually does not require treatment.[29] Exceptions include pregnancy patients and those who are to undergo transurethral prostate resection or urological instrumentation.[30,31] Preoperative screening and treatment of bacteriuria should be undertaken in those who are to undergo urological procedures in which mucosal bleeding is anticipated.[32] There is no benefit to treating asymptomatic bacteriuria in cases of spinal cord injury or disease with bladder stasis, in elderly patients, or in those with diabetes mellitus or an indwelling urinary catheter.[29] There are no recommendations for treatment of asymptomatic bacteriuria in renal transplant recipients.[29]

PREVENTION

Modifiable factors that might predispose to UTI should be corrected as practicable. Indwelling catheters should not

---

Future Considerations

- Probiotics such as *Lactobacillus* to prevent recurrent UTI
- Colonization with nonpathogenic bacteria to prevent UTIs with chronic indwelling urinary catheters or chronic bladder stasis
- Anti-adhesin vaccines

---

be used for longer than necessary. Obstructing renal stones should be treated. Drugs that may impair bladder emptying should be avoided. Cranberry products (juice and tablets) have been widely used to prevent recurrent UTIs. A meta-analysis of randomized controlled trials suggested that they reduce recurrent UTIs over 1 year in women but there were significant rates of noncompliance.[33] Cranberry juice does not prevent UTIs in the hospitalized elderly.[34] Cranberry extract capsules do not reduce bacteriuria or pyuria in patients with spinal cord injury and neurogenic bladder.[35] A substantial drug interaction between warfarin and cranberry juice occurs, causing an elevated international normalized ratio (INR).[36] Cranberry products do not dramatically reduce the incidence of UTIs, but, if they are used, close INR monitoring should be done during oral warfarin anticoagulation.

Probiotics to prevent UTI is an area of research. Specific *Lactobacillus* products reduce UTI recurrences in women, but without regulation it is difficult to determine whether a particular marketed and advertised product has any efficacy.[37] Serious infections due to *Lactobacillus* can occcur.[38,39] In children with *Lactobacillus* bacteremia, typing studies have shown the lactobacilli strains in blood to be indistinguishable from the probiotic strains ingested.[40,41] Most serious *Lactobacillus* infections occur in people with serious underlying illness.[42] The challenge with probiotics is less a concern for safety than the ability to determine efficacy. Other preventive approaches being evaluated are avirulent strains of *E. coli* to colonize the bladder, preventing colonization with virulent strains, and attempts to produce anti-adhesin vaccines[22] (see "Future Considerations").

REFERENCES

1. Hagberg L, Jodal U, Korhonen TK, et al. Adhesion, hemagglutination, and virulence of *Escherichia coli* causing urinary tract infections. Infect Immun 1981;31:564-570.
2. Kallenius G, Mollby R, Winberg J. In vitro adhesion of uropathogenic *Escherichia coli* to human periurethral cells. Infect Immun 1980;28:972-980.
3. Aronson M, Medalia O, Schori L, et al. Prevention of colonization of the urinary tract of mice with *Escherichia coli* by blocking of bacterial adherence with methyl alpha-D-mannopyranoside. J Infect Dis 1979;139:329-332.
4. Keith BR, Maurer L, Spears PA, Orndorff PE. Receptor-binding function of type 1 pili effects bladder colonization by a clinical isolate of *Escherichia coli*. Infect Immun 1986;53:693-696.
5. Iwahi T, Abe Y, Nakao M, et al. Role of type 1 fimbriae in the pathogenesis of ascending urinary tract infection induced by *Escherichia coli* in mice. Infect Immun 1983;39:1307-1315.
6. Hultgren SJ, Porter TN, Schaeffer AJ, Duncan JL. Role of type 1 pili and effects of phase variation on lower urinary tract infections produced by *Escherichia coli*. Infect Immun 1985;50:370-377.
7. Duguid JP, Clegg S, Wilson MI. The fimbrial and non-fimbrial haemagglutinins of *Escherichia coli*. J Med Microbiol 1979;12:213-227.
8. Krogfelt KA, Bergmans H, Klemm P. Direct evidence that the FimH protein is the mannose-specific adhesin of *Escherichia coli* type 1 fimbriae. Infect Immun 1990;58:1995-1998.
9. Sokurenko EV, Chesnokova V, Dykhuizen DE, et al. Pathogenic adaptation of *Escherichia coli* by natural variation of the FimH adhesin. Proc Natl Acad Sci U S A 1998;95:8922-8926.

10. Korhonen TK, Vaisanen V, Saxen H, et al. P-antigen-recognizing fimbriae from human uropathogenic *Escherichia coli* strains. Infect Immun 1982; 37:286-291.

11. Ofek I, Goldhar J, Eshdat Y, Sharon N. The importance of mannose specific adhesins (lectins) in infections caused by *Escherichia coli*. Scand J Infect Dis Suppl 1982;33:61-67.

12. Martensson E. Neutral glycolipids of human kidney: Isolation, identification, and fatty acid composition. Biochim Biophys Acta 1966;116:296-308.

13. Roberts JA, Kaack B, Kallenius G, et al. Receptors for pyelonephritogenic *Escherichia coli* in primates. J Urol 1984;131:163-168.

14. Svenson SB, Kallenius G, Korhonen TK, et al. Initiation of clinical pyelonephritis: The role of P-fimbriae-mediated bacterial adhesion. Contrib Nephrol 1984;39:252-272.

15. Roberts JA, Hardaway K, Kaack B, et al. Prevention of pyelonephritis by immunization with P-fimbriae. J Urol 1984;131:602-607.

16. Frendeus B, Wachtler C, Hedlund M, et al. *Escherichia coli* P fimbriae utilize the Toll-like receptor 4 pathway for cell activation. Mol Microbiol 2001; 40:37-51.

17. Hedlund M, Frendeus B, Wachtler C, et al. Type 1 fimbriae deliver an LPS- and TLR4-dependent activation signal to CD14-negative cells. Mol Microbiol 2001;39:542-552.

18. Godaly G, Proudfoot AE, Offord RE, et al. Role of epithelial interleukin-8 (IL-8) and neutrophil IL-8 receptor A in *Escherichia coli*-induced transuroepithelial neutrophil migration. Infect Immun 1997;65:3451-3456.

19. Hang L, Frendeus B, Godaly G, Svanborg C. Interleukin-8 receptor knockout mice have subepithelial neutrophil entrapment and renal scarring following acute pyelonephritis. J Infect Dis 2000;182:1738-1748.

20. Godaly G, Hang L, Frendeus B, Svanborg C. Transepithelial neutrophil migration is CXCR1 dependent in vitro and is defective in IL-8 receptor knockout mice. J Immunol 2000;165:5287-5294.

21. Frendeus B, Godaly G, Hang L, et al. Interleukin 8 receptor deficiency confers susceptibility to acute experimental pyelonephritis and may have a human counterpart. J Exp Med 2000;192:881-890.

22. Stamm WE, Norrby SR. Urinary tract infections: Disease panorama and challenges. J Infect Dis 2001;183(Suppl 1):S1-S4.

23. Ronald A. The etiology of urinary tract infection: Traditional and emerging pathogens. Am J Med 2002;113(Suppl 1A):14S-19S.

24. Trautner BW, Darouiche RO. Role of biofilm in catheter-associated urinary tract infection. Am J Infect Control 2004;32:177-183.

25. Thysell H. Evaluation of chemical and microscopical methods for mass detection of bacteriuria. Acta Med Scand 1969;185:393-400.

26. Warren JW, Abrutyn E, Hebel JR, et al. Guidelines for antimicrobial treatment of uncomplicated acute bacterial cystitis and acute pyelonephritis in women. Infectious Diseases Society of America (IDSA). Clin Infect Dis 1999;29:745-758.

27. Gupta K, Scholes D, Stamm WE. Increasing prevalence of antimicrobial resistance among uropathogens causing acute uncomplicated cystitis in women. JAMA 1999;281:736-738.

28. Talan DA, Stamm WE, Hooton TM, et al. Comparison of ciprofloxacin (7 days) and trimethoprim-sulfamethoxazole (14 days) for acute uncomplicated pyelonephritis pyelonephritis in women: A randomized trial. JAMA 2000; 283:1583-1590.

29. Nicolle LE, Bradley S, Colgan R, et al. Infectious Diseases Society of America guidelines for the diagnosis and treatment of asymptomatic bacteriuria in adults. Clin Infect Dis 2005;40:643-654.

30. Smaill F. Antibiotics for asymptomatic bacteriuria in pregnancy. Cochrane Database Syst Rev 2001;(2):CD000490.

31. Grabe M, Forsgren A, Hellsten S. The effect of a short antibiotic course in transurethral prostatic resection. Scand J Urol Nephrol 1984;18:37-42.

32. Rao PN, Dube DA, Weightman NC, et al. Prediction of septicemia following endourological manipulation for stones in the upper urinary tract. J Urol 1991;146:955-960.

33. Jepson RG, Mihaljevic L, Craig J. Cranberries for preventing urinary tract infections. Cochrane Database Syst Rev 2004;(2):CD001321.

34. McMurdo ME, Bissett LY, Price RJ, et al. Does ingestion of cranberry juice reduce symptomatic urinary tract infections in older people in hospital? A double-blind, placebo-controlled trial. Age Ageing 2005;34:256-261.

35. Waites KB, Canupp KC, Armstrong S, DeVivo MJ. Effect of cranberry extract on bacteriuria and pyuria in persons with neurogenic bladder secondary to spinal cord injury. J Spinal Cord Med 2004;27:35-40.

36. Rindone JP, Murphy TW. Warfarin-cranberry juice interaction resulting in profound hypoprothrombinemia and bleeding. Am J Ther 2006;13:283-284.

37. Reid G, Bruce AW. Probiotics to prevent urinary tract infections: The rationale and evidence. World J Urol 2006;24:28-32.

38. Husni RN, Gordon SM, Washington JA, Longworth DL. *Lactobacillus* bacteremia and endocarditis: Review of 45 cases. Clin Infect Dis 1997; 25:1048-1055.

39. Cannon JP, Lee TA, Bolanos JT, Danziger LH. Pathogenic relevance of *Lactobacillus:* A retrospective review of over 200 cases. Eur J Clin Microbiol Infect Dis 2005;24:31-40.

40. Kunz A, Farichok MP. Two cases of *Lactobacillus* bacteremia during probiotic treatment of short gut syndrome: The authors' reply. J Pediatr Gastroenterol Nutr 2004;39:437.

41. Land MH, Rouster-Stevens K, Woods CR, et al. *Lactobacillus* sepsis associated with probiotic therapy. Pediatrics 2005;115:178-181.

42. Hammerman C, Bin-Nun A, Kaplan M. Safety of probiotics: Comparison of two popular strains. BMJ 2006;333:1006-1008.

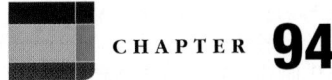

CHAPTER **94**

Health Care–Acquired Infections

Jennie Johnstone and A. Mark Joffe

K E Y   P O I N T S

- Infections are commonly acquired in health care settings and account for considerable morbidity and mortality.

- Pneumonia is the second most common nosocomial infection and is the leading cause of death due to health care–acquired infection.

- Catheter-associated urinary tract infections (CAUTIs) are the most common type of health care–acquired infection.

- Central venous catheter (CVC)-related bloodstream infection should be considered in any patient with a CVC and a fever.

- *Clostridium difficile* is the most common cause of infectious diarrhea among hospitalized patients.

Infection prevention and control as a formal discipline was introduced in the 1950s. The landmark Study on the Efficacy of Nosocomial Infection Control (SENIC) provided evidence for infection surveillance and reporting as cost-effective strategies for reducing hospital-acquired infections (see Chapter 92).[1] Health care–acquired infections are still a problem. In December 2004, the Institute of Healthcare Improvement launched the "100,000 Lives Campaign" in the United States in an effort to save lives by improving the safety and efficacy of health care.[2] Three of the six proposed interventions focused on decreasing hospital-related infections (i.e., prevention of central-line infections, surgical site infections, and ventilator-associated pneumonia). Hospital-acquired infections are increasingly viewed as potentially preventable markers of quality of care and patient safety.[3]

People who are being cared for in palliative care units or in a hospice or who require interaction with health care facilities for disease or symptom management are at risk for health care–acquired infections because of their underlying disease, its therapy, or need for supportive technologies and devices. These infections have associated morbidity and mortality and may cause additional unnecessary strain on patients, their families, their health care providers, and the health care system. Few studies have examined the incidence and nature of infections in palliative medicine, but the limited data suggest that the scope of infections and organisms afflicting the terminally ill resemble those of other hospitalized populations.[4-7]

NOSOCOMIAL PNEUMONIA

The term *nosocomial pneumonia* encompasses various disorders including hospital-acquired pneumonia (HAP), ventilator-associated pneumonia (VAP), and health care–

associated pneumonia (HCAP) (Fig. 94-1). The American Thoracic Society published guidelines for their management in adults in 2005.[8] HAP is defined as a pneumonia that occurs 48 hours or more after admission and was not incubating at the time of admission, whereas VAP is a pneumonia that arises after 48 to 72 hours of mechanical ventilation. In contrast, HCAP includes pneumonia in any patient who was hospitalized in an acute care hospital for 2 or more days within 90 days of the pneumonia, resided in a nursing home or long-term care facility, or spent any time receiving care (e.g., parenteral antibiotics, chemotherapy, hemodialysis, wound care) within 30 days of the pneumonia. Patients receiving palliative care may be at risk for the entire spectrum of nosocomial pneumonia.

Epidemiology and Prevalence

Nosocomial pneumonia is the second most common nosocomial infection and the leading cause of death from health care–acquired infection. There are 5 to 10 cases per 1000 hospital admissions, and the mortality rate is 30% to 50%.[8] The excess cost associated with the increased length and complexity of stay is about $40,000 per patient.[8]

The etiology of HAP, VAP, and HCAP is typically bacterial and includes gram-positive organisms such as *Staphylococcus aureus* and gram-negatives such as *Pseudomonas aeruginosa*, *Escherichia coli*, and *Klebsiella pneumoniae*. Polymicrobial infections are common. Nosocomial pneumonia due to multidrug-resistant pathogens is problematic (Box 94-1). Viral pneumonias are uncommon, although

Box 94-1 Multidrug-Resistant Pathogens: Special Considerations

Increasing use of antibiotics, together with lax infection control strategies, has favored the emergence of multidrug-resistant (MDR) bacteria. Rates of methicillin-resistant *Staphylococcus aureus* (MRSA), vancomycin-resistant enterococci (VRE), and multidrug-resistant gram-negative bacteria (MDR-GNB) are on the rise. Frequent and prolonged contact with hospitals or with the health care system is a risk factor for colonization with MDR bacteria. Risk factors for MDR pathogens causing nosocomial pneumonia are outlined in Table 94-3. The prevalence of MDR pathogens varies according to patient population and local epidemiology. Therefore, knowing institution-specific rates of problem pathogens and their antimicrobial susceptibility patterns is extremely useful in deciding on appropriate local empirical choices.

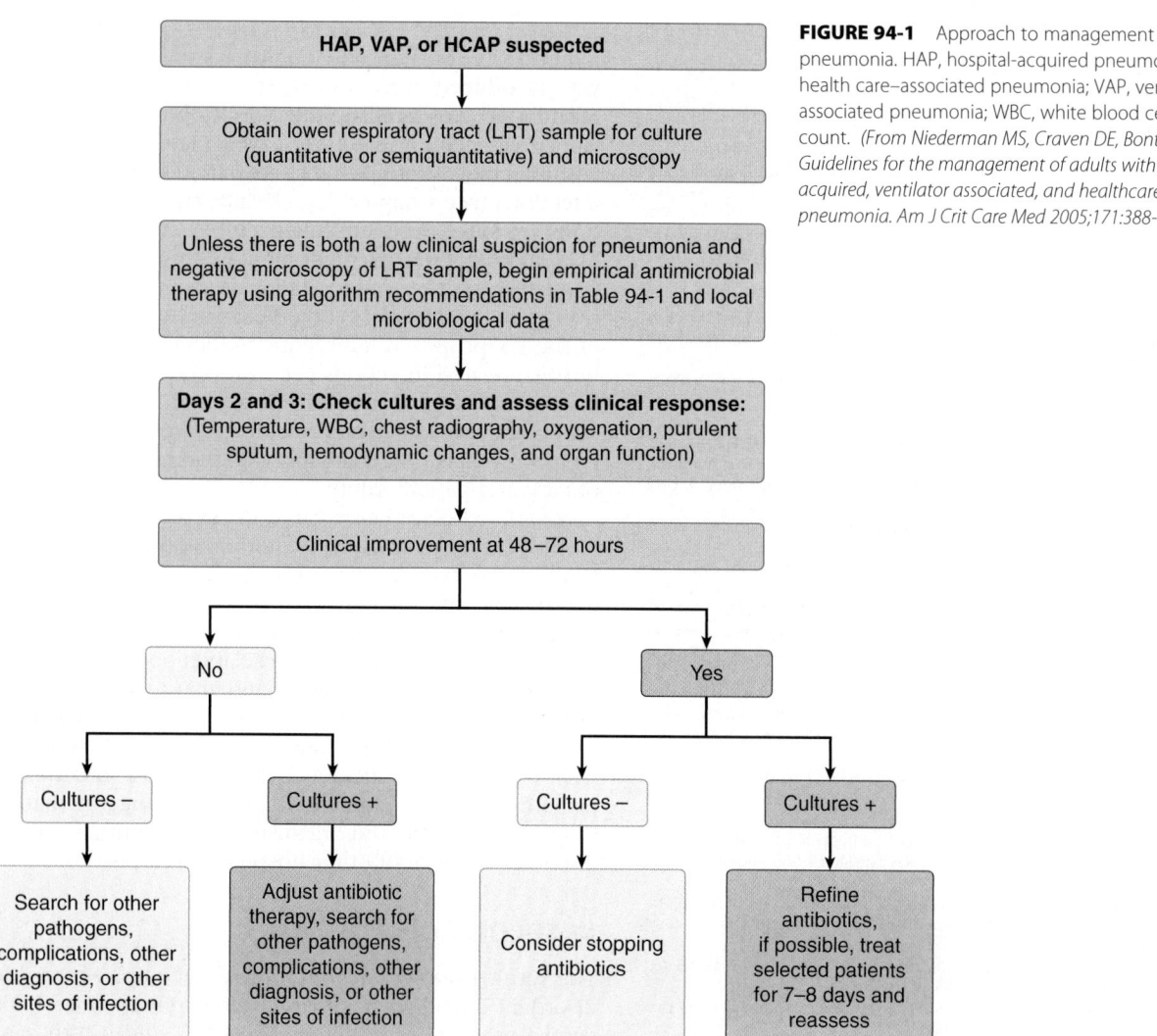

FIGURE 94-1 Approach to management of nosocomial pneumonia. HAP, hospital-acquired pneumonia; HCAP, health care–associated pneumonia; VAP, ventilator-associated pneumonia; WBC, white blood cell count. *(From Niederman MS, Craven DE, Bonten MJ, et al. Guidelines for the management of adults with hospital acquired, ventilator associated, and healthcare associated pneumonia. Am J Crit Care Med 2005;171:388-416.)*

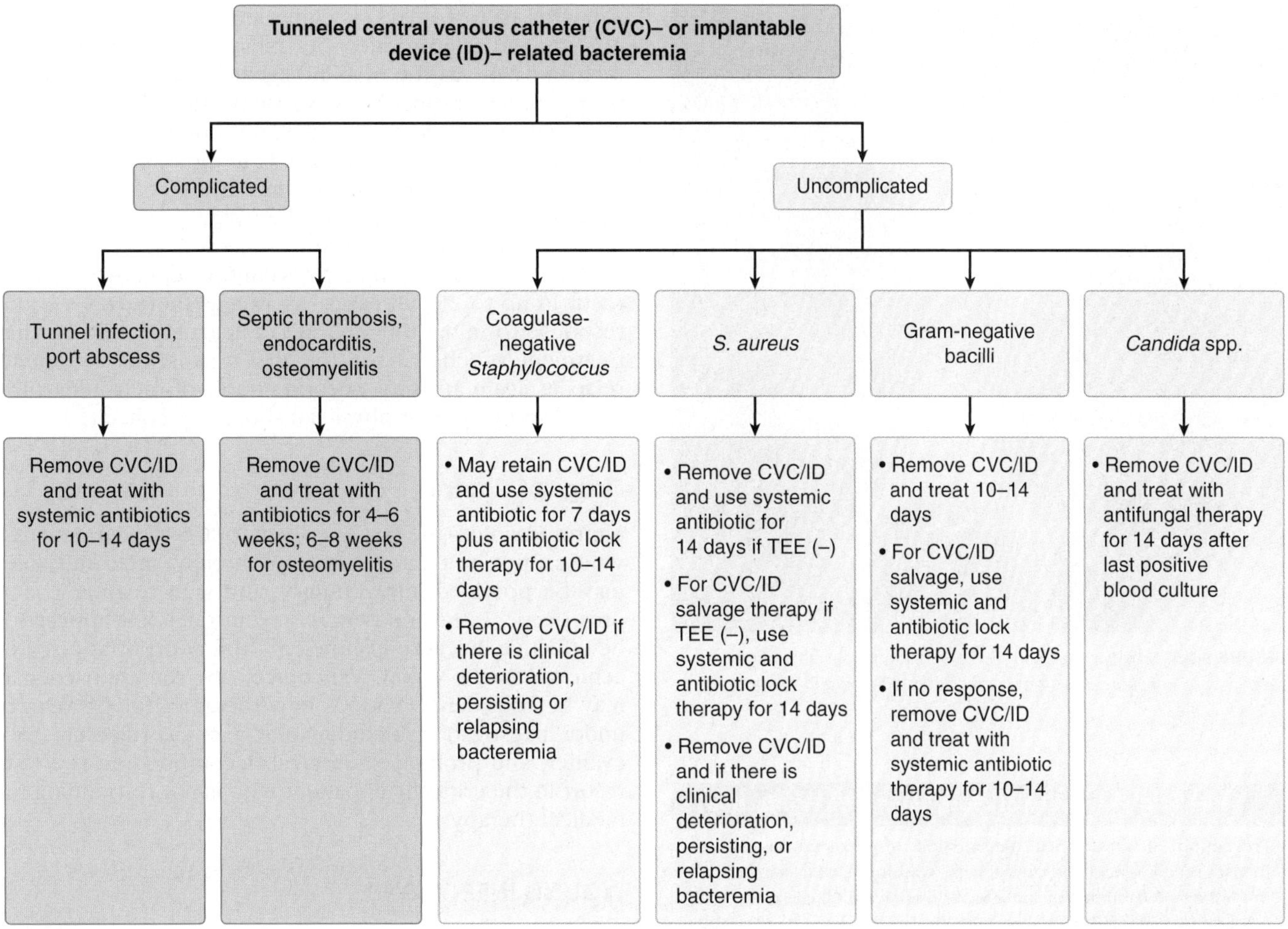

```
              ┌─────────────────────────────────────────┐
              │ Tunneled central venous catheter (CVC)– or implantable │
              │          device (ID)– related bacteremia           │
              └─────────────────────────────────────────┘
```

Complicated	Uncomplicated

Tunnel infection, port abscess	Septic thrombosis, endocarditis, osteomyelitis	Coagulase-negative *Staphylococcus*	*S. aureus*	Gram-negative bacilli	*Candida* spp.
Remove CVC/ID and treat with systemic antibiotics for 10–14 days	Remove CVC/ID and treat with antibiotics for 4–6 weeks; 6–8 weeks for osteomyelitis	• May retain CVC/ID and use systemic antibiotic for 7 days plus antibiotic lock therapy for 10–14 days • Remove CVC/ID if there is clinical deterioration, persisting or relapsing bacteremia	• Remove CVC/ID and use systemic antibiotic for 14 days if TEE (–) • For CVC/ID salvage therapy if TEE (–), use systemic and antibiotic lock therapy for 14 days • Remove CVC/ID and if there is clinical deterioration, persisting, or relapsing bacteremia	• Remove CVC/ID and treat 10–14 days • For CVC/ID salvage, use systemic and antibiotic lock therapy for 14 days • If no response, remove CVC/ID and treat with systemic antibiotic therapy for 10–14 days	• Remove CVC/ID and treat with antifungal therapy for 14 days after last positive blood culture

FIGURE 94-3 Management of bacteremia related to tunneled or surgically placed catheters. CVC, central venous catheter; ID, implantable device; TEE, transesophageal echocardiography. *(From Mermel LA, Farr BM, Sheretz RJ, et al. Guidelines for the management of intravascular catheter-related infections. Clin Infect Dis 2001;32:1249-1272.)*

pose a risk. Cephalosporin and ampicillin have been implicated most frequently, but recent virulent outbreaks of CDAD appear to be linked to newer fluoroquinolones.[21] Colonization of the colon with toxin-producing strains of *C. difficile*, in a susceptible host, may be followed by symptomatic disease. *C. difficile* produces at least two toxins, A and B, which stimulate fluid secretion, local inflammation, and mucosal injury. The inflammation forms typical pseudomembranes observed by sigmoidoscopy or colonoscopy and on biopsy (Fig. 94-4). Effects of toxin production may be mitigated by a vigorous antibody response.

Clinical Manifestations

Symptoms of CDAD can vary from mild diarrhea to septic shock with a perforated colon. Classically, symptoms include profuse watery diarrhea, abdominal pain, fever, anorexia, and general malaise. In contrast to viral diarrhea, vomiting is rare. In *C. difficile*-related ileus, diarrhea may not be seen. In those who develop toxic megacolon, mortality can be high (30%) from colonic perforation and peritonitis.[20] Abdominal radiography should be performed for those in whom *C. difficile* is suspected (Fig. 94-5).

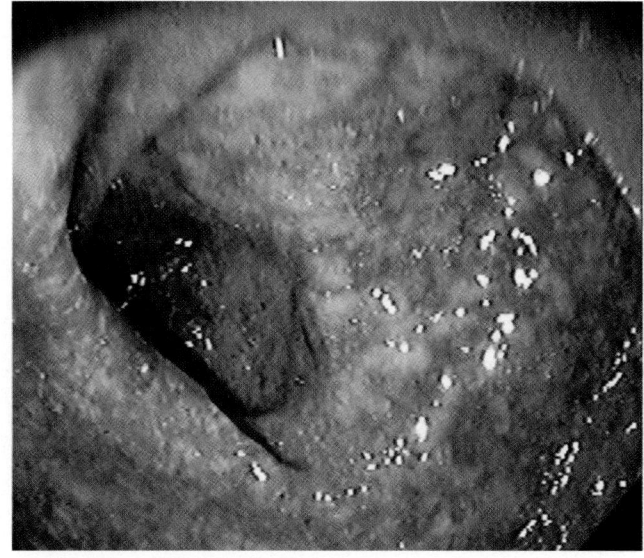

FIGURE 94-4 Pseudomembranous colitis secondary to infection with *Clostridium difficile. (Photograph courtesy of Dr. Clarence Wong.)*

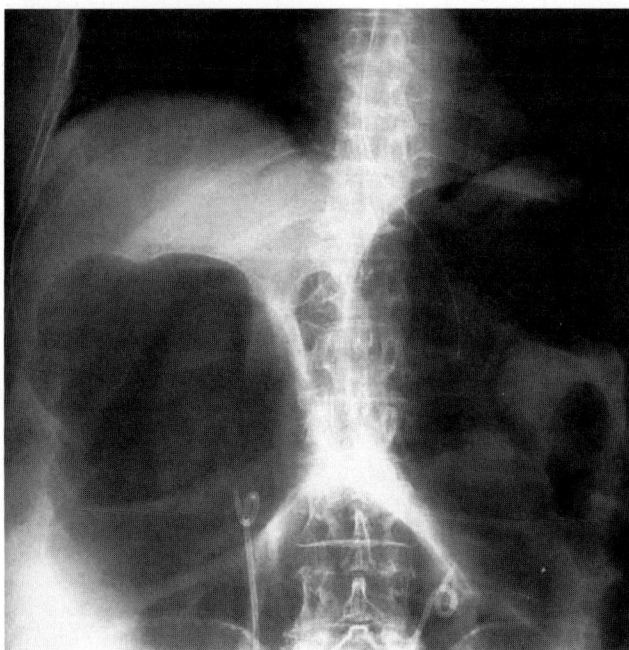

FIGURE 94-5 Toxic megacolon seen on an abdominal radiograph secondary to infection with *Clostridium difficile*. (*Photograph courtesy of Dr. Mark Joffe.*)

Box 94-4 Prevention of *Clostridium difficile* Infection

Prevention of nosocomial transmission of *Clostridium difficile* focuses on consistent and careful hand washing as well as institution of contact precautions for the affected individual (single room with consistent gown and glove use). Health care workers' hands, clothing, and equipment have been implicated in propagating outbreaks, and attention to these precautions and meticulous hand hygiene are critical. Some reports suggest that *Clostridium* spores may be more effectively killed with soap and water rather than alcohol hand wash, although this remains controversial. Thorough cleaning of affected rooms and equipment before occupation by a new patient is also important. Appropriate use of antimicrobials also has a role in preventing the development of *C. difficile*–associated diarrhea (CDAD), and restriction of implicated antibiotics (especially clindamycin) has proved to be an effective strategy for reducing outbreaks.

Leukocytosis even without toxic megacolon is common and can be impressive.

Differential Diagnosis

All hospitalized patients with diarrhea should have stool sent for detection of *C. difficile* toxin. Other possible causes of nosocomial diarrhea include viruses (e.g., norovirus, rotavirus) and bacterial pathogens (e.g., *Salmonella*). Noninfectious causes of diarrhea should also be considered, including medications, tube feedings, and fecal overflow (Box 94-4).

Treatment

First-line therapy for CDAD includes oral metronidazole, either 250 mg four times a day or 500 mg three times a day for 10 to 14 days. Oral vancomycin (125 mg four times a day for 10 to 14 days) is equivalent to metronidazole in efficacy and relapse rates, but most experts recommend metronidazole as the first-line agent because of cost and the potential for vancomycin-resistant enterococci (VRE).[20] The inciting antibiotic should be discontinued if possible, and supportive therapy such as hydration and electrolyte replacement should be given. Antidiarrheal agents should be avoided, because they may precipitate toxic megacolon.

Even when proper therapy is employed, *C. difficile* can recur in up to 25% of cases. As long as there was a good response to initial therapy, metronidazole should be the treatment of choice for the first relapse. If a patient relapses again after the second course of metronidazole, an infectious disease physician should be consulted.

Drugs of Choice

Metronidazole is the first-line agent for CDAD. For patients who cannot be treated with oral therapy, metronidazole may be provided intravenously, although treatment failures occur. Intravenous vancomycin does not appear to be effective, because insufficient drug concentrations are achieved in the colon. Vancomycin by retention enema may be considered. Various new therapies for CDAD are under investigation, including nitazoxanide, rifaximin, tolevamer, and probiotics. Surgical decompression is a last resort in the critically ill patient who is not responding to medical therapy.

WOUND INFECTIONS

Ulcers (malignant, pressure, arterial, venous, or neuropathic) need to be considered as a potential source of infection in a hospitalized patient who has a fever. Physical examination should include inspection of all pressure points in bedridden or deconditioned patients. If surgical sites are present, they should be considered as a potential source of infection and carefully inspected.

REFERENCES

1. Haley R, Culver DH, White JW, et al. The efficacy of infection surveillance and control programs in preventing nosocomial infections in US hospitals. Am J Epidemiol 1985;121:182-205.
2. Berwick DM, Calkins DR, McCannon CJ, Hackbarth AD. The 100,000 lives campaign. JAMA 2006;295:324-327.
3. Gerberding J. Hospital-onset infections: A patient safety issue. Ann Intern Med 2002;137:665-670.
4. White PH, Kuhlenschmidt HL, Vancura BG, Navari RM. Antimicrobial use in patients with advanced cancer receiving hospice care. J Pain Symptom Manage 2003;25:438-443.
5. Clayton J, Fardell B, Hutton-Potts J, et al. Parenteral antibiotics in a palliative care unit: Prospective analysis of current practice. Palliat Med 2003;17:44-48.
6. Vitetta L, Kenner D, Sali A. Bacterial infections in terminally ill hospice patients. J Pain Symptom Manage 2000;20:326-334.
7. Pereira J, Watanabe S, Wolch G. A retrospective review of the frequency of infections and patterns of antibiotic utilization on a palliative care unit. J Pain Symptom Manage 1998;16:374-381.
8. Niederman MS, Craven DE, Bonten MJ, et al. Guidelines for the management of adults with hospital acquired, ventilator associated, and healthcare associated pneumonia. Am J Crit Care Med 2005;171:388-416.
9. Falsey AR, Walsh EE. Viral pneumonia in older adults. Clin Infect Dis 2006;42:518-524.
10. Boivin G, De Serres G, Hamelin M, et al. An outbreak of severe respiratory tract infection due to human metapneumovirus in a long-term care facility. Clin Infect Dis 2007;44:1152-1158.
11. Bagshaw SM, Laupland KB. Epidemiology of intensive care unit-acquired urinary tract infections. Curr Opin Infect Dis 2006;19:67-71.
12. Trautner BW, Hull RA, Darouiche RO. Prevention of catheter-associated urinary tract infection. Curr Opin Infect Dis 2005;18:37-41.

13. Maki DG, Tambyah PA. Engineering out the risk of infection with urinary catheters. Emerg Infect Dis 2001;7:1-6.
14. Johnson JR., Kuskowski MA, Wilt TJ. Systematic review: Antimicrobial urinary catheters to prevent catheter-associated urinary tract infection in hospitalized patients. Ann Intern Med 2006;144:116-126.
15. Mermel LA, Farr BM, Sheretz RJ, et al. Guidelines for the management of intravascular catheter-related infections. Clin Infect Dis 2001;32:1249-1272.
16. Bearman MS. Bacteremias: A leading cause of death. Arch Med Res 2005;36:646-659.
17. Wisplinghoff H, Bischoff T, Tallent SM, et al. Nosocomial bloodstream infections in US hospitals: Analysis of 24,179 cases from a prospective nationwide surveillance study. Clin Infect Dis 2004;39:309-317.
18. O'Grady NP, Alexander M, Gerberding JL, et al. Guidelines for the prevention of intravascular catheter-related infections. MMWR 2002;51(RR-10):1.
19. Pronovost P, Needham D, Berenholtz S, et al. An intervention to decrease catheter-related bloodstream infections in the ICU. N Engl J Med 2006;355:2725-2732.
20. Poutanen SM, Simor AE. Clostridium difficile-associated diarrhea in adults. Can Med Assoc J 2004;171:51-58.
21. Pepin J, Saheb N, Coulombe MA, et al. Emergence of fluoroquinolones as the predominant risk factor for Clostridium difficile-associated diarrhea: A cohort study during an epidemic in Quebec. Clin Infect Dis 2005;41:1254-1260.

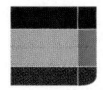

CHAPTER **95**

Fatal and Fulminant Infections

Erika Vlieghe, Karen Frame, and Robert Colebunders

K E Y   P O I N T S

- The range of (potentially) fatal infections is large and heterogeneous.

- Trying to cure the infection is usually the first goal.

- Depending on the prognosis, the role of palliation may become more prominent.

- Health care workers caring for these patients are often mentally and physically affected.

- Necessary infection control measures can increase suffering and isolation.

What is a fatal infection? A broad range of infections have the potential to become fatal if inadequately treated or if they occur in a vulnerable person. The scope is wide, from ordinary cellulitis or urinary tract infection to disseminated invasive aspergillosis. Rare infectious diseases exist with high intrinsic mortality despite the best therapy. For some of these diseases, targeted antimicrobial therapy exists but may be insufficient to overcome massive organ destruction caused by inflammation or necrosis. This result may be related to potent virulence factors of the causal microorganism (e.g., meningococcal sepsis and meningitis, necrotizing fascitis) or to a weak immune system (e.g., invasive aspergillosis, mucormycosis). For other diseases, mostly viral, no treatment exists except supportive care (e.g., Ebola and other viral hemorrhagic fevers, rabies).

The World Health Organization advocates that palliative care improve the quality of life of patients and families facing life-threatening illness through the prevention, assessment, and treatment of pain and other physical, psychosocial, and spiritual problems.[1] The role of palliative care in fulminant and often fatal infections is complex and ambiguous. With modern antimicrobial therapies, the conviction among practitioners has grown that an infection is potentially curable and that withdrawing adequate treatment would be unethical. On the other hand, treating someone who has a less than 10% survival rate for weeks or months, sometimes in seemingly "inhumane" conditions of isolation, unavoidably elicits questions about "therapeutic futility" and "dying in dignity." These questions often arise first from nurses and caregivers. Finally, certain infection control measures and fear within communities affected by outbreaks can contribute to taboo, stigmatization, and removal of the patient from caregivers and relatives, leading to a death in isolation. There is a vulnerable balance between cure and care.

BASIC SCIENCE AND EPIDEMIOLOGY

Mortality from Infectious Diseases

Common fulminant and fatal infections (Table 95-1) are a heterogeneous group, ranging from rare, localized epidemics with a invariably high case/fatality ratio, such as Ebola, to ubiquitous infections whose behavior is host dependent. The burden of infectious diseases in resource-poor areas is still high.[2,3] Most are potentially and easily curable (malaria, diarrheal and respiratory infections, tuberculosis), but they still kill millions of children and adults annually due to absent or dysfunctional health services, poverty, and malnutrition. HIV/AIDS is to date incurable, but it is treatable with preserved health for a sustained period for those with access to treatment (see Part IV, Section E). Viral hemorrhagic fevers are notorious and feared infectious killers, but casualties are low in absolute numbers, and these diseases are rare in time and place. Rabies is the main infection with an almost invariable 100% killing capacity.

Fatalities due to infections in the industrialized world are rarer but are increasing with a more aged, vulnerable population. Among the vulnerable are the growing group of individuals who are immunocompromised due to hematological or oncological disease and its treatment, those who have undergone organ transplantation, those taking immunosuppressant drugs for autoimmune illnesses, and an even larger population with diabetes, liver cirrhosis, or renal dialysis. Sepsis, nosocomial pneumonia, and rare fungal and opportunistic infections are the most common causes of infectious mortality in these settings.

New and worldwide emerging infections such as severe acute respiratory syndrome (SARS) and avian influenza H5N1 are known and feared for their fulminant clinical course and potential to spread quickly. Although this has not yet happened on a large scale, there is the potential for epidemics of such diseases in the future.

Pathophysiology

Infections can become fatal for several reasons: lack of an effective antimicrobial therapy (e.g., most fatal viral and

TABLE 95-1   Overview of Common Fulminant and Fatal Infections

INFECTION	AVERAGE MORTALITY RATE WITH BEST MEDICAL CARE (%)	ETIOLOGICAL THERAPY EXISTS?	AT-RISK POPULATION	REMARKS
VIRAL				
Rabies	100	No	Worldwide	
Viral hemorrhagic fever*	15-90	No	Rare, self-limited epidemics	Stringent isolation measures; supportive care
Viral encephalitis[†]	25	No	Worldwide	
SARS		No	Self-limited epidemic	Stringent isolation measures
Influenza H5N1	60?	±	Rare	Stringent isolation measures
CMV		Yes	Immune compromised	Meningoencephalitis, myocarditis
Herpes B	90?	±	Rare, after monkey bite	Myelitis
BACTERIAL				
Tetanus (*Clostridium tetani*)	Neonatal: 90 Adult severe: 60	±	Poor population	Preventable; supportive care can reduce mortality
Gas gangrene (*Clostridium perfringens*)	25 (100 if >48 hr)	Yes	War, cancer	Aggressive surgery; hyperbaric oxygen
Necrotizing fasciitis (streptococcal or polymicrobial)	20-47	Yes		Aggressive surgery
Septicemia: *Pseudomonas aeruginosa, Staphylococcus aureus, Neisseria meningitidis, Streptococcus pneumoniae*	30-60	Yes		
Endocarditis: *P. aeruginosa, S. aureus*	25?	Yes		
Meningitis				
Community-acquired	33	Yes		
Nosocomial	35			
S. aureus	14-77			
Leptospirosis (Weil's disease)	5-40	Yes		
Plague septicemia	33			
FUNGAL				
Invasive aspergillosis	Lung: 50-60 Brain: 100	Yes	Most frequent mold in developed countries	Immunocompromised
Mucormycosis	50	±	Rare	Immunocompromised
Cryptococcal meningitis	25-30	Yes	Frequent in HIV-endemic countries	Immunocompromised or HIV+
Rare molds: *Scedosporium, Fusarium*	50-80	±	Rare	Immunocompromised
PARASITIC				
Pneumocystis jiroveci pneumonia	Fulminant: 80 Overall: 30-50	Yes	Frequent in HIV+	
Naegleria/Acanthamoeba (primary amebic meningoencephalitis)	95		Rare	Ubiquitous
Plasmodium falciparum		Yes	Frequent in tropics	Preventable/treatable
Cryptosporidium	Fulminant diarrhea	±	Frequent in AIDS	Treatable with HAART; palliation is difficult
Strongyloides hyperinfestation		±	Rare	Immunocompromised

*Includes yellow fever, Ebola, Marburg, Lassa virus, dengue hemorrhagic fever, and Crimean Congo hemorrhagic fever.
[†]Includes Japanese encephalitis, St. Louis encephalitis, varicella-zoster virus, and CMV.
AIDS, acquired immunodeficiency syndrome; CMV, cytomegalovirus; HAART, highly active antiretroviral therapy; HIV, human immunodeficiency virus; SARS, severe acute respiratory syndrome.
Adapted from Mandell GL, Bennett JE, Dolin R (eds). Principles and Practices of Infectious Diseases, 5th ed. New York: Churchill Livingstone, 2000.

fungal diseases), inability to stop the deleterious effects of the disease (the pathophysiology of sepsis), and lack of a targeted and effective immune response (opportunistic infections in immunosuppressed transplant or chemotherapy recipients).

Lack of Effective Antimicrobial Therapy

Antimicrobial drugs were first developed[4] for the then important and known infections: staphylococcal and streptococcal infections, diphtheria, tuberculosis, and syphilis. With the rise of nosocomial infections, the antibiotic arsenal expanded. In recent decades, the group of multidrug-resistant (MDR) or omniresistant bacterial strains such as methicillin-resistant *Staphylococcus aureus* (MRSA), glycopeptide intermediate-resistant *S. aureus* (GISA), vancomycin-resistant enterococci (VRE), extended-spectrum β-lactamase–producing (ESBL⁺) organisms, MDR *Pseudomonas*, and MDR tuberculosis has grown steadily. In other infections, antibiotics are unable to reach the focus of infection (e.g., endocarditis, meningitis).

Advances in antiviral therapy have been made only since the 1970s, with acyclovir, and, more than 20 years later, with antiretroviral therapy in response to the epidemic of acquired immunodeficiency syndrome (AIDS). This has brought better understanding of viral disease and, consequently, antiviral therapy for other infections, such as hepatitis B virus (HBV), hepatitis C virus (HCV), and cytomegalovirus (CMV). The variations in pathogenic viruses and their diverse epidemiology worldwide have hampered universal therapeutic coverage for all important viral illnesses. In addition, most antiviral products are too expensive for many poor patients. However, many potentially fatal viral infections can be prevented by vaccination, including smallpox, yellow fever, HBV, polio, measles, and certain types of viral encephalitis. Worldwide coverage with even the cheapest vaccines is far from a reality. For the most fulminant and feared viral infections (rabies, Ebola, and other viral hemorrhagic fevers, SARS, influenza), no effective antiviral treatment exists. Postexposure vaccination exists for rabies but is often not within reach of those most at risk.[5]

Lack of an Effective Immune Response: "Walkover"

The body's immune system encompasses a complex interplay among several organs (e.g., skin and mucosa, blood and bone marrow, lymph nodes and spleen) and defense systems (e.g., humoral, cellular), coordinated by cytokines and other messenger molecules. Most people who are at risk for severe infections suffer from several "gaps" in their defenses. Those with hematological malignancies have not only insufficient bone marrow and lack of granulocytes but also severe mucositis and several indwelling devices through which organisms may enter. Often, they have already received broad-spectrum antibiotics which replace natural bacterial flora with MDR species through selective pressure. Concomitant malnutrition, immunosuppressant drugs, and organ failure (renal, hepatic, diabetes) may complete the picture.

Toxins and Cytokines

Some patients may suffer from hyperacute, life-threatening disease despite proper antimicrobial treatment and a healthy immune system. Toxins produced by microorganisms may play an important role in such infections, including tetanus, necrotizing fasciitis, staphylococcal toxic shock syndrome, cholera, and botulism. Timely antitoxin, when available, is then a cornerstone of treatment.[6]

Every infection triggers the body's inflammatory response through a complex interplay of cytokines and interleukins.[7] In some, the response may be so intense that more damage is caused by this "cytokine storm" than the original organism. These are vicious circles created by positive feedback mechanisms. Treatment tries to counteract the deleterious cascades of coagulation, free radicals, hypoxygenation, and organ dysfunction.[8]

DISCUSSION

There is a difficult balance in fulminant infections: some patients may have a chance of cure (albeit small) and could benefit from aggressive management in terms of survival, yet have a high chance of dying. There is a danger in labeling care as "palliative," because this can cause the patient to be denied "active management" and a chance of cure. Equally, a focus on cure in a person with a poor prognosis can deny the patient optimal palliative care. In fulminant disease, some unpleasant, painful diagnostic and therapeutic procedures (e.g., imaging, lumbar puncture, débridement) may be necessary for optimal treatment and survival. As the chance of survival decreases, the negative aspects of such procedures gradually outweigh the potential benefits, and the procedure will be regarded by patient and carers as futile. Alternatively, withholding such procedures may be seen as "giving up" the hope for cure and survival. An individualized, holistic approach to patients with fulminant infections, addressing physical (including symptom control), psychological, spiritual, and social and family needs together with regular re-evaluation of the therapeutic response and goals of care, is essential (see the five Case Studies presented in this chapter).

CASE STUDY

Clostridium perfringens Infection in a Metastatic Colonic Carcinoma

A 69-year-old woman with type 2 diabetes was admitted to the hospital with fever and feculent vaginal discharge. She had previously been diagnosed with locally advanced rectal carcinoma. Curative resection was impossible because of tumor invasion of pelvic structures and the sacrum. She underwent palliative stoma formation and radiotherapy but declined palliative chemotherapy and was depressed about her general condition. Soon after admission, a colovaginal fistula and a urinary tract infection were diagnosed, and she was started on amoxicillin-clavulanate. Two days later, she began complaining of severe pain in her left hip, radiating toward the knee. The pain rapidly became excruciating. Radiographs of the left hip and femur revealed air in the tissues around the femur, suggesting gas gangrene. Blood cultures grew *Clostridium clostridioforme* and *Clostridium perfringens*. Management would have involved extensive débridement and probably hemipelvectomy, hyperbaric oxygen therapy, and high-dose penicillin; even with these aggressive treatments, the prognosis was grim. She was stuporous from the infection and pain and did not have any relatives to discuss management decisions. Eventually, she was prescribed parenteral morphine for rapid pain relief, and she passed away 2 days later.

The combination of a fulminant and very painful infection with high intrinsic mortality in a patient with incurable disease who had previously declined palliative chemotherapy strongly influenced the decision not to start active treatment but to undertake a palliative approach. Communication within the health care team and with the patient and family in such situations is central to optimizing care. If a patient is confused or incompetent, difficult ethical issues may arise.

Good communication among health professionals and with the patient and family is crucial. Fulminant infections can progress rapidly; patients deteriorate quickly, so that most die during the battle for survival, when the main goal is survival. Highly contagious infectious diseases such as viral hemorrhagic fevers, SARS, and influenza necessitate stringent isolation measures which may add to marginalization and suboptimal symptom care.[10,11] Communication between the patient and his or her relatives may be difficult, incomplete, or nonexistent. Health care workers

 CASE STUDY

Necrotizing Fasciitis in a Young Woman in Uganda

A 27-year-old woman in rural Uganda was admitted with fever and pain in the right thigh. The initial examinations (complete blood count, ultrasound, and radiography of the femur) did not reveal any abnormalities. Pain increased, and necrotic bullae appeared on the overlying skin. Intravenous broad-spectrum antibiotics were started, and the doctor requested permission from the patient to perform a débridement. The woman, coming from a traditional community, considered herself unable to decide this matter and decided to await the return of her husband from the kraal 200 km away. Because no public transport was available and communication was limited, a messenger was sent to inform the husband. Despite experiencing terrible pain from a foul-smelling leg crawling with maggots, the patient and her mother continued to decline any intervention until the husband arrived (Fig. 95-1). He agreed immediately to disarticulation of the entire leg, but the patient died in septic shock soon afterward.

For cultural reasons, neither the patient nor the doctor was able to make a decision regarding active, aggressive management of the infection, which might have saved her life if started early in the illness. This meant that the patient did not receive palliative care either: she remained in a therapeutic "no man's land." The balance between care, cure, compassion, and anger was difficult and led to frustration among nursing staff.

 CASE STUDY

Rabies

A 25-year-old Ugandan farmer, father of four children, was admitted to a hospital with severe agitation, confusion, and fever after suffering a dog bite 2 weeks earlier. The dog had been noticed to become sick and lethargic the day after the dog bite and was thought to have rabies. A diagnosis of rabies was made.

Few treatment options exist for rabies other than postexposure treatment, which was not available in this resource-limited setting and was unlikely to help once the patient was symptomatic. Despite a mortality rate of almost 100%, rare recoveries feed the dilemma between hope for a (very unlikely) cure or care. Long-term care requires large amounts of much human and material resources. Symptom management would include sedation.[9]

 CASE STUDY

Endocarditis Caused by Mucormycosis in a Hematology Patient

A 35-year-old woman with recurrent non-Hodgkin's lymphoma was admitted after her first cycle of third-line chemotherapy with neutropenia, fever, and shock. Transthoracic echocardiography revealed large vegetations on the pulmonary and tricuspid valves; computed tomography of the chest suggested multiple septic emboli in the lungs. She was requiring full inotropic and ventilatory support. Blood cultures grew mucormycosis. She was started on intravenous amphotericin B. She developed acute respiratory distress syndrome (ARDS) and a necrotic facial lesion.

Theoretical treatment options exist but would have involved mutilating facial excision surgery. Survival chances (both short and long term) are low. Palliative care in a sedated, ventilated patient with an extremely limited prognosis would probably focus on communication with and counseling of relatives and progressive withdrawal of therapy while ensuring pain and symptom control together with sedation.

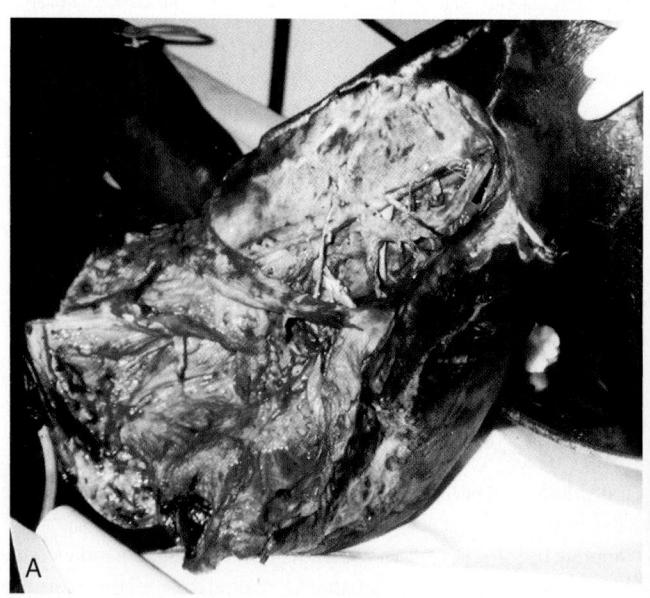
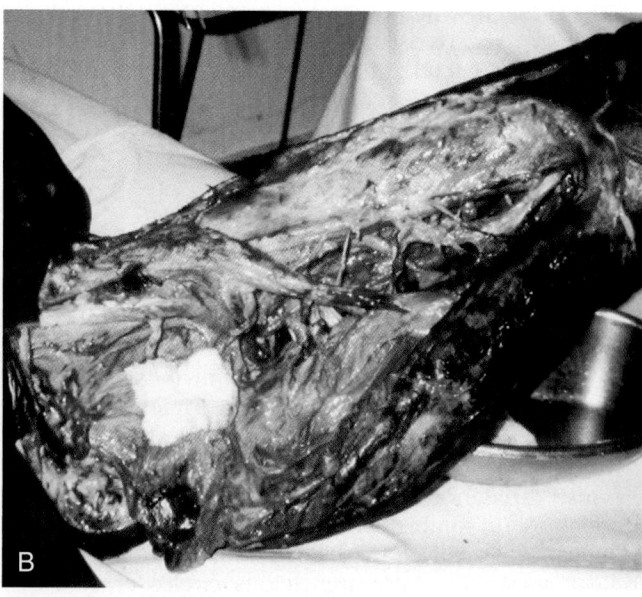

FIGURE 95-1   A and **B**, Necrotizing fasciitis in a young woman in Uganda.

CASE STUDY

Ebola Hemorrhagic Fever

A 35-year-old Ugandan soldier was admitted with a febrile illness after caring for a colleague who had died with fever and hemorrhage. Malaria slides were negative, and 2 days later he started vomiting blood and went into shock. Serological studies from the colleague confirmed Ebola hemorrhagic fever. The patient was isolated, later complained of severe abdominal pain with persistent vomiting, and became confused and agitated, pulling out intravenous lines. Local radio stations advocated shooting the patient, his family, and the health care workers caring for him to prevent the spread of Ebola. Hospital workers were not served in local markets or shops. Relatives were prevented from visiting the patient for infection control purposes. The patient was frightened and was nursed by health care workers wearing gowns and masks. Administration of parenteral medication for pain and symptom control was required, but concerns were raised because of the patient's agitation and the risk of a needlestick injury. A health worker (Fig. 95-2) was able to pray with the patient, but he was unable to receive last rites. He died in isolation with no family members around. Infection control measures required that the body be buried in a communal grave rather than at the patient's ancestral home, culturally considered a prerequisite for a good death and afterlife.

Ebola and other hemorrhagic fevers have high mortality rates, and treatment is limited to supportive care. Patients complain of abdominal pain and vomiting; confusion and agitation also occurs and can be difficult to manage. Pain and symptom control in such patients is important. Management of agitation and confusion can reduce the risk to health care workers, but parenteral medication brings with it the risk of needlestick injury. Stigma and fear are common during outbreaks, affecting both patients and those caring for them. To die in isolation, in pain, terrified, cared for by people in "bubble suits," and unable to have family or religious support is not "a good death." Cultural burial practices, even though they are important expectations of patients and their families and are believed to ensure a happy afterlife, may also have to be dispensed with, adding to family grief. Family members may often be contacts themselves, and may be monitored to see whether they become ill. A holistic approach by health care workers in such situations is essential.

themselves may also be mentally and/or physically affected by an ongoing epidemic.[12,13] In some infections, protection of health care workers and family members from acquiring the disease is also a moral obligation, yet infection control measures can result in the patient's dying in isolation. This may be at odds with cultural norms surrounding palliative care and burial practices, resulting in distress. We must judge on a case-by-case basis the role of palliative care within a comprehensive approach toward fulminant infection (see "Future Considerations").

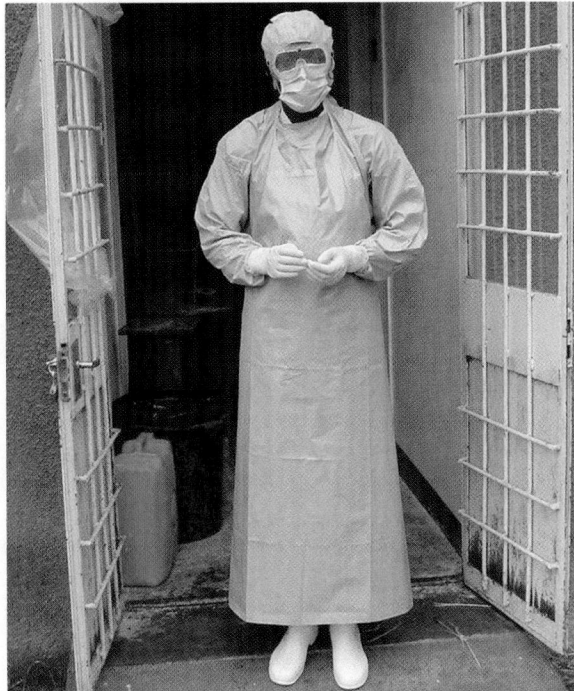

FIGURE 95-2   Ebola outfit. *(Courtesy of Dr. Larry Pepper.)*

Future Considerations

- When to stop: how low is "no chance of survival"?
- Does palliative care mean that active management should stop?
- Communication with and between patients and relatives: when, how?
- Culturally and socially sensitive, effective infection control measures: are they feasible?
- Caring for the carers: how should this best be provided (peer support?)

REFERENCES

1. World Health Organization. Palliative Care, 2002. Available at http://www.who.int/hiv/topics/palliative/care/en (accessed April 11, 2008).
2. Armstrong GL, Conn LA, Pinner RW. Trends in infectious disease mortality in the United States during the 20th century. JAMA 1999;281:61-66.
3. Lopez AD, Mathers CD, et al. Global and regional burden of disease and risk factors, 2001: Systematic analysis of population health data. Lancet 2006;367:1747-1757.
4. Porter R (ed). Drug treatment and the rise in pharmacology. In Porter R (ed). The Cambridge Illustrated History of Medicine. Cambridge: Cambridge University Press, 1996, Chapter 7.
5. World Health Organization. Rabies vaccines. Weekly Epidemiological Record 2002;77(14):109-120. Available at www.who.int/wer (accessed November 2, 2007).
6. Sobel J. Botulism. Clin Infect Dis 2005;41:1167-1173.
7. Hotchkiss RS. The pathophysiology and treatment of sepsis. N Engl J Med 2003;348:138-150.
8. Russell JA. Management of sepsis. N Engl J Med 2006;355:1699-1713.
9. Jackson AC, Warrell MJ, et al. Management of rabies in humans. Clin Infect Dis 2003;36:60-63.
10. Leong IY, Lee AO, et al. The challenge of providing holistic care in a viral epidemic: Opportunities for palliative care. Palliat Med 2004;18:12-18.
11. Bitekyerezo M, Kyobutungi C, Kizza R, et al. The outbreak and control of Ebola viral hemorrhagic fever in a Ugandan medical school. Trop Doct 2002;32:10-15.
12. Hewlett BL, Hewlett BS. Providing care and facing death: Nursing during Ebola outbreaks in Central Africa. J Transcult Nurs 2005;16(4):289-297.
13. Chan AO, Huak CY. Psychological impact of the 2003 severe acute respiratory syndrome outbreak on health care workers in a medium size regional general hospital in Singapore. Occup Med 2004;54:190-196.

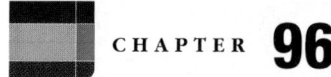

CHAPTER **96**

Antimicrobial Use in the Dying

Thomas G. Fraser

KEY POINTS

- The dying patient is at risk for infection.
- Goals of antibiotic treatment need to be defined before therapy commences.
- Efficacy of antibiotics to control symptoms is not firmly established.
- Complex clinical conditions can make rational antibiotic selection challenging.
- Decreasing antimicrobial susceptibility limits antibiotic choices.

Patients with terminal illnesses are at risk for infections and are commonly prescribed antibiotics. The incidence of symptomatic infection in hospice patients ranges from 36% to 55%.[1-4] Systemic antibiotics are commonly prescribed for dying patients in acute care hospitals.[5] The decision to use an anti-infective agent may appear straightforward, but scrutiny finds such decisions to be more complex. The major issues include the diagnosis, functional status of the patient, and available resources balanced against the severity and reversibility of the infectious syndrome. The prevalence of resistant pathogens, particularly in the heath care–experienced patient, also affects the selection of an anti-infective agent.

PATIENT FACTORS

Not all dying patients with infections are alike. The specifics of their illnesses put them at risk for infections but also affect their ability to recover from infection. For example, a patient with advanced dementia may not be able to cough; this not only increases the risk of aspiration but also prevents effective clearance of pneumonia. Metastatic cancer may lead to obstructive uropathy, predisposing to urinary tract infections. If the obstruction is not relieved, the infection will most likely not be controlled. Such interventions escalate the level of care. The prognosis and functional status may also affect treatment. For example, percutaneous intervention to relieve urinary tract obstruction may be reasonable for someone who is currently functional yet has an untreatable malignancy. Immune status must also be considered. Previous treatments or the underlying disease may cause defects in cellular or humoral immunity.

TREATMENT GOALS

Before prescribing an antibiotic for a dying patient, treatment goals need to be determined. Is one attempting to eradicate the infection? Is symptom control the primary indication? For people with limited prognosis, the level of medical intervention acceptable to the patient and family must be determined. This influences the therapeutic approach. For example, urosepsis (see Chapter 93) is theoretically reversible but requires inpatient supportive care and prompt administration of antibiotics for successful treatment. Antibiotics alone would be of limited value in such a rapid-onset, severe infection if the goal of therapy is to eradicate the infection and return the patient to his or her premorbid health level.

The efficacy of antibiotics as symptom relief in the terminally ill varies. Available data indicate that antibiotic treatment of symptomatic urinary tract infections can result in resolution of irritative voiding symptoms, but the response to respiratory tract, skin, and soft tissue infections and bacteremia is unreliable.[1-3] Of note, the uropathogens in these studies reviewed were mostly susceptible to first-line agents. In advanced dementia, one study showed that antibiotics as part of the approach to a new fever did not help this symptom.[6] One nonrandomized study of antibiotic use in demented patients with presumed pneumonia demonstrated significant discomfort from the illness, and those given antibiotics had less discomfort. Interpretation of this study is difficult, however, because those not treated were more likely to be severely demented and to have more discomfort at baseline.[7] A small series of advanced head and neck tumors in patients who presented with increased pain responded to therapy for presumed superinfection; the specifics of the antibiotic regimen were not provided[8] (Fig. 96-1).

INFECTION-SPECIFIC FACTORS

There is a clinical difference between a symptomatic urinary tract infection or bronchitis and a significant parenchymal infection such as lobar pneumonia or a deep organ space infection. The degree to which antibiotics can be expected to be successful also influences the decision to treat. The data presented earlier suggest that symptomatic urinary tract infection is one instance in which antibiotics may be expected to help. Many infections, such as abdominal or pelvic abscesses, require drainage procedures to be effectively treated. If the patient is deemed not to be a surgical candidate, antibiotics should also be questioned, because the chance for a successful outcome is then poor.

Chronic infection may develop as a complication of therapy for a fatal illness (e.g., hematological malignancy with an invasive fungal infection). Infections such as these are not curable without successful treatment of the underlying disease, and continued therapy in these circumstances may be unreasonable.

Finally, a dying patient may have an infection that, if left untreated, would pose a community threat. An example is a patient with pulmonary tuberculosis whose life expectancy is shorter than the usual length of therapy. Use of antituberculosis medications would be justified, because, if the infection is left untreated, it would pose a risk to the patient's family and other close contacts (including health care workers). Similarly, if an institution in which a patient is hospitalized experiences an influenza outbreak, prophylactic antiviral medication may help control the outbreak and prevent further disease transmission.

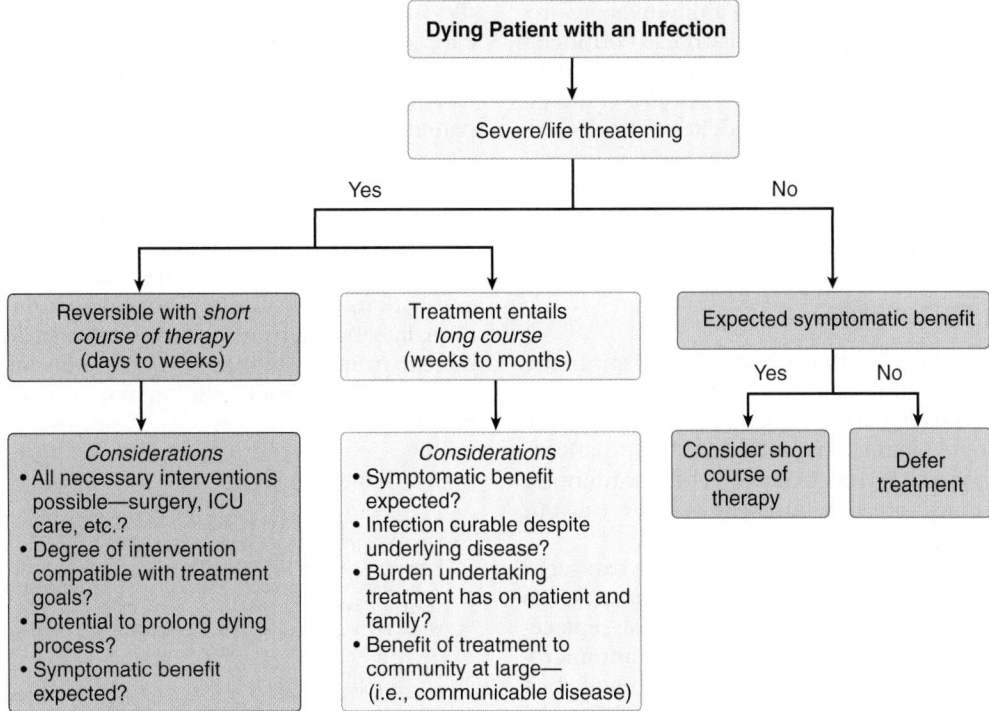

FIGURE 96-1 Management algorithm for the dying patient with an infection.

Box 96-1 Considerations for Antibiotic Selection

- Choose the agent with the narrowest possible spectrum.
- Pathogen-directed therapy is favored over empirical therapy.
- Use oral therapy whenever possible.
- Dose is based on renal and hepatic function.
- Choose empirical agents based on local susceptibility patterns.

Box 96-2 Unintended Consequences of Antibiotic Therapy in the Dying

- Burden on patient and caregivers—time and finances
- Allergic reactions
- Drug interactions
- Nausea, vomiting, diarrhea, *Clostridium difficile*-associated diarrhea
- Infusion-related complications of intravenous therapy

ANTIBIOTIC SELECTION

Once the decision has been made to initiate antibiotic therapy, the choice of agent is dictated by numerous clinical factors. Pathogen-directed therapy is favored over empirical therapy. Establishing a microbiological diagnosis requires appropriate specimens for culture, and obtaining these may be unacceptably invasive in the terminally ill.

Oral antibiotics are preferred but this may be impossible if the patient is unable to swallow. Use of intravenous antibiotics requires reliable venous access. For homebound patients, this method of drug delivery requires a commitment by the patient and family of time, effort, and often money. There are limited resources in many areas for home antibiotic infusions.

People with complicated medical problems that are in the end stage of life commonly have impaired renal and hepatic function. These issues affect the dose and administration schedule. Lack of attention to these details increases the risk of adverse drug effects (Box 96-1).

For the health care–experienced patient, decreased antibiotic susceptibility among pathogens is one of the most significant issues affecting antibiotic selection. Prior antibiotic exposure is an important historical feature that must be incorporated into antibiotic choice for many common syndromes.[9] Bacterial susceptibility patterns vary based on practice location, but several trends are widespread. There has been a significant decrease in susceptibility among uropathogens to trimethoprim-sulfamethoxazole.[10] Methicillin resistance among *Staphylococcus aureus* isolates is common in health care–experienced patients.[11] Fluoroquinolone resistance among Enterobacteriaceae and *Pseudomonas aeruginosa* is increasing.[12,13] Certain patient populations have nonsusceptible *Streptococcus pneumoniae* present with a prevalence greater than 25%.[14] The likelihood has decreased that an inexpensive, well-tolerated oral antibiotic will provide effective, empirical therapy.

The cost of antimicrobials also influences decision making, particularly if patients are enrolled in hospice or if they have no prescription drug coverage. These costs can be prohibitive if intravenous therapy is prescribed. These issues are not uncommon given the need to choose broad-spectrum agents because of increased antimicrobial resistance.

There are also unintended consequences to the use of antibiotics, particularly when the objective benefits of therapy are unclear (Box 96-2). There is a chance of allergic reaction with any antibiotic. Drug interactions can also cause dangerous adverse effects. Oral antibiotics are frequently associated with nausea and diarrhea. Peripheral or central venous access for parenteral therapy risks thrombophlebitis or deep vein thrombosis and catheter-related superinfection. A patient with delirium or dementia may require restraints to maintain venous access. Finally, *Clostridium difficile*–associated diarrhea may be endemic in some institutions and can be a devastating complication of antibiotics.[15]

ETHICAL CONSIDERATIONS

A central question for any ethical discussion of antibiotic use in the terminally ill is whether antibiotics are "usual care."[16] The opinions of patients, their families, and physicians vary.[17] Some studies suggest that both patients and families, if asked, are less likely to refuse antibiotics; physician opinions are inconsistent (see "Current Controversies").

The decision as to whether to use antibiotics can seem less important when compared to larger decisions such as whether to use mechanical ventilation or renal replacement therapy. From an infectious disease and antimicrobial stewardship perspective, however, prescribing habits do have impacts beyond the proximate situation. The use of antibiotics can lead to the development of resistant pathogens, which, in turn, may cause superinfection in treated individuals. It is difficult to quantify the risk, but it is reasonable to assume that a dying patient with a chronic illness is predisposed to further infectious morbidity. Continued use of antibiotics to treat infections as they arise (when the underlying illness cannot be affected) will most likely lead, ultimately, to fewer antibiotic choices. Antibiotics will be also more difficult to provide, with a less assured successful outcome. These medicines also tend to be more expensive. In a capitated hospice system, this may result in unreasonable costs for all as a consequence of pursuing a secondary issue when the overall outcome cannot be changed.

Practicing physicians have a duty not only to their primary patient but also to the health care population. Indiscriminate antibiotic use can foster resistance in individual patients. This poses a risk to the individual, but, in addition, someone who is colonized with resistant bacteria can serve as a reservoir for cross-transmission to others in the same health care setting. This issue is of most concern in an inpatient setting providing either acute or long-term care.

Aggressive antimicrobial treatment regimens for an infection also entail other unintended consequences. Treatment of the infection can draw focus away from the central issue—the underlying condition. This could delay

the transition to hospice and more appropriate terminal care. Another ethical consideration is whether antibiotics prolong dying and are incompatible with overall goals of care. If one successfully treats lobar pneumonia in a dying patient, does the incremental increased life expectancy also entail incremental increase in suffering from the terminal illness? Examples from other complications in the course of the dying process illustrate this point.[16] For instance, hypercalcemia as a complication of metastatic malignancy can be readily treated with bisphosphonates and hydration but is often not pursued in a person dying of malignancy. Given the lack of clearly defined symptom benefit from antibiotics, is treating an infection substantially different from treating hypercalcemia in a dying patient?

REFERENCES

1. Vitetta L, Kenner D, Sali A. Bacterial infections in terminally ill hospice patients. J Pain Symptom Manage 2000;20:326-334.
2. Reinbolt R, Shenk AM, White PH, et al. Symptomatic treatment of infections in patients with advanced cancer receiving hospice care. J Pain Symptom Manage 2005;30:175-182.
3. White PH, Kuhlenschmidt HL, Vancura BG, et al. Antimicrobial use in patients with advanced cancer receiving hospice care. J Pain Symptom Manage 2003;25:438-443.
4. Pereira J, Watanabe S, Wolch G. A retrospective review of the frequency of infections and patterns of antibiotic utilization on a palliative care unit. J Pain Symptom Manage 1998;16:374-381.
5. Ahronheim JC, Morrison S, Baskin SA, et al. Treatment of the dying in the acute care hospital. Arch Intern Med 1996;156:2094-2100.
6. Fabiszewski KJ, Volicer B, Volicer L. Effect of antibiotic treatment on outcome of fevers in institutionalized Alzheimer patients. JAMA 1990;263:3168-3172.
7. van der Steen JT, Ooms ME, van der Wal G, et al. Pneumonia: The demented patient's best friend? Discomfort after starting or withholding antibiotic treatment. J Am Geriatr Soc 2002;50:1681-1688.
8. Breuers E, MacDonald N. Intractable pain in patients with advanced head and neck tumors: A possible role of local infection. Cancer Treat Rep 1986;70:691-692.
9. Guidelines for the management of adults with hospital-acquired, ventilator-associated, and healthcare-associated pneumonia. Am J Respir Crit Care Med 2005;171:388-416.
10. Hooton TM, Besser R, Foxman B, et al. Acute uncomplicated cystitis in an era of increasing antibiotic resistance: A proposed approach to empirical therapy. Clin Infect Dis 2004;39:75-80.
11. Friedman ND, Kaye KS, Stout JE, et al. Health care-associated bloodstream infections in adults: A reason to change the accepted definition of community-acquired infections. Ann Intern Med 2002;137:791-797.
12. Fridkin SK, Hill HA, Volkova NV, et al. Temporal trends in prevalence of antimicrobial resistance in 23 U.S. hospitals. Emerg Infect Dis 2002;8:697-701.
13. National Nosocomial Infections Surveillance (NNIS) System report. Am J Infection Control 2001;29:404-421.
14. Doern GV, Heilmann KP, Huynh HK, et al. Antimicrobial resistance among clinical isolates of Streptococcus pneumoniae in the United States during 1999-2000, including a comparison of resistance rates since 1994-1995. Antimicrob Agents Chemother 2001;45:1721-1729.
15. McDonald LC, Kilgore GE, Thompson A, et al. An epidemic, toxin gene-variant strain of *Clostridium difficile*. N Engl J Med 2005;353:2433-2441.
16. Ford PJ, Fraser TG, Davis MP, et al. Anti-infective therapy at end of life: Ethical decision-making in hospice-eligible patients. Bioethics 2005;19:379-392.
17. Marcus EL, Clarfield AM, Moses AE. Ethical issues relating to the use of antimicrobial therapy in older adults. Clin Infect Dis 2001;33:1697-1705.

SUGGESTED READING

Ford PJ, Fraser TG, Davis MP, et al. Anti-infective therapy at end of life: Ethical decision-making in hospice-eligible patients. Bioethics 2005;19:379-392.

Marcus EL, Clarfield AM, Moses AE. Ethical issues relating to the use of antimicrobial therapy in older adults. Clin Infect Dis 2001;33:1697-1705.

Reinbolt R, Shenk AM, White PH, et al. Symptomatic treatment of infections in patients with advanced cancer receiving hospice care. J Pain Symptom Manage 2005;30:175-182.

White PH, Kuhlenschmidt HL, Vancura BG, et al. Antimicrobial use in patients with advanced cancer receiving hospice care. J Pain Symptom Manage 2003;25:438-443.

Current Controversies

- Efficacy of antibiotics in ameliorating symptoms
- Impact of a capitated system to provide antimicrobial therapy as part of end-of-life care
- Are antibiotics part of usual care in a dying patient?
- Are physicians willing to not treat an acute infection in a dying patient?

Procedures and Devices

CHAPTER **97**

Palliative Surgery

Geoffrey P. Dunn

Palliative surgery is one of the major enterprises of a new field of humanistic scientific initiative referred to as surgical palliative care.[1] It is evolving from a poorly defined set of procedures to an evidence-based approach to the surgical means of relieving suffering and promoting quality of life that may include cure or remission of the underlying disease.

PRINCIPLES OF SURGICAL PALLIATIVE CARE AND PALLIATIVE SURGERY

The primary principles of surgical palliative care, deeply rooted in surgical tradition, are (1) nonabandonment and (2) preservation of hope. The social expression of these principles has had a major impact on the practice of surgery. The impetus for the founding of the American College of Surgeons in 1913 (when almost all successful surgery was palliative) was the need to address the wrong of itinerant surgery (a less obvious form of abandonment) and to incorporate scientific principles into surgical practice, freeing the patient from the tyrannies of devastating illnesses and surgeons' anecdotal and often paternalistic judgments. The principles of *surgical palliative care* are fundamentally no different from those for all surgical care.

A consensus definition by oncological surgeons for *palliative surgery* states: "Palliative surgery is limited to operations performed to relieve symptoms. The operations may be inclusive of treating the disease process with curative intent, but in all cases the management of symptoms should be an element of intervention. Specifically, operations with curative intent in asymptomatic patients that result in residual disease or positive margins should be considered noncurative, not palliative."[2] Therefore, an asymptomatic patient cannot be palliated, but a symptomatic patient can be palliated and/or cured. The American College of Surgeons Surgical Palliative Care Task Force has written a more limited definition of palliative surgery: "any invasive procedure used for treatment when the major goal of treatment is relief or the prevention of symptoms to improve quality of life for patients with incurable illness. This treatment may or may not prolong life, but that is not the primary goal of the procedure."[3]

GENERAL CONSIDERATIONS

Resolution of symptoms is a measurable outcome generic to all palliative interventions. However, for invasive interventions, additional outcomes must be given more weight when planning treatment. These include the durability of symptom control, the morbidity and mortality of the procedure, and the anticipated survival.

Surgical mortality is defined as patient death occurring during and up to 30 days after a procedure. This can be a potent disincentive for surgeons to operate on patients with limited life expectancy, even for good indications. There is no consensus about what shorter duration of life expectancy would contraindicate surgery. Among 823 patients undergoing palliative operations at Memorial Sloan Kettering Cancer Center, 11% died within 30 days.[4]

Operative morbidity is common after palliative oncological surgery, occurring in up to 40% of patients, with 10% requiring additional surgery for the morbidity.[4] Operative morbidity can be difficult to distinguish from illness-related morbidity. The distinction is crucial, however, when considering surgery for constitutional symptoms (e.g., fatigue, fever, anorexia). Relief of bowel obstruction can renew alimentation but will not restore appetite in a patient with established anorexia/cachexia syndrome. Palliative surgery is most likely to provide benefit in pain, ulceration, bleeding, or complications of obstruction. Careful patient selection that reflects a clear understanding of patient goals is necessary given the desired outcome of durable symptom control without operative morbidity: this occurred less than one fifth of the time in the Memorial series. Additional considerations for palliative surgical procedures include (1) the personality and perceptions of patient and family, (2) patient physiology, (3) disease biology, (4) the intervention, and (5) the profile of the surgeon (Tables 97-1 and 97-2).

TABLE 97-1 Decision Making for Palliative Surgical Interventions	
ELEMENT OF DECISION MAKING	**CONSIDERATIONS**
Patient psyche	Active versus passive Mature versus panicked Realistic versus magical thinking
Patient physiology	Functional versus debilitated Actual versus chronological age Preserved nutrition versus hypoalbuminemic
Disease biology	Single disease versus multiple co-morbidities Slow-growing versus aggressive
The intervention	Evidence-based versus anecdotal experience ("N of 1") Routine versus uncommon Low versus high morbidity risk (physical, financial, social) Straightforward versus difficult One of many options versus no other option
Profile of the surgeon	Empathic healer versus technician Experienced versus inexperienced Cautious versus "cowboy" Realistic versus magical thinking or projecting Collegial versus isolated and dominating

From Cady B, Easson A, Aboulafia AJ, Ferson PF. Part 1: Surgical palliation of advanced illness. What's new, what's helpful. J Am Coll Surg 2005;200:115-127.

TABLE 97-2 Palliative Surgery: General Indications, Contraindications, and Complications	
INDICATIONS/CONTRAINDICATIONS	**COMPLICATIONS**
Indications For active symptoms that do not yield to nonoperative approaches or patients who prefer an operative approach	Distant and surgical site infection Bleeding Wound complications

Contraindications
  Lack of informed consent
  Lack of clearly defined goals
  Hemodynamic instability
  Imminent demise
  Disproportionately high anesthetic risk for extent of procedure
	Deep vein thrombosis
	Pneumonia
	Long hospitalization
	Anesthetic complications, Wrong site surgery

PREOPERATIVE EVALUATION

Should surgical palliative intervention be selected, preoperative preparation is completed by a preanesthetic assessment and plans for perioperative analgesia. This raises the question of how to draw the line between unwanted resuscitation and maintenance of homeostasis for perioperative survival. This dilemma can be mitigated, in part, by less invasive surgical procedures and anesthetics. For those with preexisting do not resuscitate (DNR) orders, "required reconsideration," a discussion between the patient or surrogate and the anesthesia team to clarify the goals and limits of care, is recommended by the American Society of Anesthesiology, the American College of Surgeons, and the Association of Operating Room Nurses. All condemn automatic discontinuation of DNR orders before anesthesia. The patient with a DNR order may suspend it for a specified time, after which the goals and limitations of care can be updated. Insistence on maintaining DNR status leads patients to abandon the idea of surgery. If a surgeon is uncomfortable with limitations on resuscitation, he or she is not obliged to perform the procedure but should offer to assist in alternative arrangements. For limitations on resuscitation, either procedure-based or goal-based directives can provide guidance. Procedure-based limitations specify what is authorized and what is not (e.g., "may intubate," "no chest compressions"). Goal-based limitations identify a clinical end point (e.g., "comfort only," "keep patient alive until spouse returns to hospital") with latitude for clinicians about the means.

PALLIATIVE PROCEDURES

The main indications for surgical and endoscopic palliative interventions are malnutrition, obstruction, hemorrhage, pain, fistula, and aesthetics. Obstruction, bleeding, and wound complications respond better to surgical management than do systemic symptoms such as fatigue and anorexia. Procedure planning requires the availability of expertise and increasingly sophisticated (and expensive) devices. Laparoscopic and endoscopic approaches are not risk free. Someone who is not a candidate for "open" surgery is also not a candidate for laparoscopic surgery. A nihilistic approach toward major surgery should not disqualify procedures normally used with intent to cure that are also effective for symptom control. Given the recent acceptance of palliation as a valid sole clinical goal, few procedures have undergone prospective randomized, controlled studies measuring quality of life outcomes.

Surgical ablative procedures encompass anatomical organ resection or amputation, nonanatomical resection (cytoreduction or "debulking"), and tumor destruction using thermal, cryogenic, or chemical means (Table 97-3). Open, laparoscopic, and percutaneous approaches are used. Indications include relief of local (pain, bleeding, odor) and relief of systemic symptoms such as fever in patients with renal cell carcinoma or hormonally mediated symptoms caused by endocrine tumors such as carcinoid.

Much surgical and other invasive palliation aims to relieve symptoms of luminal obstruction. Luminal occlusion, usually a marker for advanced disease, is often

TABLE 97-3   Ablative Procedures

PROCEDURE	COMMENTS
Anatomical resection	Recommendations are unclear because of lack of differentiation between palliative and noncurative surgery, ill-defined palliative end points, and study design problems.
	Palliative subtotal gastrectomy and even total gastrectomy may be indicated in selected highly symptomatic patients, although caution is advised because of the high morbidity that can greatly reduce remaining time without symptom treatment or treatment side effects.
Nonanatomical resection (cytoreduction)	Procedure targets tumor alone, using traditional approaches with scalpel, electrocautery, or newer modalities (laser and newer ablative techniques).
	Highly individualized approach makes prospective comparisons for palliative outcomes difficult; most commonly studied example is cytoreduction of macroscopic disease in stage 3 ovarian cancer.
Amputation—extremities	Indications in cancer are uncommon but include severe pain refractory to nonsurgical management; limb dysfunction, including pathological fracture; bleeding; fungation; infection; and impending exsanguination.
	Quality of life can be better after major amputation than with continued limb preservation.
	Lower extremity major amputations have a higher complication rate than upper extremity amputations do.
	Because of complex management and the infrequency of the problem in cancer, the procedure is best undertaken by experienced multidisciplinary teams.
	More common indications for palliative amputation are gangrenous complications of peripheral vascular occlusive disease.
Amputation—mastectomy	When palliative, the main indications are pain, hemorrhage, fungation, and infection.
	Usually entails a total mastectomy (removal of the breast and overlying skin but preservation of the pectoral muscles and avoidance of the axilla unless grossly involved).
	Palliative benefit may be enhanced by other tumoricidal therapies.
	Wound closure using autologous tissue grafting should be anticipated.
Radiofrequency ablation	Use mainly for liver tumors, but also for lung, kidney, bone, breast, and endocrine gland tumors.
	Electrodes bearing high-frequency alternating current (350-500 kHz) are inserted into or adjacent to the target percutaneously, laparoscopically, or during an open procedure.
	Inexpensive, but limited to tissue <5 cm in diameter.
	Less effective for tumors adjacent to high blood flow.
	Repeat applications are possible.
	Fewer complications than cryoablation.
Cryoablation	Used mainly for skin and liver tumors.
	Can be used for larger tumors but expensive because of general anesthesia (procedures are done laparoscopically or via laparotomy), equipment, and time consumption.
	Complications include cracking of tissue with hemorrhage, coagulopathy, thrombocytopenia, biliary leak, myoglobinuria, renal failure, and infection.
Ethanol ablation	Used for liver tumors; long-term survival reported.
	Percutaneous, laparoscopic, or at laparotomy.
	Repeat applications can be done.
	Lesions <2 cm are treated with one application.
	Inexpensive.
	Acetic acid, another agent used in the same way, has additional lytic properties that are useful.

accompanied by nutritional and immune dysfunction. These make the relatively new endoscopic and minimally invasive surgical approaches attractive as ultimate therapies or as temporizing measures for definitive management. Selection of these modalities has been not been based on evidence-based studies demonstrating positive impact on quality of life. We are beginning to move beyond morbidity and mortality to address questions such as the impact of gastrostomy on quality of life.[5] Scales such as the Gastric Outlet Obstruction Scoring System (GOOSS)[6] facilitate these studies. While evidence-based guidance for surgical improvement of quality of life accumulates, we must apply the current technology to the most pressing indications and avoid the more speculative problems of "pre-emptive palliation" even using less invasive means (Tables 97-4 and 97-5).

Surgical and invasive procedures are evolving. Stenting, the most flexible and most popular approach for proce-dure-based palliation, has become consistently available and practical for many U.S. hospitals only during the past 15 years (Table 97-6). Laparoscopic surgery has evolved more rapidly. Further innovation will require more technical skills and reassessment of outcomes: the constant will be opportunities to offer more than technical assistance. Every pain procedure is an opportunity to explore other reasons, including nonphysical reasons, for pain; every procedure to help eating is an opportunity to ask about other problems. Every surgical procedure is a "teaching moment" for patient, family, and those caring for them. The trust given to those doing invasive procedures places them in a unique position to respond to the patient's and family's wider concerns. This is a vision for the future of all surgery—what we can do when our procedures are so sophisticated that we have more time to spend with our patients (see "Future Considerations").

TABLE 97-4	Gastrostomy and Jejunostomy
PROCEDURE	**COMMENTS**
Percutaneous endoscopic gastrostomy (PEG)	Indications 　Nutritional/pharmaceutical delivery 　Drainage for obstruction or ileus 　Adjunct to other palliative intestinal procedures (e.g., access for stenting, recycling bile in externalized biliary diversion) Contraindications 　Inability to transilluminate abdominal wall 　Previous upper abdominal surgery (relative) 　Massive ascites (relative—possible if ascites drained and controlled) 　Uncorrectable coagulopathy 　Peritonitis Complications (5-13%)[7,8] 　Hemorrhage 　Gastric/bowel leakage causing peritonitis 　Localized skin necrosis 　Fistula formation 　Tube migration/malfunction/malposition 　Wound infection 　Tumor spread to abdominal wall 　Mortality is low and related to underlying disease Procedure[9] Endoscopic PEG placement can be done on an inpatient or outpatient basis in less than 30 minutes using conscious sedation and local anesthesia. The patient is NPO 8 hours before the procedure. The patient is supine and is monitored for respirations, pulse, blood pressure, and oxygen saturation. Topical anesthesia of the posterior pharynx and intravenous sedation are obtained, a forward-viewing endoscope is introduced, and the abdomen is sterilely prepared and draped. The stomach and duodenum are visualized. The light of the endoscope identifies the site where stomach and abdominal wall lie in close proximity in the left upper quadrant of the abdomen. Finger pressure on the transilluminated spot confirms this. There should be clear indentation of the stomach at the desired spot. Apposition of the anterior gastric wall to the abdominal wall is essential to prevent extravasation of gastric contents that can cause peritonitis. Bulky tumor infiltration of the abdominal wall preventing transillumination or apposition and massive ascites can interfere with this critical step. The overlying skin and fascia are infiltrated with a local anesthetic, and a needle is introduced through a 1 cm skin incision into the gastric lumen under endoscopic visualization. One of two approaches can now be used: In the first, a wire is introduced through the abdominal wall puncture, snared by the endoscope, pulled out through the mouth, and then used to pull the gastrostomy tube (20 F size) retrograde through the esophagus into the stomach. The endoscope is then introduced to confirm correct positioning of the tube within the gastric lumen. The tube is secured with a bolster applied to the gastrostomy exteriorly, at skin level, without compressing the skin; this prevents retraction of the tube inward. The second approach introduces the gastrostomy tube percutaneously under direct endoscopic vision. This is preferred for upper intestinal tumors to prevent seeding at the gastrostomy site. PEG placement can be done under fluoroscopy by an interventional radiologist. After PEG placement, feedings are usually commenced the next day. PEG placement for relief of malignant intestinal obstruction is safe and efficacious.[10] Some[11] recommend that care and long-term maintenance of PEGs be carried out by trained nutritional support specialists or wound care ostomy nurses in conjunction with the endoscopist.
Jejunostomy	Less common than PEG for both nutritional support and drainage. Can be inserted at open laparotomy, during a laparoscopic procedure, endoscopically, or percutaneously under fluoroscopic guidance. The tube used is smaller than for gastrostomy. When done as a surgical procedure, a site 15 cm distal to the ligament of Treitz is selected. Typically, a small T tube or straight red rubber catheter is used. For elemental diet formulas, an even smaller-bore Teflon or plastic catheter can be used, although these are unsuitable for drainage, administration of many medications, or administration of nonelemental feeding formulas. Complications resemble those of gastrostomy but also include obstruction from jejunal catheter balloon, intussusception, pneumatosis intestinalis, and bowel ischemia. Postpyloric feeding tube placement may decrease reflux and aspiration.[12,13]
Cecostomy	Used for mechanical and functional colonic obstruction in those who cannot tolerate or do not desire a more extensive procedure. May be used for access for cleansing enemas in conditions predisposing to chronic constipation. Can be done as an "open" operation under general, regional, or local anesthesia; percutaneously by an interventional radiologist, or as an endoscopically guided percutaneous procedure (percutaneous endoscopic cecostomy—PEC) similar to PEG. The same 20 F sized tube can be used; larger tubes are used in open surgical procedures. Cecostomy tubes must be irrigated frequently (minimum three to four times daily), using 30 mL tap water. Most common complications are abdominal wall sepsis, local wound problems, tube occlusion, and dislodgment. Cecostomy tubes can be removed later with prompt spontaneous closure of the colocutaneous fistula.

TABLE 97-5 Percutaneous Nephrostomy: Indications, Complications, and Procedure

Indications in advanced malignancy	Benign and malignant ureteral obstruction with bilateral hydronephrosis, unilateral ureteral obstruction with renal insufficiency, and pyelonephritis Prelude to other interventions (antegrade ureteral stent placement) Delivery of pharmacotherapeutics Diversion of urinary leaks and fistulas Diversion for hemorrhagic cystitis
Contraindications	Uncorrectable coagulopathy Imminent demise "Terminal" illness (controversial—not indicated in asymptomatic patients or patients with no immediate threat to renal function.)
Complications, major	Septic shock Hemorrhage Vascular injury (can require embolization, nephrectomy) Bowel perforation Pleural complications
Complications, minor	Fever Catheter dislodgement Catheter occlusion Infection
Procedure	Percutaneous nephrostomy placement can be accomplished about 99% of the time. It can be performed as an outpatient procedure in lower-risk patients using ultrasound or computed tomography. Open nephrostomy has been mostly abandoned because of its much higher mortality and morbidity rate, especially in patients with advanced neoplastic disease. Percutaneous nephrostomy can be performed using either a single- or a double-stick technique. With the single-stick technique, the kidney is punctured under ultrasound guidance. Following the Seldinger technique, the tract is dilated over a guidewire until the tract can accept an 8- to 12-F catheter. A variation of this approach, comparably safe, is the "one stab" technique, in which the kidney is punctured under ultrasonic guidance and a 6 F catheter is directly introduced.[14] The double-stick technique[15] injects the calyceal system with contrast and air under ultrasonic guidance; this is followed by a second stick, through which the posterior aspect of the contrast-identified calyceal system is then accessed with the drainage catheter.
Commentary	Mortality in multiple series is related solely to underlying disease. One retrospective study[16] demonstrated that in-hospital mortality for patients undergoing percutaneous nephrostomy was more common in patients with prostatic cancer, those older than 52 years of age, and those receiving hemodialysis before percutaneous nephrostomy (no quality of life parameters were reported). Interpretation of previous literature with respect to quality of life outcomes is difficult because only mortality, morbidity, and return of renal function are reported. Many reported series include procedures done for stone disease and treatment of complications of renal transplantation. Despite the frequency of persistent cancer-related symptoms after nephrostomy for malignant ureteral obstruction, the average survival of 5 months with frequent rehospitalizations, and the need for repeat procedures for recurrent ureteral obstruction, well-selected patients can anticipate relief from urinary incontinence, delirium, pain, and nausea. Because the presence of ureteral obstruction is so often a marker for advanced disease, the expected outcomes, risks, and benefits of this procedure should be matched carefully with the patient's overall goals of care before proceeding. Frequently, patients believe or are led to believe that renal failure inevitably leads to an agonizing death rather than the far more likely scenario of pharmacologically manageable delirium and coma. This should be specifically addressed when deciding if percutaneous nephrostomy or ureteral stenting should be done to preempt or resolve systemic symptoms.

Future Considerations

- What should be the extent of the surgeon's participation in palliative care ? Should it be limited to operative interventions, or should it involve a wider range of counseling and peer support?
- Is outcome measurement for surgical palliative care inherently different than for palliative medicine? How will metrics be determined?
- How does prognosis influence choice of intervention?
- What is appropriate aftercare by surgeons doing palliative procedures?
- How can preoperative joint planning by surgeons, anesthesia teams, and palliative care interdisciplinary teams be improved?
- For which symptoms is surgery most likely to be therapeutically effective without unacceptable social, economic, and psychological costs?

TABLE 97-6   Stenting Procedures in Advanced Malignancy

SYSTEM	COMMENTS
Tracheobronchial tree[17,18]	Stenting procedures can palliate symptoms for proximal, obstructing, or fistulous lesions of the tracheobronchial tree. It can be performed as a sole palliative procedure for extrinsic, compressing lesions or in conjunction with other endoluminal treatments (e.g., laser resection, electrocautery) when palliating intrinsic lesions. Stenting is also used when loss of cartilaginous support for airway patency is anticipated after endoluminal therapy.
	Silicone elastomer or wire mesh stents are used. Wire stents are becoming increasingly popular because they are thin walled, flexible, and less likely to migrate. They should be covered when used for palliation of malignant airway obstruction because of the propensity of tumor ingrowth to cause early recurrent obstruction. They can be placed with the use of a flexible bronchoscope, unlike silicone stents. Self-expanding and insufflatable varieties are available. Silicone stents have the advantages of lower cost and ease of repositioning or removal. Covered stents are useful for control of cough and aspiration from tracheoesophageal fistula. Multiple stents can be placed during a single session. It is important that the airway be patent distal to the stent. Stent configurations include T stents (inserted through a tracheostomy site for locally invasive recurrent thyroid carcinoma), Y stents (for carinal lesions), and straight stents (trachea and main stem bronchi).
Esophagus	Self-expanding metal stents (SEMS) have established their superiority over rigid plastic stents. Covered (silicone or polyurethane) stents have the advantage of minimizing tumor ingrowth to the ends of the stent, although they are more likely to migrate. SEMS are permanent, so their use is limited to malignant conditions. Multiple stents can be placed at one sitting. Covered stents are also useful for management of fistulas. Self-expanding plastic stents (SEPS) (PolyFlex) are now available; unlike SEMS, they can be easily removed, making them suitable for benign or temporary indications. They have been shown to be effective and safe for the management of malignant stricture, although migration rates can be higher than for SEMS.
Gastric outlet	Enteral Wallstent is approved by the U.S. Food and Drug Administration (FDA) for this indication. The procedure is best performed under fluoroscopy. Multiple stents can be placed for longer strictures. Consideration should be given to placement of a biliary stent before enteral stenting because of technical difficulties in accessing biliary tree through an enteral stent.[19] Risk of bleeding and perforation is low. In an analysis of 526 patients undergoing enteral stent placement, the mean prestenting GOOSS score was 0.4 (0 = no intake, 3 = low residue/full diet); the mean poststenting score was 2.4.[20]
Colon	Enteral Wallstent is FDA approved for use in malignant colonic obstruction. Technical and clinical success rates for colonic SEMS exceed 90%. Use of fluoroscopy during endoscopic insertion is strongly recommended. Compared with surgery, use of SEMS resulted in shorter intensive care unit and hospital stays and lower cost.[21] Stenting can be done for definitive palliation or to relieve obstruction, allowing for bowel preparation and elective resection for cure or palliation. Preoperative chemoradiation can be given after stent placement.[22]
Biliary ducts	Stenting of the bile ducts can be done percutaneously or endoscopically. Both approaches are effective but less morbid alternatives to surgical bypass. Mortality and morbidity are higher for surgical bypass, although the palliation obtained is life lasting. An additional advantage of surgical biliary bypass is the opportunity it provides to address gastric outlet obstruction and cancer-related pain management (celiac plexus block) during the same procedure and, on occasion, to proceed with attempt to cure.
	If surgical bypass or pancreaticobiliary resection is anticipated, preoperative stenting or decompression of the common bile duct can increase the technical difficulty of performing an enterobiliary anastomosis.
	Stenting can be done safely as an outpatient procedure with SEMS or plastic stents. Plastic stents are cheaper but are more likely to migrate and occlude. Average patency time for large-bore plastic stents is roughly 3 months, which makes them suitable for patients with a shorter prognosis. Occlusion is usually heralded by recurrent jaundice and signs of cholangitis. Occlusion from tumor ingrowth can occur with SEMS if noncovered stents are used, but covered stents are more likely to migrate. Endoscopic placement of biliary stents is less painful than the percutaneous approach and avoids the problem of externalized hardware which can be the sequela of percutaneous stent placement in some instances. In light of evidence that percutaneous biliary stent placement has a higher major morbidity rate than endoscopic placement and the additional considerations just described, percutaneous stent placement should be reserved for failed endoscopic attempts to stent, institutions that do not have the equipment or expertise for endoscopic placement, and pathological changes preventing endoscopic visualization of anatomical landmarks.[23]
Ureter	Retrograde stenting is the initial approach of choice when the ureteral orifice can be identified and obstruction is proximal enough in the ureter for the catheter to be directed proximally. For failed retrograde approaches, the uretral calyceal system is accessed via percutaneous nephrostomy, followed by antegrade stent placement. Stents can be completely internalized using either approach. Stenting can be done as an outpatient procedure with local sedation, spinal, or general anesthesia. Antibiotic prophylaxis is used. Stents require periodic replacement, but, in the setting of terminal illness, this is a highly individualized judgment.
Venous	The transjugular intrahepatic portosystemic shunt (TIPS) procedure, a form of venous endovascular stenting, can relieve symptoms of massive ascites caused by thrombosis of the hepatic veins (Budd-Chiari syndrome), treat variceal hemorrhage unresponsive to endoscopic and pharmacotherapeutic approaches in nonoperable candidates, provide definitive management for recurrent variceal hemorrhage in poor surgical candidates, and act as a "bridge" to liver transplantation in bleeding patients for whom first-line therapies have failed. Absolute contraindications include right-sided heart failure and polycystic liver disease. An important relative contraindication from a quality of life perspective is the presence of encephalopathy, which TIPS can worsen. TIPS requires considerable interventional radiology expertise. Shunt occlusion occurs in approximately half of patients by 1 year.
	Endovascular venous stents have been used to reduce massive edema secondary to tumor compression of the upper and lower venae cavae.

SUGGESTED READING

Baron TH, Dunn GP. Palliative gastroenterology. Gastroenterol Clin North Am 2006;35:1-228.

Dunn GP. Surgical palliative care. Surg Clin North Am 2005;85:169-398.

Dunn GP, Johnson AG. Surgical Palliative Care. Oxford: Oxford University Press, 2004, pp 1-267.

Wagman LD (ed). Palliative surgical oncology. Surg Oncol Clin North Am 2004;13(3):401-554.

REFERENCES

1. Dunn GP, Johnson AG. Surgical Palliative Care. Oxford: Oxford University Press, 2004, pp.1-267.
2. Wagman L. Preface: Palliative surgical oncology. Surg Oncol Clin North Am 2004;13(3):xi-xii.
3. Surgeon's Palliative Care Workgroup. Office of Promoting Excellence in End-of-Life Care: Surgeon's Palliative Care Workgroup report from the field. J Am Coll Surg 2003;197:660-686.
4. Cady B, Miner T, Morgentaler A. Part 2: Surgical palliation of advanced illness. What's new, what's helpful. J Am Coll Surg 2005;200:281-290.
5. McClave SA, Ritchie CS. The role of endoscopically placed feeding or decompression tubes. Gastroenterol Clin North Am 2006;35:83-100.
6. Adler DG, Baron TH. Endoscopic palliation of malignant gastric outlet obstruction using self-expanding metal stents: Experience in 36 patients. Am J Gastroenterol 2002;97:72-78.
7. Dunn GP. Palliating patients who have unresectable colorectal cancer: Creating the right framework and salient symptom management. Surg Clin North Am 2006;86:1065-1092.
8. Grant JP. Percutaneous endoscopic gastrostomy: Initial placement by single endoscopic technique and long term follow-up. Ann Surg 1993;217:168-174.
9. Fanning A, Ponsky J. Gastrointestinal endoscopy. In Souba WW, Fink MP, Kaiser LR, et al. (eds). ACS Surgery: Principles and Practice. New York: WebMD Professional Publishing, 2006, pp. 614-615.
10. Scheidbach H, Horbach T, Groital H, et al. Percutaneous endoscopic gastrostomy/jejunostomy (PEG/PEJ) for decompression in the upper gastrointestinal tract: Initial experience with palliative treatment of gastrointestinal obstruction in terminally ill patients with advanced carcinomas. Surg Endosc 1999;13:1103-1106.
11. McClave SA, Neff RL. Care and long-term maintenance of percutaneous endoscopic gastrostomy tubes. J Parenter Enteral Nutr 2006;30(1 Suppl):S27-S38.
12. Heyland DK, Drover JW, MacDonald S, et al. Effect of postpyloric feeding on gastroesophageal regurgitation and pulmonary microaspiration: Results of a randomized controlled trial. Crit Care Med 2001;29:1495-1501.
13. Heyland DK, Drover JW, Dhaliwal R, et al. Optimizing the benefits and minimizing the risks of enteral nutrition in the critically ill: Role of small bowel feeding. J Parenter Enteral Nutr 2002;26(Suppl 6):S51-S57.
14. Wah TM, Weston MJ, Irving HC. Percutaneous nephrostomy insertion: Outcome data from a prospective multi-operator study at a UK training centre. Clin Radiol 2004;59:255-261.
15. Funaki B, Vatakencherry G. Comparison of single-stick and double-stick techniques for percutaneous nephrostomy. Cardiovasc Intervent Radiol 2004;27:35-37.
16. Romero FR, Broglio M, Pires SR, et al. Indications for percutaneous nephrostomy in patients with obstructive uropathy due to malignant urogenital neoplasias. Int Braz J Urol 2005;3:117-124.
17. Cady B, Easson A, Aboulafia AJ, Ferson PF. Part 1: Surgical palliation of advanced illness. What's new, what's helpful. J Am Coll Surg 2005;200:115-127.
18. Berger A, Henry L, Goldberg M. Surgical palliation of thoracic malignancies. Surg Oncol Clin North Am 2004;13:429-453.
19. Adler DG, Merwat SN. Endoscopic approaches for palliation of luminal gastrointestinal obstruction. Gastroenterol Clin North Am 2006;35:65-82.
20. Dormann A, Meisner S, Verin N, Wenk Lang A. Self-expanding metal stents for gastroduodenal malignancies: Systemic review of their clinical effectiveness. Endoscopy 2004;36:543-550.
21. Binkert CA, Ledermann H, Jost R, et al. Acute colonic obstruction: Clinical aspects and cost effectiveness of preoperative and palliative treatment with self-expanding metallic stents—A preliminary report. Radiology 1998;206: 199-204.
22. Adler DG, Young-Fadok TM, Smyrk T, et al. Preoperative chemoradiation therapy after placement of a self-expanding metal stent in a patient with an obstructing rectal cancer: Clinical and pathological findings. Gastrointest Endosc 2002;55:435-437.
23. Baron TH. Palliation of malignant obstructive jaundice. Gastroenterol Clin North Am 2006;35:101-112.

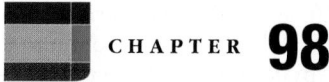

CHAPTER **98**

Gastrointestinal Endoscopy

Garret Cullen and Hugh E. Mulcahy

KEY POINTS

- Endoscopy can be a valuable tool in palliative medicine.
- Careful patient selection as part of a multidisciplinary approach is important.
- Risks of any procedure must be balanced with potential benefits and expected prognosis.
- Self-expanding metal stents are the preferred palliative treatment for malignant obstruction of the gastrointestinal tract.
- Percutaneous endoscopic gastrostomy (PEG) tube insertion can be helpful in selected patients.

Palliative gastrointestinal endoscopy has expanded over the past decade as a result of more treatments for gastrointestinal obstruction. Obstruction may manifest with nausea, vomiting, pain, jaundice, itch, and abdominal distention. It usually occurs as a complication from local extension of carcinoma of the esophagus, stomach, duodenum, pancreaticobiliary system, or colon. It can also arise from extrinsic compression by intraperitoneal metastases, especially from breast or ovarian primaries. Surgical management may be effective but has considerable morbidity and mortality. With endoscopic stenting, in particular the use of self-expanding metal stents, palliation of obstruction is now largely in the hands of endoscopists. The endoscopist can also aid nutritional support for the terminally ill patient. Percutaneous endoscopic gastrostomy (PEG) or jejunostomy (PEJ) tubes can augment nutrition in those with poor oral intake while bypassing upper gastrointestinal obstruction.

Endoscopic treatments such as photodynamic therapy, electrocautery, and even direct injection of chemotherapy agents raises the possibility of targeted local therapy aimed at reducing tumor burden and associated symptoms. It is important for the endoscopist to be aware that he or she is a member of a multidisciplinary team working to ensure patient dignity and comfort at the end of life and that, although their primary focus is on endoscopic safety and success, the treatment aim is palliative.

PATIENT SELECTION

Before any therapeutic procedure is undertaken, the endoscopist must be aware of the diagnosis and treatment plan. An untreatable malignancy is often diagnosed at endoscopy, and, when this occurs, the focus changes from cure to palliation. This situation arises frequently during endoscopic retrograde pancreatography (ERCP). A patient may be diagnosed with an unresectable cholangio-carcinoma or pancreatic cancer, necessitating definitive palliation with a metal stent. In cases of doubt, temporary measures, such as the placement of a removable plastic stent, can be employed until further investigation confirms the need for palliative treatment.

SEDATION AND ANALGESIA

As a general rule, endoscopists practice conscious sedation. For simple diagnostic procedures, small doses of short-acting benzodiazepines (e.g., midazolam) are used. Opiates are added to midazolam for more complex procedures such as ERCP or rectal stenting; newer agents such as propofol may also improve patient comfort and recovery time after the procedure. Blood pressure, pulse rate, and oxygen saturation should be monitored continuously throughout the procedure.

COMPLICATIONS

All endoscopic procedures have risks. These range from that associated with sedation and analgesia to bleeding and enteric perforation. Patients undergoing palliative endoscopy are frequently elderly with co-morbid illnesses. Both the patient and the family need to be aware of the potential benefits, risks, and treatment options before proceeding. In addition to complications, there is the potential for failure and possible need for repeated endoscopy. It is best that information be provided by, and consent obtained by, the endoscopist who will carry out the procedure.

Diagnostic endoscopy is a low-risk procedure; perforation rates are about 0.1% for gastroscopy and 0.2% for colonoscopy. Risk increases for ERCP or stent insertion but depends on the procedure and the intervention.

GASTROINTESTINAL ENDOSCOPIC PROCEDURES

Table 98-1 summarizes the indications and contraindications for gastrointestinal endoscopic procedures.

Esophagus

The incidence of esophageal adenocarcinoma is approximately 100,000 cases per annum worldwide; about 50% of these tumors are found to be unresectable at diagnosis.

TABLE 98-1 Indications and Contraindications for Gastrointestinal Endoscopy

INDICATIONS	CONTRAINDICATIONS
Symptomatic gastrointestinal tract obstruction	Unfit for sedation
Symptomatic pancreaticobiliary tract obstruction	Unfit for endoscopic procedure
Bleeding/anemia	High esophageal tumor
Malignant fistula	
Insertion of percutaneous endoscopic gastrostomy (PEG) or jejunostomy (PEJ) tube	

Self-expanding metallic stents are the main treatment option for palliation of dysphagia. They are composed of a number of metal alloys and are available in various shapes and sizes, depending on the proposed organ of placement. They expand on deployment and become embedded into the tumor and surrounding normal tissue through pressure necrosis. This anchors the stent and helps avoid stent migration. Such stents have revolutionized endoscopic management of malignant obstruction and produced a concomitant reduction in the need for surgery. Metal stents can be passed either through the scope or beside the scope over a guidewire passed under endoscopic vision, and positioned across the obstruction before being deployed. Radiological screening is not required for most esophageal stent insertions.

The procedure is well tolerated, with relief of dysphagia being attained in more than 90% of cases,[1] although stents that traverse the gastroesophageal junction may be associated with considerable reflux and regurgitation. This may be treated with proton pump inhibitors or by using stents that incorporate a one-way valve flap. Serious complications such as perforation or hemorrhage are rare (<3%), although perforation rates may be increased after previous radiotherapy or chemotherapy.[2] All metallic stents are associated with complications of bleeding, perforation, stent migration, stent malpositioning, and tumor overgrowth. The last complication can be treated with a second, overlapping stent. Alternatively, endoscopic laser therapy, electrocautery, or photodynamic therapy (PDT) can be used to treat stent occlusion. Both covered and uncovered metal stents are available. Covered stents are associated with less tumor ingrowth than uncovered stents, and they are also the treatment of choice for malignant tracheoesophageal fistulas resulting from bronchial or esophageal carcinoma.

Other treatment options for malignant esophageal obstruction include neodymium-yttrium-aluminum garnet (Nd:YAG) laser therapy, electrocautery, injection therapy, and PDT. There have been a few randomized trials comparing laser therapy to metal stents that suggest similar effectiveness for both techniques,[3] but the immediate relief of symptoms with stents and the need for repeated laser applications favor stenting in clinical practice. PDT, injection therapy, and electrocautery have yet to be validated in this setting.

Stomach and Duodenum

Primary and metastatic obstruction of the distal stomach and duodenum are late complications of pancreaticobiliary and gastrointestinal malignancies. Endoscopic enteral stents are a safe and feasible treatment option. Compared to surgery (gastrojejunostomy), endoscopic stenting results in earlier oral intake, reduced hospital stay, reduced morbidity and mortality, and reduced costs.[4] Approximately 90% of those with gastroduodenal stents improve clinically.[5] There are no data on the safety of gastroduodenal stents after chemotherapy. Patients can commence oral intake almost immediately after upper gastrointestinal stent placement but are advised to advance from liquids to solids as tolerated. In general, leafy vegetables are best avoided, because they can cause stent occlusion.

Colon and Rectum

Colorectal carcinoma manifests with acute obstruction in up to 30% of cases,[5] and emergency surgery is associated with morbidity and mortality rates of 50% and 15%, respectively.[6] Patients with extensive local or metastatic disease are often poor operative candidates, as are those with obstructions secondary to noncolonic pelvic malignancies such as bladder or ovarian carcinoma.

Endoscopic stenting for obstructing large bowel cancer was described in the 1990s and is now well established. Uncovered stents are frequently placed under fluoroscopic guidance over a guidewire with direct endoscopic vision (Fig. 98-1). Successful palliation of obstruction and avoidance of colostomy can be achieved in 85% to 100% of cases, with some stents remaining patent for longer than 1 year.[7] Most stents are placed for high rectal and sigmoid colon lesions, but they can also be placed in the right colon for an obstructing proximal cancer. Partially covered stents have also been used successfully to treat malignant colovesical and colovaginal fistulas.

Complications from colorectal stenting include colonic perforation, bleeding, stent migration, and tumor overgrowth, whereas stents in the distal rectum can cause severe tenesmus and fecal incontinence. Patients are advised to take regular stool softeners and to consume a low-residue diet after stent insertion. There are no data on the effect of concomitant chemoradiation on local complications.

Other palliative treatments that have been described include Nd:YAG laser therapy, a potentially effective treatment for obstructing rectal carcinoma. Success rates of 85% to 90% have been reported from specialist units,[8] but repeated sessions are required to maintain luminal patency, and the procedure is not widely available. Cryotherapy, PDT, electrocautery, and alcohol injection have also been used, but none of these procedures has been formally compared to either stenting or Nd:YAG laser, and all remain experimental.

Pancreaticobiliary System

Cholangiocarcinoma is the most common primary bile duct malignancy; it usually manifests at an advanced stage with biliary obstruction. Palliation can be achieved at ERCP with either plastic or metal stents, and tight strictures can be dilated before stenting with a rigid or balloon dilator. Plastic stents are predominantly used for benign obstructions, but they can be used in malignant disease to allow temporary bile duct drainage while definitive staging is awaited. However, metal stents are the preferred stenting option for palliation, because they have a lower occlusion rate,[9] are associated with fewer subsequent hospital admissions, and are more cost-effective when compared to surgical bypass.[10] Covered metal stents are used in the common bile duct, whereas lesions affecting the hilum are stented with uncovered stents to allow biliary drainage through the stent wall. There does not appear to be an increased complication rate with prior or concomitant chemoradiation.[11]

PDT is a recent development in the nonsurgical treatment of malignancies including esophageal cancer and cholangiocarcinoma. Endoscopic application has shown promise in prolonging survival of patients with advanced cholangiocarcinoma. The procedure involves intravenous administration of a nontoxic photosensitizing agent (sodium porfimer) that is preferentially taken up by malignant cells. The patient then undergoes endoscopy, during which a light-emitting probe is placed across the tumor. The light energy is absorbed by the photosensitizing agent and transferred to oxygen, producing highly reactive oxygen intermediates that cause tumor cell death. Pilot studies in unresectable cholangiocarcinoma suggest that median survival can be doubled in selected patients.[12]

Percutaneous Endoscopic Gastrostomy Feeding and Nutrition

Supplemental nutrition is frequently used in palliative care, and endoscopists usually become involved when there is a need to place an endoscopic feeding device such as a PEG tube. These devices may be helpful in head and neck cancers and untreatable dysphagia, but they do not improve quality of life or functional status, nor reduce aspiration pneumonia or help maintain skin integrity.

There are several ethical issues involving PEG tubes, but once the decision is made, the procedure is relatively straightforward. Antiplatelet agents are discontinued 1 week before the procedure, and oral anticoagulants are stopped so that coagulation times will be normal. Patients are given prophylactic antibiotics before the procedure (usually a single dose of ceftriaxone), and the sedation used is similar to that for other endoscopic procedures.

The endoscopist uses a combination of the gastroscope and external abdominal pressure to identify a suitable site for PEG placement. A small incision in the abdominal wall allows introduction of a guidewire into the stomach through a suitable needle. This guidewire is then picked up in the stomach, with the use of a biopsy forceps, and brought up the esophagus. The PEG tube is attached to the guidewire and then pulled down the esophagus and

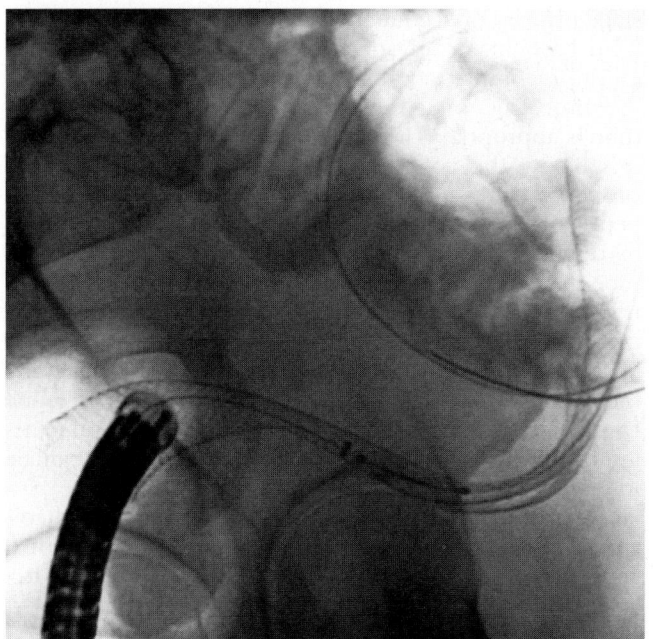

FIGURE 98-1 Overlapping colonic stents: the distal stent is being placed across the proximal stent over a guidewire.

out through the abdominal wall. A small, balloon-like device secures the PEG in the stomach. The procedure takes approximately 30 minutes and is well tolerated. Complications include failure of the procedure, infection, and bleeding. If the PEG tube becomes dislodged, it can be replaced within 12 hours without repeat endoscopy. After 12 hours, the tract that had formed will close, and a repeat endoscopic procedure will be necessary.

PEG tubes can be extended beyond gastroduodenal obstruction into the jejunum (where they are known as PEJ tubes). In addition, the endoscopist can assist in difficult placement of nasogastric or nasojejunal tubes.

FUTURE DEVELOPMENTS

Stents that emit radiation or release chemotherapeutic agents may cause tumor regression.[13,14] Endoscopic injection of cisplatin into tumor has been used to treat malignant dysphagia in esophageal carcinoma.[15]

Further data are needed on therapies such as PDT for cholangiocarcinoma. Transgastric and other forms of endoscopic surgery are new techniques that have the potential to be of benefit in the palliative treatment of selected patients.

SUMMARY

Endoscopists can contribute to the management of patients requiring palliative care. Given that these patients are frequently unsuitable for surgery or major intervention, the role of palliative endoscopy is likely to expand. As with any intervention, the potential risk of each treatment must be balanced with the expected benefit and the prognosis of the individual patient.

REFERENCES

1. Rathore O, Coss A, Patchett SE, Mulcahy HE. Direct-vision stenting: The way forward for malignant oesophageal obstruction. Endoscopy 2006;38:382-384.
2. Kinsman KJ, DeGregorio BT, Katon RM, et al. Prior radiation and chemotherapy increase the risk of life-threatening complications after insertion of metallic stents for oesophagogastric malignancy. Gastrointest Endosc 1998;47:113-120.
3. Adam A, Ellul J, Watkinson AF, et al. Palliation of inoperable oesophageal carcinoma: A prospective randomised trial of laser therapy and stent placement. Radiology 1997;202:344-348.
4. Maetani I, Tada T, Ukita T, et al. Comparison of duodenal stent placement with surgical gastrojejunostomy for palliation in patients with duodenal obstructions caused by pancreaticobiliary malignancies. Endoscopy 2004;36:73-78.
5. Mauro MA. Koehler RE, Baron TH. Advances in gastrointestinal intervention: The treatment of gastroduodenal and colorectal obstructions with metallic stents. Radiology 2000;215:659-669.
6. Deans GT, Krukowski ZH, Irwin ST. Malignant obstruction of the left colon. Br J Surg 1994;81:1270-1276.
7. Camunez F, Echenagusia A, Simo G, et al. Malignant colorectal obstruction treated by means of self-expanding metallic stents: Effectiveness before surgery and in palliation. Radiology 2000;216:492-497.
8. Mathus-Vliegan EM, Tytgat GN. Laser photocoagulation in the palliation of colorectal malignancies. Cancer 1986;57:2212-2216.
9. Rumalla A, Baron TH. Evaluation and endoscopic palliation of cholangiocarcinoma: Management of cholangiocarcinoma. Dig Dis 1999;17:194-200.
10. Martin RC, Vitale GC, Reed DN, et al. Cost comparison of endoscopic stenting vs surgical treatment for unresectable cholangiocarcinoma. Surg Endosc 2002;16:667-670.
11. Eschelman DJ, Shapiro MJ, Bonn J, at al. Malignant biliary obstruction: Long-term experience with Gianturco stents and combined-modality radiation therapy. Radiology 1996;200:717-724.
12. Harewood GC, Baron TH, Rumalla A, et al. Pilot study to asess patient outcomes following endoscopic application of photodynamic terapy for advanced cholangiocarcinoma. J Gastroenterol Hepatol 2005;20:415-420.
13. Zamora PO, Osaki S, Som P, et al. Radiolabelling brachytherapy sources with Re-188 through chelating microfilms: Stents. J Biomed Mater Res 2000;53:244-251.
14. Herdeg C, Oberhoff M, Karsch KR. Antiproliferative stent coatings: Taxol and related compounds. Semin Interv Cardiol 1998;3:197-199.
15. Harbord M, Dawes RF, Barr H, et al. Palliation of patients with dysphagia due to advanced oesophageal cancer by endoscopic injection of cisplatin/epinephrine injectable gel. Gastrointest Endosc 220;56:644-651.

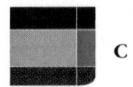

CHAPTER 99

Palliative Management of Airway Obstruction: Tracheostomy and Airway Stents

Rajeev Dhupar and Peter F. Ferson

KEY POINTS

- Symptoms of airway obstruction resulting from malignant diseases can often be relieved with a properly placed tracheostomy or an airway stent.
- In the absence of glottic obstruction, an airway stent offers better palliation than a tracheostomy.
- Placement of a silicone tracheal T-tube stent is the most versatile approach to tracheal obstruction or compression.

INDICATIONS

Few palliative procedures result in as dramatic relief as surgical airway access for airway obstruction. A person who is struggling to breathe, anxious and diaphoretic, and often agitated beyond control suddenly becomes calm and almost peaceful. Persons with symptomatic airway obstruction should be considered as candidates for surgical airway management. They may have unresectable obstructing laryngeal or pharyngeal tumors, advanced-stage primary or secondary tumors of the trachea or main stem bronchi, or advanced mediastinal metastases with extrinsic compression of the proximal airways.

For obstruction at the larynx or higher, a tracheostomy tube is appropriate. If the obstruction is several centimeters below the vocal cords, or anywhere down to the proximal main stem bronchi, an airway stent may provide better palliation.[1] Once the airway has been established by tracheostomy with a standard tracheostomy tube, the tube may be replaced with an indwelling stent, such as a tracheal T-tube stent or a T-Y stent (Boston Medical Products, Westborough, Mass.) for more extensive disease. With midtracheal obstruction, a stomal opening into the trachea may be unnecessary, because a straight silicone Dumon stent (Boston Medical Products) or a self-expanding wire stent (Boston Scientific, Natick, Mass.) can be inserted through the larynx (Fig. 99-1).

A stent has several benefits over a standard tracheostomy tube. The most obvious is that it permits normal speech, provided that the obstructing lesion is not in the larynx. It also allows the patient to breathe through the nasopharynx, bringing in humidified, filtered air. This helps prevent dry secretions within the stent, so it is easier to keep clean and patent than a tracheostomy tube.

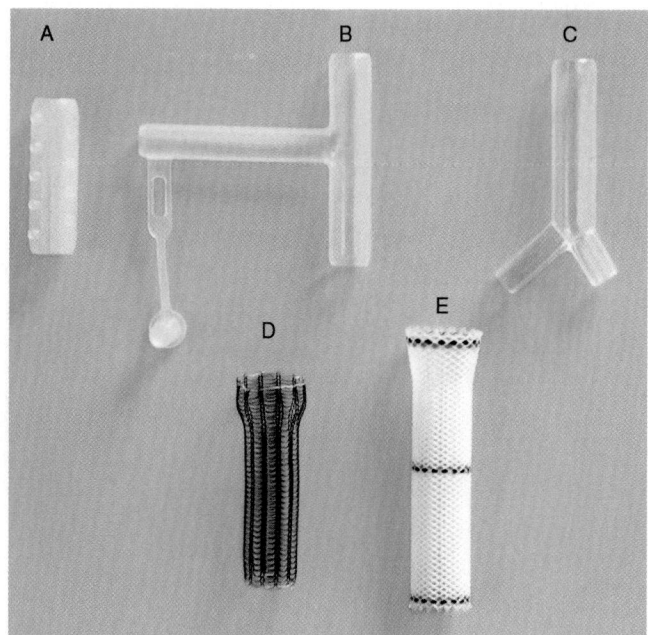

FIGURE 99-1   Airway stents. **A**, Dumon-type straight tracheal stent. **B**, Montgomery T-tube stent. **C**, Silicone Y stent for distal trachea and carina. **D**, Self-expanding wire stent. **E**, PolyFlex expandable, totally covered stent.

CLINICAL PRESENTATION AND EVALUATION

Candidates for palliative airway management are frequently, but not always, frail and emaciated with advanced cancer. The essential complaint is one of difficulty breathing, usually with increased coughing and inability to clear secretions. Depending on the degree of obstruction, the breathing pattern may show deliberate, slow, and prolonged inspiration and expiration. A wheeze may be present with forced air movement. More severe obstruction results in overt stridor and severe distress. The trachea may be deviated. Auscultation often reveals harsh breath sounds over the central airways and the neck.

A thin-slice computed tomographic scan is used to ascertain the degree of obstruction and the exact location and length. Three dimensional reconstruction in different projections can help plan intervention. Endoscopy should be done. An awake evaluation with a flexible endoscope should be performed with extreme care, because, once the bronchoscope passes the stricture, it may occlude the airway. Rigid bronchoscopy permits ventilation through the bronchoscope, even when it is passed through the stricture. This should be done with the definitive procedure, so that any bleeding or edema caused by the bronchoscope can be dealt with immediately. Observation of the degree, length, and rigidity of the stricture helps in procedure planning.

Figure 99-2A is a bronchoscopy photograph of a middle-aged woman with small cell cancer. Intraluminal tumor obstructs her right bronchus, and there is extrinsic compression of the left bronchus. She was severely dyspneic but had already received maximum radiation therapy and failed to respond to chemotherapy. Figure 99-2B shows a wire stent in her right bronchus intermedius, with patent middle and lower lobes. The distal left bronchus is also seen through the second stent. She went home and died a few weeks later with her family.

EQUIPMENT

The equipment for a standard tracheostomy tube is minimal. Simple surgical instruments and small retractors suffice. For insertion of stents, flexible and rigid bronchoscopes are required. Fluoroscopy is frequently needed.

Intraluminal Silastic stents, such as the Dumon stents which have protruding studs to help anchor the tube in place, may be used to avoid a tracheostomy. They are difficult to insert, require special inserting tubes, and cannot be cleaned except by bronchoscopy. Despite the fixation studs, they have greater risk of migration than T-tube stents, and because they fit snugly into the trachea, the proximal and distal interface tend to develop granulation tissue that may obstruct the lumen. Despite these shortcomings, these stents, when well placed, usually work well.

Self-expanding wire stents are preloaded onto an inserter system. They require fluoroscopy and flexible bronchoscopy. An array of wire stents of different lengths and diameters should be available. The central portion of such stents may be covered with an inert wrap to prevent cancer ingrowth.

DESCRIPTION OF TECHNIQUES

Tracheostomy Tube

If an airway has not been established with an endotracheal tube, local anesthesia is used.

The tracheostomy tube should be placed with a transverse skin incision, between the sternal notch and the cricoid cartilage. The trachea is exposed from the first to the fourth tracheal ring.

Various methods for incising into the trachea have been proposed (Fig. 99-3). We prefer a single vertical incision in the midline through the second and third cartilage, with extension to the fourth cartilage if necessary. This allows the lateral walls of the trachea to spread easily, so that the tracheostomy tube causes less pressure necrosis of the cartilage.

T-Tube Stent

Insertion of a T-tube stent proceeds in the same fashion as a tracheostomy tube insertion (Fig. 99-4). General anesthesia or deep sedation is necessary. Short-acting muscle relaxants, such as succinylcholine, should be used.

Like tracheostomy tubes, T-tube stents come in different sizes of diameter and length. When correctly sized, the T-tube stent ends proximally below the vocal cords and does not impair their function. Distally, it must extend beyond the stricture. The proximal and distal ends should be smaller than the diameter of the normal airway so they do not abrade the airway and cause granulations. If a stent is too long—usually proximally, which interferes with the vocal cord—the manufacturers will make custom stents quickly. Once the T-tube stent position is confirmed, anesthesia is reversed promptly.

Placement of an endotracheal tube is contraindicated when a Silastic tube is in place, because the stent can be displaced or occluded. Ventilation can be maintained via a jet ventilator or with a bag and mask.

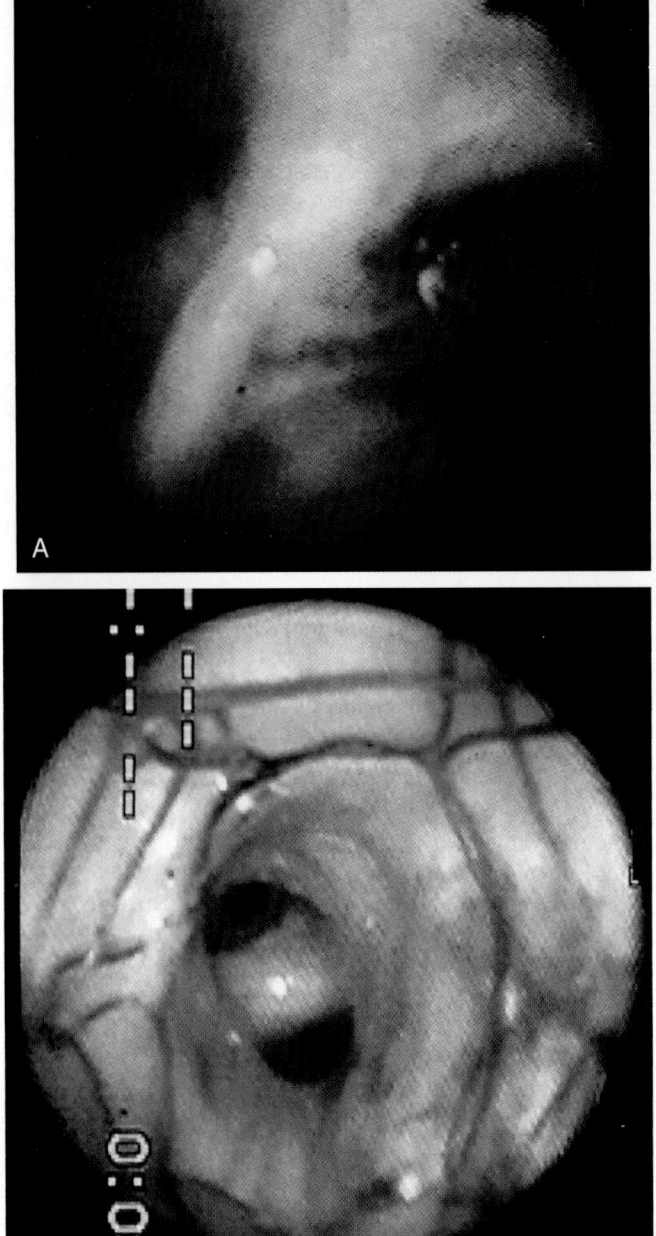

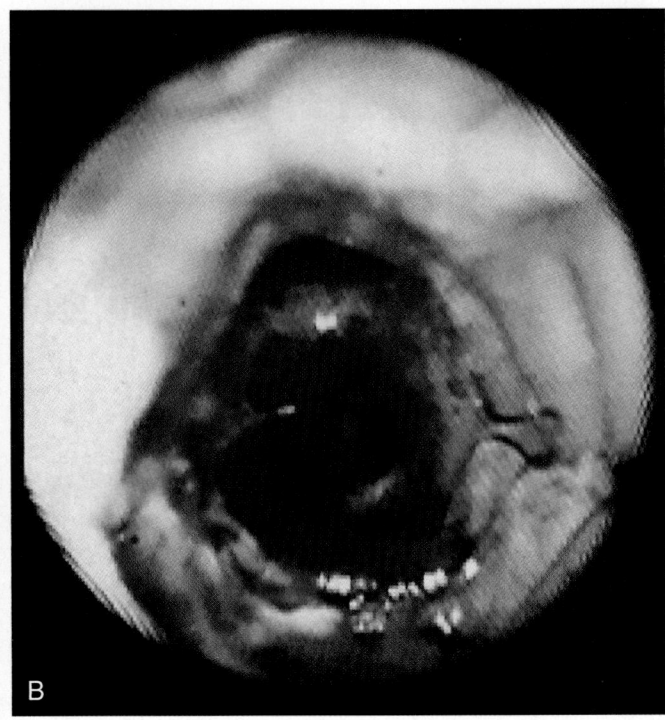

FIGURE 99-2   **A**, Bronchoscopic view of the carina. The right main stem bronchus is obstructed by tumor. The left bronchus is extrinsically compressed by tumor. **B**, After placement of wire stents, the bronchus intermedius is wide open with clearly visible orifices of the middle lobe and lower lobes. **C**, The distal left bronchus is supported, showing both upper and lower lobe bronchi.

Entirely Intraluminal Stents

Dumon stents are inserted through a rigid bronchoscope. Once the stricture has been dilated, general anesthesia with short-acting muscle relaxation is used. Like the T-tube stents, Dumon stents come in various sizes. Selection is based on measurements made during bronchoscopy. It is best to use the proprietary bronchoscope system with insertion tubes. The selected stent is loaded into the properly sized insertion tube. Fluoroscopy helps correctly position the stent, because vision is lost after the insertion tube is placed. On release of the stent, ventilation is resumed through the rigid bronchoscope, and the position of the stent is confirmed by examination with a tele-

scope or flexible bronchoscope. Anesthesia is reversed promptly.

Self-expanding wire stents are easier to insert. Local anesthesia with sedation or general anesthesia may be used. Minimal dilation is necessary. Fluoroscopy is required. A guidewire is advanced across the lesion through a flexible bronchoscope, and the proximal and distal ends of the stricture are marked fluoroscopically. The bronchoscope is withdrawn, and the stent insertion system is passed over the guidewire until the position markers align with the fluoroscopic guides. The stent is discharged from the insertion system, which is then withdrawn. Stent position is confirmed by flexible bronchos-

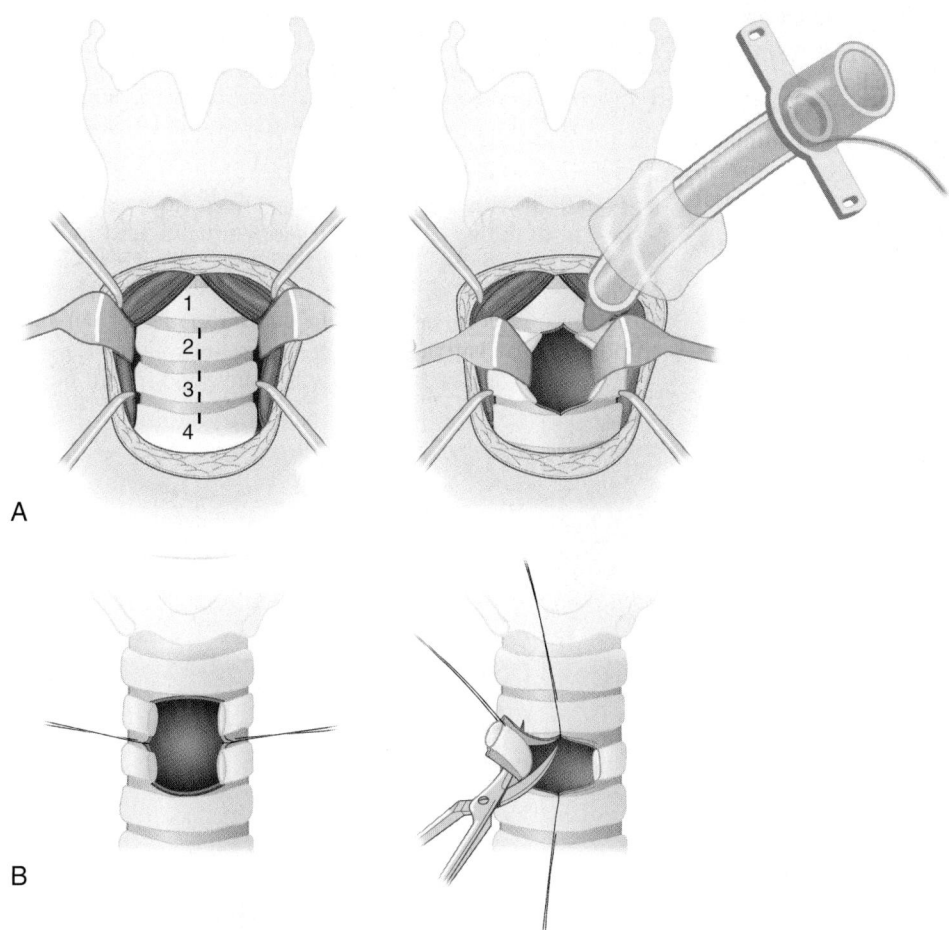

FIGURE 99-3 Two methods of opening the trachea for a standard tracheostomy. **A**, A vertical incision. **B**, Removal of a piece of cartilage. (**A,** Redrawn with permission from Grillo HC. Surgery of the Trachea and Bronchi. London: BC Decker, 2004, p 501. **B,** Redrawn with permission from Myers EN, Tracheostomy. In Myers EN [ed]. Operative Otolaryngology Head and Neck Surgery, Philadelphia: WB Saunders, 1997, p 579.)

A

B

copy. Anesthesia is reversed promptly (see "Pearls and Pitfalls").

EVIDENCE-BASED MEDICINE

The term *tracheostomy* refers to the cutting (Greek, *tomia*) of the windpipe (*trakheia*); the procedure historically was performed for upper airway obstruction. Documentation of successful procedures appears in the 16th and 17th centuries.[2] The procedure was accepted in the 19th century, during European epidemics of diphtheria, usually for temporary relief of acute airway obstruction. A more sustained palliation was directed at upper airway tumors. An early account is contained in *The Fatal Illness of Frederick the Nobel*, by Dr. Morell Mackenzie, which describes the management of laryngeal cancer in Emperor Frederick III of Prussia and Germany.[3] The major advances in perfecting the technique and safety of the procedure were made by Chevalier Jackson during the early half of the 20th century.

After the advent of endotracheal intubation, there was less need for the emergent surgical airway, and the focus turned to tracheostomies for palliation. Since then, further advances in medicine have allowed people to live longer with chronic disease, and the tracheostomy has evolved into a procedure for palliation in subacute airway obstruc-

tion. It has now become one of the most common elective operations, with a mortality rate of less than 1%.

Airway stents have not been used for as long as tracheostomies, but there is sufficient experience and literature to support their use.[46] Intraluminal silicone stents were paced in 30 patients; 27 had malignant stricture, 10 had primary lung cancer, 13 had esophageal cancer causing airway obstruction, and 4 had metastatic cancer. On a 10-point scale of dyspnea, the mean improvement was 6.1 points. The median survival time was 2 months for lung cancer and 3 months for the obstruction from esophageal cancer.[7]

Even those who require emergent intervention might benefit from airway stents. In one report, dilation and stent placement were performed to avoid "imminent asphyxia" in 10 patients with malignant stenosis of the trachea and bifurcation. All patients had long-lasting improvement. Median survival after stent insertion was 5 months for lung cancer and 8 months when esophageal cancer caused airway obstruction.[8]

Careful patient selection is necessary, because not everyone will benefit from relief of airway obstruction. Among 32 patients in an intensive care unit who had airway obstruction and underwent rigid bronchoscopy, dilation, and stenting, 14 had malignant obstruction. Nine of the 14 required mechanical ventilation after the inter-

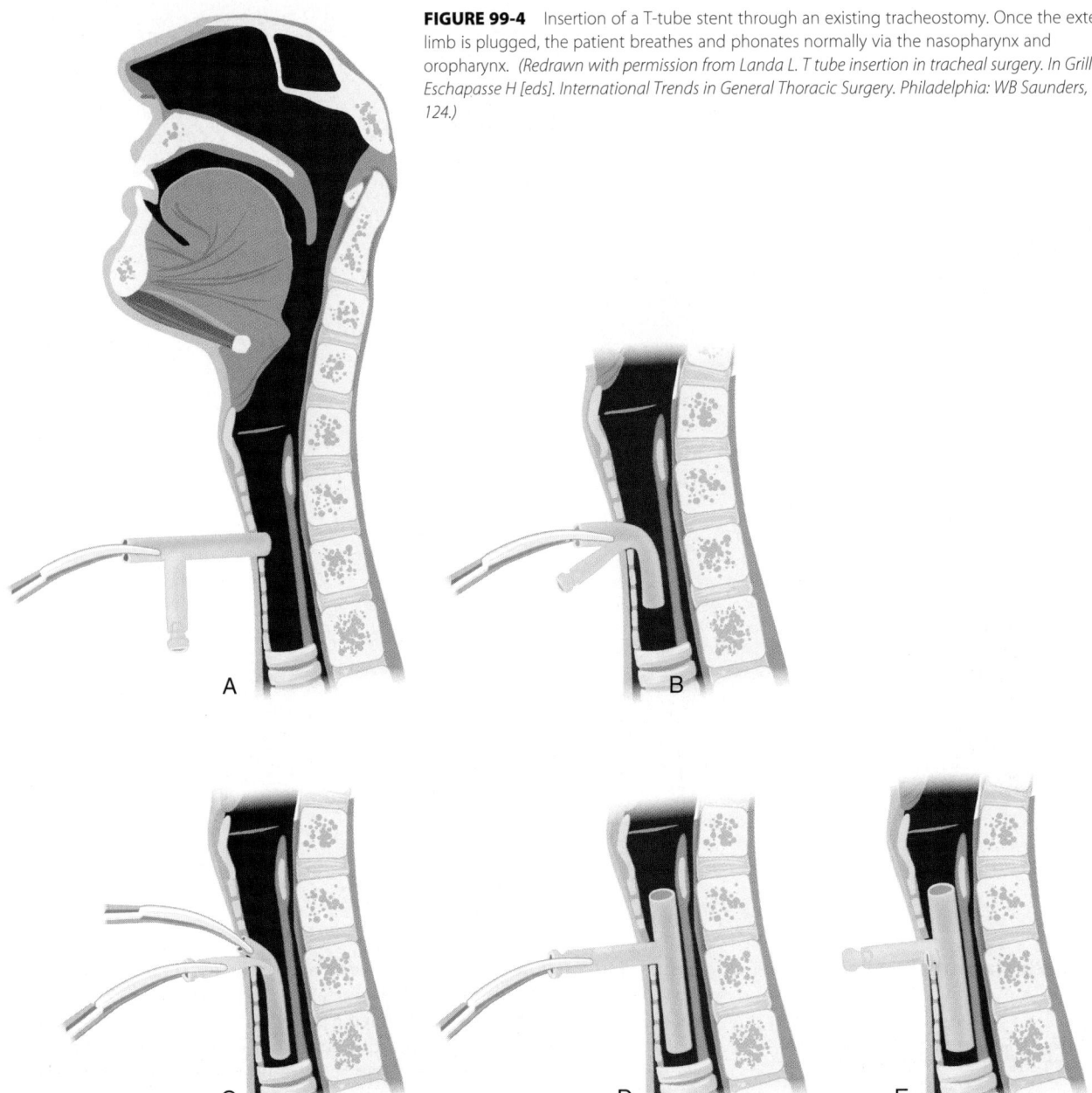

FIGURE 99-4 Insertion of a T-tube stent through an existing tracheostomy. Once the external limb is plugged, the patient breathes and phonates normally via the nasopharynx and oropharynx. *(Redrawn with permission from Landa L. T tube insertion in tracheal surgery. In Grillo HC, Eschapasse H [eds]. International Trends in General Thoracic Surgery. Philadelphia: WB Saunders, 1987, p 124.)*

vention; 7 were never extubated before death. Eleven of the 14 patients were ventilated before the intervention, and 10 of these died within 3 months.[9]

Expandable metal stents were examined in 56 patients who had symptomatic malignant airway obstruction; 77% had symptomatic improvement. Fifty-one of the 56 patients died, with a mean survival time of 77 days. At the time of the report, 5 patients were still alive, at a mean of 207 days after the procedure. In some of the patients, physiological respiratory studies and visual analogue scores for walking and breathing demonstrated significant objective and subjective improvement.[10]

An analysis in the Netherlands studied the palliative value of relieving airway obstruction in the dying. The cases of 14 patients with imminent suffocation from end-stage cancer were reviewed. Physician-assisted suicide and euthanasia are accepted practices in the Netherlands, and the authors questioned whether relief of airway obstruction merely prolonged suffering. All 14 patients expressed benefit from the stent placement. After the patients died, the researchers asked the patients' primary care physicians about the perceived benefit. Two patients had died in the hospital, but, for the other 12, the general practitioners replied that 7 procedures had been worthwhile; no evaluation was made in 4 patients, and for 1 patient the efforts were regarded as futile.[11]

CURRENT CONTROVERSIES AND FUTURE CONSIDERATIONS

Controversies concerning tracheostomy tubes themselves are few. There are some differences of opinion about

Pearls and Pitfalls

Placing a standard tracheostomy tube is a common operation. It is most often done for airway management to allow prolonged ventilatory support. These patients are already intubated and can be sedated comfortably; anesthetic management is not problematic. In contrast, a tracheostomy for airway obstruction can be fraught with technical hazards and tends to stress the surgeon, the anesthesiologist, and the patient.

If an endotracheal tube can be placed temporarily, under either direct vision or bronchoscopic guidance, tracheostomy can be easy. On the other hand, if supraglottic obstruction precludes safe placement of an endotracheal tube, the tracheostomy must be done with local anesthesia and with the patient breathing spontaneously. Once a tracheostomy tube is in place, the patient can be safely sedated, but this is usually unnecessary because of the great relief with a new airway.

Placing a stent requires more complex surgical techniques and anesthetic management. Stents are useful only if there is no laryngeal or supraglottic obstruction. If a patient is symptomatic with tracheal obstruction, this must first be cleared via bronchoscopy and either mechanical débridement, laser excision, or dilation. General anesthesia is usually required, but paralysis must be used cautiously until an adequate airway is achieved. Jet ventilation greatly facilitates rigid bronchoscopy. Hand-activated jet ventilation is acceptable for a short duration, but for anything more than the shortest procedure a mechanical jet ventilator should be used (Mistral Universal Jet Ventilator, Acutronic Medical System A.G., Hirzel, Switzerland).

Wire stents are much easier to place than silicone ones. They also have a better internal diameter than similar-sized silicone stents. They migrate less due to tissue ingrowth. This ingrowth may be a hazard, however, because these stents cannot be removed or repositioned later. The ingrowth also limits the usefulness of wire stents to persons with a short life expectancy, because overgrowth of tumor or fibroblasts may obstruct the stent in time.

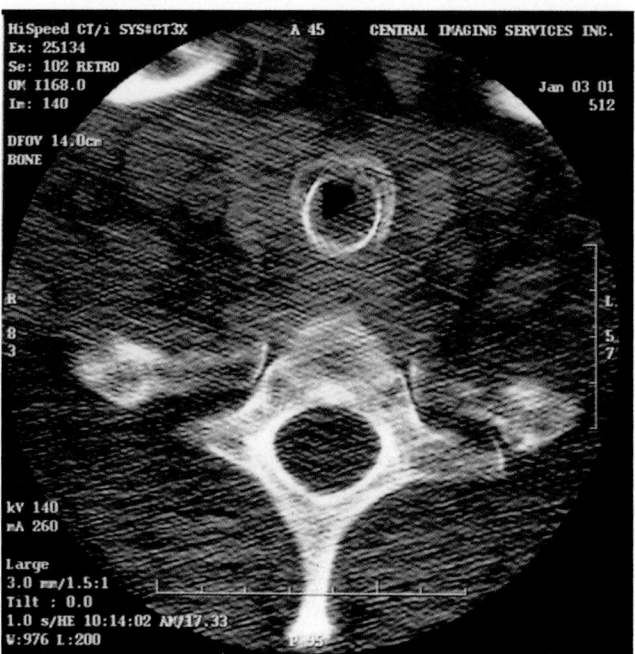

FIGURE 99-5 A computed tomographic image of a patient with a wire stent in the trachea. This stent had been placed a year previously for a benign stricture. There is marked ingrowth of fibrous tissue through the stent, occluding most of the tracheal lumen.

REFERENCES

1. Gunasekaran S, Osborn JR, Morgan A, et al. Tracheal stenting: A better method of dealing with airway obstruction due to thyroid malignancies than tracheostomy. J Laryngol Otol 2004;118:462-464.
2. Myers EN. Tracheostomy. In Operative Otolaryngology Head and Neck Surgery. Philadelphia: Saunders, 1997, pp 575-585.
3. Mackenzie M. The Fatal Illness of Frederick the Nobel. London: Sampson Low, Marston, Searle & Rivington, 1888.
4. Montgomery WW. T-tube tracheal stent. Arch Otol 1965;82:320-321.
5. Montgomery WT. Silicone tracheal T-tube. Ann Otol 1974;83:71-75.
6. Westaby S, Jackson JW, Pearson GF. A bifurcated silicone rubber stent for relief of tracheobronchial obstruction. J Thoracic Cardiovasc Surg 1982;83:414-417.
7. Abdullah V, Yim A, Wormald PJ, et al. Dumon silicone stents in obstructive tracheobronchial lesions: The Hong Kong experience. Otol Head Neck Surg 1998;118:256-260.
8. Wassermann K, Eckel HE, Michel O, et al: Emergency stenting of malignant obstruction of the upper airways: Long-term follow-up with two types of silicone prostheses. J Thoracic Cardiovasc Surg 1996;112:859-866.
9. Colt HG, Harrell JH. Therapeutic rigid bronchoscopy allows level of care changes in patients with acute respiratory failure from central airways obstruction. Chest 1997;112:202-206.
10. Wilson GE, Walshaw MJ, Hind CRK. Treatment of large airway obstruction in lung cancer using expandable metal stents inserted under direct vision via the fibreoptic bronchoscope. Thorax 1996;51:248-252.
11. Vonk-Noordegraaf A, Postmus PE, Sutedja TG. Tracheobronchial stenting in the terminal care of cancer patients with central airways obstruction. Chest 2001;120:1811-1814.

SUGGESTED READING

Colt HG, Dumon JF. Airway stents: Present and future. Clin Chest Med 1995;16:465-478.
Miyazawa T, Yamakido M, Ikeda S, et al. Implantation of Ultraflex nitinol stents in malignant tracheobronchial stenoses. Chest 2000;118:959-965.
Walser EM, Robinson B, Raza SA, et al. Clinical outcomes with airway stents for proximal versus distal malignant tracheobronchial obstructions. J Vasc Interv Rad 2004;15:471-477.

minor surgical technical issues. Most discussion centers on which type of stent to use. Silicone stents are durable and have little reaction with the airway. They are more difficult to insert, and for T tubes require a tracheal opening. Expandable wire stents are easier to insert but are troubled by tissue ingrowth, particularly with prolonged life expectancy (Fig. 99-5). They also cannot be removed. There are stents that combine expandable wire designs with the solid lining of silicone stents. One is the PolyFlex stent (Boston Scientific), which has an impervious cover over an expandable body. These stents are more difficult to insert than expandable wire stents, but they do not experience tissue ingrowth and can be removed or repositioned. However, they have a greater risk of migration.

The ideal stent for airway obstruction has not been found. Such a stent would combine ease of insertion with ease of removal. It would be impervious but also easily fixed in place and would not migrate. It would be resistant to dried secretions. Presently, for those who already have a tracheostomy opening or will require one, the silicone T-tube stent fulfills most of these qualities.

CHAPTER **100**

Pleural and Peritoneal Catheters

Timothy M. Pawlik and J. Timothy Sherwood

KEY POINTS

- Early recognition and treatment of malignant pleural effusions is essential to maximize palliation and preserve functional status.

- Initial fluid cytology may not be diagnostic, and higher-yield procedures such as thoracoscopy may be warranted if suspicion is high.

- Prolonged duration of undrained pleural effusions may lead to trapped lung parenchyma and permanent loss of function.

- Talc pleurodesis or pleural catheter placement should be strongly considered if the effusion recurs after initial thoracentesis.

- The etiology of abdominal ascites dictates the therapeutic approach.

- Ascites due to underlying liver failure or massive hepatic metastases is more amenable to diuretics than is malignant ascites. However, paracentesis is frequently needed to alleviate massive ascites regardless of the cause.

- Repeated large-volume paracentesis is safe and efficacious in malignant ascites, although the ascites frequently quickly recurs.

- Peritoneal catheters may offer a therapeutic benefit over repeated large-volume paracentesis by decreasing multiple trips to the hospital for repeat procedures and avoiding injury to visceral structures from multiple needle passes.

PLEURAL CATHETERS

Clinical Presentation and Evaluation

Pleural effusions are common and often cause significant morbidity. Disturbed cardiopulmonary anatomy and physiology, secondary to a compressive effect on the lung or a mass effect on the mediastinum, may first cause subtle symptoms such as chest discomfort, cough, or easy fatigue. More overt symptoms, such as progressive dyspnea with impaired exercise tolerance and the inability to carry out activities of daily living, may soon follow. Chronic lung collapse may also predispose to pneumonia.

Pleural effusions may be benign or malignant. Benign effusions may be transudative, commonly secondary to processes such as congestive heart failure, liver cirrhosis, hypoalbuminemia, or peritoneal dialysis. Exudative benign effusions are most often from infections (pneumonia) or pulmonary embolism. Although benign causes may be present in the palliative care setting, more commonly pleural effusions are malignant exudative processes. Up to 50% of all patients referred for investigation of a pleural effusion have malignancy.[1-3] In descending frequency, the commonly associated malignancies are lung, breast, lymphoma, ovarian, and gastric cancers. Due to the large differential diagnosis, a systematic early and aggressive

approach to pleural effusions is mandatory, because early diagnosis and treatment avoid the potential complications and impairment of quality of life that accompany their natural history.

After a thorough history and physical examination, the evaluation should begin with diagnostic imaging (Fig. 100-1). Posterior-anterior chest radiography can detect about 200 mL of pleural fluid, whereas only 50 mL is detectable on a lateral film.[4] For those who must remain predominantly supine (e.g., ventilated patients), pleural fluid can be detected radiographically as a hazy opacity that layers posteriorly while preserving vascular shadows.[5] Ultrasound and computed tomography (CT) are more accurate for estimating fluid volume.[6-8] CT may also help distinguish the effusion as malignant when nodular, mediastinal, or circumferential pleural thickening is identified.[8] In addition to diagnosis, ultrasound helps in thoracocentesis, because it can identify septations and differentiate pleural thickening from fluid.[9]

Thoracocentesis remains the first step for undiagnosed pleural effusions. Fluid should be evaluated for pH, protein, lactate dehydrogenase (LDH), glucose, cell count, Gram stain, acid-fast bacilli, microbiological culture, and cytology.[10] Light's criteria may be help differentiate transudate from exudate (Box 100-1). Malignant effusions can be diagnosed by the initial pleural fluid cytology specimen in about 60% of cases.[11,12] If second or third cytology specimens are sent, this figure increases slightly.[13] Thoracoscopy is often employed when less invasive techniques fail. The diagnostic yield is as high as 95% for malignancy.[14]

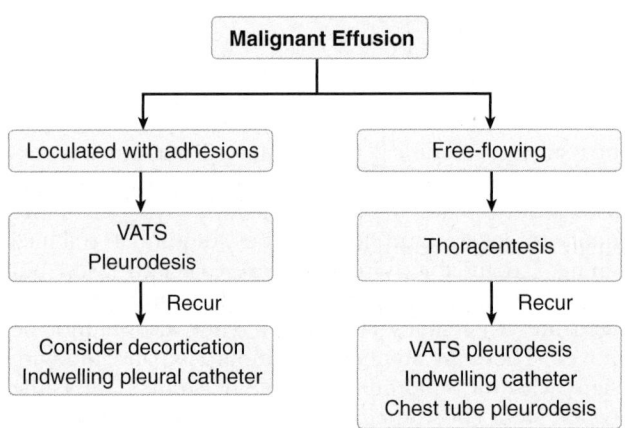

FIGURE 100-1 Treatment algorithm for patients who present with a malignant pleural effusion. VATS, video-assisted thoracoscopic surgery.

Box 100-1 Light's Criteria for Pleural Fluid

Pleural fluid is more likely to be an exudate if the fluid analysis meets one of the following criteria:

1. Ratio of pleural fluid LDH to serum LDH >0.6
2. Ratio of pleural fluid protein to serum protein >0.5
3. Pleural fluid LDH concentration greater than two-thirds of the normal serum LDH level

---

LDH, lactate dehydrogenase.
Light RW, Macgregor MI, Luchsinger PC, et al. Pleural effusions: The diagnostic separation of transudates and exudates. Ann Intern Med 1972; 77(4):507-513.

Thoracoscopy carries minimal morbidity and can be done as an outpatient procedure.

Although thoracocentesis is critical for diagnosis, its role in management pleural effusions is more limited. Malignant pleural effusions tend to be larger in volume[15] and less amenable to a single simple aspiration. Furthermore, they commonly quickly recur after simple aspiration. As such, repeat thoracocentesis is usually reserved for patients whose life expectancy is short and performance status poor.[16,17] Pleurodesis is the most effective means to manage malignant pleural effusions. Many agents can be used, including talc, quinacrine, bleomycin, tetracycline, and doxorubicin. Chemical pleurodesis can be done using either the closed technique, via tube thoracostomy, or the open technique, via video-assisted thoracoscopic surgery (VATS). Depending on the agent, efficacy ranges from 70% to 98% (Table 100-1). Successful pleurodesis relies on apposition of the visceral and parietal pleura, because the inflammatory process seals these two layers together, obliterating the potential space in which effusions form.

Many patients with pleural effusions have underlying trapped lungs, which make chemical pleurodesis untenable.[3] For this group, tunneled pleural catheters are a better option (Fig. 100-2). A useful method for determining whether the lung is trapped is lung reexpansion on chest radiography after therapeutic thoracentesis. Usually, lung trapping occurs in the lower lobes at the bases. In patients with good performance status and reasonable life expectancy, decortication should be considered.

Equipment

The equipment is dictated by the therapeutic approach (i.e., simple thoracocentesis versus closed or open pleurodesis versus indwelling catheter). The following is a general outline of the equipment that may be needed:

- Thoracocentesis tray (contains sterile gloves, povidone-iodine, local anesthetic solution, aspiration needle, syringe, guidewire, dilator, flexible catheter, suture material, and needle driver)
- Pleural fluid containers (e.g., culture bottles, specimen cups for chemistry, cell count, and cytology)
- Extension tubing with three-way stopcock
- 1-L vacuum bottles
- Indwelling catheter
- Chest tube (10 to 14 F)
- Pleurodesis agent
- Video-thoracoscopic equipment

TABLE 100-1 Relative Efficacy of Various Pleurodesis Sclerosing Agents

SCLEROSING AGENT	PERCENT RESPONSE (%)	
	MEAN	RANGE
Talc	98	72-100
Quinacrine	86	64-100
Bleomycin	64	31-85
Tetracycline	72	25-80
Doxorubicin	70	65-70

Description of Technique

Simple Thoracocentesis and Placement of Indwelling Catheter

If possible, have the patient sit upright while leaning forward on a table. Confirm the presence and extent of the pleural effusion by listening to the chest and checking for shifting dullness. If necessary, employ ultrasound to locate loculated fluid pockets. The puncture site should be 1 to 2 intercostal spaces below the upper extent of the fluid level in the posterior axillary line or posterior midclavicular line. After cleaning the area with povidone-iodine and draping the site with sterile towels, infiltrate the area with local anesthetic. Introduce the aspiration needle just above the upper edge of the rib corresponding to the previously designated entry site. Aspirate to confirm the presence of fluid. After threading the guidewire through the needle (Selinger technique), remove the introducer needle and dilate the track with the dilator over the guidewire. Thread the flexible catheter over the guidewire into the cavity. For indwelling catheters, pigtail catheters with locking mechanisms prevent accidental dislocation.[18]

To drain the effusion, connect the catheter to the connector tubing, open the three-way stopcock, and allow

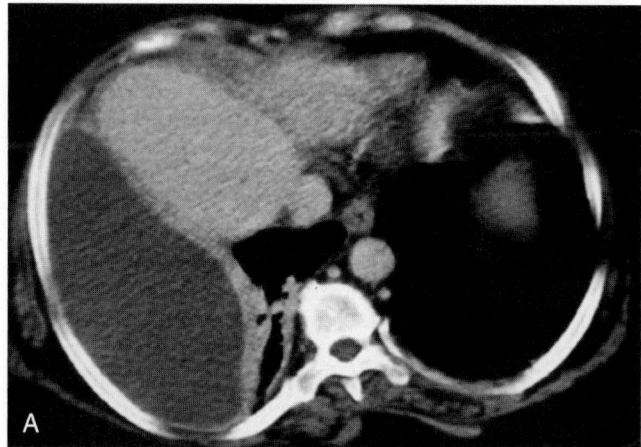

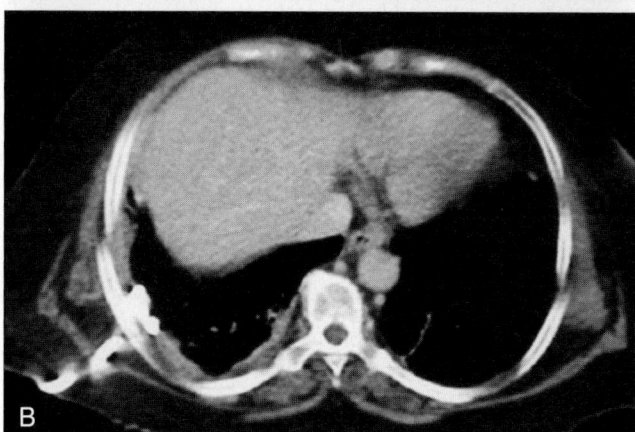

FIGURE 100-2 **A**, Computed tomogram showing loculated pleural effusion with enhancing pleura. **B**, There is almost complete resolution of the pleural effusion after placement of a pigtail catheter. (From Ozkan OS, Ozmen MN, Akhan O. Percutaneous management of parapneumonic effusions. Eur J Radiol 2005;55:311-320.)

fluid to flow into the vacuum bottles. For simple thoraco-centesis, before withdrawing the catheter, turn the stop-cock "off" so that the path to the vacuum bottle is closed, to prevent air from entering the pleural space. With indwelling catheters, the pigtail catheter should be secured, the site cleaned, and a sterile dressing applied. If a Pleurx catheter is being placed, the catheter should be tunneled through 5 cm of subcutaneous tissue before being placed through the insertion sheath. Strict attention to sterile technique is mandatory, because an infected space with a trapped lung is disastrous.

Pleurodesis

With the closed method, a chest tube is inserted to drain the pleural space. Usually, drainage is continued until the output is less than 100 mL per day. After reexpansion of the lung is confirmed radiographically, a chemical pleurodesis agent is introduced through the chest tube into the pleural space. The tube is then clamped to prevent the agent from leaking, and the patient is asked to change position about every 15 minutes for 2 hours; this pro-motes even distribution of the chemical agent in the space. In the open technique, the patient is taken to the operating room and placed under general anesthesia. A thoracic surgeon then makes a small chest incision, through which a thoracoscope is placed. Under direct vision, the pleural fluid is drained and the pleurodesis agent is inserted on the pleural surface. Modern sclerosant administration uses aerosolized talc, which allows uniform distribution on the pleural surface.

Postoperative Care

All patients should have a postprocedure chest radiograph to evaluate residual fluid, check for catheter or chest tube placement, and exclude potential complications (e.g., pneumothorax). After chest tube placement, the tube should be connected to 20 cm water suction via a closed underwater seal system. All chest tubes and indwelling catheters need to be checked routinely for patency. If the catheter or tube becomes blocked, an injection of sterile saline will usually clear it. This should not be done in a patient with a trapped lung or talc pleurodesis. In general, chest tubes can be removed when the drainage is less than 100 to 150 mL per day. After talc pleurodesis, the chest tube is placed on continuous suction for 3 to 5 days to prevent fluid pockets from forming and subsequent local failure. Those with indwelling catheters require additional teaching to care for their catheters, and fluid must be drained when they become symptomatic.

Complications

Complications after simple thoracocentesis are uncom-mon.[19] Pneumothoraces occur in 2% to 5% of patients, but many are small and asymptomatic and can be managed conservatively. Larger (>20 %) pneumothoraces and those that are symptomatic require placement of a catheter or chest tube.

Another rare but dangerous complication is reexpan-sion pulmonary edema, which occurs after rapid reexpan-sion of a chronically collapsed lung in patients with a massive pleural effusion. It usually appears immediately or within 1 hour after fluid drainage[20] and may be severe enough to cause cardiorespiratory insufficiency. Reexpan-sion pulmonary edema is rare if less than 1.5 L of fluid is removed at one time, so this should be the limit during a single thoracocentesis.

Other complications may occur from the sclerosing agents. Fever, chest pain, and even occasional episodes of acute respiratory distress syndrome (ARDS) or acute pneu-monitis occur. Complications related to chronic indwell-ing catheters include infection and catheter obstruction or malfunction. One randomized trial of Pleurx catheters demonstrated a low (<2%) risk of infection.

Evidence-Based Medicine

Two studies[21,22] reported similar success rates for pleurode-sis with small-bore (10 to 14 F) versus large-bore (24 to 38 F) chest tubes. Because tubes with smaller bores are associated with less discomfort and easier insertion, they should be favored.

Numerous studies have examined the relative efficacy of chemical pleurodesis agents. A Cochrane Review[23] that combined data from more than 300 patients revealed talc was the best agent to prevent recurrence of pleural effu-sions. Although talc has been associated with ARDS, a recent randomized trial[24] showed that the use of graded talc (small particles removed) reduces ARDS significantly, compared with mixed talc (small talc particles included). Other agents, such as tetracycline or bleomycin, are effec-tive but are fraught with significant adverse effects such as severe pain or renal failure.

Current Controversies and Future Considerations

Whether patients requiring pleurodesis should initially be managed with VATS poudrage or with chest tube pleurode-sis remains controversial. Some investigators advocate that VATS be used only after tube thoracostomy pleurodesis has failed. Other investigators[25] believe that VATS should be used as primary treatment because of the shorter dura-tion of chest tube placement and postprocedure hospital stay. One randomized trial demonstrated superior out-comes with thoracoscopic talc pleurodesis compared to tube thoracostomy when treating malignant effusions from lung or breast cancer.[26] Overall, thoracoscopy has multiple advantages over chest tube talc pleurodesis, including less pain, the ability to decorticate loculations, more uniform talc distribution, and availability of diagnostic tissue.

Another controversy involves whether indwelling cath-eters are preferable to chemical pleurodesis. Because indwelling catheters may provide for spontaneous pleurodesis in up to 40% of patients and can be performed as an outpatient procedure, some have advocated that they be used for primary management of malignant pleural effusions.

PERITONEAL CATHETERS

Clinical Presentation and Evaluation

Ascites can lead to pain, abdominal distention, respiratory difficulty, loss of appetite, nausea, and restricted mobility.

Although it can be secondary to many different processes, end-stage liver disease and malignancy are the two major causes. Approximately 50% of patients with compensated cirrhosis have ascites, and about 10% of all cases of ascites are from cancer. Those cancers most commonly associated with malignant ascites are the ovary, breast, bronchus, stomach, and pancreas cancers.[27] Up to 20% of all patients with malignant ascites have an unknown primary.[28]

On physical examination, at least 500 mL of ascitic fluid is needed before one can appreciate shifting dullness or a fluid-wave sign. Evaluation of newly diagnosed ascites should include both Doppler ultrasonography of the liver and abdomen and paracentesis (Fig. 100-3). The ultrasound can confirm the patency of hepatic and portal veins and the extent and nature of the ascites. Fluid should be sent for cell count, cultures, Gram stain, total protein, albumin, and cytology (Box 100-2).

The serum-ascites albumin gradient (SAAG) is the single best test for classifying ascites as to etiology: portal/liver (SAAG ≥ 1.1 g/dL) or nonportal/malignant (SAAG < 1.1 g/dL) (Table 100-2). The SAAG is calculated by subtracting the ascitic fluid albumin value from the serum albumin level. It is 97% accurate in the general classification of ascites. Cytology smears from paracentesis fluid are 50% to 75% sensitive in detecting malignancy.

The International Ascites Club defines refractory ascites as that which cannot be mobilized, or early recurrence of ascites that cannot be prevented by medical therapy. Ascites is also deemed to be refractory if it responds to medical therapy but the patient is intolerant of therapy due to debilitating complications (e.g., azotemia, encephalopathy, hyperkalemia). The initial management of mild to moderate ascites usually involves diuretics. Some investigators[29] have reported that the mobilization of malignant ascites with diuretics is dependent on the ascitic fluid characteristics. Specifically, although patients with massive hepatic metastases respond more like other patients with portal-derived ascites, those with peritoneal carcinomatous or malignant chylous ascites derive relatively little benefit from diuretics (Fig. 100-4). The use of a peritoneovenous shunt was popular in the past for malignant ascites, but it has fallen out of favor. One reason is that peritoneovenous shunts can be associated with potentially fatal side effects (e.g., infection, disseminated intravascular coagulation). Because of the increased risks and costs, some have suggested that this treatment should be reserved for patients with an anticipated prognosis of at least 6 months.

In a seminal study,[30] investigators showed that large-volume paracentesis for cirrhotic ascites was more effective than diuretics and had fewer complications. Other studies[31,32] corroborated the important palliative role of

---

Box 100-2 Tests That Should Be Performed on Newly Diagnosed Ascitic Fluid

1. Total protein
2. Albumin
3. Gram stain
4. Cell count
5. Culture
6. Cytology

TABLE 100-2 Differential Diagnosis of Ascites Based on Serum-Ascites Albumin Gradient (SAAG)	
SSAG < 1.1 G/DL	**SSAG ≥ 1.1 G/DL**
Peritoneal carcinomatosis	Hepatic cirrhosis
Biliary ascites	Hepatic metastases
Pancreatic ascites	Hepatocellular carcinoma
Infectious ascites	Portal vein thrombosis/Budd-Chiari syndrome
Chylous ascites	Cardiac ascites

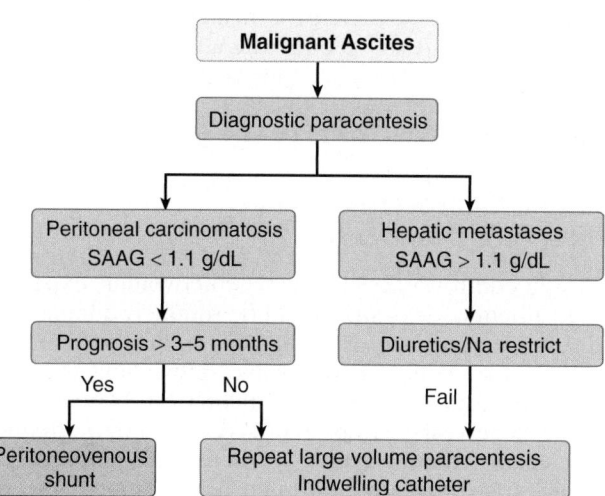

FIGURE 100-3 Treatment algorithm for patients who present with malignant ascites. SAAG, serum-ascites albumin gradient.

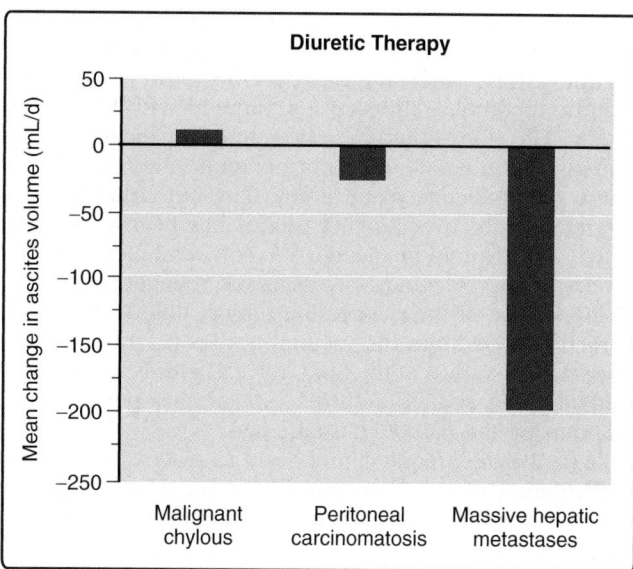

FIGURE 100-4 Although patients with massive hepatic metastases respond more like other patients with portal-derived ascites, patients with peritoneal carcinomatous or malignant chylous ascites derive relatively little benefit from diuretic therapy. (*From Pockros PJ, Esrason KT, Nguyen C, et al. Mobilization of malignant ascites with diuretics is dependent on ascitic fluid characteristics. Gastroenterology 1992;103:1302-1306.*)

paracentesis in cases of failed medical therapy. These data have been extrapolated to malignant ascites, and paracentesis has become the most popular means of managing malignant ascites. However, fluid rapidly accumulates in many patients, necessitating multiple hospital trips for repeat procedures. Repeated large-volume paracentesis can also be associated with protein loss and increased risk of injury to visceral structures due to multiple abdominal needle passes. Indwelling catheters may, therefore, be preferable to repeated large-volume paracentesis for diuretic-resistant symptomatic ascites. The median time during which these catheters remain functional is about 40 days. However, most can be revised and left in place; the incidence of tube blockage requiring removal is about 5%.

Equipment

The following is a general outline of the equipment needed to perform paracentesis and placement of an indwelling peritoneal catheter:

- Paracentesis tray (sterile gloves, povidone-iodine, local anesthetic solution, aspiration needle, syringe, guide-wire, dilator, and flexible catheter)
- Containers for ascitic fluid (e.g., culture bottles, specimen cups)
- Extension tubing with three-way stopcock
- 1-L vacuum bottles for the ascitic fluid
- Indwelling catheter (Tenckhoff or pigtail catheter; 10 to 15 F)

Description of Technique

Before the procedure, the patient should be asked to urinate so that the bladder is empty. With the patient semirecumbent, the presence and extent of the ascites should be confirmed by physical examination or ultrasonography. The preferred sites are in the midline, inferior to the umbilicus, or near either flank, away from the epigastric artery. After the site has been prepared using aseptic technique, the skin is infiltrated with local anesthetic. The skin should then be retracted caudally so that the aspiration needle does not penetrate the fascia in the same perpendicular plane as the skin, but rather forms a "Z tract." After free-flowing ascites has been confirmed with the aspiration needle, a soft catheter can be exchanged over a guidewire using the Selinger technique. With the use of the connecting tubing, fluid can then be directly drained into the vacuum bottles via the soft catheter. After removal of the fluid, the catheter is withdrawn, allowing the skin to return to its normal position and minimizing the risk of an ascitic leak.

A similar technique can be used to place a permanent indwelling catheter.[33] Specifically, a Tenckhoff or pigtail catheter is placed via a subcutaneous tunnel using a modified Selinger technique.

Postoperative Care

If a large amount of ascites is removed (>4 to 6 L), the patient may become hypovolemic. Blood pressure and pulse should be checked every 30 minutes during large-volume paracentesis and then every 6 hours thereafter. Although the routine use of albumin or other volume expanders is controversial, if there are clinical signs of hypovolemia (e.g., low urine output, tachycardia, hypotension), intravenous hydration, dextran (150 mL per liter of ascites drained), or albumin (8 g per liter ascites drained) should be considered.

Complications

Paracentesis is safe, the risk of a major complication being less than 1%.[34] Possible complications include bowel or bladder perforation, bleeding, abdominal wall hematoma, laceration of a blood vessel (e.g., epigastric), and infection. For indwelling catheters, infection can occur in up to 30% of patients, with about half of these requiring removal of the catheter.[35]

Perhaps the most common complication after paracentesis is leakage from the puncture site. In most cases, the leak stops spontaneously if the patient remains supine for a few hours with the site angled upward with a dry gauze dressing. A colostomy bag can be used to collect ascites if the leak volume is large; and, if it is persistent, a purse-string suture can be placed around the site.

An uncommon but more ominous complication of large-volume paracentesis is postparacentesis circulatory dysfunction, characterized by renal insufficiency, hypotension, and rapid recurrence of ascites. This is uncommon in malignant ascites, compared with ascites secondary to cirrhosis. As noted earlier, postparacentesis circulatory dysfunction occurs almost exclusively after more than 5 L of ascites has been removed.

Evidence-Based Medicine

There are no randomized controlled trials assessing diuretics in malignant ascites. Similarly, the choice of diuretic has not been well evaluated. There are some data suggesting that efficacy in malignant ascites depends on the ratio of the aldosterone to the renin concentration, and therefore aldosterone antagonist diuretics (e.g., spironolactone) should be considered, alone or in combination with loop diuretics.

Most data show that large-volume paracentesis is needed to manage extensive malignant ascites. Large-volume paracentesis[34] is both safe and effective. Multiple case reports have described the management of malignant ascites with long-term indwelling catheters and have reported these catheters to be safe and effective.

Current Controversies and Future Considerations

Current controversies include whether volume expanders (e.g., albumin, dextran) should be routinely administered during paracentesis of malignant ascites greater than 5 L. Another controversy involves indwelling catheters. Although they have several theoretical benefits (e.g., fewer clinic visits, less protein loss due to more frequent and smaller-volume drainage), there have not been any clinical trials evaluating repeated large-volume paracentesis versus indwelling peritoneal catheters in primary management of malignant ascites. Their role as the primary treatment of malignant ascites is controversial, because some believe there is a higher risk of peritoneal infection with an indwelling catheter.

REFERENCES

1. DiBonito L, Falconieri G, Colautti I, et al. The positive pleural effusion: A retrospective study of cytopathologic diagnoses with autopsy confirmation. Acta Cytol 1992;36:329-332.
2. Marel M, Stastny B, Melinova L, et al. Diagnosis of pleural effusions: Experience with clinical studies, 1986 to 1990. Chest 1995;107:1598-1603.
3. Bennett R, Maskell N. Management of malignant pleural effusions. Curr Opin Pulm Med 2005;11:296-300.
4. Blackmore CC, Black WC, Dallas RV, et al. Pleural fluid volume estimation: A chest radiograph prediction rule. Acad Radiol 1996;3:103-109.
5. Ruskin JA, Gurney JW, Thorsen MK, et al. Detection of pleural effusions on supine chest radiographs. AJR Am J Roentgenol 1987;148:681-683.
6. Traill ZC, Davies RJ, Gleeson FV: Thoracic computed tomography in patients with suspected malignant pleural effusions. Clin Radiol 2001;56:193-196.
7. Eibenberger KL, Dock WI, Ammann ME, et al. Quantification of pleural effusions: Sonography versus radiography. Radiology 1994;191:681-684.
8. Leung AN, Muller NL, Miller RR. CT in differential diagnosis of diffuse pleural disease. AJR Am J Roentgenol 1990;154:487-492.
9. Yang PC, Luh KT, Chang DB, et al. Value of sonography in determining the nature of pleural effusion: Analysis of 320 cases. AJR Am J Roentgenol 1992;159:29-33.
10. Medford A, Maskell N. Pleural effusion. Postgrad Med J 2005;81:702-710.
11. Nance KV, Shermer RW, Askin FB. Diagnostic efficacy of pleural biopsy as compared with that of pleural fluid examination. Mod Pathol 1991;4:320-324.
12. Prakash UB, Reiman HM. Comparison of needle biopsy with cytologic analysis for the evaluation of pleural effusion: Analysis of 414 cases. Mayo Clin Proc 1985;60:158-164.
13. Garcia LW, Ducatman BS, Wang HH. The value of multiple fluid specimens in the cytological diagnosis of malignancy. Mod Pathol 1994;7:665-668.
14. Loddenkemper R. Thoracoscopy: State of the art. Eur Respir J 1998;11:213-221.
15. Maher GG, Berger HW. Massive pleural effusion: Malignant and nonmalignant causes in 46 patients. Am Rev Respir Dis 1972;105:458-460.
16. Antunes G, Neville E, Duffy J, et al. BTS guidelines for the management of malignant pleural effusions. Thorax 2003;58(Suppl 2):ii29-ii38.
17. American Thoracic Society. Management of malignant pleural effusions. Am J Respir Crit Care Med 2000;162:1987-2001.
18. Ozkan OS, Ozmen MN, Akhan O. Percutaneous management of parapneumonic effusions. Eur J Radiol 2005;55:311-320.
19. Mynarek G, Brabrand K, Jakobsen JA, et al. Complications following ultrasound-guided thoracocentesis. Acta Radiol 2004;45:519-522.
20. Tarver RD, Broderick LS, Conces DJ Jr. Reexpansion pulmonary edema. J Thorac Imaging 1996;11:198-209.
21. Parker LA, Charnock GC, Delany DJ. Small bore catheter drainage and sclerotherapy for malignant pleural effusions. Cancer 1989;64:1218-1221.
22. Clementsen P, Evald T, Grode G, et al. Treatment of malignant pleural effusion: Pleurodesis using a small percutaneous catheter. A prospective randomized study. Respir Med 1998;92:593-596.
23. Shaw P, Agarwal R. Pleurodesis for malignant pleural effusions. Cochrane Database Syst Rev 2004;(1):CD002916.
24. Maskell NA, Lee YC, Gleeson FV, et al. Randomized trials describing lung inflammation after pleurodesis with talc of varying particle size. Am J Respir Crit Care Med 2004;170:377-382.
25. Erickson KV, Yost M, Bynoe R, et al. Primary treatment of malignant pleural effusions: Video-assisted thoracoscopic surgery poudrage versus tube thoracostomy. Am Surg 2002;68:955-959; discussion 959-960.
26. Dresler CM, Olak J, Herndon JE 2nd, et al. Phase III intergroup study of talc poudrage vs talc slurry sclerosis for malignant pleural effusion. Chest 2005;127:909-915.
27. Runyon BA. Care of patients with ascites. N Engl J Med 1994;330:337-342.
28. Ringenberg QS, Doll DC, Loy TS, et al. Malignant ascites of unknown origin. Cancer 1989;64:753-755.
29. Pockros PJ, Esrason KT, Nguyen C, et al. Mobilization of malignant ascites with diuretics is dependent on ascitic fluid characteristics. Gastroenterology 1992;87:1302-1306.
30. Gines P, Arroyo V, Quintero E, et al. Comparison of paracentesis and diuretics in the treatment of cirrhotics with tense ascites: Results of a randomized study. Gastroenterology 1987;93:234-241.
31. Appelqvist P, Silvo J, Salmela L, et al. On the treatment and prognosis of malignant ascites: Is the survival time determined when the abdominal paracentesis is needed? J Surg Oncol 1982;20:238-242.
32. Wilcox CM, Woods BL, Mixon HT. Prospective evaluation of a peritoneal dialysis catheter system for large volume paracentesis. Am J Gastroenterol 1992;87:1443-1446.
33. Barnett TD, Rubins J. Placement of a permanent tunneled peritoneal drainage catheter for palliation of malignant ascites: A simplified percutaneous approach. J Vasc Interv Radiol 2002;13:379-383.
34. Runyon BA. Paracentesis of ascitic fluid: A safe procedure. Arch Intern Med 1986;146:2259-2261.
35. Lee A, Lau TN, Yeong KY. Indwelling catheters for the management of malignant ascites. Support Care Cancer 2000;8:493-499.

SUGGESTED READING

Bennett R, Maskell N. Management of malignant pleural effusions. Curr Opin Pulm Med 2005;11:296-300.
Lee A, Lau TN, Yeong KY. Indwelling catheters for the management of malignant ascites. Support Care Cancer 2000;8:493-499.
Pockros PJ, Esrason KT, Nguyen C, et al. Mobilization of malignant ascites with diuretics is dependent on ascitic fluid characteristics. Gastroenterology 1992;103:1302-1306.
Runyon BA. Care of patients with ascites. N Engl J Med 1994;330:337-342.
Shaw P, Agarwal R. Pleurodesis for malignant pleural effusions. Cochrane Database Syst Rev 2004;(1):CD002916.

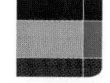

CHAPTER **101**

Interventional Radiology

Meghna Chadha and **Mark Sands**

> **K E Y   P O I N T S**
>
> - Central venous access is important in palliative care.
> - Vena cava filters can be used to prevent pulmonary embolism.
> - Transcatheter embolotherapy is used in treating in acute gastrointestinal bleeds, life-threatening hemoptysis, and primary and secondary hepatic malignancies.
> - Transjugular intrahepatic portosystemic shunts are placed in patients with variceal bleeding and ascites.

CENTRAL VENOUS ACCESS

Central venous access is an integral component in the care of malignant, infectious, and chronic diseases, and it is pivotal in much of palliative therapy. The indications for the placement of central venous catheters are expanding. The rapid growth of hemodialysis, transplantation, and oncology medicine has contributed to the need for parenteral nutrition, hemodialysis, plasmapheresis, blood transfusions, blood sampling, and long-term chemotherapy for various neoplastic and infectious diseases. Catheter materials compatible with long-term in-home use that minimize infectious and thrombotic complications have contributed to outpatient treatment and have improved patients' quality of life. Use of these materials has reduced costs and the length of hospital stay.[1,2] In some patients, central catheters are needed to manage symptoms of advanced disease that cannot be treated by less invasive routes. Central venous lines may be placed because of previous antineoplastic and supportive therapies, and they can be employed for symptom control and comfort care in patients with advanced illness. They can be requested when high-dose opioids are needed that cannot be provided by oral or subcutaneous administration for difficult pain problems and particularly for conditions such as intestinal obstruction or for optimal sedation of the dying.

Catheter and venous port placements are commonly performed interventional procedures for radiological procedures. This may be challenging when traditional venous access sites are used repeatedly because of resultant stenosis or occlusion.

There are three basic categories of venous catheters: nontunneled catheters, tunneled catheters, and implantable subcutaneous ports. The length of desired therapy and the composition and compatibility of the infusate dictate choice of device.

Nontunneled catheters are commonly placed in the central veins (i.e., subclavian and internal jugular) by blind percutaneous bedside techniques. They are primarily used for short-term access. Peripherally inserted central catheters (PICCs) are placed in the cavoatrial junction through the nondominant upper extremity vein. They may be placed at bedside through a superficial vein, or they may require imaging guidance. PICCs are composed of silicone or polyurethane. Polyurethane catheters allow a larger inner diameter for the same outer diameter. The basilic vein is preferred over the brachial and cephalic veins because there is less chance of injury to the brachial artery and nerve. The cephalic vein has the highest rate of thrombus and phlebitis. PICCs and the nontunneled, nontapered, centrally placed, silicone Hohn catheter are used for intermediate access (i.e., weeks to months).[3]

Tunneled catheters travel through a subcutaneous tract before exiting the body. They are a reasonable choice when therapy will continue for several months. They are constructed predominantly of medical-grade silicone or polyurethane materials, with a Dacron cuff bonded to the catheter. Some may have a second cuff impregnated with silver. This is positioned in the subcutaneous tunnel for stabilization. They are accessed externally and designed for long-term home use. Tunneled and nontunneled catheters are available in single, dual, or triple lumens. The numbers of ports depend on how many noncompatible medications will be infused at once. They should be kept to a bare minimum to minimize catheter-related infections. With more ports, the size of each lumen decreases, increasing the risk of catheter thrombosis[4,5] (Fig. 101-1).

Implantable ports do not exit the body but terminate in a subcutaneous device. Whenever medical therapy lasts longer than 3 months or if an external device may limit lifestyle, a port may be recommended. Implantable subcutaneous ports use the same catheter materials as tunneled catheters but are attached to a domed access reservoir (i.e., port) buried subcutaneously for stability. These devices are accessed percutaneously by a noncoring needle and intended for long-term use. They are available in single-port and dual-port configurations, which may be plastic or metal with a septum and placed on the anteromedial chest wall or the upper arm. Tunneled catheters and implantable ports are placed with the patient under conscious sedation (Fig. 101-2).

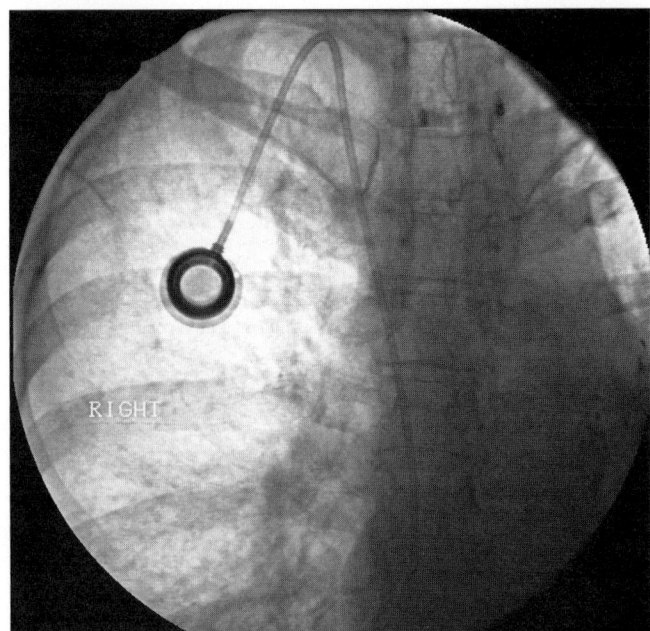

FIGURE 101-1 A 68-year-old patient with breast carcinoma. A subcutaneous implantable port is placed via the right internal jugular vein for chemotherapy.

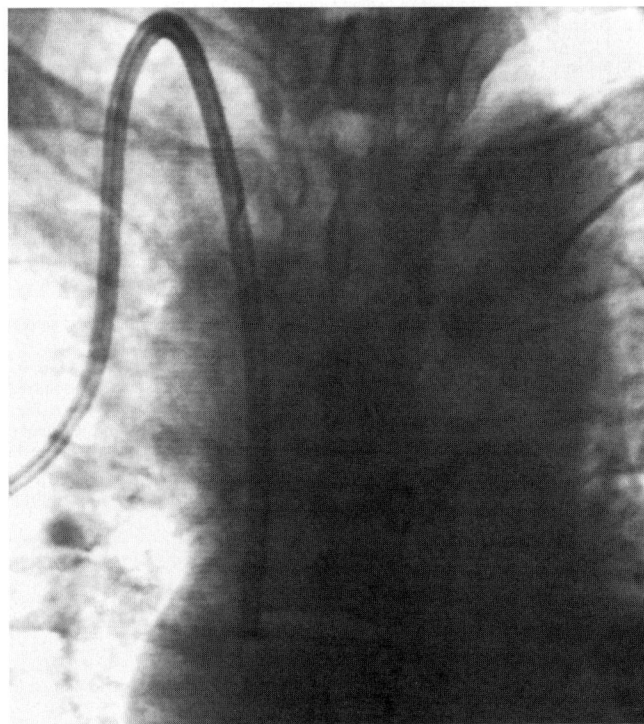

FIGURE 101-2 A 74-year-old male patient with gastric carcinoma required a triple-lumen Hickman catheter for chemotherapy, total parenteral nutrition infusion, and sampling for laboratory tests.

Hemodialysis Catheters

Hemodialysis catheters pose special challenges for long-term venous access. High-flow-rate catheters of at least 300 mL/min are needed. Access may be difficult because of central venous stenosis from many prior catheterizations. Balloon angioplasty and stent placement may be needed for ongoing access.[5,6]

Indications

Catheterization is indicated for infusion and hemodialysis. Continuous infusion is used for chemotherapy, total parenteral nutrition, patient-controlled analgesia, and continuous intravenous medication. Intermittent infusion is used for transfusion, chemotherapy, hydration, and intermittent medication. Hemodialysis is used for pheresis and blood draws.

Preprocedural Planning

The directed history and physical examination include obtaining informed consent and fasting at least 6 hours before the procedure. Questioning should determine a history of recent fever, bacteremia, or sepsis; a history of venous access problems; and the status of chest wall collateral vessels.

Laboratory tests should determine an international normalized ratio (INR) of less than 2.0 for tunneled catheters and less than 1.5 for implantable ports. The partial thromboplastin time is obtained. The platelet count should be more than 30,000 for placing tunneled catheters and more than 50,000 for implantable ports. Blood cultures should be negative for more than 48 hours.

Available images should be reviewed. Limited ultrasonography of the neck may be useful.

Antibiotic coverage for skin flora should be administered. A single dose (1 g) of intravenous cefazolin can be given, or a single dose (1 g) of intravenous vancomycin can be administered if the patient is allergic to penicillin.

Contraindications to Tunneled Catheters and Implantable Ports

Absolute contraindications include bacteremia or sepsis (i.e., hypertensive and diabetic patients are prone), infection at the insertion site, and disseminated intravascular coagulopathy. Relative contraindications include neutropenia, mild coagulopathy, and recent but resolved sepsis.[7,8] No significant difference in infectious complications are encountered in human immunodeficiency virus (HIV)–positive patients compared with the general population.[9]

Radiological Placement

Percutaneous placement requires three steps:

1. Establishment of central venous access and determination of appropriate intravascular catheter length
2. Formation of a subcutaneous tunnel or pocket
3. Placement of the catheter into the central venous system

Standard sites for central venous catheters include the internal jugular vein, external jugular vein, subclavian vein, axillary vein, brachial vein, basilic vein, and common femoral vein. Unconventional access sites include the infrarenal inferior vena cava, the suprarenal inferior vena cava (IVC), hepatic veins, and collateral veins. Long-term dialysis access through the renal vein has been reported. Nontraditional access sites may be used when conventional access sites are no longer available or impending surgeries and treatments are expected.[3,10]

Venous Access Techniques

Most operators prefer sonographic guidance for venous access, especially for nonconventional sites. This provides direct visualization of the target vessel and the soft tissue pathway to it. It also provides information concerning target vein patency at the access site and usually central to the access site. Visualization of neighboring arteries is possible, which ensures venous and not errant arterial access. After a thrombosed vein is identified, advancement of a guidewire through the occluded vessel into the central circulation may be possible. Sonographic examination of the neck may demonstrate small collateral channels that may permit catheter advancement. If significant stenosis is identified, a hydrophilic guidewire may be negotiated through the severe stenosis into the central circulation. Ultrasound allows safe venous puncture in coagulopathy, avoiding arterial puncture. Venous access using landmarks has a greater incidence of carotid and subclavian artery puncture and hematoma.

The subclavian vein has a 40% to 50% chance of thrombus formation with symptomatic thrombosis, requiring anticoagulation or catheter removal in at least 10% of patients. Long-term catheterization has been associated with stenosis or occlusions. Subclavian puncture has a high pneumothorax rate even if image guidance is used. In some, repeated trauma to the catheter in the thoracic outlet causes catheter fracture from pinch-off. With a serum creatinine level more than 3 mg/dL, arm veins should be preserved for ipsilateral fistula or graft placement.[5]

Postprocedural Management

Tunneled catheters should be flushed daily when not in use. Implantable ports should be flushed monthly. This may be done with several milliliters of heparin (100 U/mL). Maintaining patency and preventing infection are the main challenges.

Complications

Periprocedural complications include pneumothorax, hematoma, hemothorax, hemopericardium, arterial puncture, arrhythmia, air embolus, catheter kinking or malposition, brachial plexus injury, and contrast reaction (Fig. 101-3). Early (<30 days) complications include catheter tip migration, pericatheter thrombosis, catheter leakage, and sepsis. Late (>30 days) complications include catheter occlusion, venous thrombosis, superior vena cava syndrome, catheter-related infection, venous erosion, catheter tip migration, skin dehiscence, catheter fragmentation, and chylothorax (Fig. 101-4).

Complications of implantable ports include port migration or inversion due to a large pocket and Twiddler's syndrome, which is extravasation from catheter-port disconnection, septum failure, and needle dislodgment.[3,6,11] Implantable port infections may manifest as incision erythema without fever or exudate or as erythema with minimal exudate.

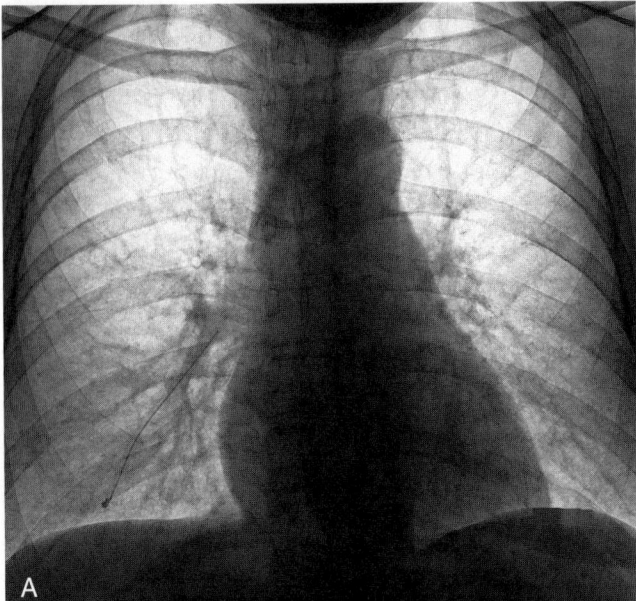

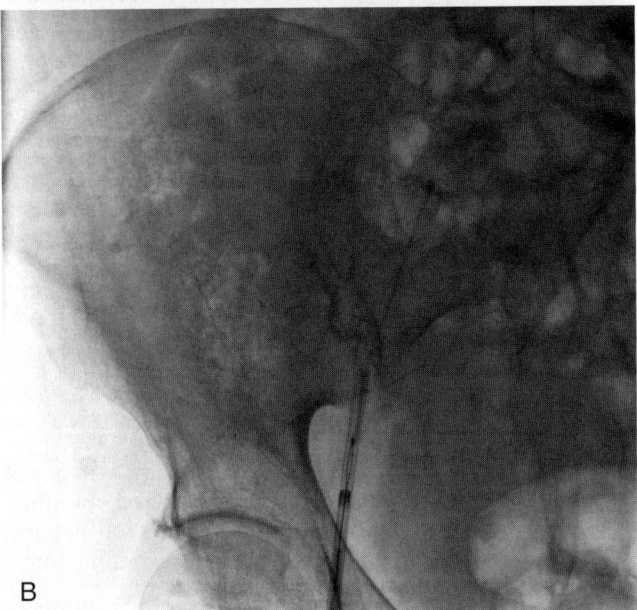

FIGURE 101-3 **A**, A 67-year-old male patient with an indwelling port for chemotherapy. During device removal, the catheter was inadvertently disconnected from the reservoir and embolized to the right lower lobe pulmonary artery. **B**, Successful transfemoral retrieval of the catheter fragment using a snare device.

Organisms most commonly identified in catheter infections are *Staphylococcus epidermidis*, *Staphylococcus aureus*, *Candida*, and *Pseudomonas* species. Catheter-related infections occur at the exit site and tunnel. Catheter-related sepsis and septic thrombus phlebitis may occur.

Repair and Device Removal

Repair kits are available for external cracks in the nondialysis catheters and the adapter kits of dialysis catheters. If repair is unsuccessful, catheter exchange is necessary.

The cuff is freed from surrounding tissues with a Kelly clamp, and the catheter is removed with progressive trac-

tion, being careful to avoid catheter breakage. Sometimes, additional fibrosis in the tunnel may need blunt dissection to free the catheter. Catheter breakage during removal often occurs at the cuff. In this case, the catheter retracts up to the tunnel. Compression should be immediately applied to prevent bleeding and embolism while preparations are made to free the catheter by high incision. Indwelling ports maybe removed in the procedure room. The catheter is isolated and clamped, the pseudocapsule around the reservoir is opened, and the port is dissected free from the pocket.[6]

VENA CAVA FILTERS

Deep vein thrombosis (DVT) with pulmonary embolism (PE) is the third leading cause of death in the United States. Between 85% and 95% of emboli arise from the iliofemoral veins. The remaining 10% to 15 % arise from the vena cava, ovarian veins, right atrium, or upper extremity thrombi. Filters do not prevent new thrombus or promote lysis of preexisting thrombus. Permanent IVC filters are not intended to be repositioned or retrieved in any manner.[12] They are reserved for patients who cannot tolerate anticoagulation, who suffer a pulmonary embolus on anticoagulation, or who have extensive thrombosis above the inguinal ligament predisposing them to significant PE despite adequate anticoagulation.

The original Greenfield filter was introduced in 1974. Percutaneous placement was first described in 1984. The filter consisted of six radiating stainless steel struts crimped and angled so the filter is cone shaped. The cone apex is directed cephalad. The rate of clinically evident recurrent PE is 4%, and the rate of caval patency is 96%. The Greenfield filter serves as the standard against which other devices are judged. Reduction in the size of introducer systems has facilitated filter delivery and has reduced procedure time and patients' blood loss. Developments in filter design and placement include retrievable devices, alternative settings, and imaging guidance for placement (Fig. 101-5).[13]

Indications

Absolute indications for vena cava filter placement include thromboembolic disease and a contraindication to anticoagulation (77%). Absolute contraindications to anticoagulation include recent stroke or neurological procedure (<2 months), recent major surgery or trauma (<2 weeks), active internal bleeding, intracranial neoplasm, recent ocular surgery, and heparin-induced thrombocytopenia. Relative contraindications for anticoagulation include recent minor trauma (<2 weeks), hematuria, occult blood in stools, peptic ulcer disease, pericarditis, bacterial endocarditis, and unstable gait.

Complications of anticoagulation occur in 5% to 60% of patients and include bleeding, heparin-induced thrombocytopenia, and warfarin-induced skin necrosis. Anticoagulation is associated with a mortality rate of up to 12%. Recurrent or progressive thromboembolic disease while adequately anticoagulated is the indication for filter placement in 3% to 27% of patients. The risk for PE with large, free-floating iliofemoral or caval thrombus is 27% to 60% despite adequate anticoagulation. This warrants place-

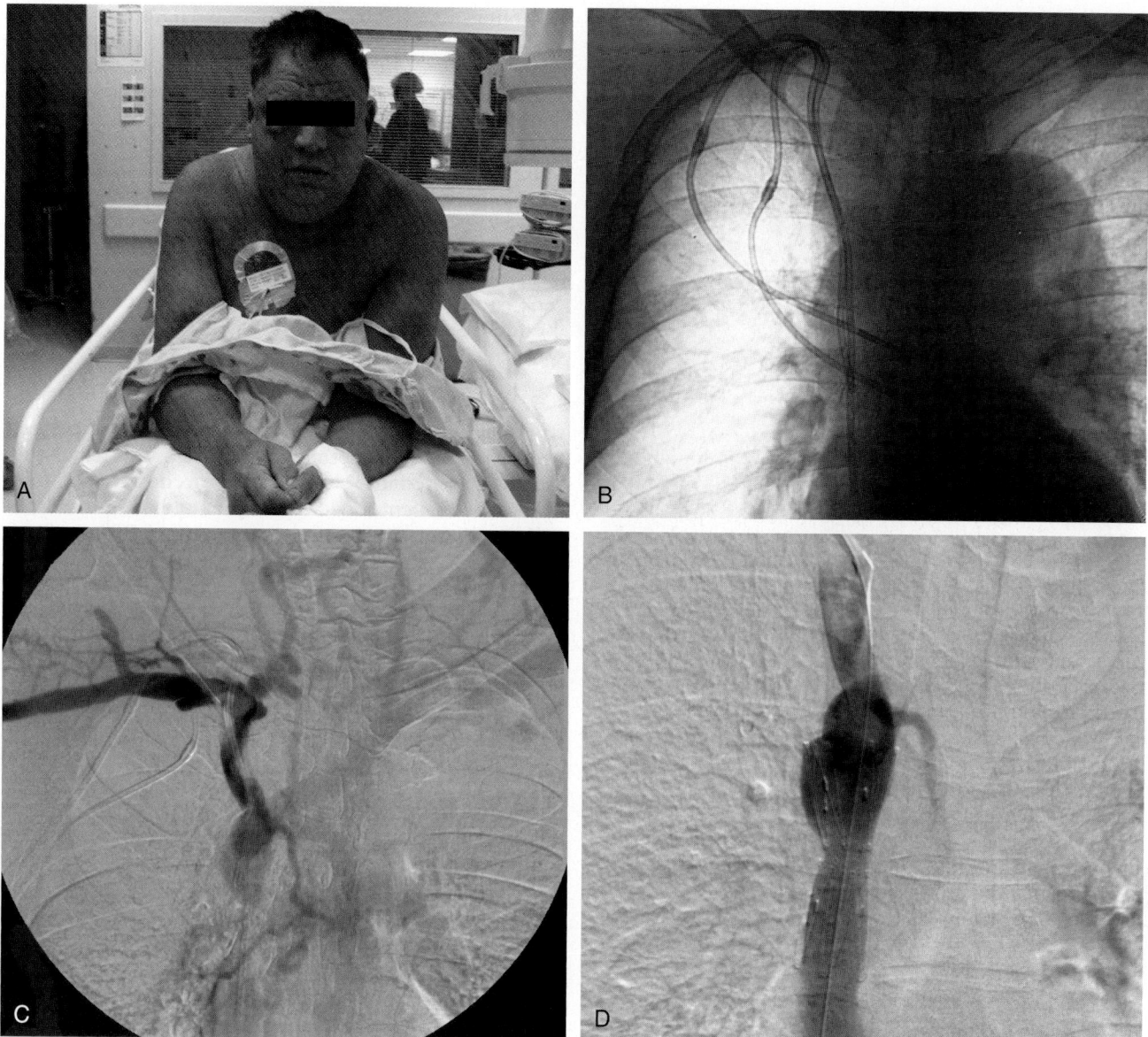

FIGURE 101-4 **A**, A 57-year-old patient with gradual swelling of the upper extremities, neck, and face. Numerous tortuous and dilated venous channels were seen over the upper chest. **B**, A long-standing tunneled catheter is seen in the right internal jugular vein. **C**, The venogram demonstrated occlusion of the superior vena cava. **D**, Successful recanalization was achieved with deployment of a Gianturco stent in the superior vena cava.

ment of an IVC filter, usually as an adjunct to anticoagulation.

Patients with relative indications for filter placement may or may not have thromboembolic disease. Prophylactic placement of a vena cava filter means placement in patients without documented thromboembolic disease but who are at significant risk, including those with poor pulmonary reserve (cardiac index <1.5 L/min/m^2), those with pulmonary or lower extremity thrombolysis or thrombectomy, surgical and trauma patients, certain orthopedic patients, and patients with malignancy. Among multitrauma patients, those at highest risk for thromboembolic disease include patients with severe brain or spinal cord injury, paraplegia or quadriplegia, long bone fracture, complex pelvic fracture, and multiple lower extremity long bone fractures.

Retrievable filters are used in many of the previously described scenarios, and indications for caval filtration can be modified and expanded in other clinical settings. Nonpermanent filters may be used when the embolism risk is time limited. This includes cases of multitrauma, temporary contraindication to anticoagulation (e.g., close to major surgery), or other situations in which indications for permanent filtration are relative (Fig. 101-6).[14,15]

Ten intracaval filter designs have been approved by the U.S. Food and Drug Administration (FDA). Filters have different sizes, designs, compositions, and introducer sizes. Filters should be assessed for rates of recurrent PE after filter placement, death from PE after filter placement, occlusion of the filter and vena cava, thrombosis of the insertion site, filter asymmetry, filter migration, potential sites of insertion, and ease of placement. An ideal vena

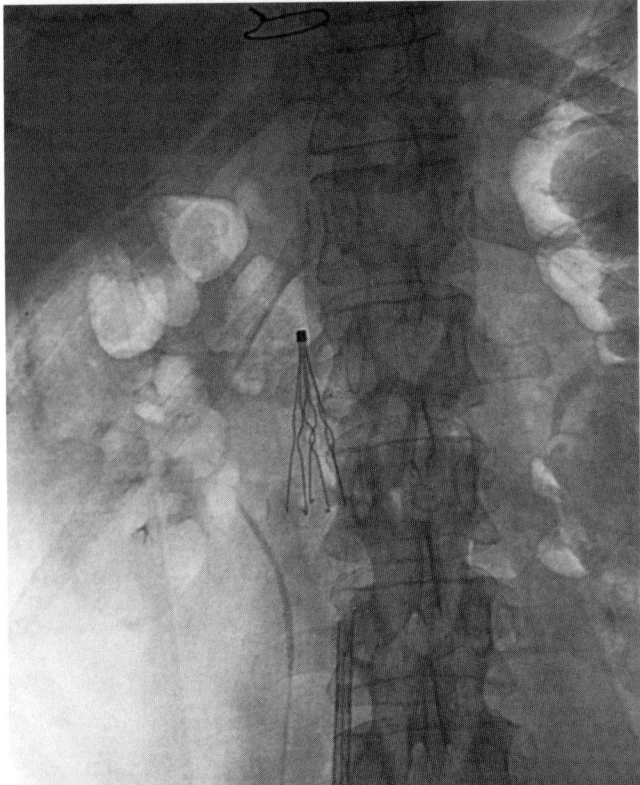

FIGURE 101-5 A Greenfield filter is identified in the infrarenal inferior vena cava of a 78-year-old man with subarachnoid hemorrhage and bilateral lower extremity deep vein thrombosis.

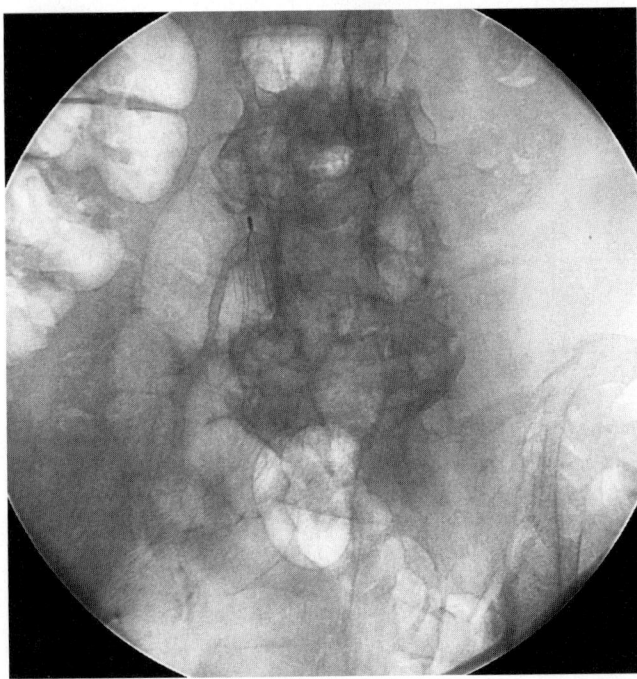

FIGURE 101-6 A retrievable filter (i.e., Bard Recovery) is seen in the infrarenal inferior vena cava.

cava filter should be biocompatible and nonthrombogenic. It should effectively filter all significant emboli, cause minimal flow disturbances, be stable in the longitudinal and transverse planes within the vena cava, and result in no injury to adjacent structures. It should be simply and safely placed, affordable, and easy retrievable.

Indications for suprarenal IVC filter placement include renal vein thrombosis, suprarenal caval thrombosis, filter placement in pregnancy, pulmonary embolism after gonadal vein thrombus, thrombosis superior to a previously placed IVC filter, and anatomic variations. Superior vena cava filters are placed for upper extremity venous thrombosis (Fig. 101-7).

Retrievable Filters

Optional filters can be retrieved or repositioned percutaneously up to a predetermined time limit, after which they are incorporated into the wall of the vena cava and function as permanent devices. They must be captured and withdrawn into the sheath to effect removal. These filters are advantageous if the clinical status may change to require a permanent device.

Absolute indications are the same as for a permanent filter when the anticipated contraindication to anticoagulation will end within the time limitations specified by the manufacturer. Relative indications include a large residual clot burden in the extremity veins, history of DVT or PE while undergoing a surgical procedure with a high risk for postoperative DVT or PE, and no DVT or PE but a high risk for thromboembolic disease.[14,15]

Filter Placement Technique

Percutaneous placement is usually achieved after access into a common femoral, internal jugular, or brachial vein. The final dilator is exchanged for a delivery sheath, which is left in the vena cava. The filter introducer system is passed through the sheath, and the filter is deployed. Imaging of the IVC is routine before filter placement to assess caval patency, anomalies, webs, or excessive narrowing of intrahepatic portions. Renal vein location must be determined to ensure proper filter position. Approximately 3% of vena cavas are oversized (>28 mm in diameter) and unsuitable for many available filters; caval diameters are measured. The gold standard for visualizing the vena cava is iodinated contrast venography performed in the angiography suite. Alternatives include carbon dioxide and gadolinium cavography. Both are safe alternatives in the critically ill, patients with renal failure, or those who have had contrast reactions.[16] Carbon dioxide cavography may underestimate caval diameter and be less sensitive for accessory renal veins. Imaging with intravascular ultrasound or duplex sonography is safe and accurate for intensive care patients who are poor candidates for hospital transport.[12,17]

Complications, Contraindications, and Follow-up

Complications include major procedural problems (<1%), access-site thromboses (2%), caval thrombus (5%), filter fracture (<1%), filter migration (<1%), filter infection

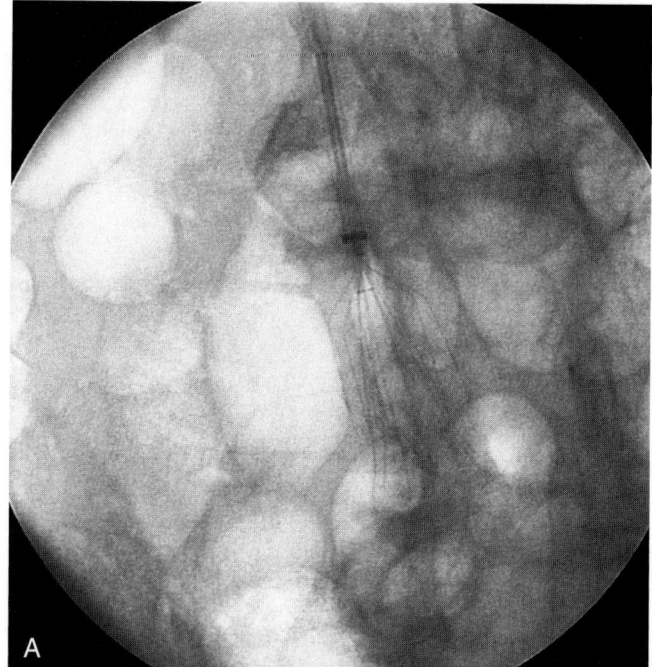

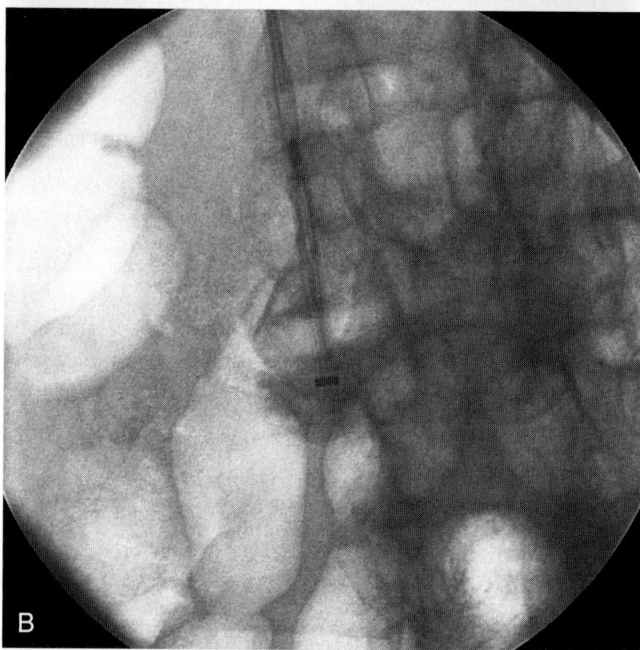

FIGURE 101-7 **A**, Retrieval of a Bard Recovery filter using a recovery cone. The cephalad aspect of the filter is engaged within the cone. **B**, The recovery sheath is advanced over the filter and then withdrawn.

TABLE 101-1	Choosing the Ideal Embolic Agent	
EMBOLIC AGENT	**SIZE**	**DURATION**
BIODEGRADABLE AGENTS		
Gelatin sponge (powder, slurry, or torpedoes)	40 μm-4 mm	2 days-6 weeks
Microfibrillar collagen	5 × 70 μm	1-8 weeks
Starch microspheres	20-70 μm	30-60 minutes
PERMANENT AGENTS		
Polyvinyl alcohol (PVA) particles	45-1180 μm	
Spherical embolics	100-1200 μm	
Spherical PVA	100-1200 μm	
Bead block	40-1200 μm	
Embospheres	40-500 μm	
Pharmaceutical embolics		
SIR-Spheres		
TheraSpheres		
Emerging agents		
Dox-Spheres		
Thermo-Spheres		
MTC-Dox spheres		
LIQUID AGENTS		
Ethanol (dehydrated)		
Iodized oil		
Glue (*n*-butyl cyanoacrylate)		
Sodium tetradecyl sulfate		
Boiling contrast		
Hypertonic glucose		

EMBOLOTHERAPY

General Principles

Highly sophisticated catheterization tools and embolic materials permit high-precision vascular occlusion.[18] Safe use of embolic materials requires understanding vascular anatomy, the disease, and the available tools to deliver the agent.

The choice of embolic agent depends on the organ, the disease, the size of the vessel to be occluded, and the goal of therapy. Large-vessel occlusion requires mechanical devices such as coils and balloons. Occlusion of higher-order branches down to the capillary level can be done with particulate or liquid embolic agents.[18]

The ideal agent is precisely sizable and nonaggregating, which avoids delivery catheter occlusion (Table 101-1). It should be transiently radiopaque to allow postprocedural and future imaging that is free of artifact and systemically nontoxic. The agent should provide reliable occlusion for the desired length of time and be nonallergenic and inexpensive. No embolic agent meets all these qualifications.[18]

Arteriographic Diagnosis and Treatment of Gastrointestinal Bleeding

Seventy-five percent of those hospitalized for gastrointestinal bleeding can be managed conservatively, with only one fourth requiring transcatheter angiography for localization and possible treatment of the bleeding vessel. Gastrointestinal bleeding may be intermittent and can originate

(<1%), and a 30-day mortality rate due to filter placement (<1%).[12]

Contraindications include total IVC thrombosis, an inability to gain IVC access, and an inability to perform imaging during filter placement. Ongoing sepsis (including septic thrombus phlebitis) is not a contraindication.

Postprocedural follow-up includes monitoring for lower extremity edema, which may indicate caval thrombus. Abdominal plain x-ray films should be obtained annually to monitor the filter position.

proximal or distal to the ligament of Treitz. The site, intermittency and rate of bleeding, and timing of the diagnostic study contribute to the potential of arteriographic diagnosis and treatment success.

The major causes of upper gastrointestinal bleeding are a Mallory-Weiss tear, peptic ulcer disease, variceal bleeds associated with portal hypertension, gastritis, neoplasia, Dieulafoy's lesion, and hemobilia.[19] Causes of lower gastrointestinal bleeding are diverticulosis, diverticulitis, angiodysplasia, colitis, colon carcinoma, inflammatory bowel disease, and polyps.[20]

Angiography can be performed on severely ill patients requiring little patient preparation or cooperation, and it may be successfully performed despite large amounts of blood in the gastrointestinal tract (Fig. 101-8). It is minimally invasive, allowing precise localization and treatment. The procedure is operator dependent and may yield false-positive results. It may be preceded by a tagged red blood cell study or a technetium 99 sulfur colloid scan when bleeding is chronic. These tests enable better patient selection for angiography and improve the diagnostic sensitivity.[18]

The angiographic appearance of bleeding may be a localized puddle of contrast material, or it may outline the source. If the lumen of the gastrointestinal tract is filled with blood clots, extravasated contrast material appears tubular like a venous structure (i.e., pseudovein sign).

Precise localization of small bowel bleeds may be delineated by injection of methylene blue by means of subselective catheterization of a superior mesenteric artery branch with a microcatheter secured at angiography, immediately before laparotomy. This may also be accomplished with intraoperative isotope scanning. Vasopressin infusion causing a sustained reduction in splanchnic blood flow may be advocated when arterial embolization is impossible or if the bleeding is diffuse.[18]

Empirical embolization may be done when there is no active contrast extravasation but endoscopy has ascertained a bleeding mucosal segment. Most commonly, the left gastric and gastroduodenal arteries are embolized empirically.

Interventional Radiology for Liver Cancer

In unresectable hepatic malignancy, whether primary HCC or metastatic disease from colorectal carcinoma, ocular melanoma, or carcinoid and islet cell tumors, systemic chemotherapy has been disappointing.[18] Chemoembolization, the simultaneous infusion of particulate and chemotherapeutic agents, has permitted higher local drug concentrations in the tumor site, increasing tumor dwell time, provoking tumor ischemia, and reducing systemic toxicity. The dual liver blood supply, relatively exclusive hepatic arterial supply of tumors, and the ease of percutaneous hepatic arterial catheterization have aided to the success of regional therapy.

The most frequent chemotherapy drugs used are doxorubicin, cisplatin, and mitomycin. These agents have high first-pass clearance, accounting for a 100-fold to 400-fold difference in liver and systemic concentrations and a high dose-response curve. The synergistic effect of polyvinyl alcohol and Lipiodol has been combined with the chemotherapeutic agent.[21]

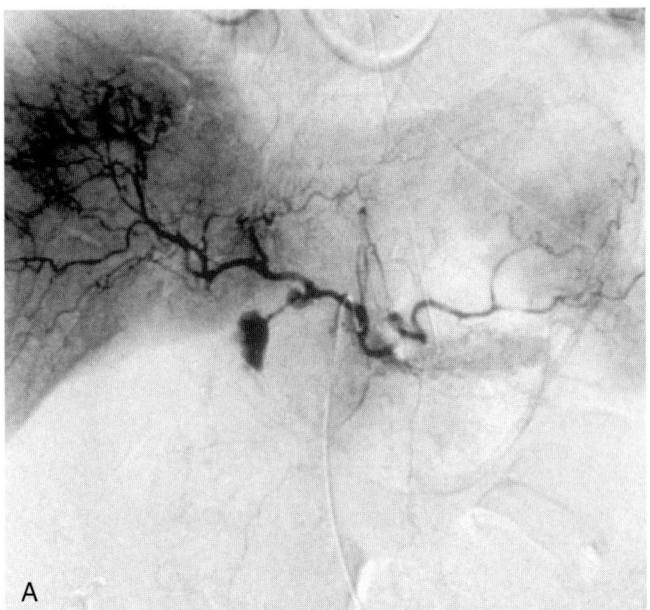

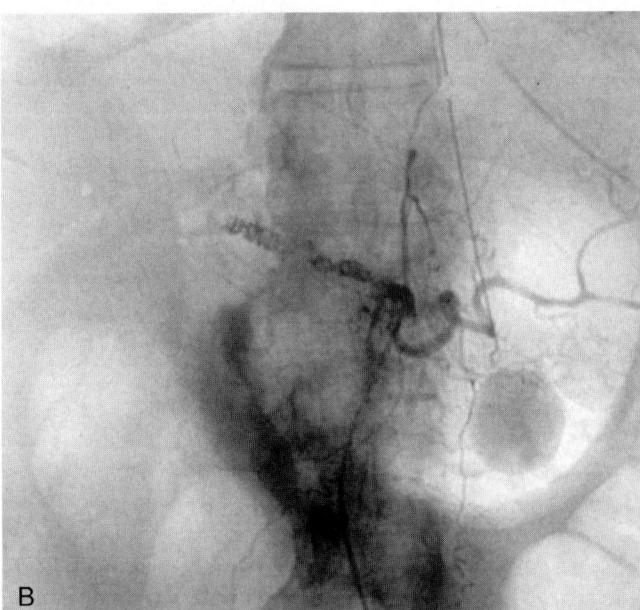

FIGURE 101-8   **A**, A 57-year-old male patient with recurrent upper gastrointestinal bleeding. Upper gastrointestinal endoscopy has demonstrated a bleeding duodenal ulcer. Active contrast extravasation is seen from the gastroduodenal artery on arteriography. **B**, Successful deployment of platinum microcoils into the bleeding vessel stops the bleeding.

Precise delineation of normal and variant hepatic arterial supply is imperative to avoid nontarget embolization. Confirmation of portal vein patency and hepatofugal flow is essential, because 39% of patients with HCC may have portal vein occlusion. If collateral flow is adequate, chemoembolization may be safely performed in patients with portal vein thrombosis. Hepatic arterial catheterization may be done with a coaxial subselective technique that uses using a 2 to 3 F microcatheter.

Common complications include postembolization syndrome, ascites, cholecystitis, intestinal ischemia, hepatic abscess, and renal failure. The results of regional chemotherapy for HCC can be evaluated by relief of symptoms, tumor shrinkage, and prolongation of survival[22] (Fig. 101-9).

Transcatheter Bronchial Artery Embolization for Hemoptysis

Severe hemoptysis most commonly occurs in patients with chronic inflammatory lung disease and in those with primary or secondary lung cancer. In patients with limited pulmonary reserve, palliative bronchial artery embolization may be better than surgical resection. In selected surgical candidates, preoperative bronchial artery embolization may reduce mortality (Table 101-2).

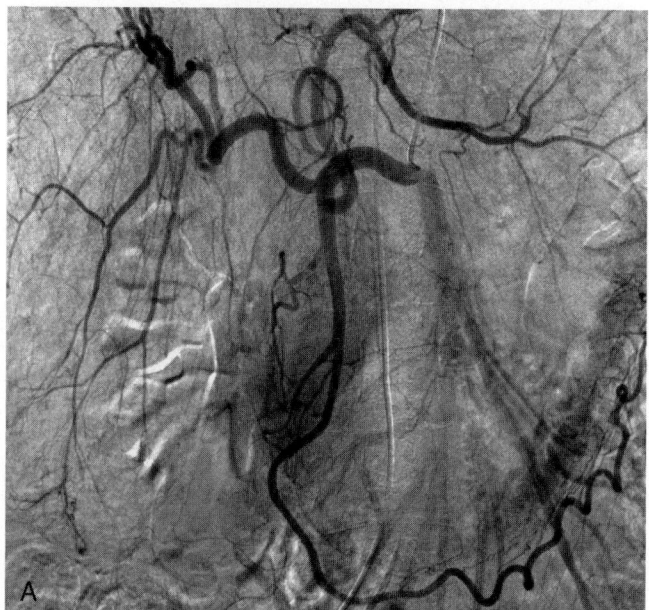

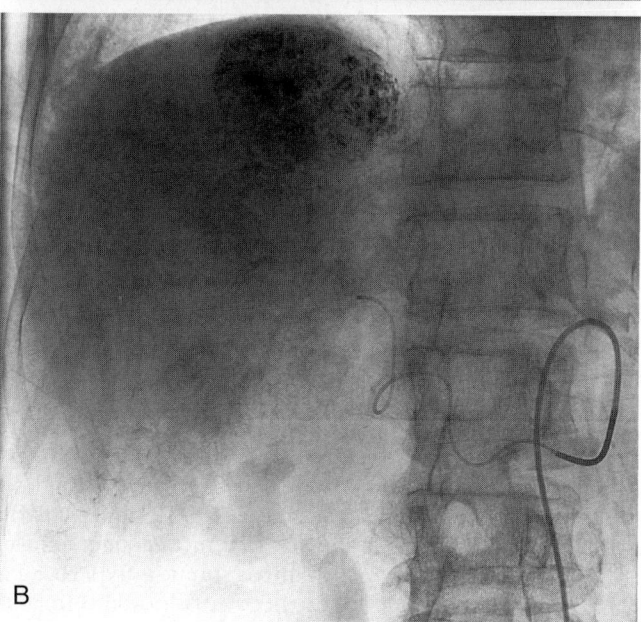

FIGURE 101-9 **A**, A 75-year-old female patient has a biopsy-proven focal mass lesion that is consistent with hepatocellular carcinoma in the right lobe of the liver. Arterial enhancement of a focal area in the right lobe of the liver suggests tumoral neovascularity. **B**, Image after successful transcatheter embolization using doxorubicin and cisplatin reconstituted with Ethiodol and polyvinyl alcohol (PVA) particles.

Variations in bronchial artery origin and extensive potential anastomotic networks between bronchial arteries and the mediastinum, spine, head, and neck should be identified, especially in cases of chronic bronchial wall inflammation. The anterior medullary branch (i.e., artery of Adamkiewicz) may arise with or receive contributions from the right intercostobronchial trunk.[23]

Cross-sectional imaging and bronchoscopy may localize the bleeding source in some patients. The goal of embolization depends on the reliability of locating a bleeding site and previous embolization procedures. Any abnormal bronchial artery supplying the site of hemorrhage should be embolized, especially the dominant bronchial artery. The most commonly used embolic agents are Gelfoam and polyvinyl alcohol particles (>250 μm in diameter to avoid neurological and tissue ischemia). Liquid embolic agents, with a potential for capillary bed occlusion and tissue infarction, should be avoided.[24]

Rates for immediate control of hemoptysis have ranged from 77% to 91%. The rate of long-term control is 70% to 80% and largely determined by progression of underlying disease process. Complications are rare but include spinal cord infarction with transverse myelitis; the latter is more common with ionic contrast media. Bronchial infarction and bronchoesophageal fistulas have been reported.[18]

Transcatheter angiography followed by embolization has been lifesaving for patients with hemoptysis from pulmonary arteriovenous malformations, premenopausal or postmenopausal bleeding from uterine leiomyomas, aortoenteric fistulas, and traumatic organ and vascular injury.[25]

TRANSJUGULAR INTRAHEPATIC PORTOSYSTEMIC SHUNT PLACEMENT

A transjugular intrahepatic portosystemic shunt (TIPS) is a percutaneously created connection within the liver between the portal and the systemic circulations. The TIPS is placed to reduce portal pressure in complications from portal hypertension. It is a less invasive alternative to surgery in end-stage liver disease. The goal is to divert portal vein flow into the hepatic vein and reduce the pressure gradient between the portal and systemic circulations. Shunt patency is maintained by an expandable metal stent across the intrahepatic tract. In experienced hands, the TIPS procedure can be successfully performed in more than 93% of patients. In addition to portal decompression to control upper gastrointestinal bleeding, TIPS may be useful for controlling ascites (Fig. 101-10).

TABLE 101-2 Hepatocellular Carcinoma: Cumulative Survival Rates with Chemoembolization

STUDY	1 YEAR	2 YEARS	3 YEARS
Nakao, 1991	88%	57%	42%
Taguchi, 1992	54%	33%	18%
Park, 1993	75%	56%	40%
Nakamura, 1994	56%	33%	18%

From Baum S, Pentecost MJ. Abrams' Angiography Interventional Radiology, 2nd ed. Philadelphia: Lippincott Williams & Wilkins, 2006. References listed in this table can be found in Chapter 27 of Baum and Pentecost.

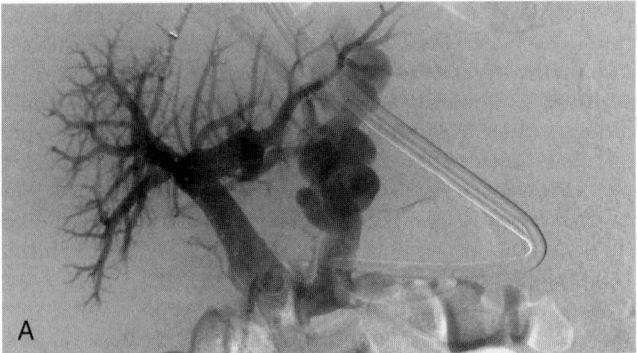

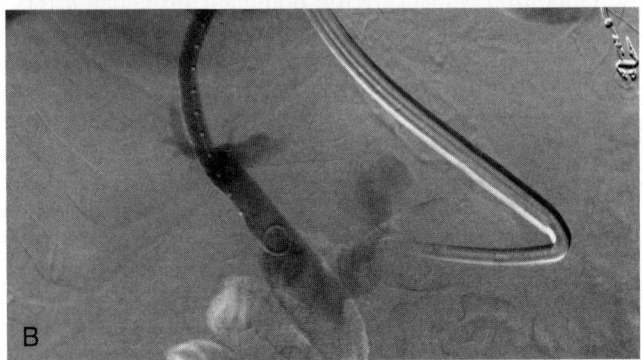

FIGURE 101-10 **A**, A 65-year-old male patient with advanced cirrhosis and recurrent upper gastrointestinal bleeding undergoing transjugular intrahepatic portosystemic shunt (TIPS). A large coronary venous varix is opacified. **B**, Successful TIPS using a 10-mm-diameter Viatorr stent-graft, resulting in diminished variceal filling.

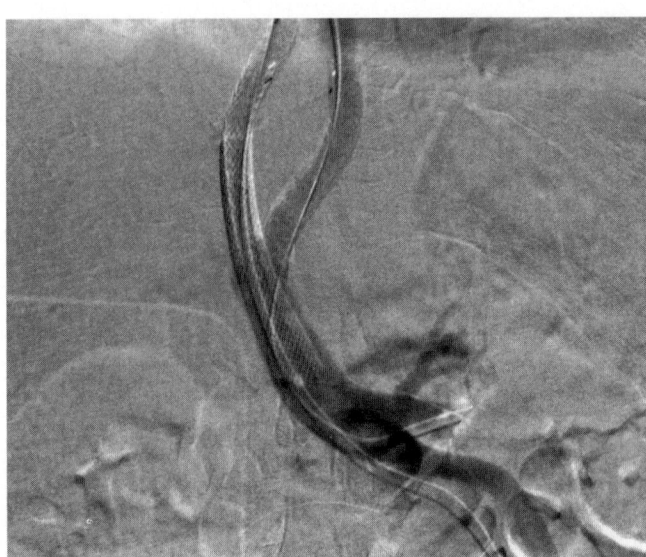

FIGURE 101-11 A 51-year-old patient with persistent symptomatic portal hypertension despite transjugular intrahepatic portosystemic shunt (TIPS) with an 8-mm graft. A second (i.e., parallel) TIPS was created with a 10-mm graft.

Indications

Recommendations for the use of TIPS are endorsed by the American Association for the Study of Liver Disease. Accepted indications include acute variceal bleeding that cannot be successfully controlled by medical treatment, including endoscopic intervention; vessel bleeding in persons intolerant or refractory to conventional medical management; ectopic variceal bleeding; refractory ascites; refractory cirrhotic hydrothorax; and Budd-Chiari syndrome.[26]

Other indications, which have not yet been confirmed, include portal hypertensive gastropathy, portal decompression in veno-occlusive disease, perihepatic renal syndrome, hepatic pulmonary syndrome, chylous fistula, thrombocytopenia, and hypersplenism.

Technique

The prototypical TIPS is created in several steps:

- Mapping a suitable hepatic vein (typically the dominant right hepatic vein)
- Passage of a long, curved needle from within the selected vein into the liver parenchyma until a suitable branch of the intrahepatic portal vein is punctured
- Passing guidewires and catheters across a liver tract into the portal system
- Mapping and performing hemodynamic assessments
- Dilating to provide a tissue bridge between the portal and hepatic veins

- Deploying the stent across this tract and enlarging it to a diameter that gives portosystemic gradient reduction to suit the specific clinical indication[27]

Contraindications

Absolute contraindications include primary prevention of variceal bleeding, congestive heart failure, multiple hepatic cysts, uncontrolled systemic infection or sepsis, unrelieved biliary obstruction, and severe pulmonary hypertension.[28]

Relative contraindications include hepatoma (especially central), obstruction of all portal veins, portal vein thrombosis, severe coagulopathy (INR > 5), thrombocytopenia (<20,000/cm³), and moderate pulmonary hypertension.

Complications

Major complications include thrombosis and stenosis (i.e., TIPS dysfunction), transcapsular rupture, hemoperitoneum, gallbladder puncture, stent malposition, hemobilia, radiation skin burn, renal failure requiring chronic dialysis, and hepatic artery injury. Minor complications include transient contrast-induced renal failure, encephalopathy (new or worse), fever, transient pulmonary edema, entrysite hematoma, and hemolysis.

Shunt insufficiency may be caused by TIPS failure. Early manifestations include stent migration, bile duct injury, slow flow from a large competitive shunt, a hypercoagulable state, intimal injury of the hepatic or portal vein, and hepatic vein stenosis. Late manifestations include pseudointimal hyperplasia and hepatic vein stenosis.

Shunt insufficiency may be managed by creation of a parallel shunt alongside the index shunt, usually from the middle or left hepatic veins to the left portal vein.[29] As the use of TIPS has increased, there has been interest in models that predict outcome. The Model for End-Stage Liver Disease (MELD) score and other models predict survival after TIPS. The modified MELD score uses serum bilirubin level, INR, and serum creatinine level. Accurate prediction of survival at 3 months and at 1 year is best determined by the MELD model.[30] The survival estimate is used to advise patients about expected outcomes and to help decide who requires referral to a liver transplantation center (Fig. 101-11).

REFERENCES

1. Hickman RO, Buckner CD, Clift RA, et al. A modified right atrial catheter for access to the venous system in marrow transplant recipients. Surg Gynecol Obstet 1979;148:871-875.
2. Funaki B. Central venous access: A primer for the diagnostic radiologist. AJR Am J Roentgenol 2002;179:309-318.
3. Baum S, Pentecost MJ. Abrams' Angiography Interventional Radiology, 2nd ed. Philadelphia: Lippincott Williams & Wilkins, 2006.
4. Jegatheeswaran A, Parmar N, Walton JM, et al. Quantitative analysis of catheter roughness induced by cutting and manipulation: A potential prothrombotic risk. Blood Coagul Fibrinolysis 2007;18531-536.
5. Sze DY, Ferral H. SIR Syllabus: Venous Interventions, 2nd ed. Society of Interventional Radiology, 2005.
6. Kandarpa K, Aruny JE. Handbook of Interventional Radiologic Procedures, 3rd ed. Philadelphia: Lippincott Williams & Wilkins, 2002.
7. Lee O, Raque JD, Lee LJ. Retrospective assessment of risk factors to predict tunneled hemodialysis catheter outcome. J Vasc Interv Radiol 2004; 15:457-461.
8. Aslam N, Lambie M, Ayub V. Use of tunneled haemodialysis catheters at the start of haemodialysis—success rates and definition of infection. Nephrol Dial Transplant 2007;22:1799-1800.
9. Dick L, Mauro MA, Jaques PF. Radiologic insertion of Hickman catheters in HIV-positive patients: Infectious complications. J Vasc Interv Radiol 1991; 3:327-329.
10. Simpson KR, Hovseian DM, Picus D. Interventional radiologic placement of chest wall ports: Results and complications in 161 consecutive placements. J Vasc Interv Radiol 1997;8:189-195.
11. Kuizon D, Colon-Otero G, Fumagalli RP. Single lumen subcutaneous ports inserted by interventional radiologists in patients undergoing chemotherapy: Incidence of infection and outcome of attempted catheter salvage. Arch Intern Med 2001;161:406-410.
12. Kandarpa K, Aruny JE. Handbook of Interventional Radiologic Procedures, 3rd ed. Philadelphia: Lippincott Williams and Wilkins, 2002.
13. Greenfeild LJ, Michana BA. Twelve-year clinical experience with the Greenfield vena caval filter. Surgery 1998;104:706-712.
14. Lorch H, Welger D, Wagner V. Current practice of temporary vena cava filter insertion: A multicenter registry. J Vasc Interv Radiol 2000;11:83-88.
15. Grande WJ, Trerotola SO, Reilly PM. Experience with the recovery filter as a retrievable inferior vena cava filter. J Vasc Interv Radiol 2005;16: 1189-1193.
16. Stoneham GW, Burbridge BE. Temporary inferior vena cava filters: In vitro comparison with permanent IVC filters. J Vasc Interv Radiol 1995;6: 731-736.
17. Kinney TB. Update on inferior vena cava filters. J Vasc Interv Radiol 2003;14:425-440.
18. Baum S, Pentecost MJ. Abrams' Angiography Interventional Radiology, 2nd ed. Philadelphia: Lippincott Williams & Wilkins, 2006.
19. Schenker MP, Duszak R, Soulen MC. Upper gastrointestinal hemorrhage and transcatheter embolotherapy: Clinical and technical factors impacting success and survival. J Vasc Interv Radiol 2001;12:1263-1271.
20. Kuo WT, Lee DE, Saad N. Superselective microcoil embolization for the treatment of lower gastrointestinal hemorrhage. J Vasc Interv Radiol 2003;14: 1503-1509.
21. Keiley JM, Rilling WS, Touzios JG. Chemoembolization in patients at high risk: Results and complications. J Vasc Interv Radiol 2006;17:47-53.
22. Ruutiainen AT, Soulen MC, Tuite CM. Chemoembolization and bland embolization of neuroendocrine tumor metastasis to the liver. J Vasc Interv Radiol 2007;18:847-855.
23. McPherson S, Routh WD, Nath H. Anomalous origin of bronchial arteries: Potential pitfall of embolotherapy for hemoptysis. J Vasc Interv Radiol 1990;1:86-88.
24. Vidal V, Therasse E, Berthiaume Y. Bronchial artery embolization in adults with cystic fibrosis: Impact on the clinical course and survival. J Vasc Interv Radiol 2006;17:953-958.
25. Mager JJ, Overtoom TCO, Blauw H. Embolotherapy of pulmonary arteriovenous malformations: Long term results in 112 patients. J Vasc Interv Radiol 2004;15:451-456.
26. Fillmore DJ, Miller FJ, Fox LF. Transjugular intrahepatic portosystemic shunt: Midterm clinical and angiographic follow-up. J Vasc Interv Radiol 1996;7:255-261.
27. Baum S, Pentecost MJ. Abrams Angiography Interventional Radiology, 2nd ed. Philadelphia: Lippincott Williams & Wilkins, 2006.
28. Ferral H, Patel NH. Selection criteria for Patients undergoing transjugular portosystemic shunt procedures: Current status. J Vasc Interv Radiol 2005; 16:49-455.
29. Redhead HA, Stanley DN, Hayes PC. The natural history of transjugular intrahepatic porto-systemic stent shunt using uncovered stents-role of host related factors. Liver Int 2006;26:572-578.
30. Montgomery A, Ferral H, Vasan R. MELD score as a predictor of early death in patients undergoing elective transjugular intrahepatic portosystemic shunt procedures. Cardiovasc Intervent Radiol 2005;28;307-312.

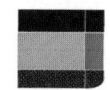

CHAPTER **102**

Durable Medical Equipment

Juliet Y. Hou, Steven I. Reger, and Vinod Sahgal

KEY POINTS

- Durable medical equipment (DME) can enhance independence and quality of life.
- The general indications of the need for DME in palliative medicine resemble those in impairments caused by other diseases.
- The goal is to find the simplest, least expensive equipment or device that best meets the individual's mobility and self-care needs. Team efforts that include the patient and caregiver for appropriate prescription, fitting, and training are important.
- Equipment needs often change as disease advances. In early stages, the equipment selection goal is to support independence; later, it is to assist the caregiver in helping the patient carry out daily activities.

Palliative care treats patients whose life expectancy is measured in months. The goal is to provide comfort, easier self-care, less family burden, and better quality of life. Important determinants of quality of life include (1) the patient's physical, cognitive, and psychological condition; (2) quality of palliative care; (3) physical environment; (4) relationships; and (5) outlook.[1] Better function and independence is clearly linked to better quality of life.

Functional decline and loss are extremely common in advanced disease, including fatigue; debility; deconditioning; motor and sensory deficits resulting from intracranial or spinal cord lesions; motor neuron disease; and cancer-, AIDS-, chemotherapy-, or radiation-induced peripheral neuropathy or myopathy. Many other factors contribute to the functional decline or loss, producing disability and handicap. The World Health Organization defines *impairment* as any loss or abnormality of physiological, psychological, or anatomical structure or function (e.g., paraplegia, pain, depression). *Disability* (activity limitation) is any restriction or lack of ability to perform an activity in the manner or within the range considered normal for a human being (e.g., self-care and ambulation dysfunction, wheelchair use). *Handicap* (participation limitation, defined by environment) reflects social barriers; it is a disadvantage for a given individual, resulting from an impairment or disability, that limits or prevents the fulfillment of a role that is normal for that individual (e.g., unable to return to previous home or work, unable to participate in leisure activities).

Durable medical equipment (DME) is designed to improve self-care and mobility, minimize primary or secondary disability or handicap, provide comfort, and preserve or restore the patient's physical function by modifying the environment and substituting for lost physical capacities. The technology may be as simple as a shoehorn or as elaborate as an environment control system operated with a mouth switch or with sound by the disabled person. A wide range of equipment is available, and new products appear every day. Information is available through vendors, insurance carriers, books, company catalogs, and the Internet. Medical providers should understand the indications, requirements, limitations, and safety precautions for commonly used equipment. Qualified physical, occupational, or speech therapists are often involved in the equipment assessment, fitting, supply, instruction, and training. The evaluation and prescription are based on physical examination, mobility and self-care skills, household activities, cognition, communication skills, and patient and family goals. Other considerations include cost, insurance coverage, and installment time. Many vendors are willing to provide equipment on temporary loan. Many private insurance carriers in the United States follow Medicare guidelines for DME reimbursement, for which patients must have deficits sufficient to impair mobility-related activities of daily living (toileting, feeding, dressing, grooming, and bathing) in the customary locations of the home. Medicare developed a nine-step qualification algorithm (Fig. 102-1) for mobility-assistive

equipment (canes, walkers, manual wheelchairs, scooters, and power wheelchairs). Keep in mind that higher technology does not guarantee higher function. Equipment needs often change as disease advances. The goal is to find the simplest, least expensive device or equipment that best meets individual mobility and self-care goals.

CLINICAL PRESENTATION AND EVALUATION

A typical sequence of equipment needs for a patient with progressive disability is described in the accompanying case study (see "Case Study: Need for Durable Medical Equipment in a Patient with Progressive Disability"). Table 102-1 lists commonly used medical equipment and clinical indications.

EQUIPMENT AND DEVICES TO ASSIST SELF-CARE

Feeding, grooming, dressing, toileting, and hygiene are basic self-care activities. These activities require a person to have a sufficient range of motion (ROM), strength, coordination, trunk control, and sitting balance. Any impairment in these abilities may cause difficulty with self-care. Adapted utensils, universal cuffs, plate guards, rocker knives, adapted cups, special handles, and straws are commonly used for self-feeding. The adapted utensil has a built-up handle to help those with weak grip hold their utensil more firmly. A bending spoon or fork shaft can accommodate persons with reduced upper-limb ROM. A universal cuff has a palm utensil, handle pocket, or cuff attached to an adjustable strap to hold various eating utensils, knives, toothbrushes, pencils, and other implements used by persons with hand weakness. An added wrist support may stabilize the wrist and prevent wrist drop during eating. Nonskid dish mats (e.g., Dycem mats) and

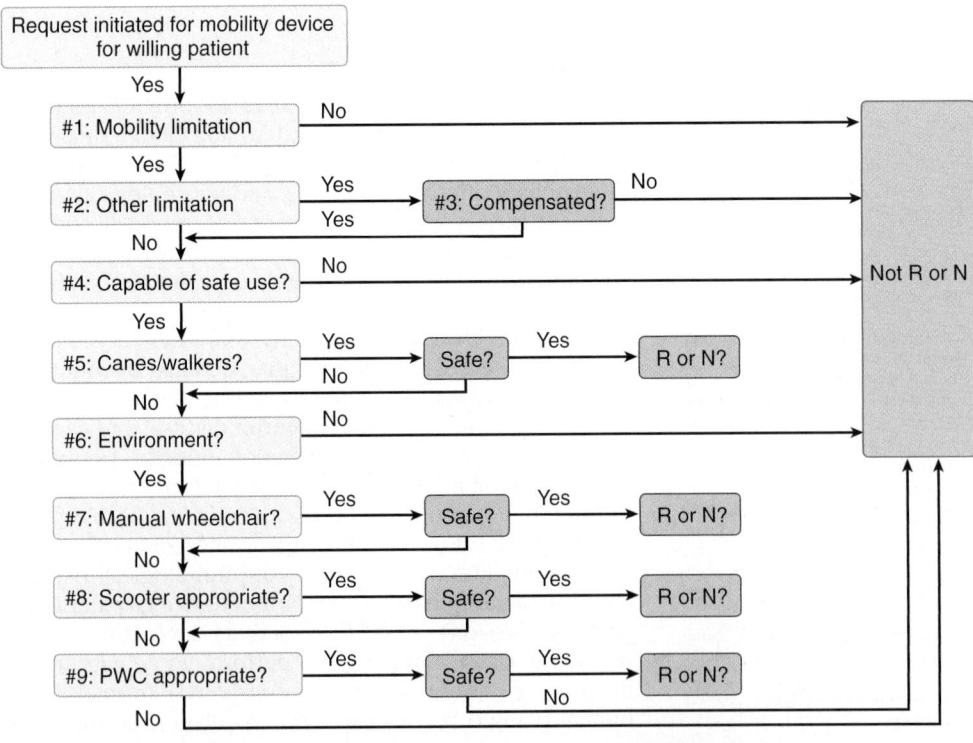

FIGURE 102-1 Clinical criteria for mobility-assistive equipment coverage. PWC, power wheelchair; R or N, rental or new.

CASE STUDY

Need for Durable Medical Equipment in a Patient with Progressive Disability

Jerry Mitchell, age 62 years, was diagnosed with amyotrophic lateral sclerosis 2 years ago. Initial weakness began in his left lower extremity. With a cane and left ankle-foot orthoses, Jerry was able to ambulate in the community without too much difficulty. When weakness spread to his right leg, he had to use crutches or a walker with a long leg brace. A power scooter helped with longer-distance travel such as for shopping, being active in the community, and saving energy to perform other daily activities. A reacher, dressing stick, sock-pulling aid, shoehorn, raised toilet seat, and shower bench assisted Jerry in self-care. Grab bars in the bathroom and a wheelchair ramp to his front door were installed.

When weakness and spasticity affected Jerry's trunk and upper extremity, caused hand/ankle deformity, and produced difficulty in self-care and ambulation, Jerry required balanced forearm orthoses attached to his wheelchair, utensil cuffs/adaptation for feeding and writing, a resting hand splint to prevent hand flexion contracture, and an ankle-foot splint to prevent foot drop contracture and heel pressure sores. An electric hospital bed, transfer board, and leg lifter helped Jerry's bed and transfer mobility. Because of difficulties transferring in and out of the power scooter and poor sitting balance, the power scooter was deemed to be inconvenient and less safe, and a power wheelchair with hand controller and proper seat cushion was supplied.

Over the next several months, Jerry's condition further declined. He went on a ventilator to support his breathing, and he depended on his wife to help with most of his daily living activities. With a Hoyer lift, his wife was able to transfer Jerry to different surfaces without injury to herself. Jerry was able to move indoors and outdoors and to perform pressure relief independently with a hand-controlled power reclining wheelchair, which promoted a positive self-image.

weighted utensils and cups are useful for those with poor coordination and hand control (tremor).

Electric shavers, electric toothbrushes, adapted brushes and combs, wash mitts, and a suction denture brush add convenience to grooming and hygiene. Reachers, button aids, zipper pulls, long-handled shoehorns, elastic shoelaces, and stocking- or sock-pulling aids assist self-dressing.

Upper limb orthoses assist functional movement, reduce pain, and prevent deformity. Static wrist-hand orthoses are commonly used to rest an injured hand, reduce pain, prevent contracture, or stretch an existing contracture. In profound upper limb weakness (e.g., C5 or some C4 spinal cord injuries), functional hand use can be achieved by combining balanced forearm orthoses and hand orthoses with a utensil attachment. The balanced forearm orthosis can be mounted on a wheelchair, table, or working surface. It consists of a forearm trough, a pivot joint, and a linkage system to support the upper limb against gravity. Patients can move the elbow and shoulder with small motions of the trunk or shoulder girdle. In the presence of hand and wrist weakness or pain, adapted

TABLE 102-1 Commonly Used Medical Equipment and Clinical Indications

TYPE OF EQUIPMENT	CLINICAL PRESENTATION
SELF-CARE/ORTHOSES	
Balanced forearm orthoses	Profound UE weakness
Long opponens splint	Wrist and hand weakness
Utensil cuff/adaptation	Hand weakness
Short opponens splint	Thumb weakness/pain or collateral ligament injury
Resting hand splint	Wrist /hand pain, spasticity, or contracture
Reacher, leg lifter, sock aide, shoehorn	LE weakness, back or hip or knee surgery
Commode chair, raised toilet seat	Paraplegia, hemiplegia, hip or knee surgery, general weakness
Rolling shower chair	Quadriplegia, general severe weakness
Electric leg-bag opener	High quadriplegia, general severe weakness
MOBILITY/FUNCTIONAL RESTORATION	
Cane	LE weakness or pain, mild weight bearing, unsteady gait
Crutch	More stable and weight bearing than cane
Walker	Most stable; LE weakness, fracture, surgery, poor balance
Platform walker	Distal UE fracture/deformity, grip weakness, elbow contracture
Hemi-walker	Hemiplegia
Manual wheelchair	Difficulty with ambulation or distance walking
Self-propelled	Must have sufficient UE strength and grip
Attendant-propelled	Poor cognition or unable to self-propel; institutional use
Pushrim-activated power-assist wheelchair	Risk of UE injury with self-propelling
Power scooter	Poor endurance (severe respiratory disorder), UE weakness or pain
Power wheelchair	General weakness, UE pain; must have sufficient cognition
Power recline or tilt-in-space wheelchair	General weakness with weight shift dependency
Transfer board	Stroke, spinal cord injury, LE amputations, non–weight bearing in both LE
Transfer lift device	Significant UE and LE weakness, transfer dependency
Hand controls for automobile	Paraplegia, hemiplegia
Hospital bed	Weakness, respiratory disorder, LE edema, traction
Van with lift	Power wheelchair user
AFO	Ankle weakness, spasticity
KAFO	Knee and ankle weakness
AFO with heel suspension	Risk of heel ulcer, foot drop contracture, or hip rotation contracture
Stair glide	Unable to climb stairs
Grab bar	Poor balance, general weakness
Wheelchair ramp	Wheelchair user

AFO, ankle-foot orthoses; KAFO, knee-ankle-foot orthoses; LE, lower extremity; UE, upper extremity.

hand or wrist-hand orthoses are often used to hold objects or stabilize joints.

BATH AND TOILET AIDS

Bathing and toileting require transfer on and off the toilet, getting in and out of the bathtub or shower, sitting, standing, clothing management, and hygiene. It can be challenging for those with impairments in sitting or standing balance, upper limb strength, coordination, or ROM. More accidents, such as slips and falls, occur in the bathroom than any other room. Grab bars placed at toileting and bathing areas or clamp-on tub rails that fit onto the tub wall, along with a nonskid safety mat inside the tub, help avoid dangerous falls.

Bathtub transfer benches or tub transfer boards allow patients to sit and scoot over to the tub instead of stepping over. The benches have a plastic seat with drainage holes, an aluminum frame with height-adjustable legs, a back support, and a handle on the left or right side. Tub and shower chairs are usually height adjustable and are placed inside the tub to allow sitting while bathing. The Versabath Seat smoothly rotates the seat 90 degrees in either direction, which helps the user get in and out of the shower safely and easily and reduces caregiver demands. For persons with limited reach or grasp, a bath mitt, a long-handled sponge, and shampoo or liquid soap pump dispensers are convenient. Bathing can be carried out with the use of a wheelchair commode or rolling shower chair (if a roll-in shower is available) or an inflatable bedbath tray in severe disability.

An aluminum height-adjustable toilet safety rail helps with occasional balance problems and can be attached to a standard toilet easily. Raised toilet seats with or without arm support add 2.5 to 4 inches to the existing toilet height, making toilet transfers easier. A bedside commode or 3-in-1 commode chair (with arm support, placed over the toilet or bedside) are height adjustable and suitable for people who have difficulty reaching the bathroom. With higher cost, an Uplift Commode Assist provides 8 to 9 inches of uplift to assist a patient in rising from the seat. This device may be used as a bedside commode or over the toilet. Bidets and urinals are often used for bedridden patients. Suppository inserters or digital stimulators provide assistance for those with hand weakness (e.g., late-stage amyotrophic lateral sclerosis [ALS], multiple sclerosis [MS]). For quadriplegics who use catheter and leg bags, helpful items include catheter inserters, various manual or electronic bag openers, and leg-bag strapping.

BED MOBILITY AND POSITIONING

Special beds and mattresses are used to prevent pressure ulcers and to assist with bed positioning and mobility. Bed mobility involves rolling from side to side, changing from supine to sitting position, and moving up and down. Patients may depend on caregivers and are highly susceptible to pressure ulcers if they have severe upper extremity weakness. Special beds are also indicated if the patient requires the head of the bed to be elevated more than 30 degrees due to congestive heart failure, chronic pulmonary disease, or aspiration; elevation of the lower extremi-

ties to reduce edema; or connection of attachments (e.g., traction), impossible with an ordinary bed.

The basic features in a hospital bed are the headboard, footboard, side rails, locking and unlocking casters, and a spring frame or metal panel to support the mattress. Adjustable components include bed height, from 20 inches in the low to 30 inches in the high position; upper body position, from supine to sitting or to a reverse Trendelenburg position; and lower extremity elevation, with or without knee flexion. Semielectronic beds combine motorized positioning of the upper body and knees with the economy of manual height adjustment. Full-electronic beds adjust upper body, knee position, and bed height all through pendant control and provide the greatest convenience for the patient and caregiver. Manual beds offer the same convenient features as electronic models but adjust manually for lower cost.

With hospital bed side rails and upper body elevation, patients can often perform bed mobility that would be difficult in a regular bed. Adjusting the bed height to match the wheelchair or commode chair height makes transfer in and out bed easier. Overhead trapeze units provide additional assistance for transfer and bed mobility for those who have lower extremity weakness but good upper extremity strength.

Serious injuries related to hospital bed use, such as injuries caused by falling out of bed or becoming caught or entrapped by the bed rail, mattress, or bed frame, have been reported.[2] Specially designed low beds without side rails feature bed height adjustment from 9.5 to 20 inches to prevent or minimize injuries caused by falling out of bed. Newer beds without large gaps, devices to close gaps, bedside floor mats, and see-through bedside bolsters serve the same purpose for those with severe cognitive impairment.

If immobility of the spine is required, a manual or power rotating bed frame that turns may be used to prevent pressure ulcers without compromising spine stability. Fracture frame and traction accessories can be added. Standing beds may be controlled manually or electronically to elevate the patient upright, which is thought to help in reducing osteoporosis and renal calculi, maintaining vascular tone, preserving a positive self-image, and providing pressure relief for some with severe weakness. Binders and elastic bandages to wrap the legs, blood pressure checking at frequent intervals, and incremental increases in the upright degrees are recommended in initial training to prevent postural hypotension.

Other devices, such as heel-suspension ankle-foot orthoses are useful for heel protection and to prevent ankle plantar flexion and hip rotation contracture. Foot waffles to prevent heel ulcers are controversial. Limited studies suggest a possible increased risk for heel ulcers with foot waffles.[3] The best heel pressure relief product has not been identified. Keeping the heels off the bed with pillows is the best-documented approach.

PRESSURE-RELIEVING BEDS AND MATTRESSES

There are many biomechanical and pathophysiological factors that contribute to pressure ulcers. External pressure has been the most frequently discussed stress factor. Other primary stress factors are shear, friction, and resulting deformation of the soft tissues. The secondary or environmental factors that are important in bed immobility are temperature, moisture, duration of the applied load, atrophy, and posture. These factors influence tissue quality by reducing the strength and the stiffness of soft tissues and increasing the coefficient of skin friction.

Various support surfaces are available for treating and preventing pressure ulcers. These either mold around the shape of the patient to distribute the patient's weight over a large area (constant low-pressure devices, or CLPs) or mechanically vary the pressure beneath the patient to reduce the duration of the pressure (alternating-pressure devices, or APs). CLP construction is usually foam, air, gel, profile foam, hammock, air suspension, water suspension, or air-particulate suspension. AP devices are air-filled cells that sequentially inflate and deflate to relieve pressure at various anatomical sites. Table 102-2[4] categorizes support surfaces according to their performance in counteracting the forces that contribute to pressure ulcers.[4] The algorithm shown in Bergstrom and colleagues guides selection of a specific support surface according to clinical condition, from low- to high-risk pressure ulcer prevention to various stages of pressure ulcer treatment.[4]

Studies[3] have shown that some high-specification foam mattresses are more effective than standard hospital foam mattresses for prevention of pressure ulcers in moderate-to high-risk patients. The relative merits of higher-tech AP and CLP support surfaces for ulcer prevention are unclear. Limited evidence suggests that low-air-loss beds reduce pressure sores in intensive care. Good evidence suggests that air-fluidized beds and low-air-loss beds are effective in pressure ulcer treatment and healing. It is difficult to choose the most effective mattress from among the available products.

TRANSFER AIDS

Transfers to the chair, bed, commode, tub, and car are essential for independent daily living.[5,6] The unassisted standing transfer requires ability to maintain the hip and knee in extension, plus sufficient shoulder depressors, adductors, elbow extensors, and hand and wrist function,

at least on one side. A long leg brace or extensor spasticity helps maintain extension if profound lower limb weakness is present. Installing grab bars, using a raised toilet seat, and adjusting the bed height to the level of the wheelchair help with wheelchair transfers.

For those who have significant weakness but are able to perform assisted standing transfer, a transfer belt provides waist support and ensures that the caregiver has a good grip on the patient without restricting the patient from using her arms. Sliding board transfer is indicated for persons who cannot stand but have sufficient upper limb strength to push and slide the buttocks and bridge the gap between two surfaces, such as paraplegics and quadriplegics (lesions at C7 or below).

In cases of extensive weakness, those who require maximum assistance of one or more persons (transfer dependent) benefit from the use of a lifter to move from one surface to another. Various electrical, hydraulic, and mechanical lift systems are effective. A properly trained small woman using these devices can lift and transfer a man more than twice her size. The mechanical and hydraulic lifts can take the form of a movable frame or a free-standing frame that hangs over the bed or on a moving track attached to the ceiling. A manual lift provides low cost and safe transfer from any position. An electrical lift makes transfer easier at higher cost. Emergency buttons allow the lifter to be switched to manual if necessary. A heavy-duty power lift features a larger weight capacity (beyond the 400-lb capacity of a regular lift).

Stair lift seats or stair glides and other, newer patient transport technologies assist in stairs transfer in those with severe weakness (e.g., late-stage Parkinson's disease, brain tumor resulting in hemiplegia, MS).

AMBULATION AIDS

Gait aids[7-9] such as canes, crutches, and walkers are most helpful for patients with unstable gait, for those whose lower limb muscles are weaker or who require decreased weight bearing on one or both legs, and for alleviating pain caused by lower limb injury, fracture, or arthritis. Ambulation aids are considered to be an extension of the upper limb. Therefore, sufficient upper extremity strength, coor-

TABLE 102-2 Support Surfaces and Characteristics						
PERFORMANCE CHARACTERISTICS	**Support Device**					
	AIR-FLUIDIZED	**LOW-AIR-LOSS**	**ALTERNATING AIR PRESSURE**	**STATIC FLOTATION, AIR OR WATER**	**FOAM**	**STANDARD MATTRESS**
↑ Support area	Yes	Yes	Yes	Yes	Yes	No
Low moisture retention	Yes	Yes	No	No	No	No
↓ Heat accumulation	Yes	Yes	No	No	No	No
Shear reduction	Yes	Yes	Yes	Yes	No	No
Pressure reduction	Yes	Yes	Yes	Yes	Yes	No
Dynamic	Yes	Yes	Yes	No	No	No
Cost per day	High	High	Moderate	Low	Low	Low
Approximate weight limit (lb)	500	400	250	No limit	400	400
Mattress type	PR	PR	POL	NPOL	NPOL	NPR

NPOL, nonpowered overlay; NPR, nonpowered replacement; POL, powered overlay; PR, powered replacement.
From Bergstrom N, Allman, RM, Alvarez, OM, et al. Treatment of Pressure Ulcers. Clinical Practice Guideline No. 15. (AHCPR Publication No. 95-0652). Rockville, MD: U.S. Department of Health and Human Services, Public Health Service, Agency for Health Care Policy and Research, 1994.

dination, and cognition are needed to master their use. The patient should be properly trained. Usually, canes are prescribed for mild to moderate impairments, and walkers for generalized weakness, minimal or no weight bearing in the lower limb, debilitating condition, or poor balance.

Although ambulation aids are safe and effective, problems can occur. Chronic walker use may cause poor posture. The repetitive forces or stress from chronic cane or walker use contributes to upper extremity tendinitis, osteoarthritis, and carpal tunnel syndrome. The relation between mobility aid use and risk of falls is less clear. Use of a mobility aid may indicate balance impairment, functional decline, or risk of falling, but some have argued that these devices may increase this risk of falls by causing tripping or disrupting balance control through other mechanisms.

Canes reduce the vertical ground reaction force on the supporting leg during standing and walking, especially in the contralateral hip abductor muscles. The cane may unload up to 20% of body weight off the affected leg when used properly. The cane should be held in the hand contralateral to the lower limb with weakness or pain, and it should be advanced with the affected limb in a three-point gait pattern. Stairs are usually ascended with the stronger lower limb first, followed by the cane and the affected limb. The affected lower limb and cane proceed down first during stair descent. Cane length is measured, with the patient standing, from the bottom of the shoe's heel to the upper border of the great trochanter. The elbow should be flexed at 20 to 30 degrees, a desirable elbow position for all ambulation aids.

Canes are made of wood or aluminum. Aluminum canes have notches and can be adjusted to fit most body heights. Standard canes can be used by patients with vestibular dysfunction, visual impairment, or sensory ataxia, because there is little or no limitation on upper extremity weight bearing. Offset canes allow weight bearing through the shaft for those with painful gait disorders. The three-or four-legged canes (quad canes) provide additional stability and weight bearing. They can stand alone, freeing the arm so that the patient can use it to assist in rising from a chair.

The disadvantages are a heavier weight than single-point canes and possibly a slower gait.

Crutches are more stable than canes because there are two points of contact with the body; they usually are prescribed for patients with greater clinical deficits than canes can assist with. Good ROM and upper limb strength are important. When used properly, a single crutch can relieve up to 50% of body weight off a lower limb. Bilateral crutches can provide 100% weight-bearing relief to a lower limb.

Axillary, Lofstrand, and platform crutches are available for various indications. Among them, the axillary crutch, which has an axillary bar and a hand grip, is most commonly prescribed. With two axillary crutches, patients can transfer 100% of body weight to the arms using swing gait. Crutch palsy, a compressive radial neuropathy reported with axillary crutch use, is rare. Prolonged body resting on the crutches and use of heavy padding on the axillary area should be avoided to reduce this risk. Forearm or Lofstrand crutches contain a forearm cuff and hand piece and are for patients who have compression neuropathy related to axillary crutch use; pressure in the axilla is avoided, and hand freedom for activity is provided. Compared with axillary crutches, forearm crutches provide less trunk support and require greater skills and trunk balance. A platform crutch has a horizontal trough and a vertical grip handle. Patients can rest their forearm and wrist on the trough. They are most appropriate for persons with coexisting arthritis or fracture of the elbow, wrist, or hand; weakness of triceps or grasp; or elbow contracture (Fig. 102-2).

Walkers provide a wider base of support and safer gait than canes and crutches. They allow up to total weight bearing off the affected lower limb when used properly. Good grasp and arm strength are essential. They are particularly useful for patients with poor balance, coordination, or lower limb strength. Slow gait, difficult maneuvering through doorways and congested areas, and poor posture are some disadvantages. The standard walker is rigid, made of aluminum, and adjustable in height. Foldable models are less durable but easier to transport. When folded, they may provide some assistance with stairs. Front-wheeled walkers

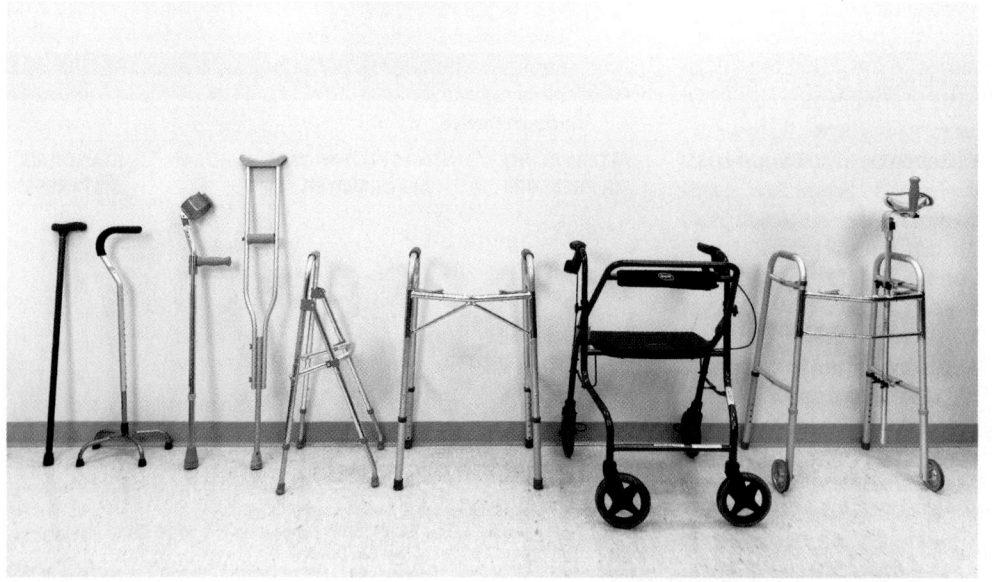

FIGURE 102-2 Compared with axillary crutches, forearm crutches provide less trunk support and require greater skills and trunk balance. A platform crutch has a horizontal trough and a vertical grip handle. Patients can rest their forearm and wrist on the trough. Platform crutches are most appropriate for persons with coexisting arthritis or fracture of the elbow, wrist, or hand; weakness of triceps or grasp; or elbow contracture.

are preferred for patients who have difficulty lifting and advancing the standard walker due to insufficient upper limb coordination or strength, severe Parkinson's disease, or moderate ataxia. They permit a smoother gait than the standard walker but provide decreased stability. Four-wheeled walkers are best used for persons with higher-functioning gait disorders who can walk longer distances with minimal weight-bearing restriction. They may be modified to provide sturdier construction, larger wheels, hand-braking systems, and seats. However, added wheels may introduce instability and danger. If the patient puts his full body weight on the four-wheeled walker, it can roll away and cause a fall. A hemi-walker provides more lateral support than a quad cane and is used in hemiplegia. Platform walkers allow weight bearing at the elbow, bypassing the hand, wrist, and part of the forearm, and are used for those with grip weakness, elbow or wrist deformities, and distal upper limb fractures.

LOWER EXTREMITY ORTHOSES

Lower extremity orthoses are not considered ambulation aids, but they provide pain reduction, joint protection, functional positioning of the joint, and supplementation of weak muscles. Many types of lower limb orthoses are available, ranging from arch supports or metatarsal pads sold over the counter to highly customized hip-knee-ankle-foot orthoses. Ankle-foot orthoses (AFOs) are the most frequently prescribed lower limb orthoses. They are usually made of plastic and/or metal. See Table 102-3 for clinical indications for AFOs. Plastic AFOs are more commonly used than the traditional metal AFOs because of their lightweight, cosmetic appearance, less cost, and interchangeability among shoes. Metal AFOs are still used for patients with fluctuating or excessive edema or insensate limb, for older patients after chronic wear, and for obese patients.

Knee-ankle-foot orthoses (KAFOs) represent the extension of plastic or metal AFOs. They have additional knee joint and thigh components, providing knee and ankle joint stability during ambulation. KAFOs may be used bilaterally or unilaterally for severe quadriceps and hamstring weakness, severe spasticity, and structural knee instability. KAFOs are often used for short-distance ambulation to complement wheelchair mobility, and they are always used in conjunction with walker or crutches during ambulation. Good trunk control and upper limb strength are therefore required. Knee orthoses may be indicated for quadriceps weakness, to prevent genu recurvatum, and to provide stability and knee immobilization after knee injuries and surgeries.

WHEELCHAIR MOBILITY

Wheelchairs offer great functional independence at home and in the community for people who are unable to walk or who can ambulate only for short distances.[5,6,10] Other goals are to maximize pulmonary function and prevent postural deformities, pain, and pressure ulcers. The home environment should be assessed before a wheelchair is prescribed. A ramp can be built or purchased to allow wheelchair access. The Americans with Disabilities Act, Titles II and III, covers access to public facilities and trans-

TABLE 102-3 Clinical Indications and Characteristics of Ankle-Foot Orthoses (AFOs)

INDICATION	CHARACTERISTICS
Over-the-counter or off-the-shelf AFO	Used on a trial basis
Foot drop	Posterior leaf spring or plastic, solid, flexible, set at 90 degrees, or double metal upright with Klenzak joint
Weak plantar flexion	Dorsiflexion stop, sole plate extends to metatarsal head
Dorsiflexion and plantar flexion weakness	Solid AFO or double metal upright with dorsiflexion and plantar flexion stop
Reduced weight bearing	Patella tendon–bearing AFO, prefabricated bivalve or custom made. Up to 50% weight-bearing reduction in affected limb. Carbon graphite inserts and rocker-bottom shoe further reduce weight bearing. Useful in tibia fracture, diabetic plantar ulcer, ankle fusion, ankle or foot avascular necrosis, and painful heel.
Ankle plantar spasticity	Solid rigid AFO or hinged with plantar flexion stop
Weak quadriceps and foot drop	Solid AFO with a few degrees of plantar flexion
Ankle instability or deformity	Solid AFO with more anterior trim line, double metal upright AFO with T-straps
Ankle pain with motion	Solid AFO

portation. These guidelines suggest that door width should be greater than 32 inches; hallways and ramps should be 36 inches or wider, and ramps should have at least 12 inches of run for each inch of rise.

Manual wheelchairs and power wheelchairs including seating systems have developed rapidly. Many styles and designs accommodate the user's mobility demands. Because of the complexity of wheelchairs, seating systems, and the requirements of various diseases and patient conditions, a team approach is important when prescribing a wheelchair, especially a power chair. The patient, family/caregivers, physician, physical therapist, occupational therapist, and sometimes the vendor are part of the team. The type of wheelchair prescribed depends on the mobility goals, method of transportation, physical and mental capabilities, home and community environment, and available funding. Rental wheelchairs for temporary use are available through most vendors.

Manual wheelchairs can be designed for attendant propulsion and self-propulsion. Individuals with paraplegia and low tetraplegia (C8 or lower level) are often capable of using manual wheelchairs efficiently. Self-propelling is a type of physical exercise to the users. However, it can cause upper limb injury and pain. Compared with power wheelchairs, manual wheelchairs are easier to transport because of their lighter weight, foldability, and low maintenance. Power wheelchairs can travel longer distances at faster speeds without user fatigue, and they preclude the upper limb repetitive injuries commonly seen in users of self-propelling manual wheelchairs. Depot or institutional wheelchairs are attendant-propelled, are inexpensive, and can accommodate variable body sizes. They are used for transportation in institutions such as hospitals, airports, and nursing facilities. They are not designed for comfort or self-propelling. For patients with severe physical or mental disability and those who are unable to propel or control a power wheelchair, a tilt-in-space attendant-propelled wheelchair is more comfortable and provides pressure relief when tilted back.

To propel a manual wheelchair, a person must have sufficient strength in bilateral upper extremities or at least one upper extremity. There are many types of self-propelling wheelchairs appropriate for various purposes. Lighter-weight wheelchairs are preferred for individuals who will propel the wheelchair for primary mobility. They are more comfortable and are easier to propel and maneuver over various surfaces such as grass, carpet, and curbs. A pushrim-activated power-assist wheelchair (PAPAW) system combines human and electric power. Human control is delivered by the arms via the pushrims, and electric power by a battery through two electric motors, providing the powered torque for mobility. The PAPAW provides intuitive control and may reduce strain or stress injuries to the upper extremities, a common secondary disabling condition among manual wheelchair users.

A hemi-wheelchair may be an option for those patients with hemiparesis caused by brain tumor, stroke, or other neurological conditions. The footrests are removed, and the seat height is lowered to allow the good arm and leg to propel and steer the chair. When the hemi-chair is used by lower limb amputees (i.e., above-the-knee or higher level), the rear axle is moved more posteriorly, to compensate for the user's more rearward center of gravity, caused by the absence of a leg. Anti-tippers are sometimes added for the same purpose.

Standing frames can be added to power or manual chairs to provide stand-up function. They allow patients to stand within the frame passively. The stand-up position provides pressure relief and weight-bearing benefits on the bone, extends body height to perform more jobs, and improves psychological outlook and bowel and bladder function. Their added cost, weight, width, and complexity may limit their use.

POWER WHEELCHAIRS

Power wheelchairs (PWC) are indicated for individuals with limited upper and lower extremity function as sequelae of brain or spinal cord lesions, neuropathy, myopathy, and other causes. They are important in restoring mobility, performing pressure relief, and minimizing social isolation and caregiver burden. To operate a PWC safely, the patient must have adequate cognitive and visual function and adequate hand or head or foot movement to operate the controls. There are many control devices to meet the needs of various motor deficits. Hand-controlled joysticks are most common. Head- or foot-operated joysticks are alternatives. For high-level quadriplegic individuals, breathing controlled sip-and-puff devices are common. Newer technologies, such as head-array sensors or chin-controlled microproportional joysticks, are available. Voice- or brain signal–activated controls are exciting developments and may be available soon.

Prevention of pressure ulcers is important in advanced disease to maintain good quality of life. Persons with good strength in their upper extremities can carry out regular weight-shifting and pressure-relief maneuvers while sitting in the wheelchair. For patients with weak upper limbs who are unable to perform pressure release maneuvers, a reclining and/or tilt-in-space PWC is frequently prescribed. The tilt-in-space wheelchair offers more advantages than the reclining wheelchair. It provides pressure relief without shear forces and reduces muscle spasm caused by the reclining motion. These additional features increase the size, cost, and weight of the wheelchair.

Cushions are another important feature of the wheelchair. When used properly, they provide pressure reduction, comfort, and good sitting position. Cushions are used for sitting and back support and are filled with foam, gel, air, or combinations of these substances. Computerized pressure mapping systems further help identify body pressure points through various cushions. In general, foam cushions are light, inexpensive, and good for posture, but they are not washable, dissipate heat poorly, and offer the least pressure relief. Gel cushions are heavier and more costly but provide better pressure relief, cleanability, heat dissipation, and posture stability. Air cushions are lightweight and washable and offer best pressure relief, but they are expensive, are poor with posture control, and require inflation maintenance. Table 102-4 summarizes various cushion performance characteristics.

TABLE 102-4 Cushion Performance and Characteristics						
FEATURE	**Cushion Type**					
	FOAM	**AIR**	**GEL**	**VISCOUS FLUID**	**FOAM/VISCOUS FLUID COMBINATION**	**FOAM/AIR COMBINATION**
Inexpensive	Yes	No	Yes	No	No	No
Easy to maintain	Yes	No	Yes	No	No	No
Easy to clean	No	Yes	Yes	No	No	No
Lightweight	Yes	Yes	Yes	No	No	Yes
Can be customized	Yes	No	No	No	Yes	Yes
Pressure distribution	Low to moderate	High	Low	Moderate to high	Moderate to high	Moderate to high
Stability	Yes	No	Yes	Yes	Yes	Yes
Heat dissipation	No	Yes	No	Yes	Yes	Yes
Shear reduction	No	Yes	No	Yes	Yes	Yes

Comb, combination; Mod, moderate; Visc, viscous.
Chart is provided by Health Aid of Ohio, Cleveland, Ohio.

Power scooters are an option for patients with cystic fibrosis, advanced chronic obstructive pulmonary disease, cardiac failure, or nonprogressive weakness. These patients can walk short distances and transfer independently but need to preserve their energy for other activities. Compared with PWCs, scooters are cheaper, are easier to transport, and have better social acceptance. However, they are less stable (some may tip over at high speed); their use requires good sitting balance, upper limb strength, and coordination, with good cognitive and visual function.

CURRENT CONTROVERSIES AND RESEARCH OPPORTUNITIES

The cost of the durable equipment increases as the patient's function declines, and disability increases along with diminishing life expectancy. The expensive equipment required for short-duration use may not be cost-effective and is sometimes controversial.

More research is needed to demonstrate the cost-effectiveness, efficiency, and safety of available DME technologies in palliative medicine. More equipment needs to be developed that can be controlled with minimal physical and mental effort. Equipment should be produced and used to decrease pain, decrease use of medications, and prevent secondary injury such pressure ulcer, contracture, or a fall.

CONCLUSION

Many types of DME are available to improve functional independence. The general DME goals for palliative care patients are similar to those for patients with impairments caused by many diseases. Team efforts that include the patient and caregiver for appropriate prescription, fitting, and training are important. Reachers, dressing sticks, long-handled sponges, upper extremity orthoses, commodes, sliding boards, tub or shower benches, hospital beds, and pressure-relieving mattresses are commonly used to assist in self-care. Canes, crutches, walkers, wheelchairs, scooters, and lower extremity orthoses help with ambulation and mobility. More research is needed to demonstrate cost-effectiveness, efficiency, and safety of available DME technologies.

REFERENCES

1. Michael K. Rehabilitation. In Ferrell BR, Coyle N (eds). Textbook of Palliative Nursing. New York: Oxford University Press, 2nd ed, 2006, 847-858.
2. Nelson A, Powell-Cope G, Gavin-Dreschnack D, et al. Technology to promote safe mobility in the elderly. Nurs Clin North Am 2004;39:649-671.
3. Cullum N, McInnes E, Bell-Syer SE, et al. Support surfaces for pressure ulcer prevention. Cochrane Database Syst Rev 2000;(2):CD001735.
4. Bergstrom N, Allman, RM, Alvarez, OM, et al. Treatment of Pressure Ulcers. Clinical Practice Guideline No. 15. (AHCPR Publication No. 95-0652). Rockville, MD: U.S. Department of Health and Human Services, Public Health Service, Agency for Health Care Policy and Research, 1994.
5. Kottke FJ, Lehmann JF. Krusen's Handbook of Physical Medicine and Rehabilitation, 4th ed. Philadelphia: WB Saunders, 1990.
6. Braddom RL, Buschbacher RM, Dumitru D. Physical Medicine and Rehabilitation, 2nd ed. Philadelphia: WB. Saunders, 2000.
7. Joyce BM, Kirby RL. Canes, crutches and walkers. Arch Am Family Physician 1991;43:535-542.
8. Bateni H, Maki BE. Assistive devices for balance and mobility: Benefits, demands, and adverse consequences. Arch Phys Med Rehabil 2005; 86:134-145.
9. Deathe AB. The biomechanics of canes, crutches and walkers. Crit Rev Phys Med Rehab 1993;5:15-29.
10. Delisa JA, Gans B, Walsh NE. Physical Medicine and Rehabilitation Principles and Practice, 4th ed. Philadelphia: Lippincott Williams & Wilkins, 2004.

CHAPTER **103**

Communication Devices

Dona Leskuski

> ### KEY POINTS
>
> - Inability to communicate causes significant social isolation.
> - Anyone who is unable to communicate by speech or writing is a potential candidate for augmentative and alternative communication (AAC) systems.
> - A thorough evaluation of the individual and situation is necessary for appropriate matching of device to user.
> - Multiple factors influence device choice.
> - Future developments present diverse opportunities for research and device design.

INDICATIONS AND CONTRAINDICATIONS

Two million Americans have communication impairments that prevent using speech or handwriting for daily communication[1] and are candidates for an augmentative and alternative communication (AAC) device. Because the population is diverse, it is impossible to use sweeping generalizations regarding device choice. The cause of impairment may be either developmental or acquired, and needs vary significantly. Persons with developmental disabilities probably have had lifelong experience with AAC devices and may have strong opinions regarding desired features.[2]

Causes of acquired communication impairments are multiple (Box 103-1). Persons with any of these causes may benefit from a communication device regardless of age, life expectancy, or duration of deficit. Those who are unwilling, unresponsive, actively dying, or without the ability to follow commands are not good candidates.

CLINICAL PRESENTATION AND EVALUATION

When considering a communication device, it is essential to conduct a thorough evaluation for a good fit between

> ### Box 103-1 Causes of Acquired Communication Interruption
>
> - Oral endotracheal tube and ventilator
> - Tracheostomy
> - Laryngectomy
> - Vocal fold paralysis or surgical alteration
> - Dysarthria
> - Speech apraxia
> - Space-occupying tumor
> - Surgical alteration of the articulators
> - Degenerative neurological condition
> - Neurological injury

the user and device. This is best accomplished by a team approach. Members can include a speech-language pathologist (SLP), physical and occupational therapists, an audiologist, a medical team or physiatrist, and, occasionally, a social worker. Assessment includes the following:

Speech-Language Pathologist

- Language and cognitive linguistic skills (see Chapter 53)
- Response consistency
- Perseveration
- Ability to learn
- Intended audience

Physical Therapist and Occupational Therapist

- Strength
- Motor coordination and targeting
- Sensation
- Visual field and scanning ability

Audiology

- Hearing

Medical Team or Physiatrist

- Projected duration of impairment
- Life expectancy
- Expectation of functional deterioration (e.g., degenerative neurological condition)

Social Worker

- Psychosocial dimensions of impaired communication
- Funding options for high-complexity devices

EQUIPMENT

Choice of equipment depends on the results of the evaluation. Persons with prior use of AAC devices may have strong opinions on desired features. They will help find the best device. Persons with newly acquired deficits may depend more on professionals for choice.[2] AAC aids are best thought of as a system and not a single entity.[1] The device does not replace all other forms of communication but supplements gestures, residual speech or writing, and facial expressions. There are two categories: low tech and high tech.

Low-tech devices do not require electricity or individualized programming.[3-5] They include the following:

1. *Communication boards*: Flexible design; may include "yes" and "no" printed on a single page, the alphabet, symbols, or phrases. Mouth pointers may be used if needed. For those with only eye movement, choices can be mounted in a square around the individual's visual field for use of gaze choice (Fig. 103-1).
2. *Palatal lift or prosthesis*: Useful after palate surgery; allows restoration of normal air flow through the articulators.
3. *One-way speaking valves*: Useful after tracheostomy to restore voice. Cuff deflation must be tolerable for their use. They can be used in line with ventilator tubing in some patients (Fig. 103-2).

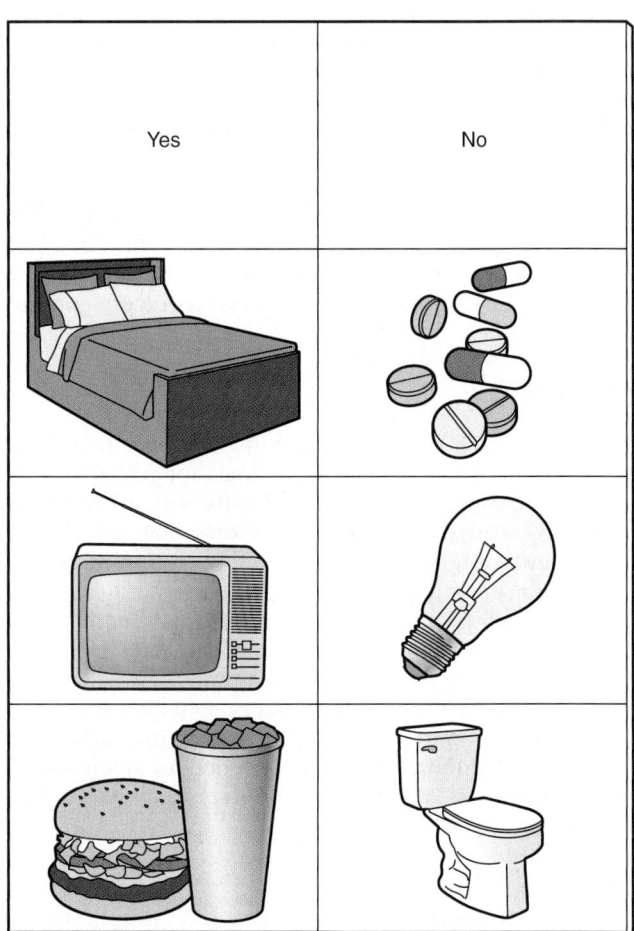

FIGURE 103-1 Symbol board.

Yes	A	B	C	D	E	F	G	H	No
Z									I
Y									J
X									K
W									L
V	U	T	S	R	Q	P	O	N	M

FIGURE 103-2 Eye gaze letter board for individuals with eye movement only.

4. *Talking tracheostomies*: Useful when cuff deflation cannot be tolerated, because they have separate fenestrated tubing that allows room air to be directed from an outside source beneath the vocal folds to restore voice. Individuals with excessive secretions may find that the fenestration gets clogged easily.

5. *Transesophageal puncture (TEP) and voice prosthesis*: Useful after laryngectomy. A surgically created tract between the trachea and esophagus allows redirection of air flow from the lungs through the prosthesis and into the esophagus to create sound through the upper esophageal sphincter.

6. *Electrolarynges*: Useful after laryngectomy for those who do not have a TEP; these devices are applied to the neck or oral cavity to create sound. Some are sophisticated, with ability to change pitch for inflection or gender and volume control for different speaking situations (Fig. 103-3).

High-tech devices include many computer-assisted modules. Depending on needs and design, they are virtually limitless in features. Many use synthesized speech in some form. The simplest add speech to communication boards. For those who require an AAC system, are cognitively intact, and have a reasonable life expectancy, the programmability and complexity of computer systems represent freedom to resume crucial life roles. Computerized models are often used; they have switches and plates that capture and utilize any movement available[6-8] (see Case Study: Use of AAC in Quadriparesis).

DESCRIPTION OF TECHNIQUES AND TRAINING

In most cases, the SLP coordinates training. SLPs may develop specialized expertise in complex AAC systems, but a general SLP can do training on most devices. Training occurs on many levels for both user and caregiver. User training focuses on consistent responses with the device. Training may be extensive, depending on endurance, cognitive-linguistic profile, and desire for success. Caregiver training focuses on facilitating device use, setup, and real-life troubleshooting. Caregivers of those who use tracheostomy speaking valves or TEP voice prostheses receive additional safety training in recognition of physical distress (Fig. 103-4).

COMPLICATIONS

Occasionally, someone finds that the device provides less than the desired result or is disinclined to continue training as disease or fatigue progresses. If this occurs, a device that worked well before may become too cumbersome. The manufacturer may be able to adapt the device to the patient's changing needs. If the system requires regular maintenance or repair, the patient may intermittently be left without the device, which may be unacceptable. All of these factors can lead to system abandonment and

C A S E   S T U D Y

Use of AAC in Quadriparesis

MP, a 49-year-old man, had sustained a spinal cord injury resulting in quadriparesis. His most functional limb was his right upper extremity, which had gross abduction and adduction of the arm along with movement of the fourth and fifth digits of the hand. He was tracheostomy dependent and required ventilator support at night. He was cared for in his home. With the aid of a customized wheelchair, he was able to venture into the community.

MP was cognitively intact and experienced extreme social isolation. Several picture and phrase boards were tried, but he found them too limiting in the number of ideas to be expressed. Alphabet boards were too slow. Eventually, MP was given a one-way tracheostomy speaking valve to achieve voicing. This met with limited success beyond the phrase level, because his respiratory support was minimal for sustaining phonation. However, when short verbal phrases were supplemented with a speech synthesizer attached to a soft-touch alphabet board, he found freedom to communicate complex ideas. A microphone attachment allowed for fair communication over the telephone. MP reported that these devices helped him return to his life and adjust to his mobility limitations.

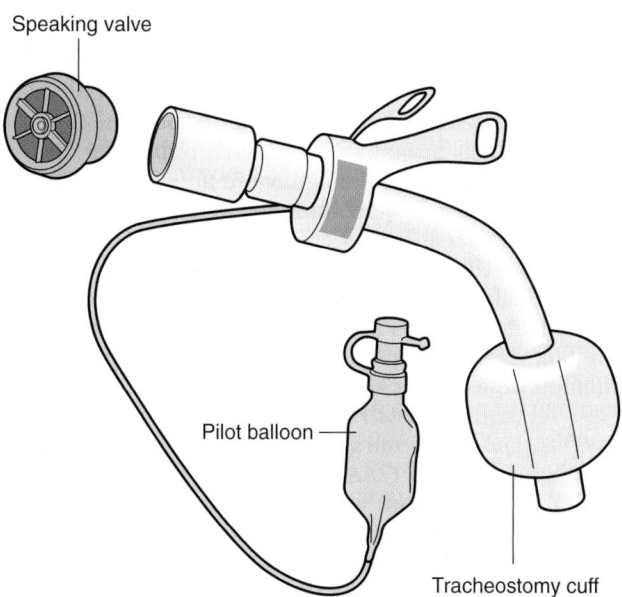

Speaking valve

Pilot balloon

Tracheostomy cuff

FIGURE 103-4 Tracheostomy speaking valve is placed on the tracheostomy hub after deflation of pilot balloon and tracheostomy cuff. The shaded area represents a one-way membrane that allows for inspiration through the speaking valve but closes during the expiratory phase, redirecting air flow through the vocal folds for phonation.

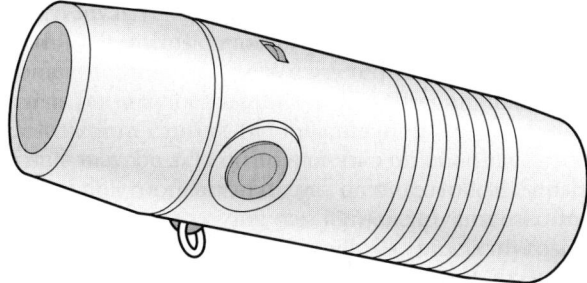

FIGURE 103-3 Electrolarynx. Shaded end is applied to the neck. Vibration is controlled by the dial on the side.

Pearls and Pitfalls

Pitfalls

- Ordering a device without thorough evaluation of individual skills
- Ordering a device without user input
- Failing to recognize that device training may take time; even simple devices are limited by motor control, sensation, endurance, and language skills.

Pearls

- Use a team approach best fit to the user.
- Plan for changes in user needs before choosing a device.
- Enlist caregivers' and users' opinions regarding device choice and troubleshooting.

Future Considerations

There are many future research opportunities in the field of augmentative and assistive communication (AAC):

- Technological advances for greater user ease
- Literacy and success with alternative communicative devices
- Quality of life studies with AAC devices
- Devices to enhance communication with patients who have low awareness
- Cost/benefit analyses of various systems
- Cost-effectiveness of AAC in limited life expectancy
- Neuroelectric and myoelectric interface of systems with users who have severe movement limitations

---

frustration as communication breaks down (see "Pearls and Pitfalls").

EVIDENCE-BASED MEDICINE

The heterogeneity of the AAC population means that randomized, controlled trials are difficult. There is much literature about usability, abandonment, language development, and behavior changes facilitated by AAC systems. Single-subject designs are one way to measure treatment effect and may add significantly to the evidence base. AAC systems are believed to have a positive effect on communication and quality of life[9,10] (see "Future Considerations").

REFERENCES

1. American Speech-Language Hearing Association. Roles and responsibilities of speech-language pathologists with respect to augmentative and alternative communication: Technical report. Rockville, MD: ASHA, January 2004. (DOI: 10.1044/policy.TR2004-00262.) Available at http://www.asha.org/policy (accessed November 15, 2007).
2. Blackstone SW, Williams MB, Joyce M. Future AAC technology needs: Consumer perspectives. Assist Technol 2002;14(1):3-16.
3. Adams L, Connolly MA. Speech Pathology for Tracheostomized and Ventilator Dependent Patients. Newport Beach, CA: Voicing!, Inc., 1993.
4. Happ MB. Communicating with mechanically ventilated patients: State of the science. AACN Clin Issues 2001;12:247-258.
5. Passy V, Baydur A, Prentice W, Darnell-Neal R. Passy-Muir tracheostomy speaking valve on ventilator-dependent patients. Laryngoscope 1993;103:653-658.
6. Happ MB, Roesch TK, Garrett K. Electronic voice-output communication aids for temporarily nonspeaking patients in a medical intensive care unit: A feasibility study. Heart Lung 2004;33:92-101.
7. Higginbotham DJ, Caves K. AAC performance and usability issues: The effect of AAC technology on the communicative process. Assist Technol 2002; 14:45-57.
8. Stern SE, Mullennix JW, Wilson SJ. Effects of perceived disability on persuasiveness of computer-synthesized speech. J Appl Psychol 2002;87:411-417.
9. Happ MB, Roesch T, Kagan SH. Communication needs, methods, and perceived voice quality following head and neck surgery: A literature review. Cancer Nurs 2004;27:1-9.
10. Lund SK, Light J. Long-term outcomes for individuals who use augmentative and alternative communication: Part I—What is a "good" outcome? Augment Altern Commun 2006;22:284-299.

SUGGESTED READING

Fox A, Pring T. The cognitive competence of speakers with acquired dysarthria: Judgements by doctors and speech and language therapists. Disabil Rehabil 2005;27:1399-1403.

Pollens R. Role of the speech-language pathologist in palliative hospice care. J Palliat Med 2004;7:694-702.

Stern SE, Mullennix JW, Wilson SJ. Effects of perceived disability on persuasiveness of computer-synthesized speech. J Appl Psychol 2002;87:411-417.

Nutrition

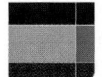

CHAPTER **104**

Physiology of Nutrition and Aging

James T. D'Olimpio

KEY POINTS

- Physiological nutritional mechanisms evolve and adapt with age and as people develop their highly individualized dietary habits. These changes range from loss of taste, smell, chewing, and digesting to diminished organ function. Biochemical systems are also involved in protein, fat, and carbohydrate assimilation, utilization, metabolism, and catabolism. Gender, cultural influences on diet and exercise, and genetic influences affect normal physiological responses to aging and disease.

- Chronic diet-induced inflammation is influenced by fat metabolism and is a contributor to chronic disease.

- Accumulation of "AGE" (advanced glycation end products) from excessive carbohydrate intake causes widespread cell damage, fibrosis, and acceleration of aging.

- Sarcopenia (muscle weakness/wasting) is an unavoidable consequence of aging but may be reduced by improved protein intake and appropriate resistance training throughout life.

An understanding of nutritional physiology is important in palliative medicine, where invariably a "goals of care" discussion includes issues related to appetite, diet, nutritive supplements, food preferences, water intake, and whether these measures improve quality of life in many clinical settings. Recent developments have led to understanding that aging is a consequence of the degree of damage done over a lifetime of exposure to excessive calories, accumulation of advanced glycation factors, loss of lean muscle mass in sarcopenia, and the important role of acute and chronic inflammation resulting from these processes. With the onset of concurrent chronic disease, the pace and severity of clinical deterioration in the sick and elderly are affected.

BASIC SCIENCE

Physiology of Appetite

Nutritional intake is a patterned response to a sensation of hunger countered by satiety. The mechanisms are complex; behaviorally, there is little correlation between food intake and cravings for specific nutrients, flavors, or tastes that are self-regulatory. Many interactions have been well characterized, and fixed physiological characteristics do change over time. For example, dysgeusia and dysosmia in the elderly increase with aging: the number of taste buds is reduced with atrophy in peripheral olfactory pathways and decreased salivary flow. Co-morbid conditions and polypharmacy affect appetite physiology. These influences are frequently multifactorial and dictate strategies to adjust taste, flavor, and smells.

Regulation of appetite involves the hypothalamus; food intake is a response produced by neuronal and hormonal afferent gut signals to the nucleus tractus solitarius, which processes additional signals from gut, omental, and subcutaneous adipose tissue.[1] These reach the first- and second-order hypothalamic neurons that regulate appetite, energy balance, and food intake. Feedback signals are then integrated from the hippocampus and amygdala. These balance hunger and satiety to reflect the net sum of these signals, which is then transmitted by the efferent pathway to the cerebral cortex. Eating patterns at the periphery are received from the autonomic nervous system, the enteric nervous system, and the endocrine-mediated hypothalamic-pituitary-adrenal axis.

Ghrelin, a 28-amino-acid peptide[2] produced in the upper gastrointestinal tract, is the major orexigenic hormone that signals hunger just before and at the start of a meal, targeting the hypothalamus.[3] The interactions among ghrelin, hypothalamic arcuate nuclear neurons, orexigenic peptides (neuropeptide Y/agouti-related protein/AGRP), and anorexigenic hormones (leptin, insulin, PYY3-36, proopiomelanocortin, α-melanocyte-stimulating hormone, and others) modulate food intake. Leptin is interesting as a nutritional mediator. It is present both peripherally in adipocytes, where increase in cell size or obese state correlates with increased levels of leptin and leptin resistance,[4] and centrally in the hypothalamus. It inhibits synthesis of hypothalamic cocaine-amphetamine related transcript (CART) and neuropeptide Y in the nonobese, leading to anorexia.[5] Changes in these homeostatic mechanisms result when disease-related upregulation and coexpression of cytokines, or either inflammatory or cancer-related constituitively produced coreceptors, modify nutrient intake and satiety patterns. These changes include chemosensory dysfunction, altered daily eating habits, food aversions, esophageal dysmotility syndromes, disrupted or abnormal digestive processes, and general polysymptomatology. Cancer anorexia is an instructive example of pathophysiological satiety. It is usually an inflammatory condition resulting from excessive stimulation of factors that disrupt hypothalamic neuronal signaling pathways[6] (Table 104-1).

TABLE 104-1   Mechanisms of Nutritional Derangement and Dysfunction

DERANGEMENT	NUTRITIONAL MEDIATOR	INTERVENTIONAL STRATEGY
Inflammation	Fat and fatty acid metabolism, ω-6 dominance	Emphasize ω-3 over ω-6 and ω-9 intake
Advanced glycation end products (AGE) and fibrosis	Carbohydrate excess (simple sugars)	Limit lifetime exposure; reversal agents in development
Sarcopenia	Protein/amino acid catabolism/proteolysis	Improve protein-calorie balance; focused resistance training throughout life

Physiology of Digestion

Macronutrients are composed of carbohydrate, protein, and fat and are differentially absorbed, broken down, and assimilated in a process that is as dependent on gut health and age as on the selection of foods. Structural elements such as the integrity of the mucosal lining and stroma, brush border, and intestinal epithelial physiology; peristalsis; and elimination play an integral role in digestion. Chronic disease, prior intra-abdominal surgery, polypharmacy, multiple co-morbidities, vascular ischemia, and parasympathetic/autonomic nervous system status undoubtedly affect digestion in sick or elderly persons.

Physiology of Carbohydrate Digestion

The average adult man consumes about 300 g of carbohydrate daily (the average woman, about 200 g), providing almost half of the total caloric intake. Although carbohydrate is a readily available and rapidly used fuel, there is little storage of carbohydrate; only 1200 calories are typically stored in liver and muscle glycogen. Proteins are closely associated with carbohydrate in foods. The mixture of simple sugars (monosaccharides and disaccharides), starches (e.g., amylose, amylopectin), and soluble and insoluble fiber dictate the pace of water absorption, binding of bile salts, and transit time through the small intestine. Dietary fiber is broken down by gut enzymes and flora to acetate, propionate, and butyrate (the primary large intestine energy sources). These stimulate colonic salt and water absorption; colonocyte proliferation and differentiation are also affected. In the small intestine brush border, enzymes such as glucoamylase, sucrase, isomaltase, and lactase hydrolyze oligosaccharides to simple sugars such as glucose. Alterations in food intake influence enzyme levels. A low-carbohydrate or carbohydrate-free diet inactivates sucrase, which can prevent efficient cleavage of short oligosaccharides such as maltose and maltotriose, leading to their malabsorption. If the brush border is compromised by bowel obstruction or damage from chemotherapy or radiotherapy, absorption can change. The enterocyte depends on a combination of facilitated diffusion and active transport to absorb monosaccharides and disaccharides; luminal or submucosal edema limits this absorptive capacity.

Physiology of Protein Digestion

Adult requirements average 0.8 g of protein per kilogram body weight per day. There are about 55,000 calories stored as protein in muscle and viscera, but only 50% is available, because depletion of more than half of total protein stores is incompatible with life.[7] Proteins accumulate in digestive juices and desquamated intestinal cells, in addition to dietary intake. About 6 to 12 g/day is excreted in feces. About 10% of amino acids that are broken down are used for protein synthesis within the enterocyte, with glutamine, glutamate, and aspartate being the primary fuel sources. Effective protein digestion depends on intraluminal hydrolysis mediated by proteases secreted by the pancreas and stomach. Enterocytes then take up amino acids, dipeptides, and tripeptides; about 90% of amino acids processed in this way appear in the portal bloodstream. The stomach produces pepsinogen and pepsin, which are dependent on stomach acidity. Enterokinase in the small intestine brush border activates pancreatic proteases. It is stimulated by the pancreatic juice trypsinogen. It also contains endopeptidases such as trypsin, which cleaves bonds between lysine and arginine. Chymotrypsin cleaves bonds from tyrosine, phenylalanine, and tryptophan, as well as elastase bonds between alanine, leucine, lycine, valine, and isoleucine. Exopeptidases (carboxypeptidase A and B) further reduce proteins with partially cleaved bonds to simpler amino acids.

Physiology of Lipid Digestion

In general, lipids need to be mixed in the mouth with carbohydrates and/or proteins and form chyme for digestion distal to the stomach; cholecystokinin (CCK) is secreted and gastric emptying is slowed to facilitate more lipid digestion. Other CCK actions include secretion of pancreatic lipase, stimulation of exocrine pancreatic bicarbonate, and stimulation of gall bladder contraction to release lecithin and bile salts. Hydrolization occurs, fatty acids are removed, lysolecithin is formed, and emulsification of fats and bile salts takes place, expanding the surface area of the oil/water interface. Because not all fats are water soluble, pancreatic lipase must break down triglycerides, helped by emulsification. Triglycerides are then cleaved to monoglycerides and two fatty acid moieties. A micelle is formed, consisting of spheres with a polar surface and a hydrophobic interior, which can also store fat-soluble vitamins. Once these reach the intestinal cell wall, the components, except for the micelle shell, are absorbed. Recombination back to triglycerides and subsequent formation of chylomicrons completes the circuit, unless the total chain length of the free fatty acid (FFA) is 10 carbon molecules or less, in which case lacteal transport to the liver takes place for direct mitochondrial oxidation. Most triglycerides are longer and require carnitine-acyltransferase for mitochondrial oxidative energy conversion.

The average Western diet includes 30% to 40% of total calories as fat. About 3% of this fat intake contains the essential linoleic acid. About 10% of total fat calories are in excess, compared with an optimal 30% of total caloric intake; this represents about 600 kcal/day not required for homeostasis. In starvation (calorie-deficit state), FFAs (by way of lipase) and glycerol are mobilized from fat stores;

vascular endothelial-based lipoprotein lipase breaks down lipoprotein/triglyceride moieties, and the released FFAs are then stored by adipocytes. Although these are constant characteristics of lipid metabolism, cholesterol homeostasis, mediated by apoprotein B, is phenotypically highly influenced by polygenic expression and variably processed during a person's lifetime.[8]

ESSENTIAL MACRONUTRIENTS: ENERGETICS, METABOLISM, AND STARVATION

Carbohydrates: Structure, Function, Glycemic Index, Glycemic Load, and Glycation

Carbohydrates are composed of monosaccharides (consisting of only one sugar molecule, such as glucose, fructose, and galactose), disaccharides (chains of two sugar molecules, including sucrose, lactose, and maltose), oligosaccharides (3- to 10-sugar chains, including raffinose and stachyose), and polysaccharides (complex starches with >10 sugar molecules, from plants and fruits). Carbohydrate stores are small and are used up after only 3 days of simple starvation, or faster in hypermetabolic or catabolic conditions. In addition to being important components of a minimally stored and immediately available energy source responsible for insulin utilization, carbohydrates affect hunger and satiety signals according to their digestive solubility. It is the relative proportion of high- and low-fiber concentrations that affects intestinal absorption and transit. This patterns the glycemic response, which promotes satiety and inhibits insulin secretion with high fibers in the gut, or stimulates hunger and decreases insulin sensitivity with low fiber concentrations. Any high load of simple sugars and refined starches promotes carbohydrate oxidation at the expense of fat oxidation.

Of equal importance is chronic hyperglycemia and the accumulation of advanced glycation end products (AGE), which is now believed responsible for many manifestations of chronic aging.[9] When AGE are formed, irreversible cross-links develop with protein/amino groups that promote fibrosis, decrease connective tissue flexibility, and alter the extracellular matrix in skin, heart, kidney, and other organs (Fig. 104-1). Atherosclerosis, cataracts, neuropathy, nephropathy, cardiomyopathy, and other end-organ "senescent" problems frequently seen with multiple co-morbidities in palliative care are often a result. These processes occur in "normal" aging but are accelerated in diabetes, chronic inflammation, cancer, and other debilitating conditions.

During decreased food intake, relative starvation takes place; adaptation starts quickly, 8 to 16 hours after a meal. Providing adequate glucose is key to fueling essential brain, nerve, and kidney functions. Insulin levels fall after glucose is mobilized from the liver via glycogenolysis and depletion of glycogen stores. Muscle, on the other hand, lacks glucose-6 phosphatase and uses alanine for conversion of glucose from hepatic gluconeogenesis.

Fats and Lipids

The lipid family includes triglycerides (fats and oils), phospholipids, and sterols. Fat in adipose tissue (typically 13.5 kg in a 70-kg man) accounts for most energy storage; about 135,000 calories are available in a nonobese individual, but long-term expansion in obesity is common. Lipolysis releases stored triglycerides into the circulation as FFAs, which increase during the first week of simple starvation. Bound to albumin, they eventually reach a plateau and are oxidized to acetoacetate and β-hydroxybutyrate in the liver. Prolonged starvation preferentially increases these fuel sources, to 25 to 100 times above baseline levels. A key feature in energy storage efficiency is fatty acid structure, typically 18 carbons in length. The location and presence of double bonds dictate the degree of saturation; for example, ω-3 fatty acids have their first double bond at carbon position 3, ω-6 have theirs at carbon position 6, and so on (Fig. 104-2).

Within food intake, it is the optimal balance of fats, proteins, and carbohydrates that dictates whether starvation or overfeeding is present. With age, the proportion of fat to muscle shifts more toward fat, and fat-free or lean body mass decreases. Fats and oils are essential, but they are less tightly regulated than proteins or carbohydrates. When excess calories are present, nonessential fats can be manufactured from other sources (carbohydrate and protein). Essential polyunsaturated fatty acids, such as linoleic and linolenic acid, must be provided in the diet. Fats store calories efficiently, with little requirement for water,

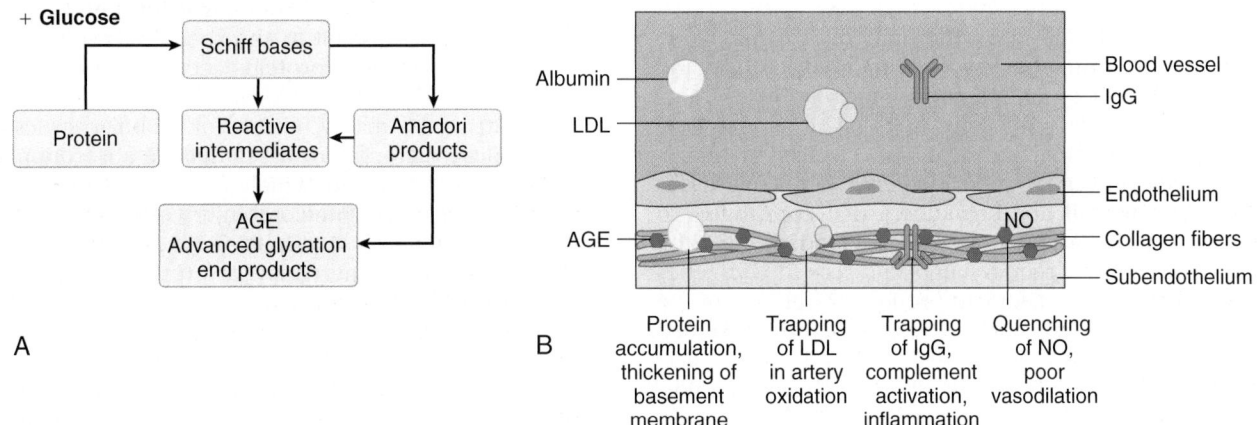

FIGURE 104-1 Schematic representations of the formation of advanced glycation end products (AGE) from protein and glucose (**A**) and their effects in the vascular system (**B**). IgG, immunoglobulin G; LDL, low-density lipoprotein; NO, nitric oxide.

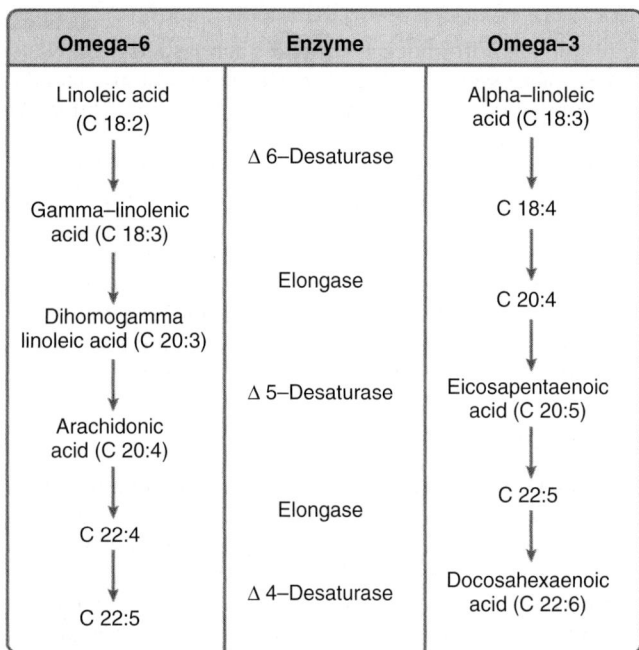

FIGURE 104-2 Pathways of fatty acid metabolism.

Omega–6	Enzyme	Omega–3
Linoleic acid (C 18:2)		Alpha–linoleic acid (C 18:3)
↓	Δ 6–Desaturase	↓
Gamma–linolenic acid (C 18:3)		C 18:4
↓	Elongase	↓
Dihomogamma linoleic acid (C 20:3)		C 20:4
↓	Δ 5–Desaturase	↓
Arachidonic acid (C 20:4)		Eicosapentaenoic acid (C 20:5)
↓	Elongase	↓
C 22:4		C 22:5
↓	Δ 4–Desaturase	↓
C 22:5		Docosahexaenoic acid (C 22:6)

TABLE 104-2 Essential, Nonessential, and Conditionally Essential Amino Acids

ESSENTIAL/CONDITIONALLY ESSENTIAL*	NONESSENTIAL
Isoleucine	Alanine
Leucine	Asparagine
Lysine	Aspartic acid
Methionine	Carnitine
Phenylalanine	Citrulline
Threonine	Cysteine
Tryptophan	Cystine
Valine	GABA
Arginine*	Glutamic acid
Glutamine*	Glutathione
Histidine*	Glycine
Taurine*	Hydroxyproline
	Ornithine
	Proline
	Serine
	Tyrosine

and yield the highest energy (9 kcal/g). Fat stores expand and contract with feeding and are "sacrificed" first during underfeeding and starvation. The ability to retain sufficient fat stores is inherited polygenetically and can have a strong environmental component.[7]

Fatty acids, especially polyunsaturated fatty acids, act as cellular signals in the modulation of inflammation-induced collagen formation and altered gene expression, especially the nuclear factor-κB (NF-κB) pathway.[10] Peroxisome proliferator–activated nuclear receptors such as PPAR-α and their target genes function together to coordinate the complex metabolic changes that serve to conserve energy during fasting and feeding. The ω-3 fatty acids are target ligands and experimentally suppress arachidonic acid–derived eicosanoid biosynthesis. They can change the gene expression and transcription activity of this pathway.[11] Nutritive physiology is profoundly affected by inflammation; in chronic illness, when cytokine production is increased, aging of vital organs is accelerated.

Proteins

Simply put, all proteins are either integral dynamic structural elements of the body involved in growth, repair, and replacement (of skin, muscle, bone, and viscera) or functional and/or signal processing units (such as enzymes, hormones, antibodies, and acid-base electrolyte regulators). The turnover of such elements is a continuous process of synthesis and breakdown that contributes to body mass and organ size and density and dictates the need for amino acid requirements and related energetics to process them. The liver can produce about 80% of the required amino acids, but the rest must be consumed (Table 104-2).

Although there exist about 80 natural amino acids, human proteins are typically composed of 21 amino acids, 9 of which are not provided by normal synthetic pathways and are "essential" (i.e., dietary derived): histidine, isoleu-

cine, leucine, lysine, methionine, phenylalanine, threonine, tryptophan, and valine. Nonessential amino acids can be made from available nitrogen and carbon skeletal sources and include alanine, asparagine, aspartic acid, carnitine, citrulline, cysteine, cystine, γ-aminobutyric acid (GABA), glutamic acid, glutamine, glutathione, glycine, hydroxyproline, ornithine, proline, serine, and tyrosine.

"Conditionally essential" amino acids, such as arginine, can be converted from other amino acids, but imbalance occurs in nature; hence, cystine and tyrosine can be converted from methionine and phenylalanine respectively, but not the other way around. Arginine is widely utilized as a substrate in endothelial-dependent physiological processes; for ammonia detoxification, hormone secretion, and immune modulation; and as a precursor for nitric oxide. Its availability can be compromised in disease and even normally during aging. All amino acids have a similar basic structure of a central carbon atom, with hydrogen, acid, and amino groups attached; some contain a sulfur. On the fourth site of the central carbon atom there is a unique side chain, which distinguishes each amino acid, with an infinite potential assembly of proteins. All amino acids, except for glycine, exist in dextro (D-) and levo (L-) forms; most are in the L-form for human consumption. The DL-forms are more difficult to absorb and digest.

It is useful to classify proteins according to chemical properties and composition (simple, compound, conjugated), nutritional quality, fibrous or globular structure, and solubility. Factors that may influence absorption are related to the degree to which carrier-mediated active transport is affected by mucosal injury or gastrointestinal dysmotility, frequently seen in the sick elderly.

The actual daily requirement of protein is variable in each individual; a macronutrient protein intake that ranges from 10% to 40% of total calories is frequently stated. Satiety depends on many factors, and proteins provide the strongest satiety signal. Insulin is the main protein regulatory hormone. Under euglycemic conditions, hyperinsulinemia inhibits proteolysis, and relative insulin deficiency leads to net protein breakdown. Plasma cortisol levels

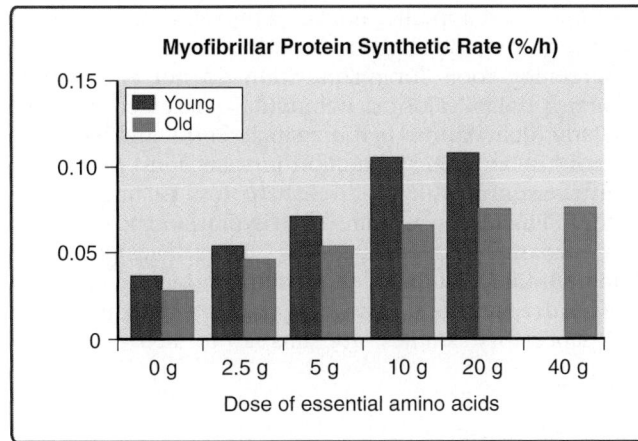

FIGURE 104-3 Amino acid/protein utilization and aging.

increase in disease and stress; they inhibit protein synthesis and accelerate breakdown. Protein conservation correlates closely with adaptive changes in lowered energy utilization and is a highly evolved process. Other hormones, such as triiodothyronine from the thyroid, are less utilized during these periods, related to overall decreased whole body lipolysis, proteolysis, and gluconeogenesis.

A nutritional consequence of aging is sarcopenia, defined as age-related loss of muscle mass, strength, and function.[12] Although sarcopenia is considered inevitable in the natural history of neuronal and neuromuscular maturation in aging, atrophy in sick and or inactive individuals begins at about age 40 years and accelerates after age 75, unless chronic muscle-wasting conditions coexist. Nevertheless, even active patients develop sarcopenia, and nutritional intervention and focused resistance training help retard or partly reverse it. The main nutritional clinical issue derives from the rate of protein synthesis in muscle. As aging occurs, changes in whole body protein turnover reflect slower synthesis rather than increased catabolism. Decreased protein synthesis results in loss of muscle mass and is further affected by decreased regenerative ability after injury, delayed wound healing, or surgery. Muscle satellite cells in the extracellular matrix and basement membrane of muscle cells decrease in number and functional capacity with age; they are sensitive to changes in dietary balance or imbalance in the quality and quantity of protein digested and assimilated. These processes are affected by hormonal changes that occur concurrently, such as decreased production of growth hormone, testosterone, and insulin-like growth factor, all of which are linked to maintenance of existing muscle or regulation of synthesis (Fig. 104-3).

CONCLUSIONS

Nutritional physiology is a dynamic science that has undergone major revisions and paradigm shifts. Common final pathological pathways are altered during aging and disease. These changes include imbalances in AGE from carbohydrate excess that lead to excessive fibrosis,[13] inflammatory states induced by fatty acid imbalance that affect immune regulation,[13] and accelerated sarcopenia seen in rates of protein synthesis and breakdown. These processes accelerate frailty, and their consideration must be incorporated into interdisciplinary nutritional interventions (see "Future Considerations").

REFERENCES

1. Schwartz MW, Woods SC, Porte D, et al. Central nervous system control of food intake. Nature 2000;404:661-671.
2. Kojima M, Hosoda H, Date Y, et al. Ghrelin is a growth hormone releasing acylated peptide from stomach. Nature 1999;402:656-660.
3. Holst B, Schwartz TW. Constitutive ghrelin receptor activity as a signaling set point in appetite regulation. Trends Pharmacol Sci 2004;25:113-117.
4. Lonnqvist F, Wennlund A, Arner P. Relationship between circulating leptin ansd peripheral fat distribution in obese subjects. Int J Obes Relat Metab Disord 1997;21:255-260.
5. Kristensen P, Judge MG, Thim L, et al. Hypothalamic CART is a new anorectic peptide regulated by leptin. Nature 1998;393:72-76.
6. Barton BE. IL-6-like cytokines and cancer cachexia: Consequences of chronic inflammation. Immunol Res 2001;23:41-58.
7. Heber D, Bowerman S. Fundamentals of human nutrition. In Heber D (ed). Nutritional Oncology, 2nd ed. Philadelphia: Elsevier, 2006, pp 1-13.
8. Galton DJ, Ferns GAA. Genetic markers to predict disease: A new problem for social genetics. QJM 1999;92:223-232.
9. Cooper M. Importance of advanced glycation end products in diabetes-associated cardiovascular and renal disease. Am J Hypertens 2004;17:31S-38S.
10. Jia Y, Turek J. Altered NF-kB gene expression and collagen formation induced by polyunsaturated fatty acids. J Nutr Biochem 2005;16:500-506.
11. Li Y, Nara TY, Nakamura M. Peroxisome proliferators-activated receptor alpha is required for feedback regulation of highly unsaturated fatty acid synthesis. J Lipid Res 2005;46:2432-2440.
12. Bross R, Javanbakht M, Bhasin S. Anabolic interventions for aging associated sarcopenia. J Clin Endocr Metab 1999;84:3420-3430.
13. Bengmark S. Impact of nutrition on ageing and disease. Curr Opin Nutr Metab Care 2006;9:2-7.

SUGGESTED READING

Bengmark S. Impact of nutrition on ageing and disease. Curr Opin Nutr Metab Care 2006;9:2-7.

Bross R, Javabakht M, Shalendr B. Anabolic interventions for aging associated sarcopenia. J Endocr Metab 1999;84:3420-3430.

Heber D, Blackburn G, Go V, Milner J (eds). Nutritional Oncology, 2nd ed. Philadelphia: Elsevier, 2006.

Konturek PC, Kontourk JW, Czesnikiewicz-Guzik M, et al. Neurohormonal control of food intake: Basic mechanisms and clinical implications. J Physiol Pharmacol 2005;56(Suppl 6):5-25.

Noll D. Restoring appetite in the elderly. Clin Geriatr 2004;12:27-32.

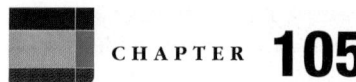

CHAPTER **105**

Determination of Nutrition and Hydration

Mellar P. Davis

The debate about hydration and nutrition in a palliative care setting has remained unsettled because of lack of evidence. Myths are commonplace, and opinion frequently is taken as fact. Nutrition and hydration are coupled but have rather different intentions, even though both involve fluid administration. Nutritional support delivers calories and micronutrients by mouth, enterally, by nasogastric tube, or through percutaneous endoscopically placed gastric tubes (PEG) or jejunal tubes (PEJ). Those without a functional gastrointestinal tract may have a central line placed and be fed by parenteral nutrition (PT) continuously infused or cycled periodically during the day. The primary purpose is to reverse caloric deprivation. On the other hand, hydration by mouth, via subcutaneous infusion (hypodermoclysis), by the intravenous route, or, rarely, by proctoclysis reverses or avoids dehydration symptoms attributable to dehydration.

Definitions of malnutrition and dehydration are not universal, and there is no grading system for either condition. *Malnutrition* can be defined as a deficiency in energy, protein, or other nutrients that leads to detrimental alterations in body function and is associated with worse outcomes than in those who are nutritionally fit. This definition purposely includes functional outcomes. Hence, interventions with meaningful outcomes must target more than simple weight gain and include improvement in function. Weight gain or increase in albumin alone is not a meaningful outcome.[1] *Cachexia* is involuntary weight loss frequently accompanied by unintended reductions in energy intake. It cannot be defined by clinically observable parameters such as weight loss, nor is it a disease, but it is assumed to be involved in severe weight loss (particularly of lean tissue). Cachexia is implicitly a more severe "malnutrition."[2] Starvation is primary caloric failure

with increased appetite; unlike cachexia, it has a distinct protein-sparing metabolism associated with it.[2]

Screening tools for malnutrition do not successfully separate primary caloric deprivation from cancer cachexia. Similarly, dehydration is not a single entity and has been taken to mean either reduction in total body water, loss of intravascular water, or selective loss of intercellular water.[3] Signs and symptoms of dehydration and malnutrition overlap with those of cancer cachexia; symptoms are commonly associated with both dehydration and malnutrition in advanced cancer. In addition, physical examination and laboratory studies are unable to separate these entities.

BASIC SCIENCE

Fat-free mass (FFM) consists of the skeleton, cartilage, tendons, extracellular water (ECW), and metabolically active body cell mass (BCM).[4] BCM determines resting energy expenditures and whole body protein turnover.[4] Protein turnover critical to nutritional assessment and replacement is measured by 24-hour urine urea nitrogen output, which indicates the degree of catabolism (when protein intake is simultaneously measured). Potassium is the major intracellular ion (98% within the BCM), and potassium radioisotopes ($^{40}K^+$) can be used to accurately measure BCM. Additional means of measuring BCM are directly, by densitometry through water dispersion (displacement), and indirectly, through electrical conductivity (bioelectrical impedance analysis, or BIA).[4,5] Anthropometric measurements such as skinfold thickness and mid-arm circumference measurement gauge fat stores and skeletal muscle mass, respectively. Total body water is found almost exclusively in FFM and consists of ECW and intracellular water (ICW). Good health is associated with a balanced distribution of ECW to ICW (ratio approximately 1:1).[6]

ICW and ECW and electrolytes conduct electronic charges. The body can be assumed to be a cylinder; impedance to an electronic current is related inversely to the cross-sectional area and directly to the length of the cylinder (Ohm's law).[7] Cell membranes hold a charge and act as capacitors. Capacitance usually adds a minor component to impedance at low frequencies.[7] Unlike the body mass index (BMI), which is calculated by dividing the weight in kilograms by the square of the height in centimeters, BIA measures total body water, ECW, ICW, lean body mass, and phase angle (a vector relationship between resistance and capacitance)—all of which can be altered by nutrition and hydration.[5,8] BIA is influenced by extremity composition, truncal fat, and water. Lean body mass contributes only a little to impedance. Compared with the BIA, isotope labeling studies better gauge BCM, but BIA measures both hydration and (indirectly) lean body mass through resistance, capacitance, and phase angle without requiring a radioisotope. Another advantage of BIA is that it is portable.[3-5] Phase angle is the vector relationship between resistance and capacitance (the arctangent of capacitance over resistance) and can be directly measured with modern BIA equipment.[9] This resistance-capacitance vector is influenced by BCM and by the relationship of ECW to ICW, both of which are critical to nutrition and hydration status.[10] Sequential determinations of phase angle from a single frequency (50 kHz) accurately measure changes in water distribution during dialysis and independently predict survival in patients with human immunodeficiency virus (HIV) infection, renal failure, and certain cancer primaries.[11,12] Expansion of ECW and reduction in body mass, typical adverse features of systemic illness, reduce the phase angle.[12]

Total body water averages 60% of body weight in young, healthy, adult men, and 50% in young, healthy, adult women. ICW accounts for one half to two thirds of total body water.[3] Aging diminishes total body water to 50% in men and 45% in women, largely through loss of ICW and, indirectly, reduced BCM.

Usual daily fluid requirements are 35 mL per kilogram of body weight. Abnormal fluid losses, gastrointestinal fistulas, diarrhea, and increased insensible loss due to fever must be considered when replacing fluids.[2] Intravascular fluid deficits reduce venous return, increase sympathetic tone and vasoconstriction, and reduce atrial natriuretic peptide. As renal perfusion decreases, both renin and angiotensin II are upregulated and released from the kidney, as well as aldosterone from the adrenal and antidiuretic hormone (ADH) from the pituitary. Aldosterone increases sodium, and ADH increases free water retention, leading to hyponatremia.

The usual energy requirements at normal resting expenditures are approximately 20 kcal per kilogram body weight per day (85 kJ/kg/day). Trauma and stress can increase resting energy expenditures to 35 to 40 kcal/kg/day (165 kJ/kg/day). The daily protein requirement is normally 0.8 g/kg but increases with stress or trauma to 1.5 g/kg. Protein needs are calculated by adding 4 to the 24-hour urine urea nitrogen in grams and multiplying by 6.25; this value helps determine total daily protein requirements.[2] A usual diet consists of 45% to 60% of calories in carbohydrates, 20% to 25% in protein, and 20% to 25% in fat, although there are significant cultural and individual differences.

Usual electrolyte needs by parenteral or enteral routes vary significantly. Replacement of minerals and vitamins is higher if parenteral nutrition is used, because vitamins and minerals are excreted by the kidneys before reaching the portal system for storage in the liver. Parenteral feeding requires more sodium, potassium, chloride, and bicarbonate than enteral feeding does, for similar reasons.[2] The normal metabolic response to caloric deprivation is a reduction in resting energy expenditures and thermogenesis.[13] Reduced resting energy expenditure minimizes weight loss during fasting. Urinary urea nitrogen excretion decreases during fasting, reflecting reduced protein catabolism. Resting energy expenditures decrease by 20% to 25% of baseline. Energy is conserved through reduction of thermogenesis.[13]

Fasting is voluntary anorexia, whereas starvation is extreme hunger, usually involuntary, associated with prolonged caloric deprivation.[14] Three metabolic phases are seen during caloric deprivation. Phase I starts immediately after the last meal and continues for several hours. Metabolism is fueled initially by glycogenolysis until liver glycogen stores are depleted. Glucose is derived from glycogen stored from the last meal. Once glycogen is depleted, fatty acids are released to provide energy for skeletal muscle and thereby reduce glucose consumption. Phase II occurs after liver glycogen stores are depleted. Glucose is temporarily made by gluconeogenesis using amino acids early in phase II. This results in a transient increase in urea nitrogen excretion. Lipolysis takes over, supplying glycerol for glucose production and sparing proteins. Ketone bodies from fatty acids begin to circulate and fuel the brain. Lipids become the main energy source during phase II, and resting energy expenditures are reduced relative to the nonfasting state. The rate of weight loss slows during this phase. Transition to overt starvation occurs at the end of phase II and the onset of phase III.[14] Phase III occurs when adipose stores are exhausted, amino acids are released, and gluconeogenesis surges again; amino acids become the main energy source, and muscle mass is rapidly depleted, leading to death.[14]

Energy expenditures during starvation are further reduced by behavioral, hormonal, and tissue changes. Behavioral changes include reduced libido, reduced physical activity, and loss of menses. Body temperature decreases, and gastrointestinal mucosa and muscle mass atrophy. The gastrointestinal tract is normally very active metabolically and accounts for 40% of the basal metabolic rate. Atrophy of the gastrointestinal tract becomes energy-saving during starvation. The mucosa atrophies to a greater extent than muscle, and cellular division within the mucosa crypts slows down. Specific dynamic action (SDA), which is the energy needed for ingestion, digestion, absorption, and assimilation of food, is dependent on gastric function. The stomach operates on a "pay-before-pumping" principle; therefore, gastroparesis becomes energy-sparing during starvation even if it causes the symptom of satiety.[14] SDA is increased with high-protein diets, whereas high carbohydrate and fat diets have reduced SDA and may be better tolerated when calories are limited.[14]

Appetite and weight are also subject to environmental and cultural conditions. Macronutrient proportions and composition vary among cultures. Carbohydrate intake can range culturally from 3% to 82% of dietary energy and fat from 6% to 54%; protein is usually kept at least to 11% of dietary energy.[15] Pronounced seasonal weight changes occur in developing countries where food availability fluctuates during the year.[15] Under normal conditions, energy and macronutrient intake follow a daily circadian rhythm. Breakfast is usually high in carbohydrates, and dinner is high in fat and protein. High-carbohydrate diets induce greater satiety than high-fat diets do.[15] Increased energy requirements usually trigger appetite and energy intake. Exceptions include anorexia after short-term exercise and at high altitudes.[15] Certain environments (e.g., cold) increase energy intake in conjunction with a twofold to threefold increase in resting energy expenditures.[15]

Appetite signals are governed by a parallel system of neuropeptide Y and pro-opiomelanocortin neurotransmitter neurons in the arcuate nucleus of the hypothalamus. Increased neuropeptide Y stimulates appetite, whereas increased pro-opiomelanocortin suppresses appetite. Negative modulators to neuropeptide Y are serotonin, leptin, and pro-inflammatory cytokines.[16] Neuropeptide Y increases parasympathetic output and reduces basal metabolic rate, whereas pro-opiomelanocortin increases sympathetic output and basal metabolic rate.[16] During the postabsorptive phase of eating (phase I), cholecystokinin is released from the duodenum and reduces gastrointestinal motility. Metabolically, during the postprandial phase, hepatocytes release glucose and insulin, and adipocytes release leptin, which downmodulates neuropeptide Y and suppresses appetite.[16]

EPIDEMIOLOGY AND PREVALENCE

Dehydration

Oral fluid intake of less than 500 mL/day occurs in 60% of those who are actively dying. However, almost 70% of hospitalized dying patients receive intravenous infusions for drug delivery and hydration.[17] Hydration (parenteral hydration) is rarely used (6% to 10%) by palliative specialists in home or inpatient hospice without a known increased symptom burden.[18] Proposed justifications for hydration at the end of life are to reduce opioid toxicity, hypercalcemia, and symptomatic dehydration and to relieve thirst. Nonmedical reasons for hydration are (1) family distress, (2) patient wishes, (3) religious choices, (4) fear of doing nothing, and (5) symbolic care.[18]

Hydration is mainly delivered through hypodermoclysis by most palliative physicians (70%) outside of the United States. Fluid volumes delivered by hypodermoclysis range from 200 to 2400 mL/day. Patients and families are reportedly involved in the decision for hydration 50% of the time, and in 90% of the cases interdisciplinary teams are involved. Patients in an acute care setting are more likely to receive intravenous fluids at high volumes and to be treated with diuretics for fluid overload. In palliative units, fluids are more likely to be administered by hypodermoclysis in small volumes (1 L/day), and diuretics are not required.[19] Fewer than 30% of surveyed medical oncologists, nursing specialists, and palliative specialists see patient improvement with hydration. Between 20% and 68% of palliative specialists notice patient deterioration with fluid overload symptoms (leg edema, ascites, and pleural effusions) when hydration is aggressively used. Between 20% and 70% of the same specialists see improvement in fluid retention symptoms with reduction or discontinuation of hydration.[20]

Thirst is assumed to be related to dehydration, yet no correlation between thirst and clinical dehydration has been demonstrated by cohort studies, nor has an association between thirst and abnormal blood chemistry values (blood urea nitrogen [BUN], sodium, and creatinine).[17,21] Half of those who stop drinking because they lack thirst have normal electrolyte levels.[22] Dehydration does not correlate with symptoms of dry mouth or respiratory secretions.[23] Dehydration in the dying appears to be less symptomatic than dehydration in normal individuals. Sixty-one percent of such patients do not complain of thirst, and those that do tend to find relief with sips of fluid and lubrication of lips rather than parenteral hydration.[23] Dehydration is not associated with an increased risk for hyperactive delirium, reduced communication capacity, increased agitation, myoclonus, or bed sores.[24] Neuropsychiatric symptoms are unchanged by hydration.[24]

Dehydration has been graded by the degree of mouth drying, lack of axillary moisture, and sunken eyes. However, these clinical signs of mucosal dehydration are frequently accompanied by fluid overload (leg edema, pleural effusion, ascites, and bronchial secretions).[25]

Signs of dehydration, but not symptoms, are more frequent in the nonhydrated dying than in hydrated patients (35% versus 14%), and fluid overload symptoms occur more frequently in the hydrated group (44% versus 29%). Symptom benefits to hydration are not proven, but symptoms of fluid overload are well documented in the dying. Third-spacing of fluids in the dying leads to the paradoxical presentation of dry mouth, dry axillae, and sunken eyes with peripheral and central fluid overload. This appears to be a part of the dying process.

Sodium, potassium, and BUN levels change independent of hydration,[24,25] and prerenal azotemia, common in the dying, does not correlate with hydration due to movement of fluid from vascular to extravascular spaces.

PATHOPHYSIOLOGY

Fluid Deficits

Fluid deficit is not a disease but a sign of an underlying disease. The terms hypovolemia, fluid depletion, and dehydration are used interchangeably but differ. Volume depletion refers to intravascular depletion of water and dehydration from losses within intercellular compartments. Extracellular sodium governs extracellular fluid, and sodium is the main determinant of osmolality. Increased sodium causes a shift of water from intercellular to extracellular spaces.[3] Hypernatremic dehydration arises from diseases of the pituitary (diabetes insipidus) and kidney that lead to greater loss of water than sodium. This is seen in up to 16% of dehydrated hospitalized patients.[3]

Hyponatremic fluid deficits arise from adrenal or kidney disease or from gastrointestinal electrolyte losses secondary to diarrhea, gastrointestinal fistulas, or vomiting. Osmotic loads, either glucose or mannitol, cause hyponatremic fluid deficits.[3]

Hyponatremic dehydration, particularly when accompanied by an elevated serum potassium concentration, should raise the suspicion of adrenal insufficiency.[3] Hyponatremic dehydration is common in patients with the acquired immunodeficiency syndrome (AIDS) and resembles the syndrome of inappropriate secretion of antidiuretic hormone (SIADH). However, AIDS-related hyponatremia is not caused by diarrhea, nausea, vomiting, or sweating. Serum creatinine is usually normal. The pathophysiology is virus-induced renal sodium wasting; it responds to normal saline and not fluid restriction.[26] The differential diagnosis of fluid deficits is presented in Table 105-1.

Dehydration in cancer may be caused by anorexia, confusion, delirium, diarrhea, dysphasia, nausea, stomatitis, vomiting, fistulas, or bowel obstruction.[3]

CLINICAL MANIFESTATIONS

No generally recognized pathognomonic symptom or sign exists for dehydration. Dehydration is claimed to cause fatigue, cognitive failure, constipation, apathy, depression, headaches, and muscle cramps, yet little evidence

TABLE 105-1 Differential Diagnosis of Fluid Deficit

GASTROINTESTINAL	RENAL	ADRENAL	PITUITARY	ELECTROLYTE ABNORMALITIES	IATROGENIC
Stomatitis	Renal tubular acidosis	Addison's disease	Diabetes insipidus	Hypercalcemia	Chemotherapy-induced tubular damage
Dysphagia	Acute tubular necrosis			Hyperglycemia	Mannitol infusions
Gastroparesis	Glomerulonephritis				Diuretics
Gastric outlet obstruction	Nephrotic syndrome				Laxatives
Small bowel obstruction					
Colitis with diarrhea					

supports these assertions.[27] Hydration in advanced cancer does not improve cognitive failure, hallucinations, or fatigue.[24] Delirium, restlessness, and myoclonus have multiple causes and do not usually respond to rehydration.[22,24] Signs of dehydration (sunken eyes, dry mouth and axillae) attributable to dehydration[24] have no association with actual volume of hydration, nor with severity of "dehydration" symptoms.[17,22] Loss of skin turgor is as much a result of loss of subcutaneous fat atrophy as of hydration status. Prerenal azotemia does not respond to hydration and co-occurs with fluid overload, probably related to fluid shifts into extravascular spaces in the dying.[24] Signs and symptoms classically attributable to dehydration in cancer are often related to other causes rather than the degree of dehydration and usually do not respond to fluids.

Because clinical evaluation of dehydration is misleading, objective measurements of fluid status, such as BIA, may help, although this has not been extensively researched. Changes in phase angle may provide a pragmatic index to hydration, but this hypothesis has not been formally tested in patients with cancer.[12] At present, a trial of hydration for symptoms should be monitored closely for improvement in target symptoms and stopped if fluid overload (increasing pleural effusions, ascites, or lower extremity edema) occurs. If target symptoms do not improve after 2 to 7 days, hydration should be discontinued.[18,19,24,25]

Cachexia/malnutrition is assessed by the degree of weight loss and BMI. Premorbid obesity hides wasting, because patients have a "normal" BMI yet significant losses of weight and lean body mass.[3] Assessment includes symptoms such as fatigue, daily activities, and quality of life. Absolute amount and rate of weight loss, dietary intake, gastrointestinal symptoms, appetite, and associated gastrointestinal symptoms, food preferences, and taste changes are part of a good nutritional history.[28] Common gastrointestinal symptoms with weight loss are early satiety, taste changes, and food aversions. The number of gastrointestinal symptoms correlates with the severity of weight loss and anorexia in patients with cancer.[3] Men lose more weight than women do.[3] Physical examination includes evaluation of subcutaneous fat, temple wasting, upper body muscle mass, ankle and sacral edema, and ascites. Weight loss occurs in most patients with advanced cancer, but BMI is abnormal in a minority. Triceps skinfold and mid-arm muscle circumference can be abnormal with a normal BMI. Gender differences occur also with cachexia:

men tend to lose more muscle mass than fat, whereas women lose fat and muscle equally.[3]

Bioelectric impedance, dual-energy x-ray absorptiometry (DEXA) scans, isotope studies, sequential magnetic resonance and computed tomography imaging for muscle and fat mass, and metabolic gas exchange (CO_2 production) for basal metabolic rate have been done for research purposes.[27] BIA composition is determined by the equations used in normal populations, so errors are significant in the readout of total body water and lean body mass. Resistance, capacitance, and phase angle are separately recorded and directly measured and may be both useful and prognostic.[7] Changes in phase angle are an indicator of altered cellular health and fluid shifts.

Certain physical findings suggest vitamin deficiencies: dry skin occurs with zinc, vitamin A, or essential fatty acid deficiencies.[3] Pleural effusions, ascites, and peripheral edema may result from low albumin; vitamin B$_{12}$, folate, iron, or riboflavin deficiencies cause cheilosis, glossitis, angular stomatitis, and atrophic papillae.[3] Low serum albumin, low prealbumin, and elevated serum C-reactive protein (CRP) concentrations suggest inflammation-related nutritional deficiency (cancer cachexia) rather than primary caloric failure. Combinations of these measurements have been used to calculate a prognostic and inflammatory nutritional index (PINI).[29] PINI is calculated as the serum α_1-acid glycoprotein plus serum CRP values divided by the serum albumin plus prealbumin. PINI is a reliable indicator of nutritional state and prognosis in noncancer inflammatory weight loss, but not in cancer in general. PINI is high in cancer due to elevated CRP, which correlates with interleukin-6 levels. CRP is prognostic in certain cancers (ovarian cancer, gastrointestinal cancers, and myeloma).[29] CRP correlates with increased basal metabolic rates and the rate of weight loss and is inversely related to serum albumin. Nonsteroidal anti-inflammatory drugs (NSAIDs) reduce CRP and basal metabolic rate, whereas corticosteroids do not. Laboratory tests are combined with a nutritional questionnaire in the Subjective Global Assessment of Nutritional Status as a screening tool for malnutrition in cancer.[28,29]

Screening by BMI and unintentional weight loss over 3 to 6 months has a low sensitivity and specificity.[30] Rates at which weight loss occur are more sensitive[3] than the absolute amounts of weight loss. A detailed screening tool, the Mini Nutritional Assessment (MNA) uses anthropometric measurements, dietary questions, global assess-

---

Box 105-1　Cancer Cachexia Differential Diagnosis

- Endocrine deficiency (hyperthyroidism, Addison's disease)
- Malabsorption caused by tumor
- Protein-losing enteropathy
- Stomatitis dysphagia
- Bowel obstruction
- Fistula
- Short gut syndrome
- Sprue
- Inflammatory bowel disease
- Whipple's disease
- Pancreatic insufficiency
- Paraneoplastic pseudo-obstruction
- Amyloid
- Pernicious anemia
- Zollinger-Ellison syndrome
- Depression

Box 105-2　Oral Therapy

1. Use oral solutions of glucose and electrolytes with less than 2 parts carbohydrate to 1 part sodium.
2. Avoid colas and apple juice in hyponatremic fluid deficit and isotonic fluid deficit.

(From Sarhill N, Mahmoud F, Walsh D, et al. Evaluation of nutritional status in advanced metastatic cancer. Support Care Cancer 2003;11:652-659.)

Box 105-3　Parenteral Treatment of Hyponatremic Fluid Deficit

1. Normal saline for asymptomatic patients with serum sodium = 120 mEq/L.
2. If serum sodium is less than 120 mEq/L and central nervous system symptoms are present, then
   a. Correct to 120 mEq/l but not > 125 mEq/L over 6 hr.
   b. Calculate the sodium deficit in mEq: ($0.6 \times$ body weight in kg $\times 140$) − plasma sodium.
   c. For acute or replacement therapy, use the following formula: (125 − serum sodium) $\times 0.6 \times$ body weight in kg = required mEq of sodium.
   d. Administer as 3% saline over 6 hr.
3. Do not fully correct serum sodium within 48 hr, to avoid pontine myelinosis.

Box 105-4　Parenteral Management of Hypernatremic Fluid Deficit

1. Treat the underlying cause.
2. Reduce sodium-containing medications (carbenicillin, ticarcillin).
3. Replace by mouth if possible.
4. Administer 5% dextrose for dehydration, normal saline for volume depletion.
5. Correct water deficit using the following formula: $0.5 \times$ body weight in kg $\times$ [(sodium/140) − 1].
6. Reduce serum sodium by only 1 mEq/L every 2 hr for the first 48 hr.
7. Use 0.9% sodium chloride or 0.45% sodium chloride infusions accordingly.
8. Avoid overhydration in cachectic terminally ill patients.

(From Sarhill N, Mahmoud F, Walsh D, et al. Evaluation of nutritional status in advanced metastatic cancer. Support Care Cancer 2003;11:652-659.)

---

ment of lifestyle, medications, mobility, and self-perceptions of health and nutrition. The MNA has high sensitivity (96%) and specificity (97%) in the elderly and is validated in cancer.[31] Both the Subjective Global Assessment Tool and the Functional Assessment of Anorexia/Cachexia Therapy appetite scale correlate with objective malnutrition in cancer and are also validated.[28] The differential diagnosis of weight loss in cancer is provided in Box 105-1.

TREATMENT

Dehydration

Oral fluid replacement should be done first. Guidelines for oral and parenteral replacement are presented in Boxes 105-2, 105-3, and 105-4. Subcutaneous hydration is underutilized in the United States. Rates of absorption for subcutaneous fluids are similar to those for intravenous fluids.[32] The half-life for absorption of subcutaneously administered fluids is 11 to 18 minutes, and bioavailability is 96%. The technique is less painful than intravenous infusion and has less risk for infection. A subcutaneous line can be maintained for 7 days without replacement, which is longer than for intravenous lines. The procedure is less expensive than intravenous infusion. Appropriate sites include the thigh, the chest in men, the lower abdomen, and the scapular area. A butterfly needle is inserted at an angle of 45 to 60 degrees to the skin surface.[32] Intermittent infusions (500 mL in 20 minutes to between 50 and 150 mL/hour over 8 hours) are commonly used. Hyaluronidase is not necessary unless more than 1 L of fluid is required over 24 hours. Hyaluronidase, 750 units, is added to the infusion or given at the skin site.[32] Recommended solutions for hypodermoclysis are 0.5% or 0.9% saline. Hypotonic solutions without electrolytes can cause shock, and hypertonic solutions result in slow absorption. Pain at the infusion site and fluid overload are the main complications associated with hypodermoclysis.[32]

Proctoclysis can be done at home. A 22-F nasogastric tube is placed in the rectum, 40 cm from the anal verge, and either normal saline or tap water is infused at an initial rate of 250 mL/hour. Side effects include pain at the time of insertion or during infusion. Infusions may induce a bowel movement.[33] Proctoclysis is the least expensive of the hydration procedures.[33]

REFERENCES

1. Coats A. Treatment goals. In Hofbauer KG (ed). Pharmacotherapy of Cachexia. Boca Raton, FL: CRC Press, Taylor and Francis Group, 2006.
2. Falconnier C, Keller U. Nutritional treatment of cachexia. In Hofbauer KG (ed). Pharmacotherapy of Cachexia. Boca Raton, FL: CRC Press, Taylor & Francis Group, 2006.
3. Sarhill N, Mahmoud F, Walsh D, et al. Evaluation of nutritional status in advanced metastatic cancer. Support Care Cancer 2003;11:652-659.
4. DiIorio BR, Scalfi L, Terracciano V, Bellizzi V. A systematic evaluation of bioelectrical impedance measurement after hemodialysis session. Kidney Int 2004;65:2435-2440.

5. Dittmar M. Reliability and variability of bioimpedance measures in normal adults: Effects of age, gender, and body mass. Am J Phys Anthropol 2003;122:361-370.
6. Vienna A, Hauser G. A qualitative approach to assessing body compartments using bioelectrical variables. Coll Antropol 1999;23:461-472.
7. Scalfi L, Di Biase G, Coltorti A, Contaldo F. Bioimpedance analysis and resting energy expenditure in undernourished and refed anorectic patients. Eur J Clin Nutr 1993;47:61-67.
8. Bauer J, Capra S. Nutrition intervention improves outcomes in patients with cancer cachexia receiving chemotherapy: A pilot study. Support Care Cancer 2004;13:270-274.
9. Zdolksek HG, Lindahl OA, Sjoberg F. Non-invasive assessment of fluid volume status in the interstitium after haemodialysis. Physiol Meas 2000;21:211-220.
10. Kuhlman MK, Zhu F, Seibert E, Levin NW. Bioimpedance, dry weight and blood pressure control: New methods and consequences. Curr Opin Nephrol Hypertens 2005;14:543-549.
11. Barbosa-Silva MC, Barros AJ, Post CL, et al. Can bioelectrical impedance analysis identify malnutrition in preoperative nutrition assessment? Nutrition 2003;19:422-426.
12. Schwenk A, Beisenherz A, Romer K, et al. Phase angle from bioelectrical impedance analysis remains an independent predictive marker in HIV infected patients in the era of highly active antiretroviral treatment. Am J Clin Nutr 2000;72:496-501.
13. Dulloo AG, Jacquet J. Adaptive reduction in basal metabolic rate in response to food deprivation in humans: A role for feedback signals from fat stores. Am J Clin Nutr 1998;68:599-606.
14. Wang T, Hung C, Randall DJ. The comparative physiology of food deprivation: From feast to famine. Annu Rev Physiol 2006;68:223-251.
15. Westerterp-Plantenga M. Effects of extreme environments on food intake in human subjects. Proc Nutr Soc 1999;58:791-798.
16. Davis MP, Dreicer R, Walsh D, et al. Appetite and cancer-associated anorexia: A review. J Clin Oncol 2004;22:1510-1517.
17. Burge F. Dehydration symptoms of palliative care cancer patients. J Pain Symptom Manage 1993;8:454-464.
18. Lanuke K, Fainsinger RL. Hydration management in palliative care settings: A survey of experts. J Palliat Care 2003;19:278-279.
19. Lanuke K, Fainsinger RL, DeMoissac D. Hydration management at the end of life. J Palliat Med 2004;7:257-263.
20. Morita T, Shima Y, Miyashita M, et al. Physician and nurse reported effects of intravenous hydration therapy on symptoms of terminally ill patients with cancer. J Palliat Med 2004;7:683-693.
21. Morita T, Teu Y, Tsunoda J, et al. Determinants of the sensation of thirst in terminally ill patients. Support Care Cancer 2001;9:177-186.
22. Ellershaw JE, Sutcliffe JM, Saunders CM. Dehydration and the dying patient. J Pain Symptom Manage 1995;10:192-197.
23. McCann RM, Hall WJ, Groth-Juncker A. Comfort care for terminally ill patients: The appropriate use of nutrition and hydration. JAMA 1994;26:1263-1266.
24. Morita T, Hyodo I, Yoshimi T, et al. Associaton between hydration volume and symptoms in terminally ill cancer patients with abdominal malignancies. Ann Oncol 2005;16:640-647.
25. Morita T, Hyodo I., Yoshimi T, et al. Artificial hydration therapy, laboratory findings, and fluid balance in terminally ill patients with abdominal malignancies. J Pain Symptom Manage 2006;31:130-139.
26. Cusano AJ, Thies HL, Siegal FP, et al. Hyponatremia in patients with acquired immune deficiency syndrome. J Acquir Immune Defic Syndr 1990;3:949-953.
27. Mattsson S, Thomas B. Development of methods for body composition studies. Physics Med Biol 2006;51:R203-R228.
28. Thoresen L, Fjeldstad I, Krogstad K, et al. Nutritional status of patients with advanced cancer: The value of using the Subjective Global Assessment of Nutritional Status as a screening tool. Palliat Med 2002;16:33-42.
29. Walsh D, Mahmoud F, Barna B. Assessment of nutritional status and prognosis in advanced cancer: Interleukin-6, C-reactive protein, and the prognostic and inflammatory nutritional index. Support Care Cancer 2003;11:60-62.
30. Bauer J, Capra S. Comparison of a malnutrition screening tool with subjective global assessment in hospitalized patients with cancer: Sensitivity and specificity. Asia Pac J Clin Nutr 2003;12:257-260.
31. Slaviero KA, Read J, Clarke SJ, Rivory LP. Baseline nutritional assessment in advanced cancer patients receiving palliative chemotherapy. Nutr Cancer 2003;46:148-157.
32. Steiner N, Bruera E. Methods of hydration in palliative care patients. J Palliat Care 1998;14:6-13.
33. Bruera E, Pruvost M, Schoeller T, et al. Proctoclysis for hydration of terminally ill cancer patients. J Pain Symptom Manage 1998;15:216-219.

CHAPTER **106**

The Anorexia-Cachexia Syndrome

Grant D. Stewart, Richard J. E. Skipworth, and Kenneth C. H. Fearon

---

KEY POINTS

- Cancer cachexia is a complex, multifactorial wasting syndrome involving loss of skeletal muscle and fat that is caused by an abnormal host response to tumor presence and tumor factors.

- Patients develop chronic negative energy and protein balance driven by reduced food intake (secondary to anorexia) and metabolic change.

- The metabolic change involves activation of the systemic inflammatory response and dysregulation of normal neurohormonal axes.

- Management requires a dedicated multidisciplinary team and is best done earlier rather than later.

- There is currently no single or combined treatment strategy that is successful in all patients. However, reversible symptoms should always be treated and nutrition optimized.

- The functional status of the patient should be as important an end point as simple weight gain.

The term *cachexia* is derived from the Greek words *kakos* and *hexis*, meaning "poor condition." Cachexia is a broad, heterogeneous syndrome. The key feature is muscle wasting that cannot be easily or completely reversed by increased food intake alone. Anorexia or loss of appetite frequently accompanies cachexia.

Cachexia is an important feature of many acute and chronic disorders (Box 106-1). Cachexia characterizes the clinical course of these conditions and leads to reduced quality of life, increased morbidity, and increased mortality. Cachexia does not have an agreed-upon definition but represents the complex metabolic process that occurs in patients with these conditions. Unlike starvation, in which fat stores alone are depleted initially, cachectic patients (Fig. 106-1) lose both skeletal muscle mass and fat.[1] Cancer is the most common cause of cachexia.

EPIDEMIOLOGY AND PREVALENCE

Cancer cachexia is common. Half of all patients with cancer lose some body weight during the course of their disease, and one third lose more than 5% of their original body weight. Weight loss is a prognostic factor in survival and renders cancer sufferers less responsive to chemoradiotherapy.[1] Up to 20% of all cancer deaths are caused directly by cachexia (through immobility, cardiac/respiratory failure).[2] Cachexia is particularly prominent in those with solid tumors of the upper gastrointestinal tract and lung (Table 106-1).[2]

Box 106-1 Conditions in Which Cachexia Occurs

- Malignancy
- Acquired immunodeficiency syndrome (AIDS)
- Chronic renal failure
- Cystic fibrosis
- Chronic obstructive pulmonary disease (COPD)
- Tuberculosis
- Heart failure
- Liver cirrhosis
- Malaria
- Thyrotoxicosis
- Rheumatoid arthritis
- Alzheimer's disease
- Severe trauma
- Major surgery
- Burn patients

TABLE 106-1	Malignancies Most Commonly Associated with Cachexia
CANCER	PERCENTAGE OF PATIENTS WITH CACHEXIA
Gastric cancer	85
Pancreatic cancer	83
Non–small cell lung cancer	61
Small cell lung cancer	57
Prostate cancer	56
Colon cancer	54
Unfavorable non-Hodgkin's lymphoma	48
Sarcoma	40
Acute nonlymphocytic leukemia	39
Breast cancer	36
Favorable non-Hodgkin's lymphoma	31

From DeWys WD, Begg C, Lavin PT, et al. Prognostic effect of weight loss prior to chemotherapy in cancer patients. Eastern Cooperative Oncology Group. Am J Med 1980;69:491-497.

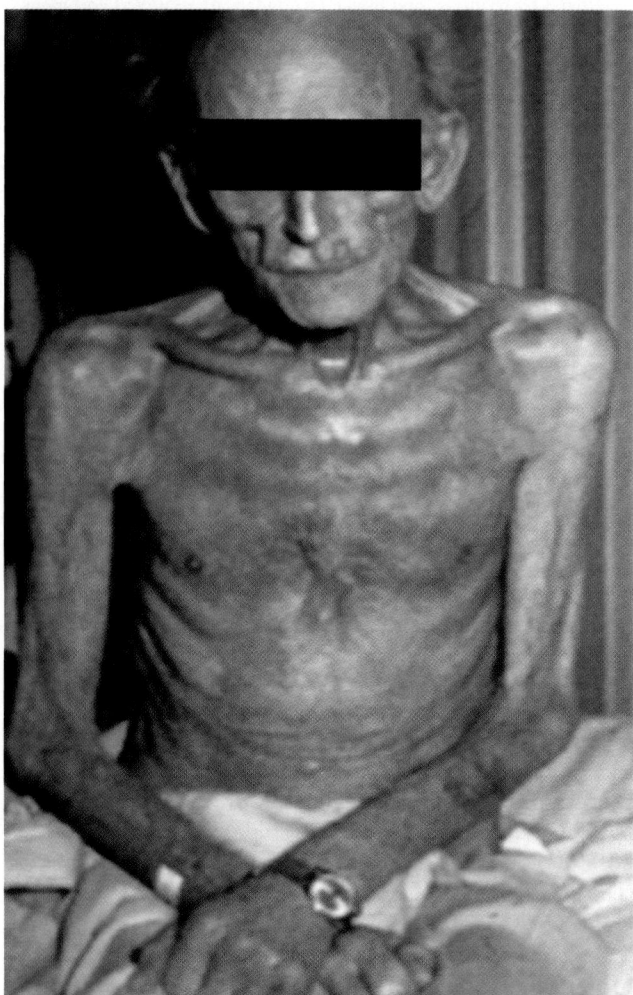

FIGURE 106-1 Cachectic patient.

Sixteen percent of patients with chronic heart failure develop cachexia during their clinical course. Mortality among cachectic heart failure patients is 50% within 18 months.[3] Malnutrition occurs in 25% to 33% of patients with moderate to severe chronic obstructive pulmonary disease (COPD) and in 40% of those with chronic renal failure.[4,5] In chronic heart failure, COPD, and chronic renal failure, there is an association between cachexia and

mortality. Human immunodeficiency virus (HIV)–related cachexia was particularly common early in the epidemic, representing the AIDS-defining diagnosis in one third of patients.[6] Since antiviral therapy became available, the incidence of wasting has declined in Western countries.

PATHOPHYSIOLOGY

Cachexia could be considered initially as a defense mechanism that aids recovery from injury and starvation by producing increased amounts of endogenous substrate. When the numerous metabolic alterations in cachexia persist chronically, the detrimental effects outweigh the benefits. Cachexia can occur without anorexia, indicating the presence of catabolic mediators produced by tumor or host cells involved in the cancer cachexia process. Catabolic mediators include pro-inflammatory cytokines, tumor-specific factors, and hormones. Figure 106-2 summarizes the pathophysiology of cachexia.

Anorexia

The anorexia component of cancer cachexia has a neuro-humoral mechanism due to disturbance of central physiological mechanisms controlling food intake. Peripheral stimuli postulated in the neurohumoral response include neuropeptide Y, melanocortin, leptin, ghrelin, malonyl coenzyme A, and serotonin (Table 106-2).[7] Secondary factors that contribute to anorexia are anxiety, depression, intestinal obstruction, nausea, vomiting, constipation, alterations in taste, and persistent pain.[2] Anorexia is not the sole cause of weight loss in cachexia, but it contributes to cachexia due through reduced oral calorie intake. The abnormal metabolic state of cachectic patients then sustains the neurochemical changes responsible for anorexia, allowing the process to continue.[1,7]

Hypermetabolism

The anorexia component of cancer cachexia reduces energy supply (by approximately 300 to 500 kcal/day), whereas hypermetabolism increases resting energy expen-

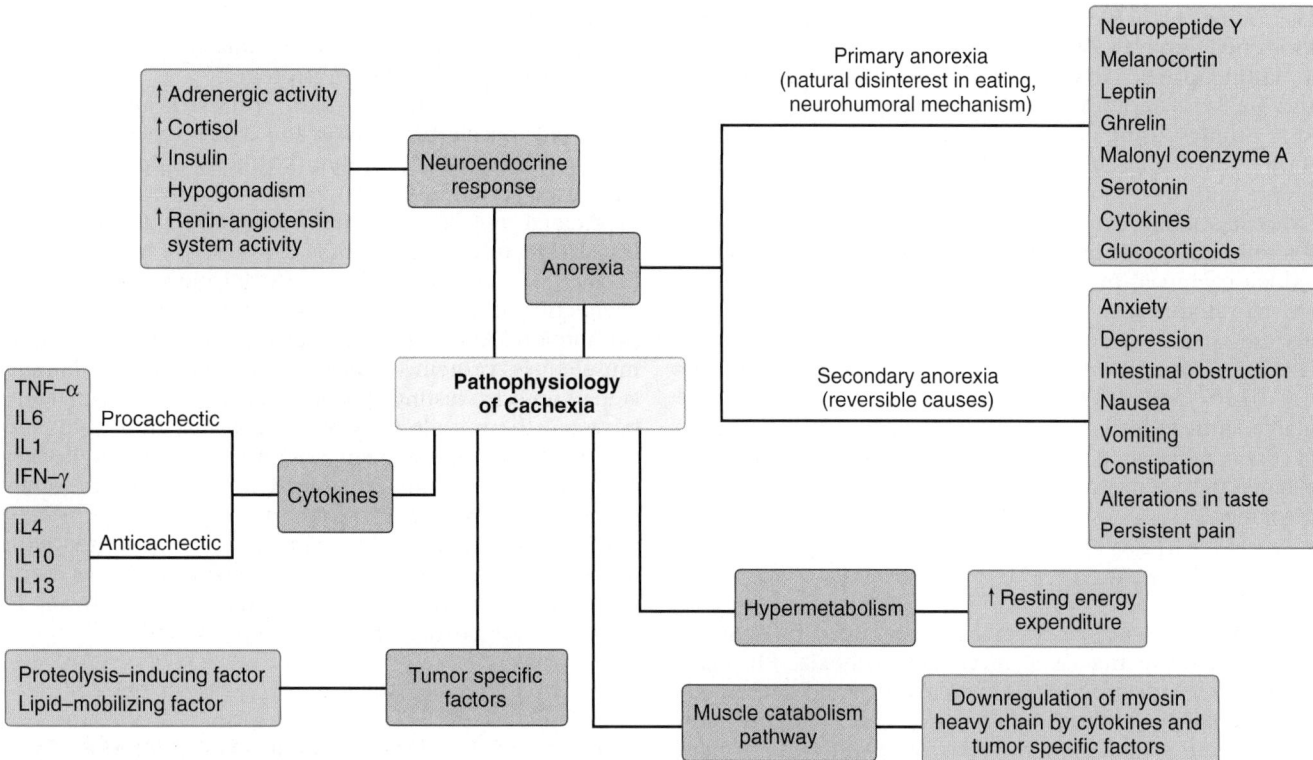

FIGURE 106-2 Pathophysiology of cachexia. IFN, interferon; IL, interleukin; TNF, tumor necrosis factor.

TABLE 106-2 Peripheral Signals Postulated to Stimulate the Hypothalamus to Release Chemicals Stimulating or Inhibiting Food Intake

FACTOR	PHYSIOLOGICAL MECHANISM	CACHEXIA MECHANISM
Neuropeptide Y (NPY)	NPY pathway stimulates energy intake	↓ NPY immunoreactive neurons exist in anorexic tumor-bearing rats
Melanocortin (α-MSH)	Associated with control of food intake	α-MSH induces anorexia via activation of MC3R and MC4R receptors in the brain.
Leptin	Produced by adipocytes, regulates appetite	↑ levels inhibit fuel intake due to blockade of NPY production
Glucocorticoids	Influence food intake	Promote leptin release by adipocytes and limit central actions of leptin
Ghrelin	Produced in the stomach, stimulates release of growth hormone and directly stimulates the hypothalamus, increasing food intake	Ghrelin is upregulated in tumor-inoculated mice, but their food intake is depressed. Plasma concentrations are high in cancer patients with cachexia; this may be a compensatory mechanism for catabolic–anabolic imbalance.
Malonyl coenzyme A	↑ levels reduce food intake by inhibition of NPY production	Mechanism may be deranged in cancer patients, resulting in anorexia.
Cytokines	Intracellular mediators in immune response	IL1, TNF-α, and IFN-γ contribute to cancer anorexia in experimental models.
Serotonin	Released from hypothalamus, leading to anorexia	Anorexic tumor-bearing rats have increased concentrations of hypothalamic serotonin. Removal of tumor returns serotonin levels and food intake to normal.

IFN, interferon; IL, interleukin; TNF, tumor necrosis factor.
From Laviano A, Meguid MM, Rossi-Fanelli F. Cancer anorexia: Clinical implications, pathogenesis, and therapeutic strategies. Lancet Oncol 2003;4:686-694.

diture (by approximately 100 to 200 kcal/day). The increased resting energy expenditure is due mainly to pro-inflammatory cytokines. These changes underlie a key paradox of cachexia: although the metabolic rate may be increased, overall (or total) energy expenditure is decreased due to a fall in physical activity.[2]

Cytokines

Experimental cachexia models suggest that pro-inflammatory cytokines such as tumor necrosis factor-α (TNF-α),

interleukin-6 (IL6), interleukin-1 (IL1), and interferon-γ (IFN-γ) all play a role. The importance of cytokines in human cachexia is less well defined. Cytokines released by tumor cells are generally not detectable in cancer patients and therefore probably act only locally to promote inflammation and activate host inflammatory cells passing through the tumor. These activated host cells then release their own cytokine cascade, which initiates the hepatic acute phase protein response (APPR).

IL6 is the main cytokine in the APPR. C-reactive protein (CRP), the prototypical acute phase reactant, has a strong association with weight loss, diminished appetite, and shortened survival. Patients receiving treatment with IL6 in antineoplastic trials report side effects of fatigue and flulike symptoms, but only some develop weight loss. Studies using incubated rat skeletal muscle have shown that IL6 has no direct effect on muscle proteolysis. TNF-α and IFN-γ induce cachexia in murine models.[8] Cytokines alone can cause the full cachexia syndrome. Therefore, it seems likely that a combination of mediators induce cachexia. In cancer, when serum cytokine levels are elevated, these levels generally correlate with the disease stage, reflecting tumor size and metastasis.[8] Other cytokines show potential as repressors of cachexia. IL4, IL10, and IL13 all have anti-inflammatory, and hence anticachectic, activity. The final wasting status of the cachectic patient depends presumably on the balance between pro-inflammatory and anti-inflammatory cytokines.[8]

Tumor-Specific Factors

Proteolysis-inducing factor (PIF) is produced by tumors and excreted in the urine in cancer cachexia. PIF may contribute to increased muscle breakdown and decreased muscle protein synthesis.[2] Cachectic cancer patients may also excrete a lipid-mobilizing factor (LMF), which may deplete adipose tissue. LMF is produced by cachexia-inducing tumors and is involved in the specific mobilization of adipose tissue.[8]

Muscle Catabolism Pathway

The mediators responsible for cancer cachexia vary among experimental models; a similar situation may occur in the human. Potential future treatments would be numerous, to target each of the various mediator systems involved in cachexia. However, there may be common elements to the catabolic signal transduction in cancer cachexia. The ubiquitin-proteasome proteolytic pathway (U-P pathway) appears to be a common proteolytic pathway in cancer-associated skeletal muscle atrophy. Reversal of the cachectic process may lie in a complete understanding of this process.[9] The U-P pathway involves a cascade of enzymes that link tags (chains of ubiquitin polypeptide [Ub]) to proteins, thereby targeting them for destruction in the proteasome, a multiunit protease complex. Activation of the U-P pathway occurs in all rodent models of cancer cachexia tested to date. Human studies show that levels of ubiquitin messenger RNA (mRNA) are twice as high in the muscle of patients with gastric cancer than in those without gastric cancer. The level of ubiquitin mRNA also correlates with disease stage.

Several cachexia factors have been identified, and mechanisms of signaling pathways have been established. However, until recently, the actual gene products targeted for downregulation during the wasting process were unknown.[10] In the basic muscle unit, the myofibril cytokines and cachexia factors (TNF-α, IFN-γ, IL6, PIF) display a high degree of selectivity for downregulation of myosin heavy chain, whereas other myofibrillar proteins are unaffected. Loss of myosin heavy chain can occur via an mRNA-dependent or a proteasome-dependent mechanism, depending on the specific cachexia factor involved.

Muscle wasting in cancer cachexia is caused by selective downregulation of key skeletal muscle gene products rather than a general loss of protein.[10]

The reduced muscle mass results from both the increased muscle proteolysis and decreased protein synthesis. The decreased protein synthesis could be due to decreased serum insulin concentrations, lower sensitivity of skeletal muscles to insulin, reduced levels of protein translation, inadequate amino acid stores, or inappropriate balance of amino acids. The reduced physical activity of cachectic patients may also play a role in reduced protein production.[1] Amino acid supplementation does not restore muscle mass protein synthesis, so it is not the rate-limiting step of muscle wasting in cancer cachexia. A potential link between the muscle wasting of muscular dystrophy and cancer cachexia has been identified. Duchenne/Becker muscular dystrophies are linked to mutations in genes encoding components of the dystrophin glycoprotein complex (DGC), a multiprotein structure associated with myofiber membranes. A positive correlation has been identified between DGC deregulation and cachexia in humans with gastroesophageal adenocarcinoma.[11]

Neurohormonal Balance

Activation of the neuroendocrine stress response is also thought to be important in cancer cachexia. Potential mediators include increased adrenergic activity, elevated cortisol, low insulin, hypogonadism, and increased activity of the renin-angiotensin system.[9] When the weight loss of cachexia starts, the body mobilizes resources. As the stress continues, there is a shift from an anabolic to a catabolic state and resistance to anabolic hormones.[12]

CLINICAL MANIFESTATIONS

Advanced cachexia (see Fig. 106-1) is easy to recognize, but early symptoms may be more subtle. An unintentional fall in weight of more than 10% with an appropriate underlying diagnosis has traditionally been used as a definition of cachexia. This neglects other relevant symptoms and, if used rigidly, delays diagnosis and treatment. Equally, with an ever-increasing tendency toward obesity in the general population, lesser degrees of weight loss are likely to identify those who, although at risk for cachexia, may still be above ideal body weight. History and examination are the most useful tools in diagnosing cachexia and assessing response to therapy (Box 106-2). Weight loss, anorexia, and fatigue are the most common symptoms reported by patients with advanced cancer. Different

---

Box 106-2 Clinical Features of Cachexia
• Weight loss
• Anorexia
• Fatigue
• Muscle wasting
• Esthesia
• Anemia
• Edema

symptoms may predominate in individual patients, and symptoms may also change with time.

Disease-associated anorexia is defined as loss of desire to eat that leads to reduced food intake. The prevalence of disease-associated anorexia ranges from 25% to 50% in cancer patients on diagnosis and greater than 60% with advanced cancer, although the higher prevalence in the latter group may be partly due to antineoplastic regimens.[7] Difficulties in clearly defining and diagnosing anorexia still exist. A visual analogue scale can be used but is unreliable if small appetite changes need to be detected. Often, the diagnosis of anorexia is made on the basis of reduced energy intake, but this could be misleading, because the reduction of ingested calories might be a consequence of dysphagia or depression rather than a sign of anorexia. To reliably assess anorexia, several symptoms that interfere with food intake and are likely to be related to changes in the control of energy intake by the central nervous system have been identified: early satiety, taste alterations, smell alterations, meat aversion, and nausea/vomiting. Patients reporting at least one of these symptoms are defined as anorectic. This diagnostic tool provides only a qualitative assessment of anorexia, so it might be advisable to quantify the extent of anorexia by a visual analogue scale.[7]

Weight and height should be recorded. Weight loss of greater than 5% suggests developing cachexia, whereas weight loss of greater than 15% suggests that the patient is well advanced into the cachectic state. The body mass index (BMI) should be calculated; a value of less than 18 indicates significant undernutrition. The World Health Organization's definition of cachexia is a BMI of 15.9 kg/m^2 or less with associated features of cachexia (see Box 106-2). Edema and ascites are common and may mask the severity of underlying weight loss. Plasma albumin concentration may be low and, if accompanied by elevated CRP or erythrocyte sedimentation rate (ESR), reflects an underlying systemic inflammatory response; this occurs in many malignancies (approximately 50% of patients with solid malignancies have an APPR on diagnosis) and contributes to the weight-losing process. There can be significant intraperson and interperson variability in CRP levels, and CRP levels can also be affected by physical activity.

DIFFERENTIAL DIAGNOSIS

Cachexia per se is rarely misdiagnosed, because the underlying disease that has caused the initiation of the cachectic process (e.g., cancer, HIV infection) is usually already known. However, "unexplained loss of weight" is a relatively common presenting symptom. This may occur secondary to diseases in which cachexia is common (e.g., malignancy), or it may result from pathology not traditionally associated with cachexia. Examples of the latter include endocrinopathies (e.g., thyrotoxicosis, diabetes mellitus), rheumatological and autoimmune diseases (e.g., polyarteritis nodosa), gastrointestinal disorders (e.g., inflammatory bowel disease, celiac disease, malabsorption), chronic infections (e.g., tuberculosis), psychiatric disturbances (e.g., anorexia nervosa), and eponymous syndromes (e.g., Parry-Romberg syndrome).

In the elderly, skeletal muscle atrophy from aging (sarcopenia) may be incorrectly diagnosed as cachexia. The chief difference between these two syndromes appears to

be the effect on fat mass. Cachexia and sarcopenia both produce decline in muscle mass, but sarcopenia, because of the relative preservation of fat mass, may not be associated with weight loss. Hypogonadism is common in elderly men (approximately 20% prevalence in men aged 60 to 80 years). Androgens are key anabolic regulators of skeletal muscle mass, and their relative lack in hypogonadal patients has been hypothesized as one cause of skeletal muscle atrophy. Aging is variably associated with cytokine system dysregulation. An overlap in the effects of proinflammatory cytokines on both sarcopenia and cachexia may represent a common pathway. An operational differentiation between these two syndromes has not yet been developed.

TREATMENT

Management should always involve repeated re-evaluation of the at-risk patient by a dedicated multidisciplinary team, including an oncologist, family physician, clinical nurse specialist, occupational therapist, and dietitian (Fig. 106-3). The purpose is to identify the cachectic process early and take prophylactic measures to attenuate it. Once a patient has become severely wasted, the primary initiating events are frequently compounded by secondary factors (e.g., prolonged bed rest), and it is often impossible to make any realistic therapeutic intervention, either practical or (given the patient's almost imminent demise) ethically advisable. This systematic approach to management is complicated by the fact that there are no agreed-upon early clinical or biochemical markers of cachexia. Current therapeutic options are limited in both scope and efficacy. The limited benefits of active management are no justification to ignore or fail to treat reversible factors associated with cachexia.

Nondrug Measures

NUTRITION

Adequate nutritional intake is paramount but is not the whole solution. In a classic study, weight-losing cancer

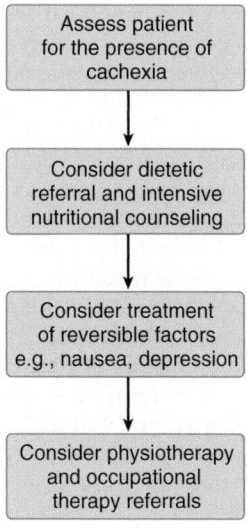

FIGURE 106-3 Management pathway for a patient recently diagnosed with a disease that causes cachexia.

patients[13] treated with enteral nutritional support demonstrated significantly less improvement in body weight, serum albumin level, creatinine/height ratio, and mid-arm muscle area, compared with weight-losing noncancer controls. There appeared to be a partial anabolic blockade to the accretion of lean tissue in advanced cancer. In contrast, gain in fat mass was the same in the wasted cancer and noncancer patients. These findings demonstrated that, although the negative energy balance in cancer cachexia can be overcome by artificial nutritional support, it is much more difficult to prevent or reverse the loss of lean body mass.

During nutritional intervention, a normal or supranormal calorie intake compensates for the anorexia associated with cachexia and slows wasting. Early and formal nutritional advice should be sought from a dietitian, followed, if necessary, by intensive nutritional counseling. Nutritional intake can be improved by small, frequent meals that are energy-dense and easy to consume (e.g., dairy products). The patient should avoid extremes of taste and smell and meals with high fat content (fat delays gastric emptying). Energy and protein-dense oral supplements can help if they are taken regularly, but compliance is often a problem.

In some patients with advanced cancer (e.g., pancreatic, esophageal), the decision may be taken to pursue artificial nutritional support (either enteral or parenteral). Recent studies of an integrated artificial nutrition approach, involving cyclooxygenase (COX) inhibitor treatment, recombinant human erythropoietin (rhEPO), and either oral nutritional support or home total parenteral nutrition (TPN), have improved patient energy balance and exercise capacity. It is important to consider the ethical balance between the benefit in quality of life (QOL) and the potential problems of artificial nutritional support (e.g., time in hospital, potential complications of central venous access for TPN).

EXERCISE REGIMENS

Physical activity is impaired in cachectic individuals for two reasons. First, wasted, cachectic muscle is likely to exhibit reduced power output and earlier fatigue than healthy muscle. Second, it has been postulated that reduced physical activity is a modulation of energy demand by the cachectic individual that serves to reduce total energy expenditure given increased resting energy expenditure.[14] Recent studies confirmed significantly lower levels of physical activity in cachectic cancer patients compared with healthy controls.[14] The levels observed in cachectic patients are comparable to those in patients with spinal cord injury living at home or in those with cerebral palsy. Levels of activity as low as this exacerbate the muscle wasting in cachexia through deconditioning. Exercise regimens, such as walking programs, may improve muscle mass and reduce subjective patient fatigue. Fatigue can be further reduced by increasing psychosocial support and limiting stress. Patients with significantly reduced energy reserves should be advised to make the most efficient use of their energy by focusing on meal times and social interaction. Input from occupational therapists and physical aids in the home may also enhance QOL. If fatigue occurs with anemia, rhEPO treatment may help, although the benefit may not solely arise from its hematopoietic effects. There is evidence for a protective role of rhEPO in experimental models of both myocardial infarction and ischemia-reperfusion injury through anti-apoptotic effects within the myocardium. There are still undefined effects of rhEPO treatment on the progression of cancer. Recent studies in anemia in head and neck cancer found that long-term rhEPO therapy significantly impaired disease control and survival.[15]

Nutritional parameters (e.g., gain in lean body mass) have been used as surrogate outcome measures in anticachexia interventions. Because physical activity is patient focused and appears to be intricately linked to QOL, there have been recent calls for its institution as a primary outcome measure.[16] Techniques to subjectively assess patient physical activity in a simple, accurate, and inexpensive fashion remain elusive.

Drugs of Choice

There have been many clinical trials assessing various pharmacological and nonpharmacological treatments for cachexia (Table 106-3). All current approved therapies (Table 106-4) and experimental treatments (Table 106-5) for cachexia interrupt the wasting process by either reducing anorexia/stimulating appetite, attenuating skeletal muscle catabolism, or stimulating muscle protein anabolism.

APPETITE STIMULANTS

In severe anorexia or early satiety, an appetite stimulant may provide symptomatic improvement. Progestational agents at high doses, such as megestrol acetate (at a starting dose of 160 mg daily, titrated up to 800 mg/day based on clinical response) or medroxyprogesterone can improve appetite in approximately 70% of cases by downregulating pro-inflammatory cytokines. Despite subjective improvement in appetite, increased food intake and induced weight gain may be observed in only about 20%. There are three further problems with this strategy. First, observed weight gain is often due to edema or increased fat deposition, rather than increased skeletal muscle. Furthermore, by reducing circulating androgen levels, progestogens may actually decrease skeletal muscle mass. This may be one reason why no definite improvement in global QOL scores has been observed in most clinical trials of progestogens. Second, the exact dose of progestogens required is unknown. Trial doses have ranged from 160 to 1600 mg/day. Third, there are significant potential side effects, including thromboembolism, hyperglycemia, hypertension, peripheral edema, alopecia, and adrenal insufficiency.

Corticosteroids can also induce a transient effect on appetite, performance status, and feeling of physical well-being, but this is usually limited to a few weeks' duration. Because of the wider side-effect profile of corticosteroids, progestogens remain the current front-line agents for cancer anorexia.

AGENTS THAT ATTENUATE SKELETAL MUSCLE CATABOLISM

The attenuation of muscle loss has long been attempted through an upstream approach, mainly based on the knowledge that pro-inflammatory cytokines are important

TABLE 106-3 Recent Clinical Trials of Cachexia Therapies*

TRIAL	N	DRUG	UNDERLYING DISEASE	OBSERVATIONS
Fuld JP et al., 2005	38	Creatine	COPD	Increases FFM, muscle strength and endurance, and health status but not exercise capacity
Marcora SM et al., 2005	10	PRT	RA	Increases FFM, total body protein, and arm and leg I BM
Storer TW et al., 2005	86	Nandrolone decanoate and rhGH	HIV	Nandrolone not significantly different from rhGH in improving LBM, FFM, BCM, ICW, and health perception
Berenstein EG and Ortiz Z, 2005—Cochrane Database System Review of 30 trials	—	MA	Cancer	Improves appetite and weight gain; insufficient data to define optimum dose
Jatoi A et al., 2005	46	Bortezomib	Cancer	Negligible favorable effects on weight loss
Persson C et al., 2005	24	Fish oil and melatonin	Cancer	No change in inflammatory mediators but weight-stabilizing effect
Gordon JN et al., 2005	50	Thalidomide	Pancreatic cancer	Attenuates loss of weight and LBM
Nagaya N et al., 2004	7	Ghrelin	CHF	Increases left ventricular function, exercise capacity, and muscle wasting
Lundholm K et al., 2004	309	Nutrition with EPO and indomethacin	Cancer	Prolongs survival, improves energy balance, increases body fat, and improves maximum exercise capacity
Burns CP et al., 2004	43	EPA	Cancer	High-dose EPA induces weight stabilization or gain in patient subset
Jatoi A et al., 2004	421	EPA and MA	Cancer	MA superior to EPA in increasing weight and appetite
Rathmacher JA et al., 2004	75	HMB	Cancer and HIV	Increases emotional profile and decreases feeling of weakness
Fearon KCH et al., 2003	200	EPA	Cancer	In post hoc dose-response analysis, increases weight and lean tissue
Khan ZH et al., 2003	11	Thalidomide	Cancer	Reverses loss of weight and LBM
Bruera E et al., 2003	60	Fish oil	Cancer	Did not significantly influence appetite, tiredness, nausea, well-being, caloric intake, nutritional status, or function
Daneryd P et al., 2003	108	Epoetin-α with indomethacin	Cancer	Increases exercise capacity and quality of life and decreases inflammatory variables
May PE et al., 2003	32	HMB	Cancer	Increases weight and FFM
Jatoi A et al., 2002	469	MA and dronabinol	Cancer	MA superior at anorexia palliation compared with combination therapy or dronabinol alone
Agteresch HJ et al., 2002	58	ATP	Lung cancer	Prevents weight loss

*Trials of cachexia therapies are often hampered by patient heterogeneity, difficulty in defining end points, limited efficacy of the tested therapies, patient attrition, and cost.
ACE, angiotensin-converting enzyme; ATP, adenosine 5′-triphosphate; BCM, body cell mass; CHF, congestive heart failure; COPD, chronic obstructive pulmonary disease; EPA, eicosapentaenoic acid; FFM, fat-free mass; HIV, human immunodeficiency virus; HMB, β-hydroxymethyl butyrate; ICW, intracellular water; LBM, lean body mass; MA, megestrol acetate; PRT, progressive resistance training; RA, rheumatoid arthritis; rhGH, recombinant human growth hormone.

humoral mediators of muscle catabolism in both human and experimental cachexia. Drugs capable of inhibiting the synthesis and/or release of cytokines (e.g., COX inhibitors, pentoxifylline, thalidomide, melatonin, statins, angiotensin-converting enzyme [ACE] inhibitors); cytokine antagonists (e.g., anticytokine antibodies, suramin); anti-inflammatory cytokines (IL12, IL15); and anti-inflammatory nutraceuticals have been extensively tested in experimental cachexia, with substantially positive results. However, clinical trials testing their efficacy in humans are limited, and only COX inhibitors and certain nutraceuticals (e.g., eicosapentaenoic acid [EPA]) represent current standard therapy. Nonsteroidal anti-inflammatory drugs (NSAIDs) with peptic ulcer prevention prolong survival of cancer patients, reduce systemic inflammation, and preserve body fat; whereas EPA, a natural ω-3 fatty acid component of fish oil, downregulates pro-inflammatory cytokines, blocks the effects of tumor-specific cachectic factors (e.g., PIF), and interacts synergistically with current cancer chemotherapeutic agents. EPA can be provided either as fish oil capsules or as part of a high-protein and high-calorie oral feeding solution (e.g., ProSure). This combination arrests nutritional decline[17] and improves physical activity.[14] A large randomized trial of EPA (N = 200) in pancreatic cancer was complicated by problems of patient compliance, but post hoc dose-response analysis demonstrated a linear relationship between plasma EPA levels and gain in lean body mass.[18]

When considering the efficacy of this upstream approach to prevent muscle catabolism, it must be remembered that the consequences of chronic impairment of the systemic inflammatory response (and the immune response) in underlying chronic disease (e.g., cancer) are unknown. Trials of IL1 receptor antagonists (e.g., anakinra) and TNF inhibitors (e.g., infliximab, etanercept) in rheumatoid arthritis have been complicated by increased opportunistic infections (particularly tuberculosis with infliximab). A more selective downstream approach would be safer and more effective at attenuating muscle loss. In this respect, direct proteasome inhibition could prove effective. Proteasome inhibition can also be achieved by pharmacological or nutritional manipulation.

TABLE 106-4 Accepted Therapies for Cachectic/Catabolic Conditions*

THERAPEUTIC CLASS/ MECHANISM OF ACTION	ACCEPTED THERAPIES	INDICATION
Appetite stimulation	Megestrol acetate	Cancer cachexia
	Cannabinoids	HIV/AIDS
Attenuation of muscle catabolism	NSAIDs	Cancer cachexia
	EPA	Cancer cachexia
	ACE inhibitors	Chronic heart failure
	β-blocker	Chronic heart failure
	TNF-α antagonist	Rheumatoid arthritis
Promotion of muscle anabolism	Testosterone	HIV/AIDS
	Nandrolone decanoate	HIV/AIDS
	Oxandrolone	HIV/AIDS and burns
	β-agonist EPO	Muscular dystrophies
Adjuvant therapy	EPO	Anemia with cancer

*Although some of these treatments are not in routine clinical use, there is a substantial body of evidence to support each of them.
ACE, angiotensin-converting enzyme; AIDS, acquired immunodeficiency syndrome; EPA, eicosapentaenoic acid; EPO, erythropoietin; HIV, human immunodeficiency virus; NSAIDs, nonsteroidal anti-inflammatory drugs; TNF, tumor necrosis factor.

TABLE 106-5 Experimental Therapies for Cachexia

EXPERIMENTAL THERAPIES	DETAILS
Anti-inflammatory cytokines (e.g., IL15)	Inhibits skeletal muscle apoptosis in rat models
Branched-chain amino acids (e.g., leucine, isoleucine, valine)	Improves protein accretion, albumin synthesis, and appetite in cancer patients
Ghrelin and ghrelin agonists	Increases food intake, induces weight gain, and improves PS in patients with COPD/CHF
Growth hormone/IGF1	Variable results in patients with burns, sepsis, trauma, CHF, and HIV/AIDS
3-hydroxymethylbutyrate (HMB)	Leucine derivative that modulates protein turnover
IL1 receptor antagonist (e.g., anakinra)	Has been trialed in rheumatoid arthritis
Myostatin antagonists	Currently being assessed in preclinical animal models
Proteasome inhibitors (e.g., bortezomib)	In phase II and III trials against various human cancers
Statins (e.g., simvastatin)	Pleiotropic effects on immune system, skeletal muscle, proteasome, and tumor
Thalidomide	Improves appetite and induces weight gain in cancer, and to a lesser degree, in HIV patients
Xanthine oxidase inhibitors (e.g., allopurinol)	Improves myocardial efficiency but not exercise capacity in CHF patients

AIDS, acquired immunodeficiency syndrome; CHF, congestive heart failure; COPD, chronic obstructive pulmonary disease; HIV, human immunodeficiency virus; IGF, insulin-like growth factor; IL, interleukin; PS, performance status.

TABLE 106-6 Reversible Symptoms of Cachexia and Their Appropriate Management

SYMPTOMS	MANAGEMENT STRATEGY
Nausea and vomiting	Antiemetic medication
Early satiety	Gastric prokinetic agents
Malabsorption	Pancreatic enzyme supplements
Constipation	Laxatives
Pain	Opiates with minimal sedation
Depression	Antidepressant medication and counseling

Experimental pharmacological agents include peptide aldehydes, lactacystin/β-lactone, vinyl sulfones, and dipeptide boronic acid analogues (e.g. bortezomib). EPA is the most widely researched nutritional proteasome inhibitor. EPA can block the U-P pathway by inhibiting the formation of certain mediators in skeletal muscle.

In cardiac cachexia, both ACE inhibitors (e.g., enalapril) and β-blockers (e.g., carvedilol, bisoprolol) on top of existing ACE-inhibitor therapy prevent (or delay) the development of weight loss in patients with congestive heart failure. The beneficial effect of β-blockers may be selective to cardiac cachexia, because β-agonists (e.g., albuterol) promote muscle anabolism in other forms of muscle atrophy.

AGENTS THAT PROMOTE SKELETAL MUSCLE ANABOLISM

Anabolic androgenic steroid administration increases mRNA expression of skeletal muscle androgen receptor, increases the intracellular utilization of amino acids derived by protein degradation, and stimulates net muscle protein synthesis, resulting in net gain of skeletal muscle mass. Testosterone, nandrolone decanoate, and oxandrolone have all been shown to be beneficial in several catabolic conditions, including severe burns, HIV infection, COPD, and sarcopenia associated with hypogonadism.

Interest has focused on the growth hormone/insulin-like growth factor 1 (IGF1) axis in the anabolic regulation of skeletal muscle mass. Despite promising results, large, randomized, placebo-controlled, multicenter trials revealed increased morbidity and mortality in critically ill intensive care patients receiving growth hormone treatment. The exact causes of the observed increased morbidity and mortality have never been elucidated. Experimental data from catabolic patients with sepsis, trauma, burns, cardiac failure, and even anorexia nervosa provide evidence that heterogeneous alterations in the somatotroph axis remain an integral part of the wasting process.

SUPPORTIVE CARE

Cachexia can be associated with many distressing, yet reversible, symptoms (Table 106-6). Efforts should be made to ameliorate these symptoms to maximize patient QOL and create an ideal background for optimization of appetite and reversal of the underlying metabolic disorder. Nausea and vomiting should be controlled with regular use of antiemetics (or surgery for mechanical obstruction); early satiety can be eased by gastric prokinetic agents; malabsorption is treated with pancreatic enzyme supplements; and constipation is relieved by laxatives. Whenever pain is significant, attempts should be made to control it with a minimum of sedation. The treatment of depression in cachectic patients with antidepressant medication, counseling, or both improves dysphoria and QOL and may also improve immune function and survival time.

REFERENCES

1. Tisdale MJ. Cachexia in cancer patients. Nat Rev Cancer 2002;2:862-871.
2. Stewart GD, Skipworth RJ, Fearon KC. Cancer cachexia and fatigue. Clin Med 2006;6:140-143.
3. Anker SD, Ponikowski P, Varney S, et al. Wasting as independent risk factor for mortality in chronic heart failure. Lancet 1997;349:1050-1053.
4. Congleton J. The pulmonary cachexia syndrome: Aspects of energy balance. Proc Nutr Soc 1999;58:321-328.
5. Kalantar-Zadeh K, Ikizler TA, Block G, et al. Malnutrition-inflammation complex syndrome in dialysis patients: Causes and consequences. Am J Kidney Dis 2003;42:864-881.
6. Weiss PJ, Wallace MR, Olson PE, et al. Changes in the mix of AIDS-defining conditions. N Engl J Med 1993;329:1962.
7. Laviano A, Meguid MM, Rossi-Fanelli F. Cancer anorexia: Clinical implications, pathogenesis, and therapeutic strategies. Lancet Oncol 2003;4:686-694.
8. Skipworth RJE, Dahele M, Fearon KCH. Diseases associated with cachexia: Cancer. In Hofbauer KG, Anker SD, Inui A, Nicholson JR (eds). Pharmacotherapy of Cachexia, 1st ed. Boca Raton, FL: CRC Press, 2006, pp 117-142.
9. MacDonald N, Easson AM, Mazurak VC, et al. Understanding and managing cancer cachexia. J Am Coll Surg 2003;197:143-161.
10. Acharyya S, Ladner KJ, Nelsen LL, et al. Cancer cachexia is regulated by selective targeting of skeletal muscle gene products. J Clin Invest 2004;114:370-378.
11. Acharyya S, Butchbach ME, Sahenk Z, et al. Dystrophin glycoprotein complex dysfunction: A regulatory link between muscular dystrophy and cancer cachexia. Cancer Cell 2005;8:421-432.
12. Clark AL. Neurohormonal factors. In Hofbauer KG, Anker SD, Inui A, Nicholson JR (eds). Pharmacotherapy of Cachexia, 1st ed. Boca Raton, FL: CRC Press, 2006, pp 71-100.
13. Nixon DW, Lawson DH, Kutner M, et al. Hyperalimentation of the cancer patient with protein-calorie undernutrition. Cancer Res 1981;41:2038-2045.
14. Moses AW, Slater C, Preston T, et al. Reduced total energy expenditure and physical activity in cachectic patients with pancreatic cancer can be modulated by an energy and protein dense oral supplement enriched with n-3 fatty acids. Br J Cancer 2004;90:996-1002.
15. Henke M, Laszig R, Rube C, et al. Erythropoietin to treat head and neck cancer patients with anaemia undergoing radiotherapy: Randomised, double-blind, placebo-controlled trial. Lancet 2003;362:1255-1260.
16. Dahele M, Fearon KC. Research methodology: Cancer cachexia syndrome. Palliat Med 2004;18:409-417.
17. Wigmore SJ, Barber MD, Ross JA, et al. Effect of oral eicosapentaenoic acid on weight loss in patients with pancreatic cancer. Nutr Cancer 2000;36:177-184.
18. Fearon KC, von Meyenfeldt MF, Moses AG, et al. Effect of a protein and energy dense N-3 fatty acid enriched oral supplement on loss of weight and lean tissue in cancer cachexia: A randomised double blind trial. Gut 2003;52:1479-1486.

SUGGESTED READING

Skipworth RJE, Dahele M, Fearon KCH. Diseases associated with cachexia: Cancer. In Hofbauer KG, Anker SD, Inui A, Nicholson JR (eds). Pharmacotherapy of Cachexia, 1st ed. Boca Raton, FL: CRC Press, 2006, pp 117-142.
Stewart GD, Skipworth RJE, Fearon KCH. Cancer cachexia and fatigue. Clin Med 2006;6:140-143.
Tisdale MJ. Cachexia in cancer patients. Nat Rev Cancer 2002;2:862-871.

CHAPTER 107

Clinical Nutrition

Jane Read and Stephen Clarke

KEY POINTS

- Malnutrition is associated with a poor quality of life, poor tolerance to treatment, and reduced survival.

- It is optimal to assess degrees of malnutrition using a valid, reliable nutrition assessment tool. Nutrition assessment and counseling should be initiated early in the palliative trajectory and reviewed on a regular basis to improve outcome.

- Invasive methods of nutrition support, such as enteral and parenteral nutrition, should be considered carefully in palliative care. One must consider the underlying disease, the patient's wishes, and the possible benefits or burdens of the intervention

- Exercise rehabilitation should be considered throughout the course of disease.

- Nutritional supplements such as eicosapentaenoic acid (EPA) and specific vitamins may have possible benefits in the palliative care setting; however, further research is required.

The goal of palliative care is to achieve and maintain optimal quality of life (QOL) in patients regardless of the response of their disease to specific treatment. Food intake and nutritional status are critical elements for QOL in palliation and must be considered in the holistic approach to care.

Malnutrition is common in palliative medicine and is now recognized as an important prognostic indicator. There are various methods for assessing nutritional status, but many have not been adequately validated. Treating malnutrition with nutrition support in palliative care has been controversial, because appropriate end points, apart from weight gain, are difficult to define. QOL outcomes are appropriate end points for nutritional interventions. New studies using nutrition and exercise interventions have focused more on QOL outcomes. Nutritional interventions have often produced positive outcomes, but larger, more rigidly controlled trials are required.

EPIDEMIOLOGY AND PREVALENCE

Malnutrition

Anorexia with subsequent weight loss and malnutrition are common in palliative care. The anorexia-cachexia syndrome is a clinically defined illness characterized by significant loss of lean body mass; it is a major source of psychological stress for patients and their families. Cachexia occurs commonly in advanced cancer, acquired immune deficiency syndrome (AIDS), chronic obstructive pulmonary disease (COPD), congestive heart failure

(CHF), dementia, chronic renal failure (CRF), and other diseases.

Up to 80% of patients with advanced cancer develop the anorexia-cachexia syndrome. The reported incidence of rapid weight loss in advanced illness varies widely. Reasons for this variability include a lack of standardized assessment; the evaluation of differing clinical populations at varying stages of disease; and inconsistencies in study design and methodology.

Weight loss may cause increased risk of morbidity, reduced response to treatment, and poorer QOL.[1,2] Those with unplanned, progressive weight loss of greater than 10% of body weight over 6 months have a worse prognosis.[3] A 5% loss of body weight may alter immune response, cardiac function, lung function, and autonomic autoregulation.[4] A trial in advanced colorectal cancer found a significant survival disadvantage in those who were malnourished according to the scored Patient-Generated Subjective Global Assessment (PGSGA) (Fig. 107-1).[5]

ASSESSMENT OF NUTRITIONAL STATUS

Most clinicians rely on body weight and rate of weight change as the major measures of nutrition. In palliative care, patients' weight may be influenced by medical issues such as ascites or edema, which may falsely elevate the measured weight. It is best to identify nutritional impairment before the patient has lost a significant amount of weight. A comprehensive nutritional assessment identifies patients who require nutritional intervention before treatment and helps detect those who are at risk for treatment-related complications. Accurate assessments of undernutrition also provide ongoing objective measures of nutritional status, which will assist clinicians in treatment decision making and in making appropriate nutritional interventions.

Nutrition screening identifies those patients who have characteristics associated with nutritional problems that may require comprehensive assessment.[6] The purpose of screening is to identify those who are malnourished or at risk of becoming malnourished. A reliable nutrition screening tool can be completed by observers of different backgrounds and is quick and easy to administer. Formal nutrition assessment provides a more comprehensive approach to nutritional status. A combination of parameters should be used, including a medical and nutrition history; list of medications; laboratory data, including serum albumin and lymphocyte count; physical examination; and anthropometric measures. A nutrition assessment tool needs to have both reliability and validity. The most useful tool is one that is sensitive enough to detect small changes over time, permitting ongoing review. The PGSGA is an example of a valid nutrition tool (Fig. 107-2; Table 107-1).[7-15] The Case Study ("Nutrition Assessment in

■ CASE STUDY

Nutrition Assessment in a Patient with Mesothelioma

Mr. SC is a 76-year-old man who has experienced a 3-month history of increasing shortness of breath, cough, right-sided chest discomfort, and loss of more than 5% of his body weight. The patient is 165 cm tall and weighs 57 kg. A chest radiograph revealed a large right-sided pleural effusion. Computed tomography of the thorax showed bilateral pleural calcification, a large right-sided pleural effusion, and extensive pleural thickening. Specific questioning provided a history of significant asbestos exposure, 30 years ago when Mr. SC was employed as a waterside worker unloading bags of asbestos. A thoracoscopic pleural drainage and biopsy confirmed a diagnosis of malignant pleural mesothelioma. A nutritional assessment using the Scored Patient-Generated Subjective Global Assessment (PGSGA) confirmed that Mr. SC was malnourished (score of 9). He was referred to a cancer dietitian for advice and began a high-protein and high-energy diet followed by regular review. He also was prescribed dexamethasone, 4 mg daily, for anabolic effect. During the next 3 weeks, Mr. SC gained 2 kg. His level of activity also improved, and he began receiving chemotherapy with pemetrexed and carboplatin, achieving a partial response after four courses of therapy. This also resulted in significant symptomatic improvement.

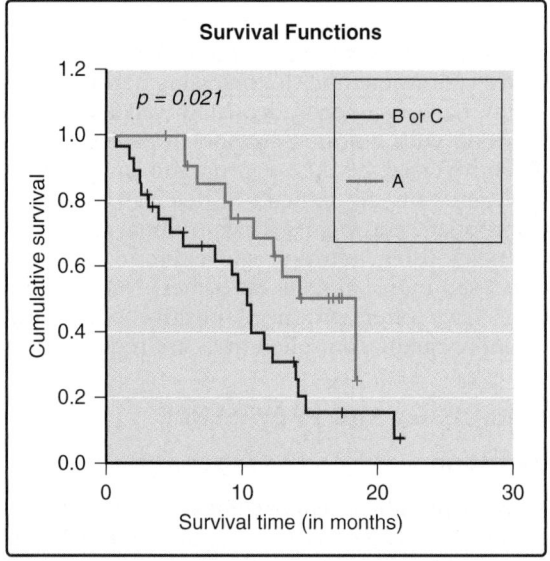

FIGURE 107-1 Survival curve stratified by the Scored Patient-Generated Subjective Global Assessment (PGSGA) group (A or B/C) in patients with advanced colorectal cancer (N = 51). *(Redrawn from Read JA, Choy ST, Beale PJ, et al. Evaluation of nutritional and inflammatory status of advanced colorectal cancer patients and its correlation with survival. Nutr Cancer 2006;55:78-85.)*

TABLE 107-1	Examples of Nutrition Screening and Assessment Tools

NUTRITION SCREENING TOOLS

Malnutrition Screening Tool (MST)[8]
Nutrition Screening Tool (NST)[9]
British Association for Parenteral and Enteral Nutrition (BAPEN) screening tool[10]

NUTRITION ASSESSMENT TOOLS

Subjective Global Assessment (SGA)[11]
Scored Patient-Generated Subjective Global Assessment (PGSGA)[7]
Malnutrition Universal Screening Tool (MUST)[12]
Mini Nutritional Assessment tool (MNA)[13,14]
Protein Energy Malnutrition Scale (PEMS)[15]

Scored Patient-Generated Subjective Global Assessment (PG-SGA)

History (Boxes 1–4 are designed to be completed by the patient.)

Patient ID Information

1. Weight (See Worksheet I)

In summary of my current and recent weight:

I currently weigh about _____ kg

I am about _____ cm tall

One month ago I weighed about _____ kg

Six months ago I weighed about _____ kg

During the past two weeks my weight has:

☐ Decreased (1)   ☐ Not changed (0)   ☐ Increased (0)

Box 1 [   ]

2. Food Intake: As compared to my normal intake, I would rate my food intake during the past month as:

☐ Unchanged (0)
☐ More than usual (0)
☐ Less than usual (1)

I am now taking:

☐ *Normal food* but less than normal amount (1)
☐ Little solid food (2)
☐ Only liquids (3)
☐ Only nutritional supplements (3)
☐ Very little of anything (4)
☐ Only tube feedings or only nutrition by vein (0)

Box 2 [   ]

3. Symptoms: I have had the following problems that have kept me from eating enough during the past two weeks (check all that apply):

☐ No problems eating (0)
☐ No appetite, just did not feel like eating (3)
☐ Nausea (1)   ☐ Vomiting (3)
☐ Constipation (1)   ☐ Diarrhea (3)
☐ Mouth sores (2)   ☐ Dry mouth (1)
☐ Things taste funny or have no taste (1)   ☐ Smells bother me (1)
☐ Problems swallowing (2)   ☐ Feel full quickly (1)
☐ Pain; where? (3)_____
☐ Other** (1) _____

**Examples: depression, money, or dental problems

Box 3 [   ]

4. Activities and Function: Over the past month, I would generally rate my activity as:

☐ Normal with no limitations (0)

☐ Not my normal self, but able to be up and about with fairly normal activities (3)

☐ Not feeling up to most things, but in bed or chair less than half the day (2)

☐ Able to do little activity and spend most of the day in bed or chair (3)

☐ Pretty much bedridden, rarely out of bed (3)

Box 4 [   ]

Additive Score of the Boxes 1–4 [   ] A

The remainder of this form will be completed by your doctor, nurse, or therapist. Thank you.

5. Disease and its relation to nutritional requirements (See Worksheet 2)

All relevant diagnoses (specify) _____

Primary disease stage (circle if known or appropriate) I II III IV Other _____

Age _____

Numerical score from Worksheet 2 [   ] B

6. Metabolic Demand (See Worksheet 3)

Numerical score from Worksheet 3 [   ] C

7. Physical (See Worksheet 4)

Numerical score from Worksheet 4 [   ] D

Global Assessment (See Worksheet 5)

☐ Well-nourished or anabolic (SGA-A)
☐ Moderate or suspected malnutrition (SGA-B)
☐ Severely malnourished (SGA-C)

Total PG-SGA score

(Total numerical score of A+B+C+D above) [   ]

(*See triage recommendations below*)

Clinician Signature _____   RD RN PA MD DO Other _____   Date _____

Nutritional Triage Recommendations: Additive score is used to define specific nutritional interventions including patient & family education, symptom management including pharmacological intervention, and appropriate nutrient intervention (food, nutritional supplements, enteral, or parenteral triage). First line nutrition intervention includes optimal symptom management.

0–1	No intervention required at this time. Re-assessment on routine and regular basis during treatment.
2–3	Patient & family education by dietitian, nurse, or other clinician with pharmacologic intervention as indicated by symptom survey (Box 3) and laboratory values as appropriate.
4–8	Requires intervention by dietitian, in conjunction with nurse or physician as indicated by symptoms survey (Box 3).
≥9	Indicates a critical need for improved symptom management and/or nutrient intervention options.

A

FIGURE 107-2 The Scored Patient-Generated Subjective Global Assessment (PGSGA). *(Redrawn from Ottery FD: Definition of standardized nutritional assessment and interventional pathways in oncology. Nutrition 1996;12(Suppl):S15-S19.)*

Boxes 1–4 of the PG-SGA are designed to be completed by the patient. The PG-SGA numerical score is determined using 1) the parenthetical points noted in boxes 1–4 and 2) the worksheets below for items not marked with parenthetical points. Scores for boxes 1 and 3 are additive within each box and scores for boxes 2 and 4 are based on the highest scored item checked off by the patient.

Worksheet 1 – Scoring Weight (Wt) Loss

To determine score, use 1 month weight data if available. Use 6 month data only if there is no 1 month weight data. Use points below to score weight change and add one extra point if patient has lost weight during the past 2 weeks. Enter total point score in Box 1 of the PG-SGA.

Wt loss in 1 month	Points	Wt loss in 6 months
10% or greater	4	20% or greater
5–9.9%	3	10–19.9%
3–4.9%	2	6–9.9%
2–2.9%	1	2–5.9%
0–1.9%	0	0–1.9%

Score for Worksheet 1= [   ]
Record in Box 1

Worksheet 2 – Scoring Criteria for Condition

Score is derived by adding 1 point for each of the conditions listed below that pertain to the patient.

Category	Points
Cancer	1
AIDS	1
Pulmonary or cardiac cachexia	1
Presence of decubitus, open wound, or fistula	1
Presence of trauma	1
Age greater than 65 years	1

Score for Worksheet 2 = [   ]
Record in Box B

Worksheet 3 – Scoring Metabolic Stress

Score for metabolic stress is determined by a number of variables known to increase protein & caloric needs. The score is additive so that a patient who has a fever of >102 degrees (3 points) and is on 10 mg of prednisone chronically (2 points) would have an additive score for this section of 5 points.

Stress	None (0)	Low (1)	Moderate (2)	High (3)
Fever	No fever	>99 and <101	≥101 and <102	≥102
Fever duration	No fever	<72 hrs	72 hrs	>72 hrs
Steroids	No steroids	Low dose (<10 mg prednisone equivalents/day)	Moderate dose (≥10 and <30 mg prednisone equivalents/day)	High dose steroids (≥30 mg prednisone equivalents/day)

Score for Worksheet 3 = [   ]
Record in Box C

Worksheet 4 – Physical Examination

Physical exam includes a subjective evaluation of 3 aspects of body composition: fat, muscle, & fluid status. Since this is subjective, each aspect of the exam is rated for degree of deficit. Muscle deficit impacts point score more than fat deficit. Definition of categories: 0 = no deficit, 1+ = mild deficit, 2+ = moderate deficit, 3+ = severe deficit. Ratings of deficit in these categories are *not* additive but are used to clinically assess the degree of deficit (or presence of excess fluid).

Fat Stores:

Orbital fat pads	0	1+	2+	3+
Triceps skin fold	0	1+	2+	3+
Fat overlying lower ribs	0	1+	2+	3+
Global fat deficit rating	**0**	**1+**	**2+**	**3+**

Fluid Status:

Ankle edema	0	1+	2+	3+
Sacral edema	0	1+	2+	3+
Ascites	0	1+	2+	3+
Global fluid status rating	**0**	**1+**	**2+**	**3+**

Muscle Status:

Temples (temporalis muscle)	0	1+	2+	3+
Clavicles (pectoralis & deltoids)	0	1+	2+	3+
Shoulders (deltoids)	0	1+	2+	3+
Interosseous muscles	0	1+	2+	3+
Scapula (latissimus dorsi, trapezius, deltoids)	0	1+	2+	3+
Thigh (quadriceps)	0	1+	2+	3+
Calf (gastrocnemius)	0	1+	2+	3+
Global muscle status rating	**0**	**1+**	**2+**	**3+**

Point score for the physical exam is determined by the overall subjective rating of total body deficit.

No deficit	score = 0 points
Mild deficit	score = 1 point
Moderate deficit	score = 2 points
Severe deficit	score = 3 points

Score for Worksheet 4 = [   ]
Record in Box D

Worksheet 5 – PG-SGA Global Assessment Categories

	Stage A	Stage B	Stage C
Category	Well-nourished	Moderately malnourished or suspected malnutrition	Severely malnourished
Weight	No wt loss **OR** Recent non-fluid wt gain	~5% wt loss within 1 month (or 10% in 6 months) **OR** No wt stabilization or wt gain (i.e., continued wt loss)	>5% wt loss in 1 month (or >10% in 6 months) **OR** No wt stabilization or wt gain (i.e., continued wt loss)
Nutrient Intake	No deficit **OR** Significant recent improvement	Definite decrease in intake	Severe deficit in intake
Nutrition Impact Symptoms	None **OR** Significant recent improvement allowing adequate intake	Presence of nutrition impact symptoms (Box 3 of PG-SGA)	Presence of nutrition impact symptoms (Box 3 of PG-SGA)
Functioning	No deficit **OR** Significant recent improvement	Moderate functional deficit **OR** Recent deterioration	Severe functional deficit **OR** Recent significant deterioration
Physical Exam	No deficit **OR** Chronic deficit but with recent clinical improvement	Evidence of mild to moderate loss of SQ fat &/or muscle mass &/or muscle tone on palpation	Obvious signs of malnutrition (e.g., severe loss of SQ tissues, possible edema)

Global PG-SGA rating (A, B, or C) = [   ]

B

FIGURE 107-2, cont'd

TABLE 107-2 Significant Weight Loss Categories

TIME PERIOD	SIGNIFICANT WEIGHT LOSS (%)	SEVERE WEIGHT LOSS (%)
1 wk	1-2	>2
1 mo	≤5	>5
3 mo	≤7.5	>7.5
6 mo	≤10	>10

Box 107-1 Symptoms That Affect the Nutritional Status of Patients in Palliative Care

- Malabsorption
- Nausea and vomiting
- Dyspepsia
- Constipation
- Diarrhea
- Depression
- Weakness
- Dysgeusia
- Xerostomia
- Mouth ulcers and oral infection
- Oral candidiasis
- Loss of appetite
- Mucositis
- Dysphagia

a Patient with Mesothelioma") provides an example of the application of these tools and subsequent nutrition therapy.

PATHOPHYSIOLOGY AND CLINICAL MANIFESTATIONS

The most clinically significant feature of malnutrition in palliative care is progressive weight loss (Table 107-2), which includes loss of both muscle and fat. This accelerated loss of skeletal muscle in the context of an inflammatory reaction is known as cachexia. Additional common features include anorexia, poor appetite, asthenia, anemia, and fatigue. Severe weight loss is defined as loss of greater than 2% of body weight in 1 week, greater than 5 % in 1 month, greater than 7.5 % in 3 months, or greater than 10% in 6 months.[16]

Most research has focused on cancer-associated cachexia. Numerous metabolic alterations occur, probably driven by tumor- or host-produced cytokines such as tumor necrosis factor (TNF) and interleukin-6 (IL6). Metabolic changes alter cellular metabolism in multiple organs, including liver, muscle, fat, and brain, leading to accelerated weight loss. Increased lipolysis and decreased lipogenesis result in a loss of adipose tissue and increased circulating triglycerides. There is increased gluconeogenesis and a reduction in insulin production, which can cause hyperglycemia. There is also loss of skeletal muscle and inability to conserve amino acids. This is associated with increased levels of proteolysis-inducing factor (PIF), which activates the ubiquitin-proteosome pathway, the principal mediator of proteolysis.[17]

In nonmalignant cachexia (e.g., in advanced cardiac disease), edema becomes a more dominant feature and may mask loss of muscle and fat. The features of cytokine-driven cachexia are the same, but fluid and salt restrictions may be required.[18] Disease-associated anorexia contributes to malnutrition by reducing oral intake. This can be exacerbated by treatment- or disease-induced nausea, vomiting, pain, dysphagia, or altered perception of food. In cancer, anorexia appears to be mediated by several cytokines, and by hormones including serotonin and hypothalamic neuropeptides[17] (Box 107-1).

TREATMENT

Dietary Recommendations

Optimal control of symptoms (Table 107-3) such as nausea and vomiting, pain, constipation, and mucosal toxicity will also enhance the ability to manage malnutrition. Appropriate medications are important for symptom management. Some symptoms result from the disease, others from the treatment.

Food plays a central role in life for everyone, including people with progressive illness. Adequate nutrition is essential, not only to meet the body's daily requirements, but also because it has social, cultural spiritual, and psychological benefits for patients and carers. Food may be a pleasurable experience; it provides comfort and a sense of normality. As a patient deteriorates, nutrition support becomes more focused on QOL and relief of symptoms, rather than active nutritional interventions aimed at improving outcome.

Early within the palliative care continuum, nutrition should be a priority. When healing is possible, good nutrition will enhance recovery. Management of nutrition needs to be consistent with the aims of palliative treatment and the patient's wishes. It is also vital for the team to be aware of disease processes and future complications. For example, a patient may be able to swallow early in the course of disease, but, as the disease progresses, swallowing may become dysfunctional, requiring alternative forms of nutrition support. In cardiac cachexia, one of the dominant factors is edema, which needs to be treated with fluid restriction, a salt-reduced diet, and replacement of water-soluble vitamins lost through increased urinary excretion and reduced absorption.

When making decisions about nutrition support, it is important to consider the diagnosis; the prognosis, current symptoms, the pathway of disease progression, treatment and possible side effects, patient comfort and social support, socioeconomic status, cultural and religious views, and ethical and legal issues. The goals of maintaining QOL must always be of utmost importance, and for this reason invasive nutrition support interventions such as enteral or parenteral feeding may not be appropriate.

Symptom management (see Table 107-3) is vital. Many drugs that alleviate one problem may provoke another, and this is where diet may help to alleviate symptoms. For example, opiates to relieve pain commonly cause constipation, but this side effect may be lessened by a diet high in fluid and fiber.

Nutrition counseling should be focused on high-calorie, high-energy meals in small portions. Patients who are unable to swallow due to conditions such as head and

TABLE 107-3 Common Symptoms and Nutritional Strategies to Provide Relief

SYMPTOM	NUTRITIONAL MANAGEMENT
Anorexia	• Consume small, high-protein and high-energy meals every 1-2 hr. • Add extra calories and protein to food (e.g., butter, skim milk powder, honey). • Take liquid supplements, soups, milk shakes, and smoothies if eating solid food is a problem. • Use snacks that contain plenty of calories and protein. • Prepare and store small portions of foods so that no preparation is required. • Try new foods; experiment with recipes, flavorings, spices, types, and consistencies of food.
Dysgeusia (change in taste)	• Rinse mouth with water before eating. • Try citrus to flavor foods. • Use plastic utensils if taste is metallic. • Zinc supplements may help to improve the return of taste.
Dry mouth	• Use moist foods with extra sauces, gravies, butter, or margarine. • Suck on hard candy or chew gum. • Eat frozen desserts. • Clean teeth (including dentures) and rinse mouth at least four times per day (after each meal and before bedtime). • Keep water handy at all times to moisten the mouth. • Avoid mouth rinses that contain alcohol. • Drink fruit nectar instead of juice.
Mouth sores	• Modify consistency of food (pureed, soft). • Add gravy and sauces to soften food. • Avoid rough, crunchy food, and cut food into small pieces. • Avoid spicy and salty foods. • Avoid highly acidic foods. • Use a straw to drink liquids. • Eat food at room temperature (not hot or cold). • Nutritional supplements may need to be considered.
Nausea	• Eat small meals several times a day. • Minimize unpleasant sensory stimulants (e.g., cooking odors). • Avoid foods that are likely to cause nausea (e.g., greasy, spicy, strong flavors), and eat bland, light foods. • Sip fluids throughout the day. • Rinse mouth before and after eating.
Constipation	• Ensure adequate fluids. • Ensure adequate fiber.
Diarrhea	• Ensure adequate fluids and fiber. • Consider probiotics if diarrhea is induced by antibiotics. • Limit vegetables that are gas-forming (e.g., cruciferous vegetables).

neck cancer or neurological disorders causing bulbar palsy, for whom there is concern about nutritional deterioration, and who otherwise have reasonable survival expectation, should be considered for enteral nutrition. Enteral feeding during the palliative phase should be carefully discussed with the patient and family. Often it is inappropriate, because it may protract suffering. In addition, in patients who are cachectic, no survival advantage is provided by standard enteral feeding. There is a risk of complications such as aspiration pneumonia and dislodgment or blockage of feeding tubes, among others.

Physical Activity

There has been little research on the effects of exercise in the palliative population, despite the fact that physical well-being has been identified as one of the most important determinants of QOL. Patients wish to remain physically independent as long as possible, so identifying and treating functional compromise is important. Despite numerous positive randomized clinical trials involving exercise in curable disease, there are few studies incorporating exercise intervention in incurable disease.

It is inappropriate to consider exercise rehabilitation only during advanced disease; rehabilitation should be considered throughout the course.[19] The benefits of exercise in palliation may depend on where the patient is in the disease trajectory. Patients who are considered to have advanced disease are now living longer, and they constitute an expanding portion of the palliative care population.

Studies in patients with advanced chronic obstructive pulmonary disease (COPD) show that exercise training produces significant improvements in exercise endurance, decreased perception of dyspnea, and lowered ventilatory requirements. Muscle biopsies of trained patients indicated that there is an increase in all enzymes responsible for oxidative muscle function.[20] However, there are few well-controlled, randomized trials assessing exercise in advanced disease. Recent phase II trials show positive results for exercise in palliative cancer patients. In one phase II trial, participation in a structured 50-minute exercise program, twice a week for 6 weeks, focusing on upper and lower limb strength, improved emotional function and reduced physical fatigue in palliative care patients.[21]

EVIDENCE FOR NUTRITION INTERVENTION

Early intervention is essential to improve patient outcome. In addition to identifying those who are malnourished, it is important to identify patients at risk of becoming malnourished and intervene early. Interventions should improve treatment tolerance, QOL, and perhaps survival. This may reduce health care costs.

Individual Dietary Counseling

Studies assessing nutrition counseling in palliative medicine are few, but previous randomized trials in cancer patients, using conventional high-energy and high-protein oral nutritional supplements to increase the oral intake, failed to show significant gains in weight and lean body mass or differences in survival, compared with controls who had no intervention.[22] The potential role of intervention was investigated in a randomized trial in colorectal cancer during radiotherapy. Patients receiving individualized dietary counseling alone had significantly improved QOL and nutritional status and reduced radiotherapy-induced morbidity, compared with those who received either nutrient-dense high-protein liquid supplements without counseling or neither counseling nor supplements.[23] Additionally, early and intense nutrition intervention in gastrointestinal and head and neck cancers during radiotherapy was beneficial in preventing deterioration in nutritional status, QOL, and physical function.[24] Compliance with a nutrition prescription of additional high-energy and high-protein nutritional supplements did not compromise or inhibit meal intake.[25]

Enteral Nutrition Support

Percutaneous endoscopic gastrostomy (PEG) tubes are the preferred device for long-term enteral nutrition for those patients who are unable to tolerate adequate nutritional intake orally. The use of PEG tubes in palliative medicine is controversial. Decisions about their use must involve assessment of the underlying disease, consideration of the patient's wishes, and evaluation of nutritional needs. In conjunction with the family, a team approach is required to assess the benefits and burdens of nutrition support.

If malnutrition is preventing further treatment, then it should be properly assessed and addressed with nutrition support strategies, including PEG feeding. If other factors are apparent that make nutrition intervention futile, then it must be approached with caution. The patient's wishes are of paramount importance, because nutritional support may add extra burden.[26]

Eicosapentaenoic Acid

There is interest in high-dose eicosapentaenoic acid (EPA) to treat cachexia and weight loss in palliative care (Table 107-4). Most studies to date have been small and nonrandomized. Nutritional supplements containing specific ω-3 fatty acids EPA and docosahexaenoic acid (DHA) helped stabilize weight and lean body mass and improved QOL in patients with advanced pancreatic cancer.[27-29] These results were duplicated in a small study of 8 patients with pancreatic or non–small cell lung cancer who were receiving chemotherapy. Significant improvements in dietary intake, nutritional status, weight, lean body mass, functional capacity, and QOL were demonstrated over an 8-week period.[30] When initial pilot studies were conducted using EPA supplements in advanced pancreatic cancer, 2 g EPA per day was sufficient to potentiate anticachectic activity. Higher doses provided no added benefit.[28,31] A randomized, controlled trial over an 8-week period compared protein- and energy-dense supplement enriched with ω-3 fatty acids to an isocaloric isonitrogenous control supplement. A dose-response analysis revealed a net gain in weight and lean body mass and improved QOL in the group taking the ω-3 enriched supplement, provided that it was taken in sufficient quantities. The quantity required was a minimum of 1.5 cans per day (237 mL in each can).[29] Other randomized trials of shorter duration, comparing high-dose fish oils in capsules (1.8 g EPA and 1.2 g DHA) with placebo found no significant effects of the fish oils on appetite, tiredness, nausea, well-being, caloric intake, nutritional status, or function.[32] The combination of EPA combined with megestrol acetate, an appetite stimulant, was found to be no better than megestrol alone. This study was conducted for about 3 months, and outcomes included QOL, weight gain (10% above baseline), and survival. The researchers did not evaluate effects on lean body mass.[33]

It has been found that ω-3 and vitamin E supplements prolong survival and have immunomodulating effects in malnourished cancer patients.[34] Despite these results, there have been few well-controlled trials, and the addition of EPA in advanced disease needs further investigation.[35]

Antioxidants and Other Vitamins

Antioxidants, including selenium and vitamins A, C, and E, are frequently used by palliative patients, especially those with cancer. They are thought to protect the body against oxidative damage. There is some evidence supporting the role of antioxidants, as well as other vitamins such as selenium and folic acid, in chemoprevention, but there are few well-designed studies in advanced disease.

Some studies have examined antioxidants in motorneuron disease, but they have been criticized for their poor design, low numbers of participants, and short duration. Although there is no clinical trial evidence to support the use of antioxidants in motor neuron disease, there is no clear contraindication.[36] There is reason for caution in taking high doses of supplements. Some clinical trials in lung cancer unexpectedly found that high-dose β-carotene increased the incidence of lung cancer.[37,38]

Nutrient supplementation in low doses is indicated only if there is nutrient deficiency (e.g., B_{12} deficiency); if nutrient intake is below recommended values; to meet public health goals; or if there are known health sequelae from therapy.[39] Interesting data have emerged on folic acid and vitamin B_{12} in patients with advanced cancer receiving the folate-based anti-cancer drug pemetrexed. Administration of 1 mg vitamin B_{12} intramuscularly every

TABLE 107-4	Randomized Controlled Trials for Nutrition Intervention in Palliative Care (Cancer Trials)			
INTERVENTION	**AUTHOR**	**PATIENTS**	**TRIAL LENGTH**	**SIGNIFICANT OUTCOMES**
EPA vs. placebo (capsules)	Bruera et al, 2003	60 patients (mixed cancer types)	2 wk	No significant results
	Gogos et al, 1995	64 patients (mixed cancer types)	40 days	Increased survival with EPA; improved performance status
	Zuijdgeest Van Leeuwen et al, 2000	17 patients	7 days	No significant results
EPA ONS vs. ONS	Fearon et al, 2003	200 patients (mixed cancer types)	8 wk	*Attenuation of LBM in both arms
EPA alone vs. EPA + Megace vs. Megace alone	Jatoi et al, 2004	421 patients (mixed cancer types)	12 wk	No significant results

EPA, eicosapentaenoic acid; LBM, lean body mass; ONS, high-energy, high-protein oral nutritional supplement (EPA ONS contains EPA).
*Post hoc analysis of the Fearon 2003 study found a significant positive correlation in the EPA arm between supplement intake and increase in body weight, LBM, and QOL, if sufficient quantity of the EPA ONS were consumed.

6 weeks with 0.5 mg/day folic acid by mouth, commencing 1 week before chemotherapy, significantly reduced myelosuppression and lethal toxicity from pemetrexed.[40] These data may prompt re-evaluation of vitamin supplementation in palliative medicine.

REFERENCES

1. Andreyev HJ, Norman AR, Oates J, et al. Why do patients with weight loss have a worse outcome when undergoing chemotherapy for gastrointestinal malignancies? Eur J Cancer 1998;34:503-509.
2. Dewys WD, Begg C, Lavin PT, et al. Prognostic effect of weight loss prior to chemotherapy in cancer patients. Eastern Cooperative Oncology Group. Am J Med 1980;69:491-497.
3. von Gunten CF, Twaddle ML. Terminal care for noncancer patients. Clin Geriatr Med 1996;12:349-358.
4. Lennard-Jones J: A positive approach to nutrition as treatment: Report from working party chair. London: King's Fund Report, 1992.
5. Read JA, Choy ST, Beale PJ, et al. Evaluation of nutritional and inflammatory status of advanced colorectal cancer patients and its correlation with survival. Nutr Cancer 2006;55:78-85.
6. American Dietitians Association. Identifying patients at risk: ADA's definitions for nutrition screening and nutrition assessment. Council on Practice (COP) Quality Management Committee. J Am Diet Assoc 1994;94:838-839.
7. Ottery FD. Definition of standardized nutritional assessment and interventional pathways in oncology. Nutrition 1996;12(Suppl):S15-S19.
8. Ferguson M, Capra S, Bauer J, et al. Development of a valid and reliable malnutrition screening tool for adult acute hospital patients. Nutrition 1999;15:458-464.
9. Weekes CE, Elia M, Emery PW. The development, validation and reliability of a nutrition screening tool based on the recommendations of the British Association for Parenteral and Enteral Nutrition (BAPEN). Clin Nutr 2004; 23:1104-1112.
10. BAPEN Malnutrition Advisory Group. Screening Tool for Adults at Risk of Malnutrition. London: British Association for Parenteral and Eneral Nutrition, 2000.
11. Detsky AS, McLaughlin JR, Baker JP, et al. What is subjective global assessment of nutritional status? JPEN J Parenter Enteral Nutr 1987;11:8-13.
12. Stratton RJ, Hackston A, Longmore D, et al. Malnutrition in hospital outpatients and inpatients: Prevalence, concurrent validity and ease of use of the "Malnutrition Universal Dcreening Tool" ("MUST") for adults. Br J Nutr 2004; 92:799-808.
13. Guigoz Y, Vellas B, Garry PJ. Mini Nutritional Assessment: A practical assessment tool for grading the nutritional state of elderly patients. Facts Res Gerontol 1994;(Suppl):15-59.
14. Guigoz Y, Vellas B, Garry PJ. Assessing the nutritional status of the elderly: The Mini Nutritional Assessment as part of the geriatric evaluation. Nutr Rev 1996;54:(1 Suppl) 59-65.
15. Linn BS. A Protein Energy Malnutrition Scale (PEMS). Ann Surg 1984; 200:747-752.
16. Blackburn GL, Bistrian BR, Maini BS, et al. Nutritional and metabolic assessment of the hospitalized patient. JPEN J Parenter Enteral Nutr 1977;1:11-22.
17. Camps C, Iranzo V, Bremnes RM, et al. Anorexia-cachexia syndrome in cancer: Implications of the ubiquitin-proteasome pathway. Support Care Cancer 2006;14:1173-1183.
18. O'Brien T, Welsh J, Dunn FG. ABC of palliative care: Non-malignant conditions. BMJ 1998;316:286-289.
19. Cheville A. Rehabilitation of patients with advanced cancer. Cancer 2001;92:1039-1048.
20. Celli BR. Pulmonary rehabilitation for patients with advanced lung disease. Clin Chest Med 1997;18:521-534.
21. Oldervoll LM, Loge JH, Paltiel H, et al. The effect of a physical exercise program in palliative care: A phase II study. J Pain Symptom Manage 2006; 31:421-430.
22. Ovesen L, Allingstrup L, Hannibal J, et al. Effect of dietary counseling on food intake, body weight, response rate, survival, and quality of life in cancer patients undergoing chemotherapy: A prospective, randomized study. J Clin Oncol 1993;11:2043-2049.
23. Ravasco P, Monteiro-Grillo I, Vidal PM, et al. Dietary counseling improves patient outcomes: A prospective, randomized, controlled trial in colorectal cancer patients undergoing radiotherapy. J Clin Oncol 2005;23:1431-1438.
24. Isenring EA, Capra S, Bauer JD. Nutrition intervention is beneficial in oncology outpatients receiving radiotherapy to the gastrointestinal or head and neck area. Br J Cancer 2004;91:447-452.
25. Bauer J, Capra S, Battistutta D, et al. Compliance with nutrition prescription improves outcomes in patients with unresectable pancreatic cancer. Clin Nutr 2005;24:998-1004.
26. McKinlay AW. Nutritional support in patients with advanced cancer: Permission to fall out? Proc Nutr Soc 2004;63:431-435.
27. Barber MD, Ross JA, Voss AC, et al. The effect of an oral nutritional supplement enriched with fish oil on weight-loss in patients with pancreatic cancer. Br J Cancer 1999;81:80-86.
28. Wigmore SJ, Barber MD, Ross JA, et al. Effect of oral eicosapentaenoic acid on weight loss in patients with pancreatic cancer. Nutr Cancer 2000;36:177-184.
29. Fearon KC, Von Meyenfeldt MF, Moses AG, et al. Effect of a protein and energy dense N-3 fatty acid enriched oral supplement on loss of weight and lean tissue in cancer cachexia: A randomised double blind trial. Gut 2003;52:1479-1486.
30. Bauer JD, Capra S. Nutrition intervention improves outcomes in patients with cancer cachexia receiving chemotherapy: A pilot study. Support Care Cancer 2005;13:270-274.
31. Wigmore SJ, Ross JA, Falconer JS, et al. The effect of polyunsaturated fatty acids on the progress of cachexia in patients with pancreatic cancer. Nutrition 1996;12:S27-S30.
32. Bruera E, Strasser F, Palmer JL, et al. Effect of fish oil on appetite and other symptoms in patients with advanced cancer and anorexia/cachexia: A double-blind, placebo-controlled study. J Clin Oncol 2003;21:129-134.
33. Jatoi A, Rowland K, Loprinzi CL, et al. An eicosapentaenoic acid supplement versus megestrol acetate versus both for patients with cancer-associated wasting: A North Central Cancer Treatment Group and National Cancer Institute of Canada collaborative effort. J Clin Oncol 2004;22:2469-2476.
34. Gogos CA, Ginopoulos P, Zoumbos NC, et al. The effect of dietary omega-3 polyunsaturated fatty acids on T-lymphocyte subsets of patients with solid tumors. Cancer Detect Prev 1995;19:415-417.
35. Dewey A, Baughan C, Dean T, et al. Eicosapentaenoic acid (EPA, an omega-3 fatty acid from fish oils) for the treatment of cancer cachexia. Cochrane Database Syst Rev 2007;(1):CD004597.
36. Orrell R, Lane R, Ross M. Antioxidant treatment for amyotrophic lateral sclerosis/motor neuron disease. Cochrane Database Syst Rev 2005;(1): CD002829.
37. The Alpha Tocopherol Beta Carotene Cancer Prevention Study Group. The effect of vitamin E and beta carotene on the incidence of lung cancer and other cancers in male smokers. N Engl J Med 1994;330:1029-1035.
38. Omenn GS, Goodman GE, Thornquist MD, et al. Effects of a combination of beta carotene and vitamin A on lung cancer and cardiovascular disease. N Engl J Med 1996;334:1150-1155.
39. Doyle C, Kushi LH, Byers T, et al. Nutrition and physical activity during and after cancer treatment: An American Cancer Society guide for informed choices. CA Cancer J Clin 2006;56:323-353.
40. Niyikiza C, Hanauske AR, Rusthoven JJ, et al. Pemetrexed safety and dosing strategy. Semin Oncol 2002;29:24-29.
41. Zuijdgeest-Van Leeuwen SD, Dagnelie PC, Wattimena JL, et al. Eicosapentaenoic acid ethyl ester supplementation in cachectic cancer patients and healthy subjects: Effects on lipolysis and lipid oxidation. Clin Nutr 2000;19:417-423.

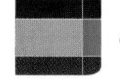

CHAPTER **108**

Principles and Management of Nutritional Support in Cancer

Federico Bozzetti and Valentina Bozzetti

KEY POINTS

- Malnutrition-cachexia adversely affects response to therapy, quality of life, and survival.

- Nutritional support partially prevents further nutritional deterioration, replenishes tissue, and may improve quality of life and survival in incurable but nonmoribund patients.

- The principles of nutritional support are similar for cancer and noncancer patients.

- Parenteral and enteral nutrition are metabolically similar; the enteral route is simpler and cheaper but less acceptable.

- The effects of nutritional support are potentiated by anticachectic agents.

- Supplements enriched with ω-3 polyunsaturated fatty acids (N-3 PUFA) are useful if tolerated.

If palliation means relief of symptoms without removing the etiological factors at their origin, as the reference to the original term *pallium* (a Roman square vest) would indicate, then artificial nutrition is infrequently palliative, because fewer than 50% of cancer patients with incurable advanced malignancy experience hunger or unmet needs for nutrition.[1,2] Focusing only on the relationship between nutritional support and quality of life (QOL) is limiting, because good nutrition is essential not only to QOL but also to survival. It is appropriate from theory and clinical practice to consider both aspects.

To properly approach the potential role of nutritional support in advanced cancer, it is important to differentiate two groups of advanced cancer patients: (1) those who are "terminal" (i.e., they have exhausted available oncological therapy), with a life expectancy of several months, and more or less symptomatic and (2) those who are "biologically terminal," with survival limited to a few weeks (or less) regardless of the stage of cancer and any further therapies. Because of the inherent ambiguity of the word "terminal," the former group could be simply defined as *incurable*, and the latter, *moribund*. This distinction, which reflects clinical status and the natural history of the disease, is fundamental because nutritional support has a role only in some incurable patients but none in the moribund. Controversies among specialists about nutritional support in advanced cancer are the result of differing interpretations of the word "terminal."

BASIC SCIENCE

Nutrition and Quality of Life

There is a cause-effect relation between nutrition and QOL,[3] derived from experimental long-term semistarvation in humans. Weight loss is associated with poor QOL in cancers of the breast, ovary, lung,[4] and gastrointestinal tract and pancreas tumors.[5,6] Weight loss plus low prealbumin levels, and abnormal anthropometric measures plus low prealbumin and albumin levels, are associated with poor QOL in surgical patients[7] and in patients with upper gastrointestinal cancers receiving home enteral nutrition.[8] We found a clear association between weight loss and fatigue, a determinant of QOL, among 1000 outpatients undergoing nutritional screening (Table 108-1).

A major study of 271 cancer patients[9] quantified the relative contributions of cancer, nutrition, and treatment to QOL. The investigators found that QOL scores were determined in 30% of the patients by cancer location, in 20% by nutrition, in 30% by weight loss, in 10% by chemotherapy, in 6% by surgery, in 3% by disease duration, and in 1% by stage of disease. In the symptom scales, only 7% and 1% of symptoms were attributed to nutrition and weight loss, respectively.

Starvation and Survival

Total starvation is incompatible with survival. Exhaustion of protein mass is the major determinant in mortality from starvation. Release of proteins may be reduced by adequate fat stores, which enables obese subjects to survive starvation for up to 1 year. As starvation progresses, continuous nitrogen loss, despite fat reserves, causes death from myofibril fragmentation and other lean mass organ depletion. In healthy adults, nitrogen loss critical for survival occurs after loss of 33% to 37% of the usual or ideal weight (i.e., after 60 to 75 days of starvation), as was demonstrated by the tragic experiences of the Leningrad siege, the Warsaw Ghetto, and the Irish hunger strikes (Table 108-2). The net nitrogen loss in cancer patients is intermediate between that of starvation and starvation with infection. Cancer patients may already be depleted at initial evaluation when they are considered for potential nutritional support.

EPIDEMIOLOGY AND PREVALENCE

Prevalence of Malnutrition and Cachexia-Related Death

The prevalence of cachexia ranges from 8% to 84%, depending on the cancer site and disease stage. Estimates of the prevalence of malnutrition in specific cancers include the following:

- Approximately 9% in urological cancer
- Up to 15% in gynecological cancer
- Up to 33% in colorectal cancer
- Up to 46% in lung cancer
- Up to 67% in head and neck cancer
- Up to 57% to 80% in esophageal or gastrointestinal cancer
- Up to 85% in pancreatic cancer

Cachexia, the main determinant of fatal outcome, ranges from 5% to 23% in advanced cancer. Decreased energy intake and weight loss predict shorter survival in advanced cancer.[10]

PATHOPHYSIOLOGY

Rationale for Nutritional Support

The progressive involuntary weight loss of cancer wasting is a complex, multifactorial syndrome that occurs through

TABLE 108-1 Weight Loss (%) in Relation to Fatigue		
FATIGUE	**MEDIAN LOSS**	**MEAN LOSS**
Absent	2.6	4.0
Mild	7.5	8.9
Moderate	13.0	13.1
Severe	15.2	15.2

TABLE 108-2 Lean Mass Depletion in Pathological Conditions			
CLINICAL CONDITION	**NITROGEN LOSS (g/DAY)**	**Time (days) Required for Loss of 30%**	
		MUSCULAR MASS	**BODY CELL MASS**
Chronic starvation	3	82	139
Infection coupled with starvation	15	10	21
Severe sepsis or trauma	20	13	20

various mechanisms associated with the tumor, host response to the tumor, and treatment. Cachexia cannot be equated with simple starvation. Recent research has identified the role of cytokines in anorexia and metabolic aberrations affecting energy and protein metabolism. These account for the poor response of weight-losing cancer patients to nutritional support. Nevertheless, provision of macronutrients and micronutrients remains essential even when anticachectic therapy is available. Patients with advanced cancer are potential candidates for artificial nutrition if they are unable to eat, or severely malnourished, or both. The importance of nutritional support and maintenance of nutritional status must be defined within the context of the symptom profile and the complexity of antitumor treatments.

Nutritional support includes both sophisticated total parenteral nutrition (TPN) and simpler enteral nutrition (EN) or through sip feeding. The more demanding, expensive, and complex a treatment is, the more specific must be the recommendations. The clinician should consider the following questions in individual cases:

1. What would change for this patient, who is currently unable to eat and malnourished or with incipient malnutrition, should nutritional status be maintained or improved by artificial nutrition? This requires an estimate of life expectancy and the impact on QOL.
2. If nutritional support is indicated, what would be the best way of administering it, and what would be the best regimen?

IMPROVED SURVIVAL AND QUALITY OF LIFE

Survival

Artificial nutrition can prolong survival only if death will occur earlier from starvation rather than tumor. Hypophagic, relatively nonsymptomatic, patients with gastrointestinal obstruction who have acceptable performance status, are without vital organ involvement, and have a life expectancy exceeding 3 months can be reasonably expected to benefit. Most candidates for TPN are those with peritoneal carcinomatosis from slow-growing tumors (ovarian tumors and some neuroendocrine, gastrointestinal, and retroperitoneal malignancies). Those suitable for EN via gastrostomy or jejunostomy are mainly affected by recurrent head and neck tumors that cause severe hypophagia or odynophagia.

Prognosis at the end of life is known to be inaccurate. Clinical prediction of survival is subjective, inherently nonreproducible, more than twice as likely to be overoptimistic rather than overpessimistic, and overestimates actual survival by a factor of 3 to 5.[11] It is also subject to the "horizon effect"—that is, short-term predictions have greater accuracy than long-term ones. Clinical prediction of survival should be used with other prognostic factors, including performance status, symptoms (e.g., anorexia, weight loss, dysphagia and xerostomia, dyspnea, cognitive impairment) and some biological factors (leucocytosis, lymphocytopenia, and C-reactive protein levels).

A systematic review[12] of eight studies (1563 patients) showed that, when clinically predicted survival was 4 months, actual survival time was about 2 months; like-

wise, when predicted survival was 6 months, only 15% of the patients survived that long. Six months is an unlikely time frame for hypophagic subjects with far-advanced cancer. Many aphagic patients with incurable cancer (i.e., with an estimated 6-month life expectancy) for whom we recommend artificial nutrition will die before 6 months due to early tumor progression. It is noteworthy that some of the relevant variables, such as anorexia, dysphagia, and weight loss, are not simply predictive but may be responsible for progressive clinical deterioration. Their effects may be counteracted by appropriate nutritional support and therefore have limited application in all potential candidates for artificial nutrition because in such conditions, they might prove to be poorly predictive of the outcome.

Quality of Life

Nutrition is an important part of daily life, because food is more than just simple intake of nutrients. It is an integral part of social, religious, and economic life, including the creation and expression of relationships. The cultural and symbolic value of nourishment, traditionally viewed as an expression of love and care for both the living and the dying, has led some clinicians (16% of internists) to consider nutrition as basic human care.[13] Physicians see nourishment as a "medical treatment" aimed at physiological objectives, but families see feeding as an "act of community."[14] Changes in nutrition have important effects on the lives of patients and their families.

Both patients and their relatives fear that inadequate food intake will lead to death by starvation: "[P]atients reported wanting and trying to eat, but being unable to do so. Family members experienced powerlessness and frustration, as they could not enable the patient to eat."[15] Moreover, patients and relatives see the possibility of parenteral nutrition at home as a relief and a positive alternative. If it is true that "quality of life is a reflection of the difference at a given moment between the hopes and the expectations of an individual and the individual's present experience,"[16] provision of nutritional support may improve QOL. Therefore, in many advanced (but not moribund) cancer patients, nutritional support must not be seen as forced nutrition of those who do not need nutritional palliation (because they are neither hungry nor thirsty), but "as a necessary prerequisite for life since patients feared wasting away when relying on their own oral intake."[15]

TREATMENT

Nutritional Regimen

If the goal of artificial nutrition is to maintain or restore nutritional status, because tumor progression is slow and the patient is asymptomatic despite the threat of malnutrition and hypophagia, then macronutrient and micronutrient requirements should be considered. Particular care must be paid to the composition of parenteral formulations, because those receiving TPN are totally dependent on the intravenously administered substrates and usually are sicker than patients who are fed enterally.

Water

Cancer patients frequently have metabolic disturbances that dictate water restriction. Water intake of about 30 mL/kg/day is appropriate, and sodium intake should not exceed 1 mmol/kg/day. The following considerations apply to determining water needs:

1. Cachexia is often associated with expansion of extracellular water volume.
2. Candidates for TPN often have peritoneal carcinomatosis and subclinical ascites, which can worsen with overzealous administration of water, glucose, and sodium. Glucose reduces renal sodium excretion and, consequently, loss of extracellular fluid. Insulin is the most probable mediator of sodium retention, perhaps through increased sympathetic activity.
3. In cancer patients, there may be excessive production of antidiuretic hormone (ADH) due to the tumor, the nausea that frequently occurs in advanced disease, or administration of morphine. The wasting syndrome associated with loss of intracellular water and solutes affects hypothalamic osmoreceptor cells to stimulate ADH release to maintain subnormal serum osmolality and serum sodium levels. Clearance of free water is decreased, additionally because the urea load to the kidney is reduced due to protein malnutrition. Synthesis of endogenous water is maintained by oxidation of carbohydrates and fats, and insensible water loss drops because of reduced physical activity.
4. It is easier to replenish a dehydrated patient than to relieve an overly hydrated patient through the use of diuretics.

Energy

Cancer patients may be hypometabolic, normometabolic, or hypermetabolic. When energy expenditure is expressed based on unit of body cell mass some are hypermetabolic. Physical activity accounts for about 25% of total energy expenditure, and dietary-induced thermogenesis about 5%. Most people affected by far-advanced malignancy are confined to bed or to a chair and are hypophagic, so an energy supply of between 20 and 30 kcal/kg/day is advised.

Because cancer patients utilize fat better than glucose (the opposite occurs in tumor cells), we prefer a fat-enriched regimen, which also has less impact on water metabolism. For instance, a regimen not exceeding 1.5 g/kg/day of fat plus 3.6 g/kg/day of glucose provides 13.5 plus 13.5 kcal/kg/day. This represents a good compromise to avoid both the side effects of glucose and the toxicity from fat overload. Medium-chain/long-chain triglyceride emulsions and those enriched with ω-3 polyunsaturated fatty acids (N3-PUFA) are preferable to reduce fat toxicity in long-term intravenous administration and overproduction of eicosanoids. The desired parenteral mixture can be easily prepared, but it may be more difficult to find the corresponding enteral formulation, so one must rely on N3-PUFA–enriched feedings.

Protein

A supply of 1 to 2 g/kg/day of protein is acceptable, provided that the blood urea nitrogen (BUN) level is normal.

Micronutrients

Micronutrients are administered in the usual doses. Concern for correcting potential deficiencies or preventing them is greater than the fear of stimulating tumor growth. Tumor growth proceeds at a high, uncontrolled rate regardless of exogenous substrates.

Choice between Enteral and Parenteral Nutrition

There is substantial nutritional equivalence between the two types of artificial nutrition. Both TPN and EN may blunt catabolic drive and promote gain of tissue, especially with coadministration of anabolic/anticatabolic agents. A common outcome, depending on cachexia severity and duration of nutritional support, is prevention of further deterioration in nutritional status. There are significant differences between TPN and EN, however.

- TPN is passive. Patients do not realize that they are receiving 1000 to 2000 or more calories per day because it may be administered in a small volume over a 24-hour period. If they have central venous catheters for other purposes, they may not know whether they are receiving therapy, nutrition, or both.
- In contrast, EN may be "forced" nutrition. Patients may not tolerate beyond a certain enteral volume due to satiety. Because the liquid enteral formula cannot be manipulated and concentrated, there is a critical volume of about 1500 mL/day to avoid deficiency of minerals and vitamins. Compliance with a feeding ostomy (or a nasogastric tube) may be less than with a central venous catheter, which appears more friendly and familiar.
- TPN can be delivered under all conditions, whereas EN requires an accessible and working gut. The concept of a working gut is broad: it means not only the capability of the gut to digest and absorb nutrients but also the ability to tolerate the desired volume in 24 hours.
- TPN is a more expensive and demanding procedure and is associated with potentially more severe complications than EN. Complications with TPN (i.e., hyperglycemia), can nevertheless be corrected without interruption more easily than with EN (i.e., if vomiting or diarrhea occurs).
- The most common approach is to use EN (especially for long-term nutritional support) and then switch to TPN if there is noncompliance or the gut is not working.

OUTCOME OF ARTIFICIAL NUTRITION

Data on the outcome of artificial nutrition mainly refer to TPN and EN administered in the home (Table 108-3; Fig. 108-1). Survival depends largely on the basic disease. However, many series mixed together patients with sequelae of cancer (radiation enteropathy, chronic surgical complications or mutilations), patients with active cancer receiving oncological therapy, and patients with incurable cancer. This makes it difficult to analyze the potential effect of home TPN and EN on survival. Nevertheless, one third to one fourth of patients survive longer with home TPN or EN than they would have with total

TABLE 108-3   Survival of Cancer Patients Receiving Home Total Parenteral Nutrition (TPN) or Home Enteral Nutrition (EN)

AUTHOR, REF. NO., AND YEAR OF PUBLICATION	PERIOD OF STUDY	NO. OF PATIENTS	SURVIVAL
HOME TPN			
Howard (1993)	1985-1990	1672	28% at 1 yr; median 6 mo; mean 4 mo
Howard et al. (1996)	1985-1992	2122	37% at 1 yr
Messing et al. (1998)	1993-1995	524	19.5% at 6 mo
Van Gossum et al. (1999)	1997	200	26% at 6-12 mo
Howard (2000)	1984-1988	1073	25% at 1 yr; median 6 mo
SINPE Register* (2004)	1980-2003	1103	20% at 1 yr; median 6 mo
HOME EN			
Howard (1993)	1985-1990	1296	32% at 1 yr; median 6 mo; mean 6 mo
Howard et al. (1996)	1989-1992	1644	41% at 1 yr
Gaggiotti et al. (2001)	1992-1999	3690	Means: head-neck, 18.3%; esophagus-stomach, 13.5%; colon-rectum, 21.8%; biliary, 16.8%; lung, 10.7%

*Courtesy of Dr. A. Palmo.
Adapted from reference 17, where full citations for all references cited in the table can be found.

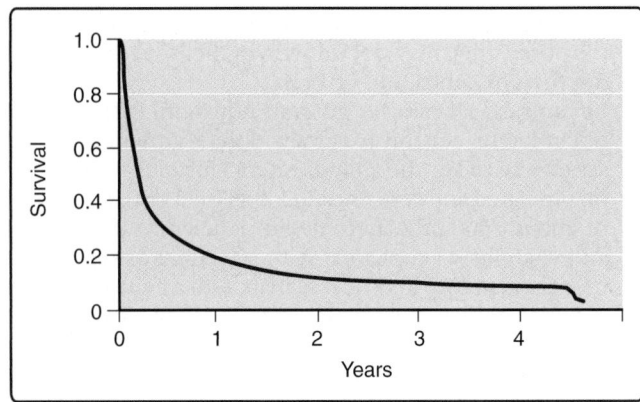

FIGURE 108-1   Survival of incurable cancer patients receiving home total parenteral nutrition.

starvation. Results are better for EN than for TPN, reflecting that those patients who can tolerate EN are, as a group, less severely ill than those fed intravenously. Data on QOL are scanty but show that it may be maintained or improved until 2 to 3 months before death.[18] The practical conclusion is that benefit in terms of survival and QOL may be expected only if the patient can survive, thanks to TPN, despite tumor progression, for longer than 3 to 4 months.

ORAL SUPPLEMENTATION WITH EICOSAPENTAENOIC ACID

Some weight-losing patients with incurable cancer can be fed by mouth. Anorexia is common in advanced disease and often precludes adequate oral nutrition. Medical oncologists refrain from treating those who are severely hypophagic; they may be supported nutritionally with oral supplements. Administration of eicosapentaenoic acid (EPA) supplements[19] is associated with increased energy and protein intake and increased lean body mass. There is a positive correlation between EPA supplementation and increased body weight and QOL. A 8-week randomized clinical trial of EPA in pancreatic cancer reported a longer median survival time (142 days) than with a standard supplement (128 days). Some benefits were not apparent in the "intention-to-treat" analysis because of poor compliance with EPA supplementation and the EPA optimal threshold dose.

CONTROVERSIES

The controversy about artificial nutrition concerns the indications. It is accepted that patients with benign intestinal failure survive "thanks to" TPN, whereas those with malignant obstruction die "despite" TPN.

Another major problem is the withdrawal of TPN. Although most ethicists have concluded that any distinction between withholding and withdrawing treatment is morally incoherent, many physicians feel ethically justified in withholding treatments they never started, but not withholding treatments already initiated. Physicians also find it easier to limit resuscitative efforts or therapies that support organs that have failed naturally (noniatrogenic), and recent interventions rather than long-standing treatments. In these cases, only open and frank dialogue with the patient and family can clarify from the beginning the expectations regarding artificial nutrition. Maintenance should occur only if outcomes meet these expectations.

PERSPECTIVES

The future goals of research in this field include the following:

- Better definition of life expectancy (duration and quality)
- Use of substrates that are not only "simple nutrients" but "metabolically cancer-specific nutrients"
- Better comprehension of the true needs of the patient with incurable cancer and tailoring of any treatment to the individual expectations

- Consideration of nutritional support in early disease. Biochemical markers of cachexia are present long before the clinical onset of symptoms.

REFERENCES

1. McCann RM, Hall WJ, Groth-Juncker A. Comfort care for terminally ill patients: The appropriate use of nutrition and hydration. JAMA 1994;272:1263-1266.
2. Morasso G, Capelli M, Viterbori P, et al. Psychological and symptom distress in terminal cancer patients with met and unmet needs. J Pain Symptom Manage 1999;17:402-409.
3. Keys A, Brozek J, Henschel A, et al. The biology of human starvation. Minneapolis: University of Minnesota Press, 1950.
4. Ovesen L, Allingstrup L, Hannibal J, et al. Effect of dietary counseling on food intake, body weight, response rate, survival, and quality of life in cancer patients undergoing chemotherapy: A prospective, randomized study. J Clin Oncol 1993;11:2043-2049.
5. Andreyev HJ, Norman AR, Oates J, Cunningham D. Why do patients with weight loss have a worse outcome when undergoing chemotherapy for gastrointestinal malignancies? Eur J Cancer 1998;34:503-509.
6. O'Gorman P, McMillan DC, McArdle CS. Impact of weight loss, appetite, and the inflammatory response on quality of life in gastrointestinal cancer patients. Nutr Cancer 1998;32:76-80.
7. Larsson J, Akerlind I, Permerth J, Hornqvist JO. The relation between nutritional state and quality of life in surgical patients. Eur J Surg 1994; 160:329-334.
8. Loeser C, von Herz U, Kuchler T, et al. Quality of life and nutritional state in patients on home enteral tube feeding. Nutrition 2003;19:605-611.
9. Ravasco P, Monteiro-Grillo I, Vidal PM, Camilo ME. Cancer: Disease and nutrition are key determinants of patients' quality of life. Support Care Cancer 2004;12:246-252.
10. Bosaeus I, Daneryd P, Lundholm K. Dietary intake, resting energy expenditure, weight loss and survival in cancer patients. J Nutr 2002;132(11 Suppl):3465S-3466S.
11. Maltoni M, Caraceni A, Brunelli C, et al.; Steering Committee of the European Association for Palliative Care. Prognostic factors in advanced cancer patients: Evidence-based clinical recommendations. A study by the Steering Committee of the European Association for Palliative Care. J Clin Oncol. 2005; 23:6240-6248.
12. Glare P, Virik K, Jones M, et al. A systematic review of physicians' survival predictions in terminally ill cancer patients. BMJ 2003;327:195.
13. Hodges MO, Tolle SW, Stocking C, Cassel CK. Tube feeding: Internists' attitudes regarding ethical obligations. Arch Intern Med 1994;154:1013-1020.
14. Miles SH. Futile tube feeding at the end of life: Family virtues and treatment decisions. Theor Med 1989;8:293-302.
15. Orrevall Y, Tishelman C, Herrington MK, Permert J. The path from oral nutrition to home parenteral nutrition: A qualitative interview study of the experiences of advanced cancer patients and their families. Clin Nutr 2004; 23:1280-1287.
16. Calman KC. Quality of life in cancer patients: An hypothesis. J Med Ethics 1984;10:124-127.
17. Bozzetti F, Bozzetti V. Efficacy of enteral and parenteral nutrition in cancer patients. In Lochs H and Thomas DR (eds). Home Care Enteral Feeding. Basel: Karger, 2004, pp 127-143.
18. Bozzetti F, Cozzaglio L, Biganzoli E, et al. Quality of life and length of survival in advanced cancer patients on home parenteral nutrition. Clin Nutr 2002;21:281-288.
19. Elia M, Van Bokhorst-de van der Schueren MA, Garvey J, et al. Enteral (oral or tube administration) nutritional support and eicosapentaenoic acid in patients with cancer: A systematic review. Int J Oncol 2006;28:5-23.

SUGGESTED READING

Bozzetti F. Total parenteral nutrition in cancer patients. Curr Opin Supp Pall Care 2007;4:281-286.

Bozzetti F. Home parenteral nutrition in cancer patient. In Bozzetti F, Staun M, Von Gossum A (eds). Home Parenteral Nutrition. Wallingford, UK: CABI Publishing, 2007.

Bozzetti F, Amadori D, Bruera E, et al. Guidelines on artificial nutrition versus hydration in terminal cancer patients. European Association for Palliative Care. Nutrition 1996;12: 163-167.

Stratton RJ, Green CJ, Elia M. Disease-related malnutrition: An evidence-based approach to treatment. Wallingford, UK: CABI Publishing, 2003.

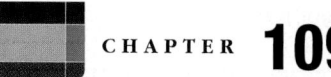

CHAPTER **109**

Nutrition in Palliative Medicine

Bart Van den Eynden, Noël Derycke, and Lucas Ceulemans

KEY POINTS

- The cancer cachexia-anorexia syndrome is a symptom complex that includes anorexia, weight loss, early satiety, anemia, asthenia, tissue wasting, and organ dysfunction.

- The aim of nutritional counseling and therapy is to improve quality of life.

- Total parenteral nutrition does not improve survival of any cancer patient and may produce net harm.

- Scientific research does not demonstrate that artificial fluid administration leads to greater comfort for advanced cancer patients or improves the functional status of patients with terminal illness.

- Hydration should always be considered in the context of the total care of a patient with advanced disease; acceptance of dehydration and administration of fluid and rehydration can be part of careful involvement in the well-being of the dying person.

- Good communication is crucial condition for high-quality food and fluid management of a cancer patient.

NUTRITION AND CANCER

The impact of cancer and antitumor treatment on nutrition can be disastrous. The *cancer cachexia-anorexia syndrome* is a symptom complex that includes anorexia, weight loss, early satiety, anemia, asthenia, tissue wasting, and organ dysfunction. It occurs most often in patients with pancreatic, gastric, and esophageal cancers and least often in those with breast cancer and non-Hodgkin's lymphomas. Cachexia in cancer patients is caused by factors such as decreased nutritional intake, increased nutritional losses, abnormalities of substrate metabolism, and effects of antitumor treatment.

Anorexia affects 80% of terminal cancer patients. Decreased nutritional intake affects patients with gastrointestinal tract malfunction, mainly those with cancers of the oral cavity, esophagus, stomach, and pancreas, and patients with psychological factors such as depression, grief, and anxiety and those with learned food aversions.

Increased nutritional loss can result from bleeding, protein losses through the intestine, diarrhea, and tumor-related catabolism. Tumor-related catabolism often is unimportant because only metabolically active tumors weighing more than 1.4 kg can consume more than 15% of daily caloric intake.[1]

Metabolic abnormalities can cause cachexia. Cancer patients often have increased energy expenditures and changes in carbohydrate, lipid, and protein metabolism. Nutrition is affected by surgery (i.e., negative nitrogen balance), chemotherapy (i.e., nausea, vomiting, and muco-esophagitis), and radiotherapy (i.e., anorexia, dysphagia, xerostomia, and colitis).

Malnutrition in the cancer patient has important consequences. Survival is shorter when there is weight loss, protein depletion, impaired immunocompetence, and poor wound healing. Death occurs when 30% to 50% of body protein stores are lost.

NUTRITIONAL ASSESSMENT

The history and physical examination are important in assessing the patient's nutritional status. The history should elicit information about the rate and extent of weight loss (>10% of body weight over 3 months suggests malnutrition); symptoms of malabsorption; food allergies; special problems such as nausea, vomiting, and swallowing problems; use of medications; alcohol consumption; and learned food aversion. During the physical examination, the clinician should pay special attention to the skin (e.g., dry, atrophic), to cheilosis and glossitis or other signs for vitamin deficiency, to muscle wasting and loss of muscle strength, and to pitting edema.

The results of laboratory tests can help determine management goals. For example, if the serum level of albumin is less than 3.4 g/dL, increased morbidity and mortality can be expected. A level of less than 3.0 g/dL indicates significant visceral protein depletion.

NUTRITIONAL THERAPY

Principles

Goals of therapy include prevention or reversal of nutritional deficits, increasing treatment response rates and survival, improving quality of life, and palliating symptoms. Factors affecting nutritional strategy include the ability to chew and swallow, ability to digest and absorb enteral nutrition, compliance, family support, and costs.

Indications for Nutritional Therapy

Nutritional therapy is indicated for malnourished cancer patients or those expected to become malnourished during their disease (e.g., chemotherapy with severe gastrointestinal dysfunction). Total parenteral nutrition decreases operative morbidity and mortality, but it does not improve survival of cancer patients and may produce net harm.[2]

Routes of Administration

The route of administration of nutritional therapy primarily is based on gastrointestinal tract functional status. If the gastrointestinal tract is normal, enteral feeding is always preferred to prevent mucosal atrophy, preserve gut flora, and maintain immune status. It is normally the most comfortable way and has fewer complications. Oral treatment is warranted for anyone unable to ingest sufficient nutrients.

The diet should deal with specific problems of oral feeding such as anorexia, nausea, changes in taste sensitivity, mucositis, xerostomia, constipation, and other distressing symptoms. For example, patients with xerostomia may use chewing gum to stimulate saliva, rinse the mouth with soda water or tea with lemon, use artificial saliva before meals, apply gravy or broth to moisten food, and avoid foods likely to cause dental caries.

The prescribed diet should reflect the pathophysiology, as in the following examples:

- Gastric resection: five or six small meals, separation of liquids from solids, restricted monocarbohydrates and lactose-containing foods, iron supplements and parenteral vitamin B_{12}
- Pancreatic insufficiency: low-fat diet, pancreatic enzymes
- Esophageal strictures and stenosis: soft diet, emphasis on liquids or high-caloric nutritional supplements

A dietician is asked to provide instructions regarding specific foods, size and frequency of meals, and other details.

Enteral feeding is indicated for people unable to ingest sufficient nutrients but whose gastrointestinal function is adequate for digestion and absorption (e.g., severe anorexia, upper gastrointestinal cancer). The routes of administration include nasogastric tubes, which are most commonly suitable for short-term use in the hospital; gastrostomy tubes placed endoscopically under local anesthesia (causes less diarrhea than a jejunostomy); and a jejunostomy tube when there is a proximal gastrointestinal obstruction or fistula. To avoid diarrhea, feeding should begin with small volumes, which are gradually increased over 3 to 4 days. Antidiarrheals are not needed.

For patients with an intact gastrointestinal tract, enteral feeding solutions requiring full digestion may be used. They contain whole proteins, fats as triglycerides, and long-chain carbohydrates. For patients with maldigestion, malabsorption, and rapid gastrointestinal transit, solutions requiring partial digestion are used. They contain lower percentages of protein and fat.

NUTRITIONAL SUPPORT FOR THE TERMINALLY ILL

Principles

There is no evidence that improving nutritional intake in patients with advanced cancer helps morbidity or mortality. The aim of nutritional counseling and therapy is to improve quality of life by maximizing enjoyment from eating (e.g., taste, social contact).

Loss of appetite is often distressing. The family members worry that "the patient is not eating enough," and the patient also may be concerned. Fears, myths, and misunderstanding often can be addressed by providing information:

- Fluid is not the same as food.
- Dehydration does not mean suffering.
- Force-feeding a dying patient only tires the patient.
- Eating does not reverse the underlying process.
- Loss of interest in food is a natural occurrence near death.
- The body takes only what it needs.
- Reduced food intake does not shorten life; it is simply a sign the body can no longer metabolize food.

Commercial nutritional supplements should be avoided because supplements suppress appetite, they are boring and unpalatable, they replace foods the patient enjoys, and there is no evidence that they improve the patient's health status. There is no place for total parenteral nutrition in managing patients with metastatic cancer and other poor-prognosis diseases.

Specific Strategies

The management team should rule out reversible causes of anorexia, such as constipation, nausea, mouth discomfort, pain, electrolyte disturbances, and depression.

Taste abnormalities may be addressed by reducing the diet urea content (e.g., less red meat, more eggs and dairy products), marinating meats before cooking and seasoning well to disguise bitter taste, serving foods at room temperature (not hot), trying tart foods, and encouraging fluids with meals.

Patients with anorexia should be given permission to eat less. Small, frequent feedings often are preferred, and smaller plates should be used for smaller helpings. The patient should be involved in menu planning, and personal food preferences should be respected. Food should be available whenever patients are hungry. For regular meals, have patients dress and sit at the table if possible. Avoid strong cooking smells at mealtimes.

Appetite stimulants may be used by patients with anorexia. The best appetite stimulant is food the patient likes, and a glass of sherry or wine may be appreciated. Multivitamin supplements and dexamethasone, megestrol acetate, medroxyprogesterone, or dronabinol (when available) may be used so stimulate appetite. For the patient with gastroparesis, a prokinetic such as metoclopramide or domperidone can help.

The management team can identify and help to remedy the social consequences of cachexia. For example, dental relining restores chewing ability and improves facial appearance. New, well-fitting clothes may be appreciated by the patient who has lost weight. These patients should not be weighed.

DEHYDRATION IN TERMINAL ILLNESS

Terminal dehydration is a negative fluid balance that occurs during the last days of life. Dehydration is clinically evident as diminished skin turgor, dry mucous membranes, shrunken eyes, tachycardia, and orthostatic hypotension that may lead to shock. Symptoms are dry mouth, thirst, apathy and lethargy, depression, confusion and delirium, headache, dysphagia, swallowing problems, nausea, vomiting, and muscle cramps. [3]

There are different kinds of dehydration: hypertonic, hypotonic, and isotonic. [4] However, in a terminal context, these types are less relevant and often unclear. Terminal hydration differs quantitatively and qualitatively from dehydration in a general clinical context. Symptoms can be a sign of dehydration or of the terminal condition.

Consequences

Dehydration causes several physiological phenomena, which may not always be negative in advanced disease. [5] Unfavorable consequences include the following:

- Severe electrolyte disturbance (e.g., acidosis, hypernatremia, hypercalcemia) that causes apathy, depression, confusion, neuromuscular hyperactivity, and muscle cramps
- Postural hypotension, increasing the risk of falls
- Hypovolemia with diminished skin blood flow and blood viscosity, increased risk for deep venous thrombosis, pulmonary embolism, and decubitus ulcers
- Lack of water causing headache, nausea, and muscle cramps
- Diminished urine production with dysuria and risk for urinary infections
- Fewer gastrointestinal secretions, with constipation, gastrointestinal pain, and discomfort

Favorable consequences [6] include the following:

- Electrolyte disturbances inducing analgesia (even lethargy and coma, considered favorable in some)
- Increased production of ketones from caloric deprivation, leading to anesthesia
- Decreased pulmonary secretions, leading to less coughing, tracheal secretion, rattle, and pulmonary edema (dyspnea decreases, and suction is needed less)
- Less urine production, reducing incontinence (in some, bladder cauterization can be avoided and less turning is needed)
- Fewer gastrointestinal secretions, diminishing nausea and vomiting
- Diminished edema peripherally and around the tumor, causing less pain and local tension
- Opioid accumulation, which helps analgesia

Management

Hypodermoclysis is an acceptable technique in palliative care. [6-8] Fluid is given subcutaneously. It is effective, simple, cheap, and comfortable for the patient, who is given 500 to 1500 mL of fluid each day. [9] Fluid administration also provides the opportunity to simultaneously administer drugs continuously or as a bolus. [10]

Electrolyte levels may be affected by rehydration. One study [12] followed blood urea levels during the last 24 hours of life. Thirteen patients received 1 to 2 L of fluid. In the treated group, the blood urea level was 151 mg/dL; in the nontreated patients, the concentration was 141 mg/dL.

The aim of rehydration is to reduce symptoms such as thirst and dry mouth. Rehydration also may be interpreted by caregivers and family as continuous care for the dying patient. Water is considered the source of all life.

Fluid and food administration in advanced disease is a delicate topic because it is about the quality of life of the dying. Because of the cognitive and symbolic significance of these acts, the feelings of the family and caregivers are also involved.

Correcting terminal dehydration is controversial. [9,10] Defenders of rehydration emphasize efficiency, symbolic meaning, and what humane care means. Opponents speak from experience about what constitutes palliative care. [11]

Symptom Control

A survey [13] recorded the complaints of 32 consecutive patients with dehydration who were mentally active and not receiving parenteral fluids. Twenty had no complaints; the complaints of the others could be controlled by small portions of food and fluid, with ice, and by keeping the lips wet. The study concluded that it was possible to relieve thirst without fluid administration (Table 109-1).

One study[11] of 52 patients with dehydration asked them to rank symptoms by using a visual analogue scale that used 0 for no complaint and 100 for the worst complaint:

- Thirst: 53.8
- Dry mouth: 60.0
- Bad taste: 46.6
- Nausea
- Fatigue: 61.8
- Pain: 33.5

Correlations between fluid intake and levels of sodium, urea concentration, and plasma osmolality were analyzed. There was no evidence for a relationship between fluid intake and the severity of symptoms and signs.

A study[14] compared mental status in states of dehydration or hydration. Hydrated patients have less agitation and somnolence, and their need for neuroleptics or sedatives was lower than for dehydrated patients. The researchers concluded that dehydration influenced mental status negatively, whereas rehydration ameliorated symptoms (Table 109-2). Only 32% of the first patient group (1988-1989) was rehydrated, compared with 73% of the second group (1991-1992). The overall finding was a significant relationship between symptoms and treatments.

Palliative Medication

In a study[15] that researched the association between symptoms and dehydration, 85% of 82 patients reported dry mouth and thirst, but there was no relationship between severity of dehydration and symptom severity. Ninety percent were also using medications (e.g., morphine, neuroleptics, spasmolytics, antidepressants) that had side effects of dry mouth and thirst.

Scientific research does not demonstrate that fluid administration leads to greater comfort. A dry mouth can be caused by medications, which is not necessarily corrected by artificial fluid administration. Thirst and dry mouth can be relieved by good, frequent mouth care and sometimes treated by giving small amounts of fluid orally.

Artificial fluid administration does not improve the functional status of a patient with a terminal illness. It may make the situation worse, because it is associated with complications such as local infection where the needle is inserted and the use of restraints. Dehydration may be a natural anesthetic to ease dying.

DECISION MAKING

Decisions about Physical Care

The cause and onset of dehydration should be considered when deciding about treatment. When there is a reversible cause (e.g., severe vomiting), temporary fluid administration can be considered.[17] When dehydration develops slowly, there will be fewer symptoms and less discomfort. Artificial fluid administration needs technical expertise, increasing the medicalization of dying. However, because of the short prognosis, some may prefer to die of disease progression rather than dehydration. A well-informed patient is a partner in making decisions about starting or stopping fluid administration.

Water is essential for survival. Administering fluid is therefore considered humane and loving care. For many caregivers, when a patient is unable to drink, it is a sign of impending death, and this evokes distressing emotions. The attitude of loved ones is also conditioned by their degree of acceptance of death. When family members insist on artificial fluid administration, it suggests they do not accept the designation of a terminal illness. In these circumstances, good communication is crucial.

We live in a society in which people believe medical science and technology will be able to overcome and cure every disease. It often is difficult to accept that nothing more can be done and that death is near. Professional and some informal caregivers are primarily directed toward treatment of diseases. Action is second nature. The transi-

---

TABLE 109-1 Controversy Surrounding Terminal Dehydration

ARGUMENTS FOR	ARGUMENTS AGAINST
Feeding and satisfying hunger is a moral duty.	Stopping feeding and offering fluid is more comfortable for terminal patients.
Dying patients have hunger and thirst.	Terminal patients are losing appetite and thirst. This is not caused by dehydration; hand dehydration causes dry mouth.
Offering food and fluid is a symbol of care.	Close contact with the patient and family and maximal comfort is better than symbolic acts.
When food and fluid are stopped in the terminally ill, it could be interpreted as discrimination because an important group of people may be labeled as unproductive or as a burden for society and systematically abandoned (i.e., slippery slope theory).	Based on experience, there is no evidence to justify administration of fluid in the terminal phase of a person's life.
Being thirsty is a serious problem (i.e., quality of life).	Dehydration has an analgesic effect and helps make dying less painful and therefore more dignified.
If people do not receive any food or fluid, they die starving and dehydrated.	

TABLE 109-2 Mental Status and Hypodermoclysis

STUDY FINDING	1988-1989	1991-1992
Hypodermoclysis	32%	73%
Agitation	26%	10%
Decreased consciousness	26%	10%
Use of haloperidol	24%	8%
Use of benzodiazepines	++	±

Data from Fainsinger RL, Bruera E. When to treat dehydration in a terminally ill patient? Support Care Cancer 1997;5:205-211.

tion from active intervention to offering comfort and support can be difficult in a climate focused on active treatment.

Each illness has unique conditions and demands. Definite recommendations about when to rehydrate or not are not possible, but some guidelines[16] can be offered:

- The patient, family, and informal caregivers should be aware that abandoning artificial fluid administration is ethically justified in some cases.
- The care team should consider the patient's wishes and viewpoints about treatment.
- Trials of hydration for a limited time are recommended when in doubt.
- When making a decision about starting or stopping fluids, the care team should not forget the emotions such a decision can evoke for the patient, family, and caregivers.
- In delirium caused by medication, temporary administration of fluid can be indicated.

The medical situation and prognosis of the patient can influence decisions about administering or stopping fluids. Factors include the kind and severity of dehydration and symptoms present; other complaints, symptoms, and signs; and electrolyte disturbances.

The care team must determine whether the cause of dehydration is reversible and whether the cause is treatable in an acceptable way, without substantial loss of quality of life. Making a decision about withholding or administering fluids should consider the effect of artificial fluid administration on the patient, determination of which symptoms may improve and which may deteriorate, incorporating the patient's wishes about prolongation of life, and understanding the psychological consequences for the patient and his or her family. After balancing the advantages and disadvantages and with agreement of the patient, family, and care team, a limited trial of rehydration may be considered, with re-evaluation scheduled in advance.

Bioethical Decisions

Management of the patient during periods of hydration or rehydration follows the same principles. For example, mouth care should be meticulous. A "last meal" should always be possible. The environment (e.g., room temperature, light) should be comfortable, and the caregivers should emphasize other aspects of physical comfort, such as touch.

The palliative care team should display an attitude of empathy, authenticity, and unconditioned acceptance of the patient. They should respect each person's dignity during the last phase of life. This takes the form of anticipating the patient's needs, providing sufficient and accurate information, offering opinions instead of advice, and respecting the patient's decisions. Patients should be able to choose autonomously, freely, and consciously.

An integral part of good palliative care is respect for patients' philosophical beliefs and their attempts to find meaning in the last phase of life. Spiritual issues often influence decisions about end-of-life care, and spiritual needs should be facilitated. The care team should maintain ethical communication with everyone involved and document decisions and discussions in the patient's chart.

CONCLUSIONS

Hydration always should be considered in the context of the total care of a patient with advanced illness. Professional caregivers should try to deliver maximal physical, psychological, moral, and existential comfort. Acceptance of dehydration can be part of authentic and caring involvement in the well-being of the dying person. Conversely, administration of fluid and rehydration also can be an expression of good care.

REFERENCES

1. Waller A, Caroline NL. Handbook of Palliative Care in Cancer, 2nd ed. London, Butterworth-Heinemann, 2000.
2. American College of Physicians. Parenteral nutrition in patients receiving cancer chemotherapy. Position paper. Ann Intern Med 1989;110:734-736.
3. Dunphy K, Finlay I, Rathbone G, et al. Rehydration in palliative and terminal care: If not—why not? Palliat Med 1995;9:221-228.
4. Billings JA. Comfort measures for the terminally ill. Is dehydration painful? J Am Geriatr Soc 1985;33:808-810.
5. Sutcliffe J, Holmes S. Dehydration: Burden or benefit to the dying patient? J Adv Nurs 1994;19:71-76.
6. Ferry M, Dardaine V, Constans T. Subcutaneous infusion or hypodermoclysis: A practical approach. J Am Geriatr Soc 1999;47:93-95.
7. Fainsinger RL, MacEachern T, Miller MJ, et al. The use of hypodermoclysis for rehydration in terminally ill cancer patients. J Pain Symptom Manage 1994;9:298-302.
8. Fainsinger R, Bruera E. The management of dehydration in terminally ill patients. J Palliat Care 1994;10:55-59.
9. Bruera E, MacDonald RN. Nutrition in cancer patients: An update and review of our experience. Issues in symptom control. Part 3. J Pain Symptom Manage 1988;3:133-140.
10. de Ridder D, Gastmans C. Terminal dehydration [in Dutch]. TVZ 1997;3:70-76.
11. Burge FI. Dehydration symptoms of palliative care cancer patients. J Pain Symptom Manage 1993;8:454-464.
12. Waller A, Adunski A, Hershkowitz M. Terminal dehydration and intravenous fluids. Lancet 1991;337:745.
13. McCann RM, Hall WJ, Groth-Juncker A. Comfort care for terminally ill patients: The appropriate use of nutrition and hydration. JAMA 1994;272:1263-1266.
14. Fainsinger RL, Bruera E. When to treat dehydration in a terminally ill patient? Support Care Cancer 1997;5:205-211.
15. Ellershaw JE, Sutcliffe JM, Saunders CM. Dehydration and the dying patients. J Pain Symptom Manag 1995;10:192-197.
16. Bozetti F, Amadori D, Bruera E, et al. Guidelines on artificial nutrition versus hydration in terminal cancer patients. European Association for Palliat Care. Nutrition 1996;12:163-167.
17. de Ridder D, Gastmans C. Dehydration among terminally ill patients: An integrated ethical and practical approach for caregivers. Nurs Ethics 1996;3:305-316.
18. Derycke N, Ceulemans L. Terminale dehydratie. Bijblijven 2006;22:48-55.

SUGGESTED READING

Bruera E, Sala R, Rico MA, et al. Effects of parenteral hydration in terminally ill cancer patients: A preliminary study. J Clin Oncol 2005;23:2366-2371.

Morita T, Bito S, Koyama H, et al. Development of a national clinical guideline for artificial hydration therapy for terminally ill cancer patients. J Palliat Med 2007;10:770-780.

Morita T, Hyodo I, Yoshimi T, et al. Artificial hydration therapy, laboratory findings, and fluid balance in terminally ill patients with abdominal malignancies. J Pain Symptom Manage 2006;31:130-139.

Morita T, Hyodo I, Yoshimi T, et al. Association between hydration volume and symptoms in terminally ill cancer patients with abdominal malignancies. Ann Oncol 2005;16:640-647.

Morita T, Shima Y, Miyashita M, et al. Physician- and nurse-reported effects of intravenous hydration therapy on symptoms of terminally ill patients with cancer. J Palliat Med 2004;7:683-693.

Morita T, Tei Y, Tsunoda J, et al. Determinants of the sensation of thirst in terminally ill cancer patients. Support Care Cancer 2001;9:177-186.

Communication

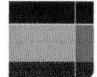

CHAPTER **110**

Good Communication: Patients, Families, and Professionals

Cathy Heaven and Claire Green

Medical interviewing is a core clinical skill. It is the medium of doctor/patient communication and relationship, the most important single source of diagnostic data, the means through which we elicit the patient's partnership and participation in the processes of care.

— LIPKIN PUTNAM & LAZARE[1] (P. IX).

Good communication is fundamental to the medical interview; it underpins the accuracy of diagnosis and allows treatment decisions tailored to the individual. Without good communication, a patient may be misdiagnosed or have problems and conditions missed. This increases the number of patient visits, length of hospital stays, number of drugs prescribed, and number of complaints received. It also creates physical and psychological distress for the individual and family.[2,3]

EVIDENCE-BASED MEDICINE

Assessment is about understanding patient needs, problems, and concerns. Between 50% and 80% of patients' concerns go undetected,[4,5] and more than half of those

suffering psychological problems are not referred for appropriate care.[6,7] Improving communication is a key factor in improving assessment.

Defining Core Principles

Patient-Centered Communication

Patient-centered medicine has it origins in the patients' rights movement of the 1960s and is codified in much of Western law. It centers on exploring patients' preferences and providing information that facilitates patient decision making.[8] Many definitions of the patient-centered approach exist.[8,9] For example, Laine and Davidoff defined it as an approach that is "closely congruent with, and responsive to patients' wants, needs and preferences."[10] Care that is patient centered identifies the wants, needs, and preferences of the individual and responds to them. Much evidence supports the value of a patient-centered approach. It is both effective and acceptable to patients and their families,[8,9] and it is associated with increased satisfaction, reduced anxiety, more accurate information recall, better treatment compliance, and better management and recovery.[8-10]

Cue-Based Communication

A cue is "a verbal or nonverbal hint which suggests an underlying unpleasant emotion and would need clarification from the health provider."[11] The Verona Sequence Analysis Group, working on behalf or the European Association of Communication in Health Care,[12] defined seven categories of patient expression classified as cues (Box 110-1). The number of cues per interview or consultation ranges from 1 or 2 to 10 or 11 per 15-minute interview.[11,13] Both the patient's emotional distress and the interviewer's cue responsiveness increase this number.[14-16]

Cue-based communication is a fundamental part of patient-centered communication. Control of the interview is shared between the patient, who gives the cues to areas of concern, and the professional, who chooses how and when to pick up the cues. What cues are heard and whether they are picked up appears to be governed by training,[13] experience, and professional cue bias.[17] Professional cue bias occurs when context-specific knowledge enables the individual clinician to limit the information needed for decision making, through filtering out irrelevant information and linking up relevant material.[17] In assessment, different physicians will attach different meanings to information gathered, filter out different cues from the patient, and make different links between pieces of information, based on the physician's life experiences, training, knowledge, and role. To communicate effec-

Box 110-1 Verona Consensus Definition of Patient Cues

Verbal Cues

- Word or phrases suggesting vague, undefined emotions (e.g., "It felt odd")
- Verbal hints to hidden concerns (e.g., "I cope with it")
- Words or phrases that describe psychological correlates or unpleasant emotional states (e.g., sleep disturbance, agitation, panic, irritability)
- Unusual or affect-loaded emphasis or repeated mentions of issues of potential importance (e.g., "hell of a day," "felt like I'd been hit by a car," use of profanity as emphasis)
- Communication of life-threatening events (e.g., "Doctor said I had cancer," "I know I am dying")

Nonverbal Cues

- Nonverbal expressions of emotion (e.g., crying)
- Nonverbal hints of emotion (e.g., signing, frowning, silence, looking away, looking uncomfortable)

Data from Del Piccolo L, Goss C, Bergvik S. The fourth meeting of the Verona Network on Sequence Analysis: Consensus finding on the appropriateness of provider responses to patient cues and concerns. Patient Educ Counsel 2006;61:473-475.

Box 110-2 Effective Interviewing Skills

- Using more eye contact at the outset of the interview
- Using open questions to get the patient talking more generally
- Using directive (closed) questions about specific problems
- Actively clarifying more about the presenting complaint
- Asking directly about feelings
- Responding to verbal and nonverbal cues
- Making supportive or empathic comments
- Asking about the impact on the home situation
- Handling interruptions well
- Coping with talkativeness

From Goldberg DP, Steele JJ, Smith C, Spivey L. Training the family doctors to recognise psychiatric illness with increased accuracy. Lancet 1980;2: 521-523.

tively, physicians must recognize and work with all types of cues, and understand their own biases, to detect and work with patients' needs most effectively. Judging when and how to do this can be difficult, especially when cues relate to sensitive or emotional areas (e.g., loss of libido). Negotiation and empathy are key skills when detecting these types of cues.

The evidence base for the value of cue-based communication is strong,[11,13] yet studies continue to report difficulties in following patient cues.[13,16] A common concern is that allowing the patient or relative to dictate the course of an interview increases its length; however, the evidence is to the contrary. Working with general practitioners, cue-based consultations were, on average, 15% shorter than when cues were missed.[18] In oncology consultations, addressing cues reduced consultation times 10% to 12%.[11]

Defining Effective Interviewing Skills

During five decades of communication research, there have been few studies of the relationship between skills and outcomes. Early studies of general practitioners highlighted the importance of some basic skills that enabled accurate identification of psychological problems[19] (Box 110-2). They showed that reading notes while a patient is talking is inhibitory. The researchers concluded that different types of questions seem important at different points in consultations; that responding to physical and emotional, verbal and nonverbal cues is important; and that showing empathy and appropriate eye contact are essential.

Validating this early work with cancer and palliative care, disclosure of key patient information, emotions, and concerns was found to be significantly promoted by core facilitative skills and inhibited by others.[20] There was a

ratio of three inhibitory skills for every facilitative skill, regardless of the interviewer's age, experience, or professional discipline. The effective interviewing skills identified (Table 110-1) now form the basis of training in the United Kingdom.[13,21,22]

In summary, effective interviewing is a proactive process that involves clarification of patients' cues. A good interviewer uses open questions to elicit cues and a combination of open and closed questions to clarify and empathically explore verbal or nonverbal cues. Effective interviewing consists of giving feedback to the patient about what the interviewer is hearing and understanding, using summary and educated guesses to check and develop understanding further, and using good but not intrusive eye contact. Furthermore, a good interviewer has an integrated approach, assessing at each stage the impact of the problems and events not only physically and practically but also emotionally, spiritually, and socially.

RECENT DEVELOPMENTS

Recent advances in conversation analysis investigated the sequence of behaviors within interviews to establish what comes before and after key moments of patient disclosure. This work validated earlier studies showing that open questions are more likely to elicit cues than closed ones,[23] that giving space by using short silences or simple facilitation (e.g., yes, right, go on) are most likely to immediately precede cues,[24] and that giving information reduces the cues being given.[25]

Importance of First Cues

If the first cue[16] of an interview is unacknowledged or not explored, then the number of cues given by the patient drops as much as 20%. This remains true even if the second cue is detected, and it becomes worse if the second cue also is missed or distanced from. The implication is that physicians must be aware of everything the patient or relative says from the very first sentences of an interaction.

Context in Which Skills Are Used

Given that so called "good skills" can be used in an inhibitory manner,[13,26,27] when an open question is linked to a cue, or used after a cue, it is 4.5 times more likely to lead

TABLE 110-1   Facilitative versus Inhibitory Interviewing Behaviors

BEHAVIOR	DESCRIPTION	EXAMPLES
FACILITATIVE BEHAVIORS		
Open directive questions	Questions that are open but directed to a particular area	How have you been since I last saw you? How has the pain been this week? How did you feel when you were told that? What is it that is bothering you about this?
Questions with a psychological focus	Eliciting information about emotions, worries, concerns, or fears	How did you feel when he told you the chemotherapy was not working? [open and psychological] Is this worrying you? What impact does the pain have on your mood?
Clarification of psychological aspects	Behavior that seeks to understand more about any emotional aspect	How strongly did you feel that? Just how low have you been? Are you able to tell me what frightens you about being here?
Empathy	A brief statement that shows a real appreciation of the patient's experience	That sounds terrible. Gosh, that must have been really hard for you. It sounds horrible.
Summarizing	Recapping two or more items previously discussed	So you had pain and nausea, and you were also confused about the tablets. You've been worrying about all sort of things—the tablets, your wife, and also about coming in here
Educated guesses	A tentative behavior in which the interviewer makes a guess or hypothesis about the situation, based on feelings or "gut reactions." The patient then confirms or refutes it. Educated guesses should be tentative in nature, because they are a guess.	I'm wondering if all these changes to your medications are worrying you. Am I right? I'm getting the impression that you are really quite unhappy about the way things are going. You know, as we talk, I am getting the feeling that even though you want to please your wife, you really don't want to go into the hospice. Would I be right?
INHIBITORY BEHAVIORS		
Leading questions	Questions that suggest or presuppose the answer	And that didn't worry you at all, did it? You are OK with those changes then, aren't you?
Physically focused questions	Questions that limit the topic to the physical experience only	How is the pain? What did the doctor tell you about your breathlessness? What physical problems have you been experiencing?
Clarifying physical aspects	Any behavior that seeks to understand more about the physical experience of the patient	Where exactly is the pain? How bad did the symptoms get? It is better or worse when you stand?
Giving advice: any information given to the patient before or after exploration of the concerns	Giving advice significantly decreases the disclosure of the patient	What you need to do is . . . . I think you ought to take things easier.

From Maguire P, Faulkner A, Booth K, et al. Helping cancer patients disclose their concerns. Eur J Cancer 1996;32A:78-81.

to patient disclosure than when it is either not linked to a cue or moves away from a cue. This finding[16] highlights the importance of a patient-focused approach to interviews. When open questions were used following the interviewer's, not the patient's, agenda, there was only a 50:50 chance of further disclosure by the patient or relative.[16]

Defining Effective Interviewing Style

Traditional approaches to medical history taking followed a systems-based approach. This approach can lead to assumptions by the patient about the types of information wanted by the physician, resulting in nondisclosure of key problems.[4,28] Comparison of the traditional medical "systems style" of medical history taking with a style that integrates both the physical and emotional modes of enquiry showed the importance of the more integrated style.[28] Integration of factual and emotional questioning significantly improved disclosure from the patient and relatives, with no loss of factual information. More physi-

cian dominance and more biomedically oriented questions were associated with less patient satisfaction, but satisfaction increased with the number of questions eliciting psychosocial information.[29]

EFFECTIVE COMMUNICATION STRATEGIES

These guidelines are not comprehensive or exhaustive and are intended to be applied flexibly. Examples are from real case histories.

Introducing the Topic of Hospice Care

Many doctors are anxious about mentioning hospice to patients because they fear the reaction it may create in the patient or relative (e.g., anger, despair, hopelessness).[4]

1. It is important to let the patient know that the conversation will be about his or her future care (*warning shot*).

2. Ask the patient to reflect on how he or she thinks things are going. Explore the patient's understanding.
3. Confirm the patient's understanding of the current situation and explore future expectations.
4. Summarize the current situation, using empathy and drawing on the evidence that things are difficult. Try to create a "case" or argument for the suggestion to come.
5. Tell the patient that you are about to suggest a solution (transition statement from listening and gathering evidence to giving a plan).
   - "What I would like to do is move on and look at what the best possible options are for you. Would that be OK?"
6. Tell the patient or relative about your plan.
   - Explain what you are offering.
   - Explain why you are offering it.
   - Explain what the advantages may be.
   - Acknowledge any disadvantages that might have already been mentioned.
7. Pause and allow your information to "go in."
8. Ask the patient or relative for their reaction.
   - "What do you think?"
   - "How do you feel about that?"
9. Explore the basis of any concerns the patient or relative may have.
   - "What is it that makes you not very keen on this plan?"
   - "What concerns you about the idea of the hospice?"
10. Empathize and respond to the patient's or relative's concerns.
    - "I guess it is hard to have to think about these things."
11. Reaffirm your view (if you still believe that hospice is the best option).
12. Be willing to change your mind if the patient's concerns or reasons make sense.

Handling Strong Emotions

Encountering strong emotions (e.g., distress, anger) is difficult and leaves many feeling uncomfortable and awkward. This often leads to physicians' employing strategies designed to keep feelings at a distance. Such strategies (discussed later) include normalizing (e.g., "You are bound to feel upset at this time") and premature reassurance (e.g., "There no need to be worried. I am sure it will be OK"). The key to working effectively with strong emotions is to allow space and time for them to be ventilated. This can feel counterintuitive and can be difficult, especially if, for example, someone is angry.

When working with strong emotions consider the following:

1. Acknowledge the emotion as soon as you are aware of it, and do not minimize or relabel it. Note that minimizing anger and referring to it as an upset can lead to escalation of the anger.
   - "I can see you are very upset."
   - "You seem angry about the situation."
2. Invite the individual to say what is making him or her feel that way (angry or upset).

- "Can you tell me what it is that is making you so tearful?"
- "What is it that's upsetting you?"
- "Can you say what particular thing went through your mind that made you cry just now?"
- "What's making you so angry?"
- "Would you like to tell me what's happened to make you so mad?"

3. Acknowledge and empathize with each aspect of the emotion.
   - "That sounds terrible, I can see now why you were so angry."
   - "It must have been awful for you"
4. Do not assume that there is only one thing driving the emotion. Having acknowledged the first aspect, screen for other things that may be worrying the person or making him or her angry. Try to build a list of all the aspects that are making up the problem.
   - "I can see that you were very upset about the words the doctor used and that it left you feeling terrible." [PAUSE . . .] "Can I check, was there something else about the situation that is also upsetting you?"
   - "So you are angry about the way your mother was left without a drink, and also about the way the nurses spoke to her. Were there any other things that happened that made you angry?"
5. Keep screening through all the concerns to ensure that you have the full list before being tempted to go further into each concern.
   - "There are clearly a lot of things we need to talk about and go through. Before we do, is there anything else about this situation that is bothering you that I need to be aware of?"
6. Take each concern and deal with it appropriately, or, if there are a number of concerns, prioritize them. Remember that ventilation may be sufficient to deal with some concerns, especially anger.
   - "You have mentioned a number of things. Perhaps I could ask you which of those seems the most pressing right now?"

Discussing Resuscitation Decisions with Patients and Relatives

Conversations about resuscitation are a common source of concern for doctors and nurses alike. Changes in health care legislation have meant these discussions are occurring more frequently, but this does not make them any easier. Guidelines for decision making on cardiopulmonary resuscitation (CPR) are available from professional bodies. Just as each patient's situation is different, each conversation about resuscitation will be different; however, the overall structure described here may help. Note that this process is synonymous with breaking bad news.

1. In the introduction, highlight to the patient or relative that the conversation is to be about how things are going.
2. Start by exploring (assessing) the patient's or relative's perception of the current situation. Your aim

is to identify whether the patient or relative is realistic or unrealistic about prognosis.

3. If the patient is unrealistic about prognosis, this issue needs addressing before do not resuscitate (DNR) orders can be discussed.

4. If the patient or relative is aware that the patient is dying, confirm that understanding.
   - *"I think you are very clear about how things are going, John. My feeling is very much like yours, that things do seem to be taking a turn for the worse, and you are deteriorating rapidly." [PAUSE and EMPATHIZE...] "Unfortunately, I'm really sorry to say you are right in thinking that it means you are dying."*

5. Introduce the topic of DNR.
   - *"Given that things have moved on, one of the things I wanted to talk to you about today, John, is in relation to what might happen if you suddenly deteriorate, or if your heart were to suddenly stop beating."*
   - Pause and allow warning shot to sink in.
   - Allow for response.

6. Allow for the patient or relative to respond, ask what you mean, or make a comment.

7. If the response does not give you a lead, then continue.
   - *"When people are getting increasingly worse, as a medical team we have to make a decision whether it would be appropriate to try to resuscitate them should their heart stop." [PAUSE and ALLOW FOR RESPONSE...] "When people have long-term illnesses, like yourself, the chance of resuscitation having any effect is, to be honest, very slight." [PAUSE and ALLOW FOR RESPONSE...].*
   - *"I don't know how you feel about this, John, but taking all things into consideration, we feel that, should something happen, the very best thing for you would not be to try and prolong your life by starting the process of resuscitation." [PAUSE.... If no response, ask,] "Do you understand what I mean, John?"*

8. Invite the patient or relative to say how it has left them feeling.
   - *"How do you feel about that, John?"*

Withdrawing Nutrition and Hydration

Withdrawal of nutrition or hydration is another difficult area to raise, because relatives and patients may see the withdrawal of nutrition and hydration as "giving up." This perception may be associated with strong emotions, such as anger, distress, or feelings of abandonment. The following suggestions are written as if talking to a relative but would also apply if talking to a patient.

1. Highlight to the relative that the conversation is about how things are going with the patient.

2. Start by exploring (assessing) the relative's perception and understanding of the patient's situation, and identify whether the relative fully understands the patient's situation and progress.
   - *"How do you feel things are going at the moment, Sarah?"*

- *"What sense are you making of it all?"*

3. If the relative is aware of how ill the patient is, confirm that understanding with empathy.
   - *"I'm so sorry, but you are right, he is getting worse."*

4. If the relative is unaware that the patient is dying, then deliver a warning shot, pause, and break the bad news about prognosis.
   - *"I'm afraid I have some very difficult news for you, Sarah. [PAUSE...] Your Dad is really very ill. [PAUSE...] He is gradually starting to get more ill. [PAUSE...] We feel that things are gradually going to continue to deteriorate now."*
   - Acknowledge any emotion shown, invite the relative to respond to the news, acknowledge any responses empathically, and elicit any concerns.
   - *"I can see that is hard to hear.... How do you feel about what I have just said?"*

5. Introduce the idea of withdrawing nutrition and hydration only after concerns about prognostic information have been dealt with.
   - *"One of the things I wanted to talk to you about was that we would like to remove your father's infusion." [PAUSE and ALLOW FOR RESPONSE...] "We feel it is no longer helping him, and it could be causing him some discomfort." [PAUSE...]*

6. Acknowledge any emotion shown, invite the relative to respond, acknowledge any responses empathically, and address any concerns.
   - *"I can see that is really hard to hear.... How do you feel about it?"*

Having Difficult Conversations with Professional Colleagues

The multidisciplinary approach has led to many benefits for patient care, as well as better working conditions for many staff, but not without difficulties. There are occasions when differences of opinion can lead to team tensions. Learning to quickly deal with these effectively reduces the emotional impact on the team and also benefits the patients and families affected.

1. Choose an appropriate time. Do not confront or challenge colleagues when you are angry or upset, because the emotion will impede your ability to listen to and to present a clear argument and will hinder resolution.

2. Make an appointment or choose a place to meet that feels comfortable and where you will not be interrupted.

3. Set the scene immediately by highlighting that the conversation is about an important issue.
   - *"I wanted to talk to you about something that is really concerning me."*

4. Set out the problem in clear and concise terms. Do not be personal or overtly critical. Try to have examples or evidence ready, and, if possible, always use the benefit of the patient as the core for your argument.
   - *"I want to talk to you about Mrs. H. Yesterday, when I spoke to her, she was really upset,*

because she felt that we (as a medical team) were giving her very mixed messages. When I talked to her, I tried to be quite honest about the seriousness of her situation, and also to give a clear warning shot that things are deteriorating. However, as we talked, it became very clear that the message that your team had given her was much more optimistic and positive. The fact that we are giving different messages is not good; it is causing Mrs. H much confusion and distress."

5. Allow the person the chance to respond and give his or her opinion of the situation.

6. Be willing to hear the colleague's viewpoint, respond to concerns and worries, but remain clear about the problem.

  - *"I appreciate that it is very difficult to tell someone bad news when they are doing so poorly. My concern, however, is that it is not in the interest of anyone, especially Mrs. H, for us to give mixed messages, or to leave false hope or raise expectations unrealistically."*

7. Do not expect an apology, but instead look for an agreement to change practice.

  - *"The most important thing is that we work together to prevent this happening again. . . . Perhaps one way forward would be to talk together about how we address things with patients. . . ."*

COMMON ERRORS

Communication often breaks down because of how physicians respond to cues; up to 58% of cues by patients may be "distanced" by the doctor.[13] Although this may be a conscious process, it may also be unconscious.[4] Behaviors that distance from the cues disclosed[13,16,20] have been identified (Table 110-2) and include things like selective atten-

TABLE 110-2	Behaviors That Distance from Cues Disclosed		
ERROR	**DESCRIPTION**	**RATIONALE**	**EXAMPLE**
Selective attention	Natural bias, developed through professional training, consciously or unconsciously affects the type of cues we "pay attention to" or hear.	This limits patients from saying more by focusing on those aspects the interviewer perceives as relevant.	*Patient:* "I was in pain, weak and tired, and was absolutely terrified that the treatment wasn't working." *Interviewer:* "Tell me about your pain. How bad was it?"
Switching the time focus	The interviewer moves the "time frame" of the interview.	This prevents patients from talking further by encouraging them to focus on a different occasion or different time frame, in which they may or may not have felt the same.	*Patient:* "It was awful. I felt so ill, and so fed up. It seemed to go on forever." *Interviewer:* "And how do you feel now?"
Switching the person focus	Focus is changed from the interviewee to a third party.	This inhibits interviewees from talking about how they feel.	*Patient:* "I felt devastated by the news. I thought I was going to die." *Interviewer:* "And how did your wife feel about it?"
Blocking	The interviewer switches the conversation topic completely; may be done unconsciously.	This inhibits patients from continuing to talk about their concern.	*Patient:* "I have been having some pain. It worries me somewhat." *Interviewer:* "How has your breathing been?"
Offering premature advice or reassurance	The interviewer offers advice or reassurance before a concern or cue has been fully explored; includes expressions that attempt to normalize the patient's concern.	Giving advice before concerns have been elicited inhibits patients from saying more, while pushing them into listening to what the professional is saying, whether relevant or not. Although giving information is sometimes relevant, it inhibits patients from talking because they are in "listening mode."	*Patient:* "I feel so shocked by the news." *Interviewer:* "You will get over that feeling, it doesn't last for too long." *Patient:* "I was really very upset when she first mentioned the word *hospice*." *Interviewer:* "Well, it's only natural that you should feel that way at first; all patients do." *Patient:* "I'm really worried about having pain. My father had so much pain, you see." *Interviewer:* "Please try not to worry about that. Not all people with cancer suffer pain, and we have made wonderful advances since your father's day. We have many, many types of pain killers available to use."
Using jargon	Interviewer or patient uses medical terms or expressions that could be misinterpreted or misunderstood.	This can be a real obstacle, and the problem is not confined to the professional; Internet access has increased patients' and relatives' use of medical terms, which may or may not be fully understood.	*Interviewer:* "The cancer is progressing, and we do not feel that you need chemotherapy any longer." *Patient:* "That's good news, that I am making progress."
Passing the buck	The interviewer, in direct response to the patient's cue or concern, advises the patient to talk to a third party.	This may be appropriate at the end of an interview, but using it immediately indicates that the interviewer does not want to hear the patient's concern.	*Patient:* "I was so upset, I just didn't know what he meant." *Interviewer:* "Clearly you need to talk to the surgeon about that, to get things clear."

tion, switching focus, and premature advice. Training significantly improves professionals' cue responses,[13] which are more often inhibitory than facilitative.[13,20]

CONTROVERSIES

Nonverbal Cues

The evidence for the relative importance of nonverbal versus verbal cues is mixed. Nonverbal cues are important indicators of patient affect, especially in depression, where verbal cues may be minimal or absent. Satisfaction increases if nonverbal cues are elicited,[30] but it is the verbal, not the nonverbal, cues that are more strongly associated with patient distress.[14] Perhaps, for professionals to improve their communication skills, they first must concentrate on facilitating verbal cues provided by the patient. If verbal cues are absent or are in opposition to the patient's nonverbal cues, then acknowledgment and exploration of the nonverbal cues becomes important. A recent review[31] concluded that appropriate acknowledgment of nonverbal cues was critical to high-quality care and that it was the nonverbal behaviors that significantly influenced the therapeutic relationship, patient satisfaction, adherence, and clinical outcomes.

Patient-Centered Approach

Although a patient-centered approach is recommended by many medical educators and researchers, there is some evidence from a randomized, controlled trial that it fails to improve medical outcome or patient satisfaction,[32] and older people prefer the traditional biomedical approach.[33]

Role of Training in Communication Skills

In both the United States and Europe, communication skills training is recognized as one way to improve health care for patients and reduce complaints.[1,2,8] There is still controversy about how these skills are acquired and assessed. Some believe that good communication skills are either innate or are learned through "osmosis" or through modeling behaviors of experienced senior colleagues.[34] However, the scientific literature supports the notion that training is highly effective in changing physicians' communication behaviors.[4,13,21,22]

CONCLUSIONS

Effective communicators are flexible in applying core principles and in using effective skills, strategies, and approaches to deal with difficult communications. The evidence supports the importance of active listening and the need to elicit, explore, and clarify not just medical facts but also the person's perceptions of events and illness. It is important to acknowledge and explore patients' and relatives' fears, needs, worries, and wishes before addressing concerns. Key skills exist; recent evidence suggests that the power of these facilitative skills is increased when they are used in a cue-based approach.

REFERENCES

1. Lipkin M Jr, Putnam SM, Lazare A (eds). The Medical Interview: Clinical Care, Education and Research. New York: Springer-Verlag, 1995.
2. National Institute for Clinical Excellence (NICE). Supportive and Palliative Care Guidelines. London, 2004. Available at http://www.nice.org.uk/guidance/index.jsp.
3. Trummer UF, Mueller P, Nowak P, et al. Does physician-patient communication that aims at empowering patients improve clinical outcomes? A case study. Patient Educ Couns 2006;61:299-306.
4. Heaven CM, Maguire P. Disclosure of concerns by hospice patients and their identification by nurses. Palliat Med 1997;11:283-290.
5. Farrell C, Heaven C, Beaver K, Maguire P. Identifying the concerns of women undergoing chemotherapy. Patient Educ Couns 2005;56:72-77.
6. Fallowfield L, Ratcliffe D, Jenkins V, Saul J. Psychiatric morbidity and its recognition by doctors in patients with cancer. Br J Cancer 2001;84:1011-1015.
7. Sharpe M, Strong V, Allen K, et al. Major depression in outpatients attending a regional cancer centre: Screening and unmet needs. Br J Cancer 2004;90:314-320.
8. Bensing JM. Bridging the gap: The separate worlds of evidence-based medicine and patient-centred medicine. Patient Educ Couns 2000;39:17-25.
9. Mead N, Bower P. Patient-centredness: A conceptual framework and review of the empirical literature. Social Sci Med 2000;51:1087-1110.
10. Laine C, Davidoff F. (1996) Patient-centred medicine: A professional evolution. JAMA 1996;275:152-156.
11. Butow PN, Dowsett S, Hagerty R, Tattersall MH. Communicating prognosis to patients with metastatic disease: What do they really want to know? Support Care Cancer 2002;10:161-168.
12. Del Piccolo L, Goss C, Bergvik S. The fourth meeting of the Verona Network on Sequence Analysis: Consensus finding on the appropriateness of provider responses to patient cues and concerns. Patient Educ Couns 2006;61:473-475.
13. Heaven C, Clegg J, Maguire P. Transfer of communication skills training from workshop to workplace: The impact of clinical supervision. Patient Educ Couns 2006;60:313-325.
14. Davenport S, Goldberg D, Miller T. How psychiatric disorders are missed during medical consultations. Lancet 1987;4:439-441.
15. Del Piccolo L, Saltini A, Zimmerman G, Dunn G. Differences in verbal behaviours of patients with and without emotional distress during primary care consultations. Psych Med 2000;30:629-643.
16. Fletcher I, Heaven C, Green C, et al. Unpublished data. Personal communication, 2006.
17. Crow R, Chase J, Lamond D. The cognitive component of nursing assessment: An analysis. J Adv Nurs 1995;22:206-212.
18. Levenson W, Horawara-Bhat R, Lamb J. A study of patient clues and physician responses in primary care and surgical settings. JAMA 2000;284:1021-1027.
19. Goldberg DP, Steele JJ, Smith C, Spivey L. Training the family doctors to recognise psychiatric illness with increased accuracy. Lancet 1980;2:521-523.
20. Maguire P, Faulkner A, Booth K, et al. Helping cancer patients disclose their concerns. Eur J Cancer 1996;32A:78-81.
21. Maguire P, Booth K, Elliot C, Jones B. Helping health professionals involved in cancer care acquire key interviewing skills: The impact of workshops. Eur J Cancer 1996;32A:1486-1489.
22. Fallowfield L, Jenkins V, Farewell V, et al. Efficacy of a Cancer Research UK communication skills training model for oncologists: A randomised controlled trial. Lancet 2002;359:650-656.
23. Zimmerman C, Del Piccolo L, Mazzi MA. Patient cues and medical interviewing in general practice: Examples of the application of sequence analysis. Epidemiologia e Psichiatria Sociale 2003;12:115-123.
24. Langewitz W, Nübling M, Weber H. A theory based approach to analysing conversation sequences. Epidemiologia e Psichiatria Sociale 2003;12:103-108.
25. Eide H, Quera V, Graugaard P, Finset A. Sequential patterns of physician-patient dialogue surrounding cancer patients' expression of concern and worry: Applying sequence analysis to RIAS. Social Sci Med 2004;59:145-155.
26. Heaven C, Maguire P, Green C. A patient centred approach to defining and assessing interviewing competency. Epidemiologia e Psichiatria Sociale 2003;12:86-91.
27. Glajchen M, Blum D, Calder K. Cancer pain management and the role of social work: Barriers and interventions. Health Social Work 1995;20:200-206.
28. Cox A, Rutter M, Holbrook D. Psychiatric interviewing—A second experimental study: Eliciting feelings. Br J Psychiatry 1988;152:64-72.
29. Bertakis D, Roter D, Putnam SM. The relationship of physician medical interview style to patients' satisfaction. J Family Practice 1991;32:175-181.
30. Di Matteo MR, Taranta A, Friedman HS, Prince LM. Predicting patient satisfaction from physicians' nonverbal communication skills. Med Care 1980;18:376-387.
31. Roter DL, Frankel RM, Hall JA, Sluyter D. The expression of emotion through nonverbal behaviour in medical visits: Mechanisms and outcomes. J Gen Intern Med 2006;21:528-534.
32. Smith RC, Lyles JS, Mettler J, et al. The effectiveness of intensive training for residents in interviewing: A randomised controlled study. Ann Intern Med 1998;128:118-126.
33. Swenson SL, Buell S, Zettler P, et al. Patient centred communication: Do patients prefer it? J Gen Intern Med 2004;19:1069-1079.
34. Langille DB, Kaufman DM, Laidlaw TA, et al. Faculty attitudes towards medical communication and their perceptions of students' communication skills training at Dalhousie University. Med Educ 2001;35:548-554.

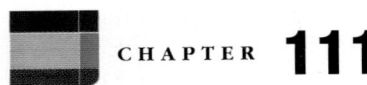

CHAPTER **111**

Telling the Truth: Bad News

Josephine M. Clayton, Phyllis N. Butow, and
Martin H. N. Tattersall

Being able to break bad news sensitively and effectively is one of the most important skills in palliative medicine. Patients with a life-limiting illness and their families commonly receive a sequence of bad news as the illness progresses. Imparting the news of a limited life span is challenging both for clinicians and for patients and their families.

TELLING THE TRUTH ABOUT A TERMINAL PROGNOSIS

Pertinent information is essential if persons with a life-limiting illness and their caregivers are to participate in decisions about their care, set realistic goals and priorities, and prepare for death and its aftermath. Clinicians need to provide information in a way that respects individual needs of patients and their families (which may be for much or little information), enhances patient and family understanding, and assists in coping and adjustment.

There are deficiencies in current practice.[1] Many health professionals (HPs) are uncomfortable in discussing prognosis and end-of-life issues.[2] Reasons include perceived lack of training, stress, insufficient time to attend to the patient's emotional needs, fear of upsetting the patient, and a feeling of inadequacy or hopelessness regarding the unavailability of curative treatment.[3-5] Discomfort can lead to avoidance of such discussions. Although some HPs believe that disclosing prognosis or introducing end-of-life issues unnecessarily upsets patients and dispels hope, evidence suggests that people can engage in such discussions with minimal stress[6] and maintain hope even when the prognosis is poor.[7]

Patients who understand their prognosis are more satisfied with their care and experience less psychological morbidity.[8,9] When cancer patients are inadequately informed about prognosis, they are more likely to choose aggressive anticancer treatments[10] and to make decisions they later regret.[11] If information is not honest and detailed, patients may perceive that HPs are withholding potentially frightening information.[12] It is therefore in the patient's best interest to be offered such information.

DISCUSSING PROGNOSIS

The dialogue about prognosis can be viewed as an ongoing conversation over time rather than a single discussion.[13] Prognostication involves more than estimating likely survival time. It also includes discussing symptoms the patient may face as the illness progresses and the likelihood of benefit from any proposed intervention. In palliative medicine, prognostic and end-of-life discussions may also include what the patient and family may experience or witness leading up to and during the actual time of dying, preferences for place of death, general preferences for care and medical treatment in the terminal phase, and what may happen or need to be done after the person dies.

Timing of Prognostic and End-of-Life Discussions

Most patients from Western countries prefer some information regarding prognosis when first diagnosed with a life-limiting illness or shortly thereafter.[14,15] They may prefer to negotiate the content and extent of this information, and some never want to discuss prognosis.[15] Patients may change their preference over time, from initially wanting much or little detail to the reverse. Information regarding prognosis should be offered, but not forced, and the option of a later discussion should be left open.[5]

Preparation for the Discussion

Prognostic discussions are never easy and may involve some technical information. Careful preparation is required. It is important to provide consistent, accurate information by reading clinical records, speaking with HPs, and consulting relevant literature for up-to-date knowledge.[16] Mentally preparing for the interview and minimizing interruptions during the discussion are important.

Relationship between the Health Professional and the Patient and Caregiver

Those who are facing a progressive, life-limiting illness place great emphasis on their relationship with their HP.[17] Attributes valued in a doctor-patient relationship include mutual trust, care, respect, honesty, empathy, support, partnership, and behavior that promotes confidence in the doctor's professional competence.[18] It is recommended that a doctor create an atmosphere of patient-centered care, wherein the patient is treated as a "whole person" and feels that the doctor is interested in and sensitive to his or her problems and feelings.[18] Even brief expressions of empathy may reduce anxiety.[19]

Who Should Be Present during the Discussion

Most patients, but not all, want a family member or friend with them[14,16] when they hear bad news, and many guidelines recommend having another HP present for additional support and continuity of care.[20] Some wish to receive prognostic information from a HP other than their doctor, or from another person, such as a priest.[5] This implies that the HP needs to negotiate who delivers the prognostic information.

How to Discuss

The first step (Box 111-1) is to clarify what the individual patient or family wants to know about prognosis. Most patients (at least from Western countries) want to know their prognosis and life expectancy.[5,14-15,17,21] A sizable minority do not want full disclosure,[22] and patients may experience conflict between wanting to know and fearing bad news.[23]

Patient and caregivers may want to know about different aspects of prognostic information, such as the likely illness trajectory, treatment options and what they may accomplish, life expectancy, likely future symptoms, and what to expect around the time of death.[14,21,23,24] Some want to know if their life span will be shortened by the illness but do not want the likely time frame.[13,15,23] These various types of prognostic and end-of-life information may be provided over a series of consultations or at different times depending on the context and the stage of illness.[15]

Some patient characteristics are associated with a greater or lesser desire for prognostic information. Younger and more educated patients commonly want more detail.[22] Patients from some cultural backgrounds prefer nondisclosure, or disclosure negotiated through the family, if life expectancy is short.[25] It is not possible to make assumptions about individuals' information needs based on their demographic characteristics or cultural background. It is important to seek patients' information preferences and tailor information to individual needs.

Checking Concerns and Responding to Emotions

Physicians cannot assume that patients will volunteer all their concerns. A substantial number of patients' concerns remain undisclosed in practice.[26,27] Hospice patients had, on average, seven concerns, but only three were disclosed to hospice nurses. Concerns disclosed most commonly related to physical issues, but "concerns about the future, appearance and loss of independence were withheld more than 80% of the time."[26] Patients may believe that psychosocial and emotional concerns are an inevitable part of illness for which nothing can be done[27]; they may perceive their concerns to be embarrassing or abnormal, or they may be apprehensive about burdening their HPs,

---

Box 111-1 Guidelines for Breaking Bad News and Discussing Prognosis in Palliative Medicine

- Prepare self and setting, and ensure uninterrupted time for discussion.
- Give patients the opportunity to have someone with them if they wish.
- Establish rapport.
- Identify the reason for this consultation and elicit patient's expectations.
- Clarify patient's understanding, and establish how much detail is wanted and about which subjects.
- Offer to discuss what to expect in the future in a sensitive manner, giving the patient the option not to discuss it.
- Explore and acknowledge patient's fears and concerns, as well as goals and wishes.
- Consider cultural and contextual factors that influence preferences for disclosure of information.
- Tailor information to patient's information preferences and concerns.
- Pace information to patient's needs, understanding, and circumstances, and ensure allocation of enough time.
- Use clear, jargon-free, understandable language.
- Be honest without being blunt or giving more detailed information than desired by the patient.
- Show empathy, care, and compassion during the entire consultation.
- Explain uncertainty and the limitations or reliability of prognostic and end-of-life information.
- Avoid being too exact with time frames except during the last few days of life.
- Reassure patients that support, treatments, and resources are available to control pain and other symptoms, but avoid premature reassurance.
- Foster hope when possible, but do not give misleading or false information in an attempt to positively influence a patient's hope.
- Facilitate realistic goals; reframe patient's and caregivers' expectations and, when appropriate, ways of coping on a day-to-day basis.
- Ensure consistency of information and approach from clinical team members.
- Foster consistency of information provision, with patient consent, to both patients and caregivers or family members.
- Consider caregivers' distinct information needs, which may require a separate meeting with caregivers (provided the patient, if mentally competent, gives consent).
- Acknowledge and respond to the patient's and caregivers' emotional concerns or distress regarding the discussion.
- Check the understanding of what has been said and whether the information provided meets the needs of the patient and/or caregiver.
- Encourage questions and requests for information clarification, and be prepared to repeat explanations.
- Leave the door open for the topic to be discussed again in the future, should the patient or caregiver wish.
- Write a summary of what has been discussed in the patient's medical record, and speak or write to other key health professionals involved in the patient's care, including the general practitioner.

---

whom they see as busy people. Patients must be encouraged to disclose all of their concerns. More concerns[28] are likely to be disclosed if the HP asks several times, "And is there anything else concerning you?" Prompting for more sensitive issues may be required. For example, the HP may say, "Many people worry about becoming dependent on others. Is that something that worries you?" HPs also need to acknowledge and respond empathically when such concerns are raised.[28]

Consideration of the Distinct or Particular Information Needs of Caregivers and Families

Providing support for families, both before and after the patient's death, is an integral component of palliative care. Families need information to feel mentally prepared, to care for their dying relative,[14,24] to be able to inform others,[29] and to prepare for their own future after the death.[30] Open discussion and provision of consistent information to patients and caregivers is important.[14,31]

Caregivers may have information needs distinct from those of the patient,[14,24,31] particularly regarding prognosis and end-of-life issues. To provide care, they may need more detailed information than the patient does about the dying process.[31] With patient consent, individual discussion allows professionals to explore caregiver concerns and information needs without the barrier of patient/caregiver protectiveness.

TRANSITION FROM A CURATIVE TO A PALLIATIVE APPROACH

Informing someone that their illness is no longer responsive to curative treatments is a challenging example of breaking bad news (see Box 111-1). In an advanced progressive and life-limiting illness, the main goals of disease-specific treatments are to improve length and quality of life. It is important that the patient understands that cure is not a treatment goal. Clinicians should be proactive for quality of life and avoid toxic treatments if little gain is likely to result.

Palliative treatments (e.g., chemotherapy) may slow progression of disease or provide symptomatic relief. If such treatments are offered, it is important that the patient has the opportunity to be as involved in decision making as desired.[32] The clinician should outline explicitly what outcomes may be improved (e.g., length of life, improvement in symptoms) and focus the discussion on the balance between potential effectiveness and potential side effects. Patients need clear information about the likely side effects, cost, and time involved, to enable informed decisions in the context of their goals.[15,33] It is essential to reassure patients that full supportive care will be provided, whether or not any disease-specific treatment is also given.[34]

The cessation of disease-specific treatment, in response to further disease progression, is another transition. It is important to sensitively explain that the disease is no longer responding and that continuing this treatment is likely to cause more side effects than benefit.[34] For example, the HP may say, "I wish that more chemotherapy would help this cancer, but unfortunately, at this stage, it will only make you sicker. It is likely that you will have a better quality of life without further chemotherapy." When ceasing disease treatments, it is important to avoid conveying that nothing more can be done but to emphasize the continued availability of supportive and symptomatic care.[35,36] For example, "As you become sicker

with this illness, we will continue to be here to provide the best available treatments to help control the symptoms and to provide support for both you and your family."

A palliative approach to care is appropriate for all patients for whom a cure is no longer possible.[37] This care may be provided by the primary health care team. For persons with more complex needs, referral to specialist palliative care services, where available, is appropriate. It is neither necessary nor desirable to wait until all disease-specific treatments have been terminated before referring the patient to specialist palliative care services, unless referral is dictated by the particular health care system or funding arrangements. Referral to specialist palliative care services may evoke fears of impending death and abandonment if the reason for referral is not communicated sensitively and effectively. The following recommendations are given for referring patients to specialist palliative care services:

- Raise the topic by being honest and open, and use the term *palliative care* (or *hospice,* depending on the country) explicitly.[38]
- Clarify and correct any misconceptions about palliative care services (e.g., that palliative care is solely for people who are dying or is associated with imminent death).[38]
- Discuss the role of the palliative care team, emphasizing expertise in symptom management, the wide range of support services available, assistance with quality of life, and support for family members.[34]
- Where feasible (to avoid a sense of abandonment), explain that patients will still be followed up by the primary health care team and/or the primary specialist (e.g., oncologist)

BALANCING HOPE AND TRUTH TELLING

Many HPs have difficulty in disclosing a limited life expectancy while maintaining the patient's hope, yet patients, caregivers, and HPs have identified hope as an integral component of the discussion of prognosis at the end of life[7,14,21,23] (Box 111-2). It is important to balance honesty with hope and empathy. Although accurate information presented in a straightforward and direct manner is often equated with honesty,[14,17] it is important that the presentation not be blunt or with too much hard, factual, or detailed information.[7]

There is a spectrum of hope,[7] from hope for a miracle cure to hope for a peaceful death; a person may simultaneously hope for a cure while acknowledging a terminal illness. Some obtain a sense of hope[21] from relationships, beliefs and faith, having symptom control, maintaining dignity, finding inner peace, enjoying a sense of humor, and thinking about meaningful life events. The following were seen by patients as hope-giving behaviors[39]: reassurance that pain will be controlled (87%); appearing to know all there is to know about the cancer (87%); being occasionally humorous (80%); offering to answer all the patient's questions (78%); saying that each day the patient survives new developments are possible (75%); and saying that the patient's will to live will affect the outcome (74%).

In some studies, patients perceived that hope could be maintained by HPs' "being there" and treating them as a whole person.[40] Others still expressed a need for hope when they knew and accepted that they were terminally ill.[14] Patients and caregivers perceived that HPs could communicate hope by "leaving the door open" (i.e., communicating in ways that allow preservation of some hope); acknowledging difficulties in prognostic estimates; presenting information about palliative care at a rate that the patient can assimilate; and respecting alternative treatments.

EVIDENCE-BASED MEDICINE

Studies informing optimal practice outlined in the previous section are descriptive, such as surveys or qualitative studies of patients' and families' views or providers' practices. Descriptive studies may be the highest level of evidence that can be collected and the most appropriate methodology for such research questions.

Some interventions may (1) enhance HPs' skills in communicating about these issues and (2) help patients assimilate information and achieve their information preferences.

Communication Skills Training for Health Professionals

HPs' communication skills do not reliably improve with experience alone. Randomized, controlled trials of communication skills training have demonstrated sustained changes in doctors' behavior. A 3-day residential communication skills course for oncologists found that partici-

pants used more focused and open questions, greater expressions of empathy, more appropriate responses to patients' cues, and fewer leading questions, both immediately after training[41] and at 12-months' follow-up.[42] Written feedback alone had little effect on objective communication outcomes of participants; active rehearsal in role-play appeared to be essential.[41]

In a small study (17 participants), a communication course for oncology fellows on breaking bad news improved participants' skills in breaking bad news, dealing with denial, and discussing end-of-life issues.[43] Further formal evaluations of communication skills training specific to palliative care, with greater emphasis on prognosis and end-of-life issues, are needed.

Audio Tapes or Written Consultation Summaries

One simple intervention to increase patients' understanding and recall of information is the use of audio tape recordings or written consultation summaries. A systematic review in oncology found that most people who received these interventions valued them.[44] In five of nine studies, audio tapes improved recall of the consultation. Patients who received an audio tape or letter were more satisfied with the information received in four of seven studies.

In one study, people who were informed of a poor prognosis at their initial oncology consultation and received a consultation audio tape[45] had worse psychological distress at 6 months' follow-up than those who did not receive a tape. Therefore, caution with audio tapes is appropriate when bad news is being delivered.[44] This may be especially relevant for palliative care, in which almost all patients have a short survival time.

Question Prompt Lists

Cancer and palliative care patients place a high value on the opportunity to ask questions of their clinicians.[17] Improved health outcomes result when patients are encouraged to ask questions during general medical consultations.[46] Some HPs encourage patients to write down their questions and bring them to medical appointments, but patients may not know what questions to ask or how to articulate their concerns.

A question prompt list (QPL)[47] is a structured list containing examples of questions for patients to ask the doctor if they wish. It is designed to encourage patient participation during medical consultation and to assist patients in acquiring information suited to their needs and at their own pace. This simple and inexpensive intervention promoted questions about prognosis in randomized studies in oncology.[47,48] Provided that the oncologist specifically addressed questions in the QPL during the consultation, those who received the prompt list were significantly less anxious immediately after the consultation and had better recall (and significantly shorter consultations).[48] This intervention appeared to allow important issues to be addressed quickly.

For patients referred to a palliative care team, suitable questions for the QPL[49] were identified in a pilot study from focus groups and individual interviews with palliative care patients, caregivers, and palliative care HPs. Many issues emerged for the QPL, including questions about the palliative care service, physical symptoms and treatment, lifestyle and quality of life, the patient's illness and what to expect in the future, support, whether the patient is concerned about his or her professional care, questions for caregivers, and end-of-life issues. The QPL for palliative care patients and their families, including 112 sample questions in a booklet form, is available at http://www.psych.usyd.edu.au/mpru/communication_tools .html (accessed November 30, 2007).

Recently, a randomized, controlled trial[50] examined the QPL in 174 patients seeing one of 15 palliative care clinicians in 10 different palliative care centers in Australia. All consultations were done in an outpatient palliative care clinic. Compared with controls, QPL patients and caregivers asked twice as many questions ($P < .0001$), and patients discussed 23% more issues covered by the QPL ($P < .0001$). QPL patients asked more prognostic questions ($P = .004$) and discussed more prognostic issues ($P = .003$) and end-of-life issues (30% versus 10%; $P = .001$). Fewer QPL patients had unmet information needs about the future ($P = .04$), the area of greatest unmet information need. QPL consultations were longer than those of controls (38 versus 31 minutes; $P = .002$). No differences between groups were observed in anxiety or in patient or physician satisfaction. A QPL and physician endorsement of its use may assist patients and their caregivers to ask questions during palliative care consultations and promote discussion about prognosis and end-of-life issues, without creating patient anxiety or impairing satisfaction.

CONCLUSIONS

Discussing bad news and prognosis is important in palliative care. Breaking bad news is difficult and distressing for HPs and for patients and their families (see "Common Errors"). We do not recommend a scripted or cookbook approach. These are complex interactions, and they often occur over time, rather than as a single discussion. Communication skills training may enhance physicians' skills to adapt their responses appropriately to the individual information and emotional needs of patients and their families. Physicians need to be aware that these needs are

likely to change throughout the illness trajectory (see "Future Considerations").

REFERENCES

1. Gysels M, Richardson A, Higginson IJ. Communication training for health professionals who care for patients with cancer: A systematic review of effectiveness. Support Care Cancer 2004;12:692-700.
2. Vandekieft G. Breaking bad news. Am Fam Physician 2001;64:1975-1978.
3. Baile WF, Lenzi R, Parker A, et al. Oncologists' attitudes toward and practices in giving bad news: An exploratory study. J Clin Oncol 2002;20:2189-2196.
4. Christakis NA, Iwashina TJ. Attitude and self-reported practice regarding prognostication in a national sample of internists. Arch Intern Med 1998;158:2389-2395.
5. Clayton JM, Butow PN, Tattersall MHN. When and how to initiate discussion about prognosis and end-of-life issues with terminally ill patients. J Pain Symptom Manage 2005;30:132-144.
6. Emanuel EJ, Fairclough DL, Wolfe P, et al. Talking with terminally ill patients and their caregivers about death, dying, and bereavement: Is it stressful? Is it helpful? Arch Intern Med 2004;164:1999-2004.
7. Clayton JM, Butow PN, Arnold RM, et al. Fostering coping and nurturing hope when discussing the future with terminally ill cancer patients and their caregivers. Cancer 2005;103:1965-1975.
8. Chochinov HM, Tataryn DJ, Wilson KG, et al. Prognostic awareness and the terminally ill. Psychosomatics 2000;41:500-504.
9. Schofield PE, Butow PN, Thompson JF, et al. Psychological responses of patients receiving a diagnosis of cancer. Ann Oncol 2003;14:48-56.
10. Weeks JC, Cook EF, O'Day SJ, et al. Relationship between cancer patients' predictions of prognosis and their treatment preferences. JAMA 1998;279:1709-1714.
11. The AM, Hak T, Koeter G, et al. Collusion in doctor-patient communication about imminent death: An ethnographic study. BMJ 2000;321:1376-1381.
12. Fallowfield LJ, Jenkins VA, Beveridge HA. Truth may hurt but deceit hurts more: Communication in palliative care. Palliat Med 2002;16:297-303.
13. Clayton JM, Butow PN, Arnold RM, et al. Discussing life expectancy with terminally ill cancer patients and their carers: A qualitative study. Support Care Cancer 2005;13:733-742.
14. Kirk P, Kirk I, Kristjanson LJ. What do patients receiving palliative care for cancer and their families want to be told? A Canadian and Australian qualitative study. BMJ 2004;328:1343-1347.
15. Hagerty RG, Butow PN, Ellis PA, et al. Cancer patient preferences for communication of prognosis in the metastatic setting. J Clin Oncol 2004;22:1721-1730.
16. Butow PN, Dowsett S, Hagerty R, et al. Communicating prognosis to patients with metastatic disease: What do they really want to know? Support Care Cancer 2002;10:161-168.
17. Wenrich MD, Curtis JR, Shannon SE, et al. Communicating with dying patients within the spectrum of medical care from terminal diagnosis to death. Arch Intern Med 2001;161:868-874.
18. Wright EB, Holcombe C, Salmon P. Doctors' communication of trust, care, and respect in breast cancer: Qualitative study. BMJ 2004;328:864-867.
19. Fogarty LA, Curbow BA, Wingard JR, et al. Can 40 seconds of compassion reduce patient anxiety? J Clin Oncol 1999;17:371-379.
20. Girgis A, Sanson-Fisher RW. Breaking bad news: Consensus guidelines for medical practitioners. J Clin Oncol 1995;13:2449-2456.
21. Greisinger AJ, Lorimor RJ, Aday LA, et al. Terminally ill cancer patients: Their most important concerns. Cancer Pract 1997;5:147-154.
22. Hagerty RG, Butow PN, Ellis PM, et al. Communicating prognosis in cancer care: A systematic review of the literature. Ann Oncol 2005;16:1005-1053.
23. Kutner JS, Steiner JF, Corbett KK, et al. Information needs in terminal illness. Soc Sci Med 1999;48:1341-1352.
24. Grbich C, Parker D, Maddocks I. Communication and information needs of care-givers of adult family members at diagnosis and during treatment of terminal cancer. Prog Palliat Care 2000;8:345-350.
25. Huang X, Butow PN, Meiser M, et al. Communicating in a multi-cultural society: The needs of Chinese cancer patients in Australia. Aust N Z J Med 1999;9:207-213.
26. Heaven CM, Maguire P. Disclosure of concerns by hospice patients and their identification by nurses. Palliat Med 1997;11:283-290.

27. Arora NK. Interacting with cancer patients: The significance of physicians' communication behaviour. Soc Sci Med 2003;57:791-806.

28. Maguire P, Faulkner A, Booth K, et al. Helping cancer patients disclose their concerns. Eur J Cancer 1996;32A:78-81.

29. Friedrichsen MJ. Justification for information and knowledge: Perceptions of family members in palliative home care in Sweden. Palliat Support Care 2003;1:239-245.

30. Steinhauser KE, Clipp EC, McNeilly M, et al. In search of a good death: Observations of patients, families, and providers. Ann Intern Med 2000;132:825-832.

31. Clayton JM, Butow PN, Tattersall MHN. The needs of terminally ill cancer patients versus those of their caregivers for information about prognosis and end-of-life issues. Cancer 2005;103:1957-1964.

32. Dowsett SM, Saul JL, Butow PN, et al. Communication styles in the cancer consultation: Preferences for a patient-centred approach. Psychooncology 2000;9:147-156.

33. Gattellari M, Voigt KJ, Butow PN, Tattersall MH. When the treatment goal is not cure: Are cancer patients equipped to make informed decisions? J Clin Oncol 2002;20:503-513.

34. Baile WF, Buckman R, Lenzi R, et al. SPIKES—A six-step protocol for delivering bad news: Application to the patient with cancer. Oncologist 2000;5:302-311.

35. Morita T, Akechi T, Ikenaga M, et al. Communication about the ending of anticancer treatment and transition to palliative care. Ann Oncol 2004;15:1551-1557.

36. Friedrichsen MJ, Strang PM, Carlsson ME. Cancer patients' interpretations of verbal expressions when given information about ending cancer treatment. Palliat Med 2002;16:323-330.

37. World Health Organization. Definition of palliative care. National cancer control guidelines: Policies and managerial guidelines. Geneva: World Health Organization, 2002.

38. Schofield P, Carey M, Love A, et al. "Would you like to talk about your future treatment options?" Discussing the transition from curative cancer treatment to palliative care. Palliat Med 2006;20:397-406.

39. Hagerty RG, Butow PN, Ellis PM, et al. Communicating with realism and hope: Incurable cancer patients' views on the disclosure of prognosis. J Clin Oncol 2005;23:1278-1288.

40. Flemming K. The imponderable: A search for meaning—The meaning of hope to palliative care cancer patients. Int J Palliat Nurs 1997;3:14-18.

41. Fallowfield L, Jenkins V, Farewell V, et al. Efficacy of a Cancer Research UK communication skills training model for oncologists: A randomised controlled trial. Lancet 2002;359:650-656.

42. Fallowfield L, Jenkins V, Farewell V, et al. Enduring impact of communication skills training: Results of a 12-month follow-up. Br J Cancer 2003;89:1445-1449.

43. Lenzi R, Baile WF, Berek J, et al. Design, conduct and evaluation of a communication course for oncology fellows. J Cancer Educ 2005;20:143-149.

44. Scott JT, Entwistle VA, Sowden AJ, et al. Recordings or summaries of consultations for people with cancer. Cochrane Database Syst Rev 2003;(2):CD001539.

45. McHugh P, Lewis S, Ford S, et al. The efficacy of audiotapes in promoting psychological well-being in cancer patients: A randomised, controlled trial. Br J Cancer 1995;71:388-392.

46. Kaplan SH, Greenfield S, Ware JE Jr. Assessing the effects of physician-patient interactions on the outcomes of chronic disease. Med Care 1989;27:S110-S127.

47. Butow PN, Dunn SM, Tattersall MH, et al. Patient participation in the cancer consultation: evaluation of a question prompt sheet. Ann Oncol 1994;5:199-204.

48. Brown RF, Butow PN, Dunn SM, et al. Promoting patient participation and shortening cancer consultations: A randomised trial. Br J Cancer 2001;85:273-279.

49. Clayton JM, Butow PN, Tattersall MHN, et al. Asking questions can help: Development and preliminary evaluation of a question prompt list for palliative care patients. Br J Cancer 2003;89:2069-2077.

50. Clayton JM, Butow PN, Devine R, et al. Randomized controlled trial of a prompt list to help advanced cancer patients and their caregivers to ask questions about prognosis and end-of-life care. J Clin Oncol 2007;25:715-723.

SUGGESTED READING

Clayton JM, Hancock K, Butow PN, et al. Clinical practice guidelines for communicating prognosis and end-of-life issues with adults in the advanced stages of a life-limiting illness, and their caregivers. Med J Australia 2007;186:S77-S108.

Hagerty RG, Butow PN, Ellis PM, et al. Communicating prognosis in cancer care: A systematic review of the literature. Ann Oncol 2005;16:1005-1053.

Schofield P, Carey M, Love A, et al. "Would you like to talk about your future treatment options?" Discussing the transition from curative cancer treatment to palliative care. Palliat Med 2006;20:397-406.

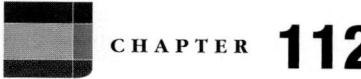

CHAPTER **112**

Problems in Communication

Katja Elbert-Avila and James A. Tulsky

KEY POINTS

- Prepare for, rather than avoid, difficult conversations.
- It is more useful to view a communication challenge as a relationship problem than to attribute it to difficult people. We can change only our own behavior.
- Manage emotions in the clinical setting.
- Further research is needed on communication problems in palliative care.

Excellent communication is an essential component of palliative care.[1-3] Chapters 10, 110, and 111 address the skills needed for successfully discussing a do not resuscitate (DNR) order, presenting palliative care, withdrawing nutrition, breaking bad news, and communicating with cultural competence. Even when these practices are applied, problems in communication occur. Patients and families facing life-threatening illness have complex medical, social, cultural, and emotional needs and perspectives, which may not be recognized by the clinicians caring for them.[2,4] Suboptimal communication is common,[5,6] and it may exacerbate the suffering of the patient and family and lead to conflict.[2,5] Conflict is common in the care of critically ill patients[7] and among families of elders with advanced chronic disease.[8] Stressful conversations and conflicts do occur in health care; attempting to avoid them may impair care and decision making.[4,9]

This chapter builds on basic communication skills by reviewing tools and strategies for clinicians to use in problem situations. These strategies are primarily derived from published expert opinion in the medical and conflict negotiation literature. There is no easily reproducible, evidence-based intervention to alleviate all of the potential communication problems clinicians may face. Although caution must be exercised when applying conceptual theories to contexts for which they were not developed,[10] considering these strategies may allow clinicians to anticipate stressful conversations, develop a greater awareness of their own responses, and prepare tools to adapt to individual situations.

COMPONENTS OF COMMUNICATION PROBLEMS

Numerous reasons exist for communication problems in palliative care. Goold and colleagues[11] suggested creating a "differential diagnosis" for conflict and evaluating potential contributing factors. Consideration of these factors, particularly those related to providers, patients and families, and provider and patient or family relationships, can offer a basis for potential solutions.

Provider Factors

Research suggests that health care providers do not fully elicit patients' concerns (particularly psychosocial concerns),[5,6] attend to affect,[5] or evaluate patients' understanding of the medical situation.[12] Physicians may not communicate frank survival estimates[13] and may avoid end-of-life issues until late in a patient's course.[4]

Several theories explain why physicians do not communicate well. Cognitive skills, not communication skills, have been emphasized in selection and training.[5] With a focus on physical health issues, many physicians may not feel responsible for or comfortable with discussing emotions.[6] Physicians' feelings and beliefs about the patient, the chronically ill, mortality, uncertainty, and their own identities as healers may influence the physician-patient relationship.[5,11] Recognizing and dealing explicitly with these emotional responses to dying patients or conflict allows them to focus more objectively on the interests of patients.[5] Physicians and other health care providers can benefit by finding the reflective time, often with colleagues, to address these issues.

Some health care providers may undervalue collaboration[4] and may lack the curiosity to learn about another person's experience and perspectives.[5] Such curiosity is considered a key ingredient in successful conversations.[14]

Patient and Family Factors

Patients and families may not fully understand the medical situation, or perceive it in the same way as health care providers. In one study, 48% of cancer patients receiving palliative care indicated cure as their goal for therapy.[15] Poor understanding may result from conflicting information sources,[11] effects of medical illness and medications, and co-morbidities.[10,16] Delirium[17] and affective disorders[18] are common in the palliative care setting, and the cognitive capacity of seriously ill hospitalized patients may be impaired,[10,19] damaging the ability to process information and to cope with strong emotions.[18] Strong emotions are common in the palliative care setting[3,18] and can affect information processing, perceptions, and decision making.[5] Patients and families may use denial and avoidance of the problem to reduce emotional distress,[2,11,18] may not be prepared to receive information, and may prefer to negotiate when information about dying is discussed.[20] Serious illness may threaten a patient's sense of identity[18] and basic needs for security, recognition, and control. Their responses to such feelings may include paranoia and distrust, overt demonstrations of involvement, perseveration about the details of care, and other behaviors seen as disruptive by health care staff.[2]

Relationship and Communication Factors

The approach to communication may itself contribute to poor communication. It is helpful to approach communication as a process that evolves over time.[2] Development of a collaborative relationship may mediate potential contributors to communication problems. If communication is approached as a discrete task and factors such as emotion, identity issues, and perception are not addressed, problems can escalate.[2] Patients, families, and clinicians may react to these problems by arguing for certain positions and missing opportunities to address underlying needs. For example, a clinician who does not assess a patient's emotions, understanding, and readiness to discuss prognosis may be surprised by a patient or family member who does not believe the diagnosis.[2] In this setting, trying to persuade the patient or family (e.g., by showing them radiological evidence) does not lead to an increased understanding of their perceptions, emotions, or needs and may contribute to distrust[2] (Table 112-1).

DIFFICULT CONVERSATIONS

Based on negotiation research, Stone[14] proposed that every difficult conversation is really three conversations and that all three need to be addressed to understand what the conversation is about (Fig. 112-1). These three conversations center on what happened, feelings, and identity. According to this model, the primary task in successful communication is not to persuade another party, but to understand what each side perceives, why they perceive it that way, how they feel, and what this means about who they are and then to use this information to reach a negotiated understanding that leaves everyone feeling heard.[14]

TABLE 112-1   Potential Contributors to Poor Communication

PATIENT OR FAMILY	PROVIDER	RELATIONSHIP
Psychosocial distress, strong emotion, grief	Psychosocial distress, strong emotion, or grief; lack of training in addressing psychosocial distress[5]	Lack of management of emotions; lack of attention to psychosocial concerns, emotions, or readiness of patient and family to consider death and dying[2,6]
Threats to role identity[11]	Threats to role identity[11]	Lack of exploration of identity issues, loss, and grief
Disadvantaged by language, culture, socioeconomic status, education level[16]	Lack of training in cultural competence[5]	Information imbalance based on conflicting perceptions, interpretations, and values
Lack of understanding of situation (e.g., effects of condition, illness, co-morbidities, conflicting sources of information, emotions)[11]	Providers not assessing for patient understanding[6]	Information imbalance
Distracted by external factors (e.g., influence of family members, perceived time pressures)	Distracted by external factors (e.g., desire to achieve an agenda, perceived time pressures)[5]	Lack of active listening; focus on positions instead of interests or values

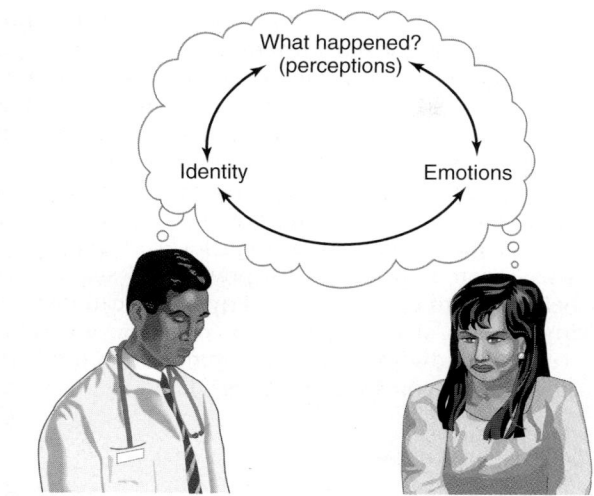

FIGURE 112-1 Difficult conversations encompass perceptions, emotions, and identity. *(Adapted from Stone D, Patton BM, Heen S. Difficult Conversations: How to discuss what matters most. New York: Viking Penguin, 1999.)*

Each side has a "what happened" story.[14] This conversation is not as much about facts as it is about interpretations, perceptions, and values.[14] Providers who do not explore these ideas may miss an opportunity to form a collaborative relationship. Using this model, providers first internally examine their own story about what has happened and their own contributions to a problem.[4,14] In discussions with the patient or family, the primary goal is to explore the patient or family's story, seeking underlying reasons for positions or interpretations. Listening with the primary purpose of understanding the other person is a way to show caring; once heard, people may be more willing to address underlying emotions and to listen.[14] A secondary goal is for the provider to express his or her views as an addition to, not a contradiction of, the views of the patient or family[21] (e.g., "You want to continue to drive, and I am concerned about your driving safety" versus "You may want to drive, but I don't think it's safe."). For this, clarity is crucial. Providers should avoid speaking in euphemisms or around the issues.[22]

Emotions are at the core of every difficult conversation; feelings should be acknowledged before problem solving is attempted.[14] Inattention to affect, the feelings and emotions associated with the content of a conversation, creates communication problems.[5] Providers should consider their own emotions and explore those of the patient and family. Handling emotions is further discussed later in this chapter.

Another aspect that makes conversations in palliative care difficult is their impact on an individual's identity.[14] The self-image as caring health professionals may not allow providers to see their contributions to the problem (e.g., attempts to "educate" a patient or family about the prognosis without acknowledging the distress this is causing). For patients, serious illness may be a threat to their identity.[18] Behaviors such as making a patient wait or interrupting the conversation to deal with other issues may further attack a patient's sense of self-worth.[22] Basic human needs for security, control over a person's life, belonging, and recognition are powerful interests in negotiations[22] and

may be threatened in the palliative care setting. For example, a patient who responds to a recommendation for increased assistance with "I can take care of myself" may perceive the recommendation as a threat to his or her self-image.[18] Rather than refuting this statement (e.g., "I don't think you can live alone."), the clinician should explore what patients mean, why it is important for them to take care of themselves, and how they perceive the recommendation. The discussion can then be reframed to address these issues (e.g., "You are someone who runs the show, and no one wants to change that. Your daughter would like to help you. I wonder if allowing her to help might make her feel needed and allow you more energy for the things you want to focus on."). Understanding a patient's self-image and the impact illness has on this can allow a clinician to better support the patient.[18]

Overcoming Disagreement

Negotiation research offers several insights into dealing with disagreement that may be useful to the health care provider. In general, experts recommend dealing explicitly with emotions, but suspending one's emotional reaction to emotional outbursts.[21,22] One technique is to slow the discussion by summarizing what the other person has said (e.g., "I want to check whether I understand what you are saying."). Negative emotions or attacks may be diffused by accepting the other person's position.[14,21,22] This is not the same as agreement; a provider can accept that a patient wishes to be cured and does not wish to be admitted to the hospital while not agreeing that both are possible (e.g., "You want a cure, and you do not want surgery. I wish there were a nonsurgical cure we could offer."). Understanding and acceptance are enhanced by active listening, paraphrasing, asking for corrections, acknowledging the patient's point, and taking the viewpoint of a nonjudgmental third party.[14,21,22] After acceptance has been expressed, the provider should reframe what has been said in a way that addresses a problem to be solved together[14,21,22] (e.g., "You are angry that your mother received pain medication without your permission. Can you tell me about your concerns?"). The goal is to build a working relationship.

Difficult People

Although patient barriers to communication exist, communication challenges are best viewed as a relationship problem instead of a problem with a difficult person.[23] By considering why a patient is challenging and including the provider's own emotional reaction, clinicians may be better able to address communication barriers and obtain useful clues about what the patient is feeling.[5,23] If the provider feels overly sad, for example, it may be a reflection of the patient's sadness. Asking the patient about this (e.g., "I wonder if you are feeling sad?") may lead to a better understanding of their emotional state.[5,23]

AN APPROACH TO HANDLING EMOTIONS

One barrier to exploring the emotions of patients and families is the concern about how to manage the response in a manner that conveys a sense of empathy.[5] Robert Smith created a mnemonic (NURS: name, understand, respect, support) to recall basic techniques in managing emotions; it has been refined further into NURSE (name, understand, respect, support, explore)[5]:

- Naming the emotion. The first step is to acknowledge the emotion. This is best done in a questioning manner (e.g., "I wonder if you feel angry.") that does not make assumptions about how the other person feels (e.g., "You are angry.").
- Expressing some sense of understanding is meant to validate the emotion. This should not presume an understanding about the other person's situation, but it acknowledges that their emotions are important and normal (e.g., "I cannot imagine what you are going through; this must be a difficult topic to discuss.").
- Respect reminds providers to praise patients and families for how they are managing a difficult situation and to acknowledge their competence and authority.
- Statements of support indicate that patients will have ongoing support for their physical and psychosocial concerns.
- Exploring patient statements and emotions (e.g., "Tell me more.") is essential in gaining a greater understanding about their concern. Anger directed at staff may reflect anger at a situation.[22] Explore potential underlying problems, such as distrust or depression.[23]

Although these techniques can be useful, it is important to remember the goal of listening to understand the other person. Careful wording cannot convey caring if the clinician is not genuinely listening.[14]

Anger

Anger at a situation, a normal response to loss or threat, may lead to expression of anger toward someone associated with that loss.[22] Providers may vary in their responses to anger, and they should reflect on their own typical response (e.g., withdrawal, defensiveness) to suspend this reaction.[21] Anger can be managed with the techniques outlined earlier for managing emotions and overcoming disagreement.

Anxiety and Denial

Denial is an inability to explicitly recognize facts because of unacceptable psychological consequences.[18,23] As a coping mechanism, this may have a positive effect by reducing anxiety,[18,23] and it may change over time or may not be complete.[18] Patients may recognize they have a terminal illness while focusing on living as if this were not the case. It usually is best not to challenge this coping mechanism.[18] A provider's attempts to persuade patients and families about the reality of a poor prognosis without paying attention to emotion are likely to lead to frustration for everyone involved.[11] Instead, acknowledging, validating, and exploring emotions and fears may allow a collaborative relationship, in which patients may better attend to information.[11,18] Denial is further explored in the Chapter 117.

Hope

Provision of hope is a challenging aspect of communication in palliative care, and it can affect decision making.[24] Patients and families want providers to balance communicating in a straightforward and honest way while maintaining hope and optimism.[1] Important aspects of hope include indications health professionals are not giving up, living normally, relationships, and reconciliation with life and death.[25,26] Patients and families can acknowledge the terminal nature of illness and still maintain hope.[26]

Physicians can respond to hope by acknowledging its importance and by assuring the patient and family that they will not be abandoned. A high level of emotional distress has been associated with physicians' statements about being able to do nothing.[3,27] Physicians can discuss the many aspects of hope and focus on achievable outcomes (e.g., "I know that you are hoping for a cure. Are there other things you are hoping for?").[5]

Role of the Spokesperson

Whether a result of the patient's preference or incapacity to make decisions, communication often occurs between clinicians and the patient's family. Patients should be involved to the extent of their capacity and desire for involvement. The law often prioritizes identification of a single decision maker.[5] This can ensure clear communication, avoid multiple stories, clarify who will provide consent or have final decision-making authority, and respect the wishes of the patient. However, overemphasis on designating a single spokesperson may exclude well-meaning people and exacerbate family conflict. For this reason, communication and decisions often involve the entire family.[5] This can create conflicts if family members disagree. One approach is to agree on a standard for decision making, such as what the patient would want.[28] This centers problem solving on something common, such as commitment to the patient's interests.[28] The communication strategies outlined in this chapter apply whether the spokesperson is the patient or family (see "Common Errors").

CONCLUSIONS, CHALLENGES, AND OPPORTUNITIES

Communication in palliative care is fraught with potential problems. Despite a large body of literature documenting

Common Errors
Avoiding or not recognizing conflict and difficult conversations[4,14]
Not eliciting the other person's understanding, perceptions, values, emotions, or intentions[4,14]
Not paying attention to emotions or affect[5]
Not assessing the readiness of the patient and family to consider death[2]
Linking palliative care with the acceptance of a short life span by framing treatment choices with statements about prognosis, such as "because we cannot cure, we will focus on comfort" (i.e., negative impact of the prognosis may affect perception of the provider's intentions)[2]
Misdiagnosing grief as denial[2]
Debating the "fact" of impending death[2] and repeatedly trying to convince the other party about medical facts or "reality"[4,14]
Presenting decisions in an impersonal manner without helping patients or families incorporate their values into decision making[2] and not making recommendations that address the other parties' interests[22]

TABLE 112-2 Trials of Communication Interventions

INTERVENTION	TRIAL DESIGN	RESULTS	STUDY
Nurse-provided information on patient preferences and prognosis to physicians	Multicenter, randomized, controlled trial	No impact on any patient outcome	SUPPORT Investigators. JAMA 1995;274:1591-1598
Proactive ethics consultation in ICU	Multicenter, randomized, controlled trial	Reduction in hospital and ICU days and life-sustaining treatment for those who did not survive to discharge; no difference in mortality	Schneiderman LJ et al. JAMA 2003;290:1166-1172
Formal family meetings in ICU	Nonrandomized, nonblinded	Decreased family nonconsensus days; reduction in resource use among those who died in the ICU	Lilly CM et al. Am J Med 2000;109:469-475
Standardized HRQL assessments in outpatient oncology clinic	Randomized, crossover	HRQL-elated issues discussed more frequently in intervention group; improved identification of patients with moderate to severe problems in several HRQL domains	Detmar SB et al. JAMA 2002;288:3027-3034
Measurement of HRQL in oncology clinic	Randomized, controlled trial	More frequent discussion of chronic, nonspecific symptoms	Velikova G et al. J Clin Oncol 2004;22:714-724
Provision of recordings or summaries of key oncology consultations	Systematic review	Five of nine studies with better recall of information and four of seven studies with increased patient satisfaction; most patients found summaries useful	Scott JT et al. Cochrane Database Syst Rev 2003;(2): CD001539

HRQL, health-related quality of life; ICU, intensive care unit.

deficiencies and proposing a variety of communication interventions (Table 112-2), many proposed interventions have not been based on empirical evidence[1] and lack evidence for efficacy and effectiveness to improve clinically important outcomes.[1,29,30] The success of required ethics consultation and family meetings in the intensive care setting suggest that a proactive approach to communication problems can improve patient care.

What type of communication should a proactive approach include? Theories developed from negotiation research may be useful to health care providers, and they suggest that attempting to understand the perceptions and values of patients and families and dealing with emotions are important features of difficult conversations and negotiations. Ultimately, these theories will need to be studied in the context of palliative care.

As research challenges in measuring the quality of life in the palliative care setting are addressed, researchers have increasing opportunities to link valid, clinically important outcomes to specific and generalizable communication interventions.[29,30] Proposals for future palliative care communication research include the following:

- Further research on patients' preferences about information,[1,3] the information and advice-giving processes,[3] and decision-making practices[3]
- The development of evidence-based, detailed, and reproducible manualized communication protocols for study and comparison in controlled trials[29,30]
- Creation of larger and more diverse standardized data sets[1]
- Improved, standardized analysis of communication data[1]
- Further research on the interdisciplinary delivery of communication interventions[3,29,30]
- Evaluation of cost-effectiveness[29,30]
- Evaluation of health service strategies to implement communication interventions in a variety of practice settings and for a variety of patient populations
- Further research on health services factors that facilitate or inhibit effective communication[10]

As the evidence base for communication interventions grows, research should also focus on communication interventions for various demographic groups, such as the elderly, or different cultural groups who may have specific communication needs and challenges. Efficient and effective ways to teach providers about communication skills should be developed.[1]

REFERENCES

1. Tulsky JA. Interventions to enhance communication among patients, providers, and families. J Palliative Med 2005;8:S95-S102.
2. Weiner JS, Roth J. Avoiding iatrogenic harm to patient and family while discussing goals of care near the end of life. J Palliative Med 2006;9:451-463.
3. de Haes H, Teunissen S. Communication in palliative care: A review of recent literature. Curr Opin Oncol 2005;17:345-350.
4. Back AL, Arnold RM. Dealing with conflict in caring for the seriously ill. JAMA 2005;293:1374-1381.
5. Tulsky JA, Arnold RM. Communication at the end of life. In Berger AM, Portney RK, Wissman DE (eds). Principles and Practices of Palliative Care and Supportive Oncology. Philadelphia: Lippincott Williams & Wilkins, 2002, pp 673-684.
6. Detmar SB, Muller MJ, Wever LDV. Patient-physician communication during outpatient palliative treatment visits. An observational study. JAMA 2001;285:1351-1357.
7. Breen CM, Abernethy AP, Abbott KH, et al. Conflict associated with decisions to limit life-sustaining treatment in intensive care units. J Gen Intern Med 2001;16:283-289.
8. Kramer BJ, Boelk AZ, Auer C. Family conflict at the end of life: Lessons learned in a model program for vulnerable older adults. J Palliat Med 2006;9:791-801.
9. Weiner JS, Cole SA. Three principles to improve clinician communication for advance care planning: Overcoming emotional, cognitive, and skill barriers. J Palliat Med 2004;7:817-829.
10. Epstein RM. Making communication research matter: What do patients notice, what do patients want, and what do patients need? Patient Educ Couns 2006;60:272-278.
11. Goold SD, Williams B, Arnold RM. Conflicts regarding decisions to limit treatment. JAMA 2000;283:909-914.
12. Gattellari, M, Voigt, K, Butow, et al. When the treatment goal is not cure: Are cancer patients equipped to make informed decisions? J Clin Oncol 2002;20:503-513.
13. Lamont EB, Christakis NA. Prognostic disclosure to patients with cancer near the end of life. Ann Intern Med 2001;134:1096-1105.
14. Stone D, Patton BM, Heen S. Difficult Conversations: How to Discuss What Matters Most. New York: Viking Penguin, 1999.
15. Petrasch S, Bauer M, Reinacher-Schick A, et al. Assessment of satisfaction with the communication process during consultation of cancer patients with potentially curable disease, cancer patients on palliative care, and HIV-positive patients. Wien Med Wochenschr 1998;148:491-499.
16. NHNRC 2004. Communicating with Patients: Advice for Medical Practitioners. Available at http://www.nhmrc.gov.au/publications/synopses/e58syn.htm (accessed April 4, 2008).

17. Spiller JA, Keen JC. Hypoactive delirium: assessing the extent of the problem for inpatient specialist palliative care. Palliat Med 2006;20:17-23.

18. Block SD.: Psychological issues in end-of-life care. J Palliat Med 2006;9: 751-772.

19. Cassell EJ, Leon AC, Kaufman SG. Preliminary evidence of impaired thinking in sick patients. Ann Intern Med 2001;134:1120-1123.

20. Hagerty RG, Butow PN, Ellis PA, et al. Cancer patient preferences for communication of prognosis in the metastatic setting. J Clin Oncol 2004;22:1721-1730.

21. Ury W. Getting Past No: Negotiating with Difficult People. New York: Bantam Books, 1993.

22. Fisher R, Ury W. Getting to Yes: Negotiating Agreement Without Giving In. New York: Penguin Books, 1983.

23. Lee SJ, Back AL, Block SD, et al. Enhancing physician-patient communication. Am Soc Hematol Educ Program 2002;464-483.

24. Grunfeld EA. Advanced breast cancer patients' perceptions of decision making for palliative chemotherapy. J Clin Oncol 2006;24:1090-1098.

25. Tattersall MHN, Butow PN, Clayton JM. Insights from cancer patient communication research. Hematol Oncol Clin North Am 2002;16:731-743.

26. Kirk P, Kirk I, Kristjanson LJ. What do patients receiving palliative care for cancer and their families want to be told? A Canadian and Australian qualitative study. BMJ 2004;328:1343.

27. Morita T, Akechi T, Ikenaga M, et al. Communication about the ending of anticancer treatment and transition to palliative care. Ann Oncol 2004;15:1551-1557.

28. Bloche MG. Managing conflict at the end of life. N Engl J Med 2005;352: 2371-2373.

29. Weiner JS, Arnold RM, Curtis JR, et al. Manualized communication interventions to enhance palliative care research and training: rigorous, testable approaches. J Palliat Med 2006;9:371-381.

30. National Institutes of Health. State-of-the-Science Conference statement: Improving end-of-life care. Presented at the State of the Science Conference, December 6-8, 2004. Available at http://www.consensus.nih.gov/2004/2004EndOfLifeCareSOS024html.htm (accessed December 13, 2007).

SUGGESTED READING

Back AL, Arnold RM. Dealing with conflict in caring for the seriously ill. JAMA 2003:293:1374-1381.

Goold SD, Williams B, Arnold RM. Conflicts regarding decisions to limit treatment: A differential diagnosis. JAMA 2000;283: 909-914.

Stone D, Patton BM, Heen S. Difficult Conversations: How to Discuss What Matters Most. New York: Viking Penguin, 1999.

Weiner JS, Roth J. Avoiding iatrogenic harm to patient and family while discussing goals of care near the end of life. J Palliat Med 2006;9:451-463.

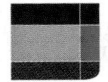

CHAPTER **113**

Counseling

David Spiegel

KEY POINTS

- Intense interpersonal closeness is experienced in being able to discuss death openly.

- Death can be discussed from the perspective of those grieving the loss of others and from that of the dying.

- Counseling provides opportunities for showing the dying how to provide wisdom, comfort, and support to those left behind.

- Existential concerns are treated as understandable, rather than as an indication of failure or weakness.

- Affective expression is encouraged, providing dimensions and means of managing it that make it less overwhelming.

Counseling may seem irrelevant or even potentially harmful in palliative care. Dying patients and their families face the end of their lives, loss of relationships, and the final limitation on their hopes and dreams. Can talking about these issues do nothing more than stir up fear and sadness? Death is a source of dread, but it is virtually impossible to comprehend. A person's pending nonexistence can be discussed in religious, existential, or biological terms, but it is often most keenly experienced as isolation and separation from loved ones. Death has a profoundly social dimension, reflecting our nature as social beings. Those who believe in life after death often focus their faith on reunion with loved ones.

Counseling, with its potential for intense emotional interaction, can address and even counter the social isolation intertwined with death anxiety. Paradoxically, intense discussion of existential concerns in a group can be reassuring in several ways. For these and other reasons, counseling is a valuable tool to support the dying.

TREATMENT INTERVENTIONS

Counseling for psychological symptoms of patients in palliative care can be determined by clarifying the nature of emotional distress (e.g., anxiety, depression, psychosis), the use of pharmacotherapy to relieve acute and chronic symptoms, and selection of appropriate psychotherapeutic interventions for problems related to anxiety, depression, existential concerns, somatic symptoms, and social and communication problems[1-3] (see Chapters 8, 54, 118, and 120). Supportive-expressive[4-6] and cognitive-behavioral models are discussed.[7]

Supportive-Expressive Psychotherapy

Common elements of psychotherapeutic intervention in palliative care, both individual and group, include social support, emotional expression, processing existential concerns, reorganizing life priorities, and living in the present[4] (Box 113-1).

Social Support

Psychotherapy, especially in groups, can provide a new social network with the common bond of facing similar problems. At a time when the illness and fear of dying and death makes a person feel removed from the flow of life and when many others withdraw because of awkwardness or fear, psychotherapeutic support provides a new and important social connection (see "Case Study: Group Support").

Emotional Expression

The expression of emotion is important in reducing social isolation and improving coping. However, patients often believe that they are controlling the psychological and physical impact of the disease by suppressing their emotional reaction to it. This attitude is often reinforced by friends and family made anxious by a display of appropriate fear or sadness in the course of dying. They often misinterpret normal anticipatory grieving as nihilism about treatment or loss of hope. Persistent negative affect (e.g., depression) often elicits anger in those involved with the

> ## Box 113-1 Supportive and Expressive Group Psychotherapy Themes
>
> - Building bonds
> - Expressing emotion
> - Detoxifying dying
> - Reordering life priorities
> - Fortifying families
> - Clarifying communication with physician
> - Symptom management

C A S E   S T U D Y

Group Support

Mary was an elegant woman who faithfully attended her supportive/expressive therapy group every week. Her hair was perfectly coiffed, and she was well dressed, even after her metastatic breast cancer had become widespread. One day, she said to the group, "You know, my husband is a banker but not a teller—he doesn't talk. I think he has had enough of my illness. I am becoming weaker, and I wonder if it isn't time for me to take steps to shorten my life."

The group could have focused on speculation about her husband, especially his lack of communication and lack of support. However, the group leader chose to focus on the here-and-now issues, viewing Mary's quandary as a question for the group as well. "I wonder if Mary is not also asking us whether we have 'had enough' of her illness and whether we would in some way feel better if she were gone?" Group members immediately gave her strong positive feedback about what an example of courage and composure she was in the face of death. She felt warmly included in the group, and she died naturally several months later. She left a provision in her will that the group would be picked up in a limousine and driven to her memorial service, where they participated in grieving her.

patient, because they seem unwilling rather than unable to modulate their feelings. However, normal anxiety and sadness related to having cancer is intermittent, and it is better managed by means of expression and working through it. Encouragement of emotional expression can enhance intimacy in families, providing opportunities for direct expression of affection and concern, and this can be effectively modeled for patient and family in psychotherapy. Psychotherapeutic setting to deal with painful affect also provides an organizing context for handling its intrusion. When unbidden thoughts involving fears of dying and death intrude, they can be better managed by patients who know that there is a time and a place during which such feelings will be expressed, acknowledged, and dealt with.

Detoxifying Dying: Processing Existential Concerns

Facing issues such as dying and death rather than exacerbating demoralization and depression, helps to reduce concerns. This approach encourages patients to face what they most fear and to find some aspect of it they can do something about (e.g., control the process of dying when

C A S E   S T U D Y

Group Psychotherapy

One group member reported, "My husband is hopeless about planning anything, and I don't want him to have to figure out what to do with my body after I die. So I called Skylawn Park (a very beautiful local cemetery overlooking the Pacific Ocean) and asked what it would cost to be buried there. They quoted me some astronomical amount of money, and I said, 'Actually, I represent a group of women looking for a place to be buried.' There was a long pause on the phone, and then the woman said, 'Skylawn Park does not offer group discounts.'" There was heartfelt laughter among the group members, who had faced the grim reality of planning for their interment and were able to laugh at the idea of obtaining a group discount at a cemetery.

death is unavoidable). Patients feel more active and less helpless, even in the face of dying.[2,4,8] Death anxiety in particular is intensified by isolation, in part because we often conceptualize death as separation from loved ones. This can be powerfully addressed by psychotherapeutic techniques that directly address such concerns.[6]

The ultimate existential concerns are death, freedom, isolation, and meaninglessness. Rather than avoiding painful or anxiety-provoking topics in an attempt to "stay positive," effective psychotherapy addresses these concerns directly with the intent of helping patients make better use of the time left. The goal is to help those facing death to see it from a new viewpoint. When worked through, life-threatening problems can be experienced as real but not overwhelming. Facing life-threatening issues directly can help patients shift from emotion-focused to problem-focused coping.[9-11]

The process of dying is often more threatening than death itself. Direct discussion of death anxiety can divide the fear of death into a series of problems: loss of control over treatment decisions, fear of separation from loved ones, anxiety about pain, and controlling the manner of dying. Discussion of these concerns can lead to means of addressing each of these issues. Even the grieving process can be reassuring while it is threatening. The patient's experience of grieving for others who have died of the same condition constitutes a deeply personal experience of the depth of loss that will be experienced by others after the patient's own death (see "Case Study: Group Psychotherapy").

Reorganizing Life Priorities and Living in the Present

The acceptance of the possibility of illness shortening life carries with it an opportunity for re-evaluating life priorities. Facing the threat of death in a way that facilitates a sense of active coping can help make the most of life.[12] This can help patients take control of the aspects of their lives they can influence while grieving and relinquishing those they cannot. For cancer patients experiencing the traumatic stressor of anticipating their imminent death and its impact on their loved ones, adjustment may be mediated by changes from past- or future-focused orientation to a present-focused orientation that is more congruent with the reality of their foreshortened future.

Enhancing Family Support

Psychotherapeutic interventions can be helpful in improving communication, identifying needs, increasing role flexibility, and adjusting to new medical, social, vocational, and financial realities.[13] Psychotherapy can be a model for clarifying communication among family and friends.

Improving Communication with Physicians

Psychotherapy can facilitate communication with physicians and other health professionals,[2,14] helping patients define issues and areas of concern that require clarification (see Chapter 111).

Symptom Control

Psychotherapy can be focused on teaching specific skills designed to control symptoms such as anxiety and pain. Techniques used include specific self-regulation skills such as self-hypnosis, meditation, biofeedback, and progressive muscle relaxation. Hypnosis is widely used for pain and anxiety control in patients with cancer to attenuate the pain experience and suffering and to allow painful emotional material to be examined while maintaining control of somatic reactions.[15] Instruction in self-hypnosis is effective in reducing pain and anxiety and for consolidating the major themes emerging from the psychotherapy.

Psychotherapeutic process goals include the following:

- Personalization to facilitate examination of here-and-now existential and other specific disease-related issues
- Affective expression to follow the affect and encourage direct expression of emotion
- Social support in the use of psychotherapy to improve communication and enhance available social support
- Active coping used in facilitating the development and use of active coping strategies in the face of dying and death

Cognitive-Behavioral Therapy

The cognitive-behavioral approach[7] assumes that previous social learning, developmental history, and significant experiences lead people to form a unique set of meanings and assumptions, or cognitive schemas, about themselves, the world, and the future. These ideas are used to organize perception and govern and evaluate behavior, and they may become maladaptive when life circumstances change. When specific schemas are activated, they directly influence a person's perceptions, interpretations, associations, and memories from a given time. Cognitive-behavioral therapy (CBT) was developed as a short-term intervention (12 to 20 sessions) for depression targeting patients' thoughts and their relation to behavior and affect.

CBT in palliative medicine features coping skills training, stress management, and an intervention to enhance cognitive and behavioral processes necessary to adjust to illness.[16] The CBT therapist identifies maladaptive cognitions, turns them into testable hypotheses, and submits them to empirical investigation, so the patient can then reject, modify, or retain them based on the evidence. Alternatively, more adaptive cognitions and behaviors are similarly examined and tested. In the early sessions, the goal is to establish a therapeutic relationship, identify primary problems, produce symptom relief, and educate the patient about psychotherapy, CBT, and the effects of thoughts, images, and beliefs on emotions and behavior.

The therapist and patient decide on the treatment goal, plan for subsequent therapy sessions, and homework assignments to augment the therapy and direct structured practice. The initial homework may require the patient to identify and record maladaptive cognitions (e.g., automatic thoughts). As therapy progresses, verbal techniques are employed to trigger automatic thoughts and associated assumptions and to reveal core beliefs, or schemas. In an environment of collaborative empiricism, the patient learns to identify, logically and empirically evaluate, and justify the usefulness of systematic biases, cognitive distortions and dysfunctional assumptions, thoughts, images, and beliefs that underlie emotional and existential distress. The therapist helps the patient challenge cognitive distortions such as overgeneralization, catastrophizing, "should" statements, magnification, minimization, dichotomous thinking, and the fallacies of control, worry, fairness, and attachment. Schemas, the complex rules and beliefs that determine the way a patient defines the self, others, and the world, are often activated during times of existential stress and are tested against the evidence as alternatives are examined. Cognitive restructuring techniques and guided discovery help the patient choose more adaptive cognitions and behaviors.

Cognitive techniques used in CBT include thought stopping, self-instruction, distraction, direct disputation, labeling distortions, and development of replacement imagery. Behavioral techniques such as activity scheduling, relaxation training, social skills training, mastery and pleasure ratings, assertiveness training, bibliotherapy, homework, behavioral rehearsal, and in vivo exposure are also employed.

The application of cognitive-behavioral principles to palliative medicine can serve as a means for discussing, coming to terms with, and improving adherence to medical treatment.[17] Kissane and colleagues[18] referred to this as cognitive-existential group therapy. They describe their approach succinctly: "Our broad therapy goals are for members to develop a supportive network, work through grief over losses, improve problem solving and develop cognitive strategies to maximize coping, enhance a sense of mastery over life, and re-evaluate priorities for the future. Specific group themes include death anxiety; fear of recurrence; living with uncertainty; understanding treatment with chemotherapy, radiotherapy, and hormone regimens; the collaborative doctor-patient relationship; body and self-image; sexuality; relationships with partner, friends, and family; surgical reconstruction; lifestyle effects; and future goals. Active coping skills are developed through teaching formal problem solving and cognitive restructuring of automatic negative thoughts" (p. 25).

EVIDENCE-BASED MEDICINE

The efficacy of psychosocial treatments for depression and anxiety in the medically ill, particularly brief psychody-

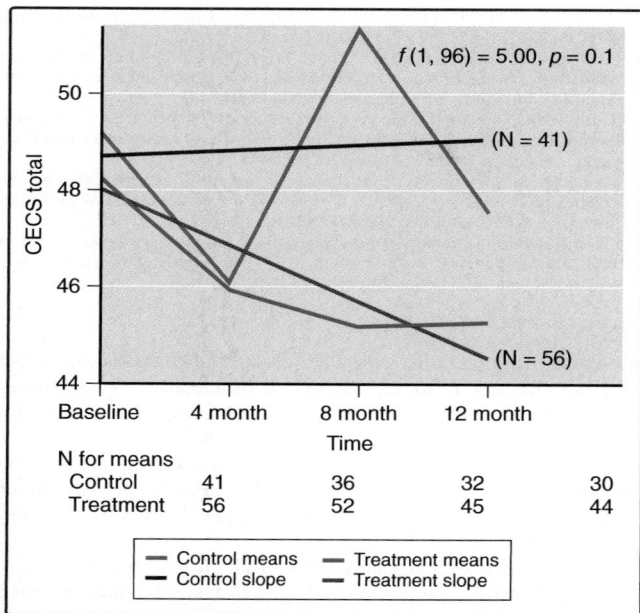

FIGURE 113-1 Effect of group therapy for metastatic breast cancer on the Courtauld Emotional Control Scale (CECS) total score. *(Adapted from Giese-Davis J, Koopman C, Butler LD, et al. Change in emotion-regulation strategy for women with metastatic breast cancer following supportive-expressive group therapy. J Consult Clin Psychol 2002;70:916-925).*

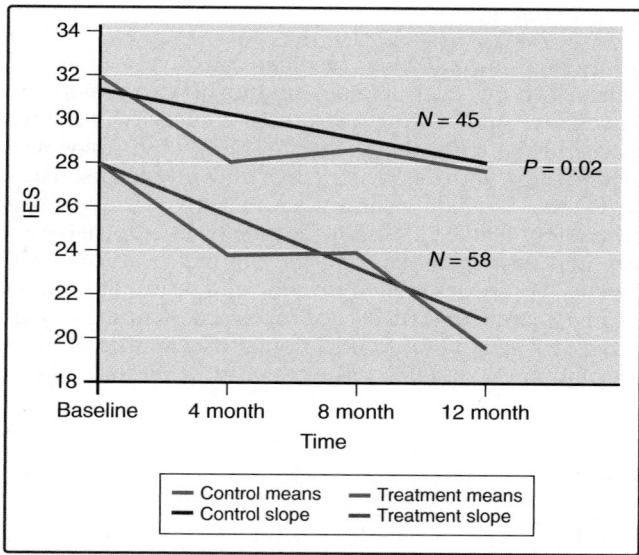

FIGURE 113-2 Effect of group therapy for metastatic breast cancer on Impact of Event Scale (IES) total score over 1 year. *(Adapted from Classen C, Butler LD, Koopman C, et al. Supportive-expressive group therapy reduces distress in metastatic breast cancer patients: A randomized clinical intervention trial. Arch Gen Psychiatry 2001;58:494-501).*

namic, educational, supportive, and interpersonal therapies; hypnosis; and behavioral and cognitive-behavioral methods, are supported by numerous outcome studies[16,19-22] (see Chapter 33).

Many of these approaches have demonstrated benefit in controlled trials. Facing the existential threat posed by cancer in the supportive-expressive model improves coping and reduces distress rather than demoralizing cancer patients.[23,24] Emotional expression facilitates resolution of long-term negative emotions.[24,25] There also is evidence of positive outcome in the related cognitive-existential model.[18,26] Progress in life goal reappraisal, reorganization of priorities, and perception of benefits may also mediate improvement in symptoms and quality of life.[27] An eight-session educational intervention providing training for advanced cancer patients in stress management, problem solving, goal setting, and assertiveness improved quality of life and specific competence in managing emotional, financial and legal problems.[28] A five-session family intervention for women with recurrent breast cancer designed to improve communication, enhance information seeking, improve coping, and manage symptoms did not affect overall quality of life, but it did reduce negative appraisal of the cancer and reduced hopelessness[29] (Figs. 113-1 and 113-2; see "Common Errors").

CONTROVERSIES AND RESEARCH OPPORTUNITIES

A systematic review of the literature that included two meta-analyses and nine well-designed, randomized, controlled trials[20] indicated that psychoeducational interventions enhance patients' knowledge about cancer and treatments but reduce depression, anxiety, nausea, and pain. One meta-analysis reported only limited effects of

Common Errors
• Ignoring or avoiding opportunities to talk directly about death and dying
• Discouraging frank expression of emotion
• Providing different prognostic information to different family members
• Failure to prepare advance directives and other planning for dying and death
• Inadequate pain control and patient control over analgesia

group therapy on improving coping skills and generally modest positive effects on distress and quality of life.[30] It employed stringent inclusion criteria, including blinding of those providing care and blinded assessment of outcome measures, which allowed inclusion of only one fourth (82 of 327) of the intervention trials, raising questions about generalizability. A different meta-analysis examining the effects of psychosocial intervention on the quality of life of cancer patients[31] found an effect size of 31, corresponding to a standardized mean difference of 65. The longer the duration of intervention (≥12 weeks), the better the outcome.

Research challenges include the following:

• Identifying components of psychotherapies that are especially effective, including emotional expression, cognitive restructuring, and enhancing social support
• Improving the match between specific patients and specific treatments
• Identifying especially helpful times in the course of palliative care to provide psychotherapy
• Better understanding the interaction between medication (including psychotropic and analgesic treatments) and facilitation of appropriate psychotherapy, analogous to the studies of psychotherapy and medication for depression

CONCLUSIONS

Counseling in palliative medicine involves enhancing social support, encouraging emotional expression and processing, confronting existential concerns, cognitive restructuring, enhancing coping skills, and improving relationships with family, friends, and physicians. These approaches include taking a more active stance about impending death. Good psychotherapists emphasize the here and now, personalizing the discussion and keeping it focused on issues related to dying and death. This direct, emotive, and supportive approach can counter death anxiety by making existential concerns a source of closeness and understanding rather than isolation.

REFERENCES

1. Rosenbaum E, Gautier H, Fobair P, et al. Cancer supportive care, improving the quality of life for cancer patients. A program evaluation report. Support Care Cancer 2004;12:293-301.
2. Spiegel D. A 43-year-old woman coping with cancer [see comments]. JAMA 1999;282:371-378.
3. Holland JC. History of psycho-oncology: Overcoming attitudinal and conceptual barriers. Psychosom Med 2002;64:206-221.
4. Spiegel D, Classen C. Group Therapy for Cancer Patients: A Research-Based Handbook of Psychosocial Care. New York: Basic Books, 2000.
5. Spiegel D, Yalom I. A support group for dying patients. Int J Group Psychother 1978;28:233-245.
6. Yalom ID. Existential Psychotherapy. New York: Basic Books, 1980.
7. Beck JS. Cognitive Therapy: Basics and Beyond. New York: Guilford Press, 1995.
8. Kissane DW, Bloch S, Smith GC, et al. Cognitive-existential group therapy for patients with primary breast cancer—techniques and themes. Psychooncology 2003;6:25-33.
9. Lazarus A, Folkman S. Stress, Appraisal, and Coping. New York: Springer, 1984.
10. Moos RH, Schaefer JA. The crisis of physical illness: An overview and conceptual approach. In Moos RH (ed). Coping with Physical Illness: New perspectives. New York: Plenum, 1987, pp 3-25.
11. Folkman S, Moskowitz J. Positive affect and the other side of coping. Am Psychol 2000;55:647-654.
12. Kinsinger DP, Penedo FJ, Antoni MH, et al. Psychosocial and sociodemographic correlates of benefit-finding in men treated for localized prostate cancer. Psychooncology 2006;15:954-961.
13. Wellisch DK. Families and cancer. Psychooncology 1998;7:1-2.
14. Fallowfield LJ, Jenkins VA, et al. Truth may hurt but deceit hurts more: Communication in palliative care. Palliat Med 2002;16:297-303.
15. Spiegel H, Spiegel D. Trance and Treatment: Clinical Uses of Hypnosis. Washington, DC: American Psychiatric Publishing, 2004.
16. Compas BE, Haaga DA, Keefe FJ, et al. Sampling of empirically supported psychological treatments from health psychology: smoking, chronic pain, cancer, and bulimia nervosa. J Consult Clin Psychol 1998;66:89-112.
17. Kissane DW, Grabsch B, Clarke DM, et al. Supportive-expressive group therapy: The transformation of existential ambivalence into creative living while enhancing adherence to anti-cancer therapies. Psychooncology 2004;13:755-768.
18. Kissane DW, Love A, Hatton A, et al. Effect of cognitive-existential group therapy on survival in early-stage breast cancer. J Clin Oncol 2004;22:4255-4260.
19. Devine EC, Westlake SK. The effects of psychoeducational care provided to adults with cancer: Meta-analysis of 116 studies. Oncol Nurs Forum 1995;22:1369-1381.
20. Barsevick AM, Sweeney C, Haney E, Chung E. A systematic qualitative analysis of psychoeducational interventions for depression in patients with cancer. Oncol Nurs Forum 2002;29:73-87.
21. Aziz NM, Rowland JH. Trends and advances in cancer survivorship research: Challenge and opportunity. Semin Radiat Oncol 2003;13:248-266.
22. Grunfeld E. Looking beyond survival: How are we looking at survivorship? J Clin Oncol 2006;24:5166-5169.
23. Spiegel D, Bloom JR, Yalom I. Group support for patients with metastatic cancer. A randomized outcome study. Arch Gen Psychiatry 1981;38:527-533.
24. Classen C, Butler LD, Koopman C, et al. Supportive-expressive group therapy reduces distress in metastatic breast cancer patients: A randomized clinical intervention study. Arch Gen Psychiatry 2001;58:494-501.
25. Giese-Davis J, Koopman C, Butler LD, et al. Change in emotion-regulation strategy for women with metastatic breast cancer following supportive-expressive group therapy. J Consult Clin Psychol 2002;70:916-925.
26. Breitbart W. Spirituality and meaning in supportive care: Spirituality- and meaning-centered group psychotherapy interventions in advanced cancer. Support Care Cancer 2002;10:272-280.
27. Andrykowski MA, Beacham AO, Schmidt JE, Harper FW. Application of the theory of planned behavior to understand intentions to engage in physical and psychosocial health behaviors after cancer diagnosis. Psychooncology 2006;15:759-771.
28. Rummans TA, Clark MM, Sloan JA, et al. Impacting quality of life for patients with advanced cancer with a structured multidisciplinary intervention: A randomized controlled trial. J Clin Oncol 2006;24:635-642.
29. Northouse L, Kershaw T, Mood E, Schafenacker A. Effects of a family intervention on the quality of life of women with recurrent breast cancer and their family caregivers. Psychooncology 2005;14:478-491.
30. Newell SA, Sanson-Fisher RW, Savolainen NJ. Systematic review of psychological therapies for cancer patients: Overview and recommendations for future research. J Natl Cancer Inst 2002;94:558-584.
31. Rehse B, Pukrop R. Effects of psychosocial interventions on quality of life in adult cancer patients: Meta-analysis of 37 published controlled outcome studies. Patient Educ Couns 2003;50:179-186.

SUGGESTED READING

Classen C, Butler LD, Koopman C, et al. Supportive-expressive group therapy reduces distress in metastatic breast cancer patients: A randomized clinical intervention trial. Arch Gen Psychiatry 2001;58:494-501.

Giese-Davis J, Koopman C, Butler LD, et al. Change in emotion-regulation strategy for women with metastatic breast cancer following supportive-expressive group therapy. J Consult Clin Psychol 2002;70:916-925.

Kissane DW, Grabsch B, Clarke DM, et al. Supportive-expressive group therapy: The transformation of existential ambivalence into creative living while enhancing adherence to anti-cancer therapies. Psychooncology 2004;13:755-768.

Spiegel D. A 43-year-old woman coping with cancer [see comments]. JAMA 1999;282:371-378.

Spiegel D, Classen C. Group Therapy for Cancer Patients: A Research-Based Handbook of Psychosocial Care. New York: Basic Books, 2000.

Yalom ID. Existential Psychotherapy. New York: Basic Books, 1980.

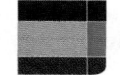

CHAPTER **114**

Public Advocacy and Community Outreach

Francesca Crippa Floriani and Elena Zucchetti

KEY POINTS

- Advocacy is an aspect of health promotion and is essential for effective health policies and programs.

- Nonprofit and voluntary organizations are important in advocating for the terminally ill. Thanks to their work, we have seen the passage from a death-denying medical culture to a culture of competent and compassionate care till the end for everybody.

- The Italian experience illustrates how nonprofit organizations can be successful in a public health approach in palliative care.

- For successful advocacy, it is fundamental to be organized: networking with similar organizations, lobbying with institutions, and building a trust relationship with the community represented.

- It is important not to be confined to a role of replacement for what the institutions do not manage to do or the market does not consider profitable; the right to quality public palliative care for all terminally ill patients still has not been reached. Advocacy is a process that never ends.

Advocacy is the process of promoting or defending the rights of a particular person or group of people.[1] More in-depth definitions that reflect the current use of the concept, include the following. Advocacy is a "partisan intervention on behalf of an individual client or identified client group . . . to secure or enhance a needed service, resource, or entitlement; to develop a new one; or to prevent or limit client involvement with a dysfunctional service system."[2] Advocacy "involves the use of tools and activities that can draw attention to an issue, gain support for it, build consensus about it, and provide arguments that will sway decision makers and public opinion to back it."[3]

The advocacy process is initiated by groups that are interested in common issues and willing to devote time, knowledge, and skills to influence decision makers to promote changes to laws and other government policies and achieve progressive changes in society.

Advocacy is an aspect of health promotion and is essential for the development and maintenance of effective health policies and programs. When applied to health, the purpose of advocacy is to advance the right of every citizen to high-quality, appropriate, and readily available health care.[4] "Health, particularly when it is threatened, is an issue of great importance to individuals and communities. So too is health care and people's relationships with professionals and systems that provide it. Needs and crises around health are common points of community mobilization and action. People have joined together to address their community's health problems, individual health problems, access to care and, ultimately, problems with health care systems."[5]

Civil society groups, nonprofit and voluntary organizations, associations, and foundations, generally defined "third sector," are important in advocating for public health.[6] For them, the needs of people are primary: They feel directly responsible to the communities they serve and are ethically bound to do all their best for the benefit of those communities. In the past, these organizations worked to repair the inefficiencies of existing services, organizing their own health care; today they are actors in a sociopolitical process for the promotion of people's rights. They are aware that working alone for a private aim is limited and that problems cannot be solved by replacing existing institutions but instead by working alongside, collaborating, and encouraging them to assume their responsibilities.

ADVOCACY AND COMMUNITY OUTREACH IN PALLIATIVE MEDICINE

People who are facing serious illness or are near death experience distressing symptoms in body, mind, and spirit, but they have the right to always receive compassionate, competent, holistic care, addressed to all aspects of their suffering: physical, emotional, spiritual, social, economical. They also have the right to full information about their condition and to participate actively in decision making about their care.

Ours is a death-denying culture, and medicine is mainly designed to cure and rehabilitate. In the past, and sometimes today, dying patients were considered to represent a failure of medical practice and were neglected by the health care system. They and their families did not get the care and services needed and experienced avoidable pain and suffering, feelings of powerlessness, loss of control, subordination, and paternalism. Despite their awareness of the inefficiencies of care, patients and families did not effectively advocate for their rights to better care and assistance. In fact, the patients, because of their particular "terminal" status, were bound to "disappear" in a limited amount of time, and families tended to distance themselves from a very painful time and soon abandoned any effort to promote better care.

Civil society found the way to express itself through the so-called "third sector." Nonprofit and voluntary organizations played an important role in detecting the problems, proposing solutions, organizing services, and fighting for the right of every person to competent and compassionate care until death.[7] Cicely Saunders, mother of the modern hospice movement, once said, referring to the time before St. Christopher's Hospice opened, that it was "imperative to move out of the formal health care system so that new knowledge and attitudes could develop."[8] Nonprofit organizations were the right direction to move in. Usually funded by independent means, they worked outside the system, were free from the interests of the ruling powers, were flexible, were open to change, and had the ability to speak out creatively where others could not because of political or economic conflict. These characteristics determined their success in giving voice to the voiceless.

THE ITALIAN EXPERIENCE: A SUCCESS STORY

The Italian experience is a good example of how the nonprofit sector has been successfully used to achieve a public health approach in palliative care. The first signs of nonprofit organizations in Italy date back to the 19th century, when many health care services were managed by religious congregations.[9] More recently, people became aware that to protect and assert their rights, charity and benevolence were not enough. People joined in organized groups and started working together to answer their needs. This meant not only organizing good services where public institutions did not succeed but also, and most importantly, working to remove the causes of malfunctioning or nonexistent services and fighting for everybody's right to receive them.

Terminal care in Italy followed this path. Until the 1970s, the care of the terminally ill by national public health services was a problem. Health care institutions did not consider the quality of care of the 250,000 persons who died every year from a terminal illness. Discussion of opioid prescriptions was taboo.

In 1977, the pioneer work of a foundation in Milan, the Fondazione Floriani, started a new course. The founder, Virgilio Floriani, a wealthy and generous philanthropist who experienced terminal cancer in his family, believed the issue was both personal and political. At first he had no training or preparation and was guided only by his sense of urgency to solve the problem of physical and psychological suffering of the terminally ill. Most health advocates begin like this,[10] but soon Floriani managed to connect to the most important international experts in the field, and with their help and expertise, together with sensitive Italian physicians, he started the spread and application of palliative care in Italy. Through the years, the Fondazione Floriani has organized home palliative care services in collaboration with public health structures; tried to find the best applications of palliative care through social, psychological, and medical research; organized professional and community educational events (meetings, congresses, and courses) for the acquisition of skills and to raise of awareness both in the general public and in local, regional, and national public bodies; and organized a specialized library in palliative care for the support of people studying or researching the subject.

The activities of the Fondazione Floriani soon inspired other groups around the country. Many other nonprofit and voluntary organizations, associations, and foundations started to work for this cause; today, they number almost 190.[11] First, they tried to answer what they considered a "social emergency"—organizing and financing their own care, research, and community and professional educational services. Subsequently, they realized that, for everybody to receive compassionate and competent care, a more widely organized approach would be more effective. In 1986, the Italian Society for Palliative Care (Società Italiana di Cure Palliative, or SICP) was established as a society of palliative care professionals. Three years later, the Italian School for Palliative Care (Scuola Italiana di Medicina e Cure Palliative, or SIMPA) was founded. In 1999, to mobilize all palliative care organizations, represent all possible aspects of palliative and terminal care, and avoid contradictory approaches, many palliative care associations joined an umbrella organization called the Federation of Palliative Care (Federazione di Cure Palliative, or FCP). The accompanying box distills the experience of these decades in terms of common errors and how to avoid them.

RECENT DEVELOPMENTS

Thanks to all this work, general public attention toward the rights of the dying intensified, and national health authorities realized that the dying had not been adequately cared for within the welfare state. Media attention to these issues grew, stimulating public interest. The final result was that Italian authorities were pushed to create guidelines and laws for the care of the dying.[12]

Some of the recent milestones in this development include the following:

- 1998: Palliative care was included as an essential part of the National Health Plan,[13,14] and the fundamental role of nonprofit organizations in developing services was recognized. In the same year, a National Commission on Palliative Care was established.
- 1999: A Palliative Care Law[15] was promulgated and provided more than 185 million euros to create, in 3 years' time, at least one hospice in every Italian region.
- 2000: The National Collective Agreement for General Practitioners[16] contained indications for the care of the dying at home and established financial incentives for general practitioners involved in home palliative care. In the same year, a decree[17] defined the minimum structural and organizational requirements for hospices.

Common Errors

All of the societies, associations, foundations, and federations involved in palliative care advocacy recognized the value of stimulating constructive changes in the health care system and in society. They engaged, initially rather spontaneously but later in an ever more organized manner, in advocacy programs such as the following:

1. *Building a trust relationship with the community*, continuously monitoring the environment to detect people's needs so as to better represent them.
2. *Offering direct care services.* Service provision shows the community that the advocacy groups are pragmatic and helps build the "trust relationship"; it also shows governmental bodies that purposes are serious and gives examples of effective affordable services.
3. *Networking with other organizations* that have the same beliefs and goals, to enhance expertise, credibility, and power.
4. *Organizing educational informational meetings* aimed at increasing the knowledge and awareness of the community about the issue of interest in all its aspects: institutional failings, people's rights, new opportunities and alternatives, and ways of affecting the institutions.
5. *Organizing formal training* for health professionals and developing a curriculum.
6. *Distributing information and educational material* through an editorial activity for lay persons (e.g., newsletters, informational booklets) and professionals (e.g., scientific journals, books, other publications).
7. *Lobbying with key public health institutions and government officials*, to advise them as to what policies need to be introduced or revised, to give assistance with the drafting of policies, and to provide examples of already organized services.

- 2001: A law on the use of opioids in pain therapy[18] broke the taboo on utilization of morphine and narcotics for the management of pain.
- 2003: An agreement between state and regional agencies defined the indicators for quality assurance in palliative care.[19]
- 2006: The Minister of Health proposed a law that simplified prescription of opioids.[20]

CONCLUSIONS

The third sector has been the driving force of palliative care. It was able to advocate for the needs of dying patients and their families, represent and effectively speak on their behalf, organize services, increase competencies among health care professionals, educate the general public, and work with governmental bodies to adopt national strategies. Its actions have led to the spread of palliative care services and availability of drugs for pain control and symptom management. But despite all this, not all tasks have been accomplished.

Today, social and health organization is going through a delicate time. The welfare state is now transforming into the welfare community. This process, because of the reduction of resources for the welfare state and the speed and creativity of civil society in filling institutional gaps, has already started and is unavoidable. The collaboration among the third (nonprofit), second (state), and the first (market) sectors must continue. The risk for the third sector is to provide only a replacement for what the insti-

Box 114-1 Research Challenges and Opportunities

1. The spread of palliative care to other groups of terminally ill patients. In the past, palliative care in Italy, and internationally, has focused mainly on cancer. There has been remarkable progress, but palliative care should be expanded to patients with other illnesses and to patient groups such as those with AIDS; those with end-stage heart, lung, and kidney diseases; pediatric patients, and patients with neurological conditions. Partnership and collaboration with advocacy groups in these fields will enable palliative care to reach more people and be more successful in changing and educating the public and influencing the thoughts of the leaders of society.[21]

2. Quality control. Palliative care for terminally ill cancer patients will soon become institutionalized. The third sector, as an advocate of patients' rights, should never abandon a critical attitude and should never stop asking questions such as the following: Why are things done like this? Do they achieve their goals? Do they satisfy patients' needs? and, Will patients benefit from them equitably?

tution has not managed to do or what the market does not consider profitable. We believe in the balance and equal dignity of the three pillars of society and are convinced that best results will be reached with their integration. Integration does not mean replacing but strengthening, supporting, promoting, collaborating, and planning of new models of care. Current research challenges are listed in Box 114-1.

Public advocacy is a long process. It requires sacrifice, patience, teamwork, flexibility, and intelligence in the choice of the best strategies to reach one's aims. Advocacy requires a strong ability to represent civil society's interests while simultaneously working with governments. One must be prepared to spend large amounts of time and energy on tasks that do not always guarantee optimal outcomes, but our experience shows that the effort is worth it and can be extremely rewarding by fueling a sense of social responsibility and contributing to a fairer society.

REFERENCES

1. Nervo G. Il volontariato di promozione e tutela dei diritti. Appunti Sulle Politiche Sociali 2004;3:152.
2. McGowan BG. Advocacy. In Encyclopedia of Social Work, vol. 1, ed. 18. Silver Spring, MD: National Association of Social Workers, 1987, pp 89-95.
3. Rice M. Advocacy and reproductive health: Successes and challenges [editorial]. Promot Educ 1999;6:2-3.
4. McCabe MS, Varricchio CG, Padberg R, et al. Women's health advocacy: Its growth and development in oncology. Semin Oncol Nurs 1995;11:137-142.
5. Bastian H. Speaking up for ourselves: The evolution of consumer advocacy in health care. Int J Technol Assess Health Care 1998;14:3-23.
6. Nathan S, Rotem A, Ritchie J. Closing the gap: Building the capacity of non-government organizations as advocates for health equity. Health Promotion Int 2002;17:69-78.
7. Fusco-Karmann C, Tinini G. A review of the volunteer movement in EAPC countries. Eur J Palliat Care 2001;8:199-202.
8. Saunders C, Summers D, Teller N. Hospice: The Living Idea. Leeds, UK: Edward Arnold, 1981.
9. Borletti I, Piazza M. Federazione non profit ONP e settore socioassistenziale. In Amadori D, De Conno F. Libro Italiano di Cure Palliative. Gaggiano (Milano), Italy: Poletto Editore, 2003, pp 517-521.
10. Avery B, Bashir S. The road to advocacy: Searching for the rainbow. Am J Public Health 2003;93:1207-1210.
11. Directory constantemente aggiornata sulle Unità di cure palliative operanti nel territorio italiano e sulle Organizzazioni non profit attive nel settore. Available at http://www.osservatoriocurepalliative.org (accessed November 30, 2007).
12. Zucco F, Welshman A. The National Health Service and the care of the dying. Eur J Palliat Care 2001;8:61-65.
13. Ministero della Sanità. Piano Sanitario Nazionale, 1998-2000. Roma: Gazzetta Ufficiale, 1998.
14. Legge di conversione N. 39. Disposizioni per assicurare interventi urgenti di attuazione del piano sanitario nazionale 1998-2000. Roma: Gazzetta Ufficiale, 1999.
15. Decreto del Ministero della Sanità. Programma Nazionale per la Realizzazione di Strutture per le Cure Palliative. Roma: Gazzetta Ufficiale, 2000.
16. Ministero della Sanità. Accordo Collettivo Nazionale per la Disciplina Dei Rapporti con i Medici di Medicina Generale. Roma: Gazzetta Ufficiale, 2000.
17. Decreto del Presidente del Consiglio dei Ministri. Atto di indirizzo e coordinamento recante requisiti strutturali, tecnologici ed organizzativi minimi per i centri residenziali di cure palliative. Roma: Gazzetta Ufficiale, 2000.
18. Legge N. 12. Norme per agevolare l'impiego dei farmaci analgesici oppiacei nella terapia del dolore. 8 Febbraio 2001.
19. Accordo sancito nella seduta della Conferenza Stato Regioni e Province autonome. 13 Marzo 2003.
20. Approvazione del Consiglio dei Ministri del disegno di legge del Ministro Livia Turco. Ottobre 2006.
21. Lee KF. Future end-of-life care: Partnership and advocacy. J Palliat Med 2002;5:329-334.

SUGGESTED READING

Chapman S. Advocacy for public health: A primer. J Epidemiol Community Health 2004;58:361-365.

Corli O. Palliative care services and non-profit organisations in Italy. Eur J Palliat Care 2003;10(1 Suppl):5-7.

Reiser SJ. The era of the patient: Using the experience of illness in shaping the missions of health care. JAMA 1993;269:1012-1017.

Zucco F, Welshman A. The National Health Service and the care for the dying. Eur J Palliat Care 2001;8:61-65.

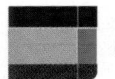

CHAPTER **115**

Telemedicine

José Pereira and Ron Spice

KEY POINTS

- Telemedicine covers many activities and technologies, and a single definition is elusive.
- Telemedicine is particularly well suited to rural and remote medicine.
- New communication technologies are opening up new possibilities in telemedicine and e-health.
- Data transmission, applicable standards, and bandwidth requirements need to be considered when adopting telemedicine.
- Several challenges, including reimbursement, licensure for cross-border consulting, and regulatory issues, need to be addressed.

New digitalized communication and information technologies are making profound changes in modern society. These technologies, led particularly by the Internet and wireless communication methods, have entered mainstream health care, where they are being used extensively, from information management to patient monitoring, clinical consultation, and education. Telemedicine supports some of this activity. It is an emerging field of expertise and has become a large industry and a focus of academic pursuit.

DEFINITIONS

Telemedicine refers to the use of communications and information technologies for the delivery or enhancement of clinical care. This generally entails delivering care at a distance. Telemedicine covers a broad spectrum of activities and can be as simple as two professionals discussing a case over the telephone, or as complex as the use of biomedical robots and devices for performing surgery at a distance. Multiple terms using the "tele-" prefix now describe various aspects of telemedicine, including teleconsulting, telenursing, teleradiology, telepsychiatry, telesurgery, telepathology, telecardiology, and telemonitoring, among others.

The terms *telemedicine, telehealth,* and *e-health* are often used interchangeably. However, *telemedicine* is more appropriately used to refer only to the provision of clinical services, whereas the term *telehealth* can refer to clinical and nonclinical services such as medical education, administration, and research conducted at a distance. The term *e-health* is increasingly being used as an umbrella term that comprises telemedicine, telehealth, and health informatics, including electronic health records. Even the term *e-health* is difficult to define; 51 unique descriptions and definitions were found in one study.[1]

PROPOSED BENEFITS OF TELEMEDICINE AND E-HEALTH

Eysenbach proposed the following benefits ("the 10 E's of e-health")[2]:

- *Efficiency* and decreased costs
- *Enhancement* of quality of care
- *Empowerment* of patients and consumers
- *Encouragement* of new and enlightened relationships between health care professionals and patients
- *Education* of patients and health professionals
- *Enabling* information exchange and communication in a standardized way between health care establishments
- *Extending* the scope of care beyond its traditional boundaries
- *Equity* by promoting equitable access to health care and health care information
- *Ethics* as an emerging set of issues
- *Evidence-base* to underscore the importance of subjecting these assertions to rigorous research and identifying the level of supporting evidence

Telemedicine appears most beneficial for populations in isolated communities and remote regions, where access to primary health care can be limited and specialized-level care is often impossible to obtain.[3] Low-cost applications are possible even in resource-limited settings.[4] Telemedicine may also enhance health care access in urban situations (e.g., home care support).

TECHNOLOGICAL CONCEPTS UNDERLYING TELEMEDICINE AND E-HEALTH

Telemedicine and e-health can be practiced either in real-time (synchronously) or asynchronously ("store-and-forward"). Real-time telemedicine involves two or more parties communicating or exchanging data simultaneously. Store-and-forward telemedicine entails acquiring medical data or images, storing them (usually on a computer), and then transmitting (forwarding) them securely to another party for later analysis or review. Store-and-forward does not require the presence of both parties at the same time. Synchronous telemedicine, on the other hand, provides immediacy and is particularly useful for emergency situations and real-time consultation.

The initial step in telemedicine requires capturing data, such as text, sound, images, and video, and converting it into electrical, digital, or optical signals for storage or transmission. The transmission medium can be wire, fiber-optic cable, radio waves, or microwaves. When a signal reaches its destination, the device on the receiving end converts or decodes the signal back into an understandable message, such as sound over a telephone or computer, images or video on a television or computer screen, and words or pictures on a computer screen.

Various devices are available to support these processes. Telecommunication through telephones, now referred to as the Plain Old Telephone System (POTS), is reliable for audio-only communication. Most telephones transmit electrical signals over the worldwide public switched telephone network (PSTN) or via radio (cellular telephone, satellite, or radiotelephone).[5] Increasingly, transmission is via the Internet using voice over internet protocol (VoIP), referred to as Internet (IP) telephone. VoIP-based calls are significantly less costly than those made on the standard telephone network, and, with sufficient broadband connection, they can also support basic one-to-one videoconferencing.

Videoteleconferencing (VTC) is one of the most common forms of synchronous telemedicine. VTC relies on digital compression of audio and video streams in real time. Video requires a large amount of data to be transmitted—the more data, the better the quality. This can be achieved through compressing the video and audio files digitally. Compression techniques have improved over the last decade, making VTC more accessible and less costly. The hardware or software that performs compression is called a *codec* (coder/decoder). The resulting digital data are then transmitted through a digital network of some kind, often via an integrated services digital network (ISDN) or an asymmetrical digital subscriber line (ADSL)—digital telephone network systems designed to allow transmission of voice and data over ordinary telephone copper wires at better quality and higher speeds. Videophones support VTC, usually on a one-to-one basis, and they are practical in that they work on regular phone lines and do not require much in terms of infrastructure. They are often used to support telehomecare. The video quality can vary, however. Special peripheral units can be added to VTC equipment to support interactive consultations, including digital cameras and microscopes, video-endoscopes, telestethoscopes, medical ultrasound imaging devices, and otoscopes.

RECENT DEVELOPMENTS

Webcams are real-time video cameras that are connected to the World Wide Web (Web), making VTC more accessible. Web-based VTC connecting multiple sites is still suboptimal but should improve soon. With the advent of improved Web-based VTC and wireless capacity that enables connection to the Internet using cellular telephone or satellite connections, high-quality home-based videoconferencing will soon be possible in more rural and remote areas where other high-speed Internet connections may not be available. Currently, such wireless capability is making mobile access to electronic health records and diagnostic imaging information possible, improving support to home care.

GENERAL APPLICATIONS OF TELEMEDICINE AND E-HEALTH

Examples of applications of telemedicine and e-health are listed in Table 115-1. The following paragraphs evaluate the success and current status of some of these applications.

Remote Consultation

Teleconsultation has been one of the most successful applications of telemedicine. It can enhance clinical deci-sion making in the community,[6,7] increase access to specialist physicians, decrease hospital admissions,[3] reduce inappropriate transfers,[8] and reduce costs across several fields, including psychiatry, emergency medicine, cardiology, pharmacy, dermatology, neurosurgery and wound care. Systematic reviews of teleconsultations generally report that, although there are some specific useful applications, particularly in support of underserviced communities, lack of conclusive evidence limits widespread use.[9]

Remote Counseling

Despite isolated success, systematic reviews of telecoun-seling have been unable to draw any conclusions because of the small number of studies, small sample sizes, and lack of randomized, controlled trial methodology.[10] Despite theoretical benefits and reports of successful use, conclusive evidence to support telephone follow-ups (TFU) after discharge from hospital is still lacking.[11]

Remote Triaging

Teletriaging may reduce unnecessary visits to health care facilities.

Remote Monitoring

Despite isolated successes, use of remote patient monitoring has not been widespread.

Remote Endoscopy

Tele-endoscopy has shown promise for remote supervision or observation of gastrointestinal and ear nose and throat endoscopic procedures by nonspecialist endoscopists, including nurses. In a rural Australian setting, it reduced travel costs for both the patient and the health care system.[12]

Remote Surgery

Urological and gastrointestinal surgeries have been conducted remotely.[13]

Distance Education

Telemedicine, particularly the use of VTC and audioconferencing, has been supporting distance learning for decades.[14]

EVIDENCE-BASES

Overall, despite numerous case reports of successes, conclusive evidence is still missing and more studies are needed to evaluate the widespread use of these technologies, particularly their cost-benefit ratios and their limitations.[15-17] Most studies indicate high levels of perceived satisfaction.[18] Unfortunately, telehealth studies to date have not used socioeconomic indicators consistently.[19] Although the benefits appear to include improved access to specialized services, continuity of care, and support for rural caregivers, challenges exist in quantifying the impact of telehealth technologies on quality of care.[20]

TABLE 115-1	Examples of Applications of Telemedicine and E-Health
DIRECT PATIENT CARE	
Teleconsultation	A specialist provides either real-time or asynchronous consultations to a health professional remotely, with or without the presence of the patient. May also involve the transmission and review of medical data, images, or videos by radiologists remotely (teleradiology).[44] Real-time consulting is essential in urgent cases such as emergency care. In other cases, telemedicine clinics can be scheduled on a regular basis (e.g., telepsychiatry clinics).
Telecounseling	Direct patient support at a distance, using either telephone or videophones.
Telemonitoring	Sensors capture and transmit biometric data such as blood pressure, heart rate, electrocardiograms, and physical activity.
Teletriaging	A typical telephone triage event might involve a call, often after hours, from a concerned family member or patient for advice. Professionals manning these services often have protocols and, increasingly, software programs to guide them through a series of questions to aid in responding appropriately.
Tele-endoscopy	Remote supervision or observation of endoscopic procedures, including gastrointestinal and ear nose and throat endoscopy.
Telesurgery	—
Symptom assessment	Handheld personal data assistants (PDAs) or tablet laptops can support real-time assessment of symptoms.
INDIRECT PATIENT CARE	
Education	—
Health informatics*	Includes electronic health records, clinical decision-making support programs, and health data management.

*Considered under e-health, and not generally under telemedicine.

APPLICATIONS IN PALLIATIVE CARE

Home Care

Home telehealth has been successfully demonstrated in palliative care, but there is limited evidence about clinical effectiveness and cost savings.[21-23] Two Canadian telehealth studies found that videophones were user friendly and generally well accepted.[22,24] Studies in the United Kingdom and United States have suggested that between 15% to 65% of home palliative care nursing visits could have been conducted through videoconferencing.[25,26] In a more recent Canadian study, Hebert and Colleagues calculated that approximately 43% of palliative care visits were appropriate for video visits.[27] The group identified four factors that may inform eligibility and decisions about a client's suitability for video visits: diagnosis (cancer versus noncancer), low Edmonton Symptom Assessment System (ESAS) symptom presence and intensity score, no caregiver present, and number and types of interventions required. Patients with a cancer diagnosis were more likely to be suitable for video visits, which suggests that disease trajectory, rather than diagnosis of "palliative," may be more influential in determining the care required and appropriateness of videophone use.

An Internet-based videophone support program provides care for families in pediatric palliative care services.[28] Some difficulties in setting up the devices and connections were reported. ISDN videophones were used in another study.[24] Patients made on average 12.5 calls per week and found the technology useful to connect with their nurses. Mixed results were found with videophones connected to elderly clients' home telephone lines.[29] Text messaging devices and videophones were used to connect veterans with a home care hospice program.[30] Patients felt an improved ability to manage their conditions at home, and there were fewer hospital admissions, emergency department visits, and bed-days of care.

After-Hours Advice Line

A pilot study suggested that an advice line may improve the provision of palliative care outside of regular office hours, by providing specialist advice.[31] The advice line was used appropriately and was not overwhelmed by calls.[32]

Consultations

In the United Kingdom, a shortage of palliative medicine consultants prompted weekly 2-hour telephone-based videoconference sessions between community-based consultant nurses and palliative care physician consultants to discuss patients with one or more unresolved symptoms or significant palliative care issues.[33] Another approach used e-mail and videoconferencing for clinical and educational support between oncologists at a referral oncology center and the oncology and palliative care unit.[34] Positive experiences have also been reported with an after-hours telephone support service for palliative care patients and their families at home.[35] Health professionals and nurses in the catchment area reported that knowing the service was there was a great security and reduced the sense of isolation predominant in rural families caring for a pallia-

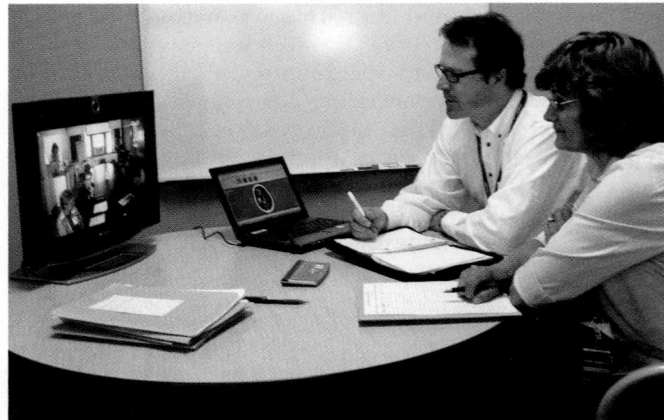

FIGURE 115-1 Teleconsulting in palliative care. A palliative care physician and nurse consultant of the Calgary Rural Palliative Care Program in Canada use a small desktop unit for video consulting with a rural-based home care team (2006). (Note the simultaneous access on the laptop computer to a secure online diagnostic imaging server relaying images of the patient's recent computed tomographic scan of the brain.)

tive care patient at home. Others reported Internet-based interactive collaborative consultation between a rural palliative care nurse practitioner and an urban medical research physician.[36] VTC provided direct patient consultations and support for home care staff and primary care physicians in rural areas (R. Spice, personal communication) (Fig. 115-1).

Symptom Assessment

Digital pen technology allows patients to self-evaluate their symptoms and transfer the results digitally over a regular mobile phone network from their home to the hospital clinic.[37] A computerized form of the McGill Pain Questionnaire can be completed using touch screen technology (PAINReportIt).[38] A PDA-based assessment tool for clinicians, called the Acute Pain Management Service (APMS), captures pain scores and drug-related side effects.[39] The digital data are also useful for clinical research.

Support of Care and Management

There are several initiatives in palliative care in Canada (Edmonton, Toronto, Victoria, Kingston) using PDA- and laptop-based technology to support clinical care, symptom assessment, and tracking of clinical activity for management and program development.

Education

VTC technology has been used to deliver continuing medical education in palliative medicine to community physicians.[40] Learners were highly satisfied, and gains in knowledge were reported. A crude cost analysis suggested cost savings. The Interactive Multimedia Palliative Care Training Project (IMPaCT) used VTC to support palliative care education across 22 sites worldwide, linking 136 professionals without the costs or time needed to travel.[41] The Pallium Project used simple telephone conferencing or POTS to link more than 110 sites across Canada for monthly 1-hour grand round sessions in which experts were interviewed using questions provided by the participants (M. Aherne and J. Pereira, personal communication) (Fig. 115-2). The sessions were recorded, saved as MP3 files, and made available for downloading in support of independent self-learning (Fig. 115-3).

Overall Vision

A broad vision of telemedicine and e-health in palliative care has been proposed based on extensive work with

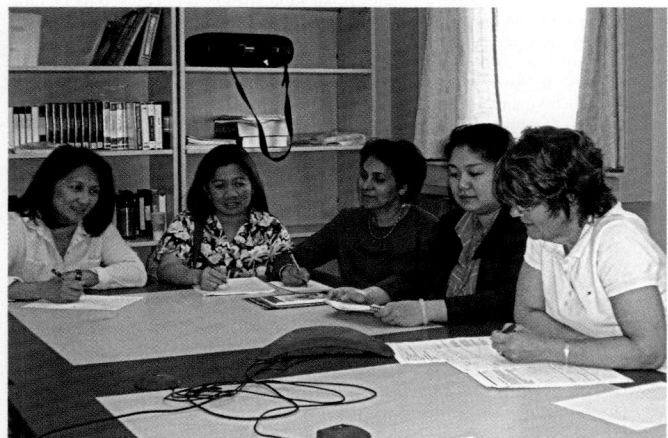

FIGURE 115-2 Community-based nurses in the Canadian Arctic (Rankin Inlet) participate in the Canadian Pallium Project's monthly telephone-based audioconference professional continuing development program in palliative care (for group-based learning), which links more than 110 sites and 260 learners across Canada (2005).

technology prototypes in palliative care.[42] This vision, called the e-Hospice, uses various telemedicine and e-health options to support palliative and hospice-based care; including electronic methods to collect symptom data and symptom profiles and broadband Internet-based VTC for patients to stay in contact with friends and family.

HEALTH INFORMATICS

Medical informatics is a large field that concerns itself with the collation, storage, and analysis of information related to public health issues, administration, program development, and patient care, among other topics. It falls outside the scope of telemedicine, but readers are encouraged to review articles on this subject, particularly concerning electronic health records and computer-based clinical support systems.

CONCLUSIONS

Telemedicine has many applications, a number of which have already been used in palliative care. Despite numerous reports of success, several issues need to be considered and addressed (see "Common Errors" and "Future Considerations"), including the need for larger studies and more consistent clinical and economic cost-benefit analyses. Successful application requires attention to several factors, including overcoming resistance to change, identifying local champions, assessing the extent to which the innovation is perceived to threaten professional work constructs concerning therapeutic relationships, and identifying potential workflow changes resulting from the technology.[43]

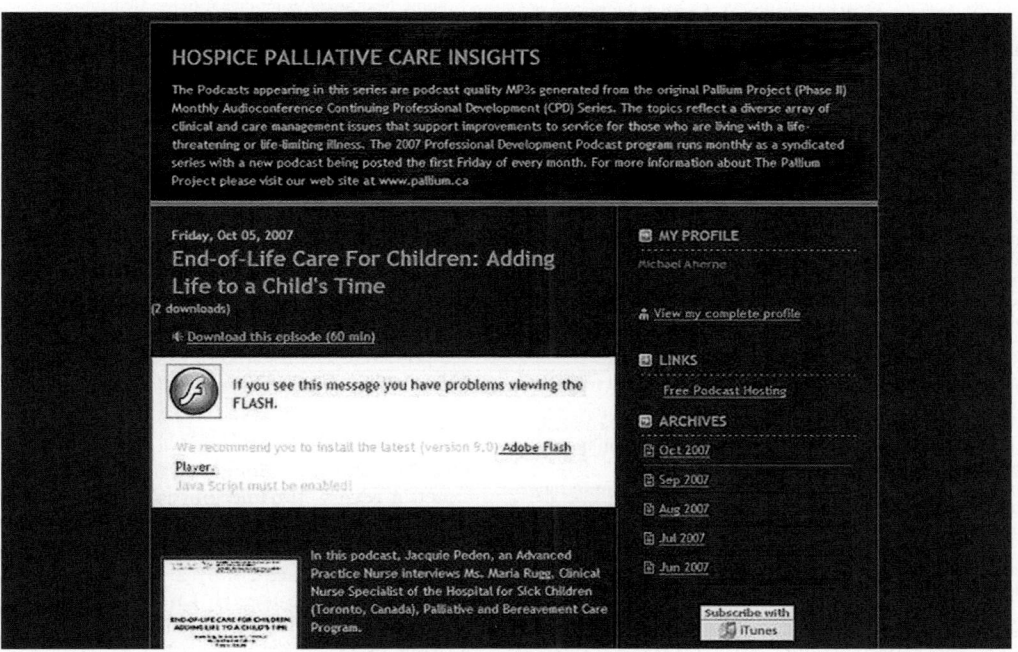

FIGURE 115-3 The Web site established by the Canadian Pallium Project has downloadable podcasts in MP3 format (for individual self-directed learning) of the monthly audioconference series (see Figure 115-2).

Common Errors

- Using technology that cannot be supported by the local informatics capacity.
- Using telehealth technology because it is available even though it is not really needed or justifiable.
- Failing to ensure confidentiality (e.g., failing to conduct videoconsultations and videoconferences in a way that protects patient information).
- Improper patient selection (e.g., videoconsultations on delirious patients).
- Improper documentation of clinical decision making done with telehealth methods.
- Making clinical decisions that should be made only with direct contact with the patient (e.g., placing too much confidence in a video image when a proper physical examination is indicated.)

Future Considerations

- Ease of use and costs.
- Legal and policy issues: Practicing across state, province, and country boundaries has medicolegal and licensure implications for health professionals and patients.
- Reimbursement: Adequate reimbursement, particularly of teleconsulting, remains a barrier.
- Standards and guidelines: The lack of widely accepted standards and guidelines is a barrier.
- Information security and privacy issues.
- Ethical issues: The blending of medicine and healthcare with e-commerce and the Internet raises many questions, as do the implications of caring for patients at a distance.
- Equity: Making health care more equitable is one of the promises of e-health, but at the same time there is a considerable threat that e-health may deepen the gap between the "haves" and the "have-nots."

REFERENCES

1. Oh H, Rizo C, Enkin M, Jadad A. What is eHealth (3): A systematic review of published definitions. J Med Internet Res 2005;7(1):e1.
2. Eysenbach G. What is e-health? J Med Internet Res 2001;3(2):e20.
3. Armstrong IJ, Haston WS. Medical decision support for remote general practitioners using telemedicine. J Telemed Telecare 1997;3(1):27-34.
4. Swinfen R. Swinfen P. Low-cost telemedicine in the developing world. J Telemed Telecare 2002;8(3):63-65.
5. Pattichis CS, Kyriacou E, Voskarides S, et al. Wireless telemedicine systems: An overview. Antennas and Propagation Magazine, IEEE. 2002;44(2):143-153.
6. Shanit D, Cheng A, Greenbaum RA. Telecardiology: Supporting the decision making process in general practice. J Telemed Telecare 1996;2(1):7-13.
7. Campbell G, Loane E, Griffiths R, et al. Comparison of teleconsultations and face-to-face consultations: Preliminary results of a United Kingdom multicentre teledermatology study. Br J Dermatol 1998;39:81-87.
8. Goh KY, Lam CK, Poon WS. The impact of teleradiology on the inter-hospital transfer of neurosurgical patients. Br J Neurosurg 1997;11:52-56.
9. Baer L, Elford DR, Cukor P. Telepsychiatry at forty: What have we learned? Harv Rev Psychiatry 1997;5:7-17.
10. Leach LS, Christensen H. A systematic review of telephone-based interventions for mental disorders. J Telemed Telecare 2006;12(3):122-129.
11. Mistiaen P, Poot E. Telephone follow-up, initiated by a hospital-based health professional, for postdischarge problems in patients discharged from hospital to home. Cochrane Database Syst Rev 2006;(4):CD004510.
12. Hughes-Anderson W, Rankin S, House J, et al. Open access endoscopy in rural and remote western Australia: Does it work? A N Z J Surg 2002;72:699-703.
13. Bowersox JC, Cornum RL. Remote operative urology using a surgical telemanipulator system: Preliminary observations. Urology 1998;52:17-22.
14. Callas PW, Ricci MA, Caputo MP. Improved rural provider access to continuing medical education through interactive videoconferencing. Telemed J E Health 2000;6:393-399.
15. Currell R, Urquhart C, Wainwright P, Lewis R. Telemedicine versus face to face patient care. Cochrane Database Syst Rev 2006;(4):CD002098.
16. Jones JF, Brennan PF. Telehealth interventions to improve clinical nursing of elders. Annu Rev Nurs Res 2002;20:293-322.
17. Miller EA. Telemedicine and doctor-patient communication: An analytical survey of the literature. J Telemed Telecare 2001;7(1):1-17.
18. Mair F, Whitten P. Systematic review of studies of patient satisfaction with telemedicine. BMJ 2000;320:1517-1520.
19. Jennett PA, Affleck Hall L, Hailey D, et al. The socio-economic impact of telehealth: A systematic review. J Telemed Telecare 2003;9(6):311-320.
20. Gagnon MP, Duplantie J, Fortin JP, Landry R. Implementing telehealth to support medical practice in rural/remote regions: What are the conditions for success? Implement Sci 2006;24:1:18.
21. De Conno F, Martini C. Video communication and palliative care at home. Eur J Palliat Care 1997;4:172-174.
22. Hebert MA, Jansen JJ, Brant R, et al. Successes and challenges in a field-based, multi-method study of home telehealth. J Telemed Telecare 2004;10(Suppl 1):41-44.
23. Hebert MA, Jansen JJ, Brant R, et al. Effectiveness of Video-Visits in Palliative Home Care: Preliminary Findings of an RCT in the Community. Proceedings of the IASTED International Conference on Telehealth, July 19-21, 2005. Calgary, Alberta: International Association of Science and Technology for Development, 2005, pp 127-130.
24. Miyazaki M, Stuart M, Liu L, et al. Use of ISDN video-phones for clients receiving palliative and antenatal home care. J Telemed Telecare 2003;9(2):72-77.
25. Allen A, Doolittle CG, Boysen DC, et al. An analysis of the suitability of home health visits for telemedicine. J Telemed Telecare 1999;5:90-96.
26. Wootton R, Loane M, Mair F, et al. A joint US-UK study of home telenursing. J Telemed Telecare 1998;4(suppl. 1):83-85.
27. Hebert MA, Paquin MJ, Whitten L. Analysis of the suitability of "video-visits" for palliative home care: Implications for practice. J Telemed Telecare 2007;13:74-78.
28. Bensink M, Armfield N, Russell T, et al. Paediatric palliative home care with Internet-based video-phones: Lessons learnt. J Telemed Telecare 2004;10(Suppl 1):10-13.
29. Guilfoyle C, Wootton R, Hassall S, et al. Videoconferencing in facilities providing care for elderly people. J Telemed Telecare 2002;8(Suppl 3):22-24.
30. Maudlin J, Keene J, Kobb R. A road map for the last journey: Home telehealth for holistic end-of-life care. Am J Hospice Palliat Med 2006;23:399-403.
31. Lloyd-Williams M. Out-of-hours palliative care advice line. Br J Gen Pract 2001;51:677.
32. Roberts D, Tayler C, MacCormack D, Barwich D. Telenursing in hospice palliative care. Can Nurse 2007;103:24-27.
33. Saysell E, Routley C. Telemedicine in community-based palliative care: Evaluation of a videolink teleconference project. Int J Palliat Nurs 2003;9:489-495.
34. Norum J, Jordhoy MS. A university oncology department and a remote palliative care unit linked together by email and videoconferencing. J Telemed Telecare 2006;12:92-96.
35. Wilkes L, Mohan S, White K, Smith H. Evaluation of an after hours telephone support service for rural palliative care patients and their families: A pilot study. Aust J Rural Health 2004;12:95-98.
36. Kuebler KK, Bruera E. Interactive collaborative consultation model in end-of-life care. J Pain Symptom Manage 2000;20:202-209.
37. Lind L, Karlsson D. A system for symptom assessment in advanced palliative home healthcare using digital pens. Med Informatics Internet Med 2004;29:199-210.
38. Wilkie DJ, Kay M, Judge M, et al. Usability of a computerized PAINReportIt in the general public with pain and people with cancer pain. J Pain Symptom Manage 2003;25:213-224.
39. Van Den Kerkhof E, Goldstein D, Rimmer M, et al. Handhelds versus paper for acute pain assessments: Time and content [abstract]. Can J Anesth 2002;49(Suppl 1):21.
40. Lynch J, Weaver L, Hall P, et al. Using telehealth technology to support CME in end-of-life care for community physicians in Ontario. Telemed J E Health 2004;10:103-107.
41. Regnard C. Using videoconferencing in palliative care. Palliat Med 2000;14:519-528.
42. Kuziemsky CE, Jahnke JH, Lau F. The e-Hospice: Beyond traditional boundaries of palliative care. Telematics Informatics 2006;23:117-133.
43. May C, Gask L, Atkinson T, et al. Resisting and promoting new technologies in clinical practice: The case of telepsychiatry. Soc Sci Med 2001;52:1889-1901.
44. Ruggiero C. Teleradiology: A review. J Telemed Telecare 1998;4:25-35.

SUGGESTED READING

Dyer KA. Ethical challenges of medicine and health on the Internet: A review [on-line journal]. J Med Internet Res 2001;3(2):e23.

Harnett B. Telemedicine systems and telecommunications. J Telemed Telecare 2006;12:4-15.

Kuziemsky CE, Jahnke JH, Lau F. The e-Hospice: Beyond traditional boundaries of palliative care. Telematics Informatics 2006;23:117-133.

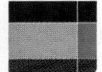

CHAPTER **116**

Making Good Decisions

Rogelio Altisent, Jacinto Bátiz, and María P. Torrubia

KEY POINTS

- Quality palliative care is composed of technical and ethical elements.
- Making good decisions is synonymous with prudent practice.
- Careful deliberation is essential to prudent decisions.
- Respecting patient autonomy is at the heart of decision making.
- Four traps in decision making exist: inertia, skepticism, lack of initiative, and failure in self-criticism.

The question about what it is to make a good decision is intuitive and frequently presents an ethical challenge. Any veteran physician can remember many situations (Box 116-1) in which there were doubts about what the best decision was. In palliative care, the decision to order a transfusion cannot be made based only on hemoglobin values. The way and the moment of informing patients and families about a bad prognosis cannot be decided only on guideline recommendations. Decisions such as withholding or withdrawing artificial feeding or transferring a patient to the hospital cannot obey only technical considerations. The total quality of clinical practice is composed of technical and ethical elements that are linked closely and demand that the trainee physician develop specific analytic capacity to make good decisions.

In palliative medicine, the issue becomes bigger when a professional who does not often face these cases must make such decisions. For example, a family doctor who has 2000 patients in 1 year does not usually encounter more than a dozen terminal patients and therefore is less trained than a palliative care expert in complex decision making. Other physicians also occasionally face difficult decisions characteristic of the palliative environment. Whatever the specialty, we should welcome the philosophy that exemplifies palliative care: to alleviate suffering.

CONCEPTS IN GOOD DECISION MAKING

Medical practice is steeped in ethics, but in palliative medicine, decisions are characteristically mixed with technical elements or even concealed by the ethical dimension. A classification of three types of ethical issues helps put the ideas in order (Box 116-2).[1]

When we think about a "good decision" in a clinical context, we are not thinking about attitudes (ethical issues type I), nor about capabilities and organizational responses (ethical issues type III). We already consider them to be resolved, at least in theory. In reality they remain, with all their indubitable moral meaning. In palliative medicine, we already accept that the main aim in terminal illness is to relieve suffering (i.e., attitude—type I), so there are no doubts when discarding measures that might be labeled "therapeutic obstinacy." It is also assumed that the physician possesses appropriate ability or training to manage pain or to communicate bad news (i.e., operational issues—type III).

The answer to ethical dilemmas—that is, difficult decision making (ethical issues type II)—is the most popular and most productive part of bioethics.[2] However, we must not lose view of types I and III, which have received less academic attention, because often they condition the type II issues that are our main interest.

Sometimes a case is in the gray area of the curative-palliative interface, such as when an aggressive treatment may cause concern or there are family pressures about sedation of a patient with moderate agitation. These are situations in which the professional cannot avoid a decision: we are guided either to action or to omission. The genuine question arises as to what is the right decision.

To complete this brief concept outline, remember that it is one thing to make a decision and another to carry it out. Starting with appropriate attitude (type I), a good resolution can occur (type II), but it may not be implemented due to organizational or personal difficulties (type III).

Attitudes are configured by education; dilemmas are solved with wisdom and training in ethics; operational issues demand capabilities, technical training, and good organization. The first case study allows thinking about the utility of this classification, which helps differentiate attitudes from operational issues, clarifying how to look for the best solution to each ethical issue (see "Case Study: Victor Gómez").

TO BE PRUDENT, NOT TO BE CERTAIN

When we are faced with making good decisions, we do not exercise theoretical reasoning, as if trying to obtain

> **Box 116-1 Examples of Difficult Decision Making in Palliative Medicine**
>
> - When do we refrain from transfusing a patient with anemia?
> - Do we have to break bad news to the patient (when, how, how much)?
> - When is it correct to withdraw artificial feeding?
> - How do we manage the clash of opinions among relatives of a terminal patient?
> - What should we do when a vital emergency occurs at home or in hospital?
> - Do we consider use of nasogastric tube feeding (or nefrostomy, colostomy, tracheotomy) as a disproportionate or an extraordinary measure?
> - At what point can we withdraw essential treatments?

> **Box 116-2 Classification of Ethical Issues**
>
> Type I. Attitudes
> Type II. Difficult decision making or dilemmas
> Type III. Operational issues (includes personal capabilities and organizational conditions)

objective scientific knowledge, but practical reasoning rooted in prudent judgment. We do not aim to make guaranteed decisions but prudent ones. A theoretical wise man can be a genius in a specialty and simultaneously imprudent when making decisions about the same matter—either extraordinarily impulsive or undecided. There are two different types of wisdom: theoretical, characteristic of the erudite, and practical, characteristic of the prudent. Appropriate knowledge is necessary, but it is not enough to make prudent decisions; rather, the first step of prudence is to ensure adequate information.

Scientific knowledge provides information, for example, on drug interactions: Can we mix medicine A with medicine B in intravenous infusions, or would a neuropathy be improved more with A or with B? Practical reasoning guides us in deciding whether it is sound to proceed to sedation of a patient with poor competence. Knowledge can be true or false, but a decision can be right (good) or wrong (bad). Scientific knowledge is examined according to the norms of experimental research, but ethical decisions cannot be verified in the same way.

RESPONSIBILITY AND PROFESSIONAL FREEDOM IN MAKING DECISIONS

Making a good decision is more than making a reasonable selection among several options: the goal is to make the best decision. We must be able to defend and justify our decision given other options, which means making a responsible decision[3] (i.e., one that can be defended).

When facing a problematic case in which we have the professional responsibility for a decision, our verdict will usually be the one that is followed. It is important to emphasize the difference between making a decision and offering guidelines that usually leave open a range of possibilities, as a substitute for the personal responsibility of the professional to whom the decision falls (see "Case Study: José Sevilla—Part 1").

CASE STUDY

Victor Gómez

Victor Gómez is a 47-year-old man with amyotrophic lateral sclerosis diagnosed 2 years ago. His wife cares for him. He is in a bed-chair for life, and he communicates by writing with the use of a slate. He presents with sialorrhea, dysphagia, and spasms and muscular pains due to rigidity and contractures.

Ethical Issue Type I

Dr. Blanco is Victor's family doctor who visits him frequently. Victor has communicated to Dr. Blanco his wish to receive only symptomatic treatment, without feeding tubes or artificial ventilation, but allowing for the control of symptoms with analgesics, relaxants, antidepressives, and hypnotics. When the end arrives, he wants to enter the hospital to receive sedation. Dr. Blanco considers that Victor has made a voluntary decision according to the rules of informed consent—that is, with personal competence, with appropriate information, and without coercion. Dr. Blanco discusses the case with the hospital neurologist, who agrees that, when the final situation takes place, Victor's wishes can be completed, carrying out a transfer to the hospital without the need of going through the emergency department.

Ethical Issue Type II

The final worsening takes place one weekend during a vacation period. Victor presents with dyspnea and confusion. His wife is very anxious, and she delegates the decisions to her brother, a medical doctor and surgeon from another city, who has come to help in these hard family circumstances. The brother calls into question the wishes communicated by Victor to Dr. Blanco; to the contrary, the relatives have the conviction that Victor had expressed his desire to fight until the end and that he should be put on artificial ventilation. Facing the dilemma, Dr. Blanco speaks in private with Victor's wife and shows her the record of the clinical history, in which Victor's decision is shown clearly.

Ethical Issue Type III

With good communication abilities, a steady emotional tone, and professional commitment, Dr. Blanco obtains the trust of Victor's wife. Victor is transferred to the hospital for the sedative treatment, in accordance with his advance directive. However, the neurologist who had previously been consulted and had agreed to this plan is on vacation, and the substitute neurologist disagrees with instituting sedation without first attempting treatment with artificial ventilation. In this way, the problem emerges again.

It is important to understand the meaning of professional freedom, joined to professional responsibility. Sometimes there have been doubts about the duty of following guidelines, predefined algorithms, or some kind of medical decision support system, as if this represented a limitation of professional freedom. The solution to the question must always respect professional freedom, remembering that, when we act following a good guide-

CASE STUDY

José Sevilla (as Told by His Family Doctor)—Part 1

José was an 82-year-old man who was my patient for more than 20 years. Several times, when he was not yet showing any cognitive deterioration because of his Alzheimer's disease, he told me of his wish to die at home. He hated hospitals and said he would go to a hospital only if it were necessary to solve a medical problem that could not be attended to at home. He insisted on not dying in a hospital bed but in his own bed, surrounded by beloved relatives. I wrote down his wishes in the medical record.

About 10 years after being diagnosed with Alzheimer's disease by a neurologist, José started to exhibit severe cognitive impairment. His condition did not allow him to decide his own treatment and medical care, but his family looked after him with love. Whenever any complication came up, such as pneumonia due to aspiration or a urinary tract infection, his family took him to the hospital for treatment. He went to the hospital several times and later came out and back to his home. Finally, in what was to be his last month of life, José experienced respiratory failure, which seriously threatened his life; in my opinion, the right treatment was symptomatic control of the dyspnea and comfort care.

His family, seeing death near, thought that the best interest for José was to die in hospital; moreover, if he died at home, it could be a bad memory for his grandchildren, who lived under the same roof. Perhaps they were expressing their fear of coping with José's death; if it happened in the hospital, the caretakers there would manage it all. I explained to the family that their father had expressed his will some years ago and had never changed his mind.

The family listened but still insisted on taking José to the hospital. I promised them my support and my dedication to caring for José at home in his last moments. I also explained to them that it was important for the family to feel satisfied that, after having cared for him during his long illness, they had also accompanied him in the death process in accordance with his desire to die at home surrounded by his dear ones.

line, it is easier to defend the decision. When, based on the circumstances of a particular case, we act outside the recommendations of guidelines, we need additional reasons to justify the decision.

Similarly, doubts have been raised about the physician's responsibility in response to a report from an ethics committee that has been consulted for advice in a difficult case. The answer from a consultant or a committee may offer one or more action courses, with justifications and analyses of consequences. But the final resolution has to be decided and assumed by the physician responsible, who can neither delegate nor share this responsibility with those who have given the advice. An exception occurs when there is a compulsory norm that requires a specific committee to proceed to the definitive verdict, rather than acting only in an advisory capacity.

RESPECTING AUTONOMY IN DECISION MAKING

Informed consent is the heart of the clinical relationship, and this implies that decision making must be shared by the competent and informed patient, following his or her values and preferences, and the patient even reserves the veto right. The responsibility for medical decisions is that of the professional, but the main character is the patient. However, professionals are also entitled to the right of a veto if they could find themselves involved in a useless or harmful decision for the patient.

Sometimes, in the academic context of bioethics, difficult decisions have been interpreted as a conflict between the beneficence principle (professional objectives) and the autonomy principle (patient preferences); quite often, a more cooperative focus on the doctor–patient relationship would lead to a better resolution, based on the interpretation that authentic beneficence cannot be reached without respecting the patient's autonomy.[4] This can be useful in palliative care, where the patient's weakness is often associated with decreased personal autonomy and competence, and with a position of vulnerability in the face of influence by external coercion.

THE WISE DECISION

Relevant characteristics of a good medical decision are that it occurs after appropriate deliberation,[5] is subjected to critical reasoning with weighing of arguments for and against, and involves appropriate consideration of the circumstances and the value of other opinions. A deliberate decision is not a personal opinion nor a brilliant insight, although these may lead to the same conclusion. We are expected to make responsible and therefore deliberate decisions. We are responsible for the means (which depend on our behavior), but not for the results (which involve factors we cannot control). What we are charged with is wisdom about making decisions, but we are not responsible for outcomes that no longer depend on us.

The professional must deliberate with calm maturity, although action may follow quickly. The purpose of the deliberation is to define well the end, the means, and the circumstances of the action. Multiple alternatives should be considered. Sometimes, a decision is not ours, but we have the responsibility to support the deliberations of the decision maker, often the patient's relatives (see "Case Study: José Sevilla—Part 2").

Usually, there are several possible good decisions in a clinical situation; for example, after a diagnosis with a bad prognosis, there are several alternatives in managing and communicating the information. But sometimes we must make a decision that cannot be postponed. In the example, a decision can be made to proceed immediately or to postpone the communication for fear of how the patient will react. In any case, we must be prepared to explain our decision as the best among all the possible ones.

In the deliberations to make good decisions, there is sound ethical justification for teamwork. The enrichment that comes from listening carefully to the various people who care for the patient, independent of their position in the team or their professional training, is a common experience. When evaluating how a treatment affects quality of life, the contribution of a relative, a voluntary caretaker, or other auxiliary staff can be important, because many times they can perceive the real needs of the patient better than the doctors can.

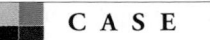

C A S E   S T U D Y

José Sevilla—Part 2

My professional duty was to facilitate the right decisions where José's wishes played a very important role. I considered that I was the one responsible for the medical decisions, but that the main character was the patient. When José was no longer competent, the family had the main responsibility in making decisions, but they could not go against the patient's will. The medical decision of solving complications in the hospital was carried out, respecting his desires, but when the final, irreversible complications appeared, I defended José's choice to not enter the hospital.

The easy thing would have been to consent to the desires of the family, but this would not have been an ethical decision. Neither was it practical or realistic to confront the family, and I decided to involve them in the deliberation. In the first place, I spoke about my understanding of the fear that generates these situations, and I explained to them other similar experiences in which the patients' relatives usually reacted in the same way. Meanwhile, I showed them my annotations in the medical recording about the patient's wish to die at home, surrounded by those dear family members who had so affectionately taken care of him. I also commented that it would not be good for the grandchildren to hide their grandfather's death from them. Finally, I used classic ethical reasoning and asked each of José's children, What would you like if you were in the same situation? At the end, they recognized that the best decision was to respect their father's wishes and to keep him at home with the appropriate control of symptoms.

This was not an easy story. I think that it finished quite well, because we achieved a good, effective, and confidential relationship thanks to many hours of dedication to José's situation. The time invested in the last deliberation with the family was decisive. I think that the best prescription for many difficult decisions of this type is heart and time—in other words, commitment and dedication.

THREE-STEP FRAMEWORK FOR APPROACHING MAKING GOOD DECISIONS

Academic bioethics has focused on[6] and produced profuse literature about sophisticated methods of solving the ethical dilemmas that often have dismayed clinicians.[7] It is necessary to offer simple approaches to aid decision making, combining technical and ethical concepts. The reasoning required to face moral dilemmas can vary in complexity. It may be useful to health professionals with limited training in ethics to provide an easy mental framework for facing such decision making (Box 116-3). We can decide at the bedside, according to the circumstances of the case (e.g., difficulties, scarcity of time, availability of resources), whether to make the decision after personal reflection (first step), after consultation with a colleague or the team (second step), or after asking the specialized opinion of a health care ethics consultant[8,9] or ethical committee (third step).

> **Box 116-3 Three-Step Framework for Making Difficult Decisions**
>
> *First*, self-reflection based on the tetrad of classic principles of bioethics (BANE):
>
> - **Beneficence:** What the professional considers best for the patient
> - **Autonomy:** What the patient (or proxy) prefers
> - **Nonmaleficence:** What must never be done
> - **Equity:** What affects the community or other persons
>
> *Second*, consultation on the problem with a colleague or with the team. This presupposes an effort to put order to the elements of the problem, explaining in a plain way and afterward reflecting about the comments received.
>
> *Third*, consultation with an ethics consultant or an ethical committee composed of members trained in a formal deliberation method that concludes with a written report.

> **Box 116-4 Four Hidden Traps in Decision Making**
>
> - Clinical inertia (concerning assessment, information, or treatment)
> - Skepticism due to moral fatigue
> - Poor initiative
> - Failure in self-criticism

HIDDEN TRAPS OF DECISION MAKING

Four common difficulties can produce camouflaged mistakes in decision making (Box 116-4). The first is the *clinical inertia* that leads to acceptance of old beliefs without criticism (e.g., the belief that dyspnea always requires treatment with oxygen). This is especially important in palliative medicine, where growing scientific knowledge has challenged tradition. We need to promote continuous improvement—on the one hand, to make correct technical decisions, evidence-based where possible; and on the other hand, to give good information to the patient in order to obtain the proper informed consent that is needed to make a good decision. Another kind of inertia   is to accept as definitive a determinate clinical setting, when continuous variation in symptoms and circumstances is a main characteristic in palliative medicine. This is why we have to review again and again.[10] Struggling against clinical inertia demands personal and professional commitment.

Skepticism due to moral fatigue is often a result of professional burnout: "I am frustrated; it is not possible to change things!" It applies to organizational issues, where there will always be problems. Sometimes this fatigue can be reflected in difficult personal relationships with patients, relatives, or colleagues. We must realize when the main problem is ourselves and not use this as an excuse to abandon the moral imperative of improving our practice and facing decisions with professionalism.

Lack of initiative, passivity, and scarce capacity to confront obstacles can produce a poor professional performance. The José Sevilla case study offers a good example. If the family doctor had adopted a passive attitude, without taking the initiative to talk with the relatives, José would have died in hospital against his will. This would have been bad decision making, caused by lack of professional initiative or perhaps by a feeling that it was easier to accept the relatives' first opinion. Promoting a process of deliberation with patients and relatives, applying teamwork, or asking for advice always demands proactive engagement. Sometimes, behind a bad decision, we can find a shortage of initiative; if this remains unnoticed, it is difficult to prevent it in the future.

The last hidden trap is *failure in self-criticism.* This occurs when inexperienced professionals are too self-reliant or experienced ones exhibit a lack of humility. Behind negligence in seeking advice about difficult dilemmas there can be temerity or pride. The best approaches to enrich the decision-making process and resolve problems were highlighted in the earlier discussion. When a person lacks some of these virtues (e.g., humility, compassion, prudence), conflicts grow.

RECENT DEVELOPMENTS

Currently, there are ethical dilemmas concerning the competence of elderly patients to make decisions about management, consent to treatment, or agree to participate in research, because of worries about cognitive incapacity.[11] Qualitative designs may help evaluate patients' decisions to refuse oncological treatment.[12] The debate about decision making and consent is couched in terms of respect for autonomy and concern for the patient's welfare.[13] Research on informing cancer patients about diagnosis and prognosis explores a sensitive area[14] that can provide good material to teach decision-making skills.

CONCLUSIONS

Clinicians have an oversophisticated view of decision making because academic bioethics is an erudite and specialized world, but this process is a daily intuitive bedside task. Some dilemmas require a methodological approach based on a framework. Prudence and personal commitment are the main factors in making good decisions, improving professional performance, and respecting patients' dignity.

REFERENCES

1. Altisent Trota R, Martín Espíldora MN, Serrat Moré D. Ética y medicina de familia. En Martín Zurro A, Cano Pérez JF (eds). Atención Primaria: Conceptos, Organización y Práctica Clínica, 5th ed. Madrid: Elsevier, 2003, pp 285-306.
2. Gracia D. Procedimientos de Decisión en Etica Clínica. Madrid: Eudema, 1991.
3. Randall F, Downie RS. Palliative Care Ethics. Oxford: Oxford University Press, 1996, pp 60-63.
4. Pellegrino ED, Thomasma DC. The Virtues in Medical Practice. Oxford: Oxford University Press, 1993, pp 57-58.
5. Gracia D. La deliberación moral: El método de la ética clínica. Med Clin (Barc) 2001;117:18-23.
6. Beauchamp TL, Childress JF. Principles of Biomedical Ethics, 4th ed. New York: Oxford University Press, 1994, pp 3-43.
7. Devettere RJ. Practical Decision Making in Health Care Ethics. Washington: Georgetown University Press, 1995, pp 76-104.
8. La Puma J, Schiedermayer D. Ethics Consultation: A Practical Guide. Boston: Jones and Bartlett, 1994.
9. Baylis FE (ed). The Health Care Ethics Consultant. Totowa, NJ: Humana Press, 1994.
10. Twycross RG, Lack SA. Therapeutics in Terminal Cancer. Edinburgh, UK: Churchill Livingstone, 1990, p 6.
11. Rosin AJ, Van Dijk Y. Subtle ethical dilemmas in geriatric management and clinical research. J Med Ethics 2005;31:355-359.
12. Van Kleffens T, Van Leeuwen E. Physicians' evaluations of patients' decisions to refuse oncological treatment. J Med Ethics 2005;31:131-136.
13. Harris J. Consent and end of life decisions. J Med Ethics 2003;29:10-15.
14. Elger BS, Harding TW. Should cancer patients be informed about their diagnosis and prognosis? Future doctors and lawyers differ. J Med Ethics 2002;28:258-265.

SUGGESTED READING

Beauchamp TL, Childress JF. Principles of Biomedical Ethics, 4th ed. New York: Oxford University Press, 1994, pp 3-43.

Gracia D. La deliberación moral: El método de la ética clínica. Med Clin (Barc) 2001;117:18-23.

Randall F, Downie RS. Palliative Care Ethics. Oxford: Oxford University Press, 1996, pp 60-79.

CHAPTER **117**

Denial and Decision-Making Capacity

Pilar Arranz and Pilar Barreto

> ## K E Y P O I N T S
>
> - Denial has implications in several aspects of complex decision making in palliative care.
> - There are two types of denial: adaptive and dysfunctional.
> - Possible determinants of denial include the patient's illness, coping style, culture, and family variables, as well as the physician–patient relationship.
> - General and specific interventions can help patients and families to face their situations.

The human species is alone in knowing it has to die, said Voltaire, but as much as we rationally know that we all die, we do not really believe it will happen to us.

COLOMBO[1]

Many people come to the end of their lives reluctantly. One factor that influences this situation is that Western society promotes denial of death. Therapeutic options must be adapted to patients' preferences in a way that respects their internal world, and this should be the main factor in decision making.

By presenting patients with information and offering them a clear choice, a decision board may enhance the power given to patients in medical encounters and help them to make decisions that are consistent with their personal values.[2] Knowing the treatment preferences of the terminally ill is critical for high-quality care. However, understanding patients' real preferences is difficult. Many factors[3] influence those preferences, with treatment outcomes being a strong determinant. Furthermore, preferences change after alterations in the treatment process. The process becomes more complicated when denial is present.

EFFECTS OF DENIAL BY THE PATIENT

Denial is a significant challenge when dealing with complex decision making. It may have repercussions in several dimensions:

1. Shared decision making refers to a process in which physicians and patients participate.
2. Patient values are important, especially in life-threatening situations when no single best treatment exists and there are tradeoffs between benefits and risks of available treatments.[2]
3. It is important to know when and how much information the patient and physician should share and whether they are promoting a sequential process or an actual shared process.
4. True shared, informed decision making is difficult, and evidence shows that it rarely happens. The understanding of options and roles is rarely explored and checked.[4] It is difficult to know whether a patient has problems understanding or is simply affected by denial.

Denial is a common psychological coping mechanism for those facing the end of life; it protects them from unpleasant realities by allowing them to refuse to perceive, acknowledge, or face these realities. It is a way of coping with anxiety, reducing tension, and restoring a sense of balance in a person's emotional experience. These mechanisms happen on an unconscious level and distort reality to make it easier for the person to deal with. When denial mechanisms are used to an extreme, they interfere with the ability to discriminate between what is real and what is not.[5]

The American Academy of Family Physicians[6] pointed out that people who face a terminal illness experience difficult emotional challenges, including loss of control, loss of roles and responsibilities, fear, anger, loneliness or isolation, and spiritual crisis. People cope with these challenges depending on their own life experience, interpersonal relationships, and coping styles; sometimes, when the threat of perception is overwhelming, denial may be the best coping strategy because of its innate protective function.

Denial seriously affects the capacity to participate in decision making because it is a barrier to information. Denial prevents patients from making decisions regarding end-of-life situations as well as those that are in the near future. The patient is unable to face reality, and competent decisions cannot be made. Denial limits the physician as regards discussing the patient's concerns and preferences.

DENIAL IN PATIENTS AND FAMILIES

Denial can be present in patients, the family, or the health team. In patients, we must differentiate adaptive from dysfunctional denial. Adaptive denial is transient in nature; information may be rejected in the process of adaptation.

If it persists, this can be problematic.[7] Dysfunctional denial is chronic and continuous; it can be produced by different etiologies.

Often, the family acts as principal decision maker on behalf of the patient, so it is crucial to identify whether the family is in denial. Denial can promote the appearance of a conspiracy of silence. Moreover, denial lessens psychological stability, effective and affective support for the patient, and collaboration with the health team. It causes complications in bereavement.

DENIAL IN PROFESSIONALS

The following points are relevant to denial among professionals:

1. There is a widespread reluctance to cope with death and dying. In this situation, the risk of inappropriate use of life-prolonging medical treatment is enhanced.
2. Society often believes that intentionally withholding life-sustaining treatment may equate with intentionally causing death.
3. More attempts are needed for linking decision making with ethical or legal concepts, because there can be a nonrecognition, or denial, of ethical consequences.[8]
4. In denial, iatrogenic influence can be the underlying agent. Intensive care units are prone to this type of denial because strong bonds are formed with patients, especially young people.
5. One of the most important consequences of professional denial is the delay of decision making to the point that the situation passes from curative to palliative.
6. In addition to delaying decision making, other negative consequences can arise, such as difficulties in the detection of symptoms or support of emotional reactions.

POSSIBLE DETERMINANTS OF DENIAL

Denial reaction can be determined by many factors, some of the most important of which are the following[9]:

- An overwhelming situation
- The experience of traumatic illness
- Previous coping style in the face of losses and threats
- Cultural variables
- Family promoters of the conspiracy of silence
- Personality
- Organic and psychopathological factors
- Contextual factors (e.g., ways of providing information, relationship with the physician)

INTERVENTIONS

The objectives in treating denial are as follows:

- To facilitate adaptation in the short, medium, and long term
- To increase care compliance to alleviate symptomatology
- To sustain emotional stability when denial is adaptive

- To promote changes, trying to open windows when denial is pathological or interferes with personal adaptation.

General Interventions

Decisive intervention when facing denial must be based on moral rationality and basic psychological knowledge. In the absence of psychopathological or organic dysfunction, patients using interpersonal denial may respond favorably to psychological intervention.[10] Moreover, most professionals state that, although patients and carers are often afraid to talk about dying, they are relieved when the topic is finally discussed.

Specific Interventions

Inevitably, for some who are in denial, a moment arrives when active treatment is no longer possible. At this point, it is important to check the individual's level of awareness. There are three possible responses:

1. The patient may realize that his or her illness cannot be cured. *Key management:* Confirm the facts and explore the resulting concerns.
2. The patient may indicate a lack of awareness and a need to deny the gravity of the illness. It can be transitory or chronic. If transitory, we are facing a reactive denial as part of a normal adaptation process (i.e., the patient does not want to or cannot be in reality).[11] *Key management:* Respect this reaction, provided the patient is coping well, accepting treatment, and not disabled by anxiety. Eventually, the patient can abandon this stance. In severe persistent anxiety, denial is probably no longer serving its defensive purpose. To be effective, treatment may have to include confrontation of the denial and other therapeutic measures such as anxiolytics.
3. Patients may oscillate in and out of awareness and denial. *Key management:* Check awareness repeatedly during subsequent consultations, and avoid making assumptions about how much information is wanted. It is important to recognize that patients sometimes need a rest from aversive stimulation.

If compelling reasons are present, it is necessary to consider challenging the denial. Denial should be confronted only if it is necessary, for example, if there is some important unfinished business or the patient is refusing treatment that might alleviate symptoms. Always do this in a way that minimizes psychological harm. The balance between negative and positive consequences must be made. If we decide on collusion, we must do it gently and use some focal open questions, such as "Have you thought about why your operation seemed so short?" (see "Common Errors").

Challenging Denial

In looking for a window on denial,[12] assess whether the denial is complete or whether there is hope that the individual can move toward some aspects of reality. Sometimes, the patient has considered that his or her life expectancy is poor. Sometimes, if the process is chronic

---

Common Errors

- Paternalist attitudes and negative communication
- Collusion without considering the patient's psychological needs
- Collusion without being emotionally prepared to cope with the fear and psychological problems that underlie denial
- Collusion without giving hope
- Biased information
- No assessment of affective/psychological components and cognitive status when competence is in doubt
- Declaration of chronic denial without checking its permanence or stability

---

Box 117-1 Interventions from Assessment to Treatment in Dealing with Denial

- Establishment of a relationship of trust is crucial in guiding patients with denial through decision making.
- It is necessary to distinguish between a problem of understanding, which is cognitive (i.e., the patient does not realize the situation), and a problem of denial, which is emotional (i.e., the patient cannot realize the situation). If it is a problem of understanding, provide information; do not make assumptions, but ask. If it is a problem of denial, determine the type of denial (adaptive or dysfunctional, transitory or chronic, organic or psychopathological).
- Explore the patient's awareness and capacity for making health care decisions. Assess the patient's emotional vulnerability, previous strategies of coping with threats, and internal resourcefulness to sustain denial.
- Respect denial unless there are compelling reasons to challenge it.
- Challenge denial only if necessary, especially when fundamental values are affected. Emotional support and counseling on knowledge and practice techniques are suitable for addressing the proposed objectives.
- Avoid confronting denial aggressively, because this can intensify denial or lead to increased anxiety.

---

and the patient is in total denial, it can be better to respect this way of coping and to wait for an opportunity such as some indication that the illness is progressing. The main objective is to guarantee the best decision through the best intermediary (if possible, one assigned by the patient); this person must be the nearest to the patient's values (Box 117-1).

RECENT DEVELOPMENTS

- There is now deeper knowledge of the components of adequate shared decision making, but there are difficulties in assessing it objectively.[2]
- Work has been done to determine the sources that influence denial status.
- The importance of health professionals' training in difficult communication, in order to avoid additional biases to the complex situation the patient is experiencing and the implication of the treatment, has been recognized.

- Improved methods for assessing autonomy and preserving the patient's competence have been developed.
- Regarding denial of impending death, a discourse analysis of the palliative care literature has been made.

CONCLUSIONS

Denial is a common coping mechanism in terminal illness. We should accommodate denial, not feed it. Denial should be recognized as a barrier to informed decision making. The best response to denial is respect, because denial is essentially protective unless it creates significant problems for the patient or relatives.

The decision to address denial can be based on how well prepared the patient is to deal with fears and all phenomena underlying them. Challenging denial must be done gently, with psychological support available, by identifying inconsistencies so that defenses will be not disrupted but awareness can be explored.[13]

We must consider that the patient, even if incompetent and a denier, in a transitory or chronic state, has not lost his or her rights. The patient's opinion can be respected based on an advance directive or through a representative. Try to guarantee the best decision through the best intermediary. This person must be the nearest to the patient's values as possible.

RESEARCH CHALLENGES

- We need more explicit assessment of patient perceptions and evaluations of treatment outcomes (including psychological states).
- A steady increase has occurred in the number of studies on preference assessment, but little research has been done on denial and decision making.
- Advance directives assume that patients can anticipate what their choices would be under future circumstances in which death is imminent. However, there is little evidence that decisions people make when they are relatively healthy predict their choices when death is imminent. Preferences for life-sustaining treatments appear to be only moderately stable, and the likelihood of choosing such treatments increases with worsening health.[14]
- The interest in death denial may be related to a larger discourse on dying in contemporary Western society. This larger discussion is reflected in palliative care, in which denial is problematic, and could invite patients to participate in planning their death while also detecting those who cannot cope with this awareness.[15]
- The assessment of the efficacy of interventions when denial is the patient's prevalent reaction is important in development of targeted research, for example, when the specific objective is denial. Given the prevalence of this reaction in clinical practice with different results, it could be useful to know which interventions best help patients and families in their adaptation to reality.
- Integration of different etiological models for a fuller understanding of denial.
- Clarify criteria to distinguish denial from confusion or difficulties in understanding.
- Denial research is linked to competence assessment; we need improved mechanisms for the objective assessment of competence, including cognitive and affective areas. The exigencies that apply when consequences are more serious for health and life need to be identified.[16]

REFERENCES

1. Colombo S. Grief in facing one's own mortality: Denial and loneliness. Med Law 2005;24:647-653.
2. Charles CA, Whelan T, Gafni A, et al. Shared treatment decision making: What does it mean to physicians? J Clin Oncol 2003;21:932-936.
3. Fried TR, Bradley EH, Towle WR, Allore H. Understanding the treatment preferences of seriously ill patients. N Engl J Med 2002;346:1061-1066.
4. Godolphin W. The role of risk communication in shared decision making. BMJ 2003;327:692-693.
5. Johnson SL. Therapist's Guide to Clinical Intervention. San Diego: Academic Press, 2004.
6. Karen Ogle. Approaching a terminally ill patient in denial: Curbside consultation. Case scenario. Am Fam Physician 1999;60:1556, 1558, 1563.
7. Rabinowitz T, Peirson R. "Nothing is wrong, doctor": Understanding and managing denial in patients with cancer. Cancer Invest 2006;24:68-76.
8. Sayers GM, Perera S. Withholding life prolonging treatment and self deception. J Med Ethics 2002;28:347-352.
9. Arranz P, Barbero J, Barreto P, Bayés R. Intervención Emocional en Cuidados Paliativos: Modelo y Protocolos, 2a ed. Barcelona:Ariel, 2005.
10. Connors SR. Denial in terminal illness: To intervene or not to intervene. Hosp J 1992;8(4):1-15.
11. Stedeford A. Facing Death: Patients, Families and Professionals. London: W Heinemann, 1984.
12. Faulkner A. Effective Interaction with Patients. New York: Churchill Livingstone, 1992.
13. Maguire P, Faulkner A. Communicate with cancer patients: 2. Handling uncertainty, collusion and denial. BMJ 1988;297:972-974.
14. Meier DE, Morrison RS. Autonomy reconsidered. N Engl J Med 2002;346:1087-1088.
15. Zimmermann C. Denial of impending death: A discourse analysis of the palliative care literature. Soc Sci Med 2004;59:1769-1780.
16. Simón P, Rodríguez JJ, Martínez A, et al. La capacidad de los pacientes para tomar decisiones. Med Clin 2001;117:419-426.

SUGGESTED READING

Clayton JM, Butow PN, Arnold RM, Tattersall MHN. Discussing end-of-life issues with terminally ill cancer patients and their carers: A qualitative study. Support Care Cancer 2005;13:589-599.

Colombo S. Grief in facing one's own mortality: Denial and loneliness. Med Law 2005;24:647-653.

Drazen JM. Decisions at the end of life. N Engl J Med 2003;349:1109-1110.

Meier DE, Morrison RS. Autonomy reconsidered. N Engl J Med 2002;346:1087-1089.

Ness DE, Ende J. Denial in the medical interview: Recognition and management. JAMA 1994;272:1777-1781.

Stiggelbout AM, de Haes JC. Patient preference for cancer therapy: An overview of measurement approaches. J Clin Oncol 2001;19:220-230.

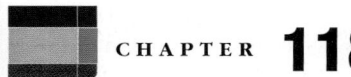

CHAPTER **118**

Evidence-Based Decision Making: Challenges and Opportunities

Amy P. Abernethy and David C. Currow

KEY POINTS

- Evidence-based practice can improve quality of care in palliative medicine.

- Decision making in palliative medicine has not always been built on research evidence, although the principles of evidence-based medicine (EBM) and palliative medicine are highly congruent.

- Barriers to evidence-based decision making in palliative medicine include lack of high-quality evidence, relative inaccessibility of available evidence, lack of critical appraisal skills on the part of practicing physicians, and a belief that these skills do not pertain to palliative care, because of either nihilism ("this person is dying") or the notion that "we know that we provide good care."

- Recent advances in clinical practice and research methodology and new information technologies have made implementation of evidence-based decision making both feasible and desirable for palliative medicine.

- EBM represents a new paradigm in medicine. Palliative medicine can showcase the application of EBM decision making in an area of medicine in which decision making involves great ambiguity and qualitative judgment.

Evidence-based medicine (EBM), also termed evidence-based practice, has ushered in an era in health care in which decision making takes center stage. Never before has the rationale for physicians' decisions been under such scrutiny. This is a result of the plethora of research evidence, of varying quality, generated over recent years. Because a large volume of data is now available to influence even routine clinical choices, accessing relevant research evidence, discerning which findings to use, and making decisions based on high-quality evidence are fast becoming essential clinical skills.

EBM is fundamentally about clinical decisions—their rationale, process, and outcomes. Though EBM is often viewed as a framework for improving cost-effectiveness, it can also be conceived of as a decision-making paradigm, one that provides a structure to enable physicians to deliver the best care. A central focus is the evaluation of best evidence as it applies to the needs, concerns, and specific situation of the individual patient; EBM is inherently about taking optimal care *of this individual*.

The evidence-based practice movement has evolved at the same time as palliative care has developed into a discrete discipline concerned with alleviation of suffering and optimization of quality of life for those with life-limiting illness. The new and important forces advancing the evolution of medicine, palliative medicine, and EBM share a common motivation—the desire to ensure best care of the individual, by utilizing up-to-date medical knowledge in conjunction with the wisdom and compassionate concern of the physician. As a new discipline, palliative medicine is unique. It has the opportunity to exemplify and demonstrate, in case method style, the incorporation of EBM methodology into a clinical realm to achieve improvement in patient-focused care.

DEFINITIONS OF EVIDENCE-BASED MEDICINE

"Evidence-based medicine is the conscientious, explicit, and judicious use of *current best evidence* in making decisions about the care of individual patients" (p. 71).[1] This definition implies the presence of an ever-evolving body of sound evidence and the integration of that evidence with professional values and ethics ("conscientious"), effective communication skills ("explicit"), and rational decision making ("judicious"), all in the context of individualized patient care. EBM has pervaded all aspects of health care over the past decade.

Despite general agreement on a good definition of EBM in principle, the reality is that the definition shifts depending upon the speaker and the audience. In health policy circles, EBM primarily represents a framework for limiting unnecessary care and thereby reducing health care waste and cost. To primary and secondary care clinicians, EBM may mean "critical appraisal skills" to adequately review an article and decide whether to apply it to patients; alternatively, these physicians may equate EBM with rigid guideline-based care. Others maintain that EBM mainly refers to data generated through clinical trials and population-based studies; despite its patient-focused definition, it may feel starkly removed from patient-centered care. This lack of consistency weakens the EBM concept and diminishes its potential to transform medicine from research to bedside care.

LACK OF EVIDENCE-BASED DECISION MAKING IN PALLIATIVE MEDICINE

The field of palliative medicine, which was formally acknowledged as a medical specialty in the United States only in 2006, is a relative late-comer to EBM. Historically, clinical decision making in palliative care has relied on qualitative judgment, anecdotal evidence, and the moral and ethical sensibilities of providers working with patients and their families. Palliative care has been provided, not because research evidence showed that it improved outcomes, diminished symptoms, or enhanced quality of life, but because it was deemed a social good ("the right thing to do") and because clinical experience suggested that bedside palliative care did yield improved patient-valued outcomes.

Such a view limits the scope of EBM, which encompasses net benefit to the patient—that is, not only the benefits but also any side effects. In palliative care, there is an added need for EBM given the time frames within which most care is provided. Which clinical pathway will provide the most predictable and timely onset of benefit in this individual or in the population being treated? Palliative care physicians base clinical decisions on considerations of compassion, understanding, kindness, and the desire to avert suffering—all of which are integral to EBM regardless of discipline. Since little research evidence of the kind usually associated with EBM (e.g., clinical trials, large observational studies) has thus far existed to support clinical decisions in palliative care, the concept of EBM has been slow to take root in this discipline.

BARRIERS TO EVIDENCE-BASED PRACTICE IN PALLIATIVE MEDICINE

Practical, philosophical, and organizational or cultural barriers have made it difficult for palliative care to embrace EBM. Most important has been the lack of a body of high-quality evidence; the challenges inherent in conducting high-quality research have impeded studies and discouraged research activity.[2] Clinical trials in palliative care research are more difficult because of opposition to randomization, recruitment difficulties, expected attrition, perceived patient burden, a wide range of (often unvalidated) outcome measures in this population, poor data management, and fragmented administrative data. A long-standing perception has held that palliative care clinical trials are not even possible. The evidence is to the contrary, with keen rates of participation when patients and caregivers are offered the opportunity to be involved in studies that improve the quality of care offered to people at the end of life.[3] To foster EBM in palliative care, strategies must be developed to overcome these research barriers.

Palliative care also lacks a shared language for generalizing results. Palliative care is practiced in many settings and manners. For example, the definition of hospice varies by culture, locale, and funding strategy. A clinical trial is conducted within the milieu of the local site and therefore within the culture of a specific palliative care service. There are no agreed methods for describing the study population that allow the populations or settings in which palliative care research is conducted to be readily compared and/or the findings to be extrapolated.

A related practical issue is that those palliative care studies that do provide quality research evidence have proved difficult for many clinicians to access. Data search strategies have historically utilized lines defined by a traditional academic discipline, such as cardiology. This query structure has complicated searches by palliative care providers, often limiting the results or requiring complex search strategies.[4] To support evidence-based decision making in palliative medicine, data-searching strategies need to recognize that palliative care crosses disciplines and that it is necessary to capture relevant palliative care data outside palliative care journals.

Philosophical resistance to the superimposition of EBM on palliative care has also slowed its acceptance. Traditionally, the ideals of palliative care include individually customized service with an emphasis on listening to the patient for information relevant to care decisions. This approach may seem incompatible with the principles and methods of EBM. Physicians may fear that EBM threatens to taint the field's pure motivation and to replace the "art" of palliative care with "cookbook" medicine. Overcoming this philosophical barrier requires a culture in which providers understand EBM as a framework for improving the quality of the care offered to individuals and as a methodology that supplements rather than supplants the judgment of the compassionate, discerning physician.

In the culture of palliative care, a perception has existed that the EBM core skills—searching the medical literature to identify articles, appraising studies, and deciding whether to apply the evidence to a specific individual—cannot be applied to the palliative care literature due to unique issues in life-limiting disease. Some studies of new interventions may consider outcomes that are pertinent to patients with a long survival time, or they may inadequately report patient-centered outcomes that are pertinent to palliative care, such as pain or near-term quality of life. When the patient's days are limited, the time required to search and appraise the literature may seem inappropriate; the clinician might instead opt to empirically "try out" an intervention to see if it works. Palliative care has defined a culture of patient-centered, hands-on, bedside care. This culture, and the philosophy underlying it, may seem inconsistent with the language of quantitative studies and population sciences. This incongruity is borne out when clinical practice guidelines ignore the unique practical aspects of caring for people with advanced life-limiting illness.

Although these practical, philosophical, and cultural barriers to evidence-based practice may seem intractable, it is incumbent on palliative medicine practitioners to critically consider the issues and devise practical solutions to overcome these obstacles. EBM is here to stay, and palliative medicine possesses the necessary elements for its adoption. Good decision making in evidence-based practice depends on motivation, competency, and overcoming barriers.[5] Cultural change and provider education will address motivation and competency; solutions to other barriers to evidence-based decision making warrant concerted attention.

BUILDING BLOCKS OF EVIDENCE-BASED DECISION MAKING

The existence and accessibility of *high-quality evidence* is a sine qua non of EBM. Evidence is "clinically relevant research, often from the basic sciences of medicine, but especially from patient centered clinical research into the accuracy and precision of diagnostic tests (including clinical examination), the power of prognostic markers, and the efficacy and safety of therapeutic, rehabilitative, and preventative regimens" (p. 71).[1]

Given a body of high-quality data, the EBM clinician must take a *systematic approach to the evidence*. This entails understanding the types of evidence, the ability to search for data and apply critical appraisal skills to make sense of it, and appropriate use of evidence-based clinical guidelines.

Evidence can be classified as primary or secondary. *Primary clinical research* includes case reports, case series, case-control studies, cohort studies, and randomized, controlled trials (RCTs) (Fig. 118-1). *Secondary research* critically summarizes and synthesizes primary research evidence; it has become critical in evidence-based practice, with meta-analysis fast gaining status as the highest form of evidence appraisal (Fig. 118-2). The concept of quantitatively pooling results from multiple studies grew out of the psychology, education, and nursing

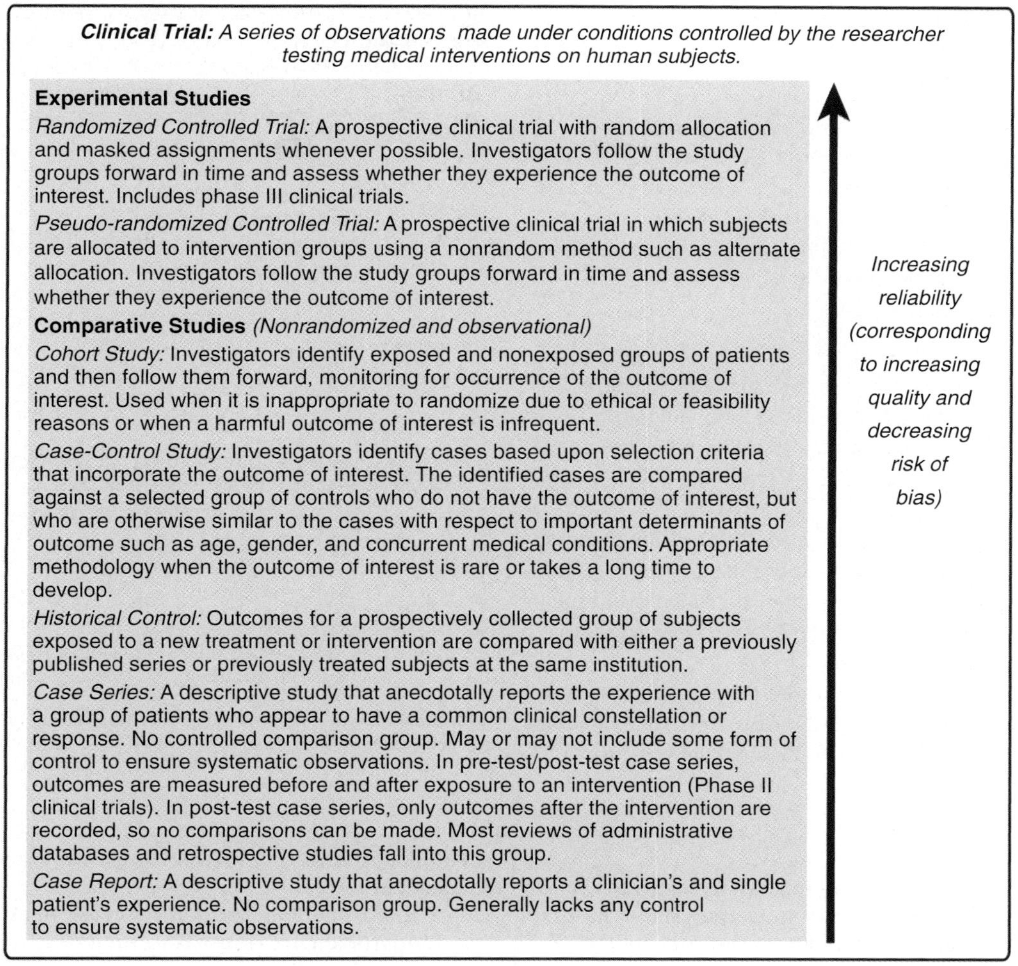

Clinical Trial: A series of observations made under conditions controlled by the researcher testing medical interventions on human subjects.

Experimental Studies

Randomized Controlled Trial: A prospective clinical trial with random allocation and masked assignments whenever possible. Investigators follow the study groups forward in time and assess whether they experience the outcome of interest. Includes phase III clinical trials.

Pseudo-randomized Controlled Trial: A prospective clinical trial in which subjects are allocated to intervention groups using a nonrandom method such as alternate allocation. Investigators follow the study groups forward in time and assess whether they experience the outcome of interest.

Comparative Studies *(Nonrandomized and observational)*

Cohort Study: Investigators identify exposed and nonexposed groups of patients and then follow them forward, monitoring for occurrence of the outcome of interest. Used when it is inappropriate to randomize due to ethical or feasibility reasons or when a harmful outcome of interest is infrequent.

Case-Control Study: Investigators identify cases based upon selection criteria that incorporate the outcome of interest. The identified cases are compared against a selected group of controls who do not have the outcome of interest, but who are otherwise similar to the cases with respect to important determinants of outcome such as age, gender, and concurrent medical conditions. Appropriate methodology when the outcome of interest is rare or takes a long time to develop.

Historical Control: Outcomes for a prospectively collected group of subjects exposed to a new treatment or intervention are compared with either a previously published series or previously treated subjects at the same institution.

Case Series: A descriptive study that anecdotally reports the experience with a group of patients who appear to have a common clinical constellation or response. No controlled comparison group. May or may not include some form of control to ensure systematic observations. In pre-test/post-test case series, outcomes are measured before and after exposure to an intervention (Phase II clinical trials). In post-test case series, only outcomes after the intervention are recorded, so no comparisons can be made. Most reviews of administrative databases and retrospective studies fall into this group.

Case Report: A descriptive study that anecdotally reports a clinician's and single patient's experience. No comparison group. Generally lacks any control to ensure systematic observations.

Increasing reliability (corresponding to increasing quality and decreasing risk of bias)

FIGURE 118-1 Types of primary clinical research studies.

Summarizes evidence about a focused clinical question	Summarizes evidence and compares outcomes about a focused clinical question	Summarizes evidence and makes recommendations about several related clinical questions
Meta-analysis	Economic analysis: • Cost-effectiveness analysis • Cost-utility analysis • Cost-benefit analysis	Evidence-based clinical practice guideline
Systematic review	Clinical decision analysis	Clinical practice guideline
Overview	Decision analysis	
Narrative review*		

Increasing reliability (corresponding to increasing quality and decreasing risk of bias)

*May not necessarily be about a focused clinical question; this is one of the causes of unreliability in narrative reviews.

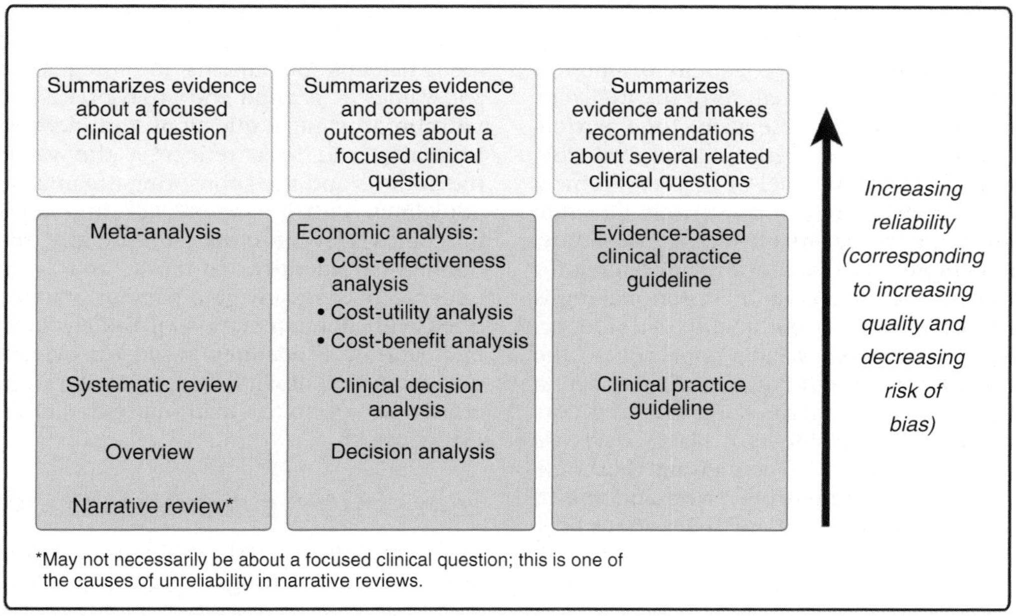

FIGURE 118-2 Types of secondary clinical research studies.

CASE STUDY

Evidence Hierarchy in Action

John is a 63-year-old retiree with a Pancoast tumor and neuropathic pain secondary to tumor infiltration and radiation injury. Fishing is his favorite pastime, but whenever he jerks his arm to set the hook he develops severe lancinating pain in his right arm. Opioids and nonsteroidal medications provide background pain relief but cannot help him deal with these unexpected breakthrough episodes. An effective adjuvant intervention is sought.

- *Meta-analysis*—A systematic review of behavioral therapies for cancer pain demonstrated that hypnosis and guided imagery improve pain control compared with placebo; other behavioral interventions studied did not lead to systematically significant improvements.[10]
- *Randomized trial*—A small, randomized trial documented the benefit of medical hypnosis in acute cancer pain.[11]
- *Case series*—Several clinicians from Sydney described their experience using medical hypnosis with their patients in a parallel session at an annual conference.
- *Anecdote*—John, the patient in this story, learned to immediately hypnotize himself whenever a fish was on his line, so that he could set the hook and gaff the fish. He returned to retired life fishing on the Florida flats.

TABLE 118-1	Levels of Evidence and Grades of Recommendations
RATING	**DESCRIPTION**
LEVELS OF EVIDENCE	
I	A systematic review of all relevant RCTs
II	At least one properly designed RCT
III-1	Well-designed pseudo-RCTs
III-2	Comparative studies (including systematic reviews of such studies) with concurrent controls and allocation not randomized, cohort studies, case-control studies, or interrupted time series with a control group
III-3	Comparative studies with historical controls, two or more single-arm studies, or interrupted time series without a parallel control group
IV	Case series, either post-test or pre-test/post-test
GRADES OF RECOMMENDATION FOR CLINICAL PRACTICE GUIDELINES AND OTHER HEALTH CARE RECOMMENDATIONS	
A1	RCTs, no heterogeneity, CIs all on one side of threshold NNT
A2	RCTs, no heterogeneity, CIs overlap threshold NNT
B1	RCTs, heterogeneity, CIs all on one side of threshold NNT
B2	RCTs, no heterogeneity, CIs overlap threshold NNT
C1	Observational studies, CIs all on one side of threshold NNT
C2	Observational studies, CIs overlap threshold NNT

CI, confidence interval; NNT, number needed to treat; RCT, randomized, controlled trial.

literatures.[6] By the mid-1980s, meta-analytic methods were applied to clinical trials,[7] and meta-analysis was first reviewed in the mainstream medical literature in 1987.[8,9]

Evidence spans a continuum from the most biased, lowest-quality research to the least biased, highest-quality studies. On the lower end of this *evidence hierarchy* are clinical anecdote and opinion; on the upper end is the RCT, the gold standard of medical research. Depending on the size of the RCT and the heterogeneity of findings within the meta-analysis, the meta-analysis or the RCT may be at the pinnacle of the evidence hierarchy for a particular clinical research topic (see Figure 118-1). Valuable information can come from any level of this hierarchy; a single case report, for instance, can powerfully illustrate a point or demonstrate an approach (see "Case Study: Evidence Hierarchy in Action"). An important concept for the clinician applying evidence-based decision making is *bias*. The degree of bias defines the quality of evidence, and that should qualify the physician's approach to the evidence presented. Improving the quality of evidence in clinical research is focused on minimizing bias and controlling potential confounding effects.[12] Biases decrease evidence quality and reliability by decreasing the confidence that the observed effect is true.[13] Nonrandomized studies are more prone to selection and assessment bias. Compared to RCTs, nonrandomized studies can dramatically underestimate or overestimate the treatment effect, most commonly indicating that the treatment is better than it really is.[14]

Practically, the evidence hierarchy and the risk of bias are often operationalized as "levels of evidence" (Table 118-1). These levels grade the various types of research evidence, classifying how strongly the conclusions should be heeded.

Clinical practice guidelines have been recommended to standardize care, improve efficiency, reduce costs, and ensure quality. Clinical practice guidelines are "systematically developed statements intended to assist practitioners and patients with decisions about appropriate health care for specific clinical circumstances" (p. 377).[15] They attempt to distill a vast amount of research into convenient readable documents and integrate it with opinions and values as needed and appropriate.[16] They often start with broad clinical questions and incorporate qualitative reasoning and bias, reflecting the value judgments of the authors and the sponsoring organization. High-quality guidelines clearly specify all important options and outcomes relevant to the clinical topic; use explicit methodology to identify, appraise, and combine evidence; undergo peer review; and present practical recommendations with documentation of the strength of the recommendations. Guidelines based on evidence have better quality and credibility than those developed from expert consensus (with or without explicit consideration of evidence).[17]

CORE SKILLS IN EVIDENCE-BASED MEDICINE

The core skills in EBM are straightforward and feasible in diverse clinical settings. They can be summarized by the tasks: ask, find, appraise, act, and evaluate. Jointly describing *critical appraisal*, these skills essentially equip the physician to (1) determine which evidence is relevant, of highest quality, and least biased, and (2) base clinical decision making on that evidence.

ACTION STEPS TO EVIDENCE-BASED DECISION MAKING IN PALLIATIVE MEDICINE

To apply evidence-based decision making, the provider must first determine the extent to which the individual wants to be involved in decision making.[18] The three principal components of shared decision making are (1) disclosure of information, (2) exploration of values about the therapy and potential health outcomes, and (3) making the actual decision.[18,19] Excellent communication skills are imperative. "To apply the results of . . . trials in clinical practice, physicians must translate the concepts and measures used to describe groups of patients into a language that can inform the decisions of an individual patient" (p. 618).[20] Formal decision aids and other forms of evidence-based patient education may help the provider communicate choices to the patient. The patient is a partner who can "learn to live with the uncertainty" (p. 548)[21] when it exists, provided that the practitioner communicates the uncertainty sensitively, in a balanced light, and according to patient communication preferences. The integration of compassion, decision making, and sensitive communication is the true art of medicine.

Application of evidence to an individual includes consideration of the generalizability and applicability of the results. *Generalizability,* or external validity, implies the extent to which findings can be extrapolated beyond the study setting and study population. *Applicability* implies the extent to which a study can be applied to an individual or group of patients. Rather than limiting application of results simply because a study's eligibility criteria and setting are inconsistent with the reality for our patient, we decide whether there is a compelling reason, based on external validity, that the results should not be applied to this individual.[22] To be relevant, the study must consider potential outcomes, harms, and costs that would be important to the individual patient. Applicability of results should be characterized in terms of the patient's underlying risk of the target event, because the benefit of an intervention increases with increasing risk of the underlying problem, whereas the risk of harm stays fixed.[23] Key elements include the individual's risk of the target disorder, the likelihood that the biology of the treatment effect will be similar in this individual, the risk of adverse effects to this individual, and local availability of the intervention.[24]

In summary, the EBM provider asks the following:

- Can the intervention be reproduced in this setting?
- Can the results be applied to this setting?
- Can the results be applied to this individual?

The physician then discusses answers to these questions with the patient, in the context of their preferences and values. Together, the clinician and patient consider:

- Were all important outcomes included?
- Are the potential benefits worth the potential harms and costs?

EVIDENCE-BASED PALLIATIVE MEDICINE

EBM defines a new conceptual paradigm in medicine. It is also a very practical approach to the clinical decisions that arise in day-to-day practice: using the least-biased evi-

---

Common Errors

- Dismissing EBM as not patient-centered or as only a way to cut health care costs.
- Failing to conscientiously and explicitly apply EBM to individualized patient care.
- Practicing evidence-supported medicine instead of evidence-based medicine—that is, making a decision and then finding an article to support that decision, rather than going through the systematic process of asking the question, finding the best available evidence, appraising the evidence, acting on the findings, and evaluating the results.
- Adopting the results of a published study before evaluating how the study was done.
- Failing to consider the external validity of the research (i.e., generalizability, applicability).

---

dence, tempered with compassion, judgment, and wisdom, to help determine the best decision for the individual patient. Many palliative medicine providers no doubt already practice EBM—but they do so at a disadvantage, compared to other disciplines, in terms of evidence availability and access, institutional support, and core skills training. By making overt the natural fit between EBM principles and practice and those of palliative medicine, and by developing EBM as the standard of care, palliative medicine will advance its fundamental mission to ensure best care of the individual. In the era of research-driven medicine, the task of improving palliative medicine can be viewed as none other than that of educating palliative care providers in the judicious, individualized application of EBM to palliative medicine (see "Common Errors").

Special Considerations in Applying Evidence-Based Decision Making to Palliative Medicine

Palliative medicine has a unique nature, distinct from that of other, curatively focused medical disciplines. Our patients are vulnerable and frail, have a high prevalence of cognitive impairment, and demonstrate changing performance status over time. Palliative medicine, far more than other disciplines, must include informal caregivers in care decisions. Leaders in palliative medicine should emphasize and address the following issues as they translate the principles and methods of EBM.

- Clinical decisions must focus on the individual.
- EBM depends on the availability and quality of data. Methods to generate meaningful palliative medicine evidence for the EBM framework are needed.
- Palliative medicine involves diverse providers. Training methods that include EBM and that teach critical appraisal skills to many kinds of providers of palliative care are needed.
- Secondary analyses, such as systematic reviews and meta-analyses, would improve the evidence basis for palliative medicine. Conduct of these studies requires synthesis of disparate data across disciplines. Although some investigators have developed robust internally held databases for this purpose, accessible databases capturing a significant breadth and number of studies for secondary research are needed.

RECENT DEVELOPMENTS IN EVIDENCE-BASED DECISION MAKING

New Methodologies to Support Clinical Trials in Palliative Care

Palliative medicine has made impressive strides in overcoming historical barriers to evidence-based practice. New clinical research methodologies make it possible to conduct previously "undoable" trials. For example, new recruitment strategies, enlightened institutional review boards, and multisite cooperation make larger clinical trials possible. The field is seeing results from international multisite clinical trials not funded by industry; international electronic data capture systems have helped make these studies feasible. Statisticians are starting to understand the realities of high attrition rates in clinical trials at the end of life and are developing plans to account for this feature. These advances will hasten the generation of sound evidence to support palliative medicine.

New Technologies Are Facilitating Evidence-Based Decision Making

Ready access to the medical literature through online resources, synthesized evidence sources, and electronic publications have made searching for research evidence much simpler. Decision making in palliative medicine relies heavily on the assessment of symptoms and on integrating this information with the evidence to determine the best course of action for the individual patient. New information technologies facilitate the challenging process of symptom assessment. E/tablets—wireless notebook-and-pen-style personal computers—are now in use in community oncology practices around the United States; e/tablets not only collect real-time patient-reported outcomes but also send patient information to a central database for research purposes. Interactive voice recognition system (IVRS) software enables physicians to longitudinally track symptoms between office visits and at home and to monitor for changes. These two technologies, alone, have the potential to transform clinical practice in palliative medicine, interdigitating symptom assessment with research evidence to support evidence-based practice. Other innovations, such as decision-support dashboards linked to evidence libraries, will no doubt complement them to enable a progressively more systematic and evidence-based approach to patient care in palliative medicine.

New Communications Strategies Help Translate Research Results to Clinical Practice

Palliative medicine is delivered across a spectrum of venues, from academic medical centers, to small community-based practices, to home visits. Discussions are underway to determine how to improve the "methods" sections of palliative care clinical research articles, so that providers can more readily assess their generalizability and applicability across varied palliative care practice settings. Others in the field plan a palliative medicine "Readers Guide to the Literature"; this will provide physicians with a practical guide on how to critically appraise the pallia-

---

Future Considerations

- Develop a common method to report the research setting and population in palliative care studies to improve generalizability and applicability.
- Improve palliative care literature search strategies to increase the number of relevant articles identified.
- Ensure that all palliative care literature is adequately cataloged.
- Enhance clinical trials methodologies and rapid dissemination of research results for practical use.

---

tive care literature, recognizing its inherent limitations (see "Future Considerations").

REFERENCES

1. Sackett DL, Rosenberg WM, Gray JA, et al. Evidence based medicine: What it is and what it isn't. BMJ 1996;312:71-72.
2. Rinck GC, van den Bos GA, Kleijnen J, et al. Methodologic issues in effectiveness research on palliative cancer care: A systematic review. J Clin Oncol 1997;15:1697-1707.
3. Mitchell GK, Abernethy AP; Investigators of the Queensland Case Conferences Trial; Palliative Care Trial. A comparison of methodologies from two longitudinal community-based randomized controlled trials of similar interventions in palliative care: What worked and what did not? J Palliat Med 2005;8:1226-1237.
4. Sladek R, Tieman J, Fazekas BS, et al. Development of a subject search filter to find palliative care information in the general medical literature. JAMA 2006;94:394-401.
5. Muir Gray JA. Evidence-Based Healthcare: How to Make Health Policy and Management Decisions, 2nd ed. Edinburgh: Churchill Livingstone, 2001.
6. Petticrew M, Roberts H. Systematic Reviews in the Social Sciences: A Practical Guide. Hoboken, NJ: John Wiley & Sons, 2005.
7. DerSimonian R, Laird N. Meta-analysis in clinical trials. Control Clin Trials 1986;7:177-188.
8. L'Abbe KA, Detsky AS, O'Rourke K. Meta-analysis in clinical research. Ann Intern Med 1987;107:224-233.
9. Sacks HS, Berrier J, Reitman D, et al. Meta-analyses of randomized controlled trials. N Engl J Med 1987;316:450-455.
10. Abernethy AP, Keefe FJ, McCrory DC, et al. Technology Assessment on the Use of Behavioral Therapies for Treatment of Medical Disorders: Part 2. Impact on Management of Patients with Cancer Pain. Report to the US Agenecy for Healthcare Research and Quality. Durham, NC: Duke Center for Clinical Health Policy Research, 2005.
11. Syrjala KL, Cummings C, Donaldson GW. Hypnosis or cognitive behavioral training for the reduction of pain and nausea during cancer treatment: A controlled clinical trial. Pain 1992;48:137-146.
12. National Health and Medical Research Council. How to Use the Evidence: Assessment and Application of Scientific Evidence. Canberra: Commonwealth of Australia, National Health and Medical Research Council, February 2000.
13. Sackett DL, Haynes RB, Guyatt GH, Tugwell P. Clinical Epidemiology: A Basic Science for Clinical Medicine, 2nd ed. Boston: Little, Brown, 1991.
14. Kunz R, Oxman AD. The unpredictability paradox: Review of empirical comparisons of randomised and non-randomised clinical trials. BMJ 1998;317:1185-1190.
15. Cook DJ, Mulrow CD, Haynes RB. Systematic reviews: Synthesis of best evidence for clinical decisions. Ann Intern Med 1997;126:376-380.
16. Hayward RS, Wilson MC, Tunis SR, et al. Users' guides to the medical literature: VIII. How to use clinical practice guidelines: A. Are the recommendations valid? The Evidence-Based Medicine Working Group. JAMA 1995;274:570-574.
17. Grol R, Dalhuijsen J, Thomas S, et al. Attributes of clinical guidelines that influence use of guidelines in general practice: Observational study. BMJ 1998;317:858-861.
18. McAlister FA, Straus SE, Guyatt GH, Haynes RB. Users' guides to the medical literature: XX. Integrating research evidence with the care of the individual patient. Evidence-Based Medicine Working Group. JAMA 2000;283:2829-2836.
19. Elwyn G, Edwards A, Gwyn R, Grol R. Towards a feasible model for shared decision making: Focus group study with general practice registrars. BMJ 1999;319:753-756.
20. Steiner JF. Talking about treatment: The language of populations and the language of individuals. Ann Intern Med 1999;130:618-622.
21. Silagy C. A view from the other side: A doctor's experience of having lymphoma. Aust Fam Physician 2001;30:547-549.
22. Guyatt GH, Sackett DL, Cook DJ. Users' guides to the medical literature: II. How to use an article about therapy or prevention: B. What were the results and will they help me in caring for my patients? Evidence-Based Medicine Working Group. JAMA 1994;271:59-63.

23. Glasziou PP, Irwig LM. An evidence based approach to individualising treatment. BMJ 1995;311:1356-1359.
24. Dans AL, Dans LF, Guyatt GH, Richardson S. Users' guides to the medical literature: XIV. How to decide on the applicability of clinical trial results to your patient. Evidence-Based Medicine Working Group. JAMA 1998;279:545-549.

SUGGESTED READING

Guyatt G, Rennie D (eds). Users' Guides to the Medical Literature: Essentials of Evidence-Based Clinical Practice. AMA Press, 2002. Available at: http://www.ama-assn.org (accessed December 4, 2007).
Muir Gray JA. Evidence-Based Healthcare: How to Make Health Policy and Management Decisions, 2nd ed. Edinburgh: Churchill Livingstone, 2001.
Sackett DL, Rosenberg WM, Gray JA, et al. Evidence based medicine: What it is and what it isn't. BMJ 1996;312:71-72.

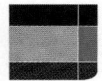

CHAPTER **119**

Determining Prognosis

Paul Glare and **Antonio Vigano**

KEY POINTS

- Prognostication is one of three cardinal clinical skills, but it is undervalued by modern medicine, compared to diagnostics and therapeutics.

- Prognosis is a branch of clinical epidemiology that is concerned with predicting outcomes of the natural history of illness.

- The growth of palliative care, specializing in care of the incurable, has renewed interest in predicting the short-term survival of the dying.

- Clinical judgment predicting survival is often inaccurate and is usually overoptimistic.

- Actuarial judgment, based on statistically derived key factors, can improve prognostic accuracy, but the factors identified have limited predictive power.

- In far-advanced cancer, tumor-related prognostic factors are less relevant than performance status, anorexia-cachexia, and some symptoms.

- Laboratory markers such as leukocytosis, lymphopenia, and acute phase reactants (C-reactive protein) are also helpful.

- Prognostic indices, nomograms, and Web-based tools are being developed for advanced cancer.

- Poor prognostication can have dire consequences in advanced cancer, as bad as choosing the wrong diagnosis or treatment.

A recent National Institutes of Health Consensus Conference on end-of-life care concluded that it is impossible to accurately predict an individual's death.[1] Despite this, predicting survival remains an important, if difficult, clinical skill to be acquired by physicians and other professionals in palliative care, for several reasons:

- To answer that most awkward question, "Doctor, how long do I have?"
- Because, in the United States, a prognosis of less than 6 months is a criterion for hospice admission.
- Because clinical decision making in far-advanced disease depends on prognosis.
- For research design and analysis.

Prognostication, along with diagnosis and therapy, has long been recognized as one of three cardinal clinical skills,[2] but it has become devalued in modern medicine due to the advances in diagnostics and therapeutics which have rendered many previously fatal illnesses curable. Modern physicians are not taught to prognosticate, and, unsurprisingly, most avoid prognosticating wherever possible.

Prognosis is a branch of clinical epidemiology that is concerned with predicting the outcomes of the natural history of an illness. There are five outcomes that can be predicted, referred to as the 5 D's:

- Death
- Disease recurrence
- Disability
- Drug toxicity
- Dollars (cost)

To these may be added a sixth D, "Derivatives," or the impact on the health of others caused by the illness.

This chapter focuses on one outcome, death, and focuses on patients with far-advanced cancer and typical survival times of less than 3 months; such patients make up most referrals to palliative care services internationally. Much of the information is also applicable to earlier-stage cancer and to other life-limiting diseases. There are two dimensions to prognosis: foreseeing, or determining the prognosis (the focus of this chapter), and foretelling, or communicating the prognosis (see Chapter 111).

SUBJECTIVE SURVIVAL PREDICTIONS

The methods used by palliative care physicians to prognosticate have not been much studied. One survey showed that only one third of doctors asked to prognosticate would offer a truthful prognosis; the rest either refused to prognosticate or predicted an outcome more optimistic than they really believed.[3] If pressed for a prediction, some physicians may become defensive and say, "I don't have a crystal ball. . . . It's up to God [or fate]!" Others may guess, rely on "intuition," or incorrectly apply population statistics such as median survival time. (Because most survival curves in advanced cancer are exponential, 90% of patients fall within the range of 0.16 to 3 to 4 times the median.)[4]

More experienced clinicians use "clinical acumen." The factors they take into account are not well understood and worthy of further research. Presumably, they take into account median survival, adjusted for how the patient appears "from the end of the bed." Accurate predictions depend on experience, reliable memory, and remaining dispassionate.

The clinical prediction of survival (CPS) is inaccurate, being overly optimistic, often by a factor of 3 or more.

The influence of the doctor's psychology cannot be ignored when subjective judgment is applied. Personal physician characteristics influence the accuracy of CPS. Older physicians and those with training in oncology or palliative care are more accurate, but a close physician–patient relationship blunts this accuracy. (A dispassionate second opinion from a senior colleague may be worthwhile if an accurate clinical survival prediction is essential.) Despite limitations, CPS is significantly correlated with actual survival and is often retained as an independent factor in multivariate analyses of prognostic factors. When it comes to measuring time to death, clinicians can discriminate but are not well calibrated.

Most subjective survival predictions are temporal, expressing the amount of remaining time in absolute terms (e.g., 2 weeks, 6 months, "hours to days"). Survival can also be predicted as the probability of being alive at a certain time point, rather than the expected time to death. Although fewer studies have been done, they suggest that such predictions are more accurate and may provide more useful information. Another approach to prognostication is to frame the question in the following terms: "Would I be surprised if this patient died within [a certain time]?"

ACTUARIAL JUDGMENT

There are many potential prognostic factors that can be analyzed to improve clinical predictions of survival. They can be conveniently categorized according to whether they are tumor-, patient- or environment-related (Table 119-1). The factors that are important in palliative care, for patients with far-advanced or terminal disease (predicted survival time <3 months) differ from those that are important earlier in the disease course.

Tumor-Related Factors

In far-advanced cancer, tumor-related factors such as size, extent of spread, and histological grade are less important and usually turn out not to be independent on multivariate analyses.

Patient-Related Factors

Patient-related factors include demographics, performance status, symptoms, laboratory parameters, psychological status, quality of life (QOL), and co-morbidities.

Demographic Factors

Factors such as age and gender are usually unimportant in far-advanced cancer.

Performance Status

Performance status is a predictor of oncological outcomes and is a reliable factor for short-term survival. Low scores predict poor survival, although high scores do not guarantee prolonged survival: those with an initially good performance status can rapidly deteriorate, usually during the final month or two of life, although a slower decline is seen in some. Unless the decline in performance status is associated with an acute, reversible problem (e.g., anemia, sepsis, side effects of treatment), it is the commencement of the terminal phase. This pattern represents the typical "death trajectory" of advanced cancer (Fig. 119-1).[5]

Many different scales have been developed for performance status, the most widely studied being the Karnofsky Performance Status Scale (KPS). Others include the scales developed by the Eastern Cooperative Oncology Group (ECOG) and the World Health Organization (WHO). A recent modification of the KPS, called the Palliative Performance Scale (PPS), was developed for physical status in hospice patients and has some utility for prognosis.[6]

Symptoms

Given that a high performance status does not guarantee good long-term survival, the prognostic challenge is to distinguish those patients about to deteriorate from those who might remain stable. The National Hospice Study showed that patients who had a good performance status but a particular symptom profile (anorexia, weight loss, xerostomia, dysphagia, dyspnea) were the ones most

TABLE 119-1 Candidate Prognostic Factors in Patients with Advanced Cancer		
TUMOR-RELATED	**HOST-RELATED**	**ENVIRONMENTAL-RELATED**
Anatomic extent	Age, gender, race	Marital status, social support
Histological grade and other features	Genetic makeup	Geography
Tumor bulk	Performance status	Access to treatment
Tumor marker level	Symptoms and signs	Expertise of oncologist
Tumor molecular biology	Psychological status	Response to treatment
Disease-free interval	Function of vital organs	Oncologist's prediction of survival
	Co-morbidities	

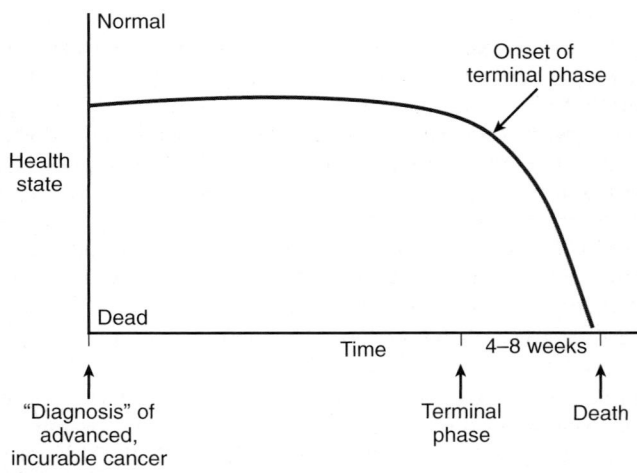

FIGURE 119-1 Typical "death trajectory" of patients with advanced cancer. *(Adapted from Lunney JR, Lynn J, Foley DJ, et al. Patterns of functional decline at the end of life. JAMA 2003;289:2387-2392.)*

likely to deteriorate.[7] People with a KPS score greater than 50 and no key symptoms had a median survival time of approximately 6 months and a small (10%) chance of living for 1.5 years, whereas those with a KPS score greater than 50 and all five symptoms had a median survival time of 2 months and a 10% chance of living for 9 months. For those with poor performance status, it made little difference whether the symptoms were present or not.

The cluster of poor performance and gastrointestinal symptoms, typically caused by the cancer cachexia syndrome, has been called the "common terminal pathway" of advanced cancer.[8] Confusion is another symptom that has been associated with a poor prognosis.[9] Pain is not usually considered predictive of poor survival in far-advanced cancer, even though pain increases in frequency and severity as cancer progresses. Episodes of severe, uncontrollable ("unendurable") pain and breathlessness are more common in the last few weeks of life.[10] Treatment with opioids does not affect survival.

Quality of Life

It is unclear whether QOL is an important determinant of survival in far-advanced cancer. The role of psychological factors in cancer survival remains controversial. Some have claimed to identify psychosocial aspects important in cancer survivorship, such as the "fighting spirit," but others have stated that the inherent biology of the disease (cancer) alone determines the prognosis. Palliative care workers can all give anecdotes of imminently dying patients who seemed to "hang on" for some important goal. Some studies in advanced cancer have found global QOL scores associated with survival, but in many studies of multidimensional QOL, only the physical symptom or physical well-being subscales appeared to correlate with survival. QOL has not been much investigated as a prognostic factor in terminal cancer. In the Therapeutic Impact Questionnaire (TIQ), only the patient-rated perception of cognitive function and global well-being had independent prognostic value. Patients had median survival times of 137, 50, and 17 days for impairment of neither, one, or both scales, respectively.[11]

Biological Parameters

Biological parameters have not been as widely investigated as clinical ones in the palliative care population, although many laboratory abnormalities have been evaluated. In both advanced and terminal cancer, leucocytosis, lymphocytopenia, low pseudocholinesterase,[12] high vitamin B_{12}, and high bilirubin and LDH have been proved significant. Other factors found to be significant in advanced cancer, such as low serum albumin and prealbumin levels, lose significance in more terminal populations. The reason is unclear but may be related to the dominance of other features of malnutrition, such as poor performance, anorexia, and weight loss. There is increasing interest in C-reactive protein as an indicator.[13]

Environmental Factors

Various environmental characteristics could be prognostic factors for advanced cancer. These include marital status, geography, and socioeconomic status. Marital status modi-

fies the effect of QOL on survival in cancer. Anticancer treatment factors (type of treatment, response to treatment) and supportive care characteristics (interventions, opioid therapy, place of care) are also candidate prognostic factors. Some multivariate analyses of prognostic factors in far-advanced cancer have incorporated these types of variables.

Co-morbidities

The impact of co-morbidities on survival in cancer has been long recognized, but few studies have investigated their importance in advanced disease; it is unclear whether they are important in far-advanced cancer.

RECENT DEVELOPMENTS

New Concept for Prognostication

A hypothetical model for the process for determining an individual's prognosis has been proposed (Fig. 119-2).[14] The diagnosis precedes and forms the basis of the generic prognosis, which is then modified for the individual by including other factors such as symptoms and co-morbidities. An important feature of prognostication, which distinguishes it from the other clinical skills, is that it is dynamic. Although the disease's prognosis is static, the patient's prognosis is dynamic and at any point of time provisional, depending on the various factors in this model. For example, a newly diagnosed cancer has a particular prognosis, which is modified depending on whether treatment is offered, the response to treatment, toxicity, and any co-morbidity.

Predictive Models

Advances in categorical data analysis and computing software have enabled identification of clinically relevant, individual prognostic factors such as performance status, symptoms, or laboratory markers. These can be weighted based on statistical parameters and combined to create predictive mathematical models; these models form the basis of prognostic indices which can then be validated

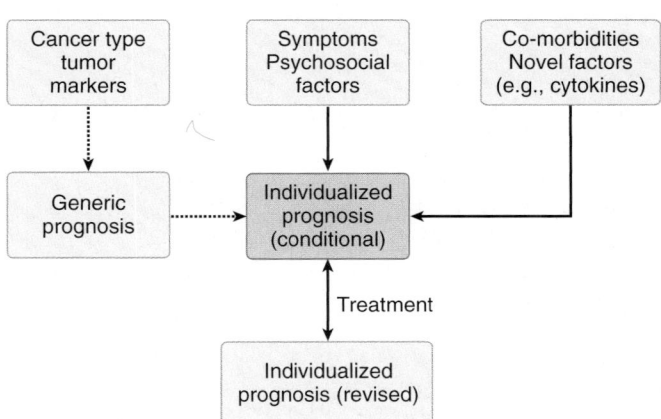

FIGURE 119-2 Conceptual model of prognostication in advanced cancer. *(Data from Mackillop WJ, Gospodorwicz M. The importance of prognosis in cancer medicine. In Gospodorwicz M, O'Sullivan B, Sobin LH (eds). Prognostic Factors in Cancer. Hoboken, NJ: Wiley-Liss, 2006, pp 3-14.)*

for widespread use. A variety of prognostic models have been developed for advanced cancer, including some for specific cancers and others for heterogeneous populations. Validated prognostic scores have also been used in terminal cancer, to identify isoprognostic subpopulations. Three such models are described here.

The Palliative Prognostic (PaP) Score[15] was built and validated in two independent, multicenter population studies of Italian home hospice cancer patients with a median survival time of 1 month. Points are awarded for symptoms (anorexia, dyspnea), poor performance status, white cell abnormalities, and the CPS (Table 119-2). These individual scores are summed for a total PaP score. Cutoff points have been developed that trisect the population into groups with high, intermediate, and low chances of surviving for the next month. This model has been validated in several countries, in various settings, and in different disease phases. A modified version includes delirium.

The Palliative Prognostic Index (PPI)[16] is a simple Japanese tool that uses performance status, two symptoms (breathlessness and delirium), and one sign (edema) to distinguish patients who have less than 3 weeks or less than 6 weeks to live. Unlike the PaP Score, it does not include CPS. The PPI is more accurate than CPS.

The Glasgow Prognostic Score (GPS)[13] combines the presence or absence of an elevated C-reactive protein concentration and hypoalbuminemia; it divides patients with lung cancer and gastrointestinal malignancies into three isoprognostic groups. It has yet to be evaluated in a heterogeneous sample.

TABLE 119-2 Calculation of the Palliative Prognostic Score (PaP) Score*

PROGNOSTIC FACTORS	DESCRIPTION	PARTIAL SCORE
Dyspnea	Absent	0
	Present	1
Anorexia	Absent	0
	Present	1.5
KPS	≥50	0
	30-40	0
	10-20	2.5
CPS (wk)	>12	0
	11-12	2.0
	9-10	2.5
	7-8	2.5
	5-6	4.5
	3-4	6.0
	1-2	8.5
Total WBC count (cells/mm³)	Normal (4800-8500)	0
	High (8501-11,000)	0.5
	Very high (>11,000)	1.5
Lymphocytes (%)	Normal (20.0-40.0)	0
	Low (12.0-19.9)	1.0
	Very low (0-11.9)	2.5

*A partial score is assigned for each of the six factors; the total of these partial scores is the PaP Score. The PaP Score determines the risk group in terms of 30-day survival probability: group A (>70% probability), score of 0 to 5.5; group B (30-70%), 5.6 to 11.0; group C (<30%), 11.1 to 17.5. CPS, clinical prediction of survival; KPS, Karnofsky Performance Score; WBC, white blood cell.

EVIDENCE-BASED MEDICINE

Evidence-based medicine is less well established for prognosis studies than for studies of therapy. Whereas the double-blind randomized, controlled trial represents the highest level of evidence for an interventional study, the hierarchy of evidence for observational data such as prognostic studies is unclear, as are the criteria for a well-designed prognostic study. One suggested hierarchy is the following:

- Level IA or IB: Meta-analysis of impact studies or cohort studies
- Level II or IIA: Randomized (±controlled) trials of the clinical benefit of a prognostic score as an aid to clinical decision making
- Level IIIA: Confirmative cohort studies to evaluate agreement between actual and predicted survival by the prospective application of indices and/or to test whether a prognostic model maintains its strength in a different patient sample
- Level IIIB: Explorative cohort studies to examine how the predictive power of a new prognostic factor relates to those factors already established and/or to estimate the magnitude of its effect
- Level IIIC: Investigative cohort studies examine the association of putative new factors with survival
- Level IV: Nonanalytic studies (case reports/case series)

Using this system, prognostication in palliative care is at level IIIA. Validated prognostic tools have been developed, but there have been no studies of these tools to aid clinical decision making in either uncontrolled (level II) or controlled (level I) studies.

Subjective Judgment: Level IIIC

Investigative cohort studies to evaluate the accuracy of doctors' survival predictions (level IIIC) in terminal cancer have been undertaken. Most have looked at the difference between predicted and actual survival after referral to palliative care or admission to a hospice. A recent systematic review,[17] involving more than 1500 predictions, showed the following:

- Predictions were more than twice as likely to be overoptimistic (median predicted survival, 6 weeks; median actual survival, 4 weeks).
- Predictions were correct to within 1 week in only 25% of cases.
- Predictions were incorrect by more than 1 month in more than 25% of cases.
- Despite inaccuracy, there was a strong correlation between predicted and actual survival, up to 6 months.
- Predictions of less than 4 weeks' survival were the most precise ("horizon effect").
- For predictions beyond 6 months, there was no relationship between predicted and actual survival.

This review showed that the CPS accounted for 50% of the variance in actual survival. This compared to 37% for the standard predictive factors (performance status, symptoms, hematology results). When the CPS and the other factors were combined, variance increased to 54%. This emphasizes the limited ability of known prognostic factors to predict survival and the need for finding novel prognostic factors in terminal cancer.

Prognostic Factors: Level IIIC

There have been several systematic reviews (Table 119-3) of level IIIC studies in far advanced cancer,[18,19] with the following results.

The association between performance status and survival, whether determined by the KPS, the ECOG scale, or some other measure of functional status, has been confirmed.

Many studies revealed an association between survival and gastrointestinal symptoms such as anorexia, weight loss, dysphagia and difficulty swallowing, and xerostomia.

There is level IIIC support for several QOL scores:

- Functional Living Index–Cancer (FLIC)
- Global health status item at the beginning of the Medical Outcome Studies Short Form–36 (SF-36)
- Symptom Distress Score
- Rotterdam Symptom Checklist
- Physical symptom subscale score of the Memorial Symptom Assessment Scale
- Spitzer Quality of Life Index
- Global European Organization for Research and Treatment of Cancer (EORTC) Core Quality of Life (QLQ-C30)

TABLE 119-3 Clinical Prognostic Factors in Patients with Advanced Cancer, According to Consistency of Evidence*

DEFINITE FACTORS	POSSIBLE FACTORS
Clinical prediction of survival (CPS)	Tumor characteristics: Primary site Secondary sites
Performance status	Patient characteristics: Age Gender Marital status
Signs and symptoms of cancer cachexia syndrome: Anorexia Weight loss Dysphagia Xerostomia	Symptoms: Pain Nausea
Other symptoms: Delirium Dyspnea	Signs: Tachycardia Fever Proteinuria
Some biological factors: Leucocytosis Lymphocytopenia C-reactive protein	Some biological factors: Anemia Hypoalbuminemia Prehypoalbuminemia Serum calcium level Serum sodium level LDH and other enzymes Co-morbidity

*Definite factors have been correlated with survival in far-advanced cancer. Possible factors have been indicated but are not confirmed, or are correlated in less-advanced disease, or have contradictory data. Additional factors have controversial indications and include multidimensional quality of life questionnaires.
LDH, lactate dehydrogenase.

Predictive Models: Level IIIA

Four studies involved construction and development of such predictive models for terminal cancer. Two have been validated (level IIIA): the PaP Score and the PPI. Prognostic factors present in all of the models were symptoms related to nutritional status (anorexia, dysphagia, weight loss, oral intake) and cognitive function (cognitive failure, delirium, confusion), whereas dyspnea and performance status were reported in two scores. One (the PaP Score), included some simple biological factors that require analysis of a blood sample. It also included the physician's subjective judgment of survival, measured up to 12 weeks, which means that the score is used *together with* rather than *instead of* clinical judgment. The original PaP Score did not include cognitive failure, which was subsequently demonstrated to subdivide each population categorized by the PaP Score into two further prognostic subgroups. None of the scores constructed so far have included psychological symptoms or QOL.

CONCLUSIONS

Many aspects of prognostication are controversial, including whether physicians should prognosticate at all. Given that prognostication is a cardinal clinical skill, a controversial issue is whether subjective CPS is useful (see "Common Errors"). The limitations of CPS were described in this chapter. The CPS has received much criticism because of these limitations and its inherent nonreproducibility. However, studies of the accuracy of CPS have found a reasonably strong correlation between CPS and actual survival and an independent prognostic effect.[21] The European Association of Palliative Care's Working Group on Prognosis provided the following recommendations on CPS[19]: (1) CPS is best used with other parameters and could be integrated into prognostic models and scores; (2) Clinicians should consider CPS combined with other prognostic factors to improve prediction accuracy.

RESEARCH CHALLENGES

There are many research challenges and opportunities in prognostication. More work can be done to improve CPS accuracy, find novel prognostic markers, and develop better prognostic models and indices. Level I and II studies of existing prognostic tools, such as the PaP Score, as clinical decision aids are needed.

New developments in biostatistics and information technology are resulting in new Web-based tools founded on algorithms and nomograms derived from large patient databases. An intriguing example is the Prognostigram,

Common Errors

- Believing that prognostication is not an important clinical skill
- Applying population-based data (e.g., median survival time) to an individual without considering the individual's symptoms, co-morbidities, or psychosocial state
- Making temporal rather than probabilistic predictions
- Giving an overly optimistic prognosis, because this may unduly influence treatment preferences[20]

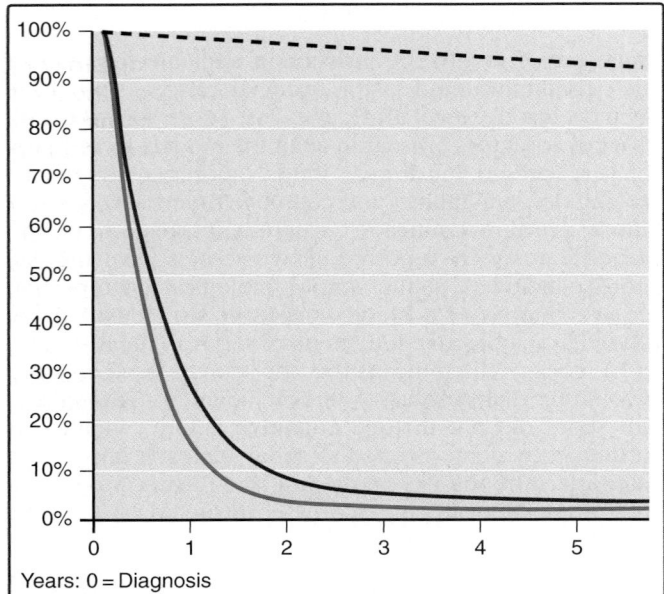

FIGURE 119-3 Prognostigram for 55- to 59-year-old white male patient with stage IV non–small cell lung cancer, showing projections without co-morbidity (*red curve*) and with severe chronic obstructive pulmonary disease (*green curve*). These curves indicate a median survival time of approximately 6 months and a 10% chance of surviving 18 months to 2 years.

which uses the Surveillance, Epidemiology and End Results (SEER) Program of the National Cancer Institute and generates individualized survival curves based on age, gender, race, primary site, extent of disease, and co-morbidities (Fig. 119-3). More information in the Prognostigram is available at http://www.cancerprognosis.org.

REFERENCES

1. National Institutes of Health. NIH State-of-the-Science Conference on Improving End-of-Life Care, Bethesda, MD, December 6-8, 2004. Final Statement.
2. Hutchinson R. Prognosis. Lancet 1934;i:697.
3. Lamont EB, Christakis NA. Prognostic disclosure to patients with cancer near the end of life. Ann Intern Med 2001;134:1096-1105.
4. Stockler MR, Tattersall MH, Boyer MJ, et al. Disarming the guarded prognosis: Predicting survival in newly referred patients with incurable cancer. Br J Cancer 2006;94:208-212.
5. Lunney JR, Lynn J, Foley DJ, et al. Patterns of functional decline at the end of life. JAMA 2003;289:2387-2392.
6. Anderson F, Downing GM, Hill J, et al. Palliative performance scale (PPS): A new tool. J Palliat Care 1996;12:5-11.
7. Reuben DB, Mor V. Clinical symptoms and length of survival in patients with terminal cancer. Arch Intern Med 1988;148:1586-1591.
8. Schonwetter R, Teasdale T, Storey P. The terminal cancer syndrome. Arch Intern Med 1989;149:965-966.
9. Caraceni A, Nanni O, Maltoni M, et al. Impact of delirium on the short term prognosis of advanced cancer patients. Italian Multicenter Study Group on Palliative Care. Cancer 2000;89:1145-1149.
10. Ventafridda V, Ripamonti C, Tamburini M, et al. Unendurable symptoms as prognostic indicators of impending death in terminal cancer patients. Eur J Cancer 1990;26:1000-1001.
11. Tamburini M, Brunelli C, Rosso S, Ventafridda V. Prognostic value of quality of life scores in terminal cancer patients. J Pain Symptom Manage 1996;11:32-41.
12. Maltoni M, Priovano M, Nanni O, et al. Biological indicies predictive of survival in 519 Italian terminally ill cancer patients. J Pain Symptom Manage 1997;13:1-9.
13. Elahi MM, McMillan DC, McArdle CS, et al. Score based on hypoalbuminemia and elevated C-reactive protein predicts survival in patients with advanced gastrointestinal cancer. Nutr Cancer 2004;48:171-173.
14. Mackillop WJ, Gospodorwicz M. The importance of prognosis in cancer medicine. In Gospodorwicz M, O'Sullivan B, Sobin LH (eds). Prognostic Factors in Cancer. Hoboken, NJ: Wiley-Liss, 2006, pp 3-14.
15. Maltoni M, Nanni O, Pirovano M, et al. Successful validation of the palliative prognostic score in terminally ill cancer patients. J Pain Symptom Manage 1999;17:240-247.
16. Morita T, Tsunoda J, Inoue S, Chihara S. Improved accuracy of physicians' survival prediction for terminally ill cancer patients using the Palliative Prognostic Index. Palliat Med 2001;15:419-424.
17. Glare P, Virik K, Jones M, et al. A systematic review of physicians' survival predictions in terminally ill cancer patients. BMJ 2003;327:195-198.
18. Vigano A, Dorgan M, Buckinham J, et al. Survival prediction in terminal cancer patients: A systematic review of the medical literature. Palliat Med 2000; 14:363-374.
19. Maltoni M, Caraceni A, Brunelli C, et al. Prognostic factors in advanced cancer patients: Evidence-based clinical recommendations. A study by the Steering Committee of the European Association for Palliative Care. J Clin Oncol 2005;23:6240-6248.
20. Weeks JC, Cook EF, O'Day SJ, et al. Relationship between cancer patients' predictions of prognosis and their treatment preferences. JAMA 1998;279:1709-1714.
21. Maltoni M, Pirovano M, Scarpi E, et al. Prediction of survival of patients terminally ill with cancer: Results of an Italian prospective multicentric study. Cancer 1995;75:2613-2622.

SUGGESTED READING

Glare P, Christakis NA (eds). Prognosis in Advanced Cancer. New York: Oxford University Press, 2008.

Gospodorwicz M, O'Sullivan B, Sobin LH (eds). Prognostic Factors in Cancer. International Union Against Cancer (UICC). Hoboken, NJ: Wiley-Liss, 2006.

Sackett D, Haynes B, Guyatt G, Tugwell P. Clinical Epidemiology: A Basic Science for Clinical Medicine, 2nd ed. Boston: Little, Brown, 1991.

Christakis N. Death Foretold: Prophecy and Prognosis in Medical Care. Chicago: University of Chicago Press, 1999.

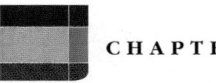

CHAPTER 120

The Plan of Care

Lucille R. Marchand

KEY POINTS

- Negotiating a plan of care requires careful assessment of the whole patient, including his or her values, an accurate diagnosis, discussion of areas of uncertainty, thoughtful prognostic information, evidence-based treatment options and their likely benefits, risks, and side effects. The clinician should share responsibility and work to empower patients and families to make the best decisions for their situation.

- An effective plan requires the clinician to listen attentively to the patient's goals and values. Patient-centered and relationship-centered care ensure that the person, and not the disease, the technology, or the clinician, is the focus.

- Negotiation of a patient-centered plan requires attention to physical, cultural, emotional, social, spiritual, and psychological issues.

- Planning includes supporting the paradox of hoping for the best while preparing for the worst.

- A successful care plan requires coordination and continuity of care among the interdisciplinary team, the family and patient, the community physician, and other relevant community health professionals and significant others.

One key issue in good palliative care is negotiating a care plan with the patient and family that has the highest likelihood of success. Family, in this context, means those who are important to the patient, such as direct family, friends, significant others, clan elders, spiritual advisors, and so on. Success means that the plan reflects the treatment goals and values of the patient and family derived through patient- and relationship-centered communication. *Patient-centered care* emphasizes the person rather than the disease as the focus, designing treatment plans and care consistent with the patient's values, needs, and preferences. This allows for shared decision making with an empowered patient who is an active rather than passive participant.[1,2] *Relationship-centered care* involves communication between the patient and the clinician to promote supportive, respectful, and effective decision making through the continuity of a trusting relationship. Patient preference may give decision-making authority to the clinician, but the initial thrust of negotiating a care plan derives from an intention to empower the patient, family, and/or significant community members in shared and informed decision making with the team of health professionals. Patient-centered care establishes a patient–clinician relationship based on empathy, trust, caring, and healing.[2]

What do patients and families want from health professionals—especially at the end of life? One study of factors identified by patients, families, and physicians for optimal end-of-life care reported the following priorities:[3]

- Achieve pain and symptom control
- Prepare for dying and have choices honored
- Have life completion
- Be touched
- Be at peace with "God"
- Have clinicians whom one can trust who listen and who are comfortable talking about dying
- Be with loved ones and relieve burdens on family
- Strengthen relationships with loved ones.

In another study, patients also wanted to avoid inappropriate prolongation of life and achieve a sense of control in dying.[4] These factors reflect the whole person, including physical, psychological, spiritual, and social well-being in the face of life-threatening illness and death.

Relationship and trust in the health care team, advance directives that are honored, preparation for dying, and optimization of relationships with loved ones are key elements for quality planning in palliative care. Integrative palliative medicine brings a holistic perspective to care planning, one that includes not only conventional treatments but alternative modalities that enhance well-being and healing and expand care options. For example, a combination of music, breath work, and analgesics can synergistically decrease pain, so that attention to relationships with loved ones is possible.

The interdisciplinary team provides coordination of care and addresses the range of patient and family needs in a terminal illness. Palliative medicine recognizes that no one person can address the complex care needed at the end of life. Through the coordinated care of the team, the physical, social, spiritual, and emotional needs of the dying patient and the family can be comprehensively and effectively addressed.

CONTINUITY AND COORDINATION OF CARE

Continuity of care requires the development of a trusting relationship among the patient, the family, and the interdisciplinary team involved. It requires the primary care physician or clinician to be at the hub of care, because this person usually has cared for the patient over time. Adding palliative medicine expertise through palliative care outpatient and inpatient services and hospice care requires careful communication and coordination among all the important health professionals, especially the primary care clinician, as well as family and significant community members in the patient's life. Effective communication includes family conferences to assist coordinated continuity of care that focuses on the patient and family goals.

COMMUNICATION AND THE FAMILY CONFERENCE

Effective communication is fundamental in formulating the plan. It requires the clinician, at times, to ask difficult questions and share uncertainty. Language is powerful, and phrases such as "Do you want everything done?" are unhelpful. Using language that is free of medical jargon and in tune with the language and values expressed by the patient is more effective.[5] The patient, family, and professionals need to do the following:

- Explore goals.
- Share information.
- Give prognostic information.
- Allow for silence and reflection as well as expression of emotion.
- Address care options (including risks and benefits).
- Assess the patient's support system and physical, psychological, and spiritual needs.
- Negotiate a treatment plan.

Communication requires ongoing discussions about treatment goals as the patient's situation changes, with modification of the plan as needed.[6,7] Steps have been identified in structured communications with patients and families that work for most end-of-life communications, such as breaking bad news, family conferences, advance care planning, decisions on withholding or withdrawing treatments.[7] These steps are

1. Prepare for the discussion.
2. Establish what the patient and family knows.
3. Determine how information is to be handled.
4. Give the information.
5. Respond to emotions.
6. Establish goals for care and treatment priorities.
7. Establish a plan.

Families are key participants in end-of-life planning and decision making.[8] The use of family conferences recognizes that the patient is a part of a larger community and that shared, patient-centered decision making requires routine communication with the family for successful planning. The genogram is an important tool in delineating important family members, family issues, and dynamics in preparation for a conference.[9]

HOLDING PARADOX: HOPE AND PREPARATION

Hoping for the best and preparing for the worst allows the physician, family, and patient to hold the paradox that hope can exist while preparing for the challenges of serious illness including death. This helps prevent abandonment of the patient if treatment does not save his or her life. The balance of hope and preparation allows for all care options and outcomes to be considered. This approach also encourages discussion of advance care planning and includes both living and dying.

Five stages appear in the evolution of this conversation[10]:

1. From the outset, discuss both hope and preparation, and take the lead from the patient as to which to discuss first.
2. Align the hopes of the patient and physician.
3. Encourage hope and preparation, but be flexible and do not impose it, because the patient may take time to reach this point.
4. Be patient and respect the patient's wishes, because the conversation evolves over time.
5. Respond to the patient's emotions, learn from your own, and respect the patient's hopes and fears.

This strategy can guide difficult conversations with patients especially at end of life or in life-threatening illness.

CULTURE

Cultural sensitivity often determines whether interventions and decision making effectively meet patient and family needs. Our society is diverse, yet truth telling and the ethical principle of autonomy in decision making, although dominant in current ethical thinking, are not universal.[11] Some cultures, such as Native American and some Asian cultures, do not speak of death, because this in itself could cause death. Even within cultural and ethnic groups, however, there are no universal preferences.[12] Through careful interviewing, the clinician can elicit the patient's and family's preferences for disclosure of information. Many families want to protect the patient from bad news. Asking patients how much information they want about their condition is one way of honoring cultural diversity. The clinician is then guided by those preferences.[13]

The desire for nondisclosure can occur for several reasons.[12] Patients and families may consider that a discussion on the plan of care is disrespectful of the patient, that it can cause undue anxiety and depression in the patient, that it can eliminate hope, and that it can cause a bad outcome through the power of speaking it. The clinician should ask about preferences, actively listen, not make assumptions about preferences, use an interpreter if needed, and demonstrate an interest in understanding the patient's and family's perspectives. A protocol is also useful in determining capacity for decision making.[14]

ADVANCE DIRECTIVES

Advance directives are not a panacea for end-of-life decision making, but they are necessary. They reflect a com-munication process, but the signed legal document is often viewed as the main outcome. Advance directives reflect decision making based on individual autonomy, but this may not be the traditional approach to decision making in many cultures. Even when advance directives are present, they may not be honored.[15-17] Activating a power of attorney for health care requires determining the patient's decision-making capacity.[12]

One notable instance of community-wide success in advance care planning is called Respecting Choices.[18] After 2 years of a community-wide educational program on advance care planning, the records of 540 decedents were audited. Eighty-five percent had advance directives, 95% of these were in the medical record, and prolongation of life at the end of life was avoided 98% of the time as desired. In a statewide initiative to apply this program across the state of Wisconsin in 2000, Life Planning 2000 produced a consumer guide for advance directives, organ donation, and "do not resuscitate" (DNR) discussions, with the legal forms included. This guide is designed to facilitate discussion concerning advance directives. Lawyers working with physicians learned that advance directives require a communication process and that the outcome of signing a form does not in itself constitute advance care planning.[17]

Cultural and social issues shape conversations about resuscitation. In interviews with patients, families, and physicians about DNR decision making, three domains were identified[19]: judging competency and capacity for patient decision making, dealing with uncertainty, and recognizing attitudes toward death. Communicating prognosis and likely outcomes of resuscitation efforts is also important. In one study, only 5% of elderly, chronically ill patients wanted resuscitation when informed that survival rates were less than 5%. Prognostic information about the success of resuscitation affected preferences for resuscitation, highlighting the need to discuss prognostic information with patients facing these decisions.[20]

In a study of African Americans older than 55 years of age, three fourths of study participants refused to fill out advance directives.[21] Factors affecting completion included spirituality, view of suffering, view of death and dying, social support networks, barriers to utilization, and mistrust of the health care system. This project used a faith-based intervention for promotion of advance directives. Prolongation of life did not necessarily translate to increased suffering, and this group did not believe that health professionals would honor advance directives. Their cultural values influenced their views that advance directives decrease hope, that planning for the unknown is irrelevant, and that only God knows when one will die.[21]

The goals and objectives for advance directives differ among physicians, patients, and families. Open, ongoing communication among these participants about goals and values, given the patient's changing health status and the differing perspectives of the family, patient, and physician, can help clarify the plan of care.[22]

RECENT DEVELOPMENTS

Recent developments in this field have included the following:

- The Capacity Assessment Tool[23]
- The CALL (Comprehensive, Adaptable, Life-affirming, Longitudinal) Palliative Care Project, a model for patient-centered continuity and coordination of care over the continuum of palliative care[24]
- The Core Process, a framework for a systematic plan of care that is patient- and family-centered and allows for continuous quality improvement by understanding care systems and recognizing and rectifying gaps in care[25]
- An excellent review of care planning for infants, children, adolescents, and their families.[26]
- A review of 22 demonstration projects, funded by the Robert Wood Johnson Foundation, called Promoting Excellence in End-of-Life Care[27]

> **Common Errors**
>
> - Failure to have an early family conference, especially at first diagnosis of a serious life-limiting illness.
> - Assuming that the clinician is the expert regarding treatment goals, options, and choices.
> - Failure to ask about and discuss advance directives, and when advance directives are known, failure to honor them.
> - Always hoping for the best or always assuming the worst, without a balance of both.
> - Limiting care to physical needs, ignoring the spiritual, psychological, social, and cultural dimensions of care.
> - Limiting care options to conventional therapies, especially when the patient is seeking alternative therapies.

EVIDENCE-BASED MEDICINE

Patient-centered communication influences health care outcomes by decreasing diagnostic tests and referrals, helping clinicians and patients find common ground in care plans, increasing emotional well-being, and reducing uncomfortable physical symptoms.[28]

In a randomized clinical trial, the PhoenixCare Intervention Program demonstrated that intensive, home-based, coordinated case management of seriously and chronically ill patients can improve outcomes in patient self-management, use of advance directives, awareness of health resources, symptom control, and well-being.[29]

In a randomized, controlled clinical trial of electronic medical record (EMR) reminders to physicians about advance directives, patients who had discussions about advance directives rated those visits as significantly more satisfying than did patients with whom advance directives were not discussed.[30]

One study of 30 elderly, English-speaking, white (90%) and African American (10%) veterans explored patients' perspectives on the essential elements of physician-patient communication regarding end-of-life care. They reported seven essential elements for medical providers[31]:

1. Engage in strategies to ensure patient understanding (mentioned by 30% of participants)
2. Communicate honestly and truthfully (27%)
3. Develop a compassionate bedside manner (27%)
4. Treat others as you would want to be treated (20%)
5. Provide empathetic care (20%)
6. Take the time needed to communicate (20%)
7. Determine patient information and decision-making preferences (17%).

Nonabandonment by health care professionals in family conferences occurring in intensive care unit settings has been studied. Expressions of nonabandonment included alleviating suffering and ensuring comfort, encouraging family members to be at the bedside of the dying patient, and being accessible to patients and families. Incorporation of these elements into family conferences at end of life needs further study.[32]

CONCLUSIONS

Effective care plans are flexible and focus on the goals of the patient and family. Patient- and relationship-centered care results in positive outcomes including greater patient and family satisfaction, increased well-being, and better symptom control. Cultural sensitivity allows the health team to be patient centered. Plans reflect the whole person and the coordinated efforts of the interdisciplinary team. Communication is essential to the planning process, and a seven-step structured process fits most end-of-life conversations. Communication allows for coordinated continuity of care, including care by the patient's primary care clinician. In planning, hoping is balanced with preparing. Including alternative and complementary modalities of care expands options for care, hope, and healing (see "Common Errors").

RESEARCH CHALLENGES

In a study on end-of-life content in treatment guidelines for nine chronic, life-threatening illnesses, only 10% of the guidelines had significant palliative care content, and 14% did not recommend palliative care interventions at all. Certainly, guideline development in treatment planning needs further attention and strengthening to reflect the state of the art palliative medicine.[33]

The EMR can assist clinicians in recognizing the need for, obtaining, and documenting advance care planning. The Henry Ford Health System reported their preliminary use of electronic advance directives. Within a health care system using the same EMR in outpatient and inpatient facilities, advance directives are available when needed.[34] Further research and evaluation data are needed to determine how the EMR can facilitate the advance directive process.

Further research and education are needed to bring together the perspectives of health professionals, patients, and families on the objectives of advance care planning and to create, evaluate, and research successful programs that can be replicated in multiple settings to achieve those objectives.[22]

REFERENCES

1. Laine C, Davidoff F. Patient-centered medicine: A professional evolution. JAMA 1996;275:152-156.
2. Stewart M, Brown JB, Weston WW, et al. Patient-Centered Medicine: Transforming the Clinical Method. Thousand Oaks, CA: Sage, 1995.
3. Steinhauser KE, Christakis NA, Clipp EC, et al. Factors considered important at the end of life by patients, family, physicians, and other care providers. JAMA 2000;284:2476-2482.
4. Singer PA, Martin DK, Kelner M. Quality end of life care: Patient perspectives. JAMA 1999;281:163-168.

5. Herbst LH, Lynn J, Mermann AC, Rhymes J. What do dying patients want and need? Patient Care 1995;29:27-39.
6. Weissman DE. Decision making at a time of crisis near the end of life. JAMA 2004;292:1738-1743.
7. Von Guten CF, Ferris FD, Emanuel LL. Ensuring competency in end-of-life care: Communication and relational skills. JAMA 2000;284:3051-3057.
8. Reust CE, Mattingly S. Family involvement in medical decision making. Fam Med 1996;28:39-45.
9. Doherty WJ, Baird MA. Family-Centered Medical Care: A Clinical Casebook. New York: Guilford, 1987.
10. Back AL, Arnold RM, Quill TE. Hope for the best, and prepare for the worst. Ann Intern Med 2003;138:439-443.
11. Candib LM. Truth telling and advance planning at the end of life: Problems with autonomy in a multicultural world. Fam Syst Health 2002;20:213-228.
12. Searight HR, Gafford J. Effect of culture on end-of-life decision making. AAHPM Bull 2005;6(4):1-4.
13. Hallenbeck J, Goldstein MK, Mebane EW. Cultural considerations of death and dying in the United States. Clin Geriatr Med 1996;12:393-407.
14. Tunzi M. Can the patient decide? Evaluating patient capacity in practice. Am Fam Physician 2001;64:299-306.
15. Hong CY, Goh LG, Lee HP. The advance directive: A review. Singapore Med J 1996;37:411-418.
16. The SUPPORT Principal Investigators. A controlled trial to improve care for seriously ill hospitalized patients. JAMA 1995;274:1591-1598.
17. Marchand L, Fowler KJ, Kokanovich O. Building successful coalitions to promote advance care planning. Am J Hospice Palliat Med 2006;23:119-126.
18. Hammes BJ, Rooney BL. Death and end of life planning in one Midwestern community. Arch Intern Med 1998;158:383-390.
19. Ventres WB. Communicating about resuscitation: Problems and prospects. J Am Board Fam Pract 1993;6:137-141.
20. Murphy DJ, Burrows D, Santilli S, et al. The influence of the probability of survival on patients' preferences regarding CPR. N Engl J Med 1994;330:545-549.
21. Bullock K. Promoting advance directives among African Americans: A faith-based model. J Pall Med 2006;9:183-195.
22. Kolarik RS, Arnold RM, Fischer GS, Tulsky JA. Objectives for advance care planning. J Palliat Med 2002;5:697-704.
23. Carney MT, Neugroschl J, Morrison RS, et al. The development and piloting of a capacity assessment tool. J Clin Ethics 2001:12:17-23.
24. London MR, McSkimming S, Drew N, et al. Evaluation of a comprehensive, adaptable, life-affirming, longitudinal (CALL) palliative care project. J Palliat Med 2005;8:1214-1225.
25. Goodlin S. Framework for improving care. AAHPM Bull 2004;5(3):1-4.
26. Himmelstein BP. Palliative care for infants, children, adolescents, and their families. J Palliat Med 2006;9:163-181.
27. Byock I, Twohig JS, Merriman M, Collins K. Promoting excellence in end-of-life care: A report on innovative models of palliative care. J Palliat Med 2006;9:137-151.
28. Stewart M, Brown JB, Donner A, et al. The impact of patient-centered care on outcomes. J Fam Pract 2000;49:796-804.
29. Aiken LS, Butner J, Lockhart CA, et al. Outcome evaluation of a randomized trial of the PhoenixCare intervention: Program of case management and coordinated care for the seriously chronically ill. J Palliat Med 2006;9:111-126.
30. Tierney WM, Dexter PR, Gramelspacher GP, et al. The effect of discussions about advance directives on patients' satisfaction with primary care. J Gen Intern Med 2001;16:32-40.
31. Rodriguez KL, Young AJ. Perspectives of elderly veterans regarding communication with medical providers about end-of-life care. J Palliat Med 2005;8:534-544.
32. West HF, Engelberg RA, Wenrich MD, Curtis JR. Expressions of non-abandonment during the intensive care unit family conferences. J Palliat Med 2005;8:797-807.
33. Mast KR, Salama M, Silverman GK, Arnold RM. End-of-life content in treatment guidelines for life-limiting diseases. J Palliat Med 2004;7:754-790.
34. Bricker LJ, Lambing A, Markey C. Enhancing communication for end of life care: An electronic advance directive process. J Palliat Med 2003;6:511-519.

SUGGESTED READING

Back AL, Arnold RM, Baile WF, et al. Approaching difficult communication tasks in oncology. CA Cancer J Clin 2005;55:164-177.

Etchells E, Darzins P, Silberfeld M, et al. Assessment of patient capacity to consent to treatment. J Gen Intern Med 1999;14:27-34.

Lang F, Quill T. Making decisions with families at the end of life. Am Fam Physician 2004;70:719-723, 725-726.

Marchand L. Integrative approach to end of life care. In Rakel D (ed). Integrative Medicine. Philadelphia: Elsevier, 2007, pp 873-875.

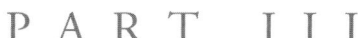

PART III

Drugs and Symptoms

Drugs

CHAPTER **121**

Principles of Pharmacology

Achiel Haemers and **Koen Augustyns**

K E Y   P O I N T S

- The final outcome of a drug application is the result of an interplay between pharmacokinetic and pharmacodynamic processes.
- Bioavailability, volume of distribution, elimination half-life, and clearance are major pharmacokinetic parameters that determine the route of application and the dosage regimen.
- Metabolic transformation can inactivate or activate the parent drug but is also an important factor in the side effect profile and the drug-drug interaction potential of a drug.
- A drug can activate or inactivate its target. The pharmacodynamic effect describes the consequence of this interaction for the body.
- Common drug targets are the receptors involved in physiological signal transduction, ion channels and ion carriers, enzymes, and functional endogenous substances such as DNA.

The final outcome of a drug application is the result of a complex interplay between the drug and the body. This interplay consists of pharmacokinetic and pharmacodynamic processes. The pharmacokinetic processes start with the absorption of the drug from its site of administration. The body considers the drug a foreign chemical substance and attempts to get rid of it by biochemical transformations and elimination strategies. These pharmacokinetic processes are highly dependent on patient-related factors such as genetic predisposition, the disease, and other variables such as age, sex, and nutritional status. The drug itself behaves as a chemical substance and interferes in one or more biochemical processes through interaction with an endogenous chemical substance called a receptor. This drug-receptor interaction is energetically driven and obeys the rules of chemical reactivity. This interaction and the consequences for the body are the pharmacodynamic processes of the drug-body interaction. These processes are also influenced by genetic and environmental factors. Pharmacogenetics is the study of the role of inheritance in interindividual variations in drug responses.

PHARMACOKINETICS

The pharmacological and clinical effects of a drug are related to the concentration of the drug at the site of action, and this is related to the drug concentration in the systemic circulation. Drug disposition is determined by a few very important parameters: bioavailability, volume of distribution, elimination half-life, and clearance.

Bioavailability

The fraction of the drug that passes into systemic circulation (expressed as a percentage) is called its *bioavailability*. The application route and the local absorption process are important factors in the extent and rate of bioavailability.

Oral ingestion is the most convenient method of drug administration. However, several factors compromise oral bioavailability, including limited membrane transport through the plasma membrane of the enterocytes, food-drug interactions, and metabolic inactivation by the mucosa, intestinal flora, or liver (first-pass effect) (Fig. 121-1). As an example, the bioavailability of oral morphine is only 25%. Bioavailability also depends on the pharmaceutical preparation: two preparations are called *bioequivalent* if they exhibit the same bioavailability.

Intravenous injection usually affords extensive and expedient bioavailability. Only the lung may serve as a temporary sink for some drugs.

Intramuscular injection affords fast and extensive bioavailability with the use of an aqueous solution. Controlled release is possible with the use of depot vehicles, such as oily preparations that provide slow release.

Subcutaneous injection affords a relatively slow but constant release of the drug. The rate is influenced by the pharmaceutical preparation and by subcutaneous fat distribution (slower release in females). The application of a vasoconstrictor, which delays diffusion of the drug, may increase its local effect.

Intrathecal injection is used when a rapid and local central nervous system (CNS) effect is necessary. Epidural and intraventricular applications are also possible.

Transdermal application provides slow but constant release. Only lipophilic drugs are able to penetrate through the skin. Controlled release is possible. Opioid analgesics such as fentanyl and buprenorphine exhibit a very strong first-pass effect after oral administration but are highly effective in transdermal therapeutic systems.

A systemic effect can also be obtained by topical application on mucous membranes (nasal, buccal).

Sublingual administration has a rapid action and a limited first-pass effect. It is applicable only for lipophilic drugs such as buprenorphine.

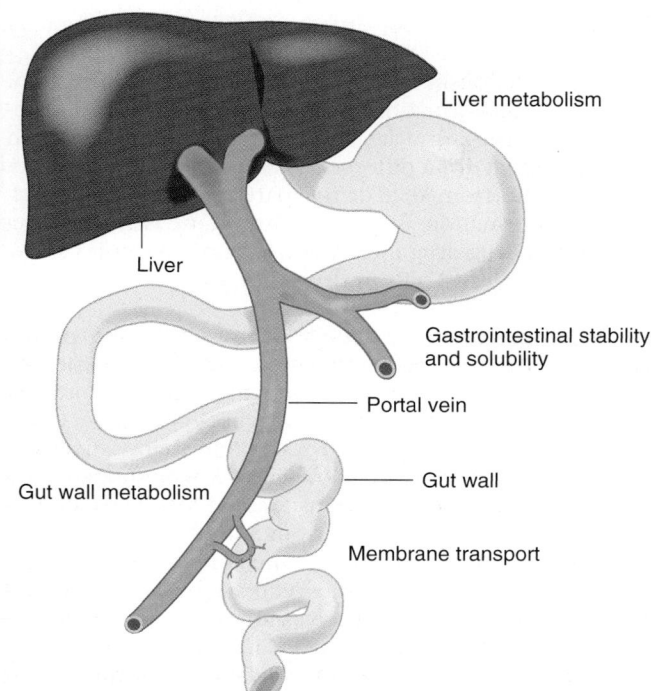

FIGURE 121-1 The term *first-pass effect* describes the inactivation of a drug in gut wall and liver. Gastrointestinal stability and solubility and limited transport through the gut wall are other factors that compromise oral drug bioavailability.

Rectal application usually shows irregular bioavailability. Half of the dosage undergoes liver first-pass metabolism.

Administration on mucous membranes (nose, lung) and skin can obtain a local effect. However, systemic side effects are possible.

Distribution

After administration and arrival into the bloodstream, a drug is distributed in the body. This process is dependent on the physicochemical properties of the drug, and the rate of distribution is influenced by cardiovascular function. Distribution into the less-perfused tissues, such as skin, fat, and viscera, may take several hours. A series of factors limit complete distribution.

A drug is partially and reversibly bound to plasma proteins such as albumin and α_1-acid glycoprotein, and only the free drug can penetrate tissues and other fluids.

Drugs can accumulate in tissues. Lipophilic drugs are stored in fat that can function as a storage site. Redistribution from the site of activity into fat may shorten the duration of action (e.g., thiopental, diazepam). The same is possible for bone tissue. Some accumulation sites are specific; for example, the accumulation of aminoglycoside antibiotics in kidney is responsible for their renal toxicity.

Transport across the cell membrane is important in drug distribution, because it is key to absorption and elimination of a drug in a given tissue. Membrane penetration may be aselective and based on passive drug diffusion. Passive diffusion depends on the lipophilicity of the drug and the degree of ionization in the pH of the surrounding liquid. Transport may be facilitated by transporters, which transfer compounds down their concentration gradient. Transport against a concentration gradient requires energy, and active transport is frequently involved in drug transport. As an example, the adenosine triphosphate (ATP)–binding cassette (ABC) transporters are important in the reverse transport of drugs out of the cell across membranes. They show ATPase activity and are not only important for the pharmacokinetic properties of a drug but also play a role in drug resistance (e.g., against several anticancer agents) and in adverse effects.

Transport into the CNS is a particular item in drug transport. The CNS is protected by the blood-brain barrier (BBB). This consists of capillary endothelial cells with tight junctions surrounded by astroglial cells. Passive transport across the BBB is possible only for lipophilic drugs. Lipophilicity also influences the rate of BBB transport. Heroin is a diacetyl ester of morphine that reaches the brain faster than its parent compounds do. Penetration is facilitated when transporters are involved: L-dopa, a hydrophilic compound, is unable to cross the BBB by diffusion but uses amino acid transporters to penetrate the brain. Moreover, ABC efflux transporters, and others, actively remove chemicals. For example, loperamide, an opioid used in diarrhea, does not show CNS morphine-like activity because of efflux by ABC transporters.

Volume of Distribution

The *volume of distribution* (V_D) is a theoretical concept describing the relationship between the total amount of drug in the body and the concentration of drug in plasma or blood. It approximates the amount of drug in the extravascular tissue and is expressed in liters. The V_D will approximate the plasma volume (about 3 L) if the drug is confined to the circulation. On the other hand, the V_D can be very high (>100 L) for drugs that accumulate in tissues. V_D is strongly dependent on age, gender, and disease state.

Clearance

As soon as the body has received a drug, it immediately starts to remove it. Clearance measures the efficiency of the body in doing this. The body usually uses the kidney and liver to clear a drug. Other clearing systems are possible: sweat, saliva, skin, and lungs. *Total clearance* is the sum of the various organ clearances and is defined as the volume of plasma from which the drug is removed in unit time, expressed in milliliters per minute per kilogram (mL/min/kg).

Renal clearance is the sum of renal filtration, active renal secretion, and reabsorption. Some drugs are cleared by excretion into the bile via hepatic clearance. Renal or hepatic disease may compromise clearance efficiency. Clearance is not only an excretion event but also includes inactivation by metabolic transformation and excretion of the resulting metabolites.

Metabolism

The renal excretion of chemical substances is compromised by their reabsorption after glomerular filtration, which is largely related to lipophilicity. Therefore, transformation into more hydrophilic structures is essential to remove drugs from the body. The same is true for hepatic excretion through bile. Decreased lipophilicity also limits the capacity of drugs to accumulate in lipophilic areas (e.g., fat tissue, brain).

The metabolic process begins in the enterocytes that line the gastrointestinal tract, where several xenobiotic-metabolizing enzymes operate. However, most drugs escape this metabolism. After absorption across the mucosa, the drug and its gastrointestinal metabolites enter the portal circulation and arrive in the liver. The liver is the most important metabolic factory, and it completes the first-pass degradation of the drug. The liver contains many diverse enzymes.

Metabolism occurs in two phases (Fig. 121-2).

Phase I Metabolism

In phase I metabolism, the xenobiotic structures are provided with hydrophilic groups such as hydroxyl and carboxylic groups, or they lose lipophilic groups such as alkyl groups. Most of the enzymes are oxygenases (adding oxygen) or dehydrogenases (removing hydrogen). Cytochrome P-450s (CYPs) and flavin monooxygenases are important superfamilies of oxidative enzymes. They interact with the drugs in the lipophilic environment of the phospholipid layers of the endoplasmic reticulum.

The human body contains about 60 CYPs, which are denoted by two numbers and one letter (e.g., CYP2D6). CYPs use a heme group, with iron as the carrier for oxygen, and are involved in the biosynthesis and metabolism of endogenous substances such as steroids and inactivation of xenobiotics. The xenobiotic-metabolizing CYPs (about 15) have a limited selectivity and use several chemical structures as substrates. One drug may be metabolized by several different CYPs. Each person has individual CYP patterns, and there are several examples of clinically relevant genetic polymorphisms. Moreover, CYP activity is strongly influenced by inducers or inhibitors from the

environment (e.g., food, drugs) and by ethnic and racial differences.

Drug metabolism does not mean drug inactivation. Metabolic transformation can activate an inactive compound (prodrug), and it can produce a metabolite with the same activity or a different pharmacological or toxicological profile from that of the parent compound. Metabolic transformation is also an important issue in drug toxicity and drug-drug interactions. A few examples show the importance of CYPs in drug therapy:

- The analgesic activity of codeine is a result of its partial (10%) oxidative demethylation into morphine by CYP2D6. About 10% of the Caucasian population lack this CYP enzyme and cannot use codeine. Asians metabolize codeine to a lesser extent than Caucasians do. CYP2D6-deficient patients need lower doses of antidepressants and are more susceptible to adverse effects such as tardive dyskinesia from antipsychotics.
- The antibiotic rifampicin and the anticonvulsant carbamazepine induce CYPs and decrease plasma levels and efficacy of oral contraceptives and of human immunodeficiency virus (HIV) protease inhibitors.
- The antibiotic erythromycin and the antifungal agent ketoconazole inhibit CYP3A enzymes and increase plasma levels and toxicity of cyclosporine and 3-hydroxy-3-methylglutaryl coenzyme A (HMG-CoA) reductase inhibitors.
- Paracetamol is partially oxidized into a quinone imine by CYP. This quinone imine is hepatotoxic but is rapidly neutralized by glutathione. Large doses of paracetamol deplete glutathione and cause fatal hepatotoxicity.

Other phase I active enzymes are reductases (e.g., nitroreductase) and hydrolases (e.g., esterases, epoxide hydrolases). Esterases are used to activate prodrugs into their active acids, such as in the group of angiotensin-converting enzyme (ACE) inhibitors.

Phase II Metabolism

In the second phase of metabolism, the drug and/or its metabolites are conjugated to very polar and hydrophilic groups such as glucuronic acid (glucuronosyltransferases), sulfuric acid (sulfotransferase), and amino acids. These conjugates are water soluble, easily excreted, and are mostly inactive. Exceptions are 6-glucuronylmorphine (which is more active than morphine) and the antihypertensive minoxidil, which is activated to minoxidil sulfate, a potassium channel opener.

Other phase II enzymes include glutathionyl-S-transferase, quenching electrophilic groups, N-acetyltransferases (NAT), and methyltransferase. These transferases are important for xenobiotic detoxification. NAT conjugates amino functions with an acetyl group. The existence of slow and rapid acetylators is the result of polymorphism in the *NAT* genes. People who are slow acetylators are more susceptible to adverse drug effects (e.g., during antituberculosis therapy with isoniazid). Glutathione-S-transferases play a role in anticancer drug resistance.

Although liver and intestines are undoubtedly the most important organs for xenobiotic metabolism, enzymes involved in metabolism are found in most tissues.

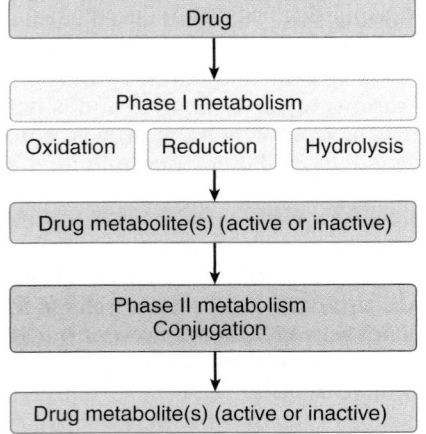

FIGURE 121-2 Drug metabolism. In the first phase, drugs are provided with polar groups by oxidation, reduction, or hydrolysis. In the second phase, these groups are conjugated to hydrophilic moieties such as glucuronic acid and sulfuric acid.

Elimination Half-Life

The *elimination half-life* is the time required to reduce the drug level in the body or in the plasma to 50% of its maximal level. This value is related to the rate of clearance (metabolism and excretion) and the V_D. The half-life of a drug is not necessarily related to its duration of action, because the half-life of major active metabolites can be different from that of the parent drug.

Dosage Regimen

An optimal therapeutic result is obtained with an optimal dosage regimen. This produces a steady-state concentration within the therapeutic window, which is the range between the adverse effect level and the minimal effective concentration. Therapeutic windows are patient related and can be large or small. Bioavailability, V_D, half-life, and clearance are important for the design of a regimen.

If a compound has a short half-life, it may be difficult to obtain a stable steady-state concentration. In such cases, controlled-release (slow-release) preparations help. The half-life of morphine is 2 to 4 hours in adults. Oral morphine must be administered 6 times in 24 hours to obtain a continuous analgesic effect. However, only two applications are needed when controlled-release tablets are used. Therapeutic monitoring is often necessary when drugs with a narrow therapeutic window, such as cyclosporine or lithium, are administered.

Figure 121-3 shows the determination of drug disposition by pharmacokinetic parameters and their controlling factors.

PHARMACODYNAMICS

A drug, traveling in the body, meets one or more chemical substances that are possible reaction partners. The interaction with these substances finally results in a pharmacodynamic and therapeutic effect. These partners, called *drug targets,* are mostly macromolecules such as proteins and nucleic acids. These targets are often, but not necessarily, ligands for endogenous substances. Most drug targets (Fig. 121-4) are proteins and can be classified into

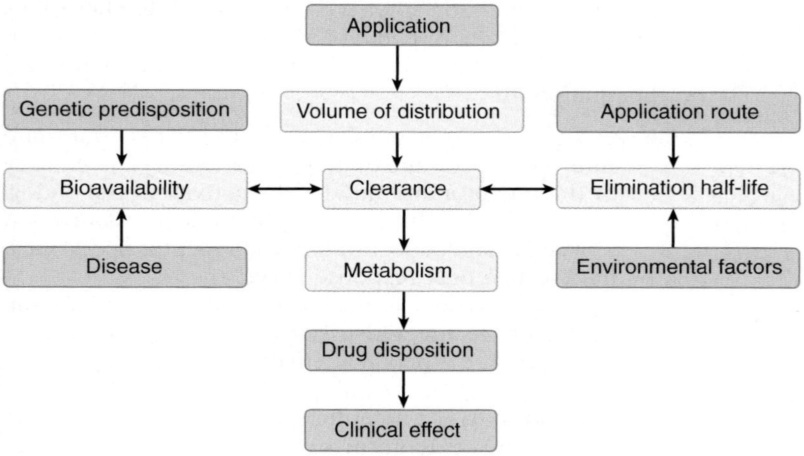

FIGURE 121-3 From application to clinical effect: important pharmacokinetic parameters and controlling factors.

FIGURE 121-4 The most important drug targets. ATPase, adenosine triphosphatase.

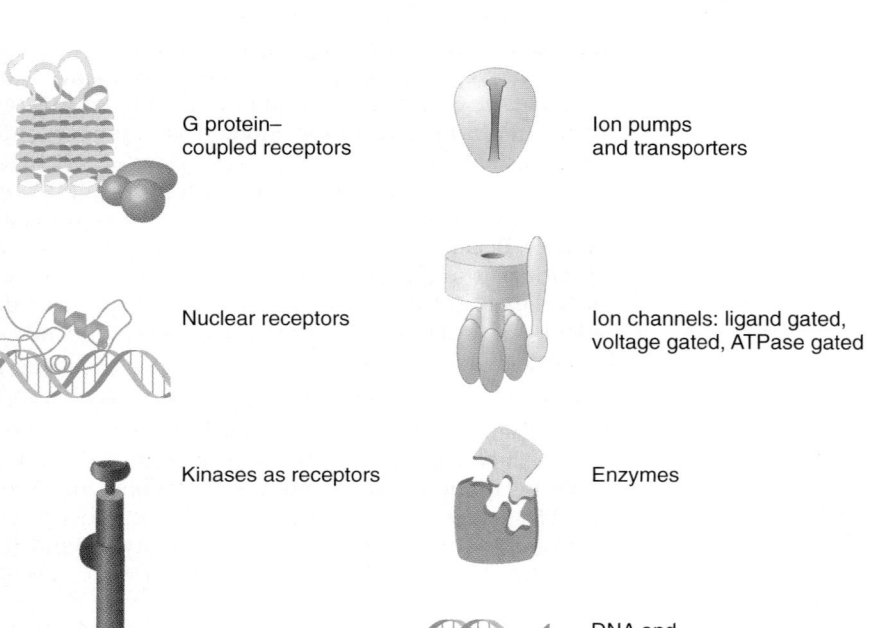

G protein–coupled receptors

Ion pumps and transporters

Nuclear receptors

Ion channels: ligand gated, voltage gated, ATPase gated

Kinases as receptors

Enzymes

DNA and protein binding

four groups: receptors involved in physiological signal transduction, ion channels, transporters, and enzymes.*

Receptors Involved in Physiological Signal Transduction

The receptors for endogenous messengers are strictly organized proteins that react with high selectivity with their ligands. These messengers include small molecules, such as epinephrine, and macromolecules, such as proteins. The receptors receive the first message and transfer it to the cell through a second messenger system, which finally activates a series of effector systems, inducing the desired cellular activity.

Receptors are classified according to their cellular localization and transduction system.

G Protein–Coupled Receptors

G protein–coupled receptors (GPCRs) are membrane receptors that are characterized by seven transmembrane α-helices and use a G protein as transducer. The "G" stands for "guanine nucleotide–binding." G proteins consists of three subunits—α, β, and γ—and are of several types. The same G protein can be associated with several different receptors, but each receptor is linked to a specific second messenger that is responsible for its downstream activity. The second messenger is an ion channel, adenylate cyclase, or phospholipase C.

GPCRs are classified according to their ligands. The ligand can function as a messenger between neuronal cells (neurotransmitter), between an organ and a cell (hormone), or between two cells (autacoid-paracrine secretion). These categories overlap.

Usually, a single ligand serves several subtypes of receptors, each with different G proteins and second messengers. Some messengers are involved in many regulatory tasks throughout the body; others are rather selective. The following messengers use clinically relevant GPCRs:

- Norepinephrine and epinephrine
- Dopamine
- Serotonin
- Histamine
- Acetylcholine
- Angiotensin II
- Endothelins
- Tachykinins
- Opioid peptides
- Hypothalamic hormones
- Parathyroid hormones
- Endogenous cannabinoids
- Somatostatin
- Leukotrienes
- Glucagon-like peptide 1
- Adenosine, ADP, and ATP
- Melatonin

A compound with pharmacological activity shows some affinity for the receptor and disturbs the ligand-

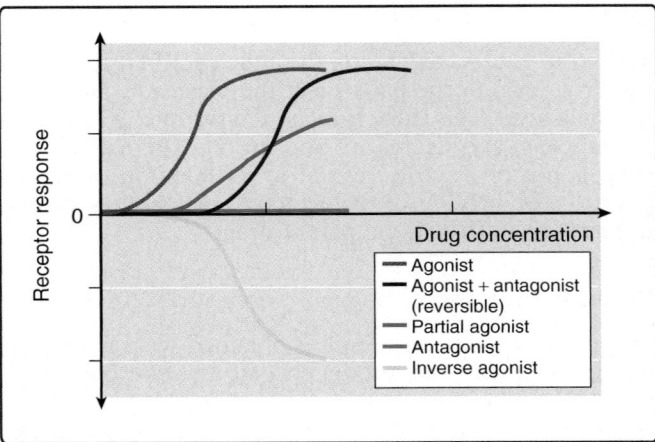

FIGURE 121-5 Response of a receptor with drugs showing affinity for different receptor conformations. The "zero" point represents the constitutive level of activity. An agonist binds to the active conformation, an inverse agonist to the inactive conformation. A partial agonist has a greater but incomplete affinity for the active conformation. An antagonist binds to both conformations and neutralizes the effect of an agonist.

receptor interaction. Such a compound can act in various ways (Fig. 121-5). A receptor exists in at least two conformations, the resting state and the active state, which are in equilibrium.

- An *agonist* binds selectively to the active state and shifts the equilibrium to it. It shows affinity and efficacy for the receptor and mimics the activity of the endogenous ligand. There is a theoretical relationship between ligand concentration and receptor occupancy, the so-called dose-response curve.
- A *partial agonist* is unable to shift the equilibrium completely to the active state. Response and efficacy are lower, and a maximal effect is not obtained.
- An *inverse agonist* exhibits selectivity for the resting state and shifts the receptor into this inactive state. The result of inverse agonism is opposite to that of agonism. Inverse agonists are pharmacologically different from antagonists. They are important in cases of constitutively active receptors. Typical inverse agonists are found in the group of antihistamine H_2–antiulcer agents, norepinephrine β-receptor antagonists, and angiotensin AT1 antagonists.
- A "real" *antagonist* shows affinity for the receptor but does not change the equilibrium. It does not show any activity. Because a receptor can bind only one molecule at a time, the antagonist competes with the endogenous ligand (or any other agonist) and neutralizes the effect of the agonist. The dose-response curve shifts to the right.

Selectivity is important in drug-receptor interactions and therapeutic activity. Endogenous ligands may show common chemical properties, such as an arylethylamine scaffold for epinephrine, serotonin, dopamine, and histamine. The same is true for the GPCRs. Moreover, one ligand often activates several receptor subtypes and has several regulatory tasks in different organs. Hence, it is not surprising that a drug never shows a "pure" activity pattern. The desired therapeutic end point will always be disturbed by adverse effects, due to occupancy of the

---

*There is some confusion as to the definition of a receptor. In the strict sense of the word, a receptor is a cellular regulatory protein that can be activated by a selective ligand. Other authors use "receptor" to refer to each drug target, including ion channels, enzymes, and carriers/transporters.

same receptor, other subtypes, or analogous GPCRs in the same or other tissues. Sometimes therapeutic efficacy is obtained through interactions with different receptors! This is the case for several antipsychotics. Altered responsiveness to drugs, due to genetic polymorphisms of receptors, has been shown for several receptors.

Receptor activity is a dynamic event. The second messenger system also sends a feedback message to the receptor. The receptor gets phosphorylated by its own second messenger system and uncouples from the effector system. On prolonged exposure to agonists, the receptors may also be taken into the cell by endocytosis. As a consequence, the effect of the drug gradually decreases when given repeatedly. Other reasons for desensitization or tolerance are exhaustion of endogenous ligands, metabolic adaptation by enzyme induction, and neutralization of the effect by a compensating physiological response. The slow disappearance of adverse effects during a continuous drug application is often the result of to this kind of drug resistance.

Receptors as Enzymes

Another family of receptors is associated with enzyme activity. The largest group of these enzymes are kinases. Kinases regulate downstream effector proteins through phosphorylation. Most of these protein phosphorylations occur on phenolic tyrosine residues. Ligands of these receptors are polypeptides such as insulin, cytokines, and growth factors that bind on the extracellular domain and activate the kinase domain at the inner face. The final goal of the interplay among the effector proteins is the activation of various transcription factors, which results in gene expression and synthesis of functional proteins. Other receptors have tyrosine phosphatase (dephosphorylation of proteins) or guanylyl cyclase (biosynthesis of cyclic guanosine monophosphate [cGMP]) activity. The atrial natriuretic peptide is a ligand for a guanylyl cyclase receptor.

Receptor enzymes can be activated pharmacologically by their ligands or analogues of those ligands. Examples are insulin (diabetes), interleukin-2 (cancer), and interferons (cancer and viral infections). More recently, inhibitors have been developed. An example of a therapeutically important tyrosine kinase inhibitor is imatinib, which selectively inhibits the kinase domain of a few tyrosine kinases, such as platelet-derived growth factor and the BCR-ABL oncogene product. The latter is associated with chronic myelocytic leukemia; imatinib is now the first-line treatment for this disease. Another receptor tyrosine kinase that is used as a target in neoplastic diseases is the epidermal growth factor (EGF) receptor.

Another strategy to neutralize ligand-receptor interactions is the use of monoclonal antibodies against the ligand or its receptor. Examples are tumor necrosis factor-α (TNF-α), interleukin (in inflammatory diseases), EGF, and vascular endothelial growth factor (in cancer). The presence or absence of EGF receptors on tumor cells is a pharmacodynamic example of the importance of pharmacogenetics in anticancer chemotherapy.

Nuclear Receptors

Nuclear receptors regulate gene transcription and control the synthesis of typical proteins and cell functions. These receptors are located in the cytosol or in the nucleus and not in the cell membrane. Ligands of these receptors are the steroid hormones (estradiol, progesterone, testosterone, aldosterone, and cortisol), thyroid hormones, the retinoids, vitamin D, and the fat metabolism–regulating peroxisome proliferator–activated receptors (PPARs). As with GPCRs, nuclear receptors may consist of several subtypes.

These lipophilic ligands cross the cell membrane, bind to the receptor, and induce conformational changes, allowing translocation to, and specific binding with, certain sequences (steroid responsive elements) of nuclear DNA. This binding, together with coactivating proteins, induces or inhibits gene expression and stimulation or inhibition of protein biosynthesis.

Drugs that activate this process are mimics of the endogenous ligands and are not necessarily specific. Because receptor and ligand structures may be similar, some drugs show nonselective activity. For example, progesterone receptor agonists derived from nortestosterone, such as norethisterone, also exhibit some androgen activity.

Antagonism of nuclear receptors is also a pharmacologically important event. The antagonists cause conformational changes in the receptor, as do the agonists, but these conformations are different and combine with corepressor proteins, resulting in an antagonistic effect. Compounds may act as agonists on one receptor and antagonists on another. Tamoxifen is an estrogen antagonist on breast cancer receptors but an agonist on endometrial receptors.

It takes hours before the impact from the activation of nuclear receptors on cellular activity becomes clear. This is much slower than the activity of GPCRs (seconds or less) or enzymes (minutes).

Ion Channels

Ion channels are important physiological regulators. These membrane-situated channels consist of several subunits. Each spans the membrane several times, with one of the transmembrane helices forming the ion channel. There are ion channels for sodium, potassium, calcium, and chloride ions. Each ion uses a series of sometimes rather different channels. These are mostly selective for one ion, but differences occur in the structure of the protein, the construction of the subunits, and the control mechanisms. Some channels are not selective for one ion. The intracellular and extracellular concentrations of these ions are crucial for cellular activity. For example, neuronal conductance depends on depolarization and polarization of the neuronal cells, which are directed by a sodium influx. Likewise, cardiac activity is completely controlled by the intracellular calcium ion concentration, which is related to the activity of the inward sodium and outward potassium currents.

The ion permeability and activity status of ion channels may be controlled by several mechanisms. Several ion channels are receptor operated (ligand gated). These receptors are situated on the channel subunits and shift the equilibrium of channel activity from less active to more active. The ligands of these receptors are the same as for the GPCRs. Important transmitters and their receptors are γ-aminobutyric acid (GABA) and its receptor, GABA$_A$; acetylcholine and the nicotinic receptors; glutamate and the *N*-methyl-D-aspartate (NMDA) receptor; and serotonin 5-HT$_3$ receptor).

Another channel activity–regulating mechanism, not associated with receptors, is the membrane potential. Ion channels that are controlled in this way are called "voltage operated." Sodium, potassium, and calcium voltage operated channels are important targets in cardiovascular therapy. Some channels, such as the pancreatic potassium channel, a target for antidiabetic drugs, are controlled by ATP.

Drugs can influence ion channels in several ways. They may activate or inhibit the receptor, but they may also react with the channel proteins themselves. Channel openers keep the channel active. Channel blockers force the channel into its resting or inactive state.

Transporters and Carriers

Ions can also be transported by carrier proteins. Examples are the transport of ions in the renal tubules and the cellular outward transport of sodium and calcium. The same is true for hydrophilic organic endogenous compounds: neurotransmitters, glucose, and amino acids cross lipophilic membranes on selective carrier proteins. Possible mechanisms, such as facilitated diffusion and energetically driven transport, were discussed earlier.

Ion pumps and several other carriers are used as drug targets. Drugs are able to react with these carriers and interfere with their activity. Ion pumps utilize ATP hydrolysis (ATPase) to create energy to move the ion against an electrochemical gradient. Of note are the gastric proton pump (H$^+$,K$^+$-ATPase) and the cardiac and renal sodium pump (Na$^+$,K$^+$-ATPase). The latter also provides energy for the renal Na$^+$,K$^+$, 2Cl$^-$ and Na$^+$,Cl$^-$ symporters (secondary active transport), both drug targets for diuretics. Gastric proton pump inhibitors are the most efficient gastric acid secretion inhibitors.

Organic compounds are transported by two superfamilies of transporters: the ABC transporters, mentioned earlier, and the solute carrier (SLC) transporters. SLC transporters are facilitated or secondary active transporters. The reuptake of aminergic neurotransmitters in presynaptic cells by SLC transporters is an example of a target for antidepressants.

Enzymes

Enzymes are biochemical catalysts. They have an essential role in biochemical and physiological processes. Almost all structural and functional elements in the body, as well as intracellular and extracellular physiological regulators, are entirely dependent on enzymatic reactions for their biosynthesis and metabolic degradation.

The activity of several drugs is associated with enzyme activity. Drugs can behave as enzyme substrates. These compounds are structural analogues of endogenous substances and are incorporated by the enzyme in functional or structural body components. The role of these components is then changed or disturbed. This therapeutic strat-

egy is used in anticancer and antiviral therapy. The application of acyclovir, for example, results in incorporation of its triphosphate in DNA, leading to chain termination.

Drugs involved in enzymatic reactions are mostly inhibitors. There are many examples of therapeutically used enzyme inhibitors that interfere in various physiological regulations.

- Enzyme inhibitors can indirectly decrease the activity of endogenous compounds by blocking their biosynthesis. Clinically important examples are aromatase (estradiol), ACE (angiotensin II), cyclooxygenase (prostaglandins), HMG-CoA reductase (cholesterol), folate reductase (tetrahydrofolate), bacterial transpeptidases (bacterial cell wall peptidoglycan), and reverse transcriptase (proviral DNA).
- Enzyme inhibitors can indirectly increase the activity of endogenous compounds by blocking their metabolic degradation. Some examples are catecholamine *O*-methyl transferase (COMT) (dopamine), monoamine oxidase (MAO) (norepinephrine, serotonin, dopamine), cholinesterase (acetylcholine), and GABA-transaminase (GABA).
- Enzyme inhibitors can interfere with cellular activity. Targets are phosphodiesterases (cyclic adenosine monophosphate [cAMP], cGMP), phosphatases, and kinases. The kinases were already discussed as transmembrane receptors, but several kinases (mostly serine-threonine phosphorylating types) are cytosolic enzymes and are important downstream physiological regulators.

In some cases, enzymes can be provided as supplements; an example is the anticoagulant plasminogen activator, tPA. The same is true for endogenous inhibitors and their analogues such as heparin. Drug target polymorphisms in the enzyme group have been shown with HMG-CoA reductase, 5-lipoxygenase, ACE, and thymidylate synthetase.

Other Drug-Targeting Strategies

Other important strategies are (1) supplementing structural or functional endogenous substances or analogues, such as prodrugs of the second messenger nitrogen oxide (e.g., nitroglycerin), and (2) direct binding of structural or functional endogenous substances, such as alkylation of DNA and binding on tubulin in cancer chemotherapy.

SUGGESTED READING

Brunton LL, Lazo SL, Parker KL (eds). Goodman and Gilman's The Pharmacological Basis of Therapeutics, 11th ed. New York: McGraw-Hill, 2006.

Rang HP, Dale MM, Ritter JM, Moore PK. Pharmacology, 5th ed. Philadelphia: Churchill Livingstone, 2003.

Page CP, Curtis MJ, Walker MJA, Hoffman BB. Integrated Pharmacology, 3rd ed. Philadelphia: Mosby Elsevier, 2006.

Walsh CT, Schwartz-Bloom RD. Levine's Pharmacology, 7th ed. New York: Taylor and Francis, 2004.

Hall IP, Pirmohamed M (eds). Pharmacogenetics. New York: Taylor and Francis, 2006.

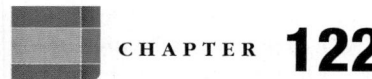

CHAPTER 122

Neuropharmacology and Psychopharmacology

Mellar P. Davis and **Leopoldo Pozuelo**

ANTIPSYCHOTIC DRUGS

The discovery in 1952 of the first antipsychotic drug, chlorpromazine, occurred by chance. Chlorpromazine

was synthesized as an antihistamine; the concept of "antipsychotics" was unknown. Chlorpromazine relieved surgical distress and was subsequently reported as treatment for schizophrenia.[1] Antipsychotics are classified by chemical structure, potency, receptor binding spectrum, and ability to cause neuropsychological ("neuroleptic") side effects. First-generation antipsychotics predate clozapine and include haloperidol, chlorpromazine, thioridazine, trifluoperazine, promethazine, and chlorpromazine. Second-generation antipsychotics are clozapine, risperidone, olanzapine, quetiapine, ziprasidone, and aripiprazole.[2,3] The term *neuroleptic* is frequently used synonymously with *antipsychotic*. Second-generation antipsychotics, particularly clozapine, have antipsychotic benefits without neuroleptic side effects; high-dose risperidone risks extrapyramidal side effects (EPS).[2]

Mechanisms of Action

All antipsychotics act on central dopamine 2 (D_2) receptors and cause depolarization blockade. D_2 receptor affinity is inversely related to the therapeutic dose.[2,3] There are six recognized dopamine receptors (D_1 through D_6); most antipsychotics block the D_2 receptor family (D_2, D_3, and D_4), and some are agonists for the D_1 receptor family (D_1 and D_5). Delirium and schizophrenia are associated with excessive mesolimbic dopamine activity leading to symptoms of delusions, hallucinations, and paranoia. Negative symptoms (anhedonia, depression, apathy) are caused by dopamine deficiencies in the mesocortical pathways[2] and alterations of serotonergic neurons. The receptor binding profiles of first- and second-generation antipsychotics are shown in Tables 122-1 and 122-2, respectively.

Blocked nigrostriatal D_2 receptors cause EPS (akathisia, parkinsonian rigidity, tremor, and tardive dyskinesia) (Fig. 122-1). Tubuloinfundibular D_2 receptor blockade causes hyperprolactinemia, galactorrhea, and loss of libido. First-generation antipsychotics have a narrow therapeutic index due to high affinity for D_2 receptors and do not discriminate between mesolimbic, mesocortical, and nigrostriatal disease pathways.[4] Second-generation antipsychotics have greater serotonin receptor affinity (5-HT_{2A}) and less affinity for the D_2 receptors. Blockade of presynaptic serotonin 5-HT_{2A} heteroreceptors increases mesocortical dopamine release, which is one mechanism by which negative schizophrenia symptoms are improved with atypical antipsy-

TABLE 122-1 Receptor Binding Profile for First-Generation Antipsychotics*

DRUG	D_2	5-HT_1	5-HT_2	α_1	α_2	H_1	M_1
Haloperidol	+++	—	+	+	—	—	—
Chlorpromazine	++	—	++	+++	—	++	++
Thioridazine	++	—	+	+++	—	++	+
Trifluoperazine	+++	—	+	+	—	+	—
Promazine	±	—	+	++	—	++	—
Prochlorperazine	+++	—	+	+	—	+	—

*—, no affinity; ±, low affinity; +, low to moderate affinity; ++, moderate to high affinity; +++, high affinity.
α, α-adrenergic receptor; D, dopamine receptor; H, histamine receptor; 5-HT, serotonin receptor; M, muscarinic receptor.

chotics (Fig. 122-2). This also decreases EPS and tardive dyskinesia and minimizes hyperprolactinemia. Several atypical antipsychotics (clozapine, ziprasidone, and aripiprazole) are also 5-HT$_{1A}$ agonists; they reduce serotonin and increase dopamine neurotransmission indirectly (see Fig. 122-2). Activation of presynaptic 5-HT$_{1A}$ receptors reduces serotonin release.[4]

Full antipsychotic benefits are not seen for up to 4 weeks, yet receptor binding occurs within hours and a steady state is reached within days (Tables 122-3 and 122-4). Long-term depolarization blockade is required to normalize downstream intracellular regulatory pathways.[3] Pharmacodynamic tolerance to antipsychotics occurs. Plasma dopamine metabolites (homovanillic acid) are initially elevated but return to normal with chronic dosing. Increased D$_2$ receptor expression and D$_2$ receptor sensitivity occur on drug withdrawal, resulting in "withdrawal" tardive dyskinesia in some patients.[2]

Neuroleptics are lipophilic and accumulate within the central nervous system (CNS). Haloperidol levels are 20 times higher than in plasma.[2] Although the serum half-life of haloperidol is 24 hours, CNS levels can be measured several days after drug discontinuation. Large interindividual variations in steady-state plasma levels produce

TABLE 122-2   Receptor Binding Profile for Second-Generation Antipsychotics*

DRUG	D$_1$	D$_2$	5-HT$_1$	5-HT$_2$	α$_1$	α$_2$	H$_1$	M$_1$
Clozapine	++	+	+	++	+	+	+++	+++
Risperidone	+	++	+	++	++	++	—	±
Olanzapine	++	++	—	++	+	±	++	++
Quetiapine	+	+	+	+	+	+	++	—
Ziprasidone	+	++	++	++	+	±	+	±

*—, no affinity; ±, low affinity; +, low to moderate affinity; ++, moderate to high affinity; +++, high affinity.
α, α-adrenergic receptor; D, dopamine receptor; H, histamine receptor; 5-HT, serotonin receptor; M, muscarinic receptor.

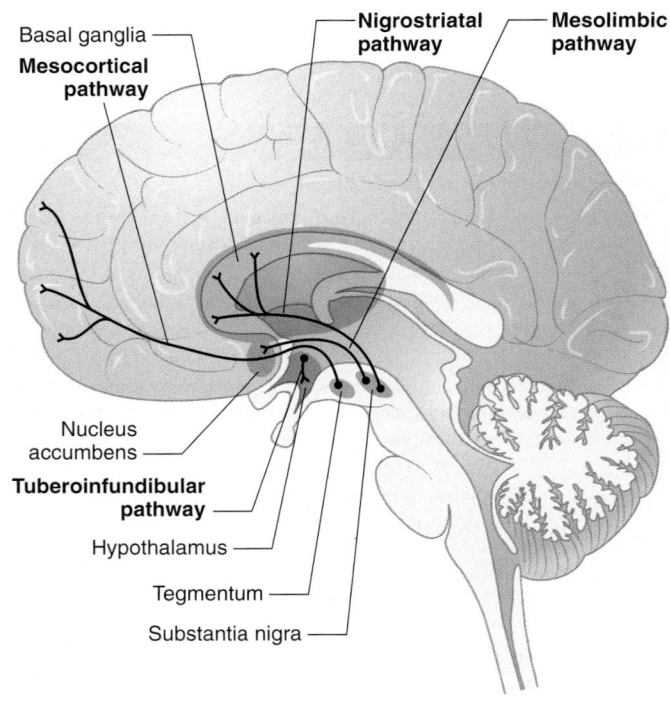

FIGURE 122-1 Dopaminergic central nervous system pathways.

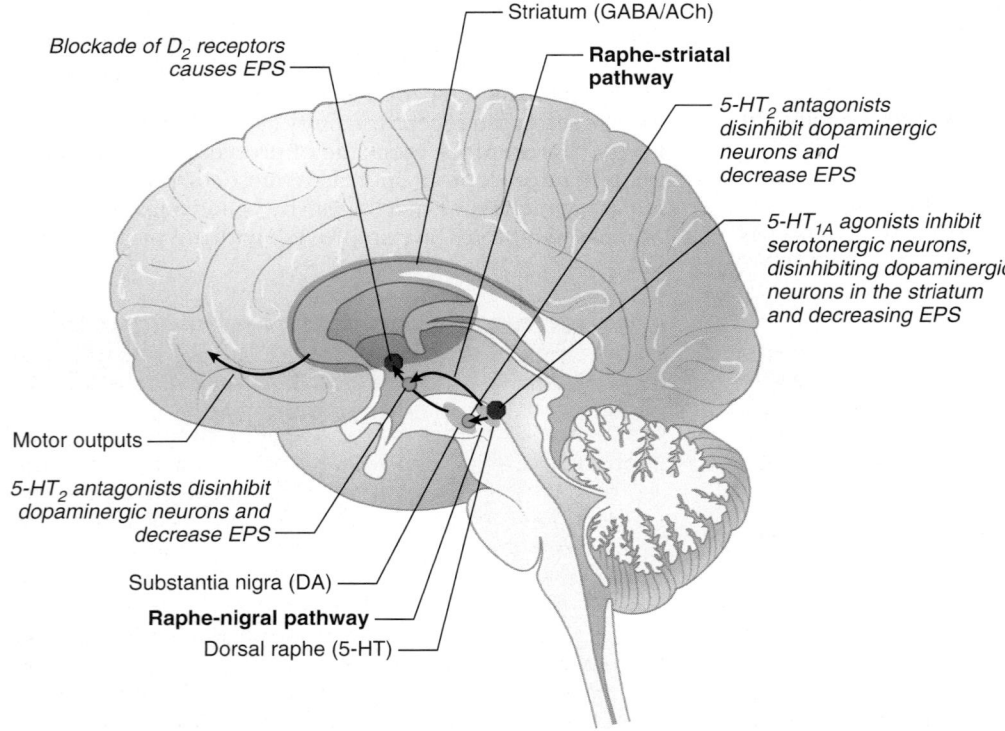

FIGURE 122-2 Mechanisms by which atypical antipsychotics reduce the extrapyramidal reactions frequently observed with classic antipsychotics. Ach, acetylcholine; D, dopamine receptor; DA, dopamine; EPS, extrapyramidal side effects; GABA, γ-aminobutyric acid; 5-HT, 5-hydroxytryptamine (serotonin) receptor.

TABLE 122-3 Pharmacokinetics of First-Generation Antipsychotics

DRUG	ABSORPTION (%)	T½ (HR)	METABOLIZING CYTOCHROMES
Haloperidol	60	12-36	CYP1A2 CYP2D6
Chlorpromazine	10-25	7-15	CYP2D6 CYP3A4
Thioridazine	4	5-26	CYP1A2 CYP2C9 CYP2D6
Trifluoperazine	?	8-12	CYP2C9 CYP2D6
Promazine	10-25	8	CYP1A2 CYP2D6
Prochlorperazine	10-25	8	CYP2C9 CYP2D6 CYP3A4

CYP, cytochrome P-450 isoenzyme; T½, half-life.

TABLE 122-5 Usual Doses for Antipsychotics

TYPICAL ANTIPSYCHOTIC	ORAL DOSAGE RANGE (MG/DAY)*
Chlorpromazine	100-300
Haloperidol	5-20
Thioridazine	30-800
Trifluoperazine	2-90
Promazine	25-1000
Prochlorperazine	15-125
Clozapine	100-900
Risperidone	1-6
Olanzapine	5-20
Quetiapine	75-800
Ziprasidone	20-160
Aripiprazole	5-30

*Dosages for delirium should be in the lower therapeutic range to start.

TABLE 122-4 Pharmacokinetics of Second-Generation Antipsychotics

ATYPICAL ANTIPSYCHOTIC	ABSORPTION	TMAX (HR)	T½ (HR)	TCSS (DAYS)	METABOLIZING CYTOCHROMES
Clozapine	Well absorbed	1-6	12	3-4	CYP1A2 CYP3A4
Risperidone	Rapid/complete	1-3	20	5-7	CYP2D6
Olanzapine	Well absorbed	5	20-70	7	CYP1A2 CYP2D6
Quetiapine	Rapid	1.5	3-7	2-3	CYP3A4
Ziprasidone	Rapid with food	3.8-5.2	5-8	1-3	CYP3A4
Aripiprazole	Not affected by food	3	25	14	CYP2D6 CYP3A4

CYP, cytochrome P-450 isoenzyme; T½, half-life; Tcss, time to steady-state concentration; Tmax, time to maximum concentration.

equivalent therapeutic responses, so therapeutic drug monitoring usually is not done. Poor correlation exists among plasma level, drug response, and toxicity. The usual doses for antipsychotics are given in Table 122-5.

Optimal striatal D_2 receptor occupancy, as determined by positron emission tomography (PET), is 60% to 80%. Occupancy of less than 60% is suboptimal, and occupancy greater than 80% is associated with EPS; higher than optimal D_2 receptor occupancy plateaus the response and increases drug side effects.[2,5]

Antipsychotics are well absorbed orally (see Tables 122-3 and 122-4) but have high first-pass hepatic clearance. A large volume of distribution results from their lipophilic nature and extensive extravascular tissue binding. Some antipsychotics have active metabolites (haloperidol, clozapine, risperidone, and aripiprazole).[2]

Major Side Effects

Dry mouth and mild tremors disappear in time or respond to dose reduction. Major side effects include EPS that are acute (dystonia, parkinsonian rigidity, and bradykinesia) (Box 122-1). Low-potency first-generation antipsychotics such as chlorpromazine and thioridazine have a lower EPS

Box 122-1 Treatment of Extrapyramidal Syndromes

- Obtain an accurate diagnosis.
- Reduce dose if possible.
- Switch from a first-generation to a second-generation antipsychotic.
- Prescribe anticholinergics or benzodiazepine for dystonia.
- Prescribe β-blockers, low-dose clonazepam, diazepam, or lorazepam for akathisia.
- Prescribe anticholinergics or amantadine for parkinsonian rigidity.

risk.[2] Akathisia can be mistaken for anxiety, resulting in inappropriate dose titration and further toxicity.[2] EPS may also be mistaken for depression with psychomotor retardation, leading to inappropriate polypharmacy. Dystonia of major muscle groups is characterized as torticollis, oculogyric crisis. The second-generation antipsychotics clozapine and quetiapine lack EPS.[2]

Tardive dyskinesia occurs with long-term use, the risk being related to potency. Tardive dyskinesia typically produces buccolinguomasticatory repetitive movements; other EPS can occur with tardive dyskinesia. Treatment consists of discontinuing the antipsychotic, switching to a second-generation antipsychotic, or starting a cholinergic agonist with a dopamine-depleting drug (reserpine or tetrabenazine).[2,6]

The neuroleptic malignant syndrome (NMS) is a hypodopaminergic hyperpyrexia syndrome consisting of the following: (1) fever greater than 40° C, (2) muscle rigidity, (3) altered consciousness, (4) fluctuating blood pressure, (5) tachypnea, (6) diaphoresis, and (7) elevated creatine phosphatase. NMS can occur with both first- and second-generation antipsychotics. Risks occur when neuroleptics are combined with dopamine-depleting agents such as reserpine or antidepressants.[2] Discontinuing amantadine while on antipsychotics or combining antipsychotics with dopamine transporter inhibitors (amphetamine or cocaine) increases the risk of NMS. Eighty percent of NMS occurs within the first 2 weeks of treatment. It evolves over 24 to 48 hours and resolves in 7 to 30 days, depending on the half-life of the antipsychotic agent.[7,8] Almost all patients with NMS have elevated creatine phosphatase, which helps differentiate it from other causes of fever[2] (Box 122-2).

Anticholinergic antipsychotics may paradoxically cause cognitive failure and also blurred vision, dry mouth, constipation, and urinary retention.[2] Certain antipsychotics (clozapine, chlorpromazine, risperidone) have significant anticholinergic activity and may cause syncope due to orthostatic hypotension. This risk is increased in the elderly. Slow titration minimizes this side effect.[2]

Antipsychotics block the cardiac potassium channels that are needed for myocyte repolarization.[9,10] Potassium channel blockade may prolong QTc intervals and precipitate ventricular arrhythmia. Antipsychotic serum levels do not correlate with the risk for arrhythmia, so therapeutic drug monitoring should not be done.[2] The risk can be genetic or related to reduced magnesium or potassium or acquired cardiac disease.[11] Medications that prolong the QTc interval should be avoided with phenothiazines or the second-generation antipsychotic ziprasidone. High-risk individuals have genetic or acquired QTc prolongation, have preexisting heart disease, or are taking high doses of antipsychotics. Drugs that reduce antipsychotic clearance or prolong QTc intervals increase the risk for arrhythmias.[11]

Routine electrocardiography (ECG) is not required unless there is (1) cardiac disease, (2) a family history of sudden death, (3) a history of syncope, or (4) congenital prolonged QTc interval. A baseline ECG study should be obtained in these instances, and repeat ECG should be done if syncope occurs. Sudden death is rare with antipsychotics, and the risk is not prohibitive.[2] A black box label has been introduced in the United States for certain antipsychotics due to the risk of ventricular arrhythmias.

Dopamine receptor blockade increases release of prolactin from pituitary lactotrophs, resulting in galactorrhea, abnormal menstruation, gynecomastia, and sexual dysfunction. Second-generation antipsychotics (except for risperidone) do not increase serum prolactin.[2] Weight gain can be substantial for certain antipsychotics (in order of prevalence): (1) clozapine and olanzapine; (2) risperidone and quetiapine; (3) ziprasidone and aripiprazole. First-generation antipsychotics cause less weight gain.[2] Both first- and second-generation antipsychotics can cause glucose intolerance in predisposed individuals. Weight gain with certain antipsychotics (clozapine and olanzapine) is associated with insulin resistance.[12] Diabetics are usually better treated with first-generation antipsychotics.[2] Hyperlipidemia is reported with clozapine and olanzapine. Risperidone and first-generation antipsychotics produce less dyslipidemia.[2] Clozapine can cause agranulocytosis, as can other antipsychotics such as chlorpromazine, to a lesser extent. Clozapine requires monitoring of the white blood cell count and absolute neutrophil count every week for 6 months, then every 2 weeks for the next 6 months, and monthly thereafter. Antipsychotics can cause cholestatic jaundice in the first few weeks, and this is often associated with eosinophilia.

Drug Interactions

Plasma levels of most antipsychotics are reduced by classic anticonvulsants and carbamazepine through induction of the cytochrome P-450 (CYP) isoenzyme CYP3A4. Haloperidol is metabolized to a neurotoxic metabolite (pyridium HPP) by CYP3A4, which is upregulated by carbamazepine. Nefazodone, trazodone, fluoxetine, and fluvoxamine delay haloperidol clearance by inhibiting CYP3A4. Other drugs that block CYP3A4, such as ketoconazole and erythromycin, do the same. In vitro studies have found that antipsychotics inhibit metabolism of tricyclic antidepressants (TCAs), and vice versa, but inhibition is minor and the clinical significance is unknown.

Pharmacodynamic interactions occur between anticholinergics and antipsychotics. Combining anticholinergics with anticholinergic antipsychotics increases the risk for delirium, dry mouth, gastroparesis, constipation, and urinary retention. Dopamine transporter blockers such as methylphenidate and dopaminergic drugs such as amantadine and bromocriptine block antipsychotic therapeutic effects. Certain antipsychotics block α_1-adrenergic receptors and potentiate antihypertensive medications, with resulting orthostatic hypotension and syncope.

Monotherapy with antipsychotics minimizes drug-drug interactions.[2] The choice of an antipsychotic is important in situations in which drug-drug interactions are a risk. Antipsychotics without antimuscarinic activity should be selected for those patients already taking antimuscarinics. If potential pharmacokinetic drug interactions are anticipated, an antipsychotic with a wide therapeutic window should be chosen.

Box 122-2 Treatment of Neuroleptic Malignant Syndrome

- Early recognition
- Antipsychotic withdrawal
- Dantrolene, 2-3 mg/kg IV, every 10-15 minutes
- Bromocriptine, 2.5-10 mg tid
- Amantadine, 200-400 mg qd
- Benzodiazepines (lorazepam)
- Combination of medications listed above
- Carbidopa, 2.5 mg, with levodopa, 100 mg, given 3-8 times per day

Evidence Base for Antipsychotics

Second-generation antipsychotics are not necessarily better antipsychotics, but they are better tolerated and have a wider therapeutic index. Certain second-generation antipsychotics have unique toxicity that requires monitoring. Side effects and symptoms influence the choice of antipsychotic medications (Boxes 122-3 and 122-4).[2]

ANTIDEPRESSANTS

Biogenic amines (norepinephrine, serotonin, and dopamine) play a principal role in depression and are the main targets for antidepressants. In the 1950s, the discovery that monoamine oxidase inhibitors (MAOIs) relieve depression led to a major paradigm shift in psychiatry. Imipramine, a chlorpromazine derivative, was the first TCA synthesized for depression.[13,14] Monoamine transporters regulate synaptic levels of monoamines, and monoamines are recycled by these presynaptic transporters.[15] Modern antidepressants act mainly as monoamine transporter inhibitors. Clinical benefits include not only improved depression but also improved attention-deficit disorders, obsessive-compulsive behavior, fatigue, and pain.[16]

Box 122-3 Research Challenges for Antipsychotic Drugs

- Comparison of clinical benefits and costs of second- versus first-generation antipsychotics in symptom management is important. Nonpsychiatric symptoms for which antipsychotics may be helpful include nausea, vomiting, anorexia, and delirium. The National Institute of Mental Health Clinical and Psychotic Trials in Intervention Effectiveness (CATIE) project is exploring prospective use of antipsychotics with the aim of providing guidelines.
- Dose-response relationships need to be established for patients who are frail, who are elderly, or who have cancer. Doses that are used in healthy populations cannot be assumed to be safe in palliative care populations.
- Choice of antipsychotics for patients with multiple symptoms needs to be explored. One drug may effectively treat multiple symptoms (e.g., nausea, vomiting, delirium, depression, and anorexia or weight loss).
- Reliable instruments and studies powered to adequate patient numbers should be able to determine differences in therapeutic benefits for targeted symptoms.

Box 122-4 Current Controversies for Antipsychotic Drugs

- Should first- or second-generation antipsychotics be used as initial therapy?
- Should first- or second-generation antipsychotics be used for medically ill patients taking multiple medications?
- Which symptoms are best treated by antipsychotics?
- What are the appropriate doses of antipsychotics in non-schizophrenic vulnerable and frail populations?

Mechanisms of Action

Monoamine neurons express monoamine transporters. Serotonin transporters (SERTs) are found in the brainstem raphe nucleus, norepinephrine transporters (NET) in the locus caeruleus, and dopamine transporters (DAT) in substantia nigra, the tegmentum area, prefrontal cortex, and cingular gyrus.[15] Transporter protein structure consists of a 12-transmembrane domain, an intracellular NH$_2$-terminal amino, and a C-terminal tail (Fig. 122-3). Between the third and fourth transmembrane sections is a large glycosylated extracellular loop that maintains the membrane surface transporter. Various segments of the transmembrane domain are important to substrate and inhibitor binding. Sodium is necessary for transport of monoamines. Ion transport differs for each transporter (one sodium and one chloride for NET and SERT, two sodium ions and one chloride for DAT). Transporters have channel-like activity, but monoamine transport can also be uncoupled from the ion conduction. Amphetamines reverse monoamine transport.[15] Transporters are downregulated through phosphorylation. Chronic antidepressants downregulate transporters without changing transporter messenger RNA (mRNA).[15] Polymorphisms of transporter structural gene and promoter gene sites are associated with attention-deficit disorders, alcoholism, compulsive-aggressive behavior, and major depression. DAT is reduced with age and in Parkinson's disease.[15]

Autoreceptors and heteroreceptors are found in perisynaptic dendrites. Autoreceptors bind the same monoamine released by the neuron, whereas heteroreceptors bind monoamines different from those produced by the neuron. For example, the heteroreceptor for norepinephrine is found on serotonin neurons and is the target for mirtazapine.[16] Autoreceptors and heteroreceptors block monoamine release via a feedback inhibition mechanism (Fig. 122-4).[17] Chronic use of selective serotonin reuptake inhibitors (SSRIs), TCAs, and dual serotonin-norepinephrine reuptake inhibitors (SNRIs) downregulates presynaptic and somatodendritic autoreceptors and heteroreceptors[16] (Figs. 122-5 and 122-6). Downregulation and desensitization of autoreceptors and heteroreceptors increases monoamine release over time[17] (Fig. 122-7). This requires 14 to 21 days. Certain antidepressants, such as mirtazapine, directly inhibit autoreceptors or heteroreceptors but not monoamine transport, which accounts for their earlier onset of activity.[16,17] The classes and usual doses of antidepressants are given in Table 122-6.

Certain antidepressants (nefazodone, trazodone, and mirtazapine) block postsynaptic serotonin 5-HT$_2$ and 5-HT$_3$ receptors (Table 122-7) This reduces serotonin side effects such as nausea, insomnia, and anxiety. 5-HT$_{2A}$ blockade secondarily increases dopamine and improves cognitive function and depression. Certain single nucleotide polymorphisms involving 5-HT$_{1B}$ autoreceptors and 5-HT$_{2A}$ and 5-HT$_{2C}$ receptors have been associated with obsessive-compulsive disorders, aggressive behavior, alcoholism, drug abuse, obesity, and schizophrenia.

Antidepressant pharmacokinetics are subject to ethnic pharmacogenetic differences and drug interactions. Twenty percent of Asians are poor metabolizers related to CYP2C19 and have delayed clearance of citalopram

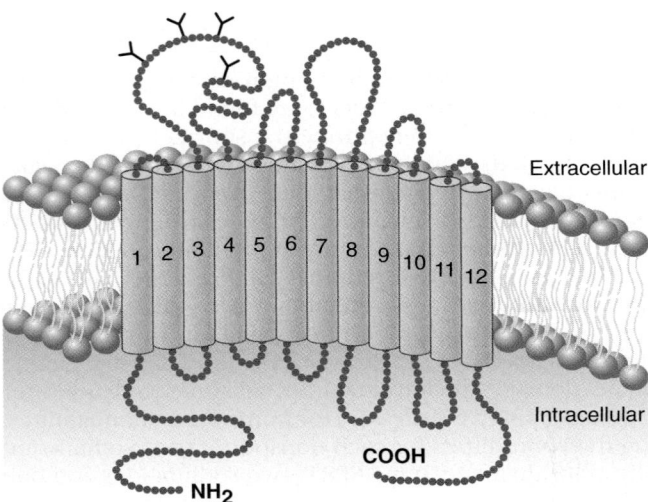

A Dopamine Transporter (DAT)

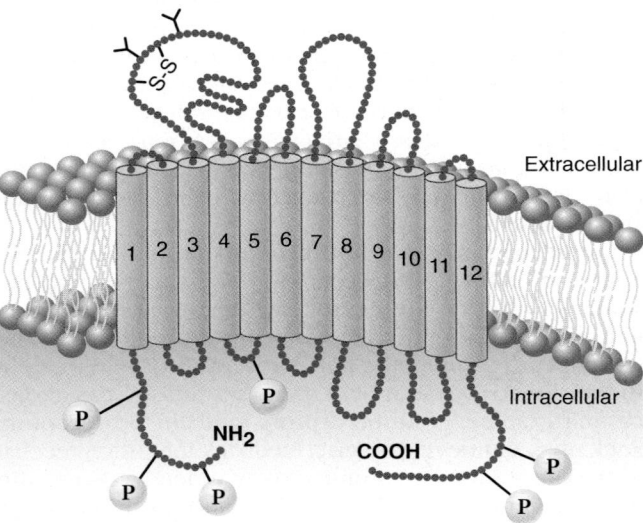

B Serotonin Transporter (SERT)

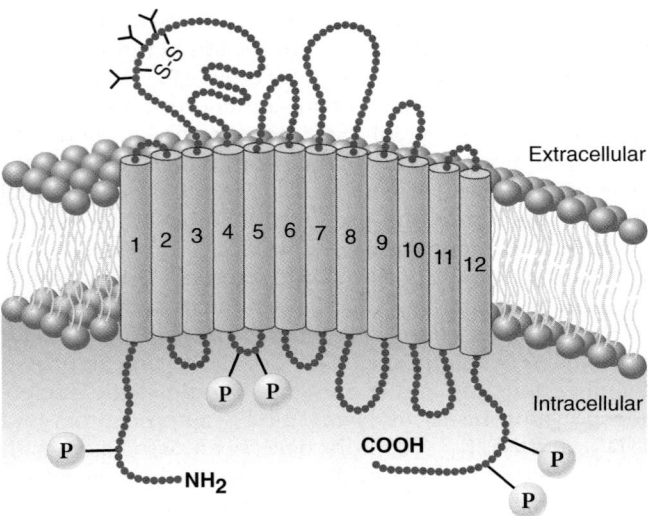

C Norepinephrine Transporter (NET)

FIGURE 122-3 Schematic appearance of monoamine transporters. COOH, carboxyl terminus; NH₂, amino terminus; P, phosphate molecule; S-S, sulfur-sulfur bond.

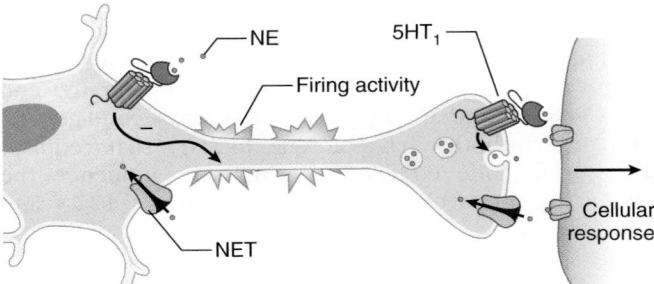

A No treatment

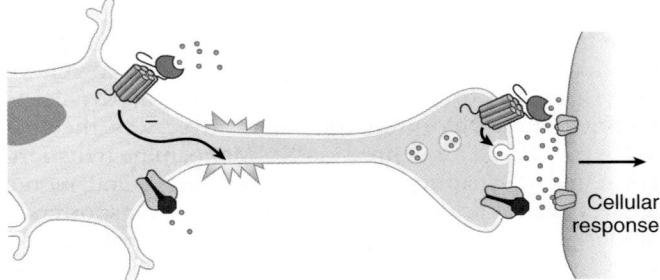

B Norepinephrine reuptake inhibitor alone

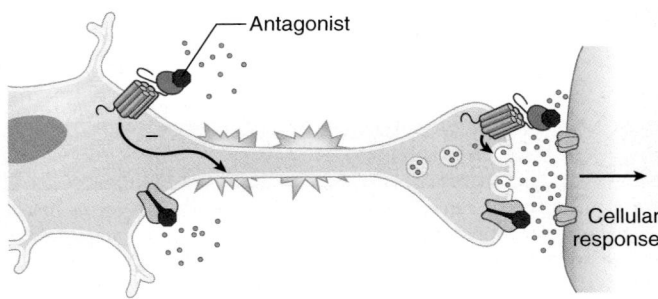

C Mechanism of antidepressant action

FIGURE 122-4 Complementary action of norepinephrine and serotonin autoreceptor blockade. Prolonged exposure of autoreceptors also causes downregulation and facilitates monoamine release. 5-HT, 5-hydroxytryptamine (serotonin); NE, norepinephrine; NET, norepinephrine transporter.

and escitalopram. Antidepressants metabolized through CYP2D6 have slow clearance in Asian and Black African populations. As a result, these patients have higher plasma levels per dose and toxicity at lower doses.[13] All SSRIs have a half-life of 15 to 30 hours, whereas fluoxetine and its active metabolite, norfluoxetine, have half-lives of 2 to 4 days and 7 to 15 days, respectively. Extended-release fluoxetine can be dosed weekly. Drug interactions are significant with fluoxetine due to inhibition of cytochromes, which markedly prolongs the half-life of this drug. Once-daily dosing for all SSRIs (except fluoxetine) is the norm.[13]

Fluoxetine and paroxetine have nonlinear pharmacokinetics due to inhibition of cytochromes that clear both drugs. Side effects resulting from dose escalation can be disproportionately increased. Citalopram, escitalopram, and sertraline have linear pharmacokinetics.[13] The plasma levels and half-life of paroxetine increase with age. Because of increased bioavailability for those older than 65 years of age, starting doses should be half of the usual doses.[13]

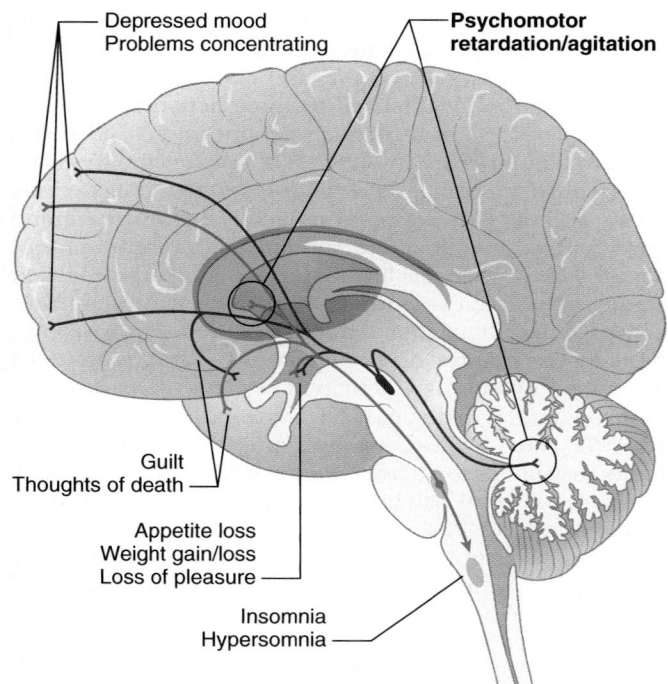

FIGURE 122-5 Central nervous system pathways that govern mood.

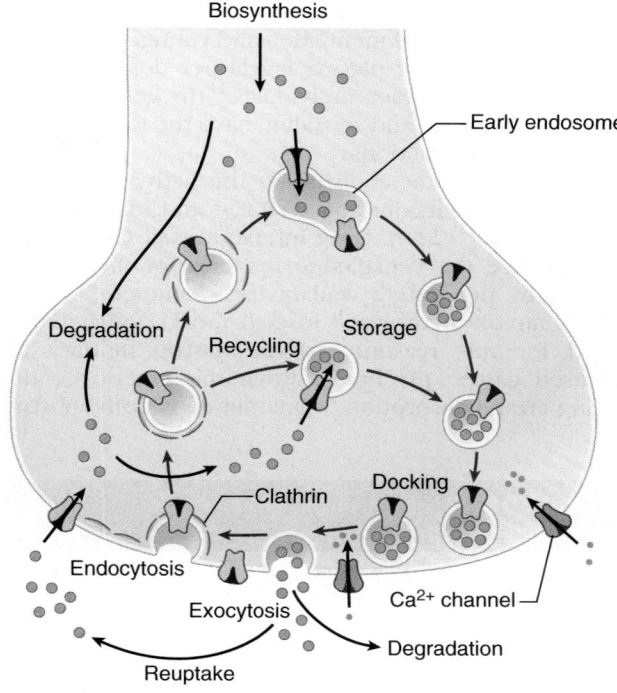

FIGURE 122-7 Cycle of monoamine neurotransmitters.

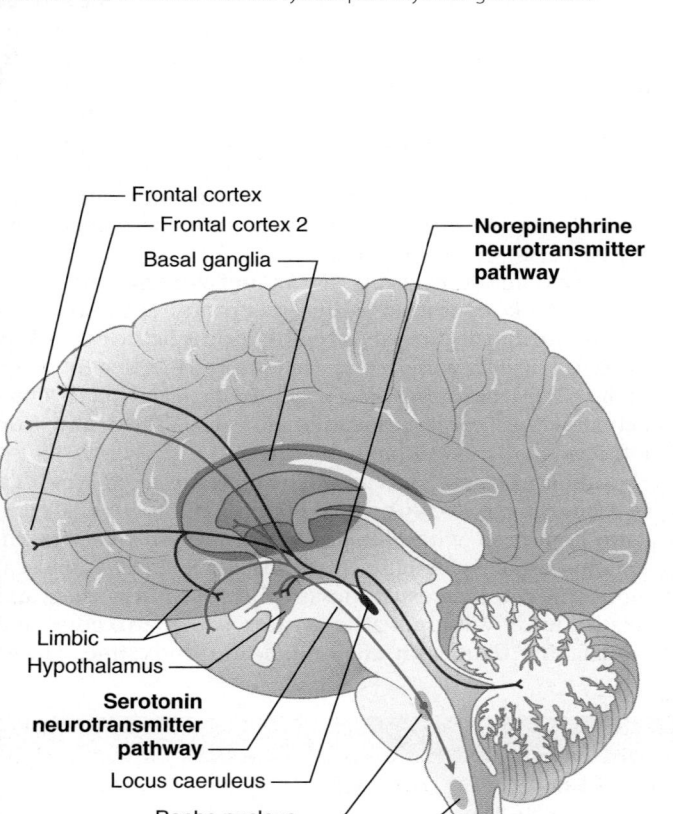

FIGURE 122-6 Pathway for serotonin and norepinephrine neurotransmission.

TABLE 122-6	Classes and Doses of Antidepressants
CLASS	**USUAL DAILY DOSE (MG)**
SSRIs	
Citalopram	20-40
Escitalopram	10-20
Fluoxetine	10-60
Paroxetine	10-50
Sertraline	50-200
SNRIs	
Duloxetine	30-60
Venlafaxine	75-225
Aminoketone	
Bupropion	150-450
Tetracyclics	
Mirtazapine	15-45
Maprotiline	25-150
Amoxapine	100-400
TCA	
Amitriptyline	75-300
Imipramine	75-300
Desipramine	75-300
Nortriptyline	75-150
MAOIs	
Isocarboxazid	40-60
Tranylcypromine	30-60
Phenelzine	48-90
Selegiline	6-12

MAOI, monoamine oxidase inhibitor; SNRI, dual serotonin-norepinephrine reuptake inhibitor; SSRI, selective serotonin reuptake inhibitor; TCA, tricyclic antidepressant.

Sertraline has age- and gender-related kinetics and does not require dose adjustment. Men and younger individuals have lower sertraline plasma levels per dose compared with women and older individuals.[13] In general, citalopram, escitalopram, and sertraline have the least potential for drug-drug interactions.

Venlafaxine is metabolized to the active metabolite, o-desmethyl venlafaxine, by CYP2D6 and inactivated by CYP3A4 (Table 122-8). Drug interactions at CYP3A4 will either reduce the venlafaxine response or increase the toxicity (by preventing venlafaxine clearance).[13] Duloxetine is rapidly hydrolyzed in acid media and is enteric coated for this reason. Delayed gastric motility and increased gastric pH break down the enteric coating, causing erratic absorption.[13] Duloxetine is both substrate and inhibitor to CYP2D6 and CYP1A2. High doses and increasing age delay clearance.[13] Duloxetine is not recommended in hepatic or renal failure.

Bupropion is metabolized to three active metabolites (hydroxybupropion, threohydroxybupropion, and erythrohydroxybupropion) by CYP2B6. These metabolites have a longer half-life than the parent drug (8 to 10 hours versus 10 to 20 hours). CYP2B6 is induced by carbamazepine and inhibited by fluoxetine, influencing bupropion clearance.[13] Mirtazapine has linear kinetics and is metabolized through multiple cytochrome enzymes and subsequently conjugated. Elimination through three cytochromes reduces the risk for drug interactions. Mirtazapine does not inhibit cytochrome activity.[13]

TCAs undergo first-pass clearance (40% to 70%) by CYP3A4 and CYP2D6. Half-life ranges from 16 to 120 hours (usually 24 to 30 hours), which allows for once-daily dosing. Prolonged half-life occurs in those who are poor metabolizers (CYP2D6) and in those with hepatic, renal, or heart failure. Imipramine is metabolized to desipramine and amitriptyline is metabolized to nortriptyline by CYP1A2, CYP2C19, and CYP3A4. Desipramine and nortriptyline account for much of the NET blockade associated with imipramine and amitriptyline, respectively.[13] Another important drug-drug interaction is with potent inhibitors of CYP2D6 (paroxetine or fluoxetine); TCA levels rise drastically when these drugs are combined with either SSRI. MAOIs undergo first-pass clearance by oxidative cytochromes and have a plasma half-life of only 2 to 4 hours. However, MAOIs irreversibly inhibit monoamine oxidase, so the biological effect is prolonged despite the brief plasma half-life. Enzyme regeneration takes weeks.[13] To avoid a serotonin syndrome, drug-free intervals of 2 to 7 weeks are required before other antidepressants (e.g., SSRIs, TCAs) can be started.[13]

Certain antidepressants (TCAs, nefazodone, and trazodone) block neurotransmitter receptors. Mirtazapine is unique in that it blocks norepinephrine heteroreceptors presynaptically and 5-HT$_2$ receptors postsynaptically. Table 122-9 describes the receptor blockade and clinical effects of antidepressants; Box 122-5 lists the side effects.

Antidepressants downregulate certain receptors that reduce side effects with chronic use.[18] Withdrawal is clinically important with SSRIs and less so with TCAs. Withdrawal results in fatigue, myalgias, loose stools, nausea, lightheadedness, restlessness, sleep disturbances, and headaches.[13] Withdrawal is greater with paroxetine and venlafaxine than with citalopram and fluoxetine. Fluox-

TABLE 122-7   Inhibition of Transporters by Antidepressants

NET/SERT INHIBITORS	NET-SELECTIVE INHIBITORS	SERT-SELECTIVE INHIBITORS
Amitriptyline	Nortriptyline	Citalopram
Imipramine	Desipramine	Fluoxetine
Nefazodone	Maprotiline	Paroxetine
Duloxetine		Sertraline
Venlafaxine		

NET, norepinephrine transporter; SERT, serotonin transporter.

TABLE 122-8   Antidepressant Pharmacokinetics: Cytochrome Metabolism

ANTIDEPRESSANT	METABOLIZING CYTOCHROMES
Citalopram	CYP2C19, CYP3A4
Escitalopram	CYP2C19, CYP3A4
Fluoxetine (norfluoxetine)	CYP2D6, CYP2C9
Paroxetine	CYP2D6 (low concentrations), CYP3A4 (higher concentrations)
Venlafaxine	CYP2D6, CYP3A4
Duloxetine	CYP1A2, CYP2D6
Bupropion	CYP2B6
Nefazodone	CYP3A4, CYP2D6
Trazodone	CYP3A4, CYP2D6
Mirtazapine	CYP1A2, CYP2D6, CYP3A4
Tricyclic antidepressants	CYP3A4, CYP1A2, CYP2D6, CYP2C19, CYP2C9

TABLE 122-9   Receptor Blockade and Clinical Effects of Antidepressants

MUSCARINIC CHOLINERGIC RECEPTOR INHIBITION	α-ADRENERGIC RECEPTOR INHIBITION	α$_2$-ADRENERGIC RECEPTOR INHIBITION	5-HT$_{2A}$ INHIBITION	D$_2$ INHIBITION
Blurred vision	Potentiation of α-blockers (prazosin) with orthostatic hypotension	Reduced depression	Reduced depression	EPS
Dry mouth	Dizziness	Blocked clonidine effects	Reduced anxiety	Hyperprolactinemia
Sinus tachycardia	Tachycardia		Improved sleep	Sexual dysfunction
Constipation			Prophylaxis for migraine	
Urinary retention			Reduced EPS (from D2-blocking drugs)	
Confusion			Reduced psychoses	

EPS, extrapyramidal side effects.

Box 122-5 Side Effects of Antidepressants

Norepinephrine Transporters (NET)

- Tremor
- Tachycardia
- Erectile and ejaculatory dysfunction
- Hypertension (when combined with sympathomimetic drugs)

Serotonin Transporters (SERT)

- Nausea
- Vomiting
- Anorexia
- Sexual dysfunction
- Anxiety (transient)
- Extrapyramidal side effects
- Serotonin syndrome (drug interactions with monoamine oxidase inhibitors, tramadol)

Dopamine Transporters (DAT)

- Psychomotor activation
- Delirium
- Confusion
- Psychoses, including paranoia

Box 122-6 Research Challenges for Antidepressants

- Development of antidepressants targeted to specific autoreceptors and heteroreceptors, to improve the onset of drug benefits, and to postsynaptic serotonin receptors, to reduce drug toxicity
- Development of transporter/autoreceptor multifunctional antidepressants
- Further studies to establish safe combinations of antidepressants and safe augmentation treatment of refractory depression
- Antidepressant switches in poor responders or in those who relapse with depression while taking antidepressants

---

Box 122-7 Current Controversies for Antidepressants

- Initial choices of antidepressants in the frail and vulnerable
- Clinically relevant factors that determine antidepressant responses
- Safe antidepressant combinations
- Drug combinations that augment antidepressant responses in poor responders
- Atypical antipsychotics in addition to antidepressants in psychotic depression
- Atypical antipsychotics in patients who are delirious
- Correlation of single nucleotide polymorphisms involving transporters and serotonin receptor responses to particular antidepressants

---

etine and its active metabolite norfluoxetine have long half-lives and fewer withdrawal symptoms. TCAs have a narrower therapeutic index (i.e., the concentration needed to harm minus the concentration needed to treat) than other antidepressants. TCAs cause cardiac electrical conduction delays and arrhythmias and impair cardiac contractility, so patients with heart failure should avoid TCA.[13] Hallucinations, loss of recent memory, confusion, and disorientation are caused by TCA anticholinergic activity. Seizures are more frequent with bupropion, amoxapine, and TCAs. TCAs and mirtazapine cause weight gain. MAOIs are generally well tolerated, although hypotension is reported. Severe MAOI reactions leading to hypertension occur with tyramine in diets and in those patients who are started on other antidepressants while taking MAOIs.[13]

Contraindications

TCAs should not be given to patients with cardiac arrhythmias, conduction defects, or systolic heart failure. Maprotiline, bupropion, and TCAs should be avoided in those with seizures, and venlafaxine in those with uncontrolled hypertension.[13]

Drug Interactions

Serious drug interactions involve the inhibition of key cytochrome enzymes (CYP3A4, CYP2D6, CYP1A2). Because fluoxetine, nefazodone, and paroxetine have nonlinear pharmacokinetics (due to autoinhibition of certain cytochrome isoenzymes), the degree of cytochrome inhibition per dose is disproportionally greater at higher doses. Paroxetine and fluoxetine have substantial drug interactions, whereas citalopram, escitalopram, and sertra-

line have fewer drug interactions.[13] SSRIs reduce dopamine release and can cause extrapyramidal reactions when combined with first-generation antipsychotics. Smoking increases duloxetine clearance (by induction of CYP1A2), whereas quinolone antibiotics and cimetidine delay it. Paroxetine and fluoxetine delay duloxetine clearance through CYP2D6. Duloxetine, on the other hand, inhibits desipramine metabolism through CYP2D6.[13] Nefazodone and trazodone are strong CYP3A4 inhibitors and therefore are not first-line antidepressants. Tricyclic pharmacodynamic adverse interactions occur with anticholinergics, antihistaminics, α_1-adrenergic agents, and antiarrhythmic drugs.[13] MAOIs have the most serious pharmacodynamic interactions. The serotonin syndrome occurs if MAOIs are combined with SSRIs, SNRIs, venlafaxine, mirtazapine, tryptophan, or certain opioid analgesics (meperidine).[13]

Evidence Base for Antidepressants

All classes of antidepressants (TCAs, SSRIs, SNRIs, autoreceptor/heteroreceptor inhibitors, and MAOIs) work equally well in depression. Differences between classes of antidepressant relate to side effects and drug interactions. The choice of antidepressants depends on clinical factors, polypharmacy, symptoms, and co-morbidities (Boxes 122-6 and 122-7).[13]

γ-AMINOBUTYRIC ACID AGONISTS

A fundamental balance between excitatory and inhibitory neurotransmitters governs neuron depolarization. γ-Aminobutyric acid (GABA) receptors are principally inhibitory receptors.[19] Many sedative drugs target GABA receptors, including bromides, benzodiazepines, barbiturates, ethanol, anesthetics, and neurosteroids.[19] Benzodiazepines are the principal GABA agonists; they account for two thirds of psychotropic prescriptions and are effective in many disorders.[20] Benzodiazepines are the most widely prescribed drugs worldwide.[21] They derive their name from the fusion of a benzene ring with a seven-member diazepine ring.[20] Tolerance, dependence, withdrawal, and fatality in overdose are concerns.[21]

Mechanisms of Action

Two GABA receptors are present in the CNS. $GABA_A$ receptors are chloride channels that hyperpolarize neurons, whereas $GABA_B$ receptors are G protein–coupled receptors that block activation of calcium and potassium channels. GABA receptors consist of pentameric structures formed from 19 different subunits transcribed by separate genes.[19,22] Clinical effects (sedation, muscle relaxation, anxiolysis) are related to the $GABA_A$ receptors subunit makeup. The benzodiazepine 1 receptors (BZ_1) contain α_1 subunits that are responsible for hypnotic effects. The benzodiazepine 2 receptors (BZ_2) contain α_2, α_3, or α_4 subunits that are responsible for anxiolysis and muscle relaxation.[23] GABA subunits differ with CNS location. Drug affinity is governed by subunit composition.[19] Benzodiazepines do not activate but positively modulate $GABA_A$ receptors; the receptor is activated only in the presence of GABA. Only barbiturates at high doses directly activate GABA chloride channels.[24] $GABA_A$ receptors are found predominantly on stellate inhibitory interneurons within the cortex and within the globus pallidus, substantia nigra, and cerebellar Purkinje cells.[21] $GABA_A$ receptors are present in abundance in the amygdala and are the site for anxiolysis.[21]

GABA is produced through glutamate decarboxylation by interneurons and subsequently packaged in synaptic vesicles and released through calcium-dependent exocytosis. GABA is taken up presynaptically by GABA transporters (GAT), similar to monoamines. Glutamate released by excitatory neurons stimulates GABA release, which in turn blocks presynaptic release of substance P and glutamate as negative feedback. Glutamate receptors rapidly become desensitized and decrease GABA release. Presynaptic autoreceptors ($GABA_B$) reduce GABA release. Certain drugs, such as tiagabine, act as indirect GABA agonists through GAT inhibition. Gabapentin and pregabalin bind to certain presynaptic $GABA_B$ receptors and prevent calcium conductance and depolarization. Both retigabine and topiramate are $GABA_A$ agonists. Vigabatrin, valproic acid, and retigabine block GABA catabolism through GABA transaminase. Cannabinoids reduce GABA reuptake. Baclofen, on the other hand, blocks GABA release via $GABA_B$ autoreceptor activation. Typical antipsychotics increase GABA release, but in the long term they down-modulate GABA receptors. Long-term use of haloperidol or clozapine also upregulates GABA transporters and reduces GABA neurotransmission. Morphine induces GABA release in the nucleus accumbens, which may play a role in rewarding effects. Overexpression of the GAT1 transporters in experimental animals reduces opioid reinforcing behavior and withdrawal.

The nonbenzodiazepine hypnotics zolpidem, zopiclone, and zaleplon (Z drugs) bind specifically to α_1 sub-units on $GABA_A$ receptors. This causes sedation but not anxiolysis or muscle relaxation.[19,23] Flumazenil allosterically blocks $GABA_A$ α_6 subunits and prevents receptor activation.[24] This site differs from the usual benzodiazepine binding site (α_1) and hence is noncompetitive.[24]

Benzodiazepines are highly lipophilic and well absorbed. The dosages and pharmacokinetics of these drugs are described in Tables 122-10 and 122-11, respectively. Plasma concentrations are proportional to oral dose, which also correlates fairly closely with drug levels at receptor sites.[20] Minimal effective concentrations (the backbone of therapeutic drug monitoring) vary greatly between individuals due to pharmacodynamic tolerance with chronic dosing; clinical response can diminish despite stable blood levels.[20] Rapidly absorbed benzodiazepines (diazepam and flurazepam) have rapid peak plasma levels and rapid intense drug effects experienced as sedation and psychological "rush." Benzodiazepines that are absorbed at a lower rate (oxazepam and temazepam) have a longer latency and a lower peak effect and are perceived as less intense.[20]

Benzodiazepines have a bimodal half-life. In single-dose studies, the alpha half-life is reached with the distribution equilibrium. In general, 95% is bound to tissues. The degree of tissue binding determines whether the benzodiazepine is long, intermediate, or short acting. Short-acting benzodiazepines have a half life of less than 5 hours, intermediate ones 6 to 12 hours, and long-acting types greater than 12 hours.[20] Benzodiazepines are also divided into

TABLE 122-10 Usual Benzodiazepine Dosages	
DRUG	**DOSAGE**
Chlordiazepoxide	10-50 mg/day
Diazepam	2-30 mg/day
Oxazepam	30-90 mg/day
Chlorazepate	30-60 mg/day
Alprazolam	0.25-2 mg/day
Temazepam	15-30 mg/day
Triazolam	0.125-0.5 mg/day
Midazolam	0.5-4 mg/hr
Clonazepam	0.5-2 mg/day

TABLE 122-11 Benzodiazepine Kinetics and Half-life		
DRUG	**METABOLIZING CYTOCHROMES**	**HALF-LIFE (HR)**
Alprazolam	CYP3A4	8-15
Chlordiazepoxide	CYP3A4	10-20
Clonazepam	CYP3A4	10-20
Chlorazepate	CYP3A4 ± CYP2D6	40-100
Diazepam	CYP2C19/CYP3A4	20-70
Midazolam	CYP3A4	1.5-3.5
Temazepam	UGT	8-12
Oxazepam	UGT	5-15
Triazolam	CYP3A4	1.5-5
Lorazepam	UGT	10-20

CYP, cytochrome P-450 isoenzyme; UGT, uridine glucuronyl transferase.

those that are conjugated and those that undergo phase I metabolism. N-Demethylation or hydroxylation by cytochromes can produce active metabolites (Table 122-12). Drug interactions accumulate with age and liver disease and are more likely in cytochrome-metabolized benzodiazepines[13] Lorazepam, oxazepam, and temazepam are conjugated benzodiazepines.

Nonbenzodiazepine GABA$_A$ Receptor Agonists

The Z drugs (zolpidem, zopiclone, and zaleplon) are selective GABA$_A$ agonists that are hypnotic only (Table 122-13).

Adverse Effects of Benzodiazepines

Sedation, the most common adverse effect of benzodiazepines, subsides after 1 week as the anxiolysis effects emerge.[13] Some patients develop disinhibition behavior characterized by hostility, aggressiveness, rage, paradoxical excitement, irritability, and behavioral dyscontrol.[13] Benzodiazepines can impair coordination, attention, and driving ability. All benzodiazepines evoke withdrawal symptoms and potentially cause psychological dependence. Short-acting benzodiazepines especially, and alprazolam in particular, cause problematic withdrawal symptoms.

Symptoms of withdrawal can be mistaken for recurrent anxiety. Benzodiazepine withdrawal can persist for months. Short-acting benzodiazepines, more than long-acting benzodiazepines, induce a persistent dependency syndrome. Tapering is necessary, especially if benzodiazepines have been taken for 1 month or longer.[13] For most benzodiazepines (except alprazolam), doses can be rapidly tapered to 50% of the dose then slowly tapered by 10% to 20% every 3 to 5 days. Alprazolam requires a very slow taper. Lorazepam may be difficult to withdraw; however, switching to diazepam or clonazepam reduces daytime craving and interdose withdrawal symptoms.

Psychotherapy for anxiety during withdrawal and the use of carbamazepine and/or valproic acid reduces withdrawal symptoms. Zolpidem at night reduces rebound insomnia from benzodiazepines.[13] Seizures are another potential problem with abrupt discontinuation. Triazolam, alprazolam, and lorazepam are particularly prone to causing withdrawal seizures. Patients with a history of a seizure and those who are on medications that reduce seizure thresholds are at greatest risk.[13]

The Z drugs can cause psychotic reactions and transient detrimental cognitive or behavioral side effects. Zaleplon does not induce rebound insomnia or withdrawal symptoms. Eszopiclone is well tolerated but can produce taste alterations and headaches.[13]

Contraindications

Benzodiazepines should be avoided in delirious or frail individuals. Fatalities with benzodiazepines alone are rare, but sedative effects and respiratory depression are potentiated by alcohol, barbiturates, TCAs, and opioids.[13]

Drug Interactions

Benzodiazepines are subject to drug interactions through cytochrome enzymes. Inhibition of CYP3A4 by nefazo-

TABLE 122-12 Benzodiazepine Dose Equivalents and Metabolites

DRUG	DOSE EQUIVALENTS (MG)	ACTIVE METABOLITE
Chlordiazepoxide	10	Yes
Diazepam	5	Yes
Oxazepam	15	No
Flurazepam	30	Yes
Chlorazepate	7.5	Yes
Triazolam	0.25	No
Lorazepam	1	No
Temazepam	30	No
Alprazolam	0.25	No
Midazolam	2	No

From Chouinard G, L.-S.K., Teboul E. Metabolism of anxiolytics and hypnotics: Benzodiazepines, buspirone, zoplicone, and zolpidem. Cell Mol Neurobiol 1999;19:533-552.

TABLE 122-13 Pharmacokinetics of Nonbenzodiazepine GABA$_A$ Receptor Agonists

DRUG	BIOAVAILABILITY (%)	T½ (HR)	METABOLIZING CYTOCHROMES	DOSE (MG/DAY)
Zolpidem	70	2-2.2	CYP3A4 CYP2C9 CYP1A2	5-20
Zaleplon	30	1	CYP3A4 Aldehyde Oxidase CYP1A2 CYP2D6	5-20
Zopiclone	80	5	CYP3A4 CYP2C8 CYP2C9	7.5
Eszopiclone	80	5	CYP3A4 CYP2C8 CYP2C9	1-3

T½, half-life.

done, macrolides (clarithromycin or erythromycin), fluoxetine, or fluvoxamine increases alprazolam levels. This is also true for triazolam, diazepam, and midazolam. Carbamazepine, phenytoin, and St. John's wort induce CYP3A4 activity and increase clearance.[25] Conjugated drugs such as lorazepam and the nitro-reduced benzodiazepines (clonazepam) do not interact with SSRIs, macrolides, or antiseizure medications.[25] Omeprazole reduces diazepam clearance, and cimetidine reduces the clearance of alprazolam, triazolam, diazepam, and midazolam by blocking CYP3A4. Grapefruit juice increases bioavailability but not clearance of CYP3A4-dependent benzodiazepines.[25] Propranolol prolongs the half-life of diazepam. Probenecid inhibits lorazepam glucuronidation.[25] Oral contraceptives inhibit triazolam and alprazolam clearance through CYP3A4.

Patients who are taking SSRIs, macrolides, or certain antiseizure medications probably should be treated with primarily glucuronidated benzodiazepines. Patients taking cytochrome-metabolized benzodiazepines should be treated with newer SSRIs such as citalopram or with venlafaxine. Antiseizure medications that do not induce CYP3A4 (gabapentin, pregabalin, valproic acid) should be used for neuropathic pain in patients who are taking benzodiazepines.

The Z drugs are subject to the same multiple drug interactions as benzodiazepines. The risk of psychological dependence is less, but falls in the elderly are still a risk.[26]

Evidence Base for Benzodiazepines

Benzodiazepines are the treatment of choice for acute anxiety and panic disorders. The lowest effective dose and shortest duration of treatment are preferred.[21] Short-acting benzodiazepines are associated with greater withdrawal effects and greater risks for seizures with discontinuation.[21] Tolerance develops to a greater extent with certain benzodiazepines than with others (Boxes 122-8 and 122-9).[21]

REFERENCES

1. Delay J, Deniker P. Neuroleptic effects of chlorpromazine in therapeutics of neuropsychiatry. J Clin Exp Psychopathol 1955;16:104-112.
2. Janicak PG, Davis JM, Preskorn SH, et al. Treatment with antipsychotics. In Janicak PG, Davis JM, Preskorn SH, et al. (eds). Principles and Practice of Psychopharmacotherapy. Philadelphia: Lippincott Williams & Wilkins, 2006, Chapter 5.
3. Dean B, Scarr E. Antipsychotic drugs: Evolving mechanisms of action with improved therapeutic benefits. Curr Drug Targets 2004;3:217-226.
4. Lieberman J. Dopamine partial agonists. CNS Drugs 2004;18:251-267.
5. Farde L, Mack RJ, Nyberg S, Halldin C. D2 occupancy, extrapyramidal side effects and antipsychotic drug treatment: A pilot study with sertindole in healthy subjects. Int Clin Psychopharmacol 1997;12(Suppl 1):S3-S7.
6. Owens D. Adverse effects of antipsychotic agents: Do newer agents offer advantages? Drugs 1996;51:895-930.
7. Keck PE, Caroff SN, McElroy SL. Neuroleptic malignant syndrome and malignant hyperthermia: End of a controversy? J Neuropsychiatry Clin Neurosci 1995;7:135-144.
8. Ananth J, Parameswaran S, Gunatilake S, et al. Neuroleptic malignant syndrome and atypical antipsychotic drugs. J Clin Psychiatry 2004;65:464-470.
9. Heist EK, Ruskin JN. Drug-induced proarrhythmia and use of QTc-prolonging agents: Clues for clinicians. Heart Rhythm 2005;2(2 Suppl):S1-S8.
10. Mackin P, Young AH. QTc interval measurement and metabolic parameters in psychiatric patients taking typical or atypical antipsychotic drugs: A preliminary study. J Clin Psychiatry 2005;66:1386-1391.
11. Titier K, Girodet PO, Verdoux H, et al. Atypical antipsychotics. Drug Safety 2005;28:35-51.
12. Newcomer J. Second-generation (atypical) antipsychotics and metabolic effects: A comprehensive literature review. CNS Drugs 2005;19:1-93.
13. Janicak PG, Davis JM, Preskorn SH, et al. Treatment with antidepressants. In Janicak PG, Davis JM, Preskorn SH, et al. (eds). Principles and Practice of Psychotherapy. Philadelphia: Lippincott Williams & Wilkins, 2006, Chapter 6.
14. Kuhn R. The treatment of depressive states with G 22355 (imipramine hydrochloride). Am J Psychiatry 1958;115:459-464.
15. Torres GE, Gainetdinov RR, Caron MG. Plasma membrane monoamine transporters: Structure, regulation and function. Nat Rev Nerosci 2003;4:13-25.
16. Briley M, Moret C. Neurobiological mechanisms involved in antidepressant therapies. Clin Neuropharmacol 1993;16:387-400.
17. Blakely RD, De Felice LJ, Hartzell HC. Molecular physiology of norepinephrine and serotonin transporters. J Exp Biol 1994;196:263-281.
18. Richelson E. Basic neuropharmacology of antidepressants relevant to the pharmacotherapy of depression. Clin Cornerstone 1999;1(4):17-30.
19. Korpi ER, Sinkkonen ST. GABA(A) receptor subtypes as targets for neuropsychiatric drug development. Pharmacol Ther 2006;109:12-32.
20. Chouinard G, Lefko-Singh K, Teboul E. Metabolism of anxiolytics and hypnotics: Benzodiazepines, buspirone, zopiclone, and zolpidem. Cell Mol Neurobiol 1999;19:533-552.
21. Janicak PG, Davis JM, Preskorn SH, et al. Treatment with antianxiety and sedative-hypnotic agents. In Janicak PG, Davis JM, Preskorn SH, et al. (eds). Principles and Practice of Psychotherapy. Philadelphia: Lippincott Williams & Wilkins, 2006, Chapter 12.
22. Mehta AK, Ticku MK. An update on GABAA receptors. Brain Res Brain Res Rev 1999;29:196-217.
23. Sanger D. The pharmacology and mechanisms of action of new generation, non-benzodiazepine hypnotic agents. CNS Drugs 2004;18:9-15.
24. Bateson A. Basic pharmacologic mechanisms involved in benzodiazepine tolerance and withdrawal. Curr Pharmaceut Design 2002;8:5-21.
25. Tanaka E. Clinically significant pharmacokinetic drug interactions with benzodiazepines. J Clin Pharm Ther 1999;24:347-355.
26. Conn DK, Madan R. Use of sleep promoting medications in nursing home residents: Risks versus benefits. Drugs Aging 2006;23:271-287.

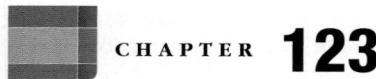

CHAPTER **123**

Prescribing

Susan Poole and Michael Dooley

QUALITY PRESCRIBING

Prescribing is the essential link between diagnosis, the decision to treat with medication, and the practical administration of the chosen therapy. It is the necessary procedure to communicate treatment decisions to other health practitioners, including pharmacists and nurses, patients, and their carers.

The principles of quality use of medicines (QUM) should be applied for optimal outcomes from prescribed medicines: select management options wisely, recognizing that the best option may not be drugs; choose suitable medicines if drugs are considered necessary; and use medicines safely and effectively.

Consideration must be given to factors associated with the disease, the patient, and the pharmacology of the selected medication.

● Disease factors—the appropriate drug or group of drugs to treat the diagnosis and obtain the desired therapeutic objective

● Patient factors—concurrent co-morbidities and organ impairment; concomitant therapies, including prescribed and over-the-counter (OTC) medications and complementary and alternative medicines; potential drug interactions; previous allergies and adverse reactions (absolute and relative contraindications); adher-

ence issues; patient and carer personal and cultural expectations; and previous experiences.

● Drug factors—efficacy, safety (adverse effects), cost, dosage, frequency, route of administration, and pharmacokinetic and pharmacodynamic properties

Quality Prescribing in Palliative Medicine

The number of symptoms that require treatment may be large, co-morbidity is common, and often the patient is elderly. Several organ systems may be impaired from advanced disease, with hepatic and renal impairment significantly affecting the ability to metabolize and eliminate medications. Polypharmacy is inevitable; the risks of adverse medication events and drug interactions are high, and there are potential adherence issues. Many therapies are outside the approved drug license, creating issues for health care providers and patients, who require information about the therapy prescribed.

The decision about any particular therapy must be made using the best available evidence and an individual approach, considering the specific characteristics that may affect therapeutic outcomes. These include co-morbidities, concurrent therapies, renal and hepatic dysfunction, and patient expectations (see Chapters 125 and 126).

Appropriate prescribing includes not only initiation of drug therapy but also integration of that therapy with existing treatments. The cornerstone is the completion of an accurate and comprehensive drug history. This must include prescription medicines, nonprescription medicines (e.g., OTC medicines), complementary and alternative therapies, previous adverse drug reactions (including allergies), and assessment of adherence (see "Medication Adherence").

The patient or carer is a key source. An effective technique is to ask patients to bring all medications with them when they come for an appointment. All medications used should be requested, including prescription, OTC, and complementary and alternative medications. If the patient is not responsible for medication administration or a reliable medication history cannot be obtained from the patient or carer, then alternative sources must be identified. These may include other health professionals, medication dispensing information, and medication lists.

Good communication is essential for effective rapport. Open-ended questions allow assessment of the knowledge and understanding of medications being used. Asking nonjudgmentally, but explicitly, how often and in what doses the patient takes the medications determines medication-taking practices, indicates the adherence to the prescribed regimen, and identifies possible medication-related adverse effects.

POLYPHARMACY

Definition of Polypharmacy

The term polypharmacy indicates concurrent use of many medications.[1] It may be associated with the use of many drugs (appropriately) or too many drugs (inappropriately).[2] So-called rational polypharmacy is a legitimate practice resulting from the range of therapeutic options for multiple concurrent illnesses and symptoms. Indiscriminate polypharmacy is a leading cause of hospitalization and adverse outcomes. Risk factors for inappropriate polypharmacy include multiple prescribers, multiple dispensing pharmacies, general frailty, and being elderly. This is complicated by the use of self-prescribed OTC medications, continuing medications prescribed for a previous illness, or taking medications prescribed for someone else. (See also Part II Section C.)

Prevalence of Polypharmacy

There is little research into polypharmacy in palliative medicine.[3,4] North American data indicate that polypharmacy is common in the elderly, with more than 40% of persons aged 65 years or older using five or more different medications each week, and 12% using 10 or more different medications.[5] Similar results were reported in Finland[6] and in Australia,[7] where an average of 3.8 and 5.2 medications, respectively, were in current use by elderly community-dwelling patients. Polypharmacy occurs even more often among hospitalized patients and inhabitants of residential care facilities.

Issues Associated with Polypharmacy

Use of a larger number of medications is associated with a higher risk of drug-drug interactions, more adverse effects due to medication, and less adherence to the intended medication regimen.[8,9] Medication-induced symptoms can produce "prescribing cascades" due to the use of additional medications.[8] The likelihood of clinically significant *drug interactions* is greatest for patients who are taking more than six medications. Twenty percent of community-dwelling palliative medicine patients and 50% of hospice inpatients were found to have received at least one pair of interacting drugs that could have caused clinically important interactions.[9,10] Vigilance is required to identify potentially serious drug interactions, even in terminal care, to ensure that therapy is not compromised, and to reduce unnecessary distress for patients and their carers.

Inappropriate polypharmacy exposes patients to unnecessary *adverse effects*. The elderly and frail are at increased risk because of their less effective metabolism and renal excretion of multiple medications. Many adverse effects are predictable and preventable,[11] and many are caused by inadequate or absent preventive measures (e.g., laxatives with opiates, or antinauseants with chemotherapy). In addition, the elderly may be more likely to suffer cognitive and sensory impairment, which can increase medication errors, a major cause of morbidity and mortality.[12]

Polypharmacy is associated with more *nonadherence* to the medication regimen and, consequently, with poor outcomes (see "Medication Adherence"). The total "tablet burden"—that is, the total number of tablets taken each day and the frequency of dosing—increases complexity, making unintentional nonadherence almost unavoidable.

Reducing the Risks of Polypharmacy

Polypharmacy—if appropriate, safe, and efficacious—is not inherently wrong. However, therapy must be tailored to the specific needs of the individual patient. Multidisciplinary interventions in which clinical pharmacists interview patients and specifically review medication outcomes and adverse events or focus on high-risk drug groups are effective in reducing polypharmacy, improving medication safety, and lowering costs.[13] Targeting high-risk drugs is more effective than a general goal of reducing polypharmacy for those patients taking multiple medications.[13] Sometimes, such reviews actually identify underutilization of appropriate medications and failure to treat, resulting in additional medication.[14] One observational study determined that, although the median number of medications prescribed before and after referral to a palliative care service was unchanged, there was more prescribing of laxatives, but no change in other regularly administered medications.[3]

Therapy rationalization and medication review may be appropriate at any time point in an illness. It is particularly pertinent at transition points in an illness and when changes in goals of care are occurring.

Several strategies may be employed to improve outcomes and reduce polypharmacy[15]:

- Ensure that a current and accurate list of all medications is obtained. Document exactly how the patient is taking each medication, with specific dosage and frequency, to identify adherence issues.
- Establish the indication and intended duration of use of each medication, including identification of the original prescriber.
- A high index of suspicion will identify any adverse drug reactions. Be aware that adverse effects may present atypically in the elderly and the frail.
- Simplify the medication regimen by targeting medications for cessation, substitution, or dose reduction. It is essential to engage the patient and carers in this process.

A plan for "deprescribing" is recommended.[15] Attention should be specifically focused on medications that present a high risk of medication misadventure and are not improving the patient's health; are causing adverse effects; are not currently being used; or are being used irregularly for non–life-threatening conditions. Deprescribing should be planned and conducted in partnership with the patient and carers. Good communication about the reasons for medication withdrawal enables the patient to give assent. In most circumstances, it is preferable to withdraw medications sequentially and gradually, especially if withdrawal effects may be anticipated.

The overall medication regimen should be examined and simplified, aiming for once- or twice-daily dosing, including the use of slow-release or controlled-release medications, where possible, to maximize adherence. Alternative routes of administration, such as the transdermal route, may be helpful. In addition, it is appropriate to critically review therapies for chronic diseases that may be unnecessary in light of realistic prognosis. Many drugs may be safely stopped near the end of life. Drugs such as statins provide little benefit for people with a very poor prognosis.

MEDICATION ADHERENCE

Adherence to (or compliance with) a medication regimen is defined as the extent to which the patient takes the medications as prescribed.[16] Long-term medication adherence for various disease conditions in various settings converges to approximately 50%.[17] Nonadherence to treatment recommendations contributes to morbidity and mortality, increased economic costs, and waste of resources.

Assessing Adherence

Patients may not readily divulge nonadherence, and many agree that they would discontinue a medication without speaking to their physician.[18] There are various techniques to estimate adherence. One of the simplest is to enter into a nonjudgmental discussion with the patient or carer about medication-taking behaviors and barriers to effective disease management. Indicators of potentially inadequate adherence include poor or inaccurate knowledge of frequency of use, excess medication remaining since last dispensing, expired medication, and inadequate therapeutic response.[15] A simple tool[19] enables the prescriber to identify adherence issues. Using the Self-Reported Medication-Taking Scale, the patient answers "Yes" (score = 0) or "No" (score = 1) to the following questions:

1. Do you ever forget to take your medication?
2. Are you careless at times about taking your medication?
3. When you feel better, do you sometimes stop taking your medication?
4. Sometimes, if you feel worse when you take the medicine, do you stop taking it?

Answering "Yes" to none of the questions indicates high adherence, answering "Yes" to one or two questions indicates moderate adherence, and answering "Yes" to three or four questions indicates low adherence. There are reliability limitations to patient or carer self-reports of adherence, due to recall bias and the social desirability to provide the response the patient perceives the clinician "wishes" to hear. More complex tools are available but are usually impractical in routine clinical practice.

Interventions to Improve Adherence

Improving adherence and consequent health outcomes in chronic disease is complex and inadequately researched. The "current methods of improving adherence . . . are mostly complex and not very effective, so that the full benefits of treatment cannot be realized."[20] Some strategies improve adherence and treatment outcomes. Simplifying the treatment regimen can be effective. Use of fewer medications and/or less frequent administration (e.g., slow-release preparations) is a successful method to improve adherence (see "Reducing the Risks of Polypharmacy"). Other adherence interventions that improve health outcomes rely on more frequent interaction with patients, with attention to adherence. Involving the patient in medical decisions and in monitoring his or her own care may enhance adherence. Appropriate education ensures understanding of the rationale for each medication, precisely how and when to take it, the expected side effects and their management, and the expected duration of treatment.[21] A frank discussion about treatment perceptions, involving family members for support and reinforcement, helps, as does use of compliance tools such as medication lists and multicompartment medication-compliance devices. Efforts to improve adherence must be maintained for as long as the treatment is needed.

OFF-LABEL AND UNLICENSED MEDICINES

Definition of Off-Label Prescribing

The term *off-label* (unlabeled or unapproved) prescribing describes the use of a medicine in a manner different from that recommended by the manufacturer in the product license (or approved product information).[22] Medications are used off-label for several reasons and may involve an unapproved indication, dose, route of administration, or patient age range. An *unlicensed* (or unregistered) medicine refers to a medicine that has not been evaluated or approved for marketing by the applicable regulatory authority.

When a product license is granted, it includes only those indications, doses, patient groups, and other specifications that were included in the manufacturer's submission and reviewed by the regulatory authority. Consequently, the regulatory approval may not encompass all evidence-based uses for the particular drug. Evidence-based uses may not be included in a product license for many reasons. There is also a significant time lag between the publication of new medical research and incorporation of this information into the license. The manufacturer may consider the cost of incorporating new information into the license to be prohibitive, especially if the market for the new use is not large, if the product is old, or if the knowledge of such new use has already been adequately promulgated.

In some areas of clinical practice, off-label, yet evidence-based, prescribing may be more appropriate than that detailed in the product license.[23] In contrast, a recent large survey of off-label prescriptions in the United States suggested that only about one quarter of off-label prescribing is justified by scientific evidence.[24]

Importantly, the licensing process regulates pharmaceutical companies and not doctors' prescribing practices. Legislation preserves a doctor's clinical freedom. Off-label prescribing is therefore legal, and medications prescribed off-label may be dispensed by pharmacists and administered by nurses. This said, when prescribing a medicine off-label, one must accept an increased level of responsibility. The prescriber must be willing to defend the practice as "reasonable" and in line with accepted practice and/or published evidence. In palliative medicine, quantitative clinical research is often lacking; in these circumstances, consensus among respected peers should be the minimum standard of evidence.

An algorithm provides a systematic approach for evaluating the appropriateness of any proposed off-label use (Fig. 123-1).[25] The decision algorithm is a structure aimed at answering the following question: "Is there high-quality evidence supporting the proposed off-label use?" In general, the rigor required to justify prescribing should resemble that used by regulatory bodies in the evaluation

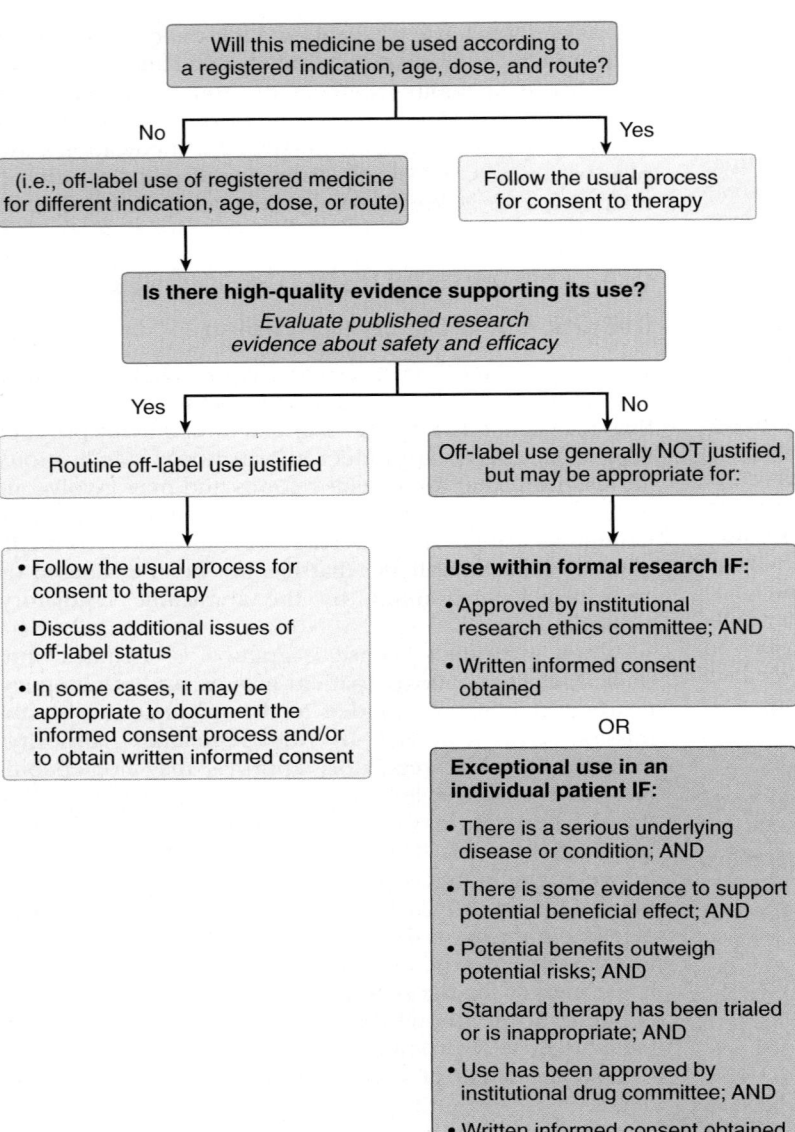

FIGURE 123-1. Algorithm to assess the appropriateness of off-label uses of medicines. *(From Gazarian M, Kelly M, McPhee J, et al. Off-label use of medicines: Consensus recommendations for evaluating appropriateness. Med J Aust 2006;185:544-548.)*

of a medicine submitted for registration approval. Routine off-label use can be justified if there is high-quality evidence supporting efficacy and sufficient evidence about safety to suggest an overall reasonable benefit-risk ratio for a given clinical context.[25] It is vital that the drug safety profile be considered, in addition to efficacy data, and then weighed against the seriousness of the condition being treated. Generally, off-label use would not be justified for "trivial" or less serious illness or if high-quality evidence were not available.[26]

Prevalence of Off-Label Use

Off-label prescribing is frequent in many areas, particularly pediatrics and psychiatric medicine, for patients with infectious diseases, in pregnancy, and in oncology and palliative medicine. There are limited data concerning off-label prescribing in palliative medicine, even though it is common. In specialist palliative care units in the United

Kingdom, approximately one quarter of medications are prescribed off-label. Medications are used for unlicensed indications in about 15% of cases and are administered by an unapproved route in approximately 11% of prescriptions.[27,28] Similar rates of off-label prescribing were identified in Australian oncology, including palliative medicine, in which 22% of prescriptions were either off-label (18%) or unlicensed (4%). Eighty-five percent of patients received at least one drug that was prescribed off-label or was unlicensed.[29] A large study in the United States revealed that 33% of chemotherapy treatments, including hormonal therapy, were off-label.[30] More than half of the patients (56%) received at least one off-label drug.

One of the frequently reported reasons for off-label prescribing in palliative medicine is the regular use of medicines by unapproved routes of administration, particularly the subcutaneous route,[27,28] and the delivery of other medications via inhalation for dyspnea or cough.[31]

Issues Associated with Off-Label and Unlicensed Drug Use

Frequent off-label prescribing in cancer therapy, and specifically in palliative care, poses added difficulties to an already complex medication regimen. Patients, particularly children, who are exposed to off-label medication use are at a higher risk of *adverse drug reactions*.[32] This may be due to the lack of systematically reviewed evidence of both safety and efficacy.

Although obtaining *informed consent* is not a legal requirement, it has been suggested that written informed consent be obtained when medications are prescribed off-label.[25] This may be impractical if off-label prescribing occurs extensively, and the process of obtaining consent may cause unnecessary alarm.[26,33]

Adequate information about medicines prescribed off-label, including indications for use and adverse effects, should be provided to patients and carers. This is particularly important because the patient information leaflet provided by the manufacturer will not contain information about unlicensed use and may contain explicit contraindications about the intended use.

Consideration must be given to the *availability and cost* of off-label and unlicensed medicines. Funding agencies, including health insurance companies and government medication funding schemes, may be reluctant to fund therapies that have not been subjected to the registration process, so cost implications to the patient must be considered.

REFERENCES

1. Finke B, Snyder K, Cantillon C, et al. Three complementary definitions of polypharmacy: Methods, application and comparison of findings in a large prescription database. Pharmacoepidemiol Drug Saf 2005;14:121-128.
2. Aronson JK. In defence of polypharmacy. Br J Clin Pharmacol 2004; 57:119-120.
3. Koh NY, Koo WH. Polypharmacy in palliative care: Can it be reduced? Singapore Med J 2002;43:279-283.
4. Twycross R, Bergl S, John S, Lewis K. Monitoring drug use in palliative care. Palliative Med 1994;8:137-143.
5. Kaufman D, Kelly J, Rosenberg L, et al. Recent patterns of medication use in the ambulatory adult population of the United States: The Slone Survey. JAMA 2002;287:337-344.
6. Linjakumpu T, Hartikainen S, Klaukka T, et al. Use of medications and polypharmacy are increasing among the elderly. J Clin Epidemiol 2002;55:809-817.
7. Atkin P, Shenfield GM. How many medications do elderly patients really take? Aust J Hosp Pharm 1993;23:109-113.
8. Rochon P, Gurwitz J. Optimising drug treatment for elderly people: The prescribing cascade. BMJ 1997;315:1096-1099.
9. Wilcock A, Thomas J, Frisby J, et al. Potential for drug interactions involving cytochrome P450 in patients attending palliative care centres: A multicentre audit. Br J Clin Pharmacol 2005;60:326-329.
10. Regnard C, Hunter A. Increased prescriber awareness of drug interactions in pall care. J Pain Symptom Manage 2005;29:219-221.
11. Lau PM, Stewart K, Dooley M. The ten most common adverse drug reactions (ADRs) in oncology patients: Do they matter to you? Support Care Cancer 2004;12:626-633.
12. Bedell S, Jabbour S, Goldberg R, et al. Discrepancies in the use of medications: Their extent and predictors in the outpatient practice. Arch Intern Med 2000;160:2129-2134.
13. Zarowitz BJ, Stebelsky LA, Muma BK, et al. Reduction of high-risk polypharmacy drug combinations in patients in a managed care setting. Pharmacotherapy 2005;25:1636-1645.
14. Sloane P, Gruber-Baldini A, Zimmerman S, et al. Medication undertreatment in assisted living settings. Arch Intern Med 2004;164:2031-2037.
15. Woodward MC. Deprescribing: Achieving better health outcomes for older people through reducing medications. J Pharm Pract Res 2003;33:323-328.
16. Osterberg L, Blaschke T. Adherence to medication. N Engl J Med 2005;353:487-497.
17. Sackett D, Snow J. The Magnitude of Compliance and Non-compliance. Baltimore: Johns Hopkins University Press, 1979.
18. Kirking D, Lee J, Ellis J, et al. Patient-reported underuse of prescription medications: A comparison of nine surveys. Med Care Res Rev 2006;63:427-446.
19. Morisky D, Green L, Levine D. Concurrent and predictive validity of a self-reported measure of medication adherence. Med Care 1986;24:67-74.
20. Haynes R, Yao X, Degani A, et al. Interventions for enhancing medication adherence (review). Cochrane Database of Systematic Reviews 2005;(4): CD000011.
21. Tarn D, Heritage J, Paterniti D, et al. Physician communication when prescribing new medications. Arch Intern Med 2006;166:1855-1862.
22. Turner S, Nunn A, Choonara I. Unlicenced drug use in children in the UK. Paed Perinatal Drug Ther 1997;1:52-55.
23. Boos J. Off label use—Label off use? Ann Oncol 2003;14:1-5.
24. Radley D, Finkelstein S, Stafford R. Off-label prescribing among office-based physicians. Arch Intern Med 2006;166:1021-1026.
25. Gazarian M, Kelly M, McPhee J, et al. Off-label use of medicines: Consensus recommendations for evaluating appropriateness. Med J Aust 2006;185: 544-548.
26. Twycross R, Wilcock A, Thorp S. Palliative Care Formulary, 1st ed. Oxford: Radcliffe Medical Press, 1998.
27. Atkinson C, Kirkham S. Unlicensed uses for medication in a palliative care unit. Palliat Med 1999;13:145-152.
28. Todd J, Davies A. Use of unlicensed medication in palliative medicine. Palliat Med 1999;13:446.
29. Poole S, Dooley M. Off-label prescribing in oncology. Support Care Cancer 2004;12:302-305.
30. Off-label Drugs: Reimbursement Policies Constrain Physicians in Their Choice of Cancer Therapies. United States General Accounting Office Report to the Chairman, Committee on Labor and Human Resources, US Senate. (GAO/PEMD-91-14). Washington, DC: GAO, September 1991.
31. Shirk M, Donahue K, Shirvani J. Unlabeled uses of nebulized medications. Am J Health Syst Pharm 2006;63:1704-1716.
32. Horen B, Montastruc J, Lapeyre-Mestre M. Adverse drug reactions and off-label drug use in paediatric outpatients. Br J Clin Pharmacol 2002;54:665-670.
33. Pavis H, Wilcock A. Prescribing of drugs for use outside their licence in palliative care: Survey of specialists in the United Kingdom. BMJ 2001;323:484-485.

SUGGESTED READING

de Vries TPGM, Henning RH, Hogerzeil HV, Fresle DA. Guide to Good Prescribing: A Practical Manual. Geneva: World Health Organization, 1994. Available at http://whqlibdoc.who.int/hq/1994/WHO_DAP_94.11.pdf (accessed December 12, 2007).

Sabate E. Adherence to Long-Term Therapies: Evidence in Action. Geneva: World Health Organization, 2003. Available at http://www.emro.who.int/ncd/Publications/adherence_report.pdf (accessed December 12, 2007).

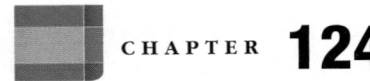

CHAPTER **124**

Interactions, Side Effects, and Management

Randy D. Miller, Kirk V. Shepard, and Edwin D. Dickerson

K E Y   P O I N T S

- Drug interactions typically result in an accentuated or diminished drug effect. Frequently, drug interactions involve increases or decreases in drug metabolism. Drug interactions may be dose dependent or dose independent and may result from a metabolite or by-product rather than from the parent compound.

- Although other drug-drug interactions may occur, most pharmacokinetic drug interactions are a result of altered metabolism by hepatic microenzymes. The cytochrome P-450 (CYP) enzymes lie on the rough and smooth endoplasmic reticula in hepatocytes and also in the intestinal mucosa (CYP3A4), brain (CYP2D6), and kidney (CYP3A5).

- A drug that inhibits the activity of a specific enzyme can block the metabolism of drugs that are substrates of that enzyme.

- Although inhibitors and inducers do not always yield clinically significant drug interactions with substrates, caution should be exercised when prescribing drugs that are known to present the possibility of a drug interaction when used concomitantly.

- There are seven desirable characteristics to consider when choosing the most appropriate drug for symptom management. These include (1) a single drug for multiple therapeutic benefits, (2) minimal drug interactions, (3) versatility with multiple routes of administration, (4) wide therapeutic window, (5) cost, (6) dosing schedule; and (7) dose response and a high to nonexistent therapeutic ceiling.

Throughout disease progression, cancer patients have on average 12 or more symptoms at any given time.[1-6] These may include anorexia, asthenia, constipation, cough, depression, dyspnea, insomnia, nausea, pain, vomiting, and xerostomia. Although the goal of symptom management in palliative care is to control, relieve, or eliminate symptoms primarily via pharmacological therapy, it is paramount to minimize polypharmacy to avoid the pharmacotherapeutic paradigm of "one symptom, one drug." It is not uncommon for patients to be taking several opioids or benzodiazepines or antiemetics at one time. Frequently, multiple antiemetics are prescribed simultaneously, although, in reality, only 33% of patients with advanced disease require more than one antiemetic.[7] The challenge to health care providers is to provide practical solutions to this growing problem.

One study of prescribing patterns in patients with advanced cancer found a median of five medications given for symptom management.[8] Another concluded that symptoms were indeed best managed with a limited number of drugs.[9] However, it is common practice for cancer patients with advanced disease to be on a regimen of up to 12 or more drugs. This may reflect of the number of corresponding symptoms these patients endure.

The percentage of patients in whom drug interactions are reported increases exponentially as the number of coadministered drugs increases. The most dramatic increase is noticed when more than five drugs are given. Reports indicate that almost all patients are at risk for drug interactions when nine or more drugs are coadministered. An estimated four different potential interactions can occur when 10 drugs are coadministered; 10 different interactions may occur when more than 12 drugs are administered together (Fig. 124-1).[10]

PRINCIPLES OF DRUG INTERACTIONS

Drug interactions occur through alterations in pharmacokinetics or pharmacodynamics of one drug when combined with a second. Although drug interactions can be beneficial, most tend to be harmful. Drug interactions typically result in an accentuated or diminished drug effect. Frequently, drug interactions involve increases or decreases in drug metabolism. Drug interactions may be dose dependent or dose independent and may result from a metabolite or by-product rather than from the parent compound. End-organ dysfunction (i.e., renal and hepatic failure) affects many end-stage cancer patients and frequently increases the risk of drug interactions. This is especially important with the use of certain drugs that have a narrow therapeutic window of efficacy. Impairment in organ function increases the risk for adverse drug reactions.

PHARMACOKINETIC DRUG INTERACTIONS

Pharmacokinetics is the movement of drugs within biological systems, including uptake, distribution, binding, elimination, and biotransformation. Before a combination of medications is prescribed, variables that potentially influence interactions must be carefully evaluated. Variables in the cancer patient population include rates of

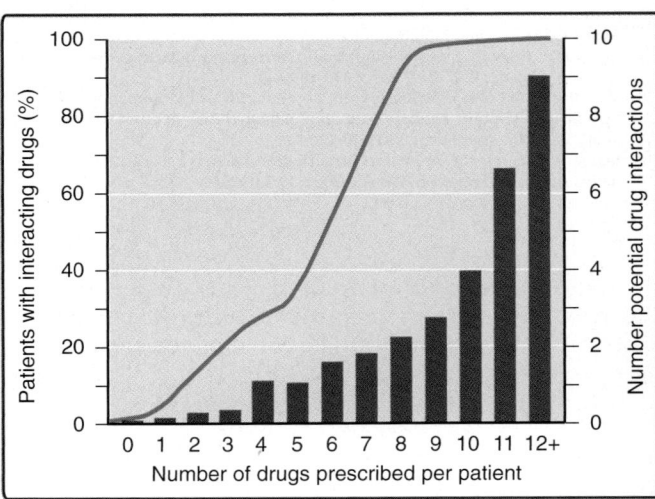

FIGURE 124-1 Drug interactions. *(From Schwartz JB. Clinical pharmacology. In Hazzard WR, Blass JP, Ettinger WH Jr, et al. [eds]. Principles of Geriatric Medicine and Gerontology, 4th ed. New York: McGraw-Hill, 1999, pp 303-331.)*

metabolism, presence of the other disease states, diet, age, race, and drug dose. Pharmacogenetic variability may influence drug metabolism. Although issues of absorption and binding have been linked to drug interactions, attention has recently shifted to the role of the drug-metabolizing enzymes in the liver and other organ sites. The cytochrome P-450 (CYP) system is the major site of most drug metabolism. As this system has been further elucidated, the potential to predict drug interactions has increased.[7]

The Cytochrome P-450 System

Although other drug-drug interactions may occur, most pharmacokinetic drug interactions are a result of altered metabolism by hepatic microenzymes. The CYP enzymes lie on the rough and smooth endoplasmic reticula in hepatocytes and also in the intestinal mucosa (CYP3A4), brain (CYP2D6), and kidney (CYP3A5).[11]

The CYP system consists of more than 20 families of isoenzymes.[11,12] Isoenzymes are a group of enzymes that catalyze the same reaction but may be differentiated by variations in physical properties, such as isoelectric point, electrophoretic mobility, kinetic parameters, or modes of regulation. More than 150 drugs are metabolized by subfamilies of the CYP system.[13] Individual drugs may be metabolized by more than one isoenzyme.[14]

The isoenzymes that are most important in drug metabolism are CYP1A2, CYP2C9, CYP2C19, CYP2D6, and CYP3A4.[14] The CYP3A4 group accounts for approximately 40% to 60% of total hepatic CYP isoenzymes and is responsible for the metabolism of several drug classes. CYP3A4 has been implicated in most CYP-450 drug interactions.[11,15-18] Certain enzymes, particularly CYP2C19 and CYP2D6, may be polymorphically expressed. This means that more than one form of the drug-metabolizing enzyme may be present in a population, a fact that has obvious potential impact on how particular drugs are metabolized within that population. For example, the CYP2D6 poor-metabolizer (PM) phenotype is found in approximately 5% to 10% of Caucasians and North Americans of African descent, and in 1% to 2% of Asians.[19] Individuals with the PM phenotype for CYP2D6 may not efficiently metabolize several important drugs, leading to a greater propensity for adverse drug interactions. Examples of drugs that might be affected by the CYP2D6 PM phenotype are amiodarone, cimetidine, haloperidol, quinidine, selective serotonin reuptake inhibitors, thioridazine, and tramadol.[20]

Over the past several years, the importance of genetic polymorphism has become increasingly apparent as scientists have discovered genetically determined variations in drug response. Because the CYP system is important in the metabolism of many drugs, a general knowledge of the major isoenzymes involved in drug metabolism is essential for optimal prescribing and monitoring of patient therapy. Exhaustive, in-depth knowledge of all of the CYP isoenzymes may not be a practical or useful goal for clinicians, because of the constant identification of new information in this dynamic and expansive area of medicine. Despite the complexity, a general understanding of the concepts can be applied to the evaluation of potential interactions that may be encountered in palliative care.

Therapeutic Effect

The substance that is acted upon and changed by an enzyme is known as a *substrate* (Table 124-1A). *Inhibitor* drugs inhibit the activity of a specific enzyme and can block the metabolism of drugs that are substrates of that enzyme (see Table 124-1B). If the body lacks other modalities to excrete these substrate drugs, they can accumulate and potentially lead to toxicity. *Inducer* drugs induce the activity of a specific enzyme and can stimulate the metabolism of drugs that are substrates of that enzyme (see Table 124-1C). This can lead to decreased blood levels of these drugs and could result in suboptimal efficacy.[19] Onset and termination of increased enzyme activity are closely related to the plasma concentration and half-life of the inducing drug.

Although inhibitors and inducers do not always yield clinically significant drug interactions with substrates, caution should be exercised when prescribing drugs that are known to present the possibility of a drug interaction when used concomitantly. For example, if a drug is administered to an extensive metabolizer, there may be undertreatment due to suboptimal drug levels. On the other hand, if a drug is administered to a slow metabolizer, there may be overtreatment due to impaired metabolism of the parent drug. This can lead to accumulation of the drug and may result in supratherapeutic or toxic levels.

As noted, drugs often influence more than one enzyme site (i.e., through the actions of the parent drug and/or its metabolites). Because patient characteristics are unique, not all patients who are given a particular drug combination will have a drug interaction. Moreover, some interactions may be mild with no dosage change needed, whereas others may be severe and require drug discontinuation. Interactions involving the CYP system are complex and multifactorial. They may be influenced by patient-specific factors such as genetics, age, nutrition, stress, and hepatic disease, as well as drug-related factors such as dose, route, duration of therapy, therapeutic index, and metabolic pathway.[21]

Knowledge in this area continues to evolve, and clinicians must attempt to stay up to date. To facilitate the identification of potential drug interactions, tables containing information on known or potential interactions involving CYP isoenzymes can be consulted (see Table 124-1). Lists of this type can serve as reference guides only and may become quickly outdated. Therefore, professional judgment and consultation with regularly updated on-line resources (e.g., MICROMEDEX, UptoDate) are recommended before clinical judgments are made in specific clinical situations.

PHARMACODYNAMIC DRUG INTERACTIONS

Pharmacodynamic drug interactions involve competition at receptor sites; however, drug metabolism remains unaltered. A common pharmacodynamic drug-drug interaction occurs between an antimuscarinic (anticholinergic) and a prokinetic drug. When these drugs are prescribed concurrently, the final pathway for the prokinetic drug (e.g., metoclopramide) is the cholinergic receptor in the myenteric plexus, but the antimuscarinic drug blocks the same receptor. Hence, the antimuscarinic drug

TABLE 124-1   Cytochrome P-450 System (CYP) Drug Interactions*

ISOENZYME	EXAMPLES
A. SUBSTRATES OF CYP ISOENZYMES	
1A2	Amitriptyline, caffeine, clomipramine, clozapine, cyclobenzaprine, grepafloxacin, imipramine, mirtazapine, olanzapine, propranolol, riluzole, ropinirole, R-warfarin, tacrine, theophylline, zileuton
2C9	Amitriptyline, carvedilol, celecoxib, diclofenac, flurbiprofen, fluvastatin, glimepiride, ibuprofen, imipramine, irbesartan, losartan, montelukast, naproxen, phenytoin, piroxicam, tolbutamide, torsemide, S-warfarin, zafirlukast
2C19	Amitriptyline, citalopram, clomipramine, diazepam, imipramine, lansoprazole, mephenytoin, omeprazole, pentamidine, phenytoin, propranolol, R-warfarin
2D6	Amitriptyline, captopril, carvedilol, chlorpromazine, clomipramine, clozapine, codeine, desipramine, dextromethorphan, dihydrocodeine, encainide, flecainide, fluoxetine, haloperidol, hydrocodone, imipramine, loratadine, maprotiline, methamphetamine, metoprolol, mexiletine, mirtazapine, nortriptyline, ondansetron, oxycodone, paroxetine, perphenazine, propafenone, propranolol, risperidone, ritonavir, sertraline, thioridazine, timolol, tolterodine, tramadol, trazodone, venlafaxine
3A4	Acetaminophen, alfentanil, alprazolam, amitriptyline, amlodipine, amprenavir, astemizole, atorvastatin, bepridil, buspirone, carbamazepine, cerivastatin, cisapride, citalopram, clarithromycin, clomipramine, cyclophosphamide, cyclosporine, dapsone, delavirdine, dexamethasone, diazepam, diltiazem, disopyramide, donepezil, doxorubicin, efavirenz, erythromycin, ethinyl estradiol, etoposide, felodipine, fentanyl, finasteride, ifosfamide, imipramine, indinavir, isradipine, itraconazole, ketoconazole, lansoprazole, lidocaine, loratadine, losartan, lovastatin, midazolam, mirtazapine, montelukast, nefazodone, nelfinavir, nicardipine, nifedipine, nimodipine, nisoldipine, paclitaxel, pimozide, prednisone, propafenone, quetiapine, quinidine, quinine, repaglinide, rifabutin, ritonavir, saquinavir, sertraline, sibutramine, sildenafil, simvastatin, sufentanil, tacrolimus, tamoxifen, terfenadine, testosterone, tolterodine, toremifene, triazolam, troleandomycin, verapamil, vinblastine, vincristine, R-warfarin, zileuton, zolpidem
B. DOCUMENTED INHIBITORS OF CYP ISOENZYMES	
1A2	Cimetidine, ciprofloxacin, diltiazem, enoxacin, erythromycin, fluoxetine, fluvoxamine, grapefruit juice, mexiletine, norfloxacin, paroxetine, sertraline, tacrine, verapamil, zileuton
2C9	Amiodarone, cimetidine, fluconazole, fluvastatin, metronidazole, miconazole, ritonavir, sulfamethoxazole, trimethoprim, zafirlukast, zileuton
2C19	Felbamate, fluoxetine, fluvoxamine, ketoconazole, omeprazole
2D6	Amiodarone, cimetidine, fluoxetine, fluvoxamine, haloperidol, paroxetine, propafenone, quinidine, sertraline, thioridazine, tramadol
3A4	Bromocriptine, cimetidine, clarithromycin, cyclosporine, danazol, diltiazem, erythromycin, ergotamine, ethinyl estradiol, fluconazole, fluoxetine, fluvoxamine, gestodene, grapefruit juice, indanivir, itraconazole, ketoconazole, miconazole, midazolam, nefazodone, nicardipine, nifedipine, omeprazole, paroxetine, progesterone, propoxyphene, quinidine, ritonavir, sertraline, testosterone, troleandomycin, verapamil, zafirlukast, zileutin
C. DOCUMENTED INDUCERS OF CYP ISOENZYMES	
1A2	Amobarbital, butabarbital, charcoal-broiled beef, cigarette smoke, cruciferous vegetables, mephobarbital, omeprazole, pentobarbital, phenobarbital, phenytoin, secobarbital
2C9	Amobarbital, butabarbital, carbamazepine, mephobarbital, pentobarbital, rifampin, rifapentine, secobarbital
2C19	Phenytoin, rifampin
2D6	None identified
3A4	Amobarbital, butabarbital, carbamazepine, dexamethasone, efavirenz, ethosuximide, griseofulvin, mephobarbital, nafcillin, pentobarbital, phenobarbital, phenytoin, primidone, rifabutin, rifampin, rifapentine, secobarbital, troglitazone

*Note that these tables represent a compilation of dynamic/changing information and can function as a guide only. Clinicians should use appropriate clinical judgment and consult recent references in the evaluation of individual cases.

competitively diminishes the therapeutic benefit of the prokinetic.[22]

Principles of Drug Therapy

The total number of drugs for symptom control should be kept to a minimum. Polypharmacy may increase the frequency of drug interactions, which may mimic the progression of the underlying disease. Ideally, one drug can be used to treat multiple symptoms, decreasing the frequency of drug-drug interactions. Limiting the number of drugs to essential drug classes while maintaining effective symptom management also improves pharmacoeconomics and cost-effectiveness.[8] In palliative care, skillful prescribing often makes the difference between poor and excellent symptom control.[23]

Portmanteau

There are seven desirable characteristics to consider when choosing the most appropriate drug for symptom management: (1) a single drug for multiple therapeutic benefits, (2) minimal drug interactions, (3) versatility with multiple routes of administration, (4) wide therapeutic window, (5) cost, (6) dosing schedule, and (7) dose response and a high to nonexistent therapeutic ceiling. Every effort should be made to use a single drug for multiple symptoms in order to minimize medications.[24] Many drugs palliate more than one symptom. Administration of such drugs is known as *portmanteau.*

In palliative medicine, a portmanteau drug is one that is used to treat several additional symptoms adjuvant to its primary intended use. Among the drugs that are considered essential in palliative care (Table 124-2),

TABLE 124-2   Twenty-Five Essential Drugs in Palliative Care

DRUG	THERAPEUTIC CLASS
Morphine (normal-release)	Opioid
Haloperidol	Antipsychotic
Metoclopramide	Antiemetic
Dexamethasone	Corticosteroid
Morphine (controlled-release)	Opioid
Amitriptyline	Antidepressant
Midazolam	Benzodiazepine
Lactulose	Laxative
Paracetamol (acetaminophen)	Nonopioid
Methadone	Opioid
Hyoscine butyl (glycopyrrolate)	Antispasmodic
Transdermal fentanyl	Opioid
Senna	Laxative
Diclofenac	Nonopioid
Clonazepam	Anticonvulsant
Megestrol acetate	Progestin
Diazepam	Benzodiazepine
Codeine	Opioid
Nystatin	Antifungal
Tramadol	Opioid
Cyclizine (meclizine)	Antihistamine
Ibuprofen	Nonopioid
Prednisone	Corticosteroid
Ranitidine	Histamine$_2$ antagonist
Docusate sodium	Laxative
Methylphenidate	Psychostimulant

Adapted from Dickerson ED. The 20 essential drugs in palliative care. Eur J Palliat Care 1999;6:130-135.

the top 7 are capable of treating 14 common symptoms.[24] Properly applied, portmanteau has the additional advantage of minimizing drug interactions and maximizing effective symptom management while improving compliance. Portmanteau reflects skilled prescribing and clinical experience. It also reduces medication errors and provides a psychological benefit by limiting the burden of multiple medications consumed by the patient.

CONCLUSION

Whereas a benchmark of five to seven drugs may be considered ideal in the treatment of symptoms associated with advanced disease, a 15% to 20% chance of a drug interaction still exists at this level of polypharmacy. As more drugs are added to the therapeutic regimen, the frequency of drug interactions also increases.

To minimize or avoid interactions of this nature, it is imperative that the clinician be well informed with regard to the pharmacokinetics and pharmacodynamics of each drug in the pharmacological regimen. Although multiple clinical case reports may provide the best early evidence that concurrent use of two drugs may have unintended or adverse consequences, reference to the CYP isoenzymes may uncover relationships between drugs and metaboliz-ing enzymes that help predict potential drug interactions. Understanding and careful attention to the complexities of the CYP system improve clinical evaluation and help optimize pharmacotherapeutic regimens.

REFERENCES

1. Twycross RG, Lack SA. Symptom Control in Advanced Cancer: Alimentary Symptoms. London: Pitman, 1986.
2. Ventafridda V, DeConno F, Ripamonti C, et al. Quality-of-life assessment during a palliative care programme. Ann Oncol 1990;1:415-420.
3. Portenoy RK, Thaler HT, Kornblith AB, et al. Symptom prevalence, characteristics and distress in a cancer population. Qual Life Res 1994;3:183-189.
4. Seamark DA, Lawrence C, Gilbert J. Characteristics of referrals to an inpatient hospice and a survey of general practioner perceptions of palliative care. J R Soc Med 1996;89:79-84.
5. Ng K, von Gunten CF. Symptoms and attitudes of 100 consecutive patients admitted to an acute hospice/palliative care unit. J Pain Symptom Manage 1998;16:307-316.
6. Walsh D, Donnelly L, Rybicki L. The symptoms of advanced cancer: Relationship to age, gender, and performance status in 1,000 patients. Support Care Cancer 2000;8:175-179.
7. Twycross R. Introducing Palliative Care, 3rd ed. Oxford: Radcliffe Medical Press, 1999, p 116.
8. Curtis EB, Walsh TD. Prescribing practices of a palliative care service. J Pain Symptom Manage 1993;8:312-316.
9. Walsh TD, West TS. Controlling symptoms in advanced cancer. BMJ 1998;296:477-481.
10. Schwartz JB. Clinical pharmacology. In Hazzard WR, Blass JP, Ettinger WH Jr, et al (eds). Principles of Geriatric Medicine and Gerontology, 4th ed. New York: McGraw-Hill, 1999, pp 303-331.
11. Ciummo P, Katz NL. Interactions and drug-metabolizing enzymes. Am Pharm 1995;35:41-52.
12. Murray M. P450 enzyme: Inhibition mechanisms, genetic regulation, and effects of liver disease. Clin Pharmacokinet 1992;23:132-146.

13. Physicians Desk Reference, 2001, 55th ed. Montvale, NJ: Medical Economics, 2001.
14. Ereshefsky L, Riesenman C, Lam YWF. Antidepressant drug interactions and the cytochrome P450 system. Clin Pharmacokinet 1995;29:10-19.
15. Slaughter RL, Edwards DJ. Recent advances: The cytochrome P450 enzymes. Ann Pharmacother 1995;29:619-624.
16. Nerbert DW, Adesnik M, Coon MJ, et al. The P450 gene superfamily: Recommended nomenclature. DNA 1987;6(1):1-11.
17. Slaughter RL. Clinical relevance of cytochrome P450 enzymes. Hosp Pharm Times 1996;7:6-15.
18. von Moltke L, Greenblatt DJ, Schmider J, et al. Metabolism of drugs by cytochrome P450 3A isoforms: Implications for drug interactions in psychopharmacology. Clin Pharmacokinet 1995;29:33-44.
19. Ritschel WA, Kearns GL. Handbook of Basic Pharmacokinetics Including Clinical Applications, 5th ed. Washington, DC: American Pharmaceutical Association, 1999, p 141.
20. Kuebler KK, Varga J, Mihelic RA. Why there is no cookbook approach to palliative care: Implications of the P450 enzyme system. Clin J Oncol Nurs 2003;7:569-572.
21. Green SM, Ables AZ, Allen JE, et al. Tarascon Pocket Pharmacopoepia 2000, Deluxe Edition. Loma Linda, CA: Tarascon Publishing, 2000.
22. Schuurkes JAJ, Helsen LFM, Ghoos ECR, et al. Stimulation of gastroduodenal motor activity: Dopaminergic and cholinergic modulation. Drug Devel Res 1986;8:233-241.
23. Kaye P. A to Z of Hospice and Palliative Care. Northampton, UK: EPL Publication, 1994, p 192.
24. Waller A, Caroline NL. Palliative Care in Cancer. Boston: Butterworth-Heinemann, 1996, p 352.

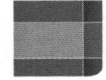

CHAPTER **125**

Drug Use in Special Populations

Paola Sacerdote

KEY POINTS

- Challenges in drug treatment in the elderly include patient-related factors such as physiological decline in organ function (renal, hepatic, immune system), altered pharmacokinetics, presence of co-morbidities, altered pharmacodynamics (increased vulnerability to adverse drug effects), and high variability in drug responses.

- Use of multiple medications in the elderly leads to a high incidence of drug interactions; the risk of undertreatment must be weighed against the risk of toxic side effects.

- The age-associated changes in body composition and organ function in children are nonlinear, and there are no broadly reliable principles for determining pediatric drug doses based on conversion from the doses used in adults.

- Drug treatment in pregnancy affects two individuals, the mother and the fetus.

- Physiological changes in the maternal compartment during pregnancy can alter pharmacokinetics and pharmacodynamics, affecting the mother's drug response.

- Knowledge of placental drug transfer and of placental and fetal metabolism is necessary to make decisions about which drugs can significantly cross to the fetus.

The proportion of the world's population older than 60 years of age doubled in the last century and will increase by twofold to threefold during the first century of this millennium.

Aging has important effects on the response to pharmacological and surgical interventions and is the major risk factor for most diseases in developed countries. The high prevalence of disease promotes frequent use of medications in older people. Polypharmacy (i.e., the use of five or more medications) occurs in 20% to 40% of this age group, and it is generally accepted that these individuals are at greater risk for adverse drug reactions. Nevertheless, it is important not to deny useful pharmacotherapy to older people simply to avoid these risks. Older people are poorly represented in clinical trials; up to 35% of published trials exclude them on the basis of age without justification. The number of older people in clinical trials needs to be increased to enhance understanding of the influences of biological processes of aging on drug actions.

Similar considerations are true also for the opposite limit of human life. Human growth and development are not linear, and fewer studies include infants and children. Therefore, a clear understanding of the disposition and actions of drugs, and the factors that affect them, is critical.

Many physiological changes that can affect drug metabolism and disposition occur in women during pregnancy. Prescribing drugs in pregnancy is an unusual risk-benefit situation. Drugs that may be of benefit or even life-saving for the mother can deform or kill the fetus. Again, clinical trials have excluded pregnant women due to practical and ethical considerations. Knowledge of how human physiology is changed during pregnancy can provide the necessary information to modify doses and schedules to ensure efficacy and minimize toxicity.

GERIATRIC CLINICAL PHARMACOLOGY

Old age is associated with impaired adaptive and homeostatic mechanisms leading to susceptibility to environmental or internal stresses with increased rates of disease and death. Almost all human physiological systems deteriorate in structure and function with age. However, older people are heterogeneous, and the differences between many older and younger people can be small. After 75 years of age, a growing proportion of this population may be frail. This is due to multiple factors including physical and mental diseases, undernutrition, and relative deprivation superimposed on the various physiological changes that occur with age alone.

Biological aging processes are linked mechanistically to altered drug handling (Box 125-1) and pharmacodynamic responses. The consequences vary accordingly to the health of the patient, the route of metabolism or drug elimination, and intrinsic drug safety.

Pharmacokinetics

The intestinal absorption of most drugs that permeate the gastrointestinal epithelium by diffusion is not reduced in the elderly in a clinically significant way. Compounds that permeate the intestine with carriers (calcium, vitamins,

---

Box 125-1 Physiological Changes in Older People That Affect Drug Disposition

- Decrease in total body mass
- Change in body composition (decreased body water and increased body fat)
- Small reduction in serum albumin
- Decreased liver size and blood flow in the liver
- Decreased renal function

---

iron) may be absorbed at lower rates. Atrophy of the epidermis and dermis is present in aging; however, the rate of transdermal drug absorption may diminish because of reduced tissue blood perfusion.[1]

Age-related changes in body composition may affect the volumes of distribution of some drugs. Body fat increases by 20% to 40 %, and body water decreases by 10% to 15 % in older people. This should increase the volume of distribution of lipophilic drugs and, conversely, decrease that of hydrophilic drugs. These changes are not considered clinically significant. The same is true for the age-related effects on protein binding. There is a reduction in blood albumin concentration of about 10%, and possibly an increase in α_1-acid glycoprotein.[1,2]

The aging of liver function plays an important role in the modification of pharmacokinetics in the elderly. The aged liver is characterized by smaller volume, less hepatic blood flow. and a reduced intrinsic enzyme capacity. Blood flow to the liver can decrease by 40% with a similar or slight reduction of liver mass. Any reduction in blood flow would be expected to cause a concomitant reduction in the clearance of drugs with high extraction fractions. There is a consistent effect of age on the clearances of flow-limited drugs, most of which are reduced by about 30% to 40%, correlating well with age-related reduction in blood flow.[1-3]

It is controversial whether a reduction of the activity of phase I enzymes occurs with aging. Despite animal literature showing a decline in cytochrome P-450 isoenzyme (CYP) content, studies in the human have not confirmed this. Even though in vitro activity, amount, and gene expression of phase I enzymes do not change with age, most drugs metabolized via phase I pathways have reduced clearance. Besides less liver blood flow, which is the main cause of the decrease, liver structural changes have been described in aging. These may interfere with oxygen availability for phase I metabolism.[1] There is no significant reduction of phase II metabolism with age, and this is consistent across studies and species. Both glutathione transferase and uridine diphosphate (UDP) glucuronyl transferase are unchanged.

A most important pharmacokinetic change is the reduction in renal drug elimination.[4,5] Glomerular filtration rate, tubular secretion, and renal blood flow are all reduced. Creatinine has been used extensively in the elderly as an index of renal function. The Cockcroft-Gault equation has been used widely to estimate the creatinine clearance (CCr) in milliliters per minute:

$$CCr = \frac{(140 - Age) \times (Weight\ in\ kg) \times (0.85\ for\ females)}{(72) \times (Serum\ creatinine\ in\ mg/dL)}$$

This formula may underestimate renal impairment, because in frail older people daily creatinine production is reduced due to decreased muscle mass, reduced exercise, and dietary meat intake.

Great heterogeneity in renal function exists in older subjects. It is difficult to separate the primary effect of aging biology on the kidney from age-related kidney disease. Increased rates of hypertension, vascular disease, and diabetes can greatly affect renal function. The prevalence of hypertension in people older than 65 years of age can negatively impact renal function.[1] It is difficult to define the specific relationship between normal aging, renal function, and altered pharmacokinetics. In healthy people, the average decline in glomerular filtration rate is probably less than 1 mL/min/year after middle age. The Cockcroft-Gault equation could be adequate to evaluate renal disease, rather than a primary age change, in older people. There exists a risk of inappropriately estimating renal function in older people, which potentially could lead to underdosing and less efficacy in some healthy old people and toxicity in other, frail old people. Acute morphine pharmacokinetics appears to be little affected by aging, but levels of glycuronide metabolites can be increased in renal-impaired older persons.[6] The importance of reducing dosage depends on the type of drug. In patients with normal age-related decline in renal function, the necessity of reducing maintenance doses of drugs with a wide therapeutic index could be questioned, but it is mandatory for agents with a narrow therapeutic index.

Pharmacodynamics

The general higher sensitivity to a given concentration of a drug in the elderly must be attributed to relevant pharmacodynamic changes.[1,2] A drug effect depends on the number of target organ receptors, the ability of the cells to respond to receptor occupation (signal transduction), and the counter-regulatory processes that preserve homeostasis. All of these phenomena are altered during aging.

Concomitant with the effect of old age on the activity and expression of many receptors, more time is required after pharmacological perturbation for counter-regulatory mechanisms to act. Reactions to drugs are generally stronger than in young individuals, and the incidence of adverse drug reactions is more common, despite the general decline in receptor number and responsivity.[7-9] Age-related changes in the cardiovascular system include β-adrenoceptor downregulation and reduced catecholamine response. A typical example of the decrease in homeostatic mechanisms is the increased susceptibility of older people to postural hypotension after administration of antihypertensive drugs. More than 11% of episodes of syncope and falls in the elderly can be attributed to drugs.

The central nervous system (CNS) is a vulnerable drug target in aging. A general neuronal loss and decrease of brain volume occurs. In the CNS, the number of dopaminergic and cholinergic receptors is decreased. The loss of dopaminergic receptors predisposes to an increased frequency and severity of extrapyramidal symptoms after dopaminergic blockade with antipsychotics and metoclopramide. The reduction of the cholinergic system predisposes to cognitive impairment and other anticholinergic effects of some antidepressants. For these reasons, nontricyclic antidepressants, such as selective serotonin reuptake inhibitors (SSRIs), must be preferred in the elderly.

Age-related changes in benzodiazepine pharmacodynamics are important. The median effective concentration (EC_{50}) for sedation after intravenous midazolam is reduced by 50% in older people, despite the lack of significant age-related changes in pharmacokinetics. Not only is sedation enhanced, but there might be confusion, ataxia, impairment of short-term memory, and various adverse behavioral effects not observed in the young. Whether these changes depend on an altered number or composition of γ-aminobutyric acid ($GABA_A$) receptors is unclear.

Pain sensitivity increases with age.[6] Opioid receptor density decreases with age, and affinity increases. Age-related decline of immune function and decreased density and proliferation of bone marrow cells increase the adverse effects of anticancer drugs and other drugs that affect the immune system and hematic homeostasis. The hematological toxicity of antiepileptic drugs, for example, is increased.

Drug Interactions

Drug-drug interactions are more likely in older people because they tend to use multiple medications.[9] The average older person may use between two and six prescribed medications, in addition to one to three nonprescription medications, routinely. The use of several medications is indicated in many recent evidence-based clinical practice guidelines, and this trend will increase further in the future.

An increased risk of potential drug interactions with increased use of medications obviously exists. The theoretical probability of a drug interaction is greater than 50% for a patient who is taking five medications, and it is up 100% if seven drugs are being administered. To reduce drug interactions, it is important that a thorough medication history be taken at each visit, including use of nonprescription drugs and herbal supplements.

Drug interactions can alter the absorption, distribution, metabolism, or excretion of a drug. Pharmacodynamic interactions (i.e., those in which one drug changes the clinical effects of another one) are particularly relevant in the elderly. The presence of disease and aging physiology may contribute to an exaggeration of the consequences that derive from drug-drug interactions. In a very elderly person who has reduced drug metabolism due to impaired liver flow, a further small inhibition of metabolism due to CYP inhibition could be deleterious and could induce serious adverse reactions. Competitive binding between two drugs at the enzyme-binding site is often responsible for inhibition of a drug's metabolism. Because approximately 50% of drugs commonly prescribed for elderly patients are metabolized by the isoform CYP3A4, increased plasma levels of two drugs metabolized by this isoenzyme are particularly dangerous in the elderly.[10]

Similarly, in elderly patients, drug-drug interactions that affect renal function are more common and potentially more significant. The glomerular filtration rate declines with advancing age, and a compensatory production of vasodilatory renal prostaglandin occurs. Chronic use of nonsteroidal anti-inflammatory drugs (NSAIDs) impairs this compensatory mechanism, leading to decreased renal function. The use of NSAIDs in association with drugs that have a narrow therapeutic range and are renally eliminated is a risk.

Conclusions: Drug Treatment in the Elderly

There is an increasing understanding of the relationship among aging, age-related diseases, and the effects of aging on pharmacology. The older population is heterogeneous, comprising an expanding number of frail older people, for whom drug adjustment is relevant. It is incorrect to consider advanced age as a general unpredictable risk factor for drug treatment, because doing so may lead to inadequate pharmacotherapy in the elderly.

DRUG TREATMENT IN CHILDREN

Special considerations also apply for drug treatment at the opposite limit of human life, in infancy and early childhood. (Challenges associated with drug treatment in relation to fetal development are discussed in the next section.)

Infants and children cannot be considered "miniature men and women." Because human growth is not linear, age-associated changes in body composition and organ function are dynamic and can be discordant during the first decade of life. Moreover, research studies infrequently include infants or young children. For these reasons, there are no broadly reliable principles or formulas for determining pediatric drug doses based on conversion from the doses used in adults. Therefore, a clear understanding of the interactions among developmental changes, ontogeny, and the disposition and actions of drugs becomes critical for safe and effective therapeutics in children.

DRUGS AND PREGNANCY

In pregnancy, numerous physiological changes alter pharmacokinetics and pharmacodynamics, affecting both the mother's response to a given drug and the amount of drug that can reach the fetus. The maternal-placental-fetal unit can be thought of as a three-compartment pharmacokinetic model with diverse properties of absorption, metabolism, and elimination.[11]

Maternal Factors

Many physiological changes that occur in pregnancy may influence drug handling and require dose adjustment (Box 125-2). The changes begin during the first trimester and become more marked during the third trimester, altering absorption, distribution, and clearance of drugs. A practical problem is the nausea and vomiting of pregnancy. Nausea is less in the evening, so it is better to prescribe dosing in the evening, if possible. Total body water increases significantly (up to 8 L), resulting in a significant increase of the volume of distribution for hydrophilic drugs. Because of hemodilution, there is a fall in the plasma albumin concentration.

Metabolism is significantly affected during pregnancy. Different CYP isoenzymes are differently modulated. Some enzymes are induced by estrogen/progesterone, resulting

> **Box 125-2 Major Considerations for Drug Handling in Pregnancy**
>
> - Drug absorption is decreased.
> - Drug elimination is increased.
> - Total plasma concentration is decreased.
> - The proportion of free drug to protein-bound drug can be altered.
> - Therapeutic drug monitoring is important.

in higher metabolism and elimination of certain drugs (e.g., phenytoin). Other isoenzymes are competitively inhibited by progesterone and estradiol, leading to impaired elimination of drugs such as theophylline. Renal blood flow is increased up to 80%, and the glomerular filtration rate rises by 50%, leading to enhanced elimination of drugs.

Considering all of these factors, it can be concluded that, in general, the volume of distribution and clearance are increased in pregnancy, lowering plasma concentrations of drugs.[12] The degree of alteration in dose schedule required depends on the magnitude of the effect for each drug and how critically therapeutic efficacy and toxicity relate to plasma concentration.[11-13]

Placental-Fetal Unit

Because drug transfer occurs mainly through passive diffusion, lipophilic drugs are more permeable than agents that are polar, ionized, and water soluble.[12,14] Protein-bound drugs do not cross the placenta. Some drugs are pumped across the placenta by active transporters. Human placenta expresses both P-glycoprotein and some members of the multidrug-resistance protein family (MRP). These transporters act bidirectionally, transporting drugs and xenobiotics from the mother to the fetus and, probably to a greater degree, from the fetus to the mother. Future studies will help clarify the role of these transport systems.[14]

The placenta itself contains enzymes that are able to metabolize drugs, such as some CYP enzymes, N-acetyltransferase, glutathione transferase, and sulfating enzymes. They may metabolize a drug as it crosses the placenta. The fetal liver has a limited ability to metabolize drugs, but some functions are present. Because most drug metabolites are polar, they might accumulate in the fetus. Moreover, fetal plasma is slightly more acidic than that of the mother, so ion trapping of basic drugs occurs. As fetal kidney function develops, the drugs and their metabolites are eliminated in the amniotic liquid. An understanding of placental transfer and metabolism of drugs has clinical significance for both maternal and fetal health.

Conclusions: Drug Treatment in Pregnancy

Over recent years, there has been a gradual rise in the use of drugs during pregnancy; analgesics, antiemetics, antibacterials, tranquilizers, and antihistamines are used most frequently. In some conditions, such as epilepsy or diabetes, the mother is continuously exposed to therapy, because it is considered that the benefit for the mother is higher than the risk to the fetus.

Specific data on how pharmacological parameters such as volume of distribution and clearance vary in pregnancy for individual drugs are limited. This is partly because of ethical and practical considerations in pharmacokinetic studies. Classically, pharmacokinetic clinical trials exclude pregnant women and women of reproductive age. Data are limited to small numbers of observations, with pooling of results from subjects at different points in the gestational sequence. Control groups vary in composition, from adult males to nonpregnant women to the same subjects 6 to 8 weeks after delivery.

CONCLUSIONS

Increased understanding of the influences of growth, development, aging processes, and age-related disease on the disposition and action of drugs is improving drug therapy at the two extremes of human life. A slight increase in the number of clinical trials with older subjects is now evident, although the heterogeneity of this population leads to great differences in responses between healthy old subjects and frail ones. Scientific progress together with an increased consciousness of the problem should lead in the near future to better use of old and new drugs in the whole population as well as for better drug utilization in palliative care.

EVIDENCE-BASED MEDICINE

The number of clinical trials leading to evidence-based approaches to prescribing, both in elderly patients and at the beginning of life, is still very low and clearly disproportionate to the amount of prescribing in these groups. Extrapolation of risk-benefit ratios from younger adults, the most represented group in clinical trials, to the geriatric population is not necessarily valid. The reasons that older people are underrepresented in clinical trials are multifactorial. Even in those studies with elderly participants, exclusion criteria may lead to the inclusion of atypically healthy older subjects.

REFERENCES

1. Mc Lean AJ, Le Couter DG. Aging biology and geriatric clinical pharmacology. Pharmacol Rev 2004;56:163-184.
2. Crome P. What's different about older people. Toxicology 2003;192:49-54.
3. Kinirons MT, O'Mahony MS. Drug metabolism and ageing. Br J Clin Pharmacol 2004;57:540-544.
4. Turnheim K. Drug therapy in the elderly. Exp Gerontol 2004;39:1731-1738.
5. Muhlberg W, Platt D. Age dependent changes of the kidneys: Pharmacological implications. Gerontology 1999;45:243-253.
6. Wilder-Smith OHG. Opioid use in the elderly. Eur J Pain 2005;9:137-140.
7. Routledge PA, Mahony MS, Woodhouse KW. Adverse drug reactions in elderly patients. Br J Clin Pharmacol 2003;57:121-126.
8. Swift GC. Pharmacodynamics: Changes in homeostatic mechanisms, receptor and target organ sensitivity in the elderly. Br J Med Bull 1990;46:36-52.
9. Delafuente JC. Understanding and preventing drug interactions in elderly patients. Crit Rev Oncol Hematol 2003;48:133-143.
10. Seymour RM, Routledge PA. Important drug-drug interactions in the elderly. Drugs Aging 1998;12:485-494.
11. Webster WS, Freeman JA. Prescription drugs and pregnancy Expert Opin Pharmacother 2003;4:949-961.
12. Dawes M, Chowienczyk PJ. Pharmacokinetics in pregnancy. Best Pract Res Clin Obstet Gynaecol 2001;15:819-826.
13. Wunsch MJ, Standard V, Schnoll S. Treatment of pain in pregnancy. Clin J Pain 2003;19:148-155.
14. Syme MR, Paxton JW, Keelan JA. Drug transfer and metabolism by the human placenta. Clin Pharmacokinet 2004;43:487-514.

SUGGESTED READING

Delafuente JC, Steward RB (eds). Therapeutics in the Elderly, 3rd ed. Cincinnati: Harvey Whitney Books, 2001.

Pickering G. Frail elderly, nutritional status and drugs. Arch Gerontol Geriatr 2004;38:174-180.

CHAPTER **126**

Kidney and Liver Disease

Wael Lasheen

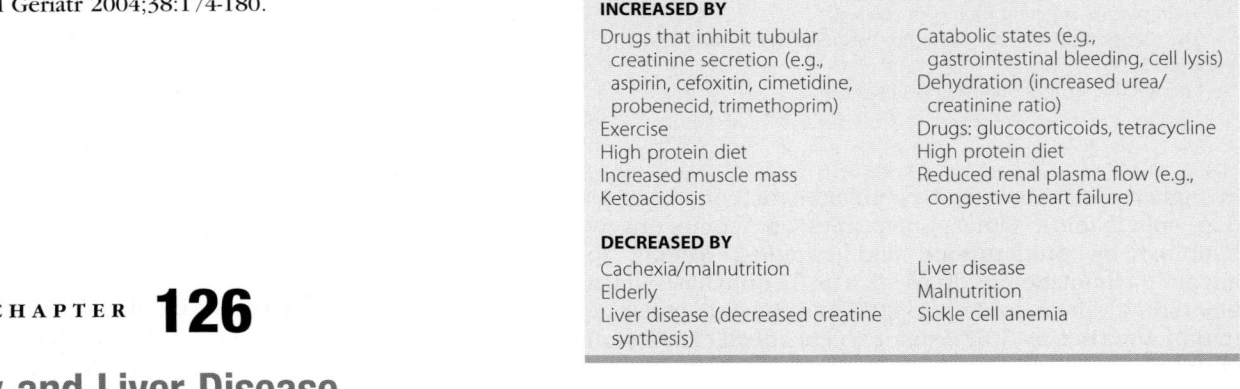

TABLE 126-1 Conditions Affecting Plasma Creatinine and Urea Levels

PLASMA CREATININE	PLASMA UREA
INCREASED BY	
Drugs that inhibit tubular creatinine secretion (e.g., aspirin, cefoxitin, cimetidine, probenecid, trimethoprim)	Catabolic states (e.g., gastrointestinal bleeding, cell lysis)
Exercise	Dehydration (increased urea/creatinine ratio)
High protein diet	Drugs: glucocorticoids, tetracycline
Increased muscle mass	High protein diet
Ketoacidosis	Reduced renal plasma flow (e.g., congestive heart failure)
DECREASED BY	
Cachexia/malnutrition	Liver disease
Elderly	Malnutrition
Liver disease (decreased creatine synthesis)	Sickle cell anemia

KEY POINTS

- Kidney and liver diseases influence the way drugs are handled and, consequently, drug actions and side effects.
- The fundamentals of kidney and liver assessment must be understood to evaluate the metabolism of drugs on these organs.
- Whatever the condition or disease, it is important to identify drugs to avoid and drugs to monitor.
- Guidelines for dosing are necessary in the treatment of kidney and liver disease.
- Unguided drug use in kidney or liver disease may result in considerable harm.

Normal absorption, distribution, elimination, and metabolism of drugs rely on intact organ functions. In kidney and liver disease, therapeutic regimens must be individualized to ensure patient safety and drug efficacy. Changes in drug dose and choice of drugs with or without drug monitoring may be necessary.

ASSESSMENT OF KIDNEY FUNCTION

The most important parameter in evaluating kidney function is the glomerular filtration rate (GFR). GFR measures how much filtrate is made by the kidney. Filtration is determined by: capillary permeability, capillary surface area, net pressure gradient, and plasma flow. The most accurate measurement method requires administration of an exogenous substance (such as inulin) and timed blood sampling. GFR is assessed in practice by estimating the creatinine clearance or by measuring the plasma urea and creatinine concentrations. Plasma creatinine levels can be misleading, because creatinine is secreted by the kidney; a decline in GFR will increase creatinine secretion, leading to overestimation of GFR. In addition, muscle mass and protein intake affect plasma creatinine. Similarly, plasma urea increases as a result of protein intake. Plasma urea underestimates GFR, because urea is partly reabsorbed in the kidneys (Table 126-1).

Estimation of the Glomerular Filtration Rate

A 24-hour collection of urine and a blood sample taken shortly after completion of the collection are commonly used to estimate the GFR. Values should be normalized for surface area, because GFR varies with body size. Incomplete urine collection frequently affects the outcome. One way to assess the completion of urine collection is to calculate the 24-hour creatinine excretion. Creatinine clearance (Ccr) is normally 120 mL/min/1.73 m² in healthy men and 100 mL/min/1.73 m² in healthy women. After the age of 40 years, the Ccr declines by 1 mL/min/year.

For rapid assessment of Ccr, the Cockcroft-Gault formula is used[1]:

$$Ccr = (140 - Age)(Weight\ in\ kg) \div (Pcr)(72)$$

where Pcr is the creatinine plasma concentration in milligrams per deciliter (mg/dL). For females, multiply the result by 0.847. This formula is inaccurate in children, in obese individuals, and in those on low-protein diets, and it should not be used if the GFR is less than 30 mL/min.

A newer formula from the Modification of Diet in Renal Disease study (MDRD) is more accurate[2,3]:

$$GFR = 170 \times (Pcr\ in\ mg/dL)^{-0.999} \times (Age\ in\ years)^{-0.176} \times SUN^{-0.17} \times ALB^{0.318}$$

where SUN is serum urea nitrogen, and ALB is serum albumin. For females, multiply by 0.762; for African Americans, multiply by 1.18.

ASSESSMENT OF LIVER FUNCTION

Liver functions are complex, and no single laboratory test can provide a complete measure of liver function (see

TABLE 126-2 Child-Pugh Classification*

PARAMETER	1 POINT	2 POINTS	3 POINTS
Total bilirubin (mg/dL)	<2	2-3	>3
Serum albumin (mg/dL)	>35	28-35	<28
Prothrombin time (INR)	<1.7	1.71-2.20	>2.20
Ascites	None	Controlled with medication	Refractory
Hepatic encephalopathy	None	Grade I-II (or controlled with medication)	Grade III-IV (or refractory)

*Points are assigned as indicated; a total score of 5-6 = class A, 7-9 = class B, and 10-15 = class C.
INR, international normalized ratio.

Chapter 84). Algorithms have been developed to assess the severity and prognosis of liver diseases. The Child-Pugh score (Table 126-2) reflects the liver synthetic function (albumin and prothrombin time) and elimination function (bilirubin), as well as major complications (ascites and encephalopathy). The Model for End-Stage Liver Disease (MELD) score includes only numerical variables that reflect liver function (prothrombin time and bilirubin level) and renal function (creatinine level). The main advantage of the MELD is that it has been validated in large populations. The Child-Pugh score is a bedside classification and is easier to perform than the MELD.[4]

MECHANISMS OF ACTION

Kidney and liver diseases influence the way drugs are handled and, consequently, drug actions and side effects. A thorough understanding of kidney and liver pathophysiology is key to safer use of medications in disease.

Kidney Dysfunction and Drug Kinetics

The kidney is the major excretory organ. Renal insufficiency and dialysis directly affect drug pharmacokinetics and pharmacodynamics. Polypharmacy and advanced age in palliative medicine populations compound the task of proper drug dosing. Impairment in kidney function may alter drug kinetics in several ways, by altering drug absorption, distribution, metabolism, and clearance.

Drug Absorption

Kidney insufficiency may alter drug absorption via multiple factors:

1. Uremic symptoms such as nausea, vomiting, and diarrhea may interfere with absorption.
2. Intestinal wall edema may hamper drug absorption. In one study the absorptive capacity of the small intestine was impaired 30% in renal failure.[5]
3. Urea conversion to ammonia by gastric urease in renal failure, or with concomitant administration of bicarbonates, citrates, or antacids, may alter pH-dependent drug absorption (e.g., ketoconazole, iron ferrous supplements) or cause drug chelation (e.g., isoniazid) and impaired absorption.

4. Delayed gastric emptying also alters drug absorption.

There are few well-controlled studies that assess kidney insufficiency and drug kinetics, and findings may be confounded by altered metabolism in the intestine or liver after drug absorption.

Altered Drug Distribution in the Body

The ratio of the administered dose of a drug to the resulting plasma concentration at equilibrium is called the *volume of distribution* (V_D). This is determined by plasma protein binding, tissue binding, and total body water. Acidic drugs (e.g., penicillins) bind mainly to albumin, and the extent of binding is reduced in kidney failure. This is commonly attributed to (1) hypoalbuminemia, (2) drug displacement by accumulating metabolites or uremic toxins, and (3) structural changes to binding sites.

Basic drugs (e.g., clindamycin) bind mainly to α_1-acid glycoprotein, an acute phase protein that can be increased twofold to threefold in kidney failure. There is little evidence that α_1-acid glycoprotein binding changes have clinical impact in renal failure. Examples of acidic and basic drugs whose protein binding decreases include barbiturates, clofibrate, diazepam, morphine, phenytoin, salicylates, and warfarin. Tissue binding changes also occur in kidney failure. Digoxin is displaced from tissue-binding sites in renal failure, decreasing V_D by 30% to 45%. Consequently, reduction in the digoxin loading dose is recommended. Fluid retention in kidney failure also alters plasma drug concentrations. Additionally, metabolic acidosis and respiratory alkalosis, common in renal failure, may cause variability in the drug tissue distribution of ionizable drugs, which is dependent on the pH differential between plasma and tissues, as well as the drug ionization constant (pKa).

Predicting the clinical consequences of V_D abnormalities is difficult. The free (unbound) drug, and not the total concentration, determines drug activity and rate of elimination. Unless kidney failure affects the unbound drug, pharmacological properties may change little. Differences in V_D for drugs with a wide therapeutic index might not be clinically important. Therefore, no test or formula can substitute for careful clinical monitoring.

Kidney Drug Metabolism

Evidence from animal studies suggests that the kidneys are more involved in drug metabolism than was previously thought. Enzymes of both phase I and phase II reactions have been identified in the human kidneys. The kidney contributes to drug biotransformation via the cytochrome P-450 (CYP)–dependent mixed-function oxidase system. These enzyme activities are less in the kidney than in the liver, except for fatty acid oxidation.[6] CYP isoforms in the kidney are different from those in the liver, with different substrate activities and different regional and stereo selectivities. For example, cyclosporine increases the total amount of CYP isoenzymes in the kidney and reduces it in the liver. In animal studies, the kidney contributes to alcohol oxidation, N-oxidation, aldehyde and ketone reduction, oxidative deamination (monoamine oxidase), and hydrolysis. In addition, the kidney contributes to several phase II (synthetic conjugation pathway) reactions, including glucuronidation, sulfation, methylation, acetylation, glutathione conjugation, mercaptopuric acid synthesis, and amino acid conjugation.[7]

Drug Excretion

Excretion of drugs in urine is governed by four processes: (1) glomerular filtration, (2) passive back-diffusion, (3) tubular secretion, and (4) tubular reabsorption.[8] Tubular secretion and reabsorption are carrier mediated, liable to saturation, and susceptible to modulation by various compounds competing for the same carriers. Tubular function is not easily assessed and not routinely measured. If the GFR is reduced, drug elimination is decreased and, usually, the plasma half-life of the drug or active drug metabolites is prolonged.

Effect of Kidney Disease on Drug Liver Metabolism

Kidney failure significantly affects drug liver metabolism. Many mechanisms have been proposed, including decreased protein synthesis in the setting of chronic renal failure, leading to reduced synthesis of metabolic enzymes. In addition, circulating serum mediators or uremic inhibitory factors may modulate the activity of CYP and other metabolic enzymes or compete with drugs for their metabolic pathways.[9]

In renal failure there are increases in (1) serum cytokines (interleukin-1, interleukin-6, and tumor necrosis factor-α), which decrease the activity of some CYP enzymes and the messenger RNAs that encode them; (2) hemoxygenase, which catalyses CYP degradation; and (3) nitric oxide, which reduces the activities of CYP1A1, CYP1A2, CYP2B1, CYP2B2, CYP2C11, and CYP3A2 and inactivates CYP2E1.[3]

Kidney failure also interferes with drug transporters such as P-glycoprotein. P-glycoprotein is an energy-dependent, nonspecific drug pump that is present in multiple organs, including the liver, and seems to play an excretory protective function.[10]

Dialysis and Drug Clearance

Dialysis relies on solute diffusion (e.g., urea) along a concentration gradient across a membrane. All dialysis techniques can potentially enhance drug clearance. Factors that influence clearance include

1. *Drug-related factors:* molecular size, water solubility, plasma protein binding, V_D, ionic charge, and rate of plasma-tissue equilibration
2. *Dialysis-specific factors:* rate of blood flow, dialysate flow rate, plasma-dialysate concentration gradient, and membrane properties
3. *Patient-related factors:* type of vascular access and degree of access recirculation

Drugs that are widely distributed in the body tissues, such as digoxin and tricyclic antidepressants, are not effectively removed by hemodialysis or peritoneal dialysis. Formulas are available to calculate the fraction of drug removed by dialysis.[2]

Liver Dysfunction and Drug Kinetics

Principles of Pharmacokinetics

Hepatic clearance of drugs depends on three variables: hepatic blood flow, the intrinsic clearance of the unbound drug, and the fraction of unbound drug in the blood. The latter two factors determine the extraction efficiency of the liver, called the *extraction coefficient* (E_H). Drugs can be categorized as having high ($E_H > 0.7$), medium ($0.3 < E_H < 0.7$), or low ($E_H < 0.3$) extraction coefficients. The hepatic clearance of highly extracted drugs is limited by the amount of drug that could be delivered to the liver *(blood flow–limited)*; it is relatively insensitive to protein binding or intrinsic enzymatic activity of the liver. On the other hand, drugs with low hepatic extraction are dependent on the hepatic intrinsic enzymatic activity and plasma protein binding *(enzyme capacity–limited)* and are relatively insensitive to blood flow. Drugs with intermediate hepatic extraction are influenced by all of these factors (Table 126-3). Although it might be expected that drug pharmacokinetics could be reliably predicted from this information, this is not the case. Extrahepatic drug metabolism, variability in drug pharmacokinetics and pharmacodynamics, and variability in disease severity complicate predictions. Nevertheless, an understanding of these fundamentals aids dose adjustments in liver disease.[11]

Liver Dysfunction and Drug Kinetics

In liver insufficiency, drug absorption and oral bioavailability can be affected in several ways. Portosystemic shunts may allow drugs to bypass the liver, increasing their bioavailability. Reduced liver metabolism may act in a similar way. In addition, cholestasis may reduce the bioavailability of fats and lipophilic drugs.

Similarly, drug distribution may be influenced by (1) reduced plasma protein binding, either from lack of plasma protein synthesis or from the circulation of plasma protein-

TABLE 126-3 Examples of Blood Flow–Limited and Enzyme Capacity–Limited Drugs

BLOOD FLOW–LIMITED ($E_H > 0.7$)	ENZYME CAPACITY–LIMITED ($E_H < 0.3$)
Alprenolol	Antipyrine
Clomethiazole	Caffeine
Dihydroergotamine	Clofibric acid
Imipramine	Diazepam
Nitrendipine	Ethosuximide
Nitroglycerin	Ketorolac
Pentazocine	Naproxen
Propofol	Phenobarbital
Propranolol	Phenytoin
Verapamil	Piroxicam
	Tolbutamide
	Valproic acid
	Vecuronium
	Warfarin

E_H, hepatic extraction coefficient.

TABLE 126-4 Inducers and Inhibitors of Cytochrome P-450 (CYP) Enzymes

ISOENZYME	INHIBITORS	INDUCERS
CYP2C9	Amiodarone	Barbiturates
	Cimetidine	Rifampin
	Cotrimoxazole	
	Fluconazole	
	Isoniazid	
CYP2C19	Fluconazole	Barbiturates
	Fluoxetine	Rifampin
	Fluvoxamine	
	Omeprazole	
CYP2D6	Amiodarone	Rifampin
	Fluoxetine	
	Haloperidol	
	Paroxetine	
	Propafenone	
	Propoxyphene	
	Quinidine	
	Thioridazine	
CYP3A4	Amiodarone	Barbiturates
	Azithromycin	Corticosteroids
	Clarithromycin	Carbamazepine
	Delavirdine	Nevirapine
	Diltiazem	Phenytoin
	Erythromycin	Rifampin
	Fluconazole	St. John's wort
	Grapefruit juice	
	Indinavir	
	Itraconazole	
	Ketoconazole	
	Nefazodone	
	Ritonavir	
	Verapamil	
	Voriconazole	

TABLE 126-5 Drugs That Require Monitoring in Patients with Kidney Failure*

AMINOGLYCOSIDES (CONVENTIONAL DOSING)†
Amikacin
Gentamycin
Tobramycin

ANTIARRHYTHMICS
Digoxin
Disopyramide
Flecainide
Lidocaine
Procainamide
Quinidine
Tocainide

ANTICONVULSANTS
Carbamazepine
Ethosuximide
Phenobarbital
Phenytoin
Primidone
Valproic acid

CYCLOSPORINE

LITHIUM

VANCOMYCIN (IV)

*Most drugs require remonitoring when dose or kidney function changes. For individual drug monitoring guidelines, consult the relevant drug chapter.

binding inhibitors (e.g., bilirubin), or (2) increased volume of distribution, as in edema or ascites.

The liver is the site for many complex metabolic pathways, and it has an important excretory role. In chronic liver disease, oxidative reactions (CYP isoenzymes) tend to be affected more than the conjugation pathways, especially glucuronidation.[11] This effect may be further complicated by the presence of inducers or inhibitors of CYP enzymes (Table 126-4); extrahepatic metabolism of drugs; biliary obstruction that impairs biliary excretion of drugs; pharmacodynamic effects of liver insufficiency on receptor binding, drug affinity, or intrinsic activity; and impaired kidney function, as in hepatorenal syndrome.[12]

DOSAGES

Kidney Dysfunction: Dosing Implications

In kidney insufficiency, drug dosage adjustment is necessary to avoid drug accumulation and adverse events while maintaining efficacy. To dose drugs in kidney insufficiency, both kidney and liver functions must first be evalu-

ated. Then a loading dose is established. Care must be taken not to reduce the dose so much that there is a delay in achieving steady state and therapeutic drug levels, which would render the patient vulnerable. Finally, a maintenance dose is determined.

Maintenance doses may be adjusted by one of two methods, both of which are based on the creatinine clearance rate (Ccr). In the *varying interval method,* the dosing interval is lengthened according to the following equation:

$$\text{Dosing interval} = \text{Normal interval} \times (\text{Normal Ccr} \div \text{Patient's Ccr})$$

Alternatively, in the *varying dose method,* the drug dosage is reduced according to the following equation:

$$\text{Dose} = \text{Normal dose} \times (\text{Patient's Ccr} \div \text{Normal Ccr})$$

Lengthening the dosing interval runs the risk of subtherapeutic drug concentrations. On the other hand, reducing the dose maintains a constant drug level but with more risk of toxicity. In all cases, close clinical observation for adverse events, drug interactions, and efficacy is required. Only a few drugs with a narrow therapeutic index require drug monitoring (Table 126-5). For

TABLE 126-6   Dosing Recommendations for Individual Drugs in Patients with Kidney Insufficiency (Percentage of Normal Dose)

DRUG	Ccr = 10-50 mL/min	Ccr < 10 mL/min	COMMENTS
Buprenorphine	ND	ND	Metabolism similar to methadone; some suggest that it is safe in KF
Codeine	75-100%	Avoid	—
Fentanyl	100%	100% ?	Care with long-term use due to effects of KF on fentanyl liver metabolism
Hydromorphone	75-100%	50%	Similar to morphine but seems safer, especially during dialysis
Meperidine	50-75%	Avoid	Normeperidine accumulates; CNS excitatory SE may not be reversible with naloxone
Methadone	100%	100%	Appears to be the safest opioid; some recommend 50% dose reduction if Ccr <10 mL/min
Morphine	75%	50%	Short-acting preparations are preferred—reduce dose and prolong dosing interval; extra dosing may be needed during or after dialysis, but beware of drug rebound due to CNS plasma re-equilibration
Oxycodone	ND	ND	Anecdotal reports of toxicity in KF
Oxymorphone	ND	ND	Accumulates in KF
Propoxyphene	100%	Avoid	Norpropoxyphene accumulation may cause CNS and cardiac toxicity
Tramadol	Dose q12h	ND	Metabolites may accumulate in KF

Ccr, creatinine clearance; CNS, central nervous system; KF, kidney failure; ND, no data; SE, side effects.

general dosing guidelines for individual drugs, see Table 126-6.[13-20]

Liver Dysfunction: Dosing Implications

In liver dysfunction, neither the type of liver damage, nor its severity, nor laboratory test results correlate with individual drug kinetics. Therefore, no general rules are available for modifying drug dosages in liver disease. In general, drugs should be dosed carefully in patients with severe liver dysfunction. Physicians must consider the following factors before starting a new drug:

1. Extent of liver disease and results of kidney function evaluation
2. Extent of drug metabolism and elimination by the liver
3. Extent of drug metabolism and elimination by extra-hepatic sites
5. Whether the drug is blood flow–limited or enzyme capacity–limited
6. Route of drug administration

Much information is available regarding the disposition of specific drugs in liver disease. Most of these data were obtained from studies of cirrhotic patients (Table 126-7).[21-23]

MAJOR SIDE EFFECTS

Unguided drug use in kidney or liver disease may result in considerable harm. Accumulation of a drug or its metabolites increases toxicity. For example, accumulation of morphine, morphine-3-glucuronate, and morphine-6-glucuronate in kidney failure can cause excessive sedation and respiratory depression. Additionally, drug accumulation may prove toxic to various organs (see Chapter 82, Chapter 84, and all of Part III, Section A).

CONTRAINDICATIONS

Drug prescribing requires careful assessment of benefits and risks. Unlike routine practice, in palliative medicine, short-term comfort may supersede long-term risks and drugs may be administered accordingly. Nevertheless, drugs that are known to be hepatotoxic or nephrotoxic (Tables 126-8 and 126-9)[24,25] must be given with care, especially in the presence of kidney and/or liver dysfunction. Certain medications may cause generalized toxic syndromes that are hard to diagnose. Phenytoin, for example, may produce fever, rash, and adenopathy.

DRUG INTERACTIONS

Impaired metabolism and/or excretion of drugs inevitably leads to increased drug interactions, even with proper dosing. This is of particular importance in palliative medicine, because polypharmacy is common. A thorough knowledge of drug interactions is vital to aid physicians in avoiding and recognizing such complications.

RESEARCH CHALLENGES

Many factors, such as obesity, smoking, concurrent drug intake, age, and alcohol use, alter drug metabolism and excretion. These factors need to be controlled in clinical trials evaluating effects of kidney and liver diseases on drugs in the human body. In addition, patients in palliative care are especially vulnerable. This creates several ethical and technical barriers to research and a dearth of well-controlled clinical trials.

There is a lack of validated measures for severity of liver disease in general, and in particular in palliative medicine; this makes dosing recommendation difficult. Moreover, there are few well-controlled clinical trials that evaluate medications in organ failure. The poorly understood causes of interpersonal variability in drug handling make universal guidelines problematic.

TABLE 126-7 Dosing Recommendations for Individual Drugs in Patients with Liver Insufficiency (Percentage of Normal Dose)

DRUG	DOSE ADJUSTMENT AND COMMENTS
OPIOID ANALGESICS	
Buprenorphine	ND
Fentanyl	NC
Hydromorphone	ND; probably similar to morphine
Meperidine	Avoid
Methadone	NC; some recommend dose reduction in severe LD
Morphine	Reduce dose and/or frequency
Oxycodone	Reduce dose or avoid
Oxymorphone	ND
Propoxyphene	Avoid; increases sedation in LF
Tramadol	Reduce dose (start at 50 mg bid); better avoided
NON-NARCOTIC ANALGESICS	
Acetaminophen	Avoid chronic use
Aspirin	NC
Ibuprofen	NC; decrease in severe LD
Naproxen	Reduce dose by >50%
BENZODIAZEPINES ND; PROLONGED HALF-LIFE	
Alprazolam	ND; prolonged half-life
Clonazepam	Avoid (but useful in terminal care)
Diazepam	Avoid
Lorazepam	NC
Midazolam	Reduce dose; prolongs sedation
Oxazepam	NC in Child-Pugh class A or B; caution in class C
Temazepam	NC
ANTICONVULSANTS	
Carbamazepine	Avoid in LF
Phenobarbital	Reduce in severe LD
Valproic acid	Reduce dose
ANTIDEPRESSANTS	
Amitriptyline	NC
Fluoxetine	Reduce dose by 50%
Paroxetine	Initial low dose
ANTIEMETICS	
Cyclizine	ND
Haloperidol	ND
Metoclopramide	NC
Ondansetron	Dose not to exceed 8 mg/day in Child-Pugh class C
ANTIBIOTICS	
Ampicillin	NC
Ceftriaxone	NC
Cefuroxime	NC
Ciprofloxacin	NC
Erythromycin	Reduce dose in moderate or severe LD
Metronidazole	Reduce dose in severe LD
MISCELLANEOUS DRUGS	
Cimetidine	Reduce dose in severe LD
Famotidine	NC
Frusemide	NC
Hydrochlorothiazide	NC
Omeprazole	NC
Prednisone	Avoid
Prednisolone	Reduce dose
Ranitidine	NC
Verapamil	Reduce dose by 50% in severe LD
Warfarin	NC

LD, liver disease; LF, liver failure; NC, no change; ND, no data.

TABLE 126-8 Drugs with Hepatotoxic Potential

Acetaminophen	Methyldopa
Allopurinol	Methyltestosterone
Aminosalicylic acid	Monoamine oxidase inhibitors
Antibiotics, various	Niacin
Antineoplastics, various	Nitrofurantoin (some trade names)
Arsenic compounds	Oral contraceptives
Aspirin	Phenothiazines (e.g., chlorpromazine)
C17-Alkylated steroids	Phenylbutazone
Diclofenac	Phenytoin
Erythromycin	Phosphorus
Halothane-related anesthetics	Propylthiouracil
HMG-CoA reductase inhibitors (statins)	Quinidine
	Sulfonamides
Indomethacin	Tetracycline
Iron	Tricyclic antidepressants
Isoniazid	Valproate
Methotrexate	Vitamin A

HMG CoA, 3-hydroxy-3-methylglutaryl coenzyme A.

TABLE 126-9 Drugs Most Implicated in Nephrotoxicity

DRUGS	COMMENTS
ACE inhibitors and ATRAs	In the setting of kidney failure, initiation of ACE inhibitors or ATRAs may worsen kidney failure or precipitate acute function failure
Antibiotics	Aminoglycosides, sulfonamides, acyclovir, and indinavir are best avoided
Intravenous contrast dyes	Can cause severe vasospasm in the afferent arteriole and acute kidney failure in susceptible individuals
NSAIDs	May lead to acute-on-chronic liver failure; the effect is dose dependent and usually reversible; acetaminophen is a safer alternative

ACE, angiotensin-converting enzyme; ATRA, all-trans-retinoic acid; NSAIDs, nonsteroidal anti-inflammatory drugs.

REFERENCES

1. European Best Practice Guidelines Expert Group on Hemodialysis, European Renal Association. Section I: Measurement of renal function, when to refer and when to start dialysis. Nephrol Dial Transplant 2002;17(Suppl 7):7-15.
2. Masaru H, Orita Y, Fukunaga M. Assessment of renal function. In Johnson RJ, Feehally J (eds). Comprehensive Clinical Nephrology, 2nd ed. New York: Mosby, 2003, pp 27-34.
3. Levey AS, Bosch JP, Lewis JB, et al; Modification of Diet in Renal Disease Study Group. A more accurate method to estimate glomerular filtration rate from serum creatinine: A new prediction equation. Ann Intern Med 1999;130:461-470.
4. Durand F, Valla D. Assessment of the prognosis of cirrhosis: Child-Pugh versus MELD. J Hepatol 2005;42(Suppl 1):S100-S107.
5. Craig RM, Murphy P, Gibson TP, et al. Kinetic analysis of D-xylose absorption in normal subjects and in patients with chronic renal failure. J Lab Clin Med 1983;101:496-506.
6. Oliw EH. Oxygenation of polyunsaturated fatty acids by cytochrome P-450 monooxygenases. Prog Lipid Res 1994;33:329-354.
7. Lohr JW, Willsky GR, Acara MA. Renal drug metabolism. Pharmacol Rev 1998;50:107-141.
8. van Ginneken CA, Russel FG. Saturable pharmacokinetics in the renal excretion of drugs. Clin Pharmacokinet 1989;16:38-54.
9. Korashy HM, Elbekai RH, El-Kadi AO. Effects of renal diseases on the regulation and expression of renal and hepatic drug-metabolizing enzymes: A review. Xenobiotica 2004;34:1-29.
10. Nolin TD, Frye RF, Matzke GR. Hepatic drug metabolism and transport in patients with kidney disease. Am J Kidney Dis 2003;42:906-925.

11. Verbeeck RK, Horsmans Y. Effect of hepatic insufficiency on pharmacokinetics and drug dosing. Pharm World Sci 1998;20(5):183-192.
12. Delco F, Tchambaz L, Schlienger R, et al. Dose adjustment in patients with liver disease. Drug Saf. 2005;28:529-545.
13. Razaq M, Balicas M, Mankan N. Use of hydromorphone (Dilaudid) and morphine for patients with hepatic and renal impairment. Am J Therapeutics 2007;14:414-416.
14. Broadbent A, Khor K, Heaney A. Palliation and chronic renal failure: Opioid and other palliative medications—Dosage guidelines. Prog Palliat Care 2003;11:183-190.
15. Fitzgerald J. Narcotic analgesics in renal failure. Conn Med 1991;55:701-704.
16. Hair PI, Curran MP, Keam SJ. Tramadol extended-release tablets. Drugs 2006;66:2017-2027; discussion 2028-2030.
17. Davis MP. Buprenorphine in cancer pain. Support Care Cancer 2005; 13:878-887.
18. Power BM, Forbes AM, van Heerden PV, Ilett KF. Pharmacokinetics of drugs used in critically ill adults. Clin Pharmacokinet 1998;34:25-56.
19. Peter W, Halstenson C. Pharamacologic approach in patients with renal failure. In Chernow B (ed). The Pharmacologic Approach to the Critically Ill Patient, 3rd ed. Baltimore, MD: Williams & Wilkins, 1994, pp 41-79.
20. Dean M. Opioids in renal failure and dialysis patients. J Pain Symptom Manage 2004;28:497-504.
21. Rhee C, Broadbent AM. Palliation and liver failure: Palliative medications dosage guidelines. J Palliat Med 2007;10:677-685.
22. Tegeder I, Lotsch J, Geisslinger G. Pharmacokinetics of opioids in liver disease. Clin Pharmacokinet 1999;37:17-40.
23. Kubisty C, Arns P, Wedlund P, Branch R. Adjustment of medications in liver failure. In Chernow B (ed). The Pharmacologic Approach to the Critically Ill Patient, 3rd ed. Baltimore, MD: Williams & Wilkins, 1994, pp 95-113.
24. Quinton A, Latry P, Biour M. Hepatox: Database on hepatotoxic drugs. Gastroenterol Clin Biol 1993;17:116-120.
25. Hewlett T. Just the berries: Nephrotoxic drugs. Can Fam Physician 2004;50:709-711.

SUGGESTED READING

Chernow B (ed). The Pharmacologic Approach to the Critically Ill Patient, 3rd ed. Baltimore, MD: Williams & Wilkins, 1994.

Johnson RJ, Feehally J (ed). Comprehensive Clinical Nephrology, 2nd ed. New York: Mosby, 2003.

Zakim D, Boyer TD (eds). Hepatology: A Textbook of Liver Disease, 4th ed. Philadephia: Saunders, 2003.

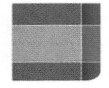

CHAPTER **127**

Routes of Administration

Marie Twomey

KEY POINTS

- Clinicians must be aware of the alternative routes of administration and understand the indications and limitations of the different routes.
- The factors that affect stability and compatibility of admixtures must be appreciated.
- Awareness of the role of parenteral routes (intravenous, intramuscular, subcutaneous) is important.
- The clinician must understand the indications and complications of intraspinal routes.

Most patients with advanced cancer suffer from several symptoms at the same time, such as pain, weakness, anorexia, nausea, vomiting, restlessness, and anxiety.[1] Often, several drugs need to be given simultaneously for optimal symptom control. Medications can also be given by various routes.

ORAL ROUTE

The most commonly used route of drug administration is the oral route, and it is the route recommended by the World Health Organization (WHO) for giving opioids to cancer patients.[2] It has the advantage of acceptability and simplicity for the patient, and it is also noninvasive.

Most medications for symptom relief can be administered orally, and often they are available in both liquid and solid formulations. Some, such as opioids, are available in immediate-release and sustained-release preparations. Immediate-release preparations provide analgesia within 20 to 30 minutes and relief for up to 4 hours. Sustained-release preparations have prolonged absorption and are useful for round-the-clock analgesia. Opioids are subject to extensive first-pass metabolism. This explains why larger doses are required with oral than with parenterally administered opioids (see Chapter 138).

Oral administration of medications may be impossible in some patients. In these cases, portable infusion pumps offer continuous parenteral drug administration, which, compared with intermittent injections, gives a more constant plasma concentration and is less painful.[3]

BUCCAL AND SUBLINGUAL ADMINISTRATION

Absorption from the oral cavity, which is rich in blood vessels, is rapid and brings the drug directly into the systemic circulation. This route also circumvents first-pass metabolism. Buccal or sublingual administration is limited by drug availability and may be inappropriate in patients with dry mouth, oral cavity injuries, or cognitive impairment.

Oral transmucosal fentanyl citrate is a "lozenge on a stick" that contains fentanyl in a hard, sweet matrix. Fentanyl is lipophilic, which means that it is absorbed rapidly through the buccal mucosa, with 25% reaching the systemic circulation. Onset of pain relief is in 5 to 10 minutes, and the duration of action is 1 to 3.5 hours.[4] The rest of the drug is swallowed and absorbed more slowly. Dosing starts at 200 μg, titrated up to 1600 μg; plasma concentration increases linearly with increasing doses. The main clinical indication is episodic (breakthrough) pain during regular strong opioid therapy.

Sublingual buprenorphine also provides rapid analgesia (15 to 20 minutes) due to its high lipid solubility. The duration of action is 6 to 9 hours. Vomiting is a common side effect with sublingual buprenorphine.

Buccal midazolam is as effective as rectal diazepam for continuous seizures in children and adolescents.[5] Administration via the mouth is more socially acceptable for patients and staff and is a useful alternative in the community setting. Midazolam given via the buccal route was used to treat 40 seizures in 14 children, and rectal diazepam was used for 39 seizures in 14 children. Midazolam stopped 30 (75%) of 40 seizures, and diazepam stopped

23 (59%) of 39 (P = .16). Time from administration to the end of the seizure did not differ between the two medications.

NASOGASTRIC AND ENTERAL FEEDING TUBES

Enteral feeding tubes may be inserted orally, nasally, or percutaneously, and feeds may be infused into the stomach, duodenum, or jejunum. Administration of drugs via feeding tubes is generally unlicensed. There are few data, and most recommendations are theoretical or based on local policy. The type of tube, location in the gastrointestinal tract, and site of drug absorption must all be considered when administering medications via enteral tubes. Bioavailability of medications with extensive first-pass metabolism (e.g., opioids, tricyclics, nitrates) may increase with intrajejunal administration. An alternative, licensed route may be preferable, such as a rectal or parenteral formulation.

For accurate dosing, the drug must be in a form that does not clog the tube but retains the absorption characteristics of the original product. Liquid formulations, if readily available, are the first choice for enteral use. Many commercial liquids have osmolalities greater than 1000 mOsm/kg. The osmolality of gastrointestinal secretions is 100 to 400 mOsm/kg. Diarrhea, cramping, abdominal distention, and vomiting may occur with administration of hyperosmolar products through the feeding tube.[6] Diluting medications with 10 to 30 mL of sterile water before delivery may help.

Injectable formulations can sometimes be appropriate via this route. Solid drug formulations may be crushed and/or dissolved in water. Simple compressed tablets and some capsules are suitable for enteral delivery. The feeding tube should be flushed with at least 30 mL of water before and after administration to clear residual medication. Advice should be sought locally when considering these options.

Extended-release products in general should not be crushed, because this affects their sustained-release properties. Crushing them may result in dose-dumping, in which the entire dose intended for a prolonged period becomes available quickly.[7] This can cause acute toxicity. Consideration must be given to the drug's physical and chemical compatibility with the enteral feed. Some medications, such as metoclopramide liquid, form precipitates when administered with enteral formulas and clog the tube. To reduce interactions, it may be necessary to stop enteral feeding for 1 to 2 hours before and after administration of a drug. Feeding rates may need to be adjusted to make up for the lost time.

RECTAL ROUTE

The rectal route can be effective in those patients who are unable to take oral medications. Its main advantage is simplicity, which allows caregivers to administer medication to the patient by this route. Several opioids are available in suppository forms. Absorption of drugs from the rectum can be extremely variable. Absorption may be affected by stool in the rectum. Defecation before complete drug absorption can also cause inadequate pain relief, as can involuntary expulsion of the drug.

Anatomical differences in hemorrhoidal venous drainage of the rectum may substantially influence the systemic drug level achieved. Drugs administered high in the rectum (drained by the superior rectal veins) are usually carried directly to the liver and, thus, are subject to first-pass metabolism. Drugs administered low in the rectum are delivered systemically by the inferior and middle rectal veins before passing through the liver. In practice, the ratio of the use of oral versus rectal opioid is 1:1, although careful assessment of the effectiveness and side effects must be used to determine efficacy.

Drugs are not always evenly distributed throughout a suppository. Most of the drug is contained in the tip. Therefore, cutting a suppository in half to reduce the dose is ineffectual. If the suppository dose needs to be reduced and there is no alternative, it should be cut lengthwise. Long-term use of the rectal route can cause rectal mucosal irritation. In the presence of diarrhea, hemorrhoids, anal fissures, or neutropenia, the rectal route should be avoided.

TRANSDERMAL ROUTE

Certain medications can be absorbed through the skin. Formulations have been designed either to produce local effects or to be absorbed and produce systemic effects. Absorption is limited by physical characteristics of the epidermis and is increased by epidermal damage. The absorption rate is increased if the skin is warm and vasodilated, as during fever.

Transdermal fentanyl and buprenorphine formulations have been developed for chronic pain. These drugs are highly lipid soluble, so they are suitable for transdermal delivery. Two different transdermal fentanyl formulations are available: a reservoir patch (fentanyl release controlled by a rate-limiting membrane from a reservoir) and a matrix patch (fentanyl embedded evenly in a drug matrix, with release controlled by the matrix physical characteristics). Patches are usually changed every 72 hours, making this a convenient alternative route. Buprenorphine is also available as a matrix patch in two formulations, delivering 5, 10, or 20 µg/hr over 7 days or 35, 52.5, or 70 µg/hr over 4 days.

PARENTERAL ROUTES

Parenteral administration involves three routes: intravenous, intramuscular, and subcutaneous. It is generally assumed that medications given by parenteral routes are completely absorbed into the systemic circulation and have a bioavailability of almost 100%. The absorption of many drugs may be complete within 30 minutes. In general, intramuscular or subcutaneous injection produces more rapid drug action than does oral administration, but this is not always the case. Some drugs are not well absorbed after intramuscular injection and even less well absorbed subcutaneously. Diazepam is a common example: oral administration is more predictable and has a more rapid effect than intramuscular injection. Parenteral routes do not undergo presystemic (first-pass) metabolism. This fact needs to be considered when calculating equivalent doses of medications (especially when converting opioids from oral to parenteral routes) if the route of administration is changed.

Intramuscular Route

Intramuscular administration is painful, especially in cachexia. Cachexia is present in 60% of patients with advanced malignancies, and intramuscular injections should be avoided in these patients if possible. This route is generally only useful when a drug is too irritating to be given subcutaneously and the intravenous route is not available.

Intravenous Route

Both intravenous and subcutaneous routes are effective in delivering opioids and other medications in the inpatient or home setting. For patients who do not have a preexisting access port or catheter, intermittent or continuous subcutaneous administration provides a painless and effective route of delivery. Pain control and side effect profiles for the two routes are quite similar and acceptable.[8] Intravenous dosing allows rapid titration and bolus dosing for breakthrough pain. However, repeated intravenous injections can produce widely fluctuating plasma opioid levels. An intravenous infusion provides a constant plasma level, avoiding trough levels and breakthrough pain. For someone with an established central venous catheter, this route is an ideal alternative. The main disadvantage is mechanical problems with the pump, which can be problematic in the home. Medications designed for subcutaneous infusion can also be used for intravenous administration.

Subcutaneous Route

The development of subcutaneous infusion by a portable, battery-operated syringe driver was a major step forward in symptom control. Syringe pumps were cumbersome, had to be plugged in, were expensive, and were suitable only for bedridden patients in the past. Small, battery-operated pumps for delivery of small volumes were then developed. These were initially used for the subcutaneous administration of desferrioxamine in the treatment of thalassemia. Intermittent bolus injections can also be given by this route.

The subcutaneous route was first described in 1979 for opioids, and is now in widespread use for subcutaneous infusions in palliative medicine. Small volumes are delivered over a long period, so the surface-to-volume ratio is large. Absorption is efficient, and there is little discomfort from tissue stretching. There is steady background control of pain and other symptoms, increasing the patient's comfort.

To avoid the use of different intravenous or subcutaneous needles, it may be beneficial to mix an opioid with other drugs, such as an opioid with an antiemetic in a single infuser. Then, a subcutaneous syringe driver allows symptom control to continue, providing comfortable parenteral treatment of pain and other cancer-related symptoms. This is convenient for pain management, particularly in the home, but it also has advantages for hospitalized patients. Subcutaneous infusions have other advantages as well (Box 127-1).

Subcutaneous infusion involves placing a butterfly needle into the anterior chest wall, abdominal wall, or thigh. The drugs are infused over a set period of time, usually 24 hours. If the patient is distressed or agitated,

---

Box 127-1 Advantages of Subcutaneous Infusions
• Relatively simple to establish
• Less painful than intravenous or intramuscular routes
• Low incidence of infection
• Control of multiple symptoms with a combination of drugs
• Plasma drug concentrations are maintained
• Pumps are usually lightweight and portable

---

placement near the scapula reduces the likelihood of accidental removal.[9] The subcutaneous site is changed if there are signs of swelling, erythema, blood in the infusion tubing, or leakage from the tubing. Infusion sites usually last 1 to 7 days.[10]

Few studies detailing the factors that affect duration of subcutaneous sites are available. One study that investigated the histopathology of subcutaneous infusion sites found that local reactions probably represent a chemical reaction to the infusion formulation.[11] Mixture pH and osmolality may have a major role in skin irritation.[12] Solutions that are too acidic or too basic are more likely to cause skin irritation. Solution isotonicity also reduces the risk of irritation. Drugs such as diazepam and prochlorperazine, which are irritants, are more likely to cause site reactions and can cause sterile abscesses. Site reactions may also be caused by a reaction to the needle. Metal needles or Teflon cannulas may be used to administer drugs. Teflon cannulas have a median life span twice that of metal butterfly needles and are a cost-effective alternative for subcutaneous infusions in the terminally ill.[13] The addition of 1 mg of dexamethasone to the syringe driver significantly extends the viability of subcutaneous cannulation sites.[14]

Drugs given subcutaneously are absorbed mainly via capillary diffusion, avoiding hepatic first-pass effects. There are no significant differences in drug absorption, adverse reactions, or analgesic outcome, compared with the intravenous route. Several factors can affect subcutaneous absorption. Absorption rate is dependent on the capillary membranes at the absorption site, drug solubility, molecular weight, drug concentration, and the volume of the solution.[15] There are limitations to the volume that can be injected subcutaneously (compared with the intramuscular route) because of the more superficial site. Absorption is also affected by body habitus, particularly the volume of subcutaneous fat. This can be a problem in severe cachexia with reduced absorption.

The subcutaneous infusion rate affects the rate of absorption. Infusion rates of less than 5 mL/hr are well tolerated. Higher infusion rates are used for rehydration with replacement fluids; this is a safe and effective technique. The subcutaneous blood flow affects the rate of absorption. Very occasionally, shut down of the patient's peripheral circulation in the terminal phase may cause unreliable absorption, requiring more frequent review and appropriate dose adjustments to prevent distress. Other patients who may experience absorption problems are those with lymphedema or severe peripheral edema. Subcutaneous administration should be avoided in edematous sites, not only because of poor absorption but also because of the increased risk of skin infection.[13]

Medication Compatibility and Stability

Subcutaneous infusions may be used for antiemetics, analgesics, anticholinergics, and sedatives. Clinical situations routinely arise that require combinations of two to three drugs in the same syringe. Opioids and adjuvant medications are mixed together in varying doses and combinations, with an infinite number of possible combinations. These mixtures each have different physical and chemical compositions, which can affect their compatibility and stability. In a survey published on palliative care practice in the United Kingdom and Ireland, a total of 19 different drugs were used in different numbers, doses, and concentrations within a single syringe; 90 different combinations were reported.[16] There have been concerns about chemical compatibility and stability of mixtures used in palliative medicine, but little research has been done. Despite extensive palliative care experience with the subcutaneous route, most of these drugs are not licensed for this route.

Drug compatibility and stability are critical to the accurate and appropriate delivery of drug therapy and in drug handling. This is especially relevant in palliative medicine, because drugs used for symptom control are often combined in concentrated forms over extended periods. The term *instability* refers to chemical reactions that are incessant and irreversible and result in the distinctly different chemical entities called *degradation products*. These can be both therapeutically inactive and possibly toxic. Visible physical changes such as precipitation, haziness, color changes, changes in viscosity, or formation of immiscible layers may occur when incompatibilities develop. Investigation of physical compatibility or stability does not guarantee chemical compatibility or drug mixture stability. Factors that affect solution stability are solution pH, drug concentration, diluents used, types of drugs, and temperature (Box 127-2). In general, drugs with similar pH are more likely to be compatible than those with widely differing pH. Infusions should contain as few drugs as possible, and in the lowest feasible concentrations.

Indications for Parental Infusions

It is worth re-emphasizing (particularly with regard to opioid analgesics) that medications administered by the subcutaneous route (or any other parenteral route) are not inherently more effective than when given orally. Intractable pain is not an indication for a syringe driver or an intravenous infusion. Additionally, use of the syringe driver should not be reserved solely for the dying. The subcutaneous route can be considered for many clinical indications that are most commonly seen in palliative medicine but are not exclusive to that field (Box 127-3).

SPINAL ROUTE

Since the 1970s, when endogenous opioids and opioid receptors were first isolated in the central nervous system, attempts have been made to optimize opioid therapy by delivering medication centrally rather than systemically. The spinal route refers to administration either into the epidural space or into the intrathecal (subarachnoid) space. All routes can be accessed with the use of temporary or permanent catheters or an implanted port. Fixed catheter systems have a longer useful life span than simple percutaneous catheters, but, because placement of fixed catheters is a surgical procedure and systems are costly, careful consideration should be given to the system chosen. Spinal drug delivery remains relatively infrequent within palliative medicine, with most units having greater experience with epidural rather than intrathecal analgesia.

Both presynaptic and postsynaptic opioid receptors within the dorsal horns of the spinal matter inhibit synaptic transmission from the peripheral afferent nociceptor to the second-order spinal neuron. Spinal administration of opioids results in a higher concentration at these receptors, and consequently more pain relief, than systemic administration. In a published series, 67% of patients reported a clinical improvement in pain relief with spinal administration, whereas 33% had no improvement.[17] Patients usually experience reduced toxicity with opioids given intraspinally at significantly lower doses than systemically.

The keys to successful spinal analgesia are appropriate patient selection, meticulous technical detail in spinal catheter placement and maintenance, and careful analgesic dose adjustment. The main indications are for those patients with opioid responsive pain who develop unacceptable side effects despite rotation of systemic opioids. Secondly, spinal analgesia is indicated for those who have inadequate pain relief despite adjuvant analgesia and escalating systemic opioid doses. Contraindications to the spinal route include active infection, concurrent anticoagulation, and cerebrospinal obstruction. Poor responders often have neuropathic pain, incident pain, or pain from mucocutaneous ulcers.

One disadvantage of epidural delivery is the need for higher drug volumes to spread more medication over several dermatomal segments to maintain analgesia. Consequently, the drug reservoir needs to be filled more fre-

---

Box 127-2 Factors That Affect Compatibility and Stability of Medications

- Order of addition of the drugs to the mixture
- Volume ratio in which the morphine solution is mixed with the drug solution
- The additives present in the morphine and the drug solution
- The temperature at which the mixture is prepared, stored, and delivered
- Diluents used
- The pH of the solutions

Box 127-3 Indications for Parenteral Infusion

- Dysphagia/odynophagia
- Inability to take oral medications due to severe weakness
- Maintenance of symptom control while the patient is unconscious
- Control of persistent nausea and vomiting
- Presence of bowel obstruction
- At the request of the patient who is taking large amounts of tablets

quently. In one study, treatment with an epidural catheter for longer than 3 weeks resulted in a complication rate of 55%, with 50% of the complications resulting from obstruction or dislocation of the catheter.[17] Other side effects include infection, postdural headache, backache, and nerve injury. The intrathecal route appears to be safer for long-term use, with fewer complications. Intrathecal lines use much smaller doses and drug volumes, allowing smaller and more portable external and implantable infusion devices. Pump refill is less frequent. Intrathecal morphine has a long safety record in postoperative pain control. Other opioids used include fentanyl, hydromorphone, and diamorphine. Only formulations specific to spinal administration should be used, because some other formulations may contain preservatives, antioxidants, and solubility enhancers that may be neurotoxic.

In animal models, high intrathecal morphine concentrations can cause aseptic intrathecal inflammatory masses.[18] Exposure to previous systemic morphine can increase the risk of intraspinal masses. The apparent dosage- or concentration-dependent risk of catheter-tip inflammatory masses suggests that physicians should respect an upper limit when titrating morphine and hydromorphone.[19] High flow rates and low drug concentrations may minimize opioid-induced inflammation.

Conventionally, the dose of intrathecal morphine is calculated as one-tenth of the epidural dose, which itself is calculated as one-tenth of the parenteral systemic dose. The calculated intrathecal morphine dose should be infused at a maximum concentration of 30 mg/mL and at a maximum dosage of 15 mg per day, if possible, to lessen the likelihood of catheter-tip inflammatory masses.[19] Intrathecal morphine with bupivacaine provides better analgesia than either drug alone. Higher-dose bupivacaine can interfere with motor or bladder function. A combination of morphine and bupivacaine or an α_2-adrenergic agonist can be used for refractory neuropathic pain. Clonidine may cause hypotension. Ziconotide in published trials has analgesic efficacy, and clinical experience is growing.

In a randomized clinical trial involving 202 patients with unrelieved pain (visual analogue scale scores of at least 5 on a scale of 0 to 10) who were receiving at least 200 mg of oral morphine or oral morphine equivalent daily, an implanted intrathecal drug delivery system (IDDS) reduced pain, significantly relieved common drug toxicities, and was associated with improved survival in refractory cancer pain.[20] Neuropathic pain and mixed neuropathic-nociceptive pain were the most common types of pain. Most patients were also taking adjuvant medications such as antidepressants, anticonvulsants, nonsteroidal anti-inflammatory drugs (NSAIDs), and, less commonly, steroids, analgesics, and neuroleptics. The IDDS resulted in statistically significant reductions in sedation, fatigue, confusion, personality changes, constipation, vomiting, and urticaria. The most common intraspinal medication used was morphine with bupivacaine (29%); hydromorphone was also used. Clonidine was added in 4%. Side effects of spinal opioids were generally less than with systemic opioids. Urinary retention and pruritus were more common; up to 46% of patients developed itch.

Other factors regarding intraspinal infusions relate to pharmacological concerns such as drug compounding in an aseptic and sterile environment. Drug-drug and drug-

<table>
<tr><td>

Future Considerations

- Development of innovative routes of drug delivery
- Continuing research into stability and compatibility of admixtures
- Awareness of catheter-tip fibrosis with higher intraspinal doses of morphine

</td></tr>
</table>

device compatibility and stability issues also arise. Morphine sulfate, bupivacaine hydrochloride, and clonidine hydrochloride are compatible for 90 days at 37° C with greater than 98% of the drugs remaining at final analysis.[21]

CONCLUSIONS

There are many route options available to the physician in administrating medications. Other routes under consideration, such as intranasal opioids, may prove useful for symptom control. Careful consideration of the pharmacodynamics of the medication should allow the physician to choose the most appropriate route for patient comfort (see "Future Considerations").

REFERENCES

1. Vainio A, Auvinen A. Prevalence of symptoms among patients with advanced cancer: An international collaborative study. Symptom Prevalence Group. J Pain Symptom Manage 1986;1: 47-55.
2. World Health Organization. Cancer Pain Relief. Geneva: WHO, 1986.
3. Bruera E. Ambulatory infusion devices in the continuing care of patients with advanced diseases. J Pain Syptom Manage 1990;5:287-296.
4. Lichtor JL, Sevario FB, Joshi GP, et al. The relative potency of oral transmucosal fentanyl citrate compared with intravenous morphine in the treatment of moderate to severe postoperative pain. Anesth Analg 1999;89:732-738.
5. Scott RC, Besag FM, Neville BG. Buccal midazolam and rectal diazepam for the treatment of prolonged seizures in childhood and adolescence: A randomised trial. Lancet 1999;353:623-626.
6. Beckwith MC, Feddema SS, Barton FG, et al. A guide to drug therapy in patients with enteral feeding tubes: Dosage from selection and administration methods. Hosp Pharm 2004;39:225-237.
7. Gilbar PJ. A guide to enteral drug administration in palliative care. J Pain Symptom Manage 1999;17:197-207.
8. Ripamonti C, Zecca E, De Conno F. Pharmacological treatment of cancer pain: Alternative routes of opioid administration. Tumori 1998;84:289-300.
9. Dickman A, Littlewood C, Varga J. The Syringe Driver, 2nd ed. New York: Oxford University Press, 2002.
10. Schneider JJ, Wilson KM, Ravenscroft PJ. A study of the osmolality and pH of subcutaneous drug infusion solutions. Aust J Hosp Pharm 1997;27:29-31.
11. Oliver DJ, Sykes NP, Carter RL. Histopathological study of subcutaneous drug infusion sites in patinets dying of cancer. Lancet 1988;1:478.
12. Sykes NP, Oliver DJ. Isotonic methotrimeprazine by continous infusion in terminal cancer care. Lancet 1987;1:393.
13. Ross JR, Saunders Y, Cochrane M, et al. A prospective, within-patient comparsion between metal butterfly needles and Teflon cannulae in subcutaneous infusion of drugs to terminally ill hospice patients. Pall Med 2002;16:13-16.
14. Reymond L, Charles MA, Bowman J, et al. The effect of dexamethasone on the longevity of syringe driver subcutaneous sites in palliative care patients. Med J Aust 2003;178:486-489.
15. Lichter I, Hunt E. Drug combinations in syringe drivers. N Z Med J 1995;108:224-226.
16. O'Doherty C, Hall EJ, Schofield L, et al. Drugs and syringe drivers: A survey of adult specialist care practice in the United Kingdom and Eire. Palliat Med 2001;15:149-154.
17. Baker L, Lee M, Regnard C. Evolving spinal analgesia practice in palliative care. Palliat Med 2004;18:507-515.
18. Yaksh TL, Horais KA, Tozier NA, et al. Chronically infused intrathecal morphine in dogs. Anesthesiology 2003;99:174-187.
19. Hassenbusch SJ, Portenory RK, Cousins M, et al. Consensus Conference 2003: An update on the management of pain by intraspinal drug delivery. Report of an expert panel. J Pain Symptom Manage 2004;27:540-563.
20. Smith TJ, Staats PS, Deer T, et al. Randomised clinical trial of an implantable drug delivery system compared with comprehensive medical management for refactory cancer pain: Impact on pain, drug releated toxicity, and survival. J Clin Oncol 2002;20:4040-4049.
21. Classen AM, Wimbish GH, Kupiec TC. Stability of admixture containing morphine sulfate, bupivacaine hydrochloride, and clonidine hydrochloride in an implantable infusion system. J Pain Sympom Manage 2004; 28:603-611.

SUGGESTED READING

Davis M, Glare P, Hardy J (eds). Opioids in Cancer Pain. New York: Oxford University Press, 2005.

Dickman A, Littlewood C, Varga J. The Syringe Driver, 2nd ed. New York: Oxford University Press, 2002.

Swarm RA, Karanikalos M, Cousins RJ. Anaesthetic techniques for pain control. In Doyle D, Hanks G, Cherny N, Calman K (eds). Oxford Textbook of Palliative Medicine, 3rd ed. New York: Oxford University Press, 2004, pp 378-396.

CHAPTER **128**

Development and Use of a Formulary

Arthur G. Lipman

KEY POINTS

- An effective formulary system requires a management committee that is normally chaired by a respected physician and staffed by a knowledgeable pharmacist.

- An effective formulary system is a consultative-teaching tool, not a restriction on which drugs can be used.

- A properly designed and maintained formulary system supports evidence-based pharmacotherapy.

- The formulary should reflect the philosophy of the professional staff of the program.

- The formulary system includes a formulary, or drug list, and policies and mechanisms for nonformulary drugs to be obtained when appropriate.

Pharmacotherapy remains the cornerstone of multimodal, interdisciplinary control of symptoms for most palliative care patients. An effective formulary is an essential patient care, teaching, consultation, and quality control tool. Used properly, a formulary provides automatic consultation on optimal drug therapy to all staff that reflects the best evidence and the most knowledgeable clinicians' views about specific drugs. An effective formulary is also invaluable for teaching health professional students and trainees about optimal pharmacotherapy. Well-conducted reviews before admission to the formulary reflect drug cost-effectiveness, so the formulary also provides economic advantages.

Formularies are as important for inpatient palliative care programs as for stand-alone home care hospices. The formulary of the host institution may not be fully applicable to palliative care. Formularies for palliative care and cure-focused care within the same health care system often do—and should—differ.

Because "formulary" has multiple meanings, it is often misunderstood. A formulary (or formulary catalog) lists drugs routinely available for use within a patient care system, but this is only one part of a system—the formulary system. Used properly, a formulary system guides clinicians in the most clinically appropriate and cost-effective pharmacotherapy in the program to which the formulary applies. An effective system helps clinicians provide optimal patient care; it is an aid—not an impediment—to practice.

Thus, although the formulary per se is a list of preferred drugs (normally with clinical information monographs appended or linked), the system is much more. Staff should know what a formulary system is and what it is not. A formulary system includes a method for evaluating and selecting suitable drug products for the formulary of an organized health care setting.[1] The system includes the formulary, which is a list of drugs (and associated information) considered by the program professionals to be most useful for patient care.[1] The formulary is a clinical tool that is developed by and belongs to the program professional. Economically driven administrative mandates to limit drug availability based on cost alone are incompatible with effective formulary systems.

It is important that medical, pharmacy, nursing, and other health professionals feel invested in the formulary system; optimally, they should feel ownership. Differences between formularies of similar palliative care programs may be appropriate and are due to variation in medical experience and expertise, patient mix, and reimbursement for drug therapy.

EVIDENCE-BASED PATIENT CARE

The formulary system should be a major force for evidence-based medicine (EBM) within the program. EBM is individualized care, not templated treatment protocols. It has been defined as the conscientious, explicit, and judicious use of current best evidence in making decisions about the care of individual patients.[2] EBM often supports the use of different medications for different patients because of patients' past reactions to pharmacotherapy.

By definition, EBM is limited to medicine, but evidence-based nursing[3] and evidence-based pharmacy[4] are increasingly being addressed. For palliative care, however, it is more appropriate to describe evidence-based patient (or palliative) care (EBPC) rather than simply EBM. EBPC is based on the best available evidence. Often, but not always the evidence is derived from randomized controlled trials (RCTs). RCTs are frequently difficult to conduct in palliative care as a result of brief and rapidly changing lengths of stay causing maturation bias, heterogeneous samples, and ethical constraints. EBM does not support selection of therapy based on anecdote (if better evidence exists), nor the common practice of clinicians simply "trying out new drugs" to "gain their own clinical experience." When new drugs are evaluated, careful observation of patient responses and formalized data collection are appropriate to optimize experiment outcomes.

Determination of the most appropriate drugs to be admitted to the formulary of a palliative care program must often be based on studies in more acute care populations. Another important factor is that most pharmacotherapy studies in palliative care environments have involved cancer patients. Today, many palliative care populations include only a minority of cancer patients, and that trend is increasing. Decision makers must determine whether it more appropriate to extrapolate results from a terminally ill cancer population to those with other advanced diseases or from acute care patients with involvement of the same organ system for which the drugs will be used.

THE FORMULARY PROCESS

The Pharmacy and Therapeutics Function

In the United States, the Pharmacy and Therapeutics (P & T) function mandated by the Joint Commission for the Accreditation of Healthcare Organizations (JCAHO) is defined in the Medical Staff (not Pharmacy) standards.[5] JCAHO accreditation is required for any American health care organization to be eligible for Medicare reimbursement. The P & T function relates to oversight of medication use policies and specific pharmacotherapy. It is required in all accredited hospitals and other JCAHO-accredited organizations. JCAHO standards do exist for home care, long-term care, and hospice programs. For hospital-based palliative care programs to be reimbursed for hospice care per se, they must be accredited by JCAHO. The accreditation requirements for and status of home care hospice programs vary from state to state.

The P & T function includes management of the organization's formulary, typically by a committee designated the P & T committee. It is normally chaired by an influential physician, and the director of pharmacy services generally serves as secretary. Committees are commonly staffed by a drug information pharmacist or other member of the pharmacy department with relevant clinical and administrative expertise. Hospital- and health system–based palliative care programs nearly always have pharmacists with the needed expertise available. Home care hospice programs that contract with traditional community pharmacists for medications may find it necessary to contact local institutional (hospital) pharmacists to assist in meeting P & T requirements.

Management of the program formulary is the major—but not only—function of the P & T committee. Pharmacy and other institutional staff typically prepare medication-related policies for approval by the P & T committee. Drug information pharmacists introduce balanced monographs on new medications suggested for admission to the formulary by any professional staff member. If the palliative care program has not yet established a formulary, doing so should be a priority for the pharmacy service.

Medications admitted to the formulary are those considered first-line drugs for patient care. Some that have particular toxicities or excessive cost or should be used only in special circumstances may be restricted in use after approval by a designated service or staff member with particular expertise in the indications for the medication. An effective formulary system recognizes when nonformulary drugs may be needed, and the program should have an efficient method to obtain such medications. In some cases it might be wise to maintain a small, restricted supply of a nonformulary drug needed on short notice. However, only drugs admitted to the formulary should be routinely available to ensure that patients normally receive the most appropriate medications.

P & T committees usually meet monthly to review medication policies, requests for formulary admission, nonformulary drug orders, and reports of adverse drug events and other matters related to drug distribution in the program. The agenda is normally prepared by the secretary and, after approval of the chair, distributed in advance to all members. Objective monographs describing drugs requested for admission to the formulary generally accompany the agenda. Although some invariably view a formulary as restrictive, the P & T committee should continually remind staff members of its true purpose—optimizing drug therapy in a cost-effective manner. The formulary admission process should be transparent, and staff who request admission of a drug to the formulary should be invited to attend the meeting to ensure that their perspectives are known and for them to see that it is a fair and balanced process. Committee members should file an annual statement listing anything perceived as producing a conflict of interest, and representatives of pharmaceutical manufacturers and other potentially biased individuals should not be part of the formulary admission process.

Resources

A pharmacist with advanced training and experience in evaluation of drug literature normally supports the P & T committee; that pharmacist (and other interested committee members) need resources to help ensure that drugs nominated for admission to the formulary are reviewed in a fair and comprehensive manner. Electronic literature abstracting and indexing services are especially useful (Box 128-1). The program should also maintain a library of peer-reviewed pain and palliative care journals (Box 128-2). Although the pharmaceutical industries in many countries publish drug-labeling monographs (including the *Physicians' Desk Reference* in the United States), they often lack objectivity, include only regulatory agency–approved indications, and frequently lack information needed for good palliative care.

Box 128-1 Some Abstracting and Indexing Services for Pain and Palliative Care Literature Searches

- MEDLINE (Index Medicus), U.S. National Library of Medicine. The leading bibliographic database of worldwide biomedical literature. It includes PubMed, which is accessible at no charge at the following Web site: http://www.ncbi.nlm.nih.gov/entrez/query.fcgi
- CINAHL (Cumulative Index to Nursing and Allied Health Literature) is another leading biomedical database that covers nursing, allied health, biomedicine, alternative/complementary medicine, consumer health, and health sciences librarianship. Originally a print index to the literature of nursing and eventually allied health information, the CINAHL database has emerged as a comprehensive and versatile guide to an exploding body of knowledge.
- EMBASE, Elsevier. With more than 9 million records, EMBASE is one of the most important biomedical bibliographic databases in the world.
- Current Contents/Clinical Medicine (CC/CM)
- Science Citation Index Expanded (SCIE)
- Google Scholar, a new service from Google, indexes only scholarly journals.

Perhaps the broadest, most authoritative and unbiased set of drug monographs, the American Hospital Formulary Service Drug Information (AHFS-DI) is published annually by the American Society of Health-System Pharmacists (ASHP).[6] This superb reference is available in several formats, including full text, online, essentials, and a personal digital assistant (PDA) format. AHFS-DI provides supporting monographs for many formulary systems. The comprehensive monographs contain information from the medical literature and expert advice from more than 500 biomedical scientists, physicians, pharmacists, pharmacologists, and other professionally qualified individuals that goes beyond Food and Drug Administration–approved labeling. Though focusing primarily on American drug use, international references are cited and medication use patterns outside the United States sometimes are discussed. The volume includes more than 40,000 medications and 100,000 drug products, off-label and labeled uses, more than 70,000 uniquely sited references, and only well-established, referenced laboratory and test inferences. Each drug monograph includes drug interactions; adverse reactions; cautions and toxicity; therapeutic perspective; specific dosage and administration information; preparations, chemistry, and stability; pharmacology and pharmacokinetics; contraindications; and more.

Specialized palliative care formularies include the *Palliative Care Formulary*, the third edition (PCF3) published in 2007.[7] It provides information on medications used in palliative care by two eminent palliative care physicians and two senior palliative care pharmacists. Drug monographs include information about indications and contraindications, pharmacokinetics, adverse effects, clinical uses, and administration with references. Drugs used for unapproved indications or administration by unapproved routes are noted. Appendices address drug compatibility in intravenous administration (including patient-controlled analgesia) pumps, drug interactions, medication administration via feeding tubes, and more. PCF3 is a valuable reference, but it is not a formulary per se. PCF3 is not a substitute for a program-specific palliative care formulary. "Program specific" reflects the opinions and judgment of the professional staff of that program, and they should feel ownership of the formulary. PCF3 has real value within a formulary system because it provides informational monographs on drugs in the program-specific formulary, and they are an essential component of a good formulary system. PCF3 reflects current drug use among knowledgeable U.K. palliative care clinicians. It is not necessarily fully evidence based. An American edition was published in October 2006 as a collaborative effort of the two lead British authors and the Hospice Education Institute in the United States.[8] The Hospice and Palliative Care Formulary–USA (HPCFusa) is available through the Hospice Education Institute.

The success of PCF led to the development of an online formulary known as PalliativeDrugs.com.[9] It provides information about drugs used in palliative care for health professionals, particularly doctors, nurses, and pharmacists in cancer care. Launched in the United Kingdom in November 2000, it has become popular and useful in the United Kingdom and in British Commonwealth countries that have similar medication use patterns. It is less applicable in the United States and other countries that have somewhat different approved drugs and use patterns. Although some of the site content is specific to the United Kingdom, it contains information useful to all practitioners. The developers have announced plans for other country-specific versions, including Australia, Canada, Holland, New Zealand, Portugal, and Sweden. The site is free to browse and use, but full access to all of its facilities requires a registration process. Registered users can access the contents and search facilities and a bulletin board to obtain and share advice with colleagues about drug-related issues. A monthly e-mail update newsletter provides the latest news about drugs used in palliative care. A German version of PCF was published in 2005, and in 2008, the Hospice and Palliative Care Formulary (HPCFusa) was published.

EVIDENCE-BASED RESOURCES

The Cochrane Collaboration

The sine qua non of EBM remains the Cochrane Library, published quarterly.[10] The Cochrane Collaboration is an international, nonprofit, independent organization dedicated to up-to-date, accurate information about health care readily available worldwide. Founded in 1993 and named for the British epidemiologist Archie Cochrane, it produces systematic reviews of health care interventions and promotes the search for evidence in clinical trials and other interventions. The major product is the *Cochrane Database of Systematic Reviews* published quarterly as part of the Cochrane Library. The Cochrane Collaboration has demonstrated and popularized tools that formulary managers find valuable. Such tools include league tables (Fig. 128-1) and Forrest plots (Fig. 128-2). The Cochrane Library consists of EBM databases updated quarterly and includes the *Cochrane Database of Systematic Reviews*—evidence-based systematic reviews prepared by the Cochrane Collaboration that provide high-quality information to people providing and receiving care and those responsible for research, teaching, funding, and administration at all levels.

There are now 50 Cochrane collaborative review groups, each preparing systematic reviews for a specific area. The Cochrane Pain, Palliative Care, and Supportive Care Group (PaPaS) focuses on prevention and treatment of pain; symptoms at the end of life; and support of patients, caregivers, and their families through the disease.[11] The editorial office for the PaPaS group is at the Pain Research Unit at Churchill Hospital in Oxford, United Kingdom. It is a valuable resource.

Another important resource for evidence-based pain management is *Bandolier*, an independent journal about evidence-based health care based at the Oxford (U.K.) Pain Research Unit. Principals in *Bandolier* include the founders and leaders of PaPaS. *Bandolier* began as a monthly publication in 1994 and has become a premier source of evidence-based health care information in the United Kingdom and worldwide for health professionals and consumers. The acclaimed electronic version of *Bandolier*[12] now has more than 1 million visitors each month from all over the world. The impetus was to find information about effectiveness (or lack of it) and put the results forward as simple bullet points of things that worked and those that did not: a bandolier with bullets. Information comes from systematic reviews, meta-analyses, randomized trials, and high-quality observational studies.

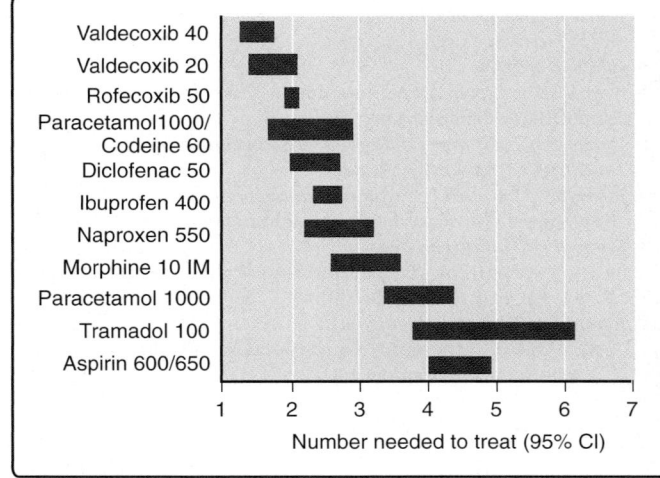

FIGURE 128-1 League table of numbers needed to treat for analgesic efficacy for some commonly used oral nonsteroidal anti-inflammatory drugs versus intramuscular morphine. *(Adapted from the number needed to treat [NNT] for at least 50% pain relief over a period of 4 to 6 hours in patients with moderate to severe pain.)*

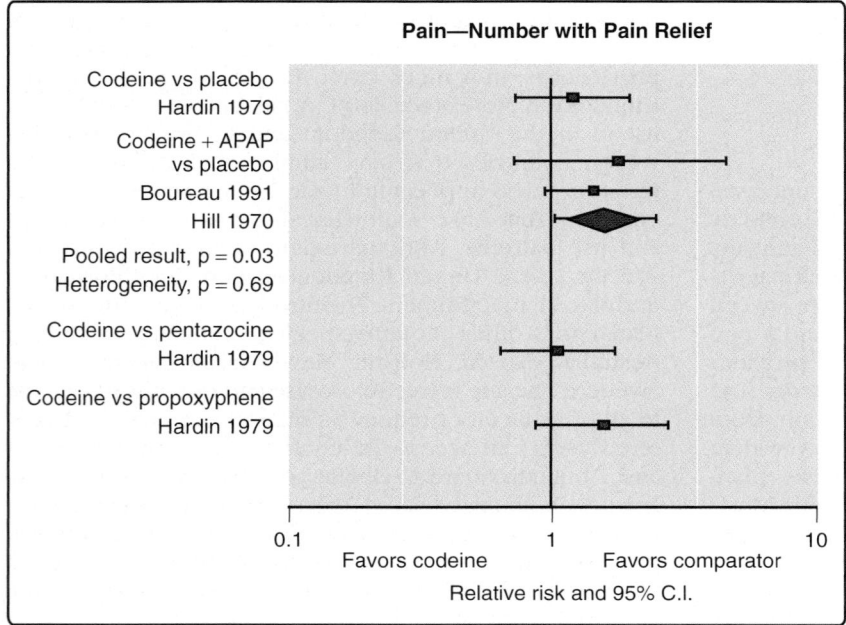

FIGURE 128-2 Forrest plot of randomized, controlled studies demonstrating lack of efficacy of codeine in the management of pain secondary to rheumatoid arthritis. Results that cross the center line lack significance. The *diamond* indicates aggregate data favoring comparator agents over codeine. APAP, acetaminophen. *(Adapted from Simon L, Lipman AG, Jacox A, et al. Guideline for the Management of Osteoarthritis, Rheumatoid Arthritis and Juvenile Chronic Arthritis Pain. Glenview, IL: American Pain Society, 2002.)*

6. McEvoy GK (ed). AHFS-Drug Information, Bethesda, MD: American Society of Health-System Pharmacists, published annually. Available at http://www.ashp.org/ahfs (accessed September 27, 2006).
7. Twycross RG, Wilcock A (eds). Palliative Care Formulary, 3rd ed. PalliativeDrugs.com, 2007.
8. Hospice Education Institute, Three Unity Square, P.O. Box 98, Machiasport, ME 04655-0098; e-mail: hospiceall.aol.com.
9. http://www.palliative drugs.com (accessed September 27, 2006).
10. http://cochrane.org (accessed September 27, 2006).
11. http://www.jr2.ox.ac.uk/Cochrane (accessed September 27, 2006).
12. http://www.ebandolier.com (accessed September 27, 2006).
13. Jacox A, Carr DB, Payne R, et al. Management of Cancer Pain. Clinical Practice Guideline (AHCPR Publication Number 94-0592). Rockville, MD: Agency for Health Care Policy and Research, U.S. Department of Health and Human Services, Public Health Service, 1994.
14. Miaskowski C, Cleary J, Burney R, et al. Guideline for the Management of Cancer Pain. Glenview, IL: American Pain Society, 2005.
15. Lipman AG, Jackson KL, Tyler LS (eds). Evidence Based Symptom Control in Palliative Care. New York: Haworth, 2000.
16. http://www.stchristophers.org.uk/page.cfm/link=13 (accessed September 27, 2006).

Clinical Practice Guidelines

The U.S. Department of Health and Human Services evidence-based clinical practice guideline *Management of Cancer Pain*, a 256-page book published in 1994, was perhaps the first modern, evidence-based guideline applicable to palliative care.[13] The American Pain Society published an update of that important document in 2005 as a 166-page book titled *Guideline for the Management of Cancer Pain in Adults and Children*.[14] A book titled *Evidence Based Symptom Control in Palliative Care* published in 2000 provides systematic reviews and validated clinical practice guidelines for 15 common problems (Box 128-3) other than pain but common in life-limiting disease.[15] It provides evidence tables, including drugs for each symptom on which literature has been published. Several chapters were subsequently rewritten in the Cochrane systematic review format and published in the Cochrane Library. A completely revised second edition has a projected publication date of 2009.

CONCLUSIONS

Palliative care has progressed greatly since the 1967 opening of what many consider the first modern palliative care program in the world, St. Christopher's Hospice in London, by the late Dame Cicely Saunders.[16] Soon after opening St. Christopher's, Dr. Saunders began a clinical research program that always had a focus on optimal pharmacotherapy. In the early 1970s, St. Christopher's included as a research fellow Dr. Robert Twycross. He remains active in advocating for palliative care formularies.[7,8] The development and maintenance of an effective formulary system should be a priority for every palliative care program. The formulary can and should be an important tool in ensuring optimal pharmacotherapy.

REFERENCES

1. American Society of Hospital Pharmacists. ASHP statement on the formulary system. Am J Hosp Pharm 1983;40:1345-1245.
2. Sackett DL, Rosenberg WM, Gray JA, et al. Evidence based medicine: What it is and what it isn't. BMJ 1996;312:71-72.
3. http://ebm.bmjjournals.com (accessed September 26, 2006).
4. Wiffen PF. Evidence-Based Pharmacy. Abindgdon, Oxon, UK: Radcliffe, 2001.
5. www.JCAHO.org (accessed September 25, 2006).

CHAPTER **129**

Antacids

Bassam Estfan

KEY POINTS

- Proton pump inhibitors (PPIs) are first-line management for the maintenance treatment of acid-related symptoms (heartburn, dyspepsia) and diseases.

- Histamine$_2$ receptor antagonists (H$_2$RAs) are useful alternatives but less efficacious in combination with nonsteroidal anti-inflammatory drugs (NSAIDs). They relieve symptoms quicker than PPIs do.

- Antacid salts are useful for quick temporary control of symptoms.

- Sucralfate is not a preferred drug alone. Its role in healing ulcers should be additive to that of other antacids.

- Prevention plus management of NSAID-induced ulcers and symptoms is best achieved with a PPI, especially when continuation of NSAIDs is necessary.

Many products have been developed for ailments caused by increased gastric acidity, including esophageal and gastroduodenal ulceration or inflammation and their associated symptoms. Simple antacids were followed by H$_2$RAs and later, by PPIs. With each new drug, use of the older classes declined, but each has a role in management and treatment. Some are available over the counter for self-prescription. Others, such as sucralfate and the prostaglandin E$_1$ derivative misoprostol, have specific indications and are infrequently used in palliative medicine.

TABLE 129-1   Indications for Use of Antacids

CONDITION	DRUG CLASS USED
Gastroesophageal reflux disorder	Antacids, H₂RA, PPI
Heartburn	Antacids, H₂RA, PPI
Dyspepsia	H₂RA, PPI, sucralfate
Indigestion	H₂RA, PPI
Peptic ulcer disease*	H₂RA, PPI, sucralfate
Prevention of drug-induced gastroduodenal ulcers	H₂RA, PPI, misoprostol
Treatment of drug-induced gastroduodenal ulcers	H₂RA, PPI
Erosive esophagitis	H₂RA, PPI
Extraesophageal acid reflux manifestations	H₂RA, PPI

*Although antacids have been shown to increase the healing rate of peptic ulcers, especially duodenal ulcers, they are nevertheless not used routinely for this indication.
H₂RA, histamine₂ receptor antagonist; PPI, proton pump inhibitor.

Antacid salts are rarely used for maintenance therapy. First of all, their effect is short-lived, and frequent administration is required for maintenance. Frequent dosing is associated with lower compliance, occasionally unacceptable side effects, or worsening of preexisting conditions such as electrolyte abnormalities. Whereas antacid salts (Table 129-1) are mainly symptomatic, H₂RAs and PPIs suppress gastric acid secretion and have a major role in treatment of disease and relief of symptoms.

Antacids in palliative medicine are used mainly for control of heartburn, dyspepsia, and other manifestations of abnormal acid exposure. Furthermore, it is important to use certain antacids to prevent or treat gastric inflammation or ulceration caused by other medications such as NSAIDs or corticosteroids.

ANTACID SALTS

The most commonly used antacid salts are aluminum hydroxide (usually combined with magnesium hydroxide), calcium carbonate, and sodium bicarbonate. They are generally used for rapid and instant relief of symptoms, such as heartburn caused by acid reflux or dyspepsia. None is superior to another, but some act more rapidly because of faster dissolution in the stomach (magnesium salts and sodium bicarbonate). Choice should be guided by side effect profile and renal function.

Mechanisms of Action

Antacids are dissolvable salts. The main mechanism of action is through a chemical reaction between the dissolved salt and gastric hydrochloric acid.[1] Aluminum salts dissolve slowly to form aluminum chloride and water. In large quantities, aluminum chloride is absorbed from the small bowel and then excreted in urine. In patients with renal insufficiency, accumulation may occur. Similarly, magnesium salts undergo a faster reaction to form magnesium chloride. When absorbed, it is also excreted through the kidney. Sodium bicarbonate quickly dissolves to form sodium chloride, carbon dioxide, and water. The sodium

content is usually high. Calcium carbonate dissolves slowly to form calcium chloride, most of which becomes insoluble and is excreted in feces.

Dosages

Antacids are generally taken on an as-needed basis and are readily available over the counter. In certain circumstances they can be taken around the clock, as in peptic ulcer disease (PUD), for the management of a persistent symptom with antacids alone. However, this practice has gone out of favor with the introduction of H₂RAs and PPIs. The usual dose of aluminum hydroxide and magnesium hydroxide is 600 to 1200 mg four times daily. The daily dosage of calcium carbonate is 1 to 2 g administered in three to four divided doses. The duration of action of antacid salts is short—up to 3 hours if taken with or after meals and up to 1 hour on an empty stomach.

Major Side Effects

Aluminum hydroxide is constipating; it also reduces blood phosphate levels and is used off-label to treat hyperphosphatemia. Excessive use in patients with renal insufficiency can lead to aluminum toxicity (dementia and severe osteomalacia). Magnesium salts cause diarrhea, and hence they are usually combined with aluminum hydroxide. Hypermagnesemia or magnesium toxicity can occur with an overdose of magnesium salts. Calcium carbonate is also constipating, and excessive use may lead to milk-alkali syndrome or hypercalcemia. Use of sodium bicarbonate can cause alkalosis and hypertension from the increased sodium load.

Contraindications

Aluminum and magnesium salts should be used with caution in patients with renal insufficiency, particularly prolonged use. Calcium carbonate is contraindicated in hypercalcemic individuals and should be used with caution in those who are at risk (e.g., multiple myeloma, and osteolytic bone metastases). Sodium bicarbonate is contraindicated in patients with congestive heart failure and those with hypertensive problems or taking a low-sodium diet.

Drug Interactions

Concurrent use of phosphate supplements with antacids greatly decreases the absorption of phosphate. Antacids affect other drugs by increasing gastric and urine pH, which may decrease intestinal absorption or increase activity as a result of decreased renal excretion of certain drugs. Absorption of ketoconazole depends on low gastric pH and thus is reduced with antacids. Absorption of some penicillins may increase with lower acidity because of their decreased degradation.

HISTAMINE₂ RECEPTOR ANTAGONISTS

H₂RAs were the first drugs that suppress gastric acid secretion. Cimetidine was the first agent in this class; others are ranitidine, famotidine, and nizatidine. Cimetidine is not as frequently used because of its major interactions with other drugs. H₂RAs work slower than antacids, but faster than PPIs in relieving symptoms. They are frequently used with PPIs for the first 4 to 5 days as a bridge to PPI maintenance therapy. In NSAID-induced gastroduodenal ulcers, H₂RAs are effective only if use of the offending drug is discontinued. Double dosing should be used to prevent ulceration in NSAID users, especially gastric ulcers, but prevention of ulcers remains inferior to that of PPIs and high-dose misoprostol.[2]

Mechanisms of Action

Control of gastric acid secretion is orchestrated by the effects of acetylcholine, gastrin, and histamine secretion on gastric parietal cells.[3] Whereas acetylcholine and gastrin are secreted in response to food or vagal stimuli, histamine seems to be constantly present. All three stimulators work synergistically to enhance acid secretion, but none is sufficient alone. H₂RAs suppress gastric acid by competitively and reversibly blocking the histamine receptors on parietal cells.[4] After oral administration, H₂RAs have a bioavailability of 50% to 70%. Most undergo minimal first-pass hepatic metabolism, except ranitidine, which has large first-pass metabolism. Protein binding for H₂RAs is 15% to 20%, but 35% for nizatidine. All H₂RAs are metabolized to inactive liver metabolites; subsequently, both drugs and their metabolites are excreted in urine. Cimetidine differs from other H₂RAs in inhibition of CYP2D6, thereby leading to various drug interactions.

Dosages

H₂RAs are taken as a single nighttime dose or as divided doses twice daily. Acid secretion at night is usually higher, so acid suppression with H₂RAs is at its best when taken before sleep.[4] The usual dose of cimetidine is 800 mg daily (maximum of 1600 mg daily). The daily dose is 300 mg for ranitidine and nizatidine and 40 mg for famotidine. The H₂RA dose should be halved in patients with renal insufficiency (creatinine clearance below 50). Parenteral formulations are available for cimetidine, ranitidine, and famotidine. Cimetidine and ranitidine are removed by hemodialysis and thus should be taken afterward. Ranitidine should be used with caution in cirrhotic patients because of increased bioavailability.

Major Side Effects

The newer H₂RAs are better tolerated than cimetidine. Side effects are infrequent but can be serious. H₂RAs may cause headache and dizziness, constipation, diarrhea, nausea, and vomiting. Acid suppressants can increase the risk for community-acquired pneumonia. Cimetidine, ranitidine, and famotidine cross the blood-brain barrier and may cause adverse effects on the central nervous system (CNS), such as confusion, delusions, or other signs of CNS toxicity, which should be considered in patients with new-onset delirium. Gynecomastia may occur with cimetidine, less so with ranitidine, because of a weak antiandrogenic effect. Hematological adverse effects can occur rarely, most notably thrombocytopenia.

Contraindications

H₂RAs are contraindicated in patients hypersensitive to the drug; additionally, because of cross-sensitivity, other drugs of the same class should not be used. With renal insufficiency, H₂RAs should be used cautiously and doses adjusted. Caution is wise in the elderly and debilitated because of CNS side effects. Ranitidine should be used with caution in patients with liver dysfunction.

Drug Interactions

H₂RAs raise gastric pH and thus affect drug absorption (e.g., ketoconazole and atazanavir). Ranitidine, famotidine, and nizatidine have few drug interactions because they do not suppress hepatic cytochrome P-450 as much as cimetidine does. Cimetidine is a CYP2D6 suppressor and inhibits drug metabolism, thereby leading to prolonged activity (phenytoin, some benzodiazepines, lidocaine, propranolol, warfarin, and theophylline).

PROTON PUMP INHIBITORS

PPIs are now more popular than antacid salts and H₂RAs. Acid suppression is more pronounced with PPIs than with H₂RAs; they are well tolerated but more expensive. PPIs are the gold standard for PUD and erosive esophagitis. They are invaluable in alleviating heartburn and functional dyspepsia. PPIs are preferred in preventing and treating NSAID-induced ulceration, especially long-term. They are most effective in dyspepsia and NSAID-induced ulceration when *Helicobacter pylori* positive.[5,6] Available PPIs include omeprazole, lansoprazole, pantoprazole, esomeprazole, and rabeprazole.

Mechanisms of Action

Acetylcholine, histamine, and gastrin activate a common pathway, the hydrogen/potassium ATPase proton pump, which results in secretion of hydrochloric acid and thus maintains gastric acidity. PPIs bind to "proton pumps" and cause prolonged blockade and more potent acid suppression than possible with histamine blockade. The original drug is transformed in the acid environment at the parietal cell to an active sulfonamide metabolite.[3] The half-life of PPIs is short, ranging from 1 to 2 hours, but their action is prolonged because of persistence of their active form at the parietal cell. All PPIs are extensively metabolized by hepatic CYP2C19 and somewhat by CYP3A4.[3] Metabolites are excreted in urine, except for lansoprazole, whose metabolites are eliminated mainly in feces.

Dosages

PPIs are acid labile, so they are enterically coated (capsules or tablets). Omeprazole suspension is combined with sodium bicarbonate to avoid disintegration of the PPI with acidity. Tablets or capsules should not be chewed or crushed. In dysphagia, capsule contents can be mixed with apple sauce and swallowed without chewing. Alternatively, omeprazole and lansoprazole suspensions can be used. Lansoprazole is also available in an orally disintegrating form that does not require swallowing. Pantoprazole is available for intravenous injection; it is successful in treating active upper gastrointestinal bleeding and suppressing acid secretion when oral use is inconvenient.

The dosage of omeprazole is 20 to 40 mg daily; lansoprazole, 15 to 30 mg daily; esomeprazole, 20 to 40 mg daily; pantoprazole, 40 to 80 mg daily; and rabeprazole, 20 mg daily. All are equally effective at equivalent dosing.[7] The preferred method of prescribing is once daily in the morning; twice-daily dosing is sometimes indicated to achieve an enhanced response. No dosage adjustment is necessary in patients with renal insufficiency, but adjustment may be needed for hepatic impairment, especially lansoprazole. Most studies have evaluated short-term use, but there is no evidence that prolonged use is associated with adverse events.

Major Side Effects

PPIs are relatively safe. Major side effects include diarrhea, constipation, flatulence, nausea, headache, and dizziness. Like H$_2$RAs, there is an increased risk for community-acquired pneumonia with acid antisecretory agents.

Contraindications

Known hypersensitivity to the drug is a contraindication, and PPIs should be used with caution in patients with liver impairment. Because omeprazole suspension is combined with sodium bicarbonate, care must be used in those with acid-base imbalances, electrolyte disturbances, or cardiovascular disease.

Drug Interactions

Drug interactions with PPIs result from suppression of gastric acid. Absorption of ketoconazole decreases with higher pH, whereas absorption of digoxin, for example, increases.

SUCRALFATE

Sucralfate is a mucosa-coating drug that protects gastric ulcers from contact with acid. Its role is unclear in nonulcerated gastric mucosa. It has no role in preventing NSAID-induced ulceration but may relieve associated dyspepsia.[8] Sucralfate is usually combined with other antacids.

Mechanisms of Action

Sucralfate is a sulfated disaccharide with no significant acid-neutralizing effect, but when bound to hydrochloric acid it forms an adhesive paste that attaches to ulcer sites.[9] This protects the ulcer from further acid and neutralizes acidity at the ulcer site, thereby promoting healing. More than 95% of sucralfate remains in the gastrointestinal tract and is excreted in feces. Sucrose sulfate, which forms on

reaction with hydrochloric acid, is also minimally absorbed and eliminated unchanged in feces.

Dosages

Sucralfate should be taken on an empty stomach at least 1 hour before meals. The usual dosage is 1 g four times a day.

Major Side Effects

Sucralfate is well tolerated. Constipation is the major side effect and is probably due to its aluminum content.

Contraindications

It should be used cautiously with other aluminum-containing drugs (e.g., antacids), especially in patients with renal insufficiency. Prolonged use in these circumstances may promote aluminum toxicity.

Drug Interactions

Fluoroquinolone blood levels decrease with concomitant use of sucralfate; a period of 2 hours should separate dosing. Sucralfate reduces absorption of ketoconazole, phenytoin, digoxin, and some H$_2$RAs. It may decrease the international normalized ratio in those taking warfarin, so separating ingestion by 2 hours is best.

EVIDENCE-BASED MEDICINE

First, in reflux esophagitis or nonerosive reflux disease, PPIs are superior to H$_2$RAs in promoting healing and heartburn control; both are better than placebo. H$_2$RAs can be used in patients intolerant of PPIs. In dyspepsia, acid suppressants have a 40% to 70% response rate, especially in ulcer- or reflux-like types (see Chapter 165). These patients may have real PUD or gastroesophageal reflux disease. In functional dyspepsia, the effect of acid suppressants is less prominent, and those with predominantly dysmotility symptoms are unlikely to benefit; their benefit over placebo is insignificant. It is controversial whether H$_2$RAs are better in dyspepsia, but the general consensus is that PPIs are more effective.

Acid suppressants are important in prevention and treatment of NSAID-induced gastroduodenal ulcers. Double doses of H$_2$RAs prevent duodenal ulcers, but less so with gastric ulcers. PPIs are superior in preventing ulcers, and such prevention seems to be greater in *H. pylori*-positive patients. In NSAID-induced ulcers, PPIs and H$_2$RAs are equally effective if use of the offending drug is stopped. Long-term PPIs should be preferred because H$_2$RAs lack effectiveness.

RESEARCH CHALLENGES

Researching antacids in the palliative population has certain challenges. Oral antacids are preferred, but in those suffering from symptoms such as dyspepsia and heartburn complicated by dysphagia, choices are limited. Some H$_2$RAs and PPIs are available parenterally, but intravenous use is inappropriate in many terminal patients; these formulations may not be available in certain countries. Rectal omeprazole may be effective in alleviating heartburn.[10] The preparation is not commercially available and requires a compound pharmacist. Antacid suppositories, if research on their pharmacokinetics and pharmacodynamics shows them to be efficacious, will solve management of symptoms in dysphagic patients and in countries in which intravenous medications and hospitalization are costly. Finally, most research involving antacids is done on a long-term basis; however, the goal in palliative and terminal patients is fast symptom control, so research should focus on prompt relief.

REFERENCES

1. Maton PN, Burton ME. Antacids revisited: A review of their clinical pharmacology and recommended therapeutic use. Drugs 1999;57:855-870.
2. Rostom A, Dube C, Wells G, et al. Prevention of NSAID-induced gastroduodenal ulcers. Cochrance Database Syst Rev 2002;(4):CD002296.
3. Robinson M. Review article: The pharmacodynamics and pharmacokinetics of proton pump inhibitors—overview and clinical implications. Aliment Pharmacol Ther 2004;20(Suppl 6):1-10.
4. Huang JQ, Hunt RH. Pharmacological and pharmacodynamic essentials of H_2-receptor antagonists and proton pump inhibitors for the practicing physician. Best Pract Res Clin Gastroenterol 2001;15:355-370.
5. Chan FKL, Sung JJY. Role of acid suppressants in prophylaxis of NSAID damage. Best Pract Res Clin Gastroenterol 2001;15:433-445.
6. Bytzer P, Talley NJ. Current indications for acid suppressants in dyspepsia. Best Pract Res Clin Gastroenterol 2001;15:385-400.
7. Caro JJ, Salas M, Ward A. Healing and relapse rates in gastroesophageal reflux disease treated with the newer proton-pump inhibitors lansoprazole, rabeprazole, and pantoprazole compared with omeprazole, ranitidine, and placebo: Evidence from randomized clinical trials. Clin Ther 2001;23:998-1017.
8. Hawkins C, Hanks GW. The gastroduodenal toxicity of nonsteroidal anti-inflammatory drugs. A review of the literature. J Pain Symptom Manage 2000;20:140-151.
9. McEvoy GK (ed). AHFS Drug information 2006. Bethesda, MD: American Society of Health-System Pharmacists, 2006.
10. Zylicz Z, van Sorge AA, Yska JP. Rectal omeprazole in the treatment of reflux pain in esophageal cancer. J Pain Symptom Manage 1998;15:144-145.
11. Walker A. The Use of subcutaneous omeprazole in the treatment of dyspepsia in palliative care patients. J Pain Symptom Manage 2004;28:529-531.
12. Komurcu S, Nelson KA, Walsh D. Gastrointestinal symptoms among inpatients with advanced cancer. Am J Hospice Palliat Med 2002;19:351-355.

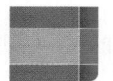

CHAPTER **130**

Antidepressants and Psychostimulants

Stephen Higgins

KEY POINTS

- Depression is underdiagnosed and undertreated in palliative medicine.
- Most antidepressants are similar in efficacy but differ in side effects.
- Psychostimulants have a quicker onset of action (days) than other antidepressants do (weeks).
- Antidepressants are more effective if accompanied by psychotherapy.
- Best practice is to start antidepressants at a low dose and titrate to the lowest effective dose.

Effective antidepressants have long been available; newer drugs are not necessarily more effective, but they may have a lower side effect profile. This lowers the threshold at which a therapeutic trial is initiated.[1] Choice can be confusing and is influenced by several factors, such as comorbid conditions, prognosis, cost, and drug interactions. Systematic evaluations of antidepressants in palliative medicine are limited, focus mostly on cancer, and do not include newer agents such as escitalopram, venlafaxine, bupropion, or mirtazapine.[2] Research in nonpalliative groups may not extrapolate well because of the numerous differences inherent in the diagnosis and treatment of depression in palliative populations. A particular difficulty lies in the often brief time scale over which response is required. Physicians should become familiar with a small number of antidepressants and seek more specialized advice when they prove ineffective or unsuitable. It is believed that antidepressants are more effective when accompanied by appropriate psychotherapy.[2]

MECHANISMS OF ACTION AND CONTRAINDICATIONS

All antidepressants act on serotonin, norepinephrine, or dopamine pathways or a combination thereof. Much is known about their pharmacodynamics, but the exact mechanism of action is often unclear. Frequently, many biological systems are affected, and it is unclear which drug action produces the antidepressant effect. A good example is the largely unexplained interval—typically several weeks—between the onset of neurotransmitter activity and clinical effect.

All antidepressants lower the seizure threshold, but neither epilepsy nor the presence of a brain tumor is an absolute contraindication. The greater concern lies with potential drug-drug interactions—usually mediated via cytochrome P-450—between antidepressants and antiepileptic agents.

Tricyclic Antidepressants

Tricyclic antidepressants (TCADs; e.g., amitriptyline, imipramine, nortriptyline, doxepin) have been widely used for many years and extensively studied. They inhibit neuronal reuptake of serotonin and norepinephrine but also have inhibitory activity at muscarinic, adrenergic, and histamine (H_1) receptors, with many side effects. TCADs are protein bound and undergo hepatic metabolism through different cytochrome P-450 pathways, with resultant interindividual variations in serum levels. These variations can be particularly significant for desipramine.[3]

In overdose they may cause fatal arrhythmias and should be avoided in patients at high risk for an overdose with suicidal intent. They are contraindicated in patients with severe liver failure, heart block, or arrhythmias or those who have recently suffered a myocardial infarction.

Selective Serotonin Reuptake Inhibitors

The selective serotonin reuptake inhibitors (SSRIs; e.g., fluoxetine, paroxetine, citalopram, escitalopram, sertraline) are the most widely used antidepressants in palliative medicine.[4] They specifically inhibit serotonin reuptake without affecting cholinergic, histaminic, or adrenergic receptors. When compared with TCADs, they have fewer side effects and are considerably safer in overdose. There is no evidence that they are more effective. For the nonspecialist they are relatively uncomplicated and thus have become widely prescribed.

Metabolism is primarily hepatic, and all SSRIs cause differing degrees of P-450 inhibition leading to significant drug-drug interactions. Sertraline, citalopram, and escitalopram are least likely to cause interactions. Fluoxetine has a long half-life and tends to not be favored in palliative medicine.

SSRIs should be used with caution in patients with renal or liver dysfunction. Depending on the metabolism of the particular agent, dose reduction may be appropriate. They should be avoided in those with severe liver or renal disease.

Serotonin-Norepinephrine Reuptake Inhibitors

Serotonin-norepinephrine reuptake inhibitors (e.g., venlafaxine, duloxetine) have a dual effect but do not significantly affect other receptors. They are well tolerated and may help relieve neuropathic pain.[5,6]

They should be used with caution in patients with cardiac disease. Dose reduction is needed in those with either liver or renal dysfunction.

Psychostimulants

Methylphenidate, dextroamphetamine, pemoline, and modafinil are examples of psychostimulants. Dextroamphetamine, methylphenidate, and pemoline interact at multiple neurotransmitters, have effects throughout the central nervous system, and thus cause generalized excitation.[7] They are well absorbed orally and elimination is renal. Pemoline can be absorbed buccally.

The onset of clinical effect is rapid, and use of psychostimulants has attracted particular attention in palliative medicine. Psychostimulants also have activity in eliminating fatigue and counteracting opioid-induced sedation.[8-11]

Modafinil is a newer psychostimulant thought to be active predominantly at the anterior hypothalamus.[12] Early reports suggest antidepressant activity without the abuse potential of other psychostimulants, but it cannot be recommended for routine use.[13]

With the exception of modafinil, the psychostimulants should be avoided in patients with unstable cardiac disease. They are also contraindicated in those with significant anxiety disorders. Pemoline is usually avoided in patients with liver disease.

Monoamine Oxidase Inhibitors

Irreversible inhibition of monoamine oxidase—a mitochondrial enzyme—leads indirectly to activation of serotonin and adrenergic receptors. Monoamine oxidase inhibitors (MAOIs; e.g., phenelzine, isocarboxazid, tranylcypromine) have a high incidence of drug-drug and drug-food interactions because of impaired tyramine handling. They are rarely used in palliative medicine and only under the careful supervision of an experienced physician.

Reversible Inhibitors of Monoamine Oxidase A

Moclobemide is a reversible inhibitor of monoamine oxidase A. It is less likely than MAOIs to cause side effects but has no clear benefit over less toxic antidepressants.[14] Moclobemide is contraindicated in patients with acute confusional states or pronounced anxiety.

Others

Mirtazapine is a presynaptic α_2-antagonist that increases central noradrenergic and serotonergic transmission. Histamine$_1$ antagonistic activity is responsible for its sedation. It has no anticholinergic activity and is not associated with cardiac side effects.

Trazodone blocks 5-HT$_2$ hydroxytryptamine receptors. It is a potent α_1-blocker and can cause significant orthostatic hypotension. Trazodone is widely used as a hypnotic—particularly in elderly populations—but its role in palliative medicine is unclear.[15,16] Contraindications are the same as for TCADs.

Bupropion is unusual because its mechanism of action involves inhibition of presynaptic dopamine and norepinephrine reuptake transporters. It undergoes hepatic metabolism to an active metabolite and has clinically significant inhibitory effects on hepatic cytochrome P4502B6. It is widely used in smoking cessation but has not been studied in palliative medicine. Early studies suggest a possible role in cancer fatigue.[17]

DOSAGES

Because of the general patient frailty in palliative medicine, antidepressants are frequently started at doses lower than in general populations (Table 130-1). Patients should be reviewed every 1 to 2 weeks at the start of treatment, and dose titration should be appropriate to the expected onset of action. Lack of response after 4 to 6 weeks should lead to consideration of switching to an alternative agent; specialists may occasionally combine agents. In all cases the lowest effective dose should be used.

Psychostimulants are an exception because clinical effects can be seen within 1 to 2 days—their main advantage. A low dose should be commenced, followed by gradual dose increases every 1 to 2 days until a therapeutic response or side effects occur or the maximum dosage is reached.[1] Tolerance may occur with prolonged use and necessitate dose adjustment.

MAJOR SIDE EFFECTS

The key differences determining prescribing patterns usually relate to side effects (Table 130-2). For many years TCADs were the first-line antidepressants; consequently, there is extensive experience with their use. They do have significant anticholinergic and sedating side effects that can amplify symptoms already present. SSRIs are now most widely prescribed—largely because of their perceived better side effect profile. MAOIs are rarely prescribed presently because of their multiple side effects and the necessary dietary restrictions.

Hyponatremia is best recognized as a side effect of SSRIs and venlafaxine. It can occur with virtually all antidepressants, particularly in the elderly. It is typically seen in the first few weeks of treatment, probably because of inappropriate antidiuretic hormone secretion. Withdrawal will lead to normalization of sodium levels in 1 to 2 weeks.

Occasionally, "side effects" may be beneficial. For example, the weight gain[18] associated with mirtazapine or trazodone may be a reason for specifically choosing these agents.

TCADs have long been recognized as helping to relieve neuropathic pain[19] and remain the best studied. Their analgesic activity often occurs at lower doses and with quicker onset than any antidepressant effect.[20] SSRIs are less effective in this regard, but early work suggests a role for venlafaxine and duloxetine.[5,6]

Current Controversies and Future Considerations
• Psychostimulants remain controversial despite their potential advantages. Further work in examining their combination with "conventional" antidepressants is needed.
• Only TCADs have been robustly examined in patients with neuropathic pain. Further study of newer agents may help define the preferred antidepressants in palliative medicine.

TABLE 130-1   Dosages and Advantages

DRUG	USUAL INITIAL DOSE (MG/DAY)	USUAL MAXIMUM DOSE (MG/DAY)	ADVANTAGES
Amitriptyline	10-50	150	Effective for neuropathic pain[19]; can have therapeutic effect at low doses; widely studied; inexpensive
Imipramine	25	200	Widely studied; effective, fewer side effects than with amitriptyline
Nortriptyline	25	150	
Fluoxetine	5-20	80	
Paroxetine	10	50	Generally well tolerated, nonsedating, safe, and effective; few drug-drug interactions, safe in cardiac disease
Sertraline	50	150	
Citalopram	10	60	
Venlafaxine	37.5	225	Generally well tolerated and safe; effective for painful diabetic neuropathy[5,6]
Duloxetine	30-60	120	
Mirtazapine	15	45	Improved appetite with or without weight gain; improves sleep
Trazodone	50-150	400	Decreases agitation, improves sleep[15]
Bupropion	150	300	May decrease fatigue[17]
Methylphenidate	5-10	30-40	Rapid onset of action; may decrease fatigue and opioid-induced sedation[9,10]; generally well tolerated
Dextroamphetamine	2.5	30-60	
Pemoline	18.75	150	No abuse potential; chewable
Phenelzine	30	60	Avoid use
Moclobemide	100-200	600	

TABLE 130-2 Major Side Effects and Drug Interactions

DRUG	MAJOR SIDE EFFECTS	DRUG INTERACTIONS
Amitriptyline	Anticholinergic (dry mouth, constipation, delirium, urinary retention), sedation, cardiotoxicity	+++
Imipramine	Less sedating than amitriptyline and fewer muscarinic side effects	+++
Nortriptyline	Less sedating than amitriptyline and fewer muscarinic side effects	
Fluoxetine	Fluoxetine—long half-life and less well tolerated	+++
Paroxetine	Nausea, vomiting, anorexia, sleep disturbance, anxiety, sexual dysfunction, hyponatremia	+++
Sertraline	Increased risk of gastrointestinal bleeding with NSAIDs	+
Citalopram	Nausea, headache, insomnia, hypertension at higher doses	+
Venlafaxine		++
Duloxetine	Nausea, headache, insomnia, hypertension at higher doses	
Mirtazapine	Sedation, constipation	++
Trazodone	Sedation, orthostatic hypotension	++
Bupropion	Anxiety, insomnia Lowers seizure threshold	++
Methylphenidate	Anxiety, insomnia, confusion, cardiac decompensation, tolerance may develop	++
Dextroamphetamine	Anxiety, insomnia, confusion, cardiac decompensation, tolerance may develop	++
Pemoline	Hepatotoxic	++
Phenelzine	Multiple drug-drug and drug-food interactions	++++
Moclobemide	Insomnia, dizziness	+++

NSAIDs, nonsteroidal anti-inflammatory drugs.

REFERENCES

1. Block SD. Assessing and managing depression in the terminally ill patient. ACP-ASIM End-of-Life Care Consensus Panel. American College of Physicians–American Society of Internal Medicine. Ann Intern Med 2000;132:209-218.
2. Rodin G, Lloyd N, Katz M, et al. The treatment of depression in cancer patients: A systematic review. Support Care Cancer 2007;15:123-136.
3. Miller KE, Adams SM, Miller MM. Antidepressant medication use in palliative care. Am J Hosp Palliat Care 2006;23:127-133.
4. Lawrie I, Lloyd-Williams M, Taylor F. How do palliative medicine physicians assess and manage depression. Palliat Med 2004;18:234-238.
5. Wernicke JF, Pritchett YL, D'Souza DN, et al. A randomized controlled trial of duloxetine in diabetic peripheral neuropathic pain. Neurology 2006;67:1411-1420.
6. Barkin RL, Barkin S. The role of venlafaxine and duloxetine in the treatment of depression with decremental changes in somatic symptoms of pain, chronic pain, and the pharmacokinetics and clinical considerations of duloxetine pharmacotherapy. Am J Ther 2005;12:431-438.
7. Homsi J, Walsh D, Nelson KA. Psychostimulants in supportive care. Support Care Cancer 2000;8:385-397.
8. Bruera E, Valero V, Driver L, et al. Patient-controlled methylphenidate for cancer fatigue: A double-blind, randomized, placebo-controlled trial. J Clin Oncol 2006;24:2073-2078.
9. Hanna A, Sledge G, Mayer ML, et al. A phase II study of methylphenidate for the treatment of fatigue. Support Care Cancer 2006;14:210-215.
10. Breitbart W, Rosenfeld B, Kaim M, Funesti-Esch J. A randomized, double-blind, placebo-controlled trial of psychostimulants for the treatment of fatigue in ambulatory patients with human immunodeficiency virus disease. Arch Intern Med 2001;161:411-420.
11. Westberg J, Gobel BH. Methylphenidate use for the management of opioid-induced sedation. Clin J Oncol Nurs 2004;8:203-205.
12. Cox JM, Pappagallo M. Modafinil: A gift to portmanteau. Am J Hosp Palliat Care 2001;18:408-410.
13. Menza MA, Kaufman KR, Castellanos A. Modafinil augmentation of antidepressant treatment in depression. J Clin Psychiatry 2000;61:378-381.
14. Papakostas GI, Fava M. A metaanalysis of clinical trials comparing moclobemide with selective serotonin reuptake inhibitors for the treatment of major depressive disorder. Can J Psychiatry 2006;51:783-790.
15. James SP, Mendelson WB. The use of trazodone as a hypnotic: A critical review. J Clin Psychiatry 2004;65:752-755.
16. Davis MP. Does trazodone have a role in palliating symptoms? Support Care Cancer 2007;15:221-224.
17. Moss EL, Simpson JS, Pelletier G, Forsyth P. An open-label study of the effects of bupropion SR on fatigue, depression and quality of life of mixed-site cancer patients and their partners. Psychooncology 2006;15:259-267.
18. Chochinov HM, Wilson KG, Enns M, Lander S. "Are you depressed?" Screening for depression in the terminally ill. Am J Psychiatry 1997;154:674-676.
19. Saarto T, Wiffen PJ. Antidepressants for neuropathic pain. Cochrane Database Syst Rev 2005;(3):CD005454.
20. Lynch ME. Antidepressants as analgesics: A review of randomized controlled trials. J Psychiatry Neurosci 2001;26:30-36.

SUGGESTED READING

Block SD. Assessing and managing depression in the terminally ill patient. ACP-ASIM End-of-Life Care Consensus Panel. American College of Physicians–American Society of Internal Medicine. Ann Intern Med 2000;132:209-218.

Miller KE, Adams SM, Miller MM. Antidepressant medication use in palliative care. Am J Hosp Palliat Care 2006;23:127-133.

Pereira J, Bruera E. Depression with psychomotor retardation: Diagnostic challenges and the use of psychostimulants. J Palliat Med 2001;4:15-21.

Rodin G, Lloyd N, Katz M, et al. The treatment of depression in cancer patients: A systematic review. Support Care Cancer 2007;15:123-136.

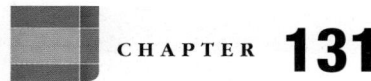

CHAPTER **131**

Antibiotics

Lukas Radbruch

K E Y   P O I N T S

- Infections are a common cause of discomfort in palliative care. Withholding antibiotic therapy may be preferred in end-stage disease.

- Potential benefit and burden should be balanced carefully for each individual, and the treatment goal should be clear. Treatment of malodor or management of other symptoms such as weakness or dyspnea may be achievable, whereas prolongation of survival often may not.

- Metronidazole and chlorophyll have been recommended for malodor from infected wounds or other bacterial contamination.

- Topical chlorophyll has been used for a long time in wound management, although little information is available in the literature.

- Metronidazole is used against anaerobic or microaerobic pathogens. Some randomized studies have shown reduction of malodor after topical and systemic application.

Infections are a frequent source of discomfort in palliative care and develop in 42% of the terminally ill in the final phase of care.[1] The diagnosis of infection does not always lead to antibiotic therapy, and only 60% to 72% of those with suspected infections are treated with antibiotics in hospice or palliative care units. Reasons for not treating infections in a Canadian palliative care unit were poor general condition and imminent death, inability to take oral antibiotics and refusal of the parenteral route, or refusal of the patient or family despite medical indication.[2]

The expense of antibiotic therapy in those with a short life expectancy should not play a part in the decision process. Antibiotics can be a major item in the budget of palliative care services, and concern has been expressed that decisions on withholding or discontinuing antibiotics could be influenced by cost. In the past year antibiotics were one of the most expensive drug classes in our own unit, requiring 12% of the pharmaceutical budget, and were surpassed only by infusions. Fear of possible legal consequences might also lead physicians to administer antibiotics, even if they are not required from a clinical standpoint.[3]

A comparison of the frequency and types of antibiotics prescribed in the last week of life in an acute care hospital, a tertiary palliative care unit, and three hospice units found marked variability in the number and type of antibiotics prescribed.[4] Antibiotics were prescribed for 58% in the acute hospital setting and for 52% in the tertiary palliative care unit, as opposed to 22% in the hospice. In the acute care and tertiary palliative care settings, the most frequent route of antibiotic administration was intravenous and, in the hospice, oral administration.

If antibiotic therapy is indicated, oral use is usually adequate for uncomplicated infections, whereas for severe infections or sepsis, intravenous application is required. For some infections local application is possible. Antibiotics (ceftriaxone) for subcutaneous administration are available only in France.[5] Intramuscular injections should not be used in palliative care patients.

Cotrimoxazole or gyrase inhibitors can be used for uncomplicated urinary tract infections (Table 131-1). Pneumonia and other infections can be treated with aminopenicillins such as amoxicillin, preferably combined with a β-lactam inhibitor such as clavulanic acid or a second-generation cephalosporin such as cefuroxime. Metronidazole administered either locally or systemically reduces unpleasant odors. Antibiotic therapy should be augmented with other drug and nondrug interventions such as fever-reducing medications and fluid substitution.

Persistent or recurrent infections will require second-line antibiotics such as aminoglycosides, macrolide antibiotics, or specific penicillins or cephalosporins. Antimycotic drugs such as fluconazole or amphotericin B may be required for mycosis of the oral cavity or the genital region, as well as rarely for other mycotic infections. Antiviral therapy with acyclovir is required for paraneoplastic herpes zoster infections. The antibiotics most frequently used in German palliative care units were amoxicillin, ciprofloxacin, and metronidazole.[6] Antibiotics were not among the ten most frequent drug classes, nor were any antibiotic drugs included in the most frequent drug list.

Little information is available on the efficacy of antibiotic therapy for control of symptoms in palliative care. In an inpatient hospice, infections were diagnosed in 31% of patients on admission, and antibiotic treatment commenced within 48 hours of admission in 60% of all patients. The overall rate of antibiotic response and control of the symptom of infection was a minimum of 40%.[7]

Antibiotics are generally well tolerated. The most frequent side effects are allergic reactions, which are usually mild and consist of fever, exanthema, or urticaria, but in some patients severe complications such as anaphylactic shock may develop. Penicillins and cephalosporins can produce neurotoxic side effects such as hallucinations, psychotic reactions, depression, or even seizures. Cephalosporins may cause nephrotoxicity, and aminoglycosides can cause ototoxicity and nephrotoxicity. Some antibiotics produce cardiac side effects, whereas others impair hepatic function. Most can cause gastrointestinal side effects, usually diarrhea, and may rarely induce pseudomembranous colitis, which has to be treated with vancomycin.

CHLOROPHYLL

Mechanisms of Action

Chlorophyll is a green pigment used by plants for the generation of energy via photosynthesis. Commercial formulations do not generally use natural chlorophyll, but chlorophyllin, a semisynthetic derivative with the magnesium atom at the center of chlorophyll replaced by a

TABLE 131-1 Classification of Antibiotic Drugs

DRUG CLASS	DRUGS	EXAMPLE
INHIBITION OF BACTERIAL CELL WALL SYNTHESIS		
Penicillins	Penicillins	Penicillin G
	Penicillinase-resistant penicillins	Oxacillin, cloxacillin, dicloxacillin
	Aminopenicillins	Ampicillin, amoxicillin
	Antipseudomonal penicillins	Carbenicillin, ticarcillin, piperacillin
Cephalosporins	First generation	Cefazolin
	Second generation	Cefuroxime, cefprozil
	Third generation	Cefotaxime, ceftriaxone
	Fourth generation	Cefepine
Carbapenems		Imipenem
Others		Clavulanic acid
INCREASING PERMEABILITY OF CELL WALLS OF MICROORGANISMS		
Polyene antifungal agents		Nystatin, amphotericin B
DISRUPTION OF FUNCTION OF RIBOSOMAL SUBUNITS TO INHIBIT PROTEIN SYNTHESIS (BACTERIOSTATIC)		
Chloramphenicol		
Tetracyclines		Doxycycline, minocycline
Macrolides		Erythromycin, clarithromycin, azithromycin
Others		Linezolid, vancomycin, clindamycin
BINDING TO RIBOSOMAL SUBUNIT TO ALTER PROTEIN SYNTHESIS (BACTERICIDAL)		
Aminoglycosides		Streptomycin, gentamicin, tobramycin, neomycin
AFFECTING BACTERIAL NUCLEIC ACID METABOLISM		
Rifamycins		Rifampicin
Quinolones		Ciprofloxacin, ofloxacin, norfloxacin
ANTIMETABOLITES		
Trimethoprim		
Sulfonamides		Sulfamethoxazole

copper atom. Unlike natural chlorophyll, chlorophyllin is water soluble.[8] The antimicrobial activity of chlorophyllin is thought to be due to its antioxidant activity, perhaps related to its ability to reduce free radicals. Older studies reported that some chlorophyllin solutions slowed the growth of anaerobic bacteria, as well as reduced malodor, probably related to blockade of bacterial proteolytic enzymes.[8]

The bioavailability of chlorophyll after oral intake seems to be nonexistent.[9] Uptake of small amounts of chlorophyllin occurs after the application of high doses, but probably only with selected components of chlorophyllin. Chlorophyll and chlorophyllin are sensitive to acidic conditions; they are degraded in the stomach to pheophytins and pyropheophytins and excreted as the predominant end product in feces. Hydrophilic chlorophyllin components or chlorophyll derivatives associated with bile salts in lipid micelles can be absorbed in small amounts by intestinal wall cells. In clinical practice, chlorophyllin is used topically. Systemic application is indicated only for internal deodorization.

Dosages

Topical application of 2.5% chlorophyll solution is recommended. Oral intake of 100 to 300 mg chlorophyllin per day reduces odor from colostomies or ileostomies or fecal odor caused by incontinence.

Major Side Effects

After oral application, green discoloration of urine or feces and yellow or black discoloration of the tongue may occur. Diarrhea is reported occasionally. Topical application may lead to mild burning or itching.[8]

Contraindications

No testing has been done in pregnant or lactating women, so chlorophyllin derivatives should be avoided.

Drug Interactions

Oral chlorophyllin may result in false-positive guaiac testing for occult blood. No drug interactions are known with chlorophyllin.

Evidence-Based Medicine

The evidence base is limited. Topical application has been shown to deodorize malodorous wounds in older studies.[10] Controlled studies with oral chlorophyll on the subjective feeling of colostomy patients[11] and on reduction of malodor in incontinent patients have shown little or no effect in comparison to placebo.

METRONIDAZOLE

Mechanisms of Action

Metronidazole belongs to the nitroimidazoles and was developed because of their trichomonacidal properties. Metronidazole is a prodrug. Anaerobic and microaerophilic pathogens such as trichomonads, *Entamoeba histolytica*, *Giardia lamblia*, and anaerobic bacteria activate the drug by reducing the nitro group.[12] The ferredoxins that these pathogens use for electron transport as part of their energy metabolism transfer single electrons to metronidazole, thereby forming a highly reactive nitro radical anion that kills susceptible organisms. Treatment of anaerobic bacteria eliminates production of the volatile fatty acids by these bacteria that cause malodor in infected wounds. Aerobic pathogens do not use ferredoxins for energy transfer and are therefore not susceptible.

Increasing oxygen levels inhibit metronidazole because oxygen competes with metronidazole for electrons. Resistance has been linked to abnormalities such as higher local oxygen concentrations or decreased ferredoxins or pyruvate ferredoxin oxidoreductase, an enzyme that indirectly catalyzes the reduction of ferredoxins, which can then transfer electrons to metronidazole.

The drug is absorbed completely after oral intake.[13] Bioavailabilty is lower with rectal (60% to 80%) or vaginal application (20% to 50%). Effective plasma concentrations are reached 20 to 60 minutes after oral application, with peak plasma concentrations achieved after 1 to 2 hours. Binding to plasma proteins is low (<20%). The volume of distribution at steady state for adults is 0.5 to 1 L/kg. Metronidazole reaches therapeutic concentrations in most tissues, including cerebrospinal fluid, but not in placental tissue.

The plasma half-life of metronidazole is 6 to 11 hours, with longer times for higher dosages. Activity for up to 24 hours has been demonstrated after the administration of 1 g of metronidazole. The drug is metabolized in the liver, with two main metabolites resulting from oxidation of the side chains, a hydroxyl derivative and an acid. The hydroxyl metabolite has about half the biological activity of the parent compound and a longer elimination half-life. Most is excreted in urine and feces, largely as metabolites, and only 12% is eliminated unchanged in urine. Renal dysfunction reduces elimination, but dosage adaptations are not required. Liver dysfunction decreases clearance, and dosages should therefore be reduced.

Tinidazole, ornidazole, and secnidazole are related nitroimidazole derivatives with similar pharmacokinetic properties. However, they are more expensive and unavailable in most countries. Tinidazole has been recommended for those unable to tolerate metronidazole.

Dosages

For anaerobic infections in palliative care, metronidazole, 400 mg orally three times daily, is recommended. Dosages should be reduced to 400 mg twice daily in elderly debilitated patients. Recurrent infections may require long-term therapy with 200 mg twice daily. Treatment recommendations also include large single oral doses of 2 g metronidazole for genital infections or 2.4 g metronidazole for 2 days for amebic liver abscess. Solutions for injection are available if oral intake is impossible, and metronidazole can be used for topical application on fungating tumors or infected wounds.

Gels or solutions are also available for topical application. However, crushed tablets in neutral gel may be used because dosages will be much higher than with commercially available products. Topical treatment will not always be sufficient for malodorous wounds, and systemic application will be more efficient in many patients.

Metronidazole, 250 to 500 mg orally three times daily for 7 to 14 days or longer, is also recommended as first-line treatment of pseudomembranous colitis caused by *Clostridium difficile* infection. Metronidazole has been used for Crohn's disease and perianal fistulas. Infections with mixed aerobic and anaerobic pathogens require metronidazole and a β-lactam antibiotic or an aminoglycoside. Metronidazole has also been used in combination regimens for *Helicobacter pylori*.

Major Side Effects

Common side effects are headache, nausea, dry mouth, and a metallic taste.[14] Neurotoxic side effects such as dizziness and vertigo are rare. More severe symptoms such as encephalopathy, convulsions, incoordination, and ataxia are rare and should lead to discontinuation of metronidazole therapy. Treatment should also be discontinued if peripheral sensory neuropathy with paresthesias or extremity numbness is reported because reversal may be slow or incomplete. Drug sensitivity can include urticaria, exanthema, flushing or pruritus, and rarely, toxic epidermal necrolysis. Dysuria and cystitis have been reported very infrequently. Darkening of urine has been reported occasionally, probably related to metabolites. Metronidazole has carcinogenic properties in animals when applied in high doses and for a prolonged period. This may be related to its mechanism of action as a radical anion.

Contraindications

Metronidazole should not be used in patients with a history of anaphylactic reactions to this drug. No information is available on the teratogenicity of metronidazole. Its use in the first trimester is not advised.

Drug Interactions

Metronidazole has an effect similar to that of disulfiram and interacts with alcohol. Abdominal distress, vomiting, flushing, or headache may occur as a result of inhibition of enzymes leading to accumulation of acetaldehyde if patients consume alcohol during or shortly after treatment with metronidazole. Metronidazole and disulfiram should not be combined because confusion or psychosis may result.

Metronidazole reduces the elimination and increases the efficacy of oral anticoagulants, phenytoin, 5-fluorouracil, and lithium. Phenytoin and phenobarbital enhance and cimetidine reduces elimination of metronidazole. The combination of lithium and metronidazole may cause lithium toxicity.

Coadministration of the anthelmintic drug mebendazole and metronidazole should be avoided because a high incidence of toxic epidermal necrolysis has been reported with this combination.

Evidence-Based Medicine

Metronidazole is included in the list of essential medicines for palliative care of the International Hospice and Palliative Care Association.[15] There is only limited evidence from controlled trials.[16] Two small trials reported a benefit with the topical application of metronidazole versus placebo,[17,18] and two other small trials reported a benefit with systemic application.[19,20]

RESEARCH CHALLENGES

Research on antibiotic therapy should concentrate on decision making more than on drug effectiveness. It is agreed that in the final phase and in the dying, antibiotic therapy should not be initiated.[17] In earlier disease stages, however, no consensus exists. Control of symptoms requires antibiotic treatment for most infections,[7] but research is needed on indications for withholding antibiotics. Poor general condition and imminent death, inability to take oral antibiotics and refusal of parenteral application, and patient or family refusal despite medical indication are reasons for withholding or discontinuing antibiotics.[2] Balancing the benefits and disadvantages of antibiotics is also influenced by side effects and complications with different drugs and routes of application. More research is needed on the tolerability of antibiotic therapy and additional burdens, such as maintenance of an intravenous line only because of antibiotic treatment.

REFERENCES

1. Nagy-Agren S, Haley H. Management of infections in palliative care patients with advanced cancer. J Pain Symptom Manage 2002;24:64-70.
2. Pereira J, Watanabe S, Wolch G. A retrospective review of the frequency of infections and patterns of antibiotic utilization on a palliative care unit. J Pain Symptom Manage 1998;16:374-381.
3. Pestinger M, Ostgathe C, Bausewein C, et al. Antibiotica in der Palliativmedizin: Ergebnisse einer Fokusgruppe. Z Palliativmedizin 2004;5:68-74.
4. Oneschuk D, Fainsinger R, Demoissac D. Antibiotic use in the last week of life in three different palliative care settings. J Palliat Care 2002;18:25-28.
5. Fonzo-Christe C, Vukasovic C, Wasilewski-Rasca AF, Bonnabry P. Subcutaneous administration of drugs in the elderly: Survey of practice and systematic literature review. Palliat Med 2005;19:208-219.
6. Nauck F, Ostgathe C, Klaschik E, et al. Drugs in palliative care: Results from a representative survey in Germany. Palliat Med 2004;18:100-107.
7. Vitetta L, Kenner D, Sali A. Bacterial infections in terminally ill hospice patients. J Pain Symptom Manage 2000;20:326-334.
8. Higdon J. Chlorophyll and Chlorophyllin. Linus Pauling Institute. Corvallis: Oregon State University, 2005.
9. Ferruzzi MG, Blakeslee J. Digestion, absorption, and cancer preventative activity of dietary chlorophyll derivatives. Nutr Res 2007;27:1-12.
10. Chernomorsky S, Segelman A, Poretz RD, et al. Effect of dietary chlorophyll derivatives on mutagenesis and tumor cell growth. Teratog Carcinog Mutagen 1999;19:313-322.
11. Christiansen SB, Byel SR, Stromsted H, et al. [Can chlorophyll reduce fecal odor in colostomy patients?] Ugeskr Laeger 1989;151:1753-1754.
12. Phillips MA, Stanley SL Jr. Chemotherapy of protozoal infections: Amebiasis, giardiasis, trichomoniasis, trypanosomiasis, leishmaniasis, and other protozoal infections. In Brunton L (ed). Goodman and Gilman's The Pharmacological Basis of Therapeutics. New York: McGraw-Hill, 2005, pp 1049-1072.
13. Lamp KC, Freeman CD, Klutman NE, Lacy MK. Pharmacokinetics and pharmacodynamics of the nitroimidazole antimicrobials. Clin Pharmacokinet 1999;36:353-373.
14. Raether W, Hanel H. Nitroheterocyclic drugs with broad spectrum activity. Parasitol Res 2003;90(Supp 1):S19-S39.
15. De Lima L. International Association for Hospice and Palliative Care list of essential medicines for palliative care. Ann Oncol 2007;18:395-399.
16. Adderley U, Smith R. Topical agents and dressings for fungating wounds. Cochrane Database Syst Rev 2007;(2):CD003948.
17. Bale S, Tebbie N, Price P. A topical metronidazole gel used to treat malodorous wounds. Br J Nurs 2004;13:S4-S11.
18. Bower M, Stein R, Evans TR, et al. A double-blind study of the efficacy of metronidazole gel in the treatment of malodorous fungating tumours. Eur J Cancer 1992;28A:888-889.
19. Ashford R, Plant G, Maher J, Teare L. Double-blind trial of metronidazole in malodorous ulcerating tumours. Lancet 1984;1:1232-1233.
20. Sparrow G, Minton M, Rubens RD, et al. Metronidazole in smelly tumours. Lancet 1980;1:1185.

SUGGESTED READING

Antibiotic Subcommittee of the Pharmacy and Therapeutics Committee of the Froedtert Hospital, 2000. MCW & FMLH Antibiotic Guide. Available at http://www.intmed.mcw.edu/AntibioticGuide.html (accessed April 20, 2007).

Lamp KC, Freeman CD, Klutman NE, Lacy MK. Pharmacokinetics and pharmacodynamics of the nitroimidazole antimicrobials. Clin Pharmacokinet 1999;36:353-373.

Nagy-Agren S, Haley H. Management of infections in palliative care patients with advanced cancer. J Pain Symptom Manage 2002;24:64-70.

Phillips MA, Stanley SL Jr. Chemotherapy of protozoal infections: Amebiasis, giardiasis, trichomoniasis, trypanosomiasis, leishmaniasis, and other protozoal infections. In Brunton L (ed). Goodman and Gilman's The Pharmacological Basis of Therapeutics. New York: McGraw-Hill, 2005, pp 1049-1072.

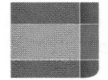

CHAPTER 132

Antiepileptic Drugs

K. Mitchell Russell

Idiopathic or cryptogenic epilepsy may be encountered as a co-morbidity in palliative medicine. Seizures may also develop from a chronic or life-limiting illness such as multiple sclerosis[1] and stroke[2] or from toxic, metabolic, or infectious causes. However, structural brain disease, including tumor and stroke, accounts for most seizures in the elderly.[3] About 20% to 40% of patients with primary brain tumors or intracerebral metastatic tumors experience seizures, as well as another 20% to 45% sometime during their illness,[4] with tumor location being the most important predictor. Those with primary brain tumors are more prone to recurrent seizures that are difficult to control pharmacologically.[5] About 15% of patients with leptomeningeal carcinomatosis have seizures,[5] but posterior fossa tumors rarely cause seizures.[6]

INDICATIONS FOR ANTIEPILEPTIC DRUGS

The goal of treating seizures in palliative medicine is to provide the best quality of life. When considering AED therapy, a balance should be found between seizure suppression, side effects, and economic and social concerns in each individual. Deciding how to achieve this goal is subject to discussion between the physician and the patient or caregiver.

DOCUMENTED SEIZURES

Accurate diagnosis plus classification of the type of seizure is essential.[7] Care must be taken to distinguish seizures from nonseizure events (e.g., myoclonus, rigors, syncope). Frequently, the event occurs outside the hospital and may be witnessed only by nonmedical caregivers, thus making diagnosis all the more difficult. Because AEDs have potential side effects, long-term AED treatment without convincing evidence of seizures is unwise.

PROPHYLAXIS OF SEIZURES

Prophylactic anticonvulsants are sometimes administered to patients with brain tumors or intracerebral metastases despite evidence that such prophylaxis does not prevent seizures.[8] Because prophylaxis with common AEDs such as benzodiazepines, carbamazepine, phenobarbital, phenytoin, and valproic acid is often associated with side effects and poor seizure control, the American Academy of Neurology has recommended that prophylactic AEDs not be used routinely in patients with newly diagnosed brain tumors.[4]

Prophylaxis after Neurosurgical Intervention

In those who have undergone a neurosurgical intervention and have not had a seizure, the anticonvulsant dose should be tapered and its use discontinued after the first postoperative week, particularly if there are side effects.[4]

MECHANISMS OF ACTION

The most commonly used first-line AEDs—carbamazepine, phenobarbital, phenytoin, and valproic acid—are all effective for partial and generalized tonic-clonic seizures,[9,10] and benzodiazepines are effective for generalized tonic-clonic seizures and status epilepticus.[11] Their mechanism of action can be categorized as either affecting ion channels, augmenting inhibitory neurotransmission, or modulating excitatory neurotransmission (Box 132-1).[12]

PHARMACOKINETICS

Pharmacokinetics (Table 132-1) can be used to help select the safest and most effective AED, particularly in palliative medicine because of frequent concomitant organ dysfunction and polypharmacy.

DOSING AND ADMINISTRATION

AEDs should be routinely administered orally if possible (Table 132-2). Administering AEDs to patients near death is challenging inasmuch as 28% experience significant dysphagia during the last 48 hours of life.[18]

Parenteral Administration

Benzodiazepines, phenobarbital, or phenytoin can be administered parenterally in the acute hospital setting for seizures or status epilepticus. The Veterans Administration cooperative trial demonstrated first-line treatment success rates of 65% for lorazepam, 58% for phenobarbital, 56% for diazepam/phenytoin, and 44% for phenytoin alone.[19] Frequently, intravenous access is limited and therefore subcutaneous access is used; however, subcutaneous administration of diazepam and lorazepam can cause irritation and hence is avoided. Midazolam has excellent bioavailability subcutaneously[20] and is well tolerated. Subcutaneous infusions of 20 to 80 mg per 24 hours can be used for seizure control or prevention near death when

---

> **Box 132-1   Mechanisms of Action**
>
> - Benzodiazepines enhance γ-aminobutyric acid (GABA)-dependent chloride conductance by binding to a $GABA_A$ receptor modulatory site, enhancing GABA-dependent chloride conductance, and hyperpolarizing and inhibiting the neuron.
> - Phenobarbital, the oldest of the commonly used AEDs, acts by prolonging inhibitory postsynaptic potentials by increasing the opening time of the chloride channel and the duration of GABA-induced bursts of neuronal activity.[13]
> - Phenytoin acts by inducing voltage- and use-dependent blockage of sodium channels, blocking the feedback that produces maximal seizure activity, and thus sparing normal brain activity.[14] This mechanism allows it to be an effective AED with minimal cognitive side effects.
> - Carbamazepine is structurally related to tricyclic antidepressants and acts by reducing sustained repetitive firing of depolarized neurons through voltage- and use-dependent blockage of sodium channels.[15]
> - Valproic acid acts by reducing sustained repetitive firing of depolarized neurons through voltage- and use-dependent blockage of sodium channels, but it probably has other mechanisms.[16]
> - The newer AEDs increase inhibitory activity as GABA analogues or enhancers, act through voltage- and use-dependent blockage of sodium channels, inhibit excitatory activity through glutamate or aspartate, and may act through other mechanisms.[17]

TABLE 132-1 Antiepileptic Drug Pharmacokinetics

DRUG	T_{MAX} (HR)	$T_{1/2}$ (HR)	TIME TO STEADY STATE (DAYS)	PROTEIN BINDING (%)	ELIMINATION
Carbamazepine	4-12	5-20	21-28 for auto-induction	40-90	Hepatic (CYP3A4)
Diazepam	0.5-2	20-80	2-3	98	Hepatic (CYP2C19, CYP3A4)
Ethosuximide	1-4	30-60	7	<10	Hepatic (CYP3A4)
Felbamate	2-6	14-23	4	25	Renal 90%
Gabapentin	2-3	5-9	1-2	0	Renal
Lamotrigine	1-3	15-60	3-10	55	Hepatic
Levetiracetam	0.6-1.3	7	2	<10	Renal
Lorazepam	2-4	10-20	2	85	Hepatic (conjugation)
Midazolam	0.5-2	1.8-6.4	1-2	97	Hepatic (CYP3A4)
Oxcarbazepine	1-2	2	2	40 (MHD)	Hepatic
Phenobarbital	0.5-4	46-136	14-21	50	Hepatic (CYP2C9, CYP2C19)
Phenytoin	2-12	10-34	7-28	90	Hepatic (CYP2C9, CYP2C19)
Pregabalin	1	9	1-2	0	Renal
Primidone	2-4	8-15	1-4	<20	Hepatic (CYP2C9, CYP2C19)
Tiagabine	1-2	2-9	1-2	96	Hepatic (oxidation and conjugation)
Topiramate	1-4	12-30	3-5	15	Renal 70%
Valproic acid	1-8	8-20	1-3	90-95	Hepatic (oxidation and conjugation)
Vigabatrin	0.5-2	5-7	2	0	Renal
Zonisamide	2-5	50-70	10-15	55	Hepatic (CYP3A4)

Adapted from Bradley WG, Daroff RB, Fenichel G, Jankovic J (eds). Neurology in Clinical Practice. Philadelphia: Elsevier, 2003; and Mosby's Drug Consult. St Louis: Elsevier/Mosby, 2005.

TABLE 132-2 Antiepileptic Drug Dosing

DRUG	USUAL INITIAL DOSE	USUAL MAXIMUM DAILY DOSE	TARGET SERUM CONCENTRATION RANGE
Carbamazepine	400 mg/day	400-2400 mg	4-14 µg/mL
Diazepam	PO: 4-40 mg IV: 5-10 mg	PO: 4-40 mg IV: 5-30 mg	100-1000 ng/mL
Ethosuximide	500 mg/day	500-2000 mg	40-80 µg/mL
Felbamate	1200 mg/day	3600 mg	40-100 µg/mL
Gabapentin	900 mg/day	4800 mg	4-16 µg/mL
Lamotrigine	25 mg every other day if taking valproic acid, 25-50 mg/day if not	100-150 mg if taking valproic acid, 300-500 mg if not	4-20 µg/mL
Levetiracetam	500-1000 mg/day	3000-4000 mg	Not defined
Lorazepam	PO: 2-6 mg IV: 0.05 mg/kg	PO: 10 mg IV: 0.044 mg/kg	10-30 ng/mL
Oxcarbazepine	300-600 mg/day	2400-3000 mg	12-30 µg/mL (MHD)
Phenobarbital	1-3 mg/kg/day	180-300 mg	10-40 µg/mL
Phenytoin	PO: 3-5 mg/kg	PO: 500-600 mg	10-20 µg/mL total 0.5-3 µg/mL unbound
Pregabalin	150 mg/day	600 mg	Not defined
Primidone	100-125 mg/day	750-2000 mg	5-10 µg/mL
Tiagabine	4-8 mg/day	80 mg	Not defined
Topiramate	25-50 mg/day	200-1000 mg	Not defined
Valproic acid	15 mg/kg (500-1000 mg)	60 mg/kg (3000-5000 mg)	50-150 µg/mL
Vigabatrin	1000 mg/day	4000 mg	Not defined
Zonisamide	100-200 mg/day	600 mg	10-40 µg/mL

MHD, 10-monohydroxy metabolite.
Adapted from DiPiro JT, Talbert RL, Yee GC, et al (eds). Pharmacotherapy, 5th ed. New York: McGraw-Hill, 2002.

oral administration is lost. Midazolam infusions may be restricted by conscious sedation policies, particularly in the United States. Alternatively, subcutaneous infusions of 180 to 300 mg phenobarbital per 24 hours may control seizures in the dying.

Rectal Administration

Rectal administration is preferred when homebound or hospice patients are unable to take oral medications.[21] Commercially prepared suppositories, tablets, or capsules should be used for routine administration. Routine rectal administration of solutions with alcohol or glycol vehicles (e.g., parenteral forms of diazepam, lorazepam, phenytoin) should be avoided because they may cause rectal irritation when used repeatedly.[21]

Diazepam, commercially available in a rectal suppository form, has excellent absorption when administered rectally, with serum drug peaks within 20 minutes sufficient to stop seizures at dosages of 0.5 mg/kg.[22] It should be considered first line for status epilepticus when the parenteral route is unavailable.

Lorazepam is often the preferred benzodiazepine for hospice because it is inexpensive, has a moderate duration of action, and exhibits relatively stable pharmacokinetics in patients with liver and kidney failure.[21] Absorption after rectal administration is about 80%, but the absorption phase is prolonged and the time to peak levels is 1 hour longer than with parenteral administration; doses to abort seizures are typically two to four times the parenteral dose.[23]

Phenobarbital also has nearly equivalent rectal and oral absorption as a suppository,[24] and phenobarbital sodium has a more rapid rate of absorption than lipophilic phenobarbital does. Either may be considered reasonable second-line treatment of status epilepticus when parenteral access is impractical and diazepam is unavailable or ineffective.

Valproic acid is a reasonable second-line rectal treatment of status epilepticus because its rectal absorption and bioavailability are comparable to that of oral administration, with early absorption in 30 minutes.[25,26]

Carbamazepine in suspension administered rectally has slower absorption, thus precluding its use in status epilepticus, but bioavailability equivalent to that of oral administration.[21] The solution must be retained in the rectum for 2 hours, which is difficult for most because it provokes the urge to defecate.[27,28]

There are few data about phenytoin absorption rectally. Parenteral phenytoin solution is poorly absorbed

TABLE 132-3 Adverse Effects of Antiepileptic Drugs

DRUG	Acute Adverse Effects		CHRONIC ADVERSE EFFECTS
	CONCENTRATION DEPENDENT	IDIOSYNCRATIC	
Benzodiazepines	Drowsiness, psychomotor incoordination, decreased concentration, cognitive deficits	Paradoxical hyperexcitability, hallucinations, sleep disturbances, blood dyscrasias, rash	Anterograde amnesia, sedation, decreased concentration
Carbamazepine	Diplopia, dizziness, drowsiness, nausea, unsteadiness, lethargy	Blood dyscrasias, rash	Hyponatremia
Ethosuximide	Ataxia, drowsiness, GI distress, unsteadiness, hiccups	Blood dyscrasias, rash	Behavior changes, headache
Felbamate	Anorexia, nausea, vomiting, insomnia, headache	Aplastic anemia, acute hepatic failure	Not established
Gabapentin	Dizziness, fatigue, somnolence, ataxia	Not established	Weight gain
Lamotrigine	Diplopia, dizziness, unsteadiness, headache	Rash	Not established
Levetiracetam	Sedation, behavioral disturbance	Not established	Not established
Oxcarbazepine	Sedation, dizziness, ataxia, nausea	Rash	Hyponatremia
Phenobarbital	Ataxia, hyperactivity, headache, unsteadiness, sedation, nausea	Blood dyscrasias, rash	Behavior changes, connective tissue disorders, intellectual blunting, metabolic bone disease, mood change, sedation
Phenytoin	Ataxia, nystagmus, behavior changes, dizziness, headache, incoordination, sedation, lethargy, cognitive impairment, fatigue, blurred vision	Blood dyscrasias, rash, immunological reaction	Behavior changes, cerebellar syndrome, connective tissue changes, skin thickening, folate deficiency, gingival hyperplasia, hirsutism, coarsening of facial features, acne, cognitive impairment, metabolic bone disease, sedation
Pregabalin	Dizziness, drowsiness, blurred vision, ataxia, tremor	Blood dyscrasias, rash	Weight gain, memory impairment
Primidone	Behavior changes, headache, nausea, sedation, unsteadiness	Blood dyscrasias, rash	Behavior change, connective tissue disorders, cognitive impairment, sedation
Tiagabine	Dizziness, fatigue, difficulty concentrating, nervousness, tremor, blurred vision, depression, weakness	Not established	Not established
Topiramate	Difficulty concentrating, psychomotor slowing, speech or language problems, somnolence, fatigue, dizziness, headache	Not established	Kidney stones
Valproic acid	GI upset, sedation, unsteadiness, tremor, thrombocytopenia	Acute hepatic failure, acute pancreatitis	Polycystic ovary–like syndrome, alopecia, weight gain, hyperammonemia
Vigabatrin	Somnolence, headache, dizziness, nervousness, blurred vision	Not established	Amnesia, depression
Zonisamide	Sedation, dizziness, cognitive impairment, nausea	Rash, oligohidrosis	Kidney stones

GI, gastrointestinal.
Adapted from DiPiro JT, Talbert RL, Yee GC, et al (eds). Pharmacotherapy, 5th ed. New York: McGraw-Hill, 2002.

rectally,[29] and capsules or tablets are probably not well absorbed either.

MAJOR SIDE EFFECTS

Adverse effects of AEDs are common and clinically important. They may be divided into acute (concentration dependent or idiosyncratic) and chronic effects (Table 132-3).

CONTRAINDICATIONS

Contraindications to AEDs are few (Table 132-4).

DRUG INTERACTIONS

Most pharmacokinetic interactions involve modification of drug metabolism.[30] Phenobarbital, phenytoin, primidone, and carbamazepine are potent inducers of the cytochrome P-450 (CYP), epoxide hydrolase, and uridine diphosphate glucuronosyltransferase (UGT) enzyme systems. Valproic acid can inhibit CYP and UGT and displace drugs from plasma albumin, which can result in clinically important drug interactions (Table 132-5). Importantly, enzyme-inducing AEDs can interact with corticosteroids, oral anticoagulants, and many cardiovascular, psychotropic, and antineoplastic drugs.[31] For example, phenobarbital induces the metabolism of corticosteroids, thus reducing their efficacy and potentially requiring dosage adjustment.

TABLE 132-4 Antiepileptic Drug Contraindications

DRUG	CONTRAINDICATION
Benzodiazepines	Acute narrow-angle glaucoma, hypersensitivity to benzodiazepines
Carbamazepine	History of bone marrow depression, hypersensitivity to tricyclic compounds, or presently taking a monoamine oxidase inhibitor
Ethosuximide	Hypersensitivity to succinimides
Felbamate	Blood dyscrasias, hepatic dysfunction, hypersensitivity to carbamates
Gabapentin	Hypersensitivity to gabapentin
Lamotrigine	Hypersensitivity to lamotrigine
Levetiracetam	Hypersensitivity to levetiracetam
Oxcarbazepine	Hypersensitivity to oxcarbazepine
Phenobarbital	History of manifest or latent porphyria, hypersensitivity to phenobarbital
Phenytoin	Sinus bradycardia, sinoatrial block, second- and third-degree atrioventricular block, Adams-Stokes syndrome, hypersensitivity to hydantoin products
Pregabalin	Hypersensitivity to pregabalin
Primidone	History of manifest or latent porphyria, hypersensitivity to phenobarbital
Tiagabine	Hypersensitivity to tiagabine
Topiramate	Hypersensitivity to topiramate
Valproic acid	Hepatic dysfunction, urea cycle disorders, hypersensitivity to valproic acid
Zonisamide	Hypersensitivity to sulfonamides, zonisamide

From Mosby's Drug Consult. St Louis, Elsevier/Mosby, 2005.

TABLE 132-5 Antiepileptic Drug Interactions

DRUG	ADDED DRUG	EFFECT	DRUG	ADDED DRUG	EFFECT
Carbamazepine (CBZ)	Felbamate	Decrease CBZ		Disulfiram	Increase PHT
	Phenobarbital	Decrease CBZ		Ethanol (acute)	Increase PHT
	Phenytoin	Decrease CBZ		Fluconazole	Increase PHT
	Cimetidine	Increase CBZ		Isoniazid	Increase PHT
	Erythromycin	Increase CBZ		Propoxyphene	Increase PHT
	Fluoxetine	Increase CBZ		Warfarin	Increase PHT
	Isoniazid	Increase CBZ		Ethanol (chronic)	Decrease PHT
	Propoxyphene	Increase CBZ		OC	Decrease OC
	Oral contraceptive (OC)	Decrease OC		Bishydroxycoumarin	Decrease anticoagulation
	Doxycycline	Decrease doxycycline		Folic acid	Decrease folic acid
				Quinidine	Decrease quinidine
	Theophylline	Decrease theophylline		Vitamin D	Decrease vitamin D
	Warfarin	Decrease warfarin	Pregabalin		No known interactions
Felbamate (FBM)	Carbamazepine	Decrease FBM		Phenytoin	Decrease PRM, increase PB
	Phenytoin	Decrease FBM		Valproic acid	Increase PRM, PB
	Valproic acid	Increase FBM		Isoniazid	Increase PRM
Gabapentin		No known interactions		Nicotinamide	Increase PRM
Lamotrigine (LTG)	Carbamazepine	Decrease LTG		Chlorpromazine	Decrease chlorpromazine
	Phenobarbital	Decrease LTG		Corticosteroids	Decrease corticosteroids
	Phenytoin	Decrease LTG		Quinidine	Decrease quinidine
	Primidone	Decrease LTG		Tricyclic antidepressants	Decrease tricyclics
	Valproic acid	Increase LTG		Furosemide	Decrease renal sensitivity to furosemide
Levetiracetam		No known interactions			
Oxcarbazepine	Carbamazepine	Decrease MHD			

TABLE 132-5   Antiepileptic Drug Interactions—cont'd

DRUG	ADDED DRUG	EFFECT	DRUG	ADDED DRUG	EFFECT
	Phenytoin	Decrease MHD	Tiagabine (TGB)	Carbamazepine	Decrease TGB
	Phenobarbital	Decrease MHD		Phenytoin	Decrease TGB
	OC	Decrease OC	Topiramate (TPM)	Carbamazepine	Decrease TPM
Phenobarbital (PB)	Felbamate	Increase PB		Phenytoin	Decrease TPM
	Phenytoin	Increase or decrease PB		Valproic acid	Decrease TMP
	Valproic acid	Increase PB		OC	Decrease OC
	Acetazolamide	Increase PB	Valproic acid (VPA)	Carbamazepine	Decrease VPA
	OC	Decrease OC		Lamotrigine	Decrease VPA
Phenytoin (PHT)	Carbamazepine	Decrease PHT		Phenobarbital	Decrease VPA
	Felbamate	Increase PHT		Primidone	Decrease VPA
	Methsuximide	Increase PHT		Phenytoin	Decrease VPA
	Phenobarbital	Increase or decrease PHT		Cimetidine	Increase VPA
				Salicylates	Increase free VPA
	Valproic acid	Decrease total PHT	Zonisamide (ZNA)	Carbamazepine	Decrease ZNA
	Vigabatrin	Decrease PHT		Phenytoin	Decrease ZNA
	Antacids	Decrease absorption of PHT		Phenobarbital	Decrease ZNA
	Cimetidine	Increase PHT			
	Chloramphenicol	Increase PHT			

Adapted from DiPiro JT, Talbert RL, Yee GC, et al (eds). Pharmacotherapy, 5th ed. New York: McGraw-Hill, 2002.

Current Controversies and Future Considerations

- Newer AEDs such as felbamate, gabapentin, lamotrigine, levetiracetam, oxcarbazepine, pregabalin, tiagabine, topiramate, vigabatrin, and zonisamide may have better pharmacokinetic profiles and less drug interactions than the classic AEDs.[32]

- Newer AEDs may be better tolerated for long-term seizure control but are more costly or have restricted availability.

REFERENCES

1. Lebrun C. [Epilepsy and multiple sclerosis.] Epileptic Disord 2004;6(Suppl 1):59-62.
2. Olsen TS. Post-stroke epilepsy. Curr Atheroscler Rep 2001;3:340-344.
3. Mahler ME. Seizures: Common causes and treatment in the elderly. Geriatrics 1987;42:73-78.
4. American Academy of Neurology. Practice parameter: Anticonvulsant prophylaxis in patients with newly diagnosed brain tumors. Available at http://www.neurology.org/cgi/content/full/54/10/1886.pdf (accessed August 2006).
5. Glantz M, Recht LD. Handbook of Clinical Neurology, vol 25. New York: Elsevier, 1997.
6. Mesiwala AH, Kuratani JD, Avellino AM, et al. Focal motor seizures with secondary generalization arising in the cerebellum. Case report and review of the literature. J Neurosurg 2002;97:190-196.
7. Brodie MJ, French JA. Management of epilepsy in adolescents and adults. Lancet 2000;356:323-329.
8. Cohen N, Strauss G, Lew R, et al. Should prophylactic anticonvulsants be administered to patients with newly-diagnosed cerebral metastases? A retrospective analysis. J Clin Oncol 1988;6:1621-1624.
9. Mattson RH, Cramer JA, Collins JF, et al. Comparison of carbamazepine, phenobarbital, phenytoin, and primidone in partial and secondarily generalized tonic-clonic seizures. N Engl J Med 1985;313:145-151.
10. Mattson RH, Cramer JA, Collins JF. A comparison of valproate with carbamazepine for the treatment of complex partial seizures and secondarily generalized tonic-clonic seizures in adults. The Department of Veterans Affairs Epilepsy Cooperative Study No. 264 Group. N Engl J Med 1992;327:765-771.
11. Henriksen O. An overview of benzodiazepines in seizure management. Epilepsia 1998;39:S2-S6.
12. DiPiro JT, Talbert RL, Yee GC, et al (eds). Pharmacotherapy, 5th ed. New York: McGraw-Hill, 2002.
13. Twyman RE, Rogers CJ, Macdonald RL. Differential regulation of gamma-aminobutyric acid receptor channels by diazepam and phenobarbital. Ann Neurol 1989;25:213-220.
14. Yaari Y, Selzer ME, Pincus JH. Phenytoin: Mechanisms of its anticonvulsant action. Ann Neurol 1986;20:171-184.
15. McLean MJ, Macdonald RL. Carbamazepine and 10,11-epoxycarbamazepine produce use- and voltage-dependent limitation of rapidly firing action potentials of mouse central neurons in cell culture. J Pharmacol Exp Ther 1986;238:727-738.
16. McLean MJ, Macdonald RL. Sodium valproate, but not ethosuximide, produces use- and voltage-dependent limitation of high frequency repetitive firing of action potentials of mouse central neurons in cell culture. J Pharmacol Exp Ther 1986;237:1001-1011.
17. White HS. Comparative anticonvulsant and mechanistic profile of the established and newer antiepileptic drugs. Epilepsia 1999;40(Suppl 5):2-10.
18. Hall P, Schroder C, Weaver L. The last 48 hours of life in long-term care: A focused chart audit. J Am Geriatr Soc 2002;50:501-506.
19. Treiman DM, Meyers PD, Walton NY, et al. A comparison of four treatments for generalized convulsive status epilepticus. Veterans Affairs Status Epilepticus Cooperative Study Group. N Engl J Med 1998;339:792-798.
20. Pecking M, Montestruc F, Marquet P, et al. Absolute bioavailability of midazolam after subcutaneous administration to healthy volunteers. Br J Clin Pharmacol 2002;54:357-362.
21. Warren DE. Practical use of rectal medications in palliative care. J Pain Symptom Manage 1996;11:378-387.
22. Remy C, Jourdil N, Villemain D, et al. Intrarectal diazepam in epileptic adults. Epilepsia 1992;33:353-358.
23. Graves NM, Kriel RL, Jones-Saete C. Bioavailability of rectally administered lorazepam. Clin Neuropharmacol 1987;10:555-559.
24. Minkov E, Lambov N, Kirchev D, et al. Biopharmaceutical investigation of rectal suppositories. Part 2(1): Pharmaceutical and biological availability of phenobarbital and phenobarbital-sodium. Pharmazie 1985;40:257-259.
25. Kanazawa O, Sengoku A, Kawai I. Treatment of childhood epilepsy with rectal valproate: Case reports and pharmacokinetic study. Brain Dev 1987;9:615-620.
26. Yoshiyama Y, Nakano S, Ogawa N. Chronopharmacokinetic study of valproic acid in man: Comparison of oral and rectal administration. J Clin Pharmacol 1989;29:1048-1052.
27. Graves NM, Kriel RL, Jones-Saete C, Cloyd JC. Relative bioavailability of rectally administered carbamazepine suspension in humans. Epilepsia 1985;26:429-433.
28. Neuvonen PJ, Tokola O. Bioavailability of rectally administered carbamazepine mixture. Br J Clin Pharmacol 1987;24:839-841.
29. Moolenaar F, Jelsma RBH, Visser J. Manipulation of rectal absorption rate of phenytoin in man. Pharmaceut Weekblad 1981;3:1051-1056.
30. Riva R, Albani F, Contin M, Baruzzi A. Pharmacokinetic interactions between antiepileptic drugs. Clinical considerations. Clin Pharmacokinet 1996;31:470-493.
31. Perucca E. Clinically relevant drug interactions with antiepileptic drugs. Br J Clin Pharmacol 2006;61:246-255.
32. Bialer M. The pharmacokinetics and interactions of new antiepileptic drugs: An overview. Ther Drug Monit 2005;27:722-726.

SUGGESTED READING

Bailer M. The pharmacokinetics and interactions of new antiepileptic drugs: An overview. Ther Drug Monit 2005;27:722-726.

Krouwer H. Management of seizures in brain tumor patients at the end of life. J Palliat Med 2000;3:465-475.

CHAPTER **133**

Cancer-Related Weight Loss

Faith D. Ottery

The major premise of optimal management of weight and nutrition in palliative medicine is proactively addressing nutritional risk or deficit in each patient from the time of diagnosis throughout the cancer care continuum.

Weight change, nutritional status, and nonobvious symptoms that affect nutrition tend to be relatively low on the priority list in a busy oncology practice. Possible exceptions include patients with cachexia and advanced disease at initial evaluation or select cancers accompanied by significant weight loss, such as non–small cell lung or pancreatic cancer or non-Hodgkin's lymphoma with "B" symptoms. Unfortunately, success in treating the advanced stages of *either* cancer or malnutrition is limited and especially compromised when they occur concomitantly.

The adverse impact of involuntary weight loss on oncological outcomes (including survival, tolerance of therapy, performance status, and quality of life) has been documented, with 5% weight loss in the previous 6 months before diagnosis or initiation of treatment being associated with decreased survival, increased toxicity, and worse quality of life.[1] Assessment of nutritional risk and deficit is complicated by constraints of time and training and the significant and growing problem of obesity. In this context, one in every three Americans could experience catabolic or involuntary weight loss of 10% to 20% and still be *overweight*. In other words, waiting until someone looks nutritionally depleted is generally too late for optimal intervention.

Importantly, disease- or cytokine-related weight loss tends to be catabolic, with progressive loss of lean tissue, and is exacerbated by decreased activity during cancer treatment or with advanced disease. Each patient will have the greatest opportunity for maintaining weight, functional status, and quality of life *throughout* the cancer course—including entry into palliative care—if attention is paid to weight loss and associated nutrition symptoms and educating patients and family about the importance of activity early in the disease or treatment process.[2]

PHARMACOLOGICAL INTERVENTION— IDENTIFICATION OF THE TREATABLE PROBLEM

Appropriate pharmacological intervention in cancer- or treatment-related weight loss demands ongoing assessment of patient signs and symptoms and consideration of evolving therapeutic goals.

Intervention may be single modality or multimodality in nature and must be customized to each patient. Several assessment tools are available for the management of symptoms.[3-5] In the Patient-Generated Subjective Global Assessment (PG-SGA), patients check off symptoms that affect their intake (referred to as nutrition impact symptoms).[5] Although these symptoms include the obvious considerations of mucositis, nausea, and vomiting or less obvious and more global symptoms such as anorexia, early satiety, or changes in taste and smell, we may fail to consider the nutritional implications of pain, fatigue, insomnia, dry mouth, presence of an ostomy, diarrhea, constipation, dental status, and finances.

The PG-SGA allows patients to self-identify, on a check-off list, symptoms that can be significant impediments to adequate nutritional intake or utilization of nutrients. Anorexia is an independent prognostic indicator in chemotherapy or multimodality therapy, and pharmacological intervention with appetite stimulants may seem to be the obvious answer.[6-9] However, if we address only appetite without addressing the other symptoms affecting nutrition, we are missing one or more interventional opportunities and potentially compromising the effectiveness of appetite stimulants. Importantly, in palliative medicine, optimal control of nutritional impact and other symptoms also contributes to better rehabilitation or palliative care.[10,11]

Generally, when pharmacological intervention of cancer-related weight loss is being considered, appetite stimulants are often the primary consideration. This includes agents specifically for appetite and treatment of weight loss or cachexia and agents such as corticosteroids, which can increase appetite and sense of well being—which in turn can lead to improved socialization and food intake.[6-9,12]

Megestrol acetate as a liquid formulation (OS or ES) is the most widely studied and commonly prescribed appetite drug with a specific appetite or weight indication.[6,7] Though commonly used off-label for appetite stimulation in oncology, megestrol is indicated for anorexia, cachexia, or unexplained significant weight loss in patients with acquired immunodeficiency syndrome (AIDS) (Table 133-1).[13]

Although the cannabinoid dronabinol is indicated for the anorexia associated with weight loss in patients with AIDS and for the nausea and vomiting associated with cancer chemotherapy in patients who have failed to

TABLE 133-1 Megestrol Acetate (OS, ES) Label Summary

DOSAGE	MAJOR SIDE EFFECTS (IN TERMS OF SEVERITY OR FREQUENCY)	CONTRAINDICATIONS	DRUG-DRUG OR DRUG-FOOD INTERACTIONS
Recommended adult dosage of OS: 400-800 mg/day (10-20 mL) Recommended adult dosage of ES: 625 mg/day (5 mL/day or one teaspoon daily)— equivalent to 800 mg or 20 mL	Thromboembolic phenomena (thrombophlebitis, pulmonary embolism, stroke) Glucose intolerance Impotence Adrenal suppression Edema Hypertension Withdrawal bleeding Insomnia	History of hypersensitivity to megestrol acetate or any component of the formulation Known or suspected pregnancy	PK studies show no significant alterations in PK parameters of zidovudine or rifabutin when MA-OS is coadministered. Effects of zidovudine or rifabutin on the PK of MA-OA, MA-ES not studied. In addition, a PK study noted in the ES PI, but not clear whether carried out in ES or OS, demonstrated that coadministration of MA and indinavir resulted in a significant decrease in PK parameters ($\approx$36% for C_{max} and $\approx$28% for AUC) of indinavir. Administration of a higher dose of indinavir should be considered when coadministered with MA. The effects of indinavir, zidovudine, or rifabutin on the PK of MA were not studied. Finally, according to ES PI, in patients who are receiving or being withdrawn from chronic Megace ES therapy, consideration should be given to the use of empirical therapy with stress doses of a rapidly acting glucocorticoid during stress or serious intercurrent illness (e.g., surgery, infection). A bioavailability study directly comparing the rate and extent of absorption of ES and OS formulations revealed that the maximum blood concentration (C_{max}) with the OS formulation was 1364 ng/mL in fed patients and 187 ng/mL in unfed patients. In contrast, the C_{max} level with ES was 1517 ng/mL in fed patients and 1041 ng/mL in unfed patients. Additionally, the study demonstrated that a lower volume of ES achieved maximum blood concentration more rapidly than the currently available OS products did.

AUC, area under the curve; MA, megestrol acetate; PI, product information; PK, pharmacokinetic.
From Megestrol acetate (oral suspension): Full prescribing information. Available at http://www.bms.com/cgi-bin/anybin.pl?sql=PI_SEQ=13 (accessed September 7, 2007); and Megestrol acetate (oral ES formulation): Full prescribing information. Available at http://www.megacees.com/PDF/Megace_ES_Portrait_PI.pdf (accessed September 7, 2007).

respond adequately to conventional antiemetics, it is used as an orexigenic agent in cancer,[14] often when a patient is experiencing both anorexia and nausea. Our understanding of endocannabinoids and cannabinoid receptors (CB1 in the central nervous system and CB1 and CB2 peripherally) has grown impressively. Potential benefits in cancer extend beyond established uses to include analgesia, antitumor effects, mood elevation, muscle relaxation, and relief from insomnia (Table 133-2).[8,9]

Use of corticosteroids in the late stages of palliative care may be appropriate, whereas earlier in the cancer course, where maintenance of body composition is important, they may be contraindicated. Corticosteroids are catabolic (i.e., increased muscle protein breakdown). In addition, they increase intake of nonprotein calories (carbohydrates and fats). Several controlled studies of various corticosteroids have been carried out in palliative medicine.[10,12,15] In general, their effects on improving appetite are short-lived (2 to 4 weeks), which may be appropriate when duration of survival is secondary. In advanced cancer, where maintenance of body composition (muscle mass) is not a major concern, administration of corticosteroids can be reasonable because of their psychogenic effect and short-lived appetite stimulation.

Oxandrolone is a testosterone derivative (anabolic steroid) indicated as adjunctive therapy for

- Weight loss after extensive surgery, chronic infections, or severe trauma
- Some who fail to gain or maintain normal weight without definite pathophysiological reasons

- Offsetting the protein catabolism associated with prolonged administration of corticosteroids
- Relief of the bone pain frequently accompanying osteoporosis[16]

Most of the published research on oxandrolone in involuntary or disease-related weight loss has involved human immunodeficiency virus (HIV) infection/AIDS, trauma/burns/wounds, growth retardation syndromes, chronic obstructive pulmonary disease, and other catabolic settings.[17,18] Pilot studies in oncology are reported in scientific meetings only, thus limiting more widespread awareness of use in oncology. Physiologically, anabolic steroids increase nitrogen retention, muscle protein synthesis, and gain in weight as lean tissue weight (Table 133-3).[17]

RESEARCH CHALLENGES

The primary research challenges include the following:

- The complex of factors that have an impact on weight and nutritional status in cancer and during cancer therapy (e.g., baseline status, disease stage at diagnosis, systemic and catabolic effects of cytokines, cancer treatment and toxicity, psychosocial variables, inactivity or bed rest, and others) can elude simplistic or single-modality approaches. Addressing one aspect in isolation significantly compromises the potential for success.

TABLE 133-2   Dronabinol Label Summary

DOSAGE	MAJOR SIDE EFFECTS (IN TERMS OF SEVERITY OR FREQUENCY)	CONTRAINDICATIONS	DRUG-DRUG OR DRUG-FOOD INTERACTIONS
Initially, 2.5 mg PO twice daily before lunch and supper. For patients unable to tolerate this 5-mg/day dosage of dronabinol, the dosage can be reduced to 2.5 mg/day administered as a single dose in the evening or at bedtime. If clinically indicated and in the absence of significant AEs, the dosage may gradually be increased to a maximum of 20 mg/day in divided doses. Caution should be exercised in escalating the dosage because of an increased frequency of dose-related AEs at higher dosages. Dosage may be increased to 2.5 mg before lunch and 5 mg before supper (or 5 mg at lunch and 5 mg after supper). Although most patients respond to 2.5 mg twice daily, 10 mg twice daily has been tolerated in ≈50% of patients.	Dose-related "high" (easy laughing, elation, and heightened awareness) in both the antiemetic (24%) and lower-dose appetite stimulant clinical trials (8%) Most frequently reported AEs in patients with AIDS during placebo-controlled clinical trials involved the CNS and were reported by 33% of patients receiving dronabinol. About 25% of patients reported a minor CNS AE during the first 2 weeks and about 4% reported such an event each week for the next 6 weeks thereafter. Side effects listed as probably causally related *Incidence rates >1%:* Generally higher with antiemetic use (in parentheses): —Palpitations, tachycardia, vasodilation/facial flush, (amnesia), anxiety/nervousness, (hallucination), (ataxia), confusion, depersonalization —Asthenia *Incidence of 3-5%:* —Dizziness, euphoria, paranoid reaction, somnolence, abnormal thinking *Incidence of 3-10%:* —Abdominal pain, nausea, vomiting *Incidence <1%:* —Hypotension, flushing, depression, nightmares, speech difficulties, tinnitus, emotional lability, tremors, fecal incontinence, diarrhea, myalgias, conjunctivitis, vision difficulties	Hypersensitivity to any cannabinoid or sesame oil	No drug-drug interactions seen during clinical trials Cannabinoids may interact with other medications through metabolic or pharmacodynamic mechanisms. Highly protein bound to plasma proteins. Although displacement has not been confirmed in vivo, HCPs should monitor for change in dosage requirements when administering dronabinol to patients receiving other highly protein-bound drugs. Published reports involving cannabinoids: —Additive tachycardia (possibly cardiotoxicity), hypertension, drowsiness with amphetamines, cocaine, sympathomimetics, anticholinergics, antihistamines, and tricyclic antidepressants —Additive or synergistic CNS effects with alcohol, sedatives, hypnotics, psychomimetics —Decreased clearance of barbiturates

AEs, adverse events; AIDS, acquired immunodeficiency syndrome; CNS, central nervous system; HCP, health care professionals.
Dronabinol: Full prescribing information. Available at http://www.marinol.com/images/pdf/MARINOLPI.pdf (accessed September 7, 2007).

TABLE 133-3   Oxandrolone Summary

DOSAGE	MAJOR SIDE EFFECTS (IN TERMS OF SEVERITY OR FREQUENCY)	CONTRAINDICATIONS	DRUG-DRUG AND DRUG–LABORATORY TEST INTERACTIONS
Adults: 2.5 to 20 mg daily in divided doses Children: total daily dose is 0.1 mg/kg or less or 0.045 mg/ lb or less. May be repeated intermittently as indicated	Caution and close monitoring in patients with COPD *Hepatic:* Cholestatic jaundice with, rarely, hepatic necrosis and death Hepatocellular neoplasms and peliosis hepatis with long-term therapy Reversible changes in liver function tests also occur and include increased bromsulfophthalein retention; increase in serum bilirubin, AST, and ALT; and changes in alkaline phosphatase In males: Prepubertal: Phallic enlargement and increased frequency or persistence of erections Postpubertal: Inhibition of testicular function, testicular atrophy and oligospermia, impotence, chronic priapism, epididymitis, and bladder irritability In females: Clitoral enlargement, menstrual irregularities *CNS:* Habituation, excitation, insomnia, depression, and changes in libido *Hematological:* Bleeding in patients receiving concomitant oral anticoagulant therapy *Breast:* Gynecomastia *Larynx:* Deepening of the voice in females	Known or suspected carcinoma of the prostate or the male breast Carcinoma of the breast in females with hypercalcemia Pregnancy Nephrosis, the nephrotic phase of nephritis Hypercalcemia	*Anticoagulants:* Anabolic steroids may increase sensitivity to oral anticoagulants. Dosage of the anticoagulant may have to be decreased to maintain desired PT. Patients receiving oral anticoagulant therapy require close monitoring, especially when anabolic steroids are started or stopped. *Warfarin:* A multidose study of oxandrolone, given as 5 or 10 mg twice daily in 15 healthy subjects concurrently treated with warfarin, resulted in a mean increase in S- warfarin half-life from 26 to 48 hours and AUC from 4.55 to 12.08 ng/hr/mL; similar increases in R-warfarin half-life and AUC were also detected. Microscopic hematuria (9/15) and gingival bleeding (1/15) were also observed. A 5.5-fold decrease in the mean warfarin dose from 6.13 to 1.13 mg/day (approximately 80-85% reduction in warfarin dose) was necessary to maintain a target INR of 1.5. When oxandrolone therapy is initiated in a patient already receiving treatment with warfarin, the INR or PT should be monitored closely and the dose of warfarin adjusted as necessary until a stable target INR or PT has been achieved. Furthermore, in patients receiving both careful monitoring of the INR or PT, adjustment of the warfarin dosage, if indicated, is recommended when the oxandrolone dose is changed or discontinued. Patients should be closely monitored for signs and symptoms of occult bleeding. *Oral hypoglycemic agents:*

TABLE 133-3 Oxandrolone Summary—cont'd

DOSAGE	MAJOR SIDE EFFECTS (IN TERMS OF SEVERITY OR FREQUENCY)	CONTRAINDICATIONS	DRUG-DRUG AND DRUG–LABORATORY TEST INTERACTIONS
	Hair: Hirsutism and male pattern baldness in females *Skin*: Acne (especially in females and prepubertal males) *Skeletal*: Premature closure of epiphyses in children *Fluid and electrolytes*: Edema, retention of serum electrolytes (sodium chloride, potassium, phosphate, calcium) *Metabolic/endocrine*: Decreased glucose tolerance, increased creatinine excretion, increased serum levels of CK and CPK, masculinization of the fetus, inhibition of gonadotropin secretion		Oxandrolone may inhibit the metabolism of oral hypoglycemic agents (e.g., known interaction with sulfonylurea oral hypoglycemic agents). *Adrenal steroids or ACTH*: In patients with edema, concomitant administration with adrenal cortical steroids or ACTH may increase the edema. *Drug–laboratory test interactions*: Anabolic steroids may decrease levels of thyroxine-binding globulin, thereby resulting in decreased total T_4 serum levels and increased resin uptake of T_3 and T_4. Free thyroid hormone levels remain unchanged. In addition, a decrease in PBI and radioactive iodine uptake may occur.

In addition to excellent management of symptoms that have an impact on nutrition and intervention with agents specifically indicated for or widely used in the treatment of cancer-related weight loss in any aspect of supportive care in cancer, there is increasing literature on the use of other alternative options.[10,15,19] See listing in Table 133-4.

ACTH, adrenocorticotropic hormone; ALT, alanine transaminase; AST, aspartate transaminase; AUC, area under the curve; CK, creatine kinase; CPK, creatine phosphokinase; INR, international normalized ratio; COPD, chronic obstructive pulmonary disease; PBI, protein-bound iodine; PT, prothrombin time; T_3, triiodothyronine; T_4, thyroxin.

From Oxandrolone. Available at http://www.savientpharma.com/oxandrinPI.pdf (accessed September 7, 2007).

TABLE 133-4 Additional Therapeutic Options

CLASS	EXAMPLES	EFFECTS ADDRESSED/DEMONSTRATED
Anticytokine agents	Thalidomide—anti-TNF	Downregulate production of TNF-α and other pro-inflammatory cytokines, inhibit the transcription factor NFκB, downregulate cyclooxygenase 2, and inhibit angiogenesis
	Monoclonal antibodies to IL6 (BE-8, CNTO 328) in multiple myeloma, renal cell carcinoma, B-cell lymphoproliferative disorders	Clinical studies of anti-IL6 antibodies—decreased C-reactive protein levels in all patients; in most, levels decreased below detectable limits; associated with decreased incidence of cancer-related anorexia and cachexia
Anti-inflammatory agents	ω-3 fatty acids, nonsteroidal anti-inflammatory drugs	Weight, lean tissue weight, cytokines, survival, and other outcomes with variable effects dependent on study design
Psychotropics	Mirtazapine, olanzapine	Anorexia, nausea, and other symptoms in patients with cancer
β-Antagonists and agonists	Antagonist: carvedilol or long-acting metoprolol Agonist: clenbuterol	Weight in cardiac cachexia Primarily studied in animal models; also in healthy patients undergoing orthopedic surgery
Complex or ill-defined mechanisms	Melatonin	Studies demonstrate a variety of effects in patients with cancer, including effects on weight and survival
Angiotensin-converting enzyme inhibitors	Imidapril	Primarily studied in cardiac cachexia but developmental studies ongoing in cancer cachexia

IL6, interleukin-6; NFκB, nuclear factor κB; TNF, tumor necrosis factor.

Data from Del Fabbro E, Dalal S, Bruera E. Symptom control in palliative care—Part II: Cachexia/anorexia and fatigue. J Palliat Med 2006;9:409-429; Elamin EM, Glass M, Camporesi E. Pharmacological approaches to ameliorating catabolic conditions. Curr Opin Clin Nutr Metab Care 2006;9:449-454; and Dewey A, Baughan C, Dean T, et al. Eicosapentaenoic acid (EPA, an omega-3 fatty acid from fish oils) for the treatment of cancer cachexia. Cochrane Database Syst Rev 2007;(1):CD004597.

- Lack of consistent, thoughtful, and standardized assessment of nutritional risk or deficit through the cancer continuum can result in reactive versus proactive intervention in both clinical and research settings. Intervention at the late stages of nutritional deficit or extremes of weight loss is not more successful than oncological intervention during late disease.
- Multiple failed single-modality or limited-modality interventional studies have led to a sense of resignation by many clinicians and researchers. The general perspective is that little can be done with pharmacological intervention that will have a positive impact on oncological outcomes, including survival, toxicity of anticancer therapy, and quality of life.

FUTURE CONSIDERATIONS

Given the well-documented adverse effects of involuntary weight loss on subjective and objective oncological outcomes, there is a critical need for randomized, prospective clinical trials.[2,10,15,20,21] Any future trials must be well designed from an oncological, physiological, and nutritional perspective and should proactively intervene in a multimodality interventional model (pharmacological, nutrient, and exercise). Only in this setting is there maximal opportunity to limit or prevent progressive weight loss and associated symptoms, thereby optimizing patient status and quality across the cancer continuum and leading to optimal status at the point that each patient enters palliative cancer care (Table 133-4).

REFERENCES

1. DeWys WD, Begg C, Lavin PT, et al. Prognostic effect of weight loss prior to chemotherapy in cancer patients. Am J Med 1980;69:491-497.
2. Baracos VE. New approaches in reversing cancer-related weight loss. Oncol Issues Nutr Cancer Update 2004;19(Suppl):5-10. Available at www.cancer.
3. Chang VT, Hwang SS, Feuerman M. Validation of the Edmonton Symptom Assessment Scale. Cancer 2000;88:2164-2171.
4. Bruera E, Kuehn N, Miller MJ, et al. The Edmonton Symptom Assessment System (ESAS): A simple method for the assessment of palliative care patients. J Palliat Care 1991;7:6-9.
5. McCallum PD. Nutrition screening and assessment in oncology. In Elliott L, Molseed LL, McCallum PD, Grant B (eds). The Clinical Guide to Oncology Nutrition, 2nd ed. Chicago: American Dietetic Association, 2006, pp 44-53.
6. Mateen F, Jatoi A. Megestrol acetate for the palliation of anorexia in advanced, incurable cancer patients. Clin Nutr 2006;25:711-715.
7. Berenstein EG, Ortiz Z. Megestrol acetate for the treatment of anorexia-cachexia syndrome. Cochrane Database of Syst Rev 2005;(2):CD004310.
8. Ben Amar M. Cannabinoids in medicine: A review of their therapeutic potential. J Ethnopharmacol 2006;105:1-25.
9. Davis M, Maida V, Daeninck P, Pergolizzi J. The emerging role of cannabinoid neuromodulators in symptom management. Support Care Cancer 2007;15:63-71.
10. Del Fabbro E, Dalal S, Bruera E. Symptom control in palliative care—Part II: Cachexia/anorexia and fatigue. J Palliat Med 2006;9:409-429.
11. Guo Y, Young BL, Hainley S, et al. Evaluation and pharmacologic management of symptoms in cancer patients undergoing acute rehabilitation in a comprehensive cancer center. Arch Phys Med Rehabil 2007;88:891-895.
12. Ottery FD, Walsh D, Strawford A. Pharmacologic management of anorexia/cachexia. Semin Oncol 1998;25(2 Suppl 6):35-44.
13. Megestrol acetate (oral ES formulation): Full prescribing information. Available at http://www.megacees.com/PDF/Megace_ES_Portrait_PI.pdf (accessed September 7, 2007); and Megestrol acetate (oral suspension): Full prescribing information. Available at http://www.bms.com/cgi-bin/anybin.pl?sql=PI_SEQ=13 (accessed September 7, 2007).
14. Dronabinol. Available at http://www.marinol.com/images/pdf/MARINOLPI.pdf (accessed September 7, 2007).
15. Elamin EM, Glass M, Camporesi E. Pharmacological approaches to ameliorating catabolic conditions. Curr Opin Clin Nutr Metab Care 2006;9:449-454.
16. Oxandrolone. Available at http://www.savientpharma.com/oxandrinPI.pdf (accessed September 7, 2007). Note: some of the more recently approved versions have an indication limited to the latter part of the original indication: "to offset the protein catabolism associated with prolonged administration of corticosteroids and for the relief of the bone pain frequently accompanying osteoporosis."
17. Orr R, Fiatarone Singh M. The anabolic androgenic steroid oxandrolone in the treatment of wasting and catabolic disorders: Review of efficacy and safety. Drugs 2004;64:725-750.
18. Wolf SE, Edelman LS, Kemalyan N, et al. Effects of oxandrolone on outcome measures in the severely burned: A multicenter prospective randomized double-blind trial. J Burn Care Res 2006;27:131-139; discussion 140-141.
19. Dewey A, Baughan C, Dean T, et al. Eicosapentaenoic acid (EPA, an omega-3 fatty acid from fish oils) for the treatment of cancer cachexia. Cochrane Database Syst Rev 2007;(1):CD004597.
20. Baracos VE. More research needed on the treatment of the cancer anorexia/cachexia syndrome. J Support Oncol 2006;4:508-509.
21. Bossola M, Pacelli F, Tortorelli A, Doglietto G. Cancer cachexia: It's time for more clinical trials. Ann Surg Oncol 2007;14:276-285.

SUGGESTED READING

Ben Amar M. Cannabinoids in medicine: A review of their therapeutic potential. J Ethnopharmacol 2006;105:1-25.

Berenstein EG, Ortiz Z. Megestrol acetate for the treatment of anorexia-cachexia syndrome. Cochrane Database Syst Rev 2005;(2):CD004310.

Del Fabbro E, Dalal S, Bruera E. Symptom control in palliative care—Part II: Cachexia/anorexia and fatigue. J Palliat Med 2006;9:409-429.

Elamin EM, Glass M, Camporesi E. Pharmacological approaches to ameliorating catabolic conditions. Curr Opin Clin Nutr Metab Care 2006;9:449-454.

Orr R, Fiatarone Singh M. The anabolic androgenic steroid oxandrolone in the treatment of wasting and catabolic disorders: Review of efficacy and safety. Drugs 2004;64:725-750.

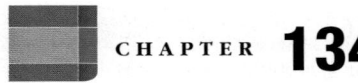

CHAPTER **134**

Anxiolytics, Sedatives, and Hypnotics

Susan B. LeGrand

KEY POINTS

- Benzodiazepines are the preferred agents for anxiety symptoms (see Chapter 151) and are still commonly used for insomnia.
- In general, they are safe but can be problematic in obstructive sleep apnea.
- Additional uses include seizure (diazepam, lorazepam, clonazepam), procedural sedation (diazepam and midazolam), alcohol withdrawal (chlordiazepoxide, lorazepam), and muscle spasm (diazepam).
- A withdrawal syndrome occurs and can include seizures, but they may be an under-recognized iatrogenic cause of delirium.
- The newer hypnosedatives, the Z-drugs, may have advantages for sleep, but the differences in patients with advanced disease may not be offset by cost concerns.

Palliative medicine patients frequently have symptoms managed with anxiolytics or sedative/hypnotics. In a 1000-patient database of individuals with advanced disease, sleep and anxiety problems occurred in 49% and 24%, respectively.[1] Sedatives, which include the benzodiazepines, have been defined as drugs that calm and decrease excitement and activity, whereas hypnotics cause drowsiness and facilitate sleep onset and maintenance.[2] The definitions overlap.

Laudanum, a mixture of alcohol and opium, was widely used in the Victorian era until the potential for addiction was recognized. Barbiturates dominated the market from the introduction of barbital in 1903 until 1960, when chlordiazepoxide was introduced. The benzodiazepines are safer alternatives and were dominant until introduction of the Z-drugs. Various alterations in the chemical structure of benzodiazepines were created in an attempt to achieve specificity for either anxiety or sleep; these alterations had only marginal pharmacological success but some commercial benefit.

BENZODIAZEPINES

Mechanisms of Action

There are many different medications within this class with similar metabolism, variable half-lives (Table 134-1), and similar actions. Selection of a given agent for a particular symptom (i.e., seizure versus insomnia) is based on differences in time to onset, lipid solubility, and the presence or absence of active metabolites rather than any true differences in effects (Table 134-2). All benzodiazepines

TABLE 134-1 Classification of Benzodiazepines and Z-Drugs by Half-Life

ULTRASHORT ACTING

Midazolam

SHORT ACTING: HALF-LIFE <6 HOURS

Clorazepate
Lorazepam
Triazolam
Zolpidem
Zopiclone
Zaleplon

INTERMEDIATE: HALF-LIFE OF 6-24 HOURS

Alprazolam
Chlordiazepoxide
Estazolam
Eszopiclone
Oxazepam
Temazepam

LONG ACTING: >24 HOURS

Clonazepam
Diazepam
Flurazepam
Quazepam

Adapted from Charney S, Mihic J, Harris RA. Hypnotics and sedatives. In Goodman and Gilman's The Pharmacological Basis of Therapeutics, 11th ed. New York: McGraw-Hill, 2005; and Dubrovsky S. Benzodiazepine receptor agonists and antagonists. In Kaplan & Sadock's Comprehensive Textbook of Psychiatry, 8th ed. Philadelphia: Lippincott Williams & Wilkins, 2005.

TABLE 134-2 Benzodiazepine Uses and Dosages

USE	ROUTES	DOSAGE
PROCEDURAL SEDATION		
Midazolam	IM, IV, SC*	Variable
Diazepam	IV	5-15 mg
Lorazepam	IV, IM	0.05 mg/kg
SEIZURE DISORDERS		
Clonazepam	Oral	Start at 1.5 mg/day; maximum, 20 mg
Diazepam (status)	IV, PR	5-10 mg; maximum, 30 mg
Lorazepam (status)	IV	0.05-0.1 mg/kg
INSOMNIA		
Estazolam	Oral	1-2 mg
Flurazepam	Oral	15-30 mg
Quazepam	Oral	7.5-15 mg
Temazepam	Oral	7.5-30 mg
Triazolam	Oral	0.125-0.25 mg
ANXIETY		
Alprazolam	Oral	0.25-0.5 mg tid; maximum, 4 mg/day
Chlordiazepoxide	Oral	5-10 mg tid-qid
Clorazepate	Oral	3.75-15 mg bid; maximum, 60 mg/day
Diazepam	Oral	2-10 mg bid-qid
Lorazepam	Oral, SL*	1 mg tid; maximum, 10 mg/day
Oxazepam	Oral	10-15 mg tid
Clonazepam	Oral	0.25 mg bid; maximum, 1-4 mg/day
ALCOHOL WITHDRAWAL		
Chlordiazepoxide		50-100 mg initially; maximum, 300-800 mg/day
Clorazepate		30 mg tid, then taper

*Anecdotal reports only, not approved by the Food and Drug Administration.
bid, two times a day; qid, four times a day; SC, subcutaneous; SL, sublingual; tid, three times a day.
Adapted from McAvoy GK (ed). AHFS Drug Information 2007. Bethesda, MD: American Society of Health System Pharmacies, 2007, 28:24.08.

interact with γ-amino butyric acid (GABA) receptors, specifically GABA$_A$.[1,2] Although barbiturates directly activate the receptor, they require the presence of GABA and then modulate its activity. This may explain their relative safety with minimal respiratory compromise unless combined with other central nervous system depressants such as alcohol. The GABA receptor is a large molecule with multiple, varying combinations of subunits[3]; many variants of these subunits alter binding of specific agents. These pharmacogenomic variations are imperfectly understood but, like opioids, undoubtedly account for much individual variation in response or tolerance to different compounds.

The principal site of activity is the central nervous system, and the benzodiazepines produce anxiolytic, anticonvulsant, and relaxation responses. Administration of midazolam and other agents before anesthesia reduces peripheral resistance with a corresponding fall in blood pressure and an increase in heart rate. Diazepam has specific cardiac effects: it increases blood flow and decreases cardiac output.[1,2] Its effects on the sleep cycle are to increase the total time slept by inducing more stage 2 sleep and decreasing all other stages, including rapid eye movement (REM) sleep. These effects do not persist after several nights. Rebound effects with a particular increase in REM sleep may occur after discontinuation.

All benzodiazepines are well absorbed orally, but clorazepate must first be decarboxylated to active drug by gastric acids. They are highly protein bound with a range of 70% (alprazolam) to 99% (diazepam); no clinically significant competition with other protein-bound drugs has been identified. Benzodiazepines are rapidly taken up in the brain and redistributed into muscle and fat with a correspondingly large volume of distribution (increased in the elderly), and most are subsequently metabolized in the liver predominantly via the cytochrome P-450 enzyme system. They are then conjugated predominantly with glucuronic acid into inactive compounds. The half-life of a particular agent depends more on whether the initial reaction inactivates it (lorazepam, midazolam, oxazepam, temazepam) or whether it creates an active metabolite (flurazepam) that may have a substantially longer half-life than the parent compound. The speed of redistribution from the brain also has an impact on use. For example, diazepam is more lipophilic than lorazepam and thus enters and leaves the brain more quickly. Consequently, lorazepam, despite a shorter elimination half-life, is preferred in status epilepticus because the effect lasts longer.

Side Effects

Side effects are typically the primary drug effect at an unacceptable level (i.e., sedation). Although the risk of respiratory depression in general is low without concomitant medications, there is concern in patients with chronic obstructive pulmonary disease (COPD) and obstructive sleep apnea. The potential for relaxation of pharyngeal musculature increasing airway collapse and a blunted response to hypercapnia is a risk. Small studies with an alternative GABA$_A$ agonist, zaleplon, have not reported respiratory toxicity, but the risk/benefit ratio has not been adequately defined.[4] Benzodiazepines have been tested in small numbers of patients with mild to moderate COPD without complications, but resting hypercapnia is a contraindication.

Cognitive and motor impairment is a major concern and can be problematic because most people underestimate the degree of impairment. Retrograde amnesia (though useful in procedural sedation) can occur with all benzodiazepines. Such amnesia may impair new learning but does not affect old memories. Motor function is typically more impaired than cognitive function. Complex sleep behavior such as sleep driving and eating has been reported, and the U.S. Food and Drug Administration (FDA) requires black box warnings for all sedative agents.[3]

Disinhibition occasionally occurs along with paradoxical and sometime bizarre behavior, including irritability, anxiety, hallucinations, hypomania, paranoia, and depression. Triazolam was recalled in the United Kingdom because of such behavior, but subsequent studies have found it to be a class effect rather than unique to one agent and uncommon.[5] These reactions may be more likely in patients with dementia.

The elderly may be particularly prone to complications with these agents, with longer-acting agents creating more falls and injury. Soft tissue injury, hip fractures, and hospital admissions may be related to benzodiazepine use, particularly at first or after an increased dose. Caution should be exercised at these times.[6]

Contraindications

There are few true contraindications other than known allergy or a previous history of unacceptable toxicity such as disinhibition. Benzodiazepines may worsen delirium[7] and are not generally recommended in this setting unless the delirium is due to drug or alcohol withdrawal. Dose reductions of at least 50% are recommended in hepatic failure. Renal failure does not affect metabolism, nor are benzodiazepines dialyzable.

Drug Interactions

Any medication metabolized by the cytochrome system has a corresponding potential for drug interactions. Plasma levels may be increased by medications that inhibit CYP3A4, such as erythromycin, ketoconazole, and many others. Enzyme inducers such as carbamazepine may lower levels. Agents such as lorazepam and oxazepam are affected less because they are directly conjugated. Unlike the barbiturates, the benzodiazepines do not induce these enzymes or affect their own metabolism.

NONBENZODIAZEPINE SEDATIVES— THE Z-DRUGS

Newer GABA-active agents specifically intended for sleep that are distinct from both benzodiazepines and each other have been introduced (Table 134-3). Eszopiclone is the *S*-isomer of zopiclone.

Mechanism of Action and Side Effects

These agents all bind GABA$_A$ receptors but have differing affinity for specific subtypes.[8] Flumazenil antagonizes their effects, thus adding support for the role of the GABA receptor. Benzodiazepines decrease the time spent in sleep stages 3, 4, and REM, which may explain some of their rebound effects. In comparison, these agents have less effect on sleep architecture and are therefore associated with less rebound insomnia.[8,9] They also appear safer in the elderly at risk for falls.[10] Their effect on memory varies. Zaleplon impairs memory only at higher than recommended dosages. Zolpidem and zopiclone affect new memory at the time of administration, but the effect resolves after 6 to 8 hours.

When choosing an agent, insomnia should be further defined as a problem of sleep initiation, sleep maintenance, or both. The short half-life of zaleplon makes it useful for problems of sleep initiation but not for maintenance. A modified-release formulation of zolpidem was created to manage both, with one layer providing rapid onset for initiation of sleep and the other providing a prolonged effect for maintenance. Zopiclone and eszopiclone have longer half-lives and therefore could be used for both. Eszopiclone has safety data extending to 12 months and is approved for chronic use in the United States. Zaleplon may be repeated for early morning awakening given its short duration of action.

These agents are generally well absorbed orally with 30% (zaleplon) to 75% (zopiclone) bioavailability. Meals high in fat may delay absorption and therefore onset. The agents are then metabolized in the liver via various cytochrome P-450 enzymes to inactive compounds (zopiclone and eszopiclone have one active metabolite that represents 11% of the total).[8] Doses should be reduced by 50% in patients with liver disease. No dose adjustments are required in those with renal failure (Table 134-4).

TABLE 134-3	Nonbenzodiazepine Sedatives (Z-Drugs)	
DRUG (BRAND NAME)	**DRUG CLASS**	**DOSE**
Zolpidem (Ambien, Ambien CR)	Imidazopyridine	10 mg (CR, 12.5 mg)—50% in the elderly
Zaleplon (Sonata)	Pyrazolopyrimidine	10 mg (range, 5-20 mg)—5 mg in the elderly
Zopiclone (Non-U.S.)	Cyclopyrrolone	5 mg (range, 3.75-7.5 mg)—3.75 mg in the elderly
Eszopiclone (Lunesta)	Cyclopyrrolone	2 mg (range, 1-3 mg)—50% in the elderly

TABLE 134-4 Pharmacokinetics of Nonbenzodiazepine Agents

DRUG	ONSET (T_{MAX})	HALF-LIFE
Zaleplon	1.4 hr	1.04 hr
Zolpidem	1.4 hr	2.1 hr
Zopiclone	1.6 hr	3.41 hr
Eszopiclone	1 hr	6 hr

Side Effects

As with the benzodiazepines, side effects are typically excess effects (i.e., sedation and early morning impairment). They are generally less of a problem than with the benzodiazepines. Retrograde amnesia has not been reported, but there are case reports of somnambulism with zolpidem. Other side effects include visual disturbances with zaleplon and zolpidem and abnormal taste with zopiclone and eszopiclone. There are rare reports of abuse with extreme doses, primarily in individuals with a previous addiction history.[11]

Drug Interactions

Because these medications are metabolized via the cytochrome system, they have the same potential for drug interactions. Inducers would decrease effects; rifampin appears to be clinically relevant. Inhibitors would increase effects, with azole antifungals probably being clinically relevant. Given their overall safety, the clinical impact of these interactions is unclear.[12] There is the potential for additive sedation with alcohol and other sedatives of abuse.

MISCELLANEOUS AGENTS

Buspirone

Buspirone is a unique agent approved for chronic anxiety disorders without apparent activity at the GABA receptor, nor does it share properties of any other anxiolytics, including benzodiazepines and barbiturates.[13] Its primary receptor activity is at 5-HT_{1A}, and it has presynaptic and partial postsynaptic agonist activity. This binding is thought to be the source of the anxiolytic effect, although the mechanism is not fully elucidated. There is also binding at dopamine receptors (D_2), but its clinical significance is unknown. Buspirone is well absorbed orally with an extensive first-pass effect. Meals do not affect absorption. Within the liver it follows two metabolic pathways and is a major substrate of CYP3A4:

1. Hydroxylation to the inactive 5-hydroxybuspirone
2. Oxidative dealkylation to the active compound 1-pyrimidinylpiperazine

Buspirone is highly protein bound (95%) but does not appear to displace other highly bound agents such as phenytoin or warfarin. Excretion is via feces and urine, with potential prolongation of the terminal half-life in patients with hepatic and renal failure; dose reductions are recommended.

There is adequate evidence to support the use of buspirone in generalized anxiety disorders, particularly if benzodiazepines have not previously been used.[14] There is no evidence of superiority. Buspirone has a delayed onset with responses in 2 weeks and then gradual further improvement. This makes it problematic in advanced disease and probably explains the reason that those previously exposed to benzodiazepines do not do as well.

Side effects are mild, with dizziness, nervousness, headache, light-headedness, and disturbed dreams reported more than with placebo. Drug interactions occur with inducers and inhibitors of CYP3A4. The potential for serotonin syndrome exists when combined with other selective serotonin reuptake inhibitors. Hypomanic episodes have been reported when used in bipolar patients. Concurrent use with monoamine oxidase inhibitors is contraindicated.

Ramelteon

A role for the pineal hormone melatonin in maintenance of circadian rhythm and sleep onset is reasonably well defined in humans.[15] Three melatonin receptors have been identified, MT_1, MT_2, MT_3, with only the first two affecting sleep. The use of melatonin itself for sleep or jet lag is controversial.[16] Studies are complicated by the lack of a uniform product because it is regulated in the United States as a supplement rather than as a medication. Ramelteon is the first melatonin receptor agonist approved by the FDA for problems with sleep initiation and for prolonged use.[17,18] Unlike the benzodiazepines and Z-drugs, it is not a controlled substance. Though well absorbed (delayed by high-fat meals), it is subject to extensive first-pass effect with oral bioavailability less than 2%. The maximum concentration is reached at 0.75 hour (T_{max}), with a half-life of 1.2 hours. Metabolism is via oxidation primarily by CYP1A2 with secondary glucuronidation. The metabolites are more active than the parent compound, with half-lives of 1 to 3 hours. Though cleared by the kidney, dose adjustment in patients with renal failure is not required. Data in patients with hepatic failure are limited, but given its relative safety, no specific recommendations exist for mild to moderate dysfunction. Side effects were no different from those in patients given placebo and included headache, somnolence, fatigue, nausea, and dizziness in less than 10%. Studies suggest a modest, yet statistically significant decreased latency to persistent sleep (i.e., improved sleep initiation). To date, no trials have compared it with other sedatives.

Others

Barbiturates are not recommended for routine use as sedatives given their potential for drug interactions, life-threatening withdrawal, and fatal overdose. With advent of the benzodiazepines and Z-drugs, their role is now primarily palliative sedation. Chloral hydrate was used as an alternative to the benzodiazepines, but tolerance develops after approximately 2 weeks. It is not recommended in patients with renal disease because it is cleared by the kidney. Chloral hydrate can cause gastric irritation and is not recommended in those with gastritis or esophagitis. Withdrawal syndromes can occur.[19]

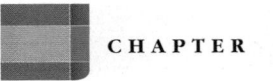

CHAPTER **135**

Nonsteroidal Anti-inflammatory Drugs

Kay Brune and Burkhard Hinz

CONCLUSIONS

Benzodiazepines are useful medications in many settings of advanced disease, although population-specific research is limited. The potential for harm is probably underappreciated. Buspirone may have a role in chronic anxiety management, but the delayed onset is problematic in advanced disease. The newer Z-drugs may contribute to management of insomnia but cannot replace the benzodiazepines for other indications. The role of ramelteon in insomnia remains to be determined.

REFERENCES

1. Charney S, Mihic J, Harris RA. Hypnotics and sedatives. In Goodman and Gilman's The Pharmacological Basis of Therapeutics, 11th ed. New York: McGraw-Hill, 2006.
2. Dubrovsky S. Benzodiazepine receptor agonists and antagonists. In Kaplan & Sadock's Comprehensive Textbook of Psychiatry, 8th ed. Philadelphia: Lippincott Williams & Wilkins, 2005.
3. McAvoy GK (ed). AHFS Drug Information 2007. Bethesda, MD: American Society of Health System Pharmacies, 2007, 28:24.08.
4. George CF. Perspectives on the management of insomnia in patients with chronic respiratory disorders. Sleep 2000;23(Suppl 1):S31-S35.
5. Jonas JM, Coleman BS, Sheridan AQ, et al. Comparative clinical profiles of triazolam versus other shorter-acting hypnotics. J Clin Psychiatry 1992; 53(Suppl):19-31.
6. Tamblyn R, Abrahamowicz M, Berger R, et al. A 5-year prospective assessment of the risk associated with individual BDZs and doses in new elderly users. J Am Geriatr Soc 2005;53:233-241.
7. Breitbart W, Marotta R, Platt MM, et al. A double-blind trial of haloperidol, chlorpromazine, and lorazepam in the treatment of delirium in hospitalized AIDS patients. Am J Psychiatry 1996;153:231-237.
8. Drover DR. Comparative pharmacokinetics and pharmacodynamics of short-acting hypnosedatives. Zaleplon, zolpidem and zopiclone. Clin Pharmacokinet 2004;43:227-238.
9. Najib J. Eszopiclone, a nonbenzodiazepine sedative-hypnotic agent for the treatment of transient and chronic insomnia. Clin Ther 2006;28:491-516.
10. Allain H, Bentue-Ferrer D, Polard E, et al. Postural instability and consequent falls and hip fractures associated with use of hypnotics in the elderly: A comparative review. Drugs Aging 2005;22:749-765.
11. Hajak G, Muller WE, Wittchen HU, et al. Abuse and dependence potential for the non-benzodiazepine hypnotics zolpidem and zopiclone: A review of case reports and epidemiological data. Addiction 2003;98:1371-1378.
12. Hesse LM, von Moltke LL, Greenblatt DJ. Clinically important drug interactions with zopiclone, zolpidem and zaleplon. CNS Drugs 2003;17:513-532.
13. Hudziak J, Waterman GS. Buspirone. In Kaplan & Sadock's Comprehensive Textbook of Psychiatry, 8th ed. Philadelphia: Lippincott Williams & Wilkins, 2005.
14. Chessick CA, Allen MH, Thase M, et al. Azapirones for generalized anxiety disorder. Cochrane Database Syst Rev 2006;(3):CD006115.
15. Turek FW, Gillette MU. Melatonin, sleep, and circadian rhythms: Rationale for development of specific melatonin agonists. Sleep Med 2004;5:523-532.
16. Buscemi N, Vandermeer B, Hooton N, et al. Efficacy and safety of exogenous melatonin for secondary sleep disorders and sleep disorders accompanying sleep restriction: Meta-analysis. BMJ 2006;332:385-393.
17. Borja N, Daniel KL. Ramelteon for the treatment of insomnia. Clin Ther 2006;28:1540-1555.
18. Morin AK, Jarvis CI, Lynch AM. Therapeutic options for sleep-maintenance and sleep-onset insomnia. Pharmacotherapy 2007;27:89-110.
19. Trevor AJ, Way WL. Sedative-hypnotic drugs. In Katzung BG (ed). Basic and Clinical Pharmacology, 10th ed. New York: McGraw-Hill, 2007.

KEY POINTS

- The most common pain is nociceptor-mediated hyperalgesia. It results from increased sensitivity of neuronal structures and is mediated by prostaglandins released in damaged inflamed (peritumorous) tissue.
- Nociceptor activation also leads to central hyperalgesia (also related to "wind up"), mediated by release of prostaglandins from cyclooxygenase 2 (COX-2) in the dorsal horn of the spinal cord.
- COX inhibition in inflamed tissue and the central nervous system (CNS) abolishes hyperalgesia and is perceived as analgesia.
- Prostaglandins are tissue hormones produced constantly and ubiquitously by COX-1. Several organ systems, including the CNS, vascular wall, heart, and kidney, constantly express COX-2. Inflamed tissue contains high COX-2 levels. COX inhibitors may cause gastrointestinal (GI) damage, a propensity for bleeding, reduced kidney function, increased blood pressure, and accelerated atherosclerosis. Limiting COX inhibition to a few organs (acidic, anti-inflammatory, nonselective COX inhibitors with a short half-life) or by enzyme selectivity (COX-2 inhibitors) reduces unwanted drug effects.
- Selection of a COX inhibitor with high enzyme and tissue selectivity, a short half-life, and dosing as low as possible for the shortest possible period is the basic principle for choice and use of selective and nonselective nonsteroidal anti-inflammatory drugs (NSAIDs). Consider the intensity, localization, and daily duration of pain!

Cancer of all types often causes serious pain.[1] The well-known pyramid of analgesic treatment in palliative medicine starts with weak analgesics,[2] which consist of drugs that interfere with production of the proalgesic mediator prostaglandin E_2 (PGE_2) via enzymes collectively called COXs.[3-5] Consequently, these most widely used drugs work by inhibiting one or several COXs and reduce hyperalgesia.[6] They are also called NSAIDs.

MECHANISMS OF ACTION

Pain results from tissue damage (hyperalgesia), destruction or impairment of pain reception neurons (neuropathic pain, allodynia), and rare neuronal disorders. The reason for pain is usually activation of nociceptors.[6] We can discriminate between peripheral[6] and central hyperalgesia.[7] The increased sensitivity of nociceptors is largely mediated by PGE_2 released via COX-2 (more than COX-1) in inflamed, traumatized, or peritumorous tissue.[6-9]

Among others, the TRPV1 receptor changes its activation profile after phosphorylation initiated via production of cyclic adenosine monophosphate from PGE_2 receptors (EP).[6] Central hyperalgesia results in increased prostaglandin production in the dorsal horn of the spinal cord via activation of COX-2 and PGE_2.[5] This process is stimulated by release of cytokine and neuronal input by sensory fibers from inflamed (damaged) tissue in the periphery.[5] The increased PGE_2 production in the dorsal horn of the spinal cord (Fig. 135-1) leads to a reduced probability of an "open" chloride channel, which is also a glycine receptor (α_3).

Reduced influx of chloride into the second neuron of pain perception causes less hyperpolarization. Inhibition of PGE_2 production via COX-2 in the spinal cord reinstates this antihyperalgesic mechanism. Peripheral and central inhibition of prostaglandin production (via COX-2) is the dominant mechanism of action of COX inhibitors (NSAIDs).[3,6,10]

Hyperalgesia may thus be waived by selective and nonselective COX-2 inhibitors. The traditional inhibitors (tNSAIDs) inhibit both enzymes; modern ones interfere only with the more important COX-2, which has relevance for side effects.[3,4,10-12] Aside from enzyme specificity, these drugs also differ in pharmacological properties.

PHARMACOLOGICAL DIFFERENCES

Both selective and nonselective COX inhibitors (Fig. 135-2) consist of molecules with different physicochemical and pharmacological characteristics (Tables 135-1 and 135-2). Two types of drugs exist: acidic and nonacidic. Nonacidic compounds are distributed almost equally throughout the body (Fig. 135-3), whereas acidic compounds accumulate and are retained in inflamed tissue (but also the central compartment, including blood, the vessel wall, the heart, and the kidney). High concentrations of these drugs are also found in the GI wall (see Fig. 135-3).

The positive aspect of this unequal tissue distribution is that clinically relevant COX inhibition occurs only at sites of high concentration, which limits the side effects of these traditional acidic compounds (tNSAIDs) to these compartments. Sequestration into inflamed tissue goes along with prolonged activity and inhibition of peripheral hyperalgesia. Fast recovery of COX activity in the central compartment (blood, heart, liver, vessel wall, and kidney) is due to fast elimination from this central compartment.[4,13]

In contrast, nonacidic compounds distribute throughout the body (see Fig. 135-3) and may cause life-threatening drug effects at high doses (e.g., acetaminophen). This risk is low with modern selective COX-2 inhibitors with a nonacidic structure (e.g., celecoxib and etoricoxib). COX-2 is expressed only in certain organs—the CNS, kidney, and vessel wall. Consequently, these compounds lack the acute lethal effects, but facilitation of atherosclerosis and kidney damage (fluid retention, hypertension) may occur.[14-16] Combining tissue selectivity and enzyme specificity may offer additional advantages. Tissue selectiv-

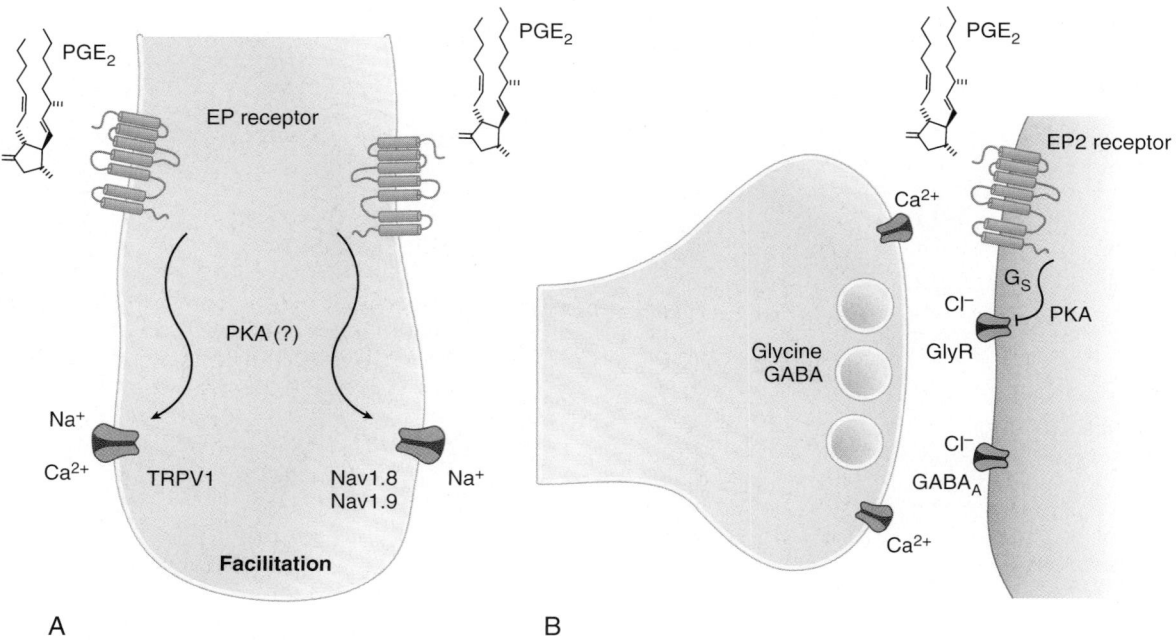

FIGURE 135-1 Molecular mechanisms of prostaglandin E_2 (PGE_2)-mediated nociceptive sensitization. **A,** Schematic representation of a polymodal (nociceptive) C fiber. PGE_2 has been shown to facilitate the activation of membrane responses to capsaicin and noxious heat, thus suggesting that the capsaicin receptor TRPV1 is a prominent target of PGE_2. TTY-resistant sodium channels (Nav1.8 and Nav1.9) may represent another target involved in peripheral sensitization processes. PKA, protein kinase A. **B,** The spinal cord dorsal horn represents a second major site of the pain-sensitizing action of PGE_2. Two possible molecular mechanisms have thus far been proposed at this site. PGE_2 reduces the action of the major inhibitory neurotransmitter glycine in the superficial layers of the dorsal horn and—at higher concentrations—leads to direct depolarization of deep dorsal horn neurons. GABA, γ-aminobutyric acid. *(Redrawn from Brune K, Zeilhofer HU. Antipyretic analgesics: Basic aspects. In McMahon SB, Koltzenburg M (eds). Wall and Melzack's Textbook of Pain, 5th ed. Philadilphia: Elsevier/Churchill Livingstone, 2006, pp 459-470.)*

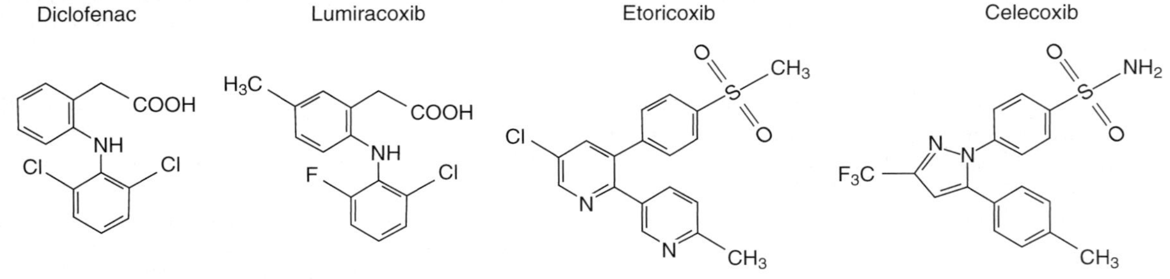

Drug				F_{oral} (%)	T_{max} (hr)	$T_{1/2}$	V_d (1/kg)

Diclofenac   Lumiracoxib   Etoricoxib   Celecoxib

	F_{oral} (%)	T_{max} (hr)	$T_{1/2}$	V_d (1/kg)
Nonspecific COX-1 plus COX-2 inhibitors [23]				
Diclofenac	>50	1–6	1–2 hr	~0.13
Ibuprofen	>90	1–6	1–2 hr	~0.13
Naproxen	>90	1–6	10–15 hr	~0.13
Piroxicam	>90	1–3	1–2 day	~0.13
Specific COX-2 inhibitors [1, 22]				
Celecoxib	20–40	3–6	4–15 hr	>1
Etoricoxib	>90	0.5–1	20–30hr	>1
Lumiracoxib	>90	1–2	2–4 hr	0.13

F_{oral} = oral bioavailability; T_{max} = time to maximum concentration;
$T_{1/2}$ = plasma half-life; V_d = volume of distribution at steady state.

FIGURE 135-2 Pharmacokinetic characteristics of antinociceptive drugs. COX, cyclooxygenase. *(Redrawn from Flower RJ. The development of COX2 inhibitors. Nat Rev Drug Discov 2003;2:179-191.)*

TABLE 135-1 Physicochemical and Pharmacological Data of Acidic Nonselective Cyclooxygenase Inhibitors

PHARMACOKINETIC/ CHEMICAL SUBCLASSES	PK_A	BINDING TO PLASMA PROTEINS	ORAL BIOAVAILABILITY	T_{MAX}*	$T_{1/2}$[†]	SINGLE DOSE (MAXIMAL DAILY DOSE) FOR ADULTS
SHORT ELIMINATION HALF-LIFE						
Salicylates						
Aspirin	3.5	50-70%	50% dose dependent	15 min	15 min	0.05-1 g[‡] (6 g)
2-Arylpropionic Acids						
Ibuprofen	4.4	99%	100%	0.5-2 hr	2 hr	200-800 mg (2.4 g)
Flurbiprofen	4.2	>99%	No data	1.5-3 hr	2.5-4 (−8) hr	50-100 mg (200 mg)
Ketoprofen	5.3	99%	90%	1-2 hr	2-4 hr	25-100 mg (200 mg)
Arylacetic/Heteroarylacetic Acids						
Diclofenac	3.9	99.7%	50% dose dependent	1-12 hr,[§] very variable	1-2 hr	25-75 mg (150 mg)
Indomethacin	4.5	99%	100%	0.5-2 hr	2-3 (−11) hr[¶], very variable	25-75 mg (200 mg)
LONG ELIMINATION HALF-LIFE						
2-Arylpropionic Acids						
Naproxen	4.2	99%	90-100%	2-4 hr	12-15 hr[¶]	250-500 mg (1.25 g)
Arylacetic Acids						
6-Methoxy-2-naphthyl-acetic acid (active metabolite of nabumetone)	4.2	99%	20-50%	3-6 hr	20-24 hr	0.5-1 g (1.5 g)
Oxicams						
Piroxicam	5.9	99%	100%	3-5 hr	14-160 hr[¶]	20-40 mg; initial dose: 40 mg
Tenoxicam	5.3	99%	100%	0.5-2 hr	25-175 hr[¶]	20-40 mg; initial dose: 40 mg
Meloxicam	4.08	99.5%	89%	7-8 hr	20 hr[§]	7.5-15 mg

*Time to reach the maximum plasma concentration after oral administration.
[†]Terminal half-life of elimination.
[‡]Single dose for inhibition of thrombocyte aggregation, 50 to 100 mg; single analgesic dose, 0.5 to 1 g.
[§]Monolithic acid-resistant tablet or similar galenic form.
[¶]Enterohepatic circulation.

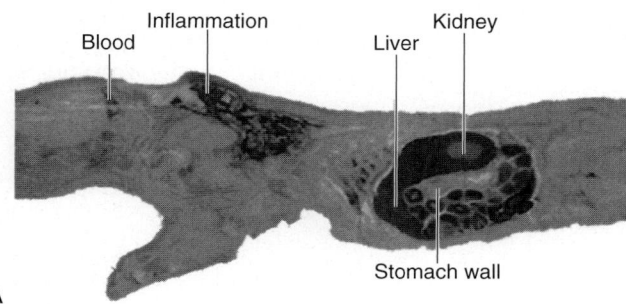

Phenylbutazone

A

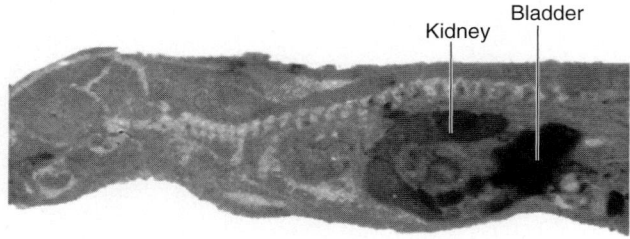

Propyphenazone

B

FIGURE 135-3 Autoradiographic localization of drugs. **A** and **B,** Autoradiographs of [^{14}C] phenylbutazone- or [^{14}C] propyphenazone-treated rats. Inflammation was elicited by subcutaneous injection of carrageenan into the neck region. The phenylbutazone-treated animal shows high radioactivity (black) in the inflamed tissue of the neck and also in the stomach wall, liver, kidney, and blood when sacrificed 5 hours after the administration of phenylbutazone and carrageenan. The brain shows little radioactivity. The rat receiving propyphenazone shows homogeneous distribution throughout the body, with high concentrations of metabolites in the kidney and bladder.

ity is less relevant at high doses of short–half-life acidic compounds or with drugs eliminated slowly from the body, including piroxicam and meloxicam ($t_{1/2}$ = 24 hours). High doses, frequent dosing, or slow elimination prevent recovery of prostaglandin production (tissue protection) in the central compartment.[13]

SELECTION OF DRUGS FOR CANCER-RELATED PAIN

One should choose nonselective inhibitors for otherwise healthy patients without GI symptoms or cardiovascular risk factors (low cost). In these patients, traditional nonsteroidals (tNSAIDs) such as diclofenac, ibuprofen, or naproxen ($t_{1/2}$ = 15 hours) should be given at the lowest meaningful dose and the longest possible dosing interval. Obviously, such treatment will lead to recovery phases. They should not be used with anticoagulants or in patients with "aspirin"-induced asthma.

Given GI risk factors, impaired blood coagulation, or a propensity for aspirin-inducible asthma, selective COX inhibitors should be used. Fluctuating pain may be best controlled with lumiracoxib (withdrawn in serveral countries because of cases of severe liver damage) as needed; mild but constant pain is treated sufficiently with celecoxib (twice daily). Serious chronic pain may

best be treated with etoricoxib once daily (at present, labeling does not include cancer pain for all these compounds).

DOSAGE

COX inhibitors interfere with proalgesic prostaglandin production in two target structures: inflamed tissue around tumor or metastases and the dorsal horn of the spinal cord. At both sites, the prevailing producer of PGE$_2$ is COX-2.[6]

Nonselective and selective drugs vary; the main differences are enzyme specificity, tissue selectivity, and overall pharmacokinetics, in particular, the elimination half-life (see Tables 135-1 and 135-2).

Treatment (see Tables 135-1 and 135-2) should be initiated with short–half-life, acidic COX inhibitors, either selective or nonselective. They are retained in peritumorous tissue and may exert long-lasting COX inhibition, whereas in the central compartments, including the heart, bloodstream (endothelium), liver, and kidney, COX activity has recovered.

MAJOR SIDE EFFECTS

Major side effects derive from the pharmacodynamic and pharmacokinetic characteristics of the drugs. As a rule of thumb, drugs that leave the body slowly (long $t_{1/2}$) show more unwanted drug effects than do those with a short half-life, provided that the latter are not administered at high doses (e.g., 2.4 g ibuprofen or ≥150 mg diclofenac) or too frequently (three and more times daily).

Selective COX-2 inhibitors are less prone to GI toxicity,[17] asthma-like reactions, and bleeding. On the other hand, they do not interfere with blood coagulation in an aspirin-like fashion.

CONTRAINDICATIONS

Specific contraindications can be derived from the mode of action (Table 135-3).

DRUG INTERACTIONS

The most important interaction is the combined activity of nonselective COX inhibitors, in particular, aspirin and naproxen, with vitamin K antagonists (see Table 135-3). The GI toxicity of all tNSAIDs is enhanced by the coadministration of glucocorticoids and selective serotonin reuptake inhibitors.

RESEARCH CHALLENGES

Selective COX-2-inhibitors compare favorably with most nonselective COX inhibitors. They may damage the cardiovascular system (proatherosclerotic)[14,18,19] and interfere with kidney function. Attempts have been made to limit inhibition of prostaglandin production to the inflamed tissue (selective inhibition of microsomal PGE synthase activity), as well as to selective PGE$_2$ (EP2) receptors (antagonists). Interference with glycinergic mechanisms, protein kinases, and other targets[20] is under investigation. For now, palliative therapy will have to rely on nonselec-

TABLE 135-2 Physicochemical and Pharmacological Data of Acidic Selective COX-2 Inhibitors

	COX-1/COX-2 RATIO*	BINDING TO PLASMA PROTEINS	VD[†]	ORAL BIOAVAILABILITY	T$_{MAX}$[‡]	T$_{1/2}$[§]	PRIMARY METABOLISM[¶] (CYTOCHROME P-450 ENZYMES)	SINGLE DOSE (MAXIMAL DAILY DOSE) FOR ADULTS
SULFONAMIDES (NONACIDIC)								
Celecoxib	30	97%	400 L	20-60%	2-4 hr	6-12 hr	Oxidation (CYP2C9, CYP3A4)[¶]	100-200 mg (400 mg) for osteoarthrosis and rheumatoid arthritis
METHYLSULFONS (NONACIDIC)								
Etoricoxib	344	92%	120 L	100%	1 hr	20-26 hr	Oxidation to 6'-hydroxymethyletoricoxib (major role: CYP3A4; ancillary role: CYP2C9, CYP2D6, CYP1A2)	60 mg (60 mg) for osteoarthrosis, 90 mg (90 mg) for rheumatoid arthritis, 120 mg (120 mg) for acute gouty arthritis
ARYLACETIC ACID (ACIDIC)								
Lumiracoxib	700	99%	13 L	74%	1-3 hr	2-6 hr	Oxidation to hydroxyllumiracoxib** (CYP2C9)	100 mg (osteoarthrosis of the hip and knee)[††]

*Ratio of 50% inhibitory concentration (IC$_{50}$) values (IC$_{50}$ COX-1/IC$_{50}$ COX-2) in the human whole blood assay.
[†]Volume of distribution.
[‡]Time to reach the maximum plasma concentration after oral administration.
[§]Terminal half-life of elimination.
[¶]All metabolites are less active than the parent compound (except parecoxib).
[¶]Compounds may inhibit CYP2D6.
**In analogy to diclofenac, the metabolism of lumiracoxib probably involves other CYP enzymes such as CYP2C8 or CYP2C19.
[††]Lumiracoxib was withdrawn in several countries in 2007-2008 because of hepatic toxicity.
Data from Brune K, Hinz B. The discovery and development of antiinflammatory drugs. Arthritis Rheum 2004;50:2391-2399.

TABLE 135-3 Major Side Effects, Drug Interactions, and Contraindications

	SIDE EFFECT	DRUG INTERACTIONS	CONTRAINDICATIONS*
NONSELECTIVE, ACIDIC DRUGS			
Aspirin[†] Diclofenac Ibuprofen Indomethacin Ketoprofen Ketorolac Naproxen[†]	Inhibition of platelet aggregation for days GI ulcerations, dyspepsia Increased BP, water retention Allergic (asthmatic) reactions Vertigo Tinnitus Numbness	Vitamin K antagonists ACE inhibitors Glucocorticoids Diuretics, lithium SSRIs Ibuprofen: reduction of low-dose aspirin cardioprotection	Hypersensitivity to the active substance or to any of the excipients Asthma, acute rhinitis, nasal polyps, angioedema, urticaria, or other allergic-type reactions after taking ASA or NSAIDs (celecoxib: sulfonamide allergy) Active peptic ulceration or GI bleeding Inflammatory bowel disease Congestive heart failure (NYHA II-IV) (etoricoxib: >NYHA I) Established ischemic heart disease, peripheral arterial disease, and/or cerebrovascular disease Moderate to severe renal dysfunction (etoricoxib: inadequate control of BP) Severe hepatic disease (Child-Pugh score ≥9; only lumiracoxib) Third trimester of pregnancy Patients younger than 18 years
Meloxicam Piroxicam	As above, but more pronounced	As above	
SELECTIVE COX-2 INHIBITORS			
Acidic			
Lumiracoxib	Increase in hepatic transaminases	—	
Nonacidic			
Celecoxib	Allergic reactions	Blocks CYP2D6	
Etoricoxib	Water retention	Reduces estrogen metabolism	
NONSELECTIVE, NONACIDIC DRUGS[‡]			
Acetaminophen	Liver damage	Not prominent	Liver damage, EtOH abuse
Phenazone	Allergic reactions	Some interactions at P-450 enzymes	Allergic reactions, pregnancy

*Harmonization by taking into account the qualitative and quantitative differences between selective and nonselective inhibitors, as well as the different drugs of a class, has been attempted by the European Medicines Evaluation Agency and the Food and Drug Administration but not completed.
[†]Only aspirin (and high doses of naproxen) inhibit platelet aggregation for days.
[‡]Relatively weak and harmless at low doses, dangerous at overdose (limited use profile).
ACE, angiotensin-converting enzyme; ASA, acetylsalicylic acid; BP, blood pressure; COX, cyclooxygenase; EtOH, ethyl alcohol; GI, gastrointestinal; NSAID, nonsteroidal anti-inflammatory drug; NYHA, New York Heart Association; SSRI, selective serotonin reuptake inhibitor.

tive and selective COX-2 inhibitors. Biochemical markers of patients at risk for cardiovascular events are under investigation.[21]

EVIDENCE-BASED MEDICINE

The therapeutic effectiveness of COX inhibitors in relieving nociceptor-mediated pain (hyperalgesia), including pain related to cancer (metastases), has been proved, but the use of selective COX-2 inhibitors in palliative medicine has not been evaluated.

REFERENCES

1. Mantyh PW. Cancer pain: Causes, consequences and therapeutic opportunities. In McMahon SB, Koltzenburg M (eds). Wall and Melzack's Textbook of Pain, 5th ed. Philadelphia: Elsevier, 2006, pp 1087-1097.
2. Hoskin PJ. Cancer pain: Treatment overview. In McMahon SB, Koltzenburg M (eds). Wall and Melzack's Textbook of Pain, 5th ed. Philadelphia: Elsevier, 2006, pp 1141-1157.
3. Flower RJ. The development of COX2 inhibitors. Nat Rev Drug Discov 2003;2:179-191.
4. Simmons DL, Botting RM, Hla T. Cyclooxygenase isozymes: The biology of prostaglandin synthesis and inhibition. Pharmacol Rev 2004;56:387-437.
5. Narumiya S, Sugimoto Y, Ushikubi F. Prostanoid receptors: Structures, properties, and functions. Physiol Rev 1999;79:1193-1226.
6. Brune K, Zeilhofer HU. Antipyretic analgesics: Basic aspects. In McMahon SB, Koltzenburg M (eds). Wall and Melzack's Textbook of Pain, 5th ed. Philadelphia: Elsevier, 2006, pp 459-470.
7. Samad TA, Moore KA, Sapirstein A, et al. Interleukin-1beta–mediated induction of Cox-2 in the CNS contributes to inflammatory pain hypersensitivity. Nature 2001;410:471-475.
8. Ahmadi S, Lippross S, Neuhuber WL, Zeilhofer HU. PGE2 selectively blocks inhibitory glycinergic neurotransmission onto rat superficial dorsal horn neurons. Nat Neurosci 2002;5:34-40.
9. Reinold H, Ahmadi S, Depner UB, et al. Spinal inflammatory hyperalgesia is mediated by prostaglandin E receptors of the EP2 subtype. J Clin Invest 2005;115:673-679.
10. Brune K, Hinz B. The discovery and development of antiinflammatory drugs. Arthritis Rheum 2004;50:2391-2399.
11. FitzGerald GA, Patrono C. The coxibs, selective inhibitors of cyclooxygenase-2. N Engl J Med 2001;345:433-442.
12. Morham SG, Langenbach R, Loftin CD, et al. Prostaglandin synthase 2 gene disruption causes severe renal pathology in the mouse. Cell 1995;83:73-82.
13. Brune K, Hinz B. Selective cyclooxygenase-2 inhibitors: Similarities and differences. Scand J Rheumatol 2004;33:1-6.
14. Kramer BK, Kammerl MC, Komhoff M. Renal cyclooxygenase-2 (COX-2). Physiological, pathophysiological, and clinical implications. Kidney Blood Press Res 2004;27:43-62.
15. Cipollone F, Rocca B, Patrono C. Cyclooxygenase-2 expression and inhibition in atherothrombosis. Arterioscler Thromb Vasc Biol 2004;24:246-255.
16. Grosser T, Fries S, FitzGerald GA. Biological basis for the cardiovascular consequences of COX-2 inhibition: Therapeutic challenges and opportunities. J Clin Invest 2006;116:4-15.
17. Schnitzer TJ, Burmester GR, Mysler E, et al. TARGET Study Group. Comparison of lumiracoxib with naproxen and ibuprofen in the Therapeutic Arthritis Research and Gastrointestinal Event Trial (TARGET), reduction in ulcer complications: Randomised controlled trial. Lancet 2004;364:665-674.
18. Cheng Y, Wang M, Yu Y, et al. Cyclooxygenases, microsomal prostaglandin E synthase-1, and cardiovascular function. J Clin Invest 2006;116:1391-1399.
19. Kearney PM, Baigent C, Godwin J, et al. Do selective cyclo-oxygenase-2 inhibitors and traditional non-steroidal anti-inflammatory drugs increase the risk of atherothrombosis? Meta-analysis of randomised trials. BMJ 2006;332:1302-1308.
20. Zeilhofer HU, Brune K. Analgesic strategies beyond the inhibition of cyclooxygenases. Trends Pharmacol Sci 2006;27:467-474.
21. Brune K, Katus HA, Moecks J, et al: High N-terminal pro-brain natriuretic peptide values predict the risk of cardiovascular adverse events from anti-inflammatory drugs: A pilot trial. Clin Chem (in press).

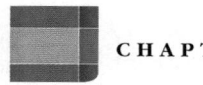

CHAPTER **136**

Diuretics

Mazen A. Hanna and Randall C. Starling

KEY POINTS

- The four major classes of diuretics commonly used are loop diuretics, thiazide diuretics, potassium-sparing diuretics, and aldosterone antagonists.
- All diuretics except aldosterone antagonists work from within the renal tubule.
- A threshold concentration of a loop diuretic must reach the tubule to achieve diuresis.
- Thiazide diuretics do not work in isolation when the glomerular filtration rate falls below 30 mL/min.
- Sequential nephron blockade with a loop and thiazide diuretic overcomes diuretic resistance.
- Appropriate use of aldosterone antagonists is necessary to avoid hyperkalemia.

Diuretics are commonly used for hypertension and heart failure. In hypertension, thiazide diuretics are first-line therapy.[1] In heart failure, they limit volume overload and symptoms of congestion. Understanding diuretic use requires knowledge of renal handling of sodium chloride and basic pharmacokinetic and pharmacodynamic principles.

MECHANISM OF ACTION

It is first important to understand how the kidney handles NaCl reabsorption. NaCl reabsorption occurs along the entire nephron at different sites and by different transporters (Fig. 136-1). Sixty percent to 65% of the filtered

Diuretics: Mechanism of Action

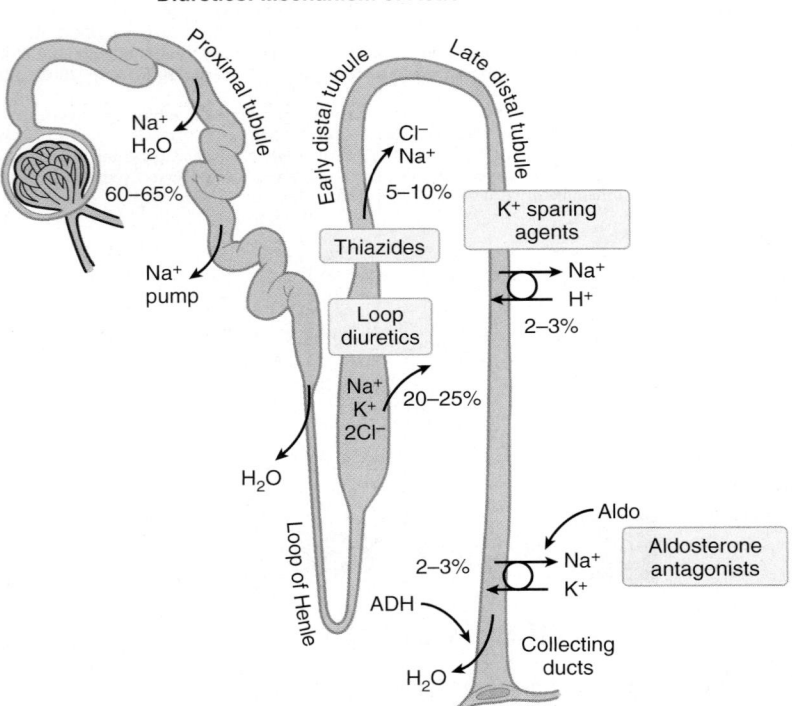

FIGURE 136-1 Reabsorption of NaCl. NaCl reabsorption occurs at different sites of the nephron by distinct transporters and mechanisms. Each class of diuretics acts at a different site of the tubule. ADH, antidiuretic hormone; Aldo, aldosterone. *(Redrawn and modified from Opie, Gersh. Drugs for the Heart, 6th ed. Philadelphia: Saunders, 2004.)*

NaCl is reabsorbed in the proximal tubule. Twenty percent to 25% of the filtered NaCl is reabsorbed in the ascending limb of the loop of Henle via the $Na^+/K^+/2Cl^-$ cotransporter. In the distal convoluted tubule, an electroneutral NaCl transporter accounts for 5% to 10%. Finally, the cortical collecting duct (under the influence of aldosterone) reabsorbs 2% to 3% in exchange for excreting potassium and hydrogen.

Most diuretics work within the tubular lumen of the nephron, except for aldosterone antagonists, which enter the basolateral membrane of cortical collecting duct cells and bind to mineralocorticoid receptors. Most diuretics that work within the tubular lumen reach their target sites by being secreted into the proximal tubule, except for osmotic diuretics, which are filtered by the glomerulus.[2] The four main diuretic classes are loop diuretics, thiazide diuretics, potassium-sparing diuretics, and aldosterone antagonists. Carbonic anhydrase inhibitors and osmotic diuretics are not discussed.

Loop Diuretics (Furosemide, Torsemide, Bumetanide)

Loop diuretics inhibit the $Na^+/K^+/2Cl^-$ cotransporter in the ascending limb of the loop of Henle (see Fig. 136-1). They are highly protein bound and not filtered by the glomerulus. Loop diuretics are actively secreted into the proximal tubule by the organic anion pathway and reach their site of action intraluminally. They also indirectly inhibit reabsorption of calcium and magnesium by their effect on transepithelial potential difference. Furosemide is the prototype. Fifty percent to 60% of an oral dose is absorbed, but the range is 10% to 90%. Bumetanide and torsemide have higher and more consistent absorption, with bioavailability approaching 90% with torsemide.[3]

Thiazide Diuretics (Hydrochlorothiazide, Chlorthalidone, Metolazone)

Similar to the loop diuretics, the thiazide diuretics are highly protein bound and secreted into the proximal tubule (via the organic acid secretory pathway). They travel intraluminally to the distal convoluted tubule, where they inhibit the electroneutral NaCl transporter by competing for the chloride site. Because this segment reabsorbs only 5% to 10% of filtered sodium, thiazide-type diuretics are less potent than loop diuretics. They are rapidly absorbed from the gastrointestinal tract and produce diuresis within 1 to 2 hours. They are longer acting than loop diuretics but work less well in patients with renal failure.[4]

Potassium-Sparing Diuretics (Amiloride, Triamterene)

Potassium-sparing diuretics directly inhibit the sodium-proton exchanger at the distal nephron and collecting duct, and their effects are independent of aldosterone. They reach their site of action both by glomerular filtration and via the proximal tubule organic base secretory pathway. Overall, these diuretics decrease sodium reabsorption and potassium excretion. They are relatively weak diuretics alone and are almost always used with thiazides. Gastrointestinal absorption is 30% with amiloride, less with triamterene.[5] Both are eliminated by the kidney.

Their major advantages are less loss of K⁺ and Mg⁺ and a mechanism of action independent of aldosterone.

Aldosterone Antagonists (Spironolactone, Eplerenone)

Aldosterone antagonists are also "potassium-sparing diuretics" but are distinct given their ability to block aldosterone. Aldosterone is secreted by the adrenal gland and reaches the cytoplasm of epithelial cells in the cortical collecting duct via the basolateral membrane. There, aldosterone forms a complex by binding to the mineralocorticoid receptor to upregulate the synthesis of new sodium channels and activate existing sodium channels.[5] The sodium is reabsorbed in exchange for potassium and hydrogen ions.

Both spironolactone and eplerenone bind competitively to mineralocorticoid receptors, thus making fewer available for aldosterone. Given that only 2% to 3% of the filtered sodium is absorbed in this segment, they are weak diuretics. Spironolactone is metabolized in the liver to the active metabolite canrenone, which has an elimination half-life of 17 hours.[5] Eplerenone is metabolized by the liver.

One of their uses is to reduce hypokalemia from loop or thiazide diuretics. More importantly, in heart failure they block the deleterious effects of aldosterone on the heart, including myocardial fibrosis and adverse remodeling.[6] They decrease mortality and sudden death in severe chronic heart failure and post–myocardial infarction left ventricular dysfunction.[7,8]

DOSAGES

Loop Diuretics (Furosemide, Torsemide, Bumetanide)

In dosing of loop diuretics, a threshold concentration must reach the renal tubule before any diuresis takes place (Table 136-1).[2] A sigmoidal dose-response curve then ensues until a ceiling effect occurs, beyond which higher doses do not produce further diuresis (Fig. 136-2). In renal failure, higher doses are required to achieve the same tubular concentration of drug because organic anions (sulfates and phosphates) compete with the loop diuretic for secretion into the proximal tubule. In heart failure, the dose-response curve is blunted and shifted to the right and absorption is slowed, thus necessitating larger doses. Oral furosemide is poorly absorbed, but oral torsemide is often effective because of better absorption when high-dose oral furosemide fails. High-dose intravenous loop diuretics may be required in both heart and renal failure for adequate diuresis (up to 160 mg furosemide intravenously)

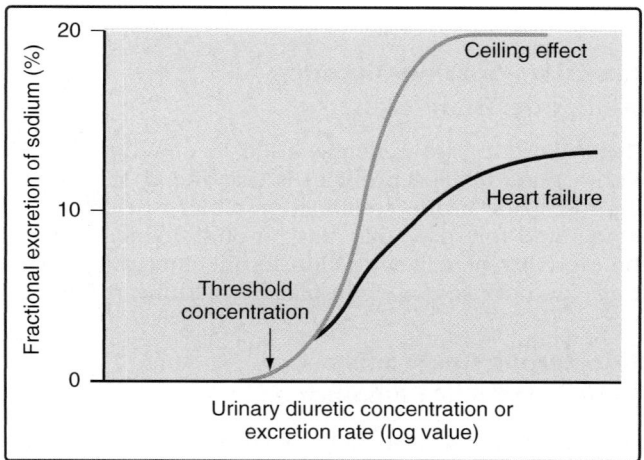

FIGURE 136-2   Dose-response curve for loop diuretics. In heart failure, the dose-response curve is blunted and shifted to the right. In renal failure, a higher serum concentration is needed to ultimately achieve the given urinary diuretic concentration desired. *(Adapted from Brater DC. Diuretic therapy. N Engl J Med 1998;339:387-395.)*

TABLE 136-1	Oral Diuretics Recommended for Use in the Treatment of Fluid Retention in Chronic Heart Failure		
DRUG	**INITIAL DAILY DOSE**	**MAXIMUM TOTAL DAILY DOSE**	**DURATION OF ACTION**
LOOP DIURETICS			
Bumetanide	0.5-1.0 mg once or twice	10 mg	4-6 hr
Furosemide	20-40 mg once or twice	600 mg	6-8 hr
Torsemide	10-20 mg once	200 mg	12-16 hr
THIAZIDE DIURETICS			
Chlorothiazide	250-500 mg once or twice	1000 mg	6-12 hr
Chlorthalidone	12.5-25 mg once	100 mg	24-72 hr
Hydrochlorothiazide	25 mg once or twice	200 mg	6-12 hr
Indapamide	2.5 mg once	5 mg	36 hr
Metolazone	2.5 mg once	20 mg	12-24 hr
POTASSIUM-SPARING DIURETICS			
Amiloride	5 mg once	20 mg	24 hr
Spironolactone	12.5-25 mg once	50 mg	2-3 days
Triamterene	50-75 mg twice	200 mg	7-9 hr
SEQUENTIAL NEPHRON BLOCKADE			
Metolazone	2.5-10 mg once plus a loop diuretic		
Hydrochlorothiazide	25-100 mg once or twice plus a loop diuretic		
Chlorothiazide (IV)	500-1000 mg once plus a loop diuretic		

when oral therapy fails. In this setting, continuous intravenous infusion can help and is possibly safer.[9,10]

Thiazide Diuretics (Hydrochlorothiazide, Chlorthalidone)

Thiazides are "low-ceiling diuretics" because maximal response is reached at low dosage. With hydrochlorothiazide, the full antihypertensive effect of 12.5 mg daily may take up to 6 weeks. Doses greater than 25 mg daily add little to therapeutic efficacy and increase side effects.[4] In congestive heart failure, higher doses are justified while monitoring serum potassium. Benefit can result from a loop diuretic with a thiazide; the thiazide blocks the nephron distally, where hypertrophy and greater sodium retention can occur during long-term loop diuretic therapy.[11-13]

Potassium-Sparing Diuretics (Amiloride, Triamterene)

These diuretics are generally used in combination pills with a thiazide. The problem is that the dose of hydrochlorothiazide in the combination tablet is usually 25 to 50 mg, and for some this may be undesirable. Based on the mortality benefit with aldosterone antagonists, these drugs are not used much in patients with heart failure.

Aldosterone Antagonists (Spironolactone, Eplerenone)

Aldosterone antagonists help avoid hyperkalemia, which can be life threatening.[14] Risk factors for hyperkalemia include diabetes, chronic kidney disease, and concomitant medications that interfere with potassium homeostasis. The challenge is to understand their pharmacology and use them safely in appropriate patients. In patients with normal renal function and normal baseline potassium, an initial dose of spironolactone of 25 mg is reasonable. In those with reduced creatinine clearance or elevated baseline potassium, a starting dose of 12.5 mg daily or every other day is best. Serum potassium should be checked 72 hours after initiating spironolactone.[15] Nonsteroidal anti-inflammatory drugs (NSAIDs), trimethoprim, and hypovolemia can all exacerbate hyperkalemia, and it is prudent to temporarily withhold the aldosterone antagonist. Those at risk for hyperkalemia should be given a low-potassium diet. In cirrhosis and ascites, high-dose spironolactone combined with a loop diuretic is recommended given the associated hyperaldosteronism. Eplerenone dosing is similar to that of spironolactone.

MAJOR SIDE EFFECTS

Major side effects derive mainly from electrolyte imbalance and reduced intravascular volume. Side effects particular to each class exist but are uncommon.

Loop Diuretics

The main side effect is hypokalemia, the risk being greatest with high intravenous doses. The mechanism involves more distal tubule delivery of Na^+, which increases urinary K^+ and H^+ excretion. This can be lessened by angiotensin-converting enzyme (ACE) inhibitors/angiotensin receptor blockers (ARBs) or potassium-sparing diuretics. Hypomagnesemia often coexists with diuretic-induced hypokalemia, and repletion of magnesium is often necessary to correct the hypokalemia. Hyponatremia is less common than with thiazides but can occur, especially with increased free water intake. Overvigorous diuresis can cause dehydration and activation of the renin-angiotensin-aldosterone system. High-dose loop diuretics given quickly can result in ototoxicity, which can be avoided by not exceeding an infusion rate of 4 mg/min.[4]

Thiazide Diuretics

Side effects resemble those of loop diuretics and are dose dependent. The main side effect is hypokalemia, which per amount of diuresis, is greater than that with loop diuretics. Hyponatremia, though uncommon, can be severe, especially in elderly women. Most of the major side effects can be avoided by using low doses. Glucose intolerance and lipid abnormalities are more likely with doses of hydrochlorothiazide above 25 mg. Decreased calcium and urate excretion occurs and can lead to mild hypercalcemia and hyperuricemia.[4]

Potassium-Sparing Diuretics

Their most dangerous adverse effect is hyperkalemia, which is rare and more likely in patients with renal disease. Concomitant NSAID use can precipitate serious hyperkalemia and should be avoided. Specific common adverse effects of amiloride are nausea, vomiting, diarrhea, and headache. Those of triamterene are nausea, vomiting, leg cramps, dizziness, and an association with interstitial nephritis and nephrolithiasis. In general, both are well tolerated but accumulate in patients with renal failure and thus are associated with an increased risk of side effects.[16]

Aldosterone Antagonists (Spironolactone, Eplerenone)

Hyperkalemia is the most serious side effect (see "Dosages"). The risk increases proportionally with renal dysfunction and is accentuated by concomitant NSAIDs, ACE inhibitors/ARBs, and trimethoprim/sulfamethoxazole. Hyperkalemia may not be manifested for several days given the long half-life of the active metabolite canrenone, and after drug discontinuation the hyperkalemic effect may persist for a few days. Avoidance of hyperkalemia requires careful dose adjustment for renal function and evaluation of electrolytes 72 hours after initiation. Because of its steroid structure, spironolactone may cause gynecomastia, impotence, decreased libido, and menstrual irregularities. Painful gynecomastia occurs in less than 10% and is dose related. Eplerenone as a selective blocker of aldosterone receptors does not cause gynecomastia and can be substituted.

12. Fliser D, Schröter M, Neubeck M, et al. Coadministration of thiazides increases the efficacy of loop diuretics even in patients with advanced renal failure. Kidney Int 1994;46:482-488.
13. Kim J, Welch WJ, Cannon J, et al. Immunocytochemical response of type A and type B intercalated cells to increases sodium delivery. Am J Physiol 1991;262:F288-F302.
14. Juurlink DN, Mamdani MM, Lee DS, et al. Rates of hyperkalemia after publication of the randomized aldactone evaluation study. N Engl J Med 2004;351: 543-551.
15. Hunt SA, Abraham WT, Chin MH, et al. ACC/AHA guideline update for the diagnosis and management of chronic heart failure in the adult. J Am Coll Cardiol 2005;46:1116-1143.
16. Gehr TWB, Sica DA, Frishman WH. Diuretic therapy in cardiovascular disease. In Frishman WH (ed). Cardiovascular Pharmacotherapeutics. New York: McGraw-Hill, 2003, pp 157-176.

CONTRAINDICATIONS

Loop Diuretics

Anuria is a contraindication, although loop diuretics have been used in an attempt to induce urine output in this setting. All loop diuretics except for ethacrynic acid are sulfonamide derivatives and must be used with caution in those with sulfa allergy. They should not be administered intravenously when electrolytes cannot be monitored.

Thiazide Diuretics

Significant hypokalemia and ventricular arrhythmias should preclude or limit the use of thiazide diuretics, especially with concomitant proarrhythmic drugs. Pregnancy is a relative contraindication.

Potassium-Sparing Diuretics and Aldosterone Antagonists

Both classes are contraindicated in patients with hyperkalemia and those at serious risk for hyperkalemia who cannot be monitored meticulously. They should be avoided when serum creatinine exceeds 2.0 to 2.5 mg/dL. Spironolactone is contraindicated in patients with peptic ulcers because it can induce gastritis, gastric bleeding, and peptic ulcers.

REFERENCES

1. Chobanian AV, Bakris GL, Black HR, et al. The Seventh Report of the Joint National Committee on Prevention, Detection, Evaluation, and Treatment of High Blood Pressure. Hypertension 2003;42:1206-1252.
2. Brater DC. Diuretic therapy. N Engl J Med 1998;339:387-395.
3. Vargo DL, Kramer WG, Black PK, et al. Bioavailabilty, pharmacokinetics, and pharmacodynamics of torsemide and furosemide in patients with congestive heart failure. Clin Pharmacol Ther 1995;57:601-609.
4. Opie LH, Kaplan NM. Diuretics. In Opie LN (ed). Drugs for the Heart, 6th ed. Philadelphia: Elsevier Saunders, 2005, pp 80-103.
5. Jackson EK. Diuretics. In Hardman JG (ed). Goodman and Gilman's The Pharmacological Basis of Therapeutics, 9th ed. New York: McGraw-Hill, 1996, pp 685-713.
6. Weber KT. Aldosterone in congestive heart failure. N Engl J Med 2001;345:1689-1697.
7. Pitt B, Zannad F, Remme WJ, et al. The effect of spironolactone on morbidity and mortality in patients with severe heart failure. N Engl J Med 1999;341:709-717.
8. Pitt B, Remme W, Zannand F, et al. Eplerenone, a selective aldosterone blocker, in patients with left ventricular dysfunction after myocardial infarction. N Engl J Med 2003;348:1309-1320.
9. Dormans TP, van Meyel JJ, Gerlag PG, et al. Diuretic efficacy of high dose furosemide in severe heart failure: Bolus injection versus continuous infusion. J Am Coll Cardiol 1996;28:376-382.
10. Rudy DW, Voelker JR, Greens PK, et al. Loop diuretics for chronic renal insufficiency: A continuous infusion is more efficacious than bolus therapy. Ann Intern Med 1991;115:360-366.
11. Wolliam GL, Tarazi RC, Bravo EL, et al. Diuretic potency of combined hydrochlorothiazide and furosemide therapy in patients with azotemia. Am J Med 1982;72:929-938.

CHAPTER **137**

Bronchodilators and Cough Suppressants

Susan B. LeGrand and Bassam Estfan

KEY POINTS

- The underlying pathology should be treated when possible, but empirical management of cough and bronchospasm is important.
- Opioid or opioid-like drugs are the most effective antitussives.
- Benzonatate is a peripheral anesthetic that may improve intractable coughing.
- Bronchodilator therapy should start with single agents and combinations used only when need is documented.
- No studies have evaluated bronchodilators in advanced disease, but unsuspected bronchospasm is common, particularly in advanced lung cancer[1]; a therapeutic trial for dyspnea is reasonable.

Bronchospasm and cough are common both as a direct effect of a life-limiting illness such as cancer or chronic obstructive lung disease (COPD) and as a common co-morbidity. Although diagnostic algorithms[2] should be followed to identify any cause that can be managed with a specific intervention, empirical therapy is essential during evaluation and may be the only therapy if no reversible cause is identified. The few effective cough remedies pose a challenge, especially in resource-poor countries where access to opioid medications may be limited or strictly regulated. Multiple bronchodilators have been approved with little evidence of substantial differences between products of the same class. Availability and preferences vary by country.

ANTITUSSIVES

Opioids

Opioids (see Chapter 138) are the mainstay of antitussive therapy (Table 137-1) and have some evidence to support their use.[3] Although codeine was one of the first opioids used for cough and is considered by some to be the gold standard, it is no more effective than placebo for cough secondary to acute upper respiratory infections.[4] Hydrocodone is a semisynthetic weak opioid that has also been widely used, most often as a syrup combined with homatropine. In a phase II nonrandomized trial in advanced cancer, 19 of 20 patients had at least 50% improvement in cough.[3] Although other opioids could theoretically be efficacious, they are rarely used.

Pharmacology

Both codeine and hydrocodone act by raising the threshold of the medullary cough centers. Codeine has good oral bioavailability (60%), with the maximum concentration being achieved in 1 to 2 hours (T_{max}) and an effective half-life of 4 hours.[5] Metabolism is via demethylation in the liver to norcodeine and morphine, which are excreted unchanged in urine. Ten percent of the metabolism is to morphine via CYP2D6. Poor metabolizers may have less benefit. Hydrocodone is also well absorbed, with T_{max} achieved at 1.3 hours and efficacy lasting 4 to 6 hours. It is metabolized by CYP2D6, with a corresponding potential for drug interactions.[5]

Dosages

The usual recommended antitussive dose of codeine is 10 to 20 mg every 4 hours as needed, with doses of up to 30 to 60 mg if response is suboptimal. Codeine is also available as a parenteral preparation with an oral-parenteral ratio of 2:1. Hydrocodone is typically dosed at 5 mg every 4 hours as needed. In a phase II trial the median daily effective dose was 10 mg in divided doses (range, 5 to 30 mg).[1] Daily doses as high as 70 mg have been used to control cough.[6] The presence of homatropine (to combat abuse) might limit dosing secondary to anticholinergic toxicity.

Side Effects

The side effects of both medications are those typical of other opioids (see Chapter 138). Constipation, nausea, and sedation are more likely with codeine than with hydrocodone.

Drug Interactions

Both have the potential for additive sedation with other central nervous system depressants and should be used with caution in these circumstances. Because hydrocodone is metabolized by CYP2D6, inhibitors of this enzyme may have decreased efficacy and inducers increased toxicity.

Dextromethorphan

Although dextromethorphan is the most widely used antitussive in the United States, there is inadequate evidence to support its use for acute cough.[4] Studies have had conflicting results, and the difference identified was of marginal clinical benefit. Its role in relieving chronic cough in patients with advanced disease has not been assessed. Dextromethorphan is an N-methyl-D-aspartate (NMDA) antagonist related to levorphanol. Unlike other opiate antitussives, it is nonsedating.

Pharmacology

The mechanism of action of dextromethorphan has not been determined. Some antitussive effect may be secondary to its syrup form, which soothes the pharynx; some suggest a role for central inhibition of the cough center through NMDA antagonism. It is well absorbed from the gut with T_{max} achieved in 15 to 30 minutes and an efficacy of 3 to 6 hours. It is primarily metabolized in the liver and excreted in urine.[5]

Dosages

The recommended daily dose is 10 to 20 mg every 4 to 6 hours, with a maximum daily dose of 120 mg.

TABLE 137-1 Antitussives					
MEDICATION	**MECHANISM**	**DOSE**	**METABOLISM**	**TOXICITY**	**INTERACTIONS**
Codeine	Increase threshold of the cough center	10-20 mg q4h	Liver—demethylation	Constipation, nausea, sedation	Addictive, sedation with CNS depressants
Hydrocodone	Increase threshold of the cough center	5 mg q4h	Liver—CYP2D6	Constipation, nausea, sedation	CYP2D6 inhibitors may decrease efficiency
Dextromethorphan	NMDA antagonism at the cough center? Syrup soothes the pharynx	10-20 mg q4h	Liver	Nausea	Fatalities with MAOI agents. Separate by 2 wk
Benzonatate	Peripheral anesthetic afferent limb of the cough reflex	100 mg q8h	Liver	Bronchospasm, laryngospasm, cardiovascular collapse if contents of capsule spill. Rare seizure with misuse	None known

CNS, central nervous system; MAOI, monoamine oxidase inhibitor; NMDA, N-methyl-D-aspartate.

Side Effects

Nausea and gastrointestinal disturbance may occur, but other side effects are rare. Dextromethorphan is nonsedating and, though not addictive, has been abused for euphoric and dissociative properties in higher doses, with some fatalities.

Drug Interactions

Dextromethorphan should not be used with monoamine oxidase inhibitors.

Benzonatate

Benzonatate is a polyethylene glycol derivative of *p*-aminobenzoic acid that is effective without opioid side effects. In a small case series it helped decrease hydrocodone-resistant cough in advanced disease.[7] Availability worldwide is limited.

Pharmacology

Benzonatate is a relative of local anesthetics such as procaine and may act peripherally by anesthetizing pulmonary stretch receptors feeding the afferent limb of the cough reflex. T_{max} is 15 minutes after ingestion, with efficacy lasting 3 to 8 hours. It is metabolized in the liver and excreted in urine.

Dosages

Benzonatate is available in capsules of 100 and 200 mg with a usual starting dose of 100 mg every 8 hours. Up to 600 mg daily can be given safely.

Side Effects

Benzonatate should be swallowed whole. Spillage of contents before ingestion numbs the oral mucosa with loss of its antitussive effect. Other serious side effects such as bronchospasm, laryngospasm, and cardiovascular collapse are related to spillage of contents or chewing on the pills. Rarely, seizures and cardiac arrest may develop with drug misuse.[5]

Drug Interactions

Benzonatate has no known drug interactions and can be used safely with concurrent medications.

Miscellaneous Antitussive Drugs

Numerous other agents have been reported in various populations and in case reports or small series (Box 137-1). Only levodropropizine, available in Europe, has been tested in cancer-related cough. It is a phenylpiperazinopropane derivative thought to work peripherally by modulating C-fiber sensitivity.[8,9] In doses of 60 to 75 mg three times daily, it was as effective as antitussive opioids, but with less somnolence.

Research Challenges

Advances in cough remedies have been limited.[10] Opioids are the main medications for symptomatic relief, and

---

Box 137-1 Miscellaneous Antitussive Agents

- Corticosteroids (systemic or inhaled)
- Levodropropizine
- Sodium cromoglycate
- Paroxetine
- Baclofen
- Diazepam

Box 137-2 Possible Future Antitussives

- Tachykinin receptor antagonists
- Vanilloid receptor antagonists
- Bradykinin receptor antagonists
- γ-Aminobutyric acid (GABA) receptor antagonists
- Selective opioid and opioid-like agonists
- Potassium channel openers
- Endogenous cannabinoids
- Serotonin agonists

---

systematic reviews question the usefulness of other agents. Despite efforts to develop effective antitussives with less toxicity, such as levocloperastine,[9] no new antitussives have been added to the market (Box 137-2). The research that does exist is focused on nonpalliative populations.

BRONCHODILATORS

Bronchodilators are commonly prescribed, but no studies have specifically evaluated their role in palliation of advanced diseases other than COPD. They are fundamental to the management of asthma and COPD, common co-morbidities in other advanced diseases. In addition, because unsuspected bronchospasm has been reported in up to 50% of lung cancer patients,[11] a trial of bronchodilators is recommended in those with related dyspnea (see Chapter 159). Bronchodilators can be divided by class: β_2-adrenergic agonists, anticholinergic agents, and methylxanthines. Within the first two classes there are also long- and short-acting preparations and combinations (Table 137-2).

Selective β_2-Adrenergic Agonist Agents

The first agents for bronchospasm, epinephrine and ephedrine, affect both α- and β-receptors with significant potential for cardiovascular complications. Isoproterenol, an agent selective for β-receptors—both β_1 and β_2—but with little affinity for α-receptors was next. Selective β_2-agents were then developed and became the medications of choice for acute asthma. They are best tolerated as inhaled agents, although some (metaproterenol, terbutaline, and albuterol) are available in oral formulations. They can be divided into groups by duration of action, with the short-acting agent isoproterenol rarely being used. Intermediate-acting agents (albuterol, terbutaline) take effect quickly and can last from 3 to 6 hours. Long-acting agents (salmeterol, formoterol) are dosed twice daily, are intended for maintenance therapy, and should never be used for

TABLE 137-2 Bronchodilators

β₂-SELECTIVE AGONISTS

Intermediate Acting

   Albuterol

   Bitolterol

   Fenoterol

   Isoetharine

   Metaproterenol

   Procaterol

   Terbutaline

   Levalbuterol

Long Acting

   Formoterol

   Salmeterol

ANTICHOLINERGIC AGENTS

   Ipratropium bromide

   Tiotropium

METHYLXANTHINES

   Aminophylline

   Theophylline

Box 137-3 Effects of β₂-Adrenergic Agonists

- Relax bronchial smooth muscle
- Suppress release of leukotrienes and histamine by mast cells
- Inhibit functional response of white blood cells
- Increase mucociliary transport

---

acute symptoms. There is significant controversy about use of the longer-acting agents in patients with asthma.[12]

Pharmacology

All increase cyclic adenosine monophosphate in cells and thereby lead to airway smooth muscle relaxation (Box 137-3). Time to effect is dependent on the route of administration and is generally 10 to 15 minutes when given by inhalation and delayed if given orally. The duration of action ranges from 3 to 6 hours for the intermediate agents to 12 hours for the long-acting ones. They are generally cleared by the liver with inactive metabolites and excreted in urine.

Dosage

Many studies have confirmed the equivalence of multi-dose inhalers and nebulized medication delivered with proper technique.[13] Dosage recommendations for palliative medicine do not exist. Treatment of COPD or acute asthma should follow established guidelines. In empirical treatment of dyspnea, dosing every 4 hours as needed with intermediate-duration agents seems reasonable, with conversion to scheduled use if helpful.

Side Effects

Toxicity is related to the dose and route. Inhalation is associated with fewer side effects than the oral or paren-

teral routes. Major side effects include cardiac palpitations and tachycardia, tremor, and sleep disturbances. Hypokalemia occurs in overdose. Levalbuterol, the *R*-enantiomer of albuterol, a racemic mixture, was marketed as having less toxicity. There is significant controversy surrounding this medication in asthma; for a hospice population it is substantially more expensive and not clearly superior.[14,15]

Drug Interactions

β-Blockers have antagonistic action with β-agonists. Non–potassium-sparing diuretics could theoretically increase the effect on potassium. There is evidence of a transient effect on digoxin levels, but the persistence of this effect is unclear.[12]

Anticholinergic Agents

Ipratropium was the first inhaled anticholinergic agent available and, in COPD, is equivalent to the β₂-selective agonists but has fewer side effects. It is recommended as the initial medication for moderate continuous symptoms. If symptoms are not adequately relieved with the single agent, combination therapy may be appropriate. The combination of ipratropium with albuterol prolongs the bronchodilator effects. Tiotropium is longer acting and has improved effects in moderate and severe disease. The palliative role of the anticholinergic agents is predominantly one of maintenance or management of exacerbations in preexisting COPD.

Pharmacology

These medications relax smooth muscle by antagonism at muscarinic receptors in airways, thereby reducing the formation of a mediator of bronchoconstriction, cyclic guanosine monophosphate. Systemic absorption is minimal after nebulizer use. Bronchodilation with ipratropium is noticeable in 15 minutes, with maximal effect occurring at 1 to 2 hours and efficacy lasting 2 to 4 hours. Tiotropium can be dosed once daily.

Side Effects

Common side effects are those seen with any anticholinergic medication, but to a lesser degree because absorption is minimal. One of the most common complaints is dry mouth, greater with tiotropium than ipratropium. Increased but not statistically significant differences occur in constipation and urinary retention.[16] A higher frequency of urinary tract infections was seen with tiotropium than with β-agonists and ipratropium. Care must be taken to avoid eye exposure with oral inhalation.

Drug Interactions

Given limited absorption, drug interactions are not significant. Concurrent use of two anticholinergic inhaled medications is not recommended.

Methylxanthines

The use of methylxanthines (theophylline and aminophylline) for asthma and COPD remains controversial. They are inexpensive, used more widely in less developed countries, and included in the guidelines for management of COPD.[17,18] Their role in the palliative management of dyspnea of other causes is unknown. There has been speculation of a role in respiratory muscle weakness, although no evidence of benefit exists.

Pharmacology

The mechanism of action is ill understood. Theophylline has anti-inflammatory and immunomodulatory effects and relaxes smooth muscle in the bronchial tree and pulmonary blood vessels.[18] It inhibits breakdown of cyclic adenosine monophosphate by inhibition of phosphodiesterases, but the effect is small and other medications with greater inhibition have no bronchodilatory effect. It also exhibits adenosine antagonism, which may explain other effects, including improved diaphragmatic contractility and increased cardiac output. A central mechanism may explain the ability to reduce central sleep apnea in heart failure.

Theophylline can be given orally or intravenously (usually as aminophylline), and sustained-release products are available. Food delays but does not prevent absorption, and the effect varies by product. The maximum concentration (C_{max}) is achieved in 1 to 2 hours, with steady-state concentrations lasting for 30 to 65 hours. The narrow therapeutic range necessitates plasma monitoring. Recommended levels are 8 to 15 μg/mL. The drug is protein bound, and therefore hepatic failure or other low-protein states can affect free drug levels and require dose reductions. It is metabolized in the liver via cytochrome P-450 (CYP) enzymes, and there is a potential for significant drug interactions. Marked interindividual differences in half-life are due to age, smoking, heart failure, liver failure, and drug interactions.

Side Effects

Overdoses of methylxanthine medications are potentially fatal because of cardiac arrhythmias. Other side effects include headaches, palpitations, dizziness, nausea and vomiting, restlessness and agitation, hypotension, and precordial pain. Seizures, both focal and generalized, have been reported with levels above 25 μg/mL. Maintenance of therapeutic levels can avoid most toxicity.

Drug Interactions

Theophylline is a major substrate of CYP3A4, with consequent effects from inducers (decreased levels) and inhibitors (increased levels). Similar effects are seen with medications that inhibit or induce CYP1A2. A search for interactions should be conducted before prescribing medications with a potential impact, and careful monitoring is required.

SUMMARY

Medications for the management of cough remain limited and marginally effective. Bronchodilators are commonly used for asthma and COPD, and their use should be maintained in the palliative setting. Their role in dyspnea in other settings is unclear, but given their minimal toxicity and commonly unrecognized bronchospasm, a therapeutic trial is reasonable. The role of methylxanthines remains speculative.

Current Controversies and Future Considerations

- New medications are needed for cough management. Many are under investigation[10] (see Box 137-2), but none are approaching availability.
- A systematic review of over-the-counter antitussives failed to show significant benefit in acute cough (including dextromethorphan and expectorants such as guaifenesin). Their use is controversial.[4]
- The role of bronchodilators in dyspnea not clearly related to bronchospasm is undefined. When, which agents, and how best to use them should be researched.
- The potential role of methylxanthines in respiratory muscle weakness should be investigated even though their use is complicated by drug interactions and monitoring requirements.

REFERENCES

1. Pratter MR, Bartter T, Akers S, DuBois J. An algorithmic approach to chronic cough. Ann Intern Med 1993;119:977-983.
2. Dudgeon D, Lertzman M. Dyspnea in the advanced cancer patient. J Pain Symptom Manage 1998;16:212-219.
3. Homsi J, Walsh D, Nelson KA, et al. A phase II study of hydrocodone for cough in advanced cancer. Am J Hosp Palliat Care 2002;19:49-56.
4. Schroeder K, Fahey T. Systematic review of randomized control trials of over the counter cough medicines for acute cough in adults. BMJ 2002;324:1-6.
5. McAvoy GK (ed). AHFS Drug Information 2006. Bethesda, MD: American Society of Health System Pharmacies, 2008, 48:08
6. Homsi J, Walsh D, Nelson KA, et al. Hydrocodone for cough in advanced cancer. Am J Hosp Palliat Care 2000;17:342-346.
7. Doona M, Walsh D. Benzonatate for opioid-resistant cough in advanced cancer. Palliat Med 1998;12:55-58.
8. Luporini G, Barni S, Marchi E, et al. Efficacy and safety of levodropropizine and dihydrocodeine on nonproductive cough in primary and metastatic lung cancer. Eur Respir J 1998;12:97-101.
9. Aliprandi P, Castelli C, Bernorio S, et al. Levocloperastine in the treatment of chronic nonproductive cough: Comparative efficacy versus standard antitussive agents. Drugs Exp Clin Res 2004;30:133-141.
10. Dicpinigaitis PV. Potential new cough therapies. Pulm Pharmacol Ther 2004;17:459-462.
11. Congleton J, Muers MK. The incidence of airflow obstruction in bronchial carcinoma, its relation to breathlessness, and response to bronchdilator therapy. Respir Med 1995;89:291-296.
12. McAvoy GK (ed). AHFS Drug Information 2006. Bethesda, MD: American Society of Health System Pharmacies, 2008, 12:12.08.12.
13. Cates CJ, Crilly JA, Rowe BH. Holding chambers (spacers) versus nebulisers for beta-agonist treatment of acute asthma. Cochrane Database Syst Rev 2006;(2):CD000052.
14. Ameredes BT, Calhoun WJ. (R)-Albuterol for asthma: Pro [a.k.a. (S)-albuterol for asthma: Con]. Am J Respir Crit Care Med 2006;174:965-969.
15. Barnes PJ. Treatment with (R)-albuterol has no advantage over racemic albuterol Am J Respir Crit Care Med 2006;174:969-972.
16. Barr RG, Bourbeau J, Camargo CA, et al. Tiotropium for stable chronic obstructive pulmonary disease. Cochrane Database Syst Rev 2005;(2):CD002876.
17. Pauwels RA, Buist AS, Calverly PM, et al. Global strategy for the diagnosis, management, and prevention of chronic obstructive pulmonary disease. NHLB/WHO Global Initiative for Chronic Obstructive Disease (GOLD) workshop summary. Am J Respir Crit Care Med 2001;163:1256-1276.
18. Undem BJ. Pharmacotherapy of asthma. In Goodman & Gilman's The Pharmacological Basis of Therapeutics, 11th ed. New York: McGraw-Hill, 2006.

CHAPTER 138

Opioids

Friedemann Nauck and Janet R. Hardy

Preparations of the opium poppy *Papaver somniferum* have been used for many hundreds of years to relieve pain. Toxic effects and addictive potential have been recognized through the ages. Morphine was isolated in 1803 and later shown to be almost entirely responsible for the analgesic activity of crude opium. The term "opiate" applies to the naturally occurring derivatives of phenanthrene, an opium alkaloid poppy extract (i.e., codeine, thebaine, and morphine). An opioid is any drug that activates the opioid receptor, thus including both opiates and synthetic and semisynthetic opioids. A "narcotic" is any drug that induces narcosis (numbness or torpor).

Morphine remains the prototypical opioid. It has a five-ringed structure with a characteristic T-shaped three-dimensional form essential for activation of the opioid receptor. Semisynthetic opioids such as hydromorphone and oxycodone have been developed by substitution of various chemical constituents of the rings. Synthetics such as fentanyl are produced by a reduction in the number of fused rings.[1]

MECHANISM OF ACTION

Our understanding of opioid pharmacology has increased markedly as a result of studies in mice lacking opioid receptors ("knockout mice") by gene targeting.[2] All opioids act through their interaction with opioid receptors located both presynaptically and postsynaptically within the CNS. The interaction of opioid and receptor leads to the release of neurotransmitters with disruption of the pain impulse.[3] The main responses mediated by the opioid receptor are analgesia, sedation, respiratory depression, emesis, reduced gastrointestinal mobility, euphoria, and dysphoria. Opioid agonists produce maximal response through binding of the opioid receptor. Antagonists have no intrinsic activity and block agonists by preventing receptor access. Partial agonists produce a submaximal receptor response.

Three distinct opioid receptors have been identified and cloned: mu, kappa, and delta. Activation of each receptor type mediates various pharmacological effects and leads to a different spectrum of activity in animal models. All opioids in common clinical use act predominantly through the mu receptor. Some may have minor activity at the other two receptors, but the clinical significance of this is unknown. Receptor subtypes have been postulated and splice variants cloned.[4] Dimerization of different opioid receptors might explain minor differences in activity between different opioids.[5]

DOSAGES

The relative binding affinities of the different opioids correlate with their analgesic potency. Several factors influence analgesia, including age, co-morbidity, end-organ function, gender, race, genetic polymorphism, and drug delivery route.[6] All commonly used opioids can be made equipotent or equianalgesic by adjusting for physicochemical and pharmacokinetic differences through correct dosage and route of administration.[1] Equianalgesic ranges between different opioids are wide, and all equianalgesic conversion tables should be used as guides only. This difficulty can generally be overcome in routine clinical practice by using conservative dose estimates, supplying breakthrough doses as required, and titrating the dose according to pain relief and side effects. The dose range necessary to control pain in different patients is great (5 mg to 5 g/day oral morphine equivalents), but in most, pain can be controlled with less than 180 mg oral morphine equivalent per day.[7]

MAJOR SIDE EFFECTS

The side effects of all opioids are similar, in keeping with their common mechanism of action and predominant activity through the mu receptor. The minor variations in side effect profile demonstrated in some controlled trials between different opioids have been attributed to differential activation of delta or kappa receptors, receptor subtypes, or dimers. There is little evidence to suggest that any one opioid has a more favorable side effect profile than any other.[8] Any difference is likely to be due to many factors affecting the pharmacodynamics and pharmacokinetics of specific drugs in individual patients. The more favorable effect of fentanyl on gut motility, for example, is more likely a result of high lipid solubility than a differential effect on opioid receptor type or subtype.

The common symptoms initially experienced when an opioid is started are nausea and drowsiness, but they generally resolve after a few days. Constipation secondary to the inhibitory effect on gut motility is universal and does not resolve with time. Less common symptoms include dry mouth, sweating, and pruritus. Delirium, confusion, hallucinations, and myoclonus suggest an excessive dose or intolerance. Respiratory depression is rare when opioids are used in controlled fashion and titrated according to pain and analgesic response.[9] Although most will become physically tolerant of long-term opioids and withdrawal symptoms are likely after sudden cessation, dependence (implying a psychological need for opioids) is rare in patients with pain.

CONTRAINDICATIONS

There are no absolute contraindications to opioids, especially when following the recommended guidelines of starting at a low dose and titrating upward according to analgesic response and side effect profile. Those metabolized largely to inactive metabolites not dependent on renal function for elimination (e.g., fentanyl and methadone) are better tolerated in renal failure.[10] Those with metabolites that do accumulate in patients with impaired renal function can still be used, however, albeit at lower doses and decreased dosing frequencies. Respiratory suppression is caused by opioid overdose. It is rarely seen when opioids are used in a controlled manner and titrated according to response and tolerability. Itching is a rare side effect. When it does occur, itching is difficult to control and is best managed by rotation to another opioid of a different class.

DRUG INTERACTIONS

The activity of opioids dependent on the cytochrome P-450 system for metabolism could theoretically be affected by other drugs known to be P-450 inducers or inhibitors. The relevance in routine clinical practice is unknown.[11] The activity of drugs metabolized primarily by glucuronidation, such as morphine and codeine, is more likely to be changed by drugs that alter hepatic blood flow. Tricyclic antidepressants can affect glucuronidation and thus the analgesic effects of morphine.

RESEARCH CHALLENGES

Research in opioid pharmacology is ongoing, and areas under investigation include the following:

- Opioid receptor heterodimerization
- Genetic polymorphism in the expression of opioid receptors
- Opioid receptor autoregulation and its relationship to tolerance and addiction
- Management of opioid-related side effects
- Opioid tolerance/intolerance
- Opioids and neuropathic pain
- Defining opioids best suited to each individual

TRAMADOL

Tramadol is a centrally acting synthetic analgesic with both opioid and nonopioid properties.[12,13] It has some affinity for the mu opioid receptor, stimulates neuronal serotonin release, and inhibits the presynaptic reuptake of both norepinephrine and serotonin. It thus influences the descending pain inhibitory system.

Tramadol has a half-life of around 6 hours after both oral and parenteral administration (Table 138-1). The time to peak plasma levels is approximately 3 hours. Its bioavailability is close to 100% after repeated oral dosing because of saturation of the liver "first-pass" effect. Tramadol shows extensive tissue binding and therefore has a large volume of distribution. The drug is predominantly excreted in urine, about a third as parent drug and two thirds as metabolites.[14] Tramadol is a racemic mixture of enantiomers that differ in their potency in inhibiting norepinephrine and serotonin uptake. Both enantiomers act in a synergistic manner for analgesia.

Tramadol is converted in the liver to two active metabolites, O-desmethyltramadol and di-N,O-desmethyltramadol. Both have greater affinity for the mu receptor than the parent drug does.[15] The importance of O-desmethyltramadol is shown in poor metabolizers of sparteine/debrisoquine. Poor metabolizers (5% to 10% of the white population in Europe) lack the isoenzyme CYP2D6, and tramadol has little or no analgesic effect in such individuals.[16] Elimination is dependent on renal function and decreased in patients with renal impairment.

TABLE 138-1	Clinical Pharmacology of Opioids				
SUBSTANCE	**BIOAVAILABILITY (% RANGE)**	**PLASMA HALF-LIFE (HR)**	**ANALGESIC DURATION OF ACTION (HR)**	**PLASMA PROTEIN-BINDING CAPACITY (%)**	**METABOLISM**
Codeine	40 (12-84)	2.0-4.5	4-6	54	Hepatic oxidative O-demethylation by CYP2D6
Tramadol	75 to >90	6	4-6	20	Demethylation by CYP2D6
Morphine	35 (15-64)	1.5-4.5	3-6	30	Hepatic glucuronidation by UDP glucuronyl transferase to M3G (60%) and M6G (10%)
Hydromorphone	37-62	2.5	4-5	8	Hepatic glucuronidation
Fentanyl	92	17	1-2	80-90	Hepatic oxidative N-dealkylation by CYP3A4
Oxycodone	75 (60-87)	3.5	4-6	40	Hepatic oxidative O-demethylation by CYP2D6, N-dealkylation by CYP3A4, and reduction
Buprenorphine	50	2.5-3	6-9	96	Dealkylation by CYP3A4) and subsequent glucuronidation
Methadone	80 (40-100)	8-75	4-5 (initial) 6-12 (steady state)	85-90	Hepatic oxidative N-dealkylation by CYP3A4

M3G, morphine-3-glucuronide; M6G, morphine-6-glucuronide; UDP, uridine diphosphate.

In palliative care units in Germany, only 6% of all patients received tramadol,[17] but it is the most frequently used "step II" analgesic worldwide. It is classified as a "weak opioid" and used to treat moderate pain. It is $1/10$ as potent as morphine. In single-dose postoperative pain studies, 50 to 150 mg tramadol was equal in analgesic efficacy to 5 to 15 mg morphine.[18] It can be administered orally, subcutaneously, intravenously, or rectally and is available in both immediate-release and slow-release oral preparations. The starting dose of the orally administered slow-release formulation is 100 mg every 8 to 12 hours. The maximum daily dose is usually quoted as 400 mg, although some have used doses up to 800 mg/day with no ill effects.[14]

Tramadol has dose-dependent opioid- and non–opioid-related (monoaminergic) side effects. The latter are characterized by headache, dizziness, and sweating. Tramadol causes less respiratory depression than other opioids do[19] and has little influence on gastric emptying or gut transit time.[19] It causes less constipation than equianalgesic doses of other strong opioids. Because of metabolism via CYP2D6, there is potential for interaction with many other drugs that are either enzyme inhibitors or inducers.

CODEINE

Codeine is a naturally occurring derivative of an opium alkaloid. It is a relatively weak analgesic with other important functions as an antitussive and antidiarrheal agent. It is less effective than paracetamol, tramadol, and non-steroidal anti-inflammatory agents.[20]

Codeine is well absorbed after oral administration but has variable bioavailability (12% to 84%). Its plasma half life is about 2.5 hours. Both the parent drug and metabolites are relatively highly protein bound. Renal clearance contributes little to overall clearance.

As with morphine, glucuronidation is the primary route of metabolism. Codeine-6-glucuronide (C6G) is the primary metabolite and accounts for greater than 80% of the parent drug. Other minor metabolites follow demethylation (i.e., norcodeine and morphine). Morphine is thought to largely be responsible for the drug's analgesic activity, as supported by the finding that those genetically deficient in the cytochrome P-450 enzyme responsible for conversion of codeine to morphine (CYP2D6) have little or no analgesic response to codeine. This is not true for extensive metabolizers, in whom morphine can readily be detected after the administration of codeine. Genetic variation in CYP2D6 activity may account for the variation in pain relief with codeine seen both between different individuals and in different racial groups.

Codeine is a relatively weak analgesic. In single-dose placebo-controlled studies, the number of patients needed to receive it at least once at a dose of 60 mg to achieve 50% pain relief was 16.7. This compares with 5.6 for paracetamol and 2.3 for diclofenac.[20] It is generally recommended that codeine be combined with a nonopioid such as aspirin or paracetamol. Several combination preparations are available commercially. Both codeine and C6G bind to the mu receptor, but the affinity is much less than with morphine. Codeine is approximately a 10th to a 12th as potent as morphine parenterally and a 3rd to a 4th as potent by mouth, although potency ratios change with repeated dosing.

The usual dose of codeine orally is 30 to 60 mg every 4 to 6 hours despite the known linear dose-response curve to at least 320 mg. The oral-to-parenteral potency ratio is around 2.3. In responders, analgesia occurs after 30 to 60 minutes and the analgesic half-life is 4 to 6 hours.

Side affects resemble those of other opioids. There is no evidence that codeine is more constipating than morphine. That it is used as an antidiarrheal agent and as an antitussive without concomitant use of laxatives may explain its unfavorable reputation in this regard. As a weak analgesic, it is the logical opioid for cough in the absence of pain. There is no evidence to suggest that it is a better antitussive agent than any other opioid, however.

MORPHINE

Morphine remains the first-line opioid of choice worldwide and is the only opioid available in many countries.[8] The great variation in the use of morphine from country to country is primarily related to cultural and legal issues. Morphine is the prototypical opioid and is composed of five interlocked rings with a characteristic T-shaped three-dimensional form thought to be essential for its interaction with the opioid receptor. Morphine is relatively water soluble and poorly lipid soluble. It shows linear pharmacokinetics not subject to autoinduction or saturation. Despite ready absorption from the gut, it has relatively poor bioavailability of about 15% to 65% with considerable interindividual variability as a result of extensive pre-systemic elimination, and about 90% of the parent drug is converted to metabolites. Its half-life depends on the route of administration: 1.5 hours after parenteral and 1.5 to 4.5 hours after oral administration.

Morphine is metabolized via glucuronidation to several metabolites, with morphine-6-glucuronide (M6G) and morphine-3-glucuronide (M3G) accounting for about 50% to 60% of each oral dose. Metabolism seems to occur primarily in the liver, but extrahepatic sites may become more important when liver function is impaired. Controversy abounds regarding M3G, but it is generally accepted to be an inactive metabolite with little or no analgesic activity. M6G is a potent mu agonist. Both morphine and M6G accumulate in renal failure patients with resultant toxicity. Morphine is well tolerated in most patients with hepatic impairment.

Morphine is available in various formulations and multiple dose sizes. It can be given orally, parenterally, rectally, and vaginally. The oral formulations come in both immediate- and delayed-release preparations. Usual teaching is to commence with a low dose of immediate-release morphine given regularly in an opioid-naïve patient and titrate according to analgesic response and toxicity. Once stable, treatment can be converted to a convenient delayed-release preparation. Dose range requirements may vary 1000-fold, but in most patients pain can be controlled with relatively low doses (≤ 200 to 300 mg/day).[21] Morphine tartrate is much more soluble than morphine sulfate and more suitable for parenteral delivery. The oral-parenteral dose equivalence is 2:1 to 3:1.

DIAMORPHINE

Diamorphine (diacetylmorphine) (heroin) is a morphine prodrug. It was originally developed as "heroin" for the treatment of chest ailments and morphine dependence. Subsequently, its abuse and addictive potential was recognized and it was banned from all countries except the United Kingdom, where it remains the opioid of choice for parenteral delivery. Diamorphine is rapidly deacetylated to 6-monoacetylmorphine and then to morphine in the liver, kidneys, brain, and blood. It is excreted mainly as conjugated morphine in urine.

It is generally accepted that there is little difference in analgesic activity or side effect profile between diamorphine and morphine. In countries in which other soluble opioids such as hydromorphone are available, it offers little advantage.

HYDROMORPHONE

Hydromorphone has a molecular structure similar to that of morphine and has similar pharmacokinetic and pharmacodynamic properties.[22] It differs from morphine in the substitution of an oxygen for the 6-hyroxyl group and in hydrogenation of the 7-8 double bond.

Hydromorphone is metabolized in the liver by 6-keto-reduction followed by glucuronidation. There is no significant cytochrome P-450 metabolism. The main metabolite is hydromorphone-3-glucuronide (H3G). This and several minor metabolites are all excreted in urine. H3G has no analgesic activity but accumulates in renal failure patients (and causes dose-dependent allodynia, myoclonus, and seizures in rats).[23] Case studies suggest increased toxicity in renal failure, but little is known about dosing in patients with renal or liver failure.

Hydromorphone is available in oral, rectal, and parenteral forms. The availability of a highly concentrated injection makes it ideal for parenteral use. There is uncertainty over the exact dose ratio of morphine and hydromorphone. Some recommend a conversion ratio of 1:7.5 (i.e., 1.3 mg of hydromorphone is equivalent to 10 mg of morphine), whereas others use a conversion ratio of 1:4 to 1:5. When converting from oral to subcutaneous hydromorphone, some use one third the oral dose and others half. Hydromorphone has typical opioid side effects. There is little difference between morphine and hydromorphone in analgesic efficacy, adverse event profile, and patient preference.[24] In the authors' opinion, it is not sufficiently unlike morphine to use as an alternative in morphine-intolerant patients.

FENTANYL

Fentanyl and the other lipophilic opioids (sufentanil, alfentanil, and remifentanil) are all 4-anilinopiperidine derivatives and have unique properties as a result of their high lipid solubility. Fentanyl is available in different formulations and is the lipophilic opioid used most widely. It is approximately 150 times more potent than morphine.

Fentanyl has a lipid solubility (octanol-water distribution coefficient) higher than 800, as opposed to 1.4 for morphine. It can pass into the CNS more readily than morphine, thus accounting for much of its potency. Fentanyl is eliminated primarily through hepatic oxidative metabolism. Up to 20% is excreted by the kidneys, but renal function does not affect pharmacokinetics. The serum half-life of 2.5 to 3.5 hours is the same in normal renal function as in end-stage renal disease, and therefore it is a drug of choice in patients with impaired renal function.

The low molecular weight, high potency, and lipid solubility of fentanyl make it ideal for the transdermal route. The transdermal therapeutic system developed commercially ("Durogesic patch") releases drug at a constant rate (12 to 100 µg/hr) over a period of 72 hours. After application of a patch, there is a delay of 17 to 48 hours before maximal concentrations are achieved. Similarly, the drug depot that accumulates in subcutaneous tissue is released for many hours after patch removal. This is ideal for chronic stable pain. Another commercial preparation using the lipophilic properties of fentanyl is oral transmucosal fentanyl citrate. Fentanyl is absorbed rapidly across the mucous membranes when the "fentanyl lozenge" is "painted" on the inside the mouth. This provides rapid analgesia with a short duration of effect and is designed for breakthrough pain. The formulation is expensive, however, and parenteral fentanyl delivered sublingually provides an alternative. Intranasal formulations have been developed to take advantage of the high intranasal bioavailability. The parenteral formulation is administered by the intravenous, epidural, intrathecal, and subcutaneous routes. Fentanyl is not licensed for subcutaneous administration, but there is much experience in palliative medicine with this route without complication. The main limiting factor is the dose–volume ratio in some preparations, which limits the dose in standard infusion systems.

There is evidence to suggest that fentanyl is less constipating than morphine. This is possibly related to its lipophilic nature, with rapid transfer into the CNS with less local effect on gastrointestinal opioid receptors. Side effects are otherwise similar to those of other opioids. Toxicity is likely if the potency of the patch formulation is underestimated; a 25-µg/hr fentanyl patch is equivalent to 60 to 90 mg/day of oral morphine. Similarly, drug continues to be released for 12 to 18 hours from skin depots after removal of the patch, which needs to be considered if converting to another opioid.

OXYCODONE

Oxycodone is a semisynthetic opioid derived from thebaine and has properties similar to those of morphine. It was originally available in low-dose combination preparations with nonopioids but is now widely administered as a single agent. It is often used as an alternative in patients intolerant of other strong opioids. Oxycodone has more consistent and greater bioavailability than morphine does (about 60%), with less first-pass metabolism. Similarly, there is less variability in plasma concentration and a more predictable pharmacokinetic profile than is the case with morphine. Oxycodone is metabolized predominately by the cytochrome P-450 system (CYP2D6). The primary metabolites, oxymorphone and noroxycodone, do not contribute significantly to the analgesic or side effects of the parent drug. The mean half-life of immediate-release oxycodone, 3.5 to 5.6 hours, is longer than that of morphine, and the drug can therefore be given every 4 to 6 hours rather than every 4 hours. Elimination of oxycodone is significantly influenced by both hepatic and renal impairment.[25]

Oxycodone is available in both immediate- and controlled-release oral preparations, rectal suppositories, and a parenteral formulation. The availability of the various formulations differs between countries. The oral dose ratio of oxycodone to morphine ranges from 1:1.5 to 1:2.0. Anecdotal reports suggest that oxycodone is better tolerated than morphine, but controlled studies have shown only minor differences between the two. An injectable formulation is available in some countries.

METHADONE

Better understanding of methadone's pharmacological and pharmacokinetic properties and equianalgesic ratios has led to its increased use as a second-line opioid for chronic cancer pain. It has no known active metabolites, is well absorbed by the oral and rectal routes, and is low in cost. There is considerable and unpredictable variation in pharmacodynamics and pharmacokinetics in different individuals and a potential for unexpected toxicity. A fundamental understanding of these unique properties plus good knowledge of how to initiate and titrate the drug and closely monitor the patient is necessary if physicians are to use it safely and effectively.

Methadone is a highly lipophilic and highly basic drug. It is absorbed rapidly after oral ingestion and has oral bioavailability of 41% to 97%. The drug undergoes extensive tissue binding in the brain, gut, kidney, liver, muscle, and lung. Although clearance is dependent on urinary pH, renal function plays little role in clearance. Methadone has a long unpredictable half-life ranging from 8 to 80 hours, which can result in accumulation and toxicity in some individuals. Clearance of methadone is unaffected by renal or hepatic impairment. Metabolism is complex. It involves several enzymes within the cytochrome P-450 family that are subject to induction, suppression, and genetic variability. As a result, clearance can vary between individuals by up to 100-fold.[26]

Methadone is a potent mu agonist with some delta opioid receptor activity. Its analgesic effect is possibly increased by its ability to bind to *N*-methyl-D-aspartate (NMDA) receptors and inhibit presynaptic serotonin reuptake.[27] Methadone is an important alternative in patients with opioid-induced side effects or insufficient pain relief. It is recommended by many for neuropathic pain, although the evidence is largely anecdotal. Switching to methadone is more complex than switching to other opioids because of the unique titration schedule, uncertainty regarding equianalgesic doses, and great variations between patients in dose response. Guidelines for conversion to methadone have been published,[27] but published conversion ratios of morphine to methadone vary.[28] Some suggest a 3:1 (morphine to methadone) ratio, but there is evidence that the ratio is dependent on the opioid dose used previously and the type of pain syndrome treated (i.e., somatic or neuro-pathic pain). This ratio may range from 5:1 for morphine equivalent doses of greater than 100 to 300 mg/day to 20:1 for doses higher than 1000 mg/day.[29]

BUPRENORPHINE

Buprenorphine is a semisynthetic opioid derived from thebaine. Its structure is similar to that of the prototype opioid. The *t*-butyl side chain substitution contributes to its unique characteristics: high lipid and water solubility, high molecular weight, and high protein binding. Buprenorphine is a partial opioid agonist. Because of the development of a transdermal preparation, it has enjoyed a resurgence in popularity.

Buprenorphine is a potent partial mu opioid receptor agonist, kappa opioid receptor antagonist, and a weak delta opioid receptor agonist.[30,31] Oral absorption is low because of gut wall metabolism and the first-pass hepatic effect. Bioavailability by the buccal and sublingual route is much higher (30% to 60%). The drug is highly protein bound and extensively sequestered in the CNS and liver. Metabolism is dependent on both dealkylation (mediated predominantly by CYP3A4) and subsequent glucuronidation in the liver and gut wall to inactive metabolites.

Buprenorphine is excreted in urine (a third) and feces (two thirds). It is probably safe in renal failure but may have to be decreased in those with hepatic impairment.[32]

As a partial agonist, buprenorphine has a ceiling effect; that is, there is a dose-related increase in analgesic efficacy in the lower dose range, with higher doses producing no greater effect. The analgesic ceiling dose for sublingual buprenorphine (about 8 to 10 mg/24 hr) is high, however, equivalent to about 480 to 600 mg/24 hr of oral morphine[31] and outside commonly used analgesic doses. The high lipid solubility has allowed it to be formulated as both sublingual tablets and transdermal patch preparations. It is also available as an injection.

Like methadone, buprenorphine has a long duration of action. It is therefore logical to use in opioid dependence programs. Because of the avidity with which it binds to the receptor, its effects are difficult to reverse with short-acting antagonists. When compared with other opioids, the development of tolerance to or dependence on buprenorphine may be reduced, perhaps because it does not induce opioid receptor internalization.[33] It has side effects similar to those of other opioids. It causes more nausea and vomiting than morphine does, but most studies comment on the low incidence of constipation.[32]

Current Controversies and Future Considerations

- Should morphine remain the worldwide opioid of first choice?
- The challenge is to develop a test to define which opioid is most suitable for each individual.
- Are opioids effective in relieving neuropathic pain?
- Should low-dose "strong opioids" be step 2 of the WHO analgesic ladder instead of "weak opioids"?
- Is the WHO analgesic ladder outdated?
- Genetic "knockout" technology has helped our understanding of opioid receptors.

REFERENCES

1. Ferrante FM. Principles of opioid pharmacotherapy: Practical implications of basic mechanisms. J Pain Symptom Manage 1996;11:265-273.
2. Kieffer BL. Opioids: First lessons from knockout mice. Trends Pharmacol Sci 1999;20:19-26.
3. Davis M, Pasternak G. Opioid receptors and opioid pharmacodynamics. In Davis M, Glare P, Hardy J (eds). Opioids in Cancer Pain. Oxford, UK: Oxford University Press, 2005, pp 11-41.
4. Pan YX. Diversity and complexity of the mu opioid receptor gene: Alternative pre-mRNA splicing and promoters. DNA Cell Biol 2005;24:736-750.
5. Gomes I, Filipovska J, Jordan BA, Devi LA. Oligomerization of opioid receptors. Methods 2002;27:358-365.
6. Davis MP. Buprenorphine in cancer pain. Support Care Cancer 2005;13: 878-887.
7. Twycross RG. Oral morphine. In Twycross RG (ed). Pain Relief in Advanced Cancer. Edinburgh: Churchill Livingstone, 1994, pp 307-333.
8. Hanks GW, Conno F, Cherny N, et al. Morphine and alternative opioids in cancer pain: The EAPC recommendations. Br J Cancer 2001;84:587-593.
9. Cherny N, Ripamonti C, Pereira J, et al. Strategies to manage the adverse effects of oral morphine: An evidence-based report. J Clin Oncol 2001;19:2542-2554.
10. Mercadante S, Arcuri E. Opioids and renal function. J Pain 2004;5:2-19.
11. Bernard SA. The interaction of medications used in palliative care. Hematol Oncol Clin North Am 2002;16:641-655.
12. Lee CR, McTavish D, Sorkin EM. Tramadol. A preliminary review of its pharmacodynamic and pharmacokinetic properties, and therapeutic potential in acute and chronic pain states. Drugs 1993;46:313-340.
13. Raffa RB, Friderichs E, Reimann W, et al. Opioid and nonopioid components independently contribute to the mechanism of action of tramadol, an "atypical" opioid analgesic. J Pharmacol Exp Ther 1992;260:275-285.
14. Leppert W, Luczak J. The role of tramadol in cancer pain treatment—a review. Support Care Cancer 2005;13:5-17.
15. Gillen C, Haurand M, Kobelt D, et al. Affinity, potency and efficacy of tramadol and its metabolites at the cloned human mu-opioid receptor. Naunyn Schmiedebergs Arch Pharmacol 2000;362:116-121.
16. Poulsen L, Arendt-Nielsen L, Brosen K, Sindrup SH. The hypoalgesic effect of tramadol in relation to CYP2D6. Clin Pharmacol Ther 1996;60:636-644.
17. Nauck F, Ostgathe C, Klaschik E, et al. Drugs in palliative care: Results from a representative survey in Germany. Palliat Med 2004;18:100-107.
18. Houmes RJ, Voets MA, Verkaaik A, et al. Efficacy and safety of tramadol versus morphine for moderate and severe postoperative pain with special regard to respiratory depression. Anesth Analg 1992;74:510-514.
19. Shipton EA. Tramadol—present and future. Anaesth Intensive Care 2000; 28:363-374.
20. McQuay H, Moore A. An Evidence-Based Resource for Pain Relief. Oxford, UK: Oxford University Press, 1998.
21. Schug SA, Zech D, Grond S, et al. A long-term survey of morphine in cancer pain patients. J Pain Symptom Manage 1992;7:259-266.
22. Sarhill N, Walsh D, Nelson KA. Hydromorphone: Pharmacology and clinical applications in cancer patients. Support Care Cancer 2001;9:84-96.
23. Babul N, Darke AC. Putative role of hydromorphone metabolites in myoclonus. Pain 1992;51:260-261.
24. Quigley C. Hydromorphone for acute and chronic pain. Cochrane Database Syst Rev 2002;(1):CD003447.
25. Kaiko RF, Benziger DP, Fitzmartin RD, et al. Pharmacokinetic-pharmacodynamic relationships of controlled release of oxycodone. Clin Pharmacol Ther 1996;59:52-61.
26. Inturrisi CE, Portenoy RK, Max MB, et al. Pharmacokinetic-pharmacodynamic relationships of methadone infusions in patients with cancer pain. Clin Pharmacol Ther 1990;47:565-577.
27. Davis M. Methadone. In Davis M, Glare P, Hardy J (eds). Opioids in Cancer Pain. Oxford, UK: Oxford University Press, 2005, pp 247-265.
28. Ripamonti C, Groff L, Brunelli C, et al. Switching from morphine to oral methadone in treating cancer pain: What is the equianalgesic dose ratio? J Clin Oncol 1998;16:3216-3221.
29. Ayonrinde OT, Bridge DT. The rediscovery of methadone for cancer pain management. Med J Aust 2000;173:536-540.
30. Rothman R. Buprenorphine: A review of the binding literature. In Cowan A, Lewis J (eds). Buprenorphine: Combatting Drug Abuse with a Unique Opioid. New York: Wiley-Liss, 1995, pp 19-29.
31. Budd K. Buprenorphine: A review. In Evidence based medicine in practice. Newmarket, UK: Hayward Medical Communications, 2002, pp 1-24. (April 2002).
32. Davis M. Opioid equianalgesia: Dynamics and kinetics. In Davis M, Glare P, Hardy J (eds). Opioids in Cancer Pain. Oxford, UK: Oxford University Press, 2005, pp 247-265.
33. Robbie DS. A trial of sublingual buprenorphine in cancer pain. Br J Clin Pharmacol 1979;7(Suppl 3):315S-317S.

SUGGESTED READING

Davis M, Glare P, Hardy J (eds). Opioids in Cancer Pain. Oxford, UK: Oxford University Press, 2005.

Twycross RG (ed). Pain Relief in Advanced Cancer. Edinburgh: Churchill Livingstone, 1994.
Twycross R, Wilcock A, Charlesworth S, Dickman A. PCF2, Palliative Care Formulary, 2nd ed. Oxford: Radcliffe Medical Press, 2002.

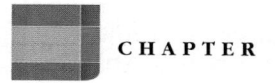

CHAPTER 139

Psychotropic Drugs

Luigi Grassi and Tiziana Antonelli

KEY POINTS

- Psychotropic drugs, such as neuroleptics and cannabinoids, have a role in palliative medicine.

- Antipsychotics, both conventional (e.g., butyrophenones and phenothiazines) and atypical (e.g., olanzapine and risperidone), can be used for the treatment of psychiatric disorders (e.g., delirium, psychotic episodes) or their symptoms (e.g., anxiety, agitation, insomnia).

- There is also evidence that antipsychotics can be used as adjuvant treatment for other symptoms (e.g., nausea, vomiting, pain) or clinical conditions (e.g., terminal restlessness).

- Attention to side effects and precautions (e.g., drug interactions, patient's clinical conditions) in the use of both antipsychotics and cannabinoids is mandatory in clinical practice.

Antipsychotics have evolved over the last 10 years, with new compounds being formulated that have fewer side effects and more specific action in disorders with psychotic symptoms, including hallucinations, thought disorders, and delusion. In palliative medicine, these disorders usually include delirium, brief psychotic reactions, psychotic depression, or psychotic disorders secondary to medical causes (e.g., brain tumors) or drugs (e.g., corticosteroids, chemotherapeutic agents). Antipsychotics include both first-generation and second-generation or atypical antipsychotics.[1-4] Both are also used for the adjuvant treatment of other symptoms such as nausea and vomiting[5] and pain resistant to conventional intervention.[6] The effectiveness of antipsychotics in palliative sedation and for severe, refractory physical symptoms in the terminally ill has been reported.[7-9]

Cannabinoids have recently come to attention for their possible use in several clinical settings, such as mood and anxiety disorders, movement disorders such as Parkinson's and Huntington's disease, neuropathic pain, multiple sclerosis and spinal cord injury, cancer, atherosclerosis, myocardial infarction, stroke, hypertension, glaucoma, obesity/metabolic syndrome, and osteoporosis.[10]

In this chapter we explore various antipsychotic agents used in palliative medicine, specifically, chlorpromazine, haloperidol, methotrimeprazine (now known as levomepromazine), and thioridazine among the conventional antipsychotics and olanzapine and risperidone among the atypical antipsychotics. We also examine the characteristics and the role of cannabinoids in palliative medicine.

CHLORPROMAZINE

Mechanism of Action

Chlorpromazine is an aliphatic phenothiazine. Its therapeutic action is related to blockade of the dopamine D_2 receptor in the brain mesolimbic dopamine pathway with a reduction in positive symptoms of psychosis (hallucinations and thought disorders). The antidopaminergic activity in the medullary chemoreceptor trigger zone areas is responsible for the antiemetic effects, whereas D_2 blockade in other regions of the brain causes the major side effects.

Chlorpromazine is readily absorbed from the gastrointestinal tract with variable bioavailability because of considerable liver first-pass metabolism. Food does not affect bioavailability consistently, but liquid concentrates may demonstrate greater bioavailability than tablets. Intramuscular (IM) administration (discouraged in palliative medicine) bypasses much of the first-pass effect, and thus higher plasma concentrations are achieved.

Chlorpromazine is highly bound to plasma proteins (>90%) and is distributed widely throughout the body; it crosses the blood-brain barrier and placenta and is distributed into milk. Its volume of distribution is about 20 L/kg. Chlorpromazine is metabolized in the liver by the cytochrome P-450 isoenzyme CYP2D6, with at least 12 different metabolites being generated; less than 1% is excreted unchanged. The terminal half-life is approximately 30 hours.

Dosage

The usual oral dose of chlorpromazine is 25 to 50 mg titrated to 75 to 150 mg in two to four divided doses. Its onset of action after oral administration is 30 to 60 minutes. Elderly and debilitated patients should start with doses at the low end of the dosage range (e.g., 25 mg daily).

The usual single parenteral dose is 25 to 50 mg/day, with elderly or debilitated patients requiring lower dosages. The IM route is used primarily when rapid action is required to control acute severe symptomatology. Chlorpromazine's onset of action after IM administration is 15 to 30 minutes. To minimize hypotension, the patient should remain recumbent for at least 30 minutes after injection.

Rectal dosing is 100 to 300 mg daily and usually takes longer to act than oral dosing.

Chlorpromazine is effective for psychotic disorders, nausea and vomiting, and delirium. A randomized controlled trial (RCT) showed efficacy (median IM dosage, 50 mg) for delirium in patients with acquired immunodeficiency syndrome (AIDS).[11]

Major Side Effects

Chlorpromazine's anti-D_2 action in the nigrostriatal pathway causes extrapyramidal reactions, including pseudoparkinsonism (e.g., motor retardation, rigidity, tremors, drooling, shuffling gait), dystonic reactions (e.g., periroral

spasms, trismus, tics, oculogyric crises, tongue protrusion, difficulty swallowing), and akathisia. Tardive dyskinesia, which may sometimes occur with long-term antipsychotic therapy, is not a major reported side effect in palliative medicine. The D_2 blockade in the mesocortical pathway can cause or worsen cognitive symptoms, and in the tuberoinfundibular pathway it increases prolactin secretion and gives rise to endocrine symptoms (gynecomastia, galactorrhea, libido disturbances).

The antihistaminergic property of chlorpromazine is related to its sedative action and other concomitant symptoms (e.g., weight gain and dizziness). Its anticholinergic properties cause several side effects, including dry mouth, blurred vision, constipation, urinary retention, and cardiovascular effects such as tachycardia. The peripheral α-adrenergic blocking activity of chlorpromazine may produce hypotension, tachycardia, fainting, and dizziness.

Chlorpromazine's direct negative inotropic and quinidine-like actions may cause prolongation of the electrocardiographic (ECG) PR and QT intervals, T-wave blunting, and ST-segment depression.

Chlorpromazine may also lower the convulsive threshold with the potential onset of seizures.

Other possible side effects include dermatological (e.g., itching, rash, erythema, photosensitivity), hematological (e.g., agranulocytosis—reported in 1 in 10,000 patients—leukopenia, granulocytopenia, eosinophilia, thrombocytopenia, anemia, aplastic anemia, pancytopenia), hepatic (e.g., cholestatic jaundice—uncommon, with an incidence of 0.1 to 4%—and related symptoms, including upper abdominal pain, nausea, fever, elevated liver enzymes, biliuria), and ophthalmological (e.g., skin-eye syndrome with progressive pigmentation of the skin or conjunctiva and discoloration of the exposed sclera and cornea).

A severe but rare complication is neuroleptic malignant syndrome (NMS), characterized by hyperpyrexia, muscle rigidity, altered mental status (including catatonic signs), autonomic instability (irregular pulse or unstable blood pressure), elevated creatine phosphokinase, myoglobinuria (rhabdomyolysis), and acute renal failure. NMS requires immediate drug discontinuation and intensive symptomatic and supportive treatment.

Contraindications

Chlorpromazine is contraindicated in comatose or depressed states secondary to central nervous system (CNS) depressants, as well as in patients with blood dyscrasias, myelosuppression, liver damage, epilepsy, or hypersensitivity to the drug. Cross-allergenicity with other phenothiazines has been reported. Chlorpromazine should be used with caution in patients with cardiovascular disorders, hypotension, impaired liver function, or a history of seizures. The risk of agranulocytosis suggests caution in the treatment of advanced medical illnesses.

Drug Interactions

The most important drug interactions include the following:

- *Anticonvulsants.* Because chlorpromazine may lower the seizure threshold, anticonvulsant therapy should be monitored closely, with adjustment of the dosage if necessary. Amphetamines may exacerbate psychotic symptoms.

- *Opioids.* Special attention is needed with administration of opioids for pain because the anticholinergic action of chlorpromazine may precipitate intestinal obstruction. Chlorpromazine may also increase the sedative effect of morphine.
- *Antihistaminics.* Concomitant administration of chlorpromazine with antihistaminics may cause additive effects on the QT interval and increase the propensity for ventricular arrhythmia.
- *Anticholinergics.* Anticholinergic agents may increase the risk for adynamic ileus (constipation, abdominal pain, and distention).
- *Tricyclic antidepressants* (TCAs). Alongside their anticholinergic properties, TCAs may increase the concentration and adverse effects of chlorpromazine.
- *CNS depressants.* Alcohol, antihistamines, general anesthetics, opiates or other narcotic analgesics, barbiturates, benzodiazepines, and other sedative/hypnotic agents may result in additive CNS depressant effects, with the risk of excessive sedation or respiratory depression.
- *Hypotensive drugs.* The combination of chlorpromazine and antihypertensive drugs may result in additive hypotensive effects and an increased risk for orthostatic hypotension or syncope.

METHOTRIMEPRAZINE (LEVOMEPROMAZINE)

Mechanism of Action

Like chlorpromazine, methotrimeprazine (also currently known as levomepromazine) is an aliphatic phenothiazine. Its antipsychotic properties, caused by anti-D_2 blockade in the brain, are less (50%) than those of chlorpromazine.

Methotrimeprazine is characterized by strong blockade of muscarinic, α_1-adrenergic, and serotonin 5-HT_{2A} receptors. Its antihistaminergic properties are moderate and its antidopaminergic (D_2 and D_3) properties weak. For these reasons it has strong sedative, tranquilizing, anxiolytic, and analgesic effects. IM levomepromazine can be used for acute pain, as a premedicant, and for postoperative analgesia.

Methotrimeprazine has incomplete oral bioavailability because it undergoes considerable first-pass liver metabolism. Its half-life is approximately 20 hours (15 to 30 hours). Maximum plasma levels occur 1 to 4 hours after oral dosing. After IM injection, maximum plasma levels are seen after 30 to 90 minutes. Its approximate distribution volume is 30 L/kg. Methotrimeprazine is lipophilic and easily crosses the blood-brain barrier and placenta, and it can also be found in breast milk. Its liquor concentration usually exceeds its plasma concentration. Methotrimeprazine is metabolized in the liver, and drug elimination is relatively slow.

Dosage

When used orally as a tranquilizer, anxiolytic, analgesic, or sedative, the starting dosage is 6 to 25 mg/day in three divided doses at mealtimes, with an increase in dosage until the optimum effect is achieved. As a sedative, a single night time dose of 10 to 25 mg is usually sufficient. In more severe conditions (e.g., psychotic disorders) or intense pain, the dosage is 50 to 75 mg/day divided into two or three daily doses, with increases until the desired effect is obtained.

Parenteral use (IM) is indicated for severe psychotic disorders or severe pain, as premedication, or for postoperative pain. Doses vary from 75 to 100 mg given as three or four deep IM injections in a large muscle. When administered as premedication or for postoperative analgesia, the average dose varies from 10 to 25 mg every 8 hours (equivalent to 20 to 40 mg orally). The last dose during premedication, given 1 hour before surgery, can be 25 to 50 mg IM.

Methotrimeprazine can be also given as an intravenous (IV) infusion during surgery at a dose of 10 to 25 mg in 500 mL of a 5% glucose solution administered at a rate of 20 to 40 drops per minute. Like chlorpromazine, it is used to treat psychotic symptoms in different clinical conditions, including organic psychosis.

In combination treatment as an adjuvant analgesic for severe or chronic pain (or both), initial doses of 30 to 75 mg daily are indicated, with slow increases to 100 to 300 mg daily. For nausea and vomiting, levomepromazine maleate may be given by mouth in a dose of 12.5 to 50 mg every 4 to 8 hours. It is also used for refractory emesis.[12] Advanced cancer patients given a minimum of 6.25 mg daily by mouth to a maximum of 25 mg via 24-hour subcutaneous infusion showed good response in ameliorating nausea and vomiting.[13] At a dosage of 25 mg/24 hr, subcutaneous levomepromazine rescue was reported to have significant effects on high-grade delayed chemotherapy-induced emesis.[14] Because of its sedative properties, levomepromazine is also used for insomnia. Doses of 25 to 50 mg 2 to 3 hours before bedtime are usual. Levomepromazine is used in palliative care for sedation, as are other phenothiazines.[15]

Major Side Effects

Side effects of methotrimeprazine resemble those of chlorpromazine, although it has half the potency and some side effects are less intense. Extrapyramidal effects are rare and usually occur only after prolonged high-dose therapy. Drowsiness is the most evident side effect early in treatment but gradually disappears during the first weeks or with adjustment in dosage. Its anticholinergic effects cause dryness of the mouth and possibly urinary retention, constipation, and tachycardia. Orthostatic hypotension may occur early when administered by the parenteral route or in high oral doses because of α_1-adrenergic blockade. Hematological (e.g., agranulocytosis), endocrine (e.g., weight gain), and gastrointestinal (e.g., cholestatic jaundice) side effects are uncommon.

Contraindications

Coma or CNS depression from alcohol, hypnotics, analgesics, or narcotics is a contraindication to the use of methotrimeprazine. It is also contraindicated in patients with blood dyscrasia, hepatic dysfunction, or sensitivity to phenothiazines. Like other phenothiazines, it can reduce the seizure threshold. Concomitant use of methotrimeprazine with opioids needs to be carefully monitored because it amplifies the therapeutic actions and side effects of opioids (the opioid dosage should be reduced by 50%). The combination of levomepromazine and tramadol should be avoided given the high risk for seizures. Likewise, combining levomepromazine with benzodiazepines or barbiturates may cause additive sedative effects and confusional states. Concomitant administration of ethanol and phenothiazines may result in additive CNS depression. TCAs and antiparkinsonian agents may increase the risk for anticholinergic activity with the possible onset of delirium, fever, and severe constipation. Caffeine, CNS stimulants, and antacids may counteract methotrimeprazine by decreasing drug absorption.

THIORIDAZINE

Mechanism of Action

Thioridazine is a piperidine phenothiazine antipsychotic like other phenothiazines and has anti-D_2 activity. Its potency is less than that of chlorpromazine. Thioridazine is rapidly and completely absorbed from the gastrointestinal tract. Maximum plasma concentrations are reached 2 to 4 hours later. Its average systemic bioavailability is 60%. Thioridazine is metabolized in the liver, with some metabolites (e.g., mesoridazine, sulforidazine) having pharmacodynamic properties similar to the parent compound. Excretion is mainly via feces (50%), but also via the kidney (<4% unchanged drug, about 30% as metabolites). Its plasma elimination half-life is between 7 and 13 hours. Thioridazine crosses the placenta and passes into breast milk.

Dosage

Thioridazine has a wide therapeutic margin. At low and medium doses it relieves tension and anxiety and is effective in treating multiple symptoms (e.g., agitation, sleep disturbance, hostility) of nonpsychotic mental disorders (25 to 50 mg). It is controversial whether antipsychotics should be used for anxiety disorders, unless resistant to other treatment, because of the lack of large, well-designed studies of antipsychotics for primary or co-morbid anxiety symptoms.[16] Daily dosages are usually given in two to four divided doses (e.g., 10 mg three times daily; 25 mg three times daily). At higher doses (100 to 600 mg), thioridazine controls symptoms of psychotic disorders, including agitation and agitated depression, hostility, and hallucinations. The maximum daily dose is 800 mg. Thioridazine has also been used for intractable pain. Its antiemetic effect is minor.

Major Side Effects

The major side effects of thioridazine are related to its anticholinergic properties. Caution is required in patients with narrow-angle glaucoma, prostatic hypertrophy, or cardiovascular disease. Prolongation of the QT interval (QTc) is more common (30 msec) than with all other antipsychotics, both conventional and atypical.[17] For these reasons and sudden unexplained death, apparently from arrhythmias or cardiac arrest, thioridazine has been with-

drawn from the market in several countries. Hypotension (usually orthostatic) may occur, especially in females, the elderly, and individuals who abuse alcohol. Given its low potency, extrapyramidal effects (including Parkinson-like symptoms), NMS, and endocrine symptoms (e.g., gynecomastia, galactorrhea) are less evident than with other antipsychotics. High doses should be avoided in those with a history of seizures. Leukopenia and agranulocytosis have been reported but are infrequent. Pigmentary retinopathy has been observed only after chronic high doses (>800 mg/day). In liver disease, regular monitoring of liver function is necessary because of possible jaundice and biliary stasis.

Contraindications

Contraindications to thioridazine include cardiovascular disease, a history of hypersensitivity to other phenothiazines, severe CNS depression, coma, bone marrow depression, and blood dyscrasia.

Drug Interactions

As other phenothiazines, thioridazine may reduce the effects of antiparkinson drugs. It may also lower the seizure threshold in epileptic patients, so adjustment of the dosage of anticonvulsant medications is necessary. Concurrent use with β-adrenergic blocking agents may increase the plasma concentration of phenothiazines. Antacids and antidiarrheal drugs may inhibit absorption of thioridazine and other phenothiazines. Thioridazine may also enhance the CNS depressant effects of alcohol, antihistamines, and other CNS depressants and the antimuscarinic effects of anticholinergic agents.

HALOPERIDOL

Mechanism of Action

Haloperidol is a conventional antipsychotic that belongs to the class of butyrophenones. It has strong anti-D_2 activity and is classified among the high-potency antipsychotics. Haloperidol is approximately 50 times more potent than chlorpromazine (haloperidol-chlorpromazine ratio, 1:50 mg), whereas its antihistaminic and anticholinergic properties are less.

Haloperidol has 60% bioavailability after oral administration. It is metabolized by liver oxidative dealkylation. Absorption via the oral route is slow, with plasma levels detectable after 60 to 90 minutes and peak levels not earlier than 4 hours. IM administration leads to peak plasma levels in 20 to 40 minutes, whereas IV injection results in peak levels in a few minutes.[2-20] When administered by slow IV infusion, its onset of action is slower but its duration is longer than after IV injection. Rectal and subcutaneous administration is also used, especially in palliative medicine. The half-life of haloperidol ranges from 12 to 36 hours. Plasma levels of 4 to 20 μg/L (up to 25 μg/L) are required for therapeutic action. Plasma levels over the therapeutic range may cause more side effects or risk haloperidol intoxication.

Dosage

Haloperidol is indicated for acute psychotic conditions, hyperactivity, and aggressive and agitated behavior, but its use in palliative care is not limited to psychosis.[18] It is the drug of choice for delirium by the American Psychiatric Association (APA)[19]; it was effective in an RCT of delirious AIDS patients.[11] Haloperidol has been also used in several trials as an antiemetic adjuvant[20] and via subcutaneous administration with tramadol for resistant pain.[21]

The dosage of haloperidol should be individualized by consideration of the severity of symptoms, age, weight, health, previous response to neuroleptics, and concomitant diseases. It is important to increase the dosage adequately until symptoms are controlled or side effects require lowering the dose or discontinuing use of the drug. When a satisfactory therapeutic response is achieved, the dosage should be gradually reduced to the lowest effective maintenance level.

For delirium, the APA guidelines suggest 1 to 2 mg for younger patients and 0.25 to 0.5 mg for elderly patients, repeated every 2 to 4 hours as needed for acute parenteral treatment. The usual doses, independent of route of administration, are 0.5 to 1 mg for mild, 2 to 5 mg for moderate, and 5 to 10 mg for severe delirium with agitation. The dose should be repeated at greater than 30-minute intervals until a clinical effect is achieved.

Haloperidol is given orally two times daily at 1 to 2 mg initially, followed by upward adjustment as tolerated until the desired effect is achieved or limiting side effects appear. It is seldom necessary to administer dosages greater than 4 to 6 mg three times daily. Thirty to 40 mg daily has been reported in severely disturbed patients or those resistant to usual doses. The safety of prolonged administration of high doses has not been established. After a therapeutic response, dosages should be gradually adjusted downward until a schedule providing adequate maintenance is reached. Maintenance dosages are commonly 1 to 2 mg three or four times daily.

In several conditions (e.g., delirium) or when symptoms are severe or rapid control is desired, IM administration of 2.5 to 5 mg may be used. Administration every 4 to 6 hours is sufficient in most, although the dosage may be repeated every hour for resistant patients if required.

Major Side Effects

Haloperidol causes extrapyramidal side effects secondary to its potent nigrostriatal D_2 blockade. The extrapyramidal reactions are usually dose related in occurrence and severity and tend to subside when the dose is reduced or use of the drug is temporarily discontinued. Tardive dyskinesia (rhythmic, involuntary movements of the tongue, face, mouth, or jaw; involuntary movements of the extremities) is not generally a problem in palliative care but can occur with long-term therapy (or after discontinuation).

Tachycardia, hypertension, and ECG changes, including prolongation of the QTc interval and changes in the ECG pattern (*torsades de pointes*), have been reported.

Endocrine side effects (e.g., gynecomastia, mastalgia) result from increased plasma prolactin. Anticholinergic side effects are rare given the low activity of haloperidol on muscarinic receptors. Hematological changes are infrequent, as are gastrointestinal effects. NMS has been reported. Moderate hypotension may occur with parenteral administration or excessive oral doses; however, vertigo and syncope are rare.

Haloperidol may lower the convulsive threshold and trigger seizures in previously controlled epileptic patients.

As with other antipsychotic agents, haloperidol should be administered cautiously to patients with severe impairment of liver or kidney function and to those with known allergies or a history of allergies to other neuroleptic drugs. Caution is also advised in pheochromocytoma and conditions predisposing to epilepsy, such as alcohol withdrawal and brain damage.

Contraindications

Haloperidol is contraindicated in patients with coma or severe intoxication from alcohol or other central depressant drugs and in those with known allergy to haloperidol, other butyrophenones, or other drug ingredients. It is contraindicated in patients with severe depression, previous spastic diseases, basal ganglia lesions, and Parkinson's syndrome (except dyskinesias secondary to levodopa), as well as in senile patients with preexisting Parkinson-like symptoms.

Drug Interactions

Haloperidol may interact with other central depressants (e.g., alcohol, opioids) and increase the side effects of these drugs (e.g., sedation, respiratory depression). Doses of concomitantly administered opioids for chronic pain can be reduced by 50%.

The therapeutic effects of levodopa may be reduced when coadministered with haloperidol, whereas use with methyldopa may increase the extrapyramidal side effects. Concomitant use with TCAs may reduce metabolism and elimination of the latter and result in increased toxicity (anticholinergic and cardiovascular side effects, lowering of the seizure threshold). Quinidine, buspirone, and fluoxetine increase plasma levels of haloperidol, whereas carbamazepine, phenobarbital, and rifampicin reduce them. Coadministration with lithium is contraindicated because of the possible onset of encephalopathy, early and late extrapyramidal side effects, other neurological symptoms, and coma. Haloperidol may also antagonize epinephrine and other sympathomimetic agents and reverse the blood pressure–lowering effects of adrenergic blocking agents such as guanethidine.

Care should be taken when using anticoagulants because of possible interference of haloperidol with these drugs.

OLANZAPINE

Mechanism of Action

Olanzapine is a thienobenzodiazepine classified among the atypical antipsychotics. Its clinical action links the selective antagonism to serotonin 5-HT_{2A} and dopamine D_1 to D_4 receptors. Its 5-HT_{2A}/D_2 antagonist properties specifically characterize olanzapine and other antipsychotics (e.g., risperidone—see later), which differentiates this class of drugs from conventional antipsychotics and defines them as atypical. This property gives rise to an antidopaminergic effect at the mesolimbic but not at the mesocortical, tuberoinfundibular, and nigrostriatal pathways. This produces a potent antipsychotic effect without significant side effects at the extrapyramidal, endocrine (e.g., increase in prolactin), and cognitive (e.g., confusion, increase in negative symptoms) levels. Antagonism at other receptors, such 5-HT$_3$, muscarinic, γ-aminobutyric acid (GABA), α_1- and β-adrenergic, and H$_1$, is weak.

Olanzapine is well absorbed and reaches peak concentrations about 6 hours after oral administration. It is eliminated by first-pass metabolism, with approximately 40% of the dose metabolized before reaching the systemic circulation. Food does not affect the rate or extent of absorption of olanzapine. Administration once daily produces steady-state concentrations in about 1 week that are approximately twice the concentration after single doses. Olanzapine is 93% bound to plasma proteins (albumin and α_1-acid glycoprotein). After IM administration, olanzapine is rapidly absorbed with peak plasma concentrations achieved within 15 to 45 minutes. Five milligrams of IM olanzapine produces a maximum plasma concentration five times higher than after oral administration of the same dosage. Olanzapine is metabolized via direct glucuronidation and cytochrome P-450 (CYP1A2 and CYP2D6)-mediated oxidation to inactive metabolites.

Dosage

Olanzapine is effective in psychotic disorders (schizophrenia, bipolar disorders in the manic phase, delirium). It is effective as a mood stabilizer. Olanzapine can be used for pain and for resistant nausea and vomiting in palliative care. One protocol consisting of 5 mg/day of oral olanzapine 2 days before chemotherapy, 10 mg the day of chemotherapy, day 1 (added to intravenous granisetron, 10 μg/kg, and dexamethasone, 20 mg), and 10 mg/day on days 2 to 4 after chemotherapy (added to dexamethasone, 8 mg orally twice daily on days 2 and 3 and 4 mg orally twice daily on day 4) gave a significant response in controlling nausea and vomiting.[22]

Olanzapine can be also administered as an IM injection for agitation in patients with acute psychotic disorders at a dose of 10 mg. Its efficacy is comparable to that of haloperidol, but with fewer extrapyramidal side effects.[23] The effect of enteral olanzapine and haloperidol is comparable in delirium, but again with fewer extrapyramidal side effects.[24] If agitation persists, a further dose of 10 mg can be administered. The safety of total daily doses greater than 30 mg or 10-mg injections given more frequently than 2 hours after the initial dose and 4 hours after the second dose has not been evaluated. IM dosages of 20 to 30 mg have been associated with orthostatic hypotension. The dosage should be lower in elderly or physically debilitated patients, even though specific data are not available.

Major Side Effects

Antagonism of muscarinic M$_1$ to M$_5$ receptors may explain its anticholinergic-like effects (e.g., dry mouth, constipation). These effects are less than those of conventional antipsychotics. Olanzapine's antagonism of histamine H$_1$ receptors is responsible for somnolence and sedation; its antagonism of α_1-adrenergic receptors may cause orthostatic hypotension. Extrapyramidal effects (especially akathisia) are rare and less potent than those encountered with conventional antipsychotics. Weight gain is significant, however. The Food and Drug Administration (FDA) now requires manufacturers of all atypical antipsychotics to include a warning about hyperglycemia and diabetes with atypical antipsychotics. There are case reports of olanzapine-induced diabetic ketoacidosis. Some studies suggest that olanzapine may decrease insulin sensitivity, increase triglyceride levels, and impair glucose metabolism. This metabolic syndrome may increase risk for cardiovascular disease.

Contraindications

Elderly patients with dementia-related psychosis treated with atypical antipsychotic drugs are at increased risk for death when compared with placebo. This finding instigated a further warning that olanzapine should be avoided in treatment of the elderly with dementia.

Drug Interaction

Interaction with other drugs has not been completely studied. Alcohol and any other centrally acting drugs should be avoided. Concomitant use of carbamazepine causes a 50% increase in clearance of olanzapine as a result of induction of CYP1A2 activity by carbamazepine. The possibility of hypotension calls for caution in the concomitant use of olanzapine and antihypertensive agents. Concurrent use of olanzapine may antagonize levodopa.

RISPERIDONE

Mechanism of Action

Risperidone is a benzisoxazole derivative and, like olanzapine, is an atypical antipsychotic. Similar to olanzapine, the mechanism of action is achieved through a combination of serotonin (5-HT$_2$) and dopamine (D$_2$) receptor antagonism. Risperidone also has low affinity for α_1- and α_2-adrenergic and histamine H$_1$ receptors and none for cholinergic, muscarinic, and β_1- and β_2-adrenergic receptors. It is well absorbed orally with a bioavailability of 70%. After oral administration, the mean peak concentration occurs in 1 hour. Risperidone is metabolized in the liver through hydroxylation (CYP2D6). Its main metabolite, 9-hydroxyrisperidone, achieves peak concentration in 3 hours. The mean half-life and that of its metabolite is about 20 hours. Risperidone and its metabolites are eliminated via urine and, to a lesser extent, via feces.

Dosage

Low doses (1 mg twice daily) should be used initially to avoid the typical first-dose effects of α-adrenoreceptor antagonists. Doses may be increased by 1 mg twice daily until a target dose of 6 mg/day (3 mg twice daily) is reached on day 3. Dosages higher than 6 mg are not usually more efficacious than lower doses, but the frequency of adverse effects increases. In elderly or debilitated patients, those with severe renal or hepatic impairment (limited ability to eliminate the drug), and those predisposed to hypotension, 0.5 mg twice daily is recommended to start, with a 0.5-mg increment twice daily until a dose of 3 mg/day (1.5 mg twice daily) is reached. Risperidone was effective for delirium in 91% of patients at a mean dose of 2.6 (±1.7 mg/day at day 3).[25] An RCT of delirious patients treated with haloperidol (starting dose, 0.5 mg twice daily) and risperidone (0.75 mg twice daily) showed that both were efficacious, with similar side effects.[26]

Major Side Effects

Risperidone may cause orthostatic hypotension with dizziness, tachycardia, and rarely syncope. Hyperglycemia, in some cases extreme and associated with ketoacidosis or hyperosmolar coma or death, also has been reported. Extrapyramidal symptoms are infrequent and in clinical trials found to be dose related (8 to 10 mg). Other side effects include nausea, anxiety, dizziness, insomnia, low blood pressure, weight gain, asthenia, and hyperpigmentation of skin.

Contraindications

Hypersensitivity to risperidone is a contraindication. Adverse cerebrovascular events (e.g., stroke, transient ischemic attack), including fatalities, are reported in elderly patients with dementia, which is the reason for a warning on the use of risperidone in this population (increased mortality in elderly patients with dementia-related psychosis). Risperidone is not approved for dementia-related psychosis.

Drug Interactions

Inhibitors of CYP2D6 interfere with conversion of risperidone to 9-hydroxyrisperidone. This occurs with quinidine, thus giving essentially all recipients a risperidone pharmacokinetic profile typical of poor metabolizers. Fluoxetine and paroxetine increase the plasma concentration of risperidone. Coadministration of carbamazepine and other known enzyme inducers (e.g., phenytoin, phenobarbital) may decrease the combined plasma concentrations of risperidone and 9-hydroxyrisperidone.

Combination with other centrally acting drugs and alcohol should be avoided. Risperidone may antagonize levodopa and dopamine agonists. Cimetidine and ranitidine increase the bioavailability of risperidone.

CANNABINOIDS
Mechanism of Action

The mechanism of action of cannabinoids is mainly related to two types of cell surface receptors in human tissue (CB1 and CB2). CB1 receptors are most abundant in mammalian brain but are also present at much lower concentration in various peripheral tissues and cells. A second cannabinoid receptor, CB2, is expressed primarily in cells of the immune and hematopoietic systems but was recently found to be present in brain, nonparenchymal cells of cirrhotic liver, endocrine pancreas, and bone. In addition to CB1 and CB2 receptors, pharmacological evidence supports the existence of one or more additional receptors for cannabinoids. Two of them have been explored: an endothelial site involved in vasodilation and endothelial cell migration.

Derivates of arachidonic acid, named anandamide and 2-arachidonoylglycerol, so-called endogenous cannabinoids, bind to the brain cannabinoid receptor with reasonably high affinity and mimic the behavioral actions of tetrahydrocannabinol (THC).

After oral administration, dronabinol is 90% to 95% absorbed; however, because of first-pass metabolism and high lipid solubility, only 10% to 20% of a dose reaches the systemic circulation. Bioavailability is slightly higher after inhalation, but with considerable interindividual variation. Peak plasma concentrations are reached a few minutes after intravenous or inhalational administration and 2 to 4 hours after oral administration. THC in plasma is bound to plasma lipoproteins (95% to 99%), less to albumin. As a lipophilic compound, THC is rapidly eliminated from plasma through distribution to highly vascularized tissue, and it crosses the blood-brain barrier. Subsequently, redistribution plus accumulation in body fat occurs. Peak effects are seen 15 to 60 minutes after the peak plasma concentration has been achieved; pharmacological effects do correlate with maximum plasma levels. The plasma half-life ranges between 28 and 57 hours because of interindividual differences in redistribution from fat tissue. Cannabinoids are metabolized by cytochrome P-450 subsystems in the liver, and metabolites are excreted in bile and urine over a period of several days with extensive enterohepatic recirculation.

Modulation of the activity of the endocannabinoid system holds therapeutic promise in many diseases and pathological conditions ranging from mood and anxiety disorders, Parkinson's and Huntington's disease, neuropathic pain, multiple sclerosis and spinal cord injury, cancer, myocardial infarction, stroke, hypertension, glaucoma, obesity/metabolic syndrome, and osteoporosis.[10,27] Use in oncology and palliative care has also been recommended in recent years,[28,29] although contradictory results and the frequency of side effects have called for caution.[30,31]

The effect of cannabinoids in palliative cancer patients has been established best for chemotherapy-induced nausea and vomiting. Capsules of Δ^9-tetrahydrocannabinol (dronabinol) and its synthetic analogue nabilone are approved for this purpose. Although the mechanism of its antiemetic action is unclear, an interaction with 5-HT$_3$ is suggested by the colocalization of CB1 and 5-HT$_3$ receptors on GABAergic neurons, where they have opposite effects on release of GABA.[32] Cannabinoids may directly inhibit 5-HT$_3$-gated ion currents by a mechanism not involving CB1 receptors.[33]

The discovery of endocannabinoids has raised the question of their potential involvement in the physiological control of appetite and energy metabolism. The first indication of a role for endocannabinoids in appetite control was the documented ability of low-dose anandamide to increase food intake when administered either systemically or into the ventromedial hypothalamus, and this effect could be due to stimulation of CB1 receptors. Sites of the orexigenic actions of endocannabinoids in both the hypothalamus and the limbic forebrain suggest their involvement in both the homeostatic and hedonic control of eating. The increased endocannabinoid activity may also contribute to obesity; its metabolic consequences were indicated by highly promising recent clinical trials with the selective CB1 receptor antagonist rimonabant.

A few studies have reported the effectiveness of THC in stimulating appetite and weight gain in cancer patients, but these effects have been more extensively documented in AIDS.[34,35] According to data from randomized trials, no significant benefit emerged from treatment with dronabinol for cancer-related anorexia-cachexia syndrome when compared with placebo or megestrol acetate.[36,37]

One of the earliest uses of cannabis was aimed at the treatment of pain. Studies have demonstrated beneficial effects of cannabinoids in animal models of pain.[38,39] In humans, the analgesic activity of THC and other cannabinoids is unclear. Randomized studies on the analgesic effect of orally administered synthetic cannabinoids in patients with postoperative, post-traumatic, cancer, or spastic pain had been reviewed in a meta-analysis.[31] Cannabinoids were not more effective than codeine in controlling pain. Modest, but clinically relevant analgesic effects have been reported in multiple sclerosis patients treated with dronabinol in a recent RCT.[40] Some studies suggest efficacy for neuropathic pain.[41] Studies regarding the effectiveness of THC or cannabis-based extracts on various forms of pain are in progress.[39]

Dosage

The starting dosage of cannabinoids for appetite stimulation is 2.5 mg orally twice daily before lunch and dinner. If adverse effects occur and do not resolve in 1 to 3 days with ongoing use, the dose may be reduced to 2.5 mg before dinner or at bedtime. If a further therapeutic effect is desired and adverse effects are absent, the dosage may be gradually increased to a maximum of 20 mg daily in divided doses. When used as an antiemetic, an initial dose of 5 mg/m^2 is administered up to 3 hours before chemotherapy and then every 2 to 4 hours after chemotherapy for a total of four to six doses per day. The dose can be titrated in increments of 2.5 mg/m^2 to a maximum of 15 mg/m^2 per dose. Side effects are more pronounced with 7 mg/m^2. Only dronabinol, not marijuana, has been approved by the Drug Enforcement Agency or the FDA for medical use.

Major Side Effects

The effects of cannabinoids are both physiological (tachycardia, hypotension, delayed gastric emptying, decreased muscle strength) and psychological (drowsiness, difficulty concentrating, and at higher doses, anxiety, delusions, and hallucinations). These symptoms are typically dose related, show considerable interpatient variability, and are more severe in the elderly. Tolerance to many of the effects of THC develops over the course of 10 to 12 days, but the orexigenic properties of the drug appear to be sustainable over study periods of up to 6 months.

Current Controversies and Future Considerations

- Randomized clinical trials of the atypical antipsychotics (e.g., olanzapine, risperidone, quetiapine, ziprasidone) for agitation and delirium are scarce in palliative medicine.
- Controversy exists about the use of cannabinoids for cancer-related anorexia-cachexia, pain, and stimulation of appetite and weight gain.

Contraindications

Dronabinol is contraindicated in patients hypersensitive to cannabinoids or sesame oil (component of the capsule).

Drug Interactions

Coadministration of ritonavir may significantly increase serum dronabinol concentrations and result in toxicity.

REFERENCES

1. Bruera E, Neumann CM. The uses of psychotropics in symptom management in advanced cancer. Psychooncology 1998;7:346-358.
2. Mazzocato C, Stiefel F, Buclin T, Berney A. Psychopharmacology in supportive care of cancer: A review for the clinician: II. Neuroleptics. Support Care Cancer 2000;8:89-97.
3. Boettger S, Breitbart W. Atypical antipsychotics in the management of delirium: A review of the empirical literature. Palliat Support Care 2005;3:227-237.
4. Lacasse H, Perreault MM, Williamson DR. Systematic review of antipsychotics for the treatment of hospital-associated delirium in medically or surgically ill patients. Ann Pharmacother 2006;40:1966-1973.
5. Skinner J, Skinner A. Levomepromazine for nausea and vomiting in advanced cancer. Hosp Med 1999;60:568-570.
6. Lussier D, Huskey AG, Portenoy RK. Adjuvant analgesics in cancer pain management. Oncologist 2004;9:571-591.
7. Kehl KA. Treatment of terminal restlessness: A review of the evidence. J Pain Palliat Care Pharmacother 2004;18:5-30.
8. Kohara H, Ueoka H, Takeyama H, et al. Sedation for terminally ill patients with cancer with uncontrollable physical distress. J Palliat Med 2005;8:20-25.
9. Cherny NI. Sedation for the care of patients with advanced cancer. Nat Clin Pract Oncol 2006;3:492-500.
10. Pacher P, Batkai S, Kunos G. The endocannabinoid system as an emerging target of pharmacotherapy. Pharmacol Rev 2006;58:389-462.
11. Breitbart W, Marotta R, Platt MM, et al. A double-blind trial of haloperidol, chlorpromazine, and lorazepam in the treatment of delirium in hospitalized AIDS patients. Am J Psychiatry 1996;153:231-237.
12. Kennett A, Hardy J, Shah S, A'Hern R. An open study of methotrimeprazine in the management of nausea and vomiting in patients with advanced cancer. Support Care Cancer 2005;13:715-721.
13. Eisenchlas JH, Garrigue N, Junin M, De Simone GG. Low-dose levomepromazine in refractory emesis in advanced cancer patients: An open-label study. Palliat Med 2005;19:71-75.
14. McCabe HL, Maraveyas A. Subcutaneous levomepromazine rescue (SLR) for high grade delayed chemotherapy-induced emesis (DCIE). Anticancer Res 2003;23:5209-5212.
15. Morita T, Bito S, Kurihara Y, Uchitomi Y. Development of a clinical guideline for palliative sedation therapy using the Delphi method. J Palliat Med 2005;8:716-729.
16. Gao K, Muzina D, Gajwani P, Calabrese JR. Efficacy of typical and atypical antipsychotics for primary and comorbid anxiety symptoms or disorders: A review. J Clin Psychiatry 2006;67:1327-1340.
17. Stollberger C, Huber JO, Finsterer J. Antipsychotic drugs and QT prolongation. Int Clin Psychopharmacol 2005;20:243-251.
18. Vella-Brincat J, Macleod AD. Haloperidol in palliative care. Palliat Med 2004;18:195-201.
19. American Psychiatric Association. Practice guideline for the treatment of patients with delirium. Am J Psychiatry 1999;156(5 Suppl):1-20.
20. Critchley P. Efficacy of haloperidol in the treatment of nausea and vomiting in the palliative patient: A systematic review. J Pain Symptom Manage 2001;22:631-634.
21. Negro S, Martin A, Azuara ML, et al. Stability of tramadol and haloperidol for continuous subcutaneous infusion at home. J Pain Symptom Manage 2005;30:192-199.
22. Navari RM, Einhorn LH, Passik SD, et al. A phase II trial of olanzapine for the prevention of chemotherapy-induced nausea and vomiting: A Hoosier Oncology Group study. Support Care Cancer 2005;13:529-534.

23. Wright P, Lindborg SR, Birkett M, et al. Intramuscular olanzapine and intramuscular haloperidol in acute schizophrenia: Antipsychotic efficacy and extrapyramidal safety during the first 24 hours of treatment. Can J Psychiatry 2003;48:716-721.

24. Skrobik YK, Bergeron N, Dumont M, Gottfried SB. Olanzapine vs haloperidol: Treating delirium in a critical care setting. Intensive Care Med 2004;30:444-449.

25. Parellada E, Baeza I, de Pablo J, Martinez G. Risperidone in the treatment of patients with delirium. J Clin Psychiatry 2004;65:348-353.

26. Han CS, Kim YK. A double-blind trial of risperidone and haloperidol for the treatment of delirium. Psychosomatics 2004;45:297-301.

27. Bagshaw SM, Hagen NA. Medical efficacy of cannabinoids and marijuana: A comprehensive review of the literature. J Palliat Care 2002;18:111-122.

28. Walsh D, Nelson KA, Mahmoud FA. Established and potential therapeutic applications of cannabinoids in oncology. Support Care Cancer 2003;11:137-143.

29. Hall W, Christie M, Currow D. Cannabinoids and cancer: Causation, remediation, and palliation. Lancet Oncol 2005;6:35-42.

30. Tramer MR, Carroll D, Campbell FA, et al. Cannabinoids for control of chemotherapy induced nausea and vomiting: Quantitative systematic review. BMJ 2001;323:16-21.

31. Campbell FA, Tramer D, Carroll D, et al. Are cannabinoids an effective and safe treatment option in the management of pain? A qualitative systematic review. BMJ 2001;323:13-16.

32. Morales M, Wang SD, Diaz-Ruiz O, Jho DH. Cannabinoid CB1 receptor and serotonin 3 receptor subunit A (5-HT3A) are co-expressed in GABA neurons in the rat telencephalon. J Comp Neurol 2004;468:205-216.

33. Barann M, Molderings G, Bruss M, et al. Direct inhibition by cannabinoids of human 5-HT3A receptors: Probable involvement of an allosteric modulatory site. Br J Pharmacol 2002;137:589-596.

34. Beal JE, Olson R, Laubenstein L, et al. Dronabinol as a treatment for anorexia with weight loss in patients with AIDS. J Pain Symptom Manage 1995;10:89-97.

35. Beal JE, Olson R, Lefkowitz L, et al. Long-term efficacy and safety of dronabinol for acquired immunodeficiency syndrome–associated anorexia. J Pain Symptom Manage 1997;14:7-14.

36. Jatoi A, Windschitl HE, Loprinzi CL, et al. Dronabinol versus megestrol acetate versus combination therapy for cancer-associated anorexia: A North Central Cancer Treatment Group study. J Clin Oncol 2002;20:567-573.

37. Cannabis-In-Cachexia-Study-Group, Strasser F, Luftner D, Possinger K, et al. Comparison of orally administered cannabis extract and delta-9-tetrahydrocannabinol in treating patients with cancer-related anorexia-cachexia syndrome: A multicenter, phase III, randomized, double-blind, placebo-controlled clinical trial from the Cannabis-In-Cachexia-Study-Group. J Clin Oncol 2006;24:3394-3400.

38. Huskey A. Cannabinoids in cancer pain management. J Pain Palliat Care Pharmacother 2006;20:43-46.

39. Ware M, Beaulieu P. Cannabinoids for the treatment of pain: An update on recent clinical trials. Pain Res Manage 2005;10(Suppl A):27A-30A.

40. Svendsen KB, Jensen TS, Bach FW. Does the cannabinoid dronabinol reduce central pain in multiple sclerosis? Randomised double blind placebo controlled crossover trial. BMJ 2004;329:253.

41. Gidal BE. New and emerging treatment options for neuropathic pain. Am J Manage Care 2006;12(9 Suppl):S269-S278.

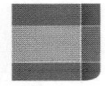

CHAPTER **140**

Laxatives

Paul J. Daeninck and **Garnet Crawford**

KEY POINTS

- Most people taking opioid analgesics will require laxatives.

- Laxatives function in different ways and are available in several formats.

- There is little evidence to support the choice of one laxative over another.

- Prevention is the preferred treatment of constipation.

- New laxatives show promise in clinical trials.

Constipation is, at best, unpleasant and inconvenient. At worst, it can be a source of suffering in and of itself and cause or exacerbate nausea, pain, delirium, dyspnea, and other symptoms. Laxatives stimulate evacuation of the bowels, and because prevention and treatment of constipation should always be primary goals, knowledge of rational laxative use is essential. Although opioids account for most constipation in palliative patients, it cannot be assumed that they are always the sole causative factor (see Chapter 154).

Normal bowel function requires coordination of gut motility, molecular transport across the bowel wall, and reflexes of defecation. Motility is mediated by the autonomic nervous system, the intrinsic nervous plexuses of the gastrointestinal tract, and hormones active in the gut. Adrenergic, muscarinic, dopaminergic, and opioid receptors all modify gut motility and transit time. Fluid and electrolyte transport across mucosal surfaces is a complex phenomenon. Opioids prolong intestinal transit time in both the small and large intestine. Prolonged bowel transit increases fluid absorption. Opioids increase anal sphincter tone and reduce awareness of rectal filling. Because both fluid absorption and prolonged transit are characteristic of constipation, therapies usually combine laxatives promoting hydration of bowel contents with those that stimulate bowel transit. Simple lifestyle measures such as diet, exercise, and hydration are also important in the prevention and treatment of constipation, although such measures become more difficult as disease progresses.

Opioids are commonly used in advanced disease and cause constipation in the majority.[1] One does not normally develop tolerance, which means that all those commencing an opioid should, unless there is a contraindication, receive a concurrent prophylactic bowel regimen. As-needed (PRN) laxatives have little place in prophylaxis. They only cause oscillation between bowel movements that are alternately hard and infrequent or loose and diarrhea-like. Neither is pleasant, and the frustration that they engender contributes to noncompliance with both analgesics and laxatives. Dosing of laxatives should be on a regular schedule and titrated according to response rather than by the opioid dose (the constipating effects of opioids are not necessarily dose dependent). Given normal bowel function despite opioids (rare), laxatives can be decreased to PRN use or discontinued. Vigilance is demanded.

Laxatives can be classified as those that soften the stool and those that stimulate intestinal motility. We have further categorized laxatives as bulk-forming agents, surfactants, stimulant laxatives, lubricants, and osmotic agents (Table 140-1). Opioid receptor antagonists specifically for use in opioid-induced bowel dysfunction (OBD) are under investigation.[2]

Bulk-forming agents work with the natural processes of the bowels to retain fluid, soften stool, and increase size, thereby enhancing gastrointestinal motility and ease of passage. Sufficient fluid intake (200 to 300 mL plus a further liter of fluid daily) is necessary concurrent with their use. They are often unsuitable for debilitated persons and usually worsen OBD. Bulk or fiber laxatives should be avoided in patients with suspected bowel obstruction.[3]

Surfactants promote fecal water retention by detergent activity. Docusate also promotes secretion of water, sodium, and chloride in the jejunum and colon.[3] Generally

TABLE 140-1　Laxative Agents for Treatment of Constipation

TYPE	ONSET OF ACTION (HR)	SIDE EFFECTS	MECHANISM OF ACTION AND COMMENTS
BULK-FORMING AGENTS			
Bran	12-24	Bloating, flatulence	Increases stool bulk, decreases transit time, increases GI motility; requires good fluid intake
Psyllium			
Methylcellulose			
Polycarbophil			
SURFACTANTS			
Docusate	12-72	Well tolerated	Detergent activity; avoid mineral oil concurrently
STIMULANTS			
Anthraquinones (senna, cascara, danthron)	6-12	Dependence with prolonged use; may cause cramping or electrolyte disturbances	Myenteric plexus stimulation increases motility; decreases absorption of fluid and electrolytes
Polyphenolics (bisacodyl, sodium phosphate)			
OSMOTIC LAXATIVES			
Lactulose/sorbitol	24-48	Very sweet; abdominal cramps and flatulence	Nonabsorbable molecules draw fluid into intestinal lumen
Mannitol	24-48		
Polyethylene glycol	0.5-1	Large volume to swallow	As for lactulose/sorbitol
LUBRICANTS			
Mineral oil	6-8	Malabsorption of fat-soluble vitamins; risk of lipid pneumonia	Lubricates and softens stool
Liquid paraffin			
SALINE LAXATIVES			
Magnesium (citrate, hydroxide, sulfate)	1-3	Electrolyte disturbances; avoid in renal insufficiency	Osmotically active particles draw fluid into colonic lumen
SUPPOSITORIES			
Glycerin	0.25-1	Rectal irritation	Induces defecation by distention of rectum. See above
Bisacodyl			
ENEMAS			
Saline	5-15 min	Rectal irritation	Large volume—useful in impaction
Phosphate	5-15 min	Hypocalcaemia	Softens impacted stool
Oil retention	6-8 min		
PROKINETIC AGENTS			
Domperidone	30-60 min	Extrapyramidal effects	Dopamine (D_2) antagonist
Metoclopramide		Confusion, extrapyramidal effects	D_2 antagonist and cholinergic agonist
OPIOID ANTAGONISTS			
Naloxone	1-3	Opioid withdrawal and loss of pain control	Orally administered. Limited use
Naltrexone			Competitive central and peripheral opioid receptor antagonists
Methylnaltrexone			
Alvimopan (ADL 8-2698)	Dose dependent	Abdominal cramping, flatulence	Acts peripherally only; not yet commercially available

well tolerated, they are ineffective if hydration is poor. Surfactants are rarely used alone, with a common regimen being a stool softener (docusate sodium or docusate calcium) combined with a stimulant laxative (e.g., senna or bisacodyl), especially when starting an opioid.

Stimulant laxatives are probably the most prescribed laxatives in North American palliative care units. They produce peristalsis by directly stimulating the intestinal myenteric plexus, thus making them a reasonable first choice for OBD. They reduce colonic electrolyte and water absorption, mainly through inhibition of Na$^+$,K$^+$-ATPase.[3] Because their onset of action is between 6 and 12 hours, bedtime dosing is logical. However, divided dosing (twice daily) may reduce abdominal cramping.

Lubricants such as paraffin or mineral oil coat the intestinal mucosa and stool surfaces and thereby reduce friction, soften the stool, and ease passage through the bowel lumen. Prolonged administration may interfere with the absorption of fat-soluble vitamins (A, D, E, K) and result in nutritional deficiency, unpleasant fecal leakage, or dangerous lung aspiration and lipid pneumonitis. Routine use of lubricant laxatives is not recommended. Some consider use of a combination of magnesium hydroxide with 25% mineral oil effective, and adverse effects are said to be minimal.[4]

The osmotically active molecules of saline laxatives such as magnesium hydroxide (milk of magnesia) or sodium phosphate (Fleet Phospho-Soda) draw water into the bowel lumen, which alters stool consistency and size and promotes reflex peristalsis by gut distention. They differ from other osmotic agents in that they are capable of systemic absorption across the bowel mucosa and can complicate preexisting conditions such as congestive heart failure, hypertension, and renal failure. Lactulose, sorbitol, mannitol, and polyethylene glycol (PEG or GoLYTELY) are indigestible synthetic molecules that work similar to the saline laxatives. Their onset of action is more delayed; patients generally do not like their sweet taste (i.e., lactulose, sorbitol) or large volumes (PEG). However, they are effective and often used as second-line agents after inadequate responses to the combination of a stimulant and softener. It is wise to increase fluid intake with any osmotic laxative. PEG-based laxatives (e.g., macrogol) have been proposed in Europe as first-line therapy for functional constipation and fecal impaction[5] and may provide long-term benefit in such patients.[6]

Rectal laxatives can be administered as either suppositories or enemas and generally work similar to the orally administered forms. They are readily accepted in Europe, but many patients in North America resist their use. The short time needed to achieve an effect makes them attractive for some patients (and staff), who may come to depend on them for relief. Suppositories are often necessary when oral laxatives cannot be used (inability to swallow or nausea and vomiting preventing oral administration) and may help stimulate anocolonic defecation reflexes. This may prevent the need for undignified and unpleasant manual disimpaction. Suppositories combining glycerin (soften and lubricate) and bisacodyl (stimulate colonic peristalsis) are often effective for hard stool low in the rectum. Bisacodyl suppositories act quickly (15 to 60 minutes versus an oral time of 6 to 12 hours) if in contact with the rectal wall because the drug will be rapidly converted to its active desacetyl form by rectal flora. Sodium phosphate is available as a rectal suppository (Carbalax), but its effectiveness is unclear.

Enemas are administered when oral laxatives and rectal suppositories are ineffective. They are unpleasant for both the patient and staff but can be administered safely in the hospital or long-term care or home setting. Commonly used enemas include the following:

- *Fleet enema*: Consisting of 150 mL sodium phosphate, Fleet enema presumably acts by releasing bound water from feces and stimulating colonic peristalsis by providing additional volume to stimulate a rectal-colic reflex. It is safe in short, intermittent courses. Prolonged use can result in hypocalcemia, hyperphosphatemia, and rectal irritation, particularly in those with hemorrhoids.
- *Saline enema*: This term is often applied to the somewhat cumbersome use of high volumes of warm saline. It may have a role in impaction if there is a long column of backed-up stool. It is safe but awkward because of placement of the enema tubing.
- *Tap water and soapsuds enema*: This enema is not recommended because of the associated risk of changes in blood volume and electrolytes. Soap is irritating to the colonic mucosa and may worsen the patient's condition rather than improve it.
- *Oil enemas (arachis oil, olive oil, mineral oil)*: Oil enemas are most commonly used as high enemas given overnight to be retained in the colon for softening and lubricating hard packed stool resistant to passage with less invasive means. Use depends on the patient's ability to retain the fluid for a prolonged period. To facilitate retention, the enema can be administered high in the descending colon with a Foley catheter and the balloon inflated for 10 to 15 minutes to minimize initial return. An oil retention enema can help patients with a large quantity of stool in the sigmoid colon and rectum, either before fecal disimpaction or immediately after, to assist in further removal of stool caught higher up in the sigmoid colon. A version of this enema, commonly known as a "POW enema," uses a mixture of equal amounts (150 mL) of hydrogen *p*eroxide, *o*il, and *w*ater. Although peroxide enemas have fallen into disuse because of potential mucosal injury, dilution with mineral oil and water creates a well-tolerated preparation that can be effective when other enemas fail.

Prevention of constipation is preferable to suffering with hard stools or infrequent bowel movements. Prokinetic agents increase peristaltic movement through the stomach and proximal small bowel, thereby reducing transit times. These effects are mediated through cholinergic activity of the bowel wall and blocked by anticholinergic drugs. Metoclopramide and domperidone are the two most commonly used agents, and they also relieve nausea (see Chapter 169) because of their dopamine receptor (D_2) antagonist activity. It is useful to combine these agents with laxatives active on the large bowel to achieve benefits throughout the entire gut. Caution should be used in prescribing them to persons with movement disorders (Parkinson's disease most commonly) or those sensitive to dopaminergic medications (extrapyramidal side effects). Domperidone acts peripherally on gut receptors and does not cross the blood-brain barrier, thus having an added level of safety, but it is not generally as effective as metoclopramide. Long-term domperidone use is associated with breast enlargement and hyperprolactinemia. Oral erythromycin has also been associated with diarrhea in up to 50% of users. It appears to exert a prokinetic effect by an interaction with motilin receptors in both the small and large bowel. Effectiveness may only last a few weeks, and it may also disrupt the balance of the gut flora, thus making it somewhat impractical.[3]

How does one use laxatives for constipation in a palliative patient? A guideline for laxative use based on evidence from randomized controlled trials would be desirable, but there have been few clinical trials. Three randomized controlled trials in palliative patients have been published since 1990,[7-9] and only one showed a difference in effectiveness.[9] Two other trials were carried

Current Controversies and Future Directions

Opioid receptor antagonists, which can quickly reverse potentially life-threatening opioid overdose, are now being studied for their role in OBD.[15] Opioid receptors exist peripherally and in the central nervous system; however, opioid action on the bowels is mediated primarily by receptors located in the gastrointestinal tract. Nonselective opioid antagonists (such as naloxone) have been used both parenterally and orally to treat constipation,[16] but there is risk of precipitating opioid withdrawal or a pain crisis, especially with parenteral use (oral naloxone has 3% systemic bioavailability and also carries the risk of withdrawal or pain, though less so).[16] Suggested dosages for oral naloxone start as low as 0.8 mg twice daily titrated up to 12 mg/day.[15] Methylnaltrexone, a quaternary derivative of naltrexone, is a peripherally acting opioid receptor antagonist under investigation for opioid-induced constipation.[2,17] It offers the advantage of targeted action on gut opioid receptors, thereby maintaining analgesia.[8] Currently, methylnaltrexone, which has received approval by health authorities in Canada, is undergoing phase III trials in North America and the preliminary results are promising. Common side effects include abdominal cramping, flatulence, nausea, and dizziness, whereas serious adverse events are equivalent to those with placebo.[18] A similar compound, alvimopan, is also in clinical trials, not only in OBD but also in postoperative patients treated with opioids.[2,19]

out in nonpalliative populations: one at a methadone maintenance program[10] and the other in healthy individuals as a model for opioid-induced constipation.[11] Little extrapolation from either study can be made to palliative patients. There have been reviews of specific drugs,[12,13] but no definitive statement about their place in constipation in palliative patients. Various algorithms have been published,[5,6] but none are based on systematic review. A Cochrane review is in process but has yet to offer a guideline because of lack of adequate trial material.[14]

A reasonable approach to laxatives would start with ruling out complete bowel obstruction, ideally with diagnostic imaging such as a simple abdominal radiograph. If any doubt about obstruction exists, only softening agents should be considered to prevent worsening of colicky pain. Hard, impacted feces will require softening with glycerin suppositories or oil enemas before expulsion. Manual disimpaction may be necessary; premedication with analgesics or sedation (or both) should be considered. A bowel full of soft feces may require treatment from above (oral stimulating laxative such as senna) and suppositories or mini-enemas. An empty rectum but full bowel may not respond to rectal laxatives and should be treated with oral preparations, including softening agents, given that the feces are probably hard and difficult to pass. Ongoing treatment to prevent further constipation would involve the use of a softener and a stimulant agent (senna and docusate, as stated earlier) or an osmotic laxative

(e.g., lactulose) with a prokinetic agent such as metoclopramide.

Maintenance of bowel function is commonly delegated by physicians to other members of the health care team despite the overwhelming prevalence of constipation in the palliative population and its significant morbidity. The clinician has many remedies to combat this often simple but unpleasant malady. Familiarity with the humble laxative is basic knowledge for any physician and most assuredly so for those caring for individuals at the end of life.

REFERENCES

1. Twycross RG, Harcourt JM. The use of laxatives at a palliative care centre. Palliat Med 1991;5:27-33.
2. Kurz A, Sessler DI. Opioid-induced bowel dysfunction. Pathophysiology and potential new therapies. Drugs 2003;63:649-671.
3. Sykes NP. Constipation and diarrhoea. In Doyle D, Hanks GWC, Cherny N, Calman K (eds). Oxford Textbook of Palliative Medicine, 3rd ed. Oxford: Oxford University Press, 2004, pp 483-496.
4. Bateman DM, Smith JM. A policy for laxatives. BMJ 1988;297:1420-1421.
5. Klaschik E, Nauck F, Ostgathe C. Constipation—modern laxative therapy. Support Care Cancer 2003;11:679-685.
6. Kamm MA. Constipation and its management. BMJ 2003;327:459-460.
7. Sykes NP. A clinical comparison of laxatives in a hospice. Palliat Med 1991;5:307-334.
8. Agra Y, Sacristan A, Gonzalez M, et al. Efficacy of senna versus lactulose in terminal cancer patients treated with opioids. J Pain Symptom Manage 1998;15:1-7.
9. Ramesh PR, Suresh Kumar K, Rajagopal MR, et al. Managing morphine-induced constipation: A controlled comparison of an Ayurvedic formulation and senna. J Pain Symptom Manage 1998;16:240-244.
10. Freedman MD, Schwartz HJ, Roby R, Fleisher S. Tolerance and efficacy of polyethylene glycol 3350/electrolyte solution versus lactulose in relieving opioid induced constipation: A double-blinded placebo-controlled trial. J Clin Pharmacol 1997;37:904-907.
11. Sykes NP. A volunteer model for the comparison of laxative in opioid-induced constipation. J Pain Symptom Manage 1997;11:363-369.
12. Hurdon V, Viola R, Schroder C. How useful is docusate in patients at risk for constipation? A systematic review of the evidence in the chronically ill. J Pain Symptom Manage 2000;19:130-136.
13. Foss JF. A review of the potential role of methylnaltrexone in opioid bowel dysfunction. Am J Surg 2001;182(Suppl 5A):19S-26S.
14. Miles CL, Fellowes D, Goodman ML, Wilkinson S. Laxatives for the management of constipation in palliative care patients. Cochrane Database Syst Rev 2006;(4):CD003448.
15. Choi YS, Billings JA. Opioid antagonists: A review of their role in palliative care, focusing on use in opioid-related constipation. J Pain Symptom Manage 2002;24;71-90.
16. Liu M, Wittbrodt E. Low-dose oral naloxone reverses opioid-induced constipation and analgesia. J Pain Symptom Manage 2002;23;48-53.
17. Yuan CS, Foss JF. Oral methylnaltrexone for opioid-induced constipation. JAMA 2000;284:1383-1384.
18. Thomas J, Lipman A, Slatkin N, et al. A phase III double-blind placebo-controlled trial of methylnaltrexone (MNTX) for opioid-induced constipation (OIC) in advanced medical illness (AMI) [abstract]. J Clin Oncol 2005; 23(Suppl):729s.
19. Taguchi A, Sharma N, Saleem RM, et al. Selective postoperative inhibitors of gastrointestinal opioid receptors. N Engl J Med 2001;345:935-940.

SUGGESTED READING

Sykes NP. Constipation and diarrhoea. In Doyle D, Hanks GWC, Cherny N, Calman K (eds). Oxford Textbook of Palliative Medicine, 3rd ed. Oxford: Oxford University Press, 2004, pp 483-496.
Yuan CS (ed). Handbook of Opioid Bowel Dysfunction. New York: Haworth, 2005.

CHAPTER **141**

Cardiac Drugs

Simon Noble and Claire Turner

GLYCERYL TRINITRATE

Glyceryl trinitrate is most commonly used for the prophylaxis and treatment of angina. It acts by smooth muscle relaxation, not only in blood vessels but also in the gastrointestinal tract, and it therefore has a role in pain secondary to smooth muscle spasm. Topically, it provides effective treatment of anal fissures, with rapid and sustained relief of pain and improving healing.[1] Nitrates provide relief from painful esophageal spasm, and glyceryl trinitrate is effective in motor dysphagia and odynophagia caused by esophagitis and esophageal spasm in advanced cancer. In such cases a trial of sublingual glyceryl trinitrate is recommended once standard measures have failed.[2,3] Glyceryl trinitrate may provide symptomatic control in biliary colic.[4] Transdermal glyceryl trinitrate prolongs the life of intravenous infusions, and it has been suggested that it could aid absorption of continuous subcutaneous infusions.[5,6]

Mechanism of Action

Glyceryl trinitrate is metabolized to nitric oxide, which stimulates guanylate cyclase. This increases guanosine monophosphate, which in turn reduces the amount of intracellular calcium available for muscle contraction. Nitric oxide relaxes all smooth muscle, including vascular, bronchial, and gastrointestinal. It seems to have a significant role in regulating distal esophageal peristalsis and relaxation of the lower esophageal sphincter.

Dosages

- Angina pectoris: 0.3 to 1 mg sublingually, repeated as required
- Anal fissure pain: 0.2% ointment applied twice daily for at least 6 weeks
- Dysphagia/odynophagia/biliary colic: 500 µg to 1 mg sublingually as needed for transient intermittent colic
- Persistent spasm: consider glyceryl trinitrate skin patches, 5 mg/24 hr, 10 mg/24 hr
- Prolonging intravenous/subcutaneous infusions: application of one 5–mg/24 hr patch daily over the infusion site

Major Side Effects

- Hypotension, facial flushing, dizziness, tachycardia, and headache

Contraindications

- Hypotension, aortic or mitral stenosis, cardiac tamponade, constrictive pericarditis, obstructive cardiomyopathy, closed-angle glaucoma, marked anemia

Drug Interactions

- Increases the hypotensive effects of other drugs
- Drugs causing dry mouth may reduce the effect of sublingual nitrates

Research Challenges

Little evidence is based on robust clinical research, and even less is available for the palliative patient population.

Evidence-Based Medicine

The evidence for using glyceryl trinitrate in patients with anal fissures is based on a double-blind, randomized, placebo-controlled trial.[1] Its use in biliary colic and in odynophagia and dysphagia is based on a few case reports.[2,4] The suggestion that transdermal glyceryl trinitrate can aid absorption of continuous subcutaneous infusions is based on its ability to prolong the life of intravenous infusions.[5,6]

DOPAMINE

Dopamine hydrochloride is a naturally occurring catecholamine that is more commonly used in the intensive care than the palliative care setting. An increasing proportion of patients receiving palliative care have nonmalignant disease, and there is a growing body of evidence that supports the use of dopamine in patients with end-stage heart failure.

Mechanism of Action

Dopamine is a sympathomimetic amine and the immediate precursor of norepinephrine. It has a combination of actions that make it useful for congestive heart failure. At very low doses, it dilates renal and mesenteric blood vessels through stimulation of specific dopaminergic receptors, which improves renal and mesenteric blood flow and sodium excretion. At higher doses, dopamine stimulates myocardial β-adrenergic receptors but induces relatively little tachycardia, whereas at still higher doses it also stimulates α-adrenergic receptors and elevates arterial pressure.

Initial research had suggested little place for dopamine in chronic cardiac disease.[7] However, several studies now suggest that parenteral dopamine given intermittently or continuously may help carefully selected patients with severe symptomatic and advanced heart failure.[8] In addition to improving heart failure symptoms, intermittent or pulsed dopamine infusions have reduced hospital admissions and emergency room visits and resulted in significant improvement on 6-minute walk test scores when compared with placebo.[9] It is possible for suitable palliative care units to give pulsed dopamine to patients with end-stage heart failure to facilitate better utilization of hospice and palliative care resources.[10]

Dosages

- Low dose (renal dose): intravenous infusion at 1 to 2 μg/kg/min
- Higher dose (cardiac inotropic dose): infusion at 2 to 5 μg/kg/min according to response

Major Side Effects

- Palpitations, tachycardia, peripheral ischemia, hypotension, hypertension, dyspnea, nausea, and headaches

Contraindications

- Tachyarrhythmia, pheochromocytoma
- Use with caution in patients with hypovolemia, acidosis, peripheral vascular disease, hypokalemia

Drug Interactions

- Monoamine oxidase inhibitors increase the effects of dopamine. Dopamine may interact with phenytoin and cause hypotension.
- The cardiac effects of dopamine are enhanced by β-blockers.

Research Challenges

Current research on inotropes in palliative care is derived from a single source. This work needs to be repeated in the broader palliative care setting with robust health and economic evaluation of its practicability in end-stage cardiac disease.

MEXILETINE

Mexiletine is a class 1B antiarrhythmic most commonly used for cardiac arrhythmias. In palliative care it is used as an adjuvant neuropathic agent and has an effect similar to that of lidocaine. Mexiletine is usually indicated only when other neuropathic agents have failed. It is often poorly tolerated because of side effects and should only be used only under specialist supervision. In particular, there is a risk for cardiac arrhythmias, so the benefit of treatment versus risk needs to be carefully evaluated. The rationale for using mexiletine over lidocaine is that it can be administered orally. A test dose of intravenous lidocaine may predict whether mexiletine will be of benefit.[11] Mexiletine is most effective for pain described as "stabbing" or "burning" or for painful sensations of heat.

Mechanism of Action

Mexiletine is a nerve membrane stabilizer. By inhibiting sodium channels it decreases excitability and slows nerve membrane conduction velocity. Mexiletine is metabolized in the liver, and significant interindividual differences in metabolism have been reported with different cytochrome P-450 CYP2D6 isoenzymes.[12]

Dosages

- A dose of 250 to 625 mg/day reduces neuropathic pain; start with 50 mg three times daily and increase by 50 mg three times daily every 3 to 7 days to a maximum of 10 mg/kg/day.
- An electrocardiogram should be obtained before and during titration.
- Tricyclic antidepressants should be stopped at least 48 hours before commencing mexiletine.

Major Side Effects

Nausea, vomiting, and constipation are most common. Others side effects include bradycardia, hypertension, cardiac arrhythmias, pulmonary infiltrates, drowsiness, tremor, confusion, convulsions, psychiatric disorders, dysarthria, ataxia, paresthesia, nystagmus, jaundice, hepatitis, and blood disorders.

Contraindications

Heart disease requiring medication and an abnormal electrocardiogram are contraindications to the use of mexiletine.

Drug Interactions

Opioids and antimuscarinics delay absorption of mexiletine. There is a risk of myocardial depression if mexiletine is used with other antiarrhythmics and a risk of arrhythmia if used with proarrhythmic drugs (e.g., tricyclic antidepressants). Mexiletine's effect is reduced by drugs causing hypokalemia (e.g., diuretics). Its plasma concentration is increased by amitriptyline but decreased by phenytoin and rifampicin.

Research Challenges

Further evaluation of mexiletine in advanced cancer pain is needed. Presently, it is used for neuropathic pain resistant to standard agents. Future research may compare its efficacy with that of other membrane stabilizers to decide whether it should be used earlier for neuropathic pain. Further research on its safety in advanced cancer is also required.

Evidence-Based Medicine

There is good evidence for use of mexiletine as a neuropathic agent in patients with diabetic neuropathy, peripheral nerve injury, and chronic pain.[13]

Two thirds of cancer patients with neuropathic pain will benefit, although no controlled trials have been conducted. Mexiletine has occasionally been used for pain caused by spinal cord injury and for central pain after stroke, although its benefit is unproven.

LIDOCAINE

Lidocaine is a local anesthetic and a class 1 antiarrhythmic. It can be administered in different ways, and this flexibility combined with its anesthetic properties means it has many uses within palliative care. Lidocaine is indicated for neuropathic pain unresponsive to opioids.[13] It is given by intravenous or subcutaneous infusion and should be administered on an inpatient basis with careful monitoring because of a risk of seizures and cardiac arrhythmias. For this reason it is generally reserved for severe intractable pain. To gain control of severe neuropathic pain, single-dose infusion can provide analgesia lasting 12 hours or longer and may predict response to oral mexiletine.[11] Lidocaine patches have also been used for neuropathic pain and have few systemic side effects. Spinal analgesia (epidural or intrathecal) combining opioids and local anesthetics may be indicated for severe neuropathic pain, such as that secondary to spinal cord compression, as well as for ischemic leg pain, tenesmic pain, muscle spasticity, and incident pain. It should be initiated by someone with specialist experience, often an anesthetist.

Lidocaine is rapidly absorbed from mucous membranes and, when applied topically as a gel, may be useful in patients with painful oral inflammation or ulceration, pressure sores, or malignant fungating wounds. It can also be used to manage dysuria or bladder spasms secondary to urinary tract infection, radiation cystitis, or bladder tumor infiltration.[14] Lidocaine ointment may relieve the pain associated with hemorrhoids and pruritus ani and, when applied before defecation, relieves the pain associated with anal fissures. For tenesmus, a rectal enema of lidocaine can be helpful.

Nebulized lidocaine has also been used for dyspnea, although its benefits are unproven. There is evidence that nebulized lidocaine may be of value in intractable cough. Because it is associated with an increased risk of aspiration secondary to pharyngeal anesthesia, patients should avoid eating for 1 hour afterward. It is recommended that a pretreatment dose of nebulized salbutamol be given because of the risk for bronchospasm.[15] Such treatment should be reserved for patients in whom other avenues have failed.

Parenteral lidocaine may help intractable itch secondary to uremia or cholestatic jaundice. Applied topically, it is absorbed somewhat and, unlike other local anesthetics, does not cause contact dermatitis. Application should be limited to short-term use only.

Mechanism of Action

Lidocaine is an amide anesthetic. It works by blocking sodium channels and hence the depolarization of nerve endings and thus produces reversible anesthesia. Nerve transmission is inhibited in all types of nerve fibers: sensory, motor, and autonomic. Other important, clinically significant pharmacological actions include smooth muscle relaxation, which can lead to vasodilation; a "quinidine-like" effect (membrane stabilization) on cardiac conduction; and mixed features of both stimulation and depression of the central nervous system, depending on the dose. Lidocaine is metabolized in the liver and should be used with caution at reduced doses in patients with liver failure.

Dosages

- Neuropathic pain: single-dose infusion of 120 mg or 2 mg/kg (6 mL of 2% lidocaine) subcutaneously or intravenously; continuous infusion initially at 20 mg/hr (24 mL of 2% lidocaine/24-hr continuous subcutaneous infusion); 5% lidocaine patch placed over the painful area
- Dysuria, bladder spasm, fungating wounds, and pressure sores: 2% lidocaine and 0.25% chlorhexidine gel
- Oral inflammation/ulceration: 2% lidocaine gel
- Tenesmus: rectal enema of 2% lidocaine gel as needed
- Cough: nebulized 2% lidocaine, 5 mL three times daily

Major Side Effects

Side effects are proportional to the plasma concentration of lidocaine. At low concentrations, light-headedness, numb tongue, metallic taste, increased blood pressure, and dizziness can occur. As the plasma concentration increases, visual and auditory disturbances, confusion, muscle twitching, and decreased blood pressure develop. At high plasma concentrations, patients are at risk for arrhythmias, convulsions, coma, and respiratory and cardiovascular system collapse. Hypersensitivity has also been reported.

Contraindications

Sinoatrial disorders, atrioventricular block, myocardial depression, and porphyria are contraindications to the use of lidocaine.

Drug Interactions

There is an increased risk of ventricular arrhythmias with concomitant administration of antipsychotics that prolong the QT interval, β-blockers, the antihistamine terfenadine, and 5-HT$_3$ antagonists. Antivirals possibly increase plasma concentrations of lidocaine. Its action is antagonized by the hypokalemia induced by loop or thiazide diuretics. Neuromuscular blockade by muscle relaxants is enhanced.

Evidence-Based Medicine

Several studies suggest lidocaine to be of benefit for neuropathic pain. Its effectiveness has been demonstrated in postherpetic neuralgia, sciatica, complex regional pain syndrome, and neuropathic cancer pain.[1-7,16] Lidocaine patches are licensed for postherpetic neuralgia but have also been reported to be of benefit for other localized peripheral neuropathic pain, particularly that in which allodynia is a prominent feature.[9,10]

In a randomized study, nebulized lidocaine had no benefit over nebulized normal saline for breathlessness in cancer patients.[11] One study investigating the efficacy of local anesthetics for cough had encouraging results, but there are unpublished anecdotal reports of its use for cough secondary to various causes.[13,17]

WARFARIN SODIUM (COUMADIN)

Warfarin is an oral anticoagulant that is generally used as the sodium salt. It is licensed for the treatment and prophylaxis of deep venous thrombosis (DVT) and pulmonary embolism (PE), and its main use in the palliative care setting is for these indications. It is also used for prevention of embolism in atrial fibrillation, in those undergoing cardioversion for atrial fibrillation, and in patients with prosthetic heart valves.

Warfarin is safe and efficacious in the general population, but less so in cancer patients. Initial warfarinization is challenging, and following standard anticoagulation protocols has produced INRs greater than 4.5 in over 60% and greater than 8 in 30%.[18] Maintaining a stable INR is similarly difficult because of

- Poor nutritional status
- Liver metastases
- Variable oral intake and drug absorption
- Drug-drug interactions

Even with strict INR monitoring, use of warfarin may be associated with bleeding in more than 50% of fully anticoagulated hospice patients.[17]

Mechanism of Action

Warfarin is an indirect antagonist of vitamin K, which is required for synthesis of the active clotting factors II (prothrombin), VII, IX, and X in the liver. Vitamin K is required for the carboxylation of specific glutamate residues in the clotting factor precursors. Warfarin acts by inhibiting vitamin K epoxide reductase, which converts vitamin K epoxide back to the reduced form.

There are two enantiomers of warfarin, the $R(+)$ and $S(-)$ forms, both of which are well absorbed. The S form is four times more potent than the R form and has a half-life of 32 hours. The R form has a half-life of 54 hours. Differences in the characteristics of the two forms are important in some drug interactions. Because the half-life of clotting factor II (prothrombin) is 60 hours, it is essential that initial anticoagulation with unfractionated heparin or low-molecular-weight heparin (LMWH) be continued for at least 5 days. Even if a therapeutic INR is achieved quickly, clotting factors with long half-lives will remain active until metabolized and excreted (Table 141-1).

Dosages

The dose will vary according to the INR. For established DVT or PE, an INR of 2.5 to 3.5 is recommended. It has been suggested that palliative care physicians aim for a lower INR to reduce the risk of bleeding. In some ways this is counterintuitive because cancer patients have a high incidence of recurrent venous thromboembolism (VTE) and lowering the INR will increase this risk.

Major Side Effects

The main side effect of warfarin is bleeding, which is increased in cancer patients even when the INR is controlled.[19] The venipunctures required to maintain stable anticoagulation have an adverse impact on quality of life.[20] Hypersensitivity, rash, alopecia, diarrhea, skin necrosis, jaundice, and hepatic dysfunction have been reported.

Contraindications

Peptic ulcer, severe hypertension, bacterial endocarditis, and pregnancy are contraindications to the use of warfarin. It should be used with caution in patients with renal or hepatic impairment, in women breastfeeding, or in those who have recently undergone surgery.

TABLE 141-1　Half-Lives of Vitamin K–Dependent Clotting Factors	
Factor II	60 hr
Factor X	40 hr
Factor IX	24 hr
Factor VII	6 hr

Drug Interactions

Many drugs interact with warfarin. Any prescribing associated with warfarin therapy should always be cross-checked for potential drug interactions. Some drugs commonly encountered in palliative care are listed in Table 141-2.

Research Challenges

Anticoagulation in advanced malignancy will continue to be controversial. Guidelines suggest that cancer patients with VTE should remain anticoagulated as long as the prothrombotic tendency is present. In patients with advanced cancer, this would imply that anticoagulation should be lifelong. It remains to be seen whether shorter anticoagulation in this group will lead to different long-term outcomes.

HEPARINS

Unfractionated heparin is a polymer with a molecular weight ranging from 6 to 40 kDa, although the average molecular weight of most commercial heparin preparations is 12 to 15 kDa. It is a member of the glycosaminoglycan family of carbohydrates (which includes the closely related molecule heparan sulfate) and consists of a variably sulfated repeating disaccharide unit.

Heparin is most commonly used for prevention or treatment of VTE. It is also used for acute coronary syndrome and atrial fibrillation. Within palliative care, LMWH is as effective as unfractionated heparin for DVT and PE and is now the initial treatment of choice.[21] LMWHs have a smaller molecular weight ranging between 3 and 7 kDa. Other advantages include a longer duration of action, which allows administration once daily and possibly a better safety profile with respect to hemorrhage, heparin-induced thrombocytopenia, and osteoporosis. Several different LMWHs are available, including

- Bemiparin (Zibor)
- Dalteparin (Fragmin)
- Enoxaparin (Clexane and Lovenox)
- Nadroparin (Fraxiparine and Fraxodil)
- Tinzaparin (Innohep)

LMWHs are administered by subcutaneous injection. They act by potentiating the inhibitory effect of antithrombin III on factor Xa and thrombin. They have a relatively higher ability to potentiate inhibition of factor Xa than to prolong the plasma clotting time, which cannot be used to guide dosage. Anti–factor Xa levels can be measured if necessary, but routine monitoring is not required because the dose is determined by body weight (Fig. 141-1).

Dosages

Primary Thromboprophylaxis

The LMWH of choice will depend on the preference of the institution. The dose used is that prescribed by the institution's formulary.

LMWH should be considered in cancer patients who are

- Undergoing surgery
- Immobile or confined to bed because of a concurrent acute medical illness
- Undertaking long-distance travel (flights longer than 6 hours)

Secondary Prophylaxis

There is now evidence to support the use of long-term LMWH in cancer-related VTE. The dose is prescribed according to body weight and administered as a daily subcutaneous injection. It is recommended that patients receive a full "treatment dose" for 1 month, followed by a reduction to 75% of this dose.[22,23] LMWH should be continued as long as the prothrombotic tendency is present (i.e., lifelong in advanced cancer).

Patients receiving LMWH who have brain or liver metastases are at higher risk for bleeding. One prospective cohort study investigated the treatment of VTE in patients

TABLE 141-2 Sampling of Drugs That Interact with Warfarin	
INCREASE INR	**DECREASE INR**
Antibacterials	Barbiturates
Cephalosporins	Carbamazepine
Trimethoprim	Vitamin K
Penicillin	Rifampicin
Macrolides	Ginseng
Metronidazole	St. John's wort
Quinolones	
Tetracycline	
Antifungals	
Fluconazole	
Itraconazole	
Ketoconazole	
Antacids	
Cimetidine	
Omeprazole	
NSAIDs	
Amiodarone	
Corticosteroids	

INR, international normalized ratio; NSAIDs, nonsteroidal anti-inflammatory drugs.

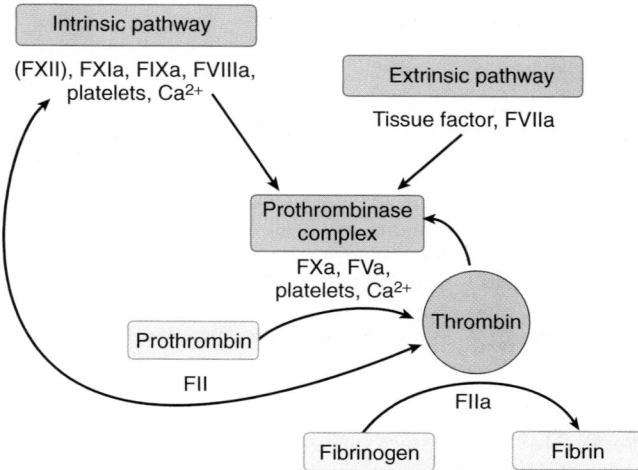

FIGURE 141-1 Site of action of warfarin.

with advanced metastatic disease and recommended the following[24]:

First week: give full-dose dalteparin according to body weight.
Subsequent weeks: give fixed-dose dalteparin, 10,000 units once daily.

There have been concerns that LMWH is too invasive in palliative care, but qualitative studies suggest it to be acceptable for primary and secondary thromboprophylaxis.[20,25]

Major Side Effects

Common (<10%, >1%): pain and bruising at the injection site, major bleeding in surgical patients receiving thromboprophylaxis and patients being treated for DVT or PE, and hematuria

---

Current Controversies and Future Considerations

Glyceryl Trinitrate

- Nitric oxide may affect the development of opioid tolerance because nitric oxide synthase inhibitors can attenuate analgesic tolerance to morphine.[16]
- Nitric oxide may therefore have a wider role to play in pain management, and this needs clarification.

Dopamine

- The use of inotropes in palliative care is a relatively new concept and is likely to require a major culture shift across the specialty. Achieving balance between perceived active and palliative treatment will be challenging.
- There may be concerns that the use of inotropes is too aggressive for palliative care and that they should be restricted to cardiology.

Mexiletine

- Despite evidence of efficacy, mexiletine is unlikely to have broad use in palliative care because of the caution in patients receiving medication for cardiac disease.
- Mexiletine's role in alleviating neuropathic pain in palliative care patients will remain unclear unless further large trials are conducted in advanced cancer.

Warfarin

- It is controversial whether warfarin should be replaced by LMWH as first-line long-term anticoagulation. Warfarin is preferred by many because it is cheaper and does not require injection.
- The benefits of LMWH are overshadowed by cost and resource allocation in those unable to self-inject. It is likely that these debates will be nullified by oral Xa inhibitors, whose efficacy in cancer patients is currently under evaluation.

Low-Molecular-Weight Heparin and Medium-Weight Heparin

- The use of LMWH is considered by some to be inappropriate in palliative care.
- LMWH has significant cost implications, and physicians are consequently reticent to prescribe it.

Uncommon (<1%, >0.1%): major bleeding in medical patients receiving thromboprophylaxis, thrombocytopenia, and spinal/epidural hematoma

Contraindications

- Active major bleeding, thrombocytopenia with a positive antiplatelet antibody test, severe renal impairment, hypersensitivity to pork

Drug Interactions

- Increased anticoagulant effect with nonsteroidal anti-inflammatory drugs, warfarin, and platelet aggregation inhibitors such as clopidogrel, dipyridamole
- Reduced anticoagulant effect with tetracycline, antihistamines, cardiac glycosides, and ascorbic acid

Research Challenges

The use of LMWH for prevention and treatment of VTE is likely to continue to be debated. Further work on the natural history of VTE in cancer is required because the true scale of the problem is unclear. Likewise, it is not known how much silent VTE contributes to symptoms such as dyspnea from PE.

REFERENCES

1. Lund J, Scholefield J. A randomized, prospective, double-blind, placebo-controlled trial of glyceryl trinitrate ointment in treatment of anal fissure. Lancet 1997;349:11-14.
2. McDonnell F, Walsh D. Treatment of odynophagia and dysphagia in advanced cancer with sublingual glyceryl trinitrate. Palliat Med 1999;13:251-252.
3. Gelfold M, Rozen P, Gilat T. Isosorbide dinitrate and nifedipine treatment of achalasia: A clinical, manumetric, and radionuclide evaluation. Gastroenterology 1982;83:963-969.
4. Hassel B. Treatment of biliary colic with nitroglycerin. Lancet 1993;342:1305.
5. Khawaja HT, Campbell MJ, Weaver PC. Effect of transdermal glyceryl trinitrate on the survival of peripheral intravenous infusions: A double-blind prospective clinical study. Br J Surg 1988;75:1212-1215.
6. Wright A, Hecker JF, Lewis GB. Use of transdermal glyceryl trinitrate to reduce failure of intravenous infusion due to phlebitis and extravasation. Lancet 1985;2:1148-1150.
7. Felker GM, O'Connor CM. Inotropic therapy for heart failure: An evidence based approach. Am Heart J 2001;142:393-401.
8. Young JB, Moen EK. Outpatient parenteral inotropic therapy for advanced heart failure. J Heart Lung Transplant 2000;19(8 Suppl):S49-S57.
9. López-Candales AL, Vora T, Gibbons W, et al. Symptomatic improvement in patients treated with intermittent infusion of inotropes: A double-blind placebo controlled pilot study. J Med 2002;33:129-146.
10. López-Candales AL, Carron C, Schwartz J. Need for hospice and palliative care services in patients with end-stage heart failure treated with intermittent infusion of inotropes. Clin Cardiol 2004;27:23-28.
11. Galer BS, Harle J, Rowbotham MC. Response to intravenous lidocaine infusion predicts subsequent response to oral mexiletine: A prospective study. J Pain Symptom Manage 1996;12:161-167.
12. Wallace MS, Magnuson S, Ridgeway B. Efficacy of oral mexiletine for neuropathic pain with allodynia: A double-blind, placebo-controlled crossover study. Reg Anaesth Pain Med 2000;25:459-467.
13. Kalso E, Tramer MR, McQuay HJ, Moore RA. Systemic local anaesthetic-type drugs in chronic pain: A systematic review. Eur J Pain 1998;2:3-14.
14. Asklin B, Cassuto J. Intravesical lidocaine in severe interstitial cystitis. Case report. Scand J Urol Nephrol 1989;23:311-312.
15. Trochtenberg S. Nebulised lidocaine in the treatment of refractory cough. Chest 1994;105:1592-1593.
16. Elliot K, Minami N, Kolesnikov YA, et al. The NMDA receptor antagonists, LY274614 and MK-801, and the nitric oxide synthase inhibitor, NG-nitro-L-arginine, attenuate analgesic tolerance to the mu-opioid morphine but not to kappa opioids. Pain 1994;56:69-75.
17. Johnson MJ. Problems of anticoagulation within a palliative care setting: An audit of hospice patients taking warfarin. Palliat Med 1997;11:306-312.
18. Noble SIR. Anticoagulation in advanced malignancy: Pitfalls, dangers and future developments [abstract]. Palliat Med 2004;18:161.

19. Hutten BA, Prins MH, Gent M, et al. Incidence of recurrent thromboembolic and bleeding complications among patients with venous thromboembolism in relation to both malignancy and achieved international normalized ratio: A retrospective analysis. J Clin Oncol 2000;18:3078-3083.
20. Noble SIR, Finlay IG. Is long-term low molecular weight heparin acceptable to palliative care patients in the treatment of cancer related venous thromboembolism? A qualitative study. Palliat Med 2005;19:197-201.
21. Prandoni P. Heparins and venous thromboembolism: Current practice and future directions. Thromb Haemost 2001;86:488-498.
22. Meyer G, Marjanovic Z, Valcke J, et al. Comparison of low-molecular-weight heparin and warfarin for the secondary prevention of venous thromboembolism in patients with cancer: A randomized controlled study. Arch Intern Med 2002;162:1729-1735.
23. Lee A, Levine MN, Baker RI, et al. Low molecular weight heparin versus a coumarin for the prevention of recurrent venous thromboembolism in patients with cancer. N Engl J Med 2003;349:146-153.
24. Monreal M, Zacharski L, Jiménez JA, et al. Fixed-dose low-molecular-weight heparin for secondary prevention of venous thromboembolism in patients with disseminated cancer: A prospective cohort study. J Thromb Haemost 2004;2:1311-1315.
25. Noble SI, Nelson A, Turner C, Finlay IG. Acceptability of low molecular weight heparin thromboprophylaxis for inpatients receiving palliative care: Qualitative study. BMJ 2006;332:577-580.

CHAPTER **142**

Local and General Anesthetics

Eric Prommer

KEY POINTS

- Abnormal input to the spinal cord as a result of peripheral nerve injury or tissue inflammation is known to be conducted via activated sodium channels. Local anesthetics can suppress these ectopic discharges by inhibiting the conformational changes that underlie channel activation.

- Each local anesthetic has a pK_a, which is the hydrogen ion concentration at which there is equilibrium between the basic uncharged form (B) and the charged cationic form (BH^+). The uncharged form is more lipophilic and penetrates nerves more efficiently.

- Systemic reactions to local anesthetics involve the central nervous system (CNS) and the cardiovascular system.

- Ketamine and propofol are two widely used general anesthetics. Further studies must be performed to confirm the benefits of ketamine in cancer pain and determine the best route, the optimal dosages, and the incidence of adverse effects. It also must be determined whether using ketamine earlier will improve outcomes.

LOCAL ANESTHETICS AND PALLIATIVE CARE

Local anesthetics are used for neuropathic pain. Important local anesthetics in palliative care are lidocaine and bupivacaine. Bupivacaine, when combined with opioids and administered intrathecally, is considered the fourth step in the World Health Organization's analgesic ladder.[1] Mexiletine is the oral cogener of lidocaine. Important general anesthetics in palliative care are ketamine and propofol. Ketamine, an *N*-methyl-D-aspartate (NMDA) receptor antagonist, is primarily used for refractory pain syndromes with a neuropathic component. Propofol is used principally for terminal sedation.

Mechanism of Action

Voltage-gated channels are responsible for propagation of nerve impulses from peripheral nociceptors along group A and dorsal root C nerve fibers into the spinal cord.[2] Conductance of nerve impulses depends on propagation of a depolarization wave along the axon by continuous coupling between excited and nonexcited membrane regions. Nerve depolarization is due to the net influx of Na^+ via Na^+ channels and slower efflux of K^+ via K^+ channels.[2] Ten different Na^+ channels have been identified and biochemically sequenced. At least four are exclusively associated with nociceptive afferent fibers.[3] Abnormal input to the spinal cord as a result of peripheral nerve injury or tissue inflammation is conducted via activated sodium channels. Local anesthetics can suppress these ectopic discharges by inhibiting the conformational changes that underlie channel activation. Local anesthetics bind in the channel's pore and occlude the path of Na^+ ions. Binding of local anesthetics is increased by membrane depolarization because more binding sites become accessible during activation (the "guarded receptor" model) and dissociation of drug from nonactivated channels is slower than from resting channels (the "modulated receptor" model).[2]

Dosage

Most local anesthetics are available as hydrochloride salts. The amino amide classes of local anesthetics (to which bupivacaine and lidocaine belong) have more stability than other classes do. The concentration of local anesthetics in blood is determined by the amount injected, the rate of absorption from the injection site, the rate of tissue distribution, and the rate of biotransformation and excretion of the specific drug. Highly perfused organs (kidneys, lungs, liver, heart, muscle) show higher concentrations of local anesthetic.[2] Local anesthetics are metabolized in the liver and excreted by the kidney. Decreased hepatic blood flow or impaired hepatic enzyme function can increase blood levels of the amino amide local anesthetics. The half-life of local anesthetics is also prolonged in congestive heart failure. Each local anesthetic has a pK_a, which is the hydrogen ion concentration at which there is equilibrium between the basic uncharged form (B) and the charged cationic form (BH^+).[2] The uncharged form is more lipophilic and penetrates nerves more efficiently. Structural modifications such as increasing the size of alkyl substituents can increase the lipophilic nature of a drug.[2]

Increasing the concentration of local anesthetic accelerates the anesthetic effect and increases plasma levels. For example, increasing the concentration of bupivacaine from 0.25% to 0.75% results in more rapid anesthetic effect. Increasing the volume of local anesthetic increases the spread of anesthesia. For example, 30 mL of 1% lidocaine in the epidural space produces anesthesia 4.3 dermatomes higher than that when 10 mL of 3% lidocaine is given.[2] Vasoconstrictors, usually epinephrine (5 μg/mL or 1:200,000), can decrease the rate of vascular absorption, thereby allowing a smaller dose and prolonged effect. The site of injection can influence the duration of activity. Bupivacaine has a longer duration of effect when given as an axillary plexus block than as an intercostal block.[2]

The effective dose range of systemic lidocaine (1.5 to 5.0 mg/kg), as a bolus or continuous infusion, is comparable among different neuropathic pain conditions.[4] A dose of 300 mg/day should not be exceeded.[5] The lidocaine test (a test dose of lidocaine) may predict response to local anesthetics (such as mexiletine).[4] The therapeutic range of lidocaine is 0.62 to 5.0 μg/mL.

Bupivacaine is started at a concentration of 0.25%, which is associated with minimal motor block.[1] The dose should not be repeated at intervals of less than 3 hours when given as a bolus. Bupivacaine can be given as a continuous infusion (bupivacaine infusion concentration ranging from 0.1% to 0.5% and infusion rates ranging from 4 to 18 mL/hr).[6] A total dosage of 400 mg in 24 hours should not be exceeded.[5] The recommended dose range of mexiletine that is reportedly effective in peripheral neuropathic pain is 400 to 1200 mg/day.[4] The mean plasma level at this range is 0.76 μg/mL.

Transdermal lidocaine patches contain 700 mg of lidocaine in an aqueous base. When applied, only 3% is absorbed.[5] Transdermal 5% lidocaine patches are applied for 12 hours and then removed.

Individual Local Anesthetics

Lidocaine

Lidocaine is an amino amide local anesthetic with a pK_a of 7.9. For neuropathic pain, lidocaine can be given intravenously, subcutaneously, and transdermally. When administered systemically (intravenously), lidocaine is distributed rapidly into highly perfused tissues (i.e., kidneys, lungs, liver, heart, muscle). Its distribution half-life is 15 to 30 minutes[5] with a volume of distribution of 1.7 L/kg, less in heart failure. Lidocaine is chiefly metabolized in the liver via de-ethylation. The cytochrome P-450 isoenzyme CYP1A2 is the primary enzyme responsible for the metabolism of lidocaine via oxidative de-ethylation and 3-hydroxylation, with lesser contribution from CYP3A4.[5] The major metabolite is monoethylglycinexylidide, similar in pharmacology and toxicity to lidocaine, but less potent.[5] Lidocaine is renally excreted, 90% as metabolites. Its elimination half-life is 1.5 to 2.0 hours. The half-life is prolonged in patients with liver but not renal failure. Protein binding is 33% to 80%[5] and depends on both plasma drug and α$_1$-acid glycoprotein concentrations. At concentrations of 1 to 4 μg/mL of free base, lidocaine is 60% to 80% protein bound.[5]

TRANSDERMAL LIDOCAINE

After application, the mean peak blood concentration of lidocaine is 0.13 μg/mL,[5] approximately $^1/_{10}$ the therapeutic concentration required to treat cardiac arrhythmias. The lidocaine concentration does not increase with daily use. The time until the maximum concentration (T$_{max}$) is achieved is approximately 11 hours.[5] Even after long-term use (several weeks) with up to three patches per day, the maximum lidocaine blood concentration does not exceed 0.13 μg/mL. The efficacy of transdermal lidocaine patches does not depend on the systemic lidocaine plasma level.[7]

Mexiletine

Mexiletine is a class IB antiarrhythmic agent and a structural analogue of lidocaine. It is administered orally with 90% oral bioavailability. Its peak effect takes place in 1.5 to 4 hours, and more than 90% of the drug is metabolized in the liver with an elimination half-life of about 6 to 17 hours.[4] Similar to lidocaine, liver disease affects elimination.

Bupivacaine

Bupivacaine is an amino amide local anesthetic with a longer duration of action than lidocaine. It has a distribution half-life of 9.1 minutes. Its volume of distribution is approximately 2.5 L/kg. Total body clearance is 0.33 to 0.52 L/min. Bupivacaine clearance depends on the serum levels of α$_1$-acid glycoprotein; clearance decreases with increased concentrations of α$_1$-acid glycoprotein.[5] Its elimination half-life is 3.5 hours. Similar to lidocaine, dose adjustments are needed in patients with liver disease. Reduced dosages should be used in elderly, young, or debilitated patients, although no specific recommendations are available.[5] It is generally accepted that concentrations greater than 4 μg/mL are excessive.

Adverse Effects

Local anesthetics are responsible for 5% to 10% of all reported adverse reactions to anesthetic drugs.[8] Systemic reactions to local anesthetics involve the CNS and the cardiovascular system, with the CNS being more susceptible than the cardiovascular system to systemically distributed local anesthetics.[8] The dose and blood level of local anesthetic required to produce CNS toxicity are lower than those that result in circulatory collapse. The symptoms of local anesthetic–induced CNS toxicity are lightheadedness and dizziness, followed frequently by visual and auditory disturbances such as difficulty focusing and tinnitus. Objective signs of CNS toxicity are usually excitatory and include shivering, muscular twitching, and tremors. If untreated, generalized seizures can occur.[8]

Cardiovascular toxicity derives from sodium channel blockade, which reduces contractility and interferes with conduction. All local anesthetics exert a dose-dependent negative inotropic action on cardiac muscle. Bupivacaine is a more potent cardiodepressant than lidocaine is. At subconvulsant doses, bupivacaine can induce ventricular arrhythmias, including fibrillation.[2] Occasionally, bupivacaine can cause a sympathetic nervous system blockade that mimics spinal cord compression.[1] CNS and cardiac toxicity is potentiated by hypoxia and hypercapnia, so acute management must minimize these conditions. Allergic reactions account for only 1% of untoward reactions. Local adverse effects such as erythema occur with the transdermal patch. Case reports describe toxicity from lidocaine patches.[7]

Drug Interactions

Lidocaine levels can be increased when retroviral agents are coadministered because of competition for CYP3A4 enzymes.[5] Coadministration of fluoroquinolones and class I antiarrhythmics can prolong the QTc interval.[5] Cimetidine, but not ranitidine can decrease lidocaine clearance by 25% to 30%.[5] Propranolol, nadolol, and metoprolol may increase lidocaine levels 20% to 30%.[5] Lidocaine and bupivacaine administration can decrease the hypnotic requirements for propofol.[5] Bupivacaine may cause bradycardia and hypotension when given with angiotensin-converting enzyme inhibitors.[5]

Contraindications

Local anesthetics are contraindicated in patients hypersensitive to local anesthetics of the amide type or any other component of the product.[5] Mexiletine is contraindicated in those with significant second- and third-degree heart block and uncompensated congestive heart failure. Spinal local anesthetics should not be given to patients with coagulation disorders, sepsis, or local infection at the proposed administration site.

Evidence-Based Medicine

Systemic administration (intravenous) of lidocaine can work in selected patients with neuropathic pain, and this effect is superior to placebo (level IA evidence).[9] There is level IB evidence of the efficacy of lidocaine in neuropathic pain (nerve injury), postherpetic neuralgia, and postamputation stump pain.[9] There is level IB evidence for infusion of lidocaine in the treatment of peripheral neuropathy.[9] One controlled study found optimal results with a dose of 5 mg/kg.[10] There is level IB evidence for the use of intrathecal bupivacaine for analgesia in patients refractory to intrathecal opioids,[6] as well as level IB evidence for mexiletine in human immunodeficiency virus-1 neuropathy, diabetic polyneuropathy, and complex regional pain syndromes (I/II).[9] There is level IB evidence for the treatment of postherpetic neuralgia with transdermal lidocaine.

Research Issues

Research questions that must be evaluated in the future include

- Identification of the sodium channel subtype important in generating painful stimuli
- Clarification of types of neuropathic pain responsive to local anesthetic
- Clarification of the role of the lidocaine test
- Determination of the effectiveness and long-term effects of mexiletine in patients with neuropathic pain
- Understanding of why a single dose of local anesthetic can provide analgesic effects beyond the duration of action of the drug

GENERAL ANESTHETICS AND PALLIATIVE CARE

Ketamine

Ketamine, a racemic phencyclidine analogue, was originally used as a general anesthetic and produced "dissociative" anesthesia whereby the patient remains awake and responds to stimuli but has a diminished sense of awareness and amnesia for events occurring while under anesthesia. When recovering from dissociative anesthesia, patients can experience reemergence phenomena such as hallucinations, floating sensations, and vivid dreams. At 10% to 20% of the general anesthetic dose, analgesia can be produced with less emergence phenomena.

Mechanism of Action

Persistent release of glutamate as a result of peripheral injury or inflammation leads to activation of NMDA receptors in supraspinal and spinal structures.[11] Activation of NMDA receptors contributes to the hyperalgesia and allodynia associated with nerve injury or inflammation. These phenomena are due to "wind-up," a state in which spinal neurons become hyperresponsive to repetitive painful stimulation. The mechanism by which the NMDA receptor contributes to neuronal wind-up involves increased intracellular calcium, generation of secondary messengers such as Ca^{+2}-sensitive protein kinase C, and production of nitric oxide.[12] In animal studies, NMDA antagonists (such as MK-801) interrupt this cycle, prevent the development and expression of wind-up phenomena, and reverse morphine tolerance.[12] The receptor is composed of two critical subunits, the NMDA R1 subunit (NR1) and the NMDA R2 subunit (NR2). The NR1 subunit is necessary for NMDA receptor–coupled channel activity, and the NR2 subunit modulates channel activity.[13] Ketamine binds to a phencyclidine site in the NR1 subunit, which inhibits the excitatory effect of glutamate. Ketamine inhibits all NMDA receptor subtypes presently cloned.[14]

Pharmacology

Ketamine is rapidly absorbed after parenteral administration but has low oral bioavailability (15%). Its plasma half-life is 2 to 4 hours. Ketamine is highly lipid soluble. It is quickly distributed into highly vascular organs, including the brain. Its distribution half-life is approximately 7 to 11 minutes. Ketamine is metabolized in the liver by N-demethylation to form norketamine, an active metabolite with analgesic potency.[5] About 90% of ketamine is excreted in urine, mostly as metabolites. Ketamine has a wide therapeutic index, so there is a low chance of lethal overdose.

Dose/Route of Administration

The most common routes of administration are the intravenous (IV)/subcutaneous (SC) and oral routes. Ketamine has been used intranasally for breakthrough pain. It is not recommended for intrathecal administration. The initial IV/SC dosage is 0.1 to 0.2 mg/kg/hr or 50 to 100 mg/day total.[15] The initial dosage is titrated if necessary every 6 hours in 25% to 30% increments until pain is relieved or adverse effects limit dose escalation. The oral ketamine dosage has been 0.5 mg/kg three times daily.[16] Ketamine has also been given in a "burst fashion" whereby the analgesic dosage is given for a few days and then stopped. When converting from the IV/SC route to the oral route, patients are often maintained at 30% to 40% of the IV/SC dosage.[17] A test dose of 2.5 mg IV/SC or 20 mg orally has been recommended (level IV evidence).[18] The use of a benzodiazepine such as midazolam, 1 mg every 6 hours, minimizes emergence phenomena.

Adverse Effects

Emergence phenomena such as floating sensations, vivid dreams, hallucinations, delirium, and excess sedation occur more commonly at anesthetic doses (6% to 35%). They are seen more frequently in the elderly and those with anxiety disorders in whom rapid infusion and increased dosages have been administered. Ketamine can cause hypertension and tachycardia, hypersalivation, increased muscle tone, and an erythematous rash on the face and neck.[5]

Contraindications

Absolute contraindications are the presence of intracranial metastasis or hydrocephalus. Relative contraindications include a seizure disorder, recent seizures, psychiatric history, labile hypertension, poorly controlled arrhythmias, and severe chronic obstructive pulmonary disease with hypercapnia.[5]

Drug Interactions

Sedative hypnotics can prolong recovery from the drug. Administration of theophylline can decrease the seizure threshold.[5]

Evidence-Based Medicine

There is level IB evidence for the use of bolus ketamine as an analgesic for pain unresponsive to opioids.[19] There is level IB evidence suggesting decreased opioid requirements when combined with ketamine.[18] There is level IV evidence for the use of burst ketamine to reverse opioid tolerance,[20] as well as level IV evidence for subcutaneous infusion of ketamine for neuropathic pain.[15] There is level IIA evidence for the use of oral ketamine as an adjuvant to oral morphine in cancer neuropathic pain.[16] There is level IB evidence for intranasal ketamine in breakthrough pain.[21] For ischemic pain, a level II study reported a potent dose-dependent analgesic effect, but with a narrow therapeutic window.[22] There is level IB evidence for low-dose ketamine (0.4-mg/kg bolus) in chronic trigeminal neuralgia.[23] There is level II evidence of reduced hyperpathia and pain relief in phantom limb pain and postherpetic neuralgia with either parenteral or oral ketamine.[23]

Research Issues

Further studies must confirm the benefits of ketamine in cancer pain and determine the best route, the optimal dosages, and the incidence of adverse effects. It also must be determined whether administering ketamine earlier will improve outcomes.

Propofol

Propofol is an IV alkyl phenol (2,6-diisopropylphenol) used for sedation and induction of anesthesia. Propofol cannot be administered as a salt because of the presence of a lone ionizable functional group, hydroxyl, which has a pK_a of 11. Propofol is miscible only in lipophilic substances or organic solvents.[24]

Mechanism of Action

Propofol is a highly lipophilic, global CNS depressant. It directly activates γ-aminobutyric acid A (GABA$_A$) receptors.

Pharmacology/Route of Administration

Propofol phosphate is enzymatically converted to propofol, formaldehyde, and inorganic phosphate. It has a large volume of distribution, and its rapid uptake and elimination from the CNS (distribution half-life, 1 to 8 minutes) result in rapid onset of action and rapid recovery when discontinued. Recovery is rapid even with prolonged use. The onset of anesthesia is approximately 10 to 50 seconds. Recovery takes place in less than 10 minutes. Protein binding is 97% to 99%. Its volume of distribution is 60 L/kg. Propofol is metabolized by glucuronide and sulfate conjugation and does not accumulate with long-term infusion. Dose reduction is not required in patients with hepatic or renal disease. CYP2B6 is the cytochrome isoform predominantly involved in the metabolism of propofol in human liver microsomes. The drug is excreted by the kidneys with an elimination half-life of 1.5 to 12.4 hours.[5]

Dosing for Palliative Sedation

No universally accepted guidelines or protocols exist. Most recommend that a bolus of 20 to 50 mg be used for emergency sedation. Propofol may be given as a continuous infusion at 10 mg/hr, with titration by 10 mg/hr every 15 to 20 minutes.[25]

Adverse Effects

Propofol can cause pain with injection. Dose-dependent hypotension is the most common complication, particularly in volume-depleted patients.[5]

Drug Interactions

Administration of propofol with local anesthetics such as bupivacaine or lidocaine is associated with an increased hypnotic effect.[5]

Contraindications

The only absolute contraindication to propofol is allergy to the drug.[5]

Evidence-Based Medicine

There is level III evidence for the use of propofol for palliative sedation.[26]

Research Issues

Research is needed to determine protocols and guidelines for administration.

REFERENCES

1. Mercadante S. Problems of long-term spinal opioid treatment in advanced cancer patients. Pain 1999;79:1-13.
2. Strichartz GR, Berde CB. Local anesthetics. In Miller RD (ed). Miller's Anesthesia, 6th ed. Philadelphia: Churchill Livingstone, 2006.
3. Lee Y, Lee CH, Oh U. Painful channels in sensory neurons. Mol Cell 2005;20:315-324.
4. Mao J, Chen LL. Systemic lidocaine for neuropathic pain relief. Pain 2000;87:7-17.
5. Micromedix Healthcare Series 2005. 2006.
6. Du Pen SL, Kharasch ED, Williams A, et al. Chronic epidural bupivacaine-opioid infusion in intractable cancer pain. Pain 1992;49:293-300.
7. Wilhelm IR, Griessinger N, Koppert W, et al. High doses of topically applied lidocaine in a cancer patient. J Pain Symptom Manage 2005;30:203-204.
8. McCaughey W. Adverse effects of local anaesthetics. Drug Saf 1992;7:178-189.
9. Tremont-Lukats IW, Challapalli V, McNicol ED, et al. Systemic administration of local anesthetics to relieve neuropathic pain: A systematic review and meta-analysis. Anesth Analg 2005;101:1738-1749.
10. Tremont-Lukats IW, Hutson PR, Backonja MM. A randomized, double-masked, placebo-controlled pilot trial of extended IV lidocaine infusion for relief of ongoing neuropathic pain. Clin J Pain 2006;22:266-271.
11. Mayer DJ, Mao J, Holt J, Price DD. Cellular mechanisms of neuropathic pain, morphine tolerance, and their interactions. Proc Natl Acad Sci U S A 1999;96:7731-7736.
12. Mao J, Price DD, Mayer DJ. Mechanisms of hyperalgesia and morphine tolerance: A current view of their possible interactions. Pain 1995;62:259-274.
13. Mao J. NMDA and opioid receptors: Their interactions in antinociception, tolerance and neuroplasticity. Brain Res Brain Res Rev 1999;30:289-304.
14. Kew JN, Kemp JA. Ionotropic and metabotropic glutamate receptor structure and pharmacology. Psychopharmacology (Berl) 2005;179:4-29.
15. Mercadante S, Lodi F, Sapio M, et al. Long-term ketamine subcutaneous continuous infusion in neuropathic cancer pain. J Pain Symptom Manage 1995;10:564-568.
16. Kannan TR, Saxena A, Bhatnagar S, Barry A. Oral ketamine as an adjuvant to oral morphine for neuropathic pain in cancer patients. J Pain Symptom Manage 2002;23:60-65.
17. Fitzgibbon EJ, Hall P, Schroder C, et al. Low dose ketamine as an analgesic adjuvant in difficult pain syndromes: A strategy for conversion from parenteral to oral ketamine. J Pain Symptom Manage 2002;23:165-170.
18. Lossignol DA, Obiols-Portis M, Body JJ. Successful use of ketamine for intractable cancer pain. Support Care Cancer 2005;13:188-193.
19. Mercadante S, Arcuri E, Tirelli W, Casuccio A. Analgesic effect of intravenous ketamine in cancer patients on morphine therapy: A randomized, controlled, double-blind, crossover, double-dose study. J Pain Symptom Manage 2000;20:246-252.
20. Mercadante S, Villari P, Ferrera P. Burst ketamine to reverse opioid tolerance in cancer pain. J Pain Symptom Manage 2003;25:302-305.
21. Carr DB, Goudas LC, Denman WT, et al. Safety and efficacy of intranasal ketamine for the treatment of breakthrough pain in patients with chronic pain: A randomized, double-blind, placebo-controlled, crossover study. Pain 2004;108:17-27.
22. Persson J, Hasselstrom J, Wiklund B, et al. The analgesic effect of racemic ketamine in patients with chronic ischemic pain due to lower extremity arteriosclerosis obliterans. Acta Anaesthesiol Scand 1998;42:750-758.
23. Rabben T, Skjelbred P, Oye I. Prolonged analgesic effect of ketamine, an N-methyl-D-aspartate receptor inhibitor, in patients with chronic pain. J Pharmacol Exp Ther 1999;289:1060-1066.
24. Sneyd JR. Recent advances in intravenous anaesthesia. Br J Anaesth 2004;93:725-736.
25. Rousseau P. Palliative sedation in the management of refractory symptoms. J Support Oncol 2004;2:181-186.
26. Lundstrom S, Zachrisson U, Furst CJ. When nothing helps: Propofol as sedative and antiemetic in palliative cancer care. J Pain Symptom Manage 2005;30:570-577.

SUGGESTED READING

Kew JN, Kemp JA. Ionotropic and metabotropic glutamate receptor structure and pharmacology. Psychopharmacology (Berl) 2005;179:4-29.

Mao J. NMDA and opioid receptors: Their interactions in antinociception, tolerance and neuroplasticity. Brain Res Brain Res Rev 1999;30:289-304.

Mao J, Chen LL. Systemic lidocaine for neuropathic pain relief. Pain 2000;87:7-17.

CHAPTER **143**

Drugs for Hypercalcemia

Jean-Jacques Body

KEY POINTS

- Tumor-induced hypercalcemia can be successfully treated in at least 90% of patients by volume repletion and bisphosphonates.
- Standard therapy consists of 4 mg zoledronic acid infused in no less than 15 minutes with concomitant rehydration; 90 mg pamidronate and 6 mg ibandronate, when available, are alternative bisphosphonate therapies.
- Calcitonin can still be useful for severe or life-threatening hypercalcemia to obtain a rapid, though transient drop in Ca levels.
- Recurrent hypercalcemia remains difficult to control, and possible intensive therapy has to consider the overall prognosis.
- Prevention of tumor-induced hypercalcemia is one of the objectives of long-term therapy with bisphosphonates for tumor bone disease. In placebo-controlled trials, bisphosphonates reduced hypercalcemic episodes by more than half.

The concentration of total extracellular Ca is normally between 8.5 and 10.3 mg/dL (or 2.12 to 2.57 mM). About half is ionized (Ca^{2+}) and the other half is protein (mainly albumin) bound or complexed with anions. Changes in serum albumin concentration can affect the total calcium concentration (every 1-g/dL change in serum albumin is roughly associated with a 0.8-mg/dL change in total calcium), which is important in cancer patients because of the high prevalence of low protein levels.

The two main causes of hypercalcemia are cancer hypercalcemia and primary hyperparathyroidism. Other causes include vitamin D intoxication, milk-alkali syndrome, hyperthyroidism, and sarcoidosis, particularly with mild or moderate and relatively stable serum Ca elevations. Besides myeloma, hypercalcemia can be observed with any type of solid tumor, but breast and lung cancer are the two most frequent.[1] Hypercalcemia occurs in 10% to 15% of people with advanced cancer, but this figure is decreasing because of earlier and prolonged use of bisphosphonates in cancer patients with bone metastases.[2] Most often, hypercalcemia complicates advanced cancer, and the median survival is 6 to 10 weeks. Breast cancer patients experience a longer median survival of 3 to 4.5 months.[1]

The diagnosis is not always clinically evident because of the lack of specificity of most symptoms. Polyuria, polydipsia, arrhythmias, nausea and vomiting, constipation, obtundation, and possibly coma in severe cases can all occur. The degree of symptomatology is more linked to the rate of increase in serum Ca than to the absolute level.

Although effective antitumor treatment is the best way to control serum Ca, a marked reduction in tumor burden is often not attainable because hypercalcemia generally complicates advanced refractory cancer. Forced saline diuresis with high-dose furosemide is risky and outdated. Volume repletion and rehydration with intravenous fluids should be part of the initial therapeutic approach for moderate or severe hypercalcemia. However, rehydration and volume repletion have only small and transient effects on serum Ca, with a median decrease of just 1 mg/dL being achieved.[3] Yet it improves clinical status and interrupts the vicious cycle of hypercalcemia by decreasing tubular calcium reabsorption. Besides volume repletion, bisphosphonates have supplanted all other drugs for tumor-induced hypercalcemia, except occasionally corticosteroids and calcitonin (see the later section "Other Drugs for Hypercalcemia").

PATHOGENESIS OF CANCER HYPERCALCEMIA AND MECHANISM OF ACTION OF BISPHOSPHONATES

Hypercalcemia can be due to bone metastases with lytic lesions or to paraneoplastic (see Chapter 233) secretion of parathyroid hormone–related peptide (PHRP). Tumor cell secretion of humoral and paracrine factors stimulates osteoclast activity and proliferation, as exemplified by increased excretion of collagen cross-links.[4] PHRP has an essential role in most cases of cancer-induced hypercalcemia. Circulating PHRP levels are high in virtually all patients with humoral hypercalcemia of malignancy and in up to two thirds with bone metastases.[5] Tubular reabsorption of calcium is enhanced because of volume depletion and the effects of PHRP on the renal tubules. Local production of PHRP and other osteolytic factors by cancer cells in bone stimulate osteoclastic bone resorption essentially through the osteoblasts. Tumor factors alter the ratio between osteoprotegerin (OPG), whose production is decreased, and RANKL (receptor activator of NFκB ligand), whose production is increased.[6] The net result of the imbalance of these regulatory factors of bone resorption is increased osteoclast proliferation and activity. Increased bone resorption is a hallmark of myeloma bone disease, and a marked increase in osteoclast-mediated bone resorption also accompanies the typical osteosclerotic disease of advanced prostate cancer. These considerations explain why bisphosphonates have been used so extensively for cancer hypercalcemia, metastatic bone pain, and prevention of the complications of bone metastases (see Chapter 222).

Bisphosphonates preferentially localize to sites of active bone remodeling. They act directly on mature osteoclasts and decrease their bone resorption activity, notably by lowering H^+ and Ca^{2+} extrusion, but they essentially act by inducing osteoclast apoptosis. Clodronate, but not the aminobisphosphonates, can be metabolized to an adenosine triphosphate analogue that is toxic to osteoclasts. On the other hand, nitrogen-containing bisphosphonates, but not clodronate, interfere with the mevalonate pathway, which is essential for cell membrane integrity. Aminobisphosphonates such as pamidronate, zoledronic acid (also named zoledronate), and ibandronate are nanomolar inhibitors of farnesyl pyrophosphate synthase. This results in inhibition of post-translational prenylation of proteins with farnesyl or geranyl isoprenoid groups. Various cellular proteins must anchor to the cell membrane via a prenyl group to become active. Most are guanosine triphosphate binding proteins, including the proteins ras and rho, and prenylated proteins are essential for osteoclast function, notably cell activity and attachment.[7] The net result, regardless of the class of bisphosphonate, is osteoclast apoptosis. Bisphosphonates can directly inhibit cancer cell growth by a combination of necrotic and apoptotic processes and inhibit the stimulatory effects of bone-derived growth factors.[8] The clinical relevance of these observations is unclear.

BISPHOSPHONATES FOR HYPERCALCEMIA

The bisphosphonates most often used are clodronate, pamidronate, and more recently, ibandronate and zoledronic acid. Others will not be reviewed because they are not as effective or have not been adequately evaluated.[1,3]

Clodronate

A single-day 1500-mg infusion of clodronate achieves normocalcemia in 50% to 80%; however, a recent dose-response study suggested no difference between doses of 600 to 1500 mg and that the overall response rate does not exceed 50%.[9] The superiority of pamidronate over clodronate has been shown in a limited but randomized study. Pamidronate was more effective but, more importantly, resulted in a longer duration of normocalcemia, with a median duration of action of 2 weeks for clodronate versus 4 weeks for pamidronate.[10] Clodronate has the advantage that it can be given subcutaneously. At a dose of 1500 mg infused over a period of 4 to 30 hours, mild site toxicity occurred in 29% of 45 infusions, and marked hypocalcemic activity was demonstrated in 12 evaluable episodes. This method should be further evaluated in the palliative setting.[11]

Pamidronate

Pamidronate is administered as a single infusion given over a 2- to 4-hour period and is viewed as the standard therapy for bone metastasis–related complications, including cancer-induced hypercalcemia.[12] A dose of 90 mg achieves normocalcemia in over 90% of unselected patients.[13] At this dose, the effects on serum Ca are not greatly influenced by the tumor type or bone metastases. There is no need to adjust the dose for initial Ca levels. The response to lower doses will be less with humoral hypercalcemia of malignancy than with bone metastases because the contributory role of PHRP on kidney calcium reabsorption will become much less evident when large bisphosphonate doses are used.[14] When hypercalcemia recurs and becomes refractory, the pathogenic and clinical importance of circulating PHRP becomes essential.[15] Pamidronate is well tolerated, with the only clinically detectable side effect being transient fever or a flulike syndrome (or both) in about 25%. To avoid renal toxicity, the duration of infusion in hypercalcemic patients cannot be less than 2 hours.

Newer and more potent bisphosphonates, such as ibandronate and zoledronic acid, have been evaluated recently and appear to be superior to pamidronate in moderate to severe cases[16] (Table 143-1). They are also more convenient to administer.

Ibandronate

A dose escalation trial of ibandronate was conducted in 147 patients with Ca levels greater than 12 mg/dL (3.0 mmol/L) after rehydration; 125 were evaluable for response. The success rate was 50% in the 2-mg group, significantly lower than that in the 4- and 6-mg dose groups, 76% and 77%, respectively. The response rate was also dependent on the initial Ca level and on tumor type, with the group with breast cancer or myeloma responding better than those with other tumors. The drug was well tolerated, the only noticeable side effect being drug-induced fever in 13%.[17]

These success rates appear to be lower than those with pamidronate, but this multicenter trial included only moderate or severe hypercalcemia. The results of a limited face-to-face comparative trial suggested that ibandronate is actually more effective than pamidronate in patients with corrected Ca levels 14 mg/dL or higher.[18]

Zoledronic Acid (Zoledronate)

Two pooled, randomized, double-blind, double-dummy trials in 275 evaluable patients with moderate or severe hypercalcemia (corrected Ca ≥ 12 mg/dL or 3 mmol/L) compared zoledronic acid, either as a 5-minute 4-mg infusion ($n = 86$) or as a 5-minute 8-mg infusion ($n = 90$), with pamidronate (90 mg infused over a 2-hour period; $n = 99$). The groups were well balanced, except that there were more patients with breast or hematological disease in the 4-mg zoledronic acid group than in the two other groups. Zoledronic acid was more efficient than pamidronate (Fig. 143-1). At day 10, success rates (Ca ≤ 10.8 mg/dL) were 88%, 87%, and 70% for the three groups, respectively. The difference was less with bone metastases (success rates of 90%, 84%, and 80%, respectively) but evident in persons without bone metastases (success rates of 87%, 90%, and 61%, respectively).

More adverse renal events occurred in the zoledronic acid than in the pamidronate group, although the incidence of elevated creatinine levels was low (5.2% in the 8-mg zoledronic acid group). The recommended dose for cancer-induced hypercalcemia is 4 mg.[18] The dose of 8 mg is no longer recommended in any condition, and to avoid renal toxicity the infusion time cannot be less than 15 minutes.

OTHER DRUGS FOR HYPERCALCEMIA

Corticosteroids are recommended only for steroid-responsive tumors (i.e., lymphoma and myeloma), for which doses vary from 40 to 100 mg of prednisone daily. Intravenous phosphate has no place in the management of hypercalcemia because of the risk of extraskeletal calcium precipitation and renal insufficiency. Calcitonin is a natural antiosteoclastic hormone whose main advantages are rapid onset of action and negligible toxicity. It is generally administered subcutaneously or intramuscularly. Calcito-

---

TABLE 143-1 Equivalent Doses of Intravenous Bisphosphonates in Moderate or Severe Hypercalcemia of Malignancy (Ca ≥ 12 mg/dL)

DRUG	COMMERCIAL NAMES	DOSE (mg)	SUCCESS RATE (%)	REFERENCE
Clodronate	Bonefos, Clastoban, Ostac	1500	50-70	9, 10
Pamidronate	Aredia or generic	90	70	16
Ibandronate	Bondronat	6	77	17
Zoledronic acid	Zometa	4	87	16
		8	88	16

Adapted from Body JJ: Hypercalcemia of malignancy. Semin Nephrol 2004;24:48-54.

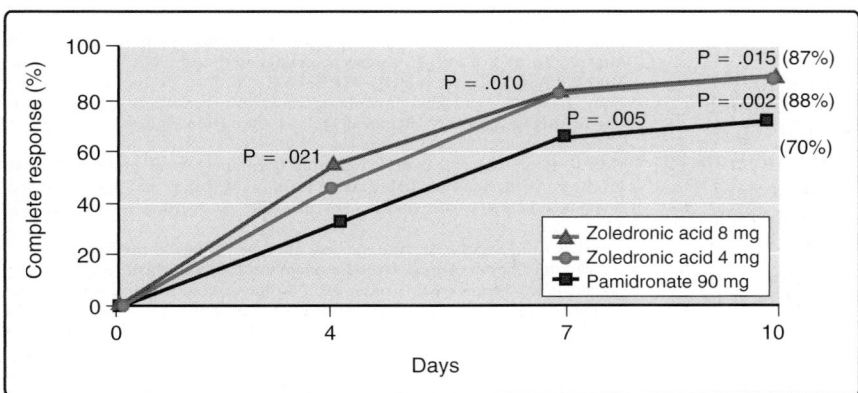

FIGURE 143-1 Comparative efficacy between zoledronic acid (4 or 8 mg) and pamidronate in 275 evaluable patients with moderate or severe tumor-induced hypercalcemia. Complete response rate was defined as normalization of corrected serum calcium to 10.8 mg/dL or lower (≥2.7 mmol/L). *(From Major P, Lortholary A, Hon J, et al. Zoledronic acid is superior to pamidronate in the treatment of hypercalcemia of malignancy: A pooled analysis of two randomized, controlled clinical trials. J Clin Oncol 2001;19:558-567.)*

nin also exerts a calciuretic effect that contributes to its hypocalcemic activity. Recommended doses vary, and a dose-response relationship has not been demonstrated. The efficacy of calcitonin is variable, partial, and transient. Serum Ca levels usually rise after a few days, and there is no further response to increased doses. Salmon calcitonin can still be recommended for 2 to 4 days at 200 to 400 IU/day for severe or life-threatening hypercalcemia because the Ca-lowering effects of bisphosphonates take 1 or 2 days (see Chapter 228). Plicamycin (or mithramycin) is another antiosteoclastic agent, but its use is limited by major toxicities, particularly when given repeatedly, and it should no longer be administered.

THE CHALLENGE OF RENAL INSUFFICIENCY

Bisphosphonates are potentially nephrotoxic, though variably.[19] There are few recommendations for treatment in patients with renal insufficiency, a classic complication of hypercalcemia.[1] A full bisphosphonate dose can be administered safely to such patients, but repeated therapy for metastatic bone disease requires a longer interval between dosing or lower doses. Improved renal function is often seen in patients with severe hypercalcemia and secondary renal failure. Pharmacokinetic data suggest that a reduction in the pamidronate dose should not be necessary in renally impaired patients.[20] In the large, previously mentioned trial that compared pamidronate and zoledronic acid, patients were excluded if their baseline serum creatinine was above 4.5 mg/dL (or 400 mmol/L), and kidney side effects seemed to be similar with both drugs.[18] Postmarketing data suggest that zoledronic acid occasionally induces acute tubular necrosis, and thus caution should be the rule, especially if myeloma is the underlying neoplasm. Current labeling guidelines recommend that zoledronic acid not be administered if creatinine clearance is less than 30 mL/min. Ibandronate is an attractive alternative because it is not nephrotoxic at the doses tested, and even loading-dose therapy does not appear to be nephrotoxic.[21] Based on ibandronate pharmacokinetics, it is recommended that the dose be reduced to 2 mg when creatinine clearance is less than 30 mL/min. Whatever the choice, attention has to be paid to the duration of bisphosphonate infusion when treating hypercalcemia with renal insufficiency.

PREVENTION OF TUMOR-INDUCED HYPERCALCEMIA

Bisphosphonates represent a major therapeutic advance for the supportive care of bone metastases (see Chapter 222). Placebo-controlled trials have established that when administered chronically by the oral route (clodronate and ibandronate) or intravenously (pamidronate, ibandronate, and zoledronic acid), bisphosphonates reduce complications linked to bone metastases by 25% to 40% in breast cancer metastatic to the skeleton.[2] In breast cancer it is recommended that treatment with bisphosphonates be initiated once osteolytic disease occurs. Because osteolysis plays a key role in progression of myeloma, it is advisable to begin bisphosphonate therapy once stage III

| **Current Controversies and Future Considerations** |

- New inhibitors of bone resorption such as an antiserum against RANKL may play a key role not only in tumor-induced hypercalcemia but also in the treatment and prevention of tumor-induced osteolysis. In two animal models of humoral hypercalcemia, the speed and duration of suppression of hypercalcemia were significantly greater with OPG than with high-dose bisphosphonates.[23] Blockade of the RANK/RANKL system could produce greater clinical efficacy than achieved with the bisphosphonates, with fewer side effects. A fully human antibody against RANKL, called denosumab, dramatically inhibits bone resorption in breast cancer with bone metastases and in myeloma.[24] The effects appear to be greater and longer in duration with denosumab than with the bisphosphonates. Comparative phase III trials between zoledronic acid and denosumab continue.
- Anti-PHRP antibodies could theoretically counteract the effects of PHRP on bone resorption and, importantly for tumor-induced hypercalcemia, counteract PHRP-induced renal Ca reabsorption. Such antibodies could be particularly useful in refractory tumor-induced hypercalcemia, the prognosis of which is currently poor.[15] They are in preclinical development.
- In patients with bone metastases undergoing prolonged bisphosphonate therapy, especially breast cancer, the development of hypercalcemia is most often an ominous sign. It often reflects resistance to bisphosphonates or the development of a major humoral component and is a difficult therapeutic challenge for which new drugs are urgently needed.

---

myeloma is diagnosed and to maintain treatment until remission. Zoledronic acid is the first bisphosphonate to have demonstrated clinically significant efficacy versus placebo in metastatic prostate cancer and other solid tumors. Bisphosphonates are thus considered in virtually all patients with metastatic bone disease to reduce bone complications.

In trials using either clodronate or pamidronate, it is estimated that the incidence of hypercalcemia was reduced by a weighted mean average of 63% in breast cancer and 37% in myeloma. These figures are higher than the reduction in frequency of other skeletal-related events[22] and are probably greater with newer, more potent bisphosphonates.

REFERENCES

1. Body JJ. Hypercalcemia of malignancy. Semin Nephrol 2004;24:48-54.
2. Body JJ. Breast cancer: Bisphosphonate therapy for metastatic bone disease. Clin Cancer Res 2006;12:6258-6263.
3. Singer F, Ritch P, Lad T, et al. Treatment of hypercalcemia of malignancy with intravenous etidronate. A controlled, multicenter study. The Hypercalcemia Study Group. Arch Intern Med 1991;151:471-476.
4. Body JJ, Delmas PD. Urinary pyridinium cross-links as markers of bone resorption in tumor-associated hypercalcemia. J Clin Endocrinol Metab 1992;74:471-475.
5. Grill V, Ho P, Body JJ, et al. Parathyroid hormone–related protein: Elevated levels in both humoral hypercalcemia of malignancy and hypercalcemia complicating metastatic breast cancer. J Clin Endocrinol Metab 1991;73:1309-1315.
6. Dunstan CR. Osteoprotegerin and osteoprotegerin ligand mediate the local regulation of bone resorption. Endocrinologist 2000;10:18-26.
7. Luckman SP, Hughes DE, Coxon FP. Nitrogen-containing bisphosphonates inhibit the mevalonate pathway and prevent post-translational prenylation of GTP-binding proteins, including ras. J Bone Miner Res 1998;13:581-589.
8. Fromigué O, Kheddoumi N, Body JJ. Bisphosphonates antagonize bone growth factors' effects on human breast cancer cells survival. Br J Cancer 2003;89:178-184.

9. Shah S, Hardy J, Rees E, et al. Is there a dose response relationship for clodronate in the treatment of tumour induced hypercalcaemia? Br J Cancer 2002;86:1235-1237.
10. Purohit O, Radstone C, Anthony C, et al. A randomised double-blind comparison of intravenous pamidronate and clodronate in the hypercalcaemia of malignancy. Br J Cancer 1995;72:1289-1293.
11. Walker P, Watanabe S, Lawlor P, et al. Subcutaneous clodronate: A study evaluating efficacy in hypercalcemia of malignancy and local toxicity. Ann Oncol 1997;8:915-916.
12. Body JJ. Bisphosphonates in oncology: Focus on clinical experience with pamidronate. Am J Cancer 2005;4:293-305.
13. Body JJ, Dumon JC. Treatment of tumour-induced hypercalcaemia with the bisphosphonate pamidronate: Dose-response relationship and influence of tumour type. Ann Oncol 1994;5:359-363.
14. Rizzoli R, Thiebaud D, Bundred N, et al. Serum parathyroid hormone–related protein levels and response to bisphosphonate treatment in hypercalcemia of malignancy. J Clin Endocrinol Metab 1999;84:3545-3550.
15. Body JJ, Louviaux I, Dumon JC. Decreased efficacy of bisphosphonates for recurrences of tumor-induced hypercalcemia. Support Care Cancer 2000;8:398-404.
16. Major P, Lortholary A, Hon J, et al. Zoledronic acid is superior to pamidronate in the treatment of hypercalcemia of malignancy: A pooled analysis of two randomized, controlled clinical trials. J Clin Oncol 2001;19:558-567.
17. Ralston SH, Thiebaud D, Herrmann Z, et al. Dose-response study of ibandronate in the treatment of cancer-associated hypercalcemia. Br J Cancer 1997;75:295-300.
18. Pecherstorfer M, Steinhauer E, Rizzoli R, et al. Efficacy and safety of ibandronate in the treatment of hypercalcemia of malignancy: A randomized multicentric comparison to pamidronate. Support Care Cancer 2003;11:539-547.
19. Body JJ. Bisphosphonates for malignancy-related bone disease: Current status, future developments. Support Care Cancer 2006;14:408-418.
20. Berenson JR, Rosen L, Vescio R, et al. Pharmacokinetics of pamidronate disodium in patients with cancer with normal or impaired renal function. J Clin Pharmacol 1997;37:285-290.
21. Body JJ, Diel IJ, Tripathy D, Bergström B. Intravenous ibandronate does not affect time to renal function deterioration in patients with skeletal metastases from breast cancer: Phase III trial results. Eur J Cancer Care 2006;15:299-330.
22. McCloskey EV, Guest JF, Kanis JA. The clinical and cost considerations of bisphosphonates in preventing bone complications in patients with metastatic breast cancer or multiple myeloma. Drugs 2001;61:1253-1274.
23. Morony S, Warmington K, Adamu S, et al. The inhibition of RANKL causes greater suppression of bone resorption and hypercalcemia compared with bisphosphonates in two models of humoral hypercalcemia of malignancy. Endocrinology 2005;146:3235-3243.
24. Body JJ, Facon T, Coleman RE, et al. A study of the biologic receptor activator of nuclear factor-κB ligand inhibitor, denosumab, in patients with multiple myeloma or bone metastases from breast cancer. Clin Cancer Res 2006;12:1221-1228.

SUGGESTED READING

Body JJ, Coleman R, Clezardin P, et al. International Society of Geriatric Oncology (SIOG) clinical practice recommendations for the use of bisphosphonates in elderly patients. Eur J Cancer 2007;43:852-858.

Fidler IJ. The pathogenesis of cancer metastasis: The 'seed and soil' hypothesis revisited. Nat Rev Cancer 2003;3:453-458.

Hillner BE, Ingle JN, Chlebowski RT, et al. American Society of Clinical Oncology 2003 update on the role of bisphosphonates and bone health issues in women with breast cancer. J Clin Oncol 2003;21:4042-4057.

Plunkett TA, Smith P, Rubens RD. Risk of complications from bone metastases in breast cancer. Implications for management. Eur J Cancer 2000;36:476-482.

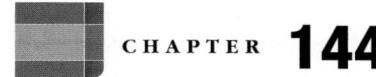

CHAPTER **144**

Antiemetic Drugs

David Dunwoodie and Paul Glare

K E Y   P O I N T S

- Nausea and vomiting are common and distressing symptoms. Thorough knowledge of the pharmacology of antiemetics, including an understanding of the emetic pathway, the neurotransmitters involved, and the mechanism of action of the different drugs, is an important part of the knowledge base of palliative care specialists.

- The main antiemetics in palliative care include prokinetic agents, dopamine antagonists, antihistamines, and corticosteroids.

- Novel agents include the cannabinoids and olanzapine.

Nausea and vomiting are common and distressing symptoms in life-limiting illnesses, so thorough knowledge of the pharmacology of antiemetics is important (see Chapter 169). Antiemetics for chemotherapy-induced emesis, such as serotonin antagonists and aprepitant, are of limited relevance to palliative care but are included here because some patients may still be undergoing chemotherapy and taking these drugs (Table 144-1). Pharmacokinetic parameters are listed in Table 144-2.

APREPITANT

Aprepitant is a selective high-affinity antagonist at human substance P neurokinin-1 receptors. It crosses the blood-brain barrier in humans to competitively bind the brain neurokinin receptor and block the effect of the natural ligand substance P in the central nervous system (CNS). Aprepitant shows little or no affinity for serotonin, dopamine, and corticosteroid receptors. It is used for the prevention of acute and delayed nausea and vomiting associated with highly and moderately emetogenic cancer chemotherapy (in combination with a serotonin 5-HT$_3$ receptor antagonist and a corticosteroid), as well as the prevention of postoperative nausea and vomiting.

Aprepitant undergoes extensive hepatic metabolism (Table 144-3), mainly via oxidation by the cytochrome P-450 isoenzyme CYP3A4 and, to a less extent, by the isoenzymes CYP1A2 and CYP2C19. It is not renally excreted.

Dose

On day 1 of chemotherapy, 125 mg is administered orally 1 hour before treatment. On days 2 and 3, the dose is

80 mg in the morning. Dosage adjustment is not required in patients with severe renal insufficiency or in those with end-stage renal disease during hemodialysis.[1] No dosage adjustment is required for mild to moderate hepatic impairment. No clinical or pharmacokinetic data are available for patients with severe hepatic insufficiency.

TABLE 144-1 Classification of Antiemetics

Prokinetics
  Metoclopramide
  Domperidone
  Cisapride
Phenothiazines
  Prochlorperazine
  Chlorpromazine
  Levomepromazine
Butyrophenones
  Haloperidol
Atypical antipsychotics
  Olanzapine
Anticholinergics
  Hyoscine butylbromide
  Hyoscine hydrobromide
Antihistamines
  Promethazine
  Cyclizine
Corticosteroids
  Dexamethasone
Benzodiazepines
  Lorazepam
5-HT$_3$ antagonists
  Ondansetron
  Granisetron
  Tropisetron
Neurokinin-1 receptor antagonists
  Aprepitant
Cannabinoids
  Nabilone
  Dronabinol
Somatostatin analogues
  Octreotide

Side Effects

The more common side effects include headache, dizziness, fatigue, constipation, diarrhea, dyspepsia, anorexia, hiccups, and eructation. Elevations in liver transaminases may occur but are usually mild and transient.

Contraindications

Contraindications include hypersensitivity to aprepitant and concomitant use of pimozide, terfenadine, astemizole, and cisapride.

Drug Interactions

Aprepitant should not be administered concurrently with pimozide, terfenadine, astemizole, or cisapride because inhibition of CYP3A4 could increase plasma concentrations of these drugs, with potentially life-threatening reactions. Concurrent administration with other drugs metabolized by CYP3A4, such as midazolam and alprazolam, may increase concentrations of these drugs. Dexamethasone is also a CYP3A4 substrate, and the manufacturer recommends reducing its dose by 50% when coadministered with aprepitant.

CHLORPROMAZINE

Chlorpromazine is a phenothiazine derivative with D$_2$, histaminic, α-adrenergic, and muscarinic receptor antagonist properties. Although both chlorpromazine and levomepromazine have broad-spectrum receptor affinity, some recommend levomepromazine over chlorpromazine because of its potent 5-HT$_2$ receptor antagonism. Phenothiazines exert their antiemetic effect primarily at the chemoreceptor trigger zone, proportionate to their antidopaminergic activity, with chlorpromazine having modest antiemetic activity. As low-potency antipsychotics, phenothiazines are more likely to cause sedation and antimuscarinic or α-adrenergic blocking effects than high-potency antipsychotics such as haloperidol are, which are more likely to cause extrapyramidal effects. There is considerable interindividual variability in oral bioavailability.[2] Chlorpromazine is extensively metabolized in the liver, with excretion in urine and bile as various active and inactive metabolites.

TABLE 144-2 Receptor Site Affinities of Commonly Used Antiemetics

DRUG	DOPAMINE ANTAGONIST	HISTAMINE ANTAGONIST	ACETYLCHOLINE ANTAGONIST	5-HT$_2$ ANTAGONIST	5-HT$_3$ ANTAGONIST	5-HT$_4$ AGONIST
Metoclopramide	++				+	++
Domperidone	++					++
Cisapride						+++
Prochlorperazine	++	+				
Levomepromazine	++	+++	++	+++		
Haloperidol	+++					
Hyoscine			+++			
Cyclizine		++	++			
Ondansetron					+++	

From Woodruff R. Palliative Medicine: Evidence Based Symptomatic and Supportive Care for Patients with Advanced Cancer, 4th ed. Melbourne, Australia, Oxford University Press, 2004.

TABLE 144-3 Pharmacokinetics of Antiemetic Drugs

DRUG	BIOAVAILABILITY (%)	ONSET (hr)	T$_{MAX}$ (hr)	T$_{\frac{1}{2}}$ (hr)	DURATION (hr)
Aprepitant	60-65		4	9-13	
Chlorpromazine	10-69[a]		PO: 2-4 IM: 0.5-1	8-35[a]	>24
Cisapride	35-40[b]	0.5-1	1-2	7-10	12-16
Cyclizine		<2	2		4-6[c]
Dexamethasone	61-86	8-24	1-2	4	36-54
Domperidone	13-17[b]	0.5	0.5	7.5-16[d]	8-16
Haloperidol	60-65	PO: >1 SC: 0.15-0.25	PO: 1.7-6 IM: 0.3-0.5	14-36	
Hyoscine butylbromide	8-10	1-2		5-6	
Hyoscine hydrobromide	N/a	SL: 0.15-0.25 SC: 0.25-0.5	0.15-0.5	5-6	0.25-10[e]
Levomepromazine	50	0.5	IM 0.5-1.5 PO: 1-3	15-30	12-24
Lorazepam	>90	SL: 0.1 PO: 0.2-0.25	SL: 1 PO: 2	12-25	6-8[f]
Metoclopramide	32-100[a]	IV: 0.01-0.05 IM: 0.15-0.25 PO: 0.5-1	<1	4-6[d]	1-2
Nabilone	85-95	1-1.5	2	2	8-12
Octreotide	N/A	?	<0.5	1.5	8-12
Olanzapine	60-80		PP: 5-8 IM: 0.25-0.75	21-54[g]	
Prochlorperazine	12.5		1.5-5	6.8-9	
Promethazine	25[h]		PO: 2-3	10-14	4-12
Serotonin antagonists					
Dolasetron	76[i]		IV: 0.6 PO: 1.4	6.6-8.8	
Granisetron	60		PO: 2	10-12[j]	
Ondansetron	60-70		IV: 0.1 PO: 0.5-2	2.5-5.4	
Palonostetron	N/A			40	
Tropisetron	60-100	PO: 1-1.3		8-40[k]	

[a]Chlorpromazine, metoclopramide: Large interindividual variation in bioavailability.
[b]Cisapride, domperidone: Food increases bioavailability.
[c]Cyclizine: Duration of action may be longer in some patients.
[d]Domperidone, metoclopramide: Half-life prolonged in renal failure.
[e]Haloperidol: Duration of action, 15 minutes for antispasmodic effect, 1 to 9 hours for antisecretory effect.
[f]Lorazepam: Duration of action does not correlate with plasma concentrations and can be up to 3 days in some patients.
[g]Olanzapine: Interindividual variability in clearance (higher in smokers, men).
[h]Promethazine: Bioavailability similar for oral and rectal administration.
[i]Dolasetron: Rapidly converted to the active metabolite hydrodolasetron, which has a bioavailability of 76%.
[j]Granisteron: Variable half-life—3 to 4 hours in the healthy, 10 to 12 hours in cancer patients.
[k]Tropisetron: Half-life variable because of CYP2D6 polymorphism, approximately 8 hours in extensive metabolizers and 30 to 40 hours in poor metabolizers.
IM, intramuscularly; IV, intravenously; PO, orally; PP, postprandially; SC, subcutaneously; SL, sublingually.

Dose

For nausea and vomiting, the usual doses are 10 to 25 mg every 4 to 6 hours orally or 25 to 50 mg every 3 to 4 hours intramuscularly. Dose reduction should be considered in patients with liver dysfunction and the elderly. In syringe drivers, chlorpromazine is usually compatible with diphenhydramine, glycopyrrolate, hydromorphone, metoclopramide, midazolam, and promethazine and usually incompatible with dexamethasone. Data are conflicting regarding compatibility with haloperidol and morphine.

Major Side Effects

Common side effects include confusion, sedation, dizziness, respiratory depression, extrapyramidal reactions,

hyperglycemia, and anticholinergic effects. Tolerance to the sedative effects occurs quickly. Other serious side effects include abnormalities in thermoregulation and neuroleptic malignant syndrome. Chlorpromazine may cause pain and irritation at the injection site, and nodule formation may occur after intramuscular administration.[6] It should be used with caution in patients with renal failure and small doses administered initially because cerebral sensitivity to antipsychotics may be increased in those with severe renal impairment. Chlorpromazine should be used with caution in people with a history of seizures because it lowers the seizure threshold.

Contraindications and Precautions

Contraindications include bone marrow depression, pheochromocytoma, hepatic failure, and known phenothiazine hypersensitivity. Precautions include prolonged use and abrupt withdrawal, epilepsy, susceptibility to anticholinergic effects, hypotension, and renal and hepatic impairment.

Drug Interactions

Most interactions with antipsychotics result from additive pharmacological effects with drugs that have similar pharmacological action, and because tolerance develops to many of these drugs, interactions are probably most important early in combination therapy. There is an increased risk for arrhythmia when antipsychotics are used with other drugs that prolong the QT interval. Chlorpromazine may cause hyperglycemia and impair glucose tolerance. It increases the miotic and sedative actions of morphine, may increase its analgesic action, and can be expected to increase the respiratory depressant actions of opioids.

CISAPRIDE

This prokinetic agent is indicated for nausea and vomiting with delayed gastric emptying unresponsive to other prokinetics and for nausea caused by selective serotonin reuptake inhibitors (SSRIs) and venlafaxine. Its antiemetic activity occurs via 5-HT$_4$ receptor agonism. Cisapride is related to metoclopramide, but it is a more potent prokinetic and increases motility of the entire gastrointestinal tract. It does not have dopamine antagonist activity. Cisapride increases release of acetylcholine in the myenteric plexus of the gut by stimulating 5-HT$_4$ receptors, which results in an increase in lower esophageal tone, accelerated gastric emptying, and increased intestinal motility. It has been withdrawn from the market because of cardiac toxicity but is still available in some countries under special access schemes. Cisapride is metabolized by CYP3A4. Use with drugs that significantly inhibit this enzyme is contraindicated because it may increase plasma concentrations of cisapride. The time to peak plasma concentration of cisapride is 1 to 2 hours, its half-life is 7 to 10 hours, and its duration of action is 12 to 16 hours.[3] Ten percent is excreted unchanged in urine.

Dose

For gastroparesis, the dosage of cisapride is 10 mg four times per day, with an increase up to 20 mg three times daily. For nausea from SSRIs, 5 mg twice daily is used. If colic or diarrhea occur, the dose should be reduced and consideration given to administering it more frequently. Cisapride should be used with caution and in reduced doses in patients with hepatic impairment. It is contraindicated in renal failure. Available preparations are 10-mg tablets and 1-mg/mL oral suspension.

Adverse Effects

The most common side effects are abdominal cramps, diarrhea, constipation, nausea, and headache. Reports of ventricular arrhythmia and QT prolongation have led to restrictions on access.

Contraindications

Cisapride is contraindicated in patients with risk factors for arrhythmia, including electrolyte disturbance, cardiac disease, renal failure, and medications that prolong the QT interval or inhibit CYP3A4. Other precautions include gastrointestinal obstruction, hemorrhage, perforation, or use immediately after surgery.

Drug Interactions

The most significant pharmacokinetic interactions involve inhibition of CYP3A4, the main route of elimination of cisapride, which results in increased plasma concentrations of cisapride and a greater risk of prolongation of the QT interval and ventricular arrhythmias.

The following drugs should not be administered concomitantly:

Macrolide antibacterials—clarithromycin, erythromycin
Azole antifungal agents—fluconazole (risk is small), itraconazole, ketoconazole
Antidepressants—nefazodone, fluvoxamine, fluoxetine
Antiretrovirals—all protease inhibitors
Others—amiodarone, cimetidine, diltiazem, verapamil, grapefruit juice, isoniazid, metronidazole, quinine

Pharmacodynamic interactions with several drugs, including various antiarrhythmics (class 1a and 3), haloperidol, phenothiazines, and tricyclic antidepressants, may further prolong the QT interval. Cisapride may increase morphine absorption and alter the absorption of other drugs.

CYCLIZINE

Cyclizine is a piperazine derivative with antihistaminic and anticholinergic properties that is used for nausea and vomiting associated with vestibular causes, raised intracranial pressure, bowel obstruction and pharyngeal stimulation, and drug-induced nausea (including opioids). Antihistamines exert their effect on the vomiting center. There is said to be no correlation between efficacy in motion sickness and antihistamine potency. Cyclizine also exerts central anticholinergic action and may have direct effects on the labyrinth and the chemoreceptor trigger zone. It is metabolized in the liver to the relatively inactive metabolite norcyclizine. Both cyclizine and norcyclizine have plasma elimination half-lives of 20 hours. Less than 1% of the oral dose is eliminated in urine in 24 hours. Subcutaneous use is unlicensed, but well tolerated, with local discomfort in 1% and erythema in 5%.[4] Local pruritus may also occur.

Doses

50 to 100 mg orally two to three times daily or 12.5 to 50 mg subcutaneously every 12 hours, with titration up to 300 mg in three divided doses, *or*
100 to 300 mg via continuous subcutaneous infusion. In syringe drivers, cyclizine may be mixed with morphine and haloperidol but is not compatible with saline.[5]

Adverse Effects

Drowsiness is typical of antihistamines, although the sedative effects of cyclizine are not marked. Excitation, insomnia, and anticholinergic effects may occur. Other less common effects include arrhythmia, hallucinations, and dystonic reactions. Cyclizine may aggravate severe heart failure and should be avoided in patients with acute myocardial infarction or severe heart failure.[5]

Contraindications

Hypersensitivity to cyclizine is a contraindication. Precautions include cardiac failure, glaucoma, bladder outlet obstruction, and chronic airflow limitation.

DEXAMETHASONE

Dexamethasone is a glucocorticoid used for nausea and vomiting and various other indications (e.g., cerebral edema, spinal cord compression, anorexia, and fatigue) in patients with life-limiting illness. It has potent glucocorticoid but minimal mineralocorticoid activity. Its mechanism of action in nausea and emesis is unknown. Several mechanisms may be operative, including reducing blood-brain barrier permeability to chemicals such as chemotherapeutic agents, depleting γ-aminobutyric acid (GABA) in the medulla, and reducing release of leu-enkephalin in the brainstem. A reduction in tumor mass as a result of the anti-inflammatory effects reducing the stimulus to emesis from peripheral autonomic stretch receptors and intracranial tumors may also contribute. Corticosteroids are metabolized mainly in the liver and excreted in urine. Apart from hydrocortisone, corticosteroids should be given once daily to minimize insomnia and maximize compliance (Table 144-4).

Doses

As an antiemetic, the dose of dexamethasone is 4 to 20 mg daily. No dose adjustment is required for renal impairment. In syringe drivers, dexamethasone is compatible with metoclopramide, morphine, and ondansetron, usually compatible with hydromorphone and glycopyrrolate, but incompatible with midazolam.

Adverse Effects

Adverse effects of dexamethasone are many and include endocrine (diabetes mellitus, hypothalamic-pituitary-adrenal axis insufficiency), psychiatric (psychoses, depression, euphoria, insomnia), musculoskeletal (osteoporosis, myopathy), gastroenterological (gastritis, peptic ulcer disease), infection (*Candida*, risk of infection, masking of sepsis), renal (hypokalemia, sodium and water retention), cardiovascular (edema, hypertension), skin and soft tissue (sweating, purpura, facial plethora, acne, striae, impaired wound healing, moon face), ocular (cataracts), and hematological (neutrophilia) effects.

Adverse reactions result from prolonged high doses or withdrawal. Adverse effects in general occur equally with all systemic corticosteroids, and the incidence increases with supraphysiological doses (approximately 7.5 mg prednisolone, 1 mg dexamethasone). Their use in patients with peptic ulcers is controversial,[7] but peptic ulceration should not be considered a contraindication. Use with nonsteroidal anti-inflammatory agents, total prednisolone doses of 10 mg equivalent or more, treatment longer than 30 days, and a history of peptic ulcer disease appear to increase the risk for peptic ulceration, and prophylactic therapy should be considered.

Patients with steroid-induced myopathy report weakness without tenderness or myalgias. There is variability in the onset of symptoms, with myopathy occurring more rapidly at higher doses. Fluorinated steroids (e.g., dexamethasone) are more likely than nonfluorinated steroids (e.g., prednisolone) to cause myopathy, and some suggest changing to a nonfluorinated steroid if myopathy develops.[8] The smallest possible dose should be used for the shortest possible period, with cessation as soon as it is apparent that it is ineffective.

Several serious psychiatric syndromes can occur with corticosteroids, including mood disorders, psychoses, and delirium. Symptoms appear to be dose related and usually develop in the first weeks of therapy. Psychiatric symptoms can occur in anyone, with no evidence that previous psychiatric disorders predispose to symptoms. Ninety percent of symptoms will be reversed with cessation of steroids, but they may recur with retreatment. Patients should be advised of the dangers of sudden cessation of steroids. Corticosteroid withdrawal or dose reduction should be considered when the maximal effect has been obtained, an adequate trial (approximately 7 to 10 days) has failed to achieve the desired effect, or side effects occur. Withdrawal can be immediate or tapered, with abrupt withdrawal being appropriate if treatment lasted less than 3 weeks and symptoms are unlikely to recur.[9]

Contraindications and Precautions

Contraindications include uncontrolled infections and known hypersensitivity to dexamethasone. Precautions include infection, diabetes, heart failure, previous peptic ulceration, psychoses, and severe affective disorder.

TABLE 144-4	Comparison of Commonly Used Corticosteroids				
DRUG	ANTI-INFLAMMATORY POTENCY	SALT RETENTION	EQUIVALENT DOSES	DURATION OF ACTION	DAILY DOSE AT WHICH ADRENAL SUPPRESSION MAY OCCUR
Hydrocortisone	1	1	20	8-12	15-30
Prednisolone	4	0.25	5	12-36	7.5-10
Dexamethasone	25	<0.01	0.5-1	36-54	1

Modified from Twycross R, Wilcock A, Charlesworth S, Dickman A. Palliative Care Formulary, 2nd ed. Oxford, Radcliffe, 2002.

Drug Interactions

Carbamazepine, phenytoin, phenobarbital, and rifampicin accelerate corticosteroid metabolism. Dexamethasone may either increase or decrease phenytoin levels. There is an increased risk for hypokalemia if taken with β_2-agonists, diuretics, and amphotericin B. The glucocorticoid effects of dexamethasone antagonize both oral hypoglycemic agents and insulin.

DOMPERIDONE

Domperidone is a benzimidazole derivative, prokinetic antiemetic that is indicated when a prokinetic effect is required with a low risk of extrapyramidal effects.[10] Its uses include nausea and vomiting from chemotherapy, antiparkinsonian medication, gastroparesis, and gastroesophageal reflux. Domperidone does not readily cross the blood-brain barrier, and its effects are due to peripheral dopamine receptor antagonism. It exerts its prokinetic effect by antagonizing the inhibitory effects of dopamine on the gastrointestinal tract (releasing the "dopamine brake"). The prokinetic effect is limited to the esophagus, stomach, and duodenum and can be blocked by antimuscarinics. Like metoclopramide, domperidone increases basal lower esophageal sphincter pressure, relaxes the pyloric sphincter, and stimulates and coordinates gastroduodenal motility. The area postrema is outside the blood-brain barrier, and domperidone can therefore antagonize dopamine-mediated activation of the chemoreceptor trigger zone.

Domperidone undergoes extensive first-pass metabolism in the gut wall and liver, with low oral bioavailability. It has no active metabolites and renal clearance is minimal. Use is limited by lack of parenteral formulations.

Doses

For delayed gastric emptying, 10 to 20 mg is taken 15 to 30 minutes before meals three or four times daily. For nausea and vomiting in parkinsonism, up to 20 mg may be taken every 4 to 8 hours. Doses may need to be reduced in patients with liver dysfunction because of extensive hepatic metabolism. Renal clearance is a minor route of elimination, so the drug would not be expected to accumulate in patients with renal failure.[10]

Adverse Reactions

Extrapyramidal side effects are rare with the recommended doses. Headache, somnolence, diarrhea, and abdominal pain have been reported.

Contraindications and Precautions

Contraindications include prolactin-releasing tumors, people in whom stimulation of gastrointestinal motility may be dangerous (e.g., bowel obstruction, perforation, or hemorrhage), administration with oral ketoconazole, and hypersensitivity to domperidone.

Drug Interactions

Concomitant administration with H_2 receptor antagonists, proton pump inhibitors, or high-dose antacids may reduce absorption. Administration should be separated by 2 hours. Combined use with anticholinergic drugs may interfere with gastrointestinal effects.

HALOPERIDOL

This butyrophenone antipsychotic is used for nausea and vomiting secondary to chemical or toxic causes (e.g., hypercalcemia; drug toxicity, including morphine; renal failure), after radiotherapy, and associated with bowel obstruction. Its other palliative uses include hyperactive delirium and hiccups. As a typical antipsychotic, haloperidol is a potent and competitive blocker of postsynaptic dopamine (D_2) receptors, with effects at the area postrema chemoreceptor trigger zone. Unlike the phenothiazines chlorpromazine and levomepromazine, it is less likely to cause sedation or hypotension but more likely to cause extrapyramidal side effects. Haloperidol has large interindividual variability in its pharmacokinetics.[11] It is extensively metabolized in the liver, with approximately 1% excreted unchanged in urine.[11]

Dose

Antiemetic doses are lower than antipsychotic doses and can be given once daily. The usual doses are 0.5 to 2.5 mg twice daily or 1 to 5 mg per 24 hours via syringe driver. Lower doses should be used in the elderly or frail. If doses of 10 mg daily are ineffective, consideration should be given to an alternative antiemetic. In syringe drivers, haloperidol is incompatible with diphenhydramine and prochlorperazine but compatible with morphine and cyclizine.

Adverse Effects

Extrapyramidal effects such as akathisia, dystonia, and parkinsonism are common. Other side effects of haloperidol include neuroleptic malignant syndrome, QT prolongation, sedation, orthostatic hypotension, abnormal liver function test results, and constipation.

Contraindications and Precautions

Haloperidol is contraindicated in patients with Parkinson's disease and other extrapyramidal disorders, prolactin-secreting tumors, and previous hypersensitivity to haloperidol. Precautions include a history of seizures (haloperidol may lower the seizure threshold), severe cardiovascular disease and QT prolongation, prolonged use, and renal or hepatic impairment.

Drug Interactions

Concomitant use of haloperidol with antiarrhythmics and other drugs known to prolong the QT interval may have additive cardiac effects. Haloperidol directly opposes the antiparkinsonian effects of levodopa and long-acting dopamine receptor agonists such as cabergoline. Concomitant use with tramadol may increase the risk for seizures. Haloperidol inhibits the metabolism of tricyclic antidepressants, which may lead to anticholinergic side effects.

HYOSCINE

Hyoscine is an antimuscarinic agent used for nausea associated with movement and bowel obstruction. Other uses in palliative care include reduction of oral and airway secretions and relief of intestinal colic. Hyoscine competitively inhibits muscarinic receptors and impairs ganglionic neural transmission, thereby resulting in decreased tone and peristalsis of gut smooth muscle and a reduction in mucosal secretory activity. It is available in two salts—hydrobromide and butylbromide. Hyoscine butylbromide is a tertiary amine that does not cross the blood-brain barrier and thus does not cause sedation or have a centrally mediated antiemetic effect. The hydrobromide form is a quaternary ammonium derivative that crosses the blood-brain barrier and may cause sedation. The duration of its antisecretory effect is highly variable. Hyoscine blocks the cholinergic pathway mediating the effect of prokinetic drugs, so this combination should be avoided.

Dose

Hyoscine hydrobromide is administered at 0.4 to 0.6 mg every 4 to 6 hours or 0.6 to 2.4 mg per 24 hours by continuous subcutaneous infusion. The dosage of hyoscine butylbromide is 20 mg subcutaneously every 4 hours or 80 to 120 mg by continuous subcutaneous infusion. It is compatible in syringe drivers with glycopyrrolate, hydromorphone, metoclopramide, midazolam, morphine, and promethazine.

Adverse Effects

Hyoscine may cause drowsiness at therapeutic doses but may also cause CNS stimulation, particularly in the presence of pain. Adverse CNS effects may be more common in the elderly and those with hepatic or renal impairment and include dizziness, drowsiness, restlessness, tremors, hallucinations, confusion, and acute psychosis or behavioral abnormalities. Other common anticholinergic side effects include hypotension, dry mouth, blurred vision, constipation, and urinary retention.

Contraindications

Patients with narrow-angle glaucoma should not take hyoscine, with caution needed in the elderly and those with a history of seizures or psychosis, impaired liver or renal function, or bladder neck obstruction.

LEVOMEPROMAZINE

Levomepromazine (previously known as methotrimeprazine) is a phenothiazine used for nausea and vomiting, terminal agitation, and pain. It is a dopamine (D_2), α_1-adrenergic, and 5-HT$_2$ receptor antagonist with anticholinergic and antihistaminic (H$_1$) properties. It is not active at the 5-HT$_3$ receptor. When compared with chlorpromazine, another phenothiazine, it has additional analgesic effects but is more sedative and more likely to cause postural hypotension.[13] Levomepromazine is no longer available in the United States. It has broad-spectrum activity and is useful in several settings, often as second-line therapy. Levomepromazine reliably produces dose-related analgesia comparable to that of opioids, with an analgesic potency ratio of approximately 3:2 (levomepromazine to morphine). The analgesic effect may be mediated through its α-adrenergic blocking properties. Some of the drug is excreted unchanged in urine, with most being excreted in urine as glucuronide and sulfoxide conjugates. The activity of these metabolites is unknown.

Dose

The usual antiemetic dose is 6.25 to 25 mg twice daily. Up to 300 mg daily has been given for other indications (e.g., pain, terminal agitation). The manufacturer has no specific dosage recommendations for renal or hepatic dysfunction. It should be administered cautiously to patients with renal or hepatic impairment because it is both metabolized in the liver and excreted in urine.

Adverse Effects

Orthostatic hypotension (dose dependent), sedation, anticholinergic effects, confusion, hallucinations, and dystonic reactions have been reported. Levomepromazine may cause skin irritation if administered subcutaneously.

Contraindications

Levomepromazine is contraindicated in patients with phenothiazine hypersensitivity, severe liver impairment, and blood dyscrasias. Precautions include orthostatic hypotension, concomitant antihypertensive medication, parkinsonism, epilepsy, myasthenia gravis, and severe cardiac or renal disease.

Drug Interactions

Although monoamine oxidase inhibitors (MAOIs) have been used safely with phenothiazines, the use of levomepromazine with MAOIs should be avoided.

LORAZEPAM

Lorazepam is a benzodiazepine with a short to intermediate duration of action that is used for anticipatory nausea because of its anxiolytic and amnestic effects. The exact mechanism of action remains unclear, but perhaps it binds to specific CNS receptors with GABA-potentiating effects. A 0.5-mg dose of lorazepam is about equipotent to 5 mg of diazepam. There are no significant differences in the time to maximum plasma concentration (T$_{max}$) after oral or sublingual administration.[14] Lorazepam is metabolized in the liver to the inactive glucuronide and is excreted both by the kidneys and in bile.

Dose

For anticipatory nausea, 1 to 2 mg is administered orally or sublingually (in addition to standard antiemetics). Up to 6 mg/day may be given for other indications. The effect of liver disease is variable. Dose reduction may be required in patients with mild to moderate hepatic impairment, but use in severe liver disease should be avoided. Lorazepam should be used with caution in patients with renal impairment.

Adverse Effects

The most common side effects include anterograde amnesia, dizziness, sedation, unsteadiness, and weakness. Other important side effects include disorientation, confusion, delirium, rebound insomnia, withdrawal seizures, depression, agitation, dysarthria, sweating, and blurred vision.

Contraindications

Contraindications include glaucoma and hypersensitivity to benzodiazepines. Lorazepam should be used cautiously in those with delirium, sleep apnea, respiratory failure, and renal and hepatic impairment and in elderly or debilitated patients; it carries the potential for abuse, dependence, and complications with abrupt withdrawal.

METOCLOPRAMIDE

Metoclopramide is a prokinetic antiemetic that is used for nausea and vomiting associated with gastric irritation, gastric stasis, incomplete bowel obstruction, chemotherapy, and radiotherapy.[15] It is also used for decreased gastrointestinal motility, gastroesophageal reflux disease, anorexia, and hiccups. It has a complex mechanism of action. In addition to both central and peripheral dopamine antagonist properties, metoclopramide facilitates release of acetylcholine from enteric neurons by antagonism of $5-HT_3$ receptors and activation of $5-HT_4$ receptors. Metoclopramide is a less potent dopamine antagonist than haloperidol and a less potent $5-HT_4$ agonist than cisapride. $5-HT_3$ antagonism occurs only at higher doses (>100 mg subcutaneously daily). Its prokinetic properties result from activation of the gut wall cholinergic system. Antimuscarinics competitively block this action, so they should not be administered together. As a D_2 receptor antagonist, metoclopramide also blocks the dopaminergic "brake" on gastric emptying induced by stress, anxiety, and nausea. Metoclopramide stimulates upper gastrointestinal tract motility, with little effect on colonic and gall bladder motility. It does not stimulate gastric, biliary, or pancreatic secretions. Bioavailability is variable (32–100%).[15] Twenty percent to 30% is excreted unchanged, with about 5% excreted in feces via bile.

Dose

For nausea caused by gastroparesis, 10 mg should be taken 30 minutes before meals and at bedtime, with increases of up to 100 mg daily. For nausea from bowel obstruction, patients should receive 10 mg every 4 to 6 hours or 40 to 60 mg/24 hr by continuous subcutaneous infusion. Metoclopramide is compatible in syringe drivers with dexamethasone, dimenhydrinate, diphenhydramine, hydromorphone, midazolam, morphine, and promethazine. A 50% dose reduction is recommended in patients with severe liver cirrhosis.[16] Clearance is significantly reduced in renal impairment, and therefore dose reductions of at least 50% are recommended in patients with moderate to severe renal impairment.[17]

Adverse Reactions

The most common side effects are restlessness, drowsiness, and fatigue. Other side effects include diarrhea, dizziness, headache, depression, delirium, insomnia, and neuroleptic malignant syndrome. Anxiety and agitation are also reported, especially after rapid injection. Metoclopramide may cause extrapyramidal symptoms, most commonly acute dystonic reactions, which are more common in children and young adults, and many symptoms occur at doses exceeding recommendations. These symptoms generally occur within a few days of starting treatment and resolve within 24 hours of cessation. Parkinsonism occurs rarely, generally during prolonged treatment in elderly patients.

Contraindications

Contraindications include concurrent intravenous administration with $5-HT_3$ antagonists, hypersensitivity to metoclopramide, and pheochromocytoma.[18] Metoclopramide should be used with caution in young adults and children. It should not be used when stimulation of muscular contractions might adversely affect the gut, such as in patients with complete bowel obstruction, gastrointestinal hemorrhage and perforation, or immediately after surgery.

Drug Interactions

Metoclopramide may alter the absorption of orally administered drugs. Absorption of drugs from the small bowel may be accelerated (e.g., paracetamol/acetaminophen), and absorption of drugs from the stomach can potentially be diminished (e.g., digoxin).

NABILONE

Nabilone is a synthetic cannabinoid used for nausea and vomiting caused by moderately emetogenic chemotherapy and unresponsive to conventional antiemetics. It is also used in palliative medicine.[19] Its mechanism of action is not fully understood. Two specific cannabinoid receptors have been isolated, CB1 and CB2, although others may exist. CB1 receptors are found mainly on neurons in the brain, spinal cord, and peripheral nerves, with CB2 receptors predominantly on immune cells.[19] Most cannabinoid effects are mediated through specific agonist or antagonist activity at these receptors, although some may be non–receptor mediated, with the antiemetic effect likely to be partly non–receptor mediated.[19] Its anxiolytic effects may also contribute to overall efficacy, and the antiemetic effect parallels the period of euphoria. Nabilone is extensively metabolized in the liver. The major excretory pathway is the biliary system, with about 65% excreted in feces and about 20% in urine. The long duration of action despite rapid metabolic elimination suggests that some effects are mediated by metabolites, which persist in the plasma for longer than 20 hours.

Dose

The initial dose for adults is 1 mg orally twice daily (increase to 2 mg twice daily if required). Nabilone should be commenced the evening before starting chemotherapy, with the second dose taken 1 to 3 hours before the first dose of chemotherapy and continued until 48 hours after the last chemotherapy dose. The dose of nabilone should not exceed 6 mg daily in three divided doses. Because of extensive metabolism in the liver, nabilone is not recommended in patients with severe hepatic impairment.

Adverse Effects

The most common adverse effects of nabilone are drowsiness and vertigo. Other effects include confusion, disorientation, euphoria, dysphoria, psychosis, hallucination, visual disturbance, depression, sleep disturbance, headache, ataxia, tremors, and dry mouth. Patients should be informed of possible mood changes and other adverse behavioral effects. Nabilone may cause less neuropsychological toxicity than dronabinol. Effects on mental state can persist for 48 to 72 hours. Tolerance to CNS effects generally develops after a few days. Because of the risk of orthostatic hypotension and reflex tachycardia, nabilone is unsuitable in those with heart failure or atrial fibrillation.

Contraindications

Nabilone is contraindicated in those with a history of psychosis and hypersensitivity to marijuana or other cannabinoids. It should be used with caution in patients with a history of psychiatric disorders or severe liver failure, in pregnant or breastfeeding women, in those with hypertension or heart disease, in the elderly, and in those younger than 18 years.

OCTREOTIDE

This somatostatin analogue is used in patients with bowel obstruction. Its other palliative uses include management of ascites, fistulas (pancreatic, enterocutaneous, buccal), severe and intractable diarrhea, and excessive respiratory secretions in the terminal phase. Octreotide acts by inhibiting secretion of insulin, glucagon, pancreatic polypeptide, gastric inhibitory polypeptide, gastrin, thyroid-stimulating hormone, and growth hormone.[20] It reduces splanchnic blood flow and inhibits gall bladder emptying. Octreotide stimulates gastric motility at low doses and accelerates emptying at moderate to high doses.[20] It diminishes pancreatic exocrine function and increases intestinal transit time. It increases absorption of water and electrolytes in the gut. Hepatic metabolism is extensive (30% to 40%). Eleven percent to 32% is excreted unchanged in urine.[20]

Dose

Dosing starts at 300 µg/day and can be increased up to 900 µg daily. Increases in dosage to greater than 1000 µg daily are unlikely to give additional benefit in bowel obstruction. Dosage adjustments may be required in patients with severe renal failure requiring dialysis and in the elderly because its half-life may be increased. The half-life may also be prolonged in cirrhosis. Octreotide is expensive, so the lowest dose that maintains control of symptoms should be used. When given as a continuous subcutaneous infusion, it should be diluted with normal saline. Octreotide can be mixed with hyoscine butylbromide, levomepromazine, metoclopramide, dexamethasone, haloperidol, and midazolam. It is incompatible with cyclizine.

Adverse Effects

The most common side effects are local skin reactions (pain, stinging, burning) and gastrointestinal effects. Other side effects include bradycardia, worsening congestive heart failure, hypertension, rash, pruritus, hot flashes, alteration in glucose metabolism, anorexia, abdominal pain, nausea, vomiting, cholelithiasis, biliary colic (on abrupt withdrawal), diarrhea, and ileus. In type 1 diabetes mellitus, octreotide decreases insulin requirements, whereas in type 2 diabetes, glucose levels are either unchanged or elevated.

Contraindications

Octreotide should not be used in those with previous hypersensitivity and with caution in patients with diabetes mellitus, renal failure, or hepatic impairment.

OLANZAPINE

Mechanism of Action

This atypical antipsychotic is used mainly for schizophrenia, agitation, and delirium but has also been reported to be effective for nausea in advanced cancer. Olanzapine has high affinity for dopamine (D_1, D_2, D_4), serotonin (5-HT_{2A}, 5-HT_{2C}, 5-HT_3), α_1-adrenergic, histamine (H_1), and five muscarinic receptor subtypes. Olanzapine's activity at multiple receptor sites is similar to that of levomepromazine. It is extensively metabolized in the liver by glucuronidation, and elimination of metabolites is both renal (60%) and fecal (30%).[21]

Dose

Olanzapine is administered at 2.5 to 10 mg/day in divided doses. Renally impaired patients have a trend toward a prolonged drug half-life, so caution is advised. Despite extensive hepatic metabolism, those with hepatic impairment (Child-Pugh class A and B) do not require dose adjustment.

Adverse Effects

The most common effects are somnolence and weight gain. Other more common side effects include dry mouth, constipation, increased appetite, agitation, bradycardia, orthostatic hypotension, and peripheral edema. Although it has fewer extrapyramidal side effects than haloperidol, including both acute and tardive syndromes, it should be used carefully in patients with Parkinson's disease. Caution is advised in those at risk of or in combination with drugs known to cause prolongation of the QT interval. Elevated blood sugar levels are relatively common, with rare reports of diabetic ketoacidosis. Monitoring for hyperglycemia is recommended.

Contraindications

Use of olanzapine is contraindicated in patients with narrow-angle glaucoma and women breastfeeding. Caution is required in the elderly and those with parkinsonism, epilepsy, diabetes, benign prostatic hyperplasia, liver disease, a history of neuroleptic malignant syndrome, breast cancer, and pituitary tumors.

Drug Interactions

Olanzapine may cause additive effects when combined with CNS depressants such as alcohol, benzodiazepines, and antidepressants. It antagonizes dopamine agonists.

PROCHLORPERAZINE

This piperazine derivative phenothiazine is used for nausea and vomiting, including that associated with migraine, as well as for vertigo. As with other phenothiazines, it acts on several neurotransmitter systems, with antagonism of D_2, muscarinic, histamine, and α-adrenergic receptors. Its antiemetic effects are mediated principally via dopamine receptor inhibition in the chemoreceptor trigger zone and vagal blockade in the gastrointestinal tract. Prochlorperazine is a more potent antiemetic than chlorpromazine. It is metabolized mainly in the liver, undergoes enterohepatic circulation, and is excreted predominantly in feces.[22,23]

Dose

When administered orally, the dose is 5 to 10 mg three or four times daily. The buccal dose is 3 to 6 mg twice daily, rectal administration is 25 mg twice daily, and the intramuscular dose is 5 to 10 mg every 3 to 4 hours to a maximum of 40 mg daily. Doses greater than these should be used only in resistant cases. Reduced doses may be required in the elderly. In syringe drivers, prochlorperazine is incompatible with midazolam, with conflicting data regarding compatibility with morphine, hydromorphone, and dexamethasone.

Adverse Effects

More common side effects include drowsiness, extrapyramidal reactions such as akathisia and parkinsonism, and anticholinergic effects such as blurred vision, dry mouth, and constipation. Prochlorperazine may cause less sedation and hypotension and fewer antimuscarinic effects than chlorpromazine, but extrapyramidal effects may be more frequent. Other important adverse reactions include hypotension, prolongation of the QT segment, neuroleptic malignant syndrome, and respiratory depression. All phenothiazines lower the seizure threshold, although they generally do not precipitate seizures without a preexisting convulsive disorder. Acute extrapyramidal reactions are

uncommon but occur more frequently in the young and may occur after a single dose.

Contraindications and Precautions

Contraindications include hypersensitivity to phenothiazines, severe hypotension, bone marrow depression, a history of blood dyscrasias, and use in children younger than 2 years. Caution is advised in patients with hepatic impairment, with consideration of dose reduction recommended. The elderly are particularly sensitive to extrapyramidal side effects, especially parkinsonism and postural hypotension. Low initial doses are recommended, with slow upward titration. Other precautions include epilepsy, a history of neuroleptic malignant syndrome, Parkinson's disease, impaired cardiac function, renal and hepatic impairment, glaucoma, prostate hypertrophy, use in children, myasthenia gravis, and those at risk for QT prolongation.

Drug Interactions

Coadministration of prochlorperazine and drugs associated with QT prolongation should be avoided. Use with levodopa and other dopamine receptor agonists should also be avoided. Concomitant use with tramadol may increase the risk for seizures.

PROMETHAZINE

Mechanism of Action

Promethazine is a phenothiazine antihistamine used for nausea and vomiting with motion, vestibular disorders, raised intracranial pressure, and sedation and itching. It is a sedating H_1 antagonist with mild antimuscarinic effects and some antiserotonergic effects. As with other antihistamines, it acts on H_1 receptors in the vomiting center and on vestibular afferents. Its oral (and rectal) bioavailability is approximately 25%.[24] Peak plasma concentrations are reached 2 to 3 hours after oral administration. Its duration of action is 4 to 12 hours, with a half-life of 10 to 14 hours. Promethazine undergoes extensive metabolism and is excreted slowly via urine and bile.

Dose

The dose of promethazine is 25 mg every 4 to 6 hours, with a maximum daily dose of 100 mg. Available data suggest no accumulation in patients with renal insufficiency, so no specific dosage adjustment appears to be necessary. In syringe drivers, promethazine is usually compatible with fentanyl, glycopyrrolate, hydromorphone, metoclopramide, and midazolam. Data regarding morphine are conflicting.

Adverse Effects

The most common side effect is sedation, although tolerance may develop over a few days. Other common side effects include dizziness, restlessness, fatigue, incoordination, headache, and anticholinergic effects. Extrapyramidal side effects are reported, but usually at higher doses. Promethazine is more sedating than cyclizine. It may lower the seizure threshold and should therefore be used with caution in those with epilepsy or when combined with other medications that lower the seizure threshold.

Contraindications and Precautions

Promethazine is contraindicated in patients with a history of an idiosyncratic reaction or hypersensitivity to promethazine or other phenothiazines, in those in whom jaundice has previously developed after taking phenothiazines, and in children younger than 2 years. Caution is required in patients with cardiovascular disease, severe hypertension, respiratory compromise, impaired hepatic function, and epilepsy.

5-HT$_3$ ANTAGONISTS

Though primarily used for nausea and vomiting after chemotherapy, radiotherapy, and surgery in palliative care, 5-HT$_3$ antagonists have been used for refractory nausea and pruritus secondary to opioids and biliary obstruction.

Serotonin (5-hydroxytryptamine, 5-HT$_3$) is found in enterochromaffin cells in the gut, where it has an important role in the regulation of gastrointestinal motility; in the CNS, where it acts as a neurotransmitter; and in platelets. Serotonin receptors have been demonstrated peripherally in enteric nervous system sensory neurons and centrally in the nucleus tractus solitarius and the chemoreceptor trigger zone, where most vagal afferents enter the brain.[25] Cytotoxic drugs or abdominal irradiation cause release of serotonin from gut enterochromaffin cells and subsequent activation of abdominal vagal afferents. Serotonin antagonists do not prevent the release of 5-HT$_3$ but appear to prevent chemotherapy-induced nausea by preventing agonism of the 5-HT$_3$ receptor by serotonin both peripherally and centrally.[25] Granisetron and dolasetron are pure 5-HT$_3$ receptor antagonists. In addition to 5-HT$_3$ receptor binding, ondansetron binds at 5-HT$_{1B}$, 5-HT$_{1c}$, α_1-adrenergic, and opioid mu receptors, and tropisetron binds to 5HT$_4$ receptors, although these differences do not translate into differences in therapeutic efficacy or adverse effect profile.[25] The duration of action of 5-HT$_3$ receptor antagonists is more strongly associated with their receptor binding than their plasma half-life.

Dolasetron

Hydrodolasetron is metabolized by CYP2D6 and CYP3A4, with 50% to 60% excreted unchanged in urine. Clearance is reduced in patients with severe hepatic (Child-Pugh category B or C) and severe renal (glomerular filtration rate <10 mL/min) impairment after oral use. After intravenous administration, clearance is reduced in those with severe renal impairment but appears to be unchanged with severe hepatic impairment.

Granisetron

Granisetron is metabolized in the liver, with less than 20% of the dose excreted unchanged in urine. Clearance is

unaffected by renal impairment but reduced by hepatic impairment and in the elderly. Less than 5% is excreted unchanged in urine, with dose adjustments considered unnecessary in renal failure.

Ondansetron

Despite a short half-life, some report that ondansetron and other 5-HT$_3$ antagonists can be effectively administered once daily.[25]

Palonosetron

Approximately 50% of administered palonosetron is metabolized, with CYP2D6 being the major enzyme involved, and approximately 80% of the dose is recovered in urine as parent drug and metabolite.

Tropisetron

Metabolism occurs predominantly in the liver. CYP2D6 is involved in the metabolism of tropisetron, and there are phenotypic populations of poor and extensive metabolizers. No active metabolites are produced. Clearance is reduced in patients with moderate to severe renal impairment and in those with cirrhosis.

Dose

- Dolasetron: Despite changes in clearance, no dose reduction is advised in patients with impaired renal or hepatic function. Dose adjustments based on age are not advised (Table 144-5).
- Granisetron: Despite reduced clearance in the elderly and in hepatic impairment, dose reductions are not advised.
- Ondansetron: Dose reduction is not recommended in the elderly. In those with severe hepatic impairment (Pugh score > 9), daily ondansetron doses should be limited to 8 mg daily. Ondansetron is compatible with dexamethasone, fentanyl, hydromorphone, and morphine in syringe drivers.
- Palonosetron: No dose adjustment is recommended in patients with any degree of renal or hepatic impairment or in elderly cancer patients.

Adverse Effects

The side effects of 5-HT$_3$ antagonists are usually mild and transient, with headache, constipation, and asthenia being the most common across the class. Other more common adverse effects include dizziness or light-headedness, sedation, abdominal pain and cramping, sensations of warmth or flushing, hiccups, elevations in liver transaminases and bilirubin, and electrocardiographic changes. Whether they have clinically significant cardiotoxicity is controversial. 5-HT$_3$ antagonists should be used cautiously with drugs that prolong the QT interval.

Drug Interactions

All 5-HT$_3$ antagonists are metabolized by cytochrome P-450 isoenzymes, although the extent of metabolism and

TABLE 144-5 Doses of 5-HT$_3$ Antagonists According to Indication

DRUG	CTIE	PREVENTION OF PONV	TREATMENT OF PONV
Dolasetron	100-200 mg*	50 mg PO or 12.5 mg IV	12.5 mg IV
Granisetron	1-3 mg[†]	1 mg IV	1 mg bid
Ondansetron	8 mg IV/IM before treatment, then 8 mg at 2-4 hr[‡]	8 mg before anesthesia, then 8 mg at 8, 16 hr	4 mg IM/IV
Palonosetron	250 µg before treatment[§]		
Tropisetron	5 mg IV before treatment, then 5 mg daily PO for 5 days	2 mg IV before induction	2 mg IV within 2 hr

*Given 1 hour before chemotherapy and continued daily for 4 to 7 days.
[†]Given 1 hour before therapy and then 2 mg daily as a single daily dose or twice-daily dosing.
[‡]A regimen for highly emetogenic chemotherapy; there are others.
[§]Repeat dosing within 7 days is not recommended.
CTIE, chemotherapy-induced emesis; PONV, postoperative nausea and vomiting.

Current Controversies and Future Considerations

Much effort has been made to describe receptor affinities of the various agents. The importance of this is challenged on two grounds. First, the emetic pathway and the neurotransmitters involved were determined for chemotherapy-induced emesis and may be irrelevant to most patients with advanced cancer. In these patients, nausea is most likely to be a feature of anorexia-cachexia syndrome (see Chapter 150), and prokinetic agents will have a key role. New agents directed against systemic inflammation (e.g., ω-3 fatty acid, thalidomide, interleukin-6 antagonists) may be important. Second, even if the various neurotransmitters are relevant to advanced cancer, the use of broad-spectrum drugs such as the various phenothiazines described earlier may make much of this information redundant.

the specific isoenzymes involved differ for each drug, with such metabolism potentially having clinically significant implications for patients receiving multiple medications and those with genetic polymorphisms. 5-HT$_3$ antagonists may decrease the efficacy of tramadol.

Contraindications and Precautions

Contraindications include previous hypersensitivity to 5-HT$_3$ receptor antagonists. They should be used with caution in patients with bowel obstruction or ileus, hepatic impairment, and cardiac conduction abnormalities, including QT prolongation.

REFERENCES

1. Dando TM, Perry CM. Aprepitant: A review of its use in the prevention of chemotherapy-induced nausea and vomiting. Drugs 2004;64:777-794.
2. Yeung PK, Hubbard JW, Korchinski ED, Midha KK. Pharmacokinetics of chlorpromazine and key metabolites. Eur J Clin Pharmacol 1993;45:563-569.
3. McCallum RW, Prakash C, Campoli-Richards DM, Goa KL. Cisapride. A preliminary review of its pharmacodynamic and pharmacokinetic properties, and therapeutic use as a prokinetic agent in gastrointestinal motility disorders. Drugs 1988;36:652-681.
4. Varma S, Deakin J, Claydon PJ. Subcutaneous cyclizine. Anaesthesia 2001;56:906-924.
5. Tan LB, Bryant S, Murray RG. Detrimental haemodynamic effects of cyclizine in heart failure. Lancet 1988;1:560-561.
6. Czock D, Keller F, Rasche FM, Haussler U. Pharmacokinetics and pharmacodynamics of systemically administered glucocorticoids. Clin Pharmacokinet 2005;44:61-98.
7. Nielsen GL, Sorensen HT, Mellemkjoer L, et al. Risk of hospitalization resulting from upper gastrointestinal bleeding among patients taking corticosteroids: A register-based cohort study. Am J Med 2001;111:541-545.
8. Batchelor TT, Taylor LP, Thaler HT, et al. Steroid myopathy in cancer patients. Neurology 1997;48:1234-1238.
9. Twycross R, Wilcock A, Charlesworth S, Dickman A. Palliative Care Formulary, 2nd ed. Oxford, Radcliffe, 2002.
10. Brogden RN, Carmine AA, Heel RC, et al. Domperidone. A review of its pharmacological activity, pharmacokinetics and therapeutic efficacy in the symptomatic treatment of chronic dyspepsia and as an antiemetic. Drugs 1982;24:360-400.
11. Kudo S, Ishizaki T. Pharmacokinetics of haloperidol: An update. Clin Pharmacokinet 1999;37:435-456.
12. Ebert U, Siepmann M, Oertel R, et al. Pharmacokinetics and pharmacodynamics of scopolamine after subcutaneous administration. J Clin Pharmacol 1998;38:720-726.
13. Skinner J, Skinner A. Levomepromazine for nausea and vomiting in advanced cancer. Hosp Med 1999;60:568-570.
14. Gram-Hansen P, Schultz A. Plasma concentrations following oral and sublingual administration of lorazepam. Int J Clin Pharmacol Ther Toxicol 1988;26:323-324.
15. Bateman DN. Clinical pharmacokinetics of metoclopramide. Clin Pharmacokinet 1983;8:523-529.
16. Magueur E, Hagege H, Attali P, et al. Pharmacokinetics of metoclopramide in patients with liver cirrhosis. Br J Clin Pharmacol 1991;31:185-187.
17. Bateman DN, Gokal R, Dodd TR, Blain PG. The pharmacokinetics of single doses of metoclopramide in renal failure. Eur J Clin Pharmacol 1981;19:437-441.
18. Plouin PF, Menard J, Corvol P. Hypertensive crisis in patient with phaeochromocytoma given metoclopramide. Lancet 1976;2:1357-1358.
19. Grotenhermen F. Pharmacokinetics and pharmacodynamics of cannabinoids. Clin Pharmacokinet 2003;42:327-360.
20. Harris AG. Somatostatin and somatostatin analogues: Pharmacokinetics and pharmacodynamic effects. Gut 1994;35(3 Suppl):S1-S4.
21. Callaghan JT, Bergstrom RF, Ptak LR, Beasley CM. Olanzapine: Pharmacokinetic and pharmacodynamic profile. Clin Pharmacokinet 1999;37:177-193.
22. Isah AO, Rawlins MD, Bateman DN. Clinical pharmacology of prochlorperazine in healthy young males. Br J Clin Pharmacol 1991;32:677-684.
23. Taylor WB, Bateman DN. Preliminary studies of the pharmacokinetics and pharmacodynamics of prochlorperazine in healthy volunteers. Br J Clin Pharmacol 1987;23:137-142.
24. Paton DM, Webster DR. Clinical pharmacokinetics of H1-receptor antagonists (the antihistamines). Clin Pharmacokinet 1985;10:477-497.
25. Gregory RE, Ettinger DS. 5-HT3 receptor antagonists for the prevention of chemotherapy-induced nausea and vomiting. A comparison of their pharmacology and clinical efficacy. Drugs 1998;55:173-189.

SUGGESTED READING

Hardman JG, Limbird LE, Gilman AG (eds). Goodman and Gilman's The Pharmacological Basis of Therapeutics, 10th ed. New York, McGraw Hill, 2001, pp 485-520.
Palliativedrugs.com.
Sweetman SC (ed). Martindale: The complete drug reference, 34th ed. London, Pharmaceutical Press, 2005.
Twycross R, Wilcock A, Charlesworth S, Dickman A. Palliative Care Formulary, 2nd ed. Oxford, Radcliffe, 2002.

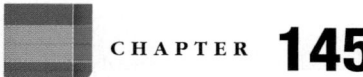

CHAPTER **145**

Corticosteroids

Louise Exton

KEY POINTS

- The widespread use of corticosteroids for palliation of advanced cancer is largely anecdotal and not evidence based.

- Most of the specific effects of corticosteroids in advanced cancer are related to glucocorticoid effects in reducing tumor-associated inflammation and edema.

- Dexamethasone is the glucocorticoid most frequently used because of its relative potency, long half-life, and minimal mineralocorticoid effects.

- Corticosteroid use is limited by well-known side effects. All patients commencing a trial of corticosteroids must have a clearly documented indication and plan for review after 5 to 7 days. If the expected benefit has not occurred, treatment should be stopped. If the patient has benefited, there must be ongoing regular review of efficacy versus toxicity.

- There is an urgent need for internationally agreed guidelines based on solid evidence to rationalize corticosteroid use in palliative medicine.

Corticosteroids are among the most commonly prescribed medications in patients with advanced cancer, with 33% to 60% of palliative care patients being prescribed corticosteroids for various specific and nonspecific indications (Table 145-1).[1-4] There is little evidence from randomized controlled trials to support such widespread use, however, although in practice they are often effective agents in controlling symptoms, at least in the short term.

Corticosteroid use is associated with many debilitating and some life-threatening side effects. Concern has been raised that palliative care patients receiving corticosteroids are not stringently monitored. All patients prescribed corticosteroids for any indication, especially those with advanced disease, who are likely to be at increased risk for toxicity, must be reviewed regularly to ensure that treatment benefits outweigh the risks.

MECHANISM OF ACTION

Corticosteroids are hormones produced by the adrenal cortex. They are divided by their actions into two classes: mineralocorticoids and glucocorticoids. The main mineralocorticoid actions involve fluid and electrolyte balance. Mineralocorticoids act on the distal convoluted tubule of the kidney to enhance reabsorption of sodium and secretion of potassium and hydrogen ions. Water is retained with sodium. The main endogenous mineralocorticoid is aldosterone. The semisynthetic compound fludrocortisone is used for replacement therapy and postural hypotension.

Glucocorticoid actions are more diverse. They bind to specific receptors in the cell cytoplasm, which then interact with DNA to modify gene transcription so that some proteins are synthesized whereas others are inhibited.[5] It is predominantly their potent anti-inflammatory effect that is beneficial in palliative medicine. Corticosteroids inhibit prostaglandin synthesis and reduce the vascular response (capillary dilation) and increased vascular permeability that cause tissue edema and swelling. They also have important metabolic effects on glucose, fat, and protein metabolism, which produces much of their toxicity. Glucocorticoids facilitate the action of many other active endogenous substances and affect cardiovascular, kidney, skeletal muscle, and central nervous system function.

Corticosteroids (Table 145-2) may be given by various routes: oral, intravenous, intramuscular, subcutaneous, and topical.[6] When given orally, they are well absorbed and rapidly distributed to all body tissues. Endogenous glucocorticoids in plasma are bound to corticosteroid-binding globulin and albumin. Synthetic steroids are less extensively protein bound and have longer half-lives. Corticosteroids are metabolized in the liver to largely inactive compounds that are excreted in urine.

TABLE 145-1 Indications for Corticosteroids in Palliative Care

SPECIFIC	NONSPECIFIC
Anticancer	Mood
Raised intracranial pressure	Fatigue/weakness
Spinal cord compression	Anorexia
Lymphangitis carcinomatosa	Pain
Bowel obstruction	Dyspnea
Superior vena cava obstruction	Nausea/vomiting
Obstructive lymphadenopathy	Fever/itching
Ureteric obstruction	Sweating
Hypercalcemia	

TABLE 145-2 Comparison of Corticosteroids

CORTICOSTEROID	SODIUM RETENTION	ANTI-INFLAMMATORY EFFICACY	DOSE EQUIVALENT (mg)	HALF-LIFE (hr)
Hydrocortisone	2	1	20	8-12
Prednisone	0.8	3.5	5	18-36
Prednisolone	0.8	4	5	18-36
Methylprednisolone	0.5	4	4	18-36
Dexamethasone	0	25-30	0.75	36-54

Adapted from Twycross RG. The risks and benefits of corticosteroids in advanced cancer. Drug Saf 1994;11:163-178.

DOSAGES

The initial dose varies according to indication and physician preference. In a palliative setting, dexamethasone (Table 145-3) is often the glucocorticoid of choice for several reasons:

- It is relatively potent when compared with other synthetic steroids.
- It has minimal mineralocorticoid effect.
- It has a long biological half-life and can be given once daily (unless restricted by tablet numbers).
- It can be given orally (2-mg and 500-μg tablets), intravenously, and subcutaneously.

MAJOR SIDE EFFECTS

Corticosteroid therapy is associated with many well-recognized side effects (Table 145-4), some of which are difficult to differentiate from progressive disease. Toxicity is traditionally associated with high doses and chronic use. Concern had been raised that side effects are underrecognized in the palliative setting and that monitoring is not as stringent as it should be. Corticosteroid-related toxicity has been reported in three large prospective surveys (Table 145-5).[1,2,4]

Hyperglycemia

Hyperglycemia is reported to affect 2% to 17% of patients in a palliative setting who are treated with corticosteroids (see Table 145-4). It is important to monitor all patients taking steroids for hyperglycemia, which can cause unpleasant symptoms and cloud the clinical picture. One regimen is to monitor nondiabetic patients taking steroids by urinalysis or blood glucose determination on day 4 and then weekly.

Gastrointestinal Toxicity

Corticosteroids alone may not significantly increase the risk for peptic ulceration. If used concurrently with nonsteroidal anti-inflammatory drug (NSAID), evidence suggests that there is a 15-fold increase in bleeding or ulceration.[7] If it is essential to combine steroids with an NSAID, gastroprotection is mandatory. Other risk factors include advanced cancer, history of peptic ulceration, and a cumulative dexamethasone dose greater than 140 mg. Some recommend gastroprotection only if two or more risk factors are present.[8]

Steroid Myopathy

Proximal myopathy is one of the most common side effects in palliative medicine and probably also the most distressing.[2] Respiratory muscle may also be affected. It can be acute or chronic:

TABLE 145-3 Corticosteroid Dosages for Common Indications in Palliative Care

INDICATION	DOSAGE
SPECIFIC	
Raised intracranial pressure	8-16 mg dexamethasone daily
Spinal cord compression	16 mg dexamethasone daily (8 mg bid)
Superior vena cava obstruction	16 mg dexamethasone daily (8 mg bid)
Bowel obstruction	8-16 mg dexamethasone daily
NONSPECIFIC	
Anorexia	4 mg dexamethasone 10-20 mg prednisolone
Nausea and vomiting	4-8 mg dexamethasone

TABLE 145-4 Side Effects of Corticosteroid Therapy

Cushingoid habitus: moon face, buffalo hump
Skin changes: striae, acne, purpura, skin fragility, poor wound healing
Proximal myopathy
Psychological disturbances: restlessness, agitation, anxiety, sleep disturbance, behavioral change, depression, psychosis
Hyperglycemia/glycosuria
Peripheral edema
Gastrointestinal toxicity
Infections: oral thrush, increased susceptibility to systemic infection
Perianal discomfort/irritation (during intravenous administration)

Osteoporosis/aseptic necrosis of bone

TABLE 145-5 Corticosteroid Toxicity in Palliative Care

SIDE EFFECT	HARDY ET AL., 2001 (N = 106)	HANKS ET AL., 1983 (N = 218)	LUNDSTROM ET AL., 2006 (N = 181)
Oral candidiasis	34%	31%	28%
Edema	34%	20%	
Cushingoid appearance	19%	18%	
Restlessness	27%	2%	
Sleeplessness	25%	2%	
Weight gain	22%	4%	
Skin changes	27%	4%	31%
Dyspepsia	19%	18%	
Proximal myopathy	24%	2%	34%
Confusion/psychosis	5%	4%	
Hyperglycemia	2%	2%	17%
Infection	1%	—	

Acute steroid myopathy is rare. Generalized muscle weakness occurs 5 to 7 days after the start of high-dose parenteral treatment (i.e., dexamethasone, 40 to 80 mg).
Chronic steroid myopathy is more readily recognized. Its onset is insidious and usually painless. The proximal muscles of the arms and legs are affected first, with the lower limbs demonstrating the earliest weakness. Patients sometimes complain of difficulty climbing stairs and rising from low chairs.

Most patients recover over a period of weeks with physiotherapy and reduction of the steroid dosage to the lowest possible level. Conversion to a nonfluorinated preparation such as prednisolone or alternate-day dosing may help.[9]

Osteoporosis

Osteoporosis is an increasingly recognized complication. A dexamethasone dose of 1 mg or higher over a 6-month period for specific indications such as cerebral tumors is a risk factor for steroid-induced osteoporosis, and preventive treatment with bisphosphonates should be considered.

Withdrawal Phenomena

Systemic corticosteroids suppress the hypothalamic-pituitary-adrenal axis. Rapid withdrawal of therapy of greater than 3 weeks' duration can cause acute adrenal insufficiency, hypotension, and death. After administration of systemic corticosteroids for more than 3 weeks, the dose should be tapered to the lowest effective dose and stopped if possible.

Gradual withdrawal of corticosteroids should be considered even after courses lasting 3 weeks or less in those with

- Repeated courses
- Other reasons for adrenocortical insufficiency (i.e., adrenal metastases)
- Daily doses greater than 40 mg prednisolone (6 mg dexamethasone)

If stress (infection, trauma, surgery) occurs within 1 week of stopping therapy, systemic corticosteroid cover should be provided. All patients taking corticosteroids should carry a treatment card warning that susceptibility to infections is increased and that treatment should never be stopped suddenly.

CORTICOSTEROIDS IN TERMINAL PHASE

In one study, 50% of patients received corticosteroids during their terminal admission; however, only 2% were switched to parenteral steroids when the oral route was lost.[10] There are disadvantages of stopping corticosteroids abruptly, even in the last days of life: loss of symptom control, withdrawal, and exacerbation of terminal restlessness. Relatives or staff may be left uncertain about whether stopping the steroid contributed to the ongoing deterioration. There is a need for greater vigilance in prescribing and monitoring corticosteroids in the terminal phase; perhaps in many patients these drugs could have been safely discontinued beforehand. Then the subgroup whose steroids should be maintained parenterally when the oral route is lost could be readily identified.

CONTRAINDICATIONS

- Contraindications: systemic infection (unless specific antimicrobial therapy is given), live virus vaccines
- Caution: diabetes mellitus, psychotic illness, peptic ulceration, concomitant NSAID treatment

DRUG INTERACTIONS

- The metabolism of corticosteroids is accelerated by several drugs, notably anticonvulsants (carbamazepine, phenytoin, phenobarbitone, and primidone) and rifampicin. This effect is more pronounced with longer-acting glucocorticoids such as dexamethasone and is clinically important with brain tumors. The dexamethasone dose may need to be increased twofold to fourfold. Alternatively, a shorter-acting glucocorticoid such as methylprednisolone could be substituted.
- Dexamethasone affects plasma phenytoin concentrations (may rise or fall), and plasma phenytoin levels should be monitored regularly.
- Corticosteroids may enhance or reduce the anticoagulant effects of warfarin, so increased monitoring is advisable, especially in patients with liver impairment.
- Corticosteroids antagonize the actions of oral hypoglycemic agents, insulin, and antihypertensives.
- There is an increased risk for hypokalemia with the concurrent use of β_2-adrenoreceptor antagonists, amphotericin, and carbenoxolone.
- Corticosteroids impair the immune response to live vaccines.

EVIDENCE-BASED MEDICINE

Corticosteroids in Palliative Care

There is little evidence to support the widespread use of corticosteroids. The evidence is derived predominantly from uncontrolled studies or case reports. Few randomized, controlled trials have been conducted. Even for specific indications such as raised intracranial pressure and spinal cord compression, the optimum dose and duration of action are inadequately established, and current practice is empirical.

Specific Indications

Raised Intracranial Pressure

Corticosteroids have been used in patients with primary and metastatic brain tumors for 50 years. They reduce tumor-associated edema and cerebral blood flow. Untreated, the median survival with cerebral metastases is about 1 month. Corticosteroids increase survival to 2 months, and additional whole brain radiotherapy increases survival to 3 to 6 months.[11] Patients with neurological deficits who were treated with corticosteroids and cranial radiotherapy had faster neurological improvement than those who underwent radiation therapy alone. There was no significant difference in overall neurological function, and corticosteroids had no independent influence on time to subsequent neurological progression or survival with concurrent cranial radiation therapy.[12]

Improvement in patients with cerebral metastases may be observed within hours of corticosteroid administration, but more commonly it occurs gradually over a period of several days. Seventy percent to 80% show significant clinical improvement.[13]

The optimal dose and duration of administration for brain tumor edema is unclear. Based on empirical clinical observations, 16 mg of dexamethasone daily in divided doses seems to be a useful schedule.[14] A two-phase, double-blind, randomized controlled trial compared 4, 8, and 16 mg of dexamethasone with respect to quality of life and toxicity in patients with metastatic brain tumors. The study found no differences between the three doses in outcome or quality of life at 1 week; however, the 4-mg dosage had to be reduced more slowly.[15] Conventional current practice uses 16 mg daily in divided doses with tapering of the dose until the end of radiation therapy. The maximum beneficial dose is not known, but doses up to 100 mg daily have been reported in those concurrently taking anticonvulsants.[16]

Spinal Cord Compression

Corticosteroids are an important initial measure in patients with spinal cord compression until definitive treatment is initiated, and their independent effect has been difficult to evaluate in clinical trials. A randomized single-blind trial of high-dose dexamethasone (96 mg intravenously followed by 96 mg orally for 3 days and then tapered in 10 days) or no corticosteroid before radiotherapy demonstrated improved gait function after corticosteroid treatment. This became statistically significant at the 6-month follow-up, with breast cancer patients deriving the most benefit.[17] The optimal dose is unclear, but because of long clinical experience in brain metastases, a similar dosing schedule has been adopted. Although up to 100-mg doses of dexamethasone have been used, current practice in the United Kingdom is to administer 16 mg/day in divided doses. This is supported by one study in which patients with metastatic spinal cord compression were randomized to receive 100 or 10 mg dexamethasone as an initial intravenous bolus followed by 16 mg orally. There was no statistical difference between the conventional and high-dose groups in terms of pain, ambulation, or bladder function.[18] A more recent review, however, suggests that there is good evidence to support high-dose dexamethasone (96 mg), but evidence for moderate-dose steroids (16 mg) is inconclusive.[19]

Bowel Obstruction

Corticosteroids act as antiemetics and coanalgesics and may therefore palliate nausea, vomiting, and pain in bowel obstruction. In addition, their anti-inflammatory activity may reduce peritumor edema and thus help resolve obstruction. A systematic review and meta-analysis of corticosteroids for malignant bowel obstruction in advanced gynecological and gastrointestinal cancer showed a trend toward resolution of bowel obstruction.[20]

Nonspecific Indications

Survey evidence suggests that many nonspecific indications improve with corticosteroids (Table 145-6).[2,4] Response is seen within 1 to 2 weeks and often persists beyond 4 weeks. This does not constitute reliable evidence of effectiveness. These studies were uncontrolled, and the second study evaluated physician clinical impression rather than the patient's.

Anorexia/Cachexia

Several randomized controlled trials have demonstrated short-term enhanced appetite in cancer patients. None have demonstrated a significant effect on nutritional status or weight gain. Other agents such as megestrol acetate, though considerably more expensive, are equally if not more efficacious and have fewer side effects.[21]

Weakness and Fatigue

There is little evidence to support the use of corticosteroids for fatigue in advanced cancer. In a placebo-controlled trial of prednisolone in patients with preterminal gastrointestinal cancer, a nonsignificant trend toward subjective improvement in strength was reported in the steroid group.[22] A larger study of 403 cancer patients randomized to methylprednisolone showed no improvement in weakness.[23]

Mood/General Well-being

Depression is common in patients with advanced cancer. Steroids are often used as a general "boost" to improve overall well-being, but there is only limited evidence to support this practice. In a controlled trial of methylprednisolone, 32 mg/day for 2 weeks, in 40 patients with terminal cancer, mood initially improved in 71%.[24] Corticosteroids have also been implicated in causing depression, but this potentially serious psychological side effect is often overlooked in clinical practice.

Pain

Corticosteroids act as adjuvant analgesics by reducing inflammation in bone, visceral pain, and edema in central nervous system tumors. They may also reduce spontane-

| | HARDY ET AL. | LUNDSTROM ET AL. | |
| | | | |
SYMPTOM	**PATIENTS "BETTER"***	**VERY GOOD**	**SOME†**
Anorexia	73%	46%	39%
Nausea and vomiting	92%	47%	40%
Pain	86%	34%	48%
Mood	59%		
Weakness	50%	33%	46%
Dyspnea	39%	25%	58%

TABLE 145-6 Symptom Response for Nonspecific Indications

*Best overall response (at any time) as reflected by improvement in a patient-rated 4-point symptom scale.
†Evaluation of treatment effect based on clinical impression of the physician/nursing staff.

ous nerve depolarization in injured nerves.[25] Several studies of their general beneficial effects in terminal cancer have reported improvement in pain and lower analgesic consumption.[24]

Nausea and Vomiting

Steroids are effective antiemetics for acute and probably delayed chemotherapy-induced emesis.[26] They are commonly used with a serotonin 5-HT$_3$ antagonist. They are also used when other antiemetics have failed, particularly in patients with liver metastases, bowel obstruction, or raised intracranial pressure, although there is little evidence to support such use.

RESEARCH CHALLENGES

There is a major need for further research to clarify the effectiveness and optimum dose and duration of use of corticosteroids in controlling both specific and nonspecific indications in palliative medicine. A key challenge to this kind of research is the numerous confounders of outcome measures because patients are commonly undergoing several treatments simultaneously to palliate a specific symptom.

REFERENCES

1. Hanks GW, Trueman T, Twycross RG. Corticosteroids in terminal cancer—a prospective analysis of current practice. Postgrad Med J 1983;59:702-706.
2. Hardy J. Corticosteroids in palliative care. Eur J Palliat Care 1998;5:46-50.
3. Needham PR, Daley AG, Lennard RF. Steroids in advanced cancer: A survey of current practice. BMJ 1992;305:999.
4. Lundstrom SH, Furst CJ. The use of corticosteroids in Swedish palliative care. Acta Oncol 2006;45:430-437.
5. Czock D, Keller F, Rasche FM, et al. Pharmacokinetics and pharmacodynamics of systemically administered glucocorticoids. Clin Pharmacokinet 2005;44:61-98.
6. Twycross RG. The risks and benefits of corticosteroids in advanced cancer. Drug Saf 1994;11:163-178.
7. Piper JM, Ray WA, Daugherty JR, et al: Corticosteroid use and peptic ulcer disease: Role of non-steroidal anti-inflammatory drugs. Ann Intern Med 1991;114:735-740.
8. Ellershaw JE, Kelly MJ. Corticosteroids and peptic ulceration. Palliat Med 1994;8:222-228.
9. Dekhuijzen PNR, Decramer M. Steroid-induced myopathy and its significance to respiratory disease: A known disease rediscovered. Eur Respir J 1992;5:997-1003.
10. Gannon C, McNamara P. A retrospective observation of corticosteroid use at the end of life in a hospice. J Pain Symptom Manage 2002;24:328-334.
11. Cairncross JG, Kim JH, Posner JB. Radiation therapy for brain metastases. Ann Neurol 1980;7:529-541.
12. Borgelt B, Gelber R, Kramer S, et al. The palliation of brain metastases; final results of the first two studies by the Radiation Therapy Oncology Group. Int J Radiat Oncol Biol Phys 1980;6:1-9.
13. Ruderman NB, Hall TC. Use of glucocorticoids in the palliative treatment of metastatic brain tumours. Cancer 1965;18:298-306.
14. French LA, Galicich JH. The use of steroids for control of cerebral oedema. Clin Neurosurg 1964;10:212-223.
15. Vecht CJ, Hovestadt A, Verbiest HBC, et al. Dose effect relationship of dexamethasone on Karnofsky performance in metastatic brain tumours: A randomised study of 4, 8 and 16 mg per day. Neurology 1994;44:675-680.
16. Renaudin J, Fewer D, Wilson CB, et al. Dose dependency of Decadron in patients with partially excised brain tumours. J Neurosurg 1973;39:302-305.
17. Sorenson PS, Helweg-Larsen S, Mouridsen H, et al. Effect of high dose dexamethasone in carcinomatous metastatic spinal cord compression treated with radiotherapy: A randomised trial. Eur J Cancer 1994;30:22-27.
18. Vecht CJ, Haaxma-Reiche H, Van Putten WL, et al. Initial bolus of conventional versus high-dose dexamethasone in metastatic spinal cord compression. Neurology 1989;39:1255-1257.
19. Loblaw DA, Laperriere. Emergency treatment of malignant extradural spinal cord compression: An evidence-based guideline. J Clin Oncol 1998;16:1613-1624.
20. Feuer DJ, Broadley KE. Systematic review and meta-analysis of corticosteroids for the resolution of malignant bowel obstruction in advanced gynaecological and gastrointestinal cancers. Ann Oncol 1999;10:1035-1041.
21. Loprinzi CL. Management of cancer anorexia/cachexia. Support Care Cancer 1995;3:120-122.
22. Moertal CG, Schmutt AJ, Reitermeier RJ, et al. Corticosteroid therapy of preterminal gastrointestinal cancer. Cancer 1974;33:1607-1609.
23. Della Cuna GR, Pellegrini A, Piazzi M. Effect of methylprednisolone sodium succinate on quality of life in pre-determined cancer patients: A placebo controlled multicenter trial. The Methylprednisolone Cancer Study Group. Eur J Cancer 1989;25:1817-1821.
24. Bruera E, Roca E, Cedaro L, et al. Action of oral methylprednisolone in terminal cancer patients: A prospective randomised double blind study. Cancer Treat Rep 1985;69:751-754.
25. Devor M, Govrin-Lippmann R, Raber P. Corticosteroids reduce neuroma hyperexcitability. In Fields HL, et al (eds). Advances in Pain Research and Therapy. New York: Raven, 1985, pp 451-455.
26. Gralla RJ, Osoba D, Kris MG, et al. Recommendations for the use of antiemetics: Evidence-based clinical practice guidelines. J Clin Oncol 1999;17:2971-2994.

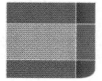

CHAPTER **146**

Drugs for Myoclonus and Tremors

Dilara Seyidova Khoshknabi

KEY POINTS

- Rationale for treatment—neurological: (1) spinal cord, (2) amyotropic lateral sclerosis, (3) multiple sclerosis; muscle spasm: (1) neurological origin, (2) muscular origin: (a) inherited, (b) acquired
- Pharmacotherapies for muscle spasms include pharmacological agents categorized by a certain mechanism of action into different groups.
- Major side effects of drugs are related to central nervous system depression.
- Contraindications vary with the medication and include hypersensitivity to the drug or any component of the formulation.
- Most antispasticity drugs cause drug interaction problems.

Spasticity is a neurological impairment of upper motor neurons. It has been described as a motor disorder characterized by a velocity-dependent decrease in the tonic stretch reflex (muscle tone) with exaggerated tendon jerks resulting from hyperexcitability of the stretch reflex as one component of the upper motor neuron syndrome.[1] Based on this definition of spasticity, the increased muscle activity (during the imposed stretching phase) results entirely from increased activity in the stretch reflex pathways with an increase in resistance to passive movement. Spasticity is also reported to result from increased stretch reflex activity (often described as "hyperexcitable" or "exaggerated").[2] However, there is insufficient evidence to support the hypothesis that abnormal activity in spasticity results exclusively from stretch reflex hyperexcitability.[1]

Spasticity is only one of the positive phenomena that may occur after an upper motor neuron lesion (Table 146-1).[3]

Somatic muscle spasms occur with lower motor neuron disease, in inherited metabolic and mitochondrial disorders, after acute extracellular volume depletion, and as a side effect of medications.[4] Muscle spasms in palliative medicine settings may be a result of co-morbid conditions and side effects of medications. Spasticity is a problem in 67% of patients with spinal cord injuries[5] and in 40% to 60% of cases of multiple sclerosis and was identified as a significant issue.[6,7]

Management is symptomatic with the goal of improving functional capability and relieving distress. The approach to treatment should be multidisciplinary and should include physical therapy and possibly surgery and pharmacotherapy.[8]

Drugs for muscle spasms include pharmacological agents categorized by a certain mechanism of action into groups such as γ-aminobutyric acid B (GABA$_B$) agonists, α_2-agonists, benzodiazepines, skeletal muscle relaxants, and botulinum toxin (Table 146-2).

MECHANISM OF ACTION

The most frequently used antispasticity drugs—baclofen, tizanidine, diazepam, and dantrolene sodium—are the only medications approved. Their main mechanism of action is through central potentiation of the inhibitory GABA effect via presynaptic interaction with GABA receptors, which potentiates the action of GABA (Box 146-1).[10]

PHARMACOKINETICS

Pharmacokinetics (Table 146-3) should be taken into account when determining the safest and most effective drugs, especially in the palliative medicine population, who often have associated organ failure and polypharmacy.

TABLE 146-2 Drugs Approved for the Treatment of Spasticity

GENERIC NAME	COMMERCIAL NAME	COMMENT
Baclofen	Lioresal	GABA$_B$ agonist
Tizanidine	Zanaflex	α_2-Agonist
Diazepam	Valium	Benzodiazepine
Dantrolene sodium	Dantrium	Skeletal muscle relaxant

Adapted from Nance PW, Young RR. Antispasticity medications. Phys Med Rehabil Clin N Am 1999;10:337-355, viii.

TABLE 146-1 Sensorimotor Signs and Symptoms after Upper Motor Neuron Lesions

POSITIVE FEATURES*	NEGATIVE FEATURES†
Increased tendon reflexes with radiation	Muscle weakness
Clonus	Loss of dexterity
Positive Babinski's sign	Fatigability
Spasticity (a velocity-dependent increase in resistance to passive movement)	
Flexor spasm	
Extensor spasm	
Mass reflex	
Dyssynergic patterns of co-contraction during movement	
Associated reactions and other dyssynergic stereotypical spastic dystonias	

*Normally characterized by increased involuntary motor activity
†Normally characterized by less voluntary motor activity.

Box 146-1 Mechanism of Action of γ-Aminobutyric Acid

- Enhanced GABA coupling to the GABA$_A$ receptor–chloride ionophore complex by binding to GABA$_A$ receptors. Such binding enhances chloride conductance and results in presynaptic inhibition in the spinal cord.
- GABA$_B$ agonists act on presynaptic and postsynaptic levels and decrease release of excitatory neurotransmitters by blocking voltage-gated calcium, which inhibits release of substance P.[9]
- α_2-Agonists are centrally acting muscle relaxants that work through α_2-adrenergic receptors and prevent release of excitatory amino acids and polysynaptic excitation of spinal cord interneurons.[10]
- Skeletal muscle relaxants reduce muscle spasms through inhibition of calcium release from the sarcoplasmic reticulum and do not directly affect the central nervous system.[10]

TABLE 146-3 Pharmacokinetics of Antispastic Agents

DRUG	T$_{MAX}$ (hr)	T$_{1/2}$ (hr)	PROTEIN BINDING (%)	METABOLISM
Baclofen	2-3	3.5	30%	Hepatic (15% of dose)
Tizanidine	3-4	2.5	30%	Hepatic (95%)
Diazepam	0.5-2	20-80	98-99%	Hepatic (CYP2C19, CYP3A4)
Dantrolene sodium	4-8	8.7	Unknown	Hepatic
Gabapentin	2-3	5-7	<3%	Renal clearance of parent drug
Dronabinol	0.4-4	20-44	97-99%	Hepatic (at least 50 metabolites)

Adapted from Meleger AL. Muscle relaxants and antispasticity agents. Phys Med Rehabil Clin N Am 2006;17:401-413; and Thomson MICROMEDEX.

DOSING AND ADMINISTRATION

Baclofen (Lioresal) is structurally related to the inhibitory neurotransmitter GABA. It reduces the excitability of primary afferent terminals, improves presynaptic inhibition, suppresses monosynaptic and polysynaptic reflex activity, reduces gamma motor neuron activity, and decreases muscle spindle sensitivity.[11] It has been used for spasticity in patients with trigeminal neuralgia.[9] Baclofen is metabolized in the liver and excreted in urine. Routes of administration include oral and intrathecal (via implanted pump) if significant adverse effects preclude systemic dose escalation.

Diazepam (Valium) is a benzodiazepine that represses behavioral arousal, agitation, and anxiety. It acts by reducing polysynaptic reflexes through GABA receptors on inhibitory neurons and has muscle relaxant, sedative, and antispasticity properties. Diazepam is metabolized in the liver and has an active metabolite, excretion of which occurs through the kidney.[10] Routes of administration include oral, rectal, injection, gel, and tablet.

Tizanidine (Zanaflex) is an imidazoline derivative that is related to the α_2-adrenergic agonist clonidine. Tizanidine binds to both α_2-adrenergic and imidazoline spinal and supraspinal receptor sites.[12] Similar to clonidine, it restores and enhances nonadrenergic presynaptic inhibition of motor units.[13] The drug is well tolerated and reduces the spasticity associated with several causes.[14] Tizanidine is administered orally and gradually titrated to avoid side effects.

Clonidine is used to treat hypotension and opioid withdrawal. It is a centrally acting α_2-adrenergic agonist that acts on the brainstem to reduce central sympathetic outflow and thereby decrease peripheral muscle resistance, blood pressure, and heart rate. Clonidine is metabolized in the liver and excreted through the kidneys. It is administered orally and transdermally.[10]

Dantrolene sodium is a hydantoin derivative that decreases release of Ca^{2+} from the sarcoplasmic reticulum; it is not a centrally acting agent. Dantrolene is metabolized in the liver and excreted through the kidneys.[9] It is administered orally and parenterally.

Gabapentin is an anticonvulsant structurally similar to GABA but with different pharmacological actions. Gabapentin blocks voltage-gated calcium channels, which prevents depolarization. It may also act on GABA receptors that contain $\alpha_2\beta$ subunits. It is not metabolized, but eliminated by renal excretion and can be hemodialyzed.[12] Gabapentin can only be given orally. Absorption is dependent on a carrier-mediated mechanism in the small bowel.

Botulinum toxin types A and B are products of the spore-forming anaerobic bacillus *Clostridium botulinum*. Toxins A, B, and F are the only neurotoxins proven effective in clinical application. They act at the neuromuscular junction and prevent calcium-dependent release of acetylcholine, thereby providing temporary drug-induced denervation. Therapeutic effect takes place in up to 1 week and can last up to 3 months, at which time repeat injections can be considered. Administration of botulinum toxin (Botox) by injection significantly decreases spasticity.[8] Repeated botulinum injections can lead to the development of antibodies and make patients resistant to its therapeutic effect.[10] In many countries, Botox has been licensed for focal spasticity. Therapeutic objectives include reduction of tonus and pain, prevention of fixed contractures, and functional improvement, in addition to relief of symptoms secondary to spasticity.[15] Physicians using Botox should be trained in the relevant topical anatomy and kinesiology because transient focal muscle paralysis begins in 24 to 72 hours, with maximal effect seen in 5 to 14 days.[8]

Use of *cannabis (Cesamet, Marinol)* as a muscle-relaxing agent may relieve some forms of spasticity, especially in patients with multiple sclerosis or spinal cord injury.[16] The duration of action of cannabis on detrusor function or muscle spasticity is unknown. Many patients smoke cannabis for the rapid relief of acute symptoms (e.g., muscle spasms) or to attenuate chronic symptoms (e.g., tremor, pain) rather than prophylaxis. This pattern of drug use is probably related to the pharmacokinetic profile of cannabinoids.[17]

MAJOR SIDE EFFECTS

Side effects vary between drugs (Table 146-4). Typical adverse effects are related to central nervous system (CNS) depression and include cognitive impairment, depression, drowsiness, fatigue, nausea, visual hallucinations, and weakness. Dry mouth, bradycardia, hypotension, constipation, and elevated liver function test results have also been reported to be common. The classic adverse effects of *baclofen* involve the CNS—depression, dizziness, drowsiness, weakness, nausea, and seizures and hallucinations caused by abrupt cessation of continuous treatment.

The side effects of *diazepam* are CNS related and include cognitive impairment, sedation, and potential for dependence.

The most commonly reported side effects of *tizanidine* are dizziness, drowsiness (54%), dry mouth (45%), visual hallucinations (3%), and elevated liver function test results when the dosage exceeds 24 mg/day. The elevated liver parameters are reversible with dosage reduction.[18]

All *benzodiazepines* generate dependence and consequently evoke withdrawal symptoms. The most frequently reported withdrawal symptoms include various gastrointestinal symptoms, diaphoresis, tremor, lethargy, dizziness, headaches, increased perception of sound and smell, restlessness, insomnia, irritability, anxiety, tinnitus, and feelings of depersonalization. Withdrawal occurs after 4 to 6 weeks of benzodiazepine administration. Symptoms may begin within 2 to 5 days of stopping treatment with benzodiazepines and persist for several weeks.[19]

Clonidine is infrequently used as a single agent for spasticity; adverse effects include bradycardia, constipation, depression, dizziness, drowsiness, dry mouth, and hypotension.

Because of the peripheral site of *dantrolene's* action, the most common side effect is weakness. Other adverse effects include drowsiness, diarrhea, and malaise.

Gabapentin is well tolerated and adverse effects include dizziness, nausea, and sedation.

Adverse effects of *botulinum toxin* include biliary colic, dizziness, edema, erythema, fever, flulike symptoms, headache, injection site pain, and nausea. Dysphagia, dry mouth, and dysphonia can be observed with injections in the cervical area.[10]

TABLE 146-4   Antispastic Drug Dosing and Side Effects

AGENT	STARTING DOSAGE	MAXIMUM RECOMMENDED DOSAGE	ADVERSE EFFECTS	MONITORING	SPECIAL ATTENTION
Baclofen	5 mg/day increasing to 15 mg/day in 3 divided doses	80 mg/day in divided doses	Muscle weakness, sedation, fatigue, dizziness, nausea	Periodic liver function tests	Abrupt cessation associated with seizures
Diazepam	2 mg/day bid or 5 mg qhs	40-60 mg/day in divided doses	Sedation, cognitive impairment, depression	Dependence potential	Withdrawal syndrome
Tizanidine	2-4 mg/day	36 mg/day in divided doses	Drowsiness, dry mouth, dizziness, reversible dose-related elevated liver transaminases	Periodic liver function tests	Not to be used with antihypertensives
Clonidine	0.1 mg/day	Not approved for spasticity; in patients with hypertension, doses as high as 2.4 mg in divided doses have been studied but rarely used; usual dose in hypertension, 0.2-0.6 mg/day	Bradycardia, hypotension, dry mouth, drowsiness, constipation, dizziness, depression		Add-on agent Hypotension may result Not to be used with tizanidine
Dantrolene	25 mg/day	400 mg/day in divided doses	Hepatotoxicity (potentially irreversible), weakness, sedation, diarrhea	Periodic liver function tests	Hepatotoxicity
Gabapentin	100 mg tid	3600 mg/day in divided doses	Stomach upset		

bid, twice daily; qhs, at bedtime; tid, three times daily.
From Kita M, Goodkin DE. Drugs used to treat spasticity. Drugs 2000;59:487-495.

TABLE 146-5   Antispasticity Drug Interactions

ANTISPASTICITY DRUGS	ADDED DRUG	EFFECT
Baclofen	Opiate analgesics, benzodiazepines, hypertensive agents	Increased effect
	CNS depressants and ethanol (sedation), tricyclic antidepressants (short-term memory loss), clindamycin (neuromuscular blockade), guanabenz (sedation), MAO inhibitors (decrease blood pressure, CNS, and respiratory effects)	Increased toxicity
Clonidine	Antipsychotics (especially low potency) or nitroprusside	Additive hypotensive effects
	β-Blockers	Potentiate bradycardia, may increase the rebound hypertension associated with withdrawal
	CNS depressants (includes barbiturates, benzodiazepines, narcotic analgesics, ethanol, and other sedative agents)	Sedative effects may be additive; monitor for increased effect
	Cyclosporine	Increases serum concentrations of cyclosporine; cyclosporine dosage adjustment may be needed
	Hypoglycemic agents	Decreases symptoms of hypoglycemia
	Levodopa	Effects may be reduced by clonidine in some patients with Parkinson's disease
	Local anesthetics	Epidural clonidine may prolong the sensory and motor blockade of local anesthetics
	Mirtazapine	Enhances the hypertensive response associated with abrupt clonidine withdrawal
	Narcotic analgesics	May potentiate the hypotensive effects of clonidine
	Tricyclic antidepressants	The antihypertensive effects of clonidine may be antagonized by tricyclic antidepressants; tricyclic antidepressants may enhance the hypertensive response associated with abrupt clonidine withdrawal
	Verapamil	Concurrent administration may be associated with hypotension and AV block in some patients (limited documentation)
Dantrolene	CYP3A4 inducers (aminoglutethimide, carbamazepine, nafcillin, nevirapine, phenobarbital, phenytoin, and rifamycin)	May decrease levels/effects of dantrolene

TABLE 146-5 Antispasticity Drug Interactions—cont'd

ANTISPASTICITY DRUGS	ADDED DRUG	EFFECT
	CYP3A4 inhibitors (azole antifungals, clarithromycin, diclofenac, doxycycline, erythromycin, imatinib, isoniazid, nefazodone, nicardipine, propofol, protease inhibitors, quinidine, telithromycin, and verapamil)	May increase levels/effects of dantrolene
	Estrogens	Hepatotoxicity
	CNS depressants	Sedation
	MAO inhibitors, phenothiazines, clindamycin	Increased neuromuscular blockade
	Verapamil, warfarin, clofibrate, and tolbutamide	Hyperkalemia and cardiac depression
	Ethanol	Increase CNS depression
	Herb/neutraceutical: avoid valerian, St. John's wort, kava kava, gotu kola	May increase CNS depression
Gabapentin	CNS depressants (includes ethanol, barbiturates, narcotic analgesics, and other sedative agents)	Additive sedative effect
Tizanidine	CYP1A2 inhibitors, including amiodarone, ciprofloxacin, fluvoxamine, ketoconazole, norfloxacin, ofloxacin, and rofecoxib	May increase levels/effects of tizanidine
	Ciprofloxacin	May increase levels/effects (e.g., hypotension) of tizanidine; concurrent use is contraindicated
	Diuretics, other α-adrenergic agonists, antihypertensives	Additive hypotensive effects may occur
	Fluvoxamine	Contraindicated, may increase levels/effects (e.g., hypotension) of tizanidine
	Oral contraceptives	May decrease clearance of tizanidine

AV, atrioventricular; CNS, central nervous system; MAO, monoamine oxidase.
Adapted from http://www.uptodateonline.com/utd/index.do

CONTRAINDICATIONS

Contraindications vary with the medication and include hypersensitivity to the drug or any component of the formulation (baclofen, diazepam, tizanidine, gabapentin, and clonidine).

Diazepam is contraindicated in those with narrow-angle glaucoma and in pregnant patients.

Tizanidine must be avoided in patients taking ciprofloxacin or fluvoxamine.

Dantrolene is not recommended in those with active hepatic disease and should not be used when spasticity helps maintain posture or balance.

DRUG INTERACTIONS

Most antispasticity drugs may cause drug interactions. Baclofen, clonidine, and dantrolene may enhance any sedative effect if prescribed with antidepressants. Concurrent administration of verapamil with clonidine may be associated with hypotension and atrioventricular block. Clinically important drug interactions are listed in Table 146-5. Antispastic drugs can interact with corticosteroids and drugs used for chemotherapy.

REFERENCES

1. Pandyan AD, Gregoric M, Barnes MP, et al. Spasticity: Clinical perceptions, neurological realities and meaningful measurement. Disabil Rehabil 2005; 27:2-6.
2. Sheean G. Neurophysiology of spasticity. In Barnes MP, Johnson GR (eds). Upper Motorneuron Syndrome and Spasticity: Clinical Management and Neurophysiology. Cambridge: Cambridge University Press, 2001, pp 12-79.
3. Barnes MP. An overview of the clinical management of spasticity. In Barnes MP, Johnson CR (eds). Upper Motorneuron Syndrome and Spasticity: Clinical Management and Neurophysiology. Cambridge: Cambridge University Press, 2001, pp 1-11.
4. Miller TM, Layzer RB. Muscle cramps. Muscle Nerve 2005;32:431-442.
5. Maynard FM, Karunas RS, Waring WP 3rd. Epidemiology of spasticity following traumatic spinal cord injury. Arch Phys Med Rehabil 1990;71:566-569.
6. Brar SP, Smith MB, Nelson LM, et al. Evaluation of treatment protocols on minimal to moderate spasticity in multiple sclerosis. Arch Phys Med Rehabil 1991;72:186-189.
7. Cervera-Deval J, Morant-Guillen MP, Fenollosa-Vasquez P, et al. Social handicaps of multiple sclerosis and their relation to neurological alterations. Arch Phys Med Rehabil 1994;75:1223-1227.
8. Kita M, Goodkin DE. Drugs used to treat spasticity. Drugs 2000;59:487-495.
9. Hwang AS, Wilcox GL. Baclofen, gamma-aminobutyric acid B receptors and substance P in the mouse spinal cord. J Pharmacol Exp Ther 1989; 248:1026-1033.
10. Meleger AL. Muscle relaxants and antispasticity agents. Phys Med Rehabil Clin N Am 2006;17:401-413.
11. Van Hemet JC. A double-blind comparison of baclofen and placebo in patients with spasticity of cerebral origin. In Feldman RG, Young, RR, Koella WP (eds). Spasticity: Disordered Motor Control. Chicago: Year Book, 1980, pp 41-49.
12. Nance PW, Young RR. Antispasticity medications. Phys Med Rehabil Clin N Am 1999;10:337-355, viii.
13. Knutsson E. Assessment of motor function in spasticity. Triangle 1982; 21:13-20.
14. Emre M. Review of clinical trials with sirdauld in spasticity. In Emre M, Benecke R (eds). Spasticity. London: Parthenon, 1989.
15. Truong DD, Jost WH. Botulinum toxin: Clinical use. Parkinsonism Relat Disord 2006;12:331-355.
16. Clifford DB. Tetrahydrocannabinol for tremor in multiple sclerosis. Ann Neurol 1983;13:669-671.
17. Brady CM, DasGupta R, Dalton C, et al. An open-label pilot study of cannabis-based extracts for bladder dysfunction in advanced multiple sclerosis. Mult Scler 2004;10:425-433.
18. United Kingdom Tizanidine Study Group. A double-blind placebo-control trial of tizanidine in the treatment of spasticity cause by multiple sclerosis. Neurology 1994;44(11 Suppl 9):S70-S79.
19. Janicak PG, Davis JM, Preskorn SH, et al. Principles and Practice of Psychopharmacotherapy, 4th ed. Philadelphia: Lippincott Williams & Wilkins, 2006.

SUGGESTED READING

Bandini F, Mazella L. Gabapentin as treatment for hemifacial spasm. Eur Neurol 1999;42:49-51.
Biering-Sørensen F, Nielsen JB, Klinge K. Spasticity—assessment: A review. Spinal Cord 2006;44:708-722.

Pandyan AD, Johnson GR, Price CI, et al. A review of the properties and limitations of the Ashworth and modified Ashworth Scales as measures of spasticity. Clin Rehabil 1999;13: 373-383.

Truong DD, Jost WH. Botulinum toxin: Clinical use. Parkinsonism Relat Disord 2006;12:331-355.

CHAPTER **147**

Drugs for Diarrhea

Catherine McVearry Kelso

KEY POINTS

- The therapeutic approach to using antidiarrheal agents is to slow intestinal transit.
- The choice of antidiarrheal therapy is based on targeting a specific known cause or applying a general nonspecific approach.
- Lomotil is the opioid antidiarrheal agent of choice.
- Loperamide is a useful agent for secretory diarrhea and management of symptoms in palliative care.
- Identify the antidiarrheal agents available to manage different types of diarrhea and their appropriate use (see Table 147-1).

Diarrhea is defined as the frequent passage or loose consistency of stool above an individual's baseline.[1] There are many potential causes in palliative medicine, including overuse of laxatives, sorbitol, infections, acquired immunodeficiency syndrome, antibiotics, chemotherapy, radiotherapy, paraneoplastic syndromes, neuroendocrine tumors, malabsorption secondary to pancreatic cancer, and bowel resection or dysfunction as a result of tumor infiltration or obstruction.[2,3] Although cancer-related diarrhea is frequent, all of the common causes of diarrhea unrelated to cancer must be considered in the palliative care population.[4,5] One of the most common reasons for "loose stools" is excess laxative use or overflow stool from fecal impaction. Diarrhea results from disordered intestinal water and electrolyte transport with an increase in transit or secretion.[6] With either mechanism, decreased absorption occurs and can lead to dehydration, malnutrition, skin breakdown, and fatigue, which adversely affect quality of life.

The basic therapeutic approach is to slow intestinal transit so that more fluid absorption can take place. In view of the different mechanisms involved, the choice of appropriate antidiarrheal therapy is directed at a known specific cause, or a general nonspecific approach is adopted. Diarrhea can often be managed by taking a general nonspecific pharmacological approach that targets slowing of gut motility. Nonpharmacological methods

need to be coupled with antidiarrheal agents to address dehydration along with appropriate gluten-free or lactose-free dietary modification (Table 147-1).

OPIOIDS

Opioid receptors are present in bowel smooth muscle and influence motility. The main mechanisms of opioid action are slower bowel transit through decreased peristalsis; inhibition of anorectal sphincter relaxation, which reduces urgency; and decreased anorectal sensitivity, which improves comfort.[2]

Loperamide

Mechanism of Action

Loperamide is the opioid antidiarrheal drug of choice because of its efficacy, potency (50 times more potent than morphine as an antidiarrheal), and lack of transmission across the blood-brain barrier.[7] It also reduces ileal calcium flux with activity independent of the opioid effect and has the highest antidiarrheal/analgesic effect among opioid-like agents.[8] Loperamide acts directly on intestinal muscles through the opioid receptor, inhibits peristalsis, and prolongs transit time. Fecal volume is reduced, which limits fluid and electrolyte loss. Anal sphincter tone increases and anorectal sensitivity decreases. Loperamide is excreted mainly in feces.

Dosage

The dosage of loperamide is 4 mg orally, followed by 2 mg after each loose stool, up to 16 mg. Loperamide should be discontinued after a 12-hour diarrhea-free interval. If symptoms have not resolved within 24 hours, loperamide, 2 mg every 2 hours, should be considered.[5,7]

Major Side Effects

Opioid-like effects may cause urinary retention at high doses.

Contraindications

Loperamide is contraindicated in individuals hypersensitive to loperamide or any component of the formulation, those with abdominal pain without diarrhea, and children younger than 2 years. Its use as primary therapy should be avoided in patients with acute dysentery, acute ulcerative colitis, bacterial enterocolitis, and pseudomembranous colitis.

Drug Interactions

The concentration of loperamide is increased when used with gemfibrozil, itraconazole, or saquinavir. Delirium may occur when used with St. John's wort or valerian.

Opium Preparations

Paregoric and Tincture of Opium

MECHANISM OF ACTION

Paregoric and tincture of opium increase smooth muscle tone in the gastrointestinal (GI) tract, decrease motility

TABLE 147-1   Drugs for Diarrhea

CLASS	DRUGS	DIARRHEA DISORDER
Opioids	Loperamide Paregoric—tincture of opium Codeine Diphenoxylate with atropine	Mild to moderate Osmotic Secretory Traveler's
Anticholinergic/antispasmodic	Atropine sulfate Dicyclomine Hyoscyamine Glycopyrrolate Diphenoxylate and atropine Belladonna and opium suppository Pyridium Plus	Mild to moderate Functional bowel disorders Irritable bowel Cramping
Bile acid sequestration	Cholestyramine	Bile induced Ileal resection
Absorbent bulk forming	Psyllium	Mild to moderate
Anti-infective/xenobiotic	Bismuth subsalicylate	Traveler's Secretory
Anti-infective	Metronidazole Vancomycin	Infectious Clostridium difficile
Anti-infective	Norfloxacin	Infectious Traveler's
Antisecretory	Clonidine Octreotide	Severe Diabetic Graft versus host Chemotherapy induced Acquired immunodeficiency syndrome Carcinoid Neuroendocrine tumor Secretory

and peristalsis, and diminish digestive secretions. The main route of excretion is renal.

DOSAGE

- Paregoric (camphorated opium tincture), 2 mg (anhydrous morphine) per 5 mL. Dose—5 to 10 mL orally one to four times a day[9]
- Tincture of opium (deodorized opium tincture), 50 mg (anhydrous morphine) per 5 mL; contains 25 times more morphine than paregoric does. Dose—0.6 mL (equivalent to 6 mg morphine) four times daily

MAJOR SIDE EFFECTS

Opium shares the side effect profile of all opiate agonists. The precautions of opiate agonist therapy should be observed, namely, central nervous system (CNS) depression and possible nausea. Opioids produce their major effects on the CNS and the bowel through mu receptors.

CONTRAINDICATIONS

- Hypersensitivity to opium or any component of the formulation

DRUG INTERACTIONS

- Increased effect/toxicity with CNS depressants (e.g., alcohol, narcotics, benzodiazepines, tricyclic antidepressants [TCAs], monoamine oxidase [MAO] inhibitors, phenothiazine)

Codeine

Mechanism of Action

Codeine is a mu receptor agonist. The analgesic effect of codeine may be due to its conversion to morphine. A 25% reduction in dosage is recommended in patients with moderate renal failure (glomerular filtration rate [GFR], 10 to 50 mL/min); in those with severe renal failure (GFR < 10 mL/min), the dosage should be reduced by 50%. A reduction in dosage is probably indicated for patients with hepatic insufficiency.

Dosage

- Oral—15 to 60 mg every 4 hours[9]

Major Side Effects

Gastrointestinal intolerance, including nausea, vomiting, and constipation, is common. Sedation occurs at higher doses as a result of opioid effects.

Contraindications

- Hypersensitivity to codeine
- Coadministration with CNS depressants (e.g., alcohol, narcotics, benzodiazepines, TCAs, MAO inhibitors, phenothiazine)

Drug Interactions

● Increased effect/toxicity with CNS depressants (e.g., alcohol, narcotics, benzodiazepines, TCAs, MAO inhibitors, phenothiazine)

Diphenoxylate Hydrochloride

Mechanism of Action

Diphenoxylate acts on the smooth muscle of the intestinal tract similar to morphine and inhibits motility. It has little to no analgesic effect. Diphenoxylate has a variable half-life (3 to 14 hours) and is excreted primarily in feces.

Dosage

● Oral—Adult dose, 5 mg four times daily[9]

Major Side Effects

● May induce nausea and vomiting

Contraindications

Diphenoxylate is contraindicated in patients with cirrhosis and jaundice. It is structurally similar to meperidine hydrochloride, so the possibility of hypertensive crisis should be considered when diphenoxylate and MAO inhibitors are used together.[9]

Drug Interactions

● Increased effect/toxicity with CNS depressants (e.g., alcohol, narcotics, benzodiazepines, TCAs, MAO inhibitors, phenothiazine)

ANTICHOLINERGICS/ANTISPASMODICS

Mechanism of Action

Anticholinergic agents bind to muscarinic cholinergic receptors and block endogenous acetylcholine. Muscarinic receptors have widespread effects, including decreasing secretions of the gastrointestinal system. They alter gut motility and dilate both the small and large intestine.[1] Antimuscarinic drugs are widely used as antiarrhythmic, antiparkinson, antiasthmatic, and antispasmodic agents.

Atropine Sulfate

Mechanism of Action

Atropine alters motility by binding to gut antimuscarinic receptors. It is metabolized in the liver and excreted in urine.

Dosage

● Oral—0.4 to 0.6 mg (range, 0.1 to 1.2) every 4 to 6 hours[9]

Major Side Effects

Adverse reactions frequently associated with antimuscarinics include dry mouth, dry skin, urinary hesitancy and retention, and constipation.

Contraindications

Antimuscarinics are contraindicated in patients with known hypersensitivity. The drugs are also contraindicated in those with angle-closure glaucoma. They should be used with caution in patients with partial obstructive uropathy and are contraindicated in those with obstructive uropathy (e.g., bladder neck obstruction caused by prostatic hypertrophy). Antimuscarinics are contraindicated in patients with myasthenia gravis. They should be administered with caution to those with known or suspected GI infections (e.g., *Clostridium difficile*-associated diarrhea and colitis) because these drugs may decrease GI motility and prolong symptoms by causing retention of the causative organism or toxin. Antimuscarinics are also contraindicated in patients with obstruction of GI tract (e.g., pyloroduodenal stenosis, achalasia), cardiospasm, paralytic ileus, or intestinal atony (especially in geriatric or debilitated patients).

Drug Interactions

Additive adverse effects from cholinergic blockade may occur when antimuscarinics are administered with phenothiazines, amantadine, antiparkinsonian drugs, glutethimide, meperidine, TCAs, muscle relaxants, antiarrhythmics with anticholinergic activity (e.g., quinidine, disopyramide, procainamide), or some antihistamines (including meclizine).[9]

Dicyclomine Hydrochloride

Mechanism of Action

Dicyclomine is used for its antispasmodic properties in those with functional disturbances in GI motility, such as irritable bowel syndrome. Elimination is through renal excretion.

Dosage

● Oral—20 mg four times daily[9]

Major Side Effects, Contraindications, Drug Interactions

● Similar to those noted with atropine

Hyoscyamine Sulfate

Mechanism of Action

Hyoscyamine is used for functional GI motility disorders such as irritable bowel syndrome. Its pharmacokinetics resemble those of atropine.

Dosage

● Oral—0.15 to 0.3 mg every 4 hours, not to exceed 1.5 mg in 24 hours[9]

Major Side Effects, Contraindications, Drug Interactions

● Similar to those noted with atropine

Glycopyrrolate

Unlike atropine or hyoscyamine (tertiary amine antimuscarinics), glycopyrrolate is a quaternary ammonium antimuscarinic with poor lipid solubility and does not readily penetrate the blood-brain barrier. It is eliminated in feces.

Dosage

- Oral—1 mg three times daily; maximum dose, 8 mg daily[9]

Major Side Effects, Contraindications, Drug Interactions

- Similar to those noted with atropine

Belladonna and Opium Suppository

Mechanism of Action

Belladonna is a naturally occurring alkaloid with antimuscarinic activity principally from its atropine content. It is used for functional GI motility disorders such as irritable bowel syndrome and neurogenic bowel disturbances. It is effective for painful bladder spasm and pelvic pain.

Dosage

- Suppository—16.2 mg every day or twice daily (belladonna extract, 0.21 mg of alkaloids of belladonna leaf, and powered opium, 30 or 60 mg)

Major Side Effects, Contraindications, Drug Interactions

- Similar to those of atropine

Phenazopyridine Hydrochloride Combination

Mechanism of Action

Phenazopyridine hydrochloride combination is used for the symptomatic relief of pain, burning, urgency, and frequency of lower urinary tract mucosa as a result of infection or trauma. One preparation consists of a combination of phenazopyridine (150 mg), butabarbital (15 mg), and hyoscyamine (0.3 mg). When combined with the barbiturate butabarbital (sedative-hypnotic), the adverse effect profile is widened. In particular, its half-life is long, 20 to 100 hours.

Dosage

- Oral—Pyridium Plus (phenazopyridine, 150 mg; butabarbital, 15 mg; hyoscyamine, 0.3 mg), three times daily for 2 days. When butabarbital sodium is used alone for routine sedation, the usual adult dosage is 15 to 30 mg three or four times daily.

Major Side Effects

Phenazopyridine has been associated with headache and mild GI disturbance. Patients should be warned that phenazopyridine will produce orange urine. Barbiturates, in addition to CNS sedation, may cause diarrhea. Hyoscyamine is an anticholinergic and has side effects similar to those of atropine.

Contraindications

Because of the barbiturate, the dosage should be reduced in geriatric or debilitated patients and those with impaired hepatic function. Phenazopyridine is contraindicated in patients with impaired renal or hepatic function.

Drug Interactions

Barbiturates may be additive or potentiate other CNS depressants, including other sedatives or hypnotics, antihistamines, tranquilizers, and alcohol.

BILE ACID RESIN

Cholestyramine

Mechanism of Action

- Bile acid sequestration

Dosage

- Oral—Oral suspension prepared from the powder, 4 g mixed with noncarbonated fluid twice daily 1 hour before meals[10]

Major Side Effect

- Constipation

Contraindications

Cholestyramine resin is ineffective and contraindicated in patients with complete biliary obstruction because no bile products reach the intestine. It is contraindicated in those hypersensitive to the drug or any ingredient in its formulation.

Drug Interactions

Because cholestyramine is an anion exchange resin, it can bind to a number of drugs in the GI tract and may delay or reduce their absorption.

ABSORBENT BULK FORMING

Psyllium

Mechanism of Action

Bulk-forming laxatives dissolve or swell in water to form an emollient gel or viscous solution. The resulting bulk in feces promotes peristalsis and reduces transit time. Bulk-forming laxatives are not generally absorbed from the GI tract. The effect of bulk formation is usually apparent within 12 to 24 hours, but the full effect may not be apparent for 2 to 3 days.

Dosage

- Oral—Mix 2 tbsp with 250 mL water, up to 30 g/day in divided doses[9]

Major Side Effects

Adverse effects are rare. Bowel or esophageal obstruction, swelling or blockage of the throat, choking, or asphyxiation have occurred when insufficient liquid was administered with such laxatives. Potentially severe hypersensitivity reactions, including acute bronchospasm and anaphylaxis, can occur in susceptible individuals after inhalation of the powder.

Contraindications

Bulk-forming laxatives should not be used in patients with esophageal obstruction or those with difficulty swallowing.

Drug Interactions

Bulk-forming agents may interfere with other medications, so they should not be taken with other medications.

ANTI-INFECTIVE AGENTS/XENOBIOTICS

Bismuth Subsalicylate

Mechanism of Action

Bismuth is one of many xenobiotics commonly used for traveler's diarrhea, nausea, and vomiting, as well as the flatus and odor associated with ileostomies and colostomies. Bismuth binds to sulfhydryl groups and decreases fecal odor through the formation of bismuth sulfide. Sulfhydryl binding is also the proposed mechanism of the antimicrobial effect of bismuth. It is used for symptomatic treatment of mild, nonspecific diarrhea and control of traveler's diarrhea (enterotoxigenic *Escherichia coli*).

Dosage

- Oral—Subsalicylate (doses based on 262 mg/15 mL liquid or 262-mg tablets): two tablets or 30 mL every 30 minutes to 1 hour as needed, up to eight doses in 24 hours[9]

Major Side Effects

Bismuth subsalicylate may cause encephalopathy. Up to 90% of the salicylate in bismuth subsalicylate is absorbed, so monitoring for overuse and possible salicylate toxicity is necessary. Discoloration of the tongue (darkening), grayish black stools, and impaction may occur in infants and debilitated patients. Monitor for hearing loss or tinnitus.

Contraindications

Hypersensitivity to bismuth or any component of the formulation is a contraindication. Subsalicylate should not be used during influenza or chickenpox because of the risk for Reye's syndrome. A history of severe GI bleeding and coagulopathy are other contraindications. It is best avoided in patients with renal impairment.

Drug Interactions

Bismuth subsalicylate tablets should be taken at least 3 hours apart from other medications. Its effect is decreased when administered with tetracyclines and uricosurics and its toxicity increased when administered with aspirin, warfarin, or hypoglycemic agents.

ANTI-INFECTIVES

Metronidazole—Oral

Mechanism of Action

Metronidazole is bactericidal and used for *C. difficile*-associated diarrhea and colitis. Eighty percent of an oral dose of metronidazole is absorbed from the GI tract. Its plasma half-life is not affected by renal function, and it may be prolonged in patients with impaired hepatic function.

Dosage

- Oral—750 mg to 2 g daily given in three or four divided doses for 7 to 14 days
- Intravenous—500 to 750 mg every 6 to 8 hours in adults when oral therapy is not feasible[10]

Major Side Effects

The most frequent adverse reaction to oral metronidazole is nausea, sometimes accompanied by headache, anorexia, dry mouth, and an unpleasant metallic taste. A furry tongue, glossitis, and stomatitis have been reported with oral metronidazole, perhaps caused by overgrowth of *Candida*.

Contraindications

Patients should be advised to avoid concurrent use of metronidazole and alcohol. Metronidazole should be used with caution and in reduced dosage in those with severe hepatic impairment. It is contraindicated if there is a history of hypersensitivity to the drug.

Drug Interactions

Metronidazole potentates oral anticoagulants by prolonging the prothrombin time. It appears to inhibit alcohol dehydrogenase and other alcohol-oxidizing enzymes and can lead to reactions such as flushing, headache, nausea, vomiting, abdominal cramps, and sweating. Because administration of disulfiram with metronidazole may lead to acute psychosis, they should not be used concomitantly.

Vancomycin—Oral

Mechanism of Action

Vancomycin is administered orally to seriously ill patients for *C. difficile*-associated diarrhea and pseudomembranous colitis or those who cannot tolerate or do not respond to oral metronidazole. Vancomycin is bactericidal, excreted renally, and requires dosage adjustment in patients with renal failure.

Dosage

- Oral—Usual adult dosage, 0.5 to 2 g daily given in three or four divided doses for 7 to 10 days[10]

Major Side Effects

- Damage to the auditory branch of the eighth cranial nerve and permanent deafness
- Unusually, "red-man syndrome," or flushing and erythema of the face and neck, with oral use

Contraindications

Vancomycin is contraindicated in patients with known hypersensitivity to the drug. Because of ototoxic and nephrotoxic effects, it should be used with caution in those with impaired renal function and avoided in individuals with previous hearing loss.

Drug Interactions

Given the possibility of additive toxicities with other ototoxic or nephrotoxic drugs (e.g., aminoglycosides, amphotericin B, bacitracin, cisplatin, colistin, polymyxin B), renal and auditory function needs to be monitored.

Norfloxacin

Mechanism of Action

Norfloxacin is a fluoroquinolone anti-infective agent. It has been effective in adults for gastroenteritis caused by susceptible enterotoxigenic *E. coli*, *Aeromonas hydrophila*, *Plesiomonas shigelloides*, *Salmonella*, *Shigella*, and *Vibrio cholerae*. Norfloxacin has been used for the short-term treatment of traveler's diarrhea. Dosage adjustment is required in patients with impaired renal function. Adults with creatinine clearance lower than 30 mL/min should receive 400 mg once daily.

Dosage

- Oral—400 mg orally twice daily for 3 to 5 days. Norfloxacin should be take at least 1 hour before or at least 2 hours after a meal or ingestion of dairy products (e.g., milk, yogurt).[9]

Major Side Effects

Nausea is one of the most frequent. Adverse effects resemble those of other fluoroquinolone anti-infectives (e.g., ciprofloxacin, norfloxacin). The most frequent adverse effects involve the GI tract or CNS.

Drug Interactions

Antacids containing magnesium, aluminum, or calcium may decrease absorption. Concomitant use of antiarrhythmic agents may increase the risk for prolongation of the QT interval during ofloxacin therapy. Hypoglycemia has been reported in diabetics. Concomitant administration of some other quinolones (e.g., ciprofloxacin, norfloxacin) with warfarin (Coumadin) also leads to increased prothrombin times. Concomitant use of some quinolones (e.g., norfloxacin) with cyclosporine may increase serum concentrations of cyclosporine. Concomitant use may increase theophylline levels.

ANTISECRETORY AGENTS

Clonidine

Mechanism of Action

Clonidine is an α_2-agonist used to reduce intestinal sympathetic tone in diabetic diarrhea and idiopathic secretory diarrhea. It stimulates sodium and chloride absorption and inhibits chloride and bicarbonate secretion in the small intestine and colon and decreases motility.[11]

Dosage

- Oral—0.1 to 0.2 mg three times daily[8]; maximum dose, 2.4 mg daily

Major Side Effects

The most frequent side effects are dry mouth, dizziness, drowsiness and sedation, and constipation, which appear to be dose related. Centrally mediated sedation and hypotension limit its use. Monitor for depression. It should not be abruptly discontinued because of the risk for rebound hypertension. To stop treatment, use a tapered withdrawal over a period of 2 to 4 days.

Contraindications

- Hypersensitivity and hypotension

Drug Interactions

Clonidine may be additive with or potentiate the action of other CNS depressants such as opiates or other analgesics, barbiturates or other sedatives, anesthetics, and alcohol. Because clonidine may produce bradycardia and atrioventricular (AV) block, additive effects should be considered if administered with other drugs that affect sinus node function or AV nodal conduction (e.g., guanethidine), β-adrenergic blocking agents (e.g., propranolol), calcium channel blocking agents, or cardiac glycosides.

Octreotide

Mechanism of Action

Octreotide inhibits secretory diarrhea brought about by carcinoid or other hormone-secreting tumors of the pancreas or GI tract, diarrhea associated with small cell lung cancer, and human immunodeficiency virus–related diarrhea. It slows intestinal mobility and reduces acid secretion.

Dosage

- Oral—50 to 100 µg subcutaneously or intravenously two to three times a day; maximum dose, 500 µg three times daily.[5,7] A long-acting depot formulation is available for chronic use once tolerance is demonstrated to daily injections for at least 2 weeks.
- Long-acting depot—20 to 30 mg intramuscularly monthly[12]

Major Side Effects

Transient nausea, bloating, and pain at the injection site have been reported. Long-term use can be complicated by cholelithiasis, hypoglycemia or hyperglycemia, hypothyroidism, or bradycardia. Those receiving octreotide should undergo baseline and periodic ultrasonographic examination of the gall bladder and bile ducts. Baseline and periodic monitoring of thyroid function is recommended. Because of octreotide-induced alterations in various hormones in glucose homeostasis, monitoring for hypoglycemia or hyperglycemia is required. Insulin requirements may be reduced in type 1 diabetes mellitus during octreotide therapy.

Contraindications

Certain effects of endogenous somatostatins (e.g., effects on GI and biliary function and motility, glucose tolerance, endocrine function) may be manifested as adverse effects during octreotide therapy.

REFERENCES

1. Powell DW. Approach to the patient with diarrhea. In Yamada T, Alpers DH, Kaplowitz N (eds). Textbook of Gastroenterology, 4th ed. Philadelphia: Lippincott Williams & Wilkins, 2003, p 844.
2. Mercadante S. Diarrhea in terminally ill patients: Pathophysiology and treatment. J Pain Symptom Manage 1995;10:298-309.
3. Sykes N. Constipation and diarrhoea. In Doyle D, Hanks G, Cherny NI, et al (eds). Oxford Textbook of Palliative Medicine, 3rd ed. New York: Oxford University Press, 2004, p 483.
4. Ippoliti C. Antidiarrheal agents for the management of treatment-related diarrhea in cancer patients. Am J Health Syst Pharm 1998;55:1573-1580.
5. Benson AB 3rd, Ajani JA, Catalano RB, et al. Recommended guidelines for the treatment of cancer treatment–induced diarrhea. J Clin Oncol 2004;22:2918-2926.
6. Pasricha PJ. Treatment of disorders of bowel motility and water flux; antiemetic agents used in biliary and pancreatic disease. In Brunton LL, Lazo JS, Parker KL (eds). Goodman and Gillman's The Pharmacological Basis of Therapeutics, 11th ed. New York: McGraw-Hill, 2006.
7. Kornblau S, Benson AB, Catalano R, et al. Management of cancer treatment-related diarrhea: Issues and therapeutic strategies. J Pain Symptom Manage 2000;19:118-129.
8. Mercadante S. Diarrhea, malabsorption, and constipation. In Berger AM, Portenoy RK, Weissman DE (eds). Principles & Practice of Palliative Care & Supportive Oncology, 2nd ed. Philadelphia: Lippincott Williams & Wilkins, 2002, p 233.
9. Mcvoy G, Snow EK, Kester L (eds). AHFS Drug Information—2007. Bethesda, MD: American Society of Health-System Pharmacists, 2007.
10. McQuaid KR. Drugs used in the treatment of gastrointestinal disease. In Katzung BG (ed). Basic and Clinical Pharmacology, 10th ed. New York: McGraw-Hill, 2007.
11. Fedorak RN. Short bowel syndrome. In Yamada T, Alpers DH, Kaplowitz N (eds). Textbook of Gastroenterology, 4th ed. Philadelphia: Lippincott Williams & Wilkins, 2003, p 1625.
12. Matulonis UA, Seiden MV, Roche M, et al. Long-acting octreotide for the treatment and symptomatic relief of bowel obstruction in advanced ovarian cancer. J Pain Symptom Manage 2005;30:563-569.
13. Hirata T, Funatsu T, Keto Y, et al. Pharmacological profile of ramosetron, a novel therapeutic agent for IBS. Inflammopharmacology 2007;15:5-9.
14. Crentsil V. Will corticosteroids and other anti-inflammatory agents be effective for diarrhea-predominant irritable bowel syndrome? Med Hypotheses 2005; 65:97-102.
15. Verkman AS, Lukacs GL, Galietta LJ. CFTR chloride channel drug discovery—inhibitors as antidiarrheals and activators for therapy of cystic fibrosis. Curr Pharm Des 2006;12:2235-2247.
16. Farthing MJ. Novel targets for the pharmacotherapy of diarrhoea: A view for the millennium. J Gastroenterol Hepatol 2000;15(Suppl):G38-G45.
17. Salazar-Lindo E, Santisteban-Ponce J, Chea-Woo E, et al. Racecadotril in the treatment of acute watery diarrhea in children. N Engl J Med 2000;343:463-467.

SUGGESTED READING

Alderman J. Diarrhea in palliative care. J Palliat Med 2005;8:449-450.

Benson AB, Ajani JA, Catalano RB, et al. Recommended guidelines for the treatment of cancer treatment–induced diarrhea. J Clin Oncol 2004;22:2918-2924.

Kornblau S, Benson, AB, Catalano R, et al. Management of cancer treatment–related diarrhea: Issues and therapeutic strategies. J Pain Symptom Manage 2000;19:118-129.

Symptom Control

CHAPTER **148**

Principles of Symptom Control

Terence L. Gutgsell

KEY POINTS

- Patients with advanced illnesses have many symptoms of moderate to severe intensity that worsen if left untreated or undertreated.

- The symptom experience is multidimensional, requiring a holistic interdisciplinary approach.

- When possible, the underlying mechanism should be treated.

- Treatment must be individualized; there is no cookie-cutter approach.

- Faith and trust in the physician and team, created by excellence in communication and care, are the foundation of palliative treatment.

THE PRIMACY OF THE SYMPTOM

In traditional medical practice, symptoms are primarily markers or indicators of an illness and especially pathophysiology of disease. The sudden onset of a productive cough, fever, chills, sweats, and pleuritic chest pain in an otherwise well and ambulatory individual prompts a clinician to consider several possible diagnoses, with community-acquired pneumonia chief among them. The next step is to consider which diagnostic studies to order, and if the diagnosis is confirmed, the physician decides on a treatment to prescribe to cure the illness. The empathetic and compassionate physician also considers what treatments can reduce the symptoms experienced by the suffering individual. In this case, the physician may prescribe expectorants or cough suppressants. A nonsteroidal anti-inflammatory drug (NSAID) may reduce the chest pain from the inflammatory response of pleuritis. If the pain is severe, perhaps an opioid and acetaminophen combination product may be prescribed. However, more often than not, the physician may overlook the intensity of the symptoms and focus on disease-oriented care to cure of the underlying condition and thereby resolve the secondary symptoms. A disease-oriented approach, although appropriate for disease eradication, often results in

someone enduring more pain and suffering than necessary. The pain and suffering experienced may prolong the illness or slow healing (Fig. 148-1).

A clinician with palliative care sensitivity emphasizes the experience of the illness as much as the disease. For that physician, a symptom is an important component of the disease process itself. The first component of good palliative care is the awareness that symptoms are the patient's experience of the illness, and the clinician has the obligation to relieve those symptoms while treating the underlying disease. Treatment of symptoms relieves suffering and often improves the rate of recovery.

For someone with a life-limiting illness that is incurable, unrelieved suffering is demoralizing and demeaning. The suffering patient may lose the will to live, become depressed and withdrawn, and decline more rapidly than would occur if his or her symptoms were well controlled. In this situation, optimal treatment of the symptoms becomes the optimal treatment of the disease. Symptoms should not be considered mere markers of disease or pathophysiology; they should share equal footing with disease management, especially in those for whom treatment of the underlying illness is of limited benefit.

PREVALENCE OF SYMPTOMS IN ADVANCED DISEASE

Several studies have demonstrated that symptoms become more frequent and severe as the patient approaches death. Among 1000 cancer patients seen by a palliative care consultation service, the median number of symptoms per patient was 11 (Fig. 148-2), with a range of 1 to 27 symptoms.[1] The 10 most common symptoms, in descending frequency, were pain, fatigue, weakness, anorexia, cachexia (>10% of premorbid weight lost), low energy, xerostomia, constipation, dyspnea, and early satiety. Generally, all symptoms were graded as moderate or severe in intensity; however, the more prevalent the symptom, the more severe was that symptom.

Symptoms are common in advanced illness[2] whether they were caused by cancer or a noncancer disease (Table 148-1). The number, prevalence, and severity of symptoms (i.e., symptom burden) increases as the patient progresses toward death (see "Case Study: Managing the Symptom Burden").

CLINICAL MANIFESTATIONS: EVALUATION AND ASSESSMENT

Whenever possible, the underlying pathophysiology and mechanism of the symptom should be identified. Symptoms may have several causes:

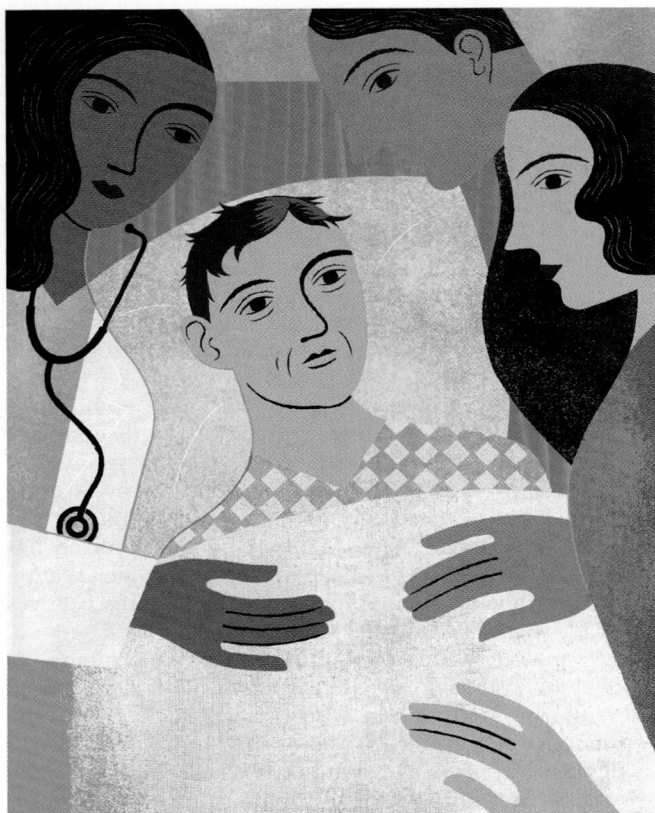

FIGURE 148-1   The physician must always be wholly compassionate toward his or her patients and their families. (From Improving End-of-Life Care. NIH Consens State Sci Statements 2004;21[3]:1-28.)

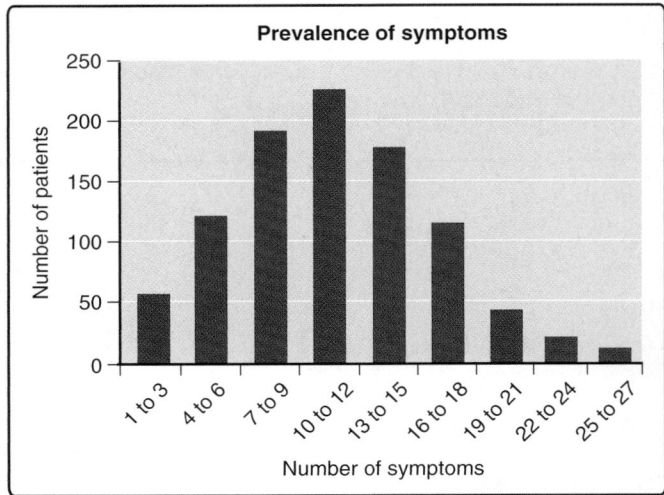

FIGURE 148-2   Prevalence of symptoms in advanced disease.

CASE STUDY

Managing the Symptom Burden

ML is a 48-year-old woman with an 8-year history of progressive cervical cancer. She is admitted to the hospital with fever, abdominal distention, constipation, nausea, and pain in the abdomen, lower back, and bilateral proximal legs. During the past 8 years, she has survived multiple abdominal operations, rounds of chemotherapy, and radiation therapy. Her examination reveals abdominal distention but no fluid wave or shifting dullness. She is moderately tender on palpation of the abdomen but has no rebound tenderness. Bowel sounds are present, but they are somewhat high pitched and come in rushes. There is 3+ lower extremity edema but no calf tenderness, erythema, or warmth. She has groin adenopathy and edema of her external genitalia. A flat plate and upright radiograph of the abdomen reveals air-fluid levels and copious amounts of stool. A urinalysis and culture reveal an infection of the urinary tract. The blood urea nitrogen and creatinine levels are 53 and 2.3, respectively.

She is treated by means of nasogastric suctioning, intravenous fluid administration, antibiotics, and laxatives. She is initially given small doses of intravenous morphine but remains in moderate to severe pain. Computed tomography demonstrates multiple intra-abdominal abscesses. Exploratory surgery is performed in an

attempt to drain the abscesses. Antibiotics are adjusted according to culture and sensitivity results.

In the postoperative period, she continues to have unabated pain. Intermittent morphine is discontinued, and continuous-infusion morphine is initiated. The rate of infusion is rapidly increased over the next 3 days. Pain worsens rather than improves. She begins to hallucinate and becomes progressively more anxious and tearful. She is having generalized motor twitches that appear to be extremely painful to her. Her husband, who is a Christian minister, and daughters tell her that she can be healed if she has faith. They are very anxious and tearful.

A palliative medicine consultation is ordered. The palliative care team immediately recognizes that the patient is suffering from a combination of opioid-induced neurotoxicity (e.g., hallucinations, myoclonus, allodynia, hyperalgesia), postoperative abdominal pain, and neuropathic pain related to sacral plexopathy injury caused by locally advanced disease and radiation injury. The morphine infusion is discontinued, and a hydromorphone infusion is started at a dose that is 75% less than the equianalgesic dose of the previously infused morphine. All potentially nephrotoxic medications are discontinued, and renal function is optimized with judicious intravenous fluid administration. A low-dose ketamine infusion is started to combat the neurogenic pain, and regularly scheduled doses of lorazepam are administered to treat the painful myoclonic episodes.

Over the next 24 to 48 hours, there is rapid improvement. The hallucinations, anxiety, and myoclonus abate. The pain diminishes to acceptable levels. Bowel function begins to improve, and the fever resolves.

The palliative care chaplain comforts the patient, husband, and family and begins to reframe hope in ways other than physical healing. The palliative care social worker begins conversation with the family about hospice support in the home after discharge. The palliative care physician continues to adjust medications for optimal symptom control and to communicate regularly with the family and attending physician regarding all palliative care treatments and goals. The palliative care nurse coordinates the efforts of the team.

TABLE 148-1 Frequency of Symptoms in Advanced Illness

SYMPTOM	CANCER (%)	CAD (%)	DEMENTIA (%)	AIDS (%)
Pain	60	60	65	60
Dyspnea	40	50	—	10
Nausea, vomiting	40	45	—	20
Insomnia	50	—	—	—
Confusion	30	40	60	30
Fatigue, weakness	50	—	80	60
Depression	45	60	60	—
Anorexia	60	40	60	40
Constipation	50	30	—	20
Incontinence	40	—	70	—
Anxiety	40	—	—	—

AIDS, acquired immunodeficiency syndrome; CAD, coronary artery disease.

- Progression or complication of the underlying disease process
- Complications of the treatment for the disease
- Side effects of the palliative treatment for another symptom
- Unrelated conditions

The clinician should obtain a careful history with special emphasis on the review of systems. A targeted physical examination coupled with appropriate laboratory and radiological investigations usually confirms the history. Mindlessly ordering routine diagnostic studies or ordering tests for clinical curiosity is not acceptable practice. Any intervention may impose considerable burden and increase the suffering of these vulnerable patients. Diagnostic procedures are ordered only if the information obtained may be acted on or change the treatment approach. Evaluations may need to be repeated frequently as the condition changes.

Tools to assess pain and other symptoms have been developed to standardize and improve clinical evaluations and provide valid and reliable guides for audits and research. Clinicians should routinely use brief assessment tools to ask patients about pain, depression, and fatigue and to initiate evidence-based treatments.[3] The most widely used validated tools for general symptom assessment of patients with palliative care needs are the Edmonton Symptom Assessment Scale (ESAS) (Fig. 148-3) and the Memorial Symptom Assessment Scale (MSAS). The original MSAS has been shortened (MSAS-SF); it is valid and reliable and can be completed in 2 to 4 minutes (Fig. 148-4). The ESAS has been well received by nursing staff in a dedicated palliative care unit.[4] It is an effective monitoring tool in long-term care facilities.[5] The Missoula-VITAS Quality of Life Index–Revised (MVQOLI-R) has been demonstrated to be effective for monitoring physical, psychosocial, and spiritual quality of life in long-term care facilities and outpatient clinics.[6] There are various assessment tools for specific symptoms, such as pain,[7] fatigue,[8] dyspnea,[9] depression,[10-11] and delirium.[12] Resources for assessment tools may be found on the Internet (http://www.promotingexcellence.org, http://www. hospicecare.com/resources/pain-research.htm, http://www.npcrc.org/).

TREATMENT

Some symptoms are hard to manage and require high-tech, complex interventions, but about 90% can be controlled with low-tech, simple interventions requiring basic medical knowledge. The key to best symptom control is the application of principles that incorporate factual medical knowledge, technical expertise, and communication skill.[13] All palliative care clinicians should apply certain principles when caring for their patients: anticipation of complications, treating underlying mechanisms of symptoms, providing individualized and holistic care, providing information and obtaining consultations, and ensuring continuity of care.

Anticipation

Most terminal conditions have complications that are predictable and can be anticipated. Awareness of them allows physicians to prevent or treat a complication at the first possible moment and thereby reduce the intensity or duration of the accompanying symptom. For example, patients with colorectal cancer are prone to bowel obstruction, and special emphasis on laxative regimens and avoidance of high-fiber diets are good choices for preventative palliative medicine for this group. Persons with gynecologic cancers may develop sacral plexopathy pain, and awareness of this painful condition may allow earlier and more successful treatment. Patients with head and neck cancers may have sudden exsanguination. Preparation of the family for this possibility is essential. If the family cannot bear the thought of such an event in the home, admission to the inpatient hospice unit at the first sign of excessive bleeding may be planned.

Palliative treatments often are associated with complications that are best prevented or treated quickly. Examples include the use of corticosteroids, which can make patients susceptible to the oropharyngeal complication of candidiasis. The clinician should institute frequent oral examinations and provide treatment at the first sign of oral thrush. Opioids have the well-known complications of constipation, nausea, sedation, and delirium. Anticipation and treatment of these problems should be routine. Less frequently recognized is the symptom complex of opioid-induced neurotoxicity (i.e., hyperalgesia, allodynia, delirium, and worsening pain). Awareness and anticipation of this possibility may prevent devastating consequences.

Psychosocial difficulties can result in poor responses to treatments. Patients with poor home support may be unable to follow complex treatment regimens. Low-income families may not be able to afford expensive medicines. Anticipation of these problems and early involvement of social services can result in better treatment strategies and outcomes.

Treating the Symptom's Underlying Mechanism

Treatment of a symptom may depend on the mechanism. For example, there are differences in the treatment of

Edmonton Symptom Assessment System:
Numerical Scale
Regional Palliative Care Program

Please circle the number that best describes:

No pain	0	1	2	3	4	5	6	7	8	9	10	Worst possible pain
Not tired	0	1	2	3	4	5	6	7	8	9	10	Worst possible tiredness
Not nauseated	0	1	2	3	4	5	6	7	8	9	10	Worst possible nausea
Not depressed	0	1	2	3	4	5	6	7	8	9	10	Worst possible depression
Not anxious	0	1	2	3	4	5	6	7	8	9	10	Worst possible anxiety
Not drowsy	0	1	2	3	4	5	6	7	8	9	10	Worst possible drowsiness
Best appetite	0	1	2	3	4	5	6	7	8	9	10	Worst possible appetite
Best feeling of well-being	0	1	2	3	4	5	6	7	8	9	10	Worst possible feeling of well-being
No shortness of breath	0	1	2	3	4	5	6	7	8	9	10	Worst possible shortness of breath
Other problem	0	1	2	3	4	5	6	7	8	9	10	

Patient's name _____

Date _____ Time _____

Completed by (check one)
☐ Patient
☐ Caregiver
☐ Caregiver assisted

Body diagram on reverse page

A

FIGURE 148-3 A, Edmonton Symptom Assessment System.

nausea associated with hypercalcemia, gastroparesis, increased intra-cranial pressure, monilial esophagitis, opioid use, or constipation. Reflex prescribing of promethazine for nausea in a terminally ill patient without considering the underlying cause is never appropriate unless the person is near death. Is the patient's abdominal pain caused by constipation, disease progress with involvement of a nerve plexus, or impending bowel obstruction? All are treated differently. Is the restlessness observed by the family or nurse caused by a distended bladder, impacted rectum, hypercalcemia, or opioid induced delirium? The appropriate use of lorazepam or haloperidol depends on the underlying mechanism and goals of care.

When someone is close to death, decisions about treatment of the underlying mechanism are more difficult. A large pleural effusion resulting from lung cancer in a patient with an estimated prognosis of 3 to 6 weeks provides such a dilemma. Should the treatment for a malignant effusion consist of a chest tube and pleurodesis, repeated thoracentesis, or only opioids and sedatives? The decision cannot be made without the involvement of the patient and family and their assessment of the benefit-burden analysis in the context of the goals of care.

Holistic Care

A patient's symptoms are experienced within the context of a life history, a family, and a community. Events that have occurred or are occurring play a significant role in the manifestation of symptoms. Cicely Saunders often spoke about "total suffering" or "total pain" as the complex interplay of symptoms in the physical, emotional, social, and spiritual domains of the patient's life.[14] Pain that may be intractable to all treatment modalities may be physical pain complicated by guilt, depression, anxiety, worry, and other psychosocial stressors. Until all the domains of personhood are explored and cared for, we may never arrive at good pain control. The role of the interdisciplinary team in this holistic approach is invaluable.

Explanation and Information

Most patients want to know what is happening in and to their bodies and with their lives. However, it is presumptuous of us to force information on patients who may not want it. Before sharing information, patients should be asked what they would like to know about their

Please mark on these pictures where it is you hurt.

FIGURE 148-3, cont'd B, Edmonton Symptom Assessment System–Pain Sites.

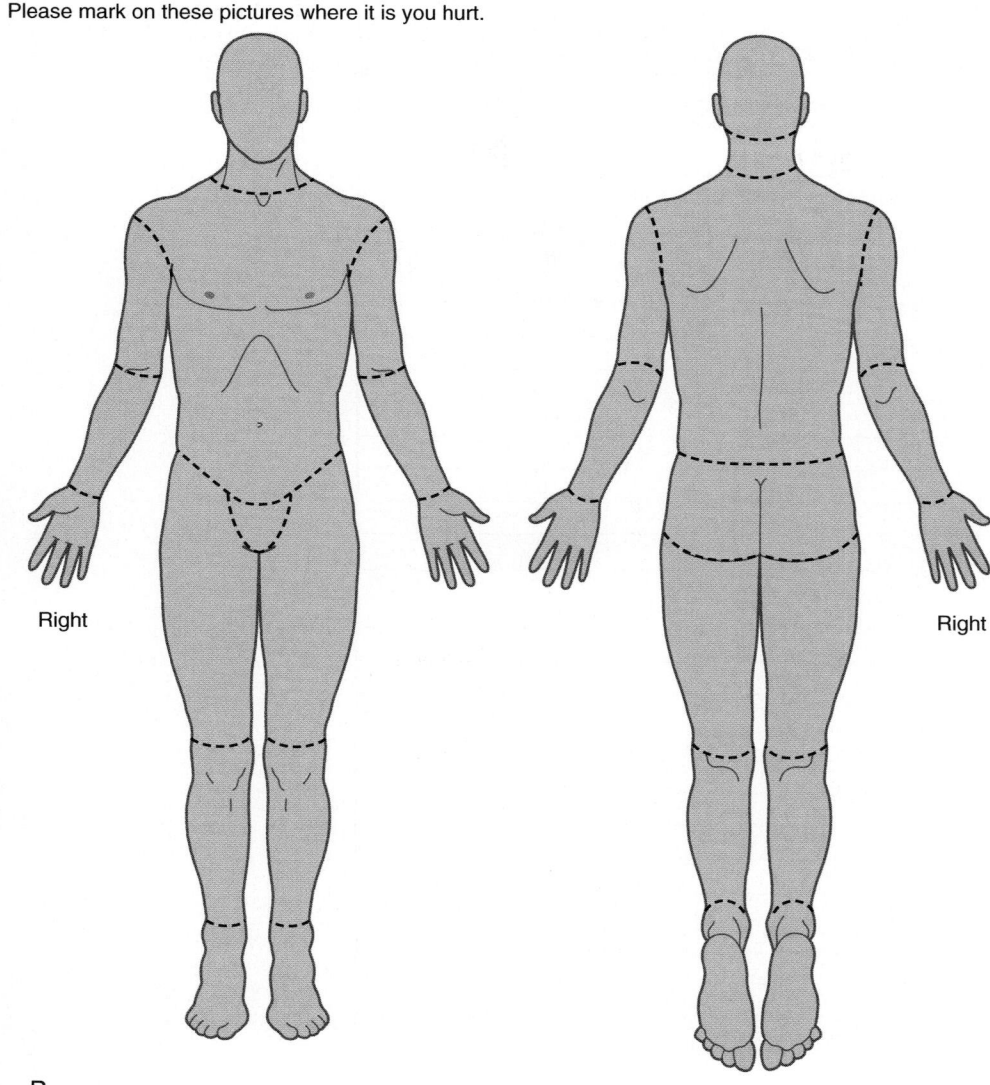

Right

Right

B

condition (e.g., illness, symptom, situation). If the patient does not wish to know, the next step is to determine who would want to know the information and whether he or she will be making decisions for the patient. Explaining the diagnosis, treatments, benefits, burdens, potential complications of treatments, and prognosis allows the patient and family to set goals for care and treatment. Giving this information and explaining its ramifications enables honest and open communication between the physician and patient, which promotes a trusting relationship and a context in which further conversations and decisions can occur.

Sharing information demystifies much of what previously was not understood. It provides the patient and family with a sense of control and security even in the face of serious illness. This sense of control and security is a form of symptom management in itself because the outcome is decreased anxiety, worry, and family distress. These conversations may need to be held on many occasions. The clinician should consider providing the patient

and family with a written summary of what was discussed and the decisions made. A tape recording of the meeting for the use of the patient and family may also be considered.

Individualized Treatment

"No one shoe fits all" should be a mantra of palliative care. Even though a terminal illness may have predictable symptoms, complications, timeline, treatments, and prognosis, each person's experience with this illness is uniquely his or hers. Most patients experience surgery, chemotherapy, radiation therapy, and the usual symptom-directed treatments, but the exact timing of treatments, responses to treatment, and emotional and physical responses to the illness are distinctively their own.

Ultimately, the patient's goals of care drive decisions about symptom treatment. For some, clarity of mind is more important than optimal pain control, in which case

FIGURE 148-4   A, Memorial Symptom Assessment Scale–Short Form (MSAS-SF).

Memorial Symptom Assessment Scale—Short Form (MSAS–SF)

I. *Instructions:* Below is a list of symptoms. If you had the symptom *during the past week,* please check *Yes*. If you did have the symptom, please check the box that tells us how much the symptom *distressed* or *bothered* you.

Check *all* the symptoms you have had during the *past week.*	Yes ✓	Not at all [0]	A little bit [1]	Some-what [2]	Quite a bit [3]	Very much [4]
	→ → *If Yes:* How much did it *distress* or *bother* you?					
Difficulty concentrating						
Pain						
Lack of energy						
Cough						
Changes in skin						
Dry mouth						
Nausea						
Feeling drowsy						
Numbness/tingling in hands and feet						
Difficulty sleeping						
Feeling bloated						
Problems with urination						
Vomiting						
Shortness of breath						
Diarrhea						
Sweats						
Mouth sores						
Problems with sexual interest or activity						
Itching						
Lack of appetite						
Dizziness						
Difficulty swallowing						
Change in the way food tastes						
Weight loss						

A

the patient may suffer more pain than the treatment team would prefer. For others, sleeping and rest as a respite from prolonged suffering is more important than alertness and social interaction, which results in a request for more sedative medicines than the treatment team would ordinarily consider appropriate. Treatment of dehydration with intravenous fluids or hypodermoclysis[15] to maintain life for several more days to allow the patient to see the birth of a grandchild may be a driving need. In another situation, terminal dehydration may be desired to prevent excess pulmonary secretions, avoid frequent urination, and lessen peripheral edema. Occasionally, people may have an exquisite sensitivity or fear of a certain medicine that would normally be the treatment of choice for a particular symptom. In this situation, an alternative medication would be chosen.

Re-evaluation and Attention to Detail

Terminal illnesses are acute illnesses with rapidly changing clinical situations. The care of these patients has been likened to hitting a moving target. Treatment strategies regarding the primary problem usually are in flux. Complications may occur at any time. Symptom-directed care may introduce its own set of problems. Responses of the patient and family to the illness may change drastically depending on their degree of denial, depression, anxiety, or acceptance of the illness. The financial status of the patient and family may be greatly and suddenly affected by the illness.

These changing situations require frequent reassessments. If the patient is in the hospital, reassessments may occur several times each day. In an inpatient hospice unit,

FIGURE 148-4, cont'd
B, Questionnaire.

Patient's Name _____ Date ___/___/___ ID # _____

Memorial Symptom Assessment Scale—
Short Form (MSAS–SF)

I. *Instructions:* Below is a list of symptoms. If you had the symptom *during the past week,* please check *Yes.* If you did have the symptom, please check the box that tells us how much the symptom *distressed* or *bothered* you.

Check *all* the symptoms you have had during the *past week.*	→ → *If Yes:* How much did it *distress* or *bother* you?					
	Yes ✓	Not at all [0]	A little bit [1]	Some-what [2]	Quite a bit [3]	Very much [4]
Hair loss						
Constipation						
Swelling of arms or legs						
"I don't look like myself"						
If you had *any other* symptoms during the *past week,* please list them below, and indicate how much the symptom *distressed* or *bothered* you. 1.						
2.						

II. Below are other commonly listed symptoms. Please indicate if you have had the symptom *during the past week,* and if so, *how often* it occurred.

Check *all* the symptoms you have had during the *past week.*	→ → *If Yes:* How *often* did it occur?				
	Yes ✓	Rarely [1]	Occasionally [2]	Frequently [3]	Almost constantly [4]
Feeling sad					
Worrying					
Feeling irritable					
Feeling nervous					

B

the patient may be continuously monitored by the treatment team as he or she is moving into an actively dying status. A homebound patient may require several visits each week by his or her hospice team. An ambulatory palliative care patient may need weekly or biweekly office visits and frequent telephone calls. This intensity of re-evaluation of the patient and family requires the involvement of an interdisciplinary team. At a minimum, the team should consist of a physician and a case management nurse. For a hospice patient or a palliative care patient admitted to the hospital, the interdisciplinary team may consist of a physician, nurse, social worker, chaplain, and certified nursing assistant. Other members of an interdisciplinary team may include a physical therapist, occupational therapist, dietitian, pharmacist, psychologist, complementary therapist, and volunteer, depending on availability and need. The presence of the interdisciplinary team allows for the attention to detail to all four domains of the human suffering experience—physical, emotional, social, and spiritual.

Consultation

Some clinical situations require the skill and expertise of clinicians outside of the interdisciplinary team. Patients with impending pathologic fractures in weight-bearing bones require the help of an orthopedic surgeon. Complex pain syndromes may benefit from the care of an interventional pain specialist to perform nerve blocks, place epidural or intrathecal catheters, and perform other procedures. Radiation oncology colleagues may be needed to irradiate painful metastases or a bleeding bronchus. Physical and occupational therapists can provide life-enhancing suggestions to improve ambulation skills, activities of daily living, or safe transfers.

These patients have complex needs that typically require more knowledge and techniques than one physician or even one interdisciplinary team can muster. The involvement of skilled experts is not an admission of weakness; it is an acknowledgment of the many needs of the suffering patient.

Continuity of Care

For ambulatory or homebound patients, a system of support that provides continuity and security is an essential component of excellent symptom management. Providing the patient and family with written instructions is essential. Oral instructions are quickly forgotten or misconstrued. Preprinted forms that list the names of scheduled and "as needed" medications, doses, times of administration, and the reasons for the drugs are easy to devise and use in a busy clinic setting.[16]

Relationship between the Palliative Care Team and the Patient and Family

The most important ingredient in the mix of principles for excellent symptom management in palliative care is the relationship between the palliative care team and the patient and family. The compassionate team brings to the bedside openness, compassion, and a desire to be of help that is transparent to the patient and family. This is a visible and metaphorical posture informed by the physical, emotional, mental, and spiritual aspects of the team. The team's attitudes and actions engender a relationship of trust and hopefulness that strengthens all aspects of the care provided and improves the response of the patient and family. The compassionate relationship between team and patient energizes and transforms all the other principles of compassionate care. The excellent team should do everything possible to cultivate this sense of compassion and helpfulness (Fig. 148-5).

DEVELOPMENTS AND CONTROVERSIES IN PALLIATIVE CARE

Evidence-based medical guidelines for palliative care are lacking. Conducting randomized, double-blind, placebo-controlled trials enrolling patients with advanced disease is almost impossible. Even establishing the nomenclature for research and practice is difficult. For example, the use of the word *palliative* in the context of chemotherapy may be interpreted differently by oncologists and palliative medicine clinicians, leading to miscommunication and subsequent confusion in physician-patient communications.

Although there is strong scientific evidence regarding the appropriate use of artificially provided nutrition, cultural, religious, and emotional factors often complicate decision-making even when using the best multidisciplinary team and communication techniques. Palliative sedation for existential suffering remains a controversial topic, and a consensus among experts in palliative medicine and bioethics has not been reached.

During the past 10 years, palliative care services in hospitals, clinics, long-term care facilities, and the home have

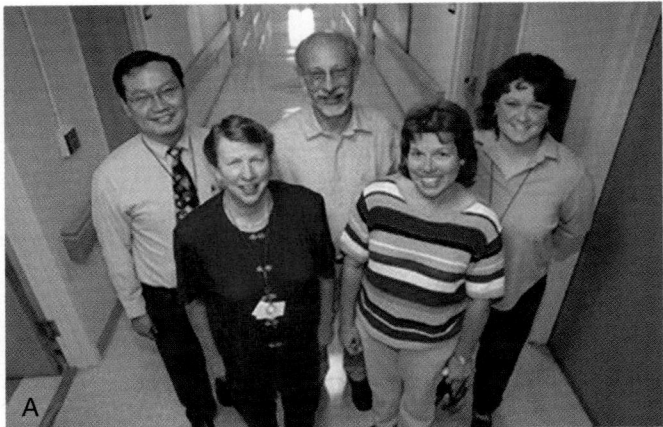

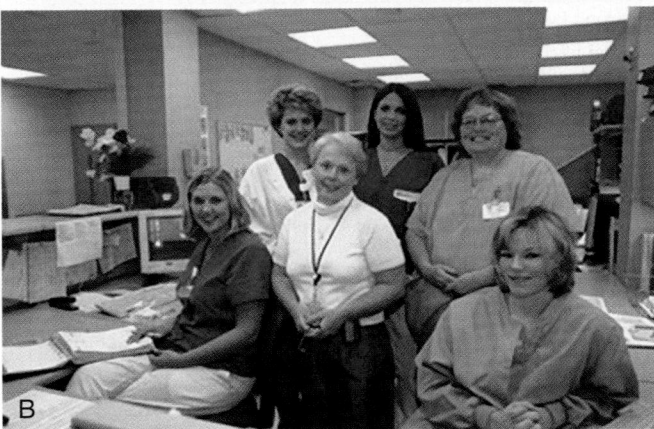

FIGURE 148-5 **A**, Palliative care team of the Palliative Care Center of the Bluegrass, Central Baptist Hospital, Lexington, Kentucky. **B**, Palliative care unit of the Central Baptist Hospital, Nursing Staff, Lexington, Kentucky.

grown and received acceptance. Training programs to meet these personnel demands continue to expand rapidly. Formal specialty status for palliative medicine has been achieved in many developed countries of the world, including the United States, and the discipline will undoubtedly continue to gain in recognition around the globe.

REFERENCES

1. Donnelly S, Walsh D: The symptoms of advanced cancer. Semin Oncol 1995;22(Suppl 3):67-72.
2. Faul C, Woof R. Physical symptom control: How to do it well. In Faul C, Woof R (eds). Palliative Care—Oxford Core Text. Oxford, UK: Oxford University Press, 2002, pp 63-71.
3. Patrick DL, Ferketich SL, Frame PS, et al. National Institutes of Health State-of-the-Science Conference Statement: Symptom management in cancer: Pain, depression, and fatigue, July 15-17, 2002. J Natl Cancer Inst Monogr 2004;32:9-16.
4. Wantanabe S, McKinnon S, Macmillan K, Hanson J. Palliative care nurses; perceptions of the Edmonton Symptom Assessment Scale: A pilot survey. Int J Palliat Nurs 2006;12:11-14.
5. Brechtl JR, Murshed S, Homel P, Bookbinder M. Monitoring symptoms in patients with advanced illness in long-term care: A pilot study. J Pain Symptom Manage 2006;32:168-174.
6. Schwartz CE, Merriman MP, Reed G, Byock I. Evaluation of the Missoula-VITAS Quality of Life Index-revised: Research tool or clinical tool? J Palliat Med 2005;8:121-135.
7. Cleeland CS, Ryan KM. Pain assessment: Global use of the Brief Pain Inventory. Ann Acad Med Singapore 1994;23:129-138.
8. Jacobsen PB. Assessment of fatigue in cancer patients. J Natl Cancer Inst Monogr 2004;32:93-97.
9. Farncombe M. Dyspnea: Assessment and treatment. Support Care Cancer 1997;5:94-99.

10. Lloyd-Williams M. Which depression screening tools should be used in palliative care? Palliat Med 2003;17:40-43.
11. Rao A, Harvey JC. Symptom management in the elderly cancer patient: Fatigue, pain and depression. J Natl Cancer Inst Monogr 2004;32:150-157.
12. Fayers PM, Hjermstad MJ, Ranhoff AH, et al. Which mini-mental state exam items can be used to screen for delirium and cognitive impairment? J Pain Symptom Manage 2005;30:41-50.
13. Faul C, Woof R. Physical symptom control: How to do it well. Palliative Care—Oxford Core Text. Oxford, UK: Oxford University Press, 2002, pp 63-71.
14. Saunders C. Into the valley of the shadow of death: A personal therapeutic journey. BMJ 1996;313:1599-1601.
15. Steiner N, Bruera E. Methods of hydration in palliative care patients. J Palliat Care 1998;14:6-13.
16. Waller A, Caroline N. General principles of palliative care in advanced cancer. Handbook of Palliative Care in Cancer, 2nd ed. London: Butterworth-Heinemann, 2000, pp 3-8.

SUGGESTED READING

Faul C, Woof R. Palliative Care—Oxford Core Text. Oxford, UK: Oxford University Press, 2002.

MacDonald N, Oneschuk D, Hagen N, et al. Palliative Medicine: A Case-Based Manual, 2nd ed. Oxford, UK: Oxford University Press, 2005.

Snyder L, Quill TE. Physician's Guide to End-of-Life Care. Philadelphia: American College of Physicians–American Society of Internal Medicine, 2001.

Waller A, Caroline N. Handbook of Palliative Care in Cancer, 2nd ed. London: Butterworth-Heinemann, 2000.

Woodruff R. Palliative Medicine: Evidence-Based Symptomatic and Supportive Care for Patients with Advanced Cancer, 4th ed. Oxford, UK: Oxford University Press, 2004.

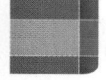

CHAPTER **149**

Symptom Epidemiology and Clusters

Jade Homsi

KEY POINTS

- Agitation, pain, shortness of breath, and delirium are the most difficult symptoms to manage for hospice nurses; pain, nausea, dysphagia, and delirium are the most difficult for general practitioners.
- Palliative medicine patients are polysymptomatic, with a median of 11 symptoms.
- Patient age, gender, performance status, primary disease, race, symptom severity and distress, and symptom assessment method influence symptom prevalence and epidemiology.
- Systematic symptom assessment that addresses physiological and psychological symptoms ideally should be used each time a patient is seen; 52% of nonvolunteered symptoms are moderate or severe, and 53% are distressing.
- Anorexia, delirium, dyspnea, dysphagia, fatigue, dry mouth, and weight loss are the symptoms most commonly reported that negatively affect survival.

In 1990, The World Health Organization defined palliative medicine as "the active total care of patients whose disease is not responsive to curative treatment. Control of pain, of other symptoms, and of psychological, social, and spiritual problems is paramount."[1] Palliative medicine patients are polysymptomatic and have a median of 11 symptoms (Table 149-1).[2,3] The symptoms may be related to the disease itself, treatment, and procedures for managing disease complications. Co-morbid conditions also may influence symptom manifestation, severity, and distress.

Managing symptoms is the reason for 79% of referrals to a palliative medicine consultation service.[4] Although 84% of palliative medicine patients report improvement in symptom control as their primary goal, symptoms are still inadequately assessed and undertreated[4] (see Chapters 148 and 181). These problems reflect the deficits in symptom research in mechanisms and pharmacologic and nonpharmacologic management, particularly for symptoms other than pain (see Chapter 30). Physicians and other professionals possess knowledge deficits and attitudinal barriers that impede effective symptom management. Pain, nausea, dysphagia, delirium, insomnia, anxiety, and depression are identified by general practitioners as difficult to deal with in palliative medicine practice.[5] Variability in measurement and methodology is common. Patients with advanced disease often may be unable to complete symptom assessments, and there is little research on the value of caregivers in the assessment and management of symptoms. This chapter discusses symptom epidemiology, important factors influencing epidemiology, the concept of symptom clusters, and the role of symptoms in predicting survival.

SYMPTOM EPIDEMIOLOGY

Seventy-two percent of patients who die in the hospital on general wards suffer at least one severe symptom. The

TABLE 149-1 Most Common Symptoms of Patients with Advanced Cancer

SYMPTOM	PATIENTS (%)	SYMPTOM	PATIENTS (%)
Pain	84	Edema	28
Easy fatigue	69	Taste change	28
Weakness	66	Hoarseness	24
Anorexia	66	Anxiety	24
Lack of energy	61	Vomiting	23
Dry mouth	57	Confusion	21
Constipation	52	Dizziness	19
Early satiety	51	Dyspepsia	19
Dyspnea	50	Dysphagia	18
Weight loss	50	Belching	18
Sleep problems	49	Bloating	18
Depression	41	Wheezing	13
Cough	38	Memory problems	12
Nausea	36	Headache	11

Adapted from Donnelly S, Walsh D. The symptoms of advanced cancer. Semin Oncol 1995;22(Suppl 3):67-72, and Walsh D, Donnelly S, Rybicki L. The symptoms of advanced cancer: Relationship to age, gender, and performance status in 1,000 patients. Support Care Cancer 2000;8:175-179.

TABLE 149-2 The Ten Symptoms Most Difficult to Manage in Hospice

SYMPTOM	HOSPICE NURSES SELECTING THE SYMPTOM (%)
Agitation	45
Pain	40
Shortness of breath	34
Confusion	33
Pressure ulcers	27
Nausea	26
Fatigue	25
Constipation	24
Depression	22
Anxiety	21

From Johnson DC, Kassner CT, Houser J, Kutner JS. Barriers to effective symptom management in hospice. J Pain Symptom Manage 2005;29:69-79.

most prevalent are anorexia, fatigue, incontinence (bladder or bowel) and dyspnea. Forty-two percent have severe pain, and less than 19% treated with analgesics enjoy good pain control.[6] There is a significant association between the desire for hastened death and pain, fatigue, loss of appetite, and feeling sad for patients with advanced cancer.[7] Most symptoms in this population are difficult to manage and sometimes are better treated in an inpatient palliative medicine unit than at home.[8] A survey of more than 850 nurses (with mean experience of more than 4 years in hospice) shows that agitation and pain are the most difficult symptoms to manage (Table 149-2).[9] The most common barriers to effective symptom management identified were inability of family care providers to implement or maintain recommended treatments, patients or families not wanting recommended treatments, and competing demands from other distressing symptoms.

Physicians who care for those with advanced disease must anticipate the likelihood of symptoms, counsel patients and families to seek medical therapy when they experience these symptoms, and intervene appropriately. Pain is the most common and widely studied symptom in patients referred early in their disease to a palliative medicine service. Fatigue and anorexia are the most common symptoms as the disease progresses and at the end of life (see Table 149-1).[2,10] Almost one half of the most frequently reported and most distressing symptoms in advanced cancer are gastrointestinal.[11] The absolute number of gastrointestinal symptoms correlates with severity of weight loss. During the final 48 hours of life, patients experience increasing weakness and immobility, loss of interest in food and drink, difficulty swallowing, and drowsiness.

Factors Influencing Symptom Epidemiology

Patient age, gender, performance status, primary disease, race, symptom severity and distress, and symptom assessment method influence symptom prevalence and epidemiology (see Chapter 63).

Age

Changes with aging organ systems include decreased gastric emptying and absorption in the gastrointestinal tract, decreased lung vital capacity and expiratory reserve volume, decreased heart rate and cardiac output, less muscle mass and strength, and other changes that negatively affect almost every system. In the general population, older women have more depression, but suicide is highest among elderly white males. Elderly cancer patients with three or more co-morbid conditions or late-stage disease are more likely to report pain or fatigue, or both, compared with those reporting neither.[12] In pain in the elderly, nociception appears unchanged with age, although perception of pain and the willingness to report it may change.[13] As age increased, more patients in pain received no analgesic drugs, in part because of underestimation or underreporting of pain.[14] This is also true for symptoms other than pain. For patients with cancer, the mean number of symptoms reported that were experienced in the last year of life decreased with age, whereas the number reported to have lasted more than 6 months increased.[15] In cancer and noncancer patients, the proportion of symptoms reported as "very distressing" decreased with age.[15] Younger patients with advanced cancer are more likely to have blackout, vomiting, pain, nausea, headache, sedation, bloating, sleep problems, anxiety, depression, and constipation (Table 149-3).[3] Although pain is more common in younger patients, no major differences are observed for pain intensity, or for incidental or neuropathic pain across different age groups.[16]

Gender

Young female cancer patients receiving palliative treatment are at greatest risk for psychological symptoms.[17] In advanced cancer, dysphagia, hoarseness, sleep problems, and weight loss are more common in men, but anxiety, early satiety, nausea, and vomiting are less common (see Table 149-3).[15] Weight loss is more common in men but more severe in women.[18] Clinically important (i.e., moderate or severe) dysphagia, dyspnea, hiccups, and hoarseness are more common in men; anxiety, nausea, vomiting, and early satiety are more common in women.[19] In hospice care, male gender is a significant risk factor for delirium.[20]

Performance Status

Performance status is a strong indicator of survival and predicts symptom prevalence. Patients with poor performance status are more likely to have confusion, sedation, blackout, hallucinations, weakness, mucositis, anorexia, memory problems, dry mouth, and constipation (see Table 149-3).[15] The use of performance status to predict symptoms is limited because it is subjective and may be influenced by acute but self-limited events.

Primary Disease

Most symptom epidemiology studies in palliative medicine are based on advanced cancer models. Comparing gastrointestinal symptoms in advanced cancer, patients with primary gastrointestinal cancers had more indigestion and hiccups than those with nongastrointestinal

TABLE 149-3 The Symptoms of Advanced Cancer: Relationship to Age, Gender, and Performance Status

MORE LIKELY IN YOUNGER PATIENTS	OR	MORE LIKELY WITH POOR PERFORMANCE STATUS	OR	LESS LIKELY WITH POOR PERFORMANCE STATUS	OR	MORE LIKELY IN MALES	OR	LESS LIKELY IN MALES	OR
Blackout	1.7	Confusion	2.2	Anxiety	0.9	Dysphagia	1.8	Early satiety	0.7
Vomiting	1.4	Sedation	2.0	Wheezing	0.8	Hoarseness	1.7	Nausea	0.6
Pain	1.3	Blackout	1.8	Pain	0.8	Weight loss	1.3	Vomiting	0.6
Nausea	1.2	Hallucinations	1.7	Itching	0.6	Sleep problems	1.3	Anxiety	0.6
Headache	1.2	Weakness	1.6						
Sedation	1.2	Mucositis	1.5						
Bloating	1.2	Anorexia	1.3						
Sleep problems	1.2	Memory problems	1.3						
Anxiety	1.2	Dry mouth	1.3						
Depression	1.2	Constipation	1.2						
Constipation	1.1								

OR, odds ratio.
From Walsh D, Donnelly S, Rybicki L. The symptoms of advanced cancer: Relationship to age, gender, and performance status in 1,000 patients. Support Care Cancer 2000;8:175-179.

cancers.[10] Clinically important (i.e., moderate or severe) dyspepsia, nausea, and vomiting occur more frequently in patients with gynecological cancers.[19] The primary cancer itself influences the symptom profile. Common symptoms in pancreatic cancer include pain (82%), anorexia (64%), early satiety (62%), xerostomia (54%), sleep problems (54%), and weight loss (51%). The most common symptoms in liver cirrhosis and hepatocellular carcinoma on admission to hospice are pain, fatigue or weakness, anorexia or vomiting, peripheral edema, cachexia, and ascites.[21]

Cancer patients have a different symptom pattern from those without cancer. On admission to hospice, 75% with heart failure report no pain, whereas 3% report chest pain, and 20% report other pains. Severe pain increases as death approaches; 41% of patient surrogates report heart failure with severe pain during the 3 days before death.[22] During the last week of life, those with heart failure have shortness of breath (60%), confusion (48%), edema (43%), and incontinence of bowel or bladder (37%).[23] Among patients with chronic obstructive pulmonary disease, 98% have shortness of breath all the time or sometimes in the last year of life; it is partly relieved in more than 50% of those treated. Other symptoms reported all or some of the time include fatigue or weakness (96%), depressed mood (77%), and pain (70%).[24]

Race

There is strong evidence that racial and ethnic minority cancer patients receive inadequate pain assessment and treatment and that these patients report more pain than white patients.[25] The biopsychosocial model of pain, ethnic differences in perception, coping, and report of pain are possible explanations. Among patients with advanced cancer, black Caribbean patients have greater symptom-related distress because of appetite loss, pain, dry mouth, nausea, vomiting, and mental confusion compared with white patients.[26]

Study participation also is influenced by ethnicity. In palliative medicine (for unknown reasons), white patients are more likely to express interest in participation in symptom research.[27]

Severity and Distress

Symptom severity and distress are two distinct variables and should be evaluated separately. Symptom severity focuses on individual symptoms rather than the patient, and distress evaluates the effect of the symptom on the patient. Symptom severity and distress may affect reported prevalence because patients seem to volunteer severe and distressing symptoms more than mild and nondistressing ones. On referral to palliative medicine, 83% of symptoms volunteered by the patient are moderate or severe, and 91% are distressing. These figures compare with 52% for moderate or severe symptoms and 53% for distressing symptoms when the symptoms are evaluated by a 48-item symptom checklist.[28] More than one half of symptoms not volunteered are moderate, severe, or distressing. Symptoms are more likely to be volunteered if they are moderate (OR: 1.7; 95% CI: 1.1 to 2.5; $P = .02$), severe (OR: 4.3; 95% CI: 2.8 to 6.7; $P < .001$), or distressing (OR: 3.8; 95% CI: 2.4 to 6; $P < .001$). In advanced cancer, when pain, anorexia, weakness, anxiety, lack of energy, easy fatigue, early satiety, constipation, and dyspnea are present, 60% to 80% of patients rated the symptoms as moderate or severe or as clinically important.[19] In the last week of life, fatigue, cachexia, anorexia, and dry mouth are the most distressful symptoms of patients with advanced cancer.[29] Caregivers and physicians underestimate symptom distress.

Symptom Assessment

Symptom assessment should rely on patients' self-reports, and repeated assessments should continue to better establish symptom prevalence. Among cancer patients, the incidence of pain ranges from 14% to 100%; depression, 1% to 42%; and fatigue, 4% to 91%. Such large ranges reflect a lack of uniform measurement and the heterogeneity of the population.[30] Cognitive impairment may also reduce self-report. Patients readily reported some symptoms more than others, influencing apparent symptom epidemiology. Patients may be unaware that treatment of certain symptoms (e.g., anorexia, dry mouth, early satiety) is possible. Education and cultural differences also influence what symptoms patients may report.

In palliative medicine, the median number of volunteered symptoms in response to open-ended questions is 1 (range, 0 to 6), whereas that when using a systematic assessment is 10 (range, 0 to 25). Some specific symptoms influence patient reporting (Table 149-4). Physicians should be careful in history taking because they may unknowingly direct what patients volunteer by preferentially asking about specific symptoms but ignoring important nonvoluntary information. All patients should at a minimum have a detailed symptom assessment at the initial consultation and periodically thereafter. Symptom assessment using a combination of volunteered reports and systematic data collection may be optimal.

SYMPTOM CLUSTERS

Concurrent related or unrelated symptoms and their effect on patient outcomes have been explored in cancer. They are referred to as *symptom clusters*. Research on symptom clusters is new, and which symptom clusters are clinically significant is unknown (see Chapter 64). A clear definition does not exist. It has been suggested that for two or three symptoms to occur concurrently is insufficient to define a cluster. Instead, at least three or more concurrent symptoms (e.g., pain, fatigue, and sleep disturbances; nausea, vomiting, and poor appetite) need to be related to each other to be called a symptom cluster.[31,32] This definition has been criticized for not specifying the meaning of "related to each other." There is no standard for what level of intensity of an individual symptom may qualify for inclusion in a cluster.

Symptom pairing is a term used for two concurrent and correlated symptoms. It is unclear whether there is a

real difference between this term and *symptom clusters*. The symptoms are not required to share the same cause.

A critical step in developing this research will be to clarify the concept of symptom clusters and determine the critical elements to establish a cluster. Symptom-related instruments need to be evaluated for their ability to provide valid and reliable data regarding many symptoms occurring concurrently.

Symptom clusters may have an adverse effect on patient outcomes and be synergistic as a predictor of morbidity. The synergistic effect of symptoms that constitute a symptom cluster remains to be determined. Clusters' associations with age, gender, ethnicity, socioeconomic status, stage of disease, and the prevalence of clinically significant symptom clusters over time also need to be determined. Research should focus on determining whether symptom severity or distress change its relationship to other symptoms within a cluster. Symptom clusters in noncancer patients need to be evaluated, because most available data are from cancer patients.

Cancer

In cancer, the cluster of pain and fatigue is associated with depression and insomnia.[33,34] Fatigue, pain, and depression are all significantly correlated with each other and with total health status. Pain, fatigue, and sleep disturbance have deleterious effects on the outcome of radiation therapy for bone metastasis, particularly depressive symptoms, functional status, and quality of life. Cancer patients who are depressed have more pain than nondepressed patients. Pain and fatigue have an independent effect on other symptoms in the elderly with cancer. The most common associated symptoms when pain and fatigue are both present or absent are weakness (62% versus 10%), dry mouth (50% versus 26%), trouble sleeping (50% versus 21%), and weight loss (50% versus 14%).[11] It is unclear whether managing these symptoms would have an important secondary effect through controlling other symptoms that occur when the patient has pain or fatigue, or both. Fatigue is an important symptom in cancer, and it can be predicted by other symptoms. Dyspnea, pain, lack of appetite, drowsiness, sadness, and irritability independently predict the presence of fatigue.[11] It has been suggested that fatigue, nausea, weakness, appetite loss, weight loss, altered taste, and vomiting form a cluster in patients with lung cancer.[35]

Advanced Cancer

Symptom clusters have not been well studied in advanced cancer. Increasing depression and anxiety are associated with fatigue,[36] and they correlate negatively with spirituality.[37] In advanced lung cancer, a cluster of dyspnea, fatigue, and anxiety[38] and interference with daily activities (with different impacts) by pain, fatigue, and dyspnea have been suggested.[39] In advanced cancer, depressive symptoms (but not age, gender, and site of cancer) at baseline predict symptom severity at 20 weeks.[40] Studies to evaluate symptom clusters in advanced cancer and differences between clusters by cancer stage are needed.

TABLE 149-4 Symptoms Likely to Be Volunteered by Patients Compared with Symptoms Assessed Systematically

SYMPTOM	ODDS RATIO*
Pain	70.3
Fatigue	8.9
Headache	8.6
Dizziness	7.5
Nausea	5.5
Diarrhea	5.5
Vomiting	5.3
Cough	4.9
Dyspnea	4.8
Anorexia	4.0
Constipation	2.5

*The study examined symptoms reported by patients after open-ended questioning and compared them (OR) with symptoms systematically assessed using a 48-question survey.
From Homsi J, Walsh D, Rivera N, et al. Symptom evaluation in palliative medicine: Patient report versus systematic assessment. Support Care Cancer 2006;14:444-453.

Symptom Clusters and Survival

Predicting survival of patients with advanced disease is a major challenge. Symptom assessment is part of the routine medical evaluation and can be an effective, inexpensive way to predict survival. Symptoms such as low fluid and food intake, general weakness, and respiratory problems or dyspnea seem most important for physicians attempting to estimate a life expectancy of 6 weeks or less in advanced disease.[41] In adult patients with a median or mean survival of less than 6 months, 16 different symptoms and the total number of symptoms have a significant negative impact on survival in univariate or multivariate analysis in prospective studies.[42] These studies are criticized as being poorly designed, including a heterogeneous population, and not using standardized symptom assessment tools validated in this or a similar population.

Anorexia, delirium, dyspnea, dysphagia, fatigue, dry mouth, and weight loss are the most commonly reported symptoms that negatively affect survival. Nausea, vomiting, peripheral edema, diarrhea, drowsiness, early satiety, fever, oliguria, pain, and restlessness affect survival to a lesser extent. Psychological symptoms such as anxiety, depression, and sadness, which are common in this population, do not affect survival. Symptom severity in cancer patients affects survival. Univariate analyses show that stronger symptoms of dyspnea, drowsiness, anorexia, and nausea are associated with shorter survival, whereas pain and depression are not.[43]

RESEARCH OPPORTUNITIES

Symptom management research should focus on evaluating multiple symptoms using longitudinal, cross-sectional studies. Evaluating relationships among multiple symptoms, specific interventions, and patient outcomes is needed. Further studies must determine whether symptom chronicity or persistence, degree of distress, patient education, or other factors influence symptom reporting.

A definition of symptom clusters does not exist. Any synergistic effect of symptoms that constitute a cluster remains to be determined. Research should examine whether levels of symptom severity or distress change associations with others within a cluster.

REFERENCES

1. World Health Organization (WHO). Cancer Pain Relief and Palliative Care. Geneva: World Health Organization, 1990.
2. Donnelly S, Walsh D. The symptoms of advanced cancer. Semin Oncol 1995;22(2 Suppl 3):67-72.
3. Walsh D, Donnelly S, Rybicki L. The symptoms of advanced cancer: Relationship to age, gender, and performance status in 1,000 patients. Support Care Cancer 2000;8:175-179.
4. Homsi J, Walsh D, Nelson KA, et al. The impact of a palliative medicine consultation service in medical oncology. Support Care Cancer 2002;10:337-342.
5. Meijler WJ, Van Heest F, Otter R, Sleijfer DT. Educational needs of general practitioners in palliative care: Outcome of a focus group study. J Cancer Educ 2005;20:28-33.
6. Toscani F, Di Giulio P, Brunelli C, et al. How people die in hospital general wards: A descriptive study. J Pain Symptom Manage 2005;30:33-40.
7. Mystakidou K, Parpa E, Katsouda E, et al. The role of physical and psychological symptoms in desire for death: A study of terminally ill cancer patients. Psychooncology 2006;15:355-360.
8. Modonesi C, Scarpi E, Maltoni M, et al. Impact of palliative care unit admission on symptom control evaluated by the Edmonton Symptom Assessment System. J Pain Symptom Manage 2005;30:367-473.
9. Johnson DC, Kassner CT, Houser J, Kutner JS. Barriers to effective symptom management in hospice. J Pain Symptom Manage 2005;29:69-79.
10. Georges JJ, Onwuteaka-Philipsen BD, et al. Symptoms, treatment and "dying peacefully" in terminally ill cancer patients: A prospective study. Support Care Cancer 2005;13:160-168.
11. Komurcu S, Nelson KA, Walsh D, et al. Gastrointestinal symptoms among inpatients with advanced cancer. Am J Hosp Palliat Care 2002t;19:351-355.
12. Given CW, Given B, Azzouz F, et al. Predictors of pain and fatigue in the year following diagnosis among elderly cancer patients. J Pain Symptom Manage 2001;21:456-466.
13. Gloth FM 3rd. Geriatric pain. Factors that limit pain relief and increase complications. Geriatrics 2000;55:46-48, 51-54.
14. Bernabei R, Gambassi G, Lapane K, et al. Management of pain in elderly patients with cancer. SAGE study group: Systematic Assessment of Geriatric Drug Use via Epidemiology. JAMA 1998;279:1877-1882.
15. Addington-Hall J, Altmann D, McCarthy M. Variations by age in symptoms and dependency levels experienced by people in the last year of life, as reported by surviving family, friends and officials. Age Ageing 1998;27:129-136.
16. Vigano A, Bruera E, Suarez-Almazor ME. Age, pain intensity, and opioid dose in patients with advanced cancer. Cancer 1998;83:1244-1250.
17. Cassileth BR, Lusk EJ, Brown LL, et al. Factors associated with psychological distress in cancer patients. Med Pediatr Oncol 1986;14:251-254.
18. Sarhill N, Mahmoud F, Walsh D, et al. Evaluation of nutritional status in advanced metastatic cancer. Support Care Cancer 2003;11:652-659.
19. Donnelly S, Walsh D, Rybicki L. The symptoms of advanced cancer: Identification of clinical and research priorities by assessment of prevalence and severity. J Palliat Care 1995;11:27-32.
20. Cobb JL, Glantz MJ, Nicholas PK, et al. Delirium in patients with cancer at the end of life. Cancer Pract 2000;8:172-177.
21. Lin MH, Wu PY, Tsai ST, et al. Hospice palliative care for patients with hepatocellular carcinoma in Taiwan. Palliat Med 2004;18:93-99.
22. Levenson JW, McCarthy EP, Lynn J, et al. The last six months of life for patients with congestive heart failure. J Am Geriatr Soc 2000;48:S101-S109.
23. Zambroski CH, Moser DK, Roser LP, et al. Patients with heart failure who die in hospice. Am Heart J 2005;149:558-564.
24. Elkington H, White P, Addington-Hall J, et al. The healthcare needs of chronic obstructive pulmonary disease patients in the last year of life. Palliat Med 2005;19:485-491.
25. Rabow MW, Dibble SL. Ethnic differences in pain among outpatients with terminal and end-stage chronic illness. Pain Med 2005;6:235-241.
26. Koffman J, Higginson IJ, Donaldson N. Symptom severity in advanced cancer, assessed in two ethnic groups by interviews with bereaved family members and friends. J R Soc Med 2003;96:10-16.
27. Crowley R, Casarett D. Patients' willingness to participate in symptom-related and disease-modifying research: Results of a research screening initiative in a palliative care clinic. Cancer 2003;97:2327-2333.
28. Homsi J, Walsh D, Rivera N, et al. Symptom evaluation in palliative medicine: Patient report versus systematic assessment. Support Care Cancer 2006;14:444-453.
29. Oi-Ling K, Man-Wah DT, Kam-Hung DN. Symptom distress as rated by advanced cancer patients, caregivers and physicians in the last week of life. Palliat Med 2005;19:228-233.
30. Patrick DL, Ferketich SL, Frame PS, et al. National Institutes of Health State-of-the-Science Conference Statement: Symptom management in cancer: Pain, depression, and fatigue, July 15-17, 2002. J Natl Cancer Inst Monogr 2004;32:9-16.
31. Dodd MJ, Miaskowski C, Lee KA. Occurrence of symptom clusters. J Natl Cancer Inst Monogr 2004;32:76-78.
32. Miaskowski C, Dodd M, Lee K. Symptom clusters: The new frontier in symptom management research. J Natl Cancer Inst Monogr 2004;32:17-21.
33. Bower J, Ganz P, Desmond K, et al. Fatigue in breast cancer survivors: Occurrence, correlates, and impact on quality of life. J Clin Oncol 2000;18:743-753.
34. Miaskowski C, Lee K. Pain, fatigue, and sleep disturbances in oncology outpatients receiving radiation therapy for bone metastasis: A pilot study. J Pain Symptom Manage 1999;17:320-332.
35. Gift AG, Jablonski A, Stommel M, Given CW. Symptom clusters in elderly patients with lung cancer. Oncol Nurs Forum 2004;31:202-212.
36. Brown DJ, McMillan DC, Milroy R. The correlation between fatigue, physical function, the systemic inflammatory response, and psychological distress in patients with advanced lung cancer. Cancer 2005;103:377-382.
37. McCoubrie RC, Davies AN. Is there a correlation between spirituality and anxiety and depression in patients with advanced cancer? Support Care Cancer 2006;14:379-385.
38. Chan CW, Richardson A, Richardson J. A study to assess the existence of the symptom cluster of breathlessness, fatigue and anxiety in patients with advanced lung cancer. Eur J Oncol Nurs 2005;9:325-333.
39. Tanaka K, Akechi T, Okuyama T, et al. Impact of dyspnea, pain, and fatigue on daily life activities in ambulatory patients with advanced lung cancer. J Pain Symptom Manage 2002;23:417-423.
40. Sherwood P, Given BA, Given CW, et al. A cognitive behavioral intervention for symptom management in patients with advanced cancer. Oncol Nurs Forum 2005;32:1190-1198.
41. Brandt HE, Deliens L, Ooms ME, et al. Symptoms, signs, problems, and diseases of terminally ill nursing home patients: A nationwide observational study in the Netherlands. Arch Intern Med 2005;165:314-320.
42. Homsi J, Luong D. Symptoms and survival in patients with advanced disease. J Palliat Med 2007;10:904-909.

43. Palmer JL, Fisch MJ. Association between symptom distress and survival in outpatients seen in a palliative care cancer center. J Pain Symptom Manage 2005;29:565-571.

SUGGESTED READING

Homsi J, Walsh D, Nelson KA, et al. The impact of a palliative medicine consultation service in medical oncology. Support Care Cancer 2002;10:337-342.

Homsi J, Walsh D, Rivera N, et al. Symptom evaluation in palliative medicine: Patient report versus systematic assessment. Support Care Cancer 2006;14:444-453.

Miaskowski C, Dodd M, Lee K. Symptom clusters: The new frontier in symptom management research. J Natl Cancer Inst Monogr 2004;32:17-21.

Patrick DL, Ferketich SL, Frame PS, et al. National Institutes of Health State-of-the-Science Conference Statement: Symptom management in cancer: Pain, depression, and fatigue, July 15-17, 2002. J Natl Cancer Inst Monogr 2004;32:9-16.

Walsh D, Donnelly S, Rybicki L. The symptoms of advanced cancer: Relationship to age, gender, and performance status in 1,000 patients. Support Care Cancer 2000;8:175-179.

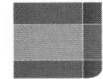

CHAPTER **150**

Anorexia and Weight Loss

Aurelius G. Omlin and **Florian Strasser**

KEY POINTS

- The anorexia-cachexia syndrome is a wasting state involving loss of muscle and fat caused by the underlying illness and mediated indirectly by secondary factors. Reduced oral intake and complex metabolic changes result in chronic negative energy and protein balance in combination with accelerated metabolism.

- Assessment requires a multidisciplinary approach at the onset.

- Secondary causes must be ruled out to identify potentially treatable conditions.

- Pharmacotherapy is only one pillar of treatment, which includes nutritional interventions, counseling, and improved physical activity.

- Effective communication with patients and their families is essential for treatment.

Anorexia-cachexia syndrome (ACS) occurs in numerous chronic end-stage disease processes, such as cancer, acquired immunodeficiency syndrome (AIDS), chronic pulmonary disease, chronic renal insufficiency, and heart failure[1] (see Chapter 106). ACS is a result of complex interactions among a chronic incurable disease, the central nervous system, and metabolic abnormalities.[2-4]

The definition is based on involuntary weight loss and loss of appetite or reduced oral intake. Various criteria are used, including symptom scales (threshold ≥3/10) or perceived burden (no threshold) for appetite, caloric intake (≤20 kcal/kg), and weight loss (>5% in 6 months or >2% in 2 months). Subjective perceptions are symptoms, whereas a syndrome includes objective variables (i.e., weight loss, caloric intake, and symptoms).[5-11]

Novel definitions are being developed, including variables of caloric intake, loss of fat and muscle mass, and chronic inflammation. It is likely that subtypes (phenotypes) will be characterized, including typical consequences such as reduced physical activity, impaired quality of life, and changes in body composition.

Working with patients suffering from ACS and their families requires careful assessment of ACS and concurrent physical and psychosocial distress, including the prognosis of a chronic incurable disease. Treatment includes counseling patients and relatives, treatment of potentially reversible secondary factors, and pharmacological and nutritional interventions (see Chapter 107). Promising pharmacological treatments have entered randomized, controlled trials. Nonpharmacological measures merit intensified future research.

BASIC SCIENCE AND PATHOPHYSIOLOGY

Differentiation between primary and secondary ACS is important. *Primary* ACS represents a metabolic status directly caused by the tumor or the chronic illness, in which complex metabolic and neuroendocrine modifications occur in an ongoing, altered inflammatory state. Catabolism is accelerated despite declining food and energy intake, and there is mobilization of peripheral proteins and lipids that maintain augmented liver synthesis of acute phase proteins. Losses of fat and body cell mass, particularly skeletal muscle, are approximately equal.[3,9,11,12] Based on animal models of primary ACS, different phenotypes exist that could be offered targeted therapy (see Chapter 106). *Secondary* ACS refers to cachexia occurring from impaired oral intake, including severe symptoms (e.g., pain, depression), concurrent catabolic states, loss of proteins, or loss of muscle tissue due to reduced physical activity (deconditioning) (Table 150-1).[8,10]

EPIDEMIOLOGY AND PREVALENCE

ACS is a silent syndrome that is easily overlooked. Early assessment and clinical suspicion seems crucial for efficient therapy[8,10] (see Chapter 63). Anorexia affects up to three fourths of cancer patients. It can occur independently of cachexia and is a poor prognostic factor.[5,10] The frequency of cachexia in patients with advanced solid tumors (except breast cancer) ranges from about 25% to more than 80% before death.[2,10] Weight loss has a significant impact on quality of life and is a poor prognostic factor.[10-13]

CLINICAL MANIFESTATIONS

ACS manifests with appetite loss, weight loss, and fatigue, often combined with chronic nausea, early satiety, and taste problems (see Chapter 169). The patient may or may not have weight loss, and edema or ascites may occur (Fig. 150-1). The family members may be distressed about the

TABLE 150-1   Checklist for Secondary Anorexia and Cachexia

MEDICAL CONDITION OR STATE	MECHANISM LEADING TO ANOREXIA OR CACHEXIA	POSSIBLE TREATMENT OPTIONS
REDUCED ORAL INTAKE FROM IMPAIRED GASTROINTESTINAL FUNCTION OR INTEGRITY		
Mouth		
Stomatitis or mucositis*	Pain, reduced taste	Topical mouth care
Xerostomia†	Reduced taste	Pilocarpin, change medication
Dysgeusia or hypogeusia†	Reduced taste	Zinc supplementation
Tooth problems†	Pain, inability to chew	Dentist
Osteonecrosis of jaw†	Pain, infection, inability to chew	Surgeon or dentist
Dysphagia or odynophagia	Pain	Depends on underlying cause
Thrush†	Pain	Antifungal medication
Upper gastrointestinal tract		
Bone metastasis of jaw	Pain, discomfort	Bisphosponates, radiation therapy
Gastroesophageal reflux†	Pain or inflammation	Proton pump inhibitors, antacids
Gastric ulcer or gastritis†	Postprandial pain	Proton pump inhibitors, antacids
Chronic nausea	Reduced oral intake	Depends on underlying cause, pharmacotherapy
Acute nausea or emesis†	Reduced oral intake	Antiemetics, counseling
Lower gastrointestinal tract		
Constipation*	Loss of appetite, nausea, early satiety	Laxatives
Bowel obstruction	Pain, nausea, emesis	Depends on underlying cause
Anal fissures or hemorrhoids†	Pain	Local therapy, depends on underlying cause
Radiation-induced esophagitis†	Pain, dysphagia	Consider total parenteral nutrition
Chronic diarrhea	Malabsorption, fear of fecal incontinence	Depends on underlying cause
REDUCED ORAL INTAKE WITH NORMAL GASTROINTESTINAL FUNCTION OR INTEGRITY		
Shortness of breath*	Reduced oral intake	Depends on underlying cause, morphine
Pain*	Anorexia, opioid-associated nausea, constipation	Analgetic therapy, depends on underlying cause
Delirium*	Reduced oral intake	Depends on underlying cause
Anxiety	Fear of fecal incontinence, fear of postprandial abdominal pain, fear of nausea	Counseling, depends on underlying cause
Fatigue	Inability to cook, shop, eat	Counseling, depends on underlying cause
Depression	Reduced appetite, anhedonia	Counseling, antidepressants
Wrong diet (e.g., too healthy, mono-item diets, Breuss hunger cure)	Inappropriate distribution of carbohydrates, proteins, and fats	Counseling
Fasting state (e.g., diagnostic tests, planned operation)	Insufficient oral intake	Consider total parenteral nutrition
Presentation of food (e.g., portions too large, unpleasant atmosphere, bad taste, social isolation, hectic ambience, bed-ridden state)	Loss of appetite, reduced oral intake	Counseling, improvement of environment
Language barrier (e.g., cannot order preferred food)	Insufficient oral intake	Counseling, translation service
Social distress (e.g., loneliness, lack of support, financial problems)	Insufficient oral intake or mono diet	Counseling, social support
Spiritual or existential distress (e.g., fear of death, unemployment)	Loss of appetite, insufficient oral intake	Counseling, support
LOSS OF PROTEINS		
Nephrotic syndrome	Protein loss	Depends on underlying cause
Frequent paracentesis or thoracentesis	Loss of proteins	Depends on underlying cause
Malabsorption or maldigestion	Loss of fat and proteins	Depends on underlying cause, pancreas enzyme substitution, slow down gut motility
Long-term cortisol therapy	Protein degradation	Depends on underlying cause
Extensive wounds	Loss of proteins	Depends on underlying cause
Bed-ridden state	Loss of physical activity, protein loss	Depends on underlying cause
Hypogonadism	Loss of muscle tissue	Hormone substitution
CATABOLIC STATES		
Hyperthyroidism	Increased catabolism, diarrhea	Depends on underlying cause
Infection or inflammation	Increased metabolism, acute phase production	Depends on underlying cause
Chronic heart, renal, or hepatic insufficiency; chronic obstructive pulmonary disease	Increased metabolism, impaired anabolism	Depends on underlying cause
Uncontrolled diabetes	Increased metabolism, impaired anabolism	Counseling, pharmacotherapy

*Very common causes of secondary anorexia or cachexia.
†Possible side effects of radiation therapy, chemotherapy, or pharmacotherapy.

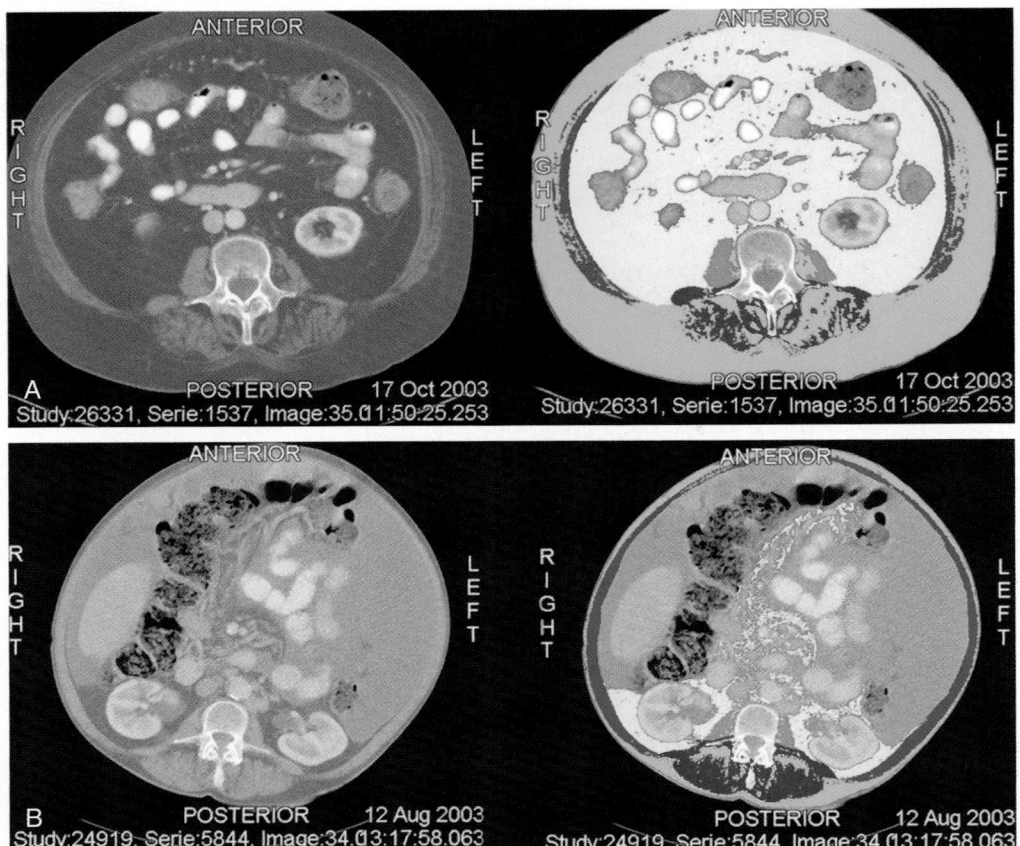

FIGURE 150-1 The clinical picture of anorexia-cachexia syndrome is complex. The two patients have a diagnosis of advanced cancer. The existence of fat hides the significant loss of muscle mass in one patient (**A**), whereas the other patient (**B**) can be directly identified as cachectic. Locations of adipose tissue are indicated by color: visceral (*yellow*), subcutaneous (*light blue*), and intramuscular (*green*). Muscle tissue also is indicated by color: paraspinal (*red*), psoas (*orange*), lateral abdominal (*dark blue*), and rectus abdominis (*purple*). (Courtesy of Professor Vickie Baracos, Department of Oncology, University of Alberta, Cross Cancer Institute, Edmonton, Alberta.)

weight loss, or they may complain about lack of concern by staff members.

EVALUATION

In clinical practice, a structured, multilevel assessment strategy seems attractive (Fig. 150-2). We propose a two-step approach with a basic assessment (level I) that includes screening for ACS and for consequences that often guide primary actions (Boxes 150-1 and 150-2). If ACS is a priority in palliative management, in-depth assessment (level II) is necessary. Level III assessments are performed in specialized settings.

Basic Assessment

Basic assessment (level I) of ACS has two parts: screening and estimation of consequences (see Box 150-1). Screening reliably and quickly determines whether the patient has ACS (see "Case Study: Managing Anorexia-Cachexia Syndrome"). ACS is likely if one of the following is identified: loss of appetite (scored as 3/10 or higher on a numeric rating or visual analogue scale), weight loss (i.e., 2% or more in 2 months or 5% or more in 6 months), reduced oral intake (≥25% less than normal by patient report), or

---

Box 150-1 Basic Assessment (Level I) for Anorexia-Cachexia Syndrome

A. Screening for anorexia-cachexia-syndrome
   1. Anorexia (≥3 of 10 on numeric rating or visual analogue scale)
      or
   2. Weight loss (2% in 2 months, 5% in 6 months)
      or
   3. Patients perceived reduction of oral intake (≥25% of normal)
B. Estimation of consequences of anorexia-cachexia syndrome
   1. Does the patient look malnourished (i.e., body composition or nutritional status)?
   2. Does the patient suffer from reduced strength or energy (i.e., physical activity or energy expenditure)?
   3. Does the patient report fatigue, early satiety, chronic nausea, bloating, tension due to edema, dry mouth, or other common symptoms (i.e., associated symptoms)?
   4. Is the patient or his or her relatives bothered by the loss of appetite or loss of weight (i.e., psychosocial-existential distress)?

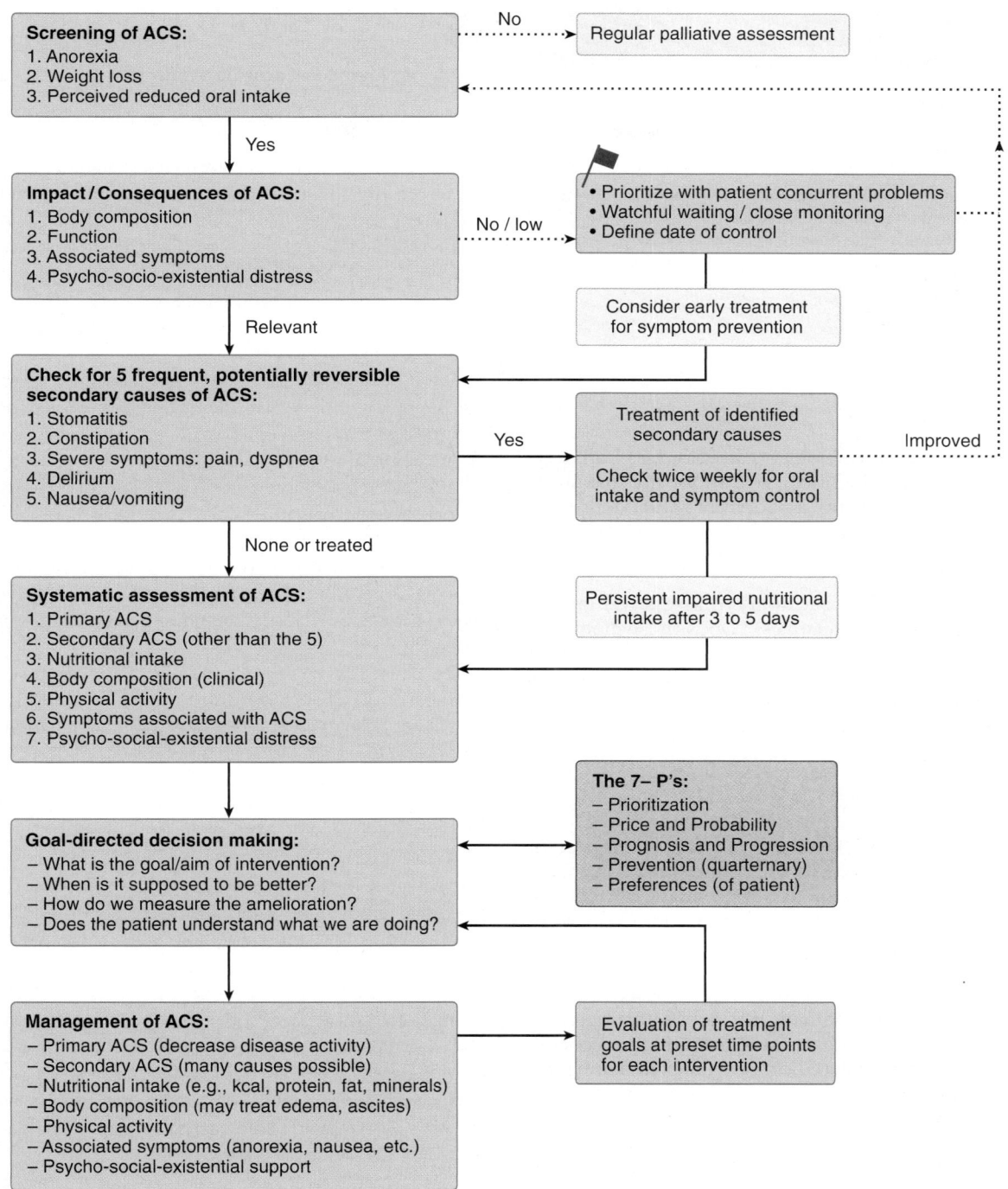

FIGURE 150-2   Flow chart for screening assessment, decision making, and management of anorexia-cachexia syndrome (ACS).

reduced intake (<20 kcal/kg). If the screening result is positive, simultaneous estimation of the impact guides further strategies.

ACS has many consequences, including nutritional status, physical function, the effects of associated symptoms, and psychosocial effects on patients and their families. ACS alters the patient's body composition and nutritional status. Bedside assessment of body composition is based on the physician's visual impression (e.g., well nourished, malnourished), an estimation of muscle

and body fat, and the clinical evaluation of edema, ascites, or pulmonary effusion.

A proxy for physical function is the Karnofsky Performance Status scale, which allows the clinician to grade patients' functioning from normal physical activity to severely disabled. A brief history allows further evaluation of activities of daily living (ADLs) or instrumental activities of daily living (IADLs).

The Edmonton Symptom Assessment Scale provides information on eight additional symptoms: pain, fatigue, nausea, depression, shortness of breath, tiredness, anxiety, and well-being. It may identify a reason for the ACS or its consequences. For example, a patient may feel depressed because of anorexia and reduced oral intake, or preexisting depression may lead to loss of appetite and reduced oral intake.

Patients may be asked questions to assess the impact of ACS on them or their relatives: "Does the weight loss bother you?" or "Are your relatives bothered by your poor appetite?" It is important to recognize patients' concerns about symptoms. Many are disturbed because anorexia and weight loss may represent tumor progression and death.

Systematic Assessment

Systematic assessment (level II) of ACS is important because findings guide individualized treatments. An algorithm combines early treatment of potentially correctable causes of secondary ACS before comprehensive assessment (see Fig. 150-2).

The first step is assessment of primary ACS, tumor dynamics, prognosis, and response to disease-oriented treatment. None of the common laboratory parameters is a reliable indicator of primary ACS. Serum albumin concentration is downregulated in chronic inflammation (serum half-life of 19 days), and it can be used to monitor long-term treatment. Prealbumin (i.e., transthyretin), with a serum half-life of 48 hours, may serve for short-term assessment.[5,8] C-reactive protein (CRP) is a nonspecific acute phase protein, and the level often is high in patients with advanced cancer or disease progression.[5] The diagnostic value, sensitivity, and specificity of proteolysis-inducing factor (PIF) and lipid-mobilizing factor (LMF) are being investigated. Further studies should clarify the role of leptin, neuropeptide Y, ghrelin, melanocortin, and other hormones and peptides. To evaluate disease dynamics (including tumor markers), the actual tumor load, tumor activity, and the expected response to antitumor therapy should be considered.

The second step is assessment of secondary, potentially reversible factors. Little information is available on the frequency and relative importance of the five common secondary factors: stomatitis, constipation, pain and dyspnea, delirium, and nausea or vomiting (see Chapters

CASE STUDY

Managing Anorexia-Cachexia Syndrome

Mr. A is a 62-year-old farmer who was diagnosed with non–small cell lung cancer with bone metastasis. After four cycles of chemotherapy, stable disease was demonstrated by computed tomography. At a routine visit 3 months later, his wife complains that he has lost weight despite all her extra cooking. Mr. A is worried because he had seen a close friend with an incurable pancreatic cancer "starve to death." Mrs. A is concerned that she is not looking after her husband's nutrition very well. Her sister told her that he should be given nutritional supplements or total parenteral nutrition.

Mr. A (initial weight of 140 pounds and height of 172 cm) has lost 28 pounds since his first visit 6 months earlier; this corresponds to a 20% loss of his premorbid weight and a change in the body mass index from 23.6 to 18.9 kg/m². The patient is distressed because of his weight loss, perceived reduced oral intake, and loss of appetite (score of 9/10).

Because the patient has lost muscle mass, he has a lack of energy and pain during movement. He has stayed at home most of the time and even stopped going for walks with his beloved dog. He expresses a fear of dying, and his wife is distressed and desperate.

The patient has no sign of stomatitis, but he reports constipation, which is confirmed on an abdominal radiograph. The patient has been using a fentanyl patch without breakthrough doses, but he was not taking laxatives. Pain for the last 24 hours was rated as 7/10, dyspnea as 3/10, and nausea as 2/10. When he achieves a (rare) bowel movement, appetite improves slightly. The patient showed no signs of cognitive impairment.

To manage the discomfort, the pain medication was adapted with adequate breakthrough dosing, adjuvant analgesics were given, and radiation therapy for the painful bone metastasis was initiated. The patient got bi-daily oral combination laxative therapy and daily enemas. Patient and spouse were educated. Pain and constipation were re-evaluated after 3 and 5 days of the new regimen. Because of persistent anorexia-cachexia syndrome (i.e., perceived oral intake only slightly better and anorexia score of 6/10), in-depth assessment was initiated by estimating primary and secondary factors, nutritional intake over 3 days, clinical body composition, symptom burden, physical function, and eating-related distress of the patient and family.

Management was agreed on with the patient, family, and interdisciplinary team. It consisted of nutritional counseling (i.e., many meals, protein-rich meals, and supplements), psychosocial counseling to enable the family to express and cope with illness-associated distress by other means than eating, home physical exercise (i.e., two sets of 10 minutes of stair climbing), intramuscular administration of testosterone, use of megestrol acetate to stimulate appetite (with re-evaluation after 2 weeks), and second-line chemotherapy (i.e., docetaxel).

169 and 232). A secondary anorexia-cachexia checklist can help identify many different causes (see Table 150-1).

Radiation therapy may cause nausea and vomiting if it is administered to the abdomen. Chemotherapy side effects (i.e., mucositis, diarrhea, or infections) can affect nutritional intake. Side effects of opioids and other pharmacological treatments are common but often unrecognized in patients with ACS.

The third step is assessment of caloric intake. Most methods depend on the patient's ability to retrospectively report what was eaten or keep a prospective dietary record over 3 days. An observer calculating or weighing food consumed at each meal improves accuracy. An approach that includes photographs of plates before and after the meal followed by calculation of caloric intake by a nutritionist has been used in research.[5,8]

The fourth step is assessment of nutritional status, body composition, conditional essential nutrients, and laboratory parameters. Measuring weight includes the history of involuntary weight loss, assessing body weight and body mass index, calculating the ideal body weight (height in centimeters – 100), and recognizing confounding conditions such as significant ascites, pleural effusion, or edema.

The subjective global assessment of a nutrition questionnaire (SGA) combines information on weight change, dietary intake, gastrointestinal symptoms, and functional impairment with information on body composition. Three groups are defined: well nourished, mildly or moderately malnourished, or severely malnourished.[5,8,10] The SGA has value mainly for the physical examination of body composition (i.e., estimation of fat and muscle mass). The secondary anorexia checklist may inform the clinical more than gastrointestinal symptoms of the SGA. Anthropometric tests (in addition to weight) include skin fold thickness (i.e., body fat) and middle upper arm circumference (i.e., indicator of muscle mass), and it can be used for longitudinal follow-up studies.

Whole-body bioimpedance analysis (BIA) is an easy to administer assessment of body composition, but body water content has to be estimated by the examiner, which may introduce a large degree of variability. Dual-photon absorptiometry or dual x-ray absorptiometry (DEXA) is reliable, but access is limited.

Measurement of muscle mass or visceral tissue mass by computed tomography (CT) or magnetic resonance imaging (MRI) is promising. This approach can take advantage of the regular monitoring of cancer patients (see Fig. 150-1).

Essential nutrients such as vitamins, amino acids, and trace elements are not routinely assessed. However, patients suffering from chronic disease may be deficient in substances such as vitamins D and E or zinc (blood levels of zinc correlate inconsistently with body reserve).

The fifth step is assessment of the patient's physical function, physical activity, and energy expenditure. Performance status (e.g., Karnofsky Performance Status, Eastern Cooperative Oncology Group [ECOG]) can approximate and monitor global function. For muscle function, grip and thigh strength monitoring is simple to administer, as is the sit-up-and-go time. Body sensors can estimate type, duration, frequency, and intensity of physical activities for indirect calculation of energy expenditure, and they may replace the laborious and expensive double-labeled water technique or indirect calorimetry.

The sixth step in the assessment of ACS is evaluation of its psychosocial impact on the patient and family members. In addition to somatic parameters, psychological characteristics, social and family concerns, and spiritual or existential distress must be included. Emotional, social, and spiritual distresses are first estimated by common symptom screening instruments. The interdisciplinary team then explores how ACS affects distress and quality of life. The Functional Assessment of Anorexia/ Cachexia Treatment (FAACT) has 12 questions that ask about pressure by family members and concerns about body appearance and weight.[10,14]

The seventh step is assessment of associated symptoms. No widely accepted symptom checklist is available for ACS symptoms, and current symptom screening lists are not designed to differentiate the consequences of ACS from concurrent symptoms, which may also cause secondary ACS. FAACT includes key symptoms but does not cover the full clinical experience. In practice, we use the Edmonton Symptom Assessment Scale, the FAACT, screening for fatigue (i.e., cognitive, emotional, and physical dimensions), and questions about eating-related distress among patients and family.

DIFFERENTIAL DIAGNOSIS

The ACS has many causes (see Fig. 150-2).

TREATMENT

Plan of Care

Five common and potentially reversible factors of secondary ACS are assessed and treated (see Fig. 150-2). Priorities should be negotiated with the patient and family, because patients' priorities often are different from those of the physicians. Treatment goals and outcome measures then are discussed with the patient, family, and interdisciplinary team. For instance, control of predominant symptoms (e.g., anorexia, chronic nausea) may be the priority for some, whereas the focus is physical activity for others.

Decision making includes the definition of an intervention goal and agreement on a re-evaluation time and symptom measurement (see Chapters 116 and 120). It is important to ensure understanding of these goals and methods by the patients and family. The 7-P model is helpful in (Box 150-3) decision making (Box 150-4).

The first step in the plan of care is to treat the primary causes of ACS. Treatment of the causative underlying illness is essential. Carefully chosen and monitored antineoplastic treatments can offer symptomatic benefit. Anti-inflammatory cytokines (e.g., tumor necrosis factor-α, interleukin-6 inhibitors, thalidomide-like agents), ghrelin, or melanocortin receptor antagonists may provide novel therapeutic approaches.[5,7,8]

The second component of the care plan is to treat the often-reversible secondary causes of ACS: stomatitis, constipation, pain and dyspnea, delirium, and nausea or vomiting. Interdisciplinary management is advisable for many secondary causes.

The third component of management is to provide appropriate nutritional support. Nutritional counseling is a cornerstone of ACS management, whereas the use of artificial nutrition in managing patients with advanced cancer is controversial. There is no evidence that increased caloric intake in all cancer patients with ACS can increase muscle mass or produce a survival advantage (see Chapters 104, 105, 108, and 109). The main reason is that primary ACS impedes effective caloric intake.[8,15] Patients with dominant starvation cachexia (i.e., most secondary ACS factors excluding catabolism) and with minimally controlled primary ACS may represent a subgroup of ACS who can profit from artificial nutrition.

Starvation is characterized as hypometabolism with reduced protein and glucose turnover but increased lipolysis without an underlying pro-inflammatory condition. Starvation is often seen in patients with bowel obstruction, those undergoing radiotherapy for head and neck cancers, and surgical patients.

Both the assessment and intervention parts of dietary counseling are essential in management (see Chapter 51). Assessment includes calculation of nutritional intake considering the relative composition of nutrients (e.g., kcal, proteins, vitamins), estimation of nutritional status to define the goals of intervention, and analysis of physical activity and underlying disease activity. Clinicians must assess eating habits, screen for family distress, and explore educational needs. Interventions include counseling to alleviate anxiety and conflict about the inability to consume a normal diet and educate cancer patients about the role of high-protein and high-fat diets (i.e., that eating "unhealthy" food is a response to their needs). Comfort-centered counseling may produce more stress reduction than achieving certain caloric and protein goals.

Enteral nutrition should be favored over parenteral nutrition, although it is important to identify the few who may profit from parenteral nutrition. Before instituting parenteral nutrition, clear time goals should be set for re-evaluation of its effectiveness and potential withdrawal.

The fourth component of the care plan is to provide measures to stabilize or improve body composition by means of combined interventions tackling nutritional intake, muscle function, and reversal of catabolism (e.g., inflammation, disease). Evidence from animal models or specific diseases suggests that vitamins, trace elements, and specific amino acids can ameliorate ACS. Extrapolation of this evidence to clinical management is controversial.

The fifth component of the management plan is to increase physical activity and exercise. Overall anabolism and especially muscle anabolism are maximized with frequent contractile exercise, particularly resistance-type activity (e.g., weightlifting) in elderly patients, and with nutritional and pharmacological support.[11] Exercise intervention studies (e.g., cancer survivors) reported improved quality of life and improved nutritional status, symptoms (e.g., nausea, fatigue, anxiety), muscle strength, and functional capacity. It is unclear which subgroups of patients with advanced incurable diseases benefit.

The sixth component of management is psychosocial-existential counseling and support. "Starving to death" is a common concern of patients with ACS and their families. Because of the high frequency and impact of eating-related distress of patients, family members, and caregivers, adequate education and counseling (including practical acts of friendship and caring) deserve high priority.

The seventh component of the care plan is treatment of associated symptoms. Associated symptoms may be the cause of ACS or may result from it. Depression may lead to reduced oral intake, and weight loss and anorexia may result in depression.

Drugs

Progestins, short-term corticosteroids, and prokinetics alleviate selected aspects of ACS. Several agents targeting appetite stimulation or secondary anorexia have been investigated with negative results. However, limited trial and preclinical data have been reported for some promising drugs (e.g., ghrelin, ATP, thalidomide, MC4-receptor antagonists, β_2-mimetics) (see Chapter 133).

Supportive Care

Evidence is growing for many pharmacological and non-pharmacological interventions. The use of progestational drugs, short-term corticosteroids, and metoclopramide for anorexia is supported by the results of randomized, controlled trials and meta-analysis.[2,5,6] However, evidence for consistent effects on weight loss or quality of life is lacking.

Studies of nutritional counseling or oral supplements have reported increased food intake, but no consistent evidence exists for improvements in body composition, function, tumor treatment response, or survival.

RESEARCH OPPORTUNITIES

Several phenotypes of primary ACS with different underlying pathophysiological mechanisms are suspected, and they should be characterized for targeted therapy. A systematic approach to assessment and classification of ACS is important for improved clinical practice.

Combined pharmacological treatments of various targets (i.e., appetite and others) and individualized interventions (e.g., nutritional support) should be evaluated. To tailor ACS treatment, research should focus on genetic variability, such as altered leptin, neuropeptide Y, melanocortin, ghrelin, and ubiquitin-proteosome pathways. The importance of the cancer cachectic factor (i.e., proteolysis-inducing factor) is controversial, but it may hold promise as a novel therapeutic target.[2,5,6,9,12]

REFERENCES

1. Morley JE, Thomas DR, Wilson MM. Cachexia: pathophysiology and clinical relevance. Am J Clin Nutr 2006;83:735-743.
2. Inui A: Cancer anorexia-cachexia syndrome: current issues in research and management. CA Cancer Clin 2002;52:72-91.
3. Davis MP, Dickerson D. Cachexia and anorexia: cancer's covert killer. Support Care Cancer 2000;8:180-187.
4. Fearon KC, Voss AC, Hustead DS, for the Cancer Cachexia Study Group. Definition of cancer cachexia: Effect of weight loss, reduced food intake, and systemic inflammation on functional status and prognosis. Am J Clin Nutr 2006;83:1345-1350.
5. Strasser F: Pathophysiology of the anorexia/cachexia syndrome. In Doyle D, Hanks G, Cherny N, Calman K (eds). Oxford Textbook of Palliative Medicine. New York: Oxford University Press, 2005.
6. Yavuzsen T, Mellar PD, Walsh D, et al. Systematic review of the treatment of cancer-associated anorexia and weight loss. J Clin Oncol 2005;85:8500-8511.
7. Strasser F: Eating-related disorders in patients with advanced cancer. Support Care Cancer 2003;11:11-20.
8. Strasser F, Bruera ED. Update on anorexia and cachexia. Hematol Oncol Clin North Am 2002;16:589-617.
9. MacDonald N, Easson AM, Mazurak VC, et al. Understanding and managing cancer cachexia. J Am Coll Surg 2003;197:143-161.
10. Strasser F, Bruera E. Cancer anorexia/cachexia syndrome: Epidemiology, pathogenesis, and assessment. In Ripamonti C, Bruera E (eds). Gastrointestinal Symptoms in Advanced Cancer Patients. New York: Oxford University Press, 2002.
11. Baracos VE. Cancer-associated cachexia and underlying biological mechanisms. Annu Rev Nutr 2006;26:435-461.
12. Giordano KF, Jatoi A: The cancer anorexia/weight loss syndrome: Therapeutic challenges. Curr Oncol Rep 2005;7:271-276.
13. Stewart GD, Skipworth RJ, Fearon KC. Cancer cachexia and fatigue. Clin Med 2006;6:140-143.
14. Strasser F, Binswanger J, Cerny T, Kesselring A. Fighting a losing battle: Eating-related distress of men with advanced cancer and their female partners. A mixed-methods study. Palliat Med 2007;21:129-137.
15. Bruera E. ABC of palliative care. Anorexia, cachexia, and nutrition. BMJ 1997;315:1219-1222.

SUGGESTED READING

Baracos VE. Cancer-associated cachexia and underlying biological mechanisms. Annu Rev Nutr 2006;26:435-461.

Inui A. Cancer anorexia-cachexia syndrome: current issues in research and management. CA Cancer Clin 2002;52:72-91.

Strasser F, Bruera ED. Update on anorexia and cachexia. Hematol Oncol Clin North Am 2002;16:589-617.

CHAPTER **151**

Anxiety

Susan B. LeGrand

KEY POINTS

- There is little specific palliative medicine evidence on the diagnosis and management of anxiety.
- The prevalence is about 25%, but it is higher among younger women.
- Anxiety may be a primary symptom, a sign of other medical illnesses or complications, or a medication side effect, and the source should be considered before initiating therapy.
- Psychotherapeutic interventions are recommended even in patients with advanced disease.
- Benzodiazepines and selective serotonin reuptake inhibitors are useful agents for treating anxiety.

Although anxiety is common in patients with advanced illness, there is little research on the symptom specific to palliative medicine. What exists is typically expert opinion extrapolated from the general psychiatric literature. *Anxiety* is defined as "the presence of fear or apprehension that is out of proportion to the context of the life situations."[1] However, for patients facing death, what is proportional to the context? As in many situations in advanced illness, the level of distress should prompt intervention rather than strict diagnostic criteria.

Anxiety may be a symptom of other conditions, and the contribution of each to the incidence of anxiety is unknown:

- A preexisting psychiatric illness exacerbated by advanced disease, such as adjustment disorders, panic disorders, depression, and generalized anxiety disorders
- A medical complication, such as sepsis, pulmonary embolus, hypoxia, delirium, or medication withdrawal
- A medication side effect, such as those of corticosteroids or metoclopramide
- Existential fears about dying or burial[2,3]

BASIC SCIENCE

Humans have the ability to react to threat by means of the neurochemical systems (e.g., cortisol, catecholamines) that govern the fight-or-flight response.. Just as an unrelieved pain stimulus may lead to long-term changes in the spinal cord and chronic pain, chronic activation of these systems and possibly early exposure to high levels of stress may fundamentally change a person, leading to chronic anxiety disorders, learned helplessness, or increased sensitivity to stress.[4]

The primary areas in the brain involved in processing stress are the locus ceruleus, hippocampus, hypothalamus, amygdala, and cerebral cortex. Many neurochemical agents increase or modulate the reactions (Table 151-1). Animal models and research in humans with anxiety states are increasing our understanding of the complex interplay of systems and the influence of genetics and experience. The lasting effect of traumas and early childhood experiences on sensitivity to stress and resilience may improve our understanding of how people approach a life-threatening situation.

EPIDEMIOLOGY AND PREVALENCE

The estimated prevalence of anxiety in the cancer population is 25%.[5] In a 1000-patient palliative medicine database, higher rates were seen for women (29% versus 20%) and those younger than 65 years (29% versus 19%).[6] Among 100 outpatients with congestive heart failure, 18% had anxiety demonstrated on a structured clinical interview for axis I disorders (SCID-I) as defined by the fourth edition of the *Diagnostic and Statistical Manual of Mental Disorders* (DSM-IV), which is considered the gold standard for diagnosis.[7] Rates of anxiety up to 70% (including combined depression with anxiety) have been reported for patients with chronic pulmonary disease.[8] Age and gender associations for these and other diseases are unknown.

CLINICAL MANIFESTATIONS

Physical symptoms of anxiety in the medically ill usually are more problematic than psychological or cognitive aspects[9] (see "Case Study: Evaluating Anxiety"). They can include tension, restlessness, autonomic hyperactivity,

 C A S E   S T U D Y

Evaluating Anxiety

Mr. S is a 65-year-old gentleman with metastatic lung cancer who was hospitalized for pain management and a spinal cord compression at T6 that has left him paralyzed. He has been successfully treated with methylphenidate for improving energy and mood.

One morning, he complained of anxiety, and the nurse requested medication for this. On evaluation, he appeared frightened and was sweating. When asked if he had other symptoms, he said that he felt short of breath. Further exploration revealed that the sudden onset of dyspnea occurred simultaneously with the severe anxiety. Spiral computed tomography confirmed the presence of a large pulmonary embolus. As demonstrated by this case, new-onset anxiety requires a search for precipitating events before or concurrent with administration of anxiolytic therapy.

TABLE 151-1	Neurotransmitters		
MEDICATION	**EFFECTS**		**LOCATION**
Norepinephrine (NE)	Increase heart rate		Locus ceruleus (LC)
	Increase startle response		
	Insomnia		
	Autonomic hyperarousal		
Hypothalamic-pituitary-adrenal (HPA) axis			
Corticotropin-releasing hormone (CRH)	Increases with stress		Extensive throughout
	Increase dehydroepiandrosterone and cortisol levels at the amygdala		
	Increases fear-related behaviors		
	Decrease food, sexual activity, growth, and reproduction		
Cortisol	Increase effect of CRH		Hippocampus
	Encode emotion-related memory		Amygdala
			Prefrontal cortex (PFC)
Neurosteroids and peptides			
Progesterone metabolites, deoxycorticosterone	Anxiolytic effects		
Arginine vasopressin (AVP)	Learning and memory		Amygdala
	Pain sensitivity		Hippocampus
	Rapid eye movement (REM) sleep		
Neuropeptide Y	Decreased memory retention		LC
	Resilience		Hypothalamus
	Vulnerability to stress		
Galanin	Modulates anxiety-related behaviors		LC
	Decrease NE release at the LC		
Serotonin	Increase anxiety ($5\text{-}HT_{2A}$)		PFC, nucleus acumens
	Decrease anxiety ($5\text{-}HT_{1A}$)		Amygdala
			Lateral hypothalamus
Cholecystokinin	Anxiogenic		Cerebral cortex
			Amygdala
			Midbrain
Opioid peptides	Decrease NE activity		

insomnia, sweating, palpitations, diarrhea, and other symptoms. Anxious individuals may repeatedly ask the same questions because they do not adequately absorb information. They may delay difficult conversations, avoid physicians, and postpone the very treatment they need.[3]

DIFFERENTIAL DIAGNOSIS

There are DSM-IV criteria for generalized anxiety disorder, anxiety disorder resulting from a medical illness, and adjustment disorder with anxiety (Table 151-2). Separating anxiety into four subsets has been proposed (Box 151-1).[10] Situational anxiety describes stress engendered by life circumstances. Psychiatric anxiety is a defined illness such as panic disorder, obsessive-compulsive disorder, or delirium. Organic anxiety is associated with metabolic disorders, medications, or medical events such as pulmonary embolus. Existential anxiety describes spiritual concerns, loss of control, or loss of dignity.

There is no uniformly accepted screening tool for anxiety in palliative medicine. The Hospital Anxiety and Depression Scale (HADS) is the most commonly used in research, but validation studies have looked more at its usefulness for identifying depression rather than anxiety.[11] The standard diagnostic tool is the DSM-IV SCID, which requires a trained individual and does not enable easy screening.

The clinician can consider an approach to diagnosis based on the time course of the symptom. New-onset anxiety in someone without a history of anxiety should prompt a careful evaluation for causative factors (Box 151-2). This does not exclude the possibility of contribut-

---

Box 151-1 Subsets of Anxiety in the Medically Ill

- Situational
- Psychiatric
- Organic
- Existential

From Stiefel F, Razavi D. Common psychiatric disorders in cancer patients. II. Anxiety and acute confusional states. Support Care Cancer 1994;2:233-237.

Box 151-2 Differential Diagnosis of Acute Anxiety

- Delirium
- Medical complications (e.g., pulmonary embolus, hypoxemia, sepsis)
- Withdrawal
- Medication side effect
- Recent bad news

TABLE 151-2 Diagnostic and Statistical Manual of Mental Disorders (DSM-IV) Criteria

GENERALIZED ANXIETY DISORDER	ADJUSTMENT DISORDERS	ANXIETY DISORDER DUE TO A MEDICAL CONDITION
A. Excessive anxiety and worry occur more days than not for at least 6 months.	A. Emotional or behavioral symptoms occur in response to one or more identifiable stressors occurring within 3 months of the onset of the stressors.	A. Prominent anxiety, panic attacks, or obsessions or compulsions predominate in the clinical picture.
B. The person finds it difficult to control the worry.	B. These symptoms or behaviors are clinically significant as evidenced by either of the following: 1. Marked distress in excess of what would be expected from exposure to the stressor 2. Significant impairment in social or occupational (academic) functioning	B. There is evidence from the history, physical examination, or laboratory findings that the disturbance is the direct physiological consequence of a general medical condition.
C. The anxiety and worry are associated with three (or more) of the following six symptoms (only one item is required for children): 1. Restlessness or feeling keyed up or on edge 2. Being easily fatigued 3. Difficulty concentrating or mind going blank 4. Irritability 5. Muscle tension 6. Sleep disturbance	C. It does not meet the criteria for another specific axis I disorder and is not merely an exacerbation of a preexisting axis I or axis II disorder.	C. It is not better accounted for by another mental disorder (e.g., adjustment disorder with anxiety, in which the stressor is a serious general medical condition).
D. The focus of the anxiety and worry is not confined to features of another psychiatric disorder (axis 1).	D. The symptoms do not represent bereavement.	D. The disturbance does not occur exclusively during the course of a delirium.
E. Causes clinically significant distress or impairment in social, occupational, or other important areas of functioning.	E. After the stressor (or its consequences) has terminated, the symptoms do not persist for more than an additional 6 months.	E. The disturbance causes clinically significant distress or impairment in social, occupational, or other important areas of functioning.
F. It is not caused by the direct physiological effects of a substance or a general medical condition.		

From Neumeister A, Bonne O, Charney DS. Anxiety disorders: Neurochemical aspects. In Sadock BJ, Sadock VA (eds). Kaplan & Sadock's Comprehensive Textbook of Psychiatry, 8th ed. New York: Lippincott Williams & Wilkins, 2005, pp 1739-1748.

ing causes in persons with a subacute or chronic history. Any change in symptoms in those individuals should warrant a search for contributing factors. Psychiatric causes are divided into specific subsets as defined in the DSM-IV (Box 151-3).[12]

TREATMENT

There have been few trials of psychotherapeutic approaches specific to anxiety. The research that exists usually looks at general psychological symptoms that include depression and anxiety. Systematic literature reviews of anxiety in cancer patients concluded that further research is required before definite recommendations can be made. Meta-analysis found good effect size favoring interventions, particularly if participants were prescreened for anxiety.[13] Brief psychotherapeutic interventions are recommended for mild to moderate anxiety and can complement medical management.[3]

Medical management of anxiety by nonpsychiatrists typically employs benzodiazepine agents (see Chapters 122 and 134). A Cochrane review concluded there were inadequate data on the efficacy of medication for palliative medicine patients to allow recommendations because none of the six trials reviewed met their criteria for inclusion.[14] General recommendations include short-acting agents such as lorazepam, alprazolam, and oxazepam, administered as needed.[15] If rebound anxiety occurs, scheduled doses of longer-acting agents such as diazepam or clonazepam can be considered. Serotonin reuptake inhibitors and buspirone, which are effective in psychiatric settings, can be considered in palliative care, but they have a delayed onset of up to 3 to 4 weeks, which is problematic in treating acute distress. For patients with a longer life expectancy, short-acting benzodiazepines combined with slower-onset agents can be considered. The major tranquilizers (see Chapter 139) are useful alternatives, particularly if they also address other symptoms. For example, someone with chronic nausea and anxiety can be managed with haloperidol or olanzapine for both symptoms.

Various complementary therapies, including music therapy[16] and aromatherapy with massage,[17] have some evidence of effectiveness in managing anxiety. Studies have shown small, transient effects. Relaxation techniques have not been independently studied in this population, but in a trial that compared alprazolam with relaxation training, both were found to be effective.[18]

CONCLUSIONS AND RESEARCH OPPORTUNITIES

Management should focus on identifying disease complications and medication toxicities in a symptomatic approach, with appropriate drug (e.g., benzodiazepines) and psychotherapeutic interventions added to the regimen as indicated.

Anxiety, although common in palliative medicine patients, has had little attention in terms of specific research. Investigations are needed in several areas:

- Anxiety-specific screening tools that incorporate a differential diagnosis
- Palliative medicine–specific treatment protocols
- Guidelines for the use of psychotherapeutic and pastoral care interventions
- Additional studies of anxiety in noncancer, advanced disease settings

REFERENCES

1. Pine ES, McClure EB. Anxiety disorders: Clinical features. In Sadock BJ, Sadock VA (eds). Kaplan & Sadock's Comprehensive Textbook of Psychiatry, 8th ed. New York: Lippincott Williams & Wilkins, 2005, pp 1768-1780.
2. Tremblay A, Breitbart W. Psychiatric dimensions of palliative care. Neurol Clin 2001;19:949-967.
3. Block SD. Psychological issues in end-of-life care. J Palliat Med 2006;9:751-772.
4. Neumeister A, Bonne O, Charney DS. Anxiety disorders: Neurochemical aspects. In Sadock BJ, Sadock VA (eds). Kaplan & Sadock's Comprehensive Textbook of Psychiatry, 8th ed. New York: Lippincott Williams & Wilkins, 2005, pp 1739-1748.
5. Donnelly S, Walsh D, Rybicki L. The symptoms of advanced cancer: Identification of clinical and research priorities by assessment of prevalence and severity. J Palliat Care 1995;11:27-32.
6. Walsh D, Donnelly S, Rybicki L. The symptoms of advanced cancer: relationship to age, gender, and performance status in 1,000 patients. Support Care Cancer 2000;8:175-179.
7. Haworth JE, Moniz-Cook E, Clark AL, et al. Prevalence and predictors of anxiety and depression in a sample of chronic heart failure patients with left ventricular systolic dysfunction. Eur J Heart Fail 2005;7:803-808.
8. Kunik ME, Roundy K, Veazey C, et al. Surprisingly high prevalence of anxiety and depression in chronic breathing disorders. Chest 2005;127:1205-1211.
9. Holland JC. Anxiety and cancer: the patient and family. J Clin Psychiatry 1989;50:20-25.
10. Stiefel F, Razavi D. Common psychiatric disorders in cancer patients. II. Anxiety and acute confusional states. Support Care Cancer 1994;2:233-237.
11. Lloyd-Williams M, Friedman T, Rudd N. An analysis of the validity of the Hospital Anxiety and Depression Scale as a screening tool in patients with advanced metastatic cancer. J Pain Symptom Manage 2001;22:990-996.
12. American Psychiatric Association: Diagnostic and Statistical Manual of Mental Disorders, 4th ed, text revision. Washington, DC: American Psychiatric Association, 2000.
13. Andrykowski MA, Manne SL. Are psychological interventions effective and accepted by cancer patients? I. Standards and levels of evidence. Ann Behav Med 2006;32:93-97.
14. Jackson KC, Lipman AG. Drug therapy for anxiety in palliative care. Cochrane Database Syst Rev (1):CD004596, 2004.
15. Breitbart WB, Jacobsen PB. Psychiatric symptom management in terminal care. Clin Geriatr Med 1996;12:329-347.
16. Gallagher LM, Lagman R, Walsh D, et al. The clinical effects of music therapy in palliative medicine. Support Care Cancer 2006;14:859-866.
17. Hadfield N. The role of aromatherapy massage in reducing anxiety in patients with malignant brain tumours. Int J Palliat Nurs 2001;7:279-285.
18. Holland JC, Morrow GR, Schmale A, et al. A randomized trial of alprazolam versus progressive muscle relaxation in cancer patients with anxiety and depressive symptoms. J Clin Oncol 1991;9:1004-1011.

CHAPTER **152**

Syncope and Blackouts

Diarmuid O'Shea and Graham Sutton

K E Y   P O I N T S

- The impact on daily life determines investigation and treatment of syncope and blackouts.

- A thorough history and physical examination helps to determine the cause.

- Simple measures, such as a medication review, rehydration, and other nonpharmacological interventions, may relieve symptoms.

- A 12-lead electrocardiogram, lying and standing blood pressures, 24-hour blood pressure, and 24-hour electrocardiogram may aid diagnosis, and conservative management reduces symptoms.

Dizziness, drowsiness, postural dizziness, and blackouts are common and often vague symptoms in everyday clinical practice. Syncope is defined as abrupt loss of consciousness associated with the loss of postural tone that may lead to a fall. The process of investigating and managing syncope in advanced disease may differ from that for someone without a terminal illness. Diagnosis and management are governed by the therapeutic goals set by the team in agreement with the patient.

Treatment is determined by the cause. No cause is found in up to 20%.[1] The key issue is how much the symptoms are affecting the patient's life. If the symptoms are causing distress, the patient and clinician must decide to what extent investigations should be carried out to identify a cause (Fig. 152-1) and, if a diagnosis is confirmed, what treatment is most appropriate (Fig. 152-2).

EPIDEMIOLOGY AND PATHOPHYSIOLOGY

The underlying causes of syncope can be divided into noncardiovascular and cardiovascular types (Table 152-1). Noncardiovascular causes include neurally mediated syncope (e.g., orthostatic hypotension, neurocardiogenic syncope, carotid hypersensitivity, and autonomic dysfunction) and seizures. Cardiovascular causes can be subdivided into arrhythmias and nonarrhythmic causes.

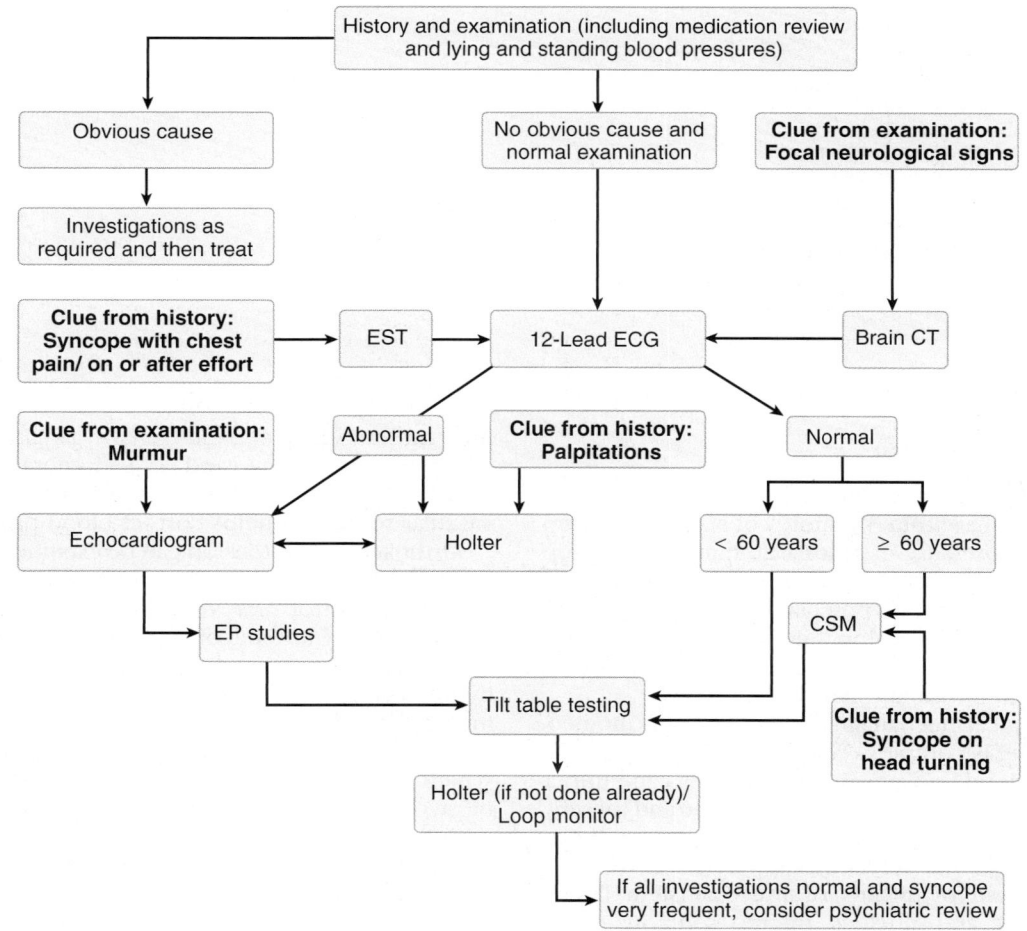

FIGURE 152-1   Guide to the history and investigation of syncope. If test results are normal, proceed to the next step. CSM, carotid sinus massage; CT, computed tomography; ECG, electrocardiogram; EP, electrophysiological testing; EST, exercise stress testing.

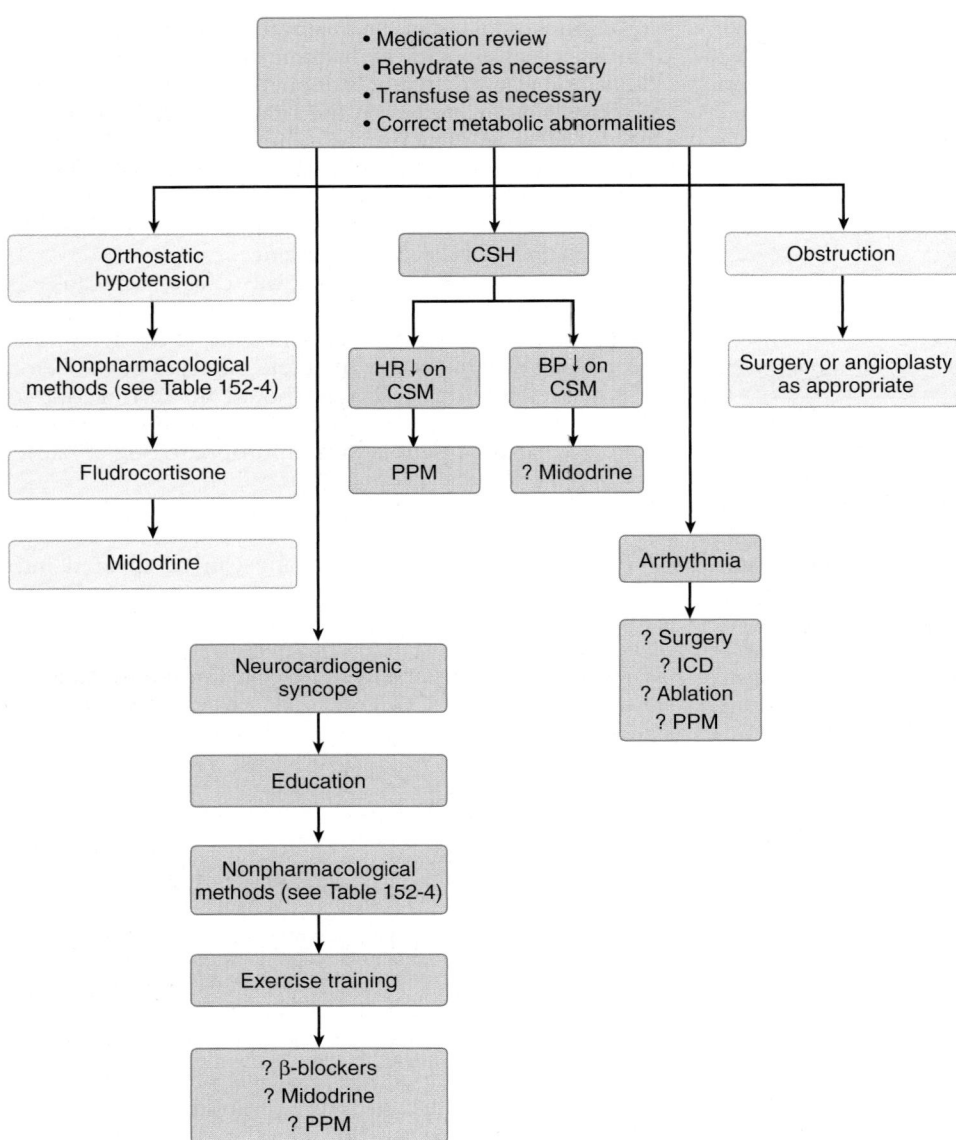

FIGURE 152-2 Guide to the treatment of syncope. BP, blood pressure; CSH, carotid sinus hypersensitivity; CSM, carotid sinus massage; HR, heart rate; ICD, implantable cardioverter-defibrillator; PPM, permanent pacemaker.

Orthostatic Hypotension

Orthostatic hypotension is defined by at least one of the following occurring within 3 minutes of standing: a drop in systolic blood pressure of at least 20 mm Hg or a drop in diastolic blood pressure of at least 10 mm Hg. The symptoms of orthostatic hypotension include dizziness, lightheadedness, blurred vision, and syncope. Symptoms are more likely in the morning and after meals, and they can be exacerbated by acute illness.

The physiological mechanism for hemodynamic homeostasis on standing is complex. When a person stands, 500 to 1000 mL of blood pools mainly in the pelvis and upper legs. This shift decreases central blood volume and thereby venous return and stroke volume. Baroreceptors and cardiopulmonary receptors detect this apparent loss of circulating volume, and by means of the brainstem lateral reticular nucleus and nucleus tractus solitarius, they increase sympathetic and decrease parasympathetic drive. Systemic vascular resistance is increased in the splanch-nic, musculoskeletal, and renal vascular beds by α_1-adrenergic receptors, and a β-adrenergic response increases heart rate. The increase in heart rate and systemic vascular resistance helps correct blood pressure.

Orthostatic hypotension can be classified by underlying cause as neurogenic or non-neurogenic (Table 152-2). Efforts to control or reverse the underlying illness may improve the symptoms of orthostatic hypotension.

Drugs are the main non-neurogenic cause of orthostatic hypotension (Table 152-3). Reducing or omitting offending medications may produce significant improvement. The α-blockers attenuate the α-adrenergic response, which increases vascular resistance and therefore should be avoided. The prevalence of orthostatic hypotension with the use of calcium antagonists ranges from 1% to 7%. The rate is low with thiazide diuretics and β-blockers, and some β-blockers with intrinsic sympathomimetic activity may improve orthostatic hypotension. Coadministration of loop diuretics with other antihypertensives increases orthostatic hypotension.[2,3]

TABLE 152-1 Classification and Clinical Features Suggesting a Specific Cause of Syncope

DIAGNOSTIC CONSIDERATION	SYMPTOM OR FINDING
NONCARDIOVASCULAR TYPE	
Carotid sinus syncope	Syncope with head rotation
Vasovagal syncope	After pain, unpleasant sight or sound
	Prolonged standing
	Athlete after exertion
Situational syncope	Micturition, cough, swallow, defecation
Orthostatic syncope	On standing
Postprandial syncope	After meals
Seizures	Witness fitting
Cerebrovascular disease	Associated with vertigo, dysarthria, diplopia or other motor and sensory symptoms of brain stem ischemia
Subclavian steal	Syncope with arm exercise
CARDIOVASCULAR TYPE	
Structural heart disease (aortic and mitral stenosis)	Syncope on exertion
Ischemic heart disease	

Modified from Kenny RA (ed). Syncope in the Older Patient: Causes, Investigations and Consequences of Syncope and Falls. London: Chapman & Hall Medical, 1996.

TABLE 152-2 Classification of Orthostatic Hypotension

NEUROGENIC CAUSES	NON-NEUROGENIC CAUSES
PRIMARY CAUSES	
Parkinsonian with autonomic failure	Volume depletion
Multiple system atrophy	Pump failure
Peripheral autonomic failure	Drugs (see Table 152-3)
	Mitral valve prolapse
	Electrolyte disturbance
SECONDARY CAUSES	
Stroke	
Brain tumor	
Multiple sclerosis	
Guillain-Barré syndrome	
Amyloidosis	
Motor neuron disease	
Diabetes	
Adrenal insufficiency	
Paraneoplastic	
Vitamin deficiencies (e.g., B_1, B_{12})	

TABLE 152-3 Drugs That May Cause Orthostatic Hypotension and Syncope

α-Adrenoceptor blockers	Antipsychotics
β-Blockers	Anti-parkinsonian agents
Calcium channel blockers	Antidepressants, especially tricyclics and MAOIs
Diuretics	Hypnotics
Nitrates	
ACE inhibitors (perhaps ARBs)	

ACE, angiotensin-converting enzyme; ARB, angiotensin receptor blocker; MAOI, monoamine oxidase inhibitor.

Neurocardiogenic Syncope

Neurocardiogenic syncope accounts for 20% to 35% of syncopal episodes.[1] Patients usually have a prodrome of diaphoresis, nausea, fatigue, and pallor. There may be a trigger, such as heat exposure or painful stimuli. Some types of neurocardiogenic syncope occur in specific circumstances (e.g., micturition, cough) because of autonomic nervous system changes.

A proposed mechanism for neurocardiogenic syncope is the Bezold-Jarisch reflex. The mechanoreceptors in the left ventricle and stretch receptors in the great veins are activated by increased pressure or volume. These activate C-fibers, which stimulate vagal afferent and efferent fibers, reducing heart rate and blood pressure and causing syncope. Vagal fibers can be activated by means of the carotid sinus reflex through carotid sinus and aortic arch baroreceptors. Central serotonergic pathways and adenosine have been linked to vasovagal syncope, but the mechanism is unclear.[4,5]

Carotid Sinus Hypersensitivity

The carotid sinus is at the bifurcation of the internal and external carotid arteries and has sensory endings in the sinus wall. Efferent fibers comprise sympathetic nerves to the heart, vasculature, and carotid vagus nerve. Carotid sinus hypersensitivity leads to exaggerated baroreceptor-mediated responses that cause hypotension or bradycardia, or both, with possible syncope. The location of the pathological lesion is unknown. Carotid sinus hypersensitivity accounts for about 1% of syncopal episodes. It is diagnosed by carotid sinus massage. Carotid sinus hypersensitivity is diagnosed if pressure there immediately leads to a pause of 3 seconds or more or a drop in systolic blood pressure of more than 50 mm Hg. Some medication, including β-blockers, rate-controlling calcium channel blockers, and digoxin, exacerbate this response. Withdrawal of the offending medication can resolve symptoms in up to 50% of patients.[6]

Seizures

Seizures are commonly considered as the possible cause of syncopal episodes because they can mimic syncope. The loss of cerebral blood flow from any cause of syncope can result in a seizure-like state. One distinguishing feature is that seizures rarely have an abrupt and complete recovery. The postictal state is also characterized by confusion and slow recovery. If there is evidence of tongue biting or many soft tissue injuries due to tonic-clonic movements, a seizure is more likely.

Arrhythmias

Arrhythmias account for approximately 15% of syncope cases.[7] An arrhythmia can occur without warning, although tachyarrhythmias may manifest with concurrent palpitations.

The most common arrhythmias include sinus bradycardia, atrioventricular (AV) nodal block, sustained ventricular tachycardia (VT), and supraventricular tachycardia (SVT). Syncope from sinus bradycardia may be caused by intrinsic sinus node disease (e.g., sick sinus syndrome, tachy-brady syndrome), drugs (e.g., β-blockers), or autonomic imbalance. The forms of AV nodal block that cause syncope are second- (type II) or third-degree AV block. Syncope from sustained VT most commonly results from structural heart disease, particularly coronary heart disease, but also is caused by dilated cardiomyopathy and right ventricular dysplasia. Torsades de pointes (a form of VT) may cause syncope in the congenital or acquired forms of the long QT syndrome. Supraventricular tachyarrhythmias, such as Wolff-Parkinson-White syndrome, have been associated with syncope.

Blood Flow Obstruction

Syncope may be caused by obstruction to blood flow because of an inability to produce a compensatory increase in cardiac output. The most common causes are aortic stenosis and hypertrophic cardiomyopathy. Less common conditions include pulmonary stenosis, idiopathic pulmonary hypertension, atrial myxomas, pulmonary embolism, and vascular steal syndromes.

CLINICAL MANIFESTATIONS

A thorough history of the patient's experiences surrounding the syncopal episodes and the medical history are essential. Information from an eyewitness can be invaluable. Clinical examination may provide clues to the diagnosis (see "Case Study: Managing Dizziness"). This should include a complete cardiovascular examination to look for structural heart disease, auscultation for carotid bruits, lying and standing blood pressures, and a neurological examination. Blood pressure should be measured after lying quietly for 5 minutes and then after 1 and 3 minutes of standing. Specific symptoms obtained from the history and the physical examination (see Fig. 152-1 and Table 152-1) guide the more appropriate diagnostic tests for the individual and include the following:

- Electrocardiogram (ECG)
- Lying and standing blood pressures
- 24-Hour ECG
- 24-Hour blood pressure
- Carotid sinus massage, supine and erect (only if negative supine)
- External loop recorder
- Electrophysiological studies
- Head-up tilt test
- Computed tomography of the head and electroencephalography if appropriate
- Implantable loop recorder

Because the first four of these tests are neither invasive nor associated with any risk, they may aid the diagnosis, conservative management, and amelioration of symptoms. They always are worth considering. The other studies have various risks and may be inappropriate for patients with advanced disease.

A 12-lead ECG should be performed, because up to 5% to 11% of patients have a diagnosis based on the results.[7] Those with a normal 12-lead ECG result (i.e., no QRS or rhythm disturbance) have a low likelihood of arrhythmia as a cause and are at low risk for sudden death.[8] If the ECG result is abnormal, a cardiac cause is more likely, and exercise stress testing, Holter monitoring, or electrophysiological testing can be pursued if appropriate. If the ECG result is normal, a neurally mediated cause is more likely, and tilt-table testing and carotid sinus massage should be considered.

TREATMENT

Management depends on the underlying cause (see Fig. 152-2). After review of a patient's medications for drugs that may contribute to syncope, rehydration, correction of any metabolic abnormality, and blood transfusion are appropriate first steps. Many medications are implicated (see Table 152-3), and stopping these should be considered.

Further management includes nonpharmacological (Table 152-4) and pharmacological treatments. Although

---

CASE STUDY

Managing Dizziness

PM, an 80-year-old man with known lung cancer, presented to the emergency department after a fall at home. He was on enalapril (10 mg daily), morphine sulfate (10 mg twice daily), aspirin (75 mg daily), atorvastatin (10 mg daily), and frusemide (40 mg daily). He had recently complained about increasing shortness of breath, worsening ankle swelling, and difficulty sleeping at night. His general practitioner had added bendrofluazide (2.5 mg daily) and nitrazepam (5 mg), to be taken at bedtime, to his drug regimen. Soon after this, he noticed lightheadedness and dizziness. These symptoms did not occur when he was lying or sitting, but he noticed them soon after he was walking around his home. Lying and standing blood pressures revealed a postural drop in his systolic blood pressure of 35 mm Hg. The electrocardiogram and blood test results were normal, and a diagnosis of orthostatic hypotension was made. After discussion with Mr. PM, the bendrofluazide was stopped, and nitrazepam was reduced to 2.5 mg, which provided some relief of his symptoms. His lightheadedness improved. He was reluctant to stop the nitrazepam completely because he had enjoyed better sleep since starting the drug.

TABLE 152-4 Nonpharmacological Management for Orthostatic Hypotension and Neurocardiogenic Syncope (Excluding Coffee or Black Liquorice)

Compression stockings	Physical countermaneuvers (e.g.,
Head up sleeping	upper leg crossing on standing,
Staged standing	gentle marching on the spot
Resting in morning and	instead of standing still)
postprandially	Black liquorice (3 g/day)
Increasing morning fluid intake by	Avoid excessive environmental
up to 2 L	temperatures
Increasing salt intake if possible	
Coffee (1 or 2 cups) after meals	

other medications have been studied, fludrocortisone and midodrine have accrued the best evidence for efficacy.

Fludrocortisone is the first-line pharmacological treatment, and it promotes a positive response in 40% to 75% of patients.[9] It has central adrenergic effects and increases arteriolar sensitivity to catecholamines and angiotensin. The starting dose is 50 μg once daily, which is increased by 25 to 50 μg every 1 to 2 weeks to alleviate symptoms without incurring side effects. Side effects include hypertension, edema, hypokalemia, depression, and headache. Electrolyte levels should be checked 1 week after starting fludrocortisone and a week after a dose change.

Midodrine, a peripheral adrenergic agonist, is second-line therapy. It can be fludrocortisone sparing when used with the mineralocorticosteroid. Side effects include scalp pruritus, tingling, and urinary urgency.

Treatment of neurocardiogenic syncope is aimed at avoiding precipitants. Education about possible presyncopal symptoms can help avert a syncopal episode by assuming a seated or supine position when possible. Exercise and tilt training have been suggested (see Table 152-4). Evidence to support medications in treating vasovagal syncope is limited. β-Blockers have been used because they were thought to be effective by decreasing mechanoreceptor activation and blocking epinephrine effects, but trials have not shown benefit over placebo. Midodrine studies have been too small or too short to show sustained benefit.[10] Although there may be a significant bradycardic response in vasovagal syncope, there is uncertainty about the role of pacemakers because of the associated vasodepressor response also found in this disorder.[11]

Treatment of carotid sinus hypersensitivity is guided by the results of the carotid sinus massage. If there is a cardioinhibitory response of more than 3 seconds with symptom reproduction and a contributory offending medication cannot be stopped, there is a role for a permanent pacemaker.[12] Although this may not prevent presyncopal symptoms, it should avert full syncope. Management of vasodepressor carotid sinus hypersensitivity is more challenging. Midodrine has been suggested by the results of one study,[13] but further research is required.

The type of arrhythmia dictates management if an arrhythmia is the cause. Treatment options for documented or inducible VTs include an implantable cardioverter-defibrillator, radiofrequency ablation, and electrophysiologically guided surgery. Although supraventricular arrhythmias can be treated with antiarrhythmic drugs, radiofrequency ablation is preferred for most. Permanent atrial or dual-chamber pacemaker implantation is indicated when sinus node dysfunction or a high-grade AV block is the cause.

Blood flow obstruction, including vascular steal syndromes, usually requires invasive or surgical correction. It can be difficult to treat.

DEVELOPMENTS AND RESEARCH OPPORTUNITIES

Implanted loop recorders seem most cost-effective for monitoring and detecting arrhythmias. The decision to consider this approach in treating advanced disease depends on discussions with the patient, palliative care team, and cardiologist.

Mobile output cardiac telemetry can help detect arrhythmias. It uses an external device that monitors the heart, and the information is available to the clinician through computer telemetry.

Combined noninvasive ambulatory ECG and hemodynamic monitoring is not available but may be soon. Impedance threshold devices (ITDs) increase intrathoracic pressure, which increases venous return. ITDs can be used in patients with severe autonomic dysfunction that causes syncope, and they may ameliorate symptoms when other conservative measures have failed.

REFERENCES

1. Soteriades ES, Evans JC, Larson MG, et al. Incidence and prognosis of syncope. N Engl J Med 2002;347: 78-88.
2. Fotherby MD, Potter JF. Orthostatic hypotension and antihypertensive therapy in the elderly. Postgrad Med J 1994;70:878-881.
3. Hajjar I. Postural blood pressure changes and orthostatic hypotension in the elderly patient. Impact of antihypertensive medications. Drugs Aging 2005; 22:56-68.
4. Grubb BP, Karas BJ: The potential role of serotonin in the pathogenesis of neurocardiogenic syncope and related autonomic disturbances. J Interv Card Electrophysiol 1998;2:325-332.
5. Sinkovec M, Grad A, Rakovec P. Role of endogenous adenosine in vasovagal syncope. Clin Auton Res 2001;11:155-161.
6. Mulcahy R, Allcock LA, O'Shea D. Timolol, carotid sinus hypersensitivity and the elderly. Lancet 1998;352:1147-1148.
7. Linzer M, Yang EH, Estes NA 3rd, et al. Diagnosing syncope. Part 1. Value of history, physical examination, and electrocardiography. Clinical Efficacy Assessment Project of the American College of Physicians. Ann Intern Med 1997;126:989-996.
8. Brignole M, Alboni P, Benditt D, et al. Guidelines on management (diagnosis and treatment) of syncope. Euro Heart J 2001;22:1256-1306.
9. Hussain RM, McIntosh SJ, Lawson J, et al. Fludrocortisone in the treatment of hypotensive disorders in the elderly. Heart 1996;76:507-509.
10. Perez-Lugones A, Schweikert R, Pavia S, et al. Usefulness of midodrine in patients with severely symptomatic neurocardiogenic syncope: a randomized control study. J Cardiovasc Electrophysiol 2001;12:935-938.
11. Kosinski DJ, Grubb BP, Wolfe DA: Permanent cardiac pacing as primary therapy for neurocardiogenic (reflex) syncope. Clin Auton Res 2004;14(Suppl 1):76-79.
12. Gregoratos G, Abrams J, Epstein AE, et al. ACC/AHA/NASPE 2002 guideline update for implantation of cardiac pacemakers and antiarrhythmia devices: summary article: A report of the American College of Cardiology/American Heart Association Task Force on Practice Guidelines (ACC/AHA/NASPE Committee to Update the 1998 Pacemaker Guidelines). Circulation 2002;106:2145-2161.
13. Moore A, Watts M, Sheehy T, et al. Treatment of vasodepressor carotid sinus syndrome with midodrine: A randomized, controlled pilot study. J Am Geriatr Soc. 2005;53:114-118.

SUGGESTED READING

Benditt DG, Blanc JJ, Brignole M, Sutton R (eds). The Evaluation and Treatment of Syncope: A Handbook for Clinical Practice. London: Blackwell Publishing, 2003.

Fall and syncope in the elderly. Clin Geriatr Med 2002;18:(2).

Kenny RA (ed). Syncope in the Older Patient: Causes, Investigations and Consequences of Syncope and Falls. New York: Chapman & Hall Medical, 1996.

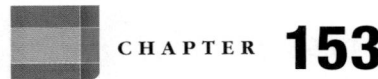

CHAPTER **153**

Airway Obstruction

Bruce H. Chamberlain

> **KEY POINTS**
>
> - Wheezing, rhonchi, and stridor are clinical observations that suggest airway obstruction.
> - Airway obstructions may be classed as reversible, resulting from bronchospasm, or fixed, resulting from destruction of lung tissue (i.e., chronic obstructive pulmonary disease) or airway impingement by a mass, scarring, or foreign bodies.
> - Treatment is based on reversing bronchospasm, reducing airway inflammation, removing or shrinking the cause of the obstruction, and managing dyspnea, cough, and anxiety.
> - Corticosteroids are the treatment of choice for airway inflammation.
> - The β_2-agonists and anticholinergics are the treatments of choice for bronchospasm.

Obstruction of the airways can occur for reasons ranging from reactive airway disease (i.e., asthma) to mechanical compression from a growing mass. Obstruction usually can be divided into two categories: reversible and fixed. Combinations of conditions may also occur because reactive and chronic obstructive airway diseases often coexist. Either or both may also be present in advanced cancer or nonmalignant causes of airway obstruction. Any obstruction to the smooth flow of air from mouth or nose to the bronchiole can cause dyspnea, cough, and anxiety and signs or physical findings such as wheezing, rhonchi, or stridor. Airway obstruction may be caused or complicated by bronchospasm and inflammation.

Treatment is based on reducing the primary obstruction, reversing bronchospasm, and treating the associated inflammation. Aggressive management of cough, dyspnea, and anxiety is discussed in other chapters (see Chapters 151, 155, and 159).

DEFINITIONS

Wheeze is a continuous, whistling or musical sound during breathing that is caused by a narrowing or obstruction somewhere in the airway. The location and timing of the wheeze may suggest the underlying cause.

Rhonchi is a term often used interchangeably with wheeze. Some reserve rhonchi to describe a coarse, lower-pitched sound rather than a more musical wheeze.

Stridor is a specific type of wheeze characterized by high-pitched, noisy breathing that indicates an airway obstruction that is usually in the trachea or larynx. Stridor that occurs only during inspiration suggests that the obstruction is in the larynx. When it occurs during both phases of breathing, it is usually in the trachea, and when it occurs only during expiration, obstruction is usually lower in the tracheal-bronchial tree.

PATHOPHYSIOLOGY AND EPIDEMIOLOGY

Wheezing and related sounds result from air moving through an airway that has become abruptly narrower. This mechanism resembles the way sound is produced by whistling or playing a wind instrument. When the obstruction is mild to moderate the airway narrowing may cause signs of wheezing; when more advanced, the obstruction may limit airflow to the degree that wheezing or other airway sounds do not occur. An obstruction that is sufficiently severe and proximal enough to severely compromise lung ventilation may result in death by suffocation.

Reversible airway obstruction is usually seen in reactive airway disease, which may be a primary condition. In palliative care, it is more often co-morbid with chronic obstructive pulmonary disease (COPD) or other lung pathology, adding a reversible component to a baseline fixed airway obstruction. In the elderly, COPD represents the most common cause of fixed airway obstruction. This is considered a disease of the lung itself or a peripheral obstruction instead of a tracheal-bronchial or central obstruction, which usually results from a mass or foreign body. In the palliative care setting, a central airway obstruction (CAO) is most often caused by tumor impingement on the airways. Tumors that originate in the trachea are unusual (600 to 700/year); however, primary lung cancer is common, and an estimated 20% to 30% develop complications of airway obstruction.[1] Nonbronchogenic cancers may also cause obstruction from direct tumor extension from cancers in adjacent tissues. Examples include esophageal and thyroid cancers and metastatic disease, most commonly renal cell, breast, and thyroid cancers. The leading nonmalignant causes of CAO are lymphadenopathy, granulation tissue, foreign bodies, and tracheal-bronchial tree scarring (Figs. 153-1 and 153-4; see "Case Study: Managing Airway Obstruction").

CLINICAL MANIFESTATIONS

The initial symptom of a CAO usually is cough from irritation of the airway, although dyspnea or hemoptysis may also be presenting symptoms. Postobstructive pneumonia may also be the initial presentation of a CAO. Wheezing and dyspnea that do not respond to aggressive management with β_2-agonists should prompt evaluation for a fixed airway obstruction. Although most obstructive processes are gradual in onset, acute events such as aspiration or sudden hemorrhage into a tumor may precipitate acute obstructive symptoms.

DIFFERENTIAL DIAGNOSIS

There are many possible causes for an airway obstruction. Some of the more common and their mechanisms are listed in Table 153-1.

TREATMENT

Treatment options vary with the underlying cause of the obstruction. An overview of available interventions based on the underlying disease is provided in Table 153-2.

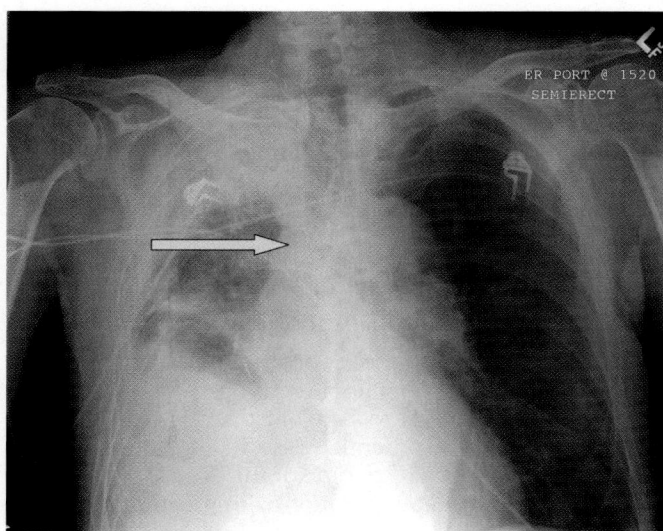

FIGURE 153-1 Patient with tumor mass causing obstruction of right main stem bronchus. The *arrow* indicates loss of the air shadow below the carina on the right. *(Courtesy of T. J. Blair, MD, PhD, Central Utah Multispecialty Clinic, Provo, UT.)*

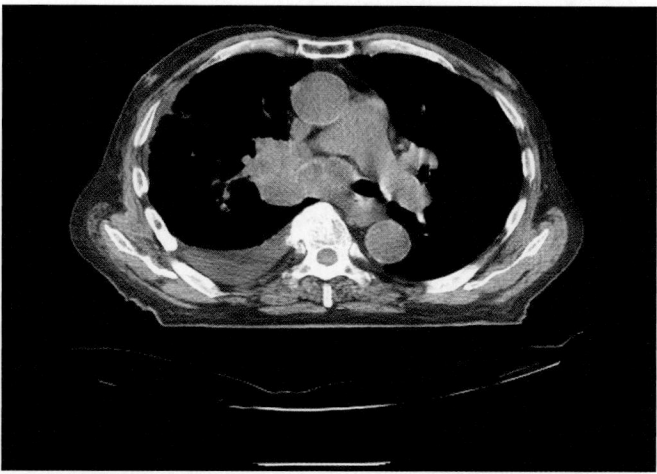

FIGURE 153-4 Computed tomography of the same patient as Figure 153-1 demonstrates complete obstruction of the right main stem bronchus by the tumor mass. *(Courtesy of T. J. Blair, MD, PhD, Central Utah Multispecialty Clinic, Provo, UT.)*

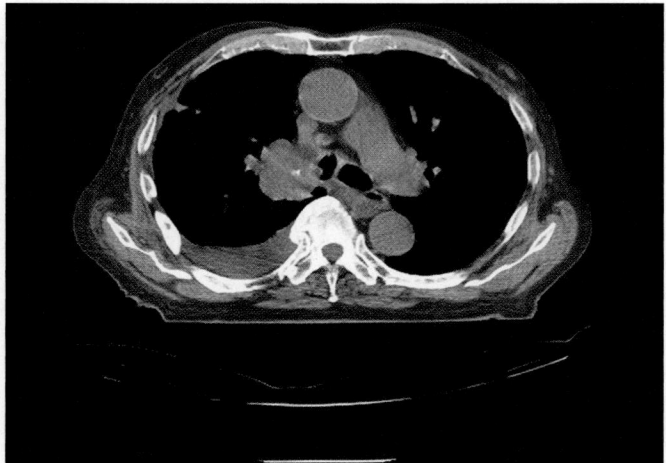

FIGURE 153-2 Computed tomography of the same patient as Figure 153-1 shows narrowing of the right main stem bronchus just below the carina. *(Courtesy of T. J. Blair, MD, PhD, Central Utah Multispecialty Clinic, Provo, UT.)*

TABLE 153-1 Causes and Mechanisms of Airway Obstruction	
CAUSE	**MECHANISM**
Asthma and allergy	Spasm of the muscles around the airways combined with inflammation of the airway
Chronic bronchitis	Excess mucus production
Chronic obstructive pulmonary disease	Loss of elastic tissue at the level of the bronchiole, allowing collapse of the airways during expiration
Foreign body	Mechanical obstruction
Tumor	Intrinsic obstruction by a tumor within the airway or extrinsic compression of the airway, resulting in a mechanical obstruction
Infection	Excess mucus production and airway inflammation
Mediastinal mass	Tumor, lymphadenopathy, blood, infection or abscess, or aortic aneurysm that compresses the airway, resulting in mechanical obstruction
Vocal cord dysfunction	Nerve damage (recurrent laryngeal) from tumor, surgery, or radiation therapy, resulting in a paralyzed vocal cord

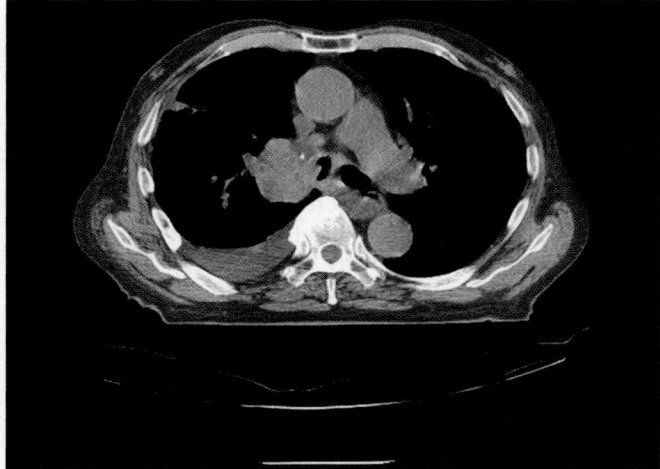

FIGURE 153-3 Computed tomography of the same patient as Figure 153-1 demonstrates further compression of the bronchus by the tumor mass. *(Courtesy of T. J. Blair, MD, PhD, Central Utah Multispecialty Clinic, Provo, UT.)*

Reversible Airway Obstruction

With reactive airway disease, the obstruction results from a combination of smooth muscle spasm and airway inflammation. The treatments of choice are bronchodilators for the muscle spasm and corticosteroids for the inflammation.

Three main classes of drugs are used for bronchodilation:

1. β_2-Adrenergic stimulants
2. Anticholinergics
3. Methylxanthines

Methylxanthine drugs (i.e., theophylines) have fallen out of favor as first-line therapy for several reasons, includ-

■■ **CASE STUDY**

Managing Airway Obstruction

RC is an 83-year-old man diagnosed with a large cell lung cancer 6 years ago. He underwent resection of two lobes of his right lung with curative intent, but the cancer recurred 4 years later with upper airway involvement. He underwent unsuccessful radiation treatment and subsequently chose palliative care rather than more aggressive, invasive interventions.

On presentation, he has severe anorexia, with a 50-lb weight loss since his diagnosis. He is constantly short of breath, which is much worse with any exertion. His voice sounds hoarse, and he has frequent cough and throat clearing, which is often productive of yellow-brown mucus but no blood. He has no significant pain. On examination, he has an audible wheeze in the inspiratory and expiratory phases of breathing. It is heard throughout the lung fields but most prominently detected in the neck. There is palpable, nontender fullness of the right anterior aspect of the neck consistent with the reported location of his tumor.

RC was started on methylprednisolone on a dose escalated to 8 mg twice each day, which provided initial improvement of his obstructive symptoms. Anxiety was managed with lorazepam (2 mg every 4 hours as needed), and pain was well managed with methadone (5 mg twice daily). He did well for 2 months but then developed an abrupt exacerbation of his symptoms, particularly swallowing difficulty, dyspnea, and agitation. He was placed on a subcutaneous morphine infusion and died comfortably 3 days later.

ing their side effects, potential for severe toxicity due to a low therapeutic index, need to monitor blood levels, and availability of safer and more effective drugs.

Anticholinergic drugs offer little to a maintenance regimen of maximal β_2-agonist therapy. However, they may have some additive effect in treating an acute exacerbation.

β_2-Agonists are the bronchodilator of first choice for managing reactive airway disease. Racemic albuterol has been the most commonly used short-acting β_2-agonist. Levalbuterol has prompted debate because of its significant cost compared with data that suggest it may be more effective and have fewer side effects than other drugs.[2] The cost-benefit ratio has been extensively discussed, but no consensus has been reached.

Corticosteroids are well-established therapy for reactive airway disease, although the mechanism by which they work is not clearly understood. They should be given as early as possible during an acute exacerbation because the effect is often delayed for up to 12 hours. Despite this delay in onset, steroids given orally or intravenously reduce the need for hospital admission during an acute exacerbation.[3]

The corticosteroids of choice are hydrocortisone, methylprednisolone, and prednisone, which is metabolized to methylprednisolone in the liver. There are various dosing protocols (e.g., 200 mg of hydrocortisone IV every 6 hours, 40 to 60 mg of methylprednisolone IV every 6 to 8 hours, 40 to 60 mg of prednisone PO every 6 to 8 hours), but the optimal dose, schedule, and duration of therapy are unclear. Treatment of an acute exacerbation, even with high doses, for less than 3 weeks does not cause adrenal suppression.

Chronic Obstructive Pulmonary Disease

Unlike the reversible airway obstruction of asthma, the fixed or partially reversible airway obstruction of stable COPD rarely responds to β_2-agonist[4] or systemic steroid therapy.[5] There are potential risks to high-dose therapy using β_2-agonists, because some of the drug is systemically absorbed and causes vasodilation with greater pulmonary ventilation-perfusion mismatch and decreased oxygen saturations.[6] Although these drugs are first-line treatment in an acute exacerbation because of their rapid onset of action, their limited efficacy and potential risks make addition of other agents necessary.

Quaternary anticholinergic agents, ipratropium and the longer-acting tiotropium, have a slower onset than β_2-agonists but produce significantly more bronchodilation, with little systemic absorption and therefore fewer side effects.[7]

Maintenance therapy with inhaled corticosteroids demonstrates no significant effect on the progressive decline in pulmonary function in COPD. Treatment does improve symptoms, reduces exacerbations, and reduces the use of health services.[8]

The recommended treatment for acute exacerbation of COPD includes antibiotics for 7 to 10 days and bronchodilators, beginning with a short-acting β_2-agonist followed by an anticholinergic agent. For a severe exacerbation, corticosteroids should be considered. They are particularly indicated if the patient is currently using a steroid (oral or inhaled), has recently completed a course of steroids, has a history of responding to steroids, or is not responding to aggressive bronchodilators.

Central Airway Obstructions

Noninvasive treatments for fixed CAO are primarily symptomatic. Airway obstructions from encroaching tumors often cause local inflammation with tissue swelling and mucus production that can result in a functional obstruction greater than the anatomical blockage. Moderate- to high-dose systemic steroids (e.g., 8 to 12 mg of dexamethasone per day with a rapid taper) to treat inflammation and mucolytics such as oral guaifenesin or normal saline by nebulizer may help.

Treatments directed at dyspnea (see Chapters 151 and 159) and anxiety are also indicated. For acute symptoms at the end of life, therapeutic sedation may offer comfort if other treatments fail or are ineffective.

Invasive or more aggressive options are available for those willing and able to tolerate the procedures. Most can be performed with a bronchoscope. For endobronchial masses, options include dilation and coring, laser

TABLE 153-2   Treatment Options for Airway Obstruction

OBSTRUCTION	INTERVENTION	EXAMPLES	COMMENTS
Reversible	β_2-Agonists	Albuterol Metaproterenol Terbutaline Formoterol Pirbuterol Salmeterol	Use a long-acting drug for maintenance and a short-acting drug for as-needed use and acute exacerbations
		Levalbuterol	More expensive but possibly fewer side effects
	Anticholinergics	Ipratropium Tiotropium	Useful in adjunct with β_2-agonist in acute exacerbations
	Methylxanthines	Theophylline	Rarely used
	Steroids, systemic	Hydrocortisone Methylprednisolone Prednisone	Primarily for acute exacerbations
	Steroids, inhaled	Fluticasone Flunisolide Mometasone Triamcinolone Budesonide Beclomethasone	Primarily for stable disease
Peripheral Fixed	β_2-Agonists	Albuterol Metaproterenol Terbutaline Formoterol Pirbuterol Salmeterol	Less effective in chronic obstructive pulmonary disease than in asthma; high doses may worsen hypoxemia
	Anticholinergics	Ipratropium Tiotropium	Effective as first-line drugs
	Steroids	Hydrocortisone Methylprednisolone Prednisone Fluticasone Flunisolide Mometasone Triamcinolone Budesonide Beclomethasone	May be helpful in an acute exacerbation under certain circumstances
Central Fixed	Invasive-Interventional	Dilation and coring Cryotherapy Electrocautery Photodynamic therapy, brachytherapy Argon plasma coagulation Laser photoresection Stenting	Higher risk but more potential for extended symptom relief
	Noninvasive, interventional	External beam radiation	
	Steroids		Reduce the swelling and inflammation associated with the obstruction
	Mucolytics	Guaifenesin Saline nebulizer treatments	Thins mucus that may be contributing to the functional obstruction

photoresection, cryotherapy, electrocautery, photodynamic therapy, brachytherapy, argon plasma coagulation, and external beam radiation. For submucosal or extrinsic masses, the options include dilation, brachytherapy, and external beam radiation.[9] Airway stents may be placed separately or in combination with several of the previously described methods.

Means of Drug Administration

Most drugs for airway obstruction may be administered by several routes. Options include metered dose inhalers (MDIs), nebulizer treatments, and oral and intravenous administration.

The MDI is the most familiar. It administers medication in an aerosol or dry powder form. This can be very effective for delivering medication, but in the geriatric and palliative care patient populations, it may be limited by the inability to correctly coordinate and administer the treatment. The use of spacers and breath-actuated inhalers can be helpful. When properly used, an MDI with a spacer is as effective as a nebulizer.[10]

Nebulizers have several possible advantages in palliative care:

1. They can be effectively used in patients too weak or otherwise unable to correctly use an MDI.
2. The machine, noise, and tubing suggest aggressive medical intervention.

3. A nebulizer can administer several other medications, such as local anesthetics for persistent cough, opiates for dyspnea (controversial but still common), and normal saline to mobilize viscous secretions.

Oral and intravenous routes are infrequently used with bronchodilators because of the risk of systemic side effects and no evidence of improved efficacy. Intravenous therapy is primarily limited to moderate- to high-dose steroids given to a patient with an acute exacerbation of symptoms.

RESEARCH OPPORTUNITIES

More information is needed on the cost and efficacy of levalbuterol compared with albuterol as first-line β_2-agonist therapy. Further research is required to determine the optimal steroid dosing protocol for acute exacerbations of obstructive symptoms and to explore the use of nebulized opioids for dyspnea and anxiety associated with obstructive disease.

REFERENCES

1. Ayers ML, Beamis JR Jr. Rigid bronchoscopy in the twenty-first century. Clin Chest Med 2001;22:355-364.
2. Truitt T, Witko J, Halpern M. Levalbuterol compared to racemic albuterol: Efficacy and outcomes in patients hospitalized with COPD or asthma. Chest 2003;123,128-135.
3. Rowe BH, Spooner C, Ducharme FM, et al. Early emergency department treatment of acute asthma with systemic corticosteroids. Cochrane Database Syst Rev 2001;(1):CD002178.
4. Braun SR, McKenzie WN, Copeland C, et al. A comparison of the effect of ipratropium and albuterol in the treatment of chronic obstructive airway disease. Arch Intern Med 1989;149:544-547.
5. Callahan CM, Dittus RS, Katz BP. Oral corticosteroid therapy for patients with stable chronic obstructive pulmonary disease: A meta-analysis. Ann Intern Med 1991;114:216-223.
6. Gross NJ, Bankwala Z: Effects of an anticholinergic bronchodilator on arterial blood gases of hypoxemic patients with chronic obstructive pulmonary disease. Comparison with beta-adrenergic agent. Am Rev Respir Dis 1987;136:1091-1094.
7. Gross NJ. Ipratropium bromide. N Engl J Med 1988; 319:486-494.
8. Alsaeedi A, Sin DD, McAlister FA. The effects of inhaled corticosteroids in chronic obstructive pulmonary disease: A systematic review of randomized placebo-controlled trials. Am J Med 2002:113:59-65.
9. Ernst A, Feller-Kopman D, Becker HD, et al. Central airway obstruction. Am J Respir Crit Care Med 2004;169:1278-1297.
10. Turner MO, Patel A, Ginsburg S, et al. Bronchodilator delivery in acute airflow obstruction: A meta-analysis. Arch Intern Med 1997; 157:1736-1744.

SUGGESTED READING

Ernst A, Feller-Kopman D, Becker HD, et al. State of the art: Central airway obstruction. Am J Respir Crit Care Med 2004;169:1278-1297.

Ernst A, Silvestri GA, Johnstone D. Interventional pulmonary procedures: Guidelines from the American College of Chest Physicians. Chest 2003;123:1693-1717.

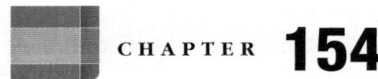

CHAPTER 154

Constipation and Diarrhea

Nigel P. Sykes

KEY POINTS

- Most ill people become constipated, and most patients on opioid analgesia require laxatives.
- Prophylactic measures are used when possible. Clinicians should anticipate the need for laxatives before constipation is established.
- Monitor the effectiveness of laxatives.
- Diarrhea is much less common in palliative medicine patients than constipation.
- Laxatives are the most common cause of diarrhea in patients receiving palliative care.
- Clinicians should look for causes that have specific treatments.
- Opioids are the most effective general oral treatment, and somatostatin analogues have a role in severe diarrhea.

CONSTIPATION

Constipation is an unglamorous symptom, but it is common and uncomfortable. About 10% of healthy individuals have constipation, and the likelihood increases with age and female gender.[1,2] Illness makes constipation worse. Hospitalized elderly people are almost three times more likely to be constipated than the same age group living at home.[3] Constipation is more common in people terminally ill with cancer than those dying of other causes.[4] About 50% of patients complain about constipation when admitted to British hospices, where it rivals or exceeds pain as a cause of distress.

Diarrhea is reported by 7% to 10% of cancer patients on admission to a hospice and 6% of similar patients in the hospital; it is far less common than constipation. Services looking after symptomatic human immunodeficiency virus (HIV)–infected patients deal with it much more frequently, for which a prevalence of 27% has been reported.[5]

Basic Science

What do we mean by *constipation*? When constipation occurs with another illness, it is a symptom, not a disease or a sign. Constipation can be defined objectively as the passage of stool infrequently or with difficulty. Individuals differ in the subjective weight they give to the components of the definition or add elements of their own.

Epidemiological studies reveal that 95%[6] of a healthy population defecate at least three times per week. These findings informed the Rome criteria,[7] which are often used in gastroenterology to define constipation (Box 154-1).

People have their own definitions of what it means to be constipated. These descriptions tend to contain the components of the Rome criteria. In my hospice unit, 85% of patients cited difficulty passing stool as a symptom of constipation and 69% mentioned reduced defecation frequency, but 45% also mentioned flatulence and abdominal bloating. There was no sense of a minimum time for these symptoms to persist.

The Rome criteria were intended to clarify the diagnosis of functional constipation in an essentially healthy population. When constipation accompanies terminal illness, the time requirement becomes less appropriate. As with other symptoms encountered in palliative medicine, constipation is primarily to be believed and relieved rather than defined.

Constipation arises from a disturbance of the rate at which food residues pass through the intestines and the balance of fluid absorption from and secretion into the gut. This prolongs the transit time from the mouth to anus and produces drier, harder bowel movements.

Intestinal Transit

Gut contents spend 2 to 4 hours in the small bowel and 24 to 48 hours in the colon. Transit may be much slower than this; almost one half of a hospice population had transit times of 4 to 12 days.[8] The small intestine responds to the pH, osmolarity, and chemical composition of the luminal contents with two patterns of activity that affect the speed of gastric emptying. The interdigestive pattern contains the migrating motor complex, in which intense rhythmic contractions of circular muscle periodically proceed distally along the gut to clear the lumen and reduce bacterial growth. Soon after eating, that pattern is replaced by the fed pattern, with ongoing contractile activity. About one half of these contractions propagate distally, so that this pattern mixes and propels the small intestinal contents.

The large bowel also displays two main types of motility but has no regular motor patterns such as the migrating motor complex. Most colonic contractile activity is segmental. This consists of irregular waves of contraction to mix the luminal contents, facilitating absorption of water and nutrients while moving the residue toward the rectum.

Less common is propagated colonic activity, which has two variants distinguished by contraction amplitude. The low-amplitude variety occurs more than 100 times per day and is associated with gut distention and passage of flatus. The high-amplitude type occurs about six times per day and corresponds to mass movements, in which large quantities of intestinal contents are propelled distally over significant distances. High-amplitude contractions are one of the major initiators of defecation.

Fluid Handling

Intestinal fluid handling is the net result of a dynamic state of absorption and secretion in the gut. About 7 L of fluid are secreted into the gut each day, to which are added at least 1.5 L of dietary fluid. Most is reabsorbed by the small bowel, especially the jejunum, but more than a liter enters the colon. Because daily stool water content is about 200 mL and the difference between constipation and diarrhea in terms of fluid excretion is about 100 mL per day, the fine tuning of fluid absorption by the colon is important in maintaining a convenient bowel habit.

Most secretion occurs as an active process from the mucosal crypt cells, whereas absorption takes place in the villous cells. Through the enteric nervous system, mechanical stimulation of mucosal sensory neurons activates secretion and stimulates blood flow and smooth muscle contraction. 5-Hydroxytryptamine, substance P, and neurokinins 1 and 2 are involved in the sensory side of the secretion reflex, and vasoactive intestinal peptide (VIP) is the secretomotor neurotransmitter. The physiological importance of this linkage is better digestion through greater mixing and dilution of luminal contents and more absorption that accompanies increased motility.

Epidemiology and Prevalence

If the prevalence of constipation is considered in palliative care, there is evidence that 61% to 63% of patients who do not take opioid analgesia require a laxative, but this rate rises to 83% to 87% if opioids are involved.[9] Because opioids are frequently used, it is not surprising that 78% of 260 palliative care inpatients were receiving a regular laxative.[10] Among 200 patients followed for 6 weeks or until death, 75% required rectal interventions (i.e., suppository, enema, or manual evacuation) during the first week after admission, and 40% continued to do so in subsequent weeks despite more laxative prescriptions.

Pathophysiology

The origins of constipation in a palliative care population are multifactorial (Box 154-2). With the exception of opioid analgesia, which is probably the most important single influence, the interplay of the different components is hard to unravel. Gut physiology indicates that three important consequences of severe illness—reduced food intake, reduced fluid intake, and reduced physical activity—likely precipitate or exacerbate constipation, and it therefore is not surprising to find frequent constipation in ill patients, even when they are not taking opioids.

The relatively infrequent mass movements of intestinal contents associated with onset of defecation occur with eating and bodily activity. It is likely that reduced appetite, through a weaker stimulus to the gastrocolic reflex, reduces high-amplitude propagated peristaltic activity. Similarly, the mass movements with the start of the daily

Box 154-2 Causes of Constipation in Medical Patients

Debilitation-Related Effects

Inadequate food intake
Low fiber diet
Weakness
Inactivity
Dehydration
Confusion
Depression
Unfamiliar toilet arrangements

Drugs

Opioids
Drugs with anticholinergic activity
    Hyoscine, glycopyrrolate
    Phenothiazines
    Tricyclic antidepressants
    Antiparkinsonian agents (particularly antimuscarinics, bro-
    mocriptine, and cabergoline)
Antacids (calcium and aluminum compounds)
Diuretics (if dehydration occurs)
Anticonvulsants (may also cause diarrhea)
Iron preparations (may also cause diarrhea)
Antihypertensive agents (particularly β-blockers, calcium channel
    blockers; angiotensin-converting enzyme inhibitors can cause
    constipation or diarrhea)
Vinca alkaloids

Malignancy

Intestinal obstruction
    Bowel wall tumor
    External compression
Damage to intrinsic or extrinsic innervation of the bowel
Hypercalcemia

Concurrent Disease

Diabetes
Hypothyroidism
Hypokalemia
Hernia
Diverticular disease
Irritable bowel syndrome
Distortion of rectal anatomy
Anorectal pain (e.g., fissure)
Colitis

Acetylcholine is the neurotransmitter for the final common pathway in the coordination of peristaltic activity, and any drugs with anticholinergic properties impair intestinal transit. However, opioids have the strongest constipating effect because of their action at endogenous opioid receptors in the gut wall. Morphine and its relatives increase sphincter tone at all gut levels from the esophagus to the anus and diminish high-amplitude propagated colonic contractions. Active fluid secretion is diminished, and fluid absorption is increased, partly because of the greater opportunity from slower transit. Rectal sensitivity is diminished, which in older patients combines with the reduced sensitivity that occurs with age and may precipitate fecal impaction. Through these many mechanisms, opioids have a marked constipating effect that is dose related (although with such scatter that the response to any dose varies greatly between individuals)[12] and to which there is little development of tolerance. Other than for transdermal fentanyl, which is somewhat less constipating,[13] there is no evidence for a difference between opioids in their constipating effects.

Clinical Manifestations

Constipation may manifest as nausea, abdominal pain, or urinary incontinence. When combined with overflow, it can masquerade as diarrhea and can mimic intestinal obstruction. A full history, abdominal examination, and unless there has been a recent full evacuation, rectal examination can avoid errors (see "Case Study: Constipation and Malignant Intestinal Obstruction" and "Case Study: Constipation and Co-morbid Disease").

Some patients rapidly experience *nausea*, with or without vomiting, in the presence of intestinal delay. Unexplained nausea or vomiting should prompt questioning and examination for constipation.

The effort of colonic muscle to propel hard feces often causes colicky *abdominal pain*. History and examination usually suggest the cause of the pain, but constipation is still sometimes treated with morphine. Such pain may be particularly marked and difficult to diagnose if abdominal or pelvic tumor coexist, perhaps because of pressure on the tumor from distended gut or partial intestinal obstruction.

Abdominal palpation may reveal fecal masses in the line of the colon, but the distinction between tumor and fecal masses can be difficult. Feces often indent if the patient can tolerate the necessary pressure and may give a crepitus-like sensation because of entrained gas. They also move, given time. An abdominal radiograph can differentiate tumor from stool (Fig. 154-1).

Fecal *impaction* is well recognized as a precipitant of *urinary incontinence* in the elderly. Recent onset of urinary incontinence should prompt abdominal and rectal examination. Impaction manifesting as diarrhea and often with incontinence occurs characteristically in the elderly, in whom inattention to the need to defecate, confusion, or rectal insensitivity leads to a large fecal mass that is impossible to pass spontaneously. Fecal material higher in the colon is broken down into semi-liquid form by bacterial action and seeps past the mass, appearing as diarrhea, and if the closing pressure of the anal sphincters has been

physical routine are lost in someone confined to bed. If drinking is diminished, the body maintains homeostasis by reabsorbing more fluid from the gut. The result is drier, harder bowel movements that are more difficult to pass.

Further indirect constipating influences of advanced illness can be intestinal narrowing by tumor and disruption of the neural coordination of peristalsis by tumor infiltration of the gut wall or paraneoplastic neuropathy affecting the intrinsic enteric nervous system or its autonomic supply.[11] Hypercalcemia of malignancy is associated with constipation, presumably as a result of the pivotal role that calcium plays in muscle contractility.

CASE STUDY

Constipation and Malignant Intestinal Obstruction

A 62-year-old woman with a history of intra-abdominal spread of ovarian cancer was admitted to a hospice inpatient unit because she had had no bowel movement for 8 days and had 3 days of persistent nausea and vomiting. Examination revealed a moderately distended abdomen with a palpable large suprapubic mass and several smaller masses in the line of the ascending and descending colon. Active bowel sounds were heard, and possible obstruction was considered. The rectum was empty. Questioning elicited a life-long tendency of constipation characterized by a stool frequency averaging two or three per week, often with straining. Small amounts of flatus were still being passed. Morphine analgesia had been commenced 3 weeks earlier, and the dose was being titrated.

The question to be settled was whether this patient had malignant intestinal obstruction—she clearly had a large pelvic tumor mass that distorted the rectum—or whether her symptoms represented an exacerbation of her long-standing constipation, perhaps by the opioids. Plain abdominal radiography showed extensive fecal loading throughout the colon as far as the pelvis but no significant fluid levels. A diagnosis of constipation possibly complicated by narrowing at the sigmoid level was made. Antiemetic medication was given subcutaneously, and initially, a predominantly softening laxative in the form of a magnesium hydroxide and liquid paraffin mixture was provided twice daily. The dose was increased on alternate administrations as long as she had no adverse effects.

She tolerated this well but had had no bowel action by the third day, when senna was added as a stimulant agent. Twenty-four hours later, after some mild colic, a repeat rectal examination showed a small amount of firm stool in the rectum. A proprietary small volume enema was administered with a moderate result. Continued upward titration of senna (up to 22.5 mg twice daily) and magnesium hydroxide plus liquid paraffin (to 30 mL three times daily) was associated with increasingly frequent evacuations of progressively softer stool and resolution of her vomiting and abdominal discomfort. She lived for several more months at home, maintaining a pattern of one bowel movement every 2 to 3 days using a combination of stimulant and softening laxatives at various doses according to response.

exceeded by the mass, it occurs as fecal leakage or incontinence. Most fecal impactions occur in the rectum and are detected by rectal examination.

Intestinal obstruction may be caused by tumor or adhesions. Known intra-abdominal malignant deposits, previous intestinal surgery, alternating constipation and diarrhea, gut colic, and nausea and vomiting combine to suggest the diagnosis of intestinal obstruction. A similar picture can, however, occur in severe constipation. The distinction is important, because attempts to clear constipation that is actually obstruction by use of stimulant laxatives can cause severe pain. Abdominal radiography may be helpful (Figs. 154-2 and 154-3).

CASE STUDY

Constipation and Co-morbid Disease

A 70-year-old woman was referred to a palliative care unit with a 5-year history of Parkinson's disease. Mobility was severely impaired, but other than mild short-term memory loss, she was cognitively intact. Constipation, for which she took a combination of lactulose and senna, had become a severe problem. She tended not to have bowel movements for several days and then, in response to titration of her laxatives, to have an urgent bowel movement resulting in incontinence and, on two occasions, rectal prolapse. It was decided to use a softening laxative alone and to precipitate defecation by use of rectal interventions when appropriate support was available. Trials showed that she preferred the use of mini-enemas to that of stimulant suppositories for this purpose.

To begin with, stimulation of a bowel movement was attempted each day. On the whole, this was successful, but the patient felt that because she usually had bowel movements only on alternate days when fit, she would rather maintain that pattern now. Accordingly, the frequency of rectal interventions was halved, and continence was largely achieved while further episodes of rectal prolapse were avoided.

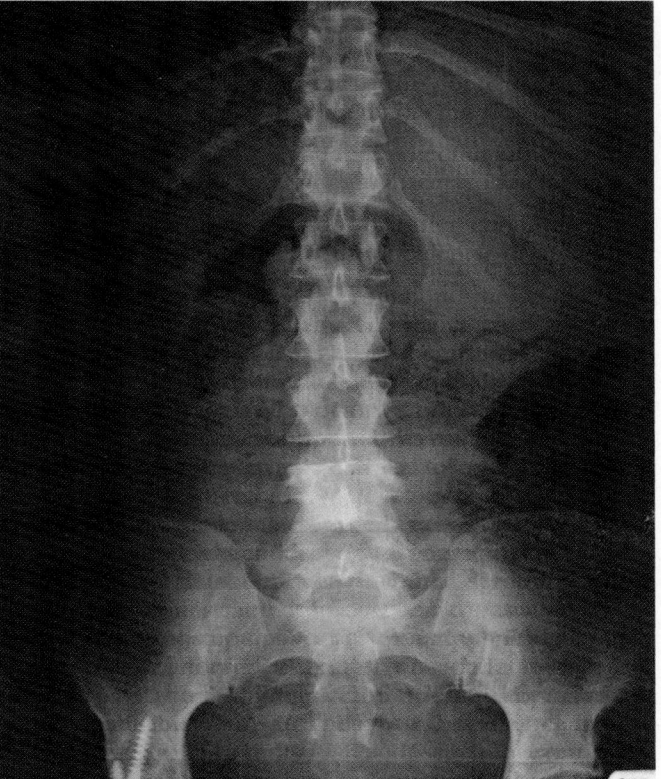

FIGURE 154-1   Plain abdominal radiograph shows extensive constipation throughout the colon.

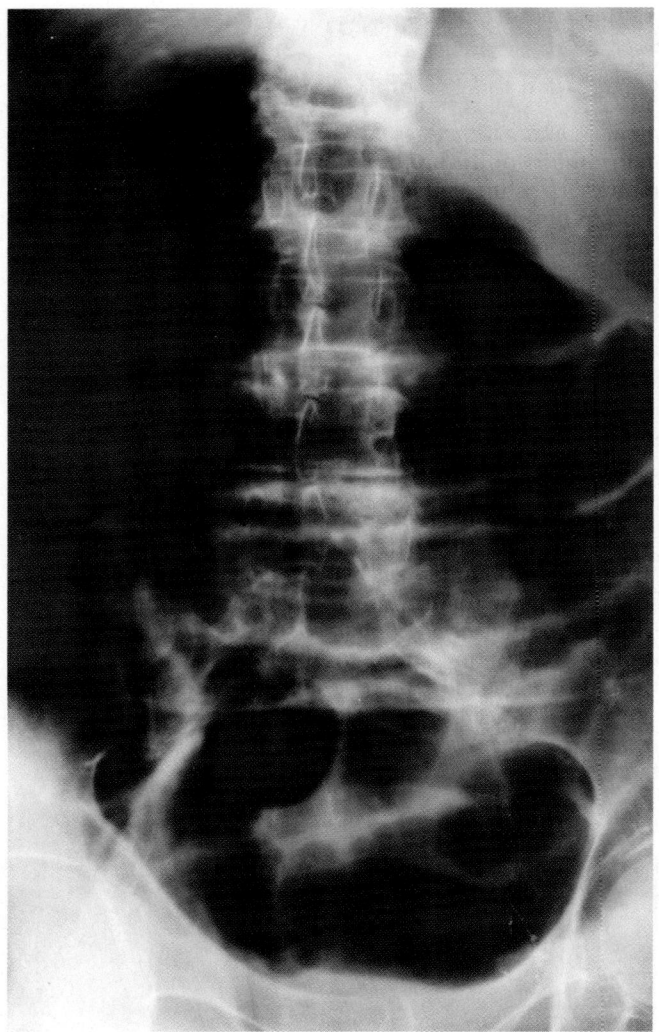

FIGURE 154-2   Plain supine abdominal radiograph shows small bowel obstruction.

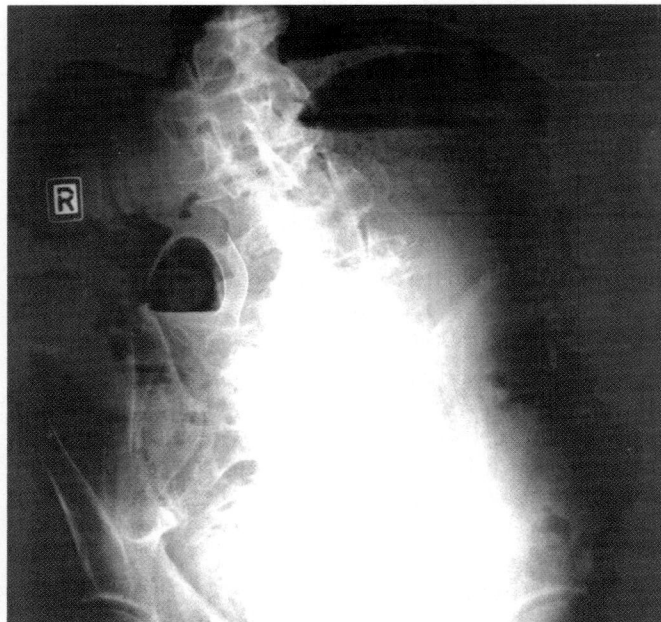

FIGURE 154-3   Erect abdominal radiograph shows fluid levels characteristic of intestinal obstruction.

Box 154-3 Constipation Prophylaxis
• Maximize general comfort
• Facilitate activity
• Encourage oral fluids
• Enhance the fiber content of the diet
• Anticipate constipating effects of drugs: alter the treatment or start a laxative prophylactically
• Create a favorable environment for elimination

Treatment

Principles

The causes of constipation in progressive disease (see Box 154-2) suggest several prophylactic measures (Box 154-3). Good general comfort should be ensured. Because of the link between colonic peristalsis and activity, patients should be encouraged and enabled to be as mobile as possible.

Constipated stools have relatively low water content, making them hard and difficult to pass, and this is worse if the patient is dehydrated. Sufficient oral fluids should be encouraged, but constipation alone rarely justifies parenteral fluids.

Ill people have small appetites, and what food they do eat tends to be low in fiber. Dietary fiber deficiency has been linked with constipation in Western societies, but in a palliative care population, the amount required to correct constipation is beyond the tolerance of ill people.[14] Although opportunities should be taken to increase the fiber content of diets, this cannot be the sole strategy, and the emphasis must be on food that is attractive to the person expected to eat it.

Clinicians should know which drugs cause constipation (see Box 154-2). They should avoid them or make a laxative available with the first prescription, without waiting until constipation is established.

Institutional lack of privacy for defecation and the use of bedpans, which impose an inappropriate posture and greatly increase the pressure required to expel a stool, are conducive to constipation. As one hospice patient said, "You can get used to anything." However, patients should be allowed privacy and the use of a bathroom, or at least a movable toilet, for defecation.

Drugs

Despite prophylaxis, most patients with advanced disease require laxatives. They are divided into agents that primarily soften the stool and those that stimulate peristalsis (Table 154-1). Most palliative care patients probably require a combination of the two types to maximize effectiveness and minimize colic,[15] but evidence for superiority of one laxative drug over another is lacking. Cost and patient preference are significant factors in the choice.

Bulking agents should be used with caution in palliative care, because if they are not taken with sufficient water,

TABLE 154-1	Commonly-Used Laxative Drugs	
EFFECT	**DRUG**	**MODE OF ACTION**
Predominantly softening	Liquid paraffin	Lubricant
	Bulk-forming agents (e.g., ispaghula)	Increase stool volume and bacterial growth
	Macrogols	Source of nonabsorbable water
	Docusate sodium, poloxamer	Surfactant: increase water penetration of the stool
	Lactulose	Osmotic: retains water in gut lumen
	Saline laxatives (e.g., magnesium hydroxide)	Osmotic; stimulates peristalsis at higher doses
Predominantly stimulant	Senna, bisacodyl, dantron	Stimulate peristalsis

they can set into a gelatinous mass that can precipitate intestinal obstruction. Liquid paraffin is not much used alone; it can cause a lipoid pneumonia if inhaled, but in some countries, is available in a proprietary combination with magnesium hydroxide that is a useful, economical, and safe softening laxative.

The use of rectal suppositories and enemas should be minimized by careful monitoring and titration of oral laxatives. Patients find suppositories less acceptable than laxatives.[16]

DIARRHEA

Epidemiology and Prevalence

Diarrhea is the passage of frequent, loose stools with urgency. It has often been defined as the passage of more than three unformed stools within a 24-hour period. Other criteria have been used, and different outcome measures create difficulty in comparing studies on occurrence and management.[19] Patients may describe diarrhea as a single, loose stool; frequent, small stools of normal or even hard consistency; or fecal incontinence. As with constipation, a complaint of diarrhea requires careful clarification.

Pathophysiology

Diarrhea persisting for over 3 weeks is said to be chronic and is often linked to serious organic disease. Most diarrhea is acute, lasting a few days, and it usually is caused by gastrointestinal infection (Box 154-4). However, the most common cause of diarrhea in palliative medicine patients is too much laxative,[10] particularly when laxative doses have been increased to clear a backlog of constipated stool. The diarrhea usually settles within 24 to 48 hours if laxatives are temporarily stopped.

Various other drugs can produce diarrhea commonly (i.e., antacids and antibiotics) or idiosyncratically (i.e., non-steroidal anti-inflammatory agents or iron preparations). Disaccharides such as sorbitol, which is used as a sweetener in some sugar-free preparations, act as osmotic laxatives and are easily overlooked as a cause. Some medications contain polyethylene glycol or propylene glycol, and they can have a similar effect.[20] Antibiotics can produce lactose intolerance, and resolution of diarrhea requires temporary withdrawal of milk products.[21]

Radiotherapy involving the abdomen or pelvis can cause diarrhea, with a peak incidence in the second or third week of therapy and continuing for some time afterward. Damage to intestinal mucosa by radiation releases prostaglandins and malabsorption of bile salts, both of which increase peristalsis. Another iatrogenic cause relevant to palliative medicine is celiac plexus blockade, which occasionally precipitates profuse, long-lasting, watery diarrhea.[22]

Steatorrheic diarrhea due to fat malabsorption may occur because of impaired secretion of pancreatic enzymes in patients with carcinoma of the pancreas or after gastrectomy or ileal resection. Gastrectomy presumably produces steatorrhea because of poor mixing of food with pancreatic and biliary secretions. However, the accompanying vagotomy causes increased fecal secretion of bile acids in some, with more water and electrolyte secretion in the colon and therefore a chologenic diarrhea, worsening the problem. Diarrhea after ileal resection is also chologenic, because the gut's ability to reabsorb bile acids is reduced. However, the picture is complex, because fat malabsorption occurs if more than about 100 cm of terminal ileum is removed. Disaccharidase deficiency is produced proportional to the length removed, leading to osmotic diarrhea from carbohydrate malabsorption.

Partial colectomy produces little or no persistent diarrhea. Total or almost total colectomy results in high-volume liquid effluent, which diminishes over 7 to 10 days but remains at 400 to 800 mL/day because of the small intestine's inability to compensate fully for the colon's water-absorbing capacity. For this reason, an ileostomy usually is fashioned. Similar symptoms can result from an enterocolic fistula caused by cancer or an operation.[23] Surgical alteration of intestinal anatomy may produce diarrhea through bacterial overgrowth.

A colonic or rectal tumor can precipitate diarrhea by causing partial intestinal obstruction, or it can loosen stools by means of increased secretion of mucus. Rarely, endocrine tumors, such as those of pancreatic islet cells or the sympathetic nervous system, cause secretory diarrhea. This can also occur with bronchogenic carcinomas from secretion of VIP, in the Zollinger-Ellison syndrome (seen with pancreatic islet cell tumors secreting gastrin), and in carcinoid tumors, in which serotonin, prostaglandins, bradykinin, and VIP secretions have been implicated.

In addition to concurrent gastrointestinal disease (see Box 154-4), dietary factors play a role in diarrhea. Excessive dietary fiber may produce diarrhea, and fruits may do so by this means and by their content of specific laxative factors.

Differential Diagnosis

Malignant intestinal obstruction and fecal impaction can cause confusion with diarrhea. Complete intestinal obstruction produces intractable constipation, but partial obstruction may manifest with diarrhea or alternating diarrhea and constipation. Fecal impaction results in fluid stool leaking past the mass, often with anal leakage or incontinence. Among hospitalized elderly patients, fecal impaction can account for 55% of instances of diarrhea,[24] demonstrating the need for careful attention to regular laxative therapy in any ill, immobile population.

Clinical Manifestations

A complaint of diarrhea demands a careful history of the frequency of defecation, the nature of the stools, and the time course of the problem. Together, these manifestations often indicate the diagnosis. Profuse, watery stools are characteristic of colonic diarrhea, whereas the pale, fatty, offensive stools of steatorrhea indicate malabsorp-

CASE STUDY

Debilitating Diarrhea

A 78-year-old man had had a partial colectomy for colonic carcinoma a few months earlier but still had progressive disease. He had re-established an acceptable bowel pattern after the operation but then developed debilitating diarrhea. He was not systemically unwell and had no history of recent antibiotic use or other significant changes in his medication. Loperamide provided improvement in stool consistency and frequency, but any attempt to withdraw the drug was associated with a relapse of the diarrhea.

A stool sample for microbiologic examination yielded no result. Nevertheless, because of his surgery and the tumor origin, there was the possibility that he could have a blind loop of bowel and a resultant overgrowth of anaerobic bacteria. An empirical trial was made of oral metronidazole. Within 3 days, it was possible to stop the loperamide without return of diarrhea.

tion due to a pancreatic or small intestinal cause. The sudden advent of diarrhea after constipation, perhaps with little warning of impending defecation, should raise the suspicion of fecal impaction (see "Case Study: Debilitating Diarrhea").

Current and recent medications should be listed. Laxatives can cause diarrhea by being given irregularly, resulting in alternating constipation and diarrhea, or given in excessive doses.

Examination should exclude fecal impaction and intestinal obstruction, and it should therefore include rectal examination and abdominal palpation for fecal masses. If there is doubt, an abdominal radiograph can make the determination.

Steatorrhea is suggested by a history of pale, greasy, floating stools. Persistent, watery diarrhea, without systemic upset that would suggest an infective cause, may be more difficult to diagnose. The differential diagnosis is between secretory diarrhea resulting from active secretion of fluid and electrolytes and osmotic diarrhea due to an additional nonabsorbed solute (e.g., a disaccharide from a medicinal solution). A clinical distinction can often be made if practicable to enforce a 24-hour fast or withdrawal of medications, because under these circumstances, osmotic diarrhea usually resolves. If in doubt, the stool osmolality and sodium and potassium concentrations should be measured. The anion gap, the difference between the stool osmolality and double the sum of the cation concentrations, is more than 50 mmol/L in osmotic diarrhea but less than 50 mmol/L in secretory diarrhea. Ileal resection produces a mixed picture, which becomes purely secretory if the patient is fasted.

For any persistent diarrhea, hematology and blood chemistry values should be checked. Diarrhea within 3 days of inpatient admission may be caused by community-acquired bacterial enteric pathogens such as *Salmonella, Shigella,* or *Campylobacter* or by a viral infection. After this point, stool culture is usually unrewarding; repeating the culture does not improve the diagnostic yield.[25] *Clostridium difficile* is the most commonly detected cause of nosocomial diarrhea, and it is identified by immunoassay of its toxins.

TREATMENT

Supportive Treatment

Other than in HIV infection, diarrhea in palliative medicine patients is rarely of sufficient degree or duration to cause a significant risk through dehydration. Ileostomy patients require an average of an extra liter of water each day and about 7 g of extra salt to compensate for their fluid and electrolyte losses, with special care needed in hot weather. If rehydration is needed, the oral route is superior to the intravenous. Proprietary rehydration solutions, which contain appropriate electrolyte concentrations and glucose to facilitate active electrolyte transport across the gut wall, are adequate for all but the most severe cases of diarrhea. Any diarrhea benefits from a diet of clear liquids, such as flat lemonade or ginger ale, and simple carbohydrates, such as toast or crackers. Milk products should be avoided in case of transient lactose intolerance. Protein and, later, fats are reintroduced gradually as diarrhea resolves.

Specific Treatment

Specific treatments exist for several causes of diarrhea (Box 154-5). Metronidazole is the first-line antibiotic for *C. difficile* diarrhea, and it can reasonably be tried when diarrhea is suspected to be caused by bacterial overgrowth.

Nonspecific antidiarrheal agents are numerous and are absorbent, adsorbent, mucosal prostaglandin inhibitors, opioids, or somatostatin derivatives (Box 154-6). These agents may make illness due to *Shigella* and *C. difficile* worse and should be used with caution if these organisms are present, there is blood in the stool, or the patient has fever.

Drugs

The opioids, usually in the form of codeine, loperamide, or diphenoxylate, are the most effective oral antidiarrheal drugs. They act by means of specific gut opioid receptors to reduce colonic peristalsis and preserve the fasting pattern of motility in the small intestine after food. In animal models, they reduce water and electrolyte secretion, but it is less clear whether this effect is present in humans at therapeutic doses. Of the three, only loperamide given orally does not reach or cross the blood-brain barrier.

The somatostatin analogues, octreotide and lanreotide, have a particular role in the management of severe diarrhea uncontrolled by opioids, such as that caused by HIV infection.

RESEARCH OPPORTUNITIES

Promising results have been obtained from the use of two quaternary derivatives of opioid antagonists, methylnaltrexone[17] and alvimopan.[18] Both drugs oppose the action of opioids at intestinal receptors but have poor systemic availability. They do not reach the central nervous system to impair analgesia.

Meta-analysis of studies of probiotics, live microbial supplements that improve the intestinal microbial balance, indicates a protective function against antibiotic-induced diarrhea.[26,27] There are also possible therapeutic effects in rotavirus diarrhea and traveler's diarrhea. Their usefulness in a palliative care population is untested.

In April 2008 methylnaltrexone by the subcutaneous route was approved by the U.S. Food and Drug Administration and by Health Canada for use in those countries and was recommended for marketing authorization by the European Medicines Agency, in each case for the treatment of opioid-induced constipation. Licensing of alvimopan is currently being sought only for the indication of postoperative ileus.

REFERENCES

1. Connell AM, Hilton C, Irvine G, et al. Variation in bowel habit in two population samples. Br Med J 1965;2:1095-1099.
2. Everhart JE, Go VL, Johannes RS, et al. A longitudinal survey of self-reported bowel habits in the United States. Dig Dis Sci 1989;34:1153-1162.
3. Wigzell FW. The health of nonagenarians. Gerontol Clin 1969;11:137-144.
4. Cartwright A, Hockey L, Anderson JL. Life before Death. London: Routledge & Kegan Paul, 1973, p 23.
5. Rolston KV, Rodriguez S, Hernandez M, Bodey GP. Diarrhoea in patients infected with HIV. Am J Med 1989;86:137-138.
6. Drossman DA, Sandler RS, McKee DC, Lovitz AJ. Bowel patterns among subjects not seeking health care. Gastroenterology 1982;83:529-534.
7. Thompson WG, Longstreth GF, Drossman DA, et al. Functional bowel disorders and functional abdominal pain. Gut 1999;45(Suppl 2):1143-1147.
8. Sykes NP. Methods of assessment of bowel function in patients with advanced cancer. Palliat Med 1990;4:287-292.
9. Twycross RG, Harcourt JM. The use of laxatives at a palliative care centre. Palliat Med 1991;5:27-33.
10. Twycross RG, Lack SA. Constipation. In Twycross RG, Lack SA (eds). Control of Alimentary Symptoms in Far Advanced Cancer. London: Churchill Livingstone, 1986, pp 166-207.
11. Jun S, Dimyan M, Jones KD, Ladabaum U. Obstipation as a paraneoplastic presentation of small cell lung cancer: Case report and literature review. Neurogasterenterol Motil 2005;17:16-22.
12. Sykes NP. The relationship between opioid use and laxative use in terminally ill cancer patients. Palliat Med 1998;12:375-382.
13. Radbruch L, Sabatowski R, Loick G, et al. Constipation and the use of laxatives: A comparison between transdermal fentanyl and oral morphine. Palliat Med 2000;14:111-119.
14. Mumford SP. Can high fibre diets improve the bowel function in patients on a radiotherapy ward? In Twycross RG, Lack SA (eds). Control of Alimentary Symptoms in Far Advanced Cancer. Edinburgh: Churchill Livingstone, 1986, p 183.
15. Sykes NP. A volunteer model for the comparison of laxatives in opioid-induced constipation. J Pain Symptom Manage 1997;11:363-369.
16. Sykes NP. A clinical comparison of laxatives in a hospice. Palliat Med 1991;5:307-314.
17. Boyd T, Yuan CS. Methylnaltrexone: Investigations in treating opioid bowel dysfunction. In Yuan CS (ed). Handbook of Opioid Bowel Dysfunction. New York: Haworth, 2005, pp 197-221.

18. Foss JF, Schmidt WK. Management of opioid-induced bowel dysfunction and post-operative ileus: Potential role of alvimopan. In Yuan CS (ed). Handbook of Opioid Bowel Dysfunction. New York: Haworth, 2005, pp 223-249.
19. Eisenberg P. An overview of diarrhea in the patient receiving enteral nutrition. Gastroenterol Nurs 2002;25:95-104.
20. Shepherd MF, Felt-Gunderson PA. Diarrhea associated with lorazepam in a tube-fed patient. Nutr Clin Pract 1996;11:117-120.
21. Noble S, Rawlinson F, Byrne A. Acquired lactose intolerance: A seldom considered cause of diarrhea in the palliative care setting. J Pain Symptom Manage 2002;23:449-450.
22. Dean AP, Reed WD. Diarrhoea—an unrecognised hazard of coeliac plexus block. Aust N Z J Med 1991;21:47-48.
23. Mercadante S. Treatment of diarrhoea due to enterocolic fistula with octreotide in a terminal cancer patient. Palliat Med 1992;6:257-259.
24. Kinnunen O, Jauhonen P, Salokannel J, Kivela SL. Diarrhoea and faecal impaction in elderly long-stay patients. Z Gerontol 1989;22:321-323.
25. Wood M. When stool cultures from adult inpatients are appropriate. Lancet 2001;357:901-902.
26. D'Souza AL, Chakravarthi R, Cooke J, Bulpitt CJ. Probiotics in prevention of antibiotic associated diarrhoea. Br Med J 2002;324:1361-1362.
27. Cremonini F, Nista EC, Bartolozzi F, et al. Meta-analysis: The effect of probiotic administration on antibiotic-associated diarrhoea. Aliment Pharmacol Ther 2002;16:1461-1467.

SUGGESTED READING

Mancini I, Bruera E. Constipation. In Ripamonti C, Bruera E (eds). Gastrointestinal Symptoms in Advanced Cancer Patients. New York: Oxford University Press, 2002, pp 193-206.

Mercadante S. Diarrhea and malabsorption. In Ripamonti C, Bruera E (eds). Gastrointestinal Symptoms in Advanced Cancer Patients. New York: Oxford University Press, 2002, pp 207-222.

Sykes NP. Constipation and diarrhoea. In Doyle D, Hanks GWC, Cherny N, Calman K (eds). Oxford Textbook of Palliative Medicine, 3rd ed. Oxford, UK: Oxford University Press, 2004, pp 483-496.

CHAPTER **155**

Cough, Hemoptysis, and Bronchorrhea

Sharon Watanabe, Yoko Tarumi, and **Pablo Amigo**

KEY POINTS

- Cough is one of the most common symptoms of lung cancer.
- Hemoptysis is a frightening symptom of lung cancer that may herald a life-ending event.
- Bronchorrhea is an uncommon but clinically significant symptom that mainly is associated with bronchioloalveolar carcinoma.
- Multiple causes may contribute to cough and hemoptysis. Reversible causes should be treated whenever possible.
- Treatment options for cough and hemoptysis include palliative radiotherapy, chemotherapy, invasive techniques, and symptomatic drug therapy. Symptom severity, disease status, and patient preference should be considered when deciding on treatment.

Cough is an important defense mechanism to help clear excess secretions and foreign material from the airways, keeping them free of obstruction and harmful substances. However, in lung cancer and other disorders, cough may become significant.

COUGH

Epidemiology and Prevalence

Cough can be categorized as acute, lasting less than 3 weeks, and chronic, lasting 3 to 8 weeks or longer; they are not mutually exclusive. Acute cough is most commonly transient, as in the common cold, but can occasionally be associated with potentially life-threatening conditions such as pulmonary embolism, congestive heart failure, and pneumonia. Chronic cough can be caused by more than one condition simultaneously. The most common causes of chronic cough (in nonsmokers not taking angiotensin-converting enzyme inhibitors [ACEIs] and a normal chest radiograph) are postnasal drip syndrome, asthma, and gastroesophageal reflux disease.[1] Other causes of chronic cough include postinfectious cough, ACEI-induced cough, bronchiectasis, psychogenic cough, interstitial lung disease, and chronic bronchitis, especially among smokers.

Cough is one of the most common symptoms of lung cancer. In a prospective, population-based survey, cough was the most common initial symptom and was the leading symptom that prompted medical attention.[2] The prevalence at diagnosis was 45% in a large, retrospective, population-based study.[3] Patients embarking on chemotherapy or radiotherapy for advanced lung cancer have cough with a frequency from 39% to more than 80%, exceeding that of pain.[4-6] The prevalence in other cancers at many stages is 22% to 37%.[7] The reported frequency in cancer patients may be influenced by prior anticancer therapies, intercurrent respiratory infections, and assessment methods. Relatively limited information is available regarding symptoms in end-stage heart failure. A comparative survey revealed that end-stage heart failure patients at a heart failure clinic had more cough than persons identified as terminally ill by a palliative care team (44% versus 26%).[8]

Pathophysiology

Cough may result from pulmonary or extrapulmonary conditions. The common link is the activation of subsets of airway sensory nerves. Respiratory disease can activate sensory nerves within the airway after release of inflammatory mediators, increased mucus secretion, or damage to the airway epithelium. Disorders of other organs that have neurons carried in the vagus (e.g., esophagus, heart) probably interact with airway neurons in higher centers to elicit the cough reflex.[9,10] In inflammatory or chronic disease, many pathological changes affect sensory nerve fibers, with increased excitability and phenotypic changes in receptor and neurotransmitter expression and sensitization of the cough reflex.[9]

Clinical Manifestations

Little is known about the impact of cough on quality of life in palliative care (see "Case Study: Cough"). A tool for cough-specific quality of life has been validated for assessing patients with chronic cough. Six domains were identified by factor analysis: physical complaint, psychosocial issues, functional abilities, emotional well-being, extreme physical complaint, and personal safety fears.[11] Another study suggested that chronic cough was associated with significant adverse effects on physical and psychosocial

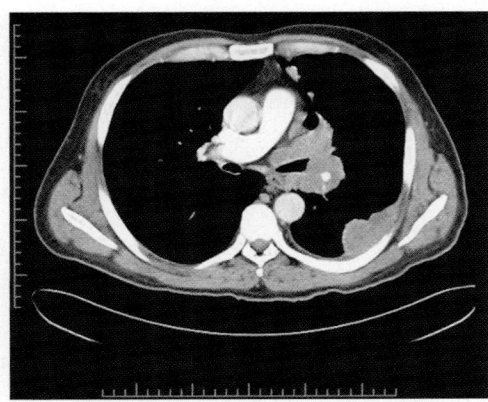

FIGURE 155-1 Computed tomography of the chest in a 54-year-old man with small cell carcinoma of the lung, who presented with shortness of breath and cough productive of blood-tinged sputum. The scan shows a left hilar mass obstructing the left upper lobe bronchus, left pleural-based masses, and a small left pleural effusion.

 C A S E   S T U D Y

Cough

A 54-year-old, male truck driver presented to the emergency room with worsening shortness of breath, back pain, and cough that occasionally produced blood-tinged sputum. He had a history of smoking 35 packs of cigarettes each year. He was recently treated with a 2-week course of antibiotics for presumed community-acquired respiratory tract infection, without improvement. Computed tomography (CT) of the chest showed a large left hilar mass, pleural effusion, multiple pleural-based masses, and lesions in the left lobe of liver (Fig. 155-1). Results of bone and CT scans of the head were negative. He underwent bronchoscopy, and pathologic analysis revealed small cell carcinoma.

Morphine was initiated for shortness of breath and cough at a dosage of 5 mg given orally every 4 hours around the clock and eventually titrated up to 15 mg given orally every 4 hours around the clock. Prednisone (30 mg daily) and inhaled salbutamol were also prescribed for chronic obstructive lung disease, which was considered a possible contributor. He received a course of chest radiotherapy, after which the cough and hemoptysis improved. He was scheduled for chemotherapy, but suddenly became short of breath and confused and began bleeding from many sites. He developed respiratory failure and died before initiation of chemotherapy.

function, particularly in the areas of ambulation, social interaction, sleep and rest, work, home management, and recreation and pastimes.[12]

Cough intensity was reported in 673 patients with stage III or IV non–small cell lung cancer with a Karnofsky performance status of 60% to 100% who were enrolled in two multicenter chemotherapy trials. Cough was documented in 86% of patients. Mean intensity for the total population was 30 on a 100-mm visual analogue scale (0 = best, 100 = worst) before chemotherapy, decreasing to 20 on day 71. In a comparison group of 63 patients with a Karnofsky performance status of 20% to 50% who did not receive chemotherapy, the mean intensity of

cough was 39 on the visual analogue scale.[6] A study of 30 patients in the last week of life showed that the degree of distress for cough was relatively low (median distress rating of 1 of 4, with 4 representing the highest distress) compared with fatigue, cachexia, and anorexia.[13] The degree of distress due to a particular symptom may vary significantly according to the stage of illness and many social factors, including culture.

Differential Diagnosis

Many factors can contribute to chronic cough in cancer patients. Causes related to the malignancy include direct mass effect, pleural effusion, cavitation, fistula, lymphangitis, pulmonary embolism, infection, or neurological damage. Studies of bronchial mucus in lung cancer documented altered rheological properties that may impair mucus clearance.[14] Debilitated patients struggle to clear their airways of secretions thickened from dehydration. Cough as a paraneoplastic manifestation of renal cell carcinoma subsided after nephrectomy.[15,16] Cancer treatments may be a factor. A longitudinal study of childhood cancer survivors suggested increased risk for chronic cough with prior chest radiotherapy, bleomycin exposure, and cyclophosphamide therapy.[17] Irinotecan and interleukin-2 have been associated with cough.[18,19] Radiotherapy may cause lymphocytic alveolitis or hypersensitivity pneumonitis associated with cough within weeks or months of therapy.[20] Table 155-1[7,21] summarizes factors that may contribute to chronic cough in cancer.

Treatment

In a cancer patient, reversible causes should be addressed. The time, effort, and adverse effects associated with investigations and treatment should be tolerable for the patient. Environmental modifications (e.g., humidification, supplementary oxygen, avoiding airway irritants such as perfumes or cigarette smoke), and proper positioning should be considered.

Palliative radiotherapy is recommended for troublesome local symptoms, most commonly cough, hemoptysis, chest pain, and breathlessness. According to a systematic review of 10 randomized, controlled trials of palliative radiotherapy for non–small cell lung cancer, there is no strong evidence that any one regimen provides greater palliation than another. Higher-dose regimens may modestly increase survival (6% at 1 year and 3% at 2 years) in carefully selected patients with good performance status, but they have more acute toxic effects, especially esophagitis. Most patients should be treated with short courses (e.g., 10 Gy/1 fraction, 16 to 17 Gy/2 fractions).[22] In a multicenter study involving 509 non–small cell lung cancer patients, cough improved in 48% and 55% at the second and third months, respectively, after two fractions of palliative radiotherapy.[23] Using hypofractionated radiotherapy for patients with symptomatic non–small cell lung cancer but poorer performance status, cough improved in 13 of the 22 patients with this symptom. Treatment was well tolerated. Only three patients were alive at 4 months of follow-up, and two of them had symptom relief.[24] Patients previously irradiated for lung cancer may benefit from repeat treatment. A retrospective study of thoracic

TABLE 155-1	Differential Diagnosis Guide: Factors Contributing to Chronic Cough in Cancer Patients		
ANATOMICAL SITE	**DIRECTLY RELATED TO CANCER**	**INDIRECTLY RELATED TO CANCER**	**UNRELATED TO CANCER**
Upper airways	Laryngeal tumor Tracheal tumor	Postirradiation tracheitis	Infection Postnasal drip
Bronchi	Primary or metastatic lung cancer Superior vena cava syndrome	Radiation-induced increased airways responsiveness Aspiration Dehydration	Chronic obstructive lung disease Infection Asthma Aspiration Perfume, cigarettes
Lung parenchyma	Lymphangitic carcinomatosis	Radiation-induced: acute lymphocytic alveolitis, acute pneumonitis, bronchiolitis obliterans organizing pneumonia, late pulmonary fibrosis Cytotoxic chemotherapy: acute idiopathic pneumonia syndrome, delayed pulmonary toxicity syndrome, interstitial pneumonitis, late pulmonary fibrosis Biological therapies: Herceptin, interleukin	Infection
Pleura	Mesothelioma Pleural effusion		
Heart	Pericardial effusion Pulmonary thromboembolism	Pulmonary congestion Pulmonary thromboembolism	Angiotensin converting-enzyme (ACE) inhibitor
Esophagus	Tracheo-esophageal fistula	Post-esophageal stent insertion	Gastroesophageal reflux
Other	Paraneoplastic syndrome		

repeat irradiation for symptomatic control in 104 lung cancer patients indicated that 65% of 37 patients with cough experienced relief. Radiation pneumonitis and radiation myelopathy were seen in three patients and one patient, respectively.[25]

Many chemotherapy trials enrolling patients with small cell lung cancer suggest cough may improve in up to 70%,[7] even those with a poor prognosis.[26] For stage IIIB and IV non–small cell cancer–related cough, the response rate in chemotherapy trials has been up to 70%.[7] One randomized trial in 169 non–small cell lung cancer patients used clinical benefit (i.e., combination of symptom score, performance status, and weight) as the primary end point; cough was relieved in 42% and 50% of those who received single-agent gemcitabine and cisplatin-based combination chemotherapy, respectively.[27]

Endobronchial approaches have been reported. In the largest prospective study of intraluminal radiotherapy, cough resolved at 6 weeks in 44% of 311 patients with inoperable lung cancer with cough.[28] In another prospective series of primary or metastatic lung cancer, the weighted symptom scores for cough in 338 patients improved 85%.[29] However, intraluminal radiotherapy has complications, including massive and mostly fatal hemorrhage, occurring in up to 32% of treated patients.[30] In a retrospective report of endobronchial cryosurgery in 521 patients with inoperable lung cancer, cough improved in 69% of 460 patients with the symptom.[31] Use of the Dumon Y-stent to palliate severe respiratory symptoms from tracheobronchial obstruction and tracheoesophageal fistula in many cancer types was described retrospectively in 86 patients, 33% of whom had cough. Eighty-four patients reported improvement of respiratory symptoms, including cough.[32]

Several mechanisms (see Fig. 155-1) are thought to be involved in controlling cough. The two major classes of therapeutic agents are centrally acting opioids and non-opioids and peripherally acting drugs. Detailed information about drugs for cough, such as bronchodilators and cough suppressants, is discussed in Chapter 137.

HEMOPTYSIS

Hemoptysis is spitting of blood derived from the lungs or bronchi. It is a frightening symptom, which may herald a life-ending event.

Epidemiology and Prevalence

The prevalence of hemoptysis in the cancer population has been documented mainly in lung cancer. In a large, retrospective, population-based study, the prevalence of hemoptysis at the diagnosis of cancer was 27%.[3] The frequency at the start of chemotherapy or radiotherapy for advanced disease ranged from 5% to 41%.[4-6] Although Twycross[33] reported a prevalence of 24% among lung cancer patients admitted to an inpatient hospice, the prevalence in the broader palliative care population is unknown. Autopsy studies suggest 3% to 5% of patients with lung cancer develop terminal, massive hemoptysis.[34,35]

Pathophysiology

The lungs receive blood from the pulmonary and bronchial arterial system. The low-pressure pulmonary system rarely produces massive hemoptysis, unless a tumor erodes the bronchial tree. The higher-systemic-pressure bronchial arteries are the most common source of profuse bleeding, accounting for 90% of massive hemoptysis.[36] Bleeding from tumors may occur from superficial mucosal invasion, erosion into blood vessels, or highly vascular lesions, usually primary bronchogenic neoplasms (metastatic lung carcinoma rarely causes hemoptysis).[37]

Clinical Manifestations

Although any hemoptysis causes great patient concern, the amount of blood dictates the diagnosis, intervention, and outcome. Hemoptysis is usually classified as nonmassive or massive based on the volume, but there is no uniform definition, although 200 to 1000 mL in 24 hours has been reported as the criterion for massive hemoptysis. Massive hemoptysis may cause hemodynamic instability and impaired alveolar gas exchange.[38]

Massive hemoptysis from malignancy has a worse prognosis than other causes. In a retrospective study of 59 patients with hemoptysis of various causes of more than 200 mL in 24 hours, the mortality rate without malignancy was 13%, and in lung cancer, other metastatic cancer, or leukemia, it was 62%, increasing to 80% if hemoptysis was more than 1000 mL in 24 hours.[39]

Differential Diagnosis

Hemoptysis should be differentiated from pseudohemoptysis (i.e., expectoration of blood originating in the nasopharynx or oropharynx) and hematemesis (i.e., vomiting of blood). Pseudohemoptysis can be diagnosed by inspection and hematemesis by other gastrointestinal symptoms and risk factors for gastrointestinal bleeding.

In palliative care, the differential diagnosis for hemoptysis includes primary or secondary neoplasm, pneumonia or other infection, pulmonary embolism, and coagulopathy. Iatrogenic hemoptysis occurs after diagnostic and therapeutic procedures. Hemoptysis may be unrelated to the malignancy. A careful history and physical examination may establish the cause.

Diagnostic tests may be indicated if identification of the causes directs specific interventions. A complete blood cell count with a differential count may help quantify blood loss, support an infectious cause, and screen for thrombocytopenia. Prothrombin time and partial thromboplastin time determinations are recommended if coagulopathy is suspected. Sputum examination may help evaluate for infection. A chest radiograph may be useful. Computed tomography or bronchoscopy, or both, may be warranted.

Treatment

Principles

Treatment should be tailored to the patient's overall status, hemoptysis severity, the underlying cause, and the wishes of the patient and family. Aggressive interventions usually described for massive hemoptysis, such as endotracheal intubation, are seldom indicated in palliative care patients.

Particular care should be exercised in communication with the patients and their families because of the emotional impact bleeding can produce. It may be necessary to mask the bleeding with dark colored towels. For patients with end-stage cancer in whom invasive diagnostic procedures and invasive management are not indicated, palliative sedation with a drug such as midazolam may be the best approach.

Treatments for malignancy-related hemoptysis include external beam radiotherapy, chemotherapy, endobronchial techniques, and bronchial artery embolization. Like cough, short-course palliative radiotherapy has been recommended for hemoptysis.[22] In a multicenter study involving 509 non–small cell lung cancer patients, hemoptysis improved in 95% at 3 months after two fractions of palliative radiotherapy.[23] In hypofractionated radiotherapy for patients with symptomatic non–small cell lung cancer and poor performance status, hemoptysis was controlled until death in all three patients with this symptom.[24] A retrospective study of thoracic repeat irradiation for symptomatic control in 104 lung cancer patients indicated that 83% of 24 patients with hemoptysis got relief.[25]

Many trials suggest chemotherapy may improve hemoptysis in up to 92% of small cell and non–small cell lung cancer patients.[7] In a randomized trial enrolling 169 non–small cell lung cancer patients in which the primary end point was clinical benefit, single-agent gemcitabine and cisplatin-based combination chemotherapy relieved hemoptysis in 69% and 59%, respectively.[27]

In the largest prospective study of intraluminal radiotherapy, resolution of hemoptysis was achieved in 89% of 254 patients with inoperable lung cancer with this symptom.[28] In another prospective series of primary or metastatic lung cancer, the weighted symptom score for hemoptysis in 226 patients improved by more than 99%.[29] A review of laser resection for palliation of tracheobronchial malignancies suggested an overall response rate for hemoptysis of 60%.[40] The use of endobronchial argon plasma coagulation was described in 56 patients with primarily cancer-related hemoptysis; control was achieved immediately in all cases, and hemoptysis did not recur at treated sites during a mean follow-up period of 97 days.[41] Endobronchial cryosurgery reportedly improved hemoptysis in 76% of 202 patients with inoperable lung cancer who had this symptom.[31] In a study evaluating the Dumon Y-stent in 86 patients with tracheobronchial obstruction or tracheoesophageal fistula associated with many cancer types, symptoms that improved included hemoptysis.[32]

Bronchial artery embolization is the most effective intervention for massive hemoptysis. Selective angiography locates the site of bleeding, after which a substance is injected into the bleeding bronchial artery. The most serious complication of bronchial artery embolization, with a reported prevalence of less than 1%, is accidental embolization of the spinal artery, causing spinal cord ischemic injury.[38] In the largest series involving lung cancer, 30 patients with nonmassive hemoptysis from advanced, inoperable disease underwent bronchial artery embolization. Bleeding stopped immediately in all, and did not recur in 47%. In 50%, bleeding recurred after a mean of 34 days. Twenty-seven percent eventually died of hemorrhage.[42]

Drugs

Pharmacological treatment should address the underlying cause whenever possible. If infection is suspected, antibiotics can be instituted. For patients with pulmonary embolism, anticoagulation with low-molecular-weight heparin may be attempted, although bleeding may worsen as a result.

Randomized, controlled trials of drugs for symptomatic relief of hemoptysis are lacking. Cough suppressants may be considered, although this may lead to accumulation of blood in the lungs and bronchi. In 16 patients with cancer-associated bleeding treated with the fibrinolytic inhibitors tranexamic acid and aminocaproic acid, hemoptysis resolved completely in the three with this symptom.[43] In another report, aerosolized vasopressin in three patients with mild to moderate hemoptysis from cancer metastatic to lung resulted in prompt resolution, without apparent adverse effect.[44]

BRONCHORRHEA

Bronchorrhea is the excess production of watery sputum (≥100 mL/day). Although it is a relatively uncommon symptom of lung malignancy, it may be clinically significant.

Basic Science

Mucus normally protects the airway epithelium from dehydration and from inhaled infectious and toxic agents. It consists of water (95%) and mucins. Mucins are glycoproteins secreted by goblet and mucous cells in the airways. They undergo hydration to form a gel with unusual viscoelastic properties that allow it to interact with cilia to effect mucociliary clearance.

The epidermal growth factor receptor (EGFR) system plays a major role in mucin production. EGFR is a membrane glycoprotein activated by ligands such as epidermal growth factor and transforming growth factor-α. EGFR expression and activation causes mucin production in airway epithelium by promoting differentiation of airway epithelial cells into goblet cells and increasing mucin synthesis. EGFR activation occurs in response to various stimuli, including bacterial products, allergens, cigarette smoke, foreign bodies, reactive oxygen species, interleukin-13, and activated neutrophils and eosinophils.[45]

Epidemiology and Prevalence

Bronchorrhea is most common as a complication of bronchioloalveolar carcinoma (BAC), which is a subtype of adenocarcinoma of the lung. It is characterized by peripheral location, intact pulmonary interstitium, and growth of malignant cells along the alveolar septa. BAC was previously considered to be rare, but studies suggest its incidence is increasing. For example, according to a pathology review of 1527 cases of lung cancer diagnosed at one American institution between 1955 and 1990, the incidence rose from 5% to 24% during the study period. The incidence of bronchorrhea in BAC is uncertain, with one review stating that it occurs in 6% of patients.[46]

Bronchorrhea has also been reported in adenocarcinoma of the colon with lymphangitic carcinomatosis, adenocarcinoma of the pancreas metastatic to lung, and adenocarcinoma of the cervix metastatic to lung.[47-49]

Pathophysiology

The pathophysiological mechanisms underlying malignancy-associated bronchorrhea are unclear. EGFR activation has been implicated because the EGFR tyrosine kinase inhibitor gefitinib suppresses mucin synthesis in mucin-secreting non–small cell lung cancer cells and reduces sputum production in BAC.[50-55] Prostaglandins may also play a role because they stimulate chloride secretion toward the airway lumen, promoting water accumulation. Upregulation of cyclooxygenase-2 and reduction in sputum production by agents that inhibit prostaglandin synthesis may occur in BAC.[56-59]

Clinical Manifestations

Bronchorrhea of up to 9 L per day, causing significant fluid and electrolyte depletion, has been reported.[60] Ventilation-perfusion mismatch, hypoxemia, and dyspnea may result from mucus filling the alveoli. The need to expectorate frequently significantly impairs quality of life.

Treatment

Principles

Treatment of bronchorrhea in palliative care patients is limited by a lack of clinical trials. Most therapies have been published as case reports and case series.

Radiotherapy is not usually an option for patients with BAC because of the disseminated lung involvement. However, one patient with metastatic BAC but limited pulmonary involvement had less bronchorrhea after local radiotherapy.[61]

Response of BAC-associated bronchorrhea to gefitinib, which is an EGFR tyrosine kinase inhibitor used in non–small cell lung cancer, was reported. In the nine cases, the improvement occurred too rapidly to be attributable to an antineoplastic effect. Rather, gefitinib appeared to directly inhibit sputum production.[51-55]

Drugs

Inhaled indomethacin reduced sputum production in a randomized, double-blind, placebo-controlled trial involving 25 patients with bronchorrhea caused by chronic bronchitis, diffuse panbronchiolitis, or bronchiectasis.[62] Two cases have been reported of BAC-associated bronchorrhea; for both patients, sputum volume decreased with inhaled indomethacin. The drug is postulated to work by inhibiting prostaglandin production.[56]

In another report,[58] sputum production decreased with high-dose corticosteroids in patients with BAC-associated bronchorrhea. Corticosteroids may reduce the airways' mucus secretion by inhibiting the gene encoding inducible cyclooxygenase and directly inhibiting glycoconjugate secretion.[58]

One report[59] described improvement in BAC after erythromycin. Possible mechanisms of action include reduction of respiratory glycoconjugate secretion, inhibition of prostaglandin synthesis, and immunomodulation.[59]

RESEARCH OPPORTUNITIES

Cough in other life-limiting disorders such as congestive heart failure requires further investigation. The effect of cough, hemoptysis, and bronchorrhea on quality of life has not been fully defined. More effective, noninvasive therapies for malignancy-related hemoptysis are needed.

Controlled clinical trials to guide treatment of bronchor-rhea are lacking.

REFERENCES

1. Irwin RS, Boulet L-P, Cloutier MM, et al. Managing cough as a defense mechanism and as a symptom. A consensus panel report of the American College of Chest Physicians. Chest 1998;114:Suppl.2, 133S-181S.
2. Koyi H, Hillerdal G, Branden E. A prospective study of a total material of lung cancer from a county in Sweden 1997-1999: Gender, symptoms, type, stage, and smoking habits. Lung Cancer 2002;36:9-14.
3. Chute CG, Greenberg ER, Baron J, et al. Presenting conditions of 1539 population-based lung cancer patients by cell type and stage in New Hampshire and Vermont. Cancer 1985;56:2107-2111.
4. Bergman B, Aaronson NK, Ahmedzai S, et al. EORTC QLQ-LC13: A modular supplement to the EORTC core quality of life questionnaire for use in lung cancer clinical trials. Eur J Cancer 1994;30A:635-642.
5. Hopwood P, Stephens RJ, on behalf of the Medical Research Council (MRC) Lung Cancer Working Party. Symptoms at presentation for treatment in patients with lung cancer: Implications for the evaluation of palliative treatment. Br J Cancer 1995;71:633-636.
6. Hollen PJ, Gralla RJ, Kris MG, et al. Normative data and trends in quality of life from the Lung Cancer Symptom Scale. Support Care Cancer 1999;7:140-148.
7. Ahmedzai SH. Cough in cancer patients. Pulm Pharmacol Ther 2004;17:415-423.
8. Anderson H, Ward C, Eardley A, et al. The concerns of patients under palliative care and a heart failure clinic are not being met. Palliat Med 2001;15:279-286.
9. Reynolds SM, Mackenzie AJ, Spina D, et al. The pharmacology of cough. Trends Pharmacol Sci 2004;25:569-576.
10. Mazzone SB. Sensory regulation of the cough reflex. Pulm Pharmacol Ther 2004;17:361-368.
11. French CT, Irwin RS, Fletcher KE, et al. Evaluation of a cough-specific quality-of-life questionnaire. Chest 2002;121:1123-1131.
12. French CL, Irwin RS, Curley FJ, et al. Impact of chronic cough on quality of life. Arch Intern Med 1998;158:1657-1661.
13. Oi-Ling K, Man-Wah DT, Kam-Hung DN. Symptom distress as rated by advanced cancer patients, caregivers and physicians in the last week of life. Palliat Med 2005;19:228-233.
14. Zayas JG, Rubin BK, York EL, et al. Bronchial mucus properties in lung cancer: Relationship with site of lesion. Canadian Respiratory J 1999;6:246-252.
15. Hagen N, Temple WJ. Cough as a systemic manifestation of cancer. J Pain Symptom Manage 1994;9:3-4.
16. Fujikawa A, Daidoh Y, Taoka Y, et al. Immediate improvement of a persistent cough after tumor embolization for renal cell carcinoma. Scand J Urol Nephrol 2002;36:393-395.
17. Mertens AC, Yasui Y, Liu Y, et al. Pulmonary complications in survivors of childhood and adolescent cancer. Cancer 2002;95:2431-2441.
18. Madarnas Y, Webstar P, Shorter AM, et al. Irinotecan-associated pulmonary toxicity. Anticancer Drugs 2000;11:709-713.
19. Eton O, Rosenblum MG, Legha SS, et al. Phase I trial of subcutaneous recombinant human interleukin-2 in patients with metastatic melanoma. Cancer 2002;95:127-134.
20. Inoue A, Kunitoh H, Sekine I, et al. Radiation pneumonitis in lung cancer patients: A retrospective study of risk factors and the long-term prognosis. Int J Radiat Oncol Biol Phys 2001;49:649-655.
21. Homsi J, Walsh D, Nelson KA. Important drugs for cough in advanced cancer. Support Care Cancer 2001;9:565-574.
22. Lester JF, Macbeth F, Toy E, et al. Palliative radiotherapy regimens for non-small cell lung cancer. Cochrane Database Syst Rev 2006;(4):CD002143.
23. Macbeth FR, Bolger JJ, Hopwood P, et al, for the Medical Research Council Lung Cancer Working Party. Randomised trial of palliative two-fraction versus more intensive 13 fraction radiotherapy for patients with inoperable non-small cell lung cancer and good performance status. Clin Oncol 1996;8:167-175.
24. Cross CK, Berman S, Buswell L, et al. Prospective study of palliative hypofractionated radiotherapy (8.5 Gy × 2) for patients with symptomatic non-small cell lung cancer. Int J Radiat Oncol Biol Phys 2004;58:1098-1105.
25. Gressen EL, Werner-Wasik M, Cohn J, et al. Thoracic reirradiation for symptomatic relief after prior radiotherapeutic management for lung cancer. Am J Clin Oncol 2000;23:160-163.
26. White SC, Lorigan P, Middleton MR, et al. Phase II study of cyclophosphamide, doxorubicin and vincristine compared with single-agent carboplatin in patients with poor prognosis small cell lung carcinoma. Cancer 2001;92:601-608.
27. Vansteenkiste J, Vandebroek J, Nackaerts K, et al. Influence of cisplatin-use, age, performance status and duration of chemotherapy on symptom control in advanced non-small cell lung cancer: Detailed symptom analysis of a randomised study comparing cisplatin-vindesine to gemcitabine. Lung Cancer 2003;40:191-199.
28. Gollins SW, Burt PA, Barber PV, et al. High dose rate intraluminal radiotherapy for carcinoma of the bronchus: Outcome of treatment of 406 patients. Radiother Oncol 1994;33:31-40.
29. Speiser BL, Spratling L. Remote afterloading brachytherapy for the local control of endobronchial carcinoma. Int J Radiat Oncol Biol Phys 1993;25:579-587.
30. Hara R, Itami J, Aruga T, et al. Risk factors for massive hemoptysis after endobronchial brachytherapy in patients with tracheobronchial malignancies. Cancer 2001;92:2623-2627.
31. Maiwand MO, Asimakopoulos G. Cryosurgery for lung cancer: Clinical results and technical aspects. Tech Cancer Res Treat 2004;3:143-150.
32. Dutau H, Toutblanc B, Lamb C, et al. Use of the Dumon Y-stent in the management of malignant disease involving the carina. Chest 2004;126:951-958.
33. Twycross RG. The terminal care of patients with lung cancer. Postgrad Med J 1973;49:732-737.
34. Cox JD, Yesner R, Mietlowski W, et al. Influence of cell type on failure pattern after irradiation for locally advanced carcinoma of the lung. Cancer 1979;44:94-98.
35. Miller RR, McGregor DH. Hemorrhage from carcinoma of the lung. Cancer 1980;46:200-205.
36. Corder R. Hemoptysis. Emerg Med Clin North Am 2003;21:421-435.
37. Reisz G, Stevens D, Boutwell C, Nair V. The causes of hemoptysis revisited. A review of the etiologies of hemoptysis between 1986 and 1995. Mo Med 1997;94:633-635.
38. Jean-Baptiste E. Clinical assessment and management of massive hemoptysis. Crit Care Med 2000;28:1642-1647.
39. Corey R, Hla KM. Major and massive hemoptysis: Reassessment of conservative management. Am J Med Sci 1987;294:301-309.
40. Hetzel MR, Smith SG. Endoscopic palliation of tracheobronchial malignancies. Thorax 1991;46:325-333.
41. Morice RC, Ece T, Ece F, et al. Endobronchial argon plasma coagulation for treatment of hemoptysis and neoplastic airway obstruction. Chest 2001;119:781-787.
42. Witt C, Schmidt B, Geisler A, et al. Value of bronchial artery embolisation with platinum coils in tumorous pulmonary bleeding. Eur J Cancer 2000;36:1949-1954.
43. Dean A, Tuffin P. Fibrinolytic inhibitors for cancer associated bleeding problems. J Pain Symptom Manage 1997;13:20-24.
44. Anwar D, Schaad N, Mazzocato C. Aerosolized vasopressin is a safe and effective treatment for mild to moderate recurrent hemoptysis in palliative care patients. J Pain Symptom Manage 2005;29:427-429.
45. Kim S, Shao MXG, Nadel JA. Mucus production, secretion, and clearance. In Mason RJ, Murray JF, Broaddus VC, Nadel JA (eds). Mason, Murray & Nadel's Textbook of Respiratory Medicine, 4th ed. Philadelphia: Elsevier, 2005, pp 330-354.
46. Barkley JE, Green MR. Bronchioloalveolar carcinoma. J Clin Oncol 1996;14:2377-2386.
47. Shimura S, Takishima T. Bronchorrhea from diffuse lymphangitic metastasis of colon carcinoma to the lung. Chest 1994;105:308-310.
48. Lembo T, Donnelly TJ. A case of pancreatic carcinoma causing massive bronchial fluid production and electrolyte abnormalities. Chest 1995;108:1161-1163.
49. Epaulard O, Moro D, Langin T, et al. Bronchorrhea revealing cervix carcinoma metastatic to the lung. Lung Cancer 2001;31:331-334.
50. Kitazaki T, Soda H, Doi S, et al. Gefitinib inhibits MUC5AC synthesis in mucin-secreting non-small cell lung cancer cells. Lung Cancer 2005;50:19-24.
51. Yano S, Kanematsu T, Miki T, et al. A report of two bronchioloalveolar carcinoma cases which were rapidly improved by treatment with the epidermal growth factor receptor tyrosine kinase inhibitor ZD1839 ("Iressa"). Cancer Sci 2003;94:453-458.
52. Kitazaki T, Fukuda M, Soda H, et al. Novel effects of gefitinib on mucin production in bronchioloalveolar carcinoma: Two case reports. Lung Cancer 2005;49:125-128.
53. Milton DT, Kris MG, Gomez JE, et al. Prompt control of bronchorrhea in patients with bronchioloalveolar carcinoma treated with gefitinib (Iressa). Support Care Cancer 2005;13:70-72.
54. Takao M, Inoue K, Watanabe F, et al. Successful treatment of persistent bronchorrhea by gefitinib in a case with recurrent bronchioloalveolar carcinoma: A case report. World J Surg Oncol 2003;1:8-10.
55. Chang GC, Yang TY, Wang NS, et al. Successful treatment of multifocal bronchioloalveolar cell carcinoma with ZD1839 (Iressa) in two patients. J Formos Med Assoc 2003;102:407-411.
56. Homma S, Kawabata M, Kishi K, et al. Successful treatment of refractory bronchorrhea by inhaled indomethacin in two patients with bronchioloalveolar carcinoma. Chest 1999;115:1465-1468.
57. Tamaoki J, Kohri K, Isono K, et al. Inhaled indomethacin in bronchorrhea in bronchioloalveolar carcinoma: Role of cyclooxygenase. Chest 2000;117:1213-1214.
58. Nakajima T, Terashima T, Nishida J, et al. Treatment of bronchorrhea by corticosteroids in a case of bronchioloalveolar carcinoma producing CA19-9. Intern Med 2002;41:225-228.
59. Hidaka N, Nagao K. Bronchioloalveolar carcinoma accompanied by severe bronchorrhea. Chest 1996;110:281-282.
60. Krawtz SM, Mehta AC, Vijayakumar S, et al. Palliation of massive bronchorrhea. Chest 1988;94:1313-1314.
61. Suga T, Sugiyama Y, Fujii T, et al. Bronchioloalveolar carcinoma with bronchorrhea treated with erythromycin. Eur Respir J 1994;7:2249-2251.
62. Tamaoki J, Chitotani A, Kobayashi K, et al. Effect of indomethacin on bronchorrhea in patients with chronic bronchitis, diffuse panbronchiolitis, or bronchiectasis. Am Rev Respir Dis 1992;145:548-552.

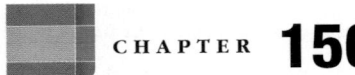

CHAPTER **156**

Delirium and Psychosis

Pierre R. Gagnon and Michel Ouellette

KEY POINTS

- Delirium is a mental disorder characterized by disturbance in consciousness and attention, as an essential feature, associated with any psychiatric symptoms, particularly cognitive, behavioral, and perceptual disturbances.
- Systematic detection, ideally using a validated instrument, is warranted because of the high prevalence of delirium among palliative care patients.
- Family members and caregivers can help to detect first signs of delirium, and they need rapid supportive interventions.
- Recognizing risk and etiologic factors is crucial, including deliriogenic medications (e.g., opioids, benzodiazepines, corticosteroids, anticholinergics).
- In addition to implementing nonpharmacological interventions and correcting underlying causes when possible, typical and atypical antipsychotics remain the mainstay of treatment.

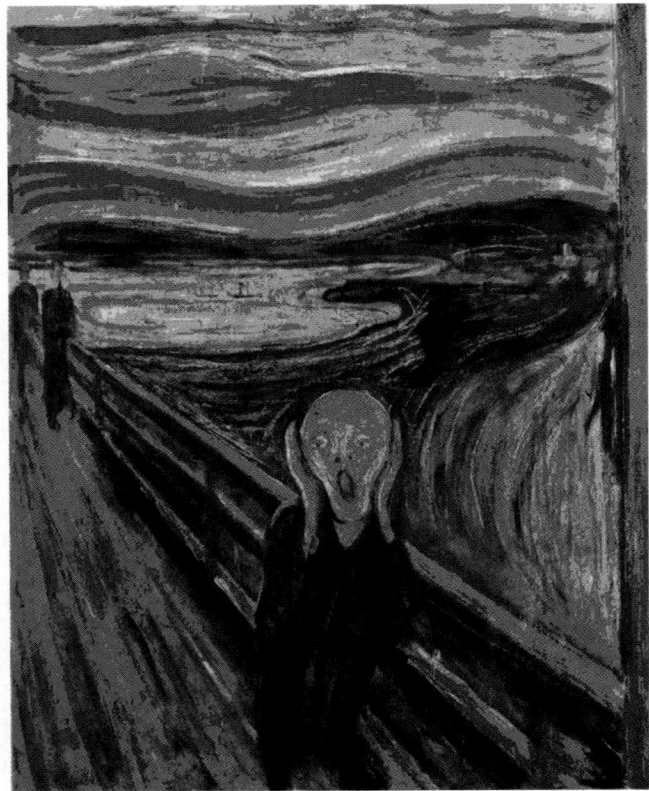

FIGURE 156-1 "The Scream" by Edvard Munch (1893).

DEFINITION

Delirium, or acute confusion, is a complex neuropsychiatric syndrome with many causes. It is characterized by alterations in consciousness and attention associated with cognitive (e.g., amnesia), behavioral (e.g., agitation), and perceptual (e.g., hallucinations) disturbances[1] (Fig. 156-1) Other clinical features include sleep-wake cycle disturbance, delusions, emotional lability, and psychomotor activity disturbance.[2,3]

Typically, delirium fluctuates during the day and cannot be accounted for by a preexisting or evolving dementia. Delirium is common among palliative care patients, particularly the terminally ill.[4] Even the hypoactive subtype[5] is highly distressing for most delirious patients, their families, and the caregivers. It negatively affects the quality of life of the patient and family members and interferes with the recognition and control of other physical and psychological symptoms.[6,7] Unfortunately, delirium is frequently underrecognized or misdiagnosed and therefore inappropriately treated or untreated (see "Common Errors"). The symptoms are diverse and sometimes mistaken for other psychiatric problems, such as mood or anxiety disorders[8] (see Chapters 66, 151, and 157).

EPIDEMIOLOGY, PREVALENCE, AND RISK FACTORS

Studies have confirmed the high prevalence of delirium in palliative care, ranging from 25% at admission to 85% in the last weeks of life.[9] Regarding delirium symptoms and formal diagnosis, a prospective study[10] using validated screening and diagnostic instruments for terminal cancer

Common Errors

- Misdiagnosis
- Differentiating delirious agitation from akathisia
- Differentiating delirious agitation from anxiety
- Hypoactive delirium versus depression
- Use of delirium worsening medication (e.g., benzodiazepine)
- Not increasing the antipsychotic according to poor response
- Not providing enough support and psycho-education to family members

patients revealed a prevalence at admission of 20% and 13%, respectively, and incidence during stay of 52% and 33%, respectively.

Risk increases with a history of delirium, severe medical illness, and poor physical functioning. Other major risk factors include brain lesions associated with a primary tumor, metastases, or other brain parenchymal lesions (e.g., meningeal carcinomatosis, abscess, hematoma). All drugs may cause delirium; the most important are narcotics, anticholinergics, sedatives, and corticosteroids.[11,12] Hydroelectrolytic and metabolic imbalances and concurrent diseases and conditions, including fecal impaction, environmental change, and sensory deprivation (i.e., hearing and vision), are other classic risk factors. Pure psychological stressors (e.g., not accepting a poor prognosis) are not sufficient to induce delirium because it is an organic encephalopathy, not a defense mechanism. However, these psychological stressors may theoretically contribute to delirium, augmenting demand on brain metabolism, although no empirical data supports this mechanism. Risk factors can be categorized according to whether they are predisposing or precipitating factors, although a combination may be present.[13] For example, urinary tract infection (i.e., precipitating factor) may cause delirium in preexisting cognitive impairment (i.e., predisposing factor) but not in the cognitively normal patient.[14] In palliative care, the putative underlying causes are limited, and it is often possible to reverse delirium by pharmacological or simpler interventions.[15]

PATHOPHYSIOLOGY

Little is known about the neuropathogenesis of delirium compared with its epidemiology, risk factors, and associated morbidity and mortality. Trepacz and Van der Mast[16] assert that certain neuroanatomical and neurotransmitter systems represent a final common neural pathway for the diverse causes of delirium. Particular brain regions, especially on the right side, are putatively implicated. Hypotheses of the central role of the hypothalamus have been posited.[17] Reduced cholinergic function, excess dopamine release, and decreased and increased serotonergic activity may underlie the different symptoms of delirium.[16] Delirium or depression may result from direct and indirect brain cytokine effects.[18]

Neuroimaging suggests that disruption to the frontal cortex, anteromedial portion of the thalamus, right basal ganglia, right posterior parietal cortex, and mesial-basal temporal-occipital cortex are important. These findings are consistent with delirium models that involve disruption of brain attentional systems, including those responsible for arousal. This final common pathway may explain core symptoms (i.e., disorientation, cognitive deficits, sleep-wake cycle disturbance, disorganized thinking, and language abnormalities), whereas others (i.e., delusions, hallucinations, illusions, and affective lability) may depend on the cause of the delirium (Fig. 156-2; see "Case Study: Delirium").

CLINICAL MANIFESTATIONS

The definition and concept of delirium lack clear boundaries,[10] but disturbance of consciousness is essential. Breitbart and Strout[19] describe prodromal symptoms (i.e., restlessness, anxiety, sleep disturbances, and irritability); a rapidly fluctuating course; affective symptoms (i.e., emotional lability, sadness, anger, or euphoria); reduced attention; increased or decreased psychomotor activity; sleep-wake cycle disruption, altered perceptions (i.e., misperceptions, illusions, or hallucinations); disorganized thinking and incoherent speech; disorientation to time, place, or person; and memory impairment. The fourth edition of the *Diagnostic and Statistical Manual of Mental Disorders,* text revision (DSM-IV-TR), criteria for delirium are provided in Box 156-1.

Three subtypes of delirium are based on arousal levels and psychomotor behavior.[3,4] Hyperactive delirium (i.e., agitated or hyperalert) manifests with hallucinations, agitation, delusions, and disorientation, and it is readily discernible. In contrast, the hypoactive type (i.e., lethargic or hypoalert) is characterized by decreased consciousness with somnolence, which may be mistaken for retarded depression.[20] The mixed form also may be difficult to recognize, with alternating features of the agitated and quiet

CASE STUDY

Delirium

A 74-year-old man is admitted for acute behavioral changes, lack of judgment, depressive features, and irritability after chemotherapy for lung cancer. He has no psychiatric history and does not drink alcohol. The mental examination reveals no agitation, and he is oriented to time, place, and person. Attention and concentration show some deficits; he is not able to tell the months backward or count from 20 to 0 without stopping and forgetting the task. He can recall one of five items after 2 minutes. He cannot explain why he is in the hospital. He does not feel at ease in the hospital and complains that his pain is not under control. His affect is anxious and his mood dysphoric; he maintains that he would rather die than go through this situation. He knows he has a cancer with a poor prognosis. His speech is slightly rambling and disorganized. He thinks he heard someone talking about him in the corridor, and he did not like it.

A diagnosis of delirium is made. He is started on haloperidol (1 mg at 5 PM and 2 mg at bedtime, in addition to 2 mg SC as needed every hour if agitated). Because there is no adequate surveillance by the family or the unit staff, a companion is recommended for the first 24 hours to avoid involuntary injury through lack of judgment or suicidal gesture. Opioid rotation is undertaken to improve pain management and delirium.

Computed tomography reveals multiple brain metastases. Dexamethasone is started to reduce brain edema. Haloperidol was increased to 5 mg at 5 PM and 10 mg at bedtime, in addition to 5 mg given subcutaneously as needed every hour if he is agitated, by day 3. The delirium improved. He felt calmer and less dysphoric, and he had better thinking processes. Pain was controlled by day 5. On day 7, he became agitated, and akathisia was diagnosed. Because the delirium was resolved, haloperidol was stopped, and lorazepam and propranolol were added to manage the akathisia. On day 12, although he reported being more comfortable physically and the akathisia was reduced by 80%, the staff complained that he had become irritable, wandered in the hospital, and stated that he was cured and that some nurses offered to go out with him. He had a clear sensorium with no significant attentional deficit; he was oriented but grandiose and delusional. A diagnosis of mania with psychotic features resulting from dexamethasone and brain metastases was made. A 24-hour companion was recommended. Quetiapine (started at 25 mg twice daily, titrated up to 300 mg within a week) was started to avoid a recurrence of akathisia with other antipsychotics, and lorazepam and propranolol were tapered off. He improved before developing severe dyspnea and died a few days later.

types. As suggested by Ross,[21] each of the subtypes may be related to particular causes.

SCREENING: DIAGNOSTIC INSTRUMENTS

Delirium Screening

In clinical practice, screening and brief cognitive function instruments are more often used than formal diagnostic instruments, which require specific training and which are

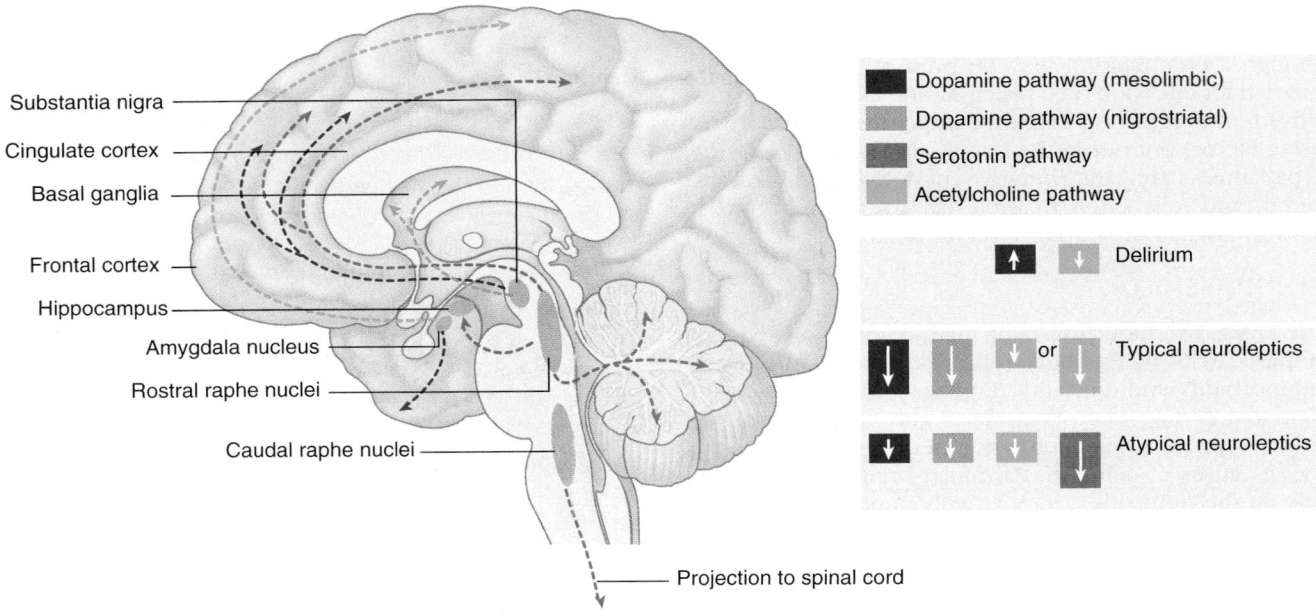

Substantia nigra
Cingulate cortex
Basal ganglia
Frontal cortex
Hippocampus
Amygdala nucleus
Rostral raphe nuclei
Caudal raphe nuclei

Dopamine pathway (mesolimbic)
Dopamine pathway (nigrostriatal)
Serotonin pathway
Acetylcholine pathway

Delirium

Typical neuroleptics

Atypical neuroleptics

Projection to spinal cord

FIGURE 156-2 Pathophysiology and treatment of delirium.

Box 156-1 Diagnostic Criteria for Delirium

Delirium due to a general medical condition (F05.0 [293.00])*

A. Disturbance of consciousness (i.e., reduced clarity of awareness of the environment) with reduced ability to focus, sustain, or shift attention
B. A change in cognition (e.g., memory deficit, disorientation, language disturbance) or the development of a perceptual disturbance that is not better accounted for by a preexisting, established, or evolving dementia
C. The disturbance develops over a short period (usually hours to days) and tends to fluctuate during the course of the day.
D. There is evidence of history, physical examination, or laboratory findings that the disturbance is caused by the direct physiological consequences of a general medical condition.

*DSM-IV-TR codes.
From American Psychiatric Association (APA). Diagnostic and Statistical Manual of Mental Disorders, 4th ed, text revision. Washington, DC: American Psychiatric Association, 2000.

more cumbersome to use. The Mini-Mental State Examination (MMSE)[22] has become one of the most frequently used neuropsychological tests in clinical evaluation of delirium. The "Blessed Orientation Memory Concentration" test (BOMC)[23] is much more convenient to use in palliative care settings than the MMSE and has equivalent psychometric properties.[24] The Confusion Rating Scale (CRS)[25] evaluates the presence and intensity of four distinct symptoms (disorientation, inappropriate behavior, inappropriate communication, illusions or hallucinations) potentially indicative of delirium, using a numerical scale ranging from 0 (no symptom) to 2 (symptom present and pronounced). The Nursing Delirium Screening Scale (Nu-DESC)[26] is a five-item scale based on the CRS, taking into account psychological and psychomotor retardation in order to also detect hypo-

active delirium. These instruments are easy to integrate into busy clinical practice and are validated with cancer patients.[10,26] The sensitivity and specificity of the Nu-DESC are 86% and 87%, respectively. Other screening instruments include NEECHAM Confusion Scale[27] and the Delirium Observation Screening Scale (DOSS)[28] for screening high-risk elderly hospitalized patients.

Diagnostic Instruments

The Confusion Assessment Method (CAM) is an instrument often used in clinical research. It is easy to use, although it may require adaptation to palliative care patients.[29] The Confusion Assessment Method for the Intensive Care Unit (CAM-ICU)[30] can detect delirium reliably and with high sensitivity and specificity. It is easy to use, takes only 2 to 3 minutes to perform, and requires minor training. The Delirium Rating Scale (DRS)[31] is easy to administer and is one of the most frequently used instruments for the assessment of delirium. The DRS also rates symptom severity.[31] The Memorial Delirium Assessment Scale (MDAS)[32] is a brief interview (approximately 10 minutes) by a trained rater and permits repeated administration within 24 hours and severity rating.

DIFFERENTIAL DIAGNOSIS

In palliative care, dementia is less prevalent but usually easily diagnosed based on a history of gradual cognitive decline and absence of clouding of consciousness or attention deficit (see Chapter 204). Dementia predisposes to delirium, which is phenomenologically similar in patients with or without dementia (although demented patients may have more symptoms).[33]

Agitated depression may have cognitive disturbance, delusion, poor concentration, and fitful sleep; retarded depression may mimic hypoactive delirium, with slowed thinking, decreased concentration and memory impair-

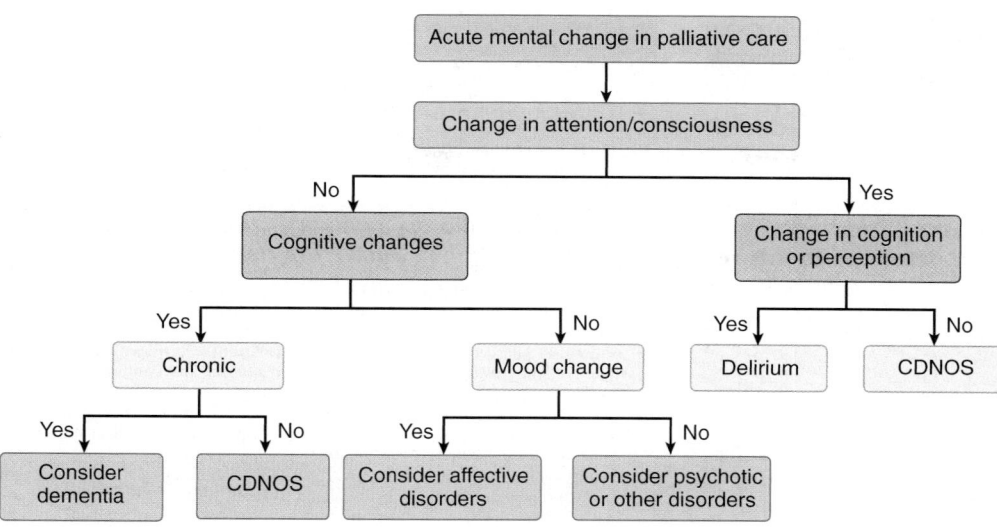

FIGURE 156-3 Diagnosis of delirium according to the *Diagnostic and Statistical Manual of Mental Disorders* (DSM-IV-TR). CDNOS, cognitive disorder not otherwise specified.

ment. In depression, the clues are previous episodes and a predominance of depressive feeling.[34] Manic episodes share some features with delirium, particularly the hyperactive or mixed subtype.

Early delirium can be misdiagnosed as psychosis, anxiety, or anger.[35] For the major functional psychoses, such as schizophrenia or bipolar disorder, the history is crucial. Organic psychosis, often resulting from the same causes as delirium, manifests with prominent delusions or hallucinations without clouding of consciousness or attentional deficit, the essential feature of delirium. The psychosis can be a substance-induced psychotic disorder with delusions (DSM-IV code 292.11) or with hallucinations (292.12), specifying whether onset was during intoxication or during withdrawal or caused by a general medical condition with delusions (293.81) or with hallucinations (293.82). A functional brief psychotic disorder (298.9) is also possible when an organic factor cannot be identified.

Delirium should be considered in anyone showing cognitive function disturbances, altered attention, fluctuating consciousness, or acute agitation.[3] Electrophysiology can be useful in borderline cases, for which a clearly abnormal electroencephalogram (e.g., diffuse slowing) suggests delirium and an organic cause (Fig. 156-3).

TREATMENT

The mainstay of therapy remains the diagnosis and treatment of conditions precipitating or perpetuating the delirium. Medications, particularly opioids, benzodiazepines, anticholinergics, and corticosteroids, should be reduced or discontinued when possible.[34,36] Nonpharmacologic interventions, such as a structured and familiar environment that helps reduce anxiety and disorientation, are essential but often neglected (Fig. 156-4).[37] Antipsychotics should be prescribed routinely, because even in hypoactive delirium, they may reduce cognitive dysfunction,[38] diminish psychological suffering, and prevent a hyperactive form.

Drugs

Antipsychotic drugs should be given in the lowest doses necessary to improve mental status. Central nervous

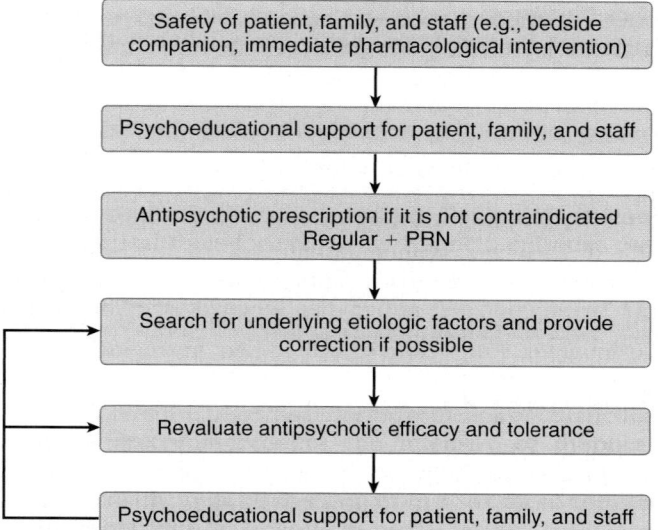

FIGURE 156-4 Management of delirium symptoms.

system depressant drugs (e.g., benzodiazepines, barbiturates) should be avoided to manage symptoms because they can worsen delirium; they are useful in alcohol or benzodiazepine withdrawal. They are sometimes used in emergencies when the goal is sedation and the antipsychotic response is slow. The choice of a neuroleptic is often made by considering prominent symptoms and the side effect profile and possible routes of administration. Empirical data are lacking to support one medication over the others. Many case series on atypical neuroleptics have been published, but the impossibility or lack of experience with the subcutaneous route limits their use. Medications useful in delirium are listed in Table 156-1.

Antipsychotics can be given once daily at bedtime, although the total dose in Table 156-1 can also be divided during the day according to the circadian variation of symptoms. Because symptoms often start during the evening and worsen at night, a common practice is to administer one third of the dose at dinner and two thirds at bedtime. Treat-

TABLE 156-1 Medication Useful in Managing Delirium in Patients with Advanced Disease

GENERIC NAME	APPROXIMATE DAILY DOSAGE RANGE	ROUTE
TYPICAL NEUROLEPTICS		
Haloperidol	0.5-20 mg	PO, IV, SC, IM
Chlorpromazine	12.5-100 mg	PO, IV, IM
Methotrimeprazine	12.5-100 mg	PO, SC, IM, IV
ATYPICAL NEUROLEPTICS		
Olanzapine	2.5-20 mg	PO, IM
Risperidone	1-6 mg	PO
Quetiapine	25-400 mg	PO
BENZODIAZEPINES		
Lorazepam	0.5-8.0 mg	PO, IV, IM, SC, SL
Midazolam	30-100 mg	IV, SC
ANESTHETICS		
Propofol	10-70 mg every hour up to 200-400 mg/H	IV

Data from References 8, 9, 40-42.

ment usually is initiated with a high-potency, dopamine-blocking agent (e.g., haloperidol, risperidone, olanzapine), which is titrated according to response and tolerance. When reaching maximum dosage, one option is to add or to switch to a more sedative antipsychotic (e.g., quetiapine, methotrimeprazine) rather than a benzodiazepine, which may worsen the cognitive deficit.

Supportive Care

Delirium often leads to a significant family distress. These caregivers can help detect early symptoms and warn medical staff so rapid supportive interventions can be made to improve their competence and lessen their burden. Such an intervention, based on psychological education by bedside nurses with a brochure explaining delirium, has been developed and tested.[39] Coordination with other team members and the support and education of staff are crucial.

CONTROVERSIES AND RESEARCH OPPORTUNITIES

Treatment is still largely based on information from case series and individual experience, with a lack of randomized, placebo-controlled trials. The role of nonpharmacological interventions in palliative care required further delineation.

Research is needed to determine whether different delirium subtypes or causes are responsive to different treatments. More should be known about which preventive interventions are effective for palliative care patients.

REFERENCES

1. Lipowski ZJ. Delirium (acute confusional states). JAMA 1987;258:1789-1792.
2. American Psychiatric Association (APA). Diagnostic and Statistical Manual of Mental Disorders, 4th ed, text revision (DSM-IV-TR). Washington, DC: American Psychiatric Association, 2000.
3. Lipowski ZJ. Delirium: Acute Confusional States. New York: Oxford University Press, 1990.
4. Trepacz PT, Teague GB, Lipowski ZJ. Delirium and other organic mental disorders in a general hospital. Gen Hosp Psychiatry 1985;7:101-106.
5. Breitbart W. Spirituality and meaning-centered group psychotherapy interventions in advanced cancer. Support Care Cancer 2001;10:272-280.
6. Bruera E, Fainsinger RL, Miller MJ, Kuehn N. The assessment of pain intensity in patients with cognitive failure: A preliminary report. J Pain Symptom Manage 1992;7:267-270.
7. Coyle N, Breitbart W, Weaver S, Portenoy R. Delirium as a contributing factor to "crescendo" pain: Three case reports. J Pain Symptom Manage 1994;9:44-47.
8. Breitbart W, Cohen K. Delirium in the terminally ill. In Chochinov HM, Breitbart W (eds). Handbook of Psychiatry in Palliative Medicine. New York: Oxford University Press, 2000, pp 75-90.
9. Massie MJ, Holland J, Glass E. Delirium in terminally ill cancer patients. Am J Psychiatry 1983;140:1048-1050.
10. Gagnon P, Allard P, Masse B, DeSerres M. Delirium in terminal cancer: A prospective study using daily screening, early diagnosis, and continuous monitoring. J Pain Symptom Manage 2000;19:412-426.
11. Han L, McCusker J, Cole M, et al. Use of medications with anticholinergic effect predicts clinical severity of delirium symptoms in older medical inpatients. Arch Intern Med 2001;161:1099-1105.
12. Gaudreau JD, Gagnon P, Roy MA, et al. Association between psychoactive medications and delirium in hospitalized patients: A critical review. Psychosomatics 2005;46:302-316.
13. Inouye SK, Bogardus ST Jr, Charpentier PA, et al. A multicomponent intervention to prevent delirium in hospitalized older patients. N Engl J Med 1999;340:669-676.
14. Burns A, Gallagley A, Byrne J. Delirium. J Neurol Neurosurg Psychiatry 2004;75:362-367.
15. Lawlor PG, Gagnon P, Mancini IL, et al. Occurrence, causes, and outcome of delirium in patients with advanced cancer: A prospective study. Arch Intern Med 2000;160:786-794.
16. Trepacz PT, Van der Mast RC. Pathophysiology of delirium. In Rockwood JL, MacDonald A (eds). Delirium in Old Age. Oxford, UK: Oxford University Press, 2002, pp 51-90.
17. Gaudreau JD, Gagnon P. Psychotogenic drugs and delirium pathogenesis: The central role of the thalamus. Med Hypotheses 2005;64:471-475.
18. Broadhurst C, Wilson K. Immunology of delirium: New opportunities for treatment and research. Br J Psychiatry 2001;179:288-289.
19. Breitbart W, Strout D. Delirium in the terminally ill. Clin Geriatr Med 2000;16:357-372.
20. Casarett DJ, Inouye SK. Diagnosis and management of delirium near the end of life. Ann Intern Med 2001;135:32-40.
21. Ross CA. CNS arousal systems: Possible role in delirium. Int Psychogeriatr 1991;3:353-371.
22. Folstein MF, Folstein SE, McHugh PR. "Mini-mental state." A practical method for grading the cognitive state of patients for the clinician. J Psychiatr Res 1975;12:189-198.
23. Katzman R, Brown T, Fuld P, et al. Validation of a short Orientation-Memory-Concentration Test of cognitive impairment. Am J Psychiatry 1983;140:734-739.
24. Fillenbaum GG, Heyman A, Wilkinson WE, Haynes CS. Comparison of two screening tests in Alzheimer's disease. The correlation and reliability of the Mini-Mental State Examination and the modified Blessed test. Arch Neurol 1987;44:924-927.
25. Williams MA. Delirium/acute confusional states: Evaluation devices in nursing. Int Psychogeriatr 1991;3:301-308.
26. Gaudreau JD, Gagnon P, Harel F, et al. Fast, systematic, and continuous delirium assessment in hospitalized patients: The nursing delirium screening scale. J Pain Symptom Manage 2005;29:368-375.
27. Neelon VJ, Champagne MT, Carlson J, Funk S. The NEECHAM Confusion Scale: Construction, validation and clinical testing. Nurs Res 1996;45:324-330.
28. Schuurmans MJ, Shortridge-Bagget LM, Duursma SA. The Delirium Observation Screening Scale: A screening instrument for delirium. Res Theory Nurs Pract 2003;17:31-50.
29. Inouye SK, van Dyck CH, Alessi CA, et al. Clarifying confusion: The confusion assessment method. A new method for detection of delirium. Ann Intern Med 1990;113:941-948.
30. Ely EW, Margolin R, Francis J, et al. Evaluation of delirium in critically ill patients: Validation of the Confusion Assessment Method for the Intensive Care Unit (CAM-ICU). Crit Care Med 2001;29:1370-1379.
31. Trepacz PT, Baker RW, Greenhouse J. A symptom rating scale for delirium. Psychiatry Res 1988;23:89-97.
32. Breitbart W, Rosenfeld B, Roth A, et al. The Memorial Delirium Assessment Scale. J Pain Symptom Manage 1997;13:128-137.
33. Cole MG, McCusker J, Dendukuri N, Han L. Symptoms of delirium among elderly medical inpatients with or without dementia. J Neuropsychiatry Clin Neurosci 2002;14:167-175.
34. Cole MG. Delirium in elderly patients. Am J Geriatr Psychiatry 2004;12:7-21.
35. Breitbart W, Chochinov HM, Passik SD. Psychiatric aspects of palliative care. In Doyle D, Hanks GWC, MacDonald N (eds). Oxford Handbook of Palliative Medicine, 2nd ed. New York: Oxford University Press, 1998, pp 933-954.

36. Friedlander MM, Brayman Y, Breitbart W. Delirium in palliative care. Oncology 2004;18:1541-1550.
37. Winell J, Roth AJ. Psychiatric assessment and symptom management in elderly cancer patients. Oncology 2005;19:1479-1490.
38. Platt MM, Breitbart W, Smith M, et al. Efficacy of neuroleptics for hypoactive delirium. J Neuropsychiatry Clin Neurosci 1994;6:66-67.
39. Gagnon P, Charbonneau C, Allard P, et al. Delirium in advanced cancer: A psychoeducational intervention for family caregivers. J Palliat Care 2002; 18:253-261.
40. Breitbart W, Marotta R, Platt MM, et al. A double-blind trial of haloperidol, chlorpromazine, and lorazepam in the treatment of delirium in hospitalized AIDS patients. Am J Psychiatry 1996;153:231-237.
41. Fleishman SB, Lesko LM, Breitbart W. Treatment of organic mental disorders in cancer patients. In Breitbart W, Holland JC (eds). Psychiatric Aspects of Symptom Management in Cancer Patients. Washington, DC: American Psychiatric Press, 1993.
42. Sipahimalani A, Masand PS. Olanzapine in the treatment of delirium. Psychosomatics 1998;39:422-429.

SUGGESTED READING

Caraceni A, Grassi L. Diagnostic assessment. In Caraceni A, Grassi L (eds). Delirium: Acute Confusional States in Palliative Medicine. New York: Oxford University Press, 2003.

Smith MJ, Breitbart WS, Platt MM. A critique of instruments and methods to detect, diagnose, and rate delirium. J Pain Symptom Manage 1995;10:35-77.

Trepacz PT, Van der Mast RC. Pathophysiology of delirium. In Rockwood JL, MacDonald A (eds). Delirium in Old Age. Oxford, UK: Oxford University Press, 2002, pp 51-90.

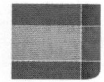

CHAPTER **157**

Depression

Susan E. McClement and Harvey Max Chochinov

KEY POINTS

- The diagnosis and treatment of depression in the terminally ill poses unique challenges.

- The sadness and anticipatory mourning experienced in a terminal illness may obfuscate the clinician's ability to differentiate existential distress from clinical depression.

- Concern about medication side effects in the severely ill may cause clinicians to be conservative in prescribing antidepressants.

- Psychological and pharmacological interventions are effective and should be combined.

- The patient's relationship with the primary medical caregiver may be the most important psychotherapeutic tool for many depressed patients.

Depression is a common problem in palliative care patients, and it tends to be underdiagnosed and undertreated.[1] Sadness and anticipatory mourning in a patient with a terminal illness may obfuscate the clinician's ability to differentiate existential distress from clinical depression. Because depression can undermine quality of life and fracture the capacity for pleasure, meaning, and connection, clinicians must be skilled in this important area (see Chapters 8 and 12). This chapter describes depression in

palliative care populations, aiming to increasing clinicians' competence and confidence in managing this prevalent issue.

BASIC SCIENCE

Structures within the limbic system such as the hypothalamus, amygdala, and hippocampus probably regulate emotions and behavior.[2] Neurotransmitters denote neurochemical messages, which convey reactions and emotions by means of neurons from one cell to another. When received by certain receptors, these neurotransmitters stop or are changed into electrical impulses. In both instances, neurotransmitters are released from their receptor sites and float back into the synapse.[2] After reuptake, they are catabolized by monoamine oxidase. The major brain neurotransmitters believed to regulate emotions and stress reaction and that are linked to depression include serotonin, norepinephrine, and dopamine.[2]

EPIDEMIOLOGY AND PREVALENCE

Variable rates of depression in palliative care settings range from 3.7% to 58%,[3] with the best estimate of prevalence of operationally defined major depression at 15%.[4] The variability has been attributed to heterogeneity in the definitions used and the populations examined.[4] Although palliative care has historically centered on patients with advanced cancer, there is increasing recognition of the need for palliative services for patients with diseases other than cancer. The rates of depression experienced by people with other types of life-limiting illnesses are given in Table 157-1.[5]

GENETICS

Evidence supports the heritability of lifetime major depression,[6] with recurrence and early age at onset characterizing those at greatest familial risk.[1] Epidemiological studies suggest response to environmental insults such as stress is moderated by genetic makeup.[7] Genetic influences may be more important in women than in men.[1,6]

PATHOPHYSIOLOGY

The exact mechanisms of depression are not understood. Altered synaptic transmission is implicated. Nerves com-

TABLE 157-1 Prevalence of Depression Associated with Various Disorders and Diseases

DISEASE OR DISORDER	PREVALENCE OF DEPRESSION
Cancer	1.5-50% of patients
Coronary artery disease	16-23% of patients
Parkinson's disease	Up to 50% of patients
Alzheimer's dementia	20-32% of patients
Stroke	19% among hospitalized patients; 23% among ambulatory patients
Multiple sclerosis	Up to 50% of patients
Huntington's disease	Up to 32% of patients
Diabetes (type 1 and 2)	15-32% of patients

Adapted from Rodin GM, Nolan RP, Katz MR. Depression. In Levenson JL (ed). Textbook of Psychosomatic Medicine. Washington, DC: American Psychiatric Publishing, 2005, pp 193-217.

municate with one another through neurotransmitter synthesis, storage, release, and induction of cellular responses. Disrupted function anywhere in this chemical process may underlie depression.[8]

The monoamine hypothesis postulates that depression occurs because of functional deficiencies of the brain's monoaminergic transmitters (e.g., norepinephrine, dopamine, 5-hydroxytryptamine [5-HT]). Research findings for monoamine transmitters in postmortem brain tissue and bodily fluids, reduced 5-HT function, and monoamine depletion have been inconsistent, suggesting the pathophysiology is not linked solely to monoamine mechanisms.[8]

The neurogenesis hypothesis postulates a link between low rates of neuronal regeneration in the hippocampus and depression. Adult neurogenesis fluctuates with environmental factors, including chronic stress, which correlates with altered hippocampal morphology. Antidepressants increase neurogenesis in the hippocampus, suggesting they act through reversal or prevention of decreased neurogenesis.[8]

Cytokines have been implicated in depression in cancer patients. Research suggests associations among inflammatory cytokines, cachexia, and depressive symptoms, although the mechanism requires further explication[9] (see "Case Study: Managing Depression").

CLINICAL MANIFESTATIONS

Laboratory tests may determine whether depression is caused by endocrine or other physical disorders. However, no specific laboratory test exists; there is no standardized tool for diagnosing or treating depression. Risk factors for depression include a history of depression, age (i.e., young adult), female gender, impaired functional status, perceived inadequate social support, uncontrolled pain, and stress.[1,6] In oncology palliative care populations, certain malignancies (e.g., brain tumors, head and neck cancers, retroperitoneal tumors) and medications (e.g., steroids vincristine, interferon, interleukin, intrathecal methotrexate) are also thought to be risk factors[10] (Fig 157-1).

 C A S E   S T U D Y

Managing Depression

Jane was 37 years old when she first presented to her physician with what was thought to be an ectopic pregnancy. Emergency surgery, however, revealed the unexpected diagnosis of ovarian cancer. Extensive gynecological surgery—including a bilateral oophorectomy and hysterectomy—left her feeling emotionally and physically depleted. Over several weeks, her mood shifted into persistent sadness, with sleep and appetite disturbances, suicidal ideation, and several serious suicide attempts. A marked feature was prominent self-deprecation. She felt she was unworthy of the time people were taking offering her psychiatric care, and she was focused on giving away her worldly possessions in preparation for her self-inflicted death.

Jane's history and extensive treatment were complex and included inpatient compulsory psychiatric hospitalization, electroconvulsive therapy, and a combination of antidepressants that put her depression into remission. Her treatment for the gynecological malignancy was successful, and depression never recurred.

Standard screening instruments such as the self-report Hospital Anxiety and Depression Scale (HADS) for mood disorder and the Mini-Mental State Examination (MMSE) or Mental Status Schedule (MSS) for cognitive impairment help screen for depression and establish baseline information to measure progress.[1,3-5] Because of the lack of sensitivity and specificity, these instruments should not replace assessment by interview, which remains the gold standard for detection.[3] The single-item screening question (Are you depressed most of the time?) evaluated by Chochinov and colleagues[11] in a cohort of terminally ill cancer patients is a reliable and accurate screen and brief enough for routine administration to the medically ill.

For diagnosis of major depression, the fourth edition of the *Diagnostic and Statistical Manual of Mental Disorders* (DSM-IV)[12] requires five of nine symptoms for 2 consecutive weeks that represent a change in the person's previous level of functioning (Table 157-2). One of the symptoms must be loss of interest or pleasure (anhedonia) or depressed mood.

To address the confounding influence of somatic symptoms in the medically ill when diagnosing depression, substitutive criteria have been proposed,[10] in which somatic symptoms from the DSM-IV criteria are removed and replaced with psychological features of depression, such as brooding, pessimism, and depressed appearance.

ASSOCIATED MEDICAL CONDITIONS

Depression has been associated with several medical conditions.[10] This relationship appears to be bidirectional, with many medical conditions believed to increase the risk, and depression increasing the risk of certain medical conditions (Table 157-3). Conditions to be considered in the differential diagnosis are described in Table 157-4.[13]

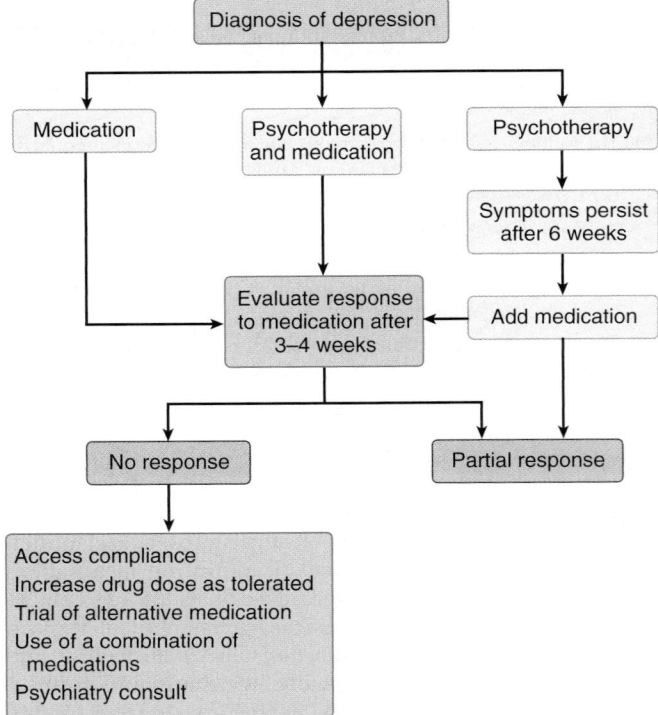

FIGURE 157-1 Diagnosis of depression.

TABLE 157-2   Diagnostic Features of Depression

CRITERIA FOR MAJOR DEPRESSIVE EPISODE

A. Five (or more) of the following symptoms have been present during the same 2-week period and represent a change from previous functioning; at least one of the symptoms is either (1) depressed mood or (2) loss of interest or pleasure

Note: Do not include symptoms that are clearly due to a general medical condition, or mood-incongruent delusions or hallucinations.

1. Depressed mood most of the day, nearly every day, as indicated by either subjective report (e.g., feels sad or empty) or observation made by others (e.g., appears tearful). **Note**: In children and adolescents, can be irritable mood.
2. Markedly diminished interest or pleasure in all, or almost all, activities most of the day, nearly every day (as indicated by either subjective account or observation made by others).
3. Significant weight loss when not dieting or weight gain (e.g., a change of more than 5% of body weight in a month), or decrease or increase in appetite nearly every day. **Note**: In children, consider failure to make expected weight gains.
4. Insomnia or hypersomnia nearly every day.
5. Psychomotor agitation or retardation nearly every day (observable by others, not merely subjective feelings of restlessness or being slowed down).
6. Fatigue or loss of energy nearly every day.
7. Feelings of worthlessness or excessive or inappropriate guilt (which may be delusional) nearly every day (not merely self-reproach or guilt about being sick).
8. Diminished ability to think or concentrate, or indecisiveness, nearly every day (either by subjective account or as observed by others).
9. Recurrent thoughts of death (not just fear of dying), recurrent suicidal ideation without a specific plan, or a suicide attempt or a specific plan for committing suicide.

B. The symptoms do not meet criteria for a Mixed Episode.
C. The symptoms cause clinically significant distress or impairment in social, occupational, or other important areas of functioning.
D. The symptoms are not due to the direct physiological effects of a substance (e.g., a drug of abuse, a medication) or a general medical condition (e.g., hypothyroidism).
E. The symptoms are not better accounted for by Bereavement, i.e., after the loss of a loved one, the symptoms persist for longer than 2 months or are characterized by marked functional impairment, morbid preoccupation with worthlessness, suicidal ideation, psychotic symptoms, or psychomotor retardation.

Reprinted with permission from American Psychiatric Association. Diagnostic and Statistical Manual of Mental Disorders, 4th ed. Washington, DC: American Psychiatric Association, 2000.

TABLE 157-3   Medical Conditions Associated with Depression

Endocrine abnormalities	Hyperthyroidism Hypothyroidism Adrenal dysfunction	Acromegaly Insulinoma Hypopituitarism
Neurological abnormalities	Parkinson's disease Alzheimer's disease Huntington's disease	Multiple sclerosis Cerebrovascular disorders
Metabolic disorders	Electrolyte disturbances Uremia	Wilson's disease Pernicious anemia
Cancers	Oat cell carcinoma Pancreatic carcinoma Central nervous system tumors	Leukemia Lymphoma
Infectious diseases	Infectious mononucleosis Hepatitis Tuberculosis Acquired immunodeficiency syndrome (AIDS)	Influenza Syphilis Encephalitis
Collagen vascular diseases	Systemic lupus erythematosus Giant cell arteritis	Rheumatoid arthritis

Adapted from Skakum K, Chochinov HM: Anxiety and depression. In MacDonald N, Oneschuk D, Hagen N, Doyle D (eds). Palliative Medicine: A Case-Based Manual. Oxford, UK: Oxford University Press, 2005.

TABLE 157-4   Differential Diagnosis of Depression

SOURCE OF DEPRESSION	EXAMPLES
Psychiatric disorder	Bereavement, adjustment disorders with depressed mood, bipolar disorder, anxiety disorder, somatization disorder, post-traumatic stress
Organic mental disorder	Delirium, neuroleptic-induced Parkinsonism, subcortical dementias, frontal lobe dysfunction
Neurologic disorder	Stroke, Parkinson's disease, multiple sclerosis, early dementia, sleep apnea, post-concussive syndrome
Neoplastic disorder	Disseminated carcinomatosis, pancreatic cancer
Medication	Steroids, metoclopramide, contraceptives, reserpine, alpha-methyldopa, anticholinesterases, insecticides, cimetidine, ranitidine, indomethacin, phenothiazine, thallium mercury, cyclosporin, vincristine, vinblastine, disulfiram
Drug withdrawal	Cocaine, amphetamines
Infection	Acquired immunodeficiency syndrome (AIDS), tuberculosis, viral pneumonia, viral hepatitis, infectious mononucleosis, tertiary syphilis
Endocrine or metabolic disorder	Hyperthyroidism, hypothyroidism, hyperparathyroidism, Cushing's syndrome, adrenal insufficiency
Collagen vascular disease	Fibromyalgia, systemic lupus erythematosus, rheumatoid arthritis
Nutritional disorder	Folate, niacin, thiamine, vitamin C and B_{12} deficiencies

From Cleveland Clinic. Available at http://www.clevlandclinicmeded.com/medicalpubs/diseasemanagement/psychiatry/delirium/delirium.htm (accessed April 5, 2006).

TREATMENT

Treatment of depressed patients with advanced illnesses usually consists of a combination of antidepressants and supportive psychotherapy.[1,3,5,10,14,15] Electroconvulsive therapy (ECT) is less commonly used. A flow chart for management is given in Figure 157-2.

Therapeutics

Pharmacological treatment should be based on available research regarding medication effectiveness, tolerability, and safety profile to minimize side effects and avoid drug interactions.[13] Antidepressants for use in patients with advanced disease and their side effects are described in Table 157-5.[16] Because of a better side effect profile, selective serotonin reuptake inhibitors (SSRIs), serotonin-norepinephrine reuptake inhibitors (SNRIs), and reversible inhibitors of monoamine oxidase A (RIMAs) are probably best suited for depressed palliative care patients[1,15] (Fig. 157-3).

Clinical Trials

Few randomized, controlled trials of interventions for depression in patients with advanced disease have been undertaken. Evidence on treatment efficacy must be extrapolated from research in those with less severe conditions and from expert opinion.[15,17] Future research needs to focus on the evaluation of pharmacological and psychotherapeutic interventions in palliative care populations.

Alternative Therapies and Common Errors

In addition to mainstream care, a plethora of therapies have emerged. Although not exhaustive, a list of alternative therapies frequently published in the literature is provided in Table 157-6.[18] Most have not been rigorously evaluated in randomized, controlled trials, and their potentials for harm or benefit are not fully understood.

Impeccable management of depression requires clinicians avoid common errors (see "Common Errors").

Nonpharmacological Measures and Supportive Care

Nonpharmacological psychotherapeutic interventions must be considered. The patient's relationship with the primary medical caregiver has been identified as the most important psychotherapeutic tool for many depressed patients, and it should not be underestimated.[5] Psychotherapeutic interventions aim to help patients understand and work through their feelings related to their disease and to help promote active coping strategies to maintain functional status.[1] These aims may be realized with group or mutual supportive therapy, and they may be augmented with techniques such as relaxation and guided imagery.[1]

EVIDENCE-BASED MEDICINE AND RESEARCH OPPORTUNITIES

Palliative care patients experiencing depression should be cared for according to the best available evidence. Within

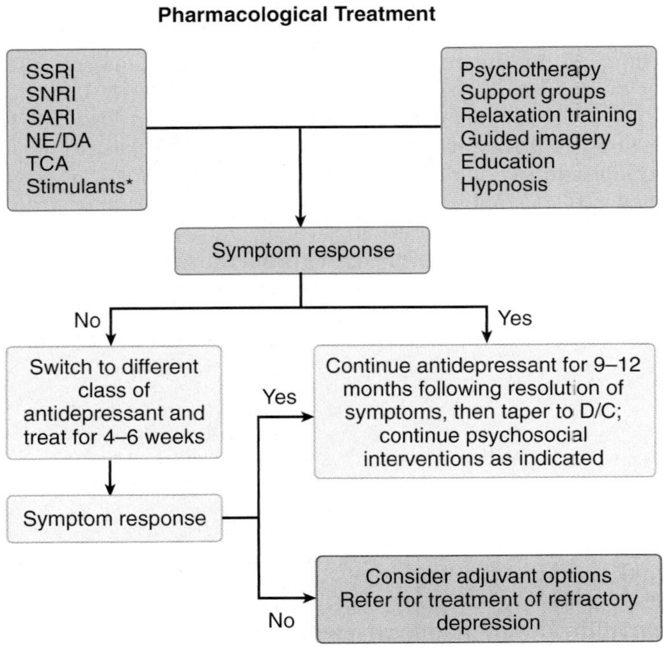

Pharmacological Treatment

```
┌─────────────┐                          ┌──────────────────┐
│ SSRI        │                          │ Psychotherapy    │
│ SNRI        │                          │ Support groups   │
│ SARI        │──────────────────────────│ Relaxation training │
│ NE/DA       │                          │ Guided imagery   │
│ TCA         │                          │ Education        │
│ Stimulants* │                          │ Hypnosis         │
└─────────────┘                          └──────────────────┘
                    │
            ┌───────────────────┐
            │ Symptom response  │
            └───────────────────┘
         No │                │ Yes
┌─────────────────┐   ┌─────────────────────────┐
│ Switch to       │   │ Continue antidepressant │
│ different class │Yes│ for 9–12 months         │
│ of antidepressant│──▶│ following resolution of │
│ and treat for   │   │ symptoms, then taper to │
│ 4–6 weeks       │   │ D/C; continue psychosocial│
└─────────────────┘   │ interventions as indicated│
         │            └─────────────────────────┘
┌─────────────────┐
│ Symptom response│
└─────────────────┘
         │ No
   ┌──────────────────────────┐
   │ Consider adjuvant options│
   │ Refer for treatment of   │
   │ refractory depression    │
   └──────────────────────────┘
```

*May be earlier consideration for patients with advanced disease

FIGURE 157-2   Management flow chart. D/C, therapy discontinued; NE/DA, norepinephrine or dopamine; SARI, serotonin antagonist reuptake inhibitors; SNRI, serotonin-norepinephrine reuptake inhibitor; SSRI. selective serotonin reuptake inhibitor; TCA, tricyclic antidepressants. *(Adapted from Abeloff MD, Armitage JO, Lichter AS, Niederhuber J. Clinical Oncology. 2nd ed. New York: Churchill Livingstone, 2000.)*

Common Errors

- Reluctance to inquire about presence of depression because of clinician's lack of time and skill and desire for emotional self-protection.
- Selective attention directed to physical versus psychological disclosures and concerns.
- Failing to recognize that the process of coping with a life-threatening illness may include anxiety, sadness, and grief and that these are normal responses and part of the adjustment process.
- Assuming emotional distress is inevitable and untreatable.
- Failure to ensure management of pain and other distressing symptoms.
- Failure to "start low and go slow" when prescribing antidepressant medications.

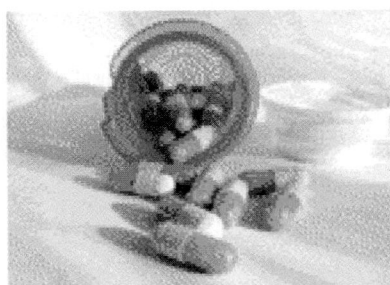

FIGURE 157-3   When planning the pharmacological management of depression, providers should consider medications' effectiveness, tolerability, and safety profile to minimize side effects and avoid drug interactions.

TABLE 157-5 Antidepressants Suggested for Use in Patients with Advanced Disease

MEDICATION	THERAPEUTIC ORAL DAILY DOSAGE (mg)	SIDE EFFECTS AND COMMENTS
Selective serotonin reuptake inhibitors (SSRIs)		SSRIs appear to have a more tolerable side effect profile than tricyclics
Fluoxetine	10-60	Long half-life of fluoxetine and potential drug-drug interactions
Fluvoxamine	50-300	Problematic (i.e., P450 enzyme system)
Paroxetine	10-60	
Sertraline	25-200	
Citalopram	10-60	
Monoamine oxidase inhibitors (MAOIs)		Orthostatic hypotension and insomnia
Isocarboxazid	20-40	In combination with opioids, may induce myoclonus and delirium
Phenelzine	30-60	Need to avoid tyramine-containing foods
Tranylcypromine	20-40	
Tricyclic antidepressants (TCAs)		Nausea, gastrointestinal upset, sexual dysfunction
Amitriptyline	25-125	Seriously ill patients may be particularly sensitive to anticholinergic effects of TCAs
Clomipramine	25-125	
Desipramine	25-125	
Doxepin	25-125	
Imipramine	25-125	
Nortriptyline	25-125	
Heterocyclic antidepressants		Extrapyramidal symptoms and tardive dyskinesia
Amoxapine	100-150	Decreased seizure threshold
Maprotiline	100-200	
Psychostimulants		Agitation, anxiety, insomnia
Dextroamphetamine	5-30	Drug of choice for those with markedly shortened life expectancy
Methylphenidate	5-30	
Pemoline	37.5-75	
Serotonin antagonist reuptake inhibitors (SARIs)		Sedation, orthostatic hypotension
Trazodone	50-200	May cause arrhythmia in patients with heart disease
Nefazodone	50-600	May cause priapism.
Norepinephrine dopamine modulators		Dry mouth, headache gastrointestinal upset, agitation, insomnia.
Bupropion	200-300	Increased risk of seizure in doses above 300 mg
Serotonin norepinephrine reuptake inhibitor (SNRI)		Headache, dry mouth, sedation, tremors
Venlafaxine	37.5-225	
Reversible inhibitors of monamine oxidase A		Dizziness, gastrointestinal upset, constipation, dry mouth, headache
Moclobemide	100-600	Cimetidine inhibits metabolism

Adapted from Lander M, Chochinov HM. Depression in the terminally ill. In Joishy S (ed). Palliative Medicine Secrets. Philadelphia: Hanley & Belfus, 1999, 181-184.

TABLE 157-6 Alternative Therapies

MEDICINES	PHYSICAL TREATMENTS	DIETARY	LIFESTYLE
Ginkgo biloba	Acupuncture	Avoidance of alcohol, sugar, and caffeine	Aromatherapy
Glutamine	Air ionization	Ingestion of omega-3 fatty acids	Bibliotherapy
Homeopathy	Light therapy		Dance and movement
Natural progesterone	Massage		Exercise
Phenylalanine			Meditation
S-adenosylmethionine (SAMe)			Music
St. John's wort			Pets
Selenium			Relaxation therapy
Tyrosine			Yoga
Folate			
B vitamins			
Vitamins D and E			

Adapted from Jorm AF, Christensen H, Griffiths KM, Rodgers B. Effectiveness of complementary and self-help treatments for depression. Med J Aust 2002;176(Suppl):S84-S96.

Box 157-1 Clinical Practice Guidelines for Quality Psychological and Psychiatric Care of Palliative Medicine Patients

- The interdisciplinary team includes professionals with patient-specific skill and training in the psychological consequences and psychiatric co-morbidities of serious illness for the patient and family, including depression, anxiety, delirium, and cognitive impairment.
- Regular, ongoing assessment of psychological reactions and psychiatric conditions occurs and is documented. Whenever possible, a validated and context-specific assessment tool should be used.
- Psychological assessment includes the patient's understanding of disease, symptoms, side effects, and their treatments and assessment of caregiving needs, capacity, and coping strategies.
- Psychological assessment includes the family's understanding of the illness and its consequences for the patient and the family and assessment of the family's caregiving capacities, needs, and coping strategies.
- The family is educated and supported to provide safe and appropriate psychological support measures to the patient.
- Pharmacological, nonpharmacological, and complementary therapies are employed in the treatment of psychological distress or psychiatric syndromes, as appropriate.
- Treatment alternatives are clearly documented and communicated and permit the patient and family to make informed choices.
- Response to symptom distress is prompt and tracked through documentation in the medical record. Regular re-evaluation of treatment efficacy occurs, and the preferences of the patient and family are documented.
- Referrals to health care professionals (e.g., psychiatrists, psychologists, social workers) with specialized skills in age-appropriate psychological and psychiatric management are made available when appropriate. Identified psychiatric co-morbidities are identified in the family or caregivers, who are referred for treatment.
- Developmentally appropriate assessment and support are provided to pediatric patients, their siblings, and the children or grandchildren of adult patients.
- Communication with children and cognitively impaired individuals occurs using verbal, nonverbal, or symbolic means appropriate to developmental stage and cognitive capacity.
- Treatment decisions are based on goals of care, assessment of risk and benefit, best evidence, and preferences of the patient and family. The goal is to address psychological needs, treat psychiatric disorders, promote adjustment, and support opportunities for emotional growth, healing, reframing, completion of unfinished business, and support through the bereavement period.
- A process for quality improvement and review of psychological and psychiatric assessment and effectiveness of treatment is documented and leads to change in clinical practice.

National Consensus Project for Quality Palliative Care. Clinical practice guidelines for quality palliative care. Brooklyn, NY: National Consensus Project for Quality Palliative Care, 2004.

TABLE 157-7 Areas of Needed Research

AREAS OF RESEARCH	EXAMPLES
Screening issues	Is training in diagnosing depression an alternative to screening instruments? How should issues that hamper uniform detection of symptom thresholds (e.g., language, personality, intraindividual or interindividual variations) be managed? How should the roles of specialized mental health professionals be defined in palliative care?
Educational issues	Given the dearth of mental health professionals in palliative care, how can education regarding detection and treatment of depression be best achieved? Who among nonpsychiatric members of the team should be trained in the management of depression, and what would be the most effective educational strategies?
Pharmacological treatment	Studies comparing pharmacological agents are limited. Factors hampering effective pharmacological treatment (i.e., physician and health care related) must be identified and targeted in intervention studies.
Nonpharmacological treatment	What constitutes success in the management of depression lacks definition. Sole reliance on quantitative approaches to evaluate psychotherapeutic interventions in existential distress may fail to capture complex care. The relative efficacy of empirically tested psychotherapeutic interventions in specific populations and cultural groups is unknown.

Adapted from Stiefel R, Die Trill M, Berney A, et al. Depression in palliative care: A pragmatic report from Expert Working Group of the European Association for Palliative Care. Support Care Cancer 2001;9:477-488.

CONCLUSIONS

Underdiagnosing and undertreating depression reduces the quality of life for terminally ill patients. Although clinical intervention cannot assuage all sadness experienced by palliative care patients, prompt recognition and proper treatment of depression can reduce suffering.

REFERENCES

1. Wilson K, Chochinov HM, de Faye BJ, et al. Diagnosis and management of depression in palliative care. In Chochinov HM, Breitbart W (eds). Handbook of Psychiatry in Palliative Medicine. Oxford, UK: Oxford University Press, 2000, pp 25-49.
2. Sadock B, Sadock VA (eds). Kaplan Sadock's Comprehensive Textbook of Psychiatry, 7th ed. Philadelphia: Lippincott Williams & Wilkins, 2000.
3. Stiefel R, Die Trill M, Berney A, et al. Depression in palliative care: A pragmatic report from Expert Working Group of the European Association for Palliative Care. Support Care Cancer 2001;9:477-488.
4. Hotopf M, Chidgey J, Addington-Hall J, Ly KL. Depression in advanced disease: A systematic review. Part 1. Prevalence and case finding. Palliat Med 2002;16:81-97.
5. Rodin GM, Nolan RP, Katz MR. Depression. In Levenson JL (ed). Textbook of Psychosomatic Medicine. Washington, DC: American Psychiatric Publishing, 2005, pp 193-217.
6. Kendler KS, Gatz M, Gardner DO, et al. A Swedish national twin study of lifetime major depression. Am J Psychiatry 2006;163:109-114.
7. Caspi A, Sugden K, Moffitt TE, et al. Influence of life stress on depression: Moderation by a polymorphism in the 5-HTT gene. Science 2003;301:386-389.
8. Bondy B. Pharmacogenomics in depression and antidepressants. Dialogoues Clin Neurosci 2005;7:223-230.

the limitations of extant data, the National Consensus Project for Quality Palliative Care[19] articulated clinical practice guidelines for the psychological and psychiatric aspects of care for these patients in 2004 (Box 157-1). Much research is needed in the areas of screening, education, and treatment (Table 157-7).

9. Illman J, Corringham R, Robinson D. Are inflammatory cytokines the common link between cancer-associated cachexia and depression? J Support Oncol 2005; 3:45-50.
10. Skakum K, Chochinov HM, Anxiety and depression. In MacDonald N, Oneschuk D, Hagen, N, Doyle D (eds). Palliative Medicine: A Case-Based Manual. Oxford, UK: Oxford University Press, 2005.
11. Chochinov HM, Wilson KG, Enns M, et al. "Are you depressed?" Screening for depression in the terminally ill. Am J Psychiatry 1997;154:674-676.
12. American Psychiatric Association. Diagnostic and Statistical Manual of Mental Disorders, 4th ed. Washington, DC: American Psychiatric Association, 1994.
13. Depression and associated medical conditions. Available at http://www.clevlandclinicmeded.com/medicalpubs/diseasemanagement/psychiatry/delirium/delirium.htm (accessed April 5, 2006).
14. Nieuwstraten C, Labris R, Holbrook A. Systematic overview of drug interactions with antidepressant medications. Can J Psychiatry 2006;51:300-315.
15. Ly KL, Chidgey J, Addington-Hall J, et al. Depression in palliative care: A systematic review. Part 2. Treatment. Palliat Med 2002;16:279-284.
16. Lander M, Chochinov HM. Depression in the terminally ill. In Joishy S (ed). Palliative Medicine Secrets. Philadelphia: Hanley & Belfus, 1999, pp 181-184.
17. McClement SE. Acquiring an evidence-base in palliative care: Challenges and future directions. Pharmacoeconomics and Outcomes Research 2006;6:37-40.
18. Jorm AF, Christensen H, Griffiths KM, Rodgers B. Effectiveness of complementary and self-help treatments for depression. Med J Aust 2002;176(Suppl):S84-S96.
19. National Consensus Project for Quality Palliative Care. Clinical practice guidelines for quality palliative care. Brooklyn, NY: National Consensus Project for Quality Palliative Care, 2004.

SUGGESTED READING

Block SD. Assessing and managing depression in the terminally ill patient. Ann Intern Med 2000;132:209-218.
Chochinov HM, Hack T, Hassard T, et al. Dignity therapy: A novel psychotherapeutic intervention for patients nearing death. J Clin Oncol 2005;23:5520-5525.
Lander M, Chochinov HM, Wilson K. Depression and the dying older patient. Clin Geriatr Med 2000;16:335-356.
MacLeod AD. Methylphenidate in terminal depression. J Pain Symptom Manage 1998;16:193-198.
Patrick DL, Ferketich SL, Frame PS, et al. National Institutes of Health State-of-the-Science Conference statement: Symptom management in cancer: Pain, depression, and fatigue. J Natl Cancer Inst Monogr 2004;32:9-16.

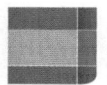

CHAPTER **158**

Dysphagia

Robin Pollens, Kathryn L. Hillenbrand, and Helen M. Sharp

KEY POINTS

- Dysphagia is a symptom of an underlying structural or neuromotor disorder, or it may be a side effect of treatment or medication.
- Because symptoms and severity often change over the course of a disease, intermittent consultation or reassessment may be needed.
- The goals of the patient and family should be part of assessment and treatment.
- Assessment identifies the source of dysphagia and evaluates treatment options.
- Dysphagia or the symptoms of dysphagia are treatable, often using several modalities.

Dysphagia is characterized by difficulty moving food from the mouth to the stomach. It can be associated with neurological, cognitive, muscular, or structural changes; with medication; or with systemic weakness. Symptoms and severity often change during disease progression, and intermittent consultation or reassessment may be needed (see Chapters 189, 192, and 232).

Although assessment and management should improve swallowing and reduce the risks of dehydration, malnutrition, and aspiration, treatment must also address the psychosocial aspects of eating (see Chapters 105 and 109). For individuals nearing the end of life, the benefits of eating are more significant than just nutrition or hydration. Given the impact of dysphagia on perceived quality of life, social relationships, nutritional status, and pulmonary safety, swallowing problems should be identified and addressed early in palliative care, with ongoing supportive consultation to meet the patient's goals and needs.

BASIC SCIENCE

The normal swallow comprises three phases: oral, pharyngeal, and esophageal. Oral manipulation of food initiates sensory impulses to the medullary reticular formation, or swallowing center, where motor responses are organized and initiated. The pharyngeal swallow provides airway protection through elevation and anterior movement of the hyoid and larynx, closure of the larynx, relaxation of the cricopharyngeal sphincter, tongue base retraction, and contraction of pharyngeal constrictors. Neuromotor control is mediated through cranial nerves V, VII, IX, X, XI, and XII.[1]

Normal changes occur with age. The swallow response gradually slows, with increased time for oral preparation and slower laryngeal and pharyngeal actions. Age-related sensory changes affect smell and taste and alter food preferences.[2]

Dysphagia occurs when there is breakdown in any of the three phases. Mechanical and sensory deficits affect the ability to maintain nutrition and hydration. When airway protection is reduced, risk increases for aspiration of secretions, foods, and liquids. Aspiration increases the risk for pneumonia, but it is not always predictive.[3] Factors that increase the risk for pneumonia include dependency for oral care, dependency for feeding, multiple medical diagnoses, being a current smoker, number of decayed teeth, number of medications, frailty or pulmonary-related diagnoses, and tube feeding.[3]

EPIDEMIOLOGY AND PREVALENCE

The prevalence of dysphagia varies with demographic variables. For example, approximately 15% of people older than 60 years who live independently have dysphagia, whereas more than 40% of residents in institutional settings (e.g., nursing homes) have dysphagia.[4] Dysphagia is common among people with disorders most often encountered in palliative care. In a retrospective study of long-term care medical records, dysphagia was recorded as one of the seven symptoms most common during the last 48 hours before death.[5] Table 158-1 describes the incidence of dysphagia according to primary medical diagnosis.

TABLE 158-1 Frequency and Predictors of Dysphagia by Disease

DISEASE	PREVALENCE OR PREDICTOR OF DYSPHAGIA
Head and neck cancer	Oral, pharyngeal, and laryngeal cancers are almost universal predictors for dysphagia. Severity varies with tumor size, location, and treatment effects.[6] Combined medical treatments may exacerbate swallowing dysfunction.
Stroke	Considerable variation occurs by site of lesion. Dysphagia occurs in 25% to 50% of patients with strokes. Dysphagia often resolves during the acute recovery period.[7]
Parkinson's disease (PD)	Significant dysphagia occurs in approximately 40% of patients with PD.[8] Speech decline and severity of tremor are predictive for dysphagia.[9]
Amyotropic lateral sclerosis (ALS)	Speech decline is most predictive of dysphagia in patients with ALS.[9]
Multiple sclerosis (MS)	Dysphagia occurs among 10% to 40% of patients with MS.[9] Cerebellar and brainstem impairments are predictive for dysphagia.[9]
Dementia	Dysphagia occurs among 50% of patients with dementia.[10] Speech decline, limb contractures, abnormal sleep-wake cycles, and loss of self-care (e.g., dressing) are predictive for dysphagia.[10]

CLINICAL MANIFESTATIONS

Patients with dysphagia demonstrate various clinically observable symptoms and complaints about eating or swallowing. Coughing, wet voice quality, and persistent throat clearing with eating are symptoms of aspiration or pharyngeal food residue after the swallow. Patients may report difficulty controlling food in their mouth, pocketing of food in their cheek, or pain with swallowing. Many show no overt symptoms of dysphagia during meals, but they develop aspiration pneumonia, decrease food intake, or lose weight[1] (see Chapters 150 and 171).

The same symptom may reflect very different underlying problems. For example, a cough may signify reduced airway protection, a tracheoesophageal fistula, pharyngeal dysfunction, cricopharyngeal dysfunction, or inadequate oral clearance. Table 158-2 provides behavioral indicators of dysphagia with a clinical example of altered eating or feeding. This summary does not offer the differential diagnosis for dysphagia, but it highlights the need to determine the underlying cause. Isolating the cause leads to treatments that address the source of the swallowing problem.

Table 158-3 summarizes the symptoms of dysphagia often observed among patients with particular chronic or progressive diseases. The dose and timing of medications also can impair swallowing. Medications can negatively affect consciousness (e.g., anticonvulsants, antidepressants, antihistamines, antispasmodics), salivary flow (e.g., antihistamines, antihypertensives, antidepressants), and

TABLE 158-2 Signs and Symptoms of Dysphagia

OBSERVATION OR COMPLAINT	DESCRIPTION*	POSSIBLE CLINICAL FINDING
Problems in feeding	Food spreads in mouth or flows out	Reduced oral sensation or control
	Does not start chewing when given a bite of food	Apraxia of swallow Impaired cognition Heightened or reduced sensation
	Food left in mouth after swallow	Reduced tongue function Reduced oral sensation
Food preference changes	Solids take too long, eats soft foods only	Reduced anteroposterior tongue movement
	Reduced intake	Reduced taste or sensation
Coughing	Coughs or chokes when drinking	Reduced tongue coordination Bolus falls over the base of tongue into airway Aspiration
	Coughs or chokes during or after eating	Reduced laryngeal closure Reduced pharyngeal peristalsis Residual material Aspiration
Voice quality changes	Hoarseness	Reduced airway closure
	Wet voice quality or throat clearing	Reduced laryngeal elevation Residue on vocal folds
Food sticking sensation	Food sticks in throat	Unilateral pharyngeal paralysis
	Food sticks at the bottom of the neck	Esophageal disorder
Physical concerns	Weight loss	Muscle fatigue resulting in poor endurance for eating
	Pain when eating	Oral thrush Dental abscess
	Fatigue while eating	Poor respiratory function or muscle fatigue
	Drooling or excessive saliva	Reduced swallow initiation Facial weakness
	Dry mouth or lack of saliva	Medication side effect

*By the patient or caregiver.
Adapted from Logemann JA. Evaluation and Treatment of Swallowing Disorders. Austin, TX: ProEd, 1998.

TABLE 158-3 Diseases Often Referred for Palliative Care and Symptoms of Dysphagia Observed in Patients with the Condition

DISEASE	CLINICAL FINDINGS	COMMON SYMPTOMS
Head and neck cancer		
After radiation treatment	Radiation effects may develop a year after radiotherapy.[1]	Reduced range of motion Reduced speed of transit Slowed pharyngeal swallow Oral pain[1]
After surgical treatment	Partial or total glossectomy decreases tongue range of motion and control. Epiglottic and supraglottic resections decrease airway protection. Total laryngectomy provides airway protection.	Reduced oral transit Oral residue Coughing, choking Often no problems Cough may reflect patent tracheoesophageal fistula
Stroke		
Brainstem	Motor cranial nerve dysfunction may be absent or preserved. Pharyngeal swallow may be delayed, weak, or absent.[1]	Coughing Absent cough with aspiration No oral or pharyngeal response to food[1]
Subcortical	Impaired coordination occurs between oral and pharyngeal phases.[1]	Coughing before or during the swallow
Cortical	Left hemisphere lesions are associated with reduced initiation and apraxia of swallow, but patient may have normal pharyngeal swallow. Right hemisphere lesions are associated with pharyngeal delays.[1]	Limited response to food in the mouth[1] Reduced oral coordination Slowed pharyngeal response Coughing, wet voice quality
Parkinson's disease	Oral, pharyngeal, or esophageal phases may be affected.[9] Swallowing function often affected by timing and dosing of Parkinson's medication[1]	Tongue rocking back and forth Delayed initiation of swallow Coughing after eating related to pharyngeal residue May report no symptoms
Amyotrophic lateral sclerosis		
Corticobulbar type	Tongue mobility is reduced.[1] Laryngeal elevation is reduced.[9]	Solid foods and thicker foods become difficult to eat Drooling and spillage Longer mealtimes Decline in calorie and fluid intake Complaints of too much saliva Respiratory fatigue Coughing or wet voice after eating
Corticospinal type	Patients may not be aware of swallowing problems.[1] If dysphagia is present, it may be related to loss of respiratory muscle support.[7]	Slow, progressive weight loss[1]
Multiple sclerosis	Patients have delayed pharyngeal swallow and reduced strength and coordination of pharyngeal wall contraction.[9]	Choking or coughing before, during, or after swallow Drink or saliva escapes lips May deny symptoms[9]
Dementia	Patients have reduced awareness of food in the mouth and reduced coordination for oral to pharyngeal transit. Symptom of underlying problem (e.g., reflux) should be sought.[10]	Food refusal Choking or coughing during or after meals Requires assistance with feeding[10]

muscle coordination (e.g., β-blockers, anticholinergics). Antineoplastics, antivirals, and some antibiotics cause stomatitis, pharyngeal ulceration, or oral candidiasis.[8] Symptoms of dysphagia also may be affected by fatigue or decreased alertness reflecting a general decline in medical status.

DIFFERENTIAL DIAGNOSIS

Figure 158-1 summarizes the typical sequence from referral for clinical evaluation to decisions about assessment. It provides management strategies described in this and later sections.

Clinical Assessment

Before evaluating swallowing, the history, medications, and current complaints or observations are reviewed. The patient is advised about the purpose of the assessment, and his or her goals for eating, nutrition, and hydration are established. The dysphagia specialist then examines the facial and oral structures, with an assessment of oral movements (e.g., tongue mobility) during speech and nonspeech tasks (see Chapter 53). Medical and dental concerns, such as reflux, oral ulcers after chemotherapy, or carious lesions, should be ruled out as causes of pain or refusal to eat.

A clinical observation of feeding and eating is conducted to evaluate the oral control of food and secretions and the ability to clear the mouth. The examiner checks behavioral aspects, such as how quickly the patient eats, fatigue, awareness of food, and ability to follow instructions. Coughing before, during, or after a swallow is a significant sign of aspiration, but 50% to 60% of those who aspirate do not cough[1] (Table 158-4).

Clinical assessment does not yield reliable information about the strength, timing, or coordination of the pharyngeal or esophageal phases. Given observable symptoms or medical signs of dysphagia, an instrumental assessment may be recommended to isolate the physiological problem

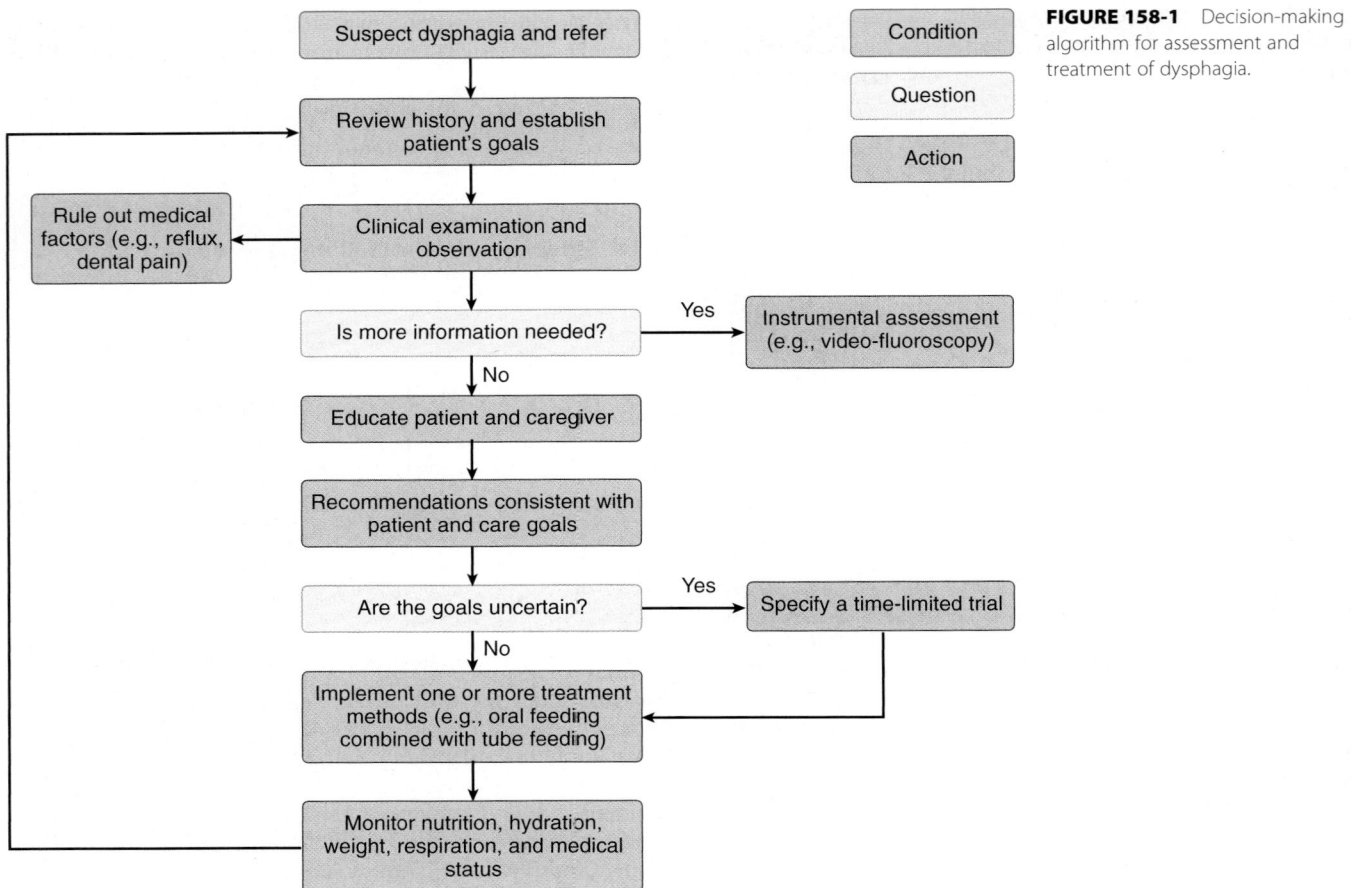

FIGURE 158-1 Decision-making algorithm for assessment and treatment of dysphagia.

| Condition |
| Question |
| Action |

Suspect dysphagia and refer

Review history and establish patient's goals

Rule out medical factors (e.g., reflux, dental pain)

Clinical examination and observation

Is more information needed? — Yes → Instrumental assessment (e.g., video-fluoroscopy)

No

Educate patient and caregiver

Recommendations consistent with patient and care goals

Are the goals uncertain? — Yes → Specify a time-limited trial

No

Implement one or more treatment methods (e.g., oral feeding combined with tube feeding)

Monitor nutrition, hydration, weight, respiration, and medical status

---

TABLE 158-4 Common Myths about the Assessment and Treatment of Dysphagia

MYTH	FACT
Presence or absence of a gag reflex indicates ability to swallow.	No data support this relationship.[1]
Swallowing evaluation is a pass/fail diagnostic tool.	Evaluation reveals the type and degree of impairment, on which treatment decisions are based.[1]
A patient who does not want tube feeding is not a candidate for swallowing intervention.	Evaluation identifies strategies to promote the safest means of oral intake.[1]

Box 158-1 Indications for an Instrumental Examination

Indications

- Assist differential diagnosis
- Confirm or determine the type and cause of the dysphagia
- Determine whether oropharyngeal dysphagia affects nutrition, hydration, or pulmonary status
- Guide management and treatment regarding the safety or efficiency of swallowing
- Update oropharyngeal function and effect of management when progression in symptoms or changed medical status occurs

Contraindications

- Patient medically unstable or unable to tolerate the procedure
- Patient unable to cooperate or voluntarily participate
- Results would not change clinical management

From American Speech-Language-Hearing Association. Clinical indicators for instrumental assessment of dysphagia. ASHA Desk Reference. Rockville, MD: ASHA, 2000.

---

and evaluate compensatory strategies (e.g., posture change). Because instrumental assessment is not always indicated, a careful clinical evaluation may eliminate additional expense and transport. Health status, level of alertness, preferences, and goals are essential components of a shared decision about instrumental assessment. Practical limitations such as transport from home may preclude instrumental assessment for frail patients. Indications for instrumental assessment are provided in Box 158-1.

Instrumental Assessment of Swallowing Function

Video-fluoroscopy and video-endoscopy are the two most commonly used methods for visualizing the swallow.[1]

Video-fluoroscopy (i.e., modified barium swallow or "cookie swallow") is the most common approach to imaging the structures and functions of swallowing. The patient swallows small amounts of barium mixed with foods and liquids, and radiographical video images document the oral, pharyngeal, and esophageal structures and coordinative functions.

Flexible endoscopic evaluation of swallowing (FEES) allows direct visualization of pharyngeal and laryngeal structures and function with swallowing. An endoscope is introduced transnasally and placed above the larynx. As the patient swallows food or liquid, the clinician can observe events before and after the swallow. The primary advantages of FEES are that assessment can be at the bedside and the patient can see the images so the technique can be used for biofeedback. FEES does not allow visualization of the oral stage nor the moment of the swallow response.[11] FEES and video-fluoroscopy require the patient's cooperation and ability to swallow voluntarily. Instrumental assessments should evaluate the effectiveness of behavioral strategies to reduce or eliminate dysphagia symptoms.[1] Treatments are developed by integrating the patient's preferences with clinical and instrumental assessments.

TREATMENT

The goal of dysphagia management in palliative care is to retain or restore safe and effective oral feeding consistent with the patient's preferences and goals (see Chapters 19 and 20). Treatments include minor modifications in the feeding approach, direct therapy, and alternative means of nutrition and hydration. These approaches should always include education of the patient and family and oral hygiene. Regardless of the treatment, swallowing function often changes, and it should be monitored.

Patient and Family Education

The patient may have preferences about continuing to eat orally, supplementing oral feeding with intravenous or tube feeding, or stopping oral feeding completely. Patients and families must be fully informed about the options, the risks, and benefits of each option. If behavioral strategies are adopted, the dysphagia specialist teaches caregivers how to implement them to retain positive interactions with family members and caregivers at mealtimes.

Compensatory Strategies

Swallowing dysfunction can often be managed through changes in the way that a patient eats or drinks. Examples include changes in posture, the size or texture of each bite of food, and the speed of food presentation. Some, such as leaning toward the stronger side of the body to encourage food propulsion through the stronger side of the pharynx, require the patient's training and cooperation, whereas others, such as the speed of food presentation, can be implemented by a caregiver.[1]

Swallowing Maneuvers

Many aspects of the swallow response can be brought under voluntary control. For example, patients can learn to hold their breath before the swallow to ensure full laryngeal closure and airway protection before swallowing. Other techniques include coughing and swallowing immediately after an initial swallow to clear pharyngeal and laryngeal residue and prevent aspiration of residue.[1]

Therapy

Therapy for swallowing includes techniques during eating and those to increase strength or range of motion of the muscles involved.[1] Techniques to increase strength or range of motion depend on the swallowing disorder and medical diagnosis. For example, range-of-motion exercises can improve speech and swallowing after surgical procedures for oral or oropharyngeal cancer,[6] but the same exercises may cause fatigue in patients with amyotrophic lateral sclerosis.[13]

Nonoral Feeding

Patients, families, and clinicians often have strong views about nonoral feeding, particularly the role of tube feeding in end-of-life care. Decisions to pursue or forgo tube feeding require active discussion and informed patient choice. The advantages and disadvantages of tube feeding are discussed in Chapters 108 and 109.

Tube feeding is often recommended as a temporary solution for severe dysphagia, and it may restore nutrition and hydration after an acute illness, such as a stroke (see Chapter 189). There is evidence-based support for alternative nutrition for patients with head and neck cancer or amyotrophic lateral sclerosis.[14] Feeding tubes are not effective in prolonging life, preventing aspiration, or improving nutrition in patients with advanced dementia.[15]

When patients with severe dysphagia forgo tube feeding but wish to continue oral feeding, it is important that they are well informed about the risks of dehydration, malnutrition, and aspiration. Swallowing and nutrition evaluations may contribute useful information about safer food consistencies and ways to obtain higher calorie and fluid intake with less effort.

Combination Approach

In most cases, more than one approach is recommended to manage dysphagia. Tube feeding is often perceived as an "all or nothing" decision, but as illustrated in the clinical case, nonoral feeding does not preclude continued eating for pleasure or social benefits (see "Case Study: Managing Dysphagia").

Drugs

There are no medications to treat specific oropharyngeal swallowing problems. However, medications may alleviate specific symptoms; for example, atropine reduces drooling.[1] Esophageal dysmotility and symptoms of gastroesophageal reflux may be amenable to pharmacological management. In patients with xerostomia, commercially available synthetic saliva may provide relief. Synthetic saliva agents include fluoride for dental benefit. Excessively thick secretions may be managed with guaifenesin, potassium iodide, or papase.[9] Although lemon-glycerin swabs are used for cleaning and lubrication, they tend to dry the mouth over time.[7] Commercially available agents are used to thicken liquids to specific consistencies (e.g., nectar, honey, pudding). Home remedies, such as rice cereal as a thickener, are also effective.

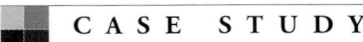

CASE STUDY

Managing Dysphagia

Susan is a 71-year-old woman who was diagnosed 3 years earlier with amyotrophic lateral sclerosis (ALS). Susan lives at home with her husband, who is her primary caregiver. She maintains an active network of friends and family through e-mail. She has changes in her motor skills, including greater dependence for daily activities, and has choking and coughing during meals. Her physician suggests a speech and swallowing evaluation. Based on the speech-language pathologist's findings, a video-fluoroscopic swallow assessment is done. To manage dysphagia, Susan is instructed in modifications such as eating softer foods, taking single sips, and tucking her chin on each swallow to improve airway protection. Susan maintains adequate nutrition and hydration using these strategies.

As her disease progresses, Susan reports that eating is no longer pleasurable and requests tube feeding. However, she expresses concern about being kept alive too long. Before placement of a percutaneous endoscopic gastrostomy (PEG) feeding tube, she and her husband have lengthy discussions to clarify her preferences about tube feeding. After 2 weeks of tube feeding, Susan notices that her energy is greater and comments that "not having to struggle to eat is one less thing to worry about." She continues to taste favorite foods at mealtimes and enjoys a glass of red wine with her husband each evening.

Nine months after PEG tube placement, Susan's respiratory status and motor skills have declined. She communicates with soft vocalizations and uses eye tracking to interface with a computer-based communication device. Susan states that she wants to continue with tube feeding, but she seeks confirmation that her family and physicians will discontinue the tube when she feels the time is right.

Supportive Care

Treatment strategies should be individualized based on the symptoms of dysphagia, the patient's medical and behavioral status, and the patient's preferences. General strategies include the following:

- Frequent, small meals to reduce fatigue and maintain caloric intake
- Upright posture for efficient swallowing function with improved airway protection
- Routine oral care and hygiene
- Modifying the rate of food presentation and size of the bolus offered
- Verbal cueing and reducing distractions during mealtime to help with cognitive and attention difficulties and to increase oral intake
- Swallowing thin liquids may be most difficult for patients with neurological deficits or disorders

DEVELOPMENTS AND RESEARCH OPPORTUNITIES

The study of oropharyngeal dysphagia is new, and specific treatment techniques have appeared in the literature over the past 25 years. Because many studies are small and specific to a particular diagnosis, their results are difficult to generalize to other populations. Over the past 10 years, larger studies have focused on the risk factors for complications of pneumonia,[3] effects of patient positioning, food temperature and viscosity, and exercise programs.[6] Current research aims to determine the optimal timing, type, and duration of treatment correlated with the specific cause of the swallowing disorder and the patient's diagnosis.[13]

Several questions warrant further consideration. Is an instrumental assessment needed when a patient aspirates? Medical and patient goals should be clear when an evaluation is requested. Assessment should identify the source of the symptom and identify the effect of behavioral strategies on reducing or eliminating symptoms of dysphagia.

Should tube feeding be recommended when aspiration is identified on instrumental assessment? Aspiration alone is not a clinical indicator for nonoral feeding. The risks of oral feeding must be balanced against the risk of aspiration and complications of tube feeding.

CONCLUSIONS

Many patients experience dysphagia as a symptom of acute, chronic, and degenerative disorders. It can be related to anatomical and physiological changes, medication side effects, or proximity to the end of life. Because of the impact on quality of life and social relationships, nutritional status, and pulmonary safety, assessment and treatment of dysphagia are important components of comprehensive palliative care. Assessment improves the education of the patient and family about options for managing the symptoms of dysphagia. Specific management approaches can reduce aspiration pneumonia risk, reduce discomfort and fatigue during eating, and improve quality of life when eating is no longer pleasurable.

REFERENCES

1. Logemann JA. Evaluation and Treatment of Swallowing Disorders. Austin, TX: ProEd, 1998.
2. Barczi SR, Sullivan PA, Robbins J. How should dysphagia care of older adults differ? Establishing optimal practice patterns. Semin Speech Lang 2000;21:347-361.
3. Langmore SE, Terpenning MS, Schork A, et al. Predictors of aspiration pneumonia: How important is dysphagia? Dysphagia 1998;13:69-81.
4. Robbins J. The current state of clinical geriatric dysphagia research (guest editorial). Department of Veterans Affairs. Available at http://www.vard.org/jour/02/39/4/guested.htm (accessed October 15, 2005).
5. Schroder H. The last 48 hours of life in long-term care: A focused chart audit. J Am Geriatr Soc 2002;50:501-506.
6. Logemann JA, Pauloski BR, Rademaker AW, et al. Speech and swallowing rehabilitation for head and neck cancer patients. Oncology 1997;11:651-663.
7. Groher M. Dysphagia: Diagnosis and Management, 3rd ed. Boston: Butterworth-Heinemann, 1997.
8. Feinberg M. The effects of medications on swallowing. In Sonies BC (ed). Dysphagia: A Continuum of Care. Gaithersburg, MD: Aspen, 1997, pp 107-120.
9. Yorkston KM, Miller RM, Strand EA. Management of Speech and Swallowing in Degenerative Diseases, 2nd ed. Austin, TX: Pro-Ed, 2004.
10. Volicer L, Seltzer B, Rheaume Y, et al. Eating difficulties in patients with probable dementia of the Alzheimer type. Geriatr Psychiatry Neurol 1989;2:188-195.
11. Langmore SE, Schatz K, Olsen N. Fiberoptic endoscopic examination of swallowing safety: A new procedure. Dysphagia 1988;2:216-219.
12. American Speech-Language-Hearing Association. Clinical Indicators for Instrumental Assessment of Dysphagia. ASHA Desk Reference. Rockville, MD: ASHA, 2000.
13. Logemann JA. The potential future of dysphagia: Population-specific diagnosis and treatment. Folio Phoniatr Logop 2000;52:136-141.

14. Haddad RY, Thomas DR. Enteral nutrition and enteral tube feeding: Review of the evidence. Clin Geriatr Med 2002;18:867-881.
15. Finucane TE, Christmas C, Travis K. Tube feeding in patients with advanced dementia: A review of the evidence. JAMA 1999;282:1365-1370.

SUGGESTED READING

American Speech-Language-Hearing Association. Dysphagia policies and ethical decision making: Policy documents and readings from ASHA. Rockville, MD: ASHA, 2002.

Pollens R. Role of the speech-language pathologist in palliative hospice care. J Palliat Med 2004;7:694-702.

Sharp HM, Bryant KN. Ethical issues in dysphagia. When patients refuse assessment or treatment. Semin Speech Lang 2003;24:285-299.

Sonies BC. Dysphagia: A continuum of care. Gaithersburg, MD: Aspen, 1997.

Sullivan PA, Guilford AM. Swallowing intervention in oncology. San Diego: Singular, 1999.

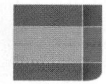

CHAPTER **159**

Dyspnea

Joshua Shadd and Deborah Dudgeon

KEY POINTS

- Tachypnea is not dyspnea.
- Dyspnea is a multidimensional, subjective experience that dramatically affects quality of life.
- Nonpharmacological interventions are important.
- Systemic opioids are the treatment of choice for patients with advanced illness.

Dyspnea is "a subjective experience of breathing discomfort that consists of qualitatively distinct sensations that vary in intensity."[1] This definition highlights three key elements of breathlessness:

1. Dyspnea is subjective. Neither its presence nor severity can be inferred from clinical or laboratory investigations[2,3]; we must ask about it.
2. Dyspnea is not merely a single sensation that varies only in intensity. The term encompasses various perceptions described by phrases such as air hunger, increased effort, chest tightness, rapid breathing, incomplete exhalation, or feeling of suffocation.
3. Like pain, dyspnea is a multidimensional, intensely personal symptom that is shaped by experiences with affective and physical components.[1]

Clinical and laboratory assessment is addressed elsewhere (see Chapters 63 and 73). Understanding the mul-

tidimensional complexity of the experience of breathlessness is crucial to relieving the symptom (Fig. 159-1). Effective symptom management must assess and address all relevant factors in the patient's experience.

EPIDEMIOLOGY AND PREVALENCE

Dyspnea is a problem in many life-limiting illnesses, and the prevalence and severity typically increase with advancing disease. Dyspnea diminishes functional status, social activities,[4] quality of life,[5] and the will to live.[6] In one international study, terminal sedation was prompted by dyspnea three times more commonly than by pain.[7]

BASIC SCIENCE AND PATHOPHYSIOLOGY

Normally an unconscious activity, respiration is managed by clusters of neurons in the medulla. They receive afferent input from several types of mechanoreceptors in respiratory muscles, airways, and lung parenchyma and chemoreceptors in aortic and carotid bodies and the medulla. Motor commands from the medulla or motor cortex by means of the medulla descend to respiratory muscles through efferent motor neurons.

Although central coordination of respiration occurs in the medulla, the conscious experience of dyspnea arises from the sensory cortex (Fig. 159-2).[8] In addition to projections from the same mechanoreceptors and chemoreceptors that inform the medullary respiratory center, the sensory cortex gets motor instructions sent to respiratory muscles from the motor cortex or medulla, or both. This confluence of sensory and motor information enables the sensory cortex to assess the effort needed to achieve the respiratory muscle function and homeostatic balance indicated by afferent mechanoreceptor and chemoreceptor signals. Dyspnea is experienced if the sensory cortex perceives a mismatch between ventilatory demand and the body's ability to respond to that demand.[9]

Clinically, dyspnea may result from impairment of mechanical ventilation by obstructive (e.g., asthma),

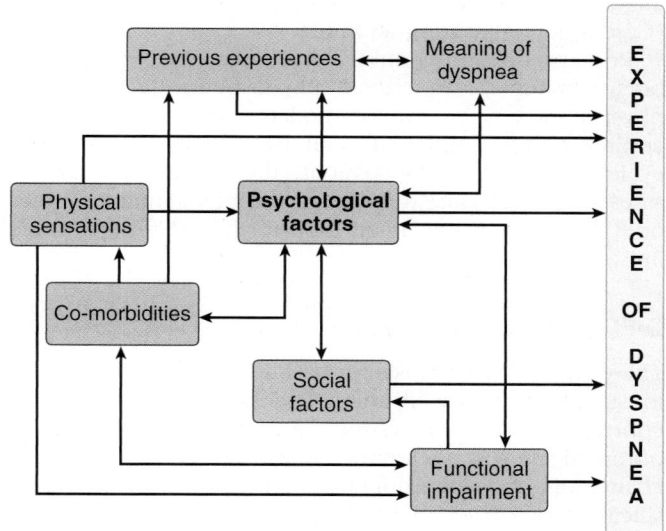

FIGURE 159-1 Many factors contribute to the experience of dyspnea.

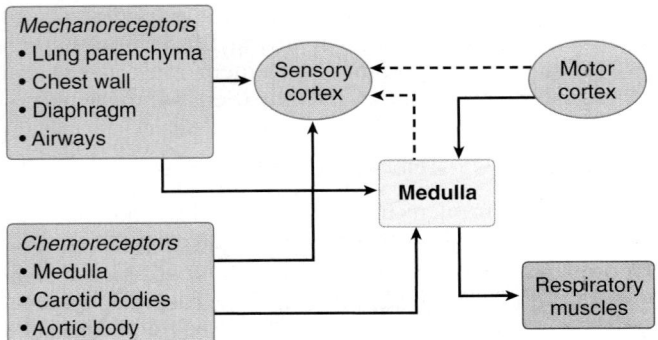

FIGURE 159-2 Neural pathways involved in the generation of dyspnea. The sensory cortex receives copies of respiratory motor commands arising from the medulla or motor cortex (*dashed lines*) and sensory information from peripheral chemoreceptors and mechanoreceptors. Dyspnea occurs if the degree of motor output required is perceived to be unsustainable or disproportionate to the sensory information received.

restrictive (e.g., neuromuscular disease), or reduced diffusion capacity (e.g., interstitial fibrosis). Alternatively, it may result from increased ventilatory demand (e.g., exercise) or occur when greater-than-normal effort is required to maintain normal ventilation (e.g., muscle weakness from cancer cachexia). In practice, dyspnea commonly is caused by many contributing physiological processes that are modified by cognitive and affective factors.

CLINICAL MANIFESTATIONS

No element of the physical examination or laboratory investigation can reliably imply the presence or intensity of dyspnea. Respiratory rate, blood gas values, and pulmonary function testing all correlate poorly with patients' reports of breathlessness. The patient's own description of his or her symptom is the only reliable indicator of dyspnea. The typical temporal pattern is one of chronic breathlessness punctuated by acute episodes, often with anxiety, pain, or a sense of impending doom. These unpredictable but expected exacerbations of dyspnea are a major source of distress for patients and their families (see "Case Study: Managing Dyspnea").

Perhaps the most important clinical manifestation of breathlessness is functional impairment. Reduction of physical activity to accommodate breathlessness is a coping strategy employed by all dyspneic patients.[4] When evaluating a breathless patient, the symptom must be assessed in the context of activity (e.g., walking 1 minute on a level surface) or in relation to the limitations it has imposed.

DIFFERENTIAL DIAGNOSIS

The differential diagnosis for breathlessness is broad, and most patients with advanced illness have many factors contributing to their dyspnea. A systematic approach to potential causes is essential because it offers the best chance of good symptom control. Box 159-1 offers a classification of causes of breathlessness. Discussion of specific causes can be found elsewhere (see Chapters 79, 80, 85, 91, 184, 185, 192, 225, 231, 236, and 239).

 C A S E   S T U D Y

Managing Dyspnea

Mr. B is a 71-year-old man with colon cancer metastatic to his liver, and his condition is followed in the palliative medicine clinic. On reviewing the symptom assessment survey he completes at every clinic visit, the provider notices that his overall well-being has worsened (rated at 7/10 on a numeric rating scale, with 0/10 representing best). Although he is still relatively active (70% on the Palliative Performance Scale), his gradually progressive dyspnea (rated 5/10) has forced him to drop out of the church choir, and he is no longer able to do his own grocery shopping.

Findings of another interview do not suggest pain, depression, anxiety, or intercurrent illness. There is no history of smoking or lung disease. Mr. B is cachectic, but results of the cardiorespiratory examination are unremarkable. Results of investigations (i.e., complete blood cell count, chest radiograph, electrocardiogram, pulmonary function tests, and pulse oximetry) are normal. The provider concludes that the most likely cause of Mr. B's dyspnea is respiratory muscle weakness from cachexia.

The multidisciplinary approach includes physiotherapy (i.e., an exercise program to counter deconditioning), occupational therapy to discuss accommodation strategies, spiritual care to address social losses and implications of progressive illness, and a dietician consultation to maximize nutrition. The fan in his room is helpful. The physician discontinues a trial of supplemental oxygen (4 L/min by nasal prongs) when he reports no significant benefit and gives him a prescription for oral morphine (5 mg every 4 hours, as needed) for dyspnea. He finds morphine beneficial, and the provider converts him to a scheduled dose with appropriate breakthrough coverage and a bowel regimen.

Box 159-1 Differential Diagnosis of Dyspnea
Thoracic Causes
Malignancies
Lung tumor (primary or metastatic)
Pleural tumor
Pleural or pericardial effusion
Major airway obstruction
Vascular occlusion
Superior vena cava obstruction
Pulmonary embolism
Multiple tumor microemboli
External compression/occlusion of pulmonary vasculature
Lymphangitic carcinomatosis
Chest wall infiltration
Phrenic nerve paralysis
Paramalignant Conditions
Pneumothorax
Pulmonary embolism
Tracheoesophageal fistula
Nonmalignant Conditions
Pneumonia
Cardiac disease
Ischemic heart disease

Congestive heart failure
Valvular disease
Arrhythmia
Pulmonary arteriovenous malformation
Obstructive lung disease
Asthma
Chronic obstructive pulmonary disease
Restrictive lung disease
Interstitial lung disease
Chest wall deformity

Treatment-Related Causes

Lung resection
Lobectomy
Pneumonectomy
Radiation-induced conditions
Radiation pneumonitis
Radiation-induced pulmonary fibrosis
Postirradiation pericarditis
Chemotherapy-induced conditions
Pulmonary toxicity (bleomycin, cyclophosphamide)
Cardiac toxicity (e.g., 5-fluorouracil, Adriamycin)
Other medications (e.g., amiodarone)

Extrathoracic Causes

Paramalignant Conditions

Respiratory muscle weakness
Paraneoplastic syndrome
Electrolyte or metabolic abnormality
Steroid myopathy
Cachexia of cancer
Anemia
Diaphragmatic paralysis
Ascites
Hepatomegaly

Nonmalignant Conditions

Metabolic acidosis
Electrolyte abnormality (e.g., hypercalcemia)
Neuromuscular disorder
Anxiety or panic attack
Hyperventilation syndrome
Obesity
Anemia
Muscle weakness, decreased aerobic efficiency due to deconditioning

TREATMENT

The ultimate goal of symptomatic treatment is to ameliorate the negative symptom experience. As with any distressing symptom, a comprehensive approach may use several strategies.

Oxygen

Supplemental oxygen is often assumed to be helpful in hypoxemia and of no benefit with normal blood oxygen levels. Neither of these holds true universally. Hypoxemic patients do not necessarily gain dyspnea relief from supplemental oxygen, highlighting a multifactorial symptom. It is impossible to predict, even on the basis of arterial oxygen saturation, who will benefit. N-of-1 trials can identify patients who respond to oxygen therapy.

Rehabilitation and Exercise Training

A rehabilitation-oriented approach (see Chapter 52) to breathlessness can decrease the production of dyspnea by respiratory muscle training, its functional impact by development of accommodation strategies, and ultimately, the symptom experience by increasing the sense of control. For ambulatory chronic obstructive pulmonary disease (COPD) patients, exercise training improves symptoms, functional status, and quality of life.[10] Although studies specific to palliative care are lacking, those most likely to benefit from exercise training are people able to participate in regular endurance exercise over several weeks.

Cognitive-Behavioral Interventions

A synopsis of the cognitive-behavioral strategies for chronic or episodic dyspnea has been published.[11] One essential intervention is assisting the patient to formulate strategies for expected but often unpredictable exacerbations. In addition to oxygen and pharmacological interventions, these may include distraction (e.g., music, guided imagery), alternative activities (e.g., a shower, a drive, praying), breathing techniques, mobilization of social supports, or contacting formal caregivers. Equipping patients with practical tools for managing dyspneic episodes can help the fear that is a central element of the suffering of breathlessness.

Air Flow

Stimulation of the trigeminal nerve by means of cutaneous or nasal receptors reduces the intensity of dyspnea. Healthy subjects reported a decrease in the intensity of experimentally induced dyspnea from a stream of cool air against the cheek.[12]

Acupuncture

Several small studies support the hypothesis that acupuncture is effective for dyspnea in various clinical conditions,[11] although results are inconsistent. Larger studies with appropriate control groups are required.

Drugs

Opioids

The primary site of action of opioids in patients with dyspnea is the medulla oblongata, although the exact mechanisms of opioids' effects on the perception of breathlessness are incompletely understood. Box 159-2 lists mechanisms by which opioids may reduce breathlessness.

There is good evidence for using systemic opioids for breathlessness in patients with advanced disease. A Cochrane collaboration systematic review of opioids for the symptomatic relief of breathlessness in terminal illness was published in 2001.[13] The report concluded that there is "statistically strong evidence for a small and probably clinically significant effect of oral and parenteral opioids in the treatment of breathlessness."[13]

The same cannot be said of nebulized opioids. Nine studies of nebulized opioids were included in the Cochrane review; not one demonstrated the superiority of nebulized opioid over placebo.[13]

After the Cochrane review, one double-blind, placebo-controlled, crossover trial of sustained-release oral morphine in dyspneic patients with mixed diagnoses demonstrated a statistically significant benefit with morphine compared with placebo (9.5 mm on a 100-mm visual analogue scale).[14] Another double-blind study observed no difference between subcutaneous and nebulized morphine in dyspneic cancer patients.[15] Unfortunately, the study was too small ($N = 11$) to produce meaningful conclusions.

Although most published trials have studied morphine, later reports of fentanyl, diamorphine, morphine-6-glucuronide, and hydromorphone for dyspnea suggest a class effect.[16] The hypothesis that standard opioid dosage equivalency calculations (developed for pain) can be reliably applied to dyspneic patients has not been formally tested.

Apprehension regarding the use of opioids for dyspnea is usually based on a perceived risk of impairing respiratory drive, thereby causing or exacerbating hypoxia or hypercapnia. Growing evidence attests to the safety of appropriately titrated opioids for dyspnea.[17,18] Measurable changes in the respiratory rate and arterial $P{CO_2}$ were seen in only a few studies, and their clinical significance is questionable.[13] The most common adverse effects experienced by those using opioids for dyspnea include constipation, nausea, and sedation. The frequency of adverse effects is similar to that of patients using opioids for pain; overall tolerability is high.

Benzodiazepines

Although benzodiazepines may have a role in combination therapy, there is no evidence they have direct benefit for breathlessness.

Combination Therapies

A small number of studies advocate the combination of a non-opioid with an opioid. A 1996 crossover study of exercise tolerance in seven men with COPD demonstrated the superiority of oral morphine (30 mg) with promethazine (25 mg) compared with placebo or oral morphine alone.[19] The study authors argue that the combination

improves exercise tolerance by decreasing the intensity of dyspnea and that it is better tolerated than higher doses of opioids alone.

Navigante[20] compared three therapeutic strategies for hospitalized advanced cancer patients with uncontrolled dyspnea: scheduled morphine (with midazolam for breakthrough), scheduled midazolam (with morphine for breakthrough), or scheduled morphine and midazolam (with morphine for breakthrough). Despite the fact that changes in dyspnea scores were almost identical in all groups, persons receiving the combination of scheduled morphine and midazolam were significantly more likely to report dyspnea relief. The study concluded that "the beneficial effects of morphine . . . could be improved with the addition of midazolam."[20]

EVIDENCE-BASED MEDICINE AND RESEARCH OPPORTUNITIES

Dyspnea is a debilitating symptom causing major functional, emotional, psychological, and social sequelae. Studies of interventions come largely from the COPD literature, and palliative care studies are small. Nonetheless, good evidence exists for systemic (but not nebulized) opioids for symptomatic relief of breathlessness in patients with advanced disease. Universal oxygen supplementation is not recommended, although some recipients can derive substantial benefit. Non-opioid medications (e.g., phenothiazines, benzodiazepines) have not been shown to have independent benefit, but they may have a role in combination therapies.

Several areas of dyspnea management need further research:

- Can dyspnea be classified (e.g., distinct causes, pathways, treatments)?
- Can drugs (e.g., anabolic steroids) reverse respiratory muscle weakness?
- What is the role for non-opioid medications in symptomatic dyspnea?
- Who should get supplemental oxygen and for how long?

REFERENCES

1. American Thoracic Society. Dyspnea. Mechanisms, assessment, and management: A consensus statement. Am J Respir Crit Care Med 1999;159:321-340.
2. Dudgeon D, Lertzman M. Dyspnea in the advanced cancer patient. J Pain Symptom Manage 1998;16:212-219.
3. Dudgeon DJ, Lertzman M, Askew GR. Physiological changes and clinical correlations of dyspnea in cancer outpatients. J Pain Symptom Manage 2001;21:373-379.
4. Brown ML, Carrieri V, Janson-Bjerklie S, et al. Lung cancer and dyspnea: The patient's perception. Oncol Nurs Forum 1986;13:19-24.
5. Roberts DK, Thorne SE, Pearson C. The experience of dyspnea in late-stage cancer. Patients' and nurses' perspectives. Cancer Nurs 1993;16:310-320.
6. Chochinov MH, Tataryn D, Clinch JJ, et al. Will to live in the terminally ill. Lancet 1999;354:816-819.
7. Fainsinger R, Waller A, Bercovici M, et al. A multicentre international study of sedation for uncontrolled symptoms in terminally ill patients. Palliat Med 2000;14:257-265.
8. Manning HL, Schwartzstein RM. Pathophysiology of dyspnea. N Engl J Med 1995;333:1547-1553.
9. Schwartzstein RM, Manning HL, Weiss JW, et al. Dyspnea: A sensory experience. Lung 1990;169:185-199.
10. Lacasse Y, Goldstein R, Lasserson TJ, Martin S. Pulmonary rehabilitation for chronic obstructive pulmonary disease. Cochrane Database Syst Rev 2006;(4): CD003793.
11. Carrieri-Kohlman V. Non-pharmacologic approaches. In Booth S, Dudgeon D (eds). Dyspnoea in advanced disease. New York: Oxford University Press, 2006, pp 171-203.

12. Schwartzstein RM, Lahive K, Pope A, et al. Cold facial stimulation reduces breathlessness induced in normal subjects. Am Rev Respir Dis 1987; 136:58-61.
13. Jennings AL, Davies AN, Higgins JPT, et al. Opioids for the palliation of breathlessness in terminal illness. Cochrane Database Syst Rev 2001;(3):CD002066.
14. Abernathy AP, Currow DC, Frith P, et al. Randomised, double blind, placebo controlled crossover trial of sustained release morphine for the management of refractory dyspnea. BMJ 2003;327:523-528.
15. Bruera E, Sala R, Spruyt O, et al. Nebulized versus subcutaneous morphine for patients with cancer dyspnea: A preliminary study. J Pain Symptom Manage 2005;29:613-618.
16. Currow DC. Pharmacological approaches to breathlessness. In Booth S, Dudgeon D (eds). Dyspnoea in advanced disease. New York: Oxford University Press, 2006, pp 237-254.
17. Allen S, Raut S, Wollard J, et al. Low dose diamorphine reduces breathlessness without causing a fall in oxygen saturation in elderly patients with end-stage idiopathic pulmonary fibrosis. Palliat Med 2005;19:128-130.
18. Hu W, Chiu T, Cheng S, et al. Morphine for dyspnea control in terminal cancer patients: Is it appropriate in Taiwan? J Pain Symptom Manage 2004;28:356-363.
19. Light RW, Stansbury DW, Webster JS. Effect of 30 mg of morphine alone or with promethazine or prochlorperazine on the exercise capacity of patients with COPD. Chest 1996;109:975-981.
20. Navigante AH, Cerchietti LC, Castro MA, et al. Midazolam as adjunct therapy to morphine in the alleviation of severe dyspnea perception in patients with advanced cancer. J Pain Symptom Manage 2006;31:38-47.

SUGGESTED READING

Booth S, Dudgeon D (eds). Dyspnoea in advanced disease: A guide to clinical management. New York: Oxford University Press, 2006.

Jennings AL, Davies AN, Higgins JPT, et al. Opioids for the palliation of breathlessness in terminal illness. Cochrane Database Syst Rev 2001;(3):CD002066.

Mahler DA, O'Donnell DE (eds). Dyspnea: Mechanisms, measurement and management, 2nd ed. Boca Raton, FL: Taylor & Francis, 2005.

Viola R, Kiteley C, Lloyd N, et al. The management of dyspnea in cancer patients. No. 13-5 in the evidence-based series from the Program in Evidence-Based Care of Cancer Care Ontario. Available at http://www.cancercare.on.ca/index_practice-Guidelines.htm (accessed January 2008).

CHAPTER **160**

Edema

Lawrence J. Clein

KEY POINTS

- Edema is distressing, disabling, and disfiguring.
- Knowledge of pathophysiology is essential for proper management.
- The cause is often multifactorial. Not knowing all the factors can make treatment difficult.
- The term *edema* is preferable to *lymphedema* in referring to the swollen body, because increased interstitial fluid due to blocked lymph nodes is only one factor.
- Removal of fluid from the interstitial space can be palliative.

Apart from actual pain and consequent insomnia, the discomfort and misery produced by the constant leaden drag of the paralyzed, inflexible, and bolster-like limb are important factors in the sum total of misery produced by the disease.

W. SAMPSON HANDLEY, 1908[1]

Sampson Handley's description of the brawny arm that develops with carcinoma of the breast, published a century ago, is still relevant. Jacques Lisfranc (1845) is reputed to have been the first to treat elephantiasis by small skin incisions. In 1879, Dr. Reginald Southey of St. Bartholomew's Hospital, London, described a fine cannula of his own design, which he used first for the drainage of a pleural effusion but subsequently for the drainage of dropsical limbs. The instrument soon came to be called Southey's tubes. Since then, numerous pharmacological, mechanical, and surgical interventions have been tried,[2-4] but severe, incapacitating edema remains a major problem.

DEFINITION

Edema refers to excess fluid in the body tissues. Most of this fluid is in the interstitial spaces, but there is usually excess fluid both in the vascular bed and within cells. Ascites and hydrothorax are sometimes considered special forms of edema, in which excess fluid accumulates in the peritoneal or pleural cavities, respectively. *Anasarca* is the name given to severe generalized edema. Cerebral edema, a specific entity, is discussed elsewhere (see Chapters 145 and 221).

BASIC SCIENCE

Water is the most abundant body component, constituting 45% to 75% of body weight. In general, total body water (TBW) is about 60% of body weight in healthy males and 50% in healthy females. TBW is inversely proportional to adipose tissue and decreases with age. TBW is distributed into two major compartments: intracellular fluid (ICF), which contains approximately 55% of TBW, and extracellular fluid (ECF), which contains 45% of TBW. The latter is subdivided into plasma (7.5% of TBW) and interstitial fluid (27.5% of TBW). Normally, there is a continuous flow of body water through the vascular system, into interstitial spaces and cells and then back again. The aim is to provide nutrition to each and every body cell and then to remove the waste products of metabolism (excretion). This continuous flow is dependent on the so-called Starling forces, named in honor of the physiologist who first demonstrated their importance.[5] They are

1. *Capillary pressure*, which is largely dependent on arterial pressure: forces fluid outward through the capillary pores at the arterial end of the capillary
2. *Interstitial fluid pressure*, which varies throughout the body: where it is negative, fluid flows into the interstitial space; where it is positive, fluid flows outward
3. *Plasma colloid osmotic pressure*, which causes, by osmosis, an inward flow through the capillary membrane

4. *Interstitial fluid colloid osmotic pressure*, which causes, by osmosis, an outward flow through the capillary membrane (opposite to the plasma colloid osmotic pressure)

When the distribution of body water changes and excess fluid accumulates in the interstitial space, edema occurs. This can result from a disturbance in several factors that together are responsible for the normal circulation and distribution of body water. Fluid can accumulate in the interstitial spaces due to abnormal leakage from capillaries or because the lymphatics are prevented from returning fluid from the interstitium back to the circulation. For further details of the physiology of body fluids, the reader is referred to a textbook of physiology.[6,7]

EPIDEMIOLOGY AND PREVALENCE

Although mild to moderate edema of the legs and lower trunk is common at the end of life, massive edema is more rare. Edema of one upper limb only is usually associated with ipsilateral carcinoma of the breast. The prevalence is related to (1) the extent of the primary disease and its involvement of the drainage of lymph nodes; (2) the type of surgery, both initially and subsequently; and (3) the adjuvant therapy employed, both radiotherapy and chemotherapy. Disease in the axilla, lymphadenectomy, and radiotherapy give rise to a 30% incidence swollen arm in these women.

Edema of one or both legs can occur; in the latter case, the genitalia are usually involved as well. This type of edema is invariably associated with pelvic malignancies (uterus, bladder, prostate, rectum). Either there is already extensive lymph node involvement or the disease has been managed by extensive surgery, lymphadenectomy, and postoperative irradiation. The incidence of edema, derived from several studies reported by Williams and colleagues, is 30% to 40%.[8]

PATHOPHYSIOLOGY

Normally, continuous circulation of body water requires the following[9]:

1. A normal heart to pump the circulation. In congestive heart failure, edema can occur. The mechanism is multifactorial and outside the scope of this chapter (see Chapter 79).
2. Normal blood vessels to allow the proper flow and diffusion of water at the capillary level. Venous obstruction resulting from thrombus or tumor pressure, or increased capillary permeability (e.g., poisons, allergy) causes edema.
3. Exchange of extracellular and intracellular water and solutes for nutrition and excretion of waste products.
4. A functioning lymphatic system for removal of protein from the interstitial space back into the vascular system. The lymph system can be blocked by cancer, infection (e.g., filariasis), surgery, irradiation, or congenital abnormality.
5. The correct body water solutes to maintain appropriate osmotic pressures between intravascular and interstitial spaces and between interstitial and intra-

cellular spaces. These solutes include electrolytes and plasma proteins. Decreased plasma proteins can occur because of loss in urine (nephrotic syndrome) or from burns and wounds or because of failure to produce proteins in liver disease or severe malnutrition. In this circumstance, the plasma colloid osmotic pressure is decreased, which leads to increased capillary filtration and excess fluid in the interstitial spaces.
6. Normal kidneys and urinary pathways to excrete unwanted water, electrolytes, and other products of metabolism.

Edema can result from a disturbance in any one or more of these factors. At the end of life, the cause is invariably multifactorial. Four case studies are provided that illustrate the symptomatic relief of leg and arm edema by the drainage technique described in this chapter.

CLINICAL MANIFESTATIONS

Clinical diagnosis is not difficult.[10] The history will reveal that an illness or its treatment has given rise to symptoms and signs of edema. The patient will report that a leg is swollen, or a shoe no longer fits. Later, when edema becomes massive, extending into the genitalia and the

CASE STUDY

Symptomatic Treatment of Leg Edema by Drainage: Early Case

A 56-year-old patient was generally healthy until diagnosed with a malignant melanoma of the left thigh 4 years ago. He refused conventional treatment apart from a local excision: there was no follow-up for almost 4 years. When seen in March of 2000, he had bilateral leg edema and had metastatic disease in the lung, liver, and inguinal regions bilaterally. In May of 2000, he was admitted to the hospital for management of ascites and edema. His liver was enlarged, and there were metastases in both groins. The skin of the scrotum showed evidence of breakdown and seepage of fluid. His lymphedema extended onto the abdomen up to the umbilicus and was massive. Various measures had been tried to treat the lymphedema, but without success. The serum albumin concentration was 22 g/L. While this patient underwent the "cat scratch treatment" to his left leg, he also agreed to small incisions under local anesthesia and sterile conditions in the lower part of his right leg to determine whether the fluid could be drained. Three superficial cutaneous incisions, approximately 0.5 cm in length, were made on the medial, front, and lateral aspects of the right lower leg, and a small piece of 1/4-inch Penrose drain was secured in each incision with a 4-0 suture. Over the next 24 hours, there was a considerable decrease in edema; the amount of fluid collected in a basin, in which the patient's right leg hung dependently, was 3775 mL. After removal of the Penrose drains, drainage continued from the leg into sterile dressings. A decrease in size of the abdomen and of the genitalia resulted in more comfort and dignity. The patient died just over 2 weeks after the commencement of drainage in the right leg.

■ CASE STUDY

Symptomatic Treatment of Leg Edema by Drainage: Needle Modification

A 64-year-old man was admitted to the palliative care unit on July 5, 2001, directly from home, where he had become completely incapacitated by swelling of the abdomen, genitalia, and legs. He was diagnosed with carcinoma of the prostate in January of 1999 and treated with a full course of radiotherapy. In April of 2000, he was noted to have bone metastases, and in October of that year, he had a craniotomy for a solitary brain metastasis. Further radiotherapy was given to the lower thoracic spine and sacrum in February of 2001. By June 2001, his legs were swelling badly. After admission to the hospital, a computed tomographic scan of the abdomen and pelvis showed extensive retroperitoneal lymphadenopathy and pelvic and mesenteric adenopathy. The serum albumin concentration was 36 g/L. Since the first application of the procedure, the treatment had been modified so that, instead of surgical incisions, no. 19 subcutaneous needles with attached plastic tubing were inserted. The plastic tubing was connected to an enclosed drainage bag (Fig. 160-1). He was treated by subcutaneous needles into both legs below the knees. Over the next week 3865 mL of fluid was drained from the right leg, and 3130 mL from the left leg. The circumferences of the thighs and calves on both sides decreased by more than 2 cm at both levels. The patient left the hospital on a 48-hour pass before discharge and stayed at home, where he lived comfortably until his death 10 days later.

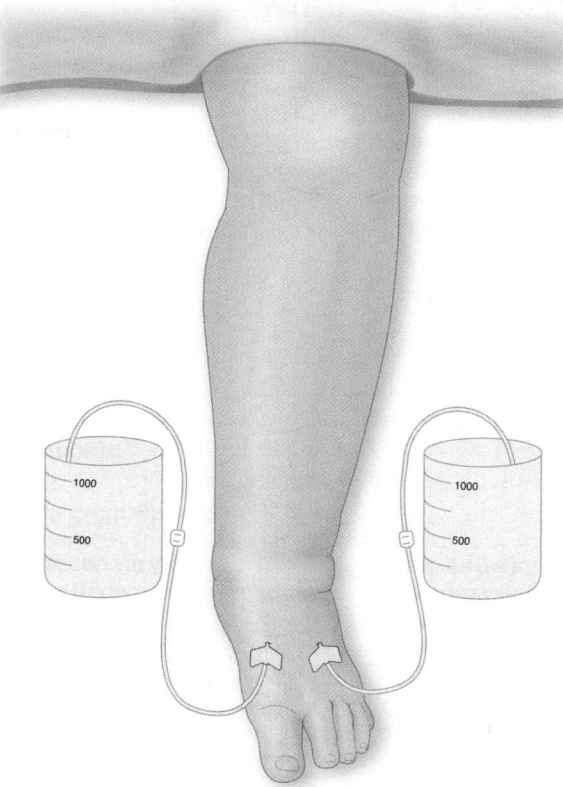

FIGURE 160-1   Ideal needle placement for subcutaneous controlled drainage. Bags lie dependent on the floor or on bed for gravity drainage.

 CASE STUDY

Symptomatic Treatment of Arm Edema by Drainage

A 68-year-old woman was diagnosed with carcinoma of the breast 10 years previously. She underwent a left mastectomy but refused other treatments. She remained in remission for 9 years. Recurrence became obvious when large supraclavicular and infraclavicular lymph nodes were found. She was noted to have marked lymphedema in her left arm. She also had brachial plexus involvement, and the left arm was painful and useless. A short course of chemotherapy and radiotherapy was given, and her pain was treated satisfactorily. However, the edema became worse. She agreed to have the fluid drained from the arm using the previously developed technique. Over 36 hours, 1500 mL of fluid was drained, and the size of the arm was reduced by about 50% (Fig. 160-2). The patient returned home and for the next several weeks kept the swelling down with an elastic bandage. When she stopped using the bandage, the swelling recurred, necessitating a second drainage 7 months later. Once again, good decompression was obtained, but her cancer progressed, and she died 5 months after the second drainage.

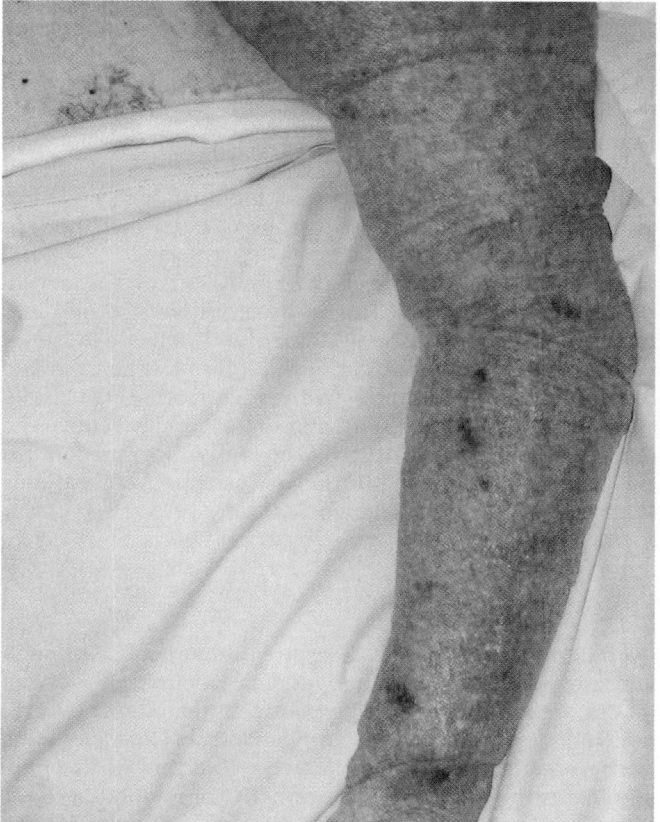

FIGURE 160-2   Same patient as in Figure 160-4 after lymph drainage procedure.

■ **C A S E   S T U D Y**

Symptomatic Treatment of Leg Edema by Drainage: Final Case

A 73-year-old man was diagnosed with carcinoma of the prostate in 1995. He was treated by radiotherapy. In March 2001, he had further radiotherapy to the pelvis for bony metastases. More bone metastases developed, and in April 2002 he was treated with strontium 89. He was first seen by the palliative care service in July 2002 for pain management. He remained comfortable for the next 6 months but had to be readmitted in February 2003 for further pain management and placement of a suprapubic catheter. He was discharged home in March 2003. A month later, he was admitted to hospice for terminal care, because he could no longer be looked after at home. At this time, he had marked swelling of both legs. Drainage was offered, and he accepted the treatment. Over the next 3 or 4 days, approximately 5 L of fluid was drained from both legs, which were reduced in size. The patient remained in the hospice. Toward the end of his life, some leg swelling recurred, but he was no longer distressed by it. The serum albumin concentration at his last admission was 33 g/L. The patient died peacefully 10 weeks later.

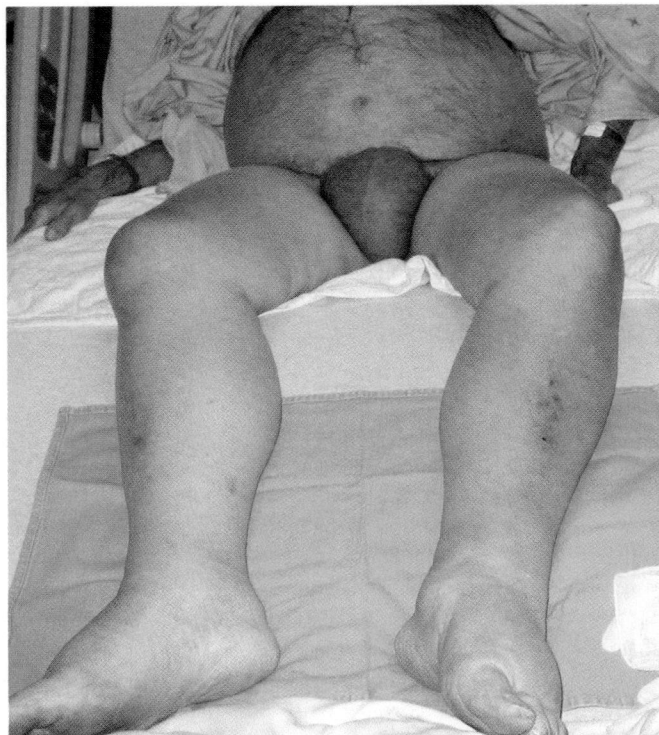

FIGURE 160-3   Massive edema of lower half of body in patient with renal cell carcinoma.

abdomen, the diagnosis is obvious (Fig. 160-3). It is often a terminal sign. The skin is taut and pitting is evident, often up to the umbilicus. Patches of redness may be apparent from extravasation of red cells through damaged capillaries or infection. "Weeping" of clear, watery fluid (lymphorrhea) sometimes occurs. The patient may complain of pain and heaviness and inability to use the limb. The patient or a caregiver may have to lift the leg onto the bed. An edematous arm secondary to breast cancer is frequently painful, heavy, and useless (Fig. 160-4).

A history of malignant melanoma or external genital cancer associated with bilateral inguinal lymphadenectomy may be associated with massive edema of the legs and genitalia.

Investigations include a determination of the serum protein concentration. This is usually low. A computed tomographic scan of the abdomen and pelvis may show compression or obstruction of the inferior vena cava and extensive retroperitoneal lymphadenopathy. Occasionally, ascites may be present, and drainage may relieve the concomitant edema in the lower limbs. Lymphadenopathy may be evident in the pelvis, especially in patients with primary pelvic malignancies.

TREATMENT

Even in mild to moderate cases, treatment may be difficult and time-consuming. When edema occurs early in an illness, treatment must be aggressive if the edema is to be controlled. The treatment is mechanical. Limb elevation is encouraged. Passive and active exercising of the limb stimulates the "muscular component" of lymphatic drainage. Simultaneously, or as soon as some reduction in limb size is obtained, compression bandages should be used. If

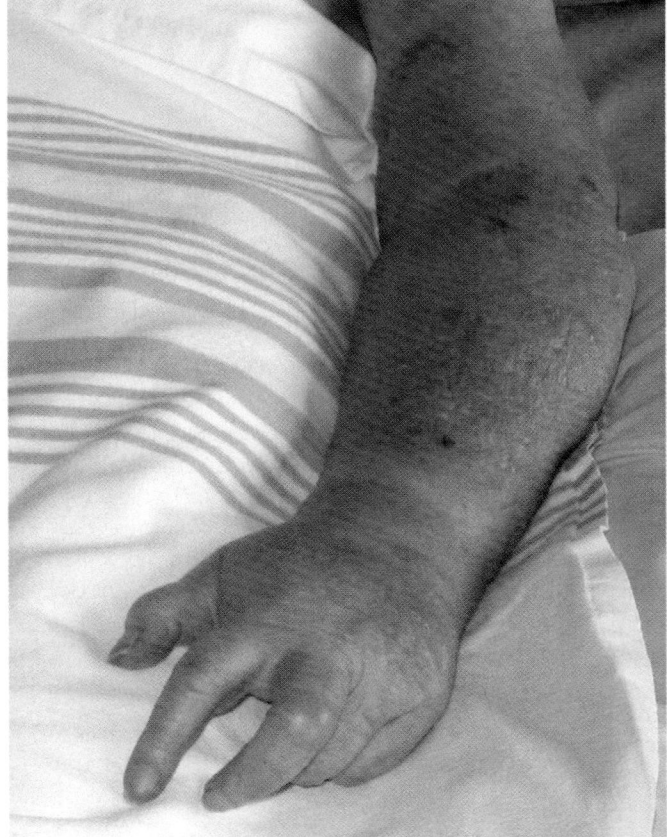

FIGURE 160-4   Swollen arm in patient with carcinoma of the left breast.

this initial therapy is unsuccessful, complete decongestive therapy (CDT) is necessary.[10,11] CDT entails massage techniques followed by bandaging and usually requires the services of expert physiotherapists specialized in this area. Many patients near the end of life are unable to tolerate CDT; moreover, if edema becomes massive, CDT is ineffective.

In my practice, I have reinvented an old technique for limb reduction.[12] Fifteen patients with massive edema, 12 of the lower extremities and 3 of the arm, have undergone this interstitial fluid drainage technique with reduction in limb size and patient satisfaction. The first attempt to drain edema involved making small incisions in the legs and keeping them open with wicks of 1/4-inch Penrose drain. Subsequent cases have been managed more simply by inserting no. 19 butterfly needles into the subcutaneous space and connecting them via tubing to a dependent drainage bag (Bardic Bile Bag, Bard Canada, Mississauga, Ontario). Large amounts of fluid have been drained, with marked reduction in swelling of the genitalia and legs; comparable results have also been achieved with arms treated similarly (see Fig. 160-4). However, this technique is suitable only for massive edema and is a palliative procedure.

Finally, there are reports suggesting that sodium selenite (selenium) is useful for severe edema, but this therapy is still experimental.[13] (See "Future Considerations.")

MANAGEMENT FLOW CHART

Figure 160-5 shows a management algorithm for the treatment of massive edema at the end of life. The following

---

Future Considerations

- If interstitial fluid cannot be returned to the general circulation, then, like pleural or peritoneal fluid, it may have to be drained.
- Subcutaneous needles in palliative care are frequently used for medication administration—a safe and minor procedure. Similar needles can drain unwanted matter from the subcutaneous (i.e., interstitial) space.
- Selenium (sodium selenite) has been recommended as an adjuvant to complete decongestive therapy (CDT) but is still investigative. Its use is mainly early in the disease. There is no evidence that it can affect the massive edema of late disease. The indications for and role of selenium remain unclear.

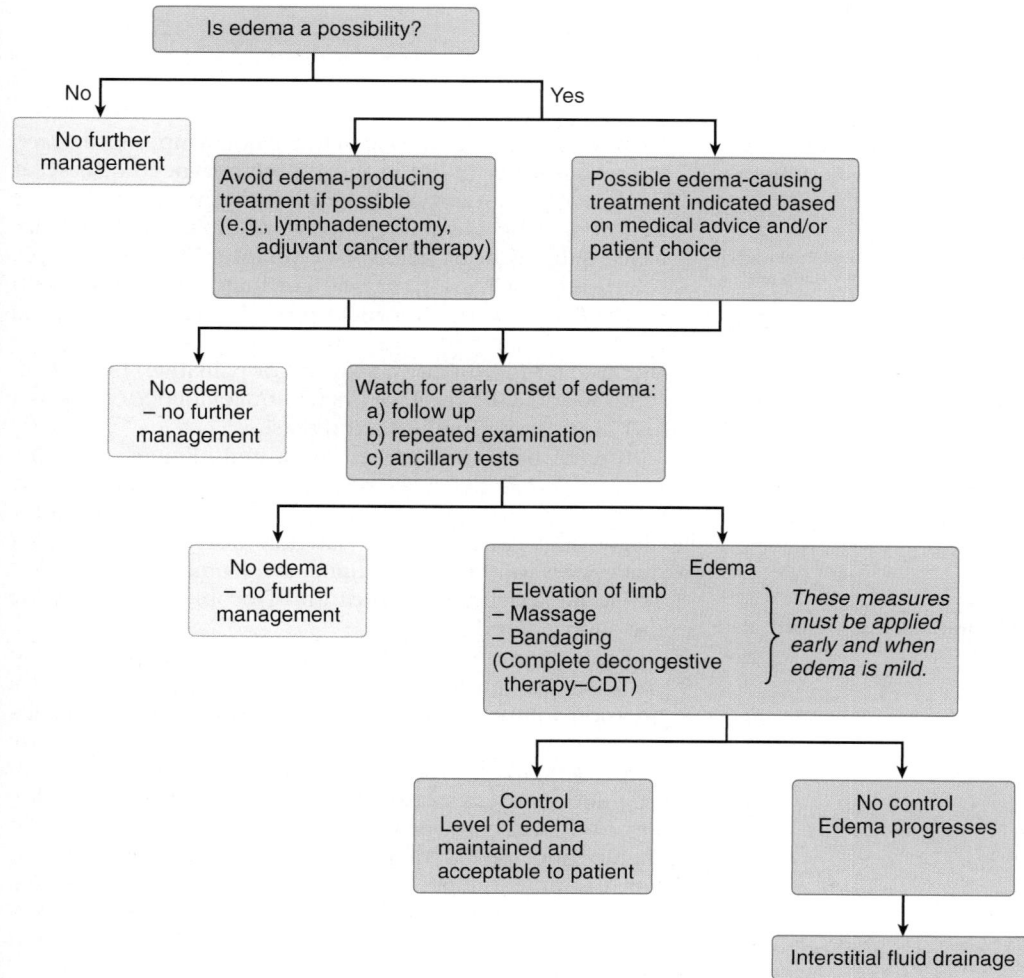

FIGURE 160-5 Algorithm for managing edema.

considerations are important in the treatment of this debilitating symptom:

1. Know which malignancies cause edema.
2. Prevention is key. For example, avoid extensive prophylactic lymphadenectomy.
3. Advise patients of risk, and encourage early reporting of symptoms.
4. Aggressive mechanical treatment (CDT) can then be instituted. This includes elevation of the limb or limbs, massage for drainage, and bandaging.
5. With the exception of congestive heart failure (for which diuretics and digitalis are indicated), there is no effective pharmacological treatment for edema. Diuretics may relieve some pressure symptoms of severe edema due to other causes, but they do not appreciably reduce the size of the limb.
6. In extreme edema at the end of life, lymph drainage (external technique) is indicated. This will reduce limb size, reduce genital swelling, improve function, and improve appearance.

REFERENCES

1. Handley WS. Lymphangioplasty: A new method for the relief of the brawny arm of breast cancer and for similar conditions of lymphatic edema. Preliminary note. Lancet 1908;1:783-785.
2. Jantet GH, Taylor GW, Kinmonth JB. Operations for primary lymphedema of the lower limbs: Results after 1-9 years. J Cardiovasc Surg 1961;2:27-36.
3. Degni M. New technique for the subcutaneous drainage of peripheral lymphedema. Lymphology 1992;25:182-183.
4. Brorson H. Complete reduction of lymphedema of the arm by liposuction after breast cancer. Scand J Plast Reconstr Hand Surg 1997;31:137-143.
5. Braunwald E: Edema. IN: Braunwald E, Fauci A, Kasper D, et al. (eds) Harrison's Principles of Internal Medicine, 15th Ed., McGraw-Hill, New York, 2001, pp. 217-222.
6. Guyton AC, Hall JE (eds). Textbook of Medical Physiology, 11th ed. Philadelphia: Saunders, 2006.
7. West JB (ed). Physiological Basis of Medical Practice, 12th ed. Philadelphia: Williams & Wilkins, 1991.
8. Williams AF, Franks PJ, Moffatt CJ. Lymphoedema: Estimating the size of the problem. Palliat Med 2005;19:300-313.
9. Stanton A. How does swelling occur? The physiology and pathophysiology of interstitial fluid formation. In Twycross R, Jenns K, Todd J (eds). Lymphedema. Oxford: Radclife Medical Press, 2000, pp. 11-21.
10. Keeley V. Clinical features of lymphoedema. In Twycross R, Jenns K, Todd J (eds). Lymphedema. Oxford: Radcliffe Medical Press, 2000, pp. 44-67.
11. Mortimer PS, Badger C. Lymphedema. In Doyle D, Hanks G, Cherny N, Calman K (eds). Oxford Textbook of Palliative Medicine, 3rd ed. New York: Oxford University Press, 2004, pp. 640-647.
12. Clein LJ, Pugachev E. Reduction of edema of lower extremities by subcutaneous, controlled drainage: Eight cases. Am J Hospice Palliat Med 2004; 21:228-232.
13. Bruns F, Schueller P. Novel treatment options in secondary lymphedema. AAHPM Q Newsl 2005;6(4):5-7.

SUGGESTED READING

Twycross R, Jenns K, Todd J (eds). Lymphedema. Oxford: Radcliffe Medical Press, 2000.

CHAPTER 161

Fatigue

Susan B. LeGrand

KEY POINTS

- Fatigue is the most common symptom in advanced disease.
- It is a multidimensional symptom that is different from the common feeling of tiredness experienced by all.
- Evaluation should include a search for reversible causes, including depression, nutritional deficits, deconditioning, organ dysfunction (particularly endocrine abnormalities), anemia, sleep disorders, and uncontrolled symptoms (particularly pain).
- Exercise treatment may help but may be difficult in advanced disease.
- There are no controlled trials of medical management, but case series, expert opinion, and anecdotal success suggest that psychostimulants (e.g., methylphenidate, modafinil) and corticosteroids may provide some symptomatic improvement.

Fatigue has emerged as one of the major symptoms detracting from quality of life in those with advanced disease. It tends to be underreported to physicians because it is believed to be inevitable and untreatable.[1] In some diseases, such as heart failure (see Chapter 79) and multiple sclerosis (see Chapter 191), fatigue may not correlate with stage of disease; but in cancer-related fatigue, it manifests in three defined settings[2]: in patients receiving chemotherapy or radiotherapy (adjuvant or palliative) (see Chapters 236 and 239), in survivors without evidence of disease, and in those with advanced disease.

Fatigue has been defined as "a multidimensional phenomenon that develops over time, diminishing energy, mental capacity, and psychologic condition."[3] Criteria for diagnosing cancer-related fatigue were adapted from guidelines for chronic fatigue syndrome (Box 161-1).[4] These demonstrate the breadth of problems covered by the simple word, "fatigue."

Fatigue related to cancer treatment follows specific patterns. Radiation therapy typically causes a slow progression followed by gradual resolution. Severity relates to fraction size and duration of treatment.[5] Chemotherapy tends to be more cyclic, with an episode of fatigue occurring shortly after treatment and lasting several days, followed by a second peak if neutropenia occurs.[6] Specific therapeutic agents may have more significant impact. For example, gemcitabine has asthenia as a potential side effect. Fatigue is prevalent, constant, and a dose-limiting toxicity in immunotherapy with interferons and interleukins.

BASIC SCIENCE

Much has been learned about pain by creating animal models—causing pain and then looking for response, blocking various receptors, and so on. But how does one identify a fatigued rat? The science has focused on (1) energy imbalance, (2) hypothalamic-pituitary-adrenal axis (HPA) abnormalities, and (3) inflammatory cytokines.[7]

There are several basic questions. Because fatigue is common in many diseases, does it have a unifying pathophysiology? Is it a central nervous system problem, a peripheral problem (neuromuscular junction), or a varying combination of both? Does one treat cause or effect (i.e., the symptom or the physiological derangement if known)? Because fatigue is often multifactorial, do all factors need to be treated for symptomatic improvement?

Energy imbalance may result from cachexia, impaired oxygen delivery, metabolic derangements, or other causes. Deconditioning could also be considered an energy imbalance, because muscles require greater effort to accomplish a task, resulting in fatigue. Correcting a particular imbalance, such as anemia, may not fully resolve fatigue, reflecting the multifactorial nature of the symptom.[8] The situation is even more complex when one realizes that some causes of energy imbalance, particularly cachexia, are cytokine induced.

The HPA axis is affected by interferon, both acutely and with long-term administration,[9] and fatigue is a dose limiting toxicity. Both hypoactivity and hyperactivity of the HPA have been proposed as causative. Hypoactivity occurs in chronic fatigue syndrome.[10] Hyperactivity is

DISEASE	PERCENTAGE	STUDY (REF. NO.)
Cancer	17-90	Cella et al, 2001 (4)
Chronic obstructive pulmonary disease	47	Mota and Pimenta, 2006 (13)
Congestive heart failure	10	National Comprehensive Cancer Network, 2006 (14)
	75	National Institute for Health and Clinical Excellence (15)
Multiple sclerosis	76-92	

TABLE 161-1 Prevalence of Fatigue

noted in chronic stress situations such as cancer. It may also cause depression, which may contribute to fatigue.[11]

Inflammatory cytokines are the most active area of research. Cytokines are messengers for the immune system. They are manufactured by T cells, macrophages, and others cells such as endothelial cells and fibroblasts. They may be locally active, or they may circulate in the bloodstream. The most commonly cited culprits are interleukin-1 (IL1), IL6, and tumor necrosis factor-α (TNF-α).[12] Many of the recombinant cytokines available for therapeutic use have fatigue as a side effect. They are also implicated in other processes that contribute to fatigue, such as anemia and cachexia.

EPIDEMIOLOGY AND PREVALENCE

The wide ranges of fatigue prevalence that have been reported (Table 161-1) reflect the varied diagnostic criteria (malignancy, multiple sclerosis) and disease stages (cancer, heart failure) addressed. One of the concerns with studies of cancer-related fatigue is the heterogeneity of the groups surveyed, which have included those with advanced disease, survivors, and individuals receiving active treatment. The lowest prevalence (17%) was reported among cancer survivors using the strictest criteria: the proposed *International Classification of Diseases and Health-Related Problems*, 10th revision (ICD-10), which requires daily fatigue for 2 weeks and 6 of 11 additional symptoms.[4] The highest numbers are reported from palliative care settings or among those undergoing active treatment, particularly immunotherapy.

Screening and diagnostic tests for fatigue are numerous, somewhat disease specific, and often not validated in other populations. They may be unidimensional, such as a visual analogue or numerical rating scale, or multidimensional (Table 161-2)[13] (see Chapter 64). For clinical practice guidelines for cancer-related fatigue, I recommend the numerical rating scale or a categorical (none/mild/moderate/severe) scale.[14] (See the two case studies on assessment and treatment of fatigue.)

CLINICAL MANIFESTATIONS

The first and most important step in diagnosis is to ask whether the patient is experiencing fatigue. Patients often suffer significantly yet fail to mention it to physicians, so

TABLE 161-2   Selection of Multidimensional Tools for Fatigue

TOOL	DISEASE
Multidimensional Fatigue Inventory (MFI)	Cancer
Profile of Mood States (POMS)	Cancer
Functional Assessment for Cancer Illness Therapy–Fatigue	Cancer
Functional Assessment of Cancer Therapy–Fatigue (FACT-F)	Cancer
Fatigue Severity State (FSS)	Multiple sclerosis
Modified Fatigue Impact Scale (MFIS)	Multiple sclerosis
Epworth Sleepiness Scale (ESS)	Multiple sclerosis
Brief Fatigue Inventory	Multiple sclerosis, cancer
Piper Fatigue Scale (PFS) and Short Form (PFS-SF)	HIV, cancer
Chalder Fatigue Scale	HIV

From Mota DD, Pimenta CA. Self-report instruments for fatigue assessment: A systematic review. Res Theory Nurs Pract 2006;20:49-78.

CASE STUDY

Assessment and Treatment of Fatigue: Nutritional Deficiency

Mrs. M was an 84-year-old woman with hormone-positive metastatic breast cancer to bone. Eighteen months earlier, she had presented with severe back pain, at which time the diagnosis was made and radiation therapy was done. Hemoglobin and hematocrit were normal at that time. She developed anemia subsequent to radiation therapy, and this had not improved despite evidence of tumor response. Her chart noted that blood work was "acceptable for current state of disease." Mrs. M, who continued to live alone, complained bitterly of fatigue and weakness that limited her ability to cook a meal or wash her dishes without needing rest before the task was complete. She was referred to the palliative medicine service for management. She denied depression and other symptoms such as pain, and she had normal organ function, with normochromic anemia as the only laboratory abnormality. Evaluation identified both iron and vitamin B_{12} deficiency. Oral iron supplementation and monthly B_{12} injections normalized her hemoglobin and resolved the fatigue.

it is imperative to assess for this symptom. National Comprehensive Cancer Network (NCCN) guidelines recommend screening on the first visit and then at "appropriate" intervals.[14] Inquiring about a symptom legitimizes it and can be both a therapeutic and an educational intervention. One of the key aspects of differential assessment is the focused history (see Chapter 61). No matter what the underlying disease, one must first be certain of its status. Does this fatigue represent the first sign of cancer or a recurrence or progression? Is it a sign of progressive cardiac failure?

One should carefully review current medications, particularly any new agents started before the onset of fatigue. In advanced disease, medications may no longer be necessary yet can cause toxicity. For example, weight loss from

CASE STUDY

Assessment and Treatment of Fatigue: Multifactorial

Mr. C was a 55-year-old man with metastatic pancreatic cancer. His cancer had recently progressed while he was receiving therapy, and he elected to enroll in hospice. His primary complaints were pain and fatigue. He was unable to attend a dinner in his honor because of fatigue. He was not sleeping well because he awakened every 2 to 3 hours needing pain medication. Laboratory values were notable for mildly elevated liver enzymes. He was referred to the palliative medicine service for management. His current pain regimen was morphine, 30 mg every 3 hours as needed. He usually waited until his pain was 7 or greater on a numerical rating scale (NRS) and achieved 75% relief within 45 to 60 minutes. His average daily morphine dose was 150 mg, with more of the breakthrough dosing occurring at night. He had been given sustained-release medication but misunderstood the plan and did not take it routinely. His intake fatigue level on an NRS was 9. He was satisfied with his current level of pain control and was worried about increasing the dose and having more fatigue. On day 1, he was prescribed sustained-release morphine, 60 mg at 8 AM and 90 mg at 8 PM, with no change in breakthrough dosing. Two days later, on phone report, his pain was better controlled and he was sleeping through the night. There was no change in his fatigue level. He was started on methylphenidate 5 mg at 8 AM and at noon, with transient improvement, and then increased to 10 mg per dose. On this regimen, his fatigue score on the NRS was 3 and he was able to go to his office for several hours. He expressed regret that he did not have this medication before his honorary dinner.

Box 161-2 Factors to Assess in Fatigue Evaluation

- Pain
- Emotional distress
- Sleep disturbance
- Anemia
- Nutrition/electrolyte assessment
- Activity level
- Co-morbidities
- Infection
- Organ dysfunction (cardiopulmonary, renal, hepatic, neurologic)
- Endocrine function

From National Comprehensive Cancer Network Practice Guidelines in Oncology, Vol. 1, 2006. Available at http://www.nice.org.uk/nicemedia/pdf/cg008guidance.pdf (accessed May 5, 2008).

cachexia can decrease the need for hypertensive medications and hypoglycemic agents. The NCCN has outlined seven factors that contribute to fatigue (Box 161-2).[14] Other diseases do not have clear guidelines. The National Institute for Health and Clinical Excellence (NICE) in the UK developed recommendations for fatigue in multiple sclerosis that include evaluation for four of the seven factors (i.e., depression, sleep, pain, and nutrition).[15] It would seem prudent to look at all seven in anyone with fatigue.

TABLE 161-3 Treatment Algorithm for Cancer-Related Fatigue

PATIENT/FAMILY EDUCATION AND COUNSELING	GENERAL STRATEGIES FOR MANAGEMENT OF FATIGUE	Specific Interventions	
		NONPHARMACOLOGIC	PHARMACOLOGIC
Information about known pattern of fatigue during and after treatment • Expected end-of-life symptom • May vary in intensity	Energy conservation • Set priorities • Delegate • Schedule activities at times of peak energy • Use labor-saving and assistive devices • Eliminate nonessential activities • Naps that do not interrupt nighttime sleep • Structured daily routine • Attend to one activity at a time • Conserve energy for valued activities Distraction (e.g., games music, reading, socializing)	Activity enhancement • Optimize level of activity • Consider referral to physical therapy/physical medicine and rehabilitation therapy as appropriate • Use caution in cases of bone metastases, immunosuppression/neutropenia, thrombocytopenia, anemia, or fever Attention-restoring therapy (e.g., nature) Nutrition consultation Sleep therapy • Consider sleep hygiene and/or sleep medication Family interaction Psychosocial interventions (category 1) • Stress management • Relaxation • Support groups	Consider psychostimulants after ruling out other causes of fatigue • Consider methylphenidate Treat for anemia as indicated Repeat evaluation

*These Guidelines are a work in progress that will be refined as often as new significant data become available.

TREATMENT

One of the guiding principles and idiomatic statements in symptom management is to treat the underlying cause whenever possible (see Chapter 148). Fixing the cause is almost always more effective than any nonspecific symptomatic intervention. For example, removing an effusion is more effective than administering morphine for dyspnea. The cause of fatigue must be sought and the contributory factors treated, knowing that the symptom itself may not fully resolve. As with many symptoms of advanced disease, the contributing factors (e.g., cachexia) may not yet have been effectively treated. One should also consider symptomatic treatment while assessment continues, as for pain management (Table 161-3).

There are no controlled trials to determine the ideal therapy. The best evidence of efficacy exists for exercise, even though most controlled trials have significant methodological problems and many were conducted in breast cancer patients, both on and off therapy. Despite these problems, there is some confidence that beginning or maintaining an exercise program is useful to prevent or treat fatigue.[16] The one attempt to study exercise in advanced disease involved 24 patients: 13 declined, and only 9 completed the intervention.[17] There was an improvement trend and a sense of satisfaction among those patients who were able to complete the study.

One of the most common recommendations for cancer patients with fatigue is energy conservation and/or activity management (ECAM). ECAM balances rest and activity by setting priorities, delegating responsibilities, pacing, and scheduling activities to reflect peaks and valleys in energy levels during the day.[18] Comprehensive educational interventions have also been tested with some benefit, often from the opportunity to talk about the symptom.[19] It is certainly reasonable to consider education for patients and families as one element of a comprehensive management strategy.

Pharmacological Interventions

In patients with limited life expectancy, medical management may be most appropriate for rapid intervention. This is not to marginalize other measures but to stress the importance of an aggressive approach in those who are suffering most. There have been only small trials of medical interventions in advanced cancer and human immunodeficiency virus (HIV) infection, and none in most other diseases except multiple sclerosis. Drug choice is often best determined by (1) other comorbid symptoms that might be addressed with the same medication (e.g., depression, fatigue, and sedation with methylphenidate), (2) life expectancy (e.g., dexamethasone for short-term use), (3) cost (e.g., modafinil).

Despite the inclusion of dexamethasone, the only study of fatigue identified evaluated its use for irinotecan-induced delayed emesis, anorexia, and fatigue. This randomized, placebo-controlled trial found benefit that approached significance for treatment-related anorexia and fatigue. Treatment in other advanced diseases is unknown. In heart failure and advanced chronic obstructive pulmonary disease, dyspnea may complicate activity and contribute to fatigue. Psychostimulants may be problematic in those who are prone to tachycardia and arrhythmias. No studies have been done to date.

SUMMARY

Fatigue is a near-universal symptoms in advanced disease and is also prevalent in less advanced chronic illness. Current knowledge is limited, and no evidence-based recommendations can be made other than the use of exercise and correction of anemia in cancer patients undergoing therapy. Management of contributing factors with nonpharmacological and/or pharmacological interventions, based on an evaluation of the patient goals of care, is recommended (see "Future Considerations").

- What is the pathophysiology?
- Is the underlying pathophysiology in different disease populations and different phases of disease the same or different?
- If different, then should studies evaluate more homogeneous populations or stratify for differences?
- What is a clinically relevant level of improvement on self-report scores?
- Is clinically relevant improvement subjective only (i.e., self-report scores improve) or quantitative (i.e., translates into improved activity level, performance status, survival, and so on)?
- Is there a preferred pharmacological therapy algorithm? Is it population specific?

REFERENCES

1. Stone P, Richardson A, Ream E, et al. Cancer-related fatigue: Inevitable, unimportant and untreatable? Results of a multi-centre patient survey. Ann Oncol 2000;11:971-975.
2. LeGrand SB. Cancer fatigue: More data, less information? Curr Oncol Rep 2002;4:275-279.
3. Portenoy RK, Itri LM. Cancer-related fatigue: Guidelines for evaluation and management. Oncologist 1999;4:1-10.
4. Cella D, Davis K, Breitbart W, Curt G; Fatigue Coalition. Cancer-related fatigue: Prevalence of proposed diagnostic criteria in a United States sample of cancer survivors. J Clin Oncol 2001;19:3385-3391.
5. Furst CJ, Ahsberg E. Dimensions of fatigue during radiotherapy: An application of the multidimensional fatigue inventory. Support Care Cancer 2001;9:355-360.
6. Berger AM. Patterns of fatigue and activity and rest during adjuvant breast cancer chemotherapy. Oncol Nurs Forum 1998;25:51-62.
7. Gutstein HB. The biologic basis of fatigue. Cancer 2001;92(6 Suppl):1678-1683.
8. Munch TN, Zhang T, Willey J, et al. The association between anemia and fatigue in patients with advanced cancer receiving palliative care. J Palliat Med 2005;8:1144-1149.
9. Malik UR, Makower DF, Wadler S. Interferon-mediated fatigue. Cancer 2001;92(6 Suppl):1664-1668.
10. Scott LV, Dinan TG. The neuroendocrinology of chronic fatigue syndrome: Focus on the hypothalamic-pituitary-adrenal axis. Funct Neurol 1999;14:3-11.
11. Checkley S. The neuroendocrinology of depression and chronic stress. Br Med Bull 1996;52:597-617.
12. Kurzrock R. The role of cytokines in cancer-related fatigue. Cancer 2001;91(6 Suppl):1684-1688.
13. Mota DD, Pimenta CA. Self-report instruments for fatigue assessment: A systematic review. Res Theory Nurs Pract 2006;20:49-78.
14. National Comprehensive Cancer Network. Clinical Practice Guidelines in Oncology, Vol. 1, 2006. Available at http://www.nccn.org/professionals/physician_gls/PDF/fatigue.pdf (accessed May 5, 2008).
15. National Institute for Health and Clinical Excellence. Published Clinical Guidelines. Available at http://www.nice.org.uk/nicemedia/pdf/cg008guidance.pdf (accessed May 5, 2008).
16. Knols R, Aaronson NK, Uebelhart D, et al. Physical exercise in cancer patients during and after medical treatment: A systematic review of randomized and controlled clinical trials. J Clin Oncol 2005;23:3830-3842.
17. Porock D, Kristjanson LJ, Tinnelly K, et al. An exercise intervention for advanced cancer patients experiencing fatigue: A pilot study. J Palliat Care 2000;16:30-36.
18. Barsevick AM, Dudley W, Beck S, et al. A randomized clinical trial of energy conservation for patients with cancer-related fatigue. Cancer 2004;100:1302-1310.
19. Ream E, Richardson A, Alexander-Dann C. Facilitating patients' coping with fatigue during chemotherapy: Pilot outcomes. Cancer Nurs 2002;25:300-308.

CHAPTER **162**

Fever and Sweats

Bart Bobb, Laurie Lyckholm, and Patrick Coyne

- Evaluation and treatment of fever and sweats must be considered in the context of burdens, benefits, and goals of care.
- Fevers and sweats should be treated only if they cause discomfort or intolerable metabolic demand.
- Antipyretics should be given on a schedule to avoid hectic fever patterns and waves of sweating.
- Ice baths, tepid sponging, and cooling blankets are uncomfortable and are best avoided.
- Universal comfort measures include treatment of thirst, fastidious oral care, attention to ambient temperature and air circulation, and provision of clean, dry clothing and bedclothes.

FEVER

Fever is defined as an oral temperature exceeding 38° C.[1] Evaluation and management must be considered in the broader context of the prognosis, the illness trajectory, and the goals of care.

Pathophysiology

The anterior hypothalamus regulates body temperature. Fever occurs when the hypothalamic "thermostat" is reset higher[1] due to pyrogens, fever-causing substances, entering the body. Exogenous pyrogens are released by pathogens (viruses, bacteria, and/or fungi). Pathogen destruction stimulates the immune system to produce endogenous pyrogens: interleukin-1 (IL1) and IL6, tumor necrosis factor (TNF), and interferons. Both exogenous and endogenous pyrogens trigger fever by increasing the hypothalamic set point.[2] The body maintains the core temperature at this new set point via shivering (skeletal muscle contraction) and nonshivering (chemical) thermogenesis, until the set point is lowered as a result of fewer pyrogens, antipyretic medications, or (misguided) nonpharmacological cooling methods such as fans, tepid baths, and cooling blankets (Fig. 162-1)[1] (see "Case Study: Treatment of Fever at the End of Life").

Clinical Manifestations

Fever usually has three phases: chill, fever, and flush.[3] The first phase, cold or chill, results from the increased hypothalamic set point, which causes the body to raise core temperature through cutaneous vasoconstriction (to prevent heat loss) and increased skeletal muscle contraction (to generate heat). The resulting symptoms are chills and rigors, respectively.[3]

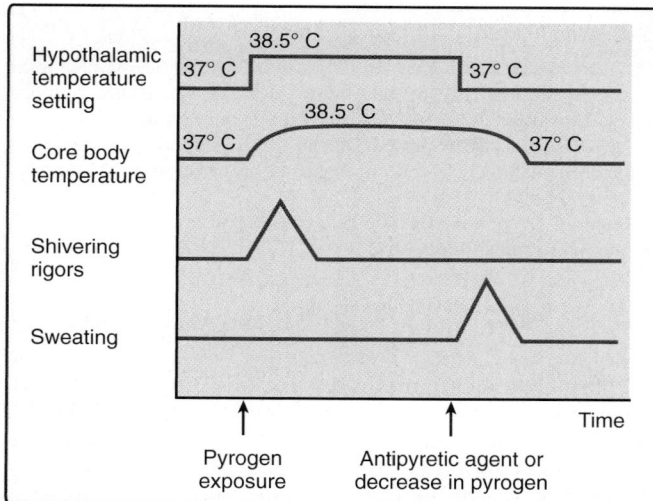

FIGURE 162-1 Physiological symptoms associated with fever and accompanying symptoms. *(From Cleary JF. Fever and sweats. In Berger AM, Portenoy RK, Weissman DE (eds). Principles and Practice of Palliative Care and Supportive Oncology, 2nd ed. Philadelphia: Lippincott, Williams & Wilkins, 2002, p 155.)*

  C A S E   S T U D Y

Treatment of Fever at the End of Life

AM, a 74-year-old patient with severe end-stage chronic obstructive pulmonary disease (COPD), was enrolled in hospice and was believed to have 2 to 4 months to live. She had a prior history of coronary artery disease and infective endocarditis and presented to the emergency room with fever and anorexia. Echocardiography revealed recurrent infective endocarditis that required valve replacement, because antibiotic therapy alone was deemed insufficient to treat the disease. Surgery, however, was not recommended due to the patient's severe COPD and overall poor prognosis. The risks of surgery simply outweighed the potential benefits. AM decided that she wished to receive comfort measures only and was admitted to the palliative care unit. Her fevers were initially low grade, and she denied discomfort associated with them; therefore, symptomatic treatment was not initiated. Plans were made to return AM home with hospice care, but her fevers suddenly escalated to greater than 103° F, she became verbally unresponsive, and it appeared that she might be actively dying. The fevers seemed to be causing distress, and acetaminophen rectal suppositories were scheduled around-the-clock. When her fevers persisted, intravenous ketorolac was scheduled every 6 hours. Her fever subsided, and she appeared more comfortable while remaining unresponsive and afebrile until she died 2 days later.

The second phase, fever, occurs when the core temperature rises to meet the newly elevated set point. Heat loss equals heat generation. Symptoms in this phase include thirst, warm and flushed skin, dehydration, lethargy, and occasionally delirium or seizures.[2]

The final phase, flush, occurs when the set point has normalized and the body uses cooling mechanisms, vasodilation and diaphoresis, to lower core temperature to the new set point.[3] Older adults often have a diminished or absent febrile response and also a lower baseline body temperature, making it difficult to diagnose fever based on body temperature.[4]

Differential Diagnosis

Common causes of fever in the palliative care setting include infection, malignancy, neurological disorders, inflammation, drugs, blood transfusions, and autoimmune diseases. Other causes include hemorrhage, constipation, and dehydration.[2]

Infections are the most common cause of fever in palliative care. Up to 90% of all new fevers from infectious pathogens are caused by bacteria, which produce endotoxins and prompt the immune system to release endogenous pyrogenic cytokines.[2] Cancer patients with neutropenia (absolute peripheral neutrophil count less than 500 cells/mL) are at high risk for infection. The exact source is not identified in 60% to 70% of the cases,[1] and 50% to 70% of those with neutropenic fever die from overwhelming sepsis if not treated within 48 hours.[2] Common sources in neutropenic patients include decubitus ulcers, surgical wounds, pneumonia, mucositis, gastrointestinal sources such as *Clostridium difficile*, urinary tract infections, vascular access devices, and nosocomial bloodstream or urine infections.[1] Fever may also occur throughout the course of infection with the human immunodeficiency virus (HIV), but it is prevalent and has more complications in the later stages.[5]

Malignancies, including solid tumors (not often considered in the context of classic "B symptoms"), may cause paraneoplastic fevers. Potential causes include production of pyrogens or cytokines, hypersensitivity reaction, and cytokine release secondary to tumor necrosis.[6]

Neurological disorders may be associated with fever in cases of central nervous system (CNS) or spinal cord infection; systemic febrile disorders (e.g., vasculitis, lupus); or primary central or peripheral neurological disorders, including spinal cord injuries above T8, hypothalamic damage secondary to head injuries, lesions, and tumors, intracranial hemorrhage without hypothalamic damage (especially intraventricular bleeding), seizures, and strokes (particularly large infarctions).[7]

Inflammation of any type may cause fever. Potential causes in palliative care include radiation therapy, aspiration pneumonia, allergic reaction, thrombophlebitis, and pulmonary embolism. Inflammatory autoimmune disorders such as systemic lupus erythematosus and rheumatoid arthritis and nonspecific vasculitides may also produce fever.

Pharmaceutical agents may cause fever via several mechanisms. Some drugs, particularly antibiotics (e.g., penicillins, cephalosporins, the antifungal agent amphotericin B) can produce an allergic response including fever. Agents used in chemotherapy (e.g., bleomycin, cisplatin) and biological therapies (e.g., interferons, growth factors) can cause fever, as can CNS drugs (e.g., phenytoin), and some cardiovascular drugs (particularly quinidine and protamine).[1] Withdrawal from certain drugs (e.g., opioids, benzodiazepines) may also cause fever.[2] Anticholinergic drugs, such as atropine, antihistamines, scopolamine, tricyclic antidepressants, phenothiazine, and butyrophenone tranquilizers, reduce heat loss through impairment of sweating.

Blood transfusions may cause fevers by various means, ranging from serious hemolytic reactions to febrile non-hemolytic reactions caused by cytokines from transfused white blood cells (WBCs) or recipient antibodies against WBC antigens. Fever due to the latter may be reduced but not prevented by filters that leukoreduce blood products. Routine acetaminophen administration could delay recognition of a serious, even lethal process such as hemolytic transfusion reaction or sepsis. No study has supported the efficacy of acetaminophen in reducing febrile, nonhemolytic reaction. Acetaminophen should be used only for uncomfortable fevers during transfusion, and careful evaluation should be performed to rule out more serious reactions.

Other causes of fever include gastrointestinal bleeding, which may manifest with a low-grade fever and sweats, as well as dehydration and severe constipation.[1]

Our challenge is not only to determine the etiology of a fever but to decide whether to do so. This involves deciding whether treatment of the underlying cause would help achieve the goals of care. For example, in cases of fever from a suspected lung infection, when the goal of care is purely comfort, defining and treating the process may not only improve fever and associated symptoms but may also improve breathing and possibly extend survival. The burdens of testing (e.g., radiography, computed tomography) and treatment with antibiotics must be weighed against the potential benefits. During palliative care, but not when a patient is actively dying, radiological testing and use of antibiotics may be indicated. Closer to the end of life, potentially uncomfortable testing (for some, even being moved to the radiology suite is painful) may be too burdensome, and empirical treatment with antibiotics and/or simple comfort measures may be best. In other instances, noninvasive methods (e.g., a urine sample to rule out urinary tract infection) may reveal an easily treatable cause, and its treatment may improve quality of life while avoiding procedures that could cause discomfort (e.g., lumbar puncture).

Treatment

Although fever may require significant evaluation to find a cause, treatment of that cause is not necessarily indicated (see "Case Study: Treatment of Fever at the End of Life"). In other cases, treatment may certainly be indicated. Antibiotics may be administered for curative or palliative purposes.[8] Fever in an adult should be treated only if it causes discomfort or severe metabolic demand, such as in severe cardiac disease. Fever itself may actually help the body's defense mechanisms. One hypothesis is that pyrogenic cytokines have beneficial effects at lower levels (in mild to moderate infections) but become harmful and accelerate death at high levels (in overwhelming infection).[9] The decision as to whether to treat fever in the palliative setting may be complex. Not all fevers, especially low grade fevers, are uncomfortable. If the patient can communicate, treatment should hinge on whether the fever is causing discomfort; if it is not, treatment is not warranted. In other cases, treating an unresponsive patient's fever may be palliative for the family.

Box 162-1 Drugs of Choice for Symptomatic Fever Treatment

- Acetaminophen, 325-650 mg by mouth (tablets, capsules, liquid, or concentrated drops [80 mg/0.8 mL] or per rectum
- NSAIDs, such as ibuprofen, 200-400 mg by mouth every 4-6 hr; naproxen, 200 mg by mouth every 8-12 hr; or ketorolac, 15-30 mg IV every 6 hr[10]
- Aspirin, 325-650 mg by mouth or per rectum every 4-6 hr
- Corticosteroids (doses vary)

NSAIDs, nonsteroidal anti-inflammatory drugs.

Pharmacological methods include acetaminophen, aspirin, and nonsteroidal anti-inflammatory drugs (NSAIDs) such as ibuprofen and naproxen, which inhibit prostaglandin synthesis and lower the hypothalamic set point. Acetaminophen is safe in most patients and is administered in tablet, suspension, concentrated drops, or suppository form. The NSAID ketorolac is available in intravenous form and is an effective antipyretic,[10] although the potential risks of gastrointestinal bleeding, renal dysfunction, and qualitative platelet dysfunction must be considered. Corticosteroids have antipyretic and anti-inflammatory properties and are appropriate if the benefit outweighs the toxicity and side effects[2] (Box 162-1).

Administration of antipyretics should be scheduled, to avoid the discomfort from waves of diaphoresis or hectic fever, patterns that result from administration on an intermittent or "PRN" basis.[11]

Nonpharmacological interventions such as sponging with tepid water and use of cooling blankets, ice packs, air conditioning, and fans may lower temperature through evaporation, radiation, convection, and conduction. They cause shivering and vasoconstriction and should be avoided, because they result in considerable discomfort for the patient. Supportive care is always indicated and includes keeping the patient's lips and mouth moist, offering cool liquids to those who can swallow, maintaining a comfortable ambient temperature, and providing clean, dry sheets and bedclothes.

SWEATS

Sweating is one of the body's methods of losing heat through evaporation to lower core body temperature during fever, exercise, or hot environments, but it is also associated with hot flashes.[5] In palliative care, patients usually suffer from either hyperhidrosis (excessive sweating) or nocturnal diaphoresis (night sweats).[12]

Pathophysiology

Both central and peripheral thermoreceptors send signals to the hypothalamus, and the autonomic nervous system (ANS) relays changes in thermoregulation to the CNS while maintaining some independent control.[2] When the body perceives a temperature above the hypothalamic set point, the hypothalamus sends signals via the ANS to effector sweat glands and the cutaneous vasculature to initiate thermal sweating, which results in generalized sweats and ultimately lowers the body's temperature.[2] Mental or emotional sweating occurs when mental excitement or stress increases the baseline rate of sweating in the palms and soles; it is controlled by both the limbic system and the hypothalamus.[12]

Differential Diagnosis

Hyperhidrosis can be classified as primary (no apparent etiology) or secondary, and as generalized or localized.[12] In palliative care, generalized hyperhidrosis may occur with various diseases, including endocrine disorders (e.g., hypoglycemia, estrogen deficiency in menopause), chronic infections (e.g., tuberculosis), and inflammatory disorders (e.g., vasculitis, sarcoidosis). It occurs in at least 5% of all cancer patients, particularly in those with lymphoid malignancies or carcinoid tumors.[2] Localized hyperhidrosis may be caused by peripheral neuropathy, or it may compensate for regional anhidrosis (loss of sweating), often confused with generalized hyperhidrosis.[12]

Clinical Manifestations

Hyperhidrosis occurs in varied patterns, including classic "night sweats," which are associated with infection or malignancy. Another clinical manifestation occurs in hot flashes with sweats due to estrogen withdrawal during menopause or hormonal treatment for breast or prostate cancer.[2] Withdrawal from certain drugs, including opiates, may produce sweats, but several drugs themselves cause excessive sweating, including opiates, certain antidepressants, acyclovir, and naproxen.[12]

Treatment

Finding and treating the underlying cause is effective. As with other symptoms in palliative care, evaluation and treatment must be undertaken in the broader context of the goals of care and the benefit-versus-burden calculus, and the patient and family must be counseled accordingly. Few treatments exist for generalized primary or localized primary hyperhidrosis. Thalidomide may reduce night sweats by blocking production of TNF-α. In a small series, four of seven patients with advanced malignancy who were given 100 mg of thalidomide at bedtime had less night sweats.[13] Localized primary hyperhidrosis may be treated with either injections of botulinum toxin or thoracic sympathectomy, which may be performed endoscopically.[12] The International Hyperhidrosis Society sponsors conferences and maintains a Web site (http://www.sweathelp.org/English/ [accessed December 22, 2007]) that provides information for people with this problem.

See Chapter 173 for an extensive discussion of the management of premature menopause and hot flashes.

CONCLUSIONS

Fever and sweats in palliative care are not dissimilar to those in other settings, but evaluation and treatment vary greatly with respect to treatment goals and the benefit-versus-burden calculus. In adults, fevers should be treated only if they cause discomfort or severe metabolic demands, and the treatment should consist of scheduled antipyretics. Overall treatment goals and the burden-versus-benefit analysis must be considered. General comfort measures always apply, including comfortable ambient temperature and circulation, fastidious mouth care, treatment of thirst, and keeping clothing and bedclothes clean and dry (see "Future Considerations").

Future Considerations
• Benefit versus harm caused by fever and implications for palliative care
• Can treatment of fever in an unresponsive patient be palliative for the family?
• Is a treatment algorithm for fever in palliative care feasible?
• Potential comfort (versus discomfort) of hydration during fevers
• The use of thalidomide for sweats

REFERENCES

1. Cleary JF. Fever and sweats. In Berger AM, Portenoy RK, Weissman DE (eds). Principles and Practice of Palliative Care and Supportive Oncology, 2nd ed. Philadelphia: Lippincott, Williams & Wilkins, 2002, pp 154-167.
2. Rhiner M, Slatkin NE. Pruritus, fever, and sweats. In Ferrell BR, Coyle N (eds). Textbook of Palliative Nursing, 2nd ed. New York: Oxford University Press, 2006, pp 345-363.
3. Dalal S, Zhukovsky DS. Pathophysiology and management of fever. J Support Oncol 2006;4:9-16.
4. Norman DC, Yoshikawa TT. Fever in the elderly. Infect Dis Clin North Am 1996;10:93-99.
5. Kemp C, Stepp L. Palliative care for patients with acquired immunodeficiency syndrome. Am J Hosp Palliat Care 1995;12:14, 17-27.
6. Zhukovsky DS. Fever and sweats in the patient with advanced cancer. Hematol Oncol Clin North Am 2002;16:579-588.
7. Powers JH, Scheld WM. Fever in neurologic diseases. Infect Dis Clin North Am 1996;10:45-66.
8. Chen LK, Chou YC, Hsu PS, et al. Antibiotic prescription for fever episodes in hospice patients. Support Care Cancer 2002;10:538-541.
9. Mackowiak PA. Fever: Blessing or curse? A unifying hypothesis. Ann Intern Med 1994;120:1037-1040.
10. Vargas R, Maneatis T, Bynum L, et al. Evaluation of the antipyretic effect of ketorolac, acetaminophen, and placebo in endotoxin-induced fever. J Clin Pharmacol 1994;34:848-853.
11. Klein NC, Cunha BA. Treatment of fever. Infect Dis Clin North Am 1996;10:211-216.
12. Pittelkow MR, Loprinzi CL. Pruritus and sweating in palliative medicine. In Doyle D, Hanks G, Cherny N, et al. (eds). Oxford Textbook of Palliative Medicine, 3rd ed. New York: Oxford University Press, 2004, pp 573-587.
13. Deaner PB. The use of thalidomide in the management of severe sweating in patients with advanced malignancy: Trial report. Palliat Med 2000;14:429-431.

SUGGESTED READING

Cleary JF. Fever and sweats. In Berger AM, Portenoy RK, Weissman DE (eds). Principles and Practice of Palliative Care and Supportive Oncology, 2nd ed. Philadelphia: Lippincott, Williams & Wilkins, 2002, pp 154-167.

Cunha BA (ed). Fever [special issue]. Infect Dis Clin North Am 1996;10(1).

Dalal S, Zhukovsky DS. Pathophysiology and management of fever. J Support Oncol 2006;4:9-16.

Mackowiak PA (ed). Fever: Basic Mechanisms and Management, 2nd ed. Philadelphia: Lippincott-Raven Publishers, 1997, pp 207-213.

Rhiner M, Slatkin NE. Pruritus, fever, and sweats. In Ferrell BR, Coyle N (eds). Textbook of Palliative Nursing, 2nd ed. New York: Oxford University Press, 2006, pp 345-363.

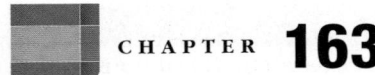

CHAPTER **163**

Hiccups

Howard S. Smith

K E Y   P O I N T S

- Hiccups are repeated, involuntary, spasmodic, diaphragmatic and inspiratory intercostal muscle contractions with early glottic closure terminating inspiration.

- There are more than 100 causes of persistent hiccups, with gastric distention and gastroesophageal reflux disease (GERD) being common etiologies.

- Numerous pharmacological agents have been utilized for the treatment of hiccups, including baclofen, gabapentin, and chlorpromazine.

- Severe intractable hiccups have led to significant detraction from quality of life, including sleep disruption, fatigue, anorexia, discomfort, and poor performance.

- Currently, treatment strategies for intractable hiccups remain empirical; no "evidence-based" approaches or valid recommendations can be derived.

Hiccups, or singultus, are repeated, involuntary, spasmodic, diaphragmatic and inspiratory intercostal muscle contractions that occur largely in irregular series, with glottic closure mediated by sensory branches of phrenic, thoracic sympathetic, and vagus nerves.[1]

Multiple phenomena occur in rapid succession to produce the characteristic hiccup. Initially, the roof of the mouth and back of the tongue lift, and this is often accompanied by a burp. Then, the diaphragm and inspiratory muscles abruptly and intensely contract, with subsequent clamping shut of the vocal cords—producing the classic "hic" sound, which is associated with a slowing of heart rate.

Usually, each individual's hiccup rate is reasonably consistent for a given hiccup episode, with a frequency of 4 to 60 hiccups per minute.[2] The frequency of hiccups is inversely related to the arterial partial pressure of carbon dioxide ($PaCO_2$); that is, as the $PaCO_2$ decreases (e.g., hyperventilation), the hiccup frequency increases. Breath holding (or breathing into a paper bag) may lead to an increase in $PaCO_2$ and, consequently, decrease in hiccup frequency. Hiccups lasting up to 48 hours are referred to as a hiccup bout and are considered acute.[3] Chronic hiccups, either persistent or recurrent, are generally considered to be pathological in nature. Hiccups lasting longer than 48 hours are referred to as persistent hiccups; if hiccups last longer than 2 months, they are considered intractable.[3]

Aside from the obvious detraction from quality of life and significant discomfort, severe intractable hiccups may affect conversation, concentration, or oral intake and can lead to fatigue, disruption of sleep,[4] and even atrioventricular asystole.[5]

There are more than 100 causes for hiccups or singultus, the most common of which are gastrointestinal. Causes may be natural or drug induced, and the same agents that are used to treat hiccups may also induce them. A wide variety of medical treatments (both nonpharmacological and pharmacological) have been used for intractable hiccups, including valproic acid, metoclopramide, chlorpromazine, prochlorperazine, promethazine, haloperidol, carbamazepine, nifedipine, phenytoin, ketamine, lidocaine, mexiletine, amitriptyline, and baclofen.[6]

BASIC SCIENCE

In 1998, Oshima and colleagues[7] found that a hiccup-like reflex could be elicited by electrical stimulation to an area in the medullary reticular formation of cats and was suppressed after an injection of baclofen in the area.[7] They hypothesized that the nucleus raphe magnus was most likely the source of the GABAergic inhibitory inputs to the hiccup reflex arc.[7] Isoflurane facilitated hiccup-like reflexes through activation of central and peripheral γ-aminobutyric acid A ($GABA_A$) receptors but suppressed them via activation of central and peripheral $GABA_B$ receptors in pentobarbital-anesthetized cats.[8] In addition to GABA receptors, dopaminergic, muscarinic, and serotonergic (e.g., 5-HT_{1A}) receptors may contribute to the pathophysiology of hiccups.

The existence of a specific discrete hiccup complex or center remains controversial; rather, an amorphous neural network coordinating various afferent inputs may function as a "hiccup center." Alternatively, rather than there being a specific hiccup-generating neural circuitry, hiccups may result largely from an imbalance between expiration and inspiration circuitry.

The hiccup reflex is thought to be composed of three major parts: an afferent limb (e.g., phrenic nerve, vagus nerve, sympathetic chain [T6-T12]), a central mediator, and an efferent limb (e.g., phrenic nerve with accessory/intercostal muscles).[9] The efferent limb also includes complex interactions among various brainstem areas, respiratory centers, phrenic nerve nuclei, medullary reticular formation, and hypothalamus.[10] The central connection between afferent and efferent limbs seems to be a nonspecific anatomic location between the cervical spine (C3-C5) and the brainstem.[10] The main efferent limb of the diaphragmatic spasms is mediated by motor fibers of the phrenic nerve.[1] The glottis closes to prevent inspiration 35 msec after electrical activity rises above the baseline in the diaphragm and respiratory muscles.[11]

EPIDEMIOLOGY AND PATHOPHYSIOLOGY

Hiccups may be up to 5 times more common in men than in women. The majority of patients evaluated in one study with hiccups were male (91%), were older than 50 years of age (range, 9 months to 80 years), and had co-morbid conditions (78%).[2]

The precise epidemiology of hiccups, and especially of severe intractable hiccups, is uncertain in the general population as well as in the palliative care population. The most common cause for hiccups among the myriad of etiologies is gastrointestinal in nature.[12] Gastric distention and gastroesophageal reflux disease (GERD) may be the most important causes.[12] A broad classification of the many causes of hiccups includes vagus and phrenic nerve irritation (e.g., intraoperative manipulation, esophagitis), central nervous system disorders (e.g., head trauma, multiple sclerosis, encephalitis), toxic-metabolic or drug-related disorders (e.g., uremia, alcohol intoxication, general anesthesia), and psychogenic factors (e.g., stress, anxiety) (Table 163-1).[5]

Pharmacological agents can induce hiccups. Thompson and Landry reported that corticosteroids and benzodiazepines are the most frequent types of drugs associated with the development of hiccups.[13] Other agents include chemotherapy drugs (e.g., cisplatin) and opioids (e.g., hydrocodone).

Agents that have been used to treat hiccups, such as antidopaminergic drugs (e.g., perphenazine) and midazolam, can also induce hiccups, and agents that have been known to induce or facilitate hiccups (e.g., anticholinergic drugs, steroids) have also seemed to be able to treat hiccups (e.g., atropine).

Bagheri and associates reported on drug-induced hiccups in France, reviewing the French pharmacological vigilance database.[14] Between 1985 and 1997, 53 cases of drug-induced hiccups were reported to the French pharmacovigilance network. Of these, 23% were related to corticosteroids, 15% to "psychiatric medications" (mainly dopaminergic anti-Parkinson agents), 12% to antibiotics (e.g., β-lactams, macrolide, fluoroquinolones), 7% to cardiovascular drugs (e.g., digoxin), 6% to analgesics (e.g., opioids), and 6% to nonsteroidal anti-inflammatory drugs. Rechallenge was positive in seven cases, with two cases considered "serious" according to the World Health Organization definition.[14]

Progesterone-induced hiccups may be caused by the glucocorticoid-like effects of progesterone. Anabolic steroid-induced hiccups occurred in an elite power lifter within 12 hours after increasing his dose. It has been proposed that progesterone, anabolic steroids, and corticosteroids may lower the threshold for synaptic transmission in the midbrain and directly stimulate the hiccup reflex arc.[15]

Nonpharmacological causes of hiccups are also numerous and are not enumerated here, but they include any subdiaphragmatic, hepatic, or other processes (e.g., tumor, infection, inflammation) that irritate the diaphragm and/or nerves to the respiratory muscles involved in the hiccup reflex arc. Causes of neurogenic hiccups include posteroventral pallidotomy, multiple sclerosis, lateral medullary infarction, medulla oblongata cavernoma, basilar artery aneurysm, and cerebellar hemangioblastoma.

TABLE 163-1	Conditions That Cause or Facilitate Hiccups	
CENTRAL/PERIPHERAL NERVOUS SYSTEM	**HEAD AND NECK**	**THORAX**
Trauma	Foreign body	Trauma/tumor
Infection	Goiter	Pneumonia
Vascular	Aneurysm	Pleuritis
Tumors (brainstem)	Pharyngitis/laryngitis	Pericarditis, myocardial infarction, or pacer malfunction
Multiple sclerosis	Tumors/cysts	Aneurysm
Phrenic/vagus nerve irritation	Membrane stimulation	Esophagitis
Ventriculoperitoneal shunts		Achalasia
Lateral medullary infarction		Esophageal stricture, injury, or obstruction
		Hiatal hernia
		Diaphragmatic eventration
		Lymphadenopathy
ABDOMEN	**METABOLIC/INFECTIOUS**	**DRUGS**
Ulcers	Hypokalemia	Steroids:
Abscess	Uremia	• Methylprednisolone
Gastritis	Hypocalcemia	• Dexamethasone
Gastric distention	Influenza	• Anabolic steroids
Pancreatitis	Herpes zoster	Barbiturates
Gastroesophageal reflux disease	Malaria	Chlordiazepoxide
Neoplasm	Tuberculosis	Methyldopa
Bowel obstruction	Alcohol	Certain antibiotics
Obstructing ureteric calculus	Diabetes mellitus	Certain chemotherapy agents
	Hypocarbia (hyperventilation)	Benzodiazepines
		Opioids
PSYCHOGENIC	**SURGICAL**	**IDIOPATHIC**
Stress/excitement	Anesthesia	
Conversion/grief reaction	Gastric distention	
Anorexia nervosa	Neck extension	
Schizophrenia	Traction on viscera	
Malingering		

Modified from Cymet TC. Retrospective analysis of hiccups in patients at a community hospital from 1995-2000. J Natl Med Assoc 2002;94:480-483, with permission.

MANAGEMENT

Treatment of hiccups should be directed at a specific cause if one can be identified. Removal of offending agents and correction of conditions or imbalances that may facilitate hiccups should constitute initial therapeutic efforts. Targeted therapy (if the cause of the hiccups is known) is the most rational approach. Hiccups secondary to GERD have resolved after treatment with proton pump inhibitors (PPIs) (e.g., lansoprazole).[16] Hiccups in a patient receiving continuous ambulatory peritoneal dialysis (CAPD) with "standard" solution improved with the use of a neutral pH dialysis solution.[17] Therefore, it is prudent to perform an appropriate history and physical examination as well as any appropriate laboratory testing, imaging, and/or endoscopic examinations. However, there are many times when the cause of the hiccups cannot be identified or addressed, and in these cases general measures or treatments should be instituted.

Pharmacological Treatment of Hiccups

Treatments for idiopathic chronic hiccups have included numerous pharmacological approaches. Baclofen, a GABA analogue that activates an inhibitory neurotransmitter, and valproic acid, which enhances GABA transmission centrally, are thought to aid in blocking the hiccup stimulus. Baclofen has been successfully used for the treatment of intractable hiccups in the palliative care population. In the study by Guelaud and colleagues,[18] 28 of 37 patients had either a complete resolution or a considerable decrease of hiccups after initiation of baclofen.

For intractable hiccups refractory to monotherapy, rational polypharmacy seems a reasonable approach. The combination of cisapride, omeprazole, and baclofen (COB) has been used for combination therapy. Because cisapride is no longer available, some clinicians have used tegaserod (also a 5-HT$_4$ receptor agonist) in its place; however, it too is now unavailable in the United States except possibly for certain patients with irritable bowel syndrome with constipation or for women younger than 55 years of age with chronic idiopathic constipation for whom no other treatment alternatives exist. Gabapentin as "add-on therapy" seems to have been occasionally successful, in the combinations of cisapride, omeprazole, and gabapentin (COG) or cisapride, omeprazole, baclofen, and gabapentin (COBG).[19] Petroianu and colleagues[20] reported the successful treatment of hiccups with COB in most of their patients (cured in 38%, alleviated in 24%). Patients with renal insufficiency (i.e., those undergoing CAPD/hemodialysis) need to be extremely cautious with baclofen therapy, because baclofen is renally eliminated. Even "low-dose" baclofen therapy in patients undergoing CAPD produced severe respiratory depression.[21]

Chlorpromazine (a dimethylamine derivative of phenothiazine) and haloperidol act centrally by dopamine antagonism in the hypothalamus. Metoclopramide may reduce the intensity of esophageal contractions and also acts as a dopamine antagonist. Nifedipine (a calcium channel blocker) may play a role in reversing abnormal depolarization in the hiccup reflex arc. Sertraline may also be beneficial.[22] Sertraline may act via effects on peripheral 5-HT$_4$ receptors in the gastrointestinal tract (reducing abnormal esophageal, gastric, or diaphragmatic mobility) or via

effects on 5-HT$_{1A}$ receptors and/or 5-HT$_2$ receptors through modulation of the autonomic nervous system, resulting in inhibition of the hiccup reflex arc.[22] Other agents and techniques that have been used for treatment of intractable chronic hiccups include nefopam (not currently available in the United States), intravenous lidocaine, short-term anesthesia, and, in anecdotal cases, quinidine, ketamine, stimulants of the central nervous system, ranitidine, dopamine agonists, clonazepam, and other anticonvulsants (e.g., phenytoin).

If a specific cause of intractable hiccups cannot be identified, I have constructed an empirical treatment algorithm (Fig. 163-1). Because relative or absolute gastric distention contributes to many cases of intractable hiccups,[23] simethicone (silica-activated dimethicone)[23] is believed to be a reasonable first-line pharmacological option. In more severe cases, or if simethicone alone is not effective, metoclopramide may be added[23]; it can be helpful as a prokinetic agent, by increasing lower esophageal tone, and thereby diminishing gastroesophageal reflux, or as a dopamine receptor antagonist. The third-

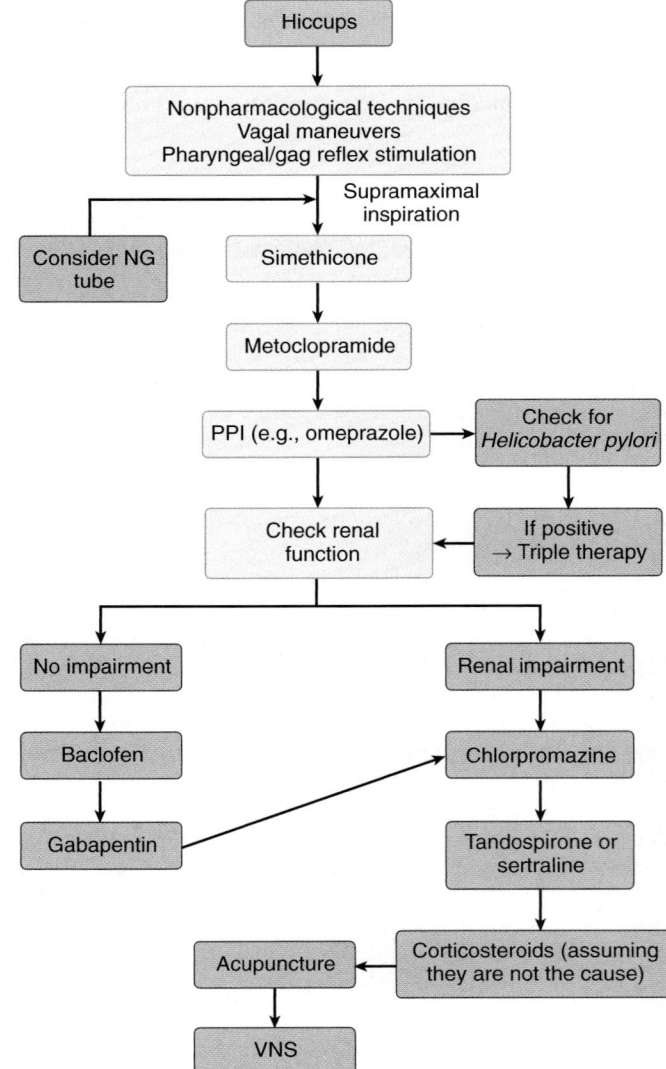

FIGURE 163-1   Empirical treatment algorithm for hiccups. NG, nasogastric; PPI, proton pump inhibitor, VNS, vagal nerve stimulation.

line pharmacological suggestion is to add baclofen, providing that renal impairment is not present. When using this treatment algorithm, the clinician should consider adding agents to existing failed agents if hiccups are not responding to therapy—rather than substituting new agents for old "failed" agents). This rationale is suggested because etiologies of the refractory singultus are not uncommonly multifactorial, and targeting several different pathways or mechanisms appears to improve therapeutic success in these challenging clinical situations.

Orr and Rowe described the case of a 35-year-old man with continuous hiccups in whom they documented moderate numbers of *Helicobacter pylori* organisms on antral gastric biopsy along with a positive urease test.[24] They believed that eradication of *H. pylori* through "triple therapy" (omeprazole, 20 mg PO twice daily; amoxicillin, 1 g PO twice daily; and clarithromycin, 500 mg PO twice daily) contributed to the complete resolution of hiccups[24]—however, this report was anecdotal.

Takahashi and colleagues described a case of continuous day and night intractable hiccups with insomnia, anorexia, and ischemic stroke in the area of the left side of the corona radiata and centrum semiovale which was refractory to many of the strategies attempted.[25] The anxiolytic agent tandospirone (a highly selective serotonin 5-HT$_{1A}$ agonist) at a dose of 30 mg/day completely abolished the hiccups.[25] 5-HT$_{1A}$ receptors are present on neurons in medullary regions that are involved in controlling respiration.[26] 5-HT$_{1A}$ agonists appear to have direct inhibitory effects on phrenic nerve activity, thereby shortening inspiratory discharges; this may be helpful in conditions such as apneusis (characterized by prolonged inspiratory discharges).[27]

Nonpharmacological Treatment of Hiccups

Nonpharmacological approaches have included physical treatments (initiating the Valsalva maneuver or counterirritation of the vagus nerve) and the use of breathing pacemakers.[28] Anecdotal physical maneuvers may be tried, such as breath holding, irritation of the nasopharynx, long and slow sips of water, compression of the nose while swallowing, intranasal ice-cold water, ice gastric lavage, prolonged pressure on the diaphragm, Heimlich maneuver, and hypnosis.[2] Pharyngeal stimulation tends to inhibit hiccups, but the effect may be only temporary.[29]

Kumar proposed that a simple technique to eliminate hiccups is to initiate the "gag reflex" by digitally depressing the base of the tongue.[30] It is conceivable that the transient arrest of respiration caused by initiation of the gag-deglutition process may restore the normal rhythmicity in the phrenic nerves.[30]

Acupuncture may be useful as a therapeutic option to combat intractable hiccups.[31,32] Payne and coworkers described a case of intractable hiccups occurring after a posterior fossa stroke which completely resolved after placement of a vagus nerve stimulator.[33]

Numerous other anecdotal treatments (e.g., cervical epidural block, cervical phrenic nerve block) have been advanced as potential treatments for intractable hiccups. There is also an anecdotal report of two cases of intractable hiccups that did not respond to "usual treatments" but were eliminated with methylcellulose (three sachets of methyl cellulose in 300 mL of warm water), the rationale being that

gastric distention may effectively eliminate the hiccup stimulus.[34] Surgical approaches to treatment of hiccups (e.g., phrenic nerve ablation) should be reserved as a last resort for only the most severe and intractable cases, because they carry a risk of pulmonary compromise.[35]

CONCLUSIONS

A myriad of treatments have been advanced to ameliorate the distressing symptom of intractable hiccups. Currently, treatment approaches remain empirical, and no "evidence-based" approaches or valid recommendations can be derived. Therefore, strategies for the treatment of intractable hiccups should be individualized and constructed on a case-by-case basis, taking into account co-morbid conditions, coexisting symptoms, and patient preferences. Intractable hiccups may have a profound effect on quality of life, potentially affecting comfort, talking, eating, sleeping, and numerous aspects of function and performance. Untreated intractable hiccups have led to poor performance, cognitive decline, exhaustion/fatigue, anorexia, weight loss, and depression/anxiety (see "Case Study: Treatment of Intractable Hiccups").

 C A S E   S T U D Y

Treatment of Intractable Hiccups

A 76-year-old man with advanced prostate cancer was admitted to the hospital with painful, bilateral, lower extremity peripheral neuropathy of uncertain etiology and painful generalized osseous metastases. His temperature was 36.5° C; heart rate, 89 beats/min; blood pressure, 140/68 mm Hg; and respiratory rate, 18 breaths/min. Pain assessment on an 11-point numerical rating scale (NRS-11) was 6, and the oxygen saturation was 96% breathing ambient air. He had guaiac-positive stool and a hematocrit of 28%. He lived alone in a small town, had smoked one pack of cigarettes per day for 50 years, and drank one beer and one glass of merlot most evenings. He never used intravenous drugs and had not previously received blood products. He was being treated with MS Contin, 90 mg PO three times daily; gabapentin, 600 mg PO three times daily; and ibuprofen, 800 mg PO three times daily for pain relief.

Three months before admission, the patient had developed early satiety and hiccups of uncertain etiology which was refractory to multiple therapies. He began being treated for hiccups with simethicone and metoclopramide, 10 mg PO every 6 hours. Omeprazole, 20 mg PO once daily, was added to his regimen, and later on, baclofen, 10 mg PO three times daily, was added. The baclofen was increased to 20 mg PO three times daily with no significant impact on the hiccups. He began to experience episodic nausea and vomiting, and, because the butyrophenone haloperidol is a more potent dopamine type 2 receptor antagonist and antiemetic than the phenothiazines (e.g., chlorpromazine) and appears to be as effective as the phenothiazines for hiccups, haloperidol, 5 mg, was given intravenously every 6 hours. At that point, the patient still had severe hiccups but was tolerating solids. A trial of sertraline, 50 mg PO once daily (subsequently increased to 100 mg PO once daily) was unsuccessfully attempted. The patient was then started on carvedilol, 6.25 mg PO four times daily, with resolution of hiccups.

Future Considerations

Future considerations for the treatment of intractable hiccups include

- Digital rectal massage*[36,37]
- 5-HT4 receptor agonists
- Carvedilol[38]
- Sertraline[22]
- Pyloric injections of botulinum toxin A[38]
- Tandospirone[25]

Dr. Frances Fesmire won the Ig Noble Prize in Medicine (bequeathed annually by the science humor journal, The Annals of Improbable Research) on October 25, 2006, for his technique to eliminate intractable hiccups.

If possible, the cause of the hiccups should be sought and targeted therapies instituted, including removal of any inciting conditions. Intractable hiccups are often found to be idiopathic or of uncertain etiology; and even if a cause is identified, they may not be amenable to removal in the palliative care population. Pharmacological approaches are often the most rational therapies for palliative care patients with intractable idiopathic hiccups.

Large, well-designed, multicenter, double-blind, randomized, placebo-controlled prospective studies are needed but are difficult to carry out, primarily because of the relatively low incidence of hiccups (see "Future Considerations").

REFERENCES

1. Heick A. [Diabolic hiccups] [Danish]. Ugeskr-Laeger 1997;159:986-988.
2. Cymet TC. Retrospective analysis of hiccups in patients at a community hospital from 1995-2000. J Natl Med Assoc 2002;94:480-483.
3. Souadjian JV, Cain JC. Intractable hiccup: Etiologic factors in 220 cases. Postgrad Med 1968;43:72-77.
4. Arnulf I, Boisteanu D, Whitelaw WA, et al. Chronic hiccups and sleep. Sleep 1996;19:227-231.
5. Malhotra S, Schwartz MJ. Atrioventricular asystole as a manifestation of hiccups. J Electrocardiol 1995;28:59-61.
6. Smith HS, Busracamwongs A. The management of hiccups in the palliative care population. Am J Hospice Palliat Care 2003;20:149-154.
7. Oshima T, Sakamoto M, Tatsuta H, et al. GABAergic inhibition of hiccup-like reflex induced by electrical stimulation in medulla of cats. Neurosci Res 1998;30:287-293.
8. Ohima T, Dohi S. Isoflurane facilitates hiccup-like reflex through gamma aminobutyric acid (GABA) A and suppresses through GABA B-receptors in pentobarbital-anesthetized cats. Anesth Analg 2004;98:346-352.
9. Samuels LA. Ten year review of anatomy, etiology and treatment. Can Med Assoc J 1952;67:315.
10. Ross J, Eledrisi M, Casner P. Persistent hiccups induced by dexamethasone. West J Med 1999;170:51-52.
11. Davis JN. An experimental study of hiccup. Brain 1970;93:851-872.
12. Friedman NL. Hiccups: A treatment review. Pharmacotherapy 1996;16:986-995.
13. Thompson DF, Landry JP. Drug-induced hiccups. Ann Pharmacother 1997;31:367-369.
14. Bagheri H, Cismondo S, Montasfruc J. [Drug-induced hiccup: A review of the France pharmacologic vigilance database.] Therapie 1999;54:35-39.
15. Dickerman RD, Jailumar S. The hiccup reflex arc and persistent hiccups with high-dose anabolic steroids: Is the brainstem the steroid-responsive locus? Clin Neuropharmacol 2001;24:62-64.
16. Saigusa H, Niimi S, Saigusa U, et al. [Laryngeal manifestations of gastroesophageal reflux disease (GERD) in pediatric patients: The usefulness of therapeutic (proton pump inhibitor [PPI] trials) [Japanese]. Nippon Jibiinkoka Gakkai Kaiho 2001;104:1025-1033.
17. La Rosa R, Giannattasio M. Hiccups in a CAPD patient treated with standard solution: Improvement with the use of a neutral pH dialysis solution. Perit Dial Int 2002;22:278-279.
18. Guelaud C, Similowski T, Bizec JL, et al. Baclofen therapy for chronic hiccup. Eur Respir J 1995;8:235-237.
19. Petroianu G, Hein G, Stegmeier-Petrianu A, et al. Gabapentin "add-on therapy" for idiopathic chronic hicchup (ICH). J Clin Gastroenterol 2000;30:321-324.
20. Petroianu G, Hein G, Petroianu A, et al. [ETICS Study: Empirical therapy of idiopathic chronic Singultus] [German]. Z Gastroenterol 1998;36:559-566.
21. Choo YM, Kim GB, Choi JY, et al. Severe respiratory depression by low-dose baclofen in the treatment of chronic hiccups in a patient undergoing CAPD. Nephron 2000;86:546-547.
22. Vaidya V. Sertraline in the treatment of hiccups. Psychosomatics 2000;41:353-355.
23. Twycross R. Baclofen for hiccups. Am J Hospice Palliat Care 2003;20:262.
24. Orr CF, Rowe DB. Helicobacter pylori hiccup. Intern Med J 2003;33:133-134.
25. Takahashi T, Murata T, Omori M, et al. Successful treatment of intractable hiccups with serotonin (5-HT) 1A receptor agonist. J Neurol 2004;251:486-487.
26. Lalley PM, Benacka R, Bischoff AM, et al. Nucleus raphe obscurus evokes 5-HT-1A receptor-mediated modulation of respiratory neurons. Brain Res 1997;747:156-159.
27. Wilken B, Lalley P, Bischoff AM, et al. Treatment of apneustic respiratory disturbance with a serotonin-receptor agonist. J Pediatr 1997;130:89-94.
28. Dobelle WH. Use of breathing pacemakers to suppress intractable hiccups of up to thirteen years duration. ASAIO J 1999;45:524-525.
29. Salem MR, Baraka A, Rattenborg CC, et al. Treatment of hiccups by pharyngeal stimulation in anesthetized and conscious subject. JAMA 1967;202:126-130.
30. Kumar A. Gag reflex for arrest of hiccups. Med Hypotheses 2005;65:206.
31. Kou S. An analysis on the therapeutic effects of auriculo-acupuncture in 38 obstinate hiccup cases of different races. J Tradit Chin Med 2005;25:7-9.
32. Liu FC, Chen CA, Yang SS, et al. Acupuncture therapy rapidly terminates intractable hiccups complicating acute myocardial infarction. South Med 2005;98:385-387.
33. Payne BR, Tiel RL, Payne MS, et al. Vagus nerve stimulation for chronic intractable hiccups: Case report. J Neurosurg 2005;102:935-937.
34. Macdonald J. Intractable hiccups. BMJ 1999;319:976.
35. Lewis JH. Hiccups: Causes and cures. J Clin Gastroenterol 1985;7:539-552.
36. Fesmire FM. Termination of intractable hiccups with digital rectal massage. Ann Emerg Med 1988;17:872.
37. Odeh M, Bassan H, Oliven A. Termination of intractable hiccups with digital rectal massage. J Intern Med 1990;227:145-146.
38. Stueber D, Swartz CM. Carvedilol suppresses intractable hiccups. J Am Board Fam Med 2006;19:418-421.

SUGGESTED READING

Smith HS, Busracamwongs A. The management of hiccups in the palliative care population. Am J Hospice Palliat Care 2003;20:149-154.
Twycross R, Regnard C. Dysphagia, dyspepsia, and hiccup. In Doyle D, Hanks GWC, MacDonald N (eds). Oxford Textbook of Palliative Medcine, 2nd ed. New York: Oxford University Press, 1998.

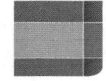

CHAPTER **164**

Incontinence: Urine and Stool

Subhasis K. Giri and Hugh D. Flood

KEY POINTS

- Urinary and fecal incontinence often share a common etiology such as immobility, dementia, or fecal impaction.
- Careful evaluation detects correctable causes, co-morbid disease, functional impairment (e.g., degree of mobility), and environmental factors such as access to toilet and/or commode.
- The priority must be to maintain and promote self-esteem and improve quality of life.
- Treatment should be directed to elimination of underlying causes.
- Treatment must include toileting assistance and scheduled toileting (prompted voiding).
- In the dying patient, placement of a catheter may help control urinary incontinence.

Urinary and fecal incontinence cause significant distress in the chronically ill. Often, they share a common etiology, such as immobility or dementia. Fifty percent or more of nursing home residents are affected, with significant morbidity and cost.[1]

URINARY INCONTINENCE

Definition and Types

Urinary incontinence (UI) is involuntary leakage of urine.[2] It predisposes to perineal rashes, pressure ulcers, urinary tract infections (UTIs), urosepsis, falls, and fractures[3] (Box 164-1).

Epidemiology

UI is common and affects quality of life (QOL) adversely. It afflicts 15% to 30% of older people at home, one third of those in acute care settings, and half of those in nursing homes.[4]

Pathophysiology

Urinary continence requires adequate control of the alternating urine storage and emptying phases of the micturition cycle by a complex interplay between the peripheral and central nervous system (Fig. 164-1). At any age, continence depends not only on the integrity of lower urinary tract function but also adequate mentation, mobility, motivation, and manual dexterity. UI in palliative medicine is commonly associated with deficits outside the urinary tract. The correctable causes include delirium, UTI, atrophic urethritis/vaginitis, drugs, excess urine output, and stool impaction (Fig. 164-2).

Detrusor overactivity (DO) and urge urinary incontinence (UUI) are common causes of UI in palliative medicine.[5] Causes of DO include intrinsic and extrinsic tumors (mechanical irritation), sacral nerve involvement, radiation cystitis, drug effects (diuretics and cyclophosphamide), UTI, central neurological causes (e.g., stroke), multiple sclerosis, dementia, and metabolic causes such as uremia, diabetes mellitus, diabetes insipidus, and hypercalcemia.

Stress urinary incontinence (SUI) is uncommon in these patients. It is caused by urethral hypermobility and/or neuromuscular defects (intrinsic sphincter deficiency). Urethral hypermobility and intrinsic sphincter deficiency may coexist. In men, SUI is usually a result of sphincter damage after radical prostatectomy for prostate cancer.

Box 164-1 Clinical Types of Urinary Incontinence

- *Urge urinary incontinence (UUI):* involuntary leakage of urine accompanied by or immediately preceded by urgency (sudden compelling desire to void that is difficult to defer).
- *Stress urinary incontinence (SUI):* involuntary leakage on effort or exertion, sneezing or coughing.
- *Mixed urinary incontinence (MUI):* combination of SUI and UUI.
- *Overflow incontinence:* leakage of urine at greater than normal bladder capacity.
- *Continuous incontinence:* continuous involuntary loss of urine.

Overflow incontinence may be caused by underactive detrusor or bladder outlet obstruction. Patients presents with retention and urine overflow, manifested most commonly as new-onset nocturnal enuresis. Bladder outlet obstruction is the most common cause of incontinence in older men and usually is caused by benign or malignant prostate enlargement. It is rare in women unless there is a large prolapse or after a bladder neck suspension or a sling procedure.

Continuous or total incontinence is associated with direct tumor invasion of urethra or bladder, causing urinary fistula. The four most common types of urinary fistula are vesicoenteric fistula, vesicovaginal, urethrocutaneous, and rectourethral (see Chapter 89). In palliative medicine, the most common causes are cancer of the cervix, bladder, and rectum, usually after radiotherapy (see "Case Study: Treatment of Urinary and Fecal Incontinence").

Clinical Manifestations

Careful evaluation is essential to detect correctable causes, co-morbid disease, functional impairment (e.g., degree of mobility), and environmental factors such as access to toilet and/or availability of commode (see Chapter

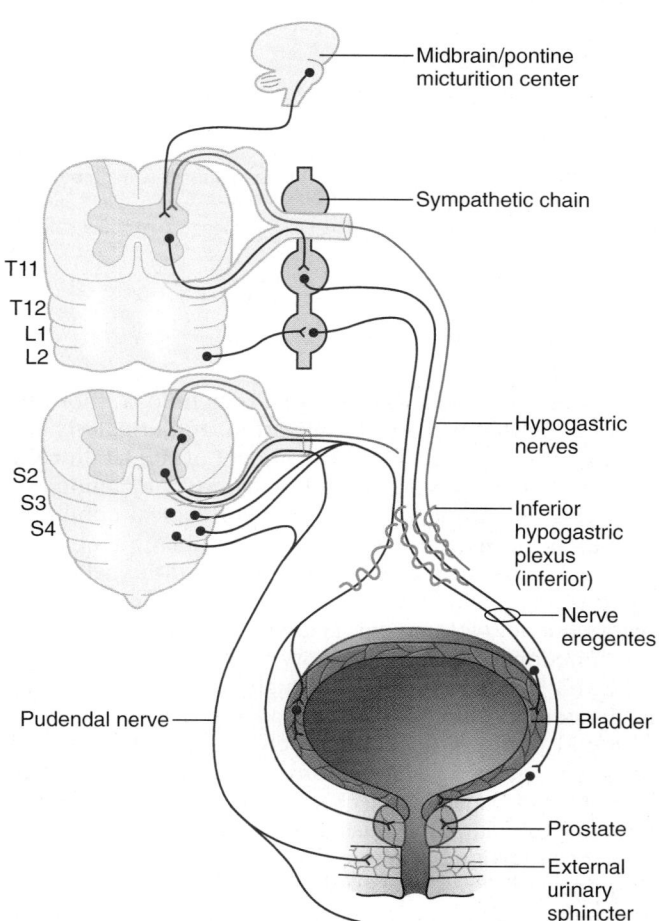

FIGURE 164-1 Schematic presentation of the neuronal control of the bladder. Micturition is partly reflex and partly a voluntary act.

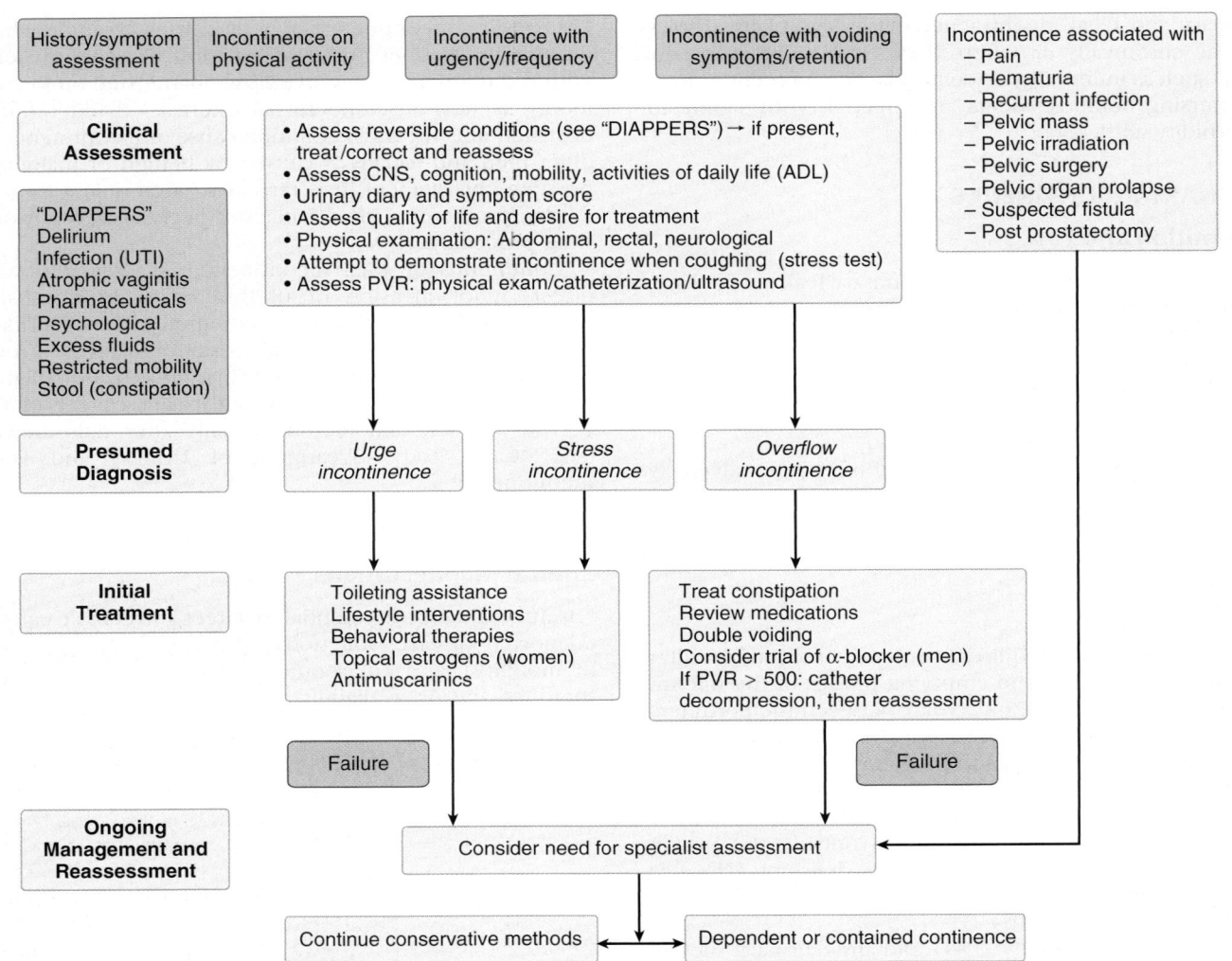

FIGURE 164-2 Management of urinary incontinence in palliative care. CNS, central nervous system; PVR, postvoid residual; UTI, urinary tract infection.

61). The initial evaluation should include a thorough history, focused physical examination, and urinalysis. It is important to enquire about the impact of the UI on QOL. The rectum and vagina should be carefully examined for any obvious pathology. Obvious neurological conditions should be noted, and a focused examination of sacral sensation and anal reflexes should be done whenever there is unexplained retention/overflow. Three- to seven-day frequency/volume charts give vital information about the functional (bladder capacity) problems experienced (Fig. 164-3). Stress testing by cough or Valsalva maneuver in the comfortably full bladder can confirm SUI.[6]

Blood urea nitrogen (BUN), creatinine, and urinalysis with or without urine culture should be performed. The postvoid residual (PVR) should be estimated in all patients by palpation, using an in-and-out catheter or bladder ultrasound scanner if available. Further investigation and specialist referral depend on the initial clinical assessment and baseline investigation. Urodynamic assessment should be considered only if it would alter therapy.

Treatment

The priority must be to maintain and promote self-esteem and improve QOL as much as possible. Treatment should be directed toward elimination of underlying causes (see Chapter 148). The detection and treatment of reversible causes, such as UTI, fecal impaction, or urinary retention, is important (see Fig. 164-2). Because many interventions depend on mobility, dexterity, and diet, a multidisciplinary approach is ideal. To reinforce advice, institute treatment (particularly behavioral modalities such as timed voiding, habit voiding, prompted voiding, and bladder training), and provide practical support, a continence adviser or nurse specialist is an essential member of an incontinence service. This professional can give simple advice regarding daily fluid requirements and caffeine and alcohol intake but also specific techniques for intermittent urinary catheterization and various external collection systems. The continence adviser and physiotherapist are vital to the success of pelvic floor training.

CASE STUDY

Treatment of Urinary and Fecal Incontinence

Mr. JR, a 75-year-old man with hormone-refractory metastatic prostatic adenocarcinoma, presented with low back pain of 2 weeks' duration and difficulty in walking for 5 days. He also complained of urinary and fecal incontinence for last 2 days. He had undergone transurethral resection of the prostate 2 years earlier. Clinical examination revealed reduced power in the lower limbs to 3/5 and sensory impairment up to the T12 dermatome. His bladder was palpable. Rectal examination revealed reduced anal tone, fecal impaction, and an enlarged, hard, irregular prostate. Plain radiography showed partial collapse of the T9, T12, and L1 vertebrae and diffuse sclerotic changes in the lumbar vertebrae and pelvis. An urgent magnetic resonance imaging study showed extensive metastatic involvement of thoracic and lumbar vertebrae with varying degrees of collapse of T9, T12, and L1 and epidural cord compression. The spinal cord compression resulted in moderate paraparesis and urinary and fecal incontinence.

Mr. JR received a course of urgent radiotherapy to the lower thoracic and upper lumbar spine and high-dose dexamethasone, which was gradually tailed off. He was mobilized with the aid of physiotherapy. His urinary incontinence was in fact caused by overflow incontinence secondary to urinary retention. Urinary retention was found to be caused, not by bladder outlet obstruction, but by an underactive detrusor. Initially, this was managed by placement of an indwelling catheter. After the patient's condition improved, the catheter was removed. Bladder emptying was managed by augmented voiding techniques (Credé maneuver—application of suprapubic pressure and Valsalva maneuvers) and by clean intermittent self-catheterization (CISC).

The patient's fecal incontinence was multifactorial in origin, caused partly by fecal impaction and partly by cord compression. Fecal impaction was treated with enema. A bowel management protocol was implemented with specific attention to appropriate stool softeners and peristaltic stimulants to prevent constipation. Incontinence episodes were reduced significantly by 2 weeks after implementation of the bowel management program. A further 2 weeks was required to achieve the goal of continence through a daily timed defecation. Staff education and reinforcement was an important part of the overall management plan. Five weeks after initiation of the program, the patient had achieved continence and reported greater self-esteem and self-control. He was able to perform CISC four times a day and was dry without wearing any pads. These regimens continued until he died 18 weeks later. In the last few days, when the patient. became unconscious, urinary incontinence was managed by condom catheter.

Palliation of symptoms and maintenance of adequate quality of life were the most important objectives in the management of this patient's incontinence. An increasing number of alternatives are available for the management of urinary and fecal incontinence, and it is important to individualize therapy for a specific patient.

TABLE 164-1	Commonly Used Anticholinergic Drugs	
ANTICHOLINERGIC DRUGS	**DOSE**	**ROUTE OF ADMINISTRATION**
Oxybutynin (immediate release)	2.5-5 mg bid-qid	Oral
Oxybutynin (extended release)	5-30 mg once daily	Oral
Oxybutynin (extended release)	36 mg twice weekly	Transdermal patch
Solifenacin	5-10 mg once daily	Oral
Tolterodine (immediate release)	2 mg bid	Oral
Tolterodine (prolonged release)	2-4 mg once daily	Oral
Trospium	20 mg bid	Oral

Detrusor Overactivity and Urge Urinary Incontinence

Simple measures, such as adjusting the timing or amount of fluid intake or providing a bedside commode or urinal, are often successful. If the patient can cooperate, bladder training extends the voiding interval.[7] Conservative measures combined with drug therapy (Table 164-1), if not contraindicated, are more effective than either approach alone. These agents have similar efficacy (70% to 75%) for decreasing incontinence episodes.[8]

Oxybutynin is a highly selective M_1 and M_3 muscarinic receptor antagonist and a direct muscle relaxant. It is the standard against which other drugs and therapies have been tested. Controlled-release preparations are just as effective but produce less dry mouth (68% versus 87%), compared with immediate-release oxybutynin. Newer preparations aim to be more selective for M_3 receptors, with a view to minimizing these adverse effects. Side effects of antimuscarinic drugs include dry mouth, constipation, blurred vision, drowsiness, nausea, vomiting, abdominal discomfort, difficulty in micturition, palpitations, headache, skin reactions, and central nervous system stimulation. Side effects can be minimized by using the once-a-day preparations and dose titration where appropriate.

Adjunctive measures, such as pads and special undergarments, are invaluable if incontinence proves refractory. Many types are now available, allowing flexibility to meet individual needs.[9] Condom catheters are helpful for men but may not be feasible for those with a small or retracted penis. Indwelling urethral catheters should be avoided for DO/UUI, because they usually exacerbate it. If they must be used (e.g., to allow healing of a pressure sore), a 14-F or 16-F, all-silicone catheter with a small balloon is preferable, to avoid leakage around the catheter.

Stress Urinary Incontinence

Conservative measures, such as adjusting fluid intake, treatment of cough, treatment of atrophic vaginitis, use of a tampon or pessary, and pelvic floor exercises, may control symptoms. Duloxetine (20 to 40 mg PO twice daily) may be helpful. Initial, transient nausea occurs in 30% of patients taking duloxetine. In mixed UI, antimuscarinics are often useful. Surgery is unlikely to be appropriate in palliative care. Palliative catheterization may be necessary in severe cases.

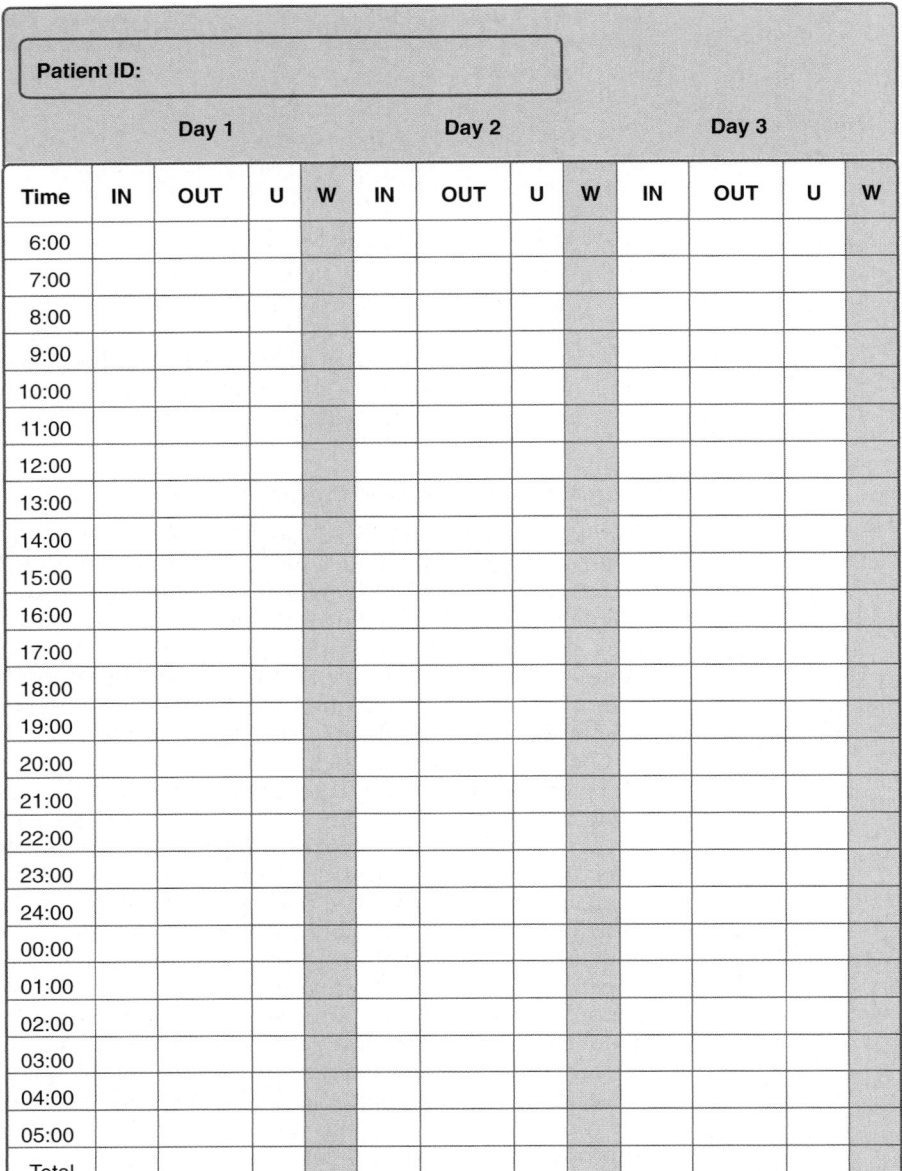

Patient ID:												
	Day 1				**Day 2**				**Day 3**			
Time	IN	OUT	U	W	IN	OUT	U	W	IN	OUT	U	W
6:00												
7:00												
8:00												
9:00												
10:00												
11:00												
12:00												
13:00												
14:00												
15:00												
16:00												
17:00												
18:00												
19:00												
20:00												
21:00												
22:00												
23:00												
24:00												
00:00												
01:00												
02:00												
03:00												
04:00												
05:00												
Total												

How to fill in this chart:
1. Record events to the nearest hour.
2. Fill in columns as outlined below:
   IN — Measure and record the amount of fluid taken in (e.g., water, tea) in mL.
   OUT — Measure and record the amount of urine passed in mL.
   U — Record each time urgency is experienced, i.e., a strong and difficult to control desire to pass urine.
   W — Record each time incontinence (involuntary leakage of urine) occurs.

FIGURE 164-3   Bladder frequency/volume chart.

Overflow Incontinence

Immediate catheterization is indicated. Definitive treatment must be individualized and may include surgical or other interventional techniques such as indwelling catheter, clean intermittent catheterization (CIC), or intraurethral stent. Overflow incontinence/retention can be a sign of spinal cord compression from metastatic prostate cancer. Specific α₁-adrenoceptor antagonists such as tamsulosin (400 µg PO once daily) or alfuzosin (2.5 to 10 mg PO once daily), followed by a voiding trial, may be useful in urinary retention due to benign prostatic enlargement. 5α-Reductase inhibitors such as finasteride (5 mg PO once daily) and dutasteride (0.5 mg PO once daily) have a longer onset of action (up to 3 months) and are inappropriate in palliative medicine. Depot formulation luteinizing hormone–releasing hormone analogues (e.g.,

triptorelin, 3-monthly IM injection; goserelin, 3-monthly SC injection) and/or oral antiandrogens (e.g., bicalutamide, 50 mg once daily; cyproterone, 100 mg twice daily) are commonly used in androgen-sensitive prostatic cancer. Transurethral prostate resection/incision is often a reasonable option even in advanced carcinoma of the prostate.

Continuous Incontinence

Use of an indwelling catheter or condom catheter in men (if the patient is not in retention) is the usual treatment. More invasive treatments should be undertaken only after consideration of life expectancy and likely QOL benefits. Vesicoenteric fistula can be managed by intestinal diversion or colostomy where appropriate. There are various options for the treatment of vesicovaginal fistula, including urethral or suprapubic catheter drainage, operative repair, and bilateral percutaneous nephrostomy. In most patients, urinary diversion via ileal conduit is required. Urethrocutaneous fistula is best managed with urinary diversion by suprapubic catheter drainage if the patient is not a candidate for definitive repair. Rectourethral fistula is usually a complication of radical prostatectomy and is best managed by temporary diversion colostomy and bladder catheterization.

FECAL INCONTINENCE

Definition

Fecal incontinence is involuntary loss of feces that causes distress for the patient.[10] Fecal incontinence, unlike urinary incontinence, soon leads to hospital admission, yet often its cause is obvious and management simple.

Epidemiology

Twenty percent of the institutionalized elderly have fecal incontinence.[11] Although the incidence in the cancer population is unknown, it is an important yet often overlooked clinical problem in the chronically ill. Fecal incontinence adversely affects self-esteem and QOL.[12]

Pathophysiology

Normal fecal continence depends on several factors: mental function, stool volume and consistency, colonic transit, rectal distensibility, anal sphincter function, anorectal sensation, and anorectal reflexes. Abnormalities of any of these factors, alone or combined, can cause incontinence.[12] The main risk factors for fecal incontinence are immobility, dementia, constipation, diarrhea, cancer, neurological disturbance of defecation, and confusional states. The most common cause, after inaccessibility to toilet, is fecal impaction with spurious diarrhea. The association of fecal incontinence and UI, known as "double incontinence," can generally be explained by the same underlying causes of poor mobility and cognitive impairment. Double incontinence may also be the result of peripheral neurological lesions (e.g., obstetric injury) or severe chronic constipation.[11] New-onset fecal incontinence in cancer, associated with other focal neurological findings such as perineal or back pain and/or motor and sensory symptoms, requires emergency medical evaluation to rule out spinal cord compression or central nervous system lesions.[13]

Clinical Manifestations

A comprehensive assessment addressing physical and mental status, previous bowel habit, dietary habits, and medications is the foundation for successful management. The initial evaluation should include a thorough history, focused physical examination, and digital rectal examination. A complete neurological examination should evaluate focal neurological abnormalities and gauge mental status. The degree to which incontinence is affecting the present illness and QOL should be established. Long-lasting (≥8 days) or permanent fecal incontinence is associated with increased mortality and is a poor prognostic marker.[11]

Laboratory tests may include a serum electrolytes and BUN. The stool should be tested for occult blood. Supine and erect abdominal radiographs can rule out impaction above the rectum. Specialized studies of the gastrointestinal tract, such as barium enema, rectal manometry, or colonoscopy, may be required in complex cases.

Treatment

The underlying cause should be treated as far as possible An algorithm outlining a possible management strategy is shown in Figure 164-4.[14] The bowel program must be individualized to meet individual needs and body functions. Consultation with a nurse who is experienced in managing fecal incontinence may be helpful before implementing the program (Box 164-2).

In fecal impaction, complete emptying of the rectum is obtained by manual disimpaction and oil-retention or tap water enemas as needed. This is followed by prevention of recurrence using laxatives such as stool softeners, saline laxatives, stimulant laxatives, and single-agent osmotic products (see Chapter 140).

If fecal incontinence is associated with diarrhea, the underlying disorders (e.g., bile salt malabsorption) should be treated if at all possible. Antidiarrheal medications, such as loperamide and diphenoxylate, or bile acid binders may help[11] (see Chapter 154).

Indications for referral to a gastroenterologist are (1) incontinence/constipation with weight loss, rectal bleeding, or anorexia; (2) high-volume diarrhea without an identified cause; and (3) a complex clinical picture or one that does not respond to standard treatment[15] (see "Future Considerations").

Box 164-2   General Measures for a Bowel Management Program

- Maintain good general symptom control
- Encourage activity and mobility
- Maintain adequate oral fluid intake
- Maximize fiber content in the diet
- Anticipate constipating drugs: alter treatment or start a laxative prophylactically
- Create a favorable environment (e.g., access to toilet or bedpan)
- Provide patient and family education and leaflet
- Review progress regularly

Future Considerations

- Injection of botulinum toxin A into the bladder is promising therapy in urge urinary incontinence (UUI) refractory to antimuscarinic therapy.
- Neuromodulation is gaining support in refractory UUI.
- Duloxetine, a combined serotonin and norepinephrine reuptake inhibitor, is of benefit in stress urinary incontinence. The usefulness of these agents in palliative medicine remains to be established.
- There is little literature addressing incontinence of urine and stool in palliative medicine.
- Trials should evaluate noninvasive interventions and improvement of urinary and fecal incontinence in chronically ill patients.

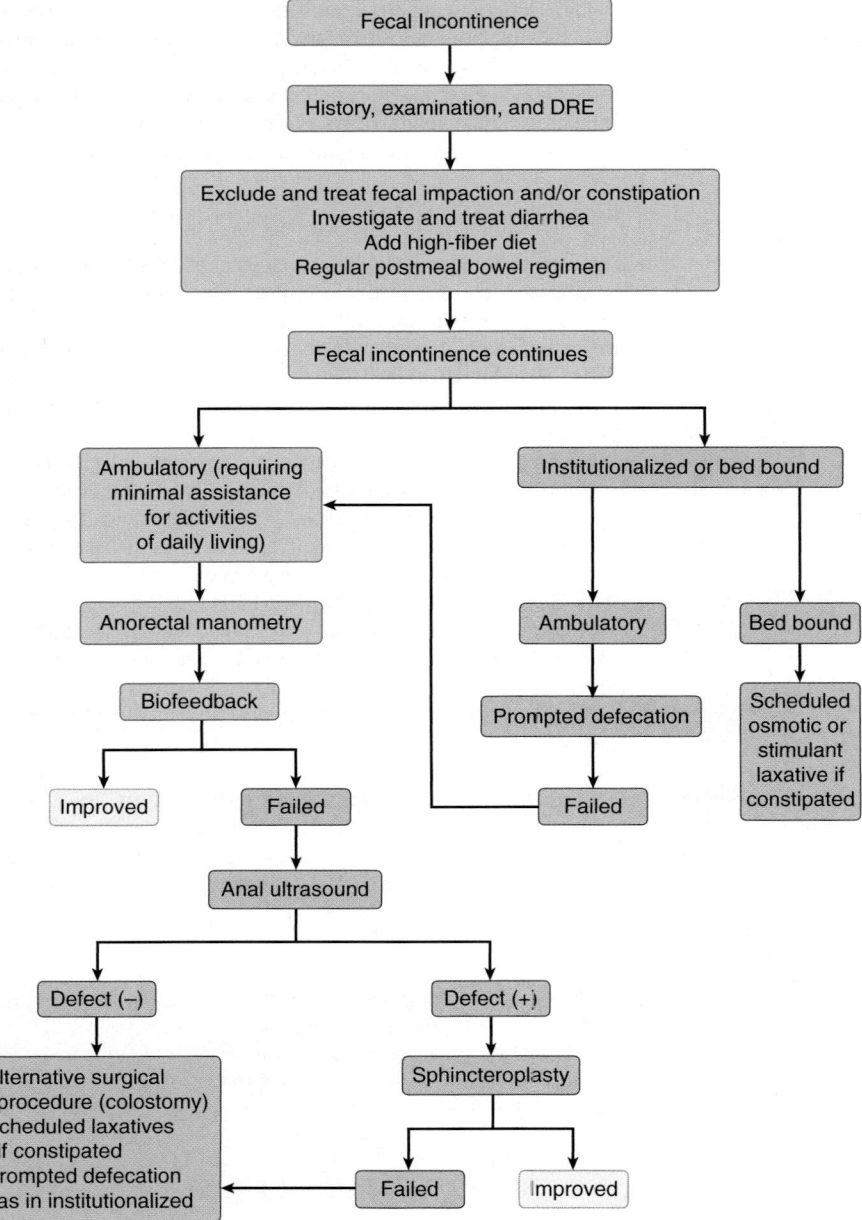

FIGURE 164-4 Algorithm for the evaluation and treatment of fecal incontinence. DRE, digital rectal examination. (*Adapted from Tariq SH, Morley JE, Prather CM. Fecal incontinence in the elderly patient. Am J Med 2003;115:22, with permission of Excerpta Medica Inc.*)

REFERENCES

1. Schnelle JF, Leung FW. Urinary and fecal incontinence in nursing homes. Gastroenterology 2004;126(Suppl 1):S41-S47.
2. Abrams P, Cardozo L, Fall M, et al; Standardisation Sub-Committee of the International Continence Society. The standardisation of terminology in lower urinary tract function: Report from the Standardisation Sub-committee of the International Continence Society. Urology 2003;61:37-49.
3. Brown JS, Vittinghoff E, Wyman JF, et al. Urinary incontinence: Does it increase risk for falls and fractures? J Am Geriatr Soc 2000;48:721-725.
4. McGrother C. Epidemiology and etiology of urinary incontinence in the elderly. World J Urol 1998;16:S3-S9.
5. Resnick NM, Baumann MM, Scott M, et al. Risk factors for incontinence in the nursing home: A multivariate study. Neurourol Urodyn 1988;7:274-276.
6. Kong TK, Morris JA, Robinson JM, et al. Predicting urodynamic dysfunction from clinical features in incontinent elderly women. Age Ageing 1990;19:257-263.
7. Burgio KL, Locher JL, Goode PS, et al. Behavioral vs drug treatment for urge urinary incontinence in older women: A randomized controlled trial. JAMA 1998;280:1995-2000.
8. Wein AJ, Rackley RR. Overactive bladder: A better understanding of pathophysiology, diagnosis and management. J Urol 2006;175:S5-S10.
9. Brink CA. Absorbent pads, garments, and management strategies. J Am Geriatr Soc 1990;38:368-373.
10. Beddar SAM, Holden-Bennett L, McCormick AM. Development and evaluation of a protocol to manage fecal incontinence in the patient with cancer. J Palliat Care 1997;13:27-38.
11. Chassagne P, Landrin I, Neveu C, et al. Fecal incontinence in the institutionalized elderly: Incidence, risk factors, and prognosis. Am J Med 1999;106:185-190.
12. Madoff RD, Williams JG, Caushaj PF: Fecal incontinence. N Engl J Med 1992;326:1002-1007.
13. Janjan NA. Radiotherapeutic management of spinal metastases. J Pain Symptom Manage. 1996;11:47-56.
14. Tariq SH, Morley JE, Prather CM. Fecal incontinence in the elderly patient. Am J Med 2003;115:217-227.
15. Romero Y, Evans JM, Fleming KC, et al. Constipation and fecal incontinence in the elderly population. Mayo Clin Proc 1996;71:81-92.

SUGGESTED READING

Basch A, Jensen L. Management of fecal incontinence. In Doughty D (ed). Urinary and Fecal Incontinence: Nursing Management. St. Louis: Mosby–Year Book, 1991, pp 235-268.

MacLeod J. Assessment of patients with fecal incontinence. In Doughty D (ed). Urinary and Fecal Incontinence: Nursing Management. St. Louis: Mosby–Year Book, 1991, pp 203-233.

Norman RW, Bailly G. Genito-urinary problems in palliative medicine. In Doyle D, Hanke G, MacDonald N (eds). Oxford Textbook of Palliative Medicine, 3rd ed. New York: Oxford University Press, 2005, pp 647-657.

Resnick NM, Yalla SV. Geriatric incontinence and voiding dysfunction. In Walsh PC, Retik AB, Vaughan ED Jr, et al. (eds). Campbell's Urology, 8th ed. Philadelphia, Saunders, 2002, pp 1218-1234.

Sykes NP. Constipation and diarrhoea. In Doyle D, Hanke G, MacDonald N (eds). Oxford Textbook of Palliative Medicine, 3rd ed. New York: Oxford University Press, 2005, pp 483-495.

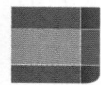

CHAPTER **165**

Indigestion

Bassam Estfan

K E Y   P O I N T S

- "Indigestion" is a vague term and encompasses many abdominal symptoms that may or may not be organic.

- Dyspepsia is functional in two thirds of cases. Acid suppressants and prokinetics are variably successful, and other means may be tried for management.

- Heartburn is a major manifestation of gastroesophageal reflux disease (GERD). It usually responds to antacids. Nonerosive reflux disease (NERD) is a distinctive cause of heartburn that may be acid independent and difficult to manage.

- Abdominal gas problems such as bloating and flatulence have various mechanisms. They can be socially disturbing. They are best treated by management of the underlying condition (e.g., irritable bowel syndrome, dyspepsia).

- Belching is a benign but bothersome phenomenon. It is associated with dyspepsia and GERD and is best managed nonpharmacologically.

"Indigestion" means lack of proper digestion. Although the term suggests a relation to food intake, symptoms are often not linked to food. Indigestion may mean heartburn or epigastric burning, acid reflux, belching, bloating, nausea, abdominal pain or discomfort, early satiety, abdominal fullness, and more.[1] These symptoms are usually referred to as indigestion when they are felt in the upper abdomen. In this case, *dyspepsia* is a more recognizable term. In the terminally ill, gastrointestinal symptoms, including indigestion, may occur from disease progression and its complications, or from drugs, but it also may be a result of functional disorders, given the prevalence of psychological disturbances. Management is pharmacologically similar to that in patients who are otherwise healthy, but unorthodox methods may be tried. Although normally such vague symptoms might dictate extensive investigation, especially if unresponsive to initial therapies, technology must be used judiciously, individualized, and guided by the goals of care in the terminally ill. Diagnosis and management of indigestion is challenging (Table 165-1).

DYSPEPSIA

Dyspepsia is pain or discomfort in the epigastrium. The Rome II definition of functional dyspepsia (FD) requires that the upper abdominal pain or discomfort has been present for at least 12 weeks in the past 12 months, without organic causes, or that it occurs in relation to defecation, changed stool consistency, or frequency. Dyspepsia can involve multiple symptoms that do not fit into other specific conditions. It has been customary to divide patients with dyspepsia into subgroups with ulcer-like versus dysmotility-like symptoms. Subgrouping may be important for research, but it is less valuable in management.

Epidemiology and Prevalence

Dyspepsia occurs in 20% to 40% of the general population and affects females more than males. Two thirds of patients have FD. Not all dyspeptic patients seek medical attention; however, because dyspepsia is a chronic problem, perhaps half of those affected will eventually seek medical attention because of secondary anxiety (e.g., worries about malignancy) or severe symptoms.[2] In patients with advanced cancer, dyspepsia was reported in 11% to 19%,[3]

TABLE 165-1	Occurrence of the Symptom of Indigestion in Selected Diseases				
DISEASE	**DYSPEPSIA**	**HEARTBURN**	**BLOATING**	**BELCHING**	**BOWEL HABIT CHANGES**
Functional dyspepsia	+	−	+	±	−
GERD	+	+	−	+	−
Irritable bowel syndrome	−	−	+	±	+
NERD	−	+	−	±	−
Peptic ulcer disease	+	±	−	−	−

GERD, gastroesophageal reflux disease; NERD, nonerosive reflux disease.

whereas another study did not report dyspepsia among those symptoms with a prevalence of greater than 10%.

Pathophysiology

Organic causes of dyspepsia, diagnosed by upper endoscopy, include gastroesophageal reflux disease (GERD), peptic ulcer disease (PUD), and gastric cancer. These affect the integrity of gastric and esophageal mucosa that protects against gastric acid. GERD and PUD are treatable. Other causes may include cholelithiasis.

Dyspepsia frequently has no organic cause; two thirds of cases are endoscopy negative and called functional.[1] However, this ratio is unclear in advanced illnesses. The pathophysiology of FD is poorly understood, and multiple mechanisms may be involved.[4] *Helicobacter pylori* infection may play a role in dyspepsia, but this is controversial. *H. pylori* eradication is superior to placebo in relieving *H. pylori*–positive dyspepsia, but this effect was suboptimal. Gastric dysmotility may contribute to dyspepsia, especially in the dysmotility-like subgroups. This may cause delayed gastric emptying, inadequate fundic relaxation, and perhaps overlap with irritable bowel syndrome (IBS). Good responses to the prokinetic drug cisapride support this theory.[5] Alcohol and smoking were not associated with an increased risk of dyspepsia.

In a palliative medicine population, several factors contribute to dyspepsia (Box 165-1), most notably medications, especially nonsteroidal anti-inflammatory drugs (NSAIDs) and corticosteroids with gastric mucosal irritation, and intra-abdominal malignancies and metastases; FD seems less significant. Many antibiotics can cause abdominal discomfort and dyspepsia. Psychological factors (anxiety, depression, and somatization) may influence the pathophysiology of FD by modulating central pain sensation (see "Case Study: Treatment of Indigestion in Palliative Care").

Clinical Manifestations

A detailed history and physical examination is likely to suggest dyspepsia. History is inaccurate in determining a cause for uninvestigated dyspepsia. If serious indicators exist (e.g., weight loss, abdominal mass, age older than 50 years, bleeding), endoscopy is essential.[6] Dyspeptic symptoms usually overlap with those of other diseases, such as IBS, GERD, and other functional bowel disorders. Symptoms of dyspepsia include belching and gastric fullness or burning; heartburn (retrosternal burning) is not a component of dyspepsia, and, if present, represents GERD. Physical examination is insignificant in FD, and abnormalities usually point to an organic etiology (masses, tenderness).

H. pylori testing is controversial, and many cases of dyspepsia are treated without investigation. Testing and treatment are more valuable if there is a high pretest infection prevalence. This is important in advanced disease, when minimizing interventions is essential. Endoscopy is important in patients with serious symptoms and if symptoms persist despite appropriate conservative management or *H. pylori* eradication. It is inappropriate in those who are debilitated or whose status is terminal unless it matches the goals of care.

Differential Diagnosis

The differential diagnosis for dyspepsia includes PUD, GERD, gastric cancer, gall bladder diseases, and irritable bowel disorder.

Treatment

An algorithm for the management of dyspepsia is presented in Figure 165-1. In the absence of organic causes, reassurance is most important. If medications are suspected, they should be stopped and/or replaced. Initial management should be acid-suppressant therapy (see Chapter 129), preferably with a proton pump inhibitor (PPI), which relieves symptoms in 40% to 70% of patients. *H. pylori* eradication is indicated with positive testing; the benefit is modest but durable. A "test-and-treat" strategy

---

Box 165-1   Dyspepsia in Advanced Illness
• *Organic causes:* peptic ulcer disease, gastroesophageal reflux disease (GERD), gastric cancer
• *Medications:* nonsteroidal anti-inflammatory drugs (NSAIDs), corticosteroids, macrolides, metronidazole, anticholinergics, opioids
• *Psychiatric conditions:* anxiety, depression, somatization disorders
• Radiotherapy to epigastric area
• *Dysmotility problems:* gastroparesis

   CASE STUDY

Treatment of Indigestion in Palliative Care

A 68-year-old man diagnosed with colon cancer metastasizing to abdominal lymph nodes and liver noticed increasing "indigestion" 3 weeks after enrolling with hospice. A home visit was scheduled to address this symptom and his family's concerns. His medications consisted of long-acting morphine for pain control, a stool softener, and methylphenidate. It appeared that this "indigestion" was of moderate severity, existed for most of the day, and was hard to describe specifically. The patient was not sure about its relation to food or the existence of new pain. Other elicited symptoms were bloating, early satiety, mild nausea, and altered taste leading to decreased appetite. He denied heartburn or melena. His family had tried over-the-counter H_2 blockers, as needed, without benefit and was now insisting on invasive investigations. Physical examination revealed an enlarged liver with normal bowel sounds. The physician met with the patient and family and discussed with them the need and burden of investigations, and the fact that the patient's symptoms were most likely multifactorial due to cancer progression locally and general effects. A metoclopramide infusion was started subcutaneously, successfully titrated until symptom relief was obtained, and then changed to pills.

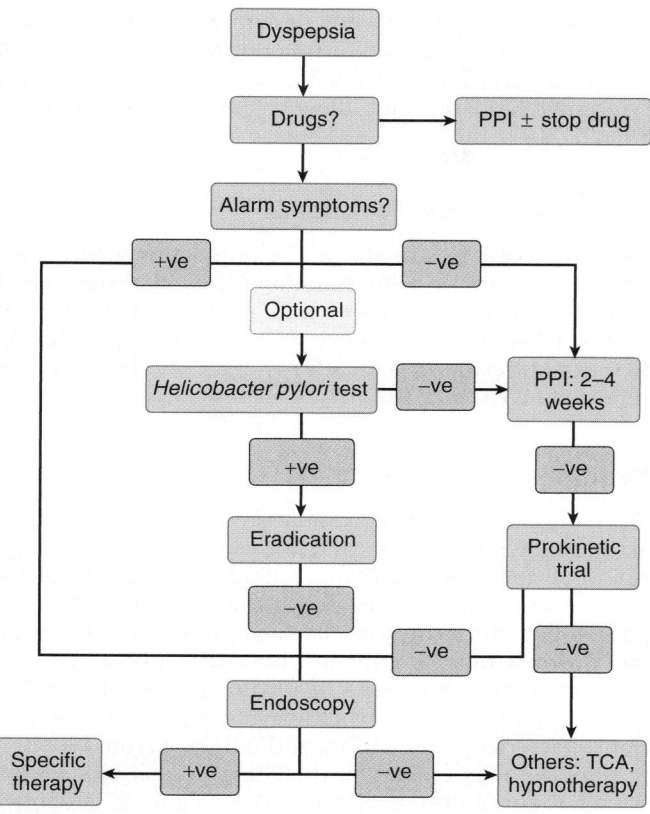

FIGURE 165-1 Dyspepsia management algorithm. −ve, negative; +ve, positive; PPI, proton pump inhibitor; TCA, tricyclic antidepressant.

is as clinically effective as, and more cost-effective, than the "test-and-scope" approach.[6]

Prokinetics are second-line management. Evidence to support the use of prokinetics is derived from cisapride studies; use is restricted because of rare fatal arrhythmogenicity. Dopamine antagonists such as metoclopramide and domperidone are alternatives, especially the latter.[7] Adjuvants such as tricyclic antidepressants (TCAs) help FD.[8] There is a good placebo response in some trials, suggesting that psychotherapy may help, although meta-analysis of psychotherapy results in dyspepsia was discouraging. Nonpharmacological approaches in FD have not been rigorously studied, but psychotherapy and hypnosis may alleviate symptoms.[9]

Evidence-Based Medicine

Several meta-analyses have been conducted of treatment methods or strategies in dyspepsia. There is no consensus on treatment. Most researchers suggest the superiority of PPI over histamine 2 receptor antagonists (H2RAs).[10] Prokinetics (cisapride and domperidone) were superior to acid suppression in some reviews, inferior in others.

HEARTBURN

Heartburn (or pyrosis) is a retrosternal burning. It is variably associated with esophageal acid reflux or regurgitation. Both symptoms are prominent in GERD. Heartburn with normal endoscopy findings and normal esophageal

acid exposure has been termed "functional." In 70% of acid reflux cases, endoscopy findings is normal; these cases are referred to as nonerosive reflux disease (NERD).[11] Heartburn must be differentiated from epigastric burning, which is a dyspeptic symptom, unless epigastric burning radiates retrosternally. Confusing terminology makes interpreting the effects of acid suppression on dyspepsia in research difficult.

Epidemiology and Prevalence

The prevalence of heartburn is 10% to 20% worldwide, with higher prevalence in westernized countries. Heartburn is reported by 44% of the general U.S. population at least once monthly, and by 20% at least once weekly. It occurs in 28% of those with advanced cancer.[12] Patients with NERD are likely to be female, thin, younger, and without hiatal hernias.

Pathophysiology

Heartburn is thought to be a result of gastroesophageal acid reflux. However, not all reflux results in heartburn, and not all heartburn is caused by reflux. In erosive reflux disease (erosive esophagitis or Barrett's esophagus), mucosal breakdown allows refluxed acid to irritate local nociceptors. Both lower esophageal sphincter (LES) relaxation and acid exposure are increased. LES pressure and acidity levels were similar or only slightly increased in NERD compared with controls. Almost half of those with heartburn have normal esophageal mucosa on endoscopy and respond poorly to acid suppressants. The mechanism of heartburn in NERD is unclear.[13] Hypersensitivity to normal acid exposure (hyperalgesia) is important in some cases. Similar responses may occur with exposures other than gastric acid (e.g., bile acids) or with mechanical distention. Prolonged esophageal contractions precede some heartburn episodes. Increased permeability of esophageal mucosa to acid may explain heartburn without mucosal damage. Psychological factors may function as perception modulators, thus facilitating heartburn.

Clinical Manifestations

History and physical examination alone are insufficient to diagnose the cause. Heartburn is different from localized gastric burning, which most likely represents dyspepsia. Heartburn, especially when it is chronic, is associated with GERD and other erosive reflux diseases that must be excluded. Esophageal spasm may cause retrosternal pain that is difficult to distinguish from heartburn. If the clinical history is suspicious, coronary artery disease should be excluded through electrocardiography or cardiac enzymes. Both conditions may respond to sublingual nitroglycerin. A diagnosis of acid-induced heartburn can be indirectly established through quick response to antacids. Lack of response does not exclude heartburn, however, because not all case of heartburn are acid-related, especially in patients without mucosal damage.

Investigations are invasive. Endoscopy is the gold standard for abnormal esophageal mucosal pathology, and biopsies may be necessary. Endoscopy is an uncomfortable and costly procedure that is best reserved for alarm symptoms (dysphagia, elderly age, upper gastrointestinal bleeding) or for those cases unresponsive to PPI. Esophageal pH monitoring with symptom recording may identify a relationship between acid reflux with a pH drop to lower than 4 and heartburn. This test is unlikely to be beneficial in NERD, because the relationship is poor, but it may help identify those at risk of future esophageal pathology. In debilitated patients or in those with advanced disease, invasive testing is inappropriate and may be replaced with empirical treatment.

Differential Diagnosis

Heartburn can occur as a result of GERD (erosive esophagitis, Barrett's esophagus) or NERD. It should not be confused with cardiac pain, which can mimic heartburn, or other with esophageal problems such as spasm.

Treatment

Heartburn, whether mucosal damage is present or not, is best treated with acid suppression. Antacid salts can be used for instant relief in those with infrequent heartburn. If heartburn is prolonged and persistent, acid suppressants are most effective. PPIs are more effective than H[2]RAs; no PPI seems superior to another at equivalent doses.[14] If the response is suboptimal, dose doubling should be tried.

Pathological features of acid reflux can heal with acid suppression, but this may not be matched by symptom response. Sixty-four percent of patients with NERD achieve full symptom control after 4 weeks of PPI therapy. For those who do not respond to acid suppression, further investigation may be needed, and treatment should be individualized. Fundoplication is not favored in NERD; its benefit is better in patients with heartburn and abnormal pH testing. Prokinetics was found to have discouraging results in heartburn or "functional heartburn." It is not known whether drugs that alter pain perception (e.g., TCAs) have any effect in resistant heartburn, but they may be worth a trial. Avoidance of foods or beverages that increase gastric acidity (e.g., fruit juices, tomato, lemon, lime) or increase relaxation of the LES (e.g., caffeinated beverages, chocolate) may help.

Evidence-Based Medicine

Randomized, controlled trials of lifestyle modifications revealed no improvement in GERD symptoms after avoiding late evening meals, sleeping with the head elevated, or losing weight.[15]

BLOATING

Bloating is the subjective feeling of abdominal fullness or excess abdominal gas, whereas abdominal distention is an objective sign representing increased abdominal girth. At least one quarter of those with bloating do not report visible abdominal distention. Bloating is frequently associated with FD, IBS, and other functional bowel disorders.

Bloating without other signs or symptoms that supports other diagnoses is called "functional bloating." Those complaining of bloating usually have moderate to severe symptoms, and bloating affects quality of life in up to 54%.[16]

Epidemiology and Prevalence

Bloating affects 10% to 30% of the population at any time, and 96% of those with functional bowel disorders. It afflicts females twice as often as males, and those with constipation more than those with diarrhea (especially in IBS). Among patients with advanced cancer, bloating was reported in 18% to 50%.[3,12]

Pathophysiology

Mechanisms remain poorly understood. Bloating is highly associated with dyspepsia and IBS, especially constipation-predominant types, and may share some mechanisms. The subjective feeling may result from varying abdominal pathologies, but many associate abdominal gas with bloating. Normal bowels contain about 200 mL of gas, the product of many processes that maintain gas balance. Gas is produced through air swallowing, gastric chemical reactions, bacterial fermentation, and diffusion from blood; it is eliminated via eructation (belching), rectal evacuation, bacterial consumption, and blood diffusion. It is controversial whether increased bowel gas volume alone causes bloating. Increased intra-abdominal content may play a role in IBS, because bloating increases with fiber bulk, including nonfermentable fibers (which are not gas producing).

Other suggested mechanisms for bloating include impaired gas handling. Gas transit is regulated by gut propulsions; foods with high fat content decrease transit, whereas local gas distention increases it. Those with bloating have impaired responses to gut distention, and an upregulated reaction to lipids obstructs gas passage. Like some other functional bowel disorders, visceral hyperalgesia or hypersensitivity may contribute to abnormal perceptions of bloating.

Those with psychiatric conditions such as depression or anxiety may have altered perceptions of bloating, but this is not strongly established. Those who believe themselves to have lactose intolerance, but do not, report bloating after consumption of dairy products but fail to do so when challenged in a placebo-controlled, blinded study. Abdominal wall weakness or failure to maintain tonicity after gas increase may cause distention more than bloating. There is no conclusive evidence about the roles of intestinal flora, female sex hormones, or food intolerances.

Clinical Manifestations

An important characteristic of bloating and distention is diurnal variation; they worsen during the day and resolve at night. They are also notable after meals, especially after a large meal or binge eating. It is important to clarify what people mean when they refer to bloating: is it the sense of excess gas, increased abdominal girth, postprandial fullness, or even the need to defecate. Good history taking will highlight other symptoms that may reveal a specific diagnosis, especially functional bowel disorders. Association with epigastric discomfort usually indicates FD, whereas relief with defecation or association with stool consistency and frequency changes suggests IBS.

Careful physical examination can detect ascites as a cause for distention, particularly with intra-abdominal malignancies. Digital rectal examination may reveal anal or rectal obstructions or signs of obstipation. Plain abdominal radiographs may show bowel obstructions or may reveal increased intraluminal gas in IBS. Abdominal scanning is more sensitive for obstructions; it is also necessary to detect ascites or intra-abdominal masses as a cause for distention, especially in the obese.

Differential Diagnosis

The most common disorders associated with bloating are FD, IBS, and functional constipation. It is also seen in malabsorption and acute diarrheal states (bacterial infections), probably secondary to increased intraluminal fluid contents. Organic diseases that may cause bloating or abdominal distention should be excluded through history, physical examination, and necessary investigations. Bowel obstruction (see Chapter 226) is common in intra-abdominal malignancies, and those afflicted may experience both bloating and distention. Ascites needs to be ruled out in patients with distention.

Treatment

Reassurance in the absence of serious organic diseases is important. Simple treatments include avoiding carbonated beverages, which increase swallowed air. Avoidance of highly flatulogenic food may relieve the flatulence frequently associated with bloating. These include beans, broccoli, cabbage, celery, radish, carrot, onion, banana, prune juice, and others.[17] Removing fiber from the diet in IBS improves bloating. Gas expulsion is quicker while standing, so immobilization can have a positive effect on bloating or distention. There may be a role for hypnotherapy in relieving bloating with IBS. Managing other conditions with bloating is likely to alleviate the symptom as well.

Pharmacological strategies for bloating are unclear. Neostigmine reduces bloating and distention through its prokinetic effect on gas transit. Another prokinetic is tegaserod, a partial agonist of the serotonin 5-HT$_4$ receptor. It is used for constipation-predominant IBS in women, with good results in both bloating and distention. Prokinetics may have a future in bloating management. Tegaserod was recently withdrawn from U.S. markets because of evidence of cardiac toxicity. Surfactants like simethicone or dimethicone alter gas bubble tension; their benefit is modest. There is no strong evidence to support activated charcoal, weight loss, or exercise as therapies for bloating. In those with excessive flatulence, the commercial product Beano (an enzymatic complex) seems to be often effective in reducing gas.

BELCHING

Belching, or eructation, is the passage of gas from the stomach or esophagus to the pharynx and then outside via the mouth or nose. It allows relief of upper abdominal discomfort and happens normally after meals.[18] Belching is not often troublesome, and literature is scarce. Occasionally, it may be significant, especially in the course of other disease entities such as GERD and FD. In GERD, acid reflux and heartburn may occur simultaneously with belching.

Epidemiology and Prevalence

Belching has been reported in 50% of those with GERD and in 18% of a palliative medicine population.[3]

Pathophysiology

Aerophagia (air swallowing) occurs normally with eating, drinking, and smoking. It causes gas accumulation and distention of the gastric fundus. This stimulates transient LES relaxation, allowing gas reflux from the stomach to the esophagus, creating a "common cavity" event. As this is formed, the gas bubble either goes back to the stomach or travels upward, depending on esophageal motility. When the movement is upward, the upper esophageal sphincter relaxes, allowing esophageopharyngeal gas passage.[19] Gastric hypersensitivity to distention in FD may increase belching with normal amounts of intragastric gas. After fundoplication, gastric belching is difficult, but belching can still occur as a result of esophageal trapping of swallowed air. Excessive belching may be psychogenic and is seen in patients with psychological distress.

Clinical Manifestations

In patients with excessive belching, the presence of GERD or FD should be investigated, in addition to a psychiatric history. Abnormal LES pressures can be investigated through manometry. There are no specific tests for belching. Gastric air bubbles on abdominal radiographs have no diagnostic value.

Differential Diagnosis

The differential diagnosis is limited to GERD, FD, and excessive belching disorder of unspecified etiology.

Treatment

Management is mainly nonpharmacological. Carbonated beverages and smoking should be stopped. Chewing gum and hard candies increase air swallowing and should be discouraged. Eating should be slow, with small boluses. When identified, associated conditions should be treated. Behavioral therapy may benefit concomitant psychiatric conditions (see "Future Considerations").

Future Considerations

- Optimal management of "indigestion" symptoms when associated with functional disorders is controversial and in need of extensive research.
- The use of empiric acid suppressants as first-line treatment is debated because of possible delayed diagnosis of uninvestigated symptoms (e.g., cancer).
- Drugs being tested for dyspepsia include serotonin agonists, cholecystokinin (CCK) antagonists, N-methyl-D-aspartate (NMDA) antagonists, neurokinin antagonists, and antidepressants; these need further research.
- Fedotozine, a κ agonist, has a promising role in functional dyspepsia with epigastric pain and may improve the bloating of irritable bowel syndrome, perhaps by decreasing visceral hypersensitivity.
- The degree to which opioids contribute to indigestion in palliative medicine patients is unclear. Nonabsorbable μ-antagonist drugs should be researched in suspected opioid-induced indigestion.

REFERENCES

1. Talley NJ, Phung N, Kalantar JS. ABC of the upper gastrointestinal tract: Indigestion—When is it functional? BMJ 2001;323:1294-1297.
2. Koloski NA, Talley NJ, Boyce PM. Predictors of health care seeking for irritable bowel disorders and nonulcer dyspepsia: A critical review of the literature on symptoms and psychosocial factors. Am J Gastroenterol 2001;96:1340-1349.
3. Walsh D, Donnelly S, Rybicki L. The symptoms of advanced cancer: Relationship to age, gender, and performance status in 1,000 patients. Support Care Cancer 2000;8:175-179.
4. Lee KJ, Kindt S, Tack J. Pathophysiology of functional dyspepsia. Best Pract Res Clin Gastroenterol 2004;18:707-716.
5. Veldhuyzen van Zanten SJ, Jones MJ, Verlinden M, et al. Efficacy of cisapride and domperidone in functional (nonulcer) dyspepsia: A metaanalysis. Am J Gastroenterol 2001;96:689-696.
6. Bytzer P. Diagnostic approach to dyspepsia. Best Pract Res Clin Gastroenterol 2004;18:681-693.
7. Cremonini F, Delgado-Aros S, Talley NJ. Functional dyspepsia: Drugs for new (and old) therapeutic targets. Best Pract Res Clin Gastroenterol 2004;18:717-733.
8. Jackson JL, O'Malley PG, Tomkins G, et al. Treatment of functional gastrointestinal disorders with antidepressant medications: A meta-analysis. Am J Med 2000;108:65-72.
9. Calvert EL, Houghton LA, Cooper P, et al. Long-term improvement in functional dyspepsia using hypnotherapy. Gastroenterology 2002;123:1778-1785.
10. Veldhuyzen van Zanten SJ, Bradette M, Chiba N, et al. Evidence-based recommendations for short- and long-term management of uninvestigated dyspepsia in primary care: An update of the Canadian Dyspepsia Working Group (CanDys) clinical management tool. Can J Gastroenterol 2005;19:285-303.
11. Papa A, Urgesi A, Grillo S, et al. Pathophysiology, diagnosis and treatment of non-erosive reflux disease (NERD). Miner Gastroenterol Dietol 2004;50:215-226.
12. Komurcu S, Nelson KA, Walsh D, et al. Gastrointestinal symptoms among in-patients with advanced cancer. Am J Hosp Palliat Care 2002;19:351-355.
13. Barlow WJ, Orlando RC. The pathogenesis of heartburn in nonerosive reflux disease: A unifying hypothesis. Gastroenterology 2005;128:771-778.
14. Devault KR. Review article: The role of acid suppression in patients with non-erosive reflux disease or functional heartburn. Aliment Pharmacol Ther 2006;23(Suppl 1):33-39.
15. Kaltenbach T, Crockett S, Gerson LB. Are lifestyle measures effective in patients with gastroesophageal reflux disease? An evidence based approach. Arch Intern Med 2006;166:965-971.
16. Houghton LA, Whorwell PJ. Towards a better understanding of abdominal bloating and distention in functional gastrointestinal disorders. Neurogastroenterol Motil 2005;17:500-511.
17. Azpiroz F, Malagelada JR. Abdominal bloating. Gastroenterology 2005;129:1060-1078.
18. Tack J, Talley NJ, Camilleri M, et al. Functional gastroduodenal disorders. Gastroenterology 2006;130:1466-1479.
19. Lin M, Triadafilopoulos G. Belching: dyspepsia or gastroesophageal reflux disease? Am J Gastroenterol 2003;98:2139-2145.

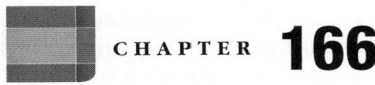

CHAPTER **166**

Pruritus

Brett Taylor Summey

KEY POINTS

- General skin care modalities should be implemented in all patients with pruritus, regardless of the cause, because xerosis and barrier impairment often contribute to the itch.
- Pruritus can occur both with and without cutaneous findings, the latter being suspicious for a systemic etiology.
- The etiology of pruritus can be classified as dermatological, systemic, neurogenic/neuropathic, psychogenic, or a hybrid.
- Unlike pain, for which several effective drugs are available, no general-purpose antipruritic drugs exist; skillful off-label use of available medications is required.
- Do not underestimate the severity of itch and the psychological toll it can inflict on quality of life.

Pruritus (itch) can be defined as an unpleasant sensation that elicits either a conscious or reflex desire to scratch. Acute pruritus serves a protective function and most likely is a sensation that developed evolutionarily to remove pruritogenic stimuli such as insects and parasites. Chronic pruritus is a nuisance and one of the most distressing physical sensations; it can lead to significant psychological disturbances and even suicide.

Pruritus is the most common symptom of dermatological diseases and is often the principal reason for consulting a dermatologist. Although itch is present in many skin diseases, it can also be secondary to an underlying systemic disorder. There is a systemic etiology in 33% to 40% of cases of diffuse itch.[1] The etiology without dermatological disease is classified into the following groups: systemic (diseases of organs other than skin), neurogenic/neuropathic (disorders of the central or peripheral nervous system or neurochemical alterations), and psychogenic (purely psychological secondary to delusions or anxiety).[2]

The neurophysiology is complex, and most of our current knowledge is derived from pain research. Recently, important mediators, receptors, and pathways of itch have been discovered. The relative paucity of research and lack of understanding of the complex pathogenesis of pruritus have hampered the development of novel therapies. Available treatments can be efficacious, but many have not been studied in controlled trials.

BASIC SCIENCE AND PATHOPHYSIOLOGY

For many years, itch was regarded as a variant of pain and was assumed to share identical neuronal pathways. Research demonstrated that increasing the intensity of pruritogenic stimuli induced increased itch but had no effect on pain. Microneurography allowed researchers to isolate distinct nerve fibers that are responsive to pruritogenic but not mechanical stimuli.[3] Currently, pruritus and pain are regarded as separate sensations, transmitted along distinct neuronal pathways.

Histamine appears to be the principal mediator of itch. Histamine activates unmyelinated C-fibers in the skin. These are itch specific, comprise 5% to10% of all afferent C-fibers in the skin, have slow conduction velocities, and have large innervation territories compared with other C-fibers.[3] Pruritogenic agents (e.g., histamine) or physical factors cause conduction of these fibers that synapse in the spinal cord dorsal horn. Neurons sensitive to histamine have been traced to the most superficial portion of the dorsal horn lamina I spinothalamic tract.[4] They cross from the dorsal horn to the contralateral side and ascend to the lateral thalamus. From the thalamus, neurons project to the anterior cingulate gyrus and sensorimotor cortex, both of which are activated in histamine-induced itch.[5]

In addition to histamine, peripheral mediators include serotonin, substance P, cytokines, proteases, prostaglandin E, opioid peptides, acetylcholine, bradykinin, and dopamine. Novel pruritogenic receptors in the skin include vanilloid receptor TRPV1, cannabinoid receptors, protease-activated receptor (PAR-2), and opioid receptors (κ and μ).[6] Opioid peptides via opioid receptors are thought to be the major mediators of central itch. Agonism of the opioid μ-receptor produces itch, whereas κ-receptor agonism inhibits itch.[7] Increased understanding of these mediators and receptors has provided targets to exploit in treatment, both in terms of currently available medications and for research into drug development (see "Case Study: Dermatological Pruritus" and "Case Study: Opiate-Induced Pruritus").

CLINICAL MANIFESTATIONS

Pruritus is challenging to gauge clinically. In pruritus secondary to dermatological diseases, the clinical appearance of the skin often helps make the diagnosis. In systemic causes, the skin examination often is normal. If xerosis is present, it may represent skin barrier impairment from the systemic disease, advancing age, or poor skin care, all of which benefit from general skin care. If a dermatological cause is not observed clinically, laboratory studies may be helpful (Box 166-1).

DIFFERENTIAL DIAGNOSIS

It is important to take a complete history and to examine the skin, mucous membranes, lymph nodes, liver, and spleen. Based on that information, the clinician should classify itch as exogenous (drug-induced or related to poor skin care), primarily dermatological, systemic, neurogenic/neuropathic, or psychogenic.[2] The differential diagnoses of dermatoses manifesting with itch are numerous, and a dermatology referral may be needed. Psychogenic pruritus should be a diagnosis of exclusion, but it should be remembered that anxiety can exacerbate other causes of pruritus. Neurogenic/neuropathic pruritus arises from disorders of the central or peripheral nervous system, such as brain tumors, multiple sclerosis, neuropathies, or nerve compression; in addition, this category overlaps with systemic causes. In the absence of a primary skin disease and recent drug addition, the etiology is likely systemic or neurogenic/neuropathic (Box 166-2).

 CASE STUDY

Opiate-Induced Pruritus

A 64-year-old woman had biliary obstruction secondary to liver metastases from gastrointestinal carcinoma. Her symptoms included mild back pain, moderate abdominal pain, and moderate generalized pruritus. Morphine was given to control the pain symptoms, but this treatment greatly increased the patient's pruritus. General measures were introduced and ondansetron was initiated in an attempt to control the opiate-induced pruritus. This was very successful, but after a few weeks the pruritus began to reappear. Mirtazapine was added at night, which was again successful in controlling the patient's itch for almost 2 months. Additional therapies considered were low-dose naltrexone (depending on patient tolerability in terms of pain and withdrawal symptoms) and subhypnotic doses of propofol. At that time, however, the patient's pain had increased significantly, requiring sedating doses of morphine. The patient died soon afterward.

 CASE STUDY

Dermatological Pruritus

A 78-year-old man entered the hospice service because of end-stage heart failure. He reported always having been an "itchy" person, but lately he had been more frequently and diffusely pruritic, most intensely at night. He had help bathing once daily with an alkaline soap and no moisturization. On physical examination, the patient was very xerotic on the extremities and back. After he began using a soap-free, lower pH cleanser and applying an emollient both after bathing and twice per day, he had near-complete itch alleviation except at night. Hydroxyzine, 25 to 50 mg at night, significantly diminished his nocturnal symptoms.

Box 166-1 Laboratory Studies in the Evaluation of Pruritus

- Complete blood count with differential
- Blood urea nitrogen, creatinine
- Liver transaminases, alkaline phosphatase, bilirubin
- Thyroid-stimulating hormone, thyroxine
- Serum iron, ferritin
- Serum glucose, calcium, phosphate
- Viral hepatitis serologies
- Stool studies (ova, parasites, occult blood)
- Chest radiography
- Human immunodeficiency virus (HIV) antibody
- Serum protein electrophoresis
- Erythrocyte sedimentation rate, C-reactive protein

TABLE 166-1 Systemic Medications for Pruritus

THERAPY	DOSAGE	CLINICAL SETTING IN WHICH THE THERAPY IS EFFECTIVE
Hydroxyzine[9]	25-100 mg q8h	Histamine-induced pruritus, nocturnal pruritus
Doxepin[7]	10-50 mg qhs	Histamine-induced pruritus, nocturnal pruritus, intractable pruritus
Paroxetine[10]	20-50 mg qd	Psychogenic itch, intractable itch in malignancy
Mirtazapine[11]	15-30 mg qhs	Nocturnal pruritus, uremic and hepatogenic pruritus
Naltrexone[12]	25-75 mg qd	Hepatogenic pruritus, uremic
Ultraviolet B phototherapy[13]	3 times per wk	Uremic pruritus, pruritus of HIV, hepatogenic pruritus
Thalidomide[14]	50-100 mg qd	Pruritus of HIV, uremic pruritus, prurigo nodularis
Gabapentin[15]	900-1800 mg qd	Neurogenic pruritus, intractable pruritus
Charcoal[16]	6 g qd	Uremic pruritus
Cholestyramine[17]	4-16 g qd	Hepatogenic pruritus, uremic pruritus
Ondansetron[18]	8 mg q4h (IV or PO)	Intractable pruritus, uremic and hepatogenic pruritus
Rifampin[19]	300-600 mg qd	Hepatogenic pruritus
Propofol[20]	10-15 mg IV bolus, then 1 mg/kg/hr IV	Hepatogenic pruritus, intractable pruritus
Butorphanol[21]	1-4 mg intranasally qd	Hepatogenic and uremic pruritus; fewer withdrawal symptoms than naltrexone

TREATMENT

The treatment of chronic or intractable pruritus can be challenging. Therapy should be geared toward nonspecific, general measures to improve pruritus. If possible, all new medications with the potential to cause pruritus should be discontinued. Lastly, systemic medications may be needed. General skin care measures should be endorsed for all patients with the symptom of itch (Box 166-3). Some believe that simple skin care can spare some patients from needing systemic therapy.[8] These measures help restore any perturbation of the epidermal barrier and prevent epidermal water loss, both important sources of itch.

Treatment in dermatological disease is based on the underlying diagnosis. Skin diseases causing itch can be as diverse as infestations (e.g., scabies), inflammatory diseases (e.g., eczema, psoriasis, mastocytosis), neoplastic disease (e.g., mycosis fungoides), and infections (e.g., tinea, varicella, folliculitis). The most important aspect of treatment is an accurate diagnosis, which often requires consultation from a dermatologist.

Treatment of systemic pruritus, including neurogenic/neuropathic causes, relies on determining the most likely etiology. Hepatogenic and nephrogenic pruritus represent most sources of systemic pruritus. Many times, medications (Table 166-1) must be used in combination, sometimes they work only transiently, and occasionally several must be tried to find an efficacious regimen (Box 166-4). All of the listed medications have been studied in small trials demonstrating some effect on decreasing pruritus. Small, localized area of pruritus can be treated topically with doxepin 5% cream three to four times per day, capsaicin 0.075% cream three to five times per day, or pramoxine 1% cream four times per day.

SUPPORTIVE CARE

A specific problem in palliative medicine involves systemic pruritus in terminal illness. Often, the itch is multifactorial, with both liver and kidney function deteriorating and increased anxiety. Systemic therapy can be toxic in such patients, which must be considered. Unfortunately, there are no studies to guide the clinician in this scenario. In multiorgan failure, mirtazapine and ondansetron can be used in low doses. In addition, opioid antagonists may not be feasible in the setting of a patient with chronic

---

Future Considerations

- New interest in the science of pruritus will lead to more research, and, in time, to more effective and specific treatments.
- Focused studies on the neurophysiology of centrally induced itch will help treat systemic pruritus.
- The specific κ opioid receptor agonist TRK-820 may be effective in systemic itch. It was shown to be valuable in uremic itch.[22]
- Vanilloid receptor overexpression may contribute to the sensation of pruritus. Vanilloid receptor antagonists could be helpful.
- Research in murine models demonstrated that certain cannabinoid receptor agonists increased the threshold of itch transmission. Studies elucidating which specific cannabinoid receptors play a role in itch transmission may provide therapeutic targets.
- Controlled trials using several of the treatment options in end-of-life palliation of itch would be beneficial.

---

pain on opiates, with the exception of butorphanol. In terminal patients with itch, the general measures mentioned in Box 166-3 are extremely important (see "Future Considerations").

REFERENCES

1. Mahboob F. Frequency and aetiology of pruritus in admitted patients in a medical ward of Mayo Hospital, Lahore. J Ayub Coll Abbottabad 2004; 16:42-43.
2. Bernhard J. Itch and pruritus: What are they and how should itches be classified? Dermatol Ther 2005;18:288-291.
3. Schmelz M, Schmidt R, Bickel A, et al. Specific C-receptors for itch in human skin. J Neurosci 1997;104:134-137.
4. Jinks S, Carstens E. Superficial dorsal horn neurons identified by intracutaneous histamine: Chemonociceptive responses and modulation by morphine. J Neurophysiol 2000;84:616-627.
5. Mochizuki H, Tashiro M, Kano M, et al. Imaging of central itch modulation in the human brain using positron emission tomography. Pain 2003;105: 339-346.
6. Steinhoff M, Bienenstock J, Schmelz M, et al. Neurophysiological, neuroimmunological, and neuroendocrine basis of pruritus. J Invest Dermatol 2006;126:1705-1718.
7. Krishnan A, Koo J. Psyche, opioids, and itch: Therapeutic consequences. Dermatol Ther 2005;18:314-322.
8. Twycross R (ed). Introducing Palliative Care, 2nd ed. Oxford: Radcliffe Medical Press, 1997.
9. O'Donoghue M, Tharp M. Antihistamines and their role as antipruritics. Dermatol Ther 2005;18:333-340.
10. Zylicz Z, Smits C, Chem D, et al. Paroxetine for pruritus of advanced cancer. J Pain Symptom Manage 1998;16:121-124.
11. Davis M, Frandsen J, Walsh D, et al. Mirtazepine for pruritus. J Pain Symptom Manage 2003;25:288-291.
12. Gilchrest B, Rowe J, Brown R. Ultraviolet phototherapy of uremic pruritus: Long-term results and possible mechanisms of action. Ann Intern Med 1979;91:17-21.
13. Wolfhagen F, Sternieri E, Hop W, et al. Oral naltrexone treatment for cholestatic pruritus: A double-blind, placebo-controlled study. Gastroenterology 1997;113:1264-1269.
14. Alfadley A, Al-Hawsawi K, Thestrup-Peterson K, et al. Treatment of prurigo nodularis with thalidomide. Int J Dermatol 2003;42:372-375.
15. Winhoven S, Coulson I, Bottomley W. Brachioradial pruritus: Response to treatment with gabapentin. Br J Dermatol 2004;150:786.
16. Giovannetti S, Barsotti G, Cupisti A, et al. Oral activated charcoal in patients with uremic pruritus. Nephron 1995;70:193-196.
17. Van Itallie T, Hashim S, Crampton R, et al. The treatment of pruritus and hypercholesterolemia of primary biliary cirrhosis with cholestyramine. N Eng J Med 1961;265:469-474.
18. Muller C, Pongratz S, Pidlich J, et al. Treatment of pruritus in chronic liver disease with the 5-hydroxytryptamine receptor type 3 antagonist ondansetron: A randomized, placebo-controlled, double-blind cross-over trial. Eur J Gastroenterol Hepatol 1998;10:865-870.
19. Tandon P, Rowe BH, Vandermeer B, et al. The efficacy and safety of bile acid binding agents, opioid antagonists, or rifampin in the treatment of cholestasis-associated pruritus. Am J Gastroenterol 2007;102:1528-1536.
20. Borgeat A, Wilder-Smith O, Mentha G, et al. Propofol and cholestatic pruritus. Am J Gastroenterol 1992;87:672-674.
21. Dawn A, Yosipovitch G. Butorphanol for treatment of intractable pruritus. J Am Acad Dermatol 2006;54:527-531.
22. Kumagai H, Saruta T. Prospects for a novel kappa-opioid receptor agonist, TRK820, in uremic pruritus. In Yosipovitch G, Greaves M (eds). Itch: Basic mechanisms and therapy. New York: Mercel Dekker, 2004, pp 279-286.

SUGGESTED READING

Ikoma A, Steinhoff M, Ständer S, et al. The neurobiology of itch. Nat Rev Neurosci 2006;7:535-547.
Summey B, Yosipovitch G. Pharmacologic advances in the systemic treatment of itch. Dermatol Ther 2005;18:328-332.
Twycross R, Wilcock A (eds). Symptom Management in Advanced Cancer, 2nd ed. Oxford: Radcliffe Medical Press, 1997.
Yosipovitch G, Greaves M, Fleischer A, et al (eds). Itch: Basic Mechanisms and Therapy. New York: Mercel Dekker, 2004.
Yosipovitch G, Greaves M, Schmelz M. Itch. Lancet 2003; 361:690-694.

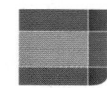

CHAPTER **167**

Memory Problems

Adam Rosenblatt

K E Y   P O I N T S

- Amnesia occurs in palliative care for numerous reasons and is caused by a disturbance in the structure or function of the brain.
- Amnesia comes in two forms: retrograde (an inability to recall past events) and anterograde (an inability to form new memories).
- Many palliative care patients have amnesia arising from a primary dementing process, such as Alzheimer's disease.
- Amnesia is also frequently a secondary manifestation of the delirious states common in palliative care, such as the delirium of hypercalcemia.
- The treatment for amnesia is resolution of delirium and conservative management. There is a pharmacopoeia for Alzheimer's disease.
- Amnestic patients may not be able to express their wishes consistently or retain the facts of their condition and prognosis.

Memory impairment, or amnesia, is caused by a disturbance in the brain structure or function and may occur in palliative care for numerous reasons. Amnesia has two main forms. *Retrograde* amnesia is a loss of ability to recall distant events, those that occurred before the onset of the brain injury. *Anterograde* amnesia is difficulty forming new memories: the patient cannot recall events that occurred after the abnormal brain state. Both types may co-occur across the spectrum of cognitive impairment. In the final stages of dying, amnesia, particularly anterograde amnesia, is not always regarded as a negative symptom by patients and families. It may render the patient unable to recall recent suffering or provide relief from anxiety about the dying process. In contrast, retrograde amnesia or severe anterograde amnesia may render the patient unable to reminisce or even to recognize family members; it may complicate end-of-life decision making and may deprive the patient of the ability to be emotionally present for friends and family members who wish to say goodbye.

EPIDEMIOLOGY

Memory problems often occur in dying elderly patients as part of a primary dementing condition, such as Alzheimer's disease or vascular dementia. Although Alzheimer's disease is associated with increased mortality and a shorter life expectancy in the elderly,[1] it is usually a contributing factor, not the primary cause of death.[2] In palliative care, preexisting dementia is common and it something the clinician must appreciate and manage to ensure the best quality of life. In other cases, those with end-stage dementing conditions may be referred to a hospice for that reason alone. Because survival in the demented varies greatly, criteria have been developed to help identify those patients with short life expectancy.[3]

Memory impairment, typically anterograde amnesia, is also part of the delirium that is common in the terminally ill.[4,5] Delirium may be caused by systemic problems such as infections, anemia, hypoxia, hypercalcemia, or other electrolyte imbalances or the effects of medications such as anticholinergics, opiates, or steroids. In some, the terminal condition may produce dementia, with associated amnesia, through its direct brain effects, in the form of cerebrovascular accident or metastatic disease.

Finally, functional or psychogenic amnesia, although not common, is sometimes found in persons who have experienced recent stressful life events and could occur in someone who has just received a grim prognosis. This type of amnesia may be distinguished by the absence of neurologic causes and its isolated retrograde nature: the individual may have no trouble forming new memories but may be densely amnestic for his or her own life history.[6]

PATHOPHYSIOLOGY

Alzheimer's disease is the most common dementia, accounting for 55% to 75% of cases.[7,8] Although the primary pathologic process is still unknown, the condition is characterized by preferential loss of cholinergic synapses and formation of amyloid plaques and neurofibrillary tangles. Vascular or multi-infarct dementia is the second most common type, accounting for 13% to 16% of cases.[7,8] It is a cognitive disorder resulting from stroke or ischemic-hypoxic brain lesions.[9] Other conditions that may cause dementia and themselves result in a terminal condition include diffuse Lewy body disease, frontotemporal dementia, Parkinson's disease, and Huntington's disease.

Memory impairment in delirium has many poorly understood mechanisms, depending on the underlying medical conditions. Some terminal conditions may cause dementia or amnesia in the absence of delirium if they have direct brain effects, by causing vascular disease, cerebral infarctions or hemorrhage, or space-occupying metastatic lesions. Hippocampal lesions are particularly associated with anterograde amnesia (see "Case Study: Memory Problems at the End of Life").

CASE STUDY

Memory Problems at the End of Life

Mr. J was an 83-year-old man with mild Alzheimer's disease. He had been living at home with his elderly wife and taking lisinopril, pravastatin, and donepezil 10 mg at bedtime for memory impairment. However, he had become more confused and listless and had lost 10 kg over a period of 2 months. An abdominal computed tomographic scanning showed a widely disseminated malignancy. At first, his family attempted to care for him at home, but he became incontinent and suffered several falls.

Mr. J was admitted to a local nursing home and enrolled in a hospice program. The decision was made discontinue his blood pressure and cholesterol-lowering drugs but not his donepezil, in the hope of maintaining his ability to communicate with his family. In fact, his memory for remote events was good, and he enjoyed reminiscing with the family about good times together. His diagnosis and prognosis were explained to him, but he could not retain this new information, asking repeatedly, "Where am I" and "What's the matter with me?" It was very painful to his family to have to tell him repeatedly that he was dying.

Two days after entering the nursing home he was awake at night, trying to get dressed and insisting that he needed to go home. He was given 1 mg of lorazepam for "anxiety." The next morning, he was unarousable during a family visit, and he did not speak until late the following night. The next day he was more alert. The PRN order for lorazepam was discontinued. A nightlight was placed in the patient's room, and the staff was instructed to take him for a brief walk down the hall and then put him back to bed if he tried to leave again. His family increased their daytime visiting hours and brought in some photographs and a dressing table from home, which he could see from his bed. When he asked, "What's the matter with me?" they told him, "You have been sick, but the doctors and nurses are taking good care of you." Over the next 2 weeks, Mr. J became progressively more obtunded, but there were moments of lucidity. He asked his daughter for a kiss and then died peacefully an hour later.

CLINICAL MANIFESTATIONS

Patients with memory problems present with inability to recall past events, those that occurred before the development of an abnormal brain state (retrograde amnesia), or inability to form new memories and recall events that occurred after the abnormal brain state (anterograde amnesia), or both. These difficulties usually arise in the context of a broader dementia syndrome, such as Alzheimer's disease, or a delirium. Those patients with focal lesions may present with purer forms of amnesia, such as the anterograde amnesia that occurs with hippocampal lesions. The memory difficulty may be detected first by visitors who notice that the patient cannot recall recent events and conversations or makes inconsistent decisions. Amnesia can make decision making and the exercise of autonomy problematic for the dying, because amnestic patients may be unable to express their wishes consistently or retain the essential facts of their condition and

TABLE 167-1 Commonly Prescribed Agents for the Dementia of Alzheimer's Disease

DRUG	INDICATION	STARTING DOSE	EFFECTIVE DOSE	MAXIMUM DOSE	SIDE EFFECTS
Donepezil	Mild to moderate AD	5 mg once daily	5 mg once daily	10 mg once daily	Nausea, vomiting, diarrhea
Rivastigmine	Mild to moderate AD, Parkinson's dementia	1.5 mg twice daily	3 mg twice daily	6 mg twice daily	Nausea, vomiting, anorexia, dizziness
Galantamine (extended-release)	Mild to moderate AD	8 mg once daily	16 mg once daily	24 mg once daily	Nausea, vomiting, anorexia, dizziness, syncope
Memantine	Moderate to severe AD	5 mg once daily	10 mg twice daily	10 mg twice daily	Dizziness, headache, confusion, constipation

AD, Alzheimer's disease.

prognosis, no matter how certain they may seem at a given, isolated point in time.

DIFFERENTIAL DIAGNOSIS

The differential diagnosis of memory impairment in the terminally ill includes delirium, global dementias, aphasia and other communication difficulties, depression, psychosis, and psychogenic amnesia. Depressed patients, in particular, may perform poorly on cognitive tests such as the Mini-Mental State Examination[10] through poor effort, often answering "I don't know" to the questions, or they may complain bitterly of amnesia and other cognitive impairment without fully demonstrating deficits on testing.

TREATMENT

The treatment for memory impairment caused by delirium is to identify the cause and attempt to rectify it (e.g., treating infections, managing metabolic disturbances, removing responsible medications). The treatment of memory impairment resulting from direct manifestations of the terminal condition, such as cerebrovascular accident or brain metastases, is usually conservative and aimed at stabilizing the patient and preventing further damage. In some, palliative radiotherapy or chemotherapy may ameliorate the memory problem by shrinking a tumor impinging on the brain.

In Alzheimer's disease, drugs (Table 167-1) modestly improve cognitive performance and forestall clinical decline.[11] These include the acetylcholinesterase inhibitors donepezil, rivastigmine, and galantamine and the N-methyl-D-aspartate (NMDA) receptor antagonist memantine, which is indicated by the U.S. Food and Drug Administration for more severe Alzheimer's disease, in contrast to the other agents. Rivastigmine has also recently received an indication for the dementia of Parkinson's disease.

In end-stage dementia, a new trial of one of these drugs would seem unlikely to be useful. Many patients come to a hospice with concurrent dementias of varying severity and taking one or more of these agents. The clinician must resist the temptation to reflexively discontinue all "unnecessary" medications. It takes only about 2 weeks for the effects of these medications to wear off, but 6 weeks or longer for them to become established. The loss of their benefits may result in worsening behavioral problems, loss of independent function, and inability to communicate with treatment providers, interact with family members,

and make decisions. The decision as to whether to discontinue such treatments must consider life expectancy, dementia severity, prior therapeutic response, and personal care goals.

SUPPORTIVE CARE

Patients with memory impairment benefit from understanding, patience, and willingness to answer repetitive questions. Keeping to a regular schedule of daytime and nighttime activities and spontaneously reorienting patients to time, place, and circumstances may help them keep their bearings, make needs known, and enjoy higher-quality interactions with family and friends. Mnemonic devices such as writing notes, keeping a journal, or displaying calendars or clocks may also help. When amnestic individuals become irritated or fixate on a faulty memory or inappropriate goal (e.g., repeatedly trying to get dressed to go to work), arguing or reasoning with them is usually unhelpful. Instead, family members and care providers should try to distract them with a pleasurable activity or a temporizing excuse (e.g., stating that the office is closed).

The use of hospice for persons with end-stage dementia is controversial, particularly given the difficulty of predicting life expectancy in these patients. The utility of long-term anti-Alzheimer's drugs is controversial. Some experts believe that these agents forestall institutionalization and functional dependency and others feel that the improvements are less clinically significant. The utility of these drugs in non-Alzheimer's dementias is not established. Amnestic patients may sometimes express strong opinions about their treatment and which interventions they would like to receive or forgo, but they may do so inconsistently. This may lead to disagreements among the family and care team. Friends and family may not want a loved one to recover from the amnesia if it is seen as protecting the person from sadness or anxiety about his or her condition.

REFERENCES

1. Larson EB, Shadlen MF, Wang L, et al. Survival after initial diagnosis of Alzheimer disease. Ann Intern Med. 2004;140:501-509.
2. Ganguli M, Dodge HH, Shen C, et al. Alzheimer disease and mortality: A 15-year epidemiological study. Arch Neurol 2005;62:779-784.
3. Luchins DJ, Hanrahan P, Murphy K. Criteria for enrolling dementia patients in hospice. J Am Geriatr Soc 1997;45:1054-1059.
4. Massie MJ, Holland J, Glass E. Delirium in terminally ill cancer patients. Am J Psychiatry 1983;140:1048-1050.

5. Casarett DJ, Inouye SK. Diagnosis and management of delirium near the end of life. Ann Intern Med 2001;135:32-40.
6. Brandt J, Van Gorp WG. Functional ("psychogenic") amnesia. Semin Neurol 2006;26:331-340.
7. Lobo A, Launer LJ, Fratiglioni L, et al. Prevalence of dementia and major subtypes in Europe: A collaborative study of population-based cohorts. Neurologic Diseases in the Elderly Research Group. Neurology 2000;54(Suppl 5):S4-S9.
8. Ebly EM, Parhad IM, Hogan DB, Fung TS. Prevalence and types of dementia in the very old: Results from the Canadian Study of Health and Aging. Neurology. 1994;44:1593-1600.
9. Roman GC, Tatemichi TK, Erkinjuntti T, et al. Vascular dementia: Diagnostic criteria for research studies. Report of the NINDS-AIREN International Workshop. Neurology 1993;43:250-260.
10. Folstein MF, Folstein SE, McHugh PR. "Min-Mental State": A practical method for grading the cognitive state of patients for the clinician. J Psychiatric Res 1975;2:189-198.
11. Ritchie CW, Ames D, Clayton T, Lai R. Meta-analysis of randomized trials of the efficacy and safety of donepezil, galantamine, and rivastigmine for the treatment of Alzheimer disease. Am J Geriatr Psychiatry 2004;12:358-369.

CHAPTER **168**

Muscle Spasms

Dilara Seyidova Khoshknabi

KEY POINTS

- Muscle spasms are quick, painful, uncontrolled contractions, often caused by involuntary repetitive firing of motor unit action potentials at high frequency, which can impair mobility and cause pain.
- Myoclonus is a brief, involuntary jerking of a muscle or group of muscles caused by neuronal discharges, often from accumulation of opioid metabolites.
- Tremor is an involuntary, rhythmic, oscillating movement of any body part caused by contractions of reciprocally innervated antagonist muscles.

MUSCLE SPASM

Muscle spasm in palliative medicine is seen often as a comorbidity or medication side effects. Muscle spasms limit mobility and cause pain. Certain types of spasticity can be prevented, whereas others are best treated at onset.

Myoclonus is an involuntary jerking of a muscle or muscle groups that is caused by repetitive neuronal discharges. Myoclonus is frequently seen during the final days of life. It may progress to seizures if left untreated.

Another neurological disturbance, *tremor*, is an involuntary, rhythmic, oscillating movement of any body part caused by contraction of reciprocally innervated antagonist muscles. Tremors cause fatigue and discomfort if left untreated. It is associated with neuropathic pain or treatment for neuropathic pain and must be carefully assessed and treated.

The term *muscle spasms* or *cramps* refers to variable rapid, painful, and uncontrolled contractions that happen unexpectedly, without cause and with little muscle stimulation. Muscle spasm and pain can last several minutes and then slowly ease. Spasms occur in normal individuals under certain conditions, such as during sleep, exercise, or pregnancy or while voluntarily contracting a muscle.[1] In palliative medicine, they may arise from comorbid illness or as a medication side effect. Muscle spasm is problematic in 67% of spinal cord injuries[2] and occurs in 40% to 60% of patients with multiple sclerosis.[3,4]

Pathophysiology

The mechanism that generates muscle cramping remains unclear. In a case series, abnormal exercise-induced stiffness and muscle pain was associated with high muscle levels of myoadenylate deaminase.[5] Cramps arise from spontaneous discharges of motor units rather than from muscle. Electromyographic (EMG) recording during muscle spasm reveals involuntary, high-frequency, repetitive firing of motor unit action potentials, a characteristic that is unlikely to be a result of spontaneous muscle activity. EMG during cramps demonstrates muscle fasciculations at the beginning and end of the cramp. Loss or damage to lower motor neurons is a primary cause for cramps, but muscle diseases are not a cause. Muscle cramps can be of central origin or may arise peripherally at the neuromuscular junction.[6]

Clinical Manifestations

Cramps with No Apparent Cause

Recurrent, nocturnal leg cramps are common in the elderly but may occur at any age. The calf or foot muscles are usually affected, and sleep is frequently disturbed. Cramps are associated with exercise, especially before conditioning. Cramps during exercise are not associated with water or fluid imbalances. Between marathon runners who developed cramps and those who did not, no differences in plasma volume, serum sodium, or serum potassium levels were observed.[7]

Lower Motor Neuron Disorders

Various diseases of the lower motor neurons are associated with cramps, including amyotrophic lateral sclerosis (ALS),[8] recovering poliomyelitis,[9] multifocal motor neuropathy, peripheral nerve injury,[10] nerve root compression,[11] and polyneuropathies.[12]

Metabolic Disorders

Metabolic disorders may cause leg cramps, particularly among pregnant women in the third trimester.[13] Some endocrine disorders, including thyroid disease and hypoadrenalism, have muscle cramps as a feature.[6] Liver disease and cirrhosis are associated with cramps due to decreased intravascular volume.[14]

Acute Extracellular Volume Depletion

Muscle cramps in those patients undergoing hemodialysis is associated with volume depletion.[15]

TABLE 168-1 Pharmacologic Treatment for Cramps

DRUG	DOSE	Adverse Effects	
		SEVERE	**COMMON**
Quinine sulfate	260 mg at bedtime	Hepatotoxicity, interstitial nephritis, ototoxicity, hemolytic-uremic syndrome, disseminated intravascular syndrome, thrombocytopenia	Nausea/vomiting, headache, dysphagia, hypoglycemia, rash
Carbamazepine	100-200 mg at bedtime	Renal toxicity, hyponatremia, hypocalcemia, thrombocytopenia, bone marrow depression, congestive heart failure, atrioventricular heart block, syncope, hepatitis, Stevens-Johnson syndrome	Nausea, vomiting, drowsiness, dizziness, hypotension, hypertension, blurred vision, double vision, pruritic rash
Gabapentin	300 mg at bedtime	Stevens-Johnson syndrome (rare)	Fatigue, dizziness, somnolence, ataxia, blurred vision, diplopia, myalgia, nystagmus, tremor, peripheral edema
Dilantin	100-200 mg at bedtime	Leukopenia, thrombocytopenia, pancytopenia, liver damage, toxic hepatitis, Stevens-Johnson syndrome	Rash, dizziness, ataxia, encephalopathy, confusion, gingival hyperplasia, osteomalacia
Vitamin E	1000 units at bedtime	—	Gastrointestinal distress

Box 168-1 Nonpharmacological Treatment for Cramps

- Stretching before exercise and at bedtime
- Foot splints
- Hydration plus sodium chloride, especially before exercise

Treatment

Nonpharmacological treatment includes stretching muscles and activating the antagonist muscles to prevent cramps during exercise and to treat nocturnal leg cramps. Another option for benign nocturnal cramps is foot splints to provide passive stretch of the calf muscle. Adding sodium (50 mmol/L) with fluid replacement or adding salt to food in addition to water replaces fluid losses.

Quinine sulfate increases the muscle refractory period and decreases the excitability of motor end plates to nerve stimulation. Some studies have demonstrated decreased cramping with botulinum toxin injection into the calf and foot muscles in those with an inherited cramping syndrome. Botulinum toxin binds presynaptically at the neuromuscular junction and relaxes muscles by preventing acetylcholine release.[16] Creatine monohydrate decreases cramps by 60% in hemodialysis.[17] There are four main drugs for muscle cramps: quinine sulfate, baclofen, phenytoin, and gabapentin of which quinine sulfate is the most potent.[6] Vitamin E reduces cramps in liver disease, cirrhosis, and hemodialysis[18,19] (Table 168-1 and Box 168-1).

MYOCLONUS

Myoclonus is a brief, involuntary muscle jerk or group of muscle contractions caused by neuronal discharges that is transient and not sustained as a spasm. A single muscle discharge occurs but can reoccur in repetitive fashion.[20] Myoclonus occurs spontaneously or with sensory stimulation, arousal, or initial movement (action myoclonus).[21] Myoclonic jerks develop in patients with multiple sclerosis, Parkinson's disease, Alzheimer's disease, or Creutzfeldt-Jakob disease. They may appear as brief muscle contractions ("positive myoclonus") or may be produced by concise lapses of muscle jerk ("negative myoclonus")[22] (Table 168-2).

In palliative medicine, myoclonus is often associated with opioids. The incidence of opioid-induced myoclonus varies between 2.7% and 87%.[23] The precise mechanism is unknown.

Pathophysiology

The specific mechanisms underlying myoclonus are poorly understood. Some types of stimulus-sensitive myoclonus may involve overexcitability in parts of the brain that control movement. Motor control pathways are interconnected in a series of feedback loops called motor pathways. These facilitate and modulate communication between brain and muscle. Key elements are neurotransmitters, which carry messages from one neuron to another. Some neurotransmitters may increase receiving cell sensitivity, whereas others inhibit receiving neurons. An imbalance between inhibitory and stimulatory neurotransmission may underlie myoclonus. (See "Case Study: Myoclonus at the End of Life.")

Clinical Manifestations

Reflex Myoclonus

Reflex myoclonus is caused by visual, auditory, and somesthetic stimuli and can be focal or generalized. Generalized myoclonus is elicited by touching or tapping the face, especially the mentalis muscle zone. Visually triggered reflex myoclonus is induced by a threatening stimulus, usually a sudden flash stimulation.

Action Myoclonus

Action myoclonus is caused by voluntary movement or intention to move. It can be worsened by attempts at precise, coordinated movements. Action myoclonus is the most disabling form of myoclonus and can affect arms, legs, face, and even voice.[20] It is often caused by hypoxic brain damage.

Negative Myoclonus

Negative myoclonus is present only during active muscular contraction and is seen in combination with positive

TABLE 168-2   Classification of Myoclonus

I. PHYSIOLOGIC MYOCLONUS (NORMAL SUBJECTS)

A. Sleep jerks (hypnic jerks)

B. Anxiety induced

C. Exercise induced

D. Hiccups (singultus)

E. Benign infantile myoclonus with feeding

II. ESSENTIAL MYOCLONUS (NO KNOWN CAUSE AND NO OTHER GROSS NEUROLOGICAL DEFICIT)

A. Hereditary (autosomal dominant)

B. Sporadic

III. EPILEPTIC MYOCLONUS (SEIZURES DOMINATE AND NO ENCEPHALOPATHY, AT LEAST INITIALLY)

A. Fragments of epilepsy

  1. Isolated epileptic myoclonic jerks

  2. Epilepsia partialis continua

  3. Idiopathic stimulus-sensitive myoclonus

  4. Photosensitive myoclonus

  5. Myoclonic absences in petit mal epilepsy

B. Childhood myoclonic epilepsy

  1. Infantile spasms

  2. Myoclonic astatic epilepsy (Lennox-Gastaut)

  3. Cryptogenic myoclonus epilepsy (Aicardi)

  4. Awakening myoclonic epilepsy of Janz (juvenile myoclonic epilepsy)

C. Benign familial myoclonic epilepsy (Rabot)

D. Progressive myoclonic epilepsy: Baltic myoclonus (Unverricht-Lundborg)

IV. SYMPTOMATIC MYOCLONUS (PROGRESSIVE OR STATIC ENCEPHALOPATHY DOMINATES)

A. Storage disease

  1. Lafora body disease

  2. GM2 gangliosidosis (late infantile, juvenile)

  3. Tay-Sachs disease

  4. Gaucher's disease (noninfantile neuronopathic form)

  5. Krabbe's leukodystrophy

  6. Ceroid-lipofuscinosis (Batten)

  7. Sialidosis (cherry red spot) (types 1 and 2)

B. Spinocerebellar degenerations

  1. Ramsay Hunt syndrome

  2. Friedreich's ataxia

  3. Ataxia telangiectasia

  4. Other spinocerebellar degenerations

C. Basal ganglia degenerations

  1. Wilson's disease

  2. Torsion dystonia

  3. Hallervorden-Spatz disease

  4. Progressive supranuclear palsy

  5. Huntington's disease

  6. Parkinson's disease

  7. Multisystem atrophy

  8. Corticobasal degeneration

  9. Dentato-rubro-pallido-luysian atrophy

D. Dementias

  1. Creutzfeldt-Jakob disease

  2. Alzheimer's disease

  3. Lewy body disease

  4. Frontotemporal dementia and parkinsonism linked to chromosome 17

E. Infections/postinfectious

  1. Subacute sclerosing panencephalitis

  2. Encephalitis lethargica

  3. Arbovirus encephalitis

  4. Herpes simplex encephalitis

  5. Human T-cell lymphotropic virus (HTLV)-1

  6. Human immunodeficiency virus (HIV)

  7. Postinfectious encephalitis

  8. Malaria

  9. Syphilis

  10. *Cryptococcus*

F. Metabolic

  1. Hyperthyroidism

  2. Hepatic failure

  3. Renal failure

  4. Dialysis syndrome

  5. Hyponatremia

  6. Hypoglycemia

  7. Nonketotic hyperglycemia

  8. Multiple carboxylase deficiency

  9. Biotin deficiency

  10. Mitochondria dysfunction

G. Toxic and drug-induced syndromes

H. Physical encephalopathies

  1. Posthypoxic (Lance-Adams)

  2. Post-traumatic

  3. Heat stroke

  4. Electric shock

  5. Decompression injury

I. Focal nervous system damage

  1. Central nervous system

    a. Poststroke

    b. Post-thalamotomy

    c. Tumor

    d. Trauma

    e. Inflammation (e.g., multiple sclerosis)

  2. Peripheral nerve lesions

J. Malabsorption

  1. Celiac disease

  2. Whipple's disease

K. Eosinophilia-myalgia syndrome

L. Paraneoplastic encephalopathies

M. Opsoclonus-myoclonus syndrome

  1. Idiopathic

  2. Paraneoplastic

  3. Infectious

  4. Other

N. Exaggerated startle syndromes

  1. Hereditary

  2. Sporadic

Adapted from Marsden CD, Hallett M, Fahn S. The nosology and pathophysiology of myoclonus. In Marsden CD, Fahn S (eds). Movement Disorders. London: Butterworths, 1982, pp 196-248.

CASE STUDY

Myoclonus at the End of Life

A 61-year-old woman was admitted with abdominal pain poorly controlled with sustained-release morphine, 120 mg PO three times daily. She had colon cancer with metastases to liver, peritoneum, and lymph nodes. Additional symptoms were sedation, confusion, and myoclonus.

Her pain control regimen was changed to IV morphine, 3 mg/hr continuous infusion and 3 mg/hr as needed, and then, due to poorly controlled pain and ongoing myoclonus, to IV hydromorphone, 1 mg/hr continuous infusion and 1 mg every 2 hours as needed. Hydromorphone was discontinued on day 4 because of poorly controlled pain, sedation, and unrelieved myoclonus. She was prescribed 30 mg methadone every 8 hours and 20 mg every 4 hours as needed. Pain control was improved, and the patient was discharged to hospice at home. Twelve days later, she was readmitted with hematuria and flank pain.

On the second admission, she was found to have a temperature of 37° C, a heart rate of 85 beats/min with a regular sinus rhythm, a respiratory rate of 18 breaths/min, and blood pressure of 133/78 mm Hg. Her oxygen saturation was 97% on 2 L of oxygen via nasal cannula, and she had a partial small bowel obstruction. Neurological examination revealed myoclonus of the extremities. Myoclonus occurred two to three times each hour and occasionally woke the patient at night.

The patient felt that the myoclonus was mild, and she wanted to remain on methadone for pain control. Her methadone dose, which had previously been converted to intravenous administration, now was reduced to 4 mg/hr as a continuous infusion with 3 mg every 3 hours as needed. She used four extra doses of methadone per day. Valproic acid, 500 mg at night for neuropathic pain, was also prescribed. Later, as the patient's pain increased and methadone was titrated for pain control, her myoclonus worsened. However the myoclonus was not bothersome to her, and she remained on methadone until she died 4 weeks later.

From Sarhill N, Davis MP, Walsh D, et al. Methadone-induced myoclonus in advanced cancer. Am J Hosp Palliat Care 2001;18:51-53.

action myoclonus. Such myoclonus is presented in two clinical forms: asterixis and postural lapses.[24] Asterixis is most common; it is usually multifocal but may involve only an isolated muscle group.[25] Postural lapses usually involve axial and proximal muscles of the lower extremities.

Spontaneous Myoclonus

Spontaneous myoclonus may be focal, multifocal, or generalized and may have several manifestations. It may be sporadic, occur suddenly, or overlap with specific movements such as with nocturnal myoclonus or, in normal individuals, with early morning myoclonic epilepsy.[20]

This type of myoclonus is usually spontaneous and focal or occurring in a segmental distribution. Spinal myoclonus is the most common type. Sensory stimulus does not influence myoclonic discharge, and myoclonus can continue during sleep.

Myoclonus from Opioids

Opioids cause various movement disorders. One of the typical and most common side effects of opioids is myoclonus. There are several theories about the pathophysiology of this side effect that involve postsynaptic transmission glycine neurons in the dorsal horn neurons resembling strychnine or N-methyl-D-aspartate (NMDA) neuroexcitatory amino acid receptor activation.[26,27]

Differential Diagnosis

Myoclonus needs to be differentiated from extrapyramidal disorders such as ticks, chorea, postural tremor, dystonia, and hemifacial spasm. True myoclonus has an abrupt and shock-like beginning and end, which separates it from other movement-related disorders.

Treatment

Treatment is based on the clinical presentation and pathophysiological findings. Cortical myoclonus responds to antiseizure medications: piracetam (8 to 20 g/day), clonazepam (2 to 15 mg/day), sodium valproate (1200 to 3000 mg/day), or primidone (500 to 1000 mg/day).[27] Postanoxic myoclonus is responsive to 5-hydroxytryptophan (the metabolic precursor of serotonin) in a maximum dose of 1 to 1.5 mg/day orally, combined with carbidopa up to 400 mg/day orally.[21]

The management of opioid myoclonus depends on the patient's pain level. Pain-free patients should have their opioid dose reduced by 20% to 30% if myoclonus is mild and then be observed. Benzodiazepines may reduce myoclonus, but they often cause sedation, weakness, drowsiness, and delirium. Baclofen is an alternative.[23,28] Opioid rotation is an alternative, particularly for those patients who are in pain and have symptomatic myoclonus.[29]

TREMOR

Tremor is one of the most common extrapyramidal disorders. It is an involuntary, rhythmic, oscillating movement caused by contractions of reciprocally innervated antagonist muscles.

Epidemiology and Prevalence

Benign tremor is frequent in the elderly.[30] Five million people older than 40 years of age in the United States have tremor.[31,32]

Pathophysiology

The pathophysiology is unclear. New methodological approaches using animal models, positron emission tomography, and EMG and electroencephalographic signals have provided new insights into the mechanisms underlying specific tremors. Physiological tremor has both mechanical and central components. Psychogenic tremor is thought to be mediated by reflex mechanisms. Symptomatic palatal tremor is most likely caused by rhythmic activity of the inferior olive. Essential tremor is also generated from within the olivocerebellar circuits. Orthostatic tremor originates from unidentified brainstem nuclei. Rest tremor of Parkinson's disease arises from the basal ganglia loop, and dystonic tremor originates from within the basal ganglia. Cerebellar tremor is in part caused by a cerebellar circuit that involves feedforward control of voluntary movements. Neuropathic tremor is believed to be caused by abnormally functioning reflex pathways. Many causes underlie toxic and drug-induced tremors[33] (Fig. 168-1).

Clinical Manifestations

Tremor is categorized as resting, postural, asterixis, kinetic or intention, task-specific, or psychogenic.

Resting or static tremor takes place with the muscle at rest and is observed most often with Parkinson's disease.

Postural tremor arises during attempts to maintain posture, such as the outstretched hands. Postural tremors can be physiological, essential, caused by basal ganglia disease (also seen in Parkinson's disease), cerebellar, associated with peripheral neuropathy, post-traumatic, or alcoholic. Asterixis is described as "liver flap," often associated with liver encephalopathy and thought to be caused by abnormal ammonia metabolism.

Kinetic or intention (action) tremor occurs during purposeful movement, such as finger-to-nose testing.

Task-specific tremor appears with goal-oriented tasks such as handwriting, speaking, or standing. This group is divided into writing tremor, vocal tremor, and orthostatic tremor.

Psychogenic tremor occurs at all ages. The key feature is a dramatic lessening or disappearance of tremor when the patient is distracted.[20,21]

Differential Diagnosis

Essential tremor is often confused with Parkinson's disease, enhanced physiologic tremor, or dystonic tremor. If the tremor is asymmetrical and occurs at rest, the diagnosis is most likely Parkinson's disease. Unlike essential tremor, Parkinson's disease is associated with other extrapyramidal signs, including bradykinesia, shuffling gait, postural instability, masked facies, micrographic handwriting, pill-rolling tremor, and hypokinetic speech. Enhanced physiological tremor is a posture-related fine tremor of high frequency (8 to 12 Hz) most often associated with alcohol or drug intoxication, anxiety, and endocrine malfunction.[34] Dystonic tremor, particularly of the head, is often confused with essential tremor. The presence of a strong family history and marked reduction of tremor with alcohol intake helps distinguish essential tremor from other disorders.

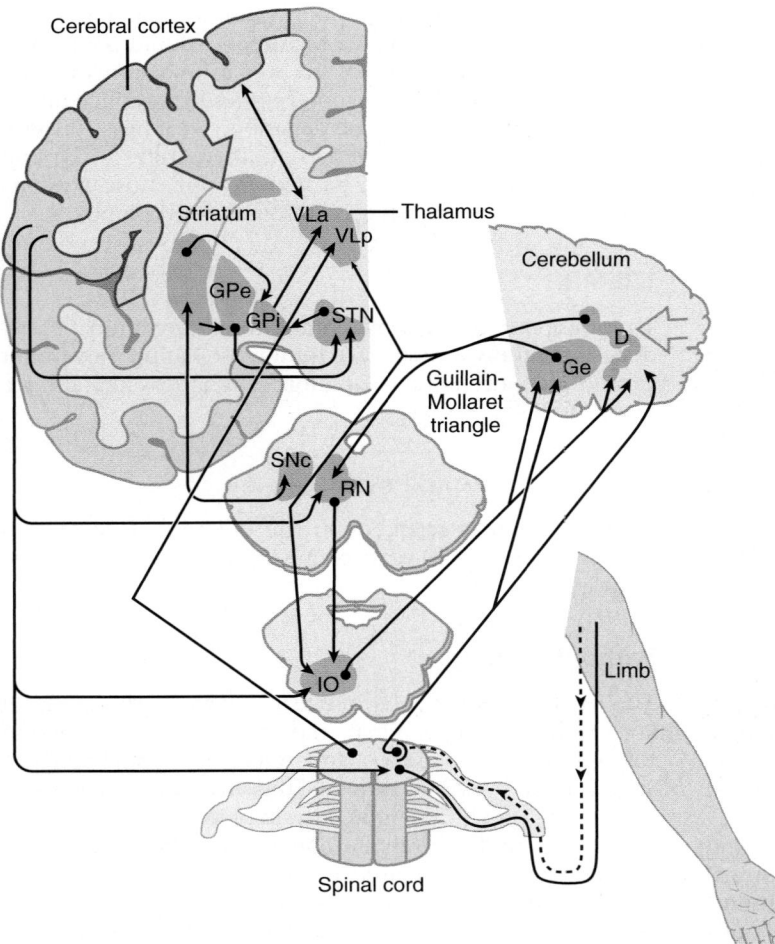

FIGURE 168-1 Schematic diagram of the pathways of various tremors. Ge, globose and emboliform nuclei; GPe and GPi globus pallidus externa and interna; IO, inferior olive; SNc, substantia nigra pars compacta; STN, subthalamic nucleus; VLa and VLp, anterior and posterior ventrolateral thalamic nuclei. (Adapted from Deuschl G, Raethjen J, Lindemann M, Krack P. The pathophysiology of tremor. Muscle Nerve 2001;24:716-735.)

TABLE 168-3 Pharmacological Treatment of Tremor

DRUG	DOSE	SIDE EFFECTS
Atenolol	50-150 mg/day	Light headedness, nausea, cough, dry mouth, sleepiness
Propranolol	60-800 mg/day	Reduced arterial BP, pulse rate, tachycardia, bradycardia, drowsiness, dizziness, exertional dyspnea, confusion, headache
Long-acting propranolol	60-800 mg/day	Same side effects as propranolol
Gabapentin	1200-1800 mg/day	Lethargy, fatigue, decreased libido, dizziness, shortness of breath, nervousness
Primidone	Up to 750 mg/day	Sedation, drowsiness, nausea, fatigue, vomiting, ataxia, unsteadiness, confusion, vertigo, acute toxic reaction
Botulinum A toxin (hand tremor)	50-100 U	Pain at injection site, stiffness, cramps, hematoma, paresthesias, reduced grip strength, hand or finger weakness
Botulinum A toxin (head tremor)	40-400 U	Postinjection pain, weakness of neck
Alprazolam	0.125-0.5 mg/day	Sedation, fatigue, potential for abuse
Nadolol	120-240 mg/day	No side effects at this dose
Sotalol	75-200 mg/day	Decreased alertness
Topiramate	Up to 40 mg/day	Difficulties with concentration, weight loss, paresthesias, anorexia, weight loss

BP, blood pressure.
Adapted from Larsen TA, Calne DB: Essential tremor. Clin Neuropharmacol 1983;6:185-206.

Treatment

The pharmacological treatment of tremor is summarized in Table 168-3. Surgical treatments include deep-brain stimulation and thalamotomy[34]; perioperative morbidity is lower with the former.[35]

REFERENCES

1. Parisi L, Pierelli F, Amabile G, et al. Muscular cramps: Proposals for a new classification. Acta Neurol Scand 2003;107:176-186.
2. Maynard FM, Karunas RS, Waring WP 3rd. Epidemiology of spasticity following traumatic spinal cord injury. Arch Phys Med Rehabil 1990;71:566-569.
3. Brar SP, Smith MB, Nelson LM, et al. Evaluation of treatment protocols on minimal to moderate spasticity in multiple sclerosis. Arch Phys Med Rehabil 1991;72:186-189.
4. Cervera-Deval J, Morant-Guillen MP, Fenollosa-Vasquez P, et al. Social handicaps of multiple sclerosis and their relation to neurological alterations. Arch Phys Med Rehabil 1994;75:1223-1227.
5. Ropper AH, Brown RH. Adams and Victor's Principles of Neurology, 8th ed. New York: McGraw-Hill, 2006.
6. Miller TM, Layzer RB. Muscle cramps. Muscle Nerve 2005;32:431-442.
7. Maughan RJ. Exercise-induced muscle cramp: A prospective biochemical study in marathon runners. J Sports Sci 1986;4:31-34.
8. Mulder DW. The clinical syndrome of amyotrophic lateral sclerosis. Mayo Clin Proc 1957;32:427-436.
9. Fetell MR, Smallberg G, Lewis LD, et al. A benign motor neuron disorder: Delayed cramps and fasciculation after poliomyelitis or myelitis. Ann Neurol 1982;11:423-427.
10. Denny-Brown D. Clinical problems in neuromuscular physiology. Am J Med 1953;15:368-390.
11. Rish BL. Nerve root compression and night cramps. JAMA 1985;254:361.
12. Hudson AJ, Brown WF, Gilbert JJ. The muscular pain-fasciculation syndrome. Neurology 1978;28:1105-1109.
13. Hertz G, Fast A, Feinsilver SH, et al. Sleep in normal late pregnancy. Sleep 1992;15:246-251.
14. Abrams GA, Concato J, Fallon MB. Muscle cramps in patients with cirrhosis. Am J Gastroenterol 1996;91:1363-1366.
15. Howe RC, Wombolt DG, Michie DD. Analysis of tonic muscle activity and muscle cramps during hemodialysis. J Dial 1978;2:85-99.
16. Bertolasi L, De Grandis D, Bongiovanni LG, et al. The influence of muscular lengthening on cramps. Ann Neurol 1993;33:176-180.
17. Chang CT, Wu CH, Yang CW, et al. Creatine monohydrate treatment alleviates muscle cramps associated with haemodialysis. Nephrol Dial Transplant 2002;17:1978-1981.
18. Konikoff F, Ben-Amitay G, Halpern Z, et al. Vitamin E and cirrhotic muscle cramps. Isr J Med Sci 1991;27:221-223.
19. Roca AO, Jarjoura D, Blend D, et al. Dialysis leg cramps. Efficacy of quinine versus vitamin E. ASAIO J 1992;38:M481-M485.
20. Watts RL, Koller WC. The nosology and pathophysiology of myoclonus. In Watts, RL, Koller WC (eds). Movement Disorders, 2nd ed. New York: McGraw-Hill, 2004, p 196.
21. Aminoff M, Greenberg D, Simon R. Clinical Neurology, 6th ed. New York: McGraw-Hill, 2005.
22. Rivest J. Myoclonus. Can J Neurol Sci 2003;30(Suppl 1):S53-S58.
23. Mercadante S. Pathophysiology and treatment of opioid-related myoclonus in cancer patients. Pain 1998;74:5-9.
24. Marsden CD, Hallett M, Fahn S. The nosology and pathophysiology of myoclonus. In Marsden CD, Fahn S (eds). Movement Disorders. London: Butterworths, 1982, pp 196-248.
25. Shibasaki H, Ikeda A, Nagamine T, et al. Cortical reflex negative myoclonus. Brain 1994;117(Pt 3):477-486.
26. Mercadante S. Opioids and akathisia. J Pain Symptom Manage 1995;10:415.
27. Darbin O, Risso JJ, Rostain JC. High pressure enhanced NMDA activity in the striatum and the globus pallidus: Relationships with myoclonia and locomotor and motor activity in rat. Brain Res 2000;852:62-67.
28. Gattera JA, Charles BG, Williams GM, et al. A retrospective study of risk factors of akathisia in terminally ill patients. J Pain Symptom Manage 1994;9:454-461.
29. Caviness JN. Myoclonus. Mayo Clin Proc 1996;71:679-688.
30. Findley LJ, Koller WC. Essential tremor: A review. Neurology 1987;37:1194-1197.
31. Larsen TA, Calne DB. Essential tremor. Clin Neuropharmacol 1983;6:185-206.
32. Rajput AH, Offord KP, Beard CM, et al. Essential tremor in Rochester, Minnesota: A 45-year study. J Neurol Neurosurg Psychiatry 1984;47:466-470.
33. Deuschl G, Raethjen J, Lindemann M, et al. The pathophysiology of tremor. Muscle Nerve 2001;24:716-735.
34. Britton TC. Essential tremor and its variants. Curr Opin Neurol 1995;8:314-319.
35. Tasker RR, Munz M, Junn FS, et al. Deep brain stimulation and thalamotomy for tremor compared. Acta Neurochir Suppl 1997;68:49-53.

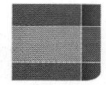

CHAPTER **169**

Nausea, Vomiting, and Early Satiety

Janet L. Abrahm and Bridget Fowler

KEY POINTS

- Prevent nausea; do not wait until it develops.
- Assess both the person and the pathophysiology.
- Minimize side effects and maximize patient control. Use cognitive techniques and drug combinations.
- With the use of tailored therapy and standard guidelines, more than 70% of those undergoing chemotherapy, surgery, or radiation therapy can be free of acute (and delayed) nausea and vomiting.

Nausea, vomiting, and early satiety seriously affect quality of life. They have physical, economic, and psychological ramifications, and they impair nutrition, socialization, and mood. Nausea is an unpleasant sensation of the need to vomit, usually referred to the throat or epigastrium; it may not lead to vomiting.[1] Vomiting is the forcible expulsion of the stomach contents due to contraction of the abdominal and chest wall musculature.[1] Early satiety is the sensation of fullness after ingestion of small amounts of liquids or solids.

PREVALENCE AND EPIDEMIOLOGY

The prevalence of early satiety is unknown; that of nausea and vomiting varies by etiology and by the extent of prevention methods used. Between 70% and 85% of pregnant women have nausea or vomiting, usually within the first 9 weeks.[2] The most severe form, hyperemesis gravidarum, occurs in up to 2%. Nausea/emesis from radiotherapy is related to the site or sites of treatment and is classified into five levels of emetogenicity.[3] Between 90% and 100% of those receiving total body irradiation will have emesis, including 60% to 80% of those undergoing abdominopelvic, upper abdominal, or mantle radiation; 30% to 60% of those receiving craniospinal irradiation; and 10% to 30% of those with irradiation to the pelvis, thorax, or head and neck. Irradiation to the breast, extremities, or brain (when also taking corticosteroids) produces only a 0% to 10% emesis risk. Between 40% and 60% of those with advanced cancer report nausea and/or vomiting, and up to 55% still have it in the last 4 weeks of life.[4-6] During chemotherapy, with adequate pre-therapy and post-therapy prophylaxis, 30% still report significant nausea but fewer than 10% have vomiting.[7] Thirty percent of postoperative patients with adequate prophylaxis also experience nausea.[8] Chemotherapy and postoperative nausea and vomiting share risk factors (Table 169-1).

PATHOPHYSIOLOGY

Nausea and vomiting result from the interplay of excitatory and inhibitory stimuli to key brain centers.[7,9] Figure 169-1 illustrates the key inputs (area postrema, vestibular nuclei, vagal afferents) and the medulla emetic center (which includes the nucleus tractus solitarius). Adjacent to this nucleus but not shown in the figure, are endogenous cannabinoid receptors, which bind exogenous and semisynthetic cannabinoids such as tetrahydrocannabinol (THC).[7]

Nausea

Drugs, metabolic imbalances, bacterial infections, and radiotherapy directly affect the area postrema on the dorsal medulla in the fourth ventricle floor. The loose blood-brain barrier there opens it to bloodstream and spinal fluid stimuli. It also receives cortical input, so that memories, conditioned responses (to sounds, sights, or smells), or anxiety can stimulate nausea and vomiting. Nausea and vomiting resulting from labyrinthine and visual activation are mediated by histamine and acetylcholine release and by stimulation of the vestibular nuclei. Gastrointestinal disorders, chemotherapy, and abdominal radiotherapy release serotonin from enterochromaffin cells. Serotonin binds 5-HT$_3$ receptors in vagal afferents that transmit signals mainly to the nucleus tractus solitarius (although some activate the area postrema). Other abdominal, thoracic, and cardiac processes activate splanchnic afferents. Pain stimuli induce nausea through afferent sympathetic neurons that synapse in the spinal cord and project to the hypothalamus; substance P activates the area postrema and the dorsal vagal complex through NK$_1$ receptors. The area postrema, vestibular nuclei, and vagal and splanchnic afferents all connect with the nucleus tractus solitarius, the central emetic pattern generator. This nucleus coordinates autonomic, gastric, and respiratory mediators of nausea and vomiting. Neurons from the nucleus project to the hypothalamic, limbic, and cortical regions.

Vomiting

Patients who retch do not actually expel gastric contents. Although gastric contents enter the esophagus, respira-

TABLE 169-1	Risk Factors for Nausea and Vomiting		
FACTOR	**CHEMOTHERAPY-RELATED**	**POSTOPERATIVE**	**PREGNANCY-RELATED**
Female sex	X	X	Fetus female
Prior nausea with event	X	X	X
Motion sickness	X	X	X
Hyperemesis gravidarum	X		X
Age <50 yr	X		
Emetogenicity of chemotherapy	X		
Low alcohol use*	X		
High expectation (+)	X		
Cytochrome P-450 isoenzyme CYP2D6	X		
Nonsmoker			X
Unplanned opioid use		X	
Multiple pregnancy			X
Migraine headaches			X

*<100 g/day alcohol.
From Hesketh PJ. Understanding the pathobiology of chemotherapy-induced nausea and vomiting: Providing a basis for therapeutic progress. Oncology 2004;18:9-14.

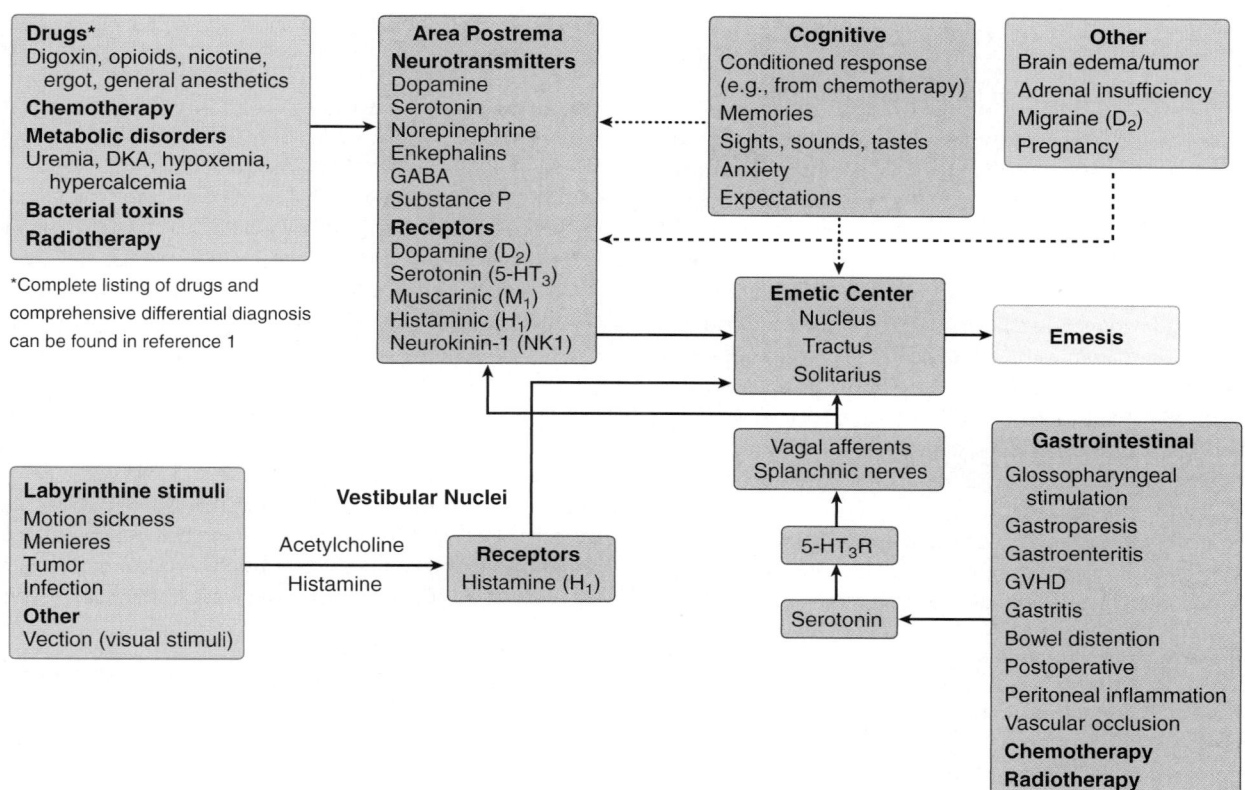

FIGURE 169-1   Pathophysiology of nausea and vomiting. The area postrema is a central processing center for various stimuli that can cause nausea and vomiting, including drugs, metabolic disorders, bacterial toxins, radiation therapy, and, to a lesser extent, cognitive and vagal inputs. Vestibular nuclei receive input from labyrinthine stimuli, and vagal afferents receive input from gastrointestinal disorders, chemotherapy, and radiotherapy. The area postrema, vestibular nuclei, vagal afferents, and cognitive stimuli all feed into the emetic center, which is the central pattern generator for initiating emesis. By understanding the various stimuli, clinicians can both treat reversible processes and select specific agents that prevent nausea and vomiting. GABA, γ-aminobutyric acid; GVHD, graft-versus-host disease; 5-HT$_3$R, serotonin (5-hydroxytryptamine 3) receptor.

tory muscles counteract abdominal muscle contraction so that food does not enter the mouth. Vomiting begins with a retrograde giant contraction from the mid-small intestine to the stomach antrum, followed by closure of the pylorus and antrum, relaxation of the lower esophageal and gastric sphincters, closure of the glottis, abdominal and respiratory muscle contraction, and cricopharyngeal contraction and subsequent relaxation.[10] The nerve pathways are poorly characterized. There is some role for vagal cholinergic nerves and substance P. There are increased levels of some hormones and neurotransmitters, but their role is unclear.[10] Of diagnostic and possibly therapeutic importance is the role of the autonomic nervous system. Persons with nausea are pale, sweating, and hypersalivating and may be hypotensive and tachycardic. They routinely have elevated parasympathetic vagal activity with increased R-R variability that peaks before nausea. Vomiting is often associated with bradycardia and hypotension.[10]

Chemotherapy-Induced Nausea and Vomiting

Chemotherapy-induced nausea and vomiting (CINV) includes three distinct syndromes: anticipatory, acute (within 24 hours after chemotherapy), and delayed. The best prevention for delayed CINV is stopping acute CINV.[11] Anticipatory nausea and vomiting (ANV) is most likely a

classic conditioned response.[12] ANV risk increases with the frequency, severity, and duration of symptoms.[12] Other possible predisposing factors include susceptibility to motion sickness, awareness of tastes or odors during infusions, younger age, lengthier infusions, greater autonomic sensitivity, and general anxiety or emotional distress.[12] The emetogenic potential of chemotherapy agents is listed in Table 169-2.

Early Satiety

Causes of early satiety include gastroparesis (the most common cause), constipation, depression, and lack of gastric motility due to external compression from tumor masses, ascites, or an enlarged liver. Gastroparesis is discussed in Chapter 226 (see "Case Study: Assessment and Treatment of Nausea and Vomiting").

DIFFERENTIAL DIAGNOSIS

Bloating, food aversion, and increased gastric acidity must be distinguished from early satiety and treated specifically.

The differential diagnosis of nausea and vomiting includes inciting factors (see Fig. 169-1). Figure 169-2 addresses assessment and diagnosis, reassessment, and treatment choices.

CASE STUDY

Assessment and Treatment of Nausea and Vomiting

Mrs. T, a 44-year-old woman with stage IV non–small cell lung cancer, had severe nausea and vomiting that necessitated hospital admission after her first chemotherapy treatment with carboplatin and taxol. She had been pretreated with dexamethasone and ondansetron and was prescribed oral ondansetron after chemotherapy but could not keep it down. Mrs. T did not drink or smoke. She had had motion sickness since childhood and had hyperemesis gravidarum with each of her three pregnancies. When she completed her family 10 years earlier, she felt great relief that she would "never have to go through that experience again." At admission, she was tearful and anxious and reported anticipatory nausea before each oncologist visit. Her mother-in-law, who was helping with the children (ages 14, 12, and 10 years), was annoyed with her and believed that she was overdramatizing her symptoms. She had told Mrs. T many times that her friends had undergone similar chemotherapy but were still able to run their households.

Initial Assessment and Treatment

Mrs. T has all the risk factors for severe nausea and vomiting after chemotherapy: (1) female gender, (2) age younger than 50 years, (3) motion sickness, (4) hyperemesis gravidarum, (5) low alcohol intake, and (6) highly emetogenic drugs that require high-level prophylaxis for both acute and delayed chemotherapy-induced nausea and vomiting (CINV). Given that her acute vomiting was not prevented, she has also developed delayed and then anticipatory nausea and vomiting (ANV).

Her quality of life may be improved by counseling, adjuvant acupuncture, cognitive-behavioral therapy, and more aggressive preventive pharmacotherapy using treatment guidelines. Counseling of Mrs. T and her family can help them to understand why she is unable to tolerate the chemotherapy and to plan for the support she needs. Acupuncture treatments have not been helpful in high-dose chemotherapy with autologous blood stem cell transplants, but they may be useful in less emetogenic therapy, such as the chemotherapy that Mrs. T received. Cognitive therapy (e.g., hypnosis) can help desensitize Mrs. T and provide strategies for her to better tolerate her treatment. For the ANV to stop, however, she will have to experience treatment unaccompanied by nausea or vomiting (i.e., uncouple the stimulus from the response).

Because she is at high risk for CINV before her first treatment, she needs prophylactic dexamethasone, aprepitant, and a 5-HT$_3$ receptor antagonist (5-HT$_3$RA) before and after chemotherapy. A benzodiazepine such as lorazepam should be added for her anxiety. Because she is unable to tolerate oral medications after chemotherapy, she might benefit from a single dose of a parenteral long-acting 5-HT$_3$RA such as palonosetron before her chemotherapy.

Second Admission

Eleven months later, Mrs. T was readmitted for nausea and vomiting and mental status changes. These symptoms were unchanged after correction of hyponatremia and dehydration. She had a normal serum calcium concentration, but a magnetic resonance imaging study revealed multiple brain metastases. Dexamethasone along with nystatin oral troches were started; her mental status improved, and the nausea and vomiting stopped. After whole-brain radiation therapy, she began a slow taper of the dexamethasone and enrolled in home hospice. Two weeks later, her hospice nurse noted that Mrs. T's nausea had returned, that food tasted strange to her, and that she had pain with swallowing. Examination revealed a red tongue without white plaques on her buccal mucosa and moon facies. She was bed bound, eating and drinking little, and complaining of painful swallowing. Her family was concerned about her increasing weakness and asked about a feeding tube.

Second Assessment and Treatment

Mrs. T's nausea and vomiting were caused initially by increased intracerebral pressure caused by her brain metastases, but the hyponatremia and dehydration resulting from the vomiting exacerbated her nausea. (Because she has non–small cell carcinoma, she might have developed hypercalcemia even without bone metastases, and this would have contributed to her symptoms and her changed mental status.) Dexamethasone reduced the swelling, eliminated the nausea and vomiting, and, together with the whole brain radiation therapy, helped her mental status. The oral nystatin eliminated the oral thrush but did not prevent esophageal candidiasis, which is now causing dysphagia. Her shiny tongue and taste abnormalities may be a result of B vitamin deficiencies. (Had she stopped taking her dexamethasone, rather than continuing the recommended taper, the ensuing adrenal insufficiency could also have caused nausea and vomiting.)

Treatment with oral fluconazole and multiple vitamins may decrease her dysphagia and taste abnormalities, but, if her anorexia is caused by disease progression, it may not improve her appetite (see Chapters 150 and 158). The oncology team, along with her home hospice team, should explore the family's concerns about Mrs. T's not eating or drinking and plans for her comfort (see Chapters 110 and 120). If she remains unable to take oral medications, custom-made dexamethasone suppositories may provide comfort, and sublingual olanzapine wafers may help the nausea and delirium that could accompany her last days.

Even in advanced disease, when the burden of diagnostic testing may outweigh the benefit, making a diagnosis or diagnoses enables clinicians to identify reversible etiologies such as gastroparesis ("I am OK until I eat or drink, and then I vomit"), obstipation, urinary tract obstruction, increased intracranial pressure, anxiety, or medication side effects. Reversal of metabolic abnormalities that are causing the symptoms (e.g., hyponatremia, hypercalcemia, adrenal insufficiency, dehydration) may be consistent with the patient's goals of care and would improve quality of life. To decide, it may help to ask patients and their families what the symptoms mean to them, how distress-

TABLE 169-2 Chemotherapy Emetogenicity

HIGH	MODERATE	LOW	MINIMAL
Cisplatin	Oxaliplatin	Paclitaxel	Bevacizumab
Mechlorethamine (nitrogen mustard)	Cytarabine (ara-C) >1000 mg/m^2	Docetaxel	Bleomycin
Streptozocin	Carboplatin	Mitoxantrone	Busulfan
Cyclophosphamide ≥1500 mg/m^2	Ifosfamide	Topotecan	2-Chlorodeoxyadenosine
Carmustine (BCNU)	Cyclophosphamide <1500 mg/m^2	Etoposide	Fludarabine
Dacarbazine (DTIC)	Doxorubicin	Pemetrexed	Rituximab
Dactinomycin	Daunorubicin	Methotrexate	Vinblastine
	Epirubicin	Mitomycin	Vincristine
	Idarubicin	Gemcitabine	Vinorelbine
	Irinotecan	Cytarabine ≤1000 mg/m^2	
		5-Flurouracil	
		Bortezomib	
		Cetuximab	
		Trastuzumab	

From American Society of Clinical Oncology; Kris MG, Hesketh PJ, Somerfield MR, et al. American Society of Clinical Oncology guideline for antiemetics in oncology: Update 2006. J Clin Oncol 2006;24:2932-2947.

ing they are, what concerns they have, and what life would be like without them.

TREATMENT

Whenever possible, reverse the underlying causes (see Fig. 169-2). Constipation is common and can be overlooked; patients assume they should not have bowel movements if not eating (see Chapter 154). For other causes, both nonpharmacological and pharmacological methods can be employed (see "Common Errors").

Nonpharmacological Measures

Nonpharmacological measures include uncovering hidden concerns and unasked questions, educating patients and families about what is happening and what is likely to happen within the patient's body, exploring patients' and families' hopes and fears, and reviewing what is possible. Helping patients sort the burdens and benefits of interventions reduces anxiety and helps nausea and even early satiety (Table 169-3). These measures are of particular benefit for palliative care patients and families, providing ways in which families can comfort their loved ones.

Patients with early satiety or nausea/vomiting from delayed gastric emptying can try a low fat diet, without non-digestible fiber, and frequent small meals. Ginger (1 g per day) and pyridoxine are superior to placebo for nausea/vomiting of early pregnancy.[14] Reports of the efficacy of ginger postoperatively have been mixed, but it helps hyperemesis gravidarum and motion sickness. In animal studies, ginger root has been effective for chemotherapy-induced emesis. One component is a 5-HT$_3$ receptor antagonist (5-HT$_3$RA).

Alternative Therapies

Alternative therapies are used alone or as adjuncts for minimizing distress and the frequency of nausea and vomiting. Those with high-quality evidence are described in Box 169-1.[15-17]

Common Errors

Assessment

- Failing to understand what the nausea, vomiting, or early satiety means to the patient and family, and failing to uncover their hidden fears and hopes
- Failing to make a nausea diagnosis: using empirical therapy when therapy specific to the cause or causes of the patient's nausea is available
- Assuming that the cause has not changed over time (someone who had postchemotherapy nausea that resolved may now have delayed gastric emptying or constipation as the cause)
- Failing to include constipation, gastritis (without pain), or adrenal insufficiency in the differential diagnosis

Therapy

- Inadequately explaining the rationale behind the therapies chosen and failing to confirm that the patient and caregiver understand
- Reserving cognitive and alternative therapies for refractory nausea or vomiting
- Failing to use all agents recommended in the CINV Guidelines, especially those that prevent delayed nausea and vomiting
- Using more than one agent from the same class of antiemetics, thereby increasing side effects without increasing the efficacy

TABLE 169-3 Nonpharmacological Treatments for Nausea and Vomiting

GINGER ROOT[14]

MEASURES TO ENHANCE GASTRIC EMPTYING AND DECREASE GASTRIC DISTENTION
Liquid diet
Frequent small meals
Foods low in lipids and fiber and high in protein

MEASURES TO MINIMIZE OTHER NOXIOUS OR ASSOCIATED STIMULI
Cool foods
Foods without odors
Foods with a pleasant appearance

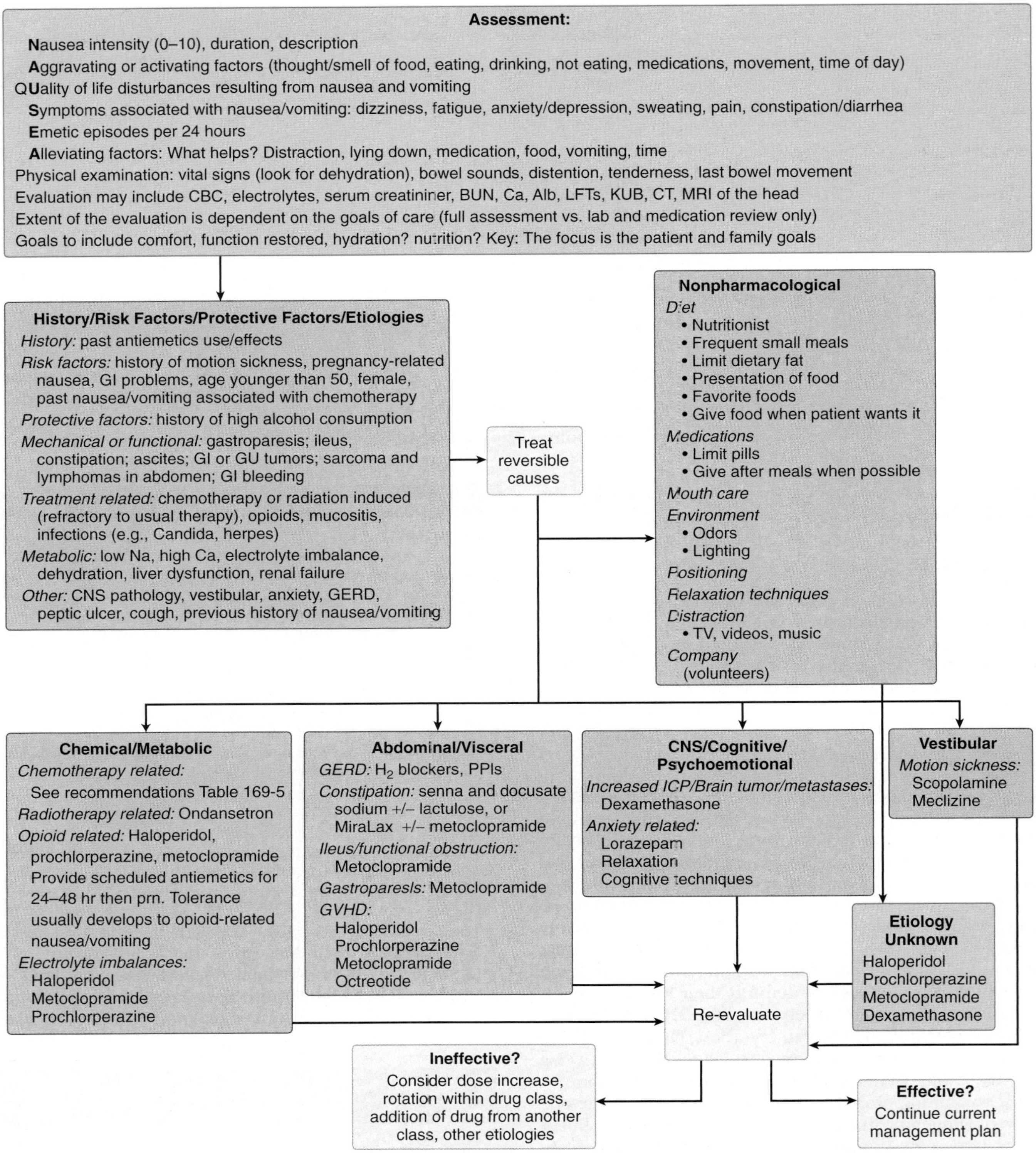

Assessment:

Nausea intensity (0–10), duration, description
Aggravating or activating factors (thought/smell of food, eating, drinking, not eating, medications, movement, time of day)
Q**U**ality of life disturbances resulting from nausea and vomiting
Symptoms associated with nausea/vomiting: dizziness, fatigue, anxiety/depression, sweating, pain, constipation/diarrhea
Emetic episodes per 24 hours
Alleviating factors: What helps? Distraction, lying down, medication, food, vomiting, time
Physical examination: vital signs (look for dehydration), bowel sounds, distention, tenderness, last bowel movement
Evaluation may include CBC, electrolytes, serum creatininer, BUN, Ca, Alb, LFTs, KUB, CT, MRI of the head
Extent of the evaluation is dependent on the goals of care (full assessment vs. lab and medication review only)
Goals to include comfort, function restored, hydration? nutrition? Key: The focus is the patient and family goals

History/Risk Factors/Protective Factors/Etiologies

History: past antiemetics use/effects
Risk factors: history of motion sickness, pregnancy-related nausea, GI problems, age younger than 50, female, past nausea/vomiting associated with chemotherapy
Protective factors: history of high alcohol consumption
Mechanical or functional: gastroparesis; ileus, constipation; ascites; GI or GU tumors; sarcoma and lymphomas in abdomen; GI bleeding
Treatment related: chemotherapy or radiation induced (refractory to usual therapy), opioids, mucositis, infections (e.g., Candida, herpes)
Metabolic: low Na, high Ca, electrolyte imbalance, dehydration, liver dysfunction, renal failure
Other: CNS pathology, vestibular, anxiety, GERD, peptic ulcer, cough, previous history of nausea/vomiting

Treat reversible causes

Nonpharmacological
Diet
- Nutritionist
- Frequent small meals
- Limit dietary fat
- Presentation of food
- Favorite foods
- Give food when patient wants it

Medications
- Limit pills
- Give after meals when possible

Mouth care
Environment
- Odors
- Lighting

Positioning
Relaxation techniques
Distraction
- TV, videos, music

Company (volunteers)

Chemical/Metabolic
Chemotherapy related:
See recommendations Table 169-5
Radiotherapy related: Ondansetron
Opioid related: Haloperidol, prochlorperazine, metoclopramide Provide scheduled antiemetics for 24–48 hr then prn. Tolerance usually develops to opioid-related nausea/vomiting
Electrolyte imbalances:
Haloperidol
Metoclopramide
Prochlorperazine

Abdominal/Visceral
GERD: H_2 blockers, PPIs
Constipation: senna and docusate sodium +/– lactulose, or MiraLax +/– metoclopramide
Ileus/functional obstruction: Metoclopramide
Gastroparesis: Metoclopramide
GVHD:
Haloperidol
Prochlorperazine
Metoclopramide
Octreotide

CNS/Cognitive/Psychoemotional
Increased ICP/Brain tumor/metastases: Dexamethasone
Anxiety related:
Lorazepam
Relaxation
Cognitive techniques

Vestibular
Motion sickness:
Scopolamine
Meclizine

Etiology Unknown
Haloperidol
Prochlorperazine
Metoclopramide
Dexamethasone

Re-evaluate

Ineffective?
Consider dose increase, rotation within drug class, addition of drug from another class, other etiologies

Effective?
Continue current management plan

FIGURE 169-2   Assessment of the patient with nausea, vomiting, or early satiety. This algorithm illustrates an assessment scheme for nausea, vomiting, or early satiety. Every attempt should be made to identify reversible causes. Alb, serum albumin concentration; BUN, blood urea nitrogen; Ca, calcium; CBC, complete blood count; CNS, central nervous system; CT, computed tomography; GERD, gastroesophageal reflux disease; GI, gastrointestinal; GU, genitourinary; GVHD, graft-versus-host disease; H_2, histamine$_2$ receptor; ICP, intracranial pressure; KUB, x-ray examinat on of the kidneys, ureters, and bladder; LFTs, liver function tests; MRI, magnetic resonance imaging; Na, sodium; PPIs, proton pump inhibitors.

Acupuncture

Acupuncture at the neiguan (pericardium 6, or P6) point produces vagal modulation typically seen with nausea and vomiting. Acupuncture is effective for chemotherapy-related and postoperative nausea/vomiting and enhances 5-HT$_3$RA efficacy.[15] Data are mixed for the efficacy of acupressure or the acustimulation wristbands for chemotherapy-related nausea, morning sickness, or motion sickness.

Cognitive-Behavioral Therapies

Cognitive-behavioral therapies can be integrated early for those at risk for early satiety or nausea and vomiting. They induce relaxation and reverse the autonomic arousal that accompanies all nausea. Progressive muscle relaxation lowers blood pressure, slows pulse and respirations, and improves subjective well-being. Progressive muscle relaxation alone does not prevent CINV, but it might do so if combined with guided imagery, emphasizing the importance of suggestion during desensitization and hypnosis. Biofeedback alone is unsuccessful. Reports of the efficacy of music therapy alone or with guided imagery are mixed.[18]

Because emetogenic stimuli are received in the cortical centers, they are exacerbated or reduced by learned responses, expectations, concomitant anxiety or depression, and misinterpretation of bodily sensations. Hypnosis and other cognitive therapies may decrease the affective response from limbic stimulation and, consequently, the frequency and intensity of nausea and vomiting. Hypnosis and systemic desensitization are effective for chemotherapy-related ANV.[10] Disturbing sensations related to memories (sights, sounds, and smells) of chemotherapy can be disassociated by systematic desensitization, using hypnosis to re-experience the challenging stimuli, sensing and controlling the autonomic reactions evoked, and removing their power to induce symptoms by blocking the ensuing cascade of events.

Patients are usually able to use hypnosis for early satiety, nausea, or vomiting if they can concentrate. Suggestions might include an opening and relaxation of swallowing and the esophagus, dissolution of any sensations of "knots," (e.g., "unwinding like a braid unwinds in the water"), followed by images of a running stream finding its bed, opening into a larger body of water which receives it easily, and then moving slowly and purposefully on, as a river meanders in a plain. Hynotherapists make tapes of sessions that the patient can later review. Suggestions for ego-strengthening and being in favorite, safe locations are often included. Hypnosis can reduce anxiety and help patients regain hope as they regain control.

Pharmacological Interventions (Table 169-4)

Initial therapy should be directed at constipation and, when consistent with the care goals, at dehydration and metabolic imbalances that cause or result from nausea and vomiting. In chronic delayed gastric emptying, replacement of minerals and vitamins may be indicated.[19]

Dopamine antagonists are often used. These include three distinct subclasses: phenothiazines (prochlorperazine, chlorpromazine, perphenazine, and thiethylperazine), butyrophenones (haloperidol and droperidol), and substituted benzamide (metoclopramide). Although structurally distinct, these agents share similar side effect profiles, which include sedation, dizziness, hypotension, and extrapyramidal symptoms. QT prolongation has been reported with haloperidol and droperidol. Droperidol is used infrequently because continuous electrocardiographic monitoring is recommended. Dopamine antagonists are used as first-line therapy in nausea and vomiting caused by opioids, electrolyte imbalances, or an unknown etiology.

Metoclopramide not only exhibits dopamine antagonism; it also increases the pressure of the lower esophageal sphincter, induces gastric promotility, and, at high doses (100 mg/m^2) has 5-HT$_3$RA activity. At usual doses (5 to 20 mg PO or IV every 6 hours), it is first-line therapy for early satiety or nausea and vomiting resulting from gastroparesis, functional obstruction, ileus, or gastroesophageal reflux disease (GERD). In those whose nausea/vomiting is refractory to intermittent metoclopramide, continuous intravenous or subcutaneous infusions at 1 to 5 mg/hr may be used.[20] However, this treatment is associated with diarrhea, dystonic reactions (more so in younger patients), and akathisia (restlessness and a feeling of anxiety, sometimes described as "ants in the pants"). Lower doses may make these side effects tolerable. Others will need a benzodiazepine. Severe akathisia requires diphenhydramine or benztropine.

Intravenous erythromycin (3 mg/kg every 8 hours) is effective for gastroparesis refractory to metoclopramide; oral erythromycin (250 mg PO three times daily) is less effective but may work in 40% of patients. Erythromycin prolongs the QT interval, and chronic use may cause deafness, pseudomembranous colitis, and overgrowth by resistant bacteria.[21]

Octreotide[22,23] may be used for severe nausea and vomiting and early satiety in gastric outlet obstruction, ileus, or partial small bowel obstruction. Doses of 50 to 300 μg subcutaneously two to three times per day reduce gastric secretion volume, eliminating the need for a nasogastric tube or venting gastrostomy. If subcutaneous therapy works, maintenance with monthly long-acting intramuscular octreotide (20 to 30 mg) is used. Octreotide slows gut motility, so it should be used with caution in reversible obstruction (see Chapter 226).

TABLE 169-4   Classes of Commonly Used Antiemetics

DRUG	DOSE/ROUTE	MAJOR SIDE EFFECTS	MANAGEMENT OF SIDE EFFECTS
SEROTONIN ANTAGONISTS			
Ondansetron (Zofran)	8-24 mg IV/PO qd	Constipation	Prophylactic laxatives
Palonosetron (Aloxi)	0.25 mg IV × 1 dose		
Granisetron (Kytril)	1 mg IV or 2 mg PO qd		
Dolasetron (Anzemet)	100 mg IV/PO qd		
SUBSTANCE P ANTAGONISTS			
Aprepitant (Emend)	125 mg on day 1 80 mg on days 2-3	Somnolence/fatigue	Nonpharmacological approaches
DOPAMINE ANTAGONISTS			
Phenothiazines			
Prochlorperazine (Compazine)	10 mg PO/PR q4-6h	EPS	Diphenhydramine, lorazepam, benztropine
Perphenazine (Trilafon)	2-4 mg PO q4-6h max 24 mg/day		
Thiethylperazine (Torecan)	10 mg PO/PR/IM qd-tid		
Substituted Benzamide			
Metoclopramide (Reglan)	10-40 mg PO/IV tid-qid	EPS, akathisia	See above
Butyrophenones			
Haloperidol (Haldol)	0.5-2 mg IV/PO q4-8h	EPS	See above
Droperidol (Inapsine)	2.5-5 mg IV q3-4h	QT prolongation	ECG monitoring required
CORTICOSTEROIDS			
Dexamethasone (Decadron)	4-20 mg PO/IV qd	Delirium, anxiety, insomnia	Re-evaluate dose/usage
Methylprednisolone (Solu-Medrol)	50-100 mg IV qd		
ANTIHISTAMINES			
Diphenhydramine (Benadryl)	25-50 mg IV/PO q4-6h	Sedation, confusion	Re-evaluate dose/usage
Dimenhydrinate (Dramamine)	50-100 mg PO/IV q4-6h		
Meclizine (Antivert)	25-50 mg PO qd		
Promethazine (Phenergan)	12.5-25 mg PO/PR/IV/IM q4h		
Trimethobenzamide (Tigan)	300 mg PO tid-qid or 200 mg PR/IM tid-qid		
ANTICHOLINERGICS			
Scopolamine (Transderm Scop)	1.5-3 mg TD q72h	Dry mouth, blurred vision	Nonpharmacological approaches
Hyoscyamine	0.125-0.25 mg SL/PO q4h		
CANNABINOIDS			
Dronabinol (Marinol)	2.5-10 mg bid-tid	Confusion, ataxia	Re-evaluate dose/usage; try single bedtime dose
Nabilone (Cesamet)	1-2 mg bid		
ANXIOLYTICS			
Lorazepam (Ativan)	0.5-2 mg PO/IV q4-6h	Confusion, sedation	Re-evaluate dose/usage
ATYPICAL ANTIPSYCHOTICS			
Olanzapine (Zyprexa)	2.5-5 mg qd-bid	Sedation	Re-evaluate dose/usage

ECG, electrocardiographic; EPS, extrapyramidal symptoms.

Ondansetron and granisetron are the best studied 5-HT$_3$RAs. This class also includes dolasetron, tropisetron, and palonosetron. Treatment guidelines view all 5-HT$_3$RAs as equivalent.[13,24] Although most data relate to CINV, these agents have been rapidly adopted in nononcology settings. They prevent postoperative emesis and emesis induced by single- or multiple-fraction radiation therapy. They are of equivalent efficacy in standard combination antiemetic regimens for chemotherapy with moderate or greater emetogenicity (see Table 169-2). They help opioid-induced nausea but promote constipation and even obstipation if adequate laxatives cannot be taken. Side effects from 5-HT$_3$RA include headache and elevated transaminases. Extrapyramidal reactions are rare; sedation, dystonic reactions, akathisia, and tardive dyskinesias do not occur.

The antiemetic mechanism of corticosteroids remains undefined. Dexamethasone and methylprednisolone are the best-studied agents, but no trials have shown superiority of one drug, although the comparative incidence of fluid retention is unknown. Megestrol acetate (400 to 800 mg PO daily), a progestational agent, is an appetite stimulant that also controls nausea. It usually works within 2 weeks. Megestrol should be used with caution in patients who are prone to deep venous thrombosis. Prolonged use followed by abrupt discontinuation can cause adrenal insufficiency.[25]

When added to a regimen of dexamethasone and a 5-HT₃RA, the neurokinin-1 (NK₁) inhibitor, aprepitant, provides significant additional protection against delayed nausea and vomiting. Aprepitant is a cytochrome P-450 isoenzyme CYP3A4 inhibitor, and it increases levels of chemotherapy agents metabolized by this route, although no clinically significant elevations have been reported. Aprepitant can reduce the effect of warfarin.

Antihistamines and anticholinergic agents help vestibular disorders causing nausea or vomiting. Scopolamine and meclizine are recommended for motion sickness and for noninfectious inner ear problems but frequently cause sedation or confusion in the elderly or medically ill.

In multiple small, randomized trials, cannabinoids have been effective antiemetics, either alone or combined with dopamine antagonists and/or corticosteroids. They have particular efficacy in nausea, vomiting, or anorexia in advanced human immunodeficiency virus (HIV) disease.[26] Cannabinoids are better tolerated by younger patients and by those with a prior positive experience with pharmaceutical cannabinoids or smoked marijuana. Starting doses as low as 2.5 to 5 mg of dronabinol two to three times daily or 1 to 2 mg of nabilone twice daily may be effective, either combined with other antiemetics or alone in those who do not tolerate or have not responded to first-line antiemetics. Starting at subtherapeutic levels, and with bedtime dosing, can enhance tolerability and titration to higher doses. Common side effects include dizziness, euphoria, somnolence, confusion, paranoia, hyperphagia, and dry mouth.

Olanzapine is an atypical antipsychotic that is effective in nausea and vomiting[27] because it binds to dopamine, serotonin, and histamine receptors. Doses of 2.5 mg to 5 mg one to two times daily, up to a maximum of 20 mg, treat nausea and vomiting caused by opioids or chemotherapy and refractory nausea in advanced cancer. Common adverse effects include somnolence, postural hypotension, constipation, dizziness, restlessness, QT prolongation, and (except in advanced cancer) weight gain.

Lorazepam has mild antiemetic activity when used alone and reduces anxiety. It is sedating but can cause paradoxical agitation and delirium, especially in older patients. Lorazepam combats akathisia and anxiety caused by metoclopramide.

Chemotherapy-Induced Nausea and Vomiting

The choice of an antiemetic agent or agents depends on the emetogenicity of the chemotherapy or radiation therapy regimen, the side effects of the agents, patient anxiety, and patient preferences. For example, younger patients have more CINV and metoclopramide-related acute dystonic reactions. Elderly patients have more extrapyramidal, anticholinergic, and sedating side effects. The 5-HT₃RAs are therefore preferred for both young and elderly patients, rather than regimens containing metoclopramide and diphenhydramine. Some do well with regimens that do not include anxiolytics; others with more anxiety may benefit from anxiolytics despite the sedation. Retrograde amnesia from benzodiazepines can reduce subsequent ANV (Table 169-5).

Alternative Routes of Drug Delivery

Continuous subcutaneous infusions of antiemetics through syringe drivers (Dickman) or portable infusion pumps are safe and effective. Dexamethasone, haloperidol, metoclopramide, lorazepam or midazolam, and hyoscine butylbromide (an anticholinergic agent used to decrease gastrointestinal fluid production and motility) are all compatible and can be used in combinations for symptom complexes. Octreotide, ondansetron, metoclopramide, and midazolam are also compatible for continuous subcutaneous infusion, as are octreotide and chlorpromazine.[28] Prochlorperazine causes subcutaneous irritation.[29]

Patients who prefer not to have infusions may benefit from commercial suppositories of chlorpromazine (50 to 100 mg) or from custom-made suppositories containing one or more of the selected antiemetics: dexamethasone, haloperidol, metoclopramide, diphenhydramine, and lorazepam.[30] Avoid combinations with overlapping side effects, such as diphenhydramine and lorazepam (sedation) or metoclopramide and haloperidol (extrapyramidal symptoms and akathisia). Useful combinations include dexamethasone and metoclopramide (for partial bowel obstruction) and dexamethasone, haloperidol, and diphenhydramine (for complete bowel obstruction and cramping).

Refractory Nausea and Vomiting

Patients for whom the burden is acceptable should be thoroughly re-evaluated to determine the cause or causes of their refractory condition (see Fig. 169-1). If no additional causes are identified, or if additional testing is desired, doses of the current medications should be maximized within the limits of adverse effects or rotated to a different drug within the same class. For instance, haloperidol, the most potent dopamine antagonist, may be substituted for prochlorperazine. Should this be ineffective, agents from different classes may be added to create a combination that minimizes the side effects from each class (see Table 169-5). Endoscopic stents (see Chapter 98) and surgical interventions (see Chapters 226 and 241) including palliative gastric pacing can help.

Treatment of Nausea, Vomiting, and Early Satiety in the Last Weeks of Life

Early satiety may be hard to distinguish from the lack of interest in eating and drinking that occurs in advanced illness.[31] As interest in food and drink wane, early satiety, nausea, and vomiting may improve in those who are not receiving supplemental nutrition or hydration. Patients receiving such support (and their families) can be asked to readdress these choices, with the hope of decreasing symptoms and improving quality of the patient's last days of life. Some may want a nasogastric tube to remain, but others may prefer occasional vomiting to leaving the tube in place. In the last weeks, testing for and reversal of metabolic abnormalities that contribute to nausea and vomiting is usually burdensome and is replaced by purely symptomatic treatment that includes the nonpharmacological and pharmacological therapies discussed in this chapter. Admission to an inpatient palliative care or hospice unit is sometimes required due to refractory

TABLE 169-5 Recommended Antiemetic Agents for Chemotherapy-Induced Nausea and Vomiting

HIGHLY EMETOGENIC POTENTIAL

Prophylaxis (each day for duration of chemotherapy):
   5-HT$_3$RA PO/IV 30 min before chemotherapy
 + Dexamethasone 12-20 mg PO/IV 30 min before chemotherapy
 ± Aprepitant 125 mg PO 1 hr before chemotherapy (use 12-mg dose of dexamethasone)

To prevent or manage delayed nausea/vomiting (for 2-5 days after chemotherapy):
   Dexamethasone 4-8 mg PO qd-bid
 ± Metoclopramide 20-40 mg PO bid-qid
 ± Aprepitant 80 mg PO in the morning on days 2 and 3

MODERATELY EMETOGENIC POTENTIAL

Prophylaxis (30 min before chemotherapy):
   5-HT$_3$RA PO/IV
 + Decadron 12 mg PO/IV

To prevent or manage delayed nausea and vomiting (for 2-3 days after chemotherapy):
   Decadron 4-8 mg PO bid
 ± Metoclopramide 20-40 mg PO bid-qid

LOW EMETOGENIC POTENTIAL

Prophylaxis (30 min before chemotherapy as needed):
   Dexamethasone 4-8 mg PO/IV
   OR Metoclopramide 10-20 mg PO/IV
   OR Compazine 10 mg PO/IV

5-HT$_3$RA, serotonin (5-hydroxytryptophan) 3 receptor antagonist.
From Flake ZA, Scalley RD, Bailey AG. Practical selection of antiemetics. Am Fam Physician 2004;69:1169-1174,1176; and National Comprehensive Cancer Network. Clinical practice guidelines in oncology: Antiemesis, version 1, 2006.

Future Considerations

- How can acupuncture, cognitive therapies, and music therapy best be integrated early into the preventive and therapeutic algorithms?
- Is systematic screening for hypnotic susceptibility, combined with cognitive therapies (see Table 169-4), an effective and efficient strategy?
- Are there genetic polymorphisms for the P6 acupuncture point? Should all patients be screened for genetic polymorphisms to maximize this modality?
- What will be the results of the National Institutes of Health trial using ginger in chemotherapy-related nausea and vomiting?
- What is the etiology of the chemotherapy-related or postoperative nausea in the 30% of patients who do not respond to available pharmacologic therapies? Should systematic dose increases of 5-HT$_3$ inhibitors be tried? What pathways remain to be identified?
- What new techniques and drugs will help in advanced disease when nausea or vomiting is unrelated to treatment or obstruction?
- Can endocannabinoid receptors be further characterized so that drugs can be designed with appetite-stimulating and antinausea properties without the cognitive effects and the ataxia that currently limit available agents?
- What will be the final clinical impact of neurokinin-1 (NK$_1$) inhibitors in prophylaxis against acute or delayed nausea and vomiting? What population will benefit most?

nausea and vomiting, but palliative sedation for this symptom is rarely needed; of patients admitted to such units, fewer than 5% required sedation[32-36] (see "Future Considerations").

REFERENCES

1. American Gastroenterological Association medical position statement: Nausea and vomiting. Gastroenterology 2001;120:261-262, 263.
2. Longstreth GF. Approach to the adult patient with nausea and vomiting. UpToDate 2005.
3. Kirkbride P. Radiation-induced emesis. In Hesketh PJ (ed). Management of Nausea and Vomiting in Cancer Treatment. Sudbury, MA: Jones and Bartlett, 2005, pp 197-210
4. Reuben DB, Mor V. Nausea and vomiting in terminal cancer patients. Arch Intern Med 1986;146:2021-2023.
5. Doyle D. Symptom relief in terminal illness. Med Pract 1983:1:694-698.
6. Coyle N, Adelhardt J, Foley KM, et al. Character of terminal illness in advanced cancer patients: Pain and other symptoms during the last 4 weeks of life. J Pain Symptom Manage 1990:5:83-93.
7. Hesketh PJ (ed). Management of Nausea and Vomiting in Cancer Treatment. Sudbury, MA: Jones and Bartlett, 2005.
8. Apfel CC, Korttila K, Abdalla M, et al. A factorial trial of six interventions for the prevention of postoperative nausea and vomiting. N Engl J Med 2004;350:2441-2451.
9. Hesketh PJ. Understanding the pathobiology of chemotherapy-induced nausea and vomiting: Providing a basis for therapeutic progress. Oncology 2004;18:9-14.
10. Hasker WL. Approach to the patient with nausea and vomiting. In Yamada T, Alpers DH, Kaplowitz N, et al. (eds). Textbook of Gastroenterology, 4th ed, 2003.
11. Mundy EA, Duhamel KN, Montgomery GH. The efficacy of behavioral interventions for cancer treatment-related side effects. Semin Clin Neuropsychiatry 2003;8:253-275.
12. Rudd JA, Andrews PLR. Mechanisms of acute, delayed, and anticipatory emesis induced by anticancer therapy. In Hesketh PJ (ed). Management of Nausea and Vomiting in Cancer Treatment. Sudbury, MA: Jones and Bartlett, 2005.
13. American Society of Clinical Oncology; Kris MG, Hesketh PJ, Somerfield MR, et al. American Society of Clinical Oncology guideline for antiemetics in oncology: Update 2006. J Clin Oncol 2006;24:2932-2947.
14. Flake ZA, Scalley RD, Bailey AG. Practical selection of antiemetics. Am Fam Physician 2004;69:1169-1174, 1176.
15. Wenger WA, Smith M, Boon H, et al. Advising patients who seek complementary and alternative medical therapies for cancer. Ann Intern Med 2003;137:889-903.
16. Pan CX, Morrison RS, Ness J, et al. Complementary and alternative medicine in the management of pain, dyspnea, and nausea and vomiting near the end of life. J Pain Symptom Manage 2000;20:374-387.
17. Vickers AJ, Cassileth BR. Unconventional therapies for cancer and for cancer-related symptoms. Lancet Oncol 2001;2:226-232.
18. Ezzone S, Baker C, Rosselet R, et al. Music as an adjunct to antiemetic therapy. Oncol Nurs Forum 1998;25:1551-1556.
19. Ogorek CP, Davidson L, Fisher RS, et al. Idiopathic gastroparesis is associated with a multiplicity of severe dietary deficiencies. Am J Gastroenterol 1991;86:423.
20. Bruera E, Seifert L, Wantanabe S, et al. Chronic nausea in advanced cancer patients: A retrospective assessment of a metoclopramide-based antiemetic regimen. J Pain Symptom Manage 1996;11:147-153.
21. Camilleri M. Treatment of delayed gastric emptying. UpToDate 2006.
22. Ripamonti C, Mercadante S. How to use octreotide for malignant bowel obstruction. J Support Oncol 2004;2:357-364.
23. Ripamonti C, Twycross R, Baines M, et al.; Expert working group of the European Association for Palliative Care (EAPC). Clinical practice recommendations for the management of bowel obstruction in patients with end-stage cancer. Support Care Cancer 2001;9:223-233.
24. National Comprehensive Cancer Network. Clinical practice guidelines in oncology: Antiemesis, Version 1, 2006. www.nccn.org
25. Abrahm JL. A Physician's Guide to Pain and Symptom Management in Cancer Patients, 2nd ed. Baltimore: Johns Hopkins University Press, 2005.
26. Beal JE, Olson R, Laugenstein L, et al. Dronabinol as a treatment for anorexia associated with weight loss in patients with AIDS. J Pain Symptom Manage 1995;10:89-97.
27. Srivastava M, Brito-Dellan N, Davis MP, et al. Olanzapine as an antiemetic in refractory nausea and vomiting in advanced cancer. J Pain Symptom Manage 2003;25:578-582.
28. Mystakidou K, Tsilika E, Kalaidopoulou O, et al. Comparison of octreotide administration vs conservative treatment in the management of inoperable bowel obstruction in patients with far advanced cancer: A randomized, double-blind, controlled clinical trial. Anticancer Res 2002;22:1187-1192.
29. Trinkle R. Compatibility of hydromorphone and prochlorperazine. Ann Pharmacol 1997;31:789-790.
30. Davis MP, Walsh D, LeGrand SB, et al. Symptom control in cancer patients: The clinical pharmacology and therapeutic role of suppositories and rectal suspensions. Support Care Cancer 2002;10:117-138.

31. Ellershaw JE, Sutcliffe JM, Saunders CM. Dehydration and the dying patient. J Pain Symptom Manage 1995;10:192-197.
32. Fainsinger R, Miller MJ, Bruera E, et al. Symptom control during the last week of life on a palliative care unit. J Palliat Care 1991;7:5-11.
33. Fainsinger RL, Landman W, Hoskings M, et al. Sedation for uncontrolled symptoms in a South African hospice. J Pain Symptom Manage 1998;16:145-152.
34. Morita T, Inoue S, Chihara S. Sedation for symptom control in Japan: The importance of intermittent use and communication with family members. J Pain Symptom Manage 1996;12:32-38.
35. Ventafridda V, Ripamonti C, DeConno F, et al. Symptom prevalence and control during cancer patient's last days of life. J Palliat Care 1990;6:7-11.
36. Cowan JD, Walsh D. Terminal sedation in palliative medicine-definition and review of the literature. Support Care Cancer 2001;9:403-407.

SUGGESTED READING

Dickman A, Schneider J, Varga J. The Syringe Driver: Continuous Subcutaneous Infusions in Palliative Care, 2nd ed. New York: Oxford University Press, 2005.

Hasker WL. Approach to the patient with nausea and vomiting. In Yamada T, Alpers DH, Kaplowitz N, et al. (eds). Textbook of Gastroenterology, 4th ed, 2003.

Hesketh PJ (ed). Management of Nausea and Vomiting in Cancer Treatment. Sudbury, MA: Jones and Bartlett, 2005.

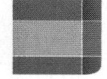

CHAPTER **170**

Nonmalignant Pain

Sharon M. Weinstein

KEY POINTS

- Nonmalignant pain (NMP) is highly prevalent.
- NMP complicates palliative care.
- It is essential to establish specific pain diagnoses.
- Palliative care providers should be familiar with the treatment of common nonmalignant painful conditions.
- Palliative care providers may best work with other clinicians as a team to optimally manage NMP in the palliative care patient.

It is important for palliative care specialists to distinguish "nonmalignant" painful conditions (NMP) from pain associated with an underlying life-threatening condition, because effective treatment strategies differ depending on the pathophysiology of the pain. Clinicians must consider the patient's preferred treatment of a long-standing painful condition and its general efficacy. Understanding a palliative care patient's psychological and physical adaptation to a long-standing painful condition will inform the care being provided to that patient and family, especially as the patient nears death.

The modifier "nonmalignant" has been used in the clinical literature to describe pain that is not associated with a life-threatening condition such as cancer. Lessons from cancer pain management have been applied to pain associated with numerous other serious conditions, such as

HIV/AIDS and sickle cell disease. Pain remains medically undertreated for several reasons. Patients' and families' concerns about opioid analgesics, lack of professional education, and professionals' fear of regulatory agency influence all contribute. Analgesic drug availability is also a significant problem. The direct costs of unrelieved pain are measured in lost productivity and in the many lives lost to suicide. Pain costs an estimated $100 billion each year in the United States alone.[1] Loss of functional status and poor quality of life are frequent, intangible costs of unrelieved pain.

Palliative care providers are strong advocates for patients' quality of life and may take on the full responsibility of providing pain management for their patients' NMP. Alternatively, palliative care providers may work within a larger team in which other professionals, such as pain specialists, provide NMP management (Box 170-1). In either case, palliative care providers should have a general understanding of NMP and its treatment.

BASIC SCIENCE

Pain is a necessary function of the nervous system. It is defined as a complex psychophysiological phenomenon, the perceptual product of complex integration of multiple brain circuits. Pain occurs when the nervous system is functioning normally to transmit the signals of tissue injury (physiological or nociceptive pain) or when there is abnormal nervous system functioning (pathological or neuropathic pain). A discrete human brain locus for conscious perception of pain has not been identified and probably does not exist.

Within the nervous system, there are endogenous mechanisms to transmit nociceptive signals, to inhibit nociception and produce analgesia, and to release analgesic mechanisms ("antianalgesia") to facilitate healing and recovery. Human pain has both sensory/discriminative and affective dimensions. The process of nociception begins when a noxious stimulus is transduced in the peripheral tissues. Nociceptive signals are transmitted over peripheral nerves to the central nervous system, where further ascending transmission and modulation occur at spinal and supraspinal levels. Pain is the final dynamic perceptual product of higher cortical processing. Neuroanatomical pathways of nociceptive processing exist, with both a human thalamic nucleus specific for pain and widely distributed cerebral cannabinoid receptors. A newly identified, widely distributed brain receptor, termed the orphan opioid receptor, and its natural ligand,

---

Box 170-1 Decision Analysis: Nonmalignant Pain (NMP) in the Palliative Care Patient

1. Establish NMP diagnosis and projected course.
2. Become familiar with NMP treatment (history and current).
3. Identify the clinician responsible for NMP treatment (e.g., pain specialist).
4. Review care options with patient and family.
5. Clarify roles and responsibilities of palliative care team and other providers regarding NMP.

"nociceptin" or "orphanin FQ," appears to facilitate pain perception in animals and may be involved in learning and memory. Many of the chemical mediators and neurotransmitters involved in transduction, transmission, modulation, and perception of nociception have been identified. Opioid receptors are widely distributed in non-neural tissues and throughout the nervous system.[2] The contribution of other neurotransmitters, such as serotonin and norepinephrine, to inhibition of pain signaling is also known.

PREVALENCE OF NONMALIGNANT PAIN

NMP is highly prevalent, and 75 million Americans suffer from chronic pain.[3] Headache and lower back pain are the most common types in developed countries. More than 25 million Americans suffer from migraines, and 9 of every 10 Americans have nonmigraine headaches each year. More than 26 million Americans between the ages of 20 and 64 years experience frequent back pain, and two thirds of American adults will have back pain during their lifetime.[4] Other common conditions include arthritis, jaw, and lower facial pain (temporomandibular dysfunction, temporomandibular joint syndrome); neuropathic pain syndromes; and fibromyalgia (a complex condition involving generalized body pain and other symptoms). Chronic painful conditions in the developing world are more likely to be related to malnutrition, infectious diseases, and trauma, including limb amputation, which affect millions of the world's inhabitants.

PATHOPHYSIOLOGY AND PAIN "DIAGNOSIS"

Advances in neuroscience research in learning, memory, and neural plasticity have begun to elucidate the pathophysiology of chronic pain. Learning and memory result from brain cellular changes. In animals, morphological changes occur from remodeling of neural arborization, creation of new circuits or strengthening old ones, formation of new active zones along existing axons, and changes in the structure of dendrites to improve the propagation of postsynaptic potentials to integrative zones. Both membrane excitability and synaptic transmission are enhanced in sensory neurons with damaged axons. Signal proteins synthesized in response to such sensitization are probably distributed throughout the neuronal arbor and thus affect structural remodeling. Perception is encoded in both anatomical structures and temporal patterns of neural activity in the brain. Long-term potentiation is one example of how neural activity itself causes changes in synaptic connectivity.

Pain is a dynamic state. The central nervous system responds to nociceptive signals acutely with activity at spinal cord, brainstem, and thalamus and with immediate alterations in cortical somatosensory synaptic patterns. Structural and functional changes occur with repeated noxious stimuli, persistent damaging stimuli, or direct injury to the nervous system itself. Chronic NMP in humans (Box 170-2) may be attributable to pathological functioning of a damaged nervous system at any level[2] (see "Case Study: Assessment of Pain and Symptoms in an Oncology Patient").

> **Box 170-2 Pathophysiological Classification of Pain**
>
> - Nociceptive pain: somatic, visceral
> - Non-nociceptive pain: neuropathic, psychogenic (rare)
> - "Unclassified" soft tissue pain syndromes: myofascial pain syndrome,* fibromyalgia syndrome

Travell J, Simons D. Myofascial Pain and Dysfunction. Baltimore: Williams & Wilkins, 1983.

 C A S E   S T U D Y

Assessment of Pain and Symptoms in an Oncology Patient

A 45-year-old woman was referred in early 2005 to the pain medicine and palliative care service for evaluation and management of pain and symptoms persisting after treatment of thyroid cancer. Her initial complaints were of generalized muscle aches, fatigue, and symptoms consistent with thermoregulatory dysfunction. She reported gradually worsening symptoms since her diagnosis of recurrent thyroid cancer and its treatment with radioactive iodine.

She characterized the pain as aching, hot, and burning. She denied stabbing pain, tingling or shock-like pain, numbness, and altered sensation. She complained of "knots in her shoulders" that extended down her back, arms, trunk, and legs, most notably her calves. She stated that the pain felt deep as opposed to superficial and that cold weather exacerbated her symptoms. The pain was worse in the evenings than the mornings. She was unable to sleep well due to pain. There was significant pain interference with activities of daily living and recreational activities. She also noted that, when resting at times she twitched and her legs were constantly in motion.

Medications on presentation included hydrocodone/acetaminophen 10/500, 1 to 2 tablets every 6 hours as needed; carisoprodol, 350 mg three times daily; acetaminophen, 500 mg 4 to 6 tablets per day; ibuprofen, 800 mg three times daily; and tramadol, 50 mg four times daily with minimal relief. She was prescribed Mirapex, 0.5 mg PO once daily; Inderal, 10 mg PO once daily; Levoxyl, 200 μg PO once daily; venlafaxine, 75 mg once daily; and lorazepam, 0.5 mg nightly at bedtime. She also was taking vitamin D, 150,000 units PO once daily; calcium, 1500 mg PO once daily; magnesium, 400 mg PO once daily; and black cohosh, 500 mg twice daily for hot flashes. Nonpharmacological treatment included hot baths and use of a heating pad daily.

Assessment and Recommendations

The patient's medical history included the following:

- 1993 Melanoma; status post surgical resection without recurrence
- 1993-1994 Multiple endocrine adenomas; surgical resection revealed thyroid cancer. The patient underwent total thyroidectomy and parathyroidectomy in 1993, with subsequent hypercalcemia. Implantation of her parathyroid glands in her left forearm did not result in function of the glands. She was treated with radioactive iodine and was without recurrence until 2004.

- 1996 Leiomyosarcoma of the vaginal wall; status post total hysterectomy and right oophorectomy
- 2003 C5-C7 cervical fusion secondary to stenosis
- 2004 Median branch blocks and facet denervation of cervical facets
- 2004 Recurrent thyroid cancer between the chin and sternal notch
- 2004 Radioactive iodine treatment
- Hypertension
- Restless legs
- Major depression

The patient's paternal grandfather died of malignant brain tumor.

The patient is married and is employed as an office manager for an ophthalmology practice. She reports no use of alcohol, tobacco, and illicit substances.

Associated symptoms include loss of appetite, laryngospasm, xerostomia; constipation treated with diet and fiber; generalized subjective muscle weakness; mood swings, anxiety, depression, and feelings of sadness related to pain and poor functional status.

The physical examination is notable for normal vital signs and complaint of generalized discomfort. Positive findings included supple neck status post thyroidectomy with trachea midline; decreased cervical spine range of motion consistent with fusion; and marked tenderness of 12/17 musculotendinous (fibromyalgia) points. Straight leg raise was negative, and the neurological examination was completely normal.

Diagnoses are fibromyalgia-like syndrome, myofascial pain syndrome, opioid-related constipation, sleep disturbance, mood disorder, and restless legs syndrome.

The following measures were recommended and instituted: (1) discontinuation of hydrocodone/acetaminophen, tramadol, and carisoprodol; (2) initiation of oxycodone, 5 to 10 mg PO every 4 hours as needed for pain (subsequently, this was titrated to oxycodone SA, 60 mg every 12 hours, and oxycodone, 10 mg PO every 4 hours as needed for breakthrough pain); (3) titration of venlafaxine to 150 mg daily; (4) topical lidocaine patches were added; (5) adjustment of the patient's bowel program; (6) continuation of other medications as prescribed; and (7) supportive counseling.

Treatment and Results

In late 2006, the patient reported painful swelling of the right leg and was referred to the sarcoma specialist for evaluation due to her history of leiomyosarcoma. Magnetic resonance imaging (MRI) with contrast of the right leg revealed no evidence of a mass lesion or abnormal fluid collection within the right leg. There was minimal vasodilatation seen within the proximal lateral leg, corresponding to skin markers. No evidence of cellulitis or myositis was found. The perifascial fluid signal seen in the medial leg with normal enhancement, overlying the medial head of the gastrocnemius and the soleus musculature, was consistent with eosinophilic fasciitis or the sequela of connective tissue disease. Subsequent clinical examinations detected no additional abnormalities; this condition was being followed.

In 2007, the patient began to complain of severe aching lower back pain. There was some referred pain into proximal lower extremities. Back pain was worse with twisting, and she had great difficulty repositioning herself in bed. No radicular symptoms or signs were present. There were no new findings on complete neurological examination.

Plain radiographs revealed severe degenerative disease at L2/L3, grade 1 retrolisthesis of L2 on L3 without abnormal motion during flexion/extension, mild degenerative lateral listhesis of L4 on L5 without evidence of abnormal motion or significant disc disease. On MRI, multilevel degenerative changes of the lumbar spine were described. Changes were worse within the L2/L3 and L4/L5 disc spaces. There was bone marrow edema and enhancement of the opposing L2/L3 end plates. Neural foramina and lateral recess narrowing were identified as described earlier. Degenerative changes were essentially unchanged when compared to the prior examination of 2006. There was a small left renal cyst. Computed tomography of the spine showed severe bony sclerosis, irregularity, osteophyte formation, and complete disc height loss at L2/L3 with mild spinal canal and bilateral neural foraminal stenosis, most likely representing chronic degenerative changes, possibly from chronic or remote osteomyelitis.

Neurosurgical consultation was obtained, and the opinion was given that collapse of the disc space at L2/L3 could be the primary source of the patient's back pain. To better localize this pain and to determine how helpful fusion at that level would be, an L2/L3 epidural steroid injection was recommended as a diagnostic procedure. Depending on that outcome, a discogram at the L2/L3 level might be considered. Pending this diagnostic evaluation, potential surgical options included L2/L3 fusion using a minimally invasive approach. The patient referred to an anesthesia pain specialist for diagnostic and therapeutic procedures.

The pain medicine and palliative care service continues to monitor the patient for medical management of her cancer-related symptoms and coordinated with other specialists to treat her nonmalignant pain.

CLINICAL MANIFESTATIONS OF COMMON CONDITIONS

A thorough evaluation of the patient with pain includes a comprehensive history, physical examination, and review of diagnostic information. The "gold standard" of pain assessment is patient self-report. The clinician may use the "PQRST" mnemonic to elicit a complete pain history (Box 170-3). Pain intensity rating scales establish a baseline against which the efficacy of analgesic interventions may be judged. Many patients must be encouraged to verbalize their pain, and most need to learn means of reporting pain intensity. When patients are unable to communicate, behavioral observations may substitute for self-report of pain intensity. Standardized tools can assess preverbal children and impaired adults. Characteristics of neuropathic pain should be elicited. Typically, patients describe burning or lancinating components. Some offer unusual complaints, such as painful numbness, itching, or crawling sensations. After amputation or evisceration, patients may complain of phantom pain referred to the lost body part. Sensations of lost visceral organs may be accompa-

P = palliative, provocative factors: What makes the pain better or worse?

Q = quality (i.e., word descriptors, such as "burning" or "stabbing")

R = region, radiation, referral: Where does it hurt? Does the pain move or travel?

S = severity (pain intensity rating scales or word descriptors)

T = temporal factors (i.e., onset, duration, daily fluctuations): When did it start? Is it constant and/or intermittent? How long does it last? Is it better or worse at certain times of the day?

nied by functional urges, such as the urge to defecate or urinate.

A psychosocial assessment should be performed, and the meaning of pain to the individual and family should be explored. Standardized pain assessment tools record the impact of pain on mood, sleep, appetite, physical activities, and social functioning. The expression of pain is influenced by an individual's prior experience and social and cultural milieu. Psychosocial circumstances and particular stressors should be elicited. Usual coping strategies should be understood. It is important to identify prior or current psychological dependency on illicit or licit drugs, including alcohol. Prior pain treatments, including prescription and nonprescription medications, and their relative efficacies should be recorded.

Physical Examination

It is important to assess the patient's general physical condition and identify physical findings to identify pain pathophysiology[5] (Box 170-4). The physiological signs of acute pain—elevated blood pressure, respiratory rate, and pulse rate—are unreliable in subacute and chronic pain. A detailed neurological examination should be performed, especially if neuropathic pain is suspected. Pain in an area of reduced sensation, allodynia (normal stimuli are painful), and hyperpathia or summation of painful stimuli indicate neural dysfunction. Complex regional pain syndrome or sympathetically maintained pain is suggested if signs of marked sympathetic dysfunction accompany diffuse burning or deep aching pain. A careful mechanical evaluation, including active and passive joint motion, weight bearing, and gait, may also reproduce the pain. In the soft tissues, one may palpate muscle spasms or discrete trigger points which, when stimulated, refer pain to another site.

The pain evaluation concludes with a review of available diagnostic imaging studies, which may be supplemented to determine the pathophysiology. Correlation should be made between clinical symptoms and signs and diagnostic, laboratory, and radiographic information. This establishes the pain "diagnosis" (Table 170-1).

Temporal features are an important part of the general pain assessment. There are different temporal patterns of NMP: constant pain, daily pain, intermittent/recurring pain that is predictable or regular, and intermittent/recurring pain that is unpredictable or irregular. Analgesic treatments vary considerably according to the temporal pattern.

Box 170-4 Physical Examination

General Inspection

- Patient's appearance and vital signs
- Evidence of abnormalities such as weight loss, muscle atrophy, deformities, trophic changes

Pain Site Assessment

- Inspect the pain sites for abnormal appearance or color of overlying skin, change of contour, visible muscle spasm
- Palpate the sites for tenderness and texture
- Use percussion to elicit, reproduce, or evaluate the pain and any tenderness on palpation
- Determine the effects of physical factors such as position, pressure, and motion

Neurological Examination

- Mental status: level of alertness, higher cognitive functions, affect
- Cranial nerves
- Sensory system: light touch and pin prick test to assess for allodynia, evoked dysesthesia, hypoesthesia/hyperesthesia, hypoalgesia/hyperalgesia, hyperpathia
- Motor system: muscle bulk and tone, abnormal movements, manual motor testing, reflexes
- Coordination, station, and gait

Musculoskeletal Examination

- Body type, posture, and overall symmetry
- Abnormal spine curvature, limb alignment, and other deformities
- Range of motion (spine, extremities)
- For muscles in neck, upper extremities, trunk, and lower extremities: observe for any abnormalities such as atrophy, hypertrophy, irritability, tenderness, and trigger points

TABLE 170-1 Diagnostic Testing for Nonmalignant Pain

TYPES OF TESTS	USES OF TESTS
Screening laboratory tests: CBC, chemistry profile (e.g., electrolytes, liver, enzymes, BUN, creatinine), urinalysis, ESR	Screen for medical illnesses, organ dysfunction
Disease-specific laboratory tests: includes autoantibodies, sickle cell test	Autoimmune disorders, SCD
Imaging studies: radiographs, CT, MRI, US, myelography	Detection of tumors, other structural abnormalities
Diagnostic procedures: lumbar puncture for CSF analysis	Detection of various central nervous system illnesses
Electrophysiologic tests: EMG (direct examination of skeletal muscle), NCV (examination of conduction along peripheral nerves)	Detection of myopathy, neuropathy, radiculopathy
Diagnostic nerve block: injection of a local anesthetic to determine the source and/or mechanism of the pain	Identification of structures responsible for the pain (e.g., sacroiliac or facet joint blocks), differentiation of pain pathophysiology

BUN, blood urea nitrogen; CBC, complete blood count; CSF, cerebrospinal fluid; CT, computed tomography; EMG, electromyography; ESR, erythrocyte sedimentation rate; MRI, magnetic resonance imaging; MS, multiple sclerosis; NCV, nerve conduction velocity; SCD, sickle cell disease; US, ultrasound.

For example, the management of headache depends not only on the intensity but also on the frequency of pain episodes. A patient diary helps establish the pattern of painful episodes.[6] Infrequent episodes may be managed with abortive treatment alone, whereas very frequent or daily headaches usually require a combination of prophylactic and abortive strategies. A complete headache management plan includes avoidance of headache triggers and maintenance of regular lifestyle habits, diet and rest, and exercise.

Lower back pain, arthritides, neuropathic pain (e.g., painful diabetic neuropathy, postherpetic neuralgia, nerve injury related),[7,8] and other conditions such as fibromyalgia often require daily management by the patient that includes physical strategies and lifestyle modifications. Published guidelines for the management of these conditions outline the proper diagnosis and combined pharmacological and nonpharmacological analgesic strategies.

DIFFERENTIAL DIAGNOSIS

Distinguishing NMP from malignant pain is important. For example, pain from spinal metastases (the most frequent site of solid tumor metastasis) must be distinguished from degenerative disc disease, which is common in adults. The clinician must carefully review the pain characteristics and correlate these with relevant diagnostic tests; that is, perform a clinicoradiographic correlation. It is strongly recommended that this be done by the clinician who has thoroughly examined the patient.[9]

TREATMENT

The steps used in the management of NMP are as follows:

1. Evaluating the patient and establishing the pain "diagnosis"
2. Identifying any curative treatment
3. Tailoring analgesic medications to the individual
4. Maximizing nonpharmacological analgesic interventions
5. Monitoring the patient for response to treatment and modifying the treatment plan accordingly.

Analgesic interventions must be integrated into the overall medical treatment plan.

Nonpharmacological Interventions

Anesthetic Procedures

Many anesthetic procedures can be done in the outpatient setting. Muscle trigger point injections and local anesthetic infiltration of painful scars are simple and carry low risk. Other neural blockades require monitoring, but not an overnight hospital stay. These include somatosensory blocks, stellate ganglion block, celiac plexus block, brachial or lumbosacral plexus block, lumbar sympathetic block, and placement of an epidural catheter. In the outpatient clinic, pain patients are evaluated for placement of intrathecal catheters for medication administration; this usually requires inpatient observation.

Neurosurgical Procedures

Pain patients may also be evaluated by the neurosurgeon to determine the indication for implanted intrathecal systems for opioid delivery, neuroaugmentation (nervous system stimulation), or neuroablative (destructive) surgical procedures. Nonpharmacological strategies using neurostimulation or neuroaugmentation techniques are being refined and offer patients relief with less medication.

Physical Treatment

Specific treatments for myofascial pain and musculoskeletal problems, such as soft tissue manipulation, may be performed in the clinic. Pain patients may be presented to physiatry staff to determine the need for rehabilitation, occupational therapy, or physical therapy programs, which may be conducted on an outpatient basis.

Psychological or Behavioral Interventions

Pain specialists work closely with psychiatrists and mental health practitioners to evaluate and treat pain and concurrent psychiatric or psychological problems. Cognitive and behavioral strategies, relaxation training, hypnosis, and individual and family psychotherapy are useful as adjunctive outpatient pain treatments. Spiritual support is a part of maintaining overall wellness, especially in the setting of life-threatening illness. Many patients with chronic NMP employ so-called complementary and alternative medicine techniques effectively for pain relief.

OUTCOMES OF PAIN MANAGEMENT

The successful management of NMP is dependent on an individualized plan of care. Clinicians working with patients on a long-term basis follow several clinical variables to judge the efficacy of the pain management plan. These include patient self-report of pain intensity, pain relief, side effects of treatment, adverse events, quality of life, and functional status. In the palliative care patient, it can be expected that, as the life-threatening disease progresses, quality of life goals will supersede functional goals of pain treatment.

DRUGS OF CHOICE

Analgesic medications have three broad effects: reducing transduction of painful peripheral stimuli, altering transmission within the central nervous system, and altering higher cortical pain perception. There are three main classes of drugs used: the nonsteroidal anti-inflammatory drugs (NSAIDs) and acetaminophen; the opioids; and an assorted group referred to as adjuvant analgesics or "co-analgesics." A special class of agents (triptans) has been developed for abortive treatment of migraine headache. Complex pharmacotherapy is the rational combination of analgesic medications that work through various mechanisms to produce pain relief. Many patients with chronic NMP are prescribed medications from more than one drug class.

NSAIDs and Acetaminophen

The NSAIDs have analgesic, antipyretic, and antiinflammatory properties (see Chapter 135). There may also be an analgesic effect on the central nervous system. No single agent has proved superior to the others as an analgesic; side effects and toxicities vary among individuals.

The mechanism of the analgesic effect of acetaminophen is uncertain; it is antipyretic, not anti-inflammatory. Side effects of acetaminophen are uncommon.

Opioid Analgesics

The oral route of administration is preferred due to convenience and costs. Modified-release or long-acting preparations are recommended to afford more even serum drug levels and to enhance patient compliance with dosing (see Chapter 138). Alternative routes of administration are considered if the oral route is unavailable, if oral dosing is impractical, or if systemic side effects are limiting. Patients may remain ambulatory with external pumps for subcutaneous, intravenous, or intraspinal (epidural, intrathecal) drug delivery. Implantable systems for intrathecal opioid and nonopioid medication administration are available. It has been demonstrated that intra-articular injection of opioid can reduce inflammatory joint pain and prevent procedural pain. For constant pain, opioids should be taken on a regular schedule, with provisions for breakthrough dosing. The dosing schedule should be selected according to the known duration of analgesic action of the particular agent.

Adjuvant Analgesics

Adjuvant analgesics are a heterogeneous class of medications. They are given to provide additive analgesic effect, to counteract the side effects of more traditional analgesics such as NSAIDs and opioids, or to treat a concurrent symptom.

Antidepressants are effective for various types of chronic pain in patients who are not depressed, and they usually should be considered, given the frequent association of pain and depression. The doses for analgesia may be much lower than those required to treat true depression. Antidepressants relieve chronic neuropathic pain. The limiting side effects of the tricyclic antidepressants, combined with opioids, demand careful titration. The sedating antidepressants may be chosen if the patient is sleep deprived due to pain.

Anticonvulsants may relieve sharp, stabbing, or lancinating neuropathic pain. Conditions in which anticonvulsants may be useful include pain due to nerve injury, postsurgical neuralgia, and tic-like pains in the head and neck. Benzodiazepines may be used as adjuncts to treat muscle spasm or myoclonus.

Hydroxyzine has analgesic, antipruritic, antiemetic, and mild sedative properties that can be beneficial. Psychostimulants can counteract opioid-induced sedation. They might also provide additive analgesia. Oral local anesthetic agents are effective in certain forms of neuropathic pain. Medications that block sympathetic nervous activity are chosen for pains that are thought to be sympathetically mediated.

Future Considerations

- Diagnostic imaging will be more applicable in defining clinical pain states.
- New pharmacological treatments for nonmalignant pain will become available.
- New nonpharmacological treatments for nonmalignant pain will become available.
- Standardized measures of clinical outcomes in pain management are being developed.

Topical agents add analgesia, sparing systemic drug burden. Capsaicin is derived from chili peppers; when applied to the skin, it depletes substance P from the neural terminals, reducing afferent nociceptive transmission. It is indicated for pain associated with peripheral nerve damage. A mixture of local anesthetics in a topical formulation prevents the pain of planned procedures such as venipuncture, bone marrow aspiration, and lumbar puncture. These are effective especially in pediatric medicine. Topical lidocaine preparations and patches relieve pain related to nerve injury. There is a growing rationale for consideration of topical opioids.

Adjuvant analgesics, when appropriately selected for specific purposes, can provide major benefit in NMP. Emerging pharmacological strategies include new formulations of opioid analgesics; new nonopioid topical, systemic, and intraspinal agents are also being actively developed.

EVIDENCE-BASED MEDICINE

Numerous professional societies and governmental agencies have developed guidelines and policies for treatment of NMP.[10-16] General policies emphasize the obligation of clinicians to properly assess and treat pain. Clinical guidelines detail management approaches and outline specific considerations for special populations, children, the elderly, and marginalized people. It is recognized that societal concern with issues of drug abuse and diversion should not outweigh patients' right to compassionate, effective pain treatment (see "Future Considerations").

CONCLUSION

Palliative care specialists have been at the forefront of advocacy for the dignity and humane treatment of those suffering from life-threatening illnesses and their families. Relief of pain, regardless of its source, is congruent with our ethic and essential to our task.

REFERENCES

1. National Institutes of Health. The NIH guide: New Directions in Pain Research I. Washington, DC: Government Printing Office, 1998.
2. Weinstein SM. Cancer pain management. Economics of Neuroscience 2002; 4:48-56.
3. Schnitzer TJ. Non-NSAID pharmacologic treatment options for the management of chronic pain. Am J Med 1998;105:45S-52S.
4. American Pain Society. Pain Facts, 2005.
5. Weinstein SM. Physical examination of the patient in pain. In Ashburn M (ed). Management of Pain. New York: Churchill Livingstone, 1998, pp 17-25.
6. Piovesan EJ, Silberstein SD. Diagnostic headache criteria and instruments. In Herndon RM (ed). Handbook of Neurologic Rating Scales, 2nd ed. New York: Demos, 2006, pp 297-345.

7. Morley-Foster P. Prevalence of neuropathic pain and need for treatment. Pain Res Manage 2006; 11(Suppl A):5A-10A.
8. Dworkin R, Backonja M, Rowbotham M, et al. Advances in neuropathic pain: diagnosis, mechanisms, and treatment recommendations. Arch Neurol 2003; 60:1524-1534.
9. Reddy S, Weinstein SM. Medical decision making in a patient with a history of cancer and chronic non-malignant pain. Clin J Pain 1995;2:242-246.
10. Koes BW, van Tulder MW, Ostelo R, et al. Clinical guidelines for the management of low back pain in primary care: An international comparison. Spine 2001;26:2504-2513.
11. American Pain Society. Guidelines for the Management of Pain in Osteoarthritis, Rheumatoid Arthritis, and Juvenile Chronic Arhtritis, 2nd ed. Skokie, IL: American Pain Society, 2002.
12. American Pain Society. Guidelines for the Management of Acute and Chronic Pain in Sickle Cell Disease. Skokie, IL: American Pain Society, 1999.
13. American Pain Society. Guidelines for the Management of Fibromyalgia Syndrome Pain in Adults and Children. Skokie, IL: American Pain Society, 2005.
14. American Pain Society. Pain Control in the Primary Care Setting. Skokie, IL: American Pain Society, 2006.
15. Howard RF. Current status of pain management in children. JAMA 2003; 290:2464-2469.
16. Model Policy for the Use of Controlled Substances for the Treatment of Pain. Dallas, TX: Federation of State Medical Boards of the United States, 2004.

SUGGESTED READING

American Pain Society: Pain Control in the Primary Care Setting. Skokie, IL: American Pain Society, 2006.

Howard RF. Current status of pain management in children. JAMA 2003;290:2464-2469.

Model Policy for the Use of Controlled Substances for the Treatment of Pain. Dallas, TX: Federation of State Medical Boards of the United States, 2004.

CHAPTER **171**

Oral Symptoms

Rajesh V. Lalla and Douglas E. Peterson

KEY POINTS

- Mouth symptoms are very common in palliative care.
- Common symptoms include dry mouth, sore mouth, and taste changes.
- Oral symptoms can be a sign of an underlying, more serious, systemic condition.
- Mouth symptoms have a significant impact on quality of life, nutrition, and cost of care.
- Many oral symptoms can be successfully managed.

Patients in palliative care settings often report mouth symptoms. Common complaints include dry mouth, a sore mouth, and taste changes. Oral symptoms can be painful (e.g., mouth sores), can result in significant functional compromise (e.g., speech impairment), and can diminish quality of life. They can also affect nutritional intake (e.g., taste changes, mouth sores), leading to malnutrition, dehydration, and wasting. Dry mouth increases

the risk of local oral infection, and mouth sores provide a pathway for systemic dissemination of infection. Oral symptoms can have a highly significant impact on the clinical course and activities of daily living in palliative care. Appropriate diagnosis and management are important and can significantly better patients' quality of life.

DRY MOUTH

Xerostomia (the patient's perception of a dry mouth) is typically but not always associated with an objective compromise in salivary production and/or flow. Salivary hypofunction causes several negative sequelae. These include difficulty in mastication, impairment of speech, compromised function of dentures, and increased risk for dental caries, periodontal disease, oral candidiasis, and other oral infections. Saliva also plays a role in delivering tastants to taste buds, so salivary deficiency can result in taste changes.

Epidemiology and Prevalence

Oral symptoms are very common in palliative care. Prevalence varies according to the specific population being studied (Table 171-1).

Pathophysiology

Secretion of saliva is controlled by the parasympathetic and sympathetic pathways of the autonomic nervous system. The secretory process is complex and involves several steps; dysfunction of any step can lead to a decrease in salivary production. The mechanistic causes of hyposalivation can be varied, ranging from frank destruction of parenchymal tissue to subtle dysfunction of the muscarinic receptors that mediate fluid secretion.[1] The most common cause of xerostomia in the elderly is side effects of medications (see "Case Study: Dry Mouth"). Although many medications can cause some salivary hypofunction, the most significant are anticholinergic, psychotropic, cardiovascular, and sympathetic agonists (Table 171-2).

TABLE 171-1	Prevalence of Dry Mouth	
STUDY	**POPULATION**	**REPORTED PREVALENCE (%)**
Karus et al., 2005	Multicenter study of HIV/AIDS patients receiving palliative care	45-62
van der Putten et al., 2003	Nursing home residents	52
Al-Nawas et al., 2006	Patients who have received radiation therapy for oral cancer	71

From Karus D, Raveis VH, Alexander C, et al. Patient reports of symptoms and their treatment at three palliative care projects servicing individuals with HIV/AIDS. J Pain Symptom Manage 2005;30:408-417; van der Putten GJ, Brand HS, Bots CP, van Nieuw Amerongen A. [Prevalence of xerostomia and hyposalivation in the nursing home and the relation with number of prescribed medication]. Tijdschr Gerontol Geriatr 2003;34:30-36; and Al-Nawas B, Al-Nawas K, Kunkel M, Grotz KA. Quantifying radioxerostomia: Salivary flow rate, examiner's score, and quality of life questionnaire. Strahlenther Onkol 2006;182:336-341.

CASE STUDY

Dry Mouth

A 63-year-old woman presented complaining of a very dry mouth, such that she had trouble chewing and speaking. Past medical history was significant for hypertension, for which she was taking hydrochlorothiazide. Clinical examination revealed a very dry-appearing oral mucosa with a fissured tongue showing atrophy of papillae. On questioning, the patient admitted to a constant dry, gritty feeling in her eyes that she had gotten used to. An unstimulated whole salivary flow test was performed and revealed a flow of 0.05 mL/min, consistent with true salivary hypofunction. The Shirmer test to measure tear secretion demonstrated a value of 2 mm, confirming a dry-eye state. Laboratory testing was positive for anti-Ro and anti-La antibodies. Biopsy of the minor salivary glands of the lower lip demonstrated multiple foci of chronic inflammatory aggregates within a 4-mm^2 area of glandular tissue. Other autoimmune diseases were ruled out, and the patient was diagnosed as having primary Sjögren's syndrome. She was prescribed pilocarpine, 5 mg by mouth, three times per day. A repeat unstimulated whole saliva flow rate performed 2 weeks later demonstrated an increased flow rate of 0.2 mL/min; the patient also reported significant improvement in her mouth and eye symptoms.

TABLE 171-2 Commonly Prescribed Xerostomia-Inducing Medications

DRUG CLASS	EXAMPLES
Anticholinergics and related drugs	Oxybutynin HCl, diphenhydramine HCl, omeprazole, famotidine, meclizine HCl
Psychotropic drugs	Trazodone HCl, diazepam, sertraline HCl, lorazepam, fluoxetine HCl, nefazodone HCl, lithium carbonate, hydroxyzine HCl, amitriptyline, desipramine HCl
Opioid analgesics	Codeine, hydromorphone, oxymorphone, fentanyl, tramadol
Cardiovascular drugs	Fosinopril, atenolol, metoprolol tartrate, diltiazem, hydrochlorothiazide, verapamil, timolol, doxazosin mesylate, felodipine, nifedipine
Sympathetic agonists	Albuterol, beclomethasone dipropionate, meta-proterenol sulfate, carbidopa-levodopa, selegiline HCl

From Janket SJ, Jones J, Rich S, et al. The effects of xerogenic medications on oral mucosa among the Veterans Dental Study participants. Oral Surg Oral Med Oral Pathol Oral Radiol Endod 2007;103:223-230.

Several systemic diseases have also been implicated in hyposalivation, especially when they are poorly controlled (Table 171-3).

Patients who have received radiation therapy to fields including the salivary glands often have significant hyposalivation. Both ductal structures and acini, particularly of the serous type, can be affected. Depending on the extent of inflammatory and degenerative changes, fibrosis may occur, resulting in lifelong salivary gland compromise. Salivary glands not within the radiation portal may become hyperplastic, partially restoring salivary volume and function.

TABLE 171-3 Diseases and Conditions Implicated with Salivary Dysfunction

SYSTEMIC DISEASES ASSOCIATED WITH HYPOSALIVATION AND/OR XEROSTOMIA

Chronic inflammatory rheumatic disorders
    Sjögren's syndrome
    Rheumatoid arthritis
    Juvenile idiopathic (rheumatoid) arthritis
    Systemic lupus erythematosus
    Systemic sclerosis (scleroderma)
    Primary biliary cirrhosis
Sarcoidosis
Diabetes mellitus
Human immunodeficiency virus (HIV)
Cytomegalovirus and other herpes viruses
Hepatitis C
Graft-versus-host disease
Ectodermal dysplasia
Depression

GENETIC OR OTHER CHRONIC DISEASES ASSOCIATED WITH SALIVARY DYSFUNCTION

Autoimmune thyroiditis
Chronic pancreatitis
Celiac disease
Cystic fibrosis
Down syndrome
Familial amyloidotic polyneuropathy
Myotonic dystrophy
Papillon-Lefèvre syndrome
Prader-Willi syndrome
Sphingolipid storage disease, Gaucher's disease
Systemic amyloidosis
Thalassemia major

CONDITIONS THAT CAUSE METABOLIC CHANGES AND ARE ASSOCIATED WITH SALIVARY HYPOFUNCTION

Dehydration
Eating disorders (anorexia/bulimia)
End-stage renal disease
Nutritional deficiencies

From von Bultzingslowen I, Sollecito TP, Fox PC, et al. Salivary dysfunction associated with systemic diseases: Systematic review and clinical management recommendations. Oral Surg Oral Med Oral Pathol Oral Radiol Endod 2007;103(Suppl):S57.e51-S57.e15.

Clinical Manifestations

Xerostomia is characterized by a sensation of oral dryness and an increased need for oral hydration. The normal unstimulated whole salivary flow rate is 0.3 to 0.5 mL/min; unstimulated whole salivary flow rates of less than 0.1 mL/min are indicative of salivary hypofunction. Patients may notice increased salivary viscosity, with resultant difficulty in swallowing foods. In addition to oral tissue dryness, oral hygiene may be compromised by the reduction in salivary lubrication and clearance. If salivary hypofunction persists for longer than 3 months, dental caries may develop due to loss of buffering capacity and decreased flow rates. Some systemic conditions that can cause hyposalivation (e.g., Sjögren's syndrome, diabetes mellitus, alcoholism, eating disorders) may be associated

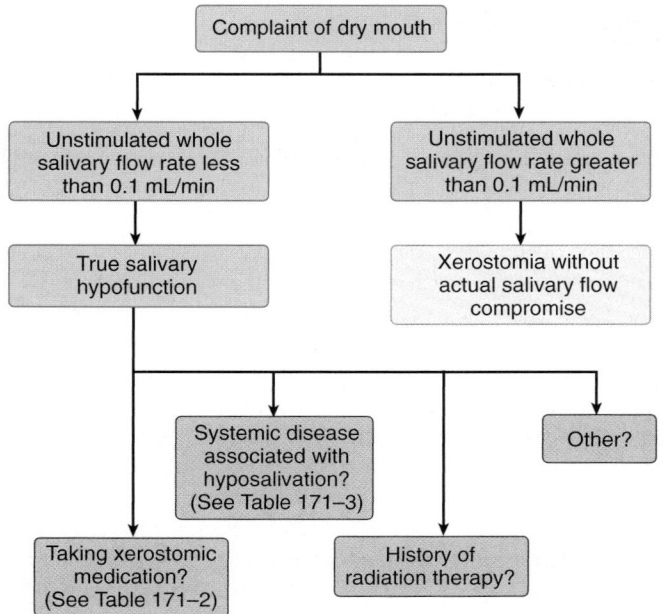

FIGURE 171-1 Diagnosis algorithm for dry mouth (xerostomia). Medications that commonly cause xerostomia are presented in Table 171-2, and systemic diseases associated with hyposalivation are listed in Table 171-3.

with a painless bilateral swelling of the major salivary glands, especially the parotid gland (Fig. 171-1).

Treatment

The first step is to determine whether a true salivary hypofunction exists. This can be accomplished by a simple measurement of whole saliva. The patient is seated upright and asked to allow all saliva to drain into a beaker by drooling or gentle spitting. The patient is instructed not to masticate, swallow, or speak. Saliva is collected for 15 minutes and then measured in a graduated syringe. The flow is expressed in milliliters per minute.[2] Unstimulated whole salivary flow of less than 0.1 mL/min is diagnostic of a true salivary hypofunction.

Management of a true salivary hypofunction depends on its cause. Hypofunction caused by use of xerostomic medications can be reversed by replacing the medication or reducing its dose, in consultation with the prescribing provider. Hypofunction resulting from systemic disease may or may not be reversible with better management of the underlying condition, depending on the amount of destruction of salivary gland tissue. Salivary hypofunction that occurs secondary to radiation therapy is dose dependent, with doses greater than 26 Gy resulting in permanent salivary hypofunction.[3] People with a true salivary hypofunction who have some functioning salivary gland tissue often respond to a systemic parasympathomimetic drug (e.g., pilocarpine, cevimeline).[1,4]

Because of the increased risk for oral infectious disease (e.g., dental caries, periodontal disease, oral candidiasis) associated with salivary hypofunction, a vigorous preventive program must be instituted to maintain adequate hydration and excellent oral hygiene (Box 171-1). Persons with cognitive impairment or neuromuscular compromise

TABLE 171-4 Prevalence of Sore Mouth/Oral Mucositis

STUDY	POPULATION	REPORTED PREVALENCE (%)
Karus et al., 2005	Multicenter study of HIV/AIDS patients receiving palliative care	2-12
Elting et al, 2003	Patients undergoing chemotherapy for solid tumors or lymphomas	30
Trotti et al., 2003	Patients receiving radiation therapy for head and neck cancer	97-100

From Karus D, Raveis VH, Alexander C, et al. Patient reports of symptoms and their treatment at three palliative care projects servicing individuals with HIV/AIDS. J Pain Symptom Manage 2005;30:408-417; Elting LS, Cooksley C, Chambers M, et al. The burdens of cancer therapy: Clinical and economic outcomes of chemotherapy-induced mucositis. Cancer 2003;98:1531-1539; and Trotti A, Bellm LA, Epstein JB, et al. Mucositis incidence, severity and associated outcomes in patients with head and neck cancer receiving radiotherapy with or without chemotherapy: A systematic literature review. Radiother Oncol 2003;66:253-262.

may need family or caregiver assistance in maintaining optimal oral hygiene and hydration.

SORE MOUTH AND STOMATODYNIA

Stomatodynia (discomfort of the oral mucosa) is a common complaint with a number of potential causes (Table 171-4).

Several oral ulcerative conditions can result in pain of the oral mucosa. Common conditions include traumatic ulcers, recurrent aphthous stomatitis (canker sores), and recurrent herpes simplex virus (HSV)–related lesions. *Oral mucositis* refers to erosive and ulcerative lesions of the oral mucosa in patients receiving chemotherapy for cancer and in patients with head and neck cancer undergoing radiation therapy to fields involving the oral cavity.

The most common oral infection causing burning of the oral mucosa is candidiasis.

Burning mouth syndrome (BMS) is characterized by a burning discomfort of the oral mucosa in the absence of any clinical signs of pathology.

Pathophysiology

Traumatic oral ulcers can be caused by various factors, including accidental biting of oral tissues, denture margins, sharp edges of teeth or dental fillings, and certain foods.

Recurrent aphthous stomatitis, also known as canker sores, is the most common oral mucosal disease in humans in all geographic regions. The pathogenesis is not understood. Some factors implicated are family history, immune disturbances, trauma, and stress. A significant body of evidence has suggested that deficiencies of various vitamins (including vitamin B_{12} and folic acid) contribute to the pathogenesis of this condition.

Recurrent lesions caused by HSV-1 most often occur at the junction of the vermilion border of the lip and the skin; they are commonly referred to as "cold sores" but do not result in soreness inside the mouth. Recurrent HSV-1 lesions can also occur intraorally. This is most often seen in immunocompromised and/or debilitated patients.

The pathophysiology of oral mucositis is multifactorial. The mechanisms involved are more complex than simply direct damage to oral epithelial cells from chemotherapy or radiation therapy. The currently accepted model for mucositis postulates five stages (Fig. 171-2). Initial initiation of tissue injury may be mediated by reactive oxygen species. This is followed by activation of second messengers that upregulate the production of proinflammatory cytokines and cause tissue injury. These cytokines further amplify the tissue injury cascade, with ulceration and secondary infection occurring. Finally, there is renewal of epithelial proliferation and differentiation, leading to healing.[5]

Oral candidiasis is most commonly caused by *Candida albicans*, which is often a part of the normal oral flora. Several factors allow the organism to cause clinical disease, including

- Hyposalivation due to medications, radiation therapy, or other causes that impairs the normal clearing function of saliva
- Use of antibiotics that alter the normal balance among the various components of the oral flora
- Use of topical or systemic steroids or other immunosuppressive agents
- Disease resulting in systemic immunosuppression (e.g., HIV/AIDS) (see "Case Study: Sore Mouth")

BMS may be classified as primary BMS, for which a local or systemic cause cannot be identified, or as secondary BMS, which may be caused by various conditions including hormonal disturbances, nutritional deficiencies, psychological changes, diabetic neuropathy, contact allergy, cranial nerve injuries, salivary hypofunction, and side effects of medications. BMS has a complex and poorly understood pathophysiology.[6] It is thought to represent an interplay of various factors, including local factors such as decreased flow and composition of saliva, peripheral nervous system alterations including taste changes, central

CASE STUDY

Sore Mouth

A 78-year-old man complained of a chronic burning sensation on his palate under his upper complete denture. He reported that the soreness persisted regardless of whether the denture was in his mouth or not. He kept his complete dentures in most of the time, including during sleep. Past medical history was significant for type II diabetes mellitus which was being treated with Glucophage. On oral examination, the hard palate surface covered by the upper complete denture was diffusely erythematous. A clear line of demarcation could be seen separating the tissues under the denture from the normal-appearing soft palate tissue. Other areas of the oral cavity appeared within normal limits. Based on clinical signs and symptoms, the patient was diagnosed as having an erythematous form of candidiasis. He was treated with 10 mg clotrimazole troches five times per day. In addition, he was instructed to keep the dentures out of his mouth except during meals. He was asked to disinfect the dentures (which contained no metal components) by immersing them for 30 minutes in a solution of 1% sodium hypochlorite, when not in use. He was further instructed to thoroughly wash the dentures before placing them in his mouth. He was also asked to apply nystatin ointment to the inner surface of the upper denture before placing it in his mouth. After 2 weeks, the patient reported a resolution of the burning sensation. Clinical examination revealed a normal pink color of the hard palate mucosa. At this point, the patient was allowed to use his dentures all day, and the antifungal agents were stopped. He was instructed to continue to keep his dentures out every night and to immerse them in a commercially available denture cleaner overnight.

nervous system abnormalities including dopamine level changes and cerebral blood flow, and psychosocial issues such as anxiety and depression.

Clinical Manifestations

Traumatic oral ulcers are found on those oral tissues that are more prone to trauma (e.g., buccal mucosa) and on sites adjacent to potential traumatic agents such as denture margins or sharp edges of teeth or dental fillings. Patients often give a history of accidental self-injury. Traumatic oral ulcers usually resolve within 2 to 4 weeks after the traumatic cause is removed or stopped. Any oral ulcer that persists for longer than 4 weeks must be biopsied to exclude malignancy.

Recurrent aphthous stomatitis typically manifests as single or multiple ulcers with a yellowish center and an erythematous border (Fig. 171-3). They usually resolve spontaneously within 10 to 14 days.

Recurrent HSV-related lesions usually occur on the outside of the lip (cold sores) but can occur intraorally, particularly in immunocompromised patients. Intraoral HSV lesions typically appear as a cluster of multiple small ulcerations on keratinized tissues such as gingiva and hard palate. Intraoral lesions in immunocompromised patients may have a prolonged course and require antiviral therapy.

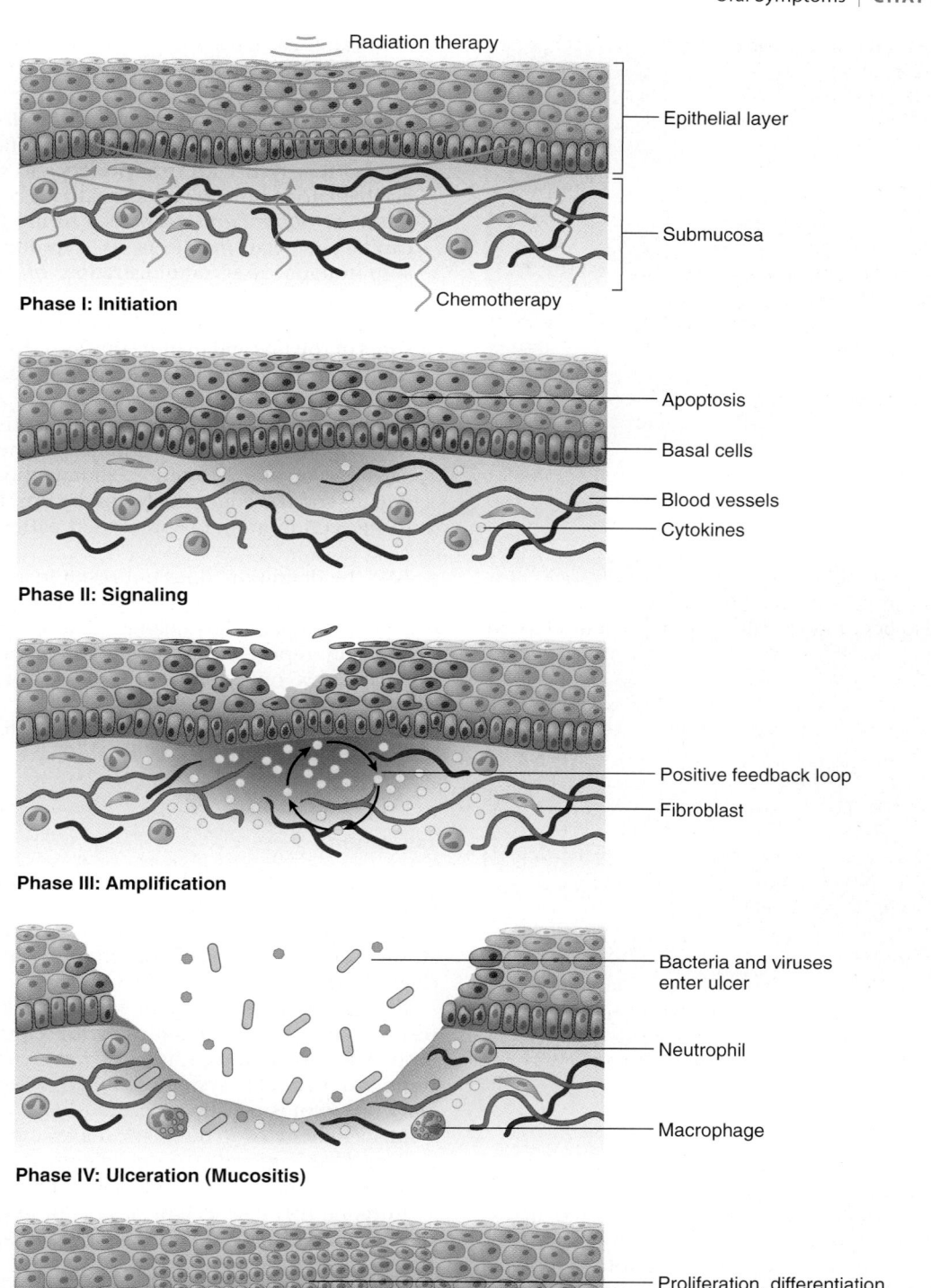

FIGURE 171-2 Five-stage model for the pathogenesis of mucositis. *(From Sonis ST. A biological approach to mucositis. J Support Oncol. 2004;2:21-32; discussion 35-26.)*

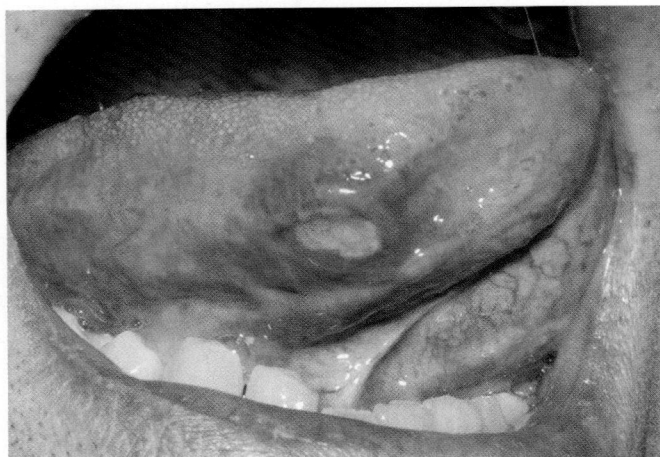

FIGURE 171-3   A lesion of recurrent aphthous stomatitis (canker sore) on the lateral tongue.

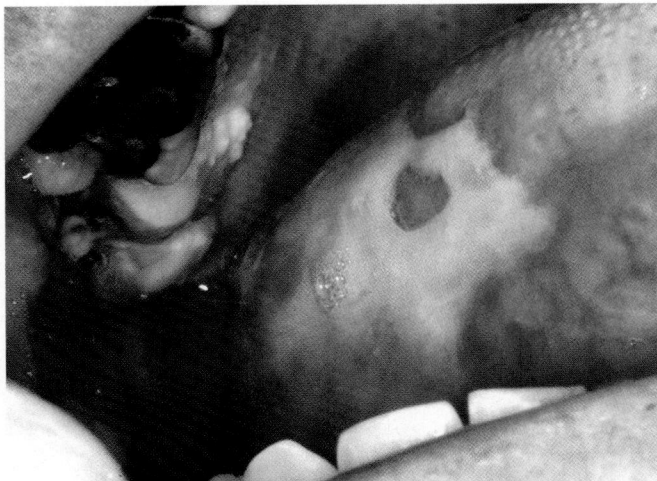

FIGURE 171-4   Oral mucositis lesion involving the right lateral and ventral tongue. This patient had received 5200 cGy of radiation therapy with concurrent chemotherapy for treatment of a squamous cell carcinoma of the right tongue.

Oral mucositis typically begins as erythema of the oral mucosa, which may be accompanied by soreness. This may progress to frank ulceration of the affected tissue, often covered by a white pseudomembrane (Fig. 171-4). Lesions can arise 1 to 2 weeks after stomatotoxic chemotherapy or after delivery of more than 30 Gy of radiation to the area. The ulcerative stage can be painful and can significantly affect nutritional intake, mouth care, and quality of life. In radiation-induced oral mucositis, lesions are limited to the tissues in the radiation field. In both chemotherapy-induced and radiation-induced oral mucositis, lesions are usually limited to nonkeratinized areas such as the buccal mucosa, lateral tongue, and soft palate. Keratinized tissues such as the gingiva, dorsal tongue, and hard palate are not usually affected. Severity of lesions is directly proportional to the chemotherapy or radiation dose. The lesions usually heal within 2 to 4 weeks after the last dose of stomatotoxic therapy has been delivered.[7]

Oral candidiasis has diverse presentations and may be associated with a burning sensation:

- *Pseudomembranous candidiasis (thrush)* shows adherent white plaques resembling cottage cheese that can be removed with firm pressure to reveal an often erythematous mucosa underneath.
- *Acute atrophic candidiasis* is a form of erythematous candidiasis that manifests as a reddened, atrophic, sore tongue after administration of broad-spectrum antibiotics.
- *Angular cheilitis* is candidiasis involving the commissures of the lips and manifesting as red, fissured lesions. It often occurs because of loss of vertical dimension in people who have lost their teeth.
- *Chronic multifocal candidiasis* is another form of erythematous candidiasis. In addition to the tongue, other sites are involved, often including the hard and soft palates and the commissures of the lips. It is more likely to be seen in immunosuppressed patients.

BMS, by definition, does not result in any clinical signs. Patients complain of a burning or scalding discomfort that may be accompanied by changes in taste and a dry mouth. Often, they report that the pain increases in intensity as the day goes on; however, it does not usually affect sleep.

An algorithm for the assessment of sore mouth is presented in Figure 171-5.

Treatment

Before primary BMS is diagnosed, potential contributing factors should be identified and managed. Topical clonazepam and cognitive behavioral therapy have the strongest evidence base for efficacy in primary BMS[6] (Fig. 171-6).

In the immunocompetent host, oral candidiasis may respond to topical therapies, with clotrimazole being more effective than nystatin. However, in immunocompromised patients, systemic therapy (e.g., fluconazole, ketoconazole) is usually needed.[8]

Management of a traumatic ulcer includes removing the traumatic agent (e.g., smoothing of a sharp tooth or denture) and follow-up to ensure healing.

Intraoral HSV lesions typically occur in an immunocompromised host and can be treated with systemic acyclovir or valacyclovir.[9]

Recurrent aphthous stomatitis usually heals spontaneously in 10 to 14 days. Topical over-the-counter anesthetic products containing benzocaine or lidocaine may reduce pain. Patients with an underlying vitamin deficiency may benefit from vitamin supplements. Large lesions or frequent episodes of recurrent aphthous stomatitis can be treated with topical steroids of varying potencies (e.g., triamcinolone acetonide, fluocinonide, dexamethasone). Rarely, systemic steroids or other agents may be needed.

Current management of oral mucositis is largely palliative and is focused on pain control (topical anesthetics and systemic analgesics), nutritional support, and good oral hygiene. A number of therapeutic agents are being studied (Table 171-5).

Patient Complaint of Sore Mouth
Obvious clinical ulceration
No obvious clinical ulceration
History of trauma
No history of trauma
Traumatic ulcer
On keratinized mucosa
On nonkeratinized mucosa
Positive HSV culture
Negative HSV culture
Recurrent HSV lesion?
Other oral ulceration (refer)
History of cancer therapy
No history of cancer therapy
Oral mucositis?
Recurrent aphthous stomatitis?
Other oral ulceration (refer)
Positive for clinical signs and fungal culture
Negative for clinical signs and fungal culture
Oral candidiasis?
Burning mouth syndrome?
Other?

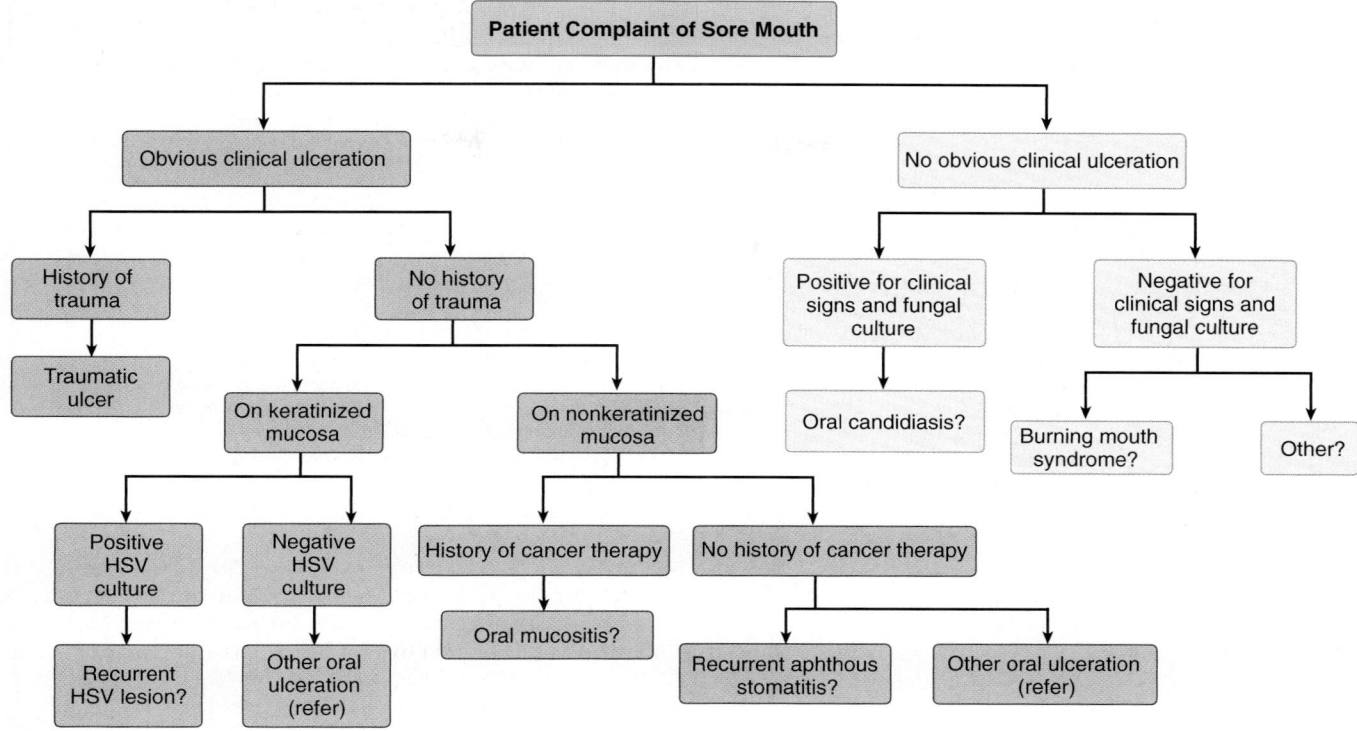

FIGURE 171-5 Diagnosis algorithm for sore mouth. HSV, herpes simplex virus.

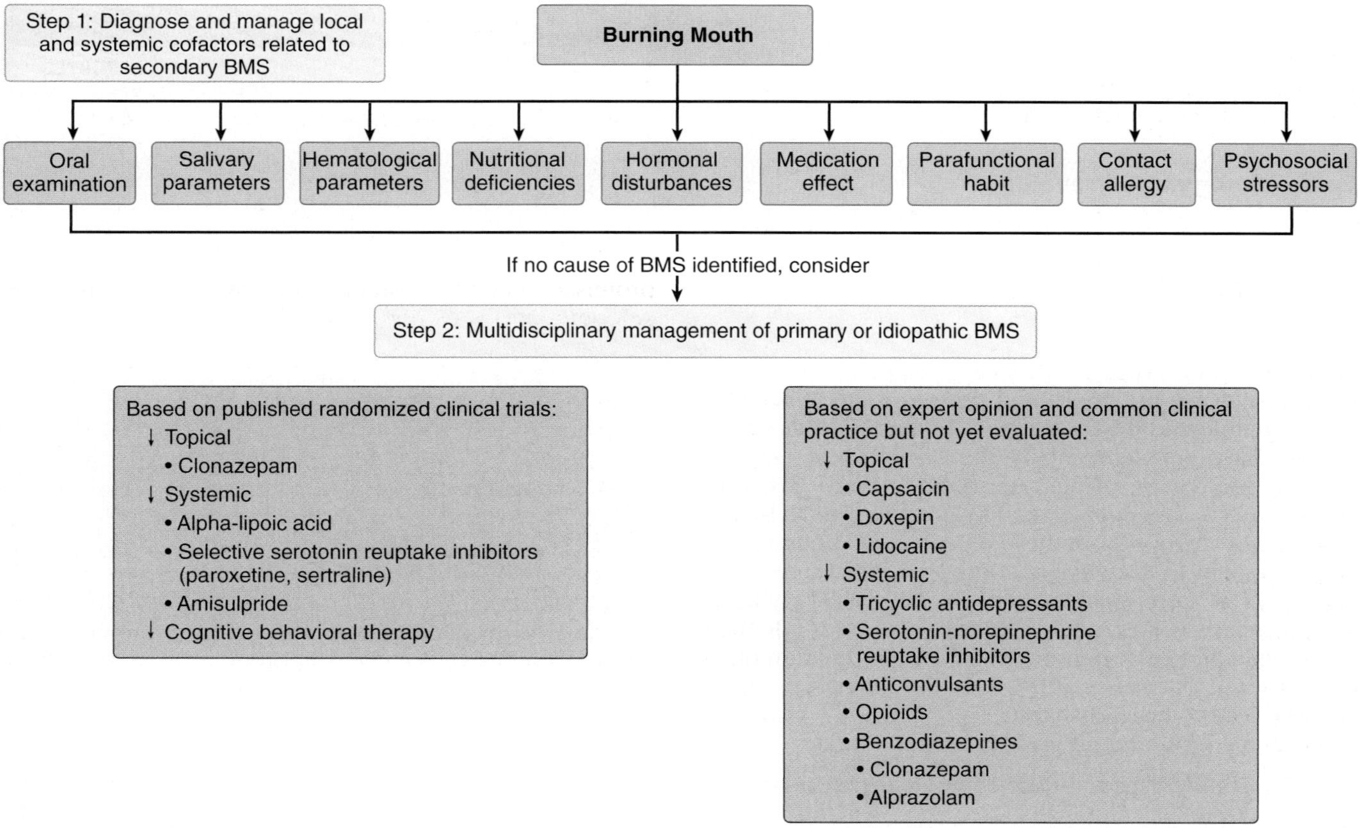

Step 1: Diagnose and manage local and systemic cofactors related to secondary BMS
Burning Mouth
Oral examination
Salivary parameters
Hematological parameters
Nutritional deficiencies
Hormonal disturbances
Medication effect
Parafunctional habit
Contact allergy
Psychosocial stressors
If no cause of BMS identified, consider
Step 2: Multidisciplinary management of primary or idiopathic BMS
Based on published randomized clinical trials:
↓ Topical
• Clonazepam
↓ Systemic
• Alpha-lipoic acid
• Selective serotonin reuptake inhibitors (paroxetine, sertraline)
• Amisulpride
↓ Cognitive behavioral therapy
Based on expert opinion and common clinical practice but not yet evaluated:
↓ Topical
• Capsaicin
• Doxepin
• Lidocaine
↓ Systemic
• Tricyclic antidepressants
• Serotonin-norepinephrine reuptake inhibitors
• Anticonvulsants
• Opioids
• Benzodiazepines
• Clonazepam
• Alprazolam

FIGURE 171-6 Algorithm for diagnosis and management of burning mouth syndrome (BMS). *(From Patton LL, Siegel MA, Benoliel R, De Laat A. Management of burning mouth syndrome: Systematic review and management recommendations. Oral Surg Oral Med Oral Pathol Oral Radiol Endod 2007;103 [Suppl]:S39.e31-S39.e13.)*

TABLE 171-5 Agents Studied for Oral Mucositis

CLASS	AGENT	CURRENT STATUS OR MASCC/ISOO GUIDELINE FOR MANAGEMENT OF ORAL MUCOSITIS
Cryotherapy	Ice chips placed in the mouth starting 5 min before chemotherapy and as needed for 30-60 min depending on half-life of agent	Recommended during administration of bolus chemotherapy with 5-fluorouracil, edatrexate, or melphalan
Growth factor	IV Keratinocyte growth factor-1 (Kepivance [Amgen])	Recommended for patients with hematological malignancies receiving high-dose chemotherapy and total body irradiation before autologous stem cell transplantation; FDA-approved in this population
Growth factor	IV Keratinocyte growth factor-2 (repifermin [HGS])	Not effective in reducing the percentage of subjects who experienced severe mucositis
Growth factor	IV Fibroblast growth factor-20 (velafermin [CuraGen])	Not effective in decreasing incidence of severe oral mucositis
Anti-inflammatory agents	Benzydamine hydrochloride mouth rinse	Recommended for patients receiving moderate-dose radiation therapy, based on previous evidence, but not FDA-approved; recent phase III trial halted due to negative results of interim analysis
Antioxidants	IV Amifostine (Ethyol [MedImmune])	No guideline; insufficient evidence of benefit for oral mucositis
Antioxidants	Topical N-acetylcysteine (RK-0202 [RxKinetix])	Currently in clinical trials
Promoters of healing	Topical L-glutamine (Saforis [MGI Pharma])	Currently in clinical trials
Antimicrobial agents	Antimicrobial lozenges	Not recommended for prevention of radiation-induced oral mucositis
Antimicrobial agents	Systemic acyclovir and analogues	Not recommended for prevention of chemotherapy-induced oral mucositis
Antimicrobial agents	Chlorhexidine mouth rinse	Not recommended for prevention of radiation-induced oral mucositis or for treatment of chemotherapy-induced oral mucositis
Topical coating agents	Topical sucralfate	Not recommended for prevention of radiation-induced oral mucositis
Laser therapy	Laser	Suggested when necessary technology and training are available

FDA, U.S. Food and Drug Administration; MASCC/ISOO, Multinational Association for Supportive Care in Cancer/International Society for Oral Oncology.

TASTE CHANGES

Taste changes can be classified as dysgeusia (altered taste), ageusia (loss of taste), hypogeusia (decreased sense of taste), or parageusia (bad taste).

Epidemiology and Prevalence

The prevalence of taste changes has been studied in various populations (Table 171-6).

Pathophysiology

Taste perception is mediated by taste receptor cells located in taste buds on the dorsal and posterior lateral surfaces of the tongue and on the palate. Chemical signals representing taste are detected by the taste receptors. This leads to the release of neurotransmitters onto gustatory afferent nerve fibers, which transmit the signal to the brain.[10] Any disruption in these receptor and neural pathways can lead to taste dysfunction. Peripheral neurological causes of taste changes include Bell's palsy, neuritis due to herpes zoster, and neoplastic processes affecting the submandibular region or the skull base. In addition, a central lesion that causes a disturbance in the taste pathway can also lead to taste changes.[11]

Many medications can lead to taste changes[12]:

- Penicillamine causes a dose-dependent partial or total loss of taste.
- Captopril has been related to a salty taste.
- Systemic griseofulvin can cause an ageusia for selected foods.

TABLE 171-6 Prevalence of Taste Changes

STUDY	POPULATION	REPORTED PREVALENCE (%)
Karus et al., 2005	Multi-center study of HIV/AIDS patients receiving palliative care	20-34
Epstein et al., 2002	Patients who have received high-dose chemotherapy as conditioning for a hematopoietic progenitor cell transplant	66
Halyard et al., 2007	Patients receiving radiation therapy for head and neck cancer	73-84

From Karus D, Raveis VH, Alexander C, et al. Patient reports of symptoms and their treatment at three palliative care projects servicing individuals with HIV/AIDS. J Pain Symptom Manage 2005;30:408-417; Epstein JB, Phillips N, Parry J, et al. Quality of life, taste, olfactory and oral function following high-dose chemotherapy and allogeneic hematopoietic cell transplantation. Bone Marrow Transplant 2002;30:785-792; Halyard MY, Jatoi A, Sloan JA, et al. Does zinc sulfate prevent therapy-induced taste alterations in head and neck cancer patients? Results of phase III double-blind, placebo-controlled trial from the North Central Cancer Treatment Group (N01C4). Int J Radiat Oncol Biol Physiol 2007;67:1318-1322.

- Bismuth has been associated with an unpleasant taste.
- Carbamazepine, phenytoin sodium, lamotrigine, baclofen, levodopa, acetazolamide, glipizide, and losartan potassium have all been associated with taste change.[11]

Taste alterations can also develop in cancer patients undergoing high-dose chemotherapy or radiation therapy to fields including the oral cavity. The etiology is probably multifactorial, including direct injury to taste receptor cells or their nerve fibers, salivary hypofunction, and secondary infection. Deficiencies of various vitamins have also been linked to taste disorders, notably vitamins A, B_6, and E (see "Case Study: Taste Changes").

Clinical Manifestations

A complaint of a change in taste may or may not be accompanied by visible clinical changes, depending on its cause.

CASE STUDY

Taste Changes

A 67-year-old man presented with a complaint of persistent taste changes such that most foods "did not taste good anymore." He denied any bad taste in his mouth when he was not eating or drinking. He stated that his mouth did not feel dry or sore but that the taste changes were very bothersome and that he had lost 8 pounds since this started, approximately 2 months earlier. He denied any history of radiation therapy or recent changes in medications. On clinical examination, the dorsal surface of the tongue showed a thick, diffuse, white coating that could be removed with some effort. The patient recalled that he had been previously treated with antifungals for this but did not receive any benefit. Other areas of the oral cavity were within normal limits; however, oral hygiene was poor. The patient reported that he brushed just once a day and sometimes forgot that too. He was asked to use an over-the-counter tongue cleaner instrument to clean the dorsal tongue of accumulated debris after each meal. Further, he was advised to brush and floss at least twice a day. At a follow-up visit 4 weeks later, the patient reported that his taste had returned to normal. Clinical examination revealed that the white coating on the dorsal tongue was greatly reduced.

Many patients present with a white coating on the dorsal tongue that interferes with the passage of tastants to the taste buds. This may be misdiagnosed as candidiasis, but it is often simply due to accumulation of food and other debris. Patients with taste changes secondary to chemotherapy or radiation therapy may show an atrophic tongue with loss of papillae, as may those with vitamin deficiencies. A dry mouth may be a contributory factor in some, because saliva carries the tastants to the taste receptors. Medication-induced taste changes typically resolve within a few weeks after discontinuation of the causative agent. By comparison, taste changes caused by high-dose radiation may take months to resolve (Fig. 171-7).

Treatment

A taste disturbance caused by a white coating of food debris covering the taste buds on the dorsum of the tongue can be easily corrected by regular use of a tongue cleaner device, available at drugstores. Taste changes caused by vitamin deficiencies resolve after correction; those that are secondary to radiation therapy may resolve spontaneously but take several months. Taste changes resulting from salivary hypofunction should resolve once salivary flow is increased. Similarly, medication-induced taste disturbances can be managed with replacement or dose reduction of the offending agent, in consultation with the prescribing provider. A taste dysfunction related to neurological causes is difficult to diagnose and treat. Zinc sulfate is often tried, despite inconsistent evidence of efficacy. A recent phase III, double-blind, placebo-controlled study did not show any benefit from zinc sulphate in taste changes secondary to radiation therapy.[13] Palliative measures such as chewing sugar-free flavored gum may be of benefit.

Taste changes may affect nutritional intake. Food preferences can lead to nutritional deficiencies and/or increased risk for dental disease. These consequences can be managed by alteration of dietary food texture and consistency, increased protein and caloric intake with snacks at mid-morning and mid-afternoon, and administration of

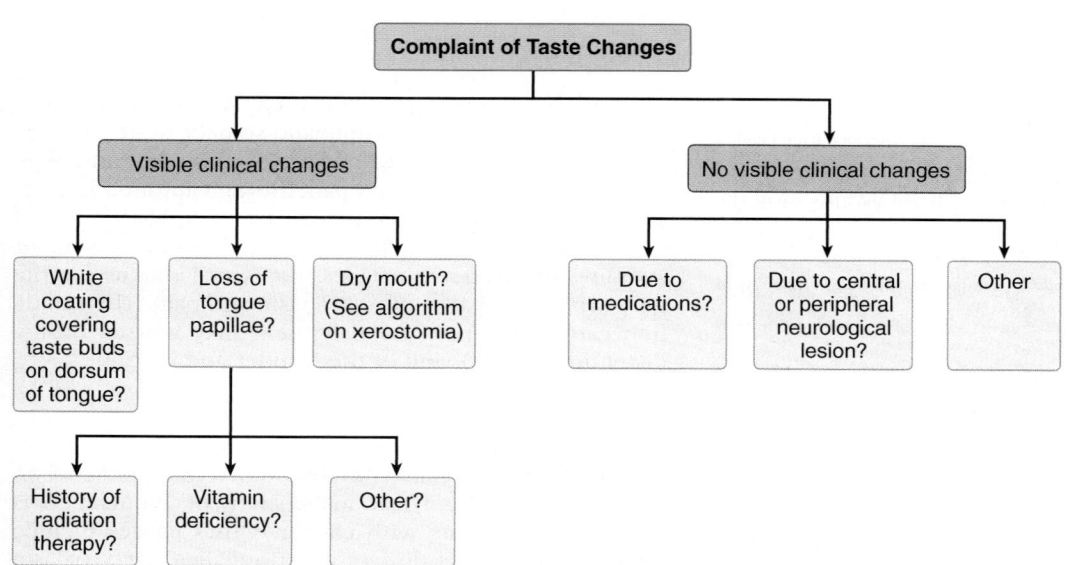

FIGURE 171-7 Diagnosis algorithm for taste changes.

Dry Mouth

Scientists at the National Institute for Dental and Craniofacial Research (NIDCR) are carrying out the first human clinical trial testing gene transfer for radiation therapy–induced dry mouth. The gene, aquaporin-1, which encodes a water channel protein, will be transferred into salivary ductal cells. Opening up of new water channels in the ductal cells is expected to result in increased salivary secretion into the mouth.

Sore Mouth

Agents currently in clinical trials for oral mucositis include growth factors, anti-inflammatory agents, antioxidants, and promoters of healing.

New topical formulations of antifungal agents are under study for oral candidiasis.

The role of nutritional deficiencies in the pathogenesis of recurrent aphthous stomatitis is being examined.

Taste Changes

The efficacy of zinc supplementation in the management of taste changes continues to be controversial and needs further study.

vitamin, mineral, and caloric supplements. Nutritional counseling may be required if the symptoms are severe or chronic.

REFERENCES

1. von Bultzingslowen I, Sollecito TP, Fox PC, et al. Salivary dysfunction associated with systemic diseases: Systematic review and clinical management recommendations. Oral Surg Oral Med Oral Pathol Oral Radiol Endod 2007;103(Suppl):S57.e51-S57.e15.
2. Speight PM, Kaul A, Melsom RD. Measurement of whole unstimulated salivary flow in the diagnosis of Sjogren's syndrome. Ann Rheum Dis 1992;51:499-502.
3. Eisbruch A, Dawson LA, Kim HM, et al. Conformal and intensity modulated irradiation of head and neck cancer: The potential for improved target irradiation, salivary gland function, and quality of life. Acta Otorhinolaryngol Belg 1999;53:271-275.
4. Shiboski CH, Hodgson TA, Ship JA, Schiodt M. Management of salivary hypofunction during and after radiotherapy. Oral Surg Oral Med Oral Pathol Oral Radiol Endod 2007;103(Suppl):S66.e61-S66.e19.
5. Sonis ST. A biological approach to mucositis. J Support Oncol 2004;2:21-32, discussion 35-26.
6. Patton LL, Siegel MA, Benoliel R, De Laat A. Management of burning mouth syndrome: Systematic review and management recommendations. Oral Surg Oral Med Oral Pathol Oral Radiol Endod 2007;103(Suppl):S39.e31-S39.e13.
7. Lalla RV, Peterson DE. Treatment of mucositis, including new medications. Cancer J 2006;12:348-354.
8. Ship JA, Vissink A, Challacombe SJ. Use of prophylactic antifungals in the immunocompromised host. Oral Surg Oral Med Oral Pathol Oral Radiol Endod 2007;103(Suppl):S6.e1-S6.e14.
9. Woo SB, Challacombe SJ. Management of recurrent oral herpes simplex infections. Oral Surg Oral Med Oral Pathol Oral Radiol Endod 2007;103(Suppl):S12.e11-S12.e18.
10. Sugita M. Taste perception and coding in the periphery. Cell Mol Life Sci 2006;63:2000-2015.
11. Heckmann JG, Heckmann SM, Lang CJ, Hummel T. Neurological aspects of taste disorders. Arch Neurol 2003;60:667-671.
12. Abdollahi M, Radfar M. A review of drug-induced oral reactions. J Contemp Dent Pract 2003;4:10-31.
13. Halyard MY, Jatoi A, Sloan JA, et al. Does zinc sulfate prevent therapy-induced taste alterations in head and neck cancer patients? Results of phase III double-blind, placebo-controlled trial from the North Central Cancer Treatment Group (N01C4). Int J Radiat Oncol Biol Physiol 2007;67:1318-1322.

SUGGESTED READING

Keefe DM, Schubert MM, Elting LS, et al. Updated clinical practice guidelines for the prevention and treatment of mucositis. Cancer 2007;109:820-831.

National Cancer Institute. Oral Complications of Chemotherapy and Head/Neck Radiation. Online document, last modified 2/20/2007. Available at http://www.cancer.gov/cancertopics/pdq/supportivecare/oralcomplications/healthprofessional (accessed December 22, 2007).
von Bultzingslowen I, Sollecito TP, Fox PC, et al. Salivary dysfunction associated with systemic diseases: Systematic review and clinical management recommendations. Oral Surg Oral Med Oral Pathol Oral Radiol Endod 2007;103(Suppl):S57.e51-S57.e15.

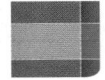

CHAPTER **172**

Tenesmus, Strangury, and Malodor

Sik Kim Ang

KEY POINTS

- Tenesmus is a constant sensation of fullness and incomplete relief during urination or bowel movement.
- Strangury is caused by bladder and urethra spasm.
- Malodor is treated by using appropriate dressings to control local wound infections and pain and to manage exudate.

TENESMUS

Tenesmus is a constant sensation of fullness or incomplete relief during urination or defecation. Patients note frequency and spastic pain in the rectum, bladder, or urethra. Pain can be poorly localized in the perineum. This condition is distressing because of the need to urinate or defecate many times daily.

Pathophysiology

The precise mechanism is not understood. The pelvis is innervated by both autonomic and somatic systems (Figs. 172-1 and 172-2). Smooth muscle contraction and pelvic organ enlargement transmit pain through autonomic afferents. During pelvic inflammation, pain impulses transmit through somatic afferents. Any tumor compressing or invading pelvic floor muscles, the sacral plexus, or the nerve roots can cause muscle spasm and pain. This condition can occur spontaneously, or it may worsen during distention or emptying of the bladder and rectum.

Differential Diagnosis

Tenesmus may be caused by the underlying pelvic disorder (Table 172-1). Local malignancy or recurrence is common in patients with cancer. Other causes include inflammatory bowel disease and proctalgia fugax (spasm

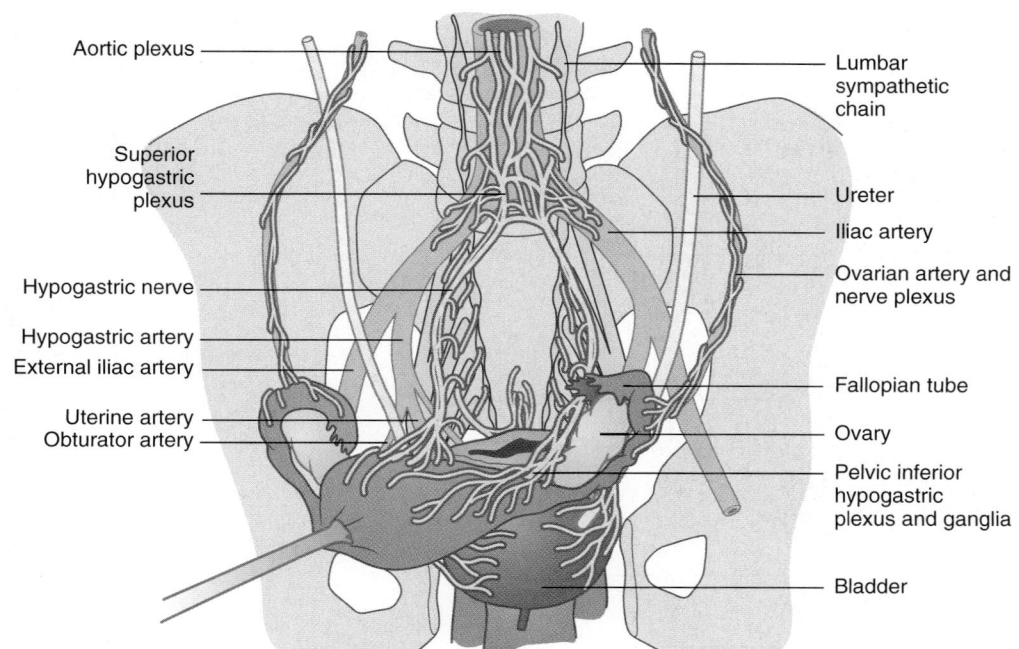

FIGURE 172-1 Nerve supply of the uterus. *(Redrawn from Bonica JJ. Principles and Practice of Obstetric Analgesia and Anesthesia. Philadelphia: FA Davis, 1967.)*

TABLE 172-1 Differential Diagnosis of Tenesmus
PELVIC MALIGNANCY
Bladder cancer
Gynecological cancer
Prostate cancer
Rectal cancer
GASTROINTESTINAL DISORDERS
Inflammatory bowel diseases
Irritable bowel disease
OTHER CONDITIONS
Radiation proctitis
Proctalgia fugax

TABLE 172-2 Treatment for Tenesmus
PHARMACOLOGICAL
Laxatives (nonstimulant)
Opioids
Calcium channel blockers (nifedipine, diltiazem)
Phenothiazines (chlorpromazine)
Chlorpromazine
Neuropathic agents (amitriptyline, nortriptyline, gabapentin, pregabalin)
Corticosteroids
Benzodiazepines
Anticholinergic drugs (belladonna alkaloids)
Miscellaneous (bupivacaine enema)
ANESTHETIC PROCEDURES
Bilateral lumbar sympathetic block
Superior hypogastric plexus block
Intrathecal infusion of opioid

of the pubococcygeus muscle). In addition, low urethral obstruction can manifest as rectal tenesmus.

Treatment

Most patients with cancer have symptom clusters; for example anxiety can worsen tenesmus. The definitive treatment is that of the underlying malignancy with either chemotherapy or radiation therapy. If this is not feasible, then the goal is to control pain and frequency. It is difficult to treat pharmacologically (Table 172-2). Opioid analgesics control pain primarily. In published case reports, nifedipine was used to reduce tenesmus frequency,[1] and methadone was administered to treat tenesmus not responding to morphine escalation.[2] Patients with neuropathic pain from tumor that is infiltrating nerves or nerve roots may benefit from corticosteroids or low-dose amitriptyline. If

the pain improves with the use of corticosteroids, patients may benefit from palliative pelvic radiotherapy. Other adjuvants such as phenothiazines, benzodiazepines, and anticholinergic drugs have been used.

In patients with intractable pain, interventional anesthesia procedures (sympathetic blocks, intrathecal opioid infusion) can be considered (see Chapter 247).[3] Bilateral lumbar sympathetic block may be effective in some patients with rectal tenesmus (Fig. 172-2). A more selective technique, superior hypogastric plexus block, may improve pelvic pain. These procedures can reduce pain intensity and opioid consumption.

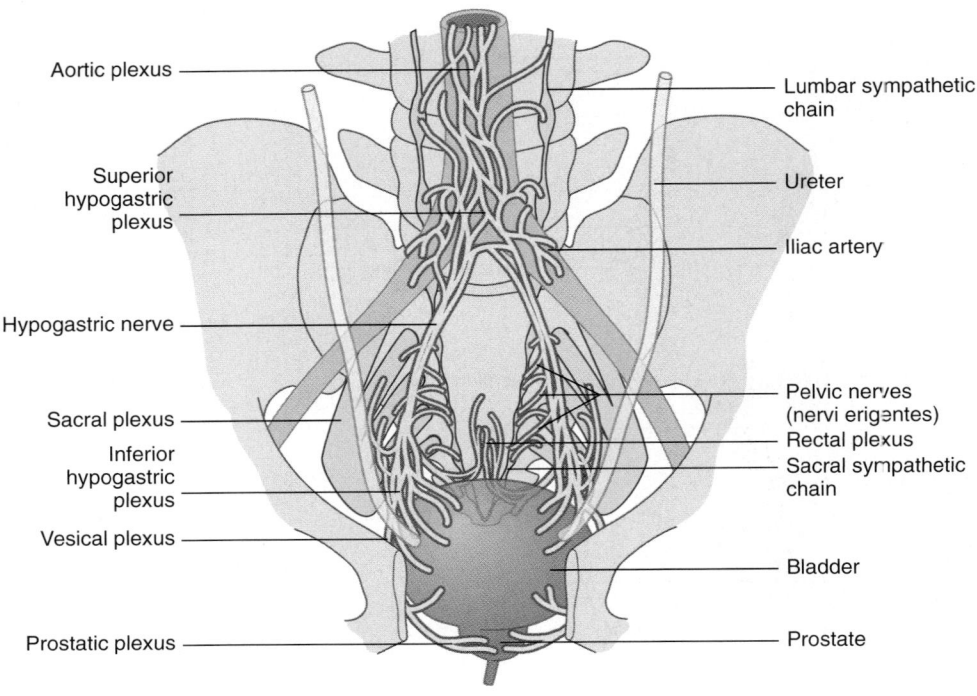

FIGURE 172-2 Anatomy of the superior and inferior hypogastric plexuses and subsidiary plexuses. *(Redrawn from Bonica JJ. The Management of Pain, 2nd ed, vol II. Philadelphia: Lea & Febiger, 1990.)*

Labels on figure:
- Aortic plexus
- Superior hypogastric plexus
- Hypogastric nerve
- Sacral plexus
- Inferior hypogastric plexus
- Vesical plexus
- Prostatic plexus
- Lumbar sympathetic chain
- Ureter
- Iliac artery
- Pelvic nerves (nervi erigentes)
- Rectal plexus
- Sacral sympathetic chain
- Bladder
- Prostate

STRANGURY

Strangury is slow, painful urination. It occurs secondary to spasm of the bladder and urethra. Strangury may manifest with abdominal hypogastric pain or symptoms suggestive of urinary tract infection such as dysuria, frequency, and urgency.

Pathophysiology

The bladder is innervated by the sympathetic, parasympathetic, and somatic nervous systems (Fig. 172-3). The parasympathetic S2, S3, and S4 provide motor function to coordinate voiding. Afferent parasympathetic fibers mediate the sensation to void, proprioception, and pain. The hypogastric plexus provides sympathetic supply to the bladder to mediate voiding, and it also fosters awareness of bladder distention and abdominal pain. Pain can originate from the bladder mucous membrane. The urethra has both motor and sensory fibers originating from the pudendal nerve. Tumor infiltrating the bladder or urethra, or any irritation of the mucous membrane, causes muscle spasm and pain.

Differential Diagnosis

It is essential to differentiate between strangury and dysuria. Abdominal examination may reveal suprapubic fullness suggesting tumor burden or urinary retention, whereas rectal examination can assess prostate size and irregularity. Treatment depends on the underlying disorder, which may need further investigation (Table 172-3).

TABLE 172-3	Investigations for Strangury
LABORATORY	
Urinalysis	
Urine cytology	
RADIOLOGY	
Plain film of the abdomen	
Ultrasound of the urinary tract	
Bladder scan	
INVASIVE PROCEDURE	
Cystoscopy	

TABLE 172-4	Differential Diagnosis of Strangury
Bladder cancer	
Bladder inflammation or cystitis	
Bladder irritation	
Tumor	
Blood clots	
Urinary catheter	
Prostate cancer	
Prostate hyperplasia	
Radiation fibrosis	
Urethral stricture	
Urinary calculus	
Urinary retention	
Urinary tract infection	

Treatment

The initial step in managing strangury is to identify any reversible or treatable causes (Table 172-4). Urinary tract infection or cystitis, irritation by urinary catheter, tumor, debris, or blood clot is managed appropriately. In some

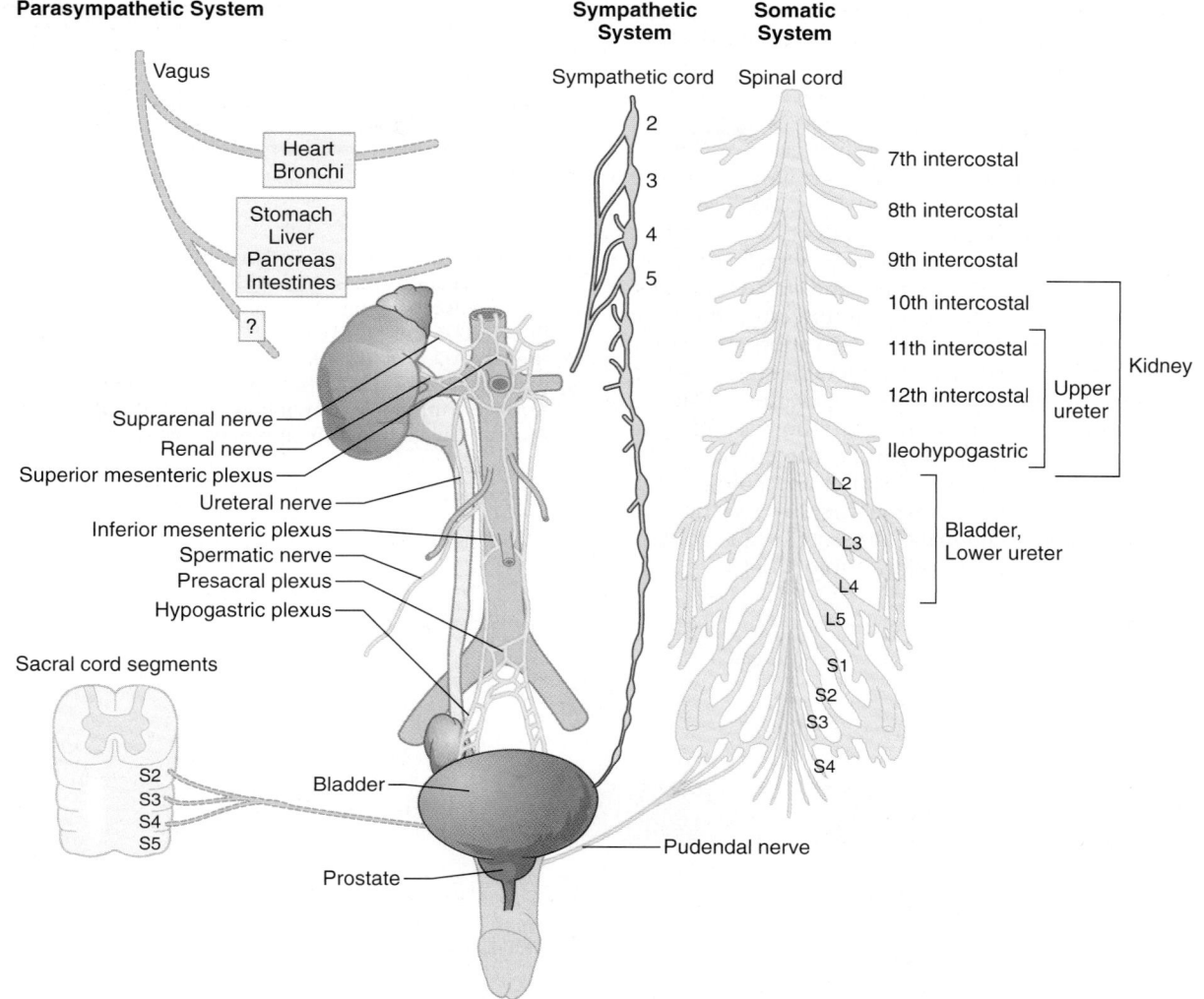

Parasympathetic System

Vagus

Heart
Bronchi

Stomach
Liver
Pancreas
Intestines

?

Suprarenal nerve
Renal nerve
Superior mesenteric plexus
Ureteral nerve
Inferior mesenteric plexus
Spermatic nerve
Presacral plexus
Hypogastric plexus

Sacral cord segments

S2
S3
S4
S5

Bladder

Prostate

Sympathetic System

Sympathetic cord

2
3
4
5

Somatic System

Spinal cord

7th intercostal
8th intercostal
9th intercostal
10th intercostal
11th intercostal
12th intercostal
Ileohypogastric

Upper ureter

Kidney

L2
L3
L4
L5
S1
S2
S3
S4

Bladder, Lower ureter

Pudendal nerve

FIGURE 172-3   Diagrammatic representation of urinary tract innervation.   *(Redrawn from Campbell MF. Urology, 2nd ed. Philadelphia: WB Saunders, 1963.)*

TABLE 172-5   Treatment for Strangury
Opium and belladonna alkaloids
Anticholinergic drugs/smooth muscle relaxants (tolterodine, oxybutynin, propantheline)
Urinary catheter (urethral, suprapubic)
Corticosteroids
Nonsteroidal anti-inflammatory drugs
Analgesic (phenazopyridine, intravesical local anesthetics, intravesical morphine)

patients, a urinary catheter (urethra or suprapubic) is necessary to relieve the symptom. Urinary catheterization can itself cause bladder irritation from excess balloon size; reducing balloon volume is sometimes sufficient.

Phenazopyridine is often used; patients should be warned their urine will turn orange. Spasm can be controlled by opium and belladonna suppositories, anticholinergic drugs, or corticosteroids (Table 172-5). Patients may not able to tolerate the side effects (dry mouth, urinary retention) of anticholinergic drugs. Responses to intravesical analgesic preparation may vary.

MALODOR

Malodor is a common complication of cutaneous or fungating wounds from tumors or pressure ulcers. This condition is offensive and distressing to patients, families, and caregivers. Malodor can lower self-esteem and cause social isolation. It is a challenging problem.

Pathophysiology

Overgrowth of organisms and colonization of aerobic and anaerobic bacteria characterize the wound. The wound produces an exudate, which is an ideal medium for bacteria colonization. The end product is the characteristic bad smell.

Treatment

It is important to use appropriate dressings to control infections, to relieve pain, and to manage the exudate. The wound should be irrigated with water during a shower to reduce bacterial counts and debris. If the wound is friable and the patient is unable to shower, an alternative is gentle irrigation with normal saline solution. The wound can be cleaned with mild soap and antibacterial cleanser, provided the cleanser does not cause burning or irritation. The ability of the patient and caregiver to participate in wound care is an important factor. Pain must be adequately treated during dressing changes. Wounds with debris may need autolytic or mechanical or surgical débridement to promote healthy tissue growth. Occlusive autolytic? dressings can worsen a bad odor. Eradication of anaerobic bacteria has a deodorizing effect.

The drug of choice is metronidazole. Oral metronidazole may cause significant nausea and taste changes, whereas topical metronidazole gel is effective for odor control and improved quality of life.[4,5] An alternative preparation is to crush metronidazole tablets in sterile water, then soak gauze in the mixture, and pack the wound. A less conventional approach is to coat the wound with yogurt or buttermilk. The rationale is that changing the pH of the wound can stop proliferation and colonization of the bacteria. In the home, aromatherapy can help to eliminate bad odors. Different dressings can contain exudate and thereby conceal odor (Table 172-6).

REFERENCES

1. McLoughlin R, McQuillan R. Using nifedipine to treat tenesmus. Palliat Med 1997;11:419-420.
2. Mercadante S, Fulfaro F, Dabbene M. Methadone in treatment of tenesmus not responding to morphine escalation. Support Care Cancer 2001;9:129-130.
3. de Leon-Casasola, OA. Neurolytic blocks of sympathetic axis for treatment of visceral pain in cancer. Curr Rev Pain 1999;3:173-177.
4. Finlay IG, Bowszyc J, Ramlau C. The effect of topical 0.75% metronidazole gel on malodorous cutaneous ulcers. J Pain Symptom Manage 1996;11:158-162.
5. Von Gruenigen VE, Coleman RL, Li AJ. Bacteriology and treatment of malodorous lower reproductive tract in gynecologic cancer patients. Obstet Gynecol 2000;96:23-27.

SUGGESTED READING

Bates-Jensen BM, Seaman S, Early L. Skin disorders: Tumor necrosis, fistula and stomas. In Ferrell BR, Coyle N (eds). Textbook of Palliative Nursing, 2nd ed. New York: Oxford University Press, 2005, pp 329-334.
Perlmutter AD, Blacklow RS. Urinary tract pain, hematuria, and pyuria. In Blacklow RS (ed). MacBryde's Sign and Symptoms: Applied Pathologic Physiology and Clinical Interpretation, 6th ed. Philadelphia: JB Lippincott, 1983.

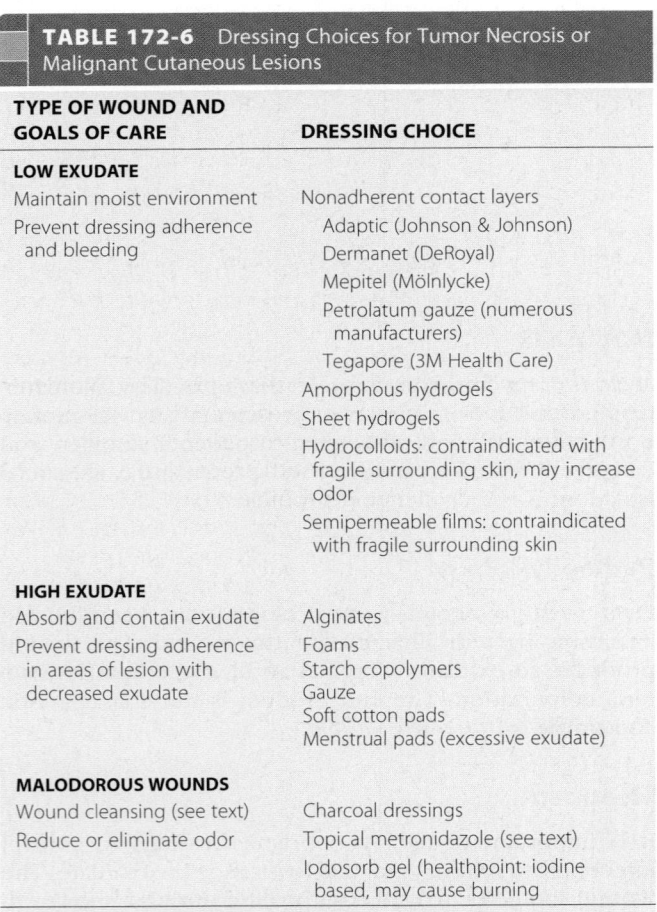

TABLE 172-6 | Dressing Choices for Tumor Necrosis or Malignant Cutaneous Lesions

TYPE OF WOUND AND GOALS OF CARE	DRESSING CHOICE
LOW EXUDATE	
Maintain moist environment	Nonadherent contact layers
Prevent dressing adherence and bleeding	Adaptic (Johnson & Johnson)
	Dermanet (DeRoyal)
	Mepitel (Mölnlycke)
	Petrolatum gauze (numerous manufacturers)
	Tegapore (3M Health Care)
	Amorphous hydrogels
	Sheet hydrogels
	Hydrocolloids: contraindicated with fragile surrounding skin, may increase odor
	Semipermeable films: contraindicated with fragile surrounding skin
HIGH EXUDATE	
Absorb and contain exudate	Alginates
Prevent dressing adherence in areas of lesion with decreased exudate	Foams
	Starch copolymers
	Gauze
	Soft cotton pads
	Menstrual pads (excessive exudate)
MALODOROUS WOUNDS	
Wound cleansing (see text)	Charcoal dressings
Reduce or eliminate odor	Topical metronidazole (see text)
	Iodosorb gel (healthpoint: iodine based, may cause burning

From Bates-Jensen BM, Seaman S, Early L. Skin disorders: Tumor necrosis, fistula and stomas. In Ferrell BR, Coyle N (eds). Textbook of Palliative Nursing, 2nd ed. New York: Oxford University Press, 2005, pp 329-334.

CHAPTER 173

Premature Menopause

Charles L. Loprinzi and Debra Barton

KEY POINTS

- Newer antidepressants decrease hot flashes.
- Gabapentin decreases hot flashes.
- Progestational agents decrease hot flashes.
- Paroxetine and other cytochrome P-450 isoenzyme CYP2D6 inhibitors should not be given to patients receiving tamoxifen.
- For vaginal dryness, local estrogen therapy relieves symptoms, but there is concern regarding its safety in women with a history of breast cancer.

Premature menopause is common in many female cancer survivors. Menopausal symptoms can be caused by surgery (e.g., bilateral oophorectomy), chemotherapy in premenopausal women, pelvic irradiation, or hormonal therapy with drugs such as tamoxifen and aromatase inhibitors. Prominent clinical problems associated with premature menopause include hot flashes, bone loss, and sexual function issues (e.g., vaginal dryness, decreased libido). These are discussed in the following sections.

PREVALENCE OF PREMATURE MENOPAUSE AND ASSOCIATED SYMPTOMS

Estimates are that 75% of women experience hot flashes, 50% have negative changes in sexual function, and almost all have bone loss as a result of aging.[1]

In the United States, the average age for menopause is 51 years.[1] For women younger than 50 years of age, treatment with chemotherapy or radiation to the pelvis can produce premature menopause. Radiation doses greater than 600 rad can cause ovarian failure.[2] Chemotherapy with alkylating agents and anthracyclines in a woman 40 years of age or older is likely to cause the ovaries to stop functioning.[3,4]

Tamoxifen increases the incidence of hot flashes. Aromatase inhibitors do not directly affect ovarian function, but they can decrease circulating estrogen and cause symptoms associated with menopause, including hot flashes, increased bone loss and a decreased libido.[5,6]

HOT FLASHES

Pathophysiology

The pathophysiology of hot flashes is not understood. Loss of normal hormonal balance, especially acutely, is the most common etiology.[7] The thermal neutral zone (i.e., the temperature zone between which one feels neither hot nor chilled) is narrowed.[7] This seems to be related to central serotonergic hypoactivity.[8]

Clinical Manifestations

Hot flashes are described as a sudden feeling of warmth, usually in the upper body.[7] They can range from mild to severe and can occur over seconds to several minutes. They may be associated with sweating. They may interrupt activities, requiring interventions to abate them.[9] At times, they are associated with substantial sweating. Nighttime hot flashes are commonly referred to as night sweats. Patients often complain that they interrupt sleep. Although some patients have only one or two hot flashes per week, others report 30 or more hot flashes in a 24-hour period.

Treatment

Table 173-1 outlines the pharmaceutical agents used to treat hot flashes and their effectiveness.

Nonmedical Therapies

Recommendations for nonmedical approaches include staying in cool environments, having fresh air available, and wearing layers of clothing.[10]

Estrogen Therapy

Estrogen has long been a standard approach. Although it is not completely effective, it is helpful in most cases. It decreases hot flashes by about 85%, compared to baseline. The effect may take 2 to 3 weeks before maximum benefit is felt. Different doses are required for different patients. The lowest dose that is effective should be selected. Premarin is standard at an initial dose of 0.625 mg per day for most patients.[11]

TABLE 173-1 Therapy for Hot Flashes

AGENT (TARGET TOTAL DAILY DOSE*)	ESTIMATED REDUCTION FROM BASELINE (%)
Placebo	20-30
Clonidine (0.1 mg)	40
Antidepressants	
Fluoxetine (20 mg)	50
Venlafaxine (75 mg)	60
Paroxetine (10 mg)	60-70
Gabapentin (900 mg)	50
Progestational agents†	85
Estrogen	85

*Lower doses of some agents are used initially, with titration upward.
†Megestrol acetate (20-40 mg/day) or a single intramuscular dose of medroxyprogesterone acetate (400-500 mg).

Some literature suggests that estrogen is safe in breast cancer survivors. A review of several phase II trials, comparing outcome with historical controls, suggested that there was no more problem with recurrent breast cancer in patients who were receiving estrogen than in those who were not.[12] Another trial, using Health Maintenance Organization (HMO) utilization data, suggested that women who received hormone replacement therapy did not have any more trouble with breast cancer recurrence than women from the same HMO plan who did not receive it.[13] In addition, a recent randomized, double-blinded, placebo-controlled Scandinavian trial, in which concomitant progesterone therapy was limited, did not demonstrate increased subsequent breast cancer among breast cancer survivors given hormone replacement therapy.[14] In addition, women in the Women's Health Initiative Trial who were randomly assigned to receive estrogen only (i.e., after hysterectomy) did not show an increased risk of breast cancer compared to those women who received placebo.[15] In fact, the breast cancer incidence was lower in those randomized to receive estrogen therapy.

Nonetheless, concerns exist about hormone replacement therapy in breast cancer survivors. The Women's Health Initiative Trial reported increased breast cancer among women who were not breast cancer survivors but who received both estrogen and progesterone.[16] A trial known as HABITS (Hormonal Replacement Therapy After Breast Cancer—Is It Safe?) reported that breast cancer survivors randomized to receive estrogen and progesterone therapy had a higher rate of recurrent breast cancer, compared with those receiving placebo.[17]

The conclusion about estrogen and/or progesterone treatment is that it is not used much, due to the risks.

Proven Nonestrogenic Therapies

CLONIDINE

Because of the concerns about estrogen replacement raised over the last couple of decades, alternatives have been investigated. One is clonidine, an older antihypertensive medication. Two large randomized, placebo-controlled trials in breast cancer survivors demonstrated that clonidine decreased hot flashes substantially more than placebo.[18,19] Placebos decreased hot flashes by 20% to 30%

from baseline, over a 4-week period.[20] Clonidine decreases hot flashes by 35% to 40%.[18,19] Clonidine has toxicities, including drowsiness, lightheadedness, and sleeping troubles, that limit its utility.

NEWER ANTIDEPRESSANTS

Newer antidepressants are helpful. In the early 1990s, it was recognized anecdotally that newer antidepressants decreased hot flashes. Pilot trials were conducted with several newer antidepressants, suggesting that they decreased hot flashes more than was expected with a placebo.[21,22] These findings led to placebo-controlled, randomized trials. Venlafaxine was the first reported.[23] At a dose of 37.5 mg/day for 1 week, escalating to 75 mg/day, hot flashes decreased by about 60% from baseline. Venlafaxine was well tolerated by most subjects, although in a subset it caused substantial nausea and vomiting. There was also a decreased appetite (which might be welcomed by some) as well as dry mouth and constipation in a minority. Two additional randomized, placebo-controlled, double-blinded clinical trials, one presented only as an abstract, also concluded that venlafaxine decreased hot flashes.[24,25]

Paroxetine, a selective serotonin reuptake inhibitor (SSRI), also decreased hot flashes more than placebo. Two randomized, placebo-controlled trials showed that it decreased hot flashes by about 60% from baseline.[26,27] Although paroxetine is relatively well tolerated by most individuals, it inhibits tamoxifen metabolism to one of tamoxifen's active metabolites[28] and is relatively contraindicated in patients receiving tamoxifen.

Fluoxetine, another SSRI, was shown in a placebo-controlled, double-blinded, crossover clinical trial to decrease hot flashes substantially more than placebo.[29] Its effect did not appear to be as great as that of venlafaxine or paroxetine. Another trial, lasting 9 months, looked at fluoxetine versus citalopram versus placebo.[30] This was presented as a negative trial. Nonetheless, the lack of a pretreatment baseline hot flash period made the study results different from those found with the other newer antidepressants.

Finally, a placebo-controlled, double-blinded trial demonstrated a trend for decreased hot flashes in women treated with sertraline, another SSRI.[31]

GABAPENTIN

Gabapentin is an antiseizure medication, different from the newer antidepressants; it anecdotally reduced hot flashes in six patients, five women and one man.[32] This led to two pilot trials, both of which suggested that gabapentin did decrease hot flashes.[33,34] Subsequently, two double-blinded, randomized clinical trials were performed. One was conducted primarily in women with breast cancer,[33] and the other was in women who did not have breast cancer.[34] Both trials reported that gabapentin, at a dose of 300 mg orally three times per day, decreased hot flashes by about 50% from baseline. This effect was sustained for the 6-week study duration in one trial and for the 12-week duration in the other.

PROGESTATIONAL AGENTS

Progestational agents, without estrogen, have also been studied. Megestrol acetate, 20 to 40 mg per day, decreases

hot flashes by about 80% over a 4-week period.[35] This effect, like that of estrogen, takes 2 to 3 weeks to fully manifest. An alternative, medroxyprogesterone acetate (Depo-Provera), also decreases hot flashes by about 85% from baseline.[36] It can be given as a single intramuscular injection. The effect is sustained for weeks to months after a single dose.[36]

OTHER STUDIED NONESTROGENIC THERAPIES

Vitamin E was studied in a placebo-controlled clinical trial with crossover.[37] The result suggested that it decreased hot flashes a little. This result has not been substantiated with a subsequent trial.[37] Nonetheless, it allows a placebo effect plus, possibly, a little more.

Soy products have been prospectively evaluated. The bulk of available information suggests that they are not any more helpful than placebo.[38,39]

Black cohosh is an alternative medicine long proposed to be helpful. Although studies in Germany suggested benefit, two well-conducted, placebo-controlled trials in the United States were unable to substantiate any greater benefit than with placebos.[40,41]

Bellergal is an old agent studied in the 1970s.[42] The reports suggested that it decreased hot flashes a little. This drug is primarily of historical interest and is not recommended.

Methyldopa has also been studied, with suggestions that it decreases hot flashes mildly.[43] Nonetheless, the toxicities observed in the single trial precluded its being recommended.

In recent years, acupuncture has been proposed and studied in pilot trials with promising results.[44,45] Prospective controlled studies continue. One completed trial, using a sham acupuncture control arm versus "medically directed" acupuncture, did not find any benefit for the medically directed acupuncture.[46] Results of further trials are awaited.

SUMMARY REGARDING TREATMENTS FOR HOT FLASHES

In summary, most women and most physicians prefer nonestrogenic therapies for hot flashes in breast cancer survivors. Progestational agents, such as intramuscular medroxyprogesterone acetate, substantially reduce hot flashes more than any other well-tested agents. Despite hypothetical concerns about progestational agents, there are no good data proving that it is detrimental in cancer patients. It is effective as short-term treatment and may reasonably be considered. In a randomized trial that prospectively compared medroxyprogesterone with venlafaxine, the former caused fewer toxicities and more substantially reduced hot flashes.[47] It also was more economical.

For physicians or patients who wish to avoid hormones altogether, newer antidepressants or gabapentin are worth trying. Venlafaxine is begun at a dose of 37.5 mg/day for 1 week and then increased to 75 mg/day. Higher doses are no better.[23] Paroxetine is used at a dose of 10 mg orally per day. Gabapentin 300 mg orally per day is recommended for a few days, increased to 300 mg twice per day for a few days, and then to 300 mg three times per day. Higher doses might be more effective[34] but have not been studied in a placebo-controlled trial.

Available data suggest that treatments that work in women are also effective in men who have hot flashes.[21,48] Therefore, despite the fact that these agents have not being evaluated nearly as thoroughly in men as in women, the same treatment recommendations are reasonable.

ONGOING STUDIES

There are several current research trials evaluating interventions in women who wish to avoid estrogen. These include studies of other new antidepressants, additional acupuncture methods, and other neuroactive agents.

BONE LOSS

Pathophysiology

Women abruptly lose bone mass at the menopause. This is caused by a loss of estrogen. For example, bone loss at the hip is about 0.5% per year after 35 years of age. However, there is an additional 5% to 7% loss associated with the menopause.[49] In breast cancer survivors, premature menopause can occur as a result of surgery, radiation therapy, and/or chemotherapy. In addition, aromatase inhibitors can potentiate bone loss in postmenopausal women.[50]

Clinical Manifestations

Bone loss is asymptomatic for a long time in most patients. Substantial chronic bone loss increases fracture risk. This can lead to pain, disability, and increased mortality.[49]

Treatment

The basic management consists of screening patients who are at risk. The American Society of Clinical Oncology (ASCO) and other groups, have developed guidelines.[51] These recommend that women at high risk receive bone mineral density screening annually.

For bone mineral density testing, T scores are commonly used to define osteopenia or osteoporosis. Osteoporosis is defined as a T score lower than −2.5 (i.e., 2.5 standard deviations below the normal maximal bone density for healthy middle-aged women). Commonly, the total bone mineral density of the lumbar spine (L2 + L3 + L4) is one measure.[49,51] The other most reliable measurement is on the femoral neck. Although measurements are done in other areas also, there is less confidence in these results.

For all women who at risk and for those with bone loss, calcium 1200 to 1500 mg per day (including dietary calcium) are recommended, along with vitamin D 400 to 800 IU/day.[49,51] In addition, weight-bearing exercise decreases bone loss. Cessation of smoking is a standard recommendation.

In osteoporosis (or osteopenia with increased risk factors), bisphosphonates are commonly recommended. These include oral bisphosphonates such as risedronate or alendronate, usually given once per week. Zoledronic acid can be given intravenously at 6- to 12-month intervals.[49,51] Bisphosphonates are well tolerated in many women, their most common clinical toxicity being heartburn. Patients should be upright for 30 minutes after taking this medication and should not eat anything during that time. A newly appreciated toxicity is osteonecrosis, which classically affects the jaw after dental procedures.[52] This can be a devastating problem, although it is uncommon (small percentage) if bisphosphonates are used for less than 2 years.

For those who cannot tolerate bisphosphonates, calcitonin is an alternative, although it is expensive and needs to be given daily.[53] Calcitonin may be less potent, with equivocal results in the hip.[49,53]

Raloxifene, a selective estrogen receptor–modifying agent like tamoxifen, has been approved by the U.S. Food and Drug Administration (FDA) for prevention of osteoporosis. Nonetheless, it is believed to be contraindicated in some cancer survivors. There are data to suggest that continued use of tamoxifen after the first 5 years may be detrimental[1]; because raloxifene is similar, it is recommended that raloxifene not be used in this group of patients. Raloxifene is also believed to be contraindicated in those who are taking aromatase inhibitors, because of the similarity of tamoxifen and raloxifene, while understanding that tamoxifen interferes with the activity of aromatase inhibitors, as was demonstrated in the Anastrozole, Tamoxifen, Alone or in Combination (ATAC) trial.[5]

Ongoing Studies

Studies continue at this time to delineate potential therapies for breast cancer survivors at risk for osteoporosis.

Understanding that premenopausal women receiving chemotherapy develop bone loss, one prospective trial randomized such women to receive either (1) calcium and vitamin D and weight-bearing exercise or (2) the same plus a bisphosphonate. It is hoped that this trial will determine whether it is appropriate to treat women prophylactically, rather than simply monitoring them closely and treating if osteoporosis develops.

Randomized trials are also evaluating women given aromatase inhibitors; women are randomly assigned to receive either calcium and vitamin D or the same plus a bisphosphonate. It does not appear to be appropriate to treat all women who are taking aromatase inhibitors with bisphosphonates, unless there is evidence of osteoporosis or marked osteopenia.

SEXUAL FUNCTION

Vaginal Dryness

Pathophysiology

The vagina contains estrogen receptors and becomes atrophic when estrogen decreases. The vaginal mucosa exhibits fewer secretions and less tissue flexibility. The vaginal lining gets thinner and pale, with decreased blood flow. The rugal folds in the vagina become less prominent. The pH of the vaginal tissue also changes, becoming more alkaline.[54,55]

Clinical Manifestations

Decreased tissue flexibility can cause pain with intercourse. Fewer secretions and smaller vaginal folds (rugae) can decrease pleasurable feelings. The thinning of the vaginal wall coupled with decreased tissue flexibility can cause trauma or bleeding with intercourse. In addition, with the higher vaginal pH, women can be more vulnerable to urinary tract infections.[54,55]

Treatment

Estrogen therapy relieves symptoms of vaginal dryness when given either systemically or locally.[56] Systemic estrogen therapy is relatively contraindicated in many women and avoided in breast cancer survivors.

Views vary with regard to local estrogen therapy. Claims have been made that little is absorbed. Nonetheless, there is evidence that vaginal estrogen therapy is systemically absorbed, regardless of the source.[57] Given the new information that suggests that depletion of all estrogen sources in postmenopausal women (i.e., with aromatase inhibitors) decreases breast cancer risk,[5] vaginal estrogen therapy is of some concern.

Nonestrogenic vaginal lubricants are available. There have been a few randomized trials involving a polycarbophil base lubricant, Replens. One study evaluated Replens against dienestrol cream,[58] another against a pectin-based lubricant,[59] a third against a placebo water-based lubricant.[60] In each study, all lubricants appeared to be effective in decreasing symptoms of dryness, dyspareunia, itching, and irritation. However, none of the nonhormonal lubricants improved the health of the vaginal tissues as well as the estrogen did.

ONGOING STUDIES

There is pilot information suggesting that pilocarpine, an agent used to treat Sjögren's syndrome, might alleviate vaginal dryness.[61] A placebo-controlled, double-blinded trial is ongoing.

Libido

Pathophysiology

Changes in sexual health, such as a decreased interest in sex or libido and inability to achieve orgasm, are common in many women as they approach middle age.[62] Many of these symptoms are probably related to hormone changes. More extensive hormonal changes and physiological effects (e.g., fatigue) resulting from treatment in cancer survivors, as well as side effects from pharmacological agents used to manage symptoms (e.g., antidepressant therapy) contribute.[63]

Nonetheless, hormonal changes are not the only issue that determines sexual health. Stress due to cancer and other life issues and body image changes related to surgery and radiation can negatively affect sexual health.[64] Relationships are also important.

Clinical Manifestations

Clinical manifestations of decreased sexual health include lack of interest, which can result not only in less frequent sexual activity but also in decreased intimacy. Other problems can include inability to have an orgasm, inability to become aroused, and decreased satisfaction with the sexual experience.[65]

Treatment

Testosterone has been the most commonly evaluated pharmacological intervention for decreased libido, orgasm, and arousal.[62] Transdermal testosterone has been tested in daily doses of 300 to 450 µg and 10 mg orally. It is thought to be safer because it bypasses first-pass liver effects and appears to have fewer side effects. Many of these studies have been done in women with bilateral oophorectomy and hypoactive sexual desire disorder. Although statistically significant differences were found for desire, orgasm, and pleasure measures in several randomized, placebo-controlled trials, the clinical significance of the differences was small and long-term safety was not established.[66,67]

Nonpharmacological interventions have also been evaluated for improving sexual health, particularly libido. The most common nonpharmacological interventions have been psychoeducational measures, including counseling and behavioral coping strategies.[62] One intervention study used a comprehensive assessment intervention for menopause-related symptom management. Outcomes included a sexual functioning scale. The intervention, which included assessing and managing hot flashes, vaginal dryness, and urinary symptoms, improved all items on the Cancer Rehabilitation Evaluation System (CARES) sexual functioning scale.[68,69] This suggests that overall sexual health can be improved by assessing and aggressively managing menopause-related symptoms.

SUMMARY

Menopause-related symptoms are prominent in cancer, as they are in women without cancer. Most problems are related to changes in hormones. Estrogen replacement therapy commonly relieves many of these complaints, but there are problems. Several nonestrogenic therapies are available for many of these symptoms. It is hoped that current studies will further refine these therapeutic options.

REFERENCES

1. Gracia CR, Freeman EW. Acute consequences of the menopausal transition: The rise of common menopausal symptoms. Endocrinol Metab Clin North Am 2004;33:675-689.
2. Burke LM. Sexual dysfunction following radiotherapy for cervical cancer. Br J Nurs 1996;5:239-244.
3. Crandall C, Petersen L, Ganz PA, et al. Association of breast cancer and its therapy with menopause-related symptoms. Menopause 2004;11:519-530.
4. Poniatowski BC, Grimm P, Cohen G. Chemotherapy-induced menopause: A literature review. Cancer Invest 2001;19:641-648.
5. Baum M, Budzar AU, Cuzick J, et al. Anastrozole alone or in combination with tamoxifen versus tamoxifen alone for adjuvant treatment of postmenopausal women with early breast cancer: First results of the ATAC randomized trial. Lancet 2002;359:2131-2139.
6. Goss PE, Ingle JN, Martino S, et al. A randomized trial of letrozole in postmenopausal women after five years of tamoxifen therapy for early-stage breast cancer. N Engl J Med 2003;349:1793-1802.
7. Shanafelt TD, Barton DL, Adjei AA, et al. Pathophysiology and treatment of hot flashes. Mayo Clin Proc 2002;77:1207-1218.
8. Berendsen HG. Hot flashes and serotonin. J Br Menopause Soc 2002;8:30-34.
9. Finck G, Barton DL, Loprinzi CL. Definitions of hot flashes in breast cancer survivors. J Pain Symptom Manage 1998;16:327-333.
10. Kronenberg F. Hot flashes: Epidemiology and physiology. Ann N Y Acad Sci 1990;592:52-86; discussion 123-133.
11. Utian WH, Shoupe D, Bachmann G. Relief of vasomotor symptoms and vaginal atrophy with lower doses of conjugated equine estrogens and medroxyprogesterone acetate. Fertil Steril 2001;75:1065-1079.
12. Col NF, Hirota LK, Orr RK, et al. Hormone replacement therapy after breast cancer: A systematic review and quantitative assessment of risk. J Clin Oncol 2001;19:2357-2363.

13. O'Meara ES, Rossing MA, Daling JR, et al. Hormone replacement after a diagnosis of breast cancer in relation to recurrence and mortality. J Natl Cancer Inst 2001;93:754-762.

14. von Schoultz E, Rutqvist LE. Menopausal hormone therapy after breast cancer: The Stockholm randomized trial. J Natl Cancer Inst 2005;97:533-535.

15. Anderson GL, Limacher M, Assaf AR, et al. Effects of conjugated equine estrogen in postmenopausal women with hysterectomy: The Women's Health Initiative randomized controlled trial. JAMA 2004;291:1701-1712.

16. Rossouw JE, Anderson GL, Prentice RL, et al. Risks and benefits of estrogen plus progestin in healthy postmenopausal women: Principal results from the Women's Health Initiative randomized controlled trial. JAMA 2002;288:321-333.

17. Homberg L, Anderson H. HABITS (Hormonal Replacement Therapy After Breast Cancer—Is It Safe?) A randomized comparison: Trial stopped. Lancet 2004;363:453-455.

18. Goldberg RM, Loprinzi CL, O'Fallon JR, et al. Transdermal clonidine for ameliorating tamoxifen-induced hot flashes. J Clin Oncol 1994;12:155-158.

19. Pandya KJ, Raubertas RF, Flynn PJ, et al. Oral clonidine in postmenopausal patients with breast cancer experiencing tamoxifen-induced hot flashes: A University of Rochester Cancer Center Community Clinical Oncology Program study. Ann Intern Med 2000;132:788-793.

20. Sloan JA, Loprinzi CL, Novotny PJ, et al. Methodologic lessons learned from hot flash studies. J Clin Oncol 2001;19:4280-4290.

21. Loprinzi CL, Pisansky TM, Fonseca R, et al. Pilot evaluation of venlafaxine hydrochloride for the therapy of hot flashes in cancer survivors. J Clin Oncol 1998;16:2377-2381.

22. Stearns V, Isaacs C, Rowland J, et al. A pilot trial assessing the efficacy of paroxetine hydrochloride (Paxil) in controlling hot flashes in breast cancer survivors. Ann Oncol 2000;11:17-22.

23. Loprinzi CL, Kugler JW, Sloan JA, et al. Venlafaxine in management of hot flashes in survivors of breast cancer: A randomised controlled trial. Lancet 2000;356:2059-2063.

24. Evans ML, Pritts E, Vittinghoff E, et al. Management of postmenopausal hot flushes with venlafaxine hydrochloride: A randomized, controlled trial. Obstet Gynecol 2005;105:161-166.

25. Kalogeropoulos S, Kampas N, Petrogiannopoulos C, et al. Long-term management of menopausal hot flashes with venlafaxine. The 11th World Congress of Gynecological Endocrinology. Gynecol Endocrinol 2004;18(Suppl 1):OP95a.

26. Stearns V, Beebe KL, Iyengar M, et al. Paroxetine controlled release in the treatment of menopausal hot flashes: A randomized controlled trial. JAMA 2003;289:2827-2834.

27. Stearns V, Slack R, Greep N, et al. Paroxetine is an effective treatment for hot flashes: Results from a prospective randomized clinical trial. J Clin Oncol 2005;23:6919-6930.

28. Stearns V, Johnson MD, Rae JM, et al. Active tamoxifen metabolite plasma concentrations after coadministration of tamoxifen and the selective serotonin reuptake inhibitor paroxetine. J Natl Cancer Inst 2003;95:1758-1764.

29. Loprinzi CL, Sloan JA, Perez EA, et al. Phase III evaluation of fluoxetine for treatment of hot flashes. J Clin Oncol 2002;20:1578-1583.

30. Suvanto-Luukkonen E, Koivunen R, Sundstrom H, et al. Citalopram and fluoxetine in the treatment of postmenopausal symptoms: A prospective, randomized, 9-month, placebo-controlled, double-blind study. Menopause 2005;12:18-26.

31. Kimmick GG, Lovato J, McQuellon R, et al. Randomized, placebo-controlled study of sertraline (Zoloft TM) for the treatment of hot flashes in women with early stage breast cancer taking tamoxifen. Proc Am Society Clin Oncol 2001;20:1585a.

32. Guttuso TJ Jr. Gabapentin's effects on hot flashes and hypothermia. Neurology 2000;54:2161-2163.

33. Pandya KJ, Morrow GR, Roscoe JA, et al. Gabapentin for hot flashes in 420 women with breast cancer: A randomised double-blind placebo-controlled trial. Lancet 2005;366:818-824.

34. Guttuso T Jr, Kurlan R, McDermott MP, et al. Gabapentin's effects on hot flashes in postmenopausal women: A randomized controlled trial. Obstet Gynecol 2003;101:337-345.

35. Loprinzi CL, Michalak JC, Quella SK, et al. Megestrol acetate for the prevention of hot flashes. N Engl J Med 1994;331:347-352.

36. Bertelli G, Venturini M, Del Mastro L, et al. Intramuscular depot medroxyprogesterone versus oral megestrol for the control of postmenopausal hot flashes in breast cancer patients: A randomized study. Ann Oncol 2002;13:883-888.

37. Barton DL, Loprinzi CL, Quella SK, et al. Prospective evaluation of vitamin E for hot flashes in breast cancer survivors. J Clin Oncol 1998;16:495-500.

38. Loprinzi CL, Quella SK, Barton D, et al. Evaluation of soy phytoestrogens for the treatment of hot flashes in breast cancer survivors: An NCCTG trial. J Clin Oncol 1999;16:495-500.

39. The role of isoflavones in menopausal health: Consensus opinion of The North American Menopause Society. Menopause 2000;7:215-229.

40. Jacobson JS, Troxel AB, Evans J, et al. Randomized trial of black cohosh for the treatment of hot flashes among women with a history of breast cancer. J Clin Oncol 2001;19:2739-2745.

41. Pockaj BA, Gallagher J, Loprinzi CL, et al. Phase III double blinded randomized trial to evaluate the use of black cohosh in the treatment of hot flashes: A NCCTG trial. (Abstract #8013.) J Clin Oncol 2005;23:732S.

42. Bergmans mg, Merkus JM, Corbey RS, et al. Effect of Bellergal Retard on climacteric complaints: A double-blind, placebo-controlled study. Maturitas 1987;9:227-234.

43. Hammond mg, Hatley L, Talbert LM. A double blind study to evaluate the effect of methyldopa on menopausal vasomotor flushes. J Clin Endocrinol Metab 1984;58:1158-1160.

44. Wyon Y, Lindgren R, Lundeberg T, et al. Effects of acupuncture on climacteric vasomotor symptoms, quality of life, and urinary excretion of neuropeptides among postmenopausal women. Menopause 1995;2:3-12.

45. Porzio G, Trapasso T, Martelli S, et al. Acupuncture in the treatment of menopause-related symptoms in women taking tamoxifen. Tumori 2002;88:128-130.

46. Vincent A, Barton D, Mandrekar J, et al. Acupuncture for hot flashes: A randomized sham-controlled clinical study. Menopause 2007;14:45-52.

47. Loprinzi C, Levitt R, Sloan JA, et al. Medroxyprogesterone acetate (MPA) versus venlafaxine for hot flashes: A North Central Cancer Treatment Group trial. (Abstract #8014.) Proc Am Soc Clin Oncol 2005;4(16S, pt I):732S.

48. Loprinzi CL, Barton DL, Carpenter LA, et al. Pilot evaluation of paroxetine for treating hot flashes in men. Mayo Clin Proc 2004;79:1247-1251.

49. Management of postmenopausal osteoporosis: Position statement of the North American Menopause Society. Menopause 2002;9:84-101.

50. Morales L, Neven P, Timmerman D, et al. Acute effects of tamoxifen and third-generation aromatase inhibitors on menopausal symptoms of breast cancer patients. Anticancer Drugs 2004;15:753-760.

51. Hillner BE, Ingle JN, Chlebowski RT, et al. American Society of Clinical Oncology 2003 update on the role of bisphosphonates and bone health issues in women with breast cancer. J Clin Oncol 2003;21:4042-4057.

52. Ruggiero SL, Mehrotra B, Rosenberg TJ, et al. Osteonecrosis of the jaws associated with the use of bisphosphonates: A review of 63 cases. J Oral Maxillofac Surg 2004;62:527-534.

53. Gur A, Colpan L, Cevik R, et al. Comparison of zinc excretion and biochemical markers of bone remodeling in the assessment of the effects of alendronate and calcitonin on bone in postmenopausal osteoporosis. Clin Biochem 2005;38:66-72.

54. SOGC Clinical Practice Guidelines: The detection and management of vaginal atrophy. Int J Gynecol Obstet 2005;88:222-228.

55. Willhite LA, O'Connell MB. Urogenital atrophy: Prevention and treatment. Pharmacotherapy 2001;21:464-480.

56. Handa VL, Bachus KE, Johnston WW, et al. Vaginal administration of low-dose conjugated estrogens: Systemic absorption and effects on the endometrium. Obstet Gynecol 1994;84:215-218.

57. Santen RJ, Pinkerton JV, Conaway M, et al. Treatment of urogenital atrophy with low-dose estradiol: Preliminary results. Menopause 2002;9:179-187.

58. Bygdeman M, Swahn ML. Replens versus dienoestrol cream in the symptomatic treatment of vaginal atrophy in postmenopausal women. Maturitas 1996;23:259-263.

59. Caswell M, Kane M. Comparison of the moisturization efficacy of two vaginal moisturizers: Pectin versus polycarbophil technologies. J Cosmet Sci 2002;53:81-87.

60. Loprinzi CL, Abu-Ghazaleh S, Sloan JA, et al. Phase III randomized double-blind study to evaluate the efficacy of a polycarbophil-based vaginal moisturizer in women with breast cancer. J Clin Oncol 1997;15:969-973.

61. Le Veque G, Hendrix S. Oral pilocarpine to treat vaginal xerosis associated with chemotherapy-induced amenorrhea in pre-menopausal women. J Clin Oncol 2004;22:749.

62. Barton D, Wilwerding M, Carpenter L, et al. Libido as part of sexuality in female cancer survivors. Oncol Nurs Forum 2004;31:599-609.

63. Greendale GA, Petersen L, Zibecchi L, et al. Factors related to sexual function in postmenopausal women with a history of breast cancer. Menopause 2001;8:111-119.

64. Gamel, C, Hengeveld M, Davis B. Informational needs about the effects of gynaecological cancer on sexuality: A review of the literature [review]. J Clin Nurs 2000;9:678-688.

65. McKee AL Jr, Schover LR. Sexuality rehabilitation. Cancer 2001;92(4 Suppl):1008-1012.

66. Shifren JL, Braunstein GD, Simon JA, et al. Transdermal testosterone treatment in women with impaired sexual function after oophorectomy. N Engl J Med 2000;343:682-688.

67. Braunstein GD, Sundwall DA, Katz M, et al. Safety and efficacy of a testosterone patch for the treatment of hypoactive sexual desire disorder in surgically menopausal women: A randomized, placebo-controlled trial. Arch Intern Med 2005;165:1582-1589.

68. Ganz PA, Greendale GA, Petersen L, et al. Managing menopausal symptoms in breast cancer survivors: Results of a randomized controlled trial. J Natl Cancer Inst 2000;92:1054-1064.

69. Zibecchi L, Greendale GA, Ganz PA. Continuing education. Comprehensive menopausal assessment: An approach to managing vasomotor and urogenital symptoms in breast cancer survivors. Oncol Nurs Forum 2003;30:393-407.

SUGGESTED READING

Barton D, Loprinzi C. Making sense of the evidence regarding nonhormonal treatments for hot flashes. Clin J Oncol Nurs 2004;8:39-42.

Hillner BE, Ingle JN, Chlebowski RT, et al. American Society of Clinical Oncology 2003 update on the role of bisphosphonates and bone health issues in women with breast cancer. J Clin Oncol 2003;21:4042-4057.

Shanafelt TD, Barton DL, Adjei AA, Loprinzi CL. Pathophysiology and treatment of hot flashes. Mayo Clin Proc 2002;77: 1207-1218.

Society of Obstetricians and Gynaecologiss of Canaca (SOGC) Clinical Practice Guidelines: The detection and management of vaginal atrophy. Int J Gynecol Obstet 2005;88:222-228.

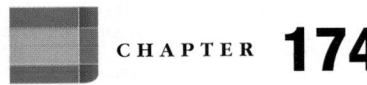

CHAPTER **174**

Death Rattle

H. Christof Müller-Busch and Thomas Jehser

KEY POINTS

- Death rattle is the breathing noise caused by the accumulation of airway secretions in the imminently dying.

- It is a strong predictor of death and is observed in about 50% of dying patients within 48 hours of death.

- It provokes more distress for the family and carers than for the dying patient and must be distinguished from dyspnea and discomfort in breathing.

- Explaining the cause to the family and friends and providing nonpharmacological measures such as positioning, fluid restriction in the final phase, and mouth care reduce the distress caused by the rattling noise in addition to specific pharmacological approaches.

- Anticholinergic drugs are effective in reducing death rattle when given early enough and before airway secretions increase.

He had difficulty in breathing and was given oxygen. . . . Mahler lay with dazed eyes: one finger was conducting on the quilt. There was a smile on his lips and twice he said: "Mozart!" His eyes were very big. I begged the doctor to give him a large dose of morphine so that he might feel nothing more. He replied in a loud voice. I seized his hands: "Talk softly, he might hear you." "He hears nothing now."

How terrible the callousness of doctors is in such moments. . . . The death-agony began. I was sent into the next room. The death-rattle lasted several hours. . . . That ghastly sound ceased suddenly at midnight of the 18th of May during a tremendous thunderstorm.[1]

The term *death rattle* describes the noisy rattling breathing that occurs in the final phase of dying. The noise is produced by oscillatory movements of secretions in the upper airway during inspiratory and expiratory phases of respiration and is accompanied by circulatory failure and lowered consciousness.[2]

The rattling noise is a strong indicator of the dying process. Death rattle should be distinguished from dyspnea, which describes the subjective feeling and per-

ception of breathlessness and the experience of respiratory effort as a "discomfort in breathing." Death rattle is often a source of distress for family members, friends, and palliative caregivers[3] in bereavement and causes concern about the quality of dying. Between 6% and 92% of dying people develop death rattle in the last days of life[4,5]; treatment success rates vary from 40% to 70%.[6]

BASIC SCIENCE

Death rattle is caused by excessive production or retention of airway secretions in patients who are too weak to expectorate or unable to swallow. It might be associated with a slight obstruction in the upper airways (hypopharynx and trachea). The accumulation of sputum in these areas usually is a result of impairment of the cough reflex, as in deep coma or near death. Airway secretions are synthesized in the salivary glands and bronchial mucosa; these structures are innervated by cholinergic nerves and are sensitive to changes in vagal tone with inhibition of secretory rate.[7] Five muscarinic receptors can be differentiated, but only the M_2 receptor on airway smooth muscle and the M_3 on glandular tissue in the salivary glands and airway mucosa produce secretions.

The distinction between the rattling noise caused by nonswallowed (or nonexpectorated) salivary and/or bronchial secretions ("real death rattle," or type 1) and the noise produced by respiratory pathology ("pseudo death rattle," or type 2) is important for treatment. Type 1 is acute and is produced by the accumulation of salivary secretions in the last hours of life in patients with reduced swallowing reflexes, whereas type 2 develops more slowly (days) in weakened patients because of increased bronchial secretions and reduced cough. Mixed cases occur in pulmonary pathology, such as lung cancer or severe pneumonia. Type 2 seems to respond less to antimuscarinics.[8]

EPIDEMIOLOGY

The reported incidence in patients with terminal disease varies from 6% to 92%[7,9,10] and may depend on pulmonary pathology and use of parenteral fluids in the terminal phase of life. Patients who were dehydrated, as measured biochemically, were less likely to develop increased respiratory tract secretions in the final phase than those who were not dehydrated.[11]

In a prospective study, death rattle was observed in 44% of hospice patients with reduced consciousness. In those with pulmonary malignancies, primary brain tumors, or brain metastases death rattle was more common.[12,13] Restriction of parenteral fluids before withdrawal of mechanical ventilation reduced the death rattle produced by excessive respiratory secretion in neurological patients.[14] In 75% of those in whom death rattle was observed, death occurred within 48 hours.[15]

PATHOPHYSIOLOGY

Airway secretions are produced by the salivary glands and bronchial mucosa muscarinic receptors. Glandular fluid production and flow rates of airway secretions vary.[16] Normally, the ciliated epithelial cells, at all levels of the respiratory tract (except the alveoli, nose, and throat), are in constant motion to propel mucus and particles up the tract to be expectorated or subconsciously swallowed.[17] Therefore, the mucociliary transport system is the primary defense mechanism for the lower respiratory tract. It prevents the entrance of viruses, bacteria, and other pathogenic substances into the body. The normal rate of approximately 2000 mL of mucus per day produced by oropharyngeal and tracheobronchial mucus glands[18] can be increased by various irritants.[19] Excessive secretions, abnormal mucus secretions inhibiting normal clearance, ciliary dysfunction, lack of swallowing, decreased or absent cough, and a supine or semirecumbent position cause pooling of secretions in the oropharynx and bronchi leading to respiratory congestion. Congestion can be stimulated by infection or inflammation, pulmonary embolism, pulmonary edema, or congestive heart failure. Bronchial secretory glands are largely innervated by vagal cholinergic nerve fibers, but stimulation of cough receptors by adrenergic nerves and inflammatory changes can produce increased secretions.[20] Respiratory congestion becomes apparent earlier if it is produced in response to infection, pulmonary edema, or aspiration of food or fluid (Fig. 174-1).

In the situation of the dying patient, increased secretion of mucus in the lower pharynx produces the noise of death rattle by turbulent airflow through or over these secretions, and its intensity is dependent on ventilatory rate and airway resistance.[21] Bennett proposed that two types of death rattles should be differentiated.[17] Type I predominantly is caused by salivary secretions that accumulate very near to death when swallowing reflexes are inhibited. Type 1 is largely unpredictable and becomes clinically significant only in the last few hours of life. Type 2 is characterized by predominantly bronchial secretions that accumulate over several days as patients deteriorate and become too weak to cough effectively (see "Case Study: Treatment of Dyspnea with Death Rattle at the End of Life").

CLINICAL MANIFESTATIONS AND DIFFERENTIAL DIAGNOSIS

Death rattle is a strong indicator that the patient is dying; it occurs within 16 to 57 hours before death and often

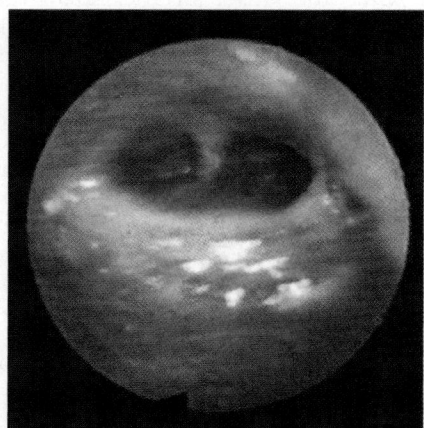

FIGURE 174-1 Fiberbronchoscopic view of accumulated secretions in the laryngeal region.

 C A S E   S T U D Y

Treatment of Dyspnea with Death Rattle at the End of Life

A 49-year-old male patient was admitted to the palliative care unit with severe dyspnea and cachexia due to hypopharyngeal carcinoma diagnosed 15 months earlier. Initial treatment consisted of high-dose radiochemotherapy with cisplatin. Second-line chemotherapy with taxol was interrupted because of local progress and pulmonary and bone metastases. With a history of heavy smoking (45 pack-years) and alcohol misuse, the patient was also suffering from chronic obstructive pulmonary disease, with permanent productive coughing, and lower leg edema caused by mixed-type cardiac disease. At admission, the patient was able to walk and speak but was too weak to expectorate effectively; he also had saliva with increased viscosity caused by poor function of the parotid glands after radiation therapy.

Treatment objectives were the relief of dyspnea and the associated fear of suffocation by instituting the following steps:

1. Inhalation of sodium chloride solution four times daily, and additional inhalation with ambroxol twice daily. Physiotherapy was added to improve breathing economy and expectoration capability
2. Intensified mouth care with citric, pineapple, and salvia extracts.
3. Antibiotics after a report of high-level colonization with *Klebsiella* species in the tracheal secretions.

After a few days, the patient improved enough to be discharged home.

Readmission became necessary after 4 weeks at home. The lymphedema had become worse and was generalized (legs, face, tongue). The patient suffered from dyspnea and was agitated and disoriented.

The treatment objectives had not changed, but different measures were undertaken:

1. In addition to medication with diuretics, spironolactone, and corticosteroids, lymph drainage massage was added to reduce lymphedema.
2. When agitated fear increased, palliative sedation with midazolam (0.5 to 3 mg/hr) was administered, which reduced the fear, ameliorated sleep, but kept up the ability to communicate with family members during the daytime.
3. For breakthrough episodes of dyspnea, the patient received morphine 2.5 mg IV four to six times daily. In addition, scopolamine, 1.4 mg/24 hr was given by continuous IV infusion.

The patient was able to respond to questions and consistently denied any fear or breathing difficulties when asked. When he reached the final stage of the dying process and was mostly somnolent, intravenous fluids were stopped while intensive mouth care by relatives and nurses was continued. No further treatment changes were necessary up to the patient's death 36 hours later.

precedes other symptoms, such as cyanosis and the clouding of consciousness. It is one of the five signs of impending death, along with reduced consciousness, breathing with mandibular movement, cyanotic extremities, and lack of radial pulse.[22] The loud gurgling, rattling noise can usually be heard without a stethoscope. Often, it is heard also from outside the patient's room and concerns neighbors and visitors.[23] Death rattle (if it developed) occurred first at a mean of 57 hours before death; other signs of impending death were found later.[4] Sometimes, the respiratory rate is increased and becomes irregular, with increased breathing efforts.

Differentiation of underlying alveolar involvement manifested by rales is difficult, if not impossible, to make by auscultation. Palpation of the chest wall can identify vibratory tremors (fremitus) in the center of the anterior chest over the trachea or more peripherally. Central vibrations suggest accumulated secretions in the trachea, whereas peripheral fremitus indicates terminal retained secretions. Additional investigations like radiographic studies or ultrasonography should be done only if an origin of the noise is suspected that might be treated with benefit.

Although similar noises may occur in patients who are not imminently dying, such as those with brain injury or with various disorders leading to increased production or decreased clearance of secretions, the possibility of imminent death should be discussed with the family.

Although death rattle is not felt as uncomfortable by most dying patients, it must be differentiated from distressing forms of dyspnea and breathing problems such as air hunger, breathlessness with panic attacks, and tachypnea, which also can occur in the dying but have different therapeutic approaches. Diminished and/or adventitious breath sounds can be a sign of pulmonary congestion.

Careful assessment of air hunger will determine whether it is treatable. Because the classic air hunger during the dying process usually does not respond to oxygen, it should not routinely be given. Dyspnea can be alleviated by opening windows and using a fan to promote air movement, which stimulates trigeminal nerve receptors in the cheek and nasopharynx, inhibiting the sensation of difficulty in breathing. Tachypnea may accompany dyspnea and should be treated with morphine (or another strong opioid). Morphine alters perceptions of breathlessness, reduces anxiety, and dilates the pulmonary vessels, thereby reducing oxygen consumption and decreasing pulmonary congestion. Symptom relief occurs before sedation, and sedation before vital signs become depressed.[24] Ordinarily, excess carbon dioxide in the blood stimulates respiration, but during the final 48 hours of life, as pulmonary congestion and poor gas exchange lead to a rise in carbon dioxide levels, the brain becomes less responsive to this signal. Breathing becomes irregular, and shallow breathing alternates with periods of apnea. Families should be made aware that this breathing pattern, known as Cheyne-Stokes respiration, is another sign of imminent death.[25]

TREATMENT

The most important aspect of care of a dying person is to reduce distress and to support the relatives in accepting and understanding the dying process. Noisy respirations almost always can be expected and, if treated appropri-

ately, should not be a concern for the family. The cause of the noisy breathing should be explained to the relatives, and they should be told that it is unlikely to be distressing for the patient. The term "death rattle" should be avoided, but communication about the sense of the noisy breathing as a sign of imminent death can reduce distressing feelings and burdening fears and perceptions.

Hydration in the terminal phase is controversial and should not concentrate on only one symptom. It must be handled individually. Reduced fluid intake can prevent the accumulation of secretions and pulmonary congestion. Parenteral and enteral infusions should be minimized; for the reduction of accumulated fluids, diuretics may be indicated. However, if a terminally ill patient exhibits agitated delirium or renal failure secondary to dehydration, artificial hydration is warranted. Fluid intake should depend on the evaluation of thirst and should be accompanied by good mouth care. When noisy breathing is observed, the patient should be positioned on the side or semiprone to facilitate postural drainage and reduce pooling of secretions. Gentle physiotherapeutic measures help when death rattle is associated with breathing problems and reduced coughing abilities.[26] In patients who are not imminently dying, a Trendelenburg maneuver may sometimes shift secretions to the oropharynx for easier removal.[27] Gentle oropharyngeal suctioning with a soft catheter can be useful, but it is often ineffective because the increased secretions encountered near death are not in the upper airway and are not easily accessible. Frequent suctioning is disturbing to both patients and relatives.

The standard of care is administration of anticholinergic drugs to block muscarinic receptors. These include the natural belladonna alkaloids (atropine, belladonna, hyoscyamine, and scopolamine) and related products. All of these agents can cause varying degrees of blurred vision, sedation, confusion, delirium, restlessness, hallucinations, palpitations, constipation, and urinary retention. The primary difference in these drugs is whether they are tertiary amines that cross the blood-brain barrier (BBB), such as scopolamine and atropine, or quaternary amines that do not, such as hyoscyamine and glycopyrrolate. Drugs that cross the BBB are apt to cause central nervous system toxicity (sedation, delirium).[28] Diuretics, dilatory drugs, opioids, and even sedatives have been used. When using anticholinergics, it seems important to administer at an early stage after the onset of the noisy respirations, although this poses difficulties. Early identification of predisposing signs can indicate the need for an anticholinergic. Sometimes, an increased dose of a currently used drug with anticholinergic properties, such as chlorpromazine or promethazine, may suffice.[29]

The most important predicting factor for treating death rattle effectively seems to be the distinction between rattle caused by nonexpectorated salivary and/or bronchial secretions and the that caused by possible underlying respiratory pathology. The distinction between salivary and bronchial secretions does not appear to play an important role.

There are no guidelines about which antisecretory drug to use and at what dose (Table 174-1). Mostly, hyoscine hydrobromide (scopolamine), hyoscyamine, or glycopyrrolate bromide (glycopyrrolate) is recommended. Hyoscine (scopolamine) is available in transdermal and

TABLE 174-1   Anticholinergic Drugs Used in Death Rattle

DRUG AND APPLICATION FORM	MECHANISM OF ACTION	SIDE EFFECTS AND PROBLEMS	DOSAGE IN ORAL TITRATION	DOSAGE IN PARENTERAL TITRATION
Hyoscine hydrobromide. (scopolamine)—tablets, ampules, drops, patch	Competitive inhibitors at postganglionic muscarinic receptor crossing BBB with direct CNS effects blocking cholinergic transmission in specific areas	Oral application is difficult in patients with swallowing problems; poor gastrointestinal absorption; skin irritation when given transdermally	Drops, tablets 0.2-0.4 mg q4-6h; titrate to symptom control	One to three transdermal patches every 3 days or 0.2-0.5 mg SC four to six times daily or 0.1 to 0.2 mg/hr by continuous IV or SC infusion
Hyoscyamine sulphate—tablets	Alkaloid of belladonna anticholinergic drug with antispasmodic properties	Oral application is difficult in patients with swallowing problems	Tablets 0.125-0.375 mg PO or SL q4-6h; titrate to symptom control	—
Glycopyrrolate—tablets, ampules	Quaternary synthetic antisecretory effects and less crossing of BBB	Xerostomia, photophobia, less CNS side effects	Start at 1 mg qd to qid; titrate to symptom control and side effects; maximum dose, 8 mg/24 hr	0.1-0.2 mg SC q4-6h or 0.4-1.2 mg/day by continuous IV or SC infusion
Atropine sulphate or hydrochloride—drops, tablets, ampules	Weaker antisecretory effects by competitive blocking muscarinic acetylcholine receptors	Confusion, hallucinations, and excitation by crossing BBB; cardiac arrhythmias	One to three drops (1%) or tablets q4-6h	0.2-0.5 mg SC or IM

BBB, blood-brain barrier; CNS, central nervous system.

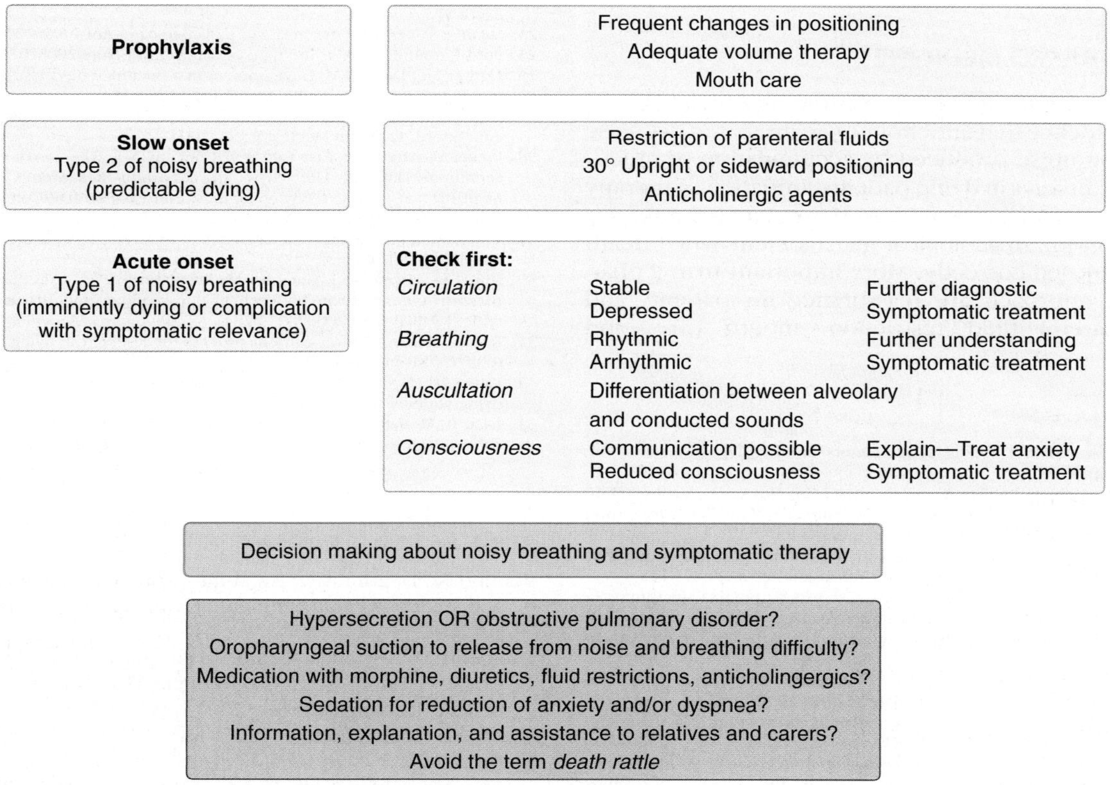

Prophylaxis	Frequent changes in positioning Adequate volume therapy Mouth care
Slow onset Type 2 of noisy breathing (predictable dying)	Restriction of parenteral fluids 30° Upright or sideward positioning Anticholinergic agents

Acute onset
Type 1 of noisy breathing
(imminently dying or complication
with symptomatic relevance)

Check first:
Circulation	Stable	Further diagnostic
	Depressed	Symptomatic treatment
Breathing	Rhythmic	Further understanding
	Arrhythmic	Symptomatic treatment
Auscultation	Differentiation between alveolary and conducted sounds	
Consciousness	Communication possible	Explain—Treat anxiety
	Reduced consciousness	Symptomatic treatment

Decision making about noisy breathing and symptomatic therapy

Hypersecretion OR obstructive pulmonary disorder?
Oropharyngeal suction to release from noise and breathing difficulty?
Medication with morphine, diuretics, fluid restrictions, anticholingergics?
Sedation for reduction of anxiety and/or dyspnea?
Information, explanation, and assistance to relatives and carers?
Avoid the term *death rattle*

FIGURE 174-2   Algorithm for assessment and decision making about noisy breathing.

parenteral formulations. Originally released to reduce motion sickness, the scopolamine patch is changed every 3 days. An alternative is intravenous or subcutaneous scopolamine, given by bolus or continuous infusion. The dosage and method of application depends on clinical experience and is not standardized. Doses range from 0.2 mg initially to 0.5 mg every 4 hours subcutaneously. Some administer 0.4 mg scopolamine subcutaneously fol-

lowed by a 1.5-mg transdermal patch. Some use atropine, 0.4 mg subcutaneously every 15 minutes, or hyoscyamine. Hyoscyamine has the advantage of not crossing the BBB and can be administered sublingually in tablet or liquid form three to four times per day.

Glycopyrrolate also does not cross the BBB and is more potent than atropine, but it is less potent than hyoscine hydrobromide. Subcutaneous bolus doses ranges from 0.2

to 0.4 mg and can be given also by continuous subcutaneous infusion.

The evidence for anticholinergic drugs remains inconclusive.[30] Subcutaneous hyoscine hydrobromide 0.4 mg is supposed to be more effective at improving symptoms at 30 minutes than glycopyrronium 0.2 mg by the same route; the duration of response is shorter for hyoscine butylbromide (1 hour) and longer for glycopyrronium (>6 hours). Randomized studies compared hyoscine hydrobromide (scopolamine) with glycopyrronium.[31] Comparative studies with hyoscine hydrobromide and glycopyrronium showed no significant clinical difference between the two.[32] One randomized study investigated the effectiveness of hyoscine hydrobromide 0.5 mg every 4 hours intravenously or subcutaneously with placebo. In addition, standardized sedatives were administered as required, and analgesic therapy was continued. Only a minimal reduction of death rattle was observed, but there was a greater incidence of pain expression and agitation in death rattle type 1.[33]

The combination of anticholinergics with prokinetic properties should be avoided. Figure 174-2 presents an algorithm for assessment and management of death rattle.

EVIDENCE-BASED MEDICINE

Evidence-based guidelines are missing, although there is empirical evidence that anticholinergic drugs can decrease the breathing noise produced by accumulation of mucus in the upper airways in dying patients. Initiation of therapy before the increased airway secretions start is important for successful pharmacological management when death rattle is diagnosed correctly. More important than a pharmacological approach are reassurance for patients and relatives, careful fluid restriction, mouth care, and positioning.

REFERENCES

1. Mahler A. Gustav Mahler: Memories and Letters. London: W. Clowes and Son, 1946.
2. Twycross R, Lichter I. The terminal phase. In Doyle D, Hanks GWC, MacDonald N (eds). Oxford Textbook of Palliative Medicine. New York: Oxford University Press, 1998, p 985.
3. Wee BL, Coleman PG, Hiller R, Holgate SH. The sound of death rattle I: Are relatives distressed by hearing the sound? Palliat Med 2006;20:171-175.
4. Morita T, Tsunoda J, Inoue S. Contributing factors to physical symptoms in terminally-ill cancer patients. J Pain Symptom Manage 1999;18:338-346.
5. Owens DA. Management of upper airway secretions at the end of life. J Hosp Palliat Nurs 2006;8:12-14.
6. Kass RM, Ellershaw J. Respiratory tract secretions in the dying patient: A retrospective study. J Pain Symptom Manage 2003;26:897-902.
7. Wildiers H, Menten J. Death rattle: Prevalence, prevention and treatment. J Pain Symptom Manage 2002;23:310-317.
8. Bennett M, Lucas V, Brennan M, et al. Using anti-muscarinic drugs in the management of death rattle: Evidence-based guidelines for palliative care. Palliat Med 2002;16:369-374.
9. Dudgeon D. Dyspnea, death rattle, and cough. In Ferrell BR, Coyle N (eds). Textbook of Palliative Nursing. New York: Oxford University Press, 2001, pp 164-174.
10. Morita T, Hyodo I, Yoshimi T, et al. Incidence and underlying etiologies of bronchial secretion in terminally ill cancer patients: A multicenter, prospective, observational study. J Pain Symptom Manage 2004;27:533-539.
11. Ellershaw JE, Sutcliffe JM, Saunders CM. Dehydration and the dying patient. J Pain Symptom Manage 1995;10:192-197.
12. Morita T, Tsunoda J, Inoue S, Chihara S. Risk factors death rattle in terminally ill cancer patients: A prospective exploratory study. Palliat Med 2000;14:19-23.
13. Voltz R, Borasio GD. Palliative therapy in the terminal stage of neurological disease. J Neurol 1997;244:2-10.
14. Kompanje EJO. The "death rattle" in the intensive care unit after withdrawal of mechanical ventilation in neurological patients. Neurocrit Care 2005;3:107-110.
15. Hallenbeck JL. Palliative Care Perspectives. New York: Oxford University Press, 2003.
16. Ship JA. Salivary glands and saliva: Diagnosing, managing, and preventing salivary gland disorders. Oral Dis 2002;8:77-89.
17. Bennett M. Death rattle: An audit of hyoscine (scopolamine) use and review of management. J Pain Symptom Manage 1996;12:229-233.
18. Elamn LB, Dubin RM, Kelley M, McCluskey L. Management of oropharyngeal and tracheobronchial secretions in patients with neurologic disease. J Palliat Med 2005;8:1150-1159.
19. Kim S, Shao MXG, Nadel J. Mucus production, secretion and and clearance. In Mason RJ, Broaddus VC, Murray JF (eds). Murray and Nadel's Textbook of Respiratory Medicine. Philadelphia: Saunders, 2005, pp 330-354.
20. Kaliner M, Shelhamer JH, Borson B, et al. Human respiratory mucous. Am Rev Respir Dis 1986;134:612-621.
21. Beach P. Treatment of respiratory congestion in patients with end-stage disease. Clin J Oncol Nurs 2003;7:153-155.
22. Morita T, Ichiki T, Tsunoda J, et al. A prospective study on the dying process in terminally ill cancer patients. Am J Hosp Palliat Care 1998;15:217-222.
23. Ellershaw J, Smith C, Overill S, et al. Care of the dying: Setting standards for symptom control in the last 48 hours of life. J Pain Symptom Manage 2001;21:12-17.
24. LaDuke S. Terminal dyspnea and palliative care. Am J Nurs 2001;101:26-31.
25. Ford Pitorak E. Care at the time of death. Am J Nurs 2003;103:42-52.
26. Corner J, O'Driscoll M. Development of a breathlessness assessment guide for use in palliative care. Palliat Med 1999;13:375-384.
27. Regnard C, Hockley J (eds). A Guide to Symptom Relief in Palliative Care, 5th ed. Oxford: Radcliffe Medical Press, 2004.
28. Bickel K, Arnold R. Fast Fact and Concept No. 109: Death Rattle and Oral Secretions. End of Life Physician Education Resource Center (EPERC). Available at http://www.eperc.mcw.edu/FastFactPDF/Concept%20109.pdf (accessed December 22, 2007).
29. Twycross R (ed). Symptom Management in Advanced Cancer, 3rd ed. Oxford: Radcliffe Medical Press, 2002.
30. Hugel H, Ellershaw J, Gambles M. Respiratory tract secretions in the dying patient: A comparison between glycopyrronium and hHyoscine hydrobromide. J Palliat Med 2006;9:279-284.
31. Rees E, Hardy J. Novel consent process for research in dying patients unable to give consent. BMJ 2003;327:198.
32. Laurey H. Hyoscine vs glycopyrronium for drying respiratory secretions in dying patients Br J Commun Nurs 2005;10:421-426.
33. Likar R, Molnar M, Rupacher E, et al. A clinical study examining the efficacy of scopolamine-hydrobromide in patients with death rattle: A randomized, double-blind, placebo-controlled study. Z Palliativmed 2002;3:15-19.

SUGGESTED READING

Bennett M. Death rattle: An audit of hyoscine (scopolamine) use and review of management. J Pain Symptom Manage 1996; 12:229-233.

Dudgeon D. Dyspnea, death rattle, and cough. In Ferrell BR, Coyle N (eds). Textbook of Palliative Nursing. New York: Oxford University Press, 2001, pp 164-174.

Twycross R, Lichter I. The terminal phase. In Doyle D, Hanks GWC, MacDonald N (eds). Oxford Textbook of Palliative Medicine. New York: Oxford University Press, 1998, p 985.

Wildiers H, Menten J. Death rattle: Prevalence, prevention and treatment. J Pain Symptom Manage 2002;23:310-317.

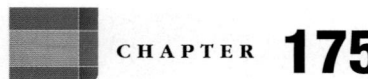

CHAPTER **175**

Seizures and Movement Disorders

Hunter Groninger and J. Cameron Muir

KEY POINTS

- Seizures are common in patients with primary or metastatic intracranial tumors.
- There is no evidence to support primary seizure prophylaxis in brain tumor patients.
- Benzodiazepines are essential for managing acute seizures but should not be used for secondary seizure prophylaxis.
- Opioid-induced myoclonus can be managed by (1) attempting to lower dosage without losing analgesia, (2) rotating to a different opioid, (3) adding a benzodiazepine.
- Neuroleptic-induced movement disorders occur in palliative populations receiving commonly used dopamine antagonists.

Neuroexcitatory symptoms are relatively common in the setting of complex cancer management. They can range from mild movement disorders to full-blown tonic-clonic seizures. Effective diagnosis and management of this array of neuroexcitatory symptoms requires a careful history and physical examination as well as a detailed review of the patient's medication profile and metabolic panel to determine potential pharmacological and/or physiological etiologies. The majority of these neuroexcitatory symptoms can be attributed to acute and/or long-term toxicities of medications. Of particular concern are the movement-related neuroexcitatory side effects (myoclonus) seen with higher-dose opioids; these symptoms are most often readily managed, and it is critically important to distinguish them from true seizure activity. This chapter reviews the common neuroexcitatory syndromes seen in the cancer setting to provide a framework for assessment and management. It also touches on some of the considerations regarding alternative routes of administration that are particularly helpful if the oral route is not possible or not feasible.

SEIZURES

Epidemiology and Prevalence

Seizures and epileptic disorders can arise from a myriad of underlying pathological conditions. A comprehensive discussion of seizure-related disorders is beyond the scope of this chapter. However, a review of tumor-related seizures is particularly relevant to palliative care practice and is discussed here.

Tumor-related seizures are a rather common symptom in patients with cancer. Seizures are the presenting symptom of brain metastases in 15% to 20% of cases, with another 10% subsequently developing seizures. In patients with primary brain tumors, 20% to 45% present with seizures, and another 15% to 30% develop them later.[1] These tumor-related seizures tend to be simple or partial complex and may result in Todd paralysis.[2]

Basic Science and Pathophysiology

The pathophysiology of tumor-related seizures is not entirely clear but most likely involves loss of γ-aminobutyric acid (GABA)–related neural inhibition.[3] In patients with gliomas, increased numbers of astrocytes may contribute to increased seizures by releasing glutamate.[2] Most seizure events are initially focal in nature, but the seizure activity quickly spreads through the cortex, leading to secondary generalization.

Clinical Manifestations

The location of the primary tumor or metastases is an important correlate of event occurrence, with temporal and frontal lobes being more common areas of seizure activity (see "Case Study: Development of Seizures in a Hospice Patient"). In this population, any type of seizure is possible: in patients with glial tumor and in those with metastatic tumors, simple partial, complex partial, and secondary generalized seizures occur in approximately equal frequencies.[1] Olfactory and gustatory phenomena are more common in patients with intracranial tumors than in patients without cancer who have seizures.[1]

Differential Diagnosis

First, one must ensure the correct diagnosis: seizures must be clinically differentiated from similar-appearing phenomena, especially syncope, falls, and myoclonus (see later discussion). Syncope near the end of life can result from any combination of etiologies including dehydration (e.g., diarrhea, vomiting, poor oral intake), hypoglycemia, generalized weakness, or medication-related hypotension. Falls also may result from generalized weakness. Myoclonus does not cause loss of consciousness and represents hyperexcitability of the nervous system. It may be caused by medications, including tricyclic antidepressants and L-dopa. In particular, myoclonus can be seen in the setting of high-dose opiates. This can be particularly problematic

---

 CASE STUDY

Development of Seizures in a Hospice Patient

Mr. Smith is a 67-year-old patient with non–small cell lung cancer who is enrolled in home hospice. At the last staging of his disease, more than 6 months ago, metastases were found in his lungs, liver, and adrenal glands. He has been relatively comfortable at home, with pain and dyspnea well controlled. Last night, his wife called the hospice to report that she came upon him lying on the living room floor, lethargic and confused. He did not recall any sudden event. The following day, the hospice nurse visits the couple. During the visit, she witnesses the sudden onset of tonic-clonic jerking, with subsequent loss of consciousness and bladder incontinence. She contacts the attending physician for instructions.

in patients who have concomitant renal insufficiency or renal failure, in whom accumulation of neuroexcitatory metabolites of morphine and meperidine (Demerol) frequently occurs. At times, differentiation of seizures from syncope, falls, or myoclonus can be difficult, especially if the patient is found unresponsive or is not a reliable historian. Many experts recommend not initiating anticonvulsant therapy until the event's cause has been more clearly determined (e.g., witness report, second event).[1]

Additionally, there are many other reasons (i.e., not explicitly tumor related) for seizures in cancer patients, and it is important to keep these in mind when evaluating a patient. These include metabolic (hypocalcemia, hypomagnesemia, hypoglycemia), hematological (hemorrhage due to disseminated intravascular coagulation or thrombocytopenia), infectious (herpes simplex virus, cryptococcal disease), and drug-induced (various chemotherapeutics, antibiotics, meperidine) causes. In these scenarios, consultation with a neurologist is recommended.

Treatment

At this time, there are no data to support primary prophylaxis of seizures in cancer patients with or without known intracerebral disease. In fact, brain tumor patients started on anticonvulsants for primary prophylaxis may experience higher rates of iatrogenic complications than other patients taking these medications.[2] Once seizures occur, however, anticonvulsant therapy should be initiated. In this setting, commonly used anticonvulsants include phenytoin, carbamazepine, valproate, and lamotrigine. Anticonvulsant drug therapy has been shown to significantly reduce the frequency of subsequent events. However, in at least one study, most patients still experienced additional seizures.[3] No data support the use of benzodiazepines for secondary seizure prophylaxis.

Because it is common for patients with advanced disease to have reduced or absent swallowing capacity, and many do not have an enteral feeding tube, administration of anticonvulsants can be challenging and requires knowledge of the various routes of administration.

Parenteral dosing necessitates either continuous infusion or repeated intravenous (phenytoin, fosphenytoin, phenobarbital, valproate), intramuscular (fosphenytoin, phenobarbital), or subcutaneous (phenobarbital) injections. (Intramuscular administration of any medication should be avoided.) Furthermore, because of vascular access challenges in the setting of advanced disease setting, none of these routes is ideal for the home-based hospice or palliative care patient. Subcutaneous infusions of phenobarbital and midazolam may be more readily utilized, but pharmacokinetic data are lacking.

Because of its simplicity, rectal administration is often the preferred route. Although the bioavailability of anticonvulsants is often unpredictable—and for a given patient may even vary from dose to dose—the bioavailability is never more than via the oral route, so a rectal dose need never be decreased. Table 175-1 shows commonly used anticonvulsants that can be rectally administered for which pharmacokinetic data exist.

To our knowledge, transdermal dosing does not yet exist, although research into this route of administration would be highly desirable.

TABLE 175-1	Rectal Bioavailability of Anticonvulsant Drugs
Phenytoin	Poor absorption*
Fosphenytoin	Not evaluated
Carbamazepine	Suspension of same total daily dose, given in multiple doses, may be used; a specially compounded suppository can also be effective—monitor serum levels[†]
Phenobarbital	Slowly but well (90%) absorbed in normal volunteers; data in patients with cancer or terminal illness are not available[‡]
Valproate	Suppositories and solutions are well absorbed—monitor serum levels[§]
Gabapentin	Poor absorption[∥]
Lamotrigine	Chewable tablets are absorbed rectally; increased dose is probably required[4]

*Chang SW, da Silva JH, Kuhl DR. Ann Pharmacother 1999;33:781-786.
[†]Graves NM, Kriel RL, Jones-Saete C, Cloyd JC. Epilepsia 1985;26:429-433.
[‡]Graves NM, Holmes GB, Kriel RL, et al. DICP 1989;23:565-568.
[§]Holmes GB, Rosenfeld WE, Graves NM, et al. Arch Neurol 1989;46:906-909.
[∥]Kriel RL, Birnbaum AK, Cloyd JC, et al. Epilepsia 1997;38:1242-1244.

Glucocorticoids are frequently a part of therapy for patients with intracerebral masses and can provide significant symptomatic improvement, especially decreased nausea and headache as well as improved appetite.[2] When managing seizures in patients taking glucocorticoids, it is important to remember that steroids can affect serum levels of anticonvulsants. Therefore, abrupt changes in steroid doses may require closer monitoring. Also, because of the beneficial effect of glucocorticoids on peritumor edema, breakthrough seizures may respond well to increasing steroid doses rather than changing or adding anticonvulsants.

For acute seizures or for status epilepticus, benzodiazepines remain the treatment of choice. Once again, the route of administration become important. Midazolam can be given via subcutaneous infusion, although data are limited in regard to this route in status epilepticus. Diazepam can be administered readily via rectal gel. Usually administered intravenously, lorazepam can also be given sublingually or nasally, but at this time no definitive guidelines exist; rectal lorazepam has a slow peak, making it a less optimal choice for managing acute seizures.

In summary, if intravenous access exists, midazolam or lorazepam is a first-line choice. If there is no intravenous access, administration of sublingual lorazepam or rectal diazepam is common practice.

MYOCLONUS

Epidemiology and Prevalence

Myoclonus is often defined as sudden, brief, involuntary movements caused by muscular contractions or disinhibitions. It is often classified by etiology as physiological (i.e., in healthy individuals), essential (benign, nonprogressive), epileptic, or symptomatic (secondary or progressive). Large epidemiological studies of myoclonus are few, but the reported data indicate a lifetime prevalence of 8.6 per 100,000 population. Generally, studies indicate that symptomatic myoclonus predominates.[5] Among this group, posthypoxic events, neurodegenerative diseases, and epilepsy constitute the greatest portion of cases. It is suggested, however, that transient syndromes such as toxic-metabolic and drug-induced myoclonus are less often reported and therefore are under-represented in medical literature.

Basic Science and Pathophysiology

The precise pathophysiology of myoclonus depends on the specific neuroanatomy involved, information that can certainly be obtained with extensive neurophysiological testing when indicated. In general, there are several categories: peripheral, spinal, subcortical-supraspinal, cortical-subcortical, and cortical.

In the palliative population, the cortical neuroanatomy group predominates and is the focus of this discussion. The cortex remains affected by progressive dementias (including Alzheimer's disease, Lewy body disorders, and Creutzfeldt-Jakob disease), posthypoxia myoclonus, and many toxic-metabolic and drug-induced etiologies. In these patients, loss of GABA neural inhibition in parts of the motor cortex seems to be greatly responsible for the twitching of hands, face, and extremities. Therefore, management depends on either treating the underlying disorder or improving this GABAergic deficiency.[5]

Clinical Manifestations

Myoclonus involves involuntary jerking movements, usually of the limbs, caused by irregular muscle activity (see "Case Study: Development of Drug-Related Myoclonus"). As noted earlier, most myoclonus is symptomatic and may be attributed to toxic-metabolic syndromes (including hepatic and renal failure), storage diseases, neurodegenerative disorders (e.g., Huntington's disease, Parkinson's disease, Alzheimer's dementia, Lewy body dementia), posthypoxic syndromes, or drug-induced myoclonus (Table 175-2). An extensive list of causes can be found in other reviews.[5]

Differential Diagnosis

The differential diagnosis of myoclonus is extensive and can be similar to that of seizures, discussed earlier in this chapter, or neuroleptic-induced movement disorders (NIMD), discussed in the next section. Again, it is important to rule out other causes of such involuntary movements and then, as much as possible, to establish the underlying cause of the myoclonus.

Treatment

In the palliative population, management of common etiologies of secondary myoclonus focuses on restoring GABAergic neural inhibition. Medications include valproic acid, benzodiazepines, and barbiturates. Clonazepam is often thought to be a most effective agent, often requiring high doses.[5] Other anticonvulsant agents have been employed but may best be used with neurology specialist expertise.

Opioid-induced myoclonus is particularly important to the palliative care practitioner. After other causes of myoclonus (e.g., renal failure) have been ruled out, three steps may be taken to manage it. If possible, the dose of the opioid should be decreased. Use of appropriate adjuvant pain medications (e.g., corticosteroids, anticonvulsants, antidepressants) may help to decrease the opiate dose while enhancing analgesia. If this cannot be done, the second option of rotating to a different opiate should be considered. Finally, benzodiazepines—particularly clonazepam (e.g., beginning at 0.5 mg twice daily)—may control the myoclonus.[6]

NEUROLEPTIC-INDUCED MOVEMENT DISORDERS

Epidemiology and Prevalence

The palliation of many symptoms requires the use of medications that block dopamine receptors. Commonly prescribed agents such as metoclopramide, haloperidol, and chlorpromazine are known to cause disorders such as acute dystonia, akathisia, parkinsonism, and tardive dyskinesia. Palliative care practitioners should be familiar with the symptoms and treatment of such NIMD.

Although the exact prevalence of NIMD in the palliative population is unclear, it is known that such disorders can be rather common. Although the incidence varies according to the drug and dosage, more potent dopamine antagonists such as haloperidol may produce symptoms of acute dystonia or akathisia in as many as 30% to 40% of

CASE STUDY

Development of Drug-Related Myoclonus

Ms. Battista, a 56-year-old woman with spindle cell sarcoma, is hospitalized for pain management. She rates her left shoulder and upper extremity pain—the site of the primary tumor—as 8/10 at rest. Also notable is her severe left upper extremity swelling. After intravenous hydromorphone is administered to control the pain, a Doppler ultrasound study shows a venous thrombus in the extremity. A hydromorphone infusion is started, with boluses administered as needed via a patient-controlled analgesia pump. Her pain is controlled the next day (2/10 at rest), but she complains of constant "twitching" and "jumping" of her arms and legs, a symptom she has never experienced before.

TABLE 175-2 Drugs Commonly Associated with Myoclonus

Tricyclic antidepressants
Selective serotonin reuptake inhibitors
Monoamine oxidase inhibitors
Lithium
Antipsychotics
Antibiotics
Opiates
Anticonvulsants
Contrast media
Calcium channel blockers
Antiarrhythmics

Data from Caviness JN, Brown P. Myoclonus: Current concepts and recent advances. Lancet Neurol 2004;3:598-607.

CASE STUDY

Development of Neuroleptic-Induced Movement Disorder

Mr. Kwon, an 82-year-old man with Alzheimer's disease, was admitted from a nursing home to an inpatient hospice facility for management of pain and agitation. His pain is managed initially with acetaminophen and parenteral opiates. To manage his agitation, the team increases his scheduled quetiapine (Seroquel). When this is not sufficient, they administer parenteral haloperidol, titrating to control of the agitation. On day 4, the nurse notes new involuntary movements in Mr. Kwon's face and neck and contacts the attending physician.

Future Considerations

Neuroexcitatory syndromes occur commonly in palliative care patient populations. These patients are usually quite debilitated as a result of one or more chronic progressive illnesses, making them vulnerable to neuroexcitatory syndromes arising from the disease processes or from disease management. Certainly, controversy may surround the management of specific syndromes, as in the case of the tardive dyskinesias. More importantly, however, few data—epidemiological and otherwise—have been gathered about these syndromes in patients receiving palliative care or hospice services. Future research should address this lack.

---

cases.[7] Rates are lower with the atypical antipsychotics, clozapine, olanzapine, risperidone, and quetiapine.[8]

Basic Science and Pathophysiology

The pathophysiology of NIMD is somewhat unclear, although hypotheses focus on the central role of the dopamine neurotransmitter. The implicated drugs block dopamine neurotransmitters, replicating to some extent the traits of Parkinson's disease (hence, "neuroleptic-induced parkinsonism"), with increased involuntary movements. In the case of acute dystonia, and to some extent tardive dyskinesia, a mechanism has been hypothesized in which the acute decrease in dopamine activity is met by a compensatory dopamine hyperfunction, leading to an imbalance in the neurotransmitter at the level of the neural synapse.[7] Notably, the development of parkinsonian-like symptoms in patients treated with neuroleptics was once a sign of adequate dosing.[7] With the development of so-called atypical antipsychotics, which generally employ a degree of intrinsic anticholinergic activity and serotonin antagonism as well as dopamine antagonism, this no longer is necessary (see "Case Study: Development of a Neuroleptic-Induced Movement Disorder").

Clinical Manifestations

Four NIMD are described here.

Acute dystonia is an involuntary, slow movement that is often described as a muscle spasm. Typical movements include torticollis, tongue protrusion, facial grimacing, and opisthotonus.

Usually developing within 2 weeks after drug initiation, *akathisia* refers to the combination of a subjective sensation of restlessness and observed purposeless movements, constantly shifting body position, or marching in place. Lying down often relieves symptoms, distinguishing akathisia from the restless legs syndrome.

Neuroleptic-induced parkinsonism tends to appear later than acute dystonia and akathisia. Clinically, it is indistinguishable from Parkinson's disease; rigidity, resting tremor, masked facies, and a dearth of purposeful movements are common findings. Again, atypical antipsychotics are less likely to cause this movement disorder.

As the name implies, *tardive dyskinesias* occur after prolonged use of dopamine-blocking agents (months to

years). Tardive dyskinesia is characterized by choreiform, athetoid, or dystonic movements, or a combination of such movements. Typically, facial, lingual, and orobuccal muscles are involved. An early sign is often dyskinetic blinking, which may be followed by repetitive chewing, jaw-clenching, blowing, grimacing, and tongue-smacking movements.

Differential Diagnosis

The differential diagnosis of NIMD includes other neuroexcitatory syndromes, such as seizures and myoclonus, which were described earlier in this chapter.

Treatment

Treatment of NIMD is relatively straightforward. Ideally, the drug dosing should be decreased or the drug changed to a different agent. Direct treatment of symptoms is best accomplished with anticholinergic agents, preferably those with M_1 subtype activity. Parenteral administration of benztropine or diphenhydramine is usually effective and should be continued for 24 to 48 hours. In mild cases, oral diphenhydramine may suffice. To treat akathisia, β-adrenergic antagonists and benzodiazepines may also be used. The beneficial mechanism of the benzodiazepines is most likely nonspecific.

Of note, L-dopa and other dopamine agonists used to treat Parkinson's disease do not help with neuroleptic-induced parkinsonism.[7] Controversy surrounds the management of tardive dyskinesia; at this time, the primary focus is on prevention. Although data are lacking, when tardive dyskinesia occurs, it is probably best to stop the offending agent. Pharmacological treatment includes dopamine presynaptic depleters such as reserpine and is best accomplished in conjunction with expert psychiatric consultation (see "Future Considerations").

REFERENCES

1. Krouwer HGJ, Pallagi JL, Graves NM. Management of seizures in brain tumor patients at the end of life. J Palliat Med 2000;3:465-475.
2. Batchelor TT, Byrne TN. Supportive care of brain tumor patients. Hematol Oncol Clin North Am 2006;20:1337-1361.
3. Hildebrand J, Lecaille C, Perennes J, Delattre JY. Neurology 2005;65:212-215.
4. Birnbaum AK, Kriel RL, Im Y, Remmel RP. Relative bioavailability of lamotrigine chewable dispersible tablets administered rectally. Pharmacotherapy 2001;21: 158-162.
5. Caviness JN, Brown P. Myoclonus: Current concepts and recent advances. Lancet Neurol 2004;3:598-607.
6. Mercadante S. Pathophysiology and treatment of opioid-related myoclonus in cancer patients. Pain 1998;74:5-9.

7. Sachdev PS. Neuroleptic-induced movement disorders: An overview. Psychiatric Clin North Am 2005;28:255-274.
8. Weintraub D, Katz IR. Pharmacologic interventions for psychosis and agitation in neurodegenerative diseases: Evidence about efficacy and safety. Psychiatr Clin North Am 2005;28:941-983.

SUGGESTED READING

Caviness JN, Brown P. Myoclonus: Current concepts and recent advances. Lancet Neurol 2004;3:598-607.

Krouwer HGJ, Pallagi JL, Graves NM. Management of seizures in brain tumor patients at the end of life. J Palliat Med 2000;3:465-475.

Sachdev PS. Neuroleptic-induced movement disorders: An overview. Psychiatric Clin North Am 2005;28:255-274.

CHAPTER **176**

Sleep Problems and Nightmares

Dilara Seyidova Khoshknabi

KEY POINTS

- Sleep problems (insomnia) is a very common and frequent symptom in patients with cancer.

- Insomnia is a multidimensional symptom that involves difficulties in falling asleep, sleep maintenance, early-morning awaking, sleep resuming, daytime fatigue, and nightmares.

- Medical causes of sleep disturbances include chronic pain, primary sleep disorders (e.g., sleep apnea, periodic limb movements, restless legs syndrome), dyspnea, pregnancy, and drug use or withdrawal.

- A potential pathological mechanism is overactivity of the hypothalamic-pituitary-adrenal (HPA) axis with excess corticotropin-releasing factors (CRF) and cortisol.

- Cognitive-behavioral therapy, nonbenzodiazepine hypnotics, sedative antihistamines, and benzodiazepines are advanced approaches to treatment.

Sleep is a natural, periodic, highly structured, and well-organized behavior. It defines an essential circadian process that is regulated by an internal hormonal process (melatonin) and light and is critical for psychophysiological health. Normal sleep consists of several stages characterized by distinct electroencephalographic (EEG) patterns. Healthy individuals enter sleep through stage I (quiet sleep), and progress through stages II through IV:

Stage I—light sleep involves slow eye movement and relaxed muscles.
Stage II—eye movements stop, and brain waves slow, with occasional bursts of rapid waves called sleep spindles.
Stage III—extremely slow brain delta waves (0.5 to 4 Hz) appear, interspersed with smaller, faster waves.
Stage IV—delta waves occur almost exclusively.

In all of these stages, there is no eye movement or muscle activity; therefore, this is defined as non–rapid eye movement (NREM) sleep. It is characterized by moderately synchronous activity on EEG. By contrast, rapid eye movement (REM) sleep is characterized by EEG activation, muscle atonia, and rapid eye movement. Stage I is replaced by REM, which repeats throughout the night and takes approximately 90 minutes to occur. In this stage, dreams occur, with vivid recall on arousal.[1]

Insomnia can be characterized as either a symptom or a clinical disorder. The symptom of insomnia refers to a subjective complaint which may include difficulty in falling asleep, trouble staying asleep, prolonged nocturnal awakenings, and early-morning awakening with inability to resume sleep. As a disorder, insomnia comprises a syndrome that includes insomnia complaints together with a specific diagnostic category (clinical or laboratory based) and significant distress or functional impairment without the presence of specific features.[2]

Insomnia is a common symptom in cancer.[3] Some studies have used quality-of-life rating systems, symptom assessment scales, and audits to determine sleep disturbances, but few have used validated instruments. Two studies examined prevalence, key causes, and management in cancer patients undergoing palliative treatment, but only one of them used a validated tool, the Pittsburgh Sleep Quality Index (PSQI).[4,5]

Subjective assessment of sleep quality and disturbances is important, because poor sleep quality and sleep disturbances can contribute to somatic or psychiatric disorders. Sleep deprivation has a detrimental physical effect on pain tolerance, immune function, mood, and physical stamina.[3,6] Psychological distress is the most prominent consequence of insomnia (or insufficient sleep), but there is evidence that subtle physiological abnormalities, such as altered immune responses or autonomic dysfunction, occur also.[6,7]

BASIC SCIENCE

Gastrointestinal hormones and neurotransmitters such as cholecystokinin (CCK) modulate many autonomic and behavioral effects, including sleep. CCK has two receptor subtypes: CCK_B, which is abundant in various brain regions, and CCK_A, which is located mainly in the gastrointestinal tract. Both are stimulated by cholecystokinin octapeptide sulfate ester (CCK-8-SE). Injection of CCK-8-SE elicits behavioral and autonomic responses such as cessation of eating, reduced exploration, social withdrawal, sleep, increased NREM sleep, and hypothermia.[8] In male Sprague-Dawley rats chronically implanted with electrodes for cortical EEG and nuchal electromyography (EMG), central injection of CCK did not induce sleep. This finding implies that CCK acts on the periphery CCK_A and CCK_B receptors that induce behaviors including the satiety syndrome and sleep.[9]

Recent research revealed a strong correlation between chronic NREM sleep and decreased insulin sensitivity. According to another theory, adenosine is important. It is a neuromodulator whose extracellular concentration increases with brain metabolism; in vitro, it inhibits basal forebrain cholinergic neurons that mediate somnogenic effects and prolonged wakefulness. Perfusion of adenosine in basal forebrain and the mesopontine inhibits cholinergic nuclei and reduces wakefulness and EEG arousal. Adenosine is a physiological sleep factor mediating the somnogenic effects of wakefulness. The duration and depth of sleep are positively modulated by adenosine.[10]

EPIDEMIOLOGY AND PREVALENCE

Incidence of insomnia varies from 10% to 50% in adults. Between 10% and 13% of the adult population suffer from chronic insomnia, and an additional 25% to 35% experience transient or occasional insomnia.[11,12] Studies of newly diagnosed cancer patients report insomnia in 30% to 50%.[13] Sleep disturbances persist in 23% to 44% of these patients for several years after treatment.[14,15]

In most prevalence studies of insomnia in cancer, patients were at various disease stages, and sleep disturbances were assessed only as part of a multisymptom assessment.[16-22] Insomnia has received limited attention as a primary cause of patient distress, and often only in the context of other symptoms or psychological illnesses. The misleading concept (pervasive among both physicians and patients) that insomnia is "normal" in cancer contributes to the lack of attention, inadequate evaluation, and poor treatment of this condition.

The prevalence of insomnia among different populations is associated with certain risk factors such as a previous history of sleep problems, increasing age, female gender, psychiatric disorders, medical disorders, impaired activities of daily living, use of anxiolytic and hypnotic medications, and lower socioeconomic status. Genetic and environmental liabilities for sleep disturbance are independent of the genetic liability for anxiety and depression. Genetic and lifestyle variables interact with genetic factors to influence the risk for insomnia.[23] In both sexes, there is a significant influence of genetics on sleep disturbance, short-sleep, and altered sleep stage associated with daytime napping and may explain the effects of sleep on personality (neuroticism and extraversion), which are known to be strongly influenced by genetic factors.[24]

PATHOPHYSIOLOGY

Two theories proposed to explain idiopathic insomnia involve either physiological or cognitive hyperarousal relative to normal sleepers.[25,26] Self-defined "poor sleepers" had higher levels of physiological activity than "good sleepers."[27] Sleep-onset insomnia is characterized by delayed sleep onset without other sleep-stage abnormalities and with increased physiological activity before sleep.[28] It is also associated with neuroticism, anxiety, and worry. In one study,[29] no difference was found in the duration of sleep after tiring physical exercise, compared with relaxation before sleep, even though physical activity significantly augmented heart rate, respiration rate, and rectal temperature before sleep. It is unlikely that physical exertion alone causes delayed sleep onset. Similarly, although evidence of increased neuroticism, anxiety, and worry is found in insomniacs, many persons experience the same symptoms but do not have difficulty sleeping. In sleep-onset insomnia,[30] sleep latency negatively correlated with scores on the Minnesota Multiphasic Personality Inventory (MMPI) and the Multiple Affect Adjective Check List (MAACL) Anxiety Scale. The relation between psycho-

pathology and delayed sleep onset is not simple. In an integrative neurobiological model of insomnia, evidence of cortical activation during sleep and sympathetic and hypothalamic-pituitary-adrenal (HPA) axis activation needs to be correlated with sleep latency delays.[31] Sleep cycles are complex and are controlled by various neurotransmitters, including noradrenaline, serotonin, acetylcholine, dopamine, histamine, γ-aminobutyric acid, the pituitary hormones, and the neurohormone melatonin, which influence sleep latency, sleep stage, and duration of sleep.[32,33] (See "Case Study: Insomnia in an Oncology Patient").

CLINICAL MANIFESTATIONS

Insomnia is precipitated by various conditions. Medical causes vary and include chronic pain, primary sleep disorders such as sleep apnea, periodic limb movements, restless legs syndrome, dyspnea, pregnancy, and drug use or withdrawal. Cancer is a potentially strong precipitating factor. Cancer patients with clinical insomnia (difficulty with falling asleep, waking up at night, getting back to sleep, early-morning awakening, and nightmares) sleep significantly fewer hours. Depression correlates with reduced sleep maintenance, nonrestorative sleep, fatigue, and nightmares. Anxiety causes more difficulty falling asleep, less restorative sleep, and nightmares. Confusion is associated with fatigue and nightmares.[5] Pain is significantly correlated with difficulty falling asleep; fatigue with difficulty falling asleep and maintaining sleep, and fewer hours of sleep; depression with early awakening; and anxiety with difficulty falling asleep and maintaining sleep and lack of restorative qualities to sleep[37] (Tables 176-1 and 176-2).

DIFFERENTIAL DIAGNOSIS

It is essential to identify causes and not to treat the problem only symptomatically, because treatment depends on cause. Assessment should include a full sleep history (from the patient and also from his or her bed partner or family, if possible), examination of mental state, and review of

---

TABLE 176-1   Diagnostic Features of Insomnia

1. Sleep disturbances, characterized by
   Difficulty falling asleep (≥30 min)
   Difficulty maintaining sleep (>30 min of nocturnal awakenings)
   Problems with resuming sleep
   Early morning awakening
   Daytime tiredness
   Naps during the day
   Nightmares
2. Sleep problems occur at least 3 nights/wk
3. Sleep disturbances impair quality of life (daytime functioning, fatigue, concentration, memory, mood)
4. Duration
   Transient or situational: ≤1 mo
   Short term or subacute: >1 mo but <6 mo
   Chronic: >6 mo

For further information, see references 2, 3, 38, and 39.

CASE STUDY

Insomnia in an Oncology Patient

A 27-year-old-man diagnosed with teratocarcinoma involving the right testis with metastases to the lungs received a regimen of cisplatin, bleomycin, and vinblastine that was administered for eight cycles. He was prescribed metoclopramide, lorazepam, and nabilone at various doses to control his emesis during the chemotherapy cycles. Insomnia had been present 2 years, since the death of a close friend. With the cancer diagnosis, discovery of metastases, and beginning of chemotherapy, his insomnia became more severe. He had stopped using sleep medications months before his cancer diagnosis due to lack of response. Frustrated with his attempts to sleep and lack of response to sleep medications, and mindful of the psychological threat of his illness, chemotherapy, and personal loss, he attempted treatment with somatic focusing[34] and imagery training.[35]

Each session started with somatic focusing, during which the patient was asked to concentrate on the tension in 16 major muscle groups, followed by relaxation through imagery, feeling his muscles becoming limp and heavy, and feeling tension give way to relaxation. Imagery training focused attention on pleasant images with closed eyes (pictures of common objects such as a book, a candle, a clock, a cup, and a bowl); these were presented as prompts and faded after visualization. Then the patient was instructed to concentrate on the specific features, colors, and movement of these images for 2 to 3 minutes. Both techniques were practiced daily at home.

The patient was asked to fill out a questionnaire during a 5-day baseline period and again in each phase of the study. The questionnaire included a record of dependent variables and latency of sleep onset, duration of sleep, and an 11-point scale of graded difficulty falling asleep, quality of sleep, tiredness, and difficulty with either maintaining pleasant thoughts or deleting unpleasant thoughts. Chemotherapy interfered with his sleeping patterns, and he needed a week to recuperate in order to revert to baseline conditions. A 2-week break occurred between cycles 3 and 4 to allow for recuperation.

This nonpharmacological approach improved the patient's sleep quality. Because he was experiencing satisfactory sleep by the end of training session 5, training treatment was terminated. Follow-up at 3, 6, and 9 months documented a continued satisfactory level of sleep. At the 12-month follow-up, only occasional use of the somatic focusing or imagery technique was necessary, because the patient's sleep had improved to the point that only certain events caused high anxiety and induced insomnia. He finished his chemotherapy treatments and had been living disease free for 10 months by the time of this case report, indicating that his insomnia was primarily acquired.[36]

medical, psychiatric, and family histories. Screening questionnaires and a sleep diary are valuable.

There are several types of insomnia. *Transient insomnia* (duration of several days) is commonplace; it may be caused by worry about an anticipated event or may be related to a family dispute, an unfamiliar sleeping environ-

ment, a brief illness, or withdrawal from hypnotic drugs. *Short-term insomnia* (several weeks) results from longer-lasting illness or worry about being ill, financial problems, or difficulties at work; from bereavement (in which case, it may become prolonged or complicated); or from psychiatric disorder; the course is fluctuating. *Chronic insomnia* (months or years) is associated with persistent psychological problems (especially stress), poor sleep hygiene (e.g., sleeping environment not conducive to sleep, snoring, restless bed partner), and excessive intake of caffeine or overuse of nicotine or alcohol, especially at night. Chronic insomnia can be triggered by physical disorders that disturb sleep (e.g., pain, respiratory disorders), psychiatric disorders (including depression, generalized anxiety, psychotic states), and medications (bronchodilators, decongestants, antidepressants, and stimulants), as well as other sleep disorders, including restless legs syndrome. *Conditioned insomnia* occurs when the original cause no longer applies but bed has become associated with being awake.[46-48]

Fatal familial insomnia (FFI), one of the inherited (autosomal dominant) neurodegenerative prion diseases, must be differentiated from sleep disorders. The chief complaints of this genetically transmitted disease are progressive severe insomnia, waking "sleep," hallucinations, autonomic disturbances (tachycardia, hypertension, hyperhidrosis, hyperthermia), a rise in circulating catecholamine levels, cognitive changes, ataxia, and endocrine manifestations with later cognitive changes resembling dementia.[49]

Insomnia should also be differentiated from the many other pathological conditions shown in Table 176-3.

Various tests are available to differentiate primary insomnia[54-56]:

1. Epworth Sleepiness Scale—a validated questionnaire that is used to assess daytime sleepiness
2. All-night polysomnography (PSG)—a test that measures activity during sleep
3. Actigraphy—a test to assess sleep-wake patterns over time (actigraphs are small, wrist-worn devices that measure movement)
4. Mental health examination for depression, anxiety, or another mental health disorder—a mental status examination, mental health history, and basic mental evaluations may be part of the initial assessment
5. Magnetic resonance imaging or other neuroimaging as indicated, to exclude structural central nervous system lesions
6. Laboratory tests to exclude medical disorders
7. Miscellaneous tests: EEG, EMG, electro-oculography, electrocardiography, airflow at nose and mouth, respiratory effort, oxygen saturation.[54-56]

TREATMENT

Management comprises various complex approaches and includes detailed documentation of sleep patterns, medical history (e.g., personal or family of psychiatric disorders or insomnia), medications, drug and alcohol use, and work-related factors (e.g., shift work), along with a survey of the sleep environment (sleep diary) and sleep-related attitudes. In palliative care, benzodiazepines are the most

TABLE 176-2   Conditions Associated with Insomnia

PREDISPOSING FACTORS	PRECIPITATING FACTORS	PERPETUATING FACTORS
Hyperarousability	Hospitalization	Excessive amount of time napping
Female gender	Radiotherapy	Sleep-interfering activities in the bedroom
Older age	Chemotherapy	Faulty beliefs and attitudes about sleep
Family history of mood or anxiety disorder	Surgery	Unrealistic sleep expectations
Personal history of mood or anxiety disorder	Bone marrow transplantation	Incorrect perceptions about sleep difficulties
Psychiatric disorder	Corticosteroids	Misattributions of daytime impairment
Co-occurrence of a psychiatric disorder	Diuretics	Misconceptions about causes of insomnia
Family history of insomnia	Neuroleptics	
Personal history of alcohol use	Biologic response modifiers (e.g., interleukins, interferons)	
Personal history of drug abuse	Menopause	
	Hormonal therapy	
	Pain	
	Delirium	
	Nausea/vomiting	

For further information, see references 40 through 45.

TABLE 176-3   Differential Diagnosis of Insomnia from Other Disorders

PSYCHIATRIC DISORDERS	MEDICAL DISORDERS	NEUROLOGIC DISORDERS	COMMON NEURODEGENERATIVE DISEASES	OTHER DISORDERS
Anxiety	Pain	Stroke	Parkinson's disease	Alcohol or illicit drug abuse
Panic attacks	Bronchial asthma	Brain tumors	Multiple-system atrophy	Sleep-wake schedule disruptions
Depression	Coronary artery disease	Causalgia	Diffuse Levzy body disease	
Stress	Peptic ulcer disease	Neuromuscular disorders	Olivopontccerebellar atrophy	
Other psychophysiological factors	Rheumatic disorders	(e.g., painful peripheral neuropathies)	Progressive supranuclear palsy	
	Inotropic	Disorders of circadian sleep rhythms	Corticobasal ganglionic degeneration	
		Narcolepsy	Fatal familial insomnia (FFI)	
		Traumatic brain injury		

For further information, see references 50 through 53.

frequently used medications.[57] However, drugs from other classes, as well as nonpharmacological therapies, should be considered (Tables 176-4 and 176-5).

Drug Side Effects

Adverse effects include various system impairments (mainly central nervous system). Benzodiazepines can have significant adverse effects such as daytime sleepiness, which is more severe with longer-acting agents (flurazepam)[61]; dose-related anterograde amnesia; impairment of other aspects of psychomotor performance (reaction time, recall, and vigilance)[62]; and increased risk of injurious falls and hip fractures in elderly people, especially with long-acting agents, high doses, multiple agents, and cognitive impairment.[63,64]

The adverse effects of antidepressants are restlessness, dizziness, insomnia, exacerbation of restless legs syndrome and periodic limb movements,[65] sedation, fatigue, anxiety, impaired cognitive function, seizure, extrapyramidal symptoms, coma, hallucinations, confusion, disorientation, impaired coordination, ataxia, headache, nightmares, and hyperpyrexia.

The side effects of antihistamines are cognitive and performance impairments.[66] The anticholinergic effects of antihistaminic medications are problematic in the elderly in terms of confusion and falls.

The adverse effects of melatonin include daytime drowsiness. Some studies suggest that melatonin affects the reproductive cycle in some mammalian species.

Drugs of Choice

Antidepressants and antipsychotic medications are frequently used for sleep disturbances in palliative medicine. Because delirium is frequent in advanced cancer, antipsychotic medications are most commonly used to manage insomnia with delirium.[80,81] Mirtazapine is attractive because of its safety and side effect profile. It has gained interest among palliative care specialists as a sedative and appetite stimulant.[82-85] Drugs commonly used but inadequately studied are the antihistamines, melatonin, valerian, and other herbal anxiolytics (e.g., kava).[86] Table 176-6 describes the outcomes of clinical trials in the pharmaceutical treatment of insomnia.

Supportive Care

Table 176-7 presents the relevant findings from reviews and clinical trials on supportive care for patients with insomnia.

TABLE 176-4 Treatment of Insomnia

GENERIC DRUG NAME (TRADE NAME)	DOSE (mg)	METABOLISM	HALF-LIFE (hr)	ADVERSE EFFECTS
BENZODIAZEPINE HYPNOTIC DRUGS				
Triazolam (Halcion)	0.125	Extensively hepatic	1.7-5	Drowsiness, anterograde amnesia
Alprazolam (Xanax)	0.5-1	Hepatic via CYP3A4	11.2	Abnormal coordination, depression, drowsiness
Lorazepam (Ativan)	0.5-4	Hepatic to inactive compounds	12.9	Sedation, respiratory depression
Temazepam (Restoril)	7.5-15	Hepatic	9.5-12.4	Confusion, dizziness, drowsiness, fatigue
Clonazepam (Klonopin)	0.5-2	Extensively hepatic	19-50	Amnesia, ataxia, coma, confusion, depression
Chlordiazepoxide (Librium)	50-100	Extensively hepatic to desmethyldiazepam	6.6-25	Drowsiness, fatigue, ataxia, lightheadedness
Diazepam (Valium)	5-10	Hepatic	20-50	Agitation, amnesia, anxiety, ataxia, confusion, depression, dizziness, drowsiness
NONBENZODIAZEPINE HYPNOTIC DRUGS				
Zalepone (Sonata)	5-10	Extensive, primarily via aldehyde oxidase	1	Chest pain, peripheral edema, amnesia, anxiety, depersonalization, depression
Zolpidem (Ambien)	5-10	Hepatic, primarily via CYP3A4	2.5-2.8	Dizziness, headache, somnolence
Zopiclone (Imovane)	5-7.5	Extensively hepatic	7	Palpitations, agitation, anterograde amnesia, anxiety, asthenia
Esopiclone (Estorra)	3	Hepatic via oxidation and demethylation (CYP2E1, CYP3A4)	6-9	Headache, chest pain, peripheral edema
ANTIDEPRESSANT DRUGS				
Amitriptyline	25-100	Hepatic to nortriptyline (active)	9-27	Restlessness, dizziness, insomnia, sedation, fatigue, anxiety, impaired cognitive function
Trazodone	25-100	Hepatic via hydroxylation and oxidation; metabolized by CYP3A4 to active metabolite, m-chlorophenylpiperazine (mCPP)	5-9	Drowsiness (20-50%), sedation, dizziness, insomnia, confusion, agitation, seizures, extrapyramidal reactions, headache, suicidal thinking and behavior
Mirtazapine	15-30	Extensively hepatic via CYP1A2, CYP2C9, CYP2D6, CYP3A4, and via demethylation and hydroxylation	20-40	Somnolence, constipation, xerostomia, increased appetite, weight gain
ANTIHISTAMINES				
Diphenhydramine	25-50	Extensively hepatic; smaller degrees in pulmonary and renal systems	2.4-9.3	Sedation, sleepiness, dizziness, disturbed coordination, headache, fatigue, nervousness
Doxylamine	25	Via multiple metabolic pathways including N-demethylation, oxidation, hydroxylation, N-acetylation to metabolites including nordoxylamine, dinordoxylamine	10-12	Dizziness, disorientation, drowsiness, headache, paradoxical CNS stimulation, vertigo
NONPRESCRIPTION MEDICATIONS				
Melatonin	0.5-6	—	—	No known toxicity or serious side effects
Valerian	200-400 (at bedtime)	—	—	May cause drowsiness or sedation
ALTERNATIVE AGENTS				
Ramelteon (Rozerem)	8 (30 min before bedtime)	Extensive first-pass effect; oxidative metabolism primarily through CYP1A2 and to a lesser extent through CYP2C and CYP3A4	1-6	CNS depression, reproductive hormonal regulation disturbances

CNS, central nervous system; CYP, cytochrome P-450 isoenzyme.
Data from references 2, 4, 48, 58, 59, and 60.

EVIDENCE-BASED MEDICINE

Longitudinal epidemiological studies demonstrate that persistent insomnia is linked to a higher incidence of depressive disorders and that chronic insomnia causes several physical health problems. Insomnia is associated with poor health, depressed mood, persistent chronic disease, physical disability, and widowhood.[87-92] Drugs and alcohol are major contributing factors.[93] These facts suggest that there is genetic vulnerability to insomnia but acquired factors are major contributors (see "Future Considerations").

TABLE 176-5	Nonpharmacological Alternative Therapies

THERAPIES	AIMS
Behavioral therapy	Decrease/change factors interfering with sleep, adaptive sleep habits, cognitive/physiological hyperarousal, and dysfunctional beliefs about sleep
Relaxation and biofeedback therapies	Target cognitive or physiological arousal that interferes with sleep (progressive muscle relaxation and biofeedback, imagery techniques, autogenic training, meditation to reduce cognitive arousal)
Sleep hygiene education	Promote environmental and lifestyle factors contributing to sleep by minimizing factors affecting sleep in negative way
Sleep restriction therapy	Decrease time in bed to maximize sleep efficiency of time spent in bed (time spent awake in bed is counterproductive and promotes insomnia)
Cognitive and multimodal therapies	Empower patient by providing a sense of control over sleep; focus on correcting dysfunctional beliefs and attitudes about insomnia
Stimulus control therapy	Recondition signals (e.g., bedroom, bedtime routine) to promote relaxation and sleep as opposed to anxiety, frustration, and wakefulness
Phototherapy	Use artificial light to adjust the timing of the sleep/wake cycle
Exercise	Increase sleep quality and slow-wave sleep, reduce sleep latency through rise in core body temperature followed by an exaggerated temperature decline during early sleep
Passive body heating	Elevate core body temperature by external body heating (immersion in hot water, ≥40° C) during the early evening to increase slow-wave sleep

Data from references 2 and 58.

TABLE 176-7	Supportive Care

REVIEWS/CLINICAL TRIALS	PRACTICE POINTS
1. Morin CM, Bootz n RR, Buysse DJ, et al. Psychological and behavioral treatment of insomnia: Update of the recent evidence (1998-2004). Sleep 2006;29:1398-1414.	Psychological and behavioral therapies produced reliable improvement in several sleep parameters in individuals with either primary insomnia or insomnia associated with medical and psychiatric disorders.
2. Morin CM, Hauri PJ, Espie CA, et al. Nonpharmacologic treatment of chronic insomnia. An American Academy of Sleep Medicine review. Sleep 1999;22:1134-1156.	Stimulus control, progressive muscle relaxation, and paradoxical intention meet APA criteria for benefits. Also, sleep restriction, biofeedback, and multifaceted CBT improve sleep.
3. Morin CM, Colecchi C, Stone J, et al. Behavioral and pharmacological therapies for late-life insomnia: A randomized controlled trial. JAMA 1999;281:991-999.	Behavioral and pharmacological approaches were effective in short-term management of insomnia in late life; sleep improvements were better sustained over time with behavioral treatment.
4. Edinger JD, Wohlgemuth WK, Radtke RA, et al. Cognitive behavioral therapy for treatment of chronic primary insomnia: A randomized controlled trial. JAMA 2001;285:1856-1364.	CBT is a viable intervention for primary sleep-maintenance insomnia. This treatment maintained clinically significant sleep improvements that lasted through 6 mo of follow-up.

APA, American Psychological Association; CBT, cognitive-behavioral therapy.

TABLE 176-6	Clinical Trials

PHARMACOLOGICAL CATEGORY	TYPE OF TRIAL	OUTCOMES
Benzodiazepines	Double-blind, placebo-controlled[61,67-69]	Demonstrated continued efficacy over a 4-5-wk period
	Single-blind[7,70]	Showed continued efficacy for 6 mo by PSG
Nonbenzodiazepine	Randomized, placebo-controlled[67]	Demonstrated efficacy for >4 wk with a hypnotic agent; the 15-mg zolpidem dosage provided no clinical advantage over 10 mg zolpidem
	Double-blind placebo-controlled[72]	Demonstrated evidence that long-term pharmacological treatment of insomnia is efficacious
Antidepressants	Double-blind[73]	Polysomnographic parameters during 4-wk trial demonstrated that trimipramine did not suppress REM sleep even in patients treated with trimipramine who had short sleep latencies during the placebo period
	Multicenter, double-blind[74]	Nefazodone was associated with greater improvement in both objective and subjective sleep
Antihistamines	Double-blind[75]	Supported the use of 50 mg diphenhydramine as an OTC sleep aid in the treatment of temporary, mild to moderate insomnia
	Randomized, double-blind, crossover trial[76]	No significant difference in tests of neurological function noted, although subjects performed more poorly, compared with placebo, on seven of eight tests while taking temazepam and on five of eight tests while taking DPH. Several instances of daytime hypersomnolence were noted in subjects taking temazepam and DPH, but none in subjects given placebo
Melatonin	Double-blind, controlled self-report[77]	Not effective in the management of psychophysiological insomnia
	Double-blind, single-crossover study[97]	Demonstrated a significant increase in total sleep time and daytime alertness compared with placebo
Valerian	Double-blind placebo-controlled[78]	Significant benefit on insomnia compared to placebo
	Questionnaires, self-rating scales, nighttime motor activity[79]	Aqueous valerian extract exerted a mild hypnotic action but did not show evidence for a change in sleep stages

DPH, diphenhydramine; OTC, over-the-counter; PSG, polysomnography; REM, rapid eye movement.

Future Considerations

Recent research provides evidence for interaction between sleep and the activation of the hypothalamic-pituitary-adrenal (HPA) axis. Hourly measurements of plasma cortisol secretion and sleep investigation in patients with severe chronic primary insomnia, compared with age- and gender-matched controls, revealed significant increases in evening and nocturnal cortisol levels. Evening cortisol levels correlated with the number of nocturnal awakenings. A significant correlation existed between sleep and the first 4 hours of nocturnal cortisol secretion. These findings suggest that changes in the HPA system influence insomnia and reflect a pathophysiological mechanism of chronic insomnia.[94]

Two major circadian processes are at work in sleep: mood function, which regulates rapid eye movement (REM) sleep and temperature,[1] and sleep-wake patterns.[2] REM stage-sleep is phase-advanced relative to the process governing sleep onset. A desynchronized shift causes REM abnormalities characteristic of depression and sleep disorders. REM sleep quality and duration affect depression. REM sleep onset and REM-related wakefulness patterns in cases of delayed/advanced sleep phase are similar to those associated with depression.[95] Melatonin suppresses REM sleep in cats, and pinealectomy in humans induces a narcoleptic-like pattern of REM sleep which remarkably resembles that of the newborn and is reversed by melatonin. Narcolepsy may be a maturation defect in the pineal gland.[96]

REFERENCES

1. Kryger M, Roth T, Dement W. Principles and Practice of Sleep Medicine, 3rd ed. Philadelphia: Sauders; 2000.
2. Buysse D, Dorsey S. Current and experimental therapeutics of Insomnia. In Davis K, Charney D, Coyle J, Nemeroff C (eds). Neuropsychopharmacology: The Fifth Generation of Progress. New York: American College of Neuropsychopharmacology; 2002. pp 1931-1944.
3. Savard J, Morin CM. Insomnia in the context of cancer: A review of a neglected problem. J Clin Oncol 2001;19:895-908.
4. Hugel H, Ellershaw JE, Cook L, et al. The prevalence, key causes and management of insomnia in palliative care patients. J Pain Symptom Manage 2004; 27:316-321.
5. Mercadante S, Girelli D, Casuccio A. Sleep disorders in advanced cancer patients: Prevalence and factors associated. Support Care Cancer 2004; 12:355-359.
6. Gislason T, Almqvist M. Somatic diseases and sleep complaints: An epidemiological study of 3,201 Swedish men. Acta Med. Scand 1987;221:475-481.
7. Kales JD, Kales A, Bixler EO, et al. Biopsychobehavioral correlates of insomnia: V. Clinical characteristics and behavioral correlates. Am J Psychiatry 1984; 141:1371-1376.
8. Antin J, Gibbs J, Holt J, et al. Cholecystokinin elicits the complete behavioral sequence of satiety in rats. J Comp Physiol Psychol 1975;89:784-790.
9. Chang HY, Kapas L. Selective activation of CCK-B receptors does not induce sleep and does not affect EEG slow-wave activity and brain temperature in rats. Physiol Behav 1997;62:175-179.
10. Porkka-Heiskanen T, Strecker RE, Thakkar M, et al. Adenosine: A mediator of the sleep-inducing effects of prolonged wakefulness. Science 1997;276:1265-1268.
11. Drake CL, Roehrs T, Roth T. Insomnia causes, consequences, and therapeutics: An overview. Depress Anxiety 2003;18:163-176.
12. Roth T. The relationship between psychiatric diseases and insomnia. Int J Clin Pract Suppl 2001;116:3-8.
13. Theobald DE. Cancer pain, fatigue, distress, and insomnia in cancer patients. Clin Cornerstone 2004;6(Suppl 1D):S15-S21.
14. Savard J, Simard S, Blanchet J, et al. Prevalence, clinical characteristics, and risk factors for insomnia in the context of breast cancer. Sleep 2001;24:583-590.
15. Davidson JR, MacLean AW, Brundage MD, Schulze K. Sleep disturbance in cancer patients. Soc Sci Med 2002;54:1309-1321.
16. Degner LF, Sloan JA. Symptom distress in newly diagnosed ambulatory cancer patients and as a predictor of survival in lung cancer. J Pain Symptom Manage 1995;10:423-431.
17. Engstrom CA, Strohl RA, Rose L, et al. Sleep alterations in cancer patients. Cancer Nurs 1999;22:143-148.
18. Ginsburg ML, Quirt C, Ginsburg AD, MacKillop WJ. Psychiatric illness and psychosocial concerns of patients with newly diagnosed lung cancer. Can Med Assoc J 1995;152:701-708.
19. Harrison LB, Zelefsky MJ, Pfister DG, et al. Detailed quality of life assessment in patients treated with primary radiotherapy for squamous cell cancer of the base of the tongue. Head Neck 1997;19:169-175.
20. Portenoy RK, Thaler HT, Kornblith AB, et al. Symptom prevalence, characteristics and distress in a cancer population. Qual Life Res 1994;3:183-189.
21. Sarna L. Correlates of symptom distress in women with lung cancer. Cancer Pract 1993;1:21-28.
22. Walsh D, Donnelly S, Rybicki L. The symptoms of advanced cancer: Relationship to age, gender, and performance status in 1,000 patients. Support. Care Cancer 2000;8:175-179.
23. Kendler KS, Heath AC, Martin NG, Eaves LJ. Symptoms of anxiety and symptoms of depression: Same genes, different environments? Arch Gen Psychiatry 1987;44:451-457.
24. Eaves LJ, Eysenck HJ, Martin NG, et al. Genes, Culture and Personality: An Empirical Approach. London: Academic Press, 1989.
25. Borkovec T. Pseudo (experiential) insomnia and idiopathic (objective) insomnia: Theoretical and therapeutic issues. Adv Behav Res Ther 1979. p. 27-55.
26. Rechtschaffen A, Monroe L. Laboratory studies of insomnia. In Kales A (ed). Sleep: Physiology and Pathology. Philadelphia: Lippincott, 1969.
27. Monroe LJ. Psychological and physiological differences between good and poor sleepers. J Abnorm Psychol 1967;72:255-264.
28. Freedman RR, Sattler HL. Physiological and psychological factors in sleep-onset insomnia. J Abnorm Psychol 1982;91:380-389.
29. Hauri P. The influence of evening activity on the onset of sleep. Psychophysiology 1969;5:426-430.
30. Freedman R, Papsdorf JD. Biofeedback and progressive relaxation treatment of sleep-onset insomnia: A controlled, all-night investigation. Biofeedback Self Regul 1976;1:253-271.
31. Drevets WC, Price JL, Simpson JR Jr, et al. Subgenual prefrontal cortex abnormalities in mood disorders. Nature 1997;386:824-827.
32. Bourne RS, Mills GH. Sleep disruption in critically ill patients: Pharmacological considerations. Anaesthesia 2004;59:374-384.
33. Dunn GP, Milch RA. Is this a bad day, or one of the last days? How to recognize and respond to approaching demise. J Am Coll Surg 2002;195:879-887.
34. Bernstein DA, Borkovec TD. Progressive Relaxation Training: A Manual for the Helping Professions. Champaign, IL: Research Press, 1973.
35. Woolfolk RL, McNulty TF. Relaxation treatment for insomnia: A component analysis. J Consult Clin Psychol 1983;51:495-503.
36. Stam HJ, Bultz BD. The treatment of severe insomnia in a cancer patient. J Behav Ther Exp Psychiatry 1986;17:33-37.
37. Sela RA, Watanabe S, Nekolaichuk CL. Sleep disturbances in palliative cancer patients attending a pain and symptom control clinic. Palliat Support Care 2005;3:23-31.
38. American Sleep Disorders Association. The International Classification of Sleep Disorders. Rochester, MN: Author, 1997.
39. American Psychiatric Association. Diagnostic and Statistical Manual of Mental Disorders. Washington DC: Author, 1994.
40. Morin CM. Insomnia: Psychological Assessment and Management. New York: The Guilford Press, 1993.
41. Jacobsen PB, Roth A, Holland J. Psycho-Oncology. In Holland JC (ed): New York: Oxford University Press, 1998, pp 257-268.
42. Omne-Ponten M, Holmberg L, Burns T, et al. Determinants of the psycho-social outcome after operation for breast cancer: Results of a prospective comparative interview study following mastectomy and breast conservation. Eur J Cancer 1992;28A:1062-1067.
43. Knobf MT, Pasacreta JV, Valentine A, et al. Chemotherapy, hormonal therapy, and immunotherapy. In Holland J (ed). Psycho-Oncology. New York: Oxford University Press, 1998, pp 277-288.
44. Cassileth PA, Lusk EJ, Torri S, et al. Antiemetic efficacy of dexamethasone therapy in patients receiving cancer chemotherapy. Arch Intern Med 1983; 143:1347-1349.
45. Ling MH, Perry PJ, Tsuang MT. Side effects of corticosteroid therapy: Psychiatric aspects. Arch Gen Psychiatry 1981;38:471-477.
46. Ancoli-Israel S. Insomnia in the elderly: A review for the primary care practitioner. Sleep 2000;23(Suppl 1):S23-S30; discussion S36-S38.
47. Edinger JD, Wohlgemuth WK. The significance and management of persistent primary insomnia: The past, present and future of behavioral insomnia therapies. Sleep Med Rev 1999;3:101-118.
48. Kupfer DJ, Reynolds CF 3rd. Management of insomnia. N Engl J Med 1997;336:341-346.
49. Montagna P, Cortelli P, Tuniper P, et al. Fatal Familial Insomnia: Inherited Prion Disease, Sleep and Thalamus. New York: Raven Press, 1994.
50. Dagan Y. Circadian rhythm sleep disorders (CRSD). Sleep Med Rev 2002; 6:45-54.
51. Earley CJ. Clinical practice: Restless legs syndrome. N Engl J Med 2003; 348:2103-2109.
52. Morin CM, Daley M, Ouellet MC. Insomnia in adults. Curr Treat Options Neurol 2001;3:9-18.
53. Reimer MA, Flemons WW. Quality of life in sleep disorders. Sleep Med Rev 2003;7:335-349.
54. Johns MW. Polysomnography at a sleep disorders unit in Melbourne. Med J Aust 1991;155:303-308.
55. Johns MW. A new method for measuring daytime sleepiness: The Epworth sleepiness scale. Sleep 1991;14:540-545.
56. Ancoli-Israel S, Cole R, Alessi C, et al. The role of actigraphy in the study of sleep and circadian rhythms. Sleep 2003;26:342-392.
57. Kvale EA, Shuster JL. Sleep disturbance in supportive care of cancer: A review. J Palliat Med 2006;9:437-450.

58. Budur K, Rodriguez C, Foldvary-Schaefer N. Advances in treating insomnia. Cleve Clin J Med 2007;74:251-252, 255-258, 261-62 passim.

59. Grunstein R. Insomnia: Diagnosis and management. Aust Fam Physician 2002;31:995-1000.

60. Sharpley AL, Cowen PJ. Effect of pharmacologic treatments on the sleep of depressed patients. Biol Psychiatry 1995;37:85-98.

61. Mitler MM, Seidel WF, van den Hoed J, et al. Comparative hypnotic effects of flurazepam, triazolam, and placebo: A long-term simultaneous nighttime and daytime study. J Clin Psychopharmacol 1984;4:2-13.

62. Tonne U, Hiltunen AJ, Vikander B, et al. Neuropsychological changes during steady-state drug use, withdrawal and abstinence in primary benzodiazepine-dependent patients. Acta Psychiatr Scand 1995;91:299-304.

63. Mustard CA, Mayer T. Case-control study of exposure to medication and the risk of injurious falls requiring hospitalization among nursing home residents. Am J Epidemiol 1997;145:738-745.

64. Neutel CI, Hirdes JP, Maxwell CJ, Patten SB. New evidence on benzodiazepine use and falls: The time factor. Age Ageing 1996;25:273-278.

65. Dorsey CM, Lukas SE, Teicher MH, et al. Effects of passive body heating on the sleep of older female insomniacs. J Geriatr Psychiatry Neurol 1996;9:83-90.

66. Meltzer EO. Antihistamine- and decongestant-induced performance decrements. J Occup Med 1990;32:327-334.

67. Scharf MB, Roth T, Vogel GW, Walsh JK. A multicenter, placebo-controlled study evaluating zolpidem in the treatment of chronic insomnia. J Clin Psychiatry 1994;12:537-549.

68. Walsh JK, Vogel GW, Scharf M, et al. A five week, polysomnographic assessment of zaleplon 10 mg for the treatment of primary insomnia. Sleep Med 2000;1:41-49.

69. Elie R, Ruther E, Farr I, et al. Sleep latency is shortened during 4 weeks of treatment with zaleplon, a novel nonbenzodiazepine hypnotic. Zaleplon Clinical Study Group. J Clin Psychiatry 1999;60:536-544.

70. Kummer J, Guendel L, Linden J, et al. Long-term polysomnographic study of the efficacy and safety of zolpidem in elderly psychiatric in-patients with insomnia. J Int Med Res 1993;21:171-184.

71. Pecknold J, Wilson R, le Morvan P. Long term efficacy and withdrawal of zopiclone: A sleep laboratory study. Int Clin Psychopharmacol 1990;5(Suppl 2):57-67.

72. Krystal AD, Walsh JK, Laska E, et al. Sustained efficacy of eszopiclone over 6 months of nightly treatment: Results of a randomized, double-blind, placebo-controlled study in adults with chronic insomnia. Sleep 2003;26:793-799.

73. Ware JC, Brown FW, Moorad PJ Jr, et al. Effects on sleep: A double-blind study comparing trimipramine to imipramine in depressed insomniac patients. Sleep 1989;12:537-549.

74. Armitage R, Yonkers K, Cole D, Rush AJ. A multicenter, double-blind comparison of the effects of nefazodone and fluoxetine on sleep architecture and quality of sleep in depressed outpatients. J Clin Psychopharmacol 1997;17:161-168.

75. Rickels K, Morris RJ, Newman H, et al. Diphenhydramine in insomniac family practice patients: A double-blind study. J Clin Pharmacol 1983;23:234-242.

76. Meuleman JR, Nelson RC, Clark RL Jr. Evaluation of temazepam and diphenhydramine as hypnotics in a nursing-home population. Drug Intell Clin Pharm 1987;21:716-720.

77. Ellis CM, Lemmens G, Parkes JD. Melatonin and insomnia. J Sleep Res 1996;5:61-65.

78. Lindahl O, Lindwall L. Double blind study of a valerian preparation. Pharmacol Biochem Behav 1989;32:1065-1066.

79. Balderer G, Borbely AA. Effect of valerian on human sleep. Psychopharmacology (Berl) 1985;87:406-409.

80. Hajak G, Rodenbeck A, Voderholzer U, et al. Doxepin in the treatment of primary insomnia: A placebo-controlled, double-blind, polysomnographic study. J Clin Psychiatry 2001;62:453-463.

81. Akechi T, Uchitomi Y, Okamura H, et al. Usage of haloperidol for delirium in cancer patients. Support. Care Cancer 1996;4:390-392.

82. Davis MP, Dickerson ED, Pappagallo M, et al. Mirtazepine: Heir apparent to amitriptyline? Am J Hosp Palliat Care 2001;18:42-46.

83. Davis MP, Khawam E, Pozuelo L, Lagman R. Management of symptoms associated with advanced cancer: Olanzapine and mirtazapine. A World Health Organization project. Expert Rev Anticancer Ther 2002;2:365-376.

84. Kast RE. Mirtazapine may be useful in treating nausea and insomnia of cancer chemotherapy. Support Care Cancer 2001;9:469-470.

85. Theobald DE, Kirsh KL, Holtsclaw E, et al. An open-label, crossover trial of mirtazapine (15 and 30 mg) in cancer patients with pain and other distressing symptoms. J Pain Symptom Manage 2002;23:442-447.

86. Glass JR, Sproule BA, Herrmann N, et al. Acute pharmacological effects of temazepam, diphenhydramine, and valerian in healthy elderly subjects. J Clin Psychopharmacol 2003;23:260-268.

87. Breslau N, Roth T, Rosenthal L, Andreski P. Sleep disturbance and psychiatric disorders: A longitudinal epidemiological study of young adults. Biol Psychiatry 1996;39:411-418.

88. Ford DE, Kamerow DB. Epidemiologic study of sleep disturbances and psychiatric disorders: An opportunity for prevention? JAMA 1989;262:1479-1484.

89. Foley DJ, Monjan AA, Izmirlian G, et al. Incidence and remission of insomnia among elderly adults in a biracial cohort. Sleep 1999;22(Suppl 2):S373-S378.

90. Roberts RE, Shema SJ, Kaplan GA, Strawbridge WJ. Sleep complaints and depression in an aging cohort: A prospective perspective. Am J Psychiatry 2000;157:81-88.

91. Heath AC, Kendler KS, Eaves LJ, Martin NG. Evidence for genetic influences on sleep disturbance and sleep pattern in twins. Sleep 1990;13:318-335.

92. McCarren M, Goldberg J, Ramakrishnan V, Fabsitz R. Insomnia in Vietnam era veteran twins: Influence of genes and combat experience. Sleep 1994;17:456-461.

93. Bastien CH, Morin CM. Familial incidence of insomnia. J Sleep Res 2000;9:49-54.

94. Rodenbeck A, Huether G, Ruther E, Hajak G. Interactions between evening and nocturnal cortisol secretion and sleep parameters in patients with severe chronic primary insomnia. Neurosci Lett 2002;324:159-163.

95. Wever RA. Influence of physical workload on free running circadian rhythms of man. Pflugers Arch 1979;381:119.

96. Sandyk R. Melatonin and maturation of REM sleep. Int J Neurosci 1992;63:105-114.

97. MacFarlare JG, Cleghorn JM, Brown GM, Steiner DL. The effects of exogenous melatonin on the total sleep time and daytime alertness of chronic insomniacs: A preliminary study. Biol Psychiatry 1991;30:371-376.

Care of the Imminently Dying

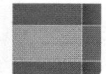

CHAPTER **177**

Diagnosis of Death and Dying

Norma O'Leary

KEY POINTS

- The diagnosis of dying is central to optimal management at the end of life.
- Altered states of consciousness may precede death, including delirium, coma, and persistent vegetative state.
- Natural death is defined by the absence of cardiorespiratory function.
- Brain death is defined as the irreversible cessation of all functions of the entire brain, including the brainstem.
- Unnatural death requires legal investigation.

Death is the inevitable and natural consequence of living. We all hope for a good death. Advances in modern medicine in the early 20th century led to the attitude that death was a medical failure, and dying patients were often neglected by health care professionals. The modern hospice movement developed in response to this situation. Dame Cicely Saunders, who pioneered palliative care as a specialty, was personally motivated to improve care for the terminally ill.[1] In the early years, palliative care was synonymous with terminal care. Although palliative care is now considered appropriate earlier in the disease trajectory of cancer, and has also broadened to include noncancer patients as well, the care of the terminal phase of life remains at the heart of the specialty.

Dying is the last phase of life before death. Recognizing that a person is entering the dying or terminal phase is critical to appropriate, responsive care planning and, possibly, a complete shift in the emphasis of care from intervention to comfort. But defining when this phase actually begins is not straightforward. Is it when the patient is in the last hours of life, or does it begin earlier, when a potentially incurable illness is diagnosed? What about patients who die suddenly? About 1 in 10 people die without any warning, with no preceding illness, and with no time for care.[2] Medical advances such as device therapy for heart failure and noninvasive ventilation for chronic obstructive pulmonary disease have revolutionized end-stage disease and made it more difficult to clearly recognize a dying phase.

Making the diagnosis of dying is essential for good end-of-life care. Barriers to the diagnosis need to be overcome (Box 177-1).[3] Failure to make the diagnosis has negative consequences, not only for the patient but also for the family and health care professionals. The patient may experience uncontrolled symptoms. Inappropriate treatment plans may be instituted, including cardiopulmonary resuscitation. Patients and relatives may get conflicting messages, potentially resulting in loss of trust, dissatisfaction, and formal complaints. Health care professionals may become disillusioned with inappropriate management of patients, causing disharmony within the team. If team members disagree, then mixed messages and opposed goals can cause poor patient management and confused communication.

In the past, health care professionals have been reluctant to make the diagnosis of dying, because it seemed akin to giving up—an admission that nothing more could be done. Such reluctance is no longer acceptable. In fact, this is the very moment when the hospice model of intensive palliative care should come into action, providing physical, psychological, social, and spiritual care for patients and their relatives (Box 177-2).

The physical moment of death can usually be recognized as the cessation of breathing and the absence of a pulse. However, the medicalization of dying has made recognition of the moment of death challenging.

CLINICAL EVALUATION

Dying

Dying is a dynamic process. The concept of a dying trajectory, first suggested in 1965, refers to the change in health status over time as death approaches.[4] The process is influenced by many factors, the most important of which is the underlying disease.[5] It is remarkable how similar dying trajectories can be for comparable diseases.

There are four prototypal death trajectories. Some people die suddenly without warning. Figure 177-1 shows the three other trajectories: steady progression and a predictable terminal phase, gradual decline punctuated by episodes of acute deterioration, and prolonged gradual decline.[6,7]

When patients are within days or weeks of death, certain signs are present. Alone, these signs could be related to potentially reversible causes. When present together, they are more likely to represent an irreversible process. The following are signs of approaching death:

Box 177-1 Barriers to the Diagnosis of Dying

- Unrealistic expectation that the patient may get better
- Disagreement within the team or with the family that the patient is dying
- No definitive diagnosis
- Lack of knowledge of the management of pain and other symptoms at the end of life
- Poor communication skills
- Concerns about withdrawing or withholding treatment
- Fear of foreshortening life
- Misinterpretation of the principle of double effect
- Concerns about resuscitation
- Cultural and spiritual barriers
- Legal complexities

Box 177-2 Goals of Care for Patients in the Dying Phase

- Use a problem-solving approach to symptom control
- Avoid unnecessary interventions
- Perform regular review of drugs and symptoms
- Address psychological and insight issues
- Provide religious and spiritual support for the patient
- Communicate with family and carers
- Update the primary health care team

- Bedridden or able to get out of bed only with great difficulty
- Profound weakness
- Little interest in food and drink
- Difficulty swallowing
- Increasingly somnolent

In the final days and hours of life, the following signs will probably be present:

- Skin gets cold, from the periphery inward
- Skin feels clammy
- Color of the skin of the extremities and around the mouth may become cyanotic
- Urine output may decrease
- Level of consciousness will diminish
- Patient may "rattle" when breathing
- Respiration is irregular and shallow—a Cheyne-Stokes pattern
- The face may look waxen
- The muscles of the face may relax, and the nose may become more prominent

Nursing staff in direct contact with the patient may be the first to recognize that the patient is dying. Patients should be assessed regularly, because the goals of care should be revised to meet the rapidly changing clinical situation.

Altered States of Consciousness That May Precede Death

Consciousness was first defined in 1890 as awareness of the self and the environment.[8] Consciousness has two

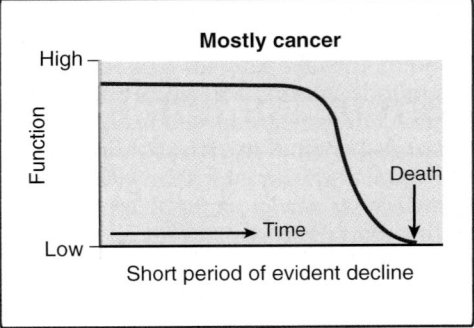

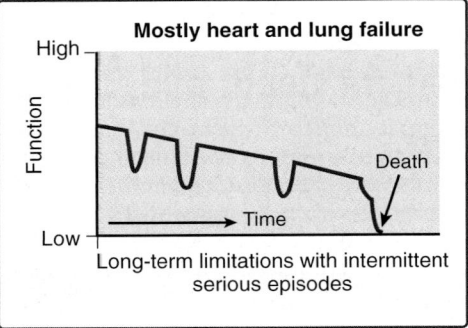

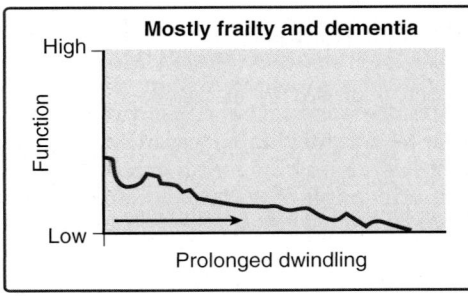

FIGURE 177-1 Death trajectories. *(Adapted from Lunney JR, Lynn J, Hogan C. Profiles of older Medicare decedents. J Am Geriatr Soc 2002;50:1108-1112.*

dimensions: wakefulness and awareness. Altered states of consciousness, from mild delirium to coma, often precede death.

Delirium

Delirium is defined as a transient organic brain syndrome that is characterized by the onset of disordered attention and cognition and is accompanied by disturbances of psychomotor behavior and perception.[9] It is observed in up to 88% of patients before death (see Chapter 156).[10]

Coma

Coma is a state in which a person is totally unaware of both self and external surroundings and is unable to respond meaningfully to external stimuli.[8] Coma results from gross impairment of both cerebral hemispheres and/or the ascending reticular activating system. Causes can be classified as either focal or diffuse brain dysfunction. The truly comatose patient is deeply unconscious, with no response to pain. If coma cannot be reversed, it will progress to irreversible brain damage and death.

Vegetative State

A *vegetative state* is a clinical condition of complete unawareness of the self and the environment in which the patient breathes spontaneously, has a stable circulation, and shows cycles of eye closure and opening that may simulate sleep and waking.[11] *Persistent* vegetative state is a vegetative state that is present 1 month after acute traumatic or nontraumatic brain injury. A *permanent* vegetative state is a vegetative state that is present for 12 months or longer.

The diagnosis of a vegetative state can be made if (1) there is no behavioral evidence of awareness of self or environment; (2) there is brain damage, usually of known cause, consistent with the diagnosis; and (3) there are no reversible causes. All available sources of information should be used when making the diagnosis; all written records, including nursing notes, should be reviewed, and staff who have cared for the patient over time should be interviewed. It is particularly important to interview family members. They may observe behavior that indicates awareness, and their opinion on the patient's level of awareness must be sought.

A patient in a vegetative state is unable to give or imply consent. The probability of recovery from a vegetative state is very low, and decisions about continuation of medical care are usually referred to the courts.[11] Any decision to withdraw feeding should be consistent with the principles of autonomy, nonmaleficence, beneficence, and justice. After artificial nutrition and hydration are withdrawn, a patient in a persistent vegetative state usually dies within 10 to 14 days.[12] The immediate cause of death is dehydration and electrolyte imbalance. Some die from intercurrent acute illnesses, such as pneumonia. Others may die from underlying cardiac or renal disease if medications are also discontinued.

The question arises whether patients in a permanent vegetative state can experience pain and suffering. The perceptions of pain and suffering are conscious experiences: unconsciousness, by definition, precludes them. It is unlikely that people in true vegetative states experience pain, but grimace-like or crying-like behaviors are common. These patterned behaviors are mediated at the subcortical level and are not manifestations of perceived pain.[13]

In rare cases, there may be uncertainty as to the diagnosis. For example, it may be difficult to distinguish a persistent vegetative state from a severe locked-in state. A locked-in syndrome is a state in which consciousness and cognition are retained but movement and communication are impossible because of severe involuntary motor paralysis.[14] The syndrome can occur with diseases of the peripheral motor nervous system such as motor neuron disease. Under such circumstances, a patient may be unable to express behavioral responses to painful stimuli, or the responses may be extremely difficult to detect; the absence of a response cannot be taken as proof of the absence of consciousness. If there is any doubt about the diagnosis and the ability of the patient to perceive pain, it is best to err on the side of caution and administer analgesia.

DEATH

Natural Death

Most people die what is called a "natural" death. *Natural death* is defined as the cessation of cardiorespiratory functioning due to a medical disease process (e.g., metastatic cancer, cerebrovascular accident). The loss of pulse and respiration is the criterion to pronounce someone dead.

Brain Death

Until the 1950s, death was recognizable by the absence of the traditional signs of life—pulse and breathing. The development of mechanical ventilation made possible the support of dead patients temporarily. The notion of death was challenged by organ donation, beginning in the 1960s.[15] Organ donation was premised on professional and public acceptance that the patient was dead. However, how could someone be perceived as dead if there was evidence of cardiopulmonary functioning, albeit mechanically supported? In 1968, a new criterion for death was defined—brain death.[16] *Brain death* is defined as the irreversible cessation of all functions of the entire brain, including the brainstem. The declaration of brain death requires that all brainstem reflexes are absent (Box 177-3)[17] and that certain preconditions and exclusions are fulfilled.[18]

Preconditions for a diagnosis of brain death:

- The patient should be in apneic coma (i.e., unresponsive and on a ventilator, with no spontaneous respiratory efforts).
- There should be no doubt that the condition is caused by irremediable structural brain damage. The diagnosis of a disorder that can lead to brainstem death (e.g., head injury, intracranial hemorrhage) should have been fully established.

Exclusions to a diagnosis of brain death:

- The possibility that unresponsive apnea is a result of poisoning, sedatives, or neuromuscular blocking agents must be excluded.
- Hypothermia must be excluded; the central body temperature should be greater than 35° C.
- There must be no significant metabolic or endocrine disturbance that could produce or contribute to coma or cause it to persist.

Box 177-3 Diagnostic Tests for the Confirmation of Brainstem Death

The following tests are used to determine that all brainstem reflexes are absent:

1. The pupils are fixed in diameter and do not respond to sharp changes in the intensity of light.
2. There is no corneal reflex.
3. The vestibulo-ocular reflexes are absent.
4. Motor responses are absent.
5. There is no gag reflex response to tracheal suctioning.
6. No respiratory movements occur when the patient is disconnected from the mechanical ventilator for long enough to ensure that the arterial carbon dioxide tension has risen above the threshold for stimulation of respiration.

- There should be no profound abnormality of the plasma electrolytes, acid-base balance, or blood glucose levels.

This clinical neurological examination remains the standard for determination of brain death by most countries.[19] There is lack of consensus internationally as to the specialty of the assessing physician and level of expertise needed, the duration of observations, and the use of confirmatory tests required to diagnose brain death.[20]

ASSESSMENT TOOLS

There are different levels of consciousness. They can be categorized on a simple coma scale (Box 177-4). The most commonly used complex coma scale, employing three groups of observations, is the Glasgow Coma Scale, which was originally suggested for head injuries (Box 177-5).

ACUTE MANAGEMENT

Chapter 178 covers the standards of care for acute management of the dying process.

COMMON ERRORS

Despite being widely accepted, the definition of brain death has been challenged. It has been challenged on a physiological level, because some persons determined to be brain dead have persistent regulated secretion of anti-

---

Box 177-4 Simple Five-point Coma Scale:

1 = Fully awake
2 = Conscious but drowsy
3 = Unconscious but responsive to pain with purposeful movement (e.g., flexion/withdrawal)
4 = Unconscious but responsive to pain by extension
5 = Unconscious and unresponsive to pain

Box 177-5 Glasgow Coma Scale

Best motor response:

6 = Moves in response to command
5 = Localizes pain
4 = Withdraws from pain
3 = Flexes in response to pain
2 = Extends in response to pain
1 = No response

Best verbal response:

5 = Fully oriented
4 = Confused
3 = Inappropriate words
2 = Incomprehensible sounds
1 = No response

Best eye response:

4 = Eyes open spontaneously
3 = Eyes open to command
2 = Eyes open in response to pain
1 = Eyes remain closed

---

diuretic hormone.[21] How can a patient be brain dead if some hypothalamic endocrine functioning is retained?

The concept of brain death also has been challenged on religious grounds. In the orthodox Jewish tradition, the majority view is that death has occurred only if there is neither breathing nor heart pulsation.[22,23] The current medical practice of withdrawing mechanical support once brain death has been pronounced may be unacceptable to some members of the Jewish community. The old practice of maintaining brain-dead patients on mechanical ventilation until asystole naturally occurs has largely ceased, yet this practice may be more acceptable to orthodox Jews.[24] In this circumstance, compromise is needed from the medical fraternity to accommodate religious beliefs that conflict with medical guidelines.

Confusion surrounding the concept of brain death can be fueled by language. Because brain-dead patients show traditional signs of life when maintained on a ventilator, it is not surprising that many people believe that brain death is a separate type of death, one that occurs before real death. This confusion is re-enforced when hospital personnel talk about "life support" being removed from such patients. We need to be consistent and clear in our language.

LINKED AREAS

Medicolegal Deaths

Medicolegal death results from some "unnatural" (unexpected, unusual, or suspicious) event such as homicide, suicide, or accident. This situation is specifically governed by legal statutes and requires legal investigation. There are broadly three systems of death investigation[25]:

1. The generic criminal investigation and judicial system examines deaths that are suspicious, in a criminal sense, through the same systems as are used to investigate suspected crime.
2. A coroner is an independent official, usually a doctor or a lawyer, who has legal responsibility for the investigation of sudden and unexplained deaths. The coroner is central to death investigation in the English legal system in Great Britain and many Commonwealth countries.
3. In the United States and Canada, many states and provinces have abolished the coroner's system and replaced it with a medical examiner's system.[26] The medical examiner systems are led by forensic pathologists and determine the cause of death but do not generally inquire into its circumstances.

Autopsy

An *autopsy* is an examination of the organs or tissues of the body after death. It is a valuable source of information, not only for the professional but also for the family. It provides answers as to the exact cause of death and may identify the etiology of previously unexplained symptoms. It can help audit medical care. It can be of therapeutic value for the grieving family by reducing uncertainty and providing answers to questions surrounding the death of a loved one. Despite these valuable roles, the rate of autopsies has dropped steeply over the last 40 years.[27] The main reason for the fall is an increased confidence in new methods of predeath diagnosis, particularly modern imaging techniques. Other reasons include doctors' discomfort in requesting permission from families, cost containment, and doubts about the value of the procedure.

Certain deaths that are considered unnatural or medicolegal require an autopsy as a mandatory part of the legal investigation of the death. Requirements for mandatory autopsies vary according to jurisdiction (Box 177-6).[25]

Verifying and Certifying Deaths

Death verification is a professional confirmation that the life has ended. *Death certification* is a formal record of the cause of death. The doctor indicates on the certificate the condition or sequence of conditions that led directly to death and any associated conditions that contributed. In most developed countries, the cause of death is registered formally. Local and national registers of deaths are a valuable source of information used to inform public health policy and health care service development.

RESEARCH CHALLENGES AND PRIORITIES

Historically, biomedical and clinical research has focused almost exclusively on the prevention, detection, or cure of disease and the prolongation of life. Recent years have seen a dramatic increase in palliative care research, broadly defined as research related to understanding and improving the quality of life at the end of life. Many challenges exist in carrying out research in the dying, including the relative vulnerability of patients, difficulty recruiting representative population samples, high attrition rates, low priority with funding agencies for research in end-of-life care, and uncertain reliability of proxy assessments.

To participate in research, patients must receive, comprehend, and retain all the information necessary to allow them to give fully informed consent.[28] Fully informed consent protects patient autonomy.[29] Many dying patients are delirious or minimally conscious, making consent difficult to obtain. Palliative care research offers a good setting for the use of advance consent.[30]

Predicting the end of life or time of death for patients is challenging because of the highly dynamic and individual nature of the dying process. And yet, "How long do I have?" is one of the questions most frequently asked of doctors. Clear prognostication can grant patients and families the time and permission to take care of unfinished

business and say goodbye. It is a valuable gift. The development of accurate prognostic models should be a research priority. Prognostic models have been proposed but are not discriminatory. The challenge is to identify disease-specific variables that predict the end of life.

Other priorities for research at the end of life include the following:

- A greater understanding of the physiological basis for terminal symptoms
- Establishing predictors of patients at high risk for suffering at the end of life
- Standardization of assessment tools at the end of life
- Caregiver needs

CONCLUSIONS

Dame Cicely Saunders said, "You matter because you are you, and you matter all the days of your life."[31] These words describe succinctly the importance of caring for patients until their life's journey has ended. Care for the dying remains the essence of what palliative care is about. Making the diagnosis of the dying phase is key to ensuring that the patient receives the best possible care and eventually experiences a good death. Although in many instances welcome medical advances have prolonged life expectancy and revolutionized the end of life experience, application of the basic principles of palliative care, pain and symptom control, and dealing with psychosocial and spiritual issues should be an automatic component of medical end-of-life care.

REFERENCES

1. Clarke D. Originating a movement: Cicely Saunders and the development of St.Christopher's Hospice, 1957-1967. Mortality 1998;3:43-63.
2. Cartwright A. Changes in life and care in the year before death 1969-1987. J Public Health Med 1987;13:81-87.
3. Ellershaw J, Ward C. Care of the dying patient: The last hours or days of life. BMJ 2003;326:30-34.
4. Glaser B, Strauss AL. Time for dying. Chicago, IL: Aldine Publishing, 1968.
5. Murray SA, Kendall M, Boyd K, et al. Illness trajectories and palliative care. BMJ 2005;330:1007-1015.
6. Lunney JR, Lynn J, Hogan C. Profiles of older Medicare decedents. J Am Geriatr Soc 2002;50:1108-1112.
7. Lunney JR, Lynn J, Foley DJ, Guralnik JM. Patterns of functional decline at the end of life. JAMA 2003;289:2387-2392.
8. Medical aspects of the persistent vegetative state: 1. The Multi-Society Task Force on PVS. N Engl J Med 1994;330:1499-1508.
9. American Psychiatric Association. Diagnostic and Statistical Manual of Mental Disorders, 4th ed. Text revision (DSM-IV-TR). Washington DC: American Psychiatric Press, 2000.
10. Lawlor, PG, Gagnon B, Mancini IL, et al. Occurence, causes and outcomes of delirium in patients with advanced cancer. Arch Intern Med 2000;160:786-794.
11. Wade DT. Ethical issues in diagnosis and management of patients in the permanent vegetative state. BMJ 2001;322:352-354.
12. Alfonso I, Lanting WA, Duenas D, et al. Discontinuation of artificial hydration and nutrition in hopelessly vegetative children. Ann Neurol 1992;32:454-455.
13. Medical aspects of the persistent vegetative state: 2. The Multi-Society Task Force on PVS. N Engl J Med 1994;330:1572-1679.
14. Position statement: Certain aspects of the care and management of profoundly and irreversibly paralysed patients with retained consciousness and cognition. Report of the Ethics and Humanities Subcommittee of the American Academy of Neurology. Neurology 1993;43:222-223.
15. Waisel DG, Truog RD. The end of life sequence. Anesthesiology 1997;87:676-686.
16. Report of the Ad Hoc Committee of the Harvard Medical School to Examine the Definition of Brain Death. A definition of irreversible coma. JAMA 1968;205:85-88.
17. Diagnosis of Brain Death. Statement issued by the Honorary Secretary of the Conference of Medical Royal Colleges and their Faculties in the United Kingdom on 11 October 1976. BMJ 1976;2:1187-1188.
18. Intensive care medicine. In Kumar P, Clark M (ed). Clinical Medicine, 5th ed. London: Saunders, 2002, pp 954-955.
19. Wijdicks EFM. The diagnosis of brain death. N EngL J Med 2001;344:16:1215-1221.

Box 177-6 Deaths That May Require Investigation

- Any violent or traumatic death
- Any death of a person detained in a prison
- Any death from a range of communicable diseases
- Any death in which occupational disease may have played a part
- Any death of a child in care
- Any death which a doctor may not certify as being from natural disease
- Any death which is the subject of significant unresolved concern or suspicion as to its cause or circumstances on the part of any family member, or any member of the public, or any health professional

20. Haupt WF. European brain death codes: A comparison of national guidelines. J Neurol 1999;246:432-437.
21. Truog RD, Fackler JC. Rethinking brain death. Crit Care Med 1992; 12:1705-1713.
22. HaLevi Wosner S. Heart transplants. In Roodyn P (ed). Pathways in Medicine. Jerusalem: Taragum Press, 1995.
23. Bleich JD. Time of death in Jewish law. New York: Z Berman, 1991.
24. Inwald D, Jakobovits I, Petros A. Brainstem death: Managing care when accepted guidelines and religious beliefs are in contrast. BMJ 2000; 320:1266-1267.
25. Death certification and investigation in England, Wales and Northern Ireland: The Report of a Fundamental Review 2003. Presented to Parliament by the Secretary of State for the Home Department by Command of Her Majesty, June 2003. CM 5831. London: The Stationery Office, 2003.
26. Milroy CM, Whitwell HL. Reforming the coroner's system. BMJ 2003; 327:175-176.
27. Bates C, Burgess H. A case for autopsy in palliative medicine. Palliat Med 2004;18:652-653.
28. Department of Health: Policy and Guidance: Consent. Available at http://www.doh.gov.uk/en/Policyandguidance/Healthandsocialcaretopics/Consent/index.htm (accessed January 27, 2008).
29. Biros MH, Lewis RJ, Olson JW, et al. Informed consent in emergency research. JAMA 1995;273:1283-1287.
30. Rees E, Hardy J. Novel consent process for research in dying patients unable to give consent. BMJ 2003;327:198-200.
31. Berger A. Palliative care in long-term facilities—a comprehensive model. J Am Geriatr Soc 1969;49:1570-1571.

SUGGESTED READING

Ellershaw J, Ward C. Care of the dying patient: The last hours or days of life. BMJ 2003;326:30-34.

Medical aspects of the persistent vegetative state: 1. The Multi-Society Task Force on PVS. N Engl J Med 1994;330: 1499-1508.

Medical aspects of the persistent vegetative state: 2. The Multi-Society Task Force on PVS. N Engl J Med 1994;330: 1572-1679.

Murray SA, Kendall M, Boyd K, et al. Illness trajectories and palliative care. BMJ 2005;330:1007-1015.

Widjicks EFM. The diagnosis of brain death. N Engl J Med 2001;344:1215-1221.

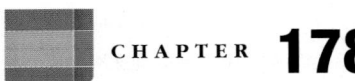

CHAPTER **178**

Standards of Care

John Ellershaw, Maureen Gambles, and Catriona Mayland

KEY POINTS

- Setting standards based on meaningful measurements in care of the dying, although challenging, is possible and worthwhile.
- Comprehensive advance care planning, based on informed decision making and incorporating regular updates, can influence choice at the end of life.
- Frameworks of care that promote cycles of review and development based on objective data can influence standards.
- Setting standards based on the views of patients and carers is vital to providing the best care.

Care of the dying is a challenging area in which to set standards. In contrast to other aspects of health care, there is no possibility of direct feedback from patients. Because medicine has become increasingly focused on cure and not care, care of the dying is not necessarily seen as important or as a priority in some settings. This chapter focuses on three areas of standard-setting: (1) anticipating care in the dying phase and putting in place specific process standards to achieve a dignified death; (2) implementing continuous quality improvement for care of the dying; and (3) using the views of bereaved relatives to set standards for care of the dying.

ANTICIPATORY PROCESS STANDARDS OF CARE FOR THE DYING

The demographics of dying is changing throughout society.[1] In developed countries, people die from chronic diseases and have predictable death trajectories. The two main elements that prevent optimal care at the end of life are lack of advance care planning (ACP) by individual patients and a health care system that is unresponsive to the changing needs of the dying and their family and carers.

Advance Care Planning by Individuals

ACP promotes patient autonomy and usually involves a discussion between individual patients and their physicians regarding their future care wishes. In some countries, ACP is encompassed within a legal framework. ACP can include the individual's concerns, important values, personal goals for care, and preferences for care in the dying phase. ACP involves sensitive communication with health care professionals so that individuals can make informed choices.[2]

When the expressed wishes of an individual are known, it enables health care personnel to support decision making into the future. It also provides guidance if the patient should become incompetent and be unable to express his or her wishes. It is important to recognize the limitations of ACP. These include ensuring that the patient makes an informed decision when the ACP is formulated and ensuring that it is updated regularly, so that changes in the patient's view or in health care treatments can be accurately represented.

When given the opportunity to express a preference, many patients express a wish to die at home, and yet many die in acute-care general hospitals.[3] Comprehensive ACP potentiates autonomy and creates a more constructive framework to enable people to die in the place of their choice.

Dying at Home

Even if patients have expressed a wish through formal ACP or direct discussion, if the health care system is unresponsive to the needs of the dying and their family and carers, it may be impossible for them to die at home. The framework of care required to enable death at home has been well documented.[4] There are key anticipatory measures a health care system must meet if a patient is to be enabled to die at home:

1. The patient has expressed a wish to die at home, and this decision is supported by the family, carers, or both.
2. There is appropriate care and support to meet the patient's needs; this may be provided by the patient's family or carers or by health care or social care workers.
3. There is appropriate care and support to meet the needs of the family and carers.
4. There is 24-hour access to nursing and medical expertise.
5. There is a robust mechanism to transmit information relating to patients dying at home between the medical and nursing staff. Out-of-hours handover forms are one mechanism.
6. There is access to drugs in the patient's home to manage symptoms in the dying phase, including pain, respiratory tract secretions, terminal agitation, dyspnea, and nausea and vomiting.
7. The patient has medication prescribed as required for symptoms in the dying phase.
8. Specific spiritual/religious needs can be met.
9. Appropriate discussions have been held with the patient and family or carers on the inappropriateness of futile interventions, including cardiopulmonary resuscitation.[5]

These anticipatory care standards can potentiate a patient's dying at home. A health care system has to be developed to ensure that these standards are established to meet an individual's request. Many of the crises that often lead to acute hospital admission in the dying phase can potentially be averted. The development of such standards enables critical review of the health care system.

CONTINUOUS QUALITY IMPROVEMENT PROGRAM FOR SETTING STANDARDS OF CARE FOR THE DYING

Continuous Quality Improvement (CQI) is a practical change management technique that implies "improvement, change, and learning."[6] It applies scientific methodology to everyday work to improve patient outcomes. It is an approach to quality management that "emphasises the organisation and systems, focuses on processes, and promotes the need for objective data to analyse and improve processes."[7]

Prerequisites for successful CQI for care of the dying include the following:

- Committed leadership
- Identification of the needs of the dying and their families
- Scrutiny of current processes of care delivery
- Ongoing education and support
- Continuous quality monitoring

The Liverpool Care Pathway Framework

The Liverpool Care Pathway (LCP) framework embodies the CQI approach to effect changes in the culture of care for the dying within individual organizations and care settings. It is recommended practice within the National Institute for Clinical Excellence (NICE) Guidance on Improving Supportive and Palliative Care[8] and is one of the frameworks being disseminated as part of the End of Life Care Initiative (EOLI). A government white paper entitled, "Our Health, Our Choice, Our Say: A New Direction for Community Services,"[9] prioritized training and recommended the LCP be applied throughout the United Kingdom. To date, approximately 254 hospitals in England, Scotland, and Northern Ireland, 121 adult inpatient hospices, 351 community-based services, and 248 Care Homes have registered with the project. In addition to the spread of the framework nationally, there are 62 registrations from 13 countries in Europe and beyond. Of these, the Netherlands has the longest association with the LCP framework.

The care pathway document itself, around which the framework is built, provides a comprehensive template of appropriate, evidence-based, multidisciplinary care for the dying. Focusing on the physical, psychological, social, spiritual/religious, and information needs of patients and carers, it is organized into three discrete sections: Initial Assessment, Ongoing Assessment, and Care after Death. The LCP replaces all other documentation at the end of life and is structured to facilitate audit of care by measuring reliable outcomes (Table 178-1).[10-12]

Initial Process

To support teams in managing cultural change in end-of-life care, a formal process for involvement with the framework (both nationally and internationally) is in place (Fig. 178-1). This provides tangible central support to participating organizations at various points.

TABLE 178-1	Initial Assessment Section—Outcomes of Care
Goal 1	Current medication assessed and nonessentials discontinued
Goal 2	PRN subcutaneous medication written up for the following indications as per protocol
	Pain—Analgesia
	Agitation—Sedative
	Respiratory tract secretions—Anticholinergic
	Nausea and vomiting—Antiemetic
	Dyspnea—Anxiolytic/muscle relaxant
Goal 3	Discontinue inappropriate interventions
Goal 3a	Decisions to discontinue inappropriate nursing interventions taken
Goal 3b	Syringe driver set up within 4 hr of doctor's orders
Goal 4	Ability to communicate in English assessed as adequate
Goal 5	Insight into condition assessed
Goal 6	Religious/spiritual needs assessed
Goal 7	Identify how family/other are to be informed of patient's impending death
Goal 8	Family/other given hospital information via facilities leaflet
Goal 9	G.P. practice is aware of patient's condition
Goal 10	Plan of care explained and discussed with
	Patient
	Family/other
Goal 11	Family/other express understanding of planned care

From the Liverpool Care Pathway for the Dying Patient, Version 11. Available at http://www.lcp-mariecurie.org.uk.

Formal registration of each site is required. Teams must identify key personnel within the organization who will undertake implementation; the written approval of the chief executive is required before formal registration. This ensures a "top down" commitment (i.e., committed leadership) to the project that underpins successful implementation.

Base review analysis (i.e., scrutiny of current care delivery) is the next step. Participating organizations are encouraged to undertake a retrospective audit (base review) of their documentation of care, the sole purpose of which is to highlight and reinforce the need for change. The base review involves identifying and evaluating 20 recent consecutive notes from within the proposed pilot area. The information within the notes is scrutinized for evidence that appropriate care has been delivered in the dying phase in light of the goals identified on the LCP. The feedback report for local dissemination (provided by the LCP central team) consists of simple charts that illustrate where the documentation of care is good and where it could be improved.

Study days, conferences, and teaching resources (ongoing education and support) are offered to participating organizations. Formal education is available in two study days. The first takes place before the implementation phase and focuses on techniques for priming the environment for change. A second, workshop-based study day brings together colleagues from different organizations facing similar issues during implementation and facilitates discussion of shared challenges and opportunities and subsequent networking.

Implementation

Successful framework implementation requires local education, mainly for generic medical and nursing colleagues. The pilot phase in any organization lasts approximately 6 months. Increasingly, a package of educational and information resources is sought to support the implementers in providing timely educational input. A project has begun within the Marie Curie Palliative Care Institute to build an Educational Toolkit for use with the LCP. This project will develop learning resources, both lectures and more informal teaching methods, to support medical and nursing colleagues in their use of the LCP.

Postimplementation analysis (i.e., continuous monitoring of quality) is the final step. Once 20 LCPs have been completed, the organization is encouraged to undertake a further practice audit of the data within the LCPs to assess any change in practice. Analysis and reporting can be facilitated by the LCP central team.

Benchmarking

One of the major challenges in effecting change is to secure and sustain that change. Benchmarking is a useful way of building regular statistical monitoring into an organization by appropriate comparison of performance with that of other, similar organizations. Benchmarking has been defined as "a continual and collaborative discipline, which involves measuring and comparing results of key processes with the best performers and adopting the best practices."[13]

Two pilot benchmarking exercises, covering populations of 2.17 and 3.1 million, respectively, were done in the northwest of England before a planned national hospital audit in 2006/2007. Data were collected in both phases: 315 patients (representing 16 organizations) in phase 1 and 394 patients (representing 24 organizations) in phase 2. For each organization, descriptive analysis illustrated the proportions of goals on the LCP that were "achieved" (i.e., met); "varianced" (not met), and "missing" (not filled in on the pathway). Data from participating organizations were then aggregated to form "benchmarks" for hospital, hospice, and community sectors. Individual organizations were able to assess their relative performance on each of the goals, compared with the benchmark for their relevant sector (Fig. 178-2). Workshops helped representatives from participating organizations to come together to discuss their performance and learn from each other, particularly from high-performing organizations.

More recently, all relevant National Health Service hospital trusts in England have been invited to provide individual hospital data from 30 LCPs for the forthcoming National Audit in Hospitals. It is hoped that the resultant benchmarks will enable robust initial data-based standards for care of the dying to emerge.

SETTING STANDARDS OF CARE FOR THE DYING: USING THE VIEWS OF BEREAVED RELATIVES

One way to set standards is to have user involvement in the evaluation of end-of-life services. This was a key recommendation in the recent NICE guidelines for supportive and palliative care.[8] By involving patients and families in defining outcomes that are important at the end of life, relevant measures can be developed to evaluate the quality of care for dying patients and their families.

Using patients to measure the quality of end-of-life care has practical and ethical difficulties. An alternative is to use instruments retrospectively with relatives and close friends during bereavement. There are several end-of-life instruments for bereaved relatives, and patients and relatives were, to some extent, involved in their development. The tools can be thought of as either domain-specific or multidimensional.

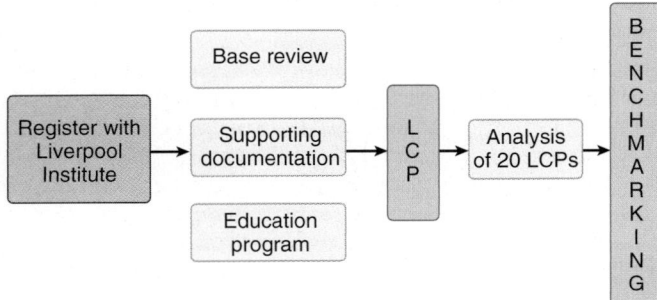

FIGURE 178-1   The Liverpool Care Pathway (LCP) continuous quality improvement process in care of the dying.

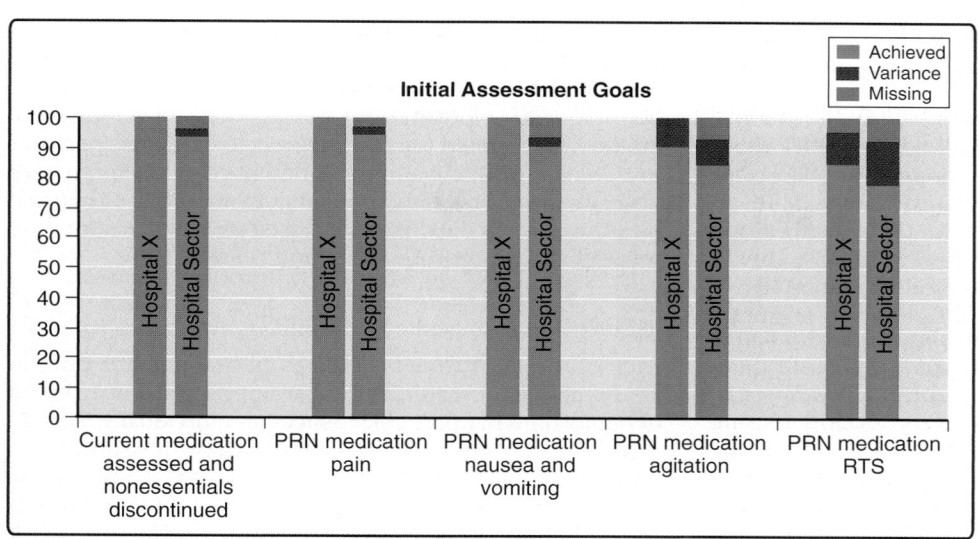

FIGURE 178-2 Example of benchmark feedback.

Domain-Specific Instruments

These two instruments specifically examine particular aspects of end-of-life care. The Family Memorial Symptom Assessment Scale Global Distress Index[14] looks at symptom prevalence, and the Care Evaluation Scale[15] analyzes the process of care.

FAMILY MEMORIAL SYMPTOM ASSESSMENT SCALE–GLOBAL DISTRESS INDEX

The Family Memorial Symptom Assessment Scale Global Distress Index, or Family MSAS-GDI, is an interviewer-administered tool that measures symptom distress experienced by a dying patient in the last week of life. It was developed in the United States. It consists of 11 items, 4 concerning psychological symptoms (worry, sadness, irritability, and nervousness) and 7 concerning physical symptoms (pain, lack of appetite, lack of energy, drowsiness, constipation, dyspnea, and dry mouth). Each item asks whether the symptom was present and uses a five-point scale to assess the frequency of each psychological symptom ("never" to "almost constantly") and the distress caused by each physical symptom ("not at all" to "very much"). There are also options for "not applicable" or "don't know," which can be used if the patient was unconscious in the last week of life. The overall score is the mean of the scores given for all of the 11 items and is regarded as the measure of "global symptom distress."[14] Testing of validity and reliability has been undertaken.

CARE EVALUATION SCALE

The Care Evaluation Scale (CES) is a postal self-completion questionnaire to evaluate the quality of the care structure and process for end-of-life care. It endeavors to identify areas of care that require improvement. The CES consists of 28 questions about the following: help with decision making, care environment, costs, coordination and consistency of care, availability of staff, relief of family burden, and physical and psycho-existential care. The questions are answered using a six-point Likert-type scale, where 1 represents "improvement not necessary" and 6 means "improvement highly necessary." There is also a "not applicable" option. Scores are adjusted so that higher scores represent a lower perception of necessity for improvement. The CES was developed in Japan[15-17] and has good validity and reliability.

Multidimensional Instruments

These five instruments examine many multidimensional aspects of care at the end of life. They can be divided into those that use "satisfaction" as the main outcome and those that use "quality" as their measure.

Tools Using "Satisfaction" as an Outcome Measure

FAMILY SATISFACTION SCALE

The Family Satisfaction Scale (FAMCARE)[18] was developed in Canada to quantify the concept of "family satisfaction with advanced cancer care."[18] It has been used as both a self-completion and an interviewer-administered questionnaire. It consists of 20 items looking at family members' satisfaction in regard to the care they and the patient received. The individual items ask about four main dimensions of care: giving of information, availability of care, psychosocial care, and physical patient care.[18] Each item has a five-point Likert-style scale on which 1 represents "very satisfied" and 5 means "very dissatisfied." The total possible score range is from 20 to 100. Preliminary measures for validity and reliability have been undertaken.

SATISFACTION SCALE FOR THE BEREAVED FAMILY RECEIVING INPATIENT PALLIATIVE CARE

The Satisfaction Scale for the Bereaved Family receiving Inpatient Palliative Care, known as the Sat-Fam-IPC,[14] is a self-completion questionnaire developed in Japan to measure carer satisfaction with an inpatient palliative care service. It is a 34-item questionnaire asking about seven different domains: nursing care, facilities, information sharing, availability of staff, family care, costs, and symptom palliation.[14] Each response option is a six-point scale on which 0 represents "very dissatisfied" and 5 means "very satisfied." Higher scores represent greater satisfaction with care. This instrument has good validity and reliability.

Tools Using "Quality" as an Outcome Measure

VIEWS OF INFORMAL CARERS—EVALUATION OF SERVICES

The Views of Informal Carers—Evaluation of Services (VOICES)[19] instrument is a self-completion postal questionnaire developed in the United Kingdom which asks about the quality of care in the last 3 months of life. It consists of 158 questions on service use, information giving and decision making, control of symptoms, unmet needs, experience of bereavement, and bereavement care. Individual questions have either "Yes/No" response options or a verbal rating scale. Completed questionnaires can be analyzed to examine specific areas in which there were issues, such as symptom control, psychosocial support, or communication. VOICES was developed using a shortened version of the interview schedule from the Regional Study of Care for the Dying (RSCD),[20] which itself was based on the methods used in the pioneering work, *Life before Death*.[21] It has been used extensively in various health care settings to evaluate the care received by patients with malignant and nonmalignant disease. It has not undergone any formal psychometric testing for validity and reliability.

TOOLKIT OF INSTRUMENTS TO MEASURE END-OF-LIFE CARE

The Toolkit of Instruments to Measure End-of-life care (TIME)[22,23] is an interviewer-administered questionnaire, developed in the United States of America, that aims to capture the family's perspective regarding the quality of care during a patient's final illness. Individual questions are categorized into eight domains of care: information and decision making, ACP, closure, coordination, achieving control and respect, family emotional support, self-efficacy, and ratings of patient-focused family care. It consists of 125 questions answered with the use of "Yes/No" response options and verbal rating scales. The information collected can be used to highlight particular issues of care, such as decision making and information, that require improvement. Development was based on the conceptual model of "patient-focused, family-centered medical care."[23] The themes arising from this approach were providing physical comfort and emotional support to the patient, promoting shared decision making, focusing on the needs and values of the individual, attending to the needs and values of family members, and coordinating health care and related services.[23] An extensive analysis of validity and reliability has been undertaken; some of the psychometric properties suggested that additional work was needed on certain domains.

QUALITY OF DYING AND DEATH

The Quality of Dying and Death (QODD) questionnaire[24,25] is a 27-item interviewer-administered instrument, developed in the United States, that assesses symptoms, experiences, and perceptions regarding the quality of the dying process. It focuses on the last week of life; however, if the patient has been unconscious, it asks the bereaved relative to reflect on the care during the last month before death. The questions address six different domains of care: symptoms and personal care, preparation for death, moment of death, family, treatment preferences, and whole person concerns. Each question begins, "How would you rate this aspect of (*patient's name*) dying experience?" The response options are scaled from 0 to 10, where 0 represents a "terrible experience" and 10 an "almost perfect experience." Higher scores indicate a better quality of dying and death.[25] The developmental model was defined as "the degree to which a person's preference for dying and the moment of death agree with observations of how the person actually died as reported by others."[24] QODD has been used in many health care settings and has good validity and reliability.

Summary

Each of these instruments creates an outcome measure to assess end-of-life care. The most appropriate instrument depends on what particular aspect an individual wishes to assess. Using the constructs within these instruments, a framework of minimal standards can be set. These can be used to compare care settings and assess interventions at the end of life. Defining and measuring quality of care for the dying provides a basis for striving to improve it.

FUTURE RESEARCH GOALS

Some of the challenges of research in standards of care at the end of life include the following:

1. To further develop robust standards for care of the dying.
2. To identify factors that enable accurate diagnosis of dying in cancer and noncancer patients.
3. To develop reliable, valid tools for reflecting bereaved relatives' direct experience and their proxy representation of the patient's experience in dying.

Future potential areas of research include prognostication, setting quality standards in palliative care, and understanding different disease trajectories.

REFERENCES

1. Davies E, Higginson IJ (eds). The Solid Facts—Palliative Care. Milan: World Health Organization, 2004.
2. Seymour J, Gott M, Bellamy G, et al. Planning for the end of life: The views of older people about advance care statements. Soc Sci Med 2004;59:57-68.
3. Higginson IJ, Sen-Gupta GJ. Place of care in advanced cancer: A qualitative systematic literature review of patient preferences. J Palliat Med 2000;3:287-300.
4. Thomas K. Caring for the Dying at Home. Oxford, UK: Radcliffe Medical Press, 2003.
5. Joint Working Party between the National Council for Palliative Care and the Ethics Committee of the Association for Palliative Medicine of Great Britain and Ireland. Ethical Decision Making: Cardiopulmonary Resuscitation (CPR) for People Who Are Terminally Ill. London: National Hospice Council, 1997.
6. Berwick DM. A primer on leading the improvement of systems. BMJ 1996;1312:619-622.
7. Graham NO. Quality in Health Care: Theory, Application and Evolution. Gaithersburg, MD: Aspen Publications, 1995.
8. National Institute for Clinical Excellence. Guidance on Cancer Services: Improving Supportive and Palliative Care for Adults with Cancer [Pamphlet]. London: NICE, 2004.
9. Department of Health. Our Health, Our Choice, Our Say: A New Direction for Community Services. London: Department of Health, 2006.
10. Ellershaw JE, Smith C, Overill S, et al. Care of the dying: Setting standards for symptom control in the last 48 hours of life. J Pain Symptom Manage 2001;21:12-17.
11. Ellershaw J, Wilkinson S (eds). A Pathway to Excellence. Oxford: Oxford University Press, 2003.
12. Liverpool Care Pathway. Available at http://www.lcp-mariecurie.org.uk.
13. Mosel D, Gift B. Collaborative benchmarking in health care. Jt Comm J Qual Improv 1994;20:239-249.
14. Hickman SE, Tilden VP, Tolle SW. Family reports of dying patients' distress: The adaptation of a research tool to assess global symptom distress in the last week of life. J Pain Symptom Manage 2001;22:565-574.

15. Morita T, Hirai K, Sakaguchi Y, et al. Measuring the quality of structure and process in end-of-life care from the bereaved family perspective. J Pain Symptom Manage 2004;27:492-501.

16. Morita T, Chihara S, Kashiwagi T. A scale to measure satisfaction of bereaved family receiving inpatient palliative care. Palliat Med 2002;16:141-150.

17. Shiozaki M, Morita T, Hirai K, et al. Why are bereaved family members dissatisfied with specialised inpatient palliative care service? A nationwide qualitative study. Palliat Med 2005;19:319-327.

18. Kristjanson LJ. Validity and reliability testing of the FAMCARE Scale: Measuring family satisfaction with advanced cancer care. Soc Sci Med 1993;36:693-701.

19. Addington-Hall J, Walker L, Jones C, et al. A randomised controlled trial of postal versus interviewer administration of a questionnaire measuring satisfaction with, and use of, services received in the year before death. J Epidemiol Community Health 1998;52:802-807.

20. Addington-Hall J, McCarthy M. Regional Study of Care for the Dying: Methods and sample characteristics. Palliat Med 1995;9:27-35.

21. Cartwright A, Hockey L, Anderson JL. Life Before Death. London: Routledge & Kegan Paul, 1973.

22. Teno JM, Clarridge B, Casey V, et al. Validation of Toolkit After-Death Bereaved Family Member Interview. J Pain Symptom Manage 2001;22:752-758.

23. Teno JM, Casey VA, Welch LC, Edgman-Levitan S. Patient-focused, family-centered end-of-life medical care: Views of the guidelines and bereaved family members. J Pain Symptom Manage 2001;22:738-751.

24. Patrick DL, Engelberg RA, Curtis JR. Evaluating the quality of dying and death. J Pain Symptom Manage 2001;22:717-726.

25. Curtis JR, Patrick DL, Engelberg RA, et al. A measure of the quality of dying and death: Initial validation using after-death interviews with family members. J Pain Symptom Manage 2002;24:17-31.

SUGGESTED READING

British Medical Association. Advance Statements about Medical Treatment. London: British Medical Association, 1995.

Ellershaw J, Wilkinson S (eds). A Pathway to Excellence. Oxford: Oxford University Press, 2003.

Gift RG, Mosel D. Benchmarking in Health Care: A Collaborative Approach. Chicago. American Hospital Association, 1994.

Steiner DL, Norman GR. Health Measurement Scales: A Practical Guide to Their Development and Use, 2nd ed. Oxford: Oxford University Press, 1995.

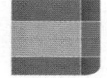

CHAPTER **179**

Palliative Sedation

John D. Cowan, Teresa Palmer, and Libby Clemens

K E Y   P O I N T S

- *Palliative sedation* is defined as medication-induced sedation that is administered, without intending to cause death, utilizing a non-opioid drug to control intolerable symptoms that are refractory in patients with advanced and incurable disease whose death is imminent (death expected in hours or days).

- *Intolerable symptoms* are those symptoms that are intolerable as defined by the patient. In a noncommunicative patient, symptoms may be assessed by the health care providers, with input from the family and caregivers.

- *Refractory symptoms* are those symptoms that remain uncontrolled after aggressive palliative treatments have been tried, for which treatment side effects are or are expected to be intolerable or for which available treatments are unlikely to provide adequate relief in an acceptable time frame, considering the patient's prognosis, life expectancy, and level of distress.

Palliative sedation (PS) is the practice of using medication-induced sedation to relieve intolerable and refractory symptoms in the terminally ill. As defined here, PS involves the use of nonopioid medications, started at low doses and titrated carefully to patient comfort, without a state of unconsciousness required. A significant body of literature over the past 20 years, using various names and definitions, has documented the provision of PS as a palliative care tool and described the efforts of providers to develop criteria and guidelines for its use.[1-14]

As death approaches, symptom control may become progressively more difficult, and for some, the goal of a peaceful death becomes elusive.[6,8,15-17] In this setting, the practice of PS has developed, with incidence varying from less than 5% to 52%[6,8,10,16-22] depending on the setting; the patient population; cultural, ethnic, and religious factors; and on the way PS is defined and applied.[6,12,15,23,24] It is provided to both cancer and noncancer patients, and most reports suggest that it is used in 15% to 30% of dying patients.[6,8,15,16,19-21]

PRINCIPLES OF ASSESSMENT AND MANAGEMENT

PS is a treatment of last resort. It is used when a patient has an advanced and incurable illness, is close to death (usually weeks or less), has intolerable and refractory symptoms, and has a do not resuscitate (DNR) order in effect.[1,4,6,17,25] Some recommend consultant corroboration that the patient requires PS.[2,8,17,25] Involvement of an interdisciplinary team including members with expertise in psychosocial and spiritual issues may be valuable in preparing the patient, family, and caregivers for PS and supporting them through the treatment and expected death.[1,4,17,26]

PS has been used for various refractory physical symptoms, with dyspnea, pain, delirium, nausea and vomiting, agitation/restlessness, seizure, and myoclonus being the most common.[2,5,7,8,18,21] Some have offered criteria for determining when a symptom is refractory.[4,6,10] The common theme is that a symptom is refractory when (1) aggressive palliative treatments have failed or have produced intolerable side effects; (2) additional treatments are unlikely to bring relief without intolerable side effects; and/or (3) the patient is likely to die before a conventional treatment could work.

Although there is no definitive list of palliative treatments that must fail before PS is appropriate, several reviews have included possible treatments for various symptoms, including pain.[4,6,10] A survey of palliative care experts reported that more than half of the patients receiving PS had greater than one qualifying symptom, and 34% received it for nonphysical symptoms.[2] Whereas most palliative care experts agree that PS is appropriate for refractory, intolerable physical and associated nonphysical suffering, its use for primarily refractory existential and/or nonphysical suffering is controversial.[4,23-29] Before PS is used to control existential or nonphysical distress, a thorough psychiatric, psychosocial, and spiritual evaluation should be performed.[6,10,25]

A careful approach to informed consent and to documentation of the PS process is recommended and helps distinguish PS from physician-assisted suicide (PAS) and euthanasia.[1,6,30] Informed consent should include documentation of discussions about PS with the patient and/or surrogate and ideally should cover, at a minimum, the following points[6]:

1. Presence of refractory symptoms requiring sedation
2. Primary goal (intent) being patient comfort
3. Patient death imminent (weeks or less)
4. No other therapeutic options
5. Notation of any professional consultations to confirm that patient is near death with refractory symptoms
6. Planned discontinuance of interventions not focused on comfort
7. Plan for hydration and nutrition during PS (clearly noting that this is a separate decision from the use of PS)
8. Anticipated risks or burdens of PS (i.e., sedation, decreased ability to communicate and take oral nourishment)

Whether there is a formal document giving consent varies by institution and locale. Including family members, caregivers, and involved health care workers in decision making is critical and can minimize misunderstandings about the intent of PS.[3,17] These discussions also should be documented in the medical record.

ETHICAL CONSIDERATIONS

PS is framed by the ethical principles of autonomy, beneficence, nonmaleficence, and justice, which are potentially in tension. Autonomy, defined as freedom to make and act on decisions, requires informed consent for PS. Autonomy may conflict with the other ethical principles when (1) patients request PS for existential or psychiatric reasons due to issues of decision-making capacity, (2) religious beliefs become involved, (3) the effects of PS on family and caregivers are considered, and (4) the interests of society are considered.[6,31]

The concept of *double effect*[4,25,26,30] is used to deal with principles of beneficence and nonmaleficence, because PS has potentially good and bad effects. Double effect analysis is used to ethically support PS as follows[6]:

1. The good effects are intended (symptom control and comfort)
2. The potential, foreseeable bad effects are not intended (decreased oral intake, potential hypotension and respiratory depression)
3. The good effects equal or outweigh the bad effects (rule of proportionality)
4. PS is morally neutral or good
5. There are no other treatments that would achieve the desired good effects without potential, foreseeable bad effects.

The use of double effect to ethically support PS has been questioned, because double effect analysis is open to personal value judgments, and determining "intent" is complex.[32-34] Further, some argue that PS is ethically indistinguishable from PAS or euthanasia.[32,33,35] Others note that intent is key, both legally and ethically,[6,14,32] and that PS is distinct from PAS and euthanasia because (1) the intent of PS is relief of suffering and not death, (2) death is not a required outcome for symptom relief with PS, and (3) it is the underlying disease process requiring PS that is the cause of death.[3,6,17,30]

ACUTE MANAGEMENT

Box 179-1 summarizes the preconditions for initiating PS and describes PS measures to be taken to control specific symptoms, as well as general measures.

General Considerations

PS should be administered in a setting that is comfortable and peaceful. It can be provided in the hospital, the home, a nursing facility, or a residential hospice.[5,7] Although PS is not an outpatient treatment, initial discussions regarding PS may be appropriate in the clinic. The idea that PS is an option for refractory symptoms may be comforting to those who express fear of dying with physical suffering.[4,17]

A skilled professional should closely monitor the patient during PS initiation until symptoms are adequately controlled, with follow-up, around-the-clock comfort monitoring provided by family, lay caregivers, and/or medical professionals educated in PS concepts. Emphasis should be placed on eye, mouth, bowel, bladder, and pressure point care.[6] Once comfort is achieved, routine monitoring of oxygen saturation, blood pressure, pulse, and heart rhythm should be stopped, because such measures do not contribute to comfort.[3,6] PS should be titrated to maximum comfort, using only the level of sedation required.[5] Formal monitoring of sedation level has been suggested,[25] but if the goal is comfort rather than level of sedation, then such monitoring is not required. Routine laboratory and imaging studies and medications not related to comfort care should be discontinued with the initiation of PS. The overall care plan should address the withdrawal of any life support measures not focused on comfort, such as mechanical ventilation, vasopressors, implanted defibrillators, blood transfusions, and artificial nutrition and hydration.[6]

Whereas artificial nutrition and hydration may not contribute to patient comfort, their withdrawal is sometimes distressing to families. Decisions on whether to continue parenteral fluids and enteral/parenteral nutrition should be made on an individual basis and distinctly from the use of PS, weighing the benefits and burdens (see Part II, Section G).[3,6,17,23,24] Most patients near death have reduced oral intake,[6,24] but patients receiving PS who are still able to take food and fluid by mouth should be offered food and drink to provide comfort, not to maintain nutrition. Although aspiration precautions should be followed, the understanding is that the benefit of pleasure to the patient from eating outweighs the risk or burden of aspiration.

Medications

Midazolam is the most frequently reported medication used for PS (>50% of PS patients),[2,5-8,14,22] but others, such as chlorpromazine, lorazepam, phenobarbital, and propofol, have documented efficacy.[2,7,8,14,22,25] The advantages and disadvantages of each should be considered beforehand (Table 179-1). Haloperidol has been reported[7,8,22] but

Box 179-1 Palliative Sedation Check List

Preparation

[ ] Patient has irreversible advanced disease.
[ ] Survival is limited to weeks or less.
[ ] A Do Not Resuscitate order is in place.
[ ] Symptom(s) are present that are refractory to therapy acceptable to the patient (examples).

Dyspnea

[ ] Provide oxygen therapy.
[ ] Maximize opioids and anxiolytic therapy.
[ ] Review the role of temporizing therapies including respiratory therapy, thoracentesis, and stents.

Pain

[ ] Maximize opioids, coanalgesics, and adjuvant analgesics including agent, route, and schedule.
[ ] Consider other therapies including invasive procedures, radiation therapy and chemotherapy, environmental changes, wound care, physical therapy, and psychotherapy.
[ ] Anticipate and aggressively manage analgesic side effects.

Delirium or Agitation/Confusion

[ ] Discontinue nonessential medications.
[ ] Change required medications to ones that are less likely to cause delirium.
[ ] Check for bladder distention and rectal impaction.
[ ] Maximize neuroleptic therapy options.
[ ] Consider role of hydration therapy.
[ ] Consider evaluation/therapy for potentially reversible processes (e.g., hypoxia, urinary infection, electrolyte imbalance).

Nausea and Vomiting

[ ] Discontinue nonessential medications.
[ ] Check for bladder distention and rectal impaction.
[ ] If specific cause is known, treat for reversible processes (e.g., brain metastases, bowel obstruction) with mediator-specific medications.
[ ] If specific cause not known or treatment is ineffective, treat with medications affecting multiple mediators.

Myoclonus

[ ] Differentiate from seizure activity.
[ ] Provide opioid rotation, clonidine, and benzodiazepines.
[ ] Consider role of hydration therapy

General Considerations

[ ] Consider a peer consultation to confirm the patient is near death with refractory symptoms.
[ ] Document the informed consent process, including refractory symptoms, treatment options, imminence of death, discontinuation of noncomfort therapies, and goals/burdens and procedure of palliative sedation.
[ ] Discontinue all treatment not focused on comfort.
[ ] Discontinue routine laboratory and imaging studies.
[ ] Discontinue medicines not needed for comfort, and adjust for ease of administration.
[ ] Discontinue unnecessary cardiopulmonary and vital sign monitoring.
[ ] Review the role of cardiac support devices and disable implanted defibrillators.
[ ] Integrate a plan to discontinue artificial life support (e.g., ventilator, dialysis).
[ ] Develop a plan for use/withdrawal of nutrition and hydration.
[ ] Identify location and staff appropriate to effectively provide palliative sedation.

Treatment Administration

[ ] Maintain aspiration precautions, eye protection, and mouth, bowel, bladder, and pressure point care.
[ ] Titrate supplemental oxygen for comfort, not for oxygen saturation.
[ ] Provide medications primarily by intravenous or subcutaneous routes.
[ ] Continue to titrate, but do not taper routine opioid therapy.
[ ] Provide sedating medication around the clock and titrate for symptom control, not level of consciousness.
[ ] Choose sedating medication based on the refractory symptom(s), provider experience, route availability, and patient location (see Table 179-1).

---

may not be as sedating as chlorpromazine, and, like chlorpromazine, it can lower the seizure threshold, exacerbate myoclonus, and be limited by extrapyramidal symptoms (EPS).[36-39] Other considerations for choosing PS medication are clinician preference and experience, route of administration, and care setting.[6] Additional medications that may be appropriate include other barbiturates,[40,41] ketamine combined with other agents,[42] and methotrimeprazine (not available in the United States).[2,7,8,22] If comfort cannot be achieved with one agent, trial of another or an additional agent with minimally overlapping disadvantages should be considered.

Intermittent or Respite Palliative Sedation

In lieu of, or as a precondition to, continuous sedation, some recommend intermittent or respite PS.[10,21,23] Considerations for deciding on the PS dose-scheduling pattern

include life expectancy, symptoms, and patient and family preferences. Intermittent PS may be attempted[10] before continuous sedation, unless symptom severity or life expectancy warrants immediate continuous PS. Some suggest that respite PS can be useful for refractory existential distress, allowing a respite with the hope that the patient will become re-energized and better able to cope.[3,10,25] Intermittent or respite PS can affect the clinician's choice of medication and the level of monitoring required during PS. For instance, phenobarbital, with its long half-life, may not be a first choice for intermittent or respite PS, and formal sedation level monitoring may be warranted if the goal is respite sedation for a defined period.

Common Errors

Opioids are inappropriate for inducing and maintaining PS because of inadequate sedation, drug tolerance, and

TABLE 179-1 Palliative Sedation Medications

MEDICATION	INITIAL OR LOADING DOSE (MG)	MAINTENANCE DOSE*(MG)	ROUTE OF ADMINISTRATION	ADVANTAGES	DISADVANTAGES
Midazolam	0.5-2	CI: 1-5/hr Higher doses reported	SQ, IV	Anticonvulsant Rapid effect Can be mixed with other drugs	Paradoxical agitation Respiratory depression Tachyphylaxis
Chlorpromazine	12.5-25	12.5-50 q 4-6 hr routine with a PRN dose	IV, PR	Helps relieve delirium and nausea Anticholinergic Inexpensive	Extrapyramidal symptoms Lowers seizure threshold Hypotension Dysphoria
Lorazepam	1-2	0.5-2 q 2-6 hr routine with a PRN dose CI: 0.5-1/hr	IV, SL, SQ	Multiple routes Anticonvulsant Anxiolytic	Paradoxical agitation Respiratory depression
Phenobarbital	60-100	60-200 q 4-6 hr routine with a PRN dose CI: 25/hr	IV, SQ	Anticonvulsant Inexpensive	Long half-life Drug interactions Tachyphylaxis Cannot be mixed with other drugs
Propofol	10	CI: 5-20/hr Titrated every 15 min for effect	IV	Short acting Rapid titration Anxiolytic Anticonvulsant	Expensive Large venous access Risk of infection Caloric load

CI, continuous infusion; IV, intravenous; PR, per rectum; PRN, as needed; SL, sublingual; SQ, subcutaneous
*Titration is often required.

potentially intolerable side effects (e.g., neurotoxicity, respiratory depression) with high doses.[3-4,6,17,37] However, most PS candidates are taking opioids[7] for pain or dyspnea or both, and they should continue taking them to avoid increased suffering or withdrawal symptoms, because the drugs in Table 179-1 are not analgesics. If the intolerable and refractory symptom is pain, the maximum tolerated dose of opioid should be reached before PS is started.[3,4,17]

In general, the intramuscular route should be avoided, and the oral, sublingual, and rectal routes are potentially problematic for PS. The intravenous (IV) route should be considered if there is a reliable, usually central, access. Often, the subcutaneous (SQ) route is best for PS regardless of setting. PS agents can be administered as continuous infusions or by bolus dosing scheduled around the clock. PRN doses are often made available.[3] PS agents usually should be started at a low dose, with careful titration until symptoms are controlled.[6,10,17,37] When PS is initiated with continuous sedation in mind, it is inadvisable to decrease the dose of the PS agent once the patient is comfortable, because doing so may cause intolerable suffering to reoccur, and the patient may die with uncontrolled symptoms.[3,4] Medications should not be increased if a patient is comfortable. Documentation of the starting dose, titration protocol,[2,5-8,10,14,22] and symptoms requiring upward titration will confirm that the intent of PS is symptom control, not death.[4,6,10,43]

Survival and Time to Death

PS, when titrated to the point of comfort, has not been proved to shorten survival.[16,22,24,31] The reported median time to death from initiation of PS is longer than 1 day,[5,7,43] with a mean ranging from 1.9 to 6.1 days[5,7,8] (see "Case Study: Palliative Sedation"). One study[18] noted no difference in survival time for palliative care patients who received sedation compared with those who did not.

CASE REPORT

Palliative Sedation

RJ was a 56-year-old man with recurrent, progressive, base of tongue cancer believed to be refractory to additional therapy by his oncologists. The patient requested a Do Not Resuscitate status and elected hospice with his goals focused on comfort. He clearly stated to his family and physicians that he did not want to return to the hospital and that he preferred to be "sleepy" rather than endure physical suffering. The patient had no other chronic medical problems but had recently had an infected central venous access line requiring removal and a bout of facial herpes zoster with postherpetic pain. No psychosocial or spiritual problems were identified. On admission to hospice, he was comfortable with his deep aching head pain and postherpetic pain well controlled on around-the-clock opioids, three adjuvant analgesics, and transdermal lidocaine. He was able to take small amounts of oral nutrition and elected to discontinue enteral nutrition.

RJ did well for about 5 weeks in home hospice care and was able to enjoy his family, but then he began having escalating head, neck, and ear pain not controlled with dose escalation of enterally provided analgesics. He reminded his caregivers that he wanted to be comfortable at home and that his goals were not being achieved. His adjuvant analgesics were escalated in dose, and his opioid was changed to a subcutaneous continuous infusion plus as-needed bolus dosing with rapid dose escalation over several days. Pain control improved initially, but the patient was somnolent. After 3 days, he developed moaning (possibly indicating uncontrolled pain) and delirium with myoclonus that was very distressful to the family. His medication regimen was simplified, adjuvant analgesics withheld, opioids rotated, transdermal clonidine and lorazepam provided for myoclonus, bowel and bladder examined for impaction/distention, electrolytes checked, urinary tract infection ruled out, oxygen therapy provided, and intravenous fluids given on a trial basis. There was no improvement in his myoclonus, and he continued to moan and cry out in apparent discomfort.

On a visit by the hospice medical director, the patient's status and options of care were discussed with his wife (health care agent) and his children. It was explained that RJ's symptoms appeared to be refractory to therapy acceptable to the patient, that parenteral fluids were not improving quality of life, that the patient wanted to die at home, that he requested sedation if necessary to control symptoms, and that survival for more than days was not expected. Use of midazolam for palliative sedation was reviewed with the family, and they requested it for patient comfort. This interaction was documented in the medical record by the medical director without the use of a formal informed consent. Opioid infusion was continued, parenteral fluids and other medications except clonidine were discontinued because they were not improving comfort, oral atropine drops for increased secretions were added, and midazolam subcutaneous infusion was started at 1 mg/hr after a 2-mg loading dose. Midazolam was titrated by 1 mg/hr by the hospice nurse until the patient was resting with minimal myoclonus and no moaning. Mouth, eye, and skin care were continued, and a Foley catheter was placed. Within 8 hours, at 5 mg/hr of midazolam, the patient was comfortable, somnolent but arousable, and requiring only extra bolus opioid dosing with repositioning. Over the next 5 days, the patient remained comfortable but somnolent and required no increase in his infusion opioid, with his final midazolam dose being 9 mg/hr. The patient died on the sixth day of palliative sedation, resting quietly with his family at the bedside.

REFERENCES

1. Braun TC, Hagen NA, Clark T. Development of a clinical practice guideline for palliative sedation. J Palliat Med 2003;6:345-350.
2. Chater S, Viola R, Paterson J, et al. Sedation for intractable distress in the dying: A survey of experts. Palliat Med 1998;12:255-269.
3. Cherny NI. The use of sedation in the management of refractory pain. Principles and Practice of Supportive Oncology Updates 2000;3:1-11.
4. Cherny NI, Portenoy RK. Sedation in the management of refractory symptoms: Guidelines for evaluation and treatment. J Palliat Care 1994;10:31-38.
5. Cowan JD, Clemens, Palmer T. Palliative sedation in a southern Appalachian community. Am J Hospice Palliat Med 2006;23:360-368.
6. Cowan JD, Palmer TW. Practical guide to palliative sedation. Curr Oncol Rep 2002;4:242-249.
7. Cowan JD, Walsh D. Terminal sedation in palliative medicine: Definition and review of the literature. Support Care Cancer 2001;9:403-407.
8. Fainsinger RL, Waller A, Bercovici M, et al. A multicentre international study of sedation for uncontrolled symptoms in terminally ill patients. Palliat Med 2000;14:257-265.
9. Kohara H, Ueoka H, Takeyama H, et al. Sedation for terminally ill patients with cancer with uncontrollable physical distress. J Palliat Med 2005;8:20-25.
10. Morita T, Bito S, Kurihara Y, et al. Development of a clinical guideline for palliative sedation therapy using the Delphi method. J Palliat Med 2005;8:716-729.
11. Morita T, Tsuneto S, Shima Y. Definition of sedation for symptom relief: A systematic literature review and a proposal of operational criteria. J Pain Symptom Manage 2002;24:447-453.
12. Rousseau P. Palliative sedation and sleeping before death: A need for clinical guidelines? J Palliat Med 2003;6:425-427.
13. Rousseau P. Palliative sedation in the control of refractory symptoms. J Palliat Med 2005;8:10-12.
14. Salacz ME, Weissman DE. Controlled sedation for refractory suffering: Parts I and II. J Palliat Med 2005;8:136-138.
15. Lichter I, Hunt E. The last 48 hours of life. J Palliat Care 1990;6:7-15.
16. Ventafridda V, Ripamonti C, de Conno F, et al. Symptom prevalence and control during cancer patients' last days of life. J Palliat Care 1990;6:7-11.
17. Wein S. Sedation in the imminently dying patient. Oncology 2000;14:585-592.
18. Chiu TY, Hu WY, Lue BH, et al. Sedation for refractory symptoms of terminal cancer patients in Taiwan. J Pain Symptom Manage 2001;21:467-472.
19. Fainsinger RL. Use of sedation by a hospital palliative care support team. J Palliat Care 1998;14:51-54.
20. Fainsinger R, Miller MJ, Bruera E. Symptom control during the last week of life on a palliative care unit. J Palliat Care 1991;7:5-11.
21. Morita T, Inoue S, Chihara S. Sedation for symptom control in Japan: The importance of intermittent use and communication with family members. J Pain Symptom Manage 1996;12:32-38.
22. Stone P, Phillips C, Spruyt O, et al. A comparison of the use of sedatives in a hospital support team and in a hospice. Palliat Med 1997;11:140-144.
23. Rousseau P. Existential suffering and palliative sedation: A brief commentary with a proposal for clinical guidelines. Am J Hosp Palliat Care 2001;18:226-228.
24. Rousseau P. The ethical validity and clinical experience of palliative sedation. Mayo Clin Proc 2000;75:1064-1069.
25. Rousseau P. Palliative sedation in the management of refractory symptoms. J Support Oncol 2004;2:181-186.
26. Krakauer EL, Penson RT, Truog RD, et al. Sedation for intractable distress of a dying patient: Acute palliative care and the principle of double effect. The Oncologist 2000;5:53-62.
27. Billings JA, Block SD. Slow euthanasia. J Palliat Care 1996;12:21-30.
28. Cherny NI, Coyle N, Foley KM. The treatment of suffering when patients request elective death. J Palliat Care 1994;10:71-79.
29. Mount B. Morphine drips, terminal sedation, and slow euthanasia: Definitions and facts, not anecdotes. J Palliat Care 1996;12:31-37.
30. Boyle J. Medical ethics and double effect: The case of terminal sedation. Theoret Med 2004;25:51-60.
31. Sykes N, Thorns A. Sedative use in the last week of life and the implications for end-of-life decision making. Arch Intern Med 2003;163:341-344.
32. Gauthier CC. Active voluntary euthanasia, terminal sedation, and assisted suicide. J Clin Ethics 2001;12:43-50.
33. Quill TE. The ambiguity of clinical intentions. N Engl J Med 1993;329:1039-1040.
34. Quill TE, Dresser R, Brock DW. The rule of double effect: A critique of its role in end-of-life decision making. N Engl J Med 1997;337:1768-1771.
35. Loewy EH. Terminal sedation, self-starvation, and orchestrating the end of life. Arch Intern Med 2001;161:329-332.
36. Dunlop RJ. Is terminal restlessness sometimes drug induced? Palliat Med 1989;3:65-66.
37. Hallenbeck J. Terminal sedation for intractable distress: Not slow euthanasia but a prompt response to suffering. West J Med 1999;171:222-223.
38. Vella-Brincat J, Macleod AD. Haloperidol in palliative care. Palliat Med 2004;18:195-201.
39. Awad AG, Voruganti LN. Neuroleptic dystonia: Revisiting the concept 50 years later. Acta Psychiatr Scand Suppl 2005;427:6-13.
40. Greene WR, Davis WH. Titrated intravenous barbiturates in the control of symptoms in patients with terminal cancer. South Med J 1991;84:332-337.
41. Truog RD, Berde CB, Mitchell C, et al. Barbiturates in the care of the terminally ill. N Engl J Med 1992;327:1678-1682.
42. Berger JM, Ryan A, Vadivelu N, et al. Ketamine-fentanyl-midazolam infusion for the control of symptoms in terminal life care. Am J Hosp Palliat Care 2000;17:127-132.
43. Muller-Busch HC, Andres I, Jehser T. Sedation in palliative care: A critical analysis of 7 years experience. BMC Palliat Care 2003;2:2-10.

SUGGESTED READING

Chater S, Viola R, Paterson J, et al. Sedation for intractable distress in the dying: A survey of experts. Palliat Med 1998;12:255-269.

Cherny NI, Portenoy RK. Sedation in the management of refractory symptoms: Guidelines for evaluation and treatment. J Palliat Care 1994;10:31-38.

Cowan JD, Walsh D. Terminal sedation in palliative medicine: Definition and review of the literature. Support Care Cancer 2001;9:403-407.

Fainsinger RL, Waller A, Bercovici M, et al. A multicentre international study of sedation for uncontrolled symptoms in terminally ill patients. Palliat Med 2000;14:257-265.

Morita T, Tsuneto S, Shima Y. Definition of sedation for symptom relief: A systematic literature review and a proposal of operational criteria. J Pain Symptom Manage 2002;24:447-453.

Rousseau P. The ethical validity and clinical experience of palliative sedation. Mayo Clin Proc 2000;75:1064-1069.

Wein S. Sedation in the imminently dying patient. Oncology 2000;14:585-592.

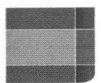

CHAPTER **180**

Care of the Dying: Hospitals and Intensive Care Units

Pamela Levack and Carol Macmillan

KEY POINTS

- Hospital culture is ambivalent to palliative care.
- Making and communicating a diagnosis that "this patient may be dying" is the key to good palliative care and a skill to be valued.
- Every referral to palliative care is an opportunity for palliative medicine (PM) and non-PM staff to discuss difficult issues and influence care.
- PM in hospital is not hospice care, nor step-down care, but a different model—using elements of hospice care integrated with acute care.
- Improved care of patients dying in hospital requires that the hospital have "ownership" of high-quality palliative care.
- PM skills have an important role in intensive care.
- Educating intensive care physicians in PM should be a priority.
- Intensive care has unique communication and clinical challenges for PM.
- The contrast between "cure" and "care" is at its most acute in the intensive care unit.
- Goals of care and forward planning are labile and flexible but essential for good intensive care PM.

Dying in the Hospital

The modern experience of dying is largely a hospital experience, usually occurring after a period of progressive disability. This has been described as a period of "chronic critical illness" in patients whose recovery after intensive care has been poor[1] or living "on thin ice" in the frail elderly.[2] Both descriptions reflect the fact that, for most people, dying in hospital is a slow process that occurs against a background of multiple chronic illnesses.[3] Medical care near death has become more intensive and more aggressive. For example, more cancer patients start new chemotherapy in the last month of life or are still receiving chemotherapy in the last 2 weeks of life.[4,5] Consequently, patients are often admitted to hospital or intensive care on an emergency basis and spend many "undesirable days," in the intensive care unit (ICU) or receiving aggressive intervention, before death.[6] Referral to hospice services may be late, serving only as "brink of death" care.

> Treatment with chemotherapy within two weeks of death is increasing (20% in USA in 1996). . . . Late referral to hospice and palliative care services is increasing.
>
> EARLE ET AL.[4]

There is tension between aggressive or life-prolonging interventions and those that focus on quality of life. The result can be conflict between the patient (or family) and health care professionals or between doctors and nurses.[7] In such circumstances, palliative care may be abrupt and late, and the needs of the patient or family unrecognized.[8] Disagreement about medical decisions between patient and staff, between relatives and staff, or among staff members is the biggest ethical issue facing the health service.[6] Continuing anticancer treatment is seen as "doing something," whereas shifting to palliative care is seen as failure of active or intensive care. Patients, not unreasonably, do not want to choose between cure and comfort care—they want both. And such simultaneous care is possible.[9]

The views of seriously ill patients[10] are clear and simple. They want

- Trust and confidence in the doctor looking after them
- Honest information about their health
- To have symptoms taken seriously and treated competently
- Not to be kept alive without hope of meaningful recovery
- To prepare for life's end by resolving conflicts and saying goodbye

These findings are similar to those reported by others,[8] with the following additions:

- To reduce the burden for the family
- To have a sense of control in their care—a voice

Unfortunately, there are numerous reports of poor care of patients dying in hospital. The perception is often that technical care is good but impersonal and basic care is poor,[11] with noisy busy environments. Even in advanced hospitals in developing countries, medical and nursing staff may have little time to devote to the dying.[12-17]

The challenges are

1. To identify the dying—not only those who will die in the next few days but also those who are likely to die during their current admission.
2. To determine which elements of palliative care can be integrated into day-to-day hospital care.[18]
3. To help medical staff understand that palliative care is not solely a nursing responsibility and that the medical role in diagnosis, decision making, and prognostication is vital.

PRINCIPLES OF ASSESSMENT AND MEASUREMENT

Many patients in hospital are actively dying, but it can be difficult to identify who they are, particularly among those with noncancer diagnoses. Shorter admissions and reduced continuity of care mean that hospital staff may not know their patients well, and the drive may be to keep "doing something" until it is patently obvious that the patient is dying. Physicians tend to be overoptimistic.[12,19] There may be no gap between aggressive or interventional palliative treatment and terminal care, and the patient and family are often unprepared for the shift from "doing everything" to "doing nothing."

> The differential diagnosis in advanced illness is as follows: this patient is seriously ill; this patient may be dying; this patient is dying.

An experienced clinician, perhaps someone not involved previously, may be best placed to diagnose whether the patient is likely to be dying, or the question may be openly raised after a formal palliative medicine consultation. It is crucial to discuss this with the responsible staff, because they need to "own the diagnosis of dying."[15] Acute-care staff may disagree, or team views may differ about the reversibility of the condition or whether further intervention may rescue the situation. Disagreement leads to mixed messages and opposing goals of care, poor patient management, and confused communications.[20]

> "Is this a patient who could die during this admission?"
> BOOKBINDER[23] AND PATTISON[3]

Palliative care clinicians prioritize the problems of advanced disease differently. Intractable nausea and pain are priorities, because people cannot understand what is happening or make decisions if they are sick or sore.

> "What is the most important thing to you at the moment?"
> "If there was one thing we could improve for you, what would it be?"

A simple rapid cycle method[21] based on rapid cycle change, has the obvious merit of asking patients and their families what would benefit them and then passing on this information for the staff to act upon. However, aggressive symptom control may be difficult, because ward staff may misconstrue effective analgesia as hastening death. Despite the lack of evidence to support this idea, these concerns are widespread.[22]

There is usually more agreement about the most appropriate approach for those who are actively dying (i.e., in their last few days or hours). A risk at this phase is that staff may withdraw from the patient, or the patient may be transferred to another place of care if the acute ward is busy. Requests for transfer to hospice are common, even when the patient is comfortable and his or her needs are being met. Comprehensive, evidence-based programs and pathways have been developed for the last 48 hours of life, to ensure high-quality care by generalists.[20,23-26] Two

criteria need to be confirmed for such pathways to be implemented:

1. All possible reversible causes for the patient's current condition have been considered.
2. The responsible team has agreed and accepted that the patient is dying.

Introduction of a new clinical pathway into a busy hospital can be resource-intensive.[27] Hospital palliative care can be very difficult if there is uncertainty or disagreement about whether the patient is or is not dying.

CLINICAL ASSESSMENT AND DIAGNOSIS

What Is the Patient's Story Up to Now?

The patient's story may be extensive and complex, and the initial meeting may be the first time the patient has had the opportunity to tell the whole story, as he or she understands it. Much will have happened, and, for the patient, trying to make sense of it is like putting together a jigsaw puzzle when some pieces may be missing. Professionals need to understand what the experience has been like for the patient and the family, and its significance; this can be learned by listening to what is said and unsaid, without premature judgment, and with minimal interruption. Fears and concerns are glimpsed, as is some idea of how much the patient and family want to be involved in decisions or discussions, and how important the pursuit of cure is.

What's Wrong?

The importance of physical examination cannot be over-estimated. It provides numerous signs that have prognostic importance in advanced disease (Table 180-1), but it also is a potent message to patients that, despite their advanced illness, they are worth examining. In addition, it is an opportunity for further, perhaps less-threatening, discussion.

Certain abnormal laboratory tests have prognostic significance (e.g., refractory hypercalcemia). A high white cell count (>8.5 cells/μL) and a low lymphocyte count (<12 cells/μL) both contribute to the Palliative Prognostic Score,[28] which can identify the probability of an individual patient's surviving for 1 month (see later discussion).

What Is the Likely Prognosis?

> "I know I have bone disease and my platelets are low—but where am I in my illness?"

If deterioration in health occurs over months, then survival is likely to be months; if over weeks, survival is likely weeks; and if over days, survival is likely to be days. Patients and their families, who may have weathered many relapses and disappointments during years of illness, may believe that recovery from the current episode will also happen. Although clinical prediction of survival is useful, it tends to be overoptimistic and for many is inaccurate.[19,29,30]

TABLE 180-1   Clinical Signs from a Palliative Medicine Perspective

Low functional status*	PPS contributes to PPI (see Table 180-2)
	KPS contributes to PaP (see Table 180-3)
	Can lead to discussion of fear of weakness, lack of independence, etc.
Cachexia (anorexia)†	Patient and family are usually blindingly aware of patient's appearance
	Can lead to discussion about "where the patient is" in his or her illness
Mouth*	Dry mouth due to reduced oral intake is common and contributes to PPI
	Thrush may lead to discussion of fluid intake, fear of being unable to drink, future wishes about fluids
Skin	Edema can be a major source of discomfort
	Poor prognostic factor in PPI
	May lead to discussion about weight loss, fluid intake, etc.
Dyspnea*†	Poor prognostic factor in PaP
Delirium*	Poor prognostic factor in PPI
Ongoing bleeding from tumor	Poor prognostic factor

KPS, Karnofsky Performance Scale; PPI, Palliative Prognostic Index; PPS, Palliative Performance Scale.
*Poor prognostic factor in PPI.
†Poor prognostic factor in PPS.
From http://www.palliative.info/teaching_material/Prognosis.pdf (accessed January 28, 2008).

TABLE 180-2   Palliative Prognostic Index (PPI)*

PARAMETER	VALUES	SCORE	MAXIMUM SCORE
PPS†	10-20	4	
	30-50	2.5	4
	≥60	0	
Oral intake	Severely reduced (mouthfuls or less)	2.5	
	Moderately reduced (more than mouthfuls)	1	2.5
	Normal	0	
Edema	Present	1	1
	Absent	0	
Dyspnea at rest	Present	3.5	3.5
	Absent	0	
Delirium	Present	4	4
	Absent	0	
Total			15

*If total PPI score is >6, estimated survival time is <3 wk.
†Palliative Performance Scale, version 2. Available at http://www.victoriahospice.org/pdfs/ppsv2.pdf (accessed January 28, 2008).
From http://www.palliative.info/teaching_material/Prognosis.pdf (accessed January 28, 2008).

> If we tell a patient he will die in a month, he is likelier to be dead in a week.
>
> ROBERTS[31]

Patients with low performance status (Palliative Performance Scale [PPS]; Karnofsky Performance Scale [KPS]) have worse survival,[28] although higher performance status does not necessarily predict long survival. Certain symptoms, such as nausea, breathlessness, and weakness, have independent value[29,30] as prognostic factors. In advanced disease (especially cancer), symptoms may be more prognostic than test results. Combining clinical prediction with other factors to produce a prognostic score gives simple, useful bedside prognostic information.[28]

Palliative Prognostic Index

The Palliative Prognostic Index (PPI)[32] is alone in estimating the probability of surviving 3 or 6 weeks using only clinical findings (Table 180-2). A combination of the clinicians' predicted survival time plus functional status (PPS) plus selected symptoms (oral intake, edema, dyspnea, and delirium) can predict the probability of surviving 3 or 6 weeks (sensitivity 80%, specificity 85%) irrespective of primary tumor site.

Palliative Prognostic Score

The Palliative Prognostic Score (PaP), which has been validated in several countries in various settings and different disease phases,[33] requires simple laboratory data in addition to clinical prediction and functional ability to

TABLE 180-3   Palliative Prognostic Score (PaP)*

PARAMETER	VALUES	SCORE
Dyspnea	Yes	1
	No	0
Anorexia	Yes	1.5
	No	0
KPS†	>30	0
	<20	2.5
Clinical predication of survival	>12	0
	11-12	2
	9-10	2.5
	7-8	2.5
	5-6	4.5
	3-4	6
	1-2	8.5
Total leukocyte count (cells ×10⁻³)	Normal	0
	High	0.5
	Very high	1.5
Lymphocytes (%)	Normal	0
	Low	1
	Very low	2.5

RISK GROUP ACCORDING TO TOTAL SCORE:

30-DAY SURVIVAL PROBABILITY	TOTAL SCORE
>70%	0-5.5
30-70%	1.6-11
<30%	11.1-17.5

*Classifies patients into three risk groups for probability of surviving 1 month.
†Karnofsky Performance Scale. Available at http://www.acsu.buffalo.edu/~drstall/karnofsky.html (accessed January 28, 2008).
From http://www.palliative.info/teaching_material/Prognosis.pdf (accessed January 28, 2008).

estimate the likelihood of surviving 4 weeks (Table 180-3). The clinicians' predicted survival time, together with KPS, symptoms (anorexia, dysphagia, dry mouth, dyspnea, delirium), and blood results (raised white cell count, reduced lymphocyte count) form a score that predicts the

70% likelihood of surviving 30 days, irrespective of primary tumor site.

What Does the Patient Understand?

There can be a large difference between the description of a patient's disease state and the patient's personal experience of his or her disease (Table 180-4).

The accompanying case study describes the experience of a patient with a rapidly growing, fatal tumor (see "Case Study: A Death in a Hospital Ward"). In this case, the goals of care in terms of symptom control were agreed on by the patient, family, oncology staff, and palliative care staff. The diagnosis of lymphoma raised the possibility of added benefit from further deep x-ray therapy. However, clinical deterioration from day to day was rapid, and treatment, although itself not painful, involved moving the patient from bed to treatment couch, which was painful. The palliative care team believed that the patient was dying but were not absolutely sure. Aggressiveness of investigation and treatment were not so easily agreed on, because there was a fear from the ward staff that use of a syringe driver in itself would accelerate death. Resolution was achieved by strong intervention on the part of the family.

Table 180-5 provides a framework for discussion of care of the dying in hospice, in the hospital, and in an intensive care unit.

MANAGEMENT

There seems little doubt that doctors do tend to take more risks in management than would patients if they were provided with the information on which to make a reasonable decision.

DUNCAN[34]

Patients expect to know, and they expect the team looking after them to know, what's happened to them, the immediate plan agreed on by everyone (goals of care), and what comes after that (future plan).

TABLE 180-4	Comparison of Description of Disease and Experience of the Patient
DISEASE	**EXPERIENCE**
Metastatic carcinoma	"It's unbelievable—I was well before Christmas."
Unknown primary	"I have a lump on my forehead but do not want to have a scar from a biopsy—I have no scars on my body."
Cord compression	"The pain in my back is bad especially when I move."
Chronic obstructive pulmonary disease	"My breathing is bad."

TABLE 180-5	Discussion Framework		
KEY ELEMENTS OF PALLIATIVE CARE	**HOSPICE**	**HOSPITAL WARD**	**INTENSIVE CARE UNIT**
1. Honest, open communication (within team and with patient and family)	Undivided attention and time available / Lines of communication open / Lots of feedback	Divided attention	Patient often incapacitated, unable to participate; relatives are surrogates / Imprecise terminology; need one main communicator
2. Basic care (time, valuing patient dignity)	Priority / Part of culture	Often hurried / Often noisy	Priority, 24 hr/day
3. Organization	Environment supports quality care / Promotes patient dignity / Focuses on family	Hugely pressured / Often target driven	Pressure on beds / Do not discharge if end of life is imminent
4. Symptom control	Expert and aggressive	Negotiated / Often challenged and consequently delayed	Often difficult to assess delivery / Rapid and potent
5. Goals of care	Accepted focus shifted from curative-palliative / Recognize that dying is likely in near future / Benefits vs burdens considered	Often delayed / May be difficult to know which patients are dying / Curative and palliative management continue in parallel	Big change in therapy, both actual and in mindset / Minimize monitoring and procedures not directly required for care
6. Future planning	A priority / Out-of-hours care planned / Preferred place of death* discussed / Attempt to resolve conflicts	Short stays mean poor planning / Discussions about death less common	Pre–intensive care discussion with patient may be possible / Must include patient's wishes if cure becomes unrealistic
7. Decision making (tests, withdrawal, treatment)	Shared if wished	Some hospital ethics committees	Burden lies with multidisciplinary team to ensure that relatives do not feel responsible for making withdrawal decision / Patient's requests, relatives' views taken into account

*For example, preferred place of care (PPC).
Adapted from National Health Services, Lancashire & South Cumbria Cancer Network. Available at http://www.cancerlancashire.org.uk/ppc (accessed January 28, 2008).

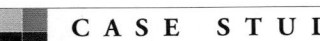

CASE STUDY

A Death in a Hospital Ward

Mrs. A was a 78-year-old, independent woman who had successfully raised three children after her husband was killed in his 40s in an accident. She had been house-bound with chronic obstructive pulmonary disease for years but was very much head of the family. She had presented 2 weeks previously with a large swelling on her forehead and increasingly severe interscapular and radicular back pain. A magnetic resonance imaging study established extradural cord compression at T6-T10, and a diagnosis of metastatic malignant lymphoma was made.

Mrs. A was admitted for pain control, deep x-ray therapy (DXT), and biopsy of frontal bone mass. She was frightened, extremely breathless, and in severe pain, especially on movement. She was treated with hydromorphone orally, and then advice for pain control was sought from the hospital palliative care team. Analgesia was converted to subcutaneous hydromorphone and dexamethasone, administered by syringe driver. As pain improved, she reflected on her life and numerous personal losses. Her breathing settled as she talked.

The medical oncologist discussed with Mrs. A and her family the fast-growing nature of the tumor and the likely diagnosis. The patient and family talked over the issues privately and decided that (1) she did not wish a biopsy and (2) she did not wish further treatment. The clinical oncologist believed that Mrs. A might well get further benefit from continuing dexamethasone and might "pick up," so she had one further treatment. The family members who stayed with the patient would not let her attend further dexamethasone treatments, because moving and lying on the hard surface was painful. She deteriorated rapidly and died comfortably 3 days later in the same ward, with her daughters present.

Communication

Communication in complex situations is difficult and is often easy for professionals to avoid. Some patients prefer not to discuss these matters, but perhaps—and this is probably more common—some professionals also prefer not to discuss end-of-life issues. Patients' wishes to do so may not be articulated or may challenge a doctor's professional autonomy[35]; on the other hand, both patient and professional may collude to restrict such discussion.[36] Talk about prognosis may thus be limited.

> The physician does and does not want to pronounce a death sentence and the patient does and does not want to hear it.
> THE AM, ET AL.[36]

Nevertheless, patients, families, and the professionals looking after them need to understand that death is a possibility before they can entertain discussions about what treatment options can be considered. Several consultations may need to take place, because people psychologically edit what they are told. Indeed, "honest information brokers" have been suggested, because it can be very hard for closely involved staff to provide such information.[5]

Communication is as much for support as for information, and palliative medicine physicians in hospitals report that discussion and rediscussion consumes most of their clinical time. Such support becomes increasingly important as the patient nears death, and it is valued and remembered by the family. It may be a simple matter of undivided attention and concern, of listening, and of speaking honestly and sensitively.

For those with advanced disease, two things happen: the patient both fights for survival and simultaneously accepts that he or she may die.[37] We must understand what worries patients most, by asking questions such as the following:

1. What's the hardest part of your illness?
2. Where do you turn for comfort when things get difficult?
3. What thing about your illness most worries you?
4. What do you see as the biggest challenge now?
5. Do you often feel depressed?
6. Do you often feel anxious?

It is not so much about direct choices, but understanding the patient's needs and allowing a solution to evolve. Once realistic goals of care and prognosis are communicated, patients often elect to avoid high technology and death-prolonging therapies, in favor of palliative goals of comfort.[38]

Symptom Control

Patients want their caregivers to take pain and symptom control seriously, and the responsibility for good symptom control rests squarely on the responsible physician. The skills of symptom control used in hospice are applicable in the acute setting, but there are barriers. Patients and professionals frequently disagree about symptom severity, or pain may be wrongly attributed to nonmalignant causes. Information volunteered by the patient may under-report symptoms by 10-fold when compared with a formal systematic symptom assessment,[39] and numerous pain control tools for hospitals are available.[40] Medical and nursing staff, patients, and families may fear that aggressive symptom control will affect the response to treatment or have adverse effects on physiology. For example, they may fear that appropriate use of opioids will shorten life,[41] despite the complete lack of data to support such a myth.[42]

Surgical teams are more comfortable with acute pain teams and standardized protocols, and they are frequently reluctant to use analgesia in advanced illness for fear of hastening death. Once the use of strong analgesia becomes unavoidable, the doses used may be larger than palliative care would initially recommend. It is also not uncommon, once a decision is made that the patient is dying, to believe that there is a specific prescription and, if an opioid is prescribed, that the dose should automatically be increased with time; this attitude may lead to overdosing and unnecessary side effects.

Basic Care and Continuity

Many patients dying in hospital do not receive basic comfort care, and contact between patients and health care professionals may be minimal. Aggressive treatment in hospital or in the ICU stresses staff.[43] The attitude of staff affects the quality of care, as does the noisy, complicated environment. Patients need to feel that they matter, to be treated with compassion,[18] and to have some personal space and privacy[44]; benchmarks for good practice have been recommended.[45]

Continuity for patients and their families means that they are confident that health professionals know what has happened before now, that they have an agreed on plan, and that they know who will care for them in the future. Unfortunately, hospitals often create discontinuity of care. Use of pathways alone is not sufficient, but time and attention paid to listening to individual patients and their families and answering their questions, even if compressed over a few days, is.

Goals of Care and Aims of Treatment

Setting and coordinating goals of care and aims of treatment is especially difficult in hospital, because it means that doctors and patients have to talk about hopes, frustrations, fears, despair, and other emotional issues in a setting where the focus is on cure.[46] Even "hospice-friendly" oncologists may have difficulties with palliative care. They may believe that reducing tumor burden equates to palliation, and it can be difficult to discuss the added value offered by palliative care, because it implies that oncological management alone is inadequate.

We need to know what specifically concerns patients, what patients understand about their illness and prognosis, and what their wishes are; this information helps the doctor decide how aggressive treatments or investigations should be. There is a considerable mismatch between what patients prefer and what treatment they actually get.[12] The SUPPORT study indicated that patients' wishes for symptom control versus invasive treatment were often ignored. There is no substitute for the physician's exploring patient preferences,[47] and discussions about goals and plans of care may occupy most of the palliative medicine physician's time (see Table 180-5).[47,48]

Research Challenges

There are several research challenges in the hospital care of the dying. The question of how to integrate palliative medicine with all hospital disciplines is paramount. In addition, we must identify which elements of palliative medicine apply to noncancer patients. Research is also needed into the science of symptoms.[49]

Dying in the Intensive Care Unit

Palliative care and intensive care may seem to have opposing aims, yet nowhere in the hospital is there such a dynamic interchange of concordant clinical strategies. Intensive care is the "techno-ward" for a hospital's sickest patients. Large, high-turnover teams of multidisciplinary and interdisciplinary skills add to the complex environment. Intensive care demands huge resources in time, money, and emotionally demanding skills of the ICU team striving for patient survival. Because the mortality rate of ICUs is approximately 40%,[50] subjecting patients and their

relatives to an ICU admission cannot be undertaken lightly. Intensivists routinely and regularly oversee "dignified" deaths of their patients; it represents a large proportion of their work. Most deaths occur after decisions to limit or withdraw treatment have been made.[51] But can we do better?

The accompanying case study describes a death occurring in the ICU (see "Case Study: A Death in an Intensive Care Unit").

CHALLENGES FOR INTENSIVE CARE

There are many challenges inherent in caring for dying patients in the ICU:

- It is the exception that the ICU team has an opportunity to meet with the patient and family before admission.
- ICU admission is usually at a point of rapid decline in the patient's condition, when informed discussions are challenging.[52]
- Rotation of medical and nursing staff make communication continuity difficult.
- There is frequently discordance between family and physician regarding how the patient is doing. Relatives' interpretations of messages about the patient's condition and prognosis may be different from what they have actually been told. Moreover, "subliminal" information is passed to the family informally at the bedside, where a nurse is always in attendance. Medical language is translated into lay terms by various team members, but in this process the emphasis or importance of each element may become skewed. For example, a patient with multiorgan failure who is making no progress overall, and therefore has a poor prognosis, may at times need a bit less oxygen or have a "better" blood pressure, but this undulating clinical course frequently ends in death; piecemeal or mixed reports may be confusing or misleading for the family. Regrettably, the desire to communicate and hear positive elements often clouds the real picture, and relatives may apportion inappropriate optimism to these snippets.
- ICU nursing care may torture patients, through the stress of endless noise and lights, sleep deprivation, thirst, painful suctioning, painful turning, and risk of pressure sores.

EDUCATION AND CONTINUING MEDICAL EDUCATION

Because there is an abundance of death and dying in the ICU, it offers opportunity for teaching and learning. The daily detailed ward rounds, in which all aspects of treatment and care are discussed system by system, is suited to including goals of care given the patient's needs and what has been discussed. The most valuable principle is that *goals of care should be the driving force for technology, not vice versa.*

Rarely do clinicians identify end-of-life care as a competency that can be improved or updated.[53] Fostering improved listening skills and getting the environment right in an otherwise impersonal technical clinical setting

◼ CASE STUDY

A Death in an Intensive Care Unit

MB, a 73-year-old woman who was a lifelong smoker, presented to the hospital on a Thursday with anorexia, fever, productive cough, weight loss, and breathlessness; on questioning, she also admitted to hemoptysis. On examination, she was cachectic, dehydrated, had heavy nicotine stains on her fingers, and had palpable craggy nodes in the left supraclavicular region. The admitting ward was extremely busy, and MB was moved to a chest ward the next day, but, because the weekend was about to begin, specific diagnostic investigations were scheduled for the following week.

From the basic results available, she had an anemia, lobar pneumonia, and enlarged hilar nodes on chest radiography. Antibiotics and oxygen therapy were commenced. *(Is this patient "not dying," "maybe dying," or "dying"?)*

The ward doctors, although anticipating a diagnosis of lung cancer, did not communicate this with the patient or family. *(Aversion to communication is often a factor, particularly when bad news is on top of the differential diagnosis.)*

On Saturday evening, MB became very tired, acutely short of breath, in pain, and distressed. Her relatives were clearly upset and wanting "something to be done." A referral to the intensive care unit (ICU) was made. *(Was there an alternative?)* No symptomatic treatment was prescribed.

The intensivists were unable to have a conversation with MB due to her symptoms, and they were themselves distressed to see her like this. *(Many patients referred to ICU are incapacitated to various degrees.)* Never having met the family before, the ICU doctor had a discussion with them outlining the clinical impression of malignancy, but without histology, and explained what admission to the ICU would involve for them and for the patient. *(Would input from a palliative care expert at this time influence goals of care and forward planning?)* Without ICU care, MB was unlikely to survive the night. The family wished everything to be done, did not want to lose their wife and mother imminently, and stated that this is what MB would want because she had "always been a fighter." *(Is there a communication failure here?)*

As MB arrived in the ICU, she suffered respiratory decompensation and underwent intubation, ventilation, placement of a nasogastric tube and a urinary catheter, attachment of noninvasive monitoring devices, and placement of an arterial line for invasive monitoring. She was sedated with benzodiazepines and opiates for endotracheal tube tolerance. *(Is this the right decision? Should a "do not resuscitate" order have been in place?)* Inotropes were initially required, and copious quantities of secretions were suctioned on a regular basis.

Bronchoscopy revealed a compressed right main bronchus and a large tumor occluding the left main bronchus, the histology of which was squamous cell carcinoma, a rapidly fatal condition even for those in "good health." *(Was a histological diagnosis really necessary?)*

The ICU consultant met with the family to convey the news. Due to ICU work patterns, he was the third ICU doctor in 24 hours to have a consultation with the family. *(Continuity in ICU is often lacking.)* The conversation was difficult, the family having been "told" that things were "better": the patient needed less oxygen, her "drugs for the blood pressure" (inotropes) had been weaned off, she was starting to pass urine, and, although drowsy and rarely able to open her eyes, she seemed to nod appropriately. *(Problems here include discomfort in conveying a poor outlook, relatives not seeing the overall picture, and the patient not spoken to about the diagnosis.)* An attempt was made to translate technical "jargon" into lay terms. *(Imprecise terminology inevitably leads to communication errors.)* MB had been in hospital less than 72 hours, and the family was exhausted and emotionally drained.

The family expressed feelings of guilt at having subjected MB to intensive care and distress at not having an opportunity "to say goodbye" properly. MB had had her death prolonged due to ICU intervention, was unable to communicate satisfactorily with her family, and had no prospect of this situation's improving (it was believed that she did not have the respiratory reserve to survive weaning from the ventilator). *(Emotional burden for the admitting ICU consultant to bear—should admission have been declined?)* Further ICU care was deemed futile and therefore not in the patient's best interests. *(Were there joint discussions with clinicians and nursing staff?)* The discussion with the family moved toward the process of treatment withdrawal and how this would be achieved. *(The decision is active extubation versus terminal wean; with the latter, the pressures delivered by the ventilator and oxygen concentration are reduced but the patient remains intubated—resulting in a longer, more controlled death.)* The comfort of MB was paramount; this, together with the necessity of ablating distress, was explained to the family, and the use of opiates and benzodiazepines in appropriately liberal doses proposed.

MB was receiving minimal ventilatory assistance—30% oxygen with pressure support. There was little to "withdraw." *(Contrast this situation with that of a patient in multiorgan failure.)* Extubation with sedation, to let events take their course, was proposed so that the final part of the dying process would be as short and natural for the family as possible. *(But it would be a very active process for the physician.)* This would allow her husband to be close to her, unimpeded by endotracheal and nasopharyngeal tubes. With her family present, MB was given adequate doses of midazolam and morphine. All monitoring had been removed. She was extubated and died peacefully over the next few minutes, without making any respiratory effort. *(What is the correct dose of opiates and benzodiazepine? Was too much administered? If the drugs are poorly judged, this can be a very distressing situation for all.)* Her husband was clearly upset but was relieved that the ordeal was over. He appreciated having his wife free of ICU paraphernalia for her final few minutes.

In the end, this death was arguably a "good death" for patient and family. The frequent experience of ICU clinicians in deciding that further treatment is futile and then making the plan to sedate and personally extubate a patient is stressful and at times lonely, despite the "team" decision.

TABLE 180-6	Keys to Improving Palliative Care in the Intensive Care Unit
TOPIC	**KEY COMMENTS**
Communication	Communicate with patient/family before ICU admission is agreed. Provide frank details regarding what ICU therapy entails. Provide a clear description of "cure" goals of care and of "comfort" forward planning strategy if it should become futile to pursue "cure."
Withholding/ withdrawing treatment	Time-limited "cure" treatment is appropriate for some—it ensures that comfort care is delivered promptly. Legally, there is no difference between withholding and withdrawing, but clinicians may have strong ethical beliefs. There is a wide range of therapies to consider.
Pain and non-pain symptoms	Observe clinical cues that may indicate pain (e.g., lacrimation, diaphoresis, tachycardia). Other symptoms may be related to nausea, thirst, turning, suctioning, and hallucinations. Diagnosing symptoms is challenging.
Bereavement support	Provide counseling. Facilitate patient groups. Offer follow-up clinics for relatives and survivors. Post-traumatic stress disorder is common among the whole family.

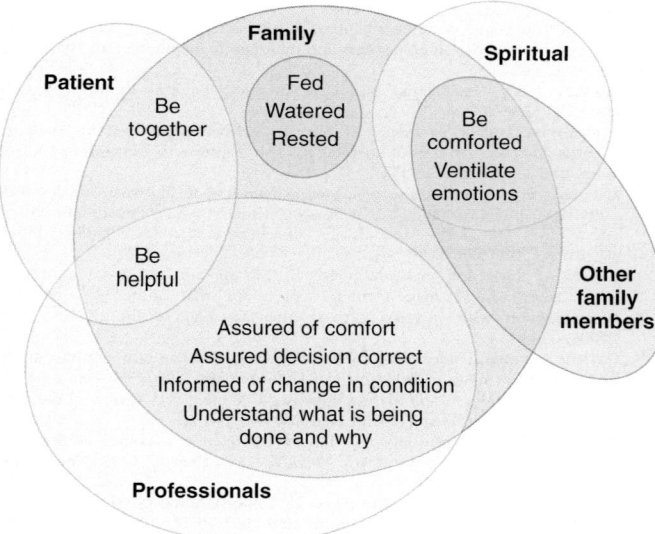

FIGURE 180-1   Complex needs and interactions of closest family members.

is a start.[54] Meetings with family should be approached with care and planning,[55] as is routine for other ICU procedures. Inviting local palliative care clinicians to participate in ward rounds and family conferences may be rewarding (Table 180-6).

FAMILY

Family beliefs and values may differ, but all family members need to have the opportunity to be with the dying person. In an ICU, this brings challenges. The dying person may not have been in the ICU for long, and relatives may not yet have had the opportunity to be at the bedside. It is an unfamiliar environment, dominated by technology, machines, and constant nursing attention, with little scope for privacy (few ICU beds in the United Kingdom are private). Even if everyone involved has had time to acclimatize, their needs are complex in this stressful situation (Fig. 180-1).[56]

ECONOMICS

The huge undersupply of intensive care facilities means, inevitably, that there is pressure to admit appropriately and discharge efficiently when this level of care is no longer required. If it becomes clear that a patient will not survive and a palliative approach is adopted, the benefits to the patient and the wider ICU community are clear. Up to 50% fewer intensive care interventions are undertaken if a palliative approach is adopted.[57] If the goals of care and time-limited therapies (e.g., trial of aggressive inotropic support for 48 hours) are discussed and based on patient response, a far shorter length of stay may be achieved without higher mortality.[58,59] To do this, the belief that we should not prolong a death must be upheld.

ETHICS: THE INCAPACITY ELEMENT

It is still rare to have advance directives, advance care plans, or the opportunity to discuss treatment limitation, withdrawal, or futility with patients while they have capacity to do so. Often these stages are reached after hours or days of critical illness deteriorating into multiorgan failure, becoming unresponsive to escalating inotropes, having a nonsurvivable diagnosis (e.g., advanced malignancy), or having no progress over many days—when care may then be deemed futile. Such patients are legally "incapacitated," and the responsibility for treatment decisions lies with the medical teams, taking cognizance of patient and family wishes whenever possible.[51] Opinions may be sought from family members, nursing staff, and other involved clinicians. At the end, the intensivist must make the call and set a plan to deliver appropriate, sensitive, respectful care that minimizes suffering for the patient, family, and carers.[60] Legally and morally, there is no distinction between treatment withdrawal and treatment limitation or nonescalation.[61] However, the practicalities are not so straightforward, and personal preference affects choices about which therapies are reduced or discontinued.

THE SWITCH FROM INTENSIVE CARE TO PALLIATION

Clinical intensive care is often practiced without diagnosis, and symptomatic physiology (e.g., low blood pressure, dyspnea) is treated without question when we are in a "cure" mode, yet this seems to be difficult when we move to a palliative phase. Perhaps the reason is that there is no specific training in when and how to switch from cure to comfort care, and intensivists are much more comfortable with the former.

Although much discussed in principle, the actual physical process of withdrawing life-sustaining treatments (Table 180-7) in ICU is rarely disclosed. Some courageous

TABLE 180-7 Therapies That Could Be Withdrawn in Palliative Care

TREATMENT CATEGORY	THERAPIES	COMMENTS
Cardiovascular	Inotropes and vasopressors Nitrates and vasodilators Ventricular assist devices Temporary pacemaker Deep venous thrombosis prophylaxis Intravenous fluids	Hypotension is the inevitable outcome
Respiratory	Oxygen Mandatory breaths Pressure support Positive end-expiratory pressure Endotracheal tube Continuous positive airway pressure Facemask/nasal oxygen	Hypoxia without hypercarbia does not cause distress
Renal	Dialysis and hemofiltration Furosemide infusion	Hyperkalemia, uremic acidosis, and fluid accumulation
Gastroenterology	Enteral feeding Parenteral feeding Peptic ulcer prophylaxis	
Neurology	Neuromuscular blockade Intracranial pressure bolt	Maintaining neuromuscular blockade may be inappropriate

TABLE 180-8 Therapies Possibly Worth Maintaining or Increasing in Palliative Care

TREATMENT CATEGORY	THERAPIES	COMMENTS
Neurology	Sedation Analgesia	Reduces anxiety, restlessness, "gasping," and fighting the ventilator*
Respiratory	Suctioning	Reduces respiratory noise; reduced incidence of endotracheal tube blockage or increased airway pressures*
General	Nicotine patch Oral hygiene Shaving and washing	Nicotine addiction Oral fetor and appearance* General comfort and care*

*Equally as important for the relatives' peace of mind.

authors have begun to challenge this taboo.[60] Other aspects of treatment may be escalated or introduced in palliative care, and these should also be considered (Table 180-8).

CONCLUSION

Modern training for intensive care medicine places the emphasis firmly on curative heroics, although the curriculum includes end-of-life care. Doctors in training in intensive care medicine must train in palliative care, and clinical integration with palliative medicine could make end-of-life care as high a priority as aggressive curative treatment

regimens. Care of the dying is distressing, both for the medical staff who bear the responsibility for changing therapeutic direction to comfort care and for the nursing staff who must carry out orders with the physicians. It is hard to keep a professional emotional distance in situations where active participation is a prerequisite. More collaboration, more research, and more discussion among the clinical community and the public should raise the profile and practice of palliative medicine in the ICU.

REFERENCES

1. Nelson JE, Meier DE, Litke A, et al. The symptom burden of chronic critical illness. Crit Care Med 2004;32:1527-1534.
2. Kinsella P. Dying without dignity. Economic and Social Research Council. Available at http://www.esrcsocietytoday.ac.uk/ESRCInfoCentre/index.aspx (accessed January 28, 2008).
3. Pattison M. Improving care through the end of life. Innovations in End-of-Life Care 2000;2(5). Available at: http://www2.edc.org/lastacts/archives.
4. Earle CC, Neville BA, Landrum MB, et al. Trends in the aggressiveness of cancer care near the end of life. J Clin Oncol 2004;22:315-321.
5. Matsuyama R, Reddy S, Smith TJ. Why do patients choose chemotherapy near the end of life? A review of the perspective of those facing death from cancer. J Clin Oncol 2006;24:3490-3496.
6. Wenger NS, Oye RK, Phillips S et al. A quantifiable adverse outcome of aggressive medical care. J Gen Intern Med 1996;11(Suppl 1):120.
7. Breslin JM, MacRae SK, Bell J, Singer PA; and the University of Toronto Joint Centre for Bioethics Clinical Ethics Group. Top 10 health care ethics challenges facing the public: Views of Toronto bioethicists. BMC Medical Ethics 2005;6:E5.
8. Singer P, Martin DK, Kelner M. Quality end-of-life care: Patients' perspectives. JAMA 1999;281:163-168.
9. Meyers FJ, Linder J, Beckett L, et al. Simultaneous care: A model approach to the perceived conflict between investigational therapy and palliative care. J Pain Symptom Manage 2004;28:548-556.
10. Heyland DK, Dodek P, Rocker G, et al. What matters most in end-of-life care: Perceptions of seriously ill patients and their family members. Can Med Assoc J 2006;174:627-641.
11. Mills M, Davies H, Macrae WA. Care of dying patients in hospital. BMJ 1994;309:583-586.
12. Hockley JM, Dunlop R, Davies RJ. Survey of distressing symptoms in dying patients and their families in hospital and the response to a symptom control team. BMJ 1988;296:1715-1717.
13. SUPPORT Principal Investigators. A controlled trial to improve care for seriously ill hospitalised patients: The Study to Understand Prognoses and Preferences for Outcomes and Risks of Treatments (SUPPORT). JAMA 1995;274:1591-1598.
14. Rogers A, Karlsen S, Addington-Hall J. "All the services were excellent. It is when the human element comes in that things go wrong": Dissatisfaction with hospital care in the last year of life. J Adv Nurs 2000;31:768-774.
15. Costello J. Nursing older dying patients: Findings from an ethnographic study of death and dying in elderly care wards. J Adv Nurs 2001;35:59-68.
16. Edmonds P, Rogers A. "If only someone had told me. . .": A review of the care of patients dying in hospital. Clin Med 2003;3:149-152.
17. Gruenewald DA, White EJ. The illness experience of older adults near the end of life: A systematic review. Anesthesiol Clin North Am 2006;24:163-180.
18. Curtis JR, Wenrich MD, Carline JD, et al. Understanding physicians' skills at providing end-of-life care. J Gen Intern Med 2001;16:41-51.
19. Glare P, Virik K, Jones M, et al. A systematic review of physician's survival predictions in terminally ill cancer patients. BMJ 2003;327:195-201.
20. Ellershaw J, Ward C. Care of the dying patient: The last hours or days of life. BMJ 2003;326:30-34.
21. Powis J, Etchells E, Martin DK, et al. Can a "good death" be made better? A preliminary evaluation of a patient-centred quality improvement strategy for severely ill in-patients. BMC Palliat Care 2004;3:2.
22. Thorns A, Sykes N. Opioid use in last week of life and implications for end-of-life decision-making. Lancet 2000;356:398-399.
23. Bookbinder M, Blank AE, Arney E, et al. Improving end-of-life care: Development and pilot-test of a clinical pathway. J Pain Symptom Manage 2005;29:529-543.
24. Bailey FA, Burgio KL, Woodby LL, et al. Improving processes of hospital care during the last hours of life. Arch Intern Med 2005;165:1722-1727.
25. Beth Israel Medical Center, Department of Pain Medicine and Palliative Care. Available at http://www.stopPain.org (assessed January 28, 2008).
26. Liverpool Care Pathways. Available at: http://www.lcp-mariecurie.org.uk.
27. Jones A, Johnstone R. Reflection on implementing a care pathway for the last days of life in nursing homes in North Wales. Int J Palliat Nurs 2004;10:507-509.
28. Maltoni M, Caraceni A, Brunelli C, et al. Prognostic factors in advanced cancer patients: Evidence-based clinical recommendations. A study by the steering

committee of the European Association for Palliative Care. J Clin Oncol 2005;23:6240-6248.

29. Vigano A, Dorgan M. Buckingham J, et al. Survival prediction in terminal cancer patients: A systematic review of the medical literature. Palliat Med 2000;14:363-374.

30. Vigano A, Donaldson N, Higginson IJ, et al. Quality of life and survival prediction in terminal cancer patients: A multicenter study. Cancer 2004; 101:1090-1098.

31. Roberts J. Describing the road to death. BMJ 2005;331:7508-7510.

32. Morita T, Tsunoda J, Inoue S, Chihara S. The Palliative Prognostic Index: A scoring system for survival prediction of terminally ill cancer patients. Support Care Cancer 1999;7:128-133.

33. Glare PA, Eychmueller S, McMahon P. Diagnostic accuracy of the palliative prognostic score in hospitalised patients with advanced cancer. J Clin Oncol 2004;22:4823-4828.

34. Duncan W. Caring or curing: Conflicts of choice. J R Soc Med 1985;78: 526-535.

35. Field D, Copp G. Communication and awareness about dying in the 1990s. Palliat Med 1999;13:459-468.

36. The AM, Hak T, Koëter G, van Der Wal G. Collusion in doctor-patient communication about imminent death: An ethnographic study. BMJ 2000;321: 1376-1381.

37. Murray SA, Kendall M, Boyd K, Sheikh A. Illness trajectories and palliative care. BMJ 2005;330:1007-1011.

38. Neuberger J. A healthy view of dying. BMJ 2003;327:207-208.

39. Homsi J, Walsh D, Rivera N, et al. Symptom evaluation in palliative medicine: Patient report vs systematic assessment. Support Care Cancer 2006;14:444-453.

40. Available at http://www.palliative.org/PC/ClinicalInfo/AssessmentTools/esas

41. Wells M, Dryden H, Guild P, et al. The knowledge and attitudes of surgical staff towards the use of opioids in cancer pain management: Can the hospital palliative care team make a difference? Eur J Cancer Care 2001;10:201-211.

42. Portenoy RK, Sibirceva U, Smout R, et al. Opioid use and survival at the end of life: A survey of a hospice population. J Pain Symptom Manage 2006;32:532-540.

43. Rady MY. Use of intensive care at the end of life in the United States. Crit Care Med 2004;32:638-643.

44. Lothian K, Philp I. Maintaining the dignity and autonomy of older people in the healthcare setting. BMJ 2001;322:668-670.

45. "Not Because They Are Old": An Independent Enquiry by the Health Advisory Service. London: HAS, 2000.

46. Willard C, Luker K. Challenges to end of life care in the acute hospital setting. Palliat Med 2006;20:611-615.

47. Rosenfield K. Palliative care assessment: What are we looking for? Gastroenterol Clin 2006;35.

48. Lo B, Quill T, Tulsky J. Discussing palliative care with patients. Ann Intern Med 1999;130:744-749.

49. Ahmedzai SH, Costa A, Blengini C, et al. A new international framework for palliative care. Eur J Cancer 2004;40:2192-2200.

50. Cook D, Rocker G, Marshall J, et al. Withdrawal of mechanical ventilation in anticipation of death in the intensive care unit. N Engl J Med 2003;349:1123-1132.

51. Prendergast TJ, Luce JM. Increasing incidence of withholding and withdrawal of life support from the critically ill. Am J Respir Crit Care Med 1997;155:15-20.

52. Rady MY, Johnson DJ. Admission to intensive care unit at the end-of-life: Is it an informed decision? Palliat Med 2004;18:705-711.

53. Danis M, Federman D, Fins JJ, et al. Incorporating palliative care into critical care education: Principles, challenges, and opportunities. Crit Care Med 1999;27:2005-2013.

54. Curtis JR, Engelberg RA, Wenrich MD, et al. Studying communication about end-of-life care during the ICU family conference: Development of a framework. J Crit Care 2002;17:147-160.

55. Curtis JR, Patrick DL, Shannon SE, et al. The family conference as a focus to improve communication about end-of-life care in the intensive care unit: Opportunities for improvement. Crit Care Med 2001;29(2 Suppl):N26-N33.

56. Truog RD, Cist AF, Brackett SE, et al. Recommendations for end-of-life care in the intensive care unit: The Ethics Committee of the Society of Critical Care Medicine. Crit Care Med 2001;29:2332-2348.

57. Campbell ML, Frank RR. Experience with an end-of-life practice at a university hospital. Crit Care Med 1997;25:197-202.

58. Lilly CM, Sonna LA, Haley KJ, et al. Intensive communication: Four-year follow-up from a clinical practice study. Crit Care Med 2003;31(5 Suppl):S394-S399.

59. Lilly CM, De Meo DL, Sonna LA, et al. An intensive communication intervention for the critically ill. Am J Med 2000;109:469-475.

60. Rubenfeld GD. Principles and practice of withdrawing life-sustaining treatments. Crit Care Clin 2000;20:435-451.

61. Brody H, Campbell ML, Faber-Langendoen K, et al. Withdrawing intensive life-sustaining treatment: Recommendations for compassionate clinical management. N Engl J Med 1997;336:652-657.

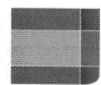

CHAPTER **181**

Comfort Care: Symptom Control in the Dying

Lesley Bicanovsky

KEY POINTS

- Symptoms must be reassessed at least daily.
- Each care plan and drug profile must be individualized.
- Active listening is part of good communication skills.
- A specific comfort care management plan needs to be implemented.
- This is the time to do, for another, what others will do for us when our time comes.

And in the end, it's not the years in your life that count. It's the life in your years.

A. LINCOLN

Medicine is more than saving lives. Dying is a unique and individual process that a person experiences only once, and it is assuredly no less miraculous than that individual's birth. The actively dying present unique challenges for a clinician. People in their final hours require careful symptom management. This is the time when we physicians must step beyond our individual skills and knowledge and do, for another, what others will do for us when the time comes.

CLINICAL EVALUATION AND DIAGNOSIS

Death is a universal part of living and should be a respectful and peaceful time. Obviously, to care for the actively dying, one must be able to diagnose dying. There are no tools specifically to diagnose dying, although changes on the Palliative Performance Scale (see Chapter 180) can indicate when death is approaching. Those in the last days of life with far advanced cancer, for example, are typically bedridden, semiconscious, and with little or no oral intake. Changes in pulse, respiration, and peripheral circulation may also be noticed (Table 181-1).

Once someone has begun the transition to an actively dying phase, the family should be brought together in a conference to discuss changing goals of care. This conversation should be undertaken in an appropriate location; it should not take place, for example, in a busy hospital hallway. It is best to document the discussion in the patient's medical chart. Physical findings of dying (see Chapter 177) should be reviewed with the family.[1] These signs and symptoms indicate that their loved one is entering an actively dying phase. The physician explains that a comfort care management plan needs to be implemented.

A "do not resuscitate" order must be negotiated and communicated to all involved. The family and physician can then review the comfort measures to be initiated. During this potentially difficult and emotional conversation, the discontinuation of vital sign assessments, intravenous hydration, pulse oximetry, any nonessential medications, and blood work should be discussed. Withdrawal of these treatments and procedures also serves to limit patient interruptions and discomfort. An oxygen mask can be changed to a nasal cannula (2-6 L) with specific orders for no further advancement of oxygen flow rates beyond those limits and no assessment of oximetry. Expert mouth care is essential (every 2 hours and as needed), and family participation is encouraged. Throughout the process, the comfort of both the family and the patient is reassessed.

SYMPTOM MANAGEMENT

Unrelieved pain, shortness of breath, and restlessness are among the most common causes of physical distress before death.[2,3] Symptoms in the actively dying must be reassessed, at a minimum of once daily, to ensure appropriate comfort care management. Unrelieved symptoms can be distressing to patients, family members, and staff. Physical distress precludes any possibility of relieving psy-

chological, social, and spiritual suffering; improving quality of remaining life; or personal closure for the patient. It also leaves a painful lasting impression on the family. Common end-stage symptoms should be anticipated and appropriate medications made readily available for efficient and effective relief (Table 181-2). The drugs used for symptom control vary from country to country, depending on availability, cost, and local preferences. The ones mentioned here are those commonly used in the United States of America.

Management Algorithm

Clinical pathways, such as the Liverpool Care Pathway, have been developed to improve the care of the dying through the use of a standardized approach (see Chapter 178). Alternatively, individualized management of symptoms and other problems can be addressed, as described here.

Pain

Pain in the dying is usually well controlled by continuing the current opioid regimen. It is often necessary to change the route of administration if the patient is unable to take medications orally. An analgesic dose given immediately before a patient is turned or moved can reduce incident pain. In the final 48 hours of life, 13% have their dose reduced, 44% have it increased, and in 48% it remains unchanged.[3] When a person is currently not having pain or pain is intermittent, then the provided dose is given only as needed. Severe unrelieved pain should be avoidable. Remember that, although unconscious people can experience pain, appropriate pain management in the dying is not just a vague order to titrate a given opioid to comfort.

Dyspnea

Dyspnea is a patient's perception of breathlessness. Many treatments that would be appropriate at an earlier stage in palliative care are no longer applicable in the actively dying patient. The incidence of dyspnea rises to 70% in the last 6 weeks of life,[4] and to 79% among those surviving less than 1 day after admission.[5] Oxygen by mask or nasal cannula and cool air from a nearby fan can reduce the sensation of breathlessness, whether or not there is a clinical hypoxia.[6] As-needed doses of an opioid can be effective. Morphine can be used, at a dose chosen based on any prior opioid exposure, and administered with a fre-

TABLE 181-1	Signs of Impending Death

Profound progressive weakness
Bed-bound state
Sleeping much of the time
Indifference to food and fluid
Difficulty swallowing
Disorientation to time, with increasingly short attention span
Low or lower blood pressure not related to hypovolemia
Urinary incontinence or retention caused by weakness
Loss of ability to close eyes
Oliguria
Hallucinations of previously deceased important individuals
References to going home or similar themes
Changes in respiratory rate and pattern (Cheyne-Stokes breathing, apneas)
Noisy breathing, airway secretions
Mottling and cooling of the skin due to vasomotor instability with venous pooling, particularly tibial
Dropping blood pressure with rising, weak pulse
Mental status changes (delirium, restlessness, agitation, coma)

TABLE 181-2	Formulary of Drugs and Doses for the Actively Dying		
SYMPTOM	**DRUG**	**ROUTE**	**INITIAL DOSE**
Pain	Morphine	IV, SQ	Naïve—0.5 mg continuous infusion with 1 mg q 1 hr as needed; prior opiate use—convert to appropriate parenteral dose
Death rattle	Glycopyrrolate	IV, SQ	0.2 mg q 6 hr as needed
	Hyoscyamine	PO, SL	2 mg q 6 hr as needed
	Scopolamine	Transdermal	0.125 mg q 6 hr as needed; one patch q 72 hr
Dyspnea	Morphine	IV, SQ	1 mg q 1 hr as needed and titrate if indicated
		PO	5 mg q 2 hr as needed and titrate if indicated
Agitation and/or restlessness	Chlorpromazine	IV, PR	25 mg q 6 hr as needed and titrate if indicated
	Phenobarbital	IV, SQ	100 mg q 3 hr as needed and titrate if indicated

quency of every hour if needed. Morphine improves dyspnea in 95% of patients with terminal cancer,[7] without causing respiratory failure.[8]

Secretions

Retained respiratory secretions can increase during the dying process, resulting in the "death rattle." This can cause much anxiety to relatives and caregivers. Aspiration of secretions is not recommended. No drug can entirely dry up secretions that have already accumulated. This symptom is usually best controlled by glycopyrrolate. The starting dose is 0.2 mg IV or SQ every 6 hours as needed. If it is not available, hyoscyamine sulfate 0.125 mg SL every 1 hour as needed can be substituted. Some use hyoscine hydrobromide. No evidence supports the choice of one drug over the other.[9,10] Fifty percent of dying patients receive hyoscine in some form in the last 48 hours of life.[11-13]

Hydration

Management of hydration in the dying is controversial.[14,15] If the potential benefits are likely to outweigh the disadvantages, then a trial of subcutaneous or intravenous fluids may be justified. Management differs based on the care setting and should be individualized. One must explain to the family that rehydration will not reverse the dying process and that it is only a time-limited trial to palliate suffering.

Restlessness and Terminal Sedation

Restlessness can be managed by chlorpromazine.[16] A starting dose of 12.5 mg to 25 mg IV every 6 hours, as needed, is initiated. Chlorpromazine can be titrated or scheduled around the clock. This is effective, and it is available in intravenous, tablet, and suppository preparations. If chlorpromazine is unavailable, benzodiazepines or phenobarbital can be used. Lorazepam can be used as 1 mg IV or PO (or SL) every 6 hours as needed. Phenobarbital is effective for palliative sedation in terminal delirium.[17-19]

Palliative sedation has aroused ethical controversy.[20] Discussion is required with the family. This centers on understanding that terminal sedation represents a conscious decision to decrease the patient's consciousness to the extent that he or she will no longer feel pain, air hunger, or other distress.[21] This sedation allows the patient to sleep through the dying process. This is not meant to expedite one's natural process of dying, but only to enhance comfort.

The family should understand that no further verbal communication will be possible with the patient. Published guidelines may help medical staff and family make a mutual decision to manage intractable distress of the dying.[22] Studies have shown that the appropriate use of sedatives results in safe relief of symptoms without shortening life.[23-25]

Vomiting

Antiemetics must be used empirically; they are given by suppository, subcutaneously, or intravenously. A nasogastric tube may be needed for intermittent aspiration to relieve recurrent large-volume vomits. Sips of water and good mouth care provide comfort. In the dying, the cause of vomiting is rarely investigated.

Bladder and Bowel Care

A Foley catheter may be needed for urinary retention, or a rectal suppository for rectal distention from constipation. Both conditions may cause distress, and both are easy to misdiagnose.

TERMINAL EMERGENCIES

Acute stridor requires immediate sedation with IV midazolam 5 to 20 mg (the dose being dependent on whether the patient recently had a dose and in what amount). Massive hemorrhage is a catastrophic event. In most cases, all that time allows is for views of the patient to be blocked by the use of a curtain. If the event is anticipated, dark towels should be readily available to make blood loss less obvious. Midazolam, 5 to 20 mg, should be available for immediate sedation.

Myoclonus is another symptom that is distressing to the family. Patients are often so ill or unconscious that they are unaware. It may be caused by dopamine antagonists, neuroleptics, high-dose opioids, or withdrawal of such drugs as benzodiazepines, barbiturates, anticonvulsants, and alcohol. Treatment should include review of all medications and dosages, sedation with midazolam, 1 to 10 mg SQ every hour until the patient is restful, and then 20 to 30 mg/day, which can be given by intermittent SC injection or by continuous IV or SC infusion as indicated. Alternatives such as rectal diazepam or clonazepam are available.

Convulsions (see Chapter 175) may require emergent treatment with midazolam, diazepam, phenobarbital, or clonazepam.

PSYCHOSOCIAL CARE

Most competent patients know how ill they are and that they will die. Hopefully, they have had the time to reflect back and to look forward. Most seek reassurance that they will not be left alone, will not suffer, and will not burden those caring for them. Before the final days to hours, it should have been agreed on by everyone, including the patient, where the process of active dying is to be spent. There are advantages and disadvantages for home, acute care hospital, and palliative care unit settings (see Chapter 180). The goal is to allow the patient to pass through the act of dying with adequate symptom management.

The emotional needs of the family are also an integral goal and must be identified, remembered, and managed. Time so spent is never wasted. The psychological needs of the dying patient, family, and loved ones are continually reassessed, and this can involve multiple members of the team (e.g., social worker, pastoral care). It must be remembered that the job is not finished at the time of death. Once a patient has died, follow-up bereavement counseling is available.

COMMON ERRORS

Diagnosing the onset of the dying process can be difficult in patients with other eventually fatal illnesses, because of the different death trajectories. In cases of end-organ failure (e.g., chronic obstructive pulmonary disease, congestive heart failure), people can be close to death but still able to respond to active treatment. For those who do not respond to treatment or for whom treatment is refused or withheld, making the diagnosis of dying is similar to making the diagnosis in cancer patients.

Some physicians are reluctant to provide adequate analgesia or sedation to people who are distressed and dying because of concerns that the drugs may inadvertently hasten death. Audits of prescribing practices in hospices have repeatedly failed to show any association between doses of morphine and death. Providing terminal sedation can also be problematic. It is generally considered that those who are dying with unrelievable physical discomfort can be offered sedation, but the situation may be less clear for people who are physically comfortable but have great psychological anguish.

RESEARCH CHALLENGES

Research in the imminently dying is challenging. There are many ethical and methodological problems. If dying patients are to be given the best possible care to respect their dignity, then we owe it to them to systematically evaluate our practices and continuously improve them. To improve symptom control in the dying, evaluation by the Plan-Do-Study-Act methodology may be a suitable alternative to traditional research designs.

CONCLUSIONS

Dying is probably the most difficult experience in the life of an individual, and it is also taxing for their family and loved ones and for the professionals providing care. Caring for an actively dying patient requires an interdisciplinary team approach. This is challenging because comfort care measures are dependent on the unique situation and symptoms of each patient and not any standardized protocol.

REFERENCES

1. Dunn GP, Milch RA. Is this a bad day or one of the last days? How to recognize and respond to approaching demise. J Am Coll Surg 2002;195:879-887.
2. Enck RE. The last few days. Am J Hosp Palliat Care 1992;9:11-13.
3. Lichter I, Hunt E. The last 48 hours of life. J Palliat Care 1990;6:7-15.
4. Ruben DB, Mor V. Dyspnea in terminally ill cancer patients. Chest 1986;89:234-236.
5. Heyse-Moore LH, Ross V, Mullee MA. How much of a problem is dyspnea in advanced cancer? Palliat Med 1991;5:20-26.
6. Spiller J, Alexander D. Domiciliary care: A comparison of the views of terminally ill patients and their care-givers. Palliat Med 1993;7:109-115.
7. Bruera E, Macmillan K, Pither J. Effects of morphine on the dyspnea of terminal cancer patients. J Pain Symptom Manage 1990;5:341-344.
8. Walsh TD. Opiates and respiratory function in advanced cancer. Recent Results Cancer Res 1994;89:115-117.
9. Lawrey H. Hyoscine vs glycopyrronium for drying respiratory secretions in dying patients. Br J Commun Nurs 2005;10:421-424.
10. Bennett M, Lucas V, Brennan M, et al.; Association for Palliative Medicine's Science Committee. Using anti-muscarinic drugs in the management of death rattle: Evidence-based guidelines for palliative care. Palliat Med 2002;16:369-374.
11. Bennet M. Death rattle: An audit of hyoscine (scopamine) use and review of management. J Pain Symptom Manage 1996;12:229-233.
12. Hughes A, Wilcock A, Corcoran R, et al. Audit of three antimuscarinic drugs for managing death rattle. J Palliat Med 2000;14:221-222.
13. Dawson HR. The use of transdermal scopolamine in the control of deathrattle. J Palliat Care 1998;5:31-33.
14. Fainsinger R, Bruera E. The management of dehydration in terminally ill patients. J Palliat Care 1994;10:55-59.
15. Fainsinger R, MacEachern T, Miller MJ, et al. The use of hypodermoclysis for rehydration in terminally ill cancer patients. J Pain Symptom Manage 1994;9:298-302.
16. McIver B, Walsh D, Nelson K. The use of chlorpromazine for symptom control in dying cancer patients. J Pain Symptom Manage 1994;9:341-345.
17. Garvin J, Chapman CR. Clinical management of dying patients. Caring for Patients at the End of Life [Special Issue]. West J Med 1995;163:268-277.
18. Stone P, Phillips C, Spruyt O, Waight C. A comparison of the use of sedatives in a hospital support team and in a hospice. Palliat Med 1997;11:140-144.
19. Fainsinger RL, Waller A, Bercovici M, et al. A multicentre international study of sedation for uncontrolled symptoms in terminally ill patients. Palliat Med 2000;14:257-265.
20. Billings JA, Block SD. Slow euthanasia. J Palliat Care 1996;12:21-30.
21. Quill TE, Dresser R, Brock DW. The rule of double effect: A critique of its role in end-of-life decision making. N Engl J Med 1997;337:1768-1771.
22. Quill TE, Byock ACP; ASIM End-Of-Life Care Consensus Panel: Responding to intractable suffering: The role of terminal sedation and voluntary refusal of foods and fluids. Ann Intern Med 2000;132:408-414.
23. Ventafridda V, Ripamonti C, De Conno F, et al. Symptom prevalence and control during cancer patients' last days of life. J Palliat Care 1990;6:7-11.
24. Sykes N, Thorns A. Sedative use in the last week of life and the implications for end-of-life decision making. Arch Intern Med 2003;163:341-344.
25. Cowen JD, Walsh D. Terminal sedation in palliative medicine: Definition and review of the literature. Support Care Cancer 2001;9:403-407.

SUGGESTED READING

AGS Ethics Committee. American Geriatrics Society (AGS) Position Statement: The Care of Dying Patients. Updated 2007. Available at http://www.americangeriatrics.org/products/positionpapers/careofd.shtml (accessed January 28, 2008).

National Comprehensive Cancer Network. NCCN Palliative Care Guidelines. Available at http://www.cancer.org/downloads/CRI/F9643.00.pdf (accessed January 28, 2008).

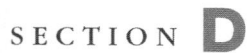
Complementary and Alternative Medicines

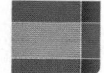

CHAPTER **182**

Integrative Medicine: Complementary Therapies

Barrie Cassileth and Jyothirmai Gubili

KEY POINTS

- Integration of evidence-based complementary therapies may enhance quality of life and improve symptom control in palliative medicine.

- Complementary therapies have proven benefit for the patient; alternative therapies may be disproved or associated with unknown risks.

- Patients should be warned that dietary supplements and vitamins are unregulated, may interact with other medications, and may be harmful.

- Acupuncture, massage, music therapy, and mind-body techniques offer significant symptomatic relief for palliative care and symptom management.

- Complementary therapies are noninvasive, pleasant, and virtually free of side effects. They are also cost effective.

Integrative medicine is the synthesis of state-of-the-art mainstream medical care and complementary therapies that help manage physical and emotional symptoms. The inclusion of effective complementary therapies in palliative care is an important response to the growing need for care that addresses patients' psychological, spiritual, and physical needs. As defined by the World Health Organization, the emphasis of palliative care is to relieve suffering.

Palliative care needs, including the needs to maintain dignity, to be free of anxiety, and to experience human interaction, have been poorly met by the health care system. The original concepts of hospice or palliative care have been resurrected and formalized, so that, along with modern pharmaceuticals and technology, the ancient mandate to relieve suffering also characterizes today's palliative medicine. The skills of nonphysician caregivers such as massage therapists, acupuncturists, and music therapists have an important role.

DEFINITIONS AND OVERVIEW

Integrative medicine is a synthesis of the best of mainstream care and adjunctive complementary therapies. It is a term applied to distinguish an evidence-based area of medical care from the realm of alternative therapies, which are nonviable approaches typically proffered for serious and end-stage illnesses. The umbrella term, "complementary and alternative medicine (CAM)," is unfortunate because it fails to distinguish between evidence-based, helpful and effective *complementary therapies* and alternative therapies, which are often falsely promoted as viable alternatives to mainstream care. We define *alternative therapies* as questionable, unproved, or disproved approaches. They can delay needed mainstream treatment and may pose danger to patients. Integrative medicine includes no questionable or disproved methods and has substantial utility throughout the course of disease, especially in the dying. Methodologically sound, randomized, controlled studies of complementary therapies and botanicals have been published in major medical journals.

The establishment of integrative medicine programs or activities in most hospitals and hospices also has stimulated solid research, enhanced the quality of clinical services, and improved patient-physician communication on the topic. Research increasingly has addressed clinical subsets of patients and symptom categories that might benefit from complementary therapies. Patients facing terminal illness are an important example. In palliative medicine, effective relief of symptoms is feasible using noninvasive complementary therapies. Palliative care professionals must understand the benefits and limitations of complementary therapies and, importantly, distinguish them from ineffective "alternatives."[1-3]

COMPLEMENTARY AND ALTERNATIVE THERAPIES IN MEDICAL PRACTICE

Although use of complementary and alternative therapies is not new, patients in the past did not discuss their interest in remedies outside of those available in mainstream clinics and hospitals but investigated them surreptitiously.[4] As the previously patriarchal doctor-patient relationship gave way to more active patient participation, patients acted on their preferences for close involvement in medical discussions and decisions.[5] Unconventional therapies became increasingly acceptable, and information about them expanded tremendously with growth of the Internet (Table 182-1).

Often, today's patients want to consider unconventional treatments. No longer uncomfortable raising the issues, patients ask their physicians for advice and expect

TABLE 182-1 Reputable Sources of Online Information on Complementary and Alternative Medicine

ORGANIZATION	WEB SITE*
National Center for Complementary and Alternative Medicine (NCCAM)	http://nccam.nih.gov
National Cancer Institute	http://www.cancer.gov/cam/index.html
Quackwatch	http://www.quackwatch.com
U.S. Department of Agriculture	http://www.nal.usda.gov/fnic
National Institutes of Health	http://dietary-supplements.info.nih.gov
U.S. Pharmacopeia	http://www.usp.org/USPVerified/dietarySupplements/faq.html
American Cancer Society	http://www.cancer.org/docroot/ETO/ETO_5.asp?sitearea = ETO
Memorial Sloan-Kettering Cancer Center	http://www.mskcc.org/aboutherbs
M. D. Anderson Cancer Center	http://www.mdanderson.org/departments/CIMER
Institute of Medicine (IOM)	http://www.iom.edu/board.asp?id = 3788

*All sites were accessed on January 26, 2008.

appropriate guidance and referrals. Because patients and family members also inquire about questionable methods, caregivers must understand both the problematic and the beneficial approaches available under the "CAM" rubric.

In the United States, depending on definitions, between 7% and 80% of cancer patients use complementary or alternative therapies.[6] The most commonly used therapies are dietary treatments, herbs, homeopathy, hypnotherapy, imagery or visualization, meditation, megavitamins, relaxation, and spiritual healing. The range is wide because of absent or variable definitions of terms, which also makes it impossible to determine, for example, whether patients used the therapies inappropriately to treat the cancer or suitably to relieve symptoms. A recent European survey found that 36% of cancer patients used "CAM," with herbal remedies predominating,[7] and a nationwide survey of cancer patients in Japan found a prevalence of 45%, most commonly herbs, mushrooms, and shark cartilage.[8] Sixty-one percent of Japanese patients used these agents without discussion with their doctors. Most U.S. physicians have learned to ask about, and patients to discuss, their use of such remedies.

ALTERNATIVE THERAPIES

Most patients with advanced cancer, pulmonary, or cardiovascular disease use complementary therapies properly, as adjuncts to mainstream care for symptom control. Disingenuous marketing misleads vulnerable patients and often draws them to nonviable "alternatives" through deceptive advertising. Hundreds of thousands of Web sites promote countless unproved and generally useless therapies to the public. Bogus products are widely available in the United States and internationally. Agents such as laetrile,[9] previously banned by the U.S. Food and Drug Administration (FDA), and interventions such as oxygen and magnetic therapies are promoted as treatments for cancer and other illnesses and are easily pursued on the Internet. Patients and family members facing terminal illness are more likely to seek unproved methods. Some popular examples are summarized in the following paragraphs.

Dietary Supplements

Dietary supplements are nonprescription items that are widely available over the counter. According to the National Nutritional Food Association, annual sales of dietary supplements reached $19.8 billion in 2003, including $4.2 billion in herbal remedies. Those most popular among cancer patients and the general public include vitamins and minerals, homeopathic remedies, herbal and other botanical remedies, antioxidants, and items promoted to enhance immune function. Two major problems exist with dietary supplements: the absence of government regulation with little quality control, and the misuse or overuse of these products with attendant negative clinical consequences. In 1994, after intense lobbying by the food supplement industry, the U.S. Congress passed legislation permitting dietary supplements to be sold over the counter without FDA review. In the United States, there is no oversight of production, standardization, packaging, or quality assurance of the multibillion-dollar dietary supplement industry.

The view that supplemental vitamins and antioxidants, typically in large quantities, are needed by cancer patients stems from the public's belief that cancer treatment depletes the body of essential building blocks, but there is no compelling evidence that ingestion of additional antioxidants is helpful.[10] Harmful interactions between antioxidants and chemotherapy are documented, and it is recommended that they be avoided during cancer treatment.[11,12]

Biological Therapies

"Biological" therapies, which use various invasive methods to detoxify the body and thus destroy disease, have remained popular for more than a century. Some have been studied and found useless, and others have been judged ineligible for careful investigation. They are the mainstay of most "alternative" clinics and spas in the United States, Europe, and elsewhere. About a dozen Tijuana clinics offer variations of the Gerson biological regimen, which aims to purify the liver with high potassium intake, coffee enemas, and large quantities of fruit and vegetable juices.[13] Other treatments are based on the use of intravenous hydrogen peroxide, oxygen, and massive vitamin doses. These are not supported by scientific data.

In the 1980s, the National Institutes of Health (NIH) supported research into so-called antineoplastons, a biological molecular therapy, after case reports suggesting that glioblastoma multiforme in children regressed with this treatment. Support for the research ended when the investigator and NIH researchers reached an impasse regarding trial design. Case reports continue, but no randomized, controlled trial of antineoplastons has been completed, and other investigators have been unable to replicate the original data.[14,15]

Shark cartilage was heavily promoted as a cancer therapy after the 1992 publication of the book, *Sharks Don't Get Cancer*. However, sharks do get cancer, and a North Central Cancer Group randomized trial of this treatment found neither survival nor quality of life differences between groups studied.[16] The anti-angiogenic properties of shark cartilage are currently under scientific investigation.

Herbs

The use of herbs is common in medical practices around the world. They are frequently used in Europe, where the prevalence of use was found to triple in people after a cancer diagnosis.[7] Some of the most powerful modern pharmaceuticals, such as paclitaxel and digoxin, are plant-derived. Herbs marketed today as adjuvants for cancer treatment or as immune-enhancers may contain harmful constituents, interfere with prescription medications, and produce serious adverse effects. Liver and kidney failure have resulted from drug-herb interactions, and many preparations are contaminated.

A prominent example is the multiherb compound called PC-SPES (PC stands for prostate cancer; SPES is Latin for "hope"). This was claimed to slow progression of prostate cancer and was extremely popular. It was found to contain diethylstilbestrol and other contaminants and was removed from the market in 2002.[17]

Essiac tea, a popular mixture of burdock, turkey rhubarb, sheep sorrel, and slippery elm, was shown by researchers from the National Cancer Institute to have no anticancer effect and, moreover, to potentially interfere with drugs metabolized via the cytochrome P-450 pathway. Popular herbs used by cancer patients can interfere with the pharmacokinetics of chemotherapeutic agents via this pathway, including ginkgo, garlic, kava, St. John's wort, and echinacea.

In addition, feverfew, garlic, ginger, and ginkgo are among the many herbs with known anticoagulant effects and should not be taken with warfarin (Coumadin) or heparin derivatives.[12]

COMPLEMENTARY THERAPIES

Complementary therapies effectively reduce anxiety, depression, pain, dyspnea, nausea, and fatigue.[2,18] Some, such as meditation and hypnosis, may be self-managed, giving patients the important opportunity to maintain a measure of independence and control over their well-being. The major supportive therapies reviewed in this chapter—acupuncture, massage therapy, music therapy, and mind-body modalities—address some of the most pervasive and difficult problems faced in palliative medicine.

Acupuncture

Acupuncture is the insertion of fine needles, for therapeutic purposes, into points on the skin. According to traditional Chinese medicine theory, these acupoints are located along channels, or meridians, that are believed to conduct "qi" or energy. Stimulation can be enhanced by heat, electrical current, or pressure.[19,20] Although anatomi-

cal structures representing meridians have not been found, some acupuncture points coincide with trigger points sensitive to pressure, indicating enriched enervation at the anatomical location (Fig. 182-1).

Recent research indicates the physiological effects of acupuncture. The stimulation of certain acupuncture points (e.g., in acupuncture treatments for chronic pain) produces demonstrable physiological change on functional magnetic resonance imaging (fMRI).[21] Acupuncture stimulates A delta fibers entering the dorsal horn of the spinal cord. These mediate segmental inhibition of pain impulses carried in slower, unmyelinated C fibers. Through neural connections in the midbrain, descending inhibition of C fiber pain impulses is also enhanced.[22] Initial interest in acupuncture and endogenous opioids was sparked by acupuncture's analgesic effects. Animal studies demonstrated that acupuncture-induced analgesia can be blocked by naloxone, a narcotic antagonist.[23,24] Mice deficient in opiate receptors showed poor acupuncture analgesia.[25]

The 1997 NIH Consensus Conference concluded that acupuncture is effective in relieving pain, nausea, and osteoarthritis. Much research shows evidence of additional benefits, and NIH supports clinical trials of acupuncture and studies of its mechanisms. In palliative care, acupuncture may be especially helpful for pain, fatigue, chemotherapy-related nausea, and xerostomia.

A meta-analysis of 33 randomized, controlled trials concluded that acupuncture was more effective in low back pain than sham acupuncture or no treatment.[26] One month of acupuncture therapy compared with physical therapy in 129 patients with low back pain found significantly less impairment in the acupuncture group, an effect that was sustained at 5 months.[27] A randomized trial in 294 patients with knee osteoarthritis showed acupuncture to be more effective than no acupuncture or minimal acupuncture.[28]

Studies of acupuncture for pain, including randomized trials and meta-analyses, have found inconsistent results, with virtually all calling for additional methodologically sound research.[29-31] When one is attempting to manage symptoms, and especially in palliative medicine, risk-benefit issues must be considered. As for most medical

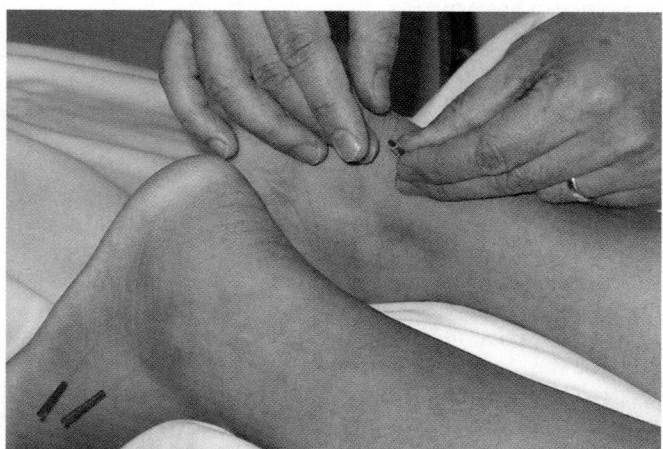

FIGURE 182-1 Acupuncture is safe and can be used to control many symptoms associated with cancer, cancer treatment, and end-stage disease.

interventions, patients do not necessarily respond identically to therapy, including acupuncture. It is effective for many, and it has the additional and rare virtues of being safe, inexpensive, and free of side effects when administered by qualified practitioners. It is worth a try.

Acupuncture helps lessen chemotherapy-induced nausea and vomiting associated with emetogenic chemotherapy, better than pharmacotherapy only.[32] The effects do not appear to result entirely from the added attention, clinician-patient interaction, or placebo effect. A meta-analysis found that acupuncture, particularly electroacupuncture, reduced chemotherapy-induced nausea and vomiting when used with standard antiemetic therapy, although the additive effects were small.[33,34]

Acupuncture may relieve xerostomia (severe dry mouth) resulting from radiotherapy for head and neck cancer. A retrospective study of 50 patients found that 70% achieved response, defined as 10% or greater improvement over baseline xerostomia inventory scores.[35] Several studies have supported acupuncture for vasomotor symptoms in postmenopausal women. It has also been investigated for vasomotor symptoms caused by androgen and estrogen ablation treatment in breast and prostate cancer. In a cohort study, 194 patients predominantly with breast cancer or prostate cancer were given four weekly acupuncture treatments; retrospective analysis showed that 79% of participants experienced a 50% or greater reduction in hot flashes after treatment.[36]

For fatigue after chemotherapy or irradiation, a major and common problem, there are few effective treatment options. The National Comprehensive Cancer Network (NCCN) guidelines list energy conservation and exercise, but these are mutually exclusive, and exercise is rarely feasible in palliative medicine. These guidelines have not lessened the severity or the prevalence of the problem.[37] Acupuncture is not physically demanding and can provide relief.[38,39] It is an empirical treatment for fatigue, given its favorable risk/benefit ratio. In an uncontrolled trial after chemotherapy, 6 weeks of acupuncture therapy reduced fatigue by 31%; among those with severe fatigue at baseline, 79% had improved fatigue scores at follow-up.[40] In contrast, fatigue was reduced in only 24% of patients during usual care.[41] Controlled studies are underway.

Massage Therapy

Massage involves the application of varying degrees of pressure on muscles and soft tissues to reduce tension and pain, improve circulation, and encourage relaxation. Swedish massage, the most common type in the United States, is gentle and comprises five basic strokes (stroking, kneading, friction, percussion, and vibration). The movement is rhythmic and free-flowing. Other variations include reflexology (foot massage), shiatsu, and tui-na (acupressure). Massage therapy requires state certification or licensure.

The effectiveness of massage therapy for symptom control has been supported by several studies.[42-44] The relative contribution of the therapist to the benefits of massage therapy is currently under study in a randomized, controlled trial. However, the importance of human touch per se is well established. Examples include the "natural experiments" of World War II and the recent experience in Eastern European orphanages, where babies who were fed and maintained in bed, but not held or given the benefit of human touch, withered and died.

Regardless of whether symptom relief stems from touch or psychological components or both, the benefits of massage therapy are well documented in palliative care.[45] Massage therapy reduces pain[46] as well as anxiety and distress.[47] In a trial that randomized hospice patients to receive 4 weeks of massage, massage plus aromatherapy, or no intervention, improvements in sleep scores and depression occurred after massage.[48] A systematic review of clinical trials showed that massage consistently reduced anxiety in cancer patients.[49]

In the largest study to date, clinically relevant improvements in symptoms were reported after the intervention, even among patients with high baseline scores. Reduced symptoms included pain, fatigue, stress/anxiety, nausea, and depression. Benefits persisted with no return toward baseline scores throughout a 48-hour follow-up period.[50] Massage therapy is currently offered at many cancer institutions for symptom control. It is also recommended by the NCCN[51] for refractory cancer pain.

Music Therapy

Music evokes deep-seated emotion. Particular types of music may hold special meaning, depending on one's life experience. Music therapy is provided by professional musicians who are also trained music therapists. They often hold professional degrees in music therapy and are adept in dealing with the psychosocial issues faced by patients and family members. Music therapy is particularly effective in palliative medicine in improving quality of life and enhancing a sense of comfort and relaxation (Fig. 182-2). Formal music therapy programs in palliative medicine exist in many major institutions. Controlled trials

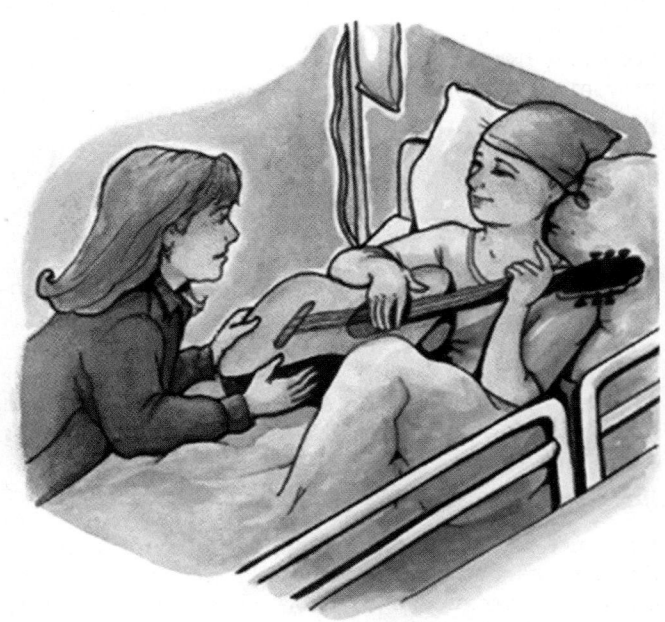

FIGURE 182-2 Music therapy reduces depression and anxiety in cancer patients.

indicate that music therapy produces emotional and physiological benefits, reducing anxiety, stress, depression, and pain. Among 80 hospice patients randomized to receive routine hospice services or services plus music therapy, there was improved quality of life in the experimental group, and the benefit improved with more music therapy over time.[52] No change in physical status or survival was observed, although other studies have shown that music therapy can significantly reduce heart rate, respiratory rate, and anxiety in hospitalized patients.[53]

Music therapy was also effective in reducing cancer pain.[54] A prospective study of 200 patients with chronic or advanced illness evaluated the effect of music therapy on anxiety, body movement, mood, facial expression, shortness of breath, and verbalizations; the results showed improvement in all of these measures ($P < .001$).[55] Music can reduce depression.[56] In a randomized, controlled trial of cancer patients undergoing autologous stem cell transplantation, anxiety, depression, and total mood disturbance scores were significantly lower in the music therapy group compared with standard-care controls.[57]

Mind-Body Therapies

Mind-body therapies in palliative medicine decrease distress and promote relaxation, but the idea that patients can influence their disease through mental or emotional work is inaccurate and can evoke guilt and inadequacy when disease continues to advance despite patients' best spiritual or mental efforts.[58] Mind-body therapies, including hypnosis, visualization, meditation, and yoga for symptom control, are more realistic and helpful. They are noninvasive and pleasant, and patients can select individual therapies according to their preferences to help manage their own care.

Hypnosis is a state of focused attention or altered consciousness in which distractions are blocked, allowing a person to concentrate on a particular subject, memory, sensation, or problem. It helps people relax and become receptive to suggestion. The suggestion, geared to effect the desired results, may come from patients themselves or from the practitioner. Hypnosis is effective in reducing many symptoms, including acute and chronic pain,[59] panic, phobias, pediatric emergencies, surgery, burns, post-traumatic stress disorder, irritable bowel syndrome, allergies, certain skin conditions, and habit control. Hypnosis is also effective for chemotherapy-related nausea and vomiting in children.[60]

Other techniques, including visualization and progressive relaxation, decrease pain and promote well-being.[61] Guided imagery, which may be considered a lighter form of hypnosis, is based on the reciprocal relationship between mind and body. It is another simple and powerful technique that directs imagination and attention in ways that produce symptom relief. Often termed "visualization" or "mental imagery," guided imagery lowers blood pressure and produces other physiological benefits, including decreased heart rate. Imagery also can relieve pain and anxiety. A study of 96 women with locally advanced breast cancer compared standard treatment with relaxation training and imagery during chemotherapy. Women in the experimental group reported increased relaxation and better quality of life.[61]

Regular meditation decreases stress and generalized anxiety, wards off bouts of chronic depression, and enables people to cope more effectively. In a randomized wait-list control study of 109 cancer patients, participation in a 7-week Mindfulness-Based Stress Reduction Program was associated with significant improvement in mood disturbance and symptoms of stress.[62] A single-arm study of breast and prostate cancer patients showed significant improvement in overall quality of life, stress, and sleep quality with regular meditation.[63] For palliative care patients who are able to try its gentle versions, yoga may be a useful way to relax. A 5000-year-old exercise regimen developed in India, yoga involves proper breathing, movement, and posture. Because its value in improving physical fitness and decreasing respiratory rate and blood pressure is documented, yoga is often part of integrative management for heart disease, asthma, diabetes, drug addiction, acquired immunodeficiency syndrome (AIDS), migraine headaches, arthritis, and cancer. In a randomized, controlled trial of 39 lymphoma patients, Tibetan yoga, which combines physical movement, breath control, and meditation, improved sleep quality.[64]

CONCLUSIONS

An increasing body of evidence supports the use of acupuncture, massage therapy, music, and mind-body interventions for symptom control. These therapies should be considered, particularly when conventional treatment produces unwarranted side effects or fails to bring satisfactory symptom relief. They also may be applied to reduce the amount of opioids or other medications required to maintain comfort. It is important to tailor complementary therapies to the needs and preferences of each patient. Given product quality control issues and potential interactions with prescription medications, physicians should be familiar with supplements commonly used by cancer patients and should refer patients to reliable sources of information.[12] There has been a concerted effort to raise awareness and encourage the use of evidence-based complementary therapies in palliative medicine and supportive oncology (see, for example, http://www.integrativeoncology.org [accessed April 21, 2008]). Complementary therapies provide a sense of patient and family empowerment, reduce troubling symptoms, and improve patient satisfaction.

REFERENCES

1. Cassileth BR, Vickers AJ. High prevalence of complementary and alternative medicine use among cancer patients: Implications for research and clinical care. J Clin Oncol 2005;23:2590-2592.
2. Deng G, Cassileth BR. Integrative oncology: Complementary therapies for pain, anxiety, and mood disturbance. CA Cancer J Clin 2005;55:109-116.
3. Weiger WA, Smith M, Boon H, et al. Advising patients who seek complementary and alternative medical therapies for cancer. Ann Intern Med 2002;137:889-903.
4. Cassileth BR, Lusk EJ, Strouse TB, et al. Contemporary unorthodox treatments in cancer medicine: A study of patients, treatments, and practitioners. Ann Intern Med 1984;101:105-112.
5. Cassileth BR, Zupkis RV, Sutton-Smith K, et al. Information and participation preferences among cancer patients. Ann Intern Med 1980;92:832-836.
6. Ernst E, Cassileth BR. The prevalence of complementary/alternative medicine in cancer: A systematic review. Cancer 1998;83:777-782.
7. Molassiotis A, Fernadez-Ortega P, Pud D, et al. Use of complementary and alternative medicine in cancer patients: A European survey. Ann Oncol 2005;16:655-663.

8. Hyodo I, Amano N, Eguchi K, et al. Nationwide survey on complementary and alternative medicine in cancer patients in Japan. J Clin Oncol 2005;23:2645-2654.

9. Cassileth BR. Sounding boards: After laetrile, what? N Engl J Med 1982;306:1482-1484.

10. Ladas EJ, Jacobson JS, Kennedy DD, et al. Antioxidants and cancer therapy: A systematic review. J Clin Oncol 2004;22:517-528.

11. D'Andrea GM. Use of antioxidants during chemotherapy and radiotherapy should be avoided. CA Cancer J Clin 2005;55:319-321.

12. Memorial Sloan-Kettering Cancer Center. About Herbs, Botanicals & Other Products. Available at http://www.mskcc.org/aboutherbs (accessed January 28, 2008).

13. Green S. A critique of the rationale for cancer treatment with coffee enemas and diet. JAMA 1992;268:3224-3227.

14. Green S. "Antineoplastons." An unproved cancer therapy. JAMA 1992;267:2924-2928.

15. Green S. Stanislaw Burzynski and "Antineoplastons." 2001. Available at http://www.quackwatch.com/01QuackeryRelatedTopics/Cancer/burzynski1.html (accessed January 28, 2008).

16. Loprinzi CL, Levitt R, Barton DL, et al. Evaluation of shark cartilage in patients with advanced cancer. Cancer 2005;104:176-182.

17. U.S. Food and Drug Administration. Safety Alert: PC SPES, SPES (BotanicLab). Available at http://www.fda.gov/medwatch/SAFETY/2002/safety02.htm#spes (accessed January 28, 2008).

18. Deng G, Cassileth BR, Yeung KS. Complementary therapies for cancer-related symptoms. J Support Oncol 2004;2:419-426; discussion 427-429.

19. Ernst E. Acupuncture: A critical analysis. J Intern Med 2006;259:125-137.

20. Sierpina VS, Frenkel MA. Acupuncture: A clinical review. South Med J 2005;98:330-337.

21. Napadow V, Kettner N, Liu J, et al. Hypothalamus and amygdala response to acupuncture stimuli in carpal tunnel syndrome. Pain 2007;130:254-266.

22. Baldry P. Acupuncture, Trigger Points and Musculoskeletal Pain. London: Churchill Livingstone, 1993.

23. Pomeranz B, Chiu D. Naloxone blockade of acupuncture analgesia: Endorphin implicated. Life Sci 1976;19:1757-1762.

24. Pomeranz B, Warma N. Electroacupuncture suppression of a nociceptive reflex is potentiated by two repeated electroacupuncture treatments: The first opioid effect potentiates a second non-opioid effect. Brain Res 1988;452:232-236.

25. Peets JM, Pomeranz B. CXBK mice deficient in opiate receptors show poor electroacupuncture analgesia. Nature 1978;273:675-676.

26. Manheimer E, White A, Berman B, et al. Meta-analysis: Acupuncture for low back pain. Ann Intern Med 2005;142:651-663.

27. Hsieh LL, Kuo CH, Lee LH, et al. Treatment of low back pain by acupressure and physical therapy: Randomised controlled trial. BMJ 2006;332:696-700.

28. Witt C, Brinkhaus B, Jena S, et al. Acupuncture in patients with osteoarthritis of the knee: A randomised trial. Lancet 2005;366:136-143.

29. Kwon YD, Pittler MH, Ernst E. Acupuncture for peripheral joint osteoarthritis: A systematic review and meta-analysis. Rheumatology (Oxford) 2006;45:1331-1337.

30. Manheimer E, Linde K, Lao L, et al. Meta-analysis: Acupuncture for osteoarthritis of the knee. Ann Intern Med 2007;146:868-877.

31. Linde K, Witt CM, Streng A, et al. The impact of patient expectations on outcomes in four randomized controlled trials of acupuncture in patients with chronic pain. Pain 2007;128:264-271.

32. Shen J, Wenger N, Glaspy J, et al. Electroacupuncture for control of myeloablative chemotherapy-induced emesis: A randomized controlled trial. JAMA 2000;284:2755-2761.

33. Ezzo J, Vickers A, Richardson MA, et al. Acupuncture-point stimulation for chemotherapy-induced nausea and vomiting. J Clin Oncol 2005;23:7188-7198.

34. Ezzo JM, Richardson MA, Vickers A, et al. Acupuncture-point stimulation for chemotherapy-induced nausea or vomiting. Cochrane Database Syst Rev 2006;(2):CD002285.

35. Johnstone PA, Niemtzow RC, Riffenburgh RH. Acupuncture for xerostomia: Clinical update. Cancer 2002;94:1151-1156.

36. Filshie J, Bolton T, Browne D, et al. Acupuncture and self acupuncture for long-term treatment of vasomotor symptoms in cancer patients: Audit and treatment algorithm. Acupunct Med 2005;23:171-180.

37. Hofman M, Ryan JL, Figueroa-Moseley CD, et al. Cancer-related fatigue: The scale of the problem. Oncologist 2007;12(Suppl 1):4-10.

38. Martin DP, Sletten CD, Williams BA, Berger IH. Improvement in fibromyalgia symptoms with acupuncture: Results of a randomized controlled trial. Mayo Clin Proc 2006;81:749-757.

39. Guo J. Chronic fatigue syndrome treated by acupuncture and moxibustion in combination with psychological approaches in 310 cases. J Tradit Chin Med 2007;27:92-95.

40. Vickers AJ, Straus DJ, Fearon B, et al. Acupuncture for postchemotherapy fatigue: A phase II study. J Clin Oncol 2004;22:1731-1735.

41. Escalante CP, Grover T, Johnson BA, et al. A fatigue clinic in a comprehensive cancer center: Design and experiences. Cancer 2001;92(6 Suppl):1708-1713.

42. Billhult A, Bergbom I, Stener-Victorin E. Massage relieves nausea in women with breast cancer who are undergoing chemotherapy. J Altern Complement Med 2007;13:53-57.

43. Mehling WE, Jacobs B, Acree M, et al. Symptom management with massage and acupuncture in postoperative cancer patients: A randomized controlled trial. J Pain Symptom Manage 2007;33:258-266.

44. Hernandez-Reif M, Ironson G, Field T, et al. Breast cancer patients have improved immune and neuroendocrine functions following massage therapy. J Psychosom Res 2004;57:45-52.

45. Wilkinson S, Aldridge J, Salmon I, et al. An evaluation of aromatherapy massage in palliative care. Palliat Med 1999;13:409-417.

46. Perlman AI, Sabina A, Williams AL, et al. Massage therapy for osteoarthritis of the knee: A randomized controlled trial. Arch Intern Med 2006;166:2533-2538.

47. Corbin L. Safety and efficacy of massage therapy for patients with cancer. Cancer Control 2005.12:158-164.

48. Soden K, Vincent K, Craske S, et al. A randomized controlled trial of aromatherapy massage in a hospice setting. Palliat Med 2004;18:87-92.

49. Fellowes D, Barnes K, Wilkinson S. Aromatherapy and massage for symptom relief in patients with cancer. Cochrane Database Syst Rev 2004;(2):CD002287.

50. Cassileth BR, Vickers AJ. Massage therapy for symptom control: Outcome study at a major cancer center. J Pain Symptom Manage 2004;28:244-249.

51. National Comprehensive Cancer Network (NCCN). Practice Guidelines in Oncology, vol.1. 2007. Available at http://www.nccn.org/professionals/physician_gls/PDF/pain.pdf (accessed January 28, 2008).

52. Hilliard RE. The effects of music therapy on the quality and length of life of people diagnosed with terminal cancer. J Music Ther 2003;40:113-137.

53. Chlan L, Evans D, Greenleaf M, et al. Effects of a single music therapy intervention on anxiety, discomfort, satisfaction, and compliance with screening guidelines in outpatients undergoing flexible sigmoidoscopy. Gastroenterol Nurs 2000;23:148-156.

54. Zimmerman L, Pozehl B, Duncan K, et al. Effects of music in patients who had chronic cancer pain. West J Nurs Res 1989;11:298-309.

55. Gallagher LM, Lagman R, Walsh D, et al. The clinical effects of music therapy in palliative medicine. Support Care Cancer 2006;14:859-866.

56. Hanser SB, Thompson LW. Effects of a music therapy strategy on depressed older adults. J Gerontol 1994;49:P265-P269.

57. Cassileth BR, Vickers AJ, Magill LA. Music therapy for mood disturbance during hospitalization for autologous stem cell transplantation: A randomized controlled trial. Cancer 2003;98:2723-2729.

58. Cassileth BR. The social implications of mind-body cancer research. Cancer Invest 1989;7:361-364.

59. Sellick SM, Zaza C. Critical review of 5 nonpharmacologic strategies for managing cancer pain. Cancer Prev Control 1998;2:7-14.

60. Zeltzer LK, Dolgin MJ, LeBaron S, et al. A randomized, controlled study of behavioral intervention for chemotherapy distress in children with cancer. Pediatrics 1991;88:34-42.

61. Walker LG, Walker MB, Ogston K, et al. Psychological, clinical and pathological effects of relaxation training and guided imagery during primary chemotherapy. Br J Cancer 1999;80:262-268.

62. Speca M, Carlson LE, Goodey E, et al. A randomized, wait-list controlled clinical trial: The effect of a mindfulness meditation-based stress reduction program on mood and symptoms of stress in cancer outpatients. Psychosom Med 2000;62:613-622.

63. Carlson LE, Speca M, Patel KD, et al. Mindfulness-based stress reduction in relation to quality of life, mood, symptoms of stress and levels of cortisol, dehydroepiandrosterone sulfate (DHEAS) and melatonin in breast and prostate cancer outpatients. Psychoneuroendocrinology 2004;29:448-474.

64. Cohen L, Warneke C, Fouladi RT, et al. Psychological adjustment and sleep quality in a randomized trial of the effects of a Tibetan yoga intervention in patients with lymphoma. Cancer 2004;100:2253-2260.

PART IV

Palliative Care and General Medicine

Complex Illnesses

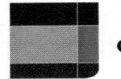

CHAPTER **183**

Organ Transplantation

Michael Herman and **Andrew P. Keaveny**

KEY POINTS

- Solid organ transplantation is a multidisciplinary effort that effectively treats organ failure.
- Transplantation demand far exceeds the available organ supply, and there are ongoing efforts to expand the donor pool.
- Careful patient selection is required; education is key.
- Long-term outcomes after transplantation will be improved by the appropriate use of immunosuppression and improved treatment of recurrent disease.
- The transplant team has an important role in the end-of-life care of transplantation candidates and recipients.

Since the first successful kidney transplantation in 1954, few areas in medicine have generated such public fascination and challenging medical, social, and ethical demands as solid organ transplantation (SOT). Replacement of a failing organ is both a dramatic medical intervention and a life-changing procedure. SOT now encompasses heart, lung, liver, kidney, pancreas, and small bowel transplants. For all these organs, successful transplantation can prolong and improve quality of life. Over the past 2 decades, advances in both surgical and medical management have improved both early and long-term results of SOT. This has produced a demand for SOT that far exceeds organ availability. Careful patient selection, organ selection and allocation, and medical care before and after surgery ensure optimal outcomes for organs used and for transplant recipients. Some patients die while awaiting SOT. Furthermore, if failure of the transplanted organ occurs, retransplantation may not be feasible. Transplantation and palliative medicine may appear to be at opposite ends of the medical spectrum, but they share important principles: a focus on the patient as a whole, including not only assessment of the physical complications of disease but also a thorough evaluation of individual psychological and social circumstances and an ongoing commitment to the patient by the professional team, who work with caregivers in support and follow-up.

EPIDEMIOLOGY AND DONOR ISSUES

There has been incremental growth in SOT over the last 30 years, with organs from both deceased and living donors being used (Fig. 183-1). In the United States, approximately 60,000 patients are currently listed for kidney transplantation, 17,000 for liver, and 3000 each for heart and lung.[1] In contrast, in 2005, just over 16,000 kidney, 6400 liver, 2000 heart, and 1400 lung transplantation procedures were performed. In 2005, the U.S. organization that coordinates transplantation, the United Network for Organ Sharing (UNOS), reported that approximately 6300 individuals were removed from the transplant waiting list because they had died, and another 1800 were too sick to undergo the procedure.[1]

Societal norms determine the acceptability of transplanting organs from deceased individuals, either after brain death or after cardiac death. In certain countries, living donor transplantation is the only realistic organ donation method, greatly limiting the potential for transplantation of organs other than liver and kidney. Surgical advances have permitted successful transplantation of lung, pancreas, and intestine from living donors.[2] Even where deceased organ donation is practiced, because of the limited supply, use of living donors may be the only means to achieve timely kidney or liver transplantation. Careful evaluation of all potential deceased donors is now undertaken, including those previously considered unsuitable, such as older donors or those with medical co-morbidities. Organs from such "extended-criteria donors" may, with careful organ and recipient matching, provide a vital SOT resource. In Europe and the United States, there is increasing emphasis on procuring organs from individuals whose heart has stopped ("donation after cardiac death"), in addition to the classic situation in which the donor is declared dead by neurological criteria.[3-6] Protocols have been developed by transplant centers to retrieve organs in such situations, thus expanding the potential pool of transplantable organs.[7]

Because live donor organs are a significant component of SOT today, with more than 6500 kidney and 323 liver transplants from living donors performed in the United States in 2005, the physical and psychosocial welfare of these donors must be carefully considered.[2,6,8,9] Critical elements in the donation process include informed consent, mechanisms to ensure that the decision to donate is voluntary, and a thorough donor evaluation. The aggregate benefits of live donation (survival, quality of life, psychological and social well-being) should outweigh the risks to the donor-recipient pair (death, medical and psychological morbidity, financial loss).[2]

In all organ donation and retrieval, a high level of regulatory oversight is desirable, for transparency, equity, and

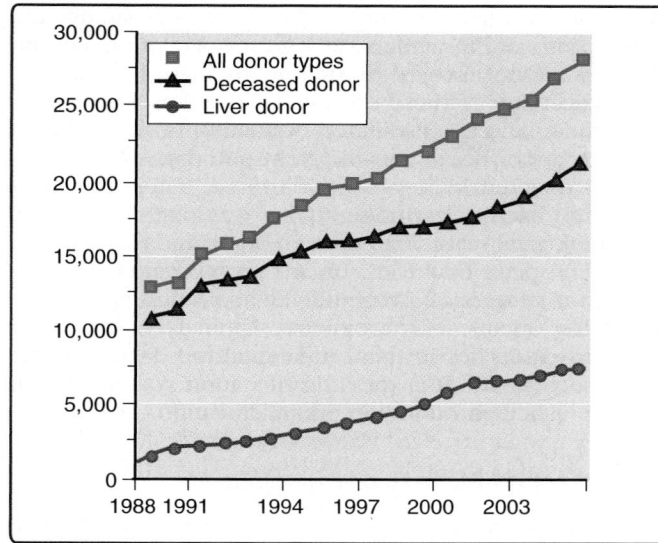

FIGURE 183-1 Growth of both deceased and living donor transplantation in the United States since 1988. *(From National Organ Procurement and Transplantation Network [OPTN] data as of January 1, 2006. Available at http://www.optn.org/data [accessed January 28, 2008].)*

TABLE 183-1 Issues of Concern during the Evaluation of Potential Recipients for Transplantation

RECIPIENT ISSUES	IMPACT ON TRANSPLANT CANDIDACY
Recipient age	Varies with organ being considered
Preexisting history of malignancy	Usually a contraindication within 2-5 yr after diagnosis and treatment, except for cutaneous nonmelanoma skin cancers
Systemic infection	Active infection usually contraindicates SOT, until treated appropriately
Untreatable advanced other organ disease, including significant organic brain disease	Contraindication for single-organ transplantation, unless multiorgan transplantation is available
Untreatable psychiatric disease, limited social support	Contraindication for SOT, because compliance and support are critical
Human immunodeficiency virus infection	Many centers no longer consider this a contraindication, if adequately controlled with antiretroviral therapy
Active alcohol or substance abuse	Contraindication; after appropriate intervention, candidacy may be reconsidered
Demonstrated inability to comply with a complex medical regimen	Contraindication; compliance and support are critical after SOT

SOT, solid organ transplantation

living donor safety. Transplantation is highly regulated within developed nations, but this does not prevent organ sharing across countries through networks such as Eurotransplant. Transparency avoids concerns about preferential treatment. An equitable system balances the tension between limited organ availability and excessive demand. Medical organizations and patient advocacy groups in Europe and the United States have collaborated with government legislators to develop organ allocation systems that reflect these aspirations. There are growing concerns about illicit trade in live organs. It is impossible to quantify this worldwide black market, but, as in many other areas of SOT, the medical community is a key factor in how nations deal with this challenge.[10,11]

RECIPIENT EVALUATION

The purpose of recipient evaluation is to determine whether someone with organ dysfunction is a suitable SOT recipient. Essential components include native organ function, exclusion of contraindications for the procedure, and education of the patient and caregivers about transplantation. A multidisciplinary team must address the complex issues ranging from disease-specific problems, co-morbid conditions, psychosocial concerns, surgical risks, and personal support (Table 183-1). Variations exist according to the candidate organs and among transplant centers regarding the emphasis placed on these issues. A unique component of the evaluation is education; specific instruction regarding the impact of transplantation on the patient lays the groundwork for postoperative care.

Once the evaluation is completed, potential recipients are presented to a multidisciplinary selection committee, where their candidacies are reviewed, management options are considered, and a decision is made regarding their suitability for transplantation now or in the future. Tools are available, such as the Model for End-Stage Liver Disease (MELD) score (a mathematical model comprising measurements of serum bilirubin, creatinine, and international normalized ratio), that can help determine optimal transplantation timing based on organ function and risk of short-term mortality.[12,13] After the candidate recipient is accepted and placed on a waiting list for SOT, regular follow-up by the transplant team is required to manage organ failure and ensure that those awaiting SOT remain suitable recipients. The option of living donation may then be explored to expedite transplantation. Coordinators in both the pretransplantation and post-transplantation settings play key roles. Unique relationships often develop and provide support during the difficult waiting period before transplantation and after surgery. The bedrock of a good transplantation program is an effective community of care, encompassing physicians, nurses, and social workers (Table 183-2).

ORGAN ALLOCATION

The principal considerations in organ allocation are justice and utility. Organs should be made available to recipients equitably, with appropriate utilization of a scarce resource. The processes by which organs are allocated vary by country and by organ in response to these concerns. There has been a significant evolution from individual surgeons' making all decisions to government-regulated nationalized allocation systems. Various levels of autonomy are assigned to transplantation centers to utilize available organs, depending on the organ offered and national policies. Complex cross-border organ-sharing networks allow the most efficient use of organs. Another factor that

TABLE 183-2 Indications for Transplantation (Main Diagnosis Categories)

ORGAN	MAJOR DISEASE CATEGORIES
Heart	Coronary artery disease Cardiomyopathy: dilated, restrictive, hypertrophic Valvular heart disease Congenital heart disease
Lung	Congenital disease, including Eisenmenger's syndrome Emphysema, chronic obstructive airways disease Cystic fibrosis Idiopathic pulmonary fibrosis Primary pulmonary hypertension α_1-Antitrypsin deficiency
Liver	Chronic hepatitis B or C infection Alcohol-related liver disease Cryptogenic cirrhosis, including NASH Cholestatic liver disease Hepatocellular carcinoma Metabolic diseases Acute liver failure
Kidney	Glomerular diseases DM Polycystic kidney disease Hypertensive nephrosclerosis Tubular and interstitial diseases Congenital, metabolic diseases
Pancreas	DM DM secondary to chronic pancreatitis, cystic fibrosis Pancreatic insufficiency secondary to cancer
Small bowel	Intestinal failure where TPN can no longer be maintained Life-threatening abdominal pathology

DM, diabetes mellitus; NASH, nonalcoholic steatohepatitis; TPN, total parenteral nutrition.
From United Network for Organ Sharing (UNOS). Available at http://www.optn.org/organDataSource (accessed January 28, 2008).

affects allocation is the ability to maintain viability of the donor organ before it is implanted in the recipient. The time from flushing and cooling of the organ in the donor (with an ice-cold preservative solution) to subsequent implantation, termed the "cold ischemia time," varies from only 4 hours for a heart to up to 24 hours for a kidney.

Rules governing waiting-list prioritization reflect each society's response to organ allocation. The U.S. Department of Health and Human Services established guidelines that emphasized standard medical criteria for patient waiting lists; medical urgency and waiting time were to be considered, with medical judgment the final determinant as to how organs should best be used. This led to the MELD scoring system, by which potential recipients were prioritized for liver transplantation. The MELD score accurately predicts short-term mortality in end-stage liver disease.[12,14] It replaced the prior system, which emphasized waiting-list time, a parameter that does not correlate with mortality while awaiting liver transplantation.

The MELD score became the first national organ allocation system to use objective data, rather than subjective criteria or SOT waiting time spent. Lung allocation in the United States is now also based on medical urgency before transplantation and the probability of success afterward. It comprises laboratory values, test results, and disease diagnosis. Neither liver nor lung allocation systems consider quality of life while awaiting transplantation; certain diseases are not favored by such mathematical modeling. The objectivity of these scoring systems has led to their acceptance and has facilitated evaluation of their impact on both donor organ and recipient outcomes. For allocation of donated kidneys in the United States, the most important factors continue to be waiting-list time and immunological matching between organ and recipient. In many European countries, organs are allocated to transplantation centers, allowing individual physicians to match particular organs with recipients. Ultimately, the art of transplantation lies in these individualized decisions; the tools, such as MELD or the lung allocation system, should further justice and utility in organ allocation.

THE TRANSPLANTATION PROCEDURE

The surgical procedure and anesthetic management for all SOT procedures has evolved to minimize morbidity and mortality. Depending on the procedure and the condition of the recipient, he or she may be transferred to a regular hospital floor immediately after surgery or may require intensive care with maximum cardiopulmonary support and hemodialysis. Advances in critical care have allowed SOT for desperately ill people with a reasonable expectation of meaningful recovery. The resources used can be formidable. Living donation is typically an elective procedure, allowing optimization of the recipient's condition before transplantation. A key component of SOT recovery is education regarding the specific medications prescribed and instructions on wound care, diet, and lifestyle. A holistic approach is essential; for example, women of childbearing age require counseling about contraception. Effective patient education greatly increases compliance and, ultimately, transplantation success.

IMMUNOSUPPRESSION

Advances in immunosuppression have been essential to SOT success. Better understanding of basic immunology, appropriate donor and recipient matching, and clinical studies of immunosuppression protocols have improved organ and recipient survival. Tolerance is defined as failure of the immune system to respond to an antigen; prevention and treatment of rejection involves relatively nonspecific immune system suppression. Because all immunosuppressive drugs have significant side effects, it is essential to tailor therapy to the individual patient. Noncompliance with medications is associated with rejection and organ failure. Tests of immune cell function are now available; in the future, functional immune assays, novel drugs, and pharmacogenetics will form the basis for immunosuppressive management. Achieving tolerance, avoiding the need for immunosuppression altogether, is an area of ongoing basic and clinical research.

Cyclosporine, a calcineurin inhibitor (CNI), brought into clinical practice in the 1980s, transformed immunosuppressive therapy (Table 183-3). Immunosuppressive drugs may be started before, during, or after the transplantation procedure. Although each solid organ has unique issues that affect the degree of immunosuppression required and the agents used, there are important recur-

TABLE 183-3	Currently Available Immunosuppressant Medications		
CLASS	**MECHANISM OF ACTION**	**COMMON SIDE EFFECTS**	**COMMON DRUG-DRUG INTERACTIONS**

Calcineurin inhibitors
  Cyclosporine
  Tacrolimus
	Inhibition of cytokine production from T cells	Renal dysfunction
		Dyslipidemia
		Hypertension
		Hirsutism
		Hyperkalemia
		Gingival hyperplasia
			Calcium channel blockers
			Antifungal agents
			Antibiotics
			Anticonvulsants
			St. John's wort

Corticosteroids	Inhibition of cytokine production from T cells and antigen-presenting cells	Hypertension Mental status changes Dyslipidemia Impaired wound healing Hyperglycemia Cushing's syndrome Myopathy Osteoporosis Fluid retention Cataracts	Phenytoin Barbiturates Carbamazepine Rifampicin Oral contraceptives

Antimetabolites
  Azathioprine
  Mycophenolate mofetil
	Antagonizes purine metabolism and/or synthesis	Nausea, vomiting, diarrhea
		Anemia
		Leukopenia
		Weight loss
		Thrombocytopenia
		Pancreatitis
			Allopurinol
			ACE inhibitors
			Methotrexate
			Tacrolimus
			Probenecid
			Antacids

Antibody induction
  Antithymocyte globulin
  Monoclonal anti–T cell antibodies (OKT-3)
  IL2 receptor antibodies (basiliximab, daclizumab)
  Alemtuzumab
	Depletes and/or modulates T-cell function	Cytokine-release syndrome
		Abdominal pain
		Leukopenia
		Thrombocytopenia
		Dyspnea
		Hypertension
		Sepsis
			—

Sirolimus	Blocks T- and B-cell activation by cytokines	Anemia Dyslipidemia Leukopenia Interstitial lung disease Thrombocytopenia Peripheral edema Impaired wound healing	Calcium channel blockers Antifungal agents Macrolide antibiotics Prokinetic agents Anticonvulsants St. John's wort

ACE, angiotensin-converting enzyme; IL2, interleukin-2.

ring management themes. Induction of immunosuppression usually involves administration of an antibody to delay the introduction of maintenance therapy and/or to help facilitate removal of an immunosuppressive agent. Recent efforts in kidney and liver transplantation have evaluated steroid minimization or steroid-free protocols. Maintenance regimens usually comprise a calcineurin inhibitor, possibly with a corticosteroid or an antimetabolite or both. Frequent monitoring of immunosuppression levels and various laboratory parameters minimizes drug toxicity. Calcineurin inhibitor–related nephrotoxicity is a concern for all cases of SOT.[15] "Renal-sparing" protocols have been developed, often including sirolimus. Many immunosuppressive agents are expensive, and lifelong monitoring adds to both direct and indirect transplantation costs.

EARLY AND LONG-TERM COMPLICATIONS

There are numerous early and long-term complications of SOT. Early complications are associated with technical surgical issues, or with the transplanted organ, or both. The first 3 months after transplantation is the highest-risk period for acute rejection, which can usually be treated successfully with appropriate changes in immunosuppressives. Bacterial, fungal, and viral infections cause significant morbidity and mortality within the first 12 months after surgery. Recurrent viral disease (hepatitis C infection of the liver, polyomavirus infection of the kidney) can cause post-transplantation organ failure. In every SOT, chronic rejection may occur. Cancer after transplantation is a particular concern: nonmelanoma skin cancer is prevalent, and there is a higher incidence of both solid organ cancers and lymphoma. Other complications include cardiovascular disease, which is the most common cause of patient death in those with a functioning kidney transplant.[16]

Monitoring of the transplanted organ includes blood tests, imaging studies, and organ biopsies, both scheduled and when changes are noted. Organ dysfunction usually necessitates adjustments in immunosuppressives and management of the complications of organ failure. Except in kidney transplantation (after which dialysis can be resumed), management options are often limited in a failed SOT. Retransplantation may be possible in some cases, but it is controversial because of the overall

Future Considerations

- Definition of optimal immunosuppressive regimens to minimize long-term complications
- Transplantation for quality of life, rather than to increase life expectancy
- Retransplantation—indications and appropriateness
- Definition and use of extended-criteria donor organs
- Optimization of organ allocation considering justice and utility
- Oversight, reimbursement, and follow-up of living donors

shortage of donor organs and worse results for retransplantation.

TRANSPLANTATION AND PALLIATIVE CARE

Although significant advances have been made in treating solid organ failure with transplantation, many patients die while awaiting SOT. The condition of those originally accepted for transplantation may deteriorate to such an extent that transplantation is no longer realistic. Organ failure after SOT is often associated with a poor prognosis. Therefore, it is important to promote advance care planning, address end-of-life issues, and identify health care proxies in the evaluation process.[17] The relationship between the transplant team, the patient, and his or her family can provide both practical and emotional support throughout the course. In terminal illness, the transplant team should ideally provide disease-specific expertise and patient knowledge that will complement the work of the palliative care services (see "Future Considerations").

REFERENCES

1. United Network for Organ Sharing (UNOS). Waiting list candidates. Available at http://www.optn.org/data (accessed January 28, 2008).
2. Pruett TL, Tibell A, Alabdulkareem A, et al. The ethics statement of the Vancouver Forum on the live lung, liver, pancreas, and intestine donor. Transplantation 2006;81:1386-1387.
3. Delmonico FL, Sheehy E, Marks WH, et al. Organ donation and utilization in the United States, 2004. Am J Transplant 2005;5:862-873.
4. Sanchez-Fructuoso AI, Marques M, Prats D, et al. Victims of cardiac arrest occurring outside the hospital: A source of transplantable kidneys. Ann Intern Med 2006;145:157-164.
5. Childress JF. How can we ethically increase the supply of transplantable organs? Ann Intern Med 2006;145:224-225.
6. Childress JF, Liverman CT (eds): Organ Donation: Opportunities for Action. Washington, DC: National Academy Press, 2006.
7. Bernat JL, D'Alessandro AM, Port FK, et al. Report of a National Conference on Donation after Cardiac Death. Am J Transplant 2006;6:281-291.
8. The consensus statement of the Amsterdam Forum on the Care of the Live Kidney Donor. Transplantation 2004;78:491-492.
9. Barr ML, Belghiti J, Villamil FG, et al. A report of the Vancouver Forum on the care of the live organ donor: Lung, liver, pancreas, and intestine data and medical guidelines. Transplantation 2006;81:1373-1385.
10. Delmonico FL. Commentary: The WHO resolution on human organ and tissue transplantation. Transplantation 2005;79:639-640.
11. Rothman SM, Rothman DJ. The hidden cost of organ sale. Am J Transplant 2006;6:1524-1528.
12. Kamath PS, Wiesner RH, Malinchoc M, et al. A model to predict survival in patients with end-stage liver disease. Hepatology 2001;33:464-470.
13. Wiesner R, Edwards E, Freeman R, et al. Model for end-stage liver disease (MELD) and allocation of donor livers. Gastroenterology 2003;124:91-96.
14. Wiesner RH, McDiarmid SV, Kamath PS, et al. MELD and PELD: Application of survival models to liver allocation. Liver Transpl 2001;7:567-580.
15. Ojo AO, Held PJ, Port FK, et al. Chronic renal failure after transplantation of a nonrenal organ. N Engl J Med 2003;349:931-940.
16. Pascual M, Theruvath T, Kawai T, et al. Strategies to improve long-term outcomes after renal transplantation. N Engl J Med 2002;346:580-590.
17. Larson AM, Curtis JR. Integrating palliative care for liver transplant candidates: "Too well for transplant, too sick for life." JAMA 2006;295:2168-2176.

CHAPTER 184

Cardiovascular Disorders

Rodney O. Tucker

KEY POINTS

- The diagnosis of advanced heart failure is a mechanical and neurohormonal syndrome with several underlying causes, including ischemic disease, valvular abnormalities, and pulmonary arterial disease.
- Cardiovascular disorders, with advanced heart failure as the leading diagnosis, constitute one of the largest categories of chronic illness in older adults.
- Advanced heart failure has a high mortality rate and is responsible for a significant portion of medical expenditures in the United States.
- Principles of palliative care include comprehensive symptom management, determination of goals of care, and advance care planning, which should be incorporated into the treatment plans for patients with cardiovascular disorders.
- Supportive and palliative care and hospice programs can provide additional support for patients and caregivers as the disease progresses.

Cardiovascular disorders describe a group of illnesses that affect the cardiopulmonary circuit and the vascular system. They include ischemic cardiomyopathy, congenital and valvular heart disease, pulmonary arterial hypertension, and diseases of the vasculature such as large-vessel and peripheral artery disease. In advanced stages, each can cause chronic heart failure (see Chapter 3). The term *advanced heart failure* describes symptoms that have progressed to New York Heart Association (NYHA) class IV or American Heart Association/American College of Cardiology (AHA/ACC) stage D.[1]

Diseases of the cardiovascular system, especially advanced heart failure, are leading causes of chronic illness and morbidity (see Chapter 79). Heart failure is responsible for most hospital admissions among the elderly population, is one of the most costly of illnesses for the U.S. Medicare system, and has a 1-year mortality rate approaching 45%.[2] Advanced cardiovascular disease is the leading noncancer diagnosis for patients admitted to hospices nationwide.[3] This underscores the importance of palliative care principles applied to patients with advanced cardiovascular disorders.

BASIC SCIENCE

Heart failure has many causes. However the advanced stage of each appears similar and shares aspects of clinical symptoms, treatment, and supportive care with the others (see Chapter 42).

Ischemic cardiomyopathy is the most common advanced cardiovascular disorder. The term usually refers to a progressive condition for which the primary cause is severe coronary artery disease with repeated or prolonged cardiac ischemia. This condition can lead to myocardial infarction, with loss of functioning cardiac muscle, scarring, and subsequent cascade of manifestations that lead to heart failure (see Chapter 72).

Valvular disease can affect any of the four valves of the heart; the most commonly affected are the mitral and aortic valves. Causes of valvular disease include congenital malformations, rheumatic fever, ischemic disease, endocarditis, calcification, and rare cases of infiltrative diseases such as systemic lupus erythematosus, and carcinoid syndrome. The underlying cause of valvular disease determines the clinical manifestations, treatment, and prognosis, although all causes can proceed to an advanced state, causing heart failure.

Pulmonary arterial hypertension has many potential causes (Table 184-1), including primary pulmonary hypertension, for which there may not be an obvious cause (see Chapter 73). The precise mechanism of primary pulmonary hypertension is unknown but likely includes problems with endothelial dysfunction, pulmonary vasoconstriction due to ion channel changes, or recurrent thrombosis in vessels. Secondary causes include conditions that lead to hypoxic vasoconstriction, including emphysema, sleep apnea, decreased vascular bed area from infiltrative diseases, chronic pulmonary embolism, or conditions leading to chronic volume or pressure overload on the heart, as occurs before congestive heart failure. Independent of the cause, right-sided heart failure can result. This more commonly occurs with valvular lesions such as mitral stenosis. Treatments for pulmonary arterial hypertension are different from those for other causes of heart failure, but the patient's symptoms are very similar in all cases.

EPIDEMIOLOGY AND PREVALENCE

More than 5 million Americans are estimated to have heart failure, with about 555,000 new cases occurring each year. The incidence approaches 10 cases per 1000 people in the general population who are 65 years or older.[4] Many series reveal that patients with advanced heart failure are increasing in terms of hospital admissions, and it is one of the leading costs for the Medicare system.[5] Heart failure disproportionately affects people older than 75 years (Fig. 184-1). In comparison, the prevalence of primary pulmonary hypertension in the general population is about 300 new cases per year according to the National Heart, Lung, and Blood Institute statistics, which is 2 cases per 1 million individuals in the general U.S. population.[6]

PATHOPHYSIOLOGY

The mechanical and neurohormonal aspects of advanced heart failure determine its clinical manifestations, symptoms, and subsequent treatment. The mechanical framework refers to the discordant relationships between pressures and blood flow in the heart and throughout the rest of the body. Whether the underlying dysfunction is abnormal filling pressure of the heart on the right or left side (e.g., valvular disease) or inadequacy of the heart muscle to pump the cardiac volume out of the heart (e.g., ischemic disease), the primary symptoms are the same.

Other changes occur under the direction of a complex neurohormonal axis, which can explain the variability in progression and severity of heart failure. The primary theory is that mechanical and volume changes may precipitate secretion of various substances and neurohormones (e.g., cytokines) that affect other organ systems, influence cardiac remodeling, and may accelerate progression of heart failure. This understanding has helped to develop new treatment modalities for heart failure.

The pathophysiology of pulmonary arterial hypertension partially depends on the many underlying causes (see Table 184-1). The main hemodynamic change in primary pulmonary hypertension is an increased resistance to blood flow in the pulmonary circuit. Progressive increases in pulmonary artery pressures with preserved cardiac output initially are replaced by reductions in cardiac output as the disease progresses. Eventually, increased

TABLE 184-1 Common Causes of Pulmonary Arterial Hypertension
Idiopathic primary hypertension
Valvular heart disease (i.e., mitral stenosis)
Pulmonary thromboembolic disease
Obstructive lung disease
Interstitial lung disease
Primary myocardial disease
Collagen vascular disease
Intravenous drug abuse
Granulomatous lung disease
Pulmonary artery stenosis
Congenital heart disease and persistent fetal circulation
Persistent or chronic arterial hypoxemia
Pulmonary venous hypertension
Sickle cell anemia

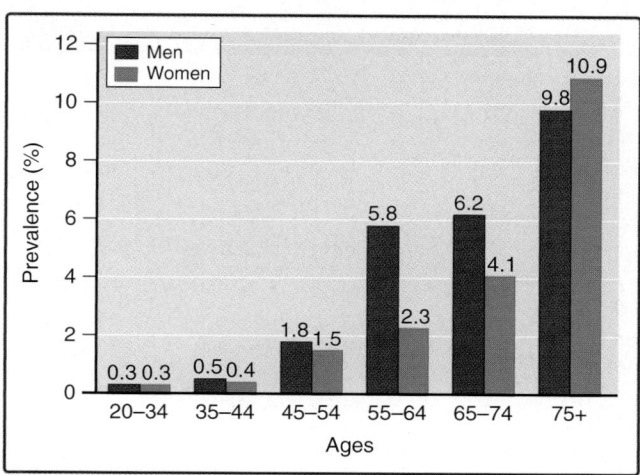

FIGURE 184-1 Prevalence of heart failure by age for men and women. *(Data from Centers for Disease Control and Prevention [CDC] and National Heart, Lung, and Blood Institute [NHLBI].)*

right heart pressure results in systemic manifestations and hypoxemia and in a restrictive pulmonary function pattern.

CLINICAL MANIFESTATIONS

Although the age of onset and severity of symptoms vary for each entity, the symptoms of advanced disease overlap (Table 184-2). There are various classification schemes for each of the disease states, such as valvular disease and pulmonary arterial hypertension. The NYHA definition of advanced heart failure is based on symptoms; patients with stage IV disease have heart failure symptoms at rest. This classification remains one of the most widely used and the most pertinent for palliative medicine and hospice care.

The clinical severity of symptoms and progression depend on the primary cause of the heart failure and response to treatment. In patients with pulmonary arterial hypertension, clinical manifestations may be negligible in the early stages, whereas someone with ischemic cardiovascular disease and a first episode of heart failure can be quite symptomatic[7] (Fig. 184-2).

On initial manifestation of ischemic disease, an individual may undergo interventional therapies (e.g., angioplasty, stents, surgery), followed by disease- and risk-modifying strategies that may provide many years of symptom-free living. With most valvular disorders, patients may be symptom free for a long time but become more symptomatic as the valvular stenosis or insufficiency worsens. Each disorder leading to heart failure can be marked by periods of variable clinical symptoms, but the overall natural course is progression of disease with time, and heart failure is likely to be the terminal diagnosis.[8]

In summary, ischemic cardiac disease, valvular disease, and pulmonary hypertension have diagnostic classes or stages. The illness trajectory depends on therapeutic responses to disease-modifying treatments.

TREATMENT

For patients with ischemic heart disease, prevention of coronary atherosclerosis is crucial to avoid myocardial ischemia and heart failure. Control of risk factors such as hypertension, diabetes, and elevated levels of low-density lipoprotein cholesterol and lifestyle modification such as weight management, smoking cessation, and regular exercise are important parts of the treatment plan. Medications such as antihypertensive drugs, lipid-lowering agents, and aspirin are commonly used. After arterial disease is diagnosed, agents such as nitrates, β-blockers, and anticoagulants may be added to the regimen. Diagnostic studies are indicated at various points in the disease trajectory if there are symptoms indicating progression. If there is evidence of progressive coronary atherosclerosis, the patient should be re-educated about risk factors and lifestyle modifications, and additional therapies should be considered.

For patients with valvular heart defects, education regarding the defect and possible symptoms and prognosis should be undertaken. Cardiac risk stratification, lifestyle modifications, and treatment of co-morbidities may be a part of management. Depending on the type and state of the valvular defect, medical regimens may include prophylaxis for endocarditis and anticoagulation. Patients should have regular follow-up examinations and periodic cardiac imaging as indicated, with re-education and treatment plan modifications in the event of disease progression.

Pulmonary arterial hypertension is a complex disease state that is progressive and that has no known cure. There has been active research into the causes and potential treatments of pulmonary hypertension, and the latest recommendations for treatment are summarized in evidence-based guidelines.[9] In general, lifestyle modification

TABLE 184-2 Common Symptoms of Patients with Advanced Cardiovascular Disorders
Shortness of breath
Lower extremity swelling
Fatigue
Cough and congestion
Dry mouth
Decreased mobility
Angina (especially in ischemic cardiovascular disease)
Noncardiac pain
Difficulty sleeping
Anxiety and depression
Loss of appetite
Loss of libido
Hemoptysis (especially in mitral stenosis)
Syncope (especially in valvular disease)
Palpitations
Confusion
Disordered breathing

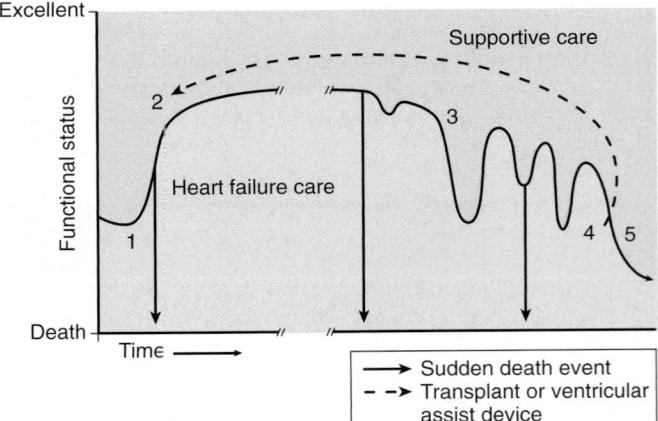

FIGURE 184-2 Schematic course of stage C and D heart failure (HF). Initial symptoms (1) of HF develop, and treatment is initiated. Plateaus of various lengths (2) may be reached with initial medical management or after mechanical support or heart transplantation. Functional status (3) declines, as evidenced by various slopes, with intermittent exacerbations of HF that respond to rescue efforts. A patient with state D HF (4) has refractory symptoms and limited function. End of life (5) may occur as sudden death at any point along the course of illness. (*Adapted from Goodlin SJ, Hauptman PJ, Arnold R, et al. Consensus statement: Palliative and supportive care in advanced heart failure. J Card Fail 2004;10:200-209.*)

that promotes overall cardiovascular conditioning without abruptly increasing the work of the heart during exertion is recommended. Loop diuretics, supplemental oxygen to maintain an oxygen saturation level more than 90%, and anticoagulation are among the mainstream treatments for pulmonary arterial hypertension. Specific treatment regimens include calcium channel blockers and single agents or combinations of medications such as prostanoids (e.g., prostacyclin), endothelin receptor antagonists (e.g., bosentan), and phosphodiesterase-5 inhibitors (e.g., sildenafil). Each has potential side effects but works differently, with the overall goal of improved oxygenation and increased functional status with fewer symptoms.[10] The role of cardiac glycosides remains unclear[11] (Table 184-3).

Advanced heart failure can be the end-stage manifestation of any of these cardiovascular disorders. Discussion of the natural history and illness trajectory with the patient should be part of the treatment plan from the time of diagnosis, with re-evaluation and re-education at various points in the disease course, depending on pivotal events. These sentinel events may include myocardial infarctions, surgery, addition of new medications, cardiovascular co-morbidities such as a cerebrovascular accident, or kidney dysfunction. Information and education about dietary restrictions, exercise, over-the-counter medication interactions, and daily weights should be included routinely for patients with heart failure at every stage.

As disease progresses, angiotensin-converting enzyme inhibitors, angiotensin receptor blockers, β-blockers, and diuretics should be incorporated. Later, inotropic therapy or vasodilators in hospitalized patients may be necessary. Electrical and mechanical devices such as pacemakers, implantable cardioverter defibrillators, and ventricular-assist devices may be part of treatment.[12]

Drugs of Choice and Evidence-Based Medicine

A periodic review of the latest information is suggested for selecting medications for each entity depending on the state or class of illness, patient preference, intolerances, potential interactions, and co-morbid conditions (see Chapter 141). The evidence base for each disease changes continually.

Supportive Care

Supportive care in advanced cardiovascular disorders takes on various meanings and emphasis, depending on the stage of the illness, acuity of the patients, and caregivers' symptom burden. Supportive care for cardiovascular illness emphasizes the educational component early in a disease course that changes over time. Patients with cardiovascular disorders usually progressively decline over many years, during which they undergo complex treatment regimens and multiple procedures. Multidrug regimens can cause psychosocial and spiritual suffering in patients as their disease progresses. Co-morbid conditions such as undertreated pain syndromes, fatigue, and depression add to the symptom burden. These symptoms may be outside the treatment range of cardiologists, who are the principal physicians involved. For example, depression is associated with a poorer prognosis and with higher rehospitalization rates for patients with nonischemic heart failure.[13] A collaborative team of primary care physicians, cardiologists, specialty care cardiac nurses, palliative care practitioners, social workers, psychologists, and complementary therapists can provide comprehensive care for patients with advancing disease.

As cardiovascular diseases progress, patients' symptom management needs and guidance through the complexities of decision making and the health care system grow. The roles of the palliative care team and hospice become more important in assisting patients and families determine their goals of care and participate in advance care planning. More patients with advanced heart failure in the United States are using hospice, a trend that is expected to continue.[3]

RESEARCH OPPORTUNITIES

More information is needed about the costs of long-term, complex medical regimens and organ transplantation. Considering the increasing demand and limited availability of organs, better guidelines are needed for comprehensive care for patients with advanced disease. Concerns about the costs and the level of care involved with the increasing use of device therapies for patients with end-stage heart failure should be considered in formulating these guidelines.

TABLE 184-3 Management Highlights		
ISCHEMIC HEART DISEASE	**VALVULAR HEART DISEASE**	**PULMONARY HYPERTENSION**
Education about risk factors	Education about the nature of the valvular defect, prognosis, and potential symptoms	Education about the nature of the illness and risk factors
Lifestyle modification	Lifestyle modification when appropriate	Lifestyle modification
Cholesterol monitoring and management	Reduction of other cardiac risk factors	Reduction of other cardiac risk factors
Blood pressure monitoring and management	Blood pressure monitoring and management	Treatment of other heart conditions, hypoxia
Diagnostic studies when appropriate	Endocarditis prophylaxis when appropriate	Periodic cardiopulmonary diagnostic studies and O_2 monitoring
Selected medications according to risk factors and state of disease	Periodic cardiac imaging according to the physician's recommendations	Selected medications according to the symptoms and state of disease
Re-education for disease progression	Selected medications according to the symptoms and state of defect	Re-education for disease progression
Discussion of long-term disease trajectory and advance planning	Re-education for progression of disease	Discussion of long-term disease trajectory and advance planning
	Discussion of long-term disease trajectory and advance planning	

REFERENCES

1. Hunt SA, Baker DW, Chin MH, et al. American College of Cardiology/American Heart Association (ACC/AHA) guidelines for the evaluation and management of chronic heart failure in the adult: Executive summary a report of the American College of Cardiology/American Heart Association Task Force on Practice Guidelines (Committee to Revise the 1995 Guidelines for the Evaluation and Management of Heart Failure): Developed in collaboration with the International Society for Heart and Lung Transplantation; endorsed by the Heart Failure Society of America. Circulation 2001;104:2996-3007.
2. Jessup M, Brozena S. Heart failure. N Engl J Med 2003;348:2007-2018.
3. National Hospice and Palliative Care Organization. Hospice Facts and Figures, 2003. Available at http://www.nhpco.org (accessed January 2008).
4. American Heart Association. Heart Disease and Stroke Statistics—2005 Update. Dallas, TX: American Heart Association, 2005.
5. Cowie MR, Fox KF, Wood DA, et al. Hospitalization of patients with heart failure: A population based study. Eur J Heart Fail 2002;23:877-885.
6. Jassal D, Sharma S, Macher B, et al. Pulmonary hypertension. eMedicine. Available at http://www.emedicine.com/RADIO/topics583.htm
7. Goodlin SJ, Hauptman PJ, Arnold R, et al. Consensus statement: Palliative and supportive care in advanced heart failure. J Card Fail 2004;10:200-209.
8. Malkin CJ, Channer KS. Life-saving or life-prolonging? Interpreting trial data and survival curves for patients with congestive heart failure. Eur J Heart Fail 2005;7:143-148.
9. American College of Chest Physicians (ACCP). Diagnosis and management of pulmonary arterial hypertension: ACCP evidence-based clinical practice guidelines. Chest 2004;126:1S-92S.
10. Lee SH, Rubin IJ. Current treatment strategies for pulmonary arterial hypertension. J Int Med 2005;258:199-215.
11. Rich S, Seidlitz M, Dodin E, et al. The short-term effects of digoxin in patients with right ventricular dysfunction from pulmonary hypertension. Chest 1998;114:787-792.
12. Tucker R, Rayburn B. Management of advanced heart failure. In Berger AM, Shuster JL, Von Roenn J. Principles and Practice of Palliative Care and Supportive Oncology. Philadelphia: Lippincott Williams & Wilkins, 2007.
13. Faris R, Purcell H, Henein MY, et al. Clinical depression is common and significantly associated with reduced survival in patients with non-ischemic heart failure. Arch Intern Med 2001;161:1849-1856.

SUGGESTED READING

American College of Chest Physicians (ACCP). Diagnosis and management of pulmonary arterial hypertension: ACCP evidence-based clinical practice guidelines. Chest 2004;126: 1S-92S.

American Heart Association. Heart Disease and Stroke Statistics—2005 Update. Dallas, TX: American Heart Association, 2005.

Goodlin SJ, Hauptman PJ, Arnold R, et al. Consensus statement: Palliative and supportive care in advanced heart failure. J Card Fail 2004;10:200-209.

Hunt SA, Baker DW, Chin MH, et al. American College of Cardiology/American Heart Association (ACC/AHA) guidelines for the evaluation and management of chronic heart failure in the adult: Executive summary a report of the American College of Cardiology/American Heart Association Task Force on Practice Guidelines (Committee to Revise the 1995 Guidelines for the Evaluation and Management of Heart Failure): Developed in collaboration with the International Society for Heart and Lung Transplantation; endorsed by the Heart Failure Society of America. Circulation 2001;104:2996-3007.

Tucker R, Rayburn B. Management of advanced heart failure. In Principles and Practice of Palliative Care and Supportive Oncology. Philadelphia: Lippincott Williams & Wilkins, 2007.

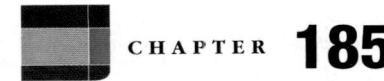

CHAPTER **185**

Respiratory Failure

Bassam Estfan

K E Y   P O I N T S

- Respiratory failure is a common pathway for many malignant and nonmalignant conditions.

- It can be classified as acute, chronic, or acute-on-chronic respiratory failure and as hypoxic or hypercapnic respiratory failure. The clinical and pathological features are often mixed.

- Therapy is management of the underlying cause. Chronic oxygen therapy is a cornerstone of management in many cases.

- Advanced planning for patients with advanced respiratory illness is the best way to prevent repeated hospitalizations and unwanted interventions.

- Supportive and aggressive care should be applied together; transition to full supportive measures must be guided by clinical judgment and the patient's wishes.

Respiratory failure or insufficiency complicates many cardiovascular, pulmonary, neuromuscular, and malignant ailments throughout the natural course of disease and when the patient is near death. Respiratory failure is a condition or a syndrome, not a disease. It can be acute, chronic, or acute-on-chronic. It is also differentiated as hypoxic, hypercapnic, or mixed respiratory failure based on blood gas values. Respiratory failure should not be confused with dyspnea, because they can exist exclusive of one another in clinical settings. It should also be differentiated from ventilatory failure, which is inadequacy of the ventilation pump represented by the neuromuscular system that generates breathing. Respiratory failure can be defined as the failure to provide adequate oxygenation to body tissues and organs or the failure to remove metabolism end products without respiratory support (e.g., oxygen therapy, mechanical ventilation).

In palliative medicine, respiratory failure is frequently encountered as a complication of malignancies, nonmalignant terminal cardiopulmonary or neuromuscular diseases, and in the final stages of any terminal disease. It is a leading cause of intensive care unit admissions, regardless of the underlying cause. Because tissue respiration is a complex process, managing the mechanical part of respiration through invasive or noninvasive ventilation may not reverse respiratory failure in severely ill patients. Invasive ventilation should be subject to appropriate medical judgment after a comprehensive evaluation of risks, benefits, and alternatives. Respiratory failure can be a major stressor for patients and their families because of the associated discomfort and the connotation respiratory failure may have, especially in acute events.

BASIC SCIENCE

The basic function of respiration is to provide adequate delivery of oxygen (O_2) for cellular use and removal of carbon dioxide (CO_2) as an end product of tissue metabolism.[1] In respiration, the pulmonary, cardiovascular, and neuromuscular systems work concomitantly to maintain gas exchange and delivery. Oxygen delivery depends on O_2 content in the atmosphere, air passage through the bronchial tree, exchange at the alveolar level, O_2 transport, and tissue uptake of O_2. Abnormalities involving any of these steps may result in respiratory failure. Ventilation pump, gas exchange, and alveolar function are also important for CO_2 elimination from the bloodstream.

Gas exchange takes place at the alveolar level, where O_2 diffuses into mixed venous blood and CO_2 diffuses into the alveoli and then into atmospheric air. The ratio of CO_2 to O_2 diffusion is roughly 20:1, which explains why hypoxia is not always associated with hypercapnia.

Breathing is regulated by the nervous and musculoskeletal systems. The breathing center is located in the brainstem, and it is regulated by inputs from two distinct systems. First, the chemosensitive area in the brainstem responds indirectly to CO_2 levels by means of the hydrogen ion concentration. Elevated CO_2 levels stimulate respiration, and decreased levels slow it. Second, the carotid bodies at the carotid bifurcations respond directly to O_2 levels and trigger respiration in response to hypoxia. In healthy persons, the CO_2 level drives breathing regulation. Efferent signals travel to the diaphragm, the principal breathing muscle, through phrenic nerves. Other supporting muscular groups include the intercostal and sternocleidomastoid muscles. Whereas inspiration is an active process, expiration is normally passive.

PATHOPHYSIOLOGY

Respiration is a process that extends beyond the act of ventilation. Abnormalities at any phase during this process may lead to respiratory failure; although ventilatory failure causes respiratory failure, not all respiratory failure is caused by ventilatory compromise. Pathologically, respiratory failure is classified as acute, chronic, or acute-on-chronic and as hypoxic, hypercapnic, or mixed.[2] These distinctions are important for management of respiratory failure and decision making. Hypoxic respiratory failure is type I, and hypercapnia is type II respiratory failure. Type I respiratory failure is defined as a PaO_2 value less than 55 mm Hg despite a fraction of inspired O_2 of 0.60 or more; clinically, hypoxia results from ventilation-perfusion mismatch at the alveolar level (Box 185-1). In type II respiratory failure, the $PaCO_2$ level rises above 45 mm Hg; hypercapnia occurs when production exceeds alveolar elimination (Box 185-2). Both frequently coexist (e.g., decreased ventilatory effort), and ventilation perfusion mismatch coexists in many cases.

CLINICAL MANIFESTATIONS

The manifestation of respiratory failure depends on its type and the rate of development. A thorough history and physical examination are essential for diagnosis and management. For patients with acute respiratory failure, a

---

Box 185-1 Factors Contributing to Hypoxia

Decreased atmospheric oxygen
  High altitudes
Airway obstruction
  Malignancy
  Bronchospasm
  Foreign bodies
  Cystic fibrosis
  Bronchiectasis
Alveolar pathology
  Flooding
    Blood (e.g., inflammatory diseases, pneumonia)
    Pus (e.g., pneumonia)
    Edema (e.g., congestive heart failure, acute respiratory distress syndrome, drugs)
  Fibrosis
    Interstitial lung diseases (e.g., idiopathic pulmonary fibrosis, asbestosis)
  Atelectasis
    Airway obstruction
    Chest wall restriction
    Deconditioning
    Pleural effusion
    Pneumothorax
  Destruction
    Chronic obstructive airway disease (e.g., chronic obstructive pulmonary disease)
Shunting of blood
  Cardiac
    Patent ductus arteriosus
    Atrial and ventricular septal defects
  Pulmonary
    Alveolar disease causing decreased gas exchange
    Pulmonary embolism decreasing blood flow to aerated alveoli
Oxygen transport
  Anemia
  Shock and hypotension
  Peripheral vascular disease
Increased oxygen demands, relative or absolute
  Thyrotoxicosis
  Febrile illnesses
  Sepsis
Failure to use oxygen at the cellular level
  Cyanide intoxication

---

focused history and evaluation should be performed, and initial attempts at management are directed at maintaining respiratory function, if clinically indicated, while awaiting identification of the cause. Symptoms may be prominent in acute respiratory failure and may include dyspnea, feeling of suffocation, anxiety, dizziness, and altered mental status. Tachypnea, cyanosis, apparent acute distress, and audible wheezing may be noticed. The pulmonary examination may reveal signs of pneumonia, pulmonary edema, or wheezing. In those with chronic respiratory failure, the clinical picture is less striking, especially in progressive neuromuscular diseases, and patients may present with subtle complaints such as sleeping problems, dyspnea on exercise and then at rest, daytime fatigue, or gradual cyanosis. With chronic hypoxia, clubbing of the nails can be seen. Dyspnea may not correlate well with the severity of respiratory failure or arterial blood gas determinations. Because most people with

Box 185-2 Factors Contributing to Hypercapnia

Increased carbon dioxide production
- Sepsis
- Exercise
- Thyrotoxicosis
- Burns
- Severe multiorgan failure

Decreased carbon dioxide elimination (i.e., ventilatory pump failure)
- Neuromuscular diseases
  - Amyotrophic lateral sclerosis
  - Guillain-Barré syndrome
  - Phrenic nerve injury
  - Drug overdose (e.g., sedatives, opioids)
  - Myasthenia gravis
  - Severe hypothyroidism
  - Malnutrition, cachexia, severe asthenia
  - Electrolyte abnormalities
  - Brainstem lesions
- Increased muscular workload
  - Bronchospasm
  - Excessive secretions
  - Hyperinflation
  - Airway obstruction
  - Kyphoscoliosis

Oxygen treatment in chronic hypercapnia

TABLE 185-1 Acute and Chronic Causes of Respiratory Failure

ACUTE CAUSES	CHRONIC CAUSES
Pneumonia	Interstitial lung diseases (e.g., idiopathic pulmonary fibrosis, asbestosis, silicosis)
Bronchitis (especially in chronic diseases)	Chronic obstructive pulmonary disease (e.g., chronic bronchitis, emphysema)
Acute myocardial infarction, acute coronary syndrome	Cystic fibrosis
Congestive heart failure	Neuromuscular diseases (e.g., amyotrophic lateral sclerosis, myasthenia gravis)
Pulmonary embolism	Progressive pleural effusion
Pneumothorax	Chronic pulmonary embolisms
Acute respiratory distress syndrome	Advanced pulmonary malignancy or metastasis
Drug overdose	Obstructive sleep apnea
Acute central nervous system injury	
Acute hemorrhage	
Shock and sepsis	
Acute pulmonary edema	

chronic respiratory failure gradually retain CO_2, symptoms of hypercapnia may not manifest classically as they would in the course of acute decompensation.

Type I respiratory failure may manifest with confusion, agitation, dyspnea, or in severe cases, with visible cyanosis. Type II respiratory failure usually manifests with somnolence, sedation, or altered mental status.

Cancer patients have many risk factors for respiratory failure such as decreased immunity and vulnerability to respiratory infection, malignant effusion, lymphangitic carcinomatosis, or progressing pulmonary metastasis. Respiratory failure may result from chemotherapy and radiation therapy.

Clinical diagnosis of respiratory failure frequently requires confirmation through invasive or noninvasive methods. Arterial blood gas (ABG) analysis is the gold standard for the diagnosis and differentiation of respiratory failure types. It is a minimally invasive test that may cause discomfort at the puncture site. Analysis can be done in minutes, and it provides an accurate reading of arterial blood pH, $PaCO_2$, PO_2, and base excess. Correct interpretation of the ABG results can determine the type of respiratory failure, its severity, whether it is acute or chronic, and whether the body is compensating adequately.[3] A less invasive method of obtaining blood gas values is the use of peripheral oximeters and capnometers; although less reliable, their values are consistent and can be practically implemented in the workup. The simultaneous evaluation of venous blood electrolytes allows further assessment of acidosis and renal compensation, especially in cases of chronic hypercapnia. Other useful laboratory tests include the thyroid-stimulating hormone (TSH) level and a complete blood cell count.

Another important test in evaluating pulmonary diseases leading to respiratory failure is the pulmonary function test (PFT) (see Chapter 73). PFT values help to differentiate causes as obstructive or restrictive. Chest radiography and computed tomography (CT) are crucial tools in the assessment of respiratory failure. They should be ordered judiciously, especially for patients with advanced disease and for whom management would not change on the basis of test results.

DIFFERENTIAL DIAGNOSIS

Management of respiratory failure depends on its type (see Boxes 185-1 and 185-2). This can be easily done with an ABG analysis or with noninvasive measures when indicated. Differential diagnosis also is based on respiratory failure acuity or chronicity (Table 185-1).

Many of the clinical diagnoses leading to respiratory failure have been discussed elsewhere in this textbook. Some chronic, nonmalignant pulmonary pathologies that can lead to respiratory failure are discussed in the following text.

Asbestosis is an environmental or occupational disease; it affects people exposed to chronic inhalation of asbestos particles. Asbestosis develops gradually over time and usually starts to manifest 10 to 15 years after the beginning of exposure. It usually manifests insidiously with dyspnea on exertion. It leads to interstitial fibrosis and a restrictive pattern seen on PFT as a decreased diffusing capacity of the lung for carbon monoxide (DLCO). Classic findings on chest radiographs include pleural plaques and a ground-glass appearance. Asbestosis predisposes to lung cancer and mesothelioma. There is no specific treatment, and it is managed empirically like many other pulmonary interstitial diseases.[4]

Cystic fibrosis (CF) is an autosomal recessive genetic disease affecting 1 in 3000 white people. It is mainly a childhood disease, but with medical advances, it has become an adult disease, with a median survival of more than 30 years. In CF, repeated infections and increased sputum retention occur, leading to bronchial tree obstruction and destruction with time. Bacterial pneumonia becomes more resistant to treatment with time, especially as *Pseudomonas aeruginosa* becomes the major colonizing bacteria in adulthood. Chest radiographs show an obstructive pattern that is followed by mucus impaction and bronchiectasis; this is more prominent on CT. An increased level of chlorine in sweat is diagnostic. Treatment is directed toward clearance of secretions through chest physical therapy and antibiotic treatment of infections. Higher doses of antibiotics are usually needed over extended periods. Mucokinetic agents are superior to mucolytics.

Chronic obstructive pulmonary disease (COPD) is one of the most common pulmonary diseases. This syndrome is subdivided into chronic bronchitis and emphysema manifesting as airway obstruction and hyperinflation, respectively, but many cases have a mixed picture. Risk factors include smoking, and α_1-antitrypsin deficiency (inherited). People with COPD experience exacerbations that cause acute respiratory compromise and, in advanced illness, the need for hospitalization, intravenous antibiotics, and possibly invasive ventilation. On PFT, there is a rapid decline in the forced expiratory volume in 1 second (FEV_1) compared with the normal population. Maintenance treatment employs bronchodilators, and systemic steroids are frequently used for exacerbations. Oxygen support is necessary for many sometime during the illness. Smoking cessation, no matter how late, slows disease progression.

Idiopathic pulmonary fibrosis is an interstitial lung disease of unknown origin. It shares many features of other pulmonary interstitial diseases, and it is a diagnosis of exclusion. It usually manifests with progressive dyspnea, cough, and inspiratory crackles heard on examination.[5] A restrictive pattern is seen on PFT, and patchy reticular opacities are seen on chest radiographs and CT scans. Idiopathic pulmonary fibrosis has a progressive course, and there is no specific therapy. Systemic corticosteroids are the cornerstone of management in addition to oxygen therapy. Cytotoxic and immunosuppressive agents can be used. Like other chronic pulmonary diseases (e.g., cystic fibrosis, COPD), the only definitive therapy is transplantation of single or double lungs.

MANAGEMENT

Treatment

The underlying cause is treated when possible. General guidelines for treatment should be followed until confirmation of the diagnosis (Fig. 185-1). Because respiratory failure can be life threatening, immediate attention should be given to the need for invasive mechanical ventilation or intensive care support. Decision making and medical judgment are the most important factors in management. Decisions consider the underlying illness and the patient's medical condition. Acute causes are usually reversible, even in the course of cancer, and deserve to be treated meticulously.

Oxygen therapy is a cornerstone of management because hypoxia usually complicates acute respiratory failure and chronic illnesses such as interstitial lung diseases. It should be used carefully at the lowest appropriate flow in those with chronic hypercapnia because of decreased sensitivity of the chemosensitive area in the brainstem to CO_2 changes; higher levels of O_2 saturation may suppress breathing under these circumstances.[6]

In those who have new-onset acute respiratory failure or an acute episode on top of chronic respiratory failure, mechanical ventilation may be needed as a bridge to pulmonary recovery and then extubation. The decision for intubation should be made in accordance with the patient's wishes. For those who have living wills or expressed prior wishes not to be resuscitated in the event of terminal diseases, resuscitation remains ethical and reasonable if the cause is deemed reversible by the treating physician and the quality of life is expected to be the same as before the event. However, cardiopulmonary resuscitation for cardiopulmonary arrest in cancer patients is futile even when it occurs in the hospital, and it should not be done routinely.

Noninvasive positive-pressure ventilation (NIPPV) has been gaining popularity as an alternative to mechanical ventilation, especially for patients with advanced chronic pulmonary diseases or advanced cancer with respiratory failure.[7,8] It is essential in managing progressive neuromuscular diseases. NIPPV can be applied temporarily in acute respiratory failure or intermittently in chronic hypercapnia or hypoxia. It improves respiratory symptoms, gas exchange, and quality of life. NIPPV works through continuous positive pressure to open the airways and assist breathing. Pressure is delivered through a tight nasal or oronasal mask; it is not designed for continuous use because it may be uncomfortable, especially if the mask is not custom made. Many patients suffer from nasal bridge pressure ulcers and discomfort. It is possible to apply NIPPV in the outpatient setting. A subset of patients cannot tolerate the pressure and find it uncomfortable.

Other invasive interventions may aid management of respiratory failure. In pleural effusion, especially of malignant origin, inserting a chest tube or a permanent drainage catheter may offer relief and prevent further accumulation. Tracheostomies may aid respiration in certain cases (see Chapter 186).

In addition to managing underlying causes, empirical symptom management is important. Correcting blood gas abnormalities usually relieves mental status changes. Dyspnea and the feeling of suffocation can be alleviated with low-dose intermittent or continuous opioids or other drugs such as chlorpromazine (see Chapter 159). Nondrug measures, such as a fan's air current directed at the face, may help. Tightness of breathing and wheezing due to bronchospasm usually respond to bronchodilators (see Chapters 137 and 153). Diuretics and cardiac inotropes are useful in managing dyspnea from pulmonary edema and decompensated congestive heart failure. Dyspnea and respiratory failure are frequently associated with increased anxiety, causing more dyspnea and thereby initiating a vicious cycle. Anxiolytics such as short- and medium-acting benzodiazepines are usually helpful in controlling the symptoms. Theophylline may promote better respiration in some with COPD or dyspnea resulting from asthe-

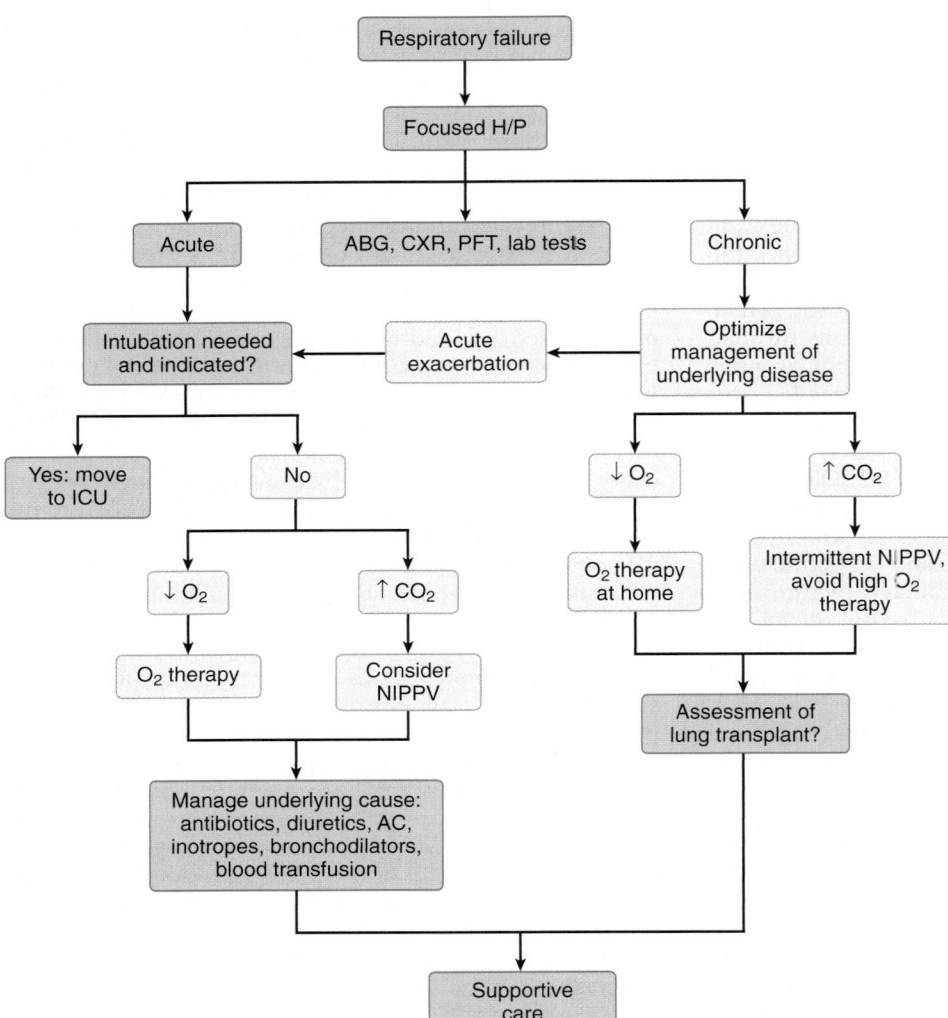

FIGURE 185-1 Algorithm for management of respiratory failure. The guidelines for treatment should be followed until confirmation of a diagnosis. ABG, arterial blood gas determinations; AC, anticoagulation; CXR, chest radiograph; H/P, history and physical examination; ICU, intensive care unit; NIPPV, noninvasive positive-pressure ventilation; PFT, pulmonary function test.

nia, but it has a narrow therapeutic window. In cases of respiratory depression caused by opioid or benzodiazepine overdose, it is appropriate to reverse the depressive effect of the drug, but not the therapeutic, by using incremental dosing of naloxone or flumazenil, respectively.

Because of the immunological vulnerability of patients with advanced cancer and pulmonary diseases, up-to-date vaccinations are important in preventing viral and bacterial pneumonias. Pneumococcal and yearly influenza vaccinations are recommended. Chest physical therapy and breathing exercises are helpful for chronic conditions.

Lung transplantation is becoming the curative measure for many chronic and advanced pulmonary diseases. Transplantation is indicated for COPD, emphysema, idiopathic pulmonary fibrosis, and cystic fibrosis. Survival after lung transplantation has improved, especially for bilateral transplant recipients, and median survival is about 5 years.[9] Those with advanced, debilitating lung diseases should be considered for lung transplantation in the absence of contraindications if the performance status is good. Nevertheless, only a few eventually undergo lung transplantation, and consideration for the surgery should not change medical management and supportive care.

Supportive Care

For most acute and chronic respiratory failure events, aggressive and targeted therapy is indicated. The extent to which these measures are applied changes with the disease course. Discussion regarding resuscitation and wishes for terminal care of patients with irreversible and terminal conditions should take place when they are in a relatively healthy state. Palliative interventions become more prominent as the disease progresses in concordance with palliative care models for life-limiting illnesses.[10]

Supportive care alone should be considered for patients with severe worsening of respiratory parameters as indicated by the PFT results, ABG analysis, and clinical picture. Repeated hospitalizations and intensive care unit stays for mechanical ventilation should trigger a discussion about the plan of care for similar events in the future. In these circumstances, the focus of care is on comfort, symptom control, and quality of life. It is important to explore patients' wishes regarding where and how they would like to spend their last days, because this may provide reasonable guidelines for future management of worsening respiratory failure.

Control of symptoms such as dyspnea, agitation, and delirium must be aggressive. In those with progressive hypercapnia, some hyperactive delirium may occur, but mostly they experience somnolence and sedation and die peacefully (see Chapter 179). Others may have an increased symptom burden that may require palliative sedation. Morphine infusion at low doses is usually sufficient to relieve the sense of dyspnea and suffocation. Titrating opioids for comfort should be done in an organized fashion based on observed symptoms, not the level of alertness. Another important measure is reduction of bronchial secretions in the dying, which helps respiration and minimizes death rattles and the family's discomfort. This is achieved by anticholinergic agents such as hyoscyamine or glycopyrrolate.

Many patients with respiratory failure are intubated and started on mechanical ventilation. Some may never be weaned off successfully and are considered terminal. The decision to withdraw life support from patients with irreversible respiratory failure is ethical and appropriate, especially if it reflects their previously stated wishes. When such decisions are made, premedication with opioids and antisecretory agents must be done, and the family should be educated regarding expectations of the patient's survival off ventilation (see Chapter 180).

Educating the families regarding respiratory failure and the predicted course of events is important for coping with death. Usually, family members detect the patient's discomfort and ask about the need for adjusting symptom management. Hospice care is an optimal service that can be offered to patients with advanced respiratory failure and their families. If care is becoming too complicated for the family, inpatient hospice units can relieve families from complex caregiving, and it allows them to be available for support.

CONTROVERSIES AND RESEARCH OPPORTUNITIES

The use of nebulized opioids has been subject to criticism regarding their effectiveness in relieving dyspnea in patients with the respiratory symptoms of advanced respiratory diseases. The use of these drugs in this patient population should be a subject for larger studies.

Empirical oxygen use in patients with respiratory failure, even when oxygen saturation levels are adequate, is controversial. Oxygen is frequently supplemented in hospice patients without evidence of hypoxia, and symptom response may be related to the air current rather than elevated O_2 levels.

Nebulized *N*-acetylcysteine and other mucolytics are commonly used for secretion management in patients with cystic fibrosis. However, this approach lacks evidence to support it.

REFERENCES

1. Guyton AC, Hall JE (eds). Textbook of Medical Physiology. Philadelphia: WB Saunders, 2000.
2. Raju P, Manthous CA. The pathology of respiratory failure. Respir Care Clin North Am 2000;6:195-212.
3. Breen PH. Arterial blood gas and pH analysis. Clinical approach and interpretation. Anesthesiol Clin North Am 2001;19:885-906.
4. Wagner GR. Asbestosis and silicosis. Lancet 1997;349:1311-1315.
5. Harari S, Caminati A. Idiopathic pulmonary fibrosis. Allergy 2005;60:421-435.
6. Ringbaek TJ. Continuous oxygen therapy for hypoxic pulmonary disease. Treat Respir Med 2005;4:397-408.
7. Nava S, Cuomo AM. Acute respiratory failure in the cancer patient: The role of non-invasive mechanical ventilation. Crit Rev Oncol Hematol 2004;51:91-103.
8. Wedzicha JA, Muir JF. Noninvasive ventilation in chronic obstructive pulmonary disease, bronchiectasis and cystic fibrosis. Eur Respir J 2002;20:777-784.
9. Studer SM, Levy RD, McNeil K, et al. Lung transplant outcomes: A review of survival, graft function, physiology, health-related quality of life and cost-effectiveness. Eur Respir J 2004;24:674-685.
10. Simonds AK. Living and dying with respiratory failure: Facilitating decision making. Chron Respir Dis 2004;1:56-59.

SUGGESTED READING

Curtis JR, Cook DJ, Sinuff T, et al. Noninvasive positive pressure ventilation in critical and palliative care settings: Understanding the goals of therapy. Crit Care Med 2007;35:932-939.

Markou NK, Myrianthefs PM, Baltopoulos GJ. Respiratory failure: An overview. Crit Care Nurse Q 2004;27:353-379.

Robinson W. Palliative care in cystic fibrosis. J Palliat Med 2000;3:187-192.

Seamark DA, Seamark CJ, Halpin DMG. Palliative care in chronic obstructive pulmonary disease: A review for clinicians. J R Soc Med 2007;100:225-233.

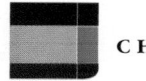

CHAPTER **186**

Respiratory Equipment

Robert E. McQuown

KEY POINTS

- Oxygen therapy is administered with the intent of treating or preventing the manifestations of hypoxia.

- Low-flow and high-flow systems are used to deliver oxygen therapy.

- Noninvasive positive-pressure ventilation (NPPV) applies positive pressure to the airway without the aid of an artificial airway device and allows patients to rest their muscles of respiration during sleep while maintaining adequate gas exchange.

- NPPV has several benefits over traditional mechanical ventilation, which continues to be used in the management of many critically ill patients.

- Mechanical ventilators are classified by the power method used (i.e., electrical, pneumatic, or fluidic), by the type of pressure delivered (i.e., positive or negative), and by the control variables used (i.e., pressure, volume, and dual).

INDICATIONS FOR OXYGEN THERAPY

Oxygen therapy involves administering oxygen at levels greater than the atmospheric composition (21%) with the intent of treating or preventing the manifestations of hypoxia.[1] Oxygen therapy is most commonly administered to patients with the diagnosis of chronic obstructive pulmonary disease (COPD) and those with hypoxemia documented as follows:

- A PaO$_2$ value of 55 mm Hg or SaO$_2$ value of 88% while breathing room air[2,3]
- A PaO$_2$ value between 56 and 59 mm Hg or SaO$_2$ value of 89% for patients presenting with clinical conditions such as cor pulmonale, congestive heart failure, or erythrocythemia (hematocrit >56%)[2,3]
- Becoming hypoxemic during mild exertion, such as ambulation
- SaO$_2$ level that falls to 88% for at least 5 minutes during sleep[3]

HIGH-FLOW AND LOW-FLOW DEVICES FOR OXYGEN DELIVERY

Devices used to deliver oxygen therapy are classified as low-flow or high-flow systems. The differences between the two are determined by the patient's inspiratory flow rate, tidal volume, and the oxygen flow rate being used. A low-flow system does not meet the patient's total inspiratory flow rate, whereas the high-flow system meets or exceeds the patient's total inspiratory flow rate (Table 186-1).

Low-Flow Systems

The nasal cannula (Fig. 186-1) is the most commonly used low-flow oxygen delivery system. Recommended flow rates between 1 and 6 L/min generate theoretical oxygen concentrations of 24% at 1 L/min and 44% at 6 L/min, increasing 4% with each 1-L increase in flow (Table 186-2). Actual values for the fraction of inspired oxygen (FIO$_2$) vary from the theoretical values because they depend on the patient's minute ventilation. A bubble humidifier

(Fig. 186-2) usually is not necessary at lower liter flows, but for flows greater than 4 L/min, a humidifier is recommended to prevent drying the nasal mucosa.[2]

Oxygen Masks

Oxygen masks (Fig. 186-3) are often used for short-term oxygen therapy. Patients tend to resist wearing the oxygen mask for long periods for several reasons:

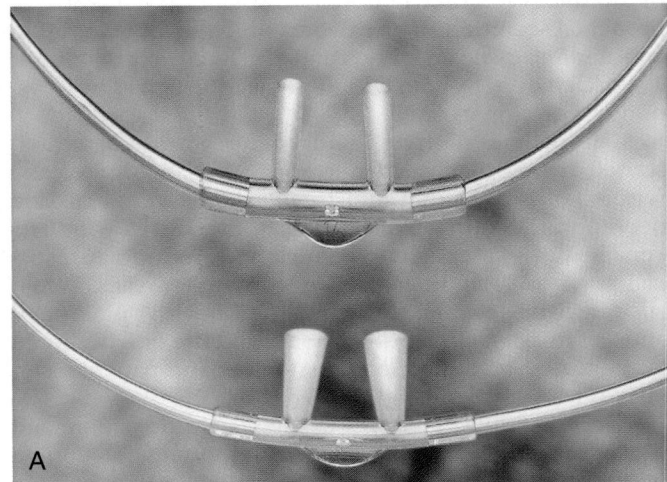

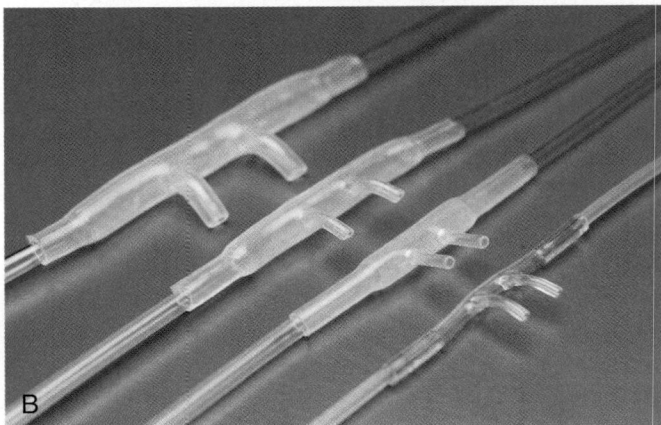

FIGURE 186-1 **A** and **B**, Nasal cannulas.

TABLE 186-1 Low-Flow and High-Flow Oxygen Delivery Systems	
LOW-FLOW SYSTEMS	**HIGH-FLOW SYSTEMS**
Nasal cannula	Air entrainment mask (e.g.. high air flow with oxygen enrichment [HAFOE] mask)
Simple oxygen mask	
Aerosol mask	
Partial and non-rebreather masks	
Transtracheal catheter	

TABLE 186-2 Theoretical Oxygen Values Using the Nasal Cannula	
FLOW RATE (L/M)	**OXYGEN CONCENTRATION (%)**
1	24
2	28
3	32
4	36
5	40
6	44

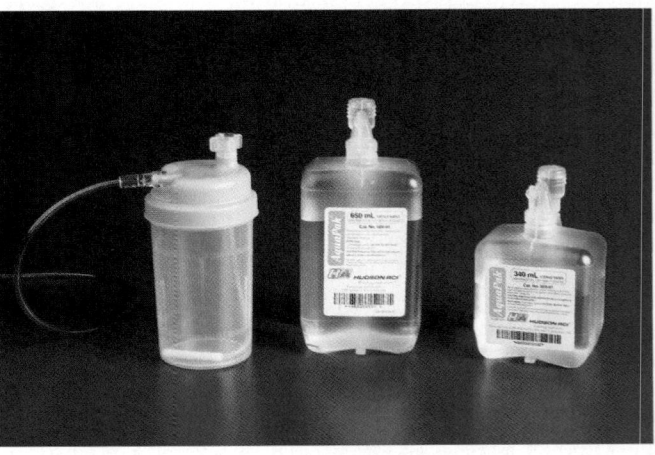

FIGURE 186-2 Bubble humidifier with sterile water containers.

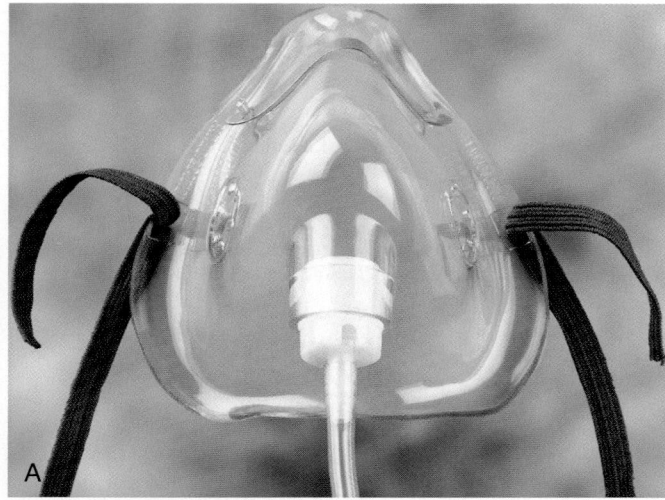

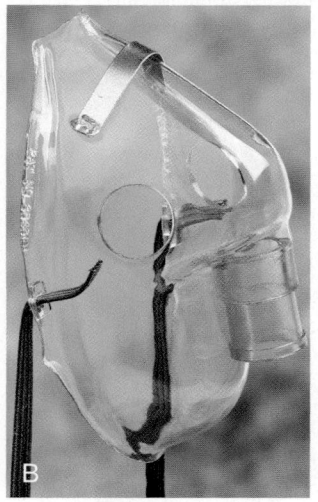

FIGURE 186-3 A and **B**, Oxygen masks.

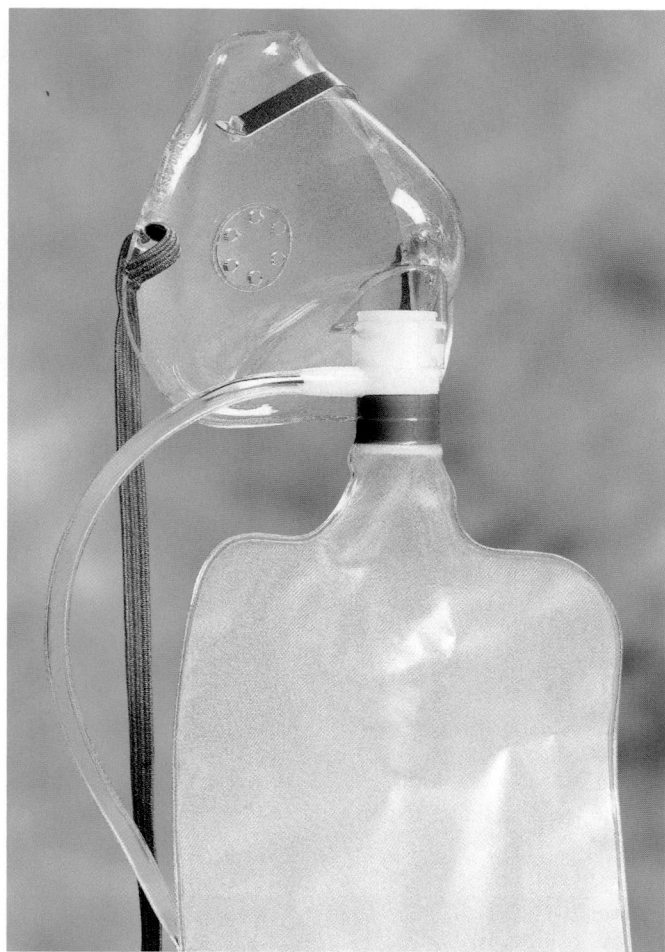

FIGURE 186-4 Partial rebreather mask.

- The mask becomes uncomfortably warm with time.
- Skin coming in contact with the mask becomes sore.
- Many patents experience feelings of claustrophobia.

Extra caution should be exercised in using oxygen masks for patients complaining about nausea, because they are at increased risk for aspiration.

Oxygen masks provide higher FIO_2 values than a nasal cannula. Recommended flow rates range from 5 to 12 L/m, and the masks deliver FIO_2 values from 0.35 to 0.70 or greater. Jensen and colleagues[4] demonstrated that a minimum flow rate of 5 L/m was needed to flush exhaled CO_2 from the oxygen mask.

The *partial-rebreather* and *non-rebreather masks* have a 600- to 800-mL reservoir bag attached. The partial rebreather mask (Fig. 186-4) captures the first one third of exhaled air into the reservoir bag. This air is high in oxygen content and is mostly composed of the end-inspired gas that previously filled the patient's anatomical dead space. The partial rebreather system is set between 6 and 10 L/min, and it delivers FIO_2 values between 0.35 and 0.60.

A series of one-way valves on the non-rebreather mask (Fig. 186-5) provides a visual and functional difference from the partial rebreather mask. These extra valves prevent exhaled air from entering the reservoir bag, thereby creating higher oxygen levels over the partial rebreather. The non-rebreather mask requires a minimum flow rate of 10 L/min, which produces FIO_2 values in the range of 0.60 to 0.80. These masks, however, do not perform consistently because they tend to leak around the area that comes into contact with the face. Because they are classified as a low-flow system, their performance continually varies in terms of FIO_2 based on the patient's ventilatory patterns.

Transtracheal Oxygen Therapy

The transtracheal catheter (Fig. 186-6) is a small-bore, distal-port, disposable tube made of kink-resistant thermoplastic polyurethane.[5] This oxygen delivery device is placed directly through the trachea between the second and third tracheal rings, with the catheter tip resting 1 to 2 cm above the patient's carina.[6] Adding oxygen directly into the airway decreases the opportunity of dilution with air, allowing oxygen flow rates to be decreased by 54% to 59% while maintaining acceptable oxygenation[6] (Box 186-1).

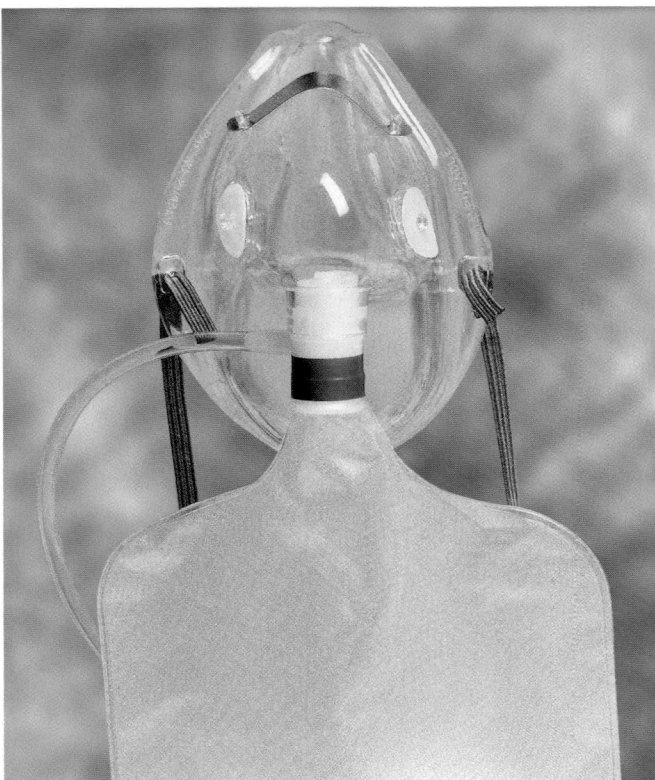

FIGURE 186-5 Non-rebreather mask.

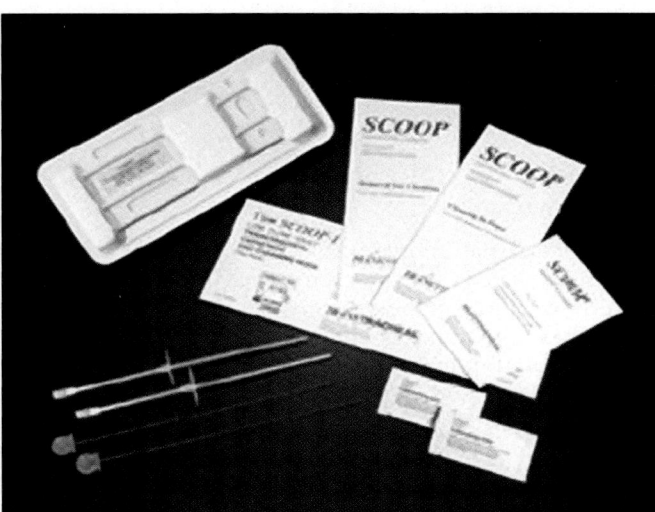

FIGURE 186-6 Transtracheal catheters.

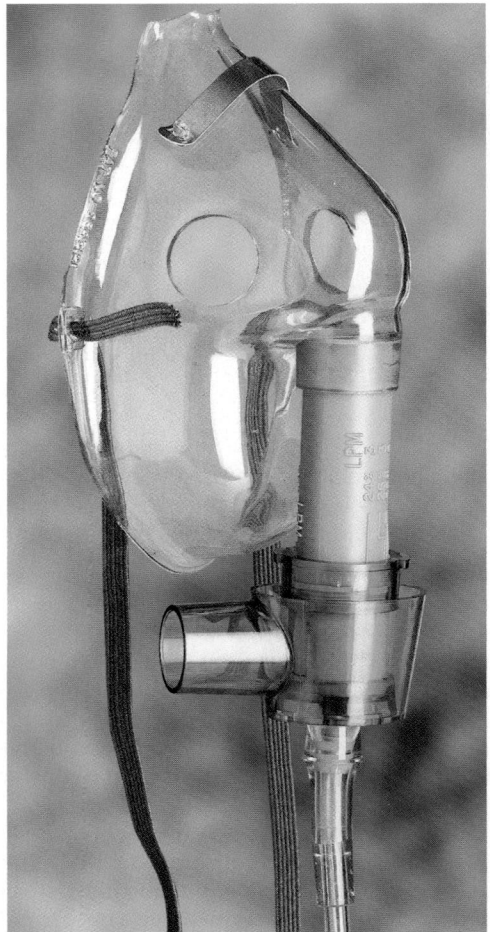

FIGURE 186-7 Air entrainment mask.

> **Box 186-1 Advantages and Disadvantages of Transtracheal Oxygen Therapy**
>
> **Advantages**
>
> - Oxygen flow rates are reduced, leading to oxygen cost savings.
> - It is less conspicuous than the nasal cannula and improves patient compliance.
> - If a problem occurs, such as an occlusion, the patient can easily revert to the nasal cannula until the problem can be corrected.
>
> **Disadvantages**
>
> - Placement of the catheter requires minor surgery, and complications (e.g., subcutaneous emphysema, infection, hemoptysis) may arise.
> - Adequate humidity and frequent cleaning are necessary to prevent mucous plugs and mucous balls from forming.
> - The catheter can be dislodged if not properly fastened in place.

High-Flow Systems

Air Entrainment Mask

The air entrainment mask (Fig.186-7) (i.e., high air flow with oxygen enrichment [HAFOE]) is classified as a high-flow system because the oxygen delivered to the patient meets or exceeds his or her inspiratory flow needs. Oxygen is forced through a restricted orifice, causing an increase in velocity that "drags" surrounding ambient air through an entrainment port.[7,8] Some styles of air entrainment mask vary the size of the restriction orifice and keep the entrainment ports consistent, whereas other styles keep the restriction constant and vary the size of the entrainment ports. Both masks perform equally well, with no distinct advantage of one style over the other. Although frequently referred to as a *Venturi mask*, the air entrainment mask (i.e., HAFOE) does not operate on the Venturi principle; it instead uses a process called *viscous shearing*.[7] At recommended liter flows, the air entrainment mask delivers precise degrees of FIO_2, with values from 0.24 to 0.50 (Table 186-3).

Noninvasive Positive-Pressure Ventilation

Noninvasive positive-pressure ventilation (NPPV) is the application of positive pressure to the airway without the aid of an artificial airway device.[7,9] Positive-pressure ventilation commonly is delivered to the patient using a nasal mask or a full facemask. Other patient interfaces range from a mouthpiece, used by the coherent patient who needs only infrequent ventilatory assistance to the total facemask, which is the largest patient interface commercially available (Fig. 186-8). NPPV has been gaining popularity over the past 15 years and has become an accepted modality in the treatment of the acutely hypoxic and chronically ill patient (Fig. 186-9).

TABLE 186-3	Air Entrainment Mask Liter Flow Table		
FIO₂ SETTING*	**RECOMMENDED FLOW (L/MIN)**	**AIR TO OXYGEN RATIO**	**TOTAL LITER FLOW (L/MIN)**
0.24	4	25:1	104
0.28	4	10:1	44
0 31	6	7:1	48
0 35	8	5:1	48
0 40	12	3:1	32
0.50	12	1.7:1	32

*Air entrainment masks differ between manufacturers, as do the recommended liter flows and fraction of inspired oxygen (FIO₂) values. The table provides values for an average air entrainment mask and its flow characteristics.

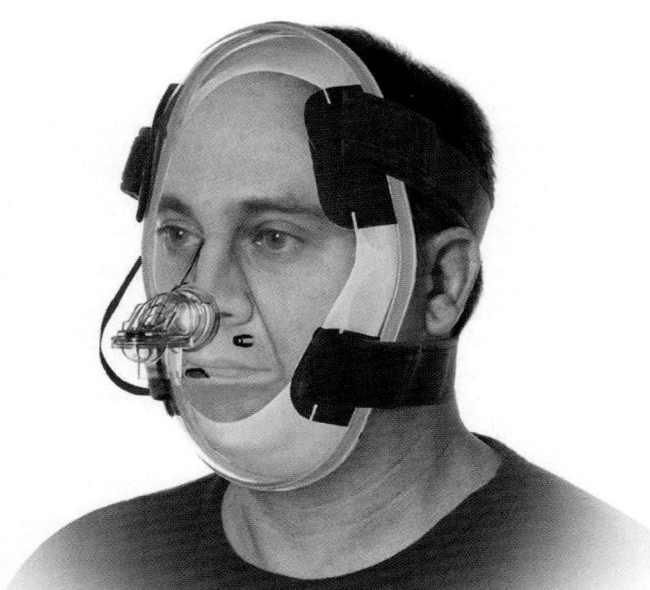

FIGURE 186-8 Total facemask.

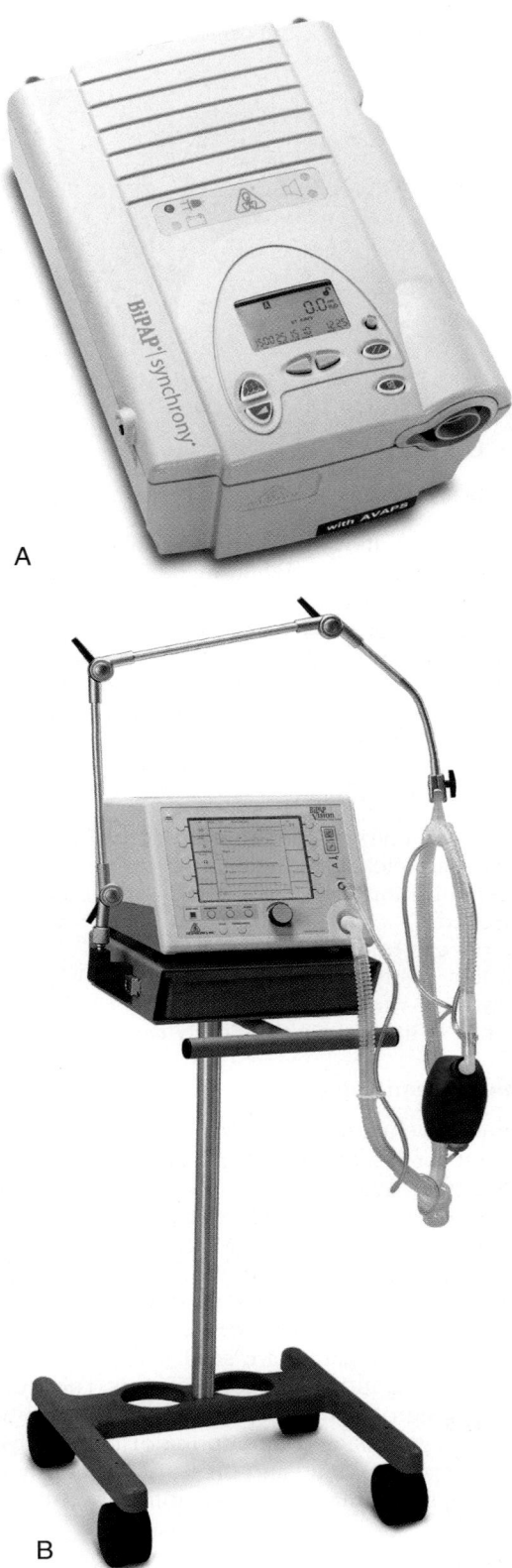

FIGURE 186-9 A-C, Three examples of machines used to provide noninvasive positive-pressure ventilation for patients.

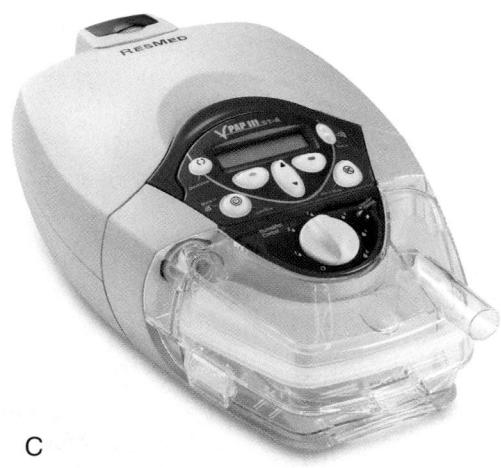

C

FIGURE 186-9, cont'd

Use of NPPV allows patients to rest their muscles of respiration during sleep while maintaining adequate gas exchange.[10] The patient retains the ability to communicate by avoiding endotracheal intubation and its associated complications. NPPV enables treatment of acute exacerbation of COPD and acute respiratory failure.[10-12] It allows weaning from mechanical ventilatory support and assists with postoperative support.[10]

The use of NPPV has several benefits over traditional mechanical ventilation:

- Incidence of airway infection is decreased.
- Mucociliary clearance mechanisms are not inhibited.
- Communication between the patient and caregivers is improved.
- Patients can orally ingest meals.
- It is less costly to provide compared with traditional mechanical ventilation.
- It is not as intimidating to family caregivers.

Mechanical Ventilation

Mechanical ventilators represent major life-sustaining equipment for the treatment or management of the critically ill patient. Ventilators are designed for treating newborns, pediatric patients, and adults, and they can be used for transport and in-home use. Modern mechanical ventilators are more sophisticated and technologically advanced compared with the machines used 10 or 15 years ago. Although many older ventilators are still in use, the later generations of ventilators are smaller and lighter, can be battery powered, and use microprocessors. These improvements in design offer volume, pressure, and flow accuracy; alarm systems; and monitoring of patient dynamics (i.e., flow, volume, time, and pressure waveforms).

Mechanical ventilators are identified by many classifications:

- By power method: electrical, pneumatic (i.e., high-pressure gas source), combined (i.e., electricity and pneumatics), and fluidic (i.e., gas flow and pressure to control other gas flows and perform logic functions)
- By pressure delivery: positive pressure (i.e., most common type of ventilator) or negative pressure (e.g., iron lung, chest cuirass)
- By control variables: pressure, volume, and dual

Robert Chatburn[8] has done extensive work to revamp and standardize the way ventilators are classified. Before his work, the American Society for Testing and Materials published the *Standard Specifications for Ventilators Intended for Use in Critical Care*, which classified ventilators in four main categories:

- Controller: a device that inflates the lungs independent of the patient's inspiratory effort
- Assister: a device designed to augment the patient's breathing, synchronizing with his or her inspiratory effort
- Assister/controller: an apparatus designed to function as an assister or, in the absence of the patient's inspiratory effort, as a controller
- Assister/controller with spontaneous breathing: a device that incorporates various modes of operation that allow the patient to breathe spontaneously at or above ambient pressure levels or with or without supplemental mandatory positive-pressure breaths

These standards of ventilator classification have since been withdrawn.

Robert Chatburn's classification[8] identifies ventilators according to the pattern of mandatory breaths:

- Control variables (i.e., pressure, volume, or dual control)
- Patterns of mandatory or spontaneous breaths (i.e., control mandatory ventilation, intermittent mandatory ventilation, and continuous spontaneous ventilation)
- Phase variables for mandatory breaths (i.e., trigger and cycle variables)
- Whether spontaneous breaths are assisted
- Conditional variables

The classifications of ventilators and the terminology used to describe them are more often determined by the manufacturer wanting to introduce a "new" mode of delivery to distinguish the product from that of the competition. The standardization of how ventilators are classified may always remain a challenge.

REFERENCES

1. American College of Chest Physicians and National Heart, Lung, and Blood Institute. National conference on oxygen therapy. Chest 1984;86:234-247.
2. American Association for Respiratory Care. AARC clinical practice guideline. Oxygen Therapy in the Home or Extended Care Facility. Respir Care 1992;37:918-922.
3. Criteria for Medicare coverage in region B, policy revision 44, June 2005. DMERC Supplier Manual. Washington, DC: Centers for Medicare and Medicaid Services, 2005, pp 3-6.
4. Jensen AG, Johnson A, Sandstedt S. Rebreathing during oxygen treatment with face mask. Acta Anaesth Scand 1991;35:289-292.
5. TransTracheal Systems. Internet resources 1999-2003. Available at www.trans-tracheal.com/products/scoop-catheters.asp (accessed January 2008).
6. Cairo JM, Pilbeam SP. Mosby's Respiratory Care Equipment, 7th ed. St. Louis: Mosby, 2004, pp 65-70.
7. Cairo JM, Pilbeam SP. Mosby's Respiratory Care Equipment, 7th ed. St. Louis: Mosby, 2004, pp 773-786.
8. Branson RD, Hess DR, Chatburn RL. Respiratory Care Equipment, 2nd ed. Philadelphia: Lippincott Williams & Wilkins, 1999.
9. White GC. Equipment Theory for Respiratory Care, 4th ed. Clifton Park, NY: Thomson Delmar Learning, 2005.
10. Hill NS. Noninvasive ventilation for chronic obstructive pulmonary disease. Respir Care 1994;49:72-87.
11. Ventilators and mechanical ventilation symposium: Part 2 [abstract 11]. Respir Care 2003;48.
12. Ventilators and mechanical ventilation symposium: Part 1 [abstract 9]. Respir Care 2003;48.

Nervous System and Musculoskeletal Disorders

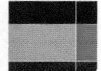

CHAPTER **187**

Congenital Intellectual Disability

Karen Ryan, Regina McQuillan, and Philip Dodd

KEY POINTS

- Worldwide, people with intellectual disabilities are disadvantaged, and their specific palliative care needs have not been widely considered.

- Those with intellectual disabilities have an increasing need for palliative care services because they are living longer and are developing age-related conditions such as cancer, cardiovascular disorders, and respiratory disease.

- Persons with intellectual disabilities have the typical palliative care needs of the general population, but they may also have additional and special needs.

- Additional and special needs may refer to issues of communication, symptom assessment, conceptualization of illness and death, truth telling, consent, and capacity.

- The intellectually disabled are at increased risk for complicated grief reactions. Staff and caregivers have traditionally underestimated the impact of loss for people with intellectual disabilities in terms of psychiatric and behavioral morbidity.

Intellectual disability is a general term, describing impairment of intelligence and social functioning. It refers to the significantly reduced ability to understand new or complex information, to learn new skills, and to cope independently. It starts before adulthood and has a lasting effect on development.[1] There is no consensus on the definitions of intelligence and social functioning, and different countries may use different synonyms for intellectual disability. These terms include *mental retardation, congenital developmental disabilities,* and *learning disabilities.*

People with intellectual disabilities commonly experience poorer access to health care services and may experience poorer outcomes while receiving services. Mistakes have been made in the provision of health care services to people with intellectual disabilities, and we should learn from them to ensure they are not repeated in palliative medicine. Palliative care professionals have a responsibility to understand the needs that result from impairment and to understand the role they can play in enabling the person. Understanding the different models of disability is an important starting point.

The classic medical or person-centered model establishes disability as an individual problem, directly caused by disease, trauma, or other health conditions. It views disability as a characteristic of the person that causes disadvantage and requires treatment. In contrast, the social model views disability as a disadvantage or restriction of activity caused by a contemporary social organization that takes little or no account of people who have physical impairments and therefore excludes them from participation in the mainstream of social activities.[2] People may have a condition (e.g., trisomy 21) that impairs their physical or mental function, but it is argued that their disability is caused by the attitudinal and physical barriers erected by society. The focus of change is therefore placed on social organizations and the environment, rather than on the individual, and the role of empowerment of people with disabilities in effecting change is emphasized.

People with intellectual disabilities are not homogeneous. Disability may be classed as mild, moderate, severe, or profound, depending on formal assessment of intelligence quotient (IQ) and social functioning, and individuals may have various co-morbid physical and sensory impairments. Individuals have heterogeneous life experiences, personalities, and attributes, and person-centered approaches to care should always be adopted when providing palliative care to anyone with an intellectual disability.

There are many more similarities between people with intellectual disabilities and the general population than there are differences. These commonalities should serve as the basis of care planning because a person with intellectual disability has the same need for control of physical symptoms and provision of psychosocial and spiritual support as any other person. The impairment or the social consequences may mean it is a challenge for palliative care staff to meet these needs, but the process can be facilitated by a partnership approach by the staff members from organizations providing services to people with intellectual disabilities.

EPIDEMIOLOGY AND PATHOPHYSIOLOGY OF INTELLECTUAL DISABILITY

The prevalence of intellectual disability is 1% to 2.5% in developed countries. Etiological agents fall into three main categories: genetic, infective, and environmental (Table 187-1). Overall, genetic causes are responsible for 40% to 50% and environmental causes for 15% to 20%. The cause remains unknown for 30% to 45%.[3]

TABLE 187-1	Causes of Intellectual Disability		
TIME OF EFFECT	**GENETIC CAUSES**	**INFECTIVE CAUSES**	**ENVIRONMENTAL CAUSES**
Antenatal	Chromosomal disorders, such as Down syndrome, Edward's syndrome, fragile-X syndrome Secondary neurological damage due to disorders of protein, lipid or mucopolysaccharide metabolism, such as phenylketonuria, Tay-Sachs, Hurler's syndrome Secondary neurological damage due to disorders of the endocrine system, such as congenital hypothyroidism	Rubella Cytomegalovirus Toxoplasmosis Human immunodeficiency virus (HIV)	Rhesus incompatibility Irradiation Drugs or toxins, such as alcohol, mercury Nutritional deficiencies, such as iodine, folate
Perinatal	Not applicable	Herpes simplex	Hypoxia, hypoglycemia, trauma
Postnatal	Not applicable	Meningitis Encephalitis Encephalopathies, such as measles	Trauma resulting in head injury Nutrition Lead

From Patja K, Molsa P, Iivanainen M. Cause-specific mortality of people with intellectual disability in a population-based, 35-year follow-up study. J Intellect Disabil Res 2001;45:30-40.

People with intellectual disabilities are living longer because of factors such as improved medical care, control of infections, and the move to community living. Age-related health problems, such as cancer and cardiovascular disease, are becoming more common. Historically, services were set up to provide care, education, and training for children and young adults, emphasizing the development of new skills and enabling individuals to lead as full and productive a life as possible. Supporting a person with declining function is less familiar and exposes new service gaps, potentially placing a strain on the staff working within these organizations.

Morbidity Associated with Intellectual Disabilities

People with intellectual disabilities have increased physical and mental health needs compared with the general population (Table 187-2). A person with intellectual disability has, on average, between five and six medical disorders,[4] and prevalence rates of psychiatric illness of 10% to 39% have been reported.[5] There has been a steady increase in the prevalence of people with severe intellectual and complex physical disabilities over the past 20 years, and this is likely to continue. These trends will inevitably have an impact on palliative care services.

Mortality Associated with Intellectual Disabilities

It is difficult to interpret the data from mortality studies, because there have been significant variations between populations sampled. Mortality patterns are significantly different for people with intellectual disabilities compared with the general population (Table 187-3). One study found the three most common causes of death for people with intellectual disabilities were vascular (36%), respiratory (22%), and neoplastic (11%) diseases.[6]

ISSUES OF CONSENT AND CAPACITY

Most of the research on the subject of decision making by and for people with intellectual disabilities has focused on

TABLE 187-2	Physical Health Problems of Adults with Intellectual Disabilities
DISORDER	**COMMENTS**
Epilepsy	Common, with incidence rates of up to 50%; frequently difficult to control, often requiring use of multiple, high-dose anticonvulsants
Visual impairments	Up to 30% have significant impairment of sight, 10% are blind or partially sighted, and 75% have refractive errors. Use of corrective lenses may pose challenges.
Hearing impairments	Prevalence of hearing impairment varies from 22% to 68%; about 7% are deaf or partially deaf.
Oral problems	Oral hygiene is a significant problem, with higher rates of untreated dental caries and periodontal disease.
Endocrine disorders	Hypothyroidism is particularly common in people with Down syndrome. Hypogonadism is more common in those with fragile-X syndrome. Type II diabetes is associated with obesity.
Nutritional disorders	Increased prevalence of the extremes of obesity or undernutrition.
Gastrointestinal disorders	Gastroesophageal disease occurs in up to 50% of institutionalized adults. Constipation is common. Disorders of swallowing and vomiting also are problematic.
Osteoporosis	Increased incidence; associated with hypogonadism, Down syndrome, and immobility.
Infectious disease	Rates of hepatitis A and B and *Helicobacter pylori* infections are increased in institutions.
Mobility disorder	Among those with severe intellectual disability, 15% have difficulty walking, and 10% are unable to walk.
Iatrogenic disorders	Incidence of side effects from medications is increased. Communication difficulties prevent early recognition of symptoms.

Adapted from Keywood K, Fovargue S, Flynn M. Best Practice? Healthcare Decision-Making by, with and for Adults with Learning Disabilities. Manchester, UK: NDT, 1999 and from Tuffrey-Wijne I. The palliative care needs of people with intellectual disabilities: A literature review. Palliat Med 2003;17:55-62.

TABLE 187-3 Mortality Patterns for People with Intellectual Disabilities	
CAUSE	**COMMENTS**
Cardiovascular disease	People with intellectual disabilities (IDs) have increased cardiovascular disease risk factors. Obesity is more common than in the general population, and people with IDs are more likely to lead sedentary lifestyles. Congenital heart disease and its sequelae are common in some groups, such as those with fragile-X, Williams', or Down syndrome.
Respiratory disease	Respiratory disorders are associated with several clinical phenotypes and account for a higher proportion of deaths of people with ID compared with the general population. Respiratory disease may develop because of congenital defects, such as musculoskeletal or cardiac abnormalities. It may also result from dysphagia, regurgitation, gastroesophageal reflux, and seizures.
Cancer	The incidences of specific cancers in people with IDs vary. There are known associations between certain syndromes and the development of different types of cancer. The link between Down syndrome and leukemia and testicular cancer is well documented. Tuberous sclerosis is associated with an increased incidence of cerebral and renal tumors. Several studies have shown an increased incidence of gastrointestinal tumors in the institutionalized population. Jancar and Jancar[15] found that 57% of cancer deaths resulted from this cause, compared with 25% in the general population. This may reflect a high infection rate for *Helicobacter pylori*.
Dementia	Dementia is increasingly recognized among older adults with IDs, particularly those with Down syndrome. The prevalence of Alzheimer's disease in people with Down syndrome increases with increasing age, and prevalence rates between 6% and 75% have been reported.[16] There appears to be no relationship between level of IDs and risk for dementia or age at onset of dementia, although the level of intellectual impairment has been associated with the rate of decline.

Adapted from tables in Meusen-van de Kerkhof R, van Brommel H, van de Wouw W, Maaskant M. Perceptions of death and management of grief in people with intellectual disability. J Policy Pract Intellect Disabil 2006;3:95-104.

general health care issues, rather than end-of-life concerns. Many adults with intellectual disabilities are not involved in decisions about their own health care, and clinicians may not offer the same treatment options to people with disabilities because of perceived difficulties in obtaining informed consent or concerns about litigation[7] (see "Case Study: Consent and Intellectual Capacity").

In law, adults are presumed to possess capacity, unless demonstrated otherwise. Capacity is a complex concept and difficult to assess. In the past, the *status approach* to capacity was used, and those with a low IQ were automatically assumed to be incompetent. Later, this approach was rejected and was replaced by the *functional approach* to capacity. It recognizes that capacity arises in a specific context, such as capacity to make a will or the ability to consent to medical treatment. It views capacity as being issue and time specific.

CASE STUDY

Consent and Intellectual Capacity

John is a 52-year-old man with Down syndrome and with a moderate intellectual disability and basic verbal ability. He was treated for depression in the past but has not required antidepressant medication recently. He lived at home until 6 years ago, when he moved into a group home in the community after the death of his father. He remains very close to his elderly mother and regularly returns to the family home to visit her. John works in a sheltered employment center and enjoys an active social life.

The care staff members notice that John has become easily fatigued and that he has lost weight. They arrange for him to visit his local physician, who finds evidence of a mass on examination of John's abdomen. Because of concern that the mass may be malignant, John is referred for further investigation. John is alarmed by the need to visit the hospital for the investigation and asks the care staff whether something is wrong. The care staff are unsure how best to reply. They do not want to worry him unnecessarily and do not feel that they have sufficient information to answer his questions correctly. They reply by reassuring him that there is nothing wrong.

Subsequent investigations confirm that John has gastric cancer. The hospital clinicians refer John's care back to his local physician because they decide that his disease is too advanced and his functional status is too poor to pursue active therapy. They do not discuss this with John but tell him that "everything will be taken care of." His physician then convenes a case conference with John's mother and the care staff to discuss how palliative care can be best provided. It is agreed that John will remain for as long as is possible in the group home. John's mother does not want him to be told about his diagnosis because she feels that the truth will be too distressing for him to cope with.

If a person is judged incompetent to make a specific decision, it is necessary for someone else to make the decision on their behalf. The laws that govern this process vary from country to country, and different jurisdictions place various degrees of emphasis on the relative importance of the *best interests* and the *substituted judgment* standards. Whichever legal framework surrounds the decision-making process, it is important that a person should not be treated as unable to make a decision unless all practicable steps to help him or her to do so have been taken.

Truth Telling and Collusion

Problems concerning truth telling are not unique to people with intellectual disabilities, because it is a natural instinct for family members to try to protect their relative from the knowledge that an illness is incurable. Caregivers are often particularly concerned about the effects such information would have on the person with intellectual disability, and they may argue that the person will not understand or that the truth is too upsetting. It is accepted that the biological reality of their own physical deterioration can result in those without intellectual disability becoming aware of their impending death, even when they are not told. The case is not as clear for a person with intellectual disability, because the lifelong treatment of death as taboo may mean that they have no models of illness or death on which to base their current experiences. Even so, case reports suggest that awareness can develop.[8]

The pressure to maintain a conspiracy of silence can be intense, and family patterns of behavior can result in the person being overprotected. However, people with intellectual disabilities often lack control and choices, and maintenance of a conspiracy of silence may result in total loss of their autonomy. Decisions about truth telling should be made in the same way as they are for the general population, and they should be grounded on ethical principles while considering individual circumstances. When considering individual circumstances, health care professionals should assess the person's levels of emotional and conceptual understanding. Family and caregivers should be involved at all stages of the process and support provided for them (see "Case Study: Truth in Communication").

Symptom Assessment

Self-report measures are considered to be the gold standard of pain management, but they pose challenges for individuals with impairments of communication. In the past, it was suggested that people with severe disabilities demonstrated pain insensitivity, but it is now recognized that an inability to verbally communicate pain does not mean it is absent. Caregivers need to be alert to the many ways people with intellectual disabilities may signal that pain is present, such as behavioral change or specific words or sounds.

The term *alternative communication* describes the nonverbal signs and behaviors people use in the place of language.[9] Research on alternative communication has focused on expression of physical pain. There are difficulties inherent in distinguishing expressions of physical pain from other causes of distress. Assessment tools, such as the Disability Distress Assessment Tool (DisDAT), should be used carefully to ensure that all expressions of distress are not treated with analgesics.[10] This involves documenting an individual's usual patterns of communication when content. Distress can then be identified if the baseline changes. After distress has been recognized, a clinical decision checklist guides caregivers in determining its cause.

People with intellectual disabilities tend to tolerate symptoms or to express them atypically as irritability, inactivity, loss of appetite, and sleep disturbance.[11] This is particularly true for symptoms of chest pain, dyspnea, dyspepsia, and micturition. This highlights the importance of remaining vigilant and avoiding the pitfall of diagnostic overshadowing, which occurs when behavioral manifestations of discomfort are mistakenly attributed to intellectual disability rather than physical illness.

Communication Skills

Many people with intellectual disabilities have limited communication or social skills, and they may have difficulty explaining their symptoms or understanding questions. They may have had negative experiences or interactions with health care professionals that affect sub-

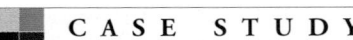

CASE STUDY

Truth in Communication

John returns to the group home, and his condition continues to deteriorate. He spends most of his time in bed. He appears distressed, and although he indicates that he has abdominal pain, he is unable to give much detail about his symptoms. He continues to ask what is wrong, and his mood appears depressed. He talks frequently about his deceased father and is afraid to go to sleep. Members of the care staff are divided; some feel that these are indications that they should engage in discussion about his illness, but others disagree.

Additional strain develops within the house when some of the other service users living in the house begin to ask questions about John's condition. Staff members are unsure how to handle issues of confidentiality and are worried that the service users will inadvertently frighten John further. A referral to the palliative care team is made to seek specialist help.

The palliative care team assesses John, concludes that he has poorly controlled nausea and abdominal pain, and recommends altering his medications. The team members feel that anxiety and fear are contributing to his distress, and they suggest that this issue be explored further. They do not feel confident in their ability to communicate effectively with John, however, and are reluctant to start the process themselves. After much discussion with John's mother and the staff from the intellectual disability service, it is agreed that the two services will work in partnership to address the issue.

A psychologist from the intellectual disability service, who worked with John when he had depression, undertakes preparatory work with John, the palliative care nurse, and John's key worker. A trusting relationship is built among all participants as John begins to review recent events and explore his feelings in the initial stages of the work. It becomes apparent that John has drawn some analogies between his own condition and that of his father before he died. As John's concerns are addressed, his distress lessens.

The team also explores John's feelings toward his fellow residents and his attitude about disclosure of information to them. John is unable to grasp the concepts of truth telling or involvement of other residents. However, it is clear that he places high value on a relationship with one particular resident and has welcomed the involvement of the other residents in his life. The team members decide in consultation with his mother that they will provide the service users with general information about John's illness to help prepare them for the changes ahead. They will also support John's ongoing relationships with his peers with the aim of maximizing his quality of life. This is successfully achieved, and John dies comfortably a few weeks later in the presence of his mother and care staff. His close friend had been at his bedside earlier that day.

sequent encounters. Interactions may therefore need to be undertaken on a gradual or staged basis, with time spent building a relationship of trust. Longer periods should be set aside for communication, and conversation should be in simple language and short sentences, appropriate to the person's developmental level. Professionals should remain sensitive to nonverbal cues and consider novel approaches to communication, such as music or art.

The usual models for breaking bad news rely on individuals having the ability to recognize a "warning shot," and this subtlety may not be recognized by people with intellectual disabilities.[12] It may instead cause distress if the individual becomes frustrated by indirect communication. People with intellectual disabilities may not understand the need to ask questions to get information, and they are also often likely to acquiesce to what they believe the health care professional wants to hear.

People with intellectual disabilities often have a short attention span, and it is helpful to recapitulate and summarize previously stated material. This also provides the opportunity to check their understanding of what has been discussed. They may have a limited ability to express emotions verbally and instead express emotions in atypical ways or through behavioral disturbance. The caregivers must recognize these nonverbal methods of communication and respond appropriately.

Conceptualization of Illness and Death

The way death and bereavement are experienced significantly depends on the intellectual and social-emotional age of the person.[13] Strategies are available (Table 187-4) that the health care professional may employ to support a person with intellectual disability who is experiencing loss.

ISSUES OF STAFF SUPPORT

Professionals working in organizations providing services for people with intellectual disabilities are frequently inexperienced in palliative care and may not be educationally or emotionally prepared to support those facing their own death or that of a peer. Nevertheless, staff members from intellectual disability services usually wish to continue in their roles as the main caregivers because of their close relationships with the individual. We need to recognize the significant nature of this relationship and be aware of a possible need to provide educational and emotional support to the staff (see "Case Study: Staff Support"). Staff members working in organizations providing services for people with intellectual disabilities report that they value collaboration with palliative care teams. They benefit from the informal support structure of the team and find it helpful to participate in funerals, remembrance services, and debriefings.

TABLE 187-4 Strategies for Dealing with Bereavement and Loss for the Person with an Intellectual Disability		
LEVEL OF INTELLECTUAL DISABILITY	**EXPERIENCE OF THE PERSON**	**SUPPORT**
Mild IQ: 50 to 70 Intellectual age: 7-12 yr	Clear realization of death Logical thought coupled to specific events Empathy exists but experienced from own perspective Grieving process comparable to general population	Engage in open communication Offer closeness: share bereavement experience and offer participation in mourning rituals Explore the feelings that lie behind reactions Engage in reminiscence
Moderate IQ: 35 to 55 Intellectual age: 4 to 8 yr	Limited realization of death Searching for logical explanations of death; growing comprehension of the irreversibility of death Basic capability of putting oneself in another person's place; projection of own feelings onto other person; feelings of guilt and fear as reactions to other people's grief Mourning reactions emerge at a later time	Provide opportunity to express grief; give logical explanations to questions, make connections visible Offer closeness: "be there" for the other person Make use of rituals, life stories, and photographs Remember the deceased person, talk about him
Severe IQ: 20 to 40 Intellectual age: 2-5 yr	Limited realization of death, death seen as temporary, magical thinking, realization of death as irreversible starts to grow as deceased person is increasingly missed Beginning of linking events such as sickness and death, understanding of death linked to concrete experiences Egocentric way of thinking Limited development of words, emotions expressed nonverbally Model behavior of others has strong influence on experience of death	Keep daily life organized and familiar; let others take over the most important patterns belonging to the deceased person Offer closeness: "be there" for the other person Make concept of death clear by answering questions on a concrete level; adjust imaginary images of death to prevent fear Watch own (model) behavior, make own emotions known, watch own language Use a variety of approaches to explore emotions, such as play, music, art Use specific (good-bye) rituals and symbols for grief management
Profound IQ: Up to 25 Intellectual age: 0-2 yr	No realization of death; loss mainly causes a disruption of bonding, security, and confidence; understanding is based on sensual (body-centered) impressions and experiences Communication is nonverbal Reactions of mourning emerge only at a later time	Offer closeness: physical contact Keep daily life organized and familiar; let others take over the most important patterns belonging to the deceased person Important resources: posture, facial expression, intonation of voice, making use of one's favorite senses, respectful touching Allow people to concretely experience change but within the space of a secure environment; offer concrete experiences to help cope with loss, enable people to feel or see what death means

◼ C A S E S T U D Y

Staff Support

John's caregivers thought that the strain that they had experienced during the course of his illness would subside after his death, but this did not happen. The staff members had feelings of guilt and felt that they "should have done more." They were preoccupied by the thought that they had in some way missed signs of his illness that might have allowed an earlier diagnosis to be made, and they were concerned that he might have suffered pain without their recognition of it. They wanted to support the other service users in grieving John's loss, but they were unsure about how to do it. The staff also felt under pressure to "return to life as normal" and to take on another service user who needed residential placement. They were torn between a professional obligation to meet the needs of the new service user and a personal feeling that it was too soon to fill John's place in the house.

BEREAVEMENT

People with intellectual disabilities are developing more varied relationships as they live longer, and the value that they place on relationships developed with peers or other members of the community should not be underestimated. The relationship between those with intellectual disability and parents remains key. Strong attachments and dependence commonly develop between elderly parents and adults with an intellectual disability who have lived together for many years. The death of a parent may be a catastrophic life event because of the loss of this relationship and because the death may result in the person experiencing the additional loss of the family home.

The preparation that a person with an intellectual disability receives for the impending death of a relative or peer is often minimal because of a tendency to withhold information about the illness. Although this may be done to protect them from anxiety, it effectively makes their grief more acute and long-term mental health problems more likely. These problems may be compounded by the exclusion of the disabled from rituals of grieving, such as funerals.

There has been little systematic research done on bereavement by people with intellectual disabilities.[14] Those who have experienced bereavement are at increased risk for mental health difficulties and aberrant behavior. People with intellectual disabilities may experience a delayed reaction to loss, and caregivers commonly do not relate subsequent behavioral disturbances to grief.

Dealing with death and bereavement is difficult, and people with intellectual disabilities are particularly disadvantaged because of social exclusion, disempowerment, and impairments of cognition, adaptive skills, and communication. It is therefore essential that caregivers engage in forward planning whenever a loss is anticipated to reduce the risk of complicated bereavement (Box 187-1).

Box 187-1 Approach to the Care of the Person with Intellectual Disability

- Everyone with an intellectual disability (ID) is a person with a distinct identity and unique life experiences, rather than a person with a label.
- Professionals should focus first on what a person with ID can do with (or without) support, rather than on what he or she cannot do.
- More than 50% of people with IDs have significant impairment of communication. They may need additional time and aides to express themselves. The involvement of a caregiver who knows the individual well can be of help in the process.
- People with IDs tend to communicate distress nonverbally. Caregivers may find the systematic use of symptom assessment tools, such as the Disability Distress Assessment Tool (DisDAT), to be helpful.
- *Challenging behavior* is a term used to describe severe problematic behavior. It has several causes, including environmental stressors, psychiatric disorders, and physical illness. It is important to find the underlying cause for the behavior to avoid the mistake of "diagnostic overshadowing."
- People with IDs are often not told about their illness or its significance. Family members and health care professionals should consider whether collusion lessens or contributes to the distress of the individual concerned, and they should act accordingly.
- The ability of people with IDs to understand the concept of illness and death is affected by their cognitive and emotional intelligence and their life experiences. These factors should be taken into consideration when communicating with a person with an ID about death and dying.
- The nature of the relationship between the person with an ID and his or her family may be complex, and family patterns of behavior may be accentuated when facing a life-limiting illness. Staff should be aware of the possible need for increased supports at this time.
- Staff working in organizations providing services for people with IDs may have their own emotional reactions to the diagnosis of a life-limiting illness. They often lack experience in the provision of palliative care to service users, and considerable support may be needed from palliative care specialists to enable the ID staff to cope.
- Palliative care specialists tend to lack confidence and experience in caring for people with IDs, and collaborative, multidisciplinary approaches to care should be undertaken.

DEVELOPMENTS AND RESEARCH OPPORTUNITIES

There is a lack of information on the palliative care needs of this population. The process of involving people with intellectual disabilities in research and service development is challenging but essential. Innovative research methodologies should be explored and encouraged.

Social services and health services traditionally operate with different types of skills, management systems, and value bases. Deficits in service provision should be addressed by a model that is patient centered and caregiver oriented and that brings palliative care and intellectual disability services into partnership. There is a growing awareness of the specific palliative care needs of this population. Knowledge deficits should be addressed with focused education and training initiatives.

Intellectual disability services characteristically show innovative approaches to partnership working, have expert communication skills, and promote advocacy and client autonomy. Palliative care services have much to gain by partnership in such an environment.

REFERENCES

1. World Health Organization (WHO). The ICD-10 Classification of Mental and Behavioural Disorders. Clinical Descriptions and Diagnostic Guidelines. Geneva: World Health Organization, 1992.
2. Union of Physically Impaired against Segregation (UPIAS). Fundamental Principles of Disability. London: UPIAS, 1976.
3. Raynham H, Gibbons R, Flint J, Higgs D. The genetic basis of mental retardation. QJM 1996;89:169-175.
4. Beange H, McElduff A, Baker W. Medical disorders of adults with mental retardation: A population study. Am J Ment Retard 1995;99:595-604.
5. Borthwick-Duffy SA. Epidemiology and prevalence of psychopathology in people with mental retardation. J Consult Clin Psychol 1994;62:17-27.
6. Patja K, Molsa P, Iivanainen M. Cause-specific mortality of people with intellectual disability in a population-based, 35-year follow-up study. J Intellect Disabil Res 2001;45:30-40.
7. Keywood K, Fovargue S, Flynn M. Best Practice? Healthcare Decision-Making by, with and for Adults with Learning Disabilities. Manchester, UK: NDT, 1999.
8. Tuffrey-Wijne I. The palliative care needs of people with intellectual disabilities: A literature review. Palliat Med 2003;17:55-62.
9. Glennen SL. Introduction to augmentative and alternative communication. In Glennen SL, DeCoste DC (eds). Handbook of Augmentative and Alternative Communication. San Diego, CA: Singular Publishing Group, 1997, pp 3-19.
10. Regnard, C, Reynolds J, Watson B, et al. Understanding distress in people with severe communication difficulties: Developing and assessing the Disability Distress Assessment Tool (DisDAT). J Intellect Disabil Res 2007;51:277-292.
11. Evenhuis HM. Medical aspects of ageing in a population with intellectual disability. III. Mobility, internal conditions and cancer. J Intellect Disabil Res 1997;41(Pt 1):8-18.
12. McEnhill L. Disability. In Oliviere D, Monroe B (eds). Death, Dying and Social Differences. Oxford, UK: Oxford University Press, 2004, pp 97-118.
13. Meeusen-van de Kerkhof R, van Bommel H, van de Wouw W, Maaskant M. Perceptions of death and management of grief in people with intellectual disability. J Policy Pract Intellect Disabil 2006;3:95-104.
14. Dodd P, Dowling S, Hollins S. A review of the emotional, psychiatric and behavioural responses to bereavement in people with intellectual disabilities. J Intellect Disabil Res 2005;49(Pt 7):537-543.
15. Jancar MP, Jancar J. Cancer and mental retardation (a forty-year review). Br Med Chirug J 1997;92:3-7.
16. Stanton LR, Coetzee RH. Down's syndrome and dementia. Adv Psy Treat 2004;10:50-58.

SUGGESTED READING

Blackman N, Todd S. Caring for People with Learning Disabilities Who Are Dying. London: Worth Publishing, 2003.

Brown H, Burns S, Flynn M. Dying Matters. London: Salomans Centre and Foundation for People with Learning Disabilities, 2005.

Hollins S, Sireling L. Books Beyond Words Series. London: St George's Mental Health Library and Royal College of Psychiatrists, 1994.

Jones A, Tuffrey-Wijne I. Positive Approaches to Palliative Care. Worcestershire, UK: British Institute for Learning Disabilities, 2004.

Read S (ed). Palliative Care for People with Learning Disabilities. London: Quay Books, 2006.

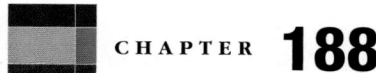

CHAPTER **188**

Musculoskeletal Disorders

Eliza Pontifex and Barry Bresnihan

KEY POINTS

- There are no disease-modifying agents for osteoarthritis, and successful management requires a multidisciplinary approach.
- Osteoporosis is underrecognized and undertreated despite the availability of many management guidelines and effective drugs.
- Biological agents have offered the best chance of achieving remission in a number of autoimmune diseases.
- A paradigm change leading to the early introduction of disease-modifying agents in inflammatory joint disease has raised an expectation for prevention of joint deformity and disability.
- There are no unequivocally effective disease-modifying agents for systemic sclerosis, and there is a clear role for palliative medicine in the later stages of the disease.

Advanced chronic musculoskeletal disorders are frequently associated with local or widespread pain that can be severe and debilitating. Major disability arising from irreversible damage to articular structures, bone, or muscle can add to the level of distress of patients and their caregivers. This chapter addresses some of the relatively common degenerative, metabolic, and inflammatory musculoskeletal disorders that are seen in rheumatology practice and in community care services.

OSTEOARTHRITIS

Basic Science

A new paradigm is emerging for the pathogenesis of osteoarthritis. Research into the early stages of this disease reveals a dynamic chondropathy with changes in adjacent bone and synovial inflammation. This challenges the traditional view of osteoarthritis as an inevitable consequence of age and wear and tear.

Epidemiology and Prevalence

Osteoarthritis is the most common type of arthritis, with a striking increase in prevalence from middle age onward. The prevalence of knee osteoarthritis alone in older populations is estimated to be up to 30%. Its natural history is progression with time, and the consequential burden on our aging society is huge, with osteoarthritis already being one of the most significant causes of disability in the elderly. Obesity is strongly associated with knee osteoarthritis and genetic factors with generalized nodal osteoarthritis, but other associations, such as occupation, are less clear.

Pathophysiology

Osteoarthritis develops when there is a loss of balance between articular cartilage synthesis and degradation. This process is multifactorial and involves biomechanical, inflammatory, and metabolic factors. Activation of chondrocytes by inflammatory mediators, mechanical stress, or other mechanisms leads to increased production of proteolytic enzymes, which breakdown cartilage extracellular matrix. The counterbalancing protective effect of tissue inhibitors of these enzymes is impaired, and the result is a net loss of cartilage. Pro-inflammatory cytokines from the synovium such as interleukin-1 (IL-1) and tumor necrosis factor-α (TNF-α) also contribute to cartilage destruction.[1] In severe cases, articular cartilage and synovial fluid quality is lost, leaving bone at the joint interface.

Clinical Manifestations

Osteoarthritis pain may originate from a bone, distended joint capsule, entheses, bursae, and muscle spasm. Typically, there is a diffuse, aching pain in the involved joint or referred area with use and relief with rest. "Crunching," "grating," or other mechanical symptoms may be described. These symptoms are caused by cartilage loss, irregularity of the joint surface, or loose bodies. In advanced cases, nocturnal joint pain may occur because of the loss of protective muscle splinting, which prevents painful range of movement during the day.

In the spine, posterior vertebral osteophytes, disc herniation, and hypertrophy of the ligamentum flavum and facet joints can cause narrowing of the spinal canal, leading to the clinical features of spinal stenosis. The latter three can cause outlet obstruction for nerve roots, producing radicular pain. Lumbar facet joint osteoarthritis causes low centralized back, buttock, and thigh pain that worsens with joint loading. Osteoarthritic joints in the elderly are susceptible to crystal arthropathies, and in debilitated patients, they can become infected in the presence of bacteremia.

Differential Diagnosis

Fractures, infection, and tumors should be excluded in cases of monoarthropathies and complicated spinal stenosis. Inflammatory, metabolic, and crystal arthropathies and polymyalgia rheumatica should be considered if joints or regions in classic distributions are affected.

The neurological differential diagnosis for radiculopathies includes peripheral entrapment neuropathies and plexopathies. Spinal stenosis can mimic the calf claudication of lower limb arterial insufficiency.

Treatment

Effective pharmacological agents for osteoarthritis have not advanced far beyond symptom relief. Outcomes are best when drug therapy is combined with multidisciplinary biopsychosocial rehabilitation, because such an approach improves function and, to a lesser degree, pain (Table 188-1). Severe osteoarthritis that has not responded satisfactorily to combined allied and medical management deserves consideration for surgical or pain unit interven-

TABLE 188-1 Nonpharmacological Measures That Improve Osteoarthritis Joint Function or Pain Outcomes
Education
Self-management program
Weight loss for load reduction on weight-bearing joints
Community social support
Physiotherapy
Lifting and reaching techniques for spinal osteoarthritis
Resistance and aerobic exercise for knee and hip osteoarthritis
Walking aids for reducing load and pain
Transcutaneous electrical nerve stimulation and thermotherapy for knee osteoarthritis
Medial knee taping for patellofemoral osteoarthritis
Occupational therapy
Functional aids for activities of daily living
Podiatry
Wedged insoles for deformity caused by knee osteoarthritis
Other therapy
Acupuncture for shoulder osteoarthritis
Avocado-soybean unsaponifiable supplements for knee osteoarthritis

tions and, failing that, palliation. In properly selected patients with severe osteoarthritis or spinal stenosis, surgical outcomes from procedures such as joint replacement or decompression surgery are superior to medical treatments in the short and long terms. Pursuit of an anatomical diagnosis of chronic low back pain using anesthetic or steroid injections of joints, sensory nerve blocks, or other procedures in a pain unit may be valuable.

Drugs of Choice

The pharmacological approach to osteoarthritis involves graduation from simple analgesics to opiates. Although the superiority of combinations over monotherapy has not been widely studied, such an approach is endorsed by the American College of Rheumatology[2] and the European League against Rheumatism.[3] Most of the simple analgesics are better than placebo in treating osteoarthritis, and topical capsaicin cream, nonsteroidal anti-inflammatory drug (NSAID) gel, and lignocaine patches may also be effective for superficial joints. Opioid or opiate patches are useful for chronic pain in osteoarthritis.

Slow-acting drugs for treating symptomatic osteoarthritis, such as glucosamine (1500 mg/day) and chondroitin sulfate (1200 mg/day), may provide superior pain relief in combination compared with placebo in moderate to severe knee osteoarthritis and may retard radiographically confirmed disease progression in mild to moderate osteoarthritis.

Supportive Care

General multidisciplinary care is described in Table 188-1. More specific recommendations are given in the following sections.

KNEE

With the use of an intra-articular steroid injection in the knee, rapid symptom relief usually occurs within 24 hours and can last for more than 2 months. No clinical feature predicts a better response, including the presence of an effusion, and the only articular contraindications are infection or surgical metal within the joint. Because of concerns about ligament and cartilage damage, intra-articular steroid injections are not recommended more often than every third month, but there is no conclusive evidence to support this practice, and palliative care patients' wishes and physicians' judgment should prevail. This applies to all osteoarthritis joints.

Intra-articular viscosupplement injections are sometimes used. However, a series of intra-articular injections of a synthetic high-molecular-weight polysaccharide is unlikely to benefit patients with severe osteoarthritis.

Tidal irrigation, arthroscopy, and débridement have been tried. There is no benefit from tidal irrigation in severe osteoarthritis, and only patients with mechanical symptoms, such as from loose cartilage fragments, and those with some remaining joint space seen on the radiograph may benefit from débridement.

SHOULDER

Suprascapular nerve block with local anesthetic or steroid done at the bedside can relieve shoulder pain with minimal motor deficit.[4]

SPINE

Because patients often have a mixed mechanical picture clinically and radiologically, the worst symptoms are the best guide to which regional measures are worth pursuing. Facet joints are symptomatic in 15% to 40% of patients with chronic low back pain. There is little evidence to support joint steroid injection, although anecdotally, some patients benefit. Radiofrequency medial branch neurotomy is carried out in pain units and may be better than placebo.

For spinal stenosis, steroid or local anesthetic injections around the gluteal, piriformis, and erector spinae muscles have anecdotally provided symptom relief in some patients. There is no benefit from injecting steroid into intervertebral discs, but newer interventional therapies such as electrotherapy to "shrink" or "seal" discs are promising for discogenic pain. Epidural corticosteroid injections at the clinically and radiologically stenosed level may improve symptoms, and caudal epidural blocks or intrathecal opioids are last resorts for intractable pain.

For patients with radiculopathy, oral pregabalin or similar drugs may improve radicular symptoms without the need for further intervention. Failing that, diagnostic or therapeutic nerve root injection with a local anesthetic or steroid can be performed for pain relief.

For chronic low back pain, various nonpharmacological therapies have been trialed. They are listed in Table 188-2.

OSTEOPOROSIS

Basic Science

Bone is a dynamic tissue. It remains under construction throughout life, with sites of resorption coupled with sites of new bone deposition. This process is driven by mechanical stress and by hormonal and metabolic mechanisms.

TABLE 188-2 Nonpharmacological Therapies for Chronic Low Back Pain

Positive results*
  Behavioral therapy
  Spinal manipulation
  Acupuncture
  Medium-firm mattress (superior to hard firm mattress)
Inconclusive results*
  Percutaneous electrical nerve stimulation
  Botulinum toxin
  Dorsal column stimulation
  Radiofrequency denervation
  Intradiscal electrotherapy
Negative results*
  Transcutaneous electrical nerve stimulation
  Biofeedback using electromyography
  Magnets
  Prolotherapy
  Orthoses, traction

*Results of studies comparing nonpharmacological therapies with placebo or no treatment for chronic low back pain of various causes.

Osteoporosis describes the net loss of bone mineral density (BMD) when bone resorption exceeds bone deposition at remodeling sites as we age. It is defined as the point at which the BMD of a postmenopausal woman or that of a man older than 50 years falls to or below 2.5 standard deviations below that of the young, healthy population as measured by dual-energy x-ray absorptiometry. This definition is controversial in clinical practice, as there are many factors in addition to BMD that affect fracture risk.

Epidemiology and Prevalence

Osteoporosis has been dubbed *the silent epidemic*, with a prevalence of one in three women and one in five men over a lifetime in the Irish population. Although more common in older age groups, particularly in postmenopausal women, the list of other risk factors and secondary causes is lengthening and includes malignancy, glucocorticoids, antiepileptic drugs, sex hormone antagonists, and immobility. A practical web-based tool developed by the World Health Organization called FRAX is now available online. It predicts an individual's 10-year risk of experiencing an osteoporotic fracture.

Pathophysiology

The precise mechanisms that lead to idiopathic osteoporosis are poorly understood. A number of age-related factors contribute, including changes in bone cell function and decreases in calcium absorption and vitamin D production, but estrogen deficiency and its early effect on accelerating imbalanced bone remodeling is the most potent.

Clinical Manifestations

A fragility fracture, one that occurs spontaneously or because of an impact from a fall from standing height, is the only clinical manifestation of osteoporosis. In the spine, the common fracture site is the thoracolumbar region, and these fractures may take up to 3 months to heal. An isolated vertebral collapse above the T7 level is unusual in idiopathic osteoporosis, and other causes should be sought. One third of acute vertebral fragility fractures are symptomatic, and of these, 75% persist as a source of chronic pain. Multiple fractures are common, and 20% of patients have further vertebral fractures within the next 12 months. The resulting kyphosis can lead to chronic neck pain from holding it in extension, muscular back pain, mechanical respiratory problems, and the painful costoiliac impingement syndrome.

Differential Diagnosis

Other causes of fragility fractures or acute bone pain include bony metastases, Paget's disease, and avascular necrosis of the femoral head.

Treatment

Professional bodies in several countries have published guidelines for the prevention and management of osteoporosis. Overall, there is general consensus for treating established osteoporosis, but guidelines for prevention in different contexts are still a matter of debate.

Drugs of Choice

For established osteoporosis, there are several therapeutic alternatives. Oral or intravenous bisphosphonates, selective estrogen receptor modulators, or androgens in deficient men are the first-line therapies used in combination with calcium and vitamin D supplementation, if not contraindicated. Although recommendations vary regionally, 1500 mg of calcium and 800 IU of vitamin D daily are suggested by the American College of Rheumatology.[5] Other agents include strontium ranelate, parathyroid hormone (PTH) analogues, and calcitonin. The latter two should not be prescribed without consultation with a specialist.

Supportive Care

Patients with and at risk for osteoporosis should be counseled about ceasing smoking, getting safe exposure to sunlight, drinking alcohol in moderation, getting 30 minutes of weight-bearing exercise three times each week, and ensuring adequate dietary sources of calcium and vitamin D.

PREVENTION

Patients taking 5 mg or more of prednisolone per day for more than 3 months should receive calcium and vitamin D supplementation, and bisphosphonate therapy or gonadal steroids (for deficient men) should be considered.[5] Bisphosphonates can prevent bone loss in patients taking androgen-deprivation therapy for prostate cancer and aromatase inhibitors for breast cancer. No professional guidelines yet exist for these regimens.

MANAGEMENT OF FRAGILITY FRACTURE

An acute fragility fracture is managed in the same way as a traumatic fracture—with orthopedic intervention if required and surgical consultation if a fractured vertebra is unstable or causing cord compression. For pain relief, simple analgesics are started, and other drug classes are added as required. Admission to the hospital may be necessary for symptom control and to ensure mobilization resumes as early as tolerated by the patient to prevent further bone loss.

There is no robust evidence that oral or intravenous bisphosphonates are effective for acute fragility fracture pain. However, nasal calcitonin (200 IU/day) was shown in one small trial to accelerate vertebral fracture pain relief compared with placebo and could be used as first-line osteoporosis therapy for 4 months after a painful fracture.[6]

Vertebroplasty and kyphoplasty have been developed to essentially replace crushed vertebral bone. Vertebroplasty involves a fluoroscopically guided injection of bone cement into the collapsed vertebra. Kyphoplasty is the insertion of an inflatable bone tamp into the collapsed vertebral body to separate the vertebral end plates before injection of bone cement. These procedures are outpatient based, are minimally invasive, and can improve spinal anatomy. Early pain relief rates have been as high as 90%,[7] but because controlled trials and long-term outcomes are lacking, patients with focal symptoms corresponding well to radiological fracture sites should be carefully selected for these procedures.

PREVENTION OF FALLS

Prevention of falls should be addressed with the assistance of allied health professionals. Mobility aids (e.g., vision assistance, rails, footwear, walking aids) and agility and resistance exercises have prolonged effects in reducing falls for the elderly. Vitamin D supplementation improves muscle strength, function, and balance. Medication can be chosen to minimize side effects such as postural hypotension, tremor, and sedation. Hip protectors are available for use.

CHRONIC INFLAMMATORY JOINT DISEASES

Basic Science

The onset of an inflammatory arthropathy is characterized by proliferation of new blood vessels in the synovium that lines the joint.[8] The activated vascular endothelium facilitates the migration of inflammatory cells into the synovium, where large amounts of cytokines, growth factors, tissue-degrading enzymes, antibodies, and other mediators are produced. The persistence and extent of these inflammatory events are determined by genetic, immunological, and environmental factors that are not fully understood. These factors also determine the phenotype of the arthritis, such as rheumatoid arthritis, ankylosing spondylitis, or undifferentiated arthritis. Rheumatoid arthritis and ankylosing spondylitis are discussed further as examples of chronic inflammatory joint diseases that are frequently associated with impaired quality of life and high levels of pain, disability, and suffering.

Epidemiology and Prevalence

Rheumatoid arthritis has an annual incidence of approximately 0.2 cases per 1000 males and 0.4 cases per 1000 females. A prevalence of 0.5% to 1.0% is reported in diverse populations worldwide. Twin studies show that rheumatoid arthritis has a heritability rate of 60%.

The annual incidence of ankylosing spondylitis is approximately 6.6 cases per 100,000 members of the white population in North American and in Europe, with a prevalence of 0.5% to 1.0%. The male-to-female ratio is 5:1. Ankylosing spondylitis is rare in African Americans. The strong association between the disease and the HLA-B27 marker is consistent in all populations.

Pathophysiology

The initiation of rheumatoid arthritis is thought to involve the presentation of a putative antigen to CD4$^+$ T lymphocytes, which then accumulate in synovial tissue. Activated T cells stimulate macrophages to secrete pro-inflammatory cytokines, including IL-1 and TNF-α, which induce secretion of tissue-degrading prostaglandin and metalloproteinase by fibroblast-like synoviocytes. These proliferating cells migrate across the surface of adjacent cartilage, forming a pannus, and subsequently, in association with other cell populations, they invade cartilage and bone, causing progressive and irreversible joint damage.

Inflammation in ankylosing spondylitis has a predilection for fibrocartilaginous sites, and subchondral bone marrow inflammation in the sacroiliac and axial joints and at peripheral sites adjacent to certain entheses is characteristic. HLA-B27 is directly involved in the pathogenesis.

Clinical Manifestations

The characteristic pattern of joint involvement in rheumatoid arthritis is symmetrical and polyarticular, affecting large and small joints of the upper and lower limbs. In advanced disease, affected joints may include the atlanto-axial joint, sometimes associated with cervical cord compression, and the temporomandibular joints, which can affect nutritional intake. Linear progression of joint damage due to partially suppressed synovial inflammation may continue for many years. This combination results in increasing disability, pain, and fatigue.

A minority of patients may develop rheumatoid arthritis–associated vasculitis, interstitial lung disease, pleurisy or pericarditis, peripheral neuropathy, and rarely, amyloidosis. Patients with chronic, long-standing rheumatoid arthritis have a higher incidence of other co-morbidities, such as Sjögren's syndrome, osteoporosis, ischemic heart disease, peripheral vascular disease, chronic leg ulcers, renal impairment, recurring infection, and peptic ulcer disease, which can further add to the levels of distress, disability, and frailty.

The first symptoms of ankylosing spondylitis include spinal pain and morning spinal stiffness, and they usually commence between the ages of 18 and 25 years. Physical examination reveals a restricted range of spinal movement that can gradually progress over many years. Persistent inflammation of the axial joints results in loss of spinal and ribcage mobility due to bony ankylosis and debilitating spinal deformities by the fifth or sixth decade of life. In established ankylosing spondylitis, quality of life may be substantially impaired, largely because of high levels of pain, often predominantly in the neck, and disability. Limited chest expansion can cause restrictive pulmonary function with distressing respiratory symptoms, including

dyspnea on minimal exertion and sleep apnea. The nonaxial joints involved include proximal large joints such as shoulders and hips. Painful enthesitis at the ischial tuberosity, tibial tubercle, or Achilles tendon insertion is also characteristic.

Differential Diagnosis

In established seropositive, erosive rheumatoid arthritis, the clinical features are characteristic and not likely to cause diagnostic uncertainty. In early rheumatoid arthritis, other causes of inflammatory arthritis, such as gout, viral and other infection-associated arthropathies, sarcoidosis, psoriatic arthritis, and systemic lupus erythematosus, may need to be considered.

Treatment

Major advances in the treatment of rheumatoid arthritis have occurred in recent years. First, a philosophical shift has resulted in prescribing effective disease-modifying antirheumatic drugs (DMARDs) early in the disease course, preferably before the development of joint damage. It is possible to suppress synovial inflammation and modify the rate of joint damage in many patients with monotherapeutic or combination DMARD regimens. Second, the introduction of targeted anticytokine therapies (i.e., biological agents) to rheumatology practice has provided possibilities for sustained suppression of disease activity, remission, and healing of joint erosions.[9] Conventional DMARDs and anti-TNF-α agents can also benefit selected patients with advanced disease who have clinical evidence of persistent inflammation. In these patients, effective suppression of inflammation can reduce pain and disability scores to a level at which any remaining symptoms are attributable to irreversible structural damage and other co-morbidities.

Conventional DMARDs are ineffective in ankylosing spondylitis. However, the anti-TNF-α agents are highly effective. When introduced during the early years of the disease, striking reductions in disease activity measures have been described. Significant benefits in long-term outcomes are likely.

Drugs of Choice

Methotrexate is the most widely used conventional DMARD for treating rheumatoid arthritis. The usual maintenance dose is 15 to 20 mg/week, administered orally or subcutaneously. It is generally well tolerated and can be continued over many years. Long-term monitoring for evidence of bone marrow suppression and hepatotoxicity is mandatory. Other DMARDs widely used in clinical practice are sulfasalazine, leflunomide, and hydroxychloroquine. Low-dose corticosteroid therapy may be appropriate in some patients with systemic manifestations of rheumatoid arthritis or with partially controlled synovitis. Biological agents that block TNF-α (e.g., infliximab, adalimumab, etanercept) or IL-1 (e.g., anakinra) may have dramatic beneficial effects in patients and may greatly improve long-term outcomes.

Infliximab is administered by intravenous infusion, and the other approved anticytokine agents are administered by subcutaneous injection. These therapies require regular monitoring by a specialist. Newer targeted therapies for rheumatoid arthritis that are available in the United States include rituximab, which results in B-cell depletion, and abatacept, which modulates T-cell activation. Symptomatic control of pain and stiffness in rheumatoid arthritis is usually achieved by NSAIDs, with or without concomitant analgesia. High doses of fish oil (approximately 10 g/day) have an anti-inflammatory effect, among other health benefits, and can reduce a patient's requirement for NSAIDs.[10] In patients with advanced rheumatoid arthritis, potent analgesia, including opiates, may be required.[11]

NSAIDs have been the mainstay of pharmacological therapy in ankylosing spondylitis. Selected patients with high levels of disease activity and high severity scores have been successfully treated with the anti-TNF-α agents infliximab, adalimumab, and etanercept.

Supportive Care

Optimal supportive care of patients with chronic inflammatory joint diseases involves a multidisciplinary team consisting of rheumatology, orthopedic, nursing, physiotherapy, and occupational therapy experts. Easy access to other health care professionals, including a pain specialist, pharmacist, medical social worker, podiatrist, dietitian, and psychologist, is recommended. Patient education and self-management programs are encouraged[12] and should include the principles of bone and joint protection, pain management, energy conservation, nutrition, footwear, and skin and dental care. An appropriate exercise regimen to maintain muscle function, posture, mobility, and independence at different disease stages is essential.

SYSTEMIC SCLEROSIS

The term *connective tissue disease* is applied to a group of chronic systemic inflammatory diseases that includes systemic lupus erythematosus, systemic sclerosis, polymyositis, and dermatomyositis. Each can affect many organ systems, including the skin, joints, muscle, heart, lungs, kidneys, central nervous system, and digestive tract. Each disease is associated with the production of specific autoantibodies that may have a role in pathogenesis that has yet to be fully defined. Among the connective tissue diseases, systemic sclerosis is the disease most likely to require palliative medicine expertise.

Basic Science

Two processes, fibrosis and microvascular occlusion, characterize the pathological appearances of the involved organs in systemic sclerosis. Genetic and environmental factors are likely to influence susceptibility and severity, but exactly what and how remains unknown. The systemic nature of the disease suggests that a circulating substance or cell type may be important. The cell types involved in systemic sclerosis include endothelial cells, interstitial fibroblasts, vascular wall smooth muscle cells, and blood leukocytes.

Epidemiology and Prevalence

The incidence of systemic sclerosis is approximately 20 cases per 1 million people each year. The prevalence is more than 150 patients per 1 million people in the general population. Systemic sclerosis has a female predominance. Patients with diffuse systemic sclerosis have a mortality rate that is four to five times greater than the general population, and the 5-year survival rate is approximately 75%.

Pathophysiology

Systemic sclerosis fibroblasts display enhanced rates of proliferation and dysregulation of matrix synthesis, leading to increased collagen biosynthesis and its deposition throughout many organ systems. Several cytokines, including IL-1, IL-17, TNF-α, platelet-derived growth factor, and connective tissue growth factor, can directly or indirectly induce these processes The second major pathophysiological process in systemic sclerosis is dysfunction of acute and chronic vascular regulatory mechanisms. Initially, there is heightened vasospastic activity that progresses to structural derangement of the microcirculation. Small arteries and arterioles develop a fibrous, concentric intimal lesion that is often associated with intravascular thrombus and lumen occlusion. Platelet activity is increased, and the fibrinolytic process is impaired. Endothelial cell injury occurs at an early stage, leading to a distorted capillary architecture and significant loss of the vascular network without a balanced increase in angiogenesis. This net catabolism results in tissue ischemia and failure. Several peptides, including platelet-derived growth factor, TNF-α, endothelin, thrombospondin-1, and vascular endothelial growth factor, have been identified as likely mediators of vascular dysregulation in systemic sclerosis.

Clinical Manifestations

Systemic sclerosis can be a disfiguring, multisystem disease that may alter every aspect of an individual's life. The clinical features at any time depend on the severity and extent of tissue replacement by collagen deposition and by the intensity of microvascular disease. Subsets of systemic sclerosis have been identified that have distinctive clinical features and outcomes. In diffuse cutaneous systemic sclerosis, extensive skin changes usually follow within 1 year of the onset of Raynaud's phenomenon. Severe Raynaud's phenomenon may result in very painful cutaneous ischemia and ulceration. Early, significant interstitial lung disease, oliguric renal failure, diffuse gastrointestinal disease, myocardial involvement, and musculoskeletal disease may develop. Progressive skin tightening causing digital contractures significantly impairs hand function and independence. There is an association between diffuse cutaneous systemic sclerosis and serum anti-topoisomerase antibodies (anti-Scl-70).

In limited cutaneous systemic sclerosis, skin involvement is usually confined to the hands, feet, and face, and sclerosis often develops years after the onset of Raynaud's phenomenon. There is a significant late incidence of pulmonary arterial hypertension, with or without interstitial lung disease.[13] There is a strong association with anticentromere antibodies. The CREST syndrome includes subcutaneous calcinosis, Raynaud's phenomenon, esophageal dysmotility, sclerodactyly (i.e., scleroderma confined to the digits), and digital or facial telangiectasia. Subcutaneous calcinosis, composed of calcium hydroxyapatite crystals, is usually confined to focal areas in the fingers and over the elbows and knees, but it can become superficial, ulcerate the skin, and lead to secondary infection.

Differential Diagnosis

The clinical characteristics of established systemic sclerosis may be readily distinguished from other connective tissue diseases. In evolving systemic sclerosis, the early clinical manifestations may suggest possible rheumatoid arthritis, systemic lupus erythematosus, polymyositis, or overlapping connective tissue diseases.

Treatment

Of the connective tissue diseases, systemic sclerosis is the most difficult to treat effectively. No putative antifibrotic or immunosuppressive agents have offered unequivocal benefit in randomized clinical trials. Effective management of some organ-based complications, such as reflux esophagitis, renal crisis, and pulmonary arterial hypertension, is beginning to emerge. Patients with systemic sclerosis should undergo regular specialist screening for cardiorespiratory and renal complications, even if they are asymptomatic.

Drugs of Choice

Raynaud's phenomenon may be modified by optimal therapeutic doses of calcium channel blockers. Iloprost, a prostanoid administered by intravenous infusion, may enhance healing of resistant digital or leg ulcers.

Symptomatic reflux esophagitis may require long-term use of proton pump inhibitors. Renal disease, especially renal crisis characterized by proteinuria, renal impairment, and severe hypertension, is associated with a poor prognosis and needs aggressive intervention, including angiotensin-converting enzyme inhibitors. High-dose corticosteroids in patients with systemic sclerosis may precipitate a renal crisis. Pulmonary arterial hypertension is associated with a poor prognosis, and vigilance is required for early detection.[14] Bosentan, an endothelin receptor antagonist, is an effective new therapy for pulmonary arterial hypertension in systemic sclerosis. Sildenafil may also be useful. Oral cyclophosphamide has been shown in clinical trials to modestly improve interstitial lung fibrosis in patients with systemic sclerosis.[15]

Supportive Care

Cigarette smoking must be avoided. It is also important to avoid cold exposure and ambient temperature changes in the home and work environment. Hand warmers and protective clothing may prevent recurrence and enhance healing of digital ulcers. Good skin care is essential. Physiotherapy and an appropriate exercise regimen may prevent or minimize limb contractures and maintain hand function and independence.

DEVELOPMENTS AND RESEARCH OPPORTUNITIES

Research into the pathogenesis of osteoarthritis continues, as does the hunt for disease-modifying agents. Trials are needed to determine the optimal combinations of analgesics and opiates for treating severe osteoarthritis. The reductionist approach to managing chronic low back pain should be investigated by pursuing an anatomical explanation with less-conventional investigations and the use of sensory nerve blocks.

For patients with osteoporosis, there is no evidence that combinations of different drug classes to increase BMD are more efficacious than PTH monotherapy. Bisphosphonates may be required to maintain and further amplify the increased BMD achieved after a PTH course is complete. Denosumab, a fully human monoclonal antibody to receptor activator of nuclear factor-κB ligand (RANKL), inhibits osteoclast function, increases BMD in clinical trials, and may be a future treatment for osteoporosis. Evidence and recommendations for primary prevention of osteoporosis and fractures in patients on sex hormone antagonists are eagerly awaited. Controlled trials and long-term data are needed to assess the benefits of vertebroplasty and kyphoplasty more thoroughly.

For patients with rheumatoid arthritis, very early introduction of effective DMARDs or biological therapies can achieve remission and prevent irreversible joint damage and functional impairment. Better trial designs are needed to demonstrate the efficacy and safety of novel compounds. Improved diagnostic, prognostic, and therapeutic biomarkers must be identified and validated. Data are needed to alleviate concerns about the long-term effects of potent immunomodulatory therapies.

For patients with systemic sclerosis, improved screening and monitoring guidelines are needed. More effective, safe antifibrotic, vasomodulatory, and immunosuppressive agents should be developed for use in patients with systemic sclerosis.

REFERENCES

1. Sarzi-Puttini P, Cimmino M, Scarpa R, et al. Osteoarthritis: An overview of the disease and its treatment strategies. Semin Arthritis Rheum 2005;35(Suppl 1):1-10.
2. Recommendations for the medical management of osteoarthritis of the hip and knee: 2000 update. American College of Rheumatology Subcommittee on Osteoarthritis Guidelines. Arthritis Rheum 2000;43:1905-1915.
3. Jordan KM, Arden NK, Doherty M, et al. EULAR recommendations 2003: An evidence based approach to the management of knee osteoarthritis: Report of a Task Force of the Standing Committee for International Clinical Studies Including Therapeutic Trials (ESCISIT). Ann Rheum Dis 2003;62:1145-1155.
4. Shanahan EM, Ahern M, Smith M, et al. Suprascapular nerve block (using bupivacaine and methylprednisolone acetate) in chronic shoulder pain. Ann Rheum Dis 2003;62:400-406.
5. Recommendations for the prevention and treatment of glucocorticoid-induced osteoporosis: 2001 update. American College of Rheumatology Ad Hoc Committee on Glucocorticoid-Induced Osteoporosis. Arthritis Rheum 2001;44:1496-1503.
6. Gennari C, Agnusdei D, Camporeale A. Use of calcitonin in the treatment of bone pain associated with osteoporosis. Calcif Tissue Int 1991;49(Suppl 2):S9-S13.
7. Hacein-Bey L, Baisden JL, Lemke DM, et al. Treating osteoporotic and neoplastic vertebral compression fractures with vertebroplasty and kyphoplasty. J Palliat Med 2005;8:931-938.
8. Bresnihan B, Tak PP. The pathogenesis and prevention of joint damage in rheumatoid arthritis: Advances from synovial biopsy and tissue analysis. Arthritis Rheum 2000;43:2619-2633.
9. van der Heide D, Landewe R, Klareskog L, et al. Presentation and analysis of data on radiographic outcome in clinical trials. Experience from the TEMPO study. Arthritis Rheum 2005;52:49-60.

10. Cleland LG, James MJ, Proudman SM. Fish oil: What the prescriber needs to know. Arthritis Res Ther 2006;8:202.
11. Borenstein D. Opioids: To use or not to use? That is the question. Arthritis Rheum 2005;52:6-10.
12. Katz P. Use of self-management behaviours to cope with rheumatoid arthritis stressors. Arthritis Rheum 2005;53:939-949.
13. Wigley FM, Lima JAC, Mayes M, et al. The prevalence of undiagnosed pulmonary arterial hypertension in subjects with connective tissue disease at the secondary health care level of community-based rheumatologists (the UNCOVER study). Arthritis Rheum 2005;52:2125-2132.
14. Steen V. Advancements in diagnosis of pulmonary arterial hypertension in scleroderma. Arthritis Rheum 2005;52:3698-3700.
15. Martinez FJ, McCune WJ. Cyclophosphamide for scleroderma lung disease. N Engl J Med 2006;354:2707-2709.

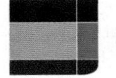

CHAPTER **189**

Stroke

Fred Frost

K E Y   P O I N T S

- Stroke is the most costly diagnosis in the hospice population.

- The most common cause of neurological disability in cancer patients is embolic, not thrombotic, stroke.

- The differential diagnosis of stroke in palliative medicine patients is broad.

- Many palliative medicine patients are eligible for thrombolytic therapy.

- Rehabilitation for stroke can improve function, even if gains in strength and endurance are impossible.

Palliative medicine physicians encounter stroke patients in various situations. Stroke is the most common disabling neurological complication, especially in patients with terminal illness or advanced cancer.[1-3] An emerging emphasis on palliative care for persons with noncancer conditions has resulted in stroke patients gaining greater access to these services. Although Medicare costs are generally lower for terminally ill patients who choose hospice care, stroke patients who choose Medicare-paid hospice benefits accrue significantly greater costs than those who retain conventional Medicare coverage.[4] Patients with the most severe strokes exhibit a flatter trajectory of health decline in their last months of life compared with patients dying of cancer, a phenomenon likely to increase the use of end-of-life medical care resources by this group.[5] Although the 5-year survival rate for stroke in the general population is about 50%, for cancer patients, stroke carries a poor prognosis, with a median survival of only 4.5 months.[6,7]

Palliative medicine providers are most likely to encounter patients who sustain a new stroke during care for other conditions. When stroke occurs in patients with advanced cancer, many diagnostic and therapeutic issues are germane to palliative care.

EPIDEMIOLOGY, PATHOPHYSIOLOGY, AND OUTCOMES

Stroke, also known as cerebrovascular accident or "brain attack," is an acute neurological injury caused by disruption of blood flow to the brain by occlusion (i.e., ischemic stroke) or rupture (i.e., hemorrhagic stroke) of a blood vessel. Stroke is a common medical condition.[8] Each year in the United States, it is estimated that 700,000 people have strokes, of which 500,000 are first attacks and 200,000 are recurrent strokes. Stroke ranks third among all causes of death after cardiovascular disease and cancer. Although hospitalization rates for stroke rose significantly between 1950 and 1980, a decline in stroke mortality rate (i.e., deaths per 100,000 people in the general population) occurred, with continued reductions through 1990. This may reflect the decreased incidence of stroke, improved overall survival among stroke patients, or a combination of both factors.[9] From the early 1970s to the early 1990s, the number of noninstitutionalized stroke survivors increased from 1.5 million to 2.4 million.[10] There are more than 4.8 million stroke survivors in the United States, making stroke the leading cause of serious long-term disability and accelerated health care costs. Since 1988, U.S. hospitalization rates for stroke have increased by almost 9%.[11]

Although the incidence of symptomatic brain infarction among terminally ill patients is unclear, it is a well-recognized cancer complication. Up to 30% of patients dying of cancer have central nervous system lesions.[12] Although most of these are metastases, autopsies identify up to one fourth as strokes.[13,14] In the general population, approximately 80% of strokes are ischemic, and 20% are hemorrhagic. As in the general population, atherosclerosis accounts for most autopsy-proven strokes in cancer patients, but symptomatic strokes are more likely to be caused by nonbacterial thrombotic endocarditis or coagulopathies, which account for more than one half of strokes with significant neurological sequelae.[15] Symptomatic, nonhemorrhagic stroke is surprisingly uncommon in cancer patients, and the reasons are unclear. Data suggest that the incidence ranges from 5% to 7%.[16] In this group, lung cancer is the most common primary tumor, followed by brain and prostate cancers. The diagnosis and management of stroke in this population is often problematic because of the multitude of special medical and social concerns surrounding their primary illnesses.

There are several well-documented risk factors for stroke. The major nonmodifiable risk factors for stroke are age, gender, race, and diabetes. The risk of stroke doubles for each successive decade after age 55 years, and stroke is more prevalent among men than women.[17] Management of modifiable risk factors reduces stroke risk. Hypertension, defined as systolic blood pressure of 140 mm Hg or greater and diastolic blood pressure of 90 mm Hg or greater, is the preeminent risk factor for ischemic and hemorrhagic strokes. Antihypertensive therapy reduces the incidence of stroke by 35% to 44%.[18] Preexisting conditions may place palliative care patients at special risk. Cigarette smoking, especially common among patients with lung cancer, doubles the ischemic stroke risk after adjusting for other risk factors, and it is associated with a twofold to fourfold increased risk for hemorrhagic stroke.[19] Atrial fibrillation occurs in 2% to 4% of the population 60 years old or older, and it is common after cancer surgery.[20-22] It is responsible for one sixth of all ischemic strokes in people older than 60 years.[23] Despite compelling evidence for anticoagulation with warfarin, it remains underused. Transient ischemic attack, defined as focal neurological deficit lasting less than 24 hours, carries a stroke risk of 20% over 90 days.[24] It is unclear whether cancer-related conditions such as hypercoagulability confer a greater risk of stroke than traditional risk factors.

In cancer patients with stroke, 94% have active systemic tumor, and 47% exhibit metastatic disease.[25] Subgroups of cancer patients are faced with special stroke risks.[26] Tamoxifen, which is used for breast cancer treatment, is associated with a statistically increased risk of subsequent stroke.[27] The effect of tamoxifen on atherogenesis and thrombosis is complex. Although these patients are at increased risk for stroke, the drug also lowers the risk for myocardial infarction. Chemotherapy with platinum-based agents has been linked to ischemic stroke, with 75% of those affected developing stroke within 10 days of their latest chemotherapy session.[28] The pathophysiology may be related to the hypomagnesemia, hyperreninemia, and hyperaldosteronemia in patients treated with these drugs.

Hypercoagulable states can be found in more than 50% of cancer patients with symptomatic strokes.[29] The level of D-dimer, a direct measurement of coagulation activity, is elevated in up to 90% of cancer patients, largely from the presence of metastatic disease. Elevated serum angiogenic factors are often identified, but they have an undetermined effect on stroke in cancer patients.[30] Establishing cause-and-effect relationships is difficult, because patients who develop symptomatic stroke may exhibit elevated D-dimer due to the stroke itself. Those with intracranial tumors harbor an additional risk of stroke, because cranial irradiation can accelerate atherosclerosis of the neck and intracranial vessels.

In an outcomes study of stroke after cancer diagnosis,[15] almost 60% exhibited neurological improvement, but only 2% returned to baseline status. Fifteen percent did not improve, and 25% died within 30 days. This contrasts with outcomes in the general population of stroke patients, for whom diminished disability is seen in almost all stroke survivors over 3 months.[31] The overall 5-year survival of 4.5 months for cancer patients with stroke is shorter than that for the general hospital population of stroke patients. In palliative medicine patients, a severe stroke may portend impending death, and disseminated cancer may limit workup and treatment.

IDENTIFICATION, DIAGNOSIS, AND TREATMENT

Although the cause of stroke is different in cancer patients and the general population, the presenting signs and symptoms are similar, including hemiparesis, aphasia, visual field deficits, and headaches. Seizures and headaches are seen in 8% of cancer patients with stroke and may indicate brain metastases, a primary brain tumor, or cerebral venous thrombosis. Many patients present with

TABLE 189-1	Differential Diagnosis of Stroke in Palliative Care Patients	
Cerebral infarction	Cerebral venous occlusion
Nonbacterial thrombotic endocarditis	Compression of cerebral vessel by tumor compression or infiltration
Cerebral intravascular coagulation	Embolization of systemic cancer
Cerebral chemotherapy injury	Tumor-associated intracerebral hemorrhage
Radiation injury	Seizures, Todd's paralysis
Fungal embolus	Complex migraine
Granulomatous angiitis	Head trauma
Metabolic encephalopathy (e.g., hypoglycemic, hepatotoxic, electrolyte disturbance)	

nonfocal neurological changes. These may be attributed to metabolic encephalopathy but can be the manifestation of a progressive thrombotic cerebral coagulopathy[32] (Table 189-1).

For the patient who sustains a stroke while under the care of palliative medicine providers, the decision-making process regarding the diagnosis and initial treatment is similar to that for other intercurrent medical complications. The patient and family are provided with as much information as possible to help them make decisions. Many issues, including underlying medical conditions, prognosis, degree of deficits, and potential for preserving function, are weighed against the risks and discomforts of treatment. For some patients, a severe stroke with major loss of brain tissue constitutes the terminal life event. In most, neurological deficits are less drastic.

Newer treatments for stroke are available that can be delivered with modest risk and discomfort. These therapies reduce the magnitude of brain tissue damage and disability. Usually, the cancer or other terminal illness is not a contraindication to treatment. Nervous system tissue is rapidly and irretrievably damaged as a stroke progresses. Diagnostic and treatment decisions must be made emergently (within minutes) for the patient to benefit from thrombolytic therapy and newer minimally invasive stroke treatments.

Unfortunately, neurological symptoms do not accurately reflect the presence or absence of infarction, and the tempo of the symptoms does not always indicate the cause of the ischemia. The initial examination of a stroke patient should be strategic rather than exhaustive. Use of a formal examination scale allows for standardization, reproducibility, and assessment of stroke severity. The National Institutes of Health Stroke Scale (NIHSS) is widely used and has been incorporated into guidelines for making decisions about thrombolytic therapy. It is an 11-item neurological examination scale that is used to evaluate the effect of acute cerebral infarction on consciousness, language, neglect, visual-field loss, extraocular movement, motor strength, ataxia, dysarthria, and sensory loss. It yields a score between 0 (i.e., no measurable deficits) and 42 (i.e., deep coma). Based on the NIHSS, stroke severity can be broadly categorized as mild (0 to 5), moderate (6 to 20), and severe (>20). Patients with NIHSS scores of more than 20 have a higher incidence of intracerebral hemorrhage when treated with emergent thrombolytic therapy.

A complete blood cell count is used to investigate possible causes of stroke, such as thrombocytosis, thrombocytopenia, polycythemia, or anemia (Table 189-2). Anticoagulants are a common cause of intracerebral hemorrhage. The prothrombin time, partial thromboplastin time, and platelet count should be checked for all those presenting with focal neurological deficits. Because of the concurrence between cardiac disease and stroke, an electrocardiogram and determination of cardiac enzymes can detect underlying atrial fibrillation and unrecognized myocardial infarction. Similarly, echocardiography is useful for cardiac lesions causing embolic strokes. Hyperglycemia augments brain injury by several mechanisms, including increased tissue acidosis from anaerobic metabolism, free radical generation, and increased blood-brain barrier permeability. Hypoglycemic focal neurological deficits, and severe hypoglycemia alone can cause neuronal injury.

Noncontrast computed tomography (CT) of the head is the principal diagnostic modality for assessing acute stroke. It is fast and highly sensitive in excluding hemorrhage, and it has the added advantage of widespread access and speed of acquisition. Early signs of infarction on CT portend poor prognosis. CT can be used to exclude thrombolytic therapy, even if care is sought within the prescribed 3-hour window. CT has been enhanced by CT angiography (CTA) and CT perfusion (CTP) imaging. CTA is sensitive for detecting occlusion in vessels around the circle of Willis, and CTP can identify irreversible ischemia. Newer magnetic resonance imaging (MRI) scanners with diffuse-weighted images can detect abnormalities from ischemia within 3 to 30 minutes of onset, when conventional MRI or CT images would still appear normal.

MANAGEMENT

Acute Stroke Treatment

Newer stroke therapies should not divert attention from the general medical issues common to critically ill stroke patients.[33] Airway protection and cardiac care remain top priorities, along with fluid management and close monitoring for elevated intracranial pressure. Many acute stroke patients present with hypertension. A target systolic blood pressure of 180 mm Hg is recommended for those with a history of hypertension. In other cases, lower blood pressure targets are appropriate (160 to 180/90 to 100 mm Hg).[34]

Timely restoration of blood flow to ischemic brain tissue is the goal of acute treatment.[35] Selected patients offered intravenous thrombolysis (IVT) with alteplase have an improved prognosis for complete or near-complete recovery at 3 months compared with placebo.[36] Alteplase is the only intravenous thrombolytic agent approved by the U.S. Food and Drug Administration. It should be administered within 3 hours from the time of stroke onset. An important aspect of the hyperacute phase of stroke assessment and management is the rapid determination of who is eligible for IVT (Table 189-3). Many palliative medicine patients qualify under these criteria.

Beyond the 3-hour window, preliminary evidence suggests that desmoteplase, a thrombolytic derived from bat saliva offers potential benefit in selected patients.[37] Intra-arterial thrombolysis (IAT) using urokinase and streptokinase has promise in better recanalization rates for middle cerebral artery stem and basilar artery occlusions. No

---

TABLE 189-3 Eligibility Criteria for the Treatment of Acute Ischemic Stroke with Recombinant Tissue Plasminogen Activator

INCLUSION CRITERIA

Clinical Criteria

Diagnosis of ischemic stroke, with onset of symptoms within 3 hours of the initiation of treatment (if the exact time of onset is unknown, it is defined as the last time the patient was known to be normal) and with a measurable neurological deficit

EXCLUSION CRITERIA

Historical Criteria

Stroke or head trauma in the prior 3 months
History of intracranial hemorrhage
Major surgery within 14 days
Gastrointestinal or genitourinary bleeding in the previous 21 days
Myocardial infarction (MI) in past 3 months
Arterial puncture (noncompressible site) within 7 days
Lumbar puncture within 7 days

Clinical Criteria

Rapidly improving stroke symptoms
Minor or isolated neurological signs
Seizure at onset of stroke with postictal residual neurological deficits
Symptoms suggesting subarachnoid hemorrhage, even if computed tomography (CT) results are normal
Clinical presentation consistent with acute MI or post-MI pericarditis
Persistent systolic blood pressure (BP) >185 mm Hg, diastolic BP > 110 mm Hg, or requiring aggressive therapy to control BP
Pregnancy or lactation
Active bleeding or acute trauma (fracture)

Laboratory Criteria

Platelets <100,000/mm^3
Serum glucose <50 mg/dL (<2.8 mmol/L) or >400 mg/dL (>22.2 mmol/L)
International normalized ratio (INR) >1.7 if on warfarin
Elevated partial thromboplastin time (PTT) if on heparin

Radiological Criteria

Evidence of hemorrhage
Evidence of major infarct signs, such as diffuse swelling of the affected hemisphere, parenchymal hypodensity, or effacement of >33% of middle cerebral artery territory

Adapted from Practice advisory: Thrombolytic therapy for acute ischemic stroke—summary statement. Report of the Quality Standards Subcommittee of the American Academy of Neurology. Neurology 1996;47:835-839; Adams HP, Adams RJ, Brott T, et al. Guidelines for the early management of patients with ischemic stroke: A scientific statement from the Stroke Council of the American Stroke Association. Stroke 2003;34:1056-1083.

TABLE 189-2 Initial Testing for a Patient with Suspected Stroke

Noncontrast computed tomography
Blood tests: complete blood cell count, platelet count, prothrombin time, partial thromboplastin time, and levels of electrolytes, glucose, cardiac enzymes, and blood urea nitrogen, creatinine
Chest radiograph
12-Lead electrocardiogram
Transesophageal echocardiography
Drug screen (e.g., Dilantin level)

studies have compared recanalization rates with outcomes after IVT and IAT, but recanalization rates for cerebrovascular occlusions averaged 70% for IAT and 34% for IVT.[38,39] Newer endovascular techniques, such as stenting, angioplasty, and mechanical clot disruption, may produce higher recanalization rates. Because these modalities are still in clinical trials, it is not possible to draw conclusions regarding their safety and efficacy in palliative medicine patients.[40]

Rehabilitation

Palliative medicine patients are frequently underserved by rehabilitation services. Funding for hospice and related programs often limits the provision of physical and occupational therapy, two disciplines central to comprehensive rehabilitation. Palliative medicine providers may not appreciate the special role therapists play in improving patients' function and quality of life. This is unfortunate, especially because rehabilitation and palliative care teams are remarkably similar in structure, culture, and emphasis on symptom management rather than cure. Physical and occupational therapists make their biggest contribution by teaching, not by serving as personal trainers or cheerleaders. Many specialize in treating patients with severe disabilities—patients who will never overcome their illness, gain strength, or improve their conditioning level. Experienced therapists teach patients and families compensatory strategies and methods of energy conservation to optimize their function and reduce the need for assistance. Therapists also play a central role in meeting adaptive equipment, assistive device, and home modification needs. If physical performance cannot be improved, the environment is adapted to augment comfort and activity. Like their palliative medicine colleagues, the rehabilitation team works with the patient and family to develop a plan that includes realistic functional goals for treatment.

Studies have documented the efficacy of rehabilitation strategies.[41-47] Speech, physical, and occupational therapy services improve functional outcomes independent of neurological recovery. In 1995, the Agency for Health Care Policy Research (AHCPR) published guidelines for rehabilitation after stroke.[48] While pointing out the value of an organized approach to rehabilitation, the AHCPR guidelines provide an outline for the medical management of stroke patients. Stroke rehabilitation services are delivered in various settings, ranging from acute hospital management to home care. Randomized trials found that functional outcomes were remarkably similar when comparing hospital with home-based services, although the stress levels and burnout rates for caregivers are significant.[49] Although they may be in the hospital or skilled nursing setting, stroke patients have many medical issues familiar to palliative medicine physicians, including problems with nutrition, hydration, skin integrity, bowel and bladder function, sleep disturbance, and depression. Regardless of the venue, the unique medical needs of this group are often best handled in consultation with specialists in physical medicine and rehabilitation, neurology, and rehabilitation nursing. Specialist consultation and engagement of the therapy team is most helpful for sensorimotor, cognitive, perceptual, swallowing, speech, and language deficits.

More than 20% of patients with stroke have impaired expressive or receptive language function.[50] Intensity of speech therapy, commencing early after stroke, has a direct correlation with improvement, and treatment by speech therapists provides superior results compared with that by trained caregivers.[51,52] Dysphagia after stroke is an independent predictor of poor functional outcome.[53] Other trials support the benefit of formal evaluation of swallowing problems by the speech pathologist and training patients and caregivers in safe swallowing techniques.[54]

Patients with moderate levels of disability from stroke often achieve significant benefit from occupational therapy that addresses feeding, dressing, bathing, grooming, and toileting.[55] For patients with hemiplegia, one-handed techniques are taught, and splinting and wheelchair support can reduce pain and disability in the affected arm. Task-oriented practice strategies add significant benefit, even in cases of a static neurological deficit.[56]

Ambulation and transfers to the bed, chair, and commode are often the focal points of patients and their families. Stroke patients who have active hip flexion and knee extension are likely to achieve some degree of ambulation.[57] Although patients with cancer or another terminal disease may not build muscle or improve endurance, improvements in efficiency and technique often come through braces and assistive devices.[58] Based on an individualized assessment, caregiver support, and the medical prognosis, the physical therapist can help palliative medicine patients and their families choose adaptive equipment and home modifications.

For some stroke patients with severe deficits, limited goals for hospital discharge, or no qualitative gains with initial treatment, therapy is not warranted. For patients with terminal illness or advanced cancer, participation is often determined by their primary disease. Even for patients with brain tumors and acute stroke, good functional outcomes and shorter hospital length of stay can be achieved with rehabilitation.[59] For patients or families who show interest and motivation, many functional goals can be met quickly and efficiently by judicious use of the rehabilitation team.

DEVELOPMENTS AND RESEARCH OPPORTUNITIES

As more noncancer patients are treated in the palliative setting, stroke care will gain importance. The optimal intensity, frequency, and duration of therapy services after stroke are being researched, but further study of thrombolytic therapies in terminal cancer patients is needed.

REFERENCES

1. American Heart Association. Heart Disease and Stroke Statistics—2004 Update. Dallas, TX: American Heart Association, 2003.
2. Lindvig K, Moller H, Mosbech J. The pattern of cancer in a large cohort of stroke patients Int J Epidemiol 1990;19:498-504.
3. Jagsi R, Griffith KA, Koelling T, et al. Stroke rates and risk factors in patients treated with radiation therapy. J Clin Oncol 2006;24:2779-2785.
4. Pyenson B, Connor S, Fitch K, et al. Medicare cost in matched hospice and non-hospice cohorts. J Pain Symptom Manage 2004;28:200-210.
5. Teno JM, Weitzen MHA, Fennell ML, et al. Dying trajectory in the last year of life. J Palliat Med 2001;4:457-464.
6. Ingall T. Stroke—incidence, mortality, morbidity and risk. J Insur Med 2004;36:143-152.
7. Brown RD, Whisnant JP, Sicks JD, et al. Stroke incidence, prevalence, and survival: Secular trends in Rochester, Minnesota, through 1989. Stroke 1996;27:373-380.

8. Feigin VL, Lawes CM, Bennett DA, Anderson CS. Stroke epidemiology: A review of population-based studies of incidence, prevalence, and case-fatality in the late 20th century. Lancet Neurol 1003;2:43-53.

9. Wolf PA, et al. In Barnett HJM, et al (eds). Stroke: Pathophysiology, Diagnosis, and Management. New York: Churchill-Livingstone, 1992, p 3.

10. Muntner P, Garrett E, Klag MJ, et al. Trends in stroke prevalence between 1973 and 1991 in the US population 25 to 74 years of age. Stroke 2002;33:1209-1213.

11. Fang J, Alderman MH. Trend of stroke hospitalization, United States, 1988-1997. Stroke 2001;32:2221-2226.

12. Iguchi Y, Kimura K, Kobayashi K, et al. Ischaemic stroke with malignancy may often be caused by paradoxical embolism. J Neurol Neurosurg Psychiatry 2006;77:1336-1339.

13. Katz JM, Segal AZ. Incidence and etiology of cerebrovascular disease in patients with malignancy. Curr Atheroscler Rep 2005;7:280-288.

14. Cestari DM, Weine DM, Panageas KS. Stroke in patients with cancer: Incidence and etiology Neurology.2004; 62: 2025-2030.

15. Rogers LR. Cerebrovascular complications in cancer patients. Neurol Clin North Am 2003;21:167-192.

16. Graus F, Rogers LR, Posner JB. Cerebrovascular complications in patients with cancer. Medicine (Baltimore) 1985;64:16-35.

17. Brown RD, Whisnant JP, Sicks JD, et al. Stroke incidence, prevalence and survival: Secular trends in Rochester, Minnesota, through 1989. Stroke.1996; 27:373-380.

18. Neal B, MacMahon S, Chapman N, for the Blood Pressure Lowering Treatment Trialists' Collaboration. Effects of ACE inhibitors, calcium antagonists, and other blood-pressure-lowering drugs: Results of prospectively designed overviews of randomized trials. Lancet 2000;356:1955-1964.

19. Kurth T, Kase CS, Berger K, et al. Smoking and risk of hemorrhagic stroke in women. Stroke. 2003;34:2792-2795.

20. Gibbs HR, Swafford J, Nguyen HD. Postoperative atrial fibrillation in cancer surgery. J Surg Oncol 1992;50:224-227.

21. Siu CW, Tung HM, Chu KW, et al. Prevalence and predictors of new onset atrial fibrillation after elective surgery for cancer. Pacing Clin Electrophysiol 2005;28(Suppl 1):120-123.

22. Roselli EE, Murthy SC, Rice TW, et al. Atrial fibrillation complicating lung cancer resection. J Thorac Cardiovasc Surg 2005;130:438-444.

23. Wolf PA, Abbott RD, Kannel WB. Atrial fibrillation as an independent risk factor for stroke: The Framingham Study. Stroke 1991;22:983-988.

24. Kernan WN, Viscoli CM, Brass LM. The stroke prognosis instrument II (SPI-II): A clinical prediction instrument for patients with transient ischemia and non-disabling ischemic stroke. Stroke 2000;31:456-462.

25. Gouin-Thibault I, Samama MM. Laboratory diagnosis of the thrombophilic state in cancer patients. Semin Thromb Haemost 1999;25:167-172.

26. Li SH, Chen WH, Tang Y, et al. Incidence of ischemic stroke post-chemotherapy: A retrospective review of 10,963 patients. Clin Neurol Neurosurg 2006;108:150-156.

27. Braithwaite RS, Chlebowski, RT, Lau J, et al. Meta-analysis of vascular and neoplastic events associated with tamoxifen. J Gen Intern Med 2003;18:937-947.

28. Shau Hsum Li.

29. ten Wolde M, Kraaijenhagen RA, Prins MH, et al. The clinical usefulness of D-dimer testing in cancer patients. Arch Intern Med 2002;162:1880-1884.

30. Dirix LY, Salgado R, Weytjens R, et al. Plasma fibrin D-dimer levels correlate with tumour volume, progression rate and survival in patients with metastatic cancer. Br J Cancer 2002;86:389-395.

31. Lai S-M 2002 in Dobkin.

32. Raizer JJ, DeAngelis LM. Cerebral sinus thrombosis diagnosed by MRI and MR venography in cancer patients. Neurology 2000;54:1222-1226.

33. Hazinski MF. Demystifying recognition and management of stroke. Curr Emerg Card Care 1996;7:8.

34. Ringleb PA, Bertram M, Keller E, Hacke W. Hypertension in patients with cerebrovascular accident. To treat or not to treat? Nephrol Dial Transplant 1998;13:2179-2181.

35. Savier JL. Time is brain: Quantified. Stroke 2006;37:263-266.

36. Tissue plasminogen activator for acute ischemic stroke. The National Institute of Neurological Disorders and Stroke rt-PA Stroke Study Group. N Engl J Med 1995;333:1581-1587.

37. Hacke W, Albers G, Al-Rawi Y, et al. The Desmoteplase in Acute Ischemic Stroke Trial (DIAS): A phase II MRI-based 9 hour window acute stroke thrombolysis trial with intravenous desmoteplase. Stroke 2005;36:66-73.

38. Furlan AJ. Acute stroke therapy: Beyond IV tPA. Cleve Clin J Med 2002;69:730-734.

39. Pessin M, del Zoppo GJ, Furlan AJ. Thrombolytic treatment in acute stroke: Review and update of selective topics. In Moskowitz MA, Caplan LR (eds): Cerebrovascular Diseases: Nineteenth Princeton Stroke Conference. Boston: Butterworth-Heinemann, 1995, pp 409-418.

40. Qureshi A. Endovascular treatment of cerebrovascular diseases and intracranial neoplasms. Lancet 2004;363:804-813.

41. Dobkin BH. The Clinical Science of Neurologic Rehabilitation. New York: Oxford University Press, 2003.

42. Gillen G, Burkhart A. Stroke Rehabilitation: A Function Based Approach. St Louis: Mosby, 2004.

43. Kalra L, Yu G, Wilson K, et al. Medical complications during stroke. Rehabil Stroke 1995;26:990-994.

44. Sivenius J, Pyorala K, Heinonen OP, et al. Significance of intensity of stroke rehabilitation. Stroke 1985;16:928-931.

45. Indredavik B, Bakke F, Solberg R, et al. Benefit of a stroke unit: A randomized controlled trial Stroke 1991;22:1026-1031.

46. Claesson L, Gosman-Hedstrom G, Fagerberg B, et al. Hospital re-admissions in relation to acute stroke unit care versus conventional care in elderly patients the first year after stroke: The Göteborg 70+ Stroke study. Age Ageing 2003;32:109-113.

47. Ma et al. 2004.

48. Gresham GE, Duncan PW, Stason, WB, et al. Post-Stroke Rehabilitation: Assessment, Referral, and Patient Management. Clinical practice guideline and quick reference guide for clinicians, no. 16. AHCPR Pub. No. 95-0663. Rockville, MD: U.S. Department of Health and Human Services, Public Health Service, and Agency for Health Care Policy and Research, May 1995.

49. Dobkin BH. Rehabilitation after stroke. N Engl J Med 2005;352:2677-2684.

50. Bhogal SK, Teasell R, Speechley M. Intensity of aphasia therapy, impact on recovery. Stroke 2003;34:987-993.

51. Robey RR. A meta-analysis of clinical outcomes in the treatment of aphasia. J Speech Lang Hear Res 1998;41:172-187.

52. Doesborgh SJ, van de Sandt-Koenderman MW, Dippel DW, et al. Effects of semantic treatment on verbal communication and linguistic processing in aphasia after stroke: A randomized controlled trial. Stroke 2004;35:141-146.

53. Smithard DG, Smeeton NC, Wolfe CD. Long-term outcome after stroke: Does dysphagia matter? Age Ageing 2007;36:90-94.

54. Legg L, Langhorne P. Rehabilitation therapy services for stroke patients living at home, systematic review of randomized trials. Lancet 2004;363:352-356.

55. Dobkin BH. Strategies for stroke rehabilitation. Lancet Neurol 2004;3:528-536.

56. Steultjens EMJ, Dekker J, Bouter LM, et al. Occupational therapy for stroke patients: A systematic review. Stroke 2003;34:676-687.

57. Glasgow Augmented Physiotherapy Study Group. Can augmented physiotherapy input enhance recovery of mobility after stroke? A randomized controlled trial. Clin Rehabil 2004;18:529-537.

58. Kwakkel G, Wagenaar RC, Koelman TW, et al. Effects of intensity of rehabilitation after stroke. Stroke 1997;28:1550-1556.

59. Greenberg E, Treger I, Ring H. Rehabilitation outcomes in patients with brain tumors and acute stroke: Comparative study of inpatient rehabilitation. Am J Phys Med Rehabil 2006;85:568-573.

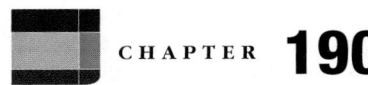

CHAPTER **190**

Parkinson's Disease

Stephen G. Reich

K E Y   P O I N T S

- Parkinson's disease (PD) is the second most common neurodegenerative disease in adults after Alzheimer's disease.

- The cardinal features of PD include slowness of movement (i.e., bradykinesia), resting tremor, and cogwheel rigidity. Patients with advanced disease have impaired balance.

- The primary defect is degeneration of the dopamine neurons of the midbrain substantia nigra. Almost all available therapies are designed to replace dopamine, and the mainstay is its precursor, levodopa.

- No therapies slow disease progression, but effective symptomatic therapy is available.

- PD can be viewed as three progressive stages. In the first stage, symptoms can be well managed with medications, and most patients function at a near-normal level. The second is characterized by a waning response to levodopa and by motor fluctuations, which can be managed effectively through polypharmacy or surgery. The third stage is complicated by disabling features that usually are unresponsive to levodopa, including imbalance with falls, dysphagia, and dementia. Not all patients reach this advanced stage.

- Nonmotor features, which are as disabling as the cardinal motor signs and are often overlooked, include sleep disturbances, dysautonomia, sensory symptoms (e.g., pain, impaired cognition, dementia), depression, anxiety, and hallucinations.

Parkinson's disease (PD) was described by James Parkinson in 1817, and little has been added to his description of the classic motor features: "Involuntary tremulous motion, with lessened muscular power, in parts not in action and even when supported; with a propensity to lean the trunk forward, and to pass from a walking to a running pace."[1] It is a common disorder, affecting about 1 in 100 persons older than 60 years.[1] The diagnosis is clinical; there are no routinely available ancillary tests to confirm the diagnosis.[1-4]

The most common presenting symptom is tremor, and at onset, PD is typically hemiparkinsonism, with a tremor at rest affecting one hand or foot. The diagnosis requires the presence of bradykinesia (i.e., slowness of movement), confirmed historically by asking if routine tasks take more time and corroborated on examination by observing the speed of finger and foot tapping, walking, arising from a chair, and looking for decreased arm swing with walking. The third feature of the clinical triad is cogwheel rigidity, which is felt as a ratchety resistance as a limb or the neck is passively moved. As the disease advances, impaired balance (with a loss of postural righting reflexes associated with falls and near falls) is confirmed on examination by observing an inability to recover balance in a step or two after being pulled backward.[1]

Although the diagnosis is typically referred to as a "waiting room diagnosis," emphasizing that it can be made at a glance, this is an overstatement. The most common misdiagnoses are essential tremor and musculoskeletal disorders. Failure to make the diagnosis often causes unnecessary testing, including spine imaging for 30% and electromyography for 22% of patients.[5] Autopsy studies reveal that more than 20% of PD cases diagnosed during life have an alternative diagnosis at autopsy, typically parkinsonian syndromes such as progressive supranuclear palsy and multiple system atrophy.[6,7]

The cause of PD remains unknown. Effective symptomatic treatment is available based on the pathological hallmark of dopamine neuron degeneration from the midbrain substantia nigra. Most therapies replace dopamine, and with treatment, most people with PD can expect a normal life span. It is useful to think about PD and its treatment in three broad, progressive, overlapping stages. However, the trajectories and manifestations differ among patients, necessitating individualized therapy.

For the first 5 to 10 years after presentation, patients respond well to most therapies and function independently, albeit with tasks taking more time and effort. In the middle stages, 5 to 15 years after onset, the effect of antiparkinsonian medications, especially levodopa, begins to wane (although levodopa does not stop working), and the initial smooth transition between dosages gives way to motor fluctuations with periods of mobility and relative ease of functioning (i.e., *on time*) punctuated by periods of worsening symptoms (i.e., *off time*) and the appearance of excessive involuntary movements known as *dyskinesias*.[8] This narrowing therapeutic window requires careful titration of antiparkinsonian medications, which can often be accomplished to maximize on time and minimize off time and dyskinesias. During this stage, deep brain surgery should be considered when fluctuations cannot be controlled with antiparkinsonian medications.

For most patients, the course evolves into a third stage dominated by motor and nonmotor symptoms and signs that are poorly responsive to dopaminergic therapies. The signs and symptoms include imbalance with falls, dysphagia, dysarthria, executive dysfunction, frank dementia, urinary bladder instability, hallucinations, and susceptibility to delirium. It is important to avoid fatalism, because many of these problems are amenable to interventions that allow an acceptable quality of life.

EPIDEMIOLOGY AND PREVALENCE

PD is found worldwide, affecting approximately 1% of people older than 60 years, and most studies suggest that men are more commonly affected.[9] In a community-based study, the prevalence of parkinsonism (i.e., including but not limited to PD) ranged from 15% among those between 65 and 74 years old to more than 50% among those 85 years and older.[10] A conservative estimate is that the number of individuals older than 50 with PD will double in the world's most populated countries by 2030, and at least 9.3 million persons will be affected.[11] The incidence increases after age 50, but as many as 5% of patients present before age 45. Reported incidence rates vary from 8 to 18 cases per 100,000 people per year.[9]

Although the cause of most cases is unknown (about 5% are monogenetic),[12] epidemiological studies suggest putative risk factors.[9] In intravenous drug abusers, the neurotoxin 1-methyl-4-phenyl-1,2,3,6-tetrahydropyridine (MPTP) selectively targets dopaminergic neurons in the substantia nigra.[12] Age is the most important risk factor, but exposure to pesticides, a rural environment, well water, and a history of head injury may also contribute. Cigarette smoking and caffeine consumption decrease the risk.[9]

PATHOPHYSIOLOGY AND BASIC SCIENCE

Most cases of PD are nongenetic or associated with only a genetic susceptibility. At least six monogenetic forms, including autosomal dominant and recessive forms, have been discovered.[13] Monogenetic forms clinically resembling sporadic PD has called into question whether what is called "PD" today will eventually give way to a more etiologically heterogeneous group of Parkinson's "diseases."[14]

Whether the cause is genetic, environmental, or yet to be discovered, the hallmark is degeneration of the dopaminergic cells in the substantia nigra pars compacta, with remaining cells containing Lewy bodies (i.e., eosinophilic, intracytoplasmic inclusions). However, this traditional concept of PD as a purely dopaminergic disorder is too simplistic.[15,16] Although dopamine replacement is the most effective treatment, many features of PD (especially nonmotor symptoms and those associated with advancing disease) are unresponsive to this approach and likely represent involvement of non-nigral areas and neurotransmitters other than dopamine.

Degeneration of the nigra may be a late stage in the pathological evolution of PD,[17] with the earliest changes occurring in the olfactory bulb and lower brainstem with spread rostrally. The clinical correlate of this shift in focus away from solely the nigra has been the concept that the earliest features of PD are nonmotor and that the cardinal motor signs are long preceded by other parkinsonian features, such as anosmia, constipation, and rapid eye movement (REM) sleep behavioral disorder.[18]

It is likely that neuronal degeneration results from a cascade of events, including inflammation, apoptosis, oxidative stress, mitochondrial dysfunction, excitotoxicity, and aggregation of abnormal proteins,[19] all of which are targets of experimental therapeutic agents. Dopamine depletion causes downstream changes in other components of the basal ganglia, which are thought to be arranged in a circuit.[4] Alterations of inhibitory and excitatory neurotransmitters within this circuit increase neuronal activity in two structures: the subthalamic nucleus (STN) and the internal segment of the globus pallidum (GPi), which is the main output of the nucleus of the basal ganglia, projecting to the motor thalamus.[4] Overactivity of these nuclei helps explain why they are the targets of surgical therapy for PD.

The three case reports correspond to each of the broad stages of PD previously described (see "Case Study: Early Stage of Parkinson's Disease," "Case Study: Middle Stage of Parkinson's Disease," and "Case Study: Advanced Stage of Parkinson's Disease").

CLINICAL MANIFESTATIONS

The clinical triad of PD is bradykinesia, rest tremor (with a "pill rolling" morphology of the fingers or pronation-supination of the forearm), and cogwheel rigidity, but tremor is absent in approximately one third of patients. Of these signs, bradykinesia is essential for the diagnosis, and it typically begins, as does resting tremor, unilaterally or at least asymmetrically. Postural instability is often listed as a key feature of PD, and although it usually develops with advancing disease, it is not present at onset and is therefore not helpful diagnostically. Postural instability, especially with falls, early in the course casts doubt on the diagnosis of PD as the cause of parkinsonism.[25] Although there are no uniformly agreed on diagnostic criteria, the U.K. Parkinson's Disease Brain Bank Criteria typically are used,[20] and they emphasize the unilateral or asymmetrical onset of symptoms and signs, a beneficial response to levodopa, and the lack of atypical features (discussed later). Additional motor features of PD are given in Box 190-1. Freezing (i.e., akinesia) refers to the inability to initiate a movement, such as taking the first step, or the sudden cessation of an ongoing movement, which usually occurs while turning, going through doorways, near obstacles, and in crowds. It is described by patients as though the feet are "glued to the floor."

 CASE STUDY

Early Stage of Parkinson's Disease

A 60-year-old man presents with a 6-month history of tremor of the dominant right hand. His handwriting has become smaller, and it is more difficult to perform fine tasks with the right hand, such as buttoning the left cuff. He has noticed a tendency to drag his right foot, and his wife pointed out that he does not swing the right arm. On examination, there is a resting tremor of the right fingers and forearm. Rapid, repetitive movements of the right hand and foot are mildly slow, and even the asymptomatic left limbs are slightly slow. His facial expression is decreased, and the voice volume is diminished. There is cogwheel rigidity at both wrists and with flexion and extension of the neck. He walks somewhat slowly with absent arm swing on the right, and the right foot is heard to scuff the floor.

This patient demonstrates typical symptoms and signs of early Parkinson's disease (PD), with the asymmetrical onset of tremor, cogwheel rigidity, and bradykinesia and no atypical signs (see Box 190-4).[1,20] At presentation, education and reassurance are the most important interventions. He should be counseled about how the diagnosis was made (i.e., clinical grounds), instructed about the need to emphasize functioning over symptoms and signs as the barometer for assessing the severity of the disease and the need for therapy, and reassured that although PD is progressive, the rate is insidious with a favorable prognosis for the near and intermediate future.

If symptoms are not affecting his functioning in a meaningful way, treatment is not necessary. If the symptoms are interfering, the treatment options include a dopamine agonist, levodopa, the MAO-B inhibitor rasagiline, and amantadine. No neuroprotective therapies are avilable.[21,22]

CASE STUDY

Middle Stage of Parkinson's Disease

A 67-year-old woman with a 7-year history of Parkinson's disease (PD) is no longer having a smooth transition between dosages of her medications. She describes the changes in her symptoms throughout the day as "like being on a roller coaster." She is taking two tablets of carbidopa plus levodopa (25/100 mg) every 4 hours along with pramipexole (1 mg three times daily). It takes at least 20 minutes for a dose of levodopa to take effect so that she can move freely. She does well for the next 2 to 3 hours, only to have parkinsonian symptoms worsen before the next dose. Sometimes, about 1 to 2 hours after a dose of levodopa, she experiences facial grimacing, head bobbing, and squirming of the limbs, which she finds embarrassing.

This patient demonstrates typical motor fluctuations, which usually surface within 5 years of initiating levodopa, including delayed onset of levodopa, end of dose wearing off, and peak-dose dyskinesias. Several options are available to smooth out the response fluctuations, including taking a lower dose of carbidopa plus levodopa more often (e.g., 1.5 tablets every 3 hours); increasing pramipexole to the maximal dose (2 mg three times daily) along with a reduction in each dose of levodopa to reduce dyskinesias; adding a catechol-*O*-methyltransferase (COMT) inhibitor or a monoamine oxidase B (MAO-B) inhibitor to extend the duration of response to levodopa along with a slight reduction in the levodopa to reduce dyskinesias; adding amantadine to help PD symptoms and attenuate dyskinesias; and consideration of deep brain stimulation if other methods are ineffective.[8,23]

CASE STUDY

Advanced Stage of Parkinson's Disease

A 76-year-old man with a 17-year history of Parkinson's disease (PD) requires assistance with almost all activities of daily living. He occasionally falls. He is often disoriented and has a poor memory. He is having visual hallucinations, seeing unfamiliar people in the home, and he is having some paranoid delusions, thinking that his pills have been poisoned. He is often agitated at night, with an exacerbation of the hallucinations. His medications include carbidopa plus levodopa (25/250 mg every 4 hours), ropinirole (5 mg three times daily), rasagiline (1 mg), amitriptyline (25 mg at bedtime, which he has taken for insomnia for many years), and tolterodine (for bladder control), in addition to drugs for hypertension, hyperlipidemia, and diabetes.

This patient's long-standing PD has become complicated by imbalance with falls, dementia, insomnia, hallucinations, and delusions. His spouse is likely exasperated and exhausted. As PD advances and particularly when dementia surfaces, many antiparkinsonian medications can be withdrawn without a major physical setback and often with improvement in cognition. Even if there is some worsening of PD, most patients and caregivers find it easier to deal with the motor than the mental complications. In all likelihood, ropinirole and rasagiline can be discontinued along with amitriptyline and tolterodine, particularly in light of their anticholinergic activity. The physician must ensure that there are no other causes of dementia, such as a subdural hematoma or metabolic disturbance, and search for possible depression. If discontinuing the medications described does not improve the psychosis, options include adding an atypical neuroleptic, such as quetiapine or clozapine.[24] Cholinesterase inhibitors have a very modest effect on Parkinson's disease dementia.[24]

Box 190-1 Other Motor Features of Parkinson's Disease

- Micrographia
- Hypomimia (i.e., decreased blink rate and facial expression)
- Soft, monotone voice (i.e., hypophonia)
- Tremor of the lips, chin, tongue, or foot
- Difficulty arising from a soft chair
- Difficulty turning in bed
- En bloc turning
- Flexed posture
- Freezing (i.e., akinesia)
- Impaired postural righting reflexes
- Falls

Box 190-2 Nonmotor Features of Parkinson's Disease

Autonomic Features

Orthostatic hypotension
Urinary bladder instability (i.e., urgency, frequency, and urge incontinence)
Erectile dysfunction
Constipation
Drooling
Dysphagia
Sweating
Thermal dysregulation (i.e., feelings of cold or hot unrelated to ambient temperature)

Sensory Features

Pain, numbness, tingling
Cramps
Akathisia
Anosmia
Frozen shoulder
Internal tremor
Fatigue

Sleep Features

Insomnia
Excessive daytime sleepiness
Restless legs syndrome
Rapid eye movement (REM) sleep behavioral disorder

Psychiatric Features

Depression
Anxiety
Panic Attacks
Delirium
Psychosis (i.e., hallucinations and delusions)
Executive dysfunction
Dementia

Although most of these features, including depression, are thought to be intrinsic features of PD, antiparkinsonian medications can cause or exacerbate nonmotor symptoms.

DIFFERENTIAL DIAGNOSIS

There is a lengthy differential diagnosis for parkinsonism (Box 190-3), but most patients presenting with parkinsonian signs and symptoms have PD. However, 20% of patients diagnosed as having PD during life will be found at autopsy to have an alternative diagnosis.[7] Of the conditions that can be confused with PD, the two most important to recognize are drug-induced parkinsonism[27] and essential tremor.[28,29]

Drug-induced parkinsonism is often unrecognized by physicians, including neurologists.[30] It is caused by drugs that block dopamine or inhibit its release, including antipsychotics and antiemetics (e.g., metoclopramide). Because drug-induced parkinsonism may take up to 1 year to resolve, all patients with parkinsonism should be asked

---

Although motor signs are the most obvious manifestations of PD, equally and often more problematic are nonmotor features (Box 190-2), and these have received increased attention during the past decade.[26] Nonmotor aspects of PD often go unrecognized by physicians despite being very disturbing for patients, and they significantly affect quality of life, often more than motor signs. Many of the nonmotor features are amenable to treatment.

Box 190-3 Differential Diagnosis of Parkinsonism

Causative Drugs or Toxins

1-Methyl-4-phenyl-1,2,3,6-tetrahydropyridine (MPTP) neurotoxin
Carbon monoxide poisoning
Manganese (Mn) intoxication (usually from industrial exposure)
Carbon disulfide poisoning (usually in solvents or pesticides)
Cyanide poisoning
Methanol poisoning

Infectious Diseases

Postencephalitic parkinsonism (i.e., encephalitis lethargica)
Human immunodeficiency virus (HIV) encephalopathy
Whipple's disease
Jakob-Creutzfeldt disease

Degenerative Diseases

Progressive supranuclear palsy
Multiple system atrophy
Corticobasal degeneration
Alzheimer's disease
Dementia with Lewy bodies
Frontotemporal dementia
Wilson's disease
Huntington's disease
Fahr's disease

Other Disorders

Vascular parkinsonism
Hydrocephalus
Post-traumatic parkinsonism
Structural lesion

Box 190-4 Clinical Features Casting Doubt on the Diagnosis of Parkinson's Disease and Suggesting a Parkinsonian Syndrome

- Little or no response to levodopa or failure to sustain an initial beneficial response
- Early-onset dysautonomia
- Early-onset bulbar dysfunction (e.g., dysarthria, dysphagia)
- Early-onset dementia or psychosis
- Early-onset imbalance and falls
- Rapid progression (e.g., use of wheelchair within 3 years of onset)
- Vertical supranuclear ophthalmoplegia or slowing of vertical saccades
- Cerebellar, pyramidal, parietal, or lower motor neuron signs
- Symmetrical onset

about past drug exposure and not just those in use at the time of presentation. The diagnosis of drug-induced parkinsonism is made retrospectively, when symptoms and signs resolve. If they do not resolve, it is safe to assume that the medication might have exacerbated a mild case of PD or had no effect.

The tremor of PD may be mistaken for essential tremor and vice versa.[31] A few key features from the history and examination often can make this distinction, but if there is any question, a consultation should be sought with a specialist in movement disorders because the implications for the natural history and treatment are distinctly different. Historically, most patients with PD who have tremor (not all patients with PD have tremor) present within months or 1 year of onset, whereas patients with essential tremor often give a history of tremor beginning years or even decades earlier. There is usually a positive family history in cases of essential tremor (i.e., autosomal dominant inheritance) and much less frequently in cases of PD. Patients with essential tremor often report temporary improvement with alcohol, unlike those with PD.

On examination, the tremor of PD typically begins unilaterally, whereas essential tremor is almost always bilateral, although it may be asymmetrical and usually of greater amplitude in the dominant hand. The PD tremor is maximal at rest, whereas essential tremor is absent at rest and activated with maintenance of posture and movement. The tremor of PD is slower (3 to 6 Hz) than essential tremor (6 to 12 Hz); the former manifests with a pill-rolling morphology of the fingers or pronation-supination of the forearm, whereas essential tremor is typically a flexion-extension movement at the wrist or shoulder. The handwriting of patients with PD is small but atremulous, and for patients with essential tremor, handwriting is normal sized with a tremor. A tremor of the head or voice suggests essential tremor, and tremor of the chin, lips, and tongue is more likely PD, although there are exceptions and overlap. Essential tremor is a monosymptomatic disorder; there are no features aside from the tremor. Patients with PD demonstrate the associated signs discussed earlier.

A complete discussion of the differential diagnosis of PD (see Box 190-3) is beyond the scope of this chapter.[32] The most common mimickers based on autopsy studies are parkinsonian syndromes,[7] also known as parkinson-plus disorders, so named because the clinical and pathological features go beyond the limits of PD. The most common parkinsonian syndromes are progressive supra-nuclear palsy (PSP)[33] and multiple system atrophy (MSA).[34] The former is characterized by early falls and vertical supranuclear ophthalmoplegia, and the latter is characterized by dysautonomia and levodopa unresponsive parkinsonism (MSA-P) or cerebellar signs (MSA-C), or both. More important than being familiar with the specific features of each parkinsonian syndrome is awareness of the red flags[35] that suggest a patient with parkinsonism does not have PD; these are listed in Box 190-4.

TREATMENT

This section provides an overview of the approach to treating PD, followed by a discussion of the drugs available in the United States with their indications and main side effects (Table 190-1), surgical treatment, and therapeutic options for selected nonmotor features of PD.

No therapies are available to slow the inexorable progression of PD,[22,36] and all available treatment is directed at alleviation of symptoms and optimizing functioning. Symptomatic treatment should commence when the symptoms begin to impact patients' activities of daily living in a way that they find meaningful. This approach

TABLE 190-1 Medications for Parkinson's Disease Available in the United States

DRUGS	AVAILABLE FORMULATIONS	USUAL THERAPEUTIC DOSE	SIDE EFFECTS
LEVODOPA			
Carbidopa and levodopa immediate release	10/100 mg 25/100 mg 25/250 mg	25/100 mg, 1-2 tablets three times daily, at least 30 minutes before meals	At initiation: nausea, orthostatic hypotension With chronic therapy: motor fluctuations, dyskinesias, hallucinations, confusion
Carbidopa and levodopa controlled release	25/100 mg 50/200 mg	1 tablet two or three times daily (approximately 4- to 6-hour dosing interval)	Same as for immediate release
Carbidopa, levodopa, and entacapone (Stalevo)	12/5/50/200 mg 25/100/200 mg 37.5/150/200 mg 50/200/200 mg	1 tablet three times daily, before meals	Same as with preparations above, plus diarrhea with entacapone
DOPAMINE AGONISTS			
Pramipexole	0.125 mg 0.25 mg 0.5 mg 0.75 mg 1 mg 1.5 mg	0.5 to 1.5 mg three times daily, 6- to 8-hour dosing interval	Nausea, vomiting, hypotension, edema, daytime sleepiness, compulsive behaviors, confusion, hallucinations
Ropinirole	0.25 mg 0.5 mg 1, 2, 3, 4, and 5 mg	2 to 8 mg three times daily, 6- to 8-hour dosing interval	Same as for pramipexole
Apomorphine	SC injection	0.2 to 0.6 mL SC as needed, 1 to 4 injections per day for off time	Nausea, hypotension, yawning, sleepiness, local site reaction
COMT INHIBITORS			
Tolcapone	100 mg 200 mg	100 to 200 mg three times daily	Exacerbation of levodopa side effects, including dyskinesias, diarrhea, rare hepatotoxicity (monitoring required)
Entacapone	200 mg	200 mg with each dose of levodopa, up to eight times per day	Exacerbation of levodopa's adverse effects, diarrhea, discolored urine (bright yellow)
MAO-B INHIBITORS			
Rasagiline	0.5 mg 1 mg	1 mg each day	Nausea, dizziness, headache, insomnia
Selegiline (also comes in an orally disintegrating tablet: Zelapar)	5 mg 1.25 mg	5 to 10 mg twice daily, breakfast and lunch 1.25 to 2.5 mg each day	Same as for rasagiline
ANTICHOLINERGICS			
Trihexyphenidyl	2.5 mg tablets	2 mg three times per day	Impaired memory, confusion, constipation, blurred vision, urinary retention, dry mouth
Benztropine	0.5-, 1-, and 2-mg tablets	0.5 to 2 mg three times per day	Same as for trihexyphenidyl
ANTIVIRALS			
Amantadine	100	100 mg two or three times per day	Livedo reticularis, hallucinations, confusion, edema

COMT, catechol-*O*-methyltransferase; MAO-B, monoamine oxidase B; SC, subcutaneous.

has several implications. First, it is not necessary to begin treatment as soon as the diagnosis is made. Second, treatment must be individualized. Third, patients need to be educated early about the goal of treatment, which is to keep them functioning at an acceptable level rather than alleviating all symptoms and signs of PD, which cannot be accomplished.

The mainstay of therapy for PD is levodopa, but unsupported concerns about it exerting a toxic effect on dopaminergic neurons and ultimately worsening the natural history of PD has caused patients and physicians to shy away from its use, a syndrome known as *levodopaphobia*.[37] An often heard claim is that the effect of levodopa "stops working after 5 years," and as such, people believe its use should be reserved as long as possible. Evidence demonstrates the fallacy of this approach and offers reassurance that levodopa is not harmful[16,38] and that it may slow the progression of early PD.[38] However, with continued use of levodopa, most patients begin to experience motor fluctuations.[8,23,39] The first to appear is caused by shortening of the duration of action of levodopa, causing symptoms to worsen before the next dose (i.e., end-of-dose wearing off), and simultaneously, there is a delay before the next dose of levodopa "kicks in." With time, these predictable fluctuations may give way to unpredictable fluctuations, known as on-off, with random swings in the control of symptoms.

Eventually, the therapeutic window of levodopa narrows, and most patients require higher dosages to achieve adequate symptom relief. At the same time, the threshold for adverse effects lowers, leading to dyskinesias, which are involuntary twisting or gyrating movements that typically coincide with peak levels of levodopa. Although dyskinesias can be unsightly, they often bother the onlooker more than the patient, who usually prefers to be dyskinetic rather than akinetic. Levodopa-induced dyskinesias can affect all parts of the body, with a predilection for head bobbing, facial grimacing, and choreiform movements of the trunk and limbs.

A few principles govern the medical management of PD. First, treatment starts with a low dose of whatever medication is chosen, and the dose is escalated gradually; similarly, withdrawal of antiparkinsonian medications should be done gradually. Second, it is best to manipulate one drug at a time. Third, the physician should have a specific goal in mind when starting a medication, focusing on improvement in functioning or minimizing fluctuations, and the patient should understand this goal of treatment. Fourth, the physician and patient should be familiar with side effects.

Pharmacological Therapy

Levodopa

Because dopamine does not cross the blood-brain barrier, it is instead replaced by its precursor levodopa, which is converted by the enzyme dopa decarboxylase to dopamine. Because conversion takes place in dopaminergic neurons and systemically, levodopa is combined with the decarboxylase inhibitor carbidopa to minimize peripheral conversion. It requires approximately 75 mg of carbidopa to inhibit dopa decarboxylase, and the 25/100-mg tablet (instead of the 10/100-mg tablet) should be used when initiating therapy. The first number refers to the amount of carbidopa and the second to levodopa. Levodopa plus carbidopa is also available in an orally dissolvable form (Parcopa). Although it is neither more effective nor more rapidly absorbed than swallowed levodopa, it has the advantage of being able to be taken without water, a convenience for some, and it can also be used if there is difficulty swallowing tablets.

Levodopa is initially dosed three times per day. The most common side effect is nausea (typically mild and short-lived) and can be minimized by starting levodopa with meals and once tolerated, shifting to at least one-half hour before meals to enhance absorption. If there is severe nausea, carbidopa can be prescribed (25-mg tablets) to further inhibit circulating dopamine, which causes nausea. If this is ineffective, levodopa can be combined with the peripheral dopamine blocker domperidone (not available in the United States).

It may take 2 to 4 weeks to reach the optimal effect. Most patients notice a dramatic effect on one-half or a

whole 25/100-mg tablet taken three times daily, but if not, the dosage can be escalated gradually, with the goal of maximizing function using the lowest dose possible. There is no absolute maximal daily dose of levodopa; in general, little additional symptom relief is achieved by taking more than 250 mg at a single dose. During the first 3 to 6 years of PD, most patients experience sufficient relief with 300 to 1000 mg per day.

Levodopa also comes in an extended-release preparation that can initially be taken twice rather than three times per day, which is not a significant advantage; it does not work for 12 hours and therefore is usually taken in the morning and early afternoon. Only 70% of levodopa in this form is absorbed, and dosing must be adjusted. There is little reason to begin extended-release levodopa, because it has no long-term advantage over regular levodopa for motor fluctuations.[40] When taken at bedtime, it can be helpful for symptoms experienced during the middle of the night, such as difficulty with turning in bed or getting out of bed and walking to the bathroom.

With time, the duration of response to each dose of levodopa shortens, necessitating a reduction in the dosing interval. If there are peak-dose dyskinesias, many patients benefit from a lower dose taken more frequently. Fluctuations are managed by careful dose titration and timing of levodopa and by combining levodopa with one or more complementary agents.[8,23]

Dopamine Agonists

Agonists work directly on dopamine receptors. There are two indications in PD: initial therapy[41,42] and as adjuncts to levodopa to reduce off time.[23] Bromocriptine is an older, ergot-type agonist that is now seldom used. It has been largely replaced by the non-ergot agonists pramipexole and ropinirole. Another ergot agonist, pergolide, was withdrawn because of its recent association with cardiac valvular disease,[43] although it was known that it and bromocriptine could cause fibrosis in the pleura, pericardium, and retroperitoneum.[44] The most recently introduced non-ergot agonist, rasagiline, is a transdermal (patch) preparation, and although not demonstrated to be more efficacious or better tolerated than oral agonists, it offers convenience and may be used for patients unable to take medications orally.[45] Because of irregularities in the delivery system, it has recently been removed from the market.

As initial therapy, agonists are much less likely than levodopa to cause motor fluctuations and dyskinesias, but only within the first 5 years of treatment.[41,42] Unsupported concerns about the "toxicity" of levodopa[16] and pharmaceutical advertising created the widespread myth that initial PD treatment must be an agonist. The treatment of PD must be individualized. Levodopa provides more symptom relief than an agonist and is better tolerated. For those in need of anything other than mild improvement of initial symptoms or for people at increased risk for side effects, such as the elderly, levodopa is preferred.

Two side effects of agonists deserve mention. The first is somnolence, which can develop with little warning and has been associated with falling asleep while driving.[46] Agonists (and most antiparkinsonian agents) should be used cautiously, if at all, in those already experiencing insomnia or excessive daytime sleepiness. Patients should be warned of this potential complication. Second, it has been recognized that patients with PD, often while taking a dopamine agonist, may experience compulsive behaviors,[47] such as pathological gambling, eating, shopping, hypersexuality (including pornography), and punding. *Punding* refers to repetitive, often purposeless motor activities such as the continual shuffling of papers or excessive non–goal-directed computer use. Because these activities are often carried out surreptitiously, patients should be queried about them and warned about the small risk of occurrence when antiparkinsonian agents, especially agonists, are prescribed.

The dopamine agonist apomorphine is available as a subcutaneous injection for the rapid (within 10 minutes) relief of off time related to fluctuations with levodopa. This is known as *rescue therapy*.[48]

Anticholinergics

Until levodopa, anticholinergics were the mainstay of treatment, but they have largely been supplanted by dopaminergic therapies and are now used infrequently. Many of their side effects, such as confusion, memory loss, dry mouth, difficulty urinating, and constipation, are poorly tolerated, especially in the elderly. Anticholinergics are often touted as more effective for tremor than other agents, but that idea is not supported by evidence. Anticholinergics are an option for initial PD treatment, but they should be used with caution, if at all, in the elderly.

Amantadine

Amantadine is an antiviral agent. It was discovered serendipitously to have a mild to modest effect on PD symptoms, although its mechanism of action has never been fully understood. Unlike most other agents, it has the advantage of requiring no titration. It can be used as initial or adjunctive therapy. A second role of amantadine, also discovered serendipitously, is that is can suppress dopamine-induced dyskinesias, an action thought to be mediated by its role as an *N*-methyl-D-aspartate (NMDA) receptor antagonist.[49]

Catechol-O-Methyl Transferase Inhibitors

The enzyme catechol-*O*-methyltransferase (COMT) catabolizes dopamine, and its inhibition therefore prolongs the elimination half-life of dopamine and extends its clinical duration of action. The two available COMT inhibitors, entacapone and tolcapone, are used as levodopa adjuncts for end-of-dose wearing off[8,23] leading to more on time. Shortly after the introduction of tolcapone, several hepatotoxicity-related deaths led to U.S. Food and Drug Administration (FDA)-mandated monitoring of liver function test results; there have been no subsequent deaths. Entacapone is available in a single preparation combined with levodopa and carbidopa. Both COMT inhibitors may exacerbate dopa-induced dyskinesias, necessitating levodopa reduction, but only if dyskinesias present a problem.

Monoamine Oxidase B Inhibitors

Inhibition of monoamine oxidase B (MAO-B) blocks catabolism and reuptake of dopamine, and like COMT inhibitors, it prolongs the duration of action of dopamine, reducing off time.[8] The two available MAO-B inhibitors are selegiline and rasagiline. Early evidence suggested that selegiline had a neuroprotective effect,[50] but that is no longer thought to be the case.[51] Both drugs are adjuncts to levodopa,[8,52] but rasagiline has a modest symptomatic effect as initial PD therapy[53] and is another option for those newly diagnosed with mild symptoms. It has the advantage of once-daily dosing. At recommended doses, selegiline and rasagiline inhibit only the B form of MAO, which occurs exclusively in the brain. They should not be associated with the cheese effect of systemic MAO inhibition (i.e., pressor effect of tyramine arising from the ingestion of cheese and the hypertensive episode produced thereby). Nevertheless, caution is recommended, and potential interactions with tricyclics, meperidine, and selective serotonin reuptake inhibitors must be considered.

Surgical Treatment

Surgical treatment has become routine, with refinements in techniques, use of imaging, advances in understanding the pathophysiology of PD, and a better appreciation for appropriate candidates. Ablative operations have largely been abandoned and replaced by deep brain stimulation (DBS), which has the advantages of avoiding destruction of the target, greater safety, and the ability to adjust the stimulation parameters to achieve the optimal effect.[54,55]

There are two indications for treating PD with DBS. It is indicated for the rare patient with disabling tremor when the thalamus ventral intermediate nucleus is the target. More common is the patient with problematic motor fluctuations, including off time and dyskinesias that cannot be managed medically; the subthalamic nucleus is the preferred target.[4]

DBS improves most of the major PD manifestations and improves quality of life, and it is superior to best medical management.[56] It is most effective for reducing the quantity and improving the quality of off time and for allowing a reduction in medication, lessening dyskinesias. To be a candidate, it is necessary to have motor fluctuations and have evidence of significant improvement with levodopa (i.e., good-quality on time). Surgery appears to be more beneficial for younger patients, but advanced age by itself is not an absolute contraindication. People with dementia and unstable psychiatric disorders, especially affective disorders and psychosis, are not good candidates. Although the benefits of DBS diminish with time as PD continues to advance, the beneficial effect is still evident at 5 years.[57]

Three main factors determine the success of DBS. The first is preoperative assessment. In addition to the characteristics previously mentioned for selecting the appropriate candidate, it is essential to ensure the diagnosis is PD and not a parkinsonian syndrome, which fails to benefit from this treatment and may worsen.[58] Patients and their families must have realistic expectations about the effects of surgery and the risks.[55] Second, the success of DBS is determined by intraoperative factors; the most important are accurate electrode placement and minimization of complications. The third determinant of success is postoperative care, primarily adjustment of the stimulation parameters and medications. Because of the complexity of DBS for PD, the procedure should be carried out in a center with a devoted team of neurologists with expertise in PD, a similarly experienced neurosurgeon, and a psychiatrist familiar with PD and DBS.

With an experienced team, complications are infrequent. The risk of intracerebral hemorrhage is 3% to 4%, and there is a 1% to 2% risk of infection. Stimulation of adjacent structures causing effects such as diplopia and tingling usually can be reversed with adjustment of the stimulating parameters.[59] The most common complications are psychiatric, including depression, hypomania, apathy, suicidal thoughts, hallucinations, and impulse-control disorders.[60] Most of these disorders are temporary and amenable to treatment, but they emphasize the importance of having a psychiatrist involved in the preoperative and postoperative care of patients undergoing DBS.

Therapy for Nonmotor Features of Parkinson's Disease

Although motor features are the most obvious signs of PD, equally prevalent and often more disabling are the many nonmotor aspects (see Box 190-3).[61,62] These features of PD were poorly characterized and poorly understood, and they often went unrecognized and underappreciated by physicians and patients, although they seriously affected quality of life. These nonmotor symptoms are intrinsic aspects of PD, derived primarily from involvement of non-dopaminergic sites within the central and peripheral nervous systems.[17,61] Many, such as daytime sleepiness, cognitive impairment, and orthostatic hypotension, are caused or exacerbated by antiparkinsonian medications, and symptoms can fluctuate with levodopa, just as the motor manifestations of PD do.

The nonmotor symptoms can be divided into several broad categories: autonomic, sensory, sleep, and psychiatric. Treatment approaches to many of the nonmotor aspects of PD (e.g., constipation, orthostatic hypotension, sexual dysfunction, restless legs syndrome) are not unique to PD.[61,63] The most important lesson regarding the non-motor aspects of PD is to be aware of them, ask patients about relevant symptoms, and appreciate that most are treatable.

Autonomic features are common in PD, and like many other nonmotor features, they worsen with advancing PD. Orthostatic hypotension is part of PD but is often exacerbated by antiparkinsonian medications and other drugs, such as antihypertensives. Nonpharmacological treatments include increased salt and water, raising the head of the bed, and use of support hose. Pharmacological options include fludrocortisone and midodrine (ProAmitine). Constipation is ubiquitous in PD and exacerbated by anticholinergic medications. Conversely, bladder dysfunction typically manifested by frequency, urgency, urge incontinence, and nocturia is often treated with anticholinergics, emphasizing the difficulty of balancing the beneficial and deleterious effects of medications in PD.

A common but frequently unvoiced symptom is sexual dysfunction affecting men and women.[64] Both may experience a change (decrease or increase) in libido and anorgasmia. Erectile dysfunction is common in men and may result from PD, its treatment, or testosterone deficiency, which may be overlooked.

Sweating in PD often occurs as an off-period symptom and frequently at night, but it may also occur when on, when on with dyskinesias, or be unrelated to motor fluctuations. If it is directly associated with motor fluctuations, treatment is directed at leveling the medication response by titrating levodopa and the use of adjunctive agents. If unsuccessful, sweating may be managed with the cautious addition of an anticholinergic. Likewise, an anticholinergic agent can reduce drooling in PD, which results from decreased frequency of swallowing, causing saliva to pool in the mouth. However, anticholinergics are often poorly tolerated, particularly by patients with advanced PD, and alternative therapies for drooling include atropine ophthalmic drops used intraorally or local injection of botulinum toxin into the salivary glands.[65]

Because PD is traditionally viewed as a motor disorder, sensory symptoms, which are common, are frequently ignored or wrongly attributed to alternative causes. There may be numbness, tingling, and pain in PD, which, like other nonmotor symptoms, may fluctuate with the timing of levodopa.[66,67] Diminished smell (i.e., anosmia) is common in PD, reflecting early involvement of the olfactory bulb.[17,67] Some patients with PD experience akathisia, which is a sensation of internal restlessness, and many experience an internal, purely subjective sensation of tremor.[68] Particularly bothersome and equally common is fatigue. It should be approached first by searching for a specific cause, such as anemia, hypothyroidism, or orthostatic hypotension. Often, no secondary cause is apparent; amantadine and ProAmitine can be tried, but there are no proven therapies for PD fatigue.

Insomnia is common in PD,[69,70] and specific causes include motor dysfunction such as tremor, stiffness, cramping, or difficulty turning, which can often be prevented by additional levodopa (often the extended-release preparation) at bedtime or on awakening to get back to sleep. Some find that satin sheets and pajamas make it easier to turn, but they also increase the risk of slipping out of bed. Restless legs syndrome and periodic limb movements of sleep are more common among patients with PD than in the general population, and both may contribute to difficulty initiating and sustaining sleep.[69,70] Everyone with insomnia should be queried about depression or anxiety.

Another common nocturnal problem is REM sleep behavioral disorder (RSBD).[69,70] Normally during REM sleep, there is muscle atony, but with an RSBD, there is paradoxically increased motor activity, taking the form of dream enactment with talking, screaming, flailing limb movements, accosting the bed partner, or jumping out of bed. Patients are rarely aware of these behaviors, and they instead affect the bed partner. If problematic or associated with fragmented sleep or daytime sleepiness, clonazepam at bedtime is often very effective.[69,70]

Insomnia from any cause is associated with daytime sleepiness, which is also a common nonmotor problem for patients with PD. Aside from sleep deprivation, other contributors to daytime sleepiness include antiparkinsonian medications, particularly dopamine agonists and anticholinergics; other drugs; and sleep apnea.[69,70] The approach to the PD patient with daytime sleepiness begins by evaluating nocturnal sleep and treating the causes of insomnia. Medications should be scrutinized carefully. If daytime sleepiness persists, consider a nocturnal and daytime sleep study. For patients with persistent somnolence, modafinil can be tried, although evidence from clinical trials suggests that it has a modest effect at best and should not be continued unless there is significant benefit.

Some nonmotor features of PD are neuropsychiatric. These diverse problems are nearly ubiquitous in PD, often more disabling than motor features for the patient and caregiver,[71] and frequently unrecognized, even by specialists in PD.[72] Depression is so common in PD that it is helpful to assume that every patient with PD is depressed until it is proved otherwise. A review concluded that aside from weak evidence supporting treatment with amitriptyline,[24] there are insufficient data to make other treatment recommendations for depression in PD, but personal experience suggests that most agents are effective. The selection depends on associated symptoms and co-morbid conditions. Anxiety also is common in PD. It may be chronic or surface in the setting of motor fluctuations when off, including panic attacks. These affective disorders and the common problem of apathy[73] are thought to reflect intrinsic components of PD itself and are not just reactive states.

Although affective disorders can occur at any time in the evolution of PD, the neuropsychiatric problems of hallucinations, psychosis, delirium, executive dysfunction, and dementia appear with advancing PD.[72] To emphasize their impact, it has been demonstrated that psychosis, including hallucinations, which affects 25% to 40% of patients with PD,[61,74] is a significant contributor, necessitating nursing home placement.[75] Patients may not spontaneously report that they experience hallucinations, and it is necessary to question all patients and caregivers about whether they are "seeing things" or having delusions that are often paranoid in nature, including delusional jealousy.

The first step in managing psychosis in PD is to reassure patients that they are not "going crazy" and that hallucinations and delusions are "the disease and medications playing a trick on your mind." For infrequent hallucinations with retained insight, no treatment is usually necessary. When psychotic symptoms are problematic, the first step is to eliminate as many medications as possible; levodopa is best tolerated at this stage of PD, used as monotherapy if possible. If medications cannot be tapered or eliminated without significantly exacerbating motor features, the hallucinations and delusions can be treated with quetiapine or clozapine, but risperidone (Risperdal), olanzapine, and traditional neuroleptics should be avoided.[24]

Hallucinations and delusions occur in the middle and advanced stages of PD, usually in the setting of cognitive impairment or frank dementia (PDD); the former typically takes the form of executive dysfunction. The prevalence of dementia varies widely based on the diagnostic criteria used and the population studied. A review suggests that about 30% of patients with PD have dementia, but when followed longitudinally, the incidence reached as high as 75% after 8 years.[76,77] Despite being an intrinsic feature of PD, reflecting involvement of nondopaminergic regions, reversible causes of dementia should still be sought, with particular attention to medications, especially those with anticholinergic activity, and pseudodementia associated with depression. Although cholinesterase inhibitors have been deemed "probably effective" for treatment of PDD and may be used, the effect is modest at best.[24]

SUPPORTIVE CARE

Although the emphasis in this discussion of the treatment for PD has been pharmacotherapy, nonpharmacological therapies, including physical, occupational, and speech therapy, can be equally effective throughout the course of the disease.[25] Patients with PD should be encouraged to remain physically and mentally active, including regular exercise. Assistance devices such as canes and walkers should be employed when there is impairment of postural righting reflexes, and useful safety equipment in the home includes tub rails and a raised toilet seat. Throughout the course of the disease and especially in advanced disease with dementia, special attention should be paid to the caregiver. Patients and caregivers should be encouraged to participate in local PD support groups and become members of patient advocacy groups, including the American Parkinson's Disease Association (http://www.apdaparkinson.org) and the National Parkinson's Foundation (http://www.parkinson.org).

EVIDENCE-BASED MEDICINE

Where applicable, the discussion of the treatment of PD in this chapter was evidence based. The American Academy of Neurology and the Movement Disorders Society have published evidence-based reviews and guidelines covering all aspects of PD, including diagnosis, initiation of therapy, management of motor fluctuations, use of alternative therapies, neuroprotection, surgical therapy, and recognition and management of the neuropsychiatric aspects of PD, including depression, dementia, and psychosis.[21,23-25,51,59,78]

REFERENCES

1. Nutt JG, Wooten GF. Diagnosis and initial management of Parkinson's disease. N Engl J Med 2005;353:1021-1027.
2. Samii A, Nutt JG, Ransom BR. Parkinson's disease. Lancet 2004;363:1783-1793.
3. Lang AE, Lozano AM. Parkinson's disease. N Engl J Med 1998;339:1044-1053.
4. Lang AE, Lozano AM. Parkinson's disease. N Engl J Med 1998;339:1130-1143.
5. Reich SG, Lederman MB, Griswold ME. Errors and delays in diagnosing Parkinson's disease. Ann Neurol 2002;52:S84.
6. Rajput AH, Rozdilsky B, Rajput A. Accuracy of clinical diagnosis in parkinsonism—a prospective study. Can J Neurol Sci 1991;18:275-278.
7. Hughes AJ, Daniel SE, Kilford L, Lees AJ. Parkinson's disease: A clinico-pathological study of 100 cases. J Neurol Neurosurg Psychiatry 1992;55:181-184.
8. Jankovic J, Stacy M. Medical management of levodopa-associated motor complications in patients with Parkinson's disease. CNS Drugs 2007;21:677-692.
9. de Lau LM, Breteler MM. Epidemiology of Parkinson's disease. Lancet Neurol 2006;5:525-35.
10. Bennett DA, Beckett LA, Murray AM, et al. Prevalence of parkinsonian signs and associated mortality in a community population of older people. N Engl J Med 1996;334:71-76.
11. Dorsey ER, Constantinescu R, Thompson JP, et al. Projected number of people with Parkinson's disease in the most populous nations, 2005 through 2030. Neurology 2007;68:384-386.
12. Klein C, Lohmann-Hedrich KL. Impact of recent genetic findings in Parkinson's disease. Curr Opin Neurol 2007;20:453-464.
13. Langston JW, Ballard P, Tetrud JW, Irwin I. Chronic parkinsonism in humans due to a product of meperidine-analog synthesis. Science 1983;219:979-980.
14. Galpern WR, Lang AE. Interface between tauopathies and synucleinopathies: A tale of two proteins. Ann Neurol 2006;59:449-458.
15. Lang AE, Obeso JA. Time to move beyond nigrostriatal dopamine deficiency in Parkinson's disease. Ann Neurol 2004;55:761-765.
16. Ahlskog JE. Beating a dead horse: Dopamine and Parkinson disease. Neurology 2007;69:1701-1711.

17. Braak H, Del Tredici K, Rüb U, et al. Staging of brain pathology related to sporadic Parkinson's disease. Neurobiol Aging 2003;24:197-211.
18. Langston JW. The Parkinson's complex: Parkinsonism is just the tip of the iceberg. Ann Neurol 2006;59:591-596.
19. Olanow CW. The pathogenesis of cell death in Parkinson's disease—2007. Movement Disorders 2007;22(Suppl 17):S355-S342.
20. Daniel SE, Lees AJ. Parkinson's Disease Society Brain Bank, London: Overview and research. J Neural Transm 1993;39:165-172.
21. Suchowersky O, Gronseth G, Perlmutter J, et al. Practice parameter: Neuroprotective strategies and alternative therapies for Parkinson's disease (an evidence-based review). Neurology 2006;66:976-982.
22. Biglan KM, Ravina B. Neuroprotection in Parkinson's disease: An elusive goal. Semin Neurol 2007;27:106-112.
23. Pahwa R, Factor SA, Lyons KE, et al, for the Quality Standards Subcommittee of the American Academy of Neurology. Practice Parameter: Treatment of Parkinson disease with motor fluctuations and dyskinesia (an evidence-based review): Report of the Quality Standards Subcommittee of the American Academy of Neurology. Neurology 2006;66:983-995.
24. Miyasaki JM, Shannon K, Voon V, et al, for the Quality Standards Subcommittee of the American Academy of Neurology. Practice Parameter: Evaluation and treatment of depression, psychosis, and dementia in Parkinson disease (an evidence-based review): Report of the Quality Standards Subcommittee of the American Academy of Neurology. Neurology 2006;66:996-1002.
25. Suchowersky O, Reich S, Perlmutter J, et al. Practice parameter: Diagnosis and prognosis of new onset Parkinson disease. Neurology 2006;66:968-975.
26. Chaudhuri KR, Healy DG, Schapira AHV. Non-motor symptoms of Parkinson's disease: Diagnosis and management. Lancet Neurol 2006;5;235-245.
27. Van Gerpen JA. Drug-induced parkinsonism. Neurologist 2002;8:363-370.
28. Reich SG. Tremor. In Slavney P, Hurko O (eds). The Primary Care Physician's Guide to Common Psychiatric and Neurologic Problems. Baltimore: Johns Hopkins University Press, 2001, pp 214-230.
29. Louis ED. Essential tremor. Lancet Neurol 2005;4:100-110.
30. Esper CD, Factor SA. Failure of recognition of drug-induced parkinsonism in the elderly. Mov Disord 2008;23:401-404.
31. Jain S, Lo SE, Louis ED. Common misdiagnosis of a common neurological disorder: How are we misdiagnosing essential tremor? Arch Neurol 2006;63:1100-1104.
32. Quinn N. Parkinsonism-recognition and differential diagnosis. Br Med J 1995;310:447-452.
33. Litvan I, Agid Y, Calne D, et al. Clinical research criteria for the diagnosis of progressive supranuclear palsy (Steele-Richardson-Olszewski syndrome): Report of the NINDS-SPSP International Workshop. Neurology 1996;47:1-9.
34. Gilman S, Low PA, Quinn N, et al. Consensus statement on the diagnosis of multiple system atrophy. J Neurol Sci 1999;163:94-98.
35. Quinn N. Multiple system atrophy—the nature of the beast. J Neurol Neurosurg Psychiatry 1989(Suppl):78-89.
36. Kieburtz K, Ravina B. Why hasn't neuroprotection worked in Parkinson's disease? Nat Clin Pract Neurol 2007;3:240-241.
37. Kurlan R. "Levodopa phobia": A new iatrogenic cause of disability in Parkinson disease. Neurology 2005;64:923-924.
38. The Parkinson Study Group. Levodopa and the progression of Parkinson's disease. N Engl J Med 2004;351:2498-2508.
39. Marsden CD, Parkes JD, Quinn NP. Fluctuations of disability in Parkinson's disease: Clinical aspects. In. Marsden CD, Fahn S, (eds). Movement Disorders. London: Butterworth, 1982, pp 96-122.
40. Block G, Liss C, Reines S, et al, for the CR First Study Group. Comparison of immediate-release and controlled release carbidopa/levodopa in Parkinson's disease. Eur Neurol 1997;37:23-27.
41. Parkinson Study Group. Pramipexole vs. levodopa as initial treatment for Parkinson's disease. JAMA 2000;284:1931-1938.
42. Rascol O, Brooks DJ, Korczyn AD, et. Al. A five-year study of the incidence of dyskinesia in patients with early Parkinson's disease who were treated with ropinirole or levodopa. N Engl J Med 2000;342:1484-1491.
43. Antonini A, Poewe W. Fibrotic heart-valve reactions to dopamine-agonist treatment in Parkinson's disease. Lancet Neurol 2007;6:826-829.
44. Tintner R, Manian P, Gauthier P, Jankovic J. Pleuropulmonary fibrosis after long-term treatment with the dopamine agonist pergolide for Parkinson disease. Arch Neurol 2005;62:1290-1295.
45. Jankovic J, Watts RL, Martin W, Boroojerdi B. Transdermal rotigotine: Double-blind, placebo-controlled trial in Parkinson disease. Arch Neurol 2007;64:676-682.
46. Frucht S, Rogers JD, Greene PE, et al. Falling asleep at the wheel: Motor vehicle mishaps in persons taking pramipexole and ropinirole. Neurology 1999;52:1908-1910.
47. Voon V, Fox SH. Medication-related impulse control and repetitive behaviors in Parkinson's disease. Arch Neurol 2007;64:1089-1096.
48. Kolls BJ, Stacy M. Apomorphine: A rapid rescue agent for the management of motor fluctuations in advanced Parkinson disease. Clin Neuropharmacol 2006;29:292-301.
49. Luginger E, Wenning GK, Bösch S, Poewe W. Beneficial effects of amantadine on L-dopa-induced dyskinesias in Parkinson's disease. Mov Disord 2000;15:873-878.
50. The Parkinson Study Group. Effect of deprenyl on the progression of disability in early Parkinson's disease. N Engl J Med 1989;321:1364-1371.
51. Miyasaki JM, Martin W, Suchowersky O, et al. Practice parameter: Initiation of treatment for Parkinson's disease: An evidence-based review: Report of the Quality Standards Subcommittee of the American Academy of Neurology. Neurology 2002;58:11-17.
52. Rascol O, Brooks DJ, Melamed E, et al, for the Largo Study Group. Rasagiline as an adjunct to levodopa in patients with Parkinson's disease and motor fluctuations (LARGO, Lasting effect in Adjunct therapy with Rasagiline Given Once daily, study): A randomised, double-blind, parallel-group trial. Lancet 2005;365:947-954.
53. Parkinson Study Group. A controlled trial of rasagiline in early Parkinson disease: The TEMPO Study. Arch Neurol 2002;59:1937-1943.
54. Volkmann J. Update on surgery for Parkinson's disease. Curr Opin Neurol 2007;20:465-469.
55. Rodriguez RL, Fernandez HH, Haq I, Okun MS. Pearls in patient selection for deep brain stimulation. Neurologist 2007;13:253-260.
56. Deuschl G, Schade-Brittinger C, Krack P, et al, for the German Parkinson Study Group, Neurostimulation Section. A randomized trial of deep-brain stimulation for Parkinson's disease. N Engl J Med 2006;355:896-908.
57. Krack P, Batir A, Van Blercom N, et al. Five-year follow-up of bilateral stimulation of the subthalamic nucleus in advanced Parkinson's disease. N Engl J Med 2003;349:1925-1934.
58. Shih LC, Tarsy D. Deep brain stimulation for the treatment of atypical parkinsonism. Mov Disord 2007;22:2149-2155.
59. Kleiner-Fisman G, Herzog J, Fisman DN, et al. Subthalamic nucleus deep brain stimulation: Summary and meta-analysis of outcomes. Mov Disord 2006;21(Suppl 14):S290-S304.
60. Voon V, Kubu C, Krack P, et al. Deep brain stimulation: Neuropsychological and neuropsychiatric issues. Mov Disord 2006;21(Suppl 14):S305-S327.
61. Chaudhuri KR, Healy DG, Schapira AH. Non-motor symptoms of Parkinson's disease: Diagnosis and management. Lancet Neurol 2006;5:235-245.
62. Shulman LM, Taback RL, Bean J, Weiner WJ. Comorbidity of the nonmotor symptoms of Parkinson's disease. Mov Disord 2001;16:507-510.
63. Pfeiffer RF, Bodis-Wollner I (eds). Parkinson's Disease and Nonmotor Dysfunction. Totowa, NJ: Humana Press, 2005.
64. Koller WC, Vetere-Overfield B, Williamson A, et al. Sexual dysfunction in Parkinson's disease. Clin Neuropharmacol 1990;13:461-463.
65. Molloy L. Treatment of sialorrhoea in patients with Parkinson's disease: Best current evidence. Curr Opin Neurol 2007;20:493-498.
66. Riley DE, Lang AE. The spectrum of levodopa-related fluctuations in Parkinson's disease. Neurology 1993;43:1459-1464.
67. Katzenschlager R, Lees AJ. Olfaction and Parkinson's syndromes: Its role in differential diagnosis. Curr Opin Neurol 2004;17:417-423.
68. Shulman LM, Singer C, Bean JA, Weiner WJ. Internal tremor in patients with Parkinson's disease. Mov Disord 1996;11:3-7.
69. Comella CL. Sleep disorders in Parkinson's disease: An overview. Mov Disord 2007;22(Suppl 17):S367-S373.
70. Comella CL. Sleep disturbances and excessive daytime sleepiness in Parkinson disease: An overview. J Neural Transm Suppl 2006;70:349-355.
71. Weintraub D, Stern MB. Psychiatric complications in Parkinson's disease. Am J Geriatr Psychiatry 2005;13:844-851.
72. Shulman LM, Taback RL, Rabinstein AA, Weiner WJ. Non-recognition of depression and other non-motor symptoms in Parkinson's disease. Parkinsonism Relat Disord 2002;8:193-197.
73. Dujardin K, Sockeel P, Devos D, et al. Characteristics of apathy in Parkinson's disease. Mov Disord 2007;22:778-784.
74. Fénelon G, Mahieux F, Huon R, Ziégler M. Hallucinations in Parkinson's disease: Prevalence, phenomenology and risk factors. Brain 2000;123(Pt 4):733-745.
75. Goetz CG, Stebbins GT. Risk factors for nursing home placement in advanced Parkinson's disease. Neurology 1993;43:2227-2229.
76. Aarsland D, Zaccai J, Brayne C. A systematic review of prevalence studies of dementia in Parkinson's disease. Mov Disord 2005;20:1255-1263.
77. Aarsland D, Andersen K, Larsen JP, et al. Prevalence and characteristics of dementia in Parkinson disease: An 8-year prospective study. Arch Neurol 2003;60:387-392.
78. Goetz CG, Poewe W, Rascol O, Sampaio C. Evidence-based medical review update: Pharmacological and surgical treatments of Parkinson's disease: 2001 to 2004. Mov Disord 2005;20:523-539.

SUGGESTED READING

Ahlskog JE. The Parkinson's Disease Treatment Book. Partnering with Your Doctor to Get the Most from Your Medications. Oxford, UK: Oxford University Press, 2005.

Factor SA, Weiner WJ (eds). Parkinson's Disease Diagnosis and Clinical Management, 2nd ed. New York: Demos, 2007.

Nutt JG, Wooten GF. Diagnosis and initial management of Parkinson's disease. N Engl J Med 2005;353:1021-1027.

Pahwa R, Lyons KE (eds). Handbook of Parkinson's Disease, 4th ed. London: Informa Healthcare, 2007.

Samii A, Nutt JG, Ransom BR. Parkinson's disease. Lancet 2004;363:1783-1793.

William WJ, Shulman LM, Lang AE. Parkinson's Disease: A Complete Guide for Patients and Families. Baltimore: Johns Hopkins, 2006.

CHAPTER **191**

Multiple Sclerosis

David A. Gruenewald and Jodie Haselkorn

K E Y   P O I N T S

- Multiple sclerosis (MS) has a pervasive effect on the lives of the affected person and his or her caregivers from early adulthood throughout an almost normal life span.

- People with MS may benefit from interdisciplinary team management to address a wide range of symptoms, including fatigue, depression, cognitive loss, visual loss, weakness, spasticity, tremors, bladder and bowel dysfunction, and acute and chronic pain syndromes.

- Symptoms considered important by health care workers may not be the most important ones for the individual with MS.

- Quality of life may be markedly affected by unpredictability of the disease course, depression, loss of social interaction, loss of autonomy, and effects of MS on family life.

Multiple sclerosis (MS) is a chronic, inflammatory, demyelinating, and axonal disorder of the brain and spinal cord. The symptoms and clinical course of MS are highly variable, and the disorder often has motor, sensory, autonomic, cognitive, and behavioral manifestations. Early symptoms may be intermittent, but in most cases, the disease eventually enters a progressive phase resulting in increasing disability and care needs.

MS often has a pervasive impact on the lives of people with MS and their families over several decades. Optimal comprehensive management of MS requires holistic, individualized care that includes disease and symptom management along with functional, psychological, social, family, economic, spiritual, and quality of life issues. This approach requires the expertise of an interdisciplinary team skilled in the management of each of these domains. The goals of care may include wellness, stabilization of disease, effective control of symptoms, maximization of function and independence, and maintenance of productivity and a meaningful place in society. The care team must be prepared to modify the goals of care and management strategies over time as the condition and priorities of the person with MS change.

PATHOPHYSIOLOGY

MS is thought to be an immune system–mediated disorder occurring in those who are genetically susceptible, but the events triggering an autoimmune response remain uncertain. MS is heterogeneous with respect to pathological, clinical, and neuroimaging findings, suggesting that many pathogenic mechanisms may be involved. The consensus is that different mechanisms lead to myelin, oligodendrocyte, and axonal injury.

The hallmark lesion is the demyelinating plaque in the brain and spinal cord of affected individuals, but the plaque's structural features vary widely between individuals. Pathogenesis of the plaque appears to involve inflammation and degeneration.[1] An initial event such as a viral infection may trigger an immune cross-reaction with an antigen such as myelin, with injury to the myelin sheath and the oligodendrocyte that produces the myelin sheath. This autoimmune response appears to involve autoreactive T cells, B cells, and macrophages and includes upregulation of various cytokines, including tumor necrosis factor-α, interleukin-2, and interferon-γ. In addition to demyelination, axonal injury occurs early in the course of inflammatory MS, and extensive injury to axons may play a key role in progressive disability. Among the factors implicated in axonal injury are cytokines, proteases, superoxides, nitric oxide, glutamate, and CD8$^+$ lymphocytes.

EPIDEMIOLOGY, PREVALENCE, AND DISEASE COURSE

MS is the most common cause of chronic neurological disability in young adults, affecting approximately 1 in 1000 people in the United States. The disease is usually diagnosed in people between 20 and 50 years old, but it may occur at any age. Twice as many women as men are affected. Whites of northern European descent have the highest incidence, but MS occurs in all races and geographical locations.

The clinical course varies widely but generally will follow one of four patterns (Table 191-1):

TABLE 191-1   Clinical Patterns of Multiple Sclerosis

MULTIPLE SCLEROSIS COURSE	PROPORTION OF CASES	CHARACTERISTICS	ASSOCIATIONS
Relapsing-remitting (RRMS)	80-85%	Acute episodes of worsening of neurological function Some recovery and no progression between episodes	Female-to-male ratio is 2:1 Younger at disease onset
Secondary progressive (SPMS)	One half of RRMS cases convert to SPMS within 10 yr Almost all convert within 25 yr	Progression of disease with increasing disability, with or without relapses	
Primary progressive (PPMS)	10%	Progressive decline in function from onset, without distinct relapses	Female-to-male ratio is 1:1 Older at disease onset
Progressive-relapsing	<5%	Progressive decline in function from onset, with acute relapses Long-term outcome similar to PPMS	

1. Relapsing-remitting MS (RRMS)
2. Primary progressive MS (PPMS)
3. Secondary progressive MS (SPMS)
4. Progressive relapsing MS

In relapsing disease, relapse is heralded by the onset of new symptoms or worsening of existing symptoms or signs that last longer than 24 hours and that are unexplained by an intercurrent illness or a hot ambient temperature. In a typical relapse, symptoms worsen over days to a few weeks and then improve or resolve over the ensuing few weeks or months. In progressive MS, symptoms or functional status worsens gradually or rapidly, without definite relapses and without recovery.

The extent of disability strongly correlates with the duration of illness. By 10 years after onset, 50% to 80% of affected persons are unable to perform usual household tasks and continue employment. After 15 years, 32% to 76% require an assistive device for ambulation, and between 11% and 29% are confined to bed. Factors associated with a poor long-term outcome are a progressive course, shorter time to disease progression, rapid onset of unremitting disability, frequent relapses in the first 2 years, multiple symptoms at onset, a short interval between the first two attacks, cerebellar symptoms at onset, and older age at onset. Overall life expectancy is decreased by 6 to 13 years compared with the general population, although excess mortality rates have improved. Severe disability is a major risk factor for death, with mortality rates approaching four times those of people without MS. More than one half eventually die of complications of MS, including pneumonias, aspiration pneumonias, pressure ulcers, and urinary tract infections (UTIs). Suicide risk is 2 to 7.5 times higher than the general population, particularly in the first few years after diagnosis. In the Netherlands, it is estimated that 5% of patients die by euthanasia or physician-assisted suicide. Assisted suicide is more likely to be considered by those who are unemployed or have multiple symptoms, experience emotional distress, are lonely, or lack social support. Those with severe physical disability are not more likely to favor assisted suicide (see "Pearls and Pitfalls").

Pearls and Pitfalls

- People with multiple sclerosis (MS) are at increased risk for suicide, especially in the first few years after the diagnosis. The physician should periodically screen for and treat depression indicated by answers to questions:
  Are you depressed?
  Have you been sad or blue most of the time lately?
  Have you recently lost interest or pleasure in things?
- People with MS are more likely than their physicians to identify nonphysical symptoms (e.g., social isolation, depression, loss of autonomy) as the most disabling manifestations of the disease.
  Person- and family-centered interdisciplinary assessment and intervention is essential.
  Clinicians should identify ways to promote choice and autonomy and should maintain the perception of reciprocity in caregiving relationships.
- People with MS often wish to be full partners in setting care goals and choosing interventions.
  Physicians should form a partnership with the person who has MS and should practice good listening and communication skills.

CLINICAL MANIFESTATIONS

The clinical signs and symptoms vary greatly and depend on the location of the central nervous system (CNS) lesions (Box 191-1). Subclinical MS may begin long before the disease manifests clinically. Over time, manifestations usually evolve and often become more severe.

Visual and sensory disturbances are among the most common symptoms of RRMS. Presenting manifestations of RRMS may include optic neuritis, weakness and clumsiness of the extremities, loss of sensation, Lhermitte's sign (i.e., paresthesias in the limbs and body elicited by flexing the neck), fatigue, cognitive dysfunction, bowel and bladder dysfunction, and ataxic gait. Individuals who enter a secondary progressive phase may develop worsening brainstem symptoms (e.g., dysarthria, dysphagia, diplopia), quadriparesis, spasticity, tremors, cognitive impairment, bladder and bowel incontinence, and other symptoms. The presenting symptoms of patients with PPMS are often weakness and gait disorders. As with SPMS, many individuals with PPMS develop other symptoms.

Overall, fatigue and depression are the most common symptoms in MS, reported by 90% and 75%, respectively. Neither fatigue nor depression correlates with disease severity. Fatigue is particularly debilitating, along with balance problems, pareses, and bladder dysfunction. Symptoms may worsen with fever, exercise, or physiological increases in body temperature (i.e., Uhthoff's symptom), sometimes suggesting the diagnosis of MS in previously undiagnosed individuals.

DIAGNOSIS AND DIFFERENTIAL DIAGNOSIS

Diagnosis is based on evidence of CNS lesions disseminated in time and space that are not better explained by

---

Box 191-1 Clinical Manifestations of Multiple Sclerosis

Motor problems
  Weakness
  Spasticity
  Cerebellar manifestations (e.g., dysarthria, ataxia, tremor)
  Dysphagia
  Diplopia
Sensory problems
  Visual loss (e.g., optic neuritis)
  Pain
    Neuropathic (e.g., dysesthesias, radicular pain, trigeminal neuralgia, Lhermitte's sign)
    Spasticity related
    Disuse related (e.g., compression fractures, complex regional pain syndrome)
  Numbness
  Dizziness and vertigo
Sexual dysfunction (e.g., erectile dysfunction, loss of libido)
Bladder dysfunction (e.g., urinary tract infections, urinary retention, urgency, incontinence)
Bowel dysfunction (e.g., constipation, fecal incontinence)
Fatigue
Heat intolerance (i.e., Uhthoff's symptom)
Depression
Emotional lability (e.g., pathological laughter, weeping)
Cognitive impairments (e.g., processing speed, memory, executive function)

an alternative diagnosis. Many presenting symptoms and an evolving clinical course suggest MS, and laboratory and imaging tests (especially magnetic resonance imaging [MRI]) may exclude other diagnoses. In cases of diagnostic uncertainty, repeat MRI scanning within 6 to 12 months may demonstrate multiple lesions of various ages. Numerous disorders in the differential diagnosis include acute disseminated encephalomyelitis, human immunodeficiency virus (HIV)–associated myelopathy, cerebrovascular disease, Behçet's syndrome, leukodystrophies, CNS sarcoidosis, and conversion disorder. Consensus criteria (i.e., McDonald criteria) for diagnosis of early MS were developed in 2001 and revised in 2005 (http://www.mult-sclerosis.org/DiagnosticCriteria.html). They are useful for patients who present with a single episode (i.e., clinically isolated syndrome), a relapsing-remitting course, or gradual symptom progression without definite attacks or remissions.

TREATMENT

The therapeutic approach may include treatments for acute relapses, disease-modifying therapies, symptom management, and rehabilitation. Evidence- and consensus-based clinical practice guidelines are available for acute relapses, disease-modifying therapies, and rehabilitation. Published guidelines are becoming available for MS symptoms such as fatigue, urinary dysfunction, and spasticity.[2]

Acute Relapses

Corticosteroids are modestly beneficial in hastening recovery from acute relapses of MS symptoms. Although the optimal dose is unknown, high-dose protocols are superior to moderate-dose regimens. Treatment is most effective soon after the onset of a relapse, although there may be some benefit even if treatment is started weeks or months afterward. There appears to be no long-term functional benefit from corticosteroid therapy for acute relapses.[3]

Disease-Modifying Therapy

Disease-modifying therapies are most effective during the relapsing-remitting phase. Treatment should begin as soon as possible after a diagnosis of RRMS is made and continued indefinitely unless there is no benefit or unacceptable side effects. Several agents reduce the number and severity of relapses, the number of new CNS lesions seen on MRI, and the progression of clinical disease on the Expanded Disability Status Scale (EDSS). Agents include interferon-β (Avonex, Betaseron, Rebif), glatiramer acetate, mitoxantrone, and natalizumab. Their overall benefit is modest (i.e., relapse rate reduced by about one third), except for natalizumab, which reduces the relapse rate by 53% to 68%. Natalizumab was withdrawn in early 2005 after three patients developed progressive multifocal leukoencephalopathy. The U.S. Food and Drug Administration reapproved natalizumab in 2006 as monotherapy, but it cannot be used with any other immunosuppressive agent and is available only through certified physicians, pharmacies, and infusion centers. Mitoxantrone has a

limited lifetime dose and is usually reserved for second-line therapy. There is no consensus about which of the other four is the agent of first choice. The choice of therapy is typically based on side effects, convenience, co-morbid illnesses, and the physician's preference.[4] Head-to-head trials of single agents and combination therapy are being conducted. Betaseron and mitoxantrone have been approved for SPMS, but it has been difficult to demonstrate reductions in rate of disease progression and long-term disability. No therapies are effective against PPMS, but rituximab is being studied.

Symptomatic Treatment

Although disease-modifying agents are changing the disease course and delaying disability, they are not effective for the associated secondary impairments. Various symptoms may adversely affect activities, social participation, and health-related quality of life.[2,5,6] Many of these symptoms are themselves disabling. Practitioners should routinely ask about symptoms and evaluate their impact on activities, social participation, and quality of life. Because many of the symptoms are common in other medical conditions, a thorough assessment is necessary. Treatment includes lifestyle modification, medical management (Table 191-2), referral to a rehabilitation professional who specializes in MS, and sometimes, surgery. People with complex disabilities may require referral to an MS specialty center for multidisciplinary assessment and management.

Fatigue

Up to 95% of people with MS experience fatigue, and for many, it is the most disabling symptom (see Chapter 161). Although the pathophysiological basis is unclear, contributing factors may include co-morbid medical illnesses such as infections, anemia, hypothyroidism, and depression; cognitive loss; sleep disturbance; deconditioning; heat exposure; and medications. In addition to potential underlying causes, management should include nonpharmacological interventions such as instruction in energy-efficiency techniques, education about and prescription of cooling devices, and an individualized aerobic exercise program.

A trial of medication is usually indicated if fatigue is severe; available agents include amantadine, acetyl-L-carnitine, and modafinil. Stimulants such as methylphenidate and dextroamphetamine are sometimes prescribed off-label (see Chapter 130).

Spasticity

Approximately 70% of people with MS have difficulty with spasticity. Spasticity may manifest as stiffness (i.e., tonic spasticity, often involving the legs and trunk) or involuntary muscle spasms (i.e., phasic spasticity). Complications include gait disorders, sleep disturbances, pain, reduced mobility, muscle and joint contractures, pressure sores, and impaired quality of life. Spasticity by itself is not harmful; if there is leg muscle weakness, some spasticity may facilitate weight bearing and assist transfers.

Triggering factors such as UTIs, constipation, skin breakdown, and other noxious stimuli should be

TABLE 191-2 First-Line Oral Medications for Multiple Sclerosis–Related Symptoms

DRUGS AND USE	DOSE	EVIDENCE-BASED RATING*	SIDE EFFECTS	PRECAUTIONS
SPASTICITY				
Baclofen	5-120 mg/day	Level A	Sedation, weakness, nausea, dizziness, dry mouth (more common with high doses)	Titrate slowly, avoid abrupt withdrawal, reduce dose with renal impairment
Tizanidine	2-36 mg/day	Level A	Sedation, dizziness, dry mouth	Titrate slowly, monitor liver function tests
TRIGEMINAL NEURALGIA				
Carbamazepine	300-1600 mg/day	Level A	Blurry vision, nystagmus, nausea, dizziness	Monitor blood cell count, liver function tests
PAINFUL TONIC SPASMS AND PAROXYSMAL DYSESTHESIAS				
Gabapentin	1200-3600 mg/day	Level U (level A for phasic spasticity)	Sedation, nausea	Titration required
CHRONIC DYSESTHESIAS				
Amitriptyline	25-150 mg/day	Level A	Dry mouth, sedation, urinary retention, constipation	Highly anticholinergic
Carbamazepine	300-1600 mg/day	Level A	Blurry vision, nystagmus, nausea, dizziness	Monitor blood count, liver function tests
Gabapentin	1200-3600 mg/day	Level A	Sedation, nausea	Titration required
FATIGUE				
Amantadine	100-200 mg/day	Level A	Usually mild; hallucinations, nausea, anxiety, insomnia	May become refractory to therapy with time
Modafinil	100-200 mg/day	Level U	Anxiety, headache, nausea, insomnia	May reduce effectiveness of hormonal contraception in women
URINARY URGENCY AND URGE INCONTINENCE				
Tolterodine	2-4 mg/day	Level A	Dry mouth, dizziness, constipation	Usually well tolerated; may cause urinary retention
Trospium chloride	20-40 mg/day	Level A	Dry mouth, dizziness, constipation	Usually well tolerated; may cause urinary retention
Oxybutynin	5-15 mg/day	Level A	Dry mouth, dizziness, constipation, somnolence	May cause urinary retention
RECURRENT BLADDER INFECTIONS				
Methenamine mandelate	1 g four times daily	Level C	Usually well-tolerated; nausea, vomiting, diarrhea, abdominal cramps	
Methenamine hippurate	1 g two times daily	Level C	Usually well-tolerated; nausea, vomiting, diarrhea, abdominal cramps	May cause transient elevations in liver transaminases
NOCTURIA AND URINARY FREQUENCY				
Desmopressin	20 μg/day intranasally	Level A	Fluid retention, hyponatremia	Caution in setting of cardiac, renal dysfunction
MEMORY PROBLEMS				
Donepezil	5-10 mg daily	Not available	Nausea, diarrhea, insomnia	Concurrent anticholinergic agents may inhibit donepezil's effects
DEPRESSION				
Sertraline	50-200 mg/day	Level U	Insomnia, somnolence, dizziness, headache, fatigue, diarrhea, dry mouth, nausea, ejaculatory dysfunction	Monitor for suicidality
Imipramine	75-300 mg/day	Level C	Dry mouth, somnolence, urinary retention, constipation, confusion, heart block	Highly anticholinergic

*Recommendations on the strength of evidence were obtained from the National Institute for Clinical Excellence (NICE). Multiple Sclerosis: Management of Multiple Sclerosis in Primary and Secondary Care. Clinical guideline 8. London: National Institute for Clinical Excellence, November 2003; from the Multiple Sclerosis Treatment Consensus Group of the German MS Society.[2] Strength of evidence recommendations are reported according to the American Academy of Neurology clinical practice guideline scheme[3] as follows:
A—Established as effective for the given condition in the specified population
B—Probably effective for the given condition in the specified population
C—Possibly effective for the given condition in the specified population
U—Data are inadequate or conflicting, and given current knowledge, treatment is unproven.

evaluated. Rehabilitation is indicated to maximize functional status and avoid disability. Active or assisted range of motion is the mainstay of a treatment program. When spasticity is associated with secondary impairments such as pain, decreased sleep, or unsafe mobility, antispasticity medications often are given with other rehabilitation measures. There is insufficient evidence to compare the effectiveness of these agents, although baclofen and tizanidine are most widely prescribed. Gabapentin may be useful for phasic spasticity and painful spasms. Dantrolene sodium is also useful, but it can cause sedation, weakness, and hepatotoxicity. Benzodiazepines relieve spasticity, but use is limited by their sedation and dependency potential. The therapeutic role of cannabinoids is uncertain. Neuromuscular blocks using botulinum toxin, phenol, or alcohol are effective for focal spasticity problems such as equinovarus deformity or adductor muscle spasticity. Intrathecal baclofen infusion using an implanted pump is indicated for lower extremity spasticity that interferes with function after oral therapy alone has failed.

Bladder Dysfunction and Infection

Bladder dysfunction occurs in up to 80% of people with MS. UTIs occur in 30% of community-dwelling people with MS presenting with bladder symptoms and must therefore be excluded. UTIs may manifest with nonspecific symptoms, including increased spasticity and pseudorelapse (i.e., worsening MS symptoms). Upper urinary tract imaging with an intravenous pyelogram or ultrasound scan may be indicated for patients with recurrent UTIs. The recurrence rate of lower UTIs may be reduced with prophylactic methenamine for urinary acidification. Long-term prophylactic antibiotics are not indicated because of the potential for selection of resistant bacteria.

Diagnostic studies indicated for bladder leakage, incontinence, or frequent UTIs include periodic checks of post-void residual urine volume. Urodynamic studies help if the diagnosis or management is difficult. Urodynamic studies can identify three common types of bladder dysfunction in MS patients:

1. Detrusor hyperreflexia with reduced bladder storage capacity
2. Bladder hyporeflexia with failure to empty
3. Detrusor-sphincter dyssynergia (i.e., failure of coordination between bladder outlet relaxation and bladder contractions)

Individuals with detrusor hyperreflexia may experience urinary urgency, frequency, and urge incontinence, and they may benefit from fluid ingestion evenly distributed throughout the day, bladder training with scheduled voiding, and avoidance of bladder irritants such as caffeine. Anticholinergic agents reduce urinary frequency and urge incontinence in people with overactive bladder. Dry mouth is less common with tolterodine and trospium chloride than with oxybutynin. Intranasal desmopressin may reduce urinary frequency and nocturia. A tricyclic antidepressant may facilitate sleep and increase bladder capacity at night.

The treatment of choice for urinary retention caused by bladder hyporeflexia or detrusor-sphincter dyssynergia is clean intermittent bladder catheterization several times daily. This may not be an option for people unable to self-catheterize. In that case, a suprapubic cystostomy and indwelling catheter may be indicated. α-Adrenergic blocking agents such as terazosin or tamsulosin may reduce bladder outlet tone in detrusor-sphincter dyssynergia, but this approach is controversial, and bladder catheterization may still be necessary.

Bowel Dysfunction

Approximately 60% of people with MS have problems with bowel function. The most common problem is constipation, which may result from neurogenic bowel dysfunction or from inadequate fluid intake, insufficient dietary fiber, medication side effects, immobility, and spasticity. Individuals with a neurogenic bowel benefit from a bowel program with timely evacuation of feces daily or every other day without incontinence (see Chapter 154). Mainstays of a bowel program include adequate fluid and dietary fiber intake; increased mobility; a daily routine for bowel elimination, usually after breakfast to take advantage of the gastrocolic reflex; adequate positioning and privacy for defecation; and medications if needed. Stool softeners may help if the stool is dry despite adequate hydration. Sennosides taken at night facilitate bowel motility. Occasionally, sorbitol or lactulose is necessary. Suppositories or mini-enemas trigger the rectocolic reflex and help trigger bowel elimination. Individuals with fecal incontinence should be assessed for stool impaction, which can manifest as leakage of liquid diarrhea. These individuals require bowel evacuation and initiation of a bowel program. Individuals who continue to have bowel incontinence despite these measures should be seen by an MS specialist.

Pain Syndromes

Two of three people with MS experience pain at some point during the disease, and for many, pain is the worst symptom (see Chapter 170). Patients may experience many acute and chronic pain problems, and careful evaluation is required. Pain may be directly from MS (e.g., trigeminal neuralgia, acute optic neuritis, chronic dysesthesias, meningeal irritation [Lhermitte's sign], muscle spasms), indirectly related (e.g., musculoskeletal pain due to contractures or poor positioning, osteoporotic compression fractures due to chronic immobility, pressure sores, urinary retention, obstipation, nerve entrapment syndromes), or unrelated to MS (e.g., degenerative arthritis).

Trigeminal neuralgia is the most common acute pain syndrome associated with MS; it occurs in up to 2% of patients. Short-term opioid use may be necessary. Long-term treatment includes carbamazepine and other antiepileptic drugs. Other paroxysmal pain syndromes such as painful tonic spasms (i.e., phasic spasticity) and paroxysmal dysesthesias seem to respond best to gabapentin or, alternatively, to lamotrigine, phenytoin, or sodium valproate. Painful optic neuritis is treated with intravenous corticosteroids.

MS-associated pain is frequently chronic and multifactorial. For some patients, medical management is relatively straightforward. For instance, chronic dysesthesias may manifest as an unpleasant burning sensation involving the limbs and trunk and can be effectively managed with tricyclic antidepressants or antiepileptic agents. Musculoskeletal pain due to poor posture, spasticity, and immobility can be managed with intensive physical and occupational therapy and appropriate medications. However, multidisciplinary assessment and management by specialists in MS and pain may be necessary for refractory pain.

Mood and Anxiety Disorders

Depression occurs in up to 90% of people with progressive MS, more commonly than in patients with other chronic medical conditions (see Chapter 157). Depression may be a consequence of MS itself, a side effect of MS treatments, or associated with secondary MS impairments. Although MS-associated mood symptoms are associated with poorer quality of life, major depression is often undertreated. People with MS are more likely than their providers to consider mental health issues important to their well-being. People with MS should periodically be screened for depression, ideally using a standardized screening tool.

Depression in people with MS is as responsive to treatment as in the general population. Psychotherapeutic and cognitive-behavioral approaches help. Tricyclic antidepressants and selective serotonin reuptake inhibitors appear effective, although well-controlled trials are lacking. Fatigue and cognitive loss can mimic depression or coexist with it. Like depression, anxiety disorders are more frequent than in the general population. Other factors such as chronic pain and social isolation, common among people with MS, can complicate assessment and management of depression. Suicidal ideation and suicide are more common than in the general population.

Tremors

Intention tremors from lesions in the cerebellum or cerebellar outflow pathways are the most common tremors in MS and one of the most difficult symptoms to treat. Anticonvulsants (e.g., carbamazepine, primidone, gabapentin, clonazepam) and intravenous ondansetron have been evaluated, but results were disappointing. Using light weights on the distal aspect of the limb or weighted utensils may produce modest functional improvement. Contralateral thalamotomy or thalamic electrostimulation may help some, but their high cost and limited availability preclude widespread use.

Cognitive Impairment

Approximately one half of people with MS develop difficulties with attention, cognitive processing speed, memory, and executive function (see Chapter 167). Cognitive impairment can occur early, although it is rarely the presenting symptom. Subjective cognitive complaints are often associated with subtle but real cognitive problems, and they should not be automatically attributed to other causes such as fatigue or depression. Memory problems are associated with increased caregiver stress.

Management should include a medication review to minimize potential adverse medication effects on cognition and an assessment for depression and fatigue. Acetylcholinesterase inhibitors such as donepezil may improve

learning and memory. Cognitive rehabilitation strategies that build on strengths and minimize weaknesses may help. Educating caregivers regarding the strengths and weaknesses of the individual with MS and how to cue to facilitate compensatory strategies may reduce interpersonal strain.

Dysphagia

Swallowing difficulty occurs in about one third of people with MS, and it often is caused by demyelinating brainstem lesions. A swallowing evaluation is indicated if there is difficulty swallowing, coughing with eating, or reports of choking. A video esophagram or barium swallow radiography may be warranted. Swallowing problems can be managed with a modified-texture diet, attention to food temperature and bite size, and swallowing precautions, including upright posture, appropriate head positioning, and minimization of distractions.

Feeding by means of a gastrostomy tube may improve symptoms and quality of life when there are repeated aspiration events or difficulty maintaining hydration and calorie targets solely by normal oral intake. Discussion with the patient and family should include specific indications for feeding tube placement, anticipated health status benefits (e.g., better hydration, fewer UTIs, less constipation), opportunities for oral intake (if any), and quality of life issues (e.g., better communication with the care partner). People should be explicitly informed that the tube can be removed at their request in the future if it is no longer compatible with their care goals. This discussion may provide an opportunity to review care goals, advance directives, and end-of-life concerns (see Chapter 105).

Respiratory Insufficiency

Respiratory complications such as aspiration pneumonia are a major cause of morbidity and mortality. In addition to weakened glottic musculature that interferes with swallowing, weak expiratory muscles cause an ineffective cough, and weak inspiratory muscles cause hypoventilation and acidosis. Expiratory muscle training, instruction in quad coughing, and an inexsufflator can manage secretions. Inspiratory muscle training may also be useful. People with advanced respiratory compromise causing oxygen desaturation can benefit from noninvasive respiratory interventions such as continuous positive-pressure ventilation, especially at night, or tracheostomy and ventilation in some patients.[6]

Rehabilitation

Interdisciplinary evaluation, coordinated treatment, education, and disease self-management are the cornerstones of MS rehabilitation, with specific interventions customized to the individual's functional status and level of social support. Issues that must be considered (in addition to disease management and symptom management) include mobility, self-care, cognition, speech, psychological adjustment, mobility, bladder and bowel function, vocational goals, leisure goals, and sexual function. Rehabilitation programs should be goal oriented, with assessments conducted by an interdisciplinary team. Progress toward these goals should be monitored using standardized instruments (e.g., Functional Independence Measure, Multiple Sclerosis Impact Scale [MSIS-29], and Modified Fatigue Impact Scale). In cases of mild disability, emphasis should be placed on maintaining wellness, strength, aerobic exercise capacity, and family and vocational roles.[7]

Several trials showed beneficial effects of outpatient and inpatient rehabilitation in the moderately disabled. Improvements in disability and participation last for approximately 6 months after rehabilitation, whereas beneficial effects on quality of life and emotional well-being may persist. Few data are available to assess potential rehabilitation benefits in severely disabled persons with MS.[7,8]

Individuals and their caregivers may face numerous challenges to acceptable quality of life, including an unpredictable disease course, impaired functioning in social and family settings, depression, symptoms, and a wide variety of unmet care needs.[9,10] For patients with advanced MS, measures of participation and quality of life validated for use in people with MS should monitor progress during rehabilitation (see Chapter 65). However, most available instruments are geared toward those less severely affected, and there is no consensus on the most appropriate measure.[9]

PALLIATIVE CARE

MS differs from most other disorders seen by palliative care specialists in that individuals with MS usually have a nearly normal life expectancy, although more than one half of affected persons ultimately die of related complications. Aside from the protracted disease course, MS shares features of other diseases that benefit from a palliative approach, including incurability; challenging symptom management; increasing physical impairment over time; emotional, psychosocial, and spiritual issues; and caregiver support. Many MS practitioners incorporate elements of palliative care into the care of people with MS, but barriers to a comprehensive palliative care approach include reluctance to offer palliative care unless death is near, the practitioner's discomfort with end-of-life discussions, difficulty recognizing the transition to terminal illness, a lack of knowledge about palliative care, and the physician's reluctance to follow people with MS who live in nursing homes. Nevertheless, people with MS and their families may have needs in the physical, emotional, psychosocial, and spiritual domains at any time during the illness, and an interdisciplinary focus on improving comfort and quality of life may be offered whenever they are receptive. Guidelines for palliative care in advanced MS are in preparation by the National Multiple Sclerosis Society.

Good communication between the provider and patient is essential (see Chapters 110 and 112). Unfortunately, unhelpful or dismissive interactions with health care professionals are often a part of the experience of living with MS.[11] No one communication strategy is successful in every case, but good communication between the provider and the person with MS may initially involve establishing a mentorship relationship with the MS patient. As people with MS gain expertise and experience with their illness, they may want the relationship to evolve from mentorship into a collaborative partnership. At this stage, the individual with MS is recognized as an expert on his or her personal experience with MS and priorities for living with MS, whereas the provider is the expert in managing issues such as symptoms, medications, and therapies. As disability becomes advanced, individuals with MS may want to address existential issues and supportive care to maintain some sense of control and autonomy.[12]

DEVELOPMENTS AND RESEARCH OPPORTUNITIES

We need to identify disease-modifying therapies that are effective in SPMS or PPMS. Research is needed to determine whether people with MS and progressive functional loss benefit from ongoing or pulsed rehabilitation interventions. We also need to identify measures of participation and quality of life that are useful in the clinical care of people with advanced MS. More work is needed to identify factors that improve the quality of dying and death of people severely affected by MS.

ACKNOWLEDGMENTS

This work was supported by the Department of Veterans Affairs.

REFERENCES

1. Frohman EM, Racke MK, Raine CS. Multiple sclerosis—the plaque and its pathogenesis. N Engl J Med 2006;354:942-955.
2. Henze T. Managing specific symptoms in people with multiple sclerosis. Int MS J 2005;12:60-68.
3. Goodin DS, Frohman EM, Garmany GP Jr, et al. Disease modifying therapies in multiple sclerosis. Neurology 2002;58:169-178.
4. Karussisa D, Biermann LD, Bohlegac S, et al. A recommended treatment algorithm in relapsing multiple sclerosis: Report of an international consensus meeting. Eur J Neurol 2006;13:61-71.
5. Krupp LB, Rizvi SA. Symptomatic therapy for underrecognized manifestations of multiple sclerosis. Neurology 2002;58(Suppl 4):S32-S39.
6. Rousseaux M, Perennou D. Comfort care in severely disabled multiple sclerosis patients. J Neurol Sci 2004;222:39-48.
7. Thompson AJ. Neurorehabilitation in multiple sclerosis: Foundations, facts and fiction. Curr Opin Neurol 2005;18:267-271.
8. Thompson AJ. Symptomatic management and rehabilitation in multiple sclerosis. J Neurol Neurosurg Psych 2001;71(Suppl 2):ii22-ii27.
9. Gruenewald DA, Higginson IJ, Vivat B, et al. Quality of life measures for the palliative care of people severely affected by multiple sclerosis: A systematic review. Mult Scler 2004;10:690-725.
10. McKeown LP, Porter-Armstrong AP, Baxter GD. The needs and experiences of caregivers of individuals with multiple sclerosis: A systematic review. Clin Rehabil 2003;17:234-248.
11. Yorkston KM, Johnson KL, Klasner ER. Taking part in life: Enhancing participation in multiple sclerosis. Phys Med Rehabil Clin North Am 2005;16:583-594.
12. Thorne S, Con A, McGuinness L, et al. Health care communication issues in multiple sclerosis: An interpretive description. Qual Health Res 2004;14:5-22.

SUGGESTED READING

Brandis M, Reitman NC, Gruenewald DA, et al. Opening doors: The Palliative Care Continuum in multiple sclerosis. New York: National Multiple, Sclerosis Society, 2008. Available at http://www.nationalmssociety.org/for-professionals/healthcare-professionals/publications/clinical_bulletins/index.aspx (accessed April 2008).
National Collaborating Centre for Chronic Conditions. Multiple Sclerosis. National Clinical Guideline for Diagnosis and Management in Primary and Secondary Care. London: National Institute for Clinical Excellence, 2004. Available at http://www.guideline.gov/summary/summary.aspx?ss=15&doc_id=5063&nbr=3547 (accessed January 2008).

National Multiple Sclerosis Society Long-Term Care Committee. Nursing Home Care of Individuals with Multiple Sclerosis: Guidelines and Recommendations for Quality Care. New York: National Multiple Sclerosis Society, 2003.

Plumb S. MS and palliative care: A guide for health and social care professionals. London: Multiple Sclerosis Society, 2006. Available at http://www.mssociety.org.uk/for_professionals/developing_services/palliative_care/index.html (accessed January 2008).

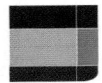

CHAPTER **192**

Amyotrophic Lateral Sclerosis

Gian Domenico Borasio

KEY POINTS

- Amyotrophic lateral sclerosis (ALS) is a paradigm for nononcological palliative care.
- Palliative care in ALS starts with the way in which the diagnosis is communicated.
- Dyspnea is the worst symptom in ALS, but it can be palliated by noninvasive home mechanical ventilation.
- Communication is often difficult and time-consuming in later disease.
- Advance care planning and end-of-life decision making are particularly important.

ALS is one of the major neurodegenerative diseases alongside Alzheimer's disease and Parkinson's disease. It is progressive, involving degeneration at all levels of the motor system. Involvement of other elements of the nervous system has been described, particularly post mortem, but motor system involvement is the most important in relation to the clinical features during life. Prominent sufferers have included the baseball star Lou Gehrig, the German philosopher Franz Rosenzweig, the physicist Stephen Hawking, and possibly Mao Tse-tung.

EPIDEMIOLOGY AND PREVALENCE

The annual incidence of ALS is 1.5 to 2 per 100,000 population, with a prevalence of 6 to 8 per 100,000. ALS accounts for approximately 0.1% of all adult deaths. ALS is rare before the age of 20 years. Most cases begin after age 40 years, and the mean age is 58 years. The incidence of ALS continues to rise with age. Men are more commonly affected than women (1.5:1 to 2:1). Approximately 5% of cases are familial, mostly with autosomal dominant inheritance. Approximately one fifth of familial cases result from mutations in the superoxide dismutase-1 gene.

BASIC SCIENCE AND PATHOPHYSIOLOGY

ALS remains poorly understood in terms of a unifying etiological hypothesis, and it may be a common end-stage pathological phenotype of diverse causes. Current work focuses largely on excitotoxicity and oxidant stress. *Excitotoxicity* is a phenomenon by which amino acid neuromodulators such as glutamate become toxic at supraphysiological concentrations. Other potential excitotoxins include α-amino-3-hydroxy-5-methyl-4-isoxazole propionic acid (AMPA) and kainate. Excitotoxins may precipitate neuronal death by triggering excessive calcium influx into the motor neuron at membrane level and thereby producing an intraneuronal cascade mechanism involving free radical intermediates that causes neuronal death. The excitotoxic and free radical theories are thus not mutually exclusive. The excitotoxic hypothesis stimulated identification of riluzole, a glutamate release inhibitor, as the first licensed disease-modifying therapy. Attempts to develop antioxidant therapies for ALS have, by contrast, been disappointing.

CLINICAL MANIFESTATIONS

Patients have clinical and pathological involvement of both upper and lower motor neurons, usually sparing the oculomotor nuclei, and the spinal Onuf nucleus, which supplies anal sphincter muscles. Most patients present with asymmetrical, distal weakness and atrophy of the arm or leg (Fig. 192-1). Bulbar onset occurs in 20% to 30%, but more than 50% of older female patients present with bulbar symptoms. The clinical hallmark is the coexistence of neurogenic atrophy, weakness, and fasciculations (resulting from lower motor neuron degeneration), with hyperactive or incongruously present deep tendon reflexes, pyramidal tract signs, and increased muscle tone from corticospinal tract involvement. Muscle cramps are

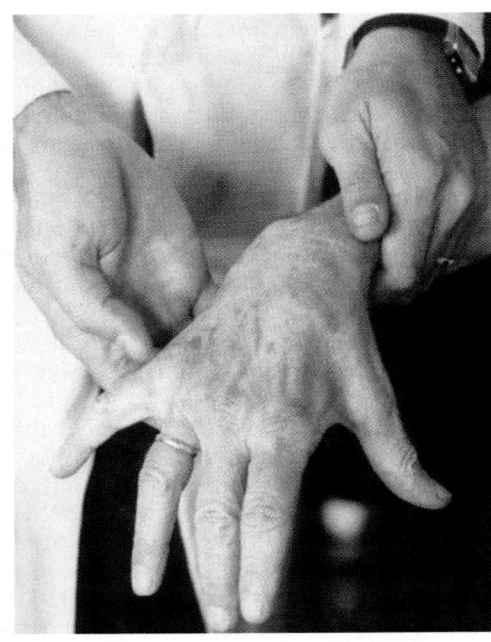

FIGURE 192-1   Muscle weakness in amyotrophic lateral sclerosis.

often present before diagnosis. Pseudobulbar affect with uncontrolled crying or laughter is common. Sensation, sphincter control, and extraocular motility are usually spared. Two percent to 3% of patients have full-fledged dementia, whereas up to 50% show mild cognitive changes related to frontotemporal dysfunction that can be detected using sensitive testing methods. Most patients retain full decision-making capacity throughout their illness. The absence of decubitus sores even when these patients are bedridden is thought to be related to biochemical skin changes.

DIAGNOSIS

The diagnosis of ALS is essentially clinical. Diagnostic criteria (the so-called El Escorial criteria) were established and have been revised.[1]

DIFFERENTIAL DIAGNOSIS

Although the classic clinical presentation leaves little diagnostic doubt, some cases can be difficult to diagnose, particularly in patients with early disease. The differential diagnosis includes physical causes (e.g., spondylotic myelopathy), immune disorders (multifocal motor neuropathy with or without antibodies to ganglioside GM1, myasthenic syndromes, inclusion body myositis, paraneoplastic syndromes), toxins (e.g., lead, organophosphates), infections (syphilis, borreliosis, Creutzfeldt-Jakob disease), metabolic disorders (e.g., diabetes, hyperthyroidism, hyperparathyroidism, porphyria), enzyme deficiencies (hexosaminidase), and other neurological disorders (motor neuropathy, myopathic syndromes, multiple sclerosis).

TREATMENT

Disease-Modifying Treatments

The antiglutamatergic agent riluzole alters the natural history and prolongs life by approximately 3 months.[2] Ten to 15% of patients discontinue treatment because of the side effects of this drug (asthenia, dizziness, gastrointestinal problems), and a few discontinue it because of significant liver enzyme elevation, which requires monitoring. It is important to tell patients in advance that riluzole has no subjective benefit, such as increased muscle strength, and that it will not stop the disease from progressing.

Alternative Therapies

Many patients turn to alternative treatments because of their dissatisfaction with available drugs. Often, this subject is not discussed with the physician because of fear of "condemnation."[3] It is best to approach this topic proactively, by offering to discuss whatever therapeutic options patients may wish to try. This avenue enables the physician to protect patients from serious financial or medical risks while preserving hope and maintaining trust in the patient-physician relationship. An example of such an alternative treatment is spurious "stem-cell therapy," offered at high cost from centers in the Ukraine or China.

Palliative Care

Even without satisfactory therapy, much can be done to alleviate suffering of patients and their families. Almost all signs and symptoms (Table 192-1) can be helped by palliative measures.[4] Palliative care starts at diagnosis (Fig. 192-2) and requires a coordinated interdisciplinary and multiprofessional approach (Table 192-2), with special attention to psychosocial and spiritual issues.

Breaking the News

Once ALS has been diagnosed, all aspects of the disease should be openly discussed with the patient and his or

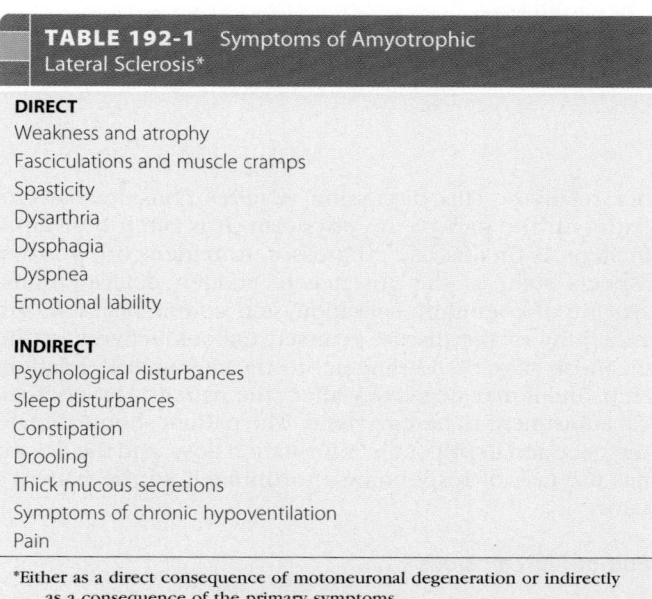

TABLE 192-1 Symptoms of Amyotrophic Lateral Sclerosis*
DIRECT
Weakness and atrophy
Fasciculations and muscle cramps
Spasticity
Dysarthria
Dysphagia
Dyspnea
Emotional lability
INDIRECT
Psychological disturbances
Sleep disturbances
Constipation
Drooling
Thick mucous secretions
Symptoms of chronic hypoventilation
Pain

*Either as a direct consequence of motoneuronal degeneration or indirectly as a consequence of the primary symptoms.

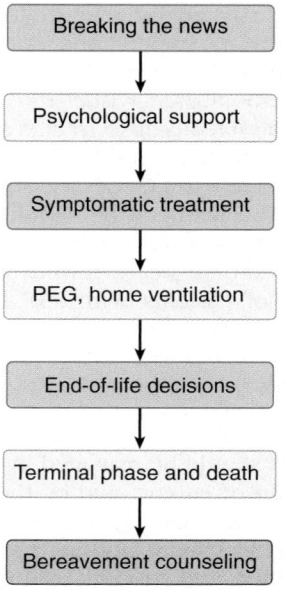

FIGURE 192-2 The course of palliative care in amyotrophic lateral sclerosis. PEG, percutaneous endoscopic gastrostomy.

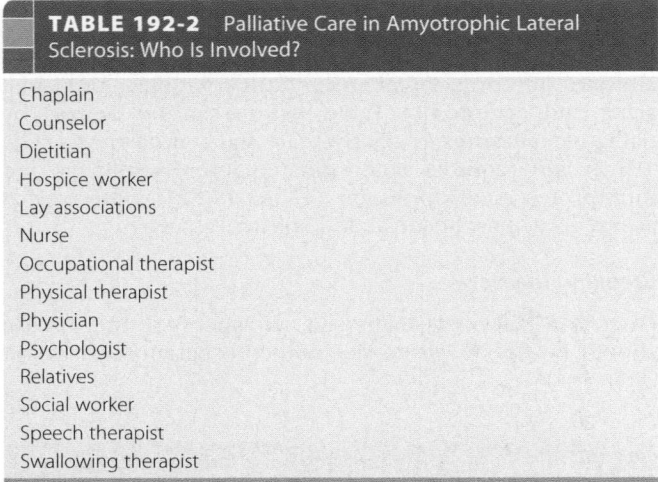

TABLE 192-2 Palliative Care in Amyotrophic Lateral Sclerosis: Who Is Involved?

Chaplain
Counselor
Dietitian
Hospice worker
Lay associations
Nurse
Occupational therapist
Physical therapist
Physician
Psychologist
Relatives
Social worker
Speech therapist
Swallowing therapist

her relatives. This discussion requires considerable empathy on the part of the physician. It is often best done in steps as the disease progresses, to underscore positive aspects such as the absence of sudden deteriorations, sparing of cognition, sensation, and continence, and the variability of the disease course.[5] Callous delivery of the diagnosis may be detrimental to the therapeutic relationship, and it may negatively affect the patient's psychological adjustment to bereavement. The patient should dictate the pace and depth of the information flow, and the doctor has the task of responding appropriately to the patient's cues.

End-of-Life Decisions

At the onset of dyspnea or chronic nocturnal hypoventilation, or when forced vital capacity drops to less than 50%, patients should be offered information about the terminal phase of ALS, because most patients fear they will "choke to death." This fear can be relieved by describing the mechanism of terminal hypercapnic coma and the resulting peaceful death during sleep.[6] At the same time, patients should be asked about their wishes in the event of terminal respiratory failure. Because tracheostomy may result in a "locked-in" syndrome and death in an intensive care unit, most patients refuse it (see "Case Study: Amyotrophic Lateral Sclerosis"). This decision should be documented in writing and incorporated into advance directives.[7] These directives should be reviewed regularly, because the preferences of patients with ALS for life-sustaining treatments change over time.

Specific Symptoms

MUSCLE WEAKNESS

Muscle weakness should be managed by regular exercise, never to the point of fatigue, and by the progressive use of proper assistive devices (e.g., cane, ankle-foot orthosis, wheelchair, aids to facilitate clothing and eating), to maximize independence and mobility. Short-term increased muscle strength may be achieved by pyridostigmine (40 to 60 mg three times daily).

CASE STUDY

Amyotrophic Lateral Sclerosis

Mrs. SL was a 72-year-old woman who had been widowed 5 years earlier. She lived with her daughter and her family, which consisted of her daughter's husband and two children aged 9 and 12 years. Mrs. SL was very active in her local church community. She had developed slurring of speech 2 years earlier. A referral had been made for speech therapy, and the speech and language therapist had asked for a neurological opinion. Further investigations had confirmed the diagnosis of amyotrophic lateral sclerosis.

In August 2005, Mrs. SL had become less mobile as a result of limb weakness. By October of that year, she required a frame, and in December, she was regularly using a wheelchair. The house in which she lived had two large rooms downstairs, and one was converted into a bedroom for Mrs. SL. The children found the loss of their television room, where they met their friends, very difficult.

Mrs. SL's speech deteriorated and was barely understandable, and she started to cough and splutter with meals. She was able to eat pureed food, although this took her daughter longer to prepare, and the family started to refuse to eat with her. After discussion, Mrs. SL was admitted for the insertion of a percutaneous endoscopic gastrostomy, and she was fed enterally at night. The grandchildren found it increasingly difficult to spend time with Mrs. SL because they could not understand her speech and felt uncomfortable with her drooling. The drooling was eased by anticholinergic medication. Mrs. SL became more breathless and chose to start noninvasive ventilation, which she tolerated quite well despite her bulbar symptoms. She made it very clear that she would not go on to invasive ventilation through a tracheostomy.

As Mrs. SL's condition deteriorated further, her friends from church continued to visit and took her to services regularly. The minister also visited and was a great support to her and her family. The local palliative care team was at the home regularly and provided practical support. The social worker met with the grandchildren and allowed them to talk about their fears and then to spend some time with their grandmother.

After 1 year on noninvasive ventilation, and 4 years into the disease, Mrs. SL decided to stop the ventilation, which she now needed almost constantly. This decision caused considerable stress to her family and her professional caregivers. The physician convened a family meeting with the social worker and the minister. The unanimous consensus was that Mrs. SL had the competence and the right to make the decision. A farewell ceremony was organized, and the family gathered at her bedside. Mrs. SL was sedated with benzodiazepines and morphine before the ventilation was discontinued, and she died peacefully at home with her family.

DYSPHAGIA

Dysphagia should first be treated by adjusting the consistency of the patient's diet (recipe books are available from many patients' associations). Specific swallowing techniques (e.g., supraglottic swallowing) can prevent aspiration. When food intake becomes intolerable because of aspiration and choking, or when oral caloric intake becomes insufficient (weight loss >10%), it is best to perform a percutaneous endoscopic gastrostomy (PEG). PEG is usually well tolerated if the patient's vital capacity is greater than 50%. A radiologically inserted gastrostomy is an alternative in patients with more advanced stages of ALS.

DYSARTHRIA

Dysarthria can lead to complete loss of oral communication. Logopedic treatment helps at first. Electronic communication devices can be a blessing in patients with advanced cases. Modern computer technology can enable even tetraplegic patients to communicate effectively. First attempts at directly exploiting brain electric currents to control computers have been encouraging.[8]

DYSPNEA

Dyspnea is the most severe symptom. At the beginning, chest physical therapy helps. Dyspnea attacks usually cause pronounced anxiety, which is best managed by short-acting benzodiazepines (lorazepam, 0.5 to 1 mg sublingually [SL]). In advanced stages, chronic nocturnal hypoventilation ensues, which may considerably hamper quality of life (Box 192-1).

Noninvasive intermittent ventilation by mask (NIV) is efficient and cost-effective in alleviating these symptoms, and it may even prolong the patient's life span.[9] NIV should be discussed with the patient and family at the onset of chronic hypoventilation, or when vital capacity drops to less than 50%.[10] The patient and family should be informed about the temporary nature of the measure, which is primarily directed toward improving quality of life, rather than prolonging it (as opposed to tracheostomy). The problem with mechanical ventilation is usually unrelated to cost or technical difficulties, but rather to the increasing care needs of ventilated patients. Slow disease progression, good communication skills, mild bulbar involvement, strong patient motivation, and a supportive family favor NIV. To be effective, NIV must be administered for at least 4 hr/day, preferably at night. It is important to reassure patients that whenever they decide to stop NIV, all necessary care and appropriate medication will ensure a peaceful death.[11] The physician has a legal and ethical duty to honor a patient's request for discontinuation of treatment.[12]

Box 192-1 Symptoms of Chronic Hypoventilation

- Daytime fatigue and sleepiness, concentration problems
- Difficulty falling asleep, disturbed sleep, nightmares
- Morning headache
- Nervousness, tremor, increased sweating, tachycardia
- Depression, anxiety
- Tachypnea, dyspnea, phonation difficulties
- Visible efforts of auxiliary respiratory muscles
- Recurrent or chronic upper respiratory tract infections
- Cyanosis, edema
- Vision disturbances, dizziness, syncope
- Reduced appetite, weight loss, recurrent gastritis
- Diffuse pain in head, neck, and extremities

PSYCHOLOGICAL SYMPTOMS

These symptoms usually consist of reactive depression, starting shortly after diagnosis. In patients with severe depression, antidepressants such as amitriptyline or the selective serotonin reuptake inhibitors may be indicated. Counseling should always be extended to family members. Despite a reportedly high interest in physician-assisted suicide among patients with ALS, suicide attempts are uncommon.[6]

SLEEP DISORDERS

Sleep disorders usually result from the patient's inability to change position during sleep. Psychological problems, muscle cramps, fasciculations, dysphagia, and dyspnea can also impair sleep. Sedatives should be used sparingly because they may impair residual muscle force.

THICK MUCOUS SECRETIONS

Such secretions result from a combination of diminished fluid intake and reduced coughing pressure. This problem is difficult to treat. N-Acetylcysteine helps a few patients. Suction is usually not fully effective unless it is performed through a tracheostomy. Both manually assisted coughing techniques and mechanical insufflation-exsufflation help to extract excess airway mucus. Physical therapy with vibration massage may be helpful, especially in the early stages of ALS.

PAIN

Up to 73% of patients with ALS have pain. Musculoskeletal pain often arises in advanced stages from atrophy and altered tone around joints. Muscle contractures and joint stiffness (e.g., frozen shoulder) may also be painful. Treatment includes physical therapy, nonsteroidal antiinflammatory drugs, and opioids. Skin pressure pain, resulting from immobility, requires special nursing attention.

PATHOLOGICAL LAUGHING OR CRYING

This condition, which occurs in up to 50% of patients, is not a mood disorder but rather an abnormal display of affect, which can be socially disturbing. It responds well to medication (Table 192-3). A combination of dextromethorphan and quinidine is effective, but further experience regarding long-term side effects and tolerability is needed.[13]

OTHER SYMPTOMS

Other symptoms that can be relieved by medication include muscle cramps, fasciculations, spasticity, and drooling (see Table 192-3). For therapy-refractory drooling, salivary gland botulinum toxin injections or radiation may be considered.

Psychosocial Care

Caregiver burden often exceeds that of patients and deserves particular attention. The physician must be sensitive to the needs and fears of the patients' children and to the importance of helping patients in their role as parents. Patient associations may provide invaluable help and assistance, and they should be involved from the moment of

TABLE 192-3 Symptomatic Medication in Amyotrophic Lateral Sclerosis (in Order of Recommendation)

SYMPTOMS	DOSAGE*
FASCICULATIONS AND MUSCLE CRAMPS	
If Mild	
Magnesium	5 mmol qd-tid
Vitamin E	400 IE bid
If Severe	
Quinine sulfate	200 mg bid
Carbamazepine	200 mg bid
Phenytoin	100 mg qd-tid
SPASTICITY	
Baclofen	10-80 mg
Tizanidine	6-24 mg
Memantine	10-60 mg
Tetrazepam	100-200 mg
DROOLING	
Amitriptyline	10-150 mg
Transdermal hyoscine patches	1-2 patches
Glycopyrrolate	0.1-0.2 mg SC/IM tid
Atropine/benztropine	0.25-0.75 mg/1-2 mg
PATHOLOGICAL LAUGHING OR CRYING	
Amitriptyline	10-150 mg
Fluvoxamine	100-200 mg
Lithium carbonate	400-800 mg
L-Dopa	500-600 mg

*Usual range of adult daily dosage; some patients may require higher doses (e.g., of antispastic medication).
bid, twice daily; IM, intramuscularly; qd, once daily; SC, subcutaneously; tid, three times daily.

Future Considerations

- Frontotemporal cognitive dysfunction has received considerable attention. Depending on instrument sensitivity, several patients exhibit subtle cognitive deficits. Although this dysfunction may slow communication, in most patients it does not significantly impair their decision-making capacity.
- Future treatment advances, possibly involving novel drug delivery strategies such as viral vectors, and multimodality regimens as in cancer, will prolong life span considerably. The transition from a rapidly fatal to a chronic progressive disease will require adaptation of the palliative approach.
- Regardless of the velocity of the disease, the dichotomy of progressive physical debilitation and largely intact cognition will always lead to situations in which patients with amyotrophic lateral sclerosis, despite optimal care, request a hastened death. Finding the most humane way to deal with these requests without endangering fundamental ethical principles of patient care is one of the great challenges of modern medicine.

diagnosis. An example is the International Alliance of ALS/MND Associations (for a worldwide list, see www.alsmndalliance.org). Referral to a tertiary care center with an interdisciplinary team may ease the neurologist's burden and may provide hope. An example is the World Federation of Neurology (a list of ALS centers worldwide can be found at www.wfnals.org).

Spiritual Care and Bereavement

Spiritual care is often underestimated. Spirituality or religious beliefs affect the use of PEG and NIV and may comfort patients.[14] Spiritual care is not limited to patients, but rather should encompass the whole family to prevent bereavement problems, which may particularly affect families dealing with ALS. The bereavement process in ALS starts at diagnosis (anticipatory grief), and callous delivery of the diagnosis may affect the psychological adjustment to bereavement.

Terminal Phase

More than 90% of patients with ALS die peacefully, mostly in their sleep. "Choking to death" is rare.[6] Without artificial ventilation, the dying process usually begins with sleep slipping into coma from increasing hypercapnia. If the patient develops restlessness or signs of dyspnea, morphine should be given, beginning with 2.5 to 5 mg orally (PO), SL, subcutaneously, or intravenously every 4 hours

(if necessary, along with chlorpromazine as an antiemetic). Because morphine is not anxiolytic, anxiety should be treated with lorazepam (beginning with 1 to 2.5 mg SL) or midazolam (beginning with 1 to 2 mg PO or SL). The dosage of morphine and anxiolytics should be increased until satisfactory symptom control is achieved. The potential of these drugs to induce respiratory depression is overestimated, and it is irrelevant in the terminal phase according to the doctrine of double effect.[11]

Most patients wish to die at home. This goal can often best be achieved through enrollment in hospice. It is advisable for the physician to initiate hospice care well in advance of the terminal phase. If death at home is impossible, inpatient hospice or palliative care units should be considered. Hospice teams can also assist caregivers during bereavement after the patient's death.

Evidence-Based Medicine

Evidence-based guidelines for the care of patients with ALS were published in 1999 by the American Academy of Neurology.[10] Several trials strengthened the evidence base for symptomatic treatment, particularly about noninvasive ventilation. The 2006 European guidelines[15] included the new evidence. More research is needed, particularly to establish the best way of attending to the psychosocial and spiritual needs of patients, families, and professional caregivers (see "Future Considerations" box).

REFERENCES

1. Brooks BR, Miller RG, Swash M, et al., World Federation of Neurology Research Group on Motor Neuron Diseases. El Escorial revisited: Revised criteria for the diagnosis of amyotrophic lateral sclerosis. Amyotroph Lateral Scler Other Motor Neuron Disord 2000;1:293-299.
2. Lacomblez L, Bensimon G, Leigh PN, et al. Dose-ranging study of riluzole in amyotrophic lateral sclerosis. Lancet 1996;347:1425-1431.
3. Wasner M, Klier H, Borasio GD. The use of alternative medicine by patients with amyotrophic lateral sclerosis. J Neurol Sci 2001;191:151-154.
4. Borasio GD, Voltz R, Miller RG. Palliative care in amyotrophic lateral sclerosis. Neurol Clin 2001;19:829-847.
5. Borasio GD, Sloan R, Pongratz DE. Breaking the news in amyotrophic lateral sclerosis. J Neurol Sci 1998;160(Suppl 1):S127-S133.
6. Neudert C, Oliver D, Wasner M, Borasio GD. The course of the terminal phase in patients with amyotrophic lateral sclerosis. J Neurol 2001;248:612-616.
7. Borasio GD, Voltz R. Advance directives. In Oliver D, Borasio GD, Walsh D (eds). Palliative Care in Amyotrophic Lateral Sclerosis: From Diagnosis to Bereavement, Oxford: Oxford University Press, 2006.

8. Kubler A, Nijboer F, Mellinger J, et al. Patients with ALS can use sensorimotor rhythms to operate a brain-computer interface. Neurology 2005;64:1775-1777.
9. Bourke S, Tomlinson T, Williams T, et al. Effects of non-invasive ventilation on survival and quality of life in patients with amyotrophic lateral sclerosis: A randomised controlled trial. Lancet Neurol 2006;5:140-147.
10. Miller RG, Rosenberg JA, Gelinas DF, et al. Practice parameter: The care of the patient with amyotrophic lateral sclerosis (an evidence-based review). Report of the Quality Standards Subcommittee of the American Academy of Neurology. Neurology 1999;52:1311-1323.
11. Borasio GD, Voltz R. Discontinuation of life support in patients with amyotrophic lateral sclerosis. J Neurol 1998;245:717-722.
12. American Academy of Neurology. Assisted suicide, euthanasia, and the neurologist: The Ethics and Humanities Subcommittee of the American Academy of Neurology. Neurology 1998;50:596-598.
13. Brooks BR, Thisted RA, Appel SH et al. Treatment of pseudobulbar affect in ALS with dextromethorphan/quinidine: A randomized trial. Neurology 2004;63:1364-1370.
14. Murphy PL, Albert SM, Weber C, et al. Impact of spirituality and religiousness on outcomes in patients with ALS. Neurology 2000;55:1581-1584.
15. Andersen PM, Borasio GD, Dengler R, et al. EFNS task force on management of amyotrophic lateral sclerosis: Guidelines for diagnosing and clinical care of patients and relatives. An evidence-based review with good practice points. Eur J Neurol 2005;12:921-938.

SUGGESTED READING

Brown R, Swash M, Pasinelli P (eds). Amyotrophic Lateral Sclerosis, 2nd ed. London: Martin Dunitz, 2006.

Mitsumoto H, Bromberg M, Johnston W, et al. Promoting excellence in end-of-life care in ALS. Amyotroph Lateral Scler Other Motor Neuron Disord 2005;6:145-154.

Mitsumoto H, Przedborski S, Gordon PH (eds). Amyotrophic Lateral Sclerosis. New York: Taylor & Francis, New York, 2006.

Oliver D, Borasio GD, Walsh D (eds). Palliative Care in Amyotrophic Lateral Sclerosis: From Diagnosis to Bereavement. Oxford: Oxford University Press, 2006.

Simmons P: Learning to Fall: The Blessings of an Imperfect Life. New York: Bantam Books, 2003.

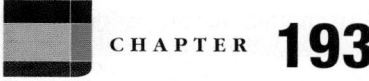

CHAPTER **193**

Quadriplegia and Paraplegia

Walter Ceranski, Bradley Buckhout, and David Oliver

KEY POINTS

- A full multidisciplinary assessment is essential to ensure that a correctable cause is excluded.
- The prevention of complications by active management is important.
- Active rehabilitation by the multidisciplinary team allows quality of life to be improved.
- Psychological aspects must be addressed to maximize recovery.
- Reassessment is essential.

The palliative care of a person with quadriplegia or paraplegia varies according to the cause. Most patients have a stable deficit and a nearly normal to normal life expectancy, but for the person with malignant spinal cord compression, the prognosis is poor, and management is different.

Regardless of the cause of the lesion, the care and management of various problems are similar. Care and management encompass both the physical features and the psychosocial aspects of coping with a severe disability. The overall aim of care is to maintain as good a quality of life as possible. It is clear that the quality of life of the patient with a spinal cord injury largely depends on that individual's focus following the injury. If patients choose to emphasize what they have lost rather than to build on what remains, their course is considerably more difficult for them and for those providing care. Early intervention from therapists (physical, occupational, and psychological) and support from family and friends are critical in this choice of direction.[1] The other keys—premorbid personality and sense of self-worth—are not alterable, although it may be possible to keep the patient's social interactions as normal as possible to reduce psychological morbidity.[2] Palliative care at the end of life may be necessary if the patient's condition deteriorates, whether from complications of the condition, from progression of the disease process causing the condition, or from other disease processes that are, in turn, influenced by the presence of paralysis.

EPIDEMIOLOGY AND PREVALENCE

The most common cause of quadriplegia or paraplegia is trauma (see the first three items in the list in the next paragraph). Most estimates place the incidence of traumatic spinal cord injury in the United States at approximately 10,000 new cases per year.[3] Prevalence stands at approximately 200,000, and male patients constitute 80% of that population. Motor vehicle accidents, falls, acts of violence, and sports injuries cause most of the trauma, factors that probably explain the preponderance of male subjects affected.

PATHOPHYSIOLOGY

The cause of quadriplegia and paraplegia is damage to the spinal cord nerves, specifically including the following:

- Direct trauma to the spinal cord
- Vascular damage, resulting from compromise of the local circulation causing ischemia or from hemorrhage
- External compression of the cord by tumor, spinal stenosis, or pressure from the spinal vertebrae, as a result of malignant infiltration
- Demyelinating disease in multiple sclerosis
- Infection: poliomyelitis
- Immune complex disorders such as Guillain-Barré syndrome

The situation progresses variably, dictated by the disease process itself. Patients with demyelinating disease have a variable course, usually with progression, whereas patients who have undergone a structural change, such as in trauma, have no further progression of the lesion. If the patient has malignant spinal cord compression, the prognosis is poor and may only be in terms of months (see Chapter 223).

Changes may lead to progression of the disability resulting from complications such as syringomyelia arising from the lesion. The aim of all management should be to minimize these changes while maximizing quality of life. This consideration dictates regular reassessment of injury level status.

The extent of the paralysis depends on the level of the lesion: (1) damage to the cervical cord leads to impairment of function (motor or sensory) of the arms, legs, pelvis, and trunk; and (2) damage to the thoracic, lumbar, or sacral cord leads to impairment of function of the trunk, legs, or pelvis, but not the arms. Ventilatory capacity may be compromised if the cervical cord is damaged, and if the lesion is higher than C4, the patient will usually be dependent on a ventilator to maintain respiration.

Spinal cord lesions may be considered to be complete or incomplete. A complete lesion leaves no sensory or motor function below the level of the lesion (see "Case Study: Quadriplegia"), whereas an incomplete lesion results in varying sensory and motor function below the lesion.

The American Spinal Injury Association (ASIA) defines this variation as follows:

- ASIA A: no sensory or motor function in S4-S5
- ASIA B: sensory preservation below the level of the lesion
- ASIA C: some motor function preserved below the level of the lesion
- ASIA D: greater preservation of motor function
- ASIA E: normal motor and sensory function[4]

CLINICAL MANIFESTATIONS

The evaluation of a patient with paralysis consists primarily of careful and thorough physical examination, to evaluate the motor and sensory impairment. The following investigations may be required to evaluate the cause and the progression of the lesion:

- Plain radiograph and bone scan for bone metastases causing malignant spinal cord compression
- Magnetic resonance imaging to show the extent of lesions
- Specific investigations for suspected diagnosis

The effects of the lesion depend on the level (Table 193-1). The symptoms that may be seen in a person with paraplegia or quadriplegia are shown in Tables 193-2[5] and 193-3.

 C A S E   S T U D Y

Quadriplegia

TR is a 36-year-old former military pilot. He was injured in an aircraft accident, which resulted in quadriplegia with a functional level of C6-C7. TR is exceptionally intelligent and analytical in his thinking. Although these would be good prognostic traits for a person with such a serious deficit, he unfortunately never accepted the recommendation that he concentrate on maximizing his remaining abilities rather than dwelling on his disabilities. As a consequence, TR presented a significant challenge to those around him. Motivating him to participate in necessary daily tasks as well as recreational activities was extremely difficult. In addition, his concern that certain activities could trigger an episode of autonomic dysreflexia had reduced his social interactions nearly to nonexistence. Here was an otherwise healthy quadriplegic patient with a stable deficit who could have been a productive person but for his psychological state. Palliative care here was primarily directed toward restoring his interest in life, while minimizing the likelihood of complications (especially those that could cause increased disability) and of episodes of autonomic dysreflexia (a source of intense anxiety).

TABLE 193-1	Injury Level and Concomitant Lesion Effects			
INJURY LEVEL	**TRANSFER**	**ADLS**	**WHEELCHAIR TYPE, IF NEEDED**	**AMBULATION**
C1-C3	Dependent	Mouth control	Power	None
C4	Dependent	Dependent	Power	Standing frame
C5	Assisted	Assisted slide board	Manual	Standing frame
C6	Independent	Independent	Manual Possible driving	Moderate assistance with frame
C7	Independent	Independent	Independent driving	Minimum assistance
C8-T1	Independent	Independent floor to wheelchair	Manual	Use of braces
T1-T4	Independent	Independent	Manual Walking with devices	Braces in parallel bars
T4-L2	Independent	Independent	Manual Walking with devices	Crutches on level
L3-L4	Independent	Independent	Manual Walking with devices	Short leg braces Crutches
L5-S1	Independent	Independent	Walking	Braces possibly needed Walking stick

ADLs, activities of daily living.
Adapted from Ceranski W. Quadriplegia and paraplegia. In Voltz R, Bernat JL, Borasio GD, Maddocks I, et al. (eds). Palliative Care in Neurology. Oxford: Oxford University Press, 2004, pp 12-134.

TABLE 193-2 Differential Diagnosis of Spinal Injuries

DISORDER	LESION OR LOCATION	CHARACTERISTICS	DIAGNOSIS
Quadriplegia	Cervical cord	Impaired breathing if above C4, motor weakness in upper and lower extremities, urinary and fecal incontinence	Meticulous history and physical examination; level of injury demonstrated by motor and sensory loss; MRI the imaging modality of choice
Paraplegia	Thoracic cord	Motor weakness in lower extremities, urinary and fecal incontinence	
Central cord syndrome	Central cord	Extremity motor weakness (upper more so than lower), sacral sensory sparing	
Brown-Séquard syndrome	Hemisection of the cord	Motor and proprioceptive loss greater on side of lesion, pain and temperature loss greater on contralateral side	
Anterior cord syndrome	Anterior cord	Motor function, pain, and temperature loss variable, intact proprioception	
Conus medullaris syndrome	Sacral cord	Loss of bladder, bowel, and lower extremity reflexes	
Cauda equina syndrome	Cauda equina	Loss of bladder, bowel, and lower extremity reflexes; injury determined to be below conus medullaris	
Vascular damage	Ischemia, infarction, hemorrhage	Anterior spinal artery occlusion, flaccid areflexic paraparesis becoming hyperreflexic, loss of pain and temperature sense but preserved position and vibration	Arteriography, MRA
External compression	Bony fragments (pathological neoplastic, infectious, or traumatic fracture), spinal stenosis, disc extrusion or herniation	Pain often at rest, neurogenic claudication, sensory and motor deficits depending on location and severity	Radiographs, CT imaging to detect disc protrusion or herniation
Demyelinating disease	White matter lesions of the brain and cord, demyelination and reactive gliosis	Variable: common at onset, paresthesias, gait disturbance, loss of abdominal reflexes, extremity hyperreflexia, dysdiadokinesis	MRI, CSF with oligoclonal bands on PEP, abnormal evoked potentials (visual, auditory, sensory)
Infection	Epidural abscess, syphilitic meningovasculitis, tuberculous meningitis, HIV vacuolar myelopathy	Fever, back pain and tenderness, pain in nerve root distribution, malaise to progressive paraparesis, sensory changes, urinary fecal retention, cord infarcts or compression	Radiographs, white blood cell nuclear scan, cultures (spinal fluid, bone, blood, adjacent soft tissue abscess), antiviral antibody titers
Immune complex disorder	Peripheral nerve demyelination	Guillain-Barré syndrome, sensory changes with paresthesias (toes and fingers) and ascending paralysis	History of recent mild upper respiratory infection or gastroenteritis, electrodiagnostic studies

CSF, cerebrospinal fluid; CT, computed tomography; MRA, magnetic resonance angiography; MRI, magnetic resonance imaging.

TABLE 193-3 Symptoms and Their Treatments

PROBLEM	PREVENTION	ASSESSMENT	TREATMENT
Autonomic dysreflexia	Minimized risk of noxious stimuli; ensuring of urinary drainage	Severe headache, sweating, anxiety, feeling of impending doom, rapid rise in blood pressure (blood pressure in quadriplegia normally ~90/50 mm Hg, so 140/90 mm Hg is high)	Identification and correction of source of noxious stimulus; consider urinary tract first; topical nitroglycerin, nifedipine puncture and sublingually
PAIN			
Neuropathic: peripheral, central	Spinal stabilization, relief of compression	Electric, sharp, burning, shooting, related to movement of spine, emanating from peripheral nerves at the injury level; deafferentation pain below the level of injury	Tricyclic antidepressants: amitriptyline, nortriptyline, carbamazepine; gabapentin, divalproate, opioids, baclofen, clonidine
Musculoskeletal	Mobility, protection and bracing of joints, HO, prevention of osteoporosis	Deep, aching dull, increased by movement and decreased by rest; radiographs	NSAIDs, steroids, opioids
Visceral	Maintenance of bowel evacuation and urine flow, avoidance of distention	Poorly localized, dull, ache, cramp; abdominal distention	Laxatives and stimulants, suppository, digital stimulation; urethral or suprapubic catheter; nonopioid and opioid analgesics
Deep vein thrombosis	Acutely: heparin-enoxaparin (Lovenox), compression socks, mobility	Unilateral swelling, erythema; Doppler ultrasound, impedance plethysmography	Heparin or enoxaparin (Lovenox) with transition to warfarin for 3-6 months, then ASA

Table continued on p. 1070

TABLE 193-3 Symptoms and Their Treatments—cont'd

PROBLEM	PREVENTION	ASSESSMENT	TREATMENT
INFECTION	Vaccinations: flu, Pneumovax		
Respiratory	Smoking cessation, secretion management	Fever, tachypnea, cough (often ineffective), poor respiratory excursions limiting physical findings; chest radiograph	Antibiotics, oxygen, chest physical therapy, small-volume nebulizers, noninvasive ventilation
Urinary	Clean intermittent self-catheter, indwelling urethral or suprapubic, with good nursing care, monthly catheter changes	Indwelling catheters are colonized! Consider treating with evidence of illness, fever, cognitive changes, abdominal symptoms	Antibiotic selection directed by culture results; catheter replacement; for recurrent episodes and sediment, consideration of catheter irrigation with Renacidin
Pressure ulcers	Frequent (2-hr) position changes to relieve pressure over bony prominences, specialty mattress (low air loss), nutrition support	Stage 1: nonblanchable erythema Stage 2: skin barrier broken to dermis Stage 3: penetration of ulcer to fat-muscle layer Stage 4: can probe to bone	Removal of all necrotic tissue for accurate staging and promotion of healing; all wounds colonized, and systemic antibiotics not indicated without evidence of osteomyelitis; wound kept moist and protected
Restricted mobility	Selection and training of most appropriate tools to maintain mobility and independence	Loss of mobility from spinal cord injury one of the most devastating in creating dependence	Appropriate mobility aid from crutches and braces to sip and puff controls on a power chair
Urinary tract or catheter obstruction	Most common cause of autonomic dysreflexia; maintenance of usual routine of catheter care and frequency of self-catheterization	Self-catheterization not done, less urine in catheter bag than usual, abdominal distention, bladder scan (bedside ultrasound)	Checking of catheter for kinks or sediment obstruction; irrigation with catheter-tipped syringe (Uroject) with lidocaine, then saline; if no result, catheter replacement, again with use of lidocaine
Bowel obstruction or infection	Aggressive bowel management with stool softeners, adequate dietary fluid and fiber, rectal stimulation with suppository or enemas	Second most common cause of autonomic dysreflexia; decreased stool output, abdominal distention, stool in rectal vault; radiography of kidneys, ureters, and bladder possibly useful	If acute, rectal instillation of dibucaine and manual stool removal; long-term increase in bowel medication regimen and hydration
Psychosocial problems	Early intervention emphasizing preserved ability	Depression screening, patient who has taken on "victim" role (often complicated by substance abuse), rather than being an active participant in care and life	Support of family and friends, consistent and compassionate care, counseling, antidepressants
Osteoporosis	Mobility with weight bearing if able, calcium and vitamin D	Dual-energy x-ray absorptiometry; suspected on plain radiographs	Bisphosphonates, adequate vitamin D and calcium
Heterotopic ossification	Mobilization	Most common in hips and thighs	NSAIDs acutely; irradiation, etidronate, surgical excision
Spasticity	Assistance of physical and occupational therapists for range of motion, bracing, standing frame	Sudden increase in spasms and rigidity possible sign of infection, fracture, or other process	Gentle range of motion; medications: diazepam, baclofen, tizanidine
Malnutrition	Assistance of dietitian for caloric needs assessment and adequacy of diet, speech therapy assessment possibly needed to assess safety of oral intake	Global evaluation: weight, height, iron and iron-binding capacity, prealbumin; suspect with poor wound, skin healing, pressure sores, infections, lassitude	Adequate calorie intake by most appropriate means; PEG tubes preferable to nasogastric tubes when swallowing impaired and unsafe
Sexual dysfunction		Erectile dysfunction	Sildenafil and other medication, vacuum assist device, intracavernous injections of alprostadil or papaverine

ASA, acetylsalicylic acid; NSAIDs, nonsteroidal anti-inflammatory drugs; PEG, percutaneous endoscopic gastrostomy.

REFERENCES

1. Manns PJ, Chad KE. Components of quality of life for persons with a quadriplegic and paraplegic spinal cord injury. Qual Health Res 2001;11:795-781.
2. Bozzacco V. Long-term psychosocial effects of spinal cord injury. Rehabil Nurs 1993;18:82-87.
3. Sekhon LHS, Fehlings MG. Epidemiology, demographics and pathophysiology of acute spinal cord injury. Spine 2001;26(Suppl):S1-S12.
4. Marino RJ. International Standards for Neurological Classification of Spinal Cord Injury, 5th ed. Chicago: American Spinal Injury Association, 2000.
5. Ceranski W. Quadriplegia and paraplegia. In Voltz R, Bernat JL, Borasio GD, Maddocks I, et al. (eds). Palliative Care in Neurology. Oxford: Oxford University Press, 2004, pp 12-134.

Pediatrics

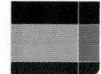

CHAPTER **194**

Neonates, Children, and Adolescents

Craig A. Hurwitz, Jeanne G. Lewandowski, and Joanne M. Hilden

KEY POINTS

- Most children who require pediatric palliative medicine services have a wide range of diagnoses including mental and physical impairments, congenital anomalies, and rare and progressive pulmonary, neurological, and metabolic diseases that are not found in the adult population.

- Parents often express dual goals for their children that seem contradictory; they continue to "hope for a miracle" and desire ongoing active therapy toward disease control and simultaneously look to maximizing comfort for their child.

- Qualitative studies suggest that children are often aware, on some level, that they may soon die, and if they are not given the opportunity to discuss their fears, children may develop feelings of isolation, anxiety, and other distress.

- A first step in caring for the child with advanced disease is to be aware of how a child's developmental stage affects his or her understanding of dying.

- Constraints on the development and implementation of pediatric palliative medicine are many and range from legal barriers, financial implications, complicated care coordination barriers, and a lack of experienced pediatric clinicians to deliver the necessary care.

Children in our society are not supposed to be born with, develop, or suffer from life-threatening and advanced illness. In short, children are not supposed to die. Not uncommonly, because the death of a child is a relatively rare event, a fatal prognosis leads to feelings of confusion and failure in health care providers. Pediatric palliative care programs can turn a potentially destructive experience into one that may strengthen bonds among family members and may remind providers that they can aggressively treat and comfort even when they cannot "cure" advanced, life-threatening conditions of childhood.

In the United States, close to 50,000 children and adolescents die each year.[1] Approximately 30% of these deaths result from accidents, homicide, or suicide. The other 70% of these deaths are from congenital and genetic diseases and other anomalies, cancer, heart disease, neurodegenerative diseases, lung disease, and infectious diseases including AIDS (Fig. 194-1).[1] Many children with severe chronic and advanced illness live much longer than previously expected because of medical, clinical, and societal advances. Children with complex chronic problems would benefit from palliative care services over months or years. Pediatric palliative medicine recognizes and anticipates the special needs of children who face life-threatening and life-limiting disease. Palliative medicine meets the needs of these children and their families. The model of care includes physicians, nurses, social workers, child life specialists, teachers, clergy, volunteers, and family care providers to provide expert pain and symptom management, assistance with medical decision making, continuity of care across health care settings, and whatever personal and family support is needed. The focus is on living as well as possible by maximizing quality of life for the child and the ongoing lives of his or her family.

ESSENTIAL ELEMENTS IN PEDIATRIC PALLIATIVE CARE

The Edmarc Experience

An early model called the Edmarc Hospice for Children was created in 1978 in rural southeastern Virginia.[2] When the hospice administrators first developed admission criteria using adult models, they anticipated that most of the patients would be children with cancer, children with less than 6 months to live, and families seeking palliation for their child, but not cure. Only 35% of pediatric patients who enrolled had cancer. The administrators quickly realized that no reference was made to remaining life expectancy in most children admitted because primary care physicians were unable to state that their patients had less than 6 months to live should the disease process take its usual course. Unlike the situation in adults, who more often than not stopped disease-oriented therapy when cure was no longer a possibility, most parents had dual goals for their children. Parents were largely unwilling to stop disease-oriented treatment even if only a remote chance existed that their child's life could be saved, but they also desired that the child's comfort be a primary focus of care. This pediatric "concurrent care" approach often resulted in more interventional care than common in dying adults.[3,4] The Edmarc experience taught that all families with seriously ill children, regardless of whether they had a "terminal" diagnosis, needed the kind of care that hospice exclusively offered. The social, emotional, spiritual, physical, and financial implications for a family raising a child with a life-threatening or life-limiting illness are just as real as those for the family of a child who will likely soon die.

Pathways to a Child's Death

The majority of deaths in childhood have four trajectories (Fig. 194-2).[1] No single model of care can be applied to

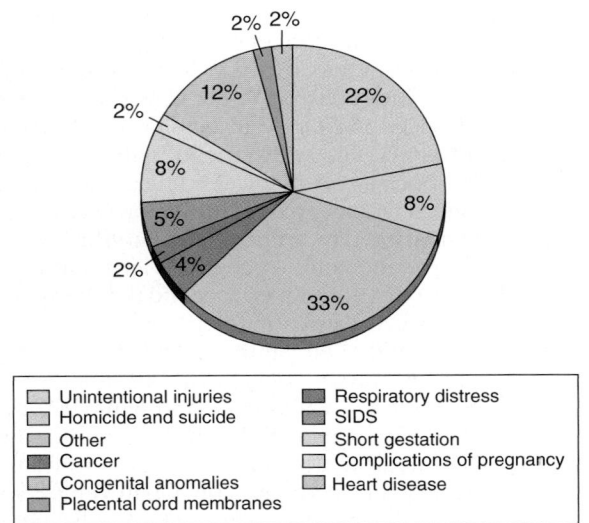

FIGURE 194-1 Percentage of total childhood deaths by major causes. SIDS, sudden infant death syndrome. *(From Reference 1.)*

all dying children and their families (Table 194-1). Children who suddenly die as a result of a tragic accident, suicide, homicide, or a condition such as sudden infant death syndrome, are unlikely to be seen by a palliative care service. They represent 30% of all pediatric deaths (see Fig. 194-1), and their families clearly need, as do their professional caregivers, assistance with memorial planning, bereavement, acute and chronic grief management, and other services offered by palliative care teams that are lacking in other health care settings.

It is a common misconception that pediatric palliative care exists primarily for children with cancer. The issues that affect children with nonmalignant chronic, advanced, or terminal disease resemble those that affect children with cancer. The following needs are common to all these groups: the need to communicate the diagnosis, to establish goals of care, to reframe hope for families, to control physical symptoms including pain, fatigue, dyspnea, and nutritional and gastrointestinal problems, to facilitate communication, to relieve psychosocial and spiritual distress, and to identify and treat depression and anxiety. Additionally, issues regarding life closure, completion, memory making, memorial planning, and grief and bereavement for children at the close of life are essential, elemental tasks that require multidisciplinary expertise (see Chapter 201).

Difference between Palliative Care for Children and for Adults

Children with life-threatening conditions and their families require palliative medicine that works concurrently with the medical team's curative goals. The American Academy of Pediatrics called for the broad incorporation

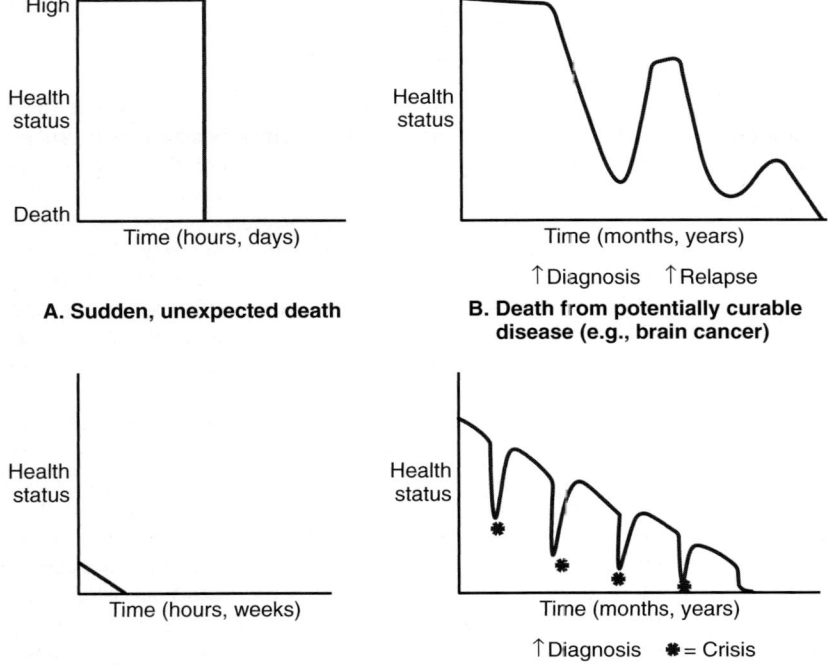

FIGURE 194-2 Prototypical trajectories of child death. *(Adapted from Reference 1.)*

A. Sudden, unexpected death

B. Death from potentially curable disease (e.g., brain cancer)

↑Diagnosis ↑Relapse

C. Death from lethal congenital anomaly

D. Death from progressive condition with intermittent crises (e.g., muscular dystrophy)

↑Diagnosis ✱= Crisis

TABLE 194-1	Indications for Pediatric Palliative Care

DIAGNOSES SUITABLE FOR CONSULTATION BY THE PEDIATRIC PALLIATIVE MEDICINE TEAM

Conditions for which curative treatment is available but may fail

Poor prognosis primary or progressive/recurrent cancer or cancer with a poor prognosis

Severe congenital or acquired heart disease

PROGRESSIVE CONDITIONS FOR WHICH TREATMENT IS EXCLUSIVELY PALLIATIVE

Chromosomal abnormalities such as trisomy 13 or trisomy 18

Progressive metabolic disorders

Severe forms of osteogenesis imperfecta

CONDITIONS REQUIRING INTENSIVE LONG-TERM TREATMENT BUT THAT ARE ULTIMATELY FATAL

Severe immunodeficiencies

Cystic fibrosis

Chronic or severe respiratory failure

Severe epidermolysis bullosa

Human immunodeficiency virus infection

Progressive renal failure for which dialysis or renal transplantation is not available or successful

Muscular dystrophy

Severe gastrointestinal disorders or malformations such as gastroschisis

CONDITIONS INVOLVING SEVERE, NONPROGRESSIVE DISABILITY AND CONSEQUENT COMPLEX MEDICAL CONDITIONS WITH COMPLICATIONS THAT MAY BE FATAL

Extreme prematurity

Severe cerebral palsy with recurrent infection

Hypoxic or anoxic brain injury

Severe neurological sequelae of infectious disease or trauma

Brain malformations such as holoprosencephaly

Complex illnesses involving multiple specialties and with challenging symptoms

Regional pain syndromes

Sickle cell disease

of palliative care into complex medical care by stating that quality pediatric service provides that "the components of palliative care are offered at diagnosis and continued throughout the course of illness, whether the outcome ends in cure or death."[5] The emphasis should be on combining life-prolonging interventions with symptom-relieving therapies to improve the child's quality and quantity of life. Most children who need palliative medicine expertise are not actively dying, but have many diagnoses including mental and physical impairments, congenital anomalies, and rare and progressive pulmonary, neurological, and metabolic diseases not found in adults. Unlike adults, the life expectancy for children with advanced pediatric illness may range from a few hours or days to years or decades. Advance care planning and expert assistance with decision making inherent in frequent reassessment of goals of care are critical in pediatric palliative care.

Serious illness creates stress and confusion for the pediatric patient and family. In addition to all the care needs engendered by serious advanced disease, the family may experience other conditions requiring evaluation, treatment, and care. Parents often become much more protective out of an overwhelming fear of losing their ill child. Siblings often lose both the physical and emotional availability of their parents as their lives change forever. They feel unable to share their concerns with already overwhelmed parents, and they have little opportunity to express their anguish for their sick brother or sister. Siblings who are not adequately informed may fear for their own health and may experience both anxiety and social isolation. They may develop feelings that range from embarrassment over the illness of their brother or sister to jealousy over the attention rendered to the sick sibling. Developmental regression, academic failure, and social withdrawal occur frequently unless siblings receive focused attention and support for their own needs, hopes, fears, and worries, both at home and at school.[6,7] Pediatric palliative care teams are expert in creatively dealing not only with the different behavioral and developmental approaches to a child's experience of his or her illness and its treatment, but also with complex family, peer, and community needs.

The Pediatric Palliative Care Team

The team must be actively involved in developing, coordinating, and implementing the individual child's care plan. This team should include professionals to address medical, nursing, social, psychological, spiritual, dietary, and environmental needs. Families may find themselves in a fast-paced, anxiety-ridden, and short-lived experience requiring intense concentration, focus, and strength, or they may have a longer, drawn-out battle with unexpected twists and turns that require endurance of mind, body, and spirit. In both situations, the team functions as adviser and teacher, by using the collective skills and wisdom of team members to guide, direct, listen, bear witness to, and be present for the family, friends, and loved ones (Fig. 194-3).[8] It is imperative that a well-functioning palliative care team recognize that patients are children with serious illnesses, not seriously ill patients who happen to be children.

The experts help to identify and clarify realistic goals of the child and family. Team members assess the understanding of medical information, especially as it affects medical decision making. They use their expertise to help accomplish these goals through ongoing communication among the child's other medical professionals and family members. Sensitive open-ended questions to identify a child's and a family's hopes, worries, fears, and concerns will offer rich and important insights to the palliative care team in their mission to sustain the entire family and each other.[9]

Supportive Environments for the Child with Advanced Illness

In caring for children with life-threatening and life-limiting disease, the setting is of paramount importance. Although the hospital may often be the most appropriate setting, the child nearing the close of life deserves the right to choose where his or her final weeks or days will be spent. It is important that the palliative care team model and advocate for a plan that will ensure that this wish is honored to the greatest extent possible.

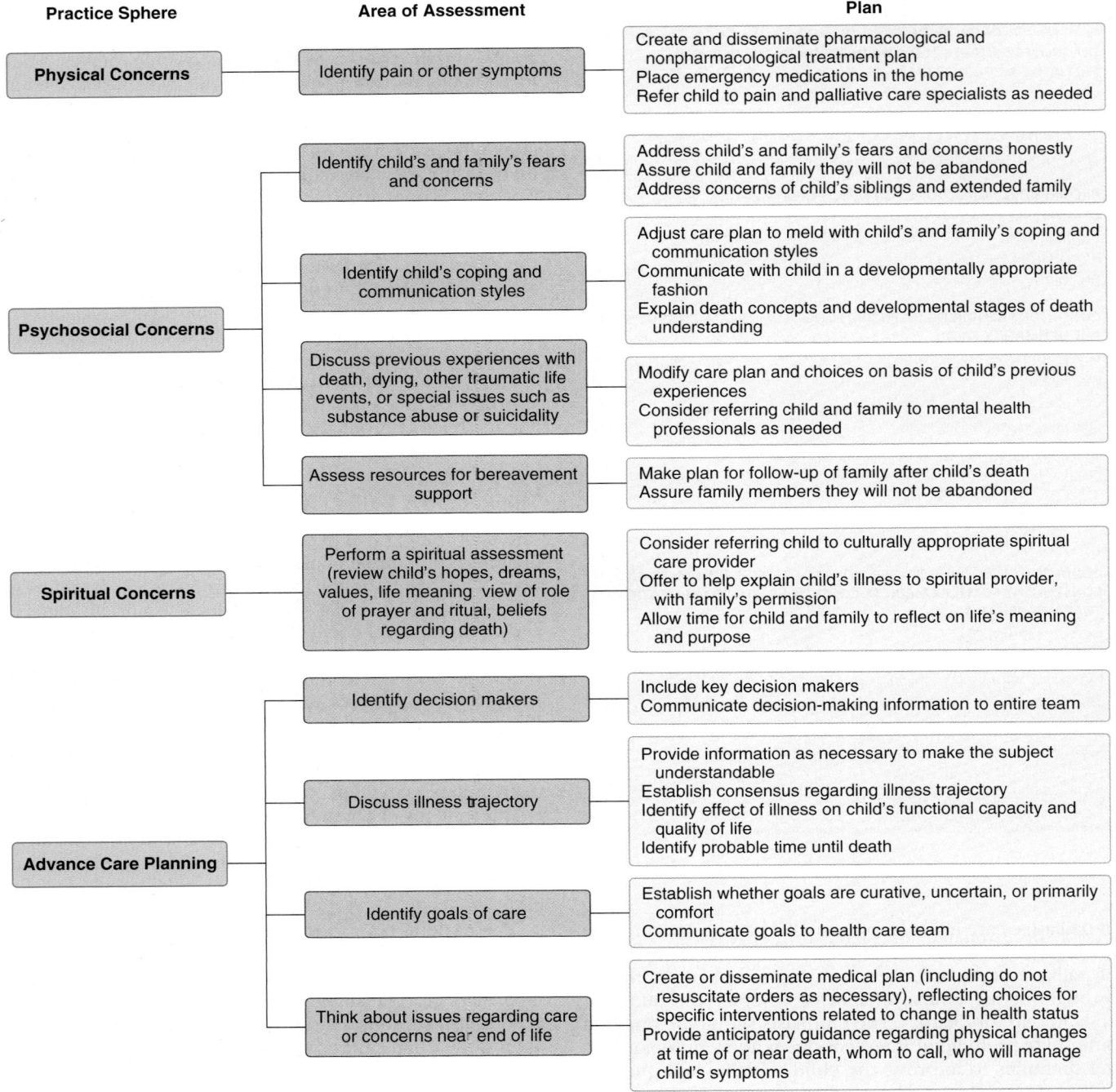

Practice Sphere	Area of Assessment	Plan

Physical Concerns → Identify pain or other symptoms →
- Create and disseminate pharmacological and nonpharmacological treatment plan
- Place emergency medications in the home
- Refer child to pain and palliative care specialists as needed

Psychosocial Concerns
- Identify child's and family's fears and concerns →
  - Address child's and family's fears and concerns honestly
  - Assure child and family they will not be abandoned
  - Address concerns of child's siblings and extended family
- Identify child's coping and communication styles →
  - Adjust care plan to meld with child's and family's coping and communication styles
  - Communicate with child in a developmentally appropriate fashion
  - Explain death concepts and developmental stages of death understanding
- Discuss previous experiences with death, dying, other traumatic life events, or special issues such as substance abuse or suicidality →
  - Modify care plan and choices on basis of child's previous experiences
  - Consider referring child and family to mental health professionals as needed
- Assess resources for bereavement support →
  - Make plan for follow-up of family after child's death
  - Assure family members they will not be abandoned

Spiritual Concerns → Perform a spiritual assessment (review child's hopes, dreams, values, life meaning view of role of prayer and ritual, beliefs regarding death) →
- Consider referring child to culturally appropriate spiritual care provider
- Offer to help explain child's illness to spiritual provider, with family's permission
- Allow time for child and family to reflect on life's meaning and purpose

Advance Care Planning
- Identify decision makers →
  - Include key decision makers
  - Communicate decision-making information to entire team
- Discuss illness trajectory →
  - Provide information as necessary to make the subject understandable
  - Establish consensus regarding illness trajectory
  - Identify effect of illness on child's functional capacity and quality of life
  - Identify probable time until death
- Identify goals of care →
  - Establish whether goals are curative, uncertain, or primarily comfort
  - Communicate goals to health care team
- Think about issues regarding care or concerns near end of life →
  - Create or disseminate medical plan (including do not resuscitate orders as necessary), reflecting choices for specific interventions related to change in health status
  - Provide anticipatory guidance regarding physical changes at time of or near death, whom to call, who will manage child's symptoms

FIGURE 194-3 Essential elements in the planning and caring for children in palliative medicine.

Although home is often the preferred place that a child nearing the end of life would choose, the decision must be made within the context of the impact of the dying child on family members. When home care for advanced illness is not feasible or possible, the medical caregivers should encourage family members to "bring home to the hospital." By being realistic, innovative, and creative, any location can become the right location for the dying child. Favorite pillows, sheets, blankets, and wall hangings can often transform a dreary hospital room into a comfortable and safe environment for the child.

School

School plays a fundamental role in the lives of children, including any seriously ill child. For the child whose disease trajectory will be measured in months to years, school may continue to give him or her the satisfaction of participating in normal school activities with peers, and of continuing to develop and reach small personal goals, and therefore should be strongly encouraged. As the ill child's disease progresses, school creates an opportunity for his or her class and teachers safely to experience changes in their classmate and thus to reassure them that

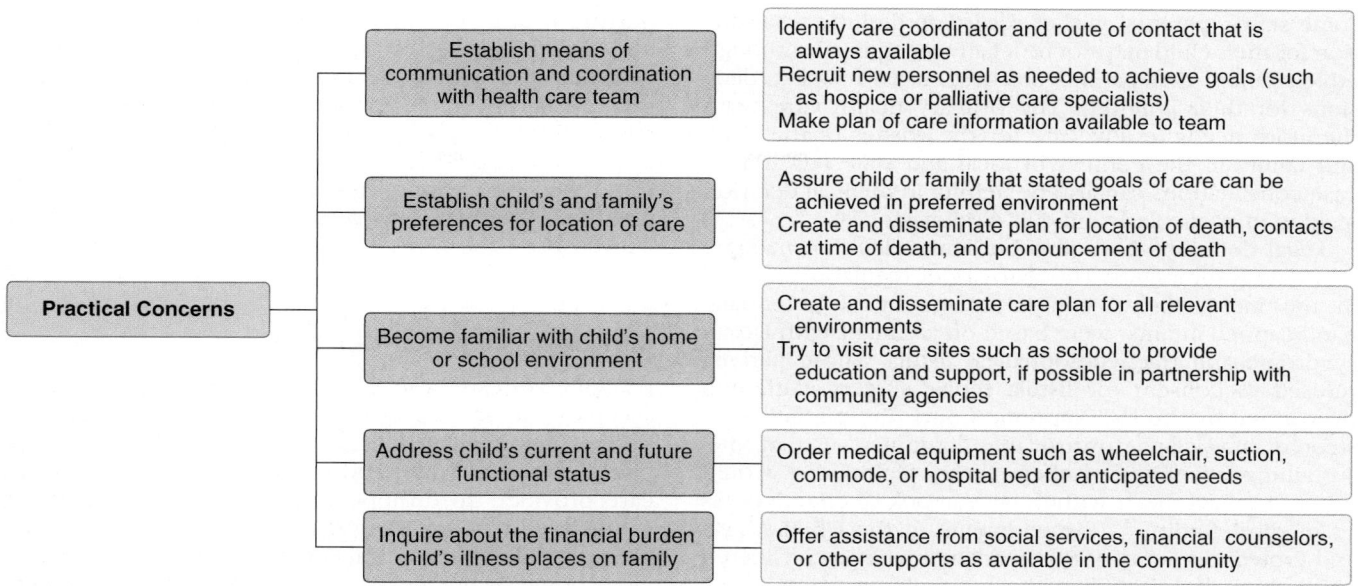

	Establish means of communication and coordination with health care team	Identify care coordinator and route of contact that is always available Recruit new personnel as needed to achieve goals (such as hospice or palliative care specialists) Make plan of care information available to team
	Establish child's and family's preferences for location of care	Assure child or family that stated goals of care can be achieved in preferred environment Create and disseminate plan for location of death, contacts at time of death, and pronouncement of death
Practical Concerns	Become familiar with child's home or school environment	Create and disseminate care plan for all relevant environments Try to visit care sites such as school to provide education and support, if possible in partnership with community agencies
	Address child's current and future functional status	Order medical equipment such as wheelchair, suction, commode, or hospital bed for anticipated needs
	Inquire about the financial burden child's illness places on family	Offer assistance from social services, financial counselors, or other supports as available in the community

FIGURE 194-3, cont'd

they are not "at risk" for the same. These "teachable opportunities" that occur for the child's school peers help friends and classmates learn to accept, understand, and participate in the special needs of their seriously ill friend.

School also plays a critical role for the siblings of a child with a progressive life-limiting illness. It often becomes the only place where siblings can be recognized as unique individuals, rather than as the brother or sister of their ill sibling. Life at home is often consumed in the care of the sick child, and little time is left for parents to tend to the other children in the family. At school, unlike home, life tends to remain consistent and predictable, and it therefore allows siblings to socialize, confide, play, and enjoy the normal activities of childhood. School allows the sibling's teachers the opportunity to observe any changes in school performance or signs of depression, anxiety, aggression, or low self-esteem, emotional signals that may need intervention.[10]

BARRIERS TO PALLIATIVE CARE IN CHILDREN

Genesis of the Chronically Ill Child

The undisputed success in improving survival rates among children with cancer, congenital heart disease, infectious diseases, and prematurity have created the unintended consequence of offering hope to parents that death can almost always be averted. Technology and medical advances (pharmaceuticals, biologicals, sterility) have contributed to the long-term survival of a new cohort of children with rare disorders and complex medical conditions who previously would have died.[11] Many such medically fragile children are prone to repeated life-threatening or life-limiting complications. Prognostication for such complex problems is challenging, and it is difficult for physicians to determine when such children may die.[4,8] Given remarkable technical advances, families (and some physicians) may view death more as a therapeutic

accident than as a natural process stemming from disease. Recognition that death is inevitable often lags behind the clinical progression and reality of the medical condition, and the result is a curative treatment approach when cure is impossible.[4] For example, a child with multiple leukemic relapses may be offered a second or third bone marrow transplantation to induce a remission or to maintain some quality of life, but with no realistic hope of cure. Parents and providers alike may reject essential palliative care services in this situation because they continue to view the procedure as potentially curative. Alternatively, health care providers may assume that a child is dying when the likelihood of recovery to a previous baseline is probable, even though that quality of life may not be perceived as reasonable by the providers. For example, we may question the use of intensive care support for a child with profound and pervasive developmental delays who develops aspiration pneumonia.

In these complex situations, palliative care may not be considered because it is perceived as tantamount to "giving up on the child," even though palliative medicine specialists can play a vital role in helping parents with medical goal setting and decision making, care management issues, continuity of care throughout the illness, symptom management, and, when necessary, memory making, anticipatory grieving, and memorial and death planning.

Legal Barriers

Complex ethical, legal, and health policy issues affect children and further complicate timely palliative care. Ethicists support the concept that children should participate in their own medical decision making when able.[12-14] Legal decisions about specific cases have supported this concept.[13] Legislative statutes often do not recognize treatment decisions or refusals of treatment by adolescents and leave all legal decision-making power with parents. In some states, parents' wishes regarding limiting resuscitation for their child may not be legally recognized, although ethicists hold that parents are best suited to make decisions for their children. The primary health care team therefore needs to advocate for the wishes of the child and family in the context of local and state law. Ethics case consultations can also be helpful in medical decision making in particularly difficult circumstances.

Legal decisions have also burdened decision making, particularly for infants. The "Baby Doe" regulations, issued in the mid-1980s to compel treatment of potentially handicapped infants, were based on an infant with Down syndrome and tracheoesophageal fistula whose parents refused to consent for fistula repair surgery. Although overturned by the U.S. Supreme Court, these regulations steered physicians toward the continued use of life-sustaining techniques when these techniques would otherwise have been withdrawn for lack of effectiveness or medical futility.[15,16] Amendments in the Child Abuse and Protection Act of 1984 broadened what is considered child abuse by classifying the withholding of medically indicated treatment for an infant with a life-threatening condition as medical neglect.[17] Regulations stipulated that handicapped infants must always receive life-sustaining treatment, except those infants in irreversible coma and except treatments that would be inhumane or futile or that would prolong dying. Although the U.S. government has yet to intervene on behalf of an allegedly medically neglected infant, these court decisions may have made some neonatologists and other pediatric specialists apprehensive about withdrawing or withholding life-sustaining therapies for dying infants.[16]

Financial Resource Implications

Many patients, both adult and pediatric, who would benefit from palliative care services do not meet eligibility criteria for community-based palliative care or hospice services. The Medicare Hospice Benefit, created by Congress in 1982, provides a per diem reimbursement for patients determined to have no longer than 6 months left to live and for whom the goal of care is purely palliative rather than curative. Unlike the situation in elderly patients, however, parents often have dual, seemingly contradictory goals for their children. They continue to "hope for a miracle" and desire ongoing active therapy toward disease control and health maintenance, and they also look to maximize comfort for their child.[3] Asking parents to choose between cure and comfort is problematic. Most palliative therapies are best applied early in an illness to maximize both the quality and the quantity of life, but making the case for such therapies with payers is often difficult.

No specific therapy is inappropriate for children with life-limiting conditions, provided it meets their goals of care. For example, one of the first acts of a parent following the birth of a child is to nourish that child. The idea of withdrawal of artificial nutrition and fluids is often inconceivable to a parent. Children with complex medical conditions may therefore have health care needs that meet these dual goals of care and may require parenteral nutrition, transfusion, assisted ventilation, or in-home nursing "shift" or "block-nursing." These services are not easily reimbursable under existing hospice insurance designed for adults.[9] Although most hospice care is provided at home, most infants and children die in hospitals. Children younger than 17 years of age make up only 0.4% of all hospice admissions.[8] Few hospices have dedicated pediatric teams, nor do they admit a sufficient number of children to achieve or maintain pediatric expertise.

Barriers to Care Coordination

Fragmented care also adversely affects children with complex medical conditions. For example, a child with severe neurological deficits who has scoliosis, chronic pain, reactive airways, and seizures may need a primary care provider, an orthopedic surgeon, a pulmonologist, a nutritionist, a neurologist, physical and occupational therapists, durable medical equipment providers, pharmacists, home health nurses, a tutor, and spiritual leaders, among others. Facilitating and coordinating care are daunting and underfinanced tasks in pediatric palliative medicine. Yet as a child's condition worsens, and as decision making and adjustments in the goals of care become necessary, families need such coordination and continuity of providers the most. Pediatric palliative medicine teams provide the care coordination sought by parents and payers alike.

Lack of Appropriate Pediatric Measures

The assessment and management of symptoms and suffering in children are difficult. Few reliable, valid, and developmentally appropriate methods are available to measure the suffering and quality of life of children with life-threatening illness. Additionally, few researchers and research dollars are devoted to studying symptom control in children.[1] A retrospective, single-institution study of the parents of children who died of cancer noted that most children suffered "a lot" or "a great deal," and treatment of symptoms was often ineffective. These findings indicated distressing symptoms similar to those in adults with cancer.[3] Substantial research studies in adult palliative medicine have helped to gauge the quality and effect of adult palliative care; these include quality of life and identification of treatment preferences and factors important in advance care planning (see Chapters 62, 65, and 120). Knowledge has also been gained about the beliefs, attitudes, and feelings of professional staff members, about the burdens that patients with chronic illnesses place on caregivers (see Chapters 50 and 51), and about management of pain and symptoms (Sections B and E). Similar studies are rare among children with life-threatening illnesses, as are measures of effectiveness of assisting parents with decision making. Multicenter studies enrolling adequate numbers of children are required to determine best practices; to establish appropriate outcome measures; to assess the current management of physical, emotional, and spiritual distress; and to learn whether current approaches to and therapies for bereaved families and children are effective.

PSYCHOSOCIAL ASPECTS OF SERIOUS ILLNESS AND DEATH IN CHILDHOOD AND ADOLESCENCE

Components of Understanding Death

As they age, children incorporate four necessary components to understanding death. These are the concepts of irreversibility, universality, nonfunctionality, and causality.[8,9] *Irreversibility* refers to the understanding that once death occurs, a person's body does not become alive again. Death is permanent, irrevocable, and final. *Universality* refers to an understanding that everyone and every living thing will die, including people known to the child, or even the child. *Nonfunctionality* connotes an understanding that, in death, all the processes and bodily functions that define life cease. Finally, the understanding that reasons, both internal and external, cause death, including suicide, defines the *causality* component to complete a mature understanding of death.

Influence of Illness on the Infant and Toddler

Treatment of serious illness in the first year of life results in forced separation from the mother, possible pain from invasive procedures, and feeding and sleeping schedules that deviate from natural cycles. Parents of an infant with a serious illness should therefore be encouraged to remain with their child as often as possible. This contact includes bathing, talking to, and feeding their child.

The major developmental goals of the toddler (1 to 3 years of age) are independence, autonomy, and self-control. These important developmental aims are often thwarted by serious illness. Because of the egocentricity characteristic of this age, death may simply mean a separation from what one treasures. Thus, the most frightening aspects of illness and hospitalization for the toddler are pain, anxiety, and separation from parents and from familiar surroundings, but not death. The most common coping method of the seriously ill toddler is regression, the loss of newly acquired developmental milestones.[18] Without consistent limitations, the toddler feels apprehensive and insecure. Parents therefore should be encouraged to maintain consistent limits. In summary, children in this developmental phase understand death as separation or abandonment. Their concerns are expressed through crying, separation anxiety, and an overwhelming need to attach to the primary caretaker. The need for physical contact in this age group is of fundamental importance.

Influence of Illness and Death on the Preschool Child

Preschool children (3 to 6 years of age) recognize death in terms of lying down and becoming immobile, but they may not understand that being dead and being alive are mutually exclusive. Death is often believed to be temporary and reversible. Children of this age have magical thinking and closely associate death with sleeping or going on a trip. They rarely appreciate the possibility of their own death, even if the close of their life is a certainty. This is the stage of development during which walking, talking, control of bodily functions, and separation from

mother take precedence. Thoughts about "bad things" or wishes for "bad things" to happen to others often lead to strong feelings of guilt and anxiety in both seriously ill children and their healthy siblings. Painful procedures, hospitalization, and separation from parents are interpreted as punishment for perceived real or imagined bad behavior.

Preschool children accept the literal meaning of words. Thus, if death has been described as "a sleeplike" state, the child may fear going to sleep and never waking up. Difficulty sleeping and frequent nightmares often occur. It is important that providers and parents allow children to express these fears. Providers are challenged to explain to parents that this will be done professionally. Books and stories that indirectly address death help to approach the subject in a nonthreatening manner.[18]

Security at this age is often derived from adhering to schedules and rules. Parents should be encouraged to maintain a normal schedule and consistent limits. Because of their association with disease as punishment, preschoolers also need repeated and gentle reassurance that nothing they did caused the illness.

Influence of Illness and Death on the School-Aged Child

As the preschooler ages, he or she will add functional considerations to the concept of death. Logical thought is beginning, and children rapidly acquire a specific and concrete understanding of death. Terminally ill school-aged children are often aware of their prognosis without being told. They are intensely aware of nonverbal clues and often understand much more than their parents or caregivers realize. These children frequently protect their parents from grief by maintaining the family's myth of curative possibility.[19] Asking these children open-ended questions about what the body is telling them about the illness, about what they think causes the way they feel, about what will happen to them in the future, and about what things are "left undone" in their lives can facilitate better family acknowledgment and understanding of just what these children know. It is imperative that honest and open communication be maintained. Open communication allows children the opportunity to discuss their fears and apprehensions. Without this opportunity, dying children bear the burden of any mistaken assumption or interpretation that is made and lose the opportunity to complete their life and say goodbye.

At this age, children also begin to worry about the integrity of their body and the loss of control. They need to have their bodies treated with respect and to be offered specific factual information if requested. This need becomes more and more important as the child ages.

Influence of Illness and Death on the Adolescent

As the child enters adolescence, thinking becomes consistent with reality, and children at this age speculate on the implications and the consequences of death. All too often, however, "adolescence" is thought of as a single stage, rather than as three distinct stages of development, each with unique characteristics. For example, an 11-year-old child experiences things in a remarkably different way from an adolescent who is 18 years old. To complicate matters in the seriously ill adolescent, some institutions may hospitalize these patients on a pediatric floor, whereas others admit adolescents to adult units and treat them as "adults."

Psychologically, early adolescence is an emotionally vulnerable period. In early adolescence, some magical thinking still exists, and the consequences of actions and behaviors are measured in a fairly distant and isolated manner. The child of this age generally remains concrete in his or her thinking.[18]

Middle adolescents (generally ages 14 to 15 years for girls and 15 to 17 years for boys) often challenge authority figures and rarely question the consequences of their behaviors. Their sense of invulnerability, evidenced by an increase in risk-taking behaviors, becomes uncomfortably apparent. Teenagers' sense of immortality makes it particularly difficult for them to deal with issues of death and loss. Adolescents at this age have a strong sense of inadequacy, and they seek peer relationships to have a sense of foundation in their lives.

By late adolescence (generally ages 16 to 19 years for girls and 17 to 19 years for boys), the young adult becomes more future oriented. These adolescents appreciate the significance and meaning of loss in a way not experienced in earlier phases of development. Teenagers begin to establish a sense of who they are, the people with whom they identify, and the type of life they want to lead.[18]

For teenagers with advanced illness, however, the difficulty of reaching even some of these critical developmental milestones may be insurmountable. Changes in appearance such as the loss of hair, the loss of a limb, delayed puberty, or the look of chronic illness may have an overwhelming effect on the self-image and self-esteem of adolescents as they become more identifiably different from their peers. Members of this age group are in the process of establishing their independence outside the family unit, but they still have strong needs to be accepted, cared for, and nurtured. Adolescents with advanced illness must simultaneously try to become dependent and to accept help in areas where they were previously independent and self-reliant. Dependence on family caregivers can ruin the adolescent's need for autonomy and can result in hostility, aggression, and even refusal of treatment. Physically handicapped and seriously ill teenagers score lower on instruments that measure social acceptance and self-worth.[20] Many young adults with chronic and progressive illnesses will not develop the cognitive skills of normal adolescence. For example, teenagers with neurodegenerative disorders may begin to decline cognitively at this age and are less likely to be permitted to experience some of the freedoms and responsibilities of their peers. Even teenagers who are cognitively intact often experience difficulty in achieving personal freedoms because of the demands of medical care or the physical limitations imposed by their disease.

Parental and medical caregiver support that focuses on promoting independence and autonomy enables the teenager to accept physical and emotional support without feeling vulnerable. The adolescent should be offered options, when possible, to foster a sense of control. Groups of peers who share similar hardships can also be invaluable to the chronically ill teenager. Such groups decrease the teenager's sense of feeling isolated and alone and provide a safe and supportive environment in which to disclose mutual emotions, experiences, and fears.

INVOLVING CHILDREN AND ADOLESCENTS IN ADVANCED CARE

School-aged children with advanced illness should have opportunities to express their fears and concerns. Otherwise, increased anxiety and feelings of isolation and alienation will prevail. These unrelieved symptoms often exacerbate pain and other symptoms, and relief of these symptoms can also lead to physical improvements.[19,21] Frequently, caregivers underestimate the dying child's awareness of his or her impending death and avoid honest communication, largely because of their own anxiety. Children of all ages should be given the opportunity to complete their lives, and communication between the child and his or her family should be encouraged within the family's ethnic, religious, and cultural value system. Children are more often afraid of isolation and abandonment than of dying. Dying children often are able to, and hoping for an opportunity to, discuss their feelings surrounding their own death. Well-trained palliative care providers can often facilitate those discussions in developmentally appropriate manners.

The adolescent is focused on the future, and acceptance of his or her death is particularly difficult. The dying process does not necessarily do away with the adolescent's need for independence. The natural and evolving disease process forces the teenager to accept dependence on family members and hospital caregivers. Even though dying involves many physical, social, and emotional losses, the typical adolescent continues to fight for independence, self-reliance, and dignity.

A growing consensus suggests that children be involved in their own goal setting to optimize outcomes consistent with their cognitive and emotional maturity and their willingness to participate.[8,11] Because of vast ethnic, cultural, and religious diversity, family values about how to approach discussions of death and a child's role must be included and respected. Active listening by medical caregivers will give teenagers a forum to express feelings of anger and loss. Hope must be maintained throughout the dying process by helping the child or adolescent to concentrate on what is left undone, to accomplish what he or she can, and to live as fully as possible, free of symptoms, for as long as possible. It is important to discuss dying openly if desired and to offer confirmation that the child is dying if requested. By simply listening, the caregiver can honor and give meaning to the child's or adolescent's experiences and can help to preserve the patient's dignity and self-respect.

SUMMARY

The delivery of palliative medicine to neonates, children, adolescents, and their families is a complicated task that requires a team with varied experience and expertise, but with the same mission: to help these children with advanced and chronic diseases live as well as possible for as long as possible. Future considerations regarding the

Future Considerations

- Palliative care and respite programs need to be developed and widely available to provide intensive symptom management and to promote the welfare of children living with a life-threatening or terminal condition.

- At the diagnosis of a life-threatening or terminal condition, it is important to offer an integrated model of palliative care that continues throughout the course of the illness, regardless of the outcome.

- Changes in the regulation and reimbursement of palliative care and hospice services are necessary to improve access for children and families in need of those services. Modifications in current regulations should include broader eligibility criteria concerning the length of expected survival and the provision of respite care and other therapies beyond those allowed by a narrow definition of "medically indicated." Adequate reimbursement should accompany those regulatory changes.

- All general and subspecialty pediatricians, family physicians, pain specialists, and pediatric surgeons need to become familiar and comfortable with the provision of palliative care to children. Residency, fellowship training, and continuing education programs should include topics such as palliative medicine, communication skills, grief and loss, managing prognostic uncertainty, decisions to forgo life-sustaining medical treatment, spiritual dimensions of life and illness, and alternative medicine. Pediatric board and subboard certifying examinations should include questions on palliative care.

- An increase in support for research into effective pediatric palliative care programming, regulation and reimbursement, pain and symptom management, and grief and bereavement counseling is necessary.

From American Academy of Pediatrics, Committee on Bioethics and Committee on Hospital Care. Palliative care for children. Pediatrics 2000;106:351-357.

way in which pediatric palliative medicine programs can serve this population most effectively were best expressed in the American Academy of Pediatrics Committee on Bioethics and Committee on Hospital Care policy statement on pediatric end-of-life care (see "Future Considerations" box).[5] Optimal pediatric palliative care requires willingness to engage the patient and family in discussions of their hopes and fears and to provide comfort and support for emotional, spiritual, and physical pain. An open-minded assessment of the patient's and family's emotional, spiritual, and physical needs and clarification of realistic goals and hopes not only improves the clinical care a patient receives, but also contributes to the satisfaction and meaning the provider gains from caring for these special children.

REFERENCES

1. Field MJ, Behrman RE (eds). When Children Die: Improving Palliative and End-of-Life Care for Children and their Families. Washington, DC: National Academies Press, 2003.
2. Sligh J. An early model of care. In Armstrong-Daley A (ed). Hospice Care for Children. New York: Oxford University Press, 1993, pp 219-230.
3. Wolfe J, Grier HE, Klar N, et al. Symptoms and suffering at the end of life in children with cancer. N Engl J Med 2000;342:326-333.
4. Wolfe J, Klar N, Grier H, et al. Understanding of prognosis among parents of children who died of cancer: Impact on treatment goals and integration of palliative care. JAMA 2000;284:2469-2475.
5. American Academy of Pediatrics, Committee on Bioethics and Committee on Hospital Care. Palliative care for children. Pediatrics 2000;106:351-357.
6. Sloper P. Experiences and support needs of siblings of children with cancer. Health Soc Care Community 2000;8:298-306.
7. Murray J. Siblings of children with cancer: A review of the literature. J Pediatr Oncol Nurs 1999;16:25-34.
8. Himelstein BP, Hilden JM, Boldt AM, et al. Pediatric palliative care. N Engl J Med 2004;350:1752-1762.
9. Hurwitz CA. Caring for the child with cancer at the close of life: "There are people who make it, and I'm hoping I'm one of them." JAMA 2004; 292:2141-2149.
10. Davies B. The grief of siblings. In Webb MB (ed). Helping Bereaved Children. New York: Guilford Press, 2002, pp 94-127.
11. Himelstein BP. Palliative care for infants, children, adolescents, and their families. J Palliat Med 2006;9:163-181.
12. Kunin H. Ethical issues in pediatric life-threatening illness: Dilemmas of consent, assent, and communication. Ethics Behav 1997;7:43-57.
13. Hartman RG. Dying young: Cues from the courts. Arch Pediatr Adolesc Med 2004;158:615-619.
14. Freyer DR. Care of the dying adolescent: Special considerations. Pediatrics 2004;113:381-388.
15. Kopelman LM. Neonatologists judge the "Baby Doe" regulations. N Engl J Med 1988;318:677-683.
16. Cuttini M, Kaminski M, Garel M. End-of-life decisions in neonatal intensive care. Lancet 2000;356:2190-2191.
17. Amendments to Child Abuse Prevention and Treatment Act. Public Law 98-457. U.S. Statute Large 1984;98(Title I, Sections 101a-312a):Unknown.
18. Gibbons MB. Psychosocial aspects of serious illness in childhood and adolescence. In Armstrong-Daley A, Goltzer SZ (eds). Hospice Care for Children. New York: Oxford University Press, 1993, pp 60-74.
19. Bluebond-Langner M. The Private Worlds of Dying Children. Princeton, NJ: Princeton University Press, 1978.
20. Hockenberry-Eaton M. Evaluation of a child's perceived self-competence during treatment for cancer. J Pediatr Oncol Nurs 1989;6:55-62.
21. Mack JW, Hilden JM, Watterson J, et al. Parent and physician perspectives on quality of care at the end of life in children with cancer. J Clin Oncol 2005; 23:9155-9161.

CHAPTER **195**

Cancer in Children

Roberto Miniero, Emanuele Castagno, and Stefano Lijoi

KEY POINTS

- More than 70% of all children with malignant disease can be cured, but cancer remains the major cause of death resulting from disease in children aged 1 to 14 years.

- Children with early-stage cancer may present with relatively nonspecific signs and symptoms that could mimic some common disorders in childhood; pain as an early symptom is rare, but it is a significant problem for most dying patients.

- Survival rate for children with malignant disease has improved dramatically since the 1970s, but the treatment has become increasingly intensive and aggressive to be more effective.

- The increasing numbers of long-term survivors have to face medical and psychosocial effects of the treatment. Secondary neoplasms may be considered the most devastating complication both physically and emotionally.

- It is important to provide all children who are considered cured with appropriate follow-up care, not only in childhood, but also into adult life, in a coordinated effort among pediatric oncologists, primary care physicians, and specialists. Parents and health professionals must be as honest as possible about diagnosis and treatment and must provide adequate information. Overprotectiveness should be avoided, so as not to compromise the children's independence.

Cancers in children are relatively uncommon and represent only about 1% of new malignant tumors in the United States (data from the Surveillance, Epidemiology, and End Results [SEER] program) and in Western Europe.[1-4] The annual incidence is 140 to 200 new cases per million children and adolescents younger than 15 years of age, so approximately 1 in 7000 children is newly diagnosed with a malignant tumor each year (Fig. 195-1). Approximately 1400 new cases occur each year in the United Kingdom, 1600 in Italy, and more than 13,000 in the United States. Since the late 1970s, a 1% to 2% increase in mean incidence of new cases per year for all malignant diseases has been observed, with a substantial year-to-year rate variation. This increase is primarily in central nervous system (CNS) tumors, neuroblastoma, and acute leukemias.[1-4]

In the United States and in Western Europe, more than 70% of all children with malignant disease can be cured (Fig. 195-2). The greatest improvement has been for leukemia, lymphomas, and CNS tumors. Despite the improved prognosis, malignant diseases remain the major cause of death from disease in children aged 1 to 14 years (~1500 deaths/year in the United States).

Pediatric cancers differ markedly from adult malignancies in the biological characteristics of the tumors and histological types. Acute lymphoblastic leukemias, CNS tumors, and sarcomas predominate in children, in whom most cancers are mesenchymal or neuroectodermal in origin. In adults, acute myeloid leukemia, chronic myeloid and lymphocytic leukemia, and carcinomas (i.e., tumors of epithelial origin) are more frequent. Many adult tumors (e.g., cancer of the breast, lung, and colon) are absent in children, whereas some tumors in children (e.g., retinoblastoma, neuroblastoma, and Wilms' tumor) are virtually absent in adults. Finally, neoplasms both in children and adults (e.g., leukemias, lymphomas, sarcomas, and CNS tumors) differ in biological, histological, and clinical presentation (Fig. 195-3).

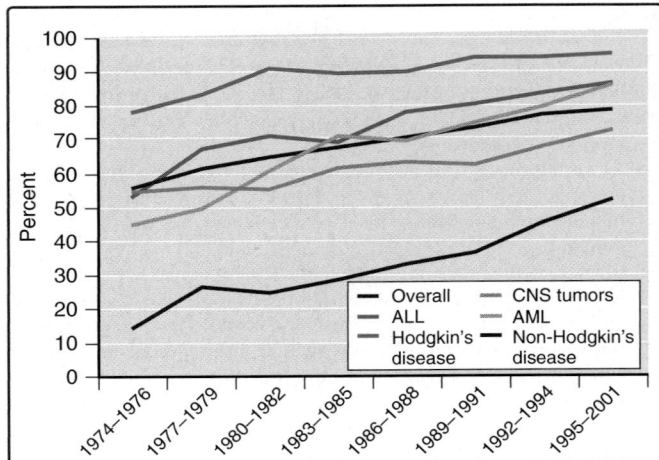

FIGURE 195-2 Trends of 5-year relative survival rates (%) by primary cancer site and year of diagnosis in children aged 0 to 14 years. ALL, acute lymphoblastic leukemia; AML, acute myeloid leukemia; CNS, central nervous system. *(Data from the Surveillance, Epidemiology, and End Results [SEER] program, National Cancer Institute. Cancer Statistics Review 1975-2002; http://www.seer.cancer.gov/.)*

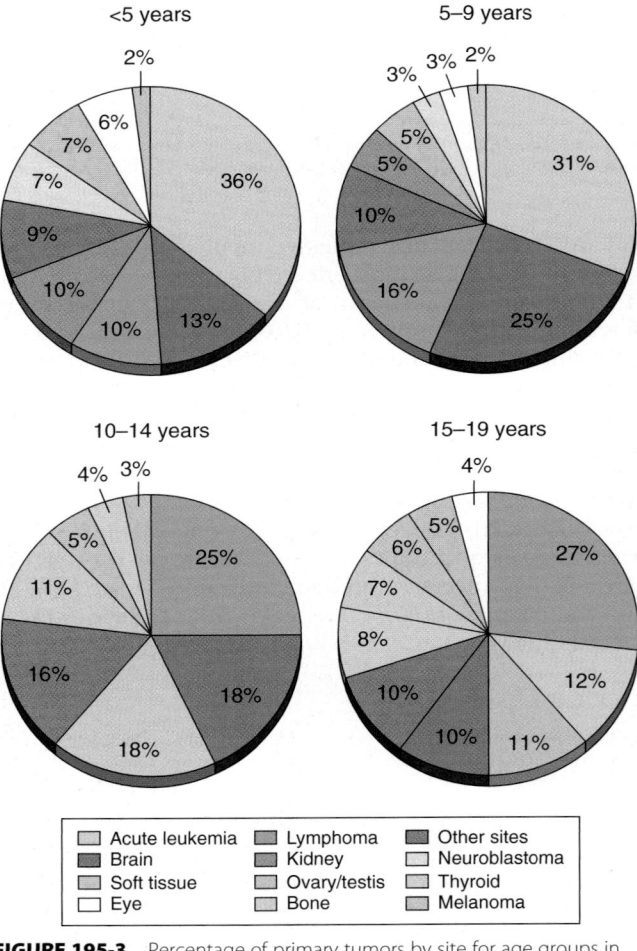

FIGURE 195-3 Percentage of primary tumors by site for age groups in childhood. *(Data from the Surveillance, Epidemiology, and End Results [SEER] program, National Cancer Institute. Monograph No. 57; http://seer.cancer.gov/.)*

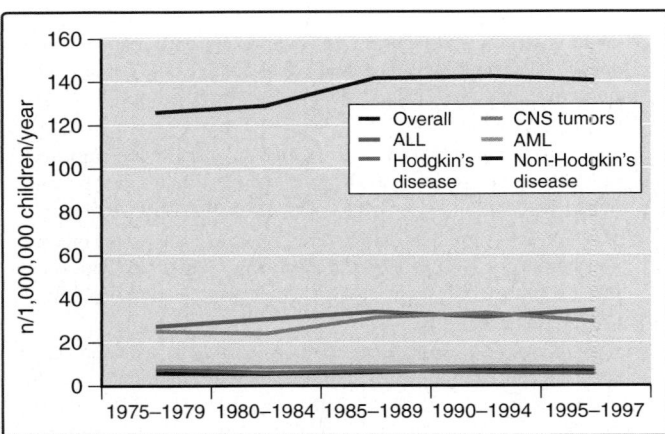

FIGURE 195-1 Trends of 5-year incidence (per 1,000,000) of the most common tumors in children aged 0 to 14 years. ALL, acute lymphoblastic leukemia; AML, acute myeloid leukemia; CNS, central nervous system. *(Data from the Surveillance, Epidemiology, and End Results [SEER] program, National Cancer Institute, for the years 1975 to 1997; http://seer.cancer.gov/.)*

ETIOLOGY

The precise causes of childhood cancer remain unclear, but they likely involve both genetic susceptibility and environmental factors. Cancer incidence is higher in the first years of life, a finding possibly reflecting embryonic origin and intrauterine oncogenesis, and then it falls to a low at the age of 10 years. Subsequently, a linear increase in incidence occurs into adulthood, but a distinction remains from common cancers in adults, in whom lifestyle and environment play major roles. The relatively short potential exposure to environmental carcinogens and the tendency of cancer in the first 2 decades of life to arise in tissues not directly exposed to the environment reflect the more important role of host factors in their origin. Childhood exposure to ionizing radiation or chemicals, parental germline exposure to them before conception, exposure to electromagnetic fields, and abnormal response to one or more common infective agents are possible risk factors.[5]

The role of infectious agents (acute leukemias, lymphomas, and CNS tumors, mainly astrocytomas) has been examined.[6,7] The paucity of exposure to infection in early childhood may condition an abnormal host response when first exposure is delayed. The Epstein-Barr virus may be implicated in Burkitt's lymphoma and Hodgkin's disease from chronic stimulation of B lymphocytes by the virus.

Genetic Factors and Inherited Predisposition to Cancer in Children

Advances in molecular genetics suggest that tumors are the result of multiple mutations in the DNA of neoplastic cells. Somatic cell DNA damage may be demonstrated in nearly all tumors; to date, more than 150 cancer-specific translocations have been identified. Despite the frequency of DNA abnormalities, childhood cancer with a truly hereditary component does not exceed 5%. The hereditary component is high for rare tumors, such as adrenocortical carcinoma (50% to 80%), optic glioma (45%), and retinoblastoma (40%), but low for more common tumors, such as CNS tumors (<3%), leukemia (2.5% to 5.0%), and Wilms' tumor (3% to 5%). Despite the low percentage caused by an inherited condition, overwhelming evidence indicates that cancer is a genetic disease in which a specific mutation is the key that causes or contributes to the disease. The hereditary predisposition hypothesis is based on epidemiological studies of familial cases, studies of associated syndromes, and molecular studies of genes involved in some tumors. More than 100 syndromes predisposing to cancer in children are reported. The genetic alteration may be passed on from parents (retinoblastoma, Li-Fraumeni syndrome) or may be a consequence of a new mutation or rearrangement in the oocyte or sperm before fertilization. This occurs, for example, in Down syndrome (~20-fold increase in risk of leukemia) and in other chromosomal abnormalities, such as trisomy 13, 13q14 deletion, monosomy X (Turner's syndrome), or extra X (Klinefelter's syndrome), that are associated with different types of cancer.

Many single gene disorders predispose to cancer in children. Most of these disorders show an autosomal dominant inheritance, with different penetrance. Retinoblas-toma represents the most carefully documented genetically determined cancer in childhood, caused by mutation of the *Rb1* gene on chromosome 13q14. In reported clusters of families, mothers of young children with soft tissue sarcoma were affected by breast cancer, leukemia, and CNS tumors. A point mutation is documented in the tumor suppressor gene *(TP53)* located at 17q12-13. In some WAGR (Wilms' tumor, aniridia, genital abnormalities, mental retardation) syndromes, involvement of the *WT1* gene on chromosome 11p13 has been observed. In adenomatous polyposis coli and Gardner's syndrome, characterized by multiple colorectal polyps in childhood and adolescence with progression to colorectal carcinoma in adulthood, the *APC* gene on chromosome 5q21 is involved. The multiple endocrine neoplasms (MEN) syndromes are autosomal dominant. Many other "cancer-prone" families have been described. Neurofibromatosis and tuberous sclerosis are autosomal inherited diseases associated with a high risk of cancer. Xeroderma pigmentosum, ataxia-telangiectasia, Fanconi's anemia, and Bloom's syndrome are autosomal recessive disorders resulting from a mutation in DNA repair mechanisms or checkpoint genes leading to increased DNA fragility.

The incidence of cancer in children with chromosomal abnormalities is higher than expected, especially during the first years of life. Moreover, some families show clustering for a particular tumor type, and other families have a higher incidence of tumors without type specificity.[8] Finally, epidemiological studies reveal an important difference in incidence for various tumors among different ethnic populations. The most striking example is Ewing's sarcoma, more common in Spain, Israel, Polynesia, and, in general, in white people, but less common in Asians and virtually absent in Africans and African Americans.

CLINICAL MANIFESTATIONS

Children with early-stage cancer may present with relatively nonspecific signs and symptoms that mimic common disorders in childhood. Because most pediatricians rarely encounter children with cancer, they should be alert to any atypical course of a common condition: *"For a pediatric oncologist the index of suspicion of cancer is high; for the primary care physician the opposite is true."*[9]

A family history of inherited diseases may be useful. The major disease categories associated with a higher childhood risk of cancer (chromosomal disorders, neurofibromatosis, von Hippel–Lindau disease, and immunodeficiencies) must be considered.

A careful clinical history must include the onset, duration, and severity of symptoms and the response to empirical treatments. Nonspecific signs and symptoms such as generalized malaise and fever are frequent in patients with leukemia, lymphomas, neuroblastoma, and sarcomas. In osteosarcoma and Ewing's sarcoma, symptoms are localized to soft tissue or bone masses; patients with sarcomas usually have persistent pain. Lymphadenopathies are common in children, and evaluation may be misleading at the onset of a neoplasm. Generally, neoplastic lymph nodes are firm, rubbery, and matted, without erythema. Evaluation of head and neck nodes is difficult because viral or bacterial infections can cause acute or chronic enlargement. Isolated enlargement of lymph nodes in other regions is more suggestive of malignancy. Persistent or increased node volume during subsequent observations is strongly suggestive of lymphomas, leukemia, neuroblastoma, and, rarely, sarcomas and thyroid cancers. Biopsy of the largest and firmest node is mandatory when lymph nodes remain enlarged after 2 to 3 weeks of observation or after antibiotic therapy or when enlarged nodes are associated with an abnormal chest radiograph or other findings.

Headache is another common symptom in pediatrics. In patients with persisting headache, a brain tumor should always be ruled out, even though it is rare. The clinical history concerning duration, severity, and location of symptoms may help the differential diagnosis, but symptoms may be misleading, especially in infants. Vomiting and headache can be observed in more than half, but approximately 95% of children with headache from a brain tumor also have an abnormal neurological examination.

Pain as an early symptom is rare and often occurs only in tumors involving primarily bone or bone marrow (e.g., leukemia, osteosarcoma) or in metastatic disease (e.g., neuroblastoma). Fifteen to 20% of children with acute lymphoblastic leukemia may have bone pain or arthralgia lasting several weeks as the only symptom, which can be mistaken for rheumatic disease.

An abdominal mass is common. Age is important for the diagnosis: in very young children, Wilms' tumor or neuroblastoma is more frequent, whereas in older children lymphoma is more likely.

Bleeding is a rare initial symptom. It occurs especially in leukemia from bone marrow involvement and secondary thrombocytopenia.

The diagnosis of childhood cancer may be difficult for nonspecialist pathologists because of unusual age-dependent varieties. Even typical childhood tumors may lack definitive morphological evidence of lineage and histogenesis, or lineage may be ambiguous. Diagnostic methodology may require techniques other than morphological studies and immunohistochemistry. Molecular genetic techniques, such as reverse transcriptase–polymerase chain reaction, in situ hybridization, cytogenetics, or DNA sequencing, are requested in most study protocols. These techniques identify genetic alterations in several human neoplasms and have become fundamental for certain childhood tumors.[10] Molecular characterization is important not only in diagnosis, but also for treatment stratification and detection of minimal residual disease. Ultimately, molecular targets will be crucial to the development of new therapeutic drugs. Genetic tests of children with cancer predisposition and prenatal or preimplantation genetic diagnosis for cancer predisposing genes represent controversies and ethical issues for the future.

PRINCIPLES OF TREATMENT

Survival has improved dramatically, but treatment has become increasingly intensive and aggressive. Unfortunately, therapy can adversely affect the patient, and the cost is measured in both acute and chronic toxicity. The success of more intensive protocols has come largely from advances in supportive care; fewer patients die of acute treatment complications, such as infections and bleeding.

The identification of risk factors allows us to stratify patients into different risk classes and to plan protocols tailored to different groups. This approach allows each patient to have more efficacious and less toxic treatment and contributes to reduced therapy-related mortality. Local therapy, such as irradiation or surgery, is a cardinal component in multimodal treatment for solid tumors, whereas chemotherapy is essential for nearly all tumors. The rationale for chemotherapy in children is no different from that in adults with leukemia or disseminated solid tumors. Furthermore, because of difficulties with surgery and radiation therapy in younger children, chemotherapy is important in reducing tumor size before surgical ablation and in preventing systemic tumor spread at diagnosis (preoperative adjuvant therapy). Chemotherapy dosages vary among different protocols and are based on the child's weight or body surface area. Recommendations for special dosage modifications in newborn and young infants are provided in therapeutic protocols. Most of these guidelines are empirical and are based on scant data. Reduced renal function, liver impairment to metabolize chemotherapeutic agents, and different body water distribution during infancy may influence plasma clearance of chemotherapeutic agents. The different absorption capacity of the gastrointestinal tract, depending on varying pH and gastric emptying time, may influence drug levels. Finally, pharmacokinetics for intrathecal administration of methotrexate and cytarabine in acute leukemia in infants is different from that at subsequent ages because of the greater capacity of these drugs to reach the CNS of infants, possibly as a result of incomplete myelination.

Surgery is critical both in diagnosis and in accurate staging. Surgical removal of the primary tumor, integrated with chemotherapy (preoperative and postoperative) and radiation therapy, offers the best chance for cure of many solid neoplasms. Through advances in the multidisciplinary approach to treatment, large resections, amputations (as in sarcomas), and enucleations (e.g., in retinoblastoma) are less frequently necessary. The surgeon also participates in central venous catheter placement in nearly all patients for administration of chemotherapy, antibiotics, blood component products, and total parenteral nutrition or to obtain blood samples, thereby avoiding repeated needle pricks.

Radiation therapy plays a major role for many patients. Because of ongoing growth and development, the sensitivity of certain structures (e.g., brain, bone, soft tissues, and lungs) is increased. The side effects are inversely related to age. Low-total dose of radiation therapy, low-dose fractional irradiation, small-volume irradiation techniques, and protraction of treatment may reduce short-term and long-term sequelae. Unfortunately, especially in younger children, sedation or general anesthesia may be required for radiation delivery and may be a stressful procedure both for the children and their parents.

Because of the nonselective mechanism of action of anticancer drugs, side effects do not differ substantially from those seen in adults. Commonly, children tolerate acute toxicity better than do adults. Furthermore, modern supportive care protocols make treatments more tolerable than before, despite being more aggressive.

Stem cell transplantation (from autologous and allogenic bone marrow, peripheral blood, or umbilical cord blood) is an important treatment option for many patients. Its role is constantly being re-evaluated by studies on histocompatibility, conditioning regimens, toxicity, control of graft-versus-host disease, and, finally, supportive therapy (Box 195-1).[11]

With more long-term survivors, these young people often face medical and psychosocial effects of treatment (Box 195-2). Much research has focused on long-term treatment effects. Growing subjects are more vulnerable than adults to the delayed adverse effects of cancer therapy. Growth impairment, infertility and gonadal disorders, neuropsychological and neurological dysfunction, cardiac and pulmonary failure, musculoskeletal disabilities, and immunity impairment are observed in 20% to 30% of young patients cured of primary tumors. Mortality

---

BOX 195-1 Supportive Care Issues in Pediatric Oncology during Treatment

- Prevention and treatment of infectious complications
- Management of fever
- Management of pain and pain-related procedures
- Prevention and monitoring of organ toxicity
- Hematological supportive care and hematopoietic cytokines
- Prevention and management of nausea and vomiting induced by chemotherapy and radiation therapy
- Mouth care
- Nutritional supportive care
- Management of central venous catheters
- Management of drug extravasation
- Treatment of oncological emergencies
- Sleep disorders, fatigue, depression, and anxiety care and psychosocial support
- Psychiatric and psychosocial support for the family
- Educational issues
- Financial and social issues for the family

BOX 195-2 Supportive Care Issue in Long-Term Survivors

- Chronic pain and rehabilitation
- Follow-up for early detection and treatment of secondary late effects
  - Impairment of normal growth (isolated growth hormone deficiency or inhibition of vertebral growth by radiation therapy)
  - Musculoskeletal disorders (e.g., scoliosis, amputation)
  - Gonadic disorders and infertility, hypothyroidism, pituitary dysfunction
- Pregnancies
- Cardiac and pulmonary function
- Gastrointestinal and liver function
- Urinary tract function
- Hematological and immunological function
- Eyes
- Teeth
- Neuropsychological and neurological function
- Late recurrence of disease and secondary malignant neoplasms
- Impairment of normal life
- Advocacy outside medical negotiation (e.g., insurance, education, employment, being allowed to adopt children)
- Alternative and complementary therapies

---

in those cured of a primary cancer in childhood is usually from recurrent tumors, secondary malignant neoplasms, or cardiac and pulmonary failure.

Physically and emotionally, secondary neoplasms may be the most devastating complication in cancer survivors. These survivors have a risk of a secondary malignant tumor that is 10 to 20 times higher compared with age-matched controls. The incidence of secondary neoplasms 20 years after diagnosis is approximately 8%. The risk and the type of secondary malignant disease differ according to the primary tumor, genetic predisposition, age at the time of first-line therapy, and therapy protocols. Acute myeloid leukemia and myelodysplastic syndromes occur within the first 10 years after treatment, whereas the risk of solid malignant tumors continues rising for 2 or more decades.[12,13]

It is important to provide all children considered cured with appropriate follow-up care, not only in childhood, but also in adult life, as a coordinated effort of pediatric oncologists, primary care physicians, and specialists. Several transition models and programs from pediatric to adult-oriented health care exist. Supportive care will not necessarily be limited to the acute disease, but rather will be extended to long-term follow-up. A comprehensive program is needed, not only for late effects, but also to help survivors overcome fear, anxiety, and depression from their vulnerability regarding late effects. Furthermore, the team may provide counseling on lifestyle and offer strategies to help both patients and their families in the battle against the issues they face with regard to education, insurance, and employment. Pediatric cancer affects not only children, but all the other members of their families as well.[14]

PALLIATIVE CARE OF THE DYING CHILD

The outlook for children with malignant disease continues to improve, and two thirds can expect to be cured. Most children who die of malignant disease do so because of progression and spread of their tumor, but a few die of treatment complications.

When a child with a malignant disease has a relapse, both the oncologist and the family must decide whether to continue with treatment against the tumor or to focus on palliative care. Many factors influence this choice, including the possibility of achieving further remission, the oncologist's personal approach, and the family's own feelings. Even when further treatment is instituted for a certain period, usually a time comes when the medical staff and the family acknowledge that the child is not going to be cured.

The symptoms that a child dying of cancer develops depend on the disease sites, both primary and metastatic. Symptoms observed terminally resemble those seen in adults, but some symptoms have greater importance because of the different range of tumors occurring in children.

In one study,[15] investigators interviewed 103 parents whose children had died of cancer. Parents reported that 89% of children suffered "a lot" and "a great deal" from at least one symptom and 51% from three or more symptoms. The most common symptoms were fatigue, pain, and dyspnea. Others included poor appetite, nausea and vomiting, constipation, and diarrhea (Fig. 195-4).

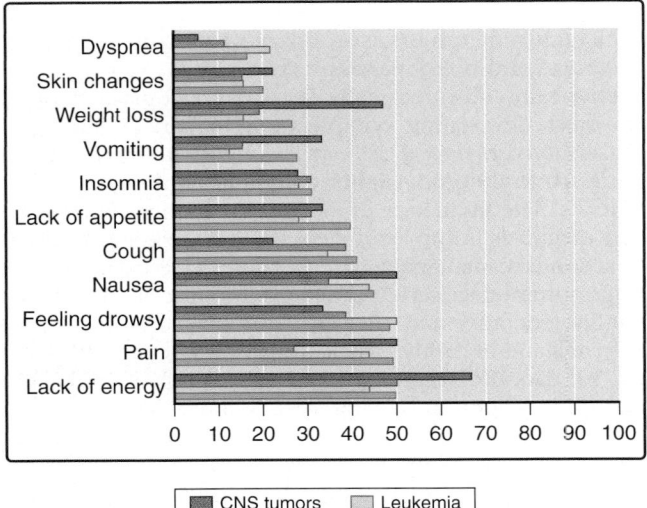

FIGURE 195-4 Prevalence (%) of symptoms associated with the most common tumors in childhood. CNS, central nervous system. *(Data from Collins JJ, Byrnes ME, Dunkel I, et al. The Memorial Symptom Assessment Scale [MSAS]: Validation study in children aged 10-18. J Pain Symptom Manage 2000;19:363-377.)*

Pain is a significant problem for most patients. Direct involvement of tissue by tumor deposits is the most common cause of bone, bone marrow, or soft tissue pain. Distention of organ capsules or obstruction of ducts may also cause pain. Sometimes, patients have nerve invasion or compression. It is possible to provide good relief of pain for most patients, although not complete relief for some.

Respiratory symptoms that may cause distress for both children and their parents include dyspnea, cough, and excessive secretions. If the cause of dyspnea either cannot be found or is not amenable to treatment, the best relief can be sought in combining drug methods with practical and supportive approaches. The sensation of breathlessness can be decreased by opioids.

Gastrointestinal symptoms, including nausea, vomiting, constipation, and sore mouth, are frequent. Careful assessment to elicit the cause is important so the most appropriate treatment can be instituted. Although anorexia often occurs, the severe cachexia seen in adults is uncommon; this finding may reflect the shorter length of terminal illnesses in children.

Brain tumors make up one fifth of all primary childhood tumors. The course of terminal disease in these children is often more prolonged. Progressive neurological deterioration with motor defects, as well as feeding and communication problems, can be distressing.

The needs of dying children are frequently neglected because emotional reactions in children are often overlooked. A difficult issue for parents is what to tell their children. Parents may try to protect their children by providing them as little upsetting information as possible. Conversely, children may sense the anxiety and upheaval in their parents and may sometimes feign ignorance in order not to upset them. All these factors heighten the child's anxiety and isolation. It is of paramount importance that parents and health professionals be as honest as possible about diagnosis and treatment and provide adequate and appropriate information, considering the child's developmental level. Discussing the ultimate diagnosis with children is even more difficult for their parents.

Children's ability to understand and recognize what death is and that death is pending depends on their developmental level. Infants have no cognitive understanding of death. Preschool-aged children understand death as temporary and reversible; they are egocentric and look at death as a punishment or wish fulfilment and may believe that they have caused their own death. School-aged children and preadolescents look at death as permanent, real, final, and universal, but sometimes they are unable to comprehend their own mortality. Adolescents have a good comprehension of the existential implications of death, especially as they gain more ability to think abstractly. Consequently, children, based on their developmental level, must be allowed to determine the pace at which they address the issue of death. It is important to allow children to lead as normal a life as possible, once the crisis of initial diagnosis and treatment has passed. Overprotectiveness should be avoided, so as not to reduce the child's independence, already limited by the illness. This means that children should resume their regular activities as much as possible: a return to school, if at all feasible, should be attempted. Care at home, with provision for education and play in accordance with their developmental level and physical abilities, gives children a vital sense of normality and continuity and a sense of purpose in their lives, and it enables them to achieve short-term goals.

Children with terminal illness have fears and fantasies about their disease and impending death, and they should be encouraged to express themselves in a setting of their choice. Some children show evidence of poor adjustment to death by behaviors such as irritability, separation anxiety and clinging, fear of the dark, noncompliance, regressive behaviors, somatic complaints, sleep and eating disturbances, decreased interest in play or other activities, poor concentration, and preoccupation with death. Imagery may play a crucial role in helping these children express their needs and fears regarding helplessness, separation from loved ones, and death.[16,17]

REFERENCES

1. Adamson P, Law G, Roman E. Assessment of trends in childhood cancer incidence. Lancet 2005;365:753.
2. Sommelet D, Clavel J, Lacour B. Contribution of national paediatric cancer registries to survey and research. Arch Pediatr 2005;12:814-816.
3. Steliarova-Foucher E, Stiller C, Kaatsch P, et al. Geographical patterns and time trends of cancer incidence and survival among children and adolescents in Europe since the 1970s. The ACCIS project: An epidemiological study. Lancet 2004;364:2097-2105.
4. Gatta G, Capoccia R, Stiller C, et al. Childhood cancer survival trends in Europe: A EUROCARE Working Group Study. J Clin Oncol 2005;23:3742-3751.
5. Cottage M, Street F, Comberton G. Childhood cancer and atmospheric carcinogens. J Epidemiol Community Health 2005;59:101-105.
6. McNally RJQ, Eden OB. An infectious aetiology for childhood acute leukemia: A review of the evidence. Br J Haematol 2004;127:243-263.
7. McNally RJQ, Eden OB, Alexander FA, et al. Is there a common aetiology for certain childhood malignancies? Results of cross-space-time clustering analyses. Eur J Cancer 2005;41:2911-2916.
8. Agha MM, Williams JI, Maret L, et al. Congenital abnormalities and childhood cancer. Cancer 2005;103:1939-1948.
9. Velez MC. Consultation with a specialist: Lymphomas. Pediatr Rev 2003;24:380-386.

10. Messahel B, Hing S, Jeffrey I, et al. Clinical features of molecular pathology of solid tumors in childhood. Lancet Oncol 2005;6:421-430.

11. Radeva JI, Van Scoyoc E, Smith FO, et al. National estimates of the use of hematopoietic stem-cell transplantation in children with cancer in the United States. Bone Marrow Transplant 2005;36:397-404.

12. Bryant R. Managing side effects of childhood cancer treatment. J Pediatr Nurs 2003;18:113-125.

13. Bhatia S. Cancer survivorship: Pediatric issues. Hematology Am Soc Hematol Educ Program 2005;507-515.

14. Langeveld NE, Stam H, Grootenhuis MA, et al. Quality of life in young adult survivors of childhood cancer. Support Care Cancer 2002;10:579-600.

15. Wolfe J, Grier HE, Klar N, et al. Symptoms and suffering at the end of life in children with cancer. N Engl J Med 2000;342:326-333.

16. Cherny NI, Hanks G. Pediatric palliative medicine. In Doyle D, Hanks G, MacDonald N (eds). Oxford Textbook of Palliative Medicine, 3rd ed. Oxford: Oxford University Press, 2005, pp 775-839.

17. Kane JR, Himelstein BP. Palliative care in pediatrics. In Berger A, Portenoy R, Weissman D (eds). Principles and Practice of Palliative Care and Supportive Oncology, 2nd ed. Philadelphia: Lippincott Williams & Wilkins, 2002, pp 1044-1061.

SUGGESTED READING

Field M, Behrman R. When Children Die. Washington, DC: National Academies Press, 2001.

Goldman A. Care of the Dying Child. Oxford: Oxford University Press, 2002.

Hindmarch C. On the Death of a Child. Abingdon, UK: Radcliffe Medical Press, 2000.

Keene N, Hobbie W, Ruccione K. Childhood Cancer Survivors. Sebastopol, CA: O'Reilly, 2000.

Pizzo PA, Poplack DG (eds). Principles and Practice of Pediatric Oncology, 6th ed. Philadelphia: Lippincott Williams & Wilkins, 2002.

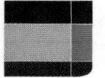

CHAPTER **196**

Psychological Adaptation of the Dying Child

Lisa N. Schum and Javier R. Kane

KEY POINTS

- Comprehensive palliative care involves attending to physical, emotional, and spiritual suffering. Referrals to mental health services (e.g., psychology, social work, pastoral care) should be made early in the dying process to facilitate optimal care.

- Treatment of psychological suffering related to pediatric terminal illness is not limited to the child. Psychological distress and the need for intervention often extend to the child's family, community, and medical team.

- Understanding death is a developmental process. From infancy through adolescence, children transition from conceptualizing death as a temporary separation to gaining an appreciation of the irreversible, final, inevitable, and causal characteristics of death. A child's experience with chronic illness or previous experience with death may influence the trajectory of his or her understanding of death concepts.

- Children often experience symptoms of emotional distress at the end of life. Existential worries, grief, and guilt are likely contributors to psychological suffering. Physical suffering, medications, and disease processes can also cause or exacerbate emotional distress in children with terminal illness.

- Assessment and diagnosis of psychological disorders at end of life are complicated by the overlap between symptoms associated with disease and treatment and symptoms attributable to emotional distress. Additionally, psychological suffering should be expected for many children with terminal illness as part of a normal grieving process. Intervention is likely to be helpful or necessary even if a dying child does not meet standard diagnostic criteria for a psychological disorder.

- Treatment of the child's psychological suffering at end of life often occurs on several levels. Reduction of physical suffering remains a priority. Additionally, providing the child with opportunities to ask questions and to discuss concerns is important. Information should be tailored to the child's developmental level of understanding and individual preferences. Formal mental health services and psychiatric medication are often indicated and should be initiated early in the dying process if necessary.

- Comprehensive palliative care involves tending to the family's suffering from the point of diagnosis through bereavement. Often, families develop close relationships with the medical team during the child's dying process. As such, some involvement with the family should extend beyond the child's death. Additionally, arranging bereavement care for the family may also be appropriate.

- Communication is a particularly difficult component of end-of-life care. Discussions about a terminal prognosis and palliative care needs should be initiated with timeliness, sensitivity, and clarity. Disclosure of end-of-life information to the child should be developmentally appropriate and sensitive to individual preferences.

- Families and children often benefit from being involved in decision-making processes regarding end-of-life care. The factors that influence end-of-life decisions often differ for children and their parents. It is recommended that special consideration be given to the preferences of the child, particularly when dissent from certain therapies may result in improvements in quality of life.

- The spiritual care of a dying child and the family is an important aspect of comprehensive end-of-life care. It is beneficial for the spiritual needs of the family to be identified early so that appropriate services and support can be available as needed throughout the dying process.

Life-threatening pediatric illness is a stressor that precipitates major physical, emotional, and spiritual distress for the sick child; the impact is not limited to the patient. Treatment of the psychological suffering related to childhood terminal illness is unique and often requires care of parents, siblings, extended family members, peers, and even the medical team. Providing psychological care and promoting effective coping for the child and family are important elements of comprehensive palliative care.

THE CHILD'S UNDERSTANDING OF ILLNESS AND DEATH

Seriously ill children learn about death from their personal experiences with disease, and many understand it better than other children their age. The level of the child's emotional and cognitive development influences how a sick child understands the realities of his or her life. From birth to 3 years of age, children grasp events at the level of feeling and action that corresponds to Piaget's sensorimotor stage of cognitive development. Children at this age may interpret death as a temporary separation or abandonment. Children at the preoperational stage of development, between the ages of 3 and 6 years, view death as a state of immobility that may be transient and reversible. During the stage of concrete operations, between 6 and 12 years of age, children begin to realize that people who die are not able to function. The four fundamental elements of death (irreversibility, finality, inevitability, and causality) are understood by most children by the age of 7 years.[1] The ability for abstract reasoning usually matures during Piaget's stage of formal operations, spanning from the age of 12 years onward. These children understand illness and death in ways similar to those of a mature adult. Given the psychological and environmental context in which serious illness unfolds, chronically ill and dying children may understand illness, death, and dying earlier than expected for their chronological age (Table 196-1). Although the steps by which children achieve sophisticated understanding of

---

TABLE 196-1 Understanding of Death According to Age

INFANT, 0-1 YR OF AGE

COGNITIVE STAGE
Sensorimotor: experiencing the world through sensory input

DEVELOPMENTAL TASK
To achieve awareness of being a separate entity from significant other

IMPACT OF ILLNESS
Distorts differentiation between self and significant other

MAJOR FEARS
Separation, strangers

CONCEPT OF DEATH
Unable to differentiate death from temporary separation or abandonment

EMOTIONAL CARE
Provide stability. Maintain consistent caregivers and routines.
Provide security. Minimize separation from parents and important caregivers. Maintain the crib as a "safe place" where no invasive procedures are performed. Encourage parents to provide physical expressions of reassurance to the infant (i.e., holding, touching).
Provide a calming environment. Infants are perceptive to the moods of their caregivers. Assist parents with reducing their own emotional distress while in the presence of the infant. Reassure parents of the adequacy of their parenting skills.
Facilitate supportive care or other mental health services for the family as needed.

SPIRITUAL CARE
Encourage and facilitate use of the spiritual support system by the family.

TODDLER, 1-2 YR OF AGE

COGNITIVE STAGE
Preoperational thought: egocentric, magical, concrete, little concept of body integrity

DEVELOPMENTAL TASK
To initiate autonomy

IMPACT OF ILLNESS
Interferes with the development of a sense of control; loss of independence

MAJOR FEARS
Separation, loss of control

CONCEPT OF ILLNESS
Phenomenism: perceiving external, unrelated, concrete phenomena as the cause of the illness through mere association (e.g., "I am sick because I don't feel well.")
Contagion: perceiving the cause of illness as the proximity between events (e.g., "I got sick because I was near you when you were sick.")

CONCEPT OF DEATH
Recognize death in terms of immobility; often viewed as reversible, temporary, or foreign.

EMOTIONAL CARE
Provide stability. Maintain consistent caregivers and routines. Explain and maintain consistent limits.
Provide security. Minimize separation from parents and important caregivers. Encourage parents to provide both physical and verbal reassurance to the child. Keep security objects at hand.
Provide a calming environment. Provide distractions (i.e., games, books, movies) when children are fussy, irritable, and clingy. Assist parents with reducing their own emotional distress while in the presence of the child. Reassure parents of the adequacy of their parenting skills.
Facilitate supportive care or other mental health services for the family as needed.

SPIRITUAL CARE
Reassure the child that the disease is not punishment from God, Higher Power, or another authority figure. Encourage and facilitate use of the spiritual support system by the family.

TABLE 196-1 Understanding of Death According to Age—cont'd

PRESCHOOL, 2-6 YR OF AGE

COGNITIVE STAGE

Preoperational thought: egocentric, magical, lacking ability to think abstractly. Children may use or repeat words that they do not understand, may translate phrases literally, or may develop their own definitions for new words or concepts.

DEVELOPMENTAL TASK

To develop of a sense of initiative

IMPACT OF ILLNESS

Disrupts or causes children to lose certain accomplishments (i.e., walking, talking, controlling body functions)

MAJOR FEARS

Loss of control, bodily injury, being left alone, the dark, the unknown

CONCEPT OF ILLNESS

Phenomenism: perceiving external, unrelated, concrete phenomena as the cause of the illness through mere association (e.g., "I am sick because I don't feel well.")

CONCEPT OF DEATH

Recognize death in terms of immobility. Often view death as reversible, temporary, or foreign. Begin to question and develop a mature concept of death.

EMOTIONAL CARE

Provide stability. Maintain consistent caregivers and routines. Explain and maintain consistent limits.
Provide security. Minimize separation from parents and important caregivers. Encourage parents to provide both physical and verbal reassurance to the child. Keep security objects at hand.
Facilitate preparation. Help the child prepare for important events by providing simple, concrete explanations. Use pictures, models, equipment, and medical play. Preparation may begin days before a major event and hours before a minor event.
Facilitate communication. Expect children to ask questions over and over again. Provide simple, concrete, consistent explanations; avoid metaphors or euphemistic language. Do not underestimate the child's level of comprehension or ability to perceive stress experienced by caregivers. Help children to label their emotions and verbalize their fears. Engage children in make-believe play; this often provides them with a safe environment to explore their thoughts or worries about illness and death.
Facilitate supportive care or other mental health services for the family as needed.

SPIRITUAL CARE

Demonstrate love, trust, respect, caring, and consistent discipline without anger. When appropriate, initiate discussions about the love and caring of the Higher Power to relieve anxiety and loneliness. Reassure the child that the disease is not punishment from God, Higher Power, or another authority figure. Encourage and facilitate use of the spiritual support system by the family.

SCHOOL AGE, 6-12 YR OF AGE

COGNITIVE STAGE

Concrete operational thought: emergence of logical thought, lingering tendency to think literally

DEVELOPMENTAL TASK

To develop a sense of industry

IMPACT OF ILLNESS

Disrupts autonomy or independence and causes feelings of inadequacy or inferiority

MAJOR FEARS

Loss of control, bodily injury, disappointing important others, death

CONCEPT OF ILLNESS

Contamination: perceiving cause of illness as a person, object, or action external to the child that is "bad" or "harmful" to the body (e.g., "I got a cold because I didn't wear a hat.")
Internalization: perceiving cause of illness as external but located inside the body (e.g., "I got a cold because I breathed in air and germs.")

CONCEPT OF DEATH

Recognize the irreversibility, inevitability, nonfunctionality, and causality

EMOTIONAL CARE

Provide stability. Maintain consistent caregivers and routines. Explain and maintain consistent limits. Encourage parents to continue enforcing family rules that remain applicable given the child's current level of functioning.
Provide security. Minimize separation from parents and important caregivers. Encourage parents to provide both physical and verbal reassurance to the child.
Facilitate communication. Encourage questions and expect repetition. Provide simple, concrete, consistent explanations; avoid metaphors or euphemistic language. Children are typically searching for reassurance that they are loved and will not be abandoned. Help children to label their emotions and to verbalize their fears.
Facilitate a normal environment. Encourage the child to participate in self-care and daily activities that are consistent with the child's age and current level of functioning (i.e., dressing self, going to school). Encourage social contact with the child's peer group. Provide diversions (i.e., games, books, movies).
Provide control. Allow the child to make choices and decisions when possible.
Facilitate supportive care or other mental health services for the family as needed.

TABLE 196-1 Understanding of Death According to Age—cont'd

SCHOOL AGE, 6-12 YR OF AGE

SPIRITUAL CARE

Demonstrate forgiveness and acceptance. Be alert to anxiety about the illness as a punishment from God, Higher Power, or another authority figure. Provide simple, concrete responses to the child's questions about spiritual beliefs. Maintain participation in spiritual rituals and contact with religious peer groups. If appropriate, promote prayer and nurturing of the child's relationship with God or Higher Power. Encourage and facilitate use of the spiritual support system by the family.

ADOLESCENT, 12-20 YR OF AGE

COGNITIVE STAGE

Formal operational thought: emergence of abstract thinking. Adolescents may maintain some magical thinking (e.g., feeling guilty for illness) and egocentrism.

DEVELOPMENTAL TASK

To develop a sense of identity

IMPACT OF ILLNESS

Disrupts newly acquired roles and responsibilities. Adolescents may resist or resent having to increase their dependence on caregivers.

MAJOR FEARS

Loss of control, altered body image, separation from peer group

CONCEPT OF ILLNESS

Physiological: perceiving cause of illness as malfunctioning organ or bodily process, explaining illness in a sequence of events
Psychophysiological: recognizing that emotions and attitudes affect health and illness

CONCEPT OF DEATH

Speculate on the implications and ramifications of death. Understand the effect of death on other people and the society as a whole. Thinking is often future oriented, thus making it difficult to understand that death is a possibility in the present.

EMOTIONAL CARE

Provide control. Allow the adolescent to be integrally involved in decision making regarding care. Allow the adolescent to make choices and decisions when possible. Facilitate productive conversations and negotiations when parents and adolescents disagree about health care decisions. Encourage the adolescent to engage in independent self-care as much as possible given his or her current level of functioning. Stress the adolescent's role in medical care, particularly the importance of cooperation and adherence.
Facilitate communication. Provide information honestly and sensitively. Adolescents often react to both the content of and the manner in which information is delivered. Be honest about treatment and consequences. Adolescents may prefer to talk about distressing issues with psychologists or social workers rather than with family members.
Facilitate a normal environment. Provide adolescents with as much privacy as possible; encourage families to respect adolescents' requests to be alone, within normal limits. Encourage the adolescent to participate in daily activities that are consistent with the child's age and current level of functioning (i.e., talking with friends, going to school). Encourage social contact with the adolescent's peer group.
Facilitate supportive care or other mental health services for the family as needed.

SPIRITUAL CARE

Provide an open, supportive environment for the adolescent to discuss illness in terms of philosophical or spiritual beliefs. Provide unbiased, honest answers. If appropriate and acceptable to the adolescent, encourage him or her to maintain participation in spiritual rituals and contact with religious peer groups. Observe and document verbalizations of patient's values and beliefs.

Data from Gibbons MB. Psychosocial aspects of serious illness in childhood and adolescence. In Armstrong-Dailey A, Zarbock Goltzer S (eds). Hospice Care for Children. New York: Oxford University Press, 1993, pp 62-63; Faulkner KW. Children's understanding of death. In Armstrong-Dailey A, Zarbock Goltzer S (eds). Hospice Care for Children. New York: Oxford University Press 1993, pp 9-21; Hart D, Schneider D. Spiritual care for children with cancer. Semin Oncol Nurs 1997;13:263-270; Thompson RJ, Gustafson KE. Developmental Changes in Conceptualizations of Health, Illness, Pain, and Death: Adaptation to Chronic Childhood Illness. Washington, DC: American Psychological Association, 1996, pp 181-195; Wood BL. A developmental biopsychosocial approach to the treatment of chronic illness in children and adolescents. In Mikesell RH, Lusterman DD, McDaniel SH (eds). Integrating Family Therapy: Handbook of Family Psychology and Systems Theory. Washington, DC: American Psychological Association, 1995, pp 437-455; and Woznick LA, Goodheart CD. Navigating the Emotional Terrain: Living with Childhood Cancer. A Practical Guide to Help Families Cope. Washington, DC: American Psychological Association, 2002, pp 9-29, 259-284.

concepts related to death and dying have been well studied,[2] less investigation has focused on effective ways to alleviate the emotional and existential suffering of terminally ill children.[3]

THE CHILD'S PSYCHOLOGICAL SUFFERING

Children nearing the end of life may experience significant emotional distress and debilitating psychological symptoms. Most parents interviewed after their child's death from cancer reported that their child experienced sadness, distress, and diminished pleasure during the last month of life.[4] Particularly during the final days, psychological suffering appears prominent. Many patients experience irritability, nervousness, worry, and sadness during the last week of life.[5] Given the high prevalence of emotional distress, it is important for practitioners to be alert to emotional and behavioral symptoms that could indicate anxiety and depression associated with terminal illness.

The source of a child's emotional distress near death may be difficult to identify. Children facing death often worry about being forgotten, leaving behind loved ones, and experiencing pain during dying.[6] Additionally, they may mourn the loss of their ability to function normally and to pursue their futures. As they contemplate death, children may struggle with adult-sized existential questions without the cognitive sophistication or life experience to resolve these issues adequately. Further, many children may carry the burden of these worries in silence, to prevent upsetting loved ones who are already distressed by the prognosis.[7]

Physical suffering is another likely contributor to emotional distress experienced by children at the end of life. Effective management of pain and other symptoms is an essential part of caring for a dying child. Indeed, aggressive symptom management may promote psychological adjustment by eliminating unnecessary physical suffering and allowing the child and family to focus on the emotional and spiritual elements of dying. In children hospitalized for cancer, 20% of psychiatric consultations identified improving pain management as a necessary treatment goal for the patients referred,[8] a finding suggesting clinically notable changes in mood and behavior when pain is poorly controlled. Additionally, the overlap of physical and psychological symptoms may exacerbate distress. For example, dyspnea, a commonly experienced symptom near death, can both induce and be caused by anxiety. Finally, psychological suffering may also be related to disease and treatment. Certain medications, central nervous system disease, endocrine dysfunction, and malnutrition are associated with mood changes.[9]

Assessment and diagnosis of psychological disorders are complicated by the overlap between symptoms associated with disease and treatment and those included in the diagnostic criteria for anxiety and depressive disorders. Dying children frequently experience fatigue, dyspnea, nausea, anorexia, insomnia, loss of appetite, and inattention,[4,5,10] which are also symptoms of anxiety and mood disorders by standard diagnostic criteria.[11] When these physical symptoms are accompanied by excessive sadness, worry, anhedonia, hopelessness, worthlessness, or suicidality, close monitoring and further assessment to rule out a psychological disorder are warranted. A comprehensive psychiatric evaluation by a trained clinician is necessary to establish the diagnosis of anxiety and mood disorders. Psychometric evaluation using standardized interviews may be too long for routine use and inappropriate for chronic illness. Symptom checklists derived from these standardized interviews can be useful screening tools.

In clinical practice, it is often difficult to differentiate between an anxiety disorder and the presence of anxiety that may be considered normal given the stressful circumstances of terminal illness. Seriously ill children may manifest symptoms of psychological distress that would benefit from intervention even if they do not meet the criteria for diagnosis of an anxiety disorder. When anxiety related to the terminal illness causes significant impairment in function, the diagnosis of an adjustment disorder with anxiety, or with mixed anxiety and depressed mood, should be considered. The clinical presentation of anxiety in younger children may consist of excessive concern about competence, need for reassurance, fear of the dark, fear of harm to self or an attachment figure, and somatic complaints. In adolescence, anxiety may manifest as unrealistic fears, excessive worry about past behavior, and self-consciousness.

Although major depression and dysthymia are relatively common in children and adolescents, most seriously ill children are not depressed. As with anxiety, depressive symptoms may occur as part of a normal grieving process. When depressive symptoms related to the terminal illness cause significant impairment in the child's functioning, the diagnosis of an adjustment disorder with depressed mood, or with mixed anxiety and depressed mood, should be considered. Grief and depressive symptoms in a child could suggest the need to explore his or her fears of death and progressive disease. The manifestations of depression vary according to the developmental stage of the child or adolescent. Younger children may show more somatic complaints, irritability, tantrums, and other behavioral problems. Older children may report low self-esteem, guilt, and hopelessness. Family function appears to be more influential than serious illness in the development of depression. Children are at increased risk of depression when their families demonstrate conflict, maltreatment, rejection, and communication problems, with little expression of positive affect and support.[12,13]

Treating the psychological distress of dying children occurs on several levels. An important starting point is to assess physical suffering and to modify symptom management, thereby reducing pain, dyspnea, and other physical symptoms likely to exacerbate emotional distress. Adjuvant drug therapy may be indicated to treat disease-related and treatment-related changes in mood and mental status.[9] An open, safe environment for the child to express concerns about illness, treatment, and death is another important task in palliative medicine. Because children's understanding of death develops as a function of their cognitive maturity and previous experience, it is important to meet children at their current level of understanding and to permit them to communicate directly about death-related worries. Children exhibiting changes in mood and behavior should be referred as early as possible for mental health services (i.e., psychology, social work, pastoral care). In particular, behavioral techniques (i.e., distraction, relaxation training, imagery) reduce anxiety and certain physical symptoms (i.e., dyspnea, muscle tension, pain) in children. Modifications to situational variables provide children and families with a sense of control.[14] This approach includes fostering social support, including the child in some level of decision making, and engaging the child in task-oriented activities. Additionally, allowing children to continue engaging in typical daily activities (i.e., school, play, social engagements), at a level commensurate with their current level of functioning, can help them meet survival goals and can maintain a relatively normal environment while possible (see Table 196-1).[15]

THE FAMILY'S PSYCHOLOGICAL SUFFERING

Learning that a child has a life-limiting illness can have a devastating impact on families. Additionally, the often prolonged, unpredictable clinical course of a child's illness can create an extended time of intense stress that places families at increased risk for problematic adjustment. For this reason, the care necessary to address the emotional needs of children and families is not restricted exclusively to any definitive span of time; instead, attention to psychological functioning of the child and family is important throughout the entire course of the illness and into bereavement.

Anticipatory grief is commonly experienced by parents and siblings awaiting a child's imminent death.[16] Parents consumed with their own grief for their dying child often find it difficult to work,[17] to attend the needs of their healthy children, and to care for their sick child.[18] Siblings often feel uninformed, worried, and confused about the dying sibling's condition and the well-being of their family.[19] After the death, even the family structure is altered. A sibling may suddenly be an only child, or a mother may find herself childless. In redefining family roles and processing grief, family members face substantial challenges after a death.

Social support is important for the adjustment of family members during a child's end-of-life care and during bereavement.[14,16,18,20] This need is complicated when families move away from home in pursuit of medical care and are thus removed from their traditional support systems. Families often find comfort in associating with other families who have experienced similar loss.[16,20] The quality of the relationships between family members and staff is also important during the dying process. Parents of children dying in hospital reported needing supportive health care providers who were readily available, emotionally expressive, and respectful of the parent-child relationship.[21]

When a child is critically ill, parents believe that they surrender control of their child's well-being to the medical team. Parents of a child with a terminal diagnosis often feel helpless, unable to protect their child from impending death, and, often, unable to control their child's physical and emotional suffering.[17,22] Helping parents to retain as much control as possible is important in the family's adjustment to the illness and death of the child. Involving parents in treatment decisions and in end-of-life planning is critical in preserving their control over their child's health and comfort.[22,23] When death is inevitable but not immediate, parents often decide to allow the child to return home. This decision is commonly considered the best choice for child and family adjustment,[24] and it provides parents with some control and a sense of normality during this difficult phase.

Many would assume that the child's death is the end point for palliative care. Often forgotten are the survivors: parents, siblings, extended family members, friends, and peers. Contact from health care providers is often noticeably absent (and missed) after the death of a child.[17,25,26] Given the intimate shared experience between the family and those health care providers involved at the bedside, it is important that contact not be terminated immediately after the death, thus leaving families feeling abandoned and forgotten.[22] Further, mental health professionals involved in the palliative care of the child should assess family members for risk factors associated with complicated bereavement, and appropriate referrals for psychological services should be made.[27]

Cognitive-behavioral therapy is effective for treating families with seriously ill children.[28] Improvement has been found in domains such as self-efficacy, self-management of disease, family functioning, psychosocial well-being, reduced isolation, social competence, hope, meaning, and pain. Additionally, family therapy is another

important intervention that can improve family functioning and support.[29] Regardless of the intervention, caregivers may facilitate coping by providing individualized care that addresses the needs of the seriously ill child as a whole person and summons available resources to help the child remain engaged in his or her preferred activities.

COMMUNICATION WITH THE CHILD AND FAMILY

Establishing accurate, effective communication with patients and families is critically important in end-of-life care, when compassionate decisions to withhold or withdraw curative or life-prolonging therapies must be made. Care of patients with end-stage disease demands effective communication related to prognosis, coping, personal life goals, self-efficacy, family cohesion, parental self-care, hope, meaning, and death. Delivery of this information can be problematic and can threaten the alliance between the family and the medical team.[22,25,26,30,31] Parents who receive information in an insensitive or inadequate manner experience significant and lasting emotional distress.[22,25] The way a child dies and the decisions parents make related to their child's end-of-life care could have lasting effects on the grieving process and on the ultimate well-being of surviving family members.[25] It is essential to develop compassionate and effective communication skills to provide parents with the information necessary to make important end-of-life decisions.

Timely delivery of news about prognosis to families is critically important in optimal palliative care. When parents and physicians agree that cure is unrealistic earlier in an illness, palliative care and a focus on alleviating suffering are implemented earlier.[31] Additionally, earlier communication about a terminal prognosis provides the family with the time they need to make preparations if they decide to take their child home to die. Without feeling secure that they have proper resources, preparation, and support, parents may feel unable to handle a home death for their child. There, timely communication about prognosis is a practical necessity. Important end-of-life communication is often delayed. Do not resuscitate orders are frequently discussed within hours of a child's death,[26] when parents are likely emotionally overwhelmed by the impending death. Additionally, parents themselves are often left with the burdensome responsibility of initiating discussions about end-of-life care with health care providers.[30]

When physicians recognize that curative therapy is no longer an option, relaying that prognosis to parents in a way that is sensitive and comprehensible is often challenging. It is important for the emotional adjustment of families that they learn of a child's terminal prognosis through compassionate communication.[25] Parents often maintain hope for cure even after learning that their child's condition is terminal.[26] When a family is pushed too aggressively toward the reality of their child's prognosis, it may cause parents to feel that the medical team no longer cares about saving their child and may lead parents to resist important treatment discussions. Psychologists and social workers may facilitate these sensitive conversations.[14,31] However, this approach is most appropriate when psychosocial professionals have been integrated into the care of the child beforehand, because parents prefer to receive bad news about their child's health from a familiar person consistently involved in their child's care.[14,20,25,32,33]

Discussing prognosis and end-of-life issues with a dying child can be a difficult and emotional task. In general, most clinicians believe that children benefit from open, honest communication about their prognosis.[34] Few empirical studies have assessed the effect of disclosure to children with terminal illness. When parents decide to disclose this information to a child, they typically assume that responsibility themselves. Some parents choose not to tell their child that he or she will die.[15,35] Many reports suggest that dying children sense that they are dying, even if the prognosis is not disclosed, and subsequently, when death-related conversation is conspicuously absent, these children feel unable to talk about their death-related fears freely.[34] One study found that parents who chose not to disclose the prognosis to their dying children experienced regret, particularly if they sensed that the child knew he or she was dying.[35]

Attempts to protect the child from difficult conversations may impose significant barriers between the child and the medical team providing care. It is important to recognize that children differ in the information they desire about their diagnosis and prognosis. Although some children find it helpful to receive detailed information about disease and treatment, others are distressed by such information. Children who demonstrate information-avoidant behavior are using a specific coping mechanism for dealing with their serious illness. Health care providers must be careful not to strip away existing coping mechanisms by providing too much information to these children and thus exposing them to further emotional suffering. Caregivers must be sensitive to the indirect clues that children give about their willingness to converse about difficult issues.[36] Young children, for example, may express separation anxiety and fear that something may happen to the parent. School-aged children may manifest regressive behavior or may show unusual fears about school or the hospital. Preadolescents may refuse to cooperate with treatment or may manifest emotional lability, tearfulness, or outbursts of anger. Adolescents may show poor compliance with the treatment plan, may express anger, or may seem overly concerned with appearance.

When delivering news about these issues to a child, it is also important to consider the child's level of understanding related to death and dying. Preparing parents and health care providers for the unanticipated questions about death that children are likely to spring on them is helpful in producing a safe, comfortable environment in which children can express and explore their concerns.[6,34] Reassure these children that they are loved, that their suffering will be treated through the entire dying process, and that they will not be abandoned by the family or the medical team. Additionally, the information needs of siblings should not be neglected. Siblings often desire clarification and more information about the dying child's disease, treatment, and prognosis[19] than they typically receive.

Little empirical evidence exists to inform recommendations for communicating with dying children about their prognosis and end-of-life issues. Although some clinicians argue that children should be told directly and honestly that death is imminent,[34] others fear that such indiscriminant delivery of potentially devastating information is not justified.[3] Without data to inform appropriate, effective communication, it remains unclear when discussions should be initiated, what information should be provided, and how this information should be delivered to dying children.[3] Further, no standardized approach exists for health care professionals to communicate with patients and their parents regarding their medical care near death. Standardized communication tools, such as the Final Stage Conference, are helpful in facilitating discussions about difficult issues, but these tools are not widely implemented.[37]

Communication with a seriously ill child requires certain skills that must be exercised long before the child is declared to have an incurable illness. Health care organizations and individual institutions promote ethical standards of practice; whether discussions with patients and families occur in a way that is goal directed, culturally sensitive, and compassionate depends primarily on the personal characteristics and communication skills of the professionals involved. The 6 Es strategy[38] may be used as a guide:

- Establish an agreement concerning open communication with parents, children, and caregivers early in the relationship.
- Engage the child at the opportune time.
- Explore what the child already knows and wants to know about the illness.
- Explain medical information according to the child's needs and age.
- Empathize with the child's emotional reactions.
- Encourage the child by reassuring him or her that you will be there to listen and be supportive.

DECISION MAKING WITH THE CHILD AND FAMILY

Overall, improved quality of life, family satisfaction, and emotional well-being may result from the provision of palliative care services that focus on effective communication, decision support, and cooperative case management with insurers.[39] Care strategies, such as the Individualized Care Planning and Coordinating Model, that provide patient-centered and family-centered care, and that support the decision making process are likely to improve the quality of care.[40] Participation of the child in decision making is particularly important. Whether the child can or should participate remains an individual decision made by the child's parents and caregivers, based on the level of the child's emotional and cognitive development. It is important to determine whether the child's participation would facilitate his or her adjustment. Many children, even as young as 6 years, are able to participate.[41] In children with cancer, patients between the ages of 10 and 20 years are often capable of participating in and understanding the consequences of their end-of-life care choices.[42] Information provided by health care providers and the avoidance of adverse side effects of treatment were the factors rated as important in the decision-making process for these patients. In contrast, their parents identified the needs to cure or prolong their child's life, to receive support from staff, and to respect their child's preferences about end-of-life care as the most important factors in their decisions. Many children and their parents reported that their concern for others was influential in their end-of-life decisions, a finding suggesting that this decision-making process is integrally connected to human relationships. The practice of directing information toward the parents, and not necessarily toward the child, perhaps reflects a more widespread culture within pediatrics. Thus, pediatric specialists may need to acquire the communication skills necessary to discuss this medical and technical information with their patients themselves.[43]

SPIRITUAL SUPPORT FOR THE CHILD AND FAMILY

Patients and their families are especially concerned with spirituality in suffering, debilitation, and dying. In a critical care unit, parents identified prayer, faith, access to and care from clergy, and the belief in the transcendent parent-child relationship that endures beyond death as important elements of pediatric end-of-life care.[44] Many clinicians agree that the key to emotional coping with serious illness and disability is frequently found within spirituality. Spirituality gives us meaning and direction and brings order into our lives. Like adults, children ask questions about spiritual issues, search for a deeper understanding of their experiences, and express their emotions in response to their own interpretation of reality.[45] They are likely to base their spirituality on the relationship with their parents or other primary caregivers, a finding suggesting that spiritual care should be offered to the patient and the family.[46] Relief of suffering may occur with a renewed sense of meaning and a restored connectedness within the child's social network.[47] Children often interpret their world in a literal, concrete way and may not possess the cognitive sophistication at young ages to think abstractly about death or spirituality. Assisting children with their processing of life experiences may require simplified language, repetition of key concepts over time, or alternative methods of communicating (i.e., play, drawing).

Identifying a child's current level of cognitive and emotional development is important in an appropriate intervention for the spiritual care of the seriously ill child.[48] Spiritual interventions in the mainstream of medical therapy help children to articulate their questions, to express their emotions, and to search for creative answers that give a sense of order.[49] Inadequate staffing, inadequate training of health care providers to detect spiritual needs, and being called to visit with patients and families too late in the illness are barriers to effective spiritual care (see Table 196-1).[50]

REFERENCES

1. Wass H. Concepts of death: A developmental perspective. In Wass H (ed). Childhood and Death. Washington, DC: Hospice Foundation of America, 1995.
2. Rushforth H. Communicating with hospitalised children: Review and application of research pertaining to children's understanding of health and illness. J Child Psychol Psychiatry 1999;40:683-691.
3. Kalnins IV. The dying child: A new perspective. J Pediatr Psychol 1977;2:39-41.
4. Wolfe J, Grier HE, Klar N, et al. Symptoms and suffering at the end of life in children with cancer. N Engl J Med 2000;342:326-333.
5. Drake R, Frost J, Collins JJ. The symptoms of dying children. J Pain Symptom Manage 2003;26:594-603.
6. Children, adolescents, and death: Myths, realities, and challenges. A statement from the Work Group on Palliative Care for Children of the International Work Group on Death, Dying, and Bereavement. Death Stud 1999;23:443-463.
7. Lewis M, Schonfeld DJ. Role of child and adolescent psychiatric consultation and liaison in assisting children and their families in dealing with death. Child Adolesc Psychiatr Clin N Am 1994;3:613-627.
8. Steif BL, Heiligenstein EL. Psychiatric symptoms of pediatric cancer pain. J Pain Symptom Manage 1989;4:191-196.
9. World Health Organization. Cancer Pain Relief and Palliative Care in Children. Geneva: World Health Organization, 1998.
10. Carter BS, Howenstein M, Gilmer MJ, et al. Circumstances surrounding the deaths of hospitalized children: Opportunities for pediatric palliative care. Pediatrics 2004;114:e361-e366.
11. American Psychiatric Association. Diagnostic and Statistical Manual of Mental Disorders, 4th ed. Washington, DC: American Psychiatric Association, 2000.
12. Birmaher B, Ryan ND, Williamson DE, et al. Childhood and adolescent depression: A review of the past 10 years. Part I. J Am Acad Child Adolesc Psychiatry 1996;35:1427-1439.
13. Birmaher B, Ryan ND, Williamson DE, et al. Childhood and adolescent depression: A review of the past 10 years. Part II. J Am Acad Child Adolesc Psychiatry 1996;35:1575-1583.
14. Tadmor CS. Preventive intervention for children with cancer and their families at the end-of-life. J Prim Prev 2004;24:311-323.
15. Freyer DR. Care of the dying adolescent: Special considerations. Pediatrics 2004;113:381-388.
16. Koocher GP. Coping with a death from cancer. J Consult Clin Psychol 1986;54:623-631.
17. James L, Johnson B. The needs of parents of pediatric oncology patients during the palliative care phase. J Pediatr Oncol Nurs 1997;14:83-95.
18. Vickers JL, Carlisle C. Choices and control: Parental experiences in pediatric terminal home care. J Pediatr Oncol Nurs 2000;17:12-21.
19. Freeman K, O'Dell C, Meola C. Childhood brain tumors: Children's and siblings' concerns regarding the diagnosis and phase of illness. J Pediatr Oncol Nurs 2003;20:133-140.
20. Goldman A. ABC of palliative care: Special problems of children. BMJ 1998; 316:49-52.
21. Meyer EC, Ritholz MD, Burns JP, Truog RD. Improving the quality of end-of-life care in the pediatric intensive care unit: Parents' priorities and recommendations. Pediatrics 2006;117:649-657.
22. Meyer EC, Burns JP, Griffith JL, Truog RD. Parental perspectives on end-of-life care in the pediatric intensive care unit. Crit Care Med 2002;30:226-231.
23. Morgan ER, Murphy SB. Care of children who are dying of cancer. N Engl J Med 2000;342:347-348.
24. Lauer ME, Mulhern RK, Wallskog JM, Camitta BM. A comparison study of parental adaptation following a child's death at home or in the hospital. Pediatrics 1983;71:107-112.
25. Contro N, Larson J, Scofield S, et al. Family perspectives on the quality of pediatric palliative care. Arch Pediatr Adolesc Med 2002;156:14-19.
26. De Graves SD, Aranda S. Exploring documentation of end-of-life care of children with cancer. Int J Palliat Nurs 2002;8:435-443.
27. Masera G, Spinetta JJ, Jankovic M, et al. Guidelines for assistance to terminally ill children with cancer: A report of the SIOP Working Committee on psychosocial issues in pediatric oncology. Med Pediatr Oncol 1999;32:44-48.
28. Barlow JH, Ellard DR. Psycho-educational interventions for children with chronic disease, parents and siblings: An overview of the research evidence base. Child Care Health Dev 2004;30:637-645.
29. Kissane DW, Bloch S, Dowe DL, et al. The Melbourne Family Grief Study: I. Perceptions of family functioning in bereavement. Am J Psychiatry 1996; 153:650-658.
30. Hilden JM, Emanuel EJ, Fairclough DL, et al. Attitudes and practices among pediatric oncologists regarding end-of-life care: Results of the 1998 American Society of Clinical Oncology survey. J Clin Oncol 2001;19:205-212.
31. Wolfe J, Klar N, Grier HE, et al. Understanding of prognosis among parents of children who died of cancer: Impact on treatment goals and integration of palliative care. JAMA 2000;284:2469-2475.
32. American Academy of Pediatrics, Committee on Bioethics and Committee on Hospital Care. Palliative care for children. Pediatrics 2000;106:351-357.
33. Tadmor CS, Postovsky S, Elhasid R, et al. Policies designed to enhance the quality of life of children with cancer at the end-of-life. Pediatr Hematol Oncol 2003;20:43-54.
34. Nitschke R, Meyer WH, Sexauer CL, et al. Care of terminally ill children with cancer. Med Pediatr Oncol 2000;34:268-270.
35. Kreicbergs U, Valdimarsdottir U, Onelov E, et al. Talking about death with children who have severe malignant disease. N Engl J Med 2004;351: 1175-1186.
36. Sourkes BM. The broken heart: Anticipatory grief in the child facing death. J Palliat Care 1996;12:56-59.
37. Nitschke R, Wunder S, Sexauer CL. The final decision on research drugs in pediatric oncology. J Pediatr Psychol 1977;2:58-64.
38. Beale EA, Baile WF, Aaron J. Silence is not golden: Communicating with children dying from cancer. J Clin Oncol 2005;23:3629-3631.
39. Hayes RM, Valentine J, Haynes G, et al. The Seattle Pediatric Palliative Care Project: Effects on family satisfaction and health-related quality of life. J Palliat Med 2006;9:716-728.

40. Baker JN, Barfield R Hinds PM, Kane J. A model to facilitate decisions in pediatric stem cell transplantation: The Individualized Care Planning and Coordination model. Biol Blood Marrow Transplant 2007;13:245-244.
41. Nitschke R, Humphrey GB, Sexauer CL, et al. Therapeutic choices made by patients with end-stage cancer. J Pediatr 1982;101:471-476.
42. Hinds PS, Drew D, Oakes LL, et al. End-of-life care preferences of pediatric patients with cancer. J Clin Oncol 2005;23:9146-9154.
43. van Dulmen AM. Children's contributions to pediatric outpatient encounters. Pediatrics 1998;102:563-568.
44. Robinson MR, Thiel MM, Backus MM, Meyer EC. Matters of spirituality at the end of life in the pediatric intensive care unit. Pediatrics 2006;118:719-2298.
45. Sommer DR. Exploring the spirituality of children in the midst of illness and suffering. ACCH Advocate 1994;1:7-12.
46. Houskamp BM, Fisher LA, Stuber ML. Spirituality in children and adolescents: Research findings and implications for clinicians and researchers. Child Adolesc Psychiatr Clin N Am 2004;13:221-230.
47. Browning D. Fragments of love: Explorations in the ethnography of suffering and professional caregiving. In Berzoff J, Silverman PR (eds). Living with Dying. New York: Columbia University Press, 2004.
48. Heilferty CM. Spiritual development and the dying child: The pediatric nurse practitioner's role. J Pediatr Health Care 2004;18:271-275.
49. Stuber ML, Houskamp BM. Spirituality in children confronting death. Child Adolesc Psychiatr Clin N Am 2004;13:127-36, viii.
50. Feudtner C, Haney J, Dimmers MA. Spiritual care needs of hospitalized children and their families: A national survey of pastoral care providers' perceptions. Pediatrics 2003;111:e67-e72.

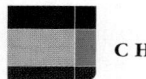

CHAPTER **197**

Family Adjustment and Support

Elaine C. Meyer and Rachel A. Tunick

KEY POINTS

- Families value honest and complete information, ready access to health care providers, and coordination of care.

- Family members can vary widely in their preferences for information, decision-making styles, and roles during a child's illness and dying process.

- Good communication and empathic relationships with health care providers are highly valued and can positively influence parental bereavement.

- Preservation and support of the parent-child relationship can foster positive bereavement adjustment, including opportunities for families to have private time, to review memories and initiate commemorative activities, and to "say goodbye" to their dying child according to their wishes.

- The social and emotional support available to families during the death and dying process and its aftermath is vitally important to coping efforts and bereavement adjustment, and it may include extended family members, friends, hospital and community health care providers, and religious personnel.

The death of a child is one of the most difficult and agonizing experiences a family can endure. The death inherently violates the expected natural order of life and has been described as "always out of season."[1] When life-threatening critical illness or traumatic injury occurs, parents who had been in charge of nearly every aspect of their child's health, education, and well-being find themselves thrust into chaos and helplessness with little preparation. Because of the circumstances, parents necessarily become dependent on hospital staff members, with whom they often have no prior relationship.[2]

Dying children and their families have special needs and considerations apart from those of adults.[1] Variable levels of cognitive and emotional development limit inferences that may be drawn about the dying child's wishes and place the burden of determining the patient's best interests principally on the parents. Families can have a staggering amount of information to assimilate and weighty health care decisions to consider.[3] To parents faced with end-of-life decision making, the most important factors are the child's quality of life, the expected neurological outcome and likelihood of improvement, the perception of pain and suffering, and the child's perceived wishes and will to live.[2,4,5] Nearly half of all parents report that they had independently considered withdrawal of life support treatment before any formal discussion with staff members.[2]

Families have identified several priorities for end-of-life care, including honest and complete information, ready access to staff, communication and coordination of care, emotional expression and support by staff, preservation of the integrity of the parent-child relationship, and faith.[6] Parents consistently emphasize that honest, complete information is vital to make some sense of seemingly incomprehensible events and to enable them to participate in decision making more fully. Practically, parents want and deserve a complete picture of relevant information, tailored to their individual needs and preferences. Most parents want to understand the "big picture" and to have a voice in their child's end-of-life care and decision making, rather than specific control over each treatment decision.[6,7] Because families vary, however, it is advisable to ask them directly about their preferences for receiving information and interacting with the team and then honor their choices.[2,6] Genuine emotional expression on the part of staff members and empathic relationships are highly valued and long remembered by families, especially given that staff members often find themselves intimately involved in what is likely one of the family's most trying, emotionally challenging times.[2,6,8,9] Caring emotional attitudes[10] by staff and a sympathetic hospital environment are associated with a healthy immediate and long-term parental bereavement outcome. Parents highly value staff efforts that preserve the integrity and sanctity of the parent-child relationship throughout the dying process and enable them to be the best parents they can be under the circumstances. Offering parents choices and support around participating in the child's care and comfort and ensuring privacy and intimate tenderness with their child are vitally important at the end of life, especially in the context of nonjudgment and nonabandonment.[6]

Parents and family members faced with their child's critical illness and death often struggle with deep existential angst and challenge.[11] It is not unusual for parents to anguish over unanswerable questions such as "Why our child?" and "Why our family?" as they grapple with and search to find meaning. The ability to resolve this search for meaning and the regaining of a sense of purpose in life are both critical to long-term bereavement adaptation.

Given the nature of the loss and the existential upheaval when a child dies, the grief of bereaved parents can be especially deep and long lasting.[1,11] The social support of family, friends, neighbors, school community, primary pediatricians, and religious support personnel are central to parents' immediate and long-term coping mechanisms.[2,10-12] Efforts should be made to identify, mobilize, and strengthen the social support network available to parents during and after the child's death.

Many families draw on their faith and spirituality to guide them in end-of-life decision making, to make meaning of the loss, and sustain them emotionally.[13,14] Despite the dominance of technology and medical discourse in the intensive care unit, many parents view their child's end of life as a spiritual journey. Staff members and chaplains are encouraged to be explicit in their hospitality to families' spirituality and religious faith, to foster a culture of acceptance and integration of spiritual perspectives, and to work collaboratively to deliver meaningful spiritual care.[13]

EPIDEMIOLOGY AND PREVALENCE

Each year, approximately 55,000 children die in the United States, just over half within the first year of life.[1] Childhood deaths account for less than 3% of total deaths annually in the United States. Beyond infancy, the most common causes are unintentional injuries, congenital anomalies, malignant neoplasms, and intentional injuries.[1,15,16] Most pediatric end-of-life care and deaths occur in acute care hospitals, typically intensive care.[17-19] Two thirds of deaths in the pediatric intensive care unit follow withdrawal of life-sustaining treatment, and removal of mechanical ventilation is the most proximate cause of death.[19]

The families of children receiving end-of-life care can present with a wide range of pragmatic, psychological, social, and spiritual needs and concerns. Broad-based assessment of the family's needs and goals is important, to support both the patient and the family most effectively through the end-of-life process and to promote optimal coping and adjustment for family members. "Case Study: Family Adjustment to the Impending Death of a Child" illustrates some of the themes that often characterize the experiences of families of children at the end of life.

CLINICAL MANIFESTATIONS

Parents who must endure the critical illness and impending death of a child have identified a range of psychosocial needs, including optimized pain control and symptom management for the child, access to medical information, and the ability to communicate freely about their own fears and feelings.[20] Individual members may manifest their particular needs and respond to end-of-life situations with similar or different emotional responses and coping styles. Siblings present with a range of emotional responses and psychosocial needs, too.

In the case study cited earlier, for example, Mrs. Richards was often tearful and was tremendously concerned that her daughter not be in pain or suffer, and she frequently asked about the effectiveness of the current pain management regimen. Mrs. Richards often lay in the bed beside her daughter and prayed in the company of other

CASE STUDY

Family Adjustment to the Impending Death of a Child

Jennifer Richards is a 16-year-old high-school sophomore who was an avid cheerleader and tennis player. A previously healthy and typically developing teenager, she was admitted to the pediatric intensive care unit (PICU) in critical condition following a motor vehicle accident; Jennifer had been the restrained front-seat passenger of a car driven by her newly licensed classmate. Jennifer was found with agonal breathing at the scene of the accident, where she was resuscitated, intubated, and transferred to the PICU at a regional children's hospital. On admission, Jennifer presented with extensive traumatic injuries including diffuse cerebral edema, pulmonary contusions, and multiple orthopedic fractures. Neurosurgical examination suggested that Jennifer's injury was not survivable, and it was likely that she would progress to brain death within the coming hours or days.

PICU staff members consulted with the unit social worker and psychologist regarding psychosocial support for Jennifer's family, which included her parents and siblings (18-year-old brother and 10-year-old sister) and several extended family members. Jennifer's parents had had multiple conversations with the staff to discuss the gravity of the situation and the grim prognosis. Family members presented as visibly distraught and overwhelmed by the suddenness and emotional intensity surrounding Jennifer's tragic accident.

family members and her parish priest; this approach seemed to provide her some solace. Meanwhile, Mr. Richards focused intently on the fluctuating monitor with Jennifer's vital signs, listened in on rounds, spoke at length with staff about the details of his daughter's medical treatment, and searched the Internet for information about traumatic brain injury. He had many questions regarding Jennifer's intracranial pressure and possible neurosurgical options. Jennifer's younger sister had been brought to the bedside briefly by her parents, but she preferred to remain in the family room to make drawings and cards for her sister under the watchful eye of extended family members. The sister seemed to be closely following the day's events by observing the emotional reactions of her relatives. Jennifer's older brother sat for some time in the family waiting room, but then asked his parents for their permission to leave the hospital to be with his girlfriend.

DIFFERENTIAL DIAGNOSES

When working with families of dying children, a broad-based assessment should be conducted to understand better the perspectives, needs, and goals of each particular family member. Approaching this issue from a systems perspective may offer valuable insights regarding the impact of the patient's experiences across the immediate and extended family that may also help to inform interventions. Within the family, historical and contextual factors to consider include individual coping style (e.g., emotion-based versus cognitive-based); information processing style; past experience with terminal illness, trauma, and loss; cultural considerations; religious preference and membership in faith community; and preexisting psychopathology. Developmental factors (e.g., age of the patient, developmental level of the siblings), the nature of the illness (e.g., chronic illness versus sudden onset), and family constellation factors (e.g., marital status, extent of involvement of extended family members) are further considerations in assessment.

Concerns about siblings are common reasons for referrals for psychosocial services in the PICU, and parents often have questions regarding sibling visitation, assistance in how to talk with siblings, and developmentally appropriate reading material.[21] Siblings of dying children, like their parents, have various emotional responses and psychosocial needs. In addition, developmental considerations, including cognitive development and its relation to children's understanding and interpretations around illness and death, are important. Preschool-aged children are prone to magical thinking and associative logic, and they may infer erroneous causal relationships around their own behaviors and their sibling's condition. Children, like adults, vary in coping styles; they may seek information, feel most comfortable when they are involved in some aspect of their sibling's care, or exhibit an avoidant coping style and prefer to be at home or with other relatives, rather than at the bedside. Temperamental and emotional factors may influence a child's experiences during this unique time and are useful for the clinician who works with the family to appreciate. Adult attention typically focuses on the sick child in these situations, and siblings may experience emotional reactions, such as jealousy, anger, and feelings of abandonment.[22]

TREATMENT

Ideally, interventions with families of dying children should be individualized based on the assessment. When planning care, families should be asked what is important to them now, and how the team may be most helpful, before setting about to address and honor the family's requests. Families need to know that what matters most to them at the end of their child's life matters to the team, and, to the greatest extent possible, the family's wishes and preferences will be honored. Perhaps most important are genuine humanness, empathy for the family, and steadfast commitment to ensure the child and family's dignity throughout the death and dying process.[6,9] Being a good listener,[23] bearing witness to the family's love for their child, making efforts to understand the child as a person, not simply a patient,[24] being flexible, and being willing to be helpful are invaluable qualities. Not only are these qualities and interventions appreciated by family members, but also such efforts, including provision of bereavement literature and proactive communication strategies, reduce symptom severity in family members, including post-traumatic stress disorder, anxiety, and depression.[25]

Many creative and meaningful supportive interventions are possible with the dying, such as offering special time together in a rocking chair, making commemorative handprints, sharing poems and books that may be helpful, having joint conversations with the health care team, discussing organ donation, where appropriate, together with organ bank personnel, mobilizing and strengthening the family's social support network, and making plans for funeral and memorial services.[26] During this time, families highly value and long remember gestures of kindness and care by staff members toward their beloved child and themselves.[2,27] Staff attendance at funerals and commemorative events is especially meaningful to parents.[27] Additional follow-up support, including sympathy cards from hospital staff involved in the dying child's care, supportive phone calls, and organized hospital-wide memorial services, may also be meaningful for bereaved families.

When withdrawal of life support is involved, families need anticipatory guidance and support. Families should be helped to establish when the withdrawal should occur and to plan who should be present, with guidance about what to expect (how the child will look, expectations for how long the child may breathe, addressing any specific questions the family may have). The family should be offered the opportunity to have private time with the child, if they wish, and if possible, staff should be available to escort the family from the hospital and make arrangements for safe travel home. The family may need help to anticipate the arrival home, and this may be eased, or not, by the presence of other family members or friends.

In the foregoing case example, Mrs. Richards may benefit from access to the pain treatment service, education, and reassurance to allay her worries that Jennifer's pain management and comfort are priorities of care. Fresh sheets and a blanket from home may make the bed more comfortable and inviting when she lies beside Jennifer. The presence and inclusion of the hospital chaplain and the family's own faith community representative, and perhaps a bedside religious service, may be appreciated and meaningful, given the solace that faith has offered to Jennifer's mother. Mr. Richards especially values accurate information, access to health care providers, and inclusion in decision making. Efforts to ensure these aspects of care may serve him well. Perhaps he may find some value in knowing that an autopsy may be conducted and that the opportunity for further follow-up will be available. These options can be discussed with the family. Given Jennifer's age and circumstances, the family may wish to invite some of her special friends or her long-time tennis coach to the bedside, depending on what they imagine Jennifer would wish. Siblings need to feel welcome and well cared for, too. Jennifer's younger sister, who loves to draw, may be offered the services and kindness of a child life specialist, who can provide art materials, age-appropriate developmental play and preparation, and children's literature. Her older brother may wish for the opportunity to participate in a family meeting to understand the circumstances better, and he may want some time with Jennifer, alone or in the company of his girlfriend or family, depending on his preference.

Taking steps such as these during the death and dying process and its aftermath, aimed at honoring preferences of families and individualizing interventions for family members in the context of a supportive, empathic, and honest relationship, may be highly valued. This approach may also optimize coping efforts and bereavement adjustment in family members long after the child's death.

Drugs of Choice

Sleep disturbances, incapacitating anxiety, and psychomotor agitation are not uncommon in family members of

Common Therapeutic Approaches

- Staff members should introduce themselves (name, role, responsibility), welcome family members, and inquire about family's preferences for how they would like to be addressed (first name or surname).
- Assess family preferences for ongoing communication (family meetings, participation on rounds, bedside consultations, telephone conversations). Promote optimal communication between family and staff members, including regular opportunities to share information, discuss treatment options, reflect on care, and approach decision making. Invite ongoing community providers (pediatrician, teacher, religious personnel) to participate in care as the family wishes.
- Reassure families that the relief of pain is a priority of the child's care and provide education about the way that pain will be assessed, monitored, and treated. Encourage family members to speak up if at any time they believe the child is in pain or is suffering.
- Provide the family access to and supportive intervention from psychosocial support and pastoral care staff members, who are integral, valued members of the team.
- Offer a variety of means to provide supportive care to families including orientation opportunities, assistance with meals, parking, and transportation, individual and family meetings, lactation support, medical language interpretation, parent and sibling groups, and parent-to-parent networking opportunities.
- Offer early referral to palliative care team and community bereavement or hospice resources to promote hospital-community continuity and to establish bridges to support families during and following the child's death.
- Invite and welcome community providers to participate in hospital-based care.
- Encourage and support staff acts of kindness and commemoration during the bereavement period.

Future Considerations

- Parental participation during rounds
- Parental presence during the child's invasive procedures and resuscitation
- Liberalization of means to enhance family-staff communication, including family meetings, journals, e-mail, and "office hours at the bedside"
- Parent advisory councils to participate in unit and hospital policy making
- Expanded interdisciplinary participation to meet the support needs of children and their families, including medicine, nursing, social work, psychology, speech and language, child life, pastoral care, alternative medicine, and parent advocacy
- Ongoing evaluation of parent perspectives and priorities to guide and improve clinical practice
- Unit-based and hospital-wide resource centers that include lending library, Internet access, patient web sites, public transportation information, local accommodation and restaurant information, relaxation and alternative medicine resources, sibling and parent social events, and hospital community bulletin board
- Early referral and integration of palliative care services during intensive care hospitalization, including in-hospital comfort care room facilities
- Partnerships between hospital-based palliative care services and community hospice programs to expand and improve services to dying children and their families, including the capacity for in-home withdrawal of life support according to the family's wishes
- Release from work duties and compensation for staff members to attend funerals and memorial services

children receiving end-of-life care. At their request, or when such symptoms interfere with their capacity to function effectively in this highly stressful and emotionally charged situation, family members can be encouraged to consult with their primary care physician regarding the advisability of psychotropic medication to address acute symptoms. In particular, antianxiety medications such as benzodiazepines may be effective in the short term.

REFERENCES

1. Field MJ, Behrman RE (eds), for the Institute of Medicine Committee on Palliative and End-of-Life Care for Children and Their Families. When Children Die: Improving Palliative and End-of-Life Care for Children and Their Families. Washington, DC: National Academies Press, 2003.
2. Meyer EC, Burns JP, Griffith JL, Truog RD. Parental perspectives on end-of-life care in the pediatric intensive care unit. Crit Care Med 2002; 30:226-231.
3. Kirchhoff KT, Walker L, Hutton A, et al. The vortex: Families' experiences with death in the intensive care unit. Am J Crit Care 2002;11:200-209.
4. Meert KL, Thurston MA, Sarnaik AP. End-of-life decision-making and satisfaction with care: Parental perspectives. Pediatr Crit Care Med 2000;1: 179-185.
5. Kirschbaum MS. Life support decisions for children: What do parents value? ANS Adv Nurs Sci 1996;19:51-71.
6. Meyer EC, Ritholz MD, Burns JP, Truog RD. Improving the quality of end-of-life care in the pediatric intensive care unit: Parents' priorities and recommendations. Pediatrics 2006;117:649-657.
7. Meyer EC, DeMaso DR, Koocher GP. Mental health consultation in the pediatric intensive care unit. Prof Psychol Res Pr 1996;27:130-136.
8. Contro N, Larson J, Scofield S, et al. Family perspectives on the quality of pediatric palliative care. Arch Pediatr Adolesc Med 2002;156:14-19.
9. Finlay I, Dallimore D. Your child is dead. BMJ 1991;302:1524-1525.
10. Meert KL, Thurston CS, Thomas R. Parental coping and bereavement outcome after the death of a child in the pediatric intensive care unit. Pediatr Crit Care Med 2001;2:324-328.
11. Rando TA. Parental loss of a child. Champaign, IL: Research Press, 1986.
12. Wolfelt A. Healing a Parent's Grieving Heart. Fort Collins, CO: Companion Press, 2002.
13. Robinson MR, Thiel MM, Backus MR, Meyer EC. Matters of spirituality at the end of life in the pediatric intensive care unit. Pediatrics 2006;118: e719-e729.
14. Meert KL, Thurston CS, Briller SH. The spiritual needs of parents at the time of their child's death in the pediatric intensive care unit and during bereavement: A qualitative study. Pediatr Crit Care Med 2005;6:420-427.
15. Guyer B, Hoyert DL, Martin JA, et al. Annual survey of vital statistics: 1998. Pediatrics 1999;104:1229-1246.
16. Feudtner C, Christakis DA, Zimmerman FJ, et al. Characteristics of deaths occurring in children's hospitals: Implications for supportive care services. Pediatrics 2002;109:887-893.
17. Crain N, Dalton H, Slonin A. End of life care for children: Bridging the gaps. Crit Care Med 2001;29:695-696.
18. McCallum DE, Byrne P, Bruera E. How children die in hospital. J Pain Symptom Manage 2000;20:417-423.
19. Burns JP, Mitchell C, Outwater KM, et al. End-of-life care in the pediatric intensive care unit after forgoing of life-sustaining treatment. Crit Care Med 2000;28:3060-3066.
20. Jones BL. Companionship, control, and compassion: A social work perspective on the needs of children with cancer and their families at the end of life. J Palliat Med 2006;9:774-788.
21. Williams J, Koocher GP. Medical crisis counseling on a pediatric intensive care unit: Case examples and clinical utility. J Clin Psychol Med Settings 1999;6: 249-258.
22. Himelstein BP. Palliative care for infants, children, adolescents, and their families. J Palliat Med 2006;9:163-181.
23. McDonagh JR, Elliott TB, Engelberg RA, et al. Family satisfaction with family conferences about end-of-life care in the intensive care unit: Increased proportion of family speech is associated with increased satisfaction. Crit Care Med 2004;32:1484-1488.
24. Curtis JR, Patrick DL, Shannon SE, et al. The family conference as a focus to improve communication about end-of-life care in the intensive care unit: Opportunities for improvement. Crit Care Med 2001;29(Suppl 2):N26-N33.
25. Lautrette A, Darmon M, Megarbane B, et al. A communication strategy and brochure for relatives of patients dying in the ICU. N Engl J Med 2007;356: 469-478.
26. Truog RD, Christ G, Browning D, Meyer EC. Sudden traumatic death in children: We did everything, but your child did not survive. JAMA 2006;295; 2646-2654.
27. Macdonald ME, Liben S, Carnevale FA, et al. Parental perspectives on hospital staff members' acts of kindness and commemoration after a child's death. Pediatrics 2005;116:884-890.

ADDITIONAL RESOURCES

Association for Children's Palliative Care (ACT) is a charity organization that aims to achieve the highest possible quality of life and care for children with life-threatening or life-limiting conditions and their families. Available at http://www.act.org.uk (accessed February 2008).

Compassionate Friends is a nonprofit support organization for bereaved families and friends following the death of a child. Their web site provides an extensive list of suggested readings. Available at http://www.compassionatefriends.com (accessed February 2008).

Initiative for Pediatric Palliative Care provides educational resources for pediatric health care providers, with aims to enhance family-centered care for children with life-threatening conditions. Available at http://www.ippcweb.org (accessed February 2008).

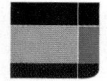 CHAPTER **198**

Pediatric Pain and Symptom Control

Christina Ullrich and Joanne Wolfe

> **KEY POINTS**
>
> - Children with life-threatening conditions frequently experience uncontrolled symptoms that can cause significant distress and may interfere with the goals of palliative care.
>
> - Symptoms should be continuously assessed, and uncontrolled symptoms should be managed intensively.
>
> - Successful symptom management relies on understanding the pathophysiology and establishing a complete differential diagnosis for the symptom.
>
> - Persistent symptoms should prompt a repeat review of the differential diagnosis.
>
> - Physical, spiritual, emotional, and existential suffering are often interrelated and should all be addressed for effective relief.

Most children with life-threatening illnesses suffer from treatable symptoms. The prevalence of unrelieved pain in children at the end of life is high (Table 198-1).[1-5] Other symptoms also cause considerable distress. A cross-sectional study of 160 children with cancer who were 10 to 18 years old found that these patients experienced multiple symptoms that caused significant physical and psychological distress.[1] Inpatients surveyed had a mean of 12.7 symptoms, and outpatients had a mean of 6.5 symptoms; the most common were lack of energy (50%), pain (48%), drowsiness (49%), nausea (45%), and cough (41%). Eighty-nine percent of children suffered "a lot" or "a great deal" from at least one symptom, and symptoms were successfully treated less than 30% of the time (Fig. 198-1).[2]

The effect of unrelieved symptoms extends beyond the mere comfort of a child with a life-threatening illness. Besides causing physical and psychological suffering, such symptoms can interfere with many palliative care goals such as attending to emotional and spiritual needs and growth and closure at the end of life. Finally, the child's illness experience will remain with the family, and memories of poorly controlled symptoms and the resulting suffering may continue to affect the family long after the child has died.[2] Meticulous symptom management is a cornerstone of effective pediatric palliative care.

SPECIAL ISSUES IN PEDIATRIC PALLIATIVE CARE

The nature of childhood death, along with its relative rarity, poses several challenges.[3] The network of care is often complex and fragmented. Other particular features are the inherent developmental differences among infants, children, and adolescents and the range of developmental capacities within each age group. Finally, death occurring during childhood runs counter to the natural order that is expected in life events. Because the death of a child seems unnatural, it may be difficult for families or care providers to focus on priorities outside of life extension for the child.[4] In the current culture of care that regards palliative care and life-extending care as mutually exclusive, the pursuit of life extension may come at the cost of optimal attention to "competing" goals such as comfort.[5]

APPROACH TO PEDIATRIC PALLIATIVE CARE

Although distinctions may be made between pediatric and adult palliative care, the basic tenets underlying symptom management are largely the same. An understanding of the goals of care is key to appropriate diagnostic and therapeutic interventions for symptoms. Active, frequent, and developmentally appropriate assessment is needed, even if the child cannot self-report because of age or developmental capacity. Once a symptom is recognized, a complete differential diagnosis should be generated, including psychological, spiritual, and existential issues that may influence the experience and expression of symptoms. Moreover, preexisting conditions (e.g., migraines or conditions not related to the life-threatening illness) can also cause symptoms. Symptoms should be targeted based on the suspected cause and the established goals of care. Uncontrolled symptoms should be treated intensively, and escalating symptoms should be considered emergencies that require immediate intervention. Once treatment is initiated, the symptom should be reassessed, and the response should be documented. Persistent symptoms should prompt a return to the differential diagnosis and possible treatment strategies.

Anticipation of symptoms that may develop in the future is also an essential feature of meticulous care. Preparedness with a plan in place and interventions at the ready can prevent troublesome symptoms from occurring or, at a minimum, escalating. Discussion with families about what symptoms to expect and how they can be addressed may provide some reassurance and a greater sense of control. Such discussions may also provide families with an opportunity to anticipate situations and decisions that may lie ahead.[6]

TABLE 198-1   Summary of Descriptive Findings Related to Unrelieved Pain and Distress in Children

REFERENCE	COUNTRY OF ORIGIN	METHODS	PROPORTION WITH PAIN AND DISTRESS BEFORE DEATH	PROPORTION OF CHILDREN WHO RECEIVED TREATMENT FOR PAIN AND DISTRESS
Drake et al., 2003[12]	Australia	Chart review and nurse interview of children who died in hospital (N = 30)	53% with pain in last week of life	NA
McCallum et al., 2000[13]	Canada	Chart review of children who died in hospital, excluding unanticipated deaths (N = 77)	65%	84% (opioids)
Sirkia et al., 1998[14]	Finland	Chart review and parent interview of children who died of cancer (N = 70)	NA	89% (NSAIDs or opioids)
Friedrichsdorf et al., 2005[15]	Germany	Provider survey of all pediatric cancer departments (N = 71)	NA	NA
Hongo et al., 2003[16]	Japan	Chart review of children who had died of cancer at a single institution	75% with pain documented in the chart	NA
Theunissen et al., 2007[17]	Netherlands	Parent survey of children who died of cancer (N = 32)	75% of parents reported that child experienced pain	25% had no improvement in pain despite treatment
Dangel, 2002[18]	Poland	Retrospective review of national databases regarding children who died with life-limiting conditions (N = 14,243)	NA	NA
Dangel, 2002[18]	Poland	Retrospective review of first cohort of children cared for by the Warsaw Hospice for Children (N = 134)	84%	NA
Henley, 2002[19]	South Africa	Chart review of inpatient deaths in children with HIV infection (N = 165)	55%	50% (paracetamol or morphine)
Jalmsell et al., 2006[2]	Sweden	Parent survey of children who died of cancer (N = 449)	45% of children with pain that could not be relieved	NA
Goldman et al, 2006[20]	United Kingdom	Survey of children with progressive cancer (N = 185)	In the last month of life, 65% with pain reported to be a "major problem," and 92% with pain	NA
Wolfe et al., 2000[5]	United States	Chart review and parent interview of children who died of cancer (N = 103)	89% with significant distress from at least one symptom in last month of life	76% treated for pain
Carter et al., 2004[21]	United States	Chart review of children who were hospitalized a minimum of 24 hr before death and died in the hospital (N = 105)	34% with physician-documented pain assessment and management in last 72 hr	90% received pain medication in the last 72 hr of life
Contro et al., 2004[22]	United States	Staff survey (N = 446) Family members of children who died (N = 68)	70% of family members reported that child experienced pain	66% of family members reported that pain was managed adequately or well

NA, not applicable; NSAIDs, nonsteroidal anti-inflammatory drugs.

CLINICAL ASSESSMENT OF SYMPTOMS

Many children 3 years of age or older are able to self-report their symptoms. Given the subjective and multidimensional nature of symptoms, self-report or parental report is the gold standard in pain assessment when it can be obtained. The responses of even young children should be heeded because some young children, particularly those who are chronically ill, may be more mature than their chronological age. Physical and behavioral signs and symptoms may also suggest discomfort, but a lack of signs does not indicate an absence of discomfort, particularly in chronically or very ill children, in whom these indicators are unreliable. Furthermore, these signs are not specific for pain and may reflect other types of distress.

Symptom assessment tools (Table 198-2) may be helpful in assessing symptoms and in measuring severity before and after interventions, but they are not validated specifically for palliative care. Another caveat to these instruments is that clinicians may underestimate a child's pain compared with the child's self-report.[7,8] A given tool (Fig. 198-2) should be used consistently with a particular child. A positive symptom should always prompt further inquiry regarding its nature (e.g., character of pain, aggravating and alleviating factors) and the meaning that the symptom holds for the child and the family. Assessment scales for nausea or vomiting, constipation, and fatigue in children with cancer, and for dyspnea in children with respiratory illnesses, and depression and delirium scales have been validated and described; however, these scales have not been widely adopted.

MANAGEMENT OF SYMPTOMS

Pain

The basic pharmacological principles guiding choice of medication, dosing, route, titration, and management of side effects in adults also apply to children. Three important differences are as follows: (1) doses in children are

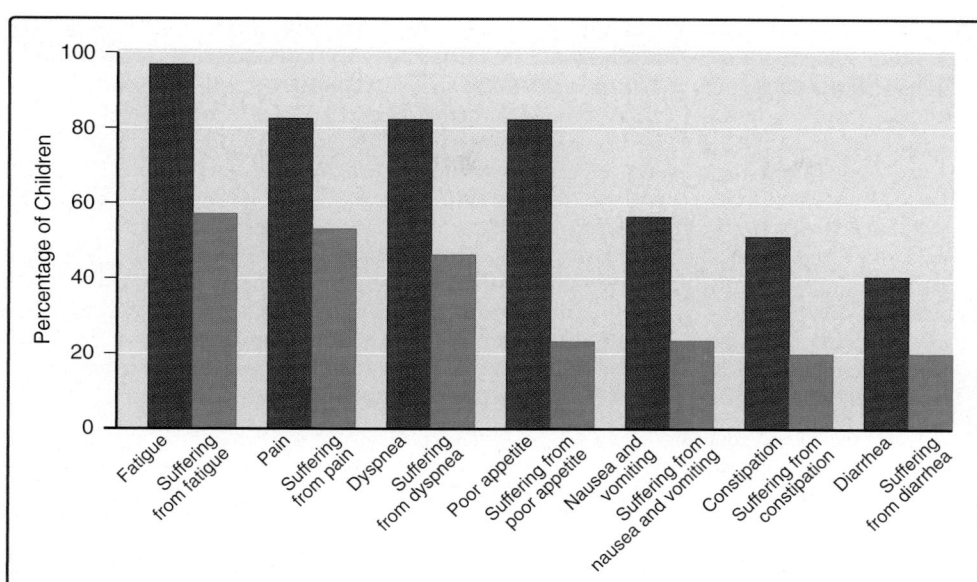

FIGURE 198-1 Symptoms, suffering, and treatment of symptoms in children with cancer at the end of life. **A**, The percentages of children who, according to parental report, experienced suffering as a result of a specific symptom. **B**, The percentages of children who, according to parental report, had "successful" treatment for a specific symptom. *(From Jalmsell L, Kreicbergs U, Onelov E, et al. Symptoms affecting children with malignancies during the last month of life: A nationwide follow-up. Pediatrics 2006;117:1314-1320.)*

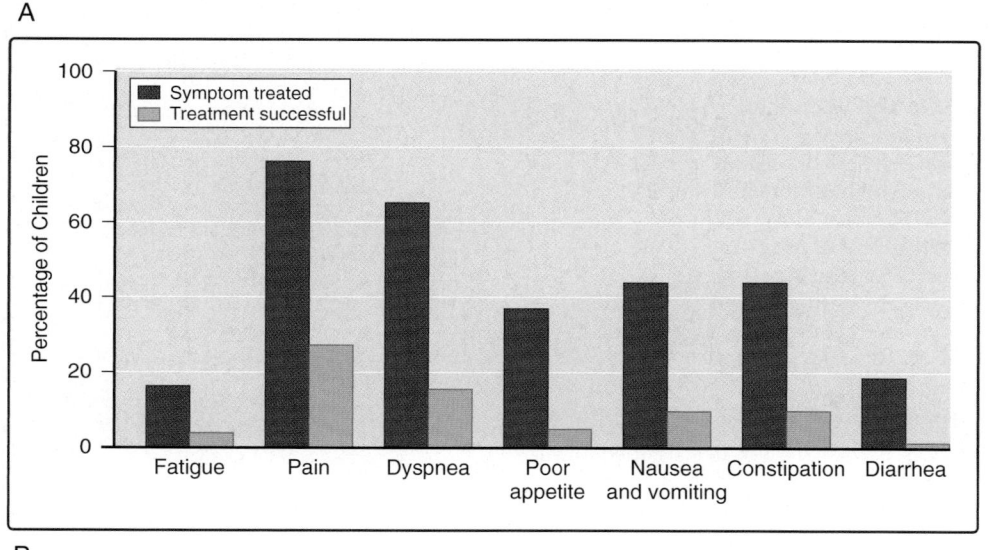

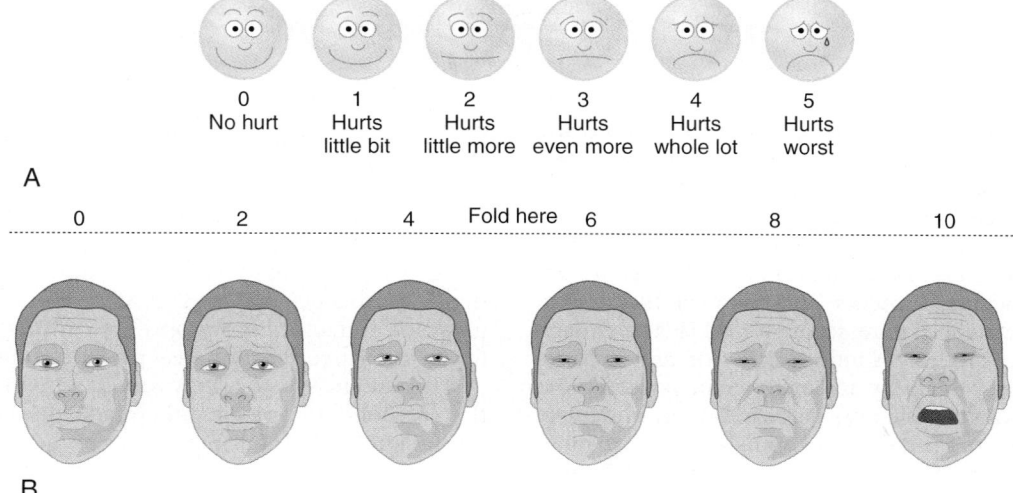

FIGURE 198-2 Faces scales. **A**, The Wong-Baker Faces Pain Rating Scale. Instructions for use in multiple languages are available at http://www.mosbysdrug-consult.com/WOW. **B**, Face Pain Scale-Revised. Instructions for use in multiple languages are available at http://painsourcebook.ca/docs/pps92.html. *(A, From Donna L, Wong D, Hockenberry-Eaton M, et al. [eds]. Wong's Essentials of Pediatric Nursing, 6th ed. St. Louis: Mosby, 2001; B, from Bieri D, Reeve R, Champion G, et al. The Faces Pain Scale for the self-assessment of the severity of pain experienced by children: Development, initial validation, and preliminary investigation for ratio scale properties. Pain 1990;41:139-150.)*

TABLE 198-2   Symptom Assessment Tools for Children

NAME AND REFERENCE	POPULATION	INDICATORS	SYMPTOM	COMMENTS
CRIES scale[23]	Full-term neonates	Based on behavioral (cry, expression, sleeplessness) and physiological (heart rate, blood pressure, need for oxygen) indicators	Pain	Designed to measure postoperative pain in neonates
FLACC[24]	Children 2 mo-7 yr old	Behavioral (face, legs, activity, crying, consolability)	Pain	Designed to score postoperative pain in children; also validated for postoperative use in children with cognitive impairment[25]
CHEOPS scale[26]	Nonverbal, regressed or cognitively impaired children	Behaviors (cry, facial expression, verbalization, torso movement, whether child touches affected site, and leg position)	Pain	Developed for postoperative pain in children
DEGR(R) scale[27]	Nonverbal, regressed cognitively impaired, 2-6 yr old	Behaviors indicating pain, anxiety	Pain	Developed to measure pain in young children with cancer and chronic pain; also used in adults with delirium or dementia
Paediatric Pain Profile[28]	Nonverbal children with severe neurological impairment	20-item behavior rating scale	Pain	Created to be a usable document for parents to assess and record their child's pain behavior
Individualized Numeric Rating Scale (INRS)[29]	Nonverbal children with neurological impairment	0-10 rating scale	Pain	Individualized markers of severity devised by parents specifically for their child
Hester's Poker Chips[30]	Verbal children ≥4 yr old	Child uses four poker chips to represent "pieces of hurt"	Pain	Any four objects of uniform appearance can be used
Wong-Baker Faces Pain Scale[31,34]	Verbal children ≥4 yr old	Limited number of faces representing degree of pain	Pain	Widely used, although faces with severe pain are crying, thus potentially confusing physical pain experienced with affective component of experience
Bieri Faces Scale[32]	Verbal children ≥4 yr old	Series of faces representing degree of pain	Pain	Other face scales exist, such as Oucher Scale (which has different ethnic versions) are available
Color Analogue Scale[26]	Verbal children ≥5 yr old	Increasing color intensity (pink to red) indicating increasing pain intensity	Pain	Developed for healthy children with recurrent headache; card has range of colors on one side and corresponding numerical equivalents on the other
Visual analogue scale[33]	Verbal children ≥7 yr old	10-cm line with ends anchored at "no pain" and "worst possible pain"	Pain	
0-10 numeric scale	Verbal children ≥7 yr old	Likert scale	Pain	Can modify range to 1-5
Memorial Symptom Assessment Scale[1,31]	Two scales available for verbal children: ages 7-12 yr and 10-18 yr	Enables children to rate severity and frequency of symptoms as well as degree of distress	Multiple symptoms	Developed for children with cancer; most children are able to complete in short time

calculated by weight in kilograms, (2) initial opioid dosing for infants *less than or equal to* 6 months of age is 25% to 33% of the usual mg/kg dose used for older children because of decreased liver and kidney function in clearing opioids, and (3) nonsteroidal anti-inflammatory drugs should be avoided in children less than 6 months of age.

Pharmacological treatments for pain (Table 198-3) should be instituted according to the World Health Organization Analgesic Ladder.[9] Administration of oral medications may require creativity to make them palatable for children. For example, mixing medications in chocolate syrup or ice cream can be useful, but it is important to ensure that the vehicle does not interact with the medication. Alternatively, medications may be given parenterally, rectally, transdermally, or transmucosally. Patient-controlled analgesia (PCA) may be used safely and effectively in children older than 6 years. In younger children, nurse-

controlled analgesia (NCA) may be used. In general, parents should not control the PCA device except in a few rare circumstances. Some children, such as those dying of cancer, may experience pain that is not well controlled even with massive doses of opioids or at the cost of sedation. In this situation, switching to an alternate opioid or regional anesthetic approaches may be considered.[10] In other situations in which refractory symptoms are causing unrelieved suffering, palliative sedation may provide comfort.[11]

The patient's history may reveal particular types of pain that respond to specific pharmacological interventions. For example, children may describe neuropathic pain as "burning" or "stabbing." Neuropathic pain is classically refractory to opioids, except for methadone, which may relieve neuropathic pain by N-methyl-D-aspartate receptor binding. Newer agents such as gabapentin (available as a liquid), pregabalin, and topical treatments such as

TABLE 198-3 Annotated Table of Medications Useful in Pediatrics

SYMPTOM	MEDICATION	STARTING DOSE	COMMENTS
Pain: mild	Acetaminophen	15 mg/kg PO q4h, max 4 g/day or 75 mg/kg/day, whichever is smaller	Available PO (including liquid), PR
	Ibuprofen	10 mg/kg PO q6h	PO (including liquid) only; avoid if risk of bleeding; use only in infants ≥6 mo; use with caution in congestive heart failure; chewable tablets contain phenylalanine
	Trilisate	10-15 mg/kg PO tid	
Pain: moderate	Codeine	0.5-1 mg/kg/dose PO q4 to max of 60 mg/dose	15-40% of children are unable to convert codeine to active form; not given IV because of significant histamine release*†
Pain: severe	Morphine, immediate-release	0.3 mg/kg PO q4h if <50 kg; 5-10 mg PO q4h	Infants <6 mo should receive 25-30% of starting dose*†
	Oxycodone	0.1 mg/kg PO q4h if <50 kg; 5-10 mg PO q4h if >50 kg	No injectable formulation*†
	Hydromorphone	0.05 mg/kg PO q4h if <50 kg; 1-2 mg PO q4h if >50 kg	Injectable form very concentrated, allowing for subcutaneous delivery*†
	Fentanyl	0.5-1.5 µg/kg IV q30min	Rapid infusion may cause chest wall rigidity*†
	Methadone	Starting dose 0.1 mg/kg PO/IV bid; recommend consultation with experienced clinician for equivalence dosing from other opioids	Only opioid with prolonged effect available as a liquid; do not adjust dose more often than q72h because prolonged biological half-life is longer than therapeutic half-life; knowledge of the pharmacokinetics of methadone is needed for converting to and from doses of other opioids; may cause QT interval prolongation, especially in adults on >200 mg/day or in those at risk for QT prolongation; interacts with several antiretrovirals†
Pain: sustained-release opioid formulations	MS Contin, Kadian (contains sustained-release pellets), Avinza (contains immediate- and extended-release beads), Oramorph	Total daily dose of MSIR divided bid	Do not crush MS Contin
	OxyContin (oxycodone)	Total daily dose of oxycodone divided bid	Do not crush†
	Duragesic (transdermal fentanyl) patch	Divide 24 hour PO morphine dose by 2 to determine starting dose of transdermal fentanyl	Smallest patch size may be too high for small children; for children >2 yr; apply to upper back in young children; patch may not be cut; typically for patients on 60 mg morphine/day or its equivalent; not appropriate when dosage changes are frequent or for opioid-naïve patients; fever >40° C causes higher serum concentrations†
Pain: neuropathic	Nortriptyline	0.5 mg/kg PO at bedtime to maximum of 150 mg/day	Fewer anticholinergic side effects than amitriptyline; may cause constipation, postural hypotension, dry mouth
	Gabapentin	Start at 5 mg/kg/day daily and gradually increase to 10-15 mg/kg/day divided tid; titrate as needed but not to exceed 2,400 mg/day	May cause neuropsychiatric events in children (aggression, emotional lability, hyperkinesia), usually mild but may require discontinuation of gabapentin; may cause dizziness or drowsiness
	Methadone	See earlier	See earlier
Dyspnea	Morphine sulfate immediate-release (MSIR)	0.1 mg/kg PO q4h PRN	†Morphine dose for dyspnea is 25-30% of morphine dose for pain
	Lorazepam	0.025 mg/kg PO/IV up to 2 mg q6h PRN	Titrate by 20-30%; may be given sublingually; avoid use in neonates
Respiratory secretions	Scopolamine patch	1.5-mg patch, change q72h	Excessive drying of secretions can cause mucus plugging of airways; good for motion-induced nausea and vomiting; handling patch and contacting eye may cause anisocoria and blurry vision; may fold patches but do not cut them
	Glycopyrrolate	0.04-0.1 mg/kg PO q4-8h	Excessive drying of secretions can cause mucus plugging of airways; anticholinergic side effects possible
	Hyoscyamine sulfate	4 gtt PO q4h PRN if <2 yr; 8 gtt PO q4h PRN if 2-12 yr; do not exceed 24 gtt/24 hr	Anticholinergic side effects including constipation, urinary retention, blurry vision are possible
Nausea	Metoclopramide	0.1-0.2 mg/kg/dose q6h, up to 10 mg/dose (prokinetic and mild nausea dosing); for chemotherapy-associated nausea, 0.5-1 mg/kg q6h PRN PO/IV/SC, give with diphenhydramine	Helpful when dysmotility an issue; may cause extrapyramidal reactions, particularly in children following IV administration of high doses; contraindicated in complete bowel obstruction or pheochromocytoma; administration with diphenhydramine reduces risk of extrapyramidal reactions
	Ondansetron	0.15 mg/kg dose q8h to max of 8 mg/dose; some institutions also use daily dosing of 0.45 mg/kg for chemotherapy	Significant experience in pediatrics; good empirical therapy for nausea in palliative care population; higher doses used with chemotherapy; oral dissolving tablet contains phenylalanine; may be prepared as oral solution

TABLE 198-3　Annotated Table of Medications Useful in Pediatrics—cont'd

SYMPTOM	MEDICATION	STARTING DOSE	COMMENTS
	Dexamethasone	if < 1 m^2: 10 mg/m^2 IV/PO daily if > 1 m^2: 10-12 mg IV/PO daily 　　max dose 10-12 mg/day	Also helpful with hepatic capsular distention, bone pain, bowel wall edema, anorexia, increased intracranial pressure; may cause mood swings or psychosis
	Lorazepam	0.025 mg/kg up to 2 mg IV/PO q6h	May be given SL; particularly helpful with anticipatory nausea; avoid use in neonates
	Dronabinol	5 mg/m^2/dose for a total of 4-6 doses per day; may increase dose in 2.5 mg/m^2 increments to a maximum of 15 mg/m^2 per dose if needed for effect; contraindicated in children < 6 yr; use with caution in children < 12 yr	Available in 2.5- and 5-mg capsules; may remove liquid contents from capsules for children who cannot swallow capsules; avoid in patients with sesame oil hypersensitivity or history of schizophrenia; may cause euphoria, dysphoria, or other mood changes; tolerance to CNS side effects usually develops in 1-3 days of continuous use; avoid in patients with depression or mania
	Scopolamine patch	1.5-mg patch, change q72h	Good for motion-induced nausea/vomiting; handling patch and contacting eye may cause anisocoria and blurry vision; may fold patches but do not cut them
Anxiety	Lorazepam	0.025 mg/kg up to 4 mg q6h IV/PO	Titrate by increase in dose by 20-30%
Agitation	Haloperidol	0.25-0.5 mg/kg PO divided tid, increase by 0.25-0.5 mg every 5-7 days (max dose 15 mg/kg/day); 0.5 mg/kg PO for acute onset, repeat q1h if needed	May cause extrapyramidal reactions, which can be reversed with diphenhydramine or Cogentin; safety not established in children <3 yr
Fatigue	Methylphenidate	0.3 mg/kg/dose up to 10 mg given qAM and noon	Rapid antidepressant effect; also improves cognition; take before meals to avoid appetite suppression; available as liquid and chewable tablet
Pruritus	Diphenhydramine	0.5-1 mg/kg q6h IV/PO (100 mg max per day)	May reverse phenothiazine-induced dystonic reactions; topical formulation on large areas of the skin or open area may cause toxic reactions; may cause paradoxical reaction in young children
	Hydroxyzine	0.5-1 mg/kg q6h IV/PO (600 mg max per day)	
Constipation	Docusate	40-150 mg/day PO in 1-4 divided doses	Stool softener available as liquid or capsule
	MiraLax (polyethylene glycol)	≤5 yr: ½ scoop (8.5 g) in 4 oz of water daily; >5 yr: 1 scoop (17 g) in 8 oz of water daily	Tasteless powder may be mixed in beverage of choice; now available over the counter
	Lactulose	5-10 mL PO up to q2h until bowel movement	Bowel stimulant; dosing q2h may cause cramping
	Senna	2.5 mL PO daily (for children >27 kg)	Bowel stimulant; available as granules
	Dulcolax (bisacodyl)	3-12 yr: 5-10 mg PO daily >12 yr 5-15 mg PO daily	Available in oral or rectal formulation
	Pediatric Fleets Enema	2.5-oz pediatric enema for children 2-11 yr; adult enema for children ≥12 yr	May repeat × 1 if needed; do not use in neutropenic patients
Muscle spasm	Diazepam	0.5 mg/kg/dose IV/PO q6h PRN; initial dose for children <5 yr is 5 mg dose; for children ≥5 yr, dose is 10 mg/dose	May be irritating if given by peripheral IV
	Baclofen	5 mg PO tid, increase by 5 mg/dose as needed	Helpful with neuropathic pain and spasticity; abrupt withdrawal may result in hallucinations and seizures; not for children <10 yr
Seizures	Lorazepam	0.1 mg/kg IV/PO/SL/PR; repeat q10min × 2	
	Diazepam	0.1 mg/kg q6h (max 5 mg/dose if <5 yr; max 10 mg/dose if >5 yr)	May be given PR as Diastat (0.2 mg/kg/dose q15min × 3 doses)
Anorexia	Megestrol acetate	10 mg/kg/day in 1-4 divided doses, up to 15 mg/kg/day or 800 mg/day	For children >10 yr; acute adrenal insufficiency may occur with abrupt withdrawal after long-term use; use with caution in patients with diabetes mellitus or history of thromboembolism; may cause photosensitivity
	Dronabinol	5 mg/m^2/dose for a total of 4-6 doses per day; may increase dose in 2.5 mg/m^2 increments to a maximum of 15 mg/m^2 per dose if needed for effect	Avoid in patients with sesame oil hypersensitivity or history of schizophrenia; may cause euphoria, dysphoria, or other mood changes; tolerance to CNS side effects usually develops in 1-3 days of continuous use; avoid in patients with depression or mania

*Breakthrough dose is 10% of 24-hr dose. See Chapter 138 for information regarding titration of opioids.
†Side effects of opioids include constipation, respiratory depression, pruritus, nausea, urinary retention, and physical dependence.
bid, twice daily; CNS, central nervous system; IV, intravenously; MSIR, morphine sulfate immediate-release; PO, by mouth; PR, rectally; PRN, as needed; q, every; SC, subcutaneously; SL, sublingually; tid, three times daily.
Data from references 35 through 38.

Lidoderm patches may be particularly helpful for this type of pain. Children may describe bone pain as "deep" or "achy" and particularly troublesome at night. Bone pain is often responsive to nonsteroidal anti-inflammatory medications and steroids.

Nausea and Vomiting

Based on the suspected origin of the nausea, an appropriate antiemetic (see Table 198-3) can be chosen. A significant difference between children and adults is the propensity for children to develop extrapyramidal side effects from certain antiemetics such as metoclopramide (in high doses) and the phenothiazines. Such reactions can be prevented or treated with diphenhydramine. Because the conditioned response of nausea develops quickly in response to a stimulus, prevention of nausea and vomiting from the start is an important strategy. For example, anxiolytics, such as lorazepam, can be helpful in preventing nausea because emotional and sensory input from the cerebral cortex can mediate anticipatory anxiety and resulting nausea.

Dyspnea

Dyspnea is a common symptom in children at the end of life. As with other symptoms, the differential diagnosis is important and may include pulmonary disease (e.g., pulmonary metastases, effusion, or pneumonia) or cardiac disease (e.g., congestive heart failure). Anxiety is a frequent component of dyspnea. The most effective pharmacological intervention is opioid administration (see Table 198-3). Other measures, such as supplemental oxygen or a fan blowing cool air, may also relieve this symptom.

Fatigue

Fatigue, the most prevalent of all cancer-related symptoms, causes significant distress and suffering (Fig. 198-3). Cancer-related fatigue can keep patients from addressing practical needs, psychosocial and spiritual distress, and opportunities for growth and closure at life's end. However, this symptom remains underappreciated and undertreated. Methylphenidate (see Table 198-3) improves fatigue and mood, pain, and cognition in adults with cancer and HIV infection regardless of the cause.

Anorexia and Cachexia

Anorexia and cachexia may be viewed as part of a natural progression in a life-threatening illness. These symptoms are also sources of distress for parents who may believe that feeding is part of their natural role. Honest and caring discussions around the meaning of feeding and the benefits and burdens of interventions to augment appetite or to provide nutrition can help. Possible interventions to improve appetite include serving small portions of the child's favorite foods and administering megestrol acetate. Although steroids can increase appetite, their multiple side effects may outweigh this benefit.

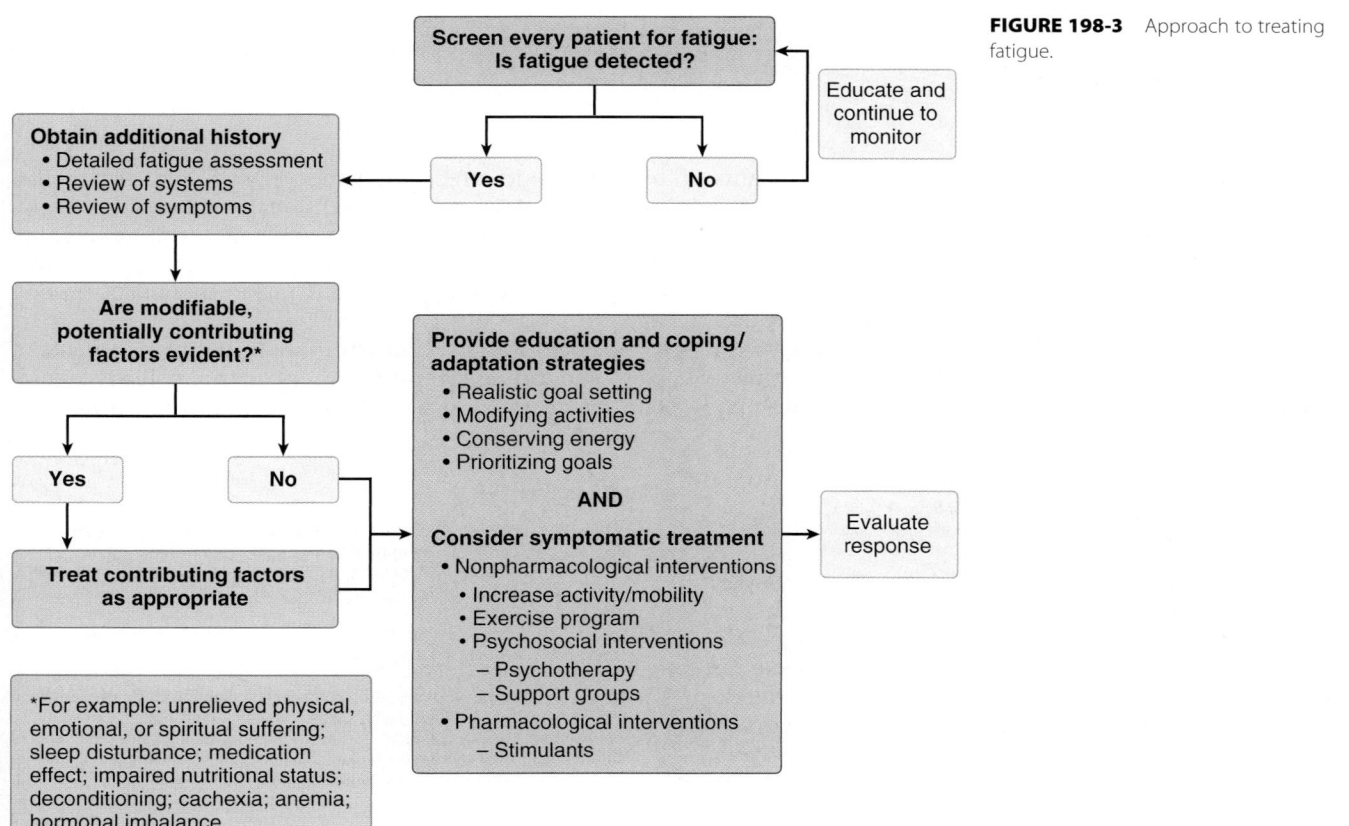

FIGURE 198-3 Approach to treating fatigue.

Box 198-1 Nonpharmacological Approaches to Symptom Management in Pediatrics

Physical

- Acupuncture may reduce pain from various causes, such as dental pain and headache in adults. It improves nausea or vomiting and acute pain in randomized, controlled trials. Few studies have evaluated acupuncture in children. Young children may be reluctant to try this technique involving needles, albeit much smaller than other needles they may have experienced.
- Massage may reduce not only pain, but also nausea, anxiety, and fatigue.
- Acupressure by Sea-Bands for nausea may help in instances beyond motion sickness, such as nausea related to chemotherapy.
- Transcutaneous electric nerve stimulation reduces pain in surgical patients.

Cognitive-Behavioral

- Hypnotherapy can be performed in children as young as 4 years.[39] Hypnosis can reduce pediatric procedural pain (e.g., bone marrow aspirate) and postoperative pain, as well as anticipatory nausea and dyspnea.
- In guided imagery, a visual image such as a pleasurable scene is used to relax the child and can reduce procedural pain and dyspnea.
- Other approaches such as distraction, breathing techniques, and art and play therapy may also be helpful, particularly for managing pain.
- Even when specific nonpharmacological techniques are not formally pursued, behavioral strategies that are easily incorporated include appropriately preparing the child, giving the child choices when possible, providing developmentally appropriate and honest explanations, using distractions, and practicing positive reinforcement.

Box 198-2 Recent Advances in Pain and Symptom Control

- Growing appreciation of the need for pediatric-specific evidence on which to base interventions for symptoms, rather than reliance on anecdotal wisdom or data from adult studies
- New agents for symptoms including neuropathic pain and nausea
- Recognition that attention to pain is a key component of high-quality medical care
- Opportunities for families with children with life-threatening illnesses to connect with one another through the Internet to share experiences, including strategies to manage symptoms

---

Future Considerations

- Assessment tools that are validated and are widely available in clinical practice, rather than limited to research
- Improved pharmacological interventions
  - Medications including opioids and benzodiazepines that are widely and consistently available from pharmacies in parenteral formulations
  - Long-acting analgesics in a wider range of doses and formulations appropriate and safe for children
  - Parenteral medications for constipation
  - Improved strategies for side effects of interventions for symptoms, such as opioid-induced pruritus
- Improved reimbursement for multidisciplinary services to alleviate spiritual or psychosocial suffering, intensive symptom-directed medical needs, and time- and effort-consuming consultations
- Medical education focused on symptom management, regardless of the trainee's intended field of study
- The option for children with extended-hour nursing already in place to enroll in hospice without losing nursing services, as well as improved respite care options for families

---

Anxiety and Depression

Selective serotonin reuptake inhibitors and stimulants are the core pharmacological interventions for depression. The physical symptoms of depression may be difficult to distinguish from those of the underlying disease. Clinicians should have a low threshold for treating depression. Because traditional antidepressants may take weeks to relieve depression, their initiation can be coupled with methylphenidate, which has a rapid antidepressant effect. As the antidepressant takes effect, methylphenidate may be tapered.

Nonpharmacological Approaches to Symptoms

Little research has been conducted to evaluate complementary and alternative medicine in pediatric symptom management. Several techniques show promise (Box 198-1). These methods may give children a sense of mastery and control over situations and may provide opportunities for family members to provide care, particularly when interventions such as disease-directed therapies have been discontinued. The traditional approach has been to treat conventional and alternative therapies as mutually exclusive. Given that many of these treatments

have few side effects, and they have potential benefits, integrating them with conventional therapies for symptoms is reasonable. Many of these therapies also exemplify the benefits of multidisciplinary care, involving psychologists, child life specialists, and music therapists, among others.

Box 198-2 lists recent advances in the management of pain and other symptoms in pediatric palliative care. Further treatment goals are addressed in the "Future Considerations" box.

REFERENCES

1. Collins JJ, Byrnes ME, Dunkel IJ, et al. The measurement of symptoms in children with cancer. J Pain Symptom Manage 2000;19:363-377.
2. Jalmsell L, Kreicbergs U, Onelov E, et al. Symptoms affecting children with malignancies during the last month of life: A nationwide follow-up. Pediatrics 2006;117:1314-1320.
3. Arias E, MacDorman MF, Strobino DM, Guyer B. Annual summary of vital statistics: 2002. Pediatrics 2003;112:1215-1230.
4. Bluebond-Langner M, Belasco JB, Goldman A, Belasco C. Understanding parents' approaches to care and treatment of children with cancer when standard therapy has failed. J Clin Oncol 2007;25:2414-2419.
5. Wolfe J, Klar N, Grier HE, et al. Understanding of prognosis among parents of children who died of cancer: Impact on treatment goals and integration of palliative care. JAMA 2000;284:2469-2475.
6. Mack JW, Hilden JM, Watterson J, et al. Parent and physician perspectives on quality of care at the end of life in children with cancer. J Clin Oncol 2005;23:9155-9161.

7. Romsing JM, Hertel S, Rasmussen M. Postoperative pain in children: Comparison between ratings of children and nurses. J Pain Symptom Manage 1996;11:42-46.
8. Beyer JE, McGrath PJ, Berde CB. Discordance between self-report and behavioral pain measures in children aged 3-7 years after surgery. J Pain Symptom Manage 1990;5:350-356.
9. World Health Organization. Cancer Pain and Relief and Palliative Care in Children. Geneva: World Health Organization, 1998.
10. Greco C, Berde C. Pain management for the hospitalized pediatric patient. Pediatr Clin North Am 2005;52:995-1027.
11. Krakauer EL, Penson RT, Truog RD, et al. Sedation for intractable distress of a dying patient: Acute palliative care and the principle of double effect. Oncologist 2000;5:53-62.
12. Drake R, Frost J, Collins JJ. The symptoms of dying children. J Pain Symptom Manage 2003;26:594-603.
13. McCallum DE, Byrne P, Bruera E. How children die in hospital. J Pain Symptom Manage 2000;20:417-423.
14. Sirkia K, Hovi L, Pouttu J, Saarinen-Pihkala UM. Pain medication during terminal care of children with cancer. J Pain Symptom Manage 1998;15:220-226.
15. Friedrichsdorf SJ, Menke A, Brun S, et al. Status quo of palliative care in pediatric oncology: A nationwide survey in Germany. J Pain Symptom Manage 2005;29:156-164.
16. Hongo T, Watanabe C, Okada S, et al. Analysis of the circumstances at the end of life in children with cancer: Symptoms, suffering and acceptance. Pediatr Int 2003;45:60-64.
17. Theunissen JMJ, Hoogerbrugge PM, van Achterberg T, et al. Symptoms in the palliative phase of children with cancer. Pediatr Blood Cancer 2007;49:160-165.
18. Dangel T. Poland: The status of pediatric palliative care. J Pain Symptom Manage 2002;24:222-224.
19. Henley LD. End of life care in HIV-infected children who died in hospital. Dev World Bioeth 2002;2:38-54.
20. Goldman A, Hewitt M, Collins GS, et al., United Kingdom Children's Cancer Study Group/Paediatric Oncology Nurses' Forum Palliative Care Working Group. Symptoms in children/young people with progressive malignant disease: United Kingdom Children's Cancer Study Group/Paediatric Oncology Nurses Forum survey. Pediatrics 2006;117:e1179-e1186.
21. Carter BS, Howenstein M, Gilmer MJ, et al. Circumstances surrounding the deaths of hospitalized children: Opportunities for pediatric palliative care. Pediatrics 2004;114:e361-e366.
22. Contro NA, Larson J, Scofield S, et al. Hospital staff and family perspectives regarding quality of pediatric palliative care. Pediatrics 2004;114:1248-1252.
23. Krechel SW, Bildner J. CRIES: A new neonatal postoperative pain measurement score. Initial testing of validity and reliability. Paediatr Anaesth 1995;5:53-61.
24. Merkel SI, Voepel-Lewis T, Shayevitz JR, Malviya S. The FLACC: A behavioral scale for scoring postoperative pain in young children. Pediatr Nurs 1997;23:293-297.
25. Voepel-Lewis T, Merkel S, Tait AR, et al. The reliability and validity of the Face, Legs, Activity, Cry, Consolability observational tool as a measure of pain in children with cognitive impairment. Anesth Analg 2002;95:1224-1229.
26. McGrath PA, Seifert CE, Speechley KN, et al. A new analogue scale for assessing children's pain: An initial validation study. Pain 1996;64:435-443.
27. Gauvain-Piquard A, Rodary C, Rezvani A, Serbouti S. The development of the DEGR(R): A scale to assess pain in young children with cancer. Eur J Pain 1999;3:165-176.
28. Hunt A, Goldman A, Seers K, et al. Clinical validation of the Paediatric Pain Profile. Dev Med Child Neurol 2004;46:9-18.
29. Solodiuk J, Curley MA. Pain assessment in nonverbal children with severe cognitive impairments: The Individualized Numeric Rating Scale (INRS). J Pediatr Nurs 2003;18:295-299.
30. Hester NK. The preoperational child's reaction to immunization. Nurs Res 1979;28:250-255.
31. Wong DL, Baker CM. Pain in children: Comparison of assessment scales. Pediatr Nurs 1988;14:9-17.
32. Bieri D, Reeve RA, Champion GD, et al. The Faces Pain Scale for the self-assessment of the severity of pain experienced by children: Development, initial validation, and preliminary investigation for ratio scale properties. Pain 1990;41:139-150.
33. Abu-Saad H. Assessing children's responses to pain. Pain 1984;19:163-171.
34. Wong DL, Whaley LF. Whaley & Wong's Essentials of Pediatric Nursing, 5th ed. St. Louis: Mosby, 1997.
35. Gordon D, Stevenson K, Griffie J, et al. Opioid equianalgesic calculations. J Palliat Med 1999;2:209-218.
36. Storey P, Knight C. UNIPAC Eight: The Hospice/Palliative Medicine Approach to Caring for Pediatric Patients. Glenview, IL: Mary Ann Liebert, 2003.
37. Storey P, Knight C. UNIPAC Three: Assessment and Treatment of Pain in the Terminally Ill. Glenview, IL: Mary Ann Liebert, 2003.
38. Taketomo C, Hodding J, Kraus D. Pediatric Dosage Handbook, 10th ed. Cleveland: Lexi-Comp, 2003.
39. Rusy L, Weisman SJ. Complementary therapies for acute pediatric pain management. Pediatr Clin North Am 2000;47:589-599.

SUGGESTED READING

Berde CB, Sethna NF. Analgesics for the treatment of pain in children. N Engl J Med 2002;347:1094-103.

Collins JJ. Cancer pain management in children. Eur J Pain 2001;5(Suppl A):37-41.

Donna L, Wong D, Hockenberry-Eaton M, et al. (eds). Wong's Essentials of Pediatric Nursing, 6th ed. St. Louis: Mosby, 2001.

Franck LS, Greenberg CS, Stevens B. Pain assessment in infants and children. Pediatr Clin North Am 2000;47:487-512.

Greco C, Berde C. Pain management for the hospitalized pediatric patient. Pediatr Clin North Am 2005;52:995-1027.

Gregoire MC, Frager G. Ensuring pain relief for children at the end of life. Pain Res Manage 2006;11:163-71.

CHAPTER **199**

Hospice and Special Services

Kevin Berger and Marcia Levetown

K E Y   P O I N T S

- Palliative and hospice care for children should be a continuum of services that address the longitudinal needs of the child and family, from the diagnosis of a potentially life-limiting condition (LLC). Palliative care should be available throughout the illness, concomitant with measures to reverse the disease when appropriate and desired.

- Children's deaths occur despite advanced technology, and they are not accepted or adequately prepared for in our society. Future program development and funding for children with LLCs should provide concurrent life-extending and palliative care, using the Medical Home model and palliative care philosophies. Palliative goals will gradually take precedence as the goals of cure or life extension become unrealistic.

- The epidemiology and demographics of death during childhood differ strikingly from adult findings. The percentage and absolute number of children who die are small, and this rarity leads to provider inexperience, fear, and even avoidance. Moreover, the causes of death among children include many unusual disorders, fraught with prognostic uncertainty.

- An understanding of child development, ethical principles, and legal concepts of assent and consent is critical to effective palliative care. The needs of the child *and* the family must be considered. It is essential that the knowing and willing child have a meaningful voice in the goals and plan of care.

- Symptoms must be managed aggressively and comprehensively throughout the illness. Procedure-related pain and anxiety, in addition to symptoms related to the illness and to treatment, must be addressed to provide the best quality of life (QOL), regardless of the final disease outcome. Fear should never prevent effective symptom management. Family outcomes improve when the child's suffering is minimized.

- Bereavement counseling is integral to care and management. Counseling specific to the loss of a child or sibling is often needed to avoid pathological grief. Many children who die do so suddenly, mainly as a result of trauma. These families should also receive palliative care through bereavement counseling.

TABLE 199-1 Demographics: Childhood Deaths in the United States in 2003

AGE (YR)	NUMBER OF DEATHS	CAUSES OF DEATH
0-1	28,428	20% congenital malformations 17% prematurity and low birth weight 8% sudden infant death syndrome 55% other
1-19	25,216	43% trauma (unintentional) 10% assault (homicide) 8.4% malignancy 4.4% congenital malformations, chromosome abnormality 3.2% cardiovascular diseases
Total	53,644	

From Hoyert D, Mathews TJ, Menacker F, et al. Annual summary of vital statistics: 2004. Pediatrics 2006;117:168-183.

Palliative care seeks to reduce or abate the discomfort related to an ailment or disease; it applies to all irreversible conditions. Physical symptom relief is the most obvious, but palliative care also encompasses emotional, spiritual, and psychosocial support for children and their families. Children with special health care needs (CSHCN), regardless of whether the condition is expected to be terminal, require care coordination to assist with activities of daily living and symptom control, and the entire family may need care to help them cope with the situation (Box 199-1). The American Academy of Pediatrics supports integrated care models in which palliative care is offered at the time of diagnosis and is continued throughout the illness, whether the outcome is cure or death.[1,2]

Palliative care should ideally be provided from the diagnosis of a disease that is a potential LLC. This care should accompany efforts to cure or reverse the process, when possible. Thus, nothing is forgone when palliative care is provided. Most children who die of nontraumatic causes are ill their entire lives. Along with the current societal lack of acceptance of childhood death, this situation creates a need for health care–related family support throughout the child's lifetime.

DECISION MAKING IN PEDIATRIC PALLIATIVE CARE

Children have unique needs based on their development, both psychologically and physiologically, and they require specialized services and knowledgeable providers. Clinical staff members must consider developmental differences in the child's preferences or ability to interpret and understand the disease process, treatment options, and prognosis.

Patient and family perceptions of QOL and the value of the offered treatment options should guide the goals of care. Health care providers should collaborate with the patient and family in judging QOL, because such determinations are heavily influenced by personal beliefs, socioeconomic status, and cultural and religious values. QOL determinations then dictate the overall goals of care.

Too often, the child's experience of suffering through treatment with advanced technologies, even when the illness is irreversible, is not acknowledged or recognized by family members and health care providers. Rather, preservation of life, despite suffering, and continued hope for cure, even if unachievable, remains the goal. This situation occurs especially when the child has no voice in the discussion and when the grief of involved adults is underrecognized and ineffectively addressed.

EPIDEMIOLOGY, PREVALENCE, AND NEED

Approximately 2.4 million adults and 53,000 children died in 2003 in the United States (Table 199-1).[3] Palliative care and hospice services are rarely designed to meet the needs of children and families. The current dominant model of palliative care in the United States is hospice. Offered only at the end of life, it is an economically parsimonious model. Hospice is offered most often as an either/or choice, requiring forgoing "curative" or life-prolonging care. This approach is rarely acceptable to a family, especially without a long-standing, trusting relationship. Few children who die access palliative care. Unnecessary suffering for the child and family often results.[4]

More than 50% of the 53,000 childhood deaths in the United States occur in the first year of life. Advances in perinatal and neonatal care have increased the short-term survival of very premature infants (22 to 25 weeks of gestation). Survival to discharge for these infants is low (1% at 22 weeks, 11% at 23 weeks, 26% at 24 weeks, and 44% at 25 weeks).[5] Most die in the neonatal intensive care unit, often after numerous painful procedures. Survivors often have significant disabilities. Palliative care programs for premature infants may enhance the willingness of caregivers and families to consider alternatives to the "technological imperative" that currently dominates their care.

Unlike in resource-poor countries, where infections such as gastroenteritis are still leading causes of death, childhood death (ages 1 to 19 years) in the United States is dominated by trauma (53%: motor vehicle accidents, drowning, child abuse, suicide, murder). Cancer accounts for only approximately 8% of deaths in childhood. Many rare fatal conditions exist, including congenital abnormalities, cardiac malformations, metabolic defects, and neurological disorders. Many children with these disorders are never recognized as terminally ill, and their families rarely benefit from a comprehensive, interdisciplinary, family-centered palliative approach that recognizes the impact of the ill child on parents and siblings.[4,6,7]

LOCATION OF DEATH: A SYMPTOM OF THE PROBLEM

Too often, chronically ill children die in a hospital, despite their preference to be at home. Sometimes a hospital death is preferred by parents, because they cannot handle their child dying at home. Often, however, a hospital death is the result of poor planning. In Washington State from 1990 to 1998, among individuals less than 25 years of age who died, 52% died in hospital,[8] 17% died at home, and 8% died in the emergency room or during transport. Among children and young adults 1 to 24 years old who died of complex chronic conditions, home deaths rose to 43%. Even among patients with chronic illnesses with more defined prognoses, such as AIDS, cystic fibrosis, muscular dystrophy, and genetic, metabolic, and congenital disorders, over half died in the hospital.

Helen House, the first pediatric hospice in England, reported 49% of deaths at home, 23% at Helen House, and only 20% in a hospital.[9] Helen House offers comprehensive palliative care, including respite services, from the time of diagnosis of a disease that is a potential LLC.

DIAGNOSTIC AND PROGNOSTIC UNCERTAINTY

Families are often given no long-term prognosis of their child's condition; this is particularly true when no diagnostic label can easily be affixed to their child's disorder. Although guidelines exist for pediatric end-of-life decision making, the process remains ambiguous. Uncertainty surrounds the assessment of QOL, and providers have a fear of prognostication. Published data may be unhelpful because survival data and rates of complications vary by community. In addition, for rare disorders, prognostic data to guide clinicians and families are limited, and many fatal conditions have subtypes with variable prognoses. In addition, clinical practice and technology are continually evolving, and these changes also affect survival (see "Future Considerations" box).

FAMILY SUPPORT

Families need information to allay their anxiety and grief, to facilitate successful adaptation, and to ensure effective

---

Future Considerations

- A need exists for improved education on ethical issues, establishing appropriate goals of care, pain management, withdrawal of medically provided nutrition and hydration, and brain death.[18]
- Financial barriers to pediatric palliative and bereavement care require comprehensive changes in policy by federal and state agencies, as well as by private insurers. These changes will require a major shift in the culture of medicine and its reimbursement.
- Developing countries face different challenges resulting from scarce resources and insufficient numbers of qualified personnel, even for illnesses that have known treatments, such as HIV infection, diseases requiring transplantation, and gastroenteritis.
- Palliative care and bereavement services must be adaptable and flexible enough to be able to serve the premature child who only has a few days to live, as well as the child who is anticipated to survive a few months to several years. These services must include also the families who are left to grieve after the sudden loss of a child as a result of trauma or acute illness.

---

planning that best meets their individualized needs. Good sources include clinicians, parents of children with similar conditions, and the literature. Families need guidance about what sources to trust on the Internet and elsewhere. They need to know about the likely course of the disease or condition and expected complications related to treatment and the illness itself. At the same time, families must understand that the information available may not reflect their child's exact course. The needs addressed by a family-centered, palliative approach include those related to financial and job choices, the effects of the illness on familial relationships, and family planning.

No better guide exists than other parents who have been through the experience themselves. It is crucial for families to find peers and parent support groups, including disease-specific national organizations and their local chapters.

LEGAL AND ETHICAL ISSUES AND THE CARE OF CHILDREN: PERMISSION, ASSENT, AND CONSENT

Children's best interests should drive health care decisions affecting them. Children should be given information appropriate to their developmental stage, to enable expression of preferences relating to testing, procedures, and treatment goals and options. This is particularly important for the mature child who has been living with a chronic illness for a long time. (For younger children, nonverbal expression may be important. Child life therapists and child psychologists can be invaluable in facilitating meaningful and effective communication.)

The American Academy of Pediatrics Committee on Bioethics[10] outlined the important concepts of informed permission, which can be granted by parents on behalf of their child, and informed assent (or dissent) of the child with the capacity or the ability to understand the options and their likely consequences and to apply his or her own values consistently to the decision. Assent is not codified in law (except when enrolling a child ≥7 years old in National Institutes of Health trials), but an ethical obligation exists to present options to the child for his or her assent or dissent. Giving the child choices that will be taken seriously affirms the child's importance, shows respect, builds trust, promotes a sense of control, and improves adherence to the mutually determined treatment plan. Although children may not always be rational and autonomous in their decision making, their concerns should be given serious consideration. Consent is a legal term that applies to an informed person who is recognized as independent under the law (often >18 years old) and who is making a decision on one's own behalf.

The United Nations Convention on the Rights of the Child of 1989 recommended that caregivers inform the child of the illness and encouraged soliciting and respecting the child's opinion.[11] Research indicates that children are infrequently informed about their condition or involved in the decisions about their care.[12] Important decisions must be family *and* child centered. Good decisions are usually arrived at after negotiation and unhurried discussions, sometimes involving extended family members and other personal advisors, such as religious leaders. Anticipating the need for and making decisions in advance of the crisis lessens family anxiety and improves the quality of the decisions and the outcomes for the child and family.[13,14]

DESIGNING AN INTEGRATED MODEL: THE MEDICAL HOME AND PEDIATRIC PALLIATIVE CARE MODEL

The American Academy of Pediatrics and the Maternal and Child Health Bureau (MCHB) of the Health Resources and Services Administration (HRSA) have promoted the Medical Home model. The term *Medical Home* refers to a partnership between the primary care physician and family to assist them in efficiently accessing and coordinating health care and community resources and support. The result should be accessible, family-centered, continuous, coordinated, compassionate, comprehensive, and culturally competent care.[15,16] Care coordination is the key goal (Fig. 199-1). The Medical Home model consists of key components similar to the basic components of the interdisciplinary palliative care model (Table 199-2).[17]

Examples of CSHCN who can benefit from palliative care include the following:

- Very premature neonates and infants
- Children with malignant disorders
- Children with congenital anomalies and genetic disorders that may be terminal, such as Tay-Sachs disease, Batten's disease, spinal muscular atrophy, muscular dystrophy, brain anomalies, trisomy 13 and 18, many forms of congenital heart disease, cystic fibrosis, and metabolic and mitochondrial disorders
- Children with severe neurological impairment and complex medical conditions, such as cerebral palsy, anoxic injury, and other head or multiple trauma

Phoenix Pediatrics, Ltd, in Phoenix, Arizona, has provided a Medical Home for CSHCN for more than 30 years. An integrated Medical Home and Palliative Care Model exists together with Hospice of the Valley. Between 2001 and 2005, there were 258 pediatric patients served by Hospice of the Valley. Of those served, 14% were

discharged from the program alive. Of those who died, the location of death was as follows: home, 69%; hospice inpatient unit, 24%; hospital, 6%; and skilled nursing facility, 1%. The average length of program stay was 63 days, with a maximum of 867 days for a child with Sanfilippo's syndrome (unpublished data). The higher number of home deaths may reflect a family's choice when such a service is available. Given opportunity and support, most families prefer the death to be at home or at a location other than the hospital.

TABLE 199-2 Similarities between the Medical Home and Pediatric Palliative Care Models

MEDICAL HOME*	PEDIATRIC PALLIATIVE CARE
Accessible	Care must be available 24 hours a day.
Family centered	Care and decision making are primarily family centered and family driven. Each family's choices should be respected.[†]
Continuous	The primary care provider is central to continuity of care.
Coordinated	This care delivery model is founded on an interdisciplinary team approach to care and addresses the whole person. Effective communication assists with medical decision making that is ethically sound, evidenced based, multidisciplinary, and family centered.[‡] The result is the provision of truthful, accurate information so patients can make decisions based on true informed consent.
Compassionate	Maintenance of a sense of autonomy, self-worth, and individuality is the focus of care.
Comprehensive	Comprehensive pain and symptom control, attention to the whole person within the context of the family.
Culturally competent	Each family's cultural, spiritual, socioeconomic, and religious differences are respected. Grief and bereavement support is provided for the individual and family.

*Sourkes B. Armfuls of Time. Montreal: McGill University Press, 1996.
[†]Committee on Hospital Care. Family centered care and the pediatrician's role. Pediatrics 2003;112:691-696.
[‡]Peabody JL, Martin GI. From how small is too small to how much is too much. Clin Perinatol 1996;23:473-89.

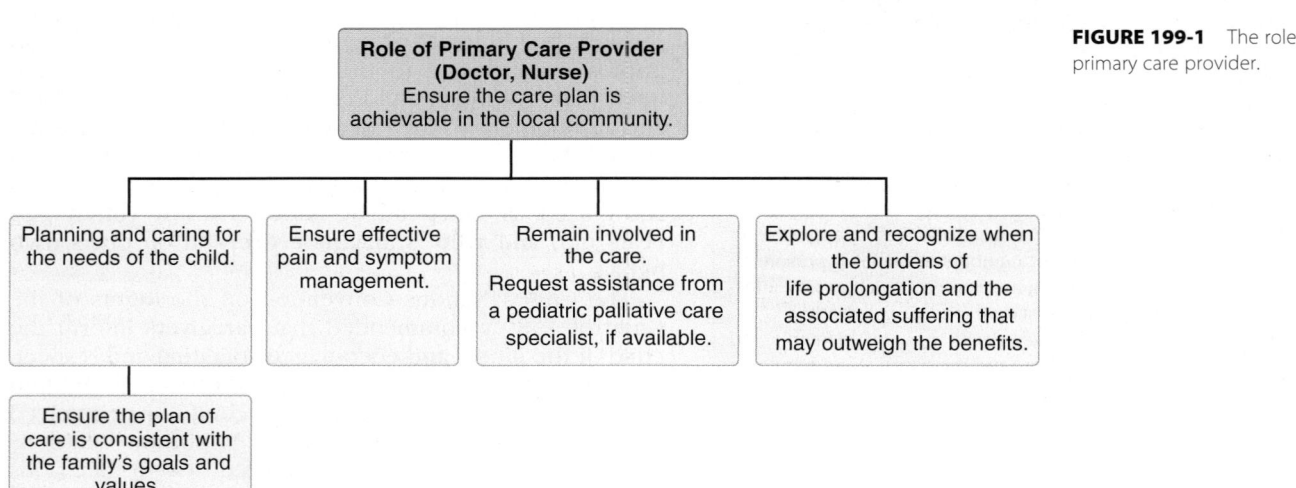

Role of Primary Care Provider (Doctor, Nurse) Ensure the care plan is achievable in the local community.

- Planning and caring for the needs of the child.
- Ensure effective pain and symptom management.
- Remain involved in the care. Request assistance from a pediatric palliative care specialist, if available.
- Explore and recognize when the burdens of life prolongation and the associated suffering that may outweigh the benefits.
- Ensure the plan of care is consistent with the family's goals and values.

FIGURE 199-1 The role of the primary care provider.

Basic Requirements and Planning for a Pediatric Palliative Care Program

The following are key elements of a pediatric palliative care program:

- Flexibility and adaptability of the care plan
- Availability in any care environment
- Continuous availability of on-call services
- Respite services
- Pediatric-specific durable medical equipment and supplies
- Pediatric-specific medications, infusions, and support services such as transfusion, radiography, and basic laboratory studies

Interdisciplinary team members in the hospice model are integral to the care and support of children and families with life-threatening conditions. Other specialists include pediatric psychologists, psychiatrists, and pain specialists. Art, music, and child life therapists can assist nonverbal children to express their needs.[17] Music therapy may be the only way to calm some neurologically impaired children. Trained volunteers can be particularly useful for the adolescent who is unable to maintain friendships because of chronic or recurrent illness and who can benefit from discussion of typical teen issues with an adolescent volunteer. Adult volunteers can take healthy siblings out and can assist families by helping with chores, for example (Fig. 199-2).

CONTINUUM OF CARE

Hospice-Based Outreach Programs

Hospice-based outreach programs typically offer psychosocial and pastoral or spiritual support for the child, siblings, and parents and assistance with problem solving, advocacy, and care coordination. Outreach or "prehospice" programs generally do not provide direct medical or nursing care, medical equipment, supplies, medications,

clinical therapy, transportation, or custodial care. Families who seek disease-directed treatments while needing hospice-style comprehensive support would be well suited to such a program. Service can also be provided by trained volunteers or self-help groups.

Grief and Bereavement

The continuum of grief starts with the loss of the healthy child, long before, and even in the absence of, the child's physical death. When the likely outcome is death, grief counseling can enable a family to embrace life, to concentrate on maximizing the QOL, and to prevent pathological grief. The grief of siblings, grandparents, close friends, and schoolmates also needs to be recognized and treated. The needs of schoolmates may need to be addressed.

Families of chronically ill children often adapt to a "new normal" when the child is alive. Many of these children survive multiple surgical procedures, recurrent bouts of pneumonia, and other complications, and their families come to expect the child to continue to overcome deterioration. Thus, even the death of the chronically ill child, like that of the trauma victim, may be perceived as "unexpected."

Professional caregiving staff members may also benefit from counseling and ongoing support. Dealing with dying is generally stressful, but it is particularly difficult and emotionally charged when the patient is a child. Support systems must be put in place to prevent professional burnout.

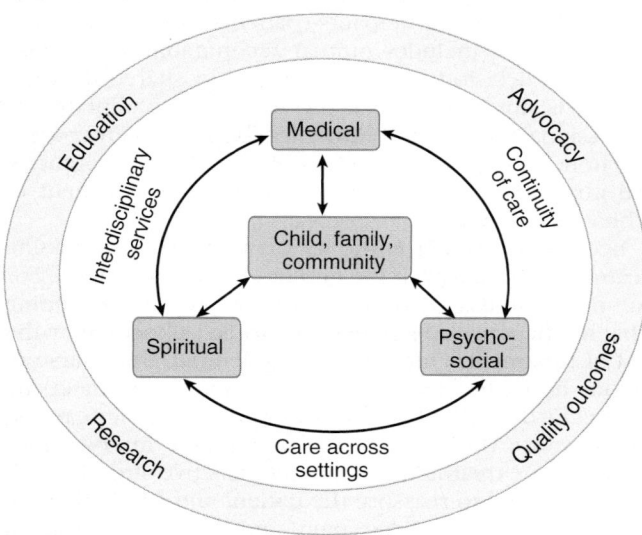

FIGURE 199-2 The interdisciplinary palliative care team. (Courtesy of Sue Huff, RN, and Marcia Levetown, MD.)

REFERENCES

1. Committee on Bioethics and Committee on Hospital Care. Palliative care for children. Pediatrics 2000;106:351-357.
2. Frager G. Palliative care and terminal care of children. Child Adolesc Psychiatr Clin N Am 1997;6:889-909.
3. Hoyert D, Mathews TJ, Menacker F, et al. Annual summary of vital statistics: 2004. Pediatrics 2006;117:168-183.
4. Williams PD et al. A community based intervention for siblings and parents of children with chronic illness or disability: The ISEE study. J Pediatr 2003;143:386-393.
5. Vohr B, Allen M. Extreme prematurity: The continuing dilemma. N Engl J Med 2005;352:71-72.
6. Mazurek Melnyk B, et al. Creating opportunities for parent empowerment: Program effects on the mental health/coping outcomes of critically ill young children and their mothers. Pediatrics 2004;113:597-607.
7. Li J, Precht DH, Mortensen PB, Olsen J. Mortality in parents after death of a child in Denmark: A nationwide follow up study. Lancet 2003;361:363-367.
8. Feudtner C, Silveira M, Christakis D. Where do children with complex chronic conditions die? Patterns in Washington State, 1980-1998. Pediatrics 2002;109:656-660.
9. Hunt A, Burne R. Medical and nursing problems of children with neurodegenerative disease. Palliat Med1995;9:19-26.
10. American Academy of Pediatrics, Committee on Bioethics. Informed consent, parental permission and assent in pediatric practice. Pediatrics 1995;95:314-317.
11. General Assembly of the United Nations. Adoption of a Convention on the Rights of the Child. New York: United Nations, 1989.
12. Wendler DS. Assent in pediatric research: Theoretical and practical considerations. J Med Ethics 2006;32:229-234.
13. Ashwal S, Perkin RM, Orr R. When too much is not enough. Pediatr Ann 1992;21:311-317.
14. Committee on Hospital Care. Family centered care and the pediatrician's role. Pediatrics 2003;112:691-696.
15. American Academy of Pediatrics, Medical Home Initiatives for Children with Special Health Care Needs Project Advisory Committee. The Medical Home. Pediatrics 2002;110:184-186.
16. Peabody JL, Martin GI. From how small is too small to how much is too much. Clin Perinatol 1996;23:473-489.
17. Sourkes B. Armfuls of Time. Montreal: McGill University Press, 1996.
18. Solomon M, Sellers D, Heller K, et al. New and lingering controversies in pediatric end-of-life care. Pediatrics 2005;116:872-883.

SUGGESTED READING

Bluebond-Langner M. The Private Worlds of Dying Children. Princeton, NJ: Princeton University Press, 1978.

Carter B, Levetown M. Palliative Care for Infants, Children, and Adolescents: A Practical Handbook. Baltimore: Johns Hopkins University Press, 2004.

Goldman A. Care of the Dying Child. Oxford: Oxford University Press, 1994.

Institute of Medicine. When Children Die: Improving Palliative and End-of-Life Care for Children and their Families. Washington, DC: National Academies Press, 2003.

Sourkes B. Armfuls of Time. Montreal: McGill University Press, 1996.

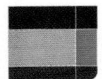

CHAPTER **200**

Pediatric Palliative Care: Interdisciplinary Support

Cynda Hylton Rushton

KEY POINTS

- A framework focused on goals of care supports integrated, holistic care for dying children and their families.

- Innovative curricula help pediatric professionals to develop the skills and knowledge they need to care for children with life-limiting conditions (and their families).

- Systematic processes, such as debriefings, rounds, and ethical consultations, help to deal with difficulties that arise in palliative medicine.

- Research has begun to document health care professional grief and moral distress.

- More research is needed on the evidence base for pediatric palliative care.

Each year, 54,000 children die in the United States, most in hospitals within critical care settings.[1] Although advances have been made in pediatric palliative care nationwide, significant gaps exist. High-quality pediatric palliative care requires that exquisite attention be paid not only to the needs of children and families, but also to the interdisciplinary team. Nurses and physicians are ill prepared to discuss palliative issues skillfully with patients or families,[2,3] and this lack of communication may cause conflicts about treatment goals and care plans. Few pediatric professionals receive training in grief and bereavement; few have access to venues where they can share their experiences and focus on their grief. In a culture where their needs are denied, pediatric professionals are frustrated and unprepared to cope with their own feelings and responses.

To develop the skills and the knowledge they need to achieve palliative care goals, pediatric professionals need interdisciplinary support systems integrated throughout the organization. In an environment where a framework focused on the goals of care is in place, these systems support professionals as they deal with the stresses of caring for dying children and their families.

GOALS OF CARE: THE FRAMEWORK

A framework that focuses on goals and outcomes, rather than on disintegrated and isolated actions, creates a shared process and language for pediatric palliative care. When palliative care and curative care are integrated, physicians and nurses move beyond serial processing to parallel processing. They no longer provide curative care first and then offer palliative care; instead, they provide both together.[4] This integration of palliative care philosophy and practices with curative interventions empowers health care professionals to focus on what can be done, rather than on what will not be done.

The goals-of-care framework illuminates the holistic needs of the child and family. It invites communication, shared decision making, and mutual goal setting to anticipate and address decision points and vulnerabilities. This approach recognizes that restoring health means more than curing an illness or eradicating a disease; it enables the child and family to respond to health, injury, and recovery in their own unique ways and to apply the knowledge and skills of practitioners to achieve shared goals. This approach acknowledges survival and cure as desirable outcomes, yet these are not the only desirable outcomes. Early integration of palliative care for children living with life-threatening conditions, particularly for those with chronic, life-limiting conditions, is desirable.[5,6] Goals such as pain and symptom relief, enhancing quality of life, creating meaningful experiences with family and friends, and achieving spiritual well-being become important.

This approach depends on respectful relationships with children, families, other professionals, and the broader community as the foundation for collaboration. Authentic collaboration respects the unique knowledge and abilities of all participants (patients, parents, and professionals) and includes mutual accountability, responsibility, and decision making. The goal of shared decision making is not to convince the patient or parent of the professional's views, but rather to discover together what will honor the patient's and family's values, preferences, and goals and what therapeutic modalities will help to achieve those goals.

Because treatment is the means to an end, discussing treatment is pointless if the end has not been defined. For the professionals, definition consists of understanding what the patient and family hopes to be or become by the end of treatment. Once the end is defined, the course of action should be clear: If the professionals can meet the goal set by the patient and family, they treat; if they cannot, they disclose the limits of the therapeutic interventions and continue treatments that meet palliative aims. In such cases, we need to reassure the patient and family that we will continue to relieve pain and symptoms, remain present, and provide support, while making it clear that sometimes children do die, despite all efforts.

Setting the goals of care requires that team members collaborate with the child and family to discover what is vital and meaningful. Together, they should explore what goals are possible for the patient and what values and preferences the patient and the family hold. The holistic answer to the question "What goals are desired by this patient and family?" goes beyond physiology and treatment to address quality of life, pain and suffering, psychosocial issues, and spirituality.

In goal setting, the care team should explore the possibility of unexpected events and anticipated illness trajectories with the child and family. We should stress that decisions may need to be reconsidered and revised after turning points in an illness trajectory. As part of ongoing goal setting, advance care planning can contribute to appreciation of the psychological, spiritual, existential, and ritual dimensions of the encounter with death. Advance care planning allows team members to get to know the patient's circle of significant others, suspend their own professional ideology of a "good death," and create healing environments.

RECENT DEVELOPMENTS

Systematic processes and structures are essential to high-quality pediatric palliative care. Adopting a goal-focused framework provides opportunities to integrate palliative care with disease-focused interventions. New interdisciplinary experiential curricula act as catalysts for cultural change; so, too, are newly developed methods that support and empower pediatric professionals.

Curricula

Innovative curricula have been developed for pediatric palliative care. Two curricula focus on essential content, while providing structure and process. The first, the pediatric End-of-Life Nursing Education Consortium (ELNEC), reflects key elements of pediatric palliative care nursing. The second, the Children's Project on Palliative/Hospice Services (ChiPPS), offers essential resources and references for pediatric palliative medicine. The third, the Initiative for Pediatric Palliative Care (IPPC), is interdisciplinary; it provides a holistic framework for family-centered pediatric care that engages parents as cofacilitators. The IPPC curriculum includes facilitation guides, videos, and educational models, designed to facilitate individual and interdisciplinary learning and to serve as a vehicle for cultural transformation.

Without institutional support, no curriculum can succeed in changing its culture to honor caregivers and intentionally create support systems. Transformation is possible only when health care professionals understand their own needs and strategies for a more supportive environment. This requires training programs that integrate self-care and renewal into the pediatric palliative curricula using experiential teaching. In the IPPC curriculum, for example, interdisciplinary health care professionals reflect on the sources of and responses to their own suffering. In the Being with Dying professional training program, health care professionals integrate contemplative practices into their work and lives and create their own self-care plans.[7]

Support Systems for Palliative Care Integration

A variety of strategies focus on the psychosocial, emotional, spiritual, and physical needs of caregivers.[8] These include daily rounds,[9] patient care conferences (PCCs), family meetings, palliative care rounds, ethics consultations, and renewal/self-care.

Daily Interdisciplinary Team Rounds

Drawing on an interdisciplinary model[9] for process improvement in critical care, the format for daily rounds can be expanded and adapted for pediatric settings. Rounds function to clarify the goals of care for individual patients; by systematically addressing questions and concerns, daily rounds make inquiry about patient and family goals and therapeutic goals explicit and routine (Box 200-1). In difficult cases, daily rounds may lead to the request for a PCC.

Patient Care Conferences

By allowing extended interdisciplinary dialogue, PCCs clarify goals for patients whose care involves multiple specialties and complex medical, psychosocial, or spiritual components. Professionals directly involved in the patient's care are invited to attend PCCs; participants include nurses, physicians, social workers, chaplains or pastoral care workers, palliative care and pain specialists, ethics consultants, hospice professionals, bereavement counselors, and case managers or advanced practice nurses who manage the process of care and coordinate discharges. PCCs serve the patient and family by giving the care team the opportunity to clarify the diagnosis,

---

Box 200-1 Proactive Identification of Patients Who Can Benefit from Palliative Interventions
• Does this patient have a disease or diagnosis that will limit his or her life span?
• Would you be surprised if this patient died in the next 6 to 12 months?
• Has the frequency of hospitalizations increased during the last 6 to 12 months?
• Has a major clinical event (e.g., relapse, need for transplant) affected this patient's condition?
• Does the patient have symptoms that have changed the frequency of clinic visits?

• Has there been a change or deterioration in the patient's
  • Pain intensity
  • Mental status
  • Energy or stamina
  • Physical or functional status
  • Respiratory function
  • Quality of life

• Does a consensus exist about the diagnosis and prognosis?
• Have concerns about the treatment plan been expressed by the patient and family?
• Does conflict exist among the family or the care team about curative or palliative goals of care?

Adapted from Rushton C, Reder E, Comello K, et al. Evaluation of the effectiveness of an interdisciplinary intervention to reduce suffering in professionals who care for dying children. J Palliat Med 2006;9:925.

prognosis, and goals with a trusted expert from within or outside the team.

Several formats are available for PCCs. Whichever format is used, a systematic process helps to create a shared language and a reliable process for communication and decision making. It can create a context for understanding patient and family values and preferences and can illuminate areas of conflict or disagreement. Some cases require PCCs at regular intervals to discuss evolving issues and goals and to address disagreements. Documenting the plan for ongoing review and revision can help to clarify expectations about treatment and to establish guideposts for decision making. One format specifies patient demographics, reason for the conference, summary of the child's illness, identification of patient, family, and staff needs and issues, creation of a palliative care plan, formulation of a discharge plan, and follow-up. Another format, the Decision Making Tool, involves a dual process: patients and families identify and communicate values, preferences, and goals with a professional who, in turn, supplies information about what is possible and feasible and makes recommendations. This approach improves patient and provider satisfaction.[10]

Family Meetings

Helping families to navigate the often uncertain process of dying involves "hoping for the best and planning for the worst." For health care professionals, it entails collecting and sharing relevant information and compassionately disclosing truthful prognosis. Uncertainty about what is in the child's best interest can create an environment where communication is ineffective and conflict arises. Framing discussions in ways that honor the hopes of the patient or family and simultaneously prepare for the possibility of death can help to neutralize conflicts. Frequent discussions with the family about the disease status can alert them to possible complications and offer evidence of clinical deterioration, can prepare them for the inevitability of death, and can support their grieving. Holding family meetings offers the opportunity to clarify goals, communicate new information and options, establish time frames, and plan care. Often family meetings are a logical next step following PCCs. In family meetings, the Decision Making Tool[10] can provide a framework to guide the discussions about goals, quality of living, treatment plans, and desired outcomes.

Palliative Care Rounds

Interdisciplinary educational sessions explore the palliative care dimensions of cases from recent or current caseloads.[8] At the Johns Hopkins Children's Center, an interdisciplinary team chooses a case that exemplifies palliative care issues, such as conflict about goals of care, pain and symptom management, or another dimension of the dying process. A physician resident or fellow presents the medical facts and the goals of care for the patient; members of the interdisciplinary team share psychosocial, emotional, and spiritual information about the patient and family. A facilitator leads the ensuing discussion of the holistic needs of the patient and engages the entire interdisciplinary team in exploring palliative issues, often even

their emotional needs. The facilitator concludes each session by summarizing the case and its implications. Participants are asked to reflect on what they have learned and how it will influence the provision of palliative care in the future.

Ethics Consultations

Quality end-of-life care needs an ethics infrastructure to support interdisciplinary professionals when concerns arise. When uncertainty, ambiguity, or disagreement exists about naming or articulating the ethical issues, about which ethics principles apply or which course of action to pursue, or about how to prioritize various ethical claims or positions, ethical consultations are particularly helpful. Although some professionals may feel that they are being accused of being unethical if a consultation is requested, such feelings are usually unwarranted and can be an obstacle to the process. Most often, the reason for consultation is a conflict in values or a tension between valid ethical positions. The very nature of ethical dilemmas is that they occur only during conflict and never during complete agreement. Thus, ethics committees give advice; they do not give "the answer." Given uncertainties, however, ethics consultations can play a critical role in proactively addressing ethical issues in the care of critically and terminally ill children.

Bereavement Debriefings

After a patient dies, professionals can benefit from access to spiritual and psychosocial resources, physical and emotional support, and, if possible, relief from responsibilities for some time. All these measures contribute to an environment for optional pediatric palliative care, as do bereavement debriefing sessions. Debriefings after deaths offer staff members the opportunity to manage their grief responses and to provide individual follow-up. HLCC adapted the traditional critical incident stress debriefing model to help professionals to realize that the physical, emotional, social, and spiritual responses after patient deaths are normal, natural responses.[8] Each session offers education about grief and recommendations for support, including strategies for coping with multiple losses, expressing grief in healthy ways, and making meaning out of grief.

Self-Care/Renewal

Optimal palliative care cannot occur without intentional and consistent attention to caregivers' needs.[11] Individuals must commit themselves to self-care, and institutions must allocate resources to programs that support it. Principles of self-care include a plan that acknowledges one's limits, recognizes practices that renew the spirit, and connects with both others and support systems.[7] These can include anything that serves the individual's well-being, from contemplation to sports, from nutrition to the arts, and more. No one way to achieve the goal exists; diverse and creative activities are individualized, such as peer-to-peer support groups, appreciative inquiry, or self-renewal activities (stress management, anger and conflict management, and emotional or spiritual rejuvenation).

Box 200-2 Common Challenges for Pediatric Palliative Care

- Miscommunication among the interdisciplinary team and with patients and families
- Holistic, interdisciplinary education curricula
- Barriers (within health care team, families, and society) to accept palliative care principles and practices and to integrate them proactively into goals of care
- Comprehensive integration of palliative care into care practices, processes, and structures
- Development of support systems and renewal for professionals
- Documentation of personal and institutional constraints that cause distress
- Access to ethics consultants and committees to assist proactive assessment and interventions to address ethical issues, particularly in situations viewed as futile
- Professional awareness and application of prominent ethical and legal guidelines

Data from references 1, 3, and 12.

Evidence-Based Medicine

The evidence to support selected interventions and to transform pediatric palliative care is limited, and systematic data are not available. Some studies in critical care and other domains address topics of concern to pediatrics, specifically caregiver grief and moral distress (Box 200-2).

Caregiver Grief and Moral Distress

When patients die, health care professionals grieve. When unrecognized, their suffering and grief can undermine the effectiveness and quality of care. The extent of grief is determined by the professional's investment in the relationship with the patient and family, expectations of professional identity and roles, and personal or social constructs.[13] These findings are consistent with studies of critical care professionals caring for adults.

Professionals struggle to balance competing professional and ethical obligations and to preserve a sense of wholeness. Their integrity can be threatened in myriad ways, including competing interests of patients, families, and other team members; the organization where they practice; and even their own behaviors and feelings. As a result, professionals may experience conflicts, dilemmas, and, in some instances, moral distress.[14] Although the sources of moral distress and threats to integrity for physicians and nurses are similar, they differ in how they perceive these issues.

A national survey of attitudes of pediatric critical care physicians and nurses on end-of-life care[15-18] revealed that more physicians (78%) than nurses (57%) agreed that withholding and withdrawing care were "ethically the same." No one in the two groups judged either practice unethical. Physicians were more likely than nurses to believe that families were well informed about the burdens and benefits of further treatment (99% versus 89%), that ethical issues were discussed well within the care team (92% versus 59%), and that ethical issues were discussed well with the family (91% versus 79%).

Moral distress occurs when clinicians are unable to translate their moral choices into moral action. It occurs when they know the ethically appropriate action to take but are prevented by obstacles, either internal or external. In such instances, acting in a manner contrary to personal and professional values undermines individual integrity and authenticity. Thirty-eight to 54% of nurses and more than half of house officers report acting against their consciences in providing care to children, but only 35% to 38% of attending physicians report this finding. Those who acted against their conscience were more likely to report concerns about overtreatment than undertreatment, particularly in critical care and non-oncology settings.[12] Symptoms of this distress may be expressed by covert actions. Unrelieved distress jeopardizes individual self-worth. Ultimately, as with all unresolved interprofessional conflicts, the quality of patient care suffers.

The moral distress experienced daily by clinicians is common, particularly among nurses and physicians in training. Regrettably, it is not uncommon for nurses, doctors, social workers, clergy, and other members of the health care team. Systematic efforts to assess the sources and intensity of the moral distress, to create systems for facilitated dialogue about situations causing the distress, and to create personal and institutional support systems to address it are essential for an ethically grounded care environment.[19]

CONCLUSIONS AND CONTROVERSIES

Despite the limitations of research to date, pediatric professionals in acute care need support systems that offer them skills and tools to help them care for dying children and their families. Communication skills training is critical for pediatric professionals, who need to be able to explore difficult issues with the patient and family through the entire dying process, beginning at diagnosis and through an unpredictable course. Clinicians need more than communication skills. They need tools and processes that foster communication, goal setting, and decision making. Family conferences early in the illness build relationships that will aid shared decision making later in the child's journey. Interdisciplinary team rounds allow all the care team members to express their concerns in ways that support holistic care.

In difficult cases, other tools prove valuable. Consultations with palliative care professionals or bioethicists can clarify issues when no clear-cut answers are possible. When consultations fail, proven methods are available for mediation and conflict resolution. Access to such resources is essential to develop a culture that supports the practice of high-quality pediatric palliative medicine.

These new practices are promising, yet the tension between high technology and palliative medicine continues in acute care settings, where children with life-limiting diseases are often treated. Until professionals are given the skills and the tools they need, they will continue to experience moral distress, grief, and suffering. This is not surprising, given that the death of a child is something no one wants to happen but may be inevitable. Health care professionals and children and their families need all the skills and tools available to help them through these tragic circumstances.

RESEARCH CHALLENGES, OPPORTUNITIES, AND ADVANCES

Research in pediatric palliative care must probe more deeply into caregiver suffering, moral distress, and ethical conflicts. According to the Institute of Medicine,[1] strategies are critically needed to help professionals to preserve their integrity and well-being. Too often, health care professionals lack the knowledge and skills to process and address their emotional responses, grief, and suffering in healthy ways.

Caregiver Grief and Moral Distress

Studies are needed to evaluate and disseminate innovative interventions that enable health care professionals to understand and address their grief when children die and their responses to the suffering of their patients and themselves. Traditional grief models have focused on disruptive symptoms and sharing feelings; understanding grief and promoting recovery require a model focused on *meaning reconstruction*. Integrating this model into interventions for professionals suggests that constructs such as burnout and compassion fatigue do not go far enough in making meaning out of tragic circumstances. Evaluation of novel interventions aimed at creating a healthy work environment and addressing and acknowledging the suffering of health care professionals are needed.

Palliative Care Curricula

Professionals may not have the requisite knowledge and skills to provide care in an ethically grounded and clinically competent manner.[1,12] Although education is improving, studies documenting the effectiveness of specific models and content are sparse. Innovative models of teaching and learning must be evaluated and disseminated. To capture the depth of impact of these methods, novel models for evaluating the impact on health care professionals and their patients and families will need to be devised. Interdisciplinary research teams that include parents can use, evaluate, and disseminate family-centered, experiential palliative care curricula such as IPPC.[20] Educational programs that offer interdisciplinary teams the opportunity to reflect on their experiences in caring for dying children and their families and to assess the effect on their own emotional and spiritual well-being and quality of care are promising. Collaborative research models are necessary to assess the impact of these interventions on important individual and patient and family outcomes.

Similar to other areas of pediatric palliative care research, interventions should be developed with preliminary data supporting their efficacy before being subjected to randomized trials. A particular challenge is to identify outcome measures that authentically reflect the lived experience of patients, families, and professionals and can capture the complex interplay of intellectual, emotional, and spiritual dynamics.

Methods for Systems Integration

Anticipating the possibility of dying for children living with life-threatening conditions is challenging. We need to develop methods for earlier integration of palliative care processes and interventions and to evaluate these interventions on key areas such as earlier pain and symptom management, ongoing communication about goals of care, advance care planning, quality of life, and holistic emotional, psychosocial, and spiritual support.[7]

REFERENCES

1. Institute of Medicine, Field MJ, Behrman DE. When Children Die: Improving Palliative and End-of-Life Care for Children and Their Families. Washington, DC: National Academies Press, 2003.
2. Browning DM, Solomon MZ. Relational learning in pediatric palliative care: Transformative education and the culture of medicine. Child Adolesc Psychiatr Clin N Am 2006;15:795-815.
3. Sahler OJ, Frager G, Levetown M, et al. Medical education about end-of-life care in the pediatric setting: Principles, challenges, and opportunities. Pediatrics 2000;105:575-584.
4. Rushton CH, Williams MA, Sabatier KH. The integration of palliative care and critical care: One vision, one voice. Crit Care Nurs Clin North Am 2002; 14:133-140.
5. Carter BS, Howenstein M, Gilmer MJ, et al. Circumstances surrounding the deaths of hospitalized children: Opportunities for pediatric palliative care. Pediatrics 2004;114:e361-e366.
6. Mack JW, Wolfe J. Early integration of pediatric palliative care: For some children, palliative care starts at diagnosis. Curr Opin Pediatr 2006;18:10-14.
7. Halifax J, Dossey B, Rushton C. Compassionate Care of the Dying: An Integral Approach. Sante Fe, NM: Prajna Mountain Publishers, 2006.
8. Rushton C, Reder E, Comello K, et al. Evaluation of the effectiveness of an interdisciplinary intervention to reduce suffering in professionals who care for dying children. J Palliat Med 2006;9:925.
9. Pronovost P, Berenholtz S, Dorman T, et al. Improving communication in the ICU using daily goals. J Crit Care 2003;18:71-75.
10. Hays RM, Haynes G, Geyer JR, Feudtner C. Communication at the end of life. In Carter B, Levetown M (eds). Palliative Care for Infants, Children, and Adolescents: A Practical Handbook. Baltimore: Johns Hopkins University Press, 2004, pp 112-140.
11. Rushton CH. The other side of caring: Caregiver suffering. In Carter B, Levetown M (eds). Palliative Care for Infants, Children, and Adolescents: A Practical Handbook. Baltimore: Johns Hopkins University Press, 2004, pp 220-243.
12. Solomon MZ, Sellers DE, Heller KS, et al. New and lingering controversies in pediatric end-of-life care. Pediatrics 2005;116:872-883.
13. Papadatou D. A proposed model of health care professionals' grieving process. Omega (Westport) 2000;31:59-77.
14. Kalvemark S, Hoglund AT, Hansson MG, et al. Living with conflicts: Ethical dilemmas and moral distress in the health care system. Soc Sci Med 2004; 58:1075-1084.
15. Burns JP, Mitchell C, Outwater KM, et al. End-of-life care in the pediatric intensive care unit after the forgoing of life-sustaining treatment. Crit Care Med 2000;28:3060-3066.
16. Burns JP, Mitchell C, Griffith JL, Truog RD. End-of-life care in the pediatric intensive care unit: Attitudes and practices of pediatric critical care physicians and nurses. Crit Care Med 2001;29:658-664.
17. Burns JP, Rushton CH. End-of-life care in the pediatric intensive care unit: Research review and recommendations. Crit Care Clin 2004;20:467-485.
18. Meyer EC, Burns JP, Griffith JL, Truog RD. Parental perspectives on end-of-life care in the pediatric intensive care unit. Crit Care Med 2002;30:226-231.
19. American Association of Critical Care Nurses. Moral Distress Position Statement. Aliso Viejo, CA: American Association of Critical Care Nurses, 2004.
20. Browning DM, Solomon MZ. The initiative for pediatric palliative care: An interdisciplinary educational approach for healthcare professionals. J Pediatr Nurs 2005;20:326-334.

SUGGESTED READING

American Association of Critical Care Nurses. AACN Standards for Establishing and Sustaining Healthy Work Environments. Aliso Viejo, CA: American Association of Critical Care Nurses, 2005.

Hanna DR. Moral distress: The state of the science. Res Theory Nurs Pract 2004;18:73-93.

Oberle K, Hughes D. Doctors' and nurses' perceptions of ethical problems in end-of-life decisions. J Adv Nurs 2001; 33:707-715.

CHAPTER **201**

Parent and Child Bereavement

Grace Christ and **Sherri Weisenfluh**

K E Y   P O I N T S

- Clinicians can play an important role in helping children to cope during a family member's terminal illness and after the death.

- Children benefit from carefully dosed information that explains what they see and hear, information that is realistic, but optimistic, especially assuring them of continued safety and care.

- Children do grieve, but differently from adults and in ways shaped by their developmental attributes.

- Children experience grief briefly (compared with adults) interspersed with play and normative activities. They may continue to revisit the loss throughout their development.

- Research supports that bereavement programs, both preparatory and after the death, may affect survivors' recovery from loss.

The death of a parent is among the most stressful events a child can face. The death of a child is a parent's worst nightmare. Research suggests that, with education and preparation, clinicians can help to support bereaved children and their surviving caregiver.

When a parent's death is expected, children are most anguished in the final weeks of the parent's life, whereas their distress declines during the year after the death.[1,2] The terminal illness can be especially stressful for children today because advances in medicine mean that a parent's "final days" may stretch to weeks, months, or even longer. This situation introduces a whole new set of challenges for families and practitioners facing bereavement. When death is expected, the goal of intervention is to reduce traumatic elements for parents and children within the terminal illness process by timely, age-appropriate information, communication, connection, and support.[1,3]

When the patient is a parent, questions often arise about how physicians and other professionals can help families to prepare for the death and how these professionals can aid families in their bereavement after the death. To guide an upcoming workshop on communication with children coping with a parent's illness, the staff of a Gilda's Club asked patients and families to submit questions about their concerns. The following represent the concerns families raise in hospice, palliative care, and active treatment settings:

- Is it normal for kids to think they will catch cancer?
- Is it normal for my child/children to withdraw or be more cautious?
- Is it normal for kids to take out their anger on the parent who doesn't have cancer?
- Is it all right to bring my child to the hospital?
- How much information do I give them about my condition?

- What if my child asks, "Is Mommy/Daddy going to die?"
- How do I know if my children are having difficulty coping?

Over the past 20 years, much research on parent and child bereavement has addressed these concerns. Through direct interviews with children about their reactions to a parent's terminal illness and through parents' reports, we have increased our understanding of the following:

- The nature of children's grief at different development levels[1,4]
- Children's reactions when the parent's death is expected and the trajectory of their recovery after the death[2,5,6]
- The risk factors that impede or slow the children's recovery and thus require evaluation[7,8]
- The protective factors used to develop interventions[9-11]

THE NATURE OF CHILDREN'S GRIEF REACTIONS

Theories of adult psychology once led us to believe that children could not grieve the loss of a parent because of cognitive and emotional immaturity. Another common belief was that the loss of a parent during childhood would likely cause depression in adulthood because of children's supposed inability to grieve in a timely way. Research, in fact, shows that the death of a parent in childhood may have a more limited effect on adult psychopathology than hypothesized.[12,13]

Children do indeed experience grief, sadness, and despair after a parent's death, but how they experience and express mourning is based largely on developmental attributes often puzzling to adults. The following characteristics of children's (versus adults') grief are common across developmental levels:

- Children experience grief intermittently and for shorter periods than adults do, and these periods are usually followed by using play or other activities to distract themselves from the pain. This back and forth is normative.
- Children do best when they receive information in careful doses over time in ways that match what they see and hear, rather than during one conversation.
- Children revisit their thoughts and feelings about the relationship with the lost parent throughout development, into adulthood, and at moments of achievement and stress.[1] This periodic reflection appears to be integrative, although children can go through periods of distress about the loss many years later.

Children experience their greatest depression and anxiety during the parent's terminal illness, rather than after the death, so it is important to intervene with the family during the terminal phase to reduce children's anxiety and to reassure them that they and the surviving parent are safe.[1,2,11]

Symptoms and Behaviors Reflecting Children's Grief

Most bereaved children show a broad range of emotional and behavioral disturbances that reflect their distress during the parent's terminal illness and after the death. These include anxiety, fears, angry outbursts, sleep disorders, social withdrawal, academic difficulties, and regression in developmental milestones. Parents and professionals often fail to recognize these signs as expressions of grief because they are shaped by the child's stage of development, and the connection between the death and the child's responses is less obvious than in adults.

Healing Children's Grief: Surviving a Parent's Death from Cancer[4] contains a comprehensive description of children's responses shaped by developmental attributes. A qualitative analysis of interviews with 88 families and 157 bereaved children revealed that much of children's behavior also reflected an effort to cope with dramatic family changes caused by illness and loss. For example, they asked, "Who will teach me math? Who will braid my hair?" Other studies found that the relationship with the surviving parent or caregiver and other aspects of the environment after the death are as important in explaining children's short-term and longer-term responses as the loss itself.[13-15]

Although bereaved children not infrequently have mild depression, most cases of depression do not reach a clinical or pathological level. The severity of bereaved children's depression is less than that in a comparison population of nonbereaved children in a psychiatric outpatient clinic. Fifteen to 20% of bereaved children across studies had symptoms requiring mental health evaluation.[5,6,16,17] Such symptoms and behaviors in bereaved children decline approximately 6 months after the death and continue improving over the next 18 months. Because children's symptoms and behaviors have not been assessed for longer than 2 years after the parent's death, later effects and delayed grief in children have not been addressed.

Concurrent Symptoms and Disorders

Concurrent symptoms and disorders, such as generalized anxiety disorder and posttraumatic stress disorder and depression, were thought uncommon in bereaved children. However, more recent studies found that these disorders are present in many children after a parent dies in traumatic circumstances, such as a terrorist attack, suicide, or homicide.[18,19] These findings highlight the importance of continued research on the impact of death circumstances on children and families and the need for effective interventions for complex and traumatic situations. Families that experience sudden loss have limited access to bereavement services, partly because they have no prior interaction with appropriate professionals who could refer them for such services. Many hospices now offer bereavement services for sudden loss as a fulfillment of their community service standard.

PSYCHOSOCIAL RISK FACTORS

Some conditions increase children's risk of adverse psychological outcomes:

- Additional previous or current stresses in the bereaved child or family are categorized as *complex bereavement*.[16] These include death by homicide or suicide, other family illnesses or deaths, previous separations or losses (e.g., divorce, adoption, a caregiver's mental illness), or preexisting mental problems in the child or adolescent. The presence of at least one of these additional substantial stresses is associated with a slower decline in children's psychological symptoms after a parent's death.
- Increased negative life events after a parent's death are associated with increased mental problems in the children.[20,21]
- Family socioeconomic status is also associated with a child's functioning. Families with limited financial resources often have additional stresses from forced changes in residence and school and from less favorable care arrangements. These changes create additional adaptive challenges for both parents and children, especially when the death further reduces a family's resources.[16]
- The child's relationship with the surviving parent or caregiver affects the child's bereavement experience.[5,8,9,22,23] Therefore, interventions that improve the surviving parent's mental health, parenting competence, and communication with the child are critical for reducing the child's symptoms.
- Parent-guidance interventions that include teaching coping skills to children improve parental function and parent-child communication.[7,10,24,25]

PSYCHOSOCIAL PROTECTIVE FACTORS

Factors that promote children's recovery after a parent's death and protect them from adverse consequences include the following (some of which are goals of bereavement interventions):

- The relationship with a surviving parent or caregiver is characterized by open communication, warmth, and positive experiences.[7,9]
- The surviving parent sustains parenting competence by learning how to recognize and respond to the children's grief, maintaining consistency in child care and in the children's environment, and supporting the children's continued development.[22,24,25]
- The child feels accepted by peers and other adults, such as relatives and teachers, and maintains self-esteem.[6,26,27]
- Adequate financial resources are available.
- Personal characteristics, such as intellectual and social competence, help.
- The opportunity to express thoughts and feelings about the deceased parent and to have them validated by others is associated with improved outcome.[7,10,25,28]
- The child or parent has no antecedent mental health factors.

BEREAVEMENT INTERVENTIONS IN PALLIATIVE MEDICINE AND HOSPICE

Children and families require two types of psychosocial intervention: (1) those during the parent or child's terminal illness and at the death and (2) those after the death.

Preparation

The goal of interventions before the death is to help parents to communicate appropriately with each child about the illness, to arrange effective and timely visits during long hospitalizations, to resolve conflicts from additional caregiving tasks, to reduce anxiety about the patient's medical condition and expected death, and to increase the family's confidence in its ability to cope. To maintain parents and children through what may be a long and crisis-filled illness, families need education, information, support, and case management. The crises and sudden changes can be traumatic for children, who cope best when (in addition to carefully designed doses of information) they are reassured about the family's support and continued care. For example, younger children may blame themselves for a disease recurrence if the cause is not clarified, or they may fear abandonment if both parents are distraught.

Preparatory interventions help parents to reduce unnecessary stress from children's misunderstandings, to reassure the children about safety, to facilitate their acceptance of the fact that one cannot control uncontrollable events, and to support their self-esteem and belief in their capacity to cope. By including children judiciously in ongoing discussions, the strength of the family circle will help them feel supported.[29] Excluding them from all such discussions is likely to make them feel shut out and alone. As one 7-year-old child said, "There are secrets in this family. I don't feel part of this family anymore. Families shouldn't have secrets."

Services during the illness should be integrated with the entity providing medical care because most families need help in coping with the patient's condition and medical treatment. Mental health professionals need to be familiar with the medical treatment and its challenges, and, conversely, medical providers benefit from close communication with mental health professionals, who provide psychosocial support. Families with young children may not use community resources because additional caregiving tasks make it difficult to find the time and emotional energy to connect to yet another community organization or system, except when such resources are needed in cases of severe mental illness.

One anticipatory intervention model for children with a terminally ill parent was evaluated within a major cancer center.[24,30] The goal of the parent-guidance intervention was to enhance parents' abilities to provide their children with support and a consistent, stable environment in which children would feel comfortable to express feelings both before and after the death. In addition, families were helped to obtain services outside the institution as needed, usually for short-term medication.

Beginning during the parent's illness, the model provided up to five low-intensity sessions with the well parent and children and up to an additional five sessions after the ill parent's death. Trends suggested that the children who participated in the program exhibited fewer mental health problems and improved self-esteem compared with children in the control group. According to children's assessments, communication with the surviving caregiver also improved significantly in the families participating in the program. Clinicians recognized families' multiple service needs and functioned at times as consultants and coordinators who could facilitate appropriate access to and use of services, while continuing to provide families with direct support, psychoeducation, consultation, and parent guidance. The intervention was well accepted by both the treating physicians and the families.

Services after the Death of a Family Member

Children who experience a family death are at risk for several negative consequences. Consequently, families also need access to bereavement and mental health services after the death.[5,8,23,31] By definition, parents with young children are likely to be young themselves. Thus, the death is untimely, and they are at risk for psychological adversity. Because the surviving caregiver is so important to children's adaptation, interventions have focused on guidance to parents in multiple family groups or to individual families.

One experimental trial of 12 concurrent group sessions included 156 families recruited from the community who had sought mental health services after a parent's death.[10] Unlike bereaved children in other samples, the children in these families exhibited severe symptoms before the study. At the end of the intervention, the investigators documented improved mental health among the girls, improved parenting, fewer negative events, and less inhibition of emotional expression among both boys and girls.

Typically, parents request and find helpful the following bereavement services:

- Repeated assessments of their children's functioning and behavior can identify needs for more intensive interventions.
- Education and counseling can help parents to understand grief in both children and adults and the impact of developmental level in children, to identify age-appropriate mourning rituals, and to understand the reactions of particular children and the possible long-term consequences of those reactions.
- Resources that will directly help the child, such as printed materials, individual and group bereavement programs, activity groups, mentoring programs, and camps, are helpful. Vital resources are often available in the schools.
- Access to resources to help them manage the family (e.g., child care, housekeeping services, and financial consultation and assistance) is useful.
- Access at various stages of recovery to referrals for ongoing counseling for themselves and for children with identified symptoms is needed.

Children are embedded in multiple social interaction systems (e.g., nuclear and extended family, school, peers, neighborhood). Therefore, services for children and adolescents should target multiple protective processes simultaneously, to increase therapeutic benefits.[32]

Increasingly, the following interventions are developed within schools and communities:

- Family loss groups often include children experiencing divorce, a parent's death, and other losses.

- Individual counseling can be a resource for a bereaved child at times of emotional distress or in need of ongoing support.
- Bereavement programs offer activity groups to educate, normalize, destigmatize, and facilitate integration.
- Community-sponsored bereavement camps offer children opportunities for normalization and destigmatization by increasing their skills in communicating the loss to other children (who have experienced the same situation) and by being encouraged to express themselves openly. Most important, the camps offer pleasurable skill-developing activities that emphasize the continuity of life and permit positive experiences during bereavement.
- Schools and community agencies may offer art and music therapy to facilitate children's grief expression.

ORGANIZATIONAL SUPPORT FOR BEREAVEMENT COUNSELING

Bereavement counseling for families is an essential component of hospice care for the first year after the death, but such services are not reimbursed through the Medicare Hospice Benefit. These programs often depend on volunteers, fund raising, donations, and memorial contributions to cover additional costs. Bereavement programs have sometimes been the "poor step-child" of hospice services. Palliative care programs and active treatment centers constantly seek fiscally viable approaches to the psychosocial support services that families are requesting more frequently during the illness and after the death.[33]

Standard and Enriched Hospice Bereavement Program Models

No state or federal standards exist in the United States for what constitutes a bereavement program in a hospice. Surveys of existing programs[34] identified the following services as those used by most hospices:

- Letters or notices about groups and meetings
- Telephone calls by bereavement personnel
- Literature or other materials about grief
- Visits by bereavement personnel
- Memorial services
- Bereavement newsletters
- Children's camps
- Support group meetings
- Holiday grief programs
- Referral to an outside therapist

Additional innovative services in individual hospice programs reflect programs tailored to specific populations, including children (P Homan, personal communication). The following are examples:

- Individual follow-up contacts and risk assessments
- Groups for newly bereaved families separate from those for families beginning 3 or 4 months after the death
- Workshops for families on bereavement-related issues (e.g., journaling, when to begin dating)
- Open groups for loss of a child
- Daytime or evening groups
- A 6-week course on bereavement and reconstitution

- Community bereavement programs for those experiencing sudden loss

SUMMARY

Because medical advances have extended the duration of many terminal illnesses, the preparation of families and the provision of follow-up bereavement care have become increasingly important. Research suggests that lack of preparation can have adverse consequences on both children and adults.[35]

Parents are increasingly concerned about the best ways to help their children to cope with the terminal illness of a family member (including the frequent medical crises), to limit their psychological risk. Although the loss of a parent or other family member is extremely difficult for families and professionals, and interventions are challenging, children can grieve and effectively reconstitute their lives with appropriate mediation and informed caregivers.

Traditionally, bereavement services in the United States have suffered financially in hospices because although such services are required by the Hospice Benefit, they are not reimbursed. Palliative care programs are eager to find effective business models that enable them to fund these much needed services. Expanding early efforts to evaluate the effectiveness of interventions is vital to develop financial support for bereavement services from terminal illness into the trajectory after the family member's death.

REFERENCES

1. Christ G, Christ A. Current approaches to helping children cope with a parent's terminal illness. CA Cancer J Clin 2006;56:197-212.
2. Siegel K, Karus D, Raveis VH. Adjustment of children facing the death of a parent due to cancer. J Am Acad Child Adolesc Psychiatry 1996;35:442-450.
3. Saldinger A, Cain A, Porterfield K. Managing traumatic stress in children anticipating parental death. Psychiatry 2003;66:168-181.
4. Christ G. Healing Children's Grief: Surviving a Parent's Death from Cancer. New York: Oxford University Press, 2000.
5. Dowdney L. Annotation: Childhood bereavement following parental death. J Child Psychol Psychiatry 2000;41:819-920.
6. Worden J. Parental death and the adjustment of school-age children. Omega 1996;29:219-230.
7. Raveis V, Siegel K, ••. Children's psychological distress following the death of a parent. J Youth Adolesc 1999;28:165-180.
8. Tremblay GC, Israel AC. Children's adjustment to parental death. Clin Psychol 1998;5:424-438.
9. Kwok OM, Haine RA, Sandler IN, et al. Positive parenting as a mediator of the relations between parental psychological distress and mental health problems of parentally bereaved children. J Clin Child Adolesc Psychol 2005;34:260-271.
10. Sandler I, Ayers T, Wolchik S, et al. The family bereavement program: Efficacy evaluation of a theory-based prevention program for parentally bereaved children and adolescents. J Consult Clin Psychol 2003;71:587-600.
11. Siegel K, Mesagno FP, Christ G. A preventive program for bereaved children. Am J Orthopsychiatry 1990;60:168-175.
12. Crook T, Eliot J. Parental death during childhood and adult depression: A critical review of the literature. Psychol Bull 1980;87:252-259.
13. Saler L, Skolnick N. Childhood parental death and depression in adulthood: Roles of surviving parent and family environment. Am J Orthopsychiatry 1992;62:504-516.
14. Elizur E, Kaffman M. Factors influencing the severity of childhood bereavement reactions. Am J Orthopsychiatry 1983;53:668-676.
15. Harris T, Brown GW, Bifulco A. Loss of parent in childhood and adult psychiatric disorder: The role of lack of adequate parental care. Psychol Med 1986;16:641-659.
16. Cerel J, Fristad MA, Verducci J, et al. Childhood bereavement: Psychopathology in the 2 years postparental death. J Am Acad Child Adolesc Psychiatry 2006;45:683-690.
17. Siegel K, Mesagno FP, Karus D, et al. Psychosocial adjustment of children with a terminally ill parent. J Am Acad Child Adolesc Psychiatry 1992;31:327-333.

18. Cerel J, Fristed MA, Weller EB, Weller RA. Suicide-bereaved children and adolescents: A controlled longitudinal examination. J Am Acad Child Adolesc Psychiatry 1999;38:672-679.

19. Pfeffer C, Altemus M, Heo M, Jiang H. Salivary cortisol and psychopathology in children bereaved by the September 11, 2001 terror attacks. Biol Psychiatry 2007;61:957-965.

20. Sandler I, Reynolds K, Kliewer W, Ramirez R. Specificity of the relation between life events and psychological symptomatology. J Clin Child Psychol 1992;21:240-248.

21. Thompson MP, Kaslow NJ, Price AN, et al. Role of secondary stressors in the parental death–child distress relation. J Abnorm Child Psychol 1998;26: 357-366.

22. Haine RA, Wolchick SA, Sandler IN, et al. Positive parenting as a protective resource for parentally bereaved children. Death Stud 2006;30:1-28.

23. Lutzke J, Ayers T. Risks and interventions for the parentally bereaved child. In Wolchik S, Sandler I (eds). Handbook of Children's Coping: Linking Theory and Intervention. New York: Plenum Press, 1997, pp 215-243.

24. Christ G, Siegel K, Raveis V, et al. Evaluation of a bereavement intervention. J Soc Work End Life Palliat Care 2005;1:57-81.

25. Siegel K, Raveis V. Patterns of communication with children when a parent has cancer. In Cooper C, Baider L, Kaplan-De-Nour A (eds). Cancer and the Family. New York: John Wiley & Sons, 1996, pp 109-128.

26. Haine RA, Ayers TS, Sandler IN, et al. Locus of control and self-esteem as stress-moderators or stress-mediators in parentally bereaved children. Death Stud 2003;27:619-640.

27. Siegel K, Raveis V. Correlates of self-esteem among children facing the loss of a parent to cancer. In Cooper C, Baider L, Kaplan-De-Nour A (eds). Cancer and the Family. Chichester, UK: John Wiley & Sons, 2000, pp 223-237.

28. Silverman P, Worden W. Children's reactions in the early months after the death of a parent. Am J Orthopsychiatry 1992;62:93-104.

29. Saldinger A, Cain AC, Porterfield K, Lohnes K. Facilitating attachment between school-aged children and a dying parent. Death Stud 2004;28:915-940.

30. Christ GH, Siegel K, Mesagno FP, Langosch D. A preventive intervention program for bereaved children: Problems of implementation. Am J Orthopsychiatry 1991;61:168-178.

31. Reinherz HZ, Giaconia R, Hauf AM, et al. Major depression in the transition to adulthood: Risks and impairments. J Abnorm Psychol 1999;108:500-510.

32. Masten A, Hubbard J, Gest SD, et al. Competence in the context of adversity: Pathways to resilience and maladaptation from childhood to late adolescence. Dev Psychopathol 1999;11:143-169.

33. Rathbun A, Denham S, McCarthy C. The Ohio hospice bereavement study: Meeting HNPCO standards. Am J Hosp Palliat Care 2003;20:448-458.

34. Demmer C. A national survey of hospice bereavement services. Omega 2003; 47:327-341.

35. Hebert R, Prigerson H, Schulz R, Arnold R. Preparing caregivers for the death of a loved one: A theoretical framework and suggestions for future research. J Palliat Med 2006;9:1167-1171.

SUGGESTED READING

Worden J. Children and Grief: When a Parent Dies. New York: Guilford Press, 1996.

Geriatrics

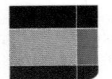

CHAPTER **202**

Demographics of Aging

Armida G. Parala

DEMOGRAPHIC TRENDS

The world's population is aging quickly. Globally, the older population (those ≥65 years of age) is growing by 2% each year, faster than the population as a whole.[1] The elderly were estimated to number 673 million worldwide in 2005 and are expected to reach 2 billion by 2050.[2] Among the older population, the oldest-old (≥85 years) is the fastest growing segment, increasing by 3.8% per year.[1] They will constitute 20% of the world's population by 2050. The number of centenarians (≥100 years) will increase from approximately 287,000 in 2006 to 3.7 million by 2050.[1]

The aging population of Europe and North America has been well reported. However, the greatest increase is in developing countries, particularly Asia, Latin America, and the Caribbean. Europe has the highest proportion of elderly, who will constitute more than 25% of its population by 2050 (Table 202-1). In the United States, the baby boomers (individuals born between 1946 and 1964) will be part of the older population by 2011, and this age group will dramatically increase through the middle of the 21st century.

In 2005, the median age worldwide was 28 years; it was predicted to reach 38 years by 2050.[2] Europe is the oldest region in the world, with a median age of 37 years, expected to increase to 47 years by 2050. The country with the oldest population in 2005 was Japan, with a median age of 43 years. However, by 2050, Asia will be the oldest region, and China will have the oldest population for a single country (Table 202-2).

LIFE EXPECTANCY

The population age is increasing due to lower birth and mortality rates worldwide. Global life expectancy is currently 66 years. People in developed countries have a higher life expectancy than those in developing regions (Fig. 202-1). In the United States, life expectancy at age 65 is 17.1 years for males and 20 years for females.[3] In the least developed countries, the life expectancies for men and women are 75 and 77 years, respectively. There are more women within the elderly population (Fig. 202-2), because their life expectancy is typically longer. Among the oldest-old, 64% are women.

DEPENDENCY RATIO

A major socioeconomic impact of population aging is the increased old-age dependency ratio. This is the number of older persons (≥65 years) per 100 working-age persons (age 15-64 years) (Fig. 202-3). Europe has the highest old-age dependency ratio—it was 23 in 2005 and is projected to reach 48 by 2050. According to the 2006 Revision of the World Population Prospects, the significant increase in the elderly population will reverse the young-to-old population ratio. Africa is the only major region where this reversal will not be evident because of the high number of young people. The age ratio reversal raises serious economic concerns; social and financial restructuring are required to prepare for the effects of the demographic shift.

MORTALITY

Death rates around the world are declining, and there is a remarkable change in mortality distribution, because most deaths now occur among the elderly.[4] The most common causes of death vary by economic regions (Table 202-3). In the United States and other developed countries, where life expectancy is high, chronic diseases and cancer are the most common killers. Alzheimer's disease is among the top 10 causes of death in high-income countries. In middle- and low-income countries, human immunodeficiency virus/acquired immunodeficiency syndrome is a common cause of mortality.

TABLE 202-1 Percentage of the Elderly Population (≥65 Years), by Region						
YEAR	**AFRICA**	**ASIA**	**EUROPE**	**LATIN AMERICA AND THE CARIBBEAN**	**NORTH AMERICA**	**OCEANIA***
1950	3.3	4.1	8.2	3.5	8.2	7.3
1975	3.2	4.1	11.5	4.2	10.3	7.3
2000	3.3	5.8	14.7	5.7	12.3	9.8
2025	4.2	10.1	20.7	10.3	18.1	15.1
2050	6.9	17.5	27.6	18.5	21.5	19.4

*Oceania includes Australia/New Zealand, Melanesia, Polynesia, and Micronesia.
From United Nations Population Division, World Population Prospects: The 2006 Revision. Available at http://www.un.org/esa/population/publications/wpp2006/WPP2006_Highlights_rev.pdf (accessed February 19, 2008).

TABLE 202-2 Countries with the Oldest Populations, 2005 and 2050

2005	2050
1. Japan	1. China, Macao SAR
2. Germany	2. Japan
3. Italy	3. Republic of Korea
4. Finland	4. Singapore
5. Bulgaria	5. Martinique
6. Croatia	6. Poland
7. Belgium	7. Bulgaria
8. Sweden	8. Slovenia
9. Slovenia	9. China, Hong Kong SAR
10. Switzerland	10. Cuba

From United Nations Population Division, World Population Prospects: The 2006 Revision. Available at http://www.un.org/esa/population/publications/wpp2006/WPP2006_Highlights_rev.pdf (accessed February 19, 2008).

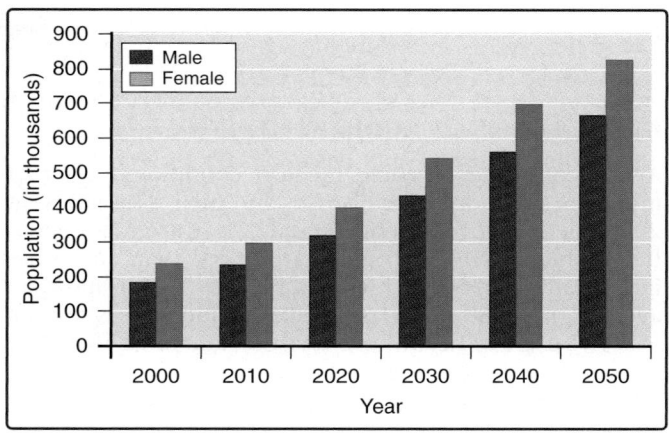

FIGURE 202-2 Global elderly population (≥65 years) by gender, 2000-2050. *(From United Nations Population Division. World Population Prospects: The 2006 Revision. Available at http://www.un.org/esa/population/publications/wpp2006/WPP2006_Highlights_rev.pdf [accessed February 19, 2008].)*

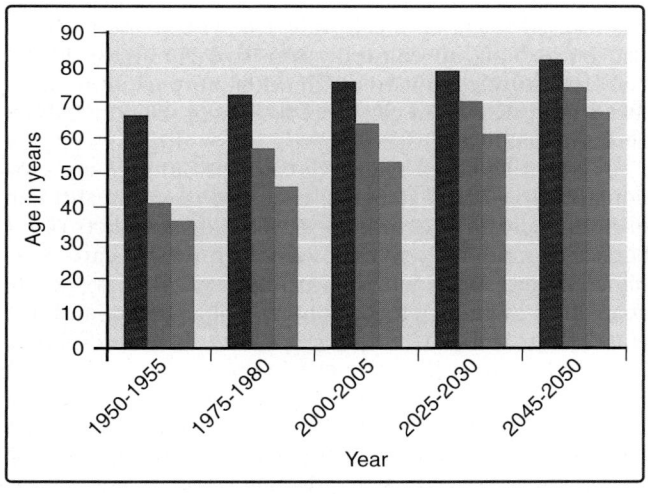

FIGURE 202-1 Life expectancy in different economic regions of the world, 1950-2050. *(From United Nations Population Division. World Population Prospects: The 2006 Revision. Available at http://www.un.org/esa/population/publications/wpp2006/WPP2006_Highlights_rev.pdf [accessed February 19, 2008].)*

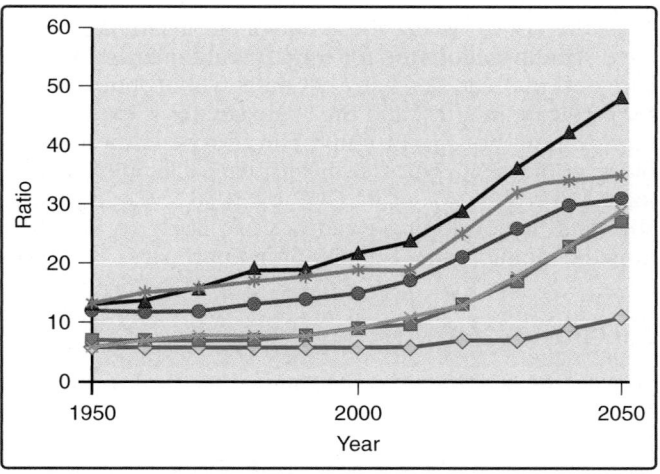
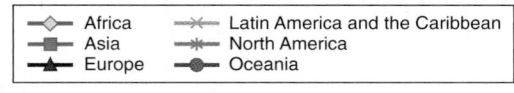

FIGURE 202-3 Old-age dependency ratio in different regions of the world. Number of older persons (age ≥65 years) per 100 working-age persons (age 15-64 years). *(From United Nations Population Division. From World Population Prospects: The 2006 Revision. Available at http://www.un.org/esa/population/publications/wpp2006/WPP2006_Highlights_rev.pdf [accessed February 19, 2008].)*

TABLE 202-3 Leading Causes of Death, by Broad Income Groups, 2002

HIGH-INCOME COUNTRIES	MIDDLE-INCOME COUNTRIES	LOW-INCOME COUNTRIES
1. Coronary heart disease	1. Stroke and other cerebrovascular diseases	1. Coronary heart disease
2. Stroke and other cerebrovascular diseases	2. Coronary heart disease	2. Lower respiratory infections
3. Trachea, bronchus, lung cancers	3. Chronic obstructive pulmonary disease	3. HIV/AIDS
4. Lower respiratory infections	4. Lower respiratory infection	4. Perinatal conditions
5. Chronic obstructive pulmonary disease	5. HIV/AIDS	5. Stroke and other cerebrovascular diseases
6. Colon and rectum cancers	6. Perinatal conditions	6. Diarrheal diseases
7. Alzheimer and other dementias	7. Stomach cancer	7. Malaria
8. Diabetes mellitus	8. Trachea, bronchus, and lung cancer	8. Tuberculosis
9. Breast cancer	9. Road traffic accidents	9. Chronic obstructive pulmonary disease
10. Stomach cancer	10. Hypertensive heart disease	10. Road traffic accidents

From World Health Organization. Fact Sheet No. 310, February 2007. Available at http://www.who.int/mediacentre/factsheets/fs310/en/ (accessed February 19, 2008).

IMPLICATIONS OF AGING IN HEALTH CARE

Age accompanies chronic medical conditions. A lot of money is spent on these diseases and their disabilities. In 2004, the U.S. government allotted 16% of its gross domestic product (GDP) to health care, more than any other industrialized nation. This amounted to $1.9 trillion, an average of $6280 per person.[5] Elderly individuals are the heaviest users of health care services, and more than 75% of U.S. health care expenditures are for treatment of chronic diseases.[6] A huge percentage of elderly health care spending is on prescription medications, physician visits, hospitalizations, and long-term care. In America, the average 75-year-old person has three chronic illnesses and is taking at least five prescription medications.[7] Chronic and degenerative conditions produce functional decline. This makes the cost of care for the elderly 3 to 5 times higher than for someone younger than 65 years of age.[8] Medical expenditures are also greater in the last year of life. Over the last 20 years, these end-of-life health care costs have steadily accounted for more than a quarter of Medicare outlays.[9] The first baby boomers will become eligible for Medicare in 2011, and the United States is expected to face a significant increase in medical expenditures for its older population. The U.S. health care allocation is projected to reach 25% of its GDP by 2030.[10] Rapidly aging societies in developing countries are likely to have the same economic issues but less time to prepare.

PALLIATIVE CARE AND AGING

Longer life expectancy and advanced medical technology have brought palliative care to the forefront in public health.[11] Technological advances in developed countries have led to delayed, expensive deaths, which have a heavy financial toll on society and individuals. In the United States, the use of expensive inpatient services has not decreased in the last year of life, even though more deaths are occurring outside of hospitals. Ironically, additional spending has not sustained life or provided a better quality of life for most frail elderly. Likewise, use of more hospital resources and physician services did not improve health or patient satisfaction.[12] Although most terminally ill patients hope for a dignified, pain-free death with their family,[13] many suffer in their last days[14] and receive futile and invasive treatments.[15] This has caused patients and their families profound suffering throughout the dying process.[14] Because quality of life and of death has now become an important societal concern, the older population needs to be educated about the choices and services available in serious illness, such as advance directives, palliative care, and hospice services.

Fundamental strides should be taken to increase awareness of the public health community about palliative care. Educating both patients and families by access to information will assist informed discourse and decisions.[10,11] Because most physicians are ill prepared,[14,16] efforts should be continued to incorporate palliative medicine education in the medical curriculum.[16] It is imperative for students to learn the importance of palliative care in the preclinical years. Postgraduate programs should also make it mandatory for trainees to learn relevant palliative medicine skills[16] and make end-of-life discussion a routine health care intervention.[17] In our ethnically diverse world, there should also be a focus on culturally sensitive communication,[11] because attitudes toward death differ among cultures, and these attitudes influence perceptions, experiences, and decision making.[18]

Discussions about palliative care are difficult, are emotionally demanding and take time; no single health care professional can successfully undertake all aspects of it.[17] Education and involvement of other health care disciplines,[19] particularly nursing, pharmacy, social work, and chaplaincy, will provide a holistic, coordinated, and integrated approach toward palliative care. Multidisciplinary, comprehensive palliative medicine programs will address the many needs of chronically ill elderly patients and their families.[20] Collaboration of palliative medicine with other medical subspecialties in the care of chronically and terminally ill patients will promote good symptom control, increased family satisfaction,[21] and lower hospital costs.[21,22]

Most chronically ill patients in developing regions experience pain and suffering when dying because they have no access to quality palliative care. In 1990, the World Health Organization (WHO) initiated a public health strategy to integrate palliative medicine into existing health systems of resource-poor countries.[23] Few coun-

Future Considerations

- Easily accessible information for patients and families
- Education and training of medical students, physicians, and other medical health professionals in palliative care
- Development and integration of palliative medicine into all health systems worldwide
- Encouragement of research and funding to improve palliative care
- Development of global public health policies and strategies to improve access, delivery, financing, and implementation of cost-effective, quality palliative medicine in both developed and developing regions

tries have successfully followed the recommendations. For the WHO strategy to be effective, governments should incorporate it at all levels of their health system, and it should be owned by the community,[24] so it can be tailored to local cultural practices, beliefs, and socioeconomic situations. Policy and system changes should be instituted to develop infrastructure, provide money, and make the necessary palliative drugs, such as opioids, affordable and available. To ensure compliance and maintain standards, the WHO should develop quality indicators and health system performance measures to monitor palliative care delivery.[25] Governmental and nongovernmental groups should work together to improve advocacy and advance palliative medicine. Further research and funding are needed to address health care gaps in care of the dying.[11,17,19,25]

Dying, just like aging, is universal. We must improve access, delivery, and financing of quality palliative care in various settings,[19,25] including hospitals, homes, and long-term care facilities, worldwide (see "Future Considerations").

REFERENCES

1. United Nations. World Ageing: 1950-2050. Available at http://www.un.org/esa/population/publications/worldageing19502050/ (accessed February 19, 2008).
2. United Nations Population Division. World Population Prospects: The 2006 Revision. Available at http://www.un.org/esa/population/publications/wpp2006/WPP2006_Highlights_rev.pdf (accessed February 19, 2008).
3. National Center for Health Statistics. Health, United States, 2007. Available at http://www.cdc.gov/nchs/hus.htm (accessed February 19, 2008).
4. World Health Organization. Fact Sheet. Available at http://www.who.int/mediacentre/factsheets/fs310.pdf
5. Smith C, Cowan C, Heffler S, et al. National health spending in 2004: Recent slowdown led by prescription drug spending. Health Aff (Millwood) 2006;25(1):186-196.
6. Hoffman C, Rice D, Sung HY. Persons with chronic conditions: Their prevalence and costs. JAMA 1996;276:1473-1479.
7. The State of Aging and Health in America 2004. Available at http://www.agingsociety.org/agingsociety/pdf/SAHA_2004.pdf (accessed February 19, 2008).
8. Centers for Disease Control and Prevention. Public health and aging: Trends in aging—United States and worldwide. MMWR Morb Mortal Wkly Rep 2003;52:101-106.
9. Hogan C, Lunney J, Gabel J, et al. Medicare beneficiaries' costs of care in the last year of life. Health Aff (Millwood) 2001;20(4):188-195.
10. Centers for Disease Control and Prevention. The State of Aging and Health in America 2007 Report. Available at http://www.cdc.gov/aging/saha.htm (accessed February 19, 2008).
11. Rao JK, Anderson LA, Smith SM. End of life is a public health issue. Am J Prev Med 2002;23:215-220.
12. The Care of Patients with Severe Chronic Illness: A Report on the Medicare Program by the Dartmouth Atlas Project. Available at http://www.dartmouthatlas.org/atlases/2006_Atlas_Exec_Summary.pdf (accessed February 19, 2008).
13. Steinhauser KE, Christakis NA, Clipp EC, et al. Factors considered important at the end of life by patients, family, physicians, and other care providers. JAMA 2000;284:2476-2482.
14. SUPPORT Principal Investigators. A controlled trial to improve care for seriously ill hospitalized patients. JAMA 1995;274:1591-1598.
15. Ahronheim JC, Morrison RS, Baskin SA, el al. Treatment of the dying in the acute care hospital: Advanced dementia and metastatic cancer. Arch Intern Med 1996;156:2094-2100.
16. Sullivan AM, Lakoma MD, Block SD. The status of medical education in end-of-life care: A national report. J Gen Intern Med 2003;18:685-695.
17. Larson DG, Tobin DR. End-of-life conversations: Evolving practice and theory. JAMA 2000;284:1573-1578.
18. Kwak J, Haley WE. Current research findings on end-of-life decision making among racially or ethnically diverse groups. Gerontologist 2005;45:634-641.
19. Reb AM. Palliative and end-of-life care: Policy analysis. Oncol Nurs Forum 2003;30:35-50.
20. Walsh D. The Harry R. Horvitz Center for Palliative Medicine (1987-1999): Development of a novel comprehensive integrated program. Am J Hosp Palliat Care 2001;18:239-250.
21. Byock I, Twohig JS, Merriman M, et al. Promoting excellence in end-of-life care: A report on innovative models of palliative care. J Palliat Med 2006;9:137-151.
22. Penrod JD, Deb P, Luhrs C, et. al. Cost and utilization outcomes of patients receiving hospital-based palliative care consultation. J Palliat Med 2006;9:855-856.
23. Stjernswärd J, Foley KM, Ferris FD. Integrating palliative care into national policies. J Pain Symptom Manage 2007;33:514-520.
24. Stjernswärd J. Palliative care: The public health strategy. J Public Health Policy 2007;28:42-55.
25. Singer PA, Bowman KW. Quality end-of-life care: A global perspective. BMC Palliat Care 2002;1:4.

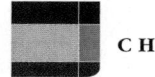

CHAPTER **203**

Biology and Physiology of Aging

Hilary Cronin and Rose Anne Kenny

K E Y   P O I N T S

- Aging results from a gradual amassing of faults in the cells and tissues that contribute to an increased risk of chronic disease and death.
- Advancing age is associated with both structural and functional changes to most systems in the body.
- Renal function decreases at a rate of 1 mL/min per year and needs to be taken into account when prescribing medication.
- Cortical atrophy of the brain has been repeatedly demonstrated with increasing age, and the prevalence of both dementia and delirium increases.

Aging theories attempt to explain why organisms grow old and to identify the processes that affect cells, organs, and biological systems. Aging occurs at multiple levels: social, psychological, physiological, morphological, cellular, and molecular. Sociological and psychological aging differ from, but are connected to, biological aging.

Aging is a subject that resonates throughout history and has been discussed by many philosophers and spiritual leaders. Biological or "pathological" aging remains a dominant research focus, particularly in wealthier countries, and the new area of study could facilitate life-extension technologies. There is no single mechanism of aging; rather, multiple mechanisms, over time, degrade general cellular function and reduce the response to stressors.

Aging results from a gradual amassing of faults in the cells and tissues that contribute to an increased risk of chronic disease and death.

TWO TYPES OF THEORIES OF AGING

(Table 203-1)

1. *Programmed theories (intrinsic):* emphasize that aging follows a biological timetable, perhaps a continuation of the one that regulates childhood growth and development.
2. *Error theories (extrinsic or "stochastic"):* emphasize environmental assaults to biological systems that gradually cause things to go wrong.

Aging is characterized by a gradual decline in organ function reserves, which reduces their ability to maintain homeostasis, especially under stress. In many organs, function loss begins at 30 to 40 years of age and proceeds at a rate of approximately 1% annually.[1] Although this decline appears continuous and irreversible, aging itself does not mean pathology. Without additional pathogenic stimuli, it will not lead to overt disease. Age-related changes pave the way for disease. Aging without disease is often referred to as "normal" or "physiological" aging. In contrast, aging associated with disease is called "abnormal" or "pathological" (Fig. 203-1).

CARDIOVASCULAR SYSTEM

Normal physiological changes occur in the cardiovascular system with advancing age. These changes affect both the structure and the function of the heart as well as the arterial system (Fig. 203-2).

TABLE 203-1	Theories of Aging
SUBTHEORY	**EXPLANATION**
PROGRAMMED THEORIES (INTRINSIC)	
Programmed longevity	Aging results from sequential switching on and off of certain genes, with senescence defined as the time at which age-associated deficits are manifested.
Endocrine theory	Biological clocks act through hormones to control the pace of aging.
Immunological theory	A programmed decline in immune system function leads to an increased vulnerability to infectious disease, aging, and death.
ERROR THEORIES (EXTRINSIC)	
Wear and tear	Cells and tissues have vital parts that wear out.
Rate of living	The greater the organism's rate of oxygen basal metabolism, the shorter its life span.
Cross linking	An accumulation of cross-linked proteins damages cells and tissues, slowing down bodily processes.
Free radicals	Accumulated damage caused by oxygen free radicals causes cells, and eventually organs, to stop functioning.
Somatic DNA damage (genetic mutations)	Genetic mutations occur and accumulate with increasing age, causing cells to deteriorate and malfunction. In particular, damage to mitochondrial DNA might lead to mitochondrial dysfunction.

Cardiac Structure

Cross-sectional echocardiography indicates that left ventricular (LV) wall thickness increases progressively with age, in both males and females, independent of cardiovascular risk factors.[2] There is a progressive loss of myocytes in both ventricles, with a reciprocal increase in myocyte volume. The aging heart has lower myocardial mass due to myocyte cell loss and reactive hypertrophy of the spared myocytes. An increase in the amount and a change in the physical properties of collagen also occur. The

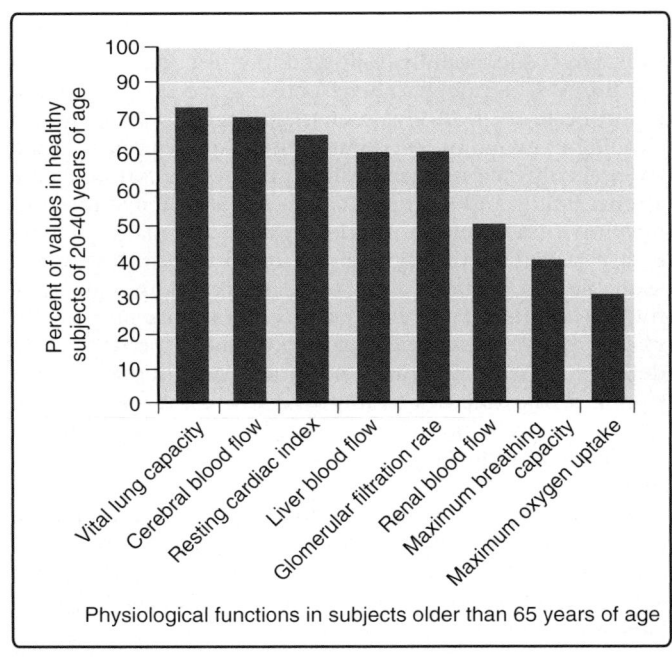

Physiological functions in subjects older than 65 years of age

FIGURE 203-1 Relationship between age and selected functional parameters. *(From Knapowski J, Wieczorowska-Tobis K, Witowski J. Pathophysiology of ageing. J Physiol Pharmacol 2002;53:135-146.)*

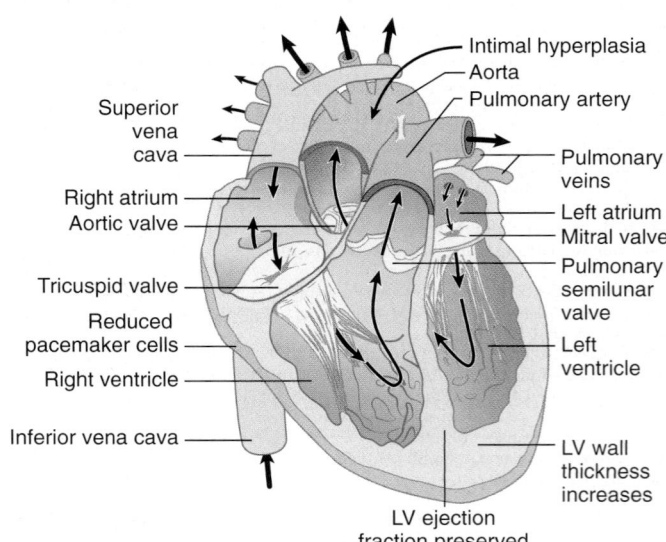

FIGURE 203-2 Cardiovascular changes with advancing age. LV, left ventricular.

number of collagen fibers increases and nonenzymatic cross-linking also increases. The myocyte-collagen ratio remains relatively unchanged, mainly because of increased myocyte size; as a result, hypertrophy rather than hyperplasia is more prominent in elderly persons. These changes increase myocardial stiffness and decrease compliance. With age, the number of pacemaker cells in the sinus node decreases.

Cardiac Function

The LV early-diastolic filling rate progressively decreases to 50% of the peak by 80 years of age. Despite slower LV filling in early diastole, more filling occurs in late diastole, due partly to a more vigorous atrial contraction, which produces an exaggerated A wave. This is accompanied by atrial hypertrophy and enlargement that is evident on auscultation as a fourth heart sound (atrial gallop). The LV end-diastolic volume does not reduce with age, but it does mildly increase while at rest and during upright exercise.

LV ejection fraction is the most common clinical measure of LV systolic function, and it is preserved. However, the maximum LV ejection fraction (the ejection fraction achieved during exhaustive upright exercise) decreases because of a dramatic reduction in ejection fraction reserve during aging. The net result in end-diastolic volume and end-systolic volume regulation during exercise is that the stroke volume index (SVI) is preserved over a wide performance range because of a greater use of the Starling mechanism.

The resting heart rate (HR) does not change with age, but the maximal achievable HR decreases; the maximal HR that an 85-year-old can achieve is about 70% of that of a 20-year-old.[2] Because the stroke volume does not change over time, the maximal cardiac output (stroke volume × HR) deceases, so the overall cardiac reserves diminish with age. The dysfunction of sympathetic modulation of the cardiovascular system with advanced age is consistent with increased spillover of catecholamine and impaired responses to α-adrenergic receptor stimulation.[2] This further reduces myocardial contractility. Aging also affects the LV afterload and vascular-ventricular load matching. This mismatch impairs LV elasticity (contractility) in response to increased afterload. In addition, diastolic pressure decreases with age, compromising myocardial perfusion and worsening overall cardiac function.

Beat-to-beat fluctuation of HR, or HR variability, is an indirect measure of autonomic function and declines steadily with age. Reduced HR variability predicts increased risk for subsequent cardiac events[3] but also increased risk for all-cause mortality.[4] The risk of atrial fibrillation dramatically increases with age; it is present in 3% to 4% of healthy volunteers older than 60 years of age, a percentage 10-fold greater than in the general adult population.[5]

Arterial Tree

Normal aging also affects the arterial system. Intimal hyperplasia and thickening, with decreased vascular compliance and increased stiffness, develop with advanced age. The intimal thickness of the carotid artery increases twofold to threefold between the ages of 20 and 90 years.[6]

Increased nonenzymatic collagen cross-linking is seen, similar to that observed in the myocardium. The elastin content in the media decreases with age. This decreases vascular elasticity (compliance) and increases stiffness. Dysfunctional endothelial vascular smooth muscle tone contributes to stiffer arterial walls independent of atherosclerotic changes.

The two main determinants of arterial blood pressure are peripheral vascular resistance and central artery stiffness. Increases in peripheral vascular resistance increase both systolic and diastolic pressure; central artery stiffness increases systolic pressure but reduces diastolic pressure.[6] Blood pressure in younger individuals is primarily dictated by peripheral vascular resistance, but with aging, central arterial stiffness becomes the main determinant of pressure.[6] Systolic blood pressure increases in adults of all ages, well into the 80s; diastolic pressure peaks in the 50s and then declines.[7] The most common hypertension in adults older than 50 years of age is isolated systolic hypertension. After allowing for hypertension, the overall effect of aging is higher systolic pressure and decreased diastolic pressure, manifested as a widened pulse pressure.

RESPIRATORY SYSTEM

The chest wall becomes increasingly rigid with advancing age. This, together with reduced respiratory muscle strength, increases closing capacity and decreases forced expiratory volume in 1 second (FEV_1). The partial pressure of oxygen also decreases progressively with age, due to a combination of age-induced mismatch between ventilation and perfusion, diffusion block, and anatomical shunt. This decrease becomes more prominent during exercise. Hypoxic and hypercapnic ventilatory drives also diminish with age. The large airways grow slightly with age, leading to more dead space.[8] The respiratory bronchioles and alveolar ducts increase in size significantly, particularly after age 60 years. The fraction of lung consisting of alveolar ducts also increases progressively over time. The cumulative surface area for gas exchange decreases by 15% by 70 years. There is progressive loss of diffusing capacity and elastic recoil with advancing age. This is mainly caused by the fusion of adjacent alveoli, which decreases surface tension forces and pulmonary elastic recoil.[8] In addition, chest wall stiffness increases with advancing age, causing a decrease in compliance. This results from a combination of factors: calcification of intercostal cartilages, arthritis of the costovertebral joints, and gradual atrophy and weakening of the intercostal muscles. With increasing age, the intercostal muscles gradually begin to atrophy and weaken, so breathing requires more from the diaphragm and abdominal muscles, but the strength of the diaphragm, as measured by the maximum transdiaphragmatic pressure, also declines with age.

Pulmonary function test changes are most affected by the age-related decreased compliance of the pulmonary system and decreased muscle strength. FEV_1 and forced vital capacity (FVC) decline progressively with age. FEV_1 decreases by 30 and 23 mL/yr in nonsmoking men and women, respectively, with an even greater decrease after 65 years. This is equivalent to an 8% to 10% decline in FEV_1 each decade. The FVC in nonsmokers decreases 15 to 30 mL/year. The vital capacity progressively decreases, and the residual volume gradually increases, leading to a relatively unchanged total lung capacity (vital capacity + residual volume). The functional residual capacity increases, although it is not as significant because of the counteraction of the increased stiffness of the chest wall. The lungs' diffusing capacity also decreases, mainly due to increased thickness of the alveolar basement membrane with advancing age, which leads to decreased gas-diffusing capabilities. The resulting ventilation-perfusion mismatch leads to higher alveolar-arterial oxygen gradients.

RENAL SYSTEM

There is a progressive decrease in the baseline kidney function after young adulthood. It remains uncertain whether these common changes reflect subclinical disease or normal aging. In most individuals, between the ages of 30 and 85 years, there is a 20% to 25% loss of renal mass, most of which is cortex. The aging kidney also exhibits hyalinization of blood vessel walls and fewer glomeruli. This process progresses to hyalinizing arteriosclerosis and scattered arteriolar obliteration, with a resultant loss of nephrons secondary to ischemia. In addition, tubular senescence is frequent in the elderly. Histologically, tubular length decreases, interstitial fibrosis is seen, and tubular basement membrane constitution and anatomical features change with age. Tubular senescence blunts reabsorption and secretion of solutes, leading to decreased capacity to reabsorb sodium and secrete potassium and hydrogen ions.

Functional changes parallel the anatomical changes. The kidneys show impaired concentrating capacity over time and a 10% decline in renal blood flow per decade after young adulthood. There is a sequential fall in the standardized glomerular filtration rate (GFR) with aging.[9] Excluding individuals with inherent renal disease, there is a 50% to 63% decline in GFR from the ages of 30 to 80 years; in other words, GFR declines by about 1 mL/min per year. Serum creatinine levels often remain normal, despite significantly reduced GFR, because of the concomitant decreased production of creatinine in elderly persons (Fig. 203-3).

Elderly persons are limited in their ability to tolerate water deprivation and, contrarily, to tolerate water boluses. Decreased maximal urinary concentration is a partial explanation of nocturia in the elderly. Antidiuretic hormone (ADH) levels are not suppressed, so failure of ADH secretion cannot account for the age-associated urinary concentrating defect. Rather, a failure of normal renal responsiveness to ADH appears to mediate this change. It is unclear whether this failure results from a decreased medullary solute gradient or a decreased tubular response to ADH at the receptor.

The hormonal regulation of fluid and electrolyte balance requires an intricate interaction among aldosterone, ADH, and atrial natriuretic peptide (ANP). Alterations in these hormones are partly responsible for changes in fluid balance with aging. ANP is produced and secreted by the cardiac atria. The concentration of ANP is increased five-fold over basal levels in the aged. The elderly exhibit an exaggerated increase in ANP in response to sodium chloride infusions. The natriuretic response to exogenous ANP is exaggerated, as is the ability to suppress aldosterone.

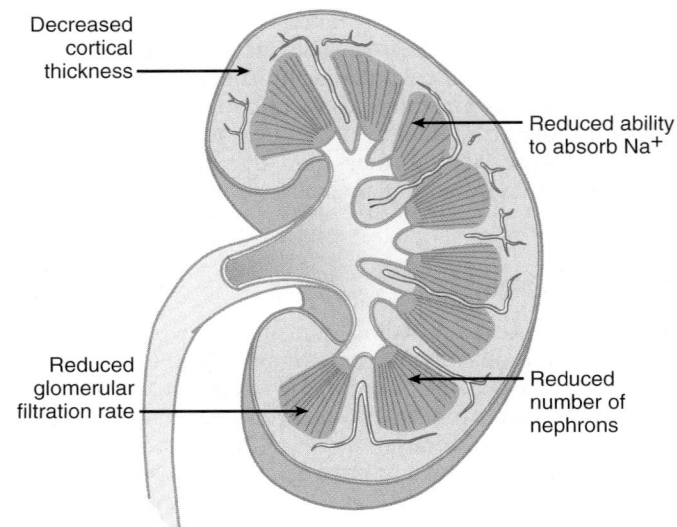

FIGURE 203-3 Cross-section of the kidney, showing changes with advancing age.

Increased ANP levels presumably cause direct suppression of renin, with a secondary decrease in angiotensin II and in aldosterone, culminating in renal loss of sodium with aging. This may help protect against volume expansion. The secretion of aldosterone is also altered. Adaptation to salt and extracellular fluid volume depletion is narrowed, with a blunted renin response to a low-sodium diet. This decreases angiotensin II and aldosterone response, with subsequent sodium loss. The clinical consequences are "salt wasting," exemplified by situations that paradoxically exaggerate clinical hypovolemia despite the body's need for maximal sodium conservation (e.g., gastrointestinal losses). The direct aldosterone response to hyperkalemia is diminished, and tubular responsiveness to aldosterone appears to be less vigorous.

GASTROINTESTINAL AND HEPATOBILIARY SYSTEMS

In the elderly, the gastrointestinal and hepatobiliary systems are affected by changes in neuromuscular function (primarily affecting the upper gastrointestinal tract), changes in the gastrointestinal tract structure (most notably in the distal colon), and changes in absorptive and secretory functions (predominantly in the small bowel and stomach, respectively).

Neuromuscular Function

Changes in the oropharynx and esophagus are primarily related to neuromuscular degeneration and changes in the ability to coordinate the complex reflexes required for successful swallowing and propulsion of food. Aberrant contraction can also be caused by muscle weakness. Failure to coordinate motility reflexes can cause numerous problems, including diffuse esophageal spasm, achalasia, and reflux. Because these age-associated problems can also be caused by primary neurological conditions, it is important to differentiate neurological deficits resulting from cerebrovascular accidents and true central nervous system degenerative processes from age-related changes.

The cricopharyngeus muscle, the primary muscle of the upper esophageal sphincter, is particularly susceptible to motility alteration; this can lead to aspiration, dysphagia, and pharyngoesophageal diverticula. Neuromuscular deficits of the lower esophagus include decreased or even absent response to normal upper esophageal peristalsis, with contraction weakness and slowing. Insufficient resting pressure in the lower esophageal sphincter can cause gastroesophageal reflux and symptoms simulating hiatal hernia and achalasia.[10]

The exact effect of aging on the stomach remains unclear. Some studies of emptying times have demonstrated increases and decreases. It has been difficult to link any alteration in gastric emptying with symptoms or pathological features.[10] These data suggest changes in the homeostatic mechanisms regulating gastric emptying in elderly persons. Neuromuscular function in the small bowel is unchanged.

Gastrointestinal Wall Structure

The upper alimentary tract does not experience significant structural changes. The oropharynx and upper esophagus musculature weakens with the development of pharyngoesophageal diverticula, causing functional problems. The gastric mucosa becomes increasingly atrophic. The primary structures affected in the small bowel are the intestinal villi. From the age of 60 years, there is a progressive decrease in their height, resulting in less surface area for absorption.[10] The normal mucosal parenchyma and smooth muscle cells become replaced by fibrous connective tissue.

The colon is most consistently affected by age-related structural alterations. Mucosal changes are noted, but they do not affect colonic absorptive capabilities.[10] The primary aging process in the colon is thickening of the muscular layers, particularly the muscularis propria and muscularis mucosa. This is caused by a buildup of elastin between myocytes in the bowel wall, not by muscle cell hyperplasia or hypertrophy. The tinea coli are affected more than the circular muscle layers, and longitudinal contraction secondary to elastin accumulation contributes to hard stool, constipation, and fecal impaction. Diverticular disease, the most common age-related colonic disease, results from concomitant weakening of the muscularis propria at locations where arteries and veins cross the bowel wall.

Secretion and Absorption

Normal aging brings significant changes in the composition and mixture of saliva, primarily a decrease in ptyalin and an increase in mucin.[11] In the elderly, saliva can become thick and viscous. Although salivation decreases with aging, it remains adequate in normal, healthy persons. Secretion of gastric acid and pepsin decline. This is more noticeable in women and becomes apparent as an attenuation of peak and basal acid secretion. Decreases in pepsin secretion correlate with the presence of age-related mucosal atrophy.[10] In the small bowel, a decrease in the height of villi and a reduction in surface area can lead to

absorption disorders. There are no significant changes in the absorptive capacity of the colon.

Several changes in liver physiology occur. The liver size decreases after 50 years, from roughly 2.5% of total body mass to just over 1.5%. Alterations in blood flow parallel this change. Although the total number of hepatocytes is decreased, there is an increase in mean cell volume, which some interpret as a cellular response to increased biological demand on the remaining cells.[10] Despite this potentially increased demand, most liver function test results remain normal. Hepatic synthesis of several proteins, including clotting factors, can be reduced, but this does not impair baseline function. Because of the larger anabolic burden on fewer hepatocytes, hepatic synthesis of these factors is unable to increase significantly beyond baseline when challenged.

No direct link of aging with major gall bladder function has been established, including absorption, mucosal physiological features, and contractile properties. There is more cholelithiasis (perhaps from an increased ratio of lipid to cholesterol in bile), but the underlying process is unclear.[10]

ENDOCRINE AND IMMUNE SYSTEMS

Men and women can expect to live one third of their lives with some hormone deficiency.[12] Numerous age-related changes occur throughout the endocrine system, the best studied being the menopause. During the first decade after menopause, women undergo rapid bone loss, most likely reflecting diminished estrogen levels. Thereafter, a slow phase of bone loss occurs, primarily from a loss of estrogen-mediated calcium homeostasis. This decreased skeletal mass occurs along with normal age-related bone loss, compounding the problems of osteoporosis and pathological bone fractures in elderly persons. In addition to bone, menopause removes estrogen's cardioprotective effect, increasing the level of low-density lipoprotein, decreasing high-density lipoprotein, and increasing atherogenesis. Low estrogen levels produce vasomotor symptoms, urogenital atrophy, increased mood swings, and loss of libido.[13] In men, levels of serum testosterone, estradiol, dehydroepiandrosterone, and dehydroepiandrosterone sulfate slowly decline, whereas sex hormone–binding globulin (SHBG), luteinizing hormone, and follicle-stimulating hormone increase.[12] Free biologically active testosterone is lowered further by increased SHBG. Hormonal changes in men are associated with changes in body mass index, osteoporosis, and sleep and mood disorders, as well as decreased libido, muscle atrophy, and possibly erectile dysfunction.[13]

Secretion of growth hormone (GH) declines with age in both experimental animals and humans. With advancing age, an increasing proportion of men and women with no clinical evidence of pituitary pathology show decreased GH secretion and decreased serum levels of insulin-like growth factor 1 (IGF1). GH has both direct and indirect actions on peripheral tissues, the indirect actions being mediated mainly by IGF1. With each decade, the GH production rate decreases by 14% and the GH half-life falls by 6%. These changes may be associated with decreased lean body and bone mass and increased body fat in aging persons. The mechanisms underlying the reduced GH secretion in animals and humans are complex. Defective pituitary function probably does not play a major role, and preserved GH secretory capacity has been demonstrated in the aged pituitary when specific hypothalamic influences were restored or toned down.

The thyroid gland in elderly persons is characterized by mild atrophy, increased fibrosis, and decreased follicular size.[14] There is less peripheral conversion of thyroxine to triiodothyronine, decreased iodine uptake, and lower levels of thyroxine and free thyroxine.[14] Whether the age-related decline in thyroid function is of clinical relevance is unclear. The neighboring parathyroid glands also undergo age-related changes. Increased parathyroid hormone levels and increased release in response to a rise in serum calcium occur in older compared with younger individuals.[15] The increased baseline levels and augmented parathyroid hormone response to stimuli have been implicated in osteoporosis and bone loss.[16] In contrast to parathyroid hormone, calcitonin levels decrease with age.

Adrenal function leads to changes in the cortisol diurnal pattern, which shifts earlier in the day, resulting in higher evening cortisols.[10] Both the pattern and the quality of sleep change. Total sleep time decreases markedly.[17] There is increased number and duration of awakenings and less deep slow-wave sleep (i.e., stages 3 and 4 of non–rapid eye movement sleep). Although baseline levels of epinephrine and norepinephrine increase, the hormonal response to stimulation is blunted.[13] The attenuated sympathetic body stress response manifests in several ways. For instance, older individuals have less cutaneous vasoconstriction in response to cold stimuli compared with younger individuals, making them more susceptible to hypothermia.[18]

Advancing age is associated with impaired glucose handling. Insulin resistance increases, with a peak at almost 80 years of age.[19] For nondiabetic individuals, progressive impairment of glucose tolerance occurs, independent of obesity and gender.[13] Overall, there is an age-related increase in fasting and postprandial glucose levels.[13] This results from a combination of anthropometric changes, environmental causes, and neurohormonal variations.

Aging is associated with less lean body mass (especially less muscle mass) and an accompanying relative increase in fat. Because muscle is the major site of glucose uptake, less muscle mass results in decreased glucose disposal. Furthermore, there is a slow, progressive redistribution of fat as intra-abdominal fat increases and subcutaneous fat on the limbs decreases. This is reflected in a decline in limb skin fold thickness.[20,21] Intra-abdominal fat is a major clinical parameter contributing to insulin resistance; it accounts for more than 50% of the variance in insulin sensitivity, whereas age per se is not associated with decreased insulin sensitivity.[21] Age-related variations in diet and physical activity also seem key.

The immune system also experiences an age-related decline. Immune system alterations are complex and pleiotropic, suggestive of remodeling or altered regulation rather than simple immune deficiency. Advanced age causes functional impairment of T lymphocyte–mediated immunity and increased susceptibility to infections. The response of T lymphocytes to interleukin-2 (IL2) also seems impaired in older individuals, as does the stress-related increase in natural killer cell activity.[13] Increased

serum inflammatory mediators are another hallmark of aging, suggestive of regulatory defects or an ongoing attack on subclinical cancer or infection. IL6, an inflammatory cytokine, has been postulated to modulate the endocrine response, with hypothalamic-pituitary-adrenal axis activation, stimulation of plasma cortisol levels, and augmentation of bone loss.[13] Qualitative changes in antibody production occur with advancing age, affecting responses to foreign antigens and prophylactic vaccines.

NEUROLOGICAL SYSTEM

Cortical atrophy of the brain has been repeatedly demonstrated with age.[22] Quantitative brain magnetic resonance imaging studies have shown that age is associated with decreased cerebral hemisphere volume, frontal region area, and temporoparietal region area. Increasing age is associated with increased volume in the lateral and third ventricles.[22] Age-related increase in peripheral cerebrospinal fluid volume is a marker of cerebral atrophy and is greater in men than in women.[22] There is minimal neuronal loss with normal aging. In contrast, neurodegenerative processes (Alzheimer's, Parkinson's, and Huntington's diseases) are strongly associated with neuronal loss. In addition to neocortical neuritic plaques and neurofibrillary tangles, Alzheimer's disease is consistently associated with severe cortical loss or atrophy,[23] with a 20% to 25% greater cortical atrophy compared with age-matched controls. Higher levels of education protect against dementia, a fact that has led to the "reserve hypothesis" of brain aging. One prediction of the reserve hypothesis is that, among elderly individuals with similar age-related brain changes (i.e., cortical atrophy), those with more education would demonstrate less cognitive impairment than those with less education.

There is evidence that normal aging is associated with alterations in cerebral hemodynamics and metabolism and structural and functional changes in various neuronal systems. During resting conditions, age-related declines in cerebral blood flow, cerebral volume, and cerebral blood flow velocity within the basal intracerebral arteries occur.[24] There is also[25] less hemodynamic response to focal brain activation (neurovascular coupling).[26] Cardiovascular risk factors significantly diminish the capability of cerebral vessels to react to increased metabolic demands or a vasodilating stimulus (e.g., carbon dioxide), thereby altering the hemodynamic response to neuronal activation.

There is a decline in all of the senses with increasing age. Smell identification progressively deteriorates even without overt medical problems.[27] Significant age-associated deterioration has been observed in taste but not in somatic sensations such as touch and burning pain in the tongue, showing that aging affects taste perception and oral somatic sensations differently. Decreased taste perception of foods may be caused primarily by perceptual loss of taste among oral sensations. The receptor cells of the retina, rods, and cones change with aging. In addition, perfusion of the optic nerve head is reduced with increasing age. Decline in visual acuity has a significant effect on memory decline.[28] Within the auditory system, there is stiffening of the tympanic membrane and sensory loss of the cochlea. A change in auditory acuity predicts change in memory performance.[29] Loss of labyrinth hair cells, nerve fibers, and vestibular ganglion cells affects the vestibulo-ocular reflex. Decreased mechanoreceptor density and sensitivity and decreased peripheral nerve conductivity decrease vibrotactile sensation.[30] In addition, decreased tactile and proprioceptive sensation has also been reported.

SUMMARY

Aging as a physiological process is associated with complex changes in all organs, and these changes occur at varying rates (Table 203-2). They affect the body's functional reserve, leading to impaired ability to maintain homeostasis and withstand stressors. Awareness of these physiological changes is an integral part of any comprehensive evaluation of the older patient.

TABLE 203-2 Summary of the Physiological Changes That Occur with Aging

ORGAN OR FUNCTION	SYMPTOMS ASSOCIATED WITH AGING
Arteries	Atherosclerosis, intimal thickening, higher blood pressure, increased risk of cardiovascular disease
Bladder	Weakened connective tissue, reduced capacity to store urine, reduced efficiency of bladder emptying
Body weight	Declining weight between ages 55 and 75 yr, due mostly to loss of lean tissue, muscle mass, water, and bone
Bones	Accelerated loss of bone cells beginning at about age 35 yr; bones become porous and brittle in the demineralizing process
Brain	Gradual loss of brain tissue, slower reaction, deterioration in memory, insomnia
Ear	Gradual loss of the ability to hear higher frequencies, starting at about age 30 yr
Endocrine	Reduced estrogen (females), reduced testosterone (males), reduced GH and IGF1, increased insulin resistance
Fat	Increased storage
Heart	Increased thickness of LV wall, reduced number of pacemaker cells, increased myocardial stiffness, and reduced compliance.
Immunity	Reduced ability to combat infection, increased autoimmune responses
Joints	Reduced synovial fluid, increased risk of osteoarthritis, destruction of cartilage, less resilience of tendons, and ligaments
Kidneys	Reduced weight and volume of the kidneys, marked reduction in functional ability, loss of nephrons, changes in electrolyte absorption and secretion
Lungs	Loss of elasticity and capacity, increasing difficulty oxygenating blood
Nose	Declining ability to smell after age 65 yr; amount of reduction varies widely among individuals
Prostate	Reduced semen making after age 60 yr; enlargement in size may cause difficulty with urination
Reaction time	Slower mental and physical responses to specific stimuli
Thermoregulation	Impaired capacity for coping with changes in environmental temperature
Tongue	Gradual decline in sense of taste
Tumors	Increased risk of malignancies

GH, growth hormone; IGF1, insulin-like growth factor 1; LV, left ventricular.

REFERENCES

1. Knapowski J, Wieczorowska-Tobis K, Witowski J. Pathophysiology of ageing. J Physiol Pharmacol 2002;53:135-146.
2. Lakatta EG, Levy D. Arterial and cardiac aging: Major shareholders in cardiovascular disease enterprises. Part II: The aging heart in health—Links to heart disease. Circulation 2003;107:346-354.
3. Tsuji H, Larson MG, Venditti FJ Jr, et al. Impact of reduced heart rate variability on risk for cardiac events. The Framingham Heart Study. Circulation 1996;94:2850-2855.
4. Tsuji H, Venditti FJ Jr, Manders ES, et al. Reduced heart rate variability and mortality risk in an elderly cohort. The Framingham Heart Study. Circulation 1994;90:878-883.
5. Furberg CD, Psaty BM, Manolio TA, et al. Prevalence of atrial fibrillation in elderly subjects (the Cardiovascular Health Study). Am J Cardiol 1994;74:236-241.
6. Lakatta EG, Levy D. Arterial and cardiac aging: Major shareholders in cardiovascular disease enterprises. Part I: Aging arteries—A "set up" for vascular disease. Circulation 2003;107:139-146.
7. Franklin SS, Gustin WT, Wong ND, et al. Hemodynamic patterns of age-related changes in blood pressure. The Framingham Heart Study. Circulation 1997;96:308-315.
8. Campbell E. Physiologic Changes in Respiratory Function. New York: Springer-Verlag, 2001.
9. Rowe JW, Andres R, Tobin JD, et al. The effect of age on creatinine clearance in men: A cross-sectional and longitudinal study. J Gerontol 1976;31:155-163.
10. Adkins R, Marshall B. Anatomic and physiologic aspects of aging. In Adkins R, Scott H (eds). Surgical Care for the Elderly, 2nd ed. Philadelphia: Lippincott-Raven, 1998.
11. Astor FC, Hanft KL, Ciocon JO. Xerostomia: A prevalent condition in the elderly. Ear Nose Throat J 1999;78:476-479.
12. Schulman C, Lunenfeld B. The ageing male. World J Urol 2002;20:4-10.
13. Perry HM 3rd. The endocrinology of aging. Clin Chem 1999;45(8 Pt 2):1369-1376.
14. Sirota DK. Thyroid function and dysfunction in the elderly: A brief review. Mt Sinai J Med 1980;47:126-131.
15. Haden ST, Brown EM, Hurwitz S, et al. The effects of age and gender on parathyroid hormone dynamics. Clin Endocrinol (Oxf) 2000;52:329-338.
16. Bilezikian JP, Silverberg SJ. Parathyroid hormone: Does it have a role in the pathogenesis of osteoporosis? Clin Lab Med 2000;20:559-567, vii.
17. Van Cauter E, Leproult R, Plat L. Age-related changes in slow wave sleep and REM sleep and relationship with growth hormone and cortisol levels in healthy men. JAMA 2000;284:861-868.
18. Smolander J. Effect of cold exposure on older humans. Int J Sports Med 2002;23:86-92.
19. Barbieri M, Rizzo MR, Manzella D, Paolisso G. Age-related insulin resistance: Is it an obligatory finding? The lesson from healthy centenarians. Diabetes Metab Res Rev 2001;17:19-26.
20. Kohrt WM, Kirwan JP, Staten MA, et al. Insulin resistance in aging is related to abdominal obesity. Diabetes 1993;42:273-281.
21. Cefalu WT, Wang ZQ, Werbel S, et al. Contribution of visceral fat mass to the insulin resistance of aging. Metabolism 1995;44:954-959.
22. Coffey CE, Lucke JF, Saxton JA, et al. Sex differences in brain aging: A quantitative magnetic resonance imaging study. Arch Neurol 1998;55:169-179.
23. Mouton PR, Martin LJ, Calhoun ME, et al. Cognitive decline strongly correlates with cortical atrophy in Alzheimer's dementia. Neurobiol Aging 1998;19:371-377.
24. Leenders KL, Perani D, Lammertsma AA, et al. Cerebral blood flow, blood volume and oxygen utilization: Normal values and effect of age. Brain 1990;113(Pt 1):27-47.
25. D'Esposito M, Deouell LY, Gazzaley A. Alterations in the BOLD fMRI signal with ageing and disease: A challenge for neuroimaging. Nat Rev Neurosci 2003;4:863-872.
26. Groschel K, Terborg C, Schnaudigel S, et al. Effects of physiological aging and cerebrovascular risk factors on the hemodynamic response to brain activation: A functional transcranial Doppler study. Eur J Neurol 2007;14:125-131.
27. Ship JA, Pearson JD, Cruise LJ, et al. Longitudinal changes in smell identification. J Gerontol A Biol Sci Med Sci 1996;51:M86-M91.
28. Anstey KJ, Luszcz MA, Sanchez L. A reevaluation of the common factor theory of shared variance among age, sensory function, and cognitive function in older adults. J Gerontol B Psychol Sci Soc Sci 2001;56:P3-P11.
29. Valentijn SA, van Boxtel MP, van Hooren SA, et al. Change in sensory functioning predicts change in cognitive functioning: Results from a 6-year follow-up in the Maastricht Aging Study. J Am Geriatr Soc 2005;53:374-380.
30. Verrillo RT. Age related changes in the sensitivity to vibration. J Gerontol. Mar 1980;35:185-193.

CHAPTER **204**

The Aging Brain and Dementia

Colm Cooney and Diarmuid O'Shea

KEY POINTS

- Patients with dementia have reduced life expectancy and complex end-of-life care needs.

- Patients with dementia invariably suffer impairment in decision making, and the palliative care approach involves close liaison between the treating multidisciplinary team and the family or next of kin.

- Discussions regarding challenging health care decisions such as provision of artificial hydration and nutrition should take place with patients and their families at the earliest appropriate opportunity.

- Attention to factors that impair the dementia sufferer's quality of life, such as pain and depression, are a central feature of the palliative care approach.

Dementia is a clinical syndrome of chronic or progressive cortical or subcortical brain dysfunction resulting in cognitive decline.[1] In most, it is a progressive terminal illness. There is an increasing recognition that dementia sufferers who are dying have care needs comparable to those of cancer patients and may benefit from a palliative approach.[2] Major challenges include addressing those who may have incapacity to make decisions regarding their care and providing adequate symptom control for patients who may be unable to articulate their distress. There is debate as to which model or setting of care is most appropriate. Specialist palliative care units for dementia have been advocated by some,[3] whereas others have emphasized the need for home-based palliative care in both developing[4] and developed countries.[5] There is a lack of systematic research to guide clinicians as to the most appropriate model of palliative care.[6]

Nevertheless, the underlying principles of the palliative care approach, with its emphasis on adequate symptom control and avoidance of unnecessary intervention, is entirely appropriate for patients with dementia in the terminal phases, whether at home or in an institution. It is an approach favored by both formal and informal carers.[7] However, any involvement of palliative care services in the terminal phase of dementia is still unusual,[8] and many receive suboptimal end-of-life care.[9]

BASIC SCIENCE AND PATHOPHYSIOLOGY

The term *dementia* refers to a clinical syndrome consisting of global cognitive impairment with clear consciousness. It is a brain disease that is usually progressive and rarely reversible.[10] The most common causes are Alzheimer's disease, which accounts for 50% of patients with

dementia[11]; vascular dementia, accounting for 10% to 20%[12]; and Lewy body dementia, accounting for 10% to 20%. Alzheimer's disease is characterized by dysfunction of multiple neurotransmitter systems, with cholinergic deficits being most prominent. Disruption of both cholinergic and glutaminergic pathways has also been documented in vascular dementia. The cholinergic deficit in Lewy body dementia is more profound than in Alzheimer's disease. These neurotransmitter abnormalities have formed the basis for drug development.

EPIDEMIOLOGY AND PREVALENCE

Substantial increases in the worldwide number of people older than 65 years of age are predicted, with a proportionate growth in the number expected to develop dementia. Meta-analyses of epidemiological studies in developing countries have established dementia prevalence rates of approximately 1.5% at age 65 years, doubling every 4 years thereafter to reach about 30% at 80 years. There appears to be some leveling off of the prevalence rate in extreme old age.[13] The greatest increase is projected to occur in developing countries, with increases in these regions from 13 million in 2000 to 84 million in 2050.

Epidemiological studies have identified older age and genetic factors as the most important causative factors for dementia in community samples.

Dementia shortens life expectancy. Early studies suggested that the average life expectancy, from the onset of illness, is approximately 8 years. The expected increase in the overall number of patients worldwide, together with the chronic and usually progressive nature of the illness, will put pose considerable challenges to services providing terminal care for these patients, who often have a protracted end stage.[14]

CLINICAL MANIFESTATIONS

The neurodegeneration causes progressive loss of function and a terminal end phase. Memory impairment is the most common early feature. Initially the short-term memory is affected, but long-term memory becomes impaired as the disease progresses, leading to the loss of significant biographical memories. Language impairment in early Alzheimer's disease is characterized by reduced verbal fluency and conversational output, with progressive motor and sensory dysphasia and eventual muteness in the later phases. However, many patients can convey and respond to emotional signals at this phase. This may assist the interpretation of distress when patients can no longer communicate verbally and are fully dependent on others for their health care needs.

The impairment of abstract thinking, judgment, and communication leads to loss of decision-making capacity, which creates challenges, particularly with regard to complex end-of-life health care decisions.

Increasing dyspraxia accompanies more severe dementia. This results in difficulty walking and eventually in immobility and impairment of eating, chewing, and swallowing. Double incontinence is invariable in the terminal stage.

In addition to the cognitive symptoms and their associated disabilities, behavioral and psychological symptoms in dementia (BPSD) also pose considerable challenges. These are more prominent as the disease progresses. Burns[15] found that aggressive behavior, defined as behavior likely to cause physical injury to others, occurred in 24% of patients with severe dementia. Mood changes are also common. Agitation occurs in up to 90% of patients at some point in the illness, increases as the dementia progresses, and may not respond to treatment.

Major depression occurs relatively frequently in Alzheimer's disease[16] but is more common with vascular dementia. Although depression occurs commonly with severe dementia, it is often unrecognized, and communication difficulties may be a major contributor. Depression manifests atypically, with dysphoria, loss of interest, apathy, and disinhibition being more common. Repetitive, noisy vocalizations are more likely with more severe dementia and may indicate pain, depression, or psychosis.

BPSD may occur either as an integral part of the illness or as an expression of other problems. Awareness of how pain may manifest in dementia is important, because there is evidence that such patients are more likely than patients with cancer to suffer pain in the last 6 months of their life. Some patients may display agitated or aggressive behavior in response to pain.[17] Many dementia sufferers do not initiate requests for analgesia but may exhibit pain by resisting help with activities of daily living. Dementia itself is a risk factor for constipation, and constipation in this context may manifest as agitated or aggressive behavior.

Dementia is an important risk factor for delirium, and patients with dementia are particularly vulnerable to delirium in response to physical stressors such as infections and iatrogenic treatments. In this situation, delirium may manifest as a sudden worsening of confusion, disturbed sleep-wake cycle, and behavioral problems such as agitation or aggression. Delirium can be very distressing for the patient in terms of increased restlessness, agitation, persecutory symptoms, and increased risk of adverse outcomes including falls and fractures.[18]

TREATMENT AND END-OF-LIFE DECISIONS IN DEMENTIA

There are a number of principles in the management of end-of-life care for patients with dementia.

Discussions with patients and their families about future health care decisions should take place as early as possible in the illness, while the patient may have decision-making capacity. This may allow patients to make informed choices about their future care and draw up advance directives. This is particularly important in anticipating difficult health care decisions such as provision of artificial hydration and nutrition. However, it often is not possible, and, if patients no longer have capacity to make decisions about their care, the palliative care approach involves collaboration between the multidisciplinary team and family members. In the absence of advance directives, family members or surrogates may contribute to such health care decisions by trying to choose decisions the patient would make if he or she had capacity. This allows for an agreed framework for future treatment, which can

be reviewed with the family during the course of the illness. These meetings can provide a forum within which to educate families regarding the natural course of dementia, discuss risk/benefit analyses of therapeutic interventions, and shift the emphasis from curative to palliative care.

Close attention by care staff to feeding, skin care, elimination, oral hygiene, and grooming are important aspects of the management of end-stage dementia.[19]

The specific issue of artificial nutrition and hydration warrants further discussion. Evidence suggests that percutaneous endoscopic gastrostomy or nasogastric tube feeding does not improve health outcomes in advanced dementia. These procedures are associated with increased morbidity and mortality. There is also some evidence that terminal dementia patients do not seem to suffer when food and fluid intake diminishes and stops, as long as they are offered water and ice chips.[20] The Alzheimer's Society, in a policy position statement on palliative care in dementia, emphasized the importance of quality rather than length of life and expressed concerns regarding the frequency of artificial feeding and hydration of dementia sufferers in the terminal phase. It seems reasonable to continue oral intake for dementia sufferers with swallowing impairment in the terminal phase of their illness. This can be facilitated using modified diet or thickened fluids, with the patient in the correct sitting posture to minimize aspiration.

The effective management of pain in terminal dementia is crucial to quality of life and, in addition, may help control behavioral problems. However, pain is often undetected and inadequately treated.[21] Pain management is a complex issue, because communication problems present significant difficulties in assessment. However, a number of scales are available that may help.[22] In addition, if a patient with end-stage dementia is unable to communicate verbally, clinical observations of facial expressions and vocalizations is accurate for assessing the presence of pain, but not its intensity.[23] One study reported low-dose opioids to be effective in reducing difficult-to-control agitation in very elderly (≥85) patients with advanced dementia.[23] However, opioids can cause significant undesirable effects in older patients with dementia, such as respiratory depression and constipation, and should be used with caution. The availability of transdermal (patch) delivery systems for analgesics allows more optimal management of pain relief in this patient group. Consultation with palliative services can be very helpful in determining the appropriate use of analgesics, including opioids.

Depression is an important cause of morbidity and mortality in dementia, and antidepressant therapy has proven benefit. Tricyclic antidepressants should be avoided because of their potential to worsen cognitive function through their anticholinergic effects. Selective serotonin reuptake inhibitors are probably the treatment of choice, and they may reduce agitation and psychosis as well as improving mood. If sleep disturbance is a problem, trazodone, an antidepressant with effects on the serotonergic system, may be helpful because of its reported efficacy in reducing symptoms of BPSD in dementia.

Psychiatrists have an important role to play in consulting with treating physicians and in educating formal and informal caregivers regarding the detection and treatment of depression in dementia.

The management of BPSD requires a thorough analysis of contributory factors to determine treatment options. This should include assessment of environmental factors contributing to the symptoms as well as attention to physical health conditions (including pain or constipation) and mental health problems such as depression or psychotic symptoms. Treatment involves a multidimensional approach that addresses underlying contributory or exacerbating factors. Nonpharmacological interventions include behavior therapies, music therapy, exercise, and assessing the impact of the environment.

Use of medications to manage BPSD should be restricted to moderate to severe symptoms that do not respond to nonpharmacological management. A wide range of medications, including antipsychotics, antidepressants, mood stabilizers, and anxiolytics are commonly used to treat BPSD. The use of antipsychotic drugs has come under particular scrutiny in view of their reported association with an increased risk of cerebrovascular events and death. The antidementia drugs, including the anticholinesterase agents and the *N*-methyl-D-aspartate receptor antagonist Memantine, may have beneficial effects on reducing BPSD and should be considered.

SUMMARY

The management of end-of-life care for people with dementia poses significant challenges to those involved. The palliative care model, with its emphasis on providing comfort rather than cure and the avoidance of iatrogenic suffering, provides a useful framework for management. The lack of systematic research in this area must be addressed to provide a platform for the development of palliative care services for these vulnerable people.

REFERENCES

1. Richie K, Lovestone S. The dementias. Lancet 2002;360:1759-1766.
2. McCarthy M, Addington-Hall J, Altmann D. The experience of dying with dementia: A retrospective study. Int J Geriatr Psychiatr 1997;12:404-409.
3. Hughes JC, Robinson L, Volicer L. Specialist palliative care in dementia. Br Med J 2005;330:57-58.
4. Sivaraman SK. Specialist palliative care in dementia [Letter]. Br Med J 2005;330:672.
5. Treloar A, Newport J, Venn-Treloar J. Specialist palliative care in dementia. Br Med J 2005;330:672.
6. Sampson EL, Ritchie CW, Lai R, et al. A systematic review of the scientific evidence for the efficacy of a palliative care approach in advanced dementia. Int Psychogeriatr 2005;17:31-40.
7. Hansen L, Salmon D, Galasko D, et al. The Lewy body variant of Alzheimer's disease: A clinical and pathological entity. Neurology 1990;40:1-8.
8. Bayer A. Death with dementia—the need for better care. Age and Ageing 2006;35:101-102.
9. Sachs GA, Shega JW, Cox-Hayley D. Barriers to end-of-life care for patients with dementia. J Gen Intern Med 2004;19:1057-1063.
10. Clarfield AM. The decreasing prevalence of reversible dementias: An updated meta-analysis. Arch Int Med 2003;163:2219-2229.
11. Cummings JL, Benson DF (eds). Dementia: Definition, prevalence, classification and approach to diagnosis. In Cummings JL, Benson D (eds). Dementia: A Clinical Approach. Boston: Butterworth-Heinemann, 1992.
12. Rocca WA, Hofman A, Brayne C, et al. The prevalence of vascular dementia in Europe: Facts and fragments from 1980-1990 studies. EURODERM. Ann Neurol 1991;30:817-824.
13. Richie K, Kildea D. Is senile dementia "age-related" or "ageing-related"? Evidence from meta-analysis of dementia prevalence in the oldest old. Lancet 1995;346:931-934.
14. Aminoff BZ, Adunsky A. Dying dementia patients: Too much suffering, too little palliation. Am J Alzheimers Dis Other Demen 2004;19:243-247.
15. Burns A, Jacoby R, Levy R. Psychiatric phenomena in Alzheimer's disease. III: Disorders of mood. Br J Psych 1990;157:81-86.
16. Burns A, O'Brien J, Ames D (eds). Dementia. London: Edward Arnold, London, 2005.
17. Buffum MD, Miaskowski C, Sands L, Brod M. A pilot study of the relationship between discomfort and agitation in patients with dementia. Geriatric Nurs 2001;22:80-85.
18. Gustafson Y, Berggren D, Brahnstrom B, et al. Acute confusional states in elderly patients treated for femoral neck fracture. J Am Geriatr Soc 1988;36:525-530.
19. Rabins, PV, Lyketsos, CG, Steele CD (eds). Practical Dementia Care, 2nd ed. New York: Oxford University Press, 2006.
20. Lloyd-Williams M. An audit of palliative care in dementia. Eur J Cancer Care 1996;5:53-55.
21. Luchins DJ, Hanrahan P. What is the appropriate level of health care for end-stage dementia patients? J Am Geriatr Soc 1993;41:25-30.
22. Krulewitch H, London MR, Skakel VJ, et al. Assessment of pain in cognitively impaired older adults: A comparison of pain assessment tools and their use by non-professional care givers. J Am Geriatr Soc 2000;48:1397-1398.
23. Manfredi PL, Breuer B, Meier DE, Libow L. Pain assessment in elderly patients with severe dementia. J Pain Symptom Manage 2003;25:48-52.

SUGGESTED READING

Agronin ME, Maletta GJ (eds). Principles and Practice of Geriatric Psychiatry, 1st ed. Philadelphia: Lippincott Williams & Wilkins, 2006.

Burns A, O'Brien J, Ames D (eds). Dementia, 3rd ed. London: Edward Arnold, 2005.

Rabins PV, Lyketsos CG, Steele CD (eds). Practical Dementia Care, 2nd ed. New York: Oxford University Press, 2006.

Rojas-Fernandez CH, Eng M, Allie ND. Pharmacologic management by clinical pharmacists of behavioural and psychological symptoms of dementia in nursing home residents: Results from a pilot study. Pharmacotherapy 2003;23:217-221.

CHAPTER **205**

The Frail Elderly

Mamta Bhatnagar and **Robert Palmer**

> **KEY POINTS**
>
> - Frailty is a process of homeostatic decline that results in reduced physiologic reserve.
> - A frail older adult is at high risk for adverse health outcomes, including hospitalization, institutionalization, and death.
> - Common manifestations of frailty are nonspecific; they include weight loss, fatigue, weakness, and decline in physical activity.
> - A functional assessment is the best available approach to help identify the frail older adult.
> - Interventions to help prevent and treat frailty can improve quality of life.

Terms such as "disablement process," slow "functional decline," or "failure to thrive" describe the presentation of the "frail" elderly patient, but a precise clinical definition of this clinical entity remains elusive. Frailty is a process of physiological decline that reduces homeostatic reserve and predisposes to organ failure. Despite the uncertainties of definition or biology, skilled clinicians can identify the frail elderly. Doing so enables clinicians to offer these patients comprehensive care and targeted interventions that improve their quality of life.

The accompanying case study illustrates many of the common features of frailty and its operational definition as a phenotype comprising five physical criteria: unintentional weight loss (10 pounds in the past year), self-reported exhaustion, weakness (e.g., as estimated by grip strength), slow walking speed, and low physical activity.[1] The occurrence of three or more of these features suggests frailty. The finding of one or two criteria identifies the individual as being at risk of frailty in an incremental fashion (see "Case Study: Frailty in an Elderly Patient").

 C A S E   S T U D Y

Frailty in an Elderly Patient

An 84-year-old woman underwent partial mastectomy for early-stage breast cancer. Her past medical history included coronary artery disease, high blood pressure, hypercholesterolemia, and generalized osteoarthritis. Two months after the surgery, she was brought by her daughter for a visit to her primary care physician. Her daughter expressed concern about her mother's decline. She reported that her mother was gradually becoming weaker, losing weight, slowing down, and appearing lethargic. The patient lived independently but required help with her laundry and cooking. During the interview the patient was slow to respond to questions. She had no specific medical symptoms. She had not been eating well and had lost 8 pounds in the past 6 months.

The examination revealed a pleasant, thin lady with orthostatic hypotension and muscle atrophy in her upper and lower extremities. On gait examination, she required the support of the arms of the chair to stand up and walked slowly, taking small strides. She was breathless after walking a short distance. The remainder of the physical examination was within normal limits. Her Mini Mental State Examination score was 26/30 (normal, ≥26), and her Geriatric Depression Scale score was 3/15 (depressed, ≥6). She was admitted to the hospital for fluid repletion. The laboratory workup revealed a hemoglobin value of 10.2 g/dL, normal red blood cell indices, an unremarkable basic metabolic panel, an erythrocyte sedimentation rate of 86 mm/hr, and a C-reactive protein concentration of 2.1 mg/dL.

The patient underwent physical rehabilitation in the hospital and was discharged home with physical therapy. Once home, however, she continued her physical decline, eating poorly and walking more slowly. She moved to her daughter's house for closer personal care. She was later readmitted to the hospital, where she developed confusion, incontinence, and weakness and required assistance with transferring to chair from bed and going to the bathroom. Physical therapy staff recommended 24-hour supervision with nursing home placement. The patient did not wish to pursue further treatment and agreed to go to her daughter's home with hospice care. She died at home 3 months later.

EPIDEMIOLOGY

Both the prevalence and the incidence of frailty in the elderly population vary with the criteria used. The frailty phenotype has been applied in research involving large elderly cohorts. Based on the phenotype, an incidence of 7% over 4 years and a point prevalence of 7% have been observed in the community-dwelling population 65 years of age and older.

CLINICAL MANIFESTATIONS

The case study illustrates the insidious, gradual, and sometimes inexplicable decline in the elderly person's physical functioning and vitality. The frailty concept underscores this gradual process of reduced homeostatic reserve and fatigue. The study patient developed weight loss with anorexia of undetermined cause and experienced an insidious decline in physical activity with weakness and exhaustion. On examination, balance and gait impairments and a loss of muscle mass were found. The loss of fat-free weight is a hallmark of frailty. Although most frail patients appear underweight, obese persons can also be frail if they manifest the physical decline and vulnerability characteristic of frailty.

Table 205-1 lists some of the assessment tools that are available for measuring frailty. Table 205-2 describes some of the pathophysiological changes associated with frailty.

Frailty: Falls and Immobility

Immobility is a common consequence of hospitalization. Physical frailty is strongly associated with a higher risk of disability after hospitalization. A concomitant illness, injury, or precipitant event, such as a fall, can dramatically increase disability independent of the presence of frailty.[2] The combination of decreased homeostatic reserve, multiple comorbidities, and physical frailty can cause severe consequences after even brief bed rest. Self-report of unsteadiness among patients admitted to a hospital places them at increased risk for in-hospital decline in independent performance of activities of daily living (ADL); moreover, those who lose ADL function immediately before admission fail to recover ADL independence.[3] The physiological changes of bed rest include decreased blood volume and cardiac output, hypoxemia, muscle atrophy, decreased muscle oxidative capacity, and generalized weakness. Visual or hearing impairment, low physical performance, and cognitive dysfunction at hospital admission increase the risk of an older adult for development of disability after protracted immobilization.[2] Medical complications of immobility include deep venous thrombosis, pressure sores, joint contractures, urinary incontinence, cardiac deconditioning, muscle weakness and falls, and pressure ulcers.

Gait disorders, balance problems, and falls are interrelated consequences of immobility. Each year, about one third of community-dwelling adults older than 65 years of age, and one half of those older than 80 years, experience a fall; 5% sustain a fracture; and about half have soft tissue injuries. More than half of the survivors from falls are discharged to a nursing home, with 50% remaining in the

TABLE 205-1 Tools for Measuring Frailty

NAME OF SCALE	DOMAINS	SCALING PROPERTIES
Clinical Global Impression of Change*	Change in 6 intrinsic domains (mobility, balance, strength, endurance, nutrition, and neuromotor performance) and 7 consequences domains (medical complexity, health care utilization, appearance, self-perceived health, ADLs, emotional status, and social status)	Each domain is scored on a 7-point scale: 7 = marked improvement 4 = no change 1 = marked worsening
Frailty Index[†]	A count of 70 deficits which include presence and severity of current diseases, ability in ADLs, and physical signs from clinical and neurologic examinations	0-7 items = mildly frail 7-13 items = moderately frail >13 = severe frailty
DSM-III-R criteria for diagnosis of frailty[‡]	History of falls, delirium, cognitive impairment or dementia	Presence of these criteria implies frailty
CSHA Function Scale[‡]	Scores a patient on each of 12 ADLs including instrumental ADLs	0 = independent 1 = needs assistance 2 = incapable
CSHA rules-based definition of frailty[‡]	Measures degree of frailty based on the presence of urinary or bowel incontinence with or without ADL dependence	Categorizes subjects as 0 (no impairment), 1, 2, or 3, with worsening impairment and dependence
CSHA Clinical Frailty Scale[†]	Tests for functionality and physical fitness	Scores range from 1 to 7; higher scores indicate dependence
Cumulative Illness Rating scale[†]	Comorbidity measure that has been validated by autopsies	Higher illness burden associated with frailty
Modified Mini Mental State examination (3MS)[†]	Adds 4 domains to the original MMSE with more grading and scoring from 0 to 100	A score of 77 or less indicates cognitive impairment
Frailty Phenotype[§]	Weight loss of >10 lb, exhaustion, level of physical activity, walk time for predetermined distance (standardized for gender and height), and grip strength (standardized for gender and body mass index)	Presence of 3 or more components suggests frailty; presence of <3 items indicates high risk of frailty

ADL, activities of daily living; CSHA, Canadian Study of Health and Aging; DSM-III-R, *Diagnostic and Statistical Manual of Mental Disorders*, Third Edition, Revised; MMSE, Mini Mental State Examination.
*Studenski S, Hayes RP, Leibowitz RQ, et al. Clinical global impression of change in physical frailty: Development of a measure based on clinical judgment. J Am Geriatr Soc 2004;52:1560-1566.
[†]Rockwood K, Song X, MacKnight C, et al. A global clinical measure of fitness and frailty in elderly people. Can Med Assoc J 2005;173:489-495.
[‡]Rockwood K, Hogan DB, MacKnight C. Conceptualisation and measurement of frailty in elderly people. Drugs Aging 2000;17:295-302.
[§]Fried LP, Tangen CM, Walston J, et al. Frailty in older adults: Evidence for a phenotype. J Gerontol A Biol Sci Med Sci 2001;56:M146-M156.

TABLE 205-2 Pathophysiology of Frailty with Aging: Musculoskeletal, Immune, and Neuroendocrine Systems

MUSCULOSKELETAL SYSTEM	IMMUNE SYSTEM (CYTOKINE CHANGES)	NEUROENDOCRINE SYSTEM
↓ Skeletal muscle mass	↓ IgG, IgA	↑ Insulin resistance
↓ Vo_2 max	↓ IL-2	↓ Growth hormone
↓ Strength and exercise tolerance	↑ IL-6	↓ IGF1
↓ Thermoregulation	↑ IL-10	↑ Cholecystokinin
↓ Energy expenditure	↓ Naïve T cells	↓ Vitamin D
↓ Resting metabolic rate	↑ Memory T cells	↓ Estrogen and testosterone
↓ Muscle innervation	↓ Mitogen response	↑ Sympathetic tone Steroid hormone dysregulation

Ig, immunoglobulin; IGF1, insulin-like growth factor 1; IL, interleukin; Vo_2 max, maximum oxygen uptake.

High-risk periods for falls include the first month after hospital discharge, periods of acute illness, and exacerbations of chronic illnesses. The use of more than four medications—especially benzodiazepines, anticonvulsants, neuroleptic agents, and tricyclic antidepressants—increases the risk. At the end of life, people are often restricted in their activities and are at risk for falls. Emphasis should be given to their prevention.

Geriatric Assessment for Frailty and Falls

The evaluation of an older adult seeks to identify individuals who are at risk of becoming frail and includes a careful search and identification of conditions that cause or trigger frailty. A comprehensive geriatric assessment is performed by a multidisciplinary team comprising a physician, nurse, and social worker. The team may also include any combination of physical and occupational therapists, speech therapists, pharmacists, or nutritionists. Comprehensive geriatric assessment is effective in identifying risk factors for functional loss, reducing the rate of functional decline in inpatient and outpatient settings, and improving quality of life.[4,5]

Assessment of physical function begins with a review of the patient's level of independence in performing both basic and instrumental ADL. The initial assessment establishes a benchmark for future comparisons and records the chronic illnesses that are responsive to therapy and can exacerbate or lead to frailty. Common examples include chronic heart failure, diabetes, thyroid diseases,

nursing home 1 year later. Most falls result from interactions between chronic or acute predisposing factors (usually intrinsic) and acute precipitating factors (usually extrinsic), such as environmental hazards. Different factors lend different weights to the risk of falling (Table 205-3). The two most important factors are lower extremity muscle weakness and a history of prior falls.[4]

In the case study, the patient had several factors predisposing to a fall, including gait deficits, muscle weakness, impaired ADL, and the use of an assistive device.

chronic infections, undiagnosed cancer, and inflammatory conditions such as temporal arteritis. Detection of dementia, depression, and delirium is included. The Mini Mental State Examination[6] evaluates cognitive function; scores of 26 or less are considered abnormal. Depression can be suspected by a positive response to the question, "Do you often feel sad or depressed?" Depressive symptoms can be further characterized by use of the Geriatric Depression Scale; scores of 6 or more on this 15-item scale are likely to indicate depression. Evaluation of the older adult includes a review of over-the-counter and prescription medications to identify side effects and drug interactions. Visual and hearing deficits are identified by asking the patient and caregiver about their presence. Vision can be examined by testing acuity or asking the patient to read the headline and the fine print of a newspaper (i.e., testing for both near and distance vision). Hearing is tested by asking the patient to repeat words whispered by the examiner when positioned behind the patient.

Critical to the evaluation of frailty, a geriatric assessment analyzes gait, physical strength, and function. Gait and mobility can be tested with the Timed Up and Go (TUG) test. The patient gets up from the arm chair, walks 10 ft (3 m) in a line, turns around, walks back to the chair, and sits down. The time required to complete this sequence is normally 10 seconds or less. Impaired balance and mobility is likely if it takes the patient longer than 20 seconds to complete the test. An abnormal test result predicts future disability. Postural stability, step height, stride length, and sway are also observed during the test. Postural stability can be assessed by walk in tandem or semitandem positions.

The most effective interventions to prevent recurrent falls are targeted at both intrinsic and extrinsic factors. Successful components include review of and adjustments in medications, balance and gait training, and muscle-strengthening exercises (see Table 205-3). Methods to reduce hip fractures from falls have also been explored. In some studies, hip protectors decrease hip fractures in frail people. However, variable results with hip protectors may be attributable to different levels of adherence to treatment or to different efficacy of different brands.

Laboratory Tests for Frailty

Laboratory tests can help detect reversible causes of frailty. The initial laboratory workup should include a complete blood count to look for anemia, with follow-up evaluation

---

TABLE 205-3   Risk Factors for Falls: Assessment and Suggested Interventions

RISK FACTOR*	ASSESSMENT	SUGGESTED INTERVENTION	EVIDENCE†
INTRINSIC FACTORS			
Muscle weakness	Proprioception and muscle strength assessment	Encourage physical activity and improve nutritional status if indicated	Resistance and strength training have been shown to be effective in active elderly people.
History of falls	Detailed history of the circumstances of previous falls	Appropriate changes in environment and activity	Assessment by a specialist, such as a physical or occupational therapist, reduces risk for falls.
Balance and gait deficits	Impaired mobility on Up and Go test; reported or observed unsteadiness of gait	Gait and strength exercises, balance training (e.g., Tai Chi Chuan); balance exercises are taught by physical therapists	Balance training is beneficial; Tai Chi is effective in well but not demented elderly people.
Use of assistive device	Observe gait with usage of device	Training in use of device (cane, walker, assistive devices)	Physical and occupational therapy improve gait and activities of daily living; hip protectors might prevent fractures from falls.
Visual acuity <20/60, ↓ depth perception, ↓ contrast sensitivity	Examine visual acuity; if reduced, consider treatable causes of impairment (glaucoma or cataracts)	Lighting without glare; visual aids; referral to an ophthalmologist; avoid multifocal glasses when walking	No randomized clinical trials are available; cataract surgery improves quality of life.
Orthostatic hypotension‡	Assess for dehydration, side effect of medications	Adequate fluid intake; slow transfers; lower extremity stockings	Community-based studies demonstrate reduced risk for falls; cardiac pacemaker implantation does not prevent falls.
EXTRINSIC FACTORS			
Medication use: psychotropic medications, class IA antiarrythmics, digoxin, diuretics	Assess for sedative-hypnotic or psychotropic drug use	Review indications for medications and look for alternatives or reduction in number of medications	Consistent risk of falls has been shown in observational studies; intervention is consistently beneficial in all settings.
Environmental hazards	A facilitated home assessment	Environmental modifications include removal of throw rugs, use of night lights, nonslip bathmats, stair rails	There is some evidence of reduced risk of falls in isolated studies, but overall benefits are not well established

*Risk factors are listed in order of decreasing odds ratios and relative risks. ADL disability, depression, cognitive impairment, age >80 years are additional risk factors for falls.
†For older adults in all health care settings, not for the palliative care population.
‡Cardiovascular symptoms such as orthostatic hypotension, carotid sinus syndrome, and vasovagal syndrome sometimes overlap with falls.
From Boult C, Boult LB, Morishita L, et al. A randomized clinical trial of outpatient geriatric evaluation and management. J Am Geriatr Soc 2001;49:351-359.

as indicated; a comprehensive metabolic panel to identify covert kidney or liver dysfunction; and measurement of inflammatory markers such as C-reactive protein and erythrocyte sedimentation rate (Box 205-1). Efforts should be made to differentiate between frailty and other causes of chronic inflammation (e.g., temporal arteritis, infections) that may be more responsive to specific therapy.

DIFFERENTIAL DIAGNOSIS: FRAILTY, DISABILITY, AND COMORBIDITY

Frailty affects physical functioning and impairs the ability to perform tasks necessary to function in society. Loss of such function in the social and personal context of the frail patient underlies the concept of disability. The frailty phenotype identifies 74% of the frail population as having comorbid disease, disability, or both; 27% have neither disability nor comorbidity.[2] Frailty confers a high risk for functional decline and disability; however, it does not presuppose concurrent disability or significant comorbidity. Most physically inactive people sustain large losses in musculoskeletal mass before they cross the disability threshold. At this threshold, patients perceive an increased effort required to complete submaximal exercise. The gradual decline in function distinguishes frailty from other acute illnesses (e.g., stroke) that produce catastrophic disability. Individual functioning can be categorized based on the performance of basic and instrumental ADL that are critical to maintaining the independence of an individual in society. ADL performance is adversely affected by the physiological changes of frailty. The patient in the case study suffered a gradual decline in physical functioning that resulted in inability to perform ADL, including transferring and toileting.

In summary, frailty has a multifactorial basis that includes age-related physiological changes and their interaction with coexistent disease states. Both acute illnesses and decompensation of long-standing chronic diseases can trigger or perpetuate the syndrome of frailty (Fig. 205-1). Co-occurrence of multiple diseases increases a person's risk of becoming frail. Social and environmental factors such as availability of medical care, rehabilitation, and external supports in the form of caregivers and structural modifications at home can alter the progression of

frailty. At its extreme, frailty ends in a "failure to thrive" that presages death.

BASIC SCIENCE AND PATHOPHYSIOLOGY

Physiological aging, an accumulation of pathological states, and environmental and social factors all contribute to frailty.

Loss of Homeostatic Reserve

Age-related decline in physiological reserve deprives an individual of the ability to respond adequately to dynamic stressors such as exercise, temperature extremes, or an acute illness (see Table 205-2). Underlying this change is a decreased range of physiological complexity within an individual. An increased vulnerability to stressors is inherent to the frailty concept. Any pathological decrement in the depleted homeostatic reserves can predispose to frailty (Fig. 205-2).

Sarcopenia

An intact musculoskeletal system is integral to independent function and performance of ADL. Skeletal muscle loss, or sarcopenia, occurs with aging and is first evident at about 35 years of age. The muscle becomes replaced with fat or fibrotic tissue. Sarcopenia decreases strength and exercise tolerance, resulting in inability to perform daily activities that ultimately leads to physical dependence on others. Sarcopenia is symmetrical in nature, and this differentiates it from cachexia, which is a loss of both fat and muscle and results from generalized wasting. The extent of sarcopenia varies with physical activity, illness burden, and medications.

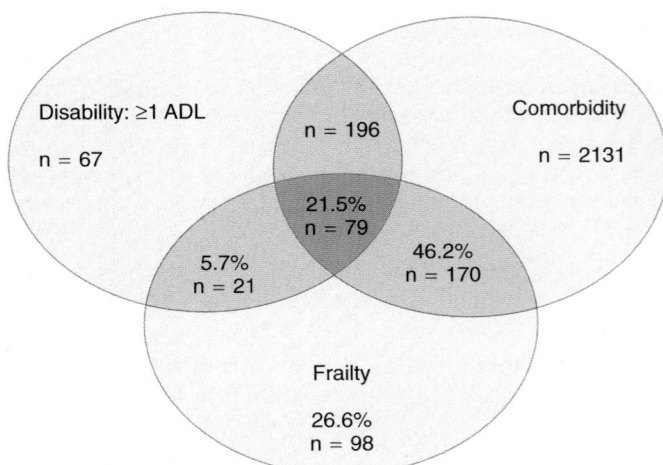

FIGURE 205-1 Overlaps between disability, frailty, and comorbidity in a community-dwelling older population. Subjects were categorized as being frail, being disabled, and/or having two or more of the following nine comorbidities: myocardial infarction, angina, congestive heart failure, claudication, arthritis, cancer, diabetes, hypertension, chronic obstructive pulmonary disease. Frailty was defined as the presence of three or more of the following five characteristics: unintentional weight loss, self-reported exhaustion, reduced grip strength, slow gait speed, low physical activity. ADL, activities of daily living.

> **Box 205-1 Common Inflammatory Conditions That Elevate Inflammatory Biomarkers**
>
> Chronic infections
> Osteomyelitis
> Infective endocarditis
> Fungal and mycobacterial infections
> Chronic heart failure
> Diabetes mellitus
> Cancers
> Chronic inflammatory diseases
> Inflammatory bowel diseases
> Soft tissue diseases (e.g., bursitis, infections)
> Collagen vascular diseases (vasculitides)
> Polymyalgia rheumatica
> Temporal arteritis (giant cell arteritis)
> Dermatomyositis/polymyositis

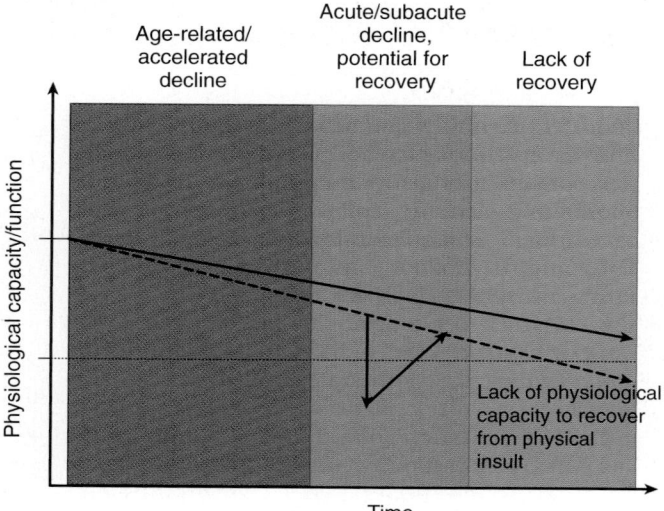

FIGURE 205-2   A hypothetical decline in physiological capacity/function with aging. Solid line represents normal aging with gradual loss of physiological reserve. Stippled line represents an accelerated decline that predisposes an individual to frailty. Superimposed on the accelerated decline, a precipitous loss in homeostatic reserve is often triggered by an event such as an infection or a fracture. If detected early, this stage can be potentially reversed with the implementation of corrective measures that enable patients to return to their premorbid state.

Neuroendocrine Dysregulation

Growth hormone and its messenger molecule, insulin-like growth factor 1 (IGF1), are responsible for the development and maintenance of lean muscle mass. With aging, IGF1 production decreases, resulting in muscle atrophy. IGF1 production is enhanced by testosterone, insulin, and vitamin D, all of which might be reduced in frail older people. The gradual fall in testosterone levels in men with aging is associated with decline in bone mineral density and lean body mass. Decline in estrogen levels in women with aging is associated with a rapid decline in bone mineral density, increased fat mass, and higher cardiovascular risk. Chronic stressors increase sympathetic tone and steroid hormone secretion, resulting in a generalized catabolic state. Vitamin D decreases hip fractures in the elderly and may help maintain muscle mass and neuromuscular function.

Immune Dysfunction and Role of Chronic Inflammation

Abnormally high peripheral levels of cytokines, inflammatory markers, and coagulation markers have been observed in the elderly, especially in the very old (≥85 years), who have the highest risk of frailty.

Cellular and Humoral Immunity

The overall number of T cells declines with age, and the ratios of the various T-cell subtypes change. An increase in memory T cells is accompanied by a disproportionately greater loss of naïve T cells. The ratio changes attenuate response to new antigens. The functioning of the memory

T cells may also become impaired, so immunization may be effective only for short periods in older individuals. There is an age-related decrease in T-cell proliferation in response to antigenic stimulation. Simultaneous activation of the humoral immune system by T cells is also decreased. The production of antibodies declines with age, and this might relate to a decline in number or function of B cells. B-cell dysfunction may also result from impairment in T-cell function. Similar to other age-related changes, the decline in immune function is variable. Immune dysfunction, as evidenced by a lower T-cell proliferative capacity, lower ratio of helper to suppressor T cells, and lower total B cell numbers, is associated with higher mortality.[7]

MOLECULAR MECHANISMS, GENETICS, AND FRAILTY

Support for a link between DNA damage and aging comes from genetic syndromes of accelerated aging. Werner's syndrome, an autosomal recessive disorder involving the helicase gene on chromosome 8, is characterized by skin and hair changes, glucose intolerance, osteoporosis, cataracts, and hypogonadism usually in the second or third decade of life. Cumulative oxygen damage to DNA from oxygen radicals generated during cellular metabolism reduces gene repair capabilities, resulting in transcription abnormalities, and unstable RNA transcripts. Replicative senescence occurs when cells become senescent after a finite number of reproductive cycles. One potential mechanism is loss of the telomere region of the chromosomes. The telomeres lost from the ends of the DNA are usually replaced by the telomerase enzyme. Age-related depletion of this enzyme results in loss of telomeres and thus exposes several gene segments to base pair loss. Cellular proteins also undergo alterations, such as glycation and oxidation, that may affect their function along critical regulatory pathways.

PHARMACOTHERAPY IN THE FRAIL ELDERLY

Frailty predisposes patients to adverse drug effects in the treatment of end-of-life symptoms. Distribution and absorption of most drugs become clinically important in the context of polypharmacy and hepatic or renal impairment (Table 205-4). Pharmacodynamic changes make the elderly more sensitive to commonly prescribed medications. For example, antihistamines such as diphenhydramine and hydroxyzine can cause anticholinergic side effects including confusion, oversedation, constipation, urinary retention, orthostatic hypotension, and falls. Nonsedating histamines, such as loratadine and fexofenadine, are reasonable alternatives. Insomnia is best treated with behavioral techniques such as sleep hygiene. When necessary, low doses of trazodone or zolpidem may be useful. Selective serotonin reuptake inhibitors are preferred for depression. If tricyclic antidepressants are required for treatment, nortriptyline and desipramine are best.

Analgesics

Aging and frailty influence the pharmacodynamics and pharmacokinetics of analgesics, narrowing their therapeutic index and increasing adverse effects and drug

TABLE 205-4	Factors Influencing Drug Metabolism and Action in the Elderly	
STEP IN DRUG PHARMACOKINETICS	**PHYSIOLOGICAL CHANGES WITH AGE**	**CLINICAL RELEVANCE**
Absorption	↓ absorptive area ↓ splanchnic blood flow ↑ gastric pH ? role of P-glycoprotein	Minimal change in absorption of most drugs May be affected by multiple drugs given simultaneously
Distribution	↓ total body water ↓ lean body mass ↑ proportion of body fat (greater in women than in men) ↓ serum albumin ↑ α_1-acid glycoprotein	Drugs in aqueous phase have higher concentrations; fat-soluble drugs have an increased V_d and a prolonged half-life Increased plasma-free fraction of highly protein-bound drugs* Free fraction of basic drugs is decreased (usually minor effect)*
Metabolism	↓ hepatic mass and blood flow ↓ phase I metabolism (CYP450) ↓ CYP3A enzyme activity No change in phase II metabolism (e.g., conjugation)	Decreased first-pass (presystemic) metabolism of drugs Decreased rate of metabolism of certain CYP450 drugs, and increased half-life of some active metabolites May require reduction in daily dosing of drugs metabolized by CYP450
Elimination	↓ renal blood flow ↓ glomerular filtration rate	Decreased clearance of drugs and their metabolites (e.g., meperidine, lithium)[†] Strong potential for drug-disease interactions and toxicity (e.g., NSAIDs and renal failure)
Alteration in pharmacodynamics: Tissue sensitivity	Alterations in receptor number and function, alterations in cellular and nuclear responses	Older patients may have increased sensitivity to certain adverse effects of commonly prescribed drugs (e.g., anticholinergic drugs, opioids)

CYP3A, cytochrome P-450 isoenzyme 3A; CYP450, cytochrome P-450 system; NSAID, nonsteroidal anti-inflammatory drugs; V_d, volume of distribution.
*Physiological changes in protein binding have no important clinical effect on free drug concentration.
[†]Renal function is often impaired by coexistent medical conditions (heart failure, arthritis) and drugs commonly used to treat those conditions (e.g., diuretics, NSAIDs).

interactions. In addition to cancer-related pain, older adults are more likely to suffer from arthritis, bone and joint disorders, and other chronic conditions, resulting in several sources of pain in the same individual. Dementia, sensory impairment, and disability in the elderly make it difficult to assess and manage pain. Both acute and continuous pain are often associated with depression, anxiety, decreased socialization, and impaired sleep and ambulation. Adequate pain treatment becomes crucial to the maintenance of quality of life of the frail patient.

Nonopioid Analgesics

For mild to moderate arthritic and musculoskeletal pain, acetaminophen alone is often effective, and, at usual therapeutic doses, it lacks acute gastrointestinal or renal side effects. Acetaminophen is safe in divided doses of up to 4000 mg/day; lower doses should be used in patients with coexistent fasting, liver disease, or regular alcohol consumption.[6] The nonsteroidal anti-inflammatory agents (NSAIDs) treat acute inflammatory pain including arthritis and soft tissue inflammation. Ibuprofen and naproxen are the usual agents. Chronic use at high doses increases adverse effects, including gastrointestinal bleeding, exacerbations of congestive heart failure and renal insufficiency, elevated blood pressure, and possibly stroke. Periodic evaluation of the frail patient's renal function and blood pressure are advisable. Nonaspirin salicylates (e.g., choline magnesium trisalicylate) are alternatives, but patients need to be monitored carefully, often through measurement of blood levels, for salicylate toxicity. Other nonopioid medications serve as adjuncts to analgesics in cases of persistent pain. Common agents include anticon-

vulsants, antidepressants, and topical analgesics, but their role in non-neuropathic pain in frail patients is not well established. Calcitonin as a nasal spray relieves pain from both cancerous and noncancerous causes (e.g., fragility fractures).

Opioids

Opioids are highly effective and are the mainstay of therapy of severe pain in frail patients. Because of frailty-related changes in drug disposition and sensitivity, opioids are started in lower than usual starting doses and are given separately from other adjuvants, to allow for independent titration of individual components. Meperidine, propoxyphene, and pentazocine are not recommended for the elderly because of central nervous system adverse effects.[8] Morphine is frequently an opioid of choice, the starting oral dosage in opioid-naïve, frail patients being 5 mg every 4 to 6 hours, with the same dose repeated every 2 hours as needed.[6] Smaller doses are initiated when morphine is given parenterally to a frail patient. The analgesic effects are titrated against the adverse effects of confusion, constipation, and nausea. Improved analgesia and patient compliance may be observed with sustained-release morphine or oxycodone.

Oxycodone is an attractive alternative to morphine for most types of pain in the elderly. Elimination of oxycodone is not as greatly affected by age, and, like morphine, its kinetics are unchanged by low protein states. Doses are lowered in liver failure, which greatly prolongs the half-life of oxycodone. Hydromorphone is as effective as morphine and can relieve the pruritus associated with morphine use but otherwise has little advantage over morphine. Codeine has no advantage over morphine and is constipating. Methadone has a long half-life in frail patients and is used cautiously, if at all, for that reason. Transdermal fentanyl patches can be introduced to frail patients who have tolerated other opioids (i.e., without respiratory depression); absorption is often delayed in the elderly patient, allowing an extended delivery time of more than 72 hours.[6] Propoxyphene and pentazocine are not recommended because of either lack of efficacy or greater incidence of side effects in the elderly.

INTERVENTIONS TO PREVENT AND TREAT FRAILTY AND ITS SEQUELAE

Hormonal Therapy

Given the hormonal changes that occur with aging and their possible roles in the development of frailty, hormonal replacement therapy with estrogen, testosterone, or growth hormone may seem reasonable. However, evidence to support their use in frail patients, especially at the end of life, is lacking. Estrogen therapy in postmenopausal women does not prolong survival or increase lean body mass. Testosterone replacement has not been studied in older men (especially those older than 85 years of age), in whom treatment includes the potential to increase prostate growth or exacerbate coronary artery disease. Growth hormone supplementation increases lean body mass, decreases fat mass, and temporarily reverses the catabolic state of disease. There is no improvement in functional status from growth hormone supplementation, and long-term risks (e.g., cardiomyopathy) are unknown. Hormone therapy has no established role for frailty.

Exercise

Both functional decline and physical inactivity reduce exercise ability in aerobic capacity, muscle strength, endurance and power, flexibility, and balance. Exercise has potential benefits for frail patients who have cardiovascular disease, hypertension, hyperlipidemia, type 2 diabetes, depression, falls, or impaired mobility. An exercise prescription promotes an active lifestyle, modifies risk factors for disability such as sarcopenia and insulin resistance, maintains and improves exercise capacity, and enhances psychosocial functioning. The response to change in activity depends on the cause and extent of disability, alterations in impairments, psychosocial factors, disease status, and other variables that are ill defined. Predicting the outcome of an exercise prescription is not straightforward.[9] Persistent pain needs to be controlled before an exercise regimen can be fully implemented. Patients who have end-stage congestive heart failure or a terminal illness, an inoperable large aortic aneurysm, or neuropsychological illness might be excluded from vigorous but not from low- to moderate-intensity exercises.

Endurance and Resistance Training

Both low-impact endurance exercises and progressive resistance exercises have established benefits in the frail elderly. Cardiovascular endurance training reduces the cardiorespiratory recruitment required to perform submaximal tasks. Included are walking, stair climbing, biking, and swimming. The frail cohort with arthritic and other musculoskeletal problems may be offered low-impact exercises such as walking and hiking or supervised water aerobics. Overall, walking bears a natural relationship to most basic ADL and is easier to integrate into lifestyle and functional tasks than most other exercise.[9] Aerobic (endurance) exercises are usually prescribed for 3 to 7 days per week with a duration of 20 to 60 minutes per session. Low- to moderate-intensity exercise shows a modest benefit in the frail elderly involving mobility tasks and cardiovascular efficacy. Loss of muscle mass is associated with aging even in older individuals who maintain a habitual form of exercise; muscle mass can be developed or maintained only by resistance exercises, such as weightlifting.[9] Progressive resistance training is usually advised for 2 to 3 days per week with 1 to 3 sets of 8 to 12 repetitions involving 8 to 10 major muscle groups. It is recommended to increase resistance (weight) progressively to maintain relative intensity. Gains in strength from resistance training are accompanied by improvements in gait, agility, aerobic capacity, and psychological responses such as improved morale and depressive symptoms and development of self-efficacy.

Balance Exercises

Balance training exercises are the least standardized of all the exercise modalities in the exercise prescription. Enhancement of balance, along with gait training and muscle strengthening exercises, form important multicomponent interventions to reduce falls in community-dwelling older people. Balance-enhancing activities are beneficial whether they are performed in a health care setting overseen by a health care professional or in the community with non–health care professionals.[10] Balance training exercises offer stressors to challenge the components of the central nervous system that maintain balance. The challenges include narrowing the base of support for the center of mass of the body; displacing the center of mass to the limits of tolerance; and removing visual, vestibular, and proprioceptive inputs to balance. Yoga and Tai Chi Chuan are two examples of formal exercises that enhance balance. Balance training can be incorporated in daily routines by asking the patient to walk tandem or sideways when crossing a room, to carry small items at arm's length, or to stand on one leg (alternating legs every 15 to 30 seconds) when standing in line or on a bus.

Structured balance training activities are often conducted in large groups by trained therapists. Tai Chi is effective in reducing falls and improving self-confidence to not fall. However, Tai Chi is most likely to reduce the risk of falls in the healthy and cognitively normal elderly. Its role in frail patients is less certain. Although the evidence for an exercise prescription in the seriously ill is sparse, the psychosocial and physical benefits of maintaining physical functioning are considerable, justifying an effort to continue an exercise regimen even in advanced disease. (See "Future Considerations.")

Future Considerations

- Standardize physical exercise prescriptions for older people.
- Systematize methods (e.g., using electronic medical health records) to detect and avoid potential adverse drug interactions.
- Explore medical and drug therapies (e.g., angiotensin-converting enzyme inhibitors) to reverse or prevent sarcopenia in older individuals.
- Identify mutable genetic markers of frailty.
- Promote public policies favoring healthy lifestyle components (e.g., weight control, smoking cessation) that help delay or prevent frailty.

REFERENCES

1. Fried LP, Tangen CM, Walston J, et al. Frailty in older adults: Evidence for a phenotype. J Gerontol A Biol Sci Med Sci 2001;56:M146-M156.
2. Gill TM, Allore HG, Holford TR, Guo Z. Hospitalization, restricted activity, and the development of disability among older persons. JAMA 2004;292:2115-2124.
3. Lindenberger EC, Landefeld CS, Sands LP, et al. Unsteadiness reported by older hospitalized patients predicts functional decline. J Am Geriatr Soc 2003;51:621-626.
4. Boult C, Boult LB, Morishita L, et al. A randomized clinical trial of outpatient geriatric evaluation and management. J Am Geriatr Soc 2001;49:351-359.
5. Cohen HJ, Feussner JR, Weinberger M, et al. A controlled trial of inpatient and outpatient geriatric evaluation and management. N Engl J Med 2002;346:905-912.
6. Davis MP, Srivastava M. Demographics, assessment and management of pain in the elderly. Drugs Aging 2003;20:23-57.
7. Morley JE, Kim MJ, Haren MT. Frailty and hormones. Rev Endocr Metab Disord 2005;6:101-108.
8. Fick DM, Cooper JW, Wade WE, et al. Updating the Beers criteria for potentially inappropriate medication use in older adults: Results of a US consensus panel of experts. Arch Intern Med 2003;163:2716-2724.
9. Singh MA. Exercise to prevent and treat functional disability. Clin Geriatr Med 2002;18:431-62, vi-vii.
10. Tinetti ME. Clinical practice: Preventing falls in elderly persons. N Engl J Med 2003;348:42-49.

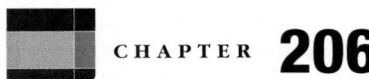

CHAPTER **206**

Caregiver Burden

Claudia Borreani and **Marcello Tamburini***

KEY POINTS

- Palliative care staff: the chronic burden
- Family caregivers: the acute burden
- The concept of vulnerability
- How to measure caregiver burden
- How to treat caregiver burden

Caring for patients with advance disease involves many concerns for caregivers. Professional and family caregivers both face the various problems of the patient, but their perspectives are different, as are the factors determining their burden. For professional caregivers, burnout and

compassion fatigue occur,[1,2] whereas family caregivers more often experience psychophysical and social distress. Collaboration among caregivers (professional and familial) is needed for good palliative care. It is important to understand how distress is generated and how to intervene to prevent or treat it.

PALLIATIVE CARE STAFF: THE CHRONIC BURDEN

Palliative care staff, because of their work with advanced disease, are at high risk for burnout from the emotional intensity of contact with death and human suffering. Every day they meet several patients and (sometimes) construct strong relations with them and their families. Every such relationship is destined to end in a relatively short time, while new ones are constructed. Often there is insufficient time to absorb these experiences. It is a chronic burden: The experience of caring does not end with the death, as it occurs for the family caregiver, but follows a continuous cycle in which the staff members pass from one case to another, often dealing simultaneously with the complexity of patients' suffering.

Chronic stress follows when a person never sees a way out of a difficult situation, when the stress of unrelenting demands and pressures extends for seemingly interminable periods of time. The worst aspect is that people get used to it; they forget about it. People are immediately aware of acute stress but ignore chronic stress because it is old, familial, and sometimes comfortable.[3]

This is not the only cause of discomfort for staff: In addition to client-related stressors in helping professions, there are job-related stressors.[4] Work overload, poor management, and resource limitations are also sources of job stress.[2] For nurses in palliative care, relationships with other health care professionals may be a particular source of stress. The team is sometimes one of the biggest stressors in the workplace, especially if role definitions are unclear or if the team environment produces uncertainty, anxiety, and frustration.

FAMILY CAREGIVERS: THE ACUTE BURDEN

In advanced disease, caregivers are needed because they provide help with activities of daily living, medications, eating, transportation, and emotional support and communicate with professionals about the patient's condition. Caring for a terminally ill family member influences multiple aspect of caregivers' lives.[5-7] Usually, caregivers are spouses (54% to 60%); 44% of them are wives. The mean patient age is 71 years, whereas caregivers are about a decade younger.[8-10]

All aspects of caregivers' quality of life may suffer, including physical, emotional, and social well-being. Caregivers often experience anxiety, depression, physical symptoms, restriction of roles and activities, and strain in marital relationships.[7,9,11] Caregiving may lead to distress from problems that began during caregiving; some, especially those who have experienced high stress while caregiving, do not show more depression after the death of the patient and may even show improvement in their health.[12,13] These observations bring about a concept of the family burden as "acute" (compared with the "chronic" burden of professional caregivers).

*Deceased.

Acute stress is common. It comes from the pressures of the recent past and anticipated demands of the near future. Acute stress is thrilling and exciting, but too much is exhausting. Because it is short-lived, it does not have enough time to do the extensive damage of long-term stress.[3]

Even if the assistance provided by relatives is long and difficult, it is finite. The discomfort ends with the death of the patient[12,13] and the bereavement process of the family members.

THE CONCEPT OF VULNERABILITY

A qualitative grounded theory study[14] explored the experiences of family members caring for a terminally ill person and the support they received from informal and professional carers. Difficulties and needs of the family members were also investigated. A core category of vulnerability was described: "Caregiving makes the family vulnerable by being more at risk of fatigue and burnout notwithstanding their courage and strength. . . . [A] continuous balance between care burden and capacity to cope [is] required, like balancing on a tightrope."[14]

Increased vulnerability occurs because of the following factors[14]:

1. Mental and physical burden
2. Restriction of normal activity
3. Fear that the beloved will have a terrible, painful death—not knowing when death will come, and in what form, may generate fear
4. Insecurity because of the frequent variations in the patient's functioning (physical and mental)

5. Loneliness resulting from caregiver protection of the patient against emotional distress, which leaves caregivers themselves isolated
6. Facing death—realizing that death is near including planning a final farewell;
7. Miscommunication from the patient if he or she does not clearly express wishes or when is dissatisfied or recalcitrant
8. Lack of support from other family members (attention paid only to the patient)
9. Poor support from health providers
10. Inadequate information

Decreased vulnerability may be achieved by the following[14]:

1. Continuing previous activities
2. Promoting hope (e.g., for a peaceful death, that the loved one will live a bit longer)
3. Keeping control and setting limits (on what one will or will not do)
4. Satisfaction about the care one has given to the patient and a positive feeling about caring
5. Good support received as caregiver

A continuous balance between care burden and capacity to cope helps avoid maladaptive consequences.

MEASUREMENT OF CAREGIVER BURDEN

Although careful clinical evaluation helps observe the described experiences, it is important to standardize measures to investigate the different factors related to the burden. Several specific tools have been developed (Table 206-1).

TABLE 206-1	Specific Tools to Measure Caregiver Burden		
INSTRUMENT	**AUTHOR AND YEAR (REF. NO.)**	**NO. OF ITEMS**	**CHARACTERISTICS**
Caregiver Strain Index (CSI)	Robinson, 1983 (15)	13	Measures objective strain and does not include subjective measures.
Cost of Care Index (CCI)	Kosberg & Cairl, 1986 (17)	20	Was constructed to identify high-risk caregivers in an Alzheimer population. Indexed items could be used for anyone caring for a sick or elderly person and can be worded as pre-caregiving and during caregiving.
Caregiver Burden Measures	Siegel et al, 1991 (18)	5	Predicts unmet needs among patients. The higher the caregiver burden, the more likely it is that a patient will report unmet needs.
The Burden Interview (BI)	Zarit et al, 1980 (19)	29	Well cited in the literature, but usually there is some modification to the original scale.
Care-giving Burden Scale (CBS)	Gerritsen & Van der Ende, 1994 (20)	26	Measures subjective burden felt by the caregiver in regard to relationship and personal consequences.
The Burden Scales	Schott-Baer et al, 1995 (21)	14	Measures the two domains of burden: subjective and objective.
Family Impact Survey	Covinsky et al, 1994 (22)	10	Measures more the objective measures of burden and not the subjective.
Caregiver Burden	Stull et al, 1994 (23)	10	Measures physical strain, social constraints, and financial strain.
Caregiver Burden Inventory (CBI)	Novak & Guest 1989 (24)	24	Measures five factors: time dependence, developmental behavior, physical burden, social burden, and emotional burden.
Caregiver Quality of Life Index—Cancer	Weitzner et al, 1999 (25)	35	Measures quality of life of the family caregiver of patients with cancer.
Screen for Caregiver Burden	Vitaliano et al, 1991 (26)	25	Measures distressing caregiver experiences.
Burden Index of Caregivers (BIC)	Miyashita et al, 2006 (27)	11	Measures five domains: time-dependent burden, emotional burden, existential burden, physical burden, and service-related burden.

TREATMENT OF CAREGIVER BURDEN

There are two methods for coping with burnout or compassion fatigue. The first is the direct approach, wherein the caregivers change what they can; the second is indirect, wherein they accept and adapt to what is impossible to change.

WORKPLACE STRESS MANAGEMENT FOR PALLIATIVE CARE WORKERS

Stress management techniques vary, from managing individual intrapersonal factors to managing the work environment to reduce external stressors. Most of the approaches described are suited for the nursing profession. Given the definition of burnout as determined by internal responses and external stressors, there are two intervention approaches[28]: personal support and environmental management.

Personal support interventions are mainly relaxation, exercise, music, education, cognitive technique, and role playing. On critical appraisal, cognitive technique appears to be effective, although the evidence is weak. Exercise, music, and relaxation are potentially effective. The benefit of social support education is debatable, and it is impossible to draw conclusions about role playing.[28]

Environmental management interventions have been based on changed nursing methods (i.e., individualized nursing care) but provided no clear evidence of effectiveness. There is more evidence for the effectiveness of personal support than environmental management in reducing workplace stress in the nursing profession.[28]

INTERVENTION TO FACILITATE FAMILY CAREGIVING

There are few data regarding interventions to relieve family distress. Interventions[29] for caregivers of patients near the end of life can consist of education, or support, or a combination of the two. Education interventions are based on programs in which nurses taught symptom management for cancer caregivers. Supportive interventions are based on counseling and teaching about coping skills and problem-solving techniques; this can be done by telephone or in face-to-face meetings.

A specific psychoeducational intervention helps increase the coping skills of caregivers in hospice care.[10] The Family COPE model is based on four components:

- Creativity (viewing problems from different perspectives to resolve them)
- Optimism (a positive but realistic attitude toward problem solving)
- Planning (setting reasonable caregiving goals and planning to reach those goals)
- Expert information

This intervention was effective in improving caregiver quality of life and reducing caregiver burden related to patients' symptoms and caregiving tasks.

REFERENCES

1. Catkins Kedel G. Burnout and compassion fatigue among hospice caregivers. Am J Hosp Palliat Care 2002;19:200-205.
2. Joinson C. Coping with compassion fatigue. Nursing 1992;22(4):116-121.
3. Miller LH, Smith AD (eds). Stress Solution: An Action Plan to Manage the Stress in Your Life. New York: Pocket Books, 1993.
4. Schaufeli W, Enzman D. The Burnout Companion to Study and Practice: A Critical Analysis. London: Taylor & Francis, 1998.
5. Wyatt G, Friedman L, Given C, et al. A profile of bereaved caregivers following provision of terminal care. J Palliat Care 1999;15:13-25.
6. Cameron J, Franche R, Cheung A, et al. Lifestyle interference and emotional distress in family caregivers of advanced cancer patients. Cancer 2002; 94:521-527.
7. Given B, Wyatt G, Given C, et al. Burden and depression among caregivers of patients with cancer at the end of life. Oncol Nurs Forum 2005;31: 1105-1117.
8. Emanuel EJ, Fairclough DL, Slutsman J, et al. Assistance from family members, friends, paid caregivers and volunteers in the care of terminally ill patients. N Engl J Med 1999;341:956-963.
9. McMillian SC, Mahon M. The impact of hospice services on the quality of life of primary caregivers. Oncol Nurse Forum 1994;21:1189-1195.
10. McMillian SC, Small BJ, Schonwetter R, et al. Impact of a coping skills intervention with family caregivers of hospice patients with cancer: A randomized clinical trial. Cancer 2006;106:214-222.
11. Nijboer C, Triemstra M, Mulder M, et al. Patterns of caregiver experiences among partners of cancer patients. Gerontologist 2000;40:738-746.
12. Shultz R, Newsom JT, Fleissner K, et al. The effects of bereavement after family caregiving. Aging Mental Health 1997;1:269-282.
13. Shultz R, Mendelsohn AB, Haley WE, et al. End of life care and the effects of bereavement among family caregivers of persons with dementia. N Engl J Med 2003;349:1936-1942.
14. Proot IM, Abu-Saad HH, Crebolder HF, et al. Vulnerability of family caregivers in terminal palliative care at home; balancing between burden and capacity. Scand J Caring Sci 2003;17:113-121.
15. Robinson BC. Validation of a caregiver strain index. J Gerontol 1983; 38:344-348.
16. Kosberg JI, Cairl R. The Cost of Care Index: A case management tool for screening informal caregivers. Gerontologist 1986;26:273-278.
17. Kosberg JI, Cairl RE, Keller DM. Components of burden: Interventive implications. Gerontologist 1990;30:236-242.
18. Siegel K, Raveis VH, Houts P, et al. Caregiver burden and unmet patient needs. Cancer 1991;68:1131-1140.
19. Zarit SH, Reever KE, Bach-Peterson J: Relatives of the impaired elderly: Correlates of feelings of burden. Gerontologist 1980;20:649-655.
20. Gerritsen JC, Van der Ende PC: The development of a care-giving burden scale. Age Aging 1994;23:483-491.
21. Schott-Baer D, Fisher L, Gregory C. Dependent care, caregiver burden, hardiness, and self-care agency of caregivers. Cancer Nurs 1995;18:299-305.
22. Covinsky KE, Goldman L, Cook EF, et al. The impact of serious illness on patients' families. JAMA 1994;272:1839-1844.
23. Stull DE, Kosloski K, Kercher K. Caregiver burden and generic well-being: Opposite sides of the same coin? Gerontologist 1994;34:88-94.
24. Novak M, Guest CI. Application of a multidimensional care-giver burden inventory. Gerontologist 1989;29:798-803.
25. Weitzner MA, Jacobsen PB, Wagner H Jr, et al. The Caregiver Quality of Life Index—Cancer (CQOLC) Scale: Development and validation of an instrument to measure quality of life of the family caregiver of patients with cancer. Qual Life Res 1999;8:55-63.
26. Vitaliano PP, Russo J, Young HM, et al. The screen for caregiver burden. Gerontologist 1991;31:76-83.
27. Miyashita M, Yamaguchi A, Kayama M, et al. Validation of the burden index of caregivers (BIC), a multidimensional short care burden scale from Japan. Health Qual Life Outcomes 2006;4:52.
28. Mimura C, Griffiths P. The effectiveness of current approaches to workplace stress management in the nursing profession: an evidence based literature review. Occup Environ Med 2003;60:10-15.
29. Mc Millian SC. Interventions to facilitate family caregiving at the end of life. J Palliat Med 2005;8:132-139.

CHAPTER **207**

Community Services

Manish Srivastava

Older patients are much more likely than the young to require community services when they are ill, especially toward the end of life. After diagnosis of a chronic disease, physicians and their staff should be able to refer patients and families to community organizations that offer educational information about the disease and direct support services such as counseling and respite services. Both patient and caregiver outcomes are significantly improved when caregiver needs are assessed and education or counseling is provided. Usually, terminally ill patients spend most of their last year of life at home being cared for by their families, without formal home care services.[1] Older patients often have chronic illnesses with multiple medical problems and slower recovery from acute illnesses, leading to increased dependence on others for activities of daily living. Many elders live alone or with a sick spouse and must seek outside assistance when unable to manage activities of daily living independently. Even though hospice care is widely available, only 20% of all adult decedents in the United States are served. Therefore, social services and community services are often needed. Most physicians are interested in community services, but unfamiliarity with the available services is a common barrier. Another barrier is the physicians' lack of time to become and remain knowledgeable about the specific services offered. Examples in this chapter refer to services available in the United States of America; availability varies greatly from country to country.

CASE MANAGEMENT

Case management is a collaborative process of assessment, planning, facilitation, and advocacy to provide quality, cost-effective care and promote optimal health outcomes. The primary goal is to identify and coordinate community services for persons who need to live at home. Case management programs typically include the following: evaluation and supervision of health, functionality, and psychosocial status; coordination of services; and consultation with physicians. A community-based case manager, commonly provided with many local and state-funded programs, not only arranges services but actively monitors those services and the patient's needs. However, case managers only rarely incorporate standard palliative care assessment and interventions in their role and functions.[2,3] Preliminary results indicate that combining palliative care with case management is a logical, feasible, and effective strategy to improve the care of seriously ill patients in the community.[4]

Agencies and organizations use various approaches for case management, ranging from simple referral services to the actual delivery of comprehensive services. The funding of case management services is neither uniform nor fair for those in need. Differences in services provided, eligibility, and levels of payment under the various reimbursement mechanisms (e.g., Medicare, Medicaid, private insurance companies) cause considerable confusion. In this environment, care management plays a crucial role. Federal, state, and private funding sources must recognize and support the valuable role of care management teams in ensuring appropriate allocation of resources, improved health care outcomes, and patient/family satisfaction.

RESPITE SERVICES

Respite care is temporary, short-term supervisory, personal, and nursing care that is provided to older adults with physical and/or mental impairments to allow the caregiver some relief or time away from caregiving responsibilities. Caregiver respite should be made a priority and should be addressed at each visit. Finding the right respite plan for the family takes time, and respite care must be modified as the patient's disease progresses. Programs may provide respite services in the person's home or at a specific site in the community (adult day services or nursing homes).

In-Home Respite Care

In-home respite care takes place in the home in which the older person lives. Depending on the caregiver's needs, in-home respite can occur on a regular or an occasional basis and during the day or the evening hours. In-home respite is most acceptable to family caregivers, because they do not have to take the older adult out of the home and also because it easily accommodates to the specific day and time the caregiver wants. However, in-home respite services can be expensive, particularly if they are used frequently for several hours per day.

Adult Day Care

Adult day services are community-based group programs that are designed to meet the needs of functionally and/or cognitively impaired adults through an individual plan of care. These structured, comprehensive programs provide various health, social, and other related support services in a protective setting during any part of a day, but less than 24-hour care. Adult day centers usually operate programs during normal business hours, 5 days a week. Some offer services in the evenings and on weekends.[5]

More than 3500 adult day centers are currently operating in the United States, and they provide care for 150,000 older Americans each day. Almost 78% of these centers are operated on a nonprofit or public basis, and the remaining 22% are for-profit. Basic services include meals, transportation, personal care, and recreation. Fifty-nine percent of participants require assistance with two or more activities of daily living (eating, bathing, dressing, toileting, or transferring); 41% require assistance in three or more areas. Daily fees for services are almost always less than a home health visit and about half the cost of a skilled nursing facility. Daily fees for adult day services vary depending on the services provided. The average cost across the country is approximately $56. An advantage of day care over in-home respite care is that it provides important peer group support and social interaction for the care receiver. For the caregiver, adult day care offers freedom from caregiving responsibilities for extended periods of time.

Day Hospices

Day hospices are common in the United Kingdom, where they are usually based in specialist palliative care units and operate similarly to day care centers in the United States. However, doctors are available to provide advice on clinical problems. In addition to assistance with bathing, wound care, and physical therapy, symptom review and management are provided in day hospices. Most patients in day hospices in the United Kingdom have cancer; other common diagnoses include AIDS, amyotrophic lateral sclerosis, and stroke.[6]

HOME CARE SERVICES

Home care provides various services that include skilled nursing, rehabilitation, social work, and personal care. The aim is to reduce the effects of disease or disability and to improve or maintain health in a home environment. Typically, home health care is begun after a lengthy hospital stay and is limited to a specified period of time. Medicare, Medicaid, and private insurance plans cover skilled services if they are medically necessary. Criteria for service receipt vary by funding source; Medicare is the most restrictive with respect to the skilled nature of care.

Services provided by home health care include skilled nursing, psychiatric nursing, physical therapy, occupational therapy, speech therapy, home health aide, and medical social services. Assistance with bathing, grooming, dressing, meals, and housekeeping for a few hours each day can make the difference between staying in the community or going to a nursing home. However, Medicare and private insurance plans, except under limited circumstances, do not reimburse this sector of home care. At least 11 million people of all ages use home care. There are at least 15,000 agencies in the United States providing these services. Agencies may be independent or affiliated with a hospital or managed care group. Most states require licensure of home health care agencies.

COMMUNITY PALLIATIVE CARE SERVICES

Community palliative care services (CPCS) originated in the United Kingdom and now have spread across Europe,

America, and Australasia. There are two models. The *comprehensive care model* is staffed by nurses and physicians who are trained in palliative care, supported by social workers, chaplains, and physical therapists. The interdisciplinary team visits the home and assists caregivers in providing basic nursing care. The extent of services offered varies from region to region. The home hospice programs based in the United States work on this model.

The *advisory model* focuses on specialist advice and support, without direct patient care. This model sets out to empower the primary physician and nurses to provide good palliative care. In the United Kingdom, many CPCS are operated by, or initially funded by, Macmillan Cancer Relief.[7]

PROGRAM OF ALL-INCLUSIVE CARE FOR THE ELDERLY

The Program of All-Inclusive Care for the Elderly (PACE) is a capitated benefit authorized by the Balanced Budget Act of 1997 (BBA) that features a comprehensive service delivery system and integrated Medicare and Medicaid financing. The program is modeled on the acute and long-term care services developed by On-Lok Senior Health Services in San Francisco, California.[8,9] The model was tested through demonstration projects of the Centers for Medicare and Medicaid Services (CMS, then called the Health Care Financing Administration, or HCFA) that began in the mid-1980s. PACE was developed to address the needs of long-term care clients, providers, and payers. For most, the comprehensive service package permits them to continue living at home while receiving services rather than be institutionalized. Capitated financing allows providers to deliver all of the services participants need rather than be limited to those services that are reimbursable under the Medicare and Medicaid fee-for-service systems.

The BBA established PACE as a permanent entity within the Medicare program and enables states to provide PACE services to Medicaid beneficiaries as a state option. Participants must be at least 55 years old, must live in the PACE service area, and must be certified as eligible for nursing home care by the appropriate state agency. The PACE program becomes the sole source of services for Medicare- and Medicaid-eligible enrollees. There are currently 33 approved PACE demonstration sites in the United States.[10]

An interdisciplinary team, consisting of professional and paraprofessional staff, assesses participants' needs, develops care plans, and delivers all services (including acute care services and, if necessary, nursing facility services). Care is integrated for a seamless provision of total care. PACE programs provide social and medical services primarily in adult day health centers, supplemented by in-home and referral services in accordance with participants' needs. The PACE service package must include all services covered by Medicare and Medicaid, as well as other services determined necessary by the interdisciplinary team for the care of the PACE participant. PACE providers receive monthly Medicare and Medicaid capitation payments for each eligible enrollee and assume the full financial risk for participants' care, without limits on amount, duration, or scope of services.

Nationally, the age range of participants is between 55 and 85 years. Although most participants have debilitating conditions, long-term prognoses vary. Certification for hospice services can be difficult because of the uncertainty of life expectancy, particularly for nonmalignant diseases such as chronic obstructive pulmonary disease, coronary artery disease, renal disease, and neurological diseases (dementia, stroke, Parkinson's disease, multiple sclerosis). Many patients with these underlying diseases who could benefit from a palliative approach are unable to access the Medicare Hospice Benefit.

Many participants in PACE programs have life-limiting illnesses, and, for this subset of PACE participants, care is guided by palliative care philosophy. These persons may have a life expectancy that is uncertain or longer than 6 months, but palliative care services can be provided outside of a traditional hospice model by the PACE program. PACE programs have developed unique ways to provide palliative care that fit with the community and the people served. This has been achieved by contracting with established hospice programs to provide services or by providing palliative care services using only PACE personnel. PACE programs are uniquely situated to provide palliative care. The multidisciplinary team is familiar with the participant's medical history, functional status, social system, and psychological needs. On enrollment, discussions about the overall goals of care are held with the participant or with a surrogate decision maker, and goals

and needs are reviewed as needed throughout the participant's stay in the program. Periodic reassessments of the participant's condition and needs are performed, enabling the team to identify the need for palliative care services and to begin services earlier than in a community-based practice. Thus, PACE programs can begin palliative care services even if the patient's prognosis is uncertain, overcoming a major limitation of the Medicare Hospice Benefit.

HOSPICE CARE IN NURSING HOMES

The Medicare Hospice Benefit was not originally established for nursing home residents, and, for the most part, Americans residing in nursing homes did not have access to the Medicare Hospice Benefit until 1986. Hospice care in nursing homes offers an opportunity to provide intensive palliative care services to dying residents without increasing nursing home staffing. Nursing homes can offer Medicare hospice care by developing working relationships (including formal contracts) with Medicare-approved hospice providers.

By electing the Medicare Hospice Benefit, nursing home residents, similar to all hospice beneficiaries, agree that the hospice has full responsibility for their plan of care. With hospice enrollment, nursing home residents and their families receive physical, psychosocial, and spiritual support and care from a hospice interdisciplinary

TABLE 207-1	Community Resources	
WEB SITE	**ORGANIZATION**	**DESCRIPTION**
www.aarp.org	AARP (formerly known as the American Association of Retired Persons)	A nonprofit membership organization dedicated to addressing the needs and interests of persons 50 years and older. Through information and education, advocacy and service, they seek to enhance the quality of life for all by promoting independence, dignity, and purpose.
www.alz.org	Alzheimer's Association	The largest national voluntary health organization dedicated to funding research into the causes, treatments, prevention, and cure of Alzheimer's disease and to providing support to the 4 million Americans with the disease, their families, and caregivers.
www.aoa.gov	Administration on Aging (AoA)	The "Elder & Families" site of this government agency contains many resources for the elderly. There is a nationwide, searchable directory of 230 national and local agencies, health associations, and organizations.
www.asaging.org	American Society on Aging (ASA)	ASA members comprise the largest multidisciplinary national community of professionals working with and on behalf of older people. The ASA has been an active and effective resource for professionals in aging and aging-related fields who want to enhance their ability to promote the well-being of aging people and their families.
www.aoa.dhhs.gov/eldfam/ How_To_Find/Agencies/Agencies.asp	Area Agencies on Aging (AAA)	Local AAAs offer information and assistance with locating a range of elder care services, including care management services, home-delivered and congregate meals, homemaker and personal care services.
www.caregiver.com	*Today's Caregiver* magazine	This site has general information on caregiving and caregivers. There are features from the current issue of the magazine on various topics in caregiving and an archive of past articles.
www.caremanager.org	National Association of Professional Geriatric Care Managers (NAPGCM)	This site answers questions about the profession and helps you find a geriatric care manager.
www.help4srs.org	H.E.L.P.	H.E.L.P. is a community-funded, nonprofit (charitable) information resource that assists older adults and their caring family and friends by providing information, planning, and problem-solving services concerning government programs and legal health care–related issues that especially affect older adults.

team, and the residents are eligible for drug coverage for medications related to their terminal illness. The nursing home continues to provide the care covered through Medicaid or private pay "room and board."

Medicare-eligible beneficiaries who live in nursing homes and have a certified terminal prognosis of 6 months or less (if disease runs its normal course) can elect hospice care if their nursing home has a contract with a Medicare-certified hospice. Medicare reimbursement policy currently disallows Medicare Part A skilled nursing facility (SNF) residents from simultaneously accessing Medicare Hospice (i.e., when the SNF care is for terminal illness); private-pay residents who elect hospice must pay privately for their nursing home care (even if eligible for Medicare SNF). Nursing homes that refer residents eligible for Medicare SNF care to hospice must forgo the higher Medicare SNF per diem and instead receive the Medicaid per diem (in most states, this is 95% of the Medicaid nursing home rate). Consequently, hospice is less likely to be accessed by residents who are eligible for SNF care under Medicare guidelines.

SPIRITUAL RESOURCES

Regardless of previous spiritual beliefs or practices, most people have spiritual or existential concerns when facing the imminent end of life. Many elderly people address these concerns in the context of an established religion, but increasing numbers do so in other contexts. The spiritual resources available to the patient become increasingly important as the disease advances. Consultations with clergy are helpful when patients and their caregivers are faced with life-prolonging options in advancing disease. Clergy can help family members address these ethical issues within the context of their own faith and culture. Spiritual care providers may be available from the patient's own tradition or from hospice programs, hospitals, and nursing facilities. Most chaplains are skilled at working with patients from diverse backgrounds and on each patient's own terms. Clergy are also able to provide grief management and bereavement care to families throughout the disease process.

COMMUNITY RESOURCE LINKS

Additional resources may be accessed through the Web sites listed in Table 207-1.

REFERENCES

1. Emanuel EJ, Fairclough DL, Slutsman J, et al. Assistance from family members, friends, paid caregivers, and volunteers in the care of terminally ill patients. N Engl J Med 1999;341:956-963.
2. Boult C, Boult L, Pacala JT. Systems of care for older populations of the future. J Am Geriat Soc 1998;46;499-505.
3. American Geriatrics Society. Case Management position statement. J Am Geriat Soc 2000;48:1338-1339.
4. Meier DE, Thar W, Jordan A, et al. Integrating case management and palliative care. J Palliat Med 2004;7:119-134.
5. National Adult Day Services Association. Available at http://www.nadsa.org (accessed February 19, 2008).
6. Mor V, Stalkewr MZ, Gralla R. Day hospital as an alternative to in-patient care for cancer patients: A random assignment trial. J Clin Epidemiol 1998; 41:771-785.
7. Clark D, Ferguson C, Nelson C. Macmillan Care Schemes in England: Results of a multi-care evaluation. Palliat Med 2000;14:129-139.
8. Eng C, Pedulla J, Eleazer GP, et al. Program of All inclusive Care for the Elderly (PACE): An innovative model of integrated geriatric care and financing J Am Geriatr Soc 1997;45:223-232.
9. Bodenheimer T. Long-term care for frail elderly people: The On-Lok Model. N Engl J Med 1999;34:1324-1328.
10. U.S. Department of Health and Human Services, Centers for Medicare and Medicaid Services. Program of All-Inclusive Care for the Elderly (PACE). Available at http://www.cms.hhs.gov/PACE/ (accessed February 19, 2008).

Acquired Immunodeficiency Syndrome

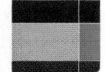

CHAPTER **208**

Acquired Immunodeficiency Syndrome: A Global Perspective

Alan J. Taege and Wendy S. Armstrong

KEY POINTS

- HIV/AIDS is a global pandemic.
- The human immunodeficiency virus (HIV) began as a zoonosis.
- HIV is transmitted via sexual contact, through contact with blood, and from mother to child.
- AIDS has the potential to decimate the developing world.
- There is a dire need for education, treatment, and a vaccine.

First described in 1981,[1] the human immunodeficiency virus (HIV), which causes the acquired immunodeficiency syndrome (AIDS), has resulted in one of the most destructive epidemics of all time (Fig. 208-1). HIV/AIDS has claimed the lives of more than 25 million people, exceeding the Black Death in the 14th century. HIV has infected another 40 million worldwide (Fig. 208-2) and has left in its path 15 million orphans, a group uniquely susceptible to infection because of their social plight. HIV is one of the most important and serious infections facing humankind in the 21st century. Currently, the global epidemic continues to outpace efforts to contain it, portending a worldwide health catastrophe.

Infections occur predominantly in young people between the ages of 14 and 49 years, during their most productive years of human life physically, biologically, and economically. The human and economic landscapes of many countries may be permanently altered by HIV/AIDS, with global implications. The impact is most profound in the developing world, where poverty, poor education, limited or no access to health care, and cultural factors make the epidemic a formidable obstacle to contain.[2] Because it is a socially stigmatizing problem, many hide their condition or refuse to be tested. This only serves to perpetuate the virus and expand the epidemic.

Genetic analysis suggests that initial transmission of HIV-1 may have occurred as early as 1930 in equatorial West Africa.[3] There is evidence to support more than one transmission from animals to humans. Subsequently, HIV spread across the globe, predominantly transmitted through sexual exposure (approximately 75% of cases), by contact with infected blood or blood products, and vertically between mother and child.

BASIC SCIENCE

HIV is a lentivirus (slow virus), a member of the retrovirus class. It is an RNA virus with a unique enzyme, reverse transcriptase, which allows the virus to produce DNA from its own RNA. The DNA is then incorporated into the host's DNA, where it may lie dormant or replicate, producing viral progeny.

After the initial acute infection with HIV, termed the *acute retroviral syndrome*, most patients experience a phase of clinical latency, during which there is little or no outward evidence of active infection. However, the virus continues to replicate and destroy CD4$^+$ T lymphocytes, despite a lack of clinical symptoms. The continued destruction of CD4$^+$ cells eventually depletes the immune system, allowing various opportunistic infections and malignancies to develop and culminating in AIDS. If allowed to progress unchecked and uncontrolled, HIV/AIDS ultimately leads to the death of the host.

EPIDEMIOLOGY

Humans are not the natural host of this class of viruses. Current evidence reveals that HIV began as a zoonosis, a disease transmitted from animals to humans.[3] Through genetic study, HIV has been linked to the simian immunodeficiency virus (SIV), which infects wild African primates (e.g., chimpanzees, mangabeys, macaques) but does not always cause disease in them. These animals are hunted for their meat, which is often sold in markets. Younger animals may be captured and kept as pets. It is thought that exposure to the blood or bites of these primates allowed SIV to cross species and infect the incidental human host, producing HIV.

There are two types of HIV: HIV-1 and HIV-2. HIV-1 appears to have arisen from SIV in chimpanzees (SIV$_{cpz}$), specifically *Pan troglodytes troglodytes*.[4,5] HIV-2 most likely crossed species from SIV in sooty mangabeys (SIV$_{sm}$). HIV-1 shares approximately 50% genetic homology with SIV$_{cpz}$, and HIV-2 has approximately 90% homology with SIV$_{sm}$. HIV-1 predominates throughout the world and is the more aggressive form of the disease. HIV-2 is less infectious and progresses more slowly than HIV-1. Thus far,

HIV-2 is geographically restricted to west central Africa, with a modest number of cases in Europe and sporadically elsewhere.

There are three groups of HIV-1: M (major), N (non-M), and O (other). More than 90% of HIV-1 is group M. Nine subtypes, or clades, are derived from strain M. They are designated A, B, C, D, F, G, H, J, and K. Various subtypes predominate in different areas of the world. For example,

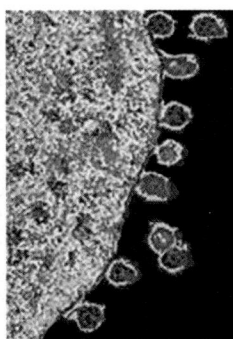

FIGURE 208-1   Electron micrograph of human immunodeficiency virus attacking a cell. *(From AVERT. Available at http://www.avert.org/photos.htm [accessed February 19, 2008].)*

subtype B dominates in Europe, the Americas, Japan, and Australia, whereas subtype C is the predominate type in eastern Africa, India, and Nepal (Fig. 208-3). Different subtypes of HIV have the ability to combine while simultaneously infecting the same host, producing a new hybrid form referred to as a *circulating recombinant form* (CRF). Marked genetic diversity exists in HIV subtypes and CRFs. This genetic diversity can make HIV difficult to treat and makes vaccine development very challenging. It may also be a factor contributing to the ability of HIV to escape immune surveillance and alter its virulence.

The global dissemination of HIV may be viewed as a series of waves of infection, with its epicenter in sub-Saharan Africa.[6] The initial ripple may have occurred coincident with the War of Liberation and Freedom between Tanzania and Uganda in 1978. HIV-1 most likely existed in the region, was acquired by soldiers during the war through sexual contact, and was then taken home, where it was further disseminated.

The arrival of HIV in the Western world during the late 1970s signaled the second wave of the epidemic. It was initially centered in the gay and bisexual population and intravenous drug users. Thereafter, it entered the blood supply, infecting recipients, particularly hemophiliacs. Eventually, children of infected women were found to

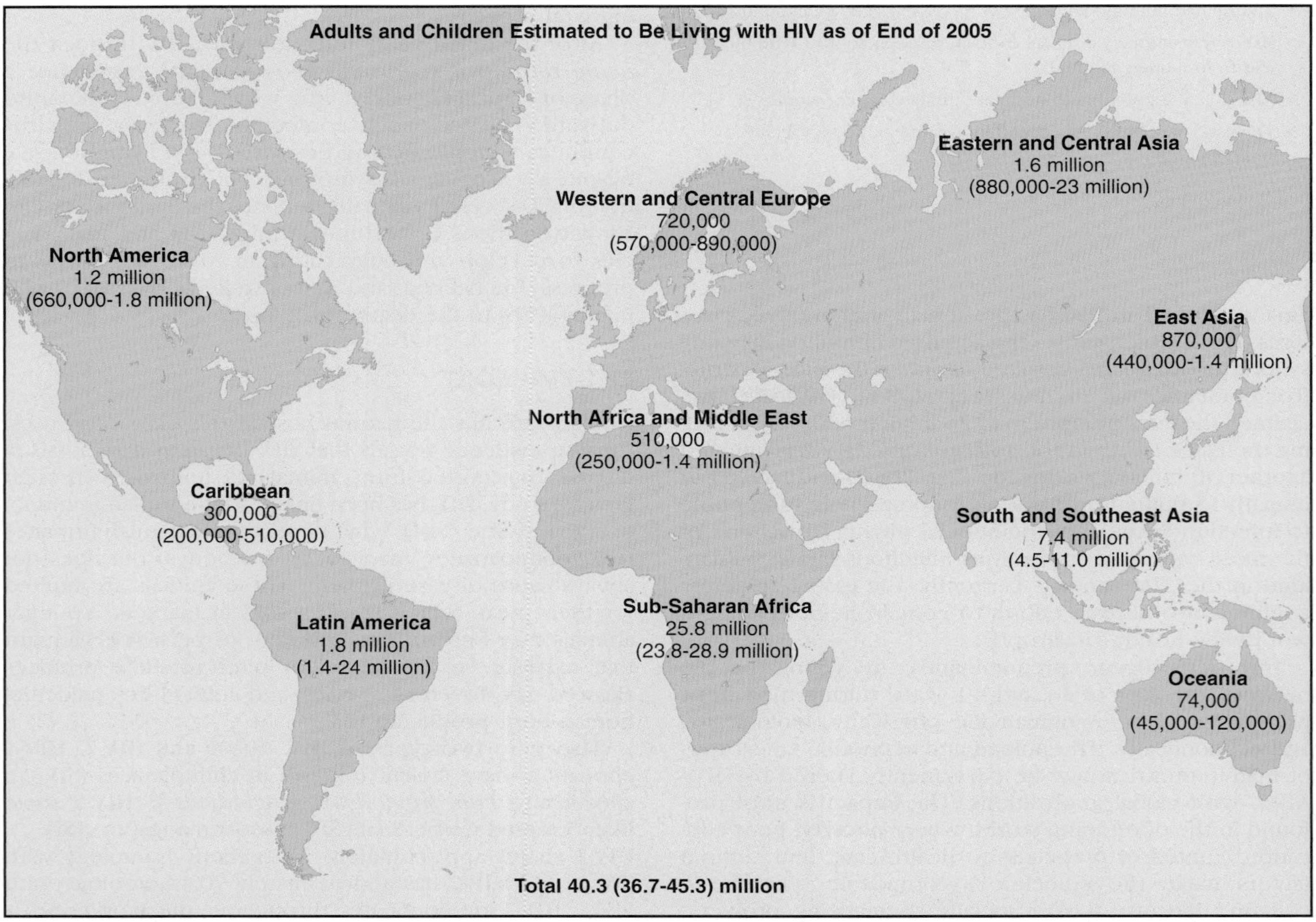

Adults and Children Estimated to Be Living with HIV as of End of 2005

Eastern and Central Asia
1.6 million
(880,000-23 million)

Western and Central Europe
720,000
(570,000-890,000)

North America
1.2 million
(660,000-1.8 million)

East Asia
870,000
(440,000-1.4 million)

North Africa and Middle East
510,000
(250,000-1.4 million)

Caribbean
300,000
(200,000-510,000)

South and Southeast Asia
7.4 million
(4.5-11.0 million)

Latin America
1.8 million
(1.4-24 million)

Sub-Saharan Africa
25.8 million
(23.8-28.9 million)

Oceania
74,000
(45,000-120,000)

Total 40.3 (36.7-45.3) million

FIGURE 208-2   Global picture of HIV, 2005. *(Redrawn from Jcint United Nations Programme on HIV/AIDS. Available at http://www.unaids.org/NetTools/Misc/ DocInfo.aspx?LANG=en&href=http://GVA-DOC-OWL/WEBcontent/Documents/pub/Topics/Epidemiology/Slides02/12-05/EpiCoreDec05Slide004_en.ppt.)*

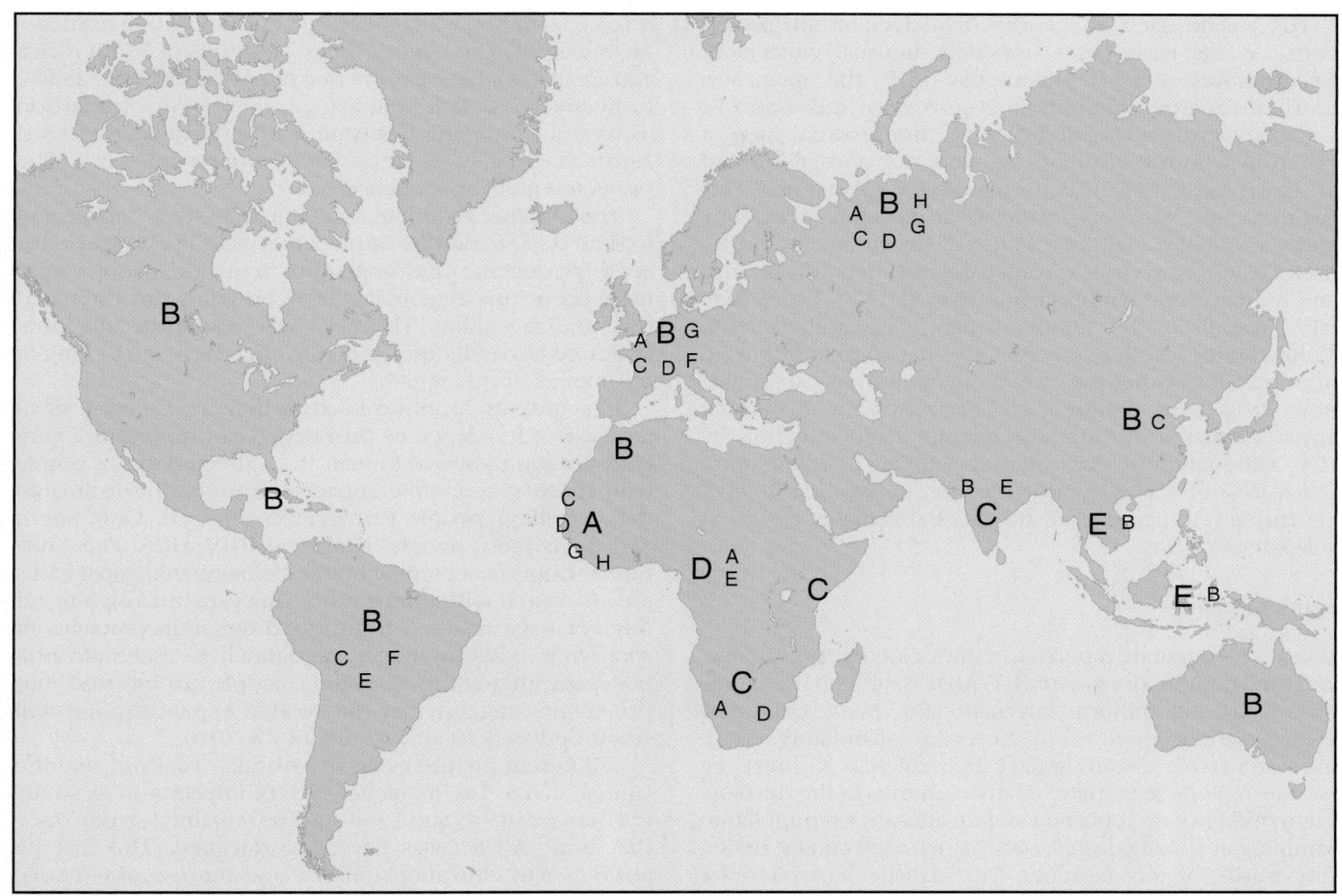

FIGURE 208-3 Global distribution of HIV-1 clades. *(Redrawn from International AIDS Vaccine Initiative. Available at http://www.iavi.org [accessed February 19, 2008].)*

have acquired HIV. During the second wave, the HIV epidemic was first described and the viral etiology was discovered.

The third wave occurred in Southeast Asia, emanating from Thailand and India. With an explosive onset in the late 1980s, the predominant groups affected were intravenous drug users and sex workers. Thailand has worked aggressively to control the epidemic, whereas progress has been much more difficult for India. The massive population at risk in India offers a frightening scenario waiting to unfold. Neighboring Pakistan and Indonesia are on the threshold of potentially serious epidemics as well.

The fourth wave struck the former Soviet Union. As in Southeast Asia, intravenous drug use provided the entry to this region, with a burgeoning secondary problem in the sex industry. Social unrest, poverty, crime, and a lack of resources are contributing to the spread of HIV and making control of the epidemic challenging.

The most recent wave has rolled into China. It may have started in rural areas through blood donation practices. Urban infections occur predominantly in intravenous drug users, but the number of cases of HIV infection is rapidly increasing.

HIV/AIDS is a global disease; however, its impact has been disproportionately experienced in the developing world, most profoundly in sub-Saharan Africa, where 10%

TABLE 208-1	Lives Lost Since the Onset of the AIDS Epidemic (Millions)	
CATEGORY	**2005**	**1981-2005**
Infections	4.9	65
Deaths	3.1	25
Living with HIV/AIDS	40.3	
Deaths in children	0.57	
Orphans		15

of the world's population live but 65% to 70% of the cases exist. Statistics compiled by the Joint United Nations Programme on HIV/AIDS (UNAIDS) for 2005 estimate that 40.3 million people are living with HIV worldwide, 25.8 million of whom reside in sub-Saharan Africa.[7] AIDS claimed 3.1 million lives in 2005, which included 570,000 children (≤15 years of age). Another 4.9 million people became infected, half of whom were younger than 24 years of age. This translates into an average of 13,500 infections and 8500 deaths daily. These figures represent a continuous upward trend over the course of the epidemic. Since the onset of the HIV epidemic, a total of 25 million lives have been lost (Table 208-1).

HIV has no age, race, gender, or socioeconomic preference. As the early cases unfolded, unusual clusters of *Pneumocystis carinii* pneumonia (PCP; the species is now designated *Pneumocystis jiroveci*) and Kaposi's sarcoma began to be described in homosexual men, a group in whom these illnesses were not normally found and for which there was no plausible explanation.[1] This "gay disease" was recognized as an immune deficiency and was initially attributed to use of sex-enhancing drugs, then Epstein-Barr virus, cytomegalovirus, hepatitis B virus, and human T-cell lymphotropic virus (HTLV). Eventually, HIV-1 was discovered simultaneously by researchers in the United States and in France.[8,9] Cases began to be reported in populations other than gay men: hemophiliacs, intravenous drug users, children, and heterosexuals. It became apparent that no group was exempt from infection by HIV. Although more males than females are infected, more than 46% of cases worldwide are in women today.[7] Seventy-seven percent of all infected females reside in sub-Saharan Africa.

PREVALENCE

Worldwide accurate reporting of the incidence, prevalence, and total number of cases of HIV/AIDS is difficult. Case definitions are not uniform internationally. Some countries, even in the developed world, do not have mandatory reporting systems (e.g., Spain) or have incomplete reporting from various regions (e.g., Italy). Many countries in the developing world have no reporting system and rely on population sampling at specified sites, such as perinatal clinics, maternity wards, or city morgues. The statistics compiled are believed to seriously underestimate the true figures. Further compounding the problem is the reluctance of many individuals to be tested. An example of the disparity can be seen in Europe, where approximately 635,000 HIV cases have been reported, but UNAIDS estimates that more than 2 million Europeans are living with HIV.

Recent trends offer hope in some areas of the world but lead to grave concern and despair in others. The prevalence of HIV in sub-Saharan Africa is 7.2%. However, it is 37.3% in Botswana—123,000 of the 330,000 residents are infected![7] The larger African countries of South Africa and Zimbabwe have prevalence rates of 21.5% and 24.6%, respectively. A stark contrast can be seen in comparison to Western and Central Europe, with a prevalence of 0.3%; North America, 0.7%; or the Caribbean region, 1.6%.[7] The projected global prevalence is 1.1%.

The rapidly expanding epidemic in Eastern Europe and Central Asia, fueled by intravenous drug use, is cause for serious concern. One quarter of a million people were infected in this region in 2005, bringing the estimated total to 1.6 million. The necessary resources and infrastructure to handle the epidemic effectively are lacking in most areas of this region.

In populous countries such as India or China, a small increase in incidence or prevalence can represent a very large total number of human lives affected and a potentially massive economic impact. Currently, it is estimated that 5 million people in India are infected. Only South Africa has more people living with HIV/AIDS. The situation in China is becoming better characterized. Most cases are associated with intravenous drug use, but a significant number have resulted from blood donation practices in rural areas. Case numbers are difficult to ascertain; estimates are that almost 1 million people are infected, but projections suggest that this total is expanding and will reach between 10 and 20 million by 2010.

A different picture exists in Australia, Thailand, and the United States. The incidence of HIV infection in Australia fell between 1985 and 1998 and has remained steady since that time; AIDS cases have also declined. This can be attributed to educational efforts and the use of effective antiretroviral therapy (ART) since 1996 in Australia. The incidence of HIV cases in Thailand fell from approximately 140,000 in 1991 to 21,000 in 2003, largely due to education, aggressive campaigns for condom use, and ART.

A dramatic drop in the number of AIDS cases and deaths was noted in the United States after ART became available. The decrease in AIDS cases and AIDS-related deaths slowed in the late 1990s, and the rates rose slightly during 2000 to 2004 (Fig. 208-4). This slight increase was

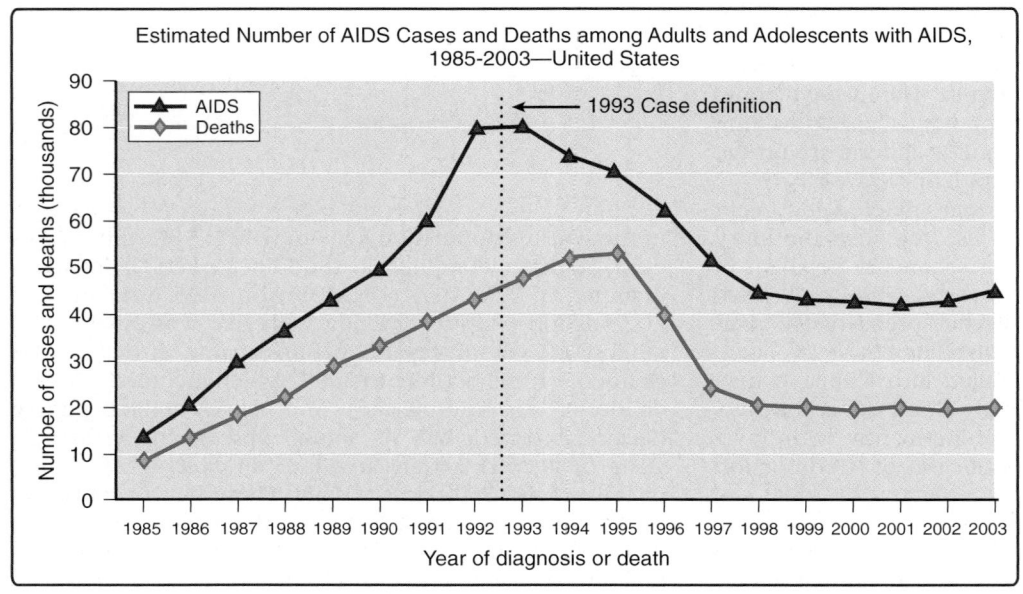

FIGURE 208-4   AIDS mortality, United States, 1985-2003. *(Redrawn from Centers for Disease Control and Prevention. AIDS Surveillance. Available at http://www.cdc.gov/hiv/graphics/surveill.htm [accessed February 19, 2008].)*

probably caused by increased numbers of people living with HIV/AIDS and living longer as a benefit of ART. This success may also be viewed as a concern. As the pool of infected people expands, it provides more potential sources for infection. Additional problems, complications of therapy, are now being encountered and include neuropathy, lipodystrophy, and coronary artery disease.

Minority populations (Blacks and Hispanics) are disproportionately affected by HIV in the United States. Overall, most cases are associated with men who have sex with men (MSM); however, rates among heterosexuals are steadily increasing. Intravenous drug users contribute a smaller but significant portion of the total cases. Approximately 1 million people are infected with HIV in the United States; 415,000 have AIDS, and more than 0.5 million have died.

Encouraging trends have been noted in Zimbabwe, with a declining adult HIV prevalence and, most notably, a 5% decrease in prevalence in pregnant women from 2002 to 2004.[7] In the capital, Harare, HIV prevalence in perinatal clinics decreased from 35% to 21% between 1999 and 2004. The prevalence rates among pregnant women in urban Kenya decreased even more dramatically, from 28% to 9% between 1999 and 2003. Education, safe sex campaigns, and condom use have been aggressively employed. Impressive success has occurred in decreasing vertical transmission from mother to child. With the use of perinatal ART prophylaxis, the rate has dropped from 24% to 8% (and lower in some instances). Similar positive findings have occurred in other African countries, in parts of the Caribbean, and in Southeast Asia.

TREATMENT AND PREVENTION

Access to ART has improved, although it is still far short of the need. The recent scale-up of therapy may have saved 250,000 to 350,000 lives in 2005.[7] Treatment coverage has expanded significantly in many areas of Latin America, reaching 80% in some countries. The United Nations "3 × 5" initiative was aimed at bringing ART to 3 million infected people by the end of 2005. The Gates Foundation, the Clinton Foundation, and the Global Fund are all working to alleviate the burden of HIV. Patent protection of some antiviral drugs has been waived to allow generic production, thereby markedly decreasing the cost and allowing therapy to be more affordable and available for areas of the developing world. An additional benefit of the increased availability of ART has been increased acceptance of HIV testing. Despite this progress, only 1 of every 10 Africans and 1 of every 7 Asians in need of ART are currently receiving it.

Recurring themes of poverty, social upheaval, social unrest, war, and inequality course through the HIV epidemic. Historically, these problems have been noted in other epidemics; they are key driving forces that must be addressed and overcome. Conquering this set of problems will vastly aid the conquest of HIV.

If there is hope of controlling the HIV epidemic, the developed world needs to assume an even larger role, assisting the developing world with access to therapy and medical technology. Extensive education must occur to overcome ignorance surrounding HIV and to foster prevention. Other areas of the world will need to adopt Thailand's aggressive condom effort. Needle exchange programs and treatment of drug addiction must become available to intravenous drug users. Further support for microbicide and vaccine development must occur, with cooperation between government and private industry. Finally, the prejudice and discrimination that continue to shroud those infected with HIV/AIDS must be overcome. If these challenges can be met, the current catastrophic global pandemic may be transformed into a chronic manageable disease with hope for a cure.

REFERENCES

1. Centers for Disease Control and Prevention. Pneumocystis pneumonia. MMWR Morb Mortal Wkly Rep 1981;30:250-252.
2. Buvé A, Bishikwabo-Nsarhaza K, Mutangadura G. The spread and effect of HIV-1 infection in sub-Saharan Africa. Lancet 2002;359:2011-2017.
3. Hahn B, Shaw G, DeCock K, Sharp P. AIDS as a zoonosis: Scientific and public health implications. Science 2000;287:607-614.
4. Gao F, Bailes E, Robertson DL, et al. Origin of HIV-1 in the chimpanzee *Pan troglodytes troglodytes*. Nature 1999;397:436-444.
5. Bailes E, Gao F, Bibollet-Ruche F, et al. Hybrid origin of SIV in chimpanzees. Science 2003;300:1713.
6. Sande M. Infection with human immunodeficiency virus, an epidemic out of control: Personal reflections. J Infect Dis 1999;179(Suppl 2):S387-S390.
7. Joint United Nations Programme on HIV/AIDS (UNAIDS). Report on the global HIV/AIDS epidemic (November 2005). Geneva: UNAIDS, 2005.
8. Gallo RC, Salahuddin SZ, Popovic M, et al. Frequent detection and isolation of cytopathic retroviruses (HTLV-III) from patients with AIDS and at risk for AIDS. Science 1984;224:500-503.
9. Barre-Sinoussi F, Chermann J, Rey F, et al. Isolation of a T-lymphotrophic retrovirus from a patient at risk for acquired deficiency syndrome (AIDS). Science 1983;220:868-871.

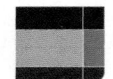

CHAPTER **209**

Biology and Natural History of Acquired Immunodeficiency Syndrome

Karen Frame, Laurence John, and Robert Colebunders

KEY POINTS

- Acquired immunodeficiency syndrome (AIDS) is caused by the human immunodeficiency virus (HIV), an RNA retrovirus.
- HIV infects and destroys CD4+ T lymphocytes, resulting in progressive deterioration of the immune response.
- Patients may remain asymptomatic for several years before developing significant immunosuppression and symptomatic disease.
- Cell-mediated immunity is impaired, resulting in increased susceptibility to opportunistic infections, caused by organisms of relatively low pathogenicity, and certain HIV-related malignancies.
- HIV targets other tissues, causing end-organ disease such as neuropathy, cardiomyopathy, and dementia.

Acquired immunodeficiency syndrome (AIDS) was first described as a clinical entity in 1981, when homosexual men were presenting to hospitals in North America and Europe with illnesses such as *Pneumocystis jiroveci* (then known as *Pneumocystis carinii*) pneumonia (PCP) and Kaposi's sarcoma.[1,2] The epidemiology of cases, and the fact that in all patients CD4[+] T lymphocytes were depleted, suggested infection by a pathogen leading to a state of immunodeficiency. The human immunodeficiency virus (HIV), an RNA retrovirus, was identified as the causative organism in 1983.[3,4] HIV causes disease through the progressive depletion of CD4[+] cells, which results in reduced cell-mediated immunity. Patients become increasingly susceptible to particular opportunistic infections and malignancies. HIV also targets specific organs such as the heart and brain, resulting in end organ damage.

BASIC SCIENCE

The Human Immunodeficiency Virus

HIV is an RNA virus belonging to the lentivirus ("slow") subfamily of Retroviridae. It is composed of an outer membrane or envelope, which is derived from the host cell membrane, and an inner core. The envelope contains two glycoproteins, gp120 and gp41, that are important for the binding and membrane fusion that are necessary for viral entry into cells (Fig. 209-1). The inner core, called the nucleocapsid, has a protein shell (p24) and contains two molecules of single-stranded viral RNA together with proteins essential for viral replication: protease, integrase, and reverse transcriptase.

The HIV genome is 9.7 kilobases (kb) in length and contains three major structural genes: *gag* (encoding core proteins), *pol* (encoding essential enzymes including protease, reverse transcriptase, and integrase), and *env* (encoding envelope proteins). These are flanked at either end by long terminal repeats (LTRs), which regulate viral RNA transcription.[5] Accessory genes *vif, vpu, tat, rev,* and *nef* interact with host cell processes to optimize viral replication.[6]

The HIV Life Cycle

HIV attaches to a host cell through an interaction between its gp120 surface glycoprotein and a combination of host cell surface receptors, including CD4 and the chemokine receptor CCR5 (Fig. 209-2). The virus then fuses with the host cell membrane, and viral RNA enters the cytoplasm. Viral RNA is transcribed to double-stranded DNA by the enzyme reverse transcriptase. This proviral DNA then enters the cell nucleus and is incorporated into the cell genome by the enzyme integrase. RNA is transcribed from the integrated proviral DNA, messenger RNA is translated into viral proteins, and new viral genomic RNA is produced for the formation of new virions. Structural viral proteins are cleaved by proteases, and a new generation of HIV virions are assembled in the cytoplasm and released, destroying the host cell. Once released, immature HIV virions undergo further maturation, facilitated by viral proteases, and then go on to infect other cells. Key enzymes and proteins involved in HIV entry and replication, such as gp41 and CCR5, reverse transcriptase, integrase, and proteases, are important targets for antiretroviral treatment (ART) (see Chapter 213).

Subtypes of HIV

There are two types of HIV virus, HIV-1 and HIV-2. HIV-2 is less common and is predominantly found in West Africa, where it is associated with a slower rate of disease progression and, importantly, a nonresponsiveness to non-

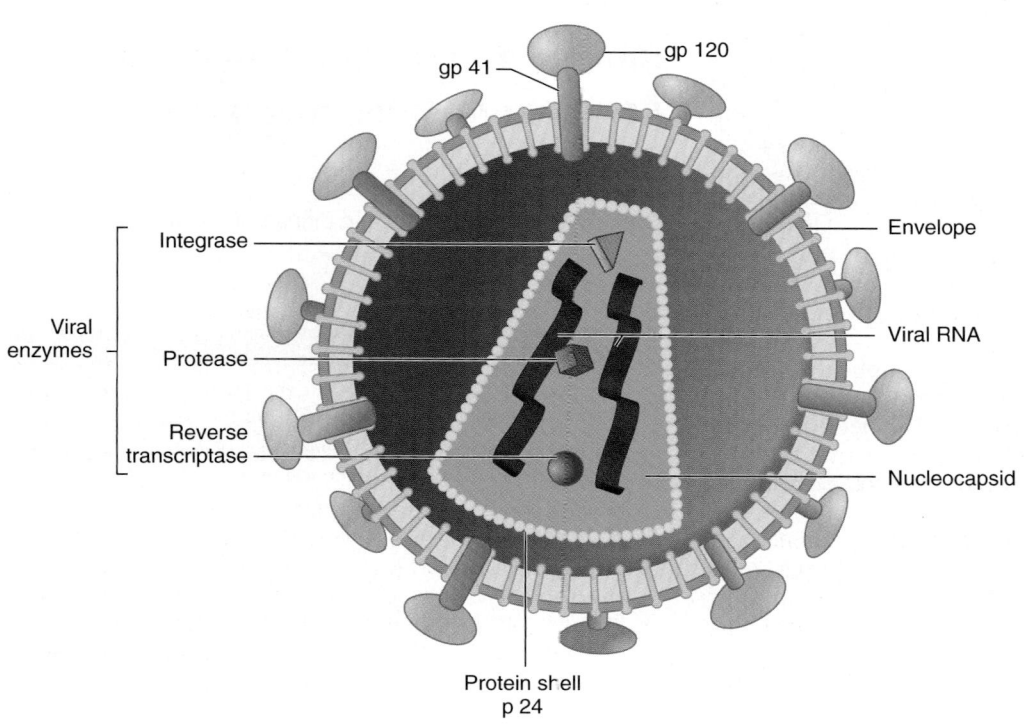

FIGURE 209-1 Schematic representation of the human immunodeficiency virus.

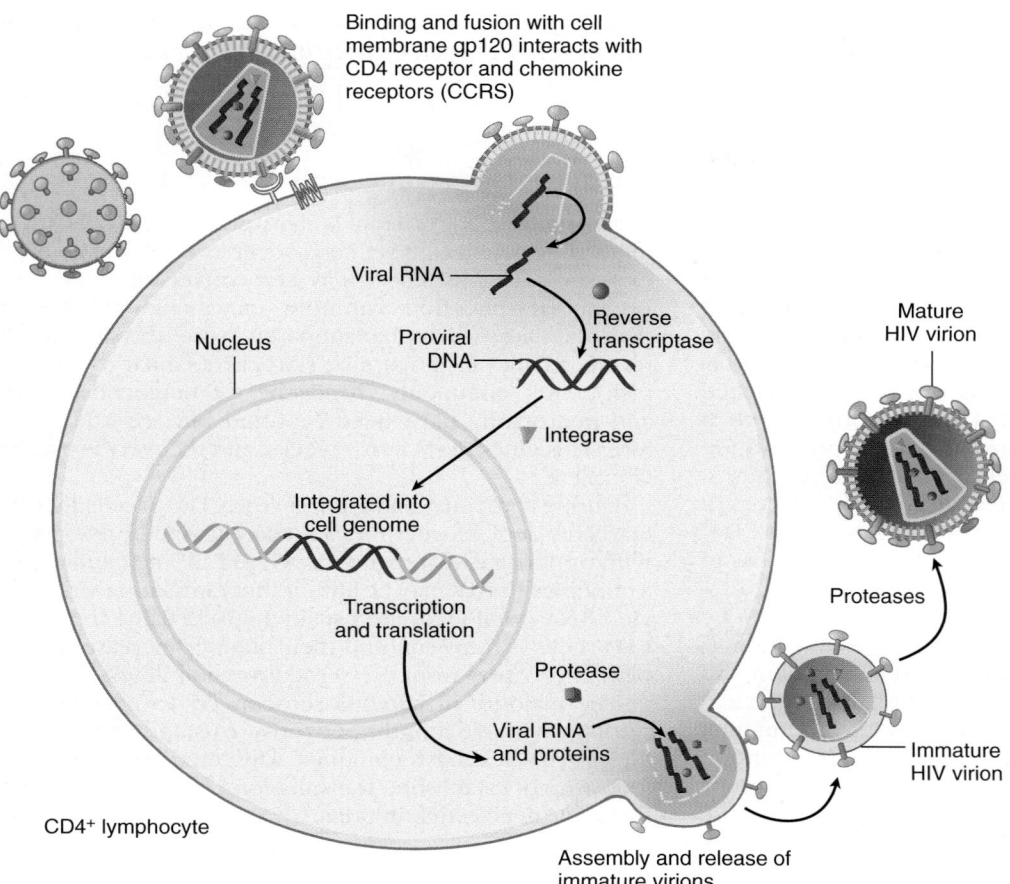

Binding and fusion with cell membrane gp120 interacts with CD4 receptor and chemokine receptors (CCRS)

Viral RNA

Reverse transcriptase

Nucleus

Proviral DNA

Integrase

Integrated into cell genome

Transcription and translation

Protease

Viral RNA and proteins

CD4⁺ lymphocyte

Assembly and release of immature virions

Mature HIV virion

Proteases

Immature HIV virion

FIGURE 209-2 Life cycle of the human immunodeficiency virus.

nucleoside–based ART. HIV-1 is classified into a number of subtypes according to the genetic sequences present in the *env* gene. The three major groups are M (main), O (outlier), and N (non-M, non-O). The M group of viruses is the major cause of AIDS worldwide. This group is further subdivided into at least nine subtypes or clades (A-K), and these are variably distributed throughout the world. In North America and Europe, the predominant clade is B, where as in sub-Saharan Africa, non–clade B viruses are more common. Although there are virological differences in the characteristics of these subtypes, the clinical implication of these differences is unclear. Certain clades may be associated with a faster progression to AIDS.[7]

Transmission of HIV

The transmission of HIV occurs during heterosexual and homosexual intercourse, through contaminated blood products or needles, and vertically from an infected mother to her newborn child (infection occurring either in utero, during birth, or from breastfeeding). During 2005, there were an estimated 4.9 million new infections; 3.2 million of these were in sub-Saharan Africa, where the majority of transmissions occurred through heterosexual intercourse.[8]

PATHOGENESIS

In infections that follow exposure via the mucosal route (e.g., sexual transmission), HIV virons bind to intraepithelial dendritic cells and macrophages. This occurs via interactions between HIV surface molecules (e.g., gp120) and host cell surface molecules (e.g., CCR5 and DC-SIGN). The virus is then transported by the dendritic cells to lymph nodes, where it is presented to CD4⁺ T cells, thus establishing infection.[9] There follows a rapid rise in viral replication, plasma viremia, and dissemination of the infection to other CD4⁺ cells, the lymphoid organs, and other tissues (e.g., central nervous system).[10]

The lymphoid tissue becomes the major reservoir of HIV infection in the body.[11] HIV-infected CD4⁺ T cells, macrophages, monocytes, and dendritic cells live in lymph nodes. Although this reservoir is less easy to quantify than the blood compartment, these cells contain the vast burden of HIV virus. A large number of resting lymphocytes are infected by the virus. These cells have an extremely long half-life (about 44 months), and, although they are, by definition, resting, they are able to become productive of infectious virus at any time, once activated in an immune response. The latent HIV provirus is not susceptible to currently available ART. HIV infection is therefore able to persist, and infected cells always have the potential to produce virus.[12] The dendritic cells and macrophages are also able to persist while harboring HIV infection; because of their mobility, they may be responsible for the ongoing dissemination of infection.[13]

The host's innate immune response to HIV infection begins within hours and includes the production of HIV inhibitory chemokines, including macrophage inflammatory protein-1α (MIP-1α), MIP-1β, and RANTES.[14] The adaptive immune response then occurs and includes both an antibody-mediated and a cell-mediated response. It is thought that the cell-mediated response is the more important component in the body's attempt at controlling HIV infection. HIV-specific cytotoxic T lymphocytes destroy virally infected cells, as part of the cell-mediated response. CD4+ T cell function is also important. A characteristic of long-term "nonprogressors" is the preservation of their HIV-specific CD4+ T-cell proliferation responses. The loss of control of HIV viral replication that occurs in late infection may be partly explained by this loss of CD4+ T-cell function, which is associated with the huge loss of CD4+ cells.[15] Antibodies against gp120 and gp41 are produced in response to infection but are not thought to be important for the control of HIV once an infection is established.[16] In addition to the fall in the CD4 count and the associated decline in CD4+ T-cell function, the virus itself plays an important part in its escape from immune control. Rapid viral replication and a high transcription error rate, characteristic of RNA viral polymerases, results in many genomic mutations occurring during the course of HIV infection. This leads to the generation of many variants of HIV within an individual; specific cytotoxic T-lymphocyte or humoral responses are eventually unable to contain all of the variant viruses, and virological escape ensues.[17]

The HIV virus causes damage to many cell types and tissues in the human body, including immune, neuronal, renal, and cardiac systems.[18] Its most important effect is on the immune system, where it particularly targets the cell-mediated immune system and therefore the ability of the body to mount an acquired immune response to HIV itself or to other infections or neoplasms.[19] CD4+ T lymphocytes are the principal target of the virus, and these crucial components of the acquired immune response are progressively destroyed by a combination of direct and indirect mechanisms. HIV damages CD4+ cells directly by causing the lysis of productively infected cells during the course of its life cycle. Infected CD4+ cells are also susceptible to destruction by cytotoxic T lymphocytes (CD8+) and syncytia formation. Destruction of noninfected CD4+ T cells is also thought to be important.[20] The number of CD4+ T-cells that are dying outnumber those that are infected.[21] Proposed mechanisms include increased immune activation of bystander cells, with a secondary increase in T-cell apoptosis (programmed cell death). The body's capacity to replace its lost CD4+ T cells is also damaged by HIV infection. There is widespread disruption to the lymphatic microenvironment,[22] and HIV also causes direct damage to the thymus, the organ responsible for maturation of bone marrow–derived progenitor lymphocytes into functional naïve CD4+ T lymphocytes. Destruction and impaired production of CD4+ cells results in progressive deterioration in immune function, which leads to increased susceptibility to opportunistic infec-

tions, impaired immunosurveillance against neoplasms, and direct end-organ damage due to HIV itself.

CLINICAL MANIFESTATIONS

Seroconversion/Primary HIV Infection

Most HIV seroconversion is asymptomatic. However, a mild, nonspecific illness may occur 6 to 8 weeks after exposure. This is known as seroconversion illness or primary HIV infection. Symptoms may include fever, joint pains, lethargy, lymphadenopathy, sore throat, mouth ulcers, a faint maculopapular skin rash (similar to measles rash), and, commonly, headache. Meningoencephalitis and neuropathy have been reported but are said to be rare. This illness lasts 2 to 3 weeks, and recovery is usually complete.

During seroconversion illness, the CD4+ T cells may be markedly depleted, at times so severely as to be associated with opportunistic infections such as PCP and candidiasis. Antibodies to HIV may be absent, but circulating virus and viral RNA (viral load) are usually high. Usually, the fall in CD4+ cells is transient, and their number increases as the patient recovers from the seroconversion illness.

The majority of patients seroconvert to positive HIV serology within 6 months of exposure using standard serological HIV testing techniques. This method is used for follow-up of established transmission events such as transfusion or needlestick injuries.

Clinical Latent Period

Most people with HIV infection are asymptomatic for a substantial (although variable) period of time during which the virus replicates, the individual remains infectious, and immune function gradually declines. Patients usually have no findings on examination except for lymphadenopathy in some.

Initially, death and replacement of CD4+ cells are in near-balance, and viral replication may be suppressed by the immune system. Therefore, a relatively steady state of cell counts and viral load may occur. As HIV infection progresses, the CD4 count falls at a rate of approximately 50 cells/mm^3 each year[23]; the immune system becomes less able to control HIV replication, and the levels of virus rise (Fig. 209-3). Immunosuppression ensues, and patients develop opportunistic infections or noninfectious complications of HIV, thus developing symptomatic disease (Table 209-1 and Figs. 209-4 through 209-7).

Symptomatic HIV Disease

Skin and mucous membrane disorders are frequently early symptoms of HIV, occurring at higher CD4 counts. Reactivation of varicella-zoster virus (shingles), prurigo (an itchy, generalized maculopapular skin rash), and fungal nail and skin infections are relatively common. Oral candida, bacterial pneumonia, tuberculosis, and some HIV-related malignancies such as Kaposi's sarcoma and non-Hodgkin's lymphoma may occur in early disease, but the risk increases as immunosuppression advances. Constitutional symptoms such as unexplained fevers and

TABLE 209-1 Complications Seen with Advancing HIV Disease

CD4⁺ COUNT (CELLS/mm³)	INFECTIOUS COMPLICATIONS	NONINFECTIOUS COMPLICATIONS
>500	Seroconversion illness	Lymphadenopathy Myopathy Guillain-Barré syndrome Aseptic meningitis
200-500	Bacterial pneumonia Pulmonary tuberculosis (within last year*) Herpes zoster Esophageal candidiasis* Kaposi's sarcoma* Oral hairy leukoplakia Acute *Cryptosporidia* diarrhea (self-limited)	Carcinoma of the cervix* Non-Hodgkin's lymphoma* Hodgkin's disease* Anemia Idiopathic thrombocytopenic purpura (ITP) Lymphocytic interstitial pneumonitis (LIP) Mononeuritis multiplex Nodular prurigo
<200	*Pneumocystis jiroveci* pneumonia (PCP)* Disseminated/chronic herpes simplex* Cerebral toxoplasmosis* Progressive multifocal leukoencephalopathy (PML)* Cryptococcal meningitis* Miliary/extrapulmonary tuberculosis* Chronic diarrhea (>1 month) due to *Cryptosporidia,* *Isospora,* or microsporidia* Disseminated histoplasmosis* Coccidioidomycosis*	Wasting* Central nervous system lymphoma* Cardiomyopathy Neuropathy HIV-associated dementia*
<50	Disseminated cytomegalovirus (CMV)* Disseminated *Mycobacterium avium-intracellulare* (MAI)*	

*AIDS-defining diagnosis.

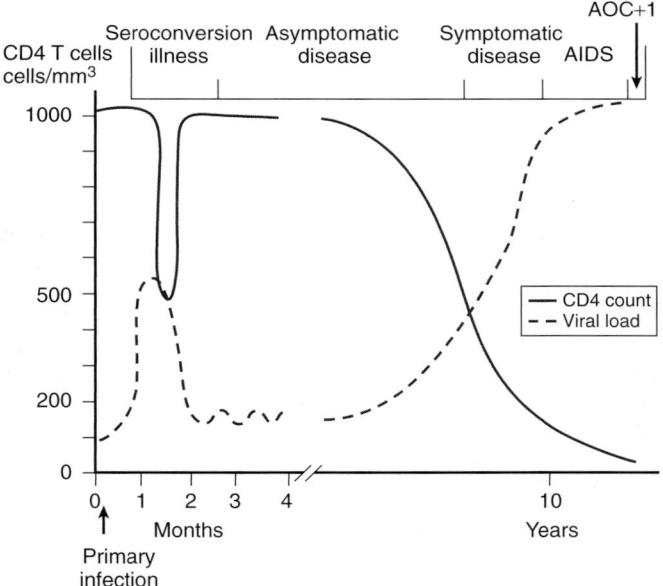

FIGURE 209-3   Natural history of HIV infection.

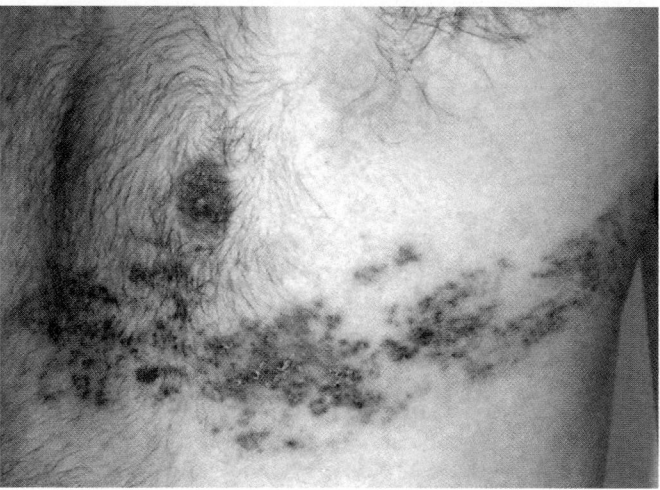

FIGURE 209-4   Herpes zoster in a patient with HIV infection.

weight loss may also occur in early symptomatic disease, although the AIDS "wasting syndrome" is usually a consequence of advanced disease.

Advanced immunosuppression (CD4 count <200 cells/mm³) results in disease caused by organisms of relatively low pathogenicity; these are known as *opportunistic infections*. Consequences of advanced immunosuppression include fungal infections such as cryptococcal meningitis, PCP, and disseminated histoplasmosis; viral infections such as cytomegalovirus (CMV), progressive

multifocal leukoencephalopathy (PML), and human herpesvirus 8 (HHV-8)–associated Kaposi's sarcoma; parasitic infections including toxoplasmosis and chronic diarrhea related to various protozoa; and the lymphomas. These result in significant symptom burden and high mortality if untreated. End-organ disease due to HIV itself, including neuropathy, cardiomyopathy, and enteropathy, are also seen in more advanced disease.

From a palliative care perspective, the underlying cause of pain and symptoms is particularly important to consider. Pain and symptoms may be caused by opportunistic infections (e.g., headache due to cryptococcal meningitis), by HIV itself (e.g., HIV enteropathy), by treatment (e.g., stavudine-related neuropathy), or by a concurrent

FIGURE 209-5 Nodular prurigo in a patient with HIV infection.

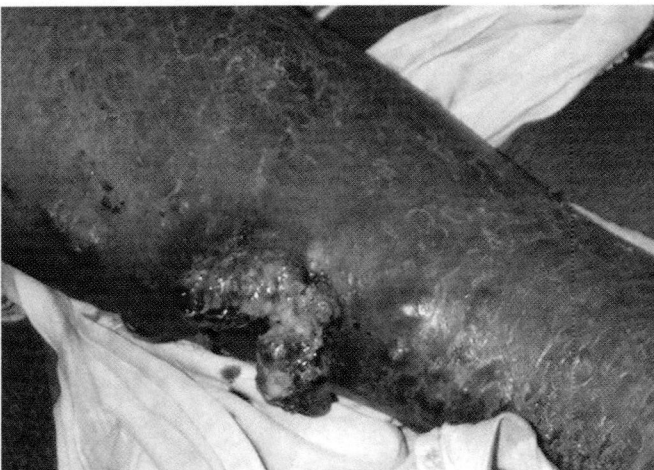

FIGURE 209-6 Kaposi's sarcoma with lymphedema in a patient with HIV infection.

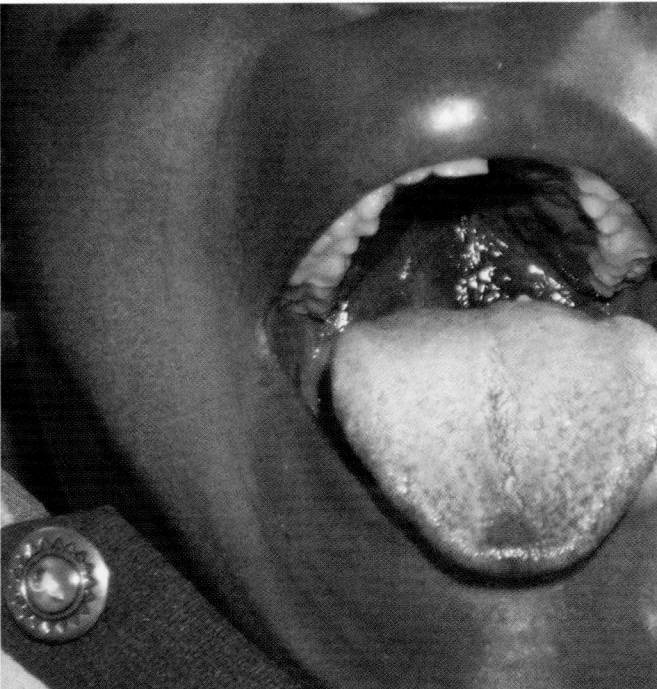

FIGURE 209-7 Oral Kaposi's sarcoma in a patient with HIV infection.

problem (e.g., arthritis). Active treatment of the underlying cause often results in improved symptom control. Pain and symptom control often goes hand-in-hand with active management, with cessation of analgesics and other symptom control measures once the opportunistic infection has been treated.

Staging of HIV Disease

There are a number of clinical staging systems, including those proposed by the U.S. Centers for Disease Control and Prevention[24] and the World Health Organization (WHO).[25] The WHO's four-stage system, which ranges from stage 1 (asymptomatic) to stage 4 (advanced disease), broadly correlates with the sequential stages of immune deficiency that develop in HIV infection.[25] The clinical syndrome of AIDS is defined by the presence of specific opportunistic infectious syndromes and/or neoplasms, the so-called *AIDS-defining events* (see Table 209-1).[24] The average time from infection to AIDS (or WHO stage 4) in Europe, North America, and Africa is 9 to 10 years.[26]

TREATMENT

HIV/AIDS is an example of a condition in which advances in treatment have dramatically changed the natural course of the disease. The advent of highly active antiretroviral treatment (HAART) (see Chapter 213) during the 1990s has transformed HIV from a fatal disease to a chronic illness for those able to access treatment. The role of palliative care in the era of HAART has also evolved as mortality in those accessing treatment has fallen. Palliative care is required in the era of HAART for those patients with pain and symptom control problems (e.g., neuropathy), for those with HIV-related cancers, for those who cannot access available treatment or access it too late, and for those in whom available treatment fails. Palliative care can help alleviate severe spiritual, social, or psychological distress and supports HAART providers in these aspects of patient care, potentially improving adherence to HAART.[27] Palliative care has been shown to improve outcomes across all stages of disease and care domains for patients with HIV/AIDS in developed countries.[28]

REFERENCES

1. Centers for Disease Control and Prevention. Kaposi's sarcoma and *Pneumocystis* pneumonia among homosexual men—New York City and California. MMWR Morb Mortal Wkly Rep 1981;30:305-308.
2. Centers for Disease Control and Prevention. *Pneumocystis* pneumonia—Los Angeles. MMWR Morb Mortal Wkly Rep 1981;30:250-252.
3. Chermann JC, Barre-Sinoussi F, Dauguet C, et al. Isolation of a new retrovirus in a patient at risk for acquired immunodeficiency syndrome. Antibiot Chemother 1983;32:48-53.
4. Gallo RC, Sarin PS, Gelmann E, et al. Isolation of human T-cell leukemia virus in acquired immune deficiency syndrome (AIDS). Science 1983;220:865-867.

5. Cleghorn FR, Reitz MS, Popovic M, et al. Human immunodeficiency viruses. In Mandell GL, Bennett JE, Dolin R (eds): Principles and Practice of Infectious Diseases, 6th ed. New York: Churchill Livingstone, 2005, pp 2119-2133.
6. Emerman M, Malim MH. HIV-1 regulatory/accessory genes: Keys to unraveling viral and host cell biology. Science 1998;280:1880-1884.
7. Kaleebu P, Ross A, Morgan D, et al. Relationship between HIV-1 Env subtypes A and D and disease progression in a rural Ugandan cohort. AIDS 2001;15:293-299.
8. Joint United Nations Programme on HIV/AIDS (UNAIDS). Report on the Global AIDS Epidemic, 2006. Available at http://www.unaids.org/en/HIV_data/2006GlobalReport/default.asp (accessed February 22, 2008).
9. Bomsel M, David V. Mucosal gatekeepers: Selecting HIV viruses for early infection. Nat Med 2002;8:114-116.
10. Grouard G, Clark EA. Role of dendritic and follicular dendritic cells in HIV infection and pathogenesis. Curr Opin Immunol 1997;9:563-567.
11. Chun TW, Carruth L, Finzi D, et al. Quantification of latent tissue reservoirs and total body viral load in HIV-1 infection. Nature 1997;387:183-188.
12. Finzi D, Blankson J, Siliciano JD, et al. Latent infection of CD4+ T cells provides a mechanism for lifelong persistence of HIV-1, even in patients on effective combination therapy. Nat Med 1999;5:512-517.
13. Clark EA. HIV: Dendritic cells as embers for the infectious fire. Curr Biol 1996;6:655-657.
14. Levy JA, Scott I, Mackewicz C, et al. Protection from HIV/AIDS: The importance of innate immunity. Clin Immunol 2003;108:167-174.
15. Rosenberg ES, Billingsley JM, Caliendo AM, et al. Vigorous HIV-1-specific CD4+ T cell responses associated with control of viremia. Science 1997;278:1447-1450.
16. Poignard P, Sabbe R, Picchio GR, et al. Neutralizing antibodies have limited effects on the control of established HIV-1 infection in vivo. Immunity 1999;10:431-438.
17. Price DA, Goulder PJ, Klenerman P, et al. Positive selection of HIV-1 cytotoxic T lymphocyte escape variants during primary infection. Proc Natl Acad Sci USA 1997;94:1890-1895.
18. Glass JD, Johnson RT. Human immunodeficiency virus and the brain. Annu Rev Neurosci 1996;19:1-26.
19. Levy JA. Pathogenesis of human immunodeficiency virus infection. Microbiol Rev 1993;57:183-289.
20. Finkel TH, Banda NK. Indirect mechanisms of HIV pathogenesis: How does HIV kill T cells? Curr Opin Immunol 1994;6:605-615.
21. Mosier DE, Gulizia RJ, MacIsaac PD, et al. Rapid loss of CD4+ T cells in human-PBL-SCID mice by noncytopathic HIV isolates. Science 1993;260:689-692.
22. Fauci A. Immunopathogenic mechanisms of human immunodeficiency virus disease: Implications for therapy. Am J Med 1995;99:59S-60S.
23. Janeway C, Travers P, Walport M, Shlomchik M. Failures of host defence mechanisms. In Janeway C (ed): Immunology: The Immune System in Health and Disease, 6th ed. New York: Garland Science, 2005, pp 491-515.
24. Centers for Disease Control and Prevention. 1993 Revised classification system for HIV infection and expanded surveillance case definition for AIDS among adolescents and adults. MMWR Recomm Rep 1993;41(RR-17):1-19.
25. World Health Organization. Proposed "World Health Organization staging system for HIV Infection and Disease": Preliminary testing by an international collaborative cross-sectional study. The WHO International Collaborating Group for the Study of the WHO Staging System. AIDS 1993;7:711-718.
26. Morgan D, Mahe C, Mayanja B, et al. HIV infection in rural Africa: Is there a difference in median time to AIDS and survival compared to that in industrialised countries? AIDS 2002;16:597-603.
27. Harding R, Higginson IJ. Palliative care in sub-Saharan Africa. Lancet 2005;365:1971-1977.
28. Harding R, Karus D, Easterbrook P, et al. Does palliative care improve outcomes for patients with HIV/AIDS? A systematic review of the evidence. Sex Transm Infect 2005;81:5-14.

CHAPTER **210**

Acquired Immunodeficiency Syndrome in Adults

Busi Mooka and Fiona Mulcahy

KEY POINTS

- Treatment of human immunodeficiency virus (HIV) infection is lifelong, and the virus cannot be eradicated from latently infected CD4+ T lymphocytes.

- All health care settings should offer routine, stigma-free, opt-out screening for HIV infection.

- As people with HIV disease live longer, management has shifted to limiting treatment side effects, malignancies, and coinfections.

- Perinatal transmission of HIV is preventable.

Human immunodeficiency virus (HIV) infections are increasing worldwide, with more than 95% of cases occurring in developing countries. Half of new infections are in females, and 40% are in people between 15 to 24 years of age.

EPIDEMIOLOGY AND PREVALENCE

In the United States, men who have sex with men account for 47% of people living with HIV, heterosexual people account for 34%, and injecting drug users account for 17%.[1] There are a disproportionate number of new diagnoses and deaths due to HIV and acquired immunodeficiency syndrome (AIDS) among minority groups, especially women. Compared with Caucasian women, African-American women are 24 times more likely to be diagnosed with AIDS, Latinas 6 times more likely, and Native American/Alaskan Native women 4.4 times more likely.[2] The prevalence of HIV in America is 0.8% (Table 210-1).

PATHOPHYSIOLOGY

In 1984, researchers discovered the human immunodeficiency virus type 1 (HIV-1), 3 years after descriptions of the clinical syndrome now known as AIDS. HIV-1 is the most common cause of AIDS worldwide. In 1986, HIV-2 was isolated in West Africa. HIV-2 immunodeficiency is milder, develops more slowly, and has less efficient vertical and heterosexual transmission.[3]

Human Immunodeficiency Virus Life Cycle

HIV is a lentivirus of the retrovirus family that primarily infects CD4+ T lymphocytes by binding to the CD4 receptor with the help of a coreceptor. The virus then fuses with the host cell's lipid bilayer, enters the cell, and

TABLE 210-1 Worldwide Prevalence of Human Immunodeficiency Virus, 2006

POPULATION	TOTAL	CHILDREN <15 YR
People living with HIV	39,500,000	2,300,000
New HIV infections	4,300,000	530,000
HIV-related deaths	2,900,000	380,000

From Joint United Nations Programme on HIV/AIDS (UNAIDS). Available at http://data.unaids.org/pub/EpiReport/2006/2006_EpiUpdate_en.pdf (accessed February 22, 2008).

TABLE 210-2 Risk of Transmission of Human Immunodeficiency Virus

EVENT	RISK OF HIV ACQUISITION PER 10,000 EVENTS
Blood transfusion	9000
Injecting drug use	67
Receptive anal intercourse	50
Needlestick injection	30
Receptive vaginal intercourse	10
Insertive anal intercourse	6.5
Insertive vaginal intercourse	5
Receptive oral intercourse	1
Insertive oral intercourse	0.5

From Varghese B, Maher JE, Peterman TA, et al. Reducing the risk of sexual HIV transmission: Quantifying the per-act risk for HIV on the basis of choice of partner, sex act, and condom use. Sex Transm Dis 2002;29:38-43.

uncoats, allowing its RNA to enter the cytoplasm (see Fig. 209-2).

The enzyme reverse transcriptase transcribes viral RNA into DNA, which is then incorporated into the host genome with the help of the integrase enzyme. Reverse transcription is a highly error-prone process. This causes considerable genetic variation in the viral progeny. Integrated into cellular DNA, HIV can remain latent for years. This is a major barrier for cure, because all current drug therapies are inactive against latent virus.

Once the cell becomes activated, the integrated DNA is transcribed into messenger RNA and translated to viral proteins, including HIV protease, which cleaves the HIV polyproteins into functional forms. Virions are assembled at the cell surface and released. The average turnover is 10 billion viral particles per day.

Within a few weeks after infection, there is an acute depletion of the bulk of gut-associated CD4$^+$ cells. This is followed by a decrease in circulating CD4$^+$ cells. Usually, the circulating CD4 count increases after the acute infection subsides. During clinical latency, the rate of loss of CD4$^+$ cells varies from patient to patient. The likelihood of opportunistic infections increases as the CD4 count declines.

Transmission of Human Immunodeficiency Virus

The risk of transmitting HIV varies by exposure. Table 210-2 describes the transmission risks associated with sexual contacts and exposure to contaminated blood or needles.[4]

Mother-to-Child Transmission

Several factors increase the risk of HIV transmission in pregnancy[5]:

- High maternal viral load (e.g., seroconversion in pregnancy)
- Premature membrane rupture (>4 hours), with or without chorioamnionitis
- Prematurity (<37 weeks' gestation)
- Invasive procedures (e.g., amniocentesis, scalp electrodes)
- Breastfeeding (increases risk by 5% to 20%)

Transmission from breastfeeding increases with breastfeeding duration, mixed feeding, breaches in the infant's oral mucosa, nipple fissures, and mastitis.

The success of prevention depends on the resources available to pregnant women and their children.[6] In the United States, there has been a 95% reduction in vertical transmission, from 945 transmissions in 1992 to 48 in 2004.

Progression of HIV Disease

Several factors contribute to the variation in rate of progression of HIV among infected individuals. These can be divided into viral factors and host factors.

Viral Factors

Replication capacity, a measure of the efficiency of the virus, influences the ability of the virus to proliferate. Certain drug-associated mutations impair viral fitness and may influence viral load and, hence, disease progression.

People infected with HIV-1 that has deletions or defects in the *nef* (*negative factor*) gene may also have slower progression of disease.

Host Factors

Human leukocyte antigen (HLA)-B alleles exert a dominant impact on viral load. The HLA class I alleles B*27 and B*57 are associated with low viral load and slower progression to symptomatic disease. However, among elite controllers (HIV RNA <50 copies/mL without therapy), fewer than half express either HLA B*27 or HLA B*57. This suggests that progression is affected by additional host genetic factors, such as polymorphisms in the ABOBEC 3G or TRIM-5α genes, or by other host factors, such as chemokine receptor polymorphisms and chemokine ligand gene duplications.

For HIV to enter cells, it usually must fuse with a chemokine receptor CCR5 on the surface of CD4$^+$ cells. The Δ32 mutation in the gene encoding the CCR5 protein results in a defective receptor site that blocks virus entry. Despite repeated HIV exposures, people who are homozygous for the mutation are resistant to most HIV infection. Heterozygotes may also be substantially resistant.

DIAGNOSIS

Who Should Be Tested

The Centers of Disease Control and Prevention (CDC) recommends routine opt-out HIV testing in all health care settings for everyone aged 13 to 64 years of age in a testing process that is simplified, free of stigma, and linked with clinical care and prevention services.[7]

Methods of Testing

Antibodies to HIV become detectable 2 to 12 weeks after infection. Antibody testing should be repeated if there is a possibility that the initial test was performed during this serological window period.

Demonstration of HIV-specific antibodies by at least two different methods is the most commonly accepted definition of a positive HIV test. The initial screening test is usually by enzyme-linked immunosorbent assay (ELISA). This screen usually looks for antibodies to the various HIV-1 subtypes and HIV-2. Screening tests have a sensitivity of at least 99.5%.

A confirmatory test using a different method is usually offered on a different blood sample. The second test is typically a Western blot assay. A conventional follow-up test should be offered 4 weeks after a positive result. The rapid test should be used, because there have been false-positive results.

The preferred preliminary method of testing in infants is polymerase chain reaction (PCR) for the first 18 months of life. Testing is typically done at 48 hours of life, again at 1 to 2 months, and then at 3 to 6 months. An infant is considered to be HIV positive if two PCR tests are positive or if the child is antibody positive after 18 months.

EVALUATION

History taking should include comorbidities, past history, mental health, family history, social and economic circumstances, substance use, and current medication. In women of childbearing age, plans and desires for children should be considered (Table 210-3).

CD4 Count

The normal absolute number of CD4+ T lymphocytes for men is 400 to 1600 cells/mm³; for women, it is 500 to 1600 cells/mm³. The count can fluctuate with acute illness, rest, pregnancy, and menstruation. The CD4 count on initial assessment should be repeated. If there is a discrepancy between the two counts, a third is recommended.[8] In pregnant women and in patients with hypersplenism, in whom the absolute CD4 count can be misleading, the CD4 percentage (often a more stable measure) may be a more useful monitoring tool.

Viral Load

Following the acute increase in HIV viral load at seroconversion, the viral load achieves a set point. Patients with a low viral set point have slower progression to symptomatic HIV disease. Quantitative HIV RNA testing monitors the response to therapy. One of the aims of therapy is to maintain the viral load below the detection level.

TABLE 210-3	Tests for Evaluation of HIV Disease Status	
TYPE OF TEST	**BASELINE TESTS IN NEW PATIENTS**	**SUBSEQUENT VISITS**
Serology	HIV antibody test	
	Syphilis	
	Hepatitis A, B, C	Assess for hepatitis vaccination
	Toxoplasma, cytomegalovirus, varicella	Repeat yearly if IgG negative
Virology	Viral load	Every 3 mo and after treatment change
	Genotypic resistance	At therapy failure
Immunology	CD4 count	Every 3-6 mo
Hematology	CBC, BUN, creatinine	Every 3-6 mo
Biochemistry	Transaminases	
	Fasting glucose, cholesterol†	
	Urinalysis	
Other	Tuberculin skin test*	
	Papanicolaou (Pap) smear	Twice in first year, then yearly
	Chlamydia, gonorrhea screen†	Repeat with partner change
	Chest radiographs†	

BUN, blood urea nitrogen; CBC, complete blood count; IgG, immunoglobulin G.

*Unless the person has a prior history of tuberculosis or a prior positive skin test.

†To be considered in all cases.

Pregnant Women

Universal routine antenatal opt-out HIV testing of pregnant women without extensive pre-test counseling or explicit written consent is recommended to detect maternal HIV infection and prevent mother-to-child transmission. Pregnant women are more likely to be tested if the test is strongly recommended or is part of a panel of routine tests.

Factors that hinder timely HIV testing in pregnant women include the following:

- Late presentation to antenatal services
- Test not offered because the provider perceived the pregnant woman to be at low risk
- Laborious consent and counseling procedure and regulations
- Communication barriers

A second HIV test should be offered in the third trimester in areas of high incidence or if there is risk of HIV seroconversion in pregnancy.

Newborn testing is recommended if maternal HIV status is undocumented after delivery. It should be done quickly to facilitate postexposure prophylaxis, which should be started within the first 12 hours of life.[7]

CLINICAL MANIFESTATIONS

Seroconversion Illness

Acute HIV seroconversion illness is symptomatic in 40% to 90% of people and lasts up to 3 weeks. Common symptoms are fever, maculopapular rash, lymphadenopathy, oral ulcers, pharyngitis, arthralgia, aseptic meningitis, malaise, weight loss, and myalgia.

Laboratory abnormalities include atypical reactive lymphocytes, lymphopenia, thrombocytopenia, abnormal transaminases, and low CD4 count. The CD4 count could drop low enough to cause AIDS-defining illnesses.

Identification during primary HIV infection could reduce the spread of HIV. Acute HIV infection can be diagnosed by detection of HIV RNA in plasma of people who have a negative or indeterminate HIV antibody test. Antiretroviral treatment for acute HIV is controversial and has not become a standard of care, because the long-term benefits have not been established. Differential diagnoses for seroconversion illness include infectious mononucleosis, influenza, acute *Toxoplasma* infection, hepatitis infection, and syphilis.

Asymptomatic Phase

After the acute seroconversion illness, there is an asymptomatic clinical latency period that may last 8 to 10 years. There is a considerable variation in the length of this period. *Long-term nonprogressors* are HIV-infected people who have high CD4 counts despite chronic HIV infection. This is an immunologically and virologically diverse group who comprise 5% of all HIV-infected people. A smaller subset, referred to as *HIV elite controllers,* maintain an HIV viral load below the limit of detection despite chronic infection.

Persistent generalized lymphadenopathy is lymphadenopathy of greater than 1 cm, occurring at two or more extrainguinal sites, for longer than 3 months in the presence of HIV without any other cause found. Persistent generalized lymphadenopathy may be found in some individuals during the latent phase. It may be associated with splenomegaly. Lymph nodes are usually mobile and nontender. Biopsy usually shows benign hyperplasia. The presence of persistent generalized lymphadenopathy does not seem to affect the rate of progression to AIDS.

Symptomatic HIV Disease

As the CD4 count declines and the HIV viral load increases, symptoms emerge. Initially, the symptoms that occur may not meet the criteria of AIDS-defining conditions.

For example:

- Bacillary angiomatosis
- Candidiasis—oropharyngeal, persistent, or poorly responsive vulvovaginal
- Cervical dysplasia (moderate or severe) or carcinoma in situ
- Herpes zoster (>1 episode or >1 dermatome)
- Idiopathic thrombocytopenic purpura
- Listeriosis
- Fever (>38.5°C) or diarrhea lasting longer than 1 month

- Oral hairy leukoplakia
- Pelvic inflammatory disease
- Peripheral neuropathy

AIDS-Defining Illnesses

AIDS is characterized by specific illnesses in people with HIV infection and CD4 counts of less than 200 cells/µL (or CD4 percentage <14%). Antiretroviral therapy has changed the significance of being diagnosed with an AIDS-defining illness.

AIDS-defining illnesses include the following:

- Candidiasis (esophagus, bronchi, trachea, lungs)
- Cervical carcinoma (invasive)
- Coccidioidomycosis (extrapulmonary or disseminated)
- Cryptococcosis (extrapulmonary)
- Cryptosporidium (chronic, intestinal lasting >1 month)
- Cytomegalovirus (CMV), other than liver, spleen, or lymph nodes; CMV retinitis
- Encephalopathy (HIV related)
- Herpes simplex (mouth ulcers for >1 month, bronchitis, pneumonitis, esophagitis)
- Histoplasmosis (extrapulmonary, disseminated)
- Isosporiasis (intestinal, lasting >1 month)
- Kaposi's sarcoma
- Lymphoma (Burkitt's, immunoblastic, primary brain)
- *Mycobacterium avium* complex, *Mycobacterium kansasii* (disseminated or extrapulmonary)
- *Pneumocystis jiroveci* pneumonia (PCP)
- Pneumonia, recurrent
- Progressive multifocal leukoencephalopathy
- *Salmonella* septicemia (recurrent)
- *Toxoplasma* (brain)
- Wasting syndrome

In the developed world, opportunistic infections have declined because of antiretroviral therapy and appropriate prophylaxis. Most people presenting with AIDS-defining illnesses in resource-rich areas are not receiving treatment for HIV, because of unknown HIV status or failure to access care. Caution should be taken when prescribing treatment and prophylaxis for opportunistic infections in pregnant women.

COINFECTION

Tuberculosis

The HIV-fueled increase in tuberculosis (TB) infections is most marked in sub-Saharan Africa, where up to 60% of HIV-infected people also have TB. Pulmonary TB can occur at any CD4 count, whereas disseminated TB occurs primarily with CD4 counts lower than 200 cells/mm³. TB recurrence is more common in HIV-positive patients.

HIV-infected patients with latent TB have a 10% annual risk of reactivating TB. The tuberculin skin test may be negative even in TB in immunosuppressed people. γ-Interferon secreted by mononuclear cells specific for TB antigens can be detected by enzyme-linked immunosorbent spot (ELISPOT). The role of this method in people with HIV infection is unclear.

In uncomplicated cases in which CD4 counts are relatively preserved, TB is treated the same way as in HIV-negative people. Directly observed therapy is recommended. If possible, it is best to defer HIV therapy for the first 8 weeks of therapy, to reduce the pill burden and the incidence of paradoxical reactions and drug interactions.

Hepatitis B

Hepatitis B is 100 times more infectious than HIV. The most common mode of transmission in the United States is sexual transmission. In the United States, 10% to 15% of HIV-infected people have chronic hepatitis B. The clinical course of hepatitis B is altered by HIV:

- Increased risk of chronicity (×5) after acute infection, compared with HIV-negative patients
- Mortality 15 times higher than in HIV-negative people, eight times higher than in hepatitis B–negative people
- More frequent reactivation (related to CD4 counts)
- Optimal duration for hepatitis B in coinfection unknown
- Less chance of seroconversion in coinfection
- Increased risk of progression to cirrhosis and death

When considering optimal treatment for people coinfected with HIV and hepatitis B, it is important not to jeopardize further HIV therapy by the drug choices made for hepatitis B. Special consideration should be made when hepatitis B–active drugs are stopped, started, or changed, because there is a risk of hepatitis flare. Similar caution should apply when starting or stopping antiretroviral therapy. The current guidelines from the U.S. Department of Health and Human Services (DHHS) advise against lamivudine, emtricitabine, or tenofovir as monotherapy in this population. Caution is advised when using adefovir, given a theoretical risk of inducing tenofovir resistance.[7]

Vaccination against hepatitis B in HIV-infected patients has a higher rate of nonresponse than in HIV-negative patients. In those who do respond, there is a need to monitor antibody levels, because protective immunity declines over time. Infants of hepatitis B coinfected women should be offered vaccination.

Hepatitis C

In the United States, 30% of HIV patients are coinfected with hepatitis C. Hepatitis C is 10 times more infectious than HIV. Although sexual transmission is less frequent than with HIV, 4% to 8% of men who have sex with men in the United States are coinfected. Sexual transmission is associated with traumatic sexual practices. Pregnant women should be offered an elective caesarean section.

When considering therapy for hepatitis C, consideration is made of the CD4 count and possible drug interactions. HIV alters the clinical course of hepatitis C infection:

- Risk of progression to cirrhosis is greater (10 to 20 years versus 30 to 40 years); other factors, such as age, alcohol, and antiretroviral therapy, also affect this progression.
- Lower response rate to hepatitis C treatment.
- Greater proportion of autoantibodies in coinfected people; their significance is not fully understood.

TREATMENT

HIV cannot be eradicated from the body, because there is a pool of latently infected CD4+ cells. Once antiretroviral therapy is started, the current recommendation is that it not be interrupted.

Four classes of antiretroviral medications are available. The choice of regimen should be tailored to the patient, considering prior antiretroviral history, resistance profile, pill burden, drug interactions, and lifestyle.

The current recommended choice of class for antiretroviral-naïve patients is a three-drug regimen: two nucleoside reverse transcriptase inhibitors with one protease inhibitor or nonnucleoside reverse transcriptase inhibitor. Care should be taken to attempt to preserve future therapeutic options when selecting regimens.

Initiation of Treatment

Current guidelines recommend that treatment of HIV should be considered after the CD4 count declines to less than 350 cells/mm^3 and before it drops to less than 200 cells/mm^3. If an opportunistic infection develops, treatment should be started promptly (regardless of CD4 count) unless there is a risk of disease flare from immune reconstitution (tuberculosis, CMV retinitis, PCP, *Toxoplasma*).

The absolute CD4 count is expected to increase on antiretroviral therapy by 50 to 100 cells/mm^3 each year until a threshold is reached. There is an accelerated CD4 response in the first 3 months of therapy. (See Chapter 211 for treatment of children with HIV infection.)

Management of HIV in Pregnancy

Alterations of drug pharmacokinetics in pregnancy change some side effect profiles. Close monitoring of transaminases, lactate levels, and hemoglobin is recommended, along with monitoring of the CD4 count and viral load. Therapeutic drug monitoring is also recommended if certain protease inhibitors are used. A resistance profile is useful to guide therapy choices. Chlamydial infection, trichomonas vaginalis, and bacterial vaginosis should be treated, because they are associated with prematurity, which increases HIV transmission.

The treatment plan depends on gestational age at diagnosis, degree of maternal immunosuppression, maternal viral load, antiretroviral history, and HIV resistance profile. A zidovudine-containing regimen is recommended for all pregnant women (antepartum and intrapartum) and their babies.[9] In women who need treatment solely for infant prophylaxis, antiretroviral treatment is discontinued after delivery.

There are four possible case scenarios:

1. HIV diagnosis in an antepartum, treatment-naïve woman
2. HIV diagnosis in an antepartum woman receiving treatment
3. HIV in a woman in labor with no antepartum treatment
4. HIV in a woman with no antiretroviral therapy before delivery

New Diagnosis of HIV Infection in a Pregnant Woman

If a woman is diagnosed in the first trimester of pregnancy, consideration should be given to deferring treatment until at least week 13 of gestation, to avoid the critical period of organogenesis. This may not be possible or desirable in severely immunosuppressed women. For women who are relatively immunologically intact, treatment is usually started at 28 weeks' gestation and stopped after delivery.

In 1994, the Pediatric AIDS Clinical Trials Group protocol 076 (PACTG 076) study showed a 70% reduction in HIV transmission when zidovudine was started between 14 and 34 weeks' gestation, continued intrapartum, and extended for 6 weeks to the infant.[9] Since the advent of highly active antiretroviral therapy (HAART) and subsequent improved survival rates, monotherapy is now considered suboptimal. In treatment-naïve patients, combination therapy is the standard of care. Monotherapy with zidovudine may be considered for women with a baseline HIV viral load of fewer than 1000 copies/mL.[10]

Pregnancy in an HIV-Positive Woman Receiving Treatment

If the pregnant woman is already taking antiretrovirals, therapy is continued without interruption in most cases. Some women may opt to stop therapy until gestational week 13 to avoid drug exposure during organogenesis.[10] Rarely, hyperemesis necessitates temporary cessation of antiretroviral therapy. In any interruption of therapy, all drugs should be stopped at once, unless the woman is taking nevirapine or efavirenz. Nevirapine and efavirenz have long half-lives and therefore must be stopped first, with the nucleoside backbone continued for 3 to 5 days longer to provide coverage during this process and reduce resistance evolution. If possible, even in treatment-experienced patients, zidovudine should be included in the regimen. Stavudine and zidovudine should not be coadministered, because they are antagonistic.[10]

The following drugs are to be avoided in pregnancy:

- Efavirenz (potential teratogenicity)
- Didanosine/stavudine combination (mitochondrial toxicity)
- Amprenavir oral solution (high alcohol levels)

The baby should get 4 to 6 weeks of zidovudine treatment.

HIV in a Laboring Woman with No Antepartum Treatment

There are several possible options for reducing transmission[11] in an HIV-positive woman in labor who has had no previous treatment:

- Intravenous zidovudine during labor, followed by 6 weeks of zidovudine in the infant
- Intravenous zidovudine with single dose nevirapine during labor, followed by up to a week of lamivudine and zidovudine to reduce the occurrence of nevirapine resistance
- Intravenous zidovudine during labor, followed by 6 weeks of zidovudine, possibly in combination with other antiviral drugs for the infant

The mother needs full staging of her HIV after delivery.

HIV in a Woman with No Antiretroviral Therapy before Delivery

Zidovudine is given to the infant for 6 weeks. Addition of other antiretrovirals for the same 6 weeks should be considered.[11]

Elective Cesarean Section

Elective section is recommended for all women who have a viral load greater than 1000 copies/mL at 36 weeks' gestation, to reduce transmission of HIV. Intravenous zidovudine should be started 3 hours before the procedure.[11]

Side Effects of Antiretrovirals in Pregnancy

NUCLEOSIDE/NUCLEOTIDE REVERSE TRANSCRIPTASE INHIBITORS

Mitochondrial toxicity is increased. The manifestations include neuropathy, myopathy, hepatic steatosis, lactic acidosis, cardiomyopathy, and pancreatitis. Lactate monitoring is useful to diagnose mitochondrial toxicity. The combination of didanosine and stavudine should be avoided, because it is associated with an increased incidence of mitochondrial toxicity. The most important differential is the HELLP syndrome (*h*emolysis, *e*levated *l*iver enzymes, and *l*ow *p*latelets).

Hemoglobin should be closely monitored in all patients taking zidovudine.

NON-NUCLEOSIDE REVERSE TRANSCRIPTASE INHIBITORS

In women with CD4 counts greater than 250 cells/mm^3, nevirapine is 9.8 times more likely to cause symptomatic hepatotoxicity, which is usually associated with a rash.[13] Women presenting in pregnancy who are already taking nevirapine may continue it, with appropriate monitoring. If nevirapine is used, transaminases should be monitored at baseline, every 2 weeks for 1 month, monthly for 4 months, and then every 1 to 3 months. Every patient with a rash needs to have her transaminases checked. With symptomatic or asymptomatic elevation of transaminases, nevirapine should be discontinued without rechallenge.[11]

PROTEASE INHIBITORS

Monitoring of glucose is recommended because of the increased risk of onset of diabetes mellitus; exacerbation of existing diabetes and diabetic ketoacidosis have also been reported. All of these conditions are also increased by pregnancy itself. There are conflicting reports regarding increased prematurity and low birth weight.

ENTRY INHIBITORS

There are only case reports of Enfuvirtide use in pregnancy, and no randomized control trials exist.

Future Considerations

- The long-term benefits of treating acute HIV infection are unclear.
- Novel antiretroviral drugs are under development (integrase inhibitors, maturation inhibitors, CCR5 inhibitors). It is challenging to treat heavily treatment-experienced patients while awaiting new drugs.
- Maintenance of a pregnancy register allows for the monitoring of all children whose mothers received antiretroviral therapy during pregnancy.
- Prevention strategies are needed to reach minority groups, especially young women.

PREVENTION

Family planning services and treatment of sexually transmitted diseases reduce the transmission of HIV. The prevalence of unprotected anal or vaginal intercourse with uninfected partners is, on average, 68% lower for HIV-infected persons who are aware of their status than for those who are infected but unaware of their status. This is particularly important in patients with high viral loads, because they are at the highest risk for transmitting HIV. Partner notification should be encouraged and reviewed at every visit.

Circumcision reduces heterosexual transmission of HIV to HIV-negative men by 50% to 60%. Condom use also reduces transmission.[14] Microbicides with various mechanisms of action are under study for protection of the vaginal mucosa against HIV infection. There are also multiple pre-exposure prophylaxis trials in progress. These methods of prevention raise multiple ethical and behavioral issues (see "Future Considerations").

REFERENCES

1. Joint United Nations Programme on HIV/AIDS and World Health Organization. AIDS Epidemic Update, December 2006. UNAIDS/06.29E. Available at http://data.unaids.org/pub/EpiReport/2006/2006_EpiUpdate_en.pdf (accessed February 22, 2008).
2. Centers for Disease Control and Prevention. HIV/AIDS Surveillance Report, Vol. 17, 2005. Estimated Numbers of Cases and Rates (per 100,000 Population) of AIDS, by Race/Ethnicity, Age Category, and Sex, 2005—50 States and the District of Columbia. Atlanta: U.S. Department of Health and Human Services, CDC, 2006, pp 1-46.
3. de Cock K, Adjorlolo G, Ekpini E, et al. Epidemiology and transmission of HIV-2: Why there is no HIV-2 pandemic. JAMA 1993;270:2083-2086.
4. Varghese B, Maher JE, Peterman TA, et al. Reducing the risk of sexual HIV transmission: Quantifying the per-act risk for HIV on the basis of choice of partner, sex act, and condom use. Sex Transm Dis 2002;29:38-43.
5. European Collaboration Study. Mother to child transmission of HIV infection in the era of highly active antiretroviral rherapy. Clin Infect Dis 2005;40:458-465.
6. Kourtis AP, Lee FK, Abrams EJ, et al. Mother to child transmission of HIV-1: Timing and implications for prevention. Lancet Infect Dis 2006;6:728-732.
7. Centers for Disease Control and Prevention. Revised recommendations for HIV testing in adults, adolescents and pregnant women in health care settings. MMWR Morb Mortal Wkly Rep 2006;55(RR-14):1-17.
8. Guidelines for the Use of Antiretroviral Agents in HIV-1 Infected Adults and Adolescents, October 10, 2006, Developed by the Panel on Clinical Practices for Treatment of HIV Infection Convened by the Department of Health and Human Services Developed by the DHHS Panel on Antiretroviral Guidelines for Adults and Adolescents—A Working Group of the Office of AIDS Research Advisory Council (OARAC). Available at http://aidsinfo.nih.gov/contentfiles/AdultandAdolescentGL.pdf (accessed February 22, 2008).
9. Connor EM, Sperling RS, Gelber R, et al. Reduction of maternal-infant transmission of human immunodeficiency virus type 1 with zidovudine treatment. N Engl J Med 1994;331:1173-1180.
10. Ioannidis JP, Abrams EJ, Ammann A, et al. Perinatal transmission of human immunodeficiency virus type 1 by pregnant women with RNA virus loads <1000 copies/ml. J Infect Dis 2001;183:539-545.
11. Public Health Service Task Force Recommendations for Use of Antiretroviral Drugs in HIV-1 Infected Pregnant Women for Maternal Health and Interventions to Reduce Perinatal Transmissions in the United States, October 12, 2006. Available at http://aidsinfo.nih.gov (accessed February 22, 2008).
12. Guay LA, Musoke P, Fleming T, et al. Intrapartum and neonatal single-dose nevirapine compared to zidovudine for prevention of mother to child transmission of HIV-1 in Kampala, Uganda: HIVNET 012 randomised trial. Lancet 1999;354:795-802.
13. Hitti J, Frental LM, Stek LM, et al. Maternal toxicity with continuous nevirapine in pregnancy. Results from PACTG 1022. J Acquir Immune Defic Syndr 2004;36:772-776.
14. Auvert B, Taljaard D, Lagarde E, et al. Randomized, controlled intervention trial of male circumcision for reduction of HIV infection risk: The ANRS 1265 trial. PLoS Med 2005;2(11):1-18.

SUGGESTED READING

Guidelines for the Use of Antiretroviral Agents in HIV-1 Infected Adults and Adolescents, October 10, 2006, Developed by the Panel on Clinical Practices for Treatment of HIV Infection Convened by the Department of Health and Developed by the DHHS Panel on Antiretroviral Guidelines for Adults and Adolescents—A Working Group of the Office of AIDS Research Advisory Council (OARAC). Available at http://aidsinfo.nih.gov/contentfiles/AdultandAdolescentGL.pdf (accessed February 22, 2008).

Public Health Service Task Force Recommendations for Use of Antiretroviral Drugs in HIV-1 Infected Pregnant Women for Maternal Health and Interventions to Reduce Perinatal Transmissions in the United States, October 12, 2006. Available at http://aidsinfo.nih.gov (accessed February 22, 2008).

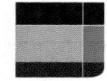

CHAPTER **211**

Palliative Care for Children and Adolescents with Human Immunodeficiency Virus/Acquired Immunodeficiency Syndrome

Elizabeth Gwyther, Michelle Meiring, Joan Marston, and Busisiwe Nkosi

KEY POINTS

- Palliative care for children with HIV/AIDS is the active total care of the child's body, mind, and spirit and also involves giving support to the family.
- Palliative care begins when illness is diagnosed and continues regardless of whether the child receives treatment directed at the disease.
- Antiretroviral treatment (ART) and early, aggressive management of opportunistic infections and other problems (e.g., malnutrition) are an essential part of good palliative care.
- ART positively influences the course of illness and quality of life of the child and family but does not effect a cure.
- Palliative care affords equal emphasis to disease-oriented care and to control of distressing symptoms.
- It is important to include the child's parents and/or carers as key members of the management team, as well as involving the child in his or her own care.

It is a challenging task, both clinically and emotionally, to work with children and adolescents who have a diagnosis of a life-threatening illness or who are dying. However, it is work that is enriching and rewarding for the health care professional who is equipped with the knowledge, skills, and attitudes to promote quality pediatric palliative care.

In the context of the HIV/AIDS pandemic, the most important role of the palliative care pediatrician is to ensure that children and adolescents who are infected with HIV (and their infected parents) have access to antiretroviral treatment (ART) according to clinical guidelines, because these drugs both improve quality and quantity of life.

DEFINITION OF PALLIATIVE CARE FOR CHILDREN

Palliative care for children represents a special field, but one that is closely related to adult palliative care. The World Health Organization (WHO) has defined palliative care appropriate for children and their families as follows[1]:

- Palliative care for children is the active total care of the child's body, mind, and spirit and also involves giving support to the family.
- Palliative care begins when illness is diagnosed and continues regardless of whether a child receives treatment directed at the disease.
- Health providers must evaluate and alleviate a child's physical, psychological, and social distress.
- Effective palliative care requires a broad, multidisciplinary approach that includes the family and makes use of available community resources; it can be successfully implemented even if resources are limited.
- Palliative care can be provided in tertiary care facilities, in community health centers, or even in homes (the child's own home, a foster home, or a residential care facility).

The WHO definition is appropriate for children with life-threatening cancer, HIV/AIDS, or a chronic illness such as cystic fibrosis, muscular dystrophy, or cerebral palsy. The extent of the HIV epidemic and the impact of this epidemic on children has increased the need for palliative care and the awareness of pediatric palliative care.

Modern pediatric care assists in the prevention and cure of many serious conditions, and the increasing access to antiretrovirals has positively affected our ability to assist many children. However, there remain children for whom cure is not possible, children who live with chronic illness or disability, and HIV-positive children who are facing life-threatening illness because of lack of access to ART or treatment failure. It is important to recognize the fact that ART does not cure AIDS. For most children, ART has the ability to turn a progressive disease that is imminently fatal into a chronic manageable condition, but there will always be a subset of children who do not have access to ART or for whom treatment has failed for whatever reason. These children and their families require

expert palliative care to "alleviate their physical, psychological, and social distress" and to provide spiritual support.

Pediatric palliative care is a specialized field that differs from adult palliative care in a number of ways. The most crucial difference is that adult palliative care "affirms life and regards dying as a normal process."[1] Although it is true that all of us will die, it is not normal that a child should die, and all feel a great sense of outrage that children should suffer and have to die. Parents often express their distress and comment that it should not be that a parent buries their child.

The Children's Issues Steering Group at the Second Global Summit of National Hospice and Palliative Care Associations, held in Korea in 2005, stated the following[2]:

- Children and adolescents with life-limiting conditions have very specific palliative care needs, which are often different from those of adults.
- If these physical, emotional, social, spiritual, and developmental needs are to be met, the carers require special knowledge and skills.
- We ask that the voices of these children and adolescents be heard, respected, and acknowledged as part of the expression of hospice care and palliative care worldwide.

As with all pediatric care, palliative care should be delivered while taking into account the child's developmental and educational needs. The functional level achieved by a child depends on the stimulation the child receives from the environment. Many HIV-infected children do not experience this stimulation, either because of illness or because of severe social deprivation in a poverty-stricken environment, with resulting developmental delay and neurological disorganization.

It is important to expose the child to regular basic sensory input to restore his or her ability to receive, process, store, and utilize information. This can be done through play, music, touch/massage, interaction with animals—the types of activity children from a privileged, affluent background take for granted. One of the important considerations for children is to be "normal," and this includes continuing with their education and play activities.[3]

Support of the Family

It is important to include the child's parents and/or carers as key members of the management team, as well as involving the child in his or her own care. Full information and respect for the parents as knowledgeable persons in the care of their child empowers the parents and engenders a sense of control that may have been lost with the impact of the diagnosis. It is also important to recognize the needs of siblings, who often are the "silent sufferers" whose own needs are superceded by the needs of the sick brother or sister, and who may be required to take on roles beyond their age and what would be considered reasonable in any other setting. This is especially true if the parents have died and either an elderly relative is caring for the orphans or the oldest child becomes the "head of the household."[4]

HIV INFECTION IN CHILDREN

Modes of Transmission

Vertical Transmission

Most children (95%) acquire HIV vertically from their mothers. Of these, 10% to 20% are infected in utero, 60% during the actual birth process, and the remaining 10% to 20% through breastfeeding.[5]

Horizontal Transmission

There are a small number of HIV-infected infants with seronegative parents. Causes such as surrogate breastfeeding and expressed breast milk have been postulated in HIV infection.

Prevention

Experience in South Africa demonstrates that, without any intervention, vertical transmission of HIV infection ranges between 19% and 36%, depending on the mother's viral load and stage of illness.[6]

Prevention of mother-to-child transmission is an important intervention to reduce the vertical transmission of the infection (Table 211-1).

HIV Awareness

The goal of HIV awareness and sex education programs is to delay the age of sexual debut in adolescents and to promote safe sex practices.

Schools may include HIV/AIDS education in their curriculum and may have school-based HIV/AIDS management and governance programs using the peer educator approach. Peer educators are trained to educate peers formally and informally with respect to HIV/AIDS and responsible behavior, to model responsible behavior, to act as referral agents for youth in need of community resources, and to become youth advocates in the community.[7]

DIAGNOSIS

If a mother is HIV-infected, her baby will test positive for HIV antibodies on the enzyme-linked immunosorbent assay (ELISA) for the first 15 months of life. In other words, the child is HIV-exposed.

To confirm HIV infection, it is necessary to test for the presence of the virus, using the HIV RNA polymerase chain reaction (PCR) test at 6 weeks of life.

Where virological tests are not available, the WHO recommends the following for presumptive diagnosis of stage 4 HIV infection (Table 211-2)[8]:

PATHOPHYSIOLOGY

Natural Course of HIV Infection in Children

Without ART, most children infected with HIV at birth will develop features of the illness by 6 months of age. Rapid progression of the disease is largely determined by the child's immature immune system. Other factors that contribute to rapid disease progression include in utero infection, maternal high viral load and low CD4 count at the time of delivery, advanced maternal illness, and maternal death from an AIDS-related cause.

Three categories of progression have been described[9]:

Category 1: rapid progression within the first year (25% to 30% of cases)
Category 2: features of infection appear early in life and disease progresses more slowly, with death occurring within 3 to 5 years (50% to 60% of cases)
Category 3: long-term survivors who live beyond 8 years of age (5% to 25% of cases)

CLINICAL MANIFESTATIONS

There are many manifestations of HIV disease. Table 211-3 lists the various conditions that make up the staging criteria for HIV in infants and children.

TREATMENT

In accordance with WHO definition of pediatric palliative care, palliative care of children with HIV infection begins when the illness is diagnosed and continues regardless of whether the child receives treatment directed at the disease. ART and early, aggressive management of opportunistic infections and other problems (e.g., malnutrition)

TABLE 211-1 UNAIDS Global Estimates of HIV Infection and AIDS in Children (<15 yr old), 2007

CATEGORY	NO. AND RANGE OF CHILDREN (MILLIONS)
Living with HIV	2.5 (2.2-2.6)
Newly infected with HIV in 2007	0.42 (0.35-0.54)
AIDS deaths in 2007	0.33 (0.31-0.38)

From Worldwide HIV & AIDS Statistics, AVERT. Available at http://www.avert.org/worldstats.htm (accessed June 6, 2008).

TABLE 211-2 WHO Recommendations for Presumptive Diagnosis of Stage 4 HIV infection

1. The infant is HIV-antibody positive (ELISA or rapid test), aged <18 mo, and symptomatic with two or more of the following:
   Oral thrush
   Severe pneumonia (requiring oxygen)
   Severe wasting/malnutrition
   Severe sepsis (requiring intravenous therapy)
2. CD4 values, if available, may be used to guide decision making; ART is required if CD4 percentage is <25%
3. Other factors that support the diagnosis of clinical stage 4 HIV infection in a seropositive infant:
   Recent HIV-related maternal death
   Advanced HIV disease in the mother
4. Confirmation of the diagnosis of HIV infection should be sought as soon as possible

ART, antiretroviral therapy; ELISA, enzyme-linked immunosorbent assay; HIV, human immunodeficiency virus; WHO, World Health Organization.
From Interim WHO Clinical Staging of HIV/AIDS and HIV/AIDS Case Definitions for Surveillance: African Region. WHO/HIV/2005.02. Available at whqlibdoc.who.int/hq/2005/WHO_HIV_2005.02.pdf (accessed February 22, 2008).

TABLE 211-3   Revised WHO Classification of HIV for Infants and Children

STAGE 1

Asymptomatic

Persistent generalized lymphadenopathy (PGL)

STAGE 2

Hepatosplenomegaly

Recurrent or chronic upper respiratory tract infections (otitis media, otorrhea, sinusitis)

Papular pruritic eruptions

Seborrheic dermatitis

Extensive human papillomavirus infection

Extensive molluscum contagiosum infection

Herpes zoster

Fungal nail infections

Recurrent oral ulcerations

Linear gingival erythema (LGE)

Angular cheilitis

Parotid enlargement

STAGE 3

Conditions in Which a Presumptive Diagnosis Can Be Made Based on Clinical Signs or Simple Investigations

Unexplained moderate malnutrition (<3rd percentile) not adequately responding to standard therapy

Unexplained persistent diarrhea (≥14 days)

Unexplained persistent fever (intermittent or constant, for >1 mo)

Oral candidiasis (outside neonatal period)

Oral hairy leukoplakia

Acute necrotizing ulcerative gingivitis/periodontitis

Pulmonary tuberculosis

Severe recurrent presumed bacterial pneumonia

Conditions in Which Confirmatory Diagnostic Testing Is Necessary

Lymphoid interstitial pneumonitis (LIP)

Unexplained anemia (<8 g/dL), neutropenia (<1000/mm³), or thrombocytopenia (<50,000/mm³) for >1 mo

Chronic HIV-associated lung disease including bronchiectasis

STAGE 4

Conditions in Which a Presumptive Diagnosis Can Be Made Based on Clinical Signs or Simple Investigations

Unexplained severe wasting or severe malnutrition not adequately responding to standard therapy (<60% of expected body weight)

Pneumocystis jiroveci pneumonia (PCP)

Recurrent severe presumed bacterial infections (e.g., empyema, pyomyositis, bone or joint infection, meningitis), excluding pneumonia

Chronic herpes simplex infection (orolabial or cutaneous for >1 mo, or visceral of any duration)

Extrapulmonary tuberculosis

Kaposi's sarcoma

Esophageal candidiasis

CNS toxoplasmosis (outside the neonatal period)

HIV encephalopathy

Conditions in Which Confirmatory Diagnostic Testing Is Necessary

CMV infection (CMV retinitis or infection of any organ other than liver, spleen, or lymph nodes, onset at age ≥1 mo)

Extrapulmonary cryptococcosis including meningitis

Any disseminated endemic mycosis (e.g., extrapulmonary histoplasmosis, coccidioidomycosis, penicilliosis)

Cryptosporidiosis

Isosporiasis

Disseminated non-tuberculous mycobacteria infection

Candidal infection of trachea, bronchi, or lungs

Acquired HIV-related rectal fistula

Cerebral or B-cell non-Hodgkin's lymphoma

Progressive multifocal leukoencephalopathy (PML)

HIV-related cardiomyopathy or HIV-related nephropathy

CMV, cytomegalovirus; CNS, central nervous system; HIV, human immunodeficiency virus; WHO, World Health Organization.
From Interim WHO Clinical Staging of HIV/AIDS and HIV/AIDS Case Definitions for Surveillance: African Region. WHO/HIV/2005.02. Available at whqlibdoc.who .int/hq/2005/WHO_HIV_2005.02.pdf (accessed February 22, 2008).

are an essential part of good palliative care. ART positively influences the course of illness and quality of life of the child and family but does not effect a cure.

The foundation of effective palliative care is good communication with the child and parents; it is patient- and family-centered care. Communication of appropriate information that is relevant to the child's age and level of understanding results in an informed patient, and this enhances adherence to treatment, whether it is ART, symptom control, nutritional care, or safe sex practices.

Antiretroviral Treatment

A number of guidelines for ART have been published. Readers should refer to their national guidelines for the management of HIV-infected children or consult with an HIV pediatrician.

Goals of Antiretroviral Therapy

The goals of ART for children[10] are to increase survival, improve quality of life, and decrease HIV-related morbidity and mortality.

Specific objectives are as follows:

- The child's CD4 count should rise above and remain above the baseline count.
- The child's viral load should become undetectable (<400 copies/mL) and remain undetectable on treatment.

Monitoring

Once ART has been initiated, patients should be monitored closely, with continuous reassessment of their response to treatment. This is achieved by monitoring

CD4 counts and viral loads. Children and their carers should be advised of the side effects of ART and should report these to their treatment providers. Routine toxicity monitoring (including liver function tests, lipase, cholesterol, glucose, and complete blood counts) is usually tailored to the child's drug regimen and done every 6 months in resource-constrained settings. Key to the success of ART is adherence. Noncompliance is the primary cause of resistance to ART and failure of highly active antiretroviral therapy (HAART) in children.

Adherence

Adherence greater than 95% ensures a good virological response and prevents the emergence of resistance. This can be achieved through regular clinic attendance and education and adherence support programs. It is recognized that adherence may decrease as time on treatment increases; for this reason, treatment support measures are of increasing importance the longer the child is on treatment.

SYMPTOM MANAGEMENT

Palliative care affords equal emphasis to disease-oriented care and to control of distressing symptoms. A traditional biomedical approach to the diagnosis and treatment of disease does not recognize the holistic care required to manage life-threatening illness, or the impact of symptoms on the person as a whole.

It is imperative in managing symptoms to achieve relief of the symptom without creating a new symptom or unwanted side effects. Specifically, in the context of pain management, it is important to relieve the pain through nonpainful interventions.

Pain Management in Children

Effective pain management depends on accurate assessment of pain. The fact that pain is both a sensory and an emotional experience and is subjective makes it challenging to assess pain and may explain the widespread undermanagement of pain.

It helps to remember Leorra Kuttner's statement that "the child's pain is real and the child is the ultimate authority on this pain."[11]

There are a number of approaches to evaluating children's pain. Wong[12] described a QUESTT mnemonic for evaluation of a child's pain:

Q = Question the child, if verbal, and question the parent or caregiver of both verbal and nonverbal children
U = Use pain rating scales
E = Evaluate behavioral and physiological changes
S = Secure parents' involvement
T = Take the cause of pain into account
T = Take action and evaluate results

In questioning the child and parent, it is important to identify the *p*recipitating and relieving factors, the *q*uality (description) of the pain, the *r*adiation of the pain, the *s*ite and *s*everity of the pain, and the *t*ime course (when it started, whether constant or intermittent). Investigation of these factors is facilitated by the mnemonic, PQRSST.

Pain rating scales, such as visual analogue scales, the Edmonton Symptom Assessment Scale, the Faces Pain Scale, or the Red Cross Children's Hospital comfort scales (which include physical, behavioral, and physiological aspects of pain) are useful for evaluating a child's response to pain management, particularly regarding pains that are difficult to control. Asking the child to draw his or her pain can also elicit the emotional aspect of the pain.

The steps taken to secure the involvement of parents or caregivers include respectfully listening to their descriptions and interpretations of the child's pain, providing a full and clear explanation of the assessment and cause of the pain, and involving them (and also the child, in an age-appropriate manner) in decision making. Encourage the parents/caregivers to have control over pain management, and assure them of the support and availability of health care professionals for obtaining advice and answers to questions.

Nondrug measures that assist in pain management for children are shown in Table 211-4.

Analgesics in Management of Pain

Pain management in children is similar to that in adults, following the WHO guidelines.[13] Pain management is administered

- By the mouth—unless the child is vomiting or has another reason for difficulty in swallowing
- By the clock—in a condition causing chronic pain, analgesics should be given regularly at a fixed dose on a fixed schedule
- By the ladder—according to the WHO analgesic ladder (Fig. 211-1).
- By the individual—the medications and dosages should be adjusted according to the child's analgesic needs, response to medication. and side effects

Adjuvant analgesics assist in control of pain when added to analgesic therapy and may allow a lower dose of the analgesic to be used (analgesic-sparing effect). Adjuvant therapies include

- Steroids—dexamethasone helps to reduce pain caused by tumor edema (e.g., raised intracranial pressure, bone pain, neuropathic pain from nerve compression or infiltration)
- Antidepressants—neuropathic pain due to nerve compression or destruction responds to tricyclic antidepressants in low doses

TABLE 211-4 Nondrug Measures for Pain Management in Children		
SENSORY	**COGNITIVE**	**COGNITIVE-BEHAVIORAL**
Thermal: heat, cold	Hypnosis	Distraction: environmental
Pressure: massage,	Imagery	stimuli, voice, music
acupressure	Intellectualization	Play therapy
Positioning:	Prayer	Biofeedback
hugging/holding,	Thought-stopping	Exercise
swaddling	Cognitive	Psychological preparation:
Sucking	restructuring	modeling, behavior
Transcutaneous	Humor	rehearsal
electrical nerve		Relaxation exercises,
stimulation (TENS)		breathing exercises

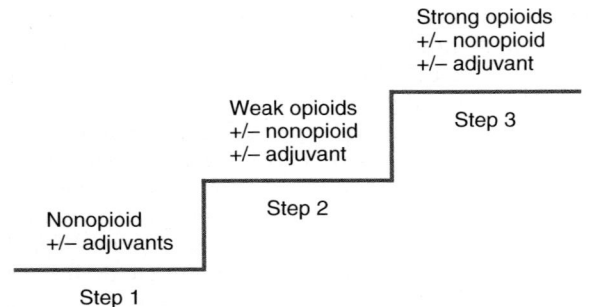

FIGURE 211-1 World Health Organization (WHO) three-step analgesic ladder with dosages for treatment of children with acquired immunodeficiency syndrome.

Nonopioids:	Paracetamol 10-15 mg/kg 4-6 hr Ibuprofen 5 mg/kg 6-8 hr to be given with meals
Weak opioids:	Codeine 0.5-1 mg/kg 4 hr Tilidine 1 mg/kg/dose 6 hr or 1 drop per 2.5 kg body mass
Opioids:	Oral morphine; <1yr: 0.1 mg/kg q4hr >1yr: 0.2-0.4 mg/kg q4hr

- Anticonvulsants—neuropathic pain from nerve damage can be modified by anticonvulsants such as carbamazepine, sodium valproate, or gabapentin.
- Ketamine is useful in resistant neuropathic pain

Anesthetic techniques for pain control include the use of intrathecal morphine, epidural analgesia, or appropriate nerve blocks.

Management of Respiratory Symptoms

It is important to ensure that the treatment for breathlessness does not frighten the child and thereby aggravate respiratory symptoms. Approaches such as explaining to an older child about the use of a nebulizer or oxygen therapy, or holding the mask slightly away from a younger child's face until he or she is used to it, assist in familiarizing the child to this form of therapy.

Dyspnea is a subjective sensation of difficulty in breathing. Preverbal children cannot describe what they are feeling, and the health care professional relies on observation to assess this symptom (Boxes 211-1 and 211-2).

Management of Dyspnea

The goal of management in dyspnea is to identify and treat the cause of dyspnea, if reversible (Table 211-5).

Nonpharmacological management of dyspnea includes the following:

- Explore psychological influences on breathlessness
- Optimal positioning
- Suctioning, if appropriate
- Relaxation techniques and breathing exercises
- Electric fan (movement of air across the face lessens the sensation of dyspnea)
- Complementary therapies

Box 211-1 Dyspnea in an Infant or Young Child—What Does Dyspnea Look Like?

- Often associated with tachypnea
- Signs of respiratory distress: poor muscle tone, nasal flaring, retraction of intercostal muscles
- Difficulty in feeding
- Restlessness due to hypoxia
- Wide-eyed, anxious look

Box 211-2 Dyspnea in Older Children and Adolescents—What Does Dyspnea Feel Like?

- Gasping or panting
- Feeling of drowning or suffocating
- Feeling of tightness in chest
- Aware of every breath
- Associated headache or lightheadedness
- Feeling frightened
- Observed signs: leaning forward and bracing (tripod position), nasal flaring, retraction of intercostal muscles

TABLE 211-5 Causes and Treatment of Dyspnea

CAUSE OF DYSPNEA	SPECIFIC TREATMENT
Hypoxia	Oxygen therapy
Infection	Antibiotics, cotrimoxazole for PCP, TB treatment
Pneumothorax, pleural effusion	Chest drain
Cardiac failure	Anti-failure treatment: diuretics, digoxin, etc.
Anemia	Hematinics, blood transfusion if appropriate
Metabolic acidosis	Depending on cause: fluids, sodium bicarbonate, insulin
Pulmonary embolism	Anticoagulant
Bronchospasm	Bronchodilatory therapy
Anxiety	Psychotherapy, relaxation techniques, benzodiazepines
Raised intracranial pressure	Dexamethasone

PCP, *Pneumocystis jiroveci* pneumonia; TB, tuberculosis.

Box 211-3 Pharmacological Treatment of Dyspnea

- Dyspnea associated with cough: saline nebulization
- Dyspnea associated with bronchospasm: bronchodilators
- Dyspnea associated with anxiety: benzodiazepines
- Dyspnea associated with excessive secretions: hyoscine butyl bromide
- To reduce the subjective sensation of dyspnea: low-dose morphine (50% of the dose used for pain management)

Pharmacological treatments are presented in Box 22-3.

Morphine has the following beneficial effects in managing dyspnea:

- Morphine decreases the sensitivity of the respiratory center to carbon dioxide and decreases the awareness of breathlessness.
- In heart failure, morphine causes vasodilatation, which decreases the load on the heart.
- At the start of morphine treatment, there is a temporary sedative effect, which reduces anxiety.
- If there is associated cough, morphine has an antitussive effect.

Management of Cough

Cough is a sudden and noisy expulsion of breath with the function of keeping the airways clear. It becomes a problem for the child and his or her carers when it interferes with sleep, rest, eating, and social functioning. Table 211-6 shows some causes and treatment of cough.

Nonpharmacological treatment of cough includes the following:

- Physiotherapy
- Humidification of air
- Postural drainage of secretions
- Hot lemon and honey/ginger drinks

Cough suppressants are indicated for the pharmacological treatment of severe cough paroxysms; they are also used when the cough is interfering with feeding or sleeping or when cough leads to exhaustion. The most appropriate cough suppressant is codeine or morphine linctus.

Gastrointestinal Symptoms

Odynophagia

The most common causes of odynophagia in children who are HIV positive are candidiasis (oral or esophageal), herpes stomatitis, and mucositis. Oral candidiasis is often related to perineal candidiasis.

Mouth Care

Mouth care is very important in children, because refusing food can rapidly lead to dehydration and to malnutrition in infants.

- The older child can use oral rinses such as saline, sodium bicarbonate, or chlorhexidine.
- Use a soft toothbrush and fluoride toothpaste.
- Clean the tongue with a soft toothbrush or gauze swab.
- Clean the lips and moisten them with petroleum jelly.
- Suck ice, lollipops, or vitamin C lozenges to encourage saliva flow.

TABLE 211-6	Causes and Treatment of Cough
CAUSE OF COUGH	**SPECIFIC TREATMENT**
Respiratory infection	Antibiotic therapy (e.g., anti-tuberculosis treatment)
Asthma	Nebulized or inhaled bronchodilators
Gastroesophageal reflux	Thickened feeds, positioning
Bronchiectasis	Physiotherapy, postural drainage, antibiotics when indicated

- Manage oral pain using local anesthetics or analgesics according to WHO guidelines.
- Avoid hot, acidic, or spicy foods.

Oral Candidiasis

Oral candidiasis may be treated with Mycostatin drops, 1 mL orally four times daily (30 minutes after feeds) for 7 to 14 days. Miconazole oral gel may be given every 4 to 6 hours (after meals) for 7 to 14 days. If infection is not clear within 2 weeks, fluconazole, 6 mg/kg, is used as a stat dose, followed by 3 mg/kg daily for 3 weeks.

Esophageal Candidiasis

Esophageal candidiasis is an AIDS-defining illness and can occur in the absence of oral candidiasis. It is treated with fluconazole, 6 mg/kg as a stat dose, followed by 3 mg/kg daily for 3 weeks. In severe cases, it may be necessary to initiate therapy intravenously.

Herpes Stomatitis

Herpes stomatitis occurs as painful ulcers on the tongue, lips, and buccal mucosa. There may be a superimposed bacterial or fungal infection. For treatment with oral acyclovir, 200 mg is given every 8 hours for 5 days in a child younger than 2 years old; in an older child, 400 mg is given every 8 hours for 5 days.

Nausea and Vomiting

Assessment is performed to identify the probable cause and mechanism of nausea and vomiting, bearing in mind that more than one cause may play a role. There are generally three pathophysiological mechanisms that cause nausea and vomiting[14]:

- Mechanical—gastric stasis, intestinal obstruction, excessive coughing, drug action on the gastrointestinal tract, gastritis, ascites, and other causes of increased intra-abdominal pressure
- "Toxic," mediated through the chemoemetic trigger zone—drugs, infections, renal failure
- Central, mediated through the vomiting center—raised intracranial pressure, anxiety, pain, vagal stimulation via mechanoreceptors in the gastrointestinal tract

Nonpharmacological measures for management of nausea include

- Adjust the environment—eliminate the smell of food or cooking.
- Offer small portions.
- Cold food may be more palatable than hot food (odor is less).
- Carers should not wear strong perfume.
- Position the patient after meals.
- Evaluate hydration regularly.

Pharmacological treatment of nausea and vomiting is shown in Table 211-7.

Management of Diarrhea

Children, and especially babies, pass stool frequently; breastfed babies may pass stool with each feeding.

TABLE 211-7	Causes and Treatment of Nausea and Vomiting	
CAUSE OF NAUSEA AND VOMITING	**FIRST-LINE TREATMENT**	**SECOND-LINE TREATMENT**
Mechanical	Metoclopramide: 100 µg/kg tid PO (**Caution**: there is a high incidence of extrapyramidal side effects of metoclopramide in children)	Dexamethascne: 1-6 mg qd
"Toxic"	Haloperidol (>12 yr): 0.5-1 mg bid to tid PO or 25-50 µg/kg/24 hr by continuous SC infusion	
Central	Cyclizine (2-12 yr): 25 mg qid PO Cyclizine (>12 yr): 50 mg tid PO	

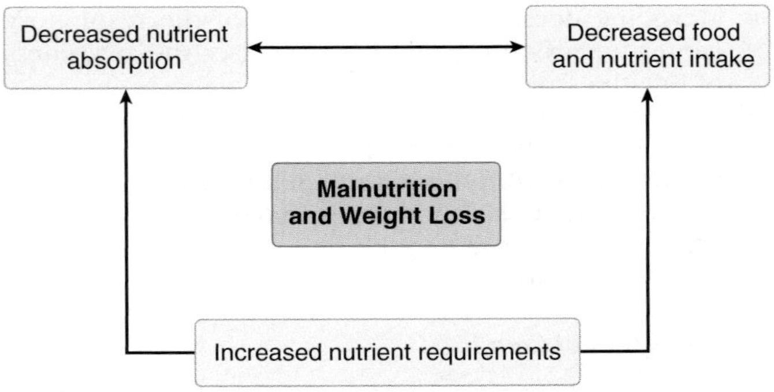

FIGURE 211-2 Malnutrition and weight loss. *(From Bekker L-G. Constitutional symptoms. In Gwyther L, Merriman A, Sebuyira LM, Schietinger H [eds]. A Clinical Guide to Supportive and Palliative Care in HIV/AIDS in Sub-Saharan Africa. Foundation for Hospices in Sub-Saharan Africa, 2006.)*

Diarrhea refers to abnormal frequency and consistency of stools. Acute diarrhea is considered as being of sudden onset, lasting 3 to 7 days; persistent diarrhea lasts more than 14 days and results in dehydration; chronic diarrhea lasts longer than 14 days but is not dehydrating.

The causes of diarrhea are evaluated according to duration, underlying disease or cause, and side effects of treatment used, including cultural practices (enemas and herbal medications).

Dehydration requires early intervention with oral rehydration solutions (ORS) or intravenous rehydration.

Milk feeds should not be stopped except when rehydrating with ORS; early refeeding decreases stool output and is comforting to the child. Temporary lactose intolerance may develop, necessitating the short-term use of soya-based milks. Solids should be started after the child is rehydrated and alert, beginning with frequent small feeds such as bananas, yogurt, pumpkin, and starchy porridge.

Pharmacological treatment in HIV-associated chronic diarrhea includes the following:

- Cholestyramine, 1 g every 6 hours PO for 5 days (half the dose for infants), plus gentamicin 50 mg/kg/day in 6 divided doses (every 4 hours) for 3 days, plus Isomil; gentamycin (*IV preparation given orally*) 50 mg/kg/day in 6 divided doses (every 4 hours) for 3 days
- Specialized milk formula for documented malabsorption
- Metronidazole
- Vitamin A and zinc
- Good nutritional support
- Antiretroviral therapy

Constitutional Symptoms

Constitutional symptoms of HIV disease include the following[15]:

Anorexia—the absence or loss of appetite for food
Cachexia—profound weight loss with associated lipolysis and loss of muscle and visceral protein due to catabolic state

Asthenia—physical and mental fatigue, easy tiring, general weakness

These constitutional symptoms are common in children infected with HIV because of the high metabolic requirements during periods of rapid growth. They cause considerable distress in family and friends because of the perception is that the child is "wasting away" or "starving to death." Because of the impact of HIV on a family's economic status, poor nutrition may be an economic consequence as well as a consequence of illness. Poor nutrition accelerates disease progression in HIV. Deficiencies of vitamins and trace elements that are essential for normal immunological function increase the risk of opportunistic infection (Fig. 211-2).

Wasting syndrome is an AIDS-defining illness characterized by the following[16]:

- Weight loss greater than 10% of baseline
- Downward crossing of at least two percentiles in a child 1 year of age or older
- Less than the 5th percentile on two consecutive measurements (>30 days apart), plus chronic diarrhea or fever lasting longer than 30 days (intermittent or constant)

Frequent, small meals of high-energy foods such as mealie meal, potato, rice, or porridge should be eaten. The nutritional value of these foods can be increased by adding 1 to 2 teaspoons of vegetable oil, margarine, or peanut butter. Additional foods to be included in the diet are

- High-protein foods such as eggs, milk (full cream), beans, lentils, meat, and fish
- High-energy drinks, if available
- Fresh fruit and vegetables (do not overcook vegetables)
- Vitamin and mineral supplements according to the recommended daily allowances (RDAs)

Skin Care

Skin conditions are common in children and adolescents with HIV infection. The following measures are recommended.

General Skin Care

Recommendations for general skin care include the following[17]:

- Bathe or shower once a day if piped water is available; use an emollient for dry or scaly skin conditions
- Use soap sparingly, or substitute a gentle cleanser; use UEA cream or another aqueous-based ointment
- Use soft, nonabrasive washcloths and towels
- Moisturize frequently with water-soluble lotion or 10% urea cream
- Encourage fluid intake
- Keep fingernails short
- Use topical antiseptic agents to prevent or treat secondary infections

Measures for specific skin conditions are shown in Table 211-8.

Pressure Sores

Pressure sores are uncommon in infants but may occur in the older, heavier child who is immobile or bedbound. Risk factors for pressure sores in the HIV-infected child/adolescent are

- Poor nutrition
- Neurological damage or sedation
- Incontinence
- Impaired healing processes: anemia, malnutrition, immunodeficiency
- Hypoxia

Measures for prevention of pressure sores include the following:

- Carers must be vigilant: inspect the skin every time the patient is moved.
- Care of the skin and pressure areas
  - The skin should be washed and dried regularly, including bed baths for the bedbound child.
  - Maintain the suppleness of the skin by regular massage with skin lotion.
  - Avoid trauma (no restraints); lift patients and do not drag when moving them in the bed.
- Perform regular positional changes every 2 to 4 hours, depending on the child's risk factors.
- Use a special mattress to distribute body weight more evenly.
- Keep the bed linen dry and free from creases.
- Keep the patient well nourished and well hydrated.
- Pain control improves mobility.

Treatment of pressure sores depends on the severity of the wound.[18]

END-OF-LIFE CARE

In the context of HIV/AIDS, especially with the increasing access to ART for children and adolescents, prognostication is inexact; a child who may look terminally ill can make a remarkable recovery for a significant period of time—many years if there is a good response to ART.[19]

It is particularly important to involve the child and family in decision making and also to consider the opinions of professionals and nonprofessionals who have been caring for the child. Consider also the timeline of the child's illness: Have there been frequent hospitalizations? Is the child's general condition deteriorating? Is there irreversible end-organ damage (e.g., cardiac failure, severe bronchiectasis)? What is the child's current and potential quality of life? What are the child's wishes for care?

If it is clear that the child's condition is deteriorating and that he or she may be in the terminal phase of illness, it is appropriate to discuss the place of death. Would the child (or family) prefer to be at home, in hospital, or in hospice at the end of life? Can the hospice staff support the family in caring for the child at home?

Even at this stage of the illness, it is important that the situation of the child or adolescent be kept as normal as possible, and that the autonomy of the child be respected. There should be someone at the child's bedside 24 hours a day, and health care professionals should be available to advise and respond to carers' concerns at all times. Effective symptom control is maintained, and feeding and oxygen is provided as appropriate. Whatever place of care is chosen, family intimacy should be encouraged. Explain to the family what to expect as the child dies and whom to call after death.

In the comprehensive provision of palliative care, bereavement care, psychosocial support, and spiritual care are also important components of care. These are covered in other chapters in this textbook. In developing countries, the HIV pandemic has affected many families and exposed children to multiple losses, often at a very early age.

TABLE 211-8	Causes and Treatment of Skin Conditions in HIV
CAUSE	**SPECIFIC TREATMENT**
Herpes zoster (shingles)	Acyclovir: 80 mg/kg/day in 3-4 divided doses for 7-10 days Pay close attention to pain control
Severe chickenpox	**Outpatient management:** Acyclovir: 80 mg/kg/day in 3-4 divided doses for 7-14 days If secondary infection develops, add amoxicillin (10-25 mg/kg q8h) AND oral flucloxacillin (12-25 mg/kg/dose q6h, maximum 500 mg/dose) **Inpatient management (for disseminated varicella):** Acyclovir: IV 500 mg/m² per dose q8h for 7-14 days or 10 mg/kg/dose in 3 divided doses for 7-14 days
Bacterial infections	Systemic antibiotics
Seborrheic dermatitis	Topical hydrocortisone 1% (for face) or Betamethasone 1% (body) bid Antihistamine (chlorphenamine)
Scabies	Topical benzyl benzoate 25% (dilute with an equal amount of water for children [12.5%] and one part with three parts of water for infants <1 yr) or gamma benzene hexachloride 1% In children <2 yr, sulphur ointment 2.5% three times daily for 3 days
Molluscum contagiosum	Responds to HAART
Papular pruritic eruptions	Topical steroids antihistamine

HAART, highly active antiretroviral therapy.

ORPHANS AND VULNERABLE CHILDREN

As well as the death of their parents, the orphaned child often has to cope with loss of income, loss of education, and loss of a home. The children may be taken into their grandmother's home, but in many cases the older child takes on the adult role as head of the household. In these situations, there is no caring adult to help a child through his or her grief and to provide the security the child needs in this distressing situation.

The planning of future care for potential orphans is an important part of providing care and comfort to a dying adult. There are a number of community initiatives focused on providing for orphaned children. Play therapy, art therapy, and/or dance therapy may assist children in expressing their grief. Memory work has proved to be a valuable tool in assisting parents who are preparing for death; it leaves a legacy for their children that preserves their sense of identity, and the parent can convey precious articles and letters to the children.

The HIV epidemic has challenged communities and clinicians to respond to the many needs of affected children and adolescents with a comprehensive and effective approach.

REFERENCES

1. Sepulveda C, Marlin A, Yoshida T, Ullrich A. WHO Definition of Palliative Care. J Pain Symptom Manage 2002;24:91-96.
2. Gelb B, Marston J, Ellis P, et al. Statement on Hospice and Palliative Care for Children. Children's Issues Steering Group, March 2005.
3. Dippennar H, Waldeck Y. Multisensory stimulation for children with life-limiting conditions. Palliative Care—Mind, Body, Spirit Conference, Hospice Palliative Care Association of South Africa, December 2005.
4. Dandridge L, Meiring M, Marcus C, et al. HPCA Paediatric Palliative Care Curriculum. Hospice Palliative Care Association of South Africa, January 2006.
5. Wilson D, Naidoo S, Bekker L-G, et al. Handbook of HIV Medicine. New York: Oxford University Press, 2002, p 250.
6. Abdool Karim S, Abdool KarimQ, Adhikari M, et al. Vertical HIV transmission in South Africa: Translating research into policy and practice. Lancet 2002;359:992-993.
7. Johnson D. Western Cape Peer Education Project. Palliative Care—Mind, Body, Spirit Conference, Hospice Palliative Care Association of South Africa, December 2005.
8. Cotton M. Classification of HIV disease in children—Towards pragmatism? S Afr J HIV Med 2005;(Nov):14-17.
9. Meyers T, Eley B, Loening W. Guidelines for the management of HIV-infected children. Department of Health, Republic of South Africa 2005 (Jacana Media), p 9.
10. Meyers T, Eley B. Guidelines for the management of HIV-infected children (National Department of Health, South Africa, 2005). S Afr J HIV Med 2005;(Nov):33-42.
11. Kuttner L. A Child in Pain: How To Help, What To Do. Point Roberts, WA: Hartley & Marks, 1996 (reprinted 2006).
12. QUESTT mnemonic. Available at http://www.fadavis.com/related_resources/27_1885_654.pdf (accessed February 22, 2008).
13. World Health Organization. Cancer Pain Relief and Palliative Care in Children. Geneva: WHO, 1998.
14. Interdisciplinary Introduction to Palliative Care 2005: Management of Symptoms in Advanced Disease. Hospice Palliative Care Association of South Africa, 2005.
15. Bruera E. Anorexia, cachexia and nutrition: ABC of Palliative Care. BMJ 1997;315:1219-1222.
16. Wilson D, Naidoo S, Bekker L-G, et al. Handbook of HIV Medicine. New York: Oxford University Press, 2002, p 312.
17. Appathurai V, Jessop S. Skin and wound care. In Gwyther L, Merriman A, Sebuyira LM, Schietinger H (eds). A Clinical Guide to Supportive and Palliative Care in HIV/AIDS in Sub-Saharan Africa. Foundation for Hospices in Sub-Saharan Africa, 2006.
18. HPCA Clinical Guidelines. Hospice Palliative Care Association of South Africa, 2006, p 27.
19. Stannard V. Paediatric Palliative care in the HIV setting. Palliative Care—Mind, Body, Spirit Conference, Hospice Palliative Care Association of South Africa, December 2005.

SUGGESTED READING

Gwyther L, Merriman A, Sebuyira LM, Schietinger H (eds). A Clinical Guide to Supportive and Palliative Care in HIV/AIDS in Sub-Saharan Africa. Foundation for Hospices in Sub-Saharan Africa, 2006.

Kuttner L. A Child in Pain: How To Help, What To Do. Point Roberts, WA: Hartley & Marks, 1996 (reprinted 2006).

Himelstein BP, Hilden JM, Morstad Boldt A, Weissman D. Pediatric palliative care. N Engl J Med 2004;350:1752-1762.

Meyers T, Eley B, Loening W. Guidelines for the Management of HIV-Infected Children. Department of Health, Republic of South Africa, 2005 (Jacana Media).

World Health Organization. Cancer Pain Relief and Palliative Care in Children. Geneva: WHO, 1998.

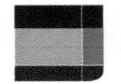

CHAPTER 212

Complications of Acquired Immunodeficiency Syndrome

Jason Faulhaber and Judith A. Aberg

KEY POINTS

- Hepatotoxicity can occur with any antiretroviral agent, but the greatest risks are with ritonavir (protease inhibitor), stavudine (nucleoside), and nevirapine (non-nucleoside).

- Dyslipidemia is associated with highly active antiretroviral therapy (HAART) and increases myocardial risk. Tenofovir decreases triglycerides and low-density lipoproteins, improving the risk profile during antiretroviral therapy.

- Initiation of HAART in the severely immunocompromised may elicit a syndrome of worsening symptomatology and progressive illness, the immune reconstitution inflammatory syndrome (IRIS).

- Other infectious or oncological diseases and treatment failure must be included in the differential diagnosis of clinical deterioration in those who recently initiated HAART, with concomitant targeted therapy against opportunistic infections.

- Palliative care is an integral component in successful management of HIV disease.

In 1987, zidovudine (AZT) was approved as the first medication to treat human immunodeficiency virus (HIV) infection. Several nucleoside analogues (e.g., lamivudine, stavudine, didanosine) soon followed. In 1996, a new class of antiretrovirals was discovered that targeted the protease enzyme. These protease inhibitors allowed development of a multidrug regimen ("cocktail") for treatment of HIV. Since then, this highly active antiretroviral treatment (HAART) regimen has become standard practice in areas where medication access is unrestricted. As a result, the originally staggering numbers of deaths from HIV/AIDS has declined, or stabilized, on a global basis, with few exceptions. People are living longer with HIV/AIDS; consequently, non-HIV–related illnesses are rising in this population, and the incidence of devastating opportunistic infections is decreasing. Whether they are from complications of therapy, metabolic dysregulation, comorbidities, or prolonged disease progression, these illnesses play a major role in the long-term management of HIV/AIDS.

Palliative care embodies the biopsychosocial approach to medicine by addressing the physical, emotional, social, and spiritual needs of patients and their supporters. The goal of palliative care is to promote quality of life. Palliative care encompasses more than the end of life; it includes the management of pain, complications of illnesses, and therapeutic agents. Despite advances in antiretroviral therapy, there is no known cure for AIDS. Therefore, end-of-life issues must be addressed before these individuals progress to a state of incapacity to make decisions, and palliative care is an integral part of comprehensive care.

BASIC SCIENCE

Antiretroviral medications can be classified based on their mechanism of action: entry inhibitors, reverse transcriptase inhibitors, integrase inhibitors, and protease inhibitors (Box 212-1).

The envelope of HIV contains two main glycoproteins, gp41 and gp120. The gp120 sits on the surface and is associated with gp41, a transmembrane protein containing four main regions. The first region anchors the protein to the viral membrane. There are two other areas which together can create a six-helix bundle, or hairpin structure. Finally, there is a fusion peptide region capable of piercing the membrane of the CD4+ T lymphocyte. Attachment of HIV to the CD4+ cell requires the interaction of gp120 and the CD4 receptor. This interaction induces a conformational change in the gp120, which allows the three gp120 subdomains to spread apart and facilitate binding to a coreceptor. The coreceptor is a chemokine receptor on the CD4+ cell membrane; it is classified as either CCR5 or CXCR4. Viruses can be either monotropic (i.e., using only one coreceptor) or dual-tropic (i.e., using both coreceptors). CXCR4-tropic viruses tend to appear later in infection and are associated with more rapid disease progression. After binding of the CD4 receptor and coreceptor, the six-helix bundle hairpin structure is formed. This forces the viral and CD4+ cell membranes to approach each other and eventually to fuse when the terminal end of the gp41 is inserted into the cell membrane. Currently, only one *entry inhibitor*, Enfuvirtide, is approved by the U.S. Food and Drug Administration (FDA). Enfuvirtide mimics part of the helical domain in gp41. When present, it inhibits the formation of the hairpin structure, preventing fusion of the HIV envelope with the CD4+ cell membrane. There are experimental drugs that block attachment and coreceptor binding. TNX-355 contains synthetic antibodies that bind to the CD4 receptors, and PRO-542 mimics the CD4 receptor itself. Both medications would prevent HIV attachment to the CD4+ cell membrane. Maraviroc and vicriviroc are experimental CCR5 antagonists that prevent coreceptor binding.

After entry, the viral RNA needs to be converted to DNA via the enzyme reverse transcriptase. Inhibitors of

---

Box 212-1 Antiretroviral Agents by Class (with Commonly Used Abbreviations)

Entry Inhibitors

- Chemokine receptor (CCR5) antagonists
  Maraviroc (MRV)
  Vicriviroc*
- Fusion inhibitor
  Enfuvirtide (ENF, T20)

Reverse Transcriptase Inhibitors

- Nucleoside (NRTIs)
  Zidovudine (AZT)
  Lamivudine (3TC)
  Stavudine (d4T)
  Didanosine (ddI)
  Zalcitabine (ddC)
  Emtricitabine (FTC)
  Abacavir (ABC)
- Nucleotide (NRTIs)
  Tenofovir (TDF)
- Non-nucleoside (NNRTIs)
  Efavirenz (EFV)
  Delavirdine (DLV)
  Nevirapine (NVP)
  Etravirine (ETR)

Integrase Inhibitors

  Raltegravir (RAL)
  Elvitegravir*

Protease Inhibitors

  Saquinavir (SQV)
  Indinavir (IDV)
  Ritonavir (RTV, r)
  Nelfinavir (NFV)
  Lopinavir (LPV)
  Atazanavir (ATV)
  Amprenavir (APV)
  Fosamprenavir (fAPV)
  Tipranavir (TPV)
  Darunavir (DRV)
- Maturation inhibitors
  Bevirimat*

Not yet approved by the U.S. Food and Drug Administration.

---

reverse transcriptase can be divided into nucleoside analogues, nucleotide analogues, and non-nucleoside analogues. Nucleoside and nucleotide analogues have structures similar to those of the normal nucleoside or nucleotide bases that are incorporated into the elongating chain of DNA. Zidovudine, lamivudine, stavudine, didanosine, zalcitabine, emtricitabine, and abacavir are the currently available *nucleoside analogues*; tenofovir is the only *nucleotide analogue* available. Non-nucleoside analogues are compounds that also inhibit reverse transcriptase, but not because they mimic the normal nucleoside bases. They bind an allosteric site on reverse transcriptase, causing a conformational change that alters the active site of the enzyme, rendering it ineffective. Efavirenz, delavirdine, and nevirapine are the currently available *non-nucleoside analogues*.

Once viral RNA has been reversely transcribed into DNA, the viral DNA needs to be integrated into the host cell's DNA. This requires the viral enzyme, integrase. No *integrase inhibitors* are currently available, but there are two investigational integrase inhibitors undergoing phase III clinical trials. As the viral DNA becomes transcribed and translated, viral proteins are formed. The protease enzyme cleaves these into smaller, functional proteins. For example, after translation, a large glycoprotein (gp160) must be cleaved by protease to form the membrane-bound proteins, gp41 and gp120. Saquinavir, indinavir, ritonavir, nelfinavir, lopinavir, atazanavir, amprenavir, fosamprenavir, tipranavir, and darunavir are the *protease inhibitors* currently available.

The HIV Gag protein must be cleaved by viral protease to produce the structural viral components that interact with other proteins. This step can be inhibited by a class of antiretrovirals called *maturation inhibitors*. The experimental drug, bevirmat (PA-457), is the prototypical example. If processing of the Gag protein is inhibited, defective, uninfectious virion particles are synthesized, preventing spread of the infection throughout the body.[1]

EPIDEMIOLOGY AND PREVALENCE

According to the World Health Organization (WHO),[1a] an estimated 33.2 million (range, 30.6 to 36.1 million) people worldwide are living with HIV infection as of December 2007. An estimated 2.5 million (range, 1.8 to 4.1 million) were newly infected with HIV, and there were an estimated 2.1 million (range, 1.9 to 2.4 million) deaths from AIDS at the end of 2007. In sub-Saharan Africa, almost all countries with population-based HIV surveys have demonstrated a decline or stability in the prevalence of HIV; the only exception was South Africa, which had a modest increase, from 18.6% to 18.8% over a 2-year period (2005-2007). In North America and Latin America, there has been little change in the epidemiology of newly acquired HIV, with men who have sex with men (MSM) and women constituting most new cases. However, there has been a demographic shift, demonstrated by an increase in the numbers of people of color and women who are infected.[2] In the United Kingdom and Europe, the numbers of new cases in women and from heterosexual transmission have increased, yet the MSM population still remains at risk.

According to data from the Centers for Disease Control and Prevention (CDC), based on 35 areas with confidential name-based HIV infection reporting, there is an increased population living with AIDS, mostly those older than 40 years of age. The most striking rise in the AIDS population over a 4-year period (2001 to 2004)—a 166% increase—occurred in people older than 60 years of age. Overall, the 12-, 24-, and 36-month survival rates after an AIDS diagnosis in 2000 were 90%, 86%, and 83%, respectively. This demonstrates that AIDS is a chronic condition, and, for this reason, complications become more significant in the course and management.[3]

In a study analyzing mortality during the period 1999 to 2004 in New York City, overall mortality in the AIDS population for both HIV-related and non–HIV-related causes decreased, but more than 75% of non–HIV-related deaths were due to substance abuse, cardiovascular disease, or cancer. Similarly, data obtained by the HIV Outpatient Study (HOPS) during 2000 to 2004 revealed an increase in non–AIDS-related deaths. As a result of prolonged survival due to effective HAART and immune system restitution, chronic comorbid conditions became more clinically relevant. Common comorbidities included liver disease (especially coinfection with hepatitis viruses), hypertension, diabetes, cardiovascular illness, pulmonary disease, and non-AIDS malignancies (e.g., lung cancer). The predominant non-AIDS causes of death included hepatic, pulmonary, and cardiovascular illnesses.[4] This underscores the need for comprehensive care, including primary care and routine screening, for people infected with HIV.

Despite widespread use of HAART in industrialized societies, there remains a strong need for palliative care. Firstly, although HAART can prolong life, it cannot cure HIV infection. Secondly, HAART is not benign; it is associated with numerous side effects, some debilitating. Thirdly, comorbidities, such as hepatitis C virus (HCV) infection and cardiovascular and cerebrovascular diseases, play a role in the long-term progression and management of HIV. Lastly, the incidence of certain HIV-related malignancies, such as non-Hodgkin's lymphoma (NHL), have not decreased in the post-HAART era.

PATHOPHYSIOLOGY

Antiretroviral Therapy

Details of the mechanisms of action of individual antiretrovirals are covered in another chapter. Combinations of certain nucleoside reverse transcriptase inhibitors (NRTIs) can cause increased toxicities or decreased efficacy or both. Zidovudine and stavudine both compete for cellular thymidine kinase, and zidovudine inhibits the phosphorylation of stavudine, rendering it less effective.[5] Similarly, lamivudine (3TC) inhibits phosphorylation of zalcitabine and emtricitabine and, therefore, should not be used in combination with these drugs. Increased toxicities occur during co-administration of stavudine and didanosine, and these agents carry warnings they should not be co-administered. The incidence of peripheral neuropathy, pancreatitis, and lactic acidosis is increased with the combination of didanosine and stavudine; zalcitabine is also associated with these toxicities. Tenofovir (TDF) increases plasma levels of didanosine, by an unidentified mechanism. This can potentiate didanosine-specific adverse reactions, such as pancreatitis and peripheral neuropathy.

NRTIs can induce mitochondrial toxicity by inhibiting human DNA polymerase γ. This was first demonstrated in muscle tissue of patients receiving zidovudine.[6] Because mitochondria are the primary energy producers of almost all cells, mitochondrial toxicity decreases aerobic energy production and increases lactate from anaerobic, mitochondria-independent metabolism. The NRTIs most commonly associated with mitochondrial toxicity are stavudine and didanosine, especially when they are used in combination. NRTIs may also contribute to dyslipidemia. Thymidine analogues (zidovudine and stavudine) appear to play a greater role than NRTIs that are not thymidine analogues. For example, one study demonstrated a significant increase in total cholesterol from baseline in a group of patients receiving a zidovudine-containing regimen, compared with a tenofovir-containing regimen.[7]

Protease inhibitors (PIs) specifically target the catalytic region of the viral protease enzyme. This region is homologous with regions of two human proteins that regulate lipid metabolism, the cytoplasmic retinoic acid–binding protein 1 (CRABP-1) and the low-density lipoprotein receptor-related protein (LRP).[8] The hypothesis is that PIs inhibit CRABP-1–mediated intracellular processes, thereby increasing the rate of apoptosis in adipocytes and preventing differentiation of preadipocytes. Ultimately, this decreases triglyceride storage and increases lipid release. The binding of PIs to LRP impairs hepatic uptake of chylomicrons and endothelial cell clearance of triglycerides. This causes hyperlipidemia and insulin resistance. PIs also increase lipoprotein (a) and inhibit glucose uptake by insulin-selective tissues.

Endocrinological Abnormalities

Adipocytes secrete a range of adipocytokines that control insulin sensitivity. One in particular, adiponectin, is involved in HIV-associated lipodystrophy.[9] In HIV-infected patients receiving HAART, adiponectin is significantly correlated with triglycerides, abdominal visceral fat, extremity fat, insulin resistance, high-density lipoprotein (HDL) levels, and NRTI use. Low adiponectin levels produce insulin resistance in liver and muscle cells.

Insulin resistance, dyslipidemia, and increased lipoprotein (a) levels are associated with higher risk of cardiovascular events due to increased atherosclerosis. Acute coronary syndrome has not been consistently linked with antiretroviral use.[10] However, the combination of unmodifiable (e.g., gender, age, genetics) and modifiable (e.g., hyperlipidemia, insulin resistance secondary to antiretroviral use) characteristics may increase the incidence of cardiovascular events.

HIV infection can decrease total cholesterol, HDL cholesterol, and low-density lipoprotein (LDL) cholesterol. Hypothesized mechanisms have included alteration in hepatic lipogenesis, manipulation of the production of cytokines, and immune dysfunction. Elevated triglycerides are caused by decreased clearance induced by the virus itself.[11] Women may be more likely than men to develop increased LDL when taking PIs, especially in combination with stavudine or lamivudine. Also, elevated LDL may be more common in black patients, whereas Hispanics may have more significant triglyceride elevations.

Lipoatrophy is the loss of fat in various body areas. It has been associated with certain antiretroviral agents as well as host factors, including older age, CD4 nadir less than 100 cells/mm³, white race, lower body weight before therapy, and prior AIDS diagnosis. NRTIs that have the greatest propensity to inhibit mitochondrial DNA polymerase γ (e.g., zalcitabine, didanosine, stavudine) are most frequently implicated.[12] The mitochondrial effect associated with specific NRTIs may be enhanced by coadministration with other antiretrovirals. It is hypothesized to cause lipoatrophy by inducing adipocyte apoptosis. A polymorphism in the tumor necrosis factor-α promoter gene has also been associated with faster onset of lipodystrophy. Hormonal mechanisms may influence lipodystro-

phy; one study found lipodystrophy was more frequent and more polymorphic in women than men.

The pathogenesis of osteopenia and consequent osteoporosis is rooted in bone remodeling, which requires a delicate balance between osteoclastic and osteoblastic activities. If osteoclasts are hyperactive, then the rate of bone destruction exceeds bone formation. Conversely, if osteoblasts are hypoactive, osteoclastic activity prevails. In animal models, indinavir inhibits osteoblast differentiation, resulting in decreased bone mineral density, and zidovudine activates osteoclastogenesis, also causing a decrease in bone mineral density. Other risk factors include duration of HIV disease, low body mass index, history of weight loss, and previous steroid use.[13]

Peripheral Neuropathy

The pathogenesis peripheral neuropathy in HIV disease has not been fully elucidated, although it is most likely multifactorial. It may be secondary to use of NRTIs or other medications such as isoniazid, ethambutol, dapsone, and vincristine.[14] It appears to be dose-dependent, especially with didanosine, zalcitabine, and stavudine. The PIs indinavir, saquinavir, and ritonavir have also been implicated in distal symmetrical polyneuropathy (DSP) through their toxic effects of inhibiting mitochondrial DNA polymerase. HIV-associated neuromuscular weakness syndrome is similar to Guillain-Barré syndrome and is characterized by hyperlactatemia, nausea, vomiting, hepatomegaly, and progressive muscle weakness. It has been linked to prolonged NRTI (especially stavudine) therapy, implicating mitochondrial toxicity; however, not all patients have hyperlactatemia at diagnosis. The role of immune-mediated mechanisms has not been excluded. Diffuse infiltrative lymphocytosis syndrome (DILS), also known as persistent CD8 lymphocytosis, develops from visceral CD8 infiltration, with involvement of salivary glands, lungs, kidneys, gastrointestinal tract, and peripheral nerves. Inflammatory demyelinating polyneuropathy (IDP) involves segmental demyelination, macrophage activation with monocytic infiltration of nerve fascicles, and endoneurial edema. Mononeuritis multiplex can appear in both early and late stages of HIV. In early HIV infection, it is often a result of a self-limited immune neuropathy or vasculitis. In late HIV infection, there has been an association with cytomegalovirus (CMV), varicella-zoster virus, and HCV infections. Progressive polyradiculopathy typically occurs in advanced HIV disease and with low CD4⁺ cell counts. It has a subacute onset, with a course lasting several days to weeks. It is typically attributed to infection with CMV[15]; however, other conditions, such as lymphoma, syphilis, mycobacterial infection, herpes simplex virus infection, and *Cryptococcus* infection have been implicated. There is widespread denervation in paraspinal muscles with normal nerve conduction velocities.

Hepatotoxicity

Several factors influence liver toxicity: direct toxicity, hypersensitivity reactions, mitochondrial toxicity, metabolic abnormalities, and immune reconstitution in patients coinfected with HCV and/or hepatitis B virus (HBV). Polymorphisms in the hepatic cytochrome pathway enzymes can cause direct toxicity from drugs that utilize that pathway. Hypersensitivity reactions are related to the host, not to the drug dosage. Typically, they appear within the first 4 to 6 weeks after initiation of the medication. Nevirapine has been linked with fatal outcome[16] in women with CD4 counts greater than 250 cells/mm[3] and in men with CD4 counts greater than 400 cells/mm[3]. A low body mass index also appears to be an independent risk factor. Mitochondrial toxicity may cause accumulation of microvesicular steatosis and mitochondrial depletion. This may evolve to macrovesicular steatosis with focal necrosis, fibrosis, cholestasis, biliary duct proliferation, and Mallory bodies, similar to alcohol-induced liver toxicity, steatosis of pregnancy, or Reye's syndrome. Insulin resistance and steatohepatitis induced by HAART may contribute to liver toxicity. Chronic infection with HCV and/or HBV can cause immune-mediated liver damage. With prolonged HIV immunosuppression, there is less inflammatory reaction in the liver. On initiation of HAART and reconstitution of the immune system, there is restoration of the immune response targeting the HCV or HBV antigens exposed on the liver cells.

Direct Complications of HIV and Other Viral Infections

There are several complications associated with HIV infection itself. There is an increased incidence of numerous malignancies, such as Kaposi's sarcoma, Hodgkin's disease, and NHL. The incidence of NHL has increased almost 200-fold in HIV disease. Despite improved survival due to HAART, the prognosis for NHL remains poor, with a median survival time of 6 months and a 2-year survival rate of 41%.[17] Almost half of all cases of HIV-associated malignancy are associated with either Epstein-Barr virus or human herpesvirus-8 (HHV-8), also called Kaposi's sarcoma–associated herpesvirus. HHV-8 has also been implicated in a subgroup of NHL known as body cavity lymphoma. Coinfection with HBV and/or HCV places patients at increased risk for hepatocellular carcinoma.

HIV, independent of antiretroviral therapy, is associated with reduced bone mineral density in both men and women.[18] Without supplementation, patients are at increased risk for osteoporosis and pathological fractures. High HIV viral loads have been associated with low testosterone levels, increasing the risk of osteopenia and coronary artery disease. HIV can be pathogenic in certain organs, such as the kidney, where it gives rise to HIV-associated nephropathy (HIVAN), with end-stage renal disease necessitating dialysis.

Cancer and Its Therapies

Because patients are living longer with chronic HIV, malignancy is a significant cause of death.[19] Kaposi's sarcoma is the most common neoplasm in HIV. Histologic evaluation of these lesions reveals a characteristic appearance of neoangiogenesis and proliferating spindle-shaped cells associated with an inflammatory infiltrate. Infection with HHV-8 has been detected in all forms of Kaposi's sarcoma. HHV-8 expresses several viral proteins, some of which are homologous to interleukin-6 and anti-apoptosis molecules of the bcl-2 family. Interleukin-6 can induce the expres-

sion of vascular endothelial growth factor, which explains the neoangiogenesis.

Most AIDS-related lymphomas exhibit B-cell derivation.[20] The WHO has delineated a three-part categorization of AIDS-related lymphomas: (1) lymphomas that also occur in the immunocompetent, such as Burkitt's lymphoma; (2) lymphomas that occur more specifically in the HIV-infected, such as primary effusion lymphoma and primary central nervous system (CNS) lymphoma; (3) lymphomas that also occur in other immunodeficiency states, such as polymorphic lymphoproliferative disorder–like B-cell lymphoma. Certain features are characteristic of AIDS-related lymphoma, compared with lymphomas in the general population: propensity for advanced disease, B symptoms, extranodal disease including in unusual locations, and prominent association with Epstein-Barr virus and HHV-8. HHV-8 has been found to be associated with body cavity lymphoma and with primary effusion lymphoma. Epstein-Barr virus is implicated in primary CNS lymphoma. Epstein-Barr virus, HIV, and other infectious agents may release various growth factors and cytokines that hyperstimulate B cells, leading to proliferation.

There is also an excess of non–AIDS-related cancers in patients with HIV infection.[21] The exact pathophysiology is unknown. For lung cancer, some factors may increase the risk similarly in both HIV-positive and HIV-seronegative people. There is a higher proportion of individuals who smoke among those with HIV infection, compared with HIV-negative individuals matched for age. In South Africa, where the incidence of HIV positivity is high but the incidence of smoking is low, no increased risk of lung cancer among HIV patients was found. However, overall there is a 2.5-fold increased risk of lung cancer among HIV infected persons compared with the general population after adjusting for smoking.

Immune Reconstitution Inflammatory Syndrome

Over the first 3 to 6 months after initiation of antiretroviral therapy, the peripheral CD4 count rises rapidly. This initial increase is primarily due to a release of memory CD4[+] cells that previously were sequestered in lymphoid tissue. This population of cells is short-lived and is replaced by a second CD4[+] population of cells that are naïve, which are released from the newly-restored thymus. It is this group of cells that allow for the "reconstitution" of the immune system. Severely immunocompromised patients may have microbial antigens present; however, given the immunological dysfunction, they are unable to mount a significant cytokine-mediated response and appear asymptomatic. With a reconstituted immune system, these new CD4[+] cells can elicit a profound immunological response. This cascade of events ultimately results in clinical deterioration. Depending on the offending pathogen, clinical manifestations may appear acutely or after prolonged immune reconstitution.[22] Mycobacterial IRIS typically arises with restoration of the cutaneous delayed-type hypersensitivity response to antigens. Because HAART improves the CD4 count and immune responsiveness, concurrent use of HAART and antimycobacterial chemotherapy may place patients at risk of IRIS. The magnitude of the rise in CD4 count does not consistently influence the development of IRIS. Also, there is individual variation in the reconstitution response; CD4 counts may remain lower than 200 cells/mm³ in 10% to 20% of advanced patients, despite having virological suppression on HAART. Several factors influence the degree of reconstitution, including older age, incomplete HIV suppression, and interruption of antiretroviral treatment (see "Case Study: Immune Reconstitution Inflammatory Syndrome").

 ## CASE STUDY

Complications Associated with Human Immunodeficiency Virus

A 23-year-old man from Mali presented to the hospital with a 2-week history of forgetfulness and bilateral weakness of the lower extremities. His past medical history was significant for HIV diagnosed 3 years previously. His most recent CD4 count, 2 months before presentation, was 23 cells/mm³ (3%), with a viral load of 1400 copies/mL. Three months ago, he was started on an HAART regimen including tenofovir, emtricitabine, and efavirenz. Physical examination revealed an afebrile man in no acute distress. Neurological examination was significant for moderate weakness without atrophy in the lower extremities bilaterally. Muscle tone was adequate. Plantar reflexes were downward bilaterally. The patient exhibited difficulty in rising from a sitting position without assistance, and he could not ambulate without assistance, secondary to loss of motor strength. Computed tomographic scan with contrast of his brain revealed several small hypodensities, some with peripheral enhancement, in a periventricular distribution without mass effect or hydrocephalus. Examination of the cerebrospinal fluid (CSF) revealed three white blood cells (all neutrophils), slightly elevated protein, and glucose appropriately normal compared with serum. A test for Jakob-Creutzfeldt disease virus via polymerase chain reaction (PCR) was positive.

The patient's clinical status deteriorated to the point of being bedridden. He remained on his antiretroviral regimen, with subsequent undetectable HIV and a rise in his CD4 count to 135 cells/mm³ (11%). He became depressed while an inpatient. He started to refuse medical therapy, including his antiretroviral regimen. He refused nutritional supplementation. He had no social support network, and his family had disavowed him. He was transferred to a rehabilitation center. He returned to the hospital 4 weeks later with fever and changed mental status. He was no longer receiving his antiretroviral therapy. CSF examination revealed significantly elevated pressure, significantly elevated protein, severe hypoglycorrhachia, and profound mononuclear pleocytosis. India ink examination of the CSF was positive for several yeast forms. Amphotericin B and flucytosine were initiated. His clinical status continued to deteriorate, necessitating intensive care. He died 4 days after therapy was begun.

The case study underscores the importance of an integrated medical approach to a severely immunocompromised individual. Given this patient's lack of social support systems, he had no assistance in managing his illness. He felt alone and consequently developed depression (or experienced worsening of preexisting depression). A multidisciplinary team should be engaged for such patients and should include members from social work, psychology, physical therapy, nutrition, HIV health education, case management, palliative care, and the medical care providers. Together, the team members can facilitate physical, emotional, and psychological improvement. These patients may experience frustration and hopelessness given their physical incapacity. Early involvement of physical therapy can benefit patients' physical and mental states. End-of-life issues can be addressed at any time during care, when patients are able to indicate whether they are ready to make those decisions. If they deny the eventuality of their condition, they can benefit from counseling, which can aid them to attain a comfortable mental awareness and, ultimately, preparedness.

CLINICAL MANIFESTATIONS

Antiretroviral Therapy

Some adverse effects are limited to specific antiretroviral agents, and some are class-wide. The most common gastrointestinal side effects are nausea, vomiting, diarrhea, and anorexia. Most antiretroviral agents cause nausea and vomiting. There should be heightened awareness with abacavir, because nausea and vomiting could be an early manifestation of hypersensitivity syndrome, a potentially life-threatening adverse reaction to abacavir. Diarrhea is common, with up to 70% of patients reporting it at some point during their illness.[23] Diarrhea is nonspecific; it may be caused by medications, infection, HIV enteropathy, or non–HIV-related conditions seen in the general population. Diarrhea can play a significant role, affecting adherence to antiretroviral therapy and quality of life. An investigation for other causes should be conducted before implicating medications.

Other gastrointestinal adverse effects include pancreatitis and hepatotoxicity. Pancreatitis is most commonly associated with didanosine or stavudine. Didanosine typically causes pancreatitis within the first 6 months of therapy, especially with CD4 counts lower than 100 cells/mm³. All antiretrovirals can cause adverse liver effects. NNRTIs and PIs are commonly implicated in medication-induced hepatotoxicity. The risk with nevirapine is greatest within the first 2 to 6 weeks of therapy; hepatotoxicity is more common in women with CD4 counts greater than 250 cells/mm³ and in men with CD4 counts greater than 400 cells/mm³. Nevirapine has been removed from the current U.S. recommendations for postexposure prophylaxis due to two cases of fulminant hepatitis and severe hepatotoxicity in otherwise healthy subjects. Medication-induced hepatotoxicity may be confounded by coinfection with HBV or HCV. Coinfection with HCV is common, occurring in up to 80% of individuals with parenterally acquired HIV. Chronic HBV infection occurs in 10% to 15% of HIV-positive individuals.[24] Hepatic steatosis, another liver-related complication, may be related to mitochondrial toxicities induced by NRTIs.

The severity of liver toxicity ranges from asymptomatic to complete liver failure. Outcomes range from spontaneous resolution to liver failure and death.[25] The scale of liver toxicity published by the National Institutes of Health (NIH) Division of Microbiology and Infectious Diseases (DMID) defines hepatotoxicity as a rise in the levels of serum glutamate pyruvate transaminase (SGPT) and/or serum glutamate oxaloacetate transaminase (SGOT) from within normal limits to above the upper limits of normal (ULN). Severity is graded from 1 to 4, based on the degree of elevation of SGPT and/or SGOT above the ULN. Nonalcoholic steatohepatitis has been reported in 16% of metabolic abnormalities associated with antiretroviral therapy, including dyslipidemia. It resembles alcoholic liver disease, with fat accumulation (steatosis) and a subsequent inflammatory response (hepatitis), but there is no history of alcohol ingestion. Stavudine increases the risk of fatty liver.

Lactic acidosis, a presumed consequence of mitochondrial toxicity, can cause various symptoms. Gastrointestinal symptoms include abdominal distention, nausea, vomiting, and diarrhea. Myalgias, cramps, fatigue, and generalized weakness are also frequently seen. Other consequences of mitochondrial toxicity include pancreatitis, peripheral neuropathy, lipoatrophy, hyperlipidemia, hyperglycemia, and osteopenia.[26]

Endocrinological Dysfunction

The term "lipodystrophy" refers to the spectrum of changes in body fat that occur with or without the metabolic syndrome, including lipid and glucose disorders associated with fat redistribution. An estimated 20% to 80% of people with HIV infection develop some form of lipodystrophy.[27] The physical features include central fat accumulation or peripheral lipoatrophy or both. Loss of buccal fat pads results in hollowing of the cheeks. Loss of subcutaneous fat of the arms and legs causes veins to become more prominent. Fat accumulation may be seen in the abdomen, the base of the neck or even the entire neck, the suprapubic area, and the breasts. Metabolic features include hyperlipidemia, insulin resistance, lactic acidosis, elevated transaminases, and type 2 diabetes mellitus. Hypertriglyceridemia can be profound with values greater than 1000 mg/dL. Such elevations may increase risk for pancreatitis and premature atherosclerosis. The HIV Outpatient Study found a strong association between PI use and myocardial infarction, even after controlling for hypertension, smoking, diabetes, age, gender, and dyslipidemia. PIs have been associated with fat accumulation in the dorsocervical region, abdomen, and breasts. NRTIs, especially stavudine, have been associated with lipoatrophy in the face and extremities. There is an increased risk of limb fat loss in patients taking PI-NRTI combinations, compared with dual PIs alone.

Osteopenia has been linked to NRTIs through asymptomatic lactic acidemia. The most common sites for bone mineral loss are the femoral and humeral heads, femoral condyles, proximal tibia, and parts of the hand and wrist.[28] One study demonstrated greater decrease in bone mineral density of the spine and hip with a tenofovir-based regimen, compared with stavudine. This difference was apparent only after initiation of antiretroviral therapy, and it appeared to level off over time. When there is an imbalance of bone resorption over formation, osteoporosis results. Osteoporosis increases the risk for fractures, although there are limited data on the long-term effects of HAART-associated osteopenia.

Peripheral Neuropathy

Peripheral neuropathy may result from use of antiretrovirals or as a direct consequence of HIV infection itself. The spectrum includes DSP, toxic neuropathy from antiretroviral drugs, DILS, IDPs, multifocal mononeuropathies, and progressive polyradiculopathy.

The most common form of neuropathy is DSP.[29] When related to HIV, DSP occurs typically in advanced HIV infection. It is diagnosed in 35% of those with AIDS and is found histologically in almost 100% of AIDS patients at autopsy. The clinical presentation is painful feet, with most patients complaining of hyperpathia in the feet. Muscle weakness is usually mild or absent. Almost 100% have depressed or absent ankle tendon reflexes. Pain and temperature sensations are impaired in the distal lower extremities.

Nerve conduction velocities are used to distinguish DSP from IDPs with length-dependent axonal polyneuropathy.[30] DILS clinically manifests as acute or subacute painful, multifocal, often symmetrical, neuropathy. There are two forms of IDP: acute and chronic. Both are characterized by evolving weakness in arms and legs, with minor sensory symptoms. Mononeuritis multiplex typically manifests as numbness and tingling in the distribution of one peripheral nerve trunk, with sequential sensory and motor involvement of other nerves occurring over weeks. The earliest symptoms of progressive polyradiculopathy include low back pain with radiation into one leg, followed by progressive leg weakness. If the condition is not identified and treated quickly, symptoms rapidly progress to flaccid paraplegia with bowel and bladder incontinence.

Cancer and Its Therapies

Kaposi's sarcoma exists in two primary settings: cutaneous and extracutaneous. Cutaneous Kaposi's sarcoma exhibits an early patch stage and a plaque stage; the latter is indicative of more advanced intradermal lesions, which can eventually become ulcerating tumors. The three main locations of extracutaneous Kaposi's sarcoma are the oral cavity, the gastrointestinal tract, and the lungs.[31] Kaposi's sarcoma is not curable with standard therapies.

AIDS-related lymphomas often manifest with persistent fevers, lymphadenopathy, and weight disturbances. These and other nonspecific constitutional symptoms are also characteristic of lymphoma in the general population. Other clinical features, such as headache or mental status change, may suggest a more specific AIDS-related lymphoma, such as primary CNS lymphoma. Radiological imaging (e.g., computed tomography) and tissue analysis provide significant assistance in diagnosis.

The incidence of non–AIDS-related cancers is increasing. According to recent New York City mortality data, lung cancer is the third most common non-AIDS cause of death among HIV-infected individuals.[31a] The median age at presentation is 40 years. The symptoms at presentation are not significantly different from those in HIV-negative patients; however, most HIV patients with lung cancer present with locally advanced or metastatic disease. A possible explanation for this is that the "typical" presenting symptoms may be confused with HIV-related opportunistic infections, delaying diagnosis. A strong association has been described between prior tuberculosis and adenocarcinoma. Scarring caused by prior tuberculosis or other opportunistic infections may increase the risk of adenocarcinoma.

Other cancers that occur more frequently in HIV-infected adults include anal cancer, Hodgkin's disease, head and neck cancer, testicular cancer, and skin cancers (basal cell, squamous cell, and melanoma). Identified risk factors for anal cancer include multiple sexual partners, receptive anal intercourse, and chronic immunosuppression. The rate of anal cancer in HIV-positive men is double that in HIV-negative men. Although there is no documented link between HIV and colorectal cancer, screening is important in an aging population receiving HAART.

Immune Reconstitution Inflammatory Syndrome

There are three primary IRIS scenarios: (1) a subclinical form consisting of "unmasking" of a previously unrecognized opportunistic infection after initiation of antiretroviral therapy, (2) an early form typified by "atypical" manifestations of an opportunistic infection with early reconstitution of the immune system, and (3) a late form manifesting months after immune reconstitution as opportunistic infections outside the range of expected CD4 counts.

A paradoxical phenomenon of worsening symptoms (e.g., high fevers, worsening lymphadenopathy, worsening pulmonary infiltrates) after initiation of antimycobacterial therapy is well described. *Mycobacterium avium* complex (MAC) IRIS may manifest with fever, painful suppurative lymphadenitis, pulmonary infiltrates, inflammatory masses, epidural abscesses, and/or osteomyelitis.[32] *Mycobacterium tuberculosis* (MTB) IRIS symptoms mimic those of MAC IRIS, with fever, pulmonary infiltrates, and lymphadenopathy. Myriad presentations of MTB IRIS have been described, including, but not limited to, hypercalcemia with pulmonary disease, cerebritis, abscesses, pleural effusions, and osteomyelitis. MAC IRIS tends to appear within the first 3 months of immune reconstitution, whereas MTB IRIS can appear as early as 1 week and as late as several months, with most cases diagnosed within the first 4 to 8 weeks. Other uncommon presentations of MAC include granulomatous masses, osteomyelitis, bursitis, Addison's disease, and skin nodules.[33] Immune-recovery uveitis and vitreitis have been described in patients with CMV IRIS. These are vision-threatening syndromes and require immediate attention. Symptoms include blurred vision and floaters. Ophthalmologic examination may reveal retinitis, vitreitis, and/or cystoid macular edema. Examination of epiretinal membranes demonstrates a predominance of T cells.

Because coinfection of HIV with HBV or HCV is not uncommon, hepatitic IRIS may manifest as "flares" after initiation of HAART. This is more common when a regimen that lacks an anti-HBV agent (e.g., lamivudine, tenofovir) is initiated. If lamivudine is part of the initial regimen, hepatitis viral resistance to lamivudine may explain the symptomatic flare. The flares cause with right upper quadrant pain, nausea, vomiting, and elevation of transaminases. Infection with a new hepatitis virus and other causes of hepatobiliary disease must be excluded. Hepatotoxicity from HAART must also be considered as a cause of elevated enzymes. A liver biopsy, if not contraindicated, may suggest hepatotoxicity due to medication, as opposed to immune reconstitution.

Clinical worsening of known progressive multifocal leukoencephalopathy (PML) and "unmasking" of subclinical PML have been associated temporally with the initiation of HAART.[34] Clinical manifestations include progressive weakness, mental clouding, and headache. Radiological worsening of lesions, including contrast enhancement and mass effect, may occur. Other CNS processes, including toxoplasmosis, lymphoma, and tuberculosis, must be excluded.

An increase in genital herpes infections within the first 6 months after initiation of HAART has been recognized as an IRIS involving herpes simplex virus. It is important to exclude acyclovir-resistant herpes simplex if there is any recurrent or persistent herpetic lesion during treatment with HAART.[35] The increase in CD8+ T cells induced by HAART has resulted in an IRIS involving varicella-zoster virus. The typical presentation is a dermatomal outbreak of herpes zoster; however, cases of transverse myelitis have been documented as a manifestation of varicella-zoster IRIS.

Cryptococcal infection may manifest as recurrent typical cryptococcal meningitis, as an atypical presentation of suppurative mediastinal lymphadenitis, or as aseptic meningitis. Typically, cryptococcal meningitis is associated with a high cerebral spinal fluid pressure, mononuclear pleocytosis of the cerebrospinal fluid, and either organismal identification via India Ink or culture or a very high titer of cryptococcal antigen. In cryptococcal IRIS, however, symptoms may be initiated by an immunological response to nonviable antigen or latent infection; therefore, the organism may not be identifiable or cultured from the cerebrospinal fluid.[36] Headache, vomiting, stiff neck, and fever still predominate as symptoms of cryptococcal meningitic IRIS. The most common time frame for cryptococcal IRIS is within 3 months after initiation of HAART.

TREATMENT

Endocrinological Abnormalities and Lipodystrophy Syndrome

Given that the etiologies of lipoatrophy and fat accumulation have not been well established, effective treatment has been difficult. Substitution of abacavir in place of stavudine or zidovudine reverses lipoatrophy.[37] However, the risk of abacavir hypersensitivity syndrome must be considered before switching regimens. There are no effective therapies for lipodystrophy. Growth hormone may reduce fat accumulation in selected individuals (notably nondiabetics); however, reaccumulation may occur with discontinuation. Insulin sensitizers, such as metformin and the thiazolidinediones, may be effective in reversing fat accumulation as well as beneficial for the cardiovascular risk profile and for improving hyperglycemia. Pioglitazone increases limb fat in HAART-treated patients with lipoatrophy. Cosmetic reconstruction (via surgery or injections with polylactic acid) has been sought by some.

Hyperlipidemia in HIV requires a two-step approach: (1) dietary control with exercise and elimination of modifiable risk factors (e.g., smoking); and (2) use of lipid-lowering agents, with or without switching antiretroviral therapy to substitute other, "lipid-friendly" antiretrovirals for the presumed offending agents. The use of fibrates (e.g., gemfibrozil, fenofibrate) is recommended for hypertriglyceridemia, especially with other cardiovascular risk factors. Alternative therapies include niacin and fish oils. Niacin raises HDL and lowers triglycerides but also has a significant side effect profile, including severe flushing, hyperglycemia, and diarrhea. Bile acid sequestrants also reduce triglycerides and increase HDL. Fish oils have been demonstrated to produce a modest reduction in triglyceride levels. There is potential for drug-drug interactions between 3-hydroxy-3-methylglutaryl coenzyme A (HMG-CoA) reductase inhibitors and most antiretrovirals. These phenomena are typically the result of inhibition of the cytochrome P-450 3A4 enzyme by the PIs. Pravastatin is minimally metabolized via this pathway and therefore is the recommended HMG-CoA reductase inhibitor to use, except with darunavir. Other options include atorvastatin, fluvastatin, and rosuvastatin.[38] Caution should be advised with any HMG-CoA reductase inhibitor and a PI, with or without efavirenz. Nevertheless, a switch in antiretroviral regimen may be considered to treat dyslipidemia. A switch that maintains virological control is paramount. The combination of tenofovir, lamivudine, and efavirenz was found to provide virological suppression comparable to stavudine, lamivudine, and efavirenz in antiretroviral therapy–naïve patients and resulted in improved lipid profiles and less lipodystrophy.[38a] In PI-mediated dyslipidemia, a switch to atazanavir may provide favorable lipid profiles.[38b]

Osteopenia and osteoporosis are treated with calcium and vitamin D supplementation and bisphosphonates. Several studies have demonstrated the benefit of bisphosphonates in patients receiving antiretrovirals.[39] In osteopenia or a history of osteoporosis, tenofovir-based regimens may worsen symptoms. Raloxifene, a selective estrogen-receptor modulator, inhibits cytochrome P-450 and can therefore interact with antiretrovirals. There have been no studies to date that investigate raloxifene with concomitant HAART in bone density restoration.

Peripheral Neuropathy

Most cases of peripheral neuropathy are treated symptomatically with nonsteroidal anti-inflammatory drugs (NSAIDs), tricyclic antidepressants, antiepileptic agents, and, if needed, narcotic analgesics. DILS responds best to antiretroviral therapy or corticosteroids or both. Acute IDP is often treated with high-dose intravenous immunoglobulin or plasmapheresis, whereas chronic IDP is initially treated with steroidal agents, with recurrences treated with high-dose intravenous immunoglobulin or plasmapheresis.[40] The treatment for mononeuritis multiplex depends on the underlying cause. If the cause is vasculitis, symptoms typically resolve with administration of corticosteroids or intravenous immunoglobulin. If CMV is involved, anti-CMV chemotherapy with ganciclovir, foscarnet, or cidofovir should be used. The most experience

in treating progressive polyradiculopathy involves intravenous ganciclovir. Successful treatment with foscarnet has been reported. Combination therapy with ganciclovir and foscarnet is recommended despite poor tolerance and decreased quality of life, both palliative care issues. The critical feature to successful therapy, however, is early diagnosis and treatment before irreversible nerve necrosis occurs.

Cancer and Its Therapies

Several therapeutic options are available for treatment of Kaposi's sarcoma. The first-line therapy is initiation of HAART, if not already prescribed. Other treatments, concomitantly administered with HAART, include interferon-α, chemotherapy, radiotherapy, intralesional chemotherapy, and cryotherapy.[41] Chemotherapeutic options include pegylated-liposomal anthracyclines, paclitaxel, vincristine, etoposide, and intramuscular bleomycin. Radiotherapy is useful if the symptoms are caused by mass effect. Intralesional chemotherapy helps those with oropharyngeal or laryngeal Kaposi's sarcoma. Thalidomide has also demonstrated moderate activity.

NHL responds to the standard chemotherapeutic regimen of cyclophosphamide, hydroxydaunomycin, Oncovin, and prednisone (CHOP) and also to the combination of cyclophosphamide, doxorubicin, and etoposide (CDE). The National Cancer Institute described a successful regimen of etoposide, vincristine, and doxorubicin for 4 days, combined with 5 days of prednisone followed by a dose of cyclophosphamide (EPOCH), adjusted according to the initial CD4 count.[42]

Hodgkin's lymphoma, although not considered an AIDS-defining malignancy, has increased recently. The three main regimens that have been studied in concurrent HAART have all demonstrated some success, albeit with serious adverse effects. The three regimens are (1) doxorubicin, bleomycin, vinblastine, and dacarbazine (ABVD); (2) bleomycin, etoposide, doxorubicin, cyclophosphamide, vincristine, procarbazine, and prednisone (BEACOPP); and (3) doxorubicin, vinblastine, mechlorethamine, etoposide, vincristine, bleomycin, prednisone, and involved field radiation for initial bulky disease (Stanford V Regimen).[43]

Aside from HAART, there are three other treatment options in primary CNS lymphoma: (1) whole-brain irradiation and corticosteroids; (2) intravenous methotrexate followed by whole-brain irradiation; and (3) methotrexate, thiotepa, and procarbazine intravenously combined with methotrexate intrathecally.[44]

Myriad side effects are associated with the use of antineoplastic agents. The treatments of these side effects are effect-specific; for example, neutropenia produced by the use of paclitaxel is treated with granulocyte colony-stimulating factor, if available. In comparison to the anthracyclines, paclitaxel is associated with more alopecia, myalgia, arthralgia, and bone marrow suppression.

The use of combination chemotherapy often is limited because of serious side effects, such as cardiotoxicity (anthracyclines), hematological toxicity, mucositis, vomiting, and alopecia.

Immune Reconstitution Inflammatory Syndrome

The most important initial step in IRIS is to eliminate other potential diagnoses, including natural progression of disease despite appropriate therapy, failure of targeted therapy (e.g., mycobacterial resistance), other infections, and cancer. In most instances, there are no definitive standards of care. To prevent IRIS, some recommend delaying antiretroviral therapy for approximately 2 months after the initiation of appropriately targeted antimicrobial chemotherapy (e.g., antituberculosis agents). For MTB and MAC IRIS, the continuation of antimycobacterial and antiretroviral therapies is recommended. In mild IRIS, NSAIDs may provide some symptomatic benefit. In more severe IRIS, a short course of corticosteroids or thalidomide may help. Drainage of large abscesses, if present, is suggested in both MTB and MAC IRIS. Corticosteroids are the cornerstone of treatment of CMV immune-recovery uveitis.

Mild hepatitic flares due to HBV may be observed without clinical intervention. With severe flares, adjusting the antiretroviral regimen to include lamivudine or emtricitabine with tenofovir may alleviate symptoms. PML IRIS is difficult to treat, because the primary treatment modality for PML is HAART. The current recommendation for PML IRIS is to continue HAART only, because corticosteroid therapy has not been of significant benefit.[45] There are no specific changes in conventional therapy for herpes simplex or varicella-zoster IRIS. Foscarnet can be used to treat acyclovir-resistant herpes simplex. The mainstay of therapy for cryptococcal IRIS is antifungal chemotherapy and maintenance of HAART. Adjunctive anti-inflammatory agents, such as corticosteroids and hydroxychloroquine, may help.[46]

Drugs of Choice

Palliative care for HIV-infected individuals is diverse; it includes prognosis, advanced care planning, and management of pain, symptoms, and drug interactions.[47] Pain can be multifactorial: it may be derived from opportunistic infections, neurotoxicity, medication toxicity, coexisting painful conditions (e.g., musculoskeletal pain), or other nonspecific entities (e.g., headache). Management of these pain symptoms may involve targeting the underlying pathology (as is the case with opportunistic infections), treating the pain through manipulation of the opioid receptors, or a combination of the two.[48] In more developed nations, where injection drug use is a significant mode of HIV transmission, pain management may require more diligence, especially if the patient has used opioid-based substances. Those who utilize a methadone maintenance program to facilitate rehabilitation require additional pain medication, because the methadone, at the maintenance dosage, does not provide analgesia.

Certain medications are metabolized through the same cytochrome pathway as analgesics and thereby may cause either insufficient analgesia (if increasing metabolism of the analgesics) or surplus analgesia (if inhibiting their metabolism). Rifampin, a medication used in the management of infections caused by mycobacteria and methicillin-resistant *Staphylococcus aureus*, increases the metabolism of methadone and other opioid analgesics by inducing the cytochrome P-450 system, thereby necessitating increasing dosages (and potentially increasing frequency) of opioids. Certain palliative medications are contraindicated with ritonavir, including benzodiazepines and histamine antagonists.

Individuals with AIDS may suffer from additional symptoms, other than pain and those caused by opportunistic infections, such as fatigue, weight loss, anxiety, depression, diarrhea, and nausea. Treatment may be disease-specific (e.g., HAART for HIV-induced fatigue and weight loss), symptom-specific (e.g., dronabinol and megestrol for weight loss and anorexia), or a combination of both.[48] Symptom-specific therapy may also improve adherence if anorexia or nausea is preventing the patient from taking every dose. The best therapy may require an individualized, multidisciplinary approach, with assessment of the risks and benefits of each type of therapy and the overall prognosis in each patient.[49]

CONCLUSIONS

Recent data have shown that individuals with HIV are experiencing more non-AIDS-related morbidities, such as cardiovascular disease, cancer, and renal disease (see "Future Considerations"). A multidisciplinary approach includes heightened screening for cardiovascular disease and cancers that typically did not afflict HIV-positive individuals before the era of HAART. Yet, even with heightened screening, patients still may present with advanced oncological disorders. Palliative care is critical. An assessment of functional status needs to be conducted, because it has been shown that impaired functional status is a strong predictor of mortality.[50] Emphasis should be placed on pain and symptom management.

Future Considerations

1. *When to start HAART and which therapy to start:* Despite all the advances and antiretroviral therapies available, we still do not know when to start HAART or which agents to use. Studies are warranted to evaluate the timing of therapy based on the immunological status of the host, long-term toxicities of therapy, and adherence issues. In addition, studies are needed to compare various therapy combinations, with end points considering safety and long-term survival.

2. *Initiation of HAART in the setting of opportunistic infections:* Given the potential for drug interactions, drug toxicities, and paradoxical worsening with the initiation of HAART at time of an acute opportunistic infection, many experts wait 1 to 2 months before starting antiretroviral therapy. However, a delay in HIV-specific therapy may lead to progression of the opportunistic infection and death.

3. *How to manage immune reconstitution inflammatory syndromes (IRIS):* Studies are warranted for exploring immune modulators and anti-inflammatory agents for IRIS.

REFERENCES

1. Li F, Goila-Gaur R, Salzwedel K, et al. PA-457: A potent HIV inhibitor that disrupts core condensation by targeting a late step in gag processing. Proc Natl Acad Sci U S A 2003;100:13555-13560.
1a. http://www.unaids.org/en/KnowledgeCentre/HIVData/EpiUpdate/EpiUpd Archive/2007/default.asp (accessed May 12, 2008).
2. 2006 Report on the Global AIDS Epidemic. Geneva: Joint United Nations Programme on HIV/AIDS, 2006.
3. Centers for Disease Control and Prevention. Epidemiology of HIV/AIDS—United States, 1981-2005. MMWR Morb Mortal Wkly Rep 2006;55:589-592.
4. Palella FJ Jr, Baker RK, Moorman AC, et al. Mortality in the highly active antiretroviral therapy era: Changing causes of death and disease in the HIV outpatient study. J AIDS 2006;43:27-34.
5. Young B. Mixing new cocktails: Drug interactions in antiretroviral regimens. AIDS Patient Care and STDs 2005;19:286-297.
6. Arnaudo E, Salakas M, Shanske S, et al. Depletion of muscle mitochondrial DNA in AIDS patients with zidovudine-induced myopathy. Lancet 1991;337:508-510.
7. Pozniak A, Gallant J, DeJesus E, et al. Superior Outcome for Tenofovir DF (TDF), Emtricitabine (FTC) and Efavirenz (EFV) Compared to Fixed-Dose Zidovudine/Lamivudine (CBV) and EFV in Antiretroviral Naïve Patients. Abstracts and Posters of the 3rd International AIDS Society Conference on HIV Pathogenesis and Treatment, Rio de Janeiro, Brazil, July 24-27, 2005. Abstract WeOa0202.
8. Carr A, Samaras K, Chisholm DJ, et al. Pathogenesis of HIV-1-protease inhibitor-associated peripheral lipodystrophy, hyperlipidaemia, and insulin resistance. Lancet 1998;351:1881-1883.
9. Vigouroux C, Maachi M, Nguyen TH, et al. Serum adipocytokines are related to lipodystrophy and metabolic disorders in HIV-infected men under antiretroviral therapy. AIDS 2003;17:1503-1511.
10. Holmberg SD, Moorman AC, Williamson JM, et al. Protease inhibitors and cardiovascular outcomes in patients with HIV-1. Lancet 2002;360:1747-1748.
11. Dube MP, Stein JH, Aberg JA, et al. Guidelines for the evaluation and management of dyslipidemia in human immunodeficiency virus (HIV)-infected adults receiving antiretroviral therapy: Recommendations of the HIV Medical Association of the Infectious Disease Society of American and the Adult AIDS Clinical Trials Group. Clin Infect Dis 2003;37:613-627.
12. Mallal SA, John M, Moore CB, et al. Contribution of nucleoside analogue reverse transcriptase inhibitors to subcutaneous fat wasting in patients with HIV infection. AIDS 2000;14:1309-1316.
13. Amorosa V, Tebas P. Bone disease and HIV infection. Clin Infect Dis 2006;42:108-114.
14. Simpson DM, Tagliati M. Nucleoside analogue-associated peripheral neuropathy in human immunodeficiency virus infection. J Acquir Immune Defic Syndr Hum Retrovirol 1995;9:153-161.
15. Behar R, Wiley C, McCutchan JA. Cytomegalovirus polyradiculopathy in acquired immune deficiency syndrome. Neurology 1987;37:557-561.
16. Stern JO, Robinson PA, Love J, et al. A comprehensive hepatic safety analysis of nevirapine in different populations of HIV infected patients. J AIDS 2003;34(Suppl 1):S21-S33.
17. Levine A, Seneviratne L, Espina BM, et al. Evolving characteristics of AIDS-related lymphoma. Blood 2000;96:4084-4090.
18. Bruera D, Luna N, David DO, et al. Decreased bone mineral density in HIV-infected patients is independent of antiretroviral therapy. J AIDS 2003;17:1917-1923.
19. Bonnet F, Lewden C, May T, et al. Malignancy-related causes of death in human immunodeficiency virus-infected patients in the era of highly active antiretroviral therapy. Cancer 2004;101:317-324.
20. Knowles DM. Etiology and pathogenesis of AIDS-related non-Hodgkin's lymphoma. Hematol Oncol Clin North Am 2003;17:785-820.
21. International Collaboration on HIV and Cancer. Highly active antiretroviral therapy and incidence of cancer in human immunodeficiency virus-infected adults. J Natl Cancer Inst 2000;92:1823-1830.
22. Lipman M, Breen R. Immune reconstitution inflammatory syndrome in HIV. Curr Opin Infect Dis 2006;19:20-25.
23. Bartlett JG, Gallant JE. 2005-6 Medical Management of HIV Infection. Baltimore: Johns Hopkins University, 2005.
24. Rockstroh J, Mocroft A, Soriano V, et al. Influence of hepatitis C on HIV disease progression and response to highly active antiretroviral therapy. J Infect Dis 2005;192:992-1002.
25. Clark S, Creighton S, Portmann B, et al. Acute liver failure associated with antiretroviral treatment for HIV: A report of six cases. J Hepatol 2002;36:295-301.
26. Carr A, Miller J, Eisman JA, et al. Osteopenia in HIV-infected men: Association with asymptomatic lactic acidemia and lower weight pre-antiretroviral therapy. AIDS 2001;15:703-709.
27. Carr A, Emery S, Law M, et al. An objective case definition of lipodystrophy in HIV-infected adults: A case-control study. Lancet 2003;361:726-735.
28. Mondy K, Tebas P. Emerging bone problems in patients infected with human immunodeficiency virus. Clin Infect Dis 2003;36(Suppl 2):S101-S105.
29. Pardo CA, McArthur JC, Griffin JW. HIV neuropathy: Insights in the pathology of HIV peripheral nerve disease. J Peripheral Nerv Sys 2001;6:21-27.
30. Cornblath DR, McArthur JC. Predominantly sensory neuropathy in patients with AIDS and AIDS-related complex. Neurology 1988;38:794-796.
31. Pantanowitz L, Dezube BJ. Kaposi's sarcoma. Ear Nose Throat J 2004;83:157.
31a. Sackoff JE, Hanna DB, Pfeiffer MR, Torian LV. Causes of death among persons with AIDS in the era of highly active antiretroviral therapy: New York City. Ann Intern Med 2006;145:397-406.
32. Phillips P, Bonner S, Gataric N, et al. Nontuberculous mycobacterial immune reconstitution syndrome in HIV-infected patients: Spectrum of disease and long-term follow-up. Clin Infect Dis 2005;41:1483-1497.
33. del Giudice P, Durant J, Counillon E, et al. Mycobacterial cutaneous manifestations: A new sign of immune restoration syndrome in patients with acquired immunodeficiency syndrome. Arch Dermatol 1999;135:1129-1130.
34. Kotecha N, George MJ, Smith TW, et al. Enhancing progressive multifocal leukoencephalopathy: An indicator of improved immune status? Am J Med 1998;105:541-543.
35. Couppie P, Sarazin F, Clyti E, et al. Increased incidence of genital herpes after HAART initiation: A frequent presentation of immune reconstitution inflammatory syndrome (IRIS) in HIV-infected patients. AIDS Patient Care STDs 2006;20:143-145.
36. Broom J, Woods M II, Allworth A. Immune reconstitution inflammatory syndrome producing atypical presentations of cryptococcal meningitis: Case report and a review of immune reconstitution-associated cryptococcal infections. Scand J Infect Dis 2006;38:219-221.
37. Carr A, Workman C, Smith DE, et al. Abacavir substitution for nucleoside analogs in patients with HIV lipoatrophy: A randomized trial. JAMA 2002;288:207-215.
38. Calza L, Colangeli V, Manfredi R, et al. Rosuvastatin for the treatment of hyperlipidemia in HIV-infected patients receiving protease inhibitors: A pilot study. AIDS 2005;19:1103-1105.
38a. Cassetti I, Madruga JV, Suleiman JM, et al. The safety and efficacy of tenofovir DF in combination with lamivudine and efavirenz through 6 years in antiretroviral-naïve HIV-1-infected patients. HIV Clin Trials 2007;8:164-172.
38b. Gatell J, Salmon-Ceron D, Lazzaria A. Efficacy and safety of atazanavir-based highly active antiretroviral therapy in patients with virologic suppression switched from a stable, boosted or unboosted protease inhibitor treatment regimen: The SWAN Study (AI424-097) 48-week results. Clin Infect Dis 2007;44:1484-1492.
39. Mondy K, Powderly W, Claxton SA, et al. Alendonate, vitamin D, and calcium for the treatment of osteopenia/osteoporosis associated with HIV infection. J AIDS 2005;38:426-431.
40. Cornblath DR. Treatment of the neuromuscular complications of human immunodeficiency virus infection. Ann Neurol 1988;23(Suppl):S88-S91.
41. Krown SE. Therapy of AIDS-associated Kaposi's sarcoma: Targeting pathogenetic mechanisms. Hematol Oncol Clin North Am 2003;17:763-783.
42. Little RF, Pittaluga S, Grant N, et al. Highly effective treatment of acquired immunodeficiency syndrome-related lymphoma with dose-adjusted EPOCH: Impact of antiretroviral therapy suspension and tumor biology. Blood 2003;101:4653-4659.
43. Levine AM, Li P, Cheung T, et al. Chemotherapy consisting of doxorubicin, bleomycin, vinblastine, and dacarbazine with granulocyte-colony-stimulating factor in HIV-infected patients with newly diagnosed Hodgkin's disease: A prospective, multi-institutional AIDS Clinical Trials Group Study (ACTG 149). J AIDS 2000;24:444-450.
44. Portegies P, Solod L, Cinque P, et al. Guidelines for the diagnosis and management of neurological complications of HIV infection. Eur J Neurol 2004;11:297-304.
45. Manzardo C, Del Mar Ortega M, Sued O, et al. Central nervous system opportunistic infections in developed countries in the highly active antiretroviral therapy era. J Neurovirol 2005;11(Suppl 3):72-82.
46. King M, Perlino C, Cinnamon J, Hernigan J. Paradoxical recurrent meningitis following therapy of cryptococcal meningitis: An immune reconstitution syndrome after the initiation of highly active antiretroviral therapy. Int J STDs AIDS 2002;13:724-726.
47. The Workgroup on Palliative and End-of-Life Care in HIV/AIDS. Integrating Palliative Care into the Continuum of HIV Care: An Agenda for Change. Promoting Excellence in End-of-Life Care, 2004.
48. Selwyn PA. Why should we care about palliative care for AIDS in the era of antiretroviral therapy. Sex Transmit Infect 2005;81:2-3.
49. Karus D, Raveis VH, Alexander C, et al. Patient reports of symptoms and their treatment at three palliative care projects servicing individuals with HIV/AIDS. J Pain Symptom Manage 2005;30:408-417.
50. Shen JM, Blank A, Selwyn PA. Predictors of mortality for patients with advanced disease in an HIV palliative care program. J AIDS 2005;40:589-592.

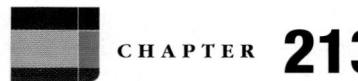

CHAPTER **213**

Treatment of Persons Infected with the Human Immunodeficiency Virus

William Powderly and Edgar Turner Overton

KEY POINTS

- Antiretroviral therapy (ART) has changed the paradigm of treatment of human immunodeficiency virus (HIV) infection.
- Resistance testing is critical for successful ART.
- Guidelines for ART are evolving.
- ART toxicities remain a critical issue with long-term suppressive ART.
- Research continues in the development of novel agents.

Since the first reports of Kaposi's sarcoma and *Pneumocystis* pneumonia in homosexual men in California and New York City in 1981 heralded the era of acquired immunodeficiency syndrome (AIDS), the scientific community has developed significant understanding of the epidemiology of the disease, its causative agent, the mechanism of immune depletion, treatment, and potential prevention.[1,2] Potent antiretroviral therapy (ART) with the capacity to inhibit viral replication and reconstitute the depleted immune system has transformed the syndrome from an inevitably terminal illness into a manageable chronic disease.

ART has changed markedly since the institution of zidovudine monotherapy in 1987. The development of combination therapy in 1996 created a new paradigm wherein viral replication could be suppressed with significant long-term benefits. The subsequent decade has seen the refinement of potent ART with newer agents that have improved efficacy, lower pill burdens, better tolerability, fewer adverse events, and better safety profiles. Additionally, recognition of the importance of viral resistance has made resistance testing a crucial component in the management of human immunodeficiency virus (HIV) disease and monitoring of the virologic response to therapy.

PRINCIPLES OF THERAPY

The goals of treatment are reduction of HIV-related morbidity and mortality, improved quality of life, restoration and improvement of immune function, and suppression of HIV viral replication to undetectable levels. These goals are inter-related and depend on the effectiveness of ART. Maximal suppression of virus replication is the crucial principle of initial treatment. This reflects the underlying replication strategies of HIV. First, HIV is characterized by extremely high viral production. Ten million lymphoid cells may be infected at any given time in an infected person, with production of as many as 10 billion viral particles daily.[3] A high level of viremia is complicated by the fact that the viral reverse transcriptase is prone to error without a correction mechanism. High viral turnover with frequent mutation in the viral genetic code leads to a diverse viral population of quasispecies. This benefits the virus as a mechanism to evade host immune responses and maintain high levels of viral replication. In partial viral suppression with only a single antiretroviral agent, the same mechanism allows the virus to selectively mutate to develop agent resistance, and this is inevitable with all available antiviral drugs.

A critical factor in the strategy to suppress HIV replication maximally and durably is the potency of the antiviral agents. Such potency requires combination therapy with three active agents from two different classes (see later discussion). This prevents the virus from developing the multiple different mutations required to evade therapy. This approach may be undermined if the virus has acquired resistance to some of the agents being used for therapy. Transmission of acquired resistant mutants is occurring with increasing frequency. It is increasingly necessary to assess resistance by baseline testing, because resistance to at least one medication is found in 10% to 20% of HIV-infected persons who are therapy naïve. If one of the agents chosen is ineffective because of preexisting resistance, a cycle of virological failure and production of a multiresistant virus may result. The regimen must be individualized for each patient, with consideration for pill burden, dosing frequency, potential drug interactions, and comorbidities such as underlying renal disease, diabetes, psychiatric illness, and coinfection with hepatitis viruses.

In cases of advanced disease, an extensive treatment history, and resistant virus, complete suppression of virus may be impossible. Then the goal is to prevent the progression to AIDS and to limit the loss of immune function while limiting further development of resistance. The latter is important, because HIV therapy is evolving, with new medications being approved almost yearly by regulatory agencies. An individual with no options today may be able to suppress the virus completely with drugs now in development.

WHEN TO START ANTIRETROVIRAL THERAPY

Before initiating ART, an HIV-infected person should undergo a complete history and physical examination and baseline laboratory studies. The purpose is to confirm HIV infection, assess ongoing risk behaviors, educate the patient about the natural history of HIV infection and preventive measures (Table 213-1), and evaluate for manifestations of AIDS or opportunistic infections and coinfections. It is important to identify comorbidities, to determine the baseline viral load and CD4+ T-lymphocyte count, and to evaluate for baseline resistance mutations that may limit therapeutic options. A vaccination history should be obtained. The initial laboratory workup should include[4]

- Baseline hematology studies
- Liver and renal function tests
- Evaluation of lipid and metabolic profile

- Assessment for hepatitis virus coinfection and other sexually transmitted diseases, including gonorrhea, chlamydia, and syphilis
- Baseline tuberculin skin test

For every patient with symptomatic HIV or a history of an AIDS-defining opportunistic infection, treatment is indicated regardless of the CD4 count. Treatment is also indicated for all persons with a CD4 count lower than 200 cells/mm³. Table 213-2 outlines the current preferred combination ART for treatment-naïve persons derived from national or international guidelines.[5-7] For the asymptomatic patient, treatment is initiated based on CD4 counts. Several observational studies and treatment interruption studies have shown treatment benefit at higher CD4 counts, and debate remains about the appropriate point at which to initiate therapy (Table 213-3). Additional studies will better inform treatment for patients with higher CD4 counts.

Regardless of these stated guidelines, therapy must be tailored to the individual, and the patient must be committed to therapy. Without excellent adherence, the regimen will fail and resistance will develop, limiting future options for viral suppression. With a higher CD4 count, the benefits and risks of initiating therapy must be carefully evaluated. Benefits for early initiation include prevention of progression to AIDS and subsequent opportunistic infections, and the possible public health benefit of limiting transmission of HIV.

TABLE 213-1 Prevention and Prophylaxis for Opportunistic Infections

CD4 COUNT (CELLS/MM³)	INTERVENTIONS
Any	Plasma viral load and CD4 count every 3-4 mo
	Baseline resistance testing
	Serology studies for *Toxoplasma gondii*
	Yearly STD screening (RPR, gonorrhea, *Chlamydia*)
	Yearly pelvic examination with Pap smear (women)
	Yearly tuberculin skin test
	Hepatitis A and B vaccination* (if indicated)
	Pneumovax* and yearly influenza vaccination
<200	Prophylaxis for PCP
<100	Prophylaxis for toxoplasmosis if serology result is positive and patient is not taking TMP-SMX
<50	Retina screening for CMV
	Prophylaxis for MAC

CMV, cytomegalovirus; MAC, *Mycobacterium avium* complex; PCP, *Pneumocystis* pneumonia; RPR, rapid plasma reagin test for syphilis; STD, sexually transmitted disease; TMP-SMX, trimethoprim-sulfamethoxazole.
*Efficacy of Pneumovax and hepatitis vaccines is poor if CD4 count is <200/mm³.

CLASSES OF ANTIRETROVIRAL DRUGS

There are currently four classes of medicines approved for the treatment of HIV infection (Table 213-4). These are identified by their mechanism of action on the different steps of the viral life cycle: nucleoside reverse transcrip-

TABLE 213-2 Recommended Regimens for Treatment-Naïve Patients*

AGENCY	RECOMMENDED TREATMENT		
	NRTI	**NNRTI**	**PI**
IAS-USA[†]			
Preferred Agent	Tenofovir/emtricitabine	Efavirenz	Atazanavir/ritonavir
	Zidovudine/lamivudine	Nevirapine	Fosamprenavir/ritonavir
	Abacavir/lamivudine		Lopinavir/ritonavir
			Saquinavir/ritonavir
DHHS[‡]			
Preferred Agent	Tenofovir/emtricitabine	Efavirenz	Atazanavir/ritonavir
	Zidovudine/lamivudine		Fosamprenavir/ritonavir bid
			Lopinavir/ritonavir bid
Alternative	Abacavir/lamivudine	Nevirapine	Atazanavir (unboosted)
	Didanosine/lamivudine		Fosamprenavir (unboosted)
			Fosamprenavir/ritonavir qd
			Lopinavir/ritonavir qd
BHIVA[§]			
Preferred Agent	Tenofovir/emtricitabine	Efavirenz	Lopinavir/ritonavir
	Zidovudine/lamivudine		
	Abacavir/lamivudine		
Alternative		Nevirapine	Atazanavir/ritonavir
			Fosamprenavir/ritonavir bid
			Atazanavir (unboosted)
			Fosamprenavir (unboosted)

NRTI, nucleoside reverse transcriptase inhibitor; NNRTI, non-nucleoside reverse transcriptase inhibitor; PI, protease inhibitor.
*All regimens combine two NRTIs with either an NNRTI or a PI (with or without ritonavir boosting).
[†]International AIDS Society-USA (IAS-USA) guidelines are created by a panel of 16 noncompensated experts who review all published clinical trial data regarding antiretroviral therapy.[5]
[‡]U.S. Department of Health and Human Services (DHHS) guidelines are developed by a working group from the Office of AIDS Research Advisory Council (OARAC), who review all drug information submitted to the U.S. Food and Drug Administration as well as research presented at conferences and published in the literature.[6]
[§]British HIV Medical Association (BHIVA) guidelines are updated by the 21-member executive committee based on critical research.[7]

TABLE 213-3 Recommendations for Initiating HAART in HIV-Infected Adults

CD4 COUNT (CELLS/MM³) OR OTHER MEASURE	IAS-USA GUIDELINES[5]	DHHS GUIDELINES[6]	BHIVA GUIDELINES[7]
Symptomatic disease	ART recommended	ART recommended	ART recommended
<200	ART recommended	ART recommended	ART recommended
>200 but <350	ART should be considered	ART should be offered	Initiate therapy in most patients
>350 with HIV RNA >100,000 copies/mL	Consider treatment with high viral loads	Treatment usually deferred; some clinicians offer ART	Defer treatment
>350 with HIV RNA <100,000 copies/mL	ART not recommended	Treatment should be deferred	Defer treatment
>350 but <500	Consider treatment in persons with rapid decline in CD4 count	See above	Defer treatment
>500	ART not recommended	See above	Defer treatment

ART, antiretroviral therapy; BHIVA, British HIV Medical Association; HAART, highly active antiretroviral therapy; IAS-USA, International AIDS Society-USA; DHHS, U.S. Department of Health and Human Services.

TABLE 213-4 Classes of Antiretroviral Agents

DRUG	ABBREVIATION	TRADE NAME	YEAR OF FDA APPROVAL
NUCLEOSIDE/NUCLEOTIDE REVERSE TRANSCRIPTASE INHIBITORS (NRTIS)			
Zidovudine	ZDV, AZT	Retrovir	1987
Didanosine	ddI	Videx, Videx EC	1991
Zalcitabine	ddC	Hivid	1992
Stavudine	d4T	Zerit	1994
Lamivudine	3TC	Epivir	1995
Abacavir	ABC	Ziagen	1998
Tenofovir	TDF	Viread	2001
Emtricitabine	FTC	Emtriva	2003
PROTEASE INHIBITORS (PIS)			
Saquinavir	SQV	Fortovase, Invirase	1995
Ritonavir	RTV	Norvir	1996
Indinavir	IDV	Crixivan	1996
Nelfinavir	NFV	Viracept	1997
Amprenavir	APV	Agenerase	1999
Lopinavir/ritonavir	LPV/r	Kaletra	2000
Atazanavir	ATV	Reyataz	2003
Fosamprenavir	FPV	Lexiva	2003
Tipranavir	TPV	Aptivus	2005
Darunavir	DRV	Prezista	2006
NON-NUCLEOSIDE REVERSE TRANSCRIPTASE INHIBITORS (NNRTIS)			
Nevirapine	NVP	Viramune	1996
Delavirdine	DLV	Rescriptor	1997
Efavirenz	EFV	Sustiva	1998
FUSION INHIBITORS (FI)			
Enfuvirtide	ENF, T20	Fuzeon	2003
FIXED-DOSE COMBINATIONS			
3TC/ZDV		Combivir	1997
3TC/ABC/ZDV		Trizivir	2000
3TC/ABC		Epzicom	2003
FTC/TDF		Truvada	2004
EFV/FTC/TDF		Atripla	2006

tase inhibitors (NRTIs), non-nucleoside reverse transcriptase inhibitors (NNRTIs), protease inhibitors (PIs), and fusion inhibitors (FIs).

Nucleoside Reverse Transcriptase Inhibitors

NRTIs inhibit viral reverse transcriptase, the enzyme that translates viral RNA into DNA in the infected cell.[8] They are also called nucleoside (or nucleotide) analogues, because their structure resembles the cellular nucleosides in DNA synthesis: the two purine nucleosides, adenosine and guanine, and the two pyrimidine nucleosides, thymidine and cytidine. NRTIs must be activated in the cell by phosphorylation in the cytoplasm. Once they are activated, the viral reverse transcriptase attempts to use them to synthesize viral DNA. They are preferentially used by the viral rather than the host reverse transcriptase because the viral enzyme lacks a corrective mechanism to identify these inhibitors. Once NRTIs are incorporated into the DNA molecule, no additional nucleotides can be added, and DNA synthesis is terminated with an incomplete and nonfunctional copy of DNA.

In most cases, two agents from this class are used as part of combination therapy, in part because they are well tolerated and many can be given in a single daily dose. Often, patients experience side effects during the first few weeks of therapy. Although these symptoms are often nonspecific, it is crucial to provide counseling and symptom treatment in the weeks after initiation of ART, particularly for the common gastrointestinal side effects. Many early-treatment adverse events related to NRTIs overlap with those related to agents from other classes (Table 213-5). Most NRTIs are excreted via the kidneys and do not have significant interactions with other drugs metabolized by the cytochrome P-450 system of the liver.

Non-nucleoside Reverse Transcriptase Inhibitors

NNRTIs reversibly bind to the reverse transcriptase enzyme and prevent its functional activity.[9] These drugs

TABLE 213-5 Toxicities of Antiretroviral Therapy

DRUG	DOSAGE	COMMON TOXICITIES	ADDITIONAL COMMENTS	RESISTANCE CONCERNS*
NUCLEOSIDE/NUCLEOTIDE REVERSE TRANSCRIPTASE INHIBITORS (NRTIS)				
Zidovudine (ZDV)	300 mg q12h	Nausea, headache, rash, anemia, leukopenia, liver toxicity, lactic acidosis, myositis	Adjust dose for renal insufficiency	69 insertion complex, Q151M Thymidine analogue mutations: M41L, D67N, K70R, L210W, T215Y/F, K219Q/E
Didanosine (ddI)	<50 kg: 250 qd >50 kg: 400 qd	GI intolerance, pancreatitis, peripheral neuropathy, lactic acidosis Should not be taken with ddC	Adjust dose for renal insufficiency	69 insertion complex, Q151M L74V, K65R
Zalcitabine (ddC)	0.75 mg q8h	Peripheral neuropathy, oral ulcers, pancreatitis Should not be taken with ddC or d4T	Adjust dose for renal insufficiency	69 insertion complex, Q151M
Stavudine (d4T)	40-60 kg: 30 mg q12h >60 kg: 40 mg q12h	Peripheral neuropathy, pancreatitis, lactic acidosis, lipoatrophy Should not be combined with ZDV or ddC	Higher rates of mitochondrial toxicity than other NRTIs Adjust dose for renal insufficiency	69 insertion complex, Q151M Thymidine analogue mutations: M41L, D67N, K70R, L210W, T215Y/F, K219Q/E
Lamivudine (3TC)	300 mg qd	GI intolerance, headache Well tolerated	Adjust dose for renal insufficiency	69 insertion complex, Q151M M184V, K65R
Abacavir (ABC)	300 mg q12h	Hypersensitivity reaction Lactic acidodis	Metabolized in liver	69 insertion complex, Q151M K65R, L74V, Y115F, M184V
Tenofovir (TDF)	300 mg qd	GI intolerance Hypophosphatemia	Adjust dose for renal insufficiency Concerns for renal toxicity Reduces levels of ATV	69 insertion complex K65R, K70E
Emtricitabine (FTC)	200 mg qd	GI intolerance, headache Hyperpigmentation Well tolerated	Adjust dose for renal insufficiency	69 insertion complex, Q151M M184V, K65R
PROTEASE INHIBITORS (PIS)				
Saquinavir (SQV)	400 mg/400 mg RTV q12h	Liver toxicity GI toxicity	Poor bioavailability if unboosted High pill burden	Major: G48V, L90M Minor: L10I/R/V, L24I, I54V/L, I63V, A71V/T, G73S, V77I, V82A/F/T/S, I84V
Ritonavir (RTV)	600 mg q12h	GI toxicity, oral paresthesias, taste perversion, headache Hypertriglyceridemia	High pill burden Most commonly used as PI booster Must be refrigerated	Not applicable
Indinavir (IDV)	800 mg q8h OR 800 mg/100 mg RTV q12h	Liver toxicity Nephrolithiasis, HTN Benign hyperbilirubinemia	Associated with fat redistribution	Major: M46I/V, V82A/F/T, I84V Minor: L10I/R/V, K20M/R, L24I, V32I, M36I, I54V/L, A71V/T, G73S/A, V77I, L90M
Nelfinavir (NFV)	1250 mg q12h	GI toxicity (diarrhea) Liver toxicity Lipid abnormalities	Favorable safety data in pregnant women Must be given with food Higher rates of failure than boosted PIs	Major: D30N, L90M Minor: L10I/R/V, M36I,M46I/L,A71V/T, V77I, V82A/F/T/S, I84V, N88D/S
Amprenavir (APV)	1200 mg q12h OR 600 mg/100 mg RTV q12h	Rash, GI toxicity Perioral paresthesias Hyperlipidemia	Has been replaced by FPV in adults	
Lopinavir/ ritonavir (LPV/r)	2 tablets q12h	GI toxicity Hypertriglyceridemia	Oral solution is available	Major: V32I, I47V/A, V82A/F/T/S Minor: L10I/R/V, K20M/R, L24I, L33F, M46I/L, I50V, F53L, I54V/L/A/M/T/S, L63P, A71V/T, G73S, I84V, L90M
Atazanavir (ATV)	400 mg qd OR 300 mg/100 mg RTV qd	Benign hyperbilirubinemia PR prolongation Rash	Less lipid abnormalities than other PIs Poor absorption if given with acid reducing agents	Major: I50L, I84V, N88S Minor: L10I/R/V, G16E, K20M/R/I/T/V, V32I, L33F, E34Q, M36I/L/V, M46I/L, G48V, F53L/Y, I54V/L/A/M/T/S, L63P, A71V/T, G73S, I85V, L90M, I93L/M
Fosamprenavir (FPV)	1400 mg bid OR 1400 mg/200 mg RTV qd OR 700 mg/100 mg RTV bid	Rash GI intolerance Liver toxicity	Better eficacy with bid than with qd dosing	Major: I50V, I84V Minor: L10I/R/V, V32I, M46I/L, I47V, I54L/V/MT/A, D60E, I62V, I64L/M/V, A71V/I/T/L, G73C/S/T/A, V82A/F/T/S, L90M
Tipranavir (TPV)	500 mg/200 mg RTV bid	Liver toxicity Rash Hyperlipidemia	Approved only for salvage therapy Rare cases of intracranial hemorrhage have been reported	Major: L33F, V82L/T, I84V Minor: L10V, I13V, K20M/R, E35G, M36I, K43T, M46L, I47V, I54A/M/V, Q58E, H69K, T74P, N83D, L90M

TABLE 213-5 Toxicities of Antiretroviral Therapy—cont'd

DRUG	DOSAGE	COMMON TOXICITIES	ADDITIONAL COMMENTS	RESISTANCE CONCERNS*
Darunavir (DRV)	600 mg /100 mg RTV bid	Rash, headache GI intolerance Liver toxicity	Approved only for salvage therapy	Major: I50V, I54M/L, L76V, I84V Minor: V11I, V32I, L33F, I47V, G73S, L89V:
NON-NUCLEOSIDE REVERSE TRANSCRIPTASE INHIBITORS (NNRTIS)				
Nevirapine (NVP)	200 mg q12h	Rash (including Stevens-Johnson syndrome) Liver toxicity	Contraindicated with CD4 counts >250 cells/mm³ (women) or 400 cells/mm³ (men)	L100I, K103N, V106A/M, V108I, Y181C/I, Y188C/L/H, G190A
Delavirdine (DLV)	400 mg q8h	Rash, headache Liver toxicity	Inferior efficacy, so uncommonly used	K103N, V106A/M, Y181C/I, Y188C/L/H, P236L
Efavirenz (EFV)	600 mg qhs	CNS effects, rash Liver toxicity	Teratogenic in nonhuman primates Contraindicated in first trimester False-positive cannabinoid test	L100I, K103N, V106A/M, V108I, Y181C/I, Y188C/L/H, G190A, P225H
FUSION INHIBITOR (FI)				
Enfuvirtide (T20)	90 mg SQ bid	Injection site reaction Hypersensitivitiy reaction	Increased risk of bacterial pneumonia	Associated with mutations in the first heptad repeat region (HR1)

CNS, central nervous system; GI, gastrointestinal; HTN, hypertensive nephropathy.
*Genetic mutations that confer resistance are identified with the following notation: a letter (which stands for the wild-type amino acid) followed by a number (which represents the location on the gene where that amino acid is encoded) followed by the amino acid mutation. The 69 insertion complex affects all NRTIs; Q151M affects all NRTIs except tenofovir. Resistance Concerns were adapted from the most recently published International AIDS Society guidelines on resistance: Johnson VA, Brun-Vezinet F, Clotet B, et al. Update of the drug resistance mutations in HIV-1: Fall 2006. Top HIV Med 2006;14:125-130.

also inhibit viral DNA synthesis. They do not require activation within the cell. Monotherapy studies were disappointing because of rapid high-level resistance resulting from a single point mutation, which made the entire class ineffective. During co-administration with two NRTIs, they are very potent at viral suppression and immune recovery. This, combined with good tolerability and simple dosing patterns (of nevirapine and efavirenz) has allowed the NNRTIs to become important components to HAART therapy.

NNRTIs are metabolized by the cytochrome P-450 system of the liver, and there are critical drug-drug interactions that must be evaluated, particularly when efavirenz is given with PIs and other agents. Although both drugs can cause hepatotoxicity, each has its own adverse events for which monitoring is required (see Table 213-5).

A hypersensitivity reaction, comprising rash and/or hepatitis, can occur early after the initiation of nevirapine. This can be life-threatening. It occurs more commonly in women and in patients initiated to therapy with higher CD4 counts (>250 cells/mm³ in women or >400 cells/mm³ in men).

Efavirenz has become the drug against which novel agents are often compared. It is a potent agent in ART in both naïve and experienced patients. Neuropsychiatric side effects such as dizziness and numbness are the most common complaints after initiation of therapy. Patients should be counseled to take the drug at bedtime, and many report vivid dreams or sleep disturbances as a consequence. These are usually transitory and resolve within 4 weeks.

Protease Inhibitors

The HIV protease is critical for the development of mature and infectious viral particles. After HIV DNA integrates into the host DNA, the host's machinery makes large pre-

cursor proteins, which are cleaved by the viral protease to yield the critical structural proteins necessary for a viable viral particle. PIs bind to the active site of the viral protease enzyme and inhibit processing of viral proteins. The viral particles subsequently released are noninfectious.

The development of PIs revolutionized HIV therapy.[10] With the addition of a PI to two NRTIs, the HIV virus could be maximally and durably suppressed. These drugs are metabolized by the cytochrome P-450 system and have numerous drug interactions, especially given the chronic nature of HIV therapy. Certain PIs are inferior to others because of either poor efficacy or toxicity, most notably full-dose ritonavir and hard-capsule saquinavir. Ritonavir, a potent inhibitor of the cytochrome P-450 system, is now used primarily to boost the levels of other PIs. When co-administered with low-dose ritonavir, other PIs have improved bioavailability, with drug levels that can inhibit even relatively resistant viruses. Regimens are less complex and have a lower pill burden, so are more tolerable. Finally, these higher, more predictable drug levels yield better results, with resistance less likely even in the event of treatment failure.

The common toxicities are gastrointestinal tolerability issues and dyslipidemia and lipodystrophy (see Table 213-5). Additionally, patients commonly report sexual dysfunction. They often have difficult drug interactions, and review of other agents cleared by the liver via the cytochrome P-450 system is crucial.

Fusion Inhibitors

Targeting of viral entry offers significant advantages over some other mechanisms of HIV inhibition. When entry is blocked, not only is the viral life cycle interrupted, but infection is prevented. Enfuvirtide, the only approved agent in this class, works by binding the viral surface protein gp41. This prevents the conformational change in the viral protein that is required for membrane fusion. Thus, viral entry is blocked.[11]

Enfuvirtide is a large peptide of 36 amino acids. It is administered subcutaneously to prevent enzymatic breakdown in the gastrointestinal tract. It is administered twice daily. The major side effect is injection site reaction. These can often be painful and can lead to injection fatigue for patients. In advanced disease, it is often difficult to identify enough sites to inject, given the significant peripheral fat wasting in AIDS. One other adverse event in clinical trials was bacterial pneumonias. This agent is very useful in advanced disease with highly resistant virus and few treatment options.

INITIAL THERAPY

With the available options, patients who are naïve to therapy usually have little difficulty suppressing the HIV virus to undetectable levels and experiencing substantial immunologic recovery. The current paradigm is to use two NRTIs combined with either an NNRTI or a boosted PI as initial therapy. The choice of NRTIs is often made easy by the fixed-dose combination pills that can be given once or twice daily. Efavirenz remains the NNRTI of choice, but there are several PIs that can be boosted by low-dose ritonavir and provide choice on the initial regimen. This initial choice should be individualized based on baseline resistance testing, comorbidities, and reproductive plans (see Table 213-2).

INITIATION OF THERAPY IN ADVANCED DISEASE

For patients who are naïve to therapy but present with advanced disease, often with an ongoing opportunistic infection, there is frequently a question as to when to initiate ART. The advantages to starting therapy center on the more rapid recovery of the immune system, which is important in long-term outcome and may improve responses for the acute opportunistic infection. Against this are the problems with increased toxicity of drugs, the possibility of drug-drug interactions, and patients' potential lack of awareness of their HIV status. Early return of immune function in an undiagnosed opportunistic infection may lead to immune-related symptoms, the so-called immune restoration inflammatory syndrome (IRIS). Currently, the approach for patients with an opportunistic infection is to treat the acute infection and then initiate ART after it is controlled. There are studies to address this issue, but treatment can be deferred until the acute illness has subsided. ART should be initiated urgently in conditions attributable to advanced HIV disease, such as HIV encephalopathy or HIV-associated nephropathy, and also in opportunistic infections, such as progressive multifocal leukoencephalopathy (PML) and cryptosporidiosis, for which no specific therapy is effective other than treating the underlying HIV infection.

Initially, it was believed that therapy in advanced disease should include a PI-based regimen combined with two NRTIs. More recent data indicate that an NNRTI regimen is as effective as a boosted-PI regimen in patients with low CD4 counts and high viral loads. Therefore, the crucial issue becomes the baseline resistance testing to identify which agents are active against a person's virus (see Table 213-2).

IRIS may complicate the management of recently initiated ART,[12] particularly in those with CD4 counts lower than 50 cells/mm[3]. In these instances, AIDS patients have a subclinical opportunistic infection that become apparent only with immune reconstitution, during the first few weeks after initiation of ART. These events have been described for mycobacterial infections (both *Mycobacterium avium* complex [MAC], and *Mycobacterium tuberculosis* [MTB]), *Pneumocystis jiroveci* pneumonia (PCP), toxoplasmosis, cryptococcal infection, histoplasmosis, and PML. An IRIS is characterized by high fever and worsening clinical manifestations of the opportunistic infection. In some cases, these syndromes are thought to reflect an immune reaction to a subclinical infection. Successful management includes continuing ART and confirming the opportunistic infection diagnosis. Initiating specific therapy for the acute infection is critical and often includes the addition of anti-inflammatory agents including corticosteroids.

RESISTANCE TO ANTIRETROVIRAL AGENTS

Resistance Testing

Resistance to ART is one of the most important challenges in the treatment of HIV infection. Among patients whose current HAART regimen is failing, up to 75% have resistance to at least one antiretroviral agent. Transmission of resistant HIV virus is documented and limits the effectiveness of therapy.[3,13] Studies evaluating resistance in HIV-infected persons presenting to care in North America and in Europe, where treatment has been most prevalent, reveal that between 9% and 20% of treatment-naïve patients have resistance to at least one medication, and 3% to 4% have multidrug resistance (resistance to two or more classes).

Two types of resistance testing are currently available: genotypic tests and phenotypic tests. Genotypic assays can be performed by sequencing the entire viral reverse transcriptase and protease genes to evaluate for mutations or by using selective probes to identify specific mutations that are well characterized as inducing resistance. Phenotypic testing is a direct measure of viral sensitivity to drugs. The virus is grown in cell culture and exposed to increasing concentrations of the antiretroviral agents. The results are compared with results from wild-type virus and the level of susceptibility of the virus to the various medications is determined. Although the interpretation of resistance tests is often complex, resistance testing is recommended before initiation of therapy in all patients to guide the selection of the antiretroviral regimen.

Principles of Management for Resistant Virus

For patients who present with advanced disease or significant past antiretroviral medicine experience or both, it is more difficult to choose an effective regimen. Nevertheless, antiretroviral drugs remain life-sustaining therapy for these patients. Many people with very advanced disease who received serial monotherapy and dual therapy in the 1990s and subsequently were treated with unboosted PIs and NNRTIs have triple-class resistance and limited options. For patients with extensive antiretroviral experience, it is critical to identify all antiretroviral agents to which the patient has been exposed and all results of previous resistance testing. In addition, repeat resistance testing may identify which agents will lack activity. Without drug pressure, the virus may revert to a "wild-type" phenotype without expression of the mutations that are archived in latent strains of the virus within that patient. That is why the history of antiretroviral use is so critical. If at least two active drugs can be identified, it may be possible to suppress the virus to undetectable levels and have immune recovery. If the patient has only one active agent available, then it may be preferable to choose a "holding regimen" to prevent further progression and minimize additional development of resistance while waiting for new agents to be developed. This last point is crucial, because novel agents and novel classes of agents are under current development.

In developing a nonsuppressive "holding regimen," the following approach should be followed. An NNRTI should not be used, because the virus rapidly develops resistance to these agents if resistance is not already present; additional NNRTI mutations will limit the utility of second generation NNRTIs currently in development, and the development of NNRTI mutations has no beneficial impact on viral fitness. Lamivudine or emtricitabine should be included in a holding regimen. These agents are well tolerated, have minimal toxicity, and lead to only the signature M184V mutation, which appears to confer a beneficial negative impact on viral fitness and also may increase the susceptibility of the virus to certain other agents (specifically, tenofovir, stavudine, zidovudine).

If possible, three active antiretrovirals should be included in the new regimen. The use of only a single new medication is unlikely to be successful and will promote resistance to the new medication. For persons without access to at least two active agents, a regimen with one of the boosted PIs and recycled NRTIs offers the best strategy for a holding regimen. This regimen should be continued until at least two new active drugs are available to develop a new suppressive regime. Patients with a viral load of less than 20,000/mm^3 have minimal progression on a nonsuppressive regimen. The use of these medicines and their role in preventing progression must be weighed against their side effects and possible toxicity. In certain circumstances, symptomatic care measures are preferable to an intolerable regimen.

Studies have evaluated the utility of structured treatment interruption for patients with very resistant virus and limited treatment options. This has proved to be a poor choice, because those patients who discontinue therapy have more rapid progression and increased morbidity and mortality. Although continued drug treatment is nonsuppressive, it may maintain a decreased viral fitness and slow progression. With removal of therapy, the virus replicates more efficiently and may cause more rapid immune decline.

TOXICITIES OF ANTIRETROVIRAL THERAPY

Toxicities are common side effects of ART. Of more than 1000 patients in a Swiss cohort, 47% reported a clinical adverse event, and 27% had a laboratory abnormality attributable to their ART.[14] There are certain expected toxicities, such as gastrointestinal intolerance with the PIs or anemia with zidovudine. Long-term toxicities have also emerged, particularly with the durable success of viral suppression. These include fat redistribution, lipid abnormalities, abnormal glucose metabolism, and an increased risk of cardiovascular disease (see Table 213-5).

Abacavir Hypersensitivity Reaction

Hypersensitivity reactions occur in about 5% of patients receiving abacavir. It usually occurs within the first 2 to 4 weeks of therapy, although reactions may occur at any time. The reaction is more common in Caucasians than those of African descent and is associated with a specific human leukocyte antigen (HLA) haplotype (HLA-B*5701). It is a multiorgan system reaction, the most common symptoms being fever, rash, gastrointestinal symptoms (nausea, vomiting, diarrhea, abdominal pain), respiratory symptoms (dyspnea, sore throat, cough), and lethargy or malaise. The multisystem nature of the reaction has led to its being misdiagnosed as an intercurrent medical illness or related to another medication. If, on evaluation, the patient does have a presentation consistent with hypersensitivity, abacavir must be permanently discontinued. Symptomatic support, such as intravenous fluids for hypotension, is advised. Once an individual has been identified as having abacavir hypersensitivity reaction, he or she should not be rechallenged with abacavir, because subsequent dosing leads to a more severe reaction and can be fatal.

Nevirapine Hepatotoxicity and Rash

The adverse events most frequently related to nevirapine are rash, fever, headache, hepatitis, and liver enzyme abnormalities. As many as 35% of patients receiving nevirapine develop a rash. Although most cases are mild and self-limited, resolving spontaneously, about 7% of persons receiving nevirapine develop a grade 3 or 4 rash necessitating drug discontinuation. A small percentage of these patients have Stevens-Johnson syndrome (SJS) and/or toxic epidermal necrolysis (TEN), life-threatening dermatoses that require hospitalization and supportive care.

Hepatotoxicity has also been identified as a common adverse event of nevirapine. Six percent of women and 2% of men develop symptomatic hepatotoxicity. Half of those with grade 3 or 4 hepatotoxicity also develop a rash. Multivariate analysis of risk factors noted an association of these toxicities with female gender and higher CD4 counts. Based on these findings, nevirapine should be given as initial therapy to women only if the CD4 count is lower than 250 cells/mm^3 (<400 cells/mm^3 in men).

Lactic Acidosis with Nucleoside Reverse Transcriptase Inhibitors

The NRTI class of antiretrovirals inhibits not only the HIV reverse transcriptase but also human mitochondrial DNA polymerase γ. In vitro, this inhibition is most pronounced with zalcitabine and didanosine, but it also occurs with stavudine and zidovudine. One probable manifestation is hyperlactatemia and severe lactic acidosis, often accompanied by hepatic steatosis. The diagnosis of lactic acidosis can be difficult, because the manifestations are nonspecific (fatigue, nausea, emesis, abdominal pain, and diarrhea). Laboratory abnormalities include an anion gap acidosis and elevated lactate levels. The lactate level should be confirmed, and arterial blood gas analysis should be performed. Discontinuation of the offending agent and symptomatic support are recommended for symptomatic patients with a lactate concentration greater than 5 mmol/L. Severe lactic acidosis in this setting has high mortality.

Peripheral Neuropathy

Peripheral neuropathy is another toxicity of certain NRTIs, specifically stavudine and didanosine. It is often difficult to absolutely attribute the neuropathy to the medications, because HIV itself causes neuropathy. The neuropathy has a stocking-glove distribution, similar to diabetic neuropathy. The neuropathy attributable to stavudine and didanosine is thought to be partially attributable to mitochondrial toxicity. It is also believed to be dose-related and partially reversible when the drug is discontinued. Neuropathy is more common in persons with advanced AIDS and low CD4 counts and in those receiving other neurotoxic agents.

LONG-TERM COMPLICATIONS OF THERAPY

A change in fat distribution is a common complaint in patients being treated for HIV infection. Both lipoatrophy (loss of fat in the face, extremities, and buttocks) and fat accumulation (increased intra-abdominal fat, enlarged dorsocervical fat pad, central adiposity, and breast enlargement in women) occur. Some patients experience both effects, although lipoatrophy is more common than fat accumulation. The thymidine analogue NRTIs (stavudine more so than zidovudine) are causally associated with fat loss, possibly related to mitochondrial toxicity in adipocytes. There are no approved interventions for lipodystrophy, but close monitoring of body changes and patient self-reporting, with alteration of HAART if changes are pronounced, is a reasonable approach. Lipoatrophy may have medical implications (insulin resistance, a proatherogenic profile) and is associated with lower quality of life in HIV-infected patients. Patients with lipoatrophy often feel stigmatized by recognizable changes easily associated with HIV. It is critical to identify such syndromes and alter therapy if possible. Prevention, through the use of alternative agents, is also appropriate.

Lipid abnormalities in HIV-infected persons are well described. Before HAART, decreased HDL and increased triglyceride levels were common in patients with advanced untreated HIV infection. HAART is associated with increased total cholesterol and triglycerides. Many of the PIs are associated with these increases, particularly ritonavir, although some of the newer PIs, such as atazanavir, are lipid neutral. The NNRTIs are associated with increases in total cholesterol and also in HDL cholesterol, with variable effects on other lipid parameters. Finally, except for the thymidine analogues (especially stavudine), which are associated with lipid abnormalities and particularly with elevated triglycerides, the NRTIs are relatively lipid neutral. Current guidelines recommend monitoring fasting lipid levels before and 4 to 6 weeks after initiation of HAART and following the National Cholesterol Education Program guidelines for lipid management.[15]

Insulin resistance is another long-term issue in ART, related in part to the direct effects of some PIs on glucose metabolism and in part to the changes in body fat, both visceral adiposity and peripheral lipoatrophy. This is of concern because of the potential development of diabetes and because of the increased cardiovascular risk and addition of medications that may interact with HIV medications. With the burgeoning diabetes epidemic, it is crucial that patients undergo routine fasting glucose evaluation and counseling on exercise and diet modification to ameliorate this complication of HIV and HAART.

FUTURE OF ANTIRETROVIRAL THERAPY

Since 2006, the FDA has approved six new agents that demonstrate the future of antiretroviral therapy. Two new PIs, tipranavir and darunavir, were developed on the basis of activity against resistant strains of virus and then found to be effective clinically in trials of patients with multi-class-resistant virus. A new NNRTI, etravirine, has activity against viruses resistant to previously available NNRTIs. Two new classes of antiretroviral agents have entered the clinical arena: a CCR5 inhibitor, maraviroc, which prevents the interaction between HIV and its cellular coreceptor and thus prevents viral entry into cells, is effective in patients with resistant virus, as is raltegravir, an integrase inhibitor, which prevents the integration of viral DNA into the host cell genome. The recently approved agent in 2006 was Atripla, a fixed-dose combination pill of efavirenz, tenofovir, and emtricitabine. This pill is novel not only because it combines drugs of different classes into one pill but also because it is a single pill taken once daily for effective and durable suppression of HIV infection. The epidemic in the developed world has clearly been changed into a manageable chronic illness.

For the foreseeable future, HAART will continue to evolve. Ongoing studies evaluate simplified regimens using the currently available boosted PIs as monotherapy. Pharmacogenomic developments are likely to provide greater insight into drug toxicities, such as the association between HLA B*5701 and abacavir hypersensitivity.[16] New targets are being explored in the search for new antiviral agents. These approaches may alter treatment strategies; however, the general principles of treatment are unlikely to change in the near future.

REFERENCES

1. Gottlieb MS, Schroff R, Schanker HM, et al. *Pneumocystis carinii* pneumonia and mucosal candidiasis in previously healthy homosexual men: Evidence of a new acquired cellular immunodeficiency. N Engl J Med 1981;305:1425.
2. Centers for Disease Control and Prevention. Twenty-five years of HIV/AIDS—United States, 1981-2006. MMWR Morb Mortal Wkly Rep 2006;55:585-589.
3. Clavel F, Hance AJ. HIV drug resistance. N Engl J Med 2004;350:1023-1035.
4. Aberg JA, Gallant JE, Anderson J, et al; HIV Medicine Association of the Infectious Diseases Society of America. Primary care guidelines for the management of persons infected with human immunodeficiency virus: Recommendations of the HIV Medicine Association of the Infectious Diseases Society of America. Clin Infect Dis 2004;39:609-629.
5. Guidelines for the Use of Antiretroviral Agents in HIV-1-Infected Adults and Adolescents, October 2006. Available at http://aidsinfo.nih.gov (accessed February 22, 2008).
6. Hammer SM, Saag MS, Schechter M, et al; International AIDS Society—USA panel. Treatment for adult HIV infection: 2006 Recommendations of the International AIDS Society—USA panel. JAMA 2006;296:827-843.

7. Gazzard B; BHIVA Writing Committee. British HIV Association (BHIVA) guidelines for the treatment of HIV-infected adults with antiretroviral therapy (2005). HIV Med 2005;6(Suppl 2):1-61.
8. Back DJ, Burger DM, Flexner CW, Gerber JG. The pharmacology of antiretroviral nucleoside and nucleotide reverse transcriptase inhibitors: Implications for once-daily dosing. J Acquir Immune Defic Syndr 2005;39(Suppl 1):S1-S23.
9. Balzarini J. Current status of the non-nucleoside reverse transcriptase inhibitors of human immunodeficiency virus type 1. Curr Top Med Chem 2004;4:921-944.
10. Flexner C. HIV-protease inhibitors. N Engl J Med 1998;338:1281-1292.
11. Manfredi R, Sabbatani S. A novel antiretroviral class (fusion inhibitors) in the management of HIV infection: Present features and future perspectives of enfuvirtide (T-20). Curr Med Chem 2006;13:2369-2384.
12. Shelburne SA, Visnegarwala F, Darcourt J, et al. Incidence and risk factors for immune reconstitution inflammatory syndrome during highly active antiretroviral therapy. AIDS 2005;19:399-406.
13. Hirsch MS, Brun-Vezinet F, Clotet B, et al. Antiretroviral drug resistance testing in adults infected with human immunodeficiency virus type 1: 2003 Recommendations of an International AIDS Society—USA Panel. Clin Infect Dis 2003;37:113-128.
14. Fellay J, Boubaker K, Ledergerber B, et al; Swiss HIV Cohort Study. Prevalence of adverse events associated with potent antiretroviral treatment: Swiss HIV Cohort Study. Lancet 2001;358:1322-1327.
15. Lundgren JD, Battegay M, Behrens G, et al. European AIDS Clinical Society (EACS) guidelines on the prevention and management of metabolic diseases in HIV. HIV Med 2008;9:72-81.
16. Mallal S, Phillips E, Carosi G, et al. HLA-B*5701 screening for hypersensitivity to abacavir. N Engl J Med 2008;358:568-579.

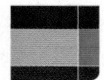

CHAPTER **214**

Symptom Management

Symptom Management in Acquired Immunodeficiency Syndrome

Jean-Michel Livrozet, Peter Selwyn, and *Marilene Filbet*

KEY POINTS

- Access to health care systems and antiretroviral drugs is a major issue affecting the prevalence of acquired immunodeficiency syndrome (AIDS) symptoms in developing countries but also in developed countries.
- Pain remains a major symptom for AIDS patients.
- Diarrhea is very common; it can be caused by many infective agents as well as antiretroviral agents.
- Weight loss is frequently a consequence of diarrhea and also of AIDS itself.
- In patients without antiretroviral agents who have a very low CD4+ T-lymphocyte count, dementia is one of the more frequent complications.

The balance between palliative and curative therapy depends on the etiology of the patient's symptoms.[1] In many cases now, curative therapies can be used for the treatment of opportunistic infections, and highly active antiretroviral therapy (HAART) is very potent for treating symptoms in patients newly diagnosed with human immunodeficiency virus (HIV) infection and restoring their immunity and level of functioning. However, even in the era of HAART, not all patients are able to benefit from these anti-HIV agents, so access to palliative care continues to be important for patients with HIV/AIDS in both the developed and the developing world.

In developed countries, patients with much treatment experience may increasingly develop mutations conferring resistance to HAART and may continue to suffer from AIDS-related events (opportunistic infections, malignancies) or other life-threatening comorbidities. In settings where HAART is available and used effectively, patients with HIV/AIDS are also surviving longer and are increasingly at risk for morbidity and mortality from end-stage liver disease, other end-organ failure, and non–AIDS-defining malignancies associated with long-term immunosuppression, such as anal, liver, and lung cancers and Hodgkin's disease. Moreover, access to the health care system and HAART may not be equal for all patients: some Central and Eastern European countries do not offer all licensed antiretroviral drugs to patients with HIV/AIDS, and in the United States the absence of universal health coverage can limit access to care for some segments of the population. Lastly, important comorbidities such as drug use, psychiatric illness, and other social and behavioral factors may pose obstacles to patients' ability to use and adhere effectively to HAART regimens.

In developing countries, many patients are still not able to access treatment, especially in South America, Asia, and Africa. Many public and private initiatives are working to provide HAART to African HIV/AIDS patients, but the drug choices are often limited and the number of treated patients is very small in comparison with the indications for treatment guided by CD4+ T-lymphocyte counts in developed countries. Very often, treatment is initiated too late and not with the best drugs available on the international market. For example, the use of protease inhibitors is very limited, and the choice is also very restricted due to costs.

In all of these situations, palliative care is important for management of HIV/AIDS, not only for dying patients, but also during the longer trajectory of chronic, progressive disease.

PAIN MANAGEMENT

Although there are many etiologies for pain in HIV/AIDS patients,[2-7] neuropathic pain occurs in at least 40% of those patients with advanced disease, including the common entity distal symmetric polyneuropathy (DSP), which can be caused by HIV infection itself. The patient experiences numbness, tingling, and a "pins and needles" sensation, especially in the distal lower extremities. In addition, some of the first-generation antiretroviral agents, such as stavudine and didanosine (zalcitabine, another implicated agent, is no longer licensed), have been associated with a clinically similar neuropathy. In the event of neuropathic symptoms, these neurotoxic agents should be changed, and their use is increasingly limited as first-line therapy.

Nociceptive pain responds both to nonopioid and opioid analgesics. The World Health Organization (WHO) analgesic ladder can be used to treat nociceptive pain, similarly to treatment in non–HIV-infected patients. Neuropathic pain often requires treatment with adjuvant medications such as antidepressants or anticonvulsants.

Because HIV-related gastrointestinal infections are common, abdominal pain from colic is frequent among HIV/AIDS patients, and antispasmodic drugs may be very useful.

Muscle spasms can be treated with benzodiazepines (diazepam or tetrazepam) or baclofen.

Corticosteroids can also be helpful in terminal care, although they may also cause or aggravate candidiasis. They improve appetite, increase energy, and can help make patients feel more comfortable.

Nonmedical interventions such as relaxation techniques and psychological, spiritual, and emotional support can also help relieve fear and anxiety in chronically ill patients[2-7] (Table 214-1).

Morphine and other opioids commonly cause side effects which can generally be prevented or treated easily through dose adjustment or other simple, symptom-specific interventions as outlined later in this chapter. Many of these symptoms lessen on their own over time. Constipation is the most frequent side effect and must be pre-

---

TABLE 214-1 Pain Management

TREATMENT	USUAL STARTING DOSE IN ADULTS	CONSIDERATIONS
MEDICAL TREATMENT*		
STEP 1: Mild Pain		
Nonopioid	Paracetamol 500-1000 mg q4-6h	Do not exceed 4 g/day. Use with careful monitoring in patients with liver disease; toxicity is dose related.
	Ibuprofen 400 mg q6h	Maximum 2.4 g/day. Contraindicated in patients with GI bleeding or bleeding disorders. Use with caution in patients with liver disease.
	Aspirin (acetylsalicylic acid) 325-500 mg q4h or 1000 mg q6h	Do not give to children <12 years old. Contraindicated in patients with GI bleeding or bleeding disorders. Use with caution in patients with liver disease.
STEP 2: Moderate Pain		
Nonopioid	Paracetamol 500-1000 mg q4-6h	Do not exceed 4 g/day. Use with careful monitoring in patients with liver disease; toxicity is dose related.
	Ibuprofen 400 mg q6h	Maximum 2.4 g/day. Contraindicated in patients with GI bleeding or bleeding disorders. Use with caution in patients with liver disease.
	Aspirin (acetylsalicylic acid) 325-500 mg q4h OR 1000 mg q6h	Do not give to children <12 years old. Contraindicated in patients with GI bleeding or bleeding disorders. Use with caution in patients with liver disease.
Opioid[†]	Codeine 25-50 mg q4h If codeine is not available, consider alternating aspirin and paracetamol. Codeine is available in fixed-dose combinations with 325-500 mg of paracetamol or aspirin and 25-60 mg of codeine Tramadol 50-100 mg q4-6h Dextropropoxyphene 27-30 mg q6h	Maximum daily dose for pain is 180-240 mg due to constipation; otherwise, switch to morphine. Prevent constipation with a stool softener and bowel stimulant; use laxatives if needed. IDUs: Use an NSAID or ibuprofen before offering codeine. Be aware of possible abuse of codeine and morphine-related drugs.
STEP 3: Severe Pain		
Nonopioid	Paracetamol 500-1000 mg q4-6h (also available in rectal suppositories)	Do not exceed 4 g/day. Use with careful monitoring in patients with liver disease; toxicity is dose related.
	Aspirin (acetylsalicylic acid) 325-500 mg q4h or 1000 mg q6h	Do not give to children <12 years old. Contraindicated in patients with GI bleeding or bleeding disorders. Use with caution in patients with liver disease.
Opioid[†]	Oral morphine[‡] 10-20 mg q3-4h in tablet or liquid form OR IV or IM morphine 5-10 mg q3-4h Dose can be increased by 50% after 24 h if severe pain persists. There is no ceiling dose.	Use 5 mg/5 mL or 50 mg/5 mL concentration, dosing according to need and rate of respiration (consider withholding if rate is <6 breaths/min). If oral morphine is not available, injectable morphine may be used rectally. Prevent constipation with a stool softener and bowel stimulant; use laxatives if needed. Severe chronic pain occurs mostly with malignancies, chronic pancreatitis, joint problems, severe neuropathy. IDUs: Same as for non-IDUs, but the needed dose is usually higher. In case of opioid substitution therapy, the substitution dose is maintained and opioid analgesics are added. Be aware of possible abuse of codeine and morphine-related drugs. Not for use in opioid-naïve patients.
	Oxycodone[‡] 5-10 mg q4h Dose can be increased by 50% after 24 h if severe pain persists.	
	Hydromorphone 2-4 mg q4h	Not for use in opioid-naive patients.
	Fentanyl transdermal patch 25-75 μg, replaced every 72 h	Not for use in opioid-naive patients.

TABLE 214-1   Pain Management—cont'd

TREATMENT	USUAL STARTING DOSE IN ADULTS	CONSIDERATIONS
SPECIAL PAIN PROBLEMS		
Neuropathic pain: burning pains, abnormal sensation pains, shooting pains, "pins and needles" sensation (common causes include HIV-related peripheral neuropathies and herpes zoster)	Use opioids ± nonopioid analgesics as above, along with one of the following adjuvants: Amitriptyline 25 mg qhs, taken at night because of side effects (e.g., fatigue), or 12.5 mg bid Gabapentin 300-800 mg tid (maximum 2.4 g/day if HAART with PI is given) Carbamazepine 200-400 mg q6h Clonazepam 0.5-1 mg bid-tid	Wait 2 wk for response, then increase gradually to 50 mg qhs or 25 mg bid; there is no sudden relief—wait at least 5 days for a response. Monitor white blood cell count, drug interactions.
Muscle spasms	Diazepam 5-10 bid-tid OR Tetrazepam 50 mg/day, up to 200 mg/day in 2 doses OR Baclofen 5 mg tid to start; increase every 3 days up to 25 mg tid	IDUs: Before administering, consider carefully the possibility of polysubstance misuse. Should be used only in the short term (maximum 6-8 wk).
In terminal care with no referral and any of the following: • Swelling around tumor • Severe esophageal candidiasis with ulceration and swallowing problems • Nerve compression • Persistent severe headache due to increased intracranial pressure	Prednisolone 15-40 mg/day for 7 days OR Dexamethasone 2-6 mg/day provided by trained health worker	Helpful in terminal care; improves appetite and makes patient feel comfortable. Reduce to lowest possible dose; withdraw if no benefit in 3 wk. Dexamethasone is about 7 times stronger than prednisolone; if prednisolone needs to be used, multiply the dexamethasone dose by 7. May cause candidiasis.
GI pain from colic	Phloroglucinol 80 mg (6 per day) OR Butylscopolamine 3-5 × 10-20 mg OR Codeine 30 mg q4h OR Trimebutine 100-200 mg tid before meals	Butylscopolamine given IV or PO has the same dosage but a different half-life (IV is more rapid). Start with IV followed by PO; if stable, use PO with IV for peaks. Codeine can cause constipation and worsening of symptoms in IDUs. Be aware of possible abuse of codeine or morphine-related drugs.
NONMEDICAL TREATMENT		
Psychological, spiritual, and/or emotional support and counseling to accompany pain medication		Pain may be more difficult to bear if accompanied by guilt, fear of dying, loneliness, anxiety, or depression. Relieve fear and anxiety by explaining events.
Relaxation techniques: physical methods (e.g., massage, breathing techniques) and cognitive methods (e.g., music)		Unless the patient is psychotic or severely depressed.

GI, gastrointestinal; HAART, highly active antiretroviral therapy; IDUs, injecting drug users; NSAID, nonsteroidal anti-inflammatory drug; PI, protease inhibitor.
*Administer only one drug from the nonopioid group and one from the opioid group at a time; aspirin every 4 hours may be given with paracetamol every 4 hours, adjusting the schedule so that one medication is given every 2 hours.
†If pain is controlled, reduce rapidly or stop morphine if it has been used for only a short time; reduce gradually if used for >2 wk.
‡Morphine and oxycodone are frequently available in long-acting (sustained-release) forms; these guidelines refer to acute pain management, which should be initiated with short-acting preparations and then, if necessary, converted to long-acting formulations if the need for chronic analgesia persists.

vented by use of a stool softener or a laxative. Occasionally, if symptoms are persistent and treatment-limiting with a particular opioid, it may be necessary to change to another opioid medication (Table 214-2).

SYMPTOM MANAGEMENT

Patients with HIV/AIDS may experience a wide range of symptoms, involving virtually every major organ system, as a result of specific infectious complications, malignancies, other comorbidities, medication toxicities, consequences of substance abuse, or HIV infection itself. Many studies from different countries[8-16] have documented a high prevalence of symptoms in patients with AIDS (Table 214-3). Whenever possible, the particular condition causing the symptom should be treated (e.g., cryptococcal meningitis causing headaches), but often it is just as important to treat the symptom itself.

Fatigue and Weakness

The fatigue and weakness observed in AIDS may often be caused by opportunistic infections, anemia due to HIV infection, or HAART toxicity, but also by lack of rest, drug or alcohol use, hormonal abnormalities (thyroid, adrenal, and sex hormones), psychological stress, and/or diet.

TABLE 214-2 Management of Side Effects of Morphine and Other Opioids

SIDE EFFECT	MANAGEMENT
Constipation	Increase fluids and fiber (fruits and vegetables or bran supplements). Give a stool softener (docusate 200-800 mg/day) at the time of prescribing, plus a stimulant (senna 7.5-8.6 mg tablets, 2 to 4 tablets bid); if no improvement, add a laxative such as macrogol (13.125 mg/dose, 1-2 doses/day) or lactulose (10-20 mL tid); if still no improvement, add bisacodyl (5-15 mg) oral tablets or rectal suppositories, as needed. Prevent by using some or all of the above measures for prophylaxis (except in chronic diarrhea).
Nausea and/or vomiting	Usually resolves in several days with an antiemetic; may need round-the-clock dosing.
Respiratory depression (rare if oral morphine is titrated against pain)	Usually no need to intervene if respiratory rate is at least 6 breaths/min. If severe, consider withholding next opioid dose, and then halve the dose.
Confusion or drowsiness (if due to the opioid)	Usually occurs at start of treatment or with increase in dose. Usually resolves within a few days. Can occur at end of life with renal failure. Halve dose or increase interval between doses.
Itching or twitching—myoclonus (if severe or present during waking hours)	With high-dose medication, consider reducing or alternating doses or using two opioids. Re-evaluate pain and treatment; pain may not be morphine responsive.
Somnolence	Extended sleep can be from exhaustion due to pain. If condition persists >2 days after starting, reduce the dose by half.
Reduction of morphine after cause of pain is controlled (common in HIV/AIDS complications)	If morphine has been used only for a short time, stop or rapidly reduce dose. If used for >2 wk, reduce gradually, watch for symptoms of withdrawal.

TABLE 214-3 Prevalence of Symptoms in Patients with AIDS*

SYMPTOMS	PREVALENCE RANGE (%)
Fatigue or lack of energy	48-45
Weight loss	37-91
Pain	29-76
Anorexia	26-51
Anxiety	25-40
Insomnia	21-50
Cough	19-60
Nausea or vomiting	17-43
Dyspnea or respiratory symptoms	15-48
Depression or sadness	15-40
Diarrhea	11-32
Constipation	10-29

*Based on available descriptive studies, predominantly in patients with late-stage disease, 1990-2002.
Data from Simpson DM. Selected peripheral neuropathies associated with human immunodeficiency virus infection and antiretroviral therapy. J Neurovirol 2002;8(Suppl 2):33-41.

TABLE 214-4 Management of Weight Loss

CONDITION	TREATMENT AND DOSE IN ADULTS	CONSIDERATIONS FOR HOME CARE
General weight loss	Encourage the sick person to eat, but do not force, because vomiting may result. Offer more frequent, smaller meals of the patient's preferred foods.	Think of reasons for weight loss (e.g., tumors, candida esophagitis, TB, atypical mycobacterium, CMV colitis, cryptosporidiosis). Avoid cooking close to the sick person. Let the sick person choose the foods he or she wants to eat from what is available. Accept that intake will decrease as the patient becomes more ill. Seek help from a trained health worker in case of rapid weight loss, consistent refusal to eat, or inability to swallow.
Anorexia and severe fatigue	Prednisolone 5-15 mg qd for up to 6 wk	To stimulate appetite
Nausea and vomiting with antiemetics	Provide antiemetics	Offer more frequent, smaller meals of the patient's preferred foods; do not force the person to eat.
Thrush or mouth ulcer	See Table 214-5.	
Diarrhea	See Table 214-7.	

CMV, cytomegalovirus; TB, tuberculosis.

Weight Loss

Weight loss is common in AIDS-associated malignancies (e.g., lymphoma, cervical cancer), and it is also a manifestation of AIDS, especially in Africa (wasting syndrome). Management is described in Table 214-4.

Mouth Ulcers or Pain on Swallowing

Mouth ulcers or painful swallowing may be caused by cytomegalovirus (CMV) ulcers of the mouth or esophagus, herpes infection, or candida esophagitis (Tables 214-5 and 214-6).

Diarrhea

Diarrhea is a symptom frequently observed in patients with terminal HIV disease and very low CD4 counts; mycobacterial infection, CMV colitis, cryptosporidiosis, microsporidiosis, giardiasis, other infective agents, and Kaposi's sarcoma may all be observed at this stage. The etiological agents may be treated with azithromycin and ethambutol (*Mycobacterium avium* complex [MAC]); with ganciclovir or valganciclovir or foscarnet (CMV); or with albendazole or other antiparasitic agents (various parasitic infections). But sometimes it is not possible to cure the gastrointestinal infection without an immune restoration of CD4+ T lymphocytes. In developing countries, and in patients without access to HAART (or with multidrug-resistant HIV) in developed countries, diarrhea is often present in dying patients. An idiopathic HIV-related enteropathy may also be observed in 25% to

50% of untreated patients. It is very important to assess both possibly treatable or reversible causes and the patient's general condition and state of hydration (Table 214-7).

Dehydration

An assessment of the state of hydration is essential in the management of chronic diarrhea. The evaluation of dehydration in adults is described in Table 214-8).

Itching

Dehydration, end-stage renal disease, and end-stage liver disease are responsible for dry skin in the same way as malnutrition. Pruritus is also often observed in fungal infections of the skin (Table 214-9).

Dementia

Dementia is a syndrome caused by disease of the brain, usually chronic or progressive, in which there is disturbance of multiple higher cortical functions, including memory, thinking, orientation, comprehension, calculation, learning capacity, language, and judgment. Consciousness is not clouded. The impairments of cognitive function are commonly accompanied, and occasionally preceded, by deterioration in emotional control, social behavior (e.g., disinhibition), or motivation.

TABLE 214-5   Management of Mouth Ulcers or Pain on Swallowing

CONDITION	TREATMENT AND DOSE IN ADULTS	CONSIDERATIONS FOR HOME CARE
General		Use soft toothbrush to gently scrub teeth, tongue, palate, and gums. Rinse mouth with diluted salt water (a pinch of salt in a glass of water) after eating and at bedtime (usually 3-4 times daily).
Candida (oral thrush)	Miconazole buccal tablets or buccal gel, 1 tablet daily for 7 days. If severe infection or no response: fluconazole 200 mg on first day, then 100 mg/day for 10-14 days or until symptoms resolve	Topical anesthetics can provide some relief. Mix 2 aspirin in water and rinse the mouth up to four times a day. Pain relief may be required (see Table 214-2). Remove food leftovers with gauze or cloth soaked in salt water. Soft foods may decrease discomfort. Textured foods and fluids may be swallowed more easily. Avoid very hot, cold, or spicy foods.
Aphthous ulcers	Prednisolone applied as crushed grains. Dexamethasone solution as mouthwash. Kenalog cream applied to sores	
Herpes simplex	Acyclovir 400 mg PO 5x/day	
Foul-smelling mouth due to oral cancer or other lesions	Metronidazole mouthwash: crush 2 tablets in water and rinse mouth	

TABLE 214-6   Management of Dry Mouth

CONDITION	TREATMENT	CONSIDERATIONS FOR HOME CARE
Dry mouth	Review medications for possible cause (side effect).	Give frequent sips of drinks. Moisten mouth regularly with water. Let the person suck on fruits such as oranges (citrus fruits should be avoided in cases of sores).
Significant lack of saliva	Refer to dentist.	

TABLE 214-7   Management of Diarrhea

CONDITION	TREATMENT AND DOSE IN ADULTS	CONSIDERATIONS FOR HOME CARE
General	Increase fluid intake to prevent dehydration. Use ORS if large volume of diarrhea. Suggest a supportive diet. Give constipating drugs (unless there is blood in stool or fever, or patient is <5 yr old or elderly): • Loperamide 4 mg to start, then 2 mg after each loose stool (maximum 12 mg/day, but some patients need more) OR • Codeine (if approved), 10 mg tid (up to 60 mg q4h) OR • Oral morphine (if approved), 2.5-5 mg q4h (if diarrhea is severe)	Encourage plenty of fluids to replace lost water (give in small amounts, frequently). Increase frequency of small amounts of food intake (e.g., rice soup, porridge, ORS, bananas, other soups). Avoid dairy, caffeine, and spicy foods. Special care for rectal area: • After the person has passed stool, clean with toilet paper or soft tissue paper • Wash the anal area three times a day with soap and water • If the patient feels pain when passing the stool, apply petroleum jelly around the anal area.
Rectal tenderness	Local anesthetic ointment or petroleum jelly	Seek the help of a trained health worker for any of the following: vomiting with fever, blood in stools, diarrhea for >5 days, increasing weakness, broken skin around the rectal area, perianal ulcers.
Incontinence	Petroleum jelly to protect perianal skin	

ORS, oral rehydration solution.

TABLE 214-8 Assessment of Dehydration in Adults

CLINICAL FEATURES	DEHYDRATION		
	MILD	**MODERATE**	**SEVERE**
General condition	Weak	Weak	Restless, irritable, cold, sweaty, peripheral cyanosis
Pulse	Normal	Slight tachycardia	Rapid, feeble
Respiration	Normal	Normal	Deep and rapid
Skin elasticity	Normal	Pinch retracts slowly	Pinch retracts very slowly
Eyes	Normal	Sunken	Deeply sunken
Mucous membranes	Slightly dry	Dry	Very dry
Urine flow	Normal amount; urine dark	Reduced amount; dark amber in color	No urine; bladder is empty

TABLE 214-9 Management of Itching

CONDITION	TREATMENT AND DOSE IN ADULTS	CONSIDERATIONS FOR HOME CARE
Scabies, prurigo, eczema, ringworm, dry itchy skin, psoriasis, icterus	Consider whether condition is a side effect of a medication. General care: • Local steroid creams may be useful if inflammation is present in the absence of infection (bacterial, fungal, or viral). • Antihistamines • Chlorpheniramine (4 or 5 mg bid), cetirizine (10 mg qd), hydroxyzine 25-50 mg tid, OR Diphenhydramine (25-50 mg qhs, or up to tid) may be useful for severe itching. For skin infections, use 0.05% chlorhexidine rinse after bathing. For itching from obstructive jaundice, try prednisolone (20 mg once daily) or haloperidol (2 × 1 mg once daily). For eczema, gently wash with warm water and dry skin; do not use soap; topical steroids may be used for short term (not on face) For ringworm, use compound benzoic and salicylic acid ointment (Whitfield's ointment) or other antifungal cream; if extensive, use fluconazole (200 mg on first day, then 100 mg once daily). Consider treatment for scabies even if no typical lesions are present: ivermectin (200 mg in one dose). For psoriasis, use coal tar ointment 5% in 2% salicylic acid; expose to sunlight 30 to 60 min/day.	Try any of the following: • Apply petroleum jelly to the itchy area. • Put one spoon of vegetable oil in 5 L of water to wash the patient. • Dilute 1 teaspoon of chlorhexidine in 1 L of water and apply after bathing. • Use warm water for bathing. Seek help from a trained heath worker for painful blisters or extensive skin infection. Medications may cause drowsiness.

Individuals with HIV may present with cognitive impairment or a dementia picture for a number of reasons. Depression and anxiety can manifest as forgetfulness and concentration difficulties, and acute infection can manifest as confusion (delirium). In addition, cognitive impairment in some people with advanced HIV and very low CD4 counts is thought to be caused by the effects of HIV on the CNS or possibly by the immune response to the virus.

The mainstay of treatment for HIV-associated dementia is HAART. In fact, with the emergence of HAART, HIV dementia has become rare. In countries where HAART is not available, HIV-associated dementia is clearly much more common.

Confusion may be a side effect of HAART regimens (e.g., efavirenz), and psychosis is a rare but significant toxic effect. AIDS-related dementia is a result of HIV infection of the central nervous system. The most effective etiological treatment is HAART (Table 214-10).

Cough or Difficulty Breathing

Cough or difficulty breathing may be caused by common opportunistic infections seen in AIDS, such as *Pneumocystis jiroveci* pneumonia (PCP), bacterial pneumonia, or tuberculosis, or by immune reconstitution syndrome, which usually is seen within 2 to 3 months after starting ART. Anti-infective therapy or antituberculosis chemotherapy are the etiology-specific treatments (Tables 214-11 and 214-12).

END-STAGE LIVER DISEASE

Access to antiretroviral treatment (HAART) and effective prophylaxis against opportunistic infections have led to prolonged survival in HIV-infected individuals. As patients live longer, liver disease has emerged as the leading cause of death in patients with HIV.[17] The most common causes of liver disease are infection with hepatitis C virus (HCV) and/or hepatitis B virus (HBV), toxicity secondary to HAART, alcohol and/or substance abuse, and hepatocellular carcinoma.

The prevalence of coinfection with HCV is greatest in areas where injection drug use is the most frequent risk factor for HIV transmission (e.g., eastern and southern European countries, North America, some Asian areas). Mortality directly attributable to liver failure in coinfected patients may be increasing for several reasons: drugs commonly used as part of HAART regimens (e.g., nevirapine) can lead to severe toxic hepatitis, which is more common

TABLE 214-10 Management of Dementia

CONDITION	TREATMENT IN ADULTS	CONSIDERATIONS FOR HOME CARE
Chronic or progressive disturbance of higher cortical functions (memory, thinking, orientation, comprehension, calculation, learning capacity, language, judgment). Consciousness is not clouded. Possible deterioration in emotional control, social behavior, or motivation. Patients with HIV may present with cognitive impairment or a dementia picture for a number of reasons: • Depression and anxiety (forgetfulness, concentration difficulties) must be excluded • Acute infection (confusion or delirium) must be excluded • Effects of HIV on the CNS (or effects of the immune response to the virus) in advanced disease	Assess for alternative explanations (e.g., depression, delirium). Assess for reversible causes (e.g., normal-pressure hydrocephalus, operable tumor, hypothyroidism, neurosyphilis, vitamin B_{12} and folate deficiencies); treat accordingly. The mainstay of treatment for HIV-associated dementia is HAART. Confusion may be a side effect of HAART regimens (e.g., efavirenz), and psychosis is a rare but significant toxic effect. If there are behavioral changes (e.g., aggression, restlessness), medication may be considered, but possible causes such as pain or fear should first be ruled out. Nonpharmacological strategies such as patient attempts at communication are preferable.	As far as possible, keep the patient in a familiar environment. • Keep things in the same place—easy to reach and see. • Keep a familiar pattern to the day's activities. • Remove dangerous objects. • Speak in simple sentences, one person at a time. • Keep noise down. • Make sure somebody is present to look after the patient. Carer support, including respite, is important. Reducing restlessness may be important because of adverse effects on the family over time.
Patients may experience paranoia, severe agitation, or distress at night	Sedatives (e.g., benzodiazepines) and antipsychotics (e.g., low-dose risperidone) are appropriate if the patient is distressed, particularly with paranoid delusions or any other psychotic symptoms. If required, due attention should be given to the increased risk of falls. Low doses are recommended (e.g., zopiclone 3.75 mg, risperidone 0.5-1 mg, haloperidol 1-2 mg), titrated up slowly as needed; benzodiazepines (e.g., lorazepam 0.5 mg, diazepam 2-5 mg) may be used acutely but are generally less effective than low-dose neuroleptics.	

CNS, central nervous system; HIV, human immunodeficiency virus.

TABLE 214-11 Management of Cough or Difficulty Breathing

CONDITION	TREATMENT AND DOSE IN ADULTS	CONSIDERATIONS FOR HOME CARE
Dyspnea with bronchospasm	Give oxygen via mask if possible. Asthma protocols: • Give bronchodilators by MDI with spacer/mask or nebulizer. • Continue until patient is not able to use them or has very shallow or labored breathing. • Prednisolone 1 mg/kg/day (usually 60 mg in one dose in the morning); wait 1 wk to assess response, then slowly reduce by 10 mg over 1 wk	For simple cough: local soothing remedies, such as honey, lemon, or steam, either plain or with eucalyptus If patient has a new productive cough for >2 wk, it may be TB; arrange with health worker to send three sputum samples for TB testing. In addition to the treatment given by a health worker: • Help the patient into the best position to ease breathing—usually sitting up. • Leaning slightly forward and resting arms on a table may help. • Use extra pillows or some back support. • Open windows to allow in fresh air. • Fan with a newspaper or clean cloth. • Give patient water frequently to loosen sputum. Safe handling and disposal of sputum: • Handle with care to avoid spreading infection. • Use a tin for spitting, and cover it. • Empty the container in the toilet and wash the tin with a detergent or clean with boiled water. Education for use of remaining lung function: • Plan activities to accommodate breathlessness. • Avoid crowding, cooking, and smoking in the patient's room.
Heart failure or excess fluid	Furosemide 40-160 mg/day, in a single or divided dose, until symptoms improve (monitor for overdiuresis)	
Cough with thick sputum	Nebulized saline If >30 mL/day of sputum, try expiratory technique ("huffing") with postural drainage. Avoid tracheal suction, which is very distressing to the patient.	
Excessive thin sputum	• Hyoscine (make use of the anticholinergic side effect) 10 mg q8h	
Pleural effusion (e.g., Karposi's sarcoma, pneumonia)	Aspirate pleural fluid if possible.	
Dry cough	Codeine 5-10 mg qid If no response, oral morphine (2.5-5 mg) as long as needed (try to reduce after 1 wk)	
New productive cough >2 wk (possible TB)	Send 3 sputum samples for AFB testing. Anti-TB chemotherapy Continue treatment to prevent transmission.	
If patient is terminal additional measures to relieve dyspnea include:	Oral morphine/tramadol in low doses. If not already taking oral morphine for pain, morphine 2.5 mg q6h (if no relief, increase dose progressively by clinical measures); treat pain and anxiety. If taking oral morphine: increase dose progressively by 25%.	

AFB, acid-fast bacillus; MDI, metered-dose inhaler; TB, tuberculosis.

TABLE 214-12 Prevention of Contractures and Stiffness

CONDITION	TREATMENT AND DOSE IN ADULTS	CONSIDERATIONS FOR HOME CARE
Stiffness and contractures Muscle spasms	Diazepam 5-10 mg bid-tid Tetrazepam 50 mg/day, up to 200 mg/day in 2 doses. Baclofen: begin with 5 mg tid, then increase every 3 days up to 25 mg tid.	Do not confine—encourage mobility. Do simple ROM exercises if patient is immobile: • Exercise limbs and joints at least twice daily. • Protect joints by holding the limb above and below and support it as much as you can. • Bend, straighten, and move joints as far as they normally go. Be gentle and move slowly without causing pain. • Stretch joints by holding as before but with firm steady pressure. • Bring the arms above the head and lift the legs to 90 degrees; let the patient do it as far as possible and then help the rest of the way. Massage the patient.

ROM, range of motion.

Future Considerations

- Physicians will need to become more familiar with side effects and interactions of both antiretroviral and palliative care medications to care for patients with HIV/AIDS.
- Access and adherence to antiretroviral regimens could improve dramatically the prevalence of dementia.
- Hepatic cirrhosis is and will become more frequent in patients coinfected with hepatitis C virus.

in patients with HCV coinfection, and the efficacy of treatment of hepatitis C may be decreased with HIV coinfection. The goals of treatment include slowing or reversal of disease progression, prevention of superimposed liver injury, prevention and treatment of complications, and, if indicated, liver transplantation.

In patients with cirrhosis, all treatment is palliative. At this time, the goals of treatment are prevention of bleeding, through reduction of hepatic portal pressure, and symptomatic treatment of hepatic encephalopathy, through standard interventions. The only cure for end-stage liver disease is transplantation in developed countries, which is not an option for many patients. This possibility may raise false hopes and lead to disappointment and frustration if it is not attainable (see "Future Considerations").

REFERENCES

1. Selwyn PA, Forstein M. Comprehensive care for late-stage HIV/AIDS: Overcoming the false dichotomy of "curative" vs. "palliative" care. JAMA 2003;290:806-814.
2. Eramova I., Matic S, Munz M (eds). Palliative Care for People Living with HIV/AIDS: Clinical Protocol for the WHO European Region. Copenhagen: World Health Organisation Regional Office for Europe, 2006.
3. Larue F, Colleau SM. Underestimation and undertreatment of pain in HIV disease: Multicentre study. BMJ 1997;314:23-28.
4. Singer JE, Fahy-Chandon B, Chi S, et al. Painful symptoms reported by ambulatory HIV-infected men in a longitudinal study. Pain 1993;54:15-19.
5. Larue F, Brasseur L, Musseault P, et al. Pain and symptoms in HIV disease: A national survey in France [Abstract]. Third Congress of the European Association for Palliative Care. J Palliative Care 1994;10:95.
6. Frich LM, Borgbjerg FM. Pain and pain treatment in AIDS patients: A longitudinal study. J Pain Symptom Manage 2000;19:339-347.
7. Wulff EA, Wang AK, Simpson DM. HIV-associated peripheral neuropathy: Epidemiology, pathophysiology and treatment. Drugs 2000;59:1251-1260.
8. Simpson DM. Selected peripheral neuropathies associated with human immunodeficiency virus infection and antiretroviral therapy. J Neurovirol 2002;8(Suppl 2):33-41.
9. Selwyn PA, Rivard M. Overview of clinical issues. In O'Neill J, Selwyn PA, Schietinger H (eds). A Clinical Guide to Supportive and Palliative Care for HIV/AIDS. Rockville, MD: Health Resources and Services Administration, 2003.
10. Moss V. Palliative care in advanced HIV disease: Presentation, problems, and palliation. AIDS 1990;4(Suppl):S235-S242.
11. Fontaine A, Larue F, Lassauniere JM. Physicians; recognition of the symptoms experienced by HIV patients: How reliable? J Pain Symptom Manage 1999;18:263-270.
12. Filbet M, Marceron V. A retrospective study of symptoms in 193 terminal inpatients with AIDS [Abstract]. Third Congress of the European Association for Palliative Care. J Palliative Care 1994;10:92.
13. Fantoni M, Ricci F, Del Borgo C, et al. Multicentre study on the prevalence of symptoms and symptomatic treatment in HIV infection. J Palliat Care 1997;13:9-13.
14. Vogl D, Rosenfeld B, Breitbart W, et al. Symptom prevalence, characteristics, and distress in AIDS outpatients. J Pain Symptom Manage 1998;18:253-262.
15. Maschke M, Kastrup O, Esser S, et al. Incidence and prevalence of neurological disorders associated with HIV since the introduction of highly active antiretroviral therapy (HAART). J Neurol Neurosurg Psychiatry 2000;69:376-380.
16. Schifitto G, McDermott MP, McArthur JC, et al; Dana Consortium on the Therapy of HIV Dementia and Related Cognitive Disorders. Incidence of and risk factors for HIV-associated distal sensory polyneuropathy. Neurology 2002;58:1764-1768.
17. Rosenthal E, Pialoux G, Bernard N; GERMIVIC Joint Study Group. Liver-related mortality in human-immunodeficiency-virus-infected patients between 1995 and 2003 in the French GERMIVIC Joint Study Group Network (MORTAVIC 2003 Study). J Viral Hepat 2007;14:183-188.

Symptom Management in Human Immunodeficiency Virus Infection in Sub-Saharan Africa

Karen Laurence, Jean-Michel Livrozet, Peter Selwyn, and Marilene Filbet

K E Y   P O I N T S

- Relief of pain and symptoms, accessible and affordable drugs, financial support and carer training and support, together with orphan support, have been identified as major needs among palliative care patients and patients with human immunodeficiency virus (HIV) infection throughout Africa.

- Hunger as a symptom needs treatment with food, not medication, and certain drugs (e.g., nonsteroidal anti-inflammatory drugs, corticosteroids) that are often required for pain and symptom control should not be taken on an empty stomach.

- The World Health Organization advocates use of the analgesic ladder for the management of both cancer and HIV-related pain, with oral morphine as the drug of choice for severe pain.

- HIV/AIDS traditionally may be considered an African illness best treated by traditional rather than Western medical treatment.
- Transport costs are a hidden barrier to accessing health and palliative care and are an important consideration in the model of palliative care service delivery.
- With increased access to antiretroviral drugs, drug interactions are becoming increasingly important considerations for palliative care providers, together with referral for antiretroviral treatment if appropriate.

In a resource-poor setting, there are immense challenges to the provision of health care, palliative care, and symptom control. There is limited access to health care services. Qualified health professionals, particularly doctors, are lacking, especially in rural areas. Drug availability is limited, as are skills in pain and symptom control. There is often a lack of awareness about palliative care and poor integration of palliative care providers with existing health services. Relief of pain and symptoms, accessible and affordable drugs, financial support and carer training and support, together with orphan support, have been identified as major needs among palliative care patients and patients with human immunodeficiency virus (HIV) infection throughout Africa.[1,2]

SYMPTOM PREVALENCE IN AFRICA

The presentation of HIV-related symptoms is influenced by a host of factors, including age, gender, genetic variability, severity of illness, culture, poverty, and available treatments, including traditional treatments.

Symptoms in people with HIV infection may be caused by HIV itself, by opportunistic infections, by AIDS-related cancers, or by side effects of treatment. Symptom prevalence is likely to be affected by the availability of treatment at a local level throughout sub-Saharan Africa. The effect of availability of antiretroviral treatment on symptom prevalence in sub-Saharan Africa is unknown. Whereas symptoms due to opportunistic infections should decrease as immunity improves, side effects of treatment are likely to increase. For example, treatment-related neuropathy is seen increasingly frequently in Uganda as a result of the cheapest antiretroviral regimen, Triomune containing stavudine (d4T).

Even in the era of antiretroviral treatment, pain and symptom control is still needed for patients with HIV-related malignancies, opportunistic infections, failure of available treatments, late presentation or inability to access care, and treatment-related side effects.

The majority of patients presenting to palliative care services in sub-Saharan Africa have more than one symptom, and pain is highly prevalent.[3-6] Hunger was found to be a severe symptom for a quarter of patients attending a home-based palliative care service in urban Uganda,[6] reflecting the underlying poverty. This highlights the need to assess local palliative care needs and symptom burden, and not to extrapolate from Western data when developing services to meet local needs. Hunger as a symptom needs treatment with food, not medication, and

certain drugs (e.g., nonsteroidal anti-inflammatory drugs, corticosteroids) that are often required for pain and symptom control should not be taken on an empty stomach. Palliative care providers in low-resource settings may need to network with other organizations to provide aspects of care that may be very different from those required in more affluent societies.

PAIN CONTROL

Supportive care without pain control is not palliative care.[7] Good pain control is possible in a resource-poor setting. The World Health Organization (WHO) advocates the use of the analgesic ladder for management of both cancer and HIV-related pain, with oral morphine as the drug of choice for severe pain. Oral morphine solution can be reconstituted from morphine powder and given every 4 hours to control pain; it is cheap and effective and can be given sublingually in a patient who is vomiting, although bioavailability via this route is variable and the dose needs to be titrated against response. Oral morphine is much cheaper than codeine and many other step 2 analgesics, and it can be started at a low dose equivalent to codeine or other weak opioids, omitting step 2 of the analgesic ladder. Unlike methadone, morphine is unaffected by enzyme inhibitors and inducers and therefore does not interact with antiretroviral drugs; it also has a less variable half-life and therefore is easier to use. In patients with AIDS-related diarrhea, the constipating side effect of morphine can be advantageous. Oral morphine is becoming available in more African countries through advocacy, although it is not yet widely available. In Uganda, nurses are undergoing specialist training to be allowed to prescribe oral morphine and other key palliative care drugs, thereby increasing availability for those in need.

With treatment of the underlying opportunistic infection, the need for medication to control pain and other symptoms is often reduced, and such drugs can be stopped. For example, patients with severe esophageal candidiasis may require opioids to enable them to swallow systemic antifungals. As the infection improves, the opioid dose can be tapered and stopped.

TRADITIONAL TREATMENTS

Traditional healers are the first port of call for health care advice for 80% of HIV patients in sub-Saharan Africa.[8] Traditional healers are often far more accessible to the rural population than governmental health services. HIV/AIDS may be considered an African illness best treated by traditional rather than Western medical treatment. Palliative care services can improve access to patients in need through training and working with traditional healers. This has resulted in successful referrals in Uganda. Traditional medicines can be useful in symptom management. They are often free, familiar to patients and their families, and grown locally. Local remedies for constipation (e.g., crushed papaya seeds) are used in Uganda and are much cheaper and often more acceptable to patients than a pharmaceutical product. Frangipani sap contains phenol derivatives and can produce local anesthesia in acute herpes zoster for up to 8 hours when painted on the lesions (Fig. 214-1).

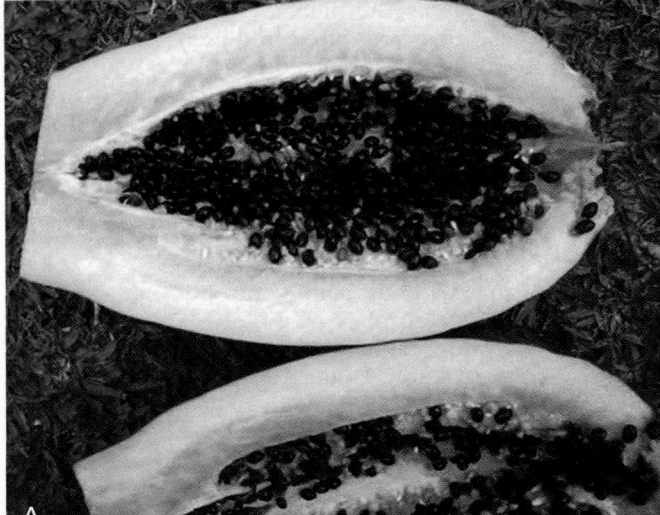

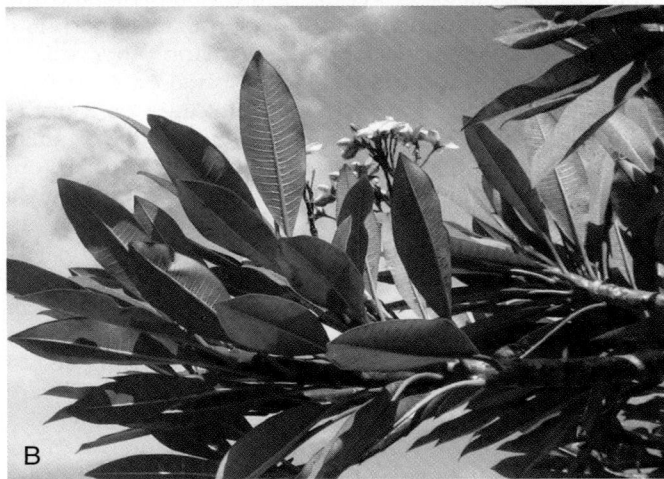

FIGURE 214-1 Use of local treatments. **A**, Papaya seeds are used for constipation. **B**, Frangipani sap is used in the treatment of herpes zoster.

TABLE 214-13	Essential Drugs for Pain and Symptom Control in Low-Resource Settings (Hospice Africa Uganda)	
GENERIC DRUG	**DOSE**	**FORM**
Amitriptyline	10, 25, 50 mg	Oral
Phenytoin	100 mg	Oral
Acetylsalicylic acid	300 mg	Oral
Diclofenac	25, 50, 75, 100 mg	Oral
	75 mg/3mL	Injection
Codeine	30 mg	Oral
Morphine	5 mg/mL, 50 mg/5 mL	Oral
Chlorpromazine	10, 25 mg	Oral/injection
Thioridazine	25, 50 mg	Oral/injection
Haloperidol	1, 2 mg	Oral
Dexamethasone	0.5, 2 mg	Oral
	8 mg/mL	Injection
Diazepam	2.5, 10 mg	Oral/injection
Furosemide	20, 40 mg	Oral/injection
Spironolactone	50, 100 mg	Oral
Ketoconazole	200 mg	Oral
Nystatin	100,000 and 500,000 U/mL	Oral
Magnesium trisilicate	1500	Oral
Metoclopramide	10 mg	Oral/injection
Metronidazole	200 mg	Tablet
Amoxicillin	250 mg	Oral
Bisacodyl	5 mg	Oral
Hyoscine butylbromide	10 mg	Oral/injection
Chlorpheniramine	4 mg	Oral

COSTS OF PALLIATIVE CARE PROVISION

Sickness arising from a background of poverty can push patients and their families into destitution. The majority of patients who are unable to work because of sickness cannot afford the basic drugs or transport costs involved in accessing palliative care.

Consideration of the cheapest regimen for treating a particular condition is important. For example, a single ibuprofen 200-mg tablet may be cheaper than a diclofenac 50-mg tablet, but the cost of eight ibuprofen tablets a day may be more than the equivalent three diclofenac tablets. Prescribing or recommending the cheapest regimen will improve compliance and symptom control. The use of drugs such as haloperidol 1.25 mg at night for nausea rather than metoclopramide 10 mg three times a day may also be more cost-effective. Essential palliative care drugs for pain and symptom control in HIV/AIDS, as advocated by Hospice Africa Uganda, are shown in Table 214-13.

Transport costs are a hidden barrier to accessing health and palliative care and are an important consideration in the model of palliative care service delivery. Transporta-tion of a sick or deceased patient may be prohibitively expensive to families. Home-based care is advocated as the most appropriate model of palliative care provision in sub-Saharan Africa, but reaching those in need is immensely challenging. Allowing relatives to report on a patient's progress, rather than bringing the patient in person for review, may be one way of facilitating continuing care, although this approach is not without its pitfalls.

DRUG INTERACTIONS WITH ANTIRETROVIRAL REGIMENS

Pharmacokinetic interactions of antiretroviral drugs, particularly the non-nucleoside reverse transcriptase inhibitors (NNRTIs), with palliative care drugs are of vital importance to palliative care providers in sub-Saharan Africa. Many palliative care drugs, particularly those useful in neuropathic pain management, are metabolized by the cytochrome P-450 system. Phenytoin, carbamazepine, ketoconazole, and cimetidine, which are frequently used in low-resource settings for symptom control because of their low cost, all have the potential to cause failure of a non-nucleoside antiretroviral-containing regimen. The mainstay of neuropathic pain management in patients receiving antiretrovirals in Africa currently is amitriptyline or another tricyclic antidepressant with opioids.

CONCLUSIONS

Symptom management in HIV/AIDS in low-resource settings is both affordable and possible with careful diagnosis of the cause of the pain and symptoms, consideration of the underlying social situation of the patient, judicious use of simple and economical medications, including traditional treatments where appropriate, and access to oral morphine. With increased access to antiretroviral drugs, drug interactions are becoming increasingly important considerations for palliative care providers, together with referral for antiretroviral treatment if appropriate.

REFERENCES

1. Sepulveda C, Habiyambere V, Amandua J, et al. Quality care at end of life in Africa. BMJ 2003;327:209-213.
2. World Health Organization. A Community Approach to Palliative Care for HIV/AIDS and/or Cancer Patients in Sub-Saharan Africa. Geneva: WHO, 2004.
3. Clipsham L, et al. Symptom Prevalence Amongst HIV/AIDS and/or Cancer Patients Attending a Palliative Care Service in Kampala, Uganda. Oral presentation to the Palliative Care in Uganda: Completing the Circle of Care conference, Palliative Care Association of Uganda, Jinja, Uganda, August 8-10, 2005.
4. Norval D. Symptoms and sites of pain experienced by AIDS patients. S Afr Med J 2004;94:450-454.
5. Sukati NA, Mndebele SC, Makoa ET, et al. HIV/AIDS symptom management in Southern Africa. J Pain Symptom Manage 2005;29:185-191.
6. Makoae L, Seboni NM, Molosiwa K, et al. The symptom experience of people living with HIV/AIDS in southern Africa. J Assoc Nurses AIDS Care 2005;16:22-32.
7. Merriman A, Kaur M. Palliative medicine in Africa: An appraisal Lancet 2005;365:1910-1911.
8. Harding R, Stewart K, Marconi K, et al. Current HIV/AIDS end of life care in Sub-Saharan Africa: A survey of models, services, challenges and priorities. BMC Public Health 2003;3:33.

PART V

Palliative Medicine in Cancer

Cancer

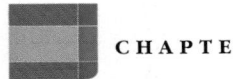

CHAPTER **215**

Biology of Cancer

Tugba Yavuzsen and **Seref Komurcu**

KEY POINTS

- Metastasis depends on interactions between metastatic cells and the microenvironment, which influence the biology of metastasis.
- The molecular basis of metastasis includes growth factors, the extracellular matrix, organ homing, matrix degradation, and cell motility.
- Cancer treatment should address metastatic cells and homeostatic factors.

The biological heterogeneity of tumor cells is the major problem in designing effective cancer treatment. Tumors with similar histological types and sizes have divergent metastatic potential and aggressive behavior.[1]

The natural history of most malignant tumors can be divided into several phases. Malignant change in the target cell, referred to as transformation; growth of the transformed cells; local invasion; and distant metastases are the main steps (Table 215-1). The transition from premalignant lesions, such as dysplasia and hyperplasia, to fully malignant, invasive tumors is a complex, multistep process defined by the ability of tumor cells.

PRINCIPLES OF TUMOR INVASION AND METASTASIS

After a cancer diagnosis is established, the important question is whether the tumor is localized or metastatic. Metastasis and tumor invasion are the major causes of cancer treatment failure. Despite better diagnosis, surgical techniques, patient care, and adjuvant treatments, most deaths from cancer are from metastatic disease. Thirty percent of patients with newly diagnosed tumors have detectable metastases. Of the remaining 70% who are clinically free of metastasis, about one half have metastatic spread detected during follow-up.[2] Metastases can be located in different organs or different regions of the same organ.

The metastatic process is not random and depends on multiple interactions between the organ's microenvironment and the tumor cells.[3] These factors include monoclonal expansion of tumor cells by genetic alterations and environmental factors such as viral infections inducing polyclonal expansion of the cells' influences on normal tissues. After accumulation of genetic alterations in a few premalignant cells, the cells convert into malignant ones. By clonal expansion, the fully malignant cells become invasive and metastatic.

Common sites of metastatic disease are lung, bone, liver, brain, and other soft tissues. The site frequency depends on the primary tumor (Table 215-2).[4] It is sometimes possible to predict the most likely primary sites from the histologic and deposition pattern of metastases.[5]

Tumor cells are biologically heterogeneous, and highly metastatic ones often require more gene alterations than nonmetastatic cells (Table 215-3).[6] Various genes are differentially expressed between metastatic and nonmetastatic clones. There are two molecular approaches for development of tumor metastases: the genetic and epigenetic models.[7,8] The genetic model is based on mutations of the genome; the epigenetic model is defined mainly as modifications of gene expression by chemokines and neurotransmitters, which do not involve changes in the DNA nucleotide sequence.[6,8] The molecular mechanism for metastasis and invasion is associated with genetic and epigenetic alterations of defined cancer cell genes. The mechanism depends on many complex interactions between metastatic cells and host homeostatic mechanisms.[9,10]

The first step in the metastatic process is penetration of the basement membrane and then invasion of the interstitial stroma by active proteolysis. Intravasation is invasion of the subendothelial basement membrane of the tumor cells, and extravasation occurs in the distant organ. Development of the malignant phenotype is also associated with tumor-induced angiogenesis, which allows tumor growth and easy hematogenous spread.[11-13] Cells eventually invade and proliferate in the distant organ, following a process similar to that at the primary site (see Table 215-1).

Angiogenesis

Angiogenesis is essential for primary tumor growth. New blood vessels form around a solid tumor,[11] and the rich vascularization increases the chance for tumor cells to reach the bloodstream and colonize secondary sites. Angiogenesis can be divided into three steps, which parallel the steps of tumor cell invasion: endothelial cell proliferation, extracellular matrix breakdown, and endothelial cell migration.[13]

TABLE 215-1   Steps in Metastasis

Transformation and growth
Vascularization (i.e., angiogenesis)
Intravasation and survival
Attachment, extravasation, and invasion
Proliferation in secondary sites

TABLE 215-2   Cancer Primary Types and Their Common Sites of Metastasis

CANCER TYPES	METASTASIS SITES
Breast cancer	Bone, lung, liver
Colorectal cancer	Lymph nodes, liver, lung, peritoneal dissemination
Esophageal cancer	Lymph nodes (i.e., anatomical skip metastasis), liver, lung
Gastric cancer	Liver, lymph nodes, peritoneal dissemination
Head and neck cancer	Lymph nodes
Lung cancer	Lymph nodes
Malignant melanoma	Lymph nodes, lung
Sarcomas	Lung, lymph nodes (e.g., epithelioid sarcoma, angiosarcoma)
Thyroid cancer	Lymph nodes

TABLE 215-3   Essential Changes in Cell Biology

Self-sufficiency in growth signals
Insensitivity to growth inhibitory (antigrowth) signals
Evasion of programmed cell death (i.e., apoptosis)
Defects in DNA repair and genomic instability
Limitless replicative potential
Sustained angiogenesis
Tissue invasion and metastasis

The main factor determining angiogenesis is tissue oxygen pressure. Oxygen can diffuse radially from blood vessels only over 150 to 200 µm. This is equivalent to a tumor mass of 2 mm³. If growth beyond 2 to 3 mm³ is to occur, it requires the formation of new blood vessels.[14] Angiogenesis is requisite for continued tumor growth and metastasis. Without vascular access, tumor cells cannot readily spread to distant sites.

Angiogenesis involves an alteration in the balance between proangiogenic and antiangiogenic molecules in the local tissue microenvironment. Tumor-associated angiogenic factors are produced by tumor cells, by the extracellular matrix, and by host cells such as macrophages that infiltrate tumors.[15,16] Vascular endothelial growth factor (VEGF) and basic fibroblast growth factor (bFGF) are the two most important tumor-associated angiogenic factors. These are commonly expressed in many tumor cells, and elevated levels are detected in the serum and urine of some cancer patients. VEGF is pivotal in developmental, physiological, and pathological angiogenesis, and it is a candidate effector molecule. VEGF stimulates endothelial cell proliferation and migration and induces expression of metalloproteinases and plasminogen activity by these cells. Overexpression of VEGF in tumor cells increases the rate of tumor growth and metastasis in animal models by stimulating vascularization (i.e., increased microvessel density).[17]

Early in their growth, most human tumors do not induce angiogenesis. Primary tumors exist in situ without a blood supply for months to years; then, some cells within the small tumor change to an angiogenic phenotype. This is the *angiogenic switch*. The molecular basis is unclear but may involve increased production of proangiogenic factors or loss of angiogenesis inhibitors. Proangiogenetic molecules may be constitutively expressed because of increased levels of certain stimulants such as activated oncogenes, cytokines, growth factors, hypoxia, low pH, signal transduction pathways, loss of tumor suppressor gene function, and tumor size.[18]

The role of the immune system is established in physiological angiogenesis, such as occurs in wound healing.[14] Inflammation-associated angiogenesis is also known as pathological angiogenesis. Cutaneous melanoma is a model of these relationships; the local inflammatory reaction correlates with an increased risk of metastasis. Tumor cells produce angiogenic molecules and induce antiangiogenesis molecules. Tumor growth is controlled by the balance of these two types of molecules. In some, wild-type tumor protein 53 (TP53) inhibits angiogenesis by inducing synthesis of the antiangiogenic molecule thrombospondin-1 and downregulating production of VEGF and hypoxia-inducible factor (HIF-1). With mutational inactivation of both *TP53* alleles (common in many cancers), the levels of thrombospondin-1 drop, VEGF levels increase, and HIF-1 production is enhanced by tumor hypoxia. Some antiangiogenesis factors, such as thrombospondin-1, may be produced by the tumor cells, whereas others, such as angiostatin, endostatin, and tumstatin, are produced in response to the tumor.

Proliferation, Cell Attachments, Invasion, and Migration

Some tumors, such as melanoma, decreasingly depend on exogenous growth factors and produce many positive growth regulators.[9] Adhesion molecules have a primary role in cellular attachment. Tumor invasion is part of the metastatic process, crossing extracellular matrix barriers of translocated tumor cells. Invasion requires lysis of matrix proteins by specific proteinases (e.g., matrix metalloproteinase [MMP], stromelysin-1).[19,20]

The motility of tumor cells is an important component of invasion. At least 11 motility factors are secreted by tumor and host cells, but only 3 are clearly defined (Table 215-4). The first group is the autocrine motility factors secreted by tumor cells. The second group is extracellular matrix proteins, which stimulate chemotaxis and haptotaxis. The third group is host-secreted growth factors. These paracrine motility factors, referred to as homing factors, cause tumor cells to move toward the organs.[9] Tumor cells colonize secondary sites (i.e., metastasis) by proliferation. Growth factors stimulate metastatic cell proliferation at secondary sites.[9] Tumor growth and survival require adequate oxygen and nutrients. Tumor cells must

TABLE 215-4 Motility Factors Secreted by Tumor or Host Cells

GROUP	FACTORS
Autocrine motility factors	Hepatocyte growth factor or scatter factor, insulin-like growth factor 2, autotoxin
Extracellular matrix proteins	Fibronectin, vitronectin, type I and IV collagens, thrombospondin
Paracrine motility factors	Insulin-like growth factor 1, interleukin-8, histamine

penetrate or attach to extracellular matrix components, which include the stroma and basement membrane, and other cells.[9]

At least three mechanisms play in role tumor cell invasion of tissue: mechanical pressure produced by rapidly proliferating cells, increased cell motility, and enzymes secreted from invasive tumor cells. Several adhesion molecules, cadherins, integrins, selectins, and immunoglobulin G superfamily members have been identified. Their synthesis and expression on the cell membrane is associated with metastatic potential. Downregulation of these adhesion molecules correlates with a greater tendency for tumor cells to detach from the primary site, but upregulation correlates with a higher potential to metastasize.[21] Integrins are transmembrane receptors that bind to extracellular matrix molecules, including collagens, fibronectin, laminin, and vitronectin. Specific integrins are important in bone metastases.[9] Cadherins, which are a family of transmembrane glycoproteins, mediate calcium-dependent cell-cell adhesion in normal tissue and various tumors. Expression correlates with tumor differentiation. E-cadherin is the most extensively studied in cancer invasion, and decreased expression is related to cancer progression.[22] It may suppress metastasis, and the loss of E-cadherin gene expression correlates with invasiveness and metastatic potential.

Matrix degradation is a critical event in the metastatic process.[15] Many proteinases degrade extracellular components, and the most important are serine proteases, cathepsins, and MMPs.[23] Tumor cells secrete proteolytic enzymes themselves or induce host cells (e.g., stromal fibroblasts, infiltrating macrophages) to elaborate proteases. Their activity is modulated by antiproteases. The MMP family of zinc-dependent extracellular proteinases influences the oncogenic signal transduction pathways that contribute to the malignant phenotype. MMP family members can be categorized in collagenase, stromelizines, gelatinase, and membrane-type MMP subfamilies.[17] A positive correlation between tumor aggressiveness and MMP expression levels has been established for most tumor types.[24-26] MMP9 and MMP2 are collagenases that cleave the type IV collagen of epithelial cells and vascular basement membranes.

Compelling evidence supports the role of MMPs in the degradation of type IV collagen, which occurs in tumor cell invasion:

1. Several invasive carcinomas, melanomas, and sarcomas produce high levels of these collagenases.

2. In situ lesions and adenomas of the breast and colon express less collagen IV–degrading collagenases than invasive tumors. MMP expression is higher in late-stage tumors.
3. Inhibition of collagenase activity by transfection with the genes for tissue inhibitors of metalloproteinases reduces metastases in animals.

Metalloproteinase inhibitors may be of value in cancer treatment. Synthetic compounds with this type of activity are being tested as therapeutic agents against some cancers.

Degradation of collagen IV exposes normally cryptic domains of the protein, which serve as important signals for angiogenesis and cell interactions. Collagen IV degradation in the basement membrane produces angiogenic stimuli and generates collagen fragments, such as endostatin and tumstatin, which are antiangiogenic. An important role of MMPs is to generate from the extracellular matrix factors that promote angiogenesis, tumor growth, and tumor cell motility. These counteract substances that inhibit angiogenesis, which also are produced by partial digestion of basement membrane components.

MMPs are inhibited by endogenous tissue inhibitors of MMP (TIMP). TIMP inhibits angiogenesis in vivo and capillary endothelial cell proliferation and migration in vitro.[26] The relationship between MMPs and TIMP reflect the balance in matrix stabilization and degradation.[19] MMP/TIMP expression may be a prognostic factor, but studies of MMP inhibitors in cancer patients showed disappointing results.[19]

Serine proteinase is a member of the plasminogen activators (PAs) family. It converts inactive plasminogen to active plasmin. There are two subgroups: tissue plasminogen activator (tPA) and urokinase plasminogen activator (uPA).[27] Both are found in breast cancer,[28] and uPA has been identified in many human cancers, including colon cancer.[29] The main role of uPA is in macrophage invasion and proteolysis during invasiveness and metastasis. Plasminogen activator function may be regulated by glycoprotein inhibitors (PAIs). The levels of PA and PAI reflect invasiveness and correlate with differentiation, stage, and metastasis of tumors. The ratio may be prognostic for some tumors, such as gastric cancer.[30]

RESEARCH CHALLENGES AND CONCLUSIONS

The outcome of cancer metastasis depends on many interactions between selected metastatic cells and homeostatic mechanisms unique to some organ microenvironments. The organ microenvironment influences the biology of cancer metastasis in several steps. Several principles form the molecular and cellular basis of site-specific tumor metastasis:

- Selective growth in the organs with the appropriate growth factors or extracellular matrix environment
- Adhesion to the endothelial surface only at the site of organ homing
- Matrix degradation and cell motility

Treatment of metastasis therefore should be aimed at metastatic tumor cells and the homeostatic factors. Advances in understanding the biological basis of cancer metastasis offer unprecedented possibilities for translating basic research into better cancer treatment.

REFERENCES

1. Fidler IJ, Hart IR. Biologic diversity in metastatic neoplasm: Origins and implications. Science 1982;217:998-1001.
2. Sugarbaker EV. Patterns of metastasis in human malignancies. Cancer Biol Rev 1981;2:235.
3. Fidler IJ. The organ microenvironment and cancer metastasis. Differentiation 2002;70:498-505.
4. Leong SP, Cady B, Jablons DM, et al. Clinical patterns of metastasis. Cancer Metastasis Rev 2006:25:221-232.
5. Horak CE, Steeg PS. Metastasis gets site specific. Cancer cell 2005;8:93-95.
6. Hanahan D, Weinberg RA. The hallmarks of cancer. Cell 2000;100:57-70.
7. Yokota J. Tumor progression and metastasis. Carcinogenesis 2000; 21:497-503.
8. Entschladen F, Drell TL, Lang K, et al. Tumour-cell migration, invasion, and metastasis: Navigation by neurotransmitters. Lancet Oncol 2004;5: 254-258.
9. Woodhouse EC, Chuaqui RF, Liotta LA. General mechanisms of metastasis. Cancer 1997;80:1529-1537.
10. Gupta GP, Massague J. Cancer metastasis. Building a framework. Cell 2006;127:679-695.
11. Folkman J. Tumor angiogenesis: Therapeutic implications. N Engl J Med 1971;285:1182-1186.
12. Folkman J, Klagsbrun M. Angiogenic factors. Science 1987;235:442-447.
13. Folkman J. Angiogenesis and metastasis. Adv Oncol 1996;12:3-7.
14. Ellis LM, Fidler IJ. Angiogenesis and metastasis. Eur J Cancer 1996; 32A:2451-2460.
15. Liotta LA, Steeg PS, Stetlet-Stevenson WG, et al. Cancer metastasis and angiogenesis: An imbalance of positive and negative regulation. Cell 1991;64: 327-336.
16. Fidler IJ, Ellis LM. The implications of angiogenesis to the biology and therapy of cancer metastasis. Cell 1994;79:185-188.
17. Wojtowicz-Prapa S. Matrix metalloproteinases. In Abeloff MD (ed). Clinical Oncology, 2nd ed. New York, Churchill Livingstone, 2000, pp 251-259.
18. Fidler IJ, Langley RR, Kerbel RS, Ellis LM. Angiogenesis. In DeVita VT Jr, Hellman S, Rosenberg SA (eds): Cancer: Principles and Practice of Oncology, 7th ed. Philadelphia, Lippincott Williams & Wilkins, 2005.
19. Fridman R. Metalloproteinase and cancer. Cancer Metastasis Rev 2006; 25:7-8.
20. Matrisian LM. Cancer biology: extracellular proteinases in malignancy. Curr Biol 1999;9:R776-R778.
21. Stetler-Stevenson WG. Invasion and metastasis. In DeVita VT Jr, Hellman S, Rosenberg SA (eds): Cancer: Principles and Practice of Oncology, 7th ed. Philadelphia, Lippincott Williams & Wilkins, 2005.
22. Busmakers MJ, Van Moorselaar RA, Giroldi RA, et al. Decreased expression of E-cadherin in the progression of rat prostatic cancer. Cancer Res 1992; 52:2916-2922.
23. Lukshev ME, Werb Z. ECM signalling, orchestrating cell behavior and misbehavior. Trends Cell Biol 1998;8:437-441.
24. Kahari VM, Saarialho-Kere U. Matrix metalloproteinases and their inhibitors in tumor growth and invasion. Ann Med 1999;31:34-45.
25. Brown PD. Clinical studies with matrix metalloproteinase inhibitors. APMIS 1999;107:174-180.
26. Schnaper HW, Grant DS, Stetler-Stevenson WG. Type IV collogenase(s) and TIMPs modulate endothelial cell morphogenesis in vitro. J Cell Physiol 1993;156:235-246.
27. Liotta LA, Kohn EC. Invasion and metastasis. In Holland JF, Kufe DW, Pollock RE, et al (eds). Holland-Frei Cancer Medicine. Hamilton, Canada, BC Decker, 2000, p 8.
28. Sherbet GV, Lakshmi MS. The genetics of cancer. London, Academic Press, 1997.
29. Boyd D, Florent D, Kim P, et al. Determination of the levels of urokinase and its receptor in human colon carcinoma cell lines. Cancer Res 1988;48:3112-3116.
30. Plebani M, Herszenyi L, Cardin R. Cysteine and serine proteases in gastric cancer. Cancer 1995;76:367-375.

SUGGESTED READING

Fidler IJ, Langley RR, Kerbel RS, Ellis LM. Angiogenesis. In DeVita VT Jr, Hellman S, Rosenberg SA (eds). Cancer: Principles and Practice of Oncology, 7th ed. Philadelphia, Lippincott Williams & Wilkins, 2005.

Liotta LA, Kohn EC. Invasion and metastasis. In Holland JF, Kufe DW, Pollock RE, et al (eds). Holland-Frei Cancer Medicine. Hamilton, Canada, BC Decker, 2000, p 8.

Stetler-Stevenson WG. Invasion and metastasis. In DeVita VT Jr, Hellman S, Rosenberg SA (eds). Cancer: Principles and Prac-

tice of Oncology, 7th ed. Philadelphia, Lippincott Williams & Wilkins, 2005.

Wojtowicz-Prapa S. Matrix metalloproteinases. In Abeloff MD (ed). Clinical Oncology, 2nd ed. New York, Churchill Livingstone, 2000, pp 251-259.

CHAPTER **216**

Epidemiology of Cancer

Kaci Osenga and James F. Cleary

K E Y   P O I N T S

- Cancer is a major cause of morbidity and death.
- There has been little impact on mortality rates in the past 30 years.
- Prolongation of survival may be achieved more by earlier detection than by true improvements in survival.
- Increasing numbers of people are living with a cancer diagnosis in developed countries.

Cancer contributes significantly to morbidity and mortality throughout the world. In 2002, the International Agency for Research on Cancer (IARC) estimated that there were 10.9 million people newly diagnosed with cancer and 6.7 million deaths related to cancer globally.[1] There were approximately 25 million persons alive with cancer (defined by the IARC as the period within 3 years of diagnosis). These figures do not include in situ cancers (i.e., breast and cervix) or the more than 1 million diagnoses of basal and squamous cell skin cancers diagnosed each year (Box 216-1).

INCIDENCE

The cancers commonly diagnosed globally are lung, breast, colorectal, stomach, and liver cancer (Table 216-1).[1] Among men, the more common types are lung, prostate, stomach, colorectal, liver, and esophageal cancers. Among women, breast, cervix, lung, colorectal, and stomach cancer are the most common. New cancer diagnoses will increase to 15 million annually by 2020, and much of this increase will occur in resource-poor countries, partly because of their increasing populations, particularly the numbers of elderly who have adopted Western lifestyles and consequent cancers from smoking, diet, and obesity. Simultaneously, there has been little progress in controlling cancers traditionally associated with poverty, such as gastric, hepatic, cervical, and esophageal cancers.

The American Cancer Society estimates that in 2007, about 1,500,000 Americans received a new diagnosis of

Box 216-1 Epidemiological Definitions for Cancer

- *Incidence* is the number of new cases occurring, expressed as an absolute number of cases per year or as a rate per 100,000 persons per year.
- *Mortality* is the number of deaths occurring, and the *mortality rate* is the number of deaths per 100,000 persons per year. Mortality is the product of the incidence and the fatality for a given cancer.
- *Fatality*, the inverse of survival, is the proportion of cancer patients who die; mortality rates therefore measure the average risk for the population of dying from a specific cancer within a specified period (usually 1 year), and fatality (1 − survival) represents the probability that an individual with cancer will die of it.
- *Prevalence* describes the number of persons alive at a particular time with the disease of interest. For comparison purposes, prevalence usually is presented as the number of persons still alive after a given number of years after the diagnosis.
- *Survival* is reported as the cumulative probability (range, 0 to 1) of survival up to a stated time after the diagnosis. *Relative survival* is the ratio of survival observed in a group of cancer patients to the survival that would be expected from general population mortality.
- *Cure* is designated if those with the disease die at the same rate as the general population.

invasive cancer (3850 people per day). The major cancer diagnoses for U.S. men are prostate, lung, colorectal, and bladder cancers and non-Hodgkin's lymphoma (Fig. 216-1). For women, the most frequent new diagnoses are breast, lung, colorectal, and cervical cancers and non-Hodgkin's lymphoma. Stomach and liver cancers are uncommon in the United States compared with the rest of the world. The incidence of breast cancer in the United States decreased in 2003, primarily among postmenopausal women.[2] The decreased incidence is thought to be associated with a decline in hormone replacement therapy. Screening has improved earlier detection and increased survival, but controversy regarding breast cancer screening continues, particularly in women younger than 50 years.[3]

In 2006, there were slightly more than 3 million new cancers diagnosed in Europe,[4] an annual increase of 300,000 since 2004.[5] Overall, lung cancer was the most common diagnosis. Among women, breast cancer was the most common cancer (29%), followed by colorectal cancer (13%) and cancer of the uterus (10%). Among men, prostate is the most frequently diagnosed cancer (20%), followed by lung (17%) and colorectal cancer (12.8%). Breast cancer is on the rise in Europe, possibly because of increased screening, whereas the rate of stomach cancer

TABLE 216-1 Global Cancer Rates

TYPE OF CANCER	MALE*			FEMALE*		
	INCIDENCE	MORTALITY	CASE-FATALITY	INCIDENCE	MORTALITY	CASE-FATALITY
Oral cavity	175.9	80.7	0.46	98.3	46.7	0.48
Nasopharynx	55.8	34.9	0.63	24.2	15.4	0.64
Other pharnyx	106.2	68	0.64	24	16	0.67
Esophagus	315.4	261.2	0.83	146.7	124.7	0.85
Stomach	603.4	446	0.74	330.5	254.3	0.77
Colorectal	550.5	278.4	0.51	472.7	250.5	0.53
Liver	442.1	416.8	0.94	184	181.4	0.99
Pancreas	124.8	119.5	0.96	107.4	107.4	1.00
Larynx	139.2	78.6	0.56	20	11.3	0.57
Lung	965.2	848	0.88	386.9	330.8	0.86
Melanoma	79	21.9	0.28	81.1	18.8	0.23
Breast				1151.3	410.7	0.36
Cervix uteri				493.2	273.5	0.55
Corpus uteri				198.8	50.3	0.25
Ovary				204.5	124.9	0.61
Prostate	679	221	0.33			
Testis	48.6	8.9	0.18			
Kidney	129.2	62.7	0.49	79.3	39.2	0.49
Bladder	273.9	108.3	0.40	82.7	36.7	0.44
Brain, CNS	108.2	80	0.74	81.3	61.6	0.76
Thyroid	37.4	11.3	0.30	103.6	24.1	0.23
NHL	175.1	98.9	0.56	125.4	73	0.58
HD	38.2	14.5	0.38	24.1	8.4	0.35
Myeloma	46.5	32.7	0.70	39.2	29.8	0.76
Leukemia	171	125.1	0.73	129.5	97.4	0.75
All sites	5801.8	3796.0	0.65	5060.7	2927.9	0.58

*Rates are given in thousands.
CNS, central nervous system; HD, Hodgkin's disease; NHL, non-Hodgkin's lymphoma.
Adapted from http://www.dep.iarc.fr/ and reference 1.

Estimated New Cases*		Estimated Deaths	
Male	**Female**	**Male**	**Female**
Prostate 218,8890 (29%)	Breast 178,480 (26%)	Lung and bronchus 89,510 (31%)	Lung and bronchus 70,880 (26%)
Lung and bronchus 114,760 (15%)	Lung and bronchus 98,620 (15%)	Prostate 27,050 (9%)	Breast 40,460 (15%)
Colon and rectum 79,130 (10%)	Colon and rectum 74,630 (11%)	Colon and rectum 26,000 (9%)	Colon and rectum 26,180 (10%)
Urinary bladder 50,040 (7%)	Uterine corpus 39,080 (6%)	Pancreas 16,840 (6%)	Pancreas 16,530 (6%)
Non-Hodgkin's lymphoma 74,200 (4%)	Non-Hodgkin's lymphoma 28,990 (4%)	Leukemia 12,320 (4%)	Ovary 15,280 (6%)
Melanoma of the skin 33,910 (4%)	Melanoma of the skin 26,030 (4%)	Liver and intrahepatic bile duct 11,280 (4%)	Leukemia 9470 (4%)
Kidney and renal pelvis 31,590 (4%)	Thyroid 25,480 (4%)	Esophagus 10,900 (4%)	Non-Hodgkin's lymphoma 9060 (3%)
Leukemia 24,800 (3%)	Ovary 22,430 (3%)	Urinary bladder 9630 (3%)	Uterine corpus 7400 (3%)
Oral cavity and pharynx 24,180 (3%)	Kidney and renal pelvis 19,600 (3%)	Non-Hodgkin's lymphoma 9600 (3%)	Brain and other nervous system 5590 (2%)
Pancreas 18,830 (2%)	Leukemia 19,440 (3%)	Kidney and renal pelvis 8080 (3%)	Liver and intrahepatic bile duct 5500 (2%)
All sites 766,860 (100%)	All sites 678,060 (100%)	All sites 289,550 (100%)	All sites 270,100 (100%)

*Excludes basal and squamous cell skin cancers and in situ carcinomas except urinary bladder.

FIGURE 216-1 Leading sites of new cancer cases and deaths: 2007 estimates. *(From the American Cancer Society, Surveillance Research, 2007, and http://www-dep.iarc.fr/.)*

is decreasing. Lung cancer is not a leading cancer diagnosis among European woman.

Tobacco is a major cause of new cancers, contributing to lung, esophageal, head and neck, and bladder cancers. Infectious agents contribute significantly to stomach, liver, cervical, and head and neck cancers and some lymphomas. In low- and middle-income countries, 26% of all cancers are attributable directly to infection; in high-income countries, the corresponding figure is only 8%.[6]

MORTALITY

Cancer is a leading cause of death worldwide and an important focus for palliative care services in most countries. For a total of 58 million deaths worldwide in 2005, cancer accounts for 7.6 million or 13% of all deaths, but it is the predominant disease referred to palliative care programs. More than 70% of all cancer deaths in 2005 occurred in low- and middle-income countries, which commonly have limited palliative care services. Deaths from cancer in the world will continue rising, with 9 million people dying each year by 2015 and 11.4 million by 2030. The main cancers leading to global cancer mortality are lung, stomach, liver, colon, breast, and esophageal cancers (Table 216-2).

More than 500,000 U.S. residents die of cancer each year (i.e., more than 1500 people per day). Although there

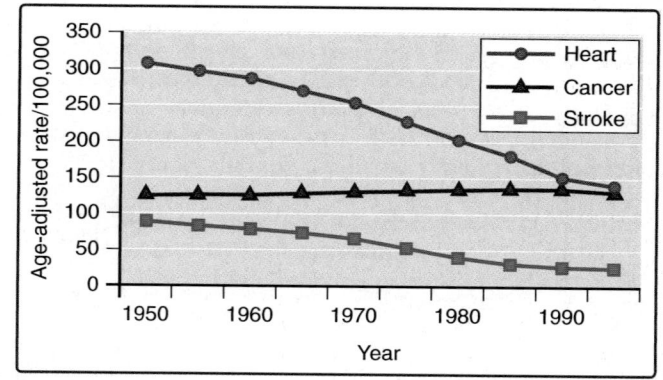

FIGURE 216-2 Age-adjusted rates for cancer cardiac mortality compared with rates for heart disease and stroke. *(From U.S. Health Department, 1996 and http://www-dep.iarc.fr/.)*

has been much celebration about declining cancer mortality rates, the decrease has been much less than for cardiovascular and cerebrovascular deaths during the past 30 years since the declaration of the "War on Cancer" (Fig. 216-2). The leading causes of cancer death for U.S. men are lung, prostate, colorectal, and pancreas cancers, followed by leukemia (see Fig. 216-1 and Table 216-2). The mortality rates for U.S. men are declining for lung (−8%),

TABLE 216-2 Global Cancer Statistics

CATEGORY	GLOBAL	BRAZIL	UNITED STATES	UNITED KINGDOM	ROMANIA	SOUTH AFRICA	KENYA	SAUDI ARABIA	INDIA	CHINA
Cancer deaths, all		190,000	579,000	142,000	45,000	41,000	18,000	12,000	826,000	1,892,000
Cancer deaths <70 yr		113,000	259,000	55,000	26,000	27,000	11,000	8,000	519,000	1,182,000
Deaths (%) in 2005		19.5	31.7	48.8	19.0	5.8	5.1	14.5	9.5	27.4
Deaths (%) in 2030		24.4	32.4	51.0	20.0	6.5	9.0	17.7	14.7	34.2

CANCER CAUSE OF DEATH BY RANK

Male

1	Lung	Lung[2]	Lung[2]	Lung[3]	Lung[1]	Lung[2]	Esophagus[2]	Liver[3]	Lung[1]	Stomach[1]
2	Prostate	Prostate[1]	Colorectal[4]	Prostate[1]	Stomach[4]	Esophagus[3]	Prostate[3]	NHL, MM[1]	H&N[2]	Lung[2]
3	Stomach	Stomach[3]	Prostate[1]	Colorectal[2]	Colorectal[3]	Prostate[1]	Stomach[4]	Lung[6]	Esophagus[3]	Liver[3]
4	Colorectal	Esophagus[5]	NHL/MM[7]	Esophagus[5]	Prostate[5]	Stomach[6]	Liver	Prostate[4]	Stomach[5]	Esophagus[4]
5	Liver	Colorectal[4]	Pancreas[9]	Stomach[7]	H&N[6]	Liver[7]	NHL. MM[5]	Bladder[5]	Prostate[4]	Colorectal[5]

Female

1	Breast	Breast[1]	Lung[2]	Breast[1]	Breast[1]	Cervix[1]	Cervix[1]	Breast[1]	Cervix[1]	Stomach[1]
2	Cervix	Lung[5]	Breast[1]	Lung[3]	Cervix[2]	Breast[2]	Breast[3]	NHL, MM[3]	Breast[2]	Lung[2]
3	Lung	Colorectal[4]	Colorectal[3]	Colorectal[2]	Colorectal[5]	Lung[6]	Stomach[6]	Colorectal[4]	NHL, MM[3]	Liver[3]
4	Colorectal	Stomach	NHL, MM[7]	Ovary[5]	Lung[7]	Esophagus[7]	NHL, MM[4]	Liver[8]	H&N[4]	Esophagus[4]
5	Stomach	Cervix[3]	Ovary[8]	NHL, MM[6]	Stomach[8]	Colorectal[5]	Liver[7]	Esophagus[9]	Esophagus[5]	Colorectal[6]

H&N, mouth and oropharynx cancers; MM, multiple myeloma; NHL, non-Hodgkin's lymphoma.

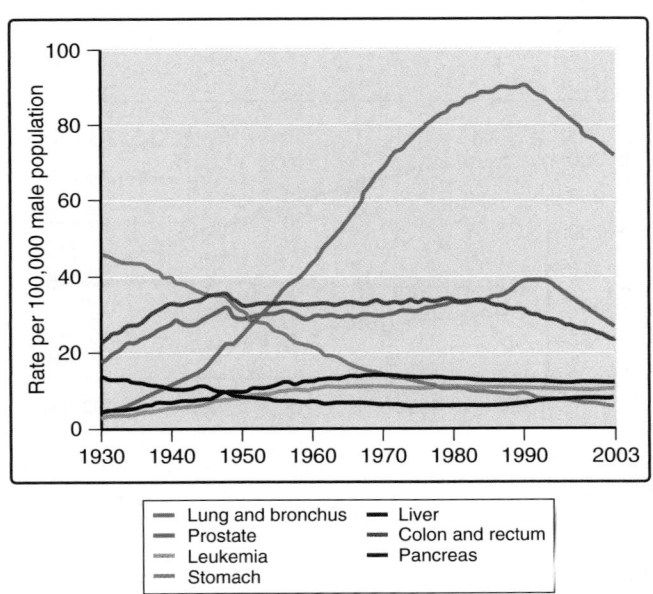

*Per 100,000 age-adjusted to the 2000 U.S. standard population.

FIGURE 216-3 Age-adjusted cancer death rates for males by anatomic site of the tumor for 1930 through 2003. *(From the American Cancer Society, Surveillance Research, 2007 and http://www-dep.iarc.fr/.)*

prostate (−18%), colorectal (−34%), and stomach cancers, whereas liver (+92%) cancer and leukemia death rates are stable or increasing (Fig. 216-3). Lung cancer is the greatest cause of cancer death among women, with almost twice the number of deaths attributed to breast cancer. Colorectal, pancreatic, and ovarian cancer are the next leading causes of cancer death among U.S. women. The mortality rate for lung cancer continues to rise for women (+133% since 1975), as do the death rates for hepatic (+57%), pancreatic (+10%), and ovarian cancers. The mortality rates for breast (−22%), colorectal (−39%), uterine, and stomach cancers are decreasing (Fig. 216-4).

In the 15 member states of the European Union, expected cancer deaths decreased by 9% from 1985 to 2000.[5] There were significant differences in cancer mortality rates between the European Union and the European Economic Area with the whole of Europe. For instance, the relative risk of death from stomach cancer for men and women was 1.71 for the whole of Europe and only 1.05 in western Europe, with a much higher risk in eastern Europe. This difference was also seen for laryngeal and lung cancer in men, although to a lesser degree. This trend was reversed for deaths from lung cancer among women, with western European women at increased risk for lung cancer, reflecting the increased smoking rate of women in western Europe. The risk of death from uterine and breast cancer was decreased among western European women. There was a slightly increased risk of death from prostate cancer in western European men and from lymphoma in both sexes.[5]

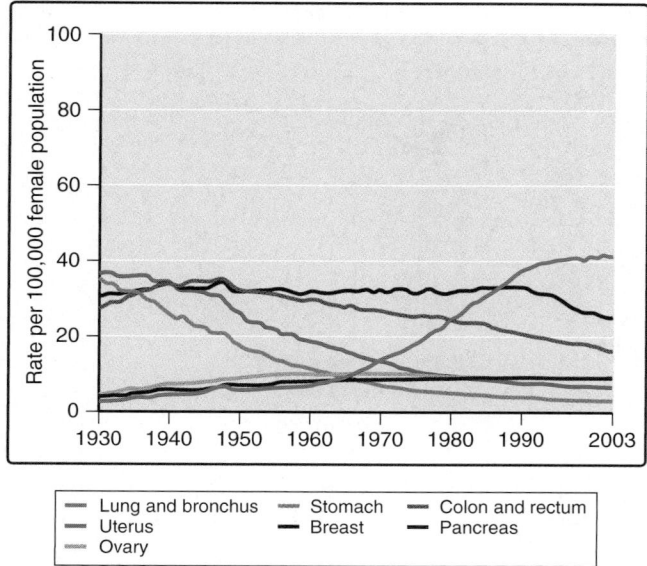

*Per 100,000 age-adjusted to the 2000 U.S. standard population. Uterus cancer death rates are for uterine cervix and uterine corpus combined.

FIGURE 216-4 Age-adjusted cancer death rates for females by anatomic site of the tumor for 1930 through 2003. *(From the American Cancer Society, Surveillance Research, 2007 and http://www-dep.iarc.fr/.)*

Common Errors

- Confusion of incidence and prevalence
- Definition of survivorship
  Anyone living with cancer as opposed to a long-term survivor
  Concept of "losing the battle" if disease recurs

The leading cause of cancer death is not always directly related to the cancer of greatest incidence. There is great variability between countries in the incidence and mortality of cancers. This is borne out by the case-fatality rate for cancers, which is the ratio of mortality to incidence each year (Fig. 216-5). Few patients with pancreatic, liver, esophageal, and lung cancers are alive at 1 year (case-fatality rate >0.8). Other common cancers, such as leukemia, myeloma, and stomach, brain, and nasopharyngeal cancer, have case-fatality rates between 60% and 80%. Colon cancer has a case-mortality rate of approximately 50%, and breast and prostate cancer approximately 30%.

PREVALENCE

The National Cancer Institute (NCI) estimates that on January 1, 2002, 10.1 million Americans were alive with a diagnosis of invasive cancer, a dramatic change over the past 30 years (see "Common Errors"). Of the 24 million people living with a cancer diagnosis approximately 3 years after the diagnosis, more than 50% live in North America and Europe, although only 40% of new cancer diagnoses occur in those continents. This situation in part reflects the earlier detection and the higher incidence of treatable tumors in those countries. Patients in resource-poor countries are more likely to develop less treatable

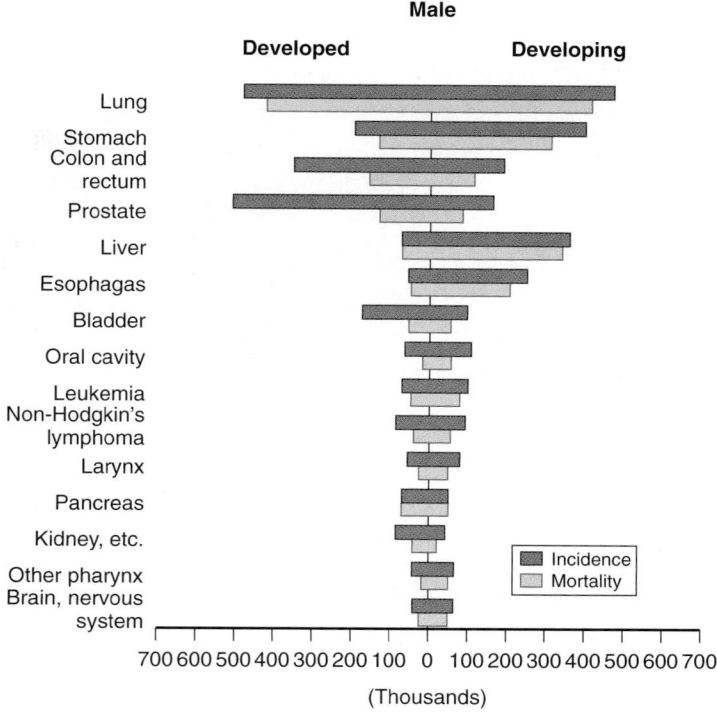

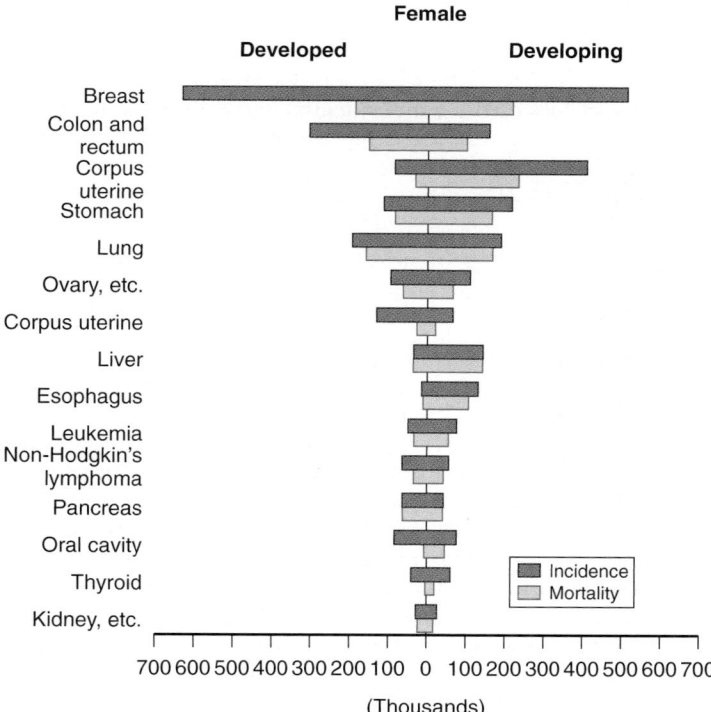

FIGURE 216-5 Ratio of mortality to incidence for various types of cancer in males and females.

cancers (i.e., hepatocellular, esophageal, and stomach cancers) and less likely to be alive at 3 years after the initial diagnosis (Fig. 216-6). This increased mortality results in differences in prevalence between regions. Although China represents approximately 20% of the world's new cancers diagnosed each year, it accounts for

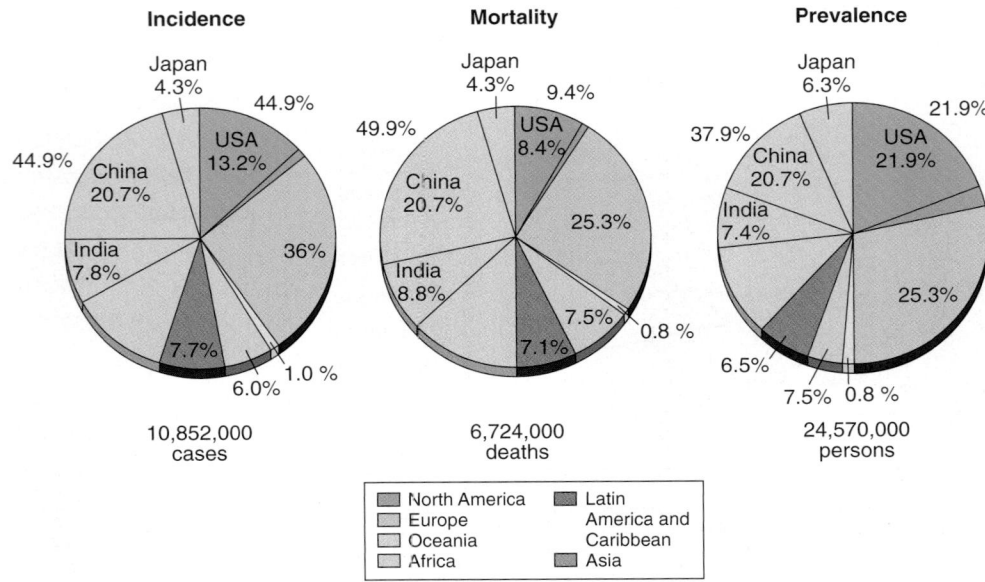

FIGURE 216-6   Worldwide distribution for the ratio of mortality to incidence of cancer.

almost 24% of the cancer deaths and only 13% of people living with a cancer diagnosis (see Fig. 216-6). North America accounts for 14% of new cancer diagnoses, 9% of deaths, and 21% of those living within 3 years of a cancer diagnosis.

SURVIVAL

For many, 5-year survival has been a measure of cure, although this does not meet the actual definition (see Box 216-1). However, 5-year survival is used to assess the impact of cancer care initiatives, showing a gradual improvement over time in many diseases, such as breast and colon cancers. U.K. data suggested that the greatest reduction in excess deaths was in uncommon cancers, whereas improvements in survival from lung, prostate, stomach, ovarian, and brain cancers were small, accounting for 33% of all cancers but only 11% of avoided deaths.[7] In the EUROCARE-3 study,[8] 5-year survival data demonstrated large differences in adult cancer survival between western and eastern Europe (Fig. 216-7), although both are lower than the rates in the U.S. Surveillance, Epidemiology, and End Results (SEER) program data. However, even within western Europe, the survival rates in the United Kingdom and Denmark for several major cancers are lower than for other western European countries. Survival is higher for women than men for most cancers. Similar statistics have been shown for specific diseases (e.g., colorectal cancer) for which the European population analyzed had a 3-year survival rate of 57% compared with the U.S. population's 3-year survival rate of 69%.[9]

DEVELOPMENTS AND CONTROVERSIES IN PALLIATIVE CARE

The increase in the number of national databases combined with better accuracy and completeness has allowed improved comparisons between countries and regional areas and analysis of influential factors. However few low- and middle-income countries have accurate or recent data about their cancer burden or major risk factors for cancer, consistent with generally poor vital and health statistics.[6] Global comparisons often rely on many assumptions in the statistical modeling that generates reports.

Cancer prevention remains the most effective method of decreasing the number of premature deaths, which is why the increased use of tobacco in resource-poor countries is a concern. Screening is another effective method. For example, screening can identify many breast cancer lesions with low malignant potential.[10]

Although some believe that cancer is not a problem in developing countries, the incidence of cancer will continue to rise in these countries with the increasing age of their populations, and common cancers will have high fatality rates.[6]

Poverty, not race, is a reason for survival differences among ethnic groups. Patients who receive equal treatment have equal survival rates.[11]

Clinically relevant improvements in cancer statistics are apparent around the world, particularly in resource-rich countries. Interpretation of these improvements requires an understanding of the terminology used. The major challenge is to bring these improvements to low- and median-resource countries.

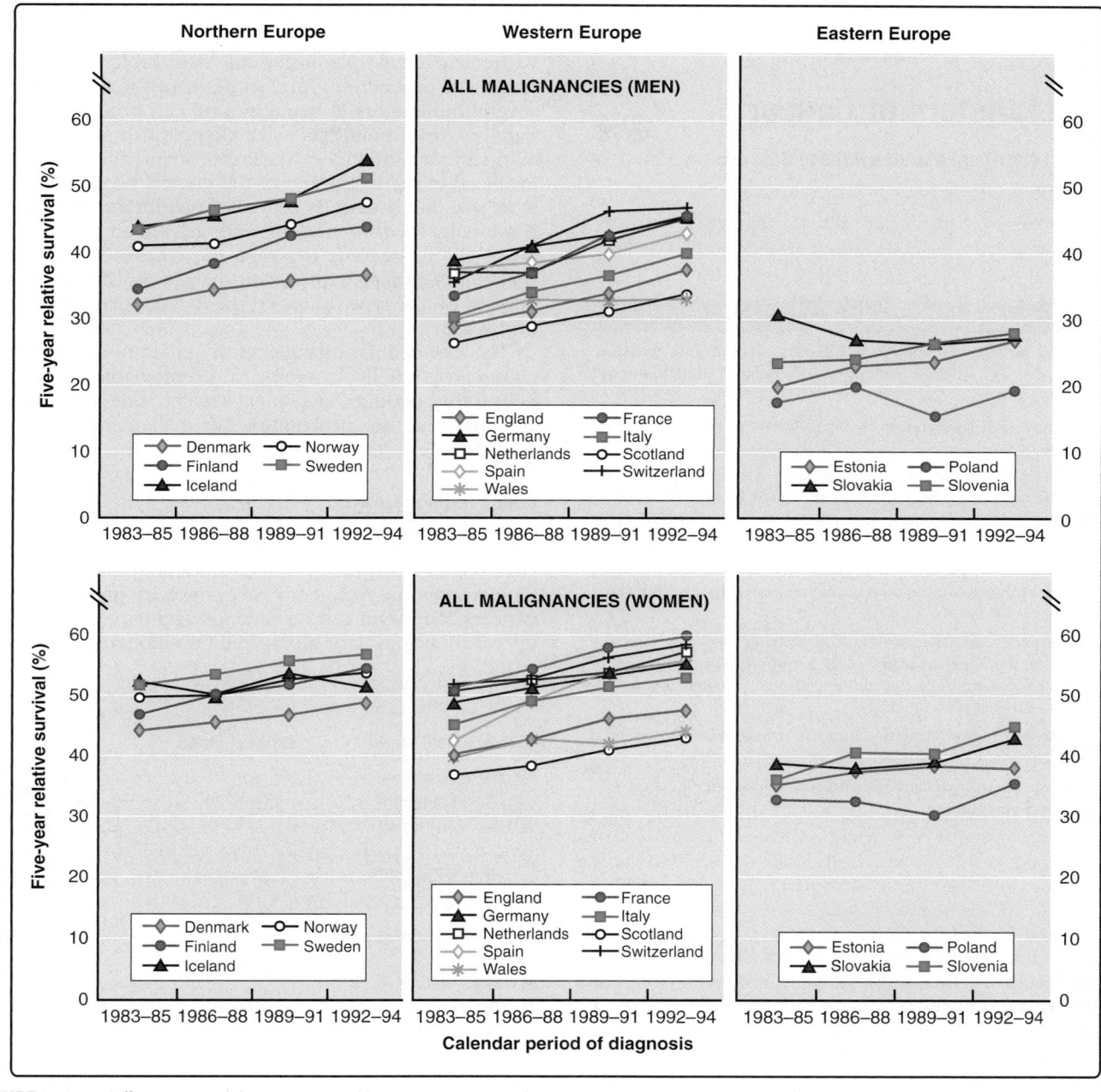

FIGURE 216-7   Differences in adult cancer survival between western and eastern European countries. *(Data from Coleman MP, Gatta G, Verdecchia A, et al. EUROCARE-3 summary: Cancer survival in Europe at the end of the 20th century. Ann Oncol 2003;14(Suppl 5):v128-v149.)*

REFERENCES

1. Parkin DM, Bray F, Ferlay J, Pisani P. Global cancer statistics, 2002. CA Cancer J Clin 2005;55:74-108.
2. Ravdin PM, Cronin KA, Howlader N, et al. The decrease in breast-cancer incidence in 2003 in the United States. N Engl J Med 2007;356:1670-1674.
3. Elmore J, Choe J. Breast cancer screening for women in their 40s: Moving from controversy about data to helping individual women. Ann Intern Med 2007;146:529-531.
4. Ferlay J, Autier P, Boniol M, et al. Estimates of the cancer incidence and mortality in Europe in 2006. Ann Oncol 2007;18:581-592.
5. Boyle P, Ferlay J. Cancer incidence and mortality in Europe, 2004. Ann Oncol 2005;16:481-488.
6. Sloan FA, Gelband H (eds). Cancer Control Opportunities in Low- and Middle-Income Countries. Washington, DC, National Academies Press, 2007.
7. Richards MA, Stockton D, Babb P, Coleman MP. How many deaths have been avoided through improvements in cancer survival? BMJ 2000;320:895-898.

8. Coleman MP, Gatta G, Verdecchia A, et al., EUROCARE-3 summary: Cancer survival in Europe at the end of the 20th century. Ann Oncol 2003;14(Suppl 5):v128-v149.
9. Ciccolallo L, Capocaccia R, Coleman MP, et al. Survival differences between European and US patients with colorectal cancer: Role of stage at diagnosis and surgery. Gut 2005;54:268-273.
10. Fryback D, Stout NK, Rosenberg MA, et al. The Wisconsin Breast Cancer Epidemiology Simulation Model. J Natl Cancer Inst Monogr 2006;36:37-47.
11. Freeman H, Chu K. Determinants of cancer disparities: Barriers to cancer screening, diagnosis, and treatment. Surg Oncol Clin North Am 2005; 14:655-669.

SUGGESTED READING

Parkin DM, Bray F, Ferlay J, Pisani P. Global cancer statistics, 2002. CA Cancer J Clin 2005;55;74-108.

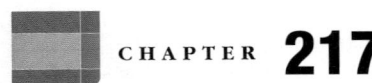

CHAPTER **217**

Natural History of Cancer

Francisco López-Lara Martín and Diego Soto de
Prado Otero

The natural history of cancer is an evolutionary process from the first significant mutation of the cell until the disease reaches its final stage. This process, which depends on the type of cancer and host factors, can last years or decades. The clonal-mutational theory of cancer posits that the genome of a stem cell is corrupted by mutations. Clonal expansion of this cell line results in changes in biological activity and the normal equilibrium of cellular growth and death.

Cancer is a multistage process that is driven by genetic and epigenetic alterations. Tumor initiation begins by mutations in cells caused by exposure to carcinogens. Two to six mutations are needed to initiate a tumor cell. Altered tumor cells may have a selective growth advantage compared with normal cells, and they may be less responsive to factors that regulate their shape and limit their growth. Accumulation of these mutated cells forms a tumor that can overcome the host's immune system and that grows locally, invading and destroying neighboring structures. Eventually, tumor cells detach, enter the lymph or bloodstream, and nest in lymph nodes or distant organs, where they reproduce the growth process of the original tumor. These new tumor foci, called secondary tumors or *metastases*, are characteristic of cancer and frequently kill the host by destroying the affected organs.

Most of the natural history of cancer is subclinical (Fig. 217-1); the tumor originates and grows for a long time without clinical manifestations detectable by ordinary diagnostic procedures. After some years, the tumor reaches several millimeters in diameter and can produce discrete signs or symptoms that make detection possible, which marks the beginning of the clinical stage. The tumor stays localized in the beginning of the clinical phase. At first, it is *in situ* and bound by the basal membrane. It expands, producing *local invasion*, and grows until it spreads regionally to become *locoregional cancer* and then *disseminated cancer* with distant metastasis. The symptoms depend on the type of tumor, the location, and the extent of disease.

The first cellular changes in the chain of events of carcinogenesis are likely simple and remediable and do not necessarily produce a clinical cancer, but as mutations accumulate, the probability of malignancy increases (Fig. 217-2).

CARCINOGENESIS

Carcinogenesis is the process of tumor development. A *carcinogen* is any factor that induces new cancers directly or increases the frequency or periodicity of spontaneous cancers. The term can be used for agents of any nature—chemical, physical, or biological. Carcinogens cause muta-

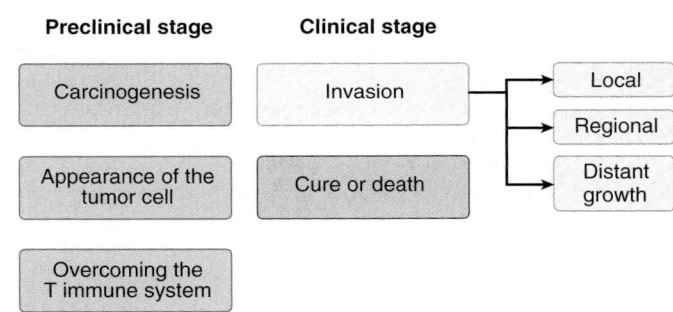

FIGURE 217-1   Stages of development of cancer.

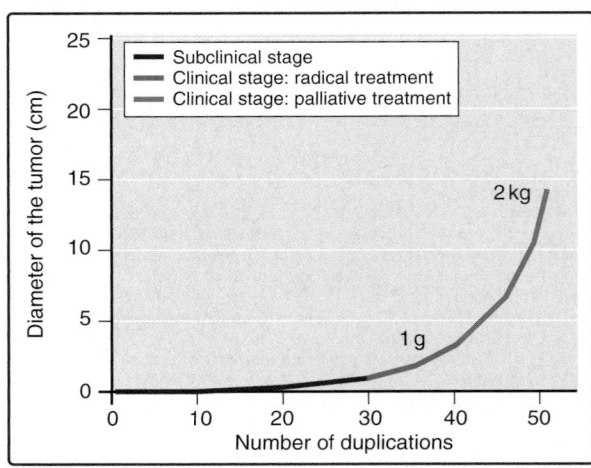

FIGURE 217-2   Growth curve of a hypothetical tumor.

tions in the base sequences of cellular DNA. The more mutations, the greater the carcinogenic effect. They are *transitions* if a pyrimidine base is changed for another or a purine base for another, *transversions* if a purine replaces a pyrimidine, *insertions* if bases are added, or *deletions* if bases are lost. These are unique changes in the DNA, but longer sequences at the genetic level also can undergo changes, which are more important. Consequences vary, but insertions and deletions usually have more drastic effects than transitions or transversions.

The first evidence that certain carcinogens could cause some cancers was provided by cases of cancers that were commonly associated with certain professions, such as cancer of the scrotum in chimney sweeps, which was described by Pott in 1775. We now recognize the carcinogenic power of many chemical, physical, and biological agents from the results of epidemiological studies that connected cancer in certain groups to exposure to agents, such as melanoma in light-skinned populations who were less protected from the effects of solar ultraviolet (UV) light. The agents that cause cancer are rarely endogenous.

Radiation

The absorption of ionizing radiation frees energy locally and causes biological damage, from punctiform mutations to DNA double-chain ruptures. The targets of ionizing radiation are the proto-oncogenes and tumor suppressor genes. The most common lesions are deletions of DNA fragments and chromosomal translocations. The risk of developing clinical cancer by radiation exposure is low because of its recessive character and little penetration, but repeated exposure and epigenetic influences can induce cancer, usually after a long latent period.

Sources of non-ionizing radiation include natural electrical and magnetic fields (e.g., thunderstorms) and artificial fields (e.g., power lines, appliances, industrial machinery). Although non-ionizing radiation has biological effects, its role as a carcinogen is controversial.

UV radiation is associated with cutaneous tumors, including melanoma and nonmelanoma cancers. It has less effect in blacks because of the protection provided by increased amounts of melanin. People who are more exposed to solar radiation, such as farmers and seamen, have a higher incidence of these cancers. The mechanism of cancer induction by UV light is direct action on DNA, where the energy forms pyrimidine dimers, which are lesions specific to this type of radiation. The cellular targets are the RAS and TP53 proteins. In addition to DNA actions, UV light has an immunosuppressant effect, especially on T-cell responses.

Chemical Agents

Genotoxic agents interact with the DNA to form stable complexes and produce mutations. Epigenetic agents facilitate cellular growth and tumor promotion. They produce *free radicals* (causing oxidative damage), and a chemical group that stimulates cellular hormonal receptors. Various pesticides, herbicides, and industrial products, such as polychlorinated biphenyls (PCBs), are chemical carcinogens.

Tobacco

Tobacco smoke contains nonvasoactive alkaloids responsible for tumors of the lung, mouth, laryngopharynx, esophagus, and bladder. The risk is related to the age smoking starts, the daily number of cigarettes, and the time that the person has been smoking. The carcinogenic alkaloids of tobacco act locally in areas of contact with the smoke (i.e., lung and upper aerodigestive tract) or become active metabolites during their elimination (i.e., bladder). Tobacco is linked to most lung cancers and is the main external risk factor. Tobacco combustion generates new carcinogens in the smoke inhaled. In heavy smokers (i.e., two or more packs per day), the risk for lung cancer is increased by a factor of 20 by the many toxic substances supplied to the lung, an organ with great absorption capacity.

Alcohol

Alcohol has mutagenic capacity that produces cancers, and the incidence of hepatocarcinoma among patients with cirrhosis of the liver is high. The risk of developing cancer increases if alcohol is combined with tobacco use, especially for cancers of the oral cavity and esophagus.

Diet

Diet is an important incidental agent because of the carcinogenic power of certain substances, such as too much fat and too many calories, and because of the absence of others, such as the lack of vegetables, which is related to colon cancer.

Asbestos

Inhalation of asbestos is associated with mesothelial and bronchial tumors. It seems that the fiber forms are responsible for the carcinogenic effects. For example, longer fibers are more carcinogenic.

Biological Agents

Viruses are responsible for many tumors in animals. Some produce human tumors when the viruses are randomly introduced in the genome of the affected cell and alter the proto-oncogenes or carry an oncogene in the viral genome. Frequently, viral infection alone is not enough to produce cancer, and other agents, such as aflatoxins, alcohol, and tobacco, are required.

The first tumor viruses discovered were the human retroviruses. Human T-lymphotropic virus types I and II (HTLV-I and HTLV-II) can cause leukemia and lymphoma; the human immunodeficiency virus (HIV) causes acquired immunodeficiency syndrome (AIDS); and human herpesvirus 8 causes tumors such as Kaposi's sarcoma. The Epstein-Barr virus predisposes infected persons to Burkitt's lymphoma and probably to nasopharyngeal carcinoma. Herpes simplex type 2 (HSV-2) is implicated in cancer of the cervix.

The hepatitis B virus (HBV), the agent that causes type B hepatitis, is implicated in hepatocarcinoma. The mechanism of transformation is indirect. The virus produces an autoimmune response that triggers hepatocellular regeneration, and the number of cells at risk for additional genetic lesions increases.

The principal human papillomaviruses (HPV) associated with cancer are types 16 and 18, which are found in 90% of cervical carcinoma cells. HPV infection also is associated with oral cancers. The carcinogenic mechanism involves interaction of gene products with cellular proteins involved in the regulation of cell division. Primary prevention is by vaccination against HPV.

Infection with *Helicobacter pylori* can contribute to the development of dyspepsia (i.e., heartburn, bloating, and nausea), gastritis (i.e., inflammation of the stomach), and ulcers in the stomach and duodenum. *H. pylori* infection is associated with stomach cancer and mucosa-associated lymphoid tissue (MALT) lymphoma. The mechanisms of cancer promotion involve enhanced production of free radicals, increased rates of host cell mutations, and alterations of host cell proteins such as adhesion molecules.

Environmental and Hereditary Factors

Epidemiological studies have shown that when people migrate to an area where a particular tumor is common, they and, more likely, the next generations are at higher risk for the tumor. Comparative population studies suggest that the new country's pattern prevails; the differences reflect lifestyle rather than ethnicity.

Oncogenes of great antiquity have been identified in certain racial groups. Hereditary cancers account for 5% to 10% of tumors in adults and a slightly higher percentage in children.

Stages of Carcinogenesis

The three consecutive stages of carcinogenesis are *initiation*, *promotion*, and *progression*. The carcinogens can be *partial* or *complete*, depending on their capacity to induce one or several stages. Two of the most common carcinogens, tobacco smoke and alcohol, are complete carcinogens. Carcinogenesis is a long, continuous, complex, and irregular process, with the tumor cell resulting from genetic instability and diverse environmental interactions.

The first event is *initiation*, which is the induction of one or several genetic mutations that favor cellular growth (Fig. 217-3). Initiation is not lethal for the cell in which it occurs, and it is induced by one or several carcinogens. Initiation is irreversible. Initiation is an obliged stage in environmental carcinogenesis, but not hereditary carcinogenesis, in which initiated cells preexist or genes are prone to increase cellular growth. In certain families, specific genes facilitate cancer, such as the oncogenes *BRCA1* and *BRCA2* in familial breast cancer. This pattern is uncommon, and more than 80% of cases are environmental in origin.

The second stage is *promotion*, in which the carcinogen acts on an initiated cell and activates latent and other mutations, which manifest as increased cellular growth. The promoting carcinogens (Tables 217-1 to 217-3) act in different ways: altering genetic expression, increasing DNA synthesis, increasing levels of superoxides and reac-

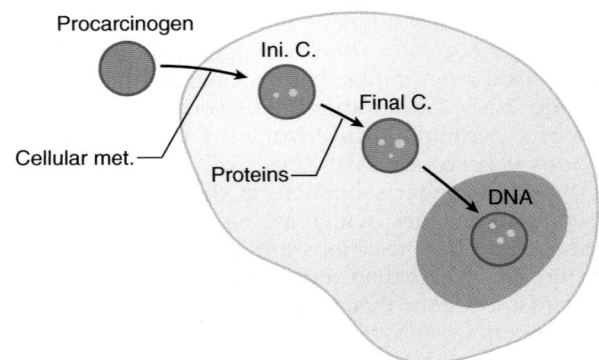

FIGURE 217-3 Initiation mechanism. Initiation is the irreversible induction of one or several cellular mutations that favor cellular growth. C., carcinogen; Ini., initial; met., metabolism.

TABLE 217-1	Chemical Carcinogens
CLASS	**EXAMPLES (EFFECT)**
LOCAL CARCINOGENS	
Polycyclic aromatic hydrocarbons	Benzanthracene (in mouse ear) Benzopyrene (in mouse ear and on skin) Methylcholanthrene (on skin)
Inorganic substances, including metals	Argon, nickel, beryllium, others
Plastics and subcutaneous metallic films	Physical carcinogens, no chemical effects
SYSTEMIC CARCINOGENS	
Azo dyes	Aminoazotoluene (caused hepatomas in rats fed with dyes) Dimethylaminoazobenzene
Heterocyclic amines	Acetylaminofluorene 2-Naphthylamine (bladder cancer in humans) Aminobiphenyl (bladder cancer in humans)
Nitrogenous compounds	Nitrosamines (industrial solvents cause hepatic and renal carcinomas in humans) Nitrites (transformation into nitrosamines and nitrosamides in the stomach, causing digestive tract cancers)
Drugs	Ethylcarbonate (sedative causes bladder cancer) Nitrogenous mustards Ethyleneamines Chloromethyl ether
Additives	Aflatoxin B1 (food preservative extracted from *Aspergillus flavus* mushroom causes hepatitis and hepatomas)
Inorganic substances, including metals	Nickel, chromium, beryllium

tive radicals, and inhibiting metabolic cooperation or the intercellular communication system. Promotion is a long and reversible stage, depending on the cellular environment, and hormones, food, and other host conditions that influence the process.

In *progression*, the cells have accumulated genetic mutations and epigenetic changes. The transformed tumor cells continue to grow and acquire the capacity for invasion and metastasizing.

TABLE 217-2 Human Carcinogens

PROMOTER	ASSOCIATED TUMOR
ENVIRONMENTAL AGENTS	
Asbestos	Bronchogenic carcinoma and mesothelioma
Halogenated hydrocarbons	Liver carcinoma
Phorbol esters	Esophageal cancer
Saccharin	Bladder cancer
Phenobarbital	Liver carcinoma
Hormones	Cancers of the breast, liver, vagina, and endometrium
CHEMICAL AGENTS	
Arsenic	Lung cancer
Asbestos	Lung cancer and mesothelioma
Aromatic amines	Bladder cancer
Benzene	Leukemia
Bis-chloromethyl ether	Lung cancer
Agents used in shoe manufacture and repair	Nasal carcinoma
Nickel refining	Lung cancer, nasal sinus carcinoma
Vinyl chloride	Hepatic angiosarcoma
Chrome and similar compounds	Lung cancer
Hematite mining (radon)	Lung cancer
Agents used in rubber industry	Leukemia, bladder cancer
Isopropyl alchohol manufacture	Paranasal sinuses carcinoma
Soot tar and oils	Skin, lung, bladder, and gastrointestinal cancers
Furniture manufacture	Nasal carcinoma
ASSOCIATED WITH LIFESTYLE	
Alcohol use	Cancers of the esophagus, liver, oropharynx, and larynx
Tobacco use	Cancers of the mouth, pharynx, larynx, lung, esophagus, and bladder
Aflatoxins	Liver cancer
Betel chewing	Oral cancers
Diet (excess fat, protein, or calories)	Cancers of the breast, colon, endometrium, prostate, and gall bladder
Late first pregnancy	Breast cancer
Low or no parity	Ovarian cancer
Sexual promiscuity	Cervical and breast cancer
ASSOCIATED WITH DIAGNOSIS OR TREATMENT	
Alkylating agents (chemotherapy)	Bladder cancer and leukemia
Inorganic arsenicals	Skin and liver cancers
Azathioprine (immunosuppressants)	Lymphoma, reticulosarcoma, skin cancer, and Kaposi's sarcoma
Chloramphenicol	Leukemia
Chlornaphazine	Bladder cancer
Diethylstilbestrol	Vaginal clear cell carcinoma
Estrogens	Hepatic carcinoma
Unopposed estrogen before and after menopause	Endometrial cancer
Prolactin	Breast adenocarcinoma
Before and after menopause	Endometrial cancer
Phenacetin	Carcinoma of the renal pelvis
Diphenylhydantoin	Lymphoma and neuroblastoma
Oxymetholone (anabolic steroids)	Liver cancer
Methoxypsoralen (plus ultraviolet light)	Skin cancer
Thorotrast	Hepatic angiosarcoma

REGULATION OF NORMAL AND TUMOR CELL GROWTH

Normal cellular proliferation occurs in a controlled manner according to the needs of the organism, from 0, as in the case of neurons that do not divide, to continuous proliferation of hematopoietic cells and intestinal epithelium. When growth is not required, the cells do not divide and stay quiescent (stage G_0). The cell cycle has four main stages:

G_1: The cell grows in size and mass from synthesis of all its components, and the stage lasts for 6 to 24 hours.
S: DNA is synthesized until duplicated, and this stage lasts for about 6 hours.
G_2: Over a period of about 3 hours, preparations are made for mitosis after replication of DNA has ended.
M: Mitosis lasts for about 1 hour.

The balance of proto-oncogenes, which are growth-promoting genes, and tumor suppressor genes determines activation or nonactivation of the cell cycle and therefore controls growth of the cell. Intercellular signals activate the proto-oncogenes and inactivate the suppressor genes if cellular growth is required, and vice versa. Other genes play a role, such as DNA repair genes, which rectify errors in nucleotides incorporated during DNA replication.

Cells do not live indefinitely. Some, such as muscle cells and neurons, have very long lives whereas others, such as hematopoietic cells, die within a few hours. Cell death can occur because of necrosis, action of toxic substances, accumulation of waste products, or other causes, but senescence is the usual cause. The number of cellular divisions has a limit. The telomeres on the ends of the chromosomes constitute a cellular clock. About 50 to 200 nucleotides are lost from the ends during each cell division, and eventually, cellular senescence occurs; this is when the programmed cell death, called *apoptosis*, occurs. Apoptosis is regulated by the *TP53* gene, which on detecting senescence or irreversible cellular damage produces tumor protein 53 (TP53), which triggers cell death. If only limited DNA damage is detected, apoptosis is not triggered by *TP53*, and the cell cycle stops in G_1, allowing the cell to repair the damage and continue the cycle.

Cell growth becomes dysregulated in tumor cells (Fig. 217-4). The mutations that deactivate the suppressor genes increase cellular proliferation. New mutations can inactivate DNA repair genes, allowing the replication errors to continue in descendent cells, and subsequent accumulated mutations transform the proto-oncogenes into growth-promoting oncogenes or produce new oncogenes, continuing the abnormal cell proliferation. If the mutations damage the TP53 system, apoptosis does not occur, and the tumor cells do not die, although they are damaged. In the late stages of progression, many tumor cells express an enzyme called telomerase, which extends the telomeres and avoids successive shortening of the chromosomes during cell division, evading apoptosis and further facilitating tumor growth.

Tumor cell growth progresses through the stages of hyperplasia, dysplasia, cancer in situ, invasive cancer, and metastasis. *Hyperplasia* occurs with the growth of apparently normal cells; in *dysplasia*, growth is transformed with the appearance of abnormal cells, caused by

TABLE 217-3 Angiogenesis Inhibitors in Clinical Trials

AGENT	CLINICAL TRIAL	MECHANISM
Marimastat	Phase III against pancreatic, breast, and lung cancer (small cells)	Synthetic inhibitor of MMPs
COL-3	Phase I/II against malignant brain tumors	Synthetic inhibitor of MMPs
Neovastat	Phase III against kidney and lung cancer	Natural inhibitor of MMPs
BMS-275291	Phase II/III, against advanced or metastatic lung cancer	Synthetic inhibitor of MMPs
Thalidomide	Phase I/II against advanced melanoma; phase II against Kaposi's sarcoma, gynecological sarcomas, glioblastoma, multiple myeloma, and liver, ovary, and prostate cancers (metastatic); phase III against lung, kidney, prostate cancer (nonmetastatic) and refractory multiple myeloma	Directly inhibits endothelial cells; unknown mechanism
Squalamine	Phase I against advanced cancers; phase II against ovary and lung cancer	Acts directly on endothelial cells, inhibiting the Na^+/H^+ exchange pump
Endostatin	Phase I against solid tumors	Direct inhibition of endothelial cells
SU5416	Phase I against advanced solid tumors of the head and neck, breast cancer (stage IIIB or IV), brain tumors (pediatric), ovarian cancer; phase I/II against acute myeloblastic leukemia; phase II against the von Hippel-Lindau disease, prostate cancer, multiple myeloma, mesothelioma; phase III against advanced colorectal cancer (metastasis)	Blocks the signal of VEGF receptors
SU6668	Phase I against advanced tumors	Blocks the signal of the VEGF, FGF, and PDGF receptors
Interferon-α	Phase II/III in pediatric patients with cancer associated with HIV, advanced multiple myeloma, recurrent and/or unresectable meningiomas, melanoma, renal carcinoma, hepatocellular carcinoma, non-Hodgkin's lymphoma, Hodgkin's disease, chronic myeloid leukemia, pancreatic adenocarcinoma	Inhibits the production of VEGF and bFGF
Anti-VEGF antibody	Phase I against solid tumors refractory to conventional treatment; phase II against metastatic renal cancer and advanced untreated colorectal cancer (combined with chemotherapy)	Monoclonal antibody directed against VEGF
EMD 121974	Phase I in HIV-positive patients with Kaposi's sarcoma; phase I/II against anaplastic glioma	Blocks integrin in endothelial cells
CAI	Phase II against ovarian and kidney cancers	Inhibits calcium influence
Interleukin-12	Phase I/II against Kaposi's sarcoma	Stimulates production of interferon-γ and IP-10
IM 862	Phase II against colon and rectal metastatic carcinoma; phase III against Kaposi's sarcoma	Unknown

FGF, fibroblast growth factor; bFGF, basic fibroblast growth factor; HIV, human immunodeficiency virus; IP-10, interferon-inducible protein 10; MMPs, matrix metalloproteinases; PDGF, platelet-derived growth factor; VEGF, vascular endothelial growth factor.
Data from the National Cancer Institute. Cancer trials. Available at http://cancertrials.nci.nih.gov (accessed March 2008).

nonrepaired degeneration and lack of maturation. The dysplastic cells proliferate and soon constitute the dominant cellular population. The accumulation of mutations turns the dysplastic cells into tumor cells. When the basal membrane contains the tumor, it is called *cancer in situ*, but when the tumor trespasses the membrane, it becomes *invasive*. The tumor becomes oblivious to the signaling system that normally inhibits growth, and it is capable of autonomously modifying the cellular environment by secreting cytokines and enzymes (e.g., proteases) that affect the basal membrane and the neighboring matrix. Changes in the tumor cell give it exceptional qualities, such as greater mobility, a capacity to adhere to matrices, or proteolytic power that favors local invasion and distant propagation. Compared with normal cells, the tumor cell has many growth and extension advantages, such as immortality, immaturity, autonomy, and the capacity to change the environment to its needs, including the formation of new blood vessels through the process of angiogenesis.

Evasion of the Cellular Immune System

The immune system is mediated by helper T lymphocytes (CD4); cytotoxic T lymphocytes (CD8), which directly lyse neoplastic cells, and natural killer (NK) cells and macrophages, which destroy tumor cells through secretion of cytokines such as interleukin-2 (IL2) and interferon-γ (IFN-γ).

In clinically detectable cancer, the tumor has escaped the immune system. Tumor evasion occurs through three mechanisms:

1. Lack of expression of tumor antigens: By reduction of their antigenic profile, or *masking*, tumor cells avoid lymphocytic recognition and tumor lysis.
2. Suppression of the immune response: Even with a competent immune system, the tumor can grow if it secretes immunosuppressant substances or induces a functional defect of the system, such as incapacity of humoral communication between T cells, lack of the appearance of specific T lymphocytes, or a defect in the secretion of cytokines.
3. High-speed tumor growth: Even if the immune system detects tumor antigens, its response can be slow compared with a fast-growing tumor.

Angiogenesis

Angiogenesis is formation of new vessels from preexisting vessels. It is a sequential process regulated by diverse

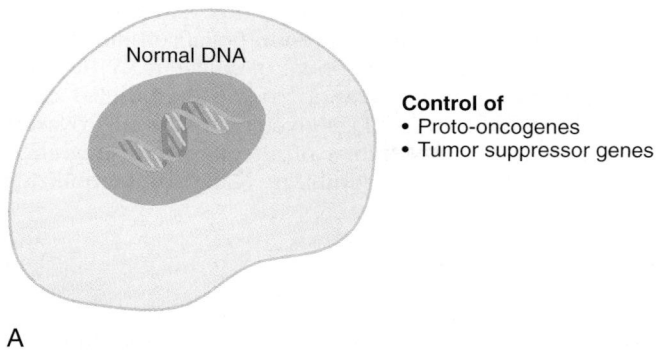

Control of
• Proto-oncogenes
• Tumor suppressor genes

A

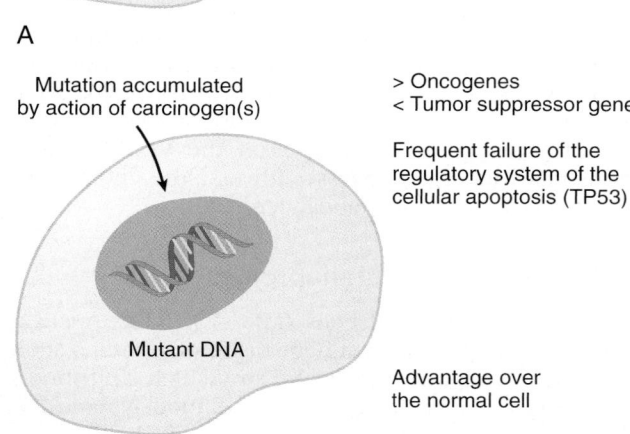

Mutation accumulated
by action of carcinogen(s)

> Oncogenes
< Tumor suppressor genes

Frequent failure of the
regulatory system of the
cellular apoptosis (TP53)

Advantage over
the normal cell

B

FIGURE 217-4   A, Regulation of the growth of a normal cell. **B,** Decontrol of growth of a tumor cell, with irreversible imbalance.

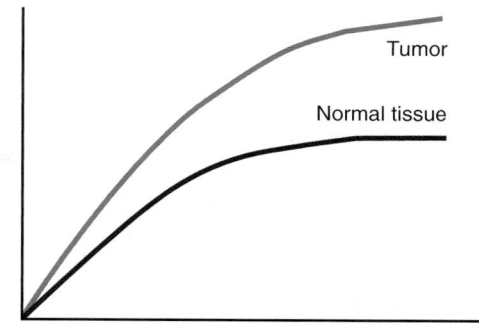

FIGURE 217-5   Gompertzian curves generated for growth of tumor and normal tissue.

factors that act on endothelial cells. After activation by proangiogenic stimuli, these cells degrade the extracellular matrix, migrate toward surrounding tissues, proliferate, and assemble to form new blood vessels. Angiogenesis is a normal mechanism in embryonic life and remains in adults in specific processes of growth and tissue recovery.

Amplified tumor growth increases the needs for waste elimination and supplies of oxygen and nutrients, which it can achieve by diffusion if the distance to the nearest capillary is small. When the tumor achieves a size of 1 mm, it needs its own vascular system. Tumor angiogenesis is necessary for tumor proliferation, local invasion and dissemination, and metastases. The process starts with secretion of tumor angiogenesis factor (TAF), which activates endothelial growth factor and the growth of new blood vessels. The neovessels have a thinner endothelium and are more permeable to tumor cells, which migrate easily through the vessels, reach the bloodstream, and nest in the capillary systems of the organs, developing metastatic growth and repeating the process of local invasion.

Various substances mediate the angiogenesis, such as certain proteases, interleukin-8 (IL8), prostaglandins, and growth factors. Some factors, such as angiostatin, inhibit angiogenesis, and the treatment of tumors with these inhibitors is being studied.

Dissemination: Development of Metastases

Cells lose their capacity for adhesion. Adhesion of cells to other cells and to the extracellular matrix is essential for

cellular differentiation, and destabilization favors dedifferentiation and invasive capacity. During this period, levels of the proteins for intercellular adhesion, such as cadherins or catenins, decrease. When normal cells lose adhesion, their growth is inhibited, but this does not happen to tumor cells. They lose the arrangement that normal cells have, instead forming irregular cellular conglomerates. The extracellular matrix is degraded. The main proteases that cause degradation of the matrix are metalloproteases (MMPs) and the serine proteases urokinase plasminogen activator (uPA) and tissue plasminogen activator (tPA).

Tumor cells can become mobile. After detaching from neighboring cells, the cells mobilize and displace to the vessels. They can move randomly (i.e., chemokinesis) or by responding to gradients (i.e., chemotaxis). The tumor cells can have amebic movement, similar to leukocytes.

Retention or extravasation of tumor cells occurs in the target organ. During metastases, the tumor cells must adhere to the vessel wall of a distant place and extravasate. Only 0.5% of the cells that reach a vessel are able to colonize, but a 1-cm tumor sends millions of cells into the bloodstream. The deposition of hematogenic metastases of various tumors is influenced by the tumor cells and by the host tissue microenvironment. For example, metastatic breast cancer cells express certain chemokines, and the main target organs for these tumor cells preferentially express their ligands.

Metastatic colonies grow. The tumor cells that settled in a distant organ start to proliferate if they receive cellular growth signals. When they grow, they must promote angiogenesis as the primary tumor did, thereby achieving local invasion and becoming capable of producing *secondary metastases*.

Macroscopic Tumor Growth

Tumor growth follows a gompertzian exponential model (Fig. 217-5). There is exponential growth in vitro and in vivo; it is fast in the beginning, and becomes slower as the tumor attains a larger size, tending to form a plateau that never completely arrives and that is fully achieved only in normal tissues. The inverse relation between the proliferative faction and tumor size characterizes this growth model. A small tumor has a large proportion of proliferative cells, and a big tumor has a small proportion of these cells. Ultimately, there is a disproportion between the

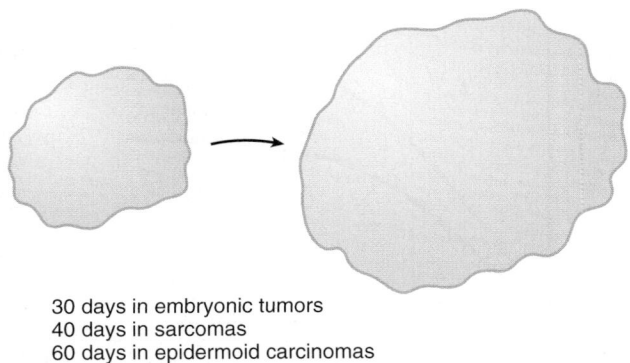

30 days in embryonic tumors
40 days in sarcomas
60 days in epidermoid carcinomas
90 days in adenocarcinomas

FIGURE 217-6 Time needed to double the tumor size.

tumor and vascular growth. In a large tumor, the smaller proliferative faction is well oxygenated because it is near the blood vessels, and the hypoxic or anoxic fraction becomes increasingly farther from the vessels as the tumor grows. Another parameter influencing tumor growth is differentiation; differentiated tumor cells grow less than undifferentiated cells, which translates into a smaller gradient on the growth curve.

The tumor duplication time is the time during which the tumor doubles in size. It is faster if the tumor is small and undifferentiated. An embryonal tumor duplicates in about 30 days, sarcomas in 40 days, epidermoid carcinomas in 60 days, and adenocarcinomas in about 90 days; these rates are approximate because the same pathological type of tumor grows at different speeds in different patients (Fig. 217-6).

Metastases grow at the same rhythm as the primary tumor but faster. They are smaller and have greater proliferative capacity, and they have survived antitumor treatments, which have selected therapy-resistant tumor clones. Tumor cells evolve through their mutations, and those surviving in clinically detectable cancer are the most resistant, impeding attempts to definitively control disseminated cancer.

DEVELOPMENTS IN TREATMENT

Angiogenesis Inhibitors

Angiogenesis plays a key role in the growth and dissemination of the malignant disease. Antiangiogenesis therapies are potential anticarcinogenic agents. In experimental animal model, inhibitors have produced impressive results in blocking the growth and dissemination of tumors, and they offer an alternative treatment for multidrug-resistant tumors that do not respond to conventional chemotherapy.

Amniogenesis inhibitors are thought to block cellular adhesion to activated endothelial cells and inhibit interactions between cellular adhesion molecules and their specific adhesion sites on the extracellular matrix. They can kill activated endothelial cells. They reduce the formation of tumor blood vessels and inhibit tumor growth and metastasis. Of the more than 300 angiogenic inhibitors, many are in clinical trials, and others are approved for clinical use (see Table 217-3).

Angiostatin, the first endogenous antiangiogenesis agent, inhibits migration of the endothelial cell and induces apoptosis. Endostatin, a fragment of collagen XVIII, inhibits proliferation and migration of the endothelial cells. Thrombospondin-1 (TSP-1), a glycoprotein of microvascular endothelial cells, inhibits proliferation and migration of the endothelial cell by inhibiting MMP-9 and mobilizing VEGF.

Growth Factor Antagonists

Growth factor antagonists act on growth factor synthesis, transport, or binding of the factor with the receptor. The only agent approved by the U.S. Food and Drug Administration (FDA) and the European Union is bevacizumab, a humanized monoclonal anti-VEGF antibody that bonds to and neutralizes all the isomorphs of the VEGF7. It has demonstrated its effectiveness with first-line chemotherapy for metastatic colorectal cancer.

Inhibitors of Matrix Metalloproteases

Microvascular endothelial cells (MECs) produce matrix, which is a complex environment made of proteins such as fibrinogen, collagen, and gelatin and which contributes to tissue support. The MEC system continuously remodels in response to physiological and pathological situations. MECs produce matrix metalloproteinases (MMPs) in response to angiogenic factors. The MMPs are a family of inducible enzymes that degrade extracellular matrix components, allowing cells to traverse connective tissue structures efficiently, and MMPs participate in MEC degradation. Specific tissue inhibitors of metalloproteinases (TIMPs) function as physiologic inhibitors of MMP activity. Several MMP inhibitors have been developed, and their effect on tumor growth and metastasis has been researched in animal models. They inhibit invasion, angiogenesis, and tumor growth, but they produce muscular and articular toxicity. In general, they act on the endothelial cell, block invasion of the MEC system, and act against the core of the primary tumor and metastatic foci.

Drugs Acting on Endothelial Cell Surface Markers

Integrins are a family of cell surface receptors expressed by activated endothelial cells, which interact with the extracellular microenvironment. They play a critical role in proliferation, regulation, migration, and survival of the cell. Disruption of integrins by monoclonal antibodies or cyclic peptides leads to TP53 activation and apoptosis of the endothelial cell. Integrin $\alpha_v\beta_3$ is important in the development and survival of the new vessels. Vitaxin, an anti-$\alpha_v\beta_3$ antibody, interferes with blood vessel formation by inducing apoptosis in newly generated endothelial cells.

Inhibitors of Signal Transduction of the Endothelial Cell

Angiogenesis is promoted by cytokines that attach to endothelial cell receptors and unleash a cascade of signals. Small molecules capable of inhibiting the transduction of endothelial cell signals have been developed. Examples include SU5416, a selective inhibitor of the KDR/Flk-1 tyrosine kinase and a potent inhibitor of tumor angiogenesis; SU101 (leflunomide), a platelet-derived growth factor receptor inhibitor; SU6668, a tyrosine kinase inhibitor of vascular endothelial growth factor receptor 2, fibroblast growth factor receptor 1, and platelet-derived growth factor receptor β; and ZD4190, an inhibitor of VEGF signaling. ZD1839 (Iressa) is an angiogenesis inhibitor that acts on the receptor of the epidermal growth factor receptor, inhibiting its phosphorylation and blocking its signal.

Other Angiogenesis Inhibitors

Several agents act on different targets from the ones previously described, and others have proven antiangiogenesis action, but their mechanism of action is unknown. Cyclooxygenase 2 (COX-2) inhibitors have aroused interest. Regular use of aspirin and other nonsteroidal anti-inflammatory drugs has been associated with decreased incidence of certain types of cancer. The cytoprotective effects of these drugs are particularly evident in colorectal cancer, with a 40% to 50% reduction in risk. NSAIDs appear to operate by inhibiting COX-2, an enzyme involved in several cancer-promoting processes. Results suggest that the effect is mediated by inhibition of angiogenesis, possibly by inhibiting production of VEFGR tyrosine kinase by endothelial cells. Other antiangiogenic agents, such as TNP-470, thalidomide, and inhibitors of angiotensin-converting enzyme, can be included in this group.

Carcinogenesis and Polymorphisms: Toward Individualized Treatment

Less than 10% of the entire human genome consists of functional DNA, composed of genes and regions implicated in transcriptional regulation and maintenance of chromosomal structure and integrity. Fifteen percent of the genome is moderately or highly repetitive, divided into repetitive DNA when individual repetition units are individually spread or satellite DNA when the units are in groups.

A polymorphic locus is a chromosome site with two or more identifiable allelic DNA sequences. The alleles or variants are such that the most common variant between them occurs in less than 99% of the total population. Polymorphisms include single nucleotide polymorphism (SNPs) and short tandem repeats (SRTs), which allow us to study specific phenotypes. The SNPs constitute the most important human genetic variant, occurring in an average density of 1 in 1000 nucleotides of a genotype in an average of 0.3 to 1 kilobase of the genome.

When polymorphisms are produced in genes that encode metabolic enzymes (e.g., cytochrome P450), proteins with different abilities to metabolize carcinogens are produced. The study of polymorphisms allows identification of genomic profiles associated with susceptibility to certain tumors. It can also predict response to drugs and help to tailor more individualized treatment. Polymorphisms serve as genetic markers; for example, microsatellites, which consist of a specific sequence of DNA bases or nucleotides that contain multiple tandem repeats, can be used in the study of families to identify genes associated with a disease.

The mapping of extensive collections of SNPs may help us perform large-scale genetic studies in humans. Genetic analyses are performed to determine the response to drugs in patients with lung cancer, colon cancer, or specific sarcomas; to individualize drug treatment; to improve therapeutic efficiency; and to minimize toxicity.

Gene Therapy: DNA Suppressor Genes

The *TP53* gene plays a fundamental role in tumor development; it is mutated in approximately 50% of tumors. It encodes the TP53 protein, a 53-kd nuclear phosphoprotein that regulates the cell cycle. The protein regulates transcription and modulates the cell cycle at the control points G_1/S and G_2/M, stopping cell growth for DNA repair or, if damage is irreparable, activating apoptosis. TP53 performs these cell cycle regulatory functions by means of p21 induction, an inhibitor of cell cycle progression, and proliferating cell nuclear antigen (PCNA) inhibition. Likewise, it induces transcription of DNA repair proteins. The protein TP53 is inactivated through kinase-dependent phosphorylation, nuclear exclusion by unknown mechanisms, and formation of complexes with the MDM-2 protein, which is encoded by a proto-oncogene inducible by the TP53. Mutation of a copy of the *TP53* gene along with deletion or inactivation of the allele causes the loss of function of the protein. The genetic mutation produces a protein with configuration changes, a longer life expectancy, and disorderly function.

Clinical trials of gene therapy using *TP53* have been promising, obtaining objective responses of 10% to 15% for tumors that are chemoresistant, such as lung cancer. Intratumoral injections of a normal *TP53* gene into these tumors use a retrovirus or adenovirus vector. These injections are being combined with chemotherapy and radiotherapy to determine whether gene therapy can increase sensitivity to conventional treatments.

CONCLUSIONS

Cancer results from a lack of control of cellular replication. One or several cells reproduce without regulation or purpose, autonomously, anarchically, uncontrollably, and accompanied by loss of apoptosis. New, pathological cells appear with the tendency to expand locally and move through the lymphatic system and bloodstream to distant sites, where this pattern of growth and expansion is repeated. The process destroys normal tissues and eventually kills the host.

The development of a malignant tumor requires complex interactions between exogenous and endogenous factors that produce genetic alterations. Advances in molecular biology have confirmed that the mutations in the genes that control cellular proliferation (i.e., proto-oncogenes, tumor suppressor genes, and DNA repair genes) cause cancer. Cancer is a genetic disease. Most cancers result from exposure to environmental agents responsible for the transforming mutations. Because of the homogeneity of the population, one individual may be 10 to several hundred times more susceptible to cancer than another, because people have different biological responses to a given dose of the causative agent. The study of DNA polymorphisms is especially important in determining the interactions between genes and exposure to external agents.

The principal exogenous carcinogens are chemicals such as alcohol, byproducts of tobacco combustion, and others found in foods and produced during industrial and occupational processes; physical promoters, such as ionizing radiation, ultraviolet light, and asbestos; and biological agents, such as viruses and *H. pylori* bacteria. The etiological agents act in multiple and sequential ways on normal cells, producing malignant transformation through a complex and progressive process of accumulation of mutations and sublethal errors that decontrol cellular growth by means of oncogenes and the inhibition of growth suppressor genes and DNA repair genes. Epigenetic factors promote expression of these alterations and proliferation of a clone of undifferentiated cells that are indifferent to apoptotic signals. The accumulation of mutations enables the tumor to modify the tissue environment to allow growth and local expansion and to gain qualities that favor dissemination. A defect in the immune system allows proliferation and continued growth until the tumor reaches a clinically detectable size.

Cancers invade surrounding tissues and develop distant metastasis. Invasion refers to direct migration and penetration of cancerous cells in neighboring tissues. Metastasis refers to the ability of cancerous cells to enter the lumens of lymphatic and blood vessels, circulate through the bloodstream, and invade normal tissues at other sites in the body. The tumor's invasive ability and metastatic ability require certain attributes, such as induction of neoangiogenesis, the capacity to adhere to and lyse the matrix, loss of intercellular unions, and cellular mobility.

Research on the mechanisms and inhibition of angiogenesis points to an important advance in cancer treatment by blocking tumor development and metastasis. The potential benefits of antiangiogenic cancer therapy demand further investigation to understand the mechanism of action, the most effective doses, and the possible secondary effects of available drugs and to develop adequate strategies to eradicate this lethal disease.

BIBLIOGRAPHY

1. Almendro V, Gascón P. Inhibitors of angiogenesis. Clin Transl Oncol 2006; 8:475-481.
2. Antonia S, Mule J, Weber J. Current developments of immunotherapy in the clinic. Current Opin Immunol 2004;16:130-136.
3. Aznar S, Lacal JC. Searching new targets for anticancer drug design The families of Ras and Rho GTPases and their effectors. Prog Nucleic Acid Res Mol Biol 2001;67:193-234.
4. Benhamou S, Sarasin A. Variability in nucleotide excision repair and cancer risk: A review. Mutat Res 2000;462:149-158.
5. Blackwood MA, Weber BL. BRCA1 and BRCA2: From molecular genetics to clinical medicine. J Clin Oncol 1998;16:1969-1977.
6. Boer J, Hoeijmakers JH. Nucleotide excision repair and human syndromes. Carcinogenesis 2000;21:453-460.
7. Canman CE, Lim DS. The role of ATM in DNA damage responses and cancer. Oncogene 1998;17:3301-3308.
8. Carnero A, Blanco C, Blanco F, et al. Exploring cellular senescence as a tumor suppressor mechanism. Rev Oncol 2003;5:249-265.
9. De Both NJ, Dinjens WN, Bosman FT. A comparative evaluation of various invasion assays testing colon carcinoma cell lines. Br J Cancer 1999; 81:934-941.
10. DeVita V, Hellman S, Rosenberg SA. Cancer: Principles and Practice of Oncology, 5th ed. Philadelphia: Lippincott-Raven, 1997.
11. DeClerck YA. Interactions between tumors cells and stromal cells and proteolytic modification of the extracellular matrix by metalloproteinases in cancer. Eur J Cancer 2000;36:1258-1268.
12. Ross DW (ed). Introduction to Oncogenes and Molecular Cancer Medicine. New York: Springer, 2003.
13. Dikic I, Szymkiewicz I, Soubeyran P. Signaling networks in the regulation of cell function. I. Cell Mol Life Sci 2003;60:1805-1827.
14. Druker BJ, Sawywers CL, Kantarjian H, et al. Activity of specific inhibitor of the Bcr-Abl tyrosine kinase in the blast crisis of chronic myeloid leukemia and acute lymphoblastic leukemia with the Philadelphia chromosome. N Engl J Med 2001;344:1038-1042.
15. Druker BJ, Talpaz M, Resta DJ, et al. Efficacy and safety of a specific inhibitor of the Bcr-Abl tyrosine kinase in chronic myeloid leukemia. N Engl J Med 2001;344:1031-1037.
16. Durker BJ, Tamura S, Buchdunger E, et al. Effects of a selective inhibitor of the Abl tyrosine kinase on growth of Bcr-Abl positive cells. Nat Med 1996; 2:561-566.
17. Evan GI, Vousden KH. Proliferation, cell cycle and apoptosis in cancer. Nature 2001;411:342-348.
18. Fearon EC. Human cancer syndromes: Clues to the origin and nature of cancer. Science 1997;278:1043-1058.
19. Fei P, El-Deiry WS. P53 and radiation responses. Oncogene 2003;22: 5774-5783.
20. Feinberg AP, Tycko B. The history of cancer epigenetics. Nat Rev Cancer 2004;4:143-153.
21. Finn O. Cancer vaccines: Between the idea and the reality. Nat Rev Immunol 2003;3:630-641.
22. Garret MD, Workman P. Discovering novel chemotherapeutic drugs for the third millennium. Eur J Cancer 1999;14:2010-2030.
23. Greten TF, Jaffee EM. Cancer vaccines. J Clin Oncol 1999;17:1047-1060.
24. Haber JE. Gatekeepers of recombination. Nature 1999;398:665-667.
25. Hellstrom K, Hellstrom I. Therapeutic vaccination with tumor cells that engage CD137. J Mol Med 2003;81:71-86.
26. Henning W, Sturzbecher HW. Homologous recombination and cell cycle checkpoints: Rad51 in tumour progression and therapy resistance.Toxicology 2003;193:91-109.
27. Holland JF, Frei E III, Bast R, et al. Cancer Medicine, 4th ed. Baltimore: Williams & Wilkins, 1997.
28. Hsu F, Caspar C, Czerwinski D, et al. Tumor specific idiotype vaccines in the treatment of patients with B-cell lymphoma—long term results of a clinical trial. Blood 1997;88:3129-3135.
29. Jaffe LF. Epigenetic theories of cancer initiation. Adv Cancer Res 2003;90:209-230.
30. Joensuu H, Roberts PJ, Sarlomo-Rikala M, et al. Effect of the tyrosine kinase inhibitor STI571 in patient with a metastatic gastrointestinal stromal tumor. N Engl J Med 2001;344:1052-1056.
31. Karran P. DNA double strand repair in mammalian cells. Curr Opin Genet Dev 2000;10:144-150.
32. Khanna K. Cancer risk and the ATM gene: A continuing debate. J Natl Cancer Inst 2000;92:795-802.
33. Khorasanizadeh S. The nucleosome: From genomic organization to genomic regulation. Cell 2004;116:259-272.
34. Lieber MR, Ma Y, Pannicke U, Schwarz K. Mechanism and regulation of human non-homologous DNA end-joining. Nat Rev Mol Cell Biol 2003;4: 712-720.
35. López-Guerrero JA. Significado oncológico y biológico de las alteraciones moleculares de p53 en cáncer humano. Oncologia 1997;20.
36. López-Lara F, Gonzalez C, Santos JA, Sanz A. Manual de Oncología Clínica. Valladolid, Spain: Secretariado de Publicaciones de la Universidad de Valladolid, 1999.
37. Ma BB, Bristow RG, Kim J, Siu LL. Combined-modality treatment of solid tumors using radiotherapy and molecular targeted agents. J Clin Oncol 2003;21:2760-2776.
38. Muñoz A. Cáncer. Genes y nuevas terapias. Madrid: Hélice, 1977.
39. Organización Panamericana de la Salud. Clasificación Estadística Internacional de Enfermedades y Problemas Relacionados con la Salud (CIE-10), 10th ed, vol 1. Publicación científica no. 554. Washington, DC: Organización Panamericana de la Salud, 1995.
40. Powell SN, Kachnic LA. Roles of BRCA1 and BRCA2 in homologous recombination, DNA replication fidelity and the cellular response to ionizing radiation. Oncogene 2003;22:5784-5791.
41. Ramirez de Molina A, Rodriguez-Gonzalez A, Lacal JC. From Ras signaling to ChoK inhibitors: A further advance in anticancer drug design. Cancer Lett 2004;206:137-148.
42. Ribas A, Butterfield L, Glaspy J, Economou J. Current developments in cancer vaccines and cellular immunotherapy. J Clin Oncol 2003;12: 2415-2432.
43. Rubin P. Oncología Clínica, 8th ed. Madrid: Elsevier España, 2002.
44. Seymour L. Novel anti-cancer agents in development: Exciting prospects and new challenges. Cancer Treat Rev 1999;25:301-312.
45. Stampfer MR, Yaswen P. Culture models of human mammary epithelial cell transformation. J Mammary Gland Biol Neoplasia 2000;5:365-378.
46. Santos-Rosa H, Caldas C. Chromatin modifier enzymes, the histone code and cancer. Eur J Cancer 2005;41:2381-402.
47. Valerie K, Povirk LF. Regulation and mechanisms of mammalian double-strand break repair. Oncogene 2003;22:5792-5812.
48. Van Oosterom AT, Judson I, Verweij J, et al. STI571, an active drug in metastatic gastrointestinal stromal tumors (GIST): An EORTC phase I study. Proc Am Soc Clin Oncol 2001;20:1a.
49. White MK, McCubrey JA. Suppression of apoptosis: Role in cell growth and neoplasia. Leucemia 2001;15:1011-1021.

50. Wierda W, Cantwell M, Woods S, et al. CD40-ligand (CD154) gene therapy for chronic lymphocytic leukemia. Blood 2001;96:2917-2924.
51. Woods CG. DNA repair disorders. Arch Dis Child 1998;78:178-184.
52. Wyllie AH. Apoptosis: An overview. Br Med Bull 1997;53:451-465.
53. Yang J, Xu ZP, Huang Y, Hamrick HE, et al. ATM and ATR: Sensing DNA damage. World J Gastroenterol 2004;10:155-156.

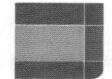

CHAPTER **218**

Principles of Medical Oncology

Imke Strohscheer

KEY POINTS

- The use of targeted therapy is a paradigm change in medical oncology.
- Knowledge of tumor biology is important for understanding chemotherapy.
- Only a few tumors can be cured when metastatic.
- Tumor staging is important for planning therapy and estimating prognosis.
- Chemotherapy can be administered in neoadjuvant, curative, and palliative settings.

TABLE 218-1 Five-Year Cancer Survival Rates for Three Periods

CANCER TYPE	1974-1976 (%)	1983-1985 (%)	1995-2001 (%)
All cancers	50	53	65
Prostate	67	75	100
Testis	79	91	96
Melanoma	80	85	92
Breast	75	78	88
Hodgkin's disease	71	79	85
Endometrium	88	83	84
Bladder	73	78	82
Cervical	69	69	73
Larynx	66	67	66
Kidney	52	56	65
Rectum	49	55	65
Colon	50	58	64
Non-Hodgkin's lymphoma	47	54	60
Leukemia	34	41	48
Ovary	37	41	45
Brain	22	27	33
Stomach	15	17	23
Lung	13	14	15
Esophagus	5	8	15
Pancreas	3	3	4

Adapted from Ozols RF, Herbst RS, Colson YL, et al. Clinical cancer advances 2006: Major research advances in cancer treatment, prevention, and screening—a report from the American Society of Clinical Oncology. J Clin Oncol 2007;1:146-162.

Cancer is one of the most common diseases in the world. More than 20 million people are living with cancer, and by 2020, there will be an estimated 30 million. In 2030, cancer is expected to be the main cause of death of people younger than 85 years in developed countries. With modern therapeutic approaches, 5-year survival rates have improved for some cancer subtypes, even as advanced and overall survival rates have increased over the past 30 years (Table 218-1). Many cancers are still associated with poor outcomes.

Oncological treatment involves surgery, radiotherapy, chemotherapy, hormone therapy, and targeted molecular therapies. Usually, these therapeutic options are combined. Despite progress in prevention and screening for cancer, more than 50% of cancer patients develop metastatic disease, and most have incurable disease. In the past 15 years, remarkable progress has been made in clinical cancer treatment. Some malignancies that have been hard to treat are responding to newer anticancer therapies. In 2005, the American Society of Clinical Oncology (ASCO) decided to publish a report every year to highlight advances in oncological therapy.[1]

BIOLOGICAL BASIS FOR CANCER TREATMENT

Tumor Growth and the Cell Cycle

To use cytotoxic drugs rationally, it is essential to understand the biological basis of cancer. Tumor growth behav-

ior correlates with cancer cell burden and depends on several parameters and changes over time. The Gompertz equation[2] describes the growth rate in relation to tumor size. The growth rate decelerates when the tumor becomes larger (II on the graph) (Fig. 218-1). Large tumors have less blood supply, resulting in cellular hypoxia and decreased nutrition. This state leads to cell death and tumor necrosis (III on the graph). The chemosensitivity of tumors is affected by the proportion of actively dividing cells, because chemotherapy is most effective against proliferating cells. This means that tumors with a high proliferation rate usually are very chemosensitive. Typical examples are high-grade lymphomas and acute leukemias. Most tumors that grow slowly are resistant to chemotherapy. According to the gompertzian model, a low tumor burden can be eliminated by cytotoxic agents.

Another important factor is the cell cycle. It is divided into five phases. G_1 phase is the first gap phase. This is necessary to produce enzymes for the DNA synthesis. The S phase is the synthesis phase, in which DNA is duplicated. The G_2 phase is the second gap phase, in which RNA and specialized proteins are synthesized. Cell division occurs in the M phase, the mitosis phase of the cell cycle. The G_0 phase is the resting phase. Cell division is not activated, but several stimuli can induce the cell to return to the cell cycle from the G_0 phase. In this phase, cells repair DNA damages.

Cytotoxic drugs are most effective against cells in the active phases of the cell cycle. In the G_0 phase, tumor cells

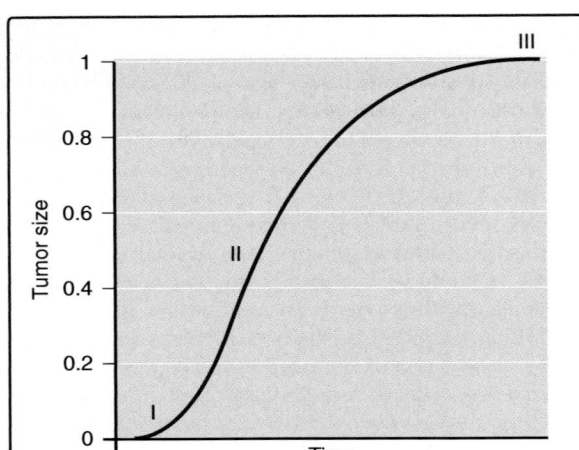

FIGURE 218-1   Gompertzian model of tumor growth in relation to tumor size. The initial growth rate (I) decelerates when the tumor becomes larger (II). Large tumors have less blood supply, resulting in cellular hypoxia and decreased nutrition, which leads to cell death and tumor necrosis (III).

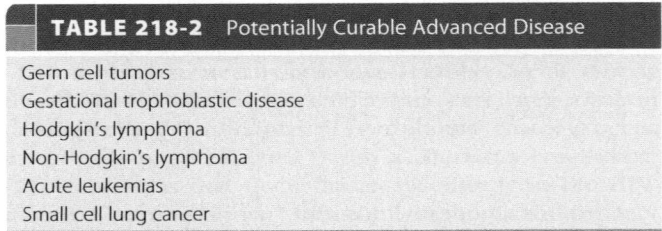

TABLE 218-2   Potentially Curable Advanced Disease
Germ cell tumors
Gestational trophoblastic disease
Hodgkin's lymphoma
Non-Hodgkin's lymphoma
Acute leukemias
Small cell lung cancer

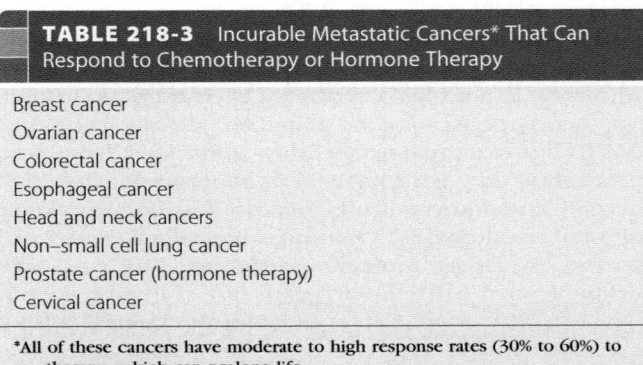

TABLE 218-3   Incurable Metastatic Cancers* That Can Respond to Chemotherapy or Hormone Therapy
Breast cancer
Ovarian cancer
Colorectal cancer
Esophageal cancer
Head and neck cancers
Non–small cell lung cancer
Prostate cancer (hormone therapy)
Cervical cancer

*All of these cancers have moderate to high response rates (30% to 60%) to therapy, which can prolong life.

are mostly insensitive to chemotherapy. The proportion of cells active in the cell cycle is the *growth fraction*. Normal tissue has a growth fraction of 20% to 30%, and most tumors have a higher growth fraction. The growth fraction is an important parameter for estimating chemosensitivity, because tumors with a high growth fraction respond better to cytotoxic agents. Bone marrow and epithelial cells typically have high growth fractions, and they are subject to the worst side effects (i.e., bone marrow suppression, mucositis, and diarrhea). Some cytotoxic drugs, such as 5-fluorouracil, cytosine-arabinoside, and methotrexate, act specifically in the S phase of the cell cycle. Etoposide, vinca alkaloids, and taxanes are active in the G_2/M phase. Some cytotoxic agents are cell cycle independent.[3]

Drug Resistance

Some types of cancer are resistant to cytotoxic drugs, and some tumors that are originally sensitive to chemotherapy develop resistance during therapy. The Goldie-Coldman random mutation hypothesis[4] suggests that one of the main reasons for developing resistance is spontaneous mutations in cancer cell lines. This depends on the tumor burden; the larger the tumor cell mass, the greater the probability for mutations. Combinations of cytotoxic agents or a change in the drug regimen can help to overcome resistance.

Pharmacological resistance mechanisms include defective cellular transport of drugs. Drug efflux can be increased by proteins (e.g., P-glycoprotein, multidrug-resistance proteins), or drug influx can be decreased (e.g., reduced levels of folate carrier). A cytoplasmic drug can be inactivated intracellularly by a multidrug-resistant protein acting as glutathione. Alterations in the target enzymes thymidylate synthase or dihydrofolate reductase are the most described resistance mechanisms for 5-fluorouracil.

Another mechanism is direct mutation of the target (e.g., tubulin, topoisomerase II). For most cytotoxic drugs,

theories about special drug resistance exist.[5] Some mechanisms are independent from the primary target or cytotoxic agent. DNA repair by proteins such as O^6-alkyl-guanine-DNA alkyltransferase, nucleotide excision repair gene, or mismatch repair occurs during the G_0 phase. One reason for unsuccessful cancer treatment is failure of programmed cell death, or *apoptosis*. Normal cell death is avoided by functional loss of the *TP53* tumor suppressor gene, and imbalances in the BCL2 family of proteins (i.e., BCL2 and BCL2L1 [formerly designated BCL-XL]) that have antiapoptotic effects.[6]

Chemosensitivity of Cancer

The response to chemotherapy correlates with the primary chemosensitivity of cancers. Chemosensitivity depends on the histological type, growth fraction, grade of tissue differentiation, tumor burden, and the various mechanisms of drug resistance. The data regarding chemosensitivity are empirical and result from clinical trials.[7] Few cancers are curable when advanced (Table 218-2). Many cancers have a moderate response to chemotherapy or hormone therapy (Table 218-3), which can prolong life. Some cancers are hard to treat, and these tumors have response rates between 10% and 30% (Table 218-4).

GENERAL PRINCIPLES OF MEDICAL ONCOLOGY

Standard of Care

The ASCO defines quality of cancer care as follows[8]:

1. Diagnosis and staging: selection and proper application of diagnostic testing and interpretation to maximize accurate diagnosis and tumor staging
2. Initial therapeutic management: selection and proper application by clinicians of treatment that optimizes outcomes

3. Management of treatment toxicity: selection and proper application by clinicians of evidence-based processes of care that minimize adverse effects from treatments

4. Referrals and coordination of care: arrangement for appropriate referrals and the timely sharing of information among involved clinicians

5. Psychosocial support: support by clinicians who are aware of the patient's significant emotional, social, or financial needs and who provide appropriate assistance or referrals

6. Patient preferences and inclusion in decision making: inclusion by clinicians who respect the patient's choices about care and who involve the patient whenever possible in choosing tests and treatment

7. Surveillance after initial therapy: selection and proper application by clinicians of diagnostic tests to detect recurrence of disease or late complications of therapy

Tumor Staging

For planning and evaluation of rational anticancer treatment, excellent tumor staging is essential. Staging is needed to evaluate tumor localization and burden to design an optimal therapeutic strategy, and staging is required to identify parameters that may influence the therapeutic response, such as tumor size, biological markers, and other biochemical factors.

Solid Tumor Staging Systems

The TNM system is most commonly used for staging solid tumors.[9] It is based on the extent of the tumor (T) for every organ system (Table 218-5), the degree of spread to the lymph nodes (N), and the presence of metastasis (M). A number is added to each letter to indicate the size or extent of the tumor and the extent of spread. Beyond these terms, each lesion is described by four classifications:

1. The clinical classification (cTNM) is based on clinical assessment before the first treatment using physical examination, radiological methods, endoscopy, biopsy, and surgical exploration.

2. The pathological classification (pT, pN, pM) provides additional data for estimating prognosis and calculating outcome.

3. The retreatment classification (rTNM) is used when relapse of malignant disease after a first treatment and a disease-free interval occurs and therapy is planned.

4. For cancer of an unknown primary (CUP), staging is based on clinical suspicion of the primary site.

Histological Classification

The World Health Organization International Histological Classification of Tumors is used to describe the histopathological type of a tumor (Fig. 218-2). The histological grade (G) is a qualitative assessment of malignant differentiation. It ranges from most differentiated (grade 1) to undifferentiated (grade 4):

TABLE 218-4 Incurable Metastatic Cancers* with Low Response Rates to Chemotherapy

Sarcoma
Gastric cancer
Hepatocellular cancer
Biliary cancer
Kidney cancer
Melanoma
Mesothelioma
Thyroid cancer
Most previously treated cancers

*All of these cancers have therapeutic response rates between 10% and 30%.

TABLE 218-5 A Primary Tumor (T)

TUMOR SIZE (T)	
TX	Primary tumor cannot be evaluated
T0	No evidence of primary tumor
Tis	Carcinoma in situ (early cancer that has not spread to neighboring tissue)
T1-T4	Size and/or extent of the primary tumor

REGIONAL LYMPH NODES (N)	
NX	Regional lymph nodes cannot be evaluated
N0	No regional lymph node involvement (no cancer found in the lymph nodes)
N1-N3	Involvement of regional lymph nodes (number and/or extent of spread)

DISTANT METASTASIS (M)	
MX	Distant metastasis cannot be evaluated
M0	No distant metastasis (cancer has not spread to other parts of the body)
M1	Distant metastasis (cancer has spread to distant parts of the body)

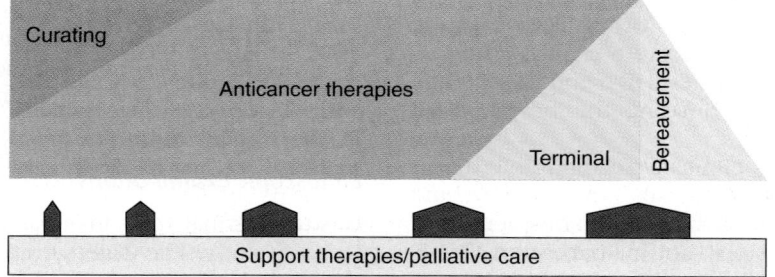

FIGURE 218-2 World Health Organization (WHO) scheme for palliative care *(From http://www.cancer.gov/cancertopics/factsheet.)*

GX: Grade cannot be assessed
G1: Well differentiated
G2: Moderately differentiated
G3: Poorly differentiated
G4: Undifferentiated

Residual Tumor Classification

After primary treatment (mainly surgery), a system exists to describe residual tumor mass:

RX: Presence of residual tumor cannot be assessed
R0: No residual tumor
R1: Microscopic residual tumor
R2: Macroscopic residual tumor

Staging of Gynecological Cancer

Gynecological tumors may be staged by the International Federation of Gynecology and Obstetrics (FIGO) system, which defines five stages. Stage 0 is carcinoma in situ. Stage 1 describes a strictly localized tumor, and stages 2 through 4 describe tumors with different degrees of extension and involvement of neighboring structures. For some cancers, the main stages are subdivided into A, B, and C classifications.

Staging of Lymphatic Cancer

Cancers of the lymphatic system (e.g., non-Hodgkin's lymphoma, Hodgkin's disease) are staged by the Ann Arbor classification:

Stage I: Involvement of a single lymph node or a single extralymphatic organ or site (IE)

Stage II: Involvement of two or more lymph node regions on the same side of the diaphragm (II) or localized involvement of an extralymphatic organ or site (IIE)

Stage III: Involvement of lymph node regions on both sides of the diaphragm (III) or localized involvement of an extralymphatic organ or site (IIIE) or spleen (IIIS), or both (IIIES)

Stage IV: Diffuse or disseminated involvement of one or more extralymphatic organs with or without associated lymph node involvement

Identification of the presence (B) or absence (A) of symptoms should be documented with each stage: A, asymptomatic; B, fever, sweats, and weight loss of more than 10% of body weight.

Clinical Assessment

Performance Status and Clinical Examination

The Eastern Cooperative Oncology Group (ECOG) scale and the Karnofsky index can be used to evaluate the performance state of a patient (Tables 218-6 and 218-7). The ECOG score is better for estimating the prognosis of patients with lung cancer.[7]

The examination reveals clinically recognizable tumor features, which include number, size, consistency, and localization of palpable lymph nodes; hepatosplenomegaly; ascites and other effusions; and palpable and visible tumor sites or malignant wounds. Clinical assessment also evaluates symptoms such as pain, weight changes, fever,

TABLE 218-6 Eastern Cooperative Oncology Group Performance Status Scale

SCORE	DESCRIPTION
0	Fully active; able to carry on all predisease activities
1	Restricted in physically strenuous activity but ambulatory and able to carry out work of a light or sedentary nature (e.g., light house work, office work)
2	Ambulatory and capable of all self-care but unable to carry out any work activities; up and about more than 50% of waking hours
3	Capable of only limited self-care; confined to bed or chair more than 50% of waking hours
4	Completely disabled; cannot perform any self-care; totally confined to bed or chair
5	Dead

TABLE 218-7 Karnofsky Performance Scale

SCORE	DESCRIPTION
100	Able to work; normal; no complaints; no evidence of disease
90	Able to carry on normal activity; minor symptoms
80	Normal activity with effort; some symptoms
70	Independent; not able to work; cares for self; unable to perform normal activities
60	Moderately disabled; dependent; requires considerable assistance and frequent care
50	Requires considerable assistance and frequent medical care
40	Disabled, dependent; requires occasional assistance; cares for most needs
30	Severely disabled; hospitalization necessary; death not imminent
20	Very sick; hospitalization necessary; active supportive treatment needed
10	Moribund; fatal processes are rapidly progressing

loss of appetite, fatigue, breathlessness, or cough. Findings should be well documented, because it can be the easiest way to evaluate the course of disease.

Radiological Studies

Radiological investigations identify the site and extension of disease or metastasis. Standard procedures are contrast-enhanced computed tomography (CT) and magnetic resonance imaging (MRI). The diagnostic value of each method depends on the cancer type and tumor localization. Sometimes, endosonographic methods are more sensitive. ^{18}F-fluorodeoxyglucose positron emission tomography (FDG-PET) reveals aspects of tumor function and enables metabolic measurements.[10] It helps to differentiate normal from malignant tissue. Radionucleotide imaging is important for identification of bone metastases and new endocrinic tumors.

Endoscopic Examinations

Gastrointestinal tract malignancies are mainly diagnosed by endoscopy. The diagnostic accuracy of gastrointestinal endoscopy is 90% to 95%. Bronchoscopy often is necessary to diagnose lung cancer.

Diagnostic Surgery and Biopsy

Because of improved radiological techniques, surgical exploration has become much less important. However, in some clinical situations (e.g., peritoneal carcinosis), patients must undergo surgical procedures. In emergencies, such as complete bowel obstruction, surgical intervention leads to a cancer diagnosis accidentally.

Intraluminal or percutaneous biopsies of suspicious lesions can reliably obtain tissue for pathohistological examination. Image guidance by sonography or CT allows safe aspiration of small lesions. The biopsy can determine the type of cancer and several prognostic features (e.g., vascular invasion, grade of differentiation, growth fraction).

Serological and Biochemical Studies

Lactate dehydrogenase and C-reactive protein levels are nonspecific parameters for tumor burden. Elevated levels of liver enzymes suggest hepatic metastasis. High alkaline phosphatase values can lead to the diagnosis of bone metastasis when a hepatic origin is excluded.

Tumor markers are biochemical substances produced by cancer cells and sometimes by normal cells. They are mainly proteins secreted by tumor cells (Table 216-8). They can be measured and are useful for evaluating some specific tumors. The concentration of tumor markers is proportional to the cancer cell burden. Because they have a short half-life, they can be used for assessing treatment response. There is no evidence to support measuring tumor markers for screening purposes (except prostate-specific antigen), because levels can be elevated in healthy people.

Hormone Receptor Status, Genetic Markers, and Cell Surface Receptors

For determining treatment decisions and prognosis for patients with breast cancer, it is essential to know whether the cancer cells express estrogen or progesterone receptors. Some tumors have specific genetic markers; for example the ERBB2/HER2 protein is overexpressed in 20% to 25% of breast cancers and up to 30% of ovarian cancers, and these tumors can be successfully targeted with therapies that include the monoclonal antibody trastuzumab. Genetic profiles have high prognostic value, especially in hematological cancers. The expression of epidermal growth factor receptors (EGFRs) or vascular endothelial growth factor receptor (VEGFR) on cancer cells can indicate the need for targeted therapy.

Tumor Response and Outcome Measures

Tumor Response

To evaluate the response to cytotoxic therapy, it is important to define outcome measures. Ongoing therapy depends on the response to chemotherapy. Three main outcome measures are used: stable disease, partial response, and complete response.

Stable disease is defined as no evidence of tumor progression in response to cytotoxic therapy. In this measure, the term *minimal response* (tumor reduction less than 50%) is included. *Partial response* is a 50% reduction or more (clinical or radiographical) in at least one dimension of the tumor mass or reduction in the level of a tumor marker. *Complete response* is complete disappearance of tumor, with no histological, radiographical, or chemical evidence of cancer.

Quality of Life Assessment

In Europe, the most widely used questionnaire for assessing quality of life in cancer patients undergoing chemotherapy is the European Organization for Research and Treatment of Cancer Quality of Life Questionnaire Core-30 (EORTC QLQ-C30). This instrument has been validated in many languages, and adaptations for several tumor types are available.[11]

TREATMENT

Chemotherapy

Anticancer drugs act on different levels against a malignant disease (Table 218-9). The first cytotoxic agent was developed from experiences with nitrogen mustard as a chemical weapon used in the World Wars. It was first administered as a single anticancer drug in the 1940s for leukemia and Hodgkin's disease. Findings that the disease rapidly relapsed after the use on a single drug led to the hypothesis that a combination of several agents could cure malignant diseases. The first trials of combination chemotherapies were initiated in the 1970s and applied particularly to breast cancer; several combination chemotherapy schemes followed. In 1974, the efficacy of cisplatin in testicular

TABLE 218-8 Common Tumor Markers

MARKER	TYPE OF CANCER
Prostate-specific antigen (PSA)	Prostate
Cancer antigen (CA) 125	Ovarian
Carcinoembryonic antigen (CEA), CA 19-9	Colorectal
α-Fetoprotein (AFP)	Hepatocellular, germ cell
CA 15-3, CEA	Breast
Human chorionic gonadotropin (β-hCG)	Germ cell
Neuron-specific enolase (NSE)	Small cell lung, neuroendocrine

TABLE 218-9 Major Classes of Anticancer Drugs

CLASS	DRUGS
Alkylating agents	Melphalan, chlorambucil, cyclophosphamide, BCNU, CCNU, procarbazine, dacarbazine, temozolomide, cisplatin, carboplatin, oxaliplatin
Antimetabolites	Methotrexate, 5-flourouracil, cytosine arabinoside, gemcitabine, pemetrexed, irinotecan, capecitabine, 6-mercaptopurine, fludarabine, 6-thioguanine, hydroxyurea
Antimicrotubule agents	Vincristine, vinblastine, vinorelbine, paclitaxel, docetaxel
Topoisomerase inhibitors	Doxorubicin, mitoxantrone, etoposide, irinotecan, topotecan

cancer was discovered, and it became possible to treat this cancer in young men with a high probability of cure. In the 1980s, paclitaxel for platinum-resistant ovarian cancer was an important advance. In 2000, targeted therapy with imatinib for chronic myelogenous leukemia and gastrointestinal stromal tumor was successful. Each year, additional anticancer drugs are approved for treatment.

Cancer patients should be treated in randomized clinical trials to produce evidence-based data on side effects and tumor response. Patients in clinical trials may have more favorable outcomes.[8] Cytotoxic chemotherapy is characterized by a low therapeutic index but high variability in therapeutic and toxic effects. In an attempt to reduce the variability, individualized dosages are given according to the body surface area (mg/m^2). Other methods include using pharmacokinetic parameters such as plasma clearance in relation to the degree of toxicity and administering dosages according to the area under the curve (AUC). This approach is effective for carboplatin.

Normally, chemotherapy is administered at 3- to 4-week intervals because it affects all body tissues and especially bone marrow, which proliferates rapidly. One side effect is suppression of leukocytes, platelets, and red blood cells. The depression of blood cells (nadir) peaks between days 10 and 14 after chemotherapy, and the cells return to normal levels between days 21 and 28. Depending on the drug or the dosage, some chemotherapy regimens are administered weekly. For incurable diseases, these concepts must be established carefully.

Many chemotherapeutic agents, such as capecitabine, vinorelbine (Navelbine), and temozolomide, are available in oral forms. This is especially beneficial for patients with advanced cancer. Some agents, such as doxorubicin and asparaginase, have been developed in pegylated liposomal forms. These chemical forms improve toxicity profiles.

To evaluate the tumor response and make a decision about further therapy, two cycles of chemotherapy are followed by assessment of the tumor burden, side effects, and improvement of symptoms. The duration of further therapy depends on the cancer subtype and response to therapy.[3,5,6]

Forms of Application

Most cytotoxic drugs require intravenous administration. Because some of these drugs can cause catastrophic tissue damage after extravasation, it is necessary to have reliable intravenous access (e.g., Port-a-Cath systems) and to have an experienced physician or a specially trained nurse give the drugs. The advantage of oral forms is that patients can take their medication as outpatients. However, careful monitoring regarding correct dosages and potential side effects is necessary.

Cutaneous metastasis and malignant lymphomas can be treated by topical miltefosine or recently developed analogues. The value of local chemotherapy using intra-arterial cytotoxic agents is unclear. Intraperitoneal chemotherapy is indicated for peritoneal carcinosis caused by ovarian cancer. For patients with pleural effusion, intrapleural cytotoxic agents can be administered after drainage of the effusion. Leptomeningeal metastasis, also known as carcinomatous meningitis, neoplastic meningitis, and neoplastic meningosis, is often treated by intrathecal che-

motherapy. Large cancer metastases or primary tumors in the liver can be treated by chemoembolization.

Combination and Dosage of Chemotherapy

A combination chemotherapy cycle includes two or more different cytotoxic drugs. In designing a therapeutic schedule for a particular cancer type, several principles are important:

- The drugs should be effective as single agents.
- They should act on different tumor mechanisms and have synergistic effects.
- Selected drugs should have different side effects and dose limitations.
- Combinations of drugs with cross-resistances should be avoided.
- Severe drug-drug interactions must be excluded.

For many cancers, the drugs exhibit a dose-response relationship. Dosages are restricted by their toxic effects on healthy tissues.

Aims of Chemotherapy

Chemotherapy has several goals. In the *neoadjuvant* setting, chemotherapy is given to patients with nonmetastatic tumors before definitive treatment, usually surgical intervention. The aim is potential shrinkage of a large, inoperable primary tumor mass to improve the likelihood of a successful complete resection or to allow less mutilating surgery (e.g., breast cancer, anal cancer, osteogenic sarcoma). Another purpose of neoadjuvant chemotherapy is to evaluate the tumor's chemosensitivity, even if it is primarily resectable, for planning further chemotherapy.

Some tumors in complete remission after first-line treatment have a high risk of recurrence. A risk profile can be used for relapse prediction. The indication for *adjuvant* therapy is defined in relation to the tumor size, number and location of involved lymph nodes, and histological, hormonal, and genetic patterns. The aim is to prevent cancer recurrence by using systemic therapy to eliminate micrometastases that can cause a relapse of the disease. Adjuvant chemotherapy has produced better long-term outcomes for patients with breast, colorectal, and non–small cell lung cancers. On average, long-term survival can be improved by 5% to 15%, but some patients derive no benefit from adjuvant chemotherapy.

Some tumor types, such as germ cell tumors or hematological malignancies, are potentially *curable* with chemotherapy alone. A curative approach includes serious side effects, such as bone marrow suppression. These patients must receive chemotherapy on fixed schedules and in full dosages, because delayed therapy and dosage reduction affect outcomes. Cytokines may be used to modulate side effects and ensure that patients will be able to receive the complete therapeutic regimen.

Most metastatic cancers are not curable with oncological treatment options. *Palliative* chemotherapy is given to prolong life, improve symptoms, and improve the quality of life of patients with incurable cancer. Chemotherapy may be given to patients with advanced cancer because they hope for cure or prolongation of life, because oncologists want to prolong life and improve the quality of life of their patients, and because prognostic uncertainty exists about the life expectancies of patients and the tumor response.[12] The potential side effects and benefits must be evaluated carefully in this situation. The decision to use palliative chemotherapy depends on the chemosensitivity of the tumor and the patient's symptoms and performance status. For some cancers, such as breast cancer, there exist recommendations for palliative therapy.[13] Most patients with an ECOG score of 2 or more or a Karnofsky index of 50 or less are unable to get chemotherapy. Sometimes, an emergency can be the indication for palliative chemotherapy, such as compression from large mediastinal mass that is a small cell lung cancer or malignant lymphoma. Tumor bleeding or refractory hypercalcemia can be an indication for palliative chemotherapy. When the cancer cells develop chemoresistance, a change of cytotoxic drugs is necessary. This phenomenon is expressed by the terms first-line and second-line chemotherapy. The first-line regimen is always the most potent chemotherapy, and the probability of a tumor response decreases after each change of therapy.[14-16]

Salvage chemotherapy is given after failure of the primary treatment (e.g., surgery, chemotherapy, radiotherapy) with curative intent. Few tumor types exist for which salvage chemotherapy is indicated.

Side Effects of Chemotherapy

Typical side effects of chemotherapy are nausea and vomiting. The likelihood of experiencing these effects has been reduced by excellent antiemetic therapy. Many common cytotoxic drugs cause alopecia. There is no appropriate prophylaxis, and especially for women, it is a burdensome side effect. Chemotherapy can also affect gonadal function in men and women. For some cytotoxic drugs, this is irreversible, and in young patients, cryoconservation should be used. After decades of successful hematological and oncological therapies, it has become evident that people undergoing curative treatment are at a high risk for long-term adverse effects, especially second cancers. These malignancies, often leukemias, have high mutation rates and often are difficult to treat. The drugs used in primary therapy must be carefully chosen to prevent second malignancies.

Other Therapeutic Approaches

Hormone therapy is indicated for treating some tumors. Several hormonal anticancer strategies are described in Table 218-10.

Targeted therapies are becoming routine. These approaches include tyrosine kinase inhibitors, monoclonal antibodies, and angiogenesis inhibitors.

For many years, metastatic renal cancer was treated with high-dose interferon-α and interleukin-2. The responses rates were low, and many side effects were reported.

Octreotide is a somatostatin analogue that is used in the palliative care of patients with carcinoid syndrome, neuroendocrine tumors, and some pancreatic cancers of neuroendocrine origin. Octreotide is highly effective, and remissions can be prolonged over months and years.

Hematological malignancies, especially multiple myeloma, have high rates of response to immunomodulatory therapies. Thalidomide was first used in treating relapsed

TABLE 218-10 Hormone Therapy

THERAPY	BREAST	OVARY	PROSTATE	THYROID
Selective estrogen receptor modulators (e.g., tamoxifen)	+	+		
Aromatase inhibitors (e.g., anastrozole, letrozole)	+	+		
Gonadorelin analogues (e.g., leuprolide acetate, goserelin)			+	
Antiandrogens (e.g., testosterone receptor antagonists, cyproterone acetate)			+	
Thyroxine				+

and refractory malignancies; it is now part of the primary therapy for myeloma. From 1956 to 1962, approximately 10,000 children were born with severe deformities, including phocomelia, because of thalidomide's teratogenic effects. Thalidomide acts on cytokine levels, has an antiangiogenic effect, and is involved in T-cell function. Lenalidomide (Revlimid), a derivative of thalidomide, has fewer side effects.

Changes in the Therapeutic Approach

Less toxic chemotherapy drugs have become available, and supportive therapy has improved. A paradigm change has occurred in the past decade regarding the aims of medical oncology. Traditionally, oncology had a disease-oriented approach, and the primary goal of oncological treatment was to cure or obtain an objective tumor response. Parameters such as quality of life, clinical benefit of response, and improvement of symptom burden are important goals, as is the treatment of elderly patients with cancer.

Changes also have taken place in the paradigm of using cytotoxic therapies. Targeted therapy means more than killing malignant cells by toxic drugs. Newer substances act in a more elegant way to eliminate cancer cells through different pathways that can better discriminate between cancer and normal cells. Strategies include antibodies against products of oncogenes or cell surface antigens, inhibitors of various kinases, and inhibitors of the angiogenesis.

ONCOLOGY AND PALLIATIVE CARE

Because more than 90% of patients receiving palliative care are cancer patients, the medical staff working in palliative care should have a basic knowledge of oncology. Patients should receive palliative therapies such as chemotherapy or radiation therapy for symptom control when there is no longer an indication for tumor-specific therapy. Although oncologists and palliative care physicians treat the same patients, the treatment goals may not overlap. The oncologist's first aim is to fight the cancer with aggressive agents. Palliative medicine practitioners can accept the limitations of advanced cancer more easily and focus effort on symptomatic therapy and psychosocial issues; this approach may seem inadequate to health care workers in other disciplines.

Progress in oncology and palliative medicine led to the conclusion that optimal treatment requires cooperation among all parties. An oncologist should understand the specialist care provided by palliative care teams. Best supportive care (BSC) is one approach being evaluated in some randomized trials of palliative chemotherapy. BSC is not defined and depends on the knowledge of the individual physician. Better cooperation between palliative care and oncology specialists may improve clinical trials.

In clinical practice, it is important to overcome the patient's perception of hopelessness and death when the oncologist refers him or her to palliative care. Many efforts have been made to develop best care models and integrate palliative care into oncological treatment in earlier disease (see Fig. 218-2). The number of institutions that integrate medical oncology and palliative care is growing every year.[17,18]

CONCLUSIONS

Despite the enormous progress in anticancer treatment, cure of metastatic cancer is unlikely. Efforts are being made to design drugs that are more effective, are specific, and have fewer side effects. The future of modern cancer therapy consists of mechanism-based treatments using the pathways of tumor origin and growth. We still need answers to many questions. Is the molecular target being modulated? Is the biochemical pathway undergoing modulation? Is the intended biological effect being achieved?[10]

The future of therapy also will include the ethical dilemma of resource allocation. Newer therapeutic approaches, tools for diagnosis, and better supportive care cost money. Anticancer agents are among the costliest in medical care. Newer drugs are substantially more expensive than conventional drugs, and the survival benefit using modern drugs is described in months.[19] Stakeholders, employers, drug and device manufacturers, private payers, patient advocates, and organizations representing medical professionals and the political structures have failed to reach a consensus about which therapeutic efforts are justifiable.[20] Physicians and other members of society need to define what is reasonable and necessary and how much money we want to spend for life prolongation of the patient with incurable diseases.

REFERENCES

1. Ozols RF, Herbst RS, Colson YL, et al. Clinical cancer advances 2006: Major research advances in cancer treatment, prevention, and screening—a report from the American Society of Clinical Oncology. J Clin Oncol 2007;1:146-162.
2. Norton L. A gompertzian model of human breast cancer growth. Cancer Res 1988;48:7067-7071.
3. Peedell C. Concise Clinical Oncology. Philadelphia: Elsevier, 2005, pp 63-85.
4. Goldie JH, Coldman AJ. A mathematical model for relating the drug sensitivity of tumours to their spontaneous mutation rate. Cancer Treat Rep 1979;63:1727-1733.
5. DeVita, VT, Hellman S, Rosenberg SA. Cancer: Principles and Practice of Oncology, 6th ed. Philadelphia: Lippincott Williams & Wilkins, 2001.
6. Brighton D, Wood M. The Royal Marsden Handbook of Cancer Chemotherapy. Philadelphia: Elsevier, 2005, pp 9 -29.
7. Ellison NM, Chevelen EM. Palliative chemotherapy. In Berger AM, Portenoy RK, Weissman DE (eds). Principles and Practice of Palliative Care and Supportive Oncology, 2nd ed. Philadelphia: Lippincott Williams & Williams, 2002, pp 698-709.
8. Schneider EC, Epstein AM, Malin JL, et al. Developing a system to assess the quality of cancer care: ASCO's national initiative on cancer care quality. J Clin Oncol 2004;22:2985-2991.
9. Greene FL, Compton CC, Fritz AG. AJCC Cancer Staging Atlas. New York: Springer, 2006.
10. Garrett MD, Workman P. Discovering novel chemotherapeutic drugs for the third millennium. Eur J Cancer 1999;35:2010-2030.
11. Aaronson NK, Ahmedzai S, Bergman B, et al. The European Organization for Research and Treatment of Cancer QLQ-C30: A quality-of-life instrument for use in international clinical trials in oncology. J Natl Cancer Inst 1993; 85:365-376.
12. Emanuel EJ, Young-Xu Y, Levinsky NG, et al. Chemotherapy use among Medicare beneficiaries at the end of life. Ann Intern Med 2003;138:639-643.
13. Beslija S, Boneterre J, Burstein H, et al. Second consensus on medical treatment of metastatic breast cancer. Ann Oncol 2007;18:215-225.
14. Browner I, Carducci MA. Palliative chemotherapy: Historical perspective, applications, and controversies. Semin Oncol 2005;32:145-155.
15. Archer VR, Billingham LJ, Culen MH. Palliative chemotherapy: No longer a contradiction in terms. Oncologist 1999;4:470-477.
16. Matsuyama R, Reddy S, Smith TJ. Why do patients choose chemotherapy near the end of life? A review of the perspective of those facing death from cancer. J Clin Oncol 2006;24:3490-3496.
17. Ahmedzai SH, Walsh TD. Palliative medicine and modern cancer care. Semin Oncol 2000;27:1-6.
18. Davis MP. Integrating palliative medicine into an oncology practice. Am J Hosp Palliat Med 2005:447-456.
19. Meropol NJ, Schulman KA. Cost of cancer care: Issues and implications. J Clin Oncol 2007;25:180-186.
20. Tunis SR. Why Medicare has not established criteria for coverage decisions. N Engl J Med 2004;350:2196-2198.

SUGGESTED READING

American Cancer Society. Information. Available at http://www.cancer.org (accessed March 2008).

Cassidy J, Bissett D, Spence RAJ. Oxford Handbook of Oncology, 2nd ed. New York: Oxford University Press, 2006.

Hoskin P, Makin W. Oncology for Palliative Medicine. New York: Oxford University Press, 2003.

National Cancer Institute (NCI). Cancer information system. Available at http://www.cis.nci.nih.gov (accessed March 2008).

Complications

CHAPTER **219**

Patterns of Metastatic Cancer

Clare Byrne and Graeme Poston

When cancer is detected, about 50% of patients have metastatic disease and probably have a high incidence of undiagnosed, occult metastases. Cancer cells detach from the primary tumor, travel to distant sites, and grow as secondary tumors. Metastases can be detected when the primary tumor is small (diameter <0.5 cm), but the primary size usually correlates with the likelihood of metastases.

Recamier first used the term *metastasis* in 1829, when he identified a brain tumor that had metastasized from a primary breast carcinoma. In 1889, Paget described distant metastases from a primary tumor as not haphazard and posited a definite pattern of metastasis for each cancer type.

BASIC SCIENCE

Beyond direct invasion, the three main routes of metastatic spread are through lymphatic vessels, through blood vessels, and across body cavities (i.e., transcelomic spread). The tumor-node-metastasis (TNM) staging system has three subgroups of metastases:

- Direct extension in relation to primary tumor size (T)
- Regional lymph nodes—usually disseminated through the lymphatic circulation (N)
- Distant sites and organs—usually through vascular dissemination (M)

Lymphatic Dissemination

Malignant tumors have different modes of spread. Squamous tumors, such as head and neck cancers, normally spread to regional lymph nodes, and only when they are more advanced do they spread to distant sites. Treatments that address regional lymph node involvement influence potential cure. Other cancers, such as breast cancer, disseminate early. Although involved lymph nodes at presentation usually correlate with distant metastases, up to 25% of breast cancers without axillary lymph node involvement have distant metastases.[1] Most solid tumors have little functional lymphatic drainage,[2] but lymphatic ingrowth into the periphery of these tumors occurs.

Vascular Dissemination

Cancer cells, like other epithelial cells, rest on a basement membrane. A crucial stage in metastasis is membrane disruption and transgression. This permits malignant cells to invade the connective tissue stroma and access capillaries and lymph vessels. Invasion requires cell motility and cell detachment from the primary tumor. These cells must be able to penetrate the vascular system and circulate (alone or as part of a tumor embolus) until stopped by adhesion to the vessel basement membrane at a distant site. For patients with breast cancer, a poor prognosis and increased likelihood of metastases are associated with the formation of new blood vessels (i.e., angiogenesis) in the primary tumor.[3] They provide nutrients to support tumor growth and allow access to the arterial circulation, promoting metastases. Cancer cells rarely penetrate the thick walls of established arteries. They enter newly formed capillaries more easily than preexisting capillaries because of defects in the new blood vessels, such as gaps between endothelial cells and a discontinuous or absent basement membrane.[4]

Peritoneal and Pleural Dissemination

Peritoneal spread usually arises from organs within the peritoneal cavity, such as the colon and ovaries. Cancer cells pass within the potential peritoneal space or by direct contact with tissues within the cavity. Metastases at the new site can shed cells and establish many disease foci by using the ascitic fluid, which provides a growth medium for cells capable of growing without anchorage. Primary and metastatic lung cancers can colonize and spread within the pleural space, causing malignant pleural effusions.

Metastatic Patterns

Two prevailing hypotheses address the variable metastatic patterns. They are the first-pass organ theory and the seed and soils theory.

First-Pass Organ Theory

The first-pass organ theory focuses on the anatomic delivery system. Secondary growth is frequently supported by the organ first encountered by vessels from a primary cancer site. Lymphatic vessels drain into lymph nodes near the affected tumor. In this way, breast cancers spread to sentinel axillary lymph nodes. Further lymphatic drainage flows through the thoracic ducts and the superior vena cava, leading to wider dissemination. The liver is the main first-pass organ for blood-borne cells in the hepatic artery and portal vein (Table 219-1). The absence of physical barriers between sinusoids and hepatocytes makes the liver accessible to establish tumor growth. In head and neck tumors, venous drainage enters the superior vena cava; because this route avoids the liver, the lungs are the main distant metastatic sites.

Selective Growth of Specific Cells at Different Sites: Seed and Soil Theory

Additional homing mechanisms and venous drainage and blood flow patterns attract certain cancers to specific sites. Although the lungs, liver, lymph nodes, bone, and brain are the most common sites, the spread of breast cancer to specific sites led Paget[5] to propose the seed and soil hypothesis. It suggests that differential tumor cell and host organ interactions occur that are favorable for metastatic development. In a review of the postmortem records of 735 patients who died of breast cancer, he found that splenic metastases occurred in only 2% of autopsies,

despite the generous arterial blood supply, but liver metastases occurred in 3% of autopsies, despite diminished arterial supply. The low rate of metastases in the spleen could not be explained by mechanical theories,[5] suggesting that cancer cells are like plant seeds that grow only in hospitable soil.

An alternative hypothesis[6] suggests that the number of metastases in an organ depends on the number of tumor cells delivered in the blood. Tumor cells are caught in the pulmonary capillary sieve and hepatic portal triads. Subsequently, hepatic or pulmonary colonies release additional cells with an affinity for a particular organ or tissue.[6]

Others[7,8] suggested that metastasis formation is related to both putative mechanisms, because circulating cancer cells need first to arrest in the small organ vessels (and extravasate through the endothelial basement membrane) but will grow only if the organ has a suitable environment for that type of tumor cell.

Genetic Predetermination

The seed and soil hypothesis is challenged by current microarray data,[9] which suggest that tumor cells may be hard-wired early on and organ specific gene expression signatures superimposed on a poor prognosis signature in the parent tumor account for the various patterns of metastasis. The identification of such genes could be a prognostic indicator in assessing which patient has synchronous metastases, and which might be vulnerable to early metachronous metastases. This knowledge should promote understanding cellular processes that influence metastasis, and help control and cure of cancer (e.g. targeted adjuvant therapies after apparently curative surgery). Whilst individual genes influence the development of metastases, metastasis remains a complex pattern, and is likely regulated by a series of genes, which when activated in a coordinated manner, result in the typical predicted behavior.

COMMON SITES OF METASTATIC SPREAD

Metastatic behavior of most common solid tumors is predictable (see Table 219-1). The most common sites are to the lungs, liver, lymph nodes, bone, and brain.

Metastatic Cancer of the Esophagus

The unique lymphatic drainage of the esophagus is a major factor in local spread (Table 219-2). Direct invasion of local structures may be facilitated by the absence of serosa, a hypothetical natural barrier, and the immediate proximity of the aorta and trachea, invasion of which contribute to a poor prognosis.

In up to 40% of patients with tumors smaller than 5 cm in diameter, disease is localized at presentation; 25% have regional nodal metastases, and 35% have distant metastases rendering the cancer incurable. For those with tumors larger than 5 cm, only 10% have localized disease, 15% have locally advanced cancer, and 75% have distant metastases. In addition to tumor size, depth of tumor invasion predicts regional lymph node status. The most common sites for distant metastases include lung, pleura, peritoneum, brain, and bone.

TABLE 219-1 Patterns of Metastatic Spread from Common Primary Tumors to Target Organs

PRIMARY TUMOR	MAIN METASTATIC SITE	OTHER METASTATIC SITES
Esophagus	Mediastinal lymph node	Lung, pleura, peritoneum, brain, bone
Stomach	Liver	Peritoneum, lymph nodes
Pancreas	Liver (85%)	Peritoneum, lymph nodes
Colorectal cancer	Intestinal lymph node (84%)	Liver, lung
Prostate	Bone (90%)	Lymph nodes
Head and neck carcinomas	Regional lymph nodes	Lung, bone
Small cell carcinoma of the lung	Thoracic lymph node (66%)	Brain, liver, bone marrow
Melanoma of the skin	Regional lymph nodes	Liver, brain, bowel
Breast	Regional lymph node (97%)	Bone, brain, adrenal, lung, liver
Ovary	Abdominal cavity (91%)	Liver, lung, pleura

Metastatic Gastric Cancer

Gastric cancers disseminate by direct extension to adjacent organs, by intramural and regional lymph nodes through lymphatic channels, by venous routes to the liver, and by transcelomic spread to the peritoneum. At diagnosis, almost 10% of early tumors and 60% to 70% of all tumors have invaded venous channels, omentum, ovaries, and elsewhere within the rectovesical pouch. Diffuse gastric cancer spreads through the submucosal and subserosal lymphatic plexuses (i.e., intramural spread). Gastric wall invasion occurs early, and after the muscular coat is invaded, lymph nodes along the lesser and greater curvatures become involved, followed by celiac axis nodes and para-aortic nodes. Intramural lymphatics support horizontal dissemination within the gastric wall from the esophagus to the duodenum. Direct extension occurs most commonly to the omentum, transverse colon, mesocolon, pancreas, and left lobe of the liver (Table 219-3).

Metastatic Pancreas Cancer

Pancreatic cancer is usually diagnosed when it is advanced and incurable. Retroperitoneal location, late presentation with the disease, multidirectional lymphatic drainage, and proximity to vital vascular structures curtail resectability with curative intent in most cases. The most common metastatic site is the liver, followed by peritoneum and lung. Venous occlusion is invariably associated with advanced metastatic disease. Other clinical signs of advanced metastatic disease include palpable liver nodules, supraclavicular lymphadenopathy, palpable abdominal mass, and peritoneal seeding in the rectovaginal or rectovesical pouch (Table 219-4).

Metastatic Colorectal Cancer

The spread of colorectal cancer is more predictable than other solid gastrointestinal malignancies. Direct invasion

---

TABLE 219-2 Metastatic Esophageal Cancer

PRESENTING SYMPTOMS	SIGNS OF METASTATIC DISEASE	DIAGNOSTIC STUDIES	DIAGNOSTIC FEATURES
Progressive dysphagia (87-95%) Weight loss (42-71%) Vomiting or regurgitation (29-45%) Pain radiating to the back (29-45%)	Hoarse voice Palpable supraclavicular nodes Malignant pleural effusion Malignant ascites Bone pain	Endoscopy and biopsy Computed tomography Endoscopic ultrasonography Laparoscopy or thoracoendoscopy	Irregular esophageal borders suggest full-thickness. penetration Lymph nodes >2 cm usually are positive for metastases. Detection of peritoneal seeding and abdominal lymph nodes

---

TABLE 219-3 Metastatic Stomach Cancer

PRESENTING SYMPTOMS	SIGNS OF METASTATIC DISEASE	DIAGNOSTIC STUDIES	DIAGNOSTIC FEATURES
Anemia Weight loss Dyspepsia Epigastric pain	Palpable epigastric lump Enlarged liver Supraclavicular lymphadenopathy Hematemesis Dysphagia	Endoscopy and biopsy Computed tomography Endoscopic ultrasonography Complete blood cell count Liver function studies	Gastric wall thickness >2 cm is an indication of transmural extension Obliteration of the perigastric fat planes indicates extragastric spread Tumor extends into the diaphragm, pancreas, gastrocolic ligament to colon, gastrohepatic ligament to liver, or gastrosplenic ligament to spleen Metastases in liver, spleen, adrenals, ovaries Detection of enlarged regional lymph nodes in left gastric, gastroepiploic, celiac, retrocrural, peripancreatic, and splenic hilar nodal chains

---

TABLE 219-4 Metastatic Pancreatic Cancer

PRESENTING SYMPTOMS	SIGNS OF METASTATIC DISEASE	DIAGNOSTIC STUDIES	DIAGNOSTIC FEATURES
Painless, obstructive jaundice Weight loss Unexplained upper abdominal or lumbar back pain	Portal hypertension Sudden onset of diabetes mellitus Idiopathic pancreatitis Unexplained steatorrhea	Computed tomography Magnetic resonance imaging Magnetic resonance cholangiopancreatography (MRCP) Endoscopic retrograde cholangiopancreatography (ERCP) Laparoscopy and fine-needle aspiration Endoscopic ultrasonography CA 19-9 tumor marker Liver function studies	Palpable liver nodules, supraclavicular lymphadenopathy, palpable abdominal mass, peritoneal seeding in rectovaginal or rectovesical pouch Obliteration of the fat planes around the pancreas Liver or lung metastases Enlarged spleen, splenic vein thrombosis, and left-sided portal hypertension Major arterial (splenic, hepatic, superior mesenteric) encasement or major venous (portal, superior mesenteric, splenic) involvement

of adjacent structures, particularly in the pelvis, occurs. Lymph node spread occurs early, and distant spread most commonly targets the liver. This ability to calculate the pattern of spread formed the basis of the first true staging system to predict prognosis after apparently curative surgery for rectal cancer. In 1932, Cuthbert Dukes produced his seminal staging system based on the degree of invasion and spread of cancer in the pathological specimen:

A: Invasion into muscularis but no farther (5-year survival rate of 90%)

B: Invasion through the muscularis but no farther and no lymph node metastases (5-year survival rate of 60%)

C: Lymph node metastases in the surgical specimen (5-year survival rate of 35%)

Dukes' system is the bedrock of all further attempts to stage colorectal cancer. Dukes described stage D (i.e., widespread disease, including the liver), because in 1932, disease beyond the possibility of surgical resection was considered incurable. With aggressive surgical strategies for resection of colorectal liver and lung metastases, we now see more patients developing late brain and bone metastases (Table 219-5).

Metastatic Prostate Cancer

Prostate cancer directly invades adjacent structures, including the perivesicular sheath, bladder, and seminal vesicles, but it rarely crosses the fascia of Denonvilliers to invade the rectum. Metastatic spread initially targets regional lymph nodes, following the internal iliac arterial chain, and then para-aortic lymph nodes. Prostate cancer is notorious for early invasion of prostatic venous plexuses, from where tumor emboli access the pelvic venous system and the systemic circulation. Visceral metastases can occur in any organ, including the lung, liver, and adrenal gland, but they most commonly seek the skeleton. Characteristically, prostate cancers produce sclerotic osteoblastic bone metastases, but osteolytic (and sometimes mixed blastic and lytic) bone lesions also occur (Table 219-6). Theories suggest these cancers disseminate in a predictable cascade: local infiltration, regional nodes, and bloodborne spread. The actual sequence is haphazard and unknown. The extent of metastatic disease and tumor burden may be proportional to the elevated level of serum prostate-specific antigen (PSA).

Metastatic Squamous Head and Neck Cancers

The common head and neck tumors arise in the squamous epithelium of the oropharynx and adjacent sinuses. Early spread is predictable, with direct invasion of adjacent structures and early lymphatic spread to the sentinel lymph node and onward to the regional lymphatic chain. Distant bloodborne spread usually targets lungs. Liver metastases occur later and are less common, possibly because of earlier presentation of patients in Western societies compared with those in Asia, where this is one of the most common tumors and one that is diagnosed at an advanced stage because medical help is delayed because of fear (Table 219-7).

Metastatic Non–Small Cell Lung Cancers

Metastatic non–small cell lung cancers account for about 80% of primary bronchus and lung cancers. They include squamous cancers, large cell cancers, and adenocarcinomas. Despite advances in understanding the cause, eradication of smoking, and increasing awareness in Western society, patients usually present with advanced and incurable cancers. At diagnosis, less than 20% are amenable to

---

TABLE 219-5 Metastatic Colorectal Cancer

PRESENTING SYMPTOMS	SIGNS OF METASTATIC DISEASE	DIAGNOSTIC STUDIES	DIAGNOSTIC FEATURES
Usually painless Liver capsule pain Weight loss Symptoms of anemia	Palpable hepatomegaly Ascites Cachexia	Deranged liver function test results (especially alkaline phosphatase) Carcinoembryonic antigen (CEA) and CA 19-9 levels elevated Liver ultrasound Computed tomography of chest, abdomen, and pelvis Magnetic resonance imaging (MRI) of the liver Combined positron emission tomography and computed tomography (PET/CT)	Elevated levels of tumor markers Hypovascular and hypervascular liver tumors on CT and MRI

TABLE 219-6 Metastatic Prostate Cancer

PRESENTING SYMPTOMS	SIGNS OF METASTATIC DISEASE	DIAGNOSTIC STUDIES	DIAGNOSTIC FEATURES
Bone pain Symptoms of anemia	Bone tenderness, pathologic fractures Cachexia	Blood levels of prostate-specific antigen (PSA) Computed tomography Magnetic resonance imaging Isotope bone scans Combined positron emission tomography and computed tomography	Sclerotic bone secondaries on plain radiographs

TABLE 219-7 Metastatic Head and Neck Cancers

PRESENTING SYMPTOMS	SIGNS OF METASTATIC DISEASE	DIAGNOSTIC STUDIES	DIAGNOSTIC FEATURES

Hoarse voice
Chronic cough
	Palpable cervical lymphadenopathy
	Cachexia
		Aspiration cytology or biopsy of lymph
		  nodes
		Chest radiograph
		Computed tomography
		Magnetic resonance imaging
		Combined positron emission
		  tomography and computed
		  tomography
			Radiologically evident pulmonary tumors
			Pleural effusion
			Liver metastases

TABLE 219-8 Metastatic Non–Small Cell Lung Cancers

PRESENTING SYMPTOMS	SIGNS OF METASTATIC DISEASE	DIAGNOSTIC STUDIES	DIAGNOSTIC FEATURES
Cough Hoarse voice Weight loss	Pancoast syndrome Virchow's node Pleural effusion Palpable hepatomegaly	Chest radiograph Lymph node cytology Liver ultrasound Computed tomography Magnetic resonance imaging Combined positron emission tomography and computed tomography	Malignant pleural effusion Liver, bone, and brain metastases

TABLE 219-9 Metastatic Malignant Melanoma

PRESENTING SYMPTOMS	SIGNS OF METASTATIC DISEASE	DIAGNOSTIC STUDIES	DIAGNOSTIC FEATURES

Weight loss	Palpable lymphadenopathy
	Palpable hepatomegaly
		Aspiration cytology or biopsy of suspicious
		  lymph nodes
		Chest radiograph
		Liver ultrasound
		Computed tomography
		Magnetic resonance imaging
		Combined positron emission tomography and
		  computed tomography
			Liver, lung, and brain metastases

potentially curative surgery. Metastases occur earlier in the large cell carcinomas and adenocarcinomas, and they usually spread to the regional lymph nodes (i.e., hilar carinal and subcarinal groups), brain, liver, adrenal glands, and bone. Squamous carcinomas metastasize more slowly, but their predilection for central sites of origin (i.e., major bronchi) may make them unresectable on anatomical grounds. However, if peripheral, they can directly invade the pleura, causing malignant pleural effusions, and if at the lung apex, they can invade adjacent neural structures, causing Pancoast's syndrome (Table 219-8).

Metastatic Malignant Melanoma

Malignant melanoma, like breast cancer, metastasizes early, and occult distant metastases may become overt many years after apparently curative surgery. Early spread occurs equally to local cutaneous tumor satellites, regional lymph nodes, and through the bloodstream to distant sites. Whether melanoma metastasizes predictably to regional sentinel lymph nodes is controversial. Melanomas

arising on the limbs are more predictable because the important lymph node basins are in the groins and axillae. Trunk melanomas are unpredictable and may metastasize simultaneously to two or more lymph node basins (i.e., neck, axilla, or groins on either side). Distant bloodborne metastases equally target the liver, lung, and brain or meninges, but melanoma also has a predilection for sites not commonly associated with metastatic spread, including distant cutaneous sites and small bowel (Table 219-9).

Metastatic Breast Cancer

Unlike melanoma, patterns of breast cancer metastases are more predictable. Lymphatic spread usually precedes blood-borne spread in early disease. The lymphatic spread occurs in the anatomical draining lymph node basin, which for lateral tumors is the ipsilateral axilla and for medial tumors may be the ipsilateral axilla and the ipsilateral internal mammary chain. Timely radical resection of these regional lymph node basins offers the chance of

TABLE 219-10	Metastatic Breast Cancer		
PRESENTING SYMPTOMS	**SIGNS OF METASTATIC DISEASE**	**DIAGNOSTIC STUDIES**	**DIAGNOSTIC FEATURES**
Weight loss Bone pain Jaundice Abdominal swelling Dyspnea	Palpable lymphadenopathy Palpable hepatomegaly Pleural effusion Ascites Pelvic mass (ovarian metastases)	Blood level of CA 50 marker Fine-needle aspiration cytology or biopsy of suspicious lymph nodes Chest radiograph Liver ultrasound Computed tomography Magnetic resonance imaging Combined positron emission tomography and computed tomography Isotope bone scan	Supraclavicular lymphadenopathy Lung and pleural disease Liver, bone, and or brain metastases

TABLE 219-11	Metastatic Ovarian Cancer		
PRESENTING SYMPTOMS	**SIGNS OF METASTATIC DISEASE**	**DIAGNOSTIC STUDIES**	**DIAGNOSTIC FEATURES**
Weight loss Abdominal swelling Dyspnea	Ascites Palpable omental mass Pleural effusion	Blood levels of CA 125, CA 72, and CA 15-3 markers Ascitic and pleural tap for cytology Chest radiograph Abdominal ultrasound Computed tomography Magnetic resonance imaging Combined positron emission tomography and computed tomography	Malignant ascites and pleural effusions Radiological evidence of peritoneal or distant disease

long-term survival. Spread to the supraclavicular fossa nodes indicates distant, incurable disease. In aggressive tumors, particularly those with vascular invasion, blood-borne spread occurs early. The frequent sites of blood-borne metastases equally include the lung, liver, brain, and bone (Table 219-10).

Metastatic Ovarian Cancer

Ovarian carcinoma has unique metastatic patterns that are completely unlike those of the male counterpart, teratoma and seminoma of the testis. Early peritoneal involvement occurs, particularly of the omentum, which can become caked in tumor. Similarly, direct invasion of adjacent structures, including the uterus and fallopian tubes, is common. Lymph node metastases (i.e., iliac and para-aortic chains) appear later and indicate distant disease, and spread to the chest is associated with malignant pleural effusion (Table 219-11).

REFERENCES

1. Cassella M, Skobe M. Lymphatic vessel activation in cancer. Ann N Y Acad Sci 2002;979:120-130.
2. Jain RK, Munn LL, Fukumuru D. Dissecting tumour pathophysiology using intravital microscopy. Nat Rev Cancer 2002;2:226-276.
3. Hasan RB, Byers R, Jayson GC. Intratumoural microvessel density in human solid tumours. Br J Cancer 2002;86:1566-1577.
4. Folkman J. Fundamental concepts of the angiogenesis process. Curr Mol Med 1993;3:643-651.
5. Paget S. The distribution of secondary growth in cancer of the breast. Lancet 1889;133:571-573.
6. Sugarbaker EV. Patterns of metastasis in human malignancies. Cancer Biol Rev 1981;2:235-278.
7. McKinnell RG, Parchment RE, Perantoni AO, Pierce GB. The Biological Basis of Cancer. New York: Cambridge University Press, 2003.
8. Khokha R, Voura E, Hill RP. Tumour progression and metastasis: Cellular, molecular and microenvironmental factors. In The Basic Science of Oncology. New York: McGraw-Hill, 2005.
9. Hess KR, Varadhachary GR, Taylor SH, et al. Metastatic patterns in adenocarcinoma. Cancer 2006;106:1624-1633.

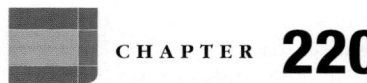

CHAPTER **220**

Neurological Complications

Yvona Griffo and Eugenie A. M. T. Obbens

KEY POINTS

- Metastatic brain tumors are complex and require a multidisciplinary approach. Potential treatment options include surgical resection, conventional radiation therapy, radiosurgery, and chemotherapy.

- Palliative relief for terminal patients with brain metastases can be obtained with anticonvulsants for seizure control, corticosteroids to combat cerebral edema, and antiemetics for nausea and vomiting.

- Most cases of epidural compression, the most common cause of spinal cord dysfunction, are caused by vertebral metastases, leading to rapid paraplegia or quadriplegia if untreated.

- High-dose steroids can relieve the pain of epidural compression and transiently improve neurological function. Urgent external beam radiation or decompressive laminectomy may avert irreversible neurological dysfunction.

- Leptomeningeal metastases affect the entire neuraxis, and despite intensive treatment with cerebrospinal fluid chemotherapy or field radiotherapy, median survival is less than 6 months.

- Plexopathy or radiculopathy in cancer results from direct compression or invasion by tumor or from radiation fibrosis, and sequelae include pain, sensory dysfunction, and weakness.

- Neuropathic pain does not respond well to opioids and requires adjuvant medications. Progressive, painless weakness can occur months to years after radiation therapy, and there is no effective treatment.

- Paraneoplastic syndromes may affect any part of the nervous system and often precede a diagnosis of cancer. They are mediated by immune responses triggered by tumors that express nervous system proteins, but antineuronal antibodies may occur without a paraneoplastic disorder.

- Treatment of paraneoplastic syndromes includes immunosuppression or immunomodulation and tumor-directed chemotherapy.

Neurological complications of cancer are common and often lead to loss of independent function[1] (Box 220-1). They may be caused by invasion of the nervous system by tumor or indirect mechanisms such as metastatic disease, autoimmune reactions, cerebrovascular and hematological abnormalities, and infections. They also may result from radiation therapy[2] and chemotherapy due to neurotoxic metabolic abnormalities, coagulopathy, immunosuppression, and infections. Fortunately, many neuro-oncological complications can be treated symptomatically and by definitive therapies that positively affect quality of life.[3]

BRAIN METASTASES

Brain metastases are the most common brain tumors (see Chapter 221). At least 100,000 patients in the United

States develop symptomatic brain metastases yearly. Approximately 10% of cancer patients develop brain metastases. Brain metastases may be single or multiple. They usually appear late in the disease, but they may be present before the primary cancer has been identified.[4] More than two thirds of patients with brain metastases have some neurological symptoms during the course of their disease. The clinical presentation of these patients is determined by the size, location, and number of lesions.[5] Most have generalized symptoms from mass effect, such as headache, altered mental status, cognitive impairment, and seizures, and focal signs and symptoms related to the anatomic location, such as hemiparesis, focal and generalized seizures, aphasia and apraxia, or visual symptoms. Approximately 15% have seizures (see Chapter 221) as a presenting symptom of the metastasis, with another 10% developing seizures later.[6] Signs and symptoms of brain metastases usually evolve over days to weeks. Sometimes, onset is acute, with a seizure or a strokelike presentation with hemiparesis caused by hemorrhage into a tumor. The latter is more common in patients with melanoma or choriocarcinoma.

The best diagnostic test for brain metastases is contrast-enhanced magnetic resonance imaging (MRI).[7] For persons presenting with suspected or proven brain metastases and no previous cancer diagnosis, the workup for systemic tumor should focus on the lungs.[8] It is reasonable to perform a mammogram and a careful skin examination for all patients. Whole-body ^{18}F-fluorodeoxyglucose positron emission tomography (FDG-PET) may reveal a primary tumor undetected by other imaging techniques.[9]

Untreated, these patients have a median survival of about 1 month.[10] Definitive treatment includes surgical resection, stereotactic radiosurgery (i.e., linear accelerator [LINAC] or Gamma Knife radiosurgery), whole-brain external radiotherapy,[11] chemotherapy, and targeted small-molecule therapy.[12] Supportive care, anticonvulsants, corticosteroids,[13] and antiemetics are also important.[14] With corticosteroids alone, median survival increases to 2 months, and with whole-brain irradiation, survival increases to 3 to 6 months.[15]

LEPTOMENINGEAL METASTASES

Leptomeningeal metastasis results in significant morbidity, and median survival is short despite therapy.[16] Overall incidence of leptomeningeal metastasis in cancer is 3% to 8%.[17] Neoplastic meningitis is common in patients with breast cancer, melanoma, non-Hodgkin's lymphoma, or small cell lung cancer.[18] It usually occurs in disseminated disease, and the risk increases with brain metastasis and posterior fossa craniotomy. Malignant cells seeding through the cerebrospinal fluid (CSF) often settle on weblike structures in stasis areas, which explains the high incidence of cranial nerve and cauda equina involvement.[19]

The clinical picture is one of multilevel neurological symptoms and signs.[20] Leptomeningeal metastasis manifests most often with headache, cranial neuropathies, painful radiculopathies, confusion, hydrocephalus, seizures, lethargy, and memory loss.[21]

The most useful laboratory test is CSF examination.[22] Many samples are often necessary. A strong tendency to adhere to nervous tissue or leptomeninges may explain why malignant cells do not appear in the CSF sample in some cases.[23] Patients with suspected leptomeningeal metastases may need one or more lumbar punctures, gadolinium-enhanced MRI of the brain and spine,[24] and a radioisotope flow study of CSF to rule out sites of blockage. If cytology results remain negative and radiological studies are not definitive, biopsy should be considered.[25] If the clinical scenario or radiological studies are highly suggestive, treatment is warranted despite persistently negative CSF cytology results.

The therapeutic approach is a combination of radiotherapy for symptomatic sites and regions of bulky disease,[26] chemotherapy, and medical management with analgesics, antiemetics, and steroids. Chemotherapy options are regional intrathecal methotrexate and cytarabine or thiotepa or systemic high-dose intravenous methotrexate, cytarabine, or thiotepa.[27] Despite intensive therapy, median survival is less than 6 months.

METASTATIC SPINAL CORD COMPRESSION

The epidural space is the most common site of spinal metastasis from solid tumors. This form of spread occurs in 5% to 10% of cases, and the thoracic spine is most frequently involved (see Chapter 222). Up to 38% of patients have several epidural metastases.[28] The associated primary tumors are those with a tendency to metastasize to vertebral bodies. Most originate from breast, lung, prostate, kidney, and gastrointestinal cancers. Spinal cord compression may be the first sign of cancer.[29] The clinical signs and symptoms are related to vertebral metastases and spinal cord and nerve root compression. Severe local back pain that gradually increases in intensity is the earliest and most common sign.[30] The pain is often more severe when the patient is supine, and it is exacerbated by increased intra-abdominal or intrathoracic pressure. Motor dysfunction occurs next. Muscle weakness, hyperactive deep tendon reflexes, spasticity, and extensor plantar responses are common. Weakness is followed by sensory abnormalities, from subjective numbness and tingling to a complete loss of all sensory modalities below the dermatome. Bladder and bowel dysfunction usually appears only after sensory changes. Early pharmacological intervention at the first sign of neurological dysfunction delays paraplegia or quadriplegia and neurological complications.

MRI is the study of choice for screening and diagnosis. MR scans demonstrate the upper and lower level of epidural metastases and the tumor's extraspinal extent.[31] The primary treatment objectives are to relieve pain and prevent spinal cord dysfunction or restore function. Cor-

ticosteroids, radiation therapy, and surgery are the main treatments.[32] Because radiation therapy is less invasive than surgical tumor removal and stabilization and has lower rates of morbidity and mortality, it is the treatment of choice for most patients. Pain must be addressed early and treated aggressively. A good bowel regimen is required because opiates and spinal autonomic dysfunction contribute to constipation. The main indications for corticosteroids are prevention of neurological deficits and analgesia. Surgical decompression is indicated when the cancer diagnosis is in doubt, the primary tumor and cell type are unknown, or the epidural tumor is in a maximally tolerated irradiation area. Major subluxation or fracture may require surgical correction.

NEOPLASIA- AND RADIATION-INDUCED PLEXOPATHIES

Plexopathy is often a disabling complication of advanced systemic cancer and may involve any of the peripheral nerve plexuses. It is characterized by severe, unrelenting pain with later weakness and sensory deficits.[33] Brachial plexopathy most commonly occurs in patients with cancer of the breast or lung.[34] Tumor invasion or compression is the most common cause of brachial plexopathy.[35] Severe pain in the involved arm, shoulder, and axilla, which often is worse with shoulder movement, is the presenting symptom. Patients also may complain of paresthesias and dysesthesias in the arm or hand. Hand weakness and atrophy and Horner's syndrome are common. In radiation-induced plexopathy, early findings are painless weakness of the arm and shoulder and progressive lymphedema.

The lumbosacral plexus usually is invaded by metastases of pelvic primary neoplasms, such as cancer of the prostate, testicle, rectum, bladder, cervix, or uterus, or by growth from metastases to regional lymph nodes or bony structures.[36] Most patients have pain followed by weakness and sensory dysfunction. The clinical diagnosis is confirmed by MRI.[37] MRI is more sensitive than computed tomography (CT) in assessing tumor plexopathy. PET scans can help detect active plexus tumor.

The most common treatment is radiotherapy. Most efforts are directed at pain relief. The multimodality approach includes opiate analgesics, local and regional blocks, sympathectomy, rhizotomy, acupuncture, nerve stimulation, tricyclic antidepressants, and anticonvulsants. Rhizotomy or cordotomy can be considered in highly selected cases. Plexopathy from radiation therapy with resulting weakness and sensory disturbances has no effective treatment.[38] Lymphedema may be treated with compressive devices and elevation.

CEREBROVASCULAR COMPLICATIONS OF CANCER

Cerebrovascular disease is the most common cause of neurological dysfunction after metastatic disease. About 15% of patients have ischemic or hemorrhagic central nervous system lesions.[39] The most common are intracerebral hematomas, and most result from bleeding into a brain metastasis or from coagulation abnormalities. The typical location of these hematomas is cerebral white matter. Hemorrhages may result in focal neurological deficits such as hemiparesis and in generalized symptoms from increased intracranial pressure, causing headache and mental status changes. Cerebral infarction is most often caused by nonbacterial thrombotic endocarditis, disseminated intravascular coagulation, or septic emboli. Central nervous system hemorrhages and infarcts are best visualized on CT scans. If the CT study is negative, MRI can reveal focal or multifocal infarctions and leptomeningeal enhancement, and magnetic resonance venography (MRV) can diagnose a venous occlusion.

Treatment and prognosis depend on the underlying cause. Treatment of tumor-related venous occlusion is typically brain radiation or chemotherapy. Corticosteroids can provide short-term benefit. Hematoma resection may be beneficial for an acute and life-threatening parenchymal intratumoral hemorrhage. Drainage of subdural fluid may be necessary if a tumor-related subdural hematoma is symptomatic.

PARANEOPLASTIC SYNDROMES

Paraneoplastic neurological disorders (see Chapter 233) are mediated by immune responses triggered by tumors that express nervous system proteins. Discrete or multifocal areas degenerate, causing diverse symptoms and deficits. These immune responses are often associated with specific antineuronal antibodies, which can be used as diagnostic markers of the paraneoplastic disorder and underlying cancer. These syndromes are nonmetastatic and not attributable to cancer therapy toxicity, cerebrovascular disease, coagulopathy, infection, or toxic and metabolic causes.[40] The incidence is highest among patients with ovarian cancer, small cell lung cancer, or Hodgkin's lymphoma. These disorders often cause severe, permanent neurological morbidity. Although they may affect any part of the nervous system, they are most commonly subsets of diffuse and multifocal paraneoplastic encephalomyelitis or paraneoplastic encephalomyeloneuritis.[41] Patients can be demented and may have cerebellar and spinal cord abnormalities, peripheral neuropathy, chaotic eye movements, ataxia, or myasthenic syndromes (Table 220-1). Several syndromes should always raise the possibility of a paraneoplastic cause, including Lambert-Eaton myasthenic syndrome, subacute cerebellar degeneration, severe sensory neuronopathy, limbic encephalopathy, and opsoclonus-myoclonus.

Investigations include CT or MRI scans of the chest, abdomen, and pelvis; mammography; and a pelvic examination. There are correlations among individual paraneoplastic syndromes, antineuronal antibody specificities, and associated tumor types. Antineuronal antibody assays have limitations. The neurological outcome varies among different disorders. Some patients have significant neurological improvements solely with treatment of the associated neoplasm. Many others are left with severe, permanent neurological disability despite tumor remission. Those with a progressive neurological disorder receiving chemotherapy should be considered for immunosuppression or immunomodulation, which may include oral or intravenous corticosteroids, intravenous immune globulin, or plasma exchange. People with progressive paraneoplastic syndromes not receiving chemotherapy should be considered for more aggressive immunosuppression, including oral or

TABLE 220-1 Neurological Paraneoplastic Disorders

CENTRAL NERVOUS SYSTEM
Multifocal encephalomyelitis
Cerebellar degeneration
Limbic encephalitis
Opsoclonus myoclonus
Extrapyramidal syndrome
Brainstem encephalitis
Myelopathy
Motor neuron disease
Stiff person syndrome

PERIPHERAL NERVOUS SYSTEM
Sensory neuronopathy
Subacute motor neuronopathy
Sensorimotor polyneuropathy
Lambert-Eaton myasthenic syndrome
Necrotizing or inflammatory myopathy
Autonomic insufficiency
Neuromyotonia
Nerve vasculitis

intravenous cyclophosphamide, tacrolimus, cyclosporin, or rituximab.

NEUROTOXICITY OF CANCER CHEMOTHERAPY

Neurotoxicity is a common side effect of many agents. It should be distinguished from other neurological complications of cancer. Any part of the peripheral or central nervous system can be affected. Each chemotherapeutic agent has potential toxicities. Diffuse encephalopathy and polyneuropathy are most common.

Sensory neuropathy is the major dose-limiting cisplatin toxicity.[42] Carboplatin is much less likely to cause neuropathy. Cytarabine in high intravenous doses is occasionally associated with peripheral neuropathy, including distal sensorimotor polyneuropathy, brachial plexopathy, or rapidly progressive, severe, ascending, demyelinating motor neuropathy resembling Guillain-Barré syndrome. High-dose etoposide causes mainly sensory polyneuropathy. Intrathecal methotrexate has been associated with lumbosacral polyradiculopathy. A predominantly sensory or sensorimotor axonal polyneuropathy is a dose-limiting toxicity of paclitaxel (Taxol) or docetaxel (Taxotere). Thalidomide may cause mainly sensory polyneuropathy. Vincristine causes dose-limiting, symmetrical, sensorimotor axonal polyneuropathy. Hepatic insufficiency is a risk factor for severe vincristine neuropathy. Myelopathy is a devastating but rare complication of intrathecal administration of methotrexate or cytarabine.

CURRENT CONTROVERSIES AND FUTURE CONSIDERATIONS

Patients with brain metastases are rarely cured, but appropriate treatment can improve the quality and duration of life. Until recently, standard treatment of brain metastases consisted of anticonvulsants, dexamethasone, and external beam radiation therapy. Newer options include surgical resection, external beam irradiation, LINAC or Gamma

Knife radiosurgery, and chemotherapy. Judicious treatment selection can effectively treat many serious symptoms of brain metastases, but poor selection may worsen quality of life. Treatment must be directed at the brain metastases and the many other symptoms limiting quality of life.

The mainstay of treatment for brain metastases has been conventional external beam irradiation. Radiation therapy can be administered after surgical resection of solitary or multiple metastatic tumors. Stereotactic radiosurgery with the LINAC or Gamma Knife can achieve similar neurological and qualitative survival for patients with multiple brain metastases compared with wholebrain irradiation.

Chemotherapy has become a better option for brain metastases. Prior reluctance to use it stemmed from concerns about the ability of chemotherapeutic agents to cross the blood-brain barrier and penetrate tumor cells, intrinsic chemoresistance of metastatic disease, and the high probability of death from systemic disease progression. Later data suggest that metastatic tumors have an impaired blood-brain barrier and that several tumors are relatively chemosensitive and may respond to chemotherapy.

REFERENCES

1. Lassman AB, De Angelis LM. Brain metastases. Neurol Clin 2003;21:1-23.
2. Chang SD, Adler JR, Hancock SL. Clinical uses of radiosurgery. Oncology 1998;12:1181-1191.
3. Berk L. An overview of radiotherapy trials for the treatment of brain metastases. Oncology 1995;9:1205-1212.
4. Posner JB, Chernik NL. Intracranial metastases from systemic cancer. Adv Neurol 1978;19:579-592.
5. Cairncross JG, Kim J-H, Posner JB. Radiation therapy of brain metastases. Ann Neurol 1980;7:529-541.
6. Posner JB. Neurologic Complications of Cancer. Philadelphia: FA Davis, 1995.
7. Delattre JY, Krol G, Thaler HT, Posner JB. Distribution of brain metastases. Arch Neurol 1988;45:741-744.
8. Vecht CJ, Haaxma-Reiche H, Noordijk EM, et al. Treatment of single brain metastasis: Radiotherapy alone or combined with neurosurgery? Ann Neurol 1993;33:583-590.
9. Schellinger PD, Meinck HM, Thron A. Diagnostic accuracy of MRI compared to CT in patient with brain metastases. J Neurol Oncol 1999;44:275-281.
10. Nussbaum ES, Djalilian HR, Chok H, Hall WA. Brain metastases: Histology, multiplicity, surgery, and survival. Cancer 1996;78:1781-1788.
11. Sneed PK, Larson DA, Wara WM. Radiotherapy for cerebral metastases. Neurosurg Clin N Am 1996;7:505-515.
12. Patchell RA. The treatment of brain metastases. Cancer Invest 1996;14:169-177.
13. Shapiro WR, Posner JB, Ushio Y, et al. Treatment of meningeal neoplasms. Cancer Treat Rep 1977;61:733-743.
14. Newton HB. Neurological complications of systemic cancer. Am Fam Physician 1999;59:878-886.
15. Newton HB. Primary brain tumors: Review of etiology, diagnosis and treatment. Am Fam Physician 1994;49:787-797.
16. Bindal RK, Sawaya R, Leavens ME, Lee JJ. Surgical treatment of multiple brain metastases. J Neurosurg 1993;79:210-216.
17. Chamberlain MC. Carcinomatous meningitis. Arch Neurol 1997;54:16-17.
18. Blam M, Hammack J. Leptomeningeal carcinomatosis. Presenting features and prognostic factors. Arch Neurol 1996;53:626-632.
19. Chamberlain MC. Combined modality treatment of leptomeningeal gliomatosis. Neurosurgery 2003;52:324-330.
20. Chamberlain MC. Neoplastic meningitis-related encephalopathy: Prognostic significance. Neurology 2003;60:A17-A18.
21. Theodore WH, Gendelman S. Meningeal carcinomatosis. Arch Neurol 1981;38:241-244.
22. Glass JP, Melamed M, Chernik NL, et al. Malignant cells in cerebrospinal fluid: The meaning of positive CSF cytology. Neurology 1999;53:382-382.
23. Grossman SA, Krabak MJ. Leptomeningeal carcinomatosis. Cancer Treat Rev 1999;25:103-119.
24. Schumacher M, Orszagh M. Imaging techniques in neoplastic meningiosis. J Neurooncol 1998;38:111-120.
25. Cheng TM, O'Neill BP, Scheithauer BW, et al. Chronic meningitis: The role of meningeal or cortical biopsy. Neurosurgery 1994;4:590-595.
26. Hildebrand J. Prophylaxis and treatment of leptomeningeal carcinomatosis in solid tumors of adulthood. J Neurooncol 1998;38:193-198.
27. De Angelis LM. Current diagnosis and treatment of leptomeningeal metastasis. J Neurooncol 1998;38:245-252.
28. Bach F, Larsen B, Rhode K, et al. Metastatic spinal cord compression: Occurrence, symptoms, clinical presentations and prognosis in 398 patients with spinal cord compression. Acta Neurochir 1990;107:37-43.
29. Arguello F, Baggs R, Duerst R, et al. Pathogenesis of vertebral metastasis and epidural spinal cord compression. Cancer 1990;65:98-106.
30. Portenoy R, Lipton R, Foley K. Back pain in the cancer patient: An algorithm for evaluation and management. Neurology 1987;37:134-138.
31. Sundaresan N, Sachdev V, Holland J. Surgical treatment of spinal cord compression from epidural metastasis. J Clin Oncol 1995;13:2330-2335.
32. Korner F, Spiegel S, Rider I, et al. Radiation therapy of metastatic spinal cord compression: Multidisciplinary team diagnosis and treatment. J Neurooncol 1999;42:85-92.
33. Kor SH, Foley KM, Posner JB. Brachial plexus lesions in patients with cancer: 100 cases. Neurology 1981;31:45-50.
34. Ampil FL. Radiotherapy for carcinomatous brachial plexopathy. Cancer 1985;56:2185-2188.
35. Glass JP. Brachial and lumbar plexopathies in cancer patients. Cancer Bull 1986;38:53-57.
36. Jaeckle KA, Young DF, Foley KM. The natural history of lumbosacral plexopathy in cancer. Neurology 1985;35:8-15.
37. Pettigrew LC, Glass JP, Maor M. Diagnosis and treatment of lumbosacral plexopathies in patients with cancer. Arch Neurol 1984;41:1282-1285.
38. Thomas JE, Cascino TL, Earle JD. Differential diagnosis between radiation and tumor plexopathy of the pelvis. Neurology 1985;35:1-7.
39. Graus F, Rogers LR, Posner JB. Cerebrovascular complications in patients with cancer. Medicine (Baltimore) 1985;64:16-35.
40. Dalman JO, Posner JB. Paraneoplastic syndromes affecting the nervous system. Semin Oncol 1997;24:318-328.
41. Rudnick SA, Dalman J. Paraneoplastic syndrome of the spinal cord, nerve, and muscle. Muscle Nerve 2000;23:1800-1818.
42. Boogerd W, Huinink WW, Dalesio O, et al. Cisplatin induced neuropathy: Central, peripheral, and autonomic nerve involvement. J Neurooncol 1990;9:255-263.

SUGGESTED READING

Ross KL, Dalman JO. Neurological complications of cancer. Semin Neurol 2004;24:347-469.

Rottenberg DA. Neurological Complications of Cancer Treatment. Boston: Butterworth-Heinemann, 1991.

Wen PY, Glantz MJ. Neurological complications of cancer [preface]. Neurol Clin 2003;21:xi-xiii.

Wiley RG. Neurological Complications of Cancer. New York: Marcel Dekker, 1995.

CHAPTER **221**

Brain Metastases

Christoph Ostgathe and **Raymond Voltz**

KEY POINTS

- The diagnosis of brain metastases often determines the transition from a curative to a palliative care approach.
- Patients with brain metastases require an interdisciplinary approach.
- Brain metastases are a major source of physical and psychosocial suffering.
- Brain edema due to metastases may provide a peaceful death in the form of sleep due to increasing cranial pressure.

In about 20% to 40% of patients with systemic malignancies, brain metastases[1] are diagnosed at some point during the illness. Life expectancy is reduced significantly, and the mean survival is 1 to 6 months, depending on the histology and the applied therapies.[2] Brain metastases often lead to serious deterioration of neurological and neurocognitive functions.[3] Treatment should aim at the best possible restoration and maintenance of quality of life by an individually tailored focus on symptoms, possibly in combination with disease-modifying treatment. The care of patients with brain metastases can be paradigmatical for an interdisciplinary medical approach that includes specialists in neurology, neuro-oncology, neurosurgery, radiotherapy, oncology, and palliative medicine. The main focus for the palliative care physician is to manage the symptoms and complications directly caused by metastases, such as focal weakness, seizures, pain, or increased intracranial pressure, and the side effects of commonly used medications, such as steroids, antiepileptics, and analgesics.

In addition to existential distress, patients with brain metastases and their families fear that the diagnosis may lead to a loss of individual control, cognition, or consciousness and a change in the patient's personality and character. This concern underlines the necessity for a multiprofessional approach that includes specialists in medicine, psychology, social work, and spiritual care.

EPIDEMIOLOGY AND PREVALENCE

The incidence of brain metastases appears to be increasing. Newer systemic treatment options increase the longevity of patients with advanced diseases, and this makes the occurrence of metastases in the central nervous system (CNS) more likely because tumor cells may "hide" behind the blood-brain barrier.[4] Improved and more broadly available imaging techniques also lead to more diagnoses.[5]

In an adult cancer population, the most frequent origins of brain metastases are lung cancer (50%), breast cancer (15% to 20%), and melanoma (10%). Renal cancer, colorectal cancer, lymphoma, and unknown primary cancer are the next most common sources. Detection of single or solitary metastases occurs more often in patients with breast, renal, or colon carcinoma, which account for one third to one fourth of diagnosed CNS metastases, whereas multiple metastases are more commonly seen in patients with melanoma or lung cancer.[6] If three or fewer metastases are detected, there may be a greater chance for successful focal therapy.[4]

Prognosis is poor for patients with brain metastases. Systemic tumor activity, the number of metastases (single or multiple), age, performance status, and response to steroids were found to be prognostic factors[7,8] (Table 221-1).

Other possible sites for metastases are the leptomeninges of the brain. Leptomeningeal metastasis, also known as carcinomatous meningitis, meningeosis carcinomatosa, neoplastic meningitis, and neoplastic meningosis, occurs in 4% to 15% of patients (in declining frequency) diagnosed with breast cancer, lung cancer, and melanoma.[9] Autopsy studies demonstrate that 19% of patients with cancer and neurological deficits have malignant involvement of the leptomeninges.[10] Up to 75% of the patients with neoplastic meningosis also suffer from brain metastases.[11]

PATHOPHYSIOLOGY

After intravasation and migration in blood or lymphatic vessels, tumor cells not destroyed by apoptosis, mechanical damage, or immunological processes have the chance to adhere in a capillary bed. Most cancers follow the patterns of venous or arterial drainage and metastasize first in a distant capillary bed. Secondary metastases can develop if the cells from the primary metastases intravasate, migrate, and arrest in a new site. This explains why brain involvement can develop rather late during the course of the disease. In some cancers (e.g., lung), the brain is a primary site for metastases. After the tumor cell arrests in the capillary bed, it must extravasate into the brain parenchyma to complete the metastatic process. The blood-brain barrier does not hinder tumor cells from extravasating, but it does provide protection for those cells against many therapeutic agents.[4]

After extravasation, surviving tumor cells grow or lie dormant. Single tumor cells or micrometastases can become dormant, a state in which proliferation and apoptosis are in balance and that may last for months or years. This explains the time between the diagnosis of the primary or apparent cure of disease and the appearance of brain metastases, which sometimes are identified years or decades later.

The pathogenesis of neoplastic meningosis is variable. The tumor cells reach the leptomeninges by hematogenous spread, by direct extension from contiguous tumor deposits, or through centripetal migration from systemic tumors along the perineural or perivascular spaces.[9] In the subarachnoid space, tumor cells can be transported and

CLASS	FACTORS	MEDIAN SURVIVAL	NO. OF METASTASES	MEDIAN SURVIVAL
I	KPS ≥70 Age <65 Controlled primary tumor *and* no extracranial disease	7.1 mo	Single Multiple	13.5 mo 6.0 mo
II	KPS ≥70 *and* age ≥65 *or* with active extracranial disease	4.2 mo	Single Multiple	8.1 mo 4.1 mo
III	KPS <70	2.3 mo		

TABLE 221-1 Prognostic Factors

KPS, Karnofsky performance score.
Data from references 7, 23, 24.

disseminated by the cerebrospinal fluid. The main foci for dissemination are the basal cisterns, the dorsal surface of the spinal chord, and the cauda equina (Fig. 221-1) (see "Case Study: Brain Metastases").

CLINICAL MANIFESTATIONS

More than 60% of patients with cerebral metastases develop some neurological symptoms during the course of their disease.[12] The most common symptoms are pain, focal weakness, cognitive dysfunction, and seizures. Symp-

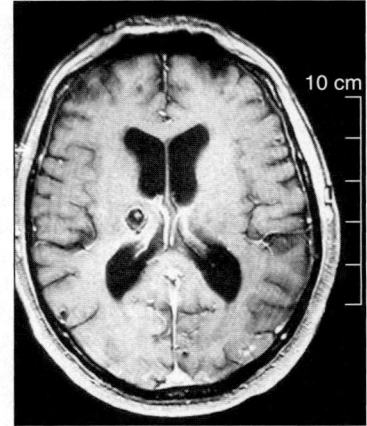

FIGURE 221-1 Noncontrast, T1-weighted magnetic resonance image of a patient with disseminated brain metastases and susceptible intralesional bleeding.

 C A S E   S T U D Y

Brain Metastases

A 57-year-old patient diagnosed with non–small cell lung cancer 18 months earlier was admitted to the medical clinic of the university hospital with acute paresis of the right arm and vertigo. Magnetic resonance imaging of his brain showed disseminated brain metastases (i.e., frontal, temporal, parietal, occipital, precentral, and postcentral lobes; cerebellum; and thalamus) up to 1.7 cm in diameter with perifocal edema and suspected bleeding within some lesions 6 months before admission and before the lung metastases were detected.

The patient received dexamethasone (24 mg daily), and whole-brain radiotherapy was started. Initially, his neurological status improved, and the patient was discharged. Radiation therapy was continued in the outpatient setting.

Five weeks later, the patient had to be readmitted to the hospital and was transferred to the palliative care unit with dyspnea and worsening neurological and neurocognitive functions, with aphasia, ataxia, continuing paresis of the arm, confusion, and cognitive deceleration. Because of the reduced functional status of the patient, management concentrated on symptom-oriented treatment. Dyspnea was controlled with 1 mg of hydromorphone every 4 hours. His nonconvulsive epileptic status was discussed, and valproic acid was prescribed. The patient deteriorated rapidly and died within 36 hours after admission.

toms and complications are closely connected to the number of lesions and the location within the CNS. Because the distribution of metastases is influenced by blood flow, most lesions are found in the cerebral hemispheres (80%), followed by the cerebellum (15%) and the brainstem (5%), preferentially at the border between gray and white matter.[3] Most patients gradually become symptomatic; in 5% to 10%, neurological changes have an acute onset, which is often caused by hemorrhage or embolic compressive infarction.[12,13] Some patients have fluctuating episodes of deterioration and improvement of orientation and behavior. Deterioration can be the sign of a nonconvulsive epileptic seizure, which must be diagnosed and treated (Table 221-2).

The mainstay of diagnosing and localizing brain metastases is gadolinium-enhanced (0.3 mmol/kg) magnetic resonance imaging (MRI), which is used far more than computed tomography (CT). In 30% of patients with single lesions detected on contrast-enhanced CT, enhanced MRI shows multiple lesions. CT can be helpful in identifying skull metastases and hemorrhage within metastases.[14]

The clinical manifestations of neoplastic meningosis vary. They can appear similar to brain metastases, with headache and mental status changes; when cranial nerves are affected, the dysfunction correlates with the function of the involved nerve (Table 221-3).

To ensure the diagnosis of neoplastic meningosis, examination of the cerebrospinal fluid is essential. A high cell count, positive cytology result, low glucose level, elevated protein level, and increased opening pressure are possible findings.

DIFFERENTIAL DIAGNOSIS

Any change in neurological and neurocognitive functions in patients with cancer should alert physicians to the possibility of malignant involvement of the CNS. The main diagnostic features can be identified on contrast-enhanced MRI or on CT. About 10% of lesions detected are not metastases, and alternative diagnoses, such as infarction, sinus vein thrombosis, hemorrhage, abscess, multiple sclerosis, or primary brain tumors such as glioblastoma, must be considered. A rare possibility is a paraneoplastic neurological disorder.[15]

TABLE 221-2 Common Symptoms and Signs of Brain Metastases

SYMPTOMS OR SIGNS	FREQUENCY	POSSIBLE CAUSE
Headache	40-50%	Increased cranial pressure, nonconvulsive status
Nausea, vomiting	20-40%	

Cognitive dysfunction
  Impaired memory
  Mood disturbances
  Confusion, hallucinations
  Disinhibition, inhibition
  Somnolence, sopor, coma
	60-70%	

Focal seizures	40%	Focal neurological symptoms
Hemiparesis		
Aphasia		
Hemianopsia	40%	
Focal weakness		

TABLE 221-3 Symptoms and Signs of Neoplastic Meningosis with a Focus on Intracranial Involvement

SYMPTOMS OR SIGNS	FREQUENCY	POSSIBLE CAUSE
Headache	30-75%	Cerebral hemisphere dysfunction
Nausea, vomiting	22-34%	
Cognitive dysfunction Lethargy Confusion Memory loss	10-25%	
Difficulty walking	27-36%	
Facial paresis	27-41%	Affection of cranial nerves
Diplopia	20-41%	
Facial numbness	8-18%	
Dysphagia	2-14%	

Adapted from Chamberlain MC. Neoplastic meningitis. Neurologist 2006;12:179-187.

MANAGEMENT

Palliative care of patients with brain metastases focuses on symptom-oriented treatment and the prophylaxis and management of side effects. However, the antineoplastic options (e.g., systemic chemotherapy, radiotherapy, stereotactic radiosurgery, and neurosurgery) must be considered on an individual basis. The palliative care specialist should be part of the decision-making process and advise the patient, family, and other health care workers about supportive measures.

Antineoplastic Treatment Options

The available evidence suggests that whole brain radiation therapy (WBRT) offers a modest survival benefit for an unselected group of patients.[2] Selection in terms of performance status (Karnofsky performance status [KPS] = 70) seems to improve the expected benefit.[2] Total doses of 30 to 37.5 Gy are suggested. Different fractionation regimens did not lead to superior overall survival; 10 fractions of 3 Gy over 2 weeks or 15 fractions of 2.5 Gy over 3 weeks are recommended.[16] In patients with a single metastasis, large lesions (>3 cm), and stable extracranial disease, surgical resection followed by WBRT is the treatment of choice.[17] Advances in techniques such as image-guided microsurgery and intraoperative functional mapping have reduced overall surgical morbidity and mortality.[18] There is no advantage for surgery with WBRT compared with WBRT alone for individuals with multiple brain metastases.[16]

As an alternative to surgery, WBRT can be reasonably combined with stereotactic radiosurgery. Stereotactic radiosurgery can deliver an effective dose of radiation to an intracranial target. It is minimally invasive, is well tolerated, and can conserve surrounding healthy tissue. No data are available that confirm a difference in outcomes between surgery and stereotactic radiosurgery. Multiple lesions, a tumor smaller than 35 mm in diameter, a minimal mass effect, metastases in or near eloquent cortex, deep lesions, and high anesthesia risk are relative indications for stereotactic radiosurgery. Relative indications for surgery include surgically accessible tumor, a mass effect, seizures, neurological deficits, and an uncertain diagnosis.[18]

Compared with other antineoplastic options, chemotherapy is inferior in the management of brain metastases. However, in contrast to the notion that the blood-brain barrier is a hindrance for chemotherapeutic agents, the regimens suited for the primary tumor can be applied to treat brain metastases, probably because the blood-brain barrier is locally destroyed. Drugs with better penetration into the CNS, such as the alkylating agent temozolomide, the small-molecule erlonitib, or the selective topoisomerase I inhibitor topotecan, are the focus of clinical trails.

Symptom-Oriented Treatment

Most symptoms of patients with brain metastases are generated by focal parenchymal changes caused by metastases or by increased intracranial pressure caused by the accompanying vasogenic edema. Treatment is mainly symptom oriented; for example, the edema may be reduced for some period. In most patients, brain metastases are only part of the general progression of the disease, and the symptom burden can be significantly aggravated by progression of the primary or metastases at other sites.

Increased Intracranial Pressure

Corticosteroids (e.g., dexamethasone) are used to reduce increased intracranial pressure. To improve patients' compliance and to reduce steroid-induced insomnia, once-daily application in the morning is possible. In patients receiving WBRT, steroids should be continued at a dosage of 4 mg/day for 1 week after irradiation and then reduced by 1 mg/day every week.[19]

Steroids have significant toxic effects (e.g., hyperglycemia, peripheral edema, myopathy, psychiatric disorders[20]), and therapy should aim for the least possible dose that can achieve symptom improvement. The starting dose for patients with increased intracranial pressure is 8 to 16 mg of dexamethasone. This should be reduced in a stepwise manner to a maintenance dose of 2 to 4 mg daily, depending on the clinical response. If no response is observed within 72 to 96 hours after initiation, steroid medication should be stopped. In case of an obvious progression of the disease with deterioration of the patient's general status, discontinuation of steroids can be considered, because brain edema due to metastases may also provide a chance of a peaceful death in the form of sleep caused by increasing cranial pressure. This decision should be discussed with the patient and the family. In case of cognitive impairment, a decision to stop or to continue steroid medication should be based on the presumed will and the medical indication. Decision making is a team process.

Seizures

Many patients with brain metastases develop epilepsy during the course of the disease. Focal or generalized seizures are the presenting symptom in 15% to 20% of these patients.[1] Patients with symptomatic epilepsy should be treated with anticonvulsants starting with the first seizure. Valproic acid (1000 to 2000 mg/day) is considered a first-line agent. The enzyme-inhibiting potential within the P450 coenzyme metabolic pathway seems to have little clinical impact. If sufficient control of epilepsy is not achieved, levetiracetam (1000 to 2000 mg/day) should be added.[21]

Prophylactic anticonvulsant treatment of patients with brain malignancies and no history of seizures is not indicated because of lack of effectiveness and possible side effects or interactions with other medications.[22] Typical side effects of antiepileptic drugs are asthenia, sleepiness, and cognitive impairment. In patients suffering from neurocognitive dysfunctions, a nonconvulsive epileptic seizure must be taken into consideration, especially in a patient with a sudden onset of the symptom or when there are rapid changes between clear and confused states.

Pain

Patients with brain metastases often suffer from headaches. Besides steroids for managing increased intracranial pressure, patients may need additional analgesics administered according to the World Health Organization pain ladder. Nonsteroidal anti-inflammatory drugs (NSAIDs) should be prescribed with caution because of the doubled gastrointestinal toxicity in combination with steroids. Neuropathic pain caused by cranial nerves involved by neoplastic meningosis can make anticonvulsant drugs (e.g., gabapentin, pregabalin, clonazepam) necessary.

Focal Neurological Deficiencies

Symptomatic treatment of focal neurological deficiencies aims to reduce focal or general edema to enhance function, at least for a limited period. Physical therapy can help to maintain patients' mobility and well-being.

Psychosocial Support

In addition to the existential distress of patients with brain metastases and their families, the diagnosis may lead to a change in or loss of individual control, cognition, or consciousness, and it may influence the patient's personality and character. Family members often feel overburdened by the situation. Besides competent medical treatment and information, psychological, social, and spiritual support should be offered to the patient and family members.

REFERENCES

1. Taillibert S, Delattre JY. Palliative care in patients with brain metastases. Curr Opin Oncol 2005;17:588-592.
2. Pease NJ, Edwards A, Moss LJ. Effectiveness of whole brain radiotherapy in the treatment of brain metastases: A systematic review. Palliat Med 2005;19:288-299.
3. Langer CJ, Mehta MP. Current management of brain metastases, with a focus on systemic options. J Clin Oncol 2005;23: 6207-6219.
4. Gavrilovic IT, Posner JB. Brain metastases: Epidemiology and pathophysiology. J Neurooncol 2005;75:5-14.
5. Richards GM, Khuntia D, Mehta MP. Therapeutic management of metastatic brain tumors. Crit Rev Oncol Hematol 2007;61:70-78.
6. Norden AD, Wen PY, Kesari S. Brain metastases. Curr Opin Neurol 2005;18:654-661.
7. Gaspar LE, Scott C, Murray K, Curran WJ. Validation of the RTOG recursive partitioning analysis (RPA) classification for brain metastases. Int J Radiat Oncol Biol Phys 2000;47:1001-1006.
8. Lagerwaard FJ, Levendag PC, Nowak PJ, et al. Identification of prognostic factors in patients with brain metastases: A review of 1292 patients, Int J Radiat Oncol Biol Phys 1999;43:795-803.
9. Chamberlain MC. Neoplastic meningitis. Neurologist 2006;12:179-187.
10. Glass JP, Melamed M, Chernik NL, Posner JB. Malignant cells in cerebrospinal fluid (CSF): The meaning of a positive CSF cytology. Neurology 1979;29: 1369-1375.
11. Ushio Y, Posner R, Kim JH, et al. Treatment of experimental spinal cord compression caused by extradural neoplasms. J Neurosurg 1977;47:380-390.
12. Oneschuk D, Bruera E. Palliative management of brain metastases. Support Care Cancer 1988;6:365-372.
13. Nutt SH, Patchell RA. Intracranial hemorrhage associated with primary and secondary tumors. Neurosurg Clin N Am 1992;3:591-599.
14. Schellinger PD, Meinck HM, Thron A. Diagnostic accuracy of MRI compared to CCT in patients with brain metastases. J Neurooncol 1999;44:275-281.
15. Voltz R, Graus F. Diagnosis and treatment of paraneoplastic neurological disorders. Onkologie 2004;27:253-258.
16. Richards GM, Khuntia D, Mehta MP. Therapeutic management of metastatic brain tumors. Crit Rev Oncol Hematol 2007;61:70-78.
17. Noordijk EM, Vecht CJ, Haaxma-Reiche H, et al. The choice of treatment of single brain metastasis should be based on extracranial tumor activity and age [see comments]. Int J Radiat Oncol Biol Phys 1994;29:711-717.
18. Vogelbaum MA, Suh JH. Resectable brain metastases. J Clin Oncol 1006;24:1289-1294.
19. Vecht CJ, Hovestadt A, Verbiest HBC, et al. Dose effect relationship of dexamethasone in metastatic brain tumors: A randomized study of doses of 4, 8, and 16 mg per day. Neurology 1994;44:675-680.
20. Hempen C, Weiss E, Hess CF. Dexamethasone treatment in patients with brain metastases and primary brain tumors: Do the benefits outweigh the side-effects? Support Care Cancer 2002;10:322-328.
21. Vecht CJ, Breemen M. Optimizing therapy of seizures in patients with brain tumors. Neurology 2006;67:S10-S13.
22. Glantz MJ, Cole BF, Forsyth PA, et al. Practice parameter: Anticonvulsant prophylaxis in patients with newly diagnosed brain tumors. Report of the Quality Standards Subcommittee of the American Academy of Neurology. Neurology 2000;54:1886-1893.
23. Lutterbach J, Bartelt S, Ostertag C. Long-term survival in patients with brain metastases. J Cancer Res Clin Oncol 2002;128:417-425.
24. Kaal EC, Taphoorn MJ, Vecht CJ. Symptomatic management and imaging of brain metastases. J Neurooncol 2005;75:15-20.

CHAPTER **222**

Bone Metastases

Aruna Mani and Charles L. Shapiro

K E Y   P O I N T S

- The skeleton is a frequent site of metastatic disease. Skeletal metastases can cause significant morbidity including pain, pathological fractures, spinal cord compression, and hypercalcemia that adversely affect quality of life.

- The normal bone microenvironment is rich in growth factors that mediate the normal dynamic balance between resorption and new bone formation. Some of these substances are also autocrine and paracrine growth factors for tumor cells. When tumors metastasize to bone, they disrupt the normal balance between bone resorption and formation so that resorption generally predominates. This causes pain, fractures, and hypercalcemia and the radiographic appearance of lytic metastases.

- Treatment of symptomatic bone metastases includes both local and systemic treatments. Local therapies include orthopedic fixation, radiation therapy, and vertebroplasty; systemic treatments include bisphosphonates and radionuclides. The best outcomes are from bone-specific treatments combined with effective anticancer therapies.

- Bisphosphonates specifically inhibit bone resorption. They reduce skeletal-related events (SREs) such as pain and pathological fracture in multiple myeloma, breast cancer, and other solid tumors.

PATHOPHYSIOLOGY

Normal bone undergoes constant resorption and new bone formation. These processes occur in discrete remodeling units mediated by two cell types: osteoclasts for bone resorption and osteoblasts for new bone formation. A dynamic balance between resorption and formation maintains bone strength and structural integrity.[1] Systemic regulation occurs through hormones such as parathyroid hormone (PTH), calcitonin, estrogens, and androgens. Cytokines and growth factors produced in the remodeling unit microenvironment regulate osteoclast and osteoblast functions.

Important examples are receptor activator of nuclear factor-κB (RANK) and RANK ligand (RANKL).[2] RANKL is expressed from osteoblasts by PTH, cytokines, and growth factors. Binding of the RANKL to RANK on osteoclast precursors differentiates them into mature osteoclasts and activates them. Osteoprotegerin (OPG) is a decoy receptor from osteoblasts in response to estrogens and other cytokines and growth factors that mimics RANK. By binding to RANKL, OPG prevents interaction of RANKL with RANK, decreases osteoclast resorption, and promotes new bone formation.

When tumor cells metastasize to bone, the normal balance between resorption and new bone formation is altered and usually causes increased osteoclastic activity. Tumor cells directly express RANKL and PTH-related protein, which increase osteoclastic activity with more resorption and cytokine and growth factor release that, in turn, stimulate tumor cell growth. This process has been termed a vicious cycle.[3-5] Metastatic prostate cancer is characterized by osteoblastic metastases; prostate cancer cells release growth factors that increase osteoblast activity.[5,6]

CLINICAL MANIFESTATIONS

The most common cancers that metastasize to bone are breast and prostate. Bone is the most frequent initial site of metastasis in women with breast cancer; 65% to 75% of patients with breast cancer will have bone metastasis. Of patients with prostate cancer, 80% to 90% will develop bone metastasis. These metastases appear either as lytic or sclerotic lesions on radiographs, depending on whether osteoclastic or osteoblastic activity predominates. Fewer than 10% of these patients will have solitary lesions. Commonly, the axial and appendicular skeleton is affected; the most common sites in breast cancer are vertebrae (70%), pelvis (40%), proximal femur (25%), and skull (14%).[7]

Up to two thirds of persons with bone metastasis have SREs including pain, pathological fracture, spinal cord compression, and hypercalcemia (see Chapter 228). The most common manifestation of bone metastasis is pain. In addition, in advanced spinal cord compression (see Chapter 223), bowel or bladder dysfunction, extremity weakness, and dermatomal sensory level deficit may occur. Early manifestations of spinal cord compression may be subtle. In any patient with cancer, either with or without known bone metastases, who presents with back pain, especially if the pain is of new onset or increased intensity, the possibility of spinal cord compression should be considered and promptly evaluated. This is because the symptoms of spinal cord compression may rapidly progress to irreversible paralysis, and outcomes directly relate to functional status at diagnosis of the compression. The symptoms of hypercalcemia (see Chapter 228) are nonspecific and may include nausea, vomiting, constipation, and confusion; if untreated, this condition may cause death.

Imaging Modalities

Imaging modalities include plain radiography, radionuclide bone scintigraphy, computed tomography (CT), magnetic resonance imaging (MRI), and positron emission tomography (PET).[1,8] The lack of sensitivity of plain radiographs limits their usefulness for detecting bone metastases. These metastases are highly specific for lytic destruction. Radionuclide bone scintigraphy (bone scan) using 99 m technetium measures osteoblastic activity, not the tumor directly.[9] Even in predominantly lytic lesions, osteoblastic overactivity is usually present, and this property is the basis for the test. Exceptions are purely lytic metastases such as in multiple myeloma, in which the bone scan may be negative.

In contrast to plain radiography, bone scanning is highly specific but lacks specificity because nonmalignant degenerative disease, infection, and other benign bone abnormalities cause focal uptake on the scan. It is common to perform the bone scan first and then plain films of areas of focal uptake. The plain film identifies either a lytic (or blastic) lesion or degenerative disease in which the focal uptake on the bone scan is clarified by the plain film. A bone scan abnormality with a normal plain radiograph merits imaging with CT or MRI to confirm bone metastasis.

PET employs fluorodeoxyglucose (FDG) or other tracers to highlight areas of increased metabolic activity. Data are conflicting about whether the overall sensitivity and specificity of PET-FDG are superior to those of bone scanning.[8] PET-FDG may be less sensitive than bone scan in prostate cancer and other tumors with predominantly sclerotic bone metastases.

The challenges of assessing therapeutic response are substantial,[8] and bone metastases are considered nonmeasurable disease by standard response assessment criteria.[10] In lytic lesions, effective treatment causes sclerosis or new bone formation. Serial skeletal radiographs may not change for up to 6 months. Scintigraphic flare is characterized by new focal lesions and increased intensity of existing lesions on serial bone scans 2 to 4 months after systemic hormone therapy in breast cancer.[11] Although scintigraphic flare often predicts subsequent treatment response, it is indistinguishable from progressive disease on the bone scan. Clinicians should be aware of this possibility and not prematurely change therapy without additional evidence suggesting disease progression, such as increasing lytic lesions.

CT and MRI scanning are not practical for evaluating therapeutic response for widespread bone metastases. PET-FDG may be useful; however, a flare is also reported, and granulocyte colony-stimulating factor may increase tracer uptake into the marrow, thereby obscuring bone metastases.[8]

Markers of bone turnover such as type I collagen telopeptides and collagen-pyridinium cross-links may act as early markers of progression in bone and may predict SREs; conversely, levels of these markers decrease after bisphosphonate therapy and may correlate with clinical benefit.[8] Although bone turnover markers seem promising, they are experimental.

TREATMENT

The goals of treatment are to palliate pain, to preserve functionality, and to reduce subsequent morbidity. Bone-specific anticancer therapies and pain medications are the mainstays of treatment. Bone metastasis may require local treatment, in addition to bone-specific systemic treatments. Local treatments include surgery for impending pathological fracture, radiation therapy, and vertebroplasty.

Orthopedic Therapy

In weight-bearing bones, orthopedic fixation of impending pathological fractures is always preferred to repairing a subsequent fracture.[12] Scoring systems based on the character of the lesion (lytic versus blastic), location, extent of cortical involvement, and pain may predict pathological fracture.[13] After orthopedic fixation, pain relief is often immediate, and patients quickly rehabilitate. Later, external beam radiation therapy to the site is usually recommended.

The decision to fix a pathological fracture also depends on additional factors such as life expectancy and functional status. In many patients, pain relief and preservation of function (e.g., walking) justify orthopedic fixation. In cancer-related spinal cord compression, surgical treatment combined with plus radiation therapy is superior to radiation therapy alone in outcomes such as the ability to walk after treatment and decreased use of opioid analgesics (see Chapter 223).[14]

Painful vertebral compression fractures may be treated with percutaneous vertebroplasty and kyphoplasty.[15,16] The procedures involve injecting bone cement directly into the affected vertebrae or inserting an inflatable bone tamp into the vertebrae and filling it with cement, respectively. Significant reductions in pain and opioid use and improvements in quality of life result, with minimal complications.

Radiation Therapy

Indications for external beam radiation therapy include *localized* pain that is poorly responsive to pain medications in an area corresponding to imaging studies that confirm bone metastases. Up to 80% of patients experience some pain relief after radiation.[9] No role exists for irradiation of asymptomatic bone metastases, and it may cause harm from compromised bone marrow function. No difference was reported in pain relief between a single large-dose fraction and standard multiple-dose fractions.[17] Patients given single fractions had higher repeat treatment rates and slightly more pathological fractures.

Systemic Therapy

Bisphosphonates are inorganic analogues of pyrophosphate and specific osteoclast inhibitors. These drugs directly inhibit osteoclastic bone resorption and recruitment of precursor cells into mature osteoclasts. Indications for the use of bisphosphonates include treatment of hypercalcemia of malignancy; reduction of pain and narcotic consumption; and decreases in subsequent SREs in patients with breast, prostate, multiple myeloma, and other solid tumors.[18-22] Oral bisphosphonates such as clodronate are less potent and bioavailable than intravenous (IV) bisphosphonates and may cause gastrointestinal toxicity.

In the United States, the three approved IV bisphosphonates are pamidronate, ibandronate, and zoledronic acid. Pamidronate (90 mg over a 2-hour infusion) and zoledronic acid (4 mg over 15 minutes), given every 3 to 4 weeks, provide similar reductions in SREs and pain relief in multiple myeloma and breast cancer.[23] By preventing SREs, bisphosphonates are cost-effective.[20] The standard schedule of IV bisphosphonates is every 3 to 4 weeks. The optimal duration and schedule are unknown, and clinical trials will address these important questions (see "Future Considerations"). This issue is important given the increasingly recognized complication of avascular osteonecrosis of the jaw (ONJ).

ONJ is a dreaded bisphosphonate complication without effective therapy, although antibiotic therapy, maintenance of good oral hygiene, and avoidance of dental surgery are recommended.[24] The cumulative hazard rate of ONJ is about 1% at 12 months and up to 11% at 4 years. Dental procedures within the past year, use of zoledronate (as opposed to pamidronate), and increasing duration of bisphosphonate treatment are predisposing factors. Caution should be used in continuing pamidronate or zoledronic acid for more than 2 years.[24]

The oral bisphosphonate clodronate may prevent bone metastases in women with early breast cancer.[25] Controlled trials of clodronate, ibandronate, and zoledronic acid will answer this important question. In prostate cancer, placebo-controlled trials of clodronate or zoledronic acid did not prevent or delay bone metastases.[21]

Radiopharmaceuticals such as strontium 89 and samarium 23 deliver localized radiation to bone metastases, as opposed to external beam radiation directed to an individual site. Radiopharmaceuticals relieve pain and decrease opioid consumption; the major toxicity is mild thrombocytopenia.[26] Radiopharmaceuticals are options for patients with multiple painful bone metastases that are poorly controlled with opioids and in whom systemic anticancer therapy is unlikely to be effective.

Future Considerations

- The optimal duration and schedule of bisphosphonate therapy are unknown. These issues are of particular importance with the increasing recognition of osteonecrosis of the jaw, which seems related to the duration of administration.
- Bone turnover markers such as telopeptides or collagen-pyridinium cross-links are promising when used to predict early response (or progression) to bisphosphonates. The use of these markers in routine clinical decision making is undefined.
- Controlled trials (although not yet reported) will establish whether bisphosphonates can prevent or delay bone metastases in women with breast cancer.

New Agents

Denosumab, a humanized monoclonal antibody directed against RANKL, led to sustained reductions in bone turnover markers (urinary and serum *N*-telopeptides) in patients with multiple myeloma and breast cancer after a single subcutaneous injection.[27] Atrasentan, an inhibitor of endothelin-1 receptor that decreases osteoblast activity, is being evaluated in metastatic prostate cancer.[28]

REFERENCES

1. Shapiro CL. Bisphosphonates in breast cancer patients with skeletal metastases. Hematol Oncol Clin North Am 1994;8:153-163.
2. Hofbauer LC, Schoppet M. Clinical implications of the osteoprotegerin/RANKL/RANK system for bone and vascular diseases. JAMA 2004;292:490-495.
3. Mundy GR. Metastasis to bone: Causes, consequences and therapeutic opportunities. Nat Rev Cancer 2002;2:584-593.
4. Kakonen SM, Mundy GR. Mechanisms of osteolytic bone metastases in breast carcinoma. Cancer 2003;97:834-839.
5. Roodman GD. Mechanisms of bone metastasis. N Engl J Med 2004;350:1655-1664.
6. Higano CS. Understanding treatments for bone loss and bone metastases in patients with prostate cancer: A practical review and guide for the clinician. Urol Clin North Am 2004;31:331-352.
7. Gainford MC, Dranitsaris G, Clemons M. Recent developments in bisphosphonates for patients with metastatic breast cancer. BMJ 2005;330:769-773.
8. Clamp A, Danson S, Nguyen H, et al. Assessment of therapeutic response in patients with metastatic bone disease. Lancet Oncol 2004;5:607-616.
9. Bagi CM. Targeting of therapeutic agents to bone to treat metastatic cancer. Adv Drug Deliv Rev 2005;57:995-1010.
10. Therasse P, Arbuck SG, Eisenhauer EA, et al. New guidelines to evaluate the response to treatment in solid tumors: European Organization for Research and Treatment of Cancer, National Cancer Institute of the United States, National Cancer Institute of Canada. J Natl Cancer Inst 2000;92:205-216.
11. Vogel CL, Schoenfelder J, Shemano I, et al. Worsening bone scan in the evaluation of antitumor response during hormonal therapy of breast cancer. J Clin Oncol 1995;13:1123-1128.
12. Katzer A, Meenen NM, Grabbe F, et al. Surgery of skeletal metastases. Arch Orthop Trauma Surg 2002;122:251-258.
13. Mirels H. Metastatic disease in long bones: A proposed scoring system for diagnosing impending pathologic fractures. 1989. Clin Orthop Relat Res 2003;415(Suppl):S4-S13.
14. Patchell RA, Tibbs PA, Regine WF, et al. Direct decompressive surgical resection in the treatment of spinal cord compression caused by metastatic cancer: A randomised trial. Lancet 2005;366:643-648.
15. Dudeney S, Lieberman IH, Reinhardt MK, et al. Kyphoplasty in the treatment of osteolytic vertebral compression fractures as a result of multiple myeloma. J Clin Oncol 2002;20:2382-2387.
16. Fourney DR, Schomer DF, Nader R, et al. Percutaneous vertebroplasty and kyphoplasty for painful vertebral body fractures in cancer patients. J Neurosurg 2003;98:21-30.
17. Sze WM, Shelley MD, Held I, et al. Palliation of metastatic bone pain: Single fraction versus multifraction radiotherapy—a systematic review of randomised trials. Clin Oncol (R Coll Radiol) 2003;15:345-352.
18. Ross JR, Saunders Y, Edmonds PM, et al. Systematic review of role of bisphosphonates on skeletal morbidity in metastatic cancer. BMJ 2003;327:469.
19. Body JJ. Bisphosphonates for malignancy-related bone disease: Current status, future developments. Support Care Cancer 2006;14:408-418.
20. Ross JR, Saunders Y, Edmonds PM, et al. A systematic review of the role of bisphosphonates in metastatic disease. Health Technol Assess 2004;8:1-176.
21. Michaelson MD, Smith MR. Bisphosphonates for treatment and prevention of bone metastases. J Clin Oncol 2005;23:8219-8224.
22. Clines GA, Guise TA. Hypercalcaemia of malignancy and basic research on mechanisms responsible for osteolytic and osteoblastic metastasis to bone. Endocr Relat Cancer 2005;12:549-583.
23. Rosen L, Gordon D, Antonio B, et al. Zoledronic acid versus pamidronate in the treatment of skeletal metastases in patients with breast cancer or osteolytic lesions of multiple myeloma: A phase III, double-blind, comparative trial. Cancer J 2001;7:377-387.
24. Bamias A, Kastritis E, Bamia C, et al. Osteonecrosis of the jaw in cancer after treatment with bisphosphonates: Incidence and risk factors. J Clin Oncol 2005;23:8580-8587.
25. Ramaswamy B, Shapiro CL. Bisphosphonates in the prevention and treatment of bone metastases. Oncology (Williston Park) 2003;17:1261-1272, 1277-1278, 1280.
26. Bauman G, Charette M, Reid R, et al. Radiopharmaceuticals for the palliation of painful bone metastasis: A systemic review. Radiother Oncol 2005;75:258-270.
27. Body JJ, Facon T, Coleman RE, et al. A study of the biological receptor activator of nuclear factor-kappaB ligand inhibitor, denosumab, in patients with multiple myeloma or bone metastases from breast cancer. Clin Cancer Res 2006;12:1221-1228.
28. Carducci MA, Jimeno A. Targeting bone metastasis in prostate cancer with endothelin receptor antagonists. Clin Cancer Res 2006;12:6296S-6300S.

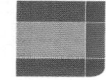

CHAPTER 223

Vertebral Metastases and Spinal Cord Compression

Nora Janjan, Edward Lin, Ian McCutcheon, George Perkins, Prajnan Das, Sunil Krishnan, Deborah Kuban, and Eric L. Chang

KEY POINTS

- Vertebral metastases are frequently associated with spinal cord compression.
- Diagnosis and management of spinal cord compression is a medical emergency.
- Early recognition is essential to good outcomes.
- Aggressive use of corticosteroids and radiation therapy is key to effective therapy.
- Focus of care is on maintaining function and palliation.

VERTEBRAL METASTASES

The issues related to the treatment of spinal cord compression from cancer present a paradigm for the treatment of metastatic disease. The profound consequence of paralysis from spinal cord compression to the patient and caregivers involves significant suffering and financial burden. Although metastatic disease is, by definition, incurable, patients greatly benefit from therapeutic strategies that prevent spinal cord compression and that diagnose and treat spinal cord compression early to maintain functional status.

Clinical Presentation

Pain Management

Pain represents a sensitive measure of cancer activity.[1-5] The limited radiation tolerance of the normal tissues, such as the spinal cord, adjacent to bone metastasis makes it impossible to administer a large dose of radiation to eradicate a measurable tumor. Palliative radiation should result in sufficient tumor regression away from critical structures to relieve symptoms. Symptoms that recur after palliative treatment most commonly result from localized tumor regrowth.

Bladder symptoms, including urinary tract infection and incontinence, result from the effects of the disease on the spinal cord because the bladder is outside the radiation field for spinal cord compression. Among 71 patients who received emergency radiation therapy during a 19-day hospitalization for metastatic spinal cord compression, urinary tract infections occurred in 12% at baseline and in 77% during hospitalization. These infections occurred among patients who received usual care while undergoing emergency radiation therapy for metastatic spinal cord compression requiring a Foley catheter and corticosteroids.[6] Once-weekly hyaluronic acid instillation with usual catheter care reduced the incidence of urinary tract infection at baseline to 0% and only 14% during hospitalization. Aggressive supportive care, like pain management, is required during palliative radiation therapy.

After bone metastases are diagnosed, the median survival rates are 12 months for breast cancer, 6 months for prostate cancer, and 3 months for lung cancer.[7-9] The distribution of bone metastases in prostate cancer has prognostic significance. Survival is significantly longer when metastases are restricted to the pelvis and lumbar spine among patients who respond to salvage hormone therapy.[10-12] Any metastatic involvement outside the pelvis and lumbar spine results in lower survival irrespective of response to salvage hormone therapy.

Unlike bone metastases in other sites, in spinal cord compression the prognostic factors are specific to functional outcome. Outcomes 1 month after treatment for spinal cord compression among 128 patients[13] revealed median survival of all patients of 59 days (range, 43 to 75 days). Thirteen percent of those treated died within a month of treatment. For ambulatory patients, median survival was 151 days (range, 80 to 222 days), median survival for those walking with assistance was 71 days (range, 46 to 96 days); 35 days (range, 26 to 44 days) for those unable to walk at diagnosis of spinal cord compression (Fig. 223-1). The median Karnofsky performance status was 50 (range, 40 to 60) but worse in lung cancer. The pace of care depended on mobility at diagnosis. Ambulatory patients generally remained at home, whereas those requiring assistance with walking and paralyzed patients generally required hospital care. Mobility and bladder function at diagnosis predicted function after radiation for spinal cord compression; only 7% of paralyzed patients regained full mobility, and only 28% of those catheterized regained full bladder function. Pain was unrelieved in 47% of patients; 18% continued to have severe pain. Quality of life measures were strongly correlated with functional status, yet only 8% of patients were anxious or depressed.

Prognosis declines rapidly with metastatic disease. Although the decline is faster in patients with visceral involvement, bone metastases still reduce survival. Spinal cord compression, which primarily results from vertebral bone metastases, portends a poor prognosis, like visceral metastases, even among patients who retain function. Care for spinal cord compression should focus on maximizing functional outcome and should address quality of life parameters through symptom control, including aggressive pain management. Prevention, early diagnosis, and treatment of spinal cord compression avoid emergency evaluations and hospitalizations and have a defined, achievable goal.

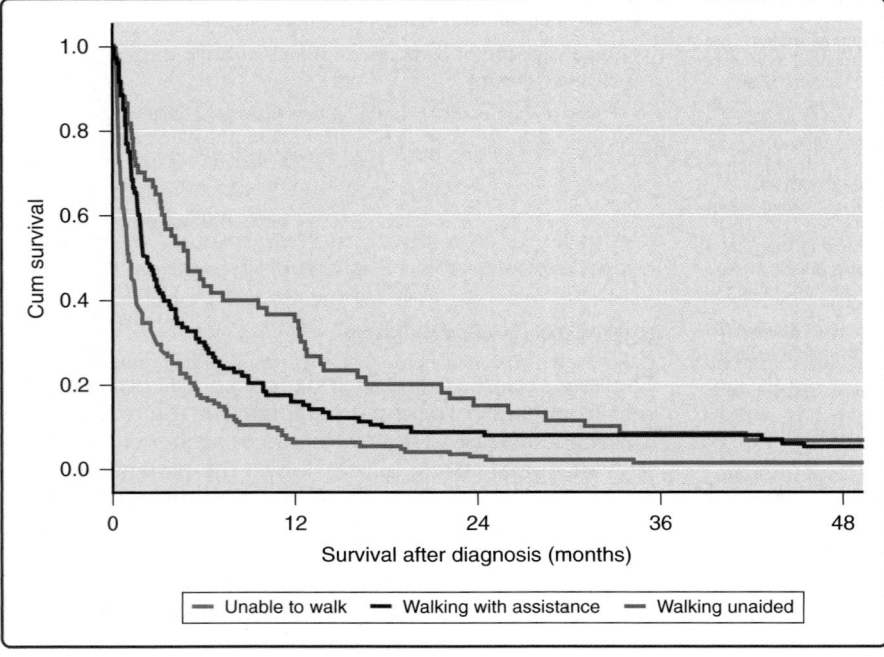

FIGURE 223-1 Survival in relation to mobility level at diagnosis of spinal cord compression. Cum, cumulative survival. *(Redrawn from Conway R, Graham J, Kidd J, et al., Scottish Cord Compression Group. What happens to people after malignant cord compression? Survival, function, quality of life, emotional well-being and place of care 1 month after diagnosis. Clin Oncol 2007;19:56-62.)*

— Unable to walk — Walking with assistance — Walking unaided

Cost-Effectiveness of Vertebral Metastases Treatment

Surgical intervention with radiation therapy, to maintain mobility with mechanical spinal instability, is cost-effective. Although 69% of patients treated with radiation alone or surgery and radiation walk at presentation, 84% of patients treated with surgery and radiation are ambulatory, compared with only 57% treated with radiation alone (Fig. 223-2). Surgery and radiation also resulted in a mean of 290 ambulatory days, with a mean 352 days of survival, compared with a mean of 91 ambulatory days, with a mean 217 days of survival. The percentage of ambulatory days relative to survival was 82% for surgery and radiation compared with 42% with radiation alone. The baseline incremental cost-effectiveness ratio (ICER) was $48 per additional day of ambulation (2003 U.S. dollars). Using survival as the measure of effectiveness resulted in an

ICER of $24,752 per life year gained.[14] Monte Carlo simulations (Fig. 223-3) that compared surgery and radiation versus radiation alone showed that savings in direct health care costs were attained 18% of the time with combined-modality therapy. When combined-modality therapy did not provide savings in health care costs, the cost of each additional day of ambulation was $242 or less ($7260/ month) 95% of the time. The cost of full-time institutional or home health care from paralysis often exceeds this amount, given the need for supplies, equipment (e.g., a wheelchair and transfer devices within the home), and a home health care provider.

Pathological Features

The potential for the development of radiation myelitis with total radiation doses that exceed 40 Gy at 2 Gy per fraction represents the limiting factor for large tumor

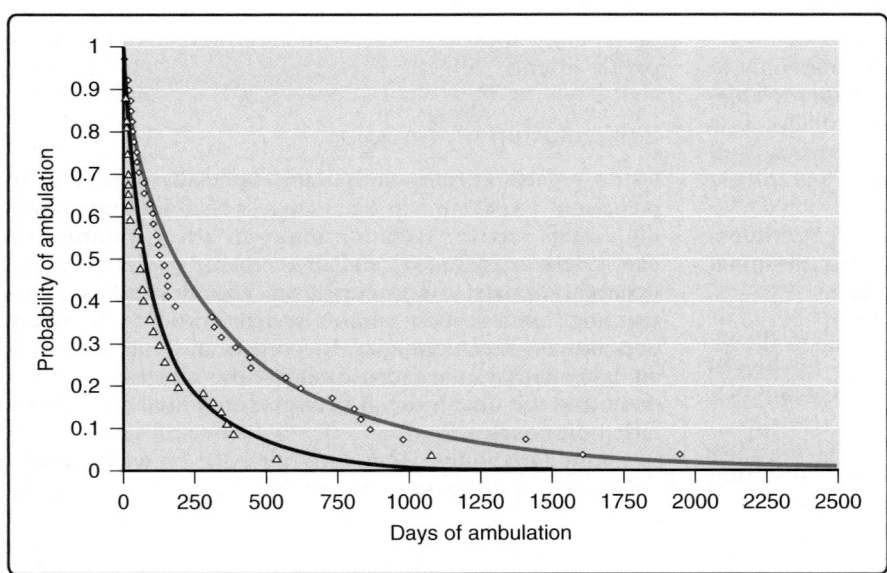

FIGURE 223-2   Kaplan-Meier versus Weibull ambulation estimates for surgery (S) with radiation (R) versus radiation alone. Kaplan-Meier days of ambulation: S + RT (diamonds); Weibull expected days of ambulation: S + RT (triangles). Kaplan-Meier days of ambulation: RT (Δ); Weibull expected days of ambulation: RT (triangles). (Redrawn from Thomas KC, Nosyk B, Fisher CG, et al. Cost-effectiveness of surgery plus radiotherapy versus radiotherapy alone for metastatic epidural spinal cord compression. Int J Radiat Oncol Biol Phys 2006;66:1212-1218.)

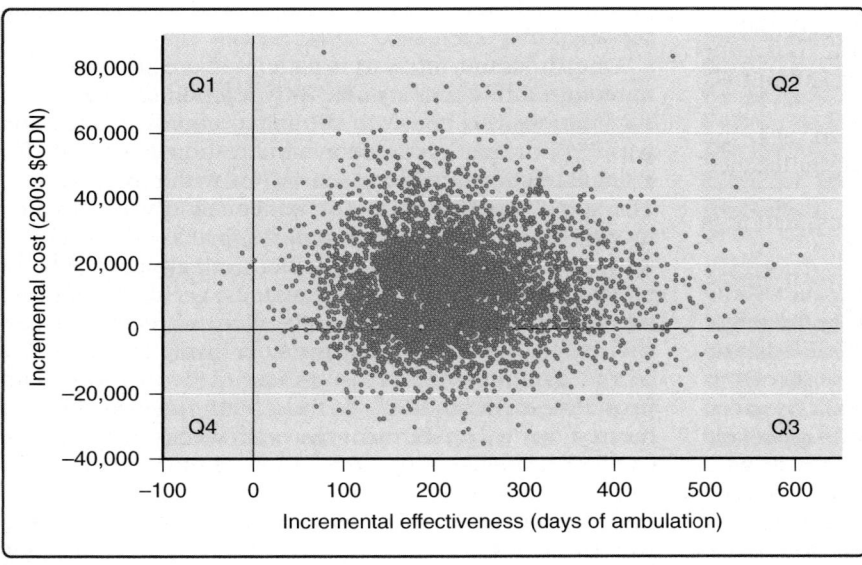

FIGURE 223-3   Scatterlot of differences in cost and days of ambulation based on Monte Carlo simulations for surgery and radiation versus radiation alone. Q1, surgery and radiation are more costly and less effective; Q2, surgery and radiation are more costly and more effective; Q3, surgery and radiation are less costly and more effective; Q4, surgery and radiation are less costly and less effective. Costs are in Canadian dollars ($CDN). (Redrawn from Thomas KC, Nosyk B, Fisher CG, et al. Cost-effectiveness of surgery plus radiotherapy versus radiotherapy alone for metastatic epidural spinal cord compression. Int J Radiat Oncol Biol Phys 2006;66:1212-1218.)

burdens near or involving the spinal canal. Furthermore, the length of spinal cord that needs to be irradiated significantly affects radiation tolerance.[15-19] Persistent pain after radiation therapy for vertebral metastases should be investigated to exclude progressive disease in or outside the radiation portal or mechanical spinal instability because of a vertebral compression fracture. Changes seen in the bone marrow on magnetic resonance imaging (MRI) scans after palliative radiation therapy initially include decreased cellularity, edema, and hemorrhage, followed by fatty replacement and fibrosis. These changes can be distinguished from progressive disease.[20-22]

Histopathological changes, experimentally observed after fractionated irradiation of the spinal cord, include white matter necrosis, massive hemorrhage, and segmental parenchymal atrophy consistently associated with abnormal neurological signs.[17] Other responses involve focal fiber loss and white matter vacuolation. Two separate mechanisms of radiation injury can occur from white matter damage and vasculopathies. White matter damage is associated with diffuse demyelination and swollen axons that can be focally necrotic and have associated glial reaction. Vascular damage has been shown experimentally to be age dependent and can result in hemorrhage, telangiectasia, and vascular necrosis.[15-19] Experimentally, low radiation doses interfere with the syringomyelia and glial scar formation that facilitate recovery of paraplegic animals.[19]

Six major types of injury have been shown experimentally from spinal column radiation. Five occur in the spinal cord, and one occurs in the dorsal root ganglia.

1. The most severe injuries occur from vascular damage and result in neurological dysfunction, including white matter necrosis, hemorrhage, and segmental parenchymal atrophy.
2. The two less severe spinal lesions are focal fiber loss and scattered white matter vacuolation resulting from glial cell damage, axons, or the vasculature. These less severe sequelae are seen with lower total radiation doses and are less likely to result in neurological dysfunction.
3. In dorsal root ganglia, radiation damage includes intracytoplasmic vacuoles and loss of neurons and satellite cells that could affect sensory function. These conditions are distinct from the posterior column demyelination in the self-limiting Lhermitte's syndrome.[16]
4. Meningeal thickening and fibrosis can also be observed after radiation, but the clinical significance of these findings is unknown.
5. Ependymal and nerve root damage from radiation is rare.

Clinical and experimental experience does not show any difference in radiosensitivity in different segments of the spinal cord.[15,18] The risk of radiation myelitis in the cervicothoracic spine is less than 5% when 6000 cGy is administered at 172 cGy per fraction (or 5000 cGy given with daily fractions of 200 cGy per fraction). Especially among patients who have received chemotherapy or who need a significant length of spinal cord irradiated, the total dose is generally limited to 4000 cGy, administered at 200 cGy per fraction, to minimize any irreversible radia-

tion injury. A steep curve based on total radiation dose predicts radiation myelopathy; a small increase in total radiation dose can result in a large increased risk of radiation myelopathy.[15,17,19] Retreatment of a previously irradiated segment of spinal cord results in a high risk of radiation-induced myelopathy because other neurological pathways cannot compensate for an injury to a specific level of the spinal cord. The radiation tolerance of the spinal cord can be compromised by prior injury. Difficulty arises in separating the pathological and radiotherapeutic causes of spinal cord compression. Vasogenic edema of the spinal cord and nerve roots can be caused by compression injury. Metastatic epidural compression results in vasogenic spinal cord edema, venous hemorrhage, loss of myelin, and ischemia. Vasogenic edema results in an increased synthesis of prostaglandin E_2, which can be inhibited by steroids or nonsteroidal anti-inflammatory agents. Other consequences of pathological compression include hemorrhage, loss of myelin, and ischemia.[15-19] Pathophysiology of disease, radiobiological factors, and technical limitations are critical determinants for radiotherapeutic approaches used and are specific to the therapeutic intent.

Reirradiation of the Spine

Issues regarding reirradiation are especially important in palliation. Experimental data suggest that acute responding tissues recover radiation injury in a few months and can tolerate additional radiation therapy. Considerable variability exists in recovery from radiation among late-reacting tissues such as the spinal cord.[23-26] Recovery depends on the technique, the organ and volume irradiated, the initial total radiation dose, the radiation fraction dose, and the time interval between the initial and second radiation courses.[24]

Limited toxicities occur with reirradiation when careful attention is paid to treatment techniques and radiobiological factors. Radiotherapeutic techniques that localize the radiation dose to the recurrent tumor and limit the dose to the surrounding normal tissues allow reirradiation of recurrent tumors. Other techniques include conformal external beam radiation (Fig. 223-4), intensity-modulated radiation therapy (IMRT) (Fig. 223-5), and proton therapy.[25,26]

One thousand fifty-seven patients were prospectively randomized to either a single 8-Gy fraction or to 24 Gy in six fractions. Response to the initial course of radiation was 73% for multiple fractions; the response was 71% for a single fraction and increased to 75% with reirradiation.[27] The spine was treated in 342 patients and was retreated in only 11% out of concern for spinal cord tolerance. Response status did not predict retreatment: 35% of patients who received single fractions, versus 8% of those who received multiple fractions, were retreated for persistent symptoms. The nonresponder group included 27% of the patients with breast cancer, 11% of those with prostate cancer, and 22% of those with lung cancer. The mean time to retreatment was 22 weeks for prostate cancer (mean pain score, 6.3), 14 weeks for breast cancer (mean pain score, 7.4), and 11 weeks for lung cancer (mean pain score, 6.5). Retreatment for nonresponders was successful in 66% of patients who received a single

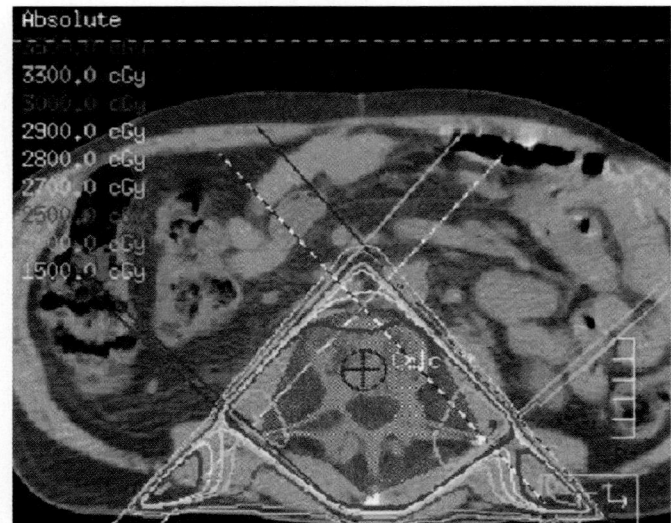

FIGURE 223-4 Conformal radiation treatment fields to vertebral metastases in the lumbar region. The isodose distribution demonstrates that less than 15 Gy is delivered to the adjacent small bowel.

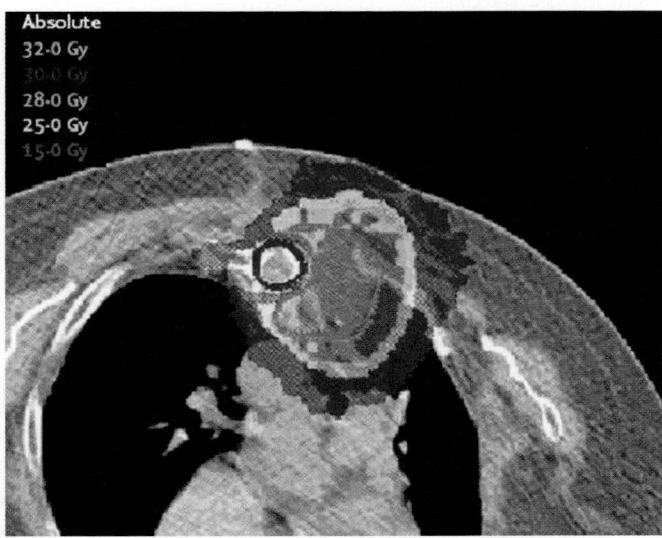

FIGURE 223-5 Intensity-modulated radiation therapy (IMRT) in the treatment of spinal cord compression. The adjacent anatomic structures receive even less radiation than with conformal radiation techniques. However, the cost of IMRT is greater than that of conformal radiation. *(From Prasad D, Schiff D. Malignant spinal cord compression. Lancet Oncol 2005;6:15-24.)*

fraction compared with 33% of those who received multiple fractions. The randomization arm of the trial, tumor type, and pain score before retreatment predicted reirradiation.

Radiobiological calculations were performed on 40 individuals who received reirradiation for spine metastases. In this model, an a/β value of 2 Gy was selected for the cervical and thoracic spine, and a value of 4 Gy was chosen for the lumbar spine; only three patients in this series received lumbar reirradiation.[26] Using a biologically effective dose (BED) calculation, BED = n, the number of fractions, × d, the dose (1 + d/2) for the cervicothoracic cord, or BED = n × d (1 + d/4) for the lumbar spine. In this model, 50 Gy delivered at 2 Gy per fraction would have a BED of 100 Gy_2 or 75 Gy_4. The median interval between the original radiation therapy and reirradiation was 20 months. The cumulative radiation doses ranged from 108 to 205 Gy_2 with a median follow-up interval of 17 months. Myelopathy developed in 11 patients 4 to 25 months (median, 11 months) after reirradiation, and it only occurred when one course of radiation was >102 Gy_2 (n = 9) or when patients were retreated within 2 months of the initial radiation. In the absence of these two risk factors, no myelopathy developed in 19 patients treated with <135.5 Gy_2 or among 7 patients treated with between 136 and 150 Gy_2. The risk of myelopathy was considered small after cumulative radiation doses <135.5 Gy_2 when the interval is at least 6 months between radiation courses and when the dose of each radiation course is <98 Gy_2.

Another series evaluated 62 patients who had received either a single 8-Gy fraction or 20 Gy delivered as five 4-Gy fractions for metastatic spinal cord compression.[28-31] Retreatment consisted of a single 8-Gy fraction, 15 Gy (five 3-Gy fractions), or 20 Gy (five 4-Gy fractions); the cumulative BED with reirradiation was 80 to 100 Gy_2. Median follow-up was 12 months (range, 4 to 42 months), and 26% survived at least 12 months after repeat irradiation. Acute radiation toxicity did not exceed grade 1 according to the Common Toxicity Criteria. Improved motor function occurred in 40% after repeat irradiation, 45% had no change, and only 15% had deterioration. Of the 16 patients who were unable to ambulate, 38% regained the ability to walk. No second in-field recurrence was observed after repeat irradiation. Myelopathy was not observed, and the outcome was not influenced by the radiation schedule.

Reirradiation has been performed among selected patients with vertebral metastases to cumulative radiation doses of 68 Gy.[24,32] Using stereotactic conformal radiation therapy and IMRT to total doses of 39 Gy, reirradiation resulted in 95% local control at 12-month follow-up.[32] Half had neurological improvement, and 13 of 16 patients had pain relief. No significant late toxicity was reported. The high cumulative radiation doses in this series were in highly selected patients with specialized techniques, and this finding does not represent the current standard of care.

SPINAL CORD COMPRESSION

Pain is the initial symptom in approximately 90% of spinal cord compressions, and spinal cord compression is associated with a poor overall prognosis. The most common primary tumor types are breast cancer, prostate cancer, and lung cancer, accounting for approximately 60% of all cases; 8% of cases result from myeloma.[33] The time from the original diagnosis to metastatic spinal disease averages 32 months, and it is 27 months from the diagnosis of skeletal metastases to spinal cord compression. Median survival in spinal cord compression ranges between 3 and 7 months, with a 36% probability of 1-year survival. For specific cancers, the mean survival time is 14 months for breast cancer, 12 months for prostate cancer, 6 months for malignant melanoma, and 3 months for lung cancer once epidural spinal cord compression is diagnosed.[34-36] From a tumor registry of 121,435 patients, the cumulative probability of at least one episode of spinal cord compression in the last 5 years of life was 2.5%.[36] The diagnosis of spinal cord compression doubled hospital time in the last year of life.

The vertebral column is involved by metastatic tumor in 40% of patients who die of cancer. Approximately 70% of vertebral metastases involve the thoracic spine, 20% involve the lumbosacral region, and 10% affect the cervical spine. Pathways include hematogenous spread, direct extension from paravertebral tumors, and cerebrospinal fluid spread.[37] Spinal cord compression can have four different causes.[33] The first and most common cause is displacement of the thecal sac by spinal epidural metastases. Second, posterior vertebral body mass extension can occur. Third, anterior extension of a mass in the dorsal elements can cause spinal canal compromise. Finally, and least frequent, an extrinsic mass can invade the vertebral foramen (Fig. 223-6).

Three classic pain syndromes result from spine metastases. Local pain, often described as an aching or gnawing pain, emanates from the segment involved by tumor.[37] Mechanical or axial back pain is aggravated with movement by increasing weight-bearing forces on the affected spinal segment. This type of pain occurs with vertebral body damage that results in spinal instability causing muscle, tendon, ligament, or joint capsule strain. Because of the mechanical abnormality, axial back pain is often refractory to analgesics and radiation therapy, and most commonly it requires spinal surgical stabilization. Radicular pain occurs when spinal metastases compress a nerve root, resulting in sharp, shooting pain. Radicular pain may radiate unilaterally or bilaterally to the upper or lower

extremities in cervical and lumbar lesions or bilaterally around the chest or upper abdomen in thoracic cord lesions.[38] Signs include depression of deep tendon reflexes, weakness, and sensory changes specific to the involved spine segment. Weakness can result in gait disorders and sensory ataxia resulting from posterior column compression; often, gait disorder and sensory ataxia can be confused with chemotherapy-related neuropathy. When the spinal cord is compressed, paresis can be flaccid, but pyramidal signs, including hyperreflexia and clonus, can occur. Dysesthetic or neuropathic pain, resulting in an intense burning sensation, also may arise from intradural extramedullary disease.[37] Sensory disturbances, such as anesthesia, hypesthesia, or paresthesia, generally occur with motor dysfunction. Back pain from extradural spinal cord compression is always progressive and may be elicited by Valsalva's maneuver. Unlike in spinal disc herniation, epidural metastases are not alleviated, and may become worse, with recumbency. Paraparesis or paraplegia occurs in more than 60% of patients, sensory loss occurs in 70% to 80%, and 14% to 77% have bladder or bowel disturbances.[31,39,40] Functional outcome is influenced by epidural mass size. Greater residual neurological impairment results from a complete spinal cord block than from a partial block.

Pain can be present for months to days before neurological dysfunction becomes manifest. Unlike in degenerative joint disease, which primarily occurs in the low cervical and low lumbar regions, pain from epidural spinal cord compression can occur anywhere in the spinal axis and is aggravated by recumbency. Any patient with cancer who has back pain, especially a patient with known metastatic involvement of the vertebral bodies, should be suspected of spinal cord compression. The risk of spinal cord

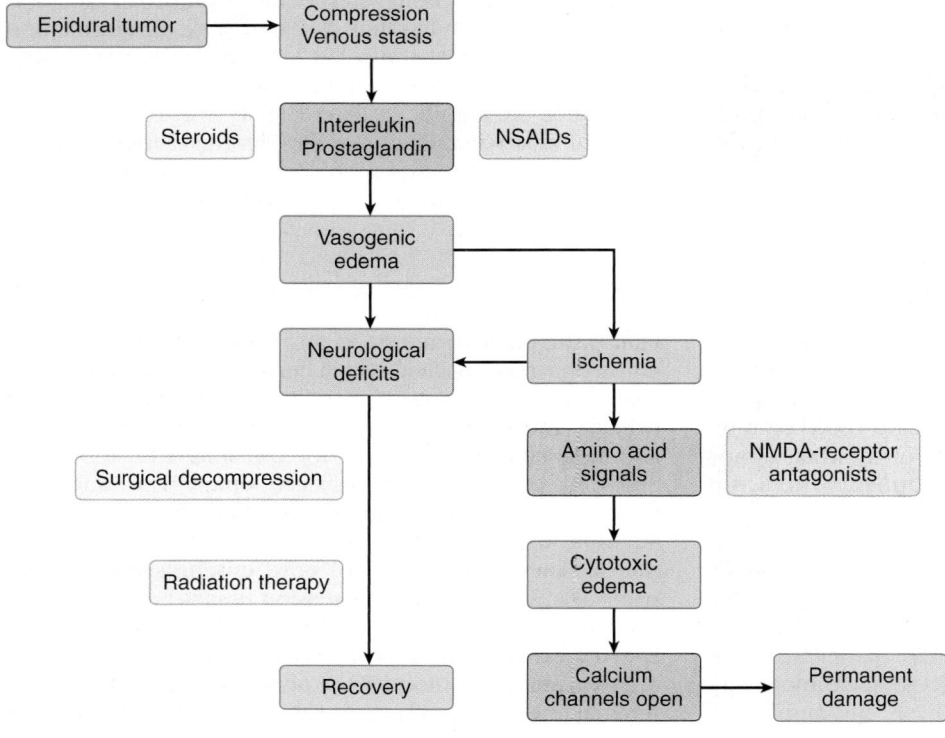

FIGURE 223-6 Pathophysiology of spinal cord compression. Progression of disease is indicated by the *blue boxes*, outcomes are shown by *green boxes*, molecular mechanisms are indicated by *violet boxes*, therapeutic options are indicated by *light tan boxes*, and experimental therapies are shown by *dark tan boxes*. NMDA, N-methyl-D-aspartate; NSAIDs, nonsteroidal anti-inflammatory drugs. *(Redrawn from Prasad D, Schiff D. Malignant spinal cord compression. Lancet Oncol 2005;6:15-24.)*

compression exceeds 60% in patients with back pain and plain film evidence of vertebral collapse from metastatic cancer.[16,40-48] Epidural spinal cord disease is documented in 17% of asymptomatic patients with an abnormal bone scan but normal plain films. When vertebral metastases are present on both on bone scan and plain film, 47% of asymptomatic patients have epidural disease.[44-46] An MRI scan to rule out spinal cord compression should be performed in symptomatic patients with osteoblastic changes on plain film even if the vertebral contour and bone scan are normal (Fig. 223-7).

Weakness can signal rapid progression of symptoms; 30% of patients with weakness become paraplegic within 1 week. Rapid weakness (<2 months) most commonly occurs in lung cancer, whereas breast and prostate cancers can progress more slowly. Neurological deficits can develop within a few hours in up to 20% of spinal cord compressions.[34,39,49-58] The rate of development of motor symptoms correlates with therapeutic improvement. Motor function improved among 86% of patients who had more than 14 days to development of symptoms. Only 29% improved when motor deficits developed 8 to 14 days before the diagnosis of spinal cord compression. Improvements occurred in only 10% when motor deficits developed over 1 to 7 days.

The severity of weakness at presentation is the most significant factor for recovery of function.[34,39,49-58] Ninety percent of patients who are ambulatory at presentation will be ambulatory after treatment. Only 13% of paraplegic patients regain function, particularly if paraplegia is present for more than 24 hours before therapy. More than 30% of patients who develop spinal cord compression are alive 1 year later, and 50% of these patients remain ambulatory with appropriate therapy. Among 102 consecutive patients with metastatic spinal cord compression, 51% were fully ambulatory at the time of radiation therapy, and 41% were ambulatory but with paraparesis. Median survival was 3.5 months; normal gait returned in 58% 2 weeks after treatment and in 71% 2 months after radiation. No paraplegic patient regained function.[49]

Among 153 consecutive cases of spinal cord compression in one study, 37% had breast cancer, 28% had prostate cancer, 18% had lung cancer, and 17% had other solid

tumors. The time between primary tumor diagnosis and spinal cord compression depended on tumor type; the shortest time was seen in lung cancer and the longest time was reported in breast cancer. Patients with lung cancer had the most severe functional deficit, with more than 50% totally paralyzed. Patients with breast cancer were ambulatory 59% of the time. More severe gait disturbances occurred when the time between the interval from primary tumor diagnosis and spinal cord compression was short. Total blockage of the spinal cord occurred in 54%, and 46% had partial blockage.[57] Total paralysis was present in 43 patients, 31 could move their legs but could not walk, 19 were able to walk with assistance, and 60 could walk unassisted. Sensory examination of the legs was normal in 34 patients, slight disturbances were present in 84, and total lack of pain perception was present in 35 patients. After radiation, 40 patients were totally paralyzed, 20 could move their legs without being able to walk, 17 were able to walk with assistance, and 76 had unassisted gait. The median survival time was 3.4 months. Survival depended on time from primary tumor diagnosis and on ambulatory function at diagnosis and after treatment.

Leptomeningeal Disease

Leptomeningeal carcinomatosis must also be considered in the diagnostic evaluation. It occurs more commonly than expected. For example, only half of patients with breast cancer who have leptomeningeal carcinomatosis are diagnosed with the leptomeningeal disease before death.[53,57-59] Lumbar puncture is a relative barrier to the diagnosis. At least three cerebral spinal fluid (CSF) samples are necessary to exclude the diagnosis of leptomeningeal disease cytologically because in 10% to 40% of patients, the initial CSF sample fails to document tumor cells.[60] MRI can identify leptomeningeal disease with normal CSF cytology and is sensitive and specific in locating nodular leptomeningeal involvement. Except in nodular leptomeningeal involvement, in which localized radiation therapy may be of benefit as an adjuvant, intrathecal chemotherapy is the treatment of choice.[53]

Imaging

Bone scans are sensitive and specific for bone metastases, but MRI is the best available technique for evaluating the bone marrow, neoplastic vertebral invasion, the central nervous system, and peripheral nerves.[44-46] Signs that differentiate osteoporosis from malignant involvement include multifocal involvement, pedicle involvement, convex cortical contour, and extraosseous soft tissue mass. In malignancy, one also notes an absence of normal fatty marrow, intravertebral fluid, fracture line, posterior angulated fragment, and fragmentation.[61]

^{18}F-fluorodeoxyglucose positron emission tomography (FDG-PET) has also found unsuspected spinal cord compression, later confirmed on MRI, in patients with melanoma.[45] Bone or other metastases rarely fail to be detected when radiographic diagnosis is pursued. When radiographic confirmation of malignancy is equivocal, bone biopsy should be considered.[46]

Radiographic determination of the involved spinal levels is critical to radiation planning. Clinical determina-

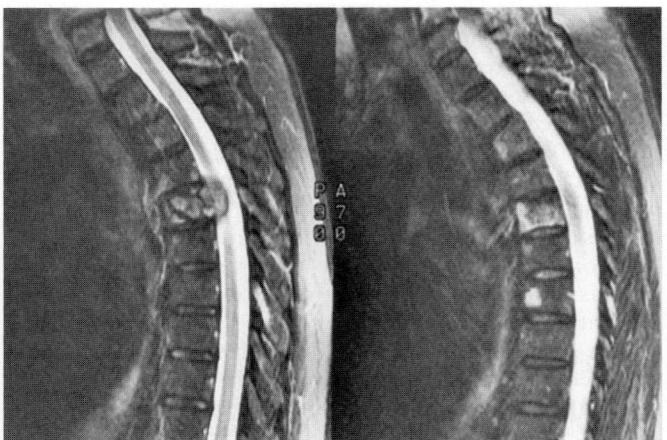

FIGURE 223-7 Magnetic resonance imaging of the spine demonstrating epidural spinal cord compression.

tion of the location of epidural spinal cord compression is incorrect in 33%.[58,62-64] Plain film radiographs show involvement of more than one spinal level in approximately one third of cases. If MRI scans, tomographic studies, and surgical findings are included, more than 85% of patients with spinal metastases have multiple sites of vertebral involvement.[40,44-46] Bone scans fail to detect bone metastases 13% of the time.[61] When bone scan shows evidence of spinal metastases, 49% have more extensive disease shown on MRI. Although spinal cord compression is caused by soft tissue epidural metastases in 75%, the remaining 25% of cases are caused by bone collapse.[54] Computed tomography (CT) finds metastases in the posterior vertebral body and shows that pedicle destruction occurs only with vertebral body involvement.[20] On plain radiographs, pedicle destruction identifies spine metastases. Osteoblastic bony expansion, common in both prostate and breast cancers, can result in spinal cord compromise and osteolytic vertebral compression fractures (Fig. 223-8).[51,54] MRI has a 93% sensitivity and a 97% specificity rate.[65] MRI findings correlate with stage of multiple myeloma, β_2-microglobulin level, type of chain, and response to therapy.[36]

Treatment

Treatment of spinal cord compression includes corticosteroids, radiation therapy, or neurosurgical intervention given on an emergency basis. Radiation therapy is the treatment of choice for most spinal cord compressions and is a radiotherapeutic emergency. Functional outcome depends on the level of symptoms when radiation is administered.[39,40,49-57] Pain relief is accomplished in 73%; the mean time to pain relief was 35 days in 108 patients with breast cancer. Recurrent symptoms at a different spinal level occurred in more than 75% within 6 months of initial treatment.[36]

Corticosteroids

Small randomized controlled trials of neurological deficits resulting from spinal cord compression have compared

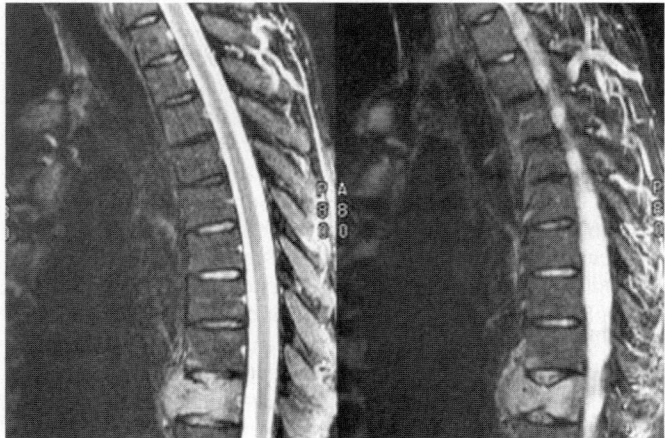

FIGURE 223-8 Osteoblastic involvement, demonstrated on magnetic resonance imaging of the spine, associated with vertebral collapse in a patient with breast cancer.

high-dose (100 mg) bolus with moderate-dose (10 mg) dexamethasone. Motor status was improved among the high-dose bolus group; adverse effects from steroids were also higher in the high-dose bolus group.[66] Corticosteroids have not been found to be necessary among patients with subclinical spinal cord compression during radiation therapy.

Surgery

A statistically significant improvement in functional outcome occurs with laminectomy and radiation therapy in epidural spinal cord compression over either modality alone for selected clinical presentations. Laminectomy promptly reduces tumor volume to relieve compression and injury of the spinal cord and to provide spinal axis stabilization. The rate of tumor regression following radiation therapy is too slow in these patients to recover lost neurological function, and radiation therapy cannot relieve compression of the spinal column from vertebral collapse. After radiation alone for partial spinal cord block, 64% of patients regain ambulation, 33% have normal sphincter tone, and 72% are pain free; median survival is 9 months.[50,51,59,63,66-69] With complete spinal cord block, only 27% of patients improve in motor function, and 42% have pain after radiation alone. In paraparetic patients who undergo laminectomy and radiation, 82% regain the ability to walk, 68% improve sphincter function, and 88% have pain relief.

Laminectomy is indicated in patients with rapid neurological deterioration, with tumor progression in a previously irradiated area, for stabilization of the spine, and in paraplegic patients with limited disease and good probability of survival, as well as for establishing a diagnosis.[14,58,62-72] Adjuvant radiation therapy is often given to treat microscopic residual disease after neurosurgical intervention.[34,58,62,68,70] Surgical restoration of the vertebral alignment may be required because of neurological compromise and pain from progressive vertebral collapse. Vertebral collapse may result from cancer or vertebral instability after cancer therapy (Fig. 223-9). Appropriate diagnostic studies and intervention should be pursued in patients with persistent pain because the neurological compromise and pain from vertebral instability can be as devastating as with epidural spinal cord metastases.[67,69]

The vertebral bodies support up to 80% of the axial load from above. Compromise of the spine load-bearing capacity is directly related to the tumor size, cross-sectional area of the remaining intact body, and bone mineral density.[37,73] Impending collapse of the vertebral body was predicted by 50% to 60% involvement of the vertebral body in the upper thoracic spine and 35% to 40% involvement in the thoracolumbar and lumbar spine.[37,74] Axial loading most commonly creates a compression fracture or a burst fracture. Although less common, invasion of the posterior spinal elements, such as the facet joints, may predispose to dislocation and translational deformity.

The surgical approach is dictated by the spine segment involved by tumor, the location of the tumor within the spine, the tumor histology, and the type of spinal reconstruction after tumor resection. The location of the tumor includes anterior, posterior, circumferential involvement, neural root encasement, and right versus left side relative

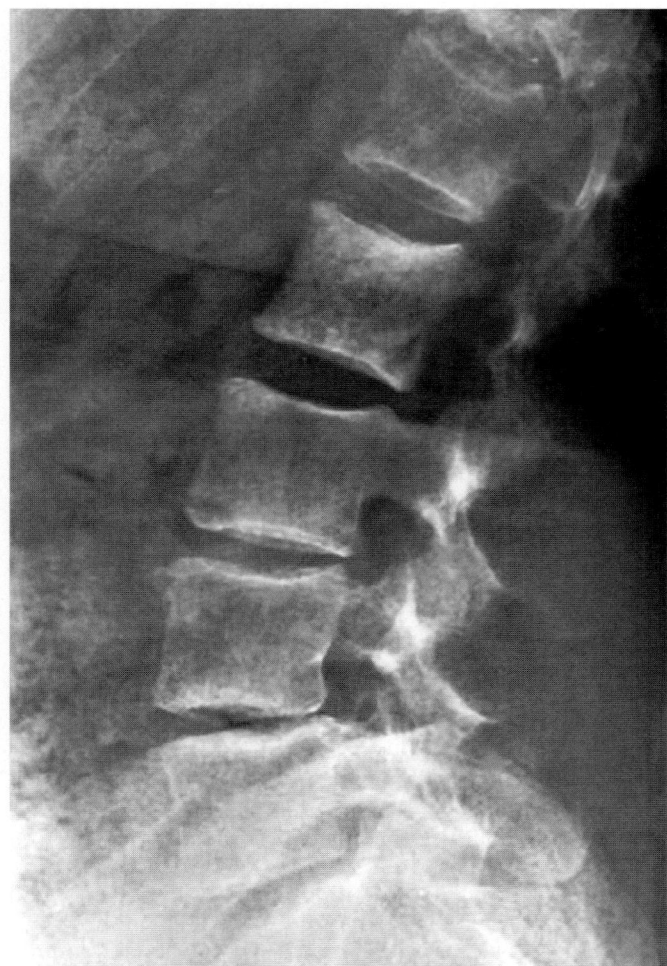

FIGURE 223-9 Compression fraction of the 12th thoracic vertebral body following an initial pain-free interval after palliative radiation. Vertebral weakness with rapid tumor regression resulting in compression fracture caused recurrent back pain from spinal instability.

to adjacent critical structures.[37] Tumor histology requires special consideration. Hypervascular tumors may require preoperative embolization (renal cell carcinoma, thyroid cancer, and hepatocellular carcinoma) to reduce intraoperative blood loss. Anterior column support can be achieved with iliac crest bone graft, cortical allograft, cage, or methylmethacrylate with supplemental plate fixation for rotational stability.[75] Posterolateral decompression followed by instrumentation allows decompression of the anterior aspect of the spinal cord and posterior decompression and stabilization of the unstable spine. Factors such as extensive bony disease may preclude stable fixation, thus exacerbating spinal instability, pain, and subsequent infection.

Percutaneous vertebroplasty is another alternative to provide biomechanical stabilization of the spine by injecting bone cement into structurally weakened vertebrae. It involves percutaneous insertion of a needle into a fractured vertebral body, under fluoroscopic guidance, typically using a transpedicular approach. Liquid methylmethacrylate is injected through the needle, and it interdigitates as it solidifies with the cancellous bone.

Vertebroplasty is often easier in osteolytic diseases such as myeloma.[76] The effect of vertebroplasty on vertebral bulge, a measure of posterior vertebral body wall motion, can be reduced up to 62%.[77,78] Tumor location affects both the vertebral bulge and axial vertebral displacement. Posterior tumor movement and tumor shape cause the greatest vertebral bulge. This procedure is an important alternative in patients with significant co-morbidities who are unable to tolerate a surgical procedure or anesthesia.

Kyphoplasty is a standard procedure for osteoporosis. It is an alternative to vertebroplasty and uses a balloon to create a space within the vertebral body that is subsequently filled with methylmethacrylate. The methylmethacrylate used in kyphoplasty is thicker and can be injected under lower pressure than that used in vertebroplasty. Among patients with cancer, kyphoplasty allows biopsy to diagnose tumor in osteoporotic patients or recurrent tumor in a previously irradiated area. In a review of 56 consecutive kyphoplasty procedures in 128 spinal segments in patients with cancer, complete or significant pain relief was accomplished in 96%, and 69% of the patients were discharged within 24 hours. The thoracic spine accounted for 65%, and the lumbar spine accounted for the remainder of the locations in which kyphoplasty was performed.[76] Exceptions to the use of kyphoplasty as a primary procedure in cancer include the following:

1. The presence of overt instability, such as bone retropulsion or subluxation
2. Clinical or radiographic evidence of spinal cord compression
3. The need for primary tumor resection and intraoperative spinal stabilization
4. Lesions above T3
5. The absence of correlating symptoms such as when pain is not mechanical and not localized to the area of fracture

Prognosis has a significant influence regarding the decision for surgical intervention of spinal cord compression. The Tokuhashi and Tomita scores accurately predict survival after surgery for patients with metastatic spinal cord compression. The six clinical parameters are as follows:

1. The Karnofsky index
2. The number of extraspinal bone metastases
3. The number of metastases in the vertebral body
4. Metastases to the major internal organs
5. The primary site of cancer
6. The severity of spinal cord palsy

A Tokuhashi score of 4 or more, or a Tomita score of 6 or less, predicted a 76% 3-month survival.[75,78,79] These findings were confirmed when postoperative outcomes were evaluated among 987 patients who underwent surgical treatment of spinal cord compression. Significant improvements in pain and quality of life were noted using the Edmonton Symptoms Assessment Scale (Fig. 223-10). Patients with primary cancers of the lung, with melanoma, and with upper gastrointestinal tumors had median survival rates of 87 days, 69.5 days, and 56 days, respectively.[75] Intermediate survivorship of 223 days and of 346 days was found for prostate cancer and breast cancer, respectively. The longest survival was in lymphoma (706 days) and myeloma (591 days). Increasing age and primary

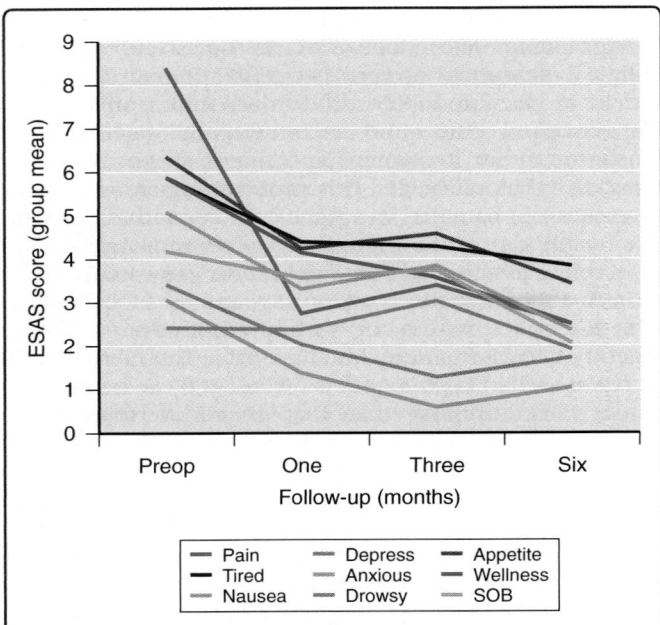

FIGURE 223-10 Trends after surgical intervention for spinal cord compression using the Edmonton Symptoms Assessment Scale (ESAS). Depress, depression; Preop, preoperative; SOB, shortness of breath. *(Redrawn from Finkelstein JA, Ford MH. Diagnosis and management of pathological fractures of the spine. Curr Orthop 2004;18:396-405.)*

lung cancer were risk factors for death within 30 days of surgery. Preoperative neurological deficits were found to be independent determinants of a worse prognosis when confounding factors were considered. Patients with preoperative neurological deficits were 19% more likely to die. When surgery was performed for persistent neurological deficits after radiation, 71% were more likely to contract a postoperative infection.

A multi-institutional nonblinded randomized trial of 101 patients compared outcomes with radiation therapy alone or surgery and radiation consisting of 30 Gy in 10 fractions. The trial was stopped early because the criterion of the predetermined early-stopping rule was met during an interim analysis. The ability to ambulate was the primary end point, and secondary end points were urinary continence, muscle strength and functional status, the need for corticosteroids and opioid analgesics, and survival time.[72] Ambulation was retained in 84% of the patients who received surgery and radiation; after radiation alone, only 57% could walk after therapy. The ability to ambulate was retained for a median of 122 days with surgery and radiation versus 13 days with radiation alone. Of the 32 patients who were unable to walk at study entry, 62% regained the ability to walk after surgery and radiation compared with only 19% with radiation alone. Ten patients (20%) in the radiation-alone group crossed over to receive surgery because of a substantial decline in motor strength; at surgery, none of these patients were ambulatory, and 30% regained the ability to walk. Median maintenance of continence was 17 days with radiation alone versus 156 days with surgery and radiation; treatment randomization and functional ability scores were determined to be significant predictors of this outcome. Use of corticosteroids and

opioid analgesics also declined in the surgery and radiation group compared with the radiation-alone group, with mean daily dexamethasone equivalent doses of 1.6 mg (range, 0.1 to 44) versus 4.2 mg (range, 0 to 50), respectively, and mean daily morphine equivalent doses of 0.4 mg (range, 0 to 44) versus 4.8 mg (range, 0 to 200), respectively. Survival was also significantly lower with radiation alone (100 days) compared with surgery and radiation (126 days); in addition to treatment randomization, predictors included primary breast cancer and lower thoracic spine level. The 30-day mortality rate was 6% for surgery and radiation and 14% for radiation alone.

Surgery often is the only available option for therapy because previously administered radiation may preclude further radiation therapy in the region of the malignant spinal cord compression. Such is often the case in lung cancer because metastases are in the thoracic spine in more than 70% of patients, and many of these patients have received mediastinal irradiation.[78] Early involvement by the radiation therapist in suspected spinal cord involvement allows time to obtain prior radiation therapy records, to determine whether further radiation is possible, and to expedite clinical decision making.

Radiation Therapy

Pooled ambulatory outcomes of patients undergoing radiation therapy in prospective studies show that 94% of ambulatory patients remain ambulatory after radiation therapy. The ability to ambulate after radiation declines to 63% among patients requiring assistance for ambulation before radiation, to 38% among paraparetic patients, and to 13% among patients paralyzed before radiation.[66]

Prognostic factors and survival were evaluated among 60 consecutive patients with metastatic spinal cord compression. Factors such as age, discharge destination, primary tumor site, other metastases, co-morbidities, and hemoglobin and albumin levels had no significant influence on survival time. Median survival time was 4.1 months once the diagnosis of metastatic spinal cord compression was made, except in gastrointestinal cancer, which had a median survival time of 0.6 months.[80] The type of primary tumor did have a direct influence, however, on the interval between the diagnosis of the primary tumor and the diagnosis of spinal cord compression resulting from metastatic disease.[39] Factors important to survival in another study, determined among 153 consecutive patients with metastatic spinal cord compression, included time from primary tumor diagnosis until spinal cord compression (although tumor type itself was not a factor) and ambulatory function at the time of diagnosis and after treatment.

Accounting for the limited prognosis, metastatic spinal cord compression has been treated either with a single 8-Gy fraction or five 4-Gy fractions. The median time to recurrence was 6 months among 62 patients (range, 2 to 40 months).[31] Retreatment consisted of another single 8-Gy fraction, or five more fractions of either 3 or 4 Gy. Motor function improved in 40% of patients, and it was stable in an additional 45%; 38% of the nonambulatory patients regained the ability to walk. This more efficient radiation treatment schedule provides sufficient tumor regression for neurological improvement.

The time under radiation needs to be considered as the opportunity cost of palliative treatment.[81] If the median survival with bone metastases is 6 months (180 days), the patient will spend 0.6% of the remaining survival time under radiation treatment when a single radiation fraction is given. If 10 radiation fractions are given, 8% of the remaining survival, and if 20 fractions are prescribed, 16% of the remaining survival, will be consumed by radiation therapy. Even if retreatment with a second single fraction is required, the patient will continue to spend about 1% of the survival time under radiation therapy. For patients with lung cancer who have a 3-month survival rate, 1% of the remaining time is spent with a single fraction of radiation as compared with 16% if 10 fractions are given or 30% if 20 fractions are prescribed.

Acute radiation toxicities are a function of the dose per fraction, the total dose, and the area and volume of tissue irradiated. If mucosal surfaces such as the upper aerodigestive tract, bowel, and bladder can be excluded from the radiation portals, acute radiation side effects can be significantly reduced whether a single fraction or multiple fractions will be prescribed. A more protracted course of radiation is still used for patients with good prognostic factors who require treatment over the spine and other critical sites.[58-60,62,63,82,83]

CLINICAL TRIALS OF RADIATION DOSE FRACTIONATION FOR SPINAL CORD COMPRESSION

One study evaluated a single 8-Gy fraction versus 20 Gy in five fractions for neuropathic pain related to bone metastases without spinal cord or cauda equina compression among 272 patients. Moderate to severe pain was noted in more than 80% before study entry, although 80% of these patients were receiving opioid analgesics.[84] Vertebral metastases, without epidural disease, accounted for approximately 90% in each treatment arm. Overcoming concerns about acute toxicity with radiation doses of greater than 3 Gy per fraction to the spine, only six patients developed acute grade 3 gastrointestinal tract or lung toxicity (three patients each). No difference was noted between treatment arms in the overall response rate (mean, 55%), complete response rate (mean, 25%), duration of complete response, or time to treatment failure.

Data exist for the efficacy of single-fraction radiation to treat metastatic disease in long bones. Radiation therapists

have been reticent to use a single fraction of radiation for spinal cord compression, as evidenced by the Trans-Tasman Radiation Oncology Group (TROG) study.[84] This study was based on concerns of efficacy and normal toxicity. The concerns of efficacy involved the risk that a single 8-Gy fraction of radiation would not result in sufficient epidural tumor regression. The risk of paralysis, with uncontrolled epidural disease, was often considered too great to conduct a clinical trial. Concerns of normal tissue toxicity with a single large radiation fraction related to the exit dose of radiation to adjacent structures such as the esophagus and stomach. Balancing these concerns against a prolonged course of radiation among patients with a poor prognosis, a few clinical trials were conducted that included usually less than 50 patients who had a poor prognosis.[85-88] A larger prospective trial of 204 patients was later performed that had randomized treatment with either a single 8-Gy fraction versus the more traditional 30 Gy in 10 fractions.[89] No difference was found in functional outcome or prognosis based on radiation schedule (Fig. 223-11). The study also demonstrated that improvement compared with no change and improvement compared with further deterioration of motor function were influenced by Eastern Cooperative Oncology Group Performance Status (ECOG-PS), the primary tumor type, ambulatory status before radiation therapy, and time between development of motor deficits and radiation therapy. Favorable tumor types included myeloma, lymphoma, small cell lung cancer, testicular seminoma; unfavorable tumors included cancer of unknown primary origin, non–small cell lung cancer, and melanoma; intermediate tumor types included all others.[89,90] No improvement in motor function occurred in patients with an unfavorable primary tumor, in those who were nonambulatory before radiation therapy, in patients who had motor deficits within 7 days before radiation therapy, and in those with an ECOG-PS of 3 to 4. Because rates of pain relief and functional outcome were comparable, it was concluded that a single 8-Gy fraction should be considered in patients with a poor survival prognosis to reduce time under treatment and patient discomfort and to lower medical and societal costs.

Based on these results, 1304 patients were evaluated in a retrospective review of five different radiation schedules for metastatic spinal cord compression. No difference was

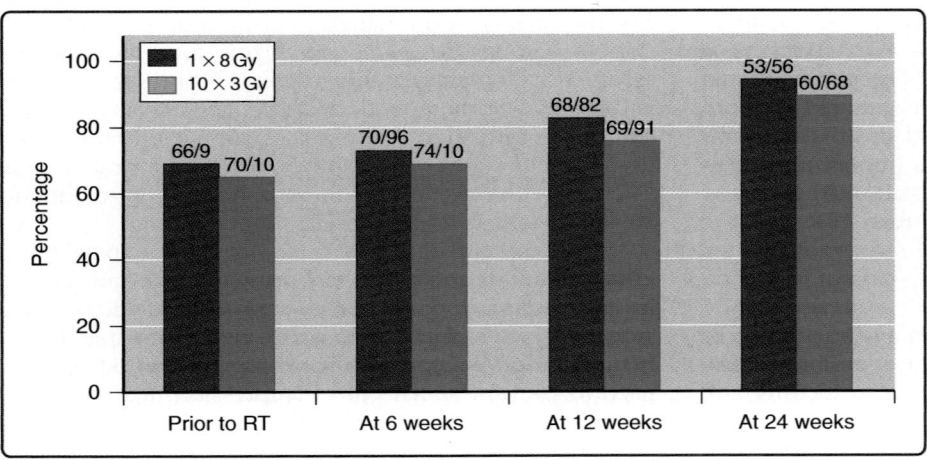

FIGURE 223-11 Comparison of ambulatory rates among 204 patients randomized either to a single 8-Gy radiation fraction or to 30 Gy in 10 fractions. Ambulatory rates were evaluated before and after radiation therapy (RT; 6 weeks, 12 weeks, and 24 weeks after RT). *(Redrawn from Rades D, Stalpers LJA, Hulshor MC, et al. Comparison of 1 × 8 Gy and 10 × 3 Gy for functional outcome in patients with metastatic spinal cord compression. Int J Radiat Oncol Biol Phys 2005;62:514-18.)*

noted among the five treatment schedules in motor function (mean, 27%) or post-treatment ambulatory rates (mean, 68%). Acute radiation toxicity was mild, and no late radiation toxicity was observed.[91] However, in-field recurrence rates at 2 years were different: 24% for 8 Gy, 26% for 20 Gy, 14% for 30 Gy, 9% for 37.5 Gy, and 7% for 40 Gy total radiation dose. No statistical difference was noted among in-field recurrence rates for 8 Gy versus 20 Gy or among 30 Gy, 37.5 Gy, or 40 Gy. Therefore, a single 8-Gy treatment is indicated for patients for spinal cord compression with poor predicted survival; dosage of 30 Gy in 10 fractions is recommended for patients with a better prognosis. In this study, favorable tumors again included lymphoma, myeloma, and seminoma, whereas unfavorable tumors included unknown primary tumors, non–small cell lung cancer, and melanoma; intermediate tumors were all other solid tumors but predominantly breast, prostate, and gastrointestinal tumors. Favorable functional outcome was related to age (≤63 years), number of involved vertebrae (fewer than four vertebrae), tumor type (favorable and intermediate), ambulatory status before radiation therapy, time between the development of motor deficits and the start of radiation (≤14 days), and interval from cancer diagnosis to the development of metastatic disease (≤24 months). Of these factors for a favorable functional outcome, ECOG-PS (≤2), type of tumor, ambulatory status before radiation, time between the development of motor deficits and the start of radiation (≤14 days), interval from cancer diagnosis to the development of metastatic disease (≤24 months), and response to radiation therapy all predicted survival. The study provided two recommendations.[91,92] Patients whose prognosis exceeds 4 to 6 months should receive 30 Gy in 10 fractions because of the lower rate of in-field recurrences and better calcification; a single 8-Gy fraction results in effective palliation in patients with survival rates of less than 4 to 6 months, reduced time under treatment, and lower cost.

Pooled ambulatory outcomes of radiation therapy in prospective studies showed that more than 96% of ambulatory patients retained ambulatory function after 30 Gy in 10 fractions, 28 Gy in 7 fractions, 15 Gy in 3 fractions or in 5 fractions, and 2 fractions of 8 Gy. For patients requiring assistance for ambulation before radiation, 75% regained ambulatory capacity after either 28 Gy in 7 fractions or 15 Gy in 3 or 5 fractions.[66] Paraparetic patients regained ambulatory status 52% of the time with 15 Gy in either 3 or 5 fractions, 50% with 30 Gy in 10 fractions, 44% with 37.5 Gy in 15 fractions, 40 Gy in 20 fractions of 2 fractions of 8 Gy, and 39% with 28 Gy in 7 fractions. Paralyzed patients regained ambulatory status 21% of the time with 28 Gy in 7 fractions and 10% of the time with 15 Gy in either 3 or 5 fractions. These pooled data demonstrate the importance of functional status over radiation dose fractionation in spinal cord compression.

SUMMARY

Spine metastases cause significant pain and can result in irreversible paralysis. Patients with known vertebral metastases require frequent clinical evaluation to identify any change in symptoms or radiographic findings suggesting risk of spinal cord compromise. Early detection of verte-

bral compromise is paramount to preventing an oncological emergency involving severe pain and neurological compromise from spinal cord compression. Emergency oncological care involves either surgical decompression or radiation therapy. Investigators continue to try, by means of systemic therapies, to prevent spinal cord compression resulting from progression of bone metastases.

Radiation remains an important modality in palliative care. Numerous clinical, prognostic, and therapeutic factors must be considered to determine the optimal treatment regimen in palliative radiation therapy in general. Symptoms that persist after palliative radiation should be evaluated. It is important to exclude disease progression in the treated area or extension of disease outside the radiation portal, especially if the patient has an associated paraspinal mass. Pain may also persist because of reduced cortical strength after treatment of spinal metastases that can result in vertebral compression or stress microfractures.

Radiation therapy is an important means of treating localized symptoms related to tumor involvement by providing a wide range of therapeutic options. Radiobiological principles, the radiation tolerance of adjacent normal tissues, and the clinical condition influence the selection of radiation technique, dose, and fraction size. Because the spinal cord is a late-reacting tissue, its radiobiological tolerance to radiation is finite. Technological advances, however, have increased our ability to treat spinal metastases with greater precision and have allowed consideration of retreatment with radiation to selected patients.

The treatment of bone metastases represents a paradigm for evaluating palliative care in terms of symptom relief, toxicities of therapy, and the financial burden to the patient, caregivers, and society. Despite enormous expenditures to treat metastases, patients continue to suffer symptoms, and they die of their disease within 24 months; the prognosis associated with the development of spinal cord compression is even more ominous. As health care resources continue to become more limited, our criteria for care must be better defined to provide care that provides effective treatment, fulfills therapeutic goals, and avoids administration of therapy with limited added benefit.

The goals of palliative therapy are very specific for patients with spinal cord compression. The treatment of spinal cord compression is a moral imperative to relieve suffering and to attempt to maintain the functional integrity and dignity of the patient. Furthermore, loss of function is among the most significant financial burdens assumed by caregivers and society. More sophisticated and costly radiotherapeutic approaches, such as IMRT and proton therapy, should be based on prognostic factors and performance status and should be reserved for more complicated clinical presentations including retreatment. Similar criteria exist for surgical intervention.

The point and types of intervention for spinal cord compression are clearer than those for prevention and early detection of spinal cord compression. Radiation and surgery, both localized therapies, are used in spinal cord compression. Systemic therapies and radiation can be used to prevent spinal cord compression. Radiation can be used to treat early vertebral or epidural involvement and thereby to prevent disease progression resulting in spinal cord compression. Radiopharmaceuticals, administered by a single injection, are an important option in patients with multifocal bone metastases who have no epidural involvement in the vertebral disease. Spinal cord compression can be prevented in patients at high risk for disease progression with limited treatment-related toxicity and time under therapy.

The development of systemic therapies, such as bisphosphonates, is important to advancing options for palliative care and to prevent the morbidity of disease progression such as spinal cord compression. Although systemic therapy with bisphosphonates has reduced the development of skeletal-related events among patients with lytic bone metastases, no analysis has specifically evaluated whether the incidence of spinal cord compression is decreased among patients with lytic bone metastases in the vertebrae at the start of bisphosphonate therapy. The 6-month period required before the full benefit of bisphosphonates is realized limits the use of bisphosphonates, because of the poor overall prognosis of these patients, after the development of spinal cord compression. Furthermore, no clear criteria guide when to start or stop bisphosphonate therapy among patients with bone metastases. The current overall financial burden and the opportunity costs, related to the frequent infusions required in bisphosphonate therapy, are high. Cost-utility analyses, which account for a broader domain of cost-effectiveness, need to be performed as part of clinical trials in every specialty, especially for palliative care end points. Clinical trials that include these criteria are critical to future practice guidelines development.

Much is accommodated during the course of cancer and its treatment. Prevention or early treatment of symptoms is often the most important care administered. The treatment of vertebral metastases and of spinal cord compression to prevent or relieve symptoms of pain and paralysis is one of the most important services rendered to patients with cancer.

REFERENCES

1. Janjan NA. Radiation for bone metastases: Conventional techniques and the role of systemic radiopharmaceuticals. Cancer 1997;80:1628-1645.
2. Liu L, Meers K, Capurso A, et al. The impact of radiation therapy on quality of life in patients with cancer. Cancer Pract 1998;6:237-242.
3. Joranson DE, Ryan KM, Gilson AM, Dahl JL. Trends in medical use and abuse of opioid analgesics. JAMA 2000;283:1710-1714.
4. Ward SE, Berry PE, Misiewicz H. Concerns about analgesics among patients and family caregivers in a hospice setting. Res Nurs Health 1996;19:205-211.
5. Weissman DE. Doctors, opioids, and the law: The effect of controlled substances regulations on cancer pain management. Semin Oncol 1993;20 (Suppl 1):53-58.
6. Mañas A, Glaría L, Peña C, et al. Prevention of urinary tract infections in palliative radiation for vertebral metastasis and spinal cord compression: A pilot study in 71 patients. Int J Radiat Oncol Biol Phys 2006;64:935-940.
7. Sherry MM, Greco FA, Johnson DH, Hainsworth JD. Breast cancer with skeletal metastases at initial diagnosis: Distinctive clinical characteristics and favorable prognosis. Cancer 1986;58:178-182.
8. Sherry MM, Greco FA, Johnson DH, Hainsworth JD. Metastatic breast cancer confined to the skeletal system. Am J Med 1986;81:381-386.
9. Plunkett TA, Smith P, Rubens RD. Risk of complications from bone metastases in breast cancer: Implications for management. Eur J Cancer 2000;36:476-462.
10. Lai PP, Perez CA, Lockett MA. Prognostic significance of pelvic recurrence and distant metastases in prostate carcinoma following definitive radiotherapy. Int J Radiat Oncol Biol Phys 1992;24:423-430.
11. Yamashita K, Denno K, Ueda T, et al. Prognostic significance of bone metastases in patients with metastatic prostate cancer. Cancer 1993;71:1297-1302.
12. Knudson G, Grinis G, Lopez-Majano V, et al. Bone scan as a stratification variable in advanced prostate cancer. Cancer 1991;68:316-320.
13. Conway R, Graham J, Kidd J, et al., Scottish Cord Compression Group. What happens to people after malignant cord compression? Survival, function,

14. Thomas KC, Nosyk B, Fisher CG, et al. Cost-effectiveness of surgery plus radiotherapy versus radiotherapy alone for metastatic epidural spinal cord compression. Int J Radiat Oncol Biol Phys 2006;66:1212-1218.
15. Jeremic B, Djuric L, Mijatovic L. Incidence of radiation myelitis of the cervical spinal cord at doses of 5500 cGy or greater. Cancer 1991;68:2138-2141.
16. Wen PY, Blanchard KL, Block CC, et al. Development of Lhermitte's sign after bone marrow transplantation. Cancer 1992;69:2262-2266.
17. Powers BE, Thames HD, Gillette SM, et al. Volume effects in the irradiated canine spinal cord: Do they exist when the probability of injury is low? Radiother Oncol 1998;46:297-306.
18. Maranzano E, Bellavita R, Floridi P, et al. Radiation induced myelopathy in long-term surviving metastatic spinal cord compression patients after hypofractionated radiotherapy: A clinical and magnetic resonance imaging analysis. Radiother Oncol 2001;60:281-288.
19. Ridet JL, Pencalet P, Belcram M, et al. Effects of spinal cord x-irradiation on the recovery of paraplegic rats. Exp Neurol 2000;161:1-14.
20. Algra PR, Heimans JJ, Valk J, et al. Do metastases in vertebrae begin in the body or the pedicles? Imaging study in 45 patients. AJR Am J Roentgenol 1992;158:1275-1279.
21. Sugimura H, Kisanuki A, Tamura S, et al. Magnetic resonance imaging of bone marrow changes after irradiation. Invest Radiol 1994;29:35-41.
22. Yankelevitz DF, Henschke C, Knapp PH, et al. Effect of radiation therapy on thoracic and lumbar bone marrow: Evaluation with MR imaging. AJR Am J Roentgenol 1991;157:87-92.
23. Hall E. Dose response relationships for normal tissues. In Radiobiology for the Radiologist, 4th ed. Philadelphia: JB Lippincott, 1994, pp 45-75.
24. Grosu AL, Andratschke N, Nieder C, Molls M. Retreatment of the spinal cord with palliative radiotherapy. Int J Radiat Oncol Biol Phys 2002;52:1288-1292.
25. Nieder C, Milas L, Ang KK. Tissue tolerance to reirradiation. Semin Radiat Oncol 2000;10:200-209.
26. Nieder C, Grosu AL, Andratschke NH, Molls M. Proposal of human spinal cord reirradiation dose based on collection of data from 40 patients. Int J Radiat Oncol Biol Phys 2005;61:851-855.
27. Morris DE. Clinical experience with retreatment for palliation. Semin Radiat Oncol 2000;10:210-221.
28. Mohiuddin M, Marks GM, Lingareddy V, Marks J. Curative surgical resection following reirradiation for recurrent rectal cancer. Int J Radiat Oncol Biol Phys 1997;39:643-649.
29. Mohiuddin M, Regine WF, Stevens J, et al. Combined intraoperative radiation and perioperative chemotherapy for unresectable cancers of the pancreas. J Clin Oncol 1995;13:2764-2768.
30. van der Linden YM, Lok JJ, Steenland E, et al., Dutch Bone Metastasis Study Group. Single fraction radiotherapy is efficacious: A further analysis of the Dutch Bone Metastasis Study controlling for the influence of retreatment. Int. J Radiat Oncol Biol Phys 2004;59:528-537.
31. Rades D, Stalpers LJA, Veninga T, Hoskin PJ. Spinal reirradiation after short-course RT for metastatic spinal cord compression. Int J Radiat Oncol Biol Phys 2005;63:872-875.
32. Milker-Zabel S, Zabel A, Thilmann C, et al. Clinical results of retreatment of vertebral bone metastases by stereotactic conformal radiotherapy and intensity-modulated radiotherapy. Int J Radiat Oncol Biol Phys 2003;55:162-167.
33. Agarwal JP, Swangsilpa T, van der Linden Y, et al. The role of external beam radiotherapy in the management of bone metastases. Clin Oncol 2006;18:747-760.
34. Boogerd W, van der Sande JJ, Kroger R. Early diagnosis and treatment of spinal metastases in breast cancer: A prospective study. J Neurol Neurosurg Psychiatry 1992;55:1188-1193.
35. Bach F, Agerlin N, Sorensen JB, et al. Metastatic spinal cord compression secondary to lung cancer. J Clin Oncol 1992;10:1781-1787.
36. Prie L, Lagarde P, Palussiere J, et al. Radiation therapy of spinal metastases in breast cancer: Retrospective analysis of 108 patients. Cancer Radiother 1997;1:234-239.
37. Sciubba DM, Gokaslan ZL. Diagnosis and management of metastatic spine disease. Surg Oncol 2006;15:141-151.
38. Spinazzè S, Caraceni A, Schrijvers D. Epidural spinal cord compression. Crit Rev Oncol Hematol 2005;56:397-406.
39. Helweg-Larsen S, Soelberg Sorensen P, Kreiner S. Prognostic factors in metastatic spinal cord compression: A prospective study using multivariate analysis of variables influencing survival and gait function in 153 patients. Int J Radiat Oncol Biol Phys 2000;46:1163-1169.
40. Altehoefer C, Ghanem N, Hogerle S, et al. Comparative detectability of bone metastases and impact on therapy of magnetic resonance imaging and bone scintigraphy in patients with breast cancer. Eur J Radiol 2001;40:16-23.
41. Barton M. Tables of equivalent dose in 2 Gy fractions: A simple application of the linear quadratic formula. Int J Radiat Oncol Biol Phys 1995;31:371-378.
42. Bates T, Yarnold JR, Blitzer P, et al. Bone metastases consensus statement. Int J Radiat Oncol Biol Phys 1992;23:215-216.
43. Bates T. A review of local radiotherapy in the treatment of bone metastases and cord compression. Int J Radiat Oncol Biol Phys 1992;23:217-221.
44. Steiner RM, Mitchell DG, Rao VM, Schweitzer ME. Magnetic resonance imaging of diffuse bone marrow disease. Radiol Clin North Am 1993;31:383-409.
45. Algra PR, Bloem JL, Tissing H, et al. Detection of vertebral metastases: Comparison between MR imaging and bone scintigraphy. Radiographics 1991;11:219-232.

46. Le Bihan DJ. Differentiation of benign versus pathologic compression fractures with diffusion-weighted MR imaging: A closer step toward the "holy grail" of tissue characterization? Radiology 1998;207:305-307.

47. Francken AB, Hong AM, Fulham MJ, et al. Detection of unsuspected spinal cord compression in melanoma patients by 18F-fluorodeoxyglucose positron emission tomography. Eur J Surg Oncol 2005;31:197-204.

48. Nielsen OS, Munro AJ, Tannock IF. Bone metastases: Pathophysiology and management policy. J Clin Oncol 1991;9:509-524.

49. Hoskin PJ, Grover A, Bhana R. Metastatic spinal cord compression: Radiotherapy outcome and dose fractionation. Radiother Oncol 2003;68:175-180.

50. Turner S, Marosszeky B, Timms I, Boyages J. Malignant spinal cord compression: A prospective evaluation. Int J Radiat Oncol Biol Phys 1993;26:141-146.

51. Wada E, Yamamoto T, Furuno M, et al. Spinal cord compression secondary to osteoblastic metastasis. Spine 1993;18:1380-1381.

52. Kim RY, Smith JW, Spencer SA, et al. Malignant epidural spinal cord compression associated with a paravertebral mass: Its radiotherapeutic outcome on radiosensitivity. Int J Radiat Oncol Biol Phys 1993;27:1079-1083.

53. Russi EG, Pergolizzi S, Gaeta M, et al. Palliative radiotherapy in lumbosacral carcinomatous neuropathy. Radiother Oncol 1993;26:172-173.

54. Saarto T, Janes R, Tenhunen M, Kouri M. Palliative radiotherapy in the treatment of skeletal metastases. Eur J Pain 2002;6:323-330.

55. Loblaw DA, Laperriere NJ, Mackillop WJ. A population-based study of malignant spinal cord compression in Ontario. Clin Oncol 2003;15:211-217.

56. Rades D, Blach M, Bremer M, et al. Prognostic significance of the time of developing motor deficits before radiation therapy in metastatic spinal cord compression: One-year results of a prospective trial. Int J Radiat Oncol Biol Phys 2000;48:1403-1408.

57. Rades D, Heidenreich F, Karstens JH. Final results of a prospective study of the prognostic value of the time to develop motor deficits before irradiation in metastatic spinal cord compression. Int J Radiat Oncol Biol Phys 2002; 53:975-979.

58. Boogerd W, van der Sande JJ. Diagnosis and treatment of spinal cord compression in malignant disease. Cancer Treat Rev 1993;19:129-150.

59. Boogerd W. Central nervous system metastasis in breast cancer. Radiother Oncol 1996;40:5-22.

60. Bach F, Bjerregaard B, Soletormos G, et al. Diagnostic value of cerebrospinal fluid cytology in comparison with tumor marker activity in central nervous system metastases secondary to breast cancer. Cancer 1993;72: 2376-2382.

61. Tehranzadeh J, Tao C. Advances in MR imaging of vertebral collapse. Semin Ultrasound CT MR 2004;25:440-460.

62. Byrne TN. Spinal cord compression from epidural metastases. N Engl J Med 1992;327:614-619.

63. Grant R, Papadopoulos SM, Greenberg HS. Metastatic epidural spinal cord compression. Neurol Clin 1991;9:825-841.

64. Hartsell WF, Scott CB, Watkins-Bruner D, et al. Randomized trial of short-versus long-course radiotherapy for palliation of painful bone metastases. J Natl Cancer Inst 2005;97:798-804.

65. Jarvik JG, Deyo RA. Diagnostic evaluation of low back pain with emphasis on imaging. Ann Intern Med 2002;137;586-597.

66. Loblaw DA, Perry J, Chambers A, Laperriere NJ. Systematic review of the diagnosis and management of malignant extradural spinal cord compression: The Cancer Care Ontario Practice Guidelines Initiative's Neuro-Oncology Disease Site Group. J Clin Oncol 2005;23:2028-2037.

67. Loblaw DA, Laperriere NJ. Emergency treatment of malignant extradural spinal cord compression: An evidence-based guideline. J Clin Oncol 1998;16:1613-1624.

68. Hatrick NC, Lucas JD, Timothy AR, Smith MA. The surgical treatment of metastatic disease of the spine. Radiother Oncol 2000;56:335-339.

69. Landmann C, Hunig R, Gratzi O. The role of laminectomy in the combined treatment of metastatic spinal cord compression. Int J Radiat Oncol Biol Phys 1992;24:627-631.

70. Maranzano E, Latini P, Checcaglini F, et al. Radiation therapy in metastatic spinal cord compression: A prospective analysis of 105 consecutive patients. Cancer 1991;67:1311-1317.

71. Janjan NA. Radiotherapeutic management of spinal metastases. J Pain Symptom Manage 1996;1:47-56.

72. Patchell RA, Tibbs PA, Regine WF, et al. Direct decompressive surgical resection in the treatment of spinal cord compression caused by metastatic cancer: A randomised trial. Lancet 2005;366:643-648.

73. Windhagen HJ, Hipp JA, Silva MJ, et al. Predicting failure of thoracic vertebrae with simulated and actual metastatic defects. Clin Orthop Relat Res 1997;344:313-319.

74. Taneichi H, Kaneda K, Takeda N, et al. Risk factors and probability of vertebral body collapse in metastases of the thoracic and lumbar spine. Spine 1997;22:239-245.

75. Finkelstein JA, Ford MH. Diagnosis and management of pathological fractures of the spine. Curr Orthop 2004;18:396-405.

76. Vrionis FD, Hamm A, Stanton N, et al. Kyphoplasty for tumor associated spinal fractures. Tech Reg Anesth Pain Manag 2005;9:35-39.

77. Tschirhart CE, Roth SE, Whyne CM. Biomechanical assessment of stability in the metastatic spine following percutaneous vertebroplasty: Effects of cement distribution patterns and volume. J Biomech 2005;38:1582-1590.

78. Tschirhart CE, Nagpurkar A, Whyne CM. Effects of tumor location, shape and surface serration on burst fracture risk in the metastatic spine. J Biomech 2004;37:653-660.

79. Tow B, Seang BT, Chong TT, Chen J. Predictors for survival in metastases to the spine. Spine J 2005;5(Suppl):73.

80. Guo Y, Young B, Palmer JL, et al. Prognostic factors for survival in metastatic spinal cord compression: A retrospective study in a rehabilitation setting. Am J Phys Med Rehabil 2003;82:665-668.

81. Chow E, Coia L, Wu J, et al. This house believes that multiple-fraction radiotherapy is a barrier to referral for palliative radiotherapy for bone metastases. Curr Oncol 2002;9:60-66.

82. Chow E, Lutz S, Beyene J. A single fraction for all, or an argument for fractionation tailored to fit the needs of each individual patient with bone metastases? Int J Radiat Oncol Biol Phys 2003;55:565-567.

83. Haddad P, Wong R, Wilson P, et al. Factors influencing the use of single versus multiple fractions of palliative radiotherapy for bone metastases: A 5-yr review and comparison to a survey. Int J Radiat Oncol Biol Phys 2003;57(Suppl): S278.

84. Roos DE, Turner SL, O'Brien PC, et al. Randomized trial of 8 Gy in 1 versus 20 Gy in 5 fractions of radiotherapy for neuropathic pain due to bone metastases (Trans-Tasman Radiation Oncology Group, TROG 96.05). Radiother Oncol 2005;75:54-63.

85. Jeremic B. Single fraction external beam radiation therapy in the treatment of localized metastatic bone pain: A review. J Pain Symptom Manage 2001; 22:1048-1058.

86. Jeremic B, Grujicic D, Cirovic V, et al. Radiotherapy of metastatic spinal cord compression. Acta Oncol 1991;30:985-986.

87. Maranzano E, Latini P, Perrucci E, et al. Short course radiotherapy (8 Gy × 2) in metastatic spinal cord compression: An effective and feasible treatment. Int J Radiat Oncol Biol Phys 1997;38:1037-1044.

88. Maranzano E, Latini P, Beneventi S, et al. Comparison of two different radiotherapy schedules for spinal cord compression in prostate cancer. Turmori 1998;84:472-477.

89. Rades D, Stalpers LJA, Hulshor MC, et al. Comparison of 1 × 8 Gy and 10 × 3 Gy for functional outcome in patients with metastatic spinal cord compression. Int J Radiat Oncol Biol Phys 2005;62:514-518.

90. Moineuse C, Kany M, Fourcade D, et al. Magnetic resonance imaging findings in multiple myeloma: Descriptive and predictive value. Joint Bone Spine 2001;68:334-344.

91. Rades D, Stalpers LJA, Veninga T, et al. Evaluation of five radiation schedules and prognostic factors for metastatic spinal cord compression. J Clin Oncol 2005;23:3366-3375.

92. Rades D, Karstens JH, Hoskin PJ, et al. Escalation of radiation dose beyond 30 Gy in 10 fractions for metastatic spinal cord compression. Int J Radiat Oncol Biol Phys 2007;67:525-531.

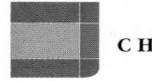

CHAPTER **224**

Malignant Ascites

Peter Demeulenaere and Bart Van den Eynden

K E Y   P O I N T S

- Ascites is an accumulation of peritoneal cavity fluids in the peritoneal cavity that can be malignant (secondary to peritoneal carcinomatosis) or nonmalignant (hepatic cirrhosis).

- Ascites is generally associated with peritoneal metastasis and obstruction of subphrenic lymphatic vessels by tumor infiltration.

- Most patients with malignancy-related ascites have a poor prognosis, and the principle of minimal disturbance should guide management, especially for those patients who are bedbound and whose life expectancy is short.

- Clinical guidelines on paracentesis related to malignancy have been published with particular attention to the need for preliminary ultrasound examination, intravenous fluid provision, and drainage time.

- Ascites secondary to chemotherapy-sensitive tumors may benefit from *chemotherapy*: a reasonable response can be expected in patients with ovarian cancer, whereas a poorer response is obtained in patients treated for gastric or colon cancer.

Normally, a healthy person has approximately 50 mL of transudate in the peritoneal cavity. Normal fluid turnover is 4 to 5 L/hour. In malignant ascites, the fluid turnover is higher than in healthy persons.

PREVALENCE AND ETIOLOGY

Ascites is accumulation of peritoneal cavity fluid that can be malignant (from peritoneal carcinomatosis) or nonmalignant (hepatic cirrhosis). Although nonmalignant conditions are more common (80% to 90%), ascites secondary to peritoneal carcinomatosis or hepatic failure resulting from metastatic disease is not uncommon (10% to 20%). Ascites occurs in 6% of patients with cancer and has a poor prognosis. Many tumors cause ascites, most frequently ovarian cancers (up to 50%), cancer of unknown origin, and gastrointestinal cancers (stomach, colon, pancreas). Ascites may be the presenting feature of cancer, of recurrence, or of metastasis. It often signifies end-stage disease. Cardiac failure, liver failure, and renal failure are common causes of nonmalignant ascites. Some tumors cause hepatic failure from massive metastatic liver involvement.

CLINICAL SYMPTOMS AND DIAGNOSIS

The most common symptoms include abdominal discomfort, difficulty in bending forward, inability to sit upright, and dyspnea. Symptoms related to gastric compression and increased intra-abdominal pressure include heartburn, nausea, vomiting, and anorexia. Peripheral edema of the legs and genitalia is common. Patients are usually symptomatic only when the abdominal wall is tense.

The diagnosis in patients with cancer is usually clinical, and investigations are usually unnecessary. The diagnosis is based on abdominal distention, shifting dullness (detects ≈500 mL), and ultrasound examination (detects 100 mL). Ultrasound may determine whether ascites is loculated by tumor adhesions. A computed tomography scan should be done to exclude bowel obstruction (use caution with oral contrast media).

PATHOGENESIS

Ascites is generally associated with peritoneal metastasis and obstruction of subphrenic lymphatic vessels by tumor infiltration. Other mechanisms include increased peritoneal permeability, increased sodium retention by hyperaldosteronism (possibly secondary to extracellular blood volume), liver metastasis leading to hypoalbuminemia, and venous obstruction (e.g., portal vein obstruction, inferior vena caval obstruction). Immune modulators, vascular permeability factors, and metalloproteinases may contribute to the condition and offer the opportunity for new therapies for malignant ascites.[1]

PROGNOSIS

When caused by cancer, ascites is associated with advanced disease. These patients have a median life expectancy of 8 to 20 weeks. In ovarian cancer, in which ascites can present early, survival of 20 to 50 weeks may occur.[2]

MANAGEMENT AND TREATMENT

Malignant ascites occurs in association with various neoplasms. It is a frequent cause of morbidity and presents significant problems, for no clear evidence-based management guidelines exist. A recent guideline for symptomatic malignant ascites is based on a systematic literature review.[3] Although paracentesis, diuretics, and shunting are commonly used, the evidence is weak. Available data show good, although temporary, effects of paracentesis on symptoms. Fluid withdrawal, flow, and concurrent intravenous hydration are insufficiently studied. Peritoneovenous (P-V) shunts can control malignant ascites, but they have to be balanced by the potential risks. The data about diuretics for malignant ascites are controversial. Diuretics should be considered in all patients, but each case should be evaluated individually.[3]

Treatment consists most effectively of removing and, if possible, preventing the return of ascites. Most people with malignancy-related ascites have a poor prognosis, and the principle of minimal disturbance should guide management, especially for patients who are bedbound and whose life expectancy is short. Although no treatment is entirely satisfactory, paracentesis generally remains the most practical effective measure.[4]

Symptomatic Treatment

Analgesia may be all that is required to overcome any discomfort or mild dyspnea, although active patients usually want the fluid drained. No randomized trials of *diuretics* in malignant ascites have been conducted. Diuretics may be effective in approximately one third of patients with malignant disease, and efficacy may be determined by plasma renin-aldosterone concentrations. Diuretics reduce malignant ascites over 2 to 3 weeks, provided high doses are used. These drugs are effective because sodium retention contributes to the ascites. Spironolactone is the key to success because it antagonizes aldosterone. Start with spironolactone, 100 to 200 mg, in addition to the loop diuretic furosemide, 40 mg (or bumetanide, 1 mg) daily; if patients tolerate these doses, double the dose after 1 week. Monitor treatment by daily abdominal girth measurement, and reduce the dose once the patient is at risk of dehydration or impaired renal function (biochemical control). Reduce diuretics to the lowest dose that controls ascites. An intravenous furosemide infusion (100 mg over 24 hours) may be an alternative to paracentesis for rapid relief of tense ascites. Patients with liver cirrhosis or liver metastasis respond better to diuretics.

Many studies on *paracentesis* in liver disease have been conducted. Removal of several liters of fluid is associated with the risk of hypotension, hypovolemia, disturbance of electrolytes, and renal impairment. Intravenous albumin reduces these risks.[5] Paracentesis is a simple, effective, and safe mechanical procedure that can provide good and immediate symptomatic relief. For an ambulatory patient, the fluid can be removed rapidly, up to 5 liters over 1 to 2 hours. In weaker patients, the fluid should be drained more slowly because hypotension can occur. The fluid reaccumulates over 1 to 3 weeks unless diuretics are used. Symptomatic benefit is maximal after the first few liters have been removed. Limit the volume of paracentesis to

5 liters maximum if renal or hepatic failure is present, if the serum albumin is less than 30 g/ L, or if the sodium concentration is lower than 125 mmol/L.[6]

Clinical guidelines on paracentesis related to malignancy have been published, with particular attention to the need for preliminary ultrasound examination, intravenous fluid provision, and drainage time.[4] The procedure is simple. Patients should have an empty bladder and should be in a semirecumbent position. The puncture site needs to be in an area without scars, tumor masses, distended bowel, bladder, liver, or inferior epigastric vessels. Stay 10 cm from the midline to avoid blood vessels. Use an aseptic technique, anesthetize the skin locally with 0.5% bupivacaine (Marcaine), and infiltrate the puncture site down to the peritoneum. Insert a large (14- to 16-gauge) intravenous cannula in the left or right iliac fossa. If fluid dribbles out of the puncture site after paracentesis, a colostomy bag can collect the fluid, which usually stops within a few hours. Warn the patient that this may occur, and reassure the patient that this leakage is harmless. If no fluid is obtained, ascites may be pocketed, so try one further puncture site or use ultrasound guidance. This procedure is contraindicated in patients with intestinal obstruction or multiple adhesions. Other contraindications include local or systemic infection and coagulopathy (platelets <40.000 or international normalized ratio >1.4).

When ascites requires frequent drainage, a permanent drainage tube may be considered. A Pleurx (Denver Biomedical) catheter with a one-way valve can be palliative; it offers convenient home drainage, and the patient does not have to wait until symptoms arise. This catheter is well tolerated, and the infection rate is low. The drain lines can be kept in place for months, until the patient's death. One study compared the safety and efficacy of two percutaneous drainage methods over 41 months: large-volume paracentesis and Pleurx catheter placement. The Pleurx catheter provided effective palliation with complications similar to those of large-volume paracentesis, and it precluded the need for frequent hospital trips for repeated percutaneous drainage.[7]

A *P-V shunt* is indicated for a relatively fit patient who is troubled by recurrent ascites. This situation arises most commonly in patients with cancer of the breast or ovary. A shunt can provide excellent control, and it should be considered early. A P-V shunt also prevents repeated paracenteses and maintains normal serum albumin concentrations. A Denver shunt or a LeVeen shunt is commonly used. It is a multiply perforated catheter that joins a one-way valve and a reservoir that can be pumped. The shunt is easily inserted using a short general anesthetic regimen. The lower abdominal end of the shunt is inserted into the hypochondrium, and the venous end is led subcutaneously to a neck incision and is inserted into the internal jugular vein. The fluid is drained into the superior vena cava; fluid flows through the shunt on inspiration. Patients should pump the reservoir to keep fluid flowing. A P-V shunt is not indicated if the fluid is blood stained or turbid (because the shunt will quickly block) or if it is loculated. Unfortunately, 30% of shunts occlude within 3 to 6 months and need to be replaced. Complications include fever, infection, shunt blockage, and coagulopathy. Facilitating hematogenous tumor spread is a theoretical disadvantage: postmortem studies showed that despite the infusion of viable malignant cells into the venous circulation, no clinically significant metastases occurred. In nonmalignant ascites, a shunt can give good palliation; blockage occurs sooner in patients with malignant disease.[8]

Chylous ascites is a rare complication of abdominal radiation or para-aortic lymph node dissection in gynecological malignant diseases. Chylous ascites in adults is a significant management problem, with high mortality from cachexia and infection or after surgical attempts at correction. A systemic approach with subcutaneous octreotide and a fat-free diet may have good results in adults. This noninvasive approach avoids surgery. Intraperitoneal corticosteroids can also be considered: 600 mg methylprednisolone at once, at the end of the tap.[9]

Etiological Treatment

Patients with ascites who have chemotherapy-sensitive tumors may benefit from *chemotherapy*: a reasonable response can be expected in ovarian cancer, although responses are less dramatic in gastric or colon cancer. Intraperitoneal chemotherapy is logical because a significantly higher drug concentration is achieved than after intravenous administration and because patients with malignant ascites have reduced peritoneal drug clearance rates. In ovarian cancer, intraperitoneal chemotherapy (cisplatin, paclitaxel) may confer a survival advantage.[10] Various other agents have been used, including bleomycin, 5-flurouracil, and thiotepa, but results with these agents are disappointing, and the use of these drugs is rarely indicated.

Laparoscopic intraperitoneal hyperthermic chemotherapy for malignant ascites is carried out at 42°C for 90 minutes, with 1.5% dextrose solution as a carrier. In one study, chemotherapeutic agents included cisplatin and doxorubicin or mitomycin, depending on the primary tumor. The drains were left in situ after surgery and were removed when perfusate drainage ceased. Ascites was controlled in all the treated cases in this study. This method benefited patients who were not candidates for cytoreductive surgery.[11]

Clinical experience with antiangiogenic agents such as the matrix metalloproteinase inhibitors and the vascular endothelial growth factor antagonists suggests that these agents may have a role in the management of malignant ascites.[12] Targeted antibody therapy (*radioimmunotherapy*) is a novel approach that has achieved useful palliation in some cases. Monoclonal antibodies to tumor antigens (detected on malignant cells in the fluid) are coupled to a radioisotope (iodine 131) and are given intraperitoneally to deliver radiation directly to tumor-bearing areas.

Cytoreductive surgery (omentectomy, debulking) should be offered to some patients with peritoneal carcinomatosis because this approach may provide significant palliation.[13] Combined treatment with intraperitoneal hyperthermic chemotherapy has shown promising survival in patients with pseudomyxoma peritonei and peritoneal dissemination of digestive tract cancer.[14]

REFERENCES

1. Aslam N, Marino CR. Malignant ascites: New concepts in pathophysiology, diagnosis and management. Arch Intern Med 2001;161:2733-2727.
2. Campbell C. Controlling malignant ascites. EJPC 2001;8:187-190.
3. Becker G, Galandi D, Blum H. Malignant ascites: Systematic review and guideline for treatment. Eur J Cancer 2006;42:589-597.
4. Stephenson J, Gilbert J. The development of clinical guidelines on paracentesis for ascites related to malignancy. Palliat Med 2002;16:213-218.
5. Wang SS, Lu CW, Chao Y, et al. Total paracentesis in non-alcoholic cirrhotics with massive ascites: Mid-term effects on systemic and hepatic haemodynamics and renal function. J Gastroenterol Hepatol 1994;9:592-596.
6. McNamara P. Paracentesis: An effective method of symptom control in the palliative care setting? Palliat Med 2000;14:62-64.
7. Rosenberg S, Courtney A, Nemcek AA Jr, Omary RA. Comparison of percutaneous management techniques for recurrent malignant ascites. J Vasc Interv Radiol 2004;15:1129-1131.
8. Zanon C, Grosso M, Apra F, et al. Palliative treatment of malignant refractory ascites by positioning of Denver peritoneovenous shunt. Tumori 2002;88:123-127.
9. Mincher L, Evans J, Jenner MW, Varney VA. The successful treatment of chylous effusions in malignant disease with octreotide. Clin Oncol 2005;17:118-121.
10. Markman M. Intraperitoneal antineoplastic drug delivery: Rationale and results. Lancet Oncol 2003;4:277-283.
11. Garofalo A, Valle M, Garcia J, Sugarbaker PH. Laparoscopic intraperitoneal hyperthermic chemotherapy for palliation of debilitating malignant ascites. Eur J Surg Oncol 2006;32:682-685.
12. Smith E, Jayson G. The current and future management of malignant ascites. Clin Oncol 2003;15:59-72.
13. Spurgeon J, Cotlar A. Cytoreductive surgery in the management of malignant ascites from adenocarcinoma of unknown primary (ACUP). Curr Surg 2005;62:500-503.
14. Glehen O, Mohamed F, Gilly FN. Peritoneal carcinomatosis from digestive tract cancer: New management by cytoreductive surgery and intraperitoneal chemohyperthermia. Lancet Oncol 2004;5:219-228.

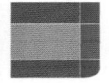

CHAPTER **225**

Pleural and Pericardial Effusions

Susan B. LeGrand

Effusions are common complications of malignant disease that cause significant distress but are also amenable to interventions that can yield significant improvement. Therapies are typically geared to drainage and prevention of reaccumulation of fluid.

BASIC SCIENCE

The fundamental cause of fluid accumulation in the pleural or pericardial space is imbalance between the amount secreted and the amount of fluid resorbed (Table 225-1).[1] Vascular endothelial growth factor (VEGF), a critical protein, is under active research in malignant disease, given the need for tumors to develop a blood supply to support growth. Cancer therapies that antagonize VEGF are already in use or are under active development. These agents typically are antibodies to the VEGF receptors (bevacizumab) or chemical inhibitors of VEGF receptor tyrosine kinase function (imatinib, sorafenib, and sunitinib). Evidence supporting the role of VEGF, originally known as vascular permeability factor, in effusions includes the following: (1) increased levels seen in pleural, pericardial, and peritoneal effusions; (2) increased levels in malignant effusions relative to benign causes; and (3) animal studies that demonstrate differences in effusion volumes with transfected genes that either increase or decrease VEGF expression.[2]

The effect of VEGF appears to be local because serum levels are not increased. Cells believed to produce VEGF in the pleural space include mesothelial, inflammatory, and infiltrating tumor cells. Although the relative contribution of inflammatory cells is unknown, their role is believed to be less important because no correlation exists between VEGF levels and inflammatory cell numbers.

Matrix metalloproteinases (MMPs) and their counterparts, tissue inhibitors of metalloproteinase (TIMPs), comprise a family of endopeptidases involved in the maintenance of the extracellular matrix.[3] Two of these substances, gelatinase A (MMP-2) and gelatinase B (MMP-9), have been identified in pleural fluid. MMP-2 has been seen in transudates and exudates, whereas MMP-9 has been seen only in exudates. Evidence includes the following: (1) correlation of the ratio of MMP-2 and MMP-9 to cause; (2) expression of MMP-2 constitutively by pleural mesothelial cells and present in all pleural effusions regardless of origin; and (3) the presence of MMP-9 only in exudative

TABLE 225-1 Mechanisms of Pleural Fluid Accumulation

MECHANISM	DISORDER
Increased hydrostatic pressure	Heart failure
Decreased oncotic pressure	Nephrotic syndrome, hypoalbuminemia
Decreased pressure in pleural space	Lung collapse
Increased permeability of microvascular circulation	Malignant disease, infection
Impaired lymphatic drainage	Malignant disease
From peritoneal space (ascites)	Malignant disease, cirrhosis

From Moores DWO. Management of malignant pleural effusion. Chest Surg Clin N Am 1994;4:481-495.

effusions, with decreasing levels seen after successful talc treatment.[4] In pericardial effusions, the reverse is seen: MMP-2 levels are higher in malignant effusions than in nonmalignant effusions or normal pleural fluid. MMP-9 was not present in normal pericardial fluid and was present in malignant and nonmalignant effusions but without significant differences in level.[5]

EPIDEMIOLOGY

Malignant effusions account for 40% of all effusions and are seen in patients with almost any type of cancer except primary brain tumors. The most common cancers associated with MPE are lung (35%), breast (23%), and lymphoma (10%). MPE may be the first presentation of malignant disease, or it may occur in advanced disease. Carcinoma of unknown primary origin is seen in 12% of patients with MPEs. In contrast, MPCEs are rarely the initial presentation and are typically seen in advanced cases of the same cancers associated with MPEs. Approximately 50% of pericardial effusions in patients with cancer may result from therapy, including radiation, graft-versus-host disease, and the retinoic acid syndrome.[6]

CLINICAL MANIFESTATIONS

Effusions may be an incidental finding on radiography or computed tomography (CT) or may manifest with severe symptoms (see "Case Study: Malignant Pleural Effusion" and "Case Study: Malignant Pericardial Effusion"). The primary symptom is dyspnea, which is usually subacute and progressive as fluid volume increases. Patients with MPE typically experience dyspnea on exertion first, and the problem worsens when they are supine. Without knowing their pathological condition, patients may determine that lying on the uninvolved side is particularly uncomfortable. Dyspnea then progresses to symptoms at rest. Cough and chest pain are also common. Physical examination is usually characteristic: decreased breath sounds, dullness to percussion, and decreased tactile fremitus are noted.

MPCE may be asymptomatic if the fluid collection is gradual enough to allow enlargement of the pericardial sac. Dyspnea, cough, chest pain, and orthopnea are common and can progress to tamponade with or without the clinical signs of jugular venous distention, pulsus paradox, muffled heart sounds, and electrical alternans. In 30 patients (8 with malignant disease), 87% had dyspnea, 3 had no signs of tamponade, and 4 had only one of the findings. In this group, 21 of 26 patients benefited from intervention, and the probability of response did not correlate with the clinical findings.[7] Concurrent pulmonary metastatic disease is common; more than 50% of patients have MPE, and more than 30% have parenchymal disease. The significance of the pericardial involvement may be unrecognized.[8]

DIFFERENTIAL DIAGNOSIS

The first step is to distinguish transudate from exudate. The original criteria—Light's—are well validated in pleural disease (Box 225-1).[9,10] Tests of documented value in pericardial disease (Table 225-2 and Fig. 225-1) have lower predictive value, and results are close to the established cutoff values. Cytology is the definitive diagnostic test, but the yield from one thoracentesis sample in pleural fluid is variable (only 47% in breast cancer).[11,12] The yield in pericardial fluid is 80%.[6] Blind pleural biopsy is not recommended because only 7% to 12% of the effusions in patients who had previously negative cytology will be correctly identified. Although CT is sensitive in detecting pericardial fluid, the test of choice for MPCE is echocardiography because it can demonstrate hemodynamic effects. Figure 225-2 illustrates the radiographic appearance of malignant pleural effusions.

 C A S E   S T U D Y

Malignant Pericardial Effusion

DM was a 61-year-old woman with metastatic breast cancer who had undergone left-sided chest wall radiation and who was receiving docetaxel chemotherapy. A routine chest radiograph suggested the possibility of a pericardial effusion. She had no symptoms other than fatigue. An echocardiogram was done, and it identified a large, circumferential pericardial effusion with collapse of the right atrium but no other evidence of tamponade. The differential diagnosis included radiation-induced effusion, docetaxel-induced effusion, and malignancy. Because chemotherapy-induced and malignant effusion would result in a change of treatment, a definitive diagnosis was needed despite the absence of symptoms. The patient was admitted for pericardiocentesis; the 850 mL of turbid fluid removed was exudative but cytologically negative. Chemotherapy was changed to paclitaxel, and she was followed up with periodic echocardiography. Four months later, fluid recurred, prompting surgical referral for creation of a subxiphoid pericardial window. At that time, involvement of the pericardium with tumor was visible, and cytology was positive. She lived an additional 3 years without further pericardial problems.

 C A S E   S T U D Y

Malignant Pleural Effusion

RS is an 86-year-old woman with a history of stage II breast cancer who was treated with adjuvant tamoxifen, lumpectomy, and radiation therapy. While caring for her dying husband, she began to lose weight and became more fatigued. She ultimately presented to an emergency room for progressive dyspnea. A right-siced pleural effusion seen on the chest radiograph, but without evidence of heart failure, prompted pulmonary referral. A diagnostic and therapeutic thoracentesis was performed, and pleural cytological findings were positive for adenocarcinoma. Other sites of metastatic disease were identified, and exemestane treatment was begun. The patient had rapid response to systemic therapy and resolved her effusion without other treatment at that time.

Box 225-1 Light's Criteria for Pleural Fluid

Ratio of pleural fluid to serum protein >0.5 or
Ratio of pleural fluid to serum LDH >0.6 or
Pleural fluid LDH concentration more than two thirds the upper limit
of normal serum LDH

LDH, lactate dehydrogenase.
From Heffner JE. Discriminating between transudates and exudates. Clin Chest Med 2006;27:241-252.

TABLE 225-2 Identifying Transudate versus Exudate in Pericardial Disease

Specific gravity >1.015
Fluid protein level >3.0 mg/dL
Ratio of fluid to serum protein >0.5
Fluid LDH value >300 U/dL
Ratio of fluid to serum LDH >0.6

LDH, lactate dehydrogenase.
From Meyers DG, Meyers RE, Prendergast TW. The usefulness of diagnostic tests on pericardial fluid. Chest 1997;111:1213-1221.

TREATMENT

Treatment must be individualized based on the underlying disease, the potential for response to systemic therapy, the performance status, and the goals of care. Dyspnea may be related to several concurrent processes such as asthenia, anemia, and pulmonary parenchymal disease. Removal of one contributing factor (e.g., the effusion) may be insufficient to provide symptomatic relief.

Fluid Removal

Thoracentesis and pericardiocentesis are successful techniques for removal of pleural and pericardial fluid. These procedures provide immediate symptom relief if the effusion is the cause. If no improvement is seen and adequate fluid has been removed (1 to 1.5 L from pleura), then further treatment will be unlikely to help. Removal of a larger volume of fluid at one time in pleural disease is associated with a risk of pulmonary edema. This approach does not constitute definitive therapy. MPE recurs in a mean of 4 days and at a rate of 98% in 30 days.[13] Repeated thoracenteses increase the risk of loculation, which is difficult to manage, as well as the risk of infection. In patients within days of death or who have a high probability of response to systemic therapy, this approach may be reasonable. In most patients, however, one diagnostic or therapeutic procedure (to confirm benefit) should be followed by definitive treatment.

Ninety percent of MPCEs will recur within 90 days of removal. Because MPCE occurs most often in advanced disease, this time frame may be adequate for some.[14] Median survival is 135 days, a finding suggesting that definitive therapy may also be needed.[15] In one study, simple pericardiocentesis was compared with prolonged catheter drainage. Patients who had prolonged catheter drainage

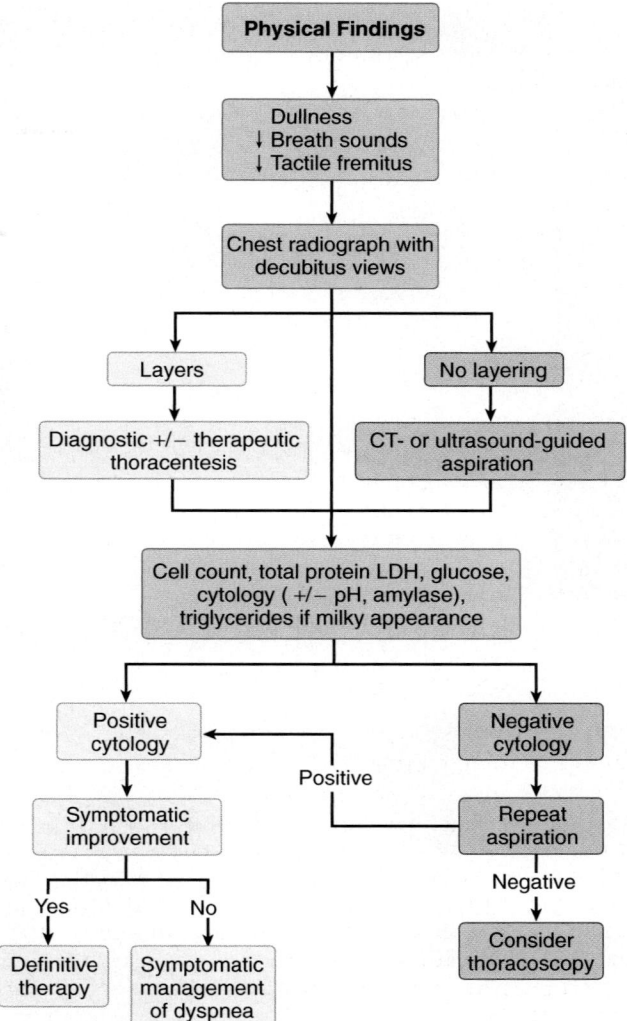

FIGURE 225-1 Diagnostic algorithm for pleural effusion. LDH, lactate dehydrogenase.

underwent fluid removal every 4 to 6 hours or as clinically indicated until drainage decreased to less than 25 to 30 mL in 24 hours. The mean duration of drainage was 3.2 ± 2.8 days. The investigators noted a significant decrease in recurrence in the group receiving prolonged drainage (36% versus 12%, *P* < .001). Recurrence after initial management was strongly predicted by simple pericardiocentesis, larger effusion size, and the urgency of the procedure.

Sclerotherapy

The goal of sclerotherapy is to create an inflammatory process within the pleural or pericardial space and thus cause fibrosis and obliteration of the space. Sclerotherapy has been the standard of care for pleural effusions; debate has been limited to which agent and by which method the sclerosing agent should be instilled.[16,17] Sclerotherapy has also been advocated for MPCE but with less evidence of benefit. In the study discussed earlier, a few of the patients in the group receiving extended catheter

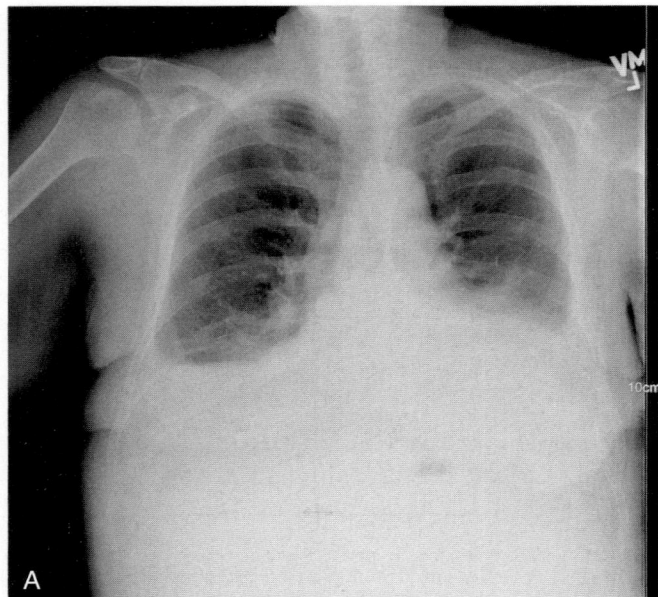

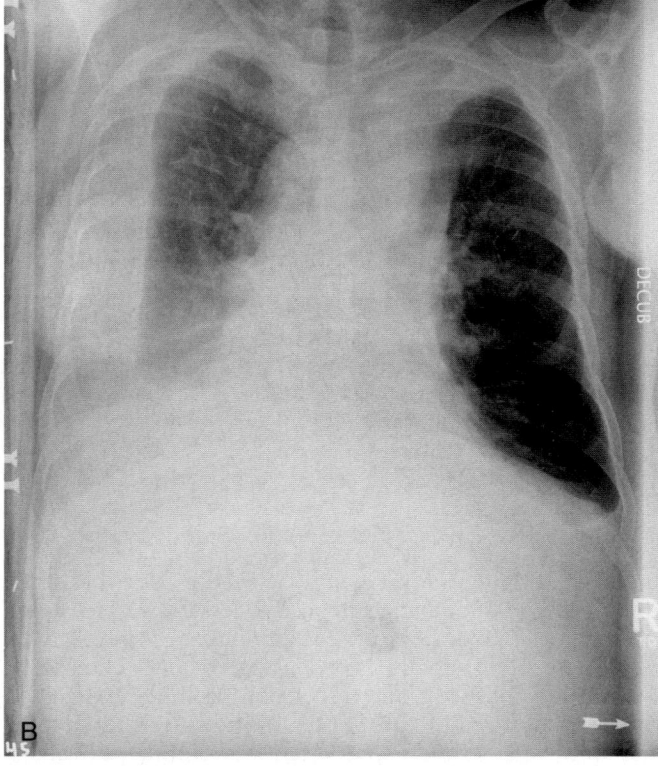

FIGURE 225-2 Posteroanterior (**A**) and lateral decubitus (**B**) images with layering of a malignant effusion.

line became unavailable, most commonly talc, as well as other tetracyclines such as doxycycline and bleomycin. Talc appears to be the sclerosant of choice.[16] Concerns expressed about the possibility that pneumonitis and acute respiratory distress syndrome may be associated with talc appear related to particle size. Large-particle talc appears to avoid this otherwise rare complication.[17]

Delivery options include bedside instillation of a talc slurry or thoracoscopic poudrage either by medical thoracoscopy or by video-assisted thoracoscopic surgery (VATS). VATS requires the use of general anesthesia with intubation and single-lung ventilation. Medical thoracoscopy uses a rigid thoracoscope and either local anesthesia or conscious sedation.[18] The thoracoscopic method seems to be associated with fewer recurrences,[16,19] but the available data included studies using both thoracoscopic methods, so no comparison can be made. VATS may not be appropriate in patients with advanced disease. Rolling of patients to ensure adequate dispersion of the talc after bedside instillation is not required.[18] Chest tubes may be removed 24 hours after instillation because prolonged drainage confers no therapeutic advantage.[18]

Indwelling Catheters

A newer approach to MPE is the use of small-bore tunneled indwelling catheters. These devices are typically inserted using local anesthesia in an outpatient setting,[20] and then the fluid is drained with vacuum bottles at home as required. One study compared chest tube thoracostomy with the tunneled indwelling catheter technique. The recurrence rate was 21% versus 13%; hospitalization lasted 6 days versus 1 day, and the infection rate was 0% versus 14%. Infections predominantly manifested as cellulitis.[21] Similar catheters have not been tested in pericardial effusions. This technique has the following advantages: (1) outpatient insertion without hospitalization, (2) patient control of symptoms, (3) use in trapped lung, (4) lasting spontaneous pleurodesis in 44% to 70% (recurrence rate, 8.7%), and (5) use in debilitated patients.[20]

Surgical Techniques

In patients with MPCE, pericardial windows can be created through subxiphoid or thoracotomy approaches, or pericardiectomy can be performed.[22] The subxiphoid approach is most common; the success rate is 91.5%, and it has a low incidence of complications. Pericardiectomy is the most definitive treatment, but it has a high mortality (13%) in patients with malignant disease. A novel approach with a percutaneous balloon through the subxiphoid approach has been reported.[22] Surgical options other than VATS are rarely indicated in MPE. Pleurectomy has significant mortality (12.5%) and morbidity, with prolonged postoperative air leaks in 10% to 20% of patients.[12]

Disease-Related Therapy

If the effusion is secondary to a chemosensitive disease such as breast cancer or hematological malignant diseases, then systemic therapy may suffice. Radiation therapy is successful to prevent recurrence of MPCE,[22] but does not have a role in MPE.

drainage also had sclerotherapy.[18,19] The relapse rate was 11% in both groups.

Drainage of the pleural space is required before or at the time of sclerotherapy, and the lung must fully re-expand for the procedure to be effective. It does not appear to matter whether drainage occurs with a large-bore tube or a small-bore tube.[18] Many agents have been tested for sclerotherapy since parenteral tetracyc-

CHAPTER **226**

Intestinal Dysfunction and Obstruction

Sebastiano Mercadante

SUMMARY

Care of patients with MPE and MPCE must be individualized based on the goals of care, disease-specific options, and life expectancy. Current treatments are focused predominantly on obliteration of the space to prevent accumulation or creation of an outlet for the fluid. In the future, therapy to prevent fluid production may become available (see "Future Considerations").

REFERENCES

1. Moores DWO. Management of malignant pleural effusion. Chest Surg Clin N Am 1994;4:481-495.
2. Grove CS, Lee YCG. Vascular endothelial growth factor: The key mediator in pleural effusion formation. Curr Opin Pulm Med 2002;8:294-301.
3. Eickelberg O, Carsten OS, Christoph W, et al. MMP and TIMP expression pattern in pleural effusions of different origins. Am J Respir Crit Care Med 1997;156:1987-1992.
4. D'Agostino P, Camemi AR, Caruso R, et al. Matrix metalloproteinases production in malignant pleural effusions after talc pleurodesis. Clin Exp Immunol 2003;134:138-142.
5. Lamparter S, Schoppet M, Christ M, et al. Matrix metalloproteinases and their inhibitors in malignant and autoreactive pericardial effusion. Am J Cardiol 2005;95:1065-1069.
6. Retter AS. Pericardial disease in the oncology patient. Heart Dis 2002;4: 387-391.
7. Cooper JP, Oliver RM, Currie P, et al. How do the clinical findings in patients with pericardial effusions influence the success of aspiration? Br Heart J 1995;73:351-354.
8. Shepard FA. Malignant pericardial effusion. Curr Opin Oncol 1997;9:170-174.
9. Light RW, MacGregor I, Luchsinger PC, et al. Pleural effusion: The diagnostic separation of transudates and exudates. Ann Intern Med 1972;77:507-513.
10. Heffner JE. Discriminating between transudates and exudates. Clin Chest Med 2006;27:241-252.
11. Meyers DG, Meyers RE, Prendergast TW. The usefulness of diagnostic tests on pericardial fluid. Chest 1997;111:1213-1221.
12. Neragi-Miandoab S. Malignant pleural effusion: Current and evolving approaches for its diagnosis and management. Lung Cancer 2006;54:1-9.
13. Anderson CB, Philpott GW, Ferguson TB. The treatment of malignant pleural effusions. Cancer 1974;33:916-922.
14. Celermajer DS, Boyer MJ, Bailey BP, Tattersall MH. Pericardiocentesis for symptomatic malignant pericardial effusion: A study of 36 patients. Med J Aust 1991;154:19-22.
15. Tsang TS, Seward JB, Barnes ME, et al. Outcomes of primary and secondary treatment of pericardial effusion in patients with malignancy. Mayo Clin Proc 2000;75:248-253.
16. Shaw P, Agarwal R. Pleurodesis for malignant pleural effusions. Cochrane Database Syst Rev 2004;(1):CD002916.
17. Janssen JP, Collier G, Astoul P, et al. Safety of pleurodesis with talc poudrage in malignant pleural effusion: A prospective cohort study. Lancet 2007; 369:1535-1539.
18. Harris RJ, Kavuru MS, Rice TW, et al. The diagnostic and therapeutic utility of thoracoscopy: A review. Chest 1995;108:828-841.
19. Tan C, Sedrakyan A, Browne J, et al. The evidence on the effectiveness of management for malignant pleural effusion: A systematic review. Eur J Cardiothorac Surg 2006;29:829-838.
20. Tremblay A, Michaud G. Single-center experience with 250 tunnelled pleural catheter insertions for malignant pleural effusion. Chest 2006;129:362-368.
21 Putman JB, Light RW, Rodriguez RM, et al. A randomized comparison of indwelling pleural catheter and doxycycline pleurodesis in the management of malignant pleural effusions. Cancer 1999;86:1992-1999.
22. Vaitkus PT, Herrmann HC, LeWinter MM. Treatment of malignant pericardial effusion. JAMA 1994;272:59-64.

KEY POINTS

- Gastroparesis is impaired transit of intraluminal contents from the stomach to the duodenum without mechanical obstruction.
- Prokinetic drugs may promote gastroduodenal contractile activity.
- Bowel obstruction may be a mode of presentation of intra-abdominal malignant disease or a feature of recurrent disease or other disorder in a patient with a history of malignant disease.
- Different levels of obstruction from specific cancers can determine different symptom patterns, can slow or accelerate progression from partial to complete occlusion, and can influence symptom presentation and intensity and hence outcome.
- Treatment of large bowel obstruction is primarily surgical; therefore, surgery should be considered in all patients with bowel obstruction and known malignant disease or a history of malignant disease.
- The palliative intent (i.e., the ability to tolerate solid food for the remaining lifetime) has been described for as many as 50% of individuals.
- Treatments with palliative intent focus on relieving bowel obstruction, preventing vomiting, and re-creating the opportunity for enteral nutrition.
- The decision to operate should be based on an accurate diagnosis, the evolution of disease, the anatomical situation and technical problems, particularly possible obstruction sites, and the general condition of the patient.

Gastrointestinal dysfunction and obstruction encompass many signs and symptoms that can occur anywhere throughout the gastrointestinal tract. These symptoms dramatically affect quality of life and typically develop in advanced cancer because such complications are often related to the site of tumor, progression of disease, and treatments, and they have a tremendous impact on the patient. Significant progress has been made in understanding the etiology and physiopathology of upper gastrointestinal motility disorders and intestinal obstruction (Fig. 226-1).

UPPER GASTROINTESTINAL DYSFUNCTION

Overall, normal gastric emptying is the culmination of complex myoelectrical and mechanical (contractile) events influenced by extrinsic (central nervous system) and intrinsic neural activity. The enteric nervous system is responsible for relaying sensory information from the stomach to the brain through the vagus nerve. It is also

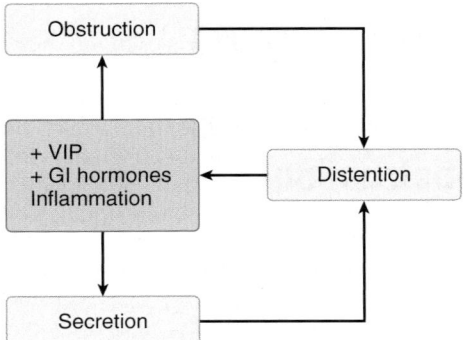

FIGURE 226-1 Physiopathology of bowel obstruction. GI, gastrointestinal; VIP, vasoactive intestinal polypeptide.

TABLE 226-1	Causes of Gastroparesis
GENERAL CATEGORY	**SPECIFIC CONDITIONS**
Neuromuscular	Diabetes
	Amyloid
	Parkinson's disease
	Shy-Drager syndrome
	Muscular (myotonic) dystrophy
	Scleroderma and other connective tissue diseases
	Hollow visceral neuropathy or myopathy
	Duchenne's muscular dystrophy
	Paraneoplastic syndromes
	Radiation
	Chronic intestinal pseudo-obstruction
Infiltrative	Malignant disease
Infectious	
Postsurgical	Vagotomy (truncal or selective)
	Partial or total gastrectomy
	Scarring or adhesions
Psychiatric	
Idiopathic	
Metabolic	Cachexia
	Hyperglycemia
	Renal insufficiency
	Thyroid dysfunction
	Parathyroid dysfunction
Medications	Anticholinergics
	Opioids
	L-Dopa
	Tricyclic antidepressants
	Phenothiazines
	Somatostatin analogues
	Calcium channel blockers
	Sympathomimetics
	Progesterone
	Cannabis
	Aluminum antacids
	Alcohol
	Sucralfate

responsible for propagation of motor impulses throughout the stomach. In addition, humoral and hormonal factors and feedback from the small intestine all play critical roles.[1]

During trituration, the pyloric sphincter is closed, and the result is retropulsion of larger food particles back into the stomach for further mixing. Food is properly broken down and mixed, and appropriate viscosity is attained. Small aliquots of liquefied food are emptied into the duodenum by gastric peristaltic contractions. This process typically occurs when food particles are small. In general, liquids always empty faster than meals with solid foods, and nonfat meals empty faster than meals high in fat content.[2]

Gastroparesis is impaired transit of intraluminal contents from the stomach to the duodenum without mechanical obstruction.[3] Gastroparesis is often idiopathic, and several factors may play a role, including diabetes and other neurological diseases or previous gastric surgical procedures. Many medications, including opioids and anticholinergic agents, may cause gastroparesis. No specific epidemiological study has been performed to investigate the frequency of this disorder in patients with advanced cancer (Table 226-1). Visceral neuropathies are less commonly reported and are difficult to diagnose. Slow intestinal transit resulting from intestinal pseudo-obstruction and prior surgical procedures involving the stomach are other possible causes.[4]

Many patients with intestinal pseudo-obstruction exhibit gastroparesis. In these circumstances, it is difficult to determine whether delayed gastric emptying is the result of direct involvement of the stomach by the same neuropathic or myopathic disorder causing the intestinal dysmotility or whether it is the result of increased gastric outlet resistance offered by the abnormal intestinal motility. Gastroparesis is also a typical sign of anorexia-cachexia syndrome (e.g., a paraneoplastic form), and it is frequently associated with poor nutritional status. Although the pathogenesis of gastroparesis is not yet completely understood, pro-inflammatory cytokines have been implicated in cachexia and dysautonomic symptoms. Data support the hypothesis that endotoxemia may be a potent trigger of systemic inflammatory response in the pathogenesis of cachexia. It can also be an expression of an autoimmune or a metabolic disorder.

Opioids affect various gastrointestinal functions, including motility, secretion, and transport of electrolyte and fluids. Moreover, opioids increase resting contractile tone in the small and large intestinal circular muscle, enhance rhythmic contractions and nonpropulsive phasic contractions in the gut, and suppress intestinal transit by acting on spinal cord and brain receptors.[5]

Different physiopathological mechanisms have been implicated in gastroparesis (Box 226-1). The most common symptoms are nausea, vomiting, early satiety, anorexia, and weight loss. Although less common, some patients only have persistent complaints of bloating or reflux symptoms that are difficult to control. Postprandial fullness and vomiting are two symptoms most likely to predict gastroparesis. Most patients have some abdominal distention and tympany.[6] Tenderness may be present in the epigastric area, and a succussion splash occasionally is heard. Because nearly all the symptoms are nonspecific, many disorders need to be considered during evaluation. Dyspepsia is one of the most common diagnoses confused with gastroparesis, and the two conditions often remain indistinguishable, although dyspepsia is not usually associated with significant nausea and vomiting. Imaging studies are rarely performed, and they include scintigraphic

Box 226-1 Mechanisms of Gastroparesis

- Impaired fundal tone, preventing or delaying the normal movement of gastric contents from the fundus into the antrum
- Antral hypomotility, prolonging trituration and delaying passage of food from the stomach into the duodenum
- Poor coordination between the antrum and duodenum, or pylorospasm, preventing normal passage of material from the stomach into the small intestine
- Gastric pacemaker dysrhythmias, leading to inefficient coupling of the electrical signal to smooth muscle cells
- Inhibitory neurohormonal feedback from the small bowel to the stomach

gastric emptying and small bowel transit studies, manometry, and use of radiopaque markers.[3]

Treatment

Diet and Glucose Control

A regimen of small, frequent meals is a mainstay of therapy. These meals should be low in fiber and fat (fat delays gastric emptying). Liquids should be emphasized over solid foods. Strict control of serum glucose concentrations is critical in diabetic patients because hyperglycemia further delays gastric emptying.

Antiemetics and Other Agents

Pharmacological treatment usually involves established drugs. Many antiemetics are used to treat nausea in gastroparesis (see Chapters 144 and 169).

Prokinetic drugs may promote gastroduodenal contractile activity. *Metoclopramide* is a substituted benzamide that peripherally acts as a cholinomimetic to release acetylcholine from intrinsic neurons in the gut. It also blocks dopamine receptors, and this effect leads to inhibition of receptive relaxation in the fundus and improves food transfer from the fundus to the antrum. Metoclopramide increases the tone and amplitude of antral contractions and peristalsis. Metoclopramide also relaxes the pylorus slightly, an effect that aids gastric emptying. In the central nervous system, antiemetic effects result from dopamine receptor blockade in the chemoreceptor trigger zone of the fourth ventricle. Starting doses of 10 mg twice daily are recommended, with a slow increase to 20 mg orally four times a day while carefully watching for side effects or adverse events. These side effects may include mild sedation or agitation, but they also involve extrapyramidal effects such as tremor, akathisia, and tardive dyskinesia, which is more likely to occur in diabetic patients than in others. The hormonal consequences of this drug induce gynecomastia, galactorrhea, mastalgia, impotence, and menstrual irregularities.

Domperidone is both a prokinetic and an antiemetic, and, like metoclopramide, it works by blocking dopamine. Domperidone does not cross the blood-brain barrier and thus does not cause central adverse effects. Domperidone is available only in an oral formulation. Starting doses of 10 mg twice a day are recommended, with a slow advance to 20 mg orally four times a day.

Erythromycin is a macrolide antibiotic that acts as a motilin agonist by increasing the number and amplitude of antral contractions. This drug is given in doses of 50 to 100 mg orally four times a day, before each of the main meals and at bedtime. Patients develop tachyphylaxis after several weeks of therapy. After a drug-free holiday, the medication can be effective again.

Tegaserod is a selective serotonin (5-hydroxytryptamine [5-HT$_4$]) agonist that is promising for use in gastroparesis. This drug increases gastric emptying and orocecal transit time without crossing the blood-brain barrier.

Preclinical and clinical studies have been conducted with two peripherally acting *opioid antagonists*, *methylnaltrexone* and *alvimopan*. Most studies focused on opioid-induced constipation (see Chapter 154).

New Treatments

Botulinum toxin inhibits acetylcholine release from synaptic vesicles at the synaptic junction and thus induces transient muscle paralysis. Botulinum toxin injection of the pylorus decreases pyloric resting tone and pylorospasm, relieves symptoms of nausea and vomiting, and improves gastric emptying in gastroparesis of different origin. Gastric electrical stimulation has been used in either idiopathic or diabetic gastroparesis. This technique employs an implantable neurostimulator that delivers a high-frequency, low-energy signal with short pulses.[3]

MALIGNANT INTESTINAL OBSTRUCTION

Gastrointestinal obstruction is a well-recognized complication and a complex problem in advanced gynecological and gastrointestinal cancer. Although it may develop any time, it occurs more often at the advanced stage; the frequency of this complication is between 5% and 51% in ovarian cancer and between 10% and 28% in primary intestinal malignant disease. Breast and lung cancers and melanoma are the most frequent extra-abdominal primary tumors causing bowel obstruction. In palliative medicine, incidences range from 3% to 15%, depending on the setting and admission criteria.[7]

Physiopathology

Bowel transit can be impeded by different mechanisms. Distal propulsion of the intestinal content is disturbed. The accumulation of secretions not absorbed determines the degree of abdominal distention and colicky activity to surmount the obstacle. The time course is variable, occurring over several days in malignant mechanical bowel obstruction. The increased uncoordinated peristaltic activity is ineffective, and a vicious circle represented by distention-secretion-motor activity worsens the clinical picture. The hypertensive state in the lumen damages intestinal epithelium with an inflammatory response enhancing the cyclooxygenase pathway and the release of prostaglandins, potent secretagogues, either by a direct effect on enterocytes or by an enteric nervous reflex. The increasing intraluminal pressure obstructs venous drainage from the blocked segment, interferes with oxygen consumption, and leads to intestinal gangrene or perforation.

The primary stimulus for vasoactive intestinal polypeptide (VIP) release seems to be hypoxia caused by intraluminal distention or, alternatively, intraluminal bacterial overgrowth. VIP is released into the portal circulation and the peripheral circulation and mediates local intestinal and systemic pathophysiological alterations accompanying small intestinal obstruction, such as hyperemia and edema of intestinal wall and accumulation of fluid in the lumen, thanks to its stimulating effects. High portal VIP levels cause hypersecretion and splanchnic vasodilatation. A disturbance of the autoregulatory local and neurohumoral control mechanisms of splanchnic flow may explain the appearance of multiple organ failure syndrome caused or worsened by systemic hypotension seen in bowel occlusion. Fluids and electrolytes are sequestered in the gut wall and its lumen in the presence of vasodilatation (third space) contributing to hypotension and leading to multiorgan system failure, the cause of death in bowel obstruction. Sepsis occurs from bacterial translocation. This phenomenon is facilitated by increased endoluminal pressure, stasis, and intestinal ischemia, conditions characteristic of bowel obstruction.[7]

Clinical Presentation and Assessment

Bowel obstruction may be a mode of presentation of intraabdominal malignant disease or a feature of recurrent disease or other disorder in a patient with a history of malignant disease. The cause may be benign, as in 10% to 48% of cases at operation (adhesions or radiation enteritis), or it may be malignant, in patients with single-site, multiple-site, or diffuse disease. Different levels of obstruction from specific cancers can determine various symptom patterns, can slow or accelerate progression from partial to complete occlusion, and can influence symptom presentation and intensity and hence outcome. Although pancreatic cancer directly involves the upper gastrointestinal tract, colon cancer mainly spreads to the small intestine, and pelvic (prostate and ovarian) cancer compresses the rectum.

The level of obstruction determines the symptoms and the severity. The higher the obstruction, the more severe are the symptoms and the fewer the signs. Continuous pain is attributable to visceral mass growth that compresses the intestine, intestinal distention, or hepatomegaly, whereas severe, superimposed colicky activity upstream from the obstruction in the small or large intestine may worsen the symptoms. Paradoxical diarrhea results from leakage of fluid stool from fecal impaction resulting from bacterial activity, generally in large bowel obstruction.

The diagnosis of intestinal obstruction is established or suspected on clinical grounds and is usually confirmed with plain abdominal radiography. Multiple air-fluid levels with distended loops of bowel are seen unless the patient has gastric outlet obstruction with frequent vomiting. Occasionally, a similar pattern is seen in paralytic ileus or pseudo-obstruction. It is often difficult to differentiate between complete and partial bowel obstruction. The computed tomography (CT) scan, which is more sensitive and specific than plain abdominal films, provides objective evaluation of the global extent of the disease, an important factor in subsequent therapeutic decision making, particularly for patients who are surgical candidates.

Treatment

Chemotherapy

Chemotherapy should be considered contraindicated in patients with bowel obstruction. Because chemotherapy generally lowers performance status and fosters maldistribution of body fluids, its toxicity is unpredictable. Many cytotoxic drugs commonly used in hormone-dependent cancers are available only in oral form and need several weeks to become effective. Chemotherapy is seldom active after second-line treatment in ovarian cancer, although chemotherapeutic agents may be considered if the tumor has not already demonstrated acquired chemoresistance. When bowel transit has been restored, chemotherapy or hormone therapy may be considered again.

Surgical Approach and Prognosis

Treatment of large bowel obstruction is primarily surgical. Therefore, surgery should be considered in all patients with bowel obstruction and known malignant disease or a history of malignant disease. A distinction should be made between patients with unconfirmed intra-abdominal malignant disease and patients with documented advanced intra-abdominal disease. In patients with unconfirmed malignant disease, conventional surgical management should be undertaken because many of these patients may have a benign obstruction.

Urgent operation is rarely necessary. Observation for up to 48 hours and even longer appears justified as long as serial x-ray films and clinical evaluation indicate improvement of the intestinal distention. A conservative approach lasting up to 5 days frequently results in resolution of the obstruction with no significant increase in mortality. Gastrointestinal intubation for removal of gases and gastrointestinal secretions is of value preoperatively and may resolve bowel obstruction in 25% of patients, especially patients with postoperative adhesions of inflammatory strictures, although many of these adhesions may become obstructed again later. Benign adhesions can occur in up to 20% of patients. Benign adhesions are more likely if the abdomen had previously been irradiated and the ileum is obstructed. In one study, gastrointestinal intubation successfully relieved 81% of small bowel obstructions resulting from postoperative adhesions.[8]

The duration of medical management remains unclear. Tube suction alone is rarely successful when the obstruction is malignant, and it is unlikely that patients with known metastatic disease will have a benign obstruction.[9] Some clinicians argue that prolonged nonoperative treatment of bowel obstruction in patients with cancer is unlikely to be successful and is fraught with complications. Partial colonic obstructions are less likely to resolve than partial small bowel obstructions. The presence of benign adhesions or a single site of obstruction may justify a relatively simple surgical procedure such as forming a loop colostomy or dividing adhesions.

Decompression of a severely distended colon may be achieved by temporary colostomy. Lysis of adhesions, resection of the obstructed bowel segment and reanastomosis, bypass of the obstructed bowel, and enterostomy are the most frequent interventions, according to the level and causes of obstruction. More than two thirds of patients have the obstruction surgically relieved and can be discharged with restored intestinal passage. Radical surgery, such as pelvic exenteration, should be considered in a few highly selected younger patients with the prospect of prolonged survival or even the possibility of cure despite extensive disease, such as patients with Hodgkin's disease.

Retrospective series, mainly uncontrolled, often suggest optimistic surgical outcomes because the selection process of these studies eliminates patients with inoperable conditions. Although operative treatment has a better outcome than nonoperative management in terms of symptom-free interval and reobstruction rates, it is has high postoperative morbidity and longer hospital stay.[8] The presence of carcinomatosis strongly influences the prognosis. Surgical intervention in patients with peritoneal carcinomatosis produces short-term success, but with significant associated morbidity and mortality.[8] Apart from obstruction, peritoneal carcinomatosis may cause motility problems because of intestinal paralysis secondary to extensive tumor involvement of the intestinal mesentery and plexuses, a situation that is not cured by surgical procedures.

The type of surgery for obstructing colorectal cancer is controversial. Two principal approaches have been used: primary resection (primary anastomosis or Hartmann's procedure) with simultaneous treatment of carcinoma and obstruction and staged resection (treatment of the obstruction before resection). Neither approach has an advantage over the other in relevant trials, and it is doubtful whether these procedures could be carried out in a timely and satisfactory way in this particular surgical context.[10]

The palliative intent (i.e., the ability to tolerate solid food for the remaining lifetime) has been described for as many as 50% of patients. This intent was confirmed in a study of short-term and long-term prognosis in 63 patients with carcinomatosis as a first presentation of cancer or after a mean disease-free interval of 15 months (from nongynecological primary tumors) in patients who underwent laparotomy. The intent was palliative, to relieve the bowel obstruction, to prevent vomiting, and to re-create the opportunity for enteral nutrition. Operative procedures included resection, bypass, gastrostomy, and colostomy. Mortality at 1 month was 21%, and the incidence of postoperative complications was high (44%). These complications included wound infections or dehiscence, sepsis, enterocutaneous fistula, further obstruction, peritoneal abscess, anastomosis dehiscence, gastrointestinal bleeding, pulmonary embolism, and deep venous thrombosis. Many patients developed intermittent symptoms of incomplete or complete obstruction until death.[8]

As would be expected from retrospective case series, wide variations exist in "control of symptoms," from 42% to more than 80%.[11] Like quality of life measurements, these variations are difficult to explore compared with standard prognostic key points such as mortality and morbidity. Small bowel obstruction, malignant disease other than colon cancer, and ascites were associated with poor palliation, whereas the type of operation, level of

obstruction, disease, and interval from diagnosis had no independent prognostic effects on survival. Only one third of patients had prolonged postoperative palliation, at a cost of significant treatment-related morbidity.[12]

Palliative surgery can improve quality of life of some patients, although it has been impossible to demonstrate prognostic factors that would allow selection of patients who could benefit from surgical palliation.[13] The decision to operate should be based on an accurate diagnosis, the evolution of disease, the anatomical situation and technical problems, particularly possible obstruction sites, and the general condition of the patient. Different points of view must be sought: medical, surgical, and anesthesiological. The surgical prognosis is generally poor because of the preoperative performance status of the patient, although perception of the prognosis depends on what the patient or relatives may expect. In advanced cancer, absolute contraindications to surgery include the following: (1) technical problems; (2) a recent laparotomy showing that surgery was technically difficult, diffuse metastatic disease, involvement of proximal stomach, or intra-abdominal diffuse carcinomatosis in a patient with severe motility problems; (3) diffuse palpable masses on physical abdominal examination; and (4) and massive ascites rapidly recurring despite drainage.[14]

Given two of these factors in ovarian cancer, the prognosis severely worsens. Palliative surgery seems more helpful in colorectal cancer, because in ovarian cancer, the response to oncological treatment is poor, morbidity and mortality are higher, and technical problems are not resolvable. Relative contraindications depend on the disease stage and the general condition of the patient, and they include extra-abdominal metastases, which may impair function (e.g., massive lung metastases), poor nutrition and general performance status with severe biochemical, immunological, and metabolic changes, advanced age, and previous radiation therapy of the abdomen or pelvis. Surgical opinion should consider the aims of the procedure, such as relief of mechanical obstruction, survival benefit, symptomatic palliation, or simply diagnosis.

Mini-Surgery

Experience is growing with minimally aggressive surgery for anatomical gastrointestinal strictures, including gastric outlet obstruction and strictures of the proximal small bowel and colon. These procedures may be useful in patients with advanced metastatic disease and those who are poor surgical risks, as well as to enable patients with coexisting medical complications to undergo later surgery (bridge operation), after staging of the disease and thorough colonic preparation.

Gastrostomy

Although nasogastric suction is the mainstay of treatment in patients with temporary bowel obstruction, this technique is poorly suited to those with complete, unresolved bowel obstruction. Patients may be troubled by the tube, and accidental or intentional dislodgment is common. Intermittent venting of a gastrostomy allows continued oral intake and enables the patient to maintain an active lifestyle without the inconvenience of a nasal tube. Gastrostomy provides the satisfaction of allowing the patient to resume oral intake of some foods, with significant psychological benefit. Gastrostomy can be inserted operatively or percutaneously, either endoscopically or by an ultrasound-guided approach. Previous surgery or massive carcinomatosis may make placement of the gastrostomy difficult or dangerous, but every effort should be made to place a gastrostomy at the time of surgical exploration if the clinical situation warrants one.

Percutaneous gastrostomy is the insertion of a tube into the stomach through the abdominal wall under fluoroscopic, ultrasound, or endoscopic guidance. Overall, this procedure controls nausea and vomiting related to bowel obstruction in 83% to 93% of patients.[15] Percutaneous gastrostomy should be avoided in patients with portal hypertension, large-volume ascites, a predisposition to bleeding, anticoagulant regimens, and active gastric ulceration. Previous surgery or extensive carcinomatosis may technically impede the gastrostomy. Although no absolute contraindications exist, ascites, previous gastric surgery, and coagulopathy are relative contraindications.

Reasons for unsuccessful percutaneous endoscopic gastrostomy include esophageal obstruction, previous gastric surgery, inability to insufflate the stomach, and colonic dislodgment. CT assistance may be useful in patients with masses compressing the stomach, with previous partial gastrectomy, and with ascites. High costs, lack of availability, and lack of real-time monitoring are the disadvantages of CT guidance. Recognized complications of gastrostomy include gastric perforation, hemorrhage, gastrocolic fistula, infection of the stoma site, and aspiration pneumonia.[15]

Stenting

Palliative stenting has expanded to include the esophagus, the gastroduodenal region, and the colon. Stent placement also serves as an adjunct to definitive surgical therapy for patients with obstructing colonic lesions, because endoscopic decompression facilitates formal bowel cleansing and subsequent single-stage elective surgery.

GASTRODUODENAL STENTS

Malignant duodenal obstruction commonly results from neoplastic invasion, more frequently from extrinsic compression from cancer of the head of the pancreas or compression by lymphadenopathy. Patients with malignant gastric outlet obstruction typically develop the condition as a result of advanced upper gastrointestinal malignant disease, although metastatic tumors to the duodenum can cause identical symptoms. The most common tumors are typically pancreatic, ampullary, or gastric in origin, although cholangiocarcinoma also has been reported.

Flexible, self-expanding metallic stents may be inserted using radiological or endoscopic techniques. Enteral stents are the mainstays of nonsurgical management of malignant gastric outlet obstruction. Metal stents can be placed across malignant gastroduodenal strictures or obstructions to provide luminal patency and thus restore oral intake.

In reported series,[13] placement was successful in 97% of patients, and clinical success (improvement in oral intake) was achieved in 89% of patients. Oral intake was possible in all successful cases, and 87% of patients could ingest at least a soft diet. The major limiting factor was the inability to pass the endoscope through the stricture. Complications of enteral stents included malpositioning, tumor ingrowth or overgrowth (17%), migration (5%), bleeding (<1%), and perforation (<1%). Tumor ingrowth and overgrowth can be treated by further stents, a technique that works well and allows one to avoid surgical intervention. Most patients can have luminal patency restored with a single stent, but for long strictures, multiple stents can be deployed in a stent-within-stent fashion.

COLONIC STENTING

These techniques allow decompression and clinical stabilization and avoidance or temporizing before surgery.[16] In patients found to have advanced or unresectable disease, endoscopic therapies can often obviate the need for any surgical intervention.

1. *Colon decompression tubes* are widely available and can be implanted with or without fluoroscopy. In patients with a residual colonic lumen, decompression tubes can be placed under direct vision. In patients with complete obstruction, guidewires and fluoroscopy can be of great value in allowing proximal colon access. Colon decompression tubes are often successful in allowing clinical decompression, and patients may be able to proceed directly to surgery.

2. *Colonic stents* have become common devices in the treatment of malignant large bowel obstruction. The use of colorectal stents, followed by single-stage bowel resection and reanastomosis, is well documented. This approach can be palliative or may serve as an adjunct to curative resection. The goal is to convert an emergency procedure to a safer, elective operation and one that can be curative. Preoperative stent placement is of additional value in patients with coexisting electrolyte imbalance, dehydration, or metabolic derangement because the stent allows the patient to be in optimal condition before surgery.[17] The tumor site influences decisions on stent placement: 70% of colon and rectal cancers are left sided and are accessible for stent placement. The stent can be inserted through the working channel of an endoscope under direct guidance, thus allowing placement in the proximal colon. Even with a small retained lumen, advancing the stent delivery system across the stricture is straightforward. Three factors should be considered before a patient is selected for an expandable metal stent in the colon: the location of the lesion, the length of the tumor, and the presence or absence of a synchronous cancer. Meticulous evaluation of the digestive tract downstream is mandatory, to avoid pointless stent placement. Two outcome measures are commonly addressed. Technical success refers to satisfactory placement of the stent across the stricture. Clinical success is defined as decompression of the obstructed large bowel, but it does *not* always include the ability to purge the colon fully. Technical and clinical success rates with colonic stents are more than 90%. Few randomized studies have compared colonic stents with surgery, but ben-

efits of stents include shorter hospitalizations and decreased costs.[18] The rate of complications, which include perforation, bleeding, and stent migration, is less than 3%; a few patients have recurrent obstruction related to tumor growth. Temporary incontinence may be observed. Normal bowel contractions can cause stent migration, especially if the stent diameter is too small, the stent is too short, or the stent is too distal in the lesion. Contraindications for a self-expanding stent are multiple stenoses and peritoneal carcinomatosis distally in the small bowel that were undiagnosed at the preprocedure radiological examination because of severe duodenal stenosis. Failure to relieve the obstruction may be secondary to an inability to cross the stricture, incomplete opening of the stent, or stent malposition that fails to traverse the entire stricture. Then it is necessary to apply additional stents across the remaining obstruction.[19]

3. *Laser therapy* is an ablative technique aimed at physically destroying malignant tissue by laser light during endoscopy to recanalize an obstructed lumen. The technique cannot be used in acute obstruction or extrinsically compressing lesions because the tumor itself must be endoscopically visible. The technique can relieve obstructive symptoms in 75% to 80% of patients. Obstructing colorectal cancer requires multiple laser treatments to maintain a patent lumen (three to four sessions during the course of the disease). Complications occur in 10% to 15% of patients and include perforation, bleeding, postprocedure pain, and fistulas or abscesses. Experience is correlated directly to better outcomes and fewer complications.[15]

Medical Management of Inoperable Malignant Bowel Obstruction

GENERAL MEASURES

Drainage of gastric fluids and replacement by intravenous fluids are still the first responses to intestinal obstruction in most clinical settings. These procedures are invasive and may cause more burden than benefit. This should be a holding measure for some days before surgery or may obviate the need for surgery temporarily or indefinitely because of resolution of the obstruction. Patients with gastric outflow obstruction or high obstruction may benefit from a nasogastric tube if nausea and vomiting cannot be controlled with medical therapy. The tube may be removed after some days of gastric decompression to continue medical therapy, if secretions are reduced.

OPIOIDS

Most patients with symptoms of bowel obstruction are receiving strong opioids, usually morphine, at diagnosis. In subsequent episodes of obstruction (to which opioids may contribute), it may be useful to choose the drug on the basis of presumed selectivity of distribution in the intestine. The oral route is precluded, and an alternative is required to facilitate the effects of symptomatic drugs.

More lipophilic drugs (e.g., methadone, fentanyl, or buprenorphine) may limit drug presence at the opioid intestinal receptors, and studies showed a more favorable ratio of constipation to analgesia with fentanyl relative to morphine. Some clinicians suggest that transdermal fentanyl and methadone may have less constipating effects or may require lower laxative doses compared with morphine. Nonsteroidal anti-inflammatory drugs are less constipating than opioids and may help patients with the opioid bowel syndrome.

HYDRATION AND PARENTERAL NUTRITION

Most patients with bowel obstruction are dehydrated because of a steal fluid syndrome of water and electrolytes in the intestine, as well as poor oral fluid intake. Dehydration may cause or worsen delirium and may trigger prerenal failure with accumulation of morphine metabolites and aggravated neurological impairment.[7] Nausea may be less severe in patients treated with moderate amounts of water (>500 mL/day), probably because of prevention of metabolic derangement associated with severe dehydration and less stimulation of the chemoreceptor trigger zone.

The theory that hydration may potentially result in more bowel secretions has never been confirmed. Administration of 1 to 1.5 L/day of solution containing electrolytes and glucose may prevent symptoms of metabolic derangement. Patients can be encouraged to eat and drink freely. Dry mouth may be treated by oral fluids, attention to mouth care, and ice cubes if anticholinergics drugs are used.

Intravenous hydration can be given through an implantable venous access site. Alternately, hydration hypodermoclysis is an easier way to administer fluids and to maintain hydration in the terminally ill patient. Most patients do not benefit from parenteral nutrition, although exceptions occur. Parenteral nutrition may prolong survival, but it can also lead to complications, further suffering, and prolonged hospitalization. This technique is often employed as a psychological measure at the insistence of relatives. In most cases, parenteral nutrition is interrupted after an appropriate explanation about the short prognosis and the lack of benefit. The routine use of parenteral nutrition should be avoided when it is designed solely to prolong life.

ANTIEMETICS

Among the antiemetics, parenteral metoclopramide has been used successfully in patients with mainly functional or incomplete obstruction with no colicky pain (rather than mechanical bowel obstruction). The combination of metoclopramide and dexamethasone has been the choice for patients with incomplete bowel obstruction.[20] This regimen is not recommended in complete mechanical bowel obstruction because it may increase colic and vomiting. Other antiemetics include haloperidol and phenothiazines. Haloperidol, in varying doses, either intravenously or subcutaneously, titrated against the effect, is a specific antidopaminergic drug that causes less sedation and has fewer anticholinergic effects compared with phenothiazines. Among the phenothiazines, methotrimeprazine, chlorpromazine, and prochlorpromazine are commonly used.

ANTISECRETIVE THERAPY FOR INOPERABLE BOWEL OBSTRUCTION

The higher the level of obstruction, the less abdominal distention is present, the greater is the vomiting, and the more difficult the condition is to manage medically. Complete obstructions are less responsive to medical management than are partial obstructions. Anticholinergics have been traditionally used as antisecretive drugs (with analgesics and antiemetics), because of their competitive inhibition of smooth muscle muscarinic receptors with impairment of ganglionic neural transmission in the bowel wall. Hyoscine butylbromide and hydrobromide and glycopyrrolate are commonly used. Hyoscine butylbromide was the first drug used in inoperable bowel obstruction. In comparison with scopolamine hydrobromide, these agents have poor central nervous system penetration and are unlikely to produce central adverse effects. They act on the myenteric cholinergic endings to reduce activity, without influencing other intestinal processes that affect the absorption and secretion of water and salts in the intestinal lumen. These agents also possess important hemodynamic and thermoregulatory effects.[7]

Octreotide, a synthetic analogue of somatostatin, with a duration of action of 8 to 12 hours, has been used for symptoms secondary to malignant bowel obstruction. It can be given by continuous subcutaneous or intravenous infusion or by bolus parenteral injection. The rationale resides in broad intestinal activity. Octreotide decreases secretion of water, sodium, and chloride of epithelial intestinal cells and increases water and electrolyte absorption. The drug also suppresses gastrointestinal and pancreatic secretions by inhibiting the stimulatory peptides, improves ion and water absorption, and inhibits carbonic anhydrase. Moreover, octreotide reduces mesenteric flow and pressure. Finally, submucosal somatostatin-containing neurons, activated by octreotide, inhibit excitatory nerves, mainly from inhibition of acetylcholine output. Relaxation occurs, thus ameliorating nonpropulsive spastic activity. These effects may result from VIP inhibition, which is increased in experimental bowel obstruction, with unfavorable effects on intestinal secretion, splanchnic flow, and peristalsis (see Chapters 144, 154, 169).[21] Doses of octreotide ranging from 0.3 to 0.6 mg/day by subcutaneous bolus or continuous subcutaneous infusion may allow removal of a gastrointestinal tube and may reduce vomiting episodes and nausea.[7]

In controlled studies with scopolamine butylbromide, octreotide significantly reduced the volume of gastrointestinal secretions within 48 hours, sufficiently that nasogastric tubes could be removed. It also promoted a faster reduction in daily episodes of vomiting and better alleviated nausea than did scopolamine butylbromide. At higher doses of octreotide and scopolamine butylbromide (0.6 to 0.8 mg/day and 80 mg/day, respectively), and chlorpromazine (5 to 25 mg/day), nausea and vomiting significantly improved with octreotide 3 days after starting the protocol. Long-acting octreotide (20 mg every 4 weeks) could be an option.[22]

Corticosteroids may reduce peritumoral inflammatory edema and may improve intestinal transit. These agents also help to resolve the obstruction, with consequent symptom relief. Steroids increase water and salt absorption and thus reduce the net balance of water and electrolytes in the intestine. Because corticosteroids are relatively inexpensive and are well tolerated, they have been largely used in palliative medicine for gastrointestinal symptoms or for resolving obstruction. Data on corticosteroids are less convincing than those on octreotide, because of the methodological weakness of existing studies.[23]

EVIDENCE-BASED DATA

All randomized trials that involved a clinical diagnosis of intestinal obstruction resulting from advanced cancer in patients treated with these drugs were analyzed in a recent systematic review.[24] Five reports fulfilled inclusion criteria, and 102 patients were identified: 52 received octreotide, 51 received hyoscine butylbromide, 37 received methylprednisolone at low and high doses, 15 received placebo, and 37 had both placebo and dexamethasone. Two studies were not blinded, and three were double blind, one with a crossover design with 5-day phases. Scarcity of retrieved data precluded any formal meta-analysis. Study duration differed among studies and ranged from 3 to 10 days. Five studies had similar entry criteria in terms of population, although different outcome measures were used, sometimes not well described. The quality score of studies was 2 to 3.

Corticosteroids were compared with placebo in two studies that showed a weak effect in relieving gastrointestinal symptoms. In one study, inclusion criteria were unclear, because some patients were included and then excluded (those with nasogastric tubes) from analysis, many drugs able to relieve gastrointestinal symptoms were allowed, timing of assessment and of outcome was uncertain, and data on different doses of methylprednisolone were summed to be compared with placebo. In the second study, the chances of resolution of bowel obstruction were largely determined by whether the patients were receiving chemotherapy. In addition, the regimen was likely to be changed during the long period between the two phases of study, these patients had relatively early-stage disease, and the investigators lacked a definition of inoperability. The use of a crossover design in such unstable patients who may have spontaneous resolution is confounding. Survival was extended compared with other controlled trials of octreotide; 25% were alive 90 days after treatment (mean survival, 75 days). Other studies have compared antisecretive drugs with different mechanisms. All these studies confirmed the superiority of octreotide over hyoscine butylbromide in 103 patients total. Nausea and vomiting improved more in patients receiving octreotide than in those receiving hyoscine butylbromide, in studies with similar designs and outcomes, at least in the short term. The population was defined more by stage and inoperability, and the patients had shorter survival compared with those receiving corticosteroids. These groups seem to be more representative of patients with advanced cancer that is often inoperable. No comparison has been done between corticosteroids and other antisecretive agents. Octreotide can be reasonably considered more effective than hyoscine butylbromide for symptoms related to inoperable bowel obstruction, whereas the role of cor-

CASE STUDY

Palliation of Malignant Intestinal Obstruction

AB, a 58-year-old woman with pancreatic cancer, was admitted for a course of chemotherapy. On admission, the patient had gastrointestinal symptoms, including nausea and vomiting, and pain related to bowel obstruction. She was transferred to the pain relief and palliative care unit. Magnetic resonance imaging showed diffuse carcinomatosis and liver metastases. The previous oral opioid regimen was switched to transdermal buprenorphine. A daily mixture of octreotide (0.3 mg) and dexamethasone (12 mg) was started intravenously, as well an initial bolus of 50 mL of amidotrizoate orally. Metoclopramide was not included in the initial regimen because of a presumed "intolerance." Two days later, the patient agreed to receive this drug, and the mixture was resumed, including metoclopramide in doses of 60 mg/day. The next day, a small amount of feces was present, and on day 4, regular intestinal passage was restored. On day 5, radiographic signs of bowel obstruction disappeared. A venous access catheter (Port-a-Cath) was inserted, and the patient was discharged home on day 7, to maintain the same regimen. She then received further treatments with gemcitabine. Subsequently, at the request of the patient, the doses of dexamethasone were reduced because of fluid accumulation, and she maintained adequate intestinal transit. Two months later, the patient is continuing the anticancer treatment and the antisecretive combination.

ticosteroids remains debatable and requires further study in a more selected population. More research is needed, possibly multicenter studies, to establish the best cost-effective treatment of nausea and vomiting.

COMBINATION OF DRUGS

A modern approach would be multimodal treatment, including different agents, particularly drugs with relatively low toxicity and different mechanisms of action. When one drug is ineffective alone, combining the two agents may reduce gastrointestinal secretions and alleviate vomiting. Treatment seems particularly effective if it is performed early and aggressively, before fecal impaction and edema render obstruction irreversible. Early intensive treatment may not only reduce gastrointestinal symptoms but may also reverse bowel transit and allow improvement in quality of life (see "Case Study: Palliation of Malignant Intestinal Obstruction"). The daily mixture includes metoclopramide (60 mg), octreotide (0.3 mg), dexamethasone (12 mg), given intravenously and then maintained as an intravenous infusion, with an initial bolus of 50 mL of amidotrizoate orally.[25]

REFERENCES

1. Lacy BE, Weiser K. Gastrointestinal motility disorders: An update. Dig Dis 2006;24:228-242.
2. Soykan I, Sivri B, Sarosiek I. Demography, clinical characteristics, psychological profiles, treatment, and long-term follow-up of patients with gastroparesis Dig Dis Sci 1998;43:2398-2404.
3. Lacy BE, Weiser K. Gastric motility, gastroparesis, and gastric stimulation. Surg Clin North Am 2005;85:967-987.
4. Mercadante S. Nausea and vomiting. In Voltz R, Bernat JL, Borasio GD, et al. (eds). Palliative Care in Neurology. New York: Oxford University Press, 2004, pp 210-220.
5. Wood JD, Galligan JJ. Function of opioids in the enteric nervous system. Neurogastroenterol Motil 2004;16(Suppl 2):17-28.
6. Davis MP, Walsh D. Gastrointestinal motility disorders. In Ripamonti C, Bruera E (eds). Gastrointestinal Symptoms in Advanced Cancer Patients. New York: Oxford University Press, 2002, pp 127-168.
7. Ripamonti C, Mercadante S. Pathophysiology and management of malignant bowel obstruction. In Doyle D, Hanks GW, McDonald N, et al. (eds). Oxford Textbook of Palliative Medicine, 3rd ed. New York: Oxford University Press, 2005, 496-506.
8. Mercadante S. Prognosis of malignant bowel obstruction. In Christakis NA, Glare P (eds). Prognosis in Advanced Cancer. New York: Oxford University press, 2008.
9. Tang E, Davis J, Silberman H. Bowel obstruction in cancer patients. Arch Surg 1995;130:832-836.
10. De Salvo GL, Gava C, Pucciarelli S, Lise M. Curative surgery for obstruction from primary left colorectal carcinoma: Primary or staged resection? Cochrane Database Syst Rev 2002;(1):CD002101.
11. Feur DJ, Broadley KE. Systematic review and metanalysis of corticosteroids for the resolution of malignant bowel obstruction in advanced gynaecological and gastrointestinal cancers. Ann Oncol 1999;10:1035-1041.
12. Blair S, Chu D, Schearz R. Outcome of palliative operations for malignant bowel obstruction in patients with peritoneal carcinomatosis from nongynecological cancer. Ann Surg Oncol 2001;8:632-637.
13. Legendre H, Vanhuyse F, Caroli-Bosc FX, Pector JC. Survival and quality of life after palliative surgery for neoplastic gastrointestinal obstruction. Eur J Surg Oncol 2001;27:364-367.
14. Ripamonti C, Twycross R, Baines M, et al. Clinical-practice recommendations for the management of bowel obstruction in patients with end-stage cancer. Support Care Cancer 2001;9:223-233.
15. Adler DG, Baron TH. Endoscopic palliation of malignant gastric outlet obstruction using self-expanding metal stents: Experience in 36 patients. Am J Gastroenterol 2002;97:72-78.
16. Balague C, Targarona EM, Sainz S, et al. Minimally invasive treatment for obstructive tumors of the left colon: Endoluminal self-expanding metal stent and laparoscopic colectomy. Preliminary results. Dig Surg 2004;21:282-286.
17. Morino M, Bertello A, Garbarini A, et al. Malignant colonic obstruction managed by endoscopic stent decompression followed by laparoscopic resections. Surg Endosc 2002;16:1483-1487.
18. Sebastian S, Johnston S, Geoghegan T, et al. Pooled analysis of the efficacy and safety of self-expanding metal stenting in malignant colorectal obstruction Am J Gastroenterol 2004;99:2051-2057.
19. Tierney W, Chuttani R, Croffie J, et al. Enteral stents. Gastrointest Endosc 2006;63:920-926.
20. Fainsinger R, Spachynski K, Hanson J, Bruera E. Symptom control in terminally ill patients with malignant bowel obstruction (MBO). J Pain Symptom Manage 1994;9:12-18.
21. Mercadante S, Maddaloni S. Octreotide in the management of inoperable gastrointestinal obstruction in terminal cancer patients. J Pain Symptom Manage 1992;7:496-498.
22. Massacesi C, Galeazzi G. Sustained release octreotide may have a role in the treatment of malignant bowel obstruction. Palliat Med 2006;20:715-716.
23. Feur DJ, Broadley KE. Systematic review and metanalysis of corticosteroids for the resolution of malignant bowel obstruction in advanced gynaecological and gastrointestinal cancers. Ann Oncol 1999;10:1035-1041.
24. Mercadante S, Casuccio A, Mangione S. Medical treatment for inoperable malignant bowel obstruction: A qualitative systematic review. J Pain Symptom Manage 2007;33:217-223.
25. Mercadante S, Ferrera P, Villari P, Marrazzo A. Aggressive pharmacological treatment for reversing bowel obstruction. J Pain Symptom Manage 2004; 28:412-416.

CHAPTER 227

Genitourinary Complications in Palliative Oncology

J. Stephen Jones

KEY POINTS

- Urinary obstruction causing renal failure is the most common serious genitourinary complication in palliative oncology.

- Discussion of end-of-life issues before relieving obstructive uropathy may allow a patient to choose to forgo repeated instrumentation and its associated morbidity.

- Spinal cord compression from metastatic disease can cause rapid onset of paraplegia or quadriplegia. Urgent external beam radiation or decompressive laminectomy can avert these irreversible sequelae.

- Hematuria is rarely life-threatening, but it can cause significant morbidity and suffering.

- Urinary tract infection in the palliative setting can be fatal as a result of obstruction, immunocompromise, or both.

People with advanced cancer can experience genitourinary complications as a result of both their primary disease and their treatments. Although many such complications may be merely symptomatic, a significant chance exists that life-threatening issues may arise or urgent intervention may be required. One of the most common late complications—azotemia—not only can be life-threatening, but also may preclude treatment options in such patients if nephrotoxicity is involved.

EPIDEMIOLOGY AND PREVALENCE

Obstruction

The most serious genitourinary complication in cancer is azotemia from obstruction. The most severe form involves acute or chronic renal failure. This complication may occur at the bladder outlet and may obstruct both systems as a result of benign prostatic hypertrophy, invasive prostate cancer, or occasionally an acontractile urinary bladder. Alternatively, one or both ureters may become obstructed by direct cancer invasion. This can occur from the primary tumor, metastasis, or, most commonly, retroperitoneal nodal disease. Azotemia may also result from nephrotoxic chemotherapy. Platinum-based regimens are frequent contributors, and dosage reduction may be required both to prevent and to avoid exacerbating azotemia.

Hematuria

Hematuria occurs when tumors involve the urinary tract primarily or secondarily. Hematuria is the hallmark of urinary tract involvement, and it occurs in most patients

with such tumors. Instrumentation is an infrequent cause of this complication. Hemorrhagic cystitis from chemotherapy drugs, particularly the oxazaphosphorine alkylating agents, may be severe. These agents can also produce urothelial cancer years after treatment, and surveillance is warranted to detect such late occurrences. Concurrent administration of mesna (sodium-2-mercaptoethane sulfonate [Uromitexan, Mesnex]) can prevent these complications, especially if it is continued for 24 to 36 hours after the last dose of chemotherapy.[1]

The final common cause of hematuria is urinary tract infection, which often occurs in patients with poorly emptying bladders, those with catheters, and the immunocompromised. Institutionalized patients are at risk of exposure to nosocomial, highly resistant organisms. Pelvic radiation may also contribute to hematuria.

CLINICAL MANIFESTATIONS

Obstruction

Obstructive uropathy most commonly manifests either with laboratory recognition of azotemia or on imaging. Metastatic evaluation for cancer surveillance often identifies unilateral or bilateral hydronephrosis. Patients infrequently present with classic symptoms of azotemia without prior recognition.

Hydronephrosis warrants rapid investigation. Unilateral hydronephrosis is typically the result of obstruction of the ipsilateral ureter by direct tumor invasion or retroperitoneal adenopathy. The associated tumor may be identified on the same radiograph (Fig. 227-1). Because most cases are identified using computed tomography, a study to demonstrate whether this is nonobstructive or obstructive uropathy is indicated. Excretory urography (intravenous

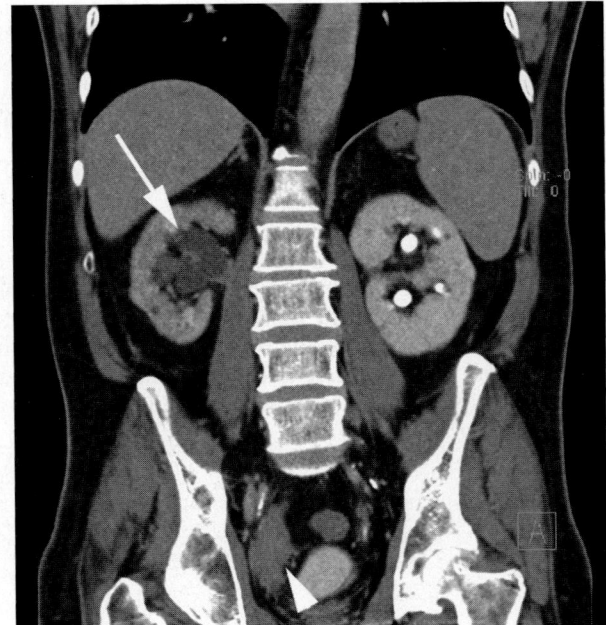

FIGURE 227-1 Computed tomography demonstrates right hydronephrosis *(dark area at the tip of the long arrow)* secondary to a pelvic tumor *(short arrow)*. *(Courtesy of Brian Herts, MD, Department of Radiology, Cleveland Clinic, Cleveland, OH.)*

pyelography) can be performed with a normal creatinine concentration, provided the patient has no known contrast allergies. A safer approach, albeit less readily accessible, is nuclear medicine diuretic renography. Furosemide is injected after the patient is administered a radioisotope such as mercaptoacetyltriglycine (MAG-3). The renal unit should experience washout of half the radioisotope activity within 10 minutes. Readings of up to 20 minutes suggest obstruction; a poorly functioning renal unit can cause a false reading. Obstruction in patients with an ileal conduit can be evaluated with a retrograde loopogram. Antibiotic coverage should be given before retrograde injection because of the risk of bacterial reflux into the collecting ducts and intravasation. However, this approach avoids the risk of a contrast allergy and nephrotoxicity.

Most patients with bilateral hydroureteronephrosis have bladder outlet obstruction. Placement of a Foley catheter can be both diagnostic and therapeutic. Failure of hydronephrosis to resolve with a Foley catheter suggests direct ureteral involvement, and upper urinary tract evaluation should then be undertaken.

Patients with advanced disease can also experience ureteral obstruction resulting from stones as a co-morbidity. In addition, rapid tissue turnover following chemotherapy can release purines and increase the risk of developing uric acid calculi.

Hematuria

The cause of hematuria should be ascertained through upper urinary tract imaging and cystoscopy unless the patient has such co-morbidity that the source would be inconsequential. Bleeding from the urinary bladder may be managed with cauterization or endoscopic resection of tumor, if identified.

Irritative Voiding Symptoms

Irritative voiding symptoms such as dysuria, nocturia, urgency, or urge incontinence (see Chapter 164) may have many causes in these patients. Tumor in the lower urinary tract, including carcinoma in situ in bladder cancer, can cause intractable irritative symptoms. Chemotherapeutic agents and other medications can cause similar difficulties, as (rarely) can neurological involvement. Neurological involvement more typically causes an atonic bladder. Cultures and cytology can assist with the diagnosis.

Spinal Cord Compression

Sudden onset of back pain or lower extremity weakness sometimes associated with loss of bowel or bladder continence suggests spinal cord invasion (Figs. 227-2 to 227-4). This complication can lead to an acute paraplegia, with catastrophic consequences. One of the most common causes is metastatic prostate cancer.

DIFFERENTIAL DIAGNOSIS

Hydronephrosis is most commonly the result of direct tumor involvement. Vesicoureteral reflux occasionally

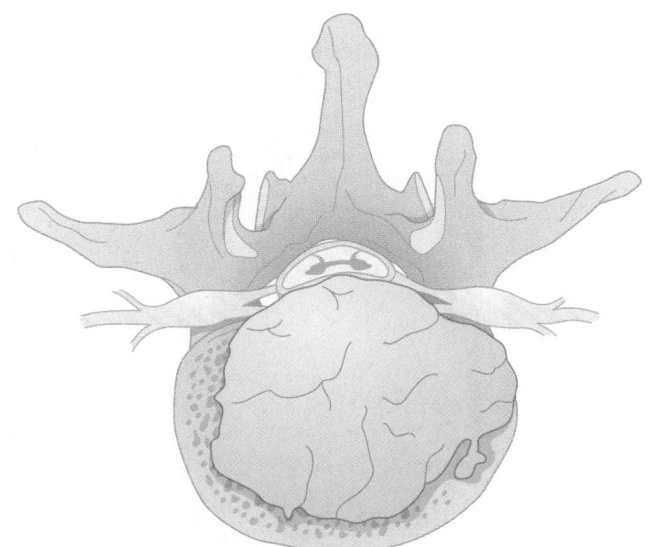

FIGURE 227-2 Tumor occupying most of the vertebral body extends into the thecal sac and compresses spinal canal contents. *(Copyright 2006, Cleveland Clinic Foundation, Cleveland, OH.)*

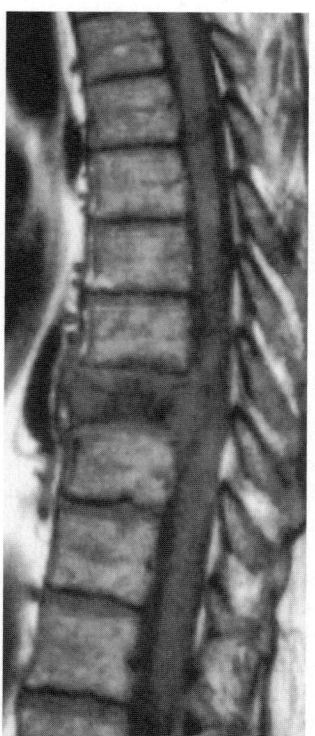

FIGURE 227-3 Sagittal T1-weighted spin echo magnetic resonance imaging scan through the lower thoracic and lumbar spine. The patchy marrow signal intensity is consistent with metastatic foci. The scan shows more diffuse replacement of the marrow signal at L2 with collapse and dorsal extension with narrowing of the spinal canal and compression of the lumbar thecal sac. *(Courtesy of Michael T. Modic, MD, Department of Radiology, Cleveland Clinic, Cleveland, OH.)*

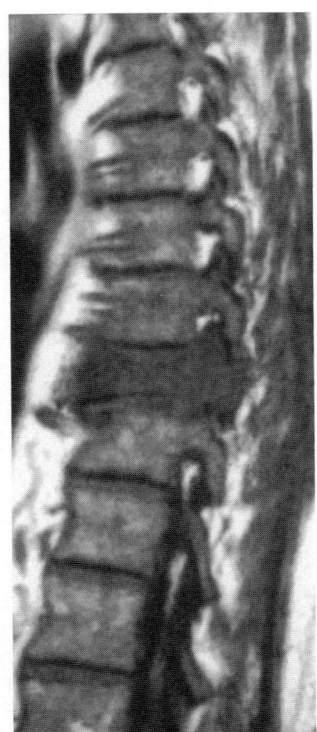

FIGURE 227-4 Midline and parasagittal T1-weighted spin echo magnetic resonance imaging scan through the thoracic spine. Abnormal marrow replacement of T9 with collapse and dorsal displacement resulted in compression of the thoracic spinal cord. *(Courtesy of Michael T. Modic, MD., Department of Radiology, Cleveland Clinic.)*

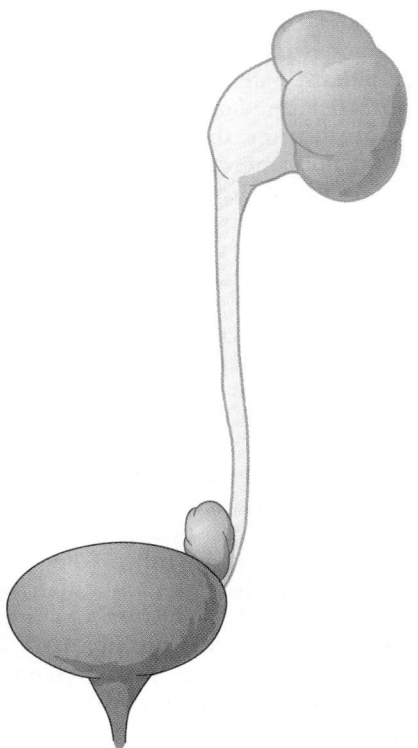

FIGURE 227-5 Left hydronephrosis secondary to a tumor obstructing the distal ureter. *(Copyright 2006, Cleveland Clinic Foundation, Cleveland, OH.)*

mimics this condition. Some patients have chronically dilated upper urinary tracts without either obstruction or reflux, so no intervention is required.

TREATMENT

Bilateral hydronephrosis is usually treated by Foley catheter placement. Patients with urinary retention may also undergo clean intermittent catheterization, ideally performed by patients themselves. This approach causes less urinary tract infection (see Chapter 93) than either urinary retention or an indwelling catheter and allows the patient to spend most of the day without a urethral catheter in place.[2] Clean intermittent catheterization can be done by clean (i.e., not sterile) technique. Occasional patients can be treated on a short-term basis with urethral stents. These stents can migrate and create long-term problems in many patients. Therefore, they are not typically used on a long-term basis, but rather are used for palliation in advanced cancer and may also enable the patient to avoid catheterization.

If the patient is a candidate for longer-term intervention, α-blockade, possibly with the addition of a 5α-reductase inhibitor, restores normal voiding in fewer than half these patients. The Medical Therapy of Prostatic Symptoms (MTOPS) study demonstrated the benefit of combined therapy in the long-term setting, although the role of this therapy in the palliative setting is unknown.[3] Prostatic obstruction from either benign prostatic hypertrophy or prostate cancer is treated with transurethral resection of the prostate (TURP) or any number of less invasive alternatives introduced more recently, including transurethral microwave therapy (TUMT), transurethral needle ablation (TUNA), and photovaporization of prostate (PVP laser). The value of these newer procedures remains controversial, and the gold standard remains the TURP.[4]

Hydronephrosis resulting from upper urinary tract obstruction can sometimes be relieved by cystoscopic ureteral stent placement. These stents are described as a "double-J" because of a curl on each end of the soft rubber tubes, which are approximately 6 to 8 French in diameter (Figs. 227-5 and 227-6). Stents may be placed without difficulty when extrinsic compression is the cause, but direct tumor involvement of the ureter can preclude placement and sometimes even visualization of the ureteral orifices. This situation is most common in prostate cancer because it directly invades the base of the bladder. I prefer to perform outpatient cystoscopy in these patients before taking them to the operating room to visualize the ureteral orifices. If the orifices are visualized, then stent placement is often feasible. Therefore, anesthetic cystoscopy with attempted stent placement has a reasonable chance of success.

If the ureteral orifices are invisible, then the likelihood of success is low enough that an attempt in the operating room is unlikely to be appropriate. In such patients, placement of a percutaneous nephrostomy tube by an interventional radiologist or urologist allows direct access to the upper urinary tract (see Chapter 102). Often, a stent may be placed through percutaneous nephrostomy access and subsequently through the obstructing tumor and into the bladder more successfully than through retrograde place-

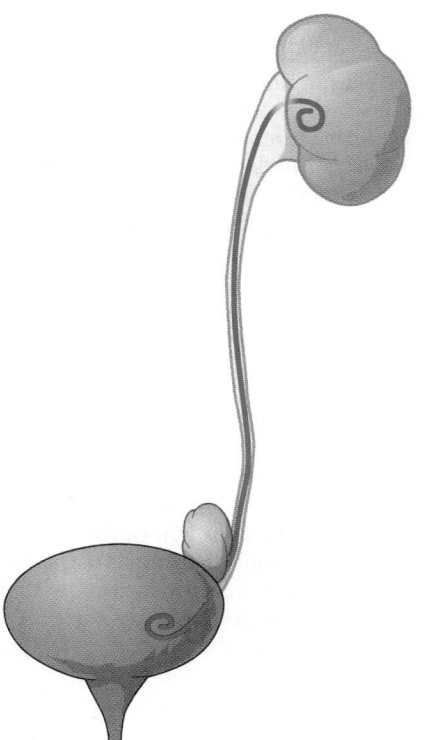

FIGURE 227-6   Resolution of hydronephrosis has resulted from bypassing the obstruction by cystoscopic placement of a ureteral "double-J" stent. *(Copyright 2006, Cleveland Clinic Foundation, Cleveland, OH.)*

Common Therapeutics

Hematuria

- Alum 1% continuous bladder irrigation (bladder irrigation should *never* be administered using an intravenous pump,* and irrigation should always be controlled through a gravity drip, to avoid the risk of urinary bladder rupture)
- Formalin 1%, 50 mL intravesically, administered under anesthesia in the operating room

Irritative Symptoms

- Tolterodine extended release (Detrol LA), 4 to 8 mg daily
- Darifenacin (Enablex), 7.5 to 15 mg orally daily
- Solifenacin (Vesicare), 5 to 10 mg daily
- Oxybutynin, 5 mg orally up to four times daily
- Oxybutynin extended release (Ditropan XL), 5 to 30 mg orally daily
- Trospium hydrochloride (Sanctura), 1 tablet twice a day
- Oxytrol patch, 3.9 mg applied to skin twice weekly

Spinal Cord Compression Resulting from Prostate Cancer Metastasis

- Ketoconazole, 400 mg intravenously three times daily (usually used with hydrocortisone, 20 mg twice daily)
- Bicalutamide (Casodex), 50 mg orally daily for the first 2 to 4 weeks after initial luteinizing hormone–releasing hormone therapy

Recommendation from Goswami AK, Mahajan RK, Nath R, Sharma SK. How safe is 1% alum irrigation in controlling intractable vesical hemorrhage? J Urol 1993;149:264-267.

ment. This often occurs several days to several weeks later, depending on the amount of bleeding at the original nephrostomy. Nephrostomy is also appropriate for patients whose stents clog frequently (more often than every 6 months). A nephrostomy tube may be irrigated with a syringe and a small amount of saline solution to keep it flowing, unlike a stent, which is completely internalized and requires an operating room trip to replace. These tubes are particularly helpful in patients with recurrent *Candida albicans* infection because of the tendency of this organism to clog the stents.

The final issue with stent placement involves the understanding that most people who develop azotemia resulting from hydronephrosis have severe, advanced disease. Long-term survival is very unlikely unless the cause is readily reversible (e.g., chemosensitive lymphoma), and patients should be informed of this prognosis before stents are placed without forethought. Azotemia is often one of the most humane causes of death, and stents and nephrostomies may create morbidity without a significant survival advantage. This factor should always be part of the decision-making process. This issue is especially important for bilateral percutaneous nephrostomies, because the tubes, which exit the flank bilaterally, make it difficult to find a comfortable position to sleep unless the patient sleeps supine, which most patients cannot comfortably do. The quality of life in this setting is typically poor. With this knowledge, many patients decline intervention. Patients with an imminent important life event such as a birthday, anniversary, graduation, or family wedding often use intervention as a temporary measure.[5]

Hematuria

Treatment of hematuria depends on the cause (see "Common Therapeutics"). Urinary tract infection is, of course, treated with antimicrobials. Empiric fluoroquinolone is often the initial treatment, although nitrofurantoin is less expensive, less likely to cause superinfection, and may be equally likely to treat isolated urinary tract infection successfully. Systemic infection is not treated adequately by nitrofurantoin, and culture-directed antibiotic coverage is appropriate. Many of these patients are immunocompromised, and urinary tract infection may quickly become life-threatening. Infection with obstruction is a medical emergency and can be rapidly fatal. Nitrofurantoin is not appropriate in the severely immunocompromised patient because it is static and not cidal to uropathogens.

When candidiasis or candiduria is the cause of hematuria (or sepsis), it is managed by systemic therapy including amphotericin B or fluconazole (Diflucan). Replacement or removal of foreign bodies such as stents or catheters that serve as a nidus of infection is appropriate, although co-morbidity may preclude use of the anesthesia required for stent replacement.

Radiation cystitis is a recalcitrant cause of hematuria resulting from urothelial microvascular proliferation. These vessels bleed easily and do not contract like normal vessels, so bleeding often persists more than with normal tissues. Fulguration using electrocautery or neodymium-yttrium-aluminum-garnet laser can be effective but requires anesthetic cystoscopy. Urinary irrigation using either normal saline solution or 1% alum for several days is often effective. Alum works as an astringent but leads to some clot precipitation and can obstruct the Foley catheter. The use of a three-way catheter with the outflow tubing pressure at least 12 to 15 cm H_2O, typically about the height of the bed rail, can minimize venous bleeding (but does not affect the less common arterial bleeding); some intravasation of irrigant is to be expected. If the irrigant is alum, then daily monitoring of prothrombin time and partial thromboplastin time will be required. Rarely, 1% formalin can be administered in the operating room. A cystogram in the operating room immediately before formalin instillation rules out reflux. If formalin refluxes, it will obliterate the ureters and, if it refluxes into the collecting ducts, destroy the function of both kidneys, an effect that could be fatal. If repeat formalin treatment is administered, a cystogram should be performed before each treatment because reflux sometimes develops from the initial formalin administration. This treatment causes severe pain, requires full anesthesia, and is an end-stage salvage option. The bladder will contract and require long-term Foley catheter placement if this treatment is administered.[6]

Hyperbaric oxygen may resolve radiation-induced hemorrhagic cystitis.[7] Multiple treatments are required, but many patients with recalcitrant bleeding experience permanent resolution. Intractable bleeding can be treated with embolization or removal of the offending organ. These patients are, without exception, major surgical risks, and the surgical mortality is high.

Hematuria in thrombocytopenia presents additional challenges. Many such patients have antiplatelet antibodies or other conditions that make platelet transfusion replacement difficult. Many patients have platelet counts lower than 5000 despite vigorous transfusion, and further efforts at normalization may be futile.

Irritative Voiding Symptoms

Irritative voiding symptoms or symptoms in patients without infection are treated with urinary topicals such as phenazopyridine, 200 mg orally three times a day, or flavoxate (Urispas), one tablet daily. Other agents include anticholinergics tolterodine extended release, darifenacin, solifenacin, oxybutynin, and trospium (see "Common Therapeutics"). A theoretical risk of urinary retention exists with these medications, although studies using tolterodine suggested than this risk even in men is no higher than that that associated with placebo.

Spinal Cord Compression

Treatment for spinal cord compression involves immediate neurology or neurosurgical consultation. Emergency external beam radiation can often shrink the tumor to avoid complete paraplegia. Swelling from radiation can occasionally exacerbate spinal cord compression, so decompressive laminectomy is required in many patients in whom muscle weakness is already present. The role of steroids is controversial.

This condition can occur in patients with almost any primary tumor. However, spinal cord compression from

prostate cancer can be managed uniquely because these patients often experience an immediate and marked response to hormonal ablation unless the cancer is hormone insensitive.[8] Hormonal ablation therapy can be most readily administered either through immediate orchiectomy or intravenous ketoconazole, which creates castrate testosterone levels within hours. Orchiectomy may be performed in the operating room, on an outpatient basis, or in the hospital ward by a urologist experienced in administration of local anesthetic.

Special precaution is required regarding administration of luteinizing hormone–releasing hormone (LH-RH) *agonists* such as leuprolide, goserelin, and newer agents. These drugs work by increasing LH-RH activity and actually increase testosterone levels for approximately the first 2 weeks. This "flare" can exacerbate any prostate cancer site for this duration, and it poses the theoretical risk of acute spinal cord compression. These agents are probably best avoided in this setting in lieu of the foregoing agents, but the concomitant administration of the antiandrogen bicalutamide (Casodex) may prevent this flare if LH-RH therapy is chosen. The LH-RH *antagonist* (as opposed to agonist discussed earlier) abarelix does not pose this risk because of its opposite effect on LH-RH.[9]

Special mention should also be made of managing prostate cancer bony metastases that do not involve spinal cord compression. Pain from bony metastases can be incapacitating in late-stage prostate cancer. Radiation therapy can reduce tumor mass and can relieve pain in days if it is localized. Complete response can be expected in 90% of patients, and another 54% achieve partial pain relief, although half these patients will ultimately have recurrent pain. The entire marrow of an involved long bone is often included in the treatment field to prevent recurrence, and these lesions in weight-bearing areas may require surgical stabilization if more than 50% of the cortex is eroded.[10] Disseminated tumors may be treated with strontium 89, which is deposited by osteoblasts near metastatic sites. This calcium analogue emits shallow-penetrating beta particles to target nearby malignant cells but limits penetration to normal tissues. Pain relief occurs over a few weeks and lasts 3 to 6 months.[11] Parenteral zoledronic acid, a

---

Future Considerations

- Management of urinary tract obstruction has not changed since the late 1970s. The newer medications for symptomatic relief such as tolterodine, solifenacin, and darifenacin do have lower side effects than their predecessors but are not more effective.

- Chemotherapeutic agents for prostate cancer have minimal impact, although the U.S. Food and Drug Administration has approved mitoxantrone and docetaxel (Taxotere) for metastatic prostate cancer. The effectiveness of these agents in the palliative setting is unknown.

- One of the most difficult decisions in late-stage prostate cancer involves hormonal ablation. Many physicians choose to discontinue the use of ablative agents in hospice patients. We recommend that these agents be maintained, based not on any belief that they will extend life, but rather because they may offer continued palliation, especially pain relief for bony metastases. No randomized controlled trials have been conducted to guide decision making in this setting.

third-generation bisphosphonate, has the potential benefit of combining pain relief with prevention of skeletal fractures by 36% in selected men treated with chronic androgen deprivation.[12] Finally, prednisone combined with docetaxel decreases pain in 35% compared with 22% of those taking the more commonly prescribed combination of prednisone and mitoxantrone.[13]

Supportive Care

Because of the risk of sepsis, many patients are treated with suppressive or prophylactic antibiotics, especially during urinary tract instrumentation such as involving stents or catheters. This practice does not reduce infection, and because of the risk of the development of resistant bacteria and superinfection, it is discouraged.

REFERENCES

1. deVries CR, Freiha FS. Hemorrhagic cystitis: A review. J Urol 1990;143:1-9.
2. Lapides J, Diokno AC, Silber SJ, Lowe BS. Clean intermittent catheterization in the treatment of urinary tract disease. J Urol 1972;107:458-461.
3. Kaplan SA, McConnell JD, Roehrborn CG, et al. Medical Therapy of Prostatic Symptoms (MTOPS) Research Group. Combination therapy with doxazosin and finasteride for benign prostatic hyperplasia in patients with lower urinary tract symptoms and a baseline total prostate volume of 25 mL or greater. J Urol 2006;175:217-20.
4. Djavan B, Madersbacher S, Klingler HC, et al. Outcome analysis of minimally invasive treatments for benign prostatic hyperplasia. Tech Urol 1999;5:12-20.
5. Jones JS. The Complete Prostate Book. Amherst, NY: Prometheus, 2005.
6. Donahue LA, Frank IN. Intravesical formalin for hemorrhagic cystitis: Analysis of therapy. J Urol 1989;141:809-812.
7. Neheman A, Nativ O, Moskovitz B, et al. Hyperbaric oxygen therapy for radiation-induced haemorrhagic cystitis. BJU Int 2005 Jul;96:107-109.
8. Nagata M, Ueda T, Komiya A, et al. Treatment and prognosis of patients with paraplegia or quadriplegia because of metastatic spinal cord compression in prostate cancer. Prostate Cancer Prostatic Dis 2003;6:169-173.
9. Weckermann D, Harzmann R. Hormone therapy in prostate cancer: LHRH antagonists versus LHRH analogues. Eur Urol 2004;46:279-284.
10. Tong D, Gillick L, Hendrickson FR. The palliation of symptomatic osseous metastases: Final results of the Study by the Radiation Therapy Oncology Group. Cancer 1982;50:893-899.
11. Brundage MD, Crook JM, Lukka H. Use of strontium-89 in endocrine-refractory prostate cancer metastatic to bone: Provincial Genitourinary Cancer Disease Site Group. Cancer Prev Control 1998;2:79-87.
12. Saad F, Gleason DM, Murray R, et al. Zoledronic Acid Prostate Cancer Study Group. A randomized, placebo-controlled trial of zoledronic acid in patients with hormone-refractory metastatic prostate carcinoma. J Natl Cancer Inst 2002;94:1458-1468.
13. Tannock IF, de Wit R, Berry WR, et al. TAX 327 Investigators. Docetaxel plus prednisone or mitoxantrone plus prednisone for advanced prostate cancer. N Engl J Med 2004;351:1502-1512.

SUGGESTED READING

Esper PS, Pienta KJ. Supportive care in the patient with hormone refractory prostate cancer. Semin Urol Oncol 1997;15:56-64.

McNamara DA, Fitzpatrick JM, O'Connell PR. Urinary tract involvement by colorectal cancer. Dis Colon Rectum 2003;46:1266-1276.

Ok JH, Meyers FJ, Evans CP. Medical and surgical palliative care of patients with urological malignancies. J Urol 2005;174:1177-1182.

Cancer-Related Syndromes

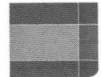

CHAPTER **228**

Hypercalcemia

Paul W. Walker

This common and life-threatening condition has variously been termed hypercalcemia of malignancy, tumor-induced hypercalcemia, and humoral hypercalcemia of malignancy. This metabolic emergency is by far the most common paraneoplastic syndrome (see Chapter 233).[1,2]

BASIC SCIENCE

Calcium homeostasis is highly regulated by a complex system of hormones in bone, kidney, and intestine.[1] This system is more effective in preventing hypocalcemia than hypercalcemia. The two major hormones that regulate calcium are parathyroid hormone (PTH) and calcitriol or $1,25\text{-}(OH)_2D_3$, the major biologically active metabolite of the vitamin D family. The 84–amino acid polypeptide PTH is secreted by the chief cells of the parathyroid glands after decreases in extracellular fluid ionized calcium concentration. This process is regulated by a simple negative feedback loop. The biological actions of PTH include the following: (1) stimulating osteoclasts to resorb bone; (2) stimulating calcium reabsorption, but inhibiting phosphate reabsorption, at the renal tubules; and (3) stimulating production of $1,25\text{-}(OH)_2D_3$ by the kidney. Calcitriol

or $1,25\text{-}(OH)_2D_3$ increases serum calcium and phosphate by increasing gut resorption, as well as by increasing bone resorption and enhancing the action of PTH to reabsorb calcium from the kidney. The role of endogenous calcitonin is uncertain and is believed to be small. Its effect is rapid, and it directly inhibits osteoclastic bone resorption.[1]

EPIDEMIOLOGY AND PREVALENCE

Table 228-1 lists the most common causes of hypercalcemia of malignancy in hospitalized patients.[3,4] The prevalence of hypercalcemia in patients with cancer ranges from 20%[5] to 30%.[6] The prevalence is low at initial diagnosis and increases with disease progression.[5] Most patients have advanced disease when hypercalcemia occurs. Survival is unusual beyond 6 months.[7,8] Underdiagnosis and undertreatment are common. Hypercalcemia is treated in less than 40% of hospitalized patients who would benefit from such treatment because of errors in diagnosis and management (see "Common Errors").[9]

PATHOPHYSIOLOGY

It is a common misconception that metastasis to bone is required to cause hypercalcemia. PTHRP is produced by cancer cells both within and outside of bone. This peptide shows 70% sequence homology with PTH over the first 13 amino acids at the N-terminal. PTHRP is larger than PTH, and three distinct isoforms have been described. It binds to the PTH receptor and shows similar biological activity to PTH.[1] Physiologically normal individuals do not have detectable circulating levels of PTHRP, whereas 80% to 90% of hypercalcemic patients with solid tumors have detectable plasma PTHRP.[10,11] In solid tumors, PTHRP plays a central role by increased bone resorption by osteoclasts and renal calcium resorption. In hematological malignancies, both tumor-produced $1,25\text{-}(OH)_2D_3$ and PTHRP have been associated with hypercalcemia.[1] Evidence indicates that other humoral factors by solid tumors (alone or with PTHRP) cause hypercalcemia through stimulation of osteoclastic bone resorption. These factors include interleukin-1 (IL-1), IL-6, transforming growth factor-α (TGF-α), tumor necrosis factor (TNF), and granulocyte colony-stimulating factor (G-CSF).[1,2] PTHRP, IL-1, IL-6, and TNF-α appear to interact with osteoblasts which upregulate osteoclast-activating factors such as receptor activator of nuclear factor-κB ligand (RANKL) and down-regulate the decoy receptor and repressor of RANKL, osteoprotegerin.

The mechanism of hypercalcemia in cancer is complicated and ranges from tumors secreting humoral factors

TABLE 228-1 Malignant Diseases Associated with Hypercalcemia

TUMOR	INCIDENCE (%)
Lung	25*-35[†]
Breast	20*-25[†]
Hematological	14[†]
Myeloma	10*
Lymphoma	3*
Head and neck	6[†]-8*
Renal/bladder (renal)	8*(3[†])
Esophagus	6*
Cervix/uterine	5*
Unknown primary	5*-7[†]
Prostate	3[†]
Colon	2*
Hepatobiliary	2*
Skin	1*
Other	6*-7[†]

*Data from Lamy O, Jenzer-Closuit A, Burckhard P. Hypercalcemia of malignancy: An undiagnosed and underrated disease. J Intern Med 2001;250:73-79.
[†]Data from Strewler GJ, Neissenson RA. Nonparathyroid hypercalcemia. Adv Intern Med 1987;32:235-258.

Common Errors

- Using serum calcium level (instead of corrected or ionized calcium)
- Not hydrating the patient before administering bisphosphonate
- Use of diuretics
- Administering phosphate
- Expecting rapid calcium normalization

TABLE 228-2 Clinical Manifestations of Hypercalcemia of Malignancy

SYSTEM	MANIFESTATIONS
Neurological	Irritability, depression, lethargy, sedation, delirium, stupor, coma
Gastrointestinal	Anorexia, nausea, vomiting, constipation
Renal	Polyuria, dehydration, decreased glomerular filtration, renal insufficiency
Cardiovascular	Bradycardia, arrhythmia, shortened QT interval, widening of T wave, prolonged PR interval

CASE STUDY

Hypercalcemia of Malignancy

AB, a 65-year-old man diagnosed with non–small cell lung cancer and two vertebral metastases, presented to the emergency department with delirium. A history of onset over approximately 1 week of nausea, decreased oral intake, fatigue, and constipation was obtained from his wife. Biochemical investigations revealed an elevated corrected calcium value of 12.5 mg/dL. A diagnosis of hypercalcemia of malignancy was made. Intravenous normal saline solution was administered vigorously, with careful attention to avoid fluid overload. Pamidronate, 90 mg intravenously, was administered as a single infusion, and calcitonin, 300 units subcutaneously, was administered every 6 hours for the first 2 days. The patient gradually improved and achieved normal serum adjusted calcium and normal cognition on day 4 of treatment.

that act at a distant site (e.g., bone and kidney) to cause hypercalcemia without bone metastasis to osteolytic disease (e.g., myeloma), in which tumor cells in bone secrete factors locally that stimulate osteoclastic bone resorption. Between these two ends of the spectrum are varying degrees of osteolytic bone destruction. It is usually unhelpful to differentiate hypercalcemia into subgroups, because the mediators appear similar, only local in one situation and systemic in another. When tumor burden is large, locally produced mediators of hypercalcemia may have systemic effects.[1]

CLINICAL MANIFESTATIONS

Calcium is important in maintaining cell membrane permeability. Hypercalcemia can therefore produce wide-ranging symptoms related to multiple organ systems (Table 228-2). Neurological symptoms range from irritability and depression to lethargy, sedation, delirium, stupor, and coma (see "Case Study: Hypercalcemia of Malignancy").[1,12] Elevated extracellular calcium levels decrease smooth muscle contractility, delay gastric emptying, and slow intestinal motility. Anorexia, nausea, vomiting, and constipation result.[13] Hypercalcemia impairs the ability of the distal nephron to concentrate urine. Polyuria may result. Compensatory polydipsia is reported; however, the anorexia, nausea, and vomiting often preclude this condition. Resulting volume contraction decreases glomerular filtration and furthers renal insufficiency. In cancer, the hypercalcemic state appears rapidly, with little opportunity for nephrolithiasis and nephrocalcinosis that can develop in primary hyperparathyroidism, in which calcium levels are chronically elevated. Cardiac manifestations may be the terminal event. Calcium ions alter cardiac electrical impulses and cause bradycardia, arrhythmia, shortened QT intervals, wide T wave, and prolonged PR intervals.[13]

The severity of symptoms at clinical presentation is related to both the rapidity of calcium elevation and the serum concentration. When symptoms are nonspecific and occur in patients with advanced cancer, it is possible erroneously to attribute the deterioration evident on presentation to end-stage disease.

DIFFERENTIAL DIAGNOSIS

Differentiation from the hypercalcemia resulting from primary hyperparathyroidism is not usually difficult. Individuals with primary hyperparathyroidism typically present with no or vague chronic symptoms. These patients are relatively well and are found to be hypercalcemic on routine laboratory screening. This situation is in contrast to hypercalcemia of malignancy, in which the individual is very ill with advanced cancer and the presentation is sudden. Occasionally, these two main causes may coexist. If necessary, an elevated PTH level can confirm primary hyperparathyroidism. Other uncommon or rare causes of hypercalcemia that may occur in palliative care include thyrotoxicosis, granulomatous diseases (sarcoidosis, tuberculosis, histoplasmosis, coccidioidomycosis), medications (vitamin D, vitamin A, thiazide diuretics, lithium, estrogen, and antiestrogens), milk-alkali syndrome, immobilization, and familial hypocalciuric hypercalcemia.[14]

Approximately 45% of plasma calcium is bound to albumin, and 10% is complexed with bicarbonate and citrate. The remaining 45% is ionized calcium, the physiologically active form. Total serum calcium is not a good indicator in patients with cancer, who often have low albumin levels and varying ionized calcium levels for a given total serum calcium.

Two methods exist to determine hypercalcemia. One is to use the total serum calcium and adjust for serum albumin (Table 228-3), an approach that is sufficient in most situations.[1] The other is to measure ionized calcium directly, and this method is thought to be a more accurate indicator.[15] This belief has been brought into question,[16] however, because errors in ionized calcium determination include methods of collection, anticoagulant use, pH changes, standard reference ranges, and, notably, significant hypoalbuminemia.[16-18]

TREATMENT

Effective antineoplastic interventions remain the best means of long-term normalization of serum calcium levels.[19] Without this therapy, what remains are strategies to normalize calcium levels for a variable duration, followed by relapses requiring repeat treatment (see "Common Therapeutics").

A key initial step is intravenous rehydration to correct volume depletion. Rehydration alone has mild and transient effects on serum calcium, but it can correct mild hypercalcemia. Normal saline solution is usually the fluid of choice. Forced diuresis with large doses of furosemide has been deemed a risky and outdated procedure.[19] Volume repletion and close monitoring of volume status without diuretics are recommended.[1]

Bisphosphonates are the mainstays of pharmacotherapy in hypercalcemia of malignancy. These drugs decrease osteoclastic bone resorption by two mechanisms, both resulting in osteoclastic apoptosis. The amino bisphosphonates (pamidronate, ibandronate, and zoledronate) are potent inhibitors of the enzyme farnesyl diphosphate syn-

thase, and they thereby block protein isoprenylation. Prenylation of small guanosine triphosphate–binding proteins is important for osteoclast structural integrity. Without it, the osteoclast undergoes apoptosis.[1] The non–nitrogen-containing bisphosphonates (e.g., clodronate) are incorporated into nonhydrolyzable adenosine triphosphate (ATP) analogues that inhibit ATP-dependent intracellular enzymes. These agents are less potent but also induce osteoclast apoptosis.[1] Evidence suggests that bisphosphonates effect osteoclastic bone resorption indirectly through osteoblasts.[1]

Oral absorption of all bisphosphonates is poor (1% oral bioavailability), so parenteral administration is indicated.[2] The mean time to normocalcemia ranges from 2 to 6 days. No study has found a significant difference between different bisphosphonates doses or times of administration and time to normocalcemia.[20] The important factors differentiating bisphosphonates include percentage of success rate in achieving normocalcemia, time to relapse, toxicity, and mode of administration.

Pamidronate is the agent most thoroughly investigated.[21] In one study, zoledronate was found to be more effective in achieving normocalcemia and in duration of normocalcemia, compared with pamidronate.[22] More renal adverse events occurred with zoledronate than with pamidronate, and this phenomenon appeared to be dose related. Ibandronate may be an alternative when concern exists about renal function because this drug has less nephrotoxicity. The renal toxicity of bisphosphonates is a class effect resulting from the formation of insoluble calcium-bisphosphonate complexes in the renal tubules. This effect may be minimized by administering the drug slowly (often over several hours) and by adequate rehydration before administration.[21] Clodronate has the advantage that it can be administered by subcutaneous infusion with minimal skin irritation and good efficacy in normalizing serum calcium.[23,24] These properties are particularly useful in the palliative hospice setting.[19] Overall toxicity with bisphosphonate use is low, and serious events are rare (Box 228-1).

Calcitonin inhibits bone resorption and renal tubular calcium reabsorption. Calcitonin has a rapid onset of action, 2 to 4 hours. This diminishes after 48 hours as a result of tachyphylaxis. The effect is partial, variable, and

---

Common Therapeutics

- Parenteral fluid rehydration (IV or SC)
  - Normal saline: 1-3 L/day or more
- Bisphosphonates
  - Clodronate: 1500 mg SC or IV (50-70%)*
  - Pamidronate: 90 mg IV (70%)*
  - Ibandronate: 4 mg IV (76%)*, 6 mg IV (77%)*
  - Zoledronate: 4 mg IV (87%)*, 8 mg IV (88%)*
- Calcitonin: 4-8 IU/kg SC q6-12h (≈300-600 IU per dose)
- Corticosteroids
  - Dexamethasone: 6-16 mg/day
  - Prednisone: 40-100 mg/day

Success rate.
IV, intravenously; SC, subcutaneously.
Adapted from Body JJ. Hypercalcemia of malignancy. Semin Nephrol 2004;24:48-54.

TABLE 228-3	Adjusted or Corrected Serum Calcium Calculation
UNITS	**FORMULA**
SI units (e.g., mmol/L)	Ca (corrected) = Total Ca (measured) + [0.02 (40 − serum albumin)]
Conventional units (e.g., mg/dL)	Ca (corrected) = Total Ca (measured) + [0.8 × (4 − serum albumin)]

Box 228-1 Side Effects of Bisphosphonates

- Hypocalcemia (common), symptomatic hypocalcemia (rare)
- Transient renal insufficiency (common), renal failure (rare)
- Acute phase response
  - Transient fever, lymphocytopenic, malaise, myalgias, flare of bone pain
  - Occurs with amino bisphosphonates only (i.e., ibandronate, pamidronate, zoledronate)
  - May be lessened with prior dosing with acetaminophen
- Ocular adverse reactions
  - Iritis, episcleritis, scleritis, and conjunctivitis (rare)
- Osteonecrosis of the jaw (rare)

Future Considerations

- Gallium nitrate
- Osteoprotegerin
- RANKL antibody (AMG-162)
- Anti–parathyroid hormone–related protein antibodies
- Integrin inhibitors
- Tyrosine kinase inhibitors
- Etiophos (WR-2721)
- Noncalcemic analogues of calcitriol

RANKL, receptor activator of nuclear factor κB.

transient. The rapid effect is useful because bisphosphonates have a delayed effect. The combined use of a bisphosphonate with calcitonin lowers serum calcium levels more effectively than the use of either agent alone.[25,26] One study reported that glucocorticoids prolonged the effective time of treatment with calcitonin by upregulating cell surface calcitonin receptors.[27] Corticosteroids effectively treat hypercalcemia in patients with steroid-responsive tumors such as lymphoma and myeloma. Recommended doses range from 40 to 100 mg of prednisone daily.[19]

Plicamycin (previously called mithramycin), formerly used to treat hypercalcemia, has considerable toxicity and should no longer be considered. In the approximately 20% of cases in which hypercalcemia is refractory to bisphosphonate administration, few clear options are present. One is a higher dose of bisphosphonate or a switch to an alternative bisphosphonate. Another option is gallium nitrate.

Gallium nitrate is highly efficacious, based on the limited studies to date.[28] Hypophosphatemia, renal toxicity, nausea, and the slow 5-day mode of administration are concerns. Further studies are necessary to determine the role of this drug.

REFERENCES

1. Clines GA, Guise TA. Hypercalcaemia of malignancy and basic research on mechanisms responsible for osteolytic and osteoblastic metastasis to bone. Endocr Relat Cancer 2005;12:549-483.
2. Hurtado J, Esbrit P. Treatment of malignant hypercalcaemia. Expert Opin Pharmacother 2002;3:521-527.
3. Strewler GJ, Neissenson RA. Nonparathyroid hypercalcemia. Adv Intern Med 1987;32:235-258.
4. Mundy GR, Martin TJ. The hypercalcemia of malignancy: Pathogenesis and management. Metabolism 1982;31:1247-1277.
5. Vassilopoalou-Sellin R, Newman BM, Taylor SH, et al. Incidence of hypercalcemia in patients with malignancy referred to a comprehensive cancer center. Cancer 1993;71:1309-1312.
6. Grill V, Martin TJ. Hypercalcemia of malignancy. Rev Endocr Metab Disord 2000;1:253-263.
7. Pecherstorfer M, Schilling T, Blind E, et al. Parathyroid hormone related protein and life expectancy in hypercalcemic cancer patients. J Clin Endocrinol Metab 1994;78:1268-1270.
8. Ralston SH, Gallacher SJ, Patel U, et al. Cancer-associated hypercalcemia: Morbidity and mortality. Clinical experience in 126 treated patients. Ann Intern Med 1990;112:499-504.
9. Lamy O, Jenzer-Closuit A, Burckhard P. Hypercalcemia of malignancy: An undiagnosed and underrated disease. J Intern Med 2001;250:73-79.
10. Burtis WJ, Brady TG, Orloff JJ, et al. Immunochemical characterization of circulating parathyroid hormone–related protein in patients with humoral hypercalcemia of cancer. N Engl J Med 1990;322:1106-1112.
11. Wimalawansa SJ. Significance of plasma PTHRP in patients with hypercalcemia of malignancy treated with bisphosphonate. Cancer 1994;73:2223-2230.
12. Leboff MS, Mikulec KH. Hypercalcemia: Clinical manifestations, pathogenesis, diagnosis, and management. In Favus MJ (ed). Primer on the Metabolic Bone Diseases and Disorders of Mineral Metabolism, 5th ed. Washington, DC: American Society for Bone and Mineral Research, 2003, pp 225-229.
13. Leyland-Jones B. Treatment of cancer-related hypercalcemia: The role of gallium nitrate. Semin Oncol 2003;30(Suppl 5):13-19.
14. Pecherstorfer M, Brenner K, Zojer N. Current management strategies for hypercalcemia. Treat Endocrinol 2003;2:273-292.
15. White TF, Farndon JR, Conceicao SC, et al. Serum calcium status in health and disease: A comparison of measured and derived parameters. Clin Chim Acta 1986;157:199-214.
16. Waterfield KE, Lee MA, Regnard CFB. Ionized calcium in isolation may not detect all cases of symptomatic hypercalcemia. Palliat Med 2005;19:431-432.
17. Butler SJ, Payne RB, Gunn IR, et al. Correlation between serum ionized calcium and serum albumin concentrations in two hospital populations. BMJ 1984;89:948-950.
18. Payne RB. Clinically significant effect of protein concentration on ion-selective electrode measurements of ionized calcium. Ann Clin Biochem 1982;19:233-237.
19. Body JJ. Hypercalcemia of malignancy. Semin Nephrol 2004;24:48-54.
20. Saunders Y, Ross JR, Broadley KE. Systematic review of bisphosphonates for hypercalcaemia of malignancy. Palliat Med 2004;18:418-431.
21. Pecherstorfer M, Brenner K, Niklas Zojer N. Current management strategies for hypercalcemia. Treat Endocrinol 2003;2:273-292.
22. Major P, Lortholary A, Hon J, et al. Zoledronic acid is superior to pamidronate in the treatment of hypercalcaemia of malignancy: A pooled analysis of two randomized, controlled clinical trials. J Clin Oncol 2001;19:558-567.
23. Walker P, Watanabe S, Lawlor P, et al. Subcutaneous clodronate: A study evaluating efficacy in hypercalcemia of malignancy and local toxicity. Ann Oncol 1997;8:915-916.
24. Roemer-Becuwe C, Vigano A, Romano F, et al. Safety of subcutaneous clodronate and efficacy in hypercalcemia of malignancy: A novel route of administration. J Pain Symptom Manage 2003;843-848.
25. Thiebaud D, Jacquet AF, Burckhardt P. Fast and effective treatment of malignant hypercalcemia: Combination of suppositories of calcitonin and a single infusion of 3-amino 1-hydroxpropylidene-1-bisphosphonate. Arch Intern Med 1990;150:2125-2128.
26. Hosking DJ, Gilson D. Comparison of the renal and skeletal actions of calcitonin in the treatment of severe hypercalcaemia of malignancy. Q J Med 1984;211:359-368.
27. Binstock ML, Mundy GR. Effect of calcitonin and glucocorticoids in combination on the hypercalcemia of malignancy. Ann Intern Med 1980;93:269-27.
28. Warrell RP, Murphy WK, Schulman P, et al. A randomized double-blind study of gallium nitrate compared with etidronate for acute control of cancer-related hypercalcemia. J Clin Oncol 1991;9:1467-1475.

CHAPTER **229**

Bone Marrow Failure

Stephen N. Makoni and Damian A. Laber

KEY POINTS

- Bone marrow failure (BMF) can be defined as reduced production of one or more hematopoietic lineages with peripheral cytopenias.

- Anemia, the most common cytopenia, occurs at some point in 50% to 80% of patients with cancer.

- Other symptoms and signs of BMF result from the underlying disease and from the side effects of chemotherapy or radiation therapy. Cancer-related pain, pathological fractures, nausea, vomiting, and muscles weakness related to hypercalcemia may bring patients to medical attention.

- Treatment should include withdrawal of offending agents if possible, such as delaying or reducing the dose of chemotherapy, supportive care, and some form of definitive therapy if possible.

- Neutropenia is the most common dose-limiting toxicity of chemotherapy and is associated with significant morbidity, including hospitalization and use of broad-spectrum antibiotics, mortality, and costs.

BMF can be defined as reduced production of one or more hematopoietic lineages with peripheral cytopenias. BMF may occur at different developmental levels of the hematopoietic cells, depending on the cause. A defect in the stem cell may cause aplastic anemia (AA), whereas a defect at a later developmental stage may cause single lineage failure.[1] BMF syndromes may occur at any age, but most are acquired and manifest in adulthood. Inherited or constitutional causes are less common and manifest in childhood to early adulthood. In malignant disease, the most common causes of cytopenias include treatment complications (chemotherapy), marrow infiltration by tumor cells with extramedullary hematopoiesis (myelophthisis), and, less frequently, autoimmunity.

EPIDEMIOLOGY AND PREVALENCE

Anemia, the most common cytopenia, occurs sometime in 50% to 80% of patients with cancer.[2] Elderly patients with cancer often have clinical symptoms of anemia at higher hemoglobin levels than do anemic patients without cancer. Pure RBC aplasia may be underdiagnosed in advanced malignant disease because anemia is so frequent that bone marrow examination is not routinely performed. Pure RBC aplasia may manifest before or after diagnosis of malignancy and follows a chronic course independent of the evolution of the underlying malignant process.

Myelophthisis occurs in less than 10% of patients with cancer who have metastatic disease.[3] Widespread infiltra-

tion of the bone marrow can occur in patients with advanced solid tumors such as lung, breast, and prostate, and it is always present in hematopoietic malignancies. The incidence and severity of chemotherapy-induced cytopenias depend on several factors, including drug characteristics (type of chemotherapy, dosing schedule, and intensity), type and duration of malignancy, and other bone marrow suppressing agents such as radiation therapy. Almost all standard chemotherapy protocols cause severe neutropenia in 10% to 40% of patients. Neutropenic fever and infections occur in less than 10%. In most patients, chemotherapy-induced cytopenias resolve in less than 1 to 2 weeks. Severe thrombocytopenia is less common, and bleeding from standard chemotherapy is rare.

Pancytopenia of mild to moderate degree is frequent in end-stage cancer because of cachexia, chemotherapy, or myelophthisis. Cytopenias may also arise from intensive chemotherapy, radiation therapy, or therapy-related myelodysplastic syndrome (MDS). The risk of therapy-related MDS is highest after exposure to alkylating agents. The estimated risk of MDS after chemotherapy and radiation therapy for Hodgkin's disease is 6% to 9%.[4] The risk of MDS following adjuvant chemotherapy for breast cancer, small cell lung cancer, testicular cancer, or ovarian cancer is low, but it may increase with use of radiation therapy. Acquired AA occurs at a rate of approximately 2 cases per million people. Of these cases, 70% to 80% are idiopathic. Most patients present between the ages of 15 and 25 years, with a smaller peak in incidence after 60 years.[5] Inherited causes of AA that present in adulthood include Fanconi's anemia (FA) and dyskeratosis congenita (DKC).[6]

PATHOPHYSIOLOGY

The pathophysiology is multifactorial. Blood loss, hemolysis, and nutritional deficiencies cause anemia by depleting iron, folate, vitamin B_{12}, and other vitamins and minerals. Cancer-related anemia, an anemia of chronic disease type, is characterized by hyporegenerative, normocytic, and normochromic anemia with reduced serum iron and transferrin saturation but elevated (or normal) ferritin levels.[7] The pathophysiology includes activation of the immune and inflammatory systems, thus leading to increased release of tumor necrosis factor, interferon-γ, and interleukin-1 (IL-1). This process impairs iron utilization, with suppression of erythroid progenitor-cell differentiation and inadequate erythropoietin production. In addition, the life span of red blood cells (RBCs) is shortened, and production cannot compensate sufficiently for the shorter survival time.

Myelosuppressive chemotherapy causes injury to all bone marrow cells, but recovery of peripheral blood counts usually occurs within weeks. Prolonged and irreversible cytopenias can result from severe damage to the hematopoietic stem cells, with transformation into leukemia or MDS. Radiation therapy may also cause severe injury to both the stem cells and the rapidly dividing progenitor cells.[1] Lymphocytes are particularly sensitive to radiation. Higher doses cause granulocytopenia, reticulocytopenia, and thrombocytopenia. Cytogenetic changes in stem cells are dose related, irreversible, and cumulative, thereby increasing the probability of leukemic transformation. Temporary functional ablation of marrow may occur even with relatively low radiation doses; however, high radiation doses should not cause significant cytopenias if the irradiated field is small. Repopulation of the bone marrow and restoration of active hematopoiesis may take several years after exposure to moderate radiation doses. With higher radiation doses, irreversible damage to the medullary stroma may be associated with permanent marrow aplasia.

Myelophthisis results from destruction of bone marrow precursor cells and their stroma, which nurture these cells to maturation and differentiation.[3] Infiltration of the marrow by cancerous cells causes release of suppressive and destructive cytokines and fibroblastic growth factors and leads to the reduction in the available bone marrow space. This situation causes pluripotent stem cells to migrate to the liver, spleen, and other organs in the body and to start extramedullary hematopoiesis. The stromal support system outside the bone marrow is not optimal for hematopoiesis, and the result is the premature release of hematopoietic cells into the circulation (leukoerythroblastosis).[3] The invading cells in chronic leukemia do not cause structural damage. The expansion volume of the pathological cells and their release of suppressor cytokines cause cytopenias.[8] Hypersplenism resulting from splenic metastases or liver disease may also contribute.

Microangiopathic hemolytic anemia is a rare complication caused by the release of procoagulants from cancer cells such as from prostate and gastrointestinal (mucin-producing) tumors.[9] Thrombocytopenia may be related to disseminated intravascular coagulopathy, especially in acute promyelocytic leukemia and in lung, breast, gastrointestinal, and urogenital malignancies (see "Case Study: Anemia in a Patient with Advanced Lung Cancer" and "Case Study: Anemia and Thrombocytopenia in a Patient with a History of Breast Cancer"). Patients with inherited diseases develop BMF because of genetic abnormalities.[5,6,10]

CLINICAL MANIFESTATIONS

Clinical manifestations depend on the underlying disease and the severity of the cytopenias. Other symptoms and signs result from the underlying disease and from the side effects of chemotherapy or radiation therapy. Cancer-related pain, pathological fractures, nausea, vomiting, and muscles weakness caused by hypercalcemia may bring patients to medical attention.[8] The clinical presentation directly related to BMF is usually proportional to peripheral blood cytopenias. All the blood elements may be depressed, or a decrease in a single cell line may dominate. Anemia is the most common hematological abnormality encountered by patients with cancer. Patients may present with fatigue, dyspnea, or signs of heart failure (see "Case Study: Anemia in a Patient with Advanced Lung Cancer"). Neutropenic patients may present with infection and sepsis. These infections are typically bacterial, including pneumonia and urinary tract infection. Invasive fungal infection is a common cause of death, especially in patients with prolonged and severe neutropenia. Bleeding is usually the most alarming presentation. Extensive hemorrhage may occur in advanced disease and is almost always associated with infections, medications such as corticosteroids, invasive procedures, complications of radiation, and erosion of tumor into major blood vessels. Bleeding may be exacerbated by platelet dysfunction in myeloproliferative disorders, multiple myeloma, and Waldenström's macroglobulinemia. These conditions may also be associated with acquired factor X deficiency in amyloidosis, a circulating heparin-like anticoagulant, fibrinolysis, and interference by myeloma protein with both fibrin polymerization and the function of other coagulation proteins. Thrombocytopenia alone seldom causes massive bleeding. It usually manifests with easy bruising and mucosal bleeding such as gum (with tooth brushing), recurrent epistaxis, and menorrhagia. During the physical examination, one must evaluate the primary malignant disease and look for splenomegaly, lymphadenopathy, skin rash, petechiae, and purpura. Inherited BMF syndromes are associated with other anomalies such as skeletal (thumb and radius) disorders, microcephaly, short stature, hypogonadism, abnormal skin pigmentation, nail dystrophy, macular or retinal hypopigmentation, and oral leukoplakia.

INVESTIGATIONS

Figure 229-1 is an algorithm for the differential diagnosis of BMF.

CASE STUDY

Anemia in a Patient with Advanced Lung Cancer

CD, a 79-year-old man, presents from hospice with severe weakness and fatigue. He spends most of the day in bed as a result of fatigue and needs assistance to ambulate. He is comfortable, has no pain, and enjoys spending time with his great-grandchildren, but he is suffering from significant fatigue. This patient was diagnosed with lung cancer 2 years ago and has extensive metastases that progressed after two different types of chemotherapeutic regimens. On examination, he is pale, without signs of hemorrhage. His hemoglobin value is 7.3 g/dL. He received 2 U of blood, and his symptoms greatly improved.

CASE STUDY

Anemia and Thrombocytopenia in a Patient with a History of Breast Cancer

EF, a 69-year-old woman, presents with progressive fatigue and easy bruising. Review of systems is unrevealing, specifically no fever, sweats, weight loss, or bleeding. She has a history of stage III breast cancer treated with mastectomy, doxorubicin (Adriamycin), cyclophosphamide, paclitaxel, and radiation therapy approximately 5 years ago. Six months ago, she had no evidence of disease. The physical examination is normal except for mild pallor. Complete blood count confirmed anemia and mild thrombocytopenia. The next tests should be bone marrow aspiration and biopsy, to evaluate for bone marrow failure from recurrent breast cancer or myelodysplastic syndrome.

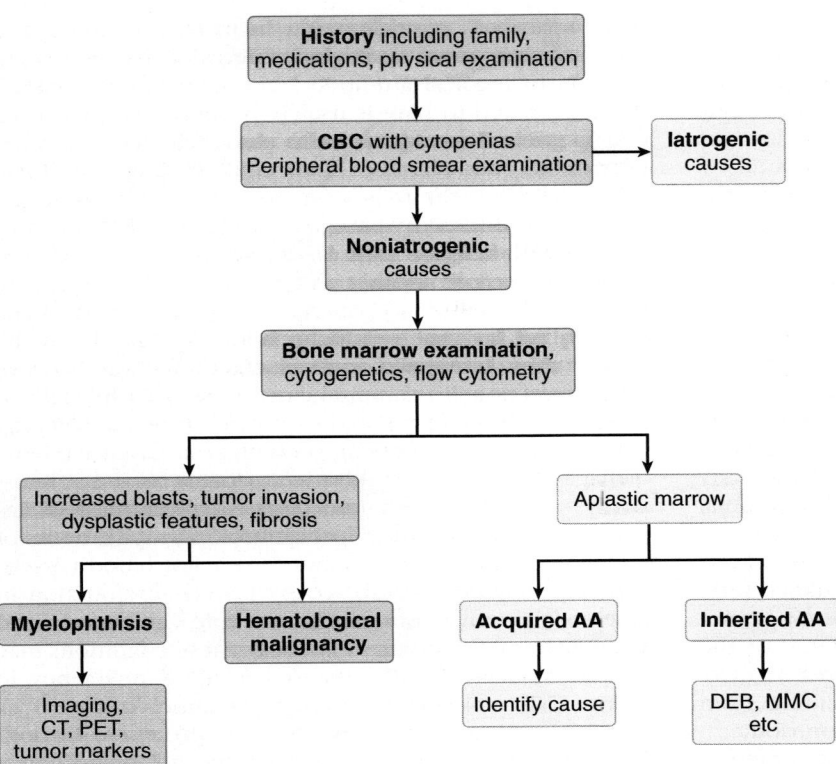

FIGURE 229-1 Differential diagnosis algorithm. AA, aplastic anemia; CBC, complete blood count; CT computed tomography; DEB, diepoxybutane; MMC, mitomycin C; PET, positron emission tomography.

Laboratory Tests

Complete Blood Count

- White blood cell differential counts
- Reticulocyte count (reflects bone marrow activity): BMF from AA, infiltrations, chemotherapy, radiation as cause of reticulocytopenia
- Hemoglobin electrophoresis: increased fetal hemoglobin in FA and DKC

Peripheral Blood Smear

- Macrocytosis suggest MDS, nutritional causes, medications, and inherited syndromes (FA, DKC, DBA).
- The leukoerythroblastic picture (tear drop form and nucleated RBCs, immature myeloid precursors, giant platelets, and thrombocytopenia)[3] is characteristic of marrow infiltration.
- Carcinocythemia (cancer cells on blood film) always indicates marrow invasion.
- Fragmented RBCs and schistocytes suggest microangiopathic hemolysis.

Other Laboratory Tests

- Serum vitamin B_{12}, folate, and iron profile
- Autoimmune profile (rare cause of AA)
- Liver function tests and viral hepatitis screen (to exclude AA after hepatitis)
- For adults less 35 years old, inherited syndromes: In FA, increased spontaneous and diepoxybutane- or mitomycin C–induced chromosomal breakages occur in cultured peripheral blood lymphocytes, and many patients

with DKC show mutations of the telomerase gene complex.[1]

Biopsy and Flow Cytometry Evaluation

Bone Marrow Aspiration and Biopsy

Bone marrow aspiration and biopsy are the gold standard diagnostic tests for any BMF syndrome. The core biopsy specimen should be at least 1 cm long. An inability to aspirate marrow (dry tap) may suggest infiltration, fibrosis, or marrow replacement. Evaluation for cellularity should be done from the core biopsy and should be at least 30% in adults. Findings are as follows:

- Hematological malignancy: increased blasts, ringed sideroblasts, Auer rods, leukemic cells
- Cancer infiltration: packed marrow and tumor clumps or nests
- Myelodysplasia: dysplastic features including megaloblastic, dyserythropoietic, or atypical megakaryocytes
- AA: increased fat infiltration with reduced cellularity (hypoplasia); residual hematopoietic cells morphologically normal; may have acquired or inherited causes
- Other findings: fibrosis, granuloma, inflammatory cells, macrophages (Gaucher's disease).
- Cytogenetic testing: may identify karyotypic abnormalities

Flow Cytometry

Flow cytometry involves the use of glycosyl phosphatidyl inositol–anchored proteins on blood cells. Deficient expression on RBCs, neutrophils, and monocytes indicates a paroxysmal nocturnal hemoglobinuria clone.

TREATMENT

Management Principles

Treatment should include withdrawal of offending agents such as delaying or reducing the dose of chemotherapy, supportive care, and some definitive therapy if possible (Fig. 229-2). In making decisions regarding dosage modifications or use of growth factors, the therapeutic goals should be considered. If the regimen has the potential for cure, the optimum dose and schedule should be maintained. If palliation is the goal, reducing doses and lengthening the interval between doses are appropriate. Individual treatment protocols should be consulted for possible modifications.

Neutropenia

Neutropenia is the most common dose-limiting toxicity of chemotherapy. This complication is associated with significant morbidity, including hospitalization and use of broad-spectrum antibiotics, mortality, and cost. The prophylactic use of myeloid growth factors after chemotherapy shortens the period of absolute neutropenia by approximately 50% compared with placebo and significantly reduces hospitalization for fever and neutropenia.[11] Guidelines recommend prophylactic use of myeloid growth factors after chemotherapy if the estimated risk of febrile neutropenia is greater than 20% when patients are receiving therapy with curative intent and to prolong survival or to improve quality of life in the palliative setting. Factors that increase the risk of chemotherapy-induced neutropenia and fever include the characteristics of the offending drug, dose intensity, extensive prior chemotherapy, history of neutropenia, concurrent radiation, advanced age, poor performance status, hematological malignancies, extensive metastatic disease, uncontrolled cancer, and bone marrow involvement. Myeloid growth factors (Box 229-1) are also beneficial in neutropenia from other causes such as chronic acquired BMF syndromes including MDS and myeloproliferative disorders, as well as in congenital BMF states.

Leukocyte transfusion can be considered under certain circumstances. The normal half-life of granulocytes in a febrile, uninfected host is 4 to 10 hours, with a daily turnover of approximately 230%. In fever or infection, the turnover can be severalfold higher. Randomized prospective trials of prophylactic leukocyte transfusion in leukopenic patients demonstrated a protective effect but no improvement in survival because of adverse effects including alloimmunization, transfusion reactions, cytomegalovirus infection, and pulmonary infiltrates. Leukocyte transfusions are not widely used in supportive care because of improvement in antibiotics and myeloid growth factors.[12]

Anemia

Anemia is present in almost all patients with end-stage cancer. Anemia also occurs in many other disorders including dementia, congestive heart failure, end-stage renal disease, and emphysema. It is one of the first signs of BMF. Therapy should maintain an adequate oxygen-carrying capacity and should minimize fatigue. Transfusion of RBCs is the quickest and most effective therapy. It is preferred for severely symptomatic patients at risk for complications from anemia such as cardiac events as well as for patients with a short life expectancy. Severe transfusion-related complications are rare; the estimated risk of fatal acute

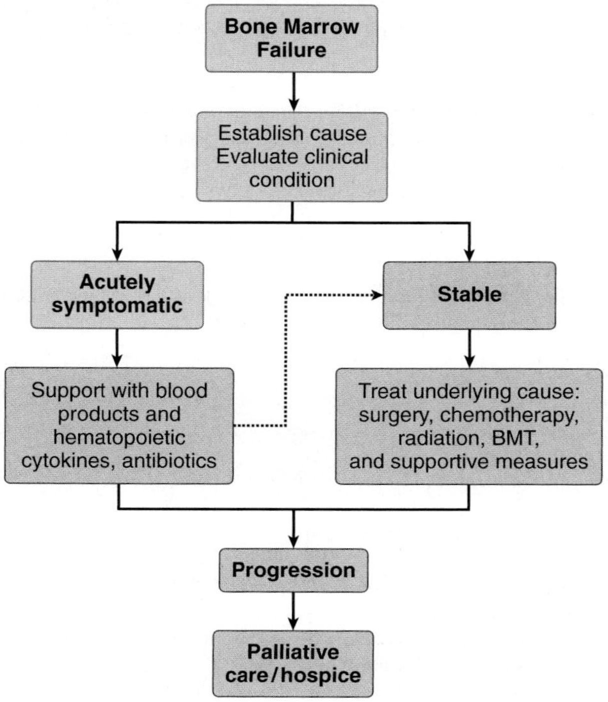

FIGURE 229-2 Management algorithm. BMT, bone marrow transplant.

Box 229-1 Myeloid Growth Factors

Filgrastim

- Daily dose of 5 μg/kg until postnadir absolute neutrophil count recovery is normal or nearly normal by laboratory standards
- Start 1 to 3 days after completion of chemotherapy and treat through postnadir recovery

Pegfilgrastim

- One dose at 6 mg per cycle of treatment
- Start 1 to 3 days after completion of chemotherapy

Sargramostim

- Used in clinical trials at a dose of 250 μg/m²/day

General Principles

- Subcutaneous route is preferred for all three agents
- Safety data appear to be similar between filgrastim and pegfilgrastim

hemolytic reactions is between 1 in 250,000 and 1 in 1 million transfusions, with 0.67 deaths per million units transfused.[13]

RBC transfusions are given for maintenance of oxygen delivery to tissues and hemodynamic homeostasis. RBC transfusions are indicated in patients with cancer who have symptomatic anemia and in whom medical necessity does not allow adequate time for correction of the underlying cause or for measures such as epoetin alfa and nutritional supplements (e.g., iron, folate, and vitamin B_{12}) to be effective. Adequate oxygen-carrying capacity to maintain minimal acceptable cardiopulmonary function can be met by a hemoglobin concentration of 7 g/dL in a healthy person. A hemoglobin level of 8 g/dL or higher is usually preferred in cancer and cancer therapy, and a level higher than 10 g/dL is preferred in patients with cardiac disease (Box 229-2).

Erythropoietin analogues can increase hemoglobin levels to prevent worsening anemia, to minimize fatigue, and to reduce the need for transfusions.[14] Clinical trials with similar end points using darbepoetin alfa showed similar results. A head-to-head randomized comparison of darbepoetin alfa (200 μg subcutaneously every 2 weeks) and epoetin alfa (40,000 U subcutaneously once a week) in 312 patients with cancer who were receiving concurrent chemotherapy revealed that more than 80% in both arms of the study achieved target hemoglobin levels. The rates of transfusions were similar and, after achievement of a hemoglobin level higher than 11 g/dL, the mean hemoglobin level was maintained at approximately 12 g/dL for the remainder of the trials in both groups.[7] Evidence-based consensus recommendations regarding erythropoietin use during chemotherapy recommend this agent for patients with a hemoglobin level lower than 10 g/dL and possibly if the hemoglobin is less than 11 g/dL.[7] Erythropoietin analogues (Table 229-1 and Box 229-3) can achieve clinically meaningful responses in anemic subjects with myeloproliferative and myelodysplastic disorders with serum erythropoietin values of less than 500 mU/mL. "Functional" iron deficiency often arises after continued erythropoietin use, and iron supplementation will be required in most patients to maintain erythropoiesis. A serum ferritin level less than 100 ng/mL is evidence of functional iron deficiency, and supplementation is warranted. Intravenous iron therapy may be superior to oral iron therapy in treating functional iron deficiency of cancer.

TABLE 229-1 Standard Erythropoietin Dosing		
RECOMMENDED INITIAL DOSING	**TITRATION IF NO RESPONSE**	**TITRATION FOR RESPONSE**
Epoetin alfa: 40,000 U once a week by subcutaneous injection	Increase dose of epoetin alfa to 60,000 U once a week by subcutaneous injection	If hemoglobin increases by >1 g/dL in a 2-wk period, dose should be reduced by 25% If hemoglobin is >12 g/dL, hold therapy Reinitiate therapy if hemoglobin falls to <12 g/dL at 25% dose reduction of the prior dose
Darbepoetin alfa: 200 μg fixed dose every 2 wk by subcutaneous injection	Increase darbepoetin alfa to ≤300 μg fixed dose every 2 wk by subcutaneous injection	

Box 229-2 Red Blood Cell Products

Whole Blood

- Rarely used
- Restores volume in setting of massive hemorrhage
- Replenishes RBCs and clotting factors in a patient deficient in both

Leukocyte-Poor RBCs

- Avoid febrile nonhemolytic transfusion reactions and alloimmunization

Washed RBCs (Plasma Removed)

- Avoidance of urticarial reactions to plasma proteins
- Useful in IgA-deficient patients with anti-IgA antibodies

Frozen Deglycerolized RBCs

- Leukocyte and plasma poor
- Useful in patients with reactions to leukocytes and plasma
- Prevents transmission of cytomegalovirus

IgA, immunoglobulin A; RBCs, red blood cells.

Box 229-3 Erythropoietin Adverse Effects

Hypertension/Seizures

- Control blood pressure before initiating therapy
- Seizures reported in patients with chronic renal failure who were receiving erythropoietin
- Monitor Hb level to reduce the risk of hypertension and seizures

Thrombosis

- Target Hb 11 to 12 g/dL to reduce the risk of arterial and venous thrombosis

Pure Red Cell Aplasia

- Evaluate all patients who develop a loss of response to erythropoietin
- Stop treatment if pure red cell aplasia is present

Survival of Patients with Cancer

- Conflicting data on reduced survival in patients receiving erythropoietin for anemia correction
- Additional clinical trials needed to determine optimal erythropoietin use in patients with cancer

Hb, hemoglobin.

Thrombocytopenia

Thrombocytopenia is a challenging complication of BMF syndromes. Platelet transfusion remains the standard of care for acute management of clinically significant thrombocytopenia. Prophylactic platelet transfusion can reduce the risk of hemorrhage when the platelet count falls to less than a predefined threshold level. This threshold for transfusion varies according to the diagnosis, clinical condition, and treatment modality.

Two types of platelet products are available. Pooled or random-donor platelets are prepared by separating platelet concentrates from a unit of donated whole blood and are pooled before administration. Because only approximately 15 mL of platelets can be collected from 1 U of whole blood and because platelets can be stored for only 5 days, platelets are a precious component of blood. Single-donor platelets are collected by plateletpheresis. During pheresis, whole blood is collected from one arm of the donor and goes into a machine called a cell separator. The blood is spun in the machine to separate the components, and a measured amount of the desired component is collected into a special bag. Then the RBCs and other components are returned to the donor. On average, 1 U of single donor is equivalent to 6 U of random-donor (pooled) platelets. Post-transfusion increments, hemostatic benefit, and side effects are similar with either product. Thus, in routine circumstances, these products can be used interchangeably; however, pooled platelets are less costly. Single-donor platelets are preferred when histocompatible platelet transfusions are needed.[15]

Randomized clinical trials reveal that a threshold platelet count of 10,000/μL was equivalent to 20,000/μL for prophylactic platelet transfusion in adults receiving therapy for acute leukemia, solid tumors, and hematopoietic cell transplantation. A higher threshold may be necessary in certain situations such as patients with clinical bleeding, high fever, leukocytosis, rapid fall of platelet count, or coagulation abnormalities (e.g., acute promyelocytic leukemia) and those undergoing invasive procedures.[15] A threshold of 20,000/μL should be considered during aggressive therapy for patients with bladder tumors and those with demonstrated necrotic tumors, owing to presumed increased risk of bleeding at these sites. Patients with chronic severe thrombocytopenia (e.g., MDS and

AA) usually have no significant bleeding despite their low platelet counts and may be observed without prophylactic transfusion, with platelet transfusions reserved for hemorrhage or during active treatment.[15]

Post-transfusion platelet counts should be obtained to assess efficacy. In an average person, a 7000 to 11,000/μL increment per unit of pooled platelet administered is expected. Patients may have a poor increment in the platelet count to a single transfusion yet have excellent increments with subsequent transfusions. A diagnosis of refractoriness to platelet transfusion should be made only when at least two ABO-compatible transfusions, stored less than 72 hours, result in poor increments. Poor survival of transfused platelets can be caused by increased consumption in sepsis, increased splenic sequestration with splenomegaly, drug-induced platelet antibodies, and recipient antibodies against donor antigens of human leukocyte antigen-A (HLA-A) and HLA-B, the ABH system, or platelet alloantigens. The incidence of alloantibody-mediated refractoriness to platelet transfusion can be decreased in acute myelogenous leukemia when both platelet and RBC products are leukoreduced by filtration before transfusion,[15] and by ultraviolet B irradiation of blood products to destroy leukocytes. It is possible that alloimmunization can also be decreased in other types of leukemia and in patients with cancer who are receiving chemotherapy.[15] Although transfusion of blood products ameliorates cytopenias, it is associated with risks (Box 229-4), the most serious of which is the potential transmission of infection.

Several thrombopoietic factors—IL-3, IL-9, IL-1β, stem cell factor, and thrombopoietin—have been tried clinically, based on preclinical thrombopoietic activity. Limited platelet recovery has been observed. A randomized placebo-controlled study of recombinant human IL-11 to prevent chemotherapy-induced thrombocytopenia in advanced breast cancer during dose-intensive chemotherapy in combination with granulocyte colony-stimulating factor demonstrated less requirement for platelet transfusions and improved time to platelet recovery to more than 50,000/μL for the IL-11 group. IL-11 (oprelvekin) is the only cytokine approved by the U.S. Food and Drug Administration for prevention and management of chemotherapy-associated thrombocytopenia.[12] Despite the positive results with platelet growth factors, these agents are not widely used because of infrequent use of dose-intensive chemotherapy, perceived cost, side effects, and short duration of thrombocytopenia.

Aplastic Anemia

Standard treatment for AA includes immunosuppression or bone marrow transplant. Patient age, availability of a matched sibling donor, and risk factors such as active infections or heavy transfusion burden are considered before choosing the best treatment. A retrospective analysis found no difference in survival between bone marrow transplant and immunosuppressive therapy (63% versus 61%) in an unselected population; however, significant differences were apparent in favor of bone marrow transplant for patients younger than 20 years (64% versus 38%).[10]

Box 229-4 Transfusion Reactions

Infection

- Viral: hepatitis A, B, C, HIV, HTLV I/II, CMV, parvovirus B19
- Bacterial contamination of RBCs and platelets

Acute Hemolytic Reactions

- Result of ABO incompatibility
- Medical emergency: stop transfusion and initiate intravenous fluids

Delayed Hemolytic Reactions

- Result of anamnestic antibody response, 2 to 10 days after transfusion
- Antibody usually of Kidd or Rh system
- Supportive measures

Anaphylactic Transfusion Reactions

- Result of the presence of IgG and anti-IgA antibodies in patients who are IgA deficient
- Stop transfusion, give epinephrine, secure airway, administer intravenous fluids

Urticarial Reactions

- Result of preexisting IgE antibodies in recipient plasma
- Can continue transfusion with diphenhydramine (Benadryl) and supportive measures

Transfusion-Related Acute Lung Injury

- Noncardiogenic pulmonary edema within 6 hours of transfusion
- Stop transfusion and give respiratory and circulatory support

Transfusion-Associated Graft-versus-Host Disease

- High-risk patients: BMT, hematological malignancies, Hodgkin's disease, NHL, ALL, AA, some solid tumors
- Irradiate blood products

Other Causes

- Circulatory overload, metabolic reactions, iron overload, post-transfusion purpura

AA, aplastic anemia; ALL, acute lymphoblastic leukemia; BMT, bone marrow transplant; CMV, cytomegalovirus; HIV, human immunodeficiency virus; HTLV, human T-cell leukemia virus; Ig, immunoglobulin; NHL, non-Hodgkin's lymphoma; RBCs, red blood cells.

Future Directions

- Decreased survival in patients with cancer who are receiving erythropoietic drugs for correction of anemia:
  - Prospective clinical trials designed and powered to measure survival in patients with cancer are needed to guide optimal use of erythropoietic agents.
- Optimal target hemoglobin when using erythropoietin analogues:
  - The risk of adverse events is higher in patients with hemoglobin values greater than 11 to 12 g/dL.
- Development of artificial blood substitutes:
  - These agents will eliminate transfusion of red blood cells and platelets and will thus reduce the risk of infectious and allergic complications.
  - They will have the advantages of universal compatibility and long shelf life.
- Novel platelet growth factors and optimal use of interleukin-11:
  - These agents are not currently not widely used for chemotherapy-induced thrombocytopenia.
- The appropriate setting for use of therapeutic granulocyte transfusion:
  - The optimal granulocyte dose is unknown.
  - Studies are needed to improve the ex vivo shelf life and in vivo survival.

REFERENCES

1. Marsh JC. Bone marrow failure syndromes. Clin Med 2005;5:332-336.
2. Harper P, Littlewood T. Anaemia of cancer: Impact on patient fatigue and long-term outcome. Oncology 2005;69(Suppl 2):2-7.
3. Makoni SN, Laber DA. Clinical spectrum of myelophthisis in cancer patients. Am J Hematol 2004;76:92-93.
4. De Angelo DJ, Stone RM. Myelodysplastic syndromes: Biology and treatment. In Hoffman R, Benz E, Shattil S (eds). Hematology: Basic Principles and Practice, 4th ed. Philadelphia: Churchill Livingstone, 2005, pp 1195-1208.
5. Brodsky RA, Jones RJ. Aplastic anaemia. Lancet 2005;365:1647-1656.
6. Freedman MH. Inherited forms of bone marrow failure. In Hoffman R, Benz E, Shattil S (eds). Hematology: Basic Principles and Practice, 4th ed. Philadelphia: Churchill Livingstone, 2005, pp 339-379.
7. Stasi R, Amadori S, Littlewood TJ, et al. Management of cancer-related anemia with erythropoietic agents: Doubts, certainties, and concerns. Oncologist 2005;10:539-554.
8. Erslev AJ. Anemia associated with marrow infiltration. In Beutler E, Lichtman MA, Coller BS, et al. (eds). Williams Hematology, 6th ed. New York: McGraw-Hill, 2001 pp 477-487.
9. Saba HI. Anemia in cancer patients: Introduction and overview. Cancer Control J 1998;5(Suppl 2).
10. Bagby GC, Lipton JM, Sloand EM, Schiffer CA. Marrow failure. Hematology Am Soc Hematol Educ Program 2004;318-336.
11. Crawford J, Ozer H, Stoller R, et al. Reduction by granulocyte colony-stimulating factor of fever and neutropenia induced by chemotherapy in patients with small-cell lung cancer. N Engl J Med 1991;325:164-170.
12. Demetri GD, Anderson KC. Disorders of blood cell production in clinical oncology. In Abeloff MD, Armitage JO, Niederhuber JE, et al. (eds). Clinical Oncology, 3rd ed. Philadelphia: Elsevier, Churchill Livingstone, 2004, p 861.
13. Goodnough LT, Brecher ME, Kanter MH, AuBuchon JP. Transfusion medicine: Blood transfusion. First of two parts. N Engl J Med 1999;340:438-447.
14. Seidenfeld J, Piper M, Flamm C, et al. Epoetin treatment of anemia associated with cancer therapy: A systematic review and meta-analysis of controlled clinical trials. J Natl Cancer Inst 2001;93:1204-1214.
15. Schiffer CA, Anderson KC, Bennett CL, et al. Platelet transfusion for patients with cancer: Clinical practice guidelines of the American Society of Clinical Oncology. J Clin Oncol 2001;19:1519-1538.

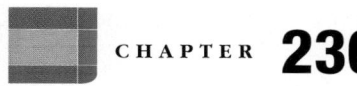

CHAPTER **230**

Bleeding and Clotting Disorders in Cancer

Nabila Bennani-Baiti and Kandice Kottke-Marchant

KEY POINTS

- Strong evidence links cancer to thrombosis and bleeding.
- A hypercoagulable state through interactions between the tumor and the hemostatic system plays a major role in cancer thrombogenesis. Tissue factor (TF), cancer procoagulant (CP), and proinflammatory cytokines are mostly implicated.
- Tumor invasion and treatment-related causes (thrombocytopenia, mucositis) are the major reasons for bleeding. Acquired coagulant factors inhibitors can also be implicated.
- Catastrophic bleeding, disseminated intravascular coagulopathy (DIC), and heparin-induced thrombocytopenia (HIT) and heparin-induced thrombocytopenia/thrombosis (HITT) are particularly feared.
- Prophylactic anticoagulation is not recommended except in high-risk patients (e.g., postoperatively). Chronic anticoagulation is the standard treatment in overt thrombotic disease.
- Low-molecular-weight heparins (LMWHs) are replacing traditional anticoagulants. Research suggests possible antineoplastic and survival benefits.
- Management of cancer-related bleeding and clotting disorders must be individualized, considering the treatment risk/burden-to-benefit ratio between the prognosis and the goals of care.

Strong evidence links cancer to an increased risk of thrombosis and bleeding. This risk is higher in palliative medicine. The relationship between cancer and coagulopathies is a two-way clinical correlation. Spontaneous bleeding and venous thromboembolism (VTE) events often precede cancer diagnosis and may be the reason to investigate for underlying malignant disease. Bleeding and clotting disorders are important causes of cancer mortality and morbidity and of increased health care costs. Oncologists and palliative medicine specialists are often faced with the challenge of managing VTE in patients with cancer, in whom the risks of recurrent thromboembolism and serious bleeding are high. Bleeding and clotting disorders cause great distress and impair the quality of life of both patients and their caregivers.

EPIDEMIOLOGY AND RISK FACTORS

Venous Thromboembolism

Epidemiology

VTE is one of the most common complications and the second most common cause of death in cancer.[1] Active malignancy increases VTE risk by a factor of 4 to 6.[1]

Approximately 15% of patients with overt cancer will develop VTE during the course of their disease. Autopsy studies show a higher prevalence of 30% to 50%.[2] The true incidence is not well determined: varying rates have been reported, probably from different diagnostic criteria.[3] Six percent of hospital admissions in medical oncology result from VTE.[1] Nine percent to 15% of patients with cancer suffer from DIC, which requires intensive intervention and is often fatal.[1] VTE events are associated with decreased survival: a 1-year survival rate of 12% versus 36% in patients with cancer with or without VTE, respectively.[4]

Risk Factors

Box 230-1 details risk factors for VTE in cancer.

TUMOR TYPE

The frequency of VTE appears to vary by cancer type.[3] The highest prevalence seems associated with mucin-producing cancers.

RECURRENT VENOUS THROMBOEMBOLISM

Patients who develop VTE before or during their disease are at increased risk of another VTE event. Cancer is an independent predictor of recurrence.[3]

EXTENT OF DISEASE AND TIMING FROM DIAGNOSIS

Advanced cancer or metastasis increases the risk of VTE.[3] A reverse relationship applies, too. Malignant diseases

---

BOX 230-1 Risk Factors for Venous Thrombosis in Cancer

Cancer Type

- Hematological
- Pancreas
- Lung
- Brain
- Gastrointestinal
- Ovary
- Breast

Extent of Disease

Recurrence of Thromboembolic Events

Timing from Diagnosis

Central Venous Catheter

Therapy-Induced Thromboembolism

- Cancer surgery
- Immobilization
- Chemotherapy
- Hormonal treatment
- Tamoxifen
- Thalidomide
- Gemtuzumab ozogamicin
- Others (anti-vascular endothelial growth factor agents, cyclooxygenase 2 inhibitors, erythropoietin)

diagnosed concurrently or shortly after VTE tend to be more advanced and have poorer prognosis.[4]

IMMOBILIZATION

Immobilization from the illness or surgery increases the risk of VTE. In patients with cancer, the risk increases twofold compared with patients who do not have cancer.[5]

INDWELLING CENTRAL VENOUS CATHETERS

Central venous catheters (CVCs) are commonly used in oncology. Despite routine flushing with heparin or saline, 41% of CVCs result in thrombosis and increased risk of infection. Only one third of these clots are symptomatic. CVC-related thrombi cause pulmonary embolism (PE) in 11% of patients. Tumor type, chemotherapy agent administered, catheter type, and insertion site influence the risk of catheter-related thrombi.[6]

THERAPY-INDUCED THROMBOEMBOLISM

The elevated risk of VTE in cancer is worsened by common therapies and interventions (see Box 230-1). Cancer surgery doubles the risk of postoperative deep vein thrombosis (DVT). The risk of fatal PE is increased by threefold compared with patients who do not have cancer. Cancer is also an independent predictor of failure of VTE prophylaxis before surgery.[1] This finding implies that a more aggressive approach needs to be taken in cancer.

With regard to systemic therapies, different cancer agents are associated with a risk of thrombosis. Cytotoxic agents (platinum compounds, high-dose fluorouracil, mitomycin), hormone therapy, thalidomide, antiangiogenic agents, and erythropoietin all increase the risk of thrombosis.[7] The risk with systemic therapy, especially chemotherapeutic and hormone therapeutic agents, has been most carefully studied in breast cancer. Regimens such as CMF (cyclophosphamide, methotrexate, and 5-fluorouracil) and CAF (cyclophosphamide, doxorubicin, and 5-fluorouracil) are linked to higher rates (2% to 15%) of both arterial and venous thrombosis.[8] This rate increases 11- to 15-fold when tamoxifen (an estrogen receptor antagonist) is given concomitantly.[9] The mechanisms by which tamoxifen increases thrombosis are unclear.

Thalidomide, an angiogenesis inhibitor, administered alone in multiple myeloma is not highly thrombogenic (1%).[10] However, in association with other chemotherapeutic agents, the risk of DVT increases to 28% compared with chemotherapy alone.[11] Suggested VTE mechanisms from thalidomide/chemotherapy combination include protein C and S deficiency, acquired activated protein C resistance, elevated factor VIII and von Willebrand's factor (vWF), and antithrombin deficiency.[7]

HIT and HITT are paradoxical complications of heparin therapy. HIT is associated with platelet activation and consequent thrombosis. Thrombosis risk (both arterial and venous) is approximately 29%. The clinical presentation may vary from limb ischemia, DVT, PE, and angina to stroke.[7]

Erythropoietin (including its long-acting form), often used in malignant disease to treat secondary anemias, is linked to a 6% increase in the risk of VTE, especially with a fast rise in hemoglobin levels or when it reaches levels greater than 12 g/dL.[7,12]

Bleeding Disorders

Bleeding occurs in 6% to 10% of patients with advanced cancer.[13] Both solid tumors and hematological malignancies are associated with bleeding disorders (Box 230-2). Some malignant diseases predispose patients to bleeding more than others. In head and neck cancer, catastrophic bleeding from blood vessel invasion is always feared. The associated mortality can be up to 40%.[13] In lung cancer,

---

BOX 230-2 Causes of Bleeding in Advanced Cancer

Cancer Invasion and Destruction

- Head and neck: risk of catastrophic bleeding
- Lung: hemoptysis
- Gastrointestinal tract (gastric, rectal, stromal tumors): chronic bleeding
- Gynecological
- Metastatic disease (renal cell carcinoma, choriocarcinoma, melanoma)

Marrow Infiltration and Thrombocytopenia

- Leukemias (acute myelocytic leukemia)
- Lymphomas
- Prostate cancer

Treatment-Related Causes

- Mucositis (chemotherapy or radiation therapy, HPCT, GVHD)
- Thrombocytopenia
- Anticoagulation (warfarin, heparin)
- NSAIDs (aspirin)

Sequestrations (All Causes of Splenomegaly)

Disseminated Intravascular Coagulopathy

- Mucin-producing cancers
- Acute promyelocytic leukemia

Nutritional Deficiencies

Advanced Liver Disease

- Hepatocellular carcinoma
- Metastatic disease
- Liver failure

Acquired Factor VIII Inhibitors

- Lymphoproliferative disease
- Multiple myeloma

Acquired Von Willebrand's Disease

- Lymphoproliferative disease
- Wilms' tumor

GVHD, graft-versus-host disease; HPCT, hematopoietic progenitor cell transplantation; NSAIDs, nonsteroidal anti-inflammatory drugs.

whereas hemoptysis can be the presenting symptom in 7% to 10%, 20% of patients suffer from hemoptysis during their disease, and in 3% it is fatal.[14]

Gastrointestinal malignant diseases are more strongly associated with chronic than acute bleeding. Gastric and rectal malignant diseases can manifest with acute bleeding, a predictor of poor prognosis.

Metastatic tumors, especially highly vascular ones such as renal cell carcinoma, melanoma, and choriocarcinoma, carry a high risk of bleeding. Hepatocellular carcinoma and metastasis to the liver are associated with hemorrhage in 5% to 15% of cases.[13] This hemorrhage is often caused by acquired factor deficiency from decreased hepatocyte factor production.

In hematological malignancies, patients with acute myelogenous leukemia are at high risk of bleeding throughout their disease. This risk is often the result of combined disorders, such as thrombocytopenia and DIC.

Thrombocytopenia is defined as a platelet count lower than 100,000/μL. Platelet activation is observed in as many as 30% of patients with cancer.[3] In a study of intensive chemotherapy regimens for solid tumors, 49% of patients required platelet transfusion.[15] Major bleeding is rare when the platelet count is greater than 20,000/μL. Bleeding incidence increases gradually between 5000 and 20,000/μL, and it is more dramatic at counts lower than 5000/μL. When hemorrhage occurs at platelet counts greater than 5000/μL, it follows a decline in platelet count. No intracranial bleeding was observed at a platelet count of more than 10,000/μL or more.[15]

PATHOPHYSIOLOGY

Hemostasis is a tightly regulated and complex physiological process (Fig. 230-1). Any imbalances can lead to either clotting or bleeding disorders (Fig. 230-2; see Chapters 85 and 86).

Pathophysiology of Cancer-Associated Thrombosis

The pathogenesis of cancer-related VTE is complex and arises from interactions between the tumor and components of the hemostatic system. Stasis, vascular injury, and hypercoagulable changes of the blood are all involved.

Pathogenesis of Cancer Hypercoagulable States

A hypercoagulable state shown by laboratory tests is found in 50% to 70% of patients with cancer.[2] Malignant cells induce abnormal activation of coagulation through molecules with procoagulant properties, such as TF, CP, and cytokines (see Fig. 230-2).[3]

TF, a 47-kDa transmembrane glycoprotein, is the principal blood coagulation activator (see Fig. 230-1; Chapter 85). TF forms a complex with activated factor VII (VIIa). This factor, in turn, activates factor X. Under normal conditions, TF is expressed only in perivascular tissues (i.e., not by endothelial cells). On vascular injury, perivascular tissue TF comes in contact with blood, which activates the TF (extrinsic and common) coagulation cascade (see Fig. 230-1). In cancer, TF expression in endothelial cells and monocytes can be induced indirectly by tumor cells through pro-inflammatory cytokines such as interleukin-1β (IL-1β) and tumor necrosis factor-α (TNF-α).[16] TF is expressed by many malignant tumors. Vascular endothelial growth factor (VEGF), a proangiogenic cytokine secreted by tumor cells, increases vascular permeability. As a result, coagulation factors may be transported to the peritumor space with consequent coagulation cascade activation.[3]

CP, a 68-kDa cysteine proteinase expressed by multiple tumors, activates factor X directly, in the absence of factor VII activation. CP also induces platelet activation.

In summary, malignant cells directly (through expression of TF and CP) and indirectly (through cytokine secretion) induce a hypercoagulable state. Changes in the

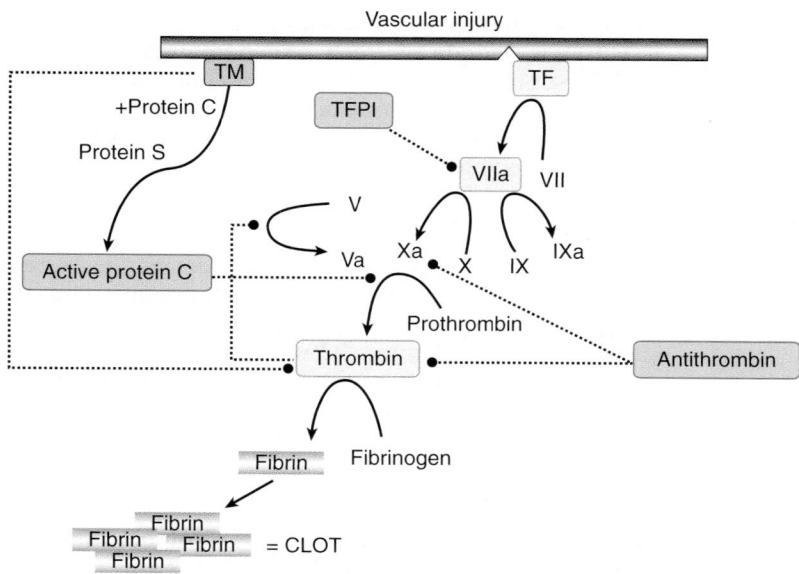

FIGURE 230-1 Tissue factor (TF; extrinsic and common) coagulation pathway. On vascular injury, TF is exposed to coagulation factors. TF forms a complex with activated factor VII, with consequent activation of factor X. Once activated, factor X induces thrombin formation, which results in fibrinogen cleavage into fibrin and clot formation. TFPI, tissue factor pathway inhibitor; TM, thrombomodulin. *Dashed lines* indicate inhibitory mechanisms. *Full arrows* indicate stimulatory and activating mechanisms.

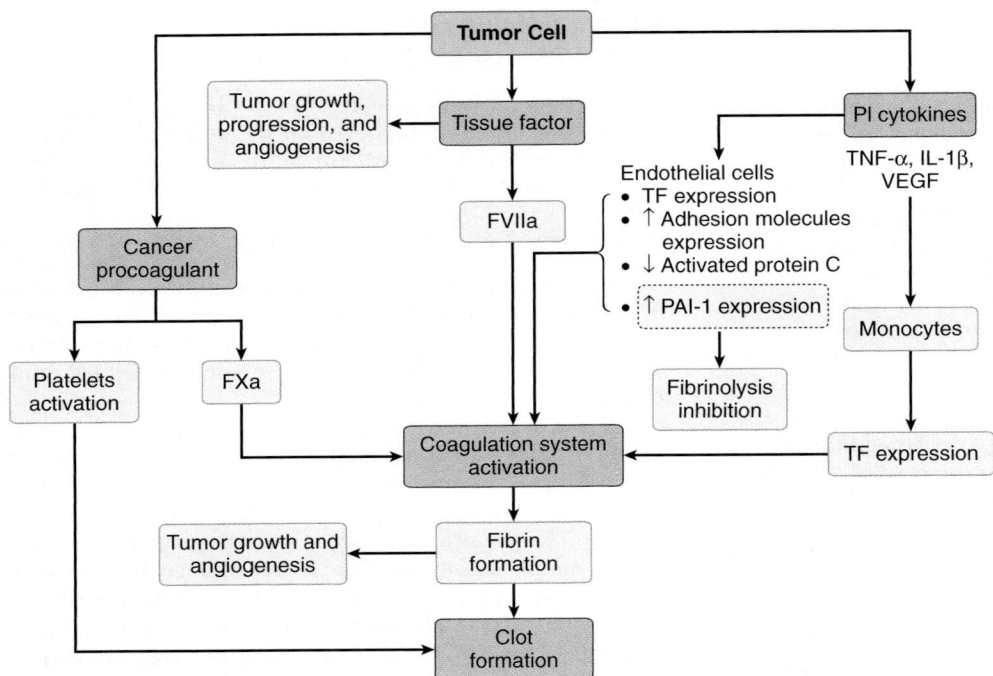

FIGURE 230-2 Pathogenesis of hypercoagulable states in cancer. FVIIa, factor VIIa; FXa, factor Xa; IL-1β, interleukin-1β; PAI-1, plasminogen activator inhibitor-1; PI, pro-inflammatory; TF, tissue factor; TNF-α, tumor necrosis factor-α; VEGF, vascular endothelial growth factor.

anticoagulant system, such as decreased activation of TF pathway inhibitor (TFPI), antithrombin, and components of the protein C pathway, could lead to abnormal termination of coagulation and hypercoagulation in patients with cancer.[17]

Stasis

Venous stasis is frequent in cancer. It can be caused by tumor expansion, with blood vessel compression, or by immobilization resulting from illness, surgery, treatment, or other complications (e.g., fractures). When venous stasis occurs, activated coagulation factors are highly concentrated in a limited area. Hypoxia from stasis induces endothelial damage and predisposes to procoagulant changes.[5]

Vascular Injury

Tumor invasion, chemotherapy, radiation therapy, intravenous catheters, and surgery induce vascular damage either directly or through induction of an inflammatory response and consequent endothelial dysfunction.

Pathophysiology of Cancer-Related Bleeding

Bleeding may result from local invasion or injury or systemic abnormalities (see Box 230-2).

Cancer Invasion and Destruction

Tumors expand through tissues of least resistance, such as blood vessels and lymphatics. Malignant tumors produce many factors to favor their growth such as angiogenesis factors (e.g., VEGF). They promote tumor neoangiogenesis and vascularization and predispose to bleeding.[13]

Treatment-Related Causes

Mucositis, a frequent adverse effect of high-dose radiation therapy or chemotherapy, is the second most frequent dose-limiting factor for some chemotherapy agents. Gastrointestinal tract mucositis of the affects up to 100% of patients who are receiving high-dose chemotherapy for hematopoietic stem cell transplantation and in 80% of patients with head and neck cancer who undergo radiation therapy.[18]

These therapeutic modalities damage the gastrointestinal tract through free radical production, with consequent inflammation and pro-inflammatory cytokine production. This process increases epithelial vascularization and vascular breakdown.[19]

Bone marrow transplantation (see Chapter 229), especially the allogenic type associated with graft-versus-host disease, may induce nonmucositis bleeding in cancer such as epistaxis, bloody diarrhea, and hemorrhagic cystitis. Graft-versus-host disease activates immune effector cells and pro-inflammatory cytokine production with multiple organ tissue damage with increased risk of a more pronounced bleeding.[13]

Thrombocytopenia

Bleeding from thrombocytopenia in cancer can be related to impaired production from myelosuppressive chemotherapy or radiation therapy or to tumor bone marrow infiltration (see Chapter 229). Thrombocytopenia in cancer may also result from splenic sequestration, immune-mediated thrombocytopenia, or increased platelet destruction related to DIC or microangiopathic anemia.

DRUG-INDUCED THROMBOCYTOPENIA

Many common drugs can induce thrombocytopenia. Heparin (particularly unfractionated heparin [UFH]), quinine, quinidine, trimethoprim-sulfamethoxazole, gold, valproic acid, thiazide diuretics, alcohol, and estrogens have all been implicated.[20]

Two types of HIT can occur. Heparin-associated thrombocytopenia (HAT) results from nonimmune mechanisms. It occurs 1 to 4 days after UFH administration, and it happens in 10% to 20% of patients. Platelets do not decrease to less than 100,000/μL, and no hemorrhagic or thrombotic complications occur. In most patients, platelets return to normal even when heparin is continued. HIT is more dramatic. It occurs in 1% to 3% of patients who receive UFH. LMWH is less likely to cause HIT as a first-line anticoagulant, but cross-reactivity with UFH-induced antibodies is nearly 100%. LMWH use in a patient who developed this complication is not recommended.[20]

Thirty percent to 80% of HIT cases manifest with thrombotic events. Fatal PE occurs in 25%. HIT results from antibody-mediated mechanisms (immunoglobulin G antibodies directed against heparin and platelet factor 4) 5 to 10 days after heparin therapy is begun. This time may be shorter in patients with previous heparin exposure. The platelet count typically decreases to less than 150,000/μL or a drop of more than 50% from baseline. It may drop as low as 50,000 to 60,000/μL.[20] The risk of bleeding from thrombocytopenia depends not only on the platelet count, but also the underlying disease, the use of drugs interfering with platelet function,[21] and complications such as fever, infection, or coagulation abnormalities.[15]

Coagulation Disturbances

In advanced cancer, bleeding can result from coagulation abnormalities associated with DIC, primary or secondary fibrinolysis, drug adverse effects, acquired coagulation factor deficiencies or inhibitors, and liver disease.

DIC arises from simultaneous increased systemic fibrin formation (hypercoagulable state), impairment of counter-regulatory anticoagulation mechanisms, and insufficient fibrinolysis. The combination results in multiple thrombi in small and midsize vessels, with consequent platelet and coagulation factor consumption. DIC can be mild (non-overt), a pure laboratory diagnosis, with slow thrombi generation and mild platelet and coagulation factor consumption. It can also be acute and dramatic, with massive thrombotic and hemostatic product consumption, possibly precipitated by sepsis, chemotherapy, and radiation therapy or disease progression. The exact mechanisms for this sudden change in DIC severity are unknown.[22]

Thrombocytopenic thrombotic purpura (TTP) results from disseminated microvascular thrombi, platelet aggregates with large amounts of vWF and little or no fibrin, which distinguish it from DIC.[22] The pathogenesis is a severe deficiency of vWF-cleaving protease ADAMTS13. Many multimers of vWF accumulate and thus induce platelet aggregation. TTP is seen in metastatic disease. Certain chemotherapy agents, particularly cyclosporine, mitomycin, cisplatin, gemcitabine, and the combination of cisplatin and bleomycin, are implicated in thrombotic microangiopathy. Drug-induced microangiopathy resembles hemolytic uremic syndrome (HUS) rather than TTP.[7,22]

Acquired factor VIII inhibitor is associated with progression of malignant disease. It is caused by an antibody against factor VIII, although the pathogenesis is still unclear.

Other Causes

In advanced cancer, nutritional deficiencies resulting from malnutrition or malabsorption and liver disease (see Chapter 84) contribute to bleeding. Patients with advanced cancer in palliative medicine are often receiving multiple medications. For a patient who is bleeding, review all medications the patient is taking. Many agents, including nonsteroidal anti-inflammatory drugs, penicillin, β-blockers, tricyclic antidepressants, and some chemotherapy agents, affect platelet function.[21] A hospice audit of anticoagulant use (warfarin [Coumadin]) showed frequent bleeding and difficulty in maintaining an international normalized ratio (INR).[13] LMWH was recommended for DVT and PE.

BASIC SCIENCE

Tumor cells can activate the coagulation system. Fibrin, the final product of clotting activation (see Fig. 230-1), may be directly involved in tumor growth, neoangiogenesis, and metastasis. Inappropriate TF expression affects tumor behavior. The tight connection between tumor behavior and hypercoagulation suggests that anticoagulants may have antineoplastic properties.

Heparins inhibit cancer metastasis. Retrospective clinical data suggest that this may be true in human cancer. Does this effect translate into an improvement in survival? Results are conflicting, with some evidence of survival benefit for heparin therapy, but no benefit with vitamin K antagonists. Of particular interest, the survival benefit was observed long after active anticoagulant administration, a finding suggesting that these drugs not only prevent and treat thrombosis, but also may affect tumor biology. Basic research (Box 230-3) suggests that heparins have antineoplastic effects, and these agents interfere with tumor cell invasion and metastasis through interaction with integrins and selectins.[1]

CLINICAL DIAGNOSIS

"Case Study: Disseminated Intravascular Coagulopathy" illustrates the clinical and laboratory features of DIC (see Chapters 85 and 86).

Thrombosis in Cancer

Symptoms

DVT and PE are the most common VTE-related cancer complications. Patients with cancer often present with typical VTE symptoms, but sometimes the clinical presentation is nonspecific because of associated cancer-related symptoms such as dyspnea with hypoxia and lymphedema (Table 230-1). Arterial thrombosis is rare compared with venous thrombosis and is often the result of nonbacterial thrombotic endocarditis or DIC.[23]

Diagnosis

Clinical symptoms and physical findings are nonspecific. Objective diagnostic testing is needed to confirm or exclude VTE. The same diagnostic paradigm in patients who do not have cancer is valid for cancer. In palliative

Basic Research: Effects of Heparins on Tumor Biology*

- The antiproliferative effects of heparins result from inhibition of proto-oncogene (c-fos, c-myc) expression by alterations in the protein kinase C pathway.
- Heparins affect leukocyte adhesion to endothelium at sites of tumor invasion.
- Heparins inhibit metastasis by rendering cancer cells more vulnerable to the cytotoxic effects of natural killer cells.
- Heparins affect angiogenesis by modulating the expression and function of angiogenic growth factors and inhibitors.
- Heparins restrain cell migration by inhibiting cell adhesion to extracellular matrix proteins.

Clinical Research: Heparins and Survival in Cancer Patient†

The following two randomized controlled trials were conducted in patients with various types of cancer but without underlying thrombosis:

- *FAMOUS study*: Effect of dalteparin on survival (N = 385). Dalteparin was associated with a modest survival advantage (not statistically significant). However, a significant increase in survival was observed in patients with a good prognosis who received dalteparin.
- *MALT study*: Effect of nadroparin on survival (N = 302). A modest but significant survival benefit was observed among patients treated with nadroparin when compared with the control group. The beneficial effect on survival was more evident among patients in whom life expectancy at entry was at least 6 months.

FAMOUS, Fragmin Advance Malignancy Outcome Study; MALT, Malignancy and LMWH Therapy Study.
**Data from Castelli R, Porro F, Torsia P. The heparins and cancer: Review of clinical trials and biological properties. Vasc Med 2004;9:205-213.*
†Data from Piccioli A, Falanga A, Baccaglini U, et al. Cancer and venous thromboembolism. Semin Thromb Hemost 2006;32:694-699.

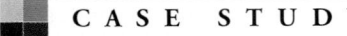

CASE STUDY

Disseminated Intravascular Coagulopathy

EF, a 61-year-old man with hormone-refractory prostate cancer and bone metastases, presented with extensive chest wall bruises, bleeding at venipuncture sites, gingival hemorrhage, and epistaxis. His platelet count was 54,000/μL (normal range, 130,000 to 400,000/μL), and his fibrinogen value was 0.09 g/L (normal range, 2 to 5 g/L). The activated partial thromboplastin time (aPTT) was 60 seconds (normal range, 28 to 38 seconds). Further studies showed a positive D-dimer test (D-dimer > 500 ng/mL). Soluble fibrin monomers were also detected. Based on these laboratory results, a diagnosis of acute disseminated intravascular coagulopathy (DIC) was made. The prostate-specific antigen level was 269 μg/L (normal range, 0 to 4 μg/L). Intravenous (IV) high-dose diethylstilbestrol diphosphate, 1 g/day for 5 days, was started. He also received packed red blood cells, platelets, and fibrinogen. The patient improved within 2 weeks of treatment, with a platelet count increase to 96,000/μL. Fibrinogen and clotting times had returned to normal. The patient received three cycles of diethylstilbestrol diphosphate. Once treatment was stopped, blood analysis suggested recurrence of DIC while the patient was clinically asymptomatic, with a platelet count of 19,000/μL, fibrinogen of 1.1 g/L and aPTT of 54 seconds. The patient responded to IV high-dose diethylstilbestrol diphosphate. However, several weeks later, he was readmitted with ecchymoses and gingival hemorrhage. Laboratory analyses confirmed recurrence of DIC. The patient was started on a new cycle of diethylstilbestrol diphosphate. Two days later, he died of cerebromeningeal bleeding.

Adapted from de la Fouchardiere C, Flechon A, Droz JP. Coagulopathy in prostate cancer. Neth J Med 2003;61:347-354

medicine, investigation is also guided by the symptom burden, performance status, and goals of care.

Contrast venography is the gold standard test; however, it has many drawbacks (cost, invasiveness, difficulty to perform and interpret, risk of further thrombosis). Duplex ultrasound is often preferred. A negative test in a highly suggestive symptomatic patient requires further evaluation with contrast venography. Duplex ultrasound is less reliable in asymptomatic, distal, and recurrent DVT.[23] Magnetic resonance angiography (MRA) is a noninvasive and accurate method for detecting thrombosis. It correlates well with contrast venography. MRA also provides more complete evaluation of central veins and blood flow, as well as adjacent structures, of great value in the differential diagnosis. If available, MRA may be preferred to contrast venography.

For diagnosis of PE, investigations include venous perfusion lung scans, venous ultrasonography, and D-dimer testing. Spiral computed tomography (CT) is specific and reliable but does not visualize subsegmental vessels. In a patient with a negative spiral CT scan but a highly suggestive history and symptoms, pulmonary arteriography is necessary.

With regard to hypercoagulation markers, high-sensitivity D-dimer assay has a high negative predictive value for DVT and PE. A negative D-dimer assay in patients with cancer is less reliable than in patients who do not have cancer.[23] Elevated fibrinogen, fibrin degradation products, fibrinopeptide A, prothrombin activation fragments 1 and 2, and thrombin antithrombin complexes are common in cancer but are not necessary for diagnosis.[2]

Specific Clinical Syndromes

UPPER EXTREMITY DEEP VEIN THROMBOSIS

Cancer is an independent predictor of upper extremity DVT. CVC use increases this risk twofold[24] and accounts for 75% of upper extremity DVT cases.[25] Swelling and extremity discomfort are the most frequent symptoms reported in upper extremity DVT. Other symptoms include erythema, a heavy and hot limb, and new visible veins at the shoulder girdle. CVC-related thrombi, however, are often asymptomatic and may be revealed only during a complication such as PE or sepsis. Physical signs are nonspecific and may occur in patients with cancer who have lymphedema, neoplastic compression of blood vessels, or postoperative muscle injury. Objective testing may be required.[26] Duplex ultrasound is the imaging test of choice. It has high sensitivity and specificity for peripheral (jugular, distal subclavian, axillary) upper extremity DVTs. False-

TABLE 230-1 Differential Diagnosis of Major Clotting and Bleeding Disorders in Cancer

DISORDER	DIFFERENTIAL DIAGNOSIS
DEEP VEIN THROMBOSIS	Localized muscle strain or contusion
	Bone fracture (metastasis, multiple myeloma)
	Baker's cyst: rupture/obstruction of popliteal vein
	Achilles tendon rupture
	Cellulitis
	Lymphedema from lymphatic obstruction
	Reflex sympathetic dystrophy
	Retroperitoneal fibrosis obstructing iliac vein or inferior vena cava
	May-Thurner syndrome: compression of left iliac vein by right common iliac artery
	Edema secondary to heart, liver, or kidney failure
PULMONARY EMBOLISM	**Cardiopulmonary Disorders**
	Dyspnea or tachypnea suggest
	Atelectasis
	Infection: pneumonia, bronchitis
	Pneumothorax
	Acute pulmonary edema
	Acute bronchial obstruction
	Pleuritic chest pain or hemoptysis suggest
	Infection: pneumonia, bronchitis, tuberculosis
	Pneumothorax
	Bronchiectasis
	Pericarditis
	Diaphragmatic inflammation
	Myositis, muscle strain
	Rib fracture
	Right-sided heart failure presentation:
	Myocardial infarction
	Myocarditis
	Cardiac tamponade
	Cardiovascular collapse suggests
	Myocardial infarction
	Acute massive hemorrhage
	Gram-negative septicemia
	Cardiac tamponade
	Spontaneous pneumothorax
DISSEMINATED INTRAVASCULAR COAGULOPATHY	Primary fibrinolysis
	Liver disease
	Vitamin K deficiency
	Sepsis
	Thrombotic thrombocytopenic purpura

negative results are possible in the subclavian artery behind the clavicle. Contrast venography may be required to confirm a highly suspicious clinical presentation of upper extremity DVT with negative duplex ultrasound. MRA may replace contrast venography. PE (36%), recurrent VTE (10%), superior vena cava syndrome, and post-thrombotic syndrome (27.3% at 2 years) are the main complications of upper extremity DVT.[24] The incidence of these complications is significantly associated with the treatment strategy used.

TROUSSEAU'S SYNDROME

Migratory superficial thrombophlebitis is a spectrum of unexplained thrombotic events ranging from thrombosis to a platelet-rich microthrombotic process that precedes diagnosis of occult visceral malignant disease.[27] It is also a manifestation of chronic DIC. This syndrome results from complex pathways leading to a hypercoagulable state. It is associated with many tumors, mainly mucin-producing carcinomas. Trousseau's syndrome is often the reason to investigate for underlying malignant disease.

BUDD-CHIARI SYNDROME

This syndrome is characterized by hepatic outflow obstruction at any level from the hepatic venules to the right atrium, regardless of the cause of obstruction. It is often associated with myeloproliferative disorders. Up to 25% of patients are asymptomatic. If the syndrome is untreated, the mortality rate is close to 80%.[28] Clinically, most patients present with hepatomegaly, right upper quadrant pain, and ascites, although the intensity of symptoms at presentation (acute and fulminate versus subacute) varies depending on the rapidity with which hepatic outflow occlusion occurs. The most common presentation is a subacute form with minimal ascites and hepatic necrosis. A subgroup may present with end-stage liver disease and portal hypertension.[28]

The diagnosis of Budd-Chiari syndrome can be made on radiological findings alone. Doppler ultrasound, CT, and magnetic resonance imaging (MRI) can all be used. Ultrasonography is the initial test of choice, but CT and MRI allow better assessment of hepatic perfusion. Radiological imaging (see Chapter 101) allows not only diagnosis, but also information used in planning therapy for patients.[29]

MARANTIC ENDOCARDITIS

This disorder is also known as nonbacterial thrombotic endocarditis. It is characterized by sterile vegetations of fibrin and platelets on the cardiac valves. Marantic endocarditis can be associated with any malignant disease (except brain tumors), especially mucin-secreting adenocarcinomas. It is believed to be part of Trousseau's syndrome, and DIC is thought to represent the underlying pathological process. The diagnosis is mainly made by echocardiography, even though this method cannot reliably differentiate the condition from infective endocarditis.[30] Proposed diagnostic criteria are as follows:

- Presence of heart murmurs
- Evidence of multiple systemic emboli
- An underlying disease known as a predisposing condition
- Echocardiographic evidence of a valvular lesion
- Serial negative blood cultures

Bleeding Disorders in Cancer

Diagnosis

It is important to identify patients at risk for bleeding and to resolve the risk factors before bleeding happens (see Box 230-2). When bleeding occurs, the severity (site, extent, and tempo) and the risk of recurrence will dictate management.

Bleeding in cancer can manifest as acute catastrophic hemorrhage, as episodic recurrent bleeding, and as chronic blood loss or low-volume oozing. Some clinical presentations can suggest the cause of the bleeding. Petechiae, ecchymoses, and mucosal bleeding suggest a platelet disorder or acquired von Willebrand's disease. Clotting factor deficiencies and inhibitors are suspected in patients with skin and muscle hematomas. Persistent venipuncture site bleeding is pathognomonic for DIC.[31] Other clinical presentations include hematochezia, melena, hemoptysis, hematuria, epistaxis, vaginal bleeding, and nonhealing ulcerated skin lesions. In frank external bleeding (e.g., hemoptysis, hematemesis), endoscopy can be both diagnostic and therapeutic (see Chapter 98). Because platelets have a life span of only 10 days, signs of thrombocytopenia are observed early. Mucosal or cutaneous bleeding with epistaxis, gingival bleeding, large bullous buccal mucosal hemorrhages, petechiae, and superficial ecchymoses can all be observed.[20]

In advanced cancer and in palliative medicine, patients are often receiving multiple medications. Determining whether thrombocytopenia is drug related and pinpointing the causative agent can be a challenge.[20]

After a careful history, physical examination, and review of medications, an initial platelet count with a peripheral blood smear can be very informative:[20]

- Schistocytes suggest microangiopathy or macroangiopathy.
- Tear drops, nucleated red blood cells, and immature granulocyte precursors suggest bone marrow replacement by abnormal tissue.

Other key laboratory studies are as follows (Table 230-2):

- A platelet function test is indicated if the platelet count is higher than 100,000/μL.
- Together, the activated thromboplastin time (aPTT) and the prothrombin time (PT) allow differentiation of TF and intrinsic pathways abnormalities. aPTT investigates the intrinsic and common coagulation pathway.
- Fibrinogen, D-dimer (or fibrin degradation products), and a clot lysis test are indicated.
- Any screening test abnormalities will prompt more specific tests:[31]
  - Bone marrow examination is used to determine the cause of thrombocytopenia.
  - Platelet aggregation tests are conducted using different agonists for abnormal platelet function.

- The mixing test to detect coagulation inhibitors differentiates clotting factor deficiency from anticoagulants. It also guides decision making about whether a transfusion will stop a hemorrhage.

Specific Clinical Presentations

DISSEMINATED INTRAVASCULAR COAGULOPATHY

DIC is a hypercoagulable state with excess consumption of platelet and coagulation factors. The diagnosis of DIC is based on a precipitating factor or disease, clinical presentation, and laboratory tests. The clinical presentation varies:[22]

- Nonovert DIC, which is asymptomatic and is diagnosed on the basis of laboratory tests alone (e.g., during anticoagulation, an impaired warfarin dose adjustment could be the first sign of underlying nonovert DIC)
- Multiple thrombotic events (i.e., Trousseau's syndrome)
- Minor perioperative bleeding
- Severe DIC with life-threatening hemorrhage, disseminated thrombi, shock, and multiple organ failure

Laboratory tests to diagnose DIC include platelet count, fibrin-related markers such as fibrin/fibrinogen-degradation products, D-dimer, PT, aPTT, and fibrinogen level (see Table 230-2).[22] Abnormal laboratory assays suggestive of DIC (see Table 230-2) are as follows:

- Thrombocytopenias usually lower than 100,000/μL
- Clotting times (PT and aPTT) prolonged in 70% and 50% of patients, respectively
- In severe DIC, decreased fibrinogen levels (50% of cases only)

Fibrinolytic activation is characterized by the following:

- Increased fibrin/fibrinogen-degradation products (85% to 100% of DIC). This test reflects both fibrin and fibrinogen degradation.
- A positive D-dimer assay. This test reflects fibrin (not fibrinogen) degradation, which makes it more reliable for DIC diagnosis.
- Other tests. Prothrombin fragments 1 + 2 and fibrinopeptide A reflect procoagulant activity; plasma antithrombin and protein C can be decreased. When

---

TABLE 230-2 Laboratory Findings in Major Cancer-Related Bleeding and Clotting Disorders

DISORDER	PLATELET COUNT	PT	aPTT	D-DIMER	FIBRINOGEN	OTHERS
Thrombotic event	−	−	−	+	−	↓ Antithrombin ↓ Protein C
DIC						
Overt	↓	↑	↑	+	↓	Schistocytes
Nonovert	↓	slight ↑	−	+	−	
TTP	↓	−	−	−		Neurological involvement ADAMTS13 ↓
HUS	↓	−	−	−		Kidney involvement

aPTT, activated partial thromboplastin time; DIC, disseminated intravascular coagulopathy; HUS, hemolytic uremic syndrome; PT, prothrombin time; TTP, thrombotic thrombocytopenic purpura.
+, positive test; ↓, decreased values; ↑, increased values; −, No change.

present, these abnormalities are highly suggestive of DIC. They predict poor prognosis; the presence of schistocytes is helpful but not essential for diagnosis.

THROMBOTIC THROMBOCYTOPENIC PURPURA

TTP is a type of thrombotic microangiopathy characterized by fever, neurological abnormalities, renal failure, thrombocytopenia, and microangiopathic hemolytic anemia.[22] Laboratory investigations confirm hemolytic anemia and thrombocytopenia and show the presence of schistocytes and elevated lactate dehydrogenase levels. In its acute form, ADAMTS13 activity is low, and antibodies to ADAMTS13 may be detected.[22]

ACQUIRED FACTOR VIII INHIBITOR

The diagnosis is suspected in patients with unexplained bleeding. Laboratory tests show prolonged aPTT and normal PT. This inhibitor is easily distinguished from DIC by a normal platelet count, normal PT, and normal fibrinogen level. Decreased factor VIII clotting activity and the presence of factor VIII inhibitors confirm the diagnosis.

HEPARIN-INDUCED THROMBOCYTOPENIA

HIT should be suspected in anyone receiving heparin who presents with a decrease of pretreatment platelet count of 50% or more compared with pretreatment values. If this decrease is before the fifth day, it is unlikely to be HIT. To detect heparin-platelet-associated antibodies, the serotonin release assay is the gold standard, although the heparin-induced platelet aggregation assay and the antiplatelet factor 4 enzyme-linked immunosorbent assay are more commonly performed because of availability and ease of use.[20]

DIFFERENTIAL DIAGNOSIS

The differential diagnosis of bleeding and clotting disorders in cancer is the same as in the general population. However, patients with cancer are often polysymptomatic (see Table 230-1 and Chapters 85 and 86).

DIC and primary fibrinolysis are differentiated based on the absence of D-dimers, normal platelet count, and antithrombin level in primary fibrinolysis. DIC is distinguished from TTP based on normal coagulation times in TTP. Unlike HUS, TTP is characterized by the predominance of neurological manifestations, whereas renal abnormalities are more predominant in HUS. ADAMTS13 level is elevated in TTP while normal in HUS.

MANAGEMENT

Management should always be oriented to the goal of care (see Chapters 85, 86, and 90).

Clotting Disorders

Management of VTE in cancer is similar to management of VTE in patients who do not have cancer. The following issues are particular to cancer:[23]

- Anticoagulation in a population with a high risk of bleeding. This issue raises the question of when to opt for inferior vena cava filters.

- Anticoagulation in patients with short survival or poor prognosis.

The benefits of anticoagulation are lower symptom burden, decreased morbidity and complications, and possibly increased survival. Benefits need to outweigh the side effects and risks of anticoagulation.

Prophylaxis

Little rationale exists to subject all patients with cancer to thromboprophylaxis (see Box 230-1) unless they have additional risks such as surgery or recurrent thrombosis.[5] On a case-to-case basis, mechanical or systemic prophylaxis is indicated. Mechanical prophylaxis involves graduated compression stockings or intermittent pneumatic compression boots. LMWH is replacing traditional anticoagulants (Fig. 230-3). In a systematic review[32] of 55 randomized controlled trials of DVT prophylaxis in patients with cancer who were undergoing surgery, higher doses of LMWH were more effective than lower doses (14% versus 8%) in preventing DVTs, with no increase in complications. Prophylaxis was discontinued because of bleeding in 3% of patients. No difference was shown between LMWH and UFH in efficacy, DVT locations, or bleeding complications. The convenience of fewer injections a day, lower risk of HIT with LMWH, less stringent monitoring, and feasibility as an outpatient treatment may justify the use of LMWH despite the drug's higher cost (Table 230-3). For prophylaxis of VTE in medical patients, the daily recommended dose of UFH is 5000 IU every 8 to 12 hours. For LMWHs, enoxaparin is recommended at 40 mg/day and dalteparin 5000 IU/day.[33]

Treatment

ACUTE TREATMENT OF VENOUS THROMBOEMBOLISM

UFH and LMWH are the treatment of choice for acute VTE (see Table 230-3). Initially, UFH may be administered as a standard bolus of 5000 IU, followed by an infusion to maintain the aPTT (aPTT is usually 2.0× control). Weight-based heparin administration uses a loading dose of 80 IU/kg with a maintenance infusion of 18 IU/kg/hour. The most widely used laboratory test for heparin therapy is the aPTT (see Table 230-3). Oral warfarin, 5 mg, can be started on day 1 after a stable dose of heparin achieves therapeutic aPTT.[33] Three LMWHs (dalteparin, enoxaparin, and tinzaparin) are currently approved for VTE in the United States.

For acute VTE in cancer, the recommended dose depends on the LMWH used. Different LMWHs are separate drugs and should not be used interchangeably:

- For dalteparin: 200 IU/kg daily for 1 month, followed by 150 IU/kg daily for 5 months
- For enoxaparin: 1.5 mg/kg daily for 6 months
- For tinzaparin: 175 IU/kg daily until the patient is adequately anticoagulated with warfarin

Despite the durations specified, patients with cancer may require indefinite anticoagulation. Although HIT is less frequent with LMWH, platelet counts must still be checked every few days. LMWH treatment may be stopped after at least 5 days of continued warfarin treatment when the INR is greater than 2.0 on two consecutive measure-

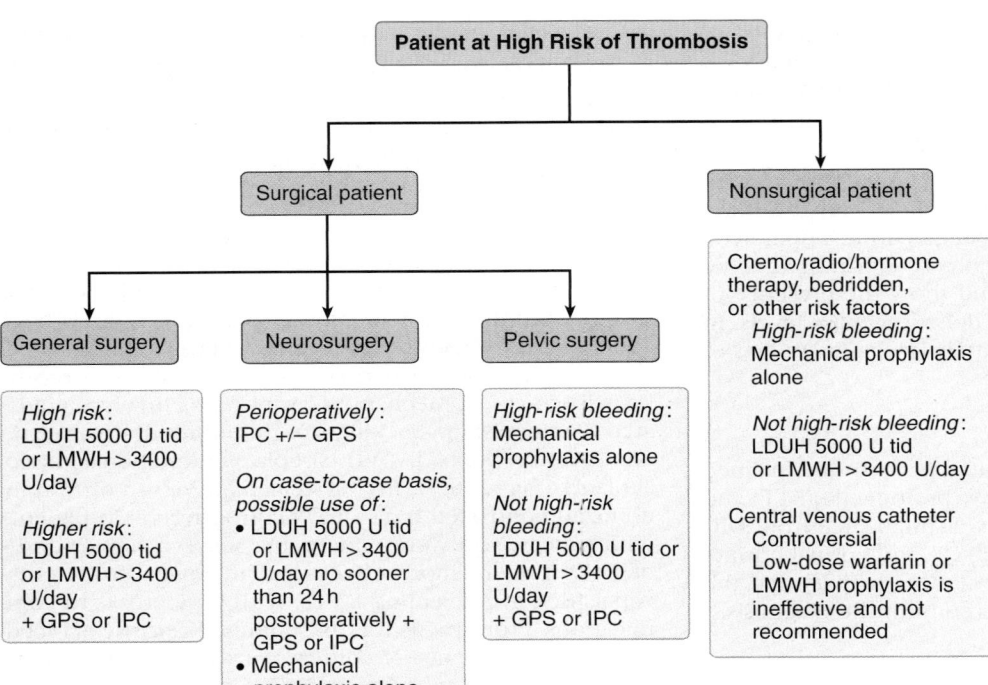

FIGURE 230-3 Evidence-based medicine of thrombosis prophylaxis in highest-risk patients with cancer. GPS, graduated compression stockings; IPC, intermittent pneumatic compression boots; LDUH, low-dose unfractionated heparin; LMWH, low-molecular-weight heparin. (*Data from Adess M, Eisner R, Nand S, et al. Thromboembolism in cancer patients: Pathogenesis and treatment. Clin Appl Thromb Hemost 2006;12:254-266.*)

TABLE 230-3 Comparison of the Main Antithrombotic Agents

AGENT	UFH	LMWH	WARFARIN
SHORT DESCRIPTION	Glycosaminoglycan MW 3-30 kDa Faster clearance and low bioavailability Anticoagulation less predictable	MW 1-10 kDa Longer clearance and bioavailability Anticoagulation more predictable	Vitamin K antagonist
MODE OF ACTION	Binds to AT Inhibits factor Xa and thrombin equally Anti-Xa to anti-IIa of 1:1 Binds to platelets: induces or inhibits aggregation	Preferentially inhibits factor Xa Anti-Xa to anti-IIa of 4:1 to 2:1	Inhibits production of functional vitamin K–dependent clotting factors
MONITORING	**aPTT** Every 6 hr initially or after dose change Once daily when stable drug level is reached Therapeutic target aPTT equivalent to anti-Xa 0.3-0.7 U/mL **Daily Platelet Count**	Platelets every few days No routine monitoring required unless kidney failure therapeutic target: anti-Xa 0.3-0.7 U/mL	INR derived from PT: 2.0-3.0 is safer
MAJOR SIDE EFFECTS AND SPECIAL CONSIDERATIONS	Higher risk of HIT High bleeding risk Osteopenia Alopecia Low cost	Lower risk of HIT Low bleeding risk Osteopenia less frequent High cost	Excessive anticoagulation with risk of bleeding Skin necrosis

aPTT, activated partial thromboplastin time; AT, antithrombin; HIT, heparin-induced thrombocytopenia; INR, international normalized ratio; LMWH, low-molecular-weight heparin; MW, molecular weight; PT, prothrombin time; UFH, unfractionated heparin.
Data from Pruemer J. Treatment of cancer-associated thrombosis: Distinguishing among antithrombotic agents. Semin Oncol 2006;33(Suppl 4):S26-S39; quiz S41-S42.

ments 24 hours apart.[33] Because of the higher risk of recurrent DVTs related to the prolonged use of inferior vena cava filters, the use of these filters is limited for individuals with a high risk of bleeding such as gastrointestinal bleeding within 2 years, central nervous system metastasis (see Chapter 221), and recent neurosurgery.[23]

LONG-TERM ANTICOAGULATION

Clinical evidence indicates that warfarin treatment maintaining an INR of 2.0 to 3.0 is sufficient for prophylaxis of VTE while minimizing the associated hemorrhagic risk observed with higher INRs.[33] For long-term therapy, this risk can be lessened by lower warfarin doses while maintaining the INR between 1.5 and 2.0. Anticoagulant treatment for at least 6 months, and often indefinitely, is indicated for patients with cancer.[33] Maintaining a therapeutic INR in a patient receiving oral anticoagulants may be difficult in cancer.[5] Long-term LMWH treatment may be preferable to warfarin because of its ease of administration and reliable anticoagulant effect (see Table 230-3).

All patients undergoing long-term anticoagulation, particularly outpatients, need to understand the implications and risks of anticoagulation. These patients must be assessed for compliance and for signs and symptoms of bleeding, and they need to have contact information should questions arise.[33] Anticoagulation should be discontinued in patients on comfort care only and in cachectic patients with risk of excessive anticoagulation.[23]

Bleeding Disorders

Bleeding management begins by full assessment of the risk of bleeding (see Box 230-2) so preventive measures can be taken. Bleeding can be very distressing to both patients and their families. Discussing the possibility of bleeding in high-risk patients and having a plan of action in case a major bleeding event happens at home may decrease anxiety. Preparing family members involves the following: using dark basins and towels to lessen the psychological distress induced by the sight of blood; if bleeding is localized, instruct caregivers how to apply pressure; in massive hemoptysis, teach the caregiver how to position the patient and provide a sedative to reduce anxiety.[13] Midazolam (2.5 to 5.0 mg), a rapidly acting anxiolytic, can be administered subcutaneously or intravenously. Bleeding management needs to be individualized depending on the underlying disease, the possibility of reversing the cause, the treatment risk-to-benefit ratio, the prognosis, and the goals of care (see Chapter 86).[34]

Measures to manage bleeding include the following:[13]

- Local measures such as packing, compression dressings, topical hemostatics, postural positioning, radiation therapy, and palliative embolization
- Systemic measures including plasma products, platelet transfusions, vitamin K, vasopressin, recombinant factor VIIa, and antifibrinolytic agents

THROMBOCYTOPENIA

Prophylactic platelet transfusion therapy is an essential part of supportive oncology. It decreases the incidence of bleeding and prolongs survival. The cutoff point for platelet transfusions is 20,000/μL, but it is not justified by evidence-based medicine. Platelet transfusions have increased to exceed red blood cell transfusions. Platelet transfusions may be lifesaving in some patients, but unnecessary transfusions have deleterious consequences: alloimmunization in patients receiving multiple transfusions, bacterial infection with transfusion-transmitted pathogens, and increased health care costs.[35]

In 2001, the American Society for Clinical Oncology[35] issued new guidelines for platelet transfusion in cancer:

1. Prophylactic platelet transfusions should be administered to patients with thrombocytopenia resulting from impaired bone marrow function when the platelet count falls to less than a predefined thresh-

old. The transfusion threshold level varies according to diagnosis, clinical condition, and treatment modality.

2. A threshold of 10,000/μL for prophylactic platelet transfusion should be used in adults receiving therapy for acute leukemia and high-dose chemotherapy with stem cell support. Transfusion at higher levels may be necessary in newborns or in patients with hemorrhage, high fever, hyperleukocytosis, rapid fall in platelet count, and coagulation abnormalities (e.g., acute promyelocytic leukemia), as well as in patients undergoing invasive procedures or circumstances in which platelet transfusions may not be readily available in emergencies.

3. For solid tumors and chemotherapy-induced thrombocytopenia, a threshold of 10,000/μL for prophylactic platelet transfusion is appropriate. However, 20,000/μL should be used during aggressive therapy for bladder tumors and for patients with demonstrated necrotic tumors.

4. Patients with chronic, stable, severe thrombocytopenia (e.g., in myelodysplasia or aplastic anemia) can be observed, and platelet transfusions can be reserved for hemorrhage or during active treatment.

5. A platelet count of 40,000 to 50,000/μL is sufficient to perform major invasive procedures in the absence of associated coagulation abnormalities. Bone marrow biopsies and aspirates are safe in patients with counts lower than 20,000/μL.

Therapeutic platelet transfusion in bleeding should be on a case-to-case basis to control symptoms. One unit of platelets increases the platelet count by approximately 6000 to 10,000/μL in adults if no splenic sequestration is present. Four to 6 U are usually required to control bleeding.[34]

HEPARIN-INDUCED THROMBOCYTOPENIA

When HIT is strongly suspected, the following steps are recommended:[36]

1. All heparin products should to be stopped immediately, without waiting for laboratory confirmation.

2. A nonheparin alternative anticoagulant can be started. In the United States, two direct thrombin inhibitors (lepirudin and argatroban) are approved for HIT. Lepirudin, a recombinant hirudin, binds irreversibly with thrombin. Because it has no antidote, this agent should be avoided in patients with renal insufficiency. At first, lepirudin is administered as a bolus (0.4 mg/kg), followed by an initial infusion at 0.15 mg/kg/hour. The aPTT needs to be monitored every 4 hours until steady state (aiming for 1.5× to 2.5×). Anaphylaxis is described after intravenous boluses. Argatroban, unlike lepirudin, is not immunogenic. The recommended dose is 2 μg/kg/minute adjusted by aPTT (aiming for 1.5× to 3.0× baseline aPTT).

3. Postpone warfarin, pending on substantial platelet count increase.

4. Avoid prophylactic platelet transfusions.

5. Test for HIT antibodies, and investigate for DVTs.

DISSEMINATED INTRAVASCULAR COAGULOPATHY

A clear-cut management paradigm is not established. Treat the precipitating factor (sepsis, progression of cancer). These factors often are unclear, and only symptomatic management is possible. Few studies have been conducted in cancer, except in patients with Trousseau's syndrome. Anticoagulation is still debated for the thrombotic component of DIC. Low-dose heparin (300 to 500 U/hour) as a continuous infusion can be used. Other proposed therapeutic options include antithrombin replacement and protein C concentrates, and some investigators have used direct thrombin inhibitors in hematological malignancies. Severity of the bleeding, the platelet count, and sometimes coagulation factor levels will determine the need for blood components. In life-threatening bleeding, fresh-frozen plasma (15 mL/kg/body weight), rather than cryoprecipitates, can be given. No evidence suggests a role for prophylactic platelets or plasma in DIC. If the platelet count is lower than 50×10^9/L and in case of an invasive procedure, platelet transfusion may be considered.[22]

THROMBOTIC THROMBOCYTOPENIC PURPURA

Management of ADAMTS13 deficiency requires plasmapheresis with fresh-frozen plasma or cryoprecipitates infusion. In patients with high titers of inhibitor who are not responding to plasma exchange, glucocorticoid administration, vincristine, or splenectomy may be used. Platelet transfusion should be avoided because of the risk of worsening intravascular thrombosis.[22]

ACQUIRED FACTOR VIII INHIBITOR

Factor replacement, immunosuppressive drugs, and plasmapheresis are therapeutic options. Immunosuppressive drugs such as steroids, cyclophosphamide, cyclosporine, and azathioprine can achieve good responses, especially with low antibody titer. In acute bleeding, human or porcine factor VIII can be required. If hemorrhage persists, additional prothrombin-complex concentrates or recombinant factor VIIa (NovoSeven) is indicated. Rituximab in combination with cytotoxic therapies was recently used for active bleeding with high-titer factor VIII inhibitors.[22]

Palliative Medicine Considerations

The goal of care should be comfort. Invasive measures and procedures should be avoided. In some patients, it is unclear whether a local or systemic measure, such as platelet transfusion or an antifibrinolytic agent, will help. Anticoagulants should be reviewed, and if the burden is greater that the benefit, these drugs should be discontinued.

CONCLUSIONS

VTE and bleeding events frequently complicate cancer. While managing patients with advanced malignant disease, it is important to keep in mind the goals of care. It is improper to expose an already fragile patient to extra procedures or therapies if life expectancy is short. In these instances, quality of life and education of patients and their families are emphasized.

REFERENCES

1. De Lorenzo F, Dotsenko O, Scully MF, et al. The role of anticoagulation in cancer patients: Facts and figures. Anticancer Agents Med Chem 2006;6:579-587.
2. Hillen HF. Thrombosis in cancer patients. Ann Oncol 2000;11(Suppl 3):273-276.
3. Winter PC. The pathogenesis of venous thromboembolism in cancer: Emerging links with tumour biology. Hematol Oncol 2006;24:126-133.
4. Sorensen HT, Mellemkjaer L, Olsen JH, et al. Prognosis of cancers associated with venous thromboembolism. N Engl J Med 2000;343:1846-1850.
5. Piccioli A, Falanga A, Baccaglini U, et al. Cancer and venous thromboembolism. Semin Thromb Hemost 2006;32:694-699.
6. Kuter DJ. Thrombotic complications of central venous catheters in cancer patients. Oncologist 2004;9:207-216.
7. Adess M, Eisner R, Nand S, et al. Thromboembolism in cancer patients: Pathogenesis and treatment. Clin Appl Thromb Hemost 2006;12:254-266.
8. Prandoni P, Piccioli A. Venous thromboembolism and cancer: A two-way clinical association. Front Biosci 1997;2:e12-e20.
9. McCaskill-Stevens W, Wilson J, Bryant J, et al. Contralateral breast cancer and thromboembolic events in African American women treated with tamoxifen. J Natl Cancer Inst 2004;96:1762-1769.
10. Barlogie B, Desikan R, Eddlemon P, et al. Extended survival in advanced and refractory multiple myeloma after single-agent thalidomide: Identification of prognostic factors in a phase 2 study of 169 patients. Blood 2001;98:492-494.
11. Zangari M, Anaissie E, Barlogie B, et al. Increased risk of deep-vein thrombosis in patients with multiple myeloma receiving thalidomide and chemotherapy. Blood 2001;98:1614-1615.
12. Nand S, Wong W, Yuen B, et al. Heparin-induced thrombocytopenia with thrombosis: Incidence, analysis of risk factors, and clinical outcomes in 108 consecutive patients treated at a single institution. Am J Hematol 1997;56:12-16.
13. Prommer E. Management of bleeding in the terminally ill patient. Hematology 2005;10:167-175.
14. Kvale PA, Simoff M, Prakash UB, et al. Lung cancer: Palliative care. Chest 2003;123:284S-311S.
15. Avvisati G, Tirindelli MC, Annibali O. Thrombocytopenia and hemorrhagic risk in cancer patients. Crit Rev Oncol Hematol 2003;48:S13-S16.
16. Gagnon B, Mancini I, Pereira J, et al. Palliative management of bleeding events in advanced cancer patients. J Palliat Care 1998;14:50-54.
17. Nijziel MR, van Oerle R, Hillen HF, et al. From Trousseau to angiogenesis: The link between the haemostatic system and cancer. Neth J Med 2006;64:403-410.
18. Rubenstein EB, Peterson DE, Schubert M, et al. Clinical practice guidelines for the prevention and treatment of cancer therapy-induced oral and gastrointestinal mucositis. Cancer 2004;100:2026-2046.
19. Peterson DE, Cariello A. Mucosal damage: A major risk factor for severe complications after cytotoxic therapy. Semin Oncol 2004;31:35-44.
20. Drews RE. Critical issues in hematology: Anemia, thrombocytopenia, coagulopathy, and blood product transfusions in critically ill patients. Clin Chest Med 2003;24:607-622.
21. Kottke-Marchant K, Corcoran G. The laboratory diagnosis of platelet disorders. Arch Pathol Lab Med 2002;126:133-146.
22. de la Fouchardiere C, Flechon A, Droz JP. Coagulopathy in prostate cancer. Neth J Med 2003;61:347-354.
23. Davis MP. Hematology in palliative medicine. Am J Hosp Palliat Care 2004;21:445-454.
24. Bernardi E, Pesavento R, Prandoni P. Upper extremity deep venous thrombosis. Semin Thromb. Hemost. 2006;32:729-736.
25. Elman EE, Kahn SR. The post-thrombotic syndrome after upper extremity deep venous thrombosis in adults: A systematic review. Thromb Res 2006;117:609-614.
26. Joffe HV, Goldhaber SZ. Upper-extremity deep vein thrombosis. Circulation 2002;106:1874-1880.
27. Varki A. Trousseau's syndrome: Multiple definitions and multiple mechanisms. Blood 2007;110:1723-1729.
28. Zimmerman MA, Cameron AM, Ghobrial RM. Budd-Chiari syndrome. Clin Liver Dis 2006;10:259-273, viii.
29. Kamath PS. Budd-Chiari syndrome: Radiologic findings. Liver Transpl 2006;12(Suppl):S21-S22.
30. Eftychiou C, Fanourgiakis P, Vryonis E, et al. Factors associated with non-bacterial thrombotic endocarditis: Case report and literature review. J Heart Valve Dis 2005;14:859-862.
31. Green D. Management of bleeding complications of hematologic malignancies. Semin Thromb Hemost 2007;33:427-434.
32. Leonardi MJ, McGory ML, Ko CY. A systematic review of deep venous thrombosis prophylaxis in cancer patients: Implications for improving quality. Ann Surg Oncol 2007;14:929-936.
33. Pruemer J. Treatment of cancer-associated thrombosis: Distinguishing among antithrombotic agents. Semin Oncol 2006;33(Suppl 4):S26-S39; quiz S41-S42.
34. Pereira J, Phan T. Management of bleeding in patients with advanced cancer. Oncologist 2004;9:561-570.
35. Benjamin RJ, Anderson KC. What is the proper threshold for platelet transfusion in patients with chemotherapy-induced thrombocytopenia? Crit Rev Oncol Hematol 2002;42:163-171.

36. Warkentin TE. Heparin-induced thrombocytopenia: Diagnosis and management. Circulation 2004;110:e454-e458.

SUGGESTED READING

Burris HA 3rd. Low-molecular-weight heparins in the treatment of cancer-associated thrombosis: A new standard of care? Semin Oncol 2006;33(Suppl 4):S3-S16; quiz S41-S42.

Frederick R, Pochet L, Charlier C, et al. Modulators of the coagulation cascade: Focus and recent advances in inhibitors of tissue factor, factor VIIa and their complex. Curr Med Chem 2005;12:397-417.

Rak J, Yu JL, Luyendyk J, Mackman N. Oncogenes, Trousseau syndrome, and cancer-related changes in the coagulome of mice and humans. Cancer Res 2006;66:10643-10646.

Schiffer CA, Anderson KC, Bennett CL, et al. Platelet transfusion for patients with cancer: Clinical practice guidelines of the American Society of Clinical Oncology. J Clin Oncol 2001; 19:1519-1538.

CHAPTER **231**

The Vena Cava Syndrome

Mario Dicato and Vincent Lens

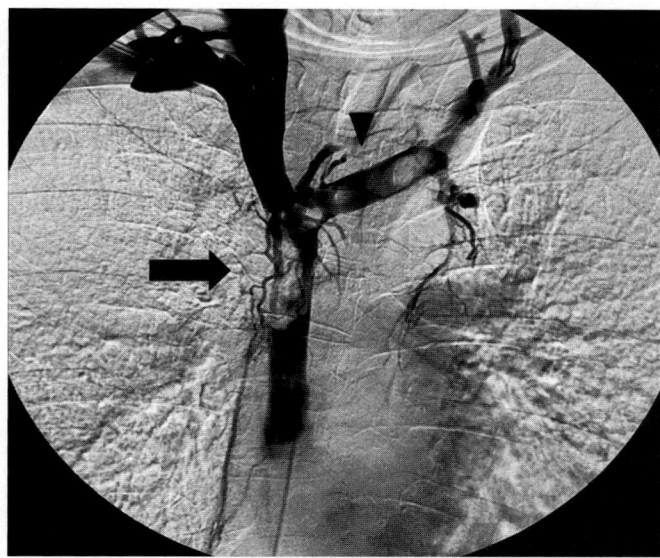

FIGURE 231-1 A 66-year-old patient with small cell lung cancer. This patient had severe superior vena cava stenosis *(arrow)* and clotting up to the left brachiocephalic vein *(arrowhead)*.

KEY POINTS

- Superior vena cava syndrome is not rare, especially in patients with lung cancer. Stenting is the treatment of choice because of rapid and excellent results in more than 90% of patients. Stenting does not preclude further therapy with chemotherapy or radiation therapy, or both.

- Superior vena cava syndrome is not an emergency, and histological diagnosis can be done before treatment is initiated.

- Thrombolysis should be considered in patients with benign superior vena cava obstruction (indwelling catheters or complication of radiation therapy).

- Stenting is also the treatment of choice for inferior vena cava obstruction.

- Approximately 90% of all vena cava syndromes are caused by lung cancer.

Superior vena cava syndrome is common in mediastinal malignant disease, especially lung cancer. Approximately 10% of patients with small cell lung cancer and approximately 2% of patients with non–small cell lung cancer will develop the syndrome (Fig. 231-1). Inferior vena cava syndrome is less frequent.

SUPERIOR VENA CAVA SYNDROME

Etiology

Benign causes include the following:

- Fibrosis
- Thrombosis, mostly from indwelling catheters.

Malignant causes are as follows:

- Compression of the cava vein by tumor or lymph nodes
- Invasion of the vena cava by tumor followed by thrombosis, most often from lung cancer, thymoma, thyroid cancer, or metastases
- Fibrosis as a late complication of radiation therapy and, occasionally, of surgery

Clinical Aspects

Symptoms of facial and upper limb edema of acute or gradual onset, acute dizziness and headache, dyspnea, and cough are the result of impaired venous blood flow. Anatomically, the azygos vein runs parallel to the vena cava. In patients with an obstruction above the azygos vein, collateral veins such as the cervical veins dilate. If the obstruction is below the azygos, blood will backflow through the azygos vein into the inferior vena cava. If the obstruction is at the level at which the azygos vein connects to the superior vena cava, small superficial thoracic veins will dilate and will become visible.

Drainage is to the inferior vena cava. Despite the sometimes dramatic and distressing clinical picture, superior vena cava obstruction is not an emergency. The diagnosis can be confirmed if obstruction is an initial clinical presentation of malignant disease and if procedures such as biopsy (transthoracic or through mediastinoscopy) can be done safely before treatment is begun.

Treatment

- Diuretics and steroids have been widely used, but these agents are not helpful.
- Standard treatment is chemotherapy or radiation therapy, or both. One can expect a response in approximately 50% to 70% of patients within 2 to 3 weeks. In

some studies, 25% of the responding patients needed more than 3 weeks to attain clinical benefit. Overall, 15% to 20% of patients will suffer a relapse, depending on how well the primary disease can be controlled. Chemotherapy and radiation therapy may be indicated in patients with malignant disease who have a good chance of rapid remission or cure.

- Open surgery is an unusual treatment approach. Studies are scarce, and the number of patients reported is small.
- Thrombolysis is most often used when the superior vena cava syndrome is related to thrombosis from an indwelling central catheter.
- Stenting is the treatment of choice.

Stenting

TECHNIQUE

Stenting is usually performed using local anesthesia, and it is always preceded by rigorous diagnostic tests. Mapping of the superior vena cava system by conventional or computed tomography venography (Fig. 231-2) is mandatory to determine the precise location of the disease and the remaining patent vessels and future position of the stent. The venous approach is usually femoral, brachial, or jugular. After having passed the obstructed area with guidewires and catheters, stenting is performed with a stiff

guidewire, with or without previous dilatation of the stenotic or occluded zone. Whatever type of stent (self-expanding or not, covered or uncovered) is used, it must be of sufficient length to cover the whole lesion, and it must have an adapted diameter to avoid migration or perforation (Fig. 231-3). When the disease involves both brachiocephalic veins, treatment of one cephalic vein is sufficient, because of the numerous collateral veins from one side to the other in the cervical region (see Fig. 231-2). The procedure is generally performed using standard monitoring and heparinization (5000 IU per procedure).

CONTRAINDICATIONS

No absolute contraindications to stenting exist. Major complications are rare and include stent migration, pulmonary emboli, superior vena cava rupture, and pericardial tamponade.

RESULTS

Various stents are available, and local habit and experience should determine the choice of stent and of the procedure. The most popular and probably most effective is the Wallstent (Boston Scientific, Natick, MA). Most studies show a success rate of nearly 100%. After stenting, symptoms resolve within 2 to 3 days and sometimes within hours. Whether anticoagulation should be given after stenting is controversial. Recurrence of the syndrome after stenting can be similar to recurrence after chemotherapy and radiation therapy, depending on the evolution of the underlying disease. Repeat stenting and placement of additional stents (depending on the anatomy) may be possible. Stenting does not influence the primary disease, and additional treatment, such as with chemotherapy or radiation therapy, or both, is usually necessary. Moreover, when treatment is purely palliative, relief of symptoms from cava obstruction can be very effective. Although no randomized studies have been conducted—

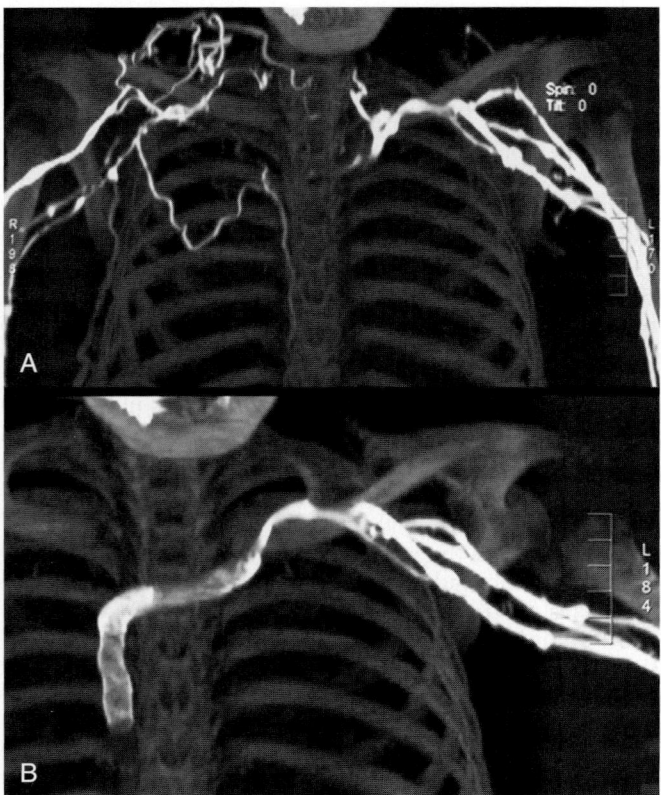

FIGURE 231-2 Mapping of the superior vena cava (SVC) system. **A**, Venogram of the superior vena cava system by computed tomography (CT) using the maximum intensity projection (MIP) reconstruction technique. As in conventional phlebography of the SVC system, simultaneous injection of contrast media in both upper limbs is done. **B**, CT MIP reconstruction image (same patient) after stenting of the SVC.

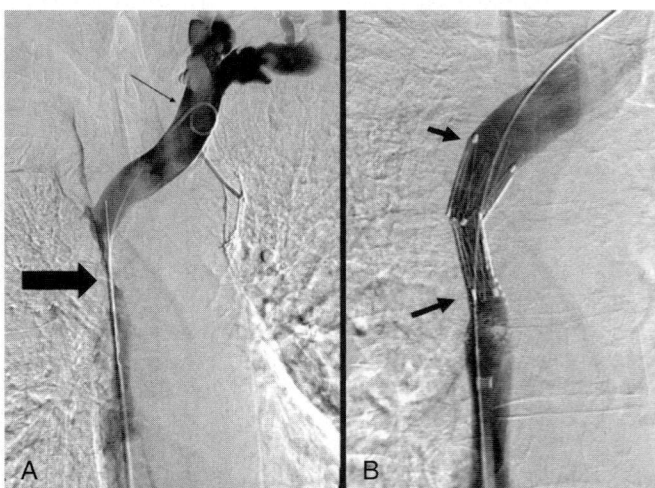

FIGURE 231-3 Superior vena cava syndrome. **A**, Superior vena cava venogram: severe stenosis *(thick arrow)*. The venogram was made after a right femoral venous approach, with insertion of the catheter *(thin arrow)* into the left brachiocephalic vein. **B**, Post-stenting venogram shows a double-Z stent in the portion of the stenotic vena cava *(arrows)*, with immediate restoration of normal blood flow.

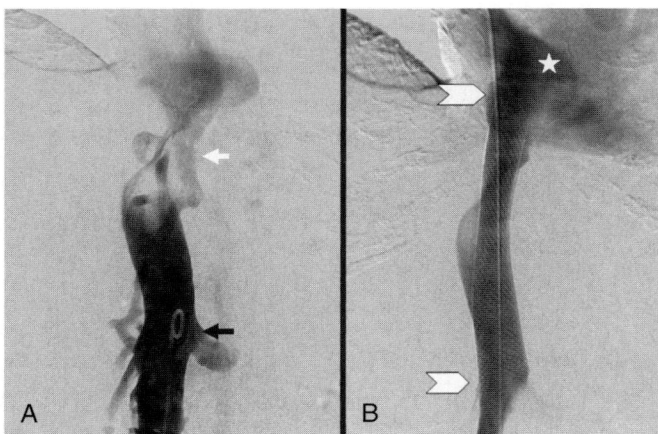

FIGURE 231-4 Inferior vena cava (IVC) syndrome resulting from liver metastasis in rectal adenocarcinoma. **A**, Severe retrohepatic IVC *(white arrow)* narrowing. The *black arrow* points to the left renal vein. **B**, Cavography after stenting with a Wallstent-type stent *(arrowheads)*; no residual compression is noted. The *star* shows the right atrium.

indeed, such studies would be ethically unacceptable, stenting has become the treatment of choice.

It appears that, at least in lung cancer, the relief of symptoms and of relapse associated with stenting is 30% better than with primary chemotherapy and radiation therapy. After stenting, many patients benefit from subsequent additional treatment. Furthermore, relief of sometimes very distressing symptoms is rapid, occasionally within hours.

INFERIOR VENA CAVA SYNDROME

Inferior vena cava syndrome is less frequent than superior vena cava syndrome, essentially because lung cancer remains the major cause of all vena cava obstructions. Clinical manifestations depend on the level of obstruction, on hepatic and renal insufficiency, and on lower body edema, mostly of the legs and scrotum. Imaging and mapping are done by computed tomography and phlebography. Stenting is the treatment of choice (Fig. 231-4).

SUGGESTED READING

de Gregorio Ariza MA, Gamboa P, Gimeno MJ, et al. Percutaneous treatment of superior vena cava syndrome using metallic stents. Eur Radiol 2003;13:853–862.

Rowell NP, Gleeson FV. Steroids, radiotherapy, chemotherapy and stents for superior vena caval obstruction in carcinoma of the bronchus: A systematic review. Clin Oncol 2002; 14:338-351.

Uberoi R. Quality assurance guidelines for superior vena cava stenting in malignant disease. Cardiovasc Intervent Radiol 2006;29:319-322.

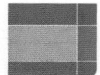

CHAPTER **232**

Oral Complications of Cancer and Its Treatment

Dorothy M. K. Keefe and Richard M. Logan

KEY POINTS

- The oral effects of cancer are mainly the result of side effects of treatment.
- Oral cancer may directly compromise vital functions by impeding eating and breathing.
- The oral side effects of cancer treatment are potentially life-threatening and compromise vital functions such as eating and breathing.
- The oral side effects of cancer treatment have a significant effect on quality of life.
- The oral side effects of cancer treatment may have negative effects on prognosis.

Apart from oral cancer itself as a direct cause of disruption of the mouth and surrounding structures (Fig. 232-1), most complications of oral cancer result from cancer treatment, particularly in patients with head and neck disease, and from high-dose chemotherapy before stem cell or bone marrow transplantation. Oral complications are common in association with all treatment modalities. These complications range from mild disturbances to debilitating, painful complications that have a marked impact on quality of life and that, in some patients, can be potentially life-threatening. Certainly, severe side effects, such as oral mucositis, markedly impair quality of life (see Chapter 65), increase the prevalence of systemic infections, and impede the ability to provide optimal treatment, thus compromising treatment effectiveness and prognosis.

CLINICAL EVALUATION

Patients should have oral evaluations and examination before, during, and after their cancer treatment. Preoperative oral assessment should include evaluations of current dental and oral health, history of dental treatment, and frequency of previous dental examinations, to gauge potential compliance with treatment. Preventive treatment is important, and thorough pretreatment assessment is important to achieve this goal, particularly in conjunction with radiation therapy or bisphosphonate administration. Because of the increased risk of osteonecrosis in these patients, and because of the unknown duration of action of bisphosphonate drugs, any teeth considered to have a poor prognosis should be extracted. If compliance is expected to be poor, the threshold for extraction may

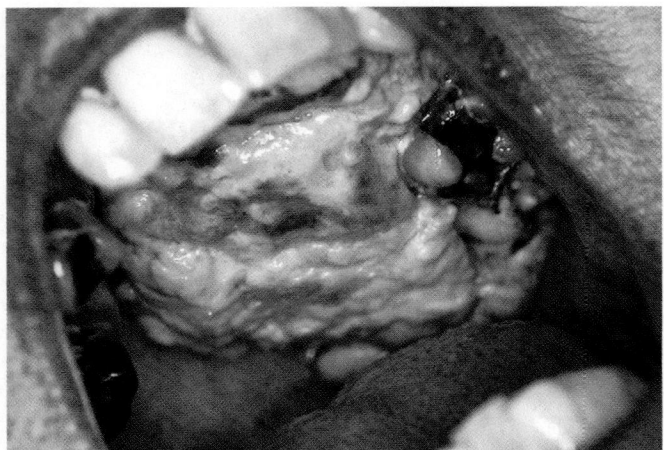

FIGURE 232-1 Squamous cell carcinoma involving the entire hard palate in a 58-year-old woman.

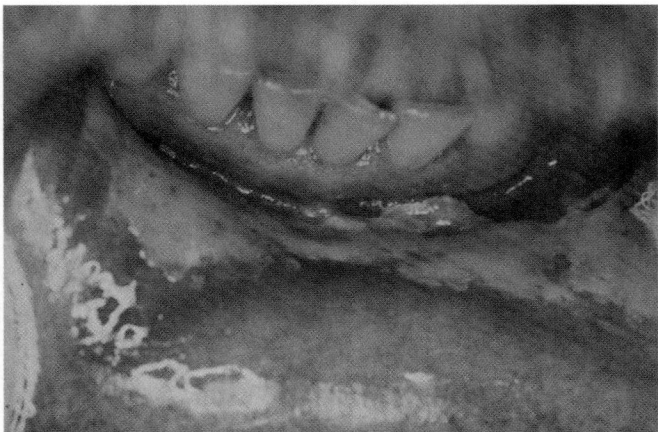

FIGURE 232-2 Radiation-induced oral mucositis in a 47-year-old man.

be lower. Following radiation therapy or bisphosphonate treatment, appropriate preventive programs should be implemented, including topical fluoride applications and reinforcement of oral hygiene protocols.

Radiographic Examination

Panoramic radiographs including the dentition and surrounding anatomy should be taken before treatment. The general state of the teeth can be assessed, and incidental findings such as retained roots, periodontal status, odontogenic infections, and other intraosseous lesions can be evaluated. Edentulous patients should also be assessed radiographically before treatment.

ORAL MUCOSITIS

Mucositis has a complex pathogenesis involving all compartments of the mucosa, rather than just the epithelium. We believe that mucositis has five overlapping stages and common features with different treatment modalities. This hypothesis suggests that transcription factors activated by chemotherapy, radiation therapy, or reactive oxygen species play a major role in triggering a biological cascade that leads to mucosal injury. In mucositis, the transcription factor nuclear factor-κB (NF-κB) is considered one of the main "drivers." Activation results in upregulation of various genes and production of pro-inflammatory cytokines, including tumor necrosis factor, interleukin-1β, and interleukin-6. This process increases tissue injury in all mucosal compartments, not exclusively epithelium. In addition, NF-κB causes upregulation of cyclooxygenase 2, which is also implicated in increasing matrix metalloproteinases, a likely mediator of tissue damage.[1] Subsequent amplification of these biological events through positive feedback loops and stimulation by bacterial cell wall products result in widespread tissue damage (i.e., ulceration). Cessation of chemotherapy or radiation therapy allows the ulceration to heal. Oral mucositis is now considered to be the "tip of the iceberg," with damage occurring in all mucosal surfaces of the body (depending on type and delivery of treatment), and gas-

TABLE 232-1	World Health Organization: Mucositis Toxicity Scale
Grade 0	No oral erythema or ulceration, normal mucosa
Grade 1	Generalized erythema and pain, patient able to maintain normal diet
Grade 2	Presence of ulceration, patient able to eat solids
Grade 3	Presence of ulceration, patient restricted to liquid diet
Grade 4	Presence of ulceration, total parenteral nutrition, alimentation not possible because of oral pain or ulceration

trointestinal mucositis is most prominent after oral mucositis.

The prevalence of oral mucositis varies according to the type of cancer treatment. For example, up to 100% of patients who undergo high-dose chemotherapy with hematopoietic stem cell transplantation develop mucositis. Similarly, up to 70% of patients receiving head and neck radiation therapy experience oral mucositis, and this percentage can be higher when regimens involve accelerated fractionation. Particular cytotoxic agents, such as 5-fluorouracil and methotrexate, are associated with a higher risk of this complication.

The clinical appearance of oral mucositis varies according to a clinical spectrum, ranging from generalized mucosal erythema to widespread ulceration that makes eating and drinking impossible (Fig. 232-2). When widespread ulceration is present, patients have a risk of developing systemic infections because this ulceration often coincides with neutropenia. It is important that the presence and severity of oral mucositis be adequately assessed. Various scales are available, and one of the most common is the World Health Organization scale (Table 232-1). This useful scale encompasses subjective, objective, and functional criteria that are easily reproducible with minimal intraobserver and interobserver variability.

Until recently, the treatment of oral mucositis was predominantly palliative, restricted to controlling pain and reducing infection. Previous guidelines often recommended what not to do.[2] However, the drug palifermin (keratinocyte growth factor) is now indicated for use in patients with hematological malignancies who are receiving high-dose chemotherapy and total body irradiation with autologous stem cell transplantation.[3] The use of palifermin in other clinical situations is under investigation because of concerns with long-term effects. In most patients, treatment of mucositis remains largely palliative, including good oral hygiene and benzydamine mouthwash; when specific cytotoxic drugs, such as 5-fluorouracil, edatrexate, and melphalan, are used, cryotherapy may be indicated.[3] Other treatment modalities such as low-level laser may help, although further clinical trials are required (see also Chapters 158, 171, 232, 236, and 239).[3]

OSTEORADIONECROSIS

Necrosis of the jaws has long been associated with radiation therapy to the head and the neck, but now it also is caused by the use of bisphosphonates. Osteonecrosis associated with radiation, or osteoradionecrosis, is well described and results when the bone in the radiation field becomes hypocellular, hypovascular, and hypoxic from radiation (Fig. 232-3). The incidence varies according to the dose of radiation and the volume of bone irradiated. The presence of teeth also increases the risk of osteoradionecrosis. Irradiated bone is less able to withstand injury, such as dental extractions, and the resulting reduction in healing capacity allows for infection from oral microflora, with subsequent exposure and sequestration of bone. Occasionally, spontaneous osteoradionecrosis occurs. Complications of osteoradionecrosis include pain, infection, and increased risk of fracture.

Bisphosphonate-associated osteonecrosis is a more recently described complication,[4] the exact mechanism of which is unknown. Bisphosphonates may disrupt of normal bone physiology, thereby affecting bone turnover and remodeling capacity. This disruption, in combination with hypovascularity, local trauma, and infection, increases the risk of osteonecrosis. Risk factors for bisphosphonate-associated osteonecrosis are ill defined, but patients receiving intravenous bisphosphonates and patients with multiple myeloma or bone metastases are at greater risk of developing bisphosphonate osteonecrosis.[4] Local factors such as dental extractions, denture trauma, oral infections, and poor oral health may also increase the risk of this complication.[4,5]

The diagnosis of osteoradionecrosis requires a thorough clinical examination demonstrating chronically exposed bone. Computed tomography scans may also demonstrate the extent of bone lesions. Often, osteoradionecrosis occurs subsequent to teeth extractions in the radiation field. When radiation therapy is planned, it is important to extract any teeth with poor prognoses, to allow adequate time for healing before treatment commences. Good preventive protocols, including topical fluoride programs, minimization of trauma from dentures or sharp dental restorations, and regular oral examinations, avoid the development of osteoradionecrosis.[6]

Established osteoradionecrosis can be managed using conservative methods or surgical intervention. Small lesions can be irrigated with saline solution with or without systemic antibiotics, and small sequestra can be gently lifted off the mucosa. When more significant surgical intervention is required, hyperbaric oxygen treatment can attempt to increase tissue oxygenation and thus promote angiogenesis (see also Chapters 171, 232, and 236).[6]

SALIVARY GLAND HYPOFUNCTION

The salivary glands are commonly affected by radiation therapy to the head and neck. Reduction in salivary flow increases the risk of dental caries (Fig. 232-4) and of oral infections and reduces taste sensation. Research has suggested that the parenchymal cells do not have a high cell turnover, and although salivary flow is diminished soon after treatment is started, salivary gland cellularity is not markedly reduced.[7,8] Radiation-induced damage to the cell plasma membrane that affects water secretion from cells may explain the changes that occur in the quantity and quality of saliva after treatment.[8] Long-term changes in the

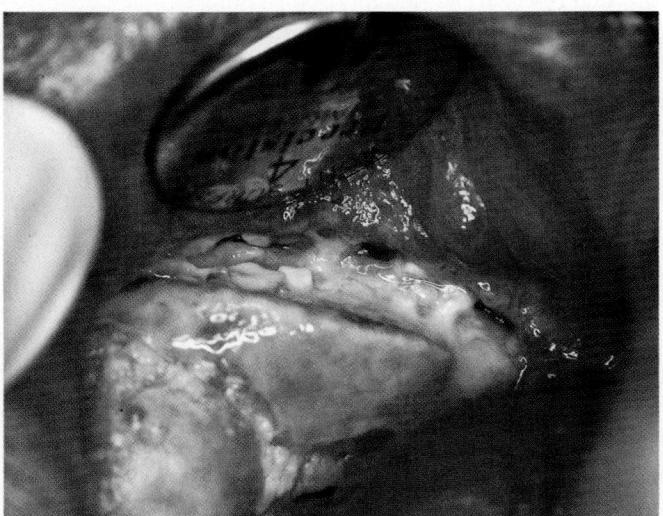

FIGURE 232-3 Osteoradionecrosis involving the lower right mandible. *(Photographs courtesy of Dr. E. Coates, Adelaide Dental Hospital.)*

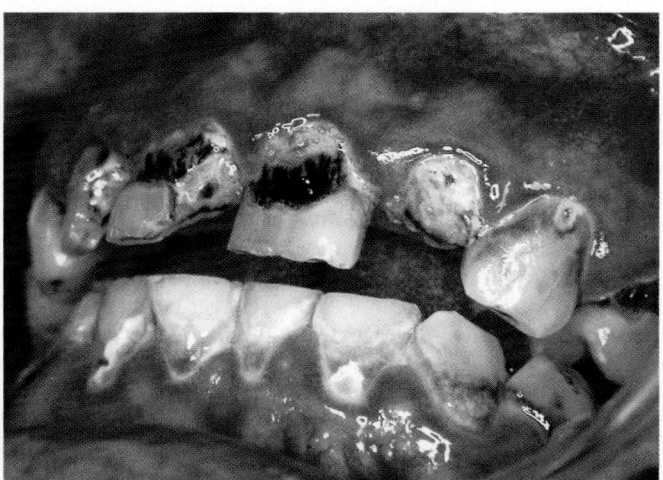

FIGURE 232-4 Rampant dental caries secondary to severe salivary hypofunction related to radiation therapy. *(Photographs courtesy of Dr. E. Coates, Adelaide Dental Hospital.)*

glands are attributed to mitotic cell death of parenchymal stem cells that reduces the capacity to replace the injured cells. The results are acinar atrophy and fibrous replacement of the gland parenchyma.

Salivary gland hypofunction is a common side effect of cancer treatment, particularly in head and neck radiation therapy, in which salivary flow can be markedly reduced after even minimal treatment. Many patients adjust to the changes in saliva subsequent to cancer treatment; however, for some patients, these changes can be debilitating and can adversely affect their quality of life. Even for patients who do not perceive a problem with their saliva, long-term problems associated with saliva quality often increase the risk of oral and dental disease. Good oral hygiene, use of topical fluoride products, and regular dental examinations are imperative. Saliva substitutes are useful in some patients, to palliate a dry mouth (see also Chapters 171 and 236).

TASTE ALTERATION

Alterations in the sensation of taste are commonly reported during cancer treatment,[9] and these changes are closely related to alterations in olfaction. These alterations can be attributed to either the tumor itself or the specific treatment modality.[10] They have important consequences in overall health because of the potential compromise in nutritional intake. Various chemotherapeutic agents are associated with taste change, including 5-fluorouracil, carboplatin, cisplatin, cyclophosphamide, and methotrexate.[10] High-dose chemotherapy before stem cell transplantation is associated with complete loss of taste.[11] Taste alterations range from complete loss of taste to hypersensitivity to specific taste sensations such as sweet or salty tastes.

Similarly, radiation therapy targets rapidly dividing cells such as those in taste and olfactory receptors. Another complicating factor in radiation therapy is the reduction in salivary flow. Saliva is important in taste by acting as a vehicle in which chemicals can be dissolved and transported to receptors. With respect to radiation therapy, taste generally returns to nearly normal levels after treatment. Because of these chronic salivary gland changes, however, minor alterations in taste may persist (see also Chapters 171, 236, and 239).

PERIODONTAL DISEASE

Cancer and cancer treatment can have various manifestations in the periodontium. Gingival tumors may appear in the mouth, and periodontal disease or changes may be the first indicators of some hematological conditions. Preexisting periodontal disease may complicate cancer treatment, particularly during neutropenia. This situation can have life-threatening implications.[12]

Assessment of periodontal health status is important before treatment for cancer. Radiation may result in avascularity and acellularity in the periodontal membrane, with widening periodontal spaces.[7,12] These changes can increase the risk of periodontal disease if good oral hygiene is not maintained. Another important aspect of periodontal disease after radiation therapy is that it is a significant risk factor for osteoradionecrosis. Patients with periodon-

tal disease who receive myelosuppressive chemotherapy are at risk of systemic infection during treatment. Elimination of potential oral sources of infection is important, and again this relates to a thorough pretreatment assessment (see also Chapter 171).

INFECTIONS

Oral infections are common during radiation therapy and chemotherapy. In radiation therapy, alteration of the oral environment from changes in salivary flow and mucosal damage increase the risk for opportunistic infections. Similarly, the immunosuppressive effect of cytotoxic drugs also increases infections both locally and systemically. The most common oral infection during or subsequent to radiation therapy or chemotherapy is oral candidiasis (Fig. 232-5).[13]

Breakdown of host defences is crucial in candidal infections. Neutropenia subsequent to cytotoxic chemotherapy can increase the risk of oral *Candida* infection. Alterations in the local oral environment also increase the risk of *Candida* infections. Reductions in salivary flow, changes in saliva quality, dentures, oral cavity tumors, surgical defects, and skin grafts all provide an environment conducive to fungal growth.

Other oral infections during cancer treatment include herpes simplex and herpes zoster infections, which again cause pain and ulceration and thus reduce the quality of life. Although these infections do not cause oral mucositis per se, they do worsen it and therefore need to be treated or prevented.[2] Often, these infections are manifestations of immunodeficiency. With respect to radiation therapy, increased shedding or reactivation of herpes simplex virus is rare.[14] The diagnosis of oral and oropharyngeal infections is made by swabbing of suspected lesions and microbiological assessment with appropriate clinical evaluation.

In immunocompromised patients, systemic antifungal agents such as fluconazole are indicated in preference to

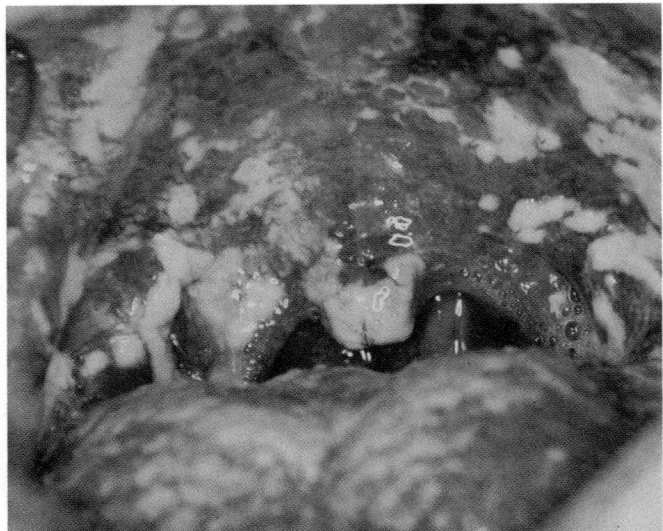

FIGURE 232-5 Pseudomembranous candidiasis involving the oropharynx subsequent to radiation therapy.

topical agents. Good oral hygiene by regular tooth brushing or, if tooth brushing is contraindicated or difficult, by using antibacterial mouthwashes such as chlorhexidine, is also important in maintaining overall oral health. In addition, good oral hygiene also reduces the carriage of fungal organisms. Thorough tooth brushing should be done at least once a day with a soft toothbrush, to minimize tissue damage. Patients who wear dentures should keep them clean because dentures can also be carriers of fungal organisms (see also Chapters 171 and 239).

CONCLUSIONS

The oral complications of cancer mainly arise from cancer treatment. These complications can have a marked effect on quality of life during treatment and, in some patients, can affect prognosis by influencing the provision of optimal cancer treatment. In most patients, prevention of problems is the best management. To achieve this goal, a multidisciplinary approach is required.

REFERENCES

1. Sonis ST. The pathobiology of mucositis. Nat Rev Cancer 2004;4:277-284.
2. Rubenstein EB, Peterson D, Schubert M, et al. Clinical practice guidelines for the prevention and treatment of cancer therapy–induced oral and gastrointestinal mucositis. Cancer 2004;100:2026-2046.
3. Keefe DMK, Schubert MM, Elting LS, et al. Updated clinical practice guidelines for the prevention and treatment of mucositis. Cancer 2007;109:820-831.
4. Migliorati CA, Casiglia J, Epstein J, et al. Managing the care of patients with bisphosphonate-associated osteonecrosis: An American Academy of Oral Medicine position paper. J Am Dent Assoc 2005;136:1658-1668.
5. Jereczek-Fossa BA, Orecchia R. Radiotherapy induced mandibular bone complications. Cancer Treat Rev 2002;28:65-74.
6. Vudiniabola S, Pirone C, Williamson J, et al. Hyperbaric oxygen in the therapeutic management of osteoradionecrosis of the facial bones. Int J Oral Maxillofac Surg 2000;29:435-438.
7. Vissink A, Jansma, J, Spijkervet FK, et al. Oral sequelae of head and neck radiotherapy. Crit Rev Oral Biol Med 2003;14:199-212.
8. Konings AWT, Coppes RP, Vissink A. On the mechanism of salivary gland radiosensitivity. Int J Rad Oncol Biol Phys 2005;62:1187-1194.
9. Comeau TB, Epstein JB, Migas C. Taste and smell dysfunction in patients receiving chemotherapy: A review of current knowledge. Support Care Cancer 2001;9:575-580.
10. Ravasco P: Aspects of taste and compliance in patients with cancer. Eur J Oncol Nurs 2005;9(Suppl):S84-S91.
11. Epstein, JB, Phillips N, Parry J, et al. Quality of life, taste, olfactory ann oral function following high-dose chemotherapy and allogeneic hematopoietic cell transplantation. Bone Marrow Transplant 2002;30:785-792.
12. Epstein JB, Stevenson-Moore P. Periodontal disease and periodontal management in patients with cancer. Oral Oncol 2001;37:613-619.
13. Soysa NS, Samaranayake LP, Ellepola ANB. Cytotoxic drugs, radiotherapy and candidiasis. Oral Oncol 2004;40:971-978.
14. Epstein JB, Gorsky M, Hancock P, et al. The prevalence of herpes simplex virus shedding and infection in the oral cavity of seropositive patients undergoing head and neck radiation therapy. Oral Surg Oral Med Oral Pathol Oral Radiol Endod 2002;94:712-716.

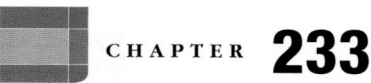

CHAPTER **233**

Paraneoplastic Syndromes

Davide Tassinari and Marco Maltoni

> ### KEY POINTS
>
> - Paraneoplastic syndromes (PNSs) are heterogeneous clinical manifestations of cancer that are not the direct result of clinical tumor extension or the side effects of treatment.
> - The main mechanisms are endocrine or paracrine tumor effects, pathological activation of homeostatic mechanisms, and pathological autoimmune responses.
> - Treatment of the tumor is the main therapeutic approach.
> - Concomitant treatment of the main resultant symptoms and physical complications is also necessary.

PNSs represent a heterogeneous group of clinical manifestations of cancer that occur in approximately 10% of patients at diagnosis and in approximately 50% during the course of the disease.[1] The real prevalence is difficult to assess because of the heterogeneous pathogenetic mechanisms and the clinical manifestations, which are not usually specific for particular cancers or a particular stage of the disease. PNSs are not caused by direct organ involvement by tumor or by side effects of treatment.[2] Some clinicians exclude endocrine tumors when considering PNSs; nevertheless, the escape from physiological homeostatic control that occurs in these tumors makes those syndromes similar to PNSs in nonendocrine tumors.

The main pathogenetic mechanisms are as follows:

- Tumor cells produce substances that directly or indirectly cause distant symptoms.
- Tumor cells help to deplete normal substances and cause a paraneoplastic manifestation.
- Host-tumor interaction results in a syndrome.

Based on these pathogenetic mechanisms, PNSs can be classified clinically into seven syndrome categories (Table 233-1):

- Endocrine
- Cutaneous
- Cardiovascular
- Neurological
- Hematological
- Paraneoplastic connectivitis
- Miscellaneous

PATHOGENETIC MECHANISMS

Figure 233-1 shows the pathogenetic classification of PNSs.

TABLE 233-1 Clinical Classification of Paraneoplastic Syndromes

ENDOCRINE SYNDROMES	CUTANEOUS SYNDROMES	CARDIOVASCULAR SYNDROMES	NEUROLOGICAL SYNDROMES	HEMATOLOGICAL SYNDROMES	PARANEOPLASTIC CONNECTIVITIS	MISCELLANEOUS
Hypercalcemia/hypocalcemia	Pigmented lesions	Migrans thrombophlebitis	Subacute sensory neuronopathy and encephalomyeloneuritis	Anemia	Dermatomyositis	Fever
Hyperglycemia/hypoglycemia	Keratoses	Nonbacterial thrombotic endocarditis	Limbic encephalitis	Erythrocytosis	Vasculitis	Lactic acidosis
Ectopic adrenocorticotropic hormone syndrome	Erythemas		Autonomic neuropathy	Granulocytosis	Amyloidosis	Protein-losing enteropathy
Gonadotropin secretion	Endocrine/metabolic lesions		Progressive cerebellar degeneration	Granulocytopenia	Hypertrophic osteoarthropathy	Anorexia-cachexia syndrome
Thyroid-stimulating hormone secretion	Bullous Lesions		Paraneoplastic vision loss	Thrombocytosis		
Prolactin, growth hormone, and human placental lactogen secretion			Opsoclonus-myoclonus	Thrombocytopenia		
Zollinger-Ellison syndrome			Paraneoplastic motor neuron disorders	Disseminated intravascular coagulopathy		
Carcinoid syndrome			Paraneoplastic peripheral neuropathies; neuromuscular junction disorders	Coagulopathies		
Syndrome of inappropriate antidiuretic hormone			Paraneoplastic muscle rigidity	Thrombophlebitis		
Oncogenous osteomalacia						

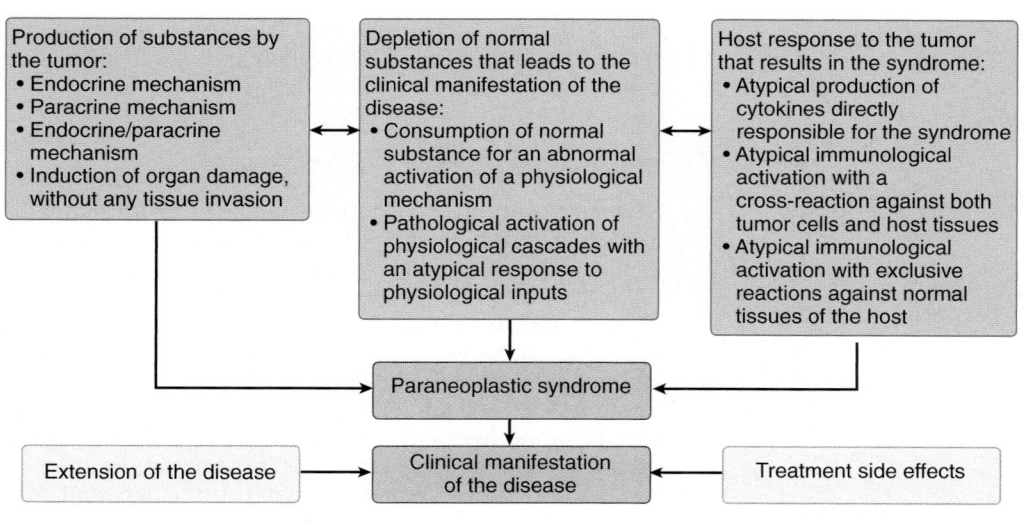

FIGURE 233-1 Pathogenetic classification of paraneoplastic syndromes and its implications in clinical practice.

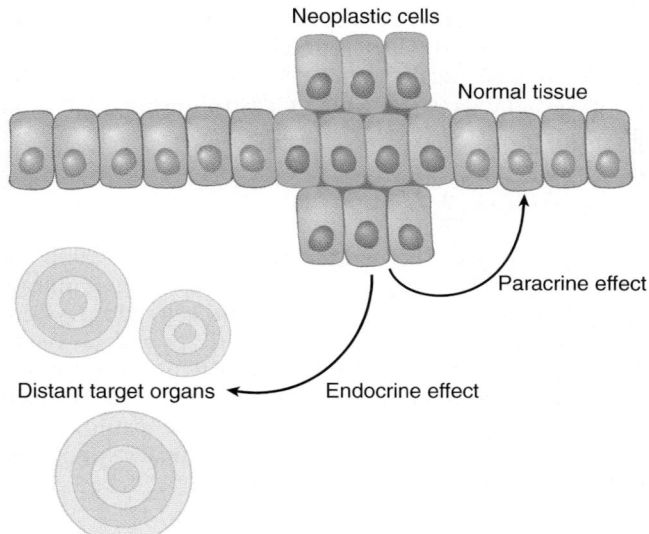

FIGURE 233-2 Tumor cells produce substances that directly or indirectly cause distant symptoms.

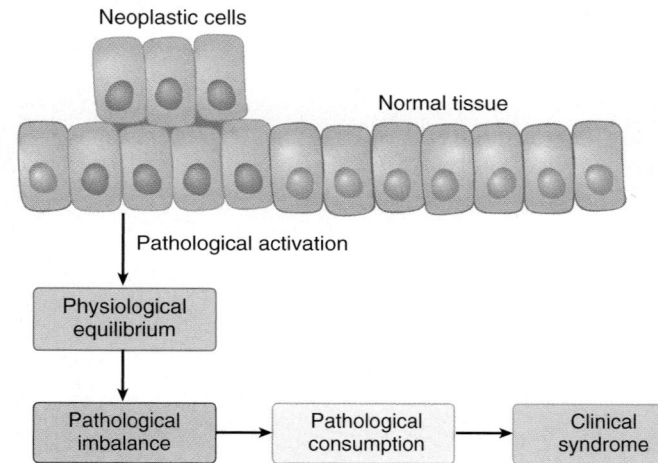

FIGURE 233-3 Tumor cells favor the depletion of normal substances that leads to a paraneoplastic manifestation.

Tumor Cells Produce Substances That Directly or Indirectly Cause Distant Symptoms

Tumor cells produce substances that act either in distant target tissues (endocrine) or in tumoral or peritumoral tissues (paracrine), or both (endocrine and paracrine effect) (Fig. 233-2). Some of these substances are natural hormones identical to their physiological counterparts. Others are hormone precursors, and some biologically active analogues. Detailed characterization of these substances is rarely useful clinically.

Tumor Cells Favor Depletion of Normal Substances and Thus Cause a Paraneoplastic Manifestation

These mechanisms are complex and are often only partly elucidated (Fig. 233-3). A typical example is disseminated

intravascular coagulopathy seen in patients with advanced solid tumors and in some acute myeloid leukemias, such as acute promyelocytic leukemia. Although the primary events are only partly known, pathological activation of the coagulation cascade and subsequent formation of microthrombi are the main pathogenetic events. The hemorrhagic syndrome results from consumption of fibrinogens or platelets.[3]

The Host Response to the Tumor Results in the Syndrome

The mechanisms are either activation of monocyte-macrophage cells that produce cytokines with endocrine or paracrine action or activation of a specific immune reaction against self with clinical signs or symptoms of autoimmune disease (Fig. 233-4). The first mechanism has been hypothesized as one responsible for the primary anorexia-cachexia syndrome and paraneoplastic anemia.[4,5] The second mechanism has been suggested for many neurological PNSs, autoimmune anemia, and thrombocytope-

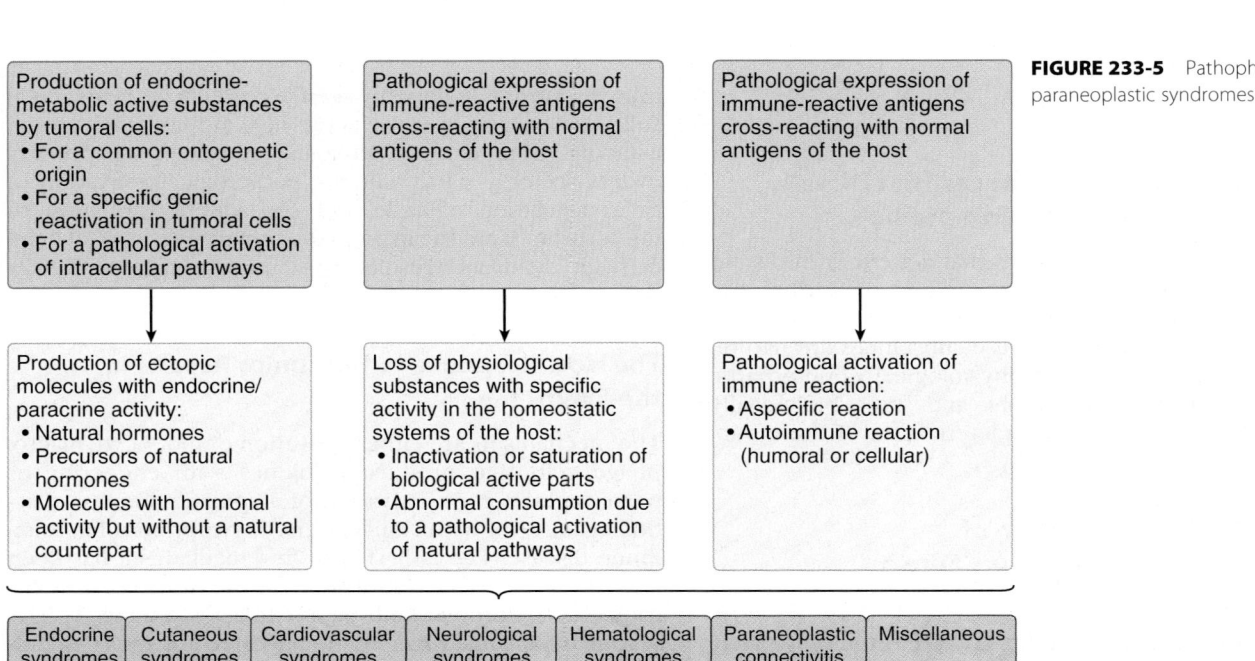

FIGURE 233-4 The host response to the tumor results in the syndrome.

TABLE 233-2	Prevalence of Paraneoplastic Syndromes
TYPE OF SYNDROME	**PREVALENCE**
Paraneoplastic syndrome as an expression of the disease at the time of diagnosis of cancer	7-10%
Paraneoplastic syndrome as an expression of the disease along the clinical history of the patient	50%
Endocrine paraneoplastic syndromes	33%
Cutaneous paraneoplastic syndromes	33%
Neurological paraneoplastic syndromes	16%
Hematological or cardiovascular expressions of a paraneoplastic syndrome	15%
Miscellaneous syndromes (gastrointestinal, immunological, or renal syndromes)	15%

nia.[6] Different mechanisms for PNSs often coexist in the same patient; similarly, more than one mechanism can cause many PNSs.

EPIDEMIOLOGY AND PREVALENCE

Seven percent to 10% of patients with cancer present with a PNS. Approximately 50% of patients with advanced cancer express signs or symptoms of a PNS during their disease course. Endocrine and cutaneous syndromes each account for about one third of PNSs (Table 233-2), and neurological, hematological or cardiovascular, and miscellaneous syndromes make up approximately 15% each (see Table 233-2). Assessing the prevalence of PNSs is complicated by their frequent coexistence with clinical evidence of the disease or side effects of treatments. Prevalence tends to be underestimated in clinical practice, and data are often inaccurate and inconclusive.

Nearly all tumors can cause a PNS. Cancer of the lung, bladder, prostate, and gastrointestinal, hematological, breast, and endocrine cancers are most frequent. Certain PNSs are associated with particular tumors, such as endocrine or neurological syndromes in lung cancer and the anorexia-cachexia syndrome in gastrointestinal or lung cancers.

PATHOPHYSIOLOGY

Common ontogenetic origin, genetic reactivation of repressed genes, expression of cross-reacting immunogenic molecules, and atypical immune activation system by neoplastic cells are credible genetic hypotheses supporting the occurrence of PNSs in particular histopathological findings; nevertheless, many aspects still remain undefined. Both the ontogenetic and the pathogenetic hypotheses help us to understand the clinical expressions of the heterogeneous PNSs (Fig. 233-5).

FIGURE 233-5 Pathophysiology of paraneoplastic syndromes.

Case Reports

"Case Study: Atypical Water Retention in Advanced Small Cell Lung Cancer," "Case Study: Somnolence and Hypercalcemia in Non–Small Cell Lung Cancer," "Case Study: Hemorrhagic Syndrome in Anemia and Thrombocytopenia in Advanced Breast Cancer," "Case Study: Progressive Ataxia in Small Cell Lung Cancer," and "Case Study: Anorexia and Weight Loss in Locally Advanced Non–Small Cell Lung Cancer" demonstrate the three mechanisms of PNSs.

CLINICAL MANIFESTATIONS

The clinical manifestations (see Table 233-1 and Figs. 233-1 and 233-5), in addition to generating suspicion of underlying cancer, often represent unique markers that allow diagnosis and follow-up during the course of the disease. Most common cutaneous or neurological PNSs do not have a laboratory or instrumental counterpart.[7,8] In the other syndromes (e.g., Cushing's syndrome from ectopic adrenocorticotropic hormone production or primary anorexia-cachexia syndrome from monocyte-macrophagic cytokine production), the identification and assessment of the substances responsible for the clinical manifestations of the syndrome play a minimal role in diagnosis and therapeutic management, and laboratory testing is unhelpful.[1,4,5]

Laboratory Findings

Although laboratory tests are fundamental in the diagnosis and follow-up of some PNSs, such tests can be superfluous in others. The identification of autoantibodies against the central or peripheral nervous system can confirm the clinical suspicion of a paraneoplastic neurological syndrome, but periodic assessment has little role in follow-up. In contrast, laboratory assessments of hypercalcemia, hyponatremia, and hyperglycemia are essential for diagnosis and follow-up during supportive treatment of those syndromes involving metabolic imbalance. In hematological syndromes and coagulopathic PNSs,[3,9] laboratory analysis (Table 233-3 and Fig. 233-6) is basic both for diagnosis and for supportive treatment.

Laboratory tests are useful in clinical practice whenever production by tumor cells of substances with or without endocrine or paracrine effects reflects extension

CASE STUDY

Atypical Water Retention in Advanced Small Cell Lung Cancer

GH, a 45-year-old man with advanced small cell lung cancer with liver, lung, and nodal involvement, had an exacerbation of anorexia, asthenia, and nausea after three courses of chemotherapy with cisplatin and etoposide. A few days later, altered mental status was noted, with frequent episodes of confusion and seizures. Brain computed tomography (CT) showed no brain metastases. CT of the thorax and abdomen showed stable disease. In addition to chemotherapy, he had received daily prednisone 25 mg. No other drugs were implicated before or during the clinical deterioration. Hyponatremia (Na$^+$ 117 mmol/L) was found, with low serum osmolarity and increased urinary osmolarity and sodium levels. Water intoxication was suspected.

Treatment with water restriction and demeclocycline, furosemide, and hypertonic saline solutions was started. The patient had rapid but incomplete resolution of his symptoms. He completed the planned chemotherapy with minimal response. Disease progression occurred 2 months later. Another course of chemotherapy was started, but the patient died 2 months later.

Comment

The syndrome of inappropriate antidiuretic hormone production occurs in 3% to 15% of patients with small cell lung cancer. This syndrome is caused by ectopic production of antidiuretic hormone with excessive renal water resorption and sodium loss. Most patients remain asymptomatic. Neurological symptoms are common when the syndrome progresses. Decreased serum osmolarity, inappropriate elevation of urine osmolarity, and increased urine sodium levels are the main laboratory findings. Water restriction, demeclocycline, furosemide, and hypertonic saline solutions are the treatment of choice during the acute phase of the syndrome, but treatment of the underlying tumor is needed for durable control of symptoms.[7]

CASE STUDY

Somnolence and Hypercalcemia in Non–Small Cell Lung Cancer

IJ, a 65-year-old man with advanced non–small cell lung cancer, reported somnolence, fatigue, asthenia, nausea, vomiting, and constipation during treatment with carboplatin and gemcitabine. Symptoms were initially attributed to chemotherapeutic side effects. The patient's condition worsened after stopping treatment. Hypercalcemia (Ca^{2+} 7.2 mEq/L) was the only abnormal biochemical finding. Treatment with fluids, furosemide, and bisphosphonates was immediately started, with a rapid response. Disease progression without bone involvement was documented during disease restaging. Second-line treatment with weekly docetaxel was started, but the patient died 3 months later of progressive disease.

Comment

Hypercalcemia is probably the most common endocrine paraneoplastic syndrome (PNS) caused by systemic hormone production with endocrine effect (mainly transforming growth factor-α or parathyroid hormone–related protein) or by production of cytokines with paracrine effect. Hypercalcemia resulting from direct bone invasion by metastatic cells is less frequent and cannot be considered a PNS. Third-generation bisphosphonates (mainly zoledronate, pamidronate, and alendronate) have modified therapy. Fluids and diuretics remain appropriate when they are used with bisphosphonates. In addition, calcitonin has a role when rapid restoration of normocalcemia is needed.[7,8]

CASE STUDY

Hemorrhagic Syndrome in Anemia and Thrombocytopenia in Advanced Breast Cancer

Spontaneous mucosal bleeding occurred in LM, a 54-year-old woman with advanced breast cancer who was treated with an aromatase inhibitor for breast cancer with bone metastases. No chemotherapy or anticoagulants had been given in the preceding weeks, and no other causes of bleeding could be identified. Laboratory findings showed thrombocytopenia, anemia, prolonged prothrombin time and partial thromboplastin time, decreased fibrinogen levels, increased fibrin degradation products, and increased D-dimer. Rapid deterioration of renal function and neurological performance occurred acutely following the hemorrhagic syndrome. A blood smear examination revealed schistocytes. The diagnosis of acute disseminated intravascular coagulopathy (DIC) was made. Plasma and platelet transfusions were given. Plasmapheresis was needed three times to control renal and neurological deterioration. Treatment with low-molecular-weight heparin was started. Chemotherapy with weekly paclitaxel was given after stopping the hormonal treatment. The patient had a rapid and progressive clinical improvement, although laboratory findings never completely returned to normal. The patient died 8 months later of progressive disease.

Comment

DIC is a rare but serious complication of advanced cancer. It may be related to the tumor (adenocarcinomas or acute myeloid leukemias) or tumor treatment (chemotherapy and hormone therapy). It can occur in an acute or a chronic form. Clinical manifestations may be thrombotic or hemorrhagic, or both forms can coexist. The primary event is disseminated microthrombotic activation that depletes fibrinogen. Thrombocytopenia, anemia, and schistocytes result from the peripheral microtrauma following the formation of thrombi. Treatment should address the reduction of thrombus formation, but anticoagulant use is frequently difficult because of ongoing hemorrhage. Plasma and platelet transfusions can help acute hemorrhagic manifestations, but treatment of the underlying disease (or stopping treatment when DIC is related to drugs) is mandatory.[3,9,10]

CASE STUDY

Progressive Ataxia in Small Cell Lung Cancer

In NP, a 55-year-old patient, progressive ataxia was the presenting feature of locally advanced small cell lung cancer; treatment with carboplatin and etoposide was immediately started. Brain involvement was excluded during disease staging, and a high titer of anti-Purkinje cell antibody (anti-Yo) suggested autoimmune paraneoplastic disease. The patient was treated with five courses of chemotherapy together with lung, mediastinal, and brain radiation therapy. Long-term treatment with prednisone was started at

diagnosis and was continued during chemotherapy. Although complete disease regression occurred after chemotherapy and radiation therapy, no neurological improvement was observed. Slow but progressive worsening of neurological performance was documented during the chemotherapy and in the relapse-free interval. This situation was not influenced by disease relapse, which occurred 18 months after first-line chemotherapy, and continued during second-line treatment and the terminal phase of the disease.

Comment

Paraneoplastic neurological syndromes are frequently autoimmune reactions initiated by the expression of cross-reactive substances by tumor cells, and they are independent of the primary tumor.[6,11] Corticosteroids are the usual treatment for neurological damage. Progression of neurological disease is frequently independent both of the underlying cancer and of any response to antineoplastic treatment.

CASE STUDY

Anorexia and Weight Loss in Locally Advanced Non–Small Cell Lung Cancer

RS, a 60-year-old patient with stage IV non–small cell lung cancer who was treated with chemotherapy, had progressive loss of appetite and body weight despite adequate nutritional intake. To increase appetite and to counter the weight loss, treatment with medroxyprogesterone acetate was started, and appetite, weight, and well-being were assessed weekly. Improved appetite and subjective well-being occurred within 2 weeks, and increased body weight was observed in the next 2 months. The progressive improvement in subjective and objective symptoms continued for approximately 4 months, after which a plateau was reached. Treatment continued for approximately 6 months. Thereafter, rapid worsening of performance status resulting from disease progression forced discontinuation of therapy.

Comment

The anorexia-cachexia syndrome is a paraneoplastic syndrome that frequently occurs in advanced non–small cell lung cancer or gastrointestinal cancer. The syndrome is caused by production of cytokines, both by the host and by the neoplasm, with endocrine and paracrine effects that influence the main metabolic processes regulating energy balance and the complex *orexiant/anorexiant* balance in the central nervous system.[4,5,12] Many trials have investigated treatments for cancer-related anorexia-cachexia. Corticosteroids and progestogens are the treatments of choice because they downregulate the cytokine cascade that induces the syndrome. The use of these agents should be determined on the basis of co-morbidities, prognostic assessment, and side effects.[13]

of the disease. Assessment can act as a surrogate index of tumor growth; in some neuroendocrine tumors, hormones or hormone-like molecules become indices of clinical response to surgical or medical treatments (Table 233-4).

TABLE 233-3 Laboratory Findings in Disseminated Intravascular Coagulopathy	
SCREENING TESTS	
Platelet count	Decreased
Prothrombin time	Increased
Partial thromboplastin time	Variable
Thrombin time	Increased
Erythrocyte morphology	Schistocytes and microspherocytes
SPECIFIC ASSAYS	
Fibrinogen	Decreased
Prothrombin	Variable
Factor V	Usually decreased
Factor VII	Variable
Factor VIIIc	Usually decreased
von Willebrand factor	Variably increased
Factor IX	Variable
Factor X	Variably decreased
Factor XI	Usually normal
Factor XIII	Usually decreased
Test of Fibrinolysis and FDP	
FDP	Increased
Plasminogen	Decreased
α_2-Antiplasmin	Variable
Plasmin	Usually increased
D-dimer	Increased
MISCELLANEOUS TESTS	
Antithrombin	Variably decreased
Protein C	Variable
Protein S	Variable

FDP, fibrin degradation product.

DIFFERENTIAL DIAGNOSIS

- A PNS can be the first sign of an underlying, unknown tumor, or the syndrome appear during the course of a known disease (Fig. 233-7).
- A PNS does not reflect the extent of disease and cannot be considered a surrogate expression of metastatic disease.
- PNS severity does not necessarily correlate with the severity of the cancer.
- A PNS is not a measure of tumor invasion of an organ.
- A PNS is not caused by treatment, nor is it a treatment side effect, although it may be mistaken for one.

TREATMENT

The therapeutic options can be classified in three main groups (Table 233-5):

- The etiological approach is primarily directed against the tumor.
- The pathogenetic approach interferes with specific physiological abnormalities.
- The symptomatic approach aims at abolishing the effects of the syndrome.

Although the etiological approach, if effective, controls both tumor growth and the clinical features of the PNS, some patients do not improve on tumor regression. The severity of some PNSs often needs a symptomatic approach, at least until tumor regression occurs.[1,10]

Etiological Approach

PNSs respond to primary tumor treatment and follow the clinical course. These include PNSs cause by syndromes of ectopic or pathological production of substances with endocrine or paracrine effects. Both surgical and chemotherapeutic or radiotherapeutic approaches can cause

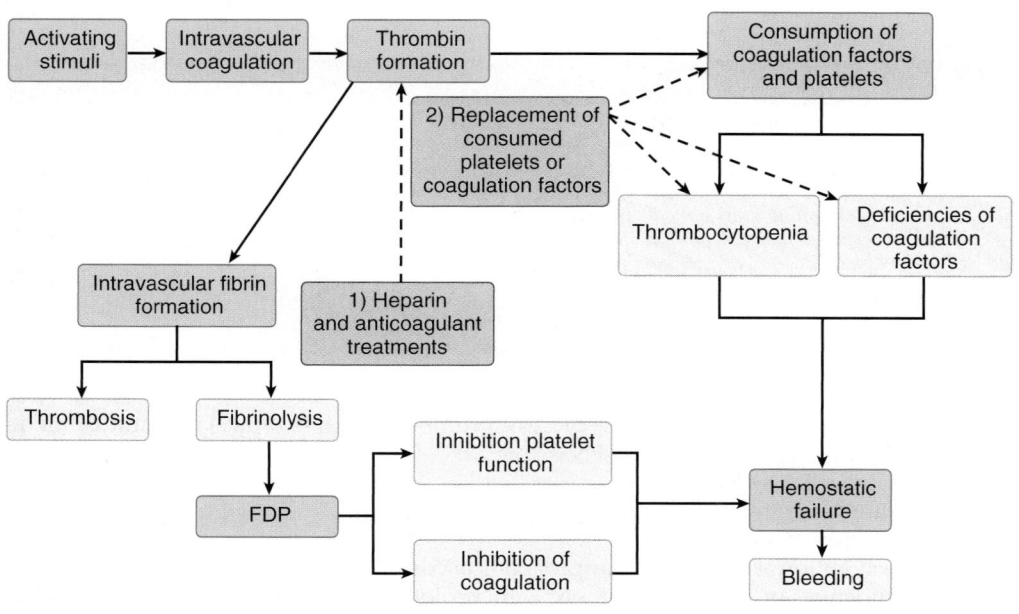

FIGURE 233-6 Pathophysiology of disseminated intravascular coagulopathy and its pathogenetic therapeutic approach (*red*). FDP, fibrin degradation product.

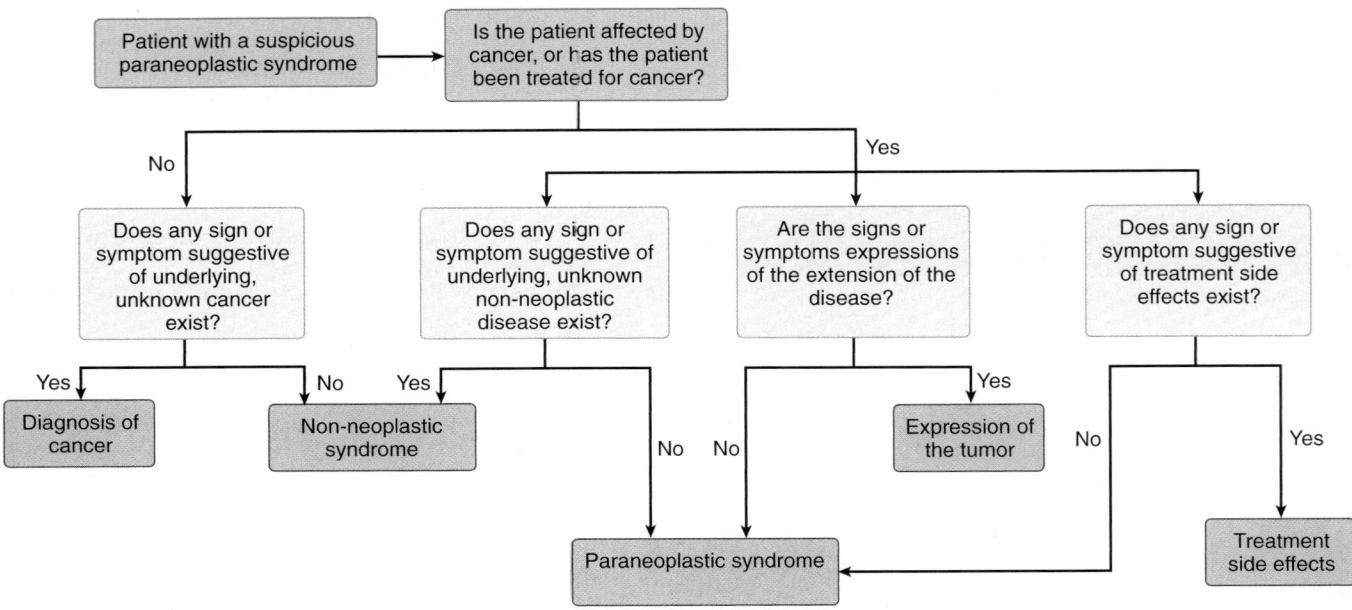

FIGURE 233-7 Differential diagnosis algorithm for paraneoplastic syndromes.

TABLE 233-4 Conditions Supporting Diagnosis and Assessment of Paraneoplastic Syndromes

CLINICAL ASSESSMENT SUFFICIENT FOR DIAGNOSIS AND FOLLOW-UP	LABORATORY FINDINGS SUPPORTIVE OF DIAGNOSIS OR FOLLOW-UP	LABORATORY FINDINGS FUNDAMENTAL FOR DIAGNOSIS AND TREATMENT
Pigmented lesions	Subacute sensory neuronopathy and encephalomyeloneuritis	Hypercalcemia/hypocalcemia
Keratoses	Limbic encephalitis	Hyperglycemia/hypoglycemia
Erythemas	Autonomic neuropathy	Zollinger-Ellison syndrome
Bullous lesions	Progressive cerebellar degeneration	Carcinoid syndrome
Anorexia-cachexia syndrome	Paraneoplastic vision loss	Anemia
Dermatomyositis	Opsoclonus-myoclonus	Erythrocytosis
Vasculitis	Paraneoplastic motor neuron disorders	Granulocytosis
Hypertrophic osteoarthropathy	Neuromuscular junction disorders	Granulocytopenia
Paraneoplastic fever	Ectopic adrenocorticotropic hormone syndrome	Thrombocytosis
Paraneoplastic peripheral neuropathies	Gonadotropin secretion	Thrombocytopenia
	Thyroid-stimulating hormone secretion	Disseminated intravascular coagulopathy
	Prolactin, growth hormone, and human placental lactogen secretion	Coagulopathies
	Syndrome of inappropriate antidiuretic hormone	Thrombophlebitis

TABLE 233-5 Therapeutic Approaches to Paraneoplastic Syndromes

ETIOLOGICAL	PATHOGENETIC	SYMPTOMATIC
Primary surgery (primary removal of neoplastic mass)	Immunosuppressive agents against autoimmune reactions (primarily corticosteroids)	Metabolic correction of fluid and electrolyte imbalance related to the syndrome (hypocalcemia/hypercalcemia, hyponatremia/ hypernatremia, hypoglycemia/hyperglycemia)
Chemotherapy and radiation therapy (primary control of tumor burden in locally advanced or metastatic disease)	Antithrombotic treatments (mainly low-molecular-weight heparins) against the prothrombotic effect of cancer	Transfusions in the acute hemorrhagic phases of coagulopathies
	Bisphosphonates against bone resorption	Rehabilitative support in neurological damage
	Octreotide in carcinoid syndrome	
	Corticosteroids or progestogens against the cytokine cascade in primary anorexia-cachexia syndrome	

regression of the PNS signs or symptoms, but clinical control of the syndrome does not necessarily imply complete regression of the disease.[1] Hematological PNSs also need control of the underlying disease to diminish clinical manifestations, and their severity often requires emergency treatment.[11] Treatment does not always allow complete control of the syndrome. Independence of the syndrome from tumor growth is typical of immune-mediated PNSs.[1,2]

Pathogenetic Approach

The approach is used in (1) treatment of autoimmune syndromes (e.g., neurological syndromes with corticosteroids

TABLE 233-6 Frequently Used Drugs for Paraneoplastic Syndromes

DRUGS	CLINICAL INDICATION
Chemotherapeutic agents	Primary treatment of locally advanced or metastatic solid tumors; primary treatment of hematological neoplasms
Corticosteroids	Pathogenetic approach to autoimmune paraneoplastic syndromes; frequently used for their anti-inflammatory effect
Progestogens	Pathogenetic treatment of anorexia-cachexia syndrome; inhibitors of main cytokines of the monocyte-macrophage system
Bisphosphonates	Drugs of choice for the hypercalcemic syndrome; helpful in reducing skeletal-related events in metastatic bone disease
Low-molecular-weight heparins	Through inhibiting factor Xa, used to reduce the extent of intravascular coagulation activation and the severity of chronic or subacute disseminated intravascular coagulopathy; must be used carefully because of the risk of exacerbating hemorrhagic manifestations of the syndrome
Transfusion	Supportive measure against acute depletion of blood elements or coagulation factors; because it replaces lost blood elements, it is only a supportive measure in hematological paraneoplastic syndromes; must be integrated with other types of treatment

Future Considerations

- Paraneoplastic syndromes (PNSs) represent a heterogeneous group of syndromes that can worsen the clinical outcome of cancer and against which no specific treatments exist.
- No biological or clinical models can predict the development of a PNS in a given disease or individual.
- Some existing models can explain the main pathogenetic events of PNSs, but little evidence supports laboratory or instrumental approaches to both diagnosis and follow-up.

or immune modulators); (2) inhibition of cytokines with endocrine or paracrine effects (e.g., treatment of cancer cachexia with progestogens or the carcinoid syndrome with octreotide); and (3) interruption of the coagulation cascade with low-molecular-weight heparin in disseminated intravascular coagulopathy. These approaches are frequently of limited value if they are not integrated with primary tumor treatment, but they remain useful when primary treatments are ineffective. A typical pathogenetic approach is treatment of hypercalcemia with bisphosphonates, whose role in interfering with bone resorption processes allows for control of hypercalcemia and reduction of skeletal complications from bone metastases.[8]

Symptomatic Approach

In addition to the foregoing, a supportive approach is often needed to control symptoms of the syndrome. A supportive (or symptomatic) approach is required in the following circumstances: (1) when symptoms are severe while the patient is waiting for primary treatments to work and (2) when a syndrome is refractory to primary treatment. The spectrum of supportive options is as heterogeneous as the spectrum of the symptoms. A symptomatic approach is never curative, although it is often rapidly effective. The most frequently used drugs are in Table 233-6. All three major approaches need to be integrated.

REFERENCES

1. Arnold SM, Lieberman FS, Foon KA. Paraneoplastic syndromes. In De Vita VT, Hellman S, Rosenberg SA (eds). Cancer: Principles and Practice of Oncology, 7th ed. Philadelphia: Lippincott Williams & Wilkins, 2005, pp 2189-2211.
2. Hall TC. Paraneoplastic syndromes: Mechanisms. Semin Oncol 1997; 24:269-276.
3. Lip GYH, Chin BSP, Blann AD. Cancer and the prothrombotic state. Lancet Oncol 2002;3:27-34.
4. Laviano A, Meguid MM, Rossi-Fanelli F. Cancer anorexia: Clinical implications, pathogenesis and therapeutic strategies. Lancet Oncol 2003;4:686-694.
5. Inui A. Cancer anorexia-cachexia syndrome: Current issues in research and management. CA Cancer J Clin 2002;52:72-91.
6. Honnorat J, Cartalat-Carel S. Advances in paraneoplastic neurological syndromes. Curr Opin Oncol 2004;16:614-620.
7. Bataller L, Dalmau JO. Paraneoplastic disorders of the central nervous system: Update on diagnostic criteria and treatment. Semin Neurol 2004;24:461-471.
8. Boyce S, Harper J. Paraneoplastic dermatoses. Dermatol Clin 2002; 20:523-532.
9. Rodgers GM. Acquired coagulation disorders. In Greer JP, Foerster J, Lukens JN, et al. (eds). Wintrobe's Clinical Hematology, 11th ed. Philadelphia: Lippincott Williams & Wilkins, 2004, pp 1669-1712.
10. Thomas L, Kwok Y, Edelman MJ. Management of paraneoplastic syndromes in lung cancer. Curr Treat Options Oncol 2004;5:51-62.
11. Staszewski H. Hematological paraneoplastic syndromes. Semin Oncol 1997;24:329-333.
12. Bruera E, Sweeney C. Cachexia and asthenia in cancer patients. Lancet Oncol 2000;1:138-147.
13. Yavuzsen T, Davis MP, Walsh D, et al. Systematic review of the treatment of cancer-associated anorexia and weight loss. J Clin Oncol 2005;23:8500-8511.

SUGGESTED READING

Bataller L, Dalmau J. Neuro-ophthalmology and paraneoplastic syndromes. Curr Opin Neurol 2004;17:3-8.
Cohen PR, Kurzrock R. Mucocutaneous paraneoplastic syndromes. Semin Oncol 1997;24:334-359.
Dalmau JO, Posner JB. Paraneoplastic syndromes affecting the nervous system. Semin Oncol 1997;24:318-328.
Maesaka JK, Mittal SK, Fishbane S. Paraneoplastic syndromes of the kidney. Semin Oncol 1997;24:373-381.
Stone SP, Buescher LS. Life-threatening paraneoplastic cutaneous syndromes. Clin Dermatol 2005;23:301-306.

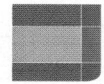

CHAPTER **234**

Autonomic Dysfunction

Maria Dietrich and Anna L. Marsland

KEY POINTS

- Secondary autonomic dysfunction from malignant disease may be common, and the cause is multifactorial.
- Autonomic dysfunction may involve the sympathetic nervous system (SNS), the parasympathetic nervous system (PNS), or the enteric nervous system (ENS).
- Gastrointestinal (GI) symptoms in cancer may be linked to autonomic dysfunction.
- Cardiovascular autonomic function testing is the core of the evaluation.
- Detailed symptom profiling and control oriented at the causes are key.

Autonomic dysfunction refers to altered function of the autonomic nervous system (ANS) that adversely affects health.[1] The specific autonomic disorder varies considerably, depending on multiple factors, including the origin, pathophysiology, site, and time course of the disorder.[1] Although it has long been known that autonomic dysfunction and neuropathy accompany many cancers, particularly in advanced stages, the pathophysiology remains unclear. Some patients with cancer develop paraneoplastic syndromes that damage the ANS.[2,3] However, it is likely that in most patients, the tumor causes more direct physical damage to the ANS. Many questions especially about pathophysiology, remain to be answered.[4]

The ANS is a division of the peripheral nervous system. It is a visceral and largely involuntary sensory and motor system that maintains links to virtually every organ system in the body (Fig. 234-1).[5] The ANS has three divisions: (a) the PNS, (b) the SNS, and (c) the ENS.

The SNS and PNS innervate cardiac muscle, smooth muscle, and glandular tissues and, when activated, produce various visceral reflexes (e.g., ocular, cardiovascular, glandular, GI, and urogenital). All divisions are tonically active. In addition, phasic SNS activation results in arousal often referred to as the fight-or-flight response, which prepares the body for action. Conversely, the PNS activates the rest-and-digest response, with a return toward homeostatic resting states. Finally, the ENS is more autonomous than the PNS and SNS and consists of the sensory and motor neurons of the GI tract, pancreas, and bladder that mediate, for example, digestive reflexes. Autonomic neurons use multiple chemical neurotransmitters. In general, sympathetic neurons release the catecholamine norepinephrine, which acts on adrenergic receptors, and parasympathetic neurons acetylcholine, which acts on cholinergic receptors.[5]

EPIDEMIOLOGY AND PREVALENCE

Autonomic dysfunction may be common among patients with cancer, particularly those with advanced disease.[3] Systematic information of prevalence is sparse.[3,6] Studies suggest that up to 50% of patients with cancer suffer

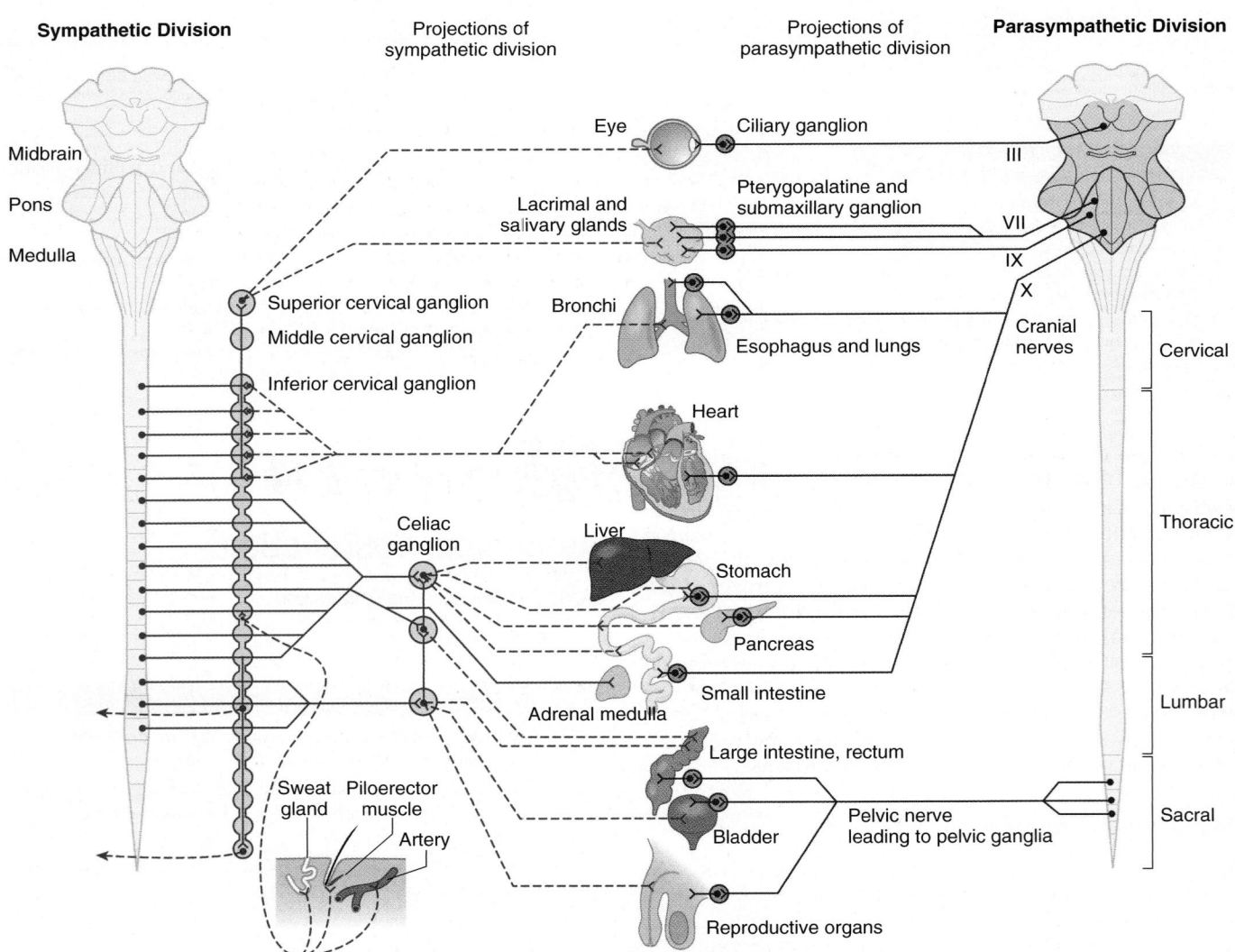

FIGURE 234-1 Sympathetic and parasympathetic divisions of the autonomic nervous system. *(From Iversen S, Iversen L, Saper CB. The autonomic nervous system and the hypothalamus. In Kandel ER, Schwartz JH, Jessell TM [eds]. Principles of Neural Science, 4th ed. New York: McGraw-Hill, 2000. Copyright © by The McGraw-Hill Companies. Used with permission.)*

symptoms of autonomic dysfunction.[6] One study found that among patients with advanced cancer, all reported signs of autonomic dysfunction, and 65% showed abnormalities on autonomic function tests.[3] Other reports suggest that autonomic neuropathy may be present in up to 28% of patients with tumor-associated paraneoplastic neuropathies[2] and in 1% to 13% of patients with multiple myeloma.[7] Paraneoplastic neuropathy occurs in only 1% of patients with cancer,[2] so this is not the only cause of autonomic dysfunction.

PATHOPHYSIOLOGY

The literature lacks specific descriptions and pathophysiological accounts of the multiple mechanisms involved.[3] Wide interindividual variability in cancer-related autonomic dysfunction suggests a complex set of disorders with multiple pathophysiological features. Autonomic dysfunction can be global or localized to a specific organ system (e.g., the GI tract).[8] It can involve preganglionic or postganglionic neurons, the SNS or the PNS, or specific neurochemical pathways, and it can originate from central or peripheral nervous system disease. With regard to autonomic subsystems affected in cancer, evidence indicates both PNS and SNS dysfunction in advanced cancer.[3] Another study found SNS, but not PNS, function significantly abnormal.[6] In addition to peripheral ANS, other investigators have found global functional impairment.[6] These studies were limited by the use of bedside measures of cardiac autonomic function, which may not provide a valid measure of global ANS status.[6]

One marker of global failure of sympathetic neurocircuitry is orthostatic hypotension. Decreased activation along sympathetic efferent pathways results in lower peripheral vascular tone, normally important in the maintenance of blood pressure (BP). Initially, compensatory mechanisms, such as the arterial baroreflex, can correct for this situation, but with time decreases in BP occur, particularly when the system makes quick adjustments, for example, following posture changes.[1] Although this is a marker of global autonomic dysfunction, the pathophysiology varies from person to person and can include lesions, denervations, or dysregulations at various sites along the sympathetic pathway. Nevertheless, evidence exists for orthostatic hypotension in advanced cancer and supports the concept of a general decline in SNS control of BP and a marker of general autonomic dysfunction.[1,9]

Some cancers involve the nervous system and result in autonomic dysfunction as a direct consequence of the disease. Multiple myeloma can infiltrate the autonomic nerves and can cause neuropathy. More often, nervous system damage results from amyloidosis. This disorder is the extracellular accumulation of amyloid that results in axonal degeneration with loss of myelinated and unmyelinated fibers.[7] In either case, depending on the location of the neural damage, the resultant neuropathy causes autonomic dysregulation or dysfunction.

GI complaints are a common concern of patients with cancer and can have a disproportionate impact on quality of life.[3,10] Autonomic dysfunction may be one explanation for the various GI symptoms that accompany advanced cancer, but the mechanisms are complex and are not understood.[11,12] It is widely suggested that GI dysmotility

and gastroparesis (delayed gastric emptying) are direct consequences of autonomic neuropathy, a hypothesis that explains common GI symptoms such as early satiety and constipation.[3,11-14]

The GI tract is controlled by all three branches of the ANS, which play important roles in gastric and intestinal motility. Activation of the SNS inhibits the GI tract, whereas the PNS is associated with stimulation of digestion. Both sympathetic dysfunction and parasympathetic dysfunction are associated with abnormal GI motility, which can result in constipation or diarrhea, respectively. Gastroparesis is typically associated with parasympathetic dysfunction. Evidence also indicates that dysfunction of all three branches of the ANS is involved in pseudo-obstruction, which causes symptoms of intestinal obstruction without verifiable obstruction.[11] Although the ANS plays an important role in these GI functions, and thus it is assumed that autonomic dysregulation is associated with GI symptoms, no study has demonstrated gastroparesis along with proven autonomic dysfunction.[3] Finally, a small subset of autonomic disorders may result from paraneoplastic syndromes. For example, anti-Hu antibodies have been linked to autonomic disturbances in small cell lung cancer.[7] The relative infrequency of these syndromes suggests that other factors account for most cases of cancer-related autonomic dysfunction.

CLINICAL MANIFESTATIONS

Several tests of autonomic function are available and have been employed in the assessment of patients with cancer. The goals of testing are (1) to evaluate the presence of autonomic dysfunction; (2) to determine the anatomic and physiological origins of any deficits (e.g., global or restricted, central or peripheral, adrenergic or cholinergic, preganglionic or postganglionic); (3) to grade the severity of any deficits; and (4) to monitor response to therapy.[8]

The assessment of cardiovascular autonomic function (Table 234-1) is the core of clinical ANS evaluation.[2,8] The most widely employed measure of autonomic function is heart rate variability (HRV). This term refers to the time-related changes in heart rate (HR) that accompany respiration (respiratory sinus arrhythmia). These high-frequency changes in HR provide a measure of parasympathetic tone. Because respiration patterns (depth and rate of breathing) alter HRV, measures are often taken during paced deep breathing.

HRV is not a good measure of sympathetic activation, for which BP responses to postural changes are the most frequent test. Orthostatic hypotension is a measure of the sympathetic control of peripheral vascular resistance.[8] In addition to these widely used clinical tests, research techniques assess cardiovascular autonomic function (see Table 234-1).[8] The advantage of these techniques is that they allow for a more direct and differentiated assessment of the pathways that contribute to autonomic dysfunction.[8]

Currently, clinical assessment is limited primarily to noninvasive *bedside* cardiovascular autonomic tests (see Table 234-1). These include the following: (1) HR responses to deep breathing, standing, and Valsalva's maneuver; and (2) BP responses to standing and static exercise.[3]

TABLE 234-1 Tests of Cardiovascular Autonomic Function: Clinical Tests and Research Techniques

CLINICAL TESTS*	RESEARCH TECHNIQUES
CARDIOVAGAL FUNCTION	
HR variability deep respiration: beat-to-beat variation in HR of three successive breathing cycles (mean of difference between maximum and minimum HR ≤15 beats/min)	Power spectral analysis
	Intraneural microneurography
	Pharmacological testing of autonomic function
HR Valsalva's maneuver: blowing through a mouthpiece at a pressure of 40 mm Hg for 10-20 sec (ratio of longest RR interval to shortest interval ≤1.20)	Assessment of baroreflex function
	Assessment of peripheral vasoconstrictor function: peripheral vascular resistance and venoarteriolar reflex
HR postural change: moving from the supine to upright posture (ratio of longest RR interval to shortest interval, also called 30:15 ratio, <1.04)	Catecholamine measures
	Assessment of venous function
	Cardiac sympathetic imaging
SYMPATHETIC ADRENERGIC FUNCTION	
BP active standing and passive tilting from the supine position (orthostatic hypotension: decrease in systolic BP of ≥20 mm Hg or a decrease in diastolic BP of ≥10 mm Hg within 3 min of standing)	
BP Valsalva's maneuver	
Isometric muscle contraction, such as sustained handgrip for 3 min at 30% of maximum effort (increase of ≤10 mm Hg)	
Cold pressor (immersion of hand into ice water for 1-3 min) or mental stress test such as mental arithmetic or Stroop color word naming test	
Prolonged tilt-table test for neurally mediated (vasovagal) syncope	
Carotid sinus massage	

*Cutoff used for determining abnormal autonomic function in parentheses.
BP, blood pressure; HR, heart rate.

Using these bedside tests, half of the patients with cancer in one study had ANS dysfunction (combination of abnormal test results).[6] When compared with a matched healthy control group, patients with cancer exhibited less of an increase in HR, a greater fall in BP on standing, and a smaller rise in BP in response to handgrip. These findings suggested SNS dysfunction. Little evidence of PNS dysfunction was reported.[6] Another study found more (65%) abnormal autonomic responses among patients with advanced cancer.[3] Most patients exhibited a smaller Valsalva ratio, an increase in HRV to deep breathing and standing, and a rise in BP in response to handgrip than normative values. In this study, however, the BP response to standing was normal for most patients. This finding is inconsistent with other findings[1,6] that postural hypotension frequently accompanies advanced cancer. The investigators attributed their failure to replicate this effect to the difficulty many of their subjects had in standing up.[6] Overall findings are consistent with regard to SNS cancer-related dysfunction and also suggest some concomitant parasympathetic dysregulation.[9]

Investigators have suggested that many frequent and distressing symptoms of advanced cancer are related to autonomic dysfunction.[3,10] Patients with advanced cancer who showed signs of abnormal autonomic function on clinical assessment also reported the following symptoms, in order of self-reported frequency: weight loss, anorexia, early satiety, weakness, nocturia, taste change, dysphagia, constipation, dry mouth, and shortness of breath.[3] Many of these are GI symptoms,[3,10] which are causally linked to autonomic dysfunction.[11,13]

DIFFERENTIAL DIAGNOSIS

Many diseases and conditions other than cancer may cause autonomic dysfunctions of varying degrees (Fig. 234-2).[1,3,9]Autonomic dysregulation among patients with

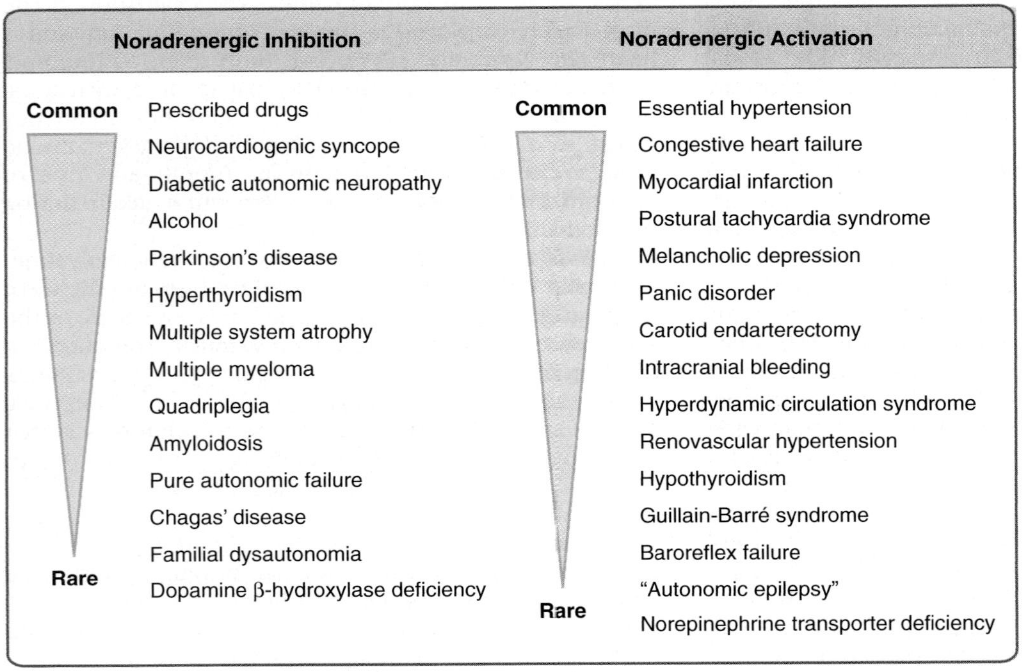

Noradrenergic Inhibition	Noradrenergic Activation
Common	**Common**
Prescribed drugs	Essential hypertension
Neurocardiogenic syncope	Congestive heart failure
Diabetic autonomic neuropathy	Myocardial infarction
Alcohol	Postural tachycardia syndrome
Parkinson's disease	Melancholic depression
Hyperthyroidism	Panic disorder
Multiple system atrophy	Carotid endarterectomy
Multiple myeloma	Intracranial bleeding
Quadriplegia	Hyperdynamic circulation syndrome
Amyloidosis	Renovascular hypertension
Pure autonomic failure	Hypothyroidism
Chagas' disease	Guillain-Barré syndrome
Familial dysautonomia	Baroreflex failure
Rare Dopamine β-hydroxylase deficiency	"Autonomic epilepsy"
	Rare Norepinephrine transporter deficiency

FIGURE 234-2 Dysautonomias featuring altered sympathetic noradrenergic function. *(From Goldstein DS. Dysautonomias: Clinical disorders of the autonomic nervous system. Ann Intern Med 2002;137:753-763. Copyright © by the American College of Physicians. Used with permission.)*

cancer may originate from conditions other than cancer.[2] Most patients with cancer are elderly and are susceptible to other age-related causes of peripheral nerve damage such as diabetes mellitus, cardiovascular disease, or nutritional deficiency.[2,3] Several studies have reported an age-related decline in HRV, one of the primary clinical measures of autonomic function.[8] Autonomic dysfunction and peripheral neuropathy may be side effects of current or past treatment. For example, chemotherapeutic agents, such as vincristine, and radiation treatment may produce autonomic dysregulation.[2,3,9,14]

Although the ANS plays a primary role in controlling the GI tract, GI symptoms can also result from many medications. For example, constipation is a frequent side effect of opioids, antidepressants, and anticholinergics.[13,15] Similarly, assessment of GI obstruction should differentiate a mechanical true obstruction from a pseudo-obstruction. In addition to autonomic dysfunction secondary to cancer, pseudo-obstructions can stem from several diseases, including connective tissue diseases (lupus, scleroderma, amyloidosis), endocrine disorders (hypoparathyroid, hypoparathyroidism, diabetes), and other primary neurological diseases that affect the ANS (Shy-Drager syndromes).[2] Finally, indirect complications of autonomic neuropathy, such as bacterial overgrowth, esophagitis, and gastritis, may contribute to symptoms and should be considered.[11]

TREATMENT

Careful assessment and a systematic treatment approach directed at the specific pathological process are necessary for effective management of autonomic dysfunction.[13] The treatment of drug-related neuropathies and associated symptoms may be easiest, by evaluating the cost-to-benefit ratio of drug withdrawal or dose reduction.[2,13] If the autonomic dysfunction is related to an underlying primary disease, treating the disease or malignancy may arrest the progression of the resultant autonomic disorder.[2] Regardless of the cause, attention should also focus on the symptoms and the comfort of patients with advanced cancer.[13] For instance, various pharmacological and behavioral options are available to treat orthostatic hypotension.[9]

Anorexia and cachexia are associated with morbidity and mortality in advanced cancer.[15,16] Treating GI symptoms in cancer is often complicated. Symptoms are concurrent, the exact pathophysiological mechanisms and interactions are not understood, and drug treatments may or may not be helpful.[13] Any medications contributing to these symptoms should be altered first, followed by medications that may relieve symptoms. For example, prokinetic agents (metoclopramide, domperidone) that increase GI motility may help if delayed gastric emptying appears to be the cause of symptoms such as constipation, early satiety, nausea, and vomiting.[13,15] Further, opioid antagonists may relieve constipation.[13,15] In addition, dietary and behavioral changes should be considered.[13] Reflecting the pervasiveness of GI symptoms in cancer, GI-related drugs account for more than half of the six top-ranked drug classes in advanced cancer, the most common being opioids, laxatives, H_2 blockers, appetite stimulants, and antiemetics.[10]

Future Considerations

- More systematic research is needed to understand the prevalence and nature of autonomic nervous system (ANS) dysregulation in cancer, to define the pathophysiology of various ANS abnormalities more accurately in patients with cancer patients, and to determine the extent to which ANS dysregulation contributes to symptoms in cancer.
- Recent neuroimaging and other research techniques will provide a better understanding of autonomic dysfunction pathophysiology.

SUMMARY

It remains to be determined to what extent autonomic dysfunction contributes to symptoms in advanced cancer. This is a fruitful area for further research. Initial findings support autonomic dysfunction in late-stage cancer, although the exact pathophysiology has yet to be determined. It is likely that this dysfunction contributes to many of the symptoms that accompany late-stage cancer. Further knowledge regarding the sites of breakdown of autonomic function would enable more focused interventions that could improve quality of life for these patients.

REFERENCES

1. Goldstein DS. Dysautonomias: Clinical disorders of the autonomic nervous system. Ann Intern Med 2002;137:753-763.
2. Corbo M, Balmaceda C. Peripheral neuropathy in cancer patients. Cancer Invest 2001;19:369-382.
3. Walsh D, Nelson KA. Autonomic nervous system dysfunction in advanced cancer. Support Care Cancer 2002;10:523-528.
4. Goldstein DS. The Autonomic Nervous System in Health and Disease. New York: Dekker, 2001.
5. Iversen S, Iversen L, Saper CB. The autonomic nervous system and the hypothalamus. In Kandel ER, Schwartz JH, Jessell TM (eds). Principles of Neural Science, 4th ed. New York: McGraw-Hill, 2000, pp 960-981.
6. Martin R, Delgado JM, Molto JM, et al. Cardiovascular reflexes in patients with malignant disease. Ital J Neurol Sci 1992;13:125-129.
7. Rudnicki SA, Dalmau J. Paraneoplastic syndromes of the peripheral nerves. Curr Opin Neurol 2005;18:598-603.
8. Freeman R. Assessment of cardiovascular autonomic function. Clin Neurophysiol 2006;117:716-730.
9. Grubb BP, Karas B. Clinical disorders of the autonomic nervous system associated with orthostatic intolerance: An overview of classification, clinical evaluation, and management. Pacing Clin Electrophysiol 1999;22:798-810.
10. Komurcu S, Nelson KA, Walsh D, et al. Gastrointestinal symptoms among inpatients with advanced cancer. Am J Hosp Palliat Care 2002;19:351-355.
11. Chelimsky G, Wszolek Z, Chelimsky TC. Gastrointestinal dysfunction in autonomic neuropathy. Semin Neurol 1996;16:259-268.
12. Nelson KA, Walsh TD, Sheehan FG, et al. Assessment of upper gastrointestinal motility in the cancer-associated dyspepsia syndrome. J Palliat Care 1993;9:27-31.
13. Komurcu S, Nelson KA, Walsh D. The gastrointestinal symptoms of advanced cancer Support Care Cancer 2000;9:32-39.
14. Sharabi Y, Dendi R, Holmes C, Goldstein DS. Baroreflex failure as a late sequela of neck irradiation. Hypertension 2003;42:110-116.
15. Lagman RL, Davis MP, LeGrand SB, Walsh D. Common symptoms in advanced cancer. Surg Clin North Am 2005;85:237-255.
16. Walsh D, Rybicki L, Nelson KA, Donnelly S. Symptoms and prognosis in advanced cancer. Support Care Cancer 2002;10:385-388.

SUGGESTED READING

Goldstein DS. The Autonomic Nervous System in Health and Disease. New York: Dekker, 2001.

Low P. Clinical Autonomic Disorders. Boston: Little, Brown, 1993.

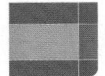

CHAPTER **235**

Radiation Principles and Techniques

John Armstrong and Aktham Sharif

K E Y   P O I N T S

- The aim is to deliver a measured dose of radiation to a defined tumor volume to eradicate the tumor and prolong survival while preserving surrounding normal tissue. Radiation therapy is also used for palliation of pain and other symptoms.

- Linear accelerators (linacs) are the main machines used, although cobalt 60 machines still have a role in palliation.

- Treatment planning traditionally uses orthogonal films in two-dimensional planning, but computed tomography (CT) three-dimensional planning is now the standard.

- Intensity-modulated radiation therapy (IMRT) and stereotactic radiosurgery (SRS) are new techniques that deliver accurate radiation doses to tumors while minimizing radiation damage to surrounding tissues.

- Radiosensitizers are chemical or pharmacological agents that increase the lethal effects of radiation when these agents are administered with it.

Radiation oncology is that discipline of human medicine dealing with the generation and dissemination of knowledge concerning the causes, prevention, and treatment of cancer and other diseases and involving special expertise in the therapeutic application of ionizing radiation.[1] Incorporating medical and nuclear physics and cellular, molecular, and cancer biology, therapeutic radiation is used alone or in conjunction with surgery and chemotherapy in malignant neoplasms and in certain benign conditions. The aims are to deliver a measured dose of radiation to a defined tumor volume and thereby eradicate the tumor and preserve the surrounding normal tissue as much as possible and to prolong survival. Radiation therapy also plays a vital role in advanced malignant disease for palliation by pain relief and symptom control.

IONIZING RADIATION, EXTERNAL BEAM RADIATION (TELETHERAPY), AND BRACHYTHERAPY

When an atom or molecule is exposed to radiation, it absorbs energy.[2] If the energy is sufficient to eject one or more orbital electrons from the atom or molecule, this is known as ionization, and that radiation is *ionizing radiation*. The most important characteristic of ionizing radiation is its ability to release very concentrated amounts of energy locally into cells. Examples of ionizing radiation are gamma rays from nuclear decay, photons, and electrons, which comprise types of x-rays. External beam radiation therapy is delivered from a distance (generally 100 cm). Brachytherapy is delivered locally from radioactive sources placed close to or within the tumor.

Linear Accelerators

A linac is the device commonly used to deliver external beam radiation for cancer.[1] The linac uses microwave technology to accelerate electrons in a part of the accelerator called the wave guide, which then allows these electrons to collide with a heavy metal target (usually tungsten). As a result, high-energy x-rays are scattered from the target. These x-rays can then be shaped to a beam and aimed at the tumor. The beam exits from a part of the linac known as the gantry, which rotates around the patient. The patient lies on a mobile table known as the couch, which can also rotate and form different angles with the gantry to deliver the treatment. The machine sits in a room called the vault, which is built with lead and concrete walls to protect the radiotherapist, who operates the machine from outside the vault, from exposure. Radiation oncologists, medical physicists, dosimetrists, and radiotherapists have specific roles in the operation, maintenance, quality control, and calibration of the linac for it to deliver the exact amount of radiation to the tumor.

Cobalt 60 Machines (Radionuclide Teletherapy)

Cobalt 60 machines, the first high-energy photon devices, were introduced in the 1950s.[3] They are being replaced by linacs; however, they remain the mainstay in developing countries. A cobalt 60 machine for palliative radiation therapy is simple to maintain, and it is practical when used for intractable pain from bony metastases, multiple brain metastases, and emergencies such as spinal cord compression, superior vena cava obstruction, and hemoptysis. The disadvantages are poor dose penetration to deep tumors and a fuzzy edge to the beam.

Cobalt machines function using a radioactive source continually undergoing nuclear decay and emitting a *beta* particle and two photons with different energies: 1.17 and 1.33 MeV. Cobalt 60 has a half-life of 5.26 years (i.e., activity is reduced by half every 5.26 years). The source needs to be changed approximately every 5 years because continuous use leads to prolonged treatment times.

SIMULATION AND TREATMENT PLANNING

Before someone begins radiation therapy, be it curative or palliative, he or she normally undergoes a simulation or treatment planning session.[4,5] Planning is usually done using x-ray fluoroscopy or a CT scanner to identify the field where the tumor lies. The patient is marked with permanent ink (tattoo) on the skin, and laser beams are used to align the patient in the same position every day. Various immobilization devices are used, depending on the treatment site. Tumor volumes are drawn either on the x-ray films or on the CT slices on a computer specially equipped with planning software for radiation therapy. Volumes of critical structures (depending on the site of the tumor) are also drawn (e.g., in brain tumors, critical structures such as the eye, optic nerve, optic chiasma, and pituitary gland) because all will receive a certain amount of radiation. Dose-volume histograms are generated to analyze the different radiation doses delivered to the tumor and adjacent critical structures. During treatment planning, decisions are made about the number and intensity of beams, patient positioning, tumor dose, and dose to adjacent normal structures. The radiation oncologist works with the dosimetrist and medical physicist to develop the optimal treatment plan to deliver an adequate dose to the tumor with minimal exposure of the normal surrounding structures. Once the plan is completed, it is checked and approved by the radiation oncologist. Further checks are made by the medical physicist. The patient is then brought in for a final session (verification), in which check films identify the treatment area from all the beams. These x-ray films display the actual shape of the treatment area, known as the *portal*. Once these images are approved, treatment can begin.

Two-Dimensional versus Three-Dimensional Planning

New techniques have evolved to identify the tumor as a target, to define its borders and to shape the radiation beam to these borders, to increase the intensity of the beam, to minimize radiation to the normal surrounding tissue, and to reduce toxicity and side effects to these tissues (Fig. 235-1).[6] Two-dimensional planning consists of orthogonal films (anterior, posterior, and lateral views) of the area of interest. Volumes are drawn on these films or CT scans. Contours of the regions of interest are made using metal wires or plaster of Paris. Larger margins around the tumor are implemented, leading to increased toxicities because of radiation exposure to normal tissues.

Three-dimensional treatment planning has revolutionized radiation therapy. Patients undergo CT scanning. Tumors are better identified in three dimensions (length, width, and depth). Intricate software leads to better tumor visualization in relation to surrounding anatomical struc-

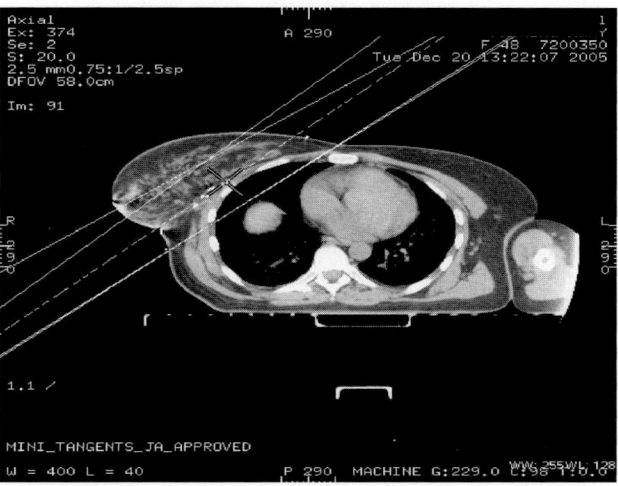

FIGURE 235-1 Virtual simulation: breast example. This approach is used in the radical treatment of breast cancer, as well as for precise focusing of beams in palliative situations.

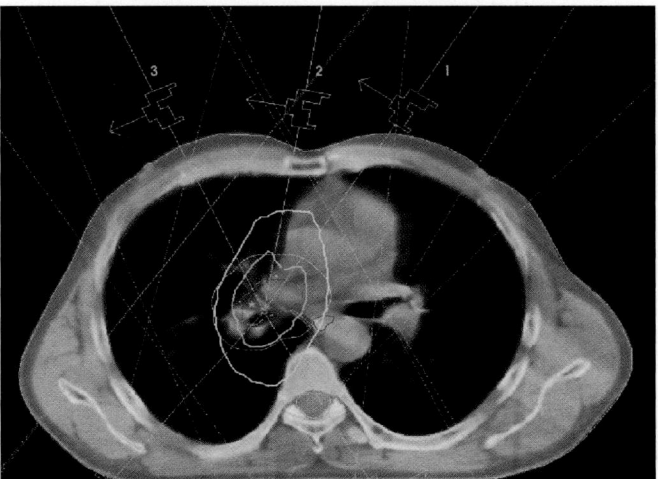

FIGURE 235-2 Lung intensity-modulated radiation therapy. This highly conformal method of radiation planning and delivery can be used for repeat treatment of tumors previously that were irradiated. The beam can be focused on the tumor and reduced to the surrounding tissues.

tures. Organ motion is analyzed, organs at risk are better identified in relation to tumor volume, and more accurate margins are drawn, thus minimizing surrounding tissue toxicity. The three-dimensional approach is now the standard method of treatment planning in radiation oncology. Two-dimensional planning is quick and inexpensive and still has its place in palliative care for treating bone and brain metastases and inoperable tumors for symptom control.

INTENSITY-MODULATED RADIATION THERAPY

IMRT is the latest advance in three-dimensional conformal radiation therapy (Fig. 235-2).[1] Small beams of radiation *(beamlets)* are aimed at the tumor from multiple angles. The radiation intensity of each beamlet can be controlled, and the shape changes many times during the treatment period, thereby delivering adequate doses to the tumor and reduced doses to the surrounding normal tissue. In this way, toxicity to normal tissues is decreased. Complex treatment planning software, CT, magnetic resonance imaging, positron emission tomography scans, and special immobilization devices are used to define tumor position accurately in relation to the healthy surrounding anatomical structures. Special head frames are used for patients with brain tumors. A computer-controlled device known as a multileaf collimator built into the linac is adjusts the size and shape of the radiation beams. The metal leaves move across the treatment area when the beam is on, thus increasing the tumor dose, blocking the beam to the normal tissue, and varying beam intensity. In the palliative setting, IMRT is particularly useful if a tumor needs repeat irradiation. The dose-sculpting ability of IMRT allows radiation to be partially diverted away from previously irradiated critical normal tissues.

Advantages of IMRT include the following:

- Reduced radiation to normal tissue
- Reduced damage to normal cells
- Increased dose to malignant cells
- Accurate radiation distribution
- Increased chance of destroying malignant cells

STEREOTACTIC RADIOSURGERY

SRS is a precise method for treating brain tumors primarily with a high dose of radiation in a focused beam to the target area (Fig. 235-3).[1] Lars Leksell, a Swedish physician and neurosurgeon, developed the *gamma knife,* the first device for treating brain abnormalities using this concept. It involves a single high dose or sometimes multiple radiation doses that converge on the brain target site or the tumor site. A specially made head device keeps the head immobile, and with highly sophisticated computer planning software, radiation is delivered stereotactically to minimize the amount of radiation delivered to healthy brain tissue. SRS is an important alternative to invasive surgery and can be used when surgical access to the tumor carries a high risk of morbidity. Randomized clinical trials are looking at the optimum dose for brain metastases and other brain lesions (e.g., arteriovenous malformations, acoustic neuromas). Comparisons among different doses for whole brain radiation therapy and SRS are being tried in which quality of life, local tumor control, and performance status are the end points.

The three basic types of SRS are as follows:

- Linac based
- Cobalt 60 based (gamma knife)
- Particle beam (proton)

The linac-based SRS is the most commonly used and widely available throughout the world. One of its main benefits is its ability to treat large tumors (>4 cm) using several sessions, an approach known as *fractionated SRS.* This machine moves around the patient and delivers the dose in increments.

The cobalt 60 gamma knife does not move during treatment. Therefore, it provides a high degree of precision within the brain. The gamma knife has been available

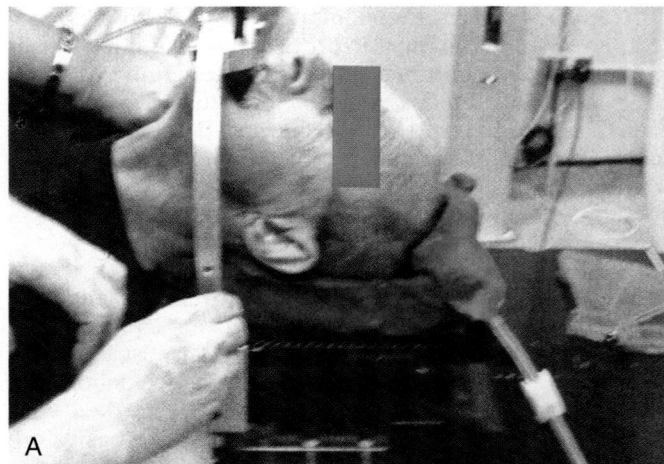

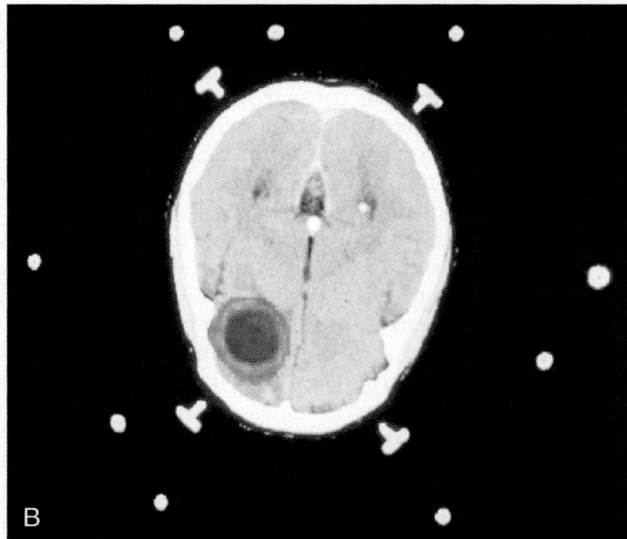

FIGURE 235-3 Frameless stereotactic radiosurgery (SRS). **A,** This outpatient procedure delivers a precisely shaped beam of very high dose to brain metastases. In selected patients, it increases survival and is equivalent to surgical resection of secondary brain tumors. SRS has also been used in other sites (e.g., spinal metastases). **B,** SRS targets.

since the 1970s and is essentially unchanged. It uses multiple radiation sources, a feature that allows for less damage to healthy tissue and better targeting. It is ideal for tumors smaller than 3.5 cm. The particle beam (proton) is in limited use in the United States. This device is extremely large and is generally used in research.

BIOLOGICAL PRINCIPLES

Overview

Following exposure of the human cell to radiation, it undergoes reactions that result in cell death. Based on its molecular structure, the cell will either die as a result of irreversible DNA damage or repair this damage and repopulate.[7,8]

Cell Cycle and DNA Damage

The cell cycle is the pattern of events that leads from one cell division to the next. The phases of the cell cycle are as follows:

- G_0: Growth and preparation of the chromosomes for replication. The cells exist in a quiescent state.
- G_1: This is the first growth phase, in which specific enzymes are formed.
- S: Synthesis of DNA. In this phase, DNA is replicated.
- G_2: In this second growth phase, the cell is prepared for the next step.
- M: Mitosis is the actual division of the cell into two daughter cells.

As the cell passes through these phases, specific proteins in the cytoplasm control this process. A "surveillance system" monitors the cell for DNA damage at certain checkpoints. This system can block progression to the next phase if it senses something wrong. The important point is that radiation interferes with the cell cycle and induces DNA damage and, eventually, cell death.

RADIOSENSITIZERS

Radiosensitizers are chemical or pharmacological agents that increase the lethal effects of radiation if they are administered with it.[9] Examples include the following:

- Halogenated primitives. 5-Iododeoxyuridine and 5-bromodeoxy uridine are similar to the normal DNA precursor thymidine. They can be incorporated into the DNA chain in place of thymidine. This process weakens the DNA chain and renders it more susceptible to radiation.
- Oxygen is an effective radiosensitizer. Research to increase the amount of oxygen and the search for compounds that mimic the ability of oxygen to sensitize cells to the effects of radiation continue.
- Certain chemotherapy agents (e.g., cisplatin, 5-fluorouracil, and gemcitabine) are used as radiosensitizers.

REFERENCES

1. Perez CA, Brady LW, Halperin EC, Schmidt-Ullrich RK. Principles and Practice of Radiation Oncology, 4th ed. Philadelphia: Lippincott Williams & Wilkins, 2003.
2. Khan FM. The Physics of Radiation Therapy, 3rd ed. Philadelphia: Lippincott, Williams & Wilkins, 2003.
3. Stanton R, Stinson D. Applied Physics for Radiation Oncology. Madison, WI: Medical Physics Publishing, 1996.
4. Bentel GC. Treatment Planning and Dose Calculation in Radiation Oncology. New York: McGraw-Hill, 1989.
5. Khan FM. Treatment Planning in Radiation Oncology, 2nd ed. Philadelphia: Lippincott Williams & Wilkins, 2006.
6. Armstrong J. Advances in radiation technology can improve survival and quality of life for cancer patients: 25th St Luke's lecture, Royal Academy of Medicine of Ireland, 7th December, 1999. Ir J Med Sci 170:63-68.
7. Percorino L. Molecular Biology of Cancer, 2nd ed. New York: Oxford University Press, 2008.
8. King RJB, Robins MW. Cancer Biology, 3rd ed. New York: Pearson Prentice-Hall, 2006.
9. Hall EJ, Amato AJ. Radiobiology for the Radiologist, 6th ed. Philadelphia: Lippincott Williams & Wilkins, 2005.

CHAPTER **236**

Complications of Radiation Therapy

John N. Staffurth

KEY POINTS

- Acute radiation effects occur during or immediately after radiation therapy and are generally discomforting but self-limiting.
- Late radiation effects continue beyond or start 90 days after radiation therapy but are considered irreversible; they may affect impact on patients' quality of life.
- The incidence and severity of toxicity depend on factors related to the patient, the tumor, and the treatment.
- For most normal tissues, the volume irradiated and the dose to which it is irradiated are most important.
- Most therapies have been developed by experience, and relatively few high-quality clinical trials have made major contributions to the field.

BASIC SCIENCE AND RADIOBIOLOGY

Radiobiology is of particular relevance to the development of toxicity. Originally, radiation therapy was delivered in single large doses (see Chapter 235). When a treatment is split into multiple daily fractions, acute normal tissue effects are reduced, with late effects spared even more. This sparing of late effects gives fractionation, now standard practice for radical therapy, a therapeutic advantage. The four radiobiological principles that explain the effects of fractionation are repair, reoxygenation, repopulation, and redistribution. A fifth factor affecting the tissue response to radiation is inherent radiosensitivity (Box 236-1).

Models that predict the effects of different fractionation schedules have been developed. The most clinically reliable is the linear-quadratic (LQ) model (Box 236-2). It uses a term called the a/β ratio, which represents sensitivity to dose and dose-squared, and represents a tissue's ability to repair radiation-induced double-stranded DNA breaks. However, this model can be modified to include the overall duration of radiation therapy. a/β ratios are now derived from clinical data, which represent whole organ outcomes such as tumor control and late toxicity, as opposed to in vitro data, which usually represent cellular events. The LQ model may allow the design of novel, optimized fractionation schedules for each tumor type.

EPIDEMIOLOGY AND PREVALENCE

The risk of developing toxicity is best considered as related to treatment or to the patient (Table 236-1).[3]

Box 236-1 Administration of Radiation Therapy and Its Effects

- Radiation therapy (RT) can be delivered in a three ways: external beam radiation therapy, brachytherapy, or injected radioisotopes. The molecular effects within irradiated cells are the same whatever the mode of delivery, but the effect on the patient depends on the tissue volume irradiated.
- Short-term effects occur during or immediately after RT. They are usually minor and, although discomforting, are self-limiting. However, in some instances, these effects may last beyond 90 days and may cause consequential late damage. RT may need to be temporarily discontinued to allow patients time to recover, but this interval allows the tumor, and normal tissue, to repopulate, and such an approach should be avoided.
- Acute effects of RT occur as the epithelial surface becomes denuded. This happens as radiation causes endothelial cell apoptosis and growth arrest of the stem cell compartment within the basal layers. Lack of replacement of the epithelial surface produces symptoms.
- Late effects start at least 90 days after RT has been completed, and the RT cannot therefore be modified. The natural history is variable; some patients experience single episodes, others have multiple episodes, and some patients have progressive symptoms. Most late effects are minor, but because many of these patients are long-term survivors, these effects can have a major impact on quality of life.
- Late effects of RT are generally irreversible, although therapies aimed at reversing chronic hypoxia may have promise. Few randomized controlled trials of preventive or therapeutic pharmaceuticals have been conducted, although this is an area of active research. So far, trials have had inconsistent results.

Box 236-2 The Linear-Quadratic Equation

Biological effective dose = Total dose (1 + [a/β ratio/dose per fraction])

TABLE 236-1 Factors Associated with the Development of Radiation Toxicity

TREATMENT-RELATED FACTORS	PATIENT-RELATED FACTORS
Total dose	Age
Dose per fraction	Prior cancer therapy
Volume irradiated	Concurrent medical conditions
Delivery technique	Social factors
Concurrent therapies	Genetics

Treatment-Related Factors

With regard to *dose-volume relationship,* the volume of irradiated normal tissue is a critical factor in late toxicity. Advanced radiation therapy techniques, such as intensity-modulated radiation therapy (IMRT), can reduce the volume of normal tissue irradiated without affecting tumor coverage. IMRT can reduce toxicity, although radiation oncologists often aim to escalate the radiation dose to improve tumor control. The precise volume of normal tissue that can safely be irradiated to different dose levels is unknown. More knowledge[4] is being acquired as three-dimensional planning and prospective collection of toxicity and quality of life data mature. Prospective data are being applied to individualized patient plans for the rectum, lung, and parotid glands, and applications will become more widespread because IMRT planning requires that radiation oncologists reconsider this issue. *Concurrent therapies* such as chemotherapy and the use of biological agents such as epidermal growth factor receptor inhibitors increase acute radiation toxicity, but their effects on late toxicity have not been fully evaluated.

Patient-Related Factors

Patient-related factors include smoking and alcohol consumption, prior radiation therapy or surgery, and general medical conditions (e.g., diabetes, acquired immunodeficiency syndrome, inflammatory bowel disease, and connective tissue diseases).[5] Patients with head and cancer who continue to smoke during radiation therapy develop more severe acute toxicity than those who discontinue smoking.[6]

GENETICS OF RADIOSENSITIVITY

Several well-defined clinical syndromes are associated with increased clinical and in vitro cellular radiosensitivity (e.g., ataxia-telangiectasia, Fanconi's anemia, Bloom's syndrome, and Nijmegan's breakage syndrome). These syndromes affect proteins in the DNA damage repair pathway. Factors governing tissue radiosensitivity are complex and involve many gene products. Abnormal gene products coded for by single nucleotide polymorphisms in critical genes influence radiosensitivity in different cell types. Studies of the DNA damage identification and repair pathways showed encouraging results implicating the *XRCC1, XRCC3, ATM,* and *TGFB1* genes.[7,8] Single-nucleotide polymorphisms in genes involved in cell-cycle checkpoints and cellular determinants of apoptosis may also be relevant. Prospective collections of high-quality data linking late toxicity, radiation therapy dosimetry, and normal tissue (and tumor) biobanks are under way (RAPPER, GENEPI).[9,10]

PATHOPHYSIOLOGY

The pathobiology of mucositis has been extensively studied.[11]

Acute Events

The acute effects of radiation (e.g., within the mucosa) progress as follows:

1. Initiation: Production of reactive oxygen species leads to the release of transforming growth factor-β (TGF-β).
2. Primary damage response: Endothelial cell apoptosis occurs through ceramide production, inflammatory cell infiltrate, and cytokine release.[12] DNA and non-DNA damage leads to activation of TP53 and nuclear factor-κB, as well as epithelial stem cell arrest.
3. Signal amplification: DNA damage repair and complex interactions of intracellular and extracel-

lular balances decide the final cell outcomes (e.g., through BCL-2, mitogen-activated protein kinase).[13]

4. Ulceration: This complication results from continued epithelial cell loss, possibly in conjunction with superinfections.

5. Healing: Stem cell recovery with accelerated proliferation. Matrix metalloproteinase and cell adhesion molecule upregulation may allow increased transit time.

Late Events

The pathophysiology of late radiation damage is not understood. It is unknown whether the critical lesions that lead to chronic changes are within the connective tissue (vasculature, inflammatory cells or extracellular matrix) or within the mucosa (stem cells). Abnormalities include loss of stem cells from all compartments, chronic hypoxia, and secondary stress events in a pro-inflammatory and pro-angiogenic microenvironment. Fibrin deposition within vessels leads to further vessel damage and to a chronic hypoxic cycle, possible mediated by TGF-β.

HISTOPATHOLOGY

The changes seen with mucosal lesions (e.g., rectum) include ulceration, atypical glandular regeneration, fibrosis, and vascular sclerosis. Simultaneous submucosal and connective tissue changes are also seen, including edema, inflammation, and dilated or sclerosed vessels. Ulceration, perforation, and strictures can all result from the combination of mucosal barrier breakdown, fibrosis, and vascular ischemia.[14]

CLINICAL MANIFESTATIONS

General Issues

Serial and Parallel Organs

- The effect on a patient may depend on other factors, such as person's functional reserve or the organ's structural and functional organization.
- Parallel organs are organized into separate subunits that function independently. Someone may have a large physiological reserve and may be asymptomatic despite areas of radiation damage (e.g., the lung).

Pearls and Pitfalls

- Recurrent aspiration pneumonia may occur as an acute or late toxicity from radiation therapy to any area from the oral cavity to the esophagus.
- Severe acute toxicities should be brought to the attention of the radiation oncologist. Possible factors include radiation sensitivity syndromes, superinfections, or treatment errors.
- Following high-dose brain radiation, deterioration in functional status is common. This effect is self-limiting and does not require an increase in steroid dose.
- Within the perineal area, severe skin reactions can be minimized by good hygiene. In frail patients, urinary and fecal incontinence should be suspected.

- Serial organs require normal functioning over each section. Minor damage may cause loss of function of the whole organ (e.g., the spinal cord).
- Many organs have both serial and parallel elements (e.g., the bowel)

Assessment, Quality of Life, and Survivorship Issues

- Survivors of cancer and of cancer treatments are increasing in number.
- Toxicity assessment has historically been retrospective.
- Multiple validated and nonvalidated clinician- and patient-completed evaluation tools are available.
- International collaborations have reduced these issues, but modifications of the tools occur regularly.
- Quality of life issues are of primary importance.
- The emphasis on curative radiation therapy is shifting from maximizing cure to quantity of life free from symptoms of disease and therapy, a concept inherent in palliative medicine for years.

Second Malignant Diseases

- Ionizing radiation is carcinogenic, and as the numbers of cancer survivors increase, so will the numbers of cancers induced by ionizing radiation. These cancers usually occur more than 10 years after therapy and affect organs that have received at least a moderate radiation dose.[15]
- The most sensitive organs are those undergoing physiological maturation (e.g., the breast in young women with Hodgkin's lymphoma).[16] These issues are especially important in children, and every attempt should be made to exclude radiation from their treatment protocol. The 1986 nuclear accident at Chernobyl in the Ukraine increased the incidence of thyroid cancers in children who were at least 3 months old in utero.[17]
- In adults, malignant diseases induced by radiation therapy affect common sites (e.g., lung and colorectal carcinomas), but bone and soft tissue sarcomas also occur. Men with prostate cancer may have an increased risk of colorectal cancers compared with men who had surgical treatment or observation. Newer radiation techniques (e.g., IMRT) increase the conformality of the high-dose region, as well as the volume of normal tissue receiving low doses, issues of concern.[18]

PREVENTIVE STRATEGIES

Three broad approaches are used prevent radiation toxicity: treatment delivery (including patient selection), general medical care, and use of molecular agents.

Radiation Techniques

Safe techniques and dose fractionation regimens have been developed that reduce severe toxicities. The aim of these technical advances is to reduce the volume of normal tissue irradiated to critical levels. These advances include improved patient selection and target volume delineation with advanced functional imaging and improved conformality of dose planning and accuracy of dose delivery using advanced delivery systems such as IMRT, image-

---

Common Errors

Acute

- Use of metal-containing topical agents during radiation therapy
- Missed diagnosis of coexisting infection (e.g., herpes zoster or moniliasis)
- Lack of awareness of deteriorating nutrition status
- Inadequate assessment of dentition before radiation therapy
- Inadequate use of systemic analgesics

Late

- Assuming that all postradiation symptoms are the result of radiation therapy
- Prolonged use of empirical therapies before formal investigations
- Delay in seeking advice from the radiation oncologist

Box 236-3 Amifostine

- Amifostine is an organic thiophosphate.
- It is a reactive oxygen species scavenger.
- Amifostine reduces pro-inflammatory cytokine production (interleukin-6 and tumor necrosis factor-α) and radiation-induced double-stranded DNA breaks.
- It preferentially spares endothelium, salivary glands, and connective tissue.
- Amifostine be delivered topically within the rectum without systemic absorption, thus avoiding toxicity and the potential for tumor radioprotection. Results of clinical trials have not been uniformly positive.
- A recent systematic review by Sasse and colleagues of 14 randomized trials including 1451 patients showed a reduced risk of toxicity and an increased rate of complete response but no difference in overall survival with radiation therapy and amifostine compared with amifostine alone.

Data from Bensadoun RJ, Schubert MM, Lalla RV, et al. Amifostine in the management of radiation-induced and chemo-induced mucositis. Support Care Cancer 2006;14:566-572; and Sasse AD, Clark LG, Sasse EC, et al. Amifostine reduces side effects and improves complete response rate during radiotherapy: Results of a meta-analysis. Int J Radiat Oncol Biol Phys 2006;64: 784-791.

guided radiation therapy, and charged particle therapy (e.g., proton therapy).

General Medical Care

Optimizing the general medical condition of the patient before radiation therapy is likely to improve tolerance to treatment. Attention to nutrition, local hygiene (oral, dental, and perineal), treatment of infections, correction of anemia, and cessation of smoking and alcohol consumption may all improve tolerance to radiation therapy. Early treatment of minor symptoms may prevent the development of more severe symptoms. Agents such as mucosal barrier agents, antibiotics, and growth factors (e.g., granulocyte-macrophage colony-stimulating factor)[19] may reduce local infection and inflammation, which likely contribute to late toxicity. For patients at high risk of toxicity in functionally essential areas, interventions to bypass these areas, such as the use of nasogastric tubes or percutaneous endoscopic gastrostomy feeding tubes, may be necessary.

Molecular Agents

Molecular agents have not entered mainstream practice, but they show promise. One pathway targeted by these agents is the release of pro-inflammatory cytokines following reactive oxygen species activation of cellular stress responses (e.g., through nuclear factor-κB). Reactive oxygen species scavengers such as amifostine were the first active agents identified (Box 236-3). Concerns have been expressed that any agents that inhibit molecular pathways in radiation damage may affect both normal tissues and tumors and thus will not have an overall benefit.

MANAGEMENT OF ACUTE TOXICITY

General Principles

Management of acute toxicity is aimed at reducing discomfort and maintaining normal function, because acute effects are generally self-limiting (Box 236-4). However,

---

Box 236-4 Summary of Principles of Acute Toxicity Management

- Identify likely toxicities and inform the patient and carers.
- Use all preventive strategies.
- Maximize nutritional status, and stop smoking and consuming alcohol.
- Maximize local hygiene, and use barrier agents and local analgesics.
- Use adequate systemic analgesia.
- Exclude secondary infections.
- Follow site-specific guidelines.

---

failure of acute effects to heal may cause permanent and consequential late damage.

The following management principles should be followed to minimize acute toxicity:

1. Identify tissues within the irradiated volume and the individual likelihood of toxicity of each tissue; consider all relevant treatment-specific and patient-specific factors.
2. Inform patients, family members, and relevant medical staff members of expected toxicities, preventive methods, and possible therapeutic interventions.
3. Reduce toxicity from epithelial tissues by maximizing hygiene, using mucosal barrier agents, and minimizing mucosal trauma.
4. Take particular care if acute skin reactions are expected, because some topical agents contain metal, which can increase the local radiation dose as a result of the formation of electrons and can worsen toxicity. When the radiation course has finished, topical agents can be used safely.
5. Minimize perineal reactions by preventing perineal urine and fecal contamination and catheterization; use of a defunctioning stoma may be necessary.

6. Ensure adequate nutrition; ideally, management involves pretherapy assessment and intervention, if necessary.
7. Ensure that topical analgesia (anesthetics, anti-inflammatory drugs, and steroids) is adequate; barrier agents are highly effective for pain.
8. Ensure adequate systemic analgesia following standard World Health Organization guidelines; anti-inflammatory drugs are often highly effective.
9. Identify and treat secondary infections early (Table 236-2 and Box 236-5).

Delayed Acute Toxicity

Two syndromes classically manifest 1 to 3 months after radiation therapy: pneumonitis and somnambulant syndrome.

Acute Pneumonitis

Following thoracic radiation, increasing shortness of breath may herald radiation pneumonitis (Table 236-3).[20,21] The risk is related to the volume of lung irradiated, the dose per fraction, and the total dose. The differential diagnosis includes pneumonia, acute respiratory distress syndrome, and cardiac failure. Chest radiographs show increased opacification with a sharp demarcation edge that does not correlate with normal lung anatomy. Computed tomography (CT) scans shows infiltrative

---

Box 236-5 Less Common Toxicities

- Hair: *Acute* and *late* effects include hair loss. This is generally temporary with low to moderate doses, but may be permanent with higher doses.
- Lymphatics: *Acute* effects are unusual. The main *late* effect is lymphedema. The risk is increased following lymphadenopathy. Nodal metastases should be excluded. Management follows standard lymphedema management.
- Nerves: *Acute* effects are unusual. Irradiation of the spinal cord can result in self-limiting Lhermitte's syndrome. *Late* effects may be catastrophic because they may result in paralysis and neuropathic pain.
- Muscles: *Late* effects include muscle wasting, which can lead to asymmetry in children.
- Gonads: *Acute* effects include azoospermia and the risk of mutagenesis. *Late* effects are infertility and hypogonadism, with reduced bone mineral density.
- Vagina: *Late* effects include vaginal dryness, vaginismus, and shortening, with reduced enjoyment from sexual intercourse. Strictures, fistulas, ulceration, and telangiectasia all occur with higher does (e.g., following brachytherapy).
- Thyroid and pituitary: Hypothyroidism and hypopituitarism can occur over time.
- Eye: Effects include cataracts, blindness, and retinal scarring.
- Larynx: Edema can lead to changes in voice quality that may become permanent. Telangiectatic vessels can result in hemoptysis. Effects are more common if smoking is continued during treatment.

TABLE 236-2 Specific Management of Acute Radiation-Induced Toxicities

ORGAN	PATHOLOGICAL FEATURES	SYMPTOMS	PREVENTIVE STRATEGIES	MANAGEMENT STRATEGIES
Skin	Erythema, desquamation, ulceration	Pain and burning	Maintain hygiene, maintain skin moisture, avoid sun exposure	Mucosal barrier agents
Swallowing apparatus	??	Reduced nutrition, aspiration pneumonia	Maintain high calorie intake	Nutritional supplements, liquidized foods, nasogastric tube or percutaneous endoscopic gastrostomy
Oral cavity	Erythema, edema, ulceration	Pain, mucositis	Reduce alcohol and smoking, use mouthwashes	Mucosal barrier agents, local and systemic analgesics and anti-inflammatory drugs, including analgesic mouthwashes
Salivary glands	Reduced production of saliva	Xerostomia, loss of taste, reduced mastication	Perform submandibular gland transfer	Artificial saliva, parasympathomimetic sialogogues
Tongue	Edema, ulceration	Reduced mastication, speech difficulties	??	Local and systemic analgesics and anti-inflammatories, antimicrobials
Esophagus	Erythema, edema, ulceration	Pain on swallowing	Reduce alcohol and smoking	Mucosal barrier agents, local and systemic analgesics
Brain	Edema and raised intracranial pressure	Headaches, vomiting, new or deteriorating preexisting neurological disorders or seizures	??	Intracranial pressure, steroids, mannitol, systemic analgesics. Seizures: initiation or increase of antiepileptics
Stomach	Edema and loss of mucosal surface	Nausea, reduced appetite, heartburn or epigastric pain	??	Antiemetics; peptic ulcer therapy, mucosal barrier agents
Small or large bowel	Edema and loss of mucosal surface	Diarrhea, urgency, abdominal bloating and pain	Implement dietary restrictions	Antidiarrheals, antispasmodics, systemic analgesics
Rectum	Edema, ulceration	Tenesmus, bleeding, urgency, frequency	??	Local and systemic analgesics and anti-inflammatory drugs
Bladder	Edema, ulceration	Dysuria, frequency, hesitancy, reduced flow rate, penile pain	??	Systemic analgesics and anti-inflammatory drugs, antispasmodics or α-blockers
Bone	Pain flare	??	??	Systemic analgesics

TABLE 236-3	Typical Features of Radiation Pneumonitis		
PATHOLOGICAL FEATURES	**SYMPTOMS**	**PREVENTIVE STRATEGIES**	**MANAGEMENT**
Mixed inflammatory cell infiltrate (resulting from increased vascular permeability and alveolar surfactant levels)	Dry cough, increasing shortness of breath, respiratory failure	Nothing	Intravenous steroids, antibiotics, oxygen and ventilatory support (condition is fatal in 33%)

pneumonitis, and single photon emission CT (SPECT) scanning shows reduced functionality. Treatment consists of general supportive care and corticosteroids. Severe radiation pneumonitis has a fatality rate up to 50%.

Somnambulant Syndrome

Somnambulant syndrome usually occurs only after high-dose brain radiation therapy (e.g., for high-grade gliomas). Neurological deterioration may be seen after stabilization or improvement. Symptoms include profound fatigue and a reduced functional level. This condition is self-limiting and does not require increased steroids. The differential diagnosis includes progressive disease.

Postradiation Rehabilitation

In most situations, acute toxicities are self-limiting, and no evidence indicates that intervention after radiation therapy reduces the severity of late effects. Possible exceptions include the following:

- Vaginal dilatation for women during and after pelvic radiation therapy may prevent vaginal stenosis and functional shortening
- Retraining of bladder filling to reduce late urinary symptoms

MANAGEMENT OF LATE TOXICITY

General Principles

Because the symptoms of late radiation-induced toxicity may not become evident until years after treatment, and because this condition is generally considered irreversible, management is aimed primarily at prevention. Recognition of less severe cases, early diagnosis, and avoidance of exacerbating clinical situations are important. Late toxicity is likely the result of a cycle of hypoxia, cytokine release, fibrosis, and increased tissue pressure. These processes may cause edema, ulceration, or tissue necrosis and may manifest as pain, stricturing, fistulation, hemorrhage, or loss of function. The following management principles should be followed for late radiation-induced toxicity (Box 236-6).

1. Exclude possible differential diagnoses, especially recurrent or secondary cancers. Avoid biopsies unless absolutely necessary.
2. Ensure adequate analgesia, both local (anesthetics, anti-inflammatory drugs, and steroids) and systemic (paracetamol, nonsteroidal anti-inflammatory drugs, and opioids).
3. Inform the radiation oncologist, and seek specialist advice from a suitable clinician with an interest in radiation toxicities.

Box 236-6 Summary of Principles of Late Toxicity Management

- Confirm the diagnosis and exclude cancer.
- Use adequate analgesia.
- Inform the radiation oncologist, and seek the advice of a specialist.
- Reverse any reversible features.
- Treat specific symptoms.
- Consider experimental therapies.

---

4. Attempt to reverse the underlying process: treat secondary infections, maximize nutritional status, use mucosal barriers, and consider temporary or permanent defunctioning ostomies.
5. Treat specific symptoms, initially conservatively, but intervention may be necessary (e.g., cautery for bleeding, surgery for fistulas, and steroids, dilatation, stenting, or surgery for strictures).
6. Consider experimental therapies for patients with severe or resistant cases.

New Therapeutic Agents for Late Toxicity

Some agents are worthy of further research:

- Hyperbaric oxygen increases the tissue oxygen concentration in hypoxic conditions.[22,23]
- Pentoxifylline allows alteration of the red blood cell membrane, to allow passage through tortuous capillaries.[24,25]

Differential Diagnosis of Late Toxicities

The signs and symptoms of late radiation toxicity are non-specific and mimic both nonmalignant and malignant conditions. As more patients become cancer survivors, it will become increasingly important to investigate fully post-therapy symptoms *and not simply assume that they are caused by radiation damage*. Investigations should be organized following consultation with the radiation oncologist or a clinician with experience in radiation-induced toxicity, because injudicious investigations (e.g., biopsy) may exacerbate the condition.

Malignancy

- Patients with locally advanced disease are at high risk of both cancer recurrence and radiation toxicity, because they often have received a higher dose or a larger treatment volume and are more likely to have received concomitant therapies.

- Environmental or genetic factors underlying the initial cancer may predispose survivors to other malignant diseases.
- Cancer is often a disease of elderly persons, in whom the incidence of many tumors is increased.
- Radiation therapy and chemotherapy are both carcinogenic.

Nonmalignant Conditions

A study of workups for gastrointestinal symptoms following pelvic radiation therapy showed that many different conditions were labeled late radiation effects. These conditions ranged from inflammatory bowel disease to hypothyroidism.[26] Other concomitant or adjuvant cancer therapies may have been used, and these can affect many different physiological features and organ systems, including the endocrine system, bone mineral density, peripheral nerves, hearing, and the heart.

Relevant Investigations

- Laboratory tests: Radiation toxicities often cause no effects other than anemia from chronic bleeding. Relevant tumor markers may help in the diagnosis of recurrent or secondary malignant diseases, Erythrocyte sedimentation rate and C-reactive protein levels may be raised in acute infections.
- Imaging: Ultrasound or CT scanning may not be able to differentiate tumor from fibrosis. Contrast-enhanced magnetic resonance imaging or positron emission tomography may be needed (e.g., for axillary masses). Radioisotope scans may be useful in exceptional cases (e.g., ProstaScint scans in prostate cancer).
- Biopsy: This procedure may be necessary, but at the risk of worsening the long-term outcome of late radiation toxicities.

Therapeutic Interventions

Figures 236-1 and 236-2 show pathways of therapeutic intervention for radiation-induced toxicities. Table 236-4 details methods for prevention and treatment of specific late complications.

Skin

- Superior hygiene should be maintained, particularly in the submammary region, groin creases, and perineal area. Skin creases often increase the local radiation dose.[27] Within the perineal region, urinary or fecal contamination can occur, and catheterization or a defunctioning colostomy may need to be considered.
- Skin moisture should be maintained with an emollient (e.g., aqueous cream). Metal-containing agents should not be used. The patient should be advised to avoid tight-fitting clothing, repeated trauma, and prolonged sun exposure, as well as prolonged exposure to water and excessive use of soaps. Aqueous cream can be used as a soap alternative.
- Desquamation is treated with topical barrier agents such as hydrogel dressings (e.g., IntraSite gel). These agents reduce pain, prevent further traumatic damage, and provide optimal conditions for healing. They can

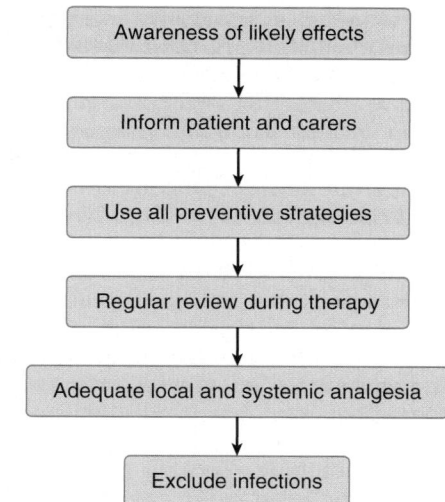

FIGURE 236-1 Management flow chart for acute effects.

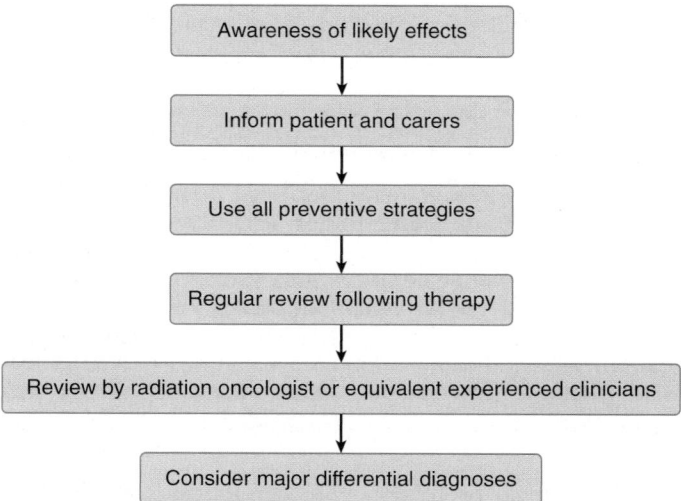

FIGURE 236-2 Management flow chart for late effects.

provide fluid to dry wounds and can facilitate autolytic débridement. These agents can be applied directly as an amorphous material (they will require a secondary cover), as a sheet, or as part of a preimpregnated gauze swab.
- Camouflage may be highly effective for some late sequelae.

Oral Cavity

- Good dental care should include a formal therapy dental assessment, fluoride mouthwashes, and corrective dental work before radiation therapy is begun. Invasive oral surgery performed after radiation therapy predisposes patients to osteoradionecrosis. Lifelong awareness of this risk is essential.
- Good oral hygiene is essential. Warm saline or antiseptic mouthwashes are recommended. Antiseptic mouthwashes may be uncomfortable, for which dilution may help.

TABLE 236-4 Specific Management of Late Radiation-Induced Toxicities

AREA	PATHOLOGICAL FEATURES	SYMPTOMS	MANAGEMENT
Skin	Telangiectasia, fibrosis, ulceration, pigment change	Pain, discomfort, distress	Mucosal barrier agents, camouflage
Swallowing apparatus	Edema, fibrosis, stricture	Poor nutrition, aspiration pneumonia	Nutritional supplements, liquidized foods, NGT or PEG, dilatation of strictures
Oral cavity	Soft tissue necrosis	Pain	Mucosal barrier agents, local and systemic analgesics and anti-inflammatory drugs, antimicrobials
Salivary glands	Reduced saliva formation	Xerostomia, loss of taste, dental caries	Artificial saliva, parasympathomimetic sialogogues
Esophagus	Hemorrhage and stricture	Bleeding and pain	Hemorrhage: cautery Stricture: liquidized food, NGT or PEG, dilatation, stenting
Brain	Necrosis	Reduced higher cognitive function, focal neurology, seizures	Antiepileptics, surgical resection of focal necrotic areas
Lung	Fibrosis	Progressive exertional dyspnea with typical radiographic changes	Symptomatic measures
Bone	Osteoradionecrosis (mandible), fractures (rib), microfractures (pelvis)	Increasing pain and tenderness, possible overlying ulcer	Prevention: (1) oral: assessment of pretherapy dentition, fluoride mouthwashes; (2) general: minimization of trauma after radiation therapy (e.g., surgery, dental work) Therapy: antimicrobials, analgesics, and surgical resection
Heart	Local or general myocardial dysfunction, constrictive pericarditis	Dyspnea, angina, cardiac failure	Prevention: consider concurrent therapies Therapy: as for comparable conditions not induced by radiation
Small or large bowel	Stricture	Diarrhea, subacute bowel obstruction	Diarrhea: antidiarrheals Subacute bowel obstruction: conservative management, laxatives, antispasmodics, steroids, stenting, surgical resection
	Fistula or perforation	Acute abdomen	Surgical resection
Bladder	Edema, ulceration, telangiectasia	Dysuria, frequency, hematuria	Frequency: antispasmodics, systemic anti-inflammatory drugs Hemorrhage: cautery; prothrombotic agents
	Constriction	Frequency, reduced capacity	Surgical resection or ureteric diversion
	Urethral stricture	Hesitancy, reduced flow rate, incontinence	α-Blockers, dilatation, stenting (catheter)
Rectum	Edema, ulceration, telangiectasia	Tenesmus, rectal bleeding, urgency, frequency, pain	Hemorrhage: local steroids, mucosal barrier agents, cautery, prothrombotic agents
	Anorectal dysfunction	Incontinence (feces or flatus)	Toileting exercises, bulking agents

NGT, nasogastric tube; PEG, percutaneous endoscopic gastrostomy

- Mechanical protection with carmellose sodium paste can cover denuded areas. Corticosteroids (e.g., triamcinolone acetonide [Kenalog in Orabase]) can be included for their anti-inflammatory effects once infections have been excluded.
- Local analgesics can be given as mouthwashes, gels, or lozenges. Mouthwashes of soluble systemic analgesics can be swallowed as part of the systemic analgesic program.
- Local anesthetic spray or direct application of ointment can be highly effective.

Salivary Glands

- These glands are highly sensitive to radiation.[28,29] Submandibular gland transplantation into low-dose areas is being investigated. Changes in the constitution of saliva may contribute to oral and dental health.
- Patients often carry a bottle of water to ease xerostomia.
- Artificial saliva preparations are available, including sprays (oral and aerosol sprays), gels, gums, liquids, and tables (lozenges and pastilles).
- Parasympathomimetic sialogogues are effective only in patients with residual functioning salivary gland tissue,

and these agents should be given 2 to 3 months to work. Agents include pilocarpine hydrochloride (5 mg three times daily with or immediately after meals, up to a maximum of 30 mg daily). Cevimeline may be an alternative (30 to 45 mg three times daily).

Lung

- Corticosteroids may reduce the severity of pneumonitis.[30]
- Any suspected cases of radiation pneumonitis should be discussed with the radiation oncologist immediately, and the patient should be referred for specialist management.
- Supportive therapy with oxygen, antibiotics, and ventilatory support should be considered in patients with severe cases of radiation pneumonitis.

Esophagus and Stomach

- Mucosal barrier agents such as oral sucralfate (1 g four times daily), antacids, and ulcer-healing drugs such as histamine H_2-antagonists or proton pump inhibitors may ease esophagitis and gastritis. Sucralfate is a complex of aluminum hydroxide and sulfated sucrose.

- Mucosal anesthetics and oral analgesics are also highly effective. Superimposed moniliasis should be considered in patients with severe or resistant cases.
- Serotonin (5-HT$_3$) antagonists are highly effective antiemetics.
- Nutritional status should be closely monitored.

Brain

- Symptoms resulting from raised intracranial pressure may respond to increased doses of systemic glucocorticoids.[31]
- Surgical bypass or intravenous mannitol may be considered in exceptional cases.
- Mannitol should be given under expert guidance.

Bowel

- Altering the diet to reduce fiber content may diminish the risk of diarrhea and should be the initial intervention once diarrhea occurs.
- Acute and chronic diarrhea responds rapidly to loperamide (4 mg as an initial dose, and then 2 mg after each loose stool).
- Antispasmodics, such as hyoscine butylbromide (10 to 20 mg four times daily by mouth), are effective for colicky abdominal pains.
- Episodes of subacute bowel obstruction should be treated conservatively, if possible: admission to hospital, nil by mouth status, nasogastric tubes, antispasmodics, systemic analgesia, and glucocorticoids. Recurrent episodes may require surgical intervention to remove strictured sections.

Rectum

- No agent can reduce the development of acute or late rectal toxicity, although amifostine and misoprostol have shown promise.[32,33]
- The most common syndrome is proctitis, characterized by urgency and frequency. This condition may respond to local steroids as either a suppository or preferably a foam enema, which provides better coverage of the distal rectum.
- Late toxicity should be thoroughly investigated by direct vision of the distal rectum at a minimum, to exclude secondary gastroenterological disease.[34]
- Supportive measures include topical and systemic analgesia, topical anti-inflammatory drugs, fecal softeners, topical mucosal barrier agents (sucralfate), and topical or systemic antibiotics.
- Rectal ulceration should be managed conservatively, and biopsies should be avoided, if possible (Fig. 236-3). Severe cases can be managed with a defunctioning colostomy (see "Case Study: Complications of Radiation Therapy" [see Fig. 236-3]).
- Telangiectatic vessels may respond to cauterization.
- Anorectal dysfunction may cause incontinence to both feces and flatus, and it has a major effect on quality of life.[35] Anorectal physiology may be diagnostic. Bulking

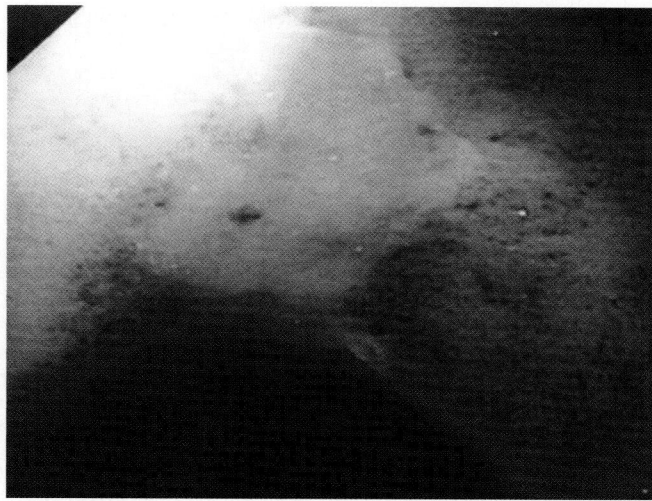

FIGURE 236-3 Rectal ulcer on the anterior rectal wall as seen on the second sigmoidoscopy in the patient in "Case Study: Complications of Radiation Therapy." This finding corresponds to the high-dose radiation region during prostate radiation therapy.

 C A S E   S T U D Y

Complications of Radiation Therapy

OP, a 68-year-old man, presented with screen-detected prostate cancer (stage T2a; Gleason score, 4 + 3; prostate-specific antigen [PSA], 5.2). Biopsies showed cancer in six of six cores on the left. Magnetic resonance imaging scan showed a tumor nodule in the left side of the prostate that extended to the apex. He was treated with neoadjuvant androgen deprivation for 5 months and three-dimensional conformal radiation therapy (74 Gy in 37 fractions). During planning, clinicians noted that a large proportion of his rectum was included in the high-dose region; the treatment margins were modified. The patient developed grade 1 acute proctitis, which was improving 3 weeks following the end of radiation therapy. However, at 6 months after treatment, he had developed grade 2 late toxicity with tenesmus and rectal bleeding. He was referred for flexible sigmoidoscopy, which confirmed radiation proctitis. The patient was initially managed conservatively with rectal steroids, foam enemas, and sterculia granules (Normacol). He was admitted for acute rectal hemorrhage and was given a blood transfusion and intravenous corticosteroids. A further sigmoidoscopy showed deterioration in appearance of the condition, and attempts to reduce blood loss were made using rectal laser coagulation. This treatment had no effect, and further sigmoidoscopy showed evidence of rectal ulceration (see Fig. 236-3). Treatment with rectal sucralfate, oral antibiotics, pentoxifylline, and vitamin E did not improve the clinical condition. The patient was started on tranexamic acid. Finally, he was referred for hyperbaric oxygen. He has received 30 fractions and has not had a dramatic improvement in his condition. This patient's final option would be a (defunctioning) colostomy. His PSA is 0.1 ng/mL.

agents (e.g., sterculia granules) or educational programs may be of help.

Bladder

- Patients should be encouraged to ensure a high fluid intake during therapy.
- Patients with severe symptoms should have urinary tract infection excluded.
- Detrusor muscle instability usually responds to an antimuscarinic agent.
- During prostate radiation therapy, urethritis may develop. It responds to selective α-blockers.[36]
- Late symptoms should be assessed and investigated in consultation with a urologist.
- Hematuria should be investigated by cystoscopy. If hematuria is the result of telangiectasia, it may respond to cauterization.
- Urethral strictures may require catheterization or dilatation.
- Uncommonly, constriction or contracture of the bladder is seen. It may respond to forced bladder expansion, but it may require cystectomy.

Evidence-Based Medicine

The following findings were reported in the *Cochrane Database of Systematic Reviews:*

Future Considerations

Factors That May Affect the Development of Toxicity

- Understanding of the cellular and whole organ effects of radiation
- Development of effective radioprotectors
- Identification of genetic factors associated with an increased risk of toxicity[10]
- Identification of molecular markers of toxicity during therapy (e.g., plasma citrulline[41])
- Increasing use of concomitant therapeutic agents (e.g., hormones, chemotherapy, biological agents[42,43])
- Description of the dose-volume relationship for acute and late toxicity (e.g., for prostate cancer[44])
- Advanced radiation therapy planning and delivery systems that provide increased normal tissue sparing and allow further dose escalation
- Individualization of the dose prescription based on patient and tumor radiogenotyping, functional and biological imaging, biological monitoring during radiation therapy, and advanced radiation therapy planning and delivery

Factors That May Affect the Management of Toxicity

- Better prospective recording of late toxicity and quality of life data
- Larger numbers of cancer survivors
- Better identification of rare radiation toxicities
- Increasing awareness and concern over radiation-induced malignant diseases
- Elucidation of the molecular processes underlying acute and late toxicity
- New drug development
- Well-designed clinical studies (currently very limited)

Nonsurgical interventions for late radiation cystitis in patients who received radical radiation therapy to the pelvis: No randomized trials were identified in this review, although 80 other studies were identified. No conclusions on comparative efficacy can be drawn.[37]

Nonsurgical interventions for late radiation proctitis after radical radiation therapy to the pelvis: Six randomized trials were identified involving a total of 184 patients. Rectal sucralfate appeared more effective than anti-inflammatory drugs, although metronidazole appeared better with anti-inflammatory drugs compared with anti-inflammatory drugs alone. Rectal hydrocortisone appeared more effective than rectal betamethasone. Short-chain fatty acid enemas were not better than placebo.[38,39]

Selenium for the side effects of chemotherapy, radiation therapy, and surgery: Two randomized trials were identified, one of which was ongoing. Preliminary results suggested an improvement in radiation induced acute diarrhea, but no data was available.[40]

REFERENCES

1. Bensadoun RJ, Schubert MM, Lalla RV, et al. Amifostine in the management of radiation-induced and chemo-induced mucositis. Support Care Cancer 2006;14:566-572.
2. Sasse AD, Clark LG, Sasse EC, et al. Amifostine reduces side effects and improves complete response rate during radiotherapy: Results of a meta-analysis. Int J Radiat Oncol Biol Phys 2006;64:784-791.
3. Lilla C, Ambrosone CB, Kropp S, et al. Predictive factors for late normal tissue complications following radiotherapy for breast cancer. Breast Cancer Res Treat 2007;106:143-150.
4. Emami B, Lyman J, Brown A, et al. Tolerance of normal tissue to therapeutic irradiation. Int J Radiat Oncol Biol Phys 1991;21:109-122.
5. Holscher T, Bentzen SM, Baumann M. Influence of connective tissue diseases on the expression of radiation side effects: A systematic review. Radiother Oncol 2006;78:123-130.
6. van der Voet JC, Keus RB, Hart AA, et al. The impact of treatment time and smoking on local control and complications in T1 glottic cancer. Int J Radiat Oncol Biol Phys 1998;42:247-255.
7. Andreassen CN, Alsner J, Overgaard J, et al. *TGFB1* polymorphisms are associated with risk of late normal tissue complications in the breast after radiotherapy for early breast cancer. Radiother Oncol 2005;75:18-21.
8. De Ruyck K, Van Eijkeren M, Claes K, et al. Radiation-induced damage to normal tissues after radiotherapy in patients treated for gynecologic tumors: Association with single nucleotide polymorphisms in *XRCC1, XRCC3,* and *OGG1* genes and in vitro chromosomal radiosensitivity in lymphocytes. Int J Radiat Oncol Biol Phys 2005;62:1140-1149.
9. West CM, McKay MJ, Holscher T, et al. Molecular markers predicting radiotherapy response: Report and recommendations from an International Atomic Energy Agency technical meeting. Int J Radiat Oncol Biol Phys 2005;62:1264-1273.
10. Burnet NG, Elliott RM, Dunning A, et al. Radiosensitivity, radiogenomics and RAPPER. Clin Oncol (R Coll Radiol) 2006;18:525-528.
11. Sonis ST. The pathobiology of mucositis. Nat Rev Cancer 2004;4:277-284.
12. Fuks Z, Kolesnick R. Engaging the vascular component of the tumor response. Cancer Cell 2005;8:89-91.
13. Belka C, Jendrossek V, Pruschy M, et al. Apoptosis-modulating agents in combination with radiotherapy-current status and outlook. Int J Radiat Oncol Biol Phys 2004;58:542-554.
14. O'Brien PC. Radiation injury of the rectum. Radiother Oncol 2001;60:1-14.
15. Suit H, Goldberg S, Niemierko A, et al. Secondary carcinogenesis in patients treated with radiation: A review of data on radiation-induced cancers in human, non-human primate, canine and rodent subjects. Radiat Res 2007;167:12-42.
16. Tward JD, Wendland MM, Shrieve DC, et al. The risk of secondary malignancies over 30 years after the treatment of non-Hodgkin lymphoma. Cancer 2006;107:108-115.
17. Moysich KB, Menezes RJ, Michalek AM. Chernobyl-related ionising radiation exposure and cancer risk: An epidemiological review. Lancet Oncol 2002;3:269-279.
18. Hall EJ. Intensity-modulated radiation therapy, protons, and the risk of second cancers. Int J Radiat Oncol Biol Phys 2006;65:1-7.
19. von Bultzingslowen I, Brennan MT, Spijkervet FK, et al. Growth factors and cytokines in the prevention and treatment of oral and gastrointestinal mucositis. Support Care Cancer 2006;14:519-527.
20. Tsoutsou PG, Koukourakis MI. Radiation pneumonitis and fibrosis: Mechanisms underlying its pathogenesis and implications for future research. Int J Radiat Oncol Biol Phys 2006;66:1281-1293.

21. Mehta V. Radiation pneumonitis and pulmonary fibrosis in non-small-cell lung cancer: Pulmonary function, prediction, and prevention. Int J Radiat Oncol Biol Phys 2005;63:5-24.

22. Dall'Era MA, Hampson NB, Hsi RA, et al. Hyperbaric oxygen therapy for radiation induced proctopathy in men treated for prostate cancer. J Urol 2006; 176:87-90.

23. Al-Waili NS, Butler GJ. Effects of hyperbaric oxygen on inflammatory response to wound and trauma: Possible mechanism of action. Sci World J 2006;6: 425-441.

24. Okunieff P, Augustine E, Hicks JE, et al. Pentoxifylline in the treatment of radiation-induced fibrosis. J Clin Oncol 2004;22:2207-2213.

25. Gothard L, Cornes P, Earl J, et al. Double-blind placebo-controlled randomised trial of vitamin E and pentoxifylline in patients with chronic arm lymphoedema and fibrosis after surgery and radiotherapy for breast cancer. Radiother Oncol 2004;73:133-139.

26. Andreyev HJ, Vlavianos P, Blake P, et al. Gastrointestinal symptoms after pelvic radiotherapy: Role for the gastroenterologist? Int J Radiat Oncol Biol Phys 2005;62:1464-1471.

27. Bolderston A, Lloyd NS, Wong RK, et al. The prevention and management of acute skin reactions related to radiation therapy: A systematic review and practice guideline. Support Care Cancer 2006;14:802-817.

28. de Castro GJ, Federico MH. Evaluation, prevention and management of radiotherapy-induced xerostomia in head and neck cancer patients. Curr Opin Oncol 2006;18:266-270.

29. Kahn ST, Johnstone PA. Management of xerostomia related to radiotherapy for head and neck cancer. Oncology (Williston Park) 2005;19:1827-1832; discussion 1832-1824, 1837-1829.

30. Kong FM, Ten Haken R, Eisbruch A, et al. Non-small cell lung cancer therapy-related pulmonary toxicity: An update on radiation pneumonitis and fibrosis. Semin Oncol 2005;32:S42-54.

31. Belka C, Budach W, Kortmann RD, et al. Radiation induced CNS toxicity: Molecular and cellular mechanisms. Br J Cancer 2001;85:1233-1239.

32. Kouloulias VE, Kouvaris JR, Pissakas G, et al. Phase II multicenter randomized study of amifostine for prevention of acute radiation rectal toxicity: Topical intrarectal versus subcutaneous application. Int J Radiat Oncol Biol Phys 2005;62:486-493.

33. Khan AM, Birk JW, Anderson JC, et al. A prospective randomized placebo-controlled double-blinded pilot study of misoprostol rectal suppositories in the prevention of acute and chronic radiation proctitis symptoms in prostate cancer patients. Am J Gastroenterol 2000;95:1961-1966.

34. Williams HR, Vlavianos P, Blake P, et al. The significance of rectal bleeding after pelvic radiotherapy. Aliment Pharmacol Ther 2005;21:1085-1090.

35. Putta S, Andreyev HJ. Faecal incontinence: A late side-effect of pelvic radiotherapy. Clin Oncol (R Coll Radiol) 2005;17:469-477.

36. Zelefsky MJ, Ginor RX, Fuks Z, et al. Efficacy of selective alpha-1 blocker therapy in the treatment of acute urinary symptoms for radiotherapy for localized prostate cancer. Int J Radiat Oncol Biol Phys 1999;45:567-570.

37. Denton AS, Clarke NW, Maher EJ. Non-surgical interventions for late radiation cystitis in patients who have received radical radiotherapy to the pelvis. Cochrane Database Syst Rev 2002;(3):CD001773.

38. Denton A, Forbes A, Andreyev J, et al. Non surgical interventions for late radiation proctitis in patients who have received radical radiotherapy to the pelvis. Cochrane Database Syst Rev 2002;(1):CD003455.

39. Denton AS, Andreyev HJ, Forbes A, et al. Systematic review for non-surgical interventions for the management of late radiation proctitis. Br J Cancer 2002;87:134-143.

40. Dennert G, Horneber M. Selenium for alleviating the side effects of chemotherapy, radiotherapy and surgery in cancer patients. Cochrane Database Syst Rev 2006;(3):CD005037.

41. Lutgens LC, Deutz N, Granzier-Peeters M, et al. Plasma citrulline concentration: A surrogate end point for radiation-induced mucosal atrophy of the small bowel. A feasibility study in 23 patients. Int J Radiat Oncol Biol Phys 2004;60:275-285.

42. Bonner JA, Harari PM, Giralt J, et al. Radiotherapy plus cetuximab for squamous-cell carcinoma of the head and neck. N Engl J Med 2006;354: 567-578.

43. Lukka H, Hirte H, Fyles A, et al. Concurrent cisplatin-based chemotherapy plus radiation for cervical cancer—a meta-analysis. Clin Oncol (R Coll Radiol) 2002;14:203-212.

44. Jackson A. Partial irradiation of the rectum. Semin Radiat Oncol 2001;11: 215-223.

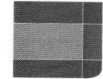

CHAPTER **237**

Palliative Radiation Therapy

Alysa Fairchild and Edward Chow

KEY POINTS

- The optimal palliative radiotherapy (RT) schedule for bone metastases (BMs), spinal cord compression (SCC), and advanced lung cancer is still controversial. This may in part be due to the existence of multiple clinical trials with conflicting results, the scarcity of strong level 1 evidence, or difficulty in the translation of evidence to general practice.

- Palliative RT is a noninvasive, effective, relatively nontoxic, cost-effective intervention for control of symptoms.

- Practice patterns in palliative RT are commonly influenced by factors other than the published literature.

- Patients' preferences in terms of RT schedules and aims have not been taken into consideration sufficiently to date.

- New modalities and sequences of modalities are showing promise in combination with external beam RT.

We show that external beam RT meets the criteria for a good palliative intervention and describe some guiding principles for ethical decision making. Published evidence is contrasted with current patterns of practice data and with the literature on patient preference for treatment of BM, SCC, and advanced lung cancer. The comparative cost-effectiveness and integration of palliative RT with other modalities is outlined. Final comments describe new developments, implications for evidenced-based medicine, and avoidance of common errors.

PRINCIPLES OF PALLIATIVE RADIATION THERAPY

A general approach to palliation in advanced cancer is to identify the cause of the symptom (while keeping in mind nonmalignant causes), treat reversible conditions such as fracture, institute pharmacological therapies, rule out iatrogenic causes and chronic pain syndromes, address nonphysical factors, and use supportive care liberally.[1,2] The general goals of palliative RT are relief of pain, preservation of mobility and function, prevention of future complications, preservation of quality of life (QOL), maintenance of skeletal integrity, and minimization of the need for both hospitalization and rehabilitation.[1,2]

A good palliative intervention should accomplish one or more of these aims and be safe, with minimal acute toxicity, a high possibility of benefit, the shortest possible time investment, minimal invasiveness, little recovery time, and cost-effectiveness. Although the possibility of long-term side effects, especially serious ones, should be considered, this is usually less of an issue in palliative patients with limited life span. The optimal palliative RT regimen is one that provides prompt and effective symptom relief with minimal toxicity and patient inconvenience; commonly, short-course palliative RT fulfills these criteria, with few contraindications.

In view of the fact that the intricacies of treatment planning are often outweighed by the complexities of decision making, Mackillop outlined 10 rules to guide the prescription of palliative RT based on well-known ethical principles (Box 237-1).[3] Among these rules are common-sense guidelines that serve as a reminder that "time is precious when life is short" and that palliative RT should consume no more resources than necessary. As he additionally articulates, treatment recommendations should be based on evidence, and if the available evidence is deficient, practitioners have an obligation to participate in the clinical research that will provide it.[3]

More than 10 years after the publication of Mackillop's article, however, controversy still exists on the optimal dose fractionation schedule for many palliative RT indications. This may be due to multiple conflicting clinical trials, the absence of strong level 1 evidence, or difficulty in translating literature results to general practice.

BONE METASTASES—TRIAL RESULTS

Approximately 25 randomized controlled trials (RCTs) investigating different dose fractionation schedules for uncomplicated BM have been published since the 1980s.[4] Although there is no specific, accepted definition of "uncomplicated," it is generally taken to mean the absence of established or impending SCC, nerve root or cauda equina compression, cranial nerve palsy, complete or impending pathological fracture, or associated soft tissue

---

Box 237-1 Ten Rules for the Practice of Palliative Radiotherapy

1.0 Palliative radiotherapy should be part of a comprehensive program of care.
2.0 The decision to recommend palliative radiotherapy should be based on a thorough assessment of the patient.
3.0 The decision to recommend palliative radiotherapy should be based on objective information.
4.0 The risk-benefit analysis should include consideration of all aspects of the patient's well-being.
5.0 The short-term risks and benefits of palliative radiotherapy are more important than those that may or may not occur in the future.
6.0 The decision to use palliative radiotherapy should be consistent with the values and preferences of the patient.
7.0 Patients should be involved in the treatment decision to the extent that they wish.
8.0 Time is precious when life is short.
  8.1 Delays in starting palliative radiotherapy should be as short as reasonably achievable.
  8.2 Courses of palliative radiotherapy should be no longer than necessary to achieve their therapeutic goal.
9.0 Palliative and curative goals should not be considered mutually exclusive.
10.0 Palliative radiotherapy should consume no more resources than necessary.

From Mackillop WJ. The principles of palliative radiotherapy: A radiation oncologist's perspective. Can J Oncol 1996;6(Suppl 1):5-11.

---

mass. More controversial is whether the presence of neuropathic pain without neurological signs or a bone lesion after surgical fixation should be included under this heading.

An updated meta-analysis reviewed 16 randomized trials that compared single-fraction (SF) and multiple-fraction (MF) schedules of palliative RT for the treatment of uncomplicated BM.[5] Studies included were published in full or abstract form and totaled 2513 randomizations to SF arms and 2487 to MF arms. The overall response rate to SF RT was 58%, and the complete response rate was 23%, which was not significantly different from the 59% and 24% experienced by patients randomized to MF RT, thus confirming the conclusions of the 2003 systematic reviews. Generally, no differences in the incidence of acute toxicity, pathological fracture, or SCC were found. After SF RT, 3.2% of patients suffered fractures versus 2.8% after MF RT ($P = .75$). SCC occurred in 2.8% of patients undergoing SF RT and 1.9% after MF RT ($P = .13$). There were significantly more retreatment episodes in the SF arm (20%) than in the MF arm (8%) ($P < .0001$), again confirming previous findings.[5]

Practice Patterns

Despite the overwhelming amount of randomized evidence and obvious patient-related, practitioner, and resource advantages, there has been reluctance to adopt SF schedules as global standard practice to date. A 2007 article reviewed surveys published between 1988 and 2006 on RT prescription patterns for BM.[4] Response rates varied from 31.2% to 82.5%. American respondents indicated an overwhelming preference for the prescription of 30 Gy in 10 daily fractions over a period of 2 weeks (30 Gy/10), and 90% to 100% of radiation oncologists (ROs) preferred MF over SF schedules. Approximately 85% of Canadians preferred MF RT, most often delivered as 20 Gy/5 over a 1-week period. MF RT was again commonly used in the United Kingdom, western Europe, Australia and New Zealand, and India; however, ROs in these countries would consider SF schedules in up to 42% of courses.[6] An international study updating patterns of practice in palliative RT is under way, with results expected to illustrate regional changes in response to recent RCTs and meta-analyses. This study will also reexamine issues taken into account in decision making to more closely pinpoint reasons behind the reluctance to use SF RT. To date, these reasons have been hypothesized to be disease related, such as the site of the bone lesion; oncologist related, such as training; and setting related, such as waiting list length.[4]

Patient Preferences

Controversy over the optimal dose fractionation has by and large ignored patient choice, with three studies to date having investigated patients' preferences for RT schedules.[7-9] In one study, 21 Australian patients with BM who had received RT between 6 weeks and 2 years previously participated in structured interviews in which they were asked to indicate the relative priority attributed to different treatment outcomes.[7] Participants generally considered medical appointments to be physically demanding and rated sustained pain relief and reduced risk of future complications their highest priorities. Convenience was acknowledged, but factors such as traveling distance and brevity of treatment were considered of secondary importance to overall QOL and treatment efficacy. Most patients favored SF RT, assuming equivalent outcomes.[7]

Patients in Singapore and Canada were studied with the same patient preference instrument, which presented differences and similarities between SF and MF RT.[8] In the Singapore study, 85% (53/62) of patients would choose extended courses of RT (24 Gy/6) over a single treatment because of lower retreatment rates and decreased fracture risk; choice did not seem to depend on age, performance status (PS), primary cancer site, cost, or pain score.

About 76% (55/72) of Canadian patients would choose a single 8-Gy session as opposed to 1 week of RT because of greater convenience.[9] Patients who chose the 1-week schedule did so largely because of the decreased likelihood of pathological fracture. Older and retired patients were more likely to select SF RT. Differences in the aforementioned three studies may be explained in part by cultural differences and potentially by differences in the decision aid instrument.

Turning the Tide?

The first indications of a shift in palliative RT prescription patterns for painful BM have started to appear. In the United Kingdom, a practice audit performed in 2003 revealed the most common schedule to be 8 to 10 Gy in a single treatment, which was used in 36% of prescriptions nationally.[10] In Sweden, a report of the results of a national audit in 2001 stated that "the principle of irradiation of skeletal metastases with a single or few fractions has been widely adopted in clinical practice" since the previous audit of 1992.[11] After the Dutch BM trial was published in 1999, "almost all Dutch institutions either changed or are planning to change their protocols to SF RT for palliation of bone metastases."[12] Finally, a recently published Scandinavian trial was terminated early because of slow recruitment, blamed on physician reluctance to randomize between SF and MF schedules.[13] We await with interest the results of the international survey, from which a rate of adoption of RCT results may be inferred.

SPINAL CORD COMPRESSION—TRIAL RESULTS

Before 2005, the results of treatment of SCC with surgery and RT did not seem to differ from RT alone, thereby resulting in surgery being largely abandoned.[14] Patchell and colleagues' trial, however, provided the first randomized evidence that surgery followed by postoperative RT was superior to RT alone for symptomatic patients with certain primary disease sites and longer than 3 months' expected survival.[15] About 30% of patients had primary genitourinary cancers. One hundred one patients were accrued before meeting early stopping criteria as a result of significantly improved outcomes in the surgery-plus-RT arm. Combined-modality patients had significantly better post-treatment ambulatory rates, median time of maintenance of ambulation, retention of continence, and maintenance of functional and motor scores, as well as lower median daily doses of steroids and analgesics. Survival

<table><tr><td>**Common Errors**</td></tr></table>

Common reasons for a suboptimal response to palliative RT for BM include the following:

- Other causes of pain can masquerade as BM in the absence of imaging studies (i.e., pain secondary to para-aortic lymphadenopathy being mistaken for spinal BM or pain referred from the hip to the knee).
- The cause of uptake on a bone scan is not metastases (e.g., arthritis, Paget's disease).
- The cause of a fracture is not metastasis (e.g., trauma, osteoporotic collapse).
- The cause of bone loss is not metastasis (e.g., deprivation of sex steroids, disuse or immobilization, systemic chemotherapy, post-radiation effect, glucocorticoids).
- The dose is too low for a relatively radioresistant histology (e.g., renal cell carcinoma).
- A geographic or marginal miss has occurred (e.g., failing to include the entire soft tissue mass).
- Subsequent disease progression or a skeletal-related event has taken place (e.g., fracture, SCC).
- Unmasking of pain has occurred (e.g., successful treatment of a dominant painful area leads to patient awareness of other painful sites).
- The end point assessment is inappropriate (e.g., failure to take into account changes in analgesic use) or takes place at an inappropriate time (e.g., during pain flare).

BM, bone metastase; RT, radiotherapy; SCC, spinal cord compression.

(126 versus 100 days), and 30-day morbidity were also better with initial surgery; 30-day mortality and length of hospital stay were no different. Ultimately, 20% of the RT-alone group crossed over to undergo surgery.[15]

Two caveats to the interpretation of this trial should be considered. Although outcomes of the surgery-plus-RT group were similar to those in the literature, outcomes of the RT-alone group were significantly worse.[14] Additionally, almost 40% of randomized patients had bone instability (pathological vertebral fracture or bone in the spinal canal), which is generally considered suboptimally treated with RT alone.[15]

Although the trial of Patchell and associates confirmed surgery to be the superior initial treatment option for a specific subgroup, the majority of patients with SCC are still treated with RT alone. As with uncomplicated BM, the most appropriate RT schedule is still being debated, probably at least partly because of the scarcity of randomized data. Patients with impending or complete SCC were excluded from 11 of the clinical trials investigating dose schedules for uncomplicated BM, as described earlier, and it was not addressed in the eligibility criteria in the remaining trials.

In the sole phase III RCT, patients with radiographically confirmed SCC, an estimated life span of less than 6 months, and no indications for primary surgery were randomized to 16 Gy/2 over a 1-week period or a split course consisting of 15 Gy/3, 4 days' rest, and then 15 Gy/5.[16] Two hundred ninety-four assessable patients were accrued, 95% of whom had back pain at entry and 6% were paraplegic. No significant differences were found in relief of back pain (56% versus 59%), ability to walk after RT (68% versus 71%), and bladder function (90% versus 89%) for short-versus split-course treatment, respectively (no *P* values given). Survival (median of 4 months) and duration of motor improvement (median of 3.5 months) were not dependent on the RT regimen, nor was toxicity. In the short-course group, 3.5% of patients had magnetic resonance imaging–documented in-field recurrence at a median of 5 months as compared with no patients in the split-course group (no *P* value given). Patients in general maintained response for the remainder of their lives.

A number of investigators have retrospectively compared different RT schedules for SCC, with a minority including patients treated with one or two fractions (Table 237-1). In the largest retrospective evaluation performed to date, data on 1852 patients who underwent RT for SCC (1992 to 2005) at multiple centers were combined.[17] Each of the contributing centers provided an unselected group of patients, usually representing two or more RT schedules. Forty-two percent received short-course RT (8 Gy/1 or 20 Gy/5), whereas the remainder received long-course RT (30 Gy/10, 35.5 Gy/15, or 40 Gy/20). Ambulatory rates before and after RT were not significantly different for the five treatment schedules, and a similar proportion of patients who were not ambulatory before RT regained the ability to walk, 28% on average (range, 26% to 31%). The 2-year in-field recurrence rate was 16% on average.[17] Significantly more in-field recurrences occurred after 8 Gy/1 (24.0%) and 20 Gy/5 (26.0%) than after greater than 20 Gy (7.0% to 9.0%), *P* < .001.[17] Acute toxicity was mild, and no late toxicity was reported. A randomized multicenter trial is under way by these investigators.

This data were reanalyzed to compare the 30-Gy/10 RT schedule received by 345 patients with the higher doses received by 577 patients.[18] Overall, motor function remained stable in 59% and improved in 21%; neither ambulation nor in-field recurrence was significantly associated with the RT dose. Likewise, after separating out treatment results in the 308 patients older than 75 years, improved functional outcome was not significantly associated with the RT schedule.[19] However, it was the only prognostic factor significant for in-field recurrence on univariate analysis.

In a study examining the outcomes of schedules with less than two fractions, 102 consecutive patients treated at a single institution between 1999 and 2001 were reviewed.[20] The RT dose was chosen by the treating RO. Motor function, continence, and pain were assessed before treatment and at 1 week, 6 weeks, and 4 months. Twenty-eight percent of patients had prostate cancer, and 85% were treated with steroids. Thirty-two percent received one to two fractions, and the rest received more than two fractions, mostly 1-week-long courses (64%). No statistically significant differences in patient characteristics or extent of SCC were found, but more patients with established paraplegia or incontinence were prescribed short fractionation. There was no difference in outcome between the two schedules despite the group receiving fewer than two fractions having worse PS, motor function, and continence at initial evaluation.

In another retrospective review of SF RT for radiologically confirmed SCC, 199 previously untreated patients received steroids, followed by 8 Gy/1 for lower extremity motor deficits.[21] Fifty-four percent had an Eastern Collaborative Oncology Group (ECOG) PS of 1 to 2, and 30% had been symptomatic for 1 week or less. Twenty-six percent (20/78) of previously nonambulatory patients regained the ability to walk after RT. Acute toxicity was limited to grade 1; no late toxicity was recorded. In-field recurrence occurred at a median interval of 5 months in 19 of 65 patients with at least 1 year of follow-up.

In summary, short- and long-course RT seem to be similarly effective with regard to functional outcome after treatment of SCC.[22] However, some studies suggest that schedules consisting of five fractions or fewer are associated with significantly more in-field recurrences. Some authors have suggested that patients with favorable histology and a long expected prognosis may therefore potentially benefit from 2 weeks of treatment; the data available, however, indicate that dose escalation past 30 Gy does not appear to be clinically useful.[18]

Practice Patterns

Two patterns-of-practice surveys have investigated management of SCC. An e-mail questionnaire concerning palliative spinal RT was sent to 200 Canadian ROs.[23] The response rate was 46% (91/200). Most respondents did not recommend SF RT for SCC, but specific numbers were not reported. The overall response rate in a two-phase survey from India was 40.5% (81/199).[24] Fifty-six percent of respondents would change their preferred MF schedule to one with more than 10 fractions in the presence of SCC. Of the 19 respondents who generally prescribe SF RT for BM, 69% would prefer an MF course in the presence of SCC.

In a survey of American ROs, Ben-Josef and colleagues described a case of impending SCC: a painful, lytic BM in T3, vertebral collapse, but no neurological deficits. Responses describing management of this case were not reported.[25] However, the same scenario was presented in a Canadian study, in which 66.9% would use 20 Gy/5,

TABLE 237-1	Comparison of Different Dose Fractionation Schedules for Spinal Cord Compression		
PATIENTS (N)	**STUDY DESIGN**	**SCHEDULE**	**RESULTS**
102	Retrospective	1-2 fractions vs. multifraction	Similar functional outcome
214	Prospective	10 × 3 Gy vs. 20 × 2 Gy	Similar functional outcome
204	Retrospective	1 × 8 Gy vs. 10 × 3 Gy	Similar functional outcome
276	Randomized	2 × 8 Gy vs. 3 × 5 Gy + 5 × 3 Gy	Similar functional outcome
1304	Retrospective	1 × 8 Gy vs. 5 × 4 Gy vs. 10 × 3 Gy vs. 15 × 2.5 Gy vs. 20 × 2 Gy	Similar functional outcome

From Agarawal J, Swangsilpa T, van der Linden Y, et al. The role of external beam radiotherapy in the management of bone metastases. Clin Oncol 2006;18:747-760.

14.1% would prescribe 30 Gy/10, and 12.9% of respondents would offer 8 Gy/1.[26] In the case of SCC, as in BM, the results of survey studies illustrate reticence to use SF schedules.

ADVANCED LUNG CANCER—TRIAL RESULTS

One systematic review of palliative thoracic RT for locally advanced or metastatic lung cancer (or both) has been published to date.[27] The authors concluded that symptom improvement was equivalent regardless of the RT dose, although higher doses were associated with more acute side effects. Any survival benefit would probably be modest and confined to patients with good PS. Neither reirradiation nor QOL end points were considered, nor was quantitative pooling performed because of the heterogeneity of studies. In 2005, three subsequent RCTs were published, with conflicting results.[28-30]

One trial accrued 148 patients to determine whether a single 10-Gy fraction was equivalent to 30 Gy/10 in patients unsuitable for radical treatment or with symptomatic local recurrence after surgery.[28] Significantly more patients randomized to MF RT (23%) than to SF RT (5%) had complete resolution of symptoms (P < .001). No significant differences were observed in overall response measured by improvement in total symptom score (TSS) (77% who received SF versus 92% who received 10 fractions improved), PS, QOL, psychological symptoms, acute toxicity, or survival. This underpowered study was published many years after trial closure and used physician assessment of symptom severity rather than patient self-assessment of individual symptoms.

Kramer and co-authors reported the results of a trial of 297 eligible patients randomized to either 16 Gy/2 over a 1-week period or 30 Gy/10.[29] Patients had either stage III lung cancer with weight loss, Stage III with ECOG of 2 or greater, or stage IV. Patient-assessed symptom and QOL questionnaires were completed. The trial showed no difference in control of symptoms over the first 9 months, but palliation over time did differ significantly (P < .001), with the 30-Gy/10 group having prolonged symptom improvement. However, patients receiving lower total doses had more rapid improvement. The 1-year survival rate was significantly better in the 30-Gy/10 group (19.6% versus 10.9%, P = .03). QOL results are to be reported separately.

One hundred symptomatic patients with locally advanced or metastatic lung cancer were randomized to either 20 Gy/5 or 16 Gy/2 over a 1-week period.[30] This trial was closed early because of slow accrual, which resulted in unequal numbers of patients in each arm. Symptom surveys were completed by patients; however, only 73% (58/80) of patients surviving longer than 2 months returned the follow-up questionnaires. The number of patients achieving symptomatic improvement, degree of response, side effects, and proportion requiring reirradiation did not differ. Median survival in the 20-Gy/5 arm was 5.3 months versus 8.0 months in the 16-Gy/2 arm (P = .016), and the RT schedule remained a significant prognostic factor for survival on multivariate analysis, with a hazard ratio of 1.65 (95% confidence interval [CI], 1.09 to 2.48; P = .017). QOL was not measured.

We have updated and expanded the Toy systematic review to include quantitative pooling of 13 RCTs investigating different RT dose fractionation schedules. A total of 3473 patients with locally advanced or metastatic lung cancer not suitable for curative-intent treatment were included. Primary objectives were to determine the RT schedule that maximized symptom palliation and survival and minimized reirradiation and toxicity. For symptom control in evaluable patients, lower-dose (LD) palliative thoracic RT was generally similar to higher-dose (HD) RT, except for the TSS: 65.5% (216/330) of LD and 77.1% (243/315) of HD patients had improvement in TSS (P = .003). A greater likelihood of symptom response was seen with schedules such as 30 Gy/10. A significant survival advantage was found for HD palliative RT, with 26.5% alive versus 21.7% at 1 year (P = .002). Survival increased with increases in dose up to 30 Gy/10, after which point no further improvements were seen. Toxicity in the form of physician-assessed dysphagia was also significantly greater in the HD arm, 20.5% versus 14.9% (P = .01). The likelihood of reirradiation was 1.22-fold higher after LD palliative RT (P = not significant [NS]).

Practice Patterns

For locally advanced, unresectable non–small cell lung cancer (NSCLC), survey results and practice audits suggest wide variation in the aim of treatment, total dose, and number of fractions prescribed, thus reflecting a lack of consensus on optimal treatment. Practice audits focusing on this area have been few in number.

In an American report on patients treated in 1984 to 1985, greater variation in fraction number and total dose was used in treating the chest and mediastinum than for any other palliative indication.[31] The modal dose was 45 Gy/25, and more than 40% of patients received a dose greater than 40 Gy/20. There was no significant correlation between treatment parameters and patient age, PS, treatment site, or primary histology, but patients without other sites of distant metastases tended to receive longer schedules. In a U.K. audit of treatment of patients with NSCLC, respondents from 26 of 54 centers typically used doses greater than 20 Gy for palliative treatment.[32] Sixty-three percent of centers used one- to two-fraction schedules versus 2% in 1988. In a follow-up U.K. audit from 2003, patients with lung cancer treated with palliative intent were predominantly prescribed 1, 5, or 10 fractions. In many instances, similar regimens were given with differing intent.[10]

The first survey study to include hypothetical cases of incurable lung cancer was published in 1989 and had a response rate of 76% (172/227).[33] For an asymptomatic man with locally advanced but nonmetastatic disease, 52% would offer RT, 14% of whom would prescribe 50 Gy/20. The remainder used 43 other treatment schedules with a median of 15 fractions. For a patient who had incurable disease with hemoptysis and cough, all 172 respondents would prescribe RT, 31% of whom would recommend 30 Gy/10 and 8% would give 20 Gy/5. The remainder suggested a further 51 different fractionation schedules with a median of ten fractions. On average for both cases, 47% of respondents were influenced in their prescription dose by training, 33% by local policy, 21% by logistical constraints, 9% by an open clinical trial, 9% by patient convenience, 5% by experience, and just 3% by trial results.

A questionnaire concerning locally advanced, unresectable, symptomatic lung cancer was sent to members of three cooperative groups; response rates were 54.9% (268/488; U.S. respondents) and 82.5% (99/120; Canadian respondents). The European response rate was not reported.[34] Nearly all would offer such a patient local RT, with the majority agreeing that the chance of cure in this situation was less than 10%. However, the intent of treatment varied: 92% of Americans would offer RT to extend life and 95% to relieve symptoms. Corresponding results were 69% and 69% for European respondents and 37% and 86% for Canadians, respectively. Canadians chose a median of 40 Gy/15; Europeans, 56 Gy/28; and Americans, 60 Gy/32. Longer RT schedules were more often prescribed by ROs who were aiming to extend life and who predicted a longer survival.

A Canadian survey study of ROs and other specialists involved in treating lung cancer proposed two hypothetical cases, one concerning asymptomatic stage IIIB disease and the other concerning high PS but symptomatic stage IV disease. Two hundred thirty-four of 330 eligible respondents (response rate of 74.1%) subspecialized in the treatment of NSCLC. For stage IIIB disease, 65% recommended RT, 17% said no active treatment, and 16% advocated RT and chemotherapy. Twenty percent recommended chemotherapy, and 80% recommended best supportive care (BSC) only for the patient with stage IV disease.[35]

Eight of 27 ROs responded to a survey in New Zealand regarding treatment of six hypothetical patients with varying stages of NSCLC.[36] For a patient with stage IIIB NSCLC and ECOG 1, 71% of ROs favored BSC and 14% preferred chemotherapy and RT. For a 46-year-old with ECOG 1 and distant metastases, 57% of ROs would recommend BSC and 14% chemotherapy and RT. The authors inferred that treatment of advanced disease was controversial.

Finally, a survey circulated to all RT departments in Australia and New Zealand requested information about current practices in treating lung cancer.[37] Twenty-four departments responded for a response rate of 63%. Again, a wide variety of palliative fractionation schedules were used: 20 for NSCLC and 15 for small cell lung cancer (SCLC). Most commonly prescribed was 20 Gy/5 (which made up 28.6% of responses for NSCLC and 34.9% for SCLC). Two-fraction schedules for NSCLC were used by 14.3% of respondents, and 11.6% used them for palliation of SCLC.

Patient Preferences

One study to date has investigated patient preference in this area, published in abstract form only.[38] Using a decision board, the pros and cons of 17 Gy/2 versus 39 Gy/13 daily fractions were presented to patients with non-metastatic but unresectable NSCLC. Ninety-two patients enrolled, with 55% choosing the longer schedule because of improved survival (90%) and local control (12%). Shorter fractionation was chosen by the remainder for reasons of shorter overall duration (80%), cost (61%), and better symptom control (20%). Fifty-six percent of patients choosing the shorter schedule were overruled by the treating RO, as opposed to only 4% choosing the longer schedule (P < .001). Interestingly, despite the suggestion of a survival benefit associated with the longer schedule, nearly half the patients believed that it was not as important as the duration of treatment and lower cost.

COST-EFFECTIVENESS

Nowhere is the need to consider economic factors in day-to-day practice more pressing than in the field of radiation oncology, where a combination of better screening, early diagnosis, improved survival as a result of systemic therapies, and innovative technology for treatment delivery mean a higher cost of delivering RT than ever before.

Bone Metastases

Several economic analyses have been performed to compare different schedules of RT or RT with another treatment modality. A cost-utility analysis was conducted prospectively within a large Dutch randomized trial in which a single 8-Gy treatment was compared with 24 Gy/6. Trial results indicated equivalent symptom palliation. When considering the estimated quality-adjusted life years (QALYs), including the effect of retreatment, SF RT provided an additional 1.7 quality-adjusted weeks and saved $1753 (U.S. dollars) over MF RT.[39]

Through the use of a Markov model, Konski estimated that SF RT was more cost-effective for painful BM than either MF RT, chemotherapy (mitoxantrone and prednisone), or analgesics (oxycodone [OxyContin] with sennosides [Senokot] bowel routine) (Table 237-2).[40] Chemotherapy had the highest expected mean total cost. MF RT resulted in only slightly more quality-adjusted life months (QALMs) than SF RT did but cost $1300 (U.S.

TABLE 237-2	Markov Model on Different Costs of Treatment of Bone Metastases				
TREATMENT	COST	INCREMENTAL COST	EFFECTIVENESS (QALM)	INCREMENTAL EFFECTIVENESS (QALM)	INCREMENTAL COST-EFFECTIVENESS ($/QALY)
Pain medication	$11,700		5.75		
SFX	$11,900	$200	6.1	0.35	$6,857
MFX	$13,200	$1,500	6.25	0.5	$36,000
Chemotherapy	$15,300	$3,600	4.93	−0.82	Dominated*

*Dominated refers to treatment providing survival inferior to that with pain medication.
MFX, multifraction; QALM, quality-adjusted life month; QALY, quality-adjusted life year; SFX, single fraction.
From Konski A. Radiotherapy is a cost-effective palliative treatment for patients with bone metastases from prostate cancer. Int J Radiat Oncol Biol Phys 2004;60:1373-1378.

dollars) more. The improved cost-effectiveness of RT in comparison to narcotic analgesics and bisphosphonates has also been reported by other investigators.[22]

Two articles have shown cost-effectiveness of the radiopharmaceutical strontium (^{89}Sr) in lifetime management costs when compared with local RT alone in patients with advanced disease.[41,42] The addition of ^{89}Sr was associated with cost savings as a result of avoidance of additional courses of RT, enough to offset its actual cost.

Most studies indicate that RT provides good value for the money when compared with other palliative treatments. From a resource perspective, SF or short-course RT should always be considered when treating pain arising from uncomplicated BM.

Advanced Lung Cancer

Two studies on the cost-effectiveness of RT for advanced NSCLC have been published. Coy and co-workers' study focused on cost-effectiveness (cost per life year gained) and cost-utility analysis (cost per QALY gained) relative to BSC, based in part on monthly patient questionnaires.[43] As a result of RT, 56.9 quality-adjusted life days were gained (95% CI, 23.6 to 81.1). The societal cost-effectiveness of palliative RT versus BSC was $12,253 (Canadian dollars) after taking into account RT costs and indirect costs such as patient travel. On a cost-utility basis, each course of RT cost $17,012 (Canadian dollars) per QALY gained.

The first economic evaluation of randomized trial data was based on the trial of Kramer and associates.[29] Quality-adjusted life expectancy was 20.0 weeks in the 30-Gy/10 arm versus 13.2 weeks in the 16-Gy/2 arm ($P = .05$).[44] Total societal costs were $16,490 (U.S. dollars) for the longer schedule and $11,164 ($P < .001$) for the shorter one after taking into consideration RT, travel costs, other medical costs, reirradiation, and indirect costs such as time away from work. Excluding all nonradiotherapy costs, the cost-utility ratio for the longer schedule versus the shorter one was $12,800 (U.S. dollars) per QALY gained. The authors concluded that 30 Gy/10 provided better value for the money, with the additional costs of the protracted schedule justified by longer survival rather than improved QOL.

INTEGRATION OF PALLIATIVE RADIOTHERAPY WITH OTHER MODALITIES

With advances in chemotherapeutics, minimally invasive surgery, and innovative radiopharmaceuticals, new combinations of modalities are being explored for additive or synergistic effects to improve clinical outcomes.

Radiotherapy and Surgery

The need for multidisciplinary, cooperative assessment is nowhere more imperative from a patient's QOL perspective than in the area of surgical intervention for SCC or pathological fracture. The SCC literature was outlined earlier.[15]

Approximately 1% of BMs fracture, 10% of which require surgical intervention. An additional proportion of patients with BM undergo prophylactic stabilization to avoid the potentially devastating consequences of frac-

ture. Postoperative RT is usually recommended after surgical stabilization to decrease pain, minimize the risk of disease progression, minimize implant failure, and reduce the risk of refracture.[45] In a review of 64 orthopedic procedures performed on 60 patients, the addition of postoperative RT increased the proportion of patients able to use the extremity, decreased revision procedures, and, interestingly, increased survival (12.4 versus 3.3 months). However, to date, no clear evidence exists on the optimal timing or schedule of postoperative RT, and prospective trials are urgently needed to clarify this issue.

Radiotherapy and Radiopharmaceuticals

Improved outcomes have been demonstrated by some studies when radioisotopes were combined with RT. For example, the multicenter Trans-Canada study compared RT with 10.8 mCi ^{89}Sr or placebo in 126 patients with BM secondary to hormone-refractory prostate cancer.[46] Forty percent of the strontium patients were pain free at 3 months as compared with 23% of the placebo patients. Seventeen percent of the patients receiving ^{89}Sr discontinued analgesics versus 2% in the placebo group. At 3 months, 59% of the strontium patients were free of new painful metastases as opposed to 34% of the placebo arm ($P < .05$), with an increased median time to further local RT of 35 weeks versus 20 weeks. QOL, pain relief, and improvement in physical activity were also statistically significantly superior in the ^{89}Sr arm.

A Norwegian randomized trial, however, reported no advantage in pain relief with the addition of ^{89}Sr to local RT.[47] All patients received 30 Gy/10 and either strontium or placebo on the first day of RT. Unfortunately, this trial was closed early because of slow accrual, with 89 patients treated as per protocol. Response rates at 3 months were 30% in the strontium group and 20% in the control group ($P =$ NS), but the addition of ^{89}Sr did decrease alkaline phosphatase at 3 months ($P = .001$). There was no difference in the number of patients with progression (41% versus 51%), progression-free survival, reported QOL, and prostate-specific antigen level. Canadian practice guidelines currently do not recommend ^{89}Sr as a routine adjuvant to local RT because of conflicting results.[48]

Radiotherapy and Chemotherapy

Whether combining RT and chemotherapy conclusively improves symptom relief or QOL in patients with advanced cancer is unknown, but trials investigating these two modalities have been undertaken in NSCLC,[49] for example, with promising results. This approach has not been prospectively investigated in the setting of BM or SCC.

RECENT DEVELOPMENTS

As our understanding of the molecular signaling mechanisms between bone cells and tumors increases, a number of targeted agents have entered clinical development. Examples include those designed for the inhibition of cathepsin K (an osteoclast-derived enzyme essential for bone resorption), src kinase (a key molecule in osteoclastogenesis), and RANKL (receptor activator of nuclear factor-κB ligand, an osteoclast differentiation and activation regulator).[50] Denosumab (AMG-162) is a fully human monoclonal antibody that binds and neutralizes RANKL with high affinity. This prevents host cells such as osteoclasts from reacting to tumor products, thereby inhibiting bone resorption. Denosumab could potentially be used to treat bone loss caused by BM, multiple myeloma, and osteoporosis.[50]

EVIDENCE-BASED MEDICINE

Both the increasing use of high-tech RT delivery and the practice patterns of ROs have contributed to the underutilization of palliative RT as a treatment modality for symptom control. Delivery of MF treatment courses to patients with uncomplicated BM despite overwhelming randomized data suggesting the equivalency of SF courses is unnecessary and contrary to the principles of evidence-based medicine. In other clinical scenarios such as SCC and locally advanced lung cancer, further investigation is required to conclusively clarify the optimal dose fractionation schedule.

RESEARCH CHALLENGES

- Establishment of the optimal RT dose fractionation schedule for SCC and after surgical stabilization of fracture requires urgent study. There have been no practice audits or patient preference studies focusing on these clinical scenarios to date.
- It is imperative that resource assessment be performed in conjunction with considerations of treatment efficacy, QOL, and toxicity when determining RT recommendations. Further comparative data are needed in this area.

CONCLUSION

It seems probable that practice variations will continue to exist until ROs critically evaluate the published literature in the context of both preferences of individual patients and considerations of resource utilization. From a commonsense perspective, the shortest possible palliative RT schedule that maximizes functional outcome seems preferable.

REFERENCES

1. British Association of Surgical Oncology Guidelines. The management of metastatic bone disease in the United Kingdom. Eur J Surg Oncol 1999;25:3-23.
2. Falkmer U, Jarhult J, Wersall P, et al. A systematic overview of radiation therapy effects in skeletal metastases. Acta Oncol 2003;42:620-633.
3. Mackillop WJ. The principles of palliative radiotherapy: A radiation oncologist's perspective. Can J Oncol 1996;6(Suppl 1):5-11.
4. Bradley NM, Husted J, Sey MS, et al. Review of patterns of practice and patients' preferences in the treatment of bone metastases with palliative radiotherapy. Support Care Cancer 2007;15:373-385.
5. Chow E, Harris K, Fan G, et al. Palliative radiotherapy trials for bone metastases: A systematic review. J Clin Oncol 2007;25:1423-1436.
6. Roos D. Continuing reluctance to use single fractions of radiotherapy for metastatic bone pain: An Australian and New Zealand practice survey and literature review. Radiother Oncol 2000;56:315-322.
7. Barton M, Dawson R, Jacob S, et al. Palliative radiotherapy of bone metastases: An evaluation of outcome measures. J Eval Clin Pract 2001;7:47-64.
8. Shakespeare TP, Lu JJ, Back MF, et al. Patient preference for radiotherapy fractionation schedule in the palliation of painful bone metastases. J Clin Oncol 2003;21:2156-2162.
9. Szumacher E, Llewellyn-Thomas H, Franssen E, et al. Treatment of bone metastases with palliative radiotherapy: Patients' treatment preferences. Int J Radiat Oncol Biol Phys 2005;61:1473-1481.
10. Williams MV, James ND, Summers ET, et al. National survey of radiotherapy fractionation practice in 2003. Clin Oncol 2006;18:3-14.
11. Moller T, Brorsson B, Ceberg J, et al. A prospective survey of radiotherapy practice in 2001 in Sweden. Acta Oncol 2003;42:387-410.
12. Van der Linden Y, Leer J. Impact of randomized trial outcome in the treatment of painful bone metastases: Pattern of practice among radiation oncologists. A matter of believers vs. non-believers? Radiother Oncol 2000;56:279-281.
13. Kaasa S, Brenne E, Lund J-A, et al. Prospective randomized multicentre trial on single fraction radiotherapy (8 Gy × 1) versus multiple fractions (3 Gy × 10) in the treatment of painful bone metastases. Radiother Oncol 2006;79:278-284.
14. Byrne TN, Borges LF, Loeffler JS. Metastatic epidural spinal cord compression: Update on management. Sem Oncol 2006;33:307-311.
15. Patchell RA, Tibbs PA, Regine WF, et al. Direct decompressive surgical resection in the treatment of spinal cord compression caused by metastatic cancer: A randomized trial. Lancet 2005;366:643-648.
16. Maranzano E, Bellavita R, Rossi R, et al. Short-course versus split-course radiotherapy in metastatic spinal cord compression: Results of a phase III, randomized, multicentre trial. J Clin Oncol 2005;23:3358-3365.
17. Rades D, Stalpers LJ, Veninga T, et al. Evaluation of five radiation schedules and prognostic factors for metastatic spinal cord compression. J Clin Oncol 2005;23:3366-3375.
18. Rades D, Karstens JH, Hoskin P, et al. Escalation of radiation dose beyond 30 Gy in 10 fractions for metastatic spinal cord compression. Int J Radiat Oncol Biol Phys 2007;67:525-531.
19. Rades D, Hoskin PJ, Karstens JH, et al. Radiotherapy of metastatic spinal cord compression in very elderly patients. Int J Radiat Oncol Biol Phys 2007;67:256-263.
20. Hoskin PJ, Grover A, Bhana R. Metastatic spinal cord compression: Radiotherapy outcome and dose fractionation. Radiother Oncol 2003;68:175-180.
21. Rades D, Stalpers LJ, Hulshof MC, et al. Effectiveness and toxicity of single-fraction radiotherapy with 1 × 8 Gy for metastatic spinal cord compression. Radiother Oncol 2005;75:70-73.
22. Agarawal J, Swangsilpa T, van der Linden Y, et al. The role of external beam radiotherapy in the management of bone metastases. Clin Oncol 2006;18:747-760.
23. Barton R, Robinson G, Gutierrez E, et al. Palliative radiation for vertebral metastases: The effect of variation in prescription parameters on the dose received at depth. Int J Radiat Oncol Biol Phys 2002;52:1083-1091.
24. Gupta T, Sarin R. Palliative radiation therapy for painful vertebral metastases: A practice survey. Cancer 2004;101:2892-2896.
25. Ben-Josef E, Shamsa F, Williams A, et al. Radiotherapeutic management of osseous metastases: A survey of current patterns of care. Int J Radiat Oncol Biol Phys 1998;40:915-921.
26. Chow E, Danjoux C, Wong R, et al. Palliation of bone metastases: A survey of patterns of practice among Canadian radiation oncologists. Radiother Oncol 2000;56:305-314.
27. Toy E, Macbeth F, Coles B, et al. Palliative thoracic radiotherapy for non–small-cell lung cancer: A systematic review. Am J Clin Oncol 2003;26:112-120.
28. Erridge SC, Gaze MN, Price A, et al. Symptom control and quality of life in people with lung cancer: a randomized trial of two palliative radiotherapy fractionation schedules. Clin Oncol 2005;17:61-67.
29. Kramer GW, Wanders SL, Noordijk EM, et al. Results of the Dutch national study of the palliative effect of irradiation using two different treatment schemes for non–small cell lung cancer. J Clin Oncol 2005;23:2962-2970.
30. Senkus-Konefka E, Dziadziuszko R, Bednaruk-Mlynski E, et al. A prospective, randomized study to compare two palliative radiotherapy schedules for non-small cell lung cancer (NSCLC). Br J Cancer 2005;92:1038-1045.
31. Coia LR, Hanks GR, Martz K, et al. Practice patterns of palliative care for the US 1984-1985. Int J Radiat Oncol Biol Phys 1988;14:1261-1269.
32. Maher J, Timothy A, Squire CJ, et al. Audit: The use of radiotherapy for NSCLC in the UK. Clin Oncol 1993;5:72-79.
33. Priestman TJ, Bullimore JA, Godden TP, et al. The Royal College of Radiologists' fractionation survey. Clin Oncol 1989;1:39-46.
34. Maher EJ, Coia L, Duncan G, et al. Treatment strategies in advanced and metastatic cancer: Differences in attitude between the USA, Canada and Europe. Int J Radiat Oncol Biol Phys 1992;23:239-244.
35. Raby B, Pater J, Mackillop W. Does knowledge guide practice? Another look at the management of non–small cell lung cancer. J Clin Oncol 1995;13:1904-1911.
36. Christmas T, Findlay M. Lung cancer treatment in New Zealand: Physicians' attitudes. N Z Med J 2004;117:1-7.
37. Holloway L. Current practice when treating lung cancer in Australasia. Australas Radiol 2007;51:62-67.
38. Tang JI, Back MF, Mukherjee R, et al. Patient preference for radiotherapy fractionation schedule in the palliation of symptomatic unresectable lung cancer [abstract 1015]. 2006;66(3 Suppl 1):S137.
39. Van den Hout WB, van der Linden YM, Steenland E, et al. Single- versus multiple-fraction radiotherapy in patients with painful bone metastases: Cost-utility analysis based on a randomized trial. J Natl Cancer Inst 2003;95:222-229.
40. Konski A. Radiotherapy is a cost-effective palliative treatment for patients with bone metastases from prostate cancer. Int J Radiat Oncol Biol Phys 2004;60:1373-1378.
41. Malmberg I, Persson U, Ask A, et al. Painful bone metastases in hormone-refractory prostate cancer: Economic costs of strontium-89 and/or external radiotherapy. Urology 1997;50:747-753.
42. McEwan AJ, Amoytte G, McGowan D, et al. A retrospective analysis of the cost effectiveness of treatment with Metastron (89-Sr chloride) in patients with prostate cancer metastatic to bone. Nucl Med Commun 1994;15:499-504.

43. Coy P, Schaafsma J, Schofield JA. The cost-effectiveness and cost-utility of high-dose palliative radiotherapy for advanced non–small cell lung cancer. Int J Radiat Oncol Biol Phys 2000;48:1025-1033.

44. Van den Hout WB, Kramer GW, Noordijk EM, et al. Cost-utility analysis of short- versus long-course palliative radiotherapy in patients with non–small cell lung cancer. J Natl Cancer Inst 2006;98:1786-1794.

45. Townsend PW, Smalley SR, Cozad SC, et al. Role of postoperative radiation therapy after stabilization of fractures caused by metastatic disease. Int J Radiat Oncol Biol Phys 1995;31:43-49.

46. Porter A, McEwan A, Powe J. Results of a randomized phase III trial to evaluate the efficacy of strontium-89 adjuvant to local field external beam irradiation in the management of endocrine resistance metastatic prostate cancer. Int J Radiat Oncol Biol Phys 1993;25:805-813.

47. Smeland S, Erikstein B, Aas M, et al. Role of strontium-89 as adjuvant to palliative external beam radiotherapy is questionable: Results of a double-blind randomized study. Int J Radiat Oncol Biol Phys 2003;56:1397-1404.

48. Bauman G, Charette M, Reid R, et al. Radiopharmaceuticals for the palliation of painful bone metastases—a systematic review. Radiother Oncol 2005;75: 258e1-258e13.

49. Michael M, Wirth A, Ball DL, et al. A phase I trial of high-dose palliative radiotherapy plus concurrent weekly vinorelbine and cisplatin in patients with locally advanced and metastatic NSCLC. Br J Cancer 2005;93:652-661.

50. Lipton A. Future treatment of bone metastases. Clin Cancer Res 2006;12(20 Suppl):6305s-6308s.

SUGGESTED READING

Agarawal J, Swangsilpa T, van der Linden Y, et al. The role of external beam radiotherapy in the management of bone metastases. Clin Oncol 2006;18:747-760.

Byrne TN, Borges LF, Loeffler JS. Metastatic epidural spinal cord compression: Update on management. Semin Oncol 2006; 33:307-311.

Chow E, Harris K, Fan G, et al. Palliative radiotherapy trials for bone metastases: A systematic review. J Clin Oncol 2007; 25:1423-1436.

Mackillop WJ. The principles of palliative radiotherapy: A radiation oncologist's perspective. Can J Oncol 1996;6(Suppl 1):5-11.

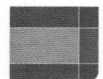

CHAPTER **238**

Principles of Modern Chemotherapy and Endocrine Therapy

Daphne Tsoi and Anna K. Nowak

KEY POINTS

- Treatment intent (curative or palliative) should be determined and discussed with the patient before therapy.

- Appropriate palliative systemic anticancer treatments in advanced cancer can alleviate cancer-related symptoms, prolong survival, and improve quality of life.

- Conventional cytotoxic chemotherapy agents exploit the more rapid proliferative cycle of cancer cells as opposed to normal cells. This nonspecificity results in a low therapeutic index and undesirable toxicity.

- Biological or targeted agents are directed toward a specific molecular target enabling cancer cell proliferation or survival. Improved specificity may result in more tolerable toxicity.

- Discontinuation of treatment should be considered if symptoms do not improve or there is significant toxicity or disease progression.

In advanced cancer, chemotherapy and endocrine therapy are almost always given for palliation rather than cure. Patients may benefit from palliative anticancer treatment through longer survival, decreased tumor volume and hence improved symptoms, and better quality of life. Potential benefit must be balanced against treatment toxicity and inconvenience. The decision to recommend palliative chemotherapy or endocrine therapy must always be individualized.

Endocrine therapy for cancer dates back a hundred years,[1] and hormonal manipulation still plays a critical role in hormone-responsive cancer. Cytotoxic chemotherapy has been the mainstay of anticancer therapy for many decades. It works primarily by killing rapidly proliferating cancer cells by targeting general cellular metabolic processes, and consequently it is not specific for malignant cells. This causes undesirable toxicity in normal tissue and gives chemotherapy a narrow therapeutic index. Recently, research has focused on molecular events and signaling pathways in the growth and proliferation of cancer cells. This approach has led to targeted therapy—well-characterized and often rationally designed agents with improved specificity for cancer cells.

TREATMENT INTENT

The intention of treatment should be determined and discussed before therapy.

Curative Intent

- *Adjuvant treatment* is systemic therapy given after local treatment (surgery or radiotherapy) for high-risk disease. It aims to eradicate putative microscopic metastases and reduce the risk of recurrence.
- *Neoadjuvant treatment* is given before local therapy. It reduces tumor bulk before surgical resection or irradiation, thereby reducing the extent of local treatment for organ preservation or improvement of local control.
- *Curative treatment of advanced cancer* is realistic in a few highly chemosensitive diseases, such as testicular cancer, high-grade lymphoma, and some leukemias.

Palliative Intent

- *Palliative chemotherapy* is used to control disease and reduce tumor volume to alleviate or prevent tumor symptoms, prolong survival, and improve quality of life. Most chemotherapy in advanced cancer is palliative.

CHEMOTHERAPY

Cytotoxic agents kill cancer cells by targeting DNA or RNA, interrupting cell division, or disrupting the chemistry of nucleic acids. They are generally classified in relation to the cell cycle (Fig. 238-1).

Phase-specific agents are effective only against the fraction of cells in a particular cell cycle phase when the drug is given.

Phase-nonspecific agents kill dividing cells at any point in the cell cycle (cycle-specific, phase-nonspecific

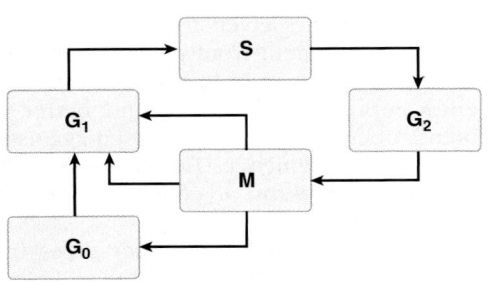

G_0 — (gap 0/resting phase) Cells are generally
      refractory to chemotherapy
G_1 — (gap 1/interphase) Protein and RNA
      synthesis for specialized cell function
S — (DNA synthesis) Doubling of DNA cellular
      content
G_2 — (gap 2) Cessation of DNA synthesis;
      production of microtubule precursors of
      mitotic spindle; continuing RNA synthesis
M — (mitosis) Segregation of genetic material
      to daughter cells. New cells enter G_0 or
      G_1 phase

FIGURE 238-1 The cell cycle.

TABLE 238-1 Common Alkylating Agents

DRUG	PROPERTY	COMMON INDICATIONS	DOSE-LIMITING TOXICITY	COMMON TOXICITY
Busulfan	Formation of carbonium ions	Chronic myeloid leukemia, myeloproliferative disorders, hematopoietic stem cell transplantation	Myelosuppression	Gastrointestinal upset, sterility
Chlorambucil	Derivative of nitrogen mustard. Only available in oral preparation	Chronic lymphocytic leukemia, indolent lymphoma, myeloma, Hodgkin's lymphoma, hairy cell leukemia, trophoblastic tumors	Myelosuppression	Gastrointestinal upset
Cyclophosphamide	Prodrug activated by hepatic cytochrome P-450 to produce nitrogen mustard	Widely used in hematologic malignancy and solid tumors—acute and chronic leukemia, lymphoma, breast and lung cancer	Myelosuppression, hemorrhagic cystitis	Alopecia, mucositis, sterility, nausea, vomiting
Dacarbazine (DTIC)	Imidazole carboxamide derivative	Hodgkin's lymphoma, malignant melanoma, sarcoma	Myelosuppression	Nausea, vomiting
Fotemustine	From nitrosourea family. Crosses blood-brain barrier	Malignant melanoma, brain cancer	Myelosuppression	Nausea, vomiting
Ifosfamide	Prodrug activated by hepatic cytochrome P-450 to produce nitrogen mustard	Lymphoma, sarcoma, relapsed testicular carcinoma	Myelosuppression, hemorrhagic cystitis (may be avoided with coadministration of mesna)	Alopecia, nausea, vomiting, neurotoxicity
Melphalan	Derivative of nitrogen mustard and phenylalanine	Multiple myeloma, some carcinomas, limb perfusion for melanoma	Myelosuppression	Anorexia, nausea, vomiting, mucositis, sterility
Nitrosoureas— lomustine (CCNU), carmustine (BCNU)	Highly lipid soluble. Cross blood-brain barrier	Brain cancer, lymphoma, myeloma, some carcinomas	Myelosuppression	Nausea, vomiting
Temozolomide	Derivative of dacarbazine. Oral preparation. Crosses blood-brain barrier	Glioblastoma, metastatic melanoma	Myelosuppression	Nausea, vomiting

drugs) or can kill nondividing cells (cycle-nonspecific drugs).

Rationale for Combination Chemotherapy

Cytotoxic agents are often used in combination. Drugs effective as single agents but with different mechanisms of action and nonoverlapping toxicity are combined at the maximum tolerated dose. The different mechanisms of action allow independent cell killing for additive or synergistic effects, thereby preventing or slowing the emergence of drug-resistant clones.

Concurrent Chemoradiotherapy

Chemotherapy can be given during radiotherapy for a radiation-sensitizing effect. Agents commonly used include cisplatin, 5-fluorouracil, and etoposide. Although they enhance the efficacy of radiation, they often potentiate toxicity. Such treatment results in improved local control and survival in various solid tumors, including anal, rectal, bladder, head and neck, esophageal, cervical, and locally advanced non–small cell lung cancer.

Alkylating Agents

Alkylating agents are the oldest class of anticancer drugs. Their primary mode of action is cross-linking of DNA strands via alkyl groups, which leads to arrest in the transition from G_1 to S and cell death (Table 238-1).

Antimetabolites

Antimetabolites work by interfering with DNA synthesis. This effect is achieved either by masquerading as structural analogues of normal molecules or by inhibiting enzymes for the synthesis of essential nucleotides (purines and pyrimidines). They are most active in the S phase of the cell cycle (Table 238-2).

Platinum Drugs

Cisplatin was the first agent in this group. It has become the most widely used anticancer drug and is efficacious in many cancers. Its use is associated with significant toxicity, however, and it is highly emetogenic. Some other toxicities resemble heavy-metal poisoning. The newer platinum agents *carboplatin* and *oxaliplatin* have similar efficacy but less toxicity.

Platinum analogues bind directly to DNA and inhibit synthesis by altering the DNA template through the formation of intrastrand cross-links (Table 238-3).

Topoisomerase Inhibitors

Topoisomerase enzymes are proteins that regulate the topology, or shape, of the DNA helix. Topoisomerase I relaxes supercoiled double-stranded DNA by making temporary single-strand breaks that are later repaired by the same enzyme. Relaxation of supercoiled DNA allows processes of replication, transcription, and recombination to take place. Topoisomerase II creates transient double-stranded breakage of DNA, thereby allowing subsequent

---

TABLE 238-2 Common Antimetabolites

DRUG	PROPERTY	INDICATIONS	DOSE-LIMITING TOXICITY	COMMON TOXICITY
FOLIC ACID ANALOGUES				
Methotrexate	Blocks dihydrofolate reductase (DHFR)	Widely used. Breast, gastrointestinal (GI), head and neck cancers; leukemia; osteogenic sarcoma; meningeal carcinomatosis	Myelosuppression, nephrotoxicity	Mucositis, nausea, vomiting
Pemetrexed	Targets multiple enzymes involved in folate metabolism	Malignant pleural mesothelioma, non–small cell lung cancer	Myelosuppression, mucositis (toxicity reduced with folic acid and vitamin B_{12} supplements)	Anorexia, GI upset
PYRIMIDINE ANALOGUES				
5-Fluorouracil (5-FU)	Blocks thymidylate synthetase	Widely used. GI malignancies (esophageal, gastric, pancreatic, colorectal, anal); breast, head and neck, ovarian cancers	Myelosuppression, mucositis, diarrhea	More common in patients with dihydropyrimidine dehydrogenase deficiency
Capecitabine	Orally active prodrug of 5-FU. Preferentially activated in tumor and liver tissue	Breast, colorectal cancer. Has the potential to replace prolonged 5-FU infusion	Hand-foot syndrome, diarrhea	GI upset
Cytarabine (ara-C)	Inhibits DNA polymerase	Acute myelogenous leukemia, non-Hodgkin's lymphoma	Myelosuppression	Nausea, vomiting, diarrhea, alopecia
Gemcitabine	Difluorinated analogue of deoxycytidine	Lung, pancreatic, breast, bladder, ovarian cancers	Myelosuppression	Flulike symptoms, nausea
PURINE ANALOGUES				
6-Mercaptopurine	Inhibits de novo purine synthesis	Maintenance therapy for acute lymphoblastic leukemia	Myelosuppression	Nausea, vomiting, anorexia
Cladribine	Deoxyadenosine analogue	Hairy cell leukemia, indolent lymphoma	Myelosuppression	Nausea, fever, chills
Fludarabine	Adenosine analogue	Chronic lymphocytic leukemia, indolent lymphoma, cutaneous T-cell lymphoma	Myelosuppression	Nausea, vomiting
Hydroxyurea	Inhibits ribonucleotide reductase	Myeloproliferative disorders, chronic myelogenous leukemia	Myelosuppression	Nausea, vomiting, rash

---

TABLE 238-3 Platinum Drugs

DRUG	INDICATIONS	DOSE-LIMITING TOXICITY	COMMON TOXICITY
Cisplatin	Widely used, including for testicular, ovarian, bladder, breast, esophageal, gastric, lung, head and neck cancers	Nephrotoxicity, peripheral neuropathy, ototoxicity	Nausea, vomiting
Carboplatin	Ovarian, lung cancer. Carboplatin may be an alternative to cisplatin in many regimens	Myelosuppression, especially thrombocytopenia	Nausea, vomiting (less severe than with cisplatin)
Oxaliplatin	Colorectal cancer. Probably active in a number of solid tumors, currently under investigation	Neutropenia, peripheral neuropathy	Stomatitis, nausea, vomiting, diarrhea

passage of a second intact DNA duplex through the break. Inhibitors targeting these enzymes disrupt normal cell replication mechanisms (Table 238-4).

Antimicrotubule Agents

Microtubules are composed of molecules of tubulin. They are the principal components of the mitotic spindle apparatus that separates the duplicate set of chromosomes during mitosis. They also help maintain cell shape and scaffolding, intracellular transport, and relay of signals between cell surface receptors and the nucleus. Microtubules are seen as highly strategic subcellular targets of anticancer agents. Vinca alkaloids and the taxanes are the main classes of antimicrotubule agents currently available, with other novel agents in development (Table 238-5).

Antitumor Antibiotics

These drugs are derived from microorganisms and act by various mechanisms. The anthracyclines, which act by

TABLE 238-4 Topoisomerase Inhibitors

DRUG	PROPERTY	INDICATIONS	DOSE-LIMITING TOXICITY	COMMON TOXICITY
TOPOISOMERASE I INHIBITORS				
Camptothecins—Plant Alkaloids (from the Oriental Yew Tree)				
Topotecan	Semisynthetic analogue of camptothecin	Ovarian, small cell lung cancers	Myelosuppression	Nausea, vomiting, anorexia
Irinotecan	SN-38 is the active metabolite	Colorectal cancer	Myelosuppression, diarrhea	Acute cholinergic-like syndrome, nausea, vomiting
TOPOISOMERASE II INHIBITORS				
Epipodophyllotoxins—Plant Alkaloids (from the Root of the May Apple or Mandrake)				
Etoposide (VP-16)	Oral preparation available	Testicular, lung cancers; lymphoma and others	Neutropenia	Nausea, vomiting, alopecia
Teniposide (VP-26)	Intravenous preparation only	Acute lymphoblastic leukemia	Neutropenia	Thrombocytopenia
ANTHRACYCLINES—ANTIBIOTICS				
Doxorubicin (Adriamycin)	14-Hydroxy derivative of daunorubicin	Widely used. Acute leukemia; breast, gastric, ovarian, bladder, thyroid cancers; neuroblastoma	Myelosuppression, cardiomyopathy	Alopecia, nausea, vomiting, stomatitis
Epirubicin	Stereoisomer of doxorubicin	Gastric, breast cancers	Myelosuppression, less cardiotoxic than doxorubicin	As above
Daunorubicin	Produced by fungus *Streptomyces peucetius*	Acute leukemia	As above	As above
Idarubicin	Daunorubicin analogue	Acute leukemia	As above	As above
Anthracycline Analogue				
Mitoxantrone	Anthracenedione compound	Prostate, breast cancers; lymphoma; acute leukemia	Bone marrow suppression	Same as anthracyclines, but milder

TABLE 238-5 Antimicrotubule Agents

DRUG	PROPERTY	INDICATIONS	DOSE-LIMITING TOXICITY	COMMON TOXICITY
VINCA ALKALOIDS				
Vinblastine	Derived from the periwinkle plant	Lymphoma, testicular cancer	Neutropenia	Alopecia, thrombocytopenia
Vincristine		Leukemia, lymphoma, small cell lung cancer, multiple myeloma	Peripheral neuropathy (dose dependent)	Alopecia, tissue necrosis if extravasated
Vinorelbine	Semisynthetic vinca alkaloid. Oral preparation available	Breast, non–small cell lung cancers	Myelosuppression	Peripheral neuropathy, constipation, nausea, vomiting
TAXANES				
Paclitaxel	Extract from bark of the Pacific yew	Breast, ovarian, non–small cell lung cancers	Neutropenia, peripheral neuropathy, hypersensitivity reaction*	Alopecia, thrombocytopenia, arthralgia, myalgia
Docetaxel	Semisynthetic taxoid. Derived from needles of the European yew	Breast, prostate, non–small cell lung cancers	Fluid retention (may be delayed with steroid premedication). Hypersensitivity reaction,* peripheral neuropathy, neutropenia	Alopecia, nail disorders, cutaneous reaction

*May be prevented with steroids and H_1 and H_2 histamine antagonist premedication.

TABLE 238-6 Antitumor Antibiotics

DRUG	PROPERTY	INDICATIONS	DOSE-LIMITING TOXICITY	COMMON TOXICITY
Bleomycin	Inhibits DNA synthesis by oxidative cleavage; inhibits DNA repair by stopping DNA ligase	Lymphoma; testicular cancer; sarcoma; squamous cell, skin, head and neck cancers	Pulmonary toxicity (pneumonitis, fibrosis), hypersensitivity reactions	Dermatological toxicity (desquamation, hyperpigmentation, pruritus), mucositis, anorexia
Dactinomycin	Intercalates between DNA base pairs and prevents RNA synthesis; inhibits topoisomerase II	Sarcoma, testicular cancer, Wilms' tumor, neuroblastoma, choriocarcinoma	Myelosuppression	Nausea, vomiting, alopecia, mucositis, diarrhea, necrosis at extravasation
Mitomycin C	Acts as an alkylating agent upon intracellular activation	Gastrointestinal, breast, lung cancers	Myelosuppression	Mild nausea and vomiting, necrosis at extravasation

inhibiting topoisomerase enzymes, are also produced by microbial fermentation (Table 238-6).

Other Agents

L-Asparaginase depletes the essential amino acid asparagine, which leads to inhibition of protein synthesis. It is used for acute leukemia. Hypersensitivity reaction is the main dose-limiting toxicity. Other common toxicities include nausea, vomiting, anorexia, cerebral dysfunction (reversible), hyperglycemia, and hepatitis.

BIOLOGICAL AND TARGETED THERAPY

Targeted therapy is rapidly evolving. The focus has been on molecularly based agents that are more specific for cancer cells. The most commonly used targeted-therapy agents are specific for the epidermal growth factor receptor (EGFR), the vascular epidermal growth factor receptor (VEGF), the HER2 receptor, and CD20 on B cells. Monoclonal antibodies in general target only a specific receptor group; the suffixes used in the World Health Organization drug nomenclature are standardized according to antibody structure. They can be murine ("omab"), chimeric ("ximab"), or humanized ("zumab") antibodies. Monoclonal antibodies are large molecules that require intravenous administration, and they usually cross the blood-brain-barrier poorly (Fig. 238-2). Tyrosine kinase inhibitors are small molecules with good bioavailability as oral preparations. They bind to the extracellular domain of the appropriate cell surface receptor and thereby inhibit the intracellular tyrosine kinase domain from initiating a cascade of events essential for cell survival (Fig. 238-3). Many tyrosine kinase inhibitors are multitargeted. The suffix "ib" denotes a small molecule inhibitor (Table 238-7).

IMMUNOTHERAPY

Cytokines are soluble proteins that mediate interactions between cells and their extracellular environment. Interferons and interleukins have been recognized for their antitumor activities.

Interferons are cytostatic and can also modulate oncogene expression and enhance the cytotoxic activity of natural killer cells, macrophages, and T cells. They have been used for various malignancies, including chronic myelogenous leukemia, hairy cell leukemia, non-Hodgkin's

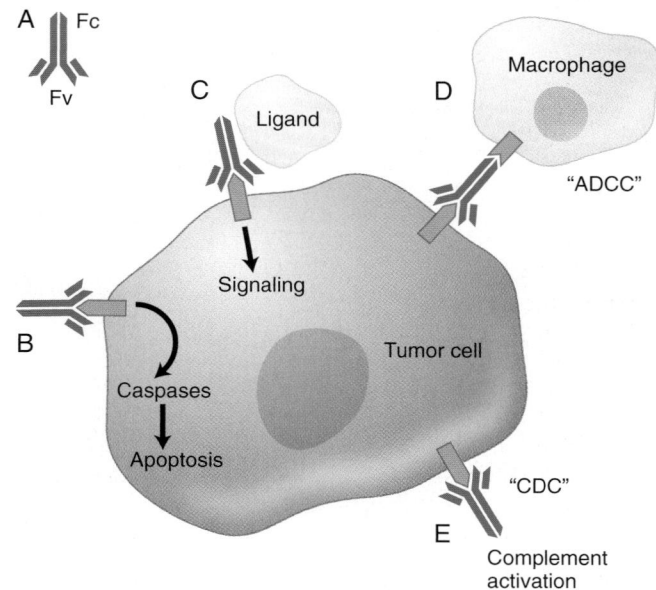

FIGURE 238-2 Mechanism of action of monoclonal antibodies. A, Specific binding region (Fv) and constant region (Fc) of monoclonal antibodies give rise to their activity. B, Binding of extracellular receptor results in signals that induce caspases and cellular apoptosis. C, Receptor binding inhibits binding of ligand, resulting in blockade of intracellular signaling. D, Recognition of Fc portion of antibody bound to antigen results in phagocytosis by macrophages with Fc receptor (antibody-dependent cellular cytotoxicity, ADCC). E, Fc portion of antibody bound to tumor antigen activates complement, resulting in cell lysis (complement-dependent cytotoxicity, CDC).

lymphoma, AIDS-related Kaposi's sarcoma, malignant melanoma, and renal cell carcinoma. The most common side effect is a flulike syndrome of fever, chill, fatigue, myalgia, anorexia, and headache. Others include nausea, myelosuppression, elevated liver enzymes, depression, and cardiac arrhythmias.

Interleukin-2 (IL2) is a major growth factor for lymphoid cells. IL2 exerts antitumor effects by stimulating host immune reactivity via the proliferation of natural killer cells, lymphokine-activated killer cells, and other cytotoxic cells based on its ability to expand the subpopulation of T cells that bear IL2 receptors. IL2 alone does not appear to exert direct antitumor activity. Melanoma and renal cell carcinoma are most responsive to IL2. Its toxicity profile resembles that of interferon and is dose dependent. Severe toxicities, including vascular leak syndrome, cardiac arrhythmia, myocardial infarction, and severe hypotension, are associated with increased mortality.

TABLE 238-7 Targeted Therapy

DRUG	TRADE NAME	TARGET	INDICATIONS	SIDE EFFECTS	COMMENTS
MONOCLONAL ANTIBODIES					
Rituximab	Rituxan	CD20	NHL	Asthenia, dizziness, headache, nausea, rash, infection, myelosuppression	1st-line treatment of DLBCL combined with chemotherapy. May have a role in 1st-line therapy for indolent lymphomas
Iodine I 131 tositumomab	Bexxar	CD20	NHL		Single course was more efficacious than "last qualifying chemotherapy" in heavily pretreated patients[2]
Yttrium Y 90 ibritumomab tiuxetan	Zevalin	CD20	NHL		Active in patients with refractory and heavily pretreated DLBCL[3]
Alemtuzumab	Campath 1H	CD52	B-cell lymphoma (relapsed, refractory, transformed), salvage B-cell chronic lymphocytic leukemia		Associated with high risk for opportunistic infection. Prophylactic antibiotic recommended
Gemtuzumab	Mylotarg	CD33	Acute myeloid leukemia		Increased risk in veno-occlusive disease
Trastuzumab	Herceptin	HER2/neu	Breast cancer (adjuvant and metastatic)	Hypersensitivity reaction, cardiotoxicity (hence not used in combination with anthracyclines)	Generally used in combination with chemotherapy. Modest activity as a single agent
Bevacizumab	Avastin	VEGF	Colorectal, renal cell carcinoma. Potential activity in head and neck cancer; NSCLC; esophageal, hepatocellular carcinoma; multiple myeloma; NHL; CML	Hypertension, proteinuria, GI perforation, impaired wound healing, diarrhea, arterial thromboembolism, hemorrhage	When combined with fluorouracil chemotherapy, has clinically meaningful benefits in metastatic colorectal cancer[4]
Cetuximab	Erbitux	EGFR	Colorectal, head and neck cancer. Activity in pancreatic cancer, NSCLC	Hypersensitivity reaction, rash	Has clinical activity given alone or in combination with irinotecan in irinotecan-refractory metastatic colorectal cancer.[5] When used in combination with radiotherapy for locoregional advanced head and neck cancer, improved clinical outcome.[6] Also has activity in advanced head and neck cancer[7]
SMALL MOLECULE INHIBITORS					
Imatinib	Gleevec	c-kit, PDGF	Bcl-Abl+ CML, c-kit+ GIST	Diarrhea, nausea, muscle cramps, fluid retention, myelosuppression	1st-line treatment of Bcl-Abl+ CML based on efficacy and toxicity profile superior to that of interferon and cytarabine.[8] Significant stable disease response in chemotherapy-refractory GIST in phase II trial[9]
Bortezomib	Velcade	Proteosome inhibitor	Refractory multiple myeloma	Malaise, fever, anorexia, diarrhea, nausea, myelosuppression	Found to be superior to high-dose dexamethasone for refractory multiple myeloma[10]
Gefitinib Erlotinib	Iressa Tarceva	EGFR	NSCLC	Skin reaction, diarrhea, nausea, anorexia, QT prolongation, interstitial lung disease (rare)	Active as single agent only. Only erlotinib has shown survival benefit in phase III trial[11]
Sunitinib	Sutent	VEGF, PDGF	Metastatic renal cell carcinoma	Fatigue, diarrhea, nausea, stomatitis, altered taste, skin reaction, hypertension, bleeding	Improved progression-free survival in comparison to interferon in 1st-line therapy in phase III study[12]
Sorafenib	Nexavar	VEGF, PDGF, Ras	Metastatic renal cell carcinoma	Rash, diarrhea, hand-foot syndrome, fatigue, hypertension	Improved progression-free survival in comparison to placebo in 2nd-line therapy after cytokines in phase III trial[13]
Temsirolimus	Torisel	mTOR	Metastatic renal cell carcinoma	Similar to sunitinib	Improved overall survival in comparison to interferon in 1st-line therapy for poor-risk group in phase III trial[14]
Lapatinib	Tykerb	EGFR/HER2	HER2+ metastatic breast cancer	Diarrhea, dyspepsia, rash	Improved progression-free survival when combined with capecitabine for trastuzumab-resistant disease in phase III trial[15]

CML, chronic myelogenous leukemia; DLBCL, diffuse large B-cell lymphoma; EGFR, epidermal growth factor receptor; GI, gastrointestinal; GIST, gastrointestinal stromal tumor; mTOR, mammalian target of rapamycin; NHL, non-Hodgkin's lymphoma; NSCLC, non–small cell lung cancer; PDGF, platelet-derived growth factor; VEGF, vascular endothelial growth factor.

TABLE 238-8 Endocrine Therapy

DRUG	MECHANISM OF ACTION	INDICATIONS	SIDE EFFECTS	COMMENTS
ESTROGEN RECEPTOR MODULATORS				
Tamoxifen	Binds to estrogen receptor and blocks the effects of endogenous estrogen. Has partial agonistic activity	Breast cancer	Hot flashes, menstrual changes, vaginal bleeding Rare: endometrial cancer, thromboembolism, retinopathy	Ovarian ablation plus tamoxifen is superior to either alone for metastatic premenopausal breast cancer[16]
Toremifene	Similar to tamoxifen. Available in the United States for metastatic breast cancer. Results equivalent to those of tamoxifen			
Fulvestrant	Estrogen receptor antagonist. "Pure antiestrogen." No agonistic activity	Metastatic breast cancer	Injection site reaction, hot flashes, nausea, headache	Available in a parenteral preparation only. Monthly intramuscular injection
PROGESTINS				
Megestrol Medroxyprogesterone	17-OH-progesterone derivatives. Exact mechanism unclear. Reported to suppress adrenal steroid synthesis, suppress estrogen receptor levels, alter tumor hormone metabolism, enhance steroid metabolism, directly kill tumor cells	Metastatic breast, endometrial, prostate cancer in palliative setting	Weight gain, fluid retention, thromboembolism	Also used for appetite stimulation in patients with anorexia
AROMATASE INHIBITORS				
Anastrozole Letrozole	Nonsteroidal competitive inhibitors of aromatase that cause inhibition of conversion of adrenal androgens to estrogens in peripheral and cancer tissues	Breast cancer (adjuvant and metastatic settings). Used in postmenopausal women only	Hot flashes, vaginal dryness, arthralgia, fatigue. Increased risk for osteoporosis and fractures	Aromatase inhibitors are superior to tamoxifen as 1st-line treatment of metastatic breast cancer in postmenopausal women
Exemestane	Steroidal aromatase inhibitor. Irreversibly binds with and permanently inactivates the enzyme	Same as anastrozole/letrozole		
ANTIANDROGENS				
Flutamide Bicalutamide Nilutamide	Nonsteroidal androgen receptor antagonists	Prostate cancer	Gynecomastia, hot flashes, impotence, nausea Rare: interstitial pneumonitis and night blindness with nilutamide. Interact with drugs metabolized by hepatic cytochrome P-450 system	Used in combination with LHRH agonists or after orchidectomy
GONADOTROPIN-RELEASING HORMONE ANALOGUES (LHRH AGONISTS)				
Goserelin Leuprolide	Inhibition of gonadotropin secretion to reduce circulating testosterone in men and estrogens in women	Metastatic prostate cancer, breast cancer in premenopausal women	Hot flashes, reduced libido, nausea	Used in combination with antiandrogens in prostate cancer to prevent initial tumor flare

LHRH, luteinizing hormone–releasing hormone.

ENDOCRINE THERAPY

Hormones have been implicated in the etiology and growth of many malignancies. Common endocrine-responsive cancers include breast, prostate, and endometrial carcinoma. The aim of endocrine cancer therapy is to deplete levels of circulating hormone or block binding of the hormone to receptors, with result being inhibition of cell proliferation and induction of apoptosis. Endocrine therapies were the first "targeted therapies" (Table 238-8).

STOPPING PALLIATIVE ANTICANCER TREATMENT

First-line palliative chemotherapy provides superior survival, symptom control, and quality of life over "best supportive care" in numerous malignancies.[17] Such benefits have also been demonstrated for second-line palliative chemotherapy in some common cancers, including non–small cell lung cancer, colon cancer, and breast cancer. New antitumor agents with less toxicity and the availabil-

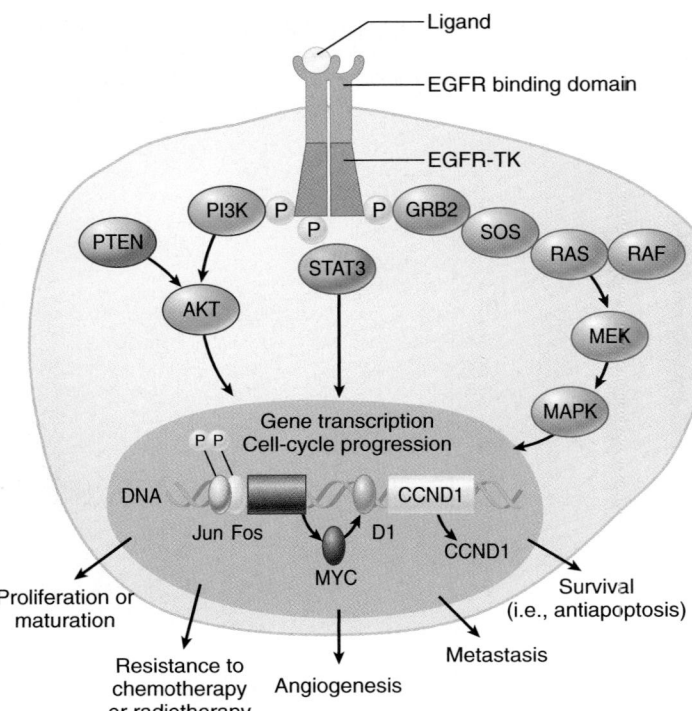

FIGURE 238-3 Epidermal growth factor receptor (EGFR) signal transduction and its biological consequences. GRB2, growth factor receptor bound protein 2; MAPK, mitogen-activated protein kinase; MEK, MAPK kinase; P, phosphorylation; PI3K, phosphatidylinositol 3'-kinase; PTEN, phosphatidylinositol-3,4,5-triphosphate3-phosphatase; SOS, son of sevenless; STAT3, signal transducer and activator of transcription 3; TK, tyrosine kinase.

ity of more effective antiemetic agents allow better management of side effects and make active anticancer treatment more acceptable. Discontinuation of treatment should be considered if there is no symptom relief, significant toxicity develops, or disease progression is noted. Patient-rated health-related quality-of-life measurements are increasingly being used as an end point in clinical trials to supplement toxicity and survival information. Many patients consider quality of life more important than survival, and clinical trial information on health-related quality of life should be discussed with patients when treatment decisions are made.

CONCLUSIONS

There have been numerous recent advances in cancer treatment. Although cytotoxic chemotherapy and endocrine therapy will play important roles in cancer management, current new drug development is focused more on targeted therapy. Ongoing research is defining the precise molecular mechanisms behind cancer development, growth, and metastasis to identify better targets for treatment. A further challenge is to identify the most effective

way of using these therapies because the high cost of new drugs places enormous economic burden on health systems worldwide. Current research is also focused on molecular predictors of treatment response to guide selection of treatment and offer individualized therapy.

REFERENCES

1. Love RR, Philips J. Oophorectomy for breast cancer: History revisited. J Natl Cancer Inst 2002;94:1433-1434.
2. Kaminski MS, Zelenetz AD, Press OW, et al. Pivotal study of iodine I 131 tositumomab for chemotherapy-refractory low-grade or transformed low-grade B-cell non-Hodgkin's lymphomas. J Clin Oncol 2001;19:3918-3928.
3. Witzig TE, Molina A, Gordon LI, et al. Long-term responses in patients with recurring or refractory B-cell non-Hodgkin lymphoma treated with yttrium 90 ibritumomab tiuxetan. Cancer 2007;109:1804-1810.
4. Hurwitz H, Fehrenbacher L, Novotny W, et al. Bevacizumab plus irinotecan, fluorouracil, and leucovorin for metastatic colorectal cancer. N Engl J Med 2004;350:2335-2342.
5. Cunningham D, Humblet Y, Siena S, et al. Cetuximab monotherapy and cetuximab plus irinotecan in irinotecan-refractory metastatic colorectal cancer. N Engl J Med 2004;351:337-345.
6. Bonner JA, Harari PM, Giralt J, et al. Radiotherapy plus cetuximab for squamous-cell carcinoma of the head and neck. N Engl J Med 2006;354:567-578.
7. Baselga J, Trigo JM, Bourhis J, et al. Phase II multicenter study of the antiepidermal growth factor receptor monoclonal antibody cetuximab in combination with platinum-based chemotherapy in patients with platinum-refractory metastatic and/or recurrent squamous cell carcinoma of the head and neck. J Clin Oncol 2005;23:5568-5577.
8. O'Brien SG, Guilhot F, Larsen RA, et al. Imatinib compared with interferon and low-dose cytarabine for newly diagnosed chronic-phase chronic myeloid leukemia. N Engl J Med 2003;348:994-1004.
9. Demetri GD, von Mehren M, Blanke CD, et al. Efficacy and safety of imatinib mesylate in advanced gastrointestinal stromal tumors. N Engl J Med 2002; 347:472-480.
10. Richardson PG, Sonneveld P, Schuster MW, et al. Bortezomib or high-dose dexamethasone for relapsed multiple myeloma. N Engl J Med 2005;352: 2487-2498.
11. Shepherd FA, Rodrigues Pereira J, Ciuleanu T, et al. Erlotinib in previously treated non–small-cell lung cancer. N Engl J Med 2005;353:123-132.
12. Motzer RJ, Hutson TE, Tomczak P, et al. Sunitinib versus interferon alfa in metastatic renal-cell carcinoma. N Engl J Med 2007;356:115-124.
13. Escudier B, Sczcylik C, Eisen T. Randomized phase III trial of the Raf kinase and VEGFR inhibitor sorafenbib (BAY 43-9006) in patients with advanced renal cell carcinoma (RCC) [abstract 4510]. J Clin Oncol 2005;23(Suppl):1093s.
14. Hudes G, Carducci M, Tomczak M. A phase III, randomized, 3-arm study of temsirolimus (TEMSR) or interferon-alpha (IFN) or the combination of TEMSR and IFN in the treatment of poor-risk patients with advanced renal cell carcinoma (adv RCC) [abstract LBA4]. J Clin Oncol 2006;24(Suppl):930s.
15. Geyer CE, Forster J, Lindquist D, et al. Lapatinib plus capecitabine for HER2-positive advanced breast cancer. N Engl J Med 2006;355:2733-2743.
16. Klijn JG, Beex LV, Mmauriac L, et al. Combined treatment with buserelin and tamoxifen in premenopausal metastatic breast cancer: A randomized study. J Natl Cancer Inst 2000;92:903-911.
17. Archer VR, Billingham IJ, Cullen MH. Palliative chemotherapy: No longer a contradiction in terms. Oncologist 1999;4:470-477.

SUGGESTED READING

Bianco R, Melisi D, Ciardiello F, Tortora G. Key cancer cell signal transduction pathways as therapeutic targets. Eur J Cancer 2006;42:290-294.
Chabner B, Longo D (eds). Cancer Chemotherapy & Biotherapy—Principles and Practice. Philadelphia: Lippincott Williams & Wilkins, 2006.
Devita V, Hellman S, Rosenberg S (eds). Cancer: Principles & Practice of Oncology. Philadelphia: Lippincott Williams & Wilkins, 2005.
Gralow JR. Optimizing the treatment of metastatic breast cancer. Breast Cancer Res Treat 2005;89(Suppl 1):S9-S15.
Krause DS, Van Etten RA. Tyrosine kinases as targets for cancer therapy. N Engl J Med 2005;353:172-187.

CHAPTER **239**

Complications of Chemotherapy

Karin Peschardt, Per Dombernowsky, and Jørn Herrstedt

Defining palliative chemotherapy is difficult. In some cases, first-line chemotherapy is given with palliative intent (e.g., advanced lung cancer), whereas in others, chemotherapy is almost always curative (e.g., testicular seminoma). In many other solid tumors, first-line chemotherapy is given with curative intent. When recurrence is diagnosed, second-line chemotherapy can prolong and increase quality of life but in most cases is unable to cure. Some live with their cancer for many years (e.g., breast cancer and prostate cancer) and undergo multiple chemotherapy or endocrine regimens (or both). Many patients have good performance status for years, and we consider them as having chronic disease.

Basic science is fundamental for the development of supportive care drugs. Many contributions to our understanding of pathophysiology in humans have come from the preclinical development of supportive care drugs, including the development of different growth factors for anemia, neutropenia, and mucositis, as well as different antiemetics. In this chapter we discuss some of the acute, subacute, and late toxicities but do not deal with complications that appear years after chemotherapy (e.g., secondary leukemia).

ALOPECIA

The most severe complications, from a patient's viewpoint, are nausea, vomiting, and hair loss.[1] Hair loss is primarily scored as a severe complication by women. Drugs such as the anthracyclines, paclitaxel, and etoposide make most people bald after one course of chemotherapy. The only successful preventive method is scalp cooling, which in six of seven randomized studies afforded significantly better hair preservation than seen in controls.[2]

GASTROINTESTINAL COMPLICATIONS

Cancer chemotherapy primarily affects cells with rapid turnover, including many cancers, but also normal cells such as epithelial cells in the gastrointestinal tract. Consequently, many complications from chemotherapy arise in the gastrointestinal tract. Such complications include mucositis, nausea, vomiting, and diarrhea.

Mucositis

Oral mucositis (see Chapters 171 and 232) develops in 10% to 40% of patients receiving conventional-dose chemotherapy (Fig. 239-1). In people irradiated for head and neck cancer, it is observed in around 90%, and with high-dose chemotherapy almost all suffer. Ulcerative mucositis is painful and a risk for systemic infection, particularly when combined with neutropenia. The pathogenesis of oral and gastrointestinal mucositis has been described in detail.[3]

Guidelines[4] for prevention of mucositis have recently been updated.[5] The most important update (Table 239-1) was based on a randomized double-blind trial[6] demonstrating prophylactic use of the recombinant human keratinocyte growth factor palifermin in patients with hematological malignant diseases undergoing fractionated whole-body irradiation and autologous stem cell transplantation.

Chemotherapy-Induced Nausea and Vomiting

Patients consider nausea and vomiting the most troublesome side effects. In particular, nausea continues to be a problem. The risk of nausea and vomiting developing depends on the chemotherapy regimen and the antiemetic

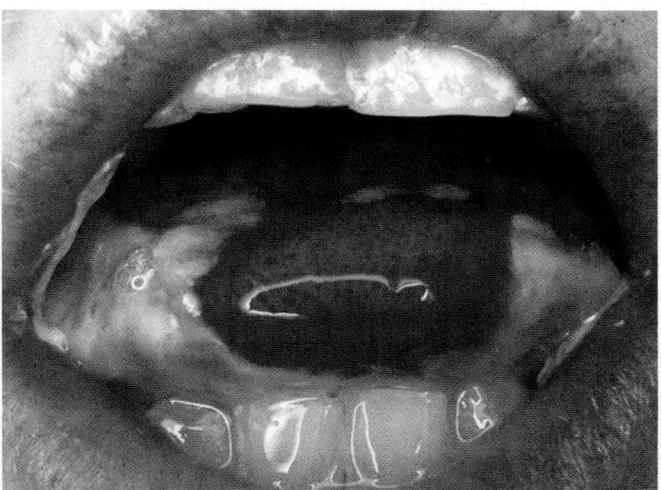

FIGURE 239-1   Patient with chemotherapy-induced oral mucositis.

TABLE 239-1 Summary of Evidence-Based Clinical Practice Guidelines* for Care of Patients with Oral and Gastrointestinal Mucositis

ORAL MUCOSITIS

Standard-Dose Chemotherapy—Prevention

The panel recommends that patients receiving bolus 5-fluorouracil (5-FU) chemotherapy undergo 30 minutes of oral cryotherapy to prevent oral mucositis.

The panel suggests that 20 to 30 minutes of oral cryotherapy be used in an attempt to decrease mucositis in patients treated with bolus doses of edatrexate.

Standard-Dose Chemotherapy—Treatment

No positive evidence-based recommendations are given.

High-Dose Chemotherapy with or without Total Body Irradiation Plus Hematopoietic Stem Cell Transplantation—Prevention

In patients with hematological malignancies receiving high-dose chemotherapy and total body irradiation with autologous stem cell transplantation, the panel recommends the use of keratinocyte growth factor-1 (palifermin) in a dose of 60 µg/kg/day for 3 days before conditioning treatment and for 3 days after transplantation for the prevention of oral mucositis.

The panel suggests the use of cryotherapy to prevent oral mucositis in patients receiving high-dose melphalan.

Low-level laser therapy (LLLT) requires expensive equipment and specialized training. Because of interoperator variability, clinical trials are difficult to conduct, and their results are difficult to compare; nevertheless, the panel is encouraged by the accumulating evidence in support of LLLT. The panel suggests that for centers able to support the necessary technology and training, LLLT be used in an attempt to reduce the incidence of oral mucositis and its associated pain in patients receiving high-dose chemotherapy or chemoradiotherapy before hematopoietic stem cell transplantation.

GASTROINTESTINAL MUCOSITIS

Standard-Dose and High-Dose Chemotherapy—Prevention

The panel recommends either ranitidine or omeprazole for the prevention of epigastric pain after treatment with cyclophosphamide, methotrexate, and 5-FU or treatment with 5-FU with or without folinic acid chemotherapy.

Standard-Dose and High-Dose Chemotherapy—Treatment

When loperamide fails to control diarrhea induced by standard-dose or high-dose chemotherapy associated with hematopoietic stem cell therapy, the panel recommends octreotide at a dose of at least 100 µg subcutaneously twice daily.

Combined Chemotherapy and Radiation Therapy—Prevention

The panel suggests that amifostine be used to reduce esophagitis induced by concomitant chemotherapy and radiotherapy in patients with non–small cell lung cancer.

*The original update of the Multinational Association for Supportive Care in Cancer/International Society of Oral Oncology (MASCC/ISOO) study group for mucositis also includes recommendations for foundations of care and radiotherapy-induced mucositis, as well as a large number of "negative" recommendations for chemotherapy-induced mucositis. These are not included in this table.

Adapted from Rubenstein EB, Peterson DE, Schubert M, et al. Clinical practice guidelines for the prevention and treatment of therapy-induced oral and gastrointestinal mucositis. Cancer 2004;100(Suppl 9):2026-2046; Keefe DM, Schubert M, Elting LS, et al. Updated clinical practice guidelines for the prevention and treatment of mucositis. Cancer 2007;109:820-831; and www.mascc.org.

prophylaxis used (see Chapters 144 and 169). Several patient-related risk factors have been identified, such as female gender, young age, previous chemotherapy with emesis, a history of motion sickness, and emesis during pregnancy. High chronic alcohol intake seems to be protective.

Antiemetics include dopamine (D_2) receptor antagonists (metoclopramide, prochlorperazine, haloperidol, metopimazine, domperidone), corticosteroids (dexamethasone, prednisolone), serotonin (5-hydroxytryptamine [5-HT_3]) receptor antagonists (ondansetron, granisetron, dolasetron, tropisetron, palonosetron), and neurokinin (NK_1) receptor antagonists (aprepitant).

Benzodiazepines have no significant effect in preventing acute or delayed emesis but are useful in some patients for anticipatory nausea and vomiting. The combination of a 5-HT_3 receptor antagonist and a corticosteroid was, until 2004, the recommended antiemetic prophylaxis for prevention of acute nausea and vomiting in patients receiving moderately or highly emetogenic chemotherapy. The NK_1 receptor antagonist aprepitant increases the effect of the aforementioned two-drug regimen with cisplatin-based chemotherapy. A single study in 866 patients showed that this effect is also observed in women with breast cancer treated with a combination of cyclophosphamide and an anthracycline.

Recommendations[7-9] depend on the emetic potential of the chemotherapy and distinguish between chemother-

apy with high (>90%), moderate (30% to 90%), low (10% to 30%), and minimal (<10%) emetic potential (Tables 239-2 and 239-3).

The 5-HT_3 and NK_1 receptor antagonists are only moderately effective in preventing nausea. Olanzapine, an antipsychotic agent, has recently demonstrated promising effects against both nausea and vomiting when added to the long-acting 5-HT_3 receptor antagonist palonosetron and dexamethasone.[10]

Chemotherapy-Induced Diarrhea

Diarrhea is most frequently caused by agents such as the fluoropyrimidines (5-fluorouracil), camptothecines (irinotecan), taxanes, and cytarabine (see Chapter 154). Other causes, including infection, food (e.g., milk, spicy food, alcohol, coffee), drugs (antibiotics, prokinetics, laxatives), and co-morbidity (e.g., inflammatory bowel disease), should be considered before treatment. 5-Fluorouracil and irinotecan cause diarrhea through different mechanisms, and therefore a combination of the two, used for colon cancer, can cause severe and sometimes life-threatening diarrhea, especially with concomitant febrile neutropenia.[11,12]

Grading of severity is difficult, and present grading scales primarily include the frequency of diarrhea but not the volume and duration. Evidence-based recommendations are therefore difficult and limited to a small number

TABLE 239-2 Emetic Risk Potential of Drugs

Minimal risk potential (<10%)	Bleomycin
	Vincristine
	Vinorelbine
	Bevacizumab
	Methotrexate (oral)
	Hydroxyurea (oral)
	Gefitinib (oral)
Low risk potential (10-30%)	Paclitaxel
	Docetaxel
	Etoposide
	Mitoxantrone
	5-Fluorouracil
	Gemcitabine
	Doxil
	Mitomycin
	Methotrexate
	Topotecan
	Pemetrexed
	Bortezomib
	Cetuximab
	Trastuzumab
	Capecitabine (oral)
Moderate risk potential (30-90%)	Cyclophosphamide (<1500 mg/m²)
	Doxorubicin
	Epirubicin
	Ifosfamide
	Carboplatin
	Irinotecan
	Cytarabine (>1 g/m²)
	Oxaliplatin
	Temozolamide (oral)
	Imatinib (oral)
	Vinorelbine (oral)
High risk potential (>90%)	Streptozocin
	Dacarbazine
	Cyclophosphamide (≥1500 mg/m²)
	Cisplatin

Modified from The Antiemetic Subcommittee of the Multinational Association of Supportive Care in Cancer (MASCC). Prevention of chemotherapy- and radiotherapy-induced emesis: Results of the 2004 Perugia International Antiemetic Consensus Conference. Ann Oncol 2006;17:20-28.

TABLE 239-3 Prophylaxis for Chemotherapy-Induced Nausea and Vomiting

EMETIC RISK GROUP	ANTIEMETICS
PROPHYLAXIS FOR ACUTE NAUSEA AND VOMITING	
High	Serotonin antagonist + dexamethasone + aprepitant
Anthracycline + cyclophosphamide (AC)	Serotonin antagonist + dexamethasone + aprepitant
Moderate (other than AC)	Serotonin antagonist + dexamethasone
Low	Dexamethasone
Minimal	No routine prophylaxis
PROPHYLAXIS FOR DELAYED NAUSEA AND VOMITING	
High	Dexamethasone + aprepitant
Anthracycline + cyclophosphamide (AC)	Aprepitant or dexamethasone
Moderate (other than AC)	Dexamethasone. A serotonin antagonist may be used as an alternative
Low	No routine prophylaxis
Minimal	No routine prophylaxis

Modified from The Antiemetic Subcommittee of the Multinational Association of Supportive Care in Cancer (MASCC). Prevention of chemotherapy- and radiotherapy-induced emesis: Results of the 2004 Perugia International Antiemetic Consensus Conference. Ann Oncol 2006;17:20-28.

of drugs (Table 239-4), such as loperamide and octreotide, in a few small trials.[11]

HEMATOLOGICAL COMPLICATIONS

Chemotherapy-induced bone marrow toxicity is most pronounced 8 to 14 days after therapy (nadir). The nitrosoureas, however, induce a delayed nadir that appears after 3 to 6 weeks. The onset and recovery of granulocytopenia, thrombocytopenia, and anemia can be predicted from the lifetime of the cells. Granulocytes live less than a day, platelets approximately 10 days, and red blood cells, in cancer patients, around 90 to 100 days. Consequently, granulocytopenia usually precedes thrombocytopenia (as does its recovery). Chemotherapy-induced anemia is rare during the first one to two courses of treatment.

Febrile Neutropenia

A granulocyte count of less than 1.0×10^9/L constitutes a significant risk for infection, and continuously decreasing values can result in a rapid and lethal course. Patients with febrile neutropenia (temperature >38.0° C and granulo-cyte count <0.5×10^9/L) should undergo a physical examination, routine blood tests, chest radiograph, and blood and urine cultures. The results of such analysis will disclose the reason for the fever and infection in less than a third of cases. Rapid administration of empirical broad-spectrum antibiotics covering both gram-negative and gram-positive bacteria is indicated and then modified according to blood culture results. In patients with solid tumors, 95% of verified infections are caused by bacteria, whereas in hematological patients, viruses and fungi should also be considered (Table 239-5).

The latest development includes oral antibiotics for low-risk patients in an outpatient setting. Risk indices defining low-risk patients are available.[13] Guidelines recommend that patients with a 20% or higher risk of febrile neutropenia receive prophylactic granulocyte colony-stimulating factor (G-CSF).[14,15] In lower-risk (10% to 20%) patients, factors such as age (>65 years), advanced-stage disease, and previous febrile neutropenia should prompt prophylactic treatment.[15] Prophylactic use of CSF is most important when dose intensity and dose density are important for survival.[15] For others, such as those receiving palliative chemotherapy, less hematotoxic chemotherapy could be considered.

Antibiotic prophylaxis in patients at high risk for febrile neutropenia is controversial. Current guidelines do not recommend its use because of antibacterial resistance and lack of survival benefit. Two large studies, one involving solid tumors or lymphomas ($N = 1565$) and the other involving acute leukemia ($N = 760$), demonstrated a significant reduction in all infection-related events in patients randomized to prophylactic treatment with a fluoroquinolone versus placebo.[16]

TABLE 239-4   Management of Chemotherapy-Induced Diarrhea

Assessment of symptoms	Grade the severity of diarrhea with Common Toxicity Criteria. Notice the duration and volume of diarrhea, fever, and dehydration
Co-morbidity	Poor performance status (PS), inflammatory bowel disease
Other causes	Consider other causes such as infection, food, and medications
Laboratory analysis	White blood cells, granulocytes, electrolytes, C-reactive protein. In the case of fever or neutropenia (or both), obtain cultures from urine, blood (including central catheters), and if indicated, feces
Treatment of uncomplicated cases (grade 1-2, PS 1-2, no dehydration/fever/neutropenia)	Loperamide up to 16 mg/24 hr.* If not resolved within 24 hours (still uncomplicated), increase the dose of loperamide to 2 mg every 2 hours and consider antibiotics. If not resolved within 48 hours (still uncomplicated), discontinue loperamide, start octreotide, and consider antibiotics
Treatment of unresolved uncomplicated or complicated cases	Discontinue chemotherapy and start intravenous fluids, antibiotics, and octreotide.

*Patients with diarrhea induced by a combination of 5-fluorouracil and irinotecan should always start treatment with high-dose loperamide (2 mg every 2 hours) directly and receive antibiotics if unresolved after 24 hours.

TABLE 239-5   Development of Empirical Antibiotic Prophylaxis in Patients with Febrile Neutropenia

1966	Risk dependent on duration and severity of febrile neutropenia
1970s	2-3 antibiotics needed for optimal prophylaxis
1980s	A cephalosporin (ceftazidime) equals the efficacy of 2-3 antibiotics
1990s	Definition of low-risk patients by the development of risk indexes. An oral antibiotic regimen can replace an intravenous regimen in low-risk patients
2000+	Validation and fine-tuning of risk indexes. Oral therapy on an outpatient basis in low-risk patients

Anemia

Chronic anemia is a problem in 30% to 50% of cancer patients. Bleeding, hemolysis, and dyshematopoiesis are the main causes, with malnutrition, infection, inflammation, radiotherapy, and chemotherapy being additional factors. Anemia can cause symptoms from nearly all organs, including fatigue, dyspnea, tachycardia, cardiac decompensation, reduced skin perfusion, fluid retention, and immune deficiency. Anemia induced by cancer is often corrected if the disease responds to therapy.

In a study of 14,520 cancer patients, 51% of those receiving chemotherapy had anemia and a hemoglobin level of less than 12 g/dL, whereas 32% of those who did not receive cancer treatment were anemic.[17] Anemia correlated with poor performance status and was treated in 39%. The mean hemoglobin level at which treatment of anemia was initiated was 9.7 g/dL, with 17% receiving epoetin, 15% transfusions, and 7% iron.[17]

TABLE 239-6   Most Important EORTC Recommendations for the Use of EPO in Anemic Patients Receiving Chemotherapy (2006 Update)

Patients whose Hb level is below 9 g/dL should be evaluated for the need for transfusions in addition to EPO.

In cancer patients receiving chemotherapy, treatment with EPO should be initiated at an Hb level of 9-11 g/dL based on anemia-related symptoms.

The target Hb concentration should not exceed 12 g/dL.

Elderly patients experience the same benefits from treatment with EPO as younger patients.

EPO may be considered in selected asymptomatic, anemic cancer patients with an Hb level <11.9 g/dL to prevent a further decline in Hb, according to individual factors (e.g., type/intensity of chemotherapy, baseline Hb) and the duration and type of further planned treatment.

Prophylactic use of EPO to prevent anemia in patients undergoing chemotherapy who have normal Hb values at the start of treatment is not recommended.

There is no evidence of increased response to EPO with the addition of oral iron supplementation. There is evidence of improved response to EPO with intravenous iron supplementation.

EORTC no longer recommends EPO for radiotherapy-induced anemia. The EORTC recommendations include a large number of "negative" recommendations. These are not included in this table.
EORTC, European Organization for Research and Treatment of Cancer; EPO, erythropoietic proteins (erythropoietin); Hb, hemoglobin.
From Bokemeyer C, Aapro MS, Courdi A, et al. EORTC guidelines for the use of erythropoietic proteins in anemic patients with cancer. Eur J Cancer 2004;40:2201-16; Bokemeyer C, Aapro MS, Courdi A, et al. EORTC guidelines for the use of erythropoietic proteins in anemic patients with cancer: 2006 update. Eur J Cancer 2007;43:258-70; and www.cancerworld.org go to SIOG.

Red blood cell transfusions have been the treatment of choice, but recombinant human erythropoietin (EPO) makes it possible to provide long-term correction of anemia.[18] Evidence-based guidelines have been published.[18,19] EPO can increase hemoglobin values, reduce the need for transfusions, and improve quality of life. Hemoglobin response rates between 28% and 75% have been reported.[19] There are no major differences in hemoglobin response between the three commercially available agents, although dose schedules differ. Darbepoietin, having the longest half-life, needs to be administered only three times per week (Table 239-6).

EPO is well tolerated, with hypertension and thromboembolic events being the most frequent adverse effects. Updated guidelines of European Organization for Research and Treatment of Cancer (EORTC) have recently been published.[20] It is debatable whether EPO has a positive or negative effect on survival when administered concomitantly with chemotherapy or radiotherapy. It is important that EPO be used only according to guidelines.[20]

Thrombocytopenia

No platelet-stimulating growth factor has yet been marketed. Current recommendations for platelet transfusions are supported by limited evidence.[21] In active bleeding, they are recommended if the platelet count is below 50 × 10⁹/L. Prophylactic transfusions are recommended in acute leukemia with a platelet count of 20 to 30 × 10⁹/L. In solid tumors, prophylactic transfusions are recommended for platelet counts below 10 × 10⁹/L (or 20 ×

10^9/L with bladder cancer or large necrotic tumors). For invasive procedures, a platelet count of 40 to 50 × 10^9/L is recommended, but minor procedures such as bone marrow aspiration can be performed with a count of 20 × 10^9/L or lower.[21]

PULMONARY TOXICITY

Pulmonary toxicity develops in less than 10% of all patients receiving established antineoplastic agents. The diagnosis depends on a history of drug exposure and exclusion of other causes such as infection, pulmonary bleeding, fluid overload, lung metastases, and concomitant cardiovascular disease.[22] *Early-onset pulmonary toxicity* (within 2 months) includes primarily interstitial pneumonitis; however, acute hypersensitivity reactions, acute noncardiogenic pulmonary edema, bronchospasm, and rarely, pleural effusions (see Case Study) and adult respiratory distress syndrome are also observed (see Chapter 73).

The drugs most frequently causing interstitial pneumonitis are bleomycin and gemcitabine. Other drugs such as methotrexate, mitomycin C, cyclophosphamide, nitrosamines, gefitinib, irinotecan, and the podophyllotoxins may also result in interstitial pneumonitis, but with low frequency. The incidence is 3% to 5% with bleomycin doses up to 250 mg/m² and rises to 20% with doses greater than 500 mg/m². Other risk factors include older age, a history of smoking, combination chemotherapy, and thoracic radiotherapy. Severity varies greatly. The condition is usually reversible but can progress to irreversible pulmonary fibrosis.

For bleomycin, the main risk factor is the cumulative dose, whereas gemcitabine-induced lung toxicity is not dose dependent. During bleomycin treatment it is recommended that regular pulmonary function testing be performed and doses adjusted accordingly. A 25% decrease in carbon monoxide diffusion capacity is an indication for withdrawal of bleomycin therapy. It is also recommended that exposure to CSF and inhalation of greater than 30% oxygen be avoided. No drug prevents chemotherapy-induced pulmonary toxicity. Management primarily includes discontinuation of the drug. High-dose steroids and diuretics can be useful in some patients.

Late-onset chemotherapy-induced lung injury (after more than 2 months) is mainly due to pulmonary fibrosis, with bleomycin, busulfan, carmustine, and mitomycin causing the highest incidence. Monoclonal antibodies and small-molecule therapeutic agents such as interleukin-2 and imatinib may cause varying degrees of acute and late pulmonary toxicity.

CASE STUDY

A 65-year-old women has small cell lung cancer complicated by pleural effusion. She is receiving three-drug combination chemotherapy, and severe grade 4 neutropenia and sepsis develop.

Comment: It is well known that malignant effusions increase the risk for adverse effects from chemotherapy, including bone marrow toxicity. The reason is that malignant effusions act as third compartments, thereby increasing the time that normal tissue is exposed to chemotherapy. Large effusions should therefore be drained before initiation of chemotherapy.

CARDIOTOXICITY

Cardiotoxicity is a rare but severe complication. Most important is congestive heart failure (CHF) from anthracyclines. Other complications include ischemic heart disease, pericarditis, cardiac arrhythmias, and hypotension or hypertension. The side effects can be acute or late and are sometimes irreversible.[23] The incidence and severity depend not only on the drugs used but also on the dose, schedule, and cumulative dose; patient factors such as older age and previous cardiac disease; and combination with other antineoplastic drugs or thoracic radiotherapy.

Congestive Heart Failure

Anthracycline-induced cardiomyopathy generally occurs within months after treatment, but sometimes years. The recommended maximum cumulative dose for doxorubicin is 450 to 500 mg/m² and that for epirubicin is 850-900 mg/m². Proposals for prevention and early detection of left ventricular (LV) dysfunction have been made (see Chapter 72). Measurement of LV ejection fraction by multiple-gated acquisition (MUGA) scanning or echocardiography is advocated, although their sensitivity for early detection of CHF is low.[24] Cardiac biopsy is the most sensitive and specific modality, but the invasive nature of the procedure limits its use. Dexrazoxane has shown some protection during treatment with anthracyclines by chelating iron and thereby preventing the formation of anthracycline-iron complexes.

Management of anthracycline-induced CHF consists of discontinuation of the drug and administration of diuretics, β-blockers, and angiotensin-converting enzyme inhibitors. In rare cases a heart transplant is necessary. Reexposure to the drug is not recommended.[23]

Trastuzumab can cause LV dysfunction and CHF.[25] Cardiac biopsies have been nonpathological, and there is no correlation with the accumulated dose. Trastuzumab may interrupt signaling pathways in myocardial cells. Combination or former treatment with anthracyclines often increases the risk.

Other Cardiovascular Complications

Damage to the coronary arteries or vasospastic effects can result in myocardial ischemia and infarction. Infusion of 5-fluoruracil can provoke an acute ischemic syndrome varying from angina pectoris to acute myocardial infarction. It is normally reversible when treatment is discontinued and relevant therapy instituted. Cardiac arrhythmias can develop from myocardial damage or indirectly as a result of anemia or electrolyte imbalance. Paclitaxel and anthracyclines may cause acute and often reversible arrhythmias during infusion.[23]

NEPHROTOXICITY

The kidneys are the elimination pathway for many chemotherapeutic agents and their metabolites and are therefore sensitive to injury. Depending on the drugs involved, the glomeruli tubules or vascular structure might be at risk varying from asymptomatic elevation of serum creatinine to acute renal failure requiring dialysis (see Chapter

82).[26,27] The doses of a number of oncology drugs are based on renal function. Caution is necessary, and renal function testing before and during treatment is recommended. Nephrotoxicity may be further aggravated by older age, hypertension, cardiac disease, diabetes, and other nephrotoxic drugs. Most frequently, nephrotoxicity is observed with platinum analogues, methotrexate, and alkylating agents.

Cisplatin-induced renal toxicity is dose related, cumulative, and manifested primarily as a decreased glomerular filtration rate (GFR). Single drug doses below 50 mg/m^2 usually result in minor or no renal damage. Higher doses or repeated daily dosing require hydration with isotonic saline and mannitol to enhance urinary output. Pathological lesions are primarily seen in the tubules, but the collecting ducts are often affected by hyponatremia and hypomagnesemia.

Carboplatin has limited nephrotoxicity when dosing is based on the GFR, and the main side effects are hematological and neurological. Oxaliplatin, a newer platinum analogue with high activity in gastrointestinal cancers, has no significant renal toxicity.

Methotrexate has no or very limited renal toxicity in conventional doses. With high-dose methotrexate plus folinic acid, renal toxicity may develop. This can be prevented by hydration and urine alkalinization, which hinder precipitation of methotrexate and its metabolites in the tubules.

Cyclophosphamide does not induce nephrotoxicity, whereas ifosfamide may produce severe renal damage. At equivalent doses, the level of the nephrotoxic metabolite chloroacetaldehyde is 40 times higher with ifosfamide. Mild to severe nephropathy develops in 5% to 30% of patients treated with ifosfamide.

NEUROTOXICITY

The nervous system can be affected by cytostatic agents through different mechanisms, and it may be difficult to differentiate such neurotoxicity from neurological manifestations of the cancer and other concomitant diseases.

Peripheral Neuropathy

Peripheral neuropathy (PNP) can be induced by several chemotherapeutic drugs, including platinum analogues, taxanes, and vinca alkaloids. The dominant symptoms are sensory, with tingling and numbness starting in the fingertips and toes and gradually spreading in a glove-and-stocking distribution. The inner ear can be damaged and often results in irreversible bilateral hearing loss or tinnitus. The motor system is rarely affected. Autonomic nervous system damage can result in constipation and colicky pain. Oxaliplatin frequently provokes muscle cramps resembling Raynaud's phenomenon and pharyngeal-laryngeal dysesthesias, which can be triggered by touching cold surfaces or drinking cold liquids.[28]

Previous or concomitant treatment with another neurotoxic drug is a risk factor. Residual PNP after first-line treatment must be considered but does not completely contraindicate treatment with other neurotoxic drugs. Coexisting neurological disease or PNP caused by alcohol or diabetes is not a contraindication to treatment.

For the platinum analogues and taxanes, PNP is often reversible, although recovery may take months to years, whereas the vinca alkaloids can provoke irreversible PNP.[29,30]

To prevent irreversible PNP, close monitoring is important, including neurological examination and frequent questioning about symptoms. If PNP reaches a certain limit, the drug should be discontinued, administered less frequently, or given in lower doses per treatment course.[31]

Different chemoprotective agents have been evaluated. The adrenocorticotropic hormone ACTH(1-9) analogue ORG2766 was effective against cisplatin-provoked PNP, but this has been questioned.[28]

Central Neurotoxicity

Ifosfamide can induce encephalopathy with symptoms ranging from dazed and light depressive periods to hallucinations, stupor, and coma. The symptoms develop during infusion or immediately after the first or second administration and disappear a few days after drug cessation. Retreatment is possible, depending on the level of side effects and the necessity of using ifosfamide. Prevention includes infusion of ifosfamide over a period of days. Metabolites such as chlorethylamine are thought to be responsible for the encephalopathy. Methylene blue, an antidote to chlorethylamine, is often used to treat ifosfamide-induced encephalopathy.

Other chemotherapeutic agents that can cause central nervous system damage include vinca alkaloids, methotrexate (high dose or administered intrathecally), and 5-fluorouracil, the latter inducing an acute reversible cerebellar syndrome consisting of slurred speech, ataxia, dizziness, and nystagmus.[29]

EXTRAVASATION

When accidental extravasation of chemotherapeutic agents occurs, a tissue reaction varying from skin irritation to necrosis of skin, connective tissue, and muscle fascia may arise.[32] Its incidence is 0.5% to 1.0%, with only a minority of cases being severe. Different drugs can cause varying damage to subcutaneous tissue, and symptoms range from pain and localized inflammation to blisters and full-thickness necrosis requiring surgical revision. The symptoms usually develop within minutes or hours and may escalate during the following weeks and months.

Based on tissue reactions, drugs are divided into three groups:

1. Vesicant (ulcerogenic) drugs causing blisters, ulcers, tissue destruction, or necrosis include anthracyclines, vinca alkaloids, dactinomycin, menogaril, mitoxantrone, and taxanes.
2. Irritant drugs causing localized pain, inflammation, or rarely, soft tissue ulcers, if large amounts are infused, include carboplatin, cisplatin, oxaliplatin, cyclophosphamide, ifosfamide, carmustine, etoposide, irinotecan, melphalan, pentostatin, streptozocin, and topotecan.
3. Nonvesicant drugs rarely causing inflammatory or necrotic reactions include methotrexate, bleomycin, fluorouracil, and gemcitabine.

TABLE 239-7 Management of Extravasation of Cytostatics

1. Stop the infusion as soon as extravasation is suspected.
2. Attempt aspiration.
3. Maintain the intravenous line initially for potential infusion of antidote. Infuse intravenously or subcutaneously (or both) around the site of the extravasation within 1 hour after occurrence and possibly repeat later.
4. Repeatedly apply local cooling (ice packs) for anthracyclines and local heating (dry heat) for vinca alkaloids.
5. Blisters and ulcers are treated with analgesics and symptomatic wound care. Plastic surgery is sometimes necessary.
6. Documentation, including photographs, is useful in follow-up.

Future Considerations

The focus on pharmacokinetics and pharmacodynamics of anti-cancer agents has led to increased interest in prediction of drug toxicity based on pharmacogenetics. Interindividual differences in toxicity can be explained by genetic variations in drug-metabolizing enzymes such as cytochrome P-450 (CYP450). These variations can lead to a reduced response (ultrarapid metabolizers) or increased toxicity (poor metabolizers) and also include potential interactions between anticancer and supportive care drugs (see Chapter 243).

The antiemetics tropisetron and ondansetron are primarily metabolized through the CYP2D6 enzyme system. In a recent trial, patients were genotyped for CYP2D6 before chemotherapy and received antiemetic treatment with tropisetron or ondansetron. Poor metabolizers had higher serum concentrations of tropisetron and ultrarapid metabolizers experienced more vomiting.[35] In ultrarapid metabolizers of CYP2D6, antiemetic therapy could be optimized by an antiemetic metabolized by another enzyme system, such as granisetron, which is metabolized via CYP3A4.

Another example of the importance of genetic variation is in patients treated with irinotecan.[36] Irinotecan is a prodrug that is metabolized to the active metabolite SN-38. UDP-glucoronosyltransferase 1A1 (UGT1A1) catalyzes the glucuronidation of SN-38. UGT1A1 variants were genotyped in patients receiving irinotecan. The UGT1A1 genotype was strongly associated with severe neutropenia. Such findings will probably enable physicians to design individualized supportive care programs based on prechemotherapy genetic analysis.

The anthracyclines bind directly to the nucleic acids in DNA and cause endocytolysis. After killing cells, the drug is absorbed into neighboring cells, which results in progressive tissue damage lasting weeks to months without intervention. Other drugs that do not bind to DNA, such as vinca alkaloids, etoposide, and taxanes, are metabolized in the tissue and therefore cause less extensive tissue damage.

Guidelines for the management of many drugs are empirical (Table 239-7). Dexrazoxane, an inhibitor of the enzyme topoisomerase II, the target of anthracyclines, is effective in managing extravasation of anthracyclines. When dexrazoxane has been infused after extravasation, surgical intervention was avoided in 98% of cases, and sequelae, including mild pain and sensory disturbances, were infrequent.[33,34] Traditionally, the antidote dimethyl sulfoxide (DMSO) was used for the extravasation of anth-racyclines, sodium thiosulfate for cisplatin, and mechlorethamine and hyaluronidase for vinca alkaloids, podophyllotoxins, and paclitaxel. The use of corticosteroids is debatable.[34] Granulocyte-macrophage colony-stimulating factor (GM-CSF) has been used in isolated cases to stimulate healing.[33]

REFERENCES

1. De Boer-Dennert M, de Wit R, Schmitz PIM, et al. Patient perceptions of the side-effects of chemotherapy: The influence of 5-HT$_3$ antagonists. Br J Cancer 1997;76:1055-1061.
2. Grevelman EG, Breed WP. Prevention of chemotherapy-induced hair loss by scalp cooling. Ann Oncol 2005;16:352-358.
3. Sonis ST, Elting LS, Keefe D, et al. Perspectives on cancer treatment–induced mucosal injury. Pathogenesis, measurement, epidemiology and consequences for patients. Cancer 2004;100(Suppl 9):1995-2025.
4. Rubenstein EB, Peterson DE, Schubert M, et al. Clinical practice guidelines for the prevention and treatment of therapy-induced oral and gastrointestinal mucositis. Cancer 2004;100(Suppl 9):2026-2046.
5. Keefe DM, Schubert M, Elting LS, et al. Updated clinical practice guidelines for the prevention and treatment of mucositis. Cancer 2007;109:820-831.
6. Spielberger R, Stiff P, Bensinger W, et al. Palifermin for oral mucositis after intensive therapy for hematologic cancers. N Engl J Med 2004;351:2590-2598.
7. The Antiemetic Subcommittee of the Multinational Association of Supportive Care in Cancer (MASCC). Prevention of chemotherapy- and radiotherapy-induced emesis: Results of the 2004 Perugia International Antiemetic Consensus Conference. Ann Oncol 2006;17:20-28.
8. Kris MG, Hesketh PJ, Sommerfield MR, et al. American Society of Clinical Oncology guideline for antiemetics in oncology: Update 2006. J Clin Oncol 2006;24:2932-2947.
9. Herrstedt J, on behalf of the ESMO Guidelines Working Group. Chemotherapy-induced nausea and vomiting: ESMO clinical recommendations for prophylaxis. Ann Oncol 2007;18(Suppl 2):ii83-ii85.
10. Navari RM, Einhorn LH, Loehrer PJ, et al. A phase II trial of olanzapine, dexamethasone and palonosetron for the prevention of chemotherapy-induced nausea and vomiting. A Hoosier Oncology Group Study. Support Care Cancer. 2007;15:1285-1291.
11. Benson AB, Ajani JA, Catalano RB, et al. Recommended guidelines for the treatment of cancer treatment–induced diarrhea. J Clin Oncol 2004;22:2918-2926.
12. Gibson RJ, Keefe DMK. Cancer chemotherapy–induced diarrhoea and constipation: Mechanism of damage and prevention strategies. Support Care Cancer 2006;14:890-900.
13. Klastersky J, Paesmans M, Rubenstein EB, et al. The Multinational Association of Supportive Care in Cancer risk index: A multinational scoring system for identifying low-risk febrile neutropenic cancer patients. J Clin Oncol 2000;18:3038-3051.
14. Smith TJ, Khatcheressian J, Lyman GH, et al. 2006 update of recommendations for the use of white blood cell growth factors: An evidence-based clinical practice guidelines. J Clin Oncol 2006;24:3187-3205.
15. Aapro MS, Cameron DA, Pettengell R, et al. EORTC guidelines for the use of granulocyte-colony stimulating factor to reduce the incidence of chemotherapy-induced febrile neutropenia in adult patients with lymphomas and solid tumours. Eur J Cancer 2006;42:2433-2453.
16. Leibovici L, Paul M, Cullen M, et al. Antibiotic prophylaxis in neutropenic patients: New evidence, practical decisions. Cancer 2006;107:1743-1751.
17. Ludwig H, Van Belle S, Barret-Lee P, et al. The European Cancer Anaemia Survey (ECAS): A large, multinational, prospective survey defining the prevalence, incidence, and treatment of anaemia in cancer patients. Eur J Cancer 2004;40:2293-2306.
18. Bokemeyer C, Aapro MS, Courdi A, et al. EORTC guidelines for the use of erythropoietic proteins in anemic patients with cancer. Eur J Cancer 2004;40:2201-2216.
19. Rizzo JD, Lichtin AE, Woolf SH, et al. Use of epoetin in patients with cancer: Evidence-based clinical practice guidelines of the American Society of Clinical Oncology and the American Society of Hematology. J Clin Oncol 2002;19:4083-4107.
20. Bokemeyer C, Aapro MS, Courdi A, et al. EORTC guidelines for the use of erythropoietic proteins in anemic patients with cancer: 2006 update. Eur J Cancer 2007;43:258-270.
21. Schiffer CA, Anderson KC, Bennet CL, et al. Platelet transfusion for patients with cancer: Clinical practice guidelines of the American Society of Clinical Oncology. J Clin Oncol 2001;19:1519-1538.
22. Limper AH. Chemotherapy induced lung disease. Clin Chest Med 2004;25:53-64.
23. Floyd JD, Nguyen DT, Lobins RL, et al. Cardiotoxicity of cancer therapy. J Clin Oncol 2005;23:7685-7696.
24. Jensen BV, Skovsgaard T, Nielsen DL. Functional monitoring of anthracycline cardiotoxicity: A prospective, blinded, long-term observational study of outcome in 120 patients. Ann Oncol 2002;13:699-709.

25. Ewer MS, Vooletich MT, Durand J-B, et al. Reversibility of trastuzumab-related cardiotoxicity: New insights based on clinical course and response to medical treatment. J Clin Oncol 2005;23:7820-7826.
26. de Jonge MAJ, Verweij J. Renal toxicities of chemotherapy. Semin Oncol 2006;33:68-73.
27. Rahman A, White RM. Cytotoxic anticancer agents and renal impairment study: The challenge remains. J Clin Oncol 2006;24:533-536.
28. Hausheer HF, Schilsky RL, Bain S, et al. Diagnosis, management and evaluation of chemotherapy-induced peripheral neuropathy. Semin Oncol 2006;33: 15-49.
29. Tuxen MK, Hansen SW. Neurotoxicity secondary to antineoplastic drugs. Cancer Treat Rev 1994;20:191-214.
30. du Bois A, Schlaich M, Lück H-J, et al. Evaluation of neurotoxicity induced by paclitaxel second-line chemotherapy. Support Care Cancer 1999;7:354-361.
31. van den Bent MJ, van Putten WLJ, Hilkens PHE, et al. Re-treatment with dose-dense weekly cisplatin after previous cisplatin chemotherapy is not complicated by significant neurotoxicity. Eur J Cancer 2002;38:387-391.
32. Ener RA, Meglathery SB, Styler M. Extravasation of systemic hemato-oncological therapies. Ann Oncol 2004;15:858-862.
33. Saghir NEI, Otrock Z, Mufarrij A. Dexrazoxane for anthracycline extravasation and GM-CSF for skin ulceration and wound healing. Lancet Oncol 2004; 5:320-321.
34. Mouridsen HT, Langer SW, Buter J, et al. Treatment of anthracycline extravasation with savene (dexrazoxane): Results from two prospective clinical multicentre studies. Ann Oncol 2007;18:546-560.
35. Kaiser R, Sezer O, Papies A, et al. Patient-tailored antiemetic treatment with 5-hydroxytryptamine type 3 receptor antagonists according to cytochrome P-450 2D6 genotypes. J Clin Oncol 2002;20:2805-2811.
36. Innocenti F, Undevia SD, Iyer L, et al. Genetic variants in the UDP-glucuronosyltransferase 1A1 gene predict the risk of severe neutropenia of irinotecan. J Clin Oncol 2004;22:1382-1388.

SUGGESTED READING

Weiss RB (guest editor). Toxicity of chemotherapy—the last decade. Semin Oncol 2006;33:1-143.

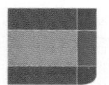

CHAPTER **240**

Palliative Chemotherapy and Corticosteroids

Davide Tassinari and **Marco Maltoni**

The role of chemotherapy in advanced or terminal cancer remains controversial.[1] The debate can be summarized as follows:

● The role of palliative chemotherapy for cancer-related symptoms is still unclear.
● It may be impossible to combine the outcomes of chemotherapy with those of a palliative approach.
● The boundary between chemotherapy and non–chemotherapy-related supportive treatments in a comprehensive treatment plan is ill-defined (see Chapter 120).
● The timing of palliative chemotherapy is unclear (when to treat and when to stop treating someone with advanced disease [see Chapter 20]).
● Which categories of patients to treat (i.e., everyone, only those with chemosensitive disease, all those with good performance status) remain undefined.

Another controversial aspect is the meaning of palliative chemotherapy within the patient-physician relationship because of differences between the patient's and physician's expectations of outcome (see Chapter 110).[2-4] Conflicting attitudes can coexist when a patient and physician have to decide on the correct comprehensive approach to the disease (Fig. 240-1).[5-8]

RECENT DEVELOPMENTS

The main developments in palliative chemotherapy have been how to translate the results of clinical research into clinical practice, how to assess quality of life outside clinical trials (see Chapter 65), and how to combine antitumor treatments with non–chemotherapy-related palliative approaches. Two improvements are identification of treatment outcomes in clinical practice and definition of the relationships between the main and surrogate efficacy end points of treatment. Overall survival and quality of life have been identified as the main outcomes of cancer treatment (*patient outcomes*). These outcomes should be the main indices of treatment efficacy, and phase III clinical trials are the best way to assess them.[9] The same paper analyzed the meaning of response rate in clinical oncology by defining it as a *cancer outcome* and an index of the activity of a treatment against the tumor (assessed in phase II clinical trials).[9] Many authors have tried to relate the main patient outcomes to cancer outcomes to identify surrogate efficacy end points for clinical research and

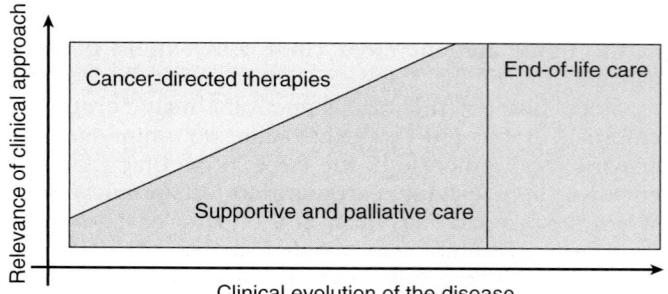

FIGURE 240-1 Cancer-directed therapies, palliative care, and end-of-life care.

practice.[10-12] Two questions merit analysis when we pass from clinical oncology to palliative care:

- How does quality of life (the main patient outcome in palliative care) relate to control of symptoms?
- Can symptom control be a surrogate end point for quality of life in palliative care that can be assessed in both clinical practice and clinical research?

Although the literature is not conclusive, control of symptoms seems to be a necessary, but insufficient surrogate for improvement in quality of life.[12,13]

EVIDENCE-BASED MEDICINE

Most of the literature tries to respond to the question of whether palliative chemotherapy actually palliates (see Chapter 118).[13-15] Some evidence supports a positive role for chemotherapy[10,13] in both control of symptoms and improvement in quality of life and overall survival in patients with metastatic breast cancer (a chemosensitive neoplasm). A more controversial debate concerns the use of palliative chemotherapy in patients with chemotherapy-resistant cancers such as metastatic pancreatic cancer, hormone-resistant prostate cancer, or primary brain tumors (see Chapter 238). Different processes may favor palliative chemotherapy if it reduces tumor mass and

- Lessens any compressive or irritative effects
- Reduces cytokine secretion by the tumor
- Supports the host's response against the tumor

Clinical evidence supporting a role of palliative chemotherapy in reducing tumor mass in chemosensitive tumors exists (e.g., small cell lung cancer, lymphomas, testicular cancer), but neither the biological process nor the clinical effects have been defined for chemoresistant neoplasms.

Definition of "Clinical Benefit"

The evidence supporting gemcitabine in metastatic pancreatic adenocarcinoma represents the most controversial aspect of palliative chemotherapy for tumor-related symptoms. Locally advanced or metastatic pancreatic cancer often causes pain, worsening performance status, and weight loss, and these symptoms are often the main cause of suffering in those with advanced disease. The so-called *clinical benefit assessment* includes pain assessment (with a visual analogue scale and morphine consumption), performance status (with the Karnofsky scale), and weight gain/loss (Fig. 240-2) (see Chapter 64).[16,17] This has been challenged as being neither a comprehensive assessment of quality of life nor a surrogate index of quality of life for clinical practice.[18] The evidence for a role of gemcitabine in advanced pancreatic cancer remains debatable.

Mitoxantrone in Hormone-Resistant Prostate Cancer

A trial that tried to demonstrate a role for mitoxantrone in hormone-resistant metastatic prostate cancer[19,20] has been challenged because it assessed pain in prostate cancer with a nonvalidated tool and compared mitoxantrone with prednisone, which is an adjuvant drug for pain and plays a limited role in the management of pain caused by bone metastases.

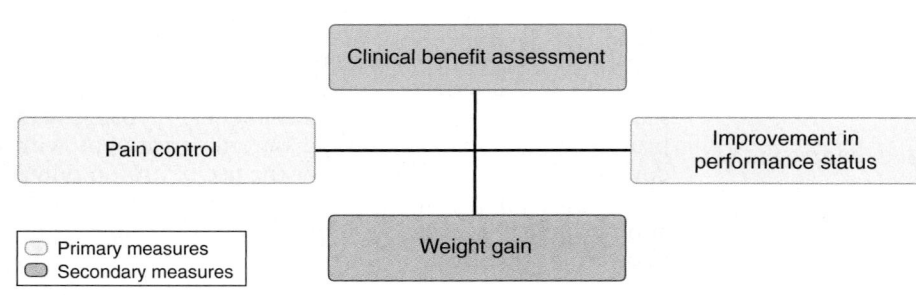

FIGURE 240-2 Clinical benefit assessment. *(Redrawn from Burris HA III, Moore MJ, Andersen J, et al. Improvements in survival and clinical benefit with gemcitabine as first-line therapy for patients with advanced pancreas cancer: A randomized trial. J Clin Oncol 1997;15:2403-2413.)*

Pain control:
- Responder: improvement of 50% or greater in pain over basal assessment via the visual analogic scale for at least 4 weeks
- Nonresponder: any worsening for at least 4 weeks
- Stable: any condition not included in the previous ones

Performance status:
- Responder: improvement of 20% or greater over basal assessment
- Nonresponder: worsening of 20% or greater over basal assessment
- Stable: any condition not included in the previous ones

Weight gain:
- Responder: improvement of 7% or greater over basal weight for at least 4 weeks
- Nonresponder: any other condition not included in the previous one

The patient is considered a responder if:
- He is a responder in the two primary measures
- He is a responder in one of the primary measures and stable in the other one
- He is stable in the two primary measures and a responder in the secondary one

Palliative Chemotherapy in Advanced Non–Small Cell Lung Cancer

Chemotherapy for advanced non–small cell lung cancer (NSCLC) has shown modest benefits in clinical practice. There is a relationship between response rate and overall survival (improvement in survival, though modest, is significant from both a statistical and clinical viewpoint),[11] and the role of chemotherapy (with or without platinum compounds) in both symptom control and symptom delay merits further investigation (see Chapter 218).[21] Trials supporting palliative chemotherapy have significant methodological limits, and neither new chemotherapeutic regimens nor modern targeted therapies have demonstrated a role in control of symptoms.[22]

Palliative Chemotherapy in Advanced Breast Cancer

Unlike the controversial results in chemotherapy-resistant tumors (pancreas, prostate, NSCLC), a role for palliative chemotherapy has been demonstrated in advanced breast cancer.[10,13] There appears to be a relationship between response rate and improvement in symptoms or survival, which supports the role of tumor shrinkage in symptom control and suggests new fields of investigation regarding chemotherapy for improvement of quality of life.

In the papers,[10,13] the authors analyzed the outcomes of about 300 women treated with anthracycline chemotherapy regimens and found that besides an improvement in symptoms during chemotherapy (see Chapter 63), an impact of chemotherapy on quality of life could be observed. It followed that despite some methodological limitations, an interesting relationship between tumor shrinkage and improvement in quality of life could be documented in this kind of patient.

Targeted Therapies in Palliation

The prototype of these new drugs (called "target molecules" for their need to have a target to act against neoplastic cells) is imatinib used for chronic myeloid leukemia.

Besides the biological and clinical roles that targeted therapies may play in clinical oncology, the controversial results in control of symptoms and improvement in quality of life merit analysis. Gefitinib is a small molecule that acts against the epithelial growth factor receptor (EGFR) tyrosine kinase and was assessed in patients with advanced NSCLC. Early evidence demonstrated that it could improve quality of life in advanced, pretreated NSCLC has not been confirmed in controlled clinical trials.[23,24] Likewise, cetuximab, a monoclonal antibody acting against EGFR, has been tested in patients with advanced, pretreated, and irinotecan-resistant colorectal cancer. Apart from interesting data on cetuximab reverting irinotecan resistance in heavily pretreated patients, one key trial did not demonstrate any palliative effect in the subset of treated patients. The improvement in response rate or time to disease progression does not support the hypothetical role of the molecule in control of symptoms or improvement in quality of life.[25]

CONCLUSIONS

Palliative chemotherapy in clinical practice remains controversial because of lack of evidence of its efficacy in controlling symptoms and improving quality of life.

Two areas need investigation:

- What is the role of palliative chemotherapy in improving quality of life in advanced disease, and how can symptom improvement be balanced against the side effects of treatment?
- When and in what type of patients should palliative chemotherapy be planned, perhaps by using a benefit predictive profile to select those to be treated?

No definitive answers exist, but a prudent approach that considers both the literature and the expectations of patients and family is appropriate when palliative chemotherapy is being considered for advanced disease.

PALLIATIVE CHEMOTHERAPY CONCLUSIONS

Corticosteroids are one of the most used classes of drugs in palliative medicine,[26] but there is little evidence for chronic treatment with corticosteroids (see Chapter 145). They are cytolytic in some hematological neoplasms (multiple myeloma and non-Hodgkin's lymphoma). Corticosteroids are used as antiemetics combined with or as an alternative to 5-hydroxytryptamine (5-HT$_3$) antagonists. They are also adjuvant drugs for pain. Corticosteroids can be used for asthenia, cancer-related fatigue, anorexia-cachexia syndrome, acute or chronic dyspnea, and intestinal subocclusive conditions.

Besides their cytolytic effect against hematological neoplastic cells, the palliative effect of corticosteroids is probably exerted through their anti-inflammatory effect. The main side effects of corticosteroids are hyperglycemia, hypertension, water and sodium retention, and gastroduodenal damage. Acute or chronic corticosteroid treatment is usually well tolerated when individualized. A controversial aspect is prevention of gastroduodenal bleeding with proton pump inhibitors during chronic treatment with corticosteroids. The evidence for the use of proton pump inhibitors during chronic treatment with nonsteroidal anti-inflammatory drugs supports a similar role during corticosteroid treatment.

Common Errors

- Treating patients nearly until death with chemotherapy, though frequent, is an index of poor quality of care and should be avoided when clinical decisions are made.
- Neither the literature nor clinical experience supports indiscriminate use of chemotherapy for tumor-related symptoms; however, some evidence supports palliative chemotherapy for chemosensitive neoplasms.
- Palliative chemotherapy is no substitute for supportive and palliative treatment, even if chemotherapy may play a role in some advanced chemosensitive tumors.
- Neither an antitumor approach nor a solely supportive and palliative one should be considered exclusively in patients with advanced cancer; instead, a comprehensive approach should be offered.

REFERENCES

1. Browner I, Carducci MA. Palliative chemotherapy: Historical perspective, applications and controversies. Semin Oncol 2005;32:145-154.
2. Earle CC, Neville BA, Landrum MB, et al. Trends in the aggressiveness of cancer care near the end of life. J Clin Oncol 2004;22:315-321.
3. Voogt E, van der Heide A, Rietjens JAC, et al. Attitudes of patients with incurable cancer toward medical treatment in the last phase of life. J Clin Oncol 2005;23:2012-2019.
4. Matsuyama R, Reddy S, Smith TJ. Why do patients choose chemotherapy near the end of life? A review of the perspective of those facing death from cancer. J Clin Oncol 2006;24:3490-3496.
5. ASCO-ESMO consensus statement on quality of cancer care. Ann Oncol 2006;17:1063-1064.
6. Lagman R, Walsh D. Integration of palliative medicine into comprehensive cancer care. Semin Oncol 2005;32:134-138.
7. Yabroff KR, Mandelblatt JS, Ingham J. The quality of medical care at the end-of-life in the USA: Existing barriers and examples of process and outcome measures. Palliat Med 2004;18:202-216.
8. Cherny NI, Catane R. Attitudes of medical oncologist toward palliative care for patients with advanced and incurable cancer. Cancer 2003;98:2502-2510.
9. ASCO Special Article. Outcomes of cancer treatment for technology assessment and cancer treatment guidelines. J Clin Oncol 1996;14:671-679.
10. Bruzzi P, Del Mastro L, Sormani MP, et al. Objective response to chemotherapy as a potential surrogate end point of survival in metastatic breast cancer patients. J Clin Oncol 2005;23:5117-5125.
11. Shanafelt TD, Loprinzi CL, Marks R, et al. Are chemotherapy response rate related to treatment-induced survival prolongations in patients with advanced cancer? J Clin Oncol 2004;22:1966-1974.
12. Tassinari D, Maltoni M, Sartori S, et al. Outcome research in palliative care: Could it represent a new dimension of clinical research or clinical practice? Support Care Cancer 2005;13:176-181.
13. Geels P, Eisenhauer E, Bezjak A, et al. Palliative effect of chemotherapy: Objective tumor response is associated with symptom improvement in patients with metastatic breast cancer. J Clin Oncol 2000;18:2395-2405.
14. Markman M. Does palliative chemotherapy palliate? J Support Oncol 2003; 1:65-67.
15. Doyle C, Crump M, Pintilie M, et al. Does palliative chemotherapy palliate? Evaluation of expectations, outcomes and costs in women receiving chemotherapy for advanced ovarian cancer. J Clin Oncol 2001;19:1266-1274.
16. Rothemberg ML, Moore MJ, Cripps MC, et al. A phase II trial of gemcitabine in patients with 5-FU refractory pancreas cancer. Ann Oncol 1996;7:347-353.
17. Burris HA III, Moore MJ, Andersen J, et al. Improvements in survival and clinical benefit with gemcitabine as first-line therapy for patients with advanced pancreas cancer: A randomized trial. J Clin Oncol 1997;15:2403-2413.
18. Tassinari D. Surrogate end points of cancer assessment: Have we really found what we are looking for? Health Qual Life Outcomes 2003;1:71.
19. Tannock IF, Osoba D, Stockler MR, et al. Chemotherapy with mitoxantrone plus prednisone or prednisone alone for symptomatic hormone-resistant prostate cancer: A Canadian randomized trial with palliative end points. J Clin Oncol 1996;14:1756-1764.
20. Osoba D, Tannock IF, Ernst DS, et al. Health-related quality of life in men with metastatic prostate cancer treated with prednisone alone or mitoxantrone and prednisone. J Clin Oncol 1999;17:1651-1653.
21. Ellison NM, Chevlen EM. Palliative chemotherapy. In Berger AM, Portenoy RK, Weissman DE (eds). Principles and Practice of Palliative Care and Supportive Oncology, 2nd ed. Philadelphia: Lippincott Williams & Wilkins, 2002, pp 698-709.
22. Tassinari D, Papi M, Fochessati F, et al. Outcomes of palliative chemotherapy in stage IV non–small-cell lung cancer. Have we found what we are looking for? Lung Cancer 2004;43:373-374.
23. Fukuoka M, Yano S, Giaccone G, et al. Multi-institutional randomized phase II trial of gefitinib for previously treated patients with advanced non–small-cell lung cancer. J Clin Oncol 2003;21:2237-2246.
24. Kris MG, Natale RB, Herbst RS, et al. Efficacy of gefitinib, an inhibitor of the epidermal growth factor receptor tyrosine kinase in symptomatic patients with non–small-cell lung cancer: A randomized trial. JAMA 2003;290:2149-2158.
25. Cunningham D, Humblet Y, Siena S, et al. Cetuximab monotherapy and cetuximab plus irinotecan in irinotecan-refractory metastatic colorectal cancer. N Engl J Med 2004;351:337-345.
26. Walsh D, Doona M, Molnar M, et al. Symptom control in advanced cancer: Important drugs and routes of administration. Semin Oncol 2000;27:69-83.

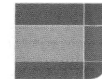

CHAPTER **241**

Principles and Practice of Surgical Oncology

Guy Hubens

KEY POINTS

- Surgical treatment of cancer is based on tumor type, localization, and stage of the disease.
- Surgical intervention should be part of a multidisciplinary team approach.
- In such an approach adjuvant and palliative surgery will become more important.
- Growing knowledge of the genetics of cancer will lead to more prophylactic cancer surgery.
- Surgical oncologists should be important participants in clinical trials.

Although the primary target of surgery in treating solid malignant tumors is still complete removal of the malignancy for cure, the role of the surgeon has changed profoundly in modern cancer treatment. In today's multidisciplinary team approach, the surgeon will be called on to obtain tissue for diagnosis, search for additional tumor deposits for staging, insert devices for administration of anticancer drugs, resect or debulk tumor for cure, or surgically treat symptoms in those incurable. To prevent tumor occurrence, a surgeon might even resect healthy organs in certain high-risk patients. All these actions should be performed in close collaboration with diagnostic radiologists, radiation and medical oncologists, pathologists, palliative medicine specialists, and others involved in the treatment of cancer.

With the growing knowledge in tumor genetics, immunology, and tumor biology, the role of surgeons will evolve, and it is their duty to continuously update their knowledge to provide optimal care. Surgical oncology has become a subspecialty, as reflected by the various national and international scientific sections and organizations devoted to surgical oncology.

DIAGNOSIS AND STAGING

Modern imaging, such as multislice computed tomography with three-dimensional reconstruction, ultrasound, magnetic resonance imaging, and nuclear medicine, still needs the ultimate proof of malignancy: examination of tissue by the pathologist. The surgeon can acquire tissue in various ways: fine-needle aspiration (FNA), core biopsy, incisional biopsy, or excisional biopsy. Each procedure has its own merits and disadvantages, and selection of the proper procedure depends on tumor location, tumor type, and subsequent therapy. These procedures are important, and the surgeon should always be aware that a poor procedure can compromise further treatment and even cure.

Fine-Needle Aspiration

In FNA, cell suspensions are obtained for cytological examination or flow cytometry, or both. This technique allows quick diagnosis but not determination of the invasiveness of the tumor. Typically, FNA was used for superficial lesions such as a thyroid nodule, breast lump, or palpable soft tissue mass. With modern endoscopic ultrasound techniques, however, the indications and possibilities of FNA have broadened. Mediastinal and intra-abdominal lesions such as pancreatic tumors and periesophageal or perigastric lymph nodes are all amenable to FNA.[1]

FNA is relatively easy to perform, requires no anesthesia, and has a high sensitivity. Other diagnostic techniques are usually necessary for optimal treatment. Tumor cell implantation along the aspiration tract may occur.[2] FNA should be performed only when the result has a direct impact on the choice of therapy.

Core Needle Biopsy

In-depth diagnosis of suspicious lesions is obtained with a core needle biopsy. It is possible to differentiate between invasive and noninvasive tumors. Under radiological guidance, more deeply situated lesions such as liver tumors are within reach. In many centers it is the procedure of choice for soft tissue masses.[3] There is debate whether core needle biopsy is superior to FNA in breast cancer.[4] For the diagnosis of lymphoma, core needle biopsy of a lymph node is insufficient.

When performing core needle biopsy it is of utmost importance that the needle be placed in an area that will be surgically removed in a subsequent operation (because the biopsy site is probably contaminated with malignant cells).

Incisional Biopsy

Incisional biopsy yields a small piece of a suspicious mass for pathological examination. It is usually undertaken when needle biopsy is inconclusive or impossible. Intra-abdominal or retroperitoneal masses beyond the reach of a needle biopsy technique are often diagnosed in this way with minimally invasive operative techniques. It has the additional advantage of detecting eventual spread of the tumor at the same intervention.

Several key technical points are important when performing incisional biopsy. For both intra-abdominal and superficial lesions, it is essential that meticulous hemostasis be achieved after the procedure to avoid hematoma and spilling of tumor cells. Biopsies on the extremities are performed along the line of the long axis of the limb, with the incision placed in an area that will be resected in the subsequent definitive operation. These precautions are aimed at preventing spilling of tumor cells and subsequent implantation outside the primary lesion.

Excisional Biopsy

Smaller skin tumors or lymph nodes are often removed in toto as an excisional biopsy. Because microscopically positive margins requiring reexcision are possible when performing an excisional biopsy of a skin tumor, it is important to orientate the specimen adequately for the pathologist.

A special, minimally invasive excisional biopsy is the sentinel lymph node (SLN) biopsy.[5-8] It is frequently used for melanomas and breast tumors. The technique is derived from the assumption that lymph node metastases follow a pathway within a lymph node basin; there is a certain lymph node that will be reached first by malignant cells (the sentinel node). By using both radioactive tracers and patent blue dye it is possible to detect this sentinel node and remove it surgically. Subsequent pathological examination will tell whether this node has been invaded by malignant cells. If negative by standard hematoxylin-eosin staining, the node can be further investigated by immunohistochemistry or reverse transcriptase polymerase chain reaction (RT-PCR). If still negative, no further lymph node dissection is usually done. Complete lymph node dissection of the involved basin will be undertaken only if tumor has metastasized to the sentinel node. Six major prospective studies on SLN biopsy in breast cancer surgery were reviewed.[7] It was concluded that the predictive power of axillary lymph node status was the same whether SLN biopsy or standard axillary lymph node dissection was used; however, SLN biopsy reduced the frequency of complications in breast surgery. It is unclear whether SLN biopsy has a positive effect on long-term survival and local control in the axilla. In melanoma, sentinel node status not only provides a reliable guide to prognosis but also allows avoidance of complete lymph node dissection in 80% to 85% of cases. Whether all patients with a positive SLN biopsy in melanoma surgery should undergo complete lymph node dissection is under investigation.

Besides breast and melanoma cancer patients, this technique is also under investigation for gastrointestinal tumors (stomach, colon, rectal cancer), gynecological tumors, head and neck cancer, and prostate cancer.[9-11]

CURATIVE SURGERY

Resection of a malignant primary tumor is considered curative when there is no evidence of distant metastases at the time of surgery and the tumor along with draining lymph nodes (if indicated) is removed with negative resection margins and no spillage of tumor cells (R0 resection). If macroscopic tumor is left behind, it is an R2 resection, and if microscopic tumor deposits are present in the resection margins, it is called R1. For every solid tumor there is a standardized surgical oncological resection technique defined for curative resection. Common surgical technical details for all these procedures are minimal tumor manipulation and early ligation of draining blood vessels.

The key in curative cancer surgery is to obtain negative resection margins for local tumor control. Traditionally, this was achieved by large and often mutilating resections. A classic example is the Halsted mastectomy for breast cancer. This procedure entailed en bloc removal of the breast with the pectoralis muscle and axillary lymph nodes. A local recurrence rate of less than 10% was achieved; before the Halsted technique it was greater than 70%. No influence on survival was noticed because advanced disease was treated at a time before screening programs.

Safe resection margins have been the issue in many clinical and histopathological studies investigating gastro-intestinal and skin cancer. For colon cancer, a proximal and distal margin of 5 cm has been accepted, whereas for rectal cancer, a 2-cm distal tumor-free margin should be obtained to minimize local recurrence. Perhaps more important than distal spread in rectal cancer is lateral spread, which has led to the concept of total mesorectal excision (TME technique).[12] With proper TME, the incidence of local rectal cancer recurrence should be less than 10%. In contrast, in melanoma cancer surgery, resection margins depend on the thickness of the primary lesion.

With surgical oncology becoming a part of the multi-disciplinary approach to cancer, the idea of wide resection for local tumor control has changed. Less extensive operations have the same or better results in controlling tumor when radiotherapy is added postoperatively. In stage I and II breast cancer, the addition of radiation therapy permitted more conservative breast surgery, with improved cosmesis and comfort. Radiation therapy can also be added locally, perioperatively as brachytherapy, such as for head and neck cancer. It should be remembered that postoperative radiotherapy can never compensate for sloppy surgery; the principles of good surgical oncology should always be the primary aim of the surgeon. Neoadjuvant radiotherapy, chemotherapy, or both, administered before surgery, has become the "gold standard" for many solid tumors. Downstaging of the primary tumor is achieved and better survival rates obtained. For instance, in esophageal cancer, neoadjuvant radio-chemotherapy has sometimes resulted in complete remission of the primary tumor, thereby rendering surgery questionable.[13]

General surgery has benefited from some technical breakthroughs in the last decades, such as minimally invasive techniques, which make surgery less traumatic. After its introduction, mainly for benign and functional pathology, malignancies were also operated on in this manner. Early studies, mainly on colon and rectal cancer, showed that resection margins and lymph node harvest could be identical to that achieved with open surgery.[14] Reports emerged of so-called port site metastases, or secondary tumor deposits at the site where the laparoscopic instruments were introduced intra-abdominally.[15] These reports caused major concern because port site metastases were deemed to be a direct consequence of the minimally invasive technique. Experimental studies demonstrated the possible effect of CO_2 pneumoperitoneum on the implantation and subsequent growth of tumor cells at trocar sites.[16] The surgeon is to be held responsible for this phenomenon because of excessive tumor manipulation and cell spillage. Large prospective trials[17] of laparoscopic treatment of colorectal cancer have shown rates of local recurrence and survival similar to those of traditional open surgery. However, because of the two-dimensional vision with laparoscopy and the limited range of motion of laparoscopic instruments, difficult surgical procedures can be awkward when performed laparoscopically.

A few years ago robotic technology was introduced. This combines the advantages of open surgery (three-dimensional vision, improved range of instruments, motion similar to the motion of the surgeon's hand) with those of minimally invasive surgery but with less patient trauma. Though originally designed for cardiac surgery, robotic surgery soon found its way into other surgical subspecialties. The largest experience in robotic oncological surgery involves radical prostatectomy for adenocarcinoma of the prostate, and now more than 3000 patients have been operated on worldwide.[18] Early reports showing promising results in both immediate postoperative complications and oncological outcome await confirmation in larger prospective trials, as is the case for smaller studies on esophageal, gastric, colon, and cervical robotic cancer surgery.[19-21]

PALLIATIVE SURGERY

Sometimes surgery is indicated for palliative reasons in advanced cancer. The most common indications are for obstruction, bleeding, infection, and to a lesser extent, pain. Pain is often a sign of invasion of a nerve plexus by tumor and is difficult to treat by surgical means.

Palliative procedures are not necessarily "small." They can involve the removal of large tumors with distant metastases to correct bleeding, debulking of tumor invasion and débridement of local septic complications, bypass procedures for obstruction, or liver resection for symptomatic metastases of neuroendocrine tumors. Planning of a palliative procedure should always involve extensive discussion between the medical, surgical, and radiation oncologist and the patient. The expected benefit should be weighted against life expectancy, procedure-associated morbidity, and other eventual treatment options for the debilitating symptoms.

SURGERY FOR METASTASES

Hematogenous metastases of various solid tumors to the liver or lung (or both) are sometimes amenable to surgical treatment, which can result in prolonged survival benefit. Numerous studies have been published on the surgical treatment of liver metastases of primary colorectal adenocarcinomas.[22] Surgical resection can be combined with other ablative procedures such as radiofrequency ablation, cryotherapy, or intratumoral alcohol injection to achieve complete destruction of metastases. Advances in surgical technique and relevant strategies such as neoadjuvant chemotherapy, portal vein embolization, and planned two-stage hepatectomy have increased the potential candidates for metastasectomy. Depending on the extent of liver involvement and the possibility of obtaining tumor-free margins, 5-year survival rates of 30% to 50% have been reported. With evolving surgical techniques and neoadjuvant therapy, the contraindications to liver surgery and prognostic factors have changed substantially.[22] Although the number of liver metastases (more than four) has traditionally been a bad prognostic sign, this has been challenged, as long as it is possible to obtain tumor-free liver margins with adequate remaining functional liver tissue. The interval between the occurrence of liver metastases and resection of the primary tumor seems to not be of major importance today. Several reports of successful treatment of synchronous liver metastases at the time of primary surgery for the colorectal cancer have been published.[22] Even extrahepatic disease is no contraindication to hepatic resection of liver secondaries. Simultaneous resection of hepatic metastases and metastases in the lung, ovaries, or hepatic lymph nodes has been reported.[22] All these studies are retrospective and need confirmation by prospective randomized controlled studies.

Not just patients with isolated colorectal liver metastases may benefit from an aggressive surgical approach. Resection of functional neuroendocrine liver metastases from a primary carcinoid tumor may result in palliation and even prolonged survival.[23] Selected patients with isolated liver secondaries from primary gynecological tumors may benefit as well.[24]

The rare patient with isolated lung metastases from a primary adenocarcinoma is also a candidate for surgical resection, with retrospective studies showing a good chance of prolonged survival.[25] Extranodal cancer deposits at the primary tumor site and the number of metastases influenced survival significantly. To improve long-term survival after lung resection for metastases, isolated lung perfusion with cytotoxic drugs as adjuvant therapy is under study,[26] an idea borrowed from isolated limb and liver perfusion for melanoma and liver metastases. Resection of lung metastases from primary osteogenic tumors and soft tissue sarcomas is more accepted.[27] If complete tumor resection is achieved, 5-year survival rates of 35% have been reported.

CANCER PREVENTION SURGERY

Rapid knowledge about inherited genetic mutations, their relationship to the development of cancer, and familial predisposition for some cancers will have an enormous impact on cancer surgery strategy. The classic "intention to treat" aspect of yesterday's surgical oncology will shift toward a more "intention to prevent" aspect in the near future. This will be even more so with decoding of the human genome and the possibility that more genes responsible for specific cancers will be identified.

Cancer prevention surgery has been performed for well-known precancerous pathologies. Examples are orchidopexy for cryptorchidism, proctocolectomy or subtotal colectomy with mucosal proctectomy and ileoanal pouch reconstruction for familial adenomatous polyposis coli syndrome or some individuals with hereditary non-polyposis colorectal carcinoma (Lynch) syndrome, and thyroidectomy in the multiple endocrine neoplasia type 2 syndrome. Detection of the *BRCA1* and *BRCA2* gene mutations implicated in hereditary breast and ovarian cancer has added prophylactic mastectomy and bilateral oophorectomy to this list.[28,29]

The potential benefits of the operation must be weighted against the morbidity and quality-of-life issues. Even if in many instances therapeutic prophylactic measures will not be surgical, it will be imperative for the oncological surgeon to have clear knowledge of the genetic changes involved in cancer development to prevent malignant disease in specific organs.

FOLLOW-UP AFTER SURGERY

If patients are included in a trial protocol, regular follow-up visits with clinical or technical investigations, or both, will be included. For others, follow-up will be determined by the type of cancer, the possibility of detecting early asymptomatic local or distant recurrences, and the treatment possibilities when such recurrences are found.

There are several theoretical reasons to include patients in a follow-up protocol. Surgeons should be on the lookout for early or late postoperative complications. Meticulous follow-up is the only possible way of evaluating the results of treatment. For certain tumors, follow-up is necessary to look for metachronous tumors such as breast and colon cancer. The search for asymptomatic early recurrence is of importance only if it has therapeutic consequences, for instance, with liver metastases in colorectal cancer and lung metastases from soft tissue sarcomas. Although a survival benefit for strict follow-up programs has never been proved, many feel reassured when seen on a regular basis. All these aspects should be discussed with the patient, and it will be more and more the case that follow-up programs will be "tailor-made" for the individual patient.

REFERENCES

1. Vander Noot MR III, Eloubeidi MA, Chen VK, et al. Diagnosis of gastrointestinal tract lesions by endoscopic ultrasound-guided fine-needle aspiration biopsy. Cancer Cytopathol 2004;102:157-163.
2. Lundstedt C, Stridbeck H, Andersson R, et al. Tumor seeding occurring after fine-needle biopsy of abdominal malignancies. Acta Radiol 1991;32:518-520.
3. Arca MJ, Biermann JS, Johnson TM, et al. Biopsy techniques for skin, soft tissue, and bone neoplasm. Surg Oncol Clin N Am 1995;17:1-11.
4. Ballo MS, Sneige N. Can core needle biopsy replace fine-needle aspiration cytology in the diagnosis of palpable breast carcinoma: A comparative study of 124 women. Cancer 1996;78:773-777.
5. Newman EA, Newman LA. Lymphatic mapping techniques and sentinel lymph node biopsy in breast cancer. Surg Clin North Am 2007;87:353-364.
6. Tangoku A, Seike J, Nakano K, et al. Current status of sentinel lymph node navigation surgery in breast and gastrointestinal tract. J Med Invest 2007; 54:1-18.
7. Sato K. Clinical trials for sentinel node biopsy in patients with breast cancer. Breast Cancer 2007;14:31-36.
8. Thompson JF, Shaw HM. Sentinel node mapping for melanoma: Results of trials and current applications. Surg Oncol Clin N Am 2007;16:35-54.
9. Kitagawa Y, Saka S, Kubo A, et al. Sentinel node for gastrointestinal malignancies. Surg Oncol Clin N Am 2007;16:71-80.
10. Kovacs AF. Head and neck squamous cell carcinoma: Sentinel node or selective dissection? Surg Oncol Clin N Am 2007;16:81-100.
11. Adib T, Barton DP. The sentinel lymph node: Relevance in gynaecological cancers. Eur J Surg Oncol 2006;32:866-874.
12. Heald RJ. Total mesorectal excision is optimal surgery for rectal cancer: A Scandinavian consensus Br J Surg 1995;82:1297-1299.
13. Fujita H, Sueyoshi S, Tanaka H, et al. Esophagectomy: Is it necessary after chemoradiotherapy for a locally advanced T4 esophageal cancer? Prospective nonrandomized trial comparing chemoradiotherapy with surgery versus without surgery. World J Surg 2005;29:25-30; discussion 30-31.
14. Martel G, Boushey RP. Laparoscopic colon surgery: Past, present and future. Surg Clin North Am 2006;86:867-897.
15. Hubens G. Port site metastases: Where are we at the beginning of the 21st century? Acta Chir Belg 2002;102:230-237.
16. Bonjer HJ, Gutt CN, Hubens G, et al. Port site metastases in laparoscopic surgery. First workshop on experimental laparoscopic surgery, Frankfurt 1997. Surg Endosc 1998;12:1102-1103.
17. Bonjer HJ, Hop WC, Nelson H, et al. Laparoscopically assisted vs open colectomy for colon cancer: Meta analysis. Arch Surg 2007;142:298-303.
18. Patel V, Chammas MF Jr, Shah S. Robotic assisted laparoscopic radical prostatectomy: A review of the current state of affairs. Int J Clin Pract 2007;61: 309-314.
19. Rawlings AL, Woodland JH, Crawford DL. Telerobotic surgery for right and sigmoid colectomies: 30 consecutive cases. Surg Endosc 2006;20:1713-1718.
20. Gutt CN, Bintintan VV, Koninger J, et al. Robotic assisted transhiatal esophagectomy. Langenbecks Arch Surg 2006;391:428-434.
21. Field JB, Benoit MF, Dinh TA, Diaz-Arrastia C. Computer-enhanced robotic surgery in gynaecologic oncology. Surg Endosc 2007;21:24-246.

22. Hao CY, Ji JF. Surgical treatment of liver metastases of colorectal cancer: Strategies and controversies in 2006. Eur J Surg Oncol 2006;32:473-483.
23. Que FG, Nagorney DM, Batts KP. Hepatic resection for metastatic neuroendocrine carcinomas. Am J Surg 1995;169:36-43.
24. Harrison LE, Brennan MF, Newman E, et al. Hepatic resection for noncolorectal, nonneuroendocrine metastases: A fifteen year experience with ninety-six patients. Surgery 1997;121:625-632.
25. McAfee MK, Allen MS, Trastek VF, et al. Colorectal lung metastases: Result of surgical excision. Ann Thorac Surg 1992;53:780-786.
26. Van Schil P (ed). Lung Metastases and Isolated Lung Perfusion. New York: Nova Science, 2005.
27. Van Geel AN, Pastorino U, Jauch KW, et al. Surgical treatment of lung metastases: The European Organisation for Research and Treatment of Cancer: Soft tissue and bone sarcoma group study of 255 patients. Cancer 1996;77:675-682.
28. Mann GB, Borgen PI. Breast cancer genes and the surgeon. J Surg Oncol 1998;67:267-274.
29. Schrag D, Kuntz KM, Garber JE, et al. Decision analysis: Effects of prophylactic mastectomy and oophorectomy on life expectancy among women with *BRCA1* or *BRCA2* mutations. N Engl J Med 1997;336:1465-1471.

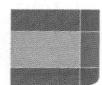

CHAPTER **242**

Palliative Orthopedic Surgery

Jason Braybrooke, Albert J. M. Yee, and Edward Chow

KEY POINTS

- With the increasing life expectancy of cancer patients and the skeleton being the third most common site for cancer metastasis, palliative orthopedic surgery is becoming an increasing part of orthopedic practice.

- Indications for surgical intervention include a painful lesion refractory to nonsurgical therapies, pathological or impending fracture, and neurological compromise, such as involvement of the spinal cord or cauda equina.

- The goals of surgery are to preserve or restore skeletal integrity or function, eliminate or prevent neurological compromise, minimize hospitalization and rehabilitation, and improve quality of life.

- Clinical and radiographic classifications have been developed to help predict metastases that are at risk of progressing to fracture. Patient outcomes appear to be improved with prophylactic nailing.

- The principles of surgical intervention for impending and pathological fractures are to provide internal stabilization of sufficient strength to allow immediate unsupported use of the limb that should last for the duration of the patient's life, stabilize the full length of the involved bone so that the chance of further surgery is minimized, and use the simplest intervention with the lowest morbidity to achieve these goals.

- The principles of surgical intervention for spinal instability and spinal cord compression are to restore the integrity of the spinal column, prevent neurological compromise, and minimize morbidity.

Palliative orthopedic surgery is becoming an increasing part of orthopedic surgery because of the increasing life expectancy of patients with cancer and the skeleton being the third most common site for metastasis (after liver and

lung). The 5-year survival rate for all known cases of cancer improved from 50% between 1974 and 1976 to 63% between 1992 and 1999.[1]

Metastases (visceral or bony) develop in two thirds of all cancer patients. Eighty percent of bone metastases arise from breast, prostate, and lung cancer.[2] Seventy percent of bone metastases occur in the axial skeleton (spine, pelvis, ribs, and skull) and 10% in the appendicular skeleton, usually the proximal ends of long bones.[3] About 1% of bone metastases fracture. The risk of fracture depends on the anatomical location, the size of the lesion, and the underlying aggressiveness of the tumor.[3,4] Forty percent of pathological fractures occur in the proximal end of the femur.[5] About 10% of bone metastases require surgical intervention.

Treatment of bone metastases is multidisciplinary,[6,7] and avoiding the potential complications of bone metastases often prompts an orthopedic assessment. Four groups of bone metastasis–related problems are recognized: impending fractures, pathological fractures, spinal instability, and spinal cord/cauda equina compression (see Chapter 241). Pain is the most common manifestation of skeletal metastasis, and radiographically detectable lesions are present in two thirds of patients.[8]

Indications for surgery are

- A painful lesion refractory to nonsurgical therapy
- Symptomatic impending fracture
- Pathological fracture
- Neurological compromise (spinal cord or cauda equina compression)

The goals of surgery are to

- Preserve/restore skeletal integrity
- Preserve/restore function
- Eliminate/prevent neurological compromise
- Minimize hospitalization/rehabilitation
- Improve quality of life

The decision-making process is based on a risk/benefit analysis that considers the risks and magnitude of the surgery and the probable postoperative prognosis of regaining function and benefiting from better pain control and quality of life. A minimum life expectancy of 6 weeks is advocated before orthopedic surgical interventions. Life expectancy is dependent on the primary cancer,[9-11] anatomical location (e.g., solid versus nonsolid organ) of the metastases,[4] burden of bone metastases,[9-11] and the presence or absence of a pathological fracture.[9,11]

Life expectancy after a pathological fracture depends on the primary tumor.[12] Mean survival is 29 months with prostate cancer, 22 months with a breast primary, and 12 and 4 months with kidney and lung cancer, respectively. These are high-risk groups to treat, and mortality rates are high. Mortality is 15% at 4 to 6 weeks and 50% 6 months after surgery.[4]

IMPENDING AND PATHOLOGICAL FRACTURES

Impending and pathological fractures are at opposite ends of the same spectrum, but the optimum time for surgically dealing with the bone lesions is controversial. An impending fracture is defined as a bony metastasis that has a significant likelihood of fracture under normal physiological loads. Clinical and radiographic classifications help predict metastases at risk for fracture. Three-dimensional imaging (see Chapters 70 and 71) coupled with computer-assisted thresholding techniques has increased accuracy in assessing three-dimensional tumor burden and the risk for fracture.[13] The incidence of long bone fractures is related to cortical involvement on plain radiographs. When 25% to 50% of the cortex is involved, the incidence of fracture was 4%; this figure rose to 61% and 79%, respectively, when 50% to 75% and 75% of the cortex was involved.[14] Another approach[15] proposed prophylactic internal fixation if the ratio of the width of the metastasis to the diameter of the bone exceeds 0.60 or there is 13 mm or greater axial cortical destruction of the femoral neck, 30 mm or greater cortical destruction of the femoral shaft, or 50% or greater cortical destruction. Another clinical scoring system grades the site, the pain, the type of lesion, and the amount of cortex affected on a 12-point scale. Patients with a score of 7 or lower should be treated by irradiation and those with a score higher than 7 by prophylactic nailing.[16] However, this score has a high false-negative rate with a specificity of 35% and sensitivity of 95%.[17] Management of impending fractures should never be based on radiographs alone. Only those that are symptomatic should be considered for surgical intervention.

The major difference between pathological and impending fractures is bone integrity. It is commonly believed that pathological fractures do not heal, but research[18] has demonstrated this view to be untrue. Thirty-five percent of pathological fractures heal at 6 weeks and 74% by 6 months. The only factor that influences bone union is patient survival because a pathological fracture adversely affects life expectancy.[9,11] This may be partly attributed to these patients having more advanced or aggressive cancer. Patient outcomes appear to improve with prophylactic nailing. Prophylactic stabilization of the femur shortens operative time, reduces complications, maintains function, and shortens hospital stay when comparing the treatment of impending versus pathological fractures.[19] Similar results were found in 184 patients treated for impending and pathological fractures. The investigators observed less blood loss, shorter hospital stay, and greater likelihood of discharge home and independent ambulation in the impending fracture group. Pathological fractures were more likely than impending fractures to require arthroplasty (i.e., joint replacement).[20]

Management of impending and pathological fractures is similar. The principles of surgery are to

- Provide internal stabilization of sufficient strength to allow immediate unsupported use of the limb for the duration of the patient's life
- Stabilize the full length of the involved bone to minimize the chance of further surgery
- Use the simplest intervention with the lowest morbidity to achieve these goals

The type of construct depends on the site of the lesion. Lesions of the axial skeleton (e.g., vertebral metastases; Fig. 242-1) and weight-bearing long bones (e.g., femur) pose the greatest risk of morbidity after fracture because of all the risks associated with prolonged bed rest (e.g., pneumonia, deep vein thrombosis and thromboembolism, and pressure sores). Newer, minimally invasive surgical strategies

allow percutaneous cannula placement to access critical bony lesions (Fig. 242-2A). Polymethyl methacrylate (PMMA) bone cement then fills metastatic deposits to strengthen bone biomechanically weakened by the tumor (see Fig. 242-2B and 2C). How contained the lesion is within bone is important to minimize extravasation of cement. This technique is straightforward and has minimal morbidity. It is particularly effective in the pelvis (i.e., cementoplasty) and the spine (i.e., vertebroplasty or kyphoplasty). Both techniques also provide mechanical support and excellent early pain relief. They can be a salvage procedure after failed radiotherapy and obviate the morbidity associated with conventional "open" surgery.[21] The risks related to vertebroplasty or kyphoplasty appear to be greater in cancer than in osteoporotic vertebral insufficiency fractures.[22,23] One study noted improvement in pain and function in 81% at a mean of 4.6 months' follow-up.[24]

The shafts of long bones are usually stabilized with intramedullary nails in impending or pathological fractures. The most common bone to be nailed is the femur, followed by the humerus. The femur generally requires a special intramedullary nail (a cephalomedullary nail). The nail has a screw that passes through it at the proximal end and into the femoral head to protect the neck from fracture because the subtrochanteric region of the femur is the most frequent site for femoral metastasis. The area may be augmented with bone cement if the bone metastasis is large. The use of intramedullary devices through smaller surgical incisions (i.e., as opposed to historical open plate fixation of femoral fractures) has enhanced surgical treatment. In a series of 30 femoral nails for pathological and impending fractures, a median survival of 6 months was obtained. There were no intraoperative complications or operative mortality.[24] Among 101 patients with femoral metastases, 92% were mobile and free of pain at a mean survival of 12 months. Fourteen died in the hospital, five had technical complications, and fat/tumor emboli developed in three.[25] Another series reported no complications after humeral nailing for pathological and impending fractures in 22 patients. All achieved full range of movement of the elbow and shoulder.[26] Using intramedullary devices in which the length of the bone is reamed has raised concern about seeding metastases. There is little evidence that internal fixation causes increased tumor spread in the same bone or beyond. In fact, internal stabilization may be associated with fewer pulmonary metastases.[27] Intramedullary reaming is often part of the surgical procedure before insertion of the intramedullary nail. Reaming creates a significant fat embolic load that can lead to systemic hypertension, oxygen desaturation, pulmonary hypertension, and occasionally cardiac arrest.[28,29] Venting (placing a hole in the distal end of the bone to allow extravasation of bone marrow during reaming) in an attempt to prevent/reduce the embolic load remains controversial.[30,31] There is no evidence that the combined effect of surgery and general anesthesia influences the overall prognosis. Endoprostheses (e.g., joint replacement components/arthroplasty) are generally used for periarticular metastases. Indications for endoprostheses are

- A solitary metastasis—in an effort to achieve a wide margin

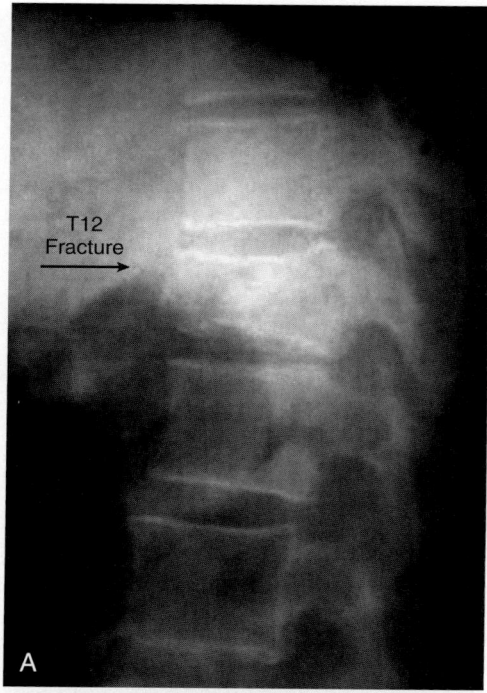

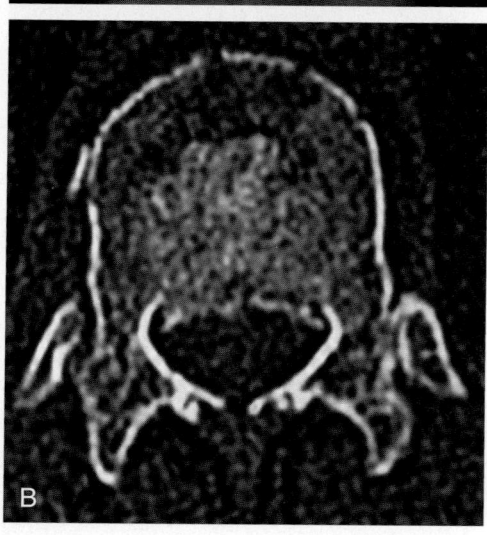

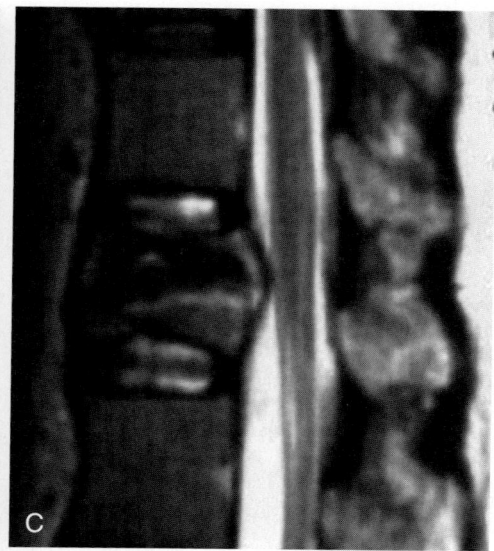

FIGURE 242-1 Vertebral body fracture after a fall from a height by an elderly osteoporotic man. **A,** Lateral radiograph depicting the fracture at thoracic level T12. **B,** Axial computed tomography scan at T12. **C,** Midsagittal T2-weighted magnetic resonance image demonstrating some retropulsion of the posterior vertebral wall into the spinal canal.

- A transcervical femoral fracture
- Metastasis/pathological fracture involving the metaphysis when conventional internal fixation is not possible
- Failure of previous internal fixation

Arthroplasty increases surgical time, complications, and morbidity. Reports on outcomes after surgery demonstrate improved function but not necessarily quality of life. Stabilization of impending/pathological fractures in 67 patients improved function but not quality of life as determined by the Short Form-36 (SF-36).[32] There was no significant reduction in pain medication. Another study demonstrated a trend toward better quality of life after surgery with the SF-36. This trend did not reach significance, however, because of a high dropout rate as a result of death and the confounding effect that adjuvant chemotherapy/radiotherapy had on quality of life.[33]

Postoperative radiotherapy is usually recommended after surgical stabilization of a pathological fracture. Those who are without visceral metastases and have a relatively long survival (e.g., >3 months) are more likely to benefit from postoperative radiotherapy. The entire bone is at risk from microscopic involvement after intramedullary nailing. The entire length of the rod used for bone stabilization should be included in the radiation field. When the radiation fields are more limited, instability of the rod, along with pain and need for reoperation, can result from recurrent osteolytic metastases outside the radiation portal. Postoperative radiation therapy is associated with patients regaining normal use of their extremity (with or without pain) and undergoing fewer reoperations at the same site.[34]

SPINAL INSTABILITY

Back pain is a common problem in metastatic cancer. The difficulty lies in deciding whether the pain is due to bone metastasis or spinal instability. Spinal instability is defined as abnormal movement between adjacent segments of

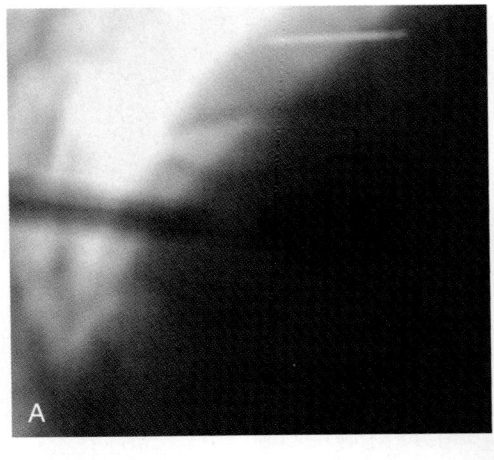

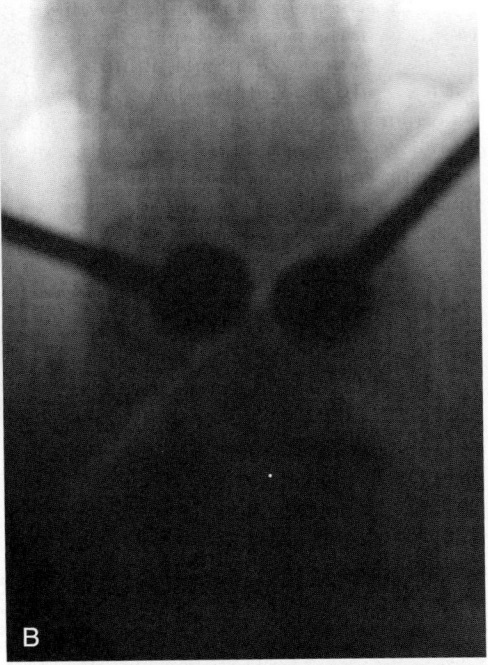

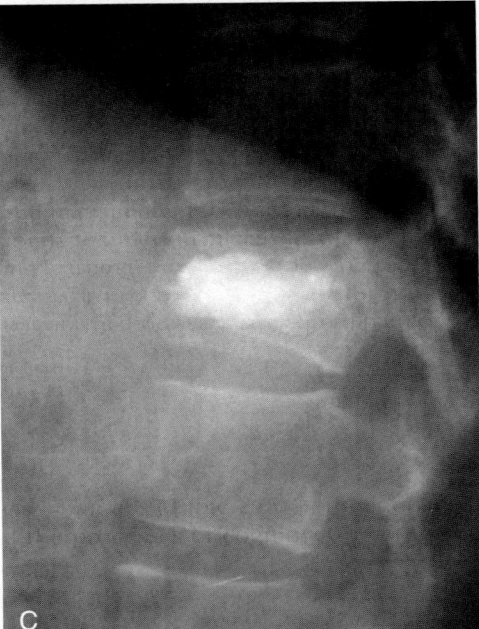

FIGURE 242-2 Vertebral body fracture treated by kyphoplasty. **A,** A cannula is inserted under radiologic guidance, after which an angiocatheter-like balloon is inflated to create a potential space for controlled filling of the vertebral body with polymethyl methacrylate. **B,** Bilateral inflation of balloons through a transpedicular approach. **C,** Radiopaque polymethyl methacrylate bone cement filling the vertebral body after the procedure (lateral plain radiograph).

the spine under normal physiological loads. In cancer it is caused by a critical level of destruction in a vertebral body leading to a pathological fracture that renders the spine unstable. This can cause a pathological burst fracture, cord compression, and paralysis. Treatment consists of stabilization of the spine with or without spinal decompression.

Similar scoring systems to predict the probability of a pathological fracture exist for spinal metastasis. One system helps predict the prognosis of metastatic spine tumors.[18] It is based on the general condition, number of extraspinal bone metastases, number of vertebral metastases, presence of visceral metastasis, the primary cancer, and the degree of spinal cord involvement. Complete

tumor excision with curettage, decompression, and stabilization is recommended for a lesion with a good prognosis (score >9) and stabilization with no or partial tumor resection for a lesion with a poor prognosis (score <5). This scoring system has been validated and revised to provide guidance on the best surgical approach.[35-37] Another system tried to predict which spinal metastases represented impending fractures[38] but has never been validated.

The principles of surgery are the same as for long bone fractures: restore the integrity of the spinal column, prevent neurological compromise, and minimize morbidity. Minimally invasive procedures such as kyphoplasty or vertebroplasty are popular means of stabilizing the spine.

Vertebroplasty involves percutaneous placement of a needle into the vertebral body (see Fig. 242-2A), followed by the injection of radiopaque PMMA under radiographic guidance (see Fig. 242-2B and 2C) to provide increased strength and decrease pain. The primary indication is usually failure of radiotherapy. It is a safe and effective way to manage pathological fractures and has minimal morbidity. There have been some reports of cement extravasation causing neurological deficits. Kyphoplasty and vertebroplasty provide pain relief in 90% and lead to complications in only 1% to 2%.[39] In 37 patients undergoing vertebroplasty, 73% had pain relief immediately and at 6 months. The procedure was complicated by cement extrusion in three cases.[40] Another study showed 95% improvement in pain and improvement in function. There were no complications from cement leakage in either the kyphoplasty or vertebroplasty group.[41]

SPINAL CORD COMPRESSION

Spinal cord compression (see Chapter 223) results from either infiltration of the bone metastasis into the spinal canal or a pathological burst fracture with or without secondary spinal deformity. In the 5 years preceding death, 2.5% of all cancer patients had at least one hospital admission for spinal cord compression, from 0.2% of patients with pancreatic cancer to 8% of those with myeloma.[42] Spinal cord compression occurs in 5% to 20% of patients with vertebral metastases.[43,44] At initial evaluation, 90% have back pain, 50% are unable to walk, and 10% to 15% have paraplegia.[45] Cord compression is an emergency condition that requires a coordinated multidisciplinary approach. To minimize treatment delays, once spinal cord compression is clinically suspected, an urgent whole-spine magnetic resonance image needs to be obtained.

Management consists of corticosteroids and surgery or radiotherapy (or both). Corticosteroids are routinely used to decrease peritumoral edema. The choice between surgery and radiotherapy should be individualized. The extent of vertebral metastatic involvement, the degree and duration of associated neurological symptoms and signs, the extent of nonbony metastatic involvement, and patient performance status are all important in decision making regarding spinal surgical intervention. Patient education regarding realistic expectations with or without surgical intervention is paramount. Radiotherapy is then delivered to the operative bed.

The strongest prognostic factor for overall survival and ambulation after treatment is pretreatment neurological status.[46] Outcome is determined by the pattern and duration of the cord compression (complete or incomplete). Patients with either incomplete cord compression, incomplete or complete paraplegia/urinary retention for less than 24 hours, or a gradual onset of cord compression lasting longer than 24 hours have a more favorable prognosis with surgical intervention. Otherwise, the prognosis is guarded with regard to bowel/bladder recovery or significant motor recovery after surgery. Preoperative neurological deficit is also associated with 19% increased mortality and a 71% increase in the incidence of postoperative wound infection.[47] In patients with an early progressive neurological deficit as a result of spinal cord

compression, surgical decompression plus stabilization is often recommended along with other postsurgical adjuvants. Whether to stabilize the spine via an anterior or posterior approach remains controversial; there is little class I evidence to guide the clinician. The decision involves consideration of several factors. Patients with disease confined to one or two vertebrae and with no cardiorespiratory co-morbidity or significant kyphotic deformity may often benefit from anterior decompression involving vertebrectomy. After adequate surgical decompression, spinal realignment can be achieved and further supported by an anterior strut (e.g., implant cage, autograft/allograft bone strut). Supplementary instrumentation either anteriorly or posteriorly is often considered as well. If the spinal deformity is not significant or if pulmonary co-morbidities preclude an anterior approach, posterior decompression using strategies adapted from the historical treatment of vertebral tuberculosis (i.e., costotransversectomy) may be useful to achieve spinal cord decompression. Conventional posterior spinal laminectomy has not been successful in treating anterior cord compression secondary to vertebral metastasis.[48] The ability to achieve multiple levels of segmental fixation posteriorly is attractive in multilevel disease, but technically difficult and often impossible anteriorly. Regarding a surgical versus nonsurgical approach, recent evidence supports the beneficial effects of surgery (with adjuvants) over radiotherapy alone. One randomized trial compared decompressive surgery followed by radiotherapy with radiotherapy alone.[49] The trial accrued 101 patients before meeting early stopping criteria because of surgical patients being more likely to retain/maintain ambulatory status than the radiotherapy-alone arm. More patients in the surgery (42/50, 84%) than the radiotherapy (29/51, 57%) group were able to walk after treatment (odds ratio, 6.2; 95% confidence interval [CI], 2.0 to 19.8; $P = .001$). Patients treated by surgery also retained the ability to walk significantly longer than those treated by radiotherapy alone (median of 122 versus 13 days, $P = .003$). Significantly more patients in the surgery than the radiation group regained the ability to walk (10/16, or 62%, versus 3/16, or 19%; $P = .01$). The need for corticosteroids and opioid analgesics was reduced in the surgical group. However, 35% in the radiotherapy arm had spinal instability, usually considered an indication for primary surgical management.[49] Improvement in quality of life after palliative spine surgery has also been reported.[50]

ADVANCES

Recent advances in minimally invasive surgical techniques and the establishment of multidisciplinary collaborative bone metastasis clinics are improving the palliative care of cancer patients.[49] In recognition of certain limitations in radiation therapy, there is increasing interest in other adjuvants that can reduce local tumor burden. Evolving strategies such as photodynamic therapy and laser-induced thermal therapy are being evaluated.[51] Coupling these advances with the ability to access critical bony lesions by minimally invasive techniques will facilitate the potential opportunity for local biological ablative therapies followed by percutaneous vertebroplasty/kyphoplasty. Altering the balance between local tumor growth and host bony repair in favor of repair while simultaneously affording mechanical stability with the currently proven strategies of percutaneous vertebroplasty/kyphoplasty is biologically attractive.

The key to good palliative orthopedic care is timely intervention to control symptoms, avoid complications, and maintain function and quality of life. This goal is facilitated by a multidisciplinary approach consisting of medical oncologists, radiation oncologists, and orthopedic surgeons. Multidisciplinary bone metastasis clinics in tertiary cancer centers are successful.[6,7]

REFERENCES

1. American Cancer Society Cancer Statistics Review 1975-2002.
2. Buckwalter JA, Brandser EA. Metastatic disease of the skeleton. Am Fam Physician 1997;55:1761-1768.
3. Hage WD, Aboulafia AJ, Aboulafia DM. Incidence, location and diagnostic evaluation of metastatic bone disease. Orthop Clin North Am 2000;31:515-528, vii.
4. Bauer HC. Controversies in the surgical management of skeletal metastases. J Bone Joint Surg Br 2005;87:608-617.
5. Sim FH. Metastatic bone disease of the pelvis and femur. Instr Course Lect 1992;41:317-327.
6. Andersson L, Chow E, Finkelstein J, et al. The ultimate one-stop for cancer patients with bone metastases: New combined bone metastases clinic. Can Oncol Nurs J 1999;9:103-104.
7. Chow E, Finkelstein J, Connolly R. New combined bone metastases clinic: The ultimate one-stop for cancer patients with bone metastases. Curr Oncol 2000;7:205-207.
8. Galasko CSB. Skeletal metastasis and mammary cancer. Ann R Coll Surg Engl 1972;50:3-28.
9. Bauer HC, Wedin R. Survival after surgery for spinal and extremity metastases. Prognostication in 241 patients. Acta Orthop Scand 1995;66:143-146.
10. Katagiri H, Takahashi M, Wakai K, et al. Prognostic factors and a scoring system for patients with skeletal metastasis. J Bone Joint Surg Br 2005;87:698-703.
11. Hansen BH, Keller J, Laitinen M, et al. The Scandinavian Sarcoma Group Skeletal Metastasis Register. Survival after surgery for bone metastases in the pelvis and extremities. Orthop Scand Suppl 2004;75:11-15.
12. Harrington KD. Impending pathologic fractures from metastatic malignancy: Evaluation and management. Instr Course Lect 1986;35:357-381.
13. Whyne CM, Hu SS, Lotz JC. Burst fracture in the metastatically involved spine: Development, validation, and parametric analysis of a three-dimensional poroelastic finite-element model. Spine 2003;28:652-660.
14. Fidler M. Incidence of fracture through metastases in long bones. Acta Orthop Scand 1981;52:623-627.
15. Menck H, Schulze S, Larsen E. Metastasis size in pathologic femoral fractures. Acta Orthop Scand 1988;59:151-154.
16. Mirels H. Metastatic disease in long bones. A proposed scoring system for diagnosing impending pathologic fractures. Clin Orthop Relat Res 1989; 249:256-264.
17. Damron TA, Morgan H, Prakash D, et al. Critical evaluation of Mirels' rating system for impending pathologic fractures. Clin Orthop Relat Res 2003; 415(Suppl):S201-S207.
18. Tokuhashi Y, Matsuzaki H, Toriyama S, et al. Scoring system for the preoperative evaluation of metastatic spine tumor prognosis. Spine 1990;15: 1110-1103.
19. Dijskstra PDS. Treatment of pathological fractures of the humeral shaft due to bone metastases: A comparison of intramedullary locking nail and plate osteosynthesis with adjunctive bone cement. Eur J Surg 1996;160:535-542.
20. Ward WG, Holsenbeck S, Dorey FJ, et al. Metastatic disease of the femur: Surgical treatment. Clin Orthop Relat Res 2003;415(Suppl):S230-S244.
21. Chow E, Holden L, Danjoux C, et al. Successful salvage using percutaneous vertebroplasty in cancer patients with painful spinal metastases or osteoporotic compression fractures. Radiother Oncol 2004;70:265-267.
22. Cheung G, Chow E, Holden L, et al. Percutaneous vertebroplasty in patients with intractable pain from osteoporotic or metastatic fractures: A prospective study using quality of life assessment. Can Assoc Radiol J 2006;57:13-21.
23. Chow E, Finkelstein J, Cheung G. Pain relief and fracture prevention in bone cancer and osteoporotic patients with percutaneous vertebroplasty/cementoplasty. Hosp News 2000;13:15.
24. Giannoudis PV, Bastawrous SS, Bunola JA, et al. Unreamed intramedullary nailing for pathological femoral fractures. Good results in 30 cases. Acta Orthop Scand 1999;70:29-32.
25. Van Doorn R, Stapert JW. Treatment of impending and actual pathological femoral fractures with the long Gamma nail in the Netherlands. Eur J Surg 2000;166:247-254.
26. Franck WM, Olivieri M, Jannasch O, et al. An expandable nailing system for the management of pathological humerus fractures. Arch Orthop Trauma Surg 2002;122:400-405.
27. Boumar WH, Multer JH, Hop WC. The influence of intramedullary nailing upon the development of metastases in the treatment of an impending pathological fracture: An experimental study. Clin Exp Metastasis 1983;1:205-212.
28. Choong PF. Cardiopulmonary complications of intramedullary fixation of long bone metastases. Clin Orthop Relat Res 2003;415(Suppl):S245-S253.
29. Gainor BJ, Buchert P. Fracture healing in metastatic bone disease. Clin Orthop Relat Res 1983;178:297-302.
30. Dalgorf D, Borkhoff CM, Stephen DJ, et al. Venting during prophylactic nailing for femoral metastases: Current orthopedic practice. Can J Surg 2003;46: 427-431.
31. Martin R, Leighton RK, Petrie D, et al. Effect of proximal and distal venting during intramedullary nailing. Clin Orthop Relat Res 1996;332:80-89.
32. Talbot M, Turcotte RE, Isler M, et al. Function and health status in surgically treated bone metastases. Clin Orthop Relat Res 2005;438:215-220.
33. Clohisy DR, Le CT, Cheng EY, et al. Evaluation of the feasibility of and results of measuring health-status changes in patients undergoing surgical treatment for skeletal metastases. J Orthop Res 2000;18:1-9.
34. Townsend P, Rosenthal H, Smalley S, et al. Impact of postoperative radiation therapy and other perioperative factors on outcomes after orthopedic stabilization of impending or pathological fractures caused by metastatic disease. J Clin Oncol 1994;12:2345-2350.
35. Enkaoua EA, Doursounian L, Chatellier G, et al. Vertebral metastases: A critical appreciation of the preoperative prognostic Tokuhashi score in a series of 71 cases. Spine 1997;22:2293-2298.
36. Tokuhashi Y, Matsuzaki H, Oda H, et al. A revised scoring system for preoperative evaluation of metastatic spine tumor prognosis. Spine 2005;30: 2186-2191.
37. Ulmar B, Richter M, Cakir B, et al. The Tokuhashi score: Significant predictive value for the life expectancy of patients with breast cancer with spinal metastases. Spine 2005;30:2222-2226.
38. Taneichi H, Kaneda K, Takeda N, et al. Risk factors and probability of vertebral body collapse in metastases of the thoracic and lumbar spine. Spine 1997;22: 239-245.
39. Hacein-Bey L, Baisden JL, Lemke DM, et al. Treating osteoporotic and neoplastic vertebral compression fractures with vertebroplasty and kyphoplasty. J Palliat Med 2005;8:931-938.
40. Weill A, Chiras J, Simon JM, et al. Spinal metastases: Indications for and results of percutaneous injection of acrylic surgical cement. Radiology 1996; 199:241-247.
41. Garfin SR, Yuan HA, Reiley MA. New technologies in spine: Kyphoplasty and vertebroplasty for the treatment of painful osteoporotic compression fractures. Spine 2001;26:1511-1515.
42. Loblaw DA, Laperriere NJ, Mackillop WJ. A population-based study of malignant spinal cord compression in Ontario. Clin Oncol (R Coll Radiol) 2003;15: 211-217.
43. Kramer J. Spinal cord compression in malignancy. Palliat Med 1992;6: 202-211.
44. DeWald RL, Bridwell KH, Prodromas C, et al. Reconstructive spinal surgery as palliation for metastatic malignancies of the spine. Spine 1985;10:21-26.
45. Sundaresan N, Galicich JH. Treatment of spinal metastases by vertebral body resection. Cancer Invest 1984;2:383-397.
46. Talcott JA, Stomper PC, Drislane FW, et al. Assessing suspected spinal cord compression: A multidisciplinary outcomes analysis of 342 episodes. Support Care Cancer 1999;7:31-38.
47. Finkelstein J, Zaveri G, Wai E, et al. A population-based study of surgery for spinal metastases. J Bone Joint Surg Br 2003;85:1045-1050.
48. Hall AJ, Mackay NN. The results of laminectomy for compression of the cord or cauda equina by extradural malignant tumour. J Bone Joint Surg Br 1973;55:497-505.
49. Patchell R, Tibbs PA, Regine F, et al. Direct decompressive surgical resection in the treatment of spinal cord compression caused by metastatic cancer: A randomized trial. Lancet 2005;366:643-648.
50. Wai EK, Finkelstein JA, Tangente RP, et al Quality of life in surgical treatment of metastatic spine disease. Spine 2003;28:508-512.
51. Burch S, Bogaards A, Siewerdsen J, et al. Photodynamic therapy for the treatment of metastatic lesions in bone: Studies in rat and porcine models. J Biomed Opt 2005;10:034011.

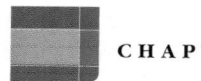

CHAPTER **243**

Modern Supportive Care in Oncology

Barry Fortner and Amy P. Abernethy

Cancer threatens expectations regarding a patient's lifetime, and as the cancer runs its deleterious course, it impinges on the quality of that life. Most antineoplastic therapies prescribed to extend life result in serious iatrogenic effects ranging from death to acute and chronic toxicities that patients and families may consider more aversive than the disease itself. When cancer treatments result in a temporary decrease in function and an increase in negative symptoms, patients have the paradoxical experience of being made "sick" by the medicine delivered to make them well.

Although the highest objective of oncology is to cure or retard the disease process, supportive care encompasses all efforts to minimize both the symptoms of cancer and the side effects of cancer treatment. The goal of supportive care is to maintain patient well-being on all human dimensions. Importantly, this includes facilitating optimal application and reception of antineoplastic interventions. Ideally, this means that surgery, radiation therapy, chemotherapy, and newer targeted agents are administered under conditions demonstrated to be effective in clinical trials. Toxicities invariably become the "dose-limiting" factor in the administration of many antineoplastic therapies; thus, prevention and alleviation of toxicities form the central objectives of supportive care. Although less toxic targeted therapies are among the greatest advances in cancer treatment, traditional chemotherapy, with or without targeted agents, will remain a mainstay of treatment during forseeable decades and supportive care will remain necessary to manage the associated toxicities.

Some of the most obvious and beneficial gains to date in the "war on cancer" have resulted from improvements in supportive care that in the context of antineoplastic agents and innovations in delivery systems, allow higher relative doses of chemotherapy and radiation therapy, combination radiation therapy and chemotherapy, and multidrug chemotherapy. Supportive care advances have also dramatically increased access to all types of cancer treatment in the outpatient and community setting. Supportive care interventions designed to combat chemotherapy-induced nausea and vomiting, neutropenia, anemia, and bone loss exemplify the relevance and effectiveness of modern supportive care.

Extending the trajectory of supportive care signifies a bright and optimistic future for oncology. Modern supportive care in oncology is and will be indelibly marked by four characteristics. First, new supportive drugs and delivery systems will be developed. Second, the emphasis on evidence-based treatment and on the quality of cancer care will place supportive care as a linchpin in quality definitions. Third, the focus on cost-effectiveness and efficiency at all levels of medical care will require evaluation and justification of supportive care on these dimensions. Fourth, dramatic enhancement and adoption of information technology will transform supportive care, beginning with already unfolding innovations in patient assessment and education.

RECENT DEVELOPMENTS

Continuation of Innovation in Drug Development

Ongoing current clinical trials presage novel agents, delivery systems, and procedures with the potential to enhance supportive care. Advances in erythropoietin-stimulating agents (ESAs), colony-stimulating factors, cytokines, and bisphosphonates serve as representative examples. ESAs are the focus of current research in chemotherapy-induced anemia and cancer-related anemia. Such research may result in clinical approaches that reduce ESA dosing frequency, incorporate oral formulations, and futher the understanding of contributing conditions, such iron deficiency and co-morbidities, that may increase the effectiveness of ESAs.

Growth colony-stimulating factors such as granulocyte colony-stimulating factor (G-CSF) and granulocyte-macrophage colony-stimulating factor (GM-CSF) are the standard of care for significant cancer-related and chemotherapy-induced issues. They are effective in reducing the risk for febrile neutropenia and decreasing hospitalization for complications of neutropenia. G-CSF also assists in the administration of several myelosuppressive chemotherapy regimens in both the outpatient and inpatient setting. The recent approval of pegfilgrastim has improved the efficiency of managing chemotherapy-induced neutropenia in that a single injection is used rather than the multiple doses indicated with filgrastim and sargramostim. Novel agents, with similar potential to enhance modern supportive care, include bisphosphonates and cytokines (see Part III, Section A: Drugs).

Evidence-Based Treatment and the Quality of Cancer Care

Virtually all areas of medicine have directed increasing attention to the availability and integrity of scientific evidence undergirding decision making. Emerging trends in oncology endorse greater adherence to guidelines, and professional societies and other consensus agencies offer clinical standards to assist providers in evidence-based medicine. With the ubiquitous development of clinical pathways by individual cancer institutions, evidence-based guidelines are being integrated into standard practice and increasingly serve as reference points for evolving payment systems. New measures of quality care[1] will undoubtedly encompass supportive agents and services rather than focusing exclusively on adherence to clinical trial–based cancer treatment guidelines and consensus statements.[2]

Requirement of Cost-Effectiveness and Efficiency

It may be surprising that supportive care drugs are among the largest overall expenditures in cancer care. Agents such as G-CSF and ESAs rank among the highest individual drug expenditures. An ongoing debate in oncology focuses on these drugs' cost-effectiveness and on the implications of cost for physician and patient choice, medical and social responsibility, and ultimately, the viability of health care. Cost-effectiveness of G-CSF models for febrile neutropenia has focused on the lofty goal of cost offset at specified risk thresholds.[3] Similar work has addressed the cost-effectiveness of novel agents for other supportive care areas, such as chemotherapy-induced nausea and vomiting[4] and chemotherapy-induced anemia.[5] Modern supportive care will require that we understand the clinical benefit of supportive care drugs and procedures in relation to the additional financial burden that add to the total cost of cancer care.

The cost of supportive care extends beyond the funds spent directly on specific drugs, procedures, or hospitalizations. Emerging research analyzes the cost of supportive care along multiple dimensions, including direct and indirect costs to the payor, provider, patient, and caregiver. Inclusion of these costs will better portray the total burden of cancer-related and chemotherapy-induced problems.

Management of chemotherapy-related toxicities, manifested as extensive fatigue, nausea, vomiting, and anemia, involves considerable human resources. A study of 400 medical professionals at 20 community oncology practices analyzed the human resource cost associated with 21-day chemotherapy regimens and approaches to managing neutropenia. The average medical encounter required 7.2 staff members, 51.8 tasks, and 4.7 events (defined as groups of related tasks); time/cost requirements for a single chemotherapy treatment ranged from 2.4 hours and $57.30 to 14.8 hours and $364.66, depending on the agent.[9] The "true cost" entailed in preparation and delivery of chemotherapy doses, both fixed (drug storage space, equipment, and information) and variable (insurance management, inventory, waste management, pharmacy staff, supplies, shipping), averaged $34.27 for a single infusion. Multiplying this by the number of infusions delivered to the Medicare population in 2003, the authors estimated total societal cost of $136.8 million for chemotherapy drug preparation alone.

A complete analysis of the cost of supportive care should also consider treatment-related costs borne by patients and their families. Cancer patients and caregivers spend much time and money arranging and preparing for medical visits, traveling to and from visits, and waiting in clinics, as well as on visits themselves. These time requirements interfere with daily activities, obligations, and routines, thereby compounding the cost of care.[6] In the future, clinicians may consider the burden that a treatment places on the patient and family/caregiver when weighing treatment options in supportive care. For example, weekly injections required for certain schedules of ESAs to alleviate chemotherapy-induced anemia may be more time-consuming and burdensome than a biweekly dosing schedule.[7] The aggregate impact of patient burden represents a substantial cost to society, one that is especially high at the end stages of cancer when supportive care is particularly important. Estimates of the cost of net patient time during the initial and final stages of cancer range from $271 (for melanoma of the skin) to $842 (for prostate cancer) during the initial phase of care and increase considerably during the final year of life, from $1509 (for melanoma of the skin) to $7799 (for gastric cancer).[8]

In the evolving cost-conscious environment of medicine, inclusive cost-effectiveness analysis will constitute a decision-making axis that with analysis of clinical outcomes, will define and maintain the quality of cancer care. One such model has been proposed by Abernethy and colleagues[10] using breakthrough pain as point of illustration. They propose that physicians will engage in better decision making if health economic data are collected and aggregated according to the nature of impact (intangible, indirect, and direct), the participants (patients, providers, and society at large), and the end points under consideration (costs, outcomes, and benefits). With increasing limits on available financial and human resources, oncology will need supportive care strategies that maximize efficient resource utilization.

Incorporation of Information Technology

In supportive care, accurate identification, description, and diagnosis of symptoms and monitoring of clinical response depend fundamentally on sound clinical assessment of patient symptoms, experiences, and functionality. Devising systematic, valid, and efficient assessment methods for these indicators is an ongoing challenge. Little change has occurred in the assessment methods used by most oncology practices. Although supportive care has made great strides in developing strategies that maintain patients' well-being in the face of life-limiting or life-altering illness, the clinical methods used to evaluate symptoms, experience of care, and quality of life (QOL) have remained virtually unchanged in essentially the form of an interview.

Much progress has been made in updating methods for assessing patient symptoms and QOL and delineating sound methods for gathering data directly from patients. These data are generally referred to as "patient-reported outcomes" (PROs) and have gained considerable attention as a new outcomes classification.[11] An umbrella term, PROs encompass a broad array of data and measures, including QOL, health-related QOL, general well-being, performance status or functionality, and life satisfaction. When collated with traditional outcomes data on disease activity and treatment efficacy, PROs provide a more complete picture of the patient's experience than typically obtained through a traditional clinical interview.

Assessment of PROs relevant to supportive care has proved problematic. In community-based settings, where most cancer patients receive treatment, providers have often neglected routine assessment of symptoms such as pain, fatigue, psychological distress, and QOL. Disruption of daily care caused by traditional paper assessment tools or the time needed for a complete symptom review[12] may account for this problem. Clinicians may also neglect assessment of PROs because of a perception that they are clinically irrelevant. PRO scales have been developed by research scientists for specific reference groups to measure a particular latent construct such as depression, hostility, or loneliness; hundreds of these scales exist, mostly to support particular research or for use in evaluating outcome in clinical trials. Most PRO measures are unsuitable for use at the point of care and do not deliver timely clinically useful information.

Oncology has witnessed an explosion of methodologies for assessing patient symptoms and experiences. These methods have the potential to transform supportive care, provide more time and space for clinician-patient communication, more quickly highlight extant patient concerns, uncover hidden patient problems, and facilitate some of the essential but sometimes mundane requirements of clinical care, such as documentation and education. Novel technologies and new applications for existing technologies are driving this transformation in assessment and, subsequently, supportive care. Electronic methods for assessing PROs occupy the forefront and carry great potential to improve supportive care. Technologies currently being developed, implemented, and studied for screening, assessing, and monitoring PROs include handheld devices (e.g., palm pilots), portable personal computers (e.g., e-tablets), and voice-response systems (e.g., interactive voice recognition systems [IVRSs]), all of which share the virtue of making routine screening and measurement of symptoms and QOL more feasible at the point of care.[12]

Despite initial concern about their reliability and useability, PROs collected by electronic methods are proving to be valid in comparison to paper-and-pencil questionnaires[13] and the traditionally "gold standard" clinician interview.[14] A recent meta-analysis that assessed the comparability of paper and electronic administration of the same questionnaires across various health and mental health contexts concluded that switching from paper to electronic administration should not require additional validation studies.[13]

New scales and measures have been developed and validated specifically to collect PROs by electronic methods. One such tool, the Cancer Care Monitor (CCM, now called the Patient Care Monitor [PCM]), a multi-

dimensional measure of symptom burden and QOL, is administered on a wireless, pen-based, notebook-sized computer called an "e-tablet" (Fig. 243-1). The CCM has been administered by e-tablet in more than 100 community oncology practices across the continental United States. CCM data correspond well to those collected by nurse-verified evaluation, with excellent agreement between CCM items and nurses' ratings on the presence or absence of symptoms and symptom severity.[14] E-tablets used to deliver the PCM can also be used in academic oncology to reliably and validly collect PROs with standard and well-recognized assessment measures such as the Functional Assessment of Cancer Therapy (FACT) subscales and the FACIT-Fatigue subscale.[15]

Evidence suggests that electronic assessment may actually yield more information relevant to quality of care than the traditional interview. Unlike clinician interviews and open-format paper-based questionnaires, electronic data collection lends itself to predefined format or checklist-type query structures. One study compared three different methods of collecting patient-reported data on adverse events. Two hundred fourteen men were randomly assigned to one of three methods in a clinical trial: checklist, open-ended questions, and open-ended defined questions. Seventy-seven percent using a checklist reported an adverse event, whereas only 14% in the open-ended questions group and 13% in the open-ended defined questions group reported adverse events.[16]

One potential advantage of electronic surveys is efficiency; this was borne out in the PCM validation. Patients took 20.83 minutes (standard deviation [SD] of 10.35) to complete the paper PCM, whereas the same patients took only 12.58 minutes (SD of 5.03) to complete the electronic PCM (paired t test (1, 37) = 4.92; $P < .001$). Moreover, the electronic CCM reduced administration time by 40%.

In an increasingly competitive environment, oncology centers will seek to increase the efficiency of practice visits without compromising the quality of patient care. Given the human resource–intensive nature of supportive care, technology solutions that improve clinicians' efficiency will offer attractive avenues for increasing effi-

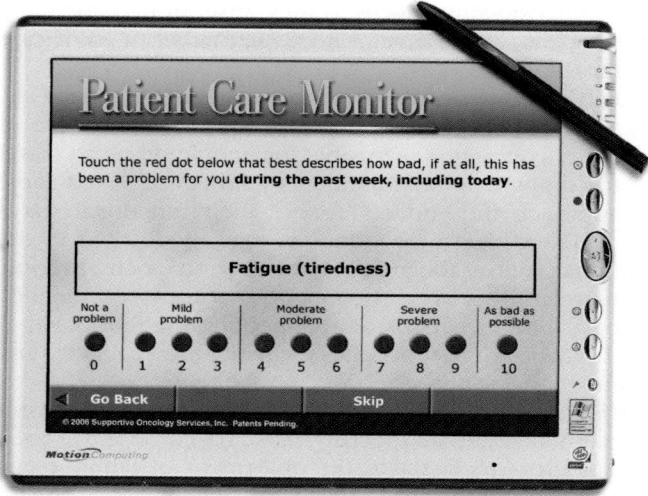

FIGURE 243-1 Patient care monitor.

■ CASE STUDY

Physicians have expressed reservations about the accuracy and reliability of PROs. Dr. T hesitated to trust an electronically administered system for collecting PROs—the Patient Care Monitor (PCM) system—until it brought to light a real and imminent danger to one of his patients. Only days after Dr. T began using the PCM system, he called his inhouse psychologist to report what he thought was a false-positive result. A cancer patient of his—a young and seemingly vibrant, optimistic college student with a ready smile and a happy demeanor—had recorded a significantly elevated score on the depression scale and had endorsed a question related to thoughts about death, which combined with other indicators of distress raises concerns about suicidal ideation. These responses did not match her personality or Dr. T's experience of illness. At Dr. T's suggestion, the young woman was evaluated to identify possible reasons for her reporting these "false-positive" scores. On interview it became apparent that she did indeed, unbeknownst to her oncologist, suffer from clinically severe depression and had even contemplated suicide. She was immediately referred for appropriate treatment. This experience, as well as many others subsequent to it, have given Dr. T a profound appreciation for the importance and relevance of PROs and for the critical role of detailed questioning about a broad range of supportive care issues.

ciency[17] and will gain traction, provided that a positive impact on quality is also demonstrated.

As palliative medicine implements new methodologies, clinical policies, and supportive care processes, we advocate the following:

- In combining technology with practice, retain a focus on patients. The ultimate goal of assessment and data collection, whatever the method, is to improve patient care, relieve suffering, and enhance QOL.
- View technology not as an end in itself but as a tool for overcoming the challenges of data collection and identifying valid patient concerns. Technology should enable providers to best target their care to and tailor it for the individual.
- Take advantage of new technologies that enable providers to routinely monitor symptoms between visits, identify patients' needs as they arise, bring patients to the clinic at the time of need, and target or tailor care for the home.
- Particularly critical for palliative medicine, tailor electronic solutions to the patient's capabilities. Use of tablet computers is feasible for people who can travel to outpatient appointments; however, as people approach the end of life and their functional status declines, electronic solutions that are feasible in the home, such as the Internet and electronic pens, become more appropriate. When incorporating a new technology, time its use for the point along the illness trajectory where it best matches the patient's capabilities and functional status.
- Use new care delivery, monitoring, and assessment methodologies—especially those based on novel technologies—to facilitate the enlistment of family members in supportive roles, for example, as proxy respondents.

- Welcome future systems in supportive care that provide robust real-time quality assurance tracking and rapid-cycle quality improvement. Such systems represent avenues for improving patient care.
- Leverage the power of future systems that generate a comprehensive picture of patients' symptoms and experiences to target collateral outcomes and thus address a fuller spectrum of patients' needs than usually encompassed in disease-specific care.

EVIDENCE-BASED MEDICINE

Without question, modern supportive care will follow the principles and practices of evidence-based medicine (EBM) (see, e.g., Chapter 118). Although supportive care has not always relied on the fundamentals of EBM—rigorous literature search, critical appraisal, evaluation, and monitoring—the novel technologies and methodological advances discussed make the application of EBM to supportive care more feasible. Evidence-based practice begins with referral to a high-quality body of research evidence; novel data technologies that capture symptoms and other PROs and make them available for both clinical and research purposes offer clinicians ready access to the body of evidence to transform supportive care and greatly improve its quality.

RESEARCH CHALLENGES

Perhaps equal to the immense potential of supportive care are the challenges that it faces as it evolves to become more patient focused, evidence based, technology facilitated, and quality enhancing.

- Drug development faces the challenge of producing novel supportive care agents that advance rather than simply match the clinical outcomes of existing agents.
- Drug developers and providers face the challenge, in a time of tightening federal budgets and a competitive medical reimbursement market, of providing supportive care options that can be defended on the basis of their cost-effectiveness at all levels of care.
- With limited financial and human resources, providers face the challenge of delivering more care with less; they will need to understand the inclusive cost of providing care in order to maintain supportive care programs that address a broad spectrum of patient concerns.
- Developers of PRO measures face the challenge of further improving the clinical meaningfulness and clinical validity of PROs, including their sensitivity (test/retest reliability), psychometric validity, and clinimetric validity.
- Clinical researchers face the challenge of carefully assessing PRO measures across the entire illness trajectory, including at the palliative care phase of illness.
- Institutions involved in supportive care face a host of regulatory issues that will emerge as PROs are routinely captured at the point of care. They will need to prepare clinical measures for audits by the Food and Drug Administration, compliance with the Health Insurance Portability and Accountability Act, medical and legal scrutiny and litigation, and pharmaceutical audits, reviews, and monitoring of clinical trials.[18]

CONCLUSIONS

In summary, newly developed drugs have vastly enhanced oncologists' power to manage and alleviate many common cancer symptoms and treatment side effects—yet this comes at significant cost to individuals, institutions, and society. The cost-effectiveness and impact of supportive care on patient outcomes and quality of care will need to be established to justify the place of supportive care in standard practice in an increasingly cost-conscious and evidence-based era. The simultaneous development of novel assessment, communication, and delivery systems that use new technologies will reduce the cost and improve the efficiency of supportive care. As PROs attain greater importance in cancer care and as both PRO and cost-effectiveness considerations earn their place in new definitions of quality care, supportive care will gain acceptance as a cornerstone of quality. There is reason for great optimism that both new technologies and new chemotherapies will facilitate the birth of a 21st century supportive care that is comprehensive, patient centered, evidence based, highest quality, and effective in improving patients' symptoms, experiences, and QOL.

REFERENCES

1. Neuss MN, Desch CE, McNiff KK, et al. A process for measuring the quality of cancer care: The Quality Oncology Practice Initiative. J Clin Oncol 2005; 23:6233-6239.
2. ASCO-ESMO consensus statement on quality cancer care. J Clin Oncol 2006;24:3498-3499.
3. Smith TJ, Khatcheressian J, Lyman GH, et al. 2006 update of recommendations for the use of white blood cell growth factors: An evidence-based clinical practice guideline. J Clin Oncol 2006;24:3187-3205.
4. Vanscoy GJ, Fortner B, Smith R, et al. Preventing chemotherapy-induced nausea and vomiting: The economic implications of choosing anti-emetics. Commun Oncol 2005;2:127-132.
5. Meehan KR, Tchekmedyian NS, Smith RE, et al. Resource utilisation and time commitment associated with correction of anaemia in cancer patients using epoetin alfa. Clin Drug Invest 2006;26:593-601.
6. Fortner BV, Tauer K, Zhu L, et al. Medical visits for chemotherapy and chemotherapy-induced neutropenia: A survey of the impact on patient time and activities. BMC Cancer 2004;4:22.
7. Fortner F, Tauer K, Zhu L, et al. The impact of medical visits for chemotherapy-induced anemia and neutropenia on the patient and caregiver: A national survey. Commun Oncol 2004;1:211-217.
8. Yabroff KR, Davis WW, Lamont EB, et al. Patient time costs associated with cancer care. J Natl Cancer Inst. 2007;99:14-23.
9. Fortner BV, Okon TA, Ahu L, et al. Costs of human resources in delivering cancer chemotherapy and managing chemotherapy-induced neutropenia in community practice. Commun Oncol 2004;1:23-28.
10. Abernethy AP, Wheeler J, Fortner B. A health economic model of breakthrough pain. Am J Manage Care 2008;14:S129-S140.
11. Wiklund I. Assessment of patient-reported outcomes in clinical trials: The example of health-related quality of life. Fundam Clin Pharmacol 2004; 18:351.
12. Fortner B, Okon T, Schwartzberg L, et al. The Cancer Care Monitor: Psychometric content evaluation and pilot testing of a computer administered system for symptom screening and quality of life in adult cancer patients. J Pain Symptom Manage 2003;26:1077-1092.
13. Gwaltney CJ, Shields A, Shiffman S. Equivalence of electronic and paper-and-pencil administration of patient reported outcome measures: A meta-analytic review. Paper presented at the Inaugural PROMIS Conference titled Building Tomorrow's Patient-Reported Outcome Measures, 2006, Gaithersburg, MD.
14. Fortner B, Baldewin S, Schwartzberg L, Houts AC. Validation of the Cancer Care Monitor items for physical symptoms and treatment side effects using expert oncology nurse evaluation. J Pain Symptom Manage 2006;31:207-214.
15. Abernethy PA, Patwardhan M, Herndon J, et al. Validation of the e-tablet as a method for delivering standard symptom and quality of life assessment scales. Manuscript submitted for publication, 2004.
16. Bent S, Padula A, Avins AL. Brief communication: Better ways to question patients about adverse medical events. Ann Intern Med 2006;144:257-261.
17. Fortner BV, Zhu L, Okon TA. The new language of community oncology. Commun Oncol 2005;4:357-362.
18. Health Insurance Portability and Accountability Act of 1996, Public Law 104-191. Fed Register 1997;62(54).

SUGGESTED READING

Bent S, Padula A, Avins AL. Brief communication: Better ways to question patients about adverse medical events. Ann Intern Med 2006;144:257-261.

Fortner B, Baldewin S, Schwartzberg L, et al. Validation of the Cancer Care Monitor items for physical symptoms and treatment side effects using expert oncology nurse evaluation. J Pain Symptom Manage 2006;31:207-214.

Fortner BV, Zhu L, Okon TA. The new language of community oncology. Commun Oncol 2005;4:357-362.

Neuss MN, Desch CE, McNiff KK, et al. A process for measuring the quality of cancer care: The Quality Oncology Practice Initiative. J Clin Oncol 2005;23:6233-6239.

Cancer Pain

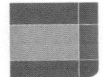

CHAPTER **244**

Pathophysiology of Cancer Pain

Catherine E. Urch

KEY POINTS

- Cancer pain shares neuropathophysiological pathways with non–cancer-related pain.
- Complex multiple neural triggers give rise to cancer pain syndromes.
- Animal models of cancer pain reveal that it has unique pain states.
- Visceral pain is poorly understood.
- Clinical treatment must be multimodal: pharmacological and nonpharmacological.

Cancer pain is often referred to as a mixed-mechanism pain. It is rarely manifested as a pure neuropathic, visceral, or somatic pain syndrome; instead, it is a complex syndrome with inflammatory, neuropathic, and ischemic components, often in multiple sites. Although the pathophysiology is complex, many cancer-induced pains are considered in terms of underlying pure pain states. The complexity is another "layer," as opposed to cancer pain being totally different and using different afferents and neurotransmitters. Thus, the neuropathic elements of cancer pain are treated with the same drugs efficacious in non–cancer-related neuropathy.

NORMAL PAIN TRANSMISSION

Normal pain transmission is the process by which peripheral noxious stimuli are transmitted to the brain rapidly and topographically to allow the appropriate and immediate response to reduce actual or potential tissue damage. Most commonly this occurs in acute pain. Aspects of this pain pathway are hard-wired, for example, Aδ and C fiber afferents, whereas others are "plastic" and dynamic and allow differential coding, attention, and response.[1]

Noxious stimuli are transmitted via lightly myelinated Aδ or virtually unmyelinated C fibers from the periphery to the dorsal horn.[1] These fibers have different thresholds below which they will not fire and varying patterns of firing depending on stimulus intensity. Stimuli need to be transduced into electrical conduction from the triggering of specific receptors, such as those for heat, chemical, or pressure (Fig. 244-1). Receptor stimulation allows direct positive ion influx and, if the threshold is achieved, rapid depolarization. The input is transmitted centrally (to the dorsal root ganglion, the cell body, and the dorsal horn) via sequential depolarizations through sodium and voltage-gated calcium channels (VDCCs). The neuronal cell body may alter receptor and neurotransmitter production and transportation, which becomes increasingly important in pathological pain.

Within the dorsal horn (see Fig. 244-1), the primary afferents terminate at synaptic junctions. Synapses allow communication and modulation of the original input. Communication occurs through the release of neurotransmitters, which can be excitatory (glutamate, glycine, substance P) or inhibitory (enkepahlins, γ-aminobutyric acid [GABA]).[2] These neurotransmitters bind to receptors and either trigger further depolarization or prevent depolarization. They can act presynaptically and postsynaptically on interneurons and non-neuronal cells (glia). The overall response transmitted to higher centers is the outcome of intense and dynamic modulation within the dorsal horn. In addition, there is a fast reflex arc that connects the dorsal and ventral horn and allows very rapid, "unconscious" withdrawal from pain stimuli.

The dorsal horn is intimately connected to the brain through several pathways (see Fig. 244-1). The spinothalamic pathways carry information to the cortical areas of the brain, which allows topographical and intensity rating of the given noxious stimuli to be consciously acknowledged. The parabrachial pathways project to brain areas responsible for the affective component of stimuli; they are nontopographical and lack intensity thresholds but are responsible for the unpleasant, aversive qualities of pain. All ascending input is extensively modulated and interconnects with memory and efferent areas of the brain, and this input can be modulated by numerous factors such as analgesia and distraction (Fig. 244-2). The brain modulates the dorsal horn via descending pathways, which can be inhibitory (noradrenergic and serotonin) or excitatory (serotonin).[3] Thus, potential feed-forward or inhibition loops can be generated entirely centrally.

Neuropathic Pain

Neuropathic pain arises from nerve damage, usually peripherally (e.g., herpes zoster pain), but it can be central (e.g., poststroke pain). The nerve damage allows a train of pathological events resulting in the classic symptoms

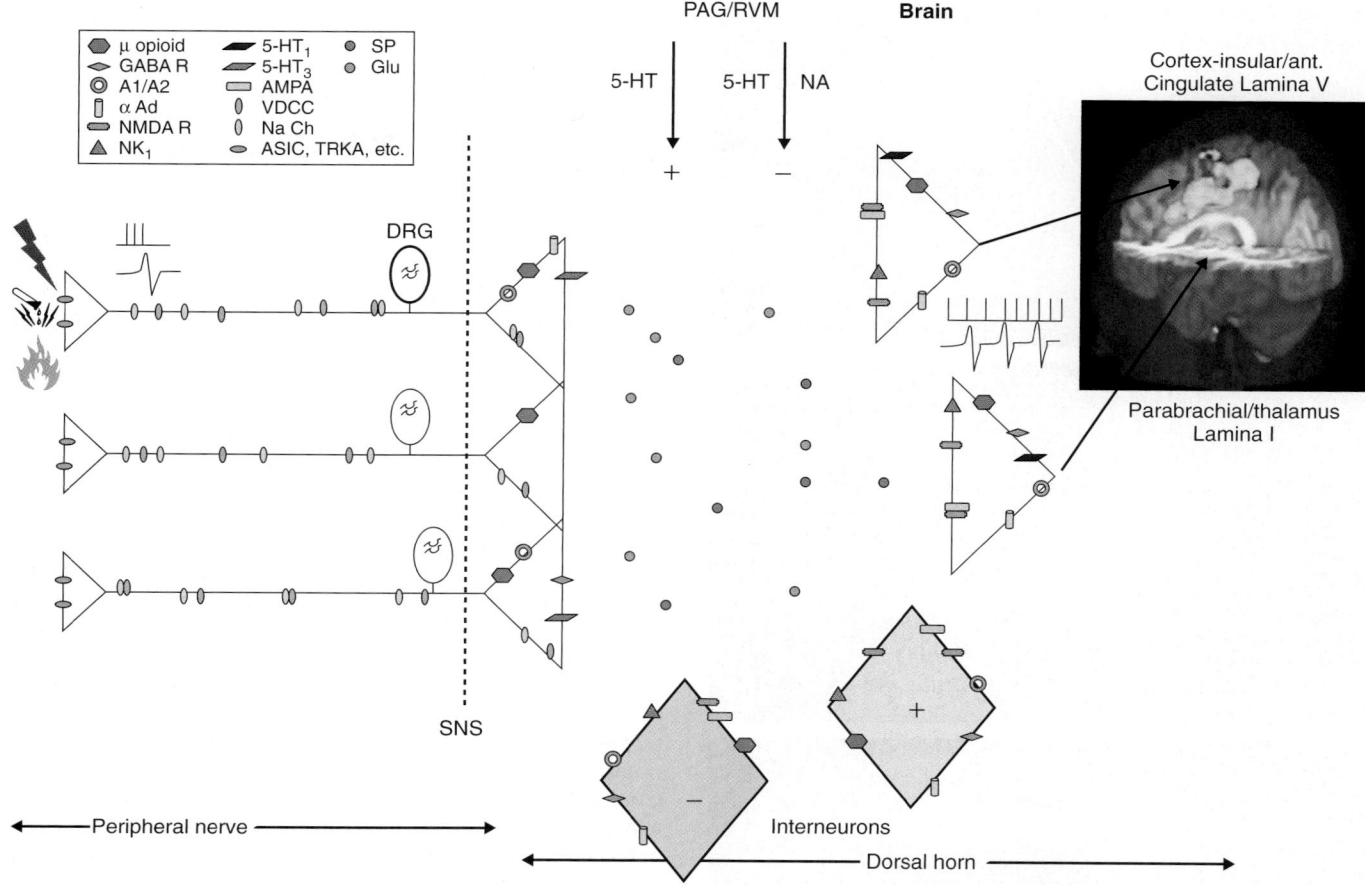

FIGURE 244-1 The diagram simplistically summarizes normal acute noxious input from the periphery through the dorsal horn to the brain. From the *left*, noxious stimuli such as heat, chemical, or mechanical injury is transduced via specific receptors, namely, temperature-coding receptors, acid-sensing ion channels (ASIC), TrkA (inflammation), or pressure receptors. Transduction allows positive ions to flow into the cell, which causes depolarization and action potentials. This is transmitted along the neuron via sodium (Na Ch) and calcium (VDCC) channels to the dorsal root ganglion (DRG) and the dorsal horn. The sympathetic nervous system (SNS) lies close to the DRG but is unaffected in acute noxious transmission. In the dorsal horn, extensive modulation of the input can occur. Neurotransmitters such as substance P (SP) or glutamate (Glu), among others, are released from the primary afferent and diffuse across the synapse. An array of receptors can be triggered, including *N*-methyl-D-aspartate (NMDA), α-amino-3-hydroxy-5-methylisoxazole-4-propionic acid (AMPA), neurokinin 1 (NK$_1$), and adenosine (A1/A2). Other neurotransmitters are also released either locally, such as enkephalins (μ-opioid receptor) and γ-aminobutyric acid (GABA), which are inhibitory, or via descending pathways, such as norepinephrine (α Ad receptor) and serotonin (5-HT$_1$ or 5-HT$_3$ receptors). The overall modulated signal (either increased as shown or decreased) is transmitted to the brain via ascending pathways, predominantly the spinothalamic from lamina V, which terminates in the cortex, and the parabrachial from lamina I, which terminates in the thalamic areas. Descending pathways arise from the brain and pass through the periaqueductal gray (PAG) and rostroventral medulla (RVM) areas before terminating in the dorsal horn.

and signs of allodynia, hyperalgesia, dysesthesia, and sensory loss (Fig. 244-3).[4]

Damage to a peripheral nerve allows persistent depolarization as a result of either abnormal stimuli of sensitized receptors or aberrant expression of fast-reacting sodium channels and VDCCs. The spontaneous and erratic discharge of the damaged neuron crosstalks to surrounding normal neurons, which causes further spread of abnormally reacting neurons. This mechanism contributes to primary and secondary hyperalgesia. The abnormal firing of the primary afferents affects the dorsal horn, so areas lack neurotransmitters, and other terminals discharge excessive and erratic neurotransmitters. The overall effect is net excitation, with recruitment of the *N*-methyl-D-aspartate (NMDA) receptor allowing massive and persistent postsynaptic depolarization. There also appears to be net loss of inhibitory pathways (both GABAergic and opioid

related). The dorsal horn excitation is mirrored in the activation of higher centers.[5] Recent functional magnetic resonance imaging (fMRI) studies suggest rewiring and hyperexcitation of cortical and afferent areas in persistent neuropathic pain.[6] A chronic pathological state of central sensitization can be maintained by central feed-forward loops with or without continued peripheral input.

Inflammatory Pain

Central hyperalgesia is produced in inflammatory pain by sensitization of the primary afferents in response to inflammatory mediators such as bradykinin, histamine, nerve growth factor (NGF), interleukins, cytokines, and adenosine triphosphate (from dying cells), among others. The neuronal response establishes a feed-forward loop with release of neurokinins (i.e., substance P) that triggers

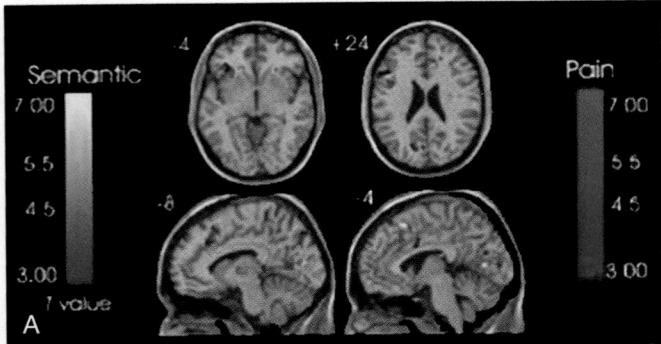

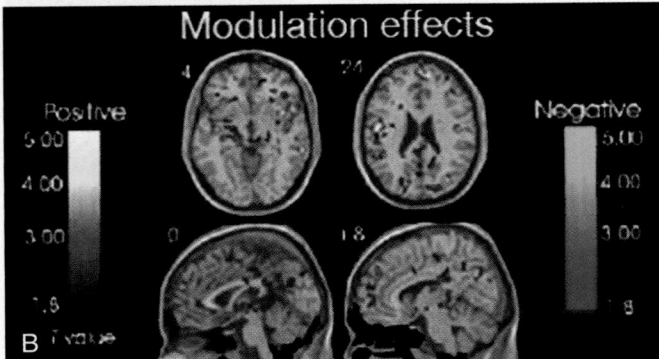

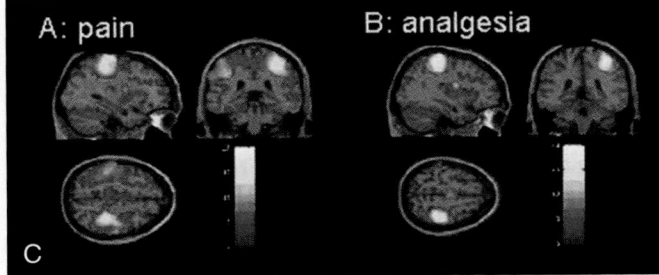

FIGURE 244-2   Functional magnetic resonance images illustrating central nervous system activity in different settings: in pain (**A** or *blue*) and modulated by analgesics (**B**) or distraction (*red*). *(From Tracey I. Functional connectivity and pain: How effectively connected is your brain? Pain 2005;116:173-174.)*

depolarization of the primary afferent. The overall effect is a reduced threshold for primary afferent depolarization and increased input to the dorsal horn.[7] Within the dorsal horn, activation of non-neuronal cells, glia and astrocytes, is essential for initiation and maintenance of central neuronal activation. Neuronal–non-neuronal communication is intricate and frequently relies on chemokines and interleukin production. In inflammatory pain there is increased cyclooxygenase 2 (COX-2) activity both peripherally and centrally. Inflammatory pain has inbuilt inhibitory loops with the coactivation of peripheral and central opioid receptors, which allows effective termination if the inflammatory stimuli are removed.

RECENT DEVELOPMENTS

Cancer-Induced Pain

Despite the clinical prevalence of visceral pain, there are few models of cancer-induced visceral pain. Indeed, even non–cancer-related visceral pain is only now being elucidated. A major problem for any animal model of cancer-induced pain is well-being of the animals. Systemic cancer or chemotherapy regimens often induce unacceptable side effects, and the pain behavior aspects are increasingly hard to interpret. More recent models of confined cancer growth within a bone or around a nerve allow detailed pathophysiology to be investigated in otherwise well animals.[8-10] The advent of animal models has revised our understanding of innervation of bone, and some unique analgesics have been developed. In therapeutic terms, animal models appear to have validity,[11] although drug efficacy is often at a lower scale when examined in humans.

Cancer-Induced Bone Pain

There are numerous models of cancer-induced bone pain, all following initial work in a mouse sarcoma model, which demonstrated evolving pain behavior and bone destruction after controlled inoculation and growth in the mouse femur.[8] The model closely parallels the clinical situation of radiologically obvious damage resulting in a pathological fracture and subsequent pain behavior of limping, limb guarding, and tenderness (Fig. 244-4). Further work established the presence of C fibers (in particular, peptidergic substance P, TrkA positive) traversing the bone trabeculae to the marrow. Nociceptive primary afferents could be triggered without periosteal damage. As the cancer invades and grows within the marrow, it induces a profound inflammatory response and activation of the osteoclast/osteoblast axis. The result is progressive bone destruction, aberrant bone remodeling, cell death, inflammation, and primary afferent destruction.[12] Triggers of primary afferents are a combination of inflammation and neuropathy occurring simultaneously. In addition, investigation of dorsal horn neuronal responses in a rat model of breast cancer (Fig. 244-5) indicated hyperalgesia different from that in neuropathic or inflammatory pain. Superficial lamina I neurons were hyperexcitable with an alteration in reactivity such that 50% of neurons now reacted to non-noxious and noxious stimuli versus only 25% in normal animals without cancer. Immunocytochemistry also suggested a unique combination of neuroreceptor activity consisting of activated glia, raised dynorphin, but a notable lack of the changes expected in neuropathic (raised NYP, galanin, etc.) or inflammatory (raised calcitonin gene–related peptide [CGRP], etc.) pain states.[8]

Attenuation of cancer-induced bone pain has been demonstrated with conventional analgesics such as opioids, albeit at doses more akin to neuropathy models, and with neuropathic agents such as gabapentin. In addition, novel targets of inhibition of bone turnover (i.e., osteoprotegerin), blocking of peripheral NGF (inflammatory) via TrkA receptor sequestering, or antagonism of the endothelin-A receptor (key in cancer cell spread and a primary afferent receptor) all significantly reduce pain behavior in animal models and in some clinical studies.

Cancer and Chemotherapy-Induced Neuropathy

Neuropathic pain in cancer patients may arise from physical compression of a nerve by the tumor or direct infiltra-

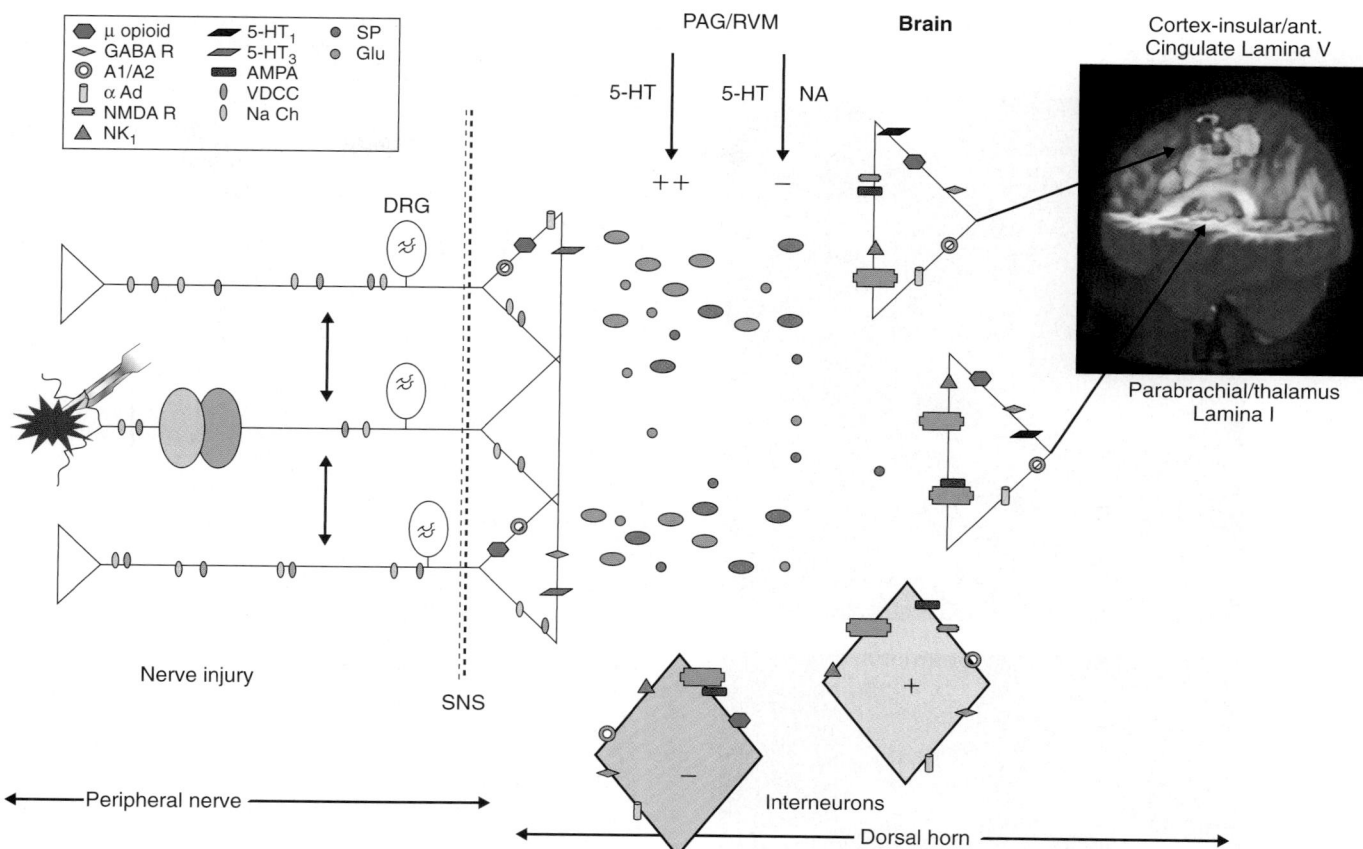

FIGURE 244-3 The same simplified diagram as in Figure 244-1 summarizes changes in the peripheral and central neuronal pathways after peripheral nerve injury (nerve transection shown) resulting in chronic neuropathy. In the periphery, the nerve distal to the injury dies and regenerates in an abnormal manner. The sodium (Na Ch) and calcium (VDCC) channels are altered in expression (more responsive) and number (increase, particularly around the area of damage). Aberrant transmission in the damaged nerve led to spontaneous discharge and epiphatic crosstalk between damaged and undamaged neurons and between the dorsal root ganglion (DRG) and sympathetic nervous system (SNS). This increases the receptive field size and spontaneous and lower-threshold discharge of neurons and can lead to aberrant excitation of the SNS. Within the dorsal horn, glutamate (Glu) and substance P (SP) are released in increased and irregular amounts (not necessarily in response to a threshold stimuli), although there may be reduced or absent release in the damaged neuron termination. Increased excitatory amino acid release results in overall excitation of the interneurons and increased transmission to the brain. Such excitation is enhanced by a reduction in inhibition by the loss of GABAergic neurons, relative inactivation of μ-opioid receptors, and facilitation of descending serotonin–5-HT$_3$ excitation pathways.

tion into the nerve, or it can be secondary to changed tissue pH (acidosis) or release of chemical algogens by the tumor, either in areas around the nerve or directly in the nerve itself after tumor infiltration. Paradoxically, neuropathy can also arise from cancer-directed therapy, either chemotherapy, radiotherapy, or surgery. Drugs such as paclitaxel, vincristine, and cisplatin produce sensory neuropathy and evoke tingling sensations, paresthesias, or numbness in the distal ends of the extremities, consistent with a glove-and-stocking distribution.

Despite a wide range of rodent neuropathy models, there are few animal models of cancer-related nerve damage. Of these, the most widely studied involve chemotherapy agents (e.g., taxol, platins) or inoculation of tumor cells adjacent to peripheral nerves (e.g., sarcoma, mammary carcinoma). In all models animals are often generally unwell. Although the originating source of pain may differ between malignant (e.g., tumor compression) and nonmalignant (diabetic neuropathy) neuropathic pain, the mechanisms and neural pathways involved in the pain state are similar, and much of the underlying pathology can be

inferred from mechanisms operating in nonmalignant neuropathic pain. For example, inoculation of Meth-A sarcoma cells in the vicinity of the mouse sciatic nerve results in growth of a tumor mass embedding the nerve.[13] Pain behavior reaches a maximum by 3 weeks after inoculation, at which time clear histological signs of nerve damage can be identified. Further immunohistochemical analysis reveals enhanced spinal expression of c-fos (a marker of neuronal activation) and neuropeptides (e.g., substance P, CGRP, dynorphin A), thus indicating enhanced pain transmission within nociceptive circuits, consistent with the behavioral findings. There is a gradual decline in pain behavior and the subsequent appearance of hyposensitivity, which may correspond to progressive motor paralysis in the animals. Evidence of nerve damage and neural infiltration by immune and malignant cells (with mild edema) suggests involvement of neuropathic and inflammatory processes in cancer-induced pain, thus highlighting the complex pathology. Models of chemotherapy-induced neuropathy are more common and indicate novel mechanisms for neuropathic pain; however, such models have

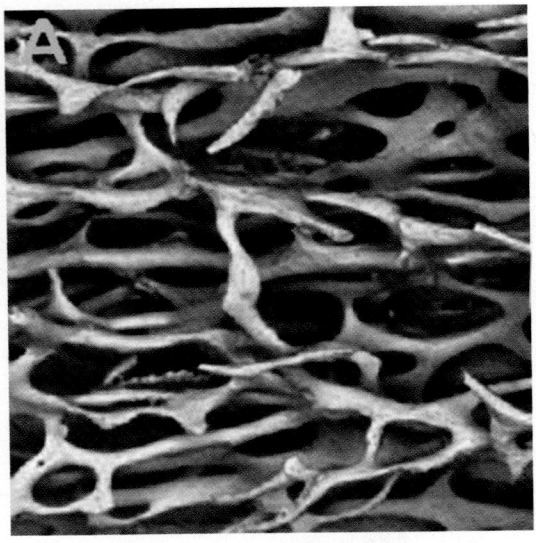

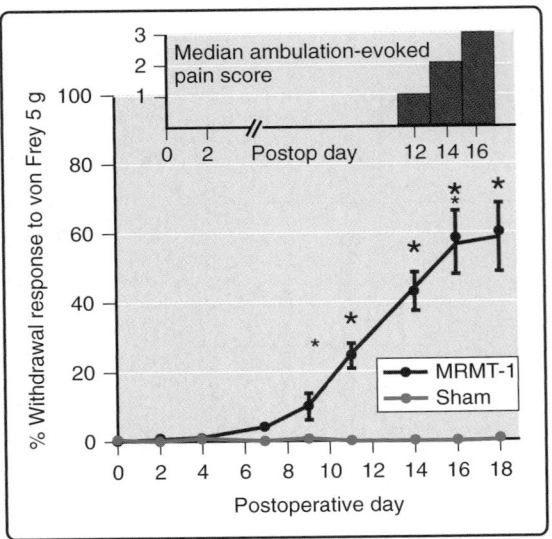

The development of mechanical hyperalgesia over time after intratibial injection of MRMT-1 (breast cancer cells)

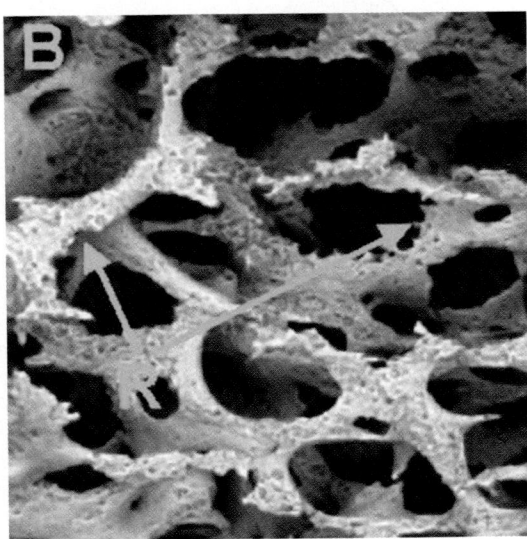

FIGURE 244-4 Radiological and behavioral changes that occur in the rat MRMT-1 model of cancer-induced bone pain (CIBP). **A,** Scanning electron micrograph of normal tibial trabeculated bone (day 0). **B,** The same bone at day 17 after injection of MRMT-1 cancer cells. The trabeculated bone is "moth-eaten" by osteoclasts and its fine structure destroyed. The graph demonstrates the behavioral changes seen after injection of MRMT-1. On the *lower* graph, the sham-injected animals remain entirely normal in response to mechanical stimuli (5-g stimulation with a von Frey filament); in contrast, the animals injected with MRMT-1 exhibit an increasing response, starting at day 9 after injection (not significant) and increasing daily until day 18 (end of the experiment). The difference in response is highly significant ($P < .0001$) by day 13 (*t* test) in the pooled number of animals at each time point 12. The *bar graph* above demonstrates another behavioral sign in the group injected with MRMT-1 only—the mean ambulatory score. From day 12 the CIBP group exhibited increased limping and then guarding of the injected tibia, which is scored 0 to 3 (increasing severity). The development of limping and ambulatory pain behavior mirrors the development of von Frey hyperalgesia. *(From Urch CE, Donovan-Rodriguez T, Gordon-Williams R, et al. Efficacy of chronic morphine in a rat model of cancer-induced bone pain: Behavior and dorsal horn pathophysiology. J Pain 2005;6:837-845.)*

difficulty reproducing the anesthesia with hyperalgesia seen in humans. In a rat model of taxol-induced neuropathy, the rat sciatic nerves revealed marked microtubular aggregation within axons, which appears to be the primary target site of this drug.[14] This interferes with microtubule dynamics by arresting cellular division and engaging apoptosis. Taxol accumulates in peripheral nerves and dorsal root ganglia.[15] In addition, neuroimmune reactions are evoked upon release of pro-inflammatory cytokines (e.g., tumor necrosis factor-α, interleukin-6). It may be that neuroimmune responses underlie the flulike symptoms experienced after therapy with taxol and could contribute to the sensory neuropathy.

Visceral Pain

There has been an increase in our understanding of visceral neurons and central processing of visceral pain. Clinical management, however, remains difficult and

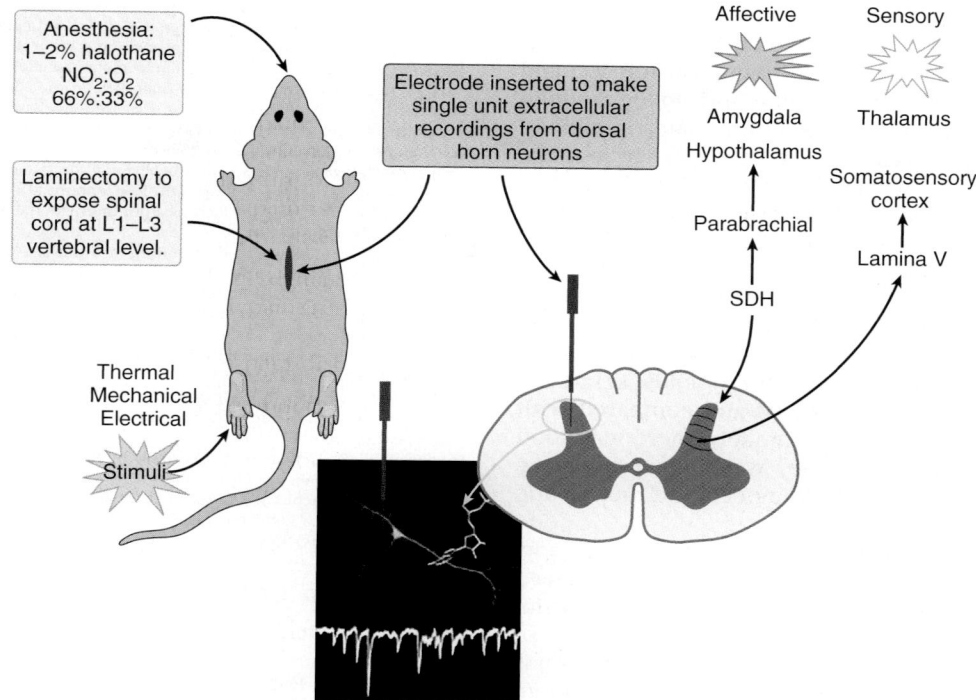

FIGURE 244-5 Experimental scheme for dorsal horn neuronal recordings from the exposed lumbar spinal cord (insertion point at the L2-L4 nerve roots). The diagram illustrates an electrode recording a single neuron (*lower panel*) in the superficial dorsal horn (enlarged section of the dorsal horn). These recordings allow differentiation between neurons by their electrical threshold (Aβ, Aδ, and C fibers) and their responses to noxious or non-noxious stimuli (applied to the dorsum of the ipsilateral hind paw). The ascending pathways from the dorsal horn are schematically shown to illustrate the integrative nature of these in vivo recordings.

unchanged.[16] Visceral pain is diffuse in nature, may be referred, and is difficult to locate, unlike somatic pain. Visceral afferents represent 10% of all spinal afferent input. They are found throughout the spinal cord and synapse with second-order neurons over several segments, which in turn receive input from several visceral and nonvisceral afferents. Each organ is innervated by two neural pathways, typically the vagus and spinal or pelvic and spinal nerve. Most visceral input is not consciously perceived; conscious perception is associated with a negative affective component of discomfort or pain. The nociceptive role of the vagus is poorly understood but appears to be predominately chemosensitive.

It is the high-threshold mechanosensitization that produces an adversive sensation. Five different classes of mechanoreceptors were identified in the lumbar spinal and pelvic nerves. Chemosensitivity has been less well studied, but it is well established that proton exposure can cause an adverse or painful response but nutrient exposure typically does not. The visceral sensory soma in the dorsal root ganglion and the more numerous (up to 80%) silent visceral nociceptors (coupled with different innovation pathways) make a more complex nociceptive pathway. From animal knockout work it appears that the acid-sensing ion channel 3 (ASIC3) is critical to mechanosensitivity in the colon whereas ASIC2 contributes an inhibitory or facilitatory function, depending on the class of neurons. In contrast to skin afferents, low-threshold mechanoreceptors also become sensitized and provide a significant increase in spinal cord input in certain conditions (e.g., inflammation).

One model of visceral cancer involves the ApcΔ716 mouse line.[17] In heterozygous mice with mutations in the gene encoding APC (adenomatous polyposis coli), multiple polyps developed spontaneously in the intestinal tract 3 weeks postnatally, thereby offering pharmacological evaluation of compounds such as COX-2 inhibitors[17] and validating it as a potential mouse model of colon cancer. The development of pain behavior in this animal model has not been reported. Further studies will assess whether such a model can be used to study cancer-induced visceral pain.

RESEARCH CHALLENGES AND ADVANCES

It is acknowledged that animal models will at best give only part of the whole story, are limited in time (most models run over a period of days or weeks, not months and years as in humans), and are unable to give higher center perceptions of suffering. Over the last 50 years animal models have allowed the exploration and interpretation of pain mechanisms, pathophysiology, and new drugs. Until a decade ago, cancer-induced bone pain was acknowledged by only a few clinicians to be a significant problem, and there was virtually no understanding of the pain mechanism. Now, with relevant animal models, the unique pathophysiology is being explored, and clinically relevant therapeutic targets are being identified for use in trials. The small but growing number of specific cancer-related animal models will shed light on previously unexplored or clinically dismissed pain states.

One common question is "just how translatable are animal model results"? Indirect evidence suggests that animal models and mechanisms of pain transmission and alteration have shaped our teaching and understanding. Relevant receptors, neurotransmitters, and modifying drugs in animals have relevance in humans. The correlation is not absolute, however, as development of the NK_1 receptor antagonists testify. In mouse models they were found to be potent analgesics but in humans, not at all (although they are good antiemetics). The reason is that humans have NK_2 and NK_3 receptors that become upregulated when the NK_1 receptor is blocked, thus nullifying the effect. In contrast, when the clinical efficacy of analgesics (e.g., amitriptyline, gabapentin, opioids, ketamine, and carbamazepine) were reviewed and compared with the efficacy predicted by animal models, there was good correlation (albeit clinical efficacy was lower), thus suggesting face value validity of both models and therapeutic development.[11]

The challenge is to make animal models clinically relevant (such as the chemotherapeutic models discussed earlier[14]), expand into difficult areas such as visceral pain, and develop an understanding of the neural networks of the central nervous system. The basic science paradigm is often reductionist and looks for a single genetic variation; however, in pain this is balanced by the need to examine these changes within a whole organism, thereby linking the molecular to the network. Enthusiasm and wonder at the results must be tempered with caution about direct clinical translation. The challenge is to raise the awareness of clinical pain states and improve diagnostics to take advantage of new clinical research from work in animal models. Alongside is the secondary issue of ensuring good analgesia, which becomes as important as disease-modifying therapies.

CONCLUSIONS

Cancer pain, despite using the same basic mechanisms of pain transmission, transduction, neurotransmitters, and receptors, is a complex pain syndrome. The multiplicity of inducers means that it is rarely a pure neuropathic, inflammatory, or visceral pain. Rather, cancer pain is unique in being the essence of interactions, modulations, and interplay from each. The ever-changing stimuli lead to complex reemergence of pain, alterations in pain balance (e.g., from visceral to neuropathic), and consequently, complex polypharmacy and non–drug-related interventions. Extrapolation from noncancer pain physiology is possible, but further work is needed to elucidate which aspects of cancer-induced pain are indeed unique.

REFERENCES

1. Besson JM. The neurobiology of pain. Lancet 1999;353:1610-1615.
2. Carpenter KJ, Dickenson AH. Molecular aspects of pain research. Pharmacogenomics J 2002;2:87-95.
3. Suzuki R, Rygh LJ, Dickenson AH. Bad news from the brain: Descending 5-HT pathways that control spinal pain processing. Trends Pharmacol Sci 2004;25:613-617.
4. Suzuki R, Dickenson AH. Neuropathic pain: Nerves bursting with excitement. Neuroreport 2000;11(12):R17-R21.
5. Bridges D, Thompson SW, Rice AS. Mechanisms of neuropathic pain. Br J Anaesth 2001;87:12-26.
6. Tracey I. Functional connectivity and pain: How effectively connected is your brain? Pain 2005;116:173-174.
7. Dickenson AH. Central acute pain mechanisms. Ann Med 1995;27:223-227.
8. Honore P, Schwei J, Rogers SD, et al. Cellular and neurochemical remodeling of the spinal cord in bone cancer pain. Prog Brain Res 2000;129:389-397.
9. Urch CE, Dickenson AH. In vivo single unit extracellular recordings from spinal cord neurones of rats. Brain Res Brain Res Protoc 2003;12:26-34.
10. Asai H, Ozaki N, Shinoda M, et al. Heat and mechanical hyperalgesia in mice model of cancer pain. Pain 2005;117:19-29.
11. Kontinen VA, Meert TF. Predictive validity of neuropathic pain models in pharmacological studies with a behavioural outcome in the rat: A systematic review. In Dotrovsky JO, Carr DB, Koltzenburg M (eds). Proceedings of the 10th World Congress on Pain. Seattle: International Association for Study of Pain, 2003, pp 489-498.
12. Mantyh PW, Clohisy DR, Koltzenburg M, Hunt SP. Molecular mechanisms of cancer pain. Nat Rev Cancer 2002;2:201-209.
13. Shimoyama M, Tanaka K, Hasue F, Shimoyama N. A mouse model of neuropathic cancer pain. Pain 2002;99:167-174.
14. Flatters SJ, Bennett GJ. Studies of peripheral sensory nerves in paclitaxel-induced painful peripheral neuropathy: Evidence for mitochondrial dysfunction. Pain 2006;122:245-257.
15. Cavaletti G, Cavalletti E, Oggioni N, et al. Distribution of paclitaxel within the nervous system of the rat after repeated intravenous administration. Neurotoxicology 2000;21:389-393.
16. Bielefeldt K, Gebhart GF. Textbook of Pain, 5th ed. Edinburgh: Churchill-Livingstone, 2005.
17. Oshima M, Dinchuk JE, Kargman SL, et al. Suppression of intestinal polyposis in Apc delta716 knockout mice by inhibition of cyclooxygenase 2 (COX-2). Cell 1996;87:803-809.

SUGGESTED READING

Marples IL, Murray P. Neuropathic pain. Lancet 1999;354:953-954.

Mercadante S, Portenoy RK. Opioid poorly-responsive cancer pain. Part 2: Basic mechanisms that could shift dose response for analgesia. J Pain Symptom Manage 2000;21:255-264.

Watkins LR, Maier SF. Beyond neurons: Evidence that immune and glial cells contribute to pathological pain states. Physiol Rev 2002;82:981-1011.

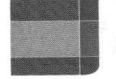

CHAPTER **245**

Psychological and Psychiatric Approaches

Holly Covington

KEY POINTS

- The perception of and response to pain is influenced by thought (cognition), mood (affect), and behavior, in addition to physiological factors.

- Early intervention to change distorted or automatic perceptions and thoughts about the pain experience can promote positive coping patterns.

- Cognitive-behavioral interventions can promote a sense of control over the pain experience.

- Inclusion of the family in early intervention will provide them with skills to help the individual with cancer manage pain toward the end of life.

- Various cognitive-behavioral techniques, along with pharmacological intervention, constitute a comprehensive approach to the management of cancer pain.

The experience of cancer pain has an impact on patients at many levels. Individuals with cancer will exhibit physical, cognitive, and emotional responses and behavioral coping. They come to treatment of cancer with many preconceived notions about pain and its management, and previous pain experiences will have a significant impact on their emotional and mental state. Based on previous cognitive awareness or understanding, the individual will bring coping skills and behavior to the illness experience that may be ineffective or inappropriate and actually self-destructive. Difficult behavior that stems from an individual's ineffective coping in response to the illness and pain experience can threaten crucial family and therapeutic relationships during a most difficult life crisis (see Chapter 8, 9, and 244).

THEORY

The Importance of Perception and the Meaning of Illness

The term "meaning" describes a central idea in several coping theories relevant to practice.[1] A cancer patient's search for meaning is a phenomenon that has gained increased attention.[2] The multidimensional process of a search for meaning in any experience involves psychological, physical, behavioral, and existential components.[3,4]

The search for meaning initially requires awareness and recognition of the event as having meaning to the individual. Situational meaning has an intrapersonal and interpersonal dimension important at the onset of a threatening event such as the diagnosis of cancer.[5] The individual gives meaning to an event as either stressful or nonstressful. Meaning is assigned as the individual assesses the experience and becomes increasingly aware or recognizes the event as important or significant.

Increased awareness releases neurotransmitters within neurocognitive networks that modulate cognition (thinking) and emotion (mood/affect). Attention, memory, and perception of past events and experiences influence thoughts (cognition) and mood (affect/emotion). Thought and mood are influenced by perception of an experience as threatening or nonthreatening based on past experience.

Physiological responses result as the individual experiences a real or perceived physical or psychological threat. Physiological threat responses involve an increase in heart rate, respiratory rate, and blood pressure. Psychological and behavioral responses are based on the meaning given to the experience event. If perceived as threatening, such as pain, individuals may respond with increased anxiety and fear. Ways of coping with the anxiety and fear of the pain experience are manifested as either effective or ineffective behavior. Some behavioral responses can be self-destructive.

Existential meaning involves a pervasive process in an individual's experience of humanness. A search for meaning in illness is an existential process to understand the current situation as it relates to one's past life and restore a sense of life order. How an individual works through this process influences and is influenced by cognitive, affective, and behavioral factors. Once understood, these factors can help the individual cope or deal with the experience positively.

The experience of pain is different for everyone, and the clinician must form a therapeutic relationship to understand each individual's cognitive, affective, and behavioral patterns. The clinician's role[6] is to create an environment that facilitates discussion about the meaning of the cancer experience. Caring presence[7] is a way of being in a relationship that involves mutual trust and sharing, transcending connectedness, and metaphysical experience. Caring presence may be one context for patients to express vulnerability and existential suffering as they search for meaning. The caring presence can provide a safe place for patients to share sensitive emotional issues or situations and to search for meaning in their cancer experience. The therapeutic relationship is an important tool in cognitive and behavioral interventions (see Case Study).

 CASE STUDY

Helen is a 52-year-old woman who was married and had no children. She lived in New York during the school year and worked as a college professor. She came home to a very small rural community, where she lived with her husband and dogs in the summer. I met her in an oncology clinic in which I worked as a nurse practitioner. She came with her husband for the first cancer treatment after a recent diagnose of multiple myeloma. She was experiencing chronic right leg and hip pain and initially had adequate pain management with opioids and antidepressants. We formed a relationship and, over time, seemed to be able to talk freely and openly about her illness, her symptoms, and possible ways to cope with the ongoing pain.

She was essentially a very warm and positive woman. When she first started coming in for treatment, her mood was fairly bright. We would talk and laugh as she made jokes or tell stories about work in New York. She had an amazing outlook on life and I loved to listen to her stories. I found her very easy to work with. We met on a regular basis to talk about how she was managing emotionally, as well as physically. She was articulate and knowledgeable about her health care needs. An open, trusting therapeutic relationship was key for Helen to feel comfortable and safe enough to talk about anything or share important sensitive personal and emotional issues. Helen expressed to me that she felt as though she were heard and understood as we worked within a nonjudgmental and therapeutic relationship of trust and caring presence. Cognitive restructuring was used during that time as an important intervention to help Helen deal with depression, negative thinking and destructive self-talk.

As her disease progressed and she started to complain of increasingly unmanageable bone pain, the staff noticed that she was becoming more and more irritable and short-tempered. She didn't want to talk about New York; in fact, it was difficult for her to talk about anything positive. She would lash out at the nurses and soon became labeled as "a difficult patient." Interventions were planned that would help Helen with the maladaptive pain behavior that had developed over time.

Beliefs and Meaning

Expert clinicians describe the concept of beliefs as being central to understanding and working with both individuals and families.[8,9] This idea is not new to clinical practice. Challenging dysfunctional beliefs and enhancing facilitative beliefs have long been at the core of cognitive restructuring therapy.[10] The search for meaning helps the adaptation process in persons with recurrent cancer.[11] Effort to understand a cancer patient's search for meaning involves talking about the meaning and purpose that the individual gives the experience and the impact that it has within a total life pattern. This integration involves reworking and redefining past meanings while simultaneously looking for meaning in the current life situation.

Past experiences are also strong determinants of how individuals respond to an illness event. Certain factors will influence both specific beliefs and the meaning that individuals attribute to events as they occur. Specifically for cancer, histories that are heard or past experiences of success or failure with the illness will influence both cognitive structures and emotional responses to diagnosis of disease. The timing of crises in the individual and family life cycle will affect the meaning of an event. Serious illness may be expected in late adulthood, and anticipation of death is a normative, universal experience. Off-time events, such as the death of a child with cancer, do not fit prevailing beliefs about the expected life trajectory and its meaning. Such events challenge existing beliefs, people's views of the controllability of life, and their ability to handle the situation.

The Pain Experience

The pain experience is multifactorial and involves psychological and behavioral components. The overall approach to management of cancer pain must include interventions that help the individual modify that overall experience to improve function at the end of life. Three intricate systems work together to produce the experience of pain:

The sensory/discriminative system
The motivational/affective system
The cognitive/evaluative system[12]

The first two are internal, whereas the third is external (Table 245-1). The sensory/discriminative system involves the part of the brain that processes pain. The motivational/affective system involves the brain area where learned responses to approaching or avoiding pain are processed. The cognitive/evaluative system incorporates the individual's experience and interpretation of pain influenced by external stimuli. The first system is primarily the focus for drugs. The second and third are the focus of cognitive and behavioral interventions that have an impact on or influence the individual's cancer pain experience. These systems can help the individual develop adaptive responses that promote positive lifestyle changes in response to the cancer pain experience.

Psychological Theory

Cognitive Theory

Cognitive therapy is based on assumptions that an individual's mood is determined by how that individual understands or views the world. The perception of pain and the thoughts and images that one has about pain have an influence on mood and behavior. The pain experience is an active process that involves internal and external stimuli. Cognitive therapy consists of four processes that help an individual develop alternative cognitive and behavioral responses (Table 245-2).[13]

Behavioral Theory

Behavioral theorists assume that behavior is the product of learning. Individuals can change their behavior based on new learning and generate changes within their environment. Clinical application of behavioral therapy is based on the conceptual view that behavior is learned and can be controlled.[14] Accordingly, an individual in pain can be taught active self-management techniques that promote self-control and ability to function in daily life. For someone with cancer pain, learning new ways to cope and deal with the pain means a potential change in the internal physical environment (the body) and an altered pain experience (see Table 245-2).

INTERVENTIONS

Cognitive Techniques

To use cognitive techniques (Table 245-3), the individual must understand the processes of cognitive therapy. The

---

TABLE 245-1 Neurological Systems That Produce Pain

INTERNAL STIMULI
Sensory/discriminative system
   Afferent fibers in the brainstem, spinal cord, and higher brain centers
Motivational/affective system
   Reticular formation, limbic system, brainstem

EXTERNAL STIMULI
Cognitive/evaluative system
   Family, culture, environment
   Individual's perception

TABLE 245-2 Cognitive Therapy Processes

PROCESS OF COGNITIVE THERAPY	EXAMPLES
Automatic thought	"Since I have cancer, I will experience unbearable pain that I can't control"
Testing thought	Help the patient examine the perceptions of pain; discuss what thoughts are exaggerations or might be inaccurate
Identifying maladaptive assumptions	Help the patient identify past patterns of behavior related to how the individual dealt or coped with the experience of pain
Testing accuracy of assumptions	Challenge the patient about thinking that the worst will always happen
Changing behavior	Discuss alternative behavioral patterns that will help the patient learn new ways of coping with the pain

clinician educates individuals about dealing with negative thinking and negative self-talk. As the interventions move toward cognitive restructuring, an explanation about the relationship between thoughts, feelings, and behavior is key. Behavioral interventions test changes in perception or responsiveness toward learning new strategies and ways of dealing with pain.[15] In addition, individuals can be helped to recognize any ineffective coping patterns from past pain experiences.

Helping the patient either visualize pain or compartmentalize the pain experience to change negative thinking may be necessary early in treatment. Helping individuals understand thought distortions, or automatic thoughts, as they relate to their worldview is key to cognitive work. Asking patients to describe evidence to support or refute their automatic thinking promotes encouragement of possible alternative viewpoints instead of focusing on the disability or illness. Teaching different thoughts, strategies, or techniques promotes a cognitive shift to provide a sense of control over the pain.

The clinician can first help the individual work through and understand automatic thoughts that involve any distortion or misrepresentation of the pain experience and the individual's emotional reaction to it. Once automatic thoughts are identified, the clinician can help the patient discard or reject an exaggeration or inaccuracy about the pain experience. In addition, it may be important to help patients recognize any ineffective patterns in past pain experiences. Once maladaptive patterns are identified, patients can develop more effective ways of regulating their pain (see Table 245-3).

Behavioral Techniques

People living with cancer pain may tend to hide or deny the pain so that life is "normal" or without the illness. Individuals may hide or deny pain because they do not want to be labeled a complainer. They usually want to keep up with others in shared activities. Denial may result from stress or fear about the pain experience and is predominantly based on past pain experiences. Trying to maintain pre-illness functioning could decrease energy stores and result in fatigue. These behavioral patterns may have developed over time and become maladaptive. Techniques or approaches to learn more adaptive measures include self-management, assertion training, and relaxation techniques (see Table 245-3).

It is imperative to assess the pain medication schedule with the patient to determine whether medication is being used for maximum effect. An individual may wait too long to take pain medication, which makes it more difficult to achieve pain control. Patients may be afraid of "becoming addicted" and not take pain medication when needed. It is important to educate patients about the importance of pain management. Education empowers them to develop a medication schedule based on time instead of need. With empowerment, more effective behavior patterns facilitate a sense of control over the pain.

Relaxation helps overcome the anxiety and fear related to the pain experience.[14] Past or present pain experience promotes anxiety and fear, which elicits a fight-or-flight response. Relaxation can produce physical responses opposite those induced by anxiety and fear. Progressive relaxation, mental or guided imagery, and deep breathing can promote physiological relaxation, reduce anxiety, and alleviate fear. Using relaxation techniques to reduce and alleviate anxiety and fear facilitates a sense of control over the pain experience.

Guided imagery can be powerful as a behavioral intervention and treatment modality. An individual takes in information from the world through the five senses. Sensory input travels to the limbic system, where images and thought, emotion, and primitive behavioral responses form.[12] Thoughts and images are formed in the individual's mind that influence the learned approach to pain avoidance behavior. These thoughts and images can also modulate the relaxation response and induce visible changes in the immune system that facilitate healing.

TABLE 245-3 Examples of Cognitive-Behavioral Techniques and Approaches

Assertion training—teaching people to express both positive and negative feelings or thoughts; positive affirmations

Self-management programs—psychoeducation and teaching the individual to take an active part in treatment; journaling thoughts and feelings

Relaxation methods
  Deep breathing
  Deep muscle relaxation
  Listening to music
  Guided or mental imagery
  Biofeedback

Systematic desensitization—reducing fear-based anxiety about pain by constructing a hierarchy of events leading to the feared situation

Reinforcement techniques—based on the principles of operant conditioning: emphasis is placed on the positive impact of relaxation, for example, or the reduction of pain

Modeling—group interventions and support to promote learning through observation and imitation

Cognitive restructuring—patient gains awareness of detrimental thought habits and learns to challenge them or substitute them with life-enhancing thoughts and beliefs

Thought stopping—inhibition of the unwanted (or irrational) thought that makes it difficult to concentrate on anything else or using distraction

Behavioral rehearsal—role-play anxiety-producing situations so that the individual can become more assertive and have an active voice in individualizing treatment

---

Common Errors

- Failure to assess individual and family current beliefs and meaning in the illness experience
- Assuming that patients will accept and are willing to use cognitive-behavioral approaches
- Waiting to implement cognitive interventions and behavioral education until pain is experienced
- Failure to include family and significant others in the cognitive-behavioral process
- Using cognitive-behavioral approaches as an alternative, as opposed to an adjunct to analgesics

RECENT DEVELOPMENTS

Cognitive-behavioral therapy (CBT) is supported by assumptions that a patient's beliefs and coping can be changed. Interventions help the individual understand and challenge false beliefs so that changes in behavior that promote positive health care outcomes can occur. Recent research reveals mixed results. Techniques such as education, relaxation, and exercise help individuals perceive the experience and gain a sense of control over pain.[14] Distracters such as relaxation, meditation, and guided imagery reduce pain intensity.[15,16] There are mixed results about the impact of CBT on pain intensity and longevity,[16] pain reduction, and mood distress.[17]

EVIDENCE-BASED MEDICINE

More research is needed on the effectiveness of psychoeducational treatments for individuals with cancer.[18] Evidence suggests that CBT and behavioral approaches are effective for cancer pain.[19,20] Relaxation-based interventions have been prevalent in the past. Cognitive restructuring, problem solving, and goal setting can reduce the experience of pain. CBT should be undertaken in conjunction with the use of analgesics. Cognitive-coping skills training can help debunk myths about the use of pain medication, including myths about tolerance and addiction.

RESEARCH CHALLENGES/OPPORTUNITIES

- Research on the relationship between CBT, the pain experience, and affective distress requires more attention.
- Assessment of the perception of pain and cognitive or behavioral interventions based on that perception spring from the theory about this process being multidimensional. This concept is essential to understanding how one perceives pain.
- A multidimensional process incorporating cognitive and behavioral interventions can restructure an individual's perceptions of pain.
- Examining the commonalities between an individual's beliefs, assumptions of the pain experience (cognitive assumptions), and pain behavior is an ongoing research challenge.
- Assisting the individual in this search may identify cognitive distortions, or automatic thoughts, that interfere with alleviation of suffering.
- Attention to individual psychophysiological characteristics is important for treatment plans that include CBT.
- Tailoring CBT to an individual's characteristics helps in coping with the experience, improves the individual's ability to engage in activities, and decreases symptom distress.[19]
- Finding time points when the individual is not overly fatigued and is consciously able to participate in therapy is a challenge.
- Important factors in the palliative setting include teaching coping skills before the onset of significant pain and how well an individual is able to focus on surrounding events toward the end of life. Teaching an individual early in the illness is another challenging factor in the use of CBT.
- Research should examine the effectiveness of cognitive behavioral interventions in advance cancer and palliative care.

CONCLUSIONS

Although cognitive-behavioral interventions are useful in early disease, more research is needed in advanced cancer and palliative care.[19] A patient with cancer[5] may draw on self-meaning and contextual meaning to bring coherence to life in the face of loss, change, and upheaval. When people experience an existential/spiritual crisis and search for meaning in the diagnosis of cancer, alleviation of suffering can come with a feeling of connection and inner peace. Clinically, we must remind ourselves to be authentically there with the individual in a relationship in which open communication and sharing promote understanding of the meaning of the pain experience. This approach will guide the use of cognitive and behavioral therapies to promote health within illness.

REFERENCES

1. Lazarus RS, Folkman S. Stress, Appraisal, and Coping. New York: Springer, 1984.
2. Luker KA, Beaver K, Leinster SJ, et al. Meaning of illness for women with breast cancer. J Adv Nurs 1996;23:1194-1202.
3. Greenstein M. The house that's on fire: Meaning-centered psychiatric treatment: A pilot study group for cancer patients. Am J Psychother 2000;54:501-512.
4. Mellon S. Comparisons between cancer survivors and family members on meaning of the illness and family quality of life. Oncol Nurs Forum 2002;29:1117-1125.
5. Fife B. The measurement of meaning in illness. Soc Sci Med 1995;40:1021-1028.
6. Richer M, Ezer H. Understanding beliefs and meaning in the experience of cancer: A concept analysis. J Adv Nurs 2000;32:1108-1115.
7. Covington H. Caring Presence: A Journey Toward a Mutual Goal [unpublished doctoral dissertation]. Denver, CO: University of Colorado Health Sciences Center, 2002.
8. Wright LM, Watson WL, Bell JM. Beliefs: The Heart of Healing in Families and Illness. New York: Basic Books, 1996.
9. Wright KB. Professional, ethical, and legal implications for spiritual care in nursing. J Nurs Schol 1996;30:81-83.
10. Beck AT, Ruch AJ, Shaw BF, et al: Cognitive Therapy of Depression. New York: Guilford Press: 1979.
11. Taylor EJ. Whys and wherefores: Adult patient perspective of the meaning of cancer. Semin Oncol Nurs 1995;11:32-40.
12. McCance KL, Huether SU (eds). Pathophysiology: The Biological Basis for Disease in Adults & Children, 4th ed. St Louis: CV Mosby, 2002.
13. Sadock BJ, Sadock VS. Kaplan & Sadock's Synopsis of Psychiatry: Behavioral Sciences/Clinical Psychiatry, 9th ed. Philadelphia: Lippincott Williams & Wilkins, 2003.
14. Turner JA, Holtzman S, Manci L. Mediators, moderators, and predictors of therapeutic change in cognitive-behavioral therapy for chronic pain. Pain 2007;127:276-286.
15. Robb KA, Williams JE, Duvivier V, et al. A pain management program for chronic cancer-treatment–related pain: A preliminary study. J Pain 2006;7:82-90.
16. Arathuzik D. Effects of cognitive-behavioral strategies on pain in cancer patients. Cancer Nurs 1994;17:207-214.
17. Tatrow K, Montgomery GH. Cognitive behavioral therapy techniques for distress and pain in breast cancer patients: A meta-analysis. J Behav Med 2006;29:17-27.
18. Devine CE. Meta-Analysis of the effect of psychoeducational interventions of pain in adults with cancer. Oncol Nurs Forum 2003;30:75-89.
19. Sherwood P, Given BA, Given CW, et al. A cognitive behavioral intervention for symptom management for patients with advanced cancer. Oncol Nurs Forum 2007;32:1190-1198.
20. Dalton JA, Keefe FJ, Carlson J, et al. Tailoring cognitive-behavioral treatment for cancer pain. Pain Manage Nurs 2004;3:3-18.

SUGGESTED READING

Breitbart W, Holland JC (eds). Psychiatric Aspects of Symptoms Management in Cancer Patients. Washington, DC: American Psychiatric Press, 1993.

Miaskowski C, Clear J, Burner R, et al. Guideline for the Management of Cancer Pain in Adults and Children. Glenview, IL: American Pain Society, 2005.

Sadock BJ, Sadock VS. Kaplan & Sadock's Synopsis of Psychiatry: Behavioral Sciences/Clinical Psychiatry, 9th ed. Philadelphia: Lippincott Williams & Wilkins, 2003.

CHAPTER **246**

Rehabilitation Approaches

Adrian Tookman and Jane Eades

KEY POINTS

- Cancer is a chronic illness and survivors may have disability.

- Services are not well equipped to deal with the issues of survivorship.

- Specialist palliative care skills are transferable to patients with rehabilitation needs.

- A well-functioning team is fundamental to a coordinated approach for effective rehabilitation.

- Noncancer patients can benefit from this approach.

- This chapter uses a broad definition of "family" in line with the United Kingdom's National Institute of Clinical Effectiveness (NICE) guidance, "including those related through committed heterosexual or same sex partnerships, birth and adoption, and others who have strong emotional and social bonds with a patient."

There have been considerable advances in oncology and palliative care. Improvements in diagnostics and treatment have led to earlier diagnosis and have had a significant influence in improving prognosis.[1,2] For a large proportion of patients, cancer is now a chronic rather than an acute illness. However, patients currently have to face multiple courses of complicated multimodality treatment; the impact of such demanding regimens has both an emotional and a physical impact on patients, and for many this results in long-term disability.

Patients now have to live with their cancer and survive with a chronic illness and its consequences. The challenge for health care professionals is to respond to the complex needs of these patients and support them throughout their cancer journey. To achieve this goal requires a paradigm shift for palliative care; we must now actively engage in the growing diversity of issues faced by patients with life-threatening illness, and the specialty has to be resilient enough to fully engage in caring for all patients with these complex needs. This will require reassessment of patient needs and an approach to delivery of services that is proactive rather than reactive. Palliative care is now an established and integral part of health care, and to maintain this

position it must recognize changing needs and respond to them—to ignore this would be detrimental to the future of the specialty and certainly not be in the best interests of patients and their families.[1,2] If palliative care does not fully embrace its responsibilities to be a full and active participant in health care, it will once again suffer loss of status and once more become relegated to a "Cinderella specialty."

A number of enlightened palliative care services have already adopted a proactive stance to managing the concurrent physical and emotional difficulties associated with progressive illness. These services use a rehabilitative approach. There is growing awareness of the suitability and value of the approach to support people who are living with cancer and surviving with disability.

Rehabilitation of cancer patients and others with advanced progressive noncancer conditions is an area in which palliative care must establish its role and define its patient population. Not only do we need to be an active participant in rehabilitative services, but we should also empower other services to assess the rehabilitative needs of patients with advanced illness. This is a significant challenge because many palliative care clinicians believe that rehabilitation is not a component of specialist palliative care. Indeed, it has been suggested that a rehabilitative approach may be detrimental to care by offering false hope and unrealistic expectations. To fully understand the potential of rehabilitation in patients with advanced and progressive illness it must be seen in the correct context. This requires practitioners to understand the key domains of the approach and develop appropriate skills.

REHABILITATION—A NEW PARADIGM FOR PALLIATIVE CARE?

To assume a rehabilitative approach in patients with "palliative needs" may seem to be a paradox, but in reality it can be highly appropriate for patients with complex, progressive illness. It provides a practical approach to management and may be applied at any stage of illness. If skilled practitioners adopt this approach to care, people can reach their maximum capacity, realize their true potential, and grow and develop when faced with a difficult situation. It is acknowledged that there are clear differences between rehabilitation in palliative care and the traditional rehabilitative approach within general medical care.[3] Rehabilitation in general medical care is typically performed for a disability that has occurred at one point in time, and there is an expectation that further deterioration is unlikely. In this situation the aim is to maximize patients' potential. Rehabilitation in this context is commonly the domain of the physiotherapist and occupational therapist, and the emphasis is on physical needs. In contrast, within the specialty of palliative care, not only are patients disabled, but they also have an advanced progressive life-threatening illness. As a result, practitioners need to apply a range of skills that combine both rehabilitative and palliative expertise. To achieve this objective it is imperative that all members of the multidisciplinary team be engaged to ensure that the complex needs of patients with advanced, progressive illness are identified and met. The scope of rehabilitation in this context is holistic in that the physical, psychological, spiritual, sexual, and social domains are addressed.

The need for support and rehabilitation of patients who have undergone treatment of cancer is well documented.[4] The literature on survivorship is substantial[5,6]; however, there is little emphasis on the practical support needed to enable individuals to manage their illness. Adjusting to the uncertainty of a life-threatening illness is, in itself, difficult. Couple this with the additional disabilities that arise from complicated and arduous therapies for cancer, and the resultant experience can be extremely traumatic for both patients and their families. Unsurprisingly, the resources available in health care to provide the necessary professional input are limited. Although a rehabilitative approach can be applied at all stages of illness, not all patients with a life-threatening illness will require access to specialist services (such as a specialist palliative care service with rehabilitation skills). Different groups of patients are appropriate for rehabilitation, and understanding this concept will enable a rational approach to planning, developing, and delivering services. The following groups of patients are appropriate for rehabilitation:

PATIENTS WHO HAVE UNDERGONE TREATMENT AND MAY BE CURED

Such patients need a range of psychological and physical therapies to enable them to recover, resocialize, and adapt to any disability that may be present. The objective is to enable patients to live as normal a life as possible. Setting time frames for recovery is important, and the aim is for the intervention to be relatively limited. On occasion, patients have long-term disabilities that require ongoing support, and the rehabilitation service will need to plan for this in either a palliative care or an alternative setting.

PATIENTS WHO HAVE UNDERGONE TREATMENT, ARE IN REMISSION, AND ARE NOT CURED

These patients may survive with disability. They are living with great uncertainty and need help to manage it. They have often undergone arduous treatments and, when their disease recurs, can feel disappointed, angry, and resentful that the treatment has not worked. They need the full range of rehabilitative resources to reframe their life and maximize their potential.

PATIENTS WITH PROGRESSIVE DISEASE

Frequently, these patients have had multiple courses of treatment and feel defeated by their cancer. They have complex physical and emotional problems and can feel cheated of a healthy future and be bitter that things did not progress as anticipated. These patients have a disease trajectory that is often one of gradual decline and progressive frailty. As care transfers more into a palliative setting, patients can feel abandoned by their oncology teams. Frail patients often "fail to thrive" and need support from a full range of rehabilitative therapies. Despite their frailty, much can be done to maximize potential, optimize control of symptoms, and reassure patients that they can have control of their future and will be supported.

PATIENTS WHO ARE CLOSE TO DEATH

Ease and solace goals to give patients a sense of control in negotiating care are important. These goals can be achieved by a rehabilitative approach to care, even at this stage of illness.

ROLE OF MEDICAL AND NURSING PRACTITIONERS AND THE WIDER TEAM IN PALLIATIVE CARE REHABILITATION

The input of allied health professionals is relatively explicit, but there is a lack of information on the roles of other key professionals. There will always be an overlap between roles and blurring of professional boundaries; however, examination of the core elements of the individual professional roles gives further insight into the essential components of successful rehabilitation and the importance of a well-functioning team.

The clinical nurse specialist is integral to the assessment process and often provides continuity of care and ongoing support of the patient. Nurses' ability to understand patients within their individual world and their skill in combining elements of care and treatment of each individual are key components of successful rehabilitation. The nursing assessment process should concentrate on exploration of the impact of illness on the patients' physical, emotional/psychological, and role function and the effects on family members/significant others. Prioritization of patients' need and goal setting are fundamental to success and should be combined with a discussion about strategies to enable achievement of goals and the appropriate time and pace for planned interventions.

The palliative medicine physician has a valuable role in rehabilitation. Although medical input could be seen to give status to physical symptoms and the sick role, the benefits of an in-depth medical assessment cannot be underestimated. Medical consultation allows confirmation of diagnoses and ensures that all treatment options for control of symptoms have been fully explored. The assumption that every patient has the correct diagnosis and has received the correct treatment on arrival at the rehabilitation service/resource is naïve; an incorrect diagnosis is often perpetuated by successive clinicians. The initial medical consultation is an invaluable opportunity to confirm the diagnoses, optimize control of symptoms, and discuss anxieties about previous diagnoses and treatments. It should provide time for patients to give a biographical account of their care, which allows uncertainties to be discussed and misperceptions corrected. A medical overview can also be invaluable in minimizing risk by assessing that the rehabilitation program is safe for the patient (Figs. 246-1 and 246-2).

Once priorities and goals have been agreed on, referral to the appropriate professionals should be made in a timely manner. To deliver care requires a coordinated approach that allows sharing of skills and expertise. The skills of members from all professional disciplines should be utilized to enable all patients to achieve their maximum potential. Some patients find that the support of social workers and counseling and complementary therapists is extremely valuable (Fig. 246-3A and B). Referral to members of the wider rehabilitation team may also be

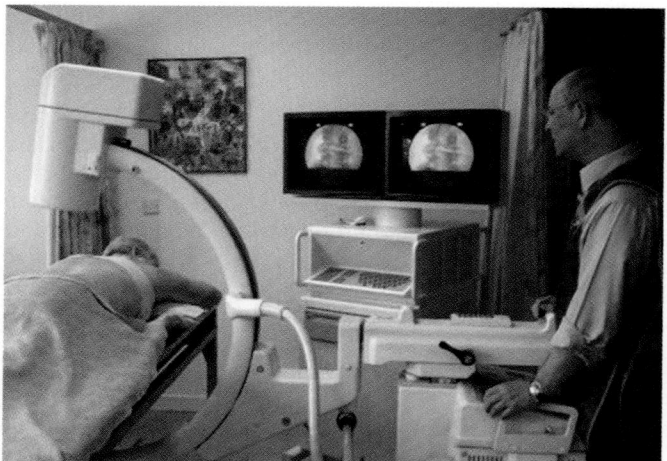

FIGURE 246-1   Investigations in a palliative care setting can be invaluable for diagnosis and treatment. Real-time radiographic imaging is being carried out in a hospice setting to screen a patient with metastatic bone disease. This helps the physiotherapy team and minimizes risk to patients. It enables appropriate therapy to be delivered and ensures them that exercise is safe.

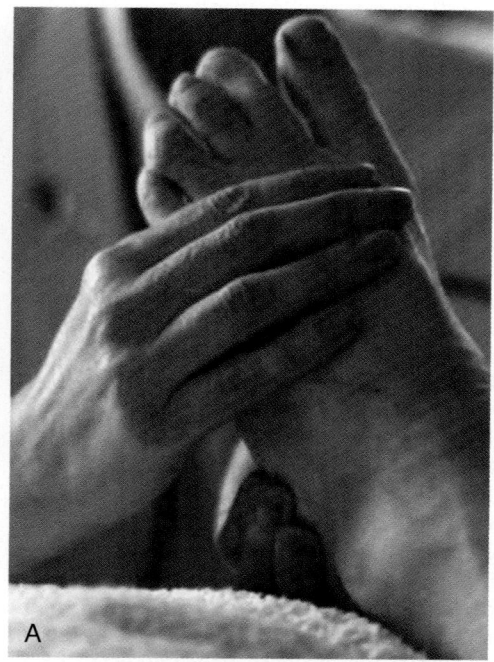

A

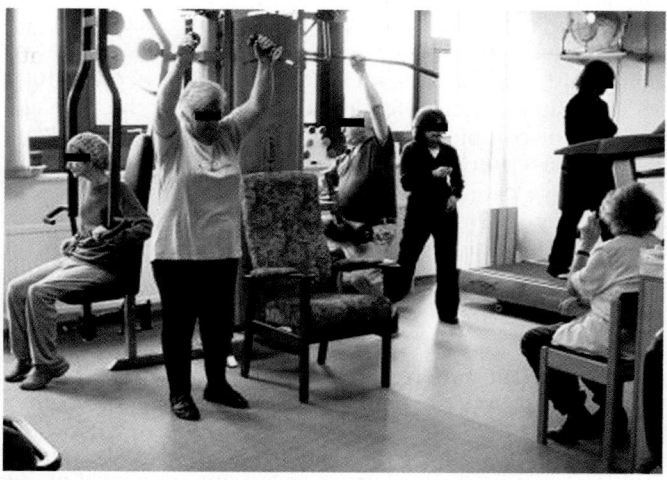

FIGURE 246-2   A rehabilitative approach allows patients to maximize their potential. An exercise program supervised by specialist physiotherapists can be structured to meet the needs of the individual. The social setting of a gym provides patients with a positive and supportive experience.

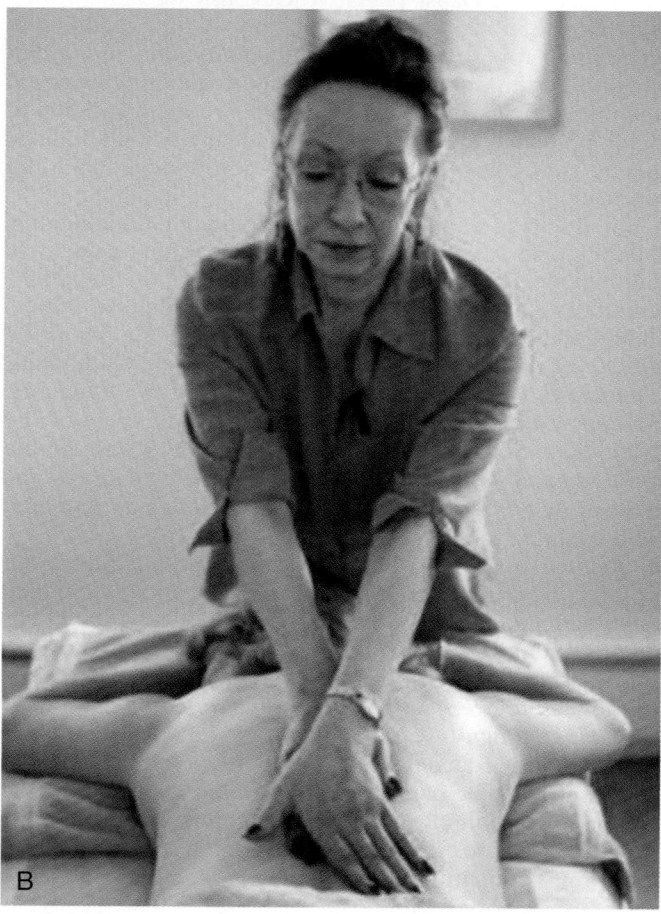

B

FIGURE 246-3   **A** and **B,** Complementary therapies. Rehabilitation is a therapeutic experience that requires a multidimensional approach to meet the physical, emotional, social, and spiritual needs of patients and their families. Teamwork is crucial, and all members of the multiprofessional team must work toward common goals. Complementary therapists are included in this approach.

suitable. This team includes appliance officers, dietitians, lymphedema therapists, physiotherapists, psychologists, stoma therapists, and the like.

To be effective, this approach to care needs to be coordinated and facilitated. This is known as delivering a complex intervention[7]; it provides a package of care in which the outcome is far greater than the sum of its component parts and is the most effective way of addressing all the needs of the patient and family. In any health care setting, when care is delivered to patients with highly complex needs, there is real strength if patients are assessed in the framework of a well-functioning, multiprofessional team.

TEAMWORK, THE REHABILITATION TEAM, AND GOAL SETTING

Effective rehabilitation is dependent on coordination of care, sharing of information, good communication, and joint decision making. Clearly, the ease with which this goal is achieved may be influenced by the care setting. Teamwork in a hospice can be comparatively easy: in a well-functioning team the members will work toward a common philosophy, and there is a good understanding of each professional's role and overlap. Multidisciplinary meetings are easy to arrange and provide a forum for information and skill sharing and the ideal opportunity to coordinate care and set goals. This may be more difficult in a hospital, where the structure of the building and traditional professional boundaries may make a coordinated and integrated approach more difficult to achieve (service delivery in the community can be similarly disjointed). Professional groups involved in the patient's care may meet rarely, which can result in a fragmented approach to care.

The rehabilitative approach within palliative care requires collaborative working if all parties are to remain consistent in their approach and enable patients to attain their goals. Specialist palliative care has well-established experience in multiprofessional teamwork. Because specialist palliative care teams in hospitals (and those that serve the community) are relatively small and composed of professionals who (theoretically) are in a position to meet regularly to discuss an individual patient's holistic needs, they can be in an ideal position to coordinate the package of care.

Goal setting is fundamental to an effective rehabilitative journey, but it is often the most difficult component to implement. The key player is the patient, whose priorities, concerns, and values should be incorporated into achievable goals. The patient's prognosis and the probable course of the illness will clearly have an impact on goals. Therefore, the goals should remain realistic, attainable, and shared between the patient and all members of the team. Achieving such objectives requires considerable professional skill, particularly when trying to overcome unrealistic goals or when goals may need to be reassessed during the latter stage of illness.

Regular review of the patient's progress is important when planning a patient's care package. The review date is influenced by prognosis and the goals agreed upon. For some patients, review will be needed within days or weeks of initiating a plan of care; for others, it may be a number of months before a review is considered beneficial.

Goal setting and regular review of palliative care patients are fundamental for effective rehabilitation; however, in some patients this approach has to be carried out in the context of an unpredictable illness and an uncertain future. Therefore, an effective rehabilitation team must remain flexible in its approach and anticipate change.

RECENT DEVELOPMENTS

It is now acknowledged that rehabilitation in cancer care is important.[4] Delivery of care requires a structure in which it is ensured that all patients are assessed for their rehabilitative needs. Within the United Kingdom, NICE guidance[2]

recommends four levels of assessment and support. The model proposed has both advantages and disadvantages; however, it does provide a helpful framework.

Level 1—A rehabilitative approach by all health care professionals delivered by generalists in all settings (home and hospital). This requires an assessment of rehabilitative needs by all professionals. To ensure that generalists can assess need, there has to be local education to raise awareness of the role of rehabilitation, as well as adequate resources to deliver the care. The specialist palliative care team will have an important role in empowering the primary care and other teams in the acute trusts (acute hospitals).

Level 2—Specific generalist interventions for specific common problems and impairments during cancer treatment (e.g., physiotherapy and dietary advice after cancer surgery). There should be care pathways and protocols for specific common rehabilitation problems. These interventions are usually delivered in an inpatient environment, commonly after surgery.

Level 3—Specialized interventions by professionals who have extensive experience, training, and education and have worked extensively with cancer patients (e.g., management of uncomplicated lymphedema). This will assume particular importance in a cancer center.

Level 4—Highly specialized interventions by advanced practitioners. This level of rehabilitation needs a fully integrated multiprofessional approach to the management of complex issues and is appropriate for patients who have undergone complex surgical procedures. In palliative care, patients often have complex needs and will benefit from a level 4 approach to rehabilitation. The full multidisciplinary team will be needed, and it is most likely to be developed in a hospice setting with close links to a cancer center/unit.

The NICE guidance provides a practical framework to understand the different levels of rehabilitation that are needed to support patients with cancer. Rehabilitation is an approach to care that can be provided by all professional groups in all settings; nonetheless, the "traditional view" that rehabilitation is primarily the domain of the physiotherapist and occupational therapist is largely supported by NICE guidance. The role of the allied health care professional in cancer care is of great importance and undervalued by the cancer team. However, to deny patients comprehensive and ongoing access to the full integrated multiprofessional team ignores the attention to detail that is needed to give optimal care to patients with complex needs. Rehabilitation needs to be owned by all professionals caring for patients with progressive illness. The skills of clinical nurse specialists, physicians, and the psychosocial team are fundamental to safe, effective, high-quality care. Any service adopting a rehabilitative approach will need to develop structures to ensure that all skills are integrated. Sadly, there are few examples of integrated multidisciplinary teamwork in the NICE guidance or published literature.

EVIDENCE-BASED MEDICINE

The success of integrated multiprofessional intervention is hard to measure. A range of tools for assessing function

Common Errors

- Assuming that palliative care is only for "end-of-life" care.
- Not responding to patients with supportive care needs—assuming that other services will deal with the complex problems in a coordinated fashion.
- Refusing to accept that noncancer patients with advanced progressive illness have needs similar to those of cancer patients and that specialist palliative care skills are transferable.
- Not developing collaborative relationships with specialists who treat noncancer patients.
- Failure to implement a systematized, integrated team approach to patients with complex needs. Working as a group of professionals rather than a team will not allow clinical synergies to develop that enhance patient care.

and daily living[8] have been used for specific conditions and by different disciplines, but they are not generally helpful for measuring the outcome of a multiprofessional approach to rehabilitation. However, because no meaningful measurement is available, it does not follow that the approach is ineffective. The rehabilitative approach is a complex intervention and should be assessed as such. The trap that many outcome measures fall into is to try to break down complex interventions into their simple component parts and assess each part individually. A complex intervention is not the sum of its parts.[7] Reducing a complex system to its component parts amounts to "irretrievable loss of what makes it a system."[9] The challenge is to acknowledge this and develop and refine our approach so that a highly complex intervention, such as rehabilitation, can be meaningfully assessed.

CONTROVERSIES

Noncancer conditions are a challenge to palliative care clinicians, and this could be a particular issue when considering developing rehabilitation services. Services need to be developed that allow all patients with complex needs access to the support and expertise that they rightly require. The fear that palliative care clinicians do not have the knowledge to care for noncancer patients is unfounded.[10] The model of care that has been developed in cancer, in which patients receive oncology expertise from medical and clinical oncology teams in parallel with palliative care, has been highly effective. Similar models of shared care must be developed for patients with noncancer conditions; collaborative working with the appropriate specialists will ensure that patients have access to the skills necessary for optimal management.

Although there may be differences between the experiences of cancer patients and patients with progressive noncancer conditions, the two groups of patients have a similar burden of symptoms[11] and in many illnesses a similar prognosis.[12-14] Consequently, it is also appropriate to adopt a rehabilitative approach to the palliative management of patients with noncancer conditions. It is freely acknowledged that specialist palliative care cannot meet all the needs of all patients with progressive malignant and nonmalignant disease. Therefore, future service development needs to be planned carefully to ensure that care is

appropriate to the need and that capacity is adequate for the demand. The reality is that there is not a "one size fits all" approach to palliative care and rehabilitation services.

CONCLUSIONS

The concept of a "rehabilitative approach" requires a paradigm shift for palliative care clinicians. It requires the interdisciplinary team to understand that patients, when faced with a life-threatening illness, need support to look at "what they can achieve" rather than on solely "coming to terms."

It is important that patients understand the implications and limitations of serious illness and the resultant disabilities. Setting goals for the future can be challenging, especially when a patient's intellectual understanding of the illness is not always matched by the emotional capacity to acknowledge the reality. Patients often see themselves as curable despite having (and understanding that they have) advanced illness. A rehabilitative approach can support patients through this stage by helping them grow and develop strategies to cope with their disabilities and uncertain future.

This shift in paradigm requires professionals to move away from their stereotypical roles in palliative care and embrace the changing health care environment in developing services that meet an unmet palliative need. No longer can we rest on our past achievements; we must be an active and integral part of health care—indeed, this was the original philosophy of the modern hospice movement. To do so we should adapt our current best practice and develop new ways of working. We must persuade our colleagues and our organizations that they must acknowledge the inevitability of change and respond; this takes strength and courage and will require both personal and organizational resilience.

ACKNOWLEDGEMENT

We are grateful to our patients for giving permission to publish the photos in the chapter and to Sabine Tilley for her skill and expertise.

REFERENCES

1. Scottish Executive Health Department. Cancer Care in Scotland: Action for Change. Edinburgh: SEHD, 2006.
2. National Institute for Clinical Excellence. Improving Supportive and Palliative Care for Adults with Cancer. London: NICE, 2004.
3. Nocon A, Baldwin S. Trends in Rehabilitation Policy: A Review of the Literature. London: Kings Fund, 1998.
4. Calman K, Hine D. A Policy Framework for Commissioning Cancer Services: A Report by the Expert Advisory Group on Cancer to the Chief Medical Officers of England and Wales. London: Department of Health, 1995.
5. Aziz NM. Cancer survivorship research: Challenge and opportunity. J Nutr 2002;132:3494-3503.
6. Tritter JQ, Calnan M. Reconsidering categorization and exploring experience. Eur J Cancer Care 2002;11:161-165.
7. Hawe P, Shiell A, Riley T. Complex interventions: How "out of control" can a randomized controlled trial be? BMJ 2004;328:1561-1563.
8. Turner-Stokes L. Measurement of Outcome in Rehabilitation: The British Society of Rehabilitation Medicine "Basket" of Measures. London: BSRM, 2000.
9. Casti JL. Would-Be Worlds: How Simulation Is Changing the Frontiers of Science. New York: John Wiley & Sons, 1997.
10. National Council for Hospice and Specialist Palliative Care. Reaching Out: Specialist Palliative Care for Adults with Non-Malignant Diseases. London: NCHSPC, 1998.
11. Solano JP, Gomes B, Higginson I. A comparison of symptom prevalence in far advanced cancer, AIDS, heart disease, chronic obstructive pulmonary disease (COPD), and renal disease. J Pain Symptom Manage 2006;31:58-69.

12. Office of National Statistics. Cancer Survival in England and Wales 1991-2001. Available at http://www.statistics.gov.uk (accessed 2006).
13. Stewart S, MacIntyre K, Hole DJ, et al. More 'malignant' than cancer? 5 yr survival following a first admission for heart failure. Eur J Heart Failure 2001;3:315-322.
14. Vestbo J, Prescott E, Lange P, et al. Vital prognosis after hospitalization for COPD: A study of a random population sample. Respir Med 1998;92: 772-776.

SUGGESTED READING

National Council for Hospice and Specialist Palliative Care. Reaching Out: Specialist Palliative Care for Adults with Non-Malignant Diseases. London: NCHSPC, 1998.
National Council for Hospice and Specialist Palliative Care. Fulfilling Lives: Rehabilitation in Palliative Care. London: NCHSPC, 2000.
Speck P. Teamwork in Palliative Care: Fulfilling or Frustrating? Oxford, Oxford University Press, 2006.
Tookman A, Hopkins K, Scharpen-Von-Heussen K. Section 14. Rehabilitation in Palliative Medicine. In Doyle D, Hanks G, Cherny N, Calman K (eds). Oxford Textbook of Palliative Medicine, 3rd ed. Oxford: Oxford University Press, 2004.

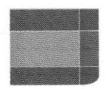

CHAPTER **247**

Cancer Pain: Anesthetic and Neurosurgical Interventions

Costantino Benedetti, James Ibinson, and Michael Adolph

KEY POINTS

- The three-step World Health Organization cancer oral pain therapy ladder is effective in alleviating cancer-related pain in up to 80% of patients. For the rest, parenteral medications and, in 5% to 10% of cancer pain patients, invasive anesthetic or neurosurgical interventions may be needed for refractory pain.

- Anesthetic or neurosurgical interventions may reduce but generally do not obliterate the need for systemic opioids. A procedure is only one component of an overall pain therapy plan that targets improved quality of life.

- Patient factors, tumor anatomy, and the availability of specialists and resources are important determinants of successful intervention.

- Neurosurgical interventions historically originated before adequate systemic opioid therapy became acceptable. Newer percutaneous approaches are viable for refractory pain. Patients must be selected carefully and the patient and family thoroughly educated regarding alternatives and anticipated outcomes before proceeding.

- A well-developed plan of care to incorporate catheters, pumps, and medication delivery must be coordinated with a willing and able home care team.

Oral analgesic therapy is the mainstay for cancer pain, and opioids are the foundation of this therapy (see Chapters 138 and 249). Up to 20% of patients will require supplementary interventions to decrease physical pain.[1] Additional forms of therapy include parenteral opioids and other analgesics such as ketamine and the more invasive anesthetic or neurosurgical techniques. Such therapy may be considered when systemic opioids fail because of inadequate pain relief, prohibitive side effects (see Chapter 250), or both. In our practice, after careful titration of oral or parenteral opioids and adjuvant medication, less than 5% of patients with cancer pain require interventional procedures. These procedures require specialists to properly perform them and appropriate supportive services. Anesthetic procedures may include peripheral nerve and ganglion blocks or spinal analgesia. Neurosurgical procedures may include ablation or creation of lesions in central nervous system structures to alter transmission of nociceptive impulses to the brain. An anesthesiologist, a neurosurgeon, or both may also perform procedures to augment endogenous analgesic mechanisms.[2] Examples include implantable pumps and intraspinal catheters positioned to deliver opioids near spinal cord receptors, an Ommaya reservoir connected to an intracerebroventricular (ICV) catheter for delivery of opioids near their receptors in the brain periaqueductal grey matter, or nerve stimulators to enhance endogenous inhibition of nociceptive impulses. Procedural interventions typically reduce the use of but may not obviate the necessity for systemic analgesics.

Interventions are one component of an overall pain therapy plan of care. Functional goals, quality of life, drug factors (such as adverse side effects), cost constraints, availability of resources, and disease considerations are included in the plan of care. Patient co-morbidities, expected outcomes, and prognosis are critical factors in the overall risk/benefit analysis for each procedure. Contraindications to anesthetic or neurosurgical interventions include coagulopathy or systemic anticoagulation, prohibitive anatomy (e.g., axial spine metastasis in someone being considered for spinal analgesia),[3] prohibitive co-morbidities, or active or impending infection.

The most frequently performed procedures include ganglion and plexus blocks, intraspinal and ICV analgesia, creation of lesions in the dorsal root entry zone (DREZ), and brain stimulation. Other neuroablative procedures are now seldom performed for pain in advanced cancer. Such procedures include cordotomy, myelotomy, tractotomy, hypophysectomy, thalamotomy, and cingulotomy (see "Suggested Reading").

CLINICAL FINDINGS AND EVALUATION

A complete history and physical examination, including the primary diagnosis, pain assessment, underlying pain mechanisms, functional status, and quality-of-life goals, are determined before considering a procedural intervention. Success or failure of previous treatments and pain therapies should be noted. If feasible, referral to a pain specialist may be considered early in a patient's course, depending on the initial complaints and the anticipated natural history of the underlying disease.

The anatomical source and distribution of the pain will guide the clinician toward potential therapeutic options with a reasonable likelihood of diminishing pain, improving function, and maximizing quality of life with an acceptable risk profile. The patient is informed of the risks and benefits, as well as available options. Written informed consent is obtained for the interventional procedure chosen.

Whenever major neurolytic blockade of sensory or sensory/motor nerves is being considered, one or two initial test blocks with local anesthetic are performed on separate occasions. This gives the patient the opportunity to experience the effects of a temporary block before a "permanent" neuroablation procedure is undertaken. On occasion, a patient will prefer avoiding a block if distressing sensations such as anesthesia or motor dysfunction occur with test injections. Invasive approaches can help manage uncontrolled pain despite the concurrent use of physical, behavioral, and drug therapies.[4]

The likelihood of pain recurring after a successful block may increase proportionally with life expectancy. A risk/benefit analysis should be considered. When a procedure is contemplated, life expectancy may be discussed with the primary oncologist before the procedure. Even when "permanent" blocks are performed, pain may return as a result of pathological or physiological nerve regeneration after any procedure, regardless of whether the neurilemma remains intact; patients should be advised accordingly. A thorough discussion of realistic goals is warranted. The patient's hopes, concerns, and individual goals should be probed with open-ended questions. For example, getting pain to zero or discontinuing all preprocedural systemic opioids may be unspoken expectations but are not usually achievable.

ANESTHETIC/ANALGESIC INTERVENTIONS

Painful somatic, visceral, neuropathic, or mixed impulses from isolated or contiguous accessible nerves may be blocked for various indications (Box 247-1). Intractable pain (see Chapter 253) can be controlled by injection of a local anesthetic or neurolytic agent in close proximity to

---

> ### Box 247-1 Rationale for Performing Nerve Blocks for Cancer Pain
>
> **Diagnostic:** To determine the source of pain in a reproducible fashion with a nondestructive injectable agent such as bupivacaine or lidocaine (e.g., somatic versus sympathetic pathways)
>
> **Prognostic:** To predict the outcome of long-lasting interventions or allow the patient to preview the effects after a permanent block (e.g., infusions, neurolysis, rhizotomy)
>
> **Therapeutic:** To treat painful conditions that respond to nerve blocks (e.g., neurolytic celiac plexus block for the pain of pancreatic cancer or anti-inflammatory corticosteroid injection to provide extended relief from nerve root compression)
>
> **Pre-emptive:** To prevent procedure-related pain

From National Cancer Institute. Pain PDQ. Available at http://www.cancer. gov/cancertopics/pdq/supportivecare/pain/HealthProfessional/page2, 2004-2006 (accessed 2/5/2006).

---

1. Peripheral nerves (for somatic pain)
2. Autonomic ganglia (for visceral pain or causalgia)
3. Spinal cord (for intrathecal or epidural analgesia)

Nondestructive agents such as local anesthetics have a short duration of action and convey helpful information after injection. Neurodestructive agents such as ethanol or phenol can be used to carry out neurolysis at sites identified by temporary local anesthetic injection as appropriate for long-term (several weeks to several months) pain relief. These agents do this by destruction of nervous system structures such as plexuses, ganglia, or nerve roots in the intrathecal space. Radiofrequency ablation (RFA) is neurodestructive by causing thermal injury. With or without image guidance, an RF handheld probe with an electrode tip emits high-frequency alternating current to generate localized frictional heat.[5]

Peripheral Nerve Blocks

Peripheral anesthetic blocks exploit the anatomical distribution of afferent nerves. Identifying the cause of the pain is helpful. Clinicians can help patients by recognizing, diagnosing, and treating common cancer pain syndromes.[6]

Ganglion and Plexus Blocks

Neurolytic Celiac Plexus Block

Pancreatic cancer may cause severe upper abdominal and midback pain. At initial evaluation, pancreatic cancer is typically advanced and often unresectable. The underlying pain mechanisms include visceral nociception (foregut organ destruction) and neuropathic nociception (involved retroperitoneal nerves). The prototype percutaneous procedure is a neurolytic celiac plexus block (NCPB). Up to 85% to 90% of patients achieve good to excellent pain relief.[7] In a randomized controlled trial of 100 patients, NCPB improved pain relief over oral opioids alone but did not affect survival or quality of life.[8]

The potential for side effects and the risk of recurrent pain have restricted NCPB to cancer patients with a limited life span. Back pain (96%), diarrhea (44%), and hypotension (38%) are the most common adverse effects. Serious complications occur after less than 2% of injections.[7] Less common are persistent lower extremity weakness and abdominal muscle weakness secondary to spillage of neurolytic agent on somatic motor nerves. To minimize serious idiosyncratic complications during NCPB, radiological localization, including computed tomography (CT), is the standard of care. Endoscopic ultrasonography-guided localization for celiac plexus neurolysis is superior to CT for localization and neurolysis of the celiac plexus.[9]

Pain control may be sustained for up to 50 days after injection, which can then be repeated. By reducing total opioid consumption, quality of life may improve by decreasing opioid-related side effects. The benefits of percutaneous neurolysis could also be obtained after open surgical neurolysis at laparotomy when unresectable pancreatic cancer is identified.[10] Intraoperative chemical splanchnicectomy was superior to placebo for pain control in a double-blinded study of 137 patients, and in some it prolonged survival.

Sympathetic Blocks

Cancers of the cervix, colon, bladder, rectum, and endometrium are the most common cancers causing pelvic and perineal pain. Pain may also be referred to the rectum, perineum, or vagina. Such pain is associated with urgency and burning; it is vague and poorly localized. Bladder spasms are frequent, and position changes exacerbate the pain. Tenesmus may be prominent. Pain that radiates to the groin is characteristic of ureteral obstruction. Local visceral pelvic pain is often complicated by impaired bowel or bladder function. Patients complain of pain, lower gastrointestinal symptoms, or gastrointestinal bleeding.

Mixed pain mechanisms are frequent with pelvic cancer pain (see Chapter 244). Somatic and autonomic symptoms and signs may overlap and create a confusing clinical picture. For severe pelvic pain, interventions may include

1. Lumbar sympathetic block
2. Superior hypogastric plexus block
3. Ganglion impar block

Lumbosacral Sympathetic Block

The sympathetic lumbosacral plexus runs on both sides of the bony vertebral bodies. To perform a lumbar sympathetic plexus block, one- and two-needle techniques have been described. Fluoroscopic guidance plus injection of contrast material confirms a good position, typically at the L2-L3 level. Neurolysis is considered after local anesthetic blocks of the sympathetic chain are effective as a temporary test measure.

Superior Hypogastric Block and Ganglion Impar Block

A superior hypogastric plexus block reduces pain scores in 70% of patients with malignant pelvic pain.[11] It is safe, and significant neurological complications rare. The ganglion impar innervates the perineum. It is located anterior to the sacrococcygeal junction and represents the end point of the left and right sympathetic chains. In one study, 8 of 16 patients achieved 100% pain relief, whereas the remainder achieved 60% or better relief on visual analogue scores.[11] A safe approach traverses the sacrococcygeal junction to avoid the underlying rectum. The advantage of this block over other neurolytic procedures for rectal pain is that bowel and bladder function is generally unaffected.

Spinal (Epidural and Intrathecal) Analgesia

Intraspinal opioids are one of the most important advances in pain therapy in the 20th century.[12-15] The relative potency of morphine injected into the intrathecal space is 10 times greater than injection into the epidural space and 100 times greater than intravenous morphine.[16] Profound analgesia is feasible without motor, sensory, or sympathetic blockade. Additional pharmacological agents such as local anesthetic or clonidine may be used to improve analgesia.

Given that hydrophilic opioids (e.g., morphine) can ascend from the lumbar site of spinal catheter placement to the cervical area, cancer pain localized not only to the abdomen or lower extremities but also to the thorax and upper extremities can be decreased with spinal analgesia.

For chronic cancer pain, intrathecal analgesia is most frequently used. Intrathecal catheters may be tunneled subcutaneously and exit the skin or be connected to a subcutaneous port. The catheter is then connected to an external pump or to a subcutaneously implanted pump. For severe pain from malignancy, we usually place an intrathecal catheter, tunnel it beneath the skin to the lateral aspect of the abdomen, and exit the skin. The catheter is attached to a continuous ambulatory drug delivery pump placed in a waist belt. The device is typically used for continuous infusion and is titrated only by the physician given the potency of intrathecal opioids.

Neurosurgical Procedures

For pain therapy, most open neurosurgical procedures were developed and popularized when experience with both systemic analgesic therapy and anesthetic procedures was limited. Although their widespread use is no longer advocated because of invasiveness, permanency, and potential complications, neurosurgical procedures can still play a role in cancer patients with pain in countries in which opioids are not readily available. Patients unable to tolerate major open neurosurgical procedures may be candidates for a percutaneous approach. Naturally, an experienced neurosurgeon and the necessary technological equipment must be available.

Intracerebroventricular Opioid Infusion

Opioids are most potent when delivered directly into the brain's cerebrospinal fluid. A catheter placed in a cerebral ventricle through a surgical burr hole and connected to an Ommaya reservoir is preferred.[17] Agents such as preservative-free morphine or hydromorphone may be delivered as a continuous infusion through an external or implantable pump or be administered intermittently (twice a day) by injection. Side effects include respiratory depression, and careful titration is warranted. Nausea and vomiting are common side effects.

Brain Stimulation

Brain stimulation is reserved for diffuse cancer pain after failure of systemic analgesic therapy and ablative techniques.[18] Up to 79% of patients achieve long-term pain control. Implantable electrode stimulation of periaqueductal and periventricular gray matter provides relief from nociceptive pain. Stimulation of the internal capsule and near the thalamus relieves neuropathic pain. Efficacy can be determined by intraoperative stimulation of an awake patient. Alternatively, electrodes can be placed in both locations to permit the patient to selectively stimulate the most effective region via an implantable stimulator.

Neurosurgical Ablative Procedures

Surgical ablation of pain pathways should, like neurolytic blockade, be considered after medical therapies are ineffective or poorly tolerated.[19] The choice of procedure is based on the location and type of pain (somatic, visceral, and neuropathic), the patient's general condition and life expectancy, and the expertise and follow-up available. Selection of patients and choice of procedure are complex (Box 247-2).

Dorsal Root Entry Zone Lesion

Creation of a lesion in the DREZ can be helpful for excruciating neuropathic pain caused by invasion of cancer into peripheral nerves or a plexus, as in Pancoast's syndrome. The sensory nerve root entry zone of the dorsal horn is ablated by laser (CO_2 or Nd-YAG) or RFA. RFA, which permits creation of a more focused lesion, reduces the risk of involving the ventral roots and producing motor weakness. Pain is reduced to acceptable levels in 60% to 70% of patients.

Other Neurosurgical Ablative Procedures

The reader is referred to the 2001 textbook *Bonica's Management of Pain* for descriptions and indications for the following neurosurgical procedures, which are seldom performed: cordotomy, myelotomy, pons or medulla tractotomy, hypophysectomy, thalamotomy, cingulotomy, trigeminal tractotomy, and mesencephalic tractotomy.

RECENT DEVELOPMENTS

Addition of a local anesthetic to opioid agents delivered by the intrathecal and epidural routes is now a well-established method of improving pain control without a significant increase in toxicity. New substances, some of which act by nonopioid mechanisms, are under development. The most recent is ziconotide, a sea snail toxin that targets neural N-type calcium channels.[20] It decreases neuropathic pain when given intrathecally. Significant systemic side effects can be minimized with slow, careful dose titration.

EVIDENCE-BASED MEDICINE

Neurolytic Celiac Plexus Block

A review of 31 studies involving 1599 patients who received 2750 celiac plexus blocks found that 85% to 90% achieved good to excellent pain relief after NCPB. The efficacy and safety of NCPB are also supported by a meta-analysis of 24 studies.[7] Only two were randomized controlled trials, however. Long-term benefit was achieved in 79% to 90% with upper abdominal pain, most frequently from pancreatic cancer. Six percent to 8% may require a second block to achieve pain control. Some suggest that the efficacy of NCPB has not been established given that pre- and post-NCPB pain assessment data are lacking in many studies.[20] There is substantial published work to validate a grade "B" recommendation based on the validity of available evidence for NCPB as a reasonable therapy for cancer pain.[8,21]

Neuraxial Opioid Administration

In a Cochrane Database comparison of the efficacy of epidural, intrathecal, and ICV opioids for cancer pain, there were no controlled trials in 72 studies published. Excellent pain relief was achieved in 73% of ICV patients, 72% of epidural patients, and 62% of intrathecal patients. Sedation, confusion, and respiratory depression were most common with ICV opioids. They concluded that pain control with ICV opioids was more effective than either epidural or intrathecal administration. However, catheter and delivery system problems were most common in ICV patients.[17] Evidence supports a grade "B" recommendation for neuraxial infusion of opioids by the ICV, epidural, and intrathecal routes for refractory cancer pain.

CONTROVERSIES

The major controversy about invasive analgesic techniques involves the threshold of their application in cancer analgesic therapy. This depends on the particular national situation. In countries in which opioids are scarce, anesthetic blocks and neurosurgical procedures may be performed more frequently than in places where the availability of opioids permits proper titration of systemic analgesics and other adjuvant medications. Invasive techniques are associated with potential complications, especially in cancer patients with a depressed immune system, which predisposes them to serious infections. Cost must also be considered. For instance, an intrathecal system, including the

---

Box 247-2 Summary of Tasker's Recommendations for Decision Making in Selecting Patients and Neurosurgical Procedures for Pain Control

1. Have simpler treatments failed?
2. Is there a reasonable chance that the proposed procedure will relieve the patient's suffering in view of the severity of the symptoms, nature of the procedure, and risk of complications?
3. Do the patient and family have a realistic understanding of the procedure's specific benefits (e.g., a procedure to decrease pain after spinal cord trauma will not affect the paraplegia)?
4. Do the patient and family acknowledge that neurosurgical procedures for pain relief have a relatively low success rate, seldom give permanent relief, and carry a risk for iatrogenic pain syndromes?
5. For nociceptive pain and the neuralgic and evoked components of neuropathic pain, interrupt the pain pathway or modulate it with morphine or deep brain stimulation.
6. For the steady causalgic dysesthetic component of neuropathic pain, induce paresthesia in the area of pain.

Data from Tasker RR: Neurostimulation and percutaneous neural destructive techniques. In Cousins MJ, Bridenbaugh PO (eds): Neural Blockade in Clinical Anesthesia and Management of Pain, 3rd ed. Philadelphia: JB Lippincott, 1998, pp 1063-1134.

Common Errors

- Inadequate effort in titrating systemic analgesia
- Late referral to a pain specialist
- Lack of a team approach

catheter and implantable pump and their placement, may cost more than $30,000 in the United States, so these procedures must be judiciously evaluated and implemented.

RESEARCH CHALLENGES/OPPORTUNITIES/ADVANCES

Intraspinal Agents

There are significant variations in how clinicians use intraspinal analgesia. Guidelines established by a consensus panel have largely focused on agents and not indications.[22] Surveys of experienced pain medicine practitioners reveal that morphine is the most popular intraspinal agent, with 62% of patients receiving morphine alone. The remaining 38% are switched to other agents or combination agents because of lack of efficacy in 80% and untoward side effects in the other 20%.[23] One group demonstrated favorable outcomes with an implanted intrathecal catheter and subcutaneous pump in cancer pain patients after a threshold of 200 mg oral morphine equivalency was reached.[24] This study is controversial, however.[25] Given the scope of practice variation, nonuniform indications, and patient variability, the future holds many opportunities to address unanswered questions about spinal analgesia.

REFERENCES

1. Meuser T, Pietruck C, Radbruch L, et al. Symptoms during cancer pain treatment following WHO-guidelines: A longitudinal follow-up study of symptom prevalence, severity and etiology. Pain 2001;93:247-257.
2. Mayer DJ, Price DD. Central nervous system mechanisms of analgesia. Pain 1976;2:379-404.
3. Appelgren L, Nordborg C, Sjoberg M, et al. Spinal epidural metastasis: Implications for spinal analgesia to treat "refractory" cancer pain. J Pain Symptom Manage 1997;13:25-42.
4. Cousins MJ, Bridenbaugh PO (eds). Neural Blockade in Clinical Anesthesia and Management of Pain. Philadelphia: JB Lippincott, 1932.
5. Goldberg SN, Gazelle GS, Halpern EF, et al. Radiofrequency tissue ablation: Importance of local temperature along the electrode tip exposure in determining lesion shape and size. Acad Radiol 1996;3:212-218.
6. National Cancer Institute. Pain PDQ. Available at http://www.cancer.gov/cancertopics/pdq/supportivecare/pain/HealthProfessional/page2, 2004-2006 (accessed 2/5/2006).
7. Eisenberg E, Carr DB, Chalmers TC. Neurolytic celiac plexus block for treatment of cancer pain: A meta-analysis. Anesth Analg 1995;80:290-295.
8. Wong GY, Schroeder DR, Carns PE, et al. Effect of neurolytic celiac plexus block on pain relief, quality of life, and survival in patients with unresectable pancreatic cancer. JAMA 2004;291:1092-1099.
9. Gress F, Schmitt C, Sherman S, et al. Endoscopic ultrasound–guided celiac plexus block for managing abdominal pain associated with chronic pancreatitis: A prospective single center experience. Am J Gastroenterol 2001;96:409-416.
10. Lillemoe KD, Cameron JL, Kaufman HS, et al. Chemical splanchnicectomy in patients with unresectable pancreatic cancer. A prospective randomized trial. Ann Surg 1993;217:447-455; discussion 456-457.
11. Plancarte R, Amescua C, Patt RB, et al. Superior hypogastric plexus block for pelvic cancer pain. Anesthesiology 1990;73:236-239.
12. Benedetti C. Intraspinal analgesia: An historical overview. Acta Anaesthesiol Scand Suppl 1987;85:17-24.
13. Wang JK. Pain relief by intrathecal injection of serotonin or morphine. Ann Anesthesiol Fr 1978;19:371-372.
14. Behar M, Magora F, Olshwang D, et al. Epidural morphine in treatment of pain. Lancet 1979;1:527-529.
15. Cousins MJ, Mather LE, Glynn CJ, et al. Selective spinal analgesia. Lancet 1979;1:1141-1142.
16. Nordberg G. Epidural versus intrathecal route of opioid administration. Int Anesthesiol Clin 1986;24:93-111.
17. Ballantyne JC, Carwood CM. Comparative efficacy of epidural, subarachnoid, and intracerebroventricular opioids in patients with pain due to cancer. Cochrane Database Syst Rev 2005;1:CD005178.
18. Wallace BA, Ashkan K, Benabid AL. Deep brain stimulation for the treatment of chronic, intractable pain. Neurosurg Clin N Am 2004;15:343-357, vii.
19. Tasker RR. Neurostimulation and percutaneous neural destructive techniques. In Cousins MJ, Bridenbaugh PO (eds). Neural Blockade in Clinical Anesthesia and Management of Pain, 3rd ed. Philadelphia: JB Lippincott, 1998, pp 1063-1134.
20. Staats PS, Yearwood T, Charapata SG, et al. Intrathecal ziconotide in the treatment of refractory pain in patients with cancer or AIDS: A randomized controlled trial. JAMA 2004;291:63-70.
21. Sharfman WH, Walsh TD. Has the analgesic efficacy of neurolytic celiac plexus block been demonstrated in pancreatic cancer pain? Pain 1990;41:267-371.
22. Oxford Centre for Evidence Based Medicine. Levels of Evidence and Grades of Recommendation. Oxford: OCEBM, 2006.
23. Bennett G, Burchiel K, Buchser E, et al. Clinical guidelines for intraspinal infusion: Report of an expert panel. PolyAnalgesic Consensus Conference 2000. J Pain Symptom Manage 2000;20:S37-S43.
24. Hassenbusch SJ, Portenoy RK. Current practices in intraspinal therapy—a survey of clinical trends and decision making. J Pain Symptom Manage 2000;20:S4-S11.
25. Smith TJ, Staats PS, Deer T, et al. Randomized clinical trial of an implantable drug delivery system compared with comprehensive medical management for refractory cancer pain: Impact on pain, drug-related toxicity, and survival. J Clin Oncol 2002;20:4040-4049.
26. Davis MP, Walsh D, Lagman R, et al. Randomized clinical trial of an implantable drug delivery system. J Clin Oncol 2003;21:2800-2801; author reply 2802-2803.

SUGGESTED READING

Benedetti C, Brock C, Cleeland C, et al. National Comprehensive Cancer Network (NCCN) practice guidelines for cancer pain. Oncology (Williston Park) 2000;14(11A):135-150.

Cousins MJ, Bridenbaugh PO. Neural Blockade in Clinical Anesthesia and Management of Pain, 2nd ed. Philadelphia: JB Lippincott, 1998.

Loeser JD, Bonica JJ (eds). Bonica's Management of Pain, 3rd ed. Philadelphia: Lippincott Williams & Wilkins, 2001.

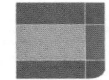

CHAPTER **248**

Acupuncture, Transcutaneous Electrical Nerve Stimulation, and Topical Analgesics

Vinod K. Podichetty and **Anantha Reddy**

KEY POINTS

- Chronic cancer pain is prevalent in patients with no adequate pain control measures.
- Complementary therapy is more common in patients with cancer than in the general population.
- Acupuncture, transcutaneous electrical nerve stimulation (TENS), and topical analgesics relieve symptoms and improve well-being when used cautiously along with mainstream care.
- Acupuncture relieves chronic cancer pain.
- Lidocaine 5% patches reduce pain in patients with postherpetic neuralgia.
- Clinical use of alternative therapies should be based on safety profile, risk/benefit ratio, and evidence.

Significant pain is experienced by 60% of individuals with any stage of cancer. Despite technological advances, they continue to face inadequate pain control. The World Health Organization (WHO) estimates that 25% of all cancer patients die with unalleviated pain.[1] Cancer pain syndromes frequently result from invasion of tissue by tumor (varying by tumor type) or pressure on the nerves. A pathophysiological classification of pain is the basis of therapeutic choice; pain can be broadly classified into

1. Nociceptive pain (ongoing tissue damage)
2. Neuropathic or non-nociceptive pain (resulting from nervous damage)
3. Psychogenic pain (somatoform pain disorder)

Identification plus treatment of the underlying lesion is imperative for both pain control and prevention of further damage. For example, epidural metastasis with impending spinal cord compression requires treatment with steroids, radiation therapy, chemotherapy, or surgical intervention. Fatigue and pain are significant target symptoms in palliative care.

Nonpharmacological approaches such as acupuncture, TENS, and topical analgesics alone or in combination with appropriate pharmacological strategies should be an integral part of care for most cancer pain. They may augment the efficacy of medications by producing fewer undesirable effects. More cancer patients are using complementary and alternative therapies to supplement their medical treatment or enhance their overall health and quality of life.[2] The number of visits and out-of-pocket expenses may exceed those for conventional medical visits. Use of alternative medicine is more common in cancer patients than in the general population.[3] Fifty-seven percent to 80% of cancer patients use one or more form of complementary and alternative medicine,[4] but not all have access to the full range of these modalities because they are rarely covered by insurance. Cancer pain can undermine the ability to fight cancer; hence, appropriate treatment based on evidence of measurable benefit should be the line of approach for improved quality of life and patient satisfaction. Chronic pain in cancer is subjugated by the neuropathic element even when associated with nociceptive pain.[5] Neuralgic and neuropathic pain is the most difficult type to treat and in general does not respond well to drugs.[6] In such conditions, complementary therapies such as acupuncture, TENS, and topical analgesics offer an alternative and conducive mode of treating pain.

ACUPUNCTURE

Background Context

Acupuncture dates back 2500 years as a traditional Chinese intervention in *The Yellow Emperor's Classic of Internal Medicine*.[7] It is a vital therapy in East Asian medicine (China, Japan, and Korea). Acupuncture has blossomed in North America, with over 40 schools, a national accrediting body, state laws regulating its practice, and a rapidly growing reputation for efficacy and effectiveness. The Food and Drug Administration (FDA) approved the use of acupuncture needles by licensed practitioners in 1996.

Acupuncture describes many procedures involving stimulation of anatomical locations on the skin by various techniques. In the most studied mechanism of stimulation of acupuncture points, the skin is penetrated by thin, solid metallic needles manipulated manually, or electrical stimulation is used. Modern acupuncture needles are fine, hairlike, stainless steel, sterile, disposable, and designed for single use. They do not resemble the hollow, stiff syringe needles used to give injections (Fig. 248-1). The needles are inserted with minimal initial sensation. Once inserted, they are manipulated to give an energetic sensation typically described as any of the following: dull and achy, heavy, tingling, spreading, distending, slightly cooling, or warming. The Chinese refer to this sensation as "*the arrival of Qi*" (pronounced "*chee*"—loosely translated as "energy"). Classic texts and modern research indicate that "arrival of the Qi" sensation greatly enhances the therapeutic effect of acupuncture and should be sought in every treatment.

How Does Acupuncture Work?

Although the exact process of action has not been elucidated, the common theory is that there are patterns of energy flow (*Qi*) throughout the body along 12 main meridians that are essential for health (Fig. 248-2). Disruptions in flow are believed to be responsible for disease.[8]

In cancer pain it has been hypothesized that acupuncture causes analgesia through the central and peripheral nervous systems. One theory is that the effects of acupuncture analgesia are partly mediated by activation of a cascade of endorphins and monoamines.[9] Evidence from magnetic resonance imaging studies in normal subjects suggests that acupuncture modulates the limbic system and subcortical gray structures of the human brain responsible for processing pain.[10] Individual therapists vary in performing the procedure, depending on convenience

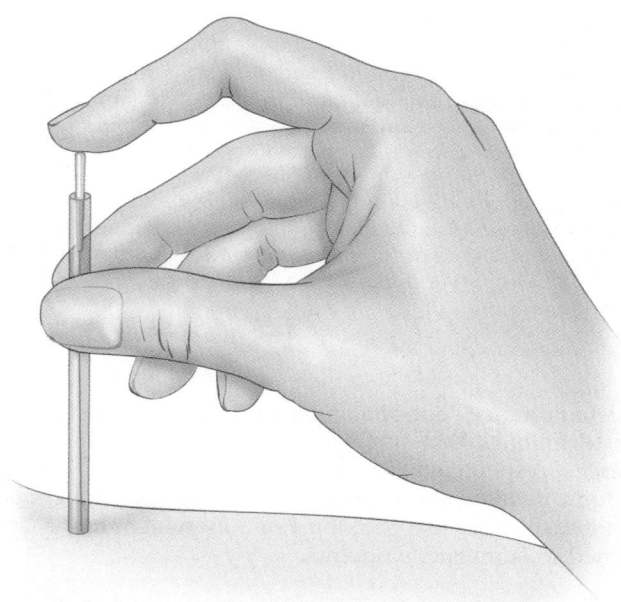

FIGURE 248-1 The classic acupuncture insertion technique (the *"tapping method"*) used by traditional therapists.

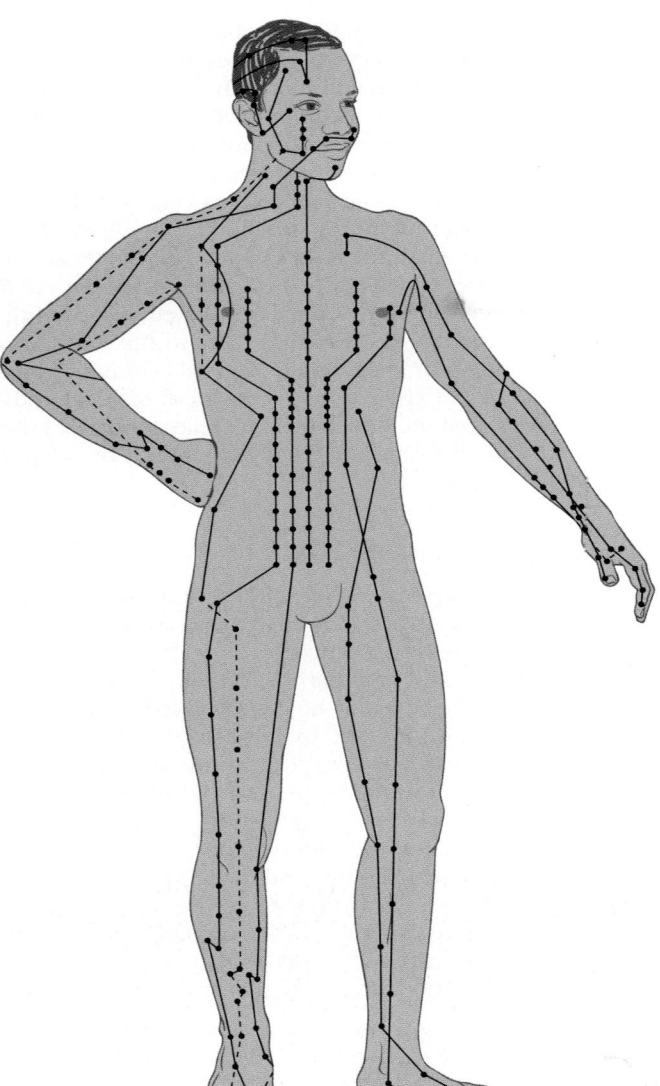

FIGURE 248-2 Location of the meridians and acupoints (acupuncture points) in the body. Meridians are invisible channels through which "*Qi*" circulates throughout the body. Patterns of energy (*Qi*) flow throughout the body along these main meridians. Specific trigger points (*acupuncture points*) are the locations where the *Qi* of the channels rises close to the surface of the body, and these point have clinical application for a specific symptom or disease. Many functional point combinations are used for management of cancer pain. There are 12 main meridians, 6 of which are *yin* and 6 are *yang*, and numerous minor ones, which form the network of energy channels.

and experience. Sonopuncture and electroacupuncture are techniques that use sound waves or tiny electrical charges, respectively, to stimulate the acupoints, with or without needles like traditional acupuncture. Some acupuncturists also use moxibustion, in which herbs are burned to stimulate acupoints.

Evidence of Support

Of all the complementary medical systems, acupuncture enjoys the most scientific credibility, including controlled trials.[11] More likely is the existence of substantial data showing that laboratory acupuncture has measurable and replicable physiological effects.[12] A 1997 National Institutes of Health consensus statement concluded that acupuncture showed promise in adult postoperative and chemotherapy-induced nausea and vomiting.[8] Numerous randomized, controlled trials and systematic reviews and meta-analyses have evaluated the clinical efficacy of acupuncture over the past 2 decades. The evidence indicates that it is effective for pain. However, the data seems to be equivocal or contradictory.[13] The conception that acupuncture may be an effective adjunctive analgesic method for cancer patients is not supported by the data currently available from most rigorous clinical trials.[14]

A recent clinical trial found that acupuncture reduced hot flashes in men after hormonal therapy for prostate cancer.[15] The analgesic effectiveness of auricular acupuncture for cancer pain has also been studied. A placebo-controlled, blinded randomized trial[16] demonstrated a clear benefit from auricular acupuncture for cancer pain despite stable analgesic treatment. Pain intensity decreased by 36% from baseline at 2 months, a statistically significant difference in comparison to controls. This study is significant because neuropathic pain is often under-responsive to conventional treatments.

Acupuncture in the Treatment of Cancer Pain

The role of acupuncture for cancer pain is to serve an adjunctive use in anesthesia, to control postoperative pain, and to aid in recovery from the side effects of various conventional therapies. Electroacupuncture controlled myeloablative chemotherapy–induced nausea and vomiting in a randomized controlled study of 104 patients with breast cancer.[17] Similar results[18] were observed with acupressure wristbands (by continuous stimulation of the PC6 point).

Acupuncture alleviates pain and, to a certain extent, controls pain in accordance with the hypothesis of the existence of specific points that should be treated in a given patient with given symptoms. Evidence suggests that it could be used to lessen local swelling postoperatively, shorten the resolution of hematoma and tissue swelling, and minimize the use of medications and their ill effects. Sonopuncture (through sound waves) and electroacupuncture (involving electrical stimulation) impart a sense of well-being and accelerate recovery. Auricular acupuncture[16] is also beneficial in select cases. It is based on the principle that clinical symptoms are projected onto the ear according to a precise somatic topography. Acupuncturists recognize these points by detection of an electrical signal that is proportional to the intensity and duration of the cancer symptoms. All cancer patients are not suitable for acupuncture. Careful selection is essential. For example, those with a low platelet count (thrombocytopenia) or a low white blood cell count (neutropenia) are at greater risk for bleeding and infection. It is imperative that the treating acupuncturist have cancer experience and take an integrated approach to the patient. Adverse events are rare but may include pain, contact dermatitis, bleeding, transient hypotension, and occasionally a retained needle.[19]

Common Errors in Acupuncture

Inadequate Treatment

- In nonresponding patients, it should not be presumed that a defined treatment regimen would relieve the problem.
- Physicians should emphasize an individual patient approach for successful treatment outcomes.

Technique Errors

- Because acupuncture has not gone through a systematic process of optimization, practice is diverse, with pain being treated by many different techniques, including but not limited to deep needling, shallow needling, insertion of thick semipermanent studs in the ear or body, laser stimulation, and electroacupuncture.
- There is also great diversity in the total number and frequency of treatment sessions, which vary in style and practice. Hence, acupuncture should be administered in accordance with the technician's training, personal experience, and preference.
- It is important to recognize the dangers and pitfalls of combining complementary and alternative therapies (acupuncture with herbs) with conventional therapy because case studies show that some complementary and alternative therapies can create potentially dangerous interactions with pharmacotherapy.

Patient-Physician Communication

- Few patients who use complementary and alternative therapies for cancer pain inform their doctors.
- Given the potential risks associated with some complementary and alternative therapies, health professionals need to adopt a more proactive role in the use of these therapies.
- Such communication could prevent adverse clinical effects and maximize the usefulness of any complementary therapy for cancer pain subsequently proved effective.
- It is an error to claim that treatment benefits are confined to particular types of patients ("subgroup effects").

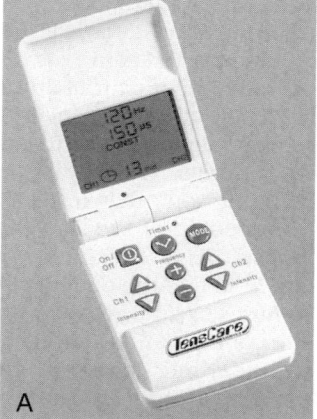

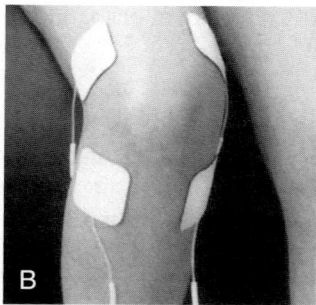

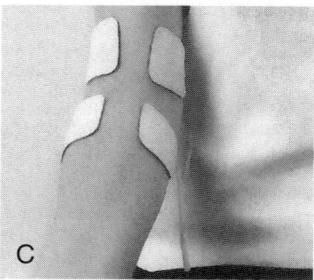

FIGURE 248-3 **A** to **C,** Transcutaneous electrical nerve stimulation (TENS) unit and electrode pads used for management of chronic, acute, and persistent pain. TENS machines deliver small electrical pulses to the body via electrodes placed on the skin, which is thought to help ease pain.

TRANSCUTANEOUS ELECTRICAL NERVE STIMULATION

TENS is a noninvasive, drug-free method for relief of pain. TENS machines deliver small electrical impulses to the body via electrodes on or near the painful area (the skin) and along the nerve fibers (Fig. 248-3A to C). The impulses suppress pain signals to the brain, and this eases the pain. In clinical studies, electrostimulation reduced perception of heat-associated pain and enhanced pain tolerance.[20] TENS also encourages the body to produce more endorphins and enkephalins. Although scientific research evidence to support the use of TENS for cancer pain is inadequate, it seems popular with patients. In many cases, stimulation greatly reduces or eliminates pain, and relief may continue for several hours after treatment. TENS is thought to work similarly to acupuncture.

Evidence of Support

Research trials of TENS for pain management have reported conflicting results. TENS is used moderately in cancer patients as an adjunct to other effective modalities because of its placebo effect. Controlled trials and a recent meta-analysis[21] concluded that TENS is not highly effective for chronic pain. Nonetheless, TENS is widely used to treat musculoskeletal pain in the elderly. So-called passive modalities such as massage, ultrasound, heat, or ice may provide temporary symptomatic relief. These modalities have the advantage of minimizing transport of older patients and low cost. These techniques may also improve exercise tolerance during rehabilitation. The outcome of TENS correlates with the origin of the intractable cancer pain. Pain from the central nervous system and autonomic pain are poorly relieved with TENS. It is most beneficial for pain from peripheral nerve lesions. Because primary true isolated metastasis in a peripheral nerve trunk is rare, TENS has a derivative role in relieving cancer pain.

How Does TENS Work?

TENS machines essentially work by interlinked processes. The *"pain gate"* control hypothesis of blocking pain is one explanation for the analgesia induced by electrical stimulation. This theory suggests that the application of varying degrees of nonpainful electrical stimuli to a painful region triggers conceptual "pain gates" to close and thereby blocks conduction of painful impulses and consequently the experience of pain. Conventional TENS use involves low-intensity, high-frequency stimulation, which primarily recruits afferent "Aαβ" fibers. TENS causes changes in sympathetic tone that result in local dilation, accompanied by reddening of the skin and a local rise in temperature.[22] Most TENS machines are ambulatory friendly and designed so that the patient can move around. TENS gives a tingling sensation to start with, which will lessen slightly (accommodation) after a few minutes, depending on the pulse rate setting of the device (Table 248-1). TENS (both high- and low-intensity stimulation) has developed into an efficient clinical tool for mild cancer pain, most typically neuropathic or musculoskeletal pain.

TOPICAL ANALGESICS

Cancer pain management should also include appropriate adjuvants such as local/topical anesthetics. The number of clinical trials that have evaluated topical analgesics for cancer pain is inadequate. Topical local anesthetics with or without corticosteroids are usually indicated for diagnostic blocks, muscle spasms, acute and chronic pain, postsurgical syndromes, and herpes zoster.[23]

Pharmacology

The lidocaine 5% patch (Lidoderm, Endo Pharmaceuticals) was approved by the FDA and launched in the United States in 1999. It is a local anesthetic that is suggested to stabilize neuronal membranes by inhibiting the ionic fluxes required for the initiation and conduction of impulses. Penetration of lidocaine into intact skin after application produces analgesia, but less than that needed to induce a complete sensory block. Topical lidocaine is applied to intact skin over the most painful area (up to three patches) and is used only once for up to 12 hours within a 24-hour period. Adjustments in drug doses are needed for the elderly, who are sensitive to analgesics and their side effects.

Efficacy in Cancer Pain

Topical lidocaine is often indicated for cancer pain. It has no systemic side effects and is well tolerated when applied on allodynic skin for up to 12 hours. An open-label prospective study demonstrated positive outcomes in postmastectomy pain (refractory neuropathic pain).[24] Double-blind, crossover clinical trials[23] comparing topical lidocaine with placebo demonstrated statistically significant differences favoring lidocaine for pain associated with postherpetic neuralgia (Table 248-2).

EVIDENCE-BASED MEDICINE

National Comprehensive Cancer Network guidelines recommend nonpharmacological modalities such as acupuncture if pain scores remain at 4 or above on a 10-point scale after re-evaluation and modification of pharmacological management.[25] In the absence of guidelines concerning when and how to incorporate complementary therapies, decisions should be based on clinical judgment, patient preference, and the risk/benefit ratio. Acupuncture is widely used for non–cancer-related pain. It relieves both acute pain, such as postoperative dental pain, and chronic pain, such as headache.[8] Whether acupuncture relieves cancer-related musculoskeletal pain is controversial.[26] It does influence the production of endogenous opioid neurotransmitters.[27] Several studies have indicated reduction of cancer pain, although lack of controls limits their conclusions. In summary, research suggests that

TABLE 248-1 TENS Machine Working Mechanism Based on the Frequency of the Electrical Current Bandwidth Unit Setting

PULSE RATE	DEVICE RANGE	MECHANISM
High (method commonly used for early cancer pain)	90-130 Hz	Triggers the "pain gates" to close, thereby blocking the pain nerve pathway to the brain
Low pulse rate	2-5 Hz	Stimulates the body to generate its own pain-easing chemicals (endorphins)

TENS, transcutaneous electrical nerve stimulation.

TABLE 248-2 Description of the Use of Acupuncture, TENS, and Topical Analgesics for Cancer Pain

MODALITY	METHODOLOGY	EFFECTS	CONJUNCTION TREATMENTS	ADVERSE EFFECTS
Acupuncture therapy	Insertion of needles along specific pathways	Analgesia, deactivation of pain processing in the brain, anti-inflammatory properties	Sonopuncture, heat, moxibustion, acupressure, or electric stimulation (TENS)	Rare, but may include exacerbation of depression, local bleeding, infection, contact dermatitis, pain
TENS	Electrical impulses	Suppression of pain signals to the brain; production of natural pain-killing chemicals	Massage, ultrasound, heat, or ice	Rare, but may include skin irritation
Topical analgesics	Pharmacokinetics	Analgesia		Sensitivity to local anesthetics, allergic reactions (rare), application site erythema, rash

TENS, transcutaneous electrical nerve stimulation.

complementary measures are valuable in certain circumstances (Table 248-3). Because strong evidence of measurable benefit for specific indications is not always available, clinical decisions should be based on the balance of evidence concerning safety and efficacy, the risk/benefit ratio, and patient preference, which will guide clinicians to make appropriate recommendations.

CONCLUSIONS

Relief of cancer-related symptoms is critical in supportive and palliative care. Complementary therapies such as acupuncture, TENS, and topical analgesics can be of assistance when conventional treatment does not bring adequate relief or causes undesirable side effects. Although a completely pain-free state is unlikely in patients with advanced disease, alternative options should be explored and tailored to the individual patient. Over the past decade, complementary and alternative therapies have become increasingly popular despite little scientific data from clinical trials. Randomized controlled trials constitute less than 1% of the published literature on cancer pain and are often of poor methodological quality. Given the widespread availability and use of these therapies, it is essential that well-designed clinical studies be conducted to assess the effectiveness or possible harm of specific modalities in defined cancer populations.

The science of complementary and alternative therapies is still inadequate to sufficiently inform physicians and patients of the benefits and potential risks. Designing well-defined protocols will be challenging, particularly for alternative therapies such as acupuncture and TENS, but such protocols are crucial to understand the effects and use of these modalities. Information about out-of-pocket expenses and insurance costs is another key factor. We need to determine how effective and safe these interventions are and whether they should be integrated into standard medical practice, as well as understand their economic and societal implications. Nonetheless, many cancer patients continue to explore complementary and alternative medicine not as an "*adjunct*" to support or palliation but as a "*cure*." In most regions of the world, many cancer patients are in advanced stages of disease when first diagnosed. In such environments, the only realistic treatment option is pain relief and palliative care.

TABLE 248-3 Common Cancer Symptoms Controlled by Acupuncture, TENS, and Topical Analgesics

ACUPUNCTURE

↓ Pain[16]

↓ Nausea and vomiting (postoperative and chemotherapy induced)[8,18]

↓ Hot flashes in men (experienced after hormonal therapy for prostate cancer)[15]

↓ Postoperative dental pain

↓ Headache

↓ Chemotherapy-induced fatigue

↓ Xerostomia (dry mouth) (caused by radiotherapy for head and neck cancer)

TENS

↓ Pain (by ↑ in endorphin and encephalin production)

↓ Heat and pain perception and ↑ pain tolerance[20]

TOPICAL LIDOCAINE

↓ Acute and chronic pain conditions[23] (by ↓ in ionic fluxes required for initiation and conduction of impulses)

↓ Refractory neuropathic pain (postmastectomy pain)[24]

TENS, transcutaneous electrical nerve stimulation.

Future Considerations

- The WHO estimates that a quarter of all cancer patients die with unrelieved pain.
- Careful selection of patients and supervision of complementary practitioners throughout disease management are essential.
- Avoid inappropriate referrals for alternative treatments.
- Jointly agreed protocols and guidelines are needed for an integrated approach between complementary and conventional practitioners.
- The National Comprehensive Cancer Network believes that the best management of any cancer patient is achieved in a clinical trial. Participation is especially encouraged.

REFERENCES

1. The World Health Organization. Putting Evidence about Cancer Pain into Practice: The Role of Clinical Guidelines, nos. 2 and 3, vol 18. Geneva, The World Health Organization, 2005.
2. Einsenberg DM, Davis RB, Ettner SL, et al. Trends in alternative medicine use in the United States, 1990-1997: Results of a follow-up national survey. JAMA 1998;280:1569-1575.
3. DiGianni LM, Garber JE, Winer EP. Complementary and alternative medicine use among women with breast cancer. J Clin Oncol 2002;20:34s-38s.
4. Richardson MA, Sanders T, Palmer JL, et al. Complementary/alternative medicine use in a comprehensive cancer center and the implications for oncology. J Clin Oncol 2000;18:2505-2514.
5. Caraceni A, Portenoy RK. A working group of the IASP Task Force on Cancer Pain. An international survey of cancer pain characteristics and syndromes. Pain 1999;82:263-274.
6. Filshie J. The non-drug treatment of neuralgic and neuropathic pain of malignancy. Cancer Surv 1988;7:161-193.
7. The Yellow Emperor's Classic of Internal Medicine. Berkeley: University of California Press, 1993, p 2002.
8. NIH Consensus Development Panel on Acupuncture. JAMA 1998;280:1518-1524.
9. Sims J. The mechanism of acupuncture analgesia: A review. Complement Ther Med 1997;5:102-111.
10. Hui KK, Liu J, Marina O, et al. The integrated response of the human cerebro-cerebellar and limbic systems to acupuncture stimulation at ST 36 as evidenced by fMRI. Neuroimage 2005;27:479-496.
11. Pomeranz B, Stux G (eds). Scientific Bases of Acupuncture. New York: Springer-Verlag, 1989.
12. Astin JA, Narie A, Pelletier R, et al. A review of the incorporation of complementary and alternative medicine by mainstream physicians. Arch Internal Med 1998;158:2303-2310.
13. Kaptchuk TJ. Acupuncture: Theory, efficacy, and practice. Ann Intern Med 2002;136:374-383.
14. Lee H, Schmidt K, Ernst E. Acupuncture for the relief of cancer-related pain—a systematic review. Eur J Pain 2005;9:437-444.
15. Hammar M, Frisk J, Grimas O, et al. Acupuncture treatment of vasomotor symptoms in men with prostatic carcinoma: A pilot study. J Urol 1999;161:853-856.
16. Alimi D, Rubino C, Pichard-Leandri E, et al. Analgesic effect of auricular acupuncture for cancer pain: A randomized, blinded, controlled trial. J Clin Oncol 2003;21:4120-4126.
17. Shen J, Wenger N, Glaspy J, et al. Electroacupuncture for control of myeloablative chemotherapy–induced emesis: A randomized controlled trial. JAMA 2000;284:2755-2761.
18. Melchart D, Ihbe-Heffinger A, Leps B, et al. Acupuncture and acupressure for the prevention of chemotherapy-induced nausea—a randomised cross-over pilot study. Support Care Cancer 2006;14:878-882.
19. Vickers A, Zollman C. Acupuncture. BMJ 1999;319:973-976.
20. Marchand S, Bushnell MC, Duncan GH. Modulation of heat pain perception by high frequency transcutaneous electrical nerve stimulation (TENS). Clin J Pain 1991;7:122-129.

21. Podichetty V, Mazanec DJ, Biscup RS. Chronic non-malignant musculoskeletal pain in older adult: Clinical issues and opioid intervention. Postgrad Med J 2003;79:627-633.
22. Abram SE, Asiddao CB, Reynolds AC. Increased skin temperature during transcutaneous electrical nerve stimulation. Anesth Analg 1980;59:22-25.
23. Galer BS, Rowbotham MC, Perander J, Friedman E. Topical lidocaine patch relieves postherpetic neuralgia more effectively than a vehicle topical patch: Results of an enriched enrollment study. Pain 1999;80:533-538.
24. Devers A, Galer BS. Topical lidocaine patch relieves a variety of neuropathic pain conditions: An open-label study. Clin J Pain 2000;16:205-208.
25. Benedetti C, Brock C, Cleeland C, et al. NCCN practice guidelines for cancer pain. Oncology (Huntingt) 2000;14:135-150.
26. Ernst E, Pittler MH. The effectiveness of acupuncture in treating acute dental pain: A systematic review. Br Dent J 1998;184:443-447.
27. Guo HF, Tian J, Wang X, et al. Brain substrates activated by electroacupuncture of different frequencies (I): Comparative study on the expression of oncogene c-fos and genes coding for three opioid peptides. Brain Res Mol Brain Res 1996;43:157-166.

SUGGESTED READING

American Pain Society. Principles of Analgesic Use in the Treatment of Acute Pain and Cancer Pain, 5th ed. Skokie, IL: American Pain Society, 2003.

Bonica JJ: Treatment of cancer pain: Current status and future needs. In Fields HL, et al (eds). Advances in Pain Research and Therapy, vol 9. New York: Raven Press, 1985, pp 589-616.

Chapman CR, Gunn CC. Acupuncture. In Bonica JJ (ed). The Management of Pain, vol 2. Philadelphia: Lea & Febiger, 1990, pp 1805-1821.

Doyle D, Hanks G, Cherny NI, et al (eds). Oxford Textbook of Palliative Medicine, 3rd ed. New York: Oxford University Press, 2005.

Duke M. Acupuncture. New York: Pyramid House, 1972.

Fulder S. The Handbook of Alternative and Complementary Medicine, 3rd ed. Oxford: Oxford University Press, 1996

Merskey H, Loeser JD, Dubner R (eds). The Paths of Pain 1975-2005. International Association for the Study of Pain. Seattle, WA: IASP Press, 2005.

Meyerson BA. Electrostimulation procedures: Effects, presumed rationale, and possible mechanisms. In Bonica JJ, Lindblom U, Iggo A, et al (eds). Advances in Pain Research and Therapy, vol 5. New York: Raven Press, 1983, pp 495-534.

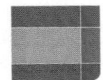

CHAPTER **249**

Opioids for Cancer Pain

Janet R. Hardy and **Friedemann Nauck**

KEY POINTS

- Morphine remains the international opioid of choice.
- Many alternative opioids available in various formulations are available.
- Some opioids are more suited to certain individuals than others, for multiple reasons.
- The oral route remains the preferred route for opioid delivery.
- The World Health Organization (WHO) analgesic ladder is recommended worldwide as a simple step-by-step guide to pain control.
- Opioid rotation can improve pain control with less toxicity in some patients.

Most patients with cancer develop pain at some stage of their illness, and most of these patients will require opioids for pain.[1] In the Western world, we are "spoiled for choice" and have a range of different opioids and opioid formulations available. The universal undertreatment of pain is widespread and well recognized.[2] This undertreatment results in part from fear of opioids and in part from misunderstandings about these drugs and how they work. It is said that nothing would have a greater impact on improving the treatment of cancer pain than implementation of existing knowledge.[3]

RECENT DEVELOPMENTS

Choice of Drug

Morphine remains the opioid of choice worldwide,[3] not because of any demonstrated superiority over any other opioid, but primarily because of its known effectiveness, familiarity, and relatively low cost (Fig. 249-1).[4] Morphine is available in various formulations and dose strengths and can be delivered by several different routes (oral, parenteral, rectal) (Table 249-1). It is not the ideal opioid; it has low variable bioavailability, active metabolites, high dependence on renal function for clearance, and an unpredictable dose-response relationship. Many patients fear morphine and equate it with dying.

In Western countries, multiple new opioids and opioid formulations are available (Fig. 249-2). How do we choose which opioid to give to our patients? Controlled studies reveal only minor differences among the various drugs, and no high-level evidence suggests that one drug is better than another. This finding is not surprising because all commonly used opioids exert their activity predominantly through the μ-opioid receptor, which is also responsible for most side effects. Some patients who are intolerant of the side effects of one opioid gain excellent pain relief with little toxicity from another opioid. Several factors may influence our choice. The art is to find the opioid best suited to each individual patient. That opioid is the one that produces adequate pain relief within an acceptable time frame with the least side effects.[5]

Availability

For various social, cultural, legal, political, and financial reasons, the availability of different opioids and opioid formulations varies among countries. This variation is reflected by the range in average dose of morphine per person per day in different countries.[6] In many Western countries, morphine is available within the boundaries of controlled prescribing. Diamorphine is available only in

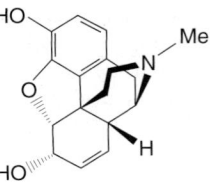

FIGURE 249-1 Chemical structure of morphine.

TABLE 249-1 Choice of Opioid

OPIOID	AVAILABILITY	POTENTIAL ADVANTAGES	POTENTIAL DISADVANTAGES
Morphine	PO (IR, MR, liquid, tablets) PR SC, IV NA	Cost Availability Familiarity Versatility Range of doses Linear kinetics	Low bioavailability Variability of dose/response relationship Active metabolites Dependence on renal function for elimination
Oxycodone	PO (IR, MR, liquid, tablets) PR SC, IV	Not recognized as morphine "Cleaner" pharmacokinetics Minimal change in kinetics with aging	Delayed clearance in hepatic failure Dose per volume restrictions for parenteral delivery
Fentanyl	TTS SC, IV SL, TM, IN NA	Transdermal formulation Probably less risk of constipation No dependence on renal function	No oral formulation Dose per volume restrictions for parenteral delivery
Methadone	PO (liquid, tablets) SC, IV	Low cost No dependence on renal function	Difficult titration Variability of dose/response relationship Long half-life Delayed toxicity Stigma of use in addiction
Diamorphine	SC, IV	Low cost Water solubility Dose per volume appropriate for SC delivery	Stigma of "heroin"
Buprenorphine	PO (tablets) SL TTS	Lipid solubility Transdermal formulation	Partial agonist property Difficulty of reversal with naloxone
Hydromorphone	PO (IR, MR, liquid, tablets) SC, IV	Water solubility Dose per volume appropriate for SC delivery	Small dose range of IR tablets

IN, intranasal; IR, immediate release; IV, intravenous; MR, modified release; NA, neuroaxial; PO, oral; PR, per rectum; SC, subcutaneous; SL, sublingual; TM, transmucosal; TTS, transdermal.

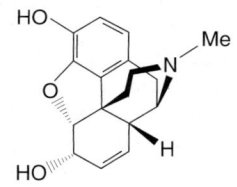

Morphine

Codeine

Thebaine

Oripavine

FIGURE 249-2 Chemical structure of opioids related to morphine.

the United Kingdom, although this drug has been shown to be no better or worse or more addictive than any other opioid.[7] Oxycodone is widely used in lower doses for mild to moderate pain in the United States, it is used as a postoperative analgesic in Finland, and it is the main opioid of choice in Scandinavia for moderate to severe pain. Until recently, transdermal fentanyl was not available in New Zealand, and parenteral oxycodone was unavailable in Australia. Similarly, parenteral formulations of the lipophilic opioids (fentanyl, alfentanil, and sufentanil) are not subsidized by the Australian government, and methadone liquid is subsidized only for use in addiction programs.

Convenience

Patients with large tablet loads may welcome the opportunity to take delayed-release preparations or opioids with long half-lives (e.g., methadone) that need to be taken only once or twice a day. Morphine, oxycodone, and hydromorphone are all available in both immediate-release and sustained-release preparations. Transdermal preparations (e.g., fentanyl, buprenorphine) are ideal for patients who have difficulty swallowing or compromised gastrointestinal tracts or who do not like the idea of carrying portable infusion devices. Opioids that can be delivered by the sublingual route (e.g., buprenorphine) offer a convenient alternative to subcutaneous injections for parenteral analgesia.

One of the advantages of morphine is the ability to use the same drug over a wide dose range and by several different routes. For example, following titration with an immediate-release formulation, the patient can be converted, when stable, to a delayed-release formulation or given parenteral morphine if the pain proves difficult to control or demands rapid titration. Until recently, parenteral oxycodone was not available; a patient previously taking oral oxycodone tablets would have to be switched to an alternative opioid if the parenteral route was indicated. Similarly, no oral formulation of fentanyl exists. Published dose conversions are inexact, and any change of opioid exposes patients to the potential risk of uncontrolled pain or drug toxicity.[8]

Tolerance

Ten percent to 30% of patients are believed to be truly intolerant of morphine.[4] These patients may benefit from a change to another opioid (see the later discussion of opioid rotation). The lipophilic opioids (e.g., fentanyl, methadone) are probably less constipating than are other opioids. These agents may be preferable in patients with severe constipation or any degree of bowel obstruction. Oxycodone has no active metabolites and "cleaner" pharmacokinetics (see Chapter 138), features that may explain why oxycodone may be better tolerated in elderly patients.

Co-morbidities and Toxicity

Morphine and its metabolites accumulate in patients with impaired renal function, with resultant toxicity. Many clinicians therefore choose opioids that are not dependent on renal function for clearance (e.g., fentanyl or methadone), although morphine can still be used (albeit in smaller doses less frequently). The elimination of oxycodone is significantly influenced by hepatic impairment. Oxycodone should therefore be used with caution in patients with end-stage liver disease. The clearance of opioids that depend on the cytochrome P-450 system for elimination (e.g., methadone, oxycodone, fentanyl) theoretically renders these drugs open to interaction with other drugs that induce or suppress enzyme activity.

Someone who has had an unfortunate past experience (e.g., uncontrolled nausea or confusion) with a particular opioid will not be willing to try that drug again. Similarly, for many patients, morphine is equated with imminent death and drug addiction. These patients are often prepared to take an opioid that does not carry the same public connotations.

Route of Delivery

The need to deliver drugs by the parenteral route (e.g., in patients with swallowing difficulties or bowel obstruction) limits the choice of opioid to some extent, although transdermal (fentanyl), sublingual (buprenorphine, fentanyl), and nasal (sufentanil) alternatives exist.

Dose Range

Many immediate-release opioids (e.g., hydromorphone) are available in low-dose formulations only. The number of tablets restricts higher dose ranges even with opioids available in delayed-release preparations. Conversely, morphine can be conveniently delivered over a wide dose spectrum because of the range of formulations available.

Type of Pain

Neuropathic pain is notoriously resistant to opioids.[9] Methadone is a weak N-methyl-D-aspartate antagonist, and anecdotal evidence suggests some advantage over morphine for neuropathic pain. Short-acting opioids (e.g., fentanyl, alfentanil) are indicated for breakthrough or incident pain of short duration, whereas opioids with long half-lives (e.g., methadone) are not.

Cost

Morphine, diamorphine, and methadone are inexpensive drugs. Many of the newer semisynthetic opioids, especially those in formulations other than oral tablets (e.g., transdermal and transbuccal preparations), remain prohibitively expensive in some countries. Opioid cost and relative cost to income are higher in developing countries.[10]

Choice of Route

The oral route is the route of choice for opioids.[11] The benefits of oral medications include ease of administration and patient convenience. The choice of an alternative route depends on such factors as the patient's ability to take oral medications, the need for rapid titration in severe pain, and the patient's preference. Some clinicians believe that a change in route, rather than a change of opioid, is the most logical means of instigating an opioid rotation to improve pain control or to lessen toxicity.[12]

If a patient is unable to take drugs orally, the rectum offers an alternative route, especially when subcutaneous administration would be difficult. The rectum is very vascular, and drugs are generally well absorbed by this route. The relative potency of oral morphine to rectal morphine is 1:1.[11] Vaginal morphine administration has been reported, but no data have been published.

Parenteral opioid administration offers a shorter time to peak analgesic effect and is therefore ideal for patients with severe or unstable pain because this route facilitates rapid titration. The ability to deliver many drugs by the subcutaneous route has revolutionized palliative medicine. Few drugs are licensed for this mode of delivery, but much experience exists worldwide in the use of opioids by this route. Diamorphine, hydromorphone, and morphine tartrate are water soluble and therefore are suitable for parenteral delivery. Morphine sulfate is less soluble and is impractical for a standard infusion device. It is difficult to deliver fentanyl through a standard Graseby subcutaneous infusion device because of the limited dose per standard ampule. More potent alternatives (alfentanil and sufentanil) do not pose volume problems but have more limited availability (Fig. 249-3). In the United States, most patients have indwelling intravenous ports that allow these drugs to be delivered intravenously. No indication exists to administer any opioid intramuscularly for chronic pain because subcutaneous administration is simpler and less painful.

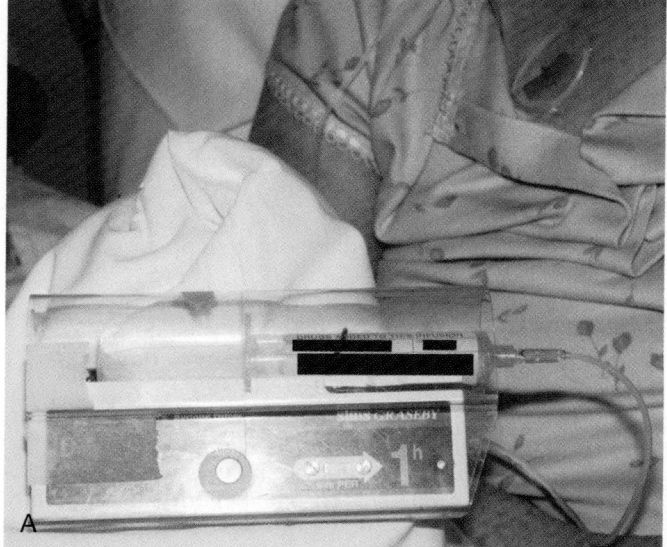

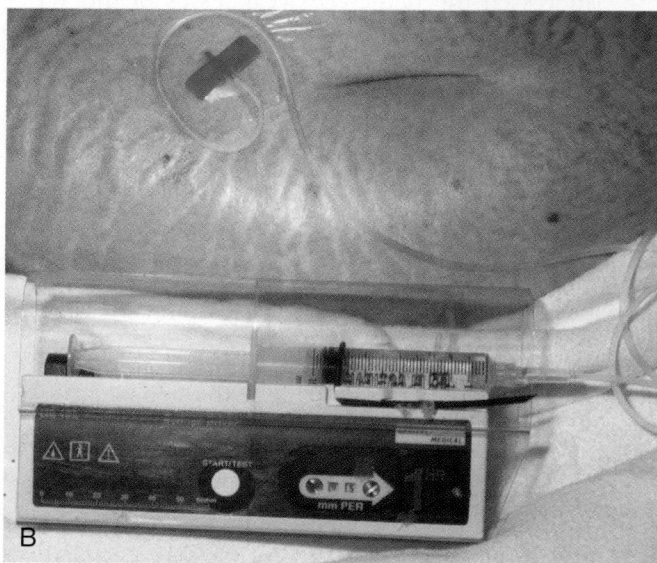

FIGURE 249-3 **A** and **B,** Syringe driver for the subcutaneous delivery of opioids.

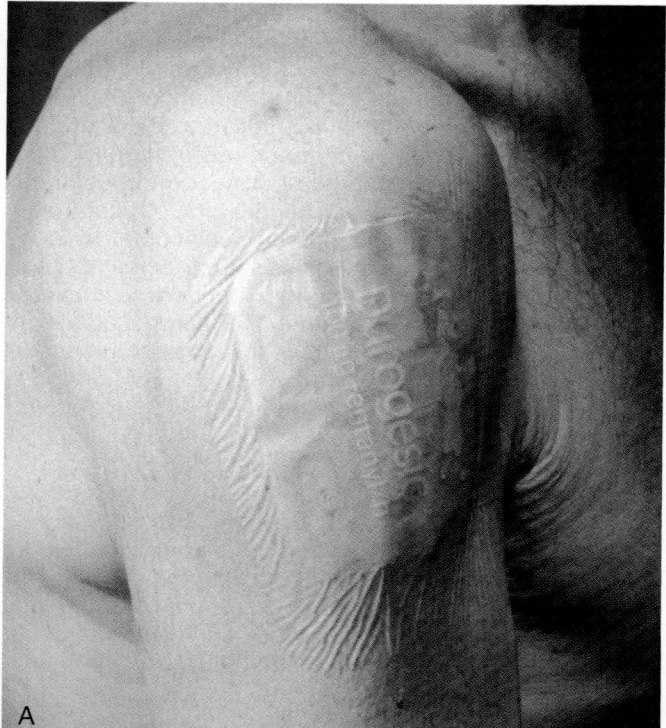

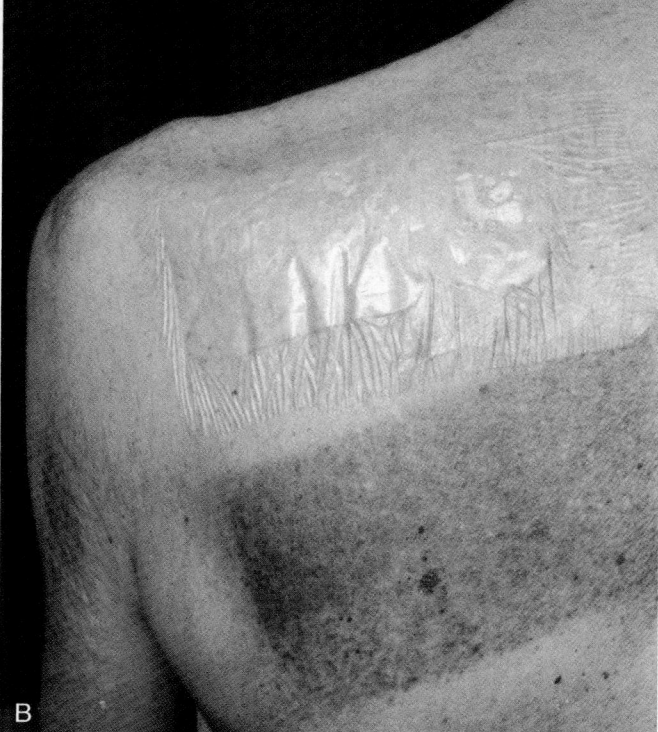

FIGURE 249-4 **A** and **B,** Patient with fentanyl patch for transdermal delivery.

Because of high lipid solubility, delayed-release fentanyl and buprenorphine preparations have been developed for transdermal administration. This route offers a convenient means of delivering these drugs at a constant rate through a rate-limiting membrane (Fig. 249-4). Failure of the patch to adhere to the skin (especially in hot, humid climates) and skin irritation have posed problems, but modern transdermal therapeutic systems have addressed these concerns.

Lipid-soluble opioids are also ideal for transmucosal or buccal delivery (Fig. 249-5). An oral transmucosal fentanyl citrate formulation is available commercially. It gives rapid analgesia and is effective for breakthrough pain.[13] Fentanyl, alfentanil, and sufentanil have all been administered intranasally.

Spinal opioids are recommended for uncontrolled pain despite maximal treatment with systemic opioids and adjuvant therapy.[4] The aim is to deliver a smaller opioid dose directly to the central nervous system opioid receptors, to improve analgesia while reducing toxicity. The choice of route (epidural or intrathecal) depends primarily on the expertise and experience of the anesthetist or pain specialist and on the facilities available. The potential for opioid toxicity and catheter complications (e.g., bleeding, infection, cerebrospinal fluid leak, catheter displacement) is high. In Western countries, the frequency of spinal opioid use often depends on the availability of a specialist pain service. When comfort and not function is the ultimate goal of care, it may be more appropriate to use a drug by an epidural or intrathecal route, even though this may restrict patients to institutional care.[5] Uncontrolled studies suggest that intracerebroventricular opioid therapy is at least as effective against pain as other neuraxial treatments and may be successful for patients whose cancer pain is resistant to other treatments.[14] Spinal opioids are used more commonly in countries that do not have access to multiple analgesics.

Dosing Strategies

The WHO analgesic ladder remains the recommended opioid dosing strategy worldwide (Fig. 249-6). It uses a few drugs and has the advantages of simplicity and transferability to many settings. It is based on the premise that drugs of increasing potency be used for pain of increasing severity in a stepwise manner while encouraging the use of adjuvants or co-analgesics at each stage as appropriate.

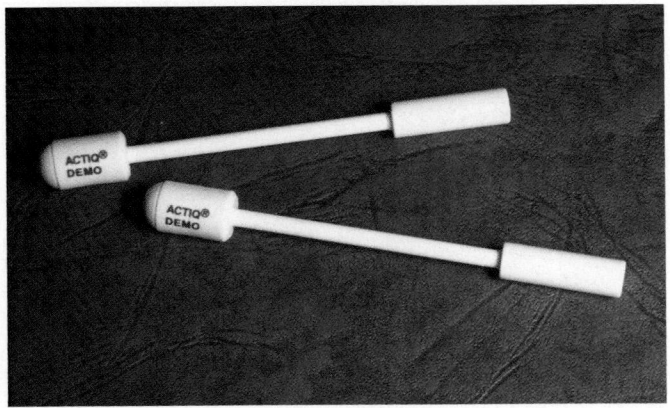

FIGURE 249-5 Fentanyl lozenge (Actiq) for delivery by the sublingual route.

Although much experience has been gained with the WHO analgesic ladder, high-level evidence to support its effectiveness is sparse.[15]

Criticisms of the ladder include the following:

1. The drugs recommended for step 2 of the ladder (e.g., codeine, dihydrocodeine) are less efficacious than some of those for step 1 (e.g., nonsteroidal anti-inflammatory drugs and paracetamol) when used alone. Therefore, more recent recommendations are as follows:
   a. Use "weak" opioids only in combination with a nonopioid (e.g., paracetamol plus codeine).
   b. Use low doses of the "stronger" opioids (e.g., morphine or oxycodone) at step 2.
2. The ladder is not mechanistic (i.e., it does not incorporate the cause of the pain).
3. The guidelines do not include dosing strategies for temporal changes in pain severity. The Agency for Healthcare Policy and Research guidelines[16] addressed the perceived weaknesses of the WHO ladder by making numerous recommendations, including those pertaining to breakthrough medication and the use of alternate opioids.
4. Morphine is nominated as the opioid of choice despite its known limitations (see earlier).
5. The ladder focuses on the pharmacological management of pain and ignores the psychosocial, educational, and supportive approaches to total pain control.

Certain alternative approaches to pain management have been proposed, including the pyramid-plus-ribbon approach[4,16] (Fig. 249-7) and the "Sydney stickman."[17] The pyramid-plus-ribbon approach depicts a hierarchy of pain management strategies from the least to the most invasive and incorporates nonpharmacological strategies such as radiation therapy and chemotherapy. The Sydney stickman approach stresses a multidimensional patient assessment and individualized treatment modalities.

Dose Titration

Published guidelines on the use of morphine recommend that all patients be commenced on a low dose of an

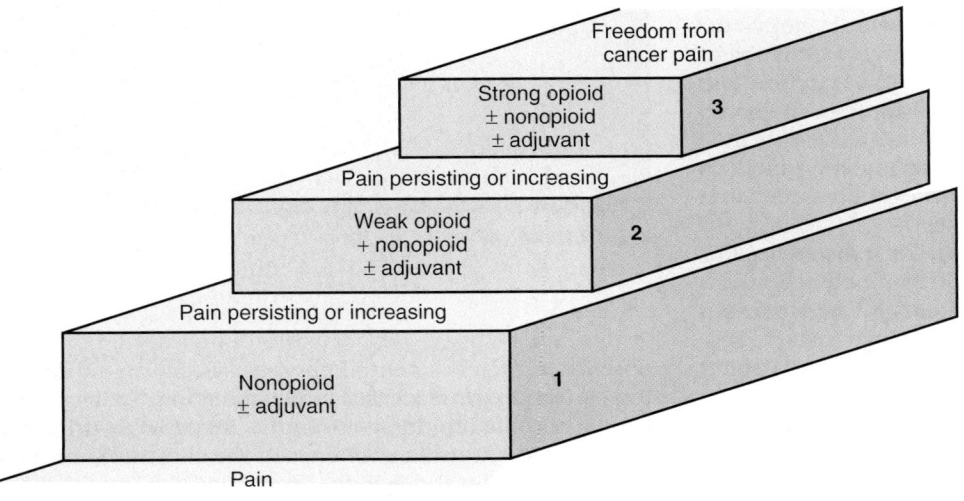

FIGURE 249-6 World Health Organization analgesic ladder.

Freedom from cancer pain

Strong opioid ± nonopioid ± adjuvant **3**

Pain persisting or increasing

Weak opioid + nonopioid ± adjuvant **2**

Pain persisting or increasing

Nonopioid ± adjuvant **1**

Pain

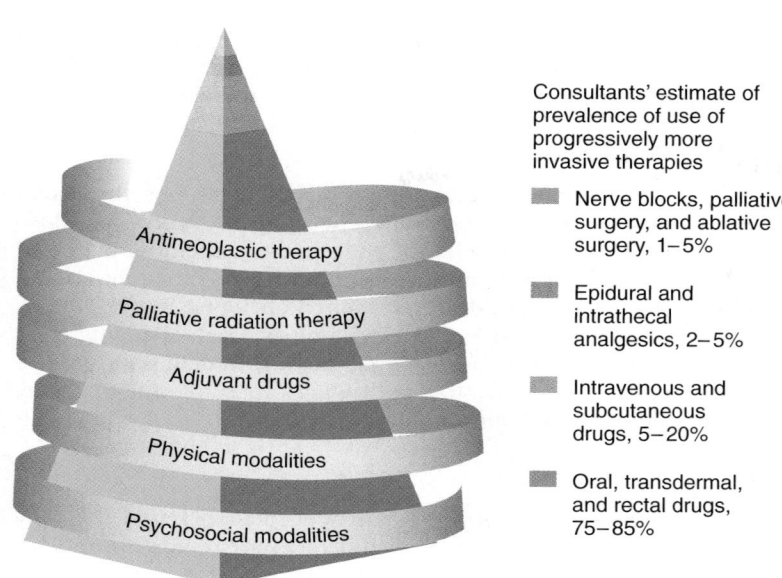

FIGURE 249-7   Pyramid-plus-ribbon approach to pain management. *(Redrawn from Jacox A, Carr D, Payne R (eds). Management of Cancer Pain. Clinical Practice Guideline no. 9. Agency for Healthcare Policy and Research publication no. 94-0592. Washington, DC: U.S. Department of Health and Human Services, 1994.)*

Consultants' estimate of prevalence of use of progressively more invasive therapies

▨ Nerve blocks, palliative surgery, and ablative surgery, 1–5%

▨ Epidural and intrathecal analgesics, 2–5%

▨ Intravenous and subcutaneous drugs, 5–20%

▨ Oral, transdermal, and rectal drugs, 75–85%

immediate-release preparation given regularly by the clock and by mouth if possible.[11] The dose is then titrated upward according to pain response and toxicity. The usual recommendation is to increase the dose by one third every 24 to 48 hours until the pain is controlled and to provide breakthrough or rescue medication, to be taken concurrently whenever necessary. No standard exists regarding the dose of breakthrough medication. Current practice is to give either one sixth (100% of the 4-hourly equivalent) or one twelfth (50% of the 4-hourly equivalent) of the total daily dose of regular morphine. Once the pain has been controlled, the patient can then be given the same dose of morphine in a delayed-release preparation once or twice per day (Box 249-1).

Prophylactic laxatives should always be prescribed concurrently, and antiemetics should be made available in case of nausea. Elderly patients, or those with renal impairment, may require smaller doses given at extended intervals. Most patients achieve pain relief with less than 200 mg morphine per day.[18]

This titration schema applies to all oral opioids with predictable kinetics and immediate- and extended-release preparations (e.g., morphine, oxycodone, and hydromorphone). This schema does not apply to those drugs with unique pharmacology such as methadone. Several dosing strategies have been recommended.[19] Clinicians are advised to adopt the strategy that suits their particular unit and to become familiar and expert with it. Similarly, the delayed-release functionality of transdermal fentanyl renders it more suitable for patients with chronic stable pain than for those with unstable pain requiring titration.

Patients with severe pain may require titration with parenteral opioids (see Box 249-1). An appropriate starting dose for opioid-naïve patients is 10 to 20 mg morphine per 24 hours (or equivalent dose of fentanyl or hydromorphone) given subcutaneously or intravenously. The dose can then be increased according to pain scores accessed after 12 to 24 hours. If the pain score remains greater than 7 out of 10, the dose can be increased 50% to 100%. For pain scores of 4 to 7, increase by 25% to 50%. If the pain score is less than 4 and the patient has side effects, reduce by 25%. Once again, no absolute guideline exists regarding the dose for breakthrough medication. If one uses the half-life of the drug as a guide, a logical dose of breakthrough subcutaneous morphine would be equivalent to the 4-hourly dose of morphine or a 2-hourly dose of a shorter-acting opioid such as fentanyl.

Opioid Rotation

Opioid rotation, switching, or *substitution* refers to changing one opioid for another to improve pain control, toxicity, or both. Worldwide, morphine remains the opioid of choice, but in many countries, where many opioids and opioid formulations are available, opioid switching has become common practice. It is routine care in more than 80% of pain episodes in some centers[5] and in less than 10% in others.[20]

Does any evidence indicate that opioid switching improves patient outcomes? A systematic review of the published literature found no controlled evidence to support the practice,[21] but anecdotal and uncontrolled evidence showed improvements in side effects or pain control when rotating from one opioid to another.

How may it work? Numerous theories have been put forward, as discussed in the following sections.

Incomplete Cross-Tolerance

The most commonly quoted explanation for the perceived benefit of opioid rotation is incomplete cross-tolerance. Tolerance to the analgesic benefit of opioids does develop over time, thereby necessitating an increase in dose with repeated dosing. When switching from one opioid to another, tolerance is said to be incomplete if a lower dose of the second opioid achieves the same or greater degree of pain control as the first. In other words, the analgesic tolerance that has developed for the first opioid is not seen with the second. The lower dose of the second opioid

Box 249-1 Titration of Morphine: Recommendations

- Use IR preparations to titrate (e.g., morphine liquid or tablets given every 4 hours orally).
- Start at a low dose, usually 10 mg every 4 hours (5 mg in elderly patients) in patients already receiving a step 2 analgesic. If step 2 is omitted, 5 mg every 4 hours may suffice.
- Prescribe breakthrough (PRN) IR morphine at the same dose as that given every 4 hours, as often as required (up to hourly).
- The number of extra doses that can be administered has no limit. Take the number of breakthrough doses into account when adjusting the total daily dose.
- Increase the 4-hourly dose by approximately 30% to 50% every 24 to 48 hours until pain is controlled. Suggested increments are as follows: 10-15-20-30-40-60-80-100-130 mg.
- A double dose of morphine at bedtime is not an effective substitute for a 4-hourly dose during the night. Patients should either be prescribed a dose in the middle of the night (to keep them on a 4-hourly dosing regimen) or encouraged to take a breakthrough dose if they wake.
- If a patient is already receiving a slow-release morphine preparation and is in severe pain, titrate again by converting back to an IR preparation given every 4 hours, with dose increases as described earlier until pain is controlled.
- Once the pain is adequately controlled with 4-hourly IR preparations, convert to a controlled-release morphine preparation. To convert the dose, add up the total morphine requirement, including both regular and breakthrough doses in the previous 24 hours, and either prescribe the appropriate dose of a 24-hour preparation once daily or divide by 2 and prescribe a 12-hourly preparation twice daily.
- Always co-prescribe IR morphine at the equivalent 4-hourly dose for breakthrough pain (e.g., 10 mg IR morphine for patients taking 30 mg ER morphine twice daily).
- All patients started on morphine should be prescribed laxatives prophylactically.
- If patients are unable to take morphine orally, the preferred alternative route is the SC route.
- IV infusion of opioids may be preferable in patients who already have an indwelling infusion catheter who have generalized edema, severe site reactions, coagulation disorders, or poor peripheral circulation.
- No indication exists for giving morphine intramuscularly for chronic pain because SC administration is simpler and less painful.
- Morphine tartrate and hydromorphone are preferred for parenteral administration because they are more soluble than morphine sulfate. Smaller volumes can therefore be given.
- The 24-hour dose of parenteral morphine is one half to one third the total daily oral dose of morphine.
- The IV dose of morphine is equivalent to the SC dose.
- Morphine should be prescribed for administration by 24-hour SC infusion (unless an hourly infusion pump is used).
- Breakthrough doses (equivalent to the 4-hourly parenteral dose) can be offered every 1-2 hours.
- A breakthrough dose should have a duration of action of approximately 4 hours.
- Assess the number of breakthrough doses required each day, and change the 24-hour dose accordingly.
- A few patients develop intolerable side effects to morphine. In such patients, a change to an alternative opioid should be considered.

ER, extended-release; IR, immediate-release; IV, intravenous; PRN, as required; SC, subcutaneous.

may also result in fewer side effects. Possible molecular explanations include receptor subtypes, receptor oligodimerization and heterodimerization, and autoregulation.[22]

Dose Equivalence

Considerable uncertainty remains regarding the exact dose equivalence of different opioids.[8] Moreover, dose equivalence may change with time and the dose of opioid used previously (as demonstrated with methadone),[23] and the appropriate dose ratio when changing from opioid A to opioid B may not be the same as when changing from B to A. Some clinicians argue that the benefit seen, at least with respect to toxicity, when rotating opioids, may simply reflect an opioid dose reduction.

Genetic Variation

Genetic polymorphism has been demonstrated not only within opioid receptors and receptor regulation mechanisms but also within hepatic cytochrome and conjugase systems that influence drug metabolism and clearance. A challenge for the future is determine which opioid is best suited to a particular individual according to his or her unique genetic profile.

Interindividual Difference in Pharmacology

Renal function affects the elimination of many opioids, especially morphine and probably oxycodone and hydromorphone. Therefore, people with impaired renal function are likely to suffer less toxicity if they are rotated to a drug that is not dependent on renal function (e.g., fentanyl or methadone). Similarly, oxycodone elimination depends on hepatic function, and age determines morphine metabolism. Many factors may therefore alter the pharmacokinetics and pharmacodynamics of any one drug and may well contribute to the tolerance of individual drugs in individual patients.

Common Errors

- Failure to use nonpharmacological means of pain control
- Withholding of opioids because of fear of addiction
- Withholding of opioids in patients with pain until disease is far advanced
- Failure to treat opioid-induced side effects prophylactically (e.g., constipation)
- Failure to treat opioid-induced side effects fully (e.g., nausea)
- Use of inappropriate opioid doses (too small or too large a dose) at inappropriate time intervals
- Failure to allay fears and misconceptions regarding opioids
- Failure to prescribe opioids for breakthrough pain
- Failure to determine the cause of pain and thus the best management
- Use of an opioid by an inappropriate route (e.g., oral opioids in patients with bowel obstruction or malabsorption)
- Failure to recognize deteriorating renal function as a cause of unexpected opioid toxicity
- Use of textbook opioid conversions without consideration of individual patient characteristics

---

Future Considerations

- Should morphine remain the opioid of first choice?
- What is the most effective way to determine the opioid best suited to the individual?
- What is the best titration schedule for methadone?
- Is the World Health Organization analgesic ladder outdated?
- What is the most efficacious dose of morphine for breakthrough pain?

REFERENCES

1. Foley KM. Acute and chronic pain syndromes. In Doyle D, Hanks G, Cherny N, Calman K (eds). Oxford Textbook of Palliative Medicine, 3rd ed. Oxford: Oxford University Press, 2004, pp 298-299.
2. Cleeland CS, Gonin R, Hatfield AK, et al. Pain and its treatment in outpatients with metastatic cancer. N Engl J Med 1994;330:592-596.
3. World Health Organization (WHO). Cancer Pain Relief, with a Guide to Opioid Availability, 2nd ed. Geneva: WHO, 1996.
4. Hanks G, de Conno F, Cherny N, et al. Morphine and alternative opioids in cancer pain: The EAPC recommendations. Br J Cancer 2001;95:587-593.
5. Cherny N, Chang V, Frager G, et al. Opioid pharmacotherapy in the management of cancer pain. Cancer 1995;76:1288-1293.
6. Zenz M, Willweber-Strumpf A. Opiophobia and cancer pain in Europe. Lancet 1993;341:1075-1076.
7. Hardy J. Diamorphine. In Davis M, Glare P, Hardy J (eds). Opioids in Cancer Pain. Oxford: Oxford University Press, 2005, pp 207-215.
8. Anderson R, Saiers J, Abram S, Schlicht C. Accuracy in equianalgesic dosing: Conversion dilemmas. J Pain Symptom Manage 2001;21:397-406.
9. Mercadante S, Portenoy R. Opioid poorly-responsive pain. J Pain Symptom Manage 2001;21:144-150.
10. De Lima L, Sweeney C, Palmer J, et al. Potent analgesics are more expensive for patients in developing countries: A comparative study. J Pain Palliat Care Pharmacother 2004;18:59-70.
11. Hanks G, de Conno, Ripamonti C, et al., on behalf of the Expert Working Group of the EAPC. Morphine in cancer pain: Modes of administration. BMJ 1996;312:823-826.
12. Enting R, Oldenmenger W, van der Rijt C, et al. A prospective study evaluating the response of patients with unrelieved cancer pain to parenteral opioids. Cancer 2002;94:3049-3056.
13. Zeppetella G, Ribeiro M. Opioids for the management of breakthrough (episodic) pain in cancer patients. Cochrane Database Syst Rev 2006;(1): CD004311.
14. Ballantyne J, Carwood C. Comparative efficacy of epidural, subarachnoid and intracerebroventricular opioids in patients with pain due to cancer. Cochrane Database Syst Rev 2005;(2):CD005178.
15. Jadad A, Browman G. The WHO ladder for cancer pain management. JAMA 1995;274:1870-1873.
16. Jacox A, Carr D, Payne R (eds). Management of Cancer Pain. Clinical Practice Guideline no. 9. Agency for Healthcare Policy and Research publication no. 94-0592. Washington, DC: U.S. Department of Health and Human Services, 1994.
17. Lickiss J. Approaching cancer pain relief. Eur J Pain 2001;5(Suppl):5-14.
18. Twycross R. Oral morphine. In Twycross R (ed). Pain Relief in Advanced Cancer. Edinburgh: Churchill Livingstone, 1994, pp 307-333.
19. Davis M. Methadone. In Davis M, Glare P, Hardy J (eds). Opioids in Cancer Pain. Oxford: Oxford University Press, 2005, pp 247-265.
20. Fainsinger R. Opioids, confusion and opioid rotation. Palliat Med 1998;12: 463-464.
21. Quigley C. Opioid switching to improve pain relief and drug tolerability. Cochrane Database Syst Rev 2004;(3):CD004847.
22. Davis M, Pasternak G. Opioid receptors and opioid pharmacodynamics. In Davis M, Glare P, Hardy J (eds). Opioids in Cancer Pain. Oxford: Oxford University Press, 2005, pp 11-43.
23. Ayonrinde O, Bridge D. The rediscovery of methadone for cancer pain management. Med J Aust 2000;173:536-540.

SUGGESTED READING

Cherny N, Ripamonti C, Pereira J, et al. Strategies to manage the adverse effects of oral morphine: An evidence-based report. J Clin Oncol 2001;19:2542-2554.

Davis M, Glare P, Hardy J (eds). Opioids in Cancer Pain. Oxford: Oxford University Press, 2005.

Glare P, Aggarwal G, Clark K. Ongoing controversies in the pharmacological management of pain. Int Med J 2004;34: 45-49.

Hanks G, de Conno F, Cherny N, et al. Morphine and alternative opioids in cancer pain: The EAPC recommendations. Br J Cancer 2001;95:587-593.

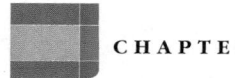

CHAPTER **250**

Opioid Side Effects and Overdose

Peter Lawlor, Michael Lucey, and Brian Creedon

KEY POINTS

- Inordinate side effect fears and a traditional stigmatized association with the terminal phase of life should not preclude judicious use of opioids.
- The main opioid side effects are gastrointestinal and neuropsychological.
- Prevention, rigorous assessment, and early intervention for side effects can facilitate dose titration and can achieve optimal analgesia for most patients.
- For unacceptable side effects such as opioid neurotoxicity, either switch the opioid or reduce the dose. A route change, mainly to subcutaneous and occasionally to intraspinal, may also be required.
- When delirium develops, look for and treat other precipitants such as dehydration and infection, in addition to making opioid adjustments.

Opioids have a pivotal role in cancer pain. In addition to their potent analgesic actions, opioids are associated with many side effects.[1-5] The most common adverse effects are gastrointestinal and neuropsychological. Neurotoxic side effects such as delirium and general neural hyperexcitability have received increasing attention.[5] The heightened recognition and reporting of such complications may relate to a more liberal use of opioids in the developed world over the past couple of decades. In turn, more liberal prescribing of opioids may well be attributable to much needed educational efforts by the World Health Organization and other national and international bodies to promote the wider use of these drugs. Such efforts aimed to dispel some of the older myths and to reduce fears surrounding opioid use in cancer pain management.

Mythical fears have surrounded the issue of opioid addiction in cancer pain management. In addition, the association of opioid use with the terminal phase of the cancer illness (see Chapters 177 to 181) has led to inordinate fears of both drowsiness and respiratory depression, which may have been mistakenly ascribed to opioid side effects. Consequently, the tendency has been for opioids to become stigmatized merely by virtue of their temporal association with this terminal phase of illness. The challenge of assessing the opioid contribution to a particular side effect, or what appears to be a side effect, is often compounded by the presence of similar effects in relation to the cancer itself, cancer treatment effects, or the effects of other medications (Fig. 250-1).[1-3] Educating physicians regarding opioid side effects and their pattern and context of development is essential to enable them to adopt proactive strategies and to intervene both promptly and appropriately, thus leading ultimately to the provision of safe and effective analgesia in patients with cancer.

Conceptually, opioid side effects may be viewed either as occurring mainly early, within the first 3 to 5 days of initial opioid treatment, or later, in which side effects are generally but not exclusively more likely to occur thereafter. This conceptual division is arbitrary in relation to some side effects such as constipation and neurotoxicity, in that they can both occur as early or late side effects (Table 250-1).

UNDERLYING CONSIDERATIONS

Therapeutic Goals and Opioid Side Effects

The standard clinical approach to cancer pain management first recognizes the interindividual variability in opioid requirements.[2] Second, it advocates opioid titration on an individual basis, with the aim to achieve the ultimate goal of a favorable balance between analgesia and side effects.[1,2] Although most patients achieve this balance, some patients experience troublesome side effects in the titration process. No specific dose triggers these adverse effects. Nonetheless, difficult pain syndromes, such as those with a neuropathic or an incident component, usually require higher doses,[6] and probably these syndromes are more strongly associated with adverse effects. For similar reasons, opioid tolerance, higher levels of psychological distress, and a prior history of substance abuse may also carry a higher risk of adverse effects, but the

evidence is largely based on case reports and case series (see Chapter 251).[5]

Renal Impairment

In renal impairment, opioid metabolites, especially those that are pharmacologically active, may accumulate and contribute to adverse effects.[2] In such cases, physicians should consider using an opioid without known active metabolites, such as fentanyl or methadone. Alternatively, the opioid dose could be reduced, and the dosing interval could be extended. Slow-release formulations should be avoided. In severe renal impairment, opioids such as morphine may need to be given only as required. The age-related decline in renal clearance should always be borne in mind when deciding on opioid doses in elderly patients.

TABLE 250-1 Opioid Side Effects: Their Temporal Association and Estimated Frequency*		
TYPE OF SIDE EFFECT OR COMPLICATION	**EARLY[†]**	**LATE[‡]**
GASTROINTESTINAL		
Dry mouth	+++	++
Nausea and vomiting	++	+
Constipation	+++	++++
RESPIRATORY		
Respiratory depression	0/+	0/+
Pulmonary edema	0/+	0/+
DERMATOLOGICAL		
Pruritus	+	+
Sweating	+	+
NEUROPSYCHOLOGICAL (SUBTLE OR MILD IMPAIRMENT)		
Sedation	++	++
Cognitive or psychomotor impairment	+	++
NEUROPSYCHOLOGICAL (FLORID OR MORE SEVERE IMPAIRMENT)		
Perceptual disturbance	+	++
Delirium	+	++
NEUROLOGICAL		
Myoclonus	+	++
Hyperalgesia/allodynia/seizures	0/+	+
MISCELLANEOUS		
Micturitional disturbance	+	+/0
Vertigo	+	+
PHARMACOLOGICAL COMPLICATIONS		
Tolerance	0/+	++
Physiological/physical dependence[§]	0/+	++++
Psychological dependence or addiction[¶]	0/+	0/+
Substance abuse or dependence disorders[¶]	0/+	0/+
Pseudoaddiction	+	+

*Estimation based on available literature data and on clinical experience in the absence of literature data.
[†]Relatively early: refers to initial 3 to 5 days of commencing opioid treatment.
[‡]Relatively later: following the initial 3 to 5 days of initial opioid treatment.
[§]Occurs in most patients receiving long-term treatment.
[¶]Rare in the absence of a prior history of substance abuse or dependence disorder.
0/+, rarely; +, occasionally; ++, often; +++, quite often; ++++, very often.

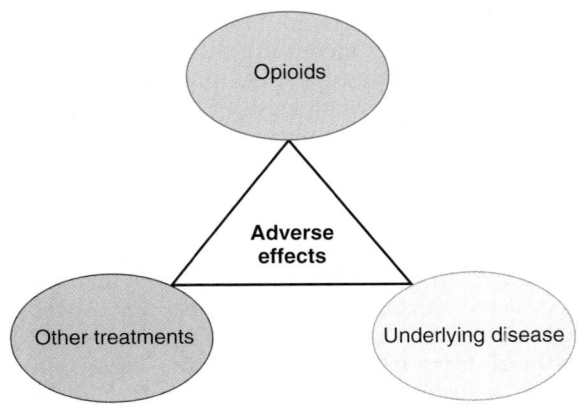

FIGURE 250-1 Adverse effects shared by opioids, other treatments, and the underlying disease.

SPECIFIC SIDE EFFECTS

Gastrointestinal Side Effects

Dry Mouth

One study suggested that dry mouth was the most frequent side effect of morphine, and its severity was positively correlated with plasma levels of both morphine and morphine-6-glucuronide.[7] Artificial saliva gels are effective but need to be applied frequently. Other medications, such as anticholinergics or antidepressants, also cause dry mouth, and their discontinuation or dose adjustment should be considered (see Chapter 171).

Nausea and Vomiting

Based on prospective studies, nausea has been observed in up to 30% of patients receiving oral morphine for cancer pain.[1,8] However, given the multidimensional nature of this symptom, it is difficult to identify the opioid contribution. Nausea and vomiting may be precipitated by input to the vomiting center in the medulla. With opioids, this input is predominantly from the chemoreceptor trigger zone through dopaminergic (D_2) and serotonin (5-HT_3) neurotransmission. Input also can occur from the vestibular apparatus through histaminergic (H_1) and cholinergic (Ach_m) neurotransmission. Gastrointestinal input to the vomiting center occurs through the vagus nerve and 5-HT_3 pathways. Opioids cause gastroparesis or delayed gastric emptying. The vomiting center also receives input from cortical areas, especially in relation to anticipatory nausea, but these pathways are less well defined, and the precise opioid contribution by this route is unclear. In the vomiting center, neurotransmission is mediated by H_1 and Ach_m pathways.

Clinical experience suggests that nausea commonly occurs with the initiation of opioid treatment but subsides, presumably from tolerance, over the first 3 to 5 days.[3] It is prudent to have at least an as-needed antiemetic available for this period. Some patients experience ongoing nausea. Careful assessment is essential to identify other causes of nausea (e.g., renal impairment).

Few head-to-head comparative studies of antiemetic use in opioid-associated nausea have been conducted. Anticholinergic medications cause sedation, as do antihistamines. The 5-HT_3 antagonists are expensive. Metoclopramide is commonly used in clinical practice because of its favorable side effect profile and its comprehensive actions: D_2 antagonism, prokinetic effect, and 5-HT_3 antagonism in higher doses.[4] One double-blind randomized placebo-controlled trial compared ondansetron (24 mg orally), placebo, and metoclopramide (10 mg orally three times daily), and found no efficacy difference in reducing opioid-associated emesis or nausea.[9]

Changing the route of administration from oral to subcutaneous, or changing the opioid itself, has been effective in small case series. Finally, opioid-related constipation must be considered a common cause of nausea (see Chapter 169).

Constipation

Chronic constipation has been observed in 20% to 70% of patients treated for chronic cancer pain.[1,8] Clinical experience suggests that tolerance to the constipating effect of opioids does not occur. No conclusive evidence indicates that the degree of constipation is opioid dose dependent. Some evidence suggests that constipation is less pronounced with methadone and fentanyl. Opioids inhibit normal peristalsis, promote fluid resorption, and inhibit secretion of fluid into the intestinal lumen. Opioids may also be associated with increased sphincter tone. Physiologically, the combination of these actions culminates in stool desiccation and diminished defecation.[4] Symptomatically, patients may complain of bloating, abdominal pain, nausea, and often overflow or spurious diarrhea (see Chapters 154 and 169).

The assessment of constipation is often neglected. The multifactorial nature of constipation should be considered. Other causes of constipation (e.g., hypercalcemia, anticholinergics, and dehydration) need to be recognized and addressed. If in doubt, plain abdominal radiographs help in the diagnosis.

Most patients receiving longer-term opioid treatment require laxatives. Most palliative care physicians prescribe laxatives prophylactically at the initiation of anticipated long-term opioid treatment. No comparative head-to-head studies of laxatives have been conducted. The usual strategy is to combine laxatives from different classes (e.g., a stimulant, an osmotic laxative, and a softener). Bulk-forming laxatives are probably best avoided in opioid-induced constipation because they rely on stretch-induced peristalsis to be effective. Given the compromised peristalsis in opioid-treated patients, bulk-forming laxatives could result in fecal impaction. Studies of orally administered peripheral opioid antagonists (e.g., alvimopan and methylnaltrexone) suggested that such agents may soon acquire a major role in opioid-induced constipation without compromising analgesia.[10]

Respiratory Side Effects

Respiratory Depression

Respiratory depression is one of the most serious side effects of opioids. It rarely occurs in cancer pain management. It is more likely at the initiation of opioid treatment, at dose titration, and sometimes after opioid switching, especially to methadone, to which a substantive degree of incomplete cross-tolerance may exist.[4] Failure to reduce the dose of methadone to account for this effect may result in respiratory depression. Finally, respiratory depression may occur after accidental overdose (see later). Elimination of the pain stimulus in situations such as progression to complete spinal cord compression or chemical neurolysis has been reported with the emergence of sedation and respiratory depression.[11]

Pulmonary Edema

Pulmonary edema has been reported. However, clinical experience suggests that this complication is rare.

Dermatological Side Effects

Pruritus

Chronic itch has been observed in up to 10% of patients receiving morphine for cancer pain. Based on the suspected mechanism of histamine release, antihistamines are commonly prescribed. Some opioids (e.g., fentanyl) are less likely to cause histamine release. Switching to a different opioid class (e.g., from morphine to fentanyl) may help, but study findings have been conflicting.

Sweating

Sweating is a common symptom in advanced cancer. However, the degree to which it can be attributed to opioids is unclear.[8] Case reports have suggested a particular association with methadone.

Neuropsychological Side Effects

Sedation and Mild Cognitive Dysfunction

Although fears of respiratory depression generally tend to be exaggerated, sedation and respiratory depression tend to occur on a continuum: increased sedation occurs before respiratory depression. Opioid-induced sedation warrants monitoring, especially at the initiation of opioid treatment and at the time of dose increments.[5]

Cognitive function refers to the acquisition, processing, storage, and retrieval of information by the brain. Cognitive deficits can occur as part of dementia, in delirium with or without baseline evidence of dementia, or occasionally in depression (depressive pseudodementia). A certain level of alertness is necessary to allow assessment of cognitive function. Not surprisingly, therefore, alertness or level of sedation and cognitive function are often assessed together both in clinical practice and in research studies. The cognitive and sedative affects of opioids have been studied mainly in volunteers and in patients receiving opioids for chronic nonmalignant pain. It is difficult to extrapolate these study findings to patients with cancer pain, in whom both sedation and cognitive impairment are common, often because of multiple contributory factors (e.g., metabolic abnormalities, other psychoactive medications, and infection). Furthermore, findings of subtle opioid-related cognitive deficits in patients who do not have cancer may either be of no clinical significance or, alternatively, more profound in patients with cancer, especially if baseline cognitive functioning is vulnerable during disease progression.[5]

Apart from a few studies on delirium, few data are available on the contribution of opioids to mild cognitive impairment or sedation specifically in patients with cancer. Although some investigators found a significant positive correlation between opioid dose and the severity of deficits, this finding was not consistent. Deficits in formal cognitive testing occur particularly with the initiation of opioid use and in association with dose increments of at least 30%.[12] Although patients reported no subjective increase in confusion, they rated drowsiness higher in association with dose increments. In a double-blind crossover study by the same group, methylphenidate administration resulted in decreased opioid-related sedation and enabled augmentation of opioid analgesia.[13]

The clinical significance and the actual level of patient distress associated with relatively mild cognitive deficits in everyday clinical practice are uncertain. However, it is possible that such deficits with or without sedation may highlight the risk of, or herald the onset of, delirium

and therefore may be precursors to more florid opioid neurotoxicity.[5]

Delirium, Perceptual Disturbance, and the "Syndrome" of Opioid-Induced Neurotoxicity

Opioid-induced neurotoxicity refers to a constellation of signs and symptoms, which by convention could be argued to constitute a syndrome (see Table 250-1).[5] Although many reports have described some or all of the phenomena associated with opioid-induced neurotoxicity, the confounding variables in advanced cancer make it difficult to determine the opioid contribution to some or all of the features of this syndrome. Investigators have speculated about the contribution of active opioid metabolites to opioid neurotoxicity; for example, much of the toxicity associated with meperidine has been attributed to its neurotoxic metabolite, normeperidine.

Delirium is a neuropsychiatric disorder characterized by a reduced level of consciousness and awareness, cognitive deficit or perceptual disturbance, acuity of onset (hours to days), fluctuating intensity, and underlying causes (see Chapter 156). Fluctuation in the intensity of presentation may even result in a lucid interval and probably partly explains why the diagnosis is frequently missed. Patients often have an accompanying disturbance of psychomotor activity, manifesting either as hypoactivity or hyperactivity, or a mixed variety. The etiological factors can include general medical conditions, medication or substance toxicity, medication or substance withdrawal, unknown causes, or perhaps more commonly multiple etiological factors. Delirium occurs frequently in advanced cancer, and most patients have delirium for hours to days before death. However, delirium can also be reversible, depending on the precipitants.

Reversible opioid related delirium has often been described. A rigorous evaluation of potential precipitants of delirium in 71 patients with advanced cancer revealed a median of 3 precipitants per episode, demonstrating its multifactorial etiology.[14] Opioids and other psychoactive medications were strongly associated with reversibility, based on defined dose reduction, medication discontinuation or switch. Dehydration frequently accompanied opioid toxicity symptoms. The typical triad of precipitants included opioid or other psychoactive medication, infection, and volume depletion or dehydration. Successful reversal typically involved treatment strategies aimed at all of these precipitants.

Some of the more florid literature reports of opioid-induced neurotoxicity also described other features such as myoclonus (jerky movements), hyperalgesia (heightened pain level), allodynia (pain on touch), and even seizures. Some or all of these features were described in patients with delirium, usually the agitated or hyperactive subtype. Many reports related to high-dose opioids, and some to patients in renal failure. Myoclonus is probably the most common neurological manifestation of opioid-induced neurotoxicity. However, it is also associated with other centrally acting medications and with renal failure. The exact pathophysiology has not been determined but clearly reflects a neuroexcitatory state (see Chapter 175).[15]

The prevalence rate of opioid-induced neurotoxicity in patients with cancer pain is unknown. However, clinical experience suggests that opioids frequently contribute to delirium in high-risk populations Many clinicians advocate routine cognitive screening to permit early detection of delirium, and consequently early intervention with treatment strategies aimed at reducing patient distress.[5] Assuming consistency with the goals of care, the treatment strategy first involves a search for identifiable and reversible causes. Second, a neuroleptic such as haloperidol is needed, especially in patients with agitation, delusions, or perceptual disturbance. Deep sedation using agents such as levomepromazine or midazolam is sometimes required, especially in patients with nonreversible delirium.

In addition to treating nonopioid causes, the opioid is commonly switched or reduced in dose. Although evidence has shown the benefits of opioid switching, the overall level of evidence remains relatively low.[1,16,17] A change to the spinal route of administration of opioid, especially in patients receiving very high doses of opioid, may be necessary (see Chapters 249 and 253).

Miscellaneous Side Effects

Vertigo

Clinical experience suggests that vertigo occurs occasionally in cancer pain management. The underlying pathophysiology is likely increased vestibular sensitivity, but this has yet to be demonstrated. Antihistamines may help.

Micturitional Disturbance

Urinary retention is a known complication of systemic opioid use, especially intrathecal administration. The precise mechanism is unclear. Urinary catheterization is usually required.

Other Miscellaneous Side Effects

Immune and endocrine side effects are discussed elsewhere.

OPIOID OVERDOSE

In cancer pain management, opioid overdose is most commonly the result of errors in pain assessment, opioid prescribing, or dose administration. Opioid overdose classically presents as sedation or respiratory depression. Sedation is a precursor to respiratory depression. However, multiple factors may contribute to sedation in advanced cancer, and determining the extent of opioid contribution can be difficult. Nonetheless, the clinical situation of coma, reduced respiratory rate, and pinpoint pupils should heighten suspicion that the status change is opioid related. In such cases, the opioid antagonist naloxone should be promptly administered.

A retrospective review of 1835 medical oncology patients admitted over a 2-year period to a university teaching hospital found that 15 (0.8%) needed naloxone (a competitive opioid antagonist) mainly for oversedation.[18] Most of the indications for naloxone were retrospectively deemed appropriate, but the doses used were judged excessive. A study from a large cancer center examined patient satisfaction and opioid-related adverse drug reactions both before and after introduction of a numerical pain treatment algorithm and found that the rate of opioid oversedation doubled following the implementation of the algorithm.[19] This finding highlights the importance of multidimensional pain assessment, rather than exclusively basing opioid treatment decisions on unidimensional numerical pain ratings.

The risk with naloxone is the precipitation of a pain crisis. However, if life-threatening respiratory depression is encountered, naloxone should be administered (Box 250-1).

CONCLUSIONS

Inordinate fears regarding opioid side effects or complications may contribute to the underuse of opioids in cancer pain. Educating patients and physicians may dispel some myths and may lead to improved awareness of side effect development. The assessment and treatment of opioid side effects warrant as much attention as opioid dose adjustment in relation to reported pain levels. Measures to prevent such side effects and their prompt effective treatment when they do occur will expand the scope for dose titration. The evaluation of these management strategies has been largely empirical, because the evidence base on which to make recommendations is weak. Controversies exist, and the research challenges are substantive (Boxes 250-2 through 250-4).[20]

Box 250-1 Opioid Overdose Management

- Administer naloxone intravenously or intramuscularly.
- Dilute an ampule of naloxone 400 µg/mL to 10 mL in 0.9% saline.
- Administer 0.5 mL (20 µg) every 2 minutes until the respiratory rate is satisfactory.
- Boluses every 30 to 60 minutes may be required in view of the short duration of action of naloxone (10 to 45 minutes). This is especially important after large doses of slow-release preparations or methadone.
- An infusion of naloxone in a syringe driver may be required.

Adapted from Quigley C. The role of opioids in cancer pain. BMJ 2005;331:825-829; and Hanks G, Cherny N, Fallon M. Opioid analgesic therapy. In Doyle D, Hanks G, Cherny N, Calman K (eds). Oxford Textbook of Palliative Medicine. Oxford: Oxford University Press, 2003.

Box 250-2 Strategies for Dealing with Opioid Side Effects

- Opioid dose reduction
- Opioid switch or rotation
- Change in route of administration
- Direct treatment of the side effect

Box 250-3 Recent Developments

- Opioid antagonists such as methylnaltrexone are used for opioid-related constipation.[10]
- Methadone is associated with the same dose escalation as morphine when it is used as a first-line opioid.[20]

Common Errors

- Inadequate pain assessment leading to inappropriate opioid use
- No objective assessment of cognition; delirium often missed
- Side effect deemed entirely opioid related; other causes missed
- Assuming that delirium is always a terminal event
- Inadequate use of laxatives
  - Nausea attributed to the opioid rather than to constipation
  - Cessation or dose reduction of laxatives in the presence of overflow diarrhea, thus worsening the situation
- Equianalgesic dose miscalculations with resultant toxicity or undertreatment of pain when switching opioid; similarly, in oral to parenteral route changes, same dose given instead of reducing by one third to two thirds

Future Considerations

- The "morphine pump" and its association with the terminal phase of life
- Determining the true opioid contribution to apparent opioid-related side effects, especially in progressive disease and other treatments
- Treating neurotoxicity: whether to change the opioid, the dose, or the route
- The contribution of opioid metabolites to side effects
- The exact role of methadone in opioid tolerance
- Conducting rigorous studies in very vulnerable patients
- Determining the true opioid contribution to apparent opioid-related side effects, especially in the presence of progressive disease and other medications
- The efficacy of opioid switching versus dose reduction for neurotoxicity
- Further evaluation of the contribution of opioid metabolites to side effects
- The safest and most effective method of switching to methadone
- Further evaluation of the role of intrathecal opioid administration
- Comparative studies in the case of both antiemetics and laxatives

REFERENCES

1. Cherny N, Ripamonti C, Pereira J, et al. Strategies to manage the adverse effects of oral morphine: An evidence-based report. J Clin Oncol 2001;19:2542-2554.
2. Quigley C. The role of opioids in cancer pain. BMJ 2005;331:825-829.
3. Hanks G, Cherny N, Fallon M. Opioid analgesic therapy. In Doyle D, Hanks G, Cherny N, Calman K (eds). Oxford Textbook of Palliative Medicine. Oxford: Oxford University Press, 2003.
4. Herndon CM, Kalauokalani DA, Cunningham AJ, et al. Anticipating and treating opioid-associated adverse effects. Expert Opin Drug Saf 2003;2:305-319.
5. Lawlor PG. The panorama of opioid-related cognitive dysfunction in patients with cancer: A critical literature appraisal. Cancer 2002;94:1836-1853.
6. Fainsinger RL, Nekolaichuk CL, Lawlor PG, et al. A multicenter study of the revised Edmonton Staging System for classifying cancer pain in advanced cancer patients. J Pain Symptom Manage 2005;29:224-237.
7. Andersen G, Sjogren P, Hansen SH, et al. Pharmacological consequences of long-term morphine treatment in patients with cancer and chronic non-malignant pain. Eur J Pain 2004;8:263-271.
8. Meuser T, Pietruck C, Radbruch L, et al. Symptoms during cancer pain treatment following WHO-guidelines: A longitudinal follow-up study of symptom prevalence, severity and etiology. Pain 2001;93:247-257.
9. Hardy J, Daly S, McQuade B, et al. A double-blind, randomised, parallel group, multinational, multicentre study comparing a single dose of ondansetron 24 mg p.o. with placebo and metoclopramide 10 mg t.d.s. p.o. in the treatment of opioid-induced nausea and emesis in cancer patients. Support Care Cancer 2002;10:231-236.
10. Choi YS, Billings JA. Opioid antagonists: A review of their role in palliative care, focusing on use in opioid-related constipation. J Pain Symptom Manage 2002;24:71-90.
11. Piquet CY, Mallaret MP, Lemoigne AH, et al. Respiratory depression following administration of intrathecal bupivacaine to an opioid-dependent patient. Ann Pharmacother 1998;32:653-655.
12. Bruera E, Macmillan K, Hanson J, MacDonald RN. The cognitive effects of the administration of narcotic analgesics in patients with cancer pain. Pain 1989;39:13-16.
13. Bruera E, Chadwick S, Brenneis C, et al. Methylphenidate associated with narcotics for the treatment of cancer pain. Cancer Treat Rep 1987;71:67-70.
14. Lawlor PG, Gagnon B, Mancini IL, et al. Occurrence, causes, and outcome of delirium in patients with advanced cancer: A prospective study. Arch Intern Med 2000;160:786-794.
15. Mercadante S. Pathophysiology and treatment of opioid-related myoclonus in cancer patients. Pain 1998;74:5-9.
16. Quigley C. Opioid switching to improve pain relief and drug tolerability. Cochrane Database Syst Rev 2004;(3):CD004847.
17. McNicol E, Horowicz-Mehler N, Fisk RA, et al. Management of opioid side effects in cancer-related and chronic noncancer pain: A systematic review. J Pain 2003;4:231-256.
18. Cleary J, Gordon DB, Hutson P, Ward S. Incidence and characteristics of naloxone administration in medical oncology patients with cancer pain. J Pharmaceutical Care Pain Symptom Control 2000;8:65-73.
19. Vila H Jr, Smith RA, Augustyniak MJ, et al. The efficacy and safety of pain management before and after implementation of hospital-wide pain management standards: Is patient safety compromised by treatment based solely on numerical pain ratings? Anesth Analg 2005;101:474-480.
20. Bruera E, Palmer JL, Bosnjak S, et al. Methadone versus morphine as a first-line strong opioid for cancer pain: A randomized, double-blind study. J Clin Oncol 2004;22:185-192.

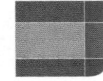

CHAPTER **251**

Opioid Use in Drug and Alcohol Abuse

Kenneth L. Kirsh, David Casper, Mindi C. Haley, and Steven D. Passik

KEY POINTS

- Aberrant drug taking does not necessarily indicate addiction, but it may be a sign that pain and other symptoms are being inadequately treated.
- Prescribing opioids to patients with cancer who have no prior history of substance abuse is unlikely to end in addiction.
- Clinicians should assess patients before opioid therapy, to manage any chance of addiction most effectively.
- Special attention should be paid to patients with a past or current history of substance abuse.
- Substance abuse and out-of-control aberrant drug taking must be addressed and managed, possibly by establishing goals. Some useful goals are ending or lowering substance abuse, requiring urine toxicology screening, making refills contingent on clinic visits, or joining 12-step programs.
- Many terminally ill patients have alcoholism. Not identifying and not treating alcoholism can lead to painful withdrawal, delirium tremens, and increased postoperative risk.

The potential exists for substance abuse in palliative medicine, although the severity of this issue varies significantly. Some patients increase drug doses without informing their physicians, or they use analgesics to treat symptoms other than those intended; other patients helpfully present with a known history of, or current addiction to, illicit drugs or prescription medications. Proper identification, assessment, and clinical management of substance-related problems are critically important for optimal patient care. Clinicians can control opioid prescriptions while continuing to prescribe controlled substances, thereby ensuring that pain is not undertreated.

EPIDEMIOLOGY

Prevalence

Approximately half the people 15 to 54 years old in the United States have used illegal drugs sometime in their lives, and 6% to 15% have a current or past substance use disorder.[1] A sharp increase in controlled prescription drug abuse has occurred in the United States; the rate has climbed by nearly 94%, from 7.8 million in 1992 to 15.1 million in 2003.[2] Given the high prevalence of substance abuse in the U.S. population and the association between drug abuse and life-threatening diseases,[3] issues related to substance abuse are commonly encountered in palliative medicine.

Within the tertiary care population with cancer, substance abuse appears uncommon. In a 6-month period in 2005, fewer than 1% of inpatient and outpatient consultations to the psychiatry service at Memorial Sloan-Kettering Cancer Center were requested for substance abuse–related issues, and only 3% of patients were subsequently diagnosed with any substance abuse disorder. This number is much lower than for substance abuse disorders in the society at large, in general medical populations, and in emergency medical departments.[4,5]

Addiction and Addiction Risk in the Medically Ill

Aberrant drug-taking behavior has several possible explanations, and pseudoaddiction must be considered if someone is reporting distress associated with unrelieved symptoms. In pseudoaddiction, behaviors such as aggressively complaints about the need for higher doses or occasional unilateral drug increases indicate desperation caused by pain, and these behaviors disappear when pain management improves.

Patients who self-medicate for anxiety, panic, depression, or even periodic dysphoria and loneliness can be viewed as aberrant drug takers. In these patients, careful diagnosis and treatment of these problems may prevent self-medication. Occasionally, aberrant drug-related behavior is the result of mild encephalopathy with confusion about the appropriate therapeutic regimen, a concern in the treatment of elderly patients. Low-dose neuroleptics, simplified drug regimens, and help in organizing medications can address such problems. Rarely do problematic behaviors indicate criminal intent (e.g., people reporting pain with the intent to sell or divert medications).

A thorough psychiatric assessment is critically important, both in the population without prior substance abuse and in known abusers, who have a high prevalence of psychiatric co-morbidity.[6] In the differential diagnosis of drug-related behavior, it is useful to consider the degree of aberrancy. Less aberrant behaviors are less likely to reflect addiction-related concerns. Conversely, more aberrant behaviors are more likely to reflect true addiction.

Opioid administration in patients with cancer who have no prior history of substance abuse is rarely associated with significant abuse or addiction.[7,8] The public and inexperienced clinicians still fear the development of addiction when cancer pain is treated with opioids. Specialists in cancer pain and palliative medicine widely believe that the major problem related to addiction is not the phenomenon itself, but rather the persistent undertreatment of pain driven by the inappropriate fear that addiction will occur. Little support exists for the view that many individuals with no personal or family history of abuse or addiction, no affiliation with a substance-abusing subculture, and no significant premorbid psychopathology will develop abuse or addiction de novo when they are given potentially abusable drugs appropriately.[9,10] Euphoria, believed common during opioid abuse, is rare after opioids are given for pain; more typically, dysphoria occurs, especially with meperidine.

Addiction Risk in Current or Remote Drug Abuse

Little information is available about the risk of abuse or addiction during or after the therapeutic administration of a potentially abusable drug to someone with a current or remote history of abuse or addiction. Anecdotal reports suggest that successful long-term opioid therapy in patients with cancer pain or chronic nonmalignant pain is possible, even if the history of abuse or addiction is remote.[11] People with pain related to acquired immunodeficiency syndrome (AIDS) have been successfully treated with morphine whether or not they were substance users or nonusers. The major group difference was that substance users required bigger morphine doses for stable pain control.[12] This finding is reassuring but does not obviate the need for caution. Although no empirical evidence indicates that short-acting drugs and the parenteral route are more likely to lead to problematic drug-related behaviors, it may be prudent to avoid them in patients with histories of substance abuse.

CLINICAL MANAGEMENT

Out-of-control aberrant drug taking in palliative medicine (in patients with or without a prior history of substance abuse) is a serious and complex clinical occurrence. The more difficult situations involve someone who is actively abusing illicit or prescription drugs or alcohol along with medical therapies. Whether the patient is an active drug abuser, has a history of substance abuse, or is not complying with the therapeutic regimen, the clinician should establish structure, control, and monitoring so that he or she can prescribe freely and without prejudice.

Multidisciplinary Approach

A multidisciplinary team approach is usually optimal for the management of substance abusers in palliative medicine. If available, mental health professionals with specialization in addictions can help team members develop strategies for management and treatment compliance. Providing care to drug-aberrant patients can cause anger and frustration among staff members. Such emotions can unintentionally compromise pain management and can contribute to feelings of patient isolation and alienation. A structured multidisciplinary approach can help the staff to understand the patient's needs better and to develop effective strategies for controlling pain and aberrant drug use simultaneously.

Assessment

The first member of the medical team to suspect problematic drug taking or a history of drug abuse should alert the palliative care team, beginning the assessment and management process.[13] A physician should assess the potential of withdrawal or other pressing concerns and should involve other staff (i.e., social work or psychiatry) in initiating and planning management strategies.

A detailed history of the duration, frequency, and desired effect of drug use is essential. Clinicians often avoid asking about substance abuse because of fear that they will anger the patient or are incorrect in their suspicion of abuse. This avoidance can contribute to continued problems. Empathic and truthful communication is always best. A careful, graduated interview can be instrumental to assess drug use. This starts the interview with broad questions about drugs (e.g., nicotine, caffeine) in the patient's life and gradually becomes more specific in focus to include illicit drugs. This approach is helpful in reducing denial and resistance.

This interviewing style may also assist in the detection of coexisting psychiatric disorders. Co-morbid psychiatric disorders can significantly contribute to aberrant drug-taking behavior. Thirty-seven percent to 62% of alcoholic patients have one or more coexisting psychiatric disorders, and the drug history may be a clue to co-morbid psychiatric disorders (e.g., drinking to quell panic symptoms). Anxiety, personality disorders, and mood disorders are most common. The assessment and treatment of co-morbid psychiatric disorders can enhance management strategies and can reduce relapse.

Development of a Treatment Plan: General Considerations

Clear treatment goals are essential for aberrant drug-related behaviors. Depending on the individual patient, complete remission of substance use problems may not be a reasonable goal. For some patients, *harm reduction* may be a better model. It aims to enhance social support, maximize treatment compliance, and contain harm done through episodic relapse.

Establishing goals of care can be very difficult, especially when poor compliance and risky behavior appear to contradict a reported desire for disease-modifying therapies. This behavior may be from the stress of coping with a life-threatening illness and the availability of prescription drugs for symptom control, which can undermine efforts to achieve abstinence.[14]

A clinician should establish goals in a relationship based on empathic listening and should accept the patient's report of distress. When possible, it is important to use nonopioid and behavioral interventions, but not as substitutes for appropriate pharmacological management. Tolerance, route of administration, and duration of action should be considered when prescribing medications for pain and symptom management. Preexisting tolerance should be taken into account for those patients who are actively abusing drugs or are maintained on methadone therapy. Failure to address tolerance can result in undermedication and can contribute to self-medication. Medications with slow onset and longer duration (e.g., fentanyl patch and sustained-release opioids) may reduce aberrant behaviors in patients with addictive disorders; people at high risk should not be given short-acting opioids for breakthrough pain. Finally, the adequacy of pain and symptom control should be frequently reassessed.

Urine Toxicology Screening

Urine toxicology screening can be a useful tool both for diagnosing potential abuse and for monitoring patients with an established abuse history. Urine toxicology screens are employed infrequently in tertiary care centers.[15] One study found that nearly 40% of the charts surveyed listed no reason for the urine toxicology screen, and the ordering physician could not be identified nearly 30% of the time.[15] Staff education efforts can address this problem and may make urine toxicology screens a vital part of treating pain in oncology patients.

The Patient with Advanced Disease

Treating addiction in advanced medical illness is labor-intensive and time-consuming. Regardless of addiction's negative impact on palliative medicine, clinicians may opt to overlook use of illicit substances or alcohol entirely and perhaps view these abuses as a last source of pleasure for the patient. Addiction behaviors may increase stress for family members, may cause family concern over misuse of medication, may potentially mask important symptoms, may lead to poor compliance with the treatment, and may diminish quality of life. Complete abstinence may not be realistic, but reduction in use can certainly have positive effects.[15]

Outpatient Management

Other strategies exist for encouraging treatment adherence in an outpatient setting. A written contract between the team and the patient structures the treatment plan, establishes clear expectations of the roles played by both parties, and outlines the consequences of aberrant drug taking. Including spot urine toxicology screens in the contract can maximize compliance. Expectations regarding clinic visits and the patient's management of medications should also be stated, such as making refills contingent on clinic attendance. The clinician should consider requiring the patient to attend 12-step programs and have the patient document attendance as a condition for ongoing prescribing. With consent, the clinician may wish to contact the patient's sponsor and make him or her aware that the patient is being treated for a chronic illness that requires medications (e.g., opioids). This approach will reduce the potential for stigmatization of the patient as being noncompliant with the ideals of the 12-step program. Finally, family members and friends should be involved to bolster social support and function. Mental health professionals should identify family members who are themselves drug abusers and who may divert the patient's medications, and these professionals should help family members with referrals to drug treatment and co-dependency groups to help the patient receive optimal medical care.

Inpatient Management

Inpatient management includes and expands on the guidelines for outpatient settings. First, drug use needs to be discussed openly. It is necessary to reassure the patient that steps will be taken to avoid adverse events such as drug or alcohol withdrawal. In some circumstances, such as preoperatively, patients should be admitted several days in advance for drug regimen stabilization. They should be provided with a private room near the nurses' station to help with monitoring and to discourage attempts to leave the hospital to purchase illicit drugs. To stem access to drugs, visitors should check in with nursing staff members before visitation, and some visitors should have their packages searched. Daily urine specimens should also be collected for random toxicology analysis.

Management should be tailored to reflect the clinician's assessment of drug abuse severity and to maintain open and honest patient communication. These guidelines may fail to curtail aberrant drug use despite repeated staff interventions. In such a case, the patient should be considered for discharge, but this approach seems necessary only in the most recalcitrant cases. The clinician should involve staff and administration about the ethical and legal implications of such a decision.

Alcohol

Alcoholism in the terminally ill patient is a serious problem. A 1995 survey in a palliative care unit observed alcohol abuse in more than 25% of patients.[16] Alcohol-dependent patients with life-threatening illnesses require careful assessment and management; such patients who are not identified and who are then admitted to hospitals can go into withdrawal, with unexpected complications. Patients at the end of life can also experience withdrawal symptoms if they decrease their alcohol intake as their physical condition declines. If the extent of the alcohol use is unknown, withdrawal symptoms may be mistaken for simple anxiety. The first symptoms of withdrawal usually begin a few hours after the cessation of alcohol intake; they often consist of tremors, agitation, and insomnia. In mild to moderate cases, these symptoms lessen within 2 days. Terminally ill patients are more likely than physically healthy persons to progress from these symptoms to delirium, characterized by autonomic hyperactivity, hallucinations, incoherence, and disorientation.[13] Delirium tremens

represents a serious medical emergency and occurs in 5% to 15% of patients in alcohol withdrawal, usually within 72 to 96 hours of withdrawal. Delirium tremens is a self-limiting condition and usually ends in 72 to 96 hours with a deep sleep. Patients have amnesia for most of what occurs during this period.

In surgical settings, alcohol withdrawal can cause up to a threefold increase in postoperative mortality when it is unrecognized and not addressed.[17] Because of poor nutrition, prior head trauma, and brain injury from excessive alcohol consumption, patients with cancer and alcoholism are already at high risk of postoperative delirium from seizures and of delirium tremens, which can be fatal.[13]

The excessive vulnerability of terminally ill patients necessitates that potential withdrawal symptoms be managed aggressively and prevented whenever possible.[17] Basic management steps (e.g., hydration, benzodiazepines, and, in some cases, neuroleptics) should be employed.[13] A vitamin-mineral solution helps to counteract the malnutrition that results from alcohol itself and from poor eating habits. Thiamine (100 mg intramuscularly or intravenously) should be administered for 3 days before switching to oral administration to prevent Korsakoff's syndrome and alcoholic dementia. A daily dose of folate (1 mg) should also be given throughout treatment.

Recovery

Depending on the recovery program (e.g., Alcoholics Anonymous, methadone maintenance programs), a patient may fear ostracism from the program's members or may experience intense fear regarding susceptibility to recurrent addiction. It is best first to explore nonopioid therapies with these patients. This approach may require referral to a pain center. Alternatives may include nonopioid or adjuvant analgesics, cognitive therapies, electrical stimulation, neural blockades, or acupuncture. When opioids are required in certain patients, it is necessary to use opioid management contracts, random urine toxicology screens, and occasional pill counts. The patient's recovery program sponsor should be included, to aid successful monitoring.

Screening Issues

Interest in predicting which patients can be maintained on opioid therapy and which patients will present management difficulty, including potential addiction, has been growing. A screening measure for chronic pain was tested.[18] The investigators identified the salient characteristics of patients with chronic pain that predict future medication misuse and developed the 24-item, self-administered Screener and Opioid Assessment for Patients with Pain (SOAPP). This test was since made into a 14-item short form that shows promise as a screening tool for substance abuse and addiction.

One study examined the relationship between aberrant drug-taking behaviors and pain outcomes during long-term treatment with opioids for nonmalignant pain.[19] A checklist tool developed from this study that may be applicable in palliative medicine. Four areas were proposed as most relevant for ongoing monitoring of patients with chronic pain who are receiving opioids. These domains are referred to as the "Four A's" (analgesia, activities of daily living, adverse side effects, and aberrant drug-taking behaviors). The monitoring of these outcomes over time should inform therapeutic decisions and should provide a framework for the clinical use of controlled drugs.

Evidence-Based Medicine

Several studies have investigated aberrant drug taking. One study examined outcomes and drug taking in 20 patients with diverse histories of drug abuse who underwent a year of long-term opioid therapy.[11] During the year of therapy, 11 patients adhered to the drug regimen, and 9 did not. Patients who did not abuse the therapy were solely abusers of alcohol (or had remote histories of polysubstance abuse), were in solid drug-free recovery, and had good social support. Patients who abused the therapy were polysubstance abusers, were not participating in 12-step programs, and had poor social support.

A major cancer center examined self-reports of aberrant drug-taking attitudes and behaviors in patients with cancer ($n = 52$) and AIDS ($n = 111$).[20] Reports of past drug use and abuse were more frequent than present reports in both groups. Current aberrant drug-related behaviors were seldom reported, but attitude items revealed that patients would consider engaging in aberrant behaviors, or would possibly excuse them in others, if pain or symptom management were inadequate.

Some behaviors are incorrectly regarded as aberrant despite limited data. For example, the patient who requests a specific pain medication or a specific route or dose is often considered suspicious by the practitioner. Other aberrant behaviors may be common in nonaddicts but have little to do with addiction; for example, many nonaddicted patients with cancer use anxiolytic medications prescribed for someone else.[20] This practice seems to reflect the undertreatment and underreporting of anxiety in oncology patients, rather than true addiction.

CONCLUSIONS

Although clinicians cannot prevent all aberrant drug-related behavior, they must recognize that virtually any drug that acts on the central nervous system, and any route of drug administration, can be abused. The problem is not the drugs themselves. Effective management of patients with pain who engage in aberrant drug-related behavior must involve a comprehensive approach that recognizes the biological, chemical, social, and psychiatric aspects of substance abuse while providing practical means to manage risk, treat pain effectively, and ensure patient safety.

Limited data relevant to risk assessment in the medically ill are available, and most data relate to the risk of serious abuse or addiction during long-term opioid treatment of chronic pain in patients with no history of substance abuse. Almost no information exists about the risk of less serious aberrant drug-related behaviors, the risk of these outcomes in patients who do have a history of abuse, or the risk associated with potentially abusable drugs other than opioids.

Research Challenges and Opportunities

Prescription drug abuse is a growing phenomenon that has been understudied. Researchers and clinicians need to create alliances to shed light on this issue and to determine the best safeguards. We need to understand the best ways to identify at-risk patients while preserving opioid use as a viable modality for all patients with pain. Early efforts to create screening instruments have been useful, but more study is needed to prove their true utility and to determine which best predicts the problematic patient. Once this information is determined, further study will need to take place regarding how best to treat this at-risk population.

REFERENCES

1. Kessler RC, Berglund P, Demler O, et al. Lifetime prevalence and age-of-onset distributions of DSM-IV disorders in the National Comorbidity Survey Replication. Arch Gen Psychiatry 2005;62:593-602.
2. National Center on Addiction and Substance Abuse at Columbia University. Under the counter: The diversion and abuse of controlled prescription drugs in the U.S., July 2005. Available at http://www.casacolumbia.org (accessed April 28, 2008).
3. Room R, Babor T, Rehm J. Alcohol and public health. Lancet 2005;365:519-530.
4. Gfoerer J, Brodsky M. The incidence of illicit drug use in the United States, 1962-1989. Br J Addiction 1992;87:1345-1351.
5. Derogatis LR, Morrow GR, Fetting J, et al. The prevalence of psychiatric disorders among cancer patients. JAMA 1983;249:751-757.
6. Gonzales GR, Coyle N. Treatment of cancer pain in a former opioid abuser: Fears of the patient and staff and their influence on care. J Pain Symptom Manage 1992;7:246-249.
7. Ad Hoc Committee on Cancer Pain of the American Society of Clinical Oncology. Cancer pain assessment and treatment curriculum guidelines. J Clin Oncol 1992;10:1976-1982.
8. Zech DF, Grond S, Lynch J, et al. Validation of the World Health Organization Guidelines for cancer pain relief: A 10 year prospective study. Pain 1995;63:65-76.
9. Meuser T, Pietruck C, Radbruch L, et al. Symptoms during cancer pain treatment following WHO guidelines: A longitudinal follow-up study of symptom prevalence, severity, and etiology. Pain 2001;93:247-257.
10. Potter JS, Hennessy G, Borrow JA, et al. Substance use histories in patients seeking treatment for controlled-release oxycodone dependence. Drug Alcohol Depend 2004;76:213-215.
11. Dunbar SA, Katz NP. Chronic opioid therapy for nonmalignant pain in patients with a history of substance abuse: Report of 20 cases. J Pain Symptom Manage 1996;11:163-171.
12. Kaplan R, Slywka J, Slagle S, et al. A titrated analgesic regimen comparing substance users and non-users with AIDS-related pain. J Pain Symptom Manage 2000;19:265-271.
13. Lundberg JC, Passik SD. Alcohol and cancer: A review for psycho-oncologists. Psychooncology 1997;6:253-266.
14. Passik SD, Portenoy RK, Ricketts PL. Substance abuse issues in cancer patients. Part 2: evaluation and treatment. Oncology (Huntingt) 1998;12:729-734.

Common Errors

- Physicians traditionally assume that cancer patients are immune to addiction or substance abuse. This misconception can lead them to have suboptimal documentation and attention placed on patients given substances such as opioids.
- The growing fear of opioid use in general is starting to become an issue even with patients with cancer. Pockets of the United States, including rural Appalachia and others hit by the growing problem of prescription opioid abuse, have seen physicians pull back from opioid use altogether.
- Physicians need to avoid either extreme and ensure due diligence in prescribing to potentially problematic patients. Good documentation of opioid prescribing should be considered an essential baseline but not necessarily sufficient for protecting the physician and the patient.

15. Passik S, Schreiber J, Kirsh KL, Portenoy RK. A chart review of the ordering and documentation of urine toxicology screens in a cancer center: Do they influence patient management? J Pain Symptom Manage 2000;19:40-44.

16. Bruera E, Moyano J, Seifert L, et al. The frequency of alcoholism among patients with pain due to terminal cancer. J Pain Symptom Manage 1995;10:599-603.

17. Maxmen JS, Ward NG. Substance-related disorders. In Essential Psychopathology and Its Treatment. New York: WW Norton, 1995, pp 132-172.

18. Butler SF, Budman SH, Fernandez K, Jamison RN. Validation of a screener and opioid assessment measure for patients with chronic pain. Pain 2004;112: 65-75.

19. Passik SD, Kirsh KL, Whitcomb LA, et al. A new tool to assess and document pain outcomes in chronic pain patients receiving opioid therapy. Clin Ther 2004;26:552-561.

20. Passik S, Kirsh, KL, McDonald M, et al. A pilot survey of aberrant drug-taking attitudes and behaviors in samples of cancer and AIDS patients. J Pain Symptom Manage 2000;19:274-286.

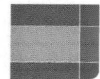

CHAPTER **252**

Nonopioid and Adjuvant Analgesics

Henry McQuay

KEY POINTS

- Antidepressants and antiepileptics are well-established treatments for neuropathic pain.

- Clinical trial evidence can be limited in both scope of neuropathic pain conditions studied and duration of treatment. Most trials are in patients with pain unrelated to cancer. This leaves palliative care prescribers to extrapolate evidence to patients with cancer.

- Lack of head-to-head comparisons results in the use of indirect comparative evidence, such as with numbers needed to treat (NNTs) derived by meta-analysis. The small numbers studied make these NNT values less robust.

- Although tricyclic antidepressants (TCAs) appear more effective than other classes of antidepressants, this increased effectiveness needs to be balanced against a higher adverse effect profile.

- League tables suggest that the character of the neuropathic pain, whether it be burning or shooting, does not determine its responsiveness to either of the drug classes.

The first reports of antiepileptic efficacy in trigeminal neuralgia go back nearly 50 years. TCA efficacy was also shown in various pain syndromes decades ago. Our concern now is not whether antidepressants and antiepileptics work in neuropathic pain (although we still have to show that effect for any new drugs), but rather how well the different drugs within the these categories work compared with each other, and indeed how well antidepressants work compared with antiepileptics. The other issue is the relative adverse effect burden within and between the two drug classes. The effectiveness of the two drug classes and the cost in adverse effects remain the focus of attention for clinicians, researchers, and patients themselves.

PHARMACOLOGY OF ANTIDEPRESSANTS AND ANTICONVULSANTS

Antidepressants

TCAs such as amitriptyline and imipramine have multimodal mechanisms of action. These drugs inhibit presynaptic uptake of serotonin and norepinephrine, interact with sodium and calcium ion channels, and block some postsynaptic histamine and muscarinic receptors. TCAs generally show nonlinear pharmacokinetics, meaning that no linear relationship exists between drug dose and steady-state serum concentration. For example, a 30-fold difference in serum concentrations has been observed with the same TCA dose in different patients. This variability can also result in significantly higher serum concentrations (and clinical effects) despite small dose changes, and vice versa. Dry mouth, drowsiness, and postural hypotension are the most frequent adverse effects, often more pronounced in elderly patients. In general, subantidepressant doses of TCAs can produce analgesic benefit; the usual starting dose of amitriptyline is 25 mg daily, titrated to a mean of approximately 75 mg.

Antiepileptics

The mechanism of action of older antiepileptic drugs, such as phenytoin and carbamazepine, was thought to occur through blockade of voltage-dependent sodium channels. More recent work suggested that carbamazepine may have additional actions by serotonergic pathways (an unsurprising finding because the drug is structurally similar to TCAs). Doses of antiepileptics used to treat neuropathic pain are similar to those used in epilepsy

EVIDENCE-BASED MEDICINE

Scope and Extrapolation

Most of the trials of neuropathic pain from which the information here was drawn were conducted in patients with postherpetic neuralgia (PHN) and painful diabetic neuropathy (PDN). These two conditions are easy to diagnose and are the test-bed for testing drug efficacy in neuropathic pain. However, most neuropathic pain is not PHN or PDN. Historically, drug remedies for PHN and PDN have been effective in other neuropathic pain syndromes and neuropathic cancer pain, but we do not know whether negative results in PHN and PDN predict a lack of efficacy in other neuropathic pain syndromes. Much of our prescribing for neuropathic pain involves extrapolation from results in other, different, pain syndromes. In palliative care, the water is muddied further if the patient has pain at multiple sites, some neuropathic and some nociceptive. On the optimistic side, historically those drugs with proven efficacy in chronic noncancer pain have also been effective in neuropathic cancer pain.

Duration

One of the major questions is how long—weeks or months—the drug should be studied for us to be certain of its efficacy. Many patients with neuropathic pain syndromes need medications for years, so the issues of efficacy and safety over the longer term are important to patients and prescribers. Most trials are of less than 8 weeks' duration, and only for more recently introduced drugs do we have information for up to 3 months of treatment. Even this information is limited in relation to the duration of the condition, and some patients whose neuropathic cancer pain results from treatment rather than from tumor may well face long-term treatment. We just do not know the proportion in whom initial drug efficacy subsequently will wane and over what period this will occur. Neither do we know the corollary, the proportion in whom initial drug efficacy is maintained without dose escalation for 1 year or indeed 5 years. Technically, neuropathic pain trials may be difficult to run because many antidepressant and antiepileptic drugs have to be titrated to the optimal dose for maximal effect and minimal adverse effects, and trial designs necessarily become complicated. The alternative (using fixed doses of these drugs) risks underdosing some patients and overdosing others, as well as underestimating efficacy and overestimating adverse effects.

Determining Relative Efficacy

Lack of Head-to-Head (Direct) Evidence

Few head-to-head comparisons of antidepressants and antiepileptics in neuropathic pain have been made, and even fewer head-to-head comparisons of different antidepressants or different antiepileptics have been reported. The small numbers of patients in these studies are surprising. For example, all the sweeping statements made about the lack of efficacy of selective serotonin reuptake inhibitors (SSRIs) in neuropathic pain are based on 81 patients in trials of good quality, and in one of those trials the SSRI did as well as the TCA. From these 81 patients, a relatively poor NNT of approximately 7 (for 50% pain relief) was calculated,[1] a value that compares poorly with the NNT quoted for TCAs of less than 3. If you exclude the trials that provided the 81 patients studied, a failed trial of fluoxetine emerges,[2] as well as a trial in which the efficacy of paroxetine was the same as a that of a TCA.[3] Reviews contain the dogma that SSRIs are ineffective in neuropathic pain.[1,4] However, we have so little evidence, so few patients have been studied, and within that small number disagreement exists. If SSRIs were to be proved effective (in a further trial or trials), then because of their adverse effect advantage over TCAs, this finding would be potentially clinically important. In the only modern head-to-head comparison, in a small study of 19 patients who crossed over between gabapentin (≤1800 mg) and amitriptyline (≤75 mg) in PDN, no significant difference was noted in pain scores with the two drugs or in global ratings of pain relief (52% with at least moderate pain relief during gabapentin and 67% during amitriptyline) ($P > .1$). Both treatments caused similar adverse events.[5]

Using Systematic Review (Indirect) Evidence

In the absence of head-to-head or direct comparisons, how are we to arrive at an assessment of the relative efficacy and tolerability of the different drugs? Earlier reviews and the most recent updates have used systematic review techniques to gather data from good-quality trials comparing antiepileptics or antidepressants with placebo, the indirect method. The efficacy of the different drugs against placebo is then calculated and expressed as the NNT. The NNT values of the different drugs may then be compared to determine the relative efficacy of the different drugs. Consider the following analogy: We want to know who is the quickest runner in the room. We could simply make everyone run 100 m and compete with each other in one race, the *direct* method. This would be the head-to-head comparison. Alternatively, we could ask each individual to run 100 m against the clock and on his or her own. We could then compare the times to calculate who was quickest. This latter *indirect* method is the equivalent of deriving relative efficacy by comparing each drug's performance against placebo. To estimate the relative efficacy of antiepileptics and antidepressants in neuropathic pain, we do not have a choice. We do not have direct comparisons, so we have to use an indirect method.

Limitations of Indirect Methods

These direct and indirect methods of assessing the efficacy of drugs for neuropathic pain produce remarkably similar estimates that support the indirect technique. However, one should be aware of the weaknesses of these methods, by far the most significant of which is size. If the performance of the drug or even the drug class is based on a small number studied, then the estimate of that performance should be treated with caution. An estimate of efficacy derived from 500 patients compared with placebo is more robust than an estimate based on just 80 patients. This concept sounds obvious and is obvious, but it is constantly forgotten. Casual mention of the NNT value for a particular treatment in neuropathic pain without reference to the size of the sample from which it was derived is misleading. Figure 252-1 shows the range of NNT values in peripheral neuropathic pain for several antidepressant and antiepileptic drugs.[1] The diameter of the point estimate for each drug is proportional to the number of patients on whom the estimate is based, and the number is printed beside the estimate.

Comparing Antidepressant Classes

For TCAs, an NNT estimate of slightly more than 2 means that roughly one patient in two treated with a TCA for peripheral neuropathic pain will achieve at least 50% pain relief. The other patient may have some relief, but not enough to pass the 50% relief mark. The estimate is based on roughly 400 patients. These patients may have been receiving different antidepressants and at different doses. The different doses should not be too much of a problem because the dose for each drug should have been optimal. If we are hypercritical and split the efficacy estimate into the individual TCAs, then we will have few data for most individual drugs. The NNT estimate with SSRI antidepressants is more than 6, meaning that just one patient in six treated with an SSRI antidepressant for peripheral neuropathic pain will achieve at least 50% pain relief, a result much worse than with TCAs. Again, the other five patients taking the SSRI may have had some relief, but they did not achieve 50% relief. The estimate is based on just 81

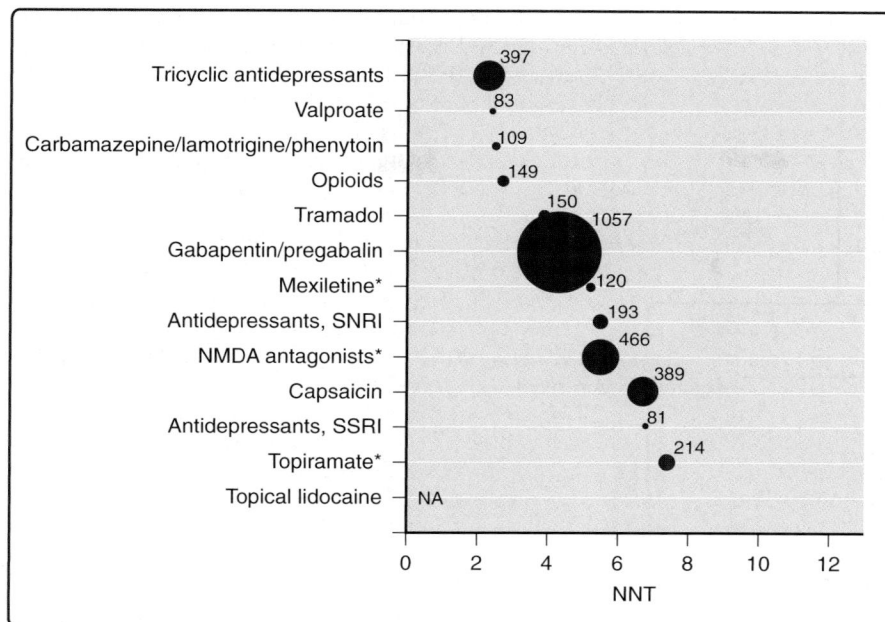

FIGURE 252-1 Range of values of numbers needed to treat (NNT) in peripheral neuropathic pain for several antidepressant and antiepileptic drugs. NMDA, *N*-methyl-D-aspartate; SNRI, serotonin norepinephrine reuptake inhibitor; SSRI, selective serotonin reuptake inhibitor. *(Redrawn from Finnerup N, Otto M, McQuay H, et al. Algorithm for neuropathic pain treatment: An evidence based proposal. Pain 2005;118:289-305.)*

patients, in stark contrast to the more than 1000 patients studied who were receiving gabapentin, with an NNT estimate of slightly higher than 4. The smaller the point estimate in the figure, the less robust is the estimate.

The Need for Clinical Trials

It is of concern we have so few data on which to base important prescribing decisions. Using antidepressants as an example, we argue that SSRIs have not been adequately tested in neuropathic pain. The potential advantage of the lower adverse effect incidence with these drugs means perhaps that we need trials of adequate size and quality to evaluate whether SSRIs do not work in neuropathic pain. The number needed to harm (NNH) for trial withdrawal related to adverse effects of TCAs compared with placebo was estimated by Finnerup and colleagues at 14.7 (10.2 to 25.2).[1] In contrast, no statistically significant difference was noted between SSRI and placebo for withdrawal related to adverse effects.

Efficacy NNT values for mixed selective norepinephrine reuptake inhibitors (SNRIs), in modern trials of high quality ($\approx$4), are similar to the NNTs for gabapentin. As with SSRIs, the adverse effect profile of the SNRIs is better than that of TCAs, with no statistically significant difference for withdrawal related to adverse effects compared with placebo. It is also possible that the favorable status of TCAs in the relative efficacy league table may result from an overestimation of benefit in older small trials, some of crossover design. Against that interpretation is the finding that in both painful polyneuropathy and PHN, the trend is toward a better effect of balanced serotonin and norepinephrine. Fresh clinical trials rather than meta-analysis are needed to examine the belief that the pharmacological multiple receptor ("shotgun") action of TCAs is more effective than that of selective ("rifle") drugs in neuropathic pain.

Using Relative Efficacy

League Tables

Diagnosing neuropathic pain is not difficult until people make it complicated. The combination of pain in an area of altered nervous system function, sometimes associated with pain on nonpainful stimulus or excessive pain in response to a not very painful stimulus, and with a muted response to conventional analgesics, leads most clinicians to think of treatment with antidepressants or antiepileptics. The choice of drug class for initial treatment and the choice of particular drug within that class are areas in which relative efficacy league tables can help. The term *league table* is used to mean a ranking of the NNT efficacy values of the different drugs, in which the lowest value is best and the highest is worst (see Fig. 252-1). The league table is based on many patients, whereas for an individual patient, the table takes little or no account of the adverse effects so important in long-term therapy. Nonetheless, the league table provides us with the probability of success and the extent of that success for the different drugs. More selective antidepressants include SSRIs such as paroxetine and fluoxetine and balanced SNRIs such as venlafaxine and the more potent duloxetine, which is licensed for PDN. Both these drug classes have virtually no blocking effects on postsynaptic receptors or ion channels, with fewer side effects. The extent to which the TCA multimodal actions contribute to their apparent superiority, and greater adverse effects, compared with SSRIs and SNRIs in neuropathic pain is controversial.

Newer antiepileptics, such as gabapentin, pregabalin, and lamotrigine, act on various receptors, including the α_2 subunit of voltage-dependent calcium channels and modulation of γ-aminobutyric acid synthesis, release, and metabolism. Adverse effects are similar for all antiepileptics, and effects most frequently reported are drowsiness, fatigue, and ataxia. Longer-term adverse effects are not

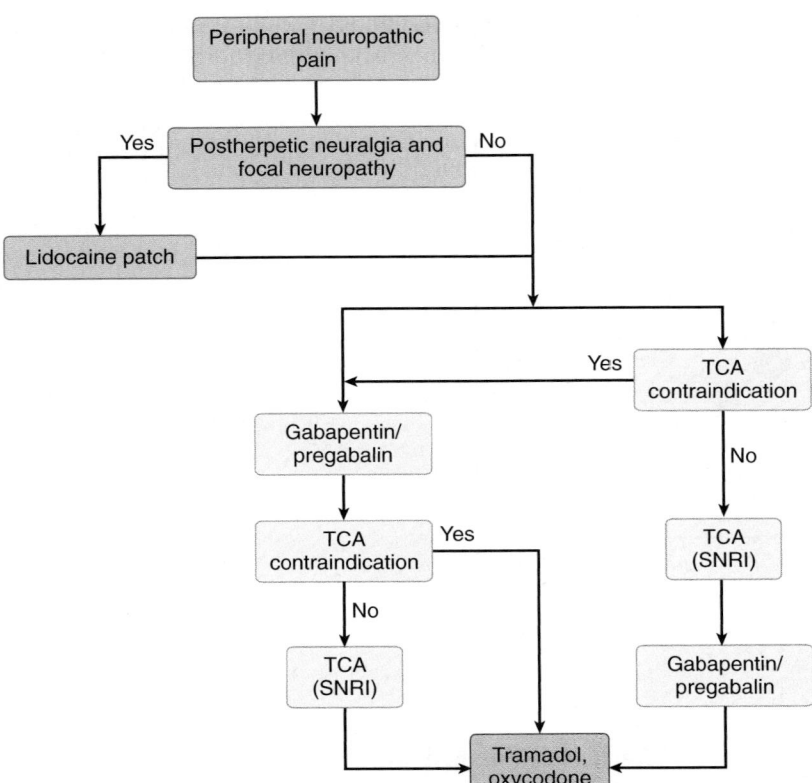

FIGURE 252-2 Algorithm in neuropathic pain. SNRI, serotonin norepinephrine reuptake inhibitor; TCA, tricyclic antidepressant.

always apparent in clinical trials of short duration; weight gain associated with gabapentin is an example.

RESEARCH CHALLENGES, OPPORTUNITIES, AND ADVANCES

A thought-provoking article suggested that current methods of classifying neuropathic pain and underlying mechanisms do not help to predict the response to different drugs.[6] Patients who did not respond to imipramine (the test TCA) tended not to respond well to the second-line drug, the antiepileptic gabapentin. Just as the character of the pain may not predict therapeutic response to one or other drug class, so for now we have one algorithm for all the different mechanisms underlying peripheral neuropathic pain.

CONCLUSIONS

The algorithm (Fig. 252-2) and the review are practical examples of where meta-analysis can take us in the management of neuropathic pain.[1,4] The algorithm attempts to encapsulate the evidence into a decision tree. The reality is that we lack the head-to-head comparison studies neces-

sary to substantiate the algorithm, and we do not know whether different mechanisms underlying various neuropathic pain syndromes mean that we should have a different algorithm for each condition. For instance, standard teaching used to be that one would use an antidepressant for a burning pain and an antiepileptic for a shooting pain. Little evidence exists to support this approach, and some evidence goes against it. These findings suggest that the character of the pain, whether it be burning or shooting, does not determine its responsiveness to either of the drug classes.

REFERENCES

1. Finnerup N, Otto M, McQuay H, et al. Algorithm for neuropathic pain treatment: An evidence based proposal. Pain 2005;118:289-305.
2. Max MB, Lynch SA, Muir J, et al. Effects of desipramine, amitriptyline, and fluoxetine on pain in diabetic neuropathy. N Engl J Med 1992;326:1250-1256.
3. Sindrup SH, Gram LF, Brosen K, et al. The selective serotonin reuptake inhibitor paroxetine is effective in the treatment of diabetic neuropathy symptoms. Pain 1990;42:135-144.
4. Attal N, Cruccu G, Haanpaa M, et al. EFNS guidelines on pharmacological treatment of neuropathic pain. Eur J Neurol 2006;13:1153-1169.
5. Morello CM, Leckband SG, Stoner CP. Randomized double-blind study comparing the efficacy of gabapentin with amitriptyline on diabetic peripheral neuropathy pain. Arch Intern Med 1999;159:1931-1937.
6. Rasmussen P, Sindrup S, Jensen T, Bach F. Therapeutic outcome in neuropathic pain: Relationship to evidence of nervous system lesion. Eur J Neurol 2004;11:545-553.

CHAPTER **253**

Challenging Pain Problems

Sebastiano Mercadante

DEFINITION OF DIFFICULT PAIN PROBLEMS

Whereas most cancer pain can be relieved with simple methods using oral analgesics, some patients may have difficult pain problems and may require more complex approaches. In 10% to 20% of patients with cancer, pain is not easily relieved.[1] Because opioids are the most commonly used drugs, and because patients with difficult problems are assumed to use this class of drugs, opioid responsiveness has been the principal focus of research. Pain poorly responsive to opioids is a clinical situation in which opioids induce severe adverse effects despite optimal symptomatic treatment, before appropriate analgesia. Thus, the ceiling doses of opioids induce adverse effects that limit further opioid dose escalation. It is impossible to predict a poor opioid response before careful drug titration, although some predictive negative factors have been identified.[2]

Neuropathic pain and incident pain have been identified as challenging situations. In several prognostic studies, they are associated with less positive outcomes. The global response to opioids, including adverse effects, is typically individual and is probably genetically determined. Clinical evidence suggests that different opioids may produce different effect profiles in individuals. Therefore, it is more appropriate to consider the response to each opioid,

rather than the general opioid response. A difficult pain problem is a clinical situation requiring specific measures and, in some cases, a high level of expertise.

INCIDENT PAIN

Incident pain limits quality of life because it interferes with daily activities.[3] Incident pain is mainly the result of movement, is commonly associated with bone metastases or fractures, and is the best-known cause of breakthrough pain. This condition is often predictable, and patients learn to limit some movements to avoid pain, which may also be absent at rest or controlled by analgesic drugs.

Other mechanisms may produce incident pain. Swallowing may induce severe incident pain in patients with extensive mucosal damage, and any skin lesion induces pain when it is touched, as a result of primary and secondary hyperalgesia. Allodynia, typically associated with nerve damage, results from touching hypersensitive skin areas.[4]

General Treatment

Attention to precipitating or alleviating factors that help to prevent or reduce pain exacerbations is paramount. The likelihood of spontaneous remission of pain after a short time may reduce the meaning of benefits attributed to specific interventions by patients. Pain induced by contact or triggering factors is a challenge. Pain induced by swallowing or speech is a frequent feature of oropharyngeal mucositis induced by chemotherapy, radiation therapy, or local infection. Other than usual mouth care (see Chapter 171), local measures may help to treat or prevent painful episodes, including local application of clonazepam, amitriptyline, ketamine, or opioids. The application of topical morphine to damaged oral mucosa has been suggested. Mouthwashes with oral rinses with 2% morphine solution have been effective in reducing swallowing-induced pain, without causing significant plasma concentration.[5] Similarly, local anesthetics and opioids have been used topically on open wounds that trigger acute episodes. Remarkable efficacy has been found with topical opioids. It is difficult to evaluate the amount absorbed locally and to determine the effective amount because of methods of preparation, concentration, dressing absorption, and local secretion. Events related to nerve damage are more commonly treated with adjuvants (see later).

Radiation therapy is an effective symptomatic treatment for local bone pain that causes transitory events. Because protracted courses of radiation therapy are difficult in patients with advanced cancer with limited life expectancy and poor performance status, single fractions may be more convenient and equally effective for pain relief. Compared with external beam radiation therapy, radioisotopes are imprecise in delivering specific doses of irradiation: advantages include less toxicity, easy administration, and effectiveness in subclinical sites of metastases (see Chapter 235). The extent of pain relief, particularly incident pain, has not been adequately quantified.[6] Rehabilitation approaches may help. Protection with orthotic devices may be useful for upper extremity bone lesions. The lower extremities are hardly amenable to orthoses because of the high degree of load. Patients with bone involvement of the lower extremities frequently lose the ability to walk. Rehabilitation approaches improve the patient's function level and compliance (see Chapter 246). Impending fractures require surgical stabilization using fixation devices or prosthetic reconstruction. Surgical stabilization of the spine and extremities may dramatically improve quality of life, decrease incident pain, and prevent complications of immobility (see Chapters 241 and 242). However, the risks should be balanced against the benefits of such interventions in patients with advanced cancer and poor performance status.

Pharmacological Treatment

Baseline pain may be absent or moderate at rest, but severe episodic pains occur with certain positions or even during deep breathing. Pain assessment is often difficult because patients try to avoid the movements that trigger the pain. Treatment response is also difficult to assess. For example, if medications are given for incident pain, this pain could also spontaneously subside before the drug shows a significant effect. Conversely, incident pain may be an expression of poor basal pain relief. It is useful to try to reduce the frequency and intensity of such episodes by increasing basal analgesic doses. Experimental models of bone cancer pain showed that metastatic bone pain could correlate with opioid responsiveness with neuropathic pain, characterized by significant peripheral and spinal neuronal excitability. On this basis, a study of incident pain showed that most patients responded to further opioid dose increases, despite having rest pain controlled.[7] Hypersensitivity to some innocuous stimulus, such as movement, probably requires pre-emptive higher doses of basal opioid medication to reduce increased pain input (see "Case Study: Optimization of Opioid Therapy for Incident Pain"), whereas the dose of opioids to maintain good analgesia at rest is insufficient during incident pain. Most increases in dose cause central toxicity, usually sedation, particularly between incident pain episodes. Methylphenidate may help opioid titration in incident pain; in one study, doubling opioid doses in 6 days achieved better pain control.[8] Patients with pain from bone metastases on weight bearing or movement may require opioid doses that cause excessive adverse effects at rest, because movement-related pain is likely to be recurrent and in some patients unpredictable.

Future Developments

Pre-emptive analgesia may include bisphosphonates. These agents are effective in reducing bone pain and in preventing skeletal events. Experimental evidence suggests a potential role for bisphosphonates in incident bone pain. Reduction in activated osteoclasts parallels attenuation of upregulation of the pro-hyperalgesic peptide dynorphin in the spinal cord. These changes reduce ongoing and movement-evoked bone cancer pain, bone destruction, and destruction of sensory nerve fibers that innervate the bone, whereas viable tumor burden remains unchanged. Similarly, some anticonvulsants, such as gabapentin, may be anti-hyperalgesic. The role of pre-emptive drugs should be better evaluated in human patients with incident pain, rather than during a general assessment of pain. The cost-

CASE STUDY

Optimization of Opioid Therapy for Incident Pain

AB, a 56-year-old man, was scheduled for a course of radiation therapy on painful bone metastases from lung cancer. However, the pain kept him from participating in simulation for radiation therapy. A pain consultation was required. The patient had severe basal pain (scored 8 on a scale from 0 to10), as well as excruciating pain on movement, caused by vertebral metastases. This pain impeded any maneuver and prevented the performance of procedures required for radiation therapy. The patient had received tramadol, ketorolac, and dexamethasone, unsuccessfully. Intravenous morphine was titrated with repeated boluses. The effective intravenous morphine dose was 8 mg. No adverse effects were recorded. He was then started with an intravenous morphine infusion of 60 mg/day. Doses were increased in the next days up to 120 mg/day, and doses were offered as needed to facilitate movements. Three days later, the patient could actively participate in the radiation therapy program, and therapy was started while the patient received 150 mg/day of intravenous morphine. Six days after starting radiation therapy, the dose of intravenous morphine was reduced at 45 mg/day because of well-controlled pain and the occurrence of somnolence, confusion, and blurred vision. These signs were interpreted as relative overdoses owing to reduction of pain intensity. The morphine dose was then slowly tapered according to pain intensity, and then it was stopped to maintain a dose of 3 mg intravenously, as needed. During his hospital stay, the patient also received chemotherapy, including carboplatin. He was discharged on the 16th day after starting radiation therapy, which was continued on an outpatient basis. Two months later, the patient was receiving nimesulide and had good pain control. Three months later, the patient was receiving 90 mg of oral morphine to maintain adequate pain control and to allow an acceptable level of activities of daily living.

to-benefit ratio should be assessed in future studies with appropriate designs.

Specific Treatments

A rescue opioid dose is traditionally used to treat incident pain in patients stabilized on a baseline opioid. The use of opioids with short half-lives such as immediate-release morphine, oxycodone, or hydromorphone is standard practice. A relationship between transient pain and the baseline dose regimen has been suggested.[1] Most oral opioids have a relatively slow onset of effect (≈30 to 45 minutes), so the pain onset may be so rapid that an oral dose could not provide prompt relief. A better result may be obtained with a parenteral rescue dose because the onset of analgesic effect is faster following parenteral than oral administration. The optimal candidates for intravenous or subcutaneous patient-controlled analgesia (PCA) are patients with an intravenous or subcutaneous access who have irregular or rapidly accelerating pain requiring immediate treatment that is not guaranteed by the slow onset of oral analgesic. This method is not always available, given that the financial burden associated with purchase of a PCA device and medication cassettes may be significant. Moreover, many patients are unable to operate a PCA device because they are overwhelmed by the technical aspects. Finally, the pump may limit patient mobility, and technical expertise is required.

Recent Developments

Oral transmucosal administration is a noninvasive approach to rapid analgesia. Highly lipophilic agents may pass rapidly through the oral mucosa, thus avoiding first-pass metabolism and achieving active plasma concentrations within minutes. Fentanyl, incorporated in a hard matrix on a handle, is rapidly absorbed. The onset of pain relief is similar to that of intravenous morphine (i.e., ≤10 minutes). When the fentanyl matrix dissolves, approximately 25% of the total fentanyl concentration crosses the buccal mucosa and enters the bloodstream. The remaining amount is swallowed, and approximately one third of this part is absorbed, with a total bioavailability of 50%.[9] Despite its longer half-life when compared with intravenous fentanyl, transmucosal fentanyl still offers a short duration of effect because of the drug's wide distribution into tissues.

SCIENTIFIC EVIDENCE

Randomized studies show clear evidence of the effectiveness of oral transmucosal fentanyl (OTFC) for breakthrough pain. OTFC produces faster relief and greater pain relief than the usual medication (i.e., oral morphine). Most controlled trials with OTFC contradicted the anecdotal assumption that the effective dose needed is a percentage of the opioid daily dose and demonstrated the lack of relationship between the effective OTFC dose and a fixed-schedule opioid regimen, regardless of the opioid used.[9-12] Dose titration is necessary for breakthrough pain, independent of the basal regimen. These studies did not specify the kind of breakthrough pain, particularly incident pain. Two thirds of episodes in patients treated with placebo did not require additional medication. This finding can be explained by the normal course of episodes, which are often relatively short-lived and improve spontaneously, or by a true placebo response. Alternately, such episodes autoresolved because of a low pain intensity of the flare. The relationship between the daily opioid basal dose and the dose for breakthrough pain was evidenced in a subsequent uncontrolled study of intravenous morphine. Intravenous morphine in doses of 20% of the daily basal regimen (after conversion with the oral route) was safe and effective in approximately 90% of episodes.[7]

FUTURE DEVELOPMENTS

The titration reported by OTFC studies complicates general practice, particularly for outpatients. Further studies should examine the dose of OTFC in patients who receive high doses of opioids, who probably could skip some titration steps. Newer delivery systems will administer opioids, principally fentanyl, as sublingual tablets or by intranasal and inhalational routes. These routes could provide more predictable absorption than the transmucosal route.

NEUROPATHIC PAIN

Neuropathic pains comprise several clinical entities with variable presentations and specific pathophysiology. The rationale for treatment directed at classifying and treating pain based on anatomy or underlying disease or mechanism has been of limited value in patients with nonmalignant pain.[13] The dynamic evolution of cancer pain syndromes is complex and unpredictable, and signs and symptoms may change during the course of disease; these observations have been confirmed by animal models.

The terms *complex regional pain syndromes (CRPS) type I (reflex sympathetic dystrophy)* and *type II (causalgia)* describe a syndrome of pain and sudomotor or vasomotor instability. These syndromes start after a noxious event, are not limited to the distribution of a single peripheral nerve, and often are disproportionate to the inciting event. Such symptoms and signs usually affect the distal part of a limb but can occasionally involve discrete regions or may spread to other body areas. Pain is burning and spontaneous in thermal or mechanically induced allodynia. The constellation of symptoms and signs of CRPS represents interrelated events sufficient to be designated a distinctive entity. What constitutes each of these events, or which are essential, is unclear, nor is the nature of the pathological changes that ensue understood. CRPS requires evidence of edema, cutaneous blood flow changes, or abnormal sudomotor activity. Whereas type I CRPS occurs after bone, joint, or soft tissue injury, type II is precipitated by nerve trunk injury. Because the pathophysiology of type I CRPS is predominantly hyperactivity of the regional sympathetic nervous system, pain management should focus on interrupting this system.

These syndromes are commonly observed in nonmalignant conditions, but they are occasionally reported in cancer. Type II CRPS consequent to nerve injury can be observed, for example, in Pancoast's syndrome, resulting from involvement of the brachial plexus and cervical sympathetic chain. Reports of treatment in type I CRPS are plagued by variable outcomes defined by changes in pain or improvements in function, as well as by inconsistent diagnostic criteria.[14] Various agents have been used for nonmalignant conditions, but no specific treatment is used in patients with cancer, so treatment overlaps that commonly used for cancer pain with a neuropathic component.

Opioid Responsiveness and Hyperalgesia

Neuropathic cancer pain is an irreversible and variegated syndrome that can follow injury to the peripheral or central nervous system. It has been described as unresponsive to opioids at usually effective doses, and it is considered a negative predictive prognostic factor in cancer pain. Neuropathic pain affects opioid response because it requires higher doses to achieve acceptable analgesia, often accompanied by greater toxicity. Although a neuropathic mechanism may reduce opioid responsiveness, it does not cause inherent resistance to opioids, and pain can still be responsive to analgesic treatment. Biochemical mechanisms underlying nerve damage may explain the need to use higher doses. Spinal cord hyperexcitation in neuropathic pain models resembles that in models of opioid-induced tolerance or hyperalgesia. Cancer pain is a more complex entity, particularly regarding analgesic response, in which numerous factors play a role. It remains unclear whether cancer pain is a unique type of pain or is merely a subtype of inflammatory or neuropathic pain. In cancer pain models, unique biochemical changes in transmitters are common in either neuropathic or inflammatory pain states.

Opioids, intended to abolish pain, can produce abnormally heightened pain sensations, characterized by lower pain threshold, commonly known as hyperalgesia. An iatrogenic syndrome may be characterized initially by declining analgesia and further opioid escalation to maintain the previous analgesia, with worsening of pain and whole-body hyperalgesia. This situation may correspond to a therapeutic paradox in which the consequence (increasing pain) is treated, thus favoring its cause (opioid escalation). Rapid tolerance and hyperalgesia, normally considered independent and unrelated phenomena, share some common biochemical mechanisms, even in acute conditions. Although extensive experimental data explain these clinical changes of opioid response, no data exist on how, when, and why these changes occur or on whether they are a simple consequence of a rapid derangement of the central nervous system, possibly in the last days of life.

Opioids should not be withheld on the assumption that the mechanism precludes a favorable response, because many patients will still respond effectively.[2] Basal treatment should include opioids appropriately titrated and eventually substituted with alternative opioids to achieve the best balance between analgesia and adverse effects. Opioid switching may provide a global opioid response improvement in more than 50% of patients presenting an inconvenient balance between analgesia and adverse effects (see Chapter 249). Switching to methadone, which would be potentially advantageous in neuropathic pain syndromes, does not offer specific benefits compared with nociceptive pain syndromes.[15]

Drugs for Neuropathic Pain: Scientific Evidence in Cancer Pain

One approach to neuropathic pain that is poorly responsive to opioids is the concurrent administration of a non-opioid analgesic. Antidepressants may improve depression, enhance sleep, and provide decreases in perception of pain (see Chapters 130 and 252). The analgesic efficacy of tricyclic antidepressants has been established in many painful disorders. The evidence supporting analgesic effects is particularly strong for amitriptyline. The analgesic effect of antidepressants is not directly related to antidepressant activity. The analgesic response is usually observed within 5 days. Common side effects include antimuscarinic effects (e.g., dry mouth, impaired visual accommodation, urinary retention, and constipation), antihistaminic effects (sedation), and anti–α-adrenergic effects (orthostatic hypotension). Alternative drugs with fewer side effects should be considered in patients predisposed to the sedative, anticholinergic, or hypotensive effects of amitriptyline. Despite the frequent use of amitriptyline in neuropathic cancer pain, the effectiveness of this drug has not been demonstrated. Small controlled studies showed that the potential benefits of amitriptyline are associated with frequent adverse effects,[16] which may

be particularly intense in people with advanced disease who are receiving opioids.

An anomaly in ion channels may play a role in molecular mechanism of neuropathic pain. Sodium channel blocking agents, such as systemic local anesthetics (e.g., mexiletine), carbamazepine, phenytoin, and open sodium channel blockers may relieve neuropathic pain. Although the exact mechanism of effect is unknown, these agents all inhibit sodium channels of hyperactive and depolarized nerves while not interfering with normal sensory function. Evidence for an analgesic effect of sodium channel blockers has been acquired in several neuropathic pain syndromes. Although patients with cancer who have neuropathic pain may benefit from lidocaine, one double-blind, crossover, placebo-controlled study failed to demonstrate any benefit from 5 mg/kg of lidocaine as an intravenous infusion over 30 minutes for neuropathic cancer pain syndromes.[17] Thus, although sodium channel blocking agents are useful for chronic neuropathic pain, no clinical study has verified these observations in cancer pain.

Anticonvulsants (e.g., carbamazepine, phenytoin, valproate, and clonazepam) may relieve pain in numerous peripheral and central neuropathic pain conditions, although variably. No measurable differences in the analgesic benefit of anticonvulsants and antidepressants were found in a systematic review of neuropathic pain. Data on cancer pain are poor. Gabapentin is promising as an adjuvant to opioid analgesia for neuropathic cancer pain. In a controlled study, the addition of gabapentin decreased the pain score and some typical sensations associated with neuropathic pain.[18]

Several studies documented the positive effects of corticosteroids on various cancer-related symptoms, including pain, appetite, energy level, food consumption, general well-being, and depression. Although analgesia in diverse pain syndromes has been reported, most of the evidence is anecdotal.

According to the plastic changes in the central nervous system associated with neuropathic pain, agents that block N-methyl-D-aspartate (NMDA) receptors may provide new tools for poorly responsive pain syndromes, particularly neuropathic syndromes. Ketamine is a noncompetitive NMDA receptor blocker that exerts its primary effect when the NMDA receptor–controlled ion channel has been opened by a nociceptive barrage. A synergistic effect between ketamine and opioids has been observed in cancer pain in patients who had lost an analgesic response to high-dose morphine. In a controlled study, ketamine reduced pain intensity in patients receiving opioids for neuropathic cancer pain.[19] Ketamine should be given at a starting dose of 100 to 150 mg daily, whereas the dose of opioids should be reduced by 50%, with the dose titrated against the effect. Responders should be selected by appropriate test dosing. Unfortunately, this drug is associated with central reactions that require careful treatment and expertise.

New Approaches

An attractive approach could focus on hyperalgesia rather than on nociception. NMDA antagonists may reduce opioid tolerance and hyperalgesia, particularly in patients with neuropathic pain. Ketamine may act predominantly by reversing morphine tolerance or opioid-induced hyperalgesia, because blockade of NMDA receptors does not change the baseline nociceptive response to painful stimulation or baseline spontaneous pain. NMDA receptor antagonists per se are unlikely to act as analgesics.[2] They are most likely to reduce the gain of pain intensity, rather than removing a normal pain response. Intermittent ketamine administration could bring more long-term reversal of central changes (see "Case Study: Anti-hyperalgesic Effect of Ketamine"). Intervals and doses remain unknown; this approach will require well-designed studies with more patients, studies that are not easy to perform. Moreover, the use of this drug is problematic and is reserved for skilled physicians.

ANESTHETIC TECHNIQUES FOR DIFFICULT PAIN

Analgesia may be achieved by regional anesthetic techniques (see Chapter 247). Because the peripheral nervous system has a significant overlap in sensory innervation, blockade of a single nerve may provide inadequate analgesia if the painful area is innervated by multiple nerves. Intermittent local anesthetic injections or continuous administration through a catheter can be helpful in some pain syndromes with breakthrough somatic and neuropathic mechanisms. Some invasive approaches have been used extensively in palliative care. For example, several methods have been proposed for pain control in the costopleural syndrome from invasion of the pleural cavity and

thoracic wall, including cervical cordotomy and subarachnoid phenol block. Percutaneous cervical cordotomy by radiofrequency has been used in patients with unilateral bone pain. It usually produces good relief for unilateral, well-localized pain of any origin except for some neuropathic pain. Analgesia tends to fade after the procedure, and some pain may persist or develop below or above the level of analgesia. The procedure risks pain exacerbation at other sites (including mirror pain), general fatigue or hemiparesis, and respiratory failure. The high rate of morbidity and mortality suggests the need for strict selection of cases.[6]

Sympathetically maintained pain may be associated with nervous system injury (e.g., in Pancoast's syndrome or lumbosacral plexopathy), which should be considered as CRPSs, or the pain may have a visceral origin. Interruption of these sympathetic or visceral afferent pathways has been applied widely in cancer pain. Unlike in somatic nerves, destruction of sympathetic nerves is not accompanied by alterations in muscle strength or sensitivity. Moreover, neuritis and deafferentation pain are not significant risks when the blocks are performed properly. Celiac pain should be considered a form of neuropathic pain, because of plexus involvement. In these cases, a splanchnic block is preferred because the invaded celiac area prevents appropriate spread of the neurolytic substances injected. When properly performed in selected patients, all these procedures may convert a patient with poorly responsive pain into one who achieves comfort with a well-tolerated dose or with less opioid consumption. Undesirable effects should be weighed against potential benefits. The choice of technique should be individualized, considering the physical status of the patient, the extent of tumor spread, and the clinician's experience. A gradual approach starting with the simplest and safest procedures is indicated.

Neuroaxial techniques are largely used in patients with cancer who are poorly responsive to systemic treatments. The analgesia obtained with spinal opioids in cancer pain is very variable. Commonly, these patients have received different systemic opioids unsuccessfully, possibly at high doses. The previous aggressive treatment with systemic opioids could leave patients unresponsive to opioids, even opioids administered by the spinal route. Neuropathic pain may be less responsive to systemic opioids or may require higher doses, and it may be equally difficult to treat with spinal opioids. Morphine remains the opioid of choice because of the most convenient systemic-to-intrathecal potency ratio compared with other opioids. The best response to spinal morphine is obtained in patients with continuous somatic or visceral pain. Neuropathic pain, somatic pain associated with bone metastases, and pain related to skin ulceration are disproportionately represented in patients in whom spinal opioids fail. Epidural opioids may have less toxicity than oral opioids in patients with plexus involvement. The advantage of epidural administration appears questionable, and intrathecal opioids may offer several advantages over epidural opioids in long-term treatment, including more satisfactory pain relief with lower doses of morphine and fewer technical problems.[20] Because of lower daily doses and volumes, intrathecal treatment is more suitable for treatment at home by continuous infusion than is epidural treatment. This is an important advantage considering the frequency

CASE STUDY

Anti-hyperalgesic Effect of Ketamine

CD, a 72-year-old woman with metastatic breast cancer, was admitted for back pain radiating to the legs as a result of lumbar metastases. The pain was aching and was exacerbated with movement. She also had bilateral knee pain. The patient had received several courses of chemotherapy, external beam radiation therapy, and different monthly cycles of pamidronate. In the past 3 years, she had received oral morphine first; the dose was slowly increased to 800 mg daily in a 2-year period. Further escalating doses of morphine produced some cognitive disturbances. The patient was then switched successfully to methadone, 90 mg daily. The dose was then increased to 240 mg daily. Bursts of intravenous ketamine, at doses of 100 mg daily for 2 days, were started with the intent to reduce or reverse the development of tolerance. The treatment was repeated monthly, to allow for a reduction in methadone dose in the subsequent months, Three months later, the patient's methadone dose was 75 mg daily, approximately 30% of the initial dose of methadone. Intermittent, rather than single-dose, administration of ketamine brought about a longer-term reversal of the central changes. It also allowed the distinction to be made between the real-time analgesic effect and the anti-hyperalgesic effect, as shown by the reduction of opioid dose that maintained analgesia, even during the intervals between ketamine treatments.

of pump recharges necessary to maintain analgesia, because even low-capacity systems may allow prolonged periods between refills. Volumes are more important when considering local anesthetics. Spinal opioids alone do not always provide adequate pain relief in difficult pain syndromes, or doses may need to be so high that specific or systemic side effects occur. Morphine-bupivacaine intrathecal treatment is highly effective and produces significant pain relief, less nonopioid analgesic and sedative consumption, and improved sleep, although gait is not significantly improved because of the location and progression of the illness and motor blockade.[21] The adverse effects must be balanced against the extent of relief of refractory pain syndromes. Personalization of the mixture obtains the best balance between analgesia and adverse effects, and it requires expertise. When the use of spinal local anesthetics is limited by their side effects, intraspinal α_2-adrenergic agonists may be effective. Epidural clonidine represents an important alternative to local anesthetics. The benefit seems restricted to neuropathic pain. Clonidine can be also administered intrathecally at convenient doses. Decreased blood pressure and heart rate, the main side effects, occur early in treatment.[22]

CONCLUSIONS

Given the complexity of difficult pain syndromes, an individual approach is recommended, and expert advice is required. Patients who do not favorably respond to opioid dose titration require more sophisticated treatment, including changes of opioid, of dose, and of route of administration, to find the best solution. Given the variability of the clinical pictures in poorly responsive patients, only skilled assessment of the opioid response and individualized treatment may address the specific issues of each patient.

REFERENCES

1. Hanks GW, Conno F, Cherny N, et al., Expert Working Group of the Research Network of the European Association for Palliative Care. Morphine and alternative opioids in cancer pain: The EAPC recommendations. Br J Cancer 2001;84:587-931.
2. Mercadante S, Portenoy RK. Opioid poorly responsive cancer pain. Part I: Clinical considerations. J Pain Symptom Manage 2001;21:144-150.
3. Portenoy RK, Payne D, Jacobsen P. Breakthrough pain: Characteristics and impact in patients with cancer pain. Pain 1999;81:129-134.
4. Mercadante S, Radbruch L, Caraceni, et al. Episodic (breakthrough pain). Cancer 2002;94:832-839.
5. Cerchietti LC, Navigante AH, Korte MW, et al. Potential utility of the peripheral analgesic properties of morphine in stomatitis-related pain: A pilot study. Pain 2003;105:265-273.
6. Mercadante S. Malignant bone pain: pathophysiology and treatment. Pain 1997;69:1-18.
7. Mercadante S, Villari P, Ferrera P, Casuccio A. Optimization of opioid therapy for preventing incident pain associated with bone metastases. J Pain Symptom Manage 2004;28:505-510.
8. Bruera E, Fainsinger R, MacEachern T, Hanson J. The use of methylphenidate in patients with incident pain receiving regular opiates: A preliminary report. Pain 1992;50:75-77.
9. Coluzzi P, Schwartzberg L, Conroy J, et al. Breakthrough cancer pain: A randomised trial comparing oral transmucosal fentanyl citrate and morphine sulphate immediate release. Pain 2001;91:123-130.
10. Christie J, Simmonds M, Patt R, et al. Dose-titration, multicenter study of oral transmucosal fentanyl citrate for the treatment of breakthrough pain in cancer patients using transdermal fentanyl for persistent pain. J Clin Oncol 1998;16:3238-3245.
11. Farrar J, Cleary J, Rauck R, et al. Oral transmucosal fentanyl citrate: Randomized, double-blinded, placebo-controlled trial for treatment of breakthrough pain in cancer patients. J Natl Cancer Inst 1998;90:611-616.
12. Portenoy R, Payne R, Coluzzi P, et al. Otransmucosal fentanyl citrate (OTFC) for the treatment of breakthrough pain in cancer patients: A controlled dose titration study. Pain 1999;79:303-312.
13. Jensen TS, Baron R. Translation of symptoms and signs into mechanisms in neuropathic pain. Pain 2003;102:1-8.
14. Kingery WS. A critical review of controlled trials for peripheral neuropathic pain and complex regional syndromes. Pain 1997;73:123-139.
15. Mercadante S, Bruera E. Opioid switching: A systemic and critical review. Cancer Treat Rev 2006;32:304-315.
16. Kalso E, Tasmuth T, Neuvonen PJ. Amitriptyline effectively relieves neuropathic pain following treatment of breast cancer. Pain 1996;64:293-302.
17. Bruera E, Ripamonti C, Brenneis C, et al. A randomized double-blind crossover trial of intravenous lidocaine in the treatment of neuropathic cancer pain. J Pain Symptom Manage 1992;7:138-140.
18. Caraceni A, Zecca E, Bonezzi C, et al. Gabapentin for neuropathic cancer pain: A randomized controlled trial from the Gabapentin Cancer Pain Study Group. J Clin Oncol 2004;22:2909-2917.
19. Mercadante S. Arcuri, E, Tirelli W, Casuccio A. The analgesic effect of ketamine in cancer patients on opioid therapy: A randomized, controlled, double-blind, cross-over, double dose study. J Pain Symptom Manage 2000;20:246-252.
20. Crul BJ, Delhaas EM. Technical complications during long-term subarachnoid or epidural administration of morphine in terminally ill cancer patients: A review of 140 cases. Reg Anesth 1991;16:209-213.
21. Mercadante S. Problems of long-term spinal opioid treatment in advanced cancer patients. Pain 1999;79:1-13.
22. Eisenach JC, DuPen S, Dubois M, et al. Epidural clonidine analgesia for intractable cancer pain. Pain 1995;61:391-399.

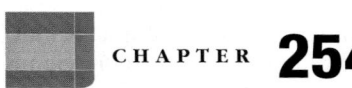

CHAPTER **254**

Pain in Cancer Survivors

Lukas Radbruch

KEY POINTS

- The prevalence of pain in cancer survivors is high. Chronic pain may persist after antineoplastic treatment, or it may appear years or even decades after cancer treatment.

- Pain from antineoplastic therapies, such as chemotherapy-induced neuropathy, or pain from radiation-related fibrosis should be treated according to the same principles and guidelines as chronic noncancer pain, considering the good prognosis and extended life expectancy of these patients.

- New pain may be an early indicator of recurrent disease, and meticulous tumor screening is required. Pain from recurrent disease should be treated according to the guidelines of cancer pain management.

- Treatment of chronic pain in cancer survivors should combine pharmacological and nonpharmacological options as required, including World Health Organization (WHO) step 3 opioids if indicated.

- Pain in cancer survivors causes considerable psychological distress, reminds the patient constantly of the malignant disease, and raises fears of disease recurrence. Persistent pain also impairs performance status and prevents complete rehabilitation.

Pain is one of the most common symptoms in cancer, and most patients report pain to be the most distressing symptom. However, even if cancer has been treated and complete remission has been achieved, pain may persist or may reappear. Even though chronic pain diminishes quality of life, impairs functional status, and prevents complete rehabilitation, patients may refrain from reporting pain to the physician. Possible barriers to disclosure include the belief that pain is a normal sequel to cancer, denial of pain as a constant reminder of the malignant disease that has been overcome, and suppression of the fear of cancer recurrence.

Caregivers should assess pain regularly in cancer survivors and should proactively ask about persistent or reappearing pain. Treatment of chronic pain in cancer survivors is mandatory to alleviate pain-related impairment of quality of life.

Two problems have to be faced. First, in many patients, treatment recommendations more closely resemble those for pain from causes other than cancer (e.g., recommendations with a significantly higher focus on patient compliance). Second, reappearing pain may always be the first sign of recurrent disease, and a high degree of suspicion has to be maintained even when tumor screening is (still) negative. These issues make pain management in cancer survivors a challenging task for the oncologists, pain specialists, and general practitioners caring for these patients.

EPIDEMIOLOGY AND PREVALENCE

Among older patients who were alive at least 5 years after the diagnosis of cancer, pain was the most frequent symptom, reported by 31%.[1] Pain was more common in breast cancer survivors (42%) than in survivors of colorectal (26%) and prostate cancer (18%). In another survey, 36% of long-term cancer survivors reported frequent pain, compared with 29% in a matched sample of persons without a history of cancer.[2]

Postmastectomy pain, defined as pain or numbness in the breast, chest wall, or axilla, has been reported in 10% to 75% of breast cancer survivors. Arm swelling or lymphedema is present in 10% to 25%. Plexopathy is less common, affecting less than 10%.[3] Pain from plexopathy is more frequent after higher-dose (>50 Gy) radiation therapy or after combined radiation therapy and chemotherapy.[4] *Intercostobrachial neuralgia,* defined as pain in the chest wall, axilla, or upper arm, ranged from 13% to 68% in different studies. Phantom pain after mastectomy was reported in 13% to 44% of survivors, and scar pain from neuroma was reported in 23% to 49% of patients.[5]

Chronic post-thoracotomy pain, defined as pain that recurs or persists along a thoracotomy scar at least 2 months following the surgical procedure, is reported in 26% to 67%. In a prospective survey, chronic pain was present in 61% of patients 1 year after thoracotomy.[6]

In a study on health-related quality of life in 143 female patients 3 to 4 years after pelvic radiation therapy for carcinoma of the endometrium and cervix, more patients reported pain in the lower back, hips, and thighs compared with pretreatment levels.[7] Breast cancer survivors suffer from continued fatigue and pain, as well as from the psychological burdens related to fear of cancer recurrence.[8] Some authors found less pain in cancer survivors. In a nationwide survey in Denmark, scores for bodily pain in the 36-item short-form quality of life questionnaire (SF-36) were lower in breast cancer survivors compared with a matched sample from the general population.[9] The

investigators concluded that a response shift may have raised the threshold in survivors.

PATHOPHYSIOLOGY

Chronic pain in cancer survivors may be caused by previous antineoplastic treatments such as chemotherapy, radiation therapy, and surgery, with either curative or palliative intent. Radiation therapy may induce fibrosis in the area of radiation that may, in turn, cause strictures and entrapments of nerve structures such as the brachiocervical plexus in breast cancer survivors. Fibrosis may appear soon after radiation therapy, but in some patients, late fibrosis has been reported, even up to 17 years after radiation therapy.[10] Chemotherapy, especially with taxane or platinum agents, causes neuropathies in many patients. Surgical procedures may damage nerve structures and may thereby cause neuropathic pain, or they may produce adhesions and scars, sometimes resulting in impaired and painful function. These lesions can aggravate cancer sequelae such as lymphedema, for example, in patients undergoing radical surgery for breast cancer.

Surgical procedures with removal of tissue may cause deafferentation pain. The loss of peripheral stimuli and the disconnection of afferent nerve fibers after surgical excision may reduce spinal feedback loops on the spinal and supraspinal level. A typical pain syndrome has been described for breast cancer survivors, who have reported pain in the distribution of the intercostobrachial nerve from a lesion of this nerve during axillary lymphadenectomy.[11] Phantom pain in the area of surgery has been described not only after the loss of limbs, but also after ablation of the breast or following excision of internal organs. Phantom pain was reported by 13% of patients after mastectomy.[12]

Chemotherapeutic agents used to treat hematological or solid cancers may damage nerve cell structures such as the axonal transport system, the myelin sheath, or the glial support system. Unlike other side effects of chemotherapy, this damage may be delayed in onset and may increase over time. Chemotherapy-induced peripheral neuropathy appears to be dose related and cumulative. Sensory, motor, and autonomic dysfunction may be present alone or in combination in up to 20% of patients following chemotherapy. Platinol agents such as oxaliplatin or cisplatin, vinca alkaloids such as vincristine, and taxanes such as paclitaxel, as well as anti-interferons and antimitotics, may cause peripheral neuropathy.[13,14]

Pain in cancer survivors can also be caused by mechanisms unrelated to antineoplastic treatment. Hypogonadism and glucocorticoid use may cause significant bone loss and osteoporosis.[15] These conditions may cause pathological fractures of vertebrae or hips, with loss of mobility and chronic pain on movement. In prostate cancer, androgen-deprivation therapy with either gonadotropin-releasing hormone (GnRH) or bilateral orchiectomy increases bone turnover, bone loss, and risk of fractures. In breast cancer survivors, estrogen deficiency resulting from age-related menopause, ovarian failure from systemic chemotherapy, or drugs such as aromatase inhibitors and GnRH analogues can cause osteoporosis.

In addition to physical causes of pain, pain in cancer survivors may be related to psychological, social, or spiritual problems, as in the concept of "total pain" by Cicely Saunders. Nonphysiological causes may include coping problems, for example, from the loss of role function with persisting disability. In addition, the experience of diagnosis and treatment as imminent threats to life can lead to psychological or spiritual pain. These issues can either aggravate nociception or cause pain by themselves.

Some cancer survivors suffer from chronic pain unrelated to cancer or its treatment. Considering the prevalence of chronic pain syndromes in the general population, many cancer survivors suffer from low back pain, osteoarthritis, and chronic tension headache (see "Case Study: Pain in a Cancer Survivor"). These pain syndromes often are diagnosed easily from the history, because patients usually can distinguish their chronic pain before the

CASE STUDY

Pain in a Cancer Survivor

CD, a 58-year-old man with Hodgkin's lymphoma, was admitted to the pain clinic because of severe diffuse pain in the pelvic region as well as in the genital and inguinal areas. He had been treated with vincristine, which had to be discontinued because of peripheral neuropathy. After remission of the lymphoma, transurethral prostatectomy was performed for chronic prostatitis. At the time of admission, no neurological deficits were detected. Oncological follow-up had found no signs of recurrent cancer. The cause of pain was not clear, and chemotherapy-induced neuropathy of pelvic nerves, neuropathic pain following prostatectomy, and psychological causes were discussed.

Pretreatment included tilidine (600 mg), in a fixed combination with naloxone (48 mg) and dipyrone (6000 mg) daily. Extensive treatment trials were performed with analgesics and co-analgesics, including oral oxycodone (≤160 mg/day), transdermal fentanyl (≤1.8 mg/day), epidural morphine (36 mg), clonidine (0.3 mg), intraspinal fentanyl (0.1 mg as a bolus), intravenous ketamine (15 mg), oral amitriptyline (75 mg), chlorprothixene (30 mg), gabapentin (1800 mg), and levomethadone, morphine, and buprenorphine. All drugs were either ineffective or caused intolerable side effects such as sedation or pruritus. The patient finally was rotated back to the previous dosage of tilidine and dipyrone.

In parallel to these treatment trials, the patient received extensive psychological counseling. Inpatient psychological treatment was suggested but rejected by the patient, who was very upset about this proposal. However, at the next follow-up visit in the outpatient clinic, the patient seemed to be relaxed and feeling much better. Asked about this change, he replied that he had just been in the oncological department, where he had been told that the last screening had found evidence of recurrent lymphoma in the pelvic region. He reported improved pain relief, even though the analgesic regimen had not been changed. Assurance of his cancer status, even though it meant life-threatening recurrence, obviously had alleviated his suffering considerably. His pain was managed with tilidine and dipyrone for the next 6 months until he died of progressive lymphoma.

cancer diagnosis from cancer pain and treatment-related pain that has developed more recently. Younger cancer patients may develop chronic noncancer pain syndromes during remission and may be worried that this pain is related to cancer.

CLINICAL MANIFESTATIONS

Pain syndromes in cancer survivors have many clinical manifestations (Table 254-1). For some tumor entities, specific pain syndromes have been described, predominantly associated with chronic neuropathic pain. Persistent nociceptive pain is rare in cancer survivors and suggests tumor recurrence. However, radiation therapy–induced fibrosis or the development of scar tissue following surgical procedures may cause chronic nociceptive pain in some patients. Adhesions may be related to visceral pain after abdominal surgery. Lymphedema is a frequent complication after radiation therapy or surgery, especially in breast cancer survivors, and it leads to painful pressure in the hand and arm.

Postmastectomy pain in the thoracic region, but even more often in the shoulder and the inner side of the upper arm (area of distribution of the intercostobrachial nerve), is another specific pain syndrome in breast cancer survivors. In a group of 134 patients, 27% reported postmastectomy pain.[16] No significant association existed between pain intensity and age at diagnosis, time after surgery, or time after treatment. Contrary to expectations, pain was found without axillary dissection, in women whose intercostobrachial nerve was spared, and women without documented postoperative complications.

Perineal pain is common after perineal resection, but also other pelvic surgical procedures. Perineal pain may be restricted to the anal region, but it may spread to adjacent areas. Peripheral neuropathy as a sequela of chemotherapy may persist after remission of cancer and may cause painful sensory deficits in hands and feet with glove-like or socklike distribution.

TABLE 254-1	Assessment of Pain in Cancer Survivors
DIAGNOSTIC FEATURES	**ASSESSMENT INSTRUMENTS**
Pain intensity	Verbal Rating Scale (VRS) Numerical Rating Scale (NRS) Visual Analogue Scale (VAS)
Pain location	Body drawing to draw location and spreading of pain
Pain type	Nociceptive Neuropathic
Treatment side effects	Sedation Nausea Vomiting Constipation Concentration difficulty Dry mouth Others
Concurrent symptoms	Anxiety Depression Fatigue Sleep disturbances Lower quality of life

Radiation therapy to the lower back or to the pelvic region may cause fibrosis and subsequent lumbosacral plexopathy, with neuropathic pain in the distribution of spinal nerve roots or nerve trunks in the plexus. Similarly, radiation therapy to chest wall, shoulder, or neck can be followed by cervicobrachial plexopathy.

Chronic pain is often accompanied by other symptoms. A high prevalence of psychological distress was found in survivors up to 11 years after curative treatment.[17] High levels of distress were found more frequently in association with pain and in patients with impaired cognitive or social function. Persistent pain may also aggravate other symptoms. In one study, more severe fatigue was reported by one third and was associated with significantly more pain, depression, and sleep disturbances.[18] In multivariate analysis, pain and depression were the strongest predictors of fatigue.

DIFFERENTIAL DIAGNOSIS

Persisting or increasing pain in cancer survivors may be an early indicator of recurrent cancer (Fig. 254-1). In a retrospective evaluation of 85 patients in a tertiary pain clinic after diagnosis of rectal carcinoma, 50 patients reported perineal pain, and in 80% of these patients, local cancer recurrence was diagnosed.[19] In 58% of patients, new pain was the first sign of the recurrence, with a median time of 5.5 months between the appearance of pain and the diagnosis of recurrence. In another 14% of patients, pelvic dissemination of cancer was considered the cause of perineal pain, and in only 6% of patients was no tumor found. Among the 35 patients with other than perineal pain, recurrent cancer was diagnosed in 54%. Pain in the distribution of the lumbosacral nerve plexus was reported much more frequently in these patients than in those without cancer recurrence.

This finding has been confirmed in other studies. In 286 patients treated with perineal resection for rectal cancer, 12% reported persistent pain over the 5-year follow-up.[20] Another 30% developed pain several months postoperatively. Late-onset pain was the highest confirmatory sign of cancer recurrence; 80% of this group died of recurrent cancer. In the group with early onset, the recurrence rate was 26%. For most patients in this group, phantom pain after rectal amputation was the cause.

In survivors of breast cancer, pain in the shoulder and arm is frequent. Differentiation of pain caused by radiation therapy–induced fibrosis of the plexus brachialis from pain related to cancer recurrence may be difficult. Both conditions may cause pain even several years after antineoplastic treatment. Severe pain with increasing intensity may be more specific for cancer recurrence, whereas radiation therapy–induced fibrosis more often produces sensory or motor dysfunction.[21]

Screening for cancer recurrence should be performed with great attention in survivors with persisting or increasing pain, and oncological follow-up has to be repeated at close intervals if screening results are negative. In a retrospective evaluation of perineal pain, computed tomography and magnetic resonance imaging initially showed negative results and confirmed cancer recurrence only much later.[19] In a case series of patients with breast cancer, neuropathic pain in the arm was thought to be caused by radiation therapy–induced fibrosis or lymphedema in 11 of 22 patients, but recurrent cancer or new metastasis was later found to be the cause in 7 of these 11 patients.[22]

TREATMENT

Pain treatment in cancer survivors should be related to the underlying pathophysiology. In recurrent cancer, analgesic therapy should follow the guidelines for cancer pain,

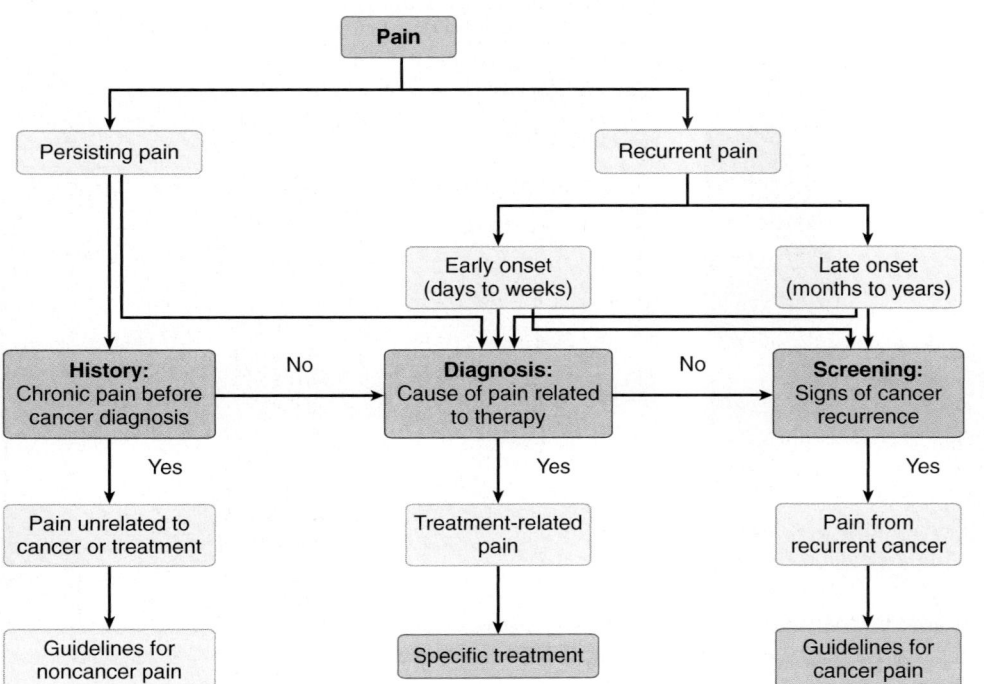

FIGURE 254-1 Algorithm for differential diagnosis and treatment.

with opioids and nonopioid analgesics as the mainstays of treatment. Opioids should be titrated up to effective dosage quickly, and doses should be increased as pain intensity increases. Antineoplastic treatment may help pain, especially radiation therapy for painful bone metastases. Steroids can decrease pain by reducing edema and inflammation around the tumor, and other co-analgesics may be effective for neuropathic pain, although in most patients only in addition to opioid therapy.

Guidelines for noncancer pain should be used for patients with chronic pain that is unrelated to cancer or cancer treatment. In these guidelines, opioids have a less clear standing than in cancer pain; controversy exists about the indication for opioids in patients with chronic noncancer pain or in defined subgroups. The treatment paradigm for some pain syndromes such as low back pain has changed considerably. The importance of pain relief has been diminished as restoration of role function has become increasingly important. Multimodal and multiprofessional treatment programs are effective, whereas drug treatment alone does not seem to make a difference. Differential diagnosis and treatment of chronic headache comprise an entire field of their own that has virtually no overlap with cancer pain management.

Persistent or recurrent treatment-related pain syndromes require careful analgesic planning. Specific therapies may be useful for some pain syndromes. Nerve blocks may be indicated for pain in the distribution of peripheral nerves such as post-thoracotomy pain or sympathetically maintained pain (Fig. 254-2). However, the duration of analgesia is moderate at most for nerve blocks with local anesthetics; prolonged series of nerve blocks are rarely feasible. Neurolytic nerve blocks with alcohol or cryotherapy aim toward long-lasting pain relief (Fig. 254-3), although they seem to work best intraoperatively. Topical lidocaine patches and capsaicin have also been used with good effect for several weeks or months.

Lymphatic drainage and complex physical therapy effectively reduce lymphedema and alleviate pressure-induced pain.[23] These regimens have to be maintained continuously because lymphedema will flare again if they are discontinued. Sometimes, surgical revision is required at the site of previous surgical procedures. Neuropathic pain related to neurinoma in the scar tissue may require surgical neurinoma excision. Adhesiolysis or removal of implanted material can be indicated in some patients.

Symptomatic analgesic therapy is necessary in most patients with treatment-related pain. In contrast to patients with advanced cancer, life expectancy is considerably longer in survivors. Consequently, treatment times of years and decades must be anticipated. This factor influences the balance of effectiveness and burden from side effects. Whereas patients with advanced cancer often bear mild to moderate side effects from analgesics for pain relief, many survivors find it difficult to tolerate even mild side effects for prolonged periods. Even less distressing side effects such as dry mouth become very aggravating when they are chronic. Opioid-related sedation is less of a burden in patients with reduced performance status who are at bed rest than in survivors who want an active lifestyle.

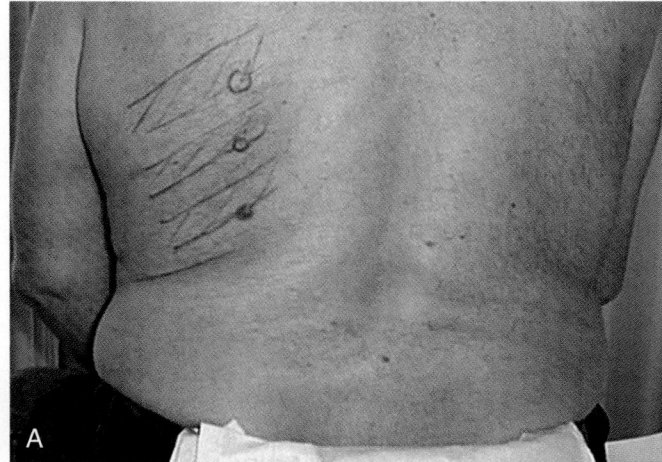

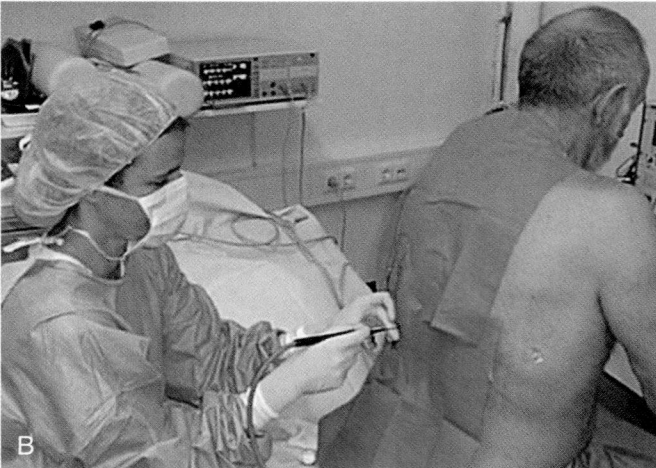

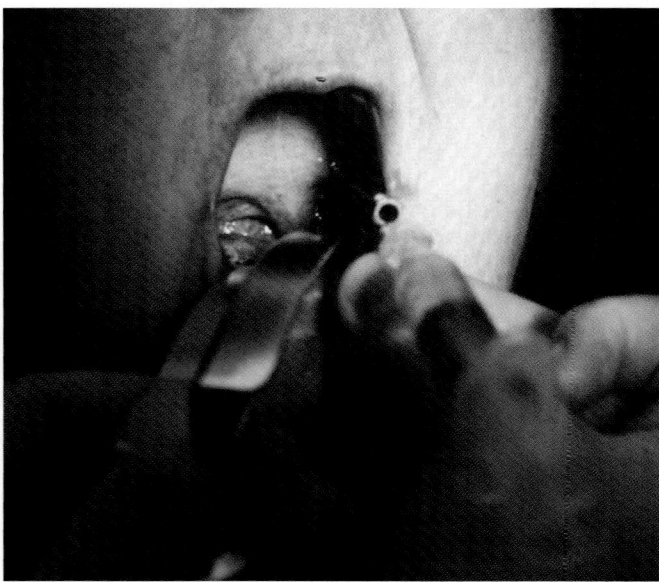

FIGURE 254-2 Ganglionic local opioid analgesia (GLOA) for sympathetically maintained pain in the area of the head and neck.

FIGURE 254-3 Neuropathic pain following thoracotomy. **A,** Injection sites are marked. **B,** Cryoanalgesia.

Future Considerations

- Most research has been done in breast cancer survivors. Little information is available on the epidemiology of pain in survivors of other cancers.
- Pain in cancer survivors may persist for decades, and little is known about the effectiveness and tolerance of analgesic treatment over prolonged periods of time.
- Trials comparing opioids, nonsteroidal anti-inflammatory drugs, antidepressants, and anticonvulsants are still missing. Effectiveness, burden from side effects, and organ toxicity or other complications influence the balance of benefit and burden and should be considered in the decision about analgesic regimens.
- The value of opioids for pain management in survivors remains unclear. The lack of organ toxicity and the adequate effectiveness of these agents are advantages of opioids, but tolerance in some patients and side effects during prolonged administration challenge the use of these drugs.

Sedation from symptomatic drug treatment may impair driving ability. Patients with progressive disease often are not able to drive because of disease-related impairment of cognitive or physical function. In cancer survivors, driving ability may have a high value, especially in rural areas. Impairment of driving ability by symptomatic treatment with opioids, benzodiazepines, or other drugs may have considerable impact on quality of life.

Long-term analgesic treatment may lead to new complications or side effects. In a controlled study with 20 male cancer survivors who chronically consumed opioids symptomatic hypogonadism correlated with depression, fatigue, and sexual dysfunction.[24]

Analgesic drugs for treatment-related pain include opioids from step 3 of the WHO analgesic ladder, nonsteroidal anti-inflammatory drugs, and other nonopioids such as dipyrone. Co-analgesic treatment with anticonvulsants, antidepressants, bisphosphonates, or steroids effectively alleviates neuropathic pain. Analgesics and co-analgesics may be used as monotherapy or in combination, often with synergistic effect. Antidepressants such as venlafaxine and amitriptyline and anticonvulsants such as gabapentin have been effective in breast cancer survivors with neuropathic pain.

Nonpharmacological treatments may provide a better balance of efficacy and side effects than analgesics and co-analgesics, and they may be used effectively for long time periods. In one report, pain in the scar area after mastectomy was treated successfully with transcutaneous nerve stimulation for 2 years, with minimal need for analgesics.[22] In another report, exercise during treatment was significantly and inversely correlated with fatigue and other symptoms, including pain, 6 months after treatment.[25]

REFERENCES

1. Deimling GT, Sterns S, Bowman KF, Kahana B. The health of older-adult, long-term cancer survivors. Cancer Nurs 2005;28:415-224.
2. Keating NL, Norredam M, Landrum MB, et al. Physical and mental health status of older long-term cancer survivors. J Am Geriatr Soc 2005;53:2145-2152.
3. Burstein HJ, Winer EP. Primary care for survivors of breast cancer. N Engl J Med 2000;343:1086-1094.
4. Pierce SM, Recht A, Lingos TI, et al. Long-term radiation complications following conservative surgery (CS) and radiation therapy (RT) in patients with early stage breast cancer. Int J Radiat Oncol Biol Phys 1992;23:915-923.
5. Jung BF, Ahrendt GM, Oaklander AL, Dworkin RH. Neuropathic pain following breast cancer surgery: Proposed classification and research update. Pain 2003;104:1-13.
6. Perttunen K, Tasmuth T, Kalso E. Chronic pain after thoracic surgery: A follow-up study. Acta Anaesthesiol Scand 1999;43:563-567.
7. Bye A, Trope C, Loge JH, et al. Health-related quality of life and occurrence of intestinal side effects after pelvic radiotherapy: Evaluation of long-term effects of diagnosis and treatment. Acta Oncol 2000;39:173-180.
8. Ferrell BR, Grant MM, Funk BM, et al. Quality of life in breast cancer survivors: Implications for developing support services. Oncol Nurs Forum 1998;25:887-895.
9. Peuckmann V, Ekholm O, Rasmussen NK, et al. Health-related quality of life in long-term breast cancer survivors: Nationwide survey in Denmark. Breast Cancer Res Treat 2007;104:39-46.
10. Strub M, Fuhr P, Kappos L. [Late manifestation of radiation injury to the plexus brachialis and plexus lumbosacralis]. Schweiz Med Wochenschr 2000;130:1407-1412.
11. Vecht CJ, Van de Brand HJ, Wajer OJ. Post-axillary dissection pain in breast cancer due to a lesion of the intercostobrachial nerve. Pain 1989;38:171-176.
12. Kroner K, Krebs B, Skov J, Jorgensen HS. [Phantom-related phenomena following mastectomy]. Ugeskr Laeger 1988;150:2233-2235.
13. Ocean AJ, Vahdat LT. Chemotherapy-induced peripheral neuropathy: Pathogenesis and emerging therapies. Support Care Cancer 2004;12:619-625.
14. Visovsky C. Chemotherapy-induced peripheral neuropathy. Cancer Invest 2003;21:439-451.
15. Hoff AO, Gagel RF. Osteoporosis in breast and prostate cancer survivors. Oncology (Williston Park) 2005;19:651-658.
16. Carpenter JS, Andrykowski MA, Sloan P, et al. Postmastectomy/postlumpectomy pain in breast cancer survivors. J Clin Epidemiol 1998;51:1285-1292.
17. Bjordal K, Kaasa S. Psychological distress in head and neck cancer patients 7-11 years after curative treatment. Br J Cancer 1995;71:592-597.
18. Bower JE, Ganz PA, Desmond KA, et al. Fatigue in breast cancer survivors: Occurrence, correlates, and impact on quality of life. J Clin Oncol 2000;18:743-753.
19. Radbruch L, Zech D, Grond S, et al. [Perineal pain and rectal cancer: Prevalence in local recurrence]. Med Klin 1991;86:180-185, 228.
20. Boas RA, Schug SA, Acland RH. Perineal pain after rectal amputation: A 5-year follow-up. Pain 1993;52:67-70.
21. Vecht CJ. Arm pain in the patient with breast cancer. J Pain Symptom Manage 1990;5:109-117.
22. Radbruch L, Zech D, Grond S, Jung H. [Therapy for symptomatic pain in advanced breast cancer]. Geburtshilfe Frauenheilkd 1992;52:404-411.
23. Moseley AL, Carati CJ, Piller NB. A systematic review of common conservative therapies for arm lymphoedema secondary to breast cancer treatment. Ann Oncol 2007;18:639-646.
24. Rajagopal A, Vassilopoulou-Sellin R, Palmer JL, et al. Symptomatic hypogonadism in male survivors of cancer with chronic exposure to opioids. Cancer 2004;100:851-858.
25. Mustian KM, Griggs JJ, Morrow GR, et al. Exercise and side effects among 749 patients during and after treatment for cancer: A University of Rochester Cancer Center Community Clinical Oncology Program Study. Support Care Cancer 2006;14:732-741.

SUGGESTED READING

Hausheer FH, Schilsky RL, Bain S, et al. Diagnosis, management, and evaluation of chemotherapy-induced peripheral neuropathy. Semin Oncol 2006;33:15-49.

INDEX

Page numbers followed by f, t, or b indicate figures, tables, or boxes, respectively.

A

AARP, 1145t
Abacavir, 1186t. *See also* Antiretroviral therapy.
  hypersensitivity reactions to, 1189
Abandonment, in hospital-based palliative care, 207,
    208b
  concerns about, 665. *See also* Advance directives.
Abatacept, for rheumatoid arthritis, 1038
ABC transporters, 669, 674
Abdomen, computed tomography of, 368-369, 369f
Abdominal distention, in bloating, 908-909
Abdominal pain
  in constipation, 848
  in dyspepsia, 905
Abscess, intra-abdominal, fistula-related, 489
Acarbose, for type 2 diabetes, 421t, 422
Access to care, 40
  ethnicity and, 52
Accreditation Council for Graduate Medical
    Education (ACGME), 119, 121-122
ACE inhibitors. *See* Angiotensin-converting enzyme
    inhibitors.
Acetaminophen, 740-745, 744t
  for fever, 892, 892b
  for pain
    in children, 1101t
    in frail elderly, 1138
    nonmalignant, 936
  for renal failure, 447, 448t
Acid-base status, determination of, 389
Acidosis
  lactic, antiretroviral therapy and, 1177, 1189-1190
  metabolic
    antiretroviral therapy and, 1177, 1189-1190
    blood pH measurement in, 389
Acquired immunodeficiency syndrome. *See* Human
    immunodeficiency virus infection.
Action myoclonus, 917
Action tremor, 920
Activities of daily living
  assessment instruments for, 359-363
  assistive aids for, 566-568, 567t. *See also* Durable
    medical equipment.
Activity, in cachexia, 592
Activity management, 889
Acupuncture, 1003-1004, 1003f, 1399-1400, 1399f,
    1400f
  common errors in, 1401
  for dyspnea, 879
  for fatigue, 1004
  for hiccups, 897
  for hot flashes, 1004
  for nausea and vomiting, 927, 1004
  for pain, 1004
    in cancer, 1400, 1402t, 1403t
  for premature menopause, 951
Acute abdomen, computed tomography of, 369, 369f
Acute care setting. *See* Hospital-based palliative care;
    Intensive care unit.
Acute leukemia. *See* Leukemia.
Acute liver failure. *See* Liver failure.
Acute palliative medicine units, 208-212

Acute phase protein response, in cachexia, 589-590
Acute respiratory failure. *See* Respiratory failure.
Acute-on-chronic liver failure, 459, 462-464, 464t.
    See also Liver failure.
Acyclovir
  for chickenpox, 1171t
  for herpes simplex infection, in HIV infection,
    1195t
  for herpes stomatitis, 1169
  for herpes zoster, 1171t
Adalimumab, for rheumatoid arthritis, 415
Addiction. *See* Substance abuse.
Adherence, in drug therapy, 689
  for pediatric HIV infection, 1167
Adhesive capsulitis, 411, 411f, 413-414
Adjuvant analgesics, 935, 936
Administration on Aging, 1145t
Adolescents, 1077-1078. *See also* Pediatric patients.
Adrenal function, age-related changes in, 1128
Adrenaline. *See* Epinephrine.
Adult day care, 1143-1144
Adult learning. *See also* Education and training.
  assessment in, 130
  competency and, 130
  conceptual frameworks for, 128-129
  determinants of, 130
  distance learning in, 131-135, 639, 639t, 640, 640f
  emerging concepts in, 129-130
  Knowles' theory of, 125-126, 126t
  learner characteristics in, 125-126
  learning styles and, 126-128
  learning theories and, 126-128
  self-directed, 131
  Web-based, 131-135
Advance care planning, 92, 98-103, 311, 662-665,
    978. *See also* Do not resuscitate orders;
    Treatment withholding/withdrawal.
  barriers to, 100
  "best practices" standard for, 100
  challenges to, 103
  "clear and convincing evidence" standard for, 100
  communication in, 101
  cultural aspects of, 103
  dementia and, 1131-1132
  dignity model for, 311, 312t
  disseminated responsibility for, 101
  essential elements of, 100-101
  evidence-based medicine and, 102
  for pediatric patients, 1091-1092
  future considerations for, 103
  history of, 98
  home care and, 223-224
  implantable cardiac defibrillators and, 108,
    430-431
  institutional factors in, 102-103
  legal issues in, 99-100
  prognosis and, 101
  rationale for, 98
  recent developments in, 101-102
Advance directives, 92, 98-103, 662-665. *See also*
    Advance care planning.
  current status of, 99-100
Advanced glycation end products (AGE), 579, 579f

Advocacy, 40, 201, 288, 634-637
Adynamic bone disease, in renal failure, 444, 446
Africa, HIV infection in, 1198-1201, 1200f, 1200t
African Americans. *See also* Cultural factors; Race/
    ethnicity.
  do not resuscitate orders and, 664
Aging. *See also* Elderly.
  advanced glycation end products and, 579
  demographics of, 1120-1123, 1121f, 1121t, 1122t
  healthy, 11
  of cardiovascular system, 1124-1125, 1124f
  of endocrine system, 1127-1128
  of gastrointestinal/hepatobiliary systems,
    1126-1127
  of immune system, 1128
  of neurological system, 1128-1129, 1130-1132
  of renal system, 1126, 1126f
  of respiratory system, 1125-1126
  physiology of, 1123-1129, 1129t
  theories of, 1123-1124, 1124t
Agitation, 287. *See also* Delirium.
  in children, 1102t
AIDS. *See* Human immunodeficiency virus infection.
Air entrainment mask, 1024-1025, 1024f, 1025t
Air hunger, 958
Airborne precautions, 511
  for tuberculosis, 511, 514
Airway clearance, in dying patients, 958, 999
Airway obstruction, 842-846
  by thick mucus
    in amyotrophic lateral sclerosis, 1065
    in children, 1101t
  case study of, 844
  causes of, 843t, 842842
  central, 842, 844-845
  clinical manifestations of, 842
  definition of, 842
  diagnosis of, 843f
  differential diagnosis of, 843t
  epidemiology of, 842
  in COPD, 842, 844, 845t
  pathophysiology of, 842
  peripheral fixed, 842, 844, 845t
  reversible, 842, 843-844, 845t
  stenting for. *See* Airway stents.
  tracheostomy for, 544-549
    technique of, 545, 547f
  treatment of, 842-846, 845t, 856
Airway secretions
  death rattle and, 956-960, 999
  removal of, 958, 999
Airway stents, 540t, 544-549, 845, 856
  advantages of, 544
  current controversies over, 548-549
  efficacy of, 547-548
  evaluation for, 545
  for cough, 856
  future considerations for, 548-549
  indications for, 544
  patient selection for, 544, 547-548
  pearls and pitfalls for, 549
  placement of, 545-547, 547f, 548f, 549
  selection of, 549